Sabiston & Spencer Surgery of the Chest

Eighth Edition
Sabiston & Spencer Surgery of the Chest
Volume 1

Frank W. Sellke, MD
Karl E. Karlson and Gloria A. Karlson
Professor of Cardiothoracic Surgery and Chief,
Division of Cardiothoracic Surgery
Alpert Medical School of Brown University
and Lifespan Hospitals
Co-director, Lifespan Heart Center
Providence, Rhode Island
Visiting Professor of Surgery
Harvard Medical School
Boston, Massachusetts

Pedro J. del Nido, MD
William E. Ladd Professor of Child Surgery
Harvard Medical School
Chief, Department of Cardiac Surgery
Children's Hospital Boston
Boston, Massachusetts

Scott J. Swanson, MD
Director of Minimally Invasive Thoracic Surgery
Division of Thoracic Surgery
Brigham and Women's Hospital
Chief Surgical Officer
Dana-Farber Cancer Institute
Harvard Medical School
Boston, Massachusetts

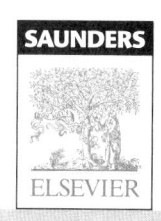

SAUNDERS
ELSEVIER

SAUNDERS
ELSEVIER

1600 John F. Kennedy Blvd.
Ste 1800
Philadelphia, PA 19103-2899

SABISTON & SPENCER SURGERY OF THE CHEST   ISBN: 978-1-4160-5225-8

Copyright © 2010, 2005, 1995, 1990, 1983, 1976, 1969, 1962 by Saunders, an imprint of Elsevier Inc.
1962 copyright renewed 1990 by John H. Gibbon, Jr. All rights reserved.

All rights reserved. No part of this publication may be reproduced or transmitted in any form or by any means, electronic or mechanical, including photocopying, recording, or any information storage and retrieval system, without permission in writing from the publisher. Details on how to seek permission, further information about the Publisher's permissions policies and our arrangements with organizations such as the Copyright Clearance Center and the Copyright Licensing Agency can be found at our website: www.elsevier.com/permissions.

This book and the individual contributions contained in it are protected under copyright by the Publisher (other than as may be noted herein).

Notices

Knowledge and best practice in this field are constantly changing. As new research and experience broaden our understanding, changes in research methods, professional practices, or medical treatment may become necessary.

Practitioners and researchers must always rely on their own experience and knowledge in evaluating and using any information, methods, compounds, or experiments described herein. In using such information or methods they should be mindful of their own safety and the safety of others, including parties for whom they have a professional responsibility.

With respect to any drug or pharmaceutical products identified, readers are advised to check the most current information provided (i) on procedures featured or (ii) by the manufacturer of each product to be administered, to verify the recommended dose or formula, the method and duration of administration, and contraindications. It is the responsibility of practitioners, relying on their own experience and knowledge of their patients, to make diagnoses, to determine dosages and the best treatment for each individual patient, and to take all appropriate safety precautions.

To the fullest extent of the law, neither the Publisher nor the authors, contributors, or editors, assume any liability for any injury and/or damage to persons or property as a matter of products liability, negligence or otherwise, or from any use of operation of any methods, products, instructions, or ideas contained in the material herein.

The Publisher

Library of Congress Cataloging-in-Publication Data
Sabiston & Spencer surgery of the chest. – 8th ed. / editor- in-chief, Frank W. Sellke; editors, Pedro J. del Nido, Scott J. Swanson.
  p. ; cm.
Includes bibliographical references and index.
ISBN 978-1-4160-5225-8
1. Chest–Surgery. 2. Heart–Surgery. I. Sabiston, David C., II. Sellke, Frank W. III. Del Nido, Pedro J.
  IV. Swanson, Scott J. V. Title: Surgery of the chest. VI. Title: Sabiston and Spencer surgery of the chest.
  [DNLM: 1. Thoracic Surgical Procedures—methods. WF 980 S116 2010]
RD536.S236 2010
617.5' 4059—dc22

2009003431

Acquisitions Editor: Judith Fletcher
Developmental Editor: Lisa Barnes
Publishing Services Manager: Tina Rebane
Senior Project Manager: Linda Lewis Grigg

Printed in USA

Last digit is the print number: 9 8 7 6 5 4 3 2 1

Working together to grow
libraries in developing countries

www.elsevier.com | www.bookaid.org | www.sabre.org

ELSEVIER   BOOK AID International   Sabre Foundation

*To my wife, Amy, who gives me love, inspiration, and unwavering support
and to our children, Michelle, Eric, Nicholas, and Amanda. They provide us with unlimited pleasure.*

FWS

To Martha, Alexander, Sara, Daniel, and Elizabeth. Thank you.

PJD

To my wife, Donna, and our children, Kate, Whit, and Maggie, who make this all worthwhile.

SJS

Contributors

Brian G. Abbott, MD, FACC, FASNC
Assistant Professor of Medicine (Clinical)
The Warren Alpert Medical School of Brown University
Division of Cardiology, Rhode Island Hospital
Medical Director, Nuclear Cardiology
Rhode Island Cardiology Center
Providence, Rhode Island
Nuclear Cardiology and Positron Emission Tomography in the Assessment of Patients with Cardiovascular Disease

David H. Adams, MD
Marie-Josée and Henry R. Kravis Professor and Chairman
Department of Cardiothoracic Surgery
Mount Sinai School of Medicine
Program Director, Mitral Valve Repair Reference Center
Mount Sinai Medical Center
New York, New York
Acquired Disease of the Mitral Valve; Ischemic Mitral Regurgitation

Lishan Aklog, MD
Chair Cardiovascular Center/Chief of Cardiovascular Surgery
Heart and Lung Institute
St. Joseph's Hospital and Medical Center
Phoenix, Arizona
Ischemic Mitral Regurgitation

Arvind K. Agnihotri, MD
Assistant Professor of Surgery
Harvard Medical School
Massachusetts General Hospital
Boston, Massachusetts
Postinfarction Ventricular Septal Defect

Louise A. Aquila Allen, PhD
Manager, Training and Clinical Support
Syncardia Systems, Inc.
Tucson, Arizona
Total Artificial Heart

Mark S. Allen, MD
Chair, Division of General Thoracic Surgery
Department of Surgery
Mayo Clinic
Rochester, Minnesota
Chest Wall Tumors

Nasser K. Altorki, MD
Professor of Cardiothoracic Surgery
Weill Cornell Medical College
Chief, Division of Thoracic Surgery
NewYork–Presbyterian Hospital
New York, New York
Screening for Lung Cancer

Robert H. Anderson, BSc, MD, FRC Path
Emeritus Professor
Institute of Child Health
University College
London, United Kingdom
Visiting Professor
Division of Pediatric Cardiology
Medical University of South Carolina
Charleston, South Carolina
Visiting Professor
Institute of Human Genetics
Newcastle University
Newcastle Upon Tyne, United Kingdom
Surgical Anatomy of the Heart

Masaki Anraku, MD, MSc
Fellow, Division of Thoracic Surgery
Toronto General Hospital/University of Toronto Faculty of Medicine
Toronto, Ontario
Canada
Lung Cancer: Surgical Treatment

Anelechi C. Anyanwu, MD
Associate Professor
Department of Cardiothoracic Surgery
Director, Heart and Heart-Lung Transplantation
Department of Cardiothoracic Surgery
Mount Sinai School of Medicine
New York, New York
Ischemic Mitral Regurgitation

Simon K. Ashiku, MD
Department of Surgery
Walnut Creek Medical Center
Walnut Creek, California
Tracheal Lesions

Erle H. Austin III, MD
Professor of Surgery
Division of Thoracic and Cardiovascular Surgery
University of Louisville School of Medicine
Chief, Congenital Cardiothoracic Surgery
Kosair Children's Hospital
Louisville, Kentucky
  Pulmonary Atresia with Intact Ventricular Septum

Eric H. Awtry, MD, FACC
Assistant Professor of Medicine
Department of Medicine
Boston University School of Medicine
Inpatient Clinical Director
Division of Cardiology
Boston Medical Center
Boston, Massachussettes
  The Pharmacologic Management of Heart Failure

Emile A. Bacha, MD, FACS
Associate Professor of Surgery
Harvard Medical School
Senior Associate in Cardiac Surgery
Children's Hospital Boston
Boston, Massachusetts
  Congenital Tracheal Disease; Ventricular Septal Defect and Double-Outlet Right Ventricle; Adult Congenital Cardiac Surgery; Image-Guided and Hybrid Surgery: Surgical Simulation

Richard Baillott, MD, FRCSC
Department of Surgery
Institut Universitaire de Cardiologie et de Pneumologie de Quebec
Laval University Faculty of Medicine
Department of Cardiac Surgery
Hôpital Laval
Quebec City, Quebec
Canada
  Deep Sternal Wound Infection

Donald S. Baim, MD
Executive VP, Chief Medical and Scientific Officer
Boston Scientific Corporation
Natick, Massachusetts
  Nonatherosclerotic Coronary Heart Disease

Leora B. Balsam, MD
Assistant Professor
Department of Cardiothoracic Surgery
New York University School of Medicine
New York, New York
  Heart Transplantation

Hendrick B. Barner, MD
Adjunct Professor of Surgery
Department of Surgery
Saint Louis University School of Medicine
Clinical Professor of Surgery
Department of Surgery
Washington University in St. Louis School of Medicine
Thoracic Surgeon
Saint Louis University Hospital
St. Louis, Missouri
  Bypass Conduit Options

David J. Barron, MD
Consultant Cardiac Surgeon
Birmingham Children's Hospital
NHS Foundation Trust
Birmingham
United Kingdom
  Surgery for Congenitally Corrected Transposition of the Great Arteries

Joseph E. Bavaria, MD
Professor of Surgery
University of Pennsylvania School of Medicine
Staff Surgeon and Vice Chief, Division of Cardiothoracic Surgery
Hospital of the University of Pennsylvania
Philadelphia, Pennsylvania
  Endovascular Therapy for Thoracic Aortic Aneurysms and Dissections

David P. Bichell, MD
Professor of Cardiac Surgery
Vanderbilt University School of Medicine
Chief, Pediatric Cardiac Surgery
Monroe Carell Jr. Children's Hospital at Vanderbilt
Nashville, Tennessee
  Atrial Septal Defect and Cor Triatriatum

Edward L. Bove, MD
Professor of Surgery
University of Michigan Medical School
Thoracic Surgeon
University of Michigan Health Systems
Ann Arbor, Michigan
  Truncus Arteriosus and Aortopulmonary Window

William J. Brawn, MD
Consultant Cardiac Surgeon
Birmingham Children's Hospital
NHS Foundation Trust
Birmingham
United Kingdom
  Surgery for Congenitally Corrected Transposition of the Great Arteries

Christian P. Brizard, MD
Associate Professor
The University of Melbourne Faculty of Medicine, Dentistry and Health Sciences School of Medicine
Cardiac Surgery Unit
Royal Children's Hospital Melbourne
Melbourne, Victoria
Australia
Congenital Anomalies of the Mitral Valve

Julie A. Brothers, MD
Assistant Professor
Department of Pediatrics
University of Pennsylvania School of Medicine
Attending, Department of Cardiology
The Children's Hospital of Philadelphia
Philadelphia, Pennsylvania
Surgery for Congenital Anomalies of the Coronary Arteries

Morgan L. Brown, MD, PhD
Resident
Department of Anesthesiology and Pain Medicine
University of Alberta
Edmonton, Alberta, Canada
Ebstein's Anomaly

Ayesha S. Bryant, MSPH, MD
Assistant Professor
Department of Surgery, Division of Cardiothoracic Surgery
University of Alabama at Birmingham School of Medicine
Birmingham, Alabama
Benign Lesions of the Lung

Harold M. Burkhart, MD
Associate Professor
Department of Surgery, Division of Cardiovascular Surgery
Mayo Clinic
Rochester, Minnesota
Congenital Lung Diseases

Christopher A. Caldarone, MD
Professor and Chair, Division of Cardiac Surgery
Department of Surgery
University of Toronto Faculty of Medicine
Staff Surgeon
Division of Cardiovascular Surgery
The Hospital for Sick Children
Toronto, Ontario
Canada
Surgical Considerations in Pulmonary Vein Anomalies

Robert M. Califf, MD
Vice Chancellor, Duke University
Professor of Medicine
Duke University School of Medicine
Director, Duke Translational Medicine Institute
Durham, North Carolina
Medical Management of Acute Coronary Syndromes

Edward Cantu III, MD
Cardiothoracic Fellow
Department of Surgery
Duke University Medical Center
Durham, North Carolina
Critical Care for the Adult Cardiac Patient

Justine M. Carr, MD
Assistant Professor
Departments of Surgery and Medicine
Harvard Medical School
Senior Director
Department of Clinical Resource Management
Beth Israel Deaconess Medical Center
Boston, Massachusetts
Clinical Quality and Safety in Cardiac Surgery

Joseph P. Carrozza, Jr., MD
Chief, Cardiovascular Division
Caritas St. Elizabeth's Medical Center
Vice President, Caritas Cardiovascular Network
Boston, Massachusetts
Interventional Cardiology

Frank Cecchin, MD
Associate Professor of Pediatrics
Department of Pediatrics
Harvard Medical School
Senior Associate in Cardiology
Children's Hospital Boston
Boston, Massachusetts
Arrhythmia and Pacemaker Surgery in Congenital Heart Disease

Robert J. Cerfolio, MD
Professor
Department of Cardiothoracic Surgery
University of Alabama at Birmingham School of Medicine
Chief, Section of Thoracic Surgery
UAB Hospital
Birmingham, Alabama
Benign Lesions of the Lung

Riya S. Chacko, MD
Cardiology Fellow
Department of Cardiology
Harvard University
Cardiology Clinical Fellow
Department of Cardiology
Beth Israel Deaconess Medical Center
Boston, Massachusetts
Interventional Cardiology

Alfred Chahine, MD, FACS, FAAP
Associate Professor of Surgery and Pediatrics
The George Washington University School of Medicine
Attending Surgeon
Department of Pediatric Surgery
Children's National Medical Center
Program Director
Department of General Surgery Residency
Georgetown University Medical Center
Washington, District of Columbia
Surgery for Congenital Lesions of the Esophagus

Vincent Chan, MD
Chief Resident
Department of Cardiac Surgery
University of Ottawa Heart Institute
Ottawa, Ontario, Canada
Coronary Artery Bypass Grafting

Frederick Y. Chen, MD, PhD
Assistant Professor of Surgery
Division of Cardiac Surgery
Harvard Medical School
Associate Surgeon
Division of Cardiac Surgery
Brigham and Women's Hospital
Boston, Massachusetts
Management of Native Valve Endocarditis

Alvin J. Chin, MD
Professor
Department of Pediatrics
University of Pennsylvania School of Medicine
Senior Physician
Division of Cardiology
Department of Pediatrics
Children's Hospital of Philadelphia
Philadelphia, Pennsylvania
Interrupted Aortic Arch

Cynthia S. Chin, MD
Assistant Professor of Surgery
Division of Cardiothoracic Surgery
Mount Sinai School of Medicine
Thoracic Surgeon
Mount Sinai Medical Center
New York, New York
Anatomy of the Thorax; Esophageal Resection and Replacement

Joanna Chikwe, MD, FRCS (CTh)
Department of Cardiothoracic Surgery
Mount Sinai School of Medicine
Associate Program Director
Department of Cardiothoracic Surgery
New York, New York
Acquired Disease of the Mitral Valve

W. Randolph Chitwood, Jr., MD
Eddie and Jo Allison Smith Distinguished Chair Professor
Department of Cardiovascular Sciences
Senior Associate Vice Chancellor for Health Sciences
East Carolina University Brody School of Medicine
Director, East Carolina Heart Institute at Pitt County
    Memorial Hospital
Greenville, North Carolina
Robotic Cardiac Surgery and Novel Visualization Systems

Karla G. Christian, MD
Associate Professor
Department of Cardiac Surgery
Vanderbilt University
Associate Chief
Department of Pediatric Cardiac Surgery
Monroe Carell, Jr. Children's Hospital at Vanderbilt
Nashville, Tennessee
Atrial Septal Defect and Cor Triatriatum

Neil A. Christie, MD
Assistant Professor of Surgery
University of Pittsburgh School of Medicine
Director, LIFE Bronchoscopy Program
Heart, Lung and Esophageal Surgery Institute
Division of Thoracic and Foregut Surgery
Member, Division of Thoracic Surgery
University of Pittsburgh Medical Center
Pittsburgh, Pennsylvania
Innovative Therapy and Technology

Joseph C. Cleveland, Jr., MD
Associate Professor of Surgery
Division of Cardiothoracic Surgery
Department of Surgery
University of Colorado Denver
Surgical Director, Adult Cardiac Transplantation/Mechanical
    Circulatory Devices
Department of Surgery, Division of Cardiothoracic Surgery
University of Colorado Hospital
Aurora, Colorado
Chief, Cardiothoracic Surgical Services
Division of Cardiothoracic Surgery
Department of Surgery
Veteran's Administration Medical Center
Denver, Colorado
*Thrombosis and Thromboembolism of Prosthetic Cardiac
Valves and Extracardiac Prostheses*

Lawrence H. Cohn, MD
Virginia and James Hubbard Professor of Cardiac Surgery
Department of Surgery
Harvard Medical School
Surgeon
Division of Cardiac Surgery
Brigham and Women's Hospital
Boston, Massachusetts
Management of Native Valve Endocarditis

William E. Cohn, MD
Associate Professor of Surgery
Baylor College of Medicine
Director
Minimally Invasive Surgical Technology
Texas Heart Institute
Adjunct Professor
Department of Bioengineering
University of Houston
Houston, Texas
Alternative Approaches to Coronary Artery Bypass Grafting

Yolanda L. Colson, MD, PhD
Associate Professor of Surgery
Harvard Medical School
Surgeon
Department of Thoracic Surgery
Brigham and Women's Hospital
Boston, Massachusetts
Interstitial Lung Diseases

Wilson S. Colucci, MD, FACC, FAHA
Thomas J. Ryan Professor of Medicine
Department of Medicine
Boston University School of Medicine
Chief, Section of Cardiovascular Medicine
Boston University Medical Center
Boston, Massachusetts
The Pharmacologic Management of Heart Failure

Andrew C. Cook, PhD
Senior Lecturer
Cardiac Unit
UCL Institute of Child Health
Great Ormond Street Hospital
NHS Foundation Trust
London, United Kingdom
Surgical Anatomy of the Heart

Joel D. Cooper, MD
Professor of Surgery
University of Pennsylvania School of Medicine
Chief, Department of Surgery
University of Pennsylvania Health System
Philadelphia, Pennsylvania
Surgery for Emphysema

Jack G. Copeland, MD
Jack G. Copeland, MD, Endowed Chair of Cardiothoracic Surgery
Professor of Surgery
University of Arizona College of Medicine
Chief, Section of Cardiothoracic Surgery
Staff Surgeon
University Medical Center
Tucson, Arizona
Total Artificial Heart

Scott W. Cowan, MD
Assistant Professor of Surgery
Department of Surgery
University of Pennsylvania
Assistant Professor of Surgery
Department of Surgery
Penn Presbyterian Medical Center
Philadelphia, Pennsylvania
Secondary Lung Tumors

Melissa Culligan, RN, BSN
Thoracic Surgery Clinical Nurse
Department of Thoracic Surgery
Penn Presbyterian Medical Center
Philadelphia, Pennsylvania
Secondary Lung Tumors

François Dagenais, MD, FRCSC
Department of Surgery
Institut Universitaire de Cardiologie et de Pneumologie de Quebec
Laval University Faculty of Medicine
Department of Cardiac Surgery
Hôpital Laval
Quebec City, Quebec
Canada
Deep Sternal Wound Infection

Ralph J. Damiano, Jr., MD
John M. Shoneberg Professor of Surgery
Vice Chairman
Department of Surgery
Washington University in St. Louis School of Medicine
Chief of Cardiac Surgery
Barnes-Jewish Hospital
St. Louis, Missouri
Surgical Treatment of Arrhythmias

Thomas A. D'Amico, MD
Professor of Surgery
Duke University School of Medicine
Section Chief and Program Director, General Thoracic Surgery
Duke University Medical Center
Director, Clinical Oncology
Duke Comprehensive Cancer Center
Durham, North Carolina
Lung Cancer: Minimally Invasive Approaches

Jonathan C. Daniel, MD
Department of Surgery
University of Arizona
Thoracic Surgeon
University Medical Center/Tucson Medical Center
Tucson, Arizona
Surgery of the Diaphragm: A Deductive Approach

Philippe G. Dartevelle, MD
Professor
Department of Thoracic and Cardiovascular Surgery
Paris Sud University
Le Kremlin–Bicêtre
Head, Department of Thoracic and Vascular Surgery and Heart-Lung Transplantation
Marie Lannelongue Hospital
Le Plessis Robinson
Paris
France
Anterior Approach to Superior Sulcus Lesions

Tirone E. David, MD, FRCSC, FACS
Professor
University of Toronto Faculty of Medicine
Head, Division of Cardiovascular Surgery
Melanie Munk Chair of Cardiovascular Surgery
Toronto General Hospital
Toronto, Ontario
Canada
Surgery of the Aortic Root and Ascending Aorta

Jonathan D'Cunha, MD, PhD
Assistant Professor
Department of Surgery
University of Minnesota Medical School
Staff Surgeon
University of Minnesota Medical Center
Fairview Health Services
Minneapolis, Minnesota
The Use of Genetic Science in Thoracic Disease

Joseph A. Dearani, MD
Professor of Surgery
Mayo Medical School College of Medicine
Division of Cardiovascular Surgery
Mayo Clinic
Rochester, Minnesota
Ebstein's Anomaly

Daniel T. DeArmond, MD
Assistant Professor
Department of Surgery
Division of Cardiothoracic Surgery
University of Texas Health Science Center at San Antonio School of Medicine
San Antonio, Texas
Congenital Lung Diseases

Pedro J. del Nido, MD
William E. Ladd Professor of Child Surgery
Harvard Medical School
Chief, Department of Cardiac Surgery
Children's Hospital Boston
Boston, Massachusetts
Surgical Approaches and Cardiopulmonary Bypass in Pediatric Cardiac Surgery; Atrioventricular Canal Defects; Transposition of the Great Arteries: Simple and Complex Forms; Image-Guided and Hybrid Surgery: Surgical Simulation

Tom R. DeMeester, MD
Professor and Chair, Department of Surgery
USC Keck School of Medicine
Los Angeles, California
Esophageal Anatomy and Function

Philippe Demers, MD
Assistant Professor of Surgery
University of Montreal
Cardiovascular Surgeon
Montreal Heart Institute and Sacre-Coeur Hospital
Montreal, Canada
Type A Aortic Dissection; Type B Aortic Dissection

Todd L. Demmy, MD
Associate Professor of Surgery and Clinical Scholar
Department of Surgery
Associate Professor of Oncology
State University of New York University of Buffalo School of Medicine and Biomedical Sciences
Chairman, Department of Thoracic Surgery
Roswell Park Cancer Institute
Buffalo, New York
Malignant Pleural and Pericardial Effusions

Eric J. Devaney, MD
Assistant Professor
Department of Surgery
University of Michigan Medical School
Cardiothoracic Surgeon
Cardiovascular Center/University of Michigan Health Systems
Ann Arbor, Michigan
Truncus Arteriosus and Aortopulmonary Window

Elisabeth U. Dexter, MD, FACS
Assistant Professor of Surgery
Department of Surgery, Section of General Thoracic Surgery
State University of New York Upstate Medical University College of Medicine
Thoracic Surgeon
Syracuse VA Medical Center
Syracuse, New York
Perioperative Care of the Thoracic Surgical Patient

Marisa Di Donato, MD
Department of Cardiac Surgery
IRCCS Istituto Policlinico San Donato
Milan
Associate Professor in Cardiology
University of Florence Faculty of Medicine and Surgery
Florence, Italy
Left Ventricular Restoration: Surgical Treatment of the Failing Heart

Christopher T. Ducko, MD
Department of Surgery
Harvard Medical School
Associate Surgeon
Department of Surgery
Brigham and Woman's Hospital
Boston, Massachusetts
Surgeon
Department of Surgery
Carney Hospital
Dorchester, Massachusetts
Surgeon
Department of Surgery
South Shore Hospital
Wymouth, Massachusetts
Pleural Tumors

Brian W. Duncan, MD
Medical Director
Cleveland Clinic
Cleveland, Ohio
Tetralogy of Fallot with Pulmonary Stenosis

Carlos M. G. Duran, MD, PhD
Chair of Cardiovascular Sciences
University of Montana College of Health Professions and Biomedical Sciences
Chairman of the Board
International Heart Institute of Montana Foundation
Missoula, Montana
Surgical Treatment of the Tricuspid Valve

Fred H. Edwards, MD
Medical Director
Department of Cardiothoracic Surgery
University of Florida
Jacksonville, Florida
Quality Improvement and Risk Stratification for Congenital Cardiac Surgery

Sitaram M. Emani, MD
Instructor in Surgery
Department of Cardiac Surgery
Harvard Medical School
Assistant in Cardiac Surgery
Department of Cardiac Surgery
Children's Hospital Boston
Boston, Massachusetts
Patent Ductus Arteriosus, Coarctation of the Aorta, and Vascular Rings; Pulmonary Atresia with Ventricular Septal Defect and Right Ventricle–to–Pulmonary Artery Conduits

Jeremy J. Erasmus, MD
Professor
Department of Diagnostic Radiology, Division of Diagnostic Imaging
The University of Texas M.D. Anderson Cancer Center
Houston, Texas
Radiologic Imaging of Thoracic Abnormalities

Dario O. Fauza, MD
Associate Professor
Department of Surgery
Harvard Medical School
Associate
Department of Surgery
Children's Hospital Boston
Boston, Massachusetts
Congenital Diaphragmatic Hernia

Felix G. Fernandez, MD
Assistant Professor
Department of Thoracic Surgery
Emory University School of Medicine
Atlanta, Georgia
Lung Transplantation

Hiran C. Fernando, MD
Associate Professor of Cardiothoracic Surgery
Boston University School of Medicine
Director of Minimally Invasive Cardiothoracic Surgery
Boston Medical Center
Boston, Massachusetts
Endoscopic Therapies for Thoracic Diseases; Innovative Therapy and Technology

Farzan Filsoufi, MD
Associate Professor
Mount Sinai Medical Center
Associate Chief Cardiac Surgery
Department of Cardiothoracic Surgery
Mount Sinai Medical Center
New York, New York
Acquired Diseases of the Mitral Valve

Michael P. Fischbein, MD, PhD
Assistant Professor of Cardiothoracic Surgery
Cardiothoracic Surgery
Stanford, California
Heart Transplantation

Rosario V. Freeman, MD, MS
Assistant Professor
Department of Internal Medicine
University of Washington School of Medicine
Acting Director, Echocardiography
Department of Medicine
University of Washington Medical Center
Seattle, Washington
Diagnostic Echocardiography (Ultrasound Imaging in Cardiovascular Diagnosis)

Joseph Friedberg, MD, FACS
Associate Professor of Surgery
Department of Surgery
University of Pennsylvania
Associate Professor of Surgery
Division of Thoracic Surgery
Department of Surgery
Penn Presbyterian Medical Center
Philadelphia, Pennsylvania
Secondary Lung Tumors

David A. Fullerton, MD
Head, Cardiothoracic Surgery
Department of Surgery
Cardiac Surgeon in Chief
Department of Surgery
University of Colorado Denver School of Medicine
Aurora, Colorado
Prosthetic Valve Endocarditis

Francis Fynn-Thompson, MD
Instructor in Surgery
Harvard Medical School
Surgical Director, Heart and Lung Transplantation
Surgical Director, Mechanical Support Program
Department of Cardiac Surgery
Children's Hospital Boston
Boston, Massachusetts
Surgical Approaches, Cardiopulmonary Bypass, and Mechanical Circulatory Support in Children; Arrhythmia and Pacemaker Surgery in Congenital Heart Disease

Lawrence A. Garcia, MD
Associate Professor of Medicine
Tufts University Medical Center
St. Elizabeth's Medical Center
Boston, Massachusetts
Coronary Angiography: Valve and Hemodynamic Assessment; Peripheral Angiography and Percutaneous Intervention

J. William Gaynor, MD
Assistant Professor of Surgery
University of Pennsylvania School of Medicine
Attending Surgeon
The Children's Hospital of Philadelphia
Philadelphia, Pennsylvania
Surgery for Congenital Anomalies of the Coronary Arteries

Tal Geva, MD
Professor of Pediatrics
Harvard Medical School
Chief, Division of Noninvasive Cardiac Imaging
Department of Cardiology
Children's Hospital Boston
Boston, Massachusetts
Diagnostic Imaging: Echocardiography and Magnetic Resonance Imaging

Sébastien Gilbert, MD
Assistant Professor of Surgery
Department of Surgery, Division of Thoracic and Foregut Surgery
University of Pittsburgh School of Medicine
Thoracic Surgeon
University of Pittsburgh Medical Center and Pittsburgh VA Medical Center
Heart, Lung and Esophageal Surgery Institute
UPMC Horizon
Pittsburgh, Pennsylvania
Endoscopic Therapies for Thoracic Diseases

A. Marc Gillinov, MD
Judith Dion Pyle Chair in Heart Valve Research
Department of Thoracic and Cardiovascular Surgery
Cleveland Clinic
Cleveland, Ohio
Tumors of the Heart

Donald D. Glower, MD
Professor
Department of Surgery
Duke University School of Medicine
Durham, North Carolina
Pericardium and Constrictive Pericarditis

Raja R. Gopaldas, MD
Thoracic Surgery Resident
Texas Heart Institute/Baylor College of Medicine
Houston, Texas
Occlusive Disease of the Brachiocephalic Vessels and Surgical Management of Simultaneous Carotid and Coronary Artery Diseases

Frederick L. Grover, MD
Department of Surgery
University of Colorado Health Sciences Center
Aurora, Colorado
Prosthetic Valve Endocarditis; Thrombosis and Thromboembolism of Prosthetic Cardiac Valves and Extracardiac Prostheses

Julius Guccione, PhD
Associate Professor of Surgery
Department of Surgery
University of California at San Francisco
Associate Professor of Surgery
VA Medical Center
San Francisco, California
Ventricular Mechanics

Constanza J. Gutierrez, MD
Director, Medical Student Education
Department of Radiology
University of Texas Health Science Center at San Antonio
San Antonio, Texas
Radiologic Imaging of Thoracic Abnormalities

John R. Guyton, MD
Associate Professor of Medicine
Assistant Professor of Pathology
Duke University School of Medicine
Director, Duke Lipid Clinic
Duke University Medical Center
Durham, North Carolina
The Coronary Circulation: Dietary and Pharmacologic Management of Atherosclerosis

John W. Hammon, MD
Professor of Surgery Emeritus
Wake Forest University School of Medicine
Department of Cardiothoracic Surgery
Wake Forest University Baptist Medical Center
Winston-Salem, North Carolina
Neuropsychological Deficits and Stroke

Zane T. Hammoud, MD
Chief of Thoracic Surgery
Henry Ford Hospital
Detroit, Michigan
The Middle Mediastinum

Thomas H. Hauser, MD, MMSc, MPH, FACC
Assistant Professor
Department of Medicine
Harvard Medical School
Director of Nuclear Cardiology
Department of Medicine
Beth Israel Deaconess Medical Center
Boston, Massachusetts
Applications of Cardiovascular Magnetic Resonance Imaging and Computed Tomography in Cardiovascular Diagnosis

Jennifer C. Hirsch, MD, MS
Lecturer
Department of Surgery
University of Michigan Medical School
Pediatric Cardiovascular Surgeon
C.S. Mott Children's Hospital Congenital Heart Center
University of Michigan Health Systems
Ann Arbor, Michigan
Truncus Arteriosus and Aortopulmonary Window

Chuong D. Hoang, MD
Assistant Professor of Surgery
Department of Cardiothoracic Surgery
Stanford University School of Medicine
Staff Surgeon
Department of Cardiothoracic Surgery
Stanford Hospital & Clinics
Stanford, California
Anterior Approach to Superior Sulcus Lesions; Anterior Mediastinal Masses

Osami Honjo, MD
Clinical Fellow, Division of Cardiovascular Surgery
The Hospital for Sick Children/University of Toronto
  Faculty of Medicine
Toronto, Ontario
Canada
Surgical Considerations in Pulmonary Vein Anomalies

Keith A. Horvath, MD
Director, Cardiothoracic Surgery Research Program
National Heart, Lung and Blood Institute
Chief, Cardiothoracic Surgery
NIH Heart Center at Suburban Hospital
Bethesda, Maryland
Transmyocardial Laser Revascularization

Jeffrey Phillip Jacobs, MD, FACS, FACC, FCCP
Clinical Professor in the Department of Surgery
University of South Florida
Surgical Director of Heart Transplantation and ECMO
The Congenital Heart Institute of Florida
All Children's Hospital
Saint Joseph's Hospital of Tampa
Saint Petersburg, Florida
Interrupted Aortic Arch; Quality Improvement and Risk Stratification for Congenital Cardiac Surgery

Marshall L. Jacobs, MD
Consultant, Department of Pediatrics and Congenital Heart
  Surgery
The Pediatrics Institute
Cleveland Clinic
Cleveland, Ohio
Interrupted Aortic Arch

Michael T. Jaklitsch, MD
Department of Thoracic Surgery
Brigham and Womens' Hospital
Boston, Massachusetts
Surgery of the Diaphragm: A Deductive Approach

Stuart W. Jamieson, MB, FRCS
Distinguished Professor of Surgery
Division of Cardiothoracic Surgery
University of California, San Diego, School of Medicine
La Jolla, California
Surgery for Pulmonary Embolism

Doraid Jarrar, MD
Staff Surgeon
Division of Cardiothoracic Surgery
Albert Einstein Medical Center
Philadelphia, Pennsylvania
Benign Lesions of the Lung

Douglas R. Johnston, MD
Staff Surgeon
Department of Thoracic and Cardiovascular Surgery
Cleveland Clinic
Cleveland, Ohio
Acquired Aortic Valve Disease

David R. Jones, MD
George R. Minor Professor of Surgery
University of Virginia School of Medicine
Chief, Division of Cardiothoracic Surgery
University of Virginia Medical Center
Charlottesville, Virginia
Other Primary Tumors of the Lung

Mark E. Josephson, MD
Department of Medicine, Cardiovascular Division
Beth Israel Deaconess Medical Center
Boston, Massachusetts
Catheter Ablation of Arrhythmias

Lilian P. Joventino, MD
Assistant Professor of Medicine
Brown University School of Medicine
Providence, Rhode Island
Staff Physician
Beth Israel Deaconess Hospital–Needham
Needham, Massachusetts
Cardiac Devices for the Treatment of Bradyarrhythmias and Tachyarrhythmias

Amy L. Juraszek, MD, FAAP, FACC
Assistant Professor of Pathology and Pediatrics
Harvard Medical School
Director, Cardiac Registry
Associate in Cardiology
Children's Hospital Boston
Boston, Massachusetts
Cardiac Embryology and Genetics

Larry R. Kaiser, MD
Alkek Williams Distinguished Professor
Department of Cardiovascular and Thoracic Surgery
University of Texas Medical School at Houston
President and Chief Executive Officer
The University of Texas Health Sciences Center at Houston
Houston, Texas
The Posterior Mediastinum

Kirk R. Kanter, MD
Professor of Surgery
Department of Surgery, Division of Cardiothoracic Surgery
Emory University School of Medicine
Chief, Pediatric Cardiac Surgery
Children's Healthcare of Atlanta at Egleston
Atlanta, Georgia
Management of Single Ventricle and Cavopulmonary Connections

Aditya K. Kaza, MD
Assistant Professor of Surgery
Section of Pediatric Cardiothoracic Surgery
Department of Surgery
University of Utah School of Medicine
Pediatric Cardiothoracic Surgeon
Primary Children's Medical Center
Congenital Cardiac Surgeon
University of Utah Hospitals
Salt Lake City, Utah
Atrioventricular Canal Defects

Steven M. Keller, MD
Chief, Department of Cardiothoracic Surgery
Montefiore Medical Center
Bronx, New York
Surgical Treatment of Hyperhidrosis

Clinton D. Kemp, MD
Senior General Surgery Resident
Department of Surgery
Johns Hopkins Medical Institutions
Baltimore, Maryland
Thoracic Trauma

Kemp H. Kernstine, MD, PhD
Clinical Professor of Surgery
University of California, San Diego, School of Medicine
La Jolla
Chief, Division of Thoracic Surgery
Director, Lung Cancer and Thoracic Oncology Program
City of Hope National Medical Center and Beckman Research Institute
Duarte, California
Congenital Lung Diseases

Shaf Keshavjee, MD, MSc, FRCSC, FACS
F.G. Pearson–R.J. Ginsberg Chair in Thoracic Surgery
Professor of Surgery
University of Toronto Faculty of Medicine
Head, Division of Thoracic Surgery
University Health Network
Toronto, Ontario
Canada
Lung Cancer: Surgical Treatment

Mark J. Krasna, MD, FACS
Medical Director
St. Joseph Medical Center–The Cancer Institute
Towson, Maryland
Neoadjuvant and Adjuvant Therapy for Esophageal Cancer

John C. Kucharczuk, MD
Assistant Professor of Surgery
University of Pennsylvania School of Medicine
Surgeon
University of Pennsylvania Health System
Philadelphia, Pennsylvania
Anterior Mediastinal Masses; Surgery for Emphysema

Alan P. Kypson, MD
Associate Professor of Surgery
Department of Cardiovascular Sciences
East Carolina Heart Institute at East Carolina University
Greenville, North Carolina
Robotic Cardiac Surgery and Novel Visualization Systems

Roger J. Laham, MD
Associate Professor of Medicine
Harvard Medical School
Research Investigator
CardioVascular Institute
Beth Israel Deaconess Medical Center
Boston, Massachusetts
Nonatherosclerotic Coronary Heart Disease

Michael J. Landzberg, MBBS
Assistant in Cardiology
Department of Cardiology and Medicine
Harvard Medical School
Harvard University
Director
Boston Adult Congenital Heart and Pulmonary Hypertension Group
Children's Hospital Boston
Brigham and Women's Hospital
Boston, Massachusetts
Adult Congenital Cardiac Surgery

Peter C. Laussen, MD
Professor
Department of Anesthesia
Harvard Medical School
Chief,
Division of Cardiovascular Critical Care
Department of Cardiology
Children's Hospital Boston
DD Hansen Chair in Pediatric Anesthesia
Department of Anesthesia
Children's Hospital Boston
Boston, Massachusetts
Surgical Approaches, Cardiopulmonary Bypass, and Mechanical Circulatory Support in Children; Pediatric Anesthesia and Critical Care

Lawrence S. Lee, MD
Resident
Department of Surgery
Brigham and Women's Hospital
Boston, Massachusetts
Management of Native Valve Endocarditis

Scott A. LeMaire, MD
Associate Professor and Director of Research
Division of Cardiothoracic Surgery
Michael E. DeBakey Department of Surgery
Baylor College of Medicine
Cardiovascular Surgery Service
The Texas Heart Institute at St. Luke's Episcopal Hospital
Houston, Texas
Occlusive Disease of the Brachiocephalic Vessels and Surgical Management of Simultaneous Carotid and Coronary Artery Diseases

Sidney Levitsky, MD
David W. and David Cheever Professor of Surgery
Harvard Medical School
Director, Cardiothoracic Surgery Care Group
Senior Vice-Chairman
Department of Surgery
Beth Israel Deaconess Medical Center
Boston, Massachusetts
Myocardial Protection

Jerrold H. Levy, MD, FAHA
Professor and Deputy Chair For Research
Anesthesiology and Critical Care
Emory University School of Medicine
Director of Cardiothoracic Anesthesiology
Anesthesiology and Critical Care
Emory Healthcare
Atlanta, Georgia
Emory University Hosptial
Atlanta, Georgia
Blood Coagulation, Transfusion, and Conservation

John R. Liddicoat, MD
Vice President/General Manager
Structural Heart Disease
Medtronic, Inc.
Minneapolis, Minnesota
Tumors of the Heart

Peter H. Lin, MD
Associate Professor
Chief, Division of Vascular Surgery and Endovascular Therapy
Michael E. DeBakey Department of Surgery
Baylor College of Medicine
Chief of Vascular Surgery
Michael E. DeBakey VA Medical Center
Houston, Texas
Occlusive Disease of the Brachiocephalic Vessels and Surgical Management of Simultaneous Carotid and Coronary Artery Diseases

Philip A. Linden, MD
Chief, Division of Thoracic and Esophageal Surgery
Case Medical Center
Cleveland, Ohio
Esophageal Resection and Replacement

John C. Lipham, MD
Assistant Professor of Surgery
Department of Surgery
University of Southern California
Keck School of Medicine
Los Angeles, California
Esophageal Anatomy and Function

Michael J. Liptay, MD
Associate Professor of Surgery
Department of Cardiovascular-Thoracic Surgery
Rush Medical College
Chief, Division of Thoracic Surgery
Rush University Medical Center
Chicago, Illinois
The Middle Mediastinum

Virginia R. Litle, MD
Assistant Professor of Surgery
Mount Sinai School of Medicine
Transplant Surgeon, Department of Cardiothoracic Surgery
Mount Sinai Medical Center
New York, New York
Staging Techniques for Carcinoma of the Esophagus

Bruce W. Lytle, MD
Chairman, Sydell and Arnold Miller Family Heart & Vascular Institute
Staff Cardiac Surgeon, Department of Thoracic and Cardiovascular Surgery
Cleveland Clinic
Cleveland, Ohio
Re-do Coronary Artery Bypass Surgery

James D. Luketich, MD
Professor of Surgery
Henry T. Bahnson Chair in Thoracic Oncology
Department of Surgery
University of Pittsburgh School of Medicine
Chief, Division of Thoracic and Foregut Surgery
Director, Thoracic Surgical Oncology
Co-Director, Lung Cancer Center
University of Pittsburgh Medical Center
Director, Heart, Lung and Esophageal Surgery Institute
UPMC Horizon
Pittsburgh, Pennsylvania
Endoscopic Therapies for Thoracic Diseases; Innovative Therapy and Technology

Michael M. Madani, MD
Associate Clinical Professor of Surgery
Division of Cardiothoracic Surgery
University of California, San Diego, School of Medicine
La Jolla, California
Surgery for Pulmonary Embolism

Michael A. Maddaus, MD
Professor of Surgery
University of Minnesota Medical School
Chief, Division of Thoracic and Foregut Surgery
Program Director, General Surgery
Co-Director, Minimally Invasive Surgery Center
Garamella Lynch Jensen Chair in Thoracic Cardiovascular Surgery
Department of Surgery
University of Minnesota Medical Center
Fairview Health Services
Minneapolis, Minnesota
The Use of Genetic Science in Thoracic Disease

Feroze Mahmood, MD
Assistant Professor
Department of Anesthesiology
Harvard Medical School
Director, Vascular Anesthesia/Perioperative Echocardiography
Department of Anesthesia Critical Care and Pain Medicine
Beth Israel Deaconess Medical Center
Boston, Massachusetts
Adult Cardiac Anesthesia

Hari R. Mallidi, MD
Instructor in Cardiothoracic Surgery
Stanford University School of Medicine
Stanford
Director, Cardiothoracic Surgery
Regional Medical Center of San Jose
San Jose, California
Heart-Lung Transplantation

Abeel A. Mangi, MD
Director, Lung and Heart Transplant
Director, Mechanical Circulation
Attending Cardiac Surgeon
Temple University Hospital
Philadelphia, Pennsylvania
Postinfarction Ventricular Septal Defect

Warren S. Manning, MD
Professor of Medicine and Radiology
Harvard Medical School
Section Chief, Non-Invasive Cardiac Imaging
Beth Israel Deaconess Medical Center
Boston, Massachusetts
Applications of Cardiovascular Magnetic Resonance Imaging and Computed Tomography in Cardiovascular Diagnosis

Edith M. Marom, MD
Professor
Department of Diagnostic Radiology, Division of Diagnostic Imaging
The University of Texas M.D. Anderson Cancer Center
Houston, Texas
Radiologic Imaging of Thoracic Abnormalities

Audrey C. Marshall, MD
Chief, Invasive Cardiology
Associate in Cardiology
Children's Hospital Boston
Department of Cardiology
Boston, Massachusetts
Cardiac Catheterization and Fetal Intervention

Christopher E. Mascio, MD
Assistant Professor of Surgery
Division of Thoracic and Cardiovascular Surgery
University of Louisville School of Medicine
Staff Surgeon, Congenital Cardiothoracic Surgery
Kosair Children's Hospital
Louisville, Kentucky
Pulmonary Atresia with Intact Ventricular Septum

David P. Mason, MD
Staff Surgeon
Department of Thoracic Surgery
Cleveland Clinic Foundation
Cleveland, Ohio
Lung Cancer: Multimodal Therapy; Spontaneous Pneumothorax

Douglas J. Mathisen, MD
Hermes H. Grillo Professor of Thoracic Surgery
Department of Surgery
Harvard Medical School
Chief, Division of Cardiothoracic Surgery
Department of Surgery
Massachusetts General Hospital
Boston, Massachusetts
Tracheal Lesions

Kenneth L. Mattox, MD
Professor and Vice Chair
Michael E. DeBakey Department of Surgery
Baylor College of Medicine
Chief of Staff/Chief of Surgery
Ben Taub General Hospital
Houston, Texas
Injury to the Heart and Great Vessels

Robina Matyal, MD
Instructor in Anesthesiology and Critical Care
Department of Anesthesia and Critical Care
Harvard Medical School
Instructor in Anesthesia and Critical Care
Department of Anesthesia and Critical Care
Beth Israel Deaconess Medical Center
Boston, Massachusetts
Adult Cardiac Anesthesia

John E. Mayer, MD
Department of Pediatric Cardiac Surgery
Children's Hospital Boston
Boston, Massachusetts
Pulmonary Atresia with Ventricular Septal Defect and Right Ventricle–to–Pulmonary Artery Conduits

James McCulley, PhD
Associate Professor of Surgery
Harvard Medical School
Director, Cardiac Surgery Research
Beth Israel Deaconess Medical Center
Boston, Massachusetts
Myocardial Protection

Doff McElhinney, MD
Assistant Professor of Pediatrics
Harvard Medical School
Associate in Cardiology
Department of Cardiology
Children's Hospital Boston
Boston, Massachusetts
Cardiac Catheterization and Fetal Intervention

Edwin C. McGee, Jr., MD
Assistant Professor in Surgery
Division of Cardiothoracic Surgery
Northwestern University Feinberg School of Medicine
Surgical Director, Heart Transplantation and Mechanical Assistance
Bluhm Cardiovascular Institute
Northwestern Memorial Hospital
Chicago, Illinois
Valve Replacement Therapy: History, Options, and Valve Type

Francis X. McGowan, Jr., MD
Professor of Anaesthesia (Pediatrics)
Harvard Medical School
Chief, Division of Cardiac Anesthesia
Director, Anesthesia/Critical Care Medicine Research Laboratory
Children's Hospital Boston
Boston, Massachusetts
Surgical Approaches and Cardiopulmonary Bypass in Pediatric Cardiac Surgery

Ciaran McNamee, MD
Instructor in Surgery
Department of Surgery
Harvard Medical School
Associate Surgeon
Department of Surgery
Brigham and Women's Hospital
Boston, Massachusetts
Pleural Tumors

Spencer J. Melby, MD
Fellow
Division of Cardiothoracic Surgery
Department of Surgery
Washington University in St. Louis
Fellow
Division of Cardiothoracic Surgery
Department of Surgery
Barnes Jewish Hospital
St. Louis, Missouri
Surgical Treatment of Arrhythmias

Lorenzo Menicanti, MD, FECTS
Department of Cardiac Surgery
IRCCS Istituto Policlinico San Donato
Milan, Italy
Left Ventricular Restoration: Surgical Treatment of the Failing Heart

Bryan F. Meyers, MD
Patrick and Joy Williamson Endowed Chair in Cardiothoracic Surgery
Professor, Surgery
Division of Cardiothoracic Surgery
Chief, Thoracic Surgery
Director, Lung Volume Reduction Program
Saint Louis, Missouri
Surgery for Emphysema; Mediastinal Anatomy and Mediastinoscopy

Carmelo A. Milano, MD
Associate Professor
Division Cardiovascular and Thoracic Surgery
Department of Surgery
Duke University School of Medicine
Durham, North Carolina
Critical Care for the Adult Cardiac Patient

D. Craig Miller, MD
Thelma and Henry Doelger Professor of Cardiovascular Surgery
Department of Cardiovascular Surgery
Stanford University School of Medicine
Stanford
Department of Cardiothoracic Surgery
Stanford University Medical Center
Palo Alto, California
Type A Aortic Dissection; Type B Aortic Dissection

Daniel L. Miller, MD
Kamal A. Mansour Professor of Surgery
Emory University School of Medicine
Chief, Section of General Thoracic Surgery
Surgical Director, Thoracic Oncology Program
The Emory Clinic
Emory Healthcare
Atlanta, Georgia
Empyema

John D. Mitchell, MD
Associate Professor of Surgery
University of Colorado–Denver School of Medicine
Chief, Section of General Thoracic Surgery
Division of Cardiothoracic Surgery
University of Colorado Hospital
Aurora
VA Eastern Colorado Healthcare System
Denver, Colorado
Infectious Lung Diseases

Jeffrey A. Morgan, MD
Associate Director,
Circulatory Assist Device Program and Cardiac Transplantation
Division of Cardiothoracic Surgery
Henry Ford Health System
Detroit, Michigan
Ventricular Assist Devices

Sudish C. Murthy, MD, PhD
Surgical Director, Center of Major Airway Disease
Department of Thoracic and Cardiovascular Surgery
Heart and Vascular Institute
Cleveland Clinic
Cleveland, Ohio
Lung Cancer: Multimodal Therapy; Surgical Treatment of Benign Esophageal Diseases

Sacha Mussot, MD, MSc
Department of Thoracic and Cardiovascular Surgery
Paris Sud University
Le Kremlin–Bicêtre
Staff Surgeon
Department of Thoracic and Vascular Surgery and Heart-Lung Transplantation
Marie Lannelongue Hospital
Le Plessis Robinson
Paris
France
Anterior Approach to Superior Sulcus Lesions

Alykhan S. Nagji, MD
Thoracic Surgery Research Resident
Department of Surgery
University Hospital and Primary Care Center
University of Virginia Health System
Charlottesville, Virginia
Other Primary Tumors of the Lung

Yoshifumi Naka, MD, PhD
Associate Professor of Surgery
Columbia University College of Physicians and Surgeons
Director, Cardiac Transplantation and Mechanical Circulatory Support Programs
NewYork–Presbyterian Hospital
New York, New York
Ventricular Assist Devices

Kurt D. Newman, MD
Professor
Departments of Surgery and Pediatrics
George Washington University School of Medicine and Health Sciences
Senior Vice President and Surgeon in Chief
Joseph E. Robert, Jr. Center for Surgical Care
Children's National Medical Center
Washington, DC
Surgery for Congenital Lesions of the Esophagus

Chukwumere Nwogu, MD
Associate Professor of Surgery
Department of Surgery
Associate Professor of Oncology
State University of New York University of Buffalo School of Medicine and Biomedical Sciences
Department of Thoracic Surgery
Roswell Park Cancer Institute
Buffalo, New York
Malignant Pleural and Pericardial Effusions

Kirsten C. Odegard, MD
Associate Professor of Anaesthesia
Harvard Medical School
Co-Clinical Director, Cardiac Anesthesia Division
Department of Anesthesia, Perioperative and Pain Medicine
Children's Hospital Boston
Boston, Massachusetts
Pediatric Anesthesia and Critical Care

Richard G. Ohye, MD
Associate Professor
Department of Surgery
University of Michigan Medical School
Director, Pediatric Cardiac Surgery
Director, Pediatric Cardiovascular Transplant Program
Program Director, Thoracic and Congenital Cardiac Surgery Residencies
University of Michigan Health Systems
Ann Arbor, Michigan
Truncus Arteriosus and Aortopulmonary Window

Mark W. Onaitis, MD
Department of Surgery, Division of Cardiovascular and Thoracic Surgery
Duke University Medical Center
Durham, North Carolina
Lung Cancer: Minimally Invasive Approaches

Catherine M. Otto, MD
J. Ward Kennedy-Hamilton Endowed Professor of Cardiology
Department of Medicine
University of Washington School of Medicine
Director, Cardiology Fellowship Programs
University of Washington Medical Center
Seattle, Washington
Diagnostic Echocardiography (Ultrasound Imaging in Cardiovascular Diagnosis)

Mehmet C. Oz, MD, FACS
Professor of Surgery
Columbia University College of Physicians and Surgeons
Staff Surgeon
Division of Thoracic Surgery
NewYork–Presbyterian Hospital
New York, New York
Ventricular Assist Devices

Bernard J. Park, MD
Assistant Attending Surgeon
Thoracic Service, Department of Surgery
Memorial Sloan-Kettering Cancer Center
New York, New York
Lung Cancer Workup and Staging

Amit N. Patel, MD
Associate Professor
Division of Cardiothoracic Surgery
Department of Surgery
University of Utah School of Medicine
Associate Professor
University of Utah Health Sciences Center
Salt Lake City, Utah
Thoracic Outlet Syndrome and Dorsal Sympathectomy

G. Alexander Patterson, MD
Evarts A. Graham Professor of Surgery
Department of Surgery, Division of Cardiothoracic Surgery
Washington University in St. Louis School of Medicine
St. Louis, Missouri
Lung Transplantation

Edward F. Patz, Jr., MD
James and Alice Chen Professor of Radiology
Department of Radiology and Department of Pharmacology and Cancer Biology
Duke University School of Medicine
Durham, North Carolina
Radiologic Imaging of Thoracic Abnormalities

Subroto Paul, MD
Assistant Professor of Cardiothoracic Surgery
Weill Cornell Medical College
Attending Surgeon, Division of Thoracic Surgery
NewYork–Presbyterian Hospital
New York, New York
Interstitial Lung Diseases

Arjun Pennathur, MD
Assistant Professor of Surgery
University of Pittsburgh School of Medicine
Heart, Lung and Esophageal Surgery Institute
University of Pittsburgh Medical Center
Pittsburgh, Pennsylvania
Innovative Therapy and Technology

Frank A. Pigula, MD
Assistant Professor of Surgery
Harvard Medical School
Associate in Cardiac Surgery
Children's Hospital Boston
Boston, Massachusetts
Surgery for Congenital Anomalies of the Aortic Valve and Root; Transposition of the Great Arteries: Simple and Complex Forms; Hypoplastic Left Heart Syndrome

Duane S. Pinto, MD
Assistant Clinical Professor of Medicine
Harvard Medical School
Director, Peripheral Angiographic Core Laboratory
CardioVascular Institute
Director, Cardiovascular Disease Fellowship Training Program
Beth Israel Deaconess Medical Center
Boston, Massachusetts
Interventional Cardiology

Marvin Pomerantz, MD
Professor of Surgery
Department of Surgery, Cardiothoracic Division
University of Colorado, Denver School of Medicine
Cardiothoracic Surgeon
University of Colorado Hospital
Aurora, Colorado
Infectious Lung Diseases

Jeffrey L. Port, MD
Associate Professor of Cardiothoracic Surgery
Weill Cornell Medical College
Associate Attending
Department of Cardiothoracic Surgery
NewYork–Presbyterian Hospital
New York, New York
Screening for Lung Cancer

Yuri B. Pride, MD
Cardiovascular Fellow
Beth Israel Deaconess Medical Center
Harvard Medical School
Boston, Massachusetts
Coronary Angiography: Valve and Hemodynamic Assessment; Peripheral Angiography and Percutaneous Intervention

Varun Puri, MD
Assistant Professor
Department of Surgery
Washington University in St. Louis School of Medicine
St. Louis, Missouri
Lung Transplantation; Mediastinal Anatomy and Mediastinoscopy

Basel Ramlawi, MD, MMSc
Attending Surgeon
Department of Cardiovascular Surgery
Methodist DeBakey Heart & Vascular Center
The Methodist Hospital
Houston, Texas
Vascular Physiology

Mark Ratcliffe, MD
Professor and Vice-Chair, Department of Surgery
University of California, San Francisco, School of Medicine
Chief of Surgery
San Francisco VA Medical Center
San Francisco, California
Ventricular Mechanics

John J. Reilly, Jr., MD
Vice Chair for Clinical Affairs
Visiting Professor of Medicine
Department of Medicine
University of Pittsburgh School of Medicine
Pittsburgh, Pennsylvania
Preoperative Evaluation of Patients Undergoing Thoracic Surgery

Bruce A. Reitz, MD
Norman E. Shumway Professor of Cardiothoracic Surgery
Department of Cardiothoracic Surgery
Stanford University School of Medicine
Stanford
Attending Surgeon
Department of Cardiothoracic Surgery
Stanford Hospital & Clinics
Palo Alto, California
Heart-Lung Transplantation

Karl G. Reyes, MD
Cardiothoracic Surgery Fellow
Department of Thoracic and Cardiovascular Surgery
Cleveland Clinic
Cleveland, Ohio
Spontaneous Pneumothorax

Thomas W. Rice, MD
Head, Section of General Thoracic Surgery
Department of Thoracic and Cardiovascular Surgery
Cleveland Clinic
Cleveland, Ohio
Lung Cancer: Multimodal Therapy Surgical Treatment of Benign Esophageal Diseases

Robert C. Robbins, MD
Department of Cardiovascular Surgery
Stanford University School of Medicine
Stanford, California
Heart Transplantation

Gaetano Rocco, MD, FRCS(Ed)
Department of Thoracic Surgery and Oncology
Division of Thoracic Surgery
National Cancer Institute, Pascale Foundation
Naples, Italy
Chylothorax

Audrey Rosinberg, MD
Vascular and Endovascular Surgeon
Assistant Program Director for Vascular Surgery
Lenox Hill Hospital
New York, New York
Nonatherosclerotic Coronary Heart Disease

Fraser Rubens, MD, MSc, FRCSC
Professor of Surgery
Department of Cardiac Surgery
University of Ottawa Faculty of Medicine
Cardiac Surgeon
University of Ottawa Heart Institute
Ottawa, Ontario
Canada
Cardiopulmonary Bypass: Technique and Pathophysiology

Marc Ruel, MD, MPH, FRCSC
Associate Professor
Department of Cardiac Surgery, Division of Cellular and Molecular Medicine
University of Ottawa Faculty of Medicine
Cardiac Surgeon and Cardiac Surgery Research Chair
Division of Cardiac Surgery
University of Ottawa Heart Institute
Ottawa, Ontario
Canada
Coronary Artery Bypass Grafting; Regenerative Cell-Based Therapy for the Treatment of Cardiac Disease

Valerie W. Rusch, MD
Professor of Surgery
Cornell Weill Medical College
Chief, Thoracic Service
Miner Chair in Intrathoracic Cancers
Department of Surgery
Memorial Sloan-Kettering Cancer Center
New York, New York
Lung Cancer Workup and Staging

Joseph F. Sabik III, MD
Chairman of Thoracic and Cardiovascular Surgery
Sydell and Arnold Miller Family Heart & Vascular Institute
Cleveland Clinic
Cleveland, Ohio
Acquired Aortic Valve Disease

Hartzell V. Schaff, MD
Chair, Division of Cardiovascular Surgery
Stuart W. Harrington Professor of Surgery
Mayo Medical School College of Medicine
Consultant, Cardiovascular Surgery
Mayo Clinic
Rochester, Minnesota
Surgical Management of Hypertrophic Cardiomyopathy

Frank W. Sellke, MD
Karl E. Karlson and Gloria A. Karlson
  Professor of Cardiothoracic Surgery and Chief,
Division of Cardiothoracic Surgery
Alpert Medical School of Brown University
  and Lifespan Hospitals
Co-director, Lifespan Heart Center
Providence, Rhode Island
Visiting Professor of Surgery
Harvard Medical School
Boston, Massachusetts
Vascular Physiology; Coronary Artery Bypass Grafting; Regenerative Cell-Based Therapy for the Treatment of Cardiac Disease

Rohit Shahani, MD, MCH, FACC
Consultant, Cardiothoracic Surgeon
Vassar Brothers Medical Center
Poughkeepsie, New York
Anatomy of the Thorax

Robert C. Shamberger, MD
Robert E. Gross Professor of Surgery
Department of Surgery
Harvard Medical School
Chief of Surgery
Department of Surgery
Children's Hospital Boston
Boston, Massachusetts
Congenital Chest Wall Deformities

Steven S. Shay, MD
Staff Physician
Department of Gastroenterology
Cleveland Clinic
Cleveland, Ohio
Surgical Treatment of Benign Esophageal Diseases

Joseph B. Shrager, MD
Professor
Department of Cardiothoracic Surgery
Stanford University School of Medicine
Stanford
Chief, Division of Thoracic Surgery
Stanford Hospital & Clinics
Staff Surgeon
Palo Alto VA Medical Center
Palo Alto, California
Anterior Mediastinal Masses

Dhruv Singhal, MD
Division of Plastic Surgery
Brigham and Women's Hospital
Boston, Massachusetts
The Posterior Mediastinum

Peter K. Smith, MD
Professor of Surgery
Duke University School of Medicine
Chief, Cardiovascular and Thoracic Surgery
Duke University Medical Center
Durham, North Carolina
Critical Care for the Adult Cardiac Patient

Richard G. Smith, MSEE
Marshall Foundation Artificial Heart Laboratory
University Medical Center
Tucson, Arizona
Total Artificial Heart

R. John Solaro, PhD
Distinguished University Professor and Head, Department
  of Physiology and Biophysics
University of Illinois at Chicago College of Medicine
Chicago, Illinois
Physiology of the Myocardium

David J. Spurlock, MD
General Surgery Resident
Department of General Surgery
Georgetown University
General Surgery Resident
Department of General Surgery
Georgetown University Hospital
Washington-District of Columbia
Surgery for Congenital Lesions of The Esophagus

Marie E. Steiner, MD, MS
Associate Professor
Department of Pediatrics, Division of Hematology-
    Oncology and Blood and Marrow Transplantation
University of Minnesota Medical School
Pediatric Critical Care Physician and Pediatric
    Hematologist-Oncologist
University of Minnesota Amplatz Children's Hospital
Fairview Health Services
Minneapolis, Minnesota
  Blood Coagulation, Transfusion, and Conservation

Matthew A. Steliga, MD
Assistant Professor
Department of Surgery, Division of Cardiothoracic Surgery
University of Arkansas for Medical Sciences College of
    Medicine
Little Rock, Arkansas
  *Lung Cancer: Surgical Strategies for Tumors Invading the
  Chest Wall*

Brendon M. Stiles, MD
Assistant Professor of Cardiothoracic Surgery
Department of Cardiothoracic Surgery, Division of Thoracic
    Surgery
Weill Cornell Medical College
Assistant Attending Cardiothoracic Surgeon
NewYork–Presbyterian Hospital
New York, New York
  Screening for Lung Cancer

Michaela Straznicka, MD, FACS
Director Thoracic Oncology Program
John Muir Medical Center
Walnut Creek, California
  *Lung Cancer: Surgical Strategies for Tumors Invading
  the Chest Wall*

David A. Stump, MD
Professor
Anesthesiology and Cardiothoracic Surgery
Wake Forest University School of Medicine
Winston Salem, North Carolina
  Neuropsychological Deficits and Stroke

David J. Sugarbaker, MD
Department of Thoracic Surgery
Brigham and Women's Hospital
Boston, Massachusetts
  Pleural Tumors

Erik J. Suuronen, PhD
Assistant Professor
Department of Surgery
University of Ottawa
Principal Investigator
Division of Cardiac Surgery
University of Ottawa Heart Institute
Ottawa, Ontario, Canada
  *Regenerative Cell-Based Therapy for the Treatment of Cardiac
  Disease*

Lars G. Svensson, MD, PhD
Professor of Surgery
Department of Thoracic and Cardiovascular Surgery
Cleveland Clinic Lerner College of Medicine of Case
    Western Reserve University
Director, Aorta Center
Director, Marfan and Connective Tissue Disorder Clinic
Director, Quality and Process Improvement for Department
    of Cardiothoracic Surgery
Cleveland Clinic
Cleveland, Ohio
  *Surgery of the Aortic Arch; Descending Thoracic and
  Thoracoabdominal Aortic Surgery*

Scott J. Swanson, MD
Director of Minimally Invasive Thoracic Surgery
Division of Thoracic Surgery
Brigham and Women's Hospital
Chief Surgical Officer
Dana-Farber Cancer Institute
Harvard Medical School
Boston, Massachusetts
  Eshophageal Resection and Replacement

Wilson Y. Szeto, MD
Assistant Professor of Surgery
Division of Cardiovascular Surgery
Department of Surgery
University of Pennsylvania Medical Center
Philadelphia, Pennsylvania
  *Endovascular Therapy for Thoracic Aortic Aneurysms
  and Dissections*

Kenichi A. Tanaka, MD, MSc
Associate Professor of Anesthesiology
Department of Anesthesiology
Emory University School of Medicine
Attending Anesthesiologist
Department of Anesthesiology
Emory University School of Medicine
Atlanta, Georgia
  Blood Coagulation, Transfusion, and Conservation

Benedict J. W. Taylor, MD
Chief Resident
University of Washington Medical Center
Department of Cardiothoracic Surgery
Seattle, Washington
Endoscopic Diagnosis of Thoracic Disease

Patricia A. Thistlethwaite, MD, PhD
Associate Professor of Surgery
Division of Cardiothoracic Surgery
University of California, San Diego, School of Medicine
La Jolla, California
Surgery for Pulmonary Embolism

Peter Tsai, MD
Assistant Professor
Michael E. DeBakey Department of Surgery
Baylor College of Medicine
Houston, Texas
Injury to the Heart and Great Vessels

Harold C. Urschel, Jr., MD
Professor of Cardiovascular and Thoracic Surgery
University of Texas Southwestern Medical School
Chair, Cardiovascular and Thoracic Surgical Research,
    Education, and Clinical Excellence
Department of Cardiovascular and Thoracic Surgery
Baylor University Medical Center
Dallas, Texas
Thoracic Outlet Syndrome and Dorsal Sympathectomy

Anne Marie Valente, MD
Instructor in Pediatrics
Harvard Medical School
Assistant in Cardiology
Children's Hospital Boston
Assistant in Cardiology
Brigham and Women's Hospital
Boston Adult Congenital Heart and Pulmonary
    Hypertension Program
Boston, Massachusetts
Adult Congenital Cardiac Surgery

Timothy L. Van Natta, MD
Associate Clinical Professor of Surgery
David Geffen School of Medicine at UCLA
Los Angeles
Staff Surgeon
Department of Surgery
Harbor-UCLA Medical Center
Torrance, California
Congenital Lung Diseases

Richard Van Praagh, MD
Professor Emeritus of Pathology
Department of Pathology
Harvard Medical School
Director Emeritus of the Cardiac Registry
Department of Pathology, Cardiology, and Cardiac Surgery
Children's Hospital Boston
Boston, Massachusetts
Segmental Anatomy

Nikolay V. Vasilyev, MD
Instructor in Surgery
Harvard Medical School
Staff Scientist
Department of Cardiac Surgery
Children's Hospital Boston
Boston, Massachusetts
Image-Guided and Hybrid Surgery: Surgical Simulation

Jeffrey B. Velotta, MD
Postdoctoral Fellow
Department of Cardiothoracic Surgery
Stanford University School of Medicine
Stanford, California
Heart Transplantation

Gus J. Vlahakes, MD
Professor of Surgery
Harvard Medical School
Chief, Division of Cardiac Surgery
Massachusetts General Hospital
Boston, Massachusetts
Valve Replacement Therapy: History, Options, and Valve Types

Pierre Voisine, MD, FRCSC
Department of Surgery
Institut Universitaire de Cardiologie et de Pneumologie
    de Quebec
Laval University Faculty of Medicine
Department of Cardiac Surgery
Hôpital Laval
Quebec City, Quebec
Canada
Deep Sternal Wound Infection

Matthew J. Wall, Jr., MD, FACS
Professor of Surgery
Michael E. DeBakey Department of Surgery
Baylor College of Medicine
Deputy Chief of Surgery; Chief of Cardiothoracic Surgery
Ben Taub General Hospital
Houston, Texas
Injury to the Heart and Great Vessels

Arthur Wallace, MD, PhD
Professor of Anesthesiology and Perioperative Care
Department of Anesthesiology and Perioperative Care
University of California, San Francisco
Attending Anesthesiologist
Department of Anesthesiology
San Francisco Veterans Affairs Medical Center
San Francisco, California
Ventricular Mechanics

Garrett L. Walsh, MD
Professor of Surgery
Department of Thoracic and Cardiovascular Surgery, Division of Surgery
The University of Texas M.D. Anderson Cancer Center
Houston, Texas
Lung Cancer: Surgical Strategies for Tumors Invading the Chest Wall

Daniel C. Weiner, MD
Resident
Brigham and Women's Hospital
Boston, Massachusetts
Surgery of the Diaphragm: A Deductive Approach

Todd S. Weiser, MD
Assistant Professor of Cardiothoracic Surgery
Mount Sinai School of Medicine
Thoracic Surgeon
Mount Sinai Medical Center
New York, New York
Tracheal Lesions

Benny Weksler, MD
Assistant Professor of Surgery
Department of Surgery
Jefferson Medical College of Thomas Jefferson University
Thoracic Surgeon
Thomas Jefferson University Hospital
Philadelphia, Pennsylvania
Endoscopic Therapies for Thoracic Diseases

Margaret V. Westfall, PhD
Associate Professor of Surgery
Department of Surgery, Cardiac Surgery Section
Staff Scientist, Westfall Research Laboratory
University of Michigan Medical School
Ann Arbor, Michigan
Physiology of the Myocardium

Benson R. Wilcox, MD
Professor of Surgery
Department of Cardiothoracic Surgery
University of North Carolina at Chapel Hill
University of North Carolina Hospital
Chapel Hill, North Carolina
Surgical Anatomy of the Heart

Jay M. Wilson, MD
Department of Surgery
Children's Hospital Boston
Boston, Massachusetts
Congenital Diaphragmatic Hernia

Joseph J. Wizorek, MD
Assistant Professor of Surgery
Department of Surgery, Division of Thoracic and Foregut Surgery
University of Pittsburgh School of Medicine
Thoracic Surgeon/Clinical Instructor
Heart, Lung and Esophageal Surgery Institute
UPMC Horizon
Greenville, Pennsylvania
Innovative Therapy and Technology

Douglas E. Wood, MD
Professor of Surgery
University of Washington School of Medicine
Associate Chief, Division of Cardiothoracic Surgery
Head, General Thoracic Surgery
University of Washington Medical Center and Seattle Cancer Care Alliance
Seattle, Washington
Endoscopic Diagnosis of Thoracic Disease

David Wrobleski, MD
Staff Electrophysiologist
Department of Cardiology
St. Vincent Hospital
Indainapolis, Indiana
Catheter Ablation of Arrhythmias

John V. Wylie, Jr., MD, FACC
Assistant Professor
Tufts Medical School
Director of Cardiac Electrophysiology
St. Elisabeth's Medical Center
Boston, Massachusetts
Catheter Ablation of Arrhythmias

Stephen C. Yang, MD, FACS, FCCP
Arthur B. and Patricia B. Modell Professor of Thoracic Surgery
Professor of Surgery and Oncology
Department of Surgery, Division of Thoracic Surgery
Johns Hopkins School of Medicine
Chief of Thoracic Surgery
Johns Hopkins Hospital and Johns Hopkins Bayview Medical Center
Baltimore, Maryland
Thoracic Trauma

Godfred Kwame Yankey, MD
Cardiothoracic Surgical Fellow
Division of Cardiothoracic Surgery
University of Maryland School of Medicine/Medical Center
Baltimore, Maryland
Neoadjuvant and Adjuvant therapy for Esophageal Cancer

Sai Yendamuri, MD
Assistant Professor of Surgery
Department of Thoracic Surgery
Assistant Professor of Oncology
State University of New York University of Buffalo School of Medicine and Biomedical Sciences
Staff Surgeon, Department of Surgery, Division of Thoracic Surgery
Roswell Park Cancer Institute
Buffalo, New York
Malignant Pleural and Pericardial Effusions

Susan B. Yeon, MD, JD
Clinical Assistant Professor in Medicine
Cardiovascular Division
Department of Medicine
Beth Israel Deaconess Medical Center
Boston, Massachusetts
Applications of Cardiovascular Magnetic Resonance Imaging and Computed Tomography in Cardiovascular Diagnosis

Barry L. Zaret, MD
Robert W. Berliner Professor of Medicine
Professor of Diagnostic Radiology
Section of Cardiovascular Medicine
Department of Internal Medicine
Yale University School of Medicine
New Haven, Connecticut
Nuclear Cardiology and Positron Emission Tomography in the Assessment of Patients with Cardiovascular Disease

Yan Zhang, MD
Doctoral Student
Department of Cellular and Molecular Medicine
University of Ottawa
Ottawa, Ontario, Canada
Regenerative Cell-Based Therapy for the Treatment of Cardiac Disease

Xiaoqin Zhao, MD
Visiting Professor
Beth Israel Deaconess Medical Center
Boston, Massachusetts
Adult Cardiac Anesthesia

Peter J. Zimetbaum, MD
Associate Professor of Medicine
Harvard Medical School
Clinical Director of Cardiology
Beth Israel Deaconess Medical Center
Boston, Massachusetts
Cardiac Devices for the Treatment of Bradyarrhythmias and Tachyarrhythmias

Hannah Zimmerman, MD
Department of Surgery
University of Arizona Medical Center
Tucson, Arizona
Total Artificial Heart

Preface

Much has evolved in the field of adult and pediatric cardiothoracic surgery since our last edition. Our new 8th edition contains the latest information on the diagnosis and treatment of disease of the thorax. Especially in such areas as stent grafting for aortic disease, intervention for congenital heart disease, thoracic imaging, minimally invasive thoracic surgery, and the surgical treatment of arrhythmias, the field has markedly transformed. Many of the same authors were asked to update their previous chapters, but some chapters have been added or eliminated, and many others have been completely re-written. We hope that the 8th edition will be received with the same enthusiasm as the 7th.

Recently, we lost one of the former editors and a giant in the field of surgery, Dr. David Sabiston. Dr. Sabiston was known not only as an innovative surgeon, having performed one of the first coronary artery bypass procedures, but also as one of the true pioneers in surgical training and education, having personally trained many of the leaders in our speciality. He edited several classic textbooks in the field, including *Sabiston & Spencer Surgery of the Chest*. We are all indebted to his innumerable contributions to the field of surgery.

Frank W. Sellke
Pedro J. del Nido
Scott J. Swanson

Contents

Volume 1

Section 1 Thoracic Surgery

Part A Evaluation and Care

Chapter 1 Anatomy of the Thorax 3
Cynthia Chin and Rohit Shahani

Chapter 2 Radiologic Imaging of Thoracic Abnormalities 25
Constanza J. Gutierrez, Edith M. Marom, Jeremy J. Erasmus, and Edward F. Patz, Jr.

Chapter 3 Preoperative Evaluation of Patients Undergoing Thoracic Surgery 39
John J. Reilly, Jr.

Chapter 4 Perioperative Care of the Thoracic Surgical Patient 47
Elisabeth U. Dexter

Part B Endoscopy

Chapter 5 Endoscopic Diagnosis of Thoracic Disease 61
Benedict J. W. Taylor and Douglas E. Wood

Chapter 6 Endoscopic Therapies for Thoracic Diseases 67
Sébastien Gilbert, Benny Weksler, Hiran C. Fernando, and James D. Luketich

Part C Trauma

Chapter 7 Thoracic Trauma 85
Clinton D. Kemp and Stephen C. Yang

Part D Trachea

Chapter 8 Tracheal Lesions 113
Todd S. Weiser, Simon K. Ashiku, and Douglas J. Mathisen

Part E Benign Lung Disease

Chapter 9 Congenital Lung Diseases 129
Kemp H. Kernstine, Timothy L. Van Natta, Harold M. Burkhart, and Daniel T. DeArmond

Chapter 10 Benign Lesions of the Lung 151
David Jarrar, Ayesha S. Bryant, and Robert J. Cerfolio

Chapter 11 Interstitial Lung Diseases 159
Subroto Paul and Yolonda L. Colson

Chapter 12 Infectious Lung Diseases 173
John D. Mitchell and Marvin Pomerantz

Chapter 13 Surgery for Emphysema 195
Bryan F. Meyers, John C. Kucharczuk, and Joel D. Cooper

Chapter 14 Lung Transplantation 207
Varun Puri, Felix G. Fernandez, and G. A. Patterson

Part F Lung Cancer

Chapter 15 Screening for Lung Cancer 231
Brendon M. Stiles, Jeffrey L. Port, and Nasser K. Altorki

Chapter 16 Lung Cancer Workup and Staging 241
Bernard J. Park and Valerie W. Rusch

Chapter 17 Lung Cancer: Surgical Treatment 253
Masaki Anraku and Shaf Keshavjee

Chapter 18 Lung Cancer: Minimally Invasive Approaches 279
Mark Onaitis and Thomas A. D'Amico

Chapter 19 Lung Cancer: Multimodal Therapy 287
Sudish C. Murthy, David P. Mason, and Thomas W. Rice

Chapter 20 Lung Cancer: Surgical Strategies for Tumors Invading the Chest Wall 295
Matthew A. Steliga, Michaela Straznicka, and Garrett L. Walsh

Chapter 21 Anterior Approach to Superior Sulcus Lesions 313
Philippe G. Dartevelle, Sacha Mussot, and Chuong D. Hoang

Part G Other Lung Malignancy

Chapter 22 Other Primary Tumors of the Lung 323
Alykhan S. Nagji and David R. Jones

Chapter 23 Secondary Lung Tumors 337
Scott Cowan, Melissa Culligan, and Joseph Friedberg

Part H Chest Wall

Chapter 24 Congenital Chest Wall Deformities 351
Robert C. Shamberger

Chapter 25 Chest Wall Tumors 379
Mark S. Allen

Chapter 26 Thoracic Outlet Syndrome and Dorsal Sympathectomy 389
Harold C. Urschel, Jr., and Amit N. Patel

Part I Pleura

Chapter 27 Spontaneous Pneumothorax 409
Karl G. Reyes and David P. Mason

Chapter 28 Empyema 413
Daniel L. Miller

Chapter 29 Chylothorax 427
Gaetano Rocco

Chapter 30 Malignant Pleural and Pericardial Effusions 431
Sai Yendamuri, Chukwumere Nwogu, and Todd L. Demmy

Chapter 31 Pleural Tumors 449
Ciaran McNamee, Christopher T. Ducko, and David J. Sugarbaker

Part J Diaphragm

Chapter 32 Surgery of the Diaphragm: A Deductive Approach 473
Daniel C. Weiner, Jonathan Daniel, and Michael T. Jaklitsch

Chapter 33 Congenital Diaphragmatic Hernia 489
Dario O. Fauza and Jay M. Wilson

Part K Esophagus—Benign Disease

Chapter 34 Eshophageal Anatomy and Function 517
John C. Lipham and Tom R. DeMeester

Chapter 35 Surgery for Congenital Lesions of the Esophagus 535
Kurt Newman, David Spurlock, and Alfred Chahine

Chapter 36 Surgical Treatment of Benign Esophageal Diseases 547
Thomas W. Rice, Steven S. Shay, and Sudish C. Murthy

Part L Esophagus—Cancer

Chapter 37 Staging Techniques for Carcinoma of the Esophagus 577
Virginia R. Litle

Chapter 38 Esophageal Resection and Replacement 589
Cynthia S. Chin, Philip A. Linden, and Scott J. Swanson

Chapter 39 Neoadjuvant and Adjuvant Therapy for Esophageal Cancer 617
G. Kwame Yankey and Mark J. Krasna

Part M Mediastinum

Chapter 40 Mediastinal Anatomy and Mediastinoscopy 623
Varun Puri and Bryan F. Meyers

Chapter 41 Anterior Mediastinal Masses 633
Chuong D. Hoang, John C. Kucharczuk, and Joseph B. Shrager

Chapter 42 The Middle Mediastinum 645
Zane T. Hammoud and Michael J. Liptay

Chapter 43 The Posterior Mediastinum 649
Larry R. Kaiser and Dhruv Singhal

Chapter 44 Surgical Treatment of Hyperhidrosis 661
Steven M. Keller

Part N The Future

Chapter 45 The Use of Genetic Science in Thoracic Disease 669
Jonathan D'Cunha and Michael A. Maddaus

Chapter 46 Innovative Therapy and Technology 683
Joseph J. Wizorek, Arjun Pennathur, Neil A. Christie, Hiran C. Fernando, and James D. Luketich

Section 2 Adult Cardiac Surgery

Part A Basic Science

Chapter 47 Surgical Anatomy of the Heart 697
Andrew C. Cook, Benson R. Wilcox, and Robert H. Anderson

Chapter 48 Vascular Physiology 711
Basel Ramlawi and Frank W. Sellke

Chapter 49 Physiology of the Myocardium 725
R. John Solaro and Margaret V. Westfall

Chapter 50 Ventricular Mechanics 739
Mark Ratcliffe, Arthur Wallace, and Julius Guccione

Chapter 51 Blood Coagulation, Transfusion, and Conservation 757
Jerrold H. Levy, Marie Steiner, and Kenichi A. Tanaka

Part B Diagnostic Procedures

Chapter 52 Coronary Angiography: Valve and Hemodynamic Assessment 775
Yuri B. Pride and Lawrence A. Garcia

Chapter 53 Applications of Cardiovascular Magnetic Resonance Imaging and Computed Tomography in Cardiovascular Diagnosis 789
Thomas H. Hauser, Susan B. Yeon, and Warren J. Manning

Chapter 54 Nuclear Cardiology and Positron Emission Tomography in the Assessment of Patients with Cardiovascular Disease 809
Brian G. Abbott and Barry L. Zaret

Chapter 55 Diagnostic Echocardiography (Ultrasound Imaging in Cardiovascular Diagnosis) 825
Rosario V. Freeman and Catherine M. Otto

Part C Medical- and Catheter-Based Treatment of Cardiovascular Disease

Chapter 56 Interventional Cardiology 847
Riya S. Chacko, Joseph P. Carrozza, Jr., and Duane S. Pinto

Chapter 57 Medical Management of Acute Coronary Syndromes 867
Robert M. Califf

Chapter 58 The Pharmacologic Management of Heart Failure 883
Eric H. Awtry and Wilson S. Colucci

Part D Perioperative and Intraoperative Care of the Cardiac Surgical Patient

Chapter 59 The Coronary Circulation: Dietary and Pharmacologic Management of Atherosclerosis 903
John R. Guyton

Chapter 60 Adult Cardiac Anesthesia 919
Feroze Mahmood, Xiaoqin Zhao, and Robina Matyal

Chapter 61 Critical Care for the Adult Cardiac Patient 933
Edward Cantu III, Carmelo A. Milano, and Peter K. Smith

Chapter 62 Cardiopulmonary Bypass: Technique and Pathophysiology 957
Fraser D. Rubens

Chapter 63 Myocardial Protection 977
Sidney Levitsky and James D. McCully

Chapter 64 Deep Sternal Wound Infection 999
Pierre Voisine, Richard Baillot, and François Dagenais

Chapter 65 Neuropsychological Deficits and Stroke 1005
John W. Hammon and David A. Stump

Chapter 66 Clinical Quality and Safety in Cardiac Surgery 1013
Justine M. Carr

Part E Surgical Management of Aortic Disease

Chapter 67 Surgery of the Aortic Root and Ascending Aorta 1021
Tirone E. David

Volume 2

Chapter 68 Surgery of the Aortic Arch 1041
Lars G. Svensson

Chapter 69 Descending Thoracic and Thoracoabdominal Aortic Surgery 1063
Lars G. Svensson

Chapter 70 Type A Aortic Dissection 1089
Philippe Demers and D. Craig Miller

Chapter 71 Type B Aortic Dissection 1115
Philippe Demers and D. Craig Miller

Chapter 72 Endovascular Therapy for Thoracic Aortic Aneurysms and Dissections 1129
Wilson Y. Szeto and Joseph E. Bavaria

Chapter 73 Occlusive Disease of the Brachiocephalic Vessels and Surgical Management of Simultaneous Carotid and Coronary Artery Diseases 1143
Raja R. Gopaldas, Peter H. Lin, and Scott A. LeMaire

Chapter 74 Peripheral Angiography and Percutaneous Intervention 1157
Yuri B. Pride and Lawrence A. Garcia

Chapter 75 Injury to the Heart and Great Vessels 1173
Peter I. Tsai, Matthew J. Wall, Jr., and Kenneth L. Mattox

Part F Surgical Management of Valvular Heart Disease

Chapter 76 Valve Replacement Therapy: History, Options, and Valve Types 1185
Edwin C. McGee, Jr., and Gus J. Vlahakes

Chapter 77 Acquired Aortic Valve Disease 1195
Douglas R. Johnston and Joseph F. Sabik III

Chapter 78 Acquired Disease of the Mitral Valve 1207
Farzan Filsoufi, Joanna Chikwe, and David H. Adams

Chapter 79 Surgical Treatment of the Tricuspid Valve *1241*
Carlos M. G. Duran

Chapter 80 Management of Native Valve Endocarditis *1259*
Lawrence S. Lee, Frederick Y. Chen, and Lawrence H. Cohn

Chapter 81 Prosthetic Valve Endocarditis *1267*
David A. Fullerton and Frederick L. Grover

Chapter 82 Thrombosis and Thromboembolism of Prosthetic Cardiac Valves and Extracardiac Prostheses *1279*
Joseph C. Cleveland, Jr., and Frederick L. Grover

Chapter 83 Robotic Cardiac Surgery and Novel Visualization Systems *1295*
Alan P. Kypson and W. Randolph Chitwood, Jr.

Part G Management of Cardiac Arrhythmias

Chapter 84 Cardiac Devices for the Treatment of Bradyarrhythmias and Tachyarrhythmias *1305*
Lilian P. Joventino and Peter J. Zimetbaum

Chapter 85 Catheter Ablation of Arrhythmias *1329*
John V. Wylie, Jr., David Wrobleski, and Mark E. Josephson

Chapter 86 Surgical Treatment of Arrhythmias *1345*
Spencer J. Melby and Ralph J. Damiano, Jr.

Part H Surgical Management of Coronary Artery Disease and Its Complications

Chapter 87 Coronary Artery Bypass Grafting *1367*
Vincent Chan, Frank W. Sellke, and Marc Ruel

Chapter 88 Alternative Approaches to Coronary Artery Bypass Grafting *1397*
William E. Cohn

Chapter 89 Bypass Conduit Options *1411*
Hendrick B. Barner

Chapter 90 Re-do Coronary Artery Bypass Surgery *1421*
Bruce W. Lytle

Chapter 91 Ischemic Mitral Regurgitation *1429*
Anelechi C. Anyanwu, Lishan Aklog, and David H. Adams

Chapter 92 Postinfarction Ventricular Septal Defect *1449*
Abeel A. Mangi and Arvind K. Agnihotri

Chapter 93 Transmyocardial Laser Revascularization *1457*
Keith A. Horvath

Chapter 94 Nonatherosclerotic Coronary Heart Disease *1467*
Audrey Rosinberg, Donald S. Baim, and Roger J. Laham

Part I Surgical Management of Heart Failure

Chapter 95 Pericardium and Constrictive Pericarditis *1479*
Donald D. Glower

Chapter 96 Surgical Management of Hypertrophic Cardiomyopathy *1493*
Hartzell Schaff

Chapter 97 Ventricular Assist Devices *1507*
Jeffrey A. Morgan, Mehmet C. Oz, and Yoshifumi Naka

Chapter 98 Total Artificial Heart *1525*
Hannah Zimmerman, Jack G. Copeland, Louise A. Aquila Allen, and Richard G. Smith

Chapter 99 Heart Transplantation *1533*
Jeffrey B. Velotta, Leora B. Balsam, Michael P. Fischbein, and Robert C. Robbins

Chapter 100 Heart–Lung Transplantation *1555*
Hari R. Mallidi and Bruce A. Reitz

Chapter 101 Left Ventricular Restoration: Surgical Treatment of the Failing Heart *1573*
Marisa Di Donato and Lorenzo Menicanti

Chapter 102 Regenerative Cell-Based Therapy for the Treatment of Cardiac Disease *1599*
Yan Zhang, Erik J. Suuronen, Frank W. Sellke, and Marc Ruel

Chapter 103 Surgery for Pulmonary Embolism *1615*
Patricia A. Thistlethwaite, Michael M. Madani, and Stuart W. Jamieson

Chapter 104 Tumors of the Heart *1633*
A. Marc Gillinov and John R. Liddicoat

Section 3 Congenital Heart Surgery

Chapter 105 Cardiac Embryology and Genetics *1641*
Amy L. Juraszek

Chapter 106 Segmental Anatomy *1651*
Richard Van Praagh

Chapter 107 Diagnostic Imaging: Echocardiography and Magnetic Resonance Imaging *1665*
Tal Geva

Chapter 108 Cardiac Catheterization and Fetal Intervention 1691
Audrey C. Marshall and Doff McElhinney

Chapter 109 Surgical Approaches and Cardiopulmonary Bypass in Pediatric Cardiac Surgery 1709
Pedro J. del Nido and Francis X. McGowan, Jr.

Chapter 110 Surgical Approaches, Cardiopulmonary Bypass, and Mechanical Circulatory Support in Children 1735
Peter C. Laussen and Francis Fynn-Thompson

Chapter 111 Pediatric Anesthesia and Critical Care 1749
Kirsten C. Odegard and Peter C. Laussen

Chapter 112 Congenital Tracheal Disease 1765
Emile A. Bacha

Chapter 113 Patent Ductus Arteriosus, Coarctation of the Aorta, and Vascular Rings 1781
Sitaram M. Emani

Chapter 114 Atrial Septal Defect and Cor Triatriatum 1797
David P. Bichell and Karla G. Christian

Chapter 115 Surgical Considerations in Pulmonary Vein Anomalies 1817
Osami Honjo and Christopher A. Caldarone

Chapter 116 Atrioventricular Canal Defects 1831
Aditya K. Kaza and Pedro J. del Nido

Chapter 117 Ventricular Septal Defect and Double-Outlet Right Ventricle 1849
Emile A. Bacha

Chapter 118 Pulmonary Atresia with Intact Ventricular Septum 1865
Christopher E. Mascio and Erle H. Austin III

Chapter 119 Tetralogy of Fallot with Pulmonary Stenosis 1877
Brian W. Duncan

Chapter 120 Pulmonary Atresia with Ventricular Septal Defect and Right Ventricle–to–Pulmonary Artery Conduits 1897
Sitaram M. Emani and John E. Mayer

Chapter 121 Truncus Arteriosus and Aortopulmonary Window 1911
Jennifer C. Hirsch, Eric J. Devaney, Richard G. Ohye, and Edward L. Bove

Chapter 122 Interrupted Aortic Arch 1927
Marshall L. Jacobs, Jeffrey P. Jacobs, and Alvin J. Chin

Chapter 123 Surgery for Congenital Anomalies of the Aortic Valve and Root 1943
Frank A. Pigula

Chapter 124 Surgery for Congenital Anomalies of the Coronary Arteries 1963
Julie A. Brothers and J. William Gaynor

Chapter 125 Transposition of the Great Arteries: Simple and Complex Forms 1981
Frank A. Pigula and Pedro J. del Nido

Chapter 126 Surgery for Congenitally Corrected Transposition of the Great Arteries 2003
William J. Brawn and David J. Barron

Chapter 127 Congenital Anomalies of the Mitral Valve 2015
Christian P. Brizard

Chapter 128 Hypoplastic Left Heart Syndrome 2025
Frank A. Pigula

Chapter 129 Management of Single Ventricle and Cavopulmonary Connections 2041
Kirk R. Kanter

Chapter 130 Ebstein's Anomaly 2055
Morgan L. Brown and Joseph A. Dearani

Chapter 131 Adult Congenital Cardiac Surgery 2069
Anne Marie Valente, Michael J. Landzberg, and Emile A. Bacha

Chapter 132 Arrhythmia and Pacemaker Surgery in Congenital Heart Disease 2083
Francis Fynn-Thompson and Frank Cecchin

Chapter 133 Image-Guided and Hybrid Surgery: Surgical Simulation 2099
Nikolay V. Vasilyev, Emile A. Bacha, and Pedro J. del Nido

Chapter 134 Quality Improvement and Risk Stratification for Congenital Cardiac Surgery 2105
Jeffrey Phillip Jacobs and Fred H. Edwards

Index i

Online Video Contents

Chapter 69 Descending Thoracic and Thoracoabdominal Aortic Surgery

    Thoracoabdominal Aortic Aneurysm Repair[1]

Chapter 83 Robotic Cardiac Surgery and Novel Visualization Systems

    Complex Robotic Mitral Valve Repair[2]

    Robotic Mitral Valve Technique Using the Haircut Technique[2]

Chapter 88 Alternative Approaches to CABG

    Off Pump Coronary Artery Bypass Grafting[3]

    Endoscopic Coronary Artery Bypass Grafting[4]

    Minimally Invasive Cardiac Surgical Coronary Artery Bypass Grafting[5]

Chapter 93 Transmyocardial Laser Revascularization

    Transmyocardial Laser Revascularization[6]

Chapter 97 Ventricular Assist Devices

    Implantation of the Heart Mate II[7]

Chapter 100 Heart–Lung Transplantation

    Heart–Lung Transplantation[8]

Chapter 101 Left Ventricular Restoration: Surgical Treatment of the Failing Heart

    Schematic representation of LV remodeling process in anterior postinfarction cardiomyopathy[9]

    Surgical reconstruction of LV inferior dilation (aneurysm) due to inferior myocardial infarction[9]

---

[1]From Lemaire S. Thoracoabdominal Aortic Aneurysm Repair. In Sellke FW (ed) Atlas of Cardiac Surgical Techniques. Philadelphia, Elsevier, 2009
[2]Courtesy of Ralph Chitwood, MD, Karen A. Gersch, MD, Michael W. Chu, MD, L.W. Nifong, MD, Jerome Fuller, MD
[3]From Puskas JD, Pusca SV. Off Pump Coronary Artery Bypass Grafting. In Sellke FW (ed) Atlas of Cardiac Surgical Techniques. Philadelphia, Elsevier, 2009.
[4]From Vassiliades TA. Endoscopic and Traditional Minimally Invasive Direct Coronary Artery Bypass. In Sellke FW (ed) Atlas of Cardiac Surgical Techniques. Philadelphia, Elsevier, 2009
[5]From Ruel M. Minimally Invasive Cardiac Surgical Coronary Artery Bypass Grafting. In Sellke FW (ed) Atlas of Cardiac Surgical Techniques. Philadelphia, Elsevier, 2009
[6]Courtesy of Keith Horvath, MD
[7]From Frazier OH. Implantation of the Heart Mate II. In Sellke FW (ed) Atlas of Cardiac Surgical Techniques. Philadelphia, Elsevier, 2009
[8]From Reitz BA, Baumgartner WA, Borkon AM, the American College of Surgeons Video Based Education Collection.
[9]Courtesy of Lorenzo Menicanti, MD, and Marisa Di Donato, MD

Section 1

Thoracic Surgery

Evaluation and Care

Endoscopy

Trauma

Trachea

Benign Lung Disease

Lung Cancer

Other Lung Malignancy

Chest Wall

Pleura

Diaphragm

Esophagus—Benign Disease

Esophagus—Cancer

Mediastinum

The Future

A. Evaluation and Care

CHAPTER 1

Anatomy of the Thorax

Cynthia Chin and Rohit Shahani

Thoracic Cage
   Thoracic Inlet
   Cervicoaxillary Canal
   Diaphragm
   The Bony Thoracic Cage
     Sternum
     Ribs

Muscles of the Thorax
   Intercostal Muscles
   Anatomy of Breathing
Surface Anatomy
Mediastinum
Tracheobronchial Tree
Lungs
Esophagus

Vessels of the Thorax
   Descending Thoracic Aorta
   Azygos Vein
   Thoracic Duct
Nerves of the Thorax
   Vagus and Recurrent Laryngeal Nerves
   Thoracic Sympathetic Chain
   Phrenic Nerves

The thorax is the upper part of the trunk, bounded by the diaphragm inferiorly, the thoracic inlet superiorly, and the thoracic cage between. Vital organs, such as the heart and lungs, reside completely within the thoracic cavity, and other, equally vital organs, such as the aorta and esophagus, extend into the abdominal cavity. The thorax can be divided into a right and left hemithorax, separated by the mediastinum. This chapter gives an overview of the anatomy of the thoracic cavity and its contents.

THORACIC CAGE

The cylindrical thoracic cage has two main purposes: it provides protection for the underlying organs, and the dynamic interactions of the bony and muscular components of the chest wall allow changes in respiratory volumes.

The bony thorax has two apertures, or openings: the superior thoracic aperture, often referred to as the thoracic inlet or cervicothoracic junction, and the inferior thoracic aperture (Fig. 1-1A).

Thoracic Inlet

The thoracic inlet is limited by the body of the first thoracic vertebra posteriorly, the first pair of ribs and their costal cartilages anterolaterally, and the superior border of the manubrium anteriorly. Many important structures travel through the cervicothoracic junction. Resection of malignancies (e.g., Pancoast's tumor) or repair of thoracic outlet syndrome requires intimate knowledge of the anatomic relationships in this area. In this kidney-shaped inlet, the trachea is midline and behind the great vessels, and the esophagus is posterior and slightly to its left. The innominate artery arises from the aortic arch and passes posterior to the manubrium and anterior to the trachea as it travels cephalad. The right and left internal jugular and subclavian veins join behind their respective sternoclavicular

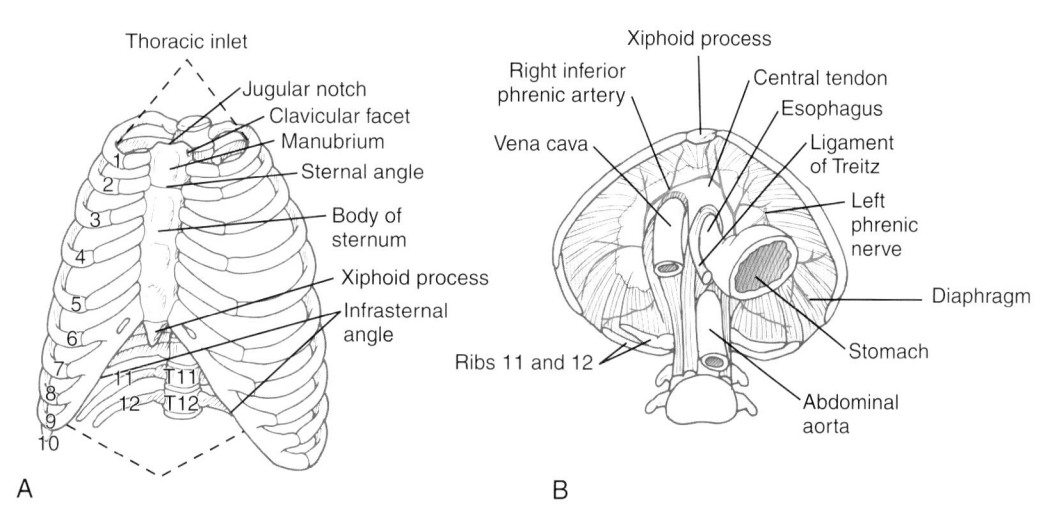

Figure 1-1
A, Bony thorax. **B,** Inferior thoracic aperture. The vena cava enters the right hemithorax through the most cranial diaphragmatic opening, located at the level of the eighth thoracic vertebra (T8). The esophagus and vagus nerves enter the abdomen at the level of the T10 vertebra. The hiatus at T12 allows the aorta, azygos vein, and thoracic duct to pass in their respective directions.

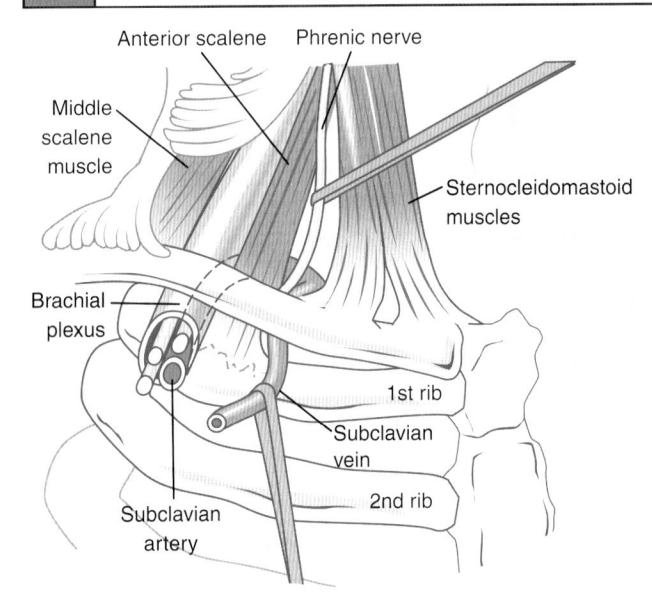

Figure 1-2
Cervicoaxillary canal and the structures that traverse this opening.

joints to form the left and right brachiocephalic veins. The left brachiocephalic vein travels right to join its counterpart to form the superior vena cava. The main muscles of this region are the sternocleidomastoid and scalene muscles, and the main nerves form the brachial plexus, but the phrenic and vagus nerves also pass through this aperture.

As the margin of the aperture slopes inferoanteriorly, the apex of each lung and its covering pleura (pleural cupola) project superiorly through the lateral parts of the thoracic inlet and are covered by a piece of cervical fascia, the suprapleural membrane (Sibson's fascia).

Cervicoaxillary Canal

The cervicoaxillary canal is bounded by the first rib inferiorly, the clavicle superiorly, and the costoclavicular ligament medially (Fig. 1-2). The structures that pass through this space include the subclavian vein and artery and the brachial plexus.

The subclavian artery passes over the first rib and goes between the scalenus anterior and scalenus middle muscles. Before passing over the first rib on its way out the cervicoaxillary canal, it gives off branches, including the thyrocervical, internal mammary, and vertebral arteries. It becomes the axillary artery after it exits from behind the pectoralis minor muscle. Compression of this artery may lead to poststenotic dilation, stenosis, aneurysmal formation, or occlusion.

The subclavian vein travels from the arm and goes behind the pectoralis minor muscle before going between the first rib and clavicle. This space is bounded medially by the costoclavicular ligament and laterally by the scalenus anterior muscles as it inserts onto the first rib. Compression of the vein occurs in this area and can lead to stenosis and occlusion.

The brachial plexus is composed of nerve roots from the C5 through the T1 vertebral foramina. These nerve roots join to form the superior trunk (C5 and C6), the middle trunk (C7), and the inferior trunk (C8 and T1). These trunks separate into anterior and posterior divisions that fuse again to form lateral, medial, and posterior cords of the brachial plexus. The plexus travels through the tunnel formed by the anterior and middle scalene muscles. It travels between the first rib and the clavicle and finally under the pectoralis minor muscle to gain access to the arm.

In the normal anatomy, there is ample room for each of these structures. There are four major areas in which the vessels or nerves can be compressed (Table 1-1). This topic will be discussed in greater detail in Chapter 26.

Diaphragm

The diaphragm, at the inferior thoracic aperture, separates the thoracic cavity from the abdominal cavity. The inferior thoracic aperture, which slopes inferoposteriorly, is limited by the 12th thoracic vertebra posteriorly, the 12th pair of ribs and costal margins anterolaterally, and the xiphisternal joint anteriorly.

The diaphragm is a curved musculotendinous sheet that is mainly convex toward the thoracic cavity. It is a continuous sheet of muscle with low posterior and lateral attachments and high anterior attachments. The central tendon is a thin but strong aponeurosis. The domes of the diaphragm descend 2 cm during quiet respiration and may travel as much as 10 cm during heightened respiratory requirements. During expiration, the right diaphragm may rise as high as the level of the nipple, whereas the left rises to a level one rib space lower. With maximal inspiration, the diaphragm flattens against the abdominal contents. The right diaphragm may flatten to the level of the 11th rib, whereas the left may flatten to the level of the 12th rib. The right diaphragm has to work against the liver, whereas the left needs to push only against the stomach and spleen. Therefore, the right diaphragm has significantly stronger fibers than the left.

The costal diaphragm receives its blood supply from the lower five intercostal and subcostal arteries, and the central portion is supplied by the phrenic arteries. The phrenic arteries may arise directly from the aorta, above the celiac axis, as a common trunk or individually. Occasionally, they arise from the celiac or renal arteries. The sole motor supply to the diaphragm is the phrenic nerve. It also supplies sensory fibers to the parietal and peritoneal pleura overlying the diaphragm. This accounts for the diaphragmatic irritation that is sometimes interpreted as ipsilateral shoulder pain.

The diaphragm has several openings through which structures can transverse from one cavity to another (see Fig. 1-1B). The inferior vena cava hiatus lies anteriorly and to the right of the midline, at the level of vertebra T8. The right phrenic nerve travels through this hiatus, and the left phrenic nerve penetrates laterally through its own opening at the same level. The esophageal aperture is at the level of the T10 vertebra, and the right and left vagal trunks that adhere to it enter the abdomen along with the esophagus.

The aortic aperture, at the T12 vertebral level, is formed by the interdigitating fibers (median arcuate ligament) of the right and left diaphragmatic crura. The azygos and hemiazygos veins and the thoracic duct also pass through this opening.

The greater and lesser splanchnic nerves gain access to the abdominal cavity via two small apertures in each of the crura, and musculophrenic branches of the internal mammary artery

Table 1–1
Sites and Structures Compressed in Thoracic Outlet Syndrome

Site	Description	Abnormalities	Structures Compressed
Sternal-costovertebral circle	This aperture can be narrowed by bony variations	Cervical first rib First rib Long transverse process	Subclavian artery Subclavian vein Brachial plexus
Scalene muscle triangle	The scalenus anterior and middle muscle insert on the first rib, creating a tunnel	Scalenus anterior and middle	Subclavian artery Brachial plexus
First rib, clavicular space	The neurovascular structures lie above the rib and below the clavicle	Costoclavicular ligament Clavicle First rib	Subclavian vein Subclavian artery Brachial plexus
Behind the pectoralis minor muscle	The neurovascular structures travel to and from the arm behind this muscle	Pectoralis minor Costocoracoid ligament	Subclavian vein Subclavian artery Brachial plexus

penetrate the diaphragm through small apertures near its connection with the costal cartilages of ribs seven to nine.

Diaphragmatic hernias can develop through known openings, such as a hiatal hernia through the esophageal hiatus, or through congenital defects. The most common congenital abnormality is a Bochdalek hernia, in which abdominal contents go through a posterolateral defect. This is seen more commonly on the left. A Morgagni hernia, on the other hand, occurs with a defect in the anterior aspect of the diaphragm just lateral to the xiphoid.

The Bony Thoracic Cage

Sternum

The sternum or breastbone is made of cancellous bone and filled with hemopoietic marrow throughout life. The main parts, the manubrium and body, are connected by a secondary cartilaginous joint that normally never ossifies and contributes to movement of the ribs.

Up to puberty, the six segments, or sternebrae, are held together by hyaline cartilage. The central four fuse to form the body of the sternum between 14 and 21 years of age. The manubrium sterni (superiorly) and the xiphoid process (inferiorly) remain separate.

The manubrium receives the sternal ends of the clavicles in a shallow concave facet. The widest portion of the manubrium has bilateral costal incisurae that articulate with the first costal cartilage to form a primary cartilaginous joint. The second costal cartilage articulates with both the lower lateral ends of the manubrium and the body of the sternum, forming separate synovial joints. The muscular attachments of the manubrium include the sternocleidomastoid muscle, the sternohyoid and the sternothyroid superiorly, and the pectoralis major muscle anterolaterally. Most of the posterior surface is bare bone, which may be in contact with the brachiocephalic vein unless thymic remnants lie between.

The gladiolus, or body of the sternum, is slanted at a steeper angle than the manubrium; its articulation with that bone forms the sternal angle. Ossification of this joint, synchondrosis, in adult life may limit normal movement at this joint. The articular facets for ribs two to seven lie along the lateral border of the body of the sternum. These make single synovial joints with the costal cartilages. The facets for the sixth and seventh costal cartilages may coalesce, especially in females. The lateral border gives attachment to the anterior intercostal membrane and the internal intercostal muscles, and the pectoralis major arises anteriorly. Weak sternopericardial ligaments pass into the fibrous pericardium.

The cartilaginous xiphoid may be bifid or perforated, is of variable length, and usually ossifies in the 4th decade. The costoxiphoid ligaments prevent its displacement during diaphragmatic contractions.

Ribs

The 12 pairs of ribs are divided into the upper seven, which that are called true ribs or vertebrosternal ribs because they form complete loops between the vertebrae and the sternum, and the lower five ribs, which fail to reach the sternum and are considered false ribs. The eighth, ninth, and 10th ribs are called vertebrocostal because each of their costal cartilages articulates with the adjacent rib cartilage. Ribs 11 and 12 are free-floating or vertebral ribs because their only articulation is with their vertebrae.

Ribs three to nine are classified as typical ribs and have a head, neck, and a shaft. The head has an upper and a lower articular facet divided by a crest for articulation with two adjacent vertebrae in synovial costovertebral joints, the lower facet articulating with the upper border of its own vertebra. The neck is flattened, with the upper border curling up into a prominent ridge—the crest. A tubercle projects posteriorly from the end of the neck and marks the junction of the neck and the body (Fig. 1-3).

The medial facet on the tubercle is covered with hyaline cartilage and makes a synovial joint with the transverse process of its own vertebra. The lateral facet receives the costotransverse ligament from the tip of its own transverse process. The shaft slopes downward and laterally for about 5 to 8 cm at an angle and then curves forward. Lateral to the angle, the lower border projects down as a sharp ridge, sheltering a costal groove. The angles of the ribs also correspond to the lateral extent of the erector spinae muscles of the back. The upper

Figure 1–3
Typical rib.

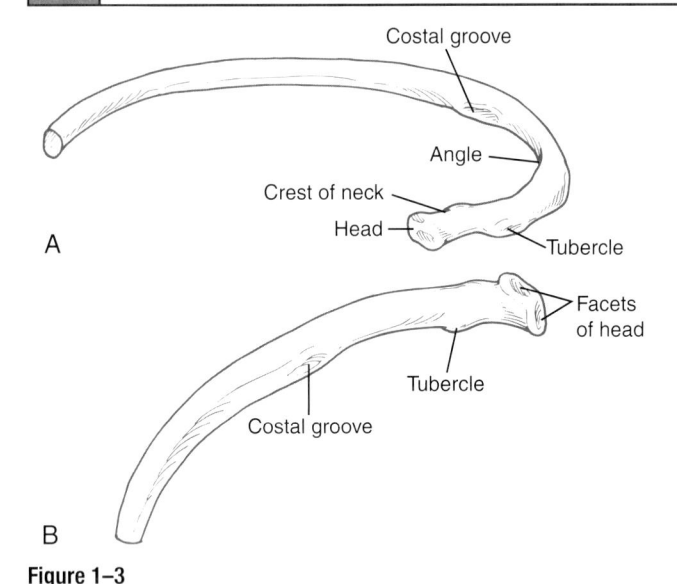

six ribs are bent into a tight curve so that the shaft has turned parallel with the neck of the rib. The lower six ribs have an opening out of the curve, which is completed by the long costal cartilages at the front of the chest. The fused cartilages of ribs seven to 10 course diagonally upward to the lower end of the sternum to form the subcostal angle. The anterior ends of the ribs have a concave fossa that is plugged by the costal cartilage in an immovable primary cartilaginous joint.

The first rib is exceptionally broad and short and very highly curved. The head is small and has a single facet for the synovial joint it makes with the upper part of the body of the T1 vertebra. The prominent tubercle is a fusion of the tubercle and the angle, and its medial facet forms a synovial joint with the first transverse process. The lateral prominent part of the tubercle receives the lateral costotransverse ligament and the costalis and longissimus parts of the erector spinae. Near the middle of the shaft, the sulci for the subclavian vessels are identified by the scalene tubercle, a spur that attaches the scalenus anterior muscle.

MUSCLES OF THE THORAX

The muscles of the chest wall serve to protect the contents of the thoracic cavity, and they assist the movements of the thorax and upper extremities (Fig. 1-4). The 17 muscles of the chest wall are not discussed in detail here, but Table 1-2 lists them with their innervations and sites of attachments. Here we focus on muscle groups that are used in chest wall reconstruction. The latissimus dorsi, pectoralis major, serratus anterior, trapezius, rectus abdominis, and external oblique are the six major muscles that are available for reconstruction (Table 1-3).

The latissimus dorsi is the largest muscle of the thorax. It originates from the lower six thoracic spinous processes and from the lumbodorsal fiber, which is attached to the lumbar and sacral vertebrae. It also has fibers originating from the iliac crest. The muscle narrows and then inserts on the intertubercle groove of the humerus. It is supplied by the thoracodorsal artery, a branch of the subscapular artery. The subscapular artery arises from the axillary artery and gives a branch to the serratus anterior muscle before supplying the latissimus dorsi. The artery can be found on the undersurface of the latissimus dorsi. The mobile arterial supply and excellent musculocutaneous collaterals allow this muscle to be moved with or without its overlying skin.

The pectoralis major muscle arises from the sternum, clavicle, and first seven ribs. It inserts on the bicipital humeral groove. It receives arterial supply from a pectoral branch of the thoracoacromial artery arising midclavicularly. It also receives some blood supply from the internal mammary, lateral intercostals, and lateral thoracic perforators. This flap is most frequently used for sternal defects.

Located between the latissimus dorsi and pectoralis major muscles is the serratus anterior muscle. This small muscle originates from the superior borders of the eighth through tenth ribs. It inserts on the tip of the scapula. Its blood supply is from a branch of the thoracodorsal artery and from the long thoracic artery. It can be used for intrathoracic purposes such as bronchial stump coverage or muscle interposition between the trachea and esophagus after a tracheo-esophageal fistula repair.

The trapezius muscle arises from the occipital bone and from the spinous process of the seventh cervical vertebra and all the thoracic vertebrae. It inserts on the lateral aspect of the clavicle, the acromion process, and the spine of the scapula. It receives its blood supply from the transverse cervical artery. Although it is a large muscle, the use of the trapezius is limited to reconstruction of the upper thoracic cavity.

Arising from the inferior borders of the fourth through twelfth ribs and inserting on the iliac crest is the external oblique muscle. It accepts blood supply from the lower thoracic intercostal arteries. Unlike the trapezius muscle, its uses are limited to the thoracic cavity below the inframammary crease.

The rectus abdominis muscle spans the entire anterior abdominal wall. It originates at the pubic crest and rises superiorly to insert on the fifth through seventh rib cartilages and xiphoid process. The superior and inferior epigastric arteries supply this vast muscle. It has been used for reconstruction of the anterior thoracic cavity, most notably after breast surgery.

Intercostal Muscles

Fibers of the intercostalis externi muscle arise from the sharp lower border of the rib above and course inferomedially (i.e., in the direction of the fingers when the hands are put into the front pockets of trousers) to the smooth upper border of the rib below. Anteriorly, it is replaced by the anterior intercostal membrane. Between the bony ribs is muscle; between the costal cartilages is membrane. In the lower spaces, the muscle interdigitates with the fibers of the external oblique (Fig. 1-5).

The intercostalis interni muscle runs from the lower costal groove of ribs one to 11, to the upper surfaces of ribs two to 12 downward and backward. Anteriorly, they extend up to the sternum but posteriorly only up to the angles of the rib. Beyond that, they are replaced by the internal intercostal membrane, which attaches to the tubercle of each rib and vertebra.

The innermost or transversus layer is divided into three groups: the innermost intercostals (anterolateral), subcostal (posterior), and transversus thoracis (anteromedial) muscles. The fibers run downward and backward, as in the internal

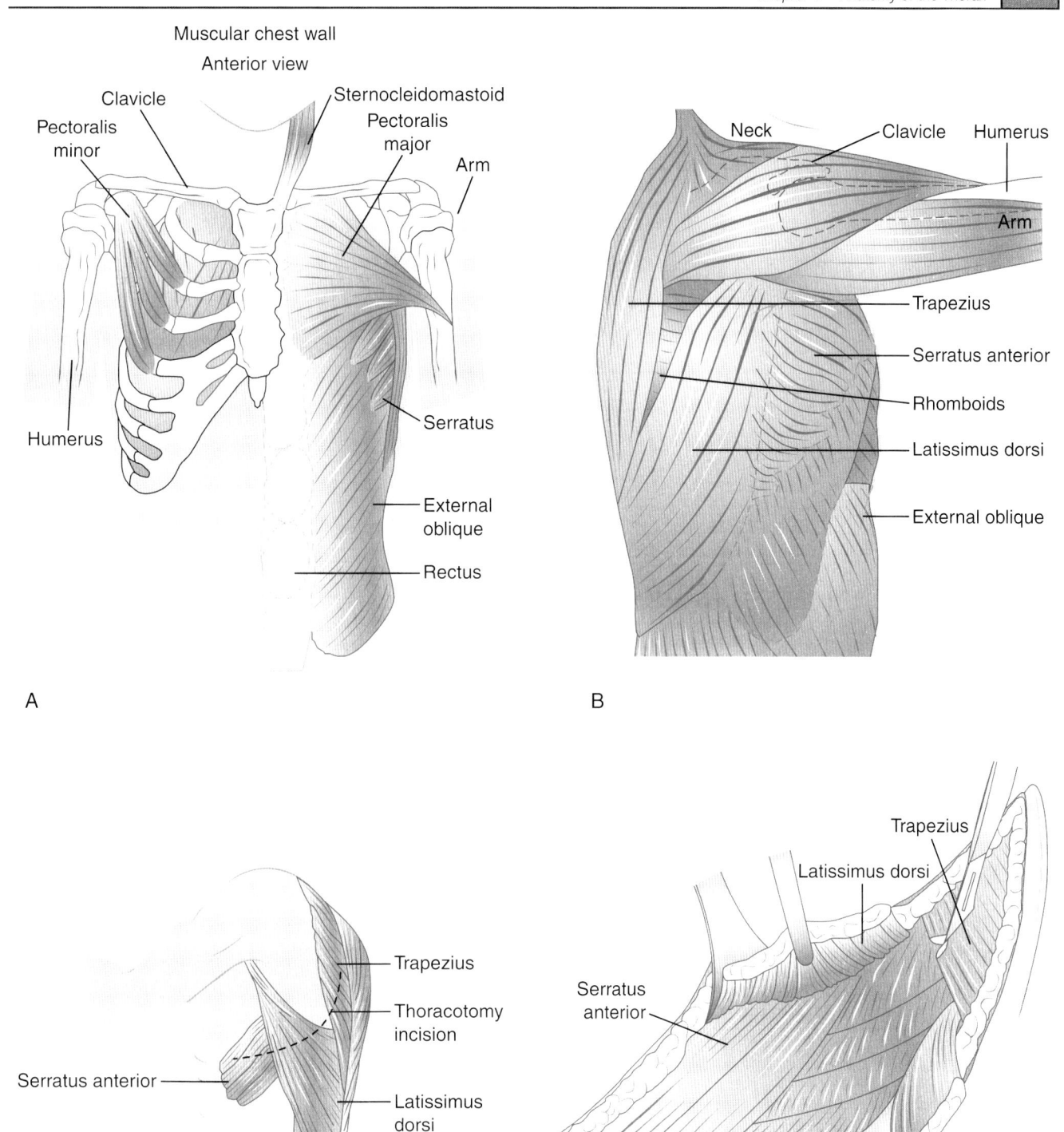

Figure 1–4
A, Anterior view of major muscles of the chest wall. **B,** Lateral view of the muscles of right hemithorax. **C,** *Dotted line* indicates placement of a standard posterolateral thoracotomy. **D,** Incisional view of muscles encountered during a posterolateral thoracotomy.

intercostal muscles. The subcostal muscles lie in the paravertebral gutter, are better developed inferiorly, and cross more than one space. The transversus thoracis was formerly called the sternocostalis, a more appropriate name. Digitations arise from the sternum bilaterally to the costal cartilages of ribs two to six.

The intercostalis intimi muscles also traverse more than one space and are better developed in the lower lateral spaces. In the plane between the innermost and outer two layers runs the neurovascular bundle. From above downward, the order is vein, artery, and nerve (mnemonic: VAN). Beyond the

Table 1–2
Attachments and Innervation of the Muscles of the Thoracic Wall

Muscle	Proximal Attachments	Distal Attachments	Innervation
Pectoralis major sternocostal head	Half of sternum, costal cartilages 1 to 6, aponeurosis of external obliquus muscle	Lateral lip of intertubercular sulcus of humerus	Medial pectoral nerve (C8-T1)
Pectoralis major clavicular head	Medial half of clavicle	Lateral lip of intertubercular sulcus of humerus	Lateral pectoral nerve (C5, 6, 7)
Pectoralis minor	Ribs 3 to 5	Coracoid process of scapula	Medial pectoral nerve
Subclavius	First rib	Medial clavicle	Nerve to subclavius (C5-6)
Deltoid	Lateral third of clavicle, acromion, and spine of scapula	Deltoid tuberosity of humerus	Axillary nerve (C5-6)
Serratus anterior	Angles of superior 10 ribs	Medial border of scapula	Long thoracic muscle nerve (C5, 6, 7)
Supraspinatus	Supraspinous fossa of the scapula, fascia of trapezius	Greater tubercle of the humerus	Suprascapular nerve (C5)
Infraspinatus	Infraspinous fossa	Greater tubercle of the humerus	Suprascapular nerve
Subscapularis	Costal surface of the scapula	Lesser tubercle of the humerus and its crest	Upper (C5-6) and lower (C5, 6, 7) subscapular nerve
Latissimus dorsi	Spinous processes of T7-12, L1-5, S1-3 vertebrae, posterior part of iliac crest, lower three to four ribs	Crest of the lesser tubercle and floor of the intertubercular groove of the humerus	Thoracodorsal nerve (C6-7)
Serratus posterior inferior	Spine of C6-T2 vertebrae	Angles of ribs 2 to 5	Segmental intercostal nerves
Serratus posterior superior	Spine of T11-L2 vertebrae	Lower border of ribs 9 to 12	Segmental intercostal nerves
Trapezius	Ligamentum nuchae, external occipital protuberance, thoracic vertebral spinous processes	Lateral one third of clavicle, acromion process along spine of scapula	Spinal accessory nerve
Levator scapulae	Transverse process of C1, C2, C3, C4 (cervical vertebrae)	Medial border of scapula, superior angle to base of scapular spine	Dorsal scapular nerve (C5)
Rhomboid major and minor	Spinous processes of C7-T5 and supraspinous ligaments	Medial border of scapula up to the inferior angle	Dorsal scapular nerve (C5)
Teres major	Lower lateral border of the scapula	Crest of the lesser tubercle of the humerus	Lower subscapular nerve (C5, 6, 7)
Teres minor	Mid to upper lateral border of the scapula	Greater tubercle of the humerus	Axillary nerve (C5-6)

Table 1–3
Arterial Supply of Muscles Used in Chest Wall Reconstruction

Muscle	Arterial Supply
Latissimus dorsi	Thoracodorsal artery
Pectoralis major	Thoracoacromial, lateral thoracic perforators, internal mammary artery, lateral intercostals artery
Serratus anterior	Thoracodorsal artery, long thoracic artery
Trapezius	Transverse cervical artery
External oblique	Lower thoracic intercostal arteries
Rectus abdominis	Superior and inferior epigastric arteries

angle of the rib posteriorly, they are protected by the downward projection of the lower border of the rib. Hence, for a thoracotomy, the periosteum is stripped off the upper half of the rib, avoiding the lower border and the neurovascular bundle (Fig. 1-6).

As in the rest of the body, the mixed spinal nerve is formed from a dorsal and a ventral root, the dorsal root being sensory and the ventral root containing somatic motor neurons. As it emerges from the intervertebral foramina, it branches into a dorsal and a ventral ramus. The dorsal ramus of the thoracic spinal nerve supplies the paravertebral back muscles and skin of the back. The ventral ramus communicates with the sympathetic chains via white rami communicantes (postganglionic fibers). Beyond this point, the true intercostal nerve lies just superficial to the parietal pleura in the endothoracic fascia. It gains the costal groove between the innermost intercostal and the internal intercostal muscles near the angle of the rib, where

Chapter 1 Anatomy of the Thorax   9

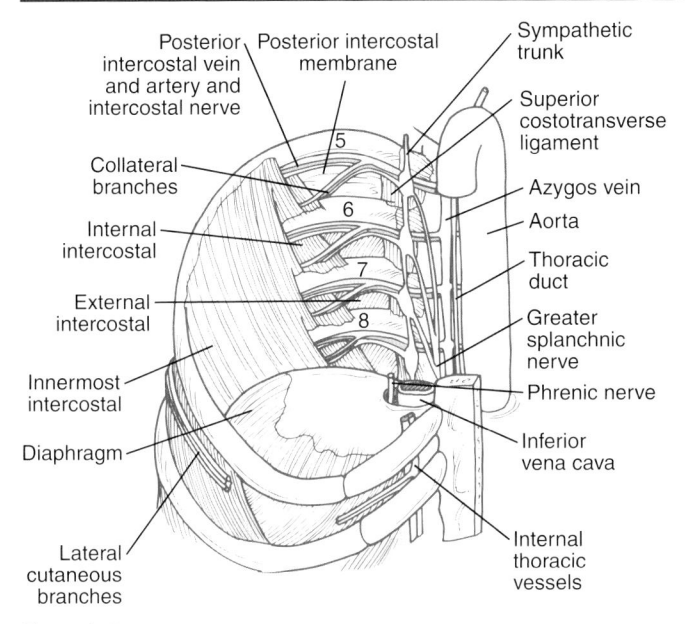

Figure 1–5
Spatial organization of the thoracic wall on the right side.

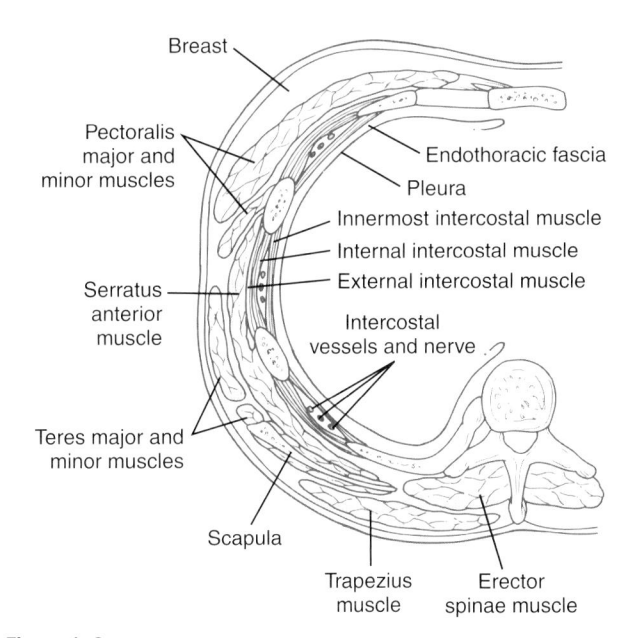

Figure 1–6
Layers of the chest wall.

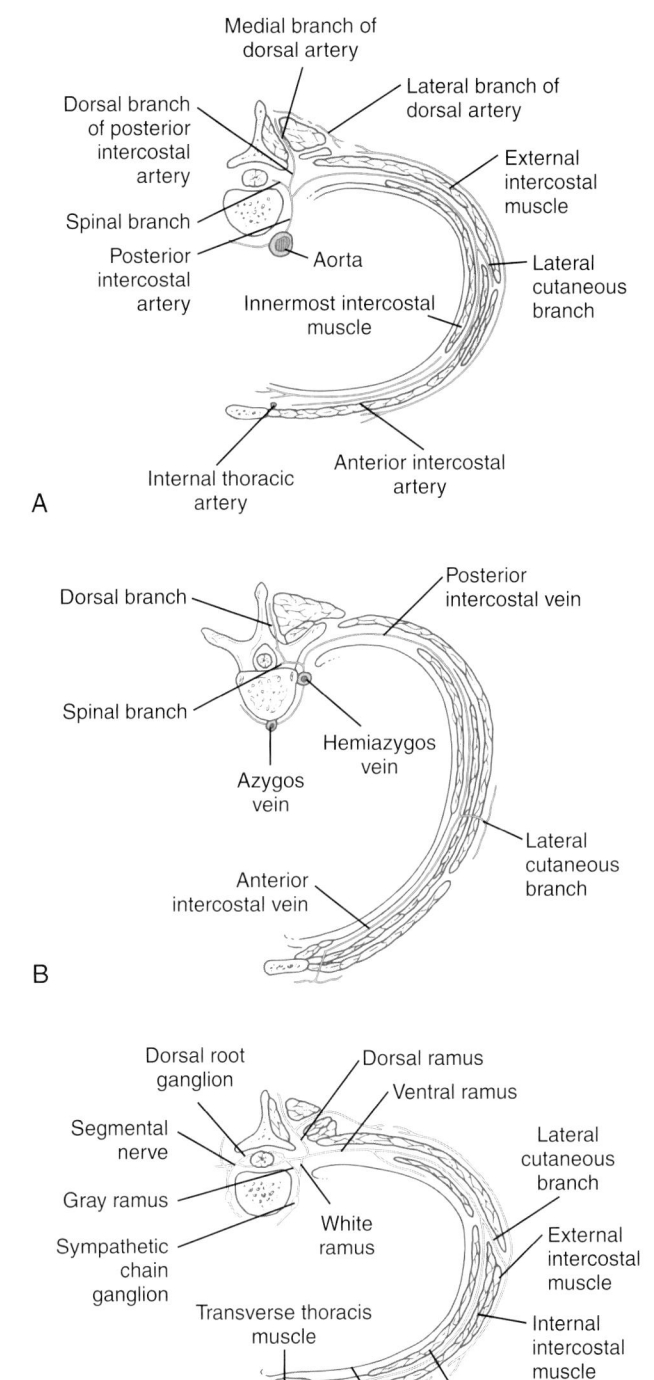

Figure 1–7
Organization of the intercostal space and the relationship of the arteries (**A**), veins (**B**), and nerves (**C**) to the muscle layers.

a collateral branch is given off. This small branch supplies the muscles of the space, the parietal pleura, and the periosteum of the rib. The main nerve itself has muscular branches, a lateral cutaneous branch, and a terminal anterior cutaneous branch. The lateral cutaneous branch given off along the midaxillary line gives off anterior and posterior branches to supply the skin over that space. Just lateral to the sternal margin, the terminal anterior cutaneous branches of the upper six nerves pierce the internal intercostal muscles, the external intercostal membrane, and the pectoralis major to reach skin. The lower five intercostal nerves slope downward behind the costal margin into the neurovascular plane of the abdominal wall. The subcostal or 12th thoracic nerve leaves the thorax by passing behind the lateral arcuate ligament and the subcostal artery and vein (Fig. 1-7). The cutaneous branches of each dermatome tend to overlap considerably; hence anesthesia after thoracic incisions is quite rare unless multiple intercostal nerves have been damaged. The first intercostal nerve is very small and supplies no skin, lacking both lateral and anterior cutaneous branches.

Two sets of intercostal arteries, the posterior and the anterior, are responsible for supplying the intercostal spaces. Their course and branching pattern closely conform to those of the intercostal nerves. The posterior intercostal arteries are branches of the descending thoracic aorta except in the first two spaces, where they are branches of the supreme intercostal artery, given off by the costocervical trunk of the second part of the subclavian artery. The aortic branches lie on the left side of the mediastinum; consequently, the right posterior intercostal arteries are longer, can be easily dissected in the left chest, and are seen best while operating on descending thoracic aortic aneurysms.

The roots of all 12 pairs of posterior intercostal arteries give rise to a dorsal branch that supplies the vertebrae, spinal cord, and deep muscles of the back. Like the nerve, the intercostal artery gives off a collateral branch, the largest muscular branch that runs along the upper border of the rib below the space. After gaining the costal groove, near the midaxillary line, it gives off the lateral cutaneous branch. The subcostal artery or the 12th thoracic posterior intercostal artery follows a similar course but has no collateral branch.

The anterior intercostal arteries are branches of the internal thoracic arteries from the first part of the subclavian artery. The internal thoracic artery runs anterior to the transversus thoracis and on the internal surface of the costal cartilages and the internal intercostal muscles. About a finger's breadth from the border of the sternum running vertically downward, it gives off two anterior intercostal arteries in each space. At the costal margin, below the sixth costal cartilage, it divides into the superior epigastric and musculophrenic arteries. The anterior intercostal arteries are smaller than the posterior intercostal arteries with which they anastomose and run predominantly along the lower border of each costal cartilage in the same fascial neurovascular plane. In the lower spaces, they are branches of the musculophrenic artery. There are no true anterior intercostal arteries in the last two spaces.

The internal thoracic arteries also give branches to the mediastinum, the thymus, the pericardium, and the sternum, and especially large perforating branches in the second to fourth space, the predominant supply to the lactating breast in females.

In each space there are one posterior and two anterior intercostal veins, designated by names identical to the arteries that they accompany. They lie above the artery and the nerve throughout their course (VAN) in the intercostal space. The anterior veins drain into the musculophrenic and internal thoracic veins. The vein of the first space or the supreme intercostal vein, posteriorly, may be a tributary of the brachiocephalic, vertebral, or superior intercostal vein. The superior intercostal vein is formed by the posterior intercostal veins of the second, third, and sometimes the fourth spaces. This drains into the azygos vein on the right side, and on the left side it arches over the aorta, superficial to the vagus and deep to the phrenic to open into the left brachiocephalic veins. Subcostal veins join the ascending lumbar veins and ascend on the left side as the hemiazygos and on the right side as the azygos vein draining the lower eight spaces. The blood in the hemiazygos vein drains across the midline, through median anastomoses into the azygos vein.

The internal thoracic vessels are part of the anastomotic chain that links the subclavian artery and brachiocephalic veins to the external iliac vessels. The intercostal vessels in turn connect to the descending aorta and azygos system of veins. In the presence of obstruction to flow, these anastomoses provide alternative channels for arterial and venous blood flow.

Anatomy of Breathing

Simple respiratory effort is attained mostly by diaphragmatic motion. The bony and muscular components of the thorax remain a stable cavity while the diaphragm acts as a piston. It flattens during inspiration to create negative intrathoracic pressure, resulting in expansion of the lungs. Once inspiration is complete, the diaphragm relaxes and the lung recoils to its original position. The intercostals muscles are important to prevent paradoxical motion during inspiration.

The thoracic cavity can change to meet increased respiratory needs. The accessory muscles of the chest wall help to increase intrathoracic volume during inspiration and decrease volume during expiration. In addition to the piston action of the diaphragm, the accessory muscles elevate the sternal body and xiphoid process anteriorly and superiorly. The lower ribs attached to the sternum follow this movement and therefore increase the diameter of the lower chest cavity. The manubrium of the sternum is relatively fixed, and the chest cavity at this level does not contribute significantly to increased respiratory needs. This dynamic response of the chest cavity helps meet increasing demands for oxygenation and ventilation.

SURFACE ANATOMY

An understanding of surface anatomy enables identification of bony and prominent structures and hence the position of deeply related structures (Fig. 1-8 and Table 1-4). The chest radiograph (Fig. 1-9) is an extension of the routine physical examination.

The suprasternal notch on the superior aspect of the manubrium is palpable between the prominent medial ends of the clavicle, and it lies at the level of the lower border of the body of the second thoracic vertebra. At the lower sternal border, the palpable xiphisternum is covered by the rectus abdominis muscles. The xiphisternal joint lies opposite the body of the ninth thoracic vertebra. The sternal angle of Louis (the junction of the manubrium with the body of the sternum) is an important landmark for the description of structures inside the chest. At this level, the second costal cartilage joins the lateral margin of the sternum. The sternal angle lies opposite the lower border of the fourth thoracic vertebral body. All other ribs are counted from this point, as the first rib is not palpable. The angle of Louis is a useful reference point for counting ribs on a computed tomography (CT) scan, and also for localizing structures in the thoracic cavity. For example, the sternomanubrial joint is an important level for many structures. At this level, the azygous crosses midline to join the superior vena cava, the thoracic duct crosses from the right hemithorax to the left hemithorax on its ascent to the left neck, the trachea bifurcates into right and left main-stem bronchus, and the aorta and pulmonary artery form the aortic pulmonary window.

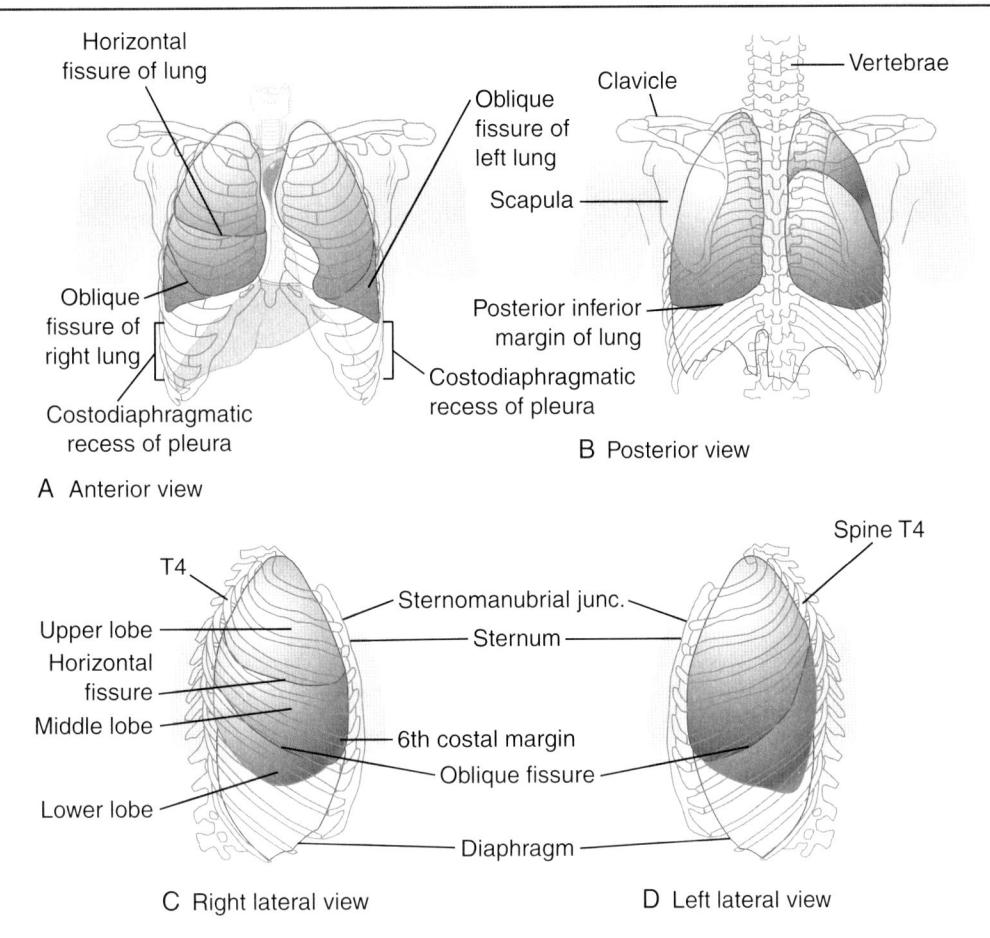

Figure 1–8
Correlation of lungs and overlying bony structures. **A**, Anterior view. **B,** Posterior view. **C,** Right lateral view. **D,** Left lateral view. The right oblique fissure courses anteriorly at the level of the fifth rib, ending near the level of the sixth rib. The posteriorly left oblique fissure is more variable, starting at a level between the third and fifth ribs. Anteriorly, it ends consistently at the level of the fifth rib. The horizontal fissure starts anteriorly at the fourth costal cartilage and joins the oblique fissure at the level of fifth rib.

The clavicle articulates with the acromion process of the scapula laterally and the sternum medially. Just below the medial joint lies the fusion of the first ribs with the lateral margin of the sternum. The costal margin is the lower boundary of the bony thorax and is formed by the cartilages of the seventh, eighth, ninth, and 10th ribs and the ends of the 11th and 12th cartilages. The lowest part of the margin is the 10th rib, and it lies at the level of the third lumbar vertebra. The lower border of the pectoralis major muscle forms the anterior axillary fold. The tendon of the latissimus dorsi forms the posterior axillary fold as it passes around the lower border of the teres major muscle.

Posteriorly, the thoracic cage is covered by muscles (trapezius, latissimus dorsi, and erector spinae) and is obscured by the scapula, but there are a few useful landmarks to the rib levels. The superior angle of the scapula lies opposite the spine of the second thoracic vertebra. The transversely running spine of the scapula is easily felt and lies at the level of the third thoracic vertebra. The lower angle of the scapula overlies the seventh rib.

The first prominent spinous process in the low midline of the neck posteriorly is that of the seventh cervical vertebra, the vertebra prominens. The tip of a spinous process of a thoracic vertebra lies posterior to the body of the next vertebra below.

The apex of the pleura extends about 3 cm above the medial third of the clavicle and behind the sternocleidomastoid muscle. It passes downward and medially behind the sternoclavicular joints. The left pleura, at the level of the fourth costal cartilage, deviates laterally for a variable distance from the cardiac notch. Both pleurae lie at the level of the eighth rib in the midclavicular line, at the level of the 10th rib in the mid-axillary line, and at the level of the 12th rib at the paravertebral level posteriorly.

The more constant right oblique fissure of the lung follows the course of the fifth rib from the midline posteriorly, more toward its lower border. Anteriorly it ends at the costochondral junction at the level of the sixth rib. The left oblique fissure has a more variable origin from the third to the fifth rib level, but anteriorly it follows a more predictable course along the fifth rib.

The transverse or horizontal fissure (present only on the right side) is marked by a horizontal line that runs backward from the fourth costal cartilage to reach the oblique fissure at the midaxillary line at the level of the fifth rib.

The pulmonary hilum lies lateral to the sternum behind the second to fourth costal cartilages and in front of the fourth to sixth vertebral bodies. The pulmonary trunk starts behind the left costal cartilage and it ascend to the level of the second costal cartilage before it bifurcates. The aorta also arises from

Table 1-4
Surface Landmarks and Correlating Intrathoracic Structures

Landmark	Underlying Structures
Sternocleidomastoid muscle (SCM)	Internal jugular vein, cupola of pleura Internal mammary artery originates between sternal and clavicular heads of the SCM and runs 2 cm from sternal edge until the sixth costal cartilage
Right manubrial border	Right brachiocephalic vein, origin of superior vena cava, brachiocephalic artery
Manubrium	Aortic arch and origin of great vessels, left brachiocephalic vein
Left manubrial border	Left common carotid and left subclavian vessels
Angle of Louis	Trachea bifurcation Level of the fourth vertebral body
Body of sternum and third to sixth costal cartilages	Heart
At the level of the angle of Louis in the right hemithorax	Azygos vein joins superior vena cava Thoracic duct crosses midline
At the level of the angle of Louis in the left hemithorax	Aortic pulmonary window
Left third costal cartilage	Origin of aorta and pulmonary artery
Right third costal cartilage	Superior vena cava empties into right atrium
Sixth costal cartilage	Level of the eighth vertebral body Inferior vena cava and right phrenic nerve pass through the diaphragm
Left seventh costal cartilage	Tenth vertebral body Esophagus and vagal trunks pass through the diaphragm
Tip of the scapula	Seventh intercostal space

the heart at the level of the left third costal cartilage. It travels superiorly to the right side of the angle of Louis before arching leftward.

The great vessels arise from the aortic arch behind the sternomanubrial joint. The brachiocephalic artery travels under the manubrium toward the right sternoclavicular joint. The left common carotid artery makes a similar ascent under the manubrium but travels toward the left sternomanubrial joint before entering the neck. The left subclavian artery travels just left of the common carotid artery. The use of surface anatomy to guide incisions and approaches for various thoracic and cardiac procedures will be discussed in later chapters.

Transcribing a chest film and a CT scan to a physical location on a patient is vital for any thoracic surgical procedure, but it is particularly important for video-assisted thoracic surgery (VATS). Often, small nodules are hard to palpate thoracoscopically unless a more localized area is identified. Anatomic landmarks can help divide and further subdivide the lung to help localize these nodules (Fig. 1-10).

MEDIASTINUM

The mediastinum is centrally located in the thoracic cavity. A pleural cavity bounds each side of the mediastinum, and its inferior and superior borders are defined by the diaphragm and the thoracic inlet, respectively. In classic descriptions, the mediastinum is divided into a superior and inferior mediastinum. The superior mediastinum lies above the plane from the sternomanubrial joint to the fourth thoracic vertebra. In the superior compartment lies the upper part of the thymus, the lower ends of the strap muscles, and the upper half of the superior vena cava, trachea, thoracic duct, and esophagus. The inferior compartment is further subdivided into anterior, middle, and posterior.

In 2000, Shields recategorized the mediastinum into three compartments: anterior, middle, and posterior. The diaphragm and bilateral pleural cavities remain the inferior and lateral borders for each of these compartments. The superior border now extends to the thoracic inlet for each compartment. The anterior compartment lies between the sternum and pericardium and great vessels. The posterior compartment lies behind the pericardium, great vessels, and tracheal bifurcation and extends to the vertebral column. The middle mediastinum is between the anterior and posterior compartments and includes the entire thoracic inlet (Table 1-5). Disease entities of the mediastinum are discussed in later chapters.

TRACHEOBRONCHIAL TREE

The trachea is a continuation of the larynx at the infracricoid level. Its average length is 11.8 cm. It has approximately 17 to 21 incomplete cartilaginous rings (4 mm wide and 1 mm thick) that maintain its elliptical shape in adults, but the shape is more circular in children. The coronal dimensions in men and women are 13 to 25 mm and 10 to 21 mm, respectively. The sagittal dimensions also differ between the sexes: 13 to 27 mm in men and 10 to 23 mm in women. With flexion of the neck, the trachea becomes almost completely an intrathoracic organ, coursing backward and downward from a subcutaneous position to rest ultimately on the esophagus and vertebral column at the level of the carina. Bearing a common embryologic origin with the esophagus, these two structures remain in intimate contact with one another, with the posterior muscular membranous wall of the trachea resting on the esophagus. The thyroid is anterior to the trachea in the neck and in the mediastinum, the thymus and parts of some of the great vessels lay anterior to the distal trachea.

The isthmus of the thyroid crosses the trachea at the second ring. The innominate artery crosses the mid trachea obliquely from right to left, and the arch of the aorta indents the esophagus slightly and appears to shift the trachea toward the right, away from its midline position. Lateral structures on the right side are predominantly venous and include the superior vena cava, azygos, and right brachiocephalic veins; lateral arterial structures on the left side include the arch of the aorta and the left common carotid artery. Both right and left vagi, along with their recurrent laryngeal nerves and the right and left sympathetic trunks, are also laterally related to the trachea. These intimate relationships of the trachea with surrounding organs are of important concern when performing cervical mediastinoscopy with lymph node biopsy.

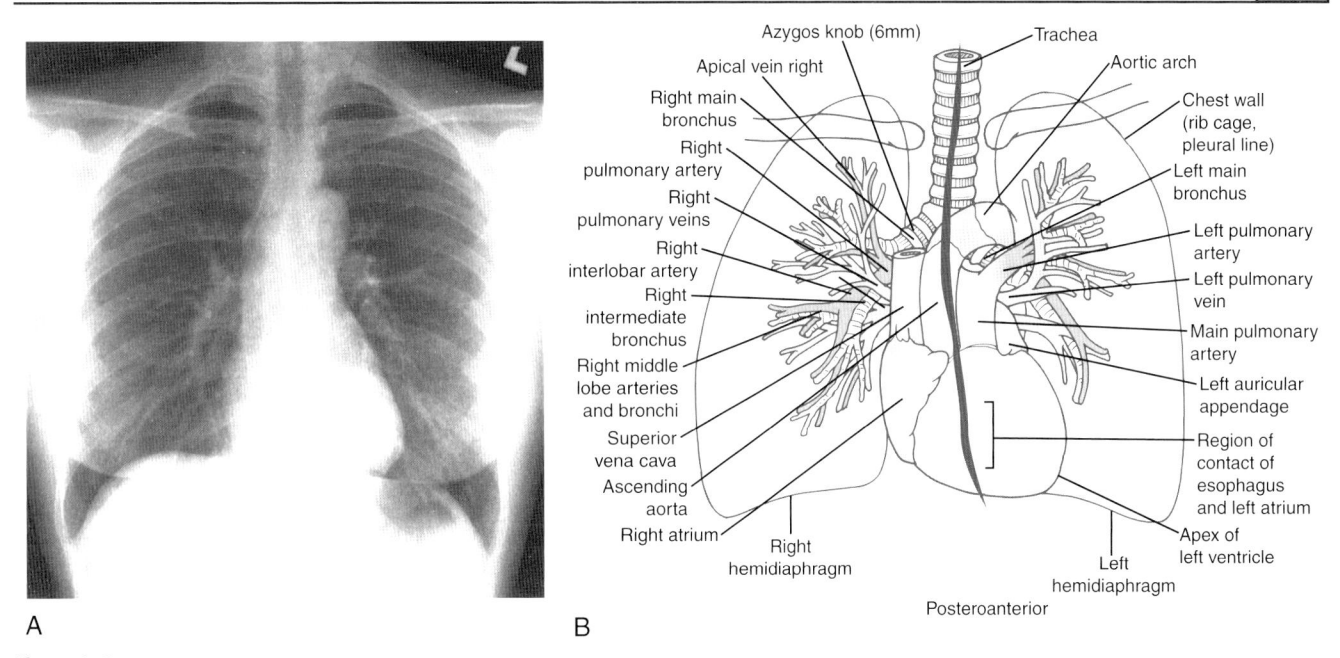

Figure 1-9
A, Posteroanterior radiograph of the chest in a normal male adult. **B,** Schematic representation of the surface projection of intrathoracic structures seen on a normal chest radiograph. *(From Butler P, Mitchell AWM, Ellis H.* Applied radiological anatomy. *Cambridge, UK: Cambridge University Press; 1999.)*

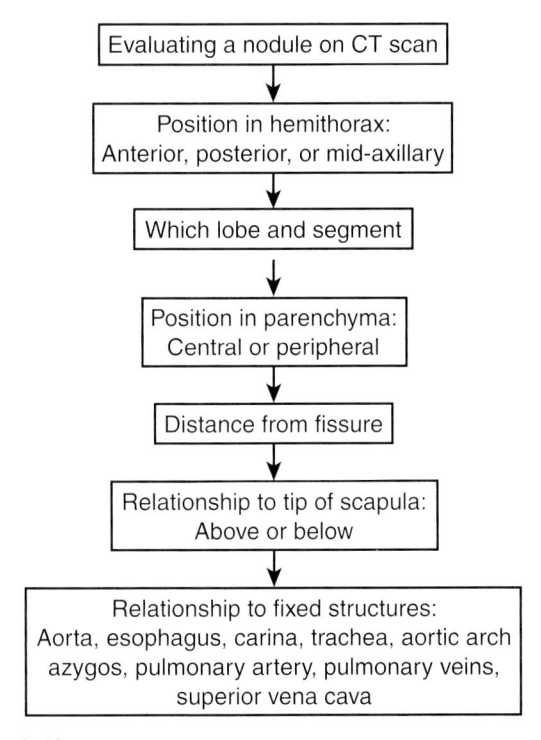

Figure 1-10
Algorithm for correlating a pulmonary nodule on CT scan to the patient during the operation.

Table 1-5
Structures in the Mediastinum

Compartment	Structures or Tissues	Pathologic Entities
Anterior	Thymus Internal mammary artery Fat Internal thoracic and prevascular lymph nodes Connective tissue Ectopic parathyroid Substernal thyroid	Thymic disease Teratoma Substernal thyroid Disease of lymph nodes Parathyroid disease Bronchogenic cysts
Middle	Heart Great vessels Trachea Proximal bronchi Vagus and phrenic nerves Esophagus Thoracic duct Proximal azygos vein Descending aorta Paratracheal lymph nodes	Lymph node disease (malignant and benign) Esophageal disease Tracheal disease Bronchogenic, pericardial, and esophageal cysts Morgagni hernia Angiomas
Posterior	Sympathetic chain Distal azygos vein Posterior paraesophageal lymph nodes	Neurogenic tumors Spinal lesions

Segmental blood supply to the trachea is from the inferior thyroid, subclavian, supreme intercostals, internal thoracic, innominate, and superior and middle bronchial arteries. This blood supply is shared with the esophagus and the main bronchi. Anastomotic arcades develop on the lateral tracheal wall and feed transverse vessels that travel between cartilaginous rings. For this reason, the trachea should not be circumferentially devascularized for a distance greater than 1 to 2 cm. The lateral arcades allow safe pretracheal dissections. Lymph drains to the posterior inferior group of deep cervical nodes and to paratracheal nodes.

The trachea bifurcates into the right and left principal bronchi (Fig. 1-11). The right principal bronchus arises in a more direct line with the trachea at an angle of about 25 degrees and passes behind the superior vena cava to reach the hilum of the lung. The left principal bronchus is slightly smaller, leaves the trachea more obliquely at an angle of about 45 degrees, passes below the arch of the aorta and the left pulmonary artery, and is almost twice as long as the right main bronchus (about 4 to 6 cm). The carinal angle can be wider in women and obese people. It can also be wider in patients with bulky subcarinal nodal disease.

The right upper lobe bronchus, also known as the eparterial bronchus, branches from the lateral wall of the right principal bronchus about 1.2 cm distal to the trachea. The upper lobe bronchus, about 1 cm in length, gives off three segmental bronchi as it makes almost a 90-degree angle with the right main bronchus and the bronchus intermedius. After a distance of approximately 1.5 to 2 cm, the middle lobe bronchus arises from the anterior surface of the bronchus intermedius. The middle lobe bronchus is 1.5 to 2.2 cm long and bifurcates into lateral and medial branches. The superior segmental bronchus to the lower lobe arises from the posterior wall of the bronchus intermedius as it terminates into the basal-stem bronchus that sends off segmental bronchi to the medial, anterior, lateral, and posterior basal segments. The medial basal segment arise anteromedially, whereas the lateral basal and posterior basal segments most often arise as a common stem.

The longer left principal bronchus bifurcates into the upper lobe bronchus that travels anterolaterally and the lower lobe bronchus that continues posteromedially. The left upper lobe bronchus divides into the superior and inferior divisions that supply the upper lobe and lingula, respectively. The superior division branches into an apical posterior segmental bronchus and an anterior segmental bronchus. The inferior or lingual bronchus, which is the equivalent of a middle lobe bronchus on the right, is 1 to 2 cm in length and divides into the superior and inferior divisions. The lower lobe bronchus on the right side gives off the superior segmental bronchus as its first branch before the basal trunk continues for about 1.5 cm as a single trunk. This then bifurcates into an anteromedial basal segmental bronchus and a common bronchial stem for the remaining basal segments.

Anatomic variations usually involve segmental bronchi arising as a common stem. Occasionally, additional bronchi may arise from the main stem and distribute to a segment that has its own bronchus. A right upper lobe bronchus originating from the trachea (a porcine tracheobronchial tree) occurs in 3% of the population. Recognizing aberrant tracheobronchial anatomy is important for placement of the double-lumen endotracheal tube as well as for performing the ensuing surgical procedure.

LUNGS

To conserve healthy tissue and to perform operations safely on the lung, the thoracic surgeon must have a thorough knowledge of the segmental bronchopulmonary anatomy. Developing

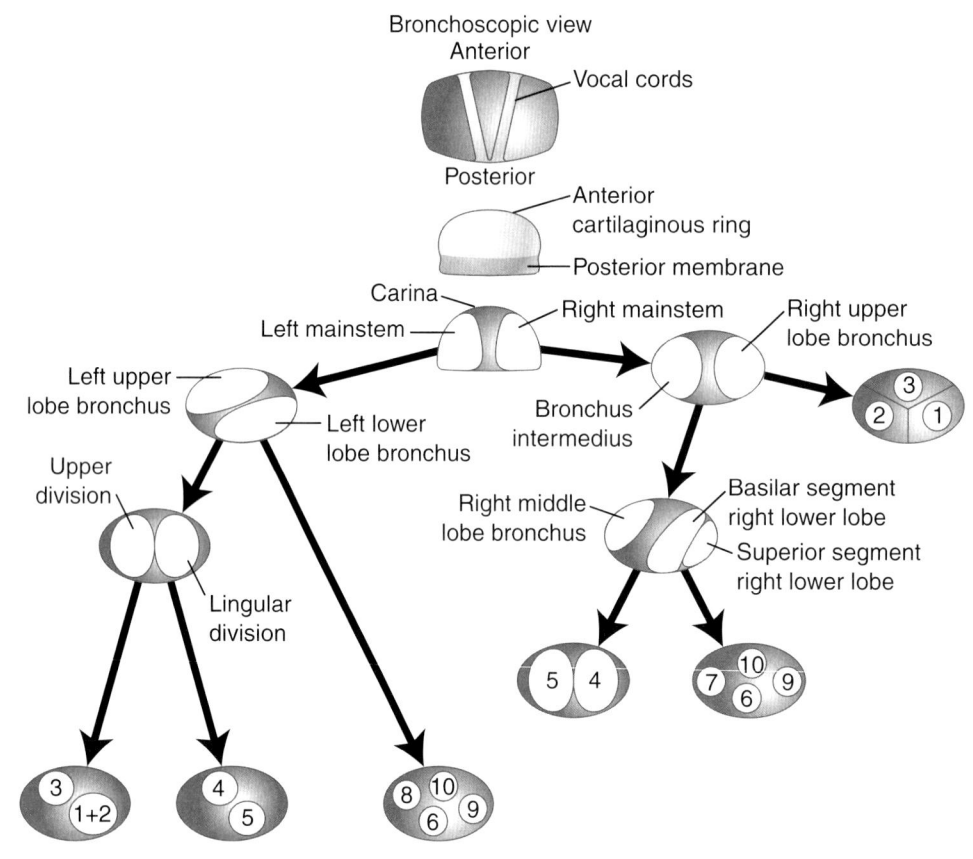

Figure 1–11
Bronchoscopic view of the tracheobronchial tree. See Figure 1-12 for names of the numbered segments.

Chapter 1 Anatomy of the Thorax

Tracheobronchial tree

Right main stem — Left main stem
Right upper lobe — Left upper lobe
Right middle lobe
Right lower lobe — Left lower lobe

Right

RUL
1. Apical segment
2. Posterior segment
3. Anterior segment

RML
4. Lateral segment
5. Medial segment

RLL
6. Superior segment
7. Medial basal segment
8. Anterior basal segment
9. Lateral basal segment
10. Posterior basal segment

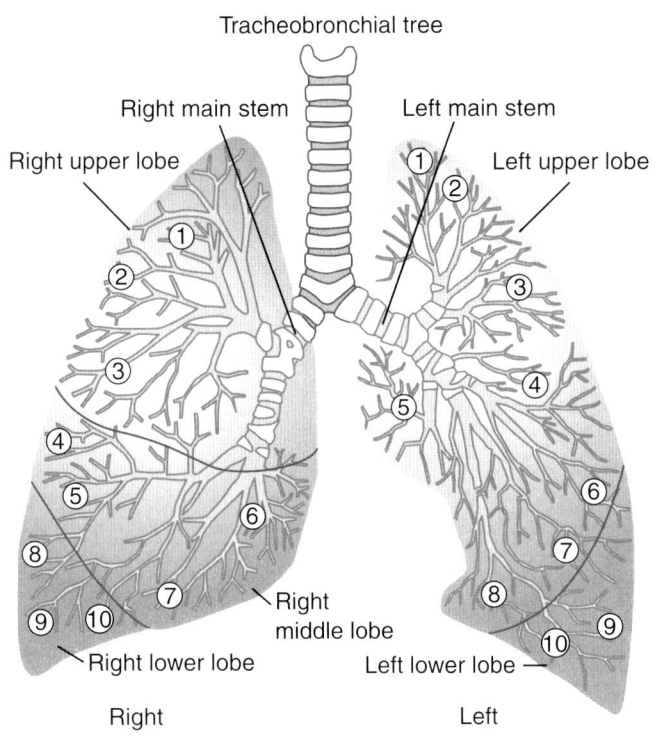

Left

1. & 2. Apical posterior segment
3. Anterior segment
4. Lingular superior segment
5. Lingular inferior segment
6. Basal superior segment
7. Lateral basal segment
8. Anterior medial basal segment
9. Lateral basal segment
10. Posterior basal segment

Figure 1–12
Segments of the right and left lung. RLL, right lower lobe; RML, right middle lobe; RUL, right upper lobe.

as outpouchings of the foregut, the ventral lung buds undergo repeated branching, to yield approximately 20 generations from the principal bronchi to the terminal alveolar sacs. With the bronchus at the center, each bronchopulmonary segment functions as an individual unit with its own pulmonary arterial and venous supply. Importantly, the pulmonary veins run in the intersegmental plane and do not accompany the bronchus and the pulmonary artery to each unit.

The lungs are free of the pleural cavity except for attachments to the heart, trachea, and inferior pulmonary ligaments. The larger right lung has three lobes—upper, middle, and lower—and is composed of 10 bronchopulmonary segments. The left lung has two lobes—upper and lower—and eight segments (Fig. 1-12). The lingula on the left side is the anatomic equivalent of the middle lobe and is incorporated into the upper lobe. The terminology proposed by Jackson and Huber for the pulmonary segments and the branches supplying them has been universally adopted. The apparent discrepancy of there being only eight segments on the left side is explained by the fact that the apical and posterior segmental bronchi of the left upper lobe and the anterior and medial segmental bronchi of the left lower lobe originate from a common stem bronchus (Fig. 1-13 and Table 1-6).

The oblique fissure on each side separates the lower lobe from the rest of the lung. Anomalous fissures of varying depth may be seen along any of the segments but are most commonly seen separating the superior segment of the lower lobe. Rarely, the apical segment of the right upper lobe may be a true tracheal lobe, with its bronchus arising directly from the trachea. The azygos lobe is not a true segment but is formed by the azygos vein cutting into the pleura and apex of the lung. Medlar evaluated 1200 lungs and found an incidence of incomplete oblique fissure on the left and right of 18% and 30%, respectively. Of these patients, 63% had an incomplete horizontal fissure.

The right and left hilum have different characteristics (Table 1-7). The right hilum exits the mediastinum below the confluence of the azygos and superior vena cava, and behind the superior vena cava and right atrial juncture. The left hilum lies below the aortic arch. The position of the pulmonary artery is somewhat different on the two sides. On the left (Fig. 1-14), the artery lies anterior and superior to the bronchus and runs in a slightly posterior direction before curving around and behind the left upper lobe bronchus. The right main-stem bronchus is the most superior and posterior of the right hilar structures, and the artery, though slightly anterior, is inferior to the bronchus (Fig. 1-15). The superior pulmonary veins are inferior and anterior to the pulmonary arteries, and the inferior pulmonary veins are even more inferior and posterior to the superior veins.

The main pulmonary artery arises to the left of the aorta and passes superiorly and to the left, anterior to the left main-stem bronchus, where it divides into the right and left main pulmonary arteries. The right pulmonary artery passes to the right behind the ascending aorta and forms the superior border of the transverse sinus. It then passes posterior to the superior vena cava and forms the superior border of the postcaval recess of Allison, whereas the right superior pulmonary vein forms the inferior border of the recess. The first branch is the truncus anterior (rarely intrapericardial); it arises superolaterally and supplies the upper lobe before the pulmonary artery enters the lung hilum (Fig. 1-16). The interlobar pulmonary artery goes between the bronchus intermedius (posterior) and superior pulmonary vein (anteriorly) and gives off the posterior ascending artery to the posterior segment of the upper lobe (Fig. 1-17). The ongoing pulmonary artery then runs behind the middle lobe bronchus. Opposite the posterior ascending artery, the middle lobe artery arise anteromedially, usually at the junction of the horizontal and oblique fissures. The arterial branch to the superior segment of the lower lobe arises posteriorly and opposite the middle lobe artery at the same level or slightly distal to it. Beyond the superior segmental artery, the common basal trunk continues in the fissure to give rise to the medial basal segmental artery, occasionally as a common branch with the anterior basal branch. The terminal branches supply the lateral and posterior basal segments.

The left pulmonary artery passes more posteriorly and superiorly than the right and is longer before giving off its first branch. Commonly, there are four branches to the left

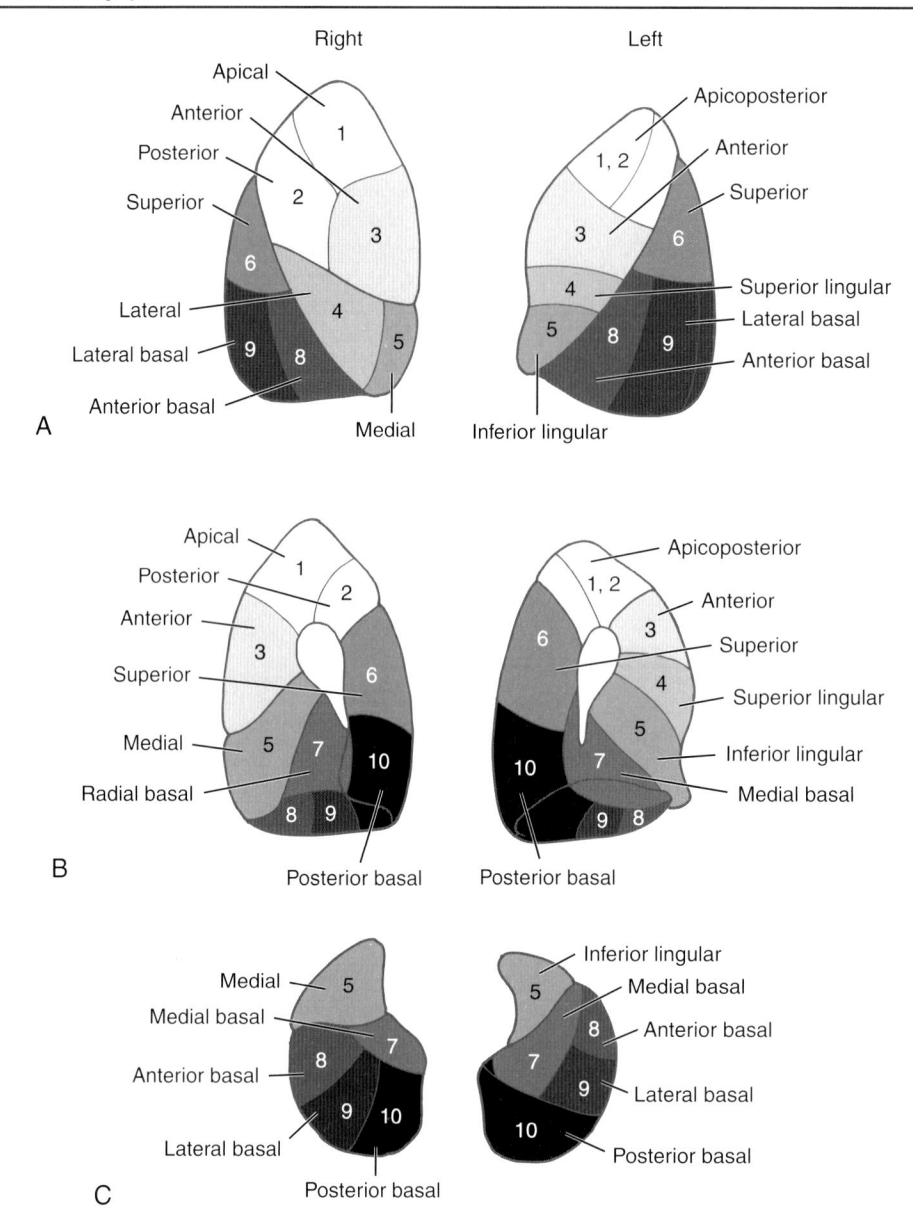

Figure 1-13
Bronchopulmonary segments. **A,** Lateral surface. **B,** Medial surface. **C,** Diaphragmatic surface.

upper lobe, but the number varies from two to seven. The first branch arises from the anterior portion of the artery and is quite short, and often its branches appear as separate vessels arising from the main artery. The second branch usually arises posterosuperiorly as the main artery passes over the left upper lobe bronchus and into the interlobar fissure, where more ascending upper lobe branches may originate (Fig. 1-18). As it enters the interlobar fissure, it gives off a branch to the superior segment of the left lower lobe and the lingular artery. Beyond the lingular branch, the common basal trunk divides into two major branches. The anterior branch supplies the anteromedial basal segments and the posterior branch supplies the lateral basal segments.

Among the common variations of the pulmonary arterial supply, the first anterior trunk on the left may be the major supply to the lingular segments. This should be suspected if a small lingular artery is found in the anterior fissure. The right side may have two major arteries that arise from the truncus anterior, which are designated the truncus anterior superior and the truncus anterior inferior.

The left superior pulmonary vein receives all the tributaries from the left upper lobe. It is closely applied to the anteroinferior portion of the pulmonary artery and makes dissection of the anterior branches quite hazardous. Its three main tributaries are apical posterior, anterior, and lingular. Occasionally, the superior and inferior lingular veins are separate. A common anomaly is drainage of the inferior lingular vein into the inferior pulmonary vein. The inferior pulmonary vein, lying more posteriorly and inferiorly, drains the entire lower lobe via two principal tributaries, the superior segmental and common basal veins. The right superior pulmonary vein is usually made up of four branches: the apical anterior, anterior-inferior, and posterior branches, which drain the upper lobe, and the inferior branch, which drains the middle lobe. Occasionally,

Table 1–6
Pulmonary Segmental Classification

Right	Left
Upper Lobe	**Upper Lobe**
1. Apical	1 and 2. Apical posterior
2. Posterior	
3. Anterior	3. Anterior
Middle Lobe	**Lingula**
4. Lateral	4. Superior lingula
5. Medial	5. Inferior lingula
Lower Lobe	**Lower Lobe**
6. Superior	6. Superior
7. Medial basal	7 and 8. Anteromedial basal
8. Anterior basal	
9. Lateral basal	9. Lateral basal
10. Posterior basal	10. Posterior basal

the middle lobe vein drains into the atrium as a separate vessel and very rarely it becomes a tributary of the inferior pulmonary vein.

The right inferior pulmonary vein is similar to the one on the left and is made up of two trunks. The common basal vein is made up of the superior basal and inferior basal tributaries, and the superior segmental vein drains the superior segment of the lower lobe. The superior and inferior pulmonary veins on the right most often enter the left atrium separately. In contrast, on the left, the two veins form a common trunk in more than 25% of the population.

The segmental branches of the pulmonary arteries usually lie on the superior or lateral surface of the segmental bronchus that they accompany and with which they branch. The venous tributaries occupy an intersegmental position, do not bear as close a relationship to the segmental bronchi, and tend to lie on their medial or inferior surfaces. Variations from the usual pattern are common: as a general rule, veins vary more than arteries, and arteries vary more than bronchi.

The systemic circulation of the lung tissues is derived from the bronchial arteries that supply the bronchi from the carina to their terminal bronchioles and that also nourish the connective tissue and visceral pleura. A single right bronchial artery usually branches from the third posterior intercostal artery, and two left bronchial arteries usually branch from the dorsal aorta, one near vertebra T5 and one inferior to the left principal bronchus. Although variations are known, most bronchial arteries arise from the anterolateral aspect of the aorta or its branches within 2 to 3 cm of the origin of the left subclavian artery and come to lie on the membranous portion of the principal bronchi. The bronchial arteries usually give off branches to the esophagus and then follow the bronchi into the lung, also giving off branches along the interalveolar connective tissue septae to the visceral pleura. There is a rich anastomosis with the pulmonary arterial supply, which is important after pulmonary transplantation.

The bronchial veins have a superficial system, with two bronchial veins on each side draining from the hilar region and visceral pleura into the azygos vein on the right and the accessory hemiazygos vein on the left. Most of the venous drainage from the deeper lung substance drains into the pulmonary venous system, accounting for the less than 100% saturation of the blood in the left atrium.

Lymphatic drainage channels run toward the hilum from subpleural vessels along the bronchi and pulmonary arteries. This flow is interrupted by multiple lymph nodes along the way, mostly situated at forking points of the bronchi. Each nodal station has a number assigned to it and is the basis of the most recent staging system for primary bronchogenic carcinoma, as proposed by Mountain and Dressler in 1997.

The most peripheral pulmonary nodes include subsegmental lymph nodes (level 14) and segmental (level 13), lobar (level 12), and interlobar (level 11) nodes in the fissures, and they are reliably removed during a lobectomy. The hilar lymph nodes (level 10), also known as bronchopulmonary nodes, are at the root of the lung and can be accessed via thoracoscopy or thoracotomy. The inferior pulmonary ligament nodes (level 9) lie in the inferior pulmonary ligament on the left and the right, and the paraesophageal nodes (level 8) lie dorsal to the posterior wall of the trachea and inferior to the carina, to the right or left of the midline esophagus (Fig. 1-19). From then on, drainage is to the central mediastinal and tracheobronchial nodes, and upward via mediastinal lymph trunks to the brachiocephalic veins (see Fig. 1-19A).

The right and left paratracheal lymph nodes (levels 2R and 2L), and the lower paratracheal lymph nodes at the tracheobronchial angle (levels 4R and 4L), and the subcarinal (level 7) lymph nodes can be identified and sampled via a standard cervical mediastinoscopy. During a right VATS or right thoracotomy, lymph nodes at levels 4R, 7, 8, and 9 can be sampled (see Fig. 1-19C,E). The Chamberlain procedure or the left VATS procedure can give access to the subaortic (level 5) and para-aortic (level 6) lymph nodes. Left VATS can also provide access to lymph nodes at levels 7, 8, and 9 (see Fig. 1-19B,D). The delphian lymph node (the highest mediastinal, pretracheal lymph node) is classified as level 1.

Thus, levels 1 through 9 are considered mediastinal lymph nodes, and metastases are classified as N2 if ipsilateral and as N3 if contralateral spread of cancer is present in these lymph node stations. Anomalies of this ipsilateral, centrally directed drainage pattern are quite common and are more likely on the left side, especially with lower lobe tumors. Up to 50% of left lower lobe tumors and 35% of left upper lobe tumors have positive contralateral (N3) mediastinal nodes, whereas contralateral metastasis is found in only 42% of right lower lobe tumors and 18% of right upper lobe tumors when N2 lymph nodes are negative for tumor. Instead of draining to hilar nodes, the left upper lobe tumors follow an alternative path to the subaortic, periaortic, and anterior mediastinal nodes in up to one third of patients.

The vagus nerve and the sympathetic plexus contribute to the poorly developed anterior pulmonary plexus around the main pulmonary arteries, and to the well-developed posterior plexus of nerves around the bronchi. The vagus nerve carries all the afferent innervation from the bronchial mucosa, sensing stretch in the alveoli and pleura, pressure in the

Table 1–7
Characteristics of Left and Right Lung and Their Lobes

Side or Lobe	Characteristics
Right lung	Hilum enters behind the superior vena cava or the right atrial juncture below the azygos nerve. Ten segments Three lobes with a horizontal and oblique fissure The most superior and posterior structure in the right hilum is the right main-stem bronchus. The right pulmonary artery is superior and slightly posterior to the right superior pulmonary vein. The right pulmonary artery is inferior and anterior to the right main-stem bronchus. Pulmonary veins most often enter heart separately.
Left lung	Hilum courses under aortic arch. Eight segments Two lobes with an oblique fissure Left pulmonary artery lies anterior and superior to the left main-stem bronchus. The left superior vein is anterior and inferior to the left pulmonary artery. Greatest variation in number and location of pulmonary artery branches Superior and inferior veins form common trunk before entering left atrium in 25% of the population.
Right upper lobe	Arterial supply from truncus anterior branch coming off right main pulmonary artery at apex of hilum and from posterior ascending artery, found posterior to superior pulmonary vein or in fissure as ongoing pulmonary artery exits lung parenchyma. Venous drainage into upper division of superior pulmonary vein Right upper lobe bronchus posterior in hilum Three segments
Right middle lobe	Arterial supply from one (45%) or two (48%) middle lobe arteries found from the right pulmonary artery at the confluences of the horizontal and oblique fissures. Middle lobe vein drains most often into superior pulmonary vein and occasionally into inferior pulmonary vein. Middle lobe bronchus from bronchus intermedius Two segments From anterior to posterior: middle lobe vein, bronchus, artery
Right lower lobe	Superior segmental artery and basilar artery are terminal branches of right pulmonary artery in the fissure. Inferior pulmonary vein Right lower lobe bronchus Five segments From anterior to posterior: inferior pulmonary vein, pulmonary artery, bronchus
Left upper lobe	Two to eight arterial branches First branch of the pulmonary artery comes off behind superior pulmonary vein. Varying number of posterior ascending arteries are given off after first branch as the pulmonary artery courses over and behind the left main-stem bronchus. Lingular artery: most anterior branch in fissure going to upper lobe Superior pulmonary vein with upper division and lingular veins Four segments Left upper lobe bronchus posterior to vein
Left lower lobe	Superior segmental artery and basilar artery are terminal branches of right pulmonary artery in the fissure. Inferior pulmonary vein Left lower lobe bronchus Four segments From anterior to posterior: inferior pulmonary vein, pulmonary artery, bronchus
Segments	Triangular parenchyma with apex toward center Bronchus runs in middle of segment Segmental artery on posterior surface of bronchus Veins in intersegmental planes Veins vary more than arteries, which vary more than bronchus Lingular and superior segmentectomies are easiest Basilar and apical segmentectomies harder Anterior segmentectomy hardest

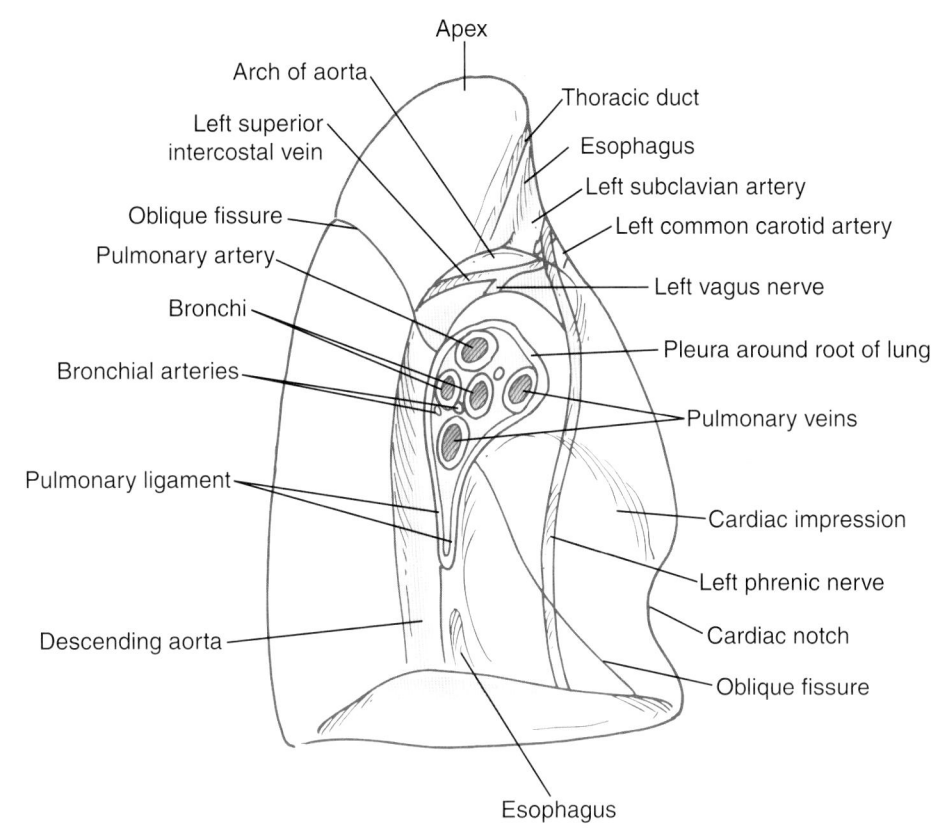

Figure 1–14
The medial surface of the left lung.

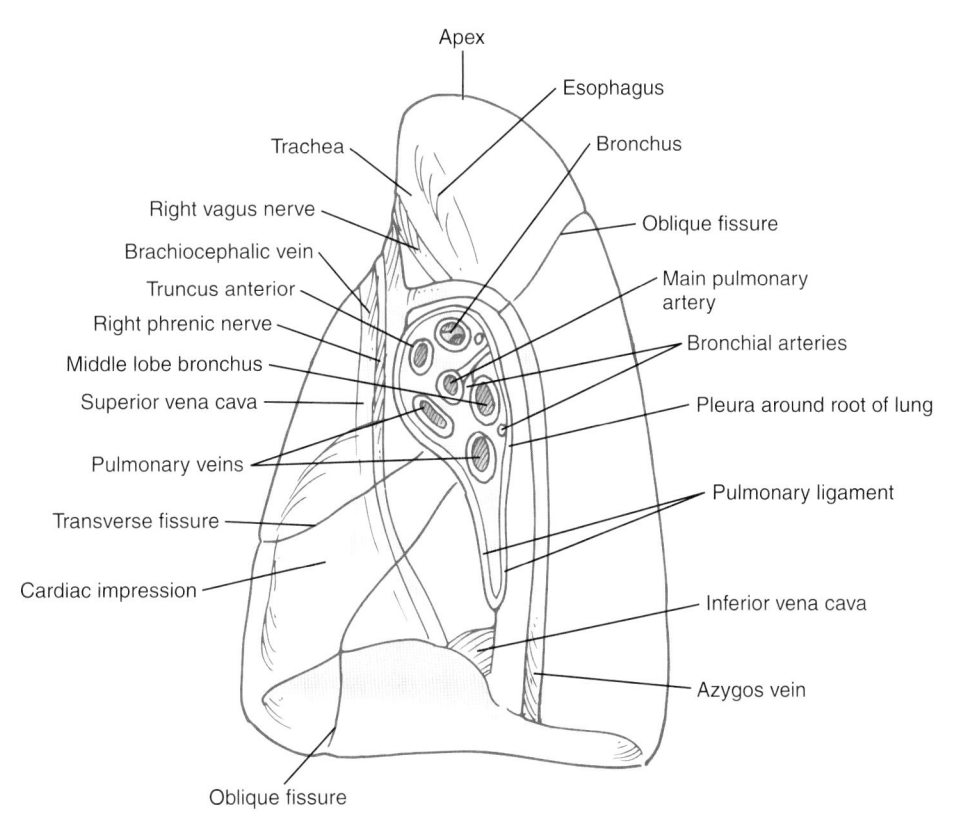

Figure 1–15
The medial surface of the right lung.

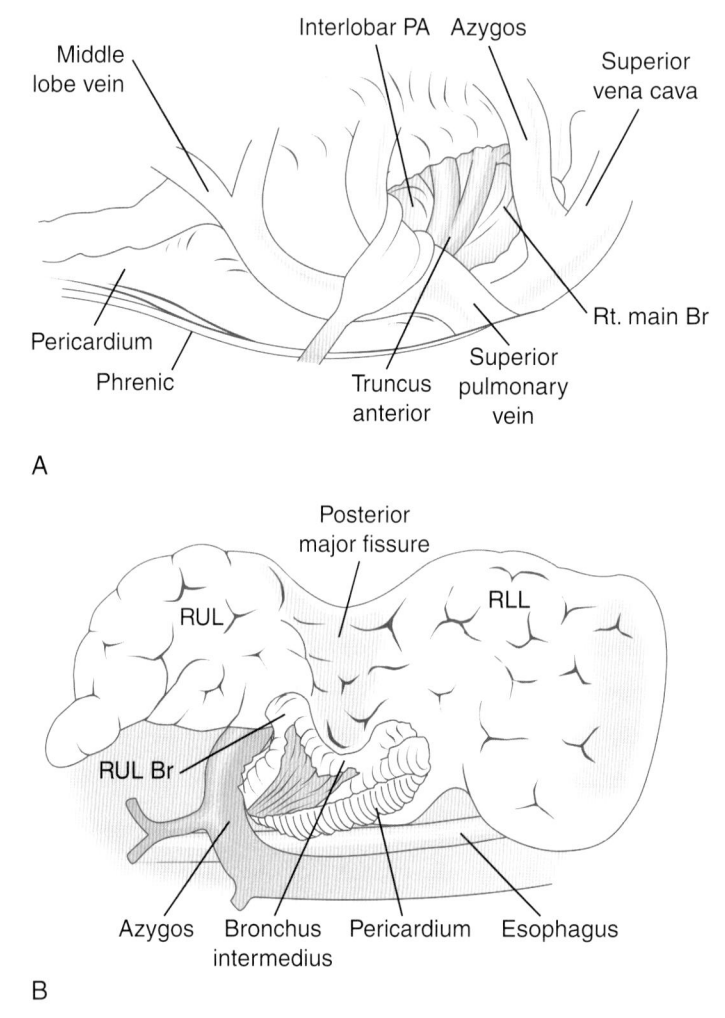

Figure 1-16
Hilum of the right lung. **A,** Anterior view. **B,** Posterior view. Br, branch; PA, pulmonary artery; RLL, right lower lobe; RUL, right upper lobe.

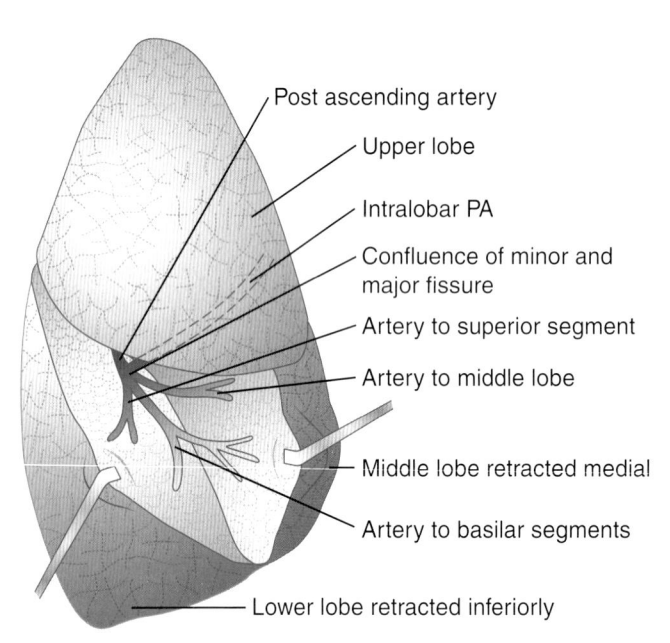

Figure 1-17
Pulmonary artery as it exits the parenchyma of the right upper lobe into the confluence of the major and minor fissures. PA, pulmonary artery.

pulmonary veins, and mediating pain. Efferent fibers in the vagus constrict the bronchi, and the sympathetic efferents are vasoconstricting to the pulmonary vessels and secretomotor to the bronchial plexus.

The left and right hemithoraces each contain a variety of other vital organs in addition to the lungs. The thoracic duct, esophagus, aorta, and azygos vein can be visualized in the right hemithorax, whereas the aortic arch, descending aorta, and distal esophagus may be seen in the left hemithorax.

ESOPHAGUS

The esophagus is a muscular tube that starts at the upper esophageal sphincter (the cricopharyngeus) and travels approximately 25 cm to the lower esophageal sphincter at the gastroesophageal junction. The cricopharyngeus is 15 cm from the incisor teeth. By endoscopy, the gastroesophageal junction is measured to be 38 to 40 cm from the incisors in men, and generally 2 cm shorter in women. The cervical esophagus is slightly left of midline as it enters the thoracic inlet in front of the body of the T1 vertebra and posterior to the trachea. After it passes the aortic arch, it inclines forward and passes in front of the descending thoracic aorta to obtain a position left of midline as it travels through the esophageal hiatus opposite

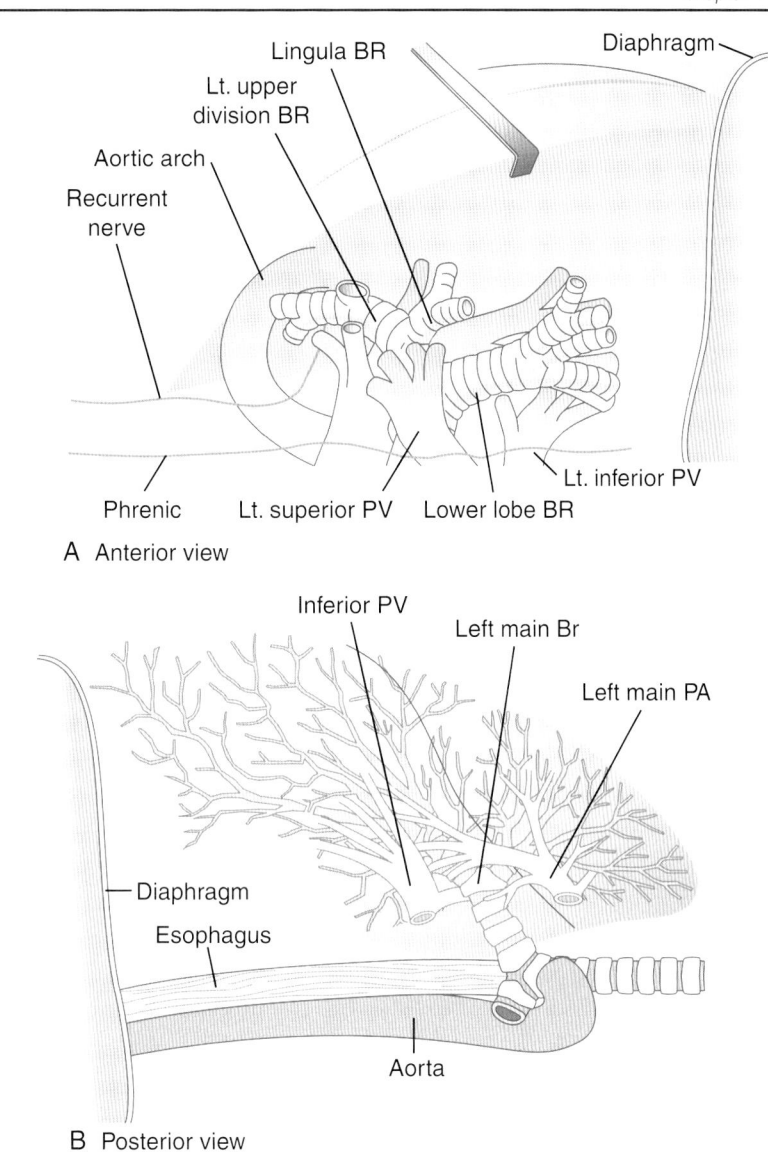

Figure 1-18
Hilum of the left lung. **A,** Anterior view. **B,** Posterior view. BR, branch; PA, pulmonary artery; PV, pulmonary vein.

the body of the 10th thoracic vertebra. At the level of the T8 vertebra, the left lateral wall of the esophagus that was covered by the aorta is in contact with the parietal pleura as the aorta goes directly behind it. This is a common site of perforation in patients with Boerhaave's syndrome. The right lateral surface of the esophagus is completely covered by parietal pleura except where the azygos vein crosses it at the level of the T4 vertebra. When choosing the side for a thoracotomy, avoiding interference from the aortic arch is the primary concern. Access to the proximal esophagus is difficult from the left hemithorax because of the overlying aortic arch.

Endoscopic examination of the esophagus reveals several constrictions on the esophageal lumen in addition to the narrowing at the upper and lower esophageal sphincters. The additional constrictions are seen endoscopically where the esophagus crosses the aortic arch at 22 to 25 cm from the incisors, and where it is crossed by the left main-stem bronchi at 27.5 cm from the incisors. These anatomic relationships may also be seen radiographically. A notch indentation is often seen in its left lateral wall on a barium swallow radiograph as the esophagus passes to the right of the aorta at the level of the tracheal bifurcation. The left main-stem bronchus may indent it slightly as it passes over the esophagus.

The blood supply of the cervical esophagus is from branches of the inferior thyroid artery. The thoracic esophagus is supplied by the esophageal branches of the aorta and the bronchial arteries. Most individuals have one right-sided and one or two left-sided bronchial arterial branches. The upper aortic esophageal branch is usually shorter and originates at the T6 or T7 vertebral level, and the lower larger branch originates at the level of the eighth or ninth thoracic vertebra. Finally, the abdominal esophagus receives its supply from branches of the left gastric and inferior phrenic arteries. In the wall of the esophagus, there is an extensive longitudinal anastomotic network in the muscular and submucosal layers, a basis for portasystemic anastomoses. The venous drainage follows the arterial supply. A submucosal plexus drains into a periesophageal venous plexus, from which the veins originate

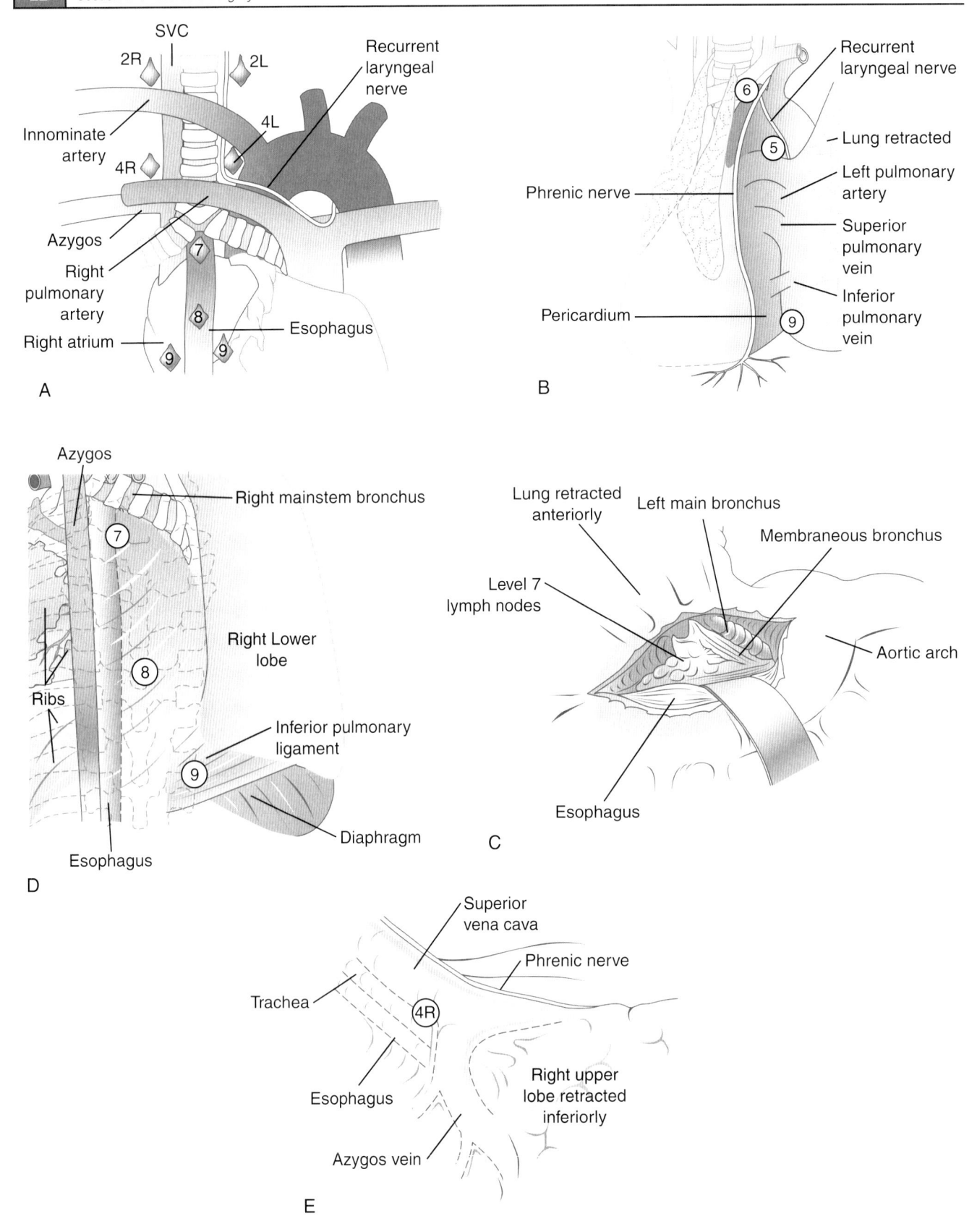

Figure 1-19
Mediastinal lymph nodes. **A,** Anterior view. **B,** Left lung retracted posteriorly to expose lymph nodes at levels 5, 6, and 9. **C,** Anterior retraction of the left lung to expose lymph nodes at level 7. **D,** Anterior retraction of right lung to expose lymph nodes at levels 7, 8, and 9. **E,** Inferior and posterior retraction of right lung to expose lymph nodes at level 4R.

and empty into the inferior thyroid, bronchial, azygos, and left gastric veins.

Two large interconnecting networks that course longitudinally form the lymphatic network of the esophagus. The mucosal network extends into the submucosal network, and flow is predominantly (6:1) longitudinal rather than segmental. These pierce the muscular wall, and ultimately lymph channels follow the arterial supply. The cervical esophagus drains into the deep cervical nodes alongside the inferior thyroid vessels, whereas the abdominal portion drains to the preaortic group of the celiac nodes along the left gastric artery. The thoracic esophagus drains into the tracheobronchial nodes superiorly and the subcarinal and paraesophageal nodes inferiorly.

After giving off their recurrent laryngeal branches, which supply the cricopharyngeal sphincter and cervical esophagus, the vagus nerves descend onto the anterior wall of the esophagus and form a complex vagal esophageal plexus, a network of interconnecting fibers that forms the preganglionic parasympathetic supply to the esophagus. These connect to the enteric ganglia in the myenteric and submucosal plexuses that are located in the wall of the esophagus. Just above the diaphragm, the plexus usually gives rise to two nerve trunks, the anterior and posterior vagal trunks. The anterior trunk contains predominantly left vagal fibers and the posterior contains mainly right, with considerable contribution from one another.

Cervical and thoracic sympathetic ganglia contribute visceral branches to the esophagus, and a few branches from the splanchnic nerves also reach the esophagus. Their effect on the esophageal muscle is unknown. The vagus nerve is the motor supply to the esophageal muscle, and the secretomotor nerve supplies the esophageal glands. Afferent pain fibers appear to run in both the vagal and vasomotor sympathetic supply; hence, esophageal pain can be referred to the neck, arm, and thoracic wall.

The mucosal lining of the esophagus is composed of nonkeratinized, stratified squamous epithelium supported by a lamina propria and a thick muscularis mucosa. The mucous membrane is thick and in the collapsed state is thrown into longitudinal folds. Mucosal glands in the submucosa are mainly found at the upper and lower ends of the esophagus. The muscular wall consists of an inner circular and an outer longitudinal layer that are visceral smooth muscle in the lower two thirds and skeletal striated muscle in the upper third. Except for the short intra-abdominal segment, the lack of a serosa in the rest of the esophagus accounts for the difficulty in suturing the esophagus.

VESSELS OF THE THORAX

Descending Thoracic Aorta

The descending thoracic aorta starts at the level of the fourth thoracic vertebra. It is a posterior mediastinal structure that arises just left of the vertebral column and travels toward the midline as it descends toward the diaphragm. When it goes through the aortic hiatus at the level of the 12th thoracic vertebra, it is anterior to the vertebral column. In the left hemithorax, anterior to the descending aorta, are the left pulmonary hilum, the pericardium, and the esophagus, and posteriorly is the vertebral column. In the right hemithorax, the esophagus is lateral to the aorta until it takes up a position anterior to the aorta near the diaphragm. The thoracic duct and azygos vein are lateral to the aorta in the right hemithorax. Branches of the descending thoracic aorta include pericardial, bronchial, mediastinal, phrenic, and posterior intercostal and subcostal arteries. The descending aorta is fixed at the origin of the left subclavian artery, which is therefore a common site for transection of the aorta during motor vehicle accidents.

Azygos Vein

The origin of the azygos vein is not constant. It typically starts from the posterior aspect of the inferior vena cava, but it may originate from a lumbar azygos vein or from the confluence of the subcostal and ascending lumbar vein. It ascends through the aortic hiatus in the diaphragm. It rises in the right hemithorax in the posterior mediastinum until the fourth vertebral body, and then it turns medially over the right pulmonary hilum to join the superior vena cava.

Thoracic Duct

The thoracic duct carries chylous material, which is rich in lipids, proteins, and lymphocytes. It begins at the confluence of the abdominal lymphatic trunks known as the cisterna chili. From its origin at the level of the 12th thoracic vertebra, the thoracic duct travels through the aortic hiatus and ascends in the right hemithorax between the descending thoracic aorta (medial) and the azygos vein (lateral) and posterior to the esophagus, until it crosses medially at the level of the fifth thoracic vertebral body. Once in the left hemithorax, it continues its ascent on the left side of the esophagus. It crosses the aortic arch anteriorly and then travels posterior to the left subclavian artery. It travels out of the thoracic inlet for 3 to 4 cm before arching and descending anterior to the medial border of the scalenus anterior and finally joining the venous system near the confluence of the left subclavian and internal jugular veins.

NERVES OF THE THORAX

Vagus and Recurrent Laryngeal Nerves

The vagus nerve passes inferiorly from the base of the skull to the thoracic inlet in the carotid sheath. On the right side, the right vagus travels behind the internal jugular vein and dives behind the sternoclavicular joint to give off the right recurrent laryngeal nerve. The right recurrent laryngeal nerve recurs on the ipsilateral subclavian artery and then ascends in the tracheoesophageal groove. The left recurrent laryngeal nerve recurs on the aortic arch and then rises in the tracheoesophageal groove. Both recurrent laryngeal nerves enter the larynx with the laryngeal branch of the inferior thyroid artery.

The right vagus continues to descend into the thoracic cavity behind the right brachiocephalic vein and then lateral to the trachea. It travels posteriorly and lies predominantly posterior to the right pulmonary hilum, where several bronchial branches are given off. The remaining vagal fibers join fibers from the left to form the posterior vagal trunk.

The left vagus enters the thorax between the common carotid and the subclavian arteries behind the left brachiocephalic vein. It crosses the left side of the aortic arch and gives off the left recurrent laryngeal nerve before descending behind the left pulmonary hilum. It also gives off bronchial branches at this level. Fibers from the left and right vagi form the anterior and posterior vagal trunks, which enter the abdomen through the esophageal hiatus.

Thoracic Sympathetic Chain

The thoracic sympathetic chain is formed by ganglia of the autonomic nervous system. The first thoracic ganglia, in the majority of patients, fuses with the inferior cervical ganglia. The thoracic sympathetic chain predominantly lies on the costal head under the pleura. The nerves interact with corresponding spinal nerves with white and gray rami. Ligation of sympathetic ganglia is performed to treat hyperhidrosis, facial blushing, Raynaud's disease, and reflex sympathetic dystrophy. When collateral nerve fibers bypass the sympathetic trunk, sympathectomy results in failure. These fibers can reach the brachial plexus without passing through the sympathetic ganglia. The nerve of Kuntz is the most described collateral nerve. Although in clinical literature, the nerve of Kuntz is reported in 10% of cases, it is reported 80% of the time in anatomic descriptions. Techniques for ligation of ganglia from T1 to T3 are discussed in later chapters.

Phrenic Nerves

The right and left phrenic nerves arise from the third, fourth, and fifth cervical rami and course inferiorly in an oblique manner on the respective anterior surfaces of the scalenus anterior muscle. At the thoracic inlet, the nerve is on the medial border of the scalenus anterior muscle, just 3 to 4 cm from the sternoclavicular joint. It then enters the thoracic inlet posterior to the subclavian vein and anterior to the internal mammary artery. Injury to the phrenic nerve may occur during surgical procedures such as a scalene node biopsy or Pancoast's tumor resection. When dissecting a pre-scalene node, which is often done for lung cancer staging or confirmation of sarcoidosis, caution should be used to avoid entering the scalenus anterior sheath in which the phrenic nerve lies. Pancoast's tumor resections require division of the first rib. The scalenus anterior muscle should be divided as close to the first rib as possible to avoid injury to the overlying phrenic nerve.

After entering the thoracic cavity, the right phrenic nerve travels inferiorly, just lateral to the brachiocephalic vein and the superior vena cava. It continues its descent over the pericardium and the underlying right atrium and inferior vena cava. Just as it goes through the diaphragm, it divides into three branches know as the anterior, posterior, and anterolateral branches.

The left phrenic nerve at the root of the neck may pass anterior to the first part of the subclavian artery and behind the thoracic duct, or it may follow the same course as the right phrenic nerve. It then crosses anterior to the internal mammary artery and travels in the groove between the left common carotid and subclavian arteries. It crosses anteromedial to the aortic arch and travels over the pericardium toward the diaphragm. In the same manner as its right-sided counterpart, it divides as it travels through the diaphragm to give off branches on the abdominal surface. The branches travel from its central position in the diaphragm to supply the sternal, crural, and posterior aspects of the diaphragm. Radial incisions in the diaphragm from the costal edge to the esophagus will lead to damage of the phrenic nerve. Peripheral circumferential incisions in the diaphragm are safest with regard to the phrenic nerve. Similar incisions in the central tendon are also safe.

SUGGESTED READING

Agur AMR, Lee MJ. *Grant's atlas of anatomy*. 10th ed. Philadelphia: Lippincott Williams & Wilkins; 1999.
Bannister LH, Berry MM, Collins P, et al. *Gray's anatomy: the anatomical basis of medicine and surgery*. 38th ed. New York: Churchill Livingstone; 1995.
Brock RC. *The anatomy of the bronchial tree: with special reference to the surgery of lung abscess*. 2nd ed. London: Oxford University Press; 1954.
Butler J. *The bronchial circulation; lung biology in health and disease*. Vol. 57. New York: Marcel Dekker; 1992.
Butler P, Mitchell AWM, Ellis H. *Applied radiological anatomy*. Cambridge, UK: Cambridge University Press; 1999.
Cho DM, Lee DY, Sung SW. Anatomical variations of rami communicantes in the upper thoracic sympathetic trunk. *Eur J Cardiothoracic Surg* 2005;**27**:320-4.
Chung IH, Oh CS, Koh KS, Kim HJ, Paik HC, Lee DY. Anatomical variations of the T2 nerve root (including the nerve of Kuntz) and their implications for sympathectomy. *J Thorac Cardiovasc Surg* 2002;**123**:498-501.
Clemente CD. *Gray's anatomy*. 30th American edition Philadelphia: Lea & Febiger; 1985.
Conley DM, Rosse C. *The digital anatomist: the interactive atlas of thoracic viscera* (CD-ROM). Seattle: University of Washington School of Medicine; 1996.
Deslauriers J. Thoracic anatomy part I. *Thorac Surg Clin* 2007;**17**:443-666.
Ehrlich E, Alexander WF. Surgical implications of upper thoracic independent sympathetic pathways. *Arch Surg* 1951;**62**:6009-14.
Funatsu T, Yoshito M, Hatakenoka R, et al. The role of mediastinoscopic biopsy in preoperative assessment of lung cancer. *J Thorac Cardiovasc Surg* 1992;**104**:1688.
Hashmonai M, Kopelman D, Kein O, Schein M. Upper thoracic sympathectomy for primary palmar hyperhidrosis: long-term follow-up. *Br J Surg* 1992;**79**:268-71.
Healy JE. *Surgical anatomy of the thorax*. Philadelphia: WB Saunders; 1970.
Jackson CL, Huber JF. Correlated applied anatomy of the bronchial tree and lungs with a system of nomenclature. *Dis Chest* 1943;**9**:319.
Lewis WH. *Gray's anatomy: the anatomical basis of medicine and surgery*. 20th ed. New York: Bartleby; 2000.
Kirgis HD, Kuntz A. Inconstant sympathetic neural pathways: their relation to sympathetic denervation of the upper extremity. *Arch Surg* 1942;**44**:95-102.
Kuntz A. Distribution of the sympathetic rami to the brachial plexus: its relation to sympathectomy affecting the upper extremity. *Arch Surg* 1927;**15**:871-7.
Liebow AA. Patterns of origin and distribution of the major bronchial arteries in man. *Am J Anat* 1965;**117**:19.
Lin TS. Video-assisted thoracoscopic "resympathicotomy" for palmar hyperhidrosis: analysis of 42 cases. *Ann Thorac Surg* 2001;**72**:895-8.
Marhold F, Izay B, Zacherl J, Tschabitscher M, Neumayer C. Thoracoscopic and anatomic landmarks of Kuntz's nerve: implications for sympathetic surgery. *Ann Thorac Surg* 2008;**86**:1653-8.
Marhold F, Neumayer C, Tschabitscher M. The sympathetic trunk and its neural pathway to the upper limb: review of the literature. *Eur Surg* 2005;**37**:114-20.
Medlar EM. Variations in interlobar fissures. *Am J Roentgenol* 1947;**57**:723-5.
Mountain CF, Dressler CM. Regional lymph node classification for lung cancer staging. *Chest* 1997;**111**:1718.
Netter FM. *The Ciba collection of medical illustrations*. Vol. 7. Summit, NJ: Ciba-Geigy; 1996.
Ramsaroop L, Partab P, Singh B, Satyapal KS. Thoracic origin of a sympathetic supply to the upper limb: the "nerve of Kuntz" revisited. *J Anat* 2001;**199**:675-82.
Ramsaroop L, Singh B, Moodley J, Partab P, Satyapal KS. Anatomical basis for a successful upper limb sympathectomy in the thoracoscopic era. *Clin Anat* 2004;**17**:294-9.
Riquet M, Manach D, Dupont P, et al. Anatomic basis of lymphatic spread of lung carcinoma to the mediastinum: Anatomo-clinical correlations. *Surg Radiol Anat* 1994;**16**:229.
Rosse C, Rosse PG. *Hollinshead's textbook of anatomy*. 5th ed. Philadelphia: Lippincott-Raven; 1997.
Roussos C. *The thorax; lung biology in health and disease, vol. 85*. New York: Marcel Dekker; 1995.
Shields TW. The mediastinum, its compartments and the mediastinal lymph nodes. *General thoracic surgery*. 5th ed. Philadelphia: Lippincott Williams & Wilkins; 2000.
Van Rhede van der Kloot E, Drukker J, Lemmens HAJ, Greep JM. The high thoracic sympathetic nerve system—its anatomic variability. *J Surg Res* 1986;**40**:112-9.
Wragg LE, Milloy FJ, Anson BJ. Surgical aspects of the pulmonary artery supply to the middle lobe and lower lobes of the lungs. *Surg Gynecol Obstet* 1968;**127**:531.

CHAPTER 2
Radiologic Imaging of Thoracic Abnormalities

Constanza J. Gutierrez, Edith M. Marom, Jeremy J. Erasmus, and Edward F. Patz, Jr.

Mediastinal Abnormalities
  Aortic Dissection
  Trauma
    Trauma: Airways and Esophagus
  Evaluation of Airways: Nontrauma
  Mediastinal Tumors

Lung Abnormalities
  Solitary Pulmonary Opacities
  Staging Lung Cancer
  Interstitial Lung Disease and Pulmonary Abscesses
Pleural and Chest Wall Abnormalities

Malignant Pleural Mesothelioma
Pleural Collections
Chest Wall Disease
Postoperative Imaging
Pulmonary Embolism
Summary

Since the late 1990s, advances in imaging technology, including digital subtraction chest radiographs, multidetector spiral computed tomography (MDCT), positron emission tomography (PET) with computer tomography (CT), and magnetic resonance imaging (MRI), have improved diagnostic accuracy and management of patients with thoracic abnormalities. These studies are routinely distributed electronically to the clinical service as digital images via a picture archiving and communication system, expediting interpretation and information transfer.

This chapter is a general overview of the advances in thoracic imaging, with a focus on imaging modalities used for the evaluation of the surgical patient. Topics reviewed include a spectrum of mediastinal, lung, pleural, and chest wall abnormalities commonly encountered by thoracic surgeons when imaging is important for diagnosis and management.

MEDIASTINAL ABNORMALITIES

Mediastinal abnormalities have a variety of causes, including congenital malformations, infections, trauma, and neoplasms. Clinical history and prior radiographs are often sufficient to determine the etiology and the necessity for further evaluation. In the absence of prior imaging studies, chest radiographs, CT, or MRI are most commonly used to establish a diagnosis, or to provide a differential diagnosis.[1]

Aortic Dissection

MDCT with intravenous contrast is the modality of choice when an aortic dissection is suspected. The sensitivity and specificity approaches 100%, with an accuracy that is superior to that of angiography.[2,3] MDCT can determine the type and extent of the dissection for management decisions. The primary diagnostic finding on CT is an intimal flap separating the true from the false lumen. Type A dissections involve the ascending aorta and originate just above the aortic valve plane, and they are usually considered for surgical repair (Fig. 2-1). Type B dissections, however, originate just below the level of the ligamentum arteriosum, and they spiral down the descending aorta. These patients are often hypertensive and are managed medically.

More recently, if a patient presents with chest pain and the diagnosis is uncertain, the rapid technologic advancement in CT scanners has allowed the use of 64-slice MDCT to image the entire thoracic volume with a high-resolution retrospective electrocardiography (ECG)-gating technique, evaluating not only the aorta but also the coronary and pulmonary arteries in a single study.[4]

When iodinated contrast agents are contraindicated, MRI or transesophageal echo (TEE) can be used to diagnose and determine the type of dissection. Although these imaging modalities are accurate, both have limitations in large patients, and the ability to perform these studies in the acute setting is not optimal.

Trauma

Patients with thoracic trauma usually require imaging evaluation, and the type of study depends on the mechanism of injury and the structures potentially involved. From a radiographic perspective, the chest radiograph is typically the first study performed and often dictates whether additional imaging is warranted. The radiographic findings suggestive of traumatic aortic injury (TAI) are an indistinct aortic arch or descending aorta, a left apical cap, tracheal displacement to the right, displacement of the nasogastric tube to the right of the T4 spinous process, mediastinal widening, and inferior displacement of the left main-stem bronchus (Fig. 2-2).[5-7] Less specific findings include a left pleural effusion and widening of the paravertebral stripe.[8,9] These features, however, are only suggestive, not indicative, of an aortic injury. In contradistinction, the negative predictive value of a normal chest radiograph for an aortic injury is 94% to 96%.[9,10] If there is a chest radiographic abnormality, MDCT is typically the next study of choice. MDCT allows the rapid acquisition of thin slices (1 to 3 mm) and three-dimensional (3D) reconstruction and is now the primary imaging method for the diagnosis of TAI if the chest radiograph is abnormal. The sensitivity for this technique is 100%, and the specificity ranges from 83%

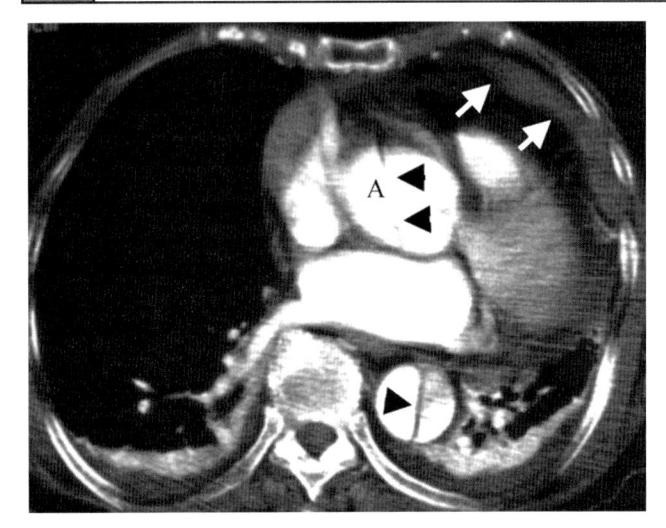

Figure 2–1
Ruptured type A aortic dissection. Axial contrast-enhanced chest CT shows pericardial fluid *(arrows)* surrounding dilated ascending aorta (A) with an intimal flap extending from the valve plane into the descending aorta *(arrowheads)*. There are small pleural effusions and basilar atelectasis.

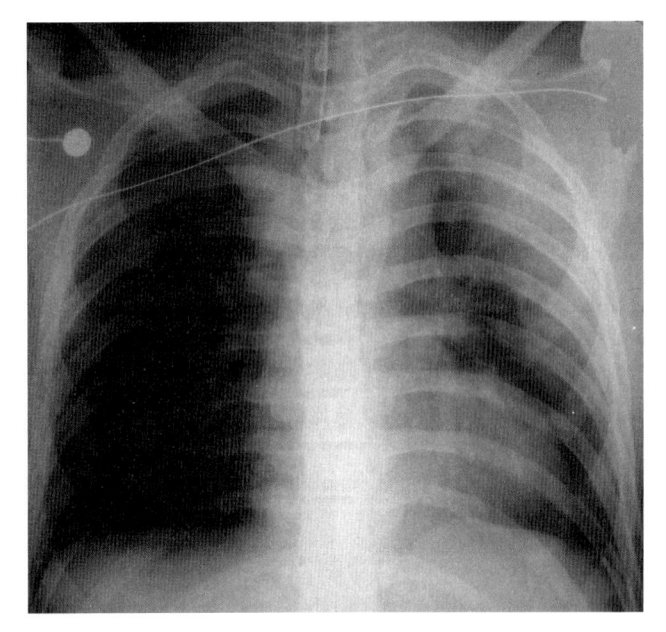

Figure 2–2
Traumatic aortic injury. Portable chest radiograph shows indistinct descending aorta, left apical cap, tracheal displacement to the right, and inferior displacement of the left main-stem bronchus.

to 99.7% (Fig. 2-3).[11-15] The absence of a periaortic abnormality and a normal-appearing aorta on MDCT has a negative predictive value of 100%.[14,15] Additional thoracic injuries can be identified at the same time, thus limiting investigation of the trauma patient to one study.[12] Indirect signs of TAI, most notably a periaortic hematoma, are found in 91% of patients with surgically proven TAI.[12] If this finding is present, further evaluation with an aortogram may be required. Aortography is safe and accurate, with a negative predictive value for TAI approaching 100%. Direct signs for TAI include a linear intraluminal filling defect, pseudoaneurysm formation, an abrupt caliber change, and active contrast extravasation.[12,16,17]

Additional thoracic abnormalities are found in only 7% of patients who do not have an aortic transection on MDCT. Such abnormalities are usually a combination of pneumothoraces, multiple rib fractures, and pulmonary contusions.[18]

Trauma: Airways and Esophagus

Tracheal and esophageal injuries are uncommon but are typically found after a motor vehicle accident or another penetrating trauma (Fig. 2-4). Many of these injuries are not recognized initially because of subtle or nonspecific clinical and radiologic findings. Delayed or missed diagnosis can result in death or severe complications such as ventilatory failure, mediastinitis, sepsis, airway stenosis, bronchiectasis, recurrent pulmonary infections, and permanent pulmonary function impairment.[19]

Chest radiographic findings of tracheobronchial and esophageal injury are nonspecific and can include pneumomediastinum, pneumothorax, and progressive subcutaneous emphysema.[19-21] MDCT is the imaging modality of choice for visualization of the airways. Patients with tracheal rupture characteristically have an abnormal air collection in the thorax, and air can occasionally be demonstrated in the soft tissues of the neck.[22] Success in visualizing the tracheal injury ranges from 71% to 94%, and multiplanar reconstructions can be useful in localizing and defining the extent of injury.[20,22] MDCT also provides information about the esophagus, although if pneumomediastinum, with or without mediastinal fluid, is found on chest radiographs or CT after trauma, a barium swallow or endoscopy is usually warranted to exclude an esophageal tear.

Evaluation of Airways: Nontrauma

Focal or diffuse lesions of the central airways are produced by a variety of diseases, including infection, malignancy, trauma, aspiration, collagen vascular disease, and idiopathic entities such as sarcoidosis or amyloidosis. Even though patients may present with significant symptoms, airway abnormalities are frequently not apparent or are overlooked on the chest radiograph. If there is a clinical suspicion of a tracheobronchial abnormality, further evaluation by CT is warranted.[23,24] MDCT using thin slices (1 to 3 mm) is preferred, as it produces excellent axial and multiplanar images of complex tracheobronchial anatomy, depicting even web-like stenosis that can easily be missed or underestimated with thicker sections (Fig. 2-5).[24,25]

Mediastinal Tumors

Mediastinal tumors, a large, diverse group of neoplasms, have historically been described radiographically according to their location in the anterior, middle, or posterior compartments. This description facilitates differential diagnosis and can aid in treatment planning.

Tumors that occur primarily in the anterior mediastinum include hemangiomas, lymphatic malformations, thymic lesions (cysts, thymolipoma, thymoma, thymic carcinoma), parathyroid adenomas, germ cell tumors, and lymphoma (Fig. 2-6). CT and MRI are particularly useful for showing local soft tissue and vascular invasion of thymomas, local invasion,

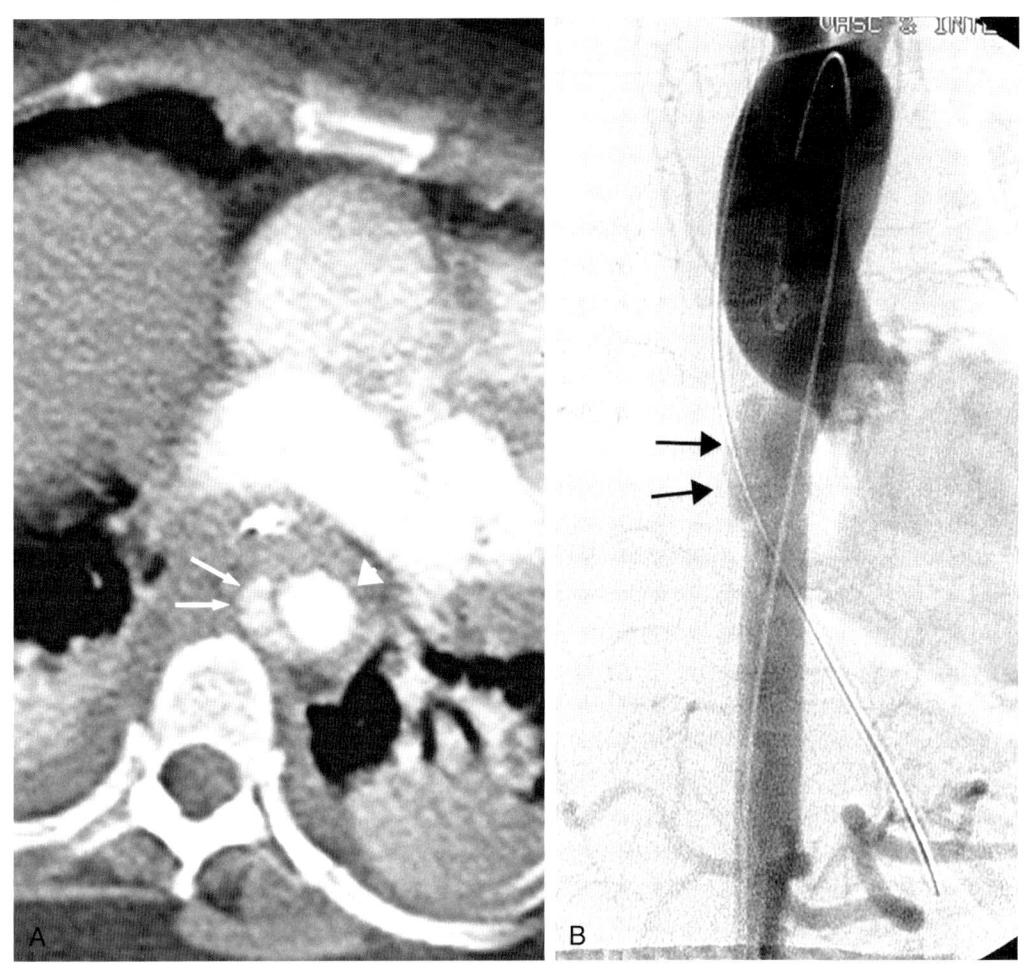

Figure 2–3
Traumatic aortic injury after motor vehicle accident. **A,** Axial contrast-enhanced chest CT demonstrates contrast located in a pouch *(arrows)* beside the descending aorta *(arrowhead)* consistent with traumatic injury and pseudoaneurysm. **B,** Aortogram confirms CT finding of aortic transection *(arrows)*.

and early dissemination to regional lymph nodes of thymic carcinomas and, because of the varying composition of soft tissue, fat, calcium, and hemorrhage in teratomas, can occasionally differentiate these tumors from thymomas and lymphomas.[26-30]

Tumors that occur primarily in the middle mediastinum are foregut malformations, pericardial cysts, and neoplasms arising from the esophagus and trachea. Bronchogenic cysts are the most common mediastinal foregut cysts and are typically located in the subcarinal or right paratracheal region. They appear on CT as a round or spherical masses of water attenuation, although many have increased attenuation from proteinaceous debris or blood.[31-33] Esophageal tumors can manifest as middle mediastinal masses, although esophageal carcinoma more frequently manifests as diffuse thickening of the esophagus. Endoscopy and endoscopic-directed ultrasound biopsy are usually used to evaluate locoregional extent and nodal metastases. CT is useful in showing the extent of involvement of adjacent structures such as the airways, aorta, pericardium, and spine, and in revealing distant nodal metastases (celiac, gastrohepatic ligament).

Tumors that occur primarily in the posterior compartment are neurogenic tumors. In fact, 20% of all adult and 35% of all pediatric mediastinal neoplasms are neurogenic tumors, and most are located in the posterior mediastinum.[34,35] Neurogenic tumors are classified as tumors of peripheral nerves (neurofibromas, schwannomas, malignant tumors of nerve sheath origin) or sympathetic ganglia (ganglioneuromas, ganglioneuroblastomas, neuroblastomas) and are optimally assessed by MRI. MRI is the preferred modality for evaluating neurogenic tumors, as it can simultaneously assess (1) intraspinal extension, (2) spinal cord abnormalities, (3) longitudinal extent of tumor, and (4) extradural extension.

LUNG ABNORMALITIES

Thoracic imaging is essential in the workup of pulmonary abnormalities, including lung nodules and focal opacities, intrathoracic malignancies, diffuse interstitial lung disease, and infection. Low-dose CT (LDCT) has also been proposed as a screening tool for lung cancer; however, no data have yet shown that this approach reduces lung cancer mortality.[36,37] The results of the National Lung Screening Trial (NLST), a randomized study comparing the effectiveness of LDCT to chest radiography in more than 50,000 participants, will, it is hoped, clarify the role of thoracic imaging in screening.

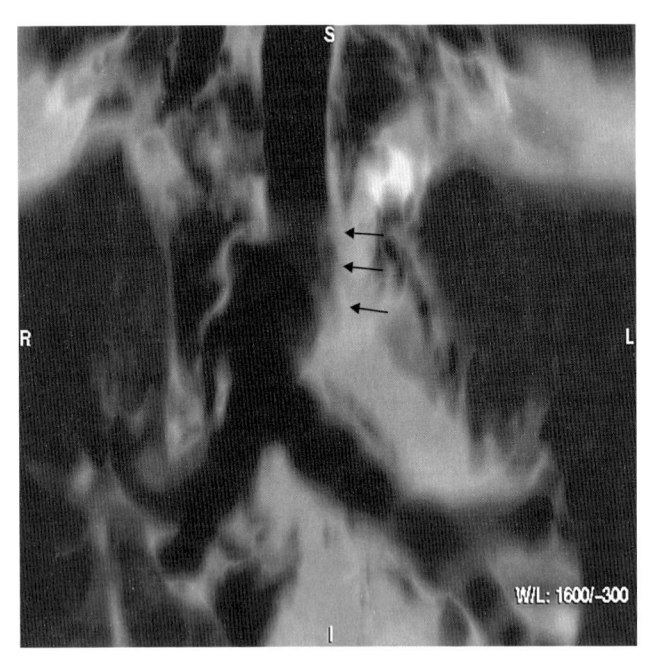

Figure 2–4
Tracheal rupture after motor vehicle accident in a patient with no respiratory symptoms and a chest radiograph demonstrating pneumomediastinum. Coronal reformations of CT (2.5-mm collimation) show pneumomediastinum and discontinuation of the trachea (arrows).

Solitary Pulmonary Opacities

Solitary pulmonary opacities are a common radiologic finding and are usually benign, but because of concern about lung cancer, further evaluation is often suggested. The goal is to differentiate malignant and benign lesions so that those patients who require surgery are correctly identified. Although morphologic features may suggest whether a nodule is benign or malignant, there is considerable overlap, and at least 20% of malignant nodules have a benign appearance.[38-40] Specific patterns of calcification and stability in size for 2 years have historically been the only reliable findings useful in determining benignity. More recently, the ability to distinguish between benign and malignant opacities has improved with assessment of perfusion using contrast-enhanced CT[41] and assessment of metabolism using PET imaging with fluorodeoxyglucose labeled with radioactive fluoride (^{18}F) (FDG).

Contrast-enhanced CT can be used to differentiate benign and malignant nodules because the intensity of enhancement is directly related to the vascularity of the nodule and to the likelihood of malignancy.[42,43] Typically, malignant nodules enhance more than 20 Hounsfield units (HU), whereas benign nodules enhance less than 15 HU (Fig. 2-7).[44] Nodule-enhancement CT has a very high negative predictive value but poor specificity. FDG-PET has a lower sensitivity but a higher specificity and may be helpful

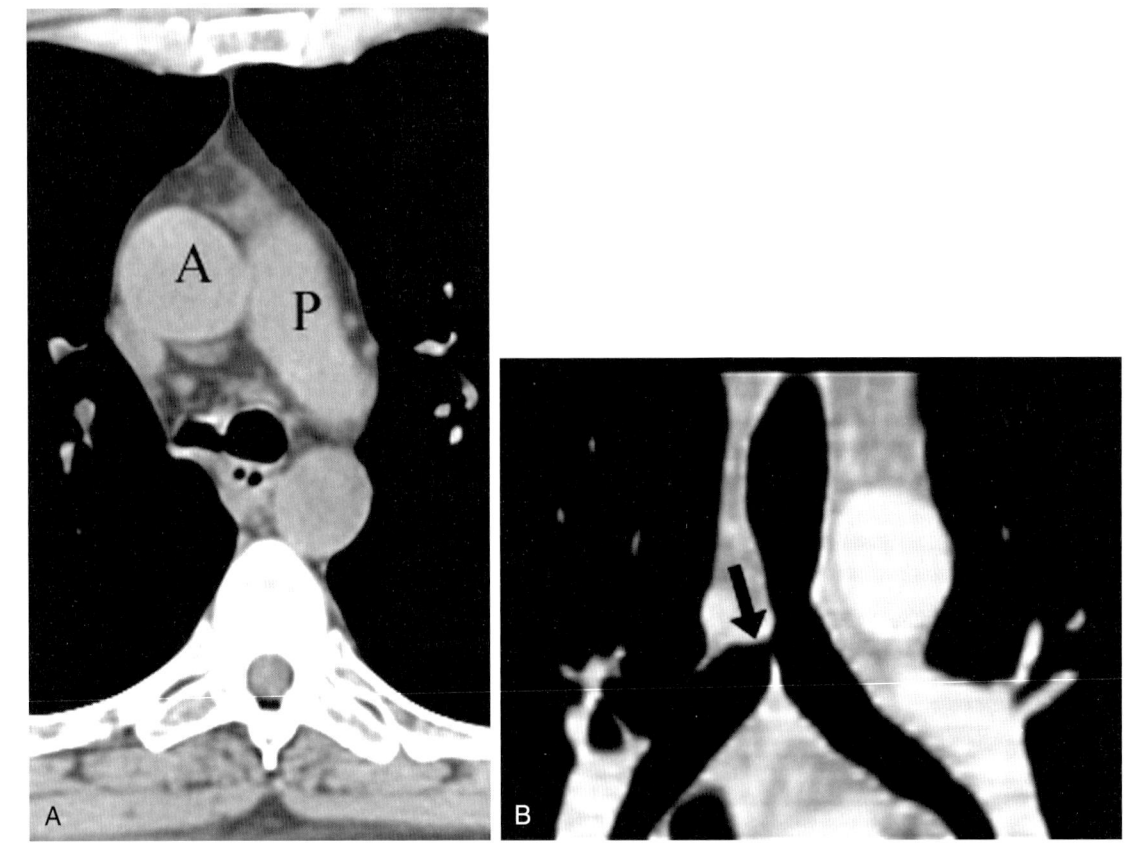

Figure 2–5
Focal stenosis of the right main-stem bronchus from invasive aspergillosis. **A,** Axial CT shows normal caliber of left main bronchus and marked concentric narrowing of right main bronchus. A, ascending aorta; P, pulmonary artery. **B,** Coronal reconstruction shows that the right main bronchus stenosis involves short focal segment (arrow).

to further evaluate a patient who has a nodule that enhances 20 HU or more on CT.[45]

PET imaging also allows differentiation of malignant and benign nodules that are indeterminate after conventional imaging (Fig. 2-8). A meta-analysis of 40 studies on the accuracy of FDG-PET reports a sensitivity of 97% and a specificity of 78% when used in the evaluation of 10-mm or larger nodules.[46] However, a recent prospective integrated PET-CT evaluation of 585 patients (496 malignant, 89 benign nodules) showed that although a high standardized uptake value (SUV) (>4.1) was associated with a 96% likelihood of malignancy, the likelihood of malignancy was still 25% when the SUV was 0 to 2.5.[47] It has been shown that the maximal SUVs on integrated FDG-PET/CT are useful in differentiating benign and malignant pulmonary nodules.[47] Furthermore, in malignant nodules that are smaller than 1 cm in diameter or have ground-glass or partially solid morphology, FDG uptake is variable and unreliable in differentiating benign from malignant nodular opacities.[48]

The Fleischner Society has guidelines for the management of small, indeterminate pulmonary nodules detected incidentally on routine chest CT.[49]

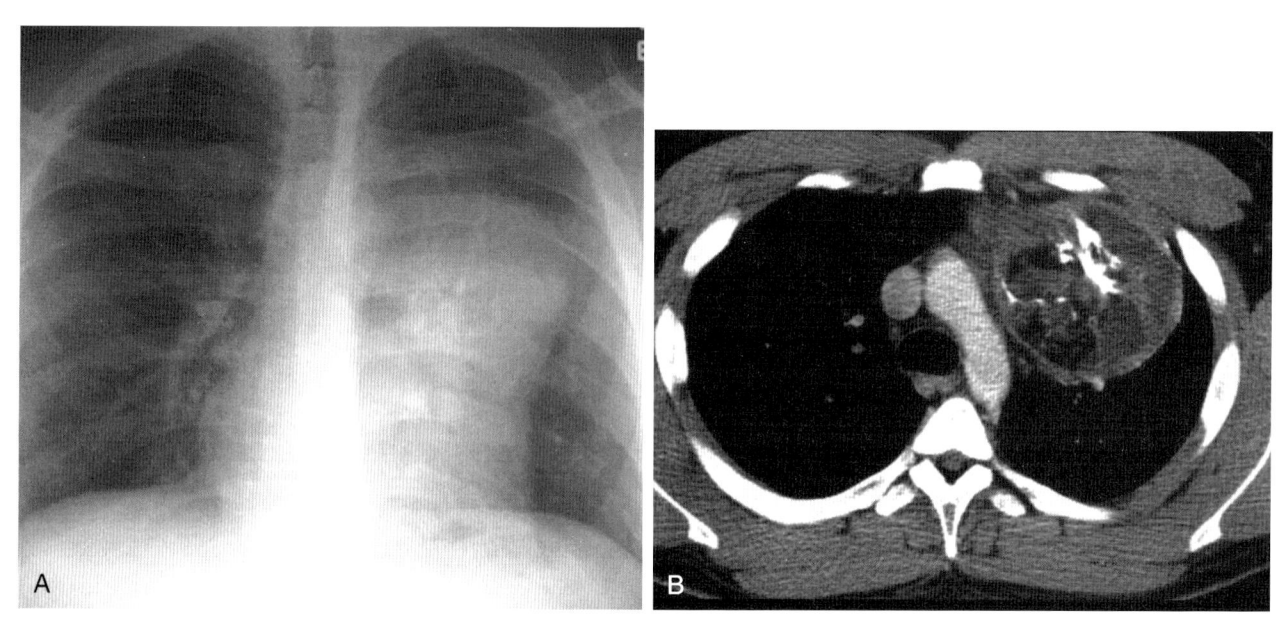

Figure 2-6
Anterior mediastinal mass. **A,** Posteroanterior chest radiograph demonstrates a smoothly marginated, left-sided anterior mediastinal mass. **B,** Axial CT image confirms the mass, with mixed heterogeneous components, including fat, soft tissue, fluid, and calcification. These findings are diagnostic of a teratoma.

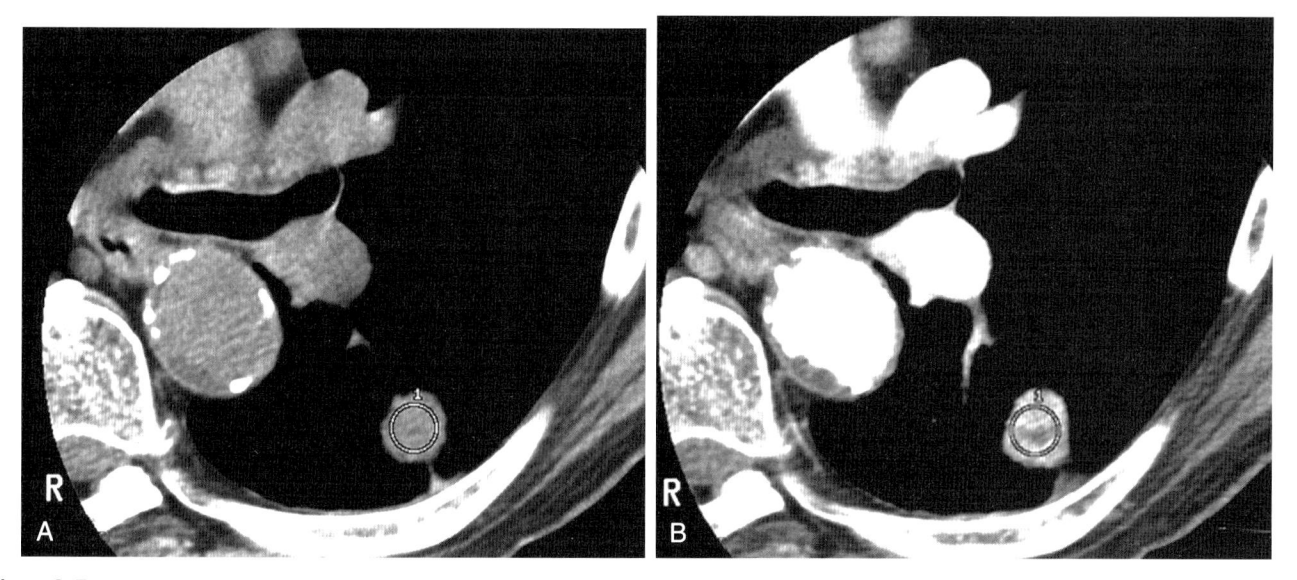

Figure 2-7
Non–small cell cancer. **A,** Noncontrast CT shows left lung nodule with attenuation value of 24 HU. **B,** Contrast CT shows nodule enhancement of 70 HU and central necrosis. Enhancement greater than 20 HU is suggestive of malignancy, and resection revealed non–small cell cancer. *(Courtesy of Tom Hartman, MD, Mayo Clinic, Rochester, MN; reprinted with permission from Haaga et al. CT and MR Imaging of the whole body. St. Louis: Mosby; 2002.)*

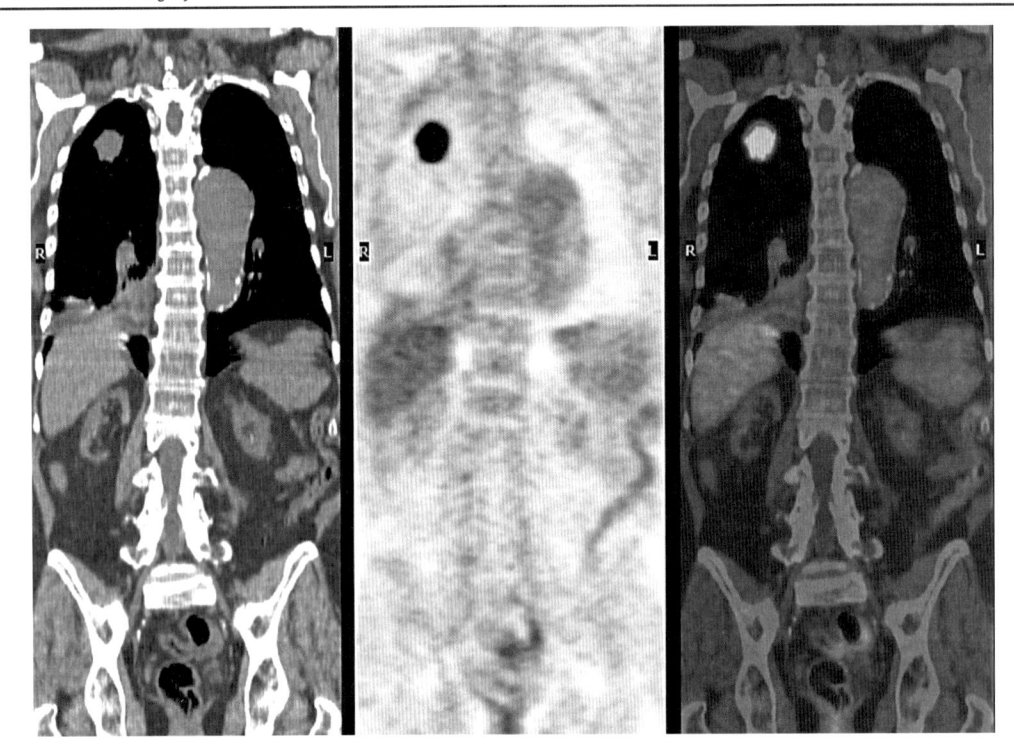

Figure 2–8
Non–small cell lung cancer. Coronal CT *(left)*, PET *(center)*, and fused CT-PET *(right)* images show small nodule in the right upper lobe with increased uptake of [^{18}F]fluorodeoxyglucose, which is consistent with malignancy. (See color plate.)

Staging Lung Cancer

Staging, the assessment of the anatomic extent of non–small cell lung cancer (NSCLC), usually determines treatment and prognosis. Clinical staging typically includes CT and, more recently, PET-CT. The current tumor (T), node (N), and metastasis (M) staging system is being modified, and the greater emphasis on the importance of the size of the primary tumor will require CT for accurate determination.[50,51] CT is also usually used to define chest wall or mediastinal invasion but is inaccurate in differentiating between anatomic contiguity and subtle invasion.[52-56] Although MRI has better soft-tissue contrast resolution than CT, the two modalities have the same limitations for assessing local disease (Fig. 2-9).[52,54,57,58]

The presence of nodal metastases and their locations are important for determining management and prognosis (Fig. 2-10).[50,59] CT is most commonly used to assess the size of nodes (>10 cm in short-axis diameter), and size is the only criterion used to suggest nodal metastases.[60] PET imaging improves the accuracy of nodal staging. In a meta-analysis of 17 studies comprising 833 patients, the overall sensitivity of PET for detecting nodal metastases was 83% and the specificity was 92%, whereas the sensitivity and specificity of chest CT were 59% and 78%, respectively.[61] Interestingly, in the presence of enlarged lymph nodes, PET and PET-CT become less specific and less accurate but more sensitive in detecting nodal metastases.[62,63]

The adrenal glands, liver, brain, bones, and lymph nodes are the most common sites of metastatic disease at presentation. However, the role of imaging these areas at presentation is not clearly defined.[27,64,65] Routine imaging of the upper abdomen is performed as part of the initial chest CT evaluation in most patients with NSCLC. However, because clinical staging of NSCLC with CT and MRI is often inaccurate, whole-body imaging with PET-CT can be performed to improve accuracy. PET has a higher sensitivity and specificity than CT in detecting metastases to the adrenal glands, bones, and extrathoracic lymph nodes. Whole-body PET imaging stages intra- and extrathoracic disease in a single study, detects occult extrathoracic metastases in up to 24% of patients selected for curative resection, and has been shown to be cost effective (Fig. 2-11).[66-70]

Metastases to the adrenal glands are detected in up to 20% of patients with NSCLC at presentation. If an adrenal mass contains fat or has an attenuation value of less than 10 HU on a noncontrast CT scan, the mass can be considered benign.[71] Lesions with attenuation values of more than 10 HU can be further evaluated with MRI using chemical shift analysis and dynamic gadolinium enhancement to determine whether they are malignant or benign.[72] FDG-PET is useful in distinguishing benign from malignant adrenal masses detected on CT, and it is particularly advocated when the adrenal mass is small. Two series with PET have shown a sensitivity of 100% and specificities of 80% to 90% in identifying adrenal metastases.[73,73a]

Routine CT or MRI of the central nervous system has been advocated because up to 18% of patients with NSCLC have brain metastases at presentation, and 10% of these patients have no associated neurologic symptoms. However, routine CT or MRI of the central nervous system remains controversial, as the yield is low for asymptomatic patients with early disease.[74] The prevailing clinical practice is to perform CT or MRI for patients who have neurologic signs or symptoms, as well for asymptomatic patients with stage III disease who are being considered for aggressive local therapy such as thoracotomy or radiation.[75,76]

Because imaging rarely reveals occult skeletal metastases in an asymptomatic patient, bone radiographs, technetium 99m

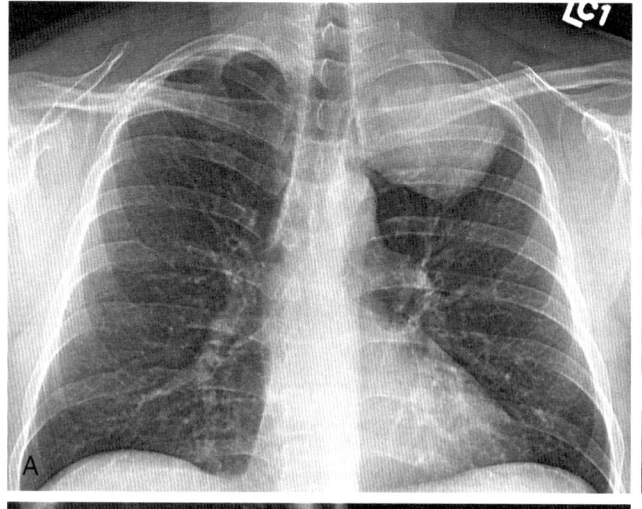

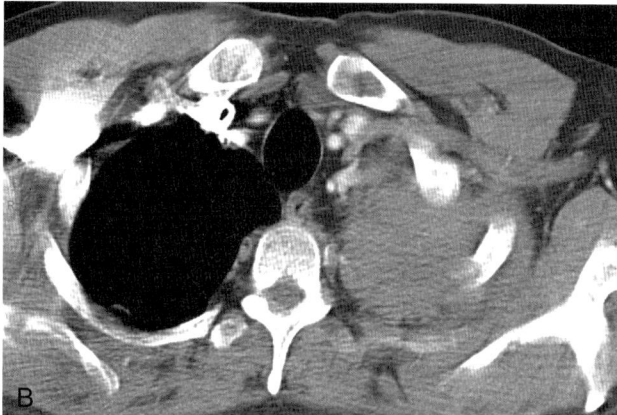

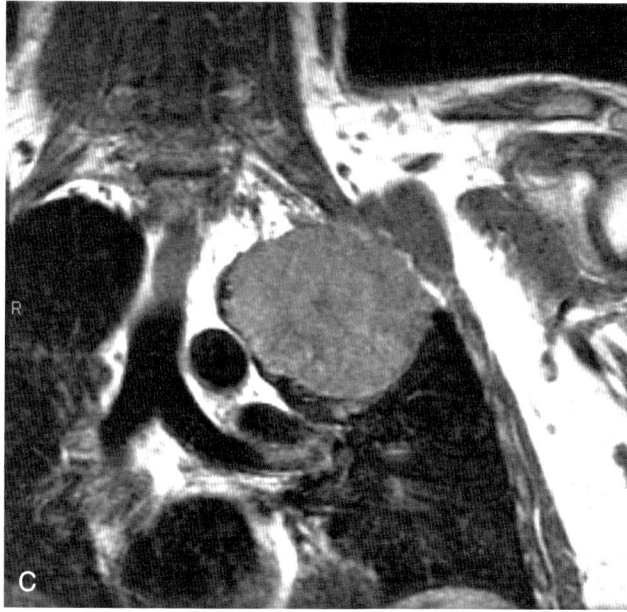

Figure 2–9
Non–small cell lung cancer. **A,** Posteroanterior chest radiograph shows large left upper lobe lung mass. **B,** CT confirms a large, well-circumscribed mass in the apex of the left thorax. Note difficulty in evaluation of local invasion on axial image. **C,** Coronal T1-weighted image shows preservation of adjacent soft tissue planes, a finding consistent with absence of mediastinal, chest wall, and brachial plexus invasion.

(99mTc)-labeled methylene diphosphonate bone scintigraphy, and MRI are generally performed only if the patient has focal bone pain or an elevated alkaline phosphatase level.[76] PET imaging has to a large extent replaced 99mTc-labeled methylene diphosphonate bone scintigraphy in the evaluation of bone metastases in patients with NSCLC. The specificity, sensitivity, negative predictive value, positive predictive value, and accuracy of PET scanning in the assessment of bone metastases has been reported to exceed 90%.[77-80]

Interstitial Lung Disease and Pulmonary Abscesses

Imaging studies are essential for determining the diagnosis in patients with pulmonary symptoms and focal or diffuse lung disease. If the diagnosis is uncertain after clinical and imaging evaluations, surgical biopsies may be requested before therapy is initiated. Radiologic studies are often very useful in determining the optimal site to biopsy, as well as the biopsy method (transbronchial or wedge biopsy) (Fig. 2-12). Lung abscesses, usually caused by aspiration of anaerobic bacteria, typically occur in patients with altered levels of consciousness, gastroesophageal dysmotility, and poor dental hygiene.

Medical therapy (systemic antibiotics, postural drainage) is the initial treatment of choice and is curative in most patients. However, lung abscesses in children less than 7 years of age typically do not drain spontaneously and are less likely to respond to medical management. Surgical or percutaneous drainage is required in the 11% to 21% of patients with lung abscesses who fail to respond to medical therapy. Drainage of an abscess is recommended when (1) the patient has persistent sepsis 5 to 7 days after initiation of antibiotic therapy, (2) the abscess is larger than 4 cm, or (3) the abscess increases in size while the patient is on medical therapy.

Percutaneous CT-guided catheter drainage has less morbidity and mortality than surgical resection, and in most cases clinical and radiologic improvement occurs rapidly after catheter drainage. Although the mean time to abscess resolution is 10 to 15 days, marked improvement of sepsis (fever, leukocytosis) usually occurs within 48 hours of drainage. Failure of percutaneous drainage can occur when the abscess (1) contains viscous, organized tissue, (2) is multiloculated, or (3) has a thick, noncollapsible wall. Potential complications of lung abscesses drainage with a percutaneous tube include bleeding, bronchopleural fistula, and empyema.[81,82]

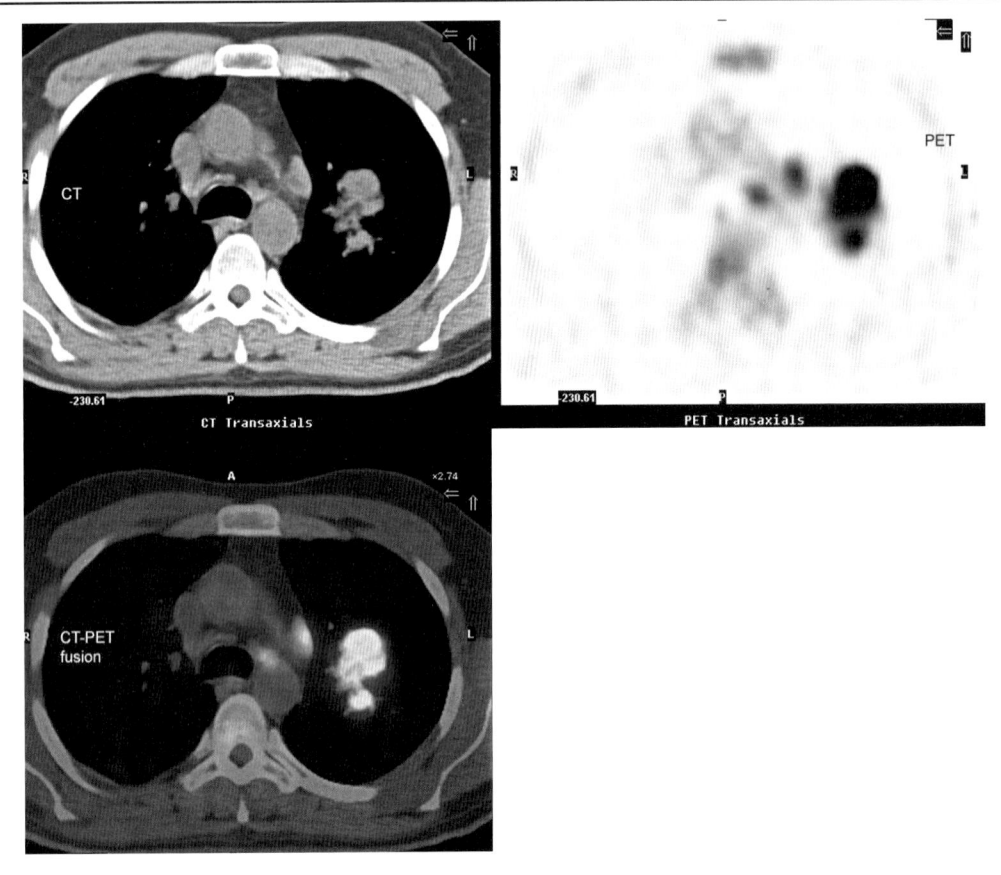

Figure 2–10
Non–small cell lung cancer. Axial CT, PET, and fused CT-PET images show left upper lobe lung malignancy with increased uptake of [18F]fluorodeoxyglucose (FDG) consistent with a malignancy. Enlarged prevascular and normal-sized left lower lobe paratracheal nodes show increased FDG uptake compared with uptake in the mediastinum, confirmed to be metastases. Note absence of FDG uptake in right lower paratracheal nodes, indicative of absence of nodal metastases. (See color version in the online edition through Expert Consult.)

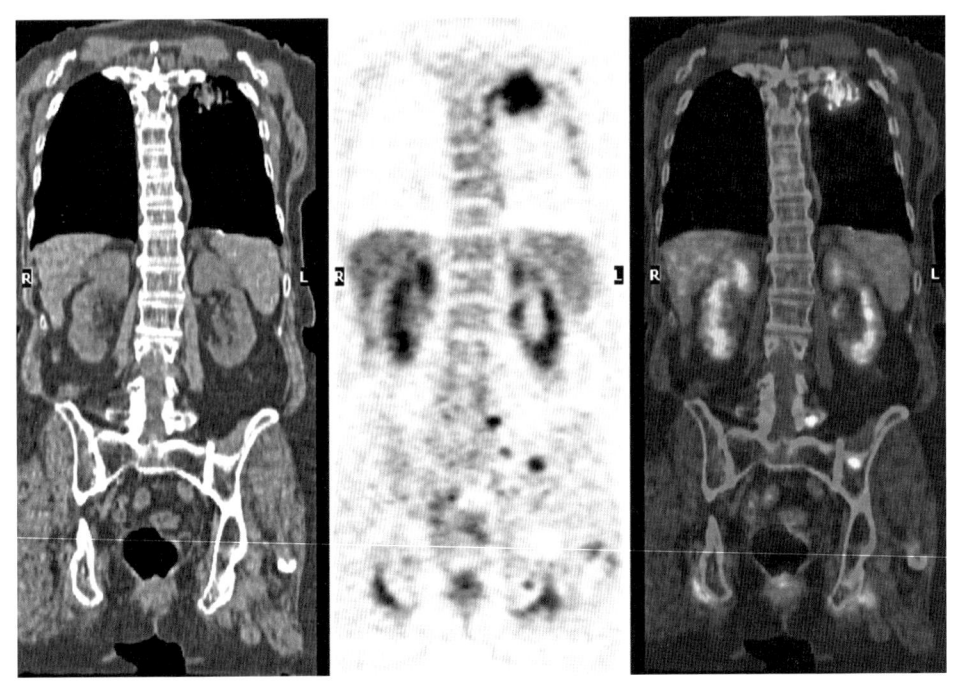

Figure 2–11
Non–small cell lung cancer. Coronal CT (left), PET (center), and fused CT-PET (right) images show left upper lobe lung malignancy with increased [18F]fluorodeoxyglucose (FDG). Note focal increased FDG uptake in lumbar spine and pelvis due to metastases. (See color version in the online edition through Expert Consult.)

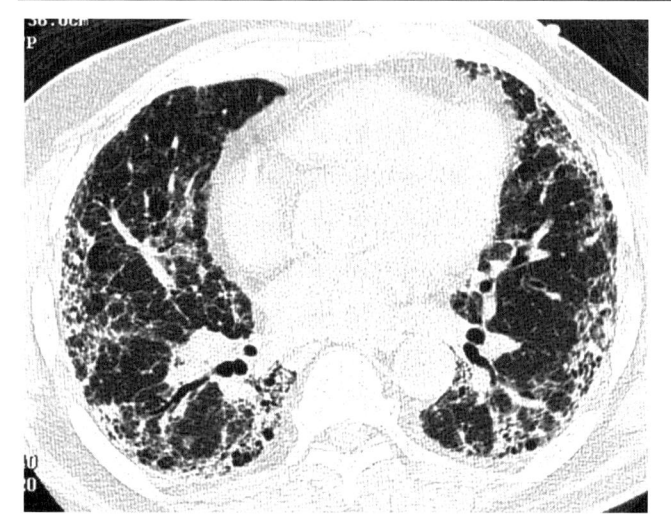

Figure 2–12
Usual interstitial pneumonitis (UIP). Axial high-resolution CT image through the bases demonstrates diffuse lung disease with area of predominantly peripheral ground-glass opacities, architectural distortion, and cystic spaces consistent with pulmonary fibrosis. Lung biopsy confirmed UIP.

PLEURAL AND CHEST WALL ABNORMALITIES
Malignant Pleural Mesothelioma

Malignant pleural mesothelioma (MPM) is an uncommon tumor that arises from mesothelial cells of the pleura and less commonly of the pericardium or peritoneum. Approximately 2000 new cases are diagnosed in the United States each year, the majority of which are associated with prior asbestos exposure.[83] Treatment options depend on the stage at presentation, with surgical resection sometimes performed in limited disease.[84,85] Primarily in an attempt to identify patients who are potentially resectable, the New International Staging System for MPM emphasizes criteria used to determine local tumor extension and regional lymph nodes status in a traditional TMN system.[86,87] The presence of advanced locoregional primary tumor (T4), N2-3 disease (mediastinal, internal mammary, and supraclavicular lymph nodes), or M1 disease precludes surgery.

MRI has historically been considered to be superior to CT in the staging of MPM. However, in a study comparing the accuracy of MRI and nonspiral CT in evaluation of MPM,[88] MRI and CT were found have nearly equivalent diagnostic accuracies (50% to 65%) in overall staging. The only significant differences were in two categories: invasion of the diaphragm (CT accuracy, 55%; MRI, 82%; $P = .01$) and invasion of endothoracic fascia or a single chest wall focus (CT accuracy, 46%; MRI, 69%; $P = .05$) (Fig. 2-13).

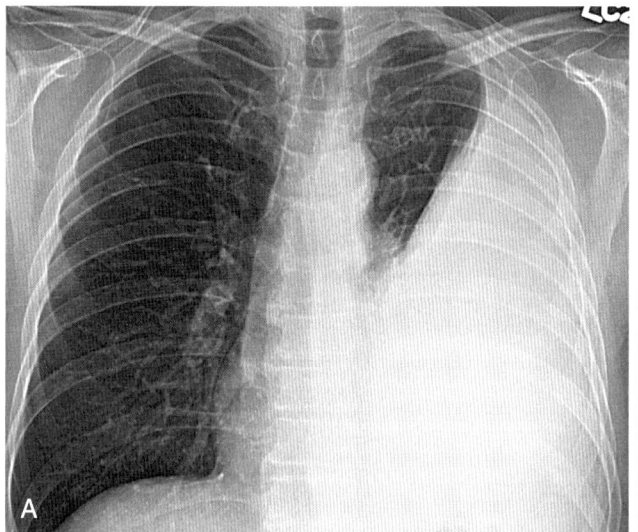

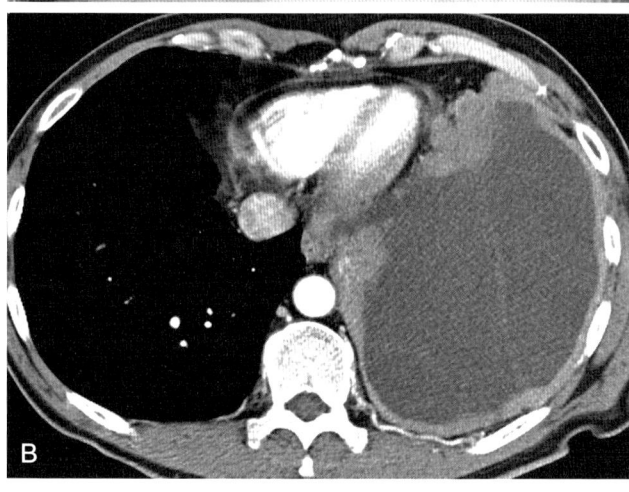

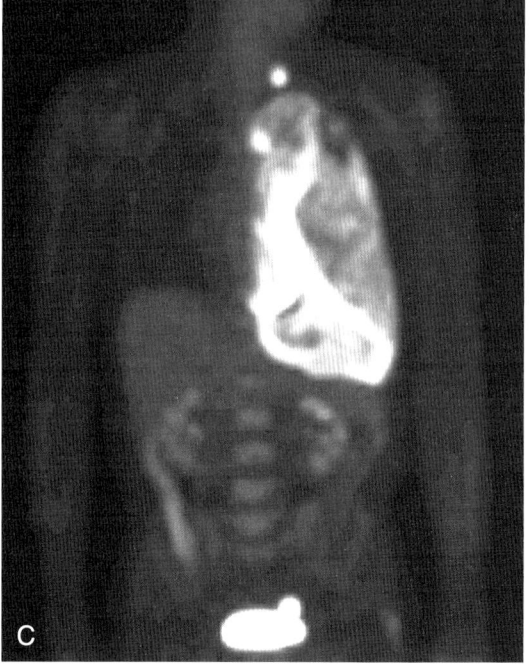

Figure 2–13
Malignant pleural mesothelioma in a patient being evaluated for extrapleural pneumonectomy. **A,** Posteroanterior chest radiograph shows large left pleural effusion. **B,** Contrast-enhanced CT shows large left effusion and a diffuse pleural mass encasing the left hemithorax. **C,** Coronal whole-body PET scan shows diffuse pleural increased [^{18}F]fluorodeoxyglucose uptake in mass and focal uptake in the neck. Biopsy of left lower neck node revealed metastatic mesothelioma, precluding resection.

PET and PET-CT imaging are also being used to evaluate patients with MPM. However, because of the poor spatial resolution of PET, the sensitivity for correct T staging using PET alone is only 19%.[89] The use of integrated PET-CT has improved the accuracy of T staging, and a sensitivity of 67% has been reported for T4 disease.[90] The sensitivity of PET for detecting nodal metastatic disease is poor (i.e., 11% for PET alone and 38% for integrated PET-CT).[89,90] PET-CT imaging is useful in detecting distant metastatic disease and has been reported to detect extrathoracic metastases that were undetected by clinical and morphologic imaging in 24% of patients with MPM.[89-91]

Pleural Collections

Fluid collections in the pleural space are caused by a variety of diseases, including infection, trauma, inflammation, and neoplasm. Although some patients can be managed conservatively, interventional procedures such as pleural fluid aspiration, with or without placement of a drainage catheter, or pleural biopsies are frequently performed for either diagnostic or therapeutic purposes. The type of intervention depends on a spectrum of clinical and imaging features, including symptoms, extent of disease, and etiology of the pleural abnormality. Imaging studies, most frequently with CT, can delineate the extent and complexity of the pleural collection.

Chest Wall Disease

Abnormalities of the chest wall are unusual and are most commonly the result of soft tissue tumors, metastatic disease, infections, iatrogenic causes, trauma, and congenital lesions. The choice of imaging modality for this spectrum of diseases often depends on the suspected etiology, but CT is usually the initial study for evaluation. Although CT can provide the requisite diagnostic information and has superb multiplanar capabilities for surgical planning, MRI is typically also performed, as its superior soft tissue contrast resolution can be useful in accurately delineating the extent of involvement of the chest wall (Fig. 2-14).

POSTOPERATIVE IMAGING

Early awareness of surgical complications is important, as timely management is associated with a decrease in mortality.[11,92,93] Chest radiographs commonly demonstrate abnormalities in patients after cardiothoracic procedures. An increase in heart size may be caused by perioperative myocardial infarction or hypervolemia, although most frequently it is the result of fluid in the pericardial sac or mediastinal fat. In some cases, the mediastinal contours appear normal on chest radiographs even though a significant amount of bleeding has occurred.[94] In other cases, the normal mediastinum may appear enlarged as a result of magnification effects on the supine, expiratory radiograph.[95] CT can be used to evaluate mediastinal widening and air collections in patients after sternotomy and can be useful in suggesting the diagnosis of mediastinitis.[96-99]

Pulmonary Embolism

Clinical signs and symptoms of pulmonary embolism (PE) are neither sensitive nor specific, because patients can present with chest pain, shortness of breath, or oxygen desaturation.

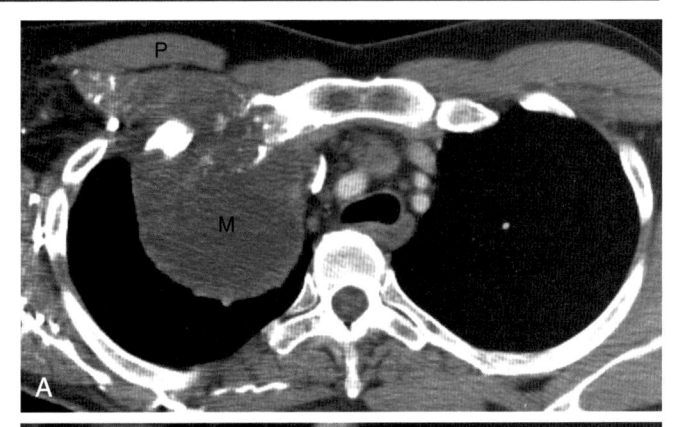

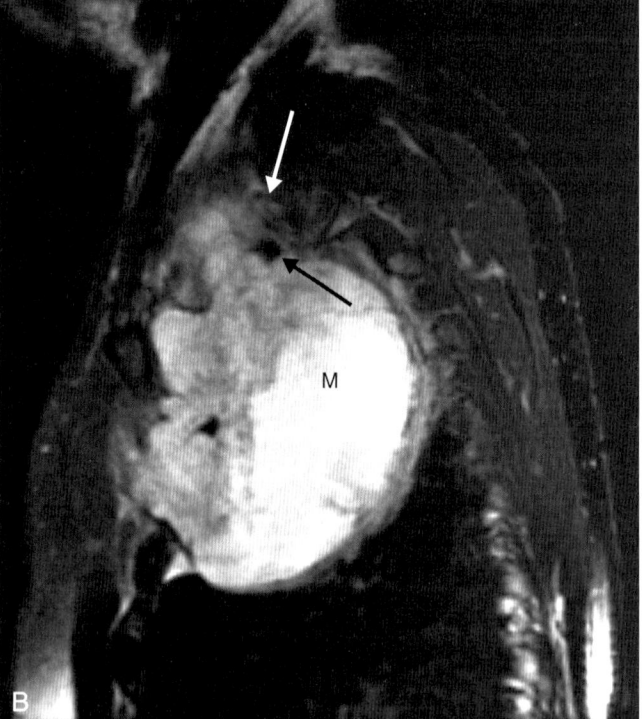

Figure 2-14
A 60-year-old man with newly diagnosed chondrosarcoma of the first rib presented with right shoulder pain. **A,** Contrast-enhanced axial chest CT shows a large mass (M) arising from the right first rib. Note that density of mass is similar to that of muscle, as compared to the right pectoralis major muscle (P). The brachial plexus cannot be visualized. **B,** T2-weighted sagittal MRI distinguishes the intensity of the mass (M) from that of surrounding soft tissues and muscles. This enabled direct visualization of the right subclavian artery *(black arrow)* and brachial plexus *(two black dots abutting tip of white arrow)*, which are surrounded by the tumor.

Initial imaging with chest radiographs is useful to search for other causes that can clinically mimic PE such as pleural effusions, pneumothorax, pneumonia, or congestive heart failure. The chest radiographic findings in patients with PE are nonspecific and include consolidation, atelectasis, pleural effusion, peripheral wedge-shaped opacities, enlargement of a pulmonary artery, and focal oligemia. However, 80% of patients with PE have a normal chest film.[100]

If a diagnosis of PE is suspected and the chest radiograph does not suggest a reasonable alternative diagnosis, other imaging modalities can be used for further evaluation. Multidetector CT angiography (CTA) is the method of choice

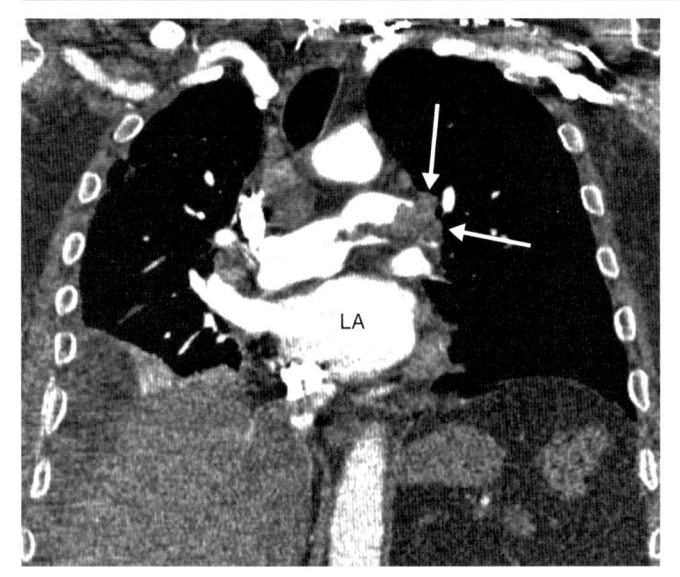

Figure 2-15
Pulmonary embolism. A 67-year-old man with metastatic non–small cell lung cancer presented with dyspnea on exertion. Contrast-enhanced multidetector CT shows a saddle embolus *(arrows)* in the left pulmonary artery. LA, left atrium.

for imaging the pulmonary vasculature when PE is suspected. CTA has a sensitivity and specificity between 83% and 100% and between 89% and 97%, respectively,[101-103] and the sensitivity for PE detection with 64-slice MDCT is expected to be better.[104] Additional advantages of using multidetector CTA to diagnose PE include the ability to quantify the obstruction to the pulmonary arterial bed[105-108] and the ability to predict 30-day mortality after acute pulmonary embolism by assessing cardiac strain as seen by an interval increase in right-left ventricular diameter ratios (Fig. 2-15).[109]

Evaluation of PE can also be performed with other imaging modalities such as conventional angiography, MRI, or ventilation-perfusion ($\dot{V}-\dot{Q}$) scans. Currently, because of the high sensitivity and specificity of CTA in detecting PE, as well as the ability to suggest alternative diagnoses, these modalities are infrequently used in the evaluation of patients with suspected PE. In this regard, a recent study that evaluated discordant CT and angiographic findings showed that CT was significantly more sensitive than angiography in the detection of pulmonary embolism.[40] $\dot{V}-\dot{Q}$ scans still have a role in the evaluation of PE disease in patients who are allergic to iodinated contrast agents or who have impaired renal function. In patients with a normal chest radiograph and a normal $\dot{V}-\dot{Q}$ scan, there is a very low probability of pulmonary embolus and no further evaluation for PE is required.[83,110] Patients with a high pretest probability of PE and a high-probability scan are likely to have pulmonary embolism, and treatment is often initiated. Unfortunately, most patients suspected of having PE have an abnormal chest radiograph and an indeterminate $\dot{V}-\dot{Q}$ scan, which then results in additional diagnostic studies, including MDCT and lower extremity ultrasound.

MRI is suboptimal in detecting emboli in segmental and subsegmental PE. A meta-analysis of studies of gadolinium-enhanced MRI for detecting acute PE reported sensitivities of 77% to 100% and specificities of 95% to 98%.[111] In the most recent study reviewed, the sensitivity of MRI was 100% for PE in the central and lobar arteries, 84% in the segmental arteries, but only 40% in the subsegmental branches.[112] In fact, identification of small emboli with MRI has subsequently been shown to be inferior to that with multidetector CTA.[113] A further limitation of MRI is that the study may be technically challenging to perform, especially in the acute setting, in the postoperative patient, or in the patient in the intensive care unit.[65,114,115] Additionally, the use of MRI contrast agents is now contraindicated in patients with impaired renal function, because of an association between gadolinium-based contrast agents and the development of nephrogenic systemic fibrosis.[116,117]

SUMMARY

Imaging plays an important role in the diagnosis and follow-up of patients with pulmonary diseases. Recent advances in imaging technologies have revolutionized evaluation of thoracic disease, with improvements in patient management. Careful selection of the appropriate imaging studies improves diagnostic accuracy, limits the number of tests performed, and decreases unnecessary surgery. It is anticipated that further improvement of existing modalities and continued development of novel imaging technologies will improve diagnostic imaging strategies and patient outcomes in the future.

REFERENCES

1. Slater EE, DeSanctis RW. The clinical recognition of dissecting aortic aneurysm. *Am J Med* 1976;**60**:625-33.
2. Bansal RC, Chandrasekaran K, Ayala K, Smith DC. Frequency and explanation of false negative diagnosis of aortic dissection by aortography and transesophageal echocardiography. *J Am Coll Cardiol* 1995;**25**:1393-401.
3. Sommer T, Fehske W, Holzknecht N, et al. Aortic dissection: a comparative study of diagnosis with spiral CT, multiplanar transesophageal echocardiography, and MR imaging. *Radiology* 1996;**199**:347-52.
4. Johnson TR, Nikolaou K, Wintersperger BJ, et al. ECG-gated 64-MDCT angiography in the differential diagnosis of acute chest pain. *AJR Am J Roentgenol* 2007;**188**:76-82.
5. Creasy JD, Chiles C, Routh WD, Dyer RB. Overview of traumatic injury of the thoracic aorta. *Radiographics* 1997;**17**:27-45.
6. Simeone JF, Deren MM, Cagle F. The value of the left apical cap in the diagnosis of aortic rupture: a prospective and retrospective study. *Radiology* 1981;**139**:35-7.
7. Stark P, Cook M, Vincent A, Smith DC. Traumatic rupture of the thoracic aorta: a review of 49 cases. *Radiologe* 1987;**27**:402-6.
8. Mirvis SE, Bidwell JK, Buddemeyer EU, Diaconis JN, Pais SO, Whitley JE. Imaging diagnosis of traumatic aortic rupture: a review and experience at a major trauma center. *Invest Radiol* 1987;**22**:187-96.
9. Woodring JH, King JG. The potential effects of radiographic criteria to exclude aortography in patients with blunt chest trauma: results of a study of 32 patients with proved aortic or brachiocephalic arterial injury. *J Thorac Cardiovasc Surg* 1989;**97**:456-60.
10. Mirvis SE, Bidwell JK, Buddemeyer EU, et al. Value of chest radiography in excluding traumatic aortic rupture. *Radiology* 1987;**163**:487-93.
11. Cheung EH, Craver JM, Jones EL, Murphy DA, Hatcher Jr CR, Guyton RA. Mediastinitis after cardiac valve operations: Impact upon survival. *J Thorac Cardiovasc Surg* 1985;**90**:517-22.
12. Cleverley JR, Barrie JR, Raymond GS, Primack SL, Mayo JR. Direct findings of aortic injury on contrast-enhanced CT in surgically proven traumatic aortic injury: a multi-centre review. *Clin Radiol* 2002;**57**:281-6.
13. Demetriades D, Gomez H, Velmahos GC, et al. Routine helical computed tomographic evaluation of the mediastinum in high-risk blunt trauma patients. *Arch Surg* 1998;**133**:1084-8.
14. Fabian TC, Davis KA, Gavant ML, et al. Prospective study of blunt aortic injury: Helical CT is diagnostic and antihypertensive therapy reduces rupture. *Ann Surg* 1998;**227**:666-76; discussion 676-677.

15. Mirvis SE, Shanmuganathan K, Buell J, Rodriguez A. Use of spiral computed tomography for the assessment of blunt trauma patients with potential aortic injury. *J Trauma* 1998;**45**:922-30.
16. Gavant ML, Flick P, Menke P, Gold RE. CT aortography of thoracic aortic rupture. *AJR Am J Roentgenol* 1996;**166**:955-61.
17. Gavant ML, Menke PG, Fabian T, Flick PA, Graney MJ, Gold RE. Blunt traumatic aortic rupture: Detection with helical CT of the chest. *Radiology* 1995;**197**:125-33.
18. Brink M, Deunk J, Dekker HM, et al. Added value of routine chest MDCT after blunt trauma: Evaluation of additional findings and impact on patient management. *AJR Am J Roentgenol* 2008;**190**:1591-8.
19. Lee RB. Traumatic injury of the cervicothoracic trachea and major bronchi. *Chest Surg Clin N Am* 1997;**7**:285-304.
20. Scaglione M, Romano S, Pinto A, Sparano A, Scialpi M, Rotondo A. Acute tracheobronchial injuries: Impact of imaging on diagnosis and management implications. *Eur J Radiol* 2006;**59**:336-43.
21. Eijgelaar A, Homan van der Heide JN. A reliable early symptom of bronchial or tracheal rupture. *Thorax* 1970;**25**:120-5.
22. Chen JD, Shanmuganathan K, Mirvis SE, Killeen KL, Dutton RP. Using CT to diagnose tracheal rupture. *AJR Am J Roentgenol* 2001;**176**:1273-80.
23. Marom EM, Goodman PC, McAdams HP. Focal abnormalities of the trachea and main bronchi. *AJR Am J Roentgenol* 2001;**176**:707-11.
24. Naidich DP, Gruden JF, McGuinness G, McCauley DI, Bhalla M. Volumetric (helical/spiral) CT (VCT) of the airways. *J Thorac Imaging* 1997;**12**:11-28.
25. Boiselle PM. Multislice helical CT of the central airways. *Radiol Clin North Am* 2003;**41**:561-74.
26. Brown LR, Aughenbaugh GL. Masses of the anterior mediastinum: CT and MR imaging. *AJR Am J Roentgenol* 1991;**157**:1171-80.
27. Lee JD, Choe KO, Kim SJ, Kim GE, Im JG, Lee JT. CT findings in primary thymic carcinoma. *J Comput Assist Tomogr* 1991;**15**:429-33.
28. Moeller KH, Rosado-de-Christenson ML, Templeton PA. Mediastinal mature teratoma: Imaging features. *AJR Am J Roentgenol* 1997;**169**:985-90.
29. Verstandig AG, Epstein DM, Miller Jr WT, Aronchik JA, Gefter WB, Miller WT. Thymoma: report of 71 cases and a review. *Crit Rev Diagn Imaging* 1992;**33**:201-30.
30. Zerhouni EA, Scott Jr WW, Baker RR, Wharam MD, Siegelman SS. Invasive thymomas: Diagnosis and evaluation by computed tomography. *J Comput Assist Tomogr* 1982;**6**:92-100.
31. Barakos JA, Brown JJ, Brescia RJ, Higgins CB. High signal intensity lesions of the chest in MR imaging. *J Comput Assist Tomogr* 1989;**13**:797-802.
32. LeBlanc J, Guttentag AR, Shepard JA, McLoud TC. Imaging of mediastinal foregut cysts. *Can Assoc Radiol J* 1994;**45**:381-6.
33. McAdams HP, Kirejczyk WM, Rosado-de-Christenson ML, Matsumoto S. Bronchogenic cyst: Imaging features with clinical and histopathologic correlation. *Radiology* 2000;**217**:441-6.
34. Azarow KS, Pearl RH, Zurcher R, Edwards FH, Cohen AJ. Primary mediastinal masses: a comparison of adult and pediatric populations. *J Thorac Cardiovasc Surg* 1993;**106**:67-72.
35. Davis Jr RD, Oldham Jr HN, Sabiston Jr DC. Primary cysts and neoplasms of the mediastinum: recent changes in clinical presentation, methods of diagnosis, management, and results. *Ann Thorac Surg* 1987;**44**:229-37.
36. Bach PB, Jett JR, Pastorino U, Tockman MS, Swensen SJ, Begg CB. Computed tomography screening and lung cancer outcomes. *JAMA* 2007;**297**:953-61.
37. Henschke CI, Yankelevitz DF, Libby DM, Pasmantier MW, Smith JP, Miettinen OS. Survival of patients with stage I lung cancer detected on CT screening. *N Engl J Med* 2006;**355**:1763-71.
38. Gurney JW, Lyddon DM, McKay JA. Determining the likelihood of malignancy in solitary pulmonary nodules with Bayesian analysis. Part II: application. *Radiology* 1993;**186**:415-22.
39. Seemann MD, Staebler A, Beinert T, et al. Usefulness of morphological characteristics for the differentiation of benign from malignant solitary pulmonary lesions using HRCT. *Eur Radiol* 1999;**9**:409-17.
40. Zwirewich CV, Vedal S, Miller RR, Muller NL. Solitary pulmonary nodule: High-resolution CT and radiologic-pathologic correlation. *Radiology* 1991;**179**:469-76.
41. Reference deleted.
42. Swensen SJ, Brown LR, Colby TV, Weaver AL. Pulmonary nodules: CT evaluation of enhancement with iodinated contrast material. *Radiology* 1995;**194**:393-8.
43. Zhang M, Kono M. Solitary pulmonary nodules: Evaluation of blood flow patterns with dynamic CT. *Radiology* 1997;**205**:471-8.
44. Swensen SJ, Viggiano RW, Midthun DE, et al. Lung nodule enhancement at CT: Multicenter study. *Radiology* 2000;**214**:73-80.

45. Christensen JA, Nathan MA, Mullan BP, Hartman TE, Swensen SJ, Lowe VJ. Characterization of the solitary pulmonary nodule: ^{18}F-FDG PET versus nodule-enhancement CT. *AJR Am J Roentgenol* 2006;**187**:1361-7.
46. Gould MK, Maclean CC, Kuschner WG, Rydzak CE, Owens DK. Accuracy of positron emission tomography for diagnosis of pulmonary nodules and mass lesions: a meta-analysis. *JAMA* 2001;**285**:914-24.
47. Bryant AS, Cerfolio RJ. The maximum standardized uptake values on integrated FDG-PET/CT is useful in differentiating benign from malignant pulmonary nodules. *Ann Thorac Surg* 2006;**82**:1016-20.
48. Nomori H, Watanabe K, Ohtsuka T, Naruke T, Suemasu K, Uno K. Evaluation of F-18 fluorodeoxyglucose (FDG) PET scanning for pulmonary nodules less than 3 cm in diameter, with special reference to the CT images. *Lung Cancer* 2004;**45**:19-27.
49. MacMahon H, Austin JH, Gamsu G, et al. Guidelines for management of small pulmonary nodules detected on CT scans: a statement from the Fleischner Society. *Radiology* 2005;**237**:395-400.
50. Mountain CF. Revisions in the International System for Staging Lung Cancer. *Chest* 1997;**111**:1710-7.
51. Goldstraw P, Crowley J, Chansky K, et al. The IASLC Lung Cancer Staging Project: Proposals for the revision of the TNM stage groupings in the forthcoming (seventh) edition of the TNM Classification of malignant tumours. *J Thorac Oncol* 2007;**2**:706-14.
52. Klein JS, Webb WR. The radiologic staging of lung cancer. *J Thorac Imaging* 1991;**7**:29-47.
53. Martini N, Heelan R, Westcott J, et al. Comparative merits of conventional, computed tomographic, and magnetic resonance imaging in assessing mediastinal involvement in surgically confirmed lung carcinoma. *J Thorac Cardiovasc Surg* 1985;**90**:639-48.
54. McLoud TC, Filion RB, Edelman RR, Shepard JA. MR imaging of superior sulcus carcinoma. *J Comput Assist Tomogr* 1989;**13**:233-9.
55. Ratto GB, Piacenza G, Frola C, et al. Chest wall involvement by lung cancer: computed tomographic detection and results of operation. *Ann Thorac Surg* 1991;**51**:182-8.
56. Yokoi K, Mori K, Miyazawa N, Saito Y, Okuyama A, Sasagawa M. Tumor invasion of the chest wall and mediastinum in lung cancer: evaluation with pneumothorax CT. *Radiology* 1991;**181**:147-52.
57. Webb WR, Sostman HD. MR imaging of thoracic disease: clinical uses. *Radiology* 1992;**182**:621-30.
58. Webb WR, Gatsonis C, Zerhouni EA, et al. CT and MR imaging in staging non-small cell bronchogenic carcinoma: report of the Radiologic Diagnostic Oncology Group. *Radiology* 1991;**178**:705-13.
59. Mountain CF, Dresler CM. Regional lymph node classification for lung cancer staging. *Chest* 1997;**111**:1718-23.
60. Glazer GM, Gross BH, Quint LE, Francis IR, Bookstein FL, Orringer MB. Normal mediastinal lymph nodes: number and size according to American Thoracic Society mapping. *AJR Am J Roentgenol* 1985;**144**:261-5.
61. Birim O, Kappetein AP, Stijnen T, Bogers AJ. Meta-analysis of positron emission tomographic and computed tomographic imaging in detecting mediastinal lymph node metastases in nonsmall cell lung cancer. *Ann Thorac Surg* 2005;**79**:375-82.
62. Al-Sarraf N, Gately K, Lucey J, Wilson L, McGovern E, Young V. Lymph node staging by means of positron emission tomography is less accurate in non-small cell lung cancer patients with enlarged lymph nodes: analysis of 1,145 lymph nodes. *Lung Cancer* 2008;**60**:62-8.
63. de Langen AJ, Raijmakers P, Riphagen I, Paul MA, Hoekstra OS. The size of mediastinal lymph nodes and its relation with metastatic involvement: a meta-analysis. *Eur J Cardiothorac Surg* 2006;**29**:26-9.
64. Remy-Jardin M, Remy J, Deschildre F, et al. Diagnosis of pulmonary embolism with spiral CT: comparison with pulmonary angiography and scintigraphy. *Radiology* 1996;**200**:699-706.
65. Rotello LC, Radin EJ, Jastremski MS, Craner D, Milewski A. MRI protocol for critically ill patients. *Am J Crit Care* 1994;**3**:187-90.
66. Reed CE, Harpole DH, Posther KE, et al. Results of the American College of Surgeons Oncology Group Z0050 trial: the utility of positron emission tomography in staging potentially operable non-small cell lung cancer. *J Thorac Cardiovasc Surg* 2003;**126**:1943-51.
67. van Tinteren H, Hoekstra OS, Smit EF, et al. Effectiveness of positron emission tomography in the preoperative assessment of patients with suspected non-small-cell lung cancer: the PLUS multicentre randomised trial. *Lancet* 2002;**359**:1388-93.
68. Lardinois D, Weder W, Hany TF, et al. Staging of non-small-cell lung cancer with integrated positron-emission tomography and computed tomography. *N Engl J Med* 2003;**348**:2500-7.
69. Verhagen AF, Bootsma GP, Tjan-Heijnen VC, et al. FDG-PET in staging lung cancer: How does it change the algorithm? *Lung Cancer* 2004;**44**:175-81.

70. Verboom P, van Tinteren H, Hoekstra OS, et al. Cost-effectiveness of FDG-PET in staging non-small cell lung cancer: the PLUS study. *Eur J Nucl Med Mol Imaging* 2003;**30**:1444-9.
71. Boland GW, Lee MJ, Gazelle GS, Halpern EF, McNicholas MM, Mueller PR. Characterization of adrenal masses using unenhanced CT: an analysis of the CT literature. *AJR Am J Roentgenol* 1998;**171**:201-4.
72. McLoud TC, Bourgouin PM, Greenberg RW, et al. Bronchogenic carcinoma: analysis of staging in the mediastinum with CT by correlative lymph node mapping and sampling. *Radiology* 1992;**182**:319-23.
73. Yun M, Kim W, Alnafisi N, Lacorte L, Jang S, Alavi A. 18F-FDG PET in characterizing adrenal lesions detected on CT or MRI. *J Nucl Med* 2001;**42**:1795-9.
73a. Erasmus JJ, Patz EF Jr, McAdams HP, et al. Evaluation of adrenal masses in patients with bronchogenic carcinoma using ^{18}F-fluorodeoxyglucose positron emission tomography. *AJR AM J Roentgenol* 1997;**168**:1357-60.
74. Yokoi K, Kamiya N, Matsuguma H, et al. Detection of brain metastasis in potentially operable non-small cell lung cancer: a comparison of CT and MRI. *Chest* 1999;**115**:714-9.
75. Pfister DG, Johnson DH, Azzoli CG, et al. American Society of Clinical Oncology treatment of unresectable non-small-cell lung cancer guideline: Update 2003. *J Clin Oncol* 2004;**22**:330-53.
76. Silvestri GA, Gould MK, Margolis ML, et al. Noninvasive staging of non-small cell lung cancer: ACCP evidenced-based clinical practice guidelines. *Chest* 2007;**132**(3 Suppl):178S-201.
77. Bury T, Barreto A, Daenen F, Barthelemy N, Ghaye B, Rigo P. Fluorine-18 deoxyglucose positron emission tomography for the detection of bone metastases in patients with non-small cell lung cancer. *Eur J Nucl Med* 1998;**25**:1244-7.
78. Hsia TC, Shen YY, Yen RF, Kao CH, Changlai SP. Comparing whole body ^{18}F-2-deoxyglucose positron emission tomography and technetium-99m methylene diophosphate bone scan to detect bone metastases in patients with non-small cell lung cancer. *Neoplasma* 2002;**49**:267-71.
79. Marom EM, McAdams HP, Erasmus JJ, et al. Staging non-small cell lung cancer with whole-body PET. *Radiology* 1999;**212**:803-9.
80. Schirrmeister H, Arslandemir C, Glatting G, et al. Omission of bone scanning according to staging guidelines leads to futile therapy in non-small cell lung cancer. *Eur J Nucl Med Mol Imaging* 2004;**31**:964-8.
81. Erasmus JJ, McAdams HP, Rossi S, Kelley MJ. Percutaneous management of intrapulmonary air and fluid collections. *Radiol Clin North Am* 2000;**38**:385-93.
82. Klein JS, Schultz S, Heffner JE. Interventional radiology of the chest: Image-guided percutaneous drainage of pleural effusions, lung abscess, and pneumothorax. *AJR Am J Roentgenol* 1995;**164**:581-8.
83. Royal HD. Radionuclide imaging of the lung. *Curr Opin Radiol* 1989;**1**:446-59.
84. Waller DA. The role of surgery in diagnosis and treatment of malignant pleural mesothelioma. *Curr Opin Oncol* 2003;**15**:139-43.
85. Zellos L, Sugarbaker DJ. Current surgical management of malignant pleural mesothelioma. *Curr Oncol Rep* 2002;**4**:354-60.
86. Patz Jr EF, Rusch VW, Heelan R. The proposed new international TNM staging system for malignant pleural mesothelioma: application to imaging. *AJR Am J Roentgenol* 1996;**166**:323-7.
87. Rusch VW. A proposed new international TNM staging system for malignant pleural mesothelioma from the International Mesothelioma Interest Group. *Lung Cancer* 1996;**14**:1-2.
88. Heelan RT, Rusch VW, Begg CB, Panicek DM, Caravelli JF, Eisen C. Staging of malignant pleural mesothelioma: comparison of CT and MR imaging. *AJR Am J Roentgenol* 1999;**172**:1039-47.
89. Flores RM, Akhurst T, Gonen M, Larson SM, Rusch VW. Positron emission tomography defines metastatic disease but not locoregional disease in patients with malignant pleural mesothelioma. *J Thorac Cardiovasc Surg* 2003;**126**:11-6.
90. Erasmus JJ, Truong MT, Smythe WR, et al. Integrated computed tomography-positron emission tomography in patients with potentially resectable malignant pleural mesothelioma: Staging implications. *J Thorac Cardiovasc Surg* 2005;**129**:1364-70.
91. Schneider DB, Clary-Macy C, Challa S, et al. Positron emission tomography with F18-fluorodeoxyglucose in the staging and preoperative evaluation of malignant pleural mesothelioma. *J Thorac Cardiovasc Surg* 2000;**120**:128-33.
92. Breyer RH, Mills SA, Hudspeth AS, Johnston FR, Cordell AR. A prospective study of sternal wound complications. *Ann Thorac Surg* 1984;**37**:412-6.
93. Rutledge R, Applebaum RE, Kim BJ. Mediastinal infection after open heart surgery. *Surgery* 1985;**97**:88-92.
94. Katzberg RW, Whitehouse GH, deWeese JA. The early radiologic findings in the adult chest after cardiopulmonary bypass surgery. *Cardiovasc Radiol* 1978;**1**:205-15.
95. Harris RS. The pre-operative chest film in relation to post-operative management: Some effects of different projection, posture and lung inflation. *Br J Radiol* 1980;**53**:196-204.
96. Goodman LR, Teplick SK. Computed tomography in acute cardiopulmonary disease. *Radiol Clin North Am* 1983;**21**:741-58.
97. Goodman LR, Kay HR, Teplick SK, Mundth ED. Complications of median sternotomy: computed tomographic evaluation. *AJR Am J Roentgenol* 1983;**141**:225-30.
98. Kay HR, Goodman LR, Teplick SK, Mundth ED. Use of computed tomography to assess mediastinal complications after median sternotomy. *Ann Thorac Surg* 1983;**36**:706-14.
99. Goodman LR. Imaging after cardiac surgery. In: Goodman LR, Putman PC, editors. *Critical care imaging*. Philadelphia: Saunders; 1992; p. 83.
100. Stein PD, Alavi A, Gottschalk A, et al. Usefulness of noninvasive diagnostic tools for diagnosis of acute pulmonary embolism in patients with a normal chest radiograph. *Am J Cardiol* 1991;**67**:1117-20.
101. Qanadli SD, Hajjam ME, Mesurolle B, et al. Pulmonary embolism detection: Prospective evaluation of dual-section helical CT versus selective pulmonary arteriography in 157 patients. *Radiology* 2000;**217**:447-55.
102. Stein PD, Fowler SE, Goodman LR, et al. Multidetector computed tomography for acute pulmonary embolism. *N Engl J Med* 2006;**354**:2317-27.
103. Winer-Muram HT, Rydberg J, Johnson MS, et al. Suspected acute pulmonary embolism: Evaluation with multi-detector row CT versus digital subtraction pulmonary arteriography. *Radiology* 2004;**233**:806-15.
104. Haidary A, Bis K, Vrachliotis T, Kosuri R, Balasubramaniam M. Enhancement performance of a 64-slice triple rule-out protocol vs 16-slice and 10-slice multidetector CT-angiography protocols for evaluation of aortic and pulmonary vasculature. *J Comput Assist Tomogr* 2007;**31**:917-23.
105. Engelke C, Rummeny EJ, Marten K. Acute pulmonary embolism on MDCT of the chest: Prediction of cor pulmonale and short-term patient survival from morphologic embolus burden. *AJR Am J Roentgenol* 2006;**186**:1265-71.
106. Mastora I, Remy-Jardin M, Masson P, et al. Severity of acute pulmonary embolism: Evaluation of a new spiral CT angiographic score in correlation with echocardiographic data. *Eur Radiol* 2003;**13**:29-35.
107. Qanadli SD, El Hajjam M, Vieillard-Baron A, et al. New CT index to quantify arterial obstruction in pulmonary embolism: comparison with angiographic index and echocardiography. *AJR Am J Roentgenol* 2001;**176**:1415-20.
108. Wu AS, Pezzullo JA, Cronan JJ, Hou DD, Mayo-Smith WW. CT pulmonary angiography: Quantification of pulmonary embolus as a predictor of patient outcome—Initial experience. *Radiology* 2004;**230**:831-5.
109. Lu MT, Cai T, Ersoy H, et al. Interval increase in right-left ventricular diameter ratios at CT as a predictor of 30-day mortality after acute pulmonary embolism: Initial experience. *Radiology* 2008;**246**:281-7.
110. Garg K, Sieler H, Welsh CH, Johnston RJ, Russ PD. Clinical validity of helical CT being interpreted as negative for pulmonary embolism: Implications for patient treatment. *AJR Am J Roentgenol* 1999;**172**:1627-31.
111. Stein PD, Woodard PK, Hull RD, et al. Gadolinium-enhanced magnetic resonance angiography for detection of acute pulmonary embolism: an in-depth review. *Chest* 2003;**124**:2324-8.
112. Oudkerk M, van Beek EJ, Wielopolski P, et al. Comparison of contrast-enhanced magnetic resonance angiography and conventional pulmonary angiography for the diagnosis of pulmonary embolism: a prospective study. *Lancet* 2002;**359**:1643-7.
113. Kluge A, Luboldt W, Bachmann G. Acute pulmonary embolism to the subsegmental level: diagnostic accuracy of three MRI techniques compared with 16-MDCT. *AJR Am J Roentgenol* 2006;**187**:W7-14.
114. Barnett GH, Ropper AH, Johnson KA. Physiological support and monitoring of critically ill patients during magnetic resonance imaging. *J Neurosurg* 1988;**68**:246-50.
115. Dunn V, Coffman CE, McGowan JE, Ehrhardt JC. Mechanical ventilation during magnetic resonance imaging. *Magn Reson Imaging* 1985;**3**:169-72.
116. Marckmann P, Skov L, Rossen K, et al. Nephrogenic systemic fibrosis: suspected causative role of gadodiamide used for contrast-enhanced magnetic resonance imaging. *J Am Soc Nephrol* 2006;**17**:2359-62.
117. Thomsen HS. Nephrogenic systemic fibrosis: a serious late adverse reaction to gadodiamide. *Eur Radiol* 2006;**16**:2619-21.

CHAPTER 3

Preoperative Evaluation of Patients Undergoing Thoracic Surgery

John J. Reilly, Jr.

Physiologic Effects of Thoracic Surgery
Patient Population Undergoing Thoracic Surgery
Most Common Complications After Thoracic Surgery
Goals of the Preoperative Evaluation
History and Physical Examination
  History

Physical Examination
Laboratory Studies
Imaging Studies
Pulmonary Function Testing
Prediction of Postoperative Lung Function
Cardiac Assessment of Patients Under Consideration for Thoracic Surgical Procedures

Assessment of Functional Capacity
Arterial Blood Gas Measurements
Pulmonary Hemodynamics
Age
Evaluation and Risk Stratification

The decision to proceed with any surgical procedure involves a careful consideration of the anticipated benefits of surgery and an assessment of the risks associated with the surgical procedure. An important component of estimating the benefit of surgery is knowledge of the natural history of the condition in question in the absence of surgery.

A popular, and inaccurate, conception of preoperative evaluation is that the evaluating physician "clears" the patient for surgery. Implicit in this terminology is the assumption that a cleared patient has a low risk for perioperative morbidity. As will be discussed in this chapter, it is more accurate to view the role of preoperative evaluation as meeting two goals: defining the morbidity and risks of surgery, both short term and long term, and identifying specific factors or conditions in patients that can be addressed to modify the patient's risk of morbidity. The formulation of an approach to accomplish these goals requires knowledge of the effects of thoracic surgery on patients.

PHYSIOLOGIC EFFECTS OF THORACIC SURGERY

Surgical procedures and the anesthesia administered to allow such procedures have significant impact on respiratory physiology that contributes to the development of postoperative pulmonary complications. Given that the incidence of pulmonary complications is directly related to the proximity of the planned procedure to the diaphragms, patients undergoing pulmonary, esophageal, or other thoracic surgical procedures fall into the category of patients at high risk for postoperative respiratory complication.[1]

The intraoperative use of inhaled volatile agents can affect gas exchange by altering diaphragmatic and chest wall function. These changes occur without corresponding alterations in blood flow, which creates low ventilation-perfusion areas, resulting in widening of the alveolar-arterial oxygen gradient.

In the postoperative period, a variety of factors contribute to the development of complications. These include an alteration in breathing pattern to one of rapid shallow breaths with the absence of periodic deep breaths (sighs) and abnormal diaphragmatic function. These result both from pain and from diaphragmatic dysfunction resulting from splanchnic efferent neural impulses arising from the manipulation of abdominal contents. This has the effect of reducing the functional residual capacity (FRC), the resting volume of the respiratory system. The FRC declines by an average of 35% after thoracotomy and lung resection and by about 30% after upper abdominal operations.[2-4] If the FRC declines sufficiently to approach closing volume, the volume at which small airway closure begins to occur, patients develop atelectasis and are predisposed to infectious complications. Closing volume is elevated in patients with underlying lung disease.

The alterations in lung volumes that occur result in a reduction in both the inspiratory capacity (the maximal inhalation volume attained starting from a given lung volume) and the expiratory reserve volume (the maximal exhalation volume from a given lung volume), contribute to a decline in the effectiveness of cough, and result in increased difficulty in clearing of pulmonary secretions.

PATIENT POPULATION UNDERGOING THORACIC SURGERY

Many patients undergoing a noncardiac thoracic surgical procedure do so because of known or suspected lung or esophageal cancer. These diseases share the common risk factor of a significant and prolonged exposure to cigarette smoking. The combination of age and prolonged cigarette smoking results in a patient population with a significant incidence of comorbid factors in addition to the primary diagnosis. Several reports use the Charlson Comorbidity Index as an indicator of comorbid conditions and predictor of postoperative complications. This index generates a score based on the presence of comorbid conditions and has been demonstrated to stratify risk of postoperative complications in thoracic surgery patients.[5,6]

In one study, the mean age of patients undergoing esophagectomy was 58.1 years; 45% of patients were older than 60 years.[7] In another Japanese study, the median age was 62.3 years; 88% were male.[8] In a study comparing transhiatal esophagectomy with transthoracic esophagectomy, the mean ages of the patients were 69 years and 64 years, with patients up to the age of 79 years included in the study.[9] In a review, 28% to 32% of patients undergoing esophagectomy in the United States were older than 75 years, and 40% had a Charlson score above 3.[10]

Similarly, patients with lung cancer tend to be older and have comorbid conditions. In a series of 344 patients, 36% were older than 70 years and 95% had a significant smoking history.[11] A review of Medicare patients undergoing thoracic surgery in the United States showed that of patients undergoing lobectomy, 32% to 35% were older than 75 years (44% women), and 32% had a Charlson score above 3.[10] In the same series, 21% to 26% of patients undergoing pneumonectomy were older than 75 years (28% women), and 56% had a Charlson score above 3.

A significant source of comorbidity in the population of patients with lung cancer is chronic obstructive pulmonary disease (COPD). The diagnosis of COPD is an independent risk factor, controlling for cigarette smoke exposure, for the development of lung cancer.

Thus, the patient population presenting for major thoracic surgical procedures tends to be older, has a high incidence of comorbid conditions, and contains a disproportionate number of patients with obstructive lung disease. The combination of these factors, plus the magnitude of the surgical procedures, presents a challenge to the clinicians evaluating such patients. The potential for perioperative morbidity and mortality is substantial, but at the same time, the lack of effective alternative therapy for the patient's malignant disease means that the consequence of not being a surgical candidate is almost certain mortality. This quandary has led Gass and Olsen[12] to ask, What is an acceptable surgical mortality in a disease with 100% mortality?

MOST COMMON COMPLICATIONS AFTER THORACIC SURGERY

These are discussed in more detail elsewhere in this book (see Chapter 4). In general, the most frequent complications after major thoracic procedures fall into the categories of respiratory and cardiovascular. Although the exact frequency varies from series to series, pneumonia, atelectasis, arrhythmias (particularly atrial fibrillation), and congestive heart failure are the most common. Myocardial infarction, prolonged air leak, empyema, and bronchopleural fistula also occur at a significant frequency.[11,13,14] It follows, therefore, that particular attention to pulmonary and cardiac reserve and risk factors should be a major component of the preoperative evaluation.

GOALS OF THE PREOPERATIVE EVALUATION

The clinicians evaluating a patient for a major thoracic surgical procedure have several goals for the evaluation process. The most obvious of these goals are to provide all parties with an assessment of the risks, both short and long term, of morbidity and mortality from the procedure in a given patient and simultaneously to identify factors that can be addressed to reduce the possibility of adverse events. Less obvious is that the comprehensive evaluation of a patient as part of the preoperative assessment allows the identification of risk factors and health issues independent of the planned surgery and facilitates the institution of interventions indicated regardless of plans for surgery.

HISTORY AND PHYSICAL EXAMINATION

Although the field of thoracic surgery has been dramatically altered by the development of new technologies in both imaging and therapeutics, the history and physical examination remain the most important components of the preoperative evaluation. There is no substitute for a careful history and examination by an experienced clinician.

History

Table 3-1 highlights the important components of the patient's history. Whereas many of the elements of the history are self-explanatory, several require some further exposition. A critical component of the preoperative evaluation is the assessment of a patient's functional status. Functional status is an important component of the decision algorithm for both the pulmonary and cardiac elements of the preoperative evaluation. A variety of approaches have been taken to determine functional capacity. These include questionnaires; tests of locomotion, such as the 6-minute walk or stair climbing; and cardiopulmonary exercise testing (discussed later). One convenient approach to use is the Duke Activity Status Index (DASI) (Table 3-2), a questionnaire that can be administered during an interview or can be self-administered.[15]

There is a rough correlation between the score on the DASI, which ranges from 0 to 58.2, and maximal oxygen uptake. In addition, the answers to this questionnaire can be used to estimate the functional capacity of the patient in metabolic equivalents (METs), as described in the section on cardiac assessment.

In addition to these considerations, patients should be asked about signs or symptoms suggesting the presence of metastatic disease. These include new headaches, focal

Table 3–1

Important Components of History in Preoperative Evaluation

Presenting symptoms and circumstances of diagnosis
Prior diagnosis of pulmonary or cardiac disease
Comorbid conditions: diabetes mellitus, liver disease, renal disease
Prior experiences with general anesthesia and surgery
Cigarette smoking: never, current, ex-smoker (if ex-smoker, when did patient stop?)
Inventory of functional capacity of patient (e.g., Duke Activity Status Index)
Medications and allergies
Alcohol use, including prior history of withdrawal syndromes

Table 3-2
Duke Activity Status Index

Question	Activity: Can you	Yes	No
1	Take care of yourself, that is, eating, dressing, bathing, or using the toilet?	2.75	0
2	Walk indoors, such as around your house?	1.75	0
3	Walk a block or two on level ground?	2.75	0
4	Climb a flight of stairs or walk up a hill?	5.50	0
5	Run a short distance?	8.00	0
6	Do light work around the house like dusting or washing dishes?	2.70	0
7	Do moderate work around the house like vacuuming, sweeping floors, or carrying in groceries?	3.50	0
8	Do heavy work around the house like scrubbing floors or lifting or moving heavy furniture?	8.00	0
9	Do yard work like raking leaves, weeding, or pushing a power mower?	4.50	0
10	Have sexual relations?	5.25	0
11	Participate in moderate recreational activities like golf, bowling, dancing, doubles tennis, or throwing a baseball or football?	6.00	0
12	Participate in strenuous sports like swimming, singles tennis, football, basketball, or skiing?	7.50	0

From Hlatky MA, Boineau RE, Higginbotham MB, et al. A brief self-administered questionnaire to determine functional capacity (the Duke Activity Status Index).

neurologic signs or symptoms, new-onset seizure disorder, bone pain, and recent fractures. Patients should also be questioned about symptoms related to paraneoplastic syndromes. These can range from the relatively subtle symptoms of hypercalcemia to more dramatic neurologic symptoms.

Physical Examination

The examination of the patient includes an assessment of general overall appearance, including signs of wasting. Respiratory rate and the use of accessory muscles of respiration are noted. Examination of the head and neck includes assessment of adenopathy and focal neurologic deficits or signs, particularly Horner's syndrome in patients with a lung mass. The pulmonary examination includes an assessment of diaphragmatic motion (by percussion) and notes any paradoxical respiratory pattern in the recumbent position. The relative duration of exhalation as well as the presence or absence of wheezing should be noted. The presence of rales should raise the possibility of pneumonia, heart failure, or pulmonary fibrosis. The cardiac examination includes assessment of a third heart sound to suggest left ventricular failure, murmurs to suggest valvular lesions, and an accentuated pulmonic component of the second heart sound suggestive of pulmonary hypertension. The heart rhythm and the absence or presence of any irregular heart beats are noted. The abdominal examination notes liver size, presence or absence of palpable masses or adenopathy, and any tenderness. The examination of extremities notes any edema, cyanosis, or clubbing. Clubbing should not be attributed to COPD and raises the possibilities of intrathoracic malignant disease or congenital heart disease. The patient's gait should be observed, both as an assessment of neurologic function and to confirm the patient's ability to participate in postoperative mobilization.

Laboratory Studies

It is reasonable practice to check electrolyte values, renal function, and clotting parameters and to obtain a complete blood count as part of the preoperative assessment. In patients with known or suspected malignant disease, liver function and serum calcium concentration should also be checked.

IMAGING STUDIES

This issue is covered in detail elsewhere in this text. For patients undergoing pulmonary parenchymal resection, review of images is essential to estimate the amount of lung that will be removed in surgery. In this setting, patients usually have a computed tomographic (CT) scan of the chest. In addition to the pathologic process for which the patient has been referred, the scan should be reviewed for signs of emphysema or pulmonary fibrosis. In general, review of images is an important component of surgical planning and determination of the extent of resection, which in turn influences the process of evaluation of the patient.

PULMONARY FUNCTION TESTING

The utility of preoperative pulmonary function testing in part depends on the type of operative procedure being planned. For patients undergoing mediastinoscopy, drainage of pleural effusions, or pleural biopsy or esophageal surgery and who have no prior history of lung disease or unexplained dyspnea, preoperative pulmonary function testing is unlikely to contribute to the preoperative evaluation.

For patients being considered for pulmonary parenchymal resection, preoperative pulmonary function testing should be performed. Although a variety of pulmonary function tests have been examined in this setting, the two that have emerged as being predictive of postoperative complications are the *forced expiratory volume in 1 second* (FEV_1) measured during spirometry and the *diffusing capacity for carbon monoxide* (DL_{CO}). Both of these values can be used to provide a rough estimate of the risk of operative morbidity and mortality. In addition, they are used to calculate the *predicted postoperative* values for FEV_1 and DL_{CO} (ppo-FEV_1 and ppo-DL_{CO}, respectively).

PREDICTION OF POSTOPERATIVE LUNG FUNCTION

Predicted postoperative lung function has been demonstrated to be an important predictor of operative risk. In general, the available methods for calculation of postoperative lung function result in an underestimate of actual measured lung function once the patient has recovered from surgery. Two approaches are commonly used for calculation of postoperative lung function: simple calculation and the regional assessment of lung function.

Simple calculation is based on the assumption of homogeneously distributed lung function and requires knowledge of the number of segments to be resected and the preoperative value. For FEV_1, the formula is ppo-FEV_1 = FEV_1 [1 − (number of segments resected × .0526)]. A similar calculation is done for DL_{CO}. For the majority of patients, this approach to calculation is sufficient and, as mentioned before, results in a postoperative predicted value that is somewhat less than what is measured after recovery.

In certain situations, simple calculation is inaccurate in predicting postoperative lung function. The clinical situations in which regional assessment of lung function is indicated are summarized in Table 3-3. A variety of approaches have been used to attempt to assess the regional distribution of lung function, including lateral position testing, bronchospirometry, quantitative radionuclide ventilation-perfusion scanning, and quantitative CT scanning. The test most frequently used currently is radionuclide scanning. Typically, the data from quantitative radionuclide ventilation-perfusion scans are reported as the percentage of function contributed by six lung regions: upper third, middle third, and lower third of each hemithorax. These data, combined with the knowledge of the preoperative lung function value and the location and planned extent of resection, allow the calculation of a predicted postoperative value. An alternative approach is the use of quantitative CT scanning, which categorizes lung tissue with an attenuation between −910 and −500 Hounsfield units as "functional lung tissue," and in a manner analogous to that used for radionuclide scanning, an estimate of remaining functional lung tissue can be made on the basis of knowledge of the extent of planned resection.[16] Comparison with radionuclide scanning suggests that quantitative CT scanning correlates with measured postoperative function as well as or better than radionuclide scanning does.[17] This approach also allows prediction of postoperative oxygen saturation, which in turn has a correlation with postoperative complications and recovery time.[18] Like other methods of predicting postoperative lung function, it may underestimate residual function in patients with COPD.[19] Despite these data and the potential advantages of using the CT scan for both anatomic definition and functional calculations, eliminating the need for the additional time and expense of a radionuclide perfusion scan, it has not been widely adopted (see Table 3-3).

CARDIAC ASSESSMENT OF PATIENTS UNDER CONSIDERATION FOR THORACIC SURGICAL PROCEDURES

The basic philosophy of cardiac assessment for surgical procedures has changed in recent years, as reflected in the recent guidelines jointly formulated by the American College of Cardiology and the American Heart Association.[20] The preoperative evaluation is now viewed as an opportunity to perform a general cardiac assessment and to initiate risk factor modification or management rather than a specific intervention centered on surgery. The practice is to institute medical management as indicated by the patient's condition, rather than specific preoperative recommendations. In keeping with this approach, current concepts are that coronary revascularization, by either catheter approach or bypass grafting, is rarely indicated solely to reduce operative risk in a particular patient.

The preoperative cardiac evaluation incorporates both the cardiac risks associated with the operation under consideration and the specific risk factors of the particular patient under consideration. In general, thoracic surgical procedures fall into the risk categories of high (cardiac risk > 5%, operations with an anticipated long procedure time, major fluid shifts, or blood loss) and intermediate (1% > cardiac risk < 5%, intrathoracic surgery).

As with the evaluation in general, the cornerstone of preoperative cardiac evaluation is a careful history and physical examination. In addition to inquiries directed at cardiac risk factors such as family history, smoking history, history of hypercholesterolemia, history of diabetes mellitus or hypertension, and history of prior cardiac disease, special attention is directed to questions to assess the patient's functional capacity. One common way is to classify a patient's functional capacity in terms of metabolic equivalents or METs. Four METs is the energy expenditure required to climb a flight of stairs, to walk up a hill or briskly on level ground, or to run a short distance (items 3 to 5 on the DASI); 1 to 4 METs are required to perform self-care, to ambulate on level ground within a residence, and to perform light housework (items 1, 2, 3, and 6 on the DASI). More than 10 METs are required to participate in strenuous sports such as singles tennis, bicycling, and basketball (item 12 on the DASI).

The combination of the classification of clinical predictors, the patient's functional capacity, and the risk of surgery then

Table 3-3
Indications for Preoperative Assessment of the Regional Distribution of Lung Function

Significant airflow obstruction on spirometry (FEV_1 < 80% predicted and FEV_1/FVC < 0.70)
Significant pleural disease
Known or suspected endobronchial obstruction
Central lung mass
History of prior lung resection

determines the approach to preoperative evaluation. Current guidelines recommend a stepwise approach to the evaluation after a comprehensive history, physical examination, and review of the electrocardiogram. If a patient has had coronary revascularization within the past 5 years and has not had a clinical change since then, or if the patient has had a cardiac evaluation within the past 2 years that did not demonstrate the patient to be at high risk, further testing is usually not indicated. If neither of these considerations applies, the next step is to classify patients according to their clinical predictors.

For patients with a history of myocardial infarction within 30 days, unstable coronary syndromes, decompensated congestive heart failure, significant arrhythmias, or severe valvular disease, delay of the procedure should be considered for all but emergency procedures. Such patients should have medical risk factor management and modification initiated, and consideration should be given to performing coronary angiography.

Patients with good functional capacity (defined as ≥4 METs) and no cardiac symptoms should proceed with the planned surgery. For patients in whom functional capacity is unknown or is limited to less than 4 METs, current recommendations are that those with a history of heart disease, history of congestive heart failure or currently compensated congestive heart failure, diabetes mellitus, renal insufficiency, or history of cerebrovascular disease may proceed with surgery with heart rate control in the perioperative setting. Of note, recent data suggest that beta-blockers may be safely used in acutely ill patients with COPD.[21] Those with none of these characteristics do not require heart rate control as part of perioperative management. Patients with one or more of the aforementioned characteristics should have noninvasive testing only if it will change management. This approach is summarized in Figure 3-1.

For all patients, any long-term issues meriting consideration of risk factor modification or therapy should be addressed in the postoperative period. Appropriate therapy is instituted when the patient is stable enough to tolerate it.

ASSESSMENT OF FUNCTIONAL CAPACITY

For patients undergoing pulmonary resection, functional capacity is an important predictor of postoperative morbidity and mortality. In addition to the role of functional capacity in determining the appropriate cardiac evaluation before surgery (see Fig. 3-1), functional capacity has predictive value for postoperative complications independent of that derived from pulmonary function testing.

In clinical practice, there are two common approaches to assessment of functional capacity: symptom-limited maximal cardiopulmonary exercise testing with expired gas analysis; and threshold testing, which requires patients to attain a certain functional goal. Among the latter, the most commonly employed test is stair climbing. Published data on stair climb testing suggest that patients with the ability to climb more than 3 flights (54 steps) are at acceptable risk for lobectomy and that patients with the ability to climb more than 4.6 to 5 flights are at acceptable risk for pneumonectomy. Conversely, patients unable to climb more than 12 m on a symptom-limited stair climbing test are at high risk for perioperative morbidity and mortality.[11,22-29] An alternative to stair climbing is the shuttle walk, in which subjects walk back and forth ("shuttle") on a 10-m course at a pace cued by an audio signal, increasing in speed every minute until the subject is too breathless to maintain the target pace. A result of less than 25 shuttles has been reported to correlate with maximal oxygen uptake (see later) of less than 10 mL/kg/min and, by inference, with prohibitive operative risk.[30]

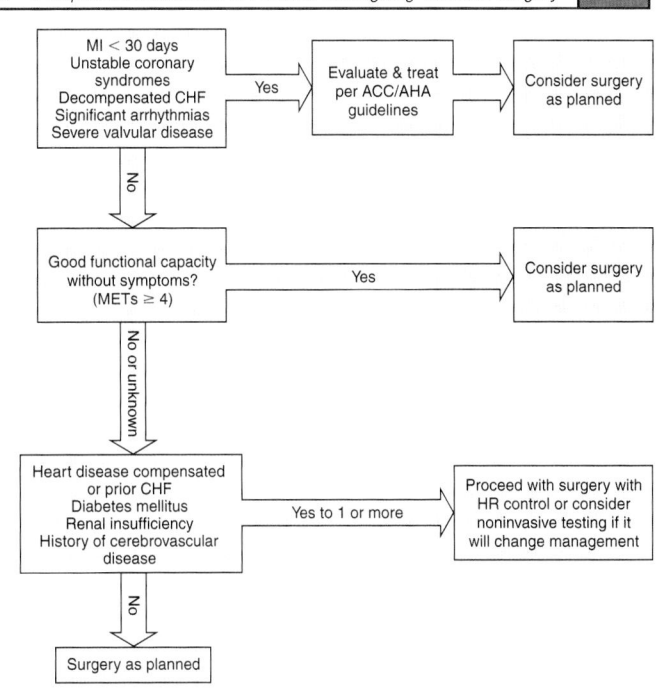

Figure 3-1
Cardiac evaluation algorithm. *(Modified from Fleisher LA, Beckman JA, Brown KA, et al. ACC/AHA 2007 Guidelines on Perioperative Cardiovascular Evaluation and Care for Noncardiac Surgery: Executive Summary.[20])*

Maximal symptom-limited cardiopulmonary testing has been studied as a mode of assessment of functional capacity. The most commonly reported result of such testing is the maximal oxygen uptake ($M\dot{V}O_2$) normalized for body mass, expressed as milliliters per kilogram per minute. Alternatively, the data are reported as a percentage of predicted value. There is good agreement that patients with an $M\dot{V}O_2$ of more than 15 to 20 mL/kg/min are at low or "acceptable" risk for perioperative complications and mortality.[31-33] Conversely, patients with an $M\dot{V}O_2$ of less than 10 to 12 mL/kg/min are at high risk for thoracic surgery.[29,34-36] In addition to these applications, the preoperative $M\dot{V}O_2$ can also be used in concert with a regional assessment of lung function to calculate a predicted postoperative $M\dot{V}O_2$ (ppo-$M\dot{V}O_2$), in a manner analogous to that described for lung function parameters.[35] The ppo-$M\dot{V}O_2$ can then be used to stratify perioperative risk.

Currently available data suggest that patients with a predicted postoperative FEV_1 or DL_{CO} of less than 40% should have additional risk stratification with a test of functional capacity. An alternative sequence of evaluation has been assessed by Bolliger and Perruchoud,[37] who advocate functional assessment in all patients with an FEV_1 or DL_{CO} below 80% predicted and reserve regional assessment of lung function for patients with a maximal oxygen uptake of 10 to 20 mL/kg/min or 40% to 75% of predicted. A synthesis of current recommendations for preoperative evaluation for pulmonary resection is presented in Figure 3-2.[38]

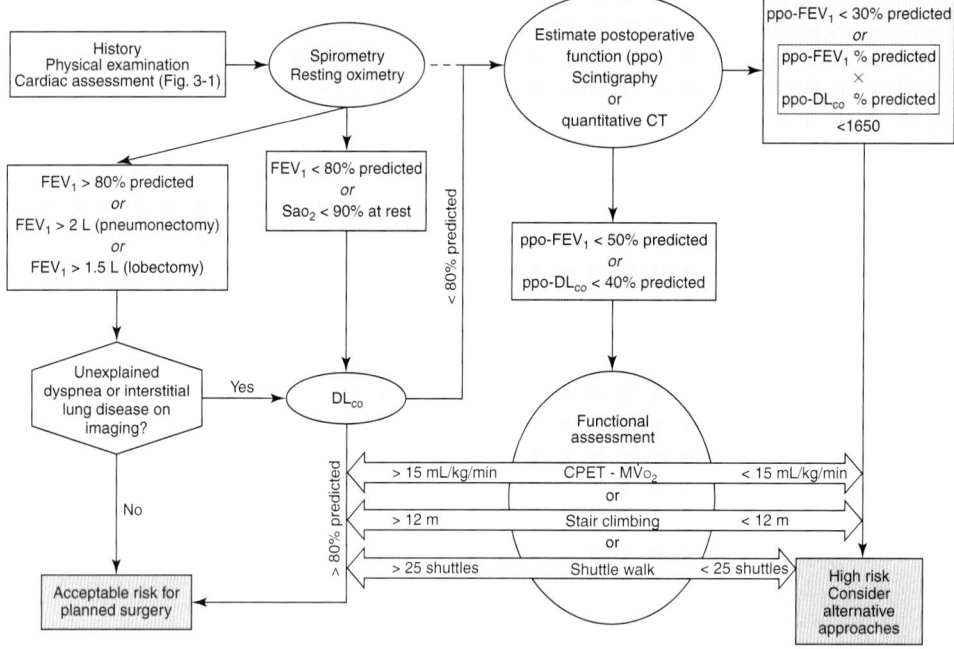

Figure 3–2
Preoperative evaluation algorithm. CPET, cardiopulmonary exercise testing.

Arterial Blood Gas Measurements

Commonly measured preoperatively, arterial blood gases have been used to attempt to stratify risk of perioperative complications. Reports on the utility of arterial oxygen saturation in preoperative evaluation are contradictory; some suggest that resting hypoxemia or exertional desaturation identifies patients at higher risk, but others fail to confirm this association.[39,40] This has led to the recommendation that patients with resting SaO_2 below 90% have further physiologic evaluation.[38] Common clinical dogma is that patients with a resting PCO_2 above 45 mm Hg are at increased risk.[31,41] Several studies, however, have demonstrated that resection may be safely undertaken in patients with resting hypercarbia in the absence of other contraindications to surgery.[14,31,42]

Pulmonary Hemodynamics

Measurements of resting pulmonary hemodynamics, pulmonary artery occlusion, or exercise hemodynamics have been studied as preoperative assessments. The data generated are contradictory and generally do not add substantially to information obtained from functional assessment and pulmonary function testing.[26]

Age

Although age has been confirmed in many series as a risk factor for perioperative complications, much of the additional risk from age results from comorbid factors. When studies control for comorbidities, patients are at mildly (approximately twofold) increased risk because of age.[43] Current consensus is that age alone, particularly in the presence of a good functional capacity, is not a contraindication to surgery.[28,38]

Table 3–4
Risk Assessment for Pulmonary Surgery

Higher Risk	Lower Risk
Age > 70 years	FEV_1: >2 L for pneumonectomy; >1.5 L for lobectomy; >0.6 L for segmentectomy
Higher extent of resection (pneumonectomy > lobectomy > wedge resection)	Predicted postoperative FEV_1 > 30%-40%
Poor exercise performance	Stair climbing: >5 flights for pneumonectomy; 3 flights for lobectomy
Low predicted postoperative FEV_1	Cycle ergometry > 83 watts
Low predicted postoperative DL_{co}	Predicted postoperative DL_{co} > 40%
Prolonged operative time	Maximal oxygen uptake > 15-20 mL/kg/min

EVALUATION AND RISK STRATIFICATION

Table 3-4 presents parameters that identify patients at higher and lower risk for complications after pulmonary surgery. Building on these parameters, various authors have attempted to create a multifactor risk assessment tool that incorporates a variety of these parameters.[44] A recommended approach to the preoperative evaluation, based on recent published consensus guidelines, is presented in Figure 3-2.[38] Patients who fall into the conventional category of high or prohibitive risk and who are candidates for lung volume reduction surgery by virtue of having severe airflow obstruction and upper lobe–predominant emphysema may be candidates for parenchymal resection if the lesion requiring resection falls within the tissue that would be resected as part of lung volume reduction. In this case, the predicted postoperative FEV$_1$ would actually be higher than that measured preoperatively, and standard prediction algorithms would not apply (see Table 3-4 and Fig. 3-2).[45-48]

REFERENCES

1. Smetana GW. Preoperative pulmonary evaluation. *N Engl J Med* 1999;**340**: 937-44.
2. Ali J, Weisel RD, Layug AB, Kripke BJ, Hechtman HB. Consequences of postoperative alterations in respiratory mechanics. *Am J Surg* 1974;**128**:376-82.
3. Craig DB. Postoperative recovery of pulmonary function. *Anesth Analg* 1981;**60**:46-52.
4. Meyers JR, Lembeck L, O'Kane H, Baue AE. Changes in functional residual capacity of the lung after operation. *Arch Surg* 1975;**110**:576-83.
5. Charlson ME, Pompei P, Ales KL, MacKenzie CR. A new method of classifying prognostic comorbidity in longitudinal studies: development and validation. *J Chronic Dis* 1987;**40**:373-83.
6. Birim O, Maat AP, Kappetein AP, van Meerbeeck JP, Damhuis RA, Bogers AJ. Validation of the Charlson comorbidity index in patients with operated primary non-small cell lung cancer. *Eur J Cardiothorac Surg* 2003;**23**:30-4.
7. Mariette C, Finzi L, Fabre S, Balon JM, Van Seuningen I, Triboulet JP. Factors predictive of complete resection of operable esophageal cancer: a prospective study. *Ann Thorac Surg* 2003;**75**:1720-6.
8. Gomi K, Oguchi M, Hirokawa Y, et al. Process and preliminary outcome of a patterns-of-care study of esophageal cancer in Japan: patients treated with surgery and radiotherapy. *Int J Radiat Oncol Biol Phys* 2003;**56**:813-22.
9. Hulscher JB, van Sandick JW, de Boer AG, et al. Extended transthoracic resection compared with limited transhiatal resection for adenocarcinoma of the esophagus. *N Engl J Med* 2002;**347**:1662-9.
10. Birkmeyer JD, Siewers AE, Finlayson EV, et al. Hospital volume and surgical mortality in the United States. *N Engl J Med* 2002;**346**:1128-37.
11. Ploeg AJ, Kappetein AP, van Tongeren RB, Pahlplatz PV, Kastelein GW, Breslau PJ. Factors associated with perioperative complications and long-term results after pulmonary resection for primary carcinoma of the lung. *Eur J Cardiothorac Surg* 2003;**23**:26-9.
12. Gass GD, Olsen GN. Preoperative pulmonary function testing to predict postoperative morbidity and mortality. *Chest* 1986;**89**:127-35.
13. Bernard A, Ferrand L, Hagry O, Benoit L, Cheynel N, Favre JP. Identification of prognostic factors determining risk groups for lung resection. *Ann Thorac Surg* 2000;**70**:1161-7.
14. Kearney DJ, Lee TH, Reilly JJ, DeCamp MM, Sugarbaker DJ. Assessment of operative risk in patients undergoing lung resection: Importance of predicted pulmonary function. *Chest* 1994;**105**:753-9.
15. Hlatky MA, Boineau RE, Higginbotham MB, et al. A brief self-administered questionnaire to determine functional capacity (the Duke Activity Status Index). *Am J Cardiol* 1989;**64**:651-4.
16. Wu MT, Chang JM, Chiang AA, et al. Use of quantitative CT to predict postoperative lung function in patients with lung cancer. *Radiology* 1994;**191**:257-62.
17. Wu MT, Pan HB, Chiang AA, et al. Prediction of postoperative lung function in patients with lung cancer: comparison of quantitative CT with perfusion scintigraphy. *AJR Am J Roentgenol* 2002;**178**:667-72.
18. Ueda K, Kaneda Y, Sudoh M, et al. Role of quantitative CT in predicting hypoxemia and complications after lung lobectomy for cancer, with special reference to area of emphysema. *Chest* 2005;**128**:3500-6.
19. Sverzellati N, Chetta A, Calabro E, et al. Reliability of quantitative computed tomography to predict postoperative lung function in patients with chronic obstructive pulmonary disease having a lobectomy. *J Comput Assist Tomogr* 2005;**29**:819-24.
20. Fleisher LA, Beckman JA, Brown KA, et al. ACC/AHA 2007 Guidelines on Perioperative Cardiovascular Evaluation and Care for Noncardiac Surgery: Executive Summary: A Report of the American College of Cardiology/American Heart Association Task Force on Practice Guidelines (Writing Committee to Revise the 2002 Guidelines on Perioperative Cardiovascular Evaluation for Noncardiac Surgery) Developed in Collaboration With the American Society of Echocardiography, American Society of Nuclear Cardiology, Heart Rhythm Society, Society of Cardiovascular Anesthesiologists, Society for Cardiovascular Angiography and Interventions, Society for Vascular Medicine and Biology, and Society for Vascular Surgery. *J Am Coll Cardiol* 2007;**50**:1707–32.
21. Dransfield MT, Rowe SM, Johnson JE, Bailey WC, Gerald LB. Use of beta blockers and the risk of death in hospitalised patients with acute exacerbations of COPD. *Thorax* 2008;**63**:301-5.
22. Brunelli A, Refai M, Xiume F, et al. Performance at symptom-limited stair-climbing test is associated with increased cardiopulmonary complications, mortality, and costs after major lung resection. *Ann Thorac Surg* 2008;**86**:240-7; discussion 7-8.
23. Brunelli A, Sabbatini A, Xiume F, et al. Inability to perform maximal stair climbing test before lung resection: a propensity score analysis on early outcome. *Eur J Cardiothorac Surg* 2005;**27**:367-72.
24. Olsen GN, Bolton JW, Weiman DS, Hornung CA. Stair climbing as an exercise test to predict the postoperative complications of lung resection. Two years' experience. *Chest* 1991;**99**:587-90.
25. Pollock M, Roa J, Benditt J, Celli B. Estimation of ventilatory reserve by stair climbing. A study in patients with chronic airflow obstruction. *Chest* 1993;**104**:1378-83.
26. Reilly JJ. Preparing for pulmonary resection: preoperative evaluation of patients. *Chest* 1997;**112**:206S-8S.
27. Reilly JJ Jr. Evidence-based preoperative evaluation of candidates for thoracotomy. *Chest* 1999;**116**:474S-6S.
28. Schuurmans MM, Diacon AH, Bolliger CT. Functional evaluation before lung resection. *Clin Chest Med* 2002;**23**:159-72.
29. Richter Larsen K, Svendsen UG, Milman N, Brenoe J, Petersen BN, Brene J. Exercise testing in the preoperative evaluation of patients with bronchogenic carcinoma. *Eur Respir J* 1997;**10**:1559-65.
30. Singh SJ, Morgan MD, Scott S, Walters D, Hardman AE. Development of a shuttle walking test of disability in patients with chronic airways obstruction. *Thorax* 1992;**47**:1019-24.
31. Morice RC, Peters EJ, Ryan MB, Putnam JB, Ali MK, Roth JA. Exercise testing in the evaluation of patients at high risk for complications from lung resection. *Chest* 1992;**101**:356-61.
32. Smith TP, Kinasewitz GT, Tucker WY, Spillers WP, George RB. Exercise capacity as a predictor of post-thoracotomy morbidity. *Am Rev Respir Dis* 1984;**129**:730-4.
33. Wang J, Olak J, Ferguson MK. Diffusing capacity predicts operative mortality but not long-term survival after resection for lung cancer. *J Thorac Cardiovasc Surg* 1999;**117**:581-6; discussion 6-7.
34. Bechard D, Wetstein L. Assessment of exercise oxygen consumption as preoperative criterion for lung resection. *Ann Thorac Surg* 1987;**44**:344-9.
35. Bolliger CT, Wyser C, Roser H, Soler M, Perruchoud AP. Lung scanning and exercise testing for the prediction of postoperative performance in lung resection candidates at increased risk for complications. *Chest* 1995;**108**(2):341-8.
36. Wang JS, Abboud RT, Evans KG, Finley RJ, Graham BL. Role of CO diffusing capacity during exercise in the preoperative evaluation for lung resection. *Am J Respir Crit Care Med* 2000;**162**:1435-44.
37. Bolliger CT, Perruchoud AP. Functional evaluation of the lung resection candidate. *Eur Respir J* 1998;**11**:198-212.
38. Colice GL, Shafazand S, Griffin JP, Keenan R, Bolliger CT. Physiologic evaluation of the patient with lung cancer being considered for resectional surgery: ACCP evidenced-based clinical practice guidelines (2nd edition). *Chest* 2007;**132**: 161S-77S.
39. Ninan M, Sommers KE, Landreneau RJ, et al. Standardized exercise oximetry predicts postpneumonectomy outcome. *Ann Thorac Surg* 1997;**64**:328-32; discussion 32-3.
40. Win T, Jackson A, Groves AM, et al. Relationship of shuttle walk test and lung cancer surgical outcome. *Eur J Cardiothorac Surg* 2004;**26**:1216-9.
41. Preoperative pulmonary function testing. American College of Physicians [comment]. *Ann Intern Med* 1990;**112**:793-4.
42. Bolliger CT. Pre-operative assessment of the lung cancer patient. *S Afr Med J* 2001;**91**:120-3.
43. Smetana GW. Preoperative pulmonary assessment of the older adult. *Clin Geriatr Med* 2003;**19**:35-55.
44. Ferguson MK, Durkin AE. A comparison of three scoring systems for predicting complications after major lung resection. *Eur J Cardiothorac Surg* 2003;**23**: 35-42.
45. McKenna RJ Jr, Fischel RJ, Brenner M, Gelb AF. Combined operations for lung volume reduction surgery and lung cancer. *Chest* 1996;**110**:885-8.
46. Allen GM, DeRose JJ Jr. Pulmonary nodule resection during lung volume reduction surgery. *AORN J* 1997;**66**:808-10, 12, 14 passim.
47. Mentzer SJ, Swanson SJ. Treatment of patients with lung cancer and severe emphysema. *Chest* 1999;**116**:477S-9S.
48. Pompeo E, De Dominicis E, Ambrogi V, Mineo D, Elia S, Mineo TC. Quality of life after tailored combined surgery for stage I non-small-cell lung cancer and severe emphysema. *Ann Thorac Surg* 2003;**76**:1821-7.

CHAPTER 4
Perioperative Care of the Thoracic Surgical Patient
Elisabeth U. Dexter

Preoperative Preparation
  Prophylaxis
    Atrial Fibrillation
    Deep Venous Thrombosis
    Stress Ulceration and Gastritis
    Infection
  Miscellaneous
Intraoperative Care
  Ventilation
  Monitoring
  Body Temperature

Positioning
Fluid Administration
Drainage
Specimen Management
Postoperative Care
  Fluid Management
  Blood Administration
  Medications
  Analgesia
  Nutrition
  Respiratory Therapy

Wound Care
Management of Drainage Tubes
Physical Therapy
Management of Complications
  Early Complications
  Late Complications
  Complications after Esophageal Surgery
  Miscellaneous
Discharge Planning

Thoracic surgical patients require careful attention in the perioperative period. Often these are older patients who have baseline abnormalities of lung function, decreased nutritional status, and other comorbid diseases. Postoperatively, factors that influence patient recovery include removal of all or a portion of a lung, painful incisions, retention of secretions, change in the shape and mechanics of the thoracic cage, and reconfiguration of gastrointestinal continuity, which result in suboptimal pulmonary function, decreased appetite, decreased mobility and strength, and increased risk of aspiration.

Perioperative care of the thoracic surgical patient requires a team approach. The surgeon is uniquely qualified to be the captain of the team because he or she is aware of the patient's functional status preoperatively, the operative findings and events, and the postoperative anatomy that will dictate each patient's needs and restrictions. Members of the team include the surgeon, anesthesiologist, pain management specialist, nurse, respiratory therapist, physical therapist, occupational therapist, speech pathologist, dietician, and social worker.

PREOPERATIVE PREPARATION

An in-depth review of preoperative assessment is covered in Chapter 3. Medical optimization for thoracotomy patients includes adjustment of medications for chronic obstructive pulmonary disease (COPD), including administration of bronchodilators and steroids and treatment of acute bronchitis or pneumonia.[1] Total resolution may not be possible if the pneumonia is caused by a postobstructive process secondary to lung mass or chronic aspiration from gastroesophageal reflux disease.

Patients with borderline pulmonary function benefit from pulmonary rehabilitation that increases their exercise tolerance and respiratory muscular strength before the resection.[2] Preoperative pulmonary rehabilitation should be a routine component for all patients undergoing lung volume reduction surgery.[3,4] Smoking cessation is of great importance. Support groups, counseling, nicotine replacement therapy, and Wellbutrin therapy are available and successful.[5] If there is no smoking cessation program associated with the provider's hospital, programs can be located by calling the local American Lung Association. Timing of smoking cessation before the operation remains debatable. Vaporciyan and colleagues showed that patients who quit smoking 4 weeks or more before surgery had a lower incidence of pulmonary complications than patients who continued to smoke or quit fewer than 4 weeks before pneumonectomy.[6] Historically, 6 weeks of smoking cessation before surgery is recommended to avoid the copious bronchorrhea that accompanies regeneration of the cilia that clear mucus between 2 and 4 weeks after smoking cessation.[7] However, Barrera and coworkers found no difference in the incidence of pulmonary complications between patients who were still smoking at the time of surgery and those who had quit fewer than 2 months before thoracotomy for lung resection.[8] Our current recommendation is that all smokers requiring lung resection should be encouraged to quit smoking, and assisted to do so, at any time period before surgery.

Additional comorbid diseases that need to be managed include coronary artery disease, diabetes mellitus, and myasthenia gravis.[1,9] The American Heart Association and the American College of Cardiology classify thoracic surgical procedures as medium risk. When there is no clinical history of risk factors for cardiac disease, no further workup is necessary if a preoperative 12-lead electrocardiogram (ECG) is normal.[10] If a patient has risk factors for cardiac disease, further testing should be done to assess the presence and degree of disease. However, revascularization for significant coronary stenosis may not be preferable to medical therapy such as β-blocker administration for preventing perioperative cardiac events.[11]

Diabetic patients should have their cardiac, renal/intravascular volume, and glucose status checked before elective surgery.[12] Electrolytes should be checked preoperatively and abnormalities treated. Baseline creatinine measurement is helpful. Acute elevation in creatinine needs to be investigated before elective thoracic surgery. Orthostatic vital signs should be also performed.

Diabetic patients optimally should have good glycemic control preoperatively. Long-acting sulfonylureas should be discontinued 48 to 72 hours before elective surgery. Shorter-acting sulfonylureas or secretagogues such as metformin can be stopped 12 hours before surgery. Long-acting insulin can be continued until the day of surgery if control has been good. If there is glucose level fluctuation, long-acting insulin should be stopped 24 to 48 hours before surgery, and sliding-scale insulin should be used with frequent glucose checks.[12]

For patients with myasthenia gravis, the goal of preoperative preparation is to reduce the risk of myasthenic crisis, which is acute respiratory muscle malfunction leading to respiratory failure. Dosages of steroids and anticholinesterase medication should be tailored to the patient's symptoms. More aggressive and rapid therapies include infusion of intravenous immune globulin and plasmapheresis.[9,13] Plasmapheresis usually requires multiple exchanges and is recommended for patients with a vital capacity of less than 2.0 L.

Prophylaxis

Atrial Fibrillation

The incidence of postoperative atrial fibrillation ranges between 3% and 30% in thoracic surgical patients.[14] It increases the risk of stroke and prolongs postoperative length of stay, thus increasing hospital cost and mortality rate.[14,15] The only consistent risk factor in surgical patients is age greater than 60 years.[16] A retrospective review of over 2900 patients revealed increased relative risks of atrial fibrillation of 3.89, 7.16, 8.91, and 2.95 for lobectomy, bi-lobectomy, pneumonectomy, and esophagectomy, respectively, compared with a single wedge resection.[14] Numerous studies on the prevention and treatment of postoperative atrial fibrillation have been done, but the majority were performed for cardiac surgical patients. There are currently no compelling data to recommend routine prophylaxis of atrial fibrillation in thoracic surgical patients.[17] Meta-analysis shows that β-blocker, D-sotalol, and amiodarone are all effective in lowering the incidence of postoperative atrial fibrillation in cardiac surgical patients. Only amiodarone had a significant decrease in length of stay (by 0.9 days).[18] However, there have been reports of acute pulmonary toxicity from amiodarone therapy in postoperative cardiothoracic surgery patients. No randomized trial has been done to study this phenomenon.[19] Digoxin has been tried for prophylaxis but is not effective.[17] Intravenous diltiazem was studied specifically in thoracic surgical patients and almost halved the incidence of postoperative atrial fibrillation (15% versus 25% for placebo patients).[16] Studies of magnesium for prophylaxis and therapy of postoperative atrial fibrillation showed mixed results.[17]

For atrial fibrillation with rapid ventricular response, rate control is the main priority. Conversion back to normal sinus rhythm is a secondary but not an immediate goal. Prophylaxis of atrial fibrillation with beta-blocker or calcium channel blocker should be considered for patients older than 60 years.

Box 4–1
Risk Factors for Venous Thromboembolism

- Surgery
- Trauma (major or lower extremity)
- Immobility, paresis
- Malignancy
- Cancer therapy (hormonal, chemotherapy, or radiotherapy)
- Previous venous thromboembolism
- Increasing age
- Pregnancy and the postpartum period
- Estrogen-containing oral contraception or hormone replacement therapy
- Selective estrogen receptor modulators
- Acute medical illness
- Heart or respiratory failure
- Inflammatory bowel disease
- Nephrotic syndrome
- Myeloproliferative disorders
- Paroxysmal nocturnal hemoglobinuria
- Obesity
- Smoking
- Varicose veins
- Central venous catheterization
- Inherited or acquired thrombophilia

Reprinted with permission from Geerts WH, Heit JA, Clagett GP, et al. Chest 2001;119(1 Suppl): 132-75S.

Deep Venous Thrombosis

Postoperatively, a majority of thoracic surgery patients are slow to move because of pain, respiratory distress, and age. A review of multiple studies estimated a 10% to 30% incidence of deep venous thrombosis in patients in medical and surgical intensive care units.[20] The current recommendations for deep venous thrombosis prophylaxis from the American College of Chest Physicians vary depending on patient risk (Box 4-1 and Table 4-1).[21] Low-dose unfractionated heparin (LDUH) use does not interfere with epidural catheter placement or removal. However, low-molecular-weight heparin (LMWH) should be held for 12 to 24 hours before epidural placement or removal, to decrease the risk of hematoma formation. Use of LMWH for 2 to 3 weeks after hospital discharge in patients undergoing major cancer surgery may reduce the incidence of asymptomatic deep venous thrombosis.[21]

Stress Ulceration and Gastritis

Stress ulceration prophylaxis is recommended in critically ill patients with coagulopathy, expected mechanical ventilation for longer than 48 hours, history of gastrointestinal bleeding or gastric ulceration in the past year, and at least two of the following: sepsis, intensive care unit stay of greater than 1 week, high-dose steroid administration, or occult bleeding lasting 6 or more days.[22] The incidence of clinically significant bleeding remains low with use of pharmacologic agents for prophylaxis. Several strategies can be used for stress ulcer

Table 4-1
Levels of Thromboembolism Risk in Surgical Patients without Prophylaxis

Level of risk	Successful prevention strategies
Low risk • Minor surgery in patients <40 yr with no additional risk factors	No specific prophylaxis; early and aggressive mobilization
Moderate risk • Minor surgery in patients with additional risk factors • Surgery in patients aged 40–60 yr with no additional risk factors	LDUH (5000 units q12h), LMWH (≤3400 U daily), GCS, or IPC
High risk • Surgery in patients >60 yr, or age 40–60 with additional risk factors (prior VTE, cancer, molecular hypercoagulability)	LDUH (5000 U q8h), LMWH (>3400 U daily), or IPC
Highest risk • Surgery in patients with multiple risk factors (age >40 yr, cancer, prior VTE) • Hip or knee arthroplasty, hip fracture surgery • Major trauma; spinal cord injury	LMWH (>3400 U daily), fondaparinux, oral vitamin K antagonists (INR, 2–3), or IPC/GCS + LDUH/LMWH

GCS, graduated pneumatic compression stockings; INR, international normalized ratio; IPC, intermittent pneumatic compression; LDUH, low-dose unfractionated heparin; LMWH, low-molecular-weight heparin; VTE, venous thromboembolism.
Reprinted with permission from Geerts WH, Heit JA, Clagett GP, et al. Chest 2001;*119*(1 Suppl):132-75S.

prophylaxis. Sucralfate decreases the risk of nosocomial pneumonia compared with the other agents.[23] There is no intravenous formulation of sucralfate, so it can be given only to patients who can have oral or intragastric medications, and it must be given four times a day.[22] There is an increased risk of aluminum toxicity if sucralfate is used for longer than 2 weeks in patients with renal insufficiency.[24] Both histamine-2 (H_2) blockers and proton pump inhibitors are effective in lowering gastric pH.[25] H_2 blockers interfere with the metabolism of medications that pass through the cytochrome P450 pathway, and dosages of other medications may need to be adjusted.[26] Eating, or, if that is not possible, enteral feeding, is also helpful for prevention of stress ulcers postoperatively.

Infection

A properly timed dose of intravenous first-generation cephalosporin is efficacious in preventing wound infections from skin pathogens.[27] For patients with β-lactam allergy, vancomycin or intravenous clindamycin are the substitutes of choice. Vancomycin administration must be started early enough to ensure that the dose is completely infused before incision is made. The prophylactic antibiotic is continued for one to two doses postoperatively. No data have supported the use of antibiotic beyond 24 hours for wound prophylaxis.

Prophylaxis for pneumonia and empyema in patients undergoing lung resection or esophageal resection is an attractive concept, as these involve clean-contaminated operative fields. Postoperative pneumonia was found in approximately 25% of patients undergoing lung resection in two different studies.[28,29] Radu and colleagues demonstrated that only 18% of the pathogens postoperatively isolated from patients with pneumonia were susceptible to first-generation cephalosporin.[28] They recommend consideration of use of prophylactic antibiotic to cover both gram-positive and gram-negative organisms.

Unfortunately, no clear data support this practice. The Surgical Care Improvement Project (SCIP)[30] is a national program sponsored by the Center for Medicare and Medicaid Services along with other health organizations (American Hospital Association, Centers for Disease Control and Prevention) to decrease the number of surgical complications. Randomized trials showing an improved outcome with use of antibiotics effective on gram-negative organisms are needed for surgeons in the United States to justify their practice. SCIP participation delineates the timing of prophylactic antibiotic administration (within 1 hour of surgical incision), the type of antibiotic (first-generation cephalosporin with exceptions for medical reasons), and the duration of prophylactic antibiotic administration (limited to 24 hours or less for all surgeries except cardiac surgery; for cardiac surgery, 48 hours).

If a patient is receiving antibiotic for a therapeutic reason, prophylactic antibiotic use does not apply.[30]

Miscellaneous

Blood products are reserved for patients who have anemia because of preoperative chemotherapy, chronic disease, phlebotomy, or bleeding. Patients having elective major thoracic surgery should be given the option of autologous blood donation, which results in decreased risks of infection, transfusion reaction, and immune modulation, and increased cost effectiveness.[31-33] Careful screening must be done to ensure there is no contraindication and there is adequate time to alleviate the iatrogenic anemia caused by autologous blood donation.[31,32] Use of erythropoietic agents has been effective in eliminating or decreasing the amount of anemia in patients with cancer who have received chemotherapy or radiation therapy. Although preoperative or postoperative use of erythropoietin or darbepoetin is an attractive idea for thoracic oncology patients, no data exist to support this practice. In addition, there are reports of increased risk of deep venous thrombosis in oncology patients given erythropoietic agents for anemia.[34]

Bowel preparation may be desired before complicated gastroesophageal operations during which colon interposition may be needed.

Warfarin therapy for patients with prosthetic heart valves should be stopped 72 hours before surgery, and intravenous unfractionated heparin should be started when the international normalized ratio (INR) is less than 2.0 for patients at high risk of thromboembolic incidents. Patients at high risk include those with mechanical heart valves in the mitral position and those with three of the following: atrial fibrillation, left ventricular dysfunction, previous thromboembolism, hypercoagulable condition, and mechanical prosthesis. For patients with prosthetic heart valves and low risk of thromboembolic incident, and for those with arrhythmia or low ejection fraction on anticoagulation, no bridge therapy is recommended.[35]

Surgery should never be delayed because of the unavailability of equipment. Hospitals often have equipment (laparoscopes/thoracoscopes, video equipment, lasers, vessel sealing devices, ultrasonic devices, radiofrequency devices, cryoablation equipment, robots, specialized retractors) that is used by several different services. Such equipment should be reserved before the surgery to ensure that it is available and functioning properly.

INTRAOPERATIVE CARE

Good communication with the anesthesiologist or anesthetist is essential. Airway management should be discussed beforehand if there are special circumstances. The entire operative team should know the plan of the operation including (1) position and position changes, (2) instrument, equipment, and medication needs (e.g., vessel sealing devices, drainage tubes, local anesthetic), (3) general length of the operation, and (4) postoperative disposition (e.g., extubation versus postoperative ventilation, ward versus intensive care).

Ventilation

Single-lung ventilation during thoracotomy or thoracoscopy is accomplished by placing a double-lumen tube, bronchial blocker, Univent tube, or, as a last resort, a single-lumen tube down the desired main-stem bronchus.[36] Use of lower intraoperative tidal volumes during single-lung ventilation has been shown to decrease the incidence of respiratory failure in pneumonectomy patients.[37] Increased peak inspiratory pressure, decreased oxygen saturation, and increased end-tidal CO_2 during the procedure without a known etiology from the surgical field lead to a differential diagnosis of retained secretions or blood, dislodgement of the endotracheal tube or blocker, or contralateral pneumothorax. Stabilization may require reinflation of the operative-side lung if increased fraction of inspired O_2 (FIO_2) administration and oxygen flow and gentle bagging by the anesthesiologist do not improve the situation. Investigations and treatments include suctioning of obstructing blood or mucus, bronchoscopy and repositioning of single-lung ventilation equipment, or decompression of the contralateral pleural space of air.

Monitoring

Different operations require different levels of monitoring.[1] ECG monitoring and continuous pulse oximetry are necessary in all cases. An arterial line is placed if there is a need for multiple blood samples. Continuous arterial pressure monitoring is useful during procedures involving mediastinal dissection, such as transhiatal esophagectomy, to gauge cardiac or great vessel compression. Temperature monitoring by bladder temperature probe or esophageal temperature probe is necessary for major procedures (see Body Temperature, next).

Intravenous access should be appropriate for the invasiveness and potential blood loss of the procedure. Anticipated blood loss is rarely enough to justify the need for large-bore central lines. However, adequate access is necessary before the procedure starts, because the arms, chest, and groin are often inaccessible for line placement during an operation done in the decubitus or prone position. In emergency situations, a large-bore line can be placed in the operative field via the subclavian vein, superior vena cava, inferior vena cava, or azygous vein.

Body Temperature

Mild hypothermia has been shown to increase wound infection, blood loss and transfusion requirements, and cardiac events including ventricular tachycardia, cardiac arrest, and myocardial infarction.[38] Heat loss through thoracotomy, sternotomy, and laparotomy incisions can be lessened by keeping the room temperature greater than 21° C, using airway heating and humidification devices, covering portions of the patient not in the operative field, and using forced-air warming blankets. Warm saline lavage intrapleurally and intraperitoneally can also be performed. Rarely are intravenous fluid warmers needed.

Positioning

Careful positioning of the patient is of utmost importance in the operating room. The surgeon needs to ensure adequate access for the planned operation as well as any potential counterincisions or chest wall resection. Use of muscle flaps often requires planning ahead to protect the vascular supply and leave adequate skin coverage. Padding to prevent neuropathy includes the use of an axillary roll for the decubitus position and padding of both arms. Stability of the patient during the operation can be achieved using a deflatable beanbag, sand bags, laminectomy rolls, and security straps or tapes. The lithotomy position also requires careful positioning to prevent postoperative neuropathy.[39]

Fluid Administration

Fluid administration during pulmonary resection is kept to a minimum. If pneumonectomy is planned, administration of 1 L of fluid during the intraoperative course has been advocated. During esophagectomy, more fluid administration may be needed because of increased blood loss and third spacing. Clear communication between surgeon and anesthesiologist regarding blood loss, hemodynamic trends, and pressor and fluid administration during the operation is crucial.

Drainage

If the planned operation is scheduled to take longer than 3 hours or if an epidural catheter is used, a bladder catheter should be placed. Orogastric or nasogastric tube drainage, or both, are important for decompression during esophageal and gastric operations. The semirigid tube can be helpful for localization during reoperation or within radiated fields with abundant scar tissue or fibrous reaction.

The viscosity of the substance being drained dictates the size and shape necessary for adequate drainage of the pleural space. Smaller anterior tubes are used to drain air. Larger posterior tubes, including preformed 90-degree-angle tubes, are useful for dependent drainage of blood, pus, chyle, or exudative fluid along the diaphragm. One pleural tube is adequate for drainage after routine lobar resection if it is positioned posterior to and to the apex of the pleural cavity to drain both fluid and air. If significant disruption of lung parenchyma is known or suspected, use of more than one pleural drainage tube is prudent to prevent formation of subcutaneous emphysema and improve the chance of pleural opposition.[40] Additional chest tubes are used for empyema or hemothorax drainage or fistula drainage.

Use of a drainage tube after pneumonectomy is controversial. Reasons cited for leaving a chest tube after pneumonectomy include ability to monitor bleeding, manipulate intrapleural pressure, and adjust mediastinal shifting by instilling or removing air. The chest tube is removed intraoperatively after the patient is placed supine, in the recovery room, or on the first postoperative day. Many surgeons leave no drainage tube after pneumonectomy and encounter no increased morbidity. It is our recommendation that no drainage tube be left after pneumonectomy unless bleeding is a significant concern. We question the sterility and advisability of adding or removing air from the postpneumonectomy pleural space.

A gastrostomy tube is useful if prolonged stomach drainage is needed. This may decrease the risk of aspiration that is theoretically present from having a tube traversing and stenting the upper esophagus or neo-esophageal conduit open. A gastrostomy tube is more comfortable for the patient than an indwelling nasoenteral tube. A jejunostomy tube is placed as access for nutrition and medicine administration if failure to thrive or a prolonged period of receiving nothing by mouth (NPO status) is anticipated.

If flaps are created, drains to prevent seroma formation are placed. If there is concern of leakage of the gastrointestinal tract, bronchopleural fistula, empyema, or chylothorax, good drainage can prevent systemic infection and allow nutritional support and time for healing.

Specimen Management

The surgeon must also ensure that sample and specimen collection is done properly. Careful labeling and delivery of frozen sections are of paramount importance in determining resection margins, resectability, and staging. Intraoperative communication with the pathologist performing frozen section may be necessary before proceeding with the next portion of an operation. If possible, orienting the specimen and viewing the frozen section with the pathologist are recommended. A recent retrospective subset analysis of the data from the American College of Surgeons Oncology Group Z0060 trial of esophageal resection revealed that more accurate accounting and assignment of lymph node station occurs when surgeons separate and label lymph nodes for analysis than when the pathologist dissects, counts, and labels the nodes.[41] Cultures for bacterial, fungal, and acid-fast bacilli need to be processed and collected in the correct specimen containers/mediums.

POSTOPERATIVE CARE

As in many other specialties, clinical pathways serve to improve the quality of care, and they have the added benefit of reducing cost.[42] Almost all thoracic surgical patients can be transferred from the recovery room to a stepdown unit or surgical ward instead of to an intensive care unit. For thymectomy, segmentectomy, lobectomy, pneumonectomy, lung volume reduction, and esophagectomy patients, telemetry and continuous pulse oximetry are recommended. The arterial line placed during surgery is transduced until the day after surgery.

Fluid Management

Fluid administration for lung resection patients must be determined on an individual basis. Vasodilation secondary to use of local anesthetic in epidural catheters, and the use of antihypertensive medications justify careful administration of fluid to maintain blood pressure and adequate end-organ perfusion. In a review of published reports of postoperative pulmonary edema, Slinger found that multiple factors were probably contributors to the formation of the edema.[43] The review gives guidelines regarding postoperative fluid management: (1) a maximum of 20 mL/kg fluid to be given intravenously for the first 24 postoperative hours, (2) acceptance of average urine output of 0.5 mL/kg/hr the first 24 hours, and (3) use of vasopressors if tissue perfusion is inadequate and the 20 mL/kg maximum of fluid has already been administered. Other manipulations such as lowering the dose of the epidural infusion or removing the local anesthetic component of the epidural infusion and leaving only narcotic may decrease sympathetic blockade and vascular vasodilation. There are no randomized trials that show a benefit of colloid administration versus crystalloid administration for fluid boluses.[44]

Blood Administration

No hemoglobin level or hematocrit has been documented as being a threshold for recommending transfusion. In critically ill patients with cardiovascular disease, a hemoglobin level of 7.0 to 9.0 g/dL is well tolerated.[45] Although intuition argues that a higher hemoglobin level provides better oxygen delivery, the increased oxygen extraction by most organs and tissues when stressed negates the need for a higher hemoglobin level. This is not true for the heart, which extracts most of the oxygen delivered under nonstressed physiologic conditions and requires increases in blood flow to increase oxygen delivery with physiologic stress. For critically ill patients with acute cardiac ischemia, increased mortality was found with a restrictive transfusion protocol.[46]

Medications

Each patient's preoperative medications should be reviewed before restarting them postoperatively. Often, antihypertensive medications need to be held for several doses until fluid shifting and equilibrium are attained to prevent continued hypotension. We recommend restarting beta-blocker therapy as soon as possible after the operation to prevent rebound tachycardia from withdrawal. This also decreases the occurrence of atrial fibrillation and of rapid ventricular response should postoperative atrial fibrillation occur.

Administration of postoperative antibiotics for more than 48 hours has not been definitively proven to decrease the amount of pneumonia or wound infection in thoracic surgical patients.[47] SCIP (see Infection, earlier) protocol requires use of a first-generation cephalosporin (unless the patient is allergic) for 24 hours or less for wound prophylaxis. Treatment of known infection precludes following SCIP protocol.[30]

Many patients suffer from nausea after general anesthesia or postoperative pain medications. Antiemetics such as metoclopramide, ondansetron, promethazine, trimethobenzamide, and prochlorperazine can help. Stress ulcer prophylaxis is now recommended for high-risk surgical patients only (see Stress Ulceration and Gastritis, earlier).[22] Esophagectomy patients have a high risk of reflux.[48-50] H_2-receptor blockers or proton pump inhibitors should be continued in patients who demonstrate reflux on barium swallow tests postoperatively, have symptoms of heartburn, or have a history of Barrett's disease. Vagotomized patients may benefit from the prokinetic effects of erythromycin or metoclopramide. However, erythromycin may cause gastrointestinal upset and metoclopramide can produce extrapyramidal symptoms. Use of low-molecular-weight heparin, low-dose unfractionated heparin, or sequential compression devices continues until the patient is reliably walking at least four times a day for patients with a low risk for deep venous thrombosis. For higher-risk patients, a combination of pharmacologic and mechanical prophylaxis should be used until the same ambulatory criteria are met (see Box 4-1 and Table 4-1).[21] The constipating effects of narcotic medications and decreased motility indicate the need for a bowel management protocol.

Analgesia

Pain control is one of the most important aspects of postoperative care for thoracic surgery patients, and the amount of literature on this subject is beyond the scope of this chapter. Studies have shown the benefit of continuous and patient-controlled epidural analgesia on pain control and the potential benefit to pulmonary function after thoracotomy.[51-53] A meta-analysis of paravertebral block versus epidural analgesia showed no difference in pain control between the methods. However, the incidence of failed block, hypotension, nausea and vomiting, and pulmonary complication was less with paravertebral block.[54]

Intravenous patient-controlled analgesia (PCA) is also effective for post-thoracotomy and laparotomy pain.[55] Supplementation of intravenous PCA narcotic with additional intravenous medication or electroacupuncture (acupuncture with an alternating current of 60 Hz applied to the needle for 30 min/session) has been suggested.[56,57] Nonsteroidal anti-inflammatory agents such as ketorolac have been effective adjuncts with either epidural or intravenous PCA.[58-60] Other methods of pain relief that have mixed reports and small study sizes include intercostal blocks,[61,62] phrenic nerve infiltration,[63] transcutaneous electrical nerve stimulation,[64] intrapleural or extrapleural nerve block,[62] and cryoanalgesia of the intercostal nerves.[65-67]

The increased use of minimally invasive surgery has resulted in an expectation that amount, duration, and invasiveness of postoperative analgesia will decrease. No multicenter randomized trials have produced data to support this hypothesis, although single-center case series have.[68-70]

Nutrition

Adequate nutrition is of paramount importance in the postoperative period.[71,72] Most lung resection patients can be started on clear liquids or a regular diet the evening of surgery. A more cautious approach may be necessary if there is concern about a difficult airway or a higher risk of respiratory failure. Nausea and vomiting are fairly common after general anesthesia, and narcotic medications may magnify the problem. If liquids are tolerated, the patient's diet can be advanced starting the day after surgery. After uneventful laparoscopic fundoplication, clear liquids can be given the evening of surgery. These patients need to be counseled preoperatively and postoperatively about taking most of their fluid between meals, eating smaller portions more frequently during the day, and avoiding foods such as dry bread, raw vegetables, large chunks of meat, and foods and fluids that increase gas production in the immediate postoperative period. Providing patients at discharge with a list of eating tips and foods to avoid is recommended. Dysphagia due to swelling of a complete fundoplication may occur after the operation. This can lead to inability to advance the diet beyond liquids for several days or weeks.[73] If this persists past several weeks and the patient is losing weight, the need for dilation or investigation for a complication such as a slipped wrap, stricture, or previously undiagnosed motility disorder must be considered.[74]

Oral intake after esophagectomy is started after a confirmatory test for leakage and blockage, such as a barium swallow test or grape juice test, is passed.[50,75] Most surgeons wait 5 to 7 days postoperatively.[76,77] Surgeon preference, problems encountered during the operation, and neoadjuvant therapy influence when the study is obtained, although recent data showed no evidence of increased anastomotic leakage when neoadjuvant treatment was given.[78] If the test results are favorable, clear liquids are started and the diet is advanced as tolerated. The patient is counseled about expected changes in eating habits, dietary intake, jejunostomy tube feeding, and weight stabilization. Placement of a jejunostomy tube during esophagectomy allows enteral feeding 24 to 48 hours after operation. Tube feedings are generally started at a low rate, such as 20 mL/hr, and advanced to a goal rate to provide total caloric and protein needs over the next 48 hours. If a jejunostomy tube is not placed, total parenteral nutrition administration until oral intake is tolerated can be considered.

Respiratory Therapy

The most common complications after thoracic surgery are related to the pulmonary system. Vigilant postoperative pulmonary care decreases the incidence of complications.[76,79] Incentive spirometry and chest physiotherapy, including clapping, postural drainage, and vibratory therapy, aid in mobilizing mucous secretions and allowing patients to clear their own secretions. Cough can be stimulated and secretions suctioned by placing a soft suction catheter through the nose and into the trachea. Studies have advocated placement of a mini-tracheostomy in high-risk patients and have shown favorable results in reducing pulmonary complications.[80] Ambulation is an excellent method of decreasing atelectasis. Nebulized albuterol is very helpful in curtailing or preventing bronchospastic episodes. If a patient has had multiple manipulations of the upper airway and there is concern about edema and stridor, intravenous and aerosolized steroids and aerosolized racemic epinephrine are effective in reducing edema.

Wound Care

Incision care is usually routine if the skin is closed. Open wounds historically are packed with gauze moistened with saline, dilute antibiotic solution, sodium hypochlorite (Dakin's) solution, acetic acid solution, or dilute Betadine solution. Newer dressings, including silicone-impregnated dressings, thin polyurethane films, hydrocolloids, alginates, polyurethane foams, and hydrogels, are available, although there are no strong data to recommend the use of one over the other or gauze.[81] Vacuum dressings can be placed in clean wounds and can speed the healing process.[82] Open chests for bronchopleural fistula are packed with gauze soaked in antibiotic solution until a decision is made about definitive closure.[83-85] If muscle or skin flaps are raised and there is the potential for seroma formation, drains may be left and binders or ace bandages can be considered. Depending on the muscle rotation used and the tautness of the closure, restriction of range of motion may be required for several days to prevent tension and dislodgement or compromise of flap vascular supply.

When tracheal resection with primary anastomosis with release procedures are done, a sturdy skin stitch from the chin to the anterior chest will remind the patient to keep the head neutral or mildly flexed to allow healing of the tracheal anastomosis with less tension.[86] For wounds that are difficult to heal, such as those in previous radiation fields, hyperbaric oxygen therapy can be considered.[87] A minimal oxygen concentration must be achieved for any benefit of this cumbersome and costly wound care alternative. No randomized, blinded studies have shown definite benefit of hyperbaric oxygen therapy for wound healing except for osteoradionecrosis.

Management of Drainage Tubes

Placement and removal of chest tubes should be standardized by protocol after lung resection. Tubes are left in as long as any air leak remains, but recent studies indicate that earlier transition from water suction to water seal is not harmful and promotes quicker resolution of parenchymal air leakage.[88-90] Fluid drainage of 300 to 400 mL or less per 24 hours is acceptable for chest tube removal after lung resection.[88] Chest tube removal after pleurodesis for malignant pleural effusion has a stricter volume requirement, as these patients are known to have problems absorbing pleural fluid normally. Chest tube removal after drainage of chylothorax or empyema must be tailored to the particular patient's course. When there is any concern about anastomotic leak in the chest or mediastinum after esophageal resection or tracheal reconstruction, tubes should be left until resolution of the leakage. Mediastinal tubes are left after median sternotomy is performed for removal of bilateral lung tumors, lung reduction surgery, or mediastinal mass resection.

A nasogastric tube is left after esophagectomy and for complicated benign esophageal operations. The tube is removed when drainage from the gastrointestinal tract is less that 300 to 500 mL/24 hr and there is no concern of anastomotic leak.

Bladder catheters are placed for drainage and as a measure of adequate end-organ perfusion in patients having operations longer than 3 hours. Patients, especially older men, who have an epidural catheter often have difficulty voiding and usually require the indwelling bladder catheter until the epidural is discontinued.

Physical Therapy

Exercise therapy after lung resection benefits patients by decreasing pulmonary complications, restoring mobility and independence, and decreasing the potential for deep venous thrombosis. Pulmonary rehabilitation is designed specifically to help patients clear secretions, strengthen respiratory muscles, and provide cardiopulmonary exercise.[2-4] A patient who requires continuous chest tube suction can exercise on a stationary bicycle in the hospital room.

Management of Complications

Early Complications

Respiratory Failure

Atelectasis/Pneumonia
The most common complication after a thoracic operation is respiratory failure. When complications are the result of atelectasis and retained secretions, treatment with aggressive pulmonary toilet, postural drainage, incentive spirometry, nasotracheal suction, ambulation, and a nebulizer will help avoid development of pneumonia. If pneumonia is suspected (fever, elevated and rising white blood cell count, purulent sputum production, no other source of infection), empiric treatment with a second-generation cephalosporin is justified, as radiographic changes of pneumonia may lag temporally.[91] Ferdinand and Shennib[91] advocate using bronchoscopy with lavage or protected brush for diagnosis of post-thoracotomy pneumonia. Antibiotic therapy can be adjusted after culture results return. The worsening spiral of need for intubation can sometimes be avoided with bronchoscopy to remove thick tenacious secretions or retained clot. The benefits of minitracheostomy have already been mentioned.[80]

Pulmonary Edema
Pulmonary edema in lobectomy patients is serious but can usually be treated with diuresis. Postpneumonectomy pulmonary edema may be fatal. Aggressive respiratory care including intubation may be necessary to manage a patient with postpneumonectomy pulmonary edema, which has a mortality rate of greater than 50%.[43] Postpneumonectomy pulmonary edema should always be considered, and avoidance of excessive fluid administration is important.[37,43,92] Other maneuvers during surgery that have been recommended to avoid postpneumonectomy pulmonary edema include using tidal volumes of only 5 to 6 mL/kg to avoid barotrauma or volutrauma to the inflated lung,[37,93] avoidance of fresh-frozen plasma transfusion,[94] and administration of steroids,[95] although data are mainly from single-institution case series and retrospective studies. Although disruption

of the lymphatic drainage resulting from lymphadenectomy has previously been implicated as a causative factor, data from the American College of Surgeons Oncology Group Z0030 trial did not support this finding.[96] Controversy still exists about whether the side of the pneumonectomy affects the risk of postpneumonectomy pulmonary edema, and whether induction chemotherapy or chemoradiotherapy increases that risk.[92-94,96-99]

Urine output should be accepted at 0.5 mL/kg/hr the night of surgery, and excess fluid administration should be avoided. Measures to keep pulmonary artery pressures low should be instituted. The patient should be given adequate FIO_2, and hypercarbia, pain that causes splinting, and atelectasis need to be avoided.[43] Routine administration of diuretic starting in the recovery room can be considered.

Acute Respiratory Distress Syndrome

Acute lung injury and acute respiratory distress syndrome (ARDS) are rare but potentially fatal complications after thoracic surgery; the reported frequency of each is 2% to 4%.[100-102] Aggressive support with reintubation if necessary and administration of positive end-expiratory pressure and adequate FIO_2 to support the patient while the lung recovers is important. No medication has been proven to improve the outcome of ARDS. Steroids can be tried for a short course.[103] Prone position, nitric oxide, and high-frequency oscillating ventilation improve arterial oxygenation, but no randomized controlled studies have been performed that show increased survival with these treatments.[104-106] Other therapies reported include prostaglandins, extracorporeal membrane oxygenation, and liquid ventilation.[104] Treatment of underlying pneumonia is necessary. Careful attention to other organ systems and nutritional support give the patient's lungs time to recover. The mortality rate for ARDS with no other organ system affected remains at 50% to 64%.[100,101]

If a patient displays signs of hypoxia and the etiologies just mentioned are not the cause, pulmonary embolism, myocardial ischemia, arrhythmia, and heart failure need to be investigated.

Cardiac Complications

Myocardial Infarction

Myocardial infarction should be treated with oxygen therapy, ECG monitoring, morphine, and aspirin if bleeding is not a great concern.[107,108] Inotropic or pressor support may be needed in the immediate postoperative period. If the patient's blood pressure cannot be adequately supported with medications, intra-aortic balloon pump placement should be considered. Patients with continuing ischemia and hemodynamic instability should be taken for cardiac catheterization to delineate significant stenosis and should undergo catheter-based therapy if indicated. Anticoagulants such as heparin or GIIb/IIIa platelet inhibitors, or both, are recommended for unstable angina, but recent surgery and risk of bleeding may preclude their use. Patients older than 75 years also benefit from early revascularization but have a higher risk of bleeding complications.[107-109] The surgeon must exercise judgment regarding the risks and benefits of these drug interventions after surgery. Arrhythmias should be treated according to advanced cardiac life support protocol if the patient is hemodynamically unstable.[110]

Atrial Fibrillation

The immediate goal of treatment of postoperative atrial fibrillation is rate control with beta-blocker or calcium channel blocker.[111] When atrial fibrillation occurs while a patient is on beta-blocker, D-sotalol, amiodarone, magnesium, or diltiazem prophylaxis, ventricular response rate is significantly lower than that with placebo.[16-18] If the patient is on one of these agents and continues to have a rapid ventricular response with hypotension, combination therapy or cardioversion, or both, may be necessary. Careful monitoring of the ECG is necessary if drug combinations are used. The shortest-acting beta-blocker available is esmolol. It requires a loading dose and administration by continuous infusion because of its short half-life. It is more costly than other beta-blockers, but it can more easily be titrated, and, should the patient develop hemodynamic instability, its effects dissipate quickly when discontinued. Digoxin can be given for rate control, but a load must be given in multiple doses over several hours to achieve an adequate serum level. It is inexpensive and has no negative inotropic or vasodilating effects. Of the calcium channel blockers, diltiazem has become favored for rate control of atrial fibrillation because it causes less vasodilation leading to hypotension.

Amiodarone has a long half-life and variable solubility and uptake when given orally. Onset of action is about 0.5 to 3 hours after an intravenous load. Oral loading can be done if started preoperatively. Magnesium is poorly absorbed orally and is usually given intravenously perioperatively. Sotalol can be given orally or intravenously for atrial fibrillation. The D-enantiomer works as a class III agent, not as a β-blocker. If preoperative time allows, all of the oral agents are safe to start before the patient enters the hospital.[17] Monitoring of pulmonary function is needed with amiodarone because of reported acute and chronic pulmonary toxicity.[19] Sotalol may need to be withdrawn because of bradycardia and hypotension. Anticoagulation shoud be instituted if the patient remains in atrial fibrillation, or is in and out of atrial fibrillation for more than 48 hours, to prevent thrombus formation and stroke. Rarely is cardioversion necessary, but if more than 48 hours has passed since the onset of atrial fibrillation, echocardiography should be performed to check for atrial thrombus. If atrial thrombus is present, cardioversion should not be performed. If there is no history of atrial fibrillation preoperatively, rate control and antiarrhythmic agents as well as anticoagulation can usually be discontinued at 3 months after surgery.

Bleeding

Postoperative bleeding is monitored by chest tube output. Sudden occurrence of large-volume, bloody drainage requires immediate reexploration to find and stop the source of bleeding. Less rapid bleeding of more than 100 mL/hr for 2 consecutive hours is also excessive after thoracic surgery. Prothrombin time, partial thromboplastin time, platelet count, and, if the patient has been on aspirin, bleeding time should be measured. If a coagulopathy exists, expeditious administration of deficient factors and keeping the patient normothermic should help slow or stop bleeding. If bleeding persists after correction of deficient factors, exploration for a bleeding source should be performed. If there is no coagulopathy or if hematoma causes significant mediastinal or lung compression, reexploration is necessary. Transfusion of packed red blood cells should be considered, depending on the patient's hemoglobin level and hemodynamic condition.

Late Complications

Pulmonary Complications

A prolonged air leak is defined as one that lasts longer than 7 postoperative days. If the patient has an emphysematous lung and the leak is small, several manipulations can be performed to encourage the leak to stop. If a pneumothorax or residual space still exists, placing the chest tube on higher suction can be tried, either by raising the water level in the suction chamber or by closing the air vent to the suction chamber and controlling the amount of suction pressure from the wall source. Pressures above 40 to 60 mm Hg are not recommended. Placement of another chest tube may help fully reexpand the lung if the air leak is substantial. If no residual space exists, placement of the chest tube to water seal or on a Heimlich valve can encourage the leak to seal. A Heimlich valve may allow the patient to leave the hospital sooner. If the tube happens to be lying against a bleb or a raw surface of the lung, pulling the tube back several centimeters (if it is possible to still leave the last side hole within the pleural cavity) and twisting the tube 180 degrees can be helpful. A blood patch can be attempted by injecting approximately 50 to 100 mL of the patient's own blood through the chest tube.[112-114] This has been shown to be effective in both partially and fully expanded lungs, but it may need to be repeated several times and may increase the risk of empyema. Talc sclerosis through the chest tube can be performed, although this will cause pleural fusion, making it difficult to reenter the chest cavity in the future.[89] If none of these works, the patient may need to be taken back to the operating room for leak closure. Air leak from the lung parenchyma can be troublesome because of friable lung tissue. Direct suturing with or without pledgets, use of fibrin sealants and glue,[115] and stapling of a leak with pericardial or polytetrafluoroethylene strips can be attempted.

Bronchopleural Fistula

If air is leaking from the bronchial stump, adequate chest tube drainage to prevent or drain empyema is necessary.[83,84] Bronchoscopy should be performed to look at the stump. If no large opening is seen, selective bronchography can be performed with 5 to 10 mL of propyliodone diluted 1:1 with saline.[116] Treatment may consist of operative closure or endobronchial closure. Multiple biological glues, adhesives, medications, and objects have been reported to successfully seal small bronchopleural fistulas in case reports.[115-118] Special catheters and deployment devices are necessary to administer the treatments through the bronchoscope to the site of the leak. Redo thoracotomy and operative closure of the leaking bronchial stump may be needed. The standard approach of Deschamps and colleagues includes trimming a long bronchial stump or débriding a poorly vascularized stump and then covering the stump with an extraskeletal muscle flap (e.g., the serratus anterior or latissimus dorsi).[83] If vascularized tissue is inadequate to primarily close a bronchopleural fistula, the extraskeletal muscle is sewn circumferentially to the stump for closure. Wide drainage to prevent unilateral empyema and contralateral soiling should be performed. This may include reopening the whole thoracotomy and performing open packing in the operating room every several days or under conscious sedation in the patient's room for several days to weeks until the cavity is clean. An Eloesser flap can be performed to facilitate open packing. Once clean, dilute antibiotic solution is instilled, and airtight chest closure is performed. Mobilization of the remaining chest wall musculature and additional rib resection may be necessary to allow chest wall closure without tension.[85] This alleviates a lifetime of packing an open chest, which predisposes to failure to thrive and recurrent bronchitis and pneumonia, and limits the patient's daily activities and lifestyle. An alternative approach involves pleural irrigation with antibiotic solution, intravenous antibiotics, and nutritional support. Gharagozloo and colleagues recommend an antibiotic solution composed of gentamicin (80 mg/L), neomycin (500 mg/L), and polymyxin B (100 mg/L), and an airtight thoracotomy closure without drainage should be instituted when pleural cultures are negative.[84] Ng and coworkers used antibiotic irrigation for 2 weeks, tailored to the organism grown in pleural culture.[119]

A persistent pleural space after lung resection can be prevented with a pleural tent if it is anticipated at the time of surgery.[120] The apical portion of the parietal pleura is dissected from the chest wall and tacked to the upper intercostal muscle of the thoracotomy. The chest tubes are placed within the pleural tent. The pleura adhere to the surface of the remaining lung and help seal over any leaking areas, and they decrease the volume of space that the remaining lung needs to fill. Either the space on top of the pleural tent in the apex fills with serous fluid, as it does after a pneumonectomy, or the lung expands to fill the whole space. This is also aided by elevation of the hemidiaphragm. Encouraging the diaphragm to rise can be accomplished by pneumoperitoneum.[121] Air can be instilled across the diaphragm with a needle during thoracotomy, or periumbilically at a later time. Care must be taken not to damage the liver, spleen, or stomach. Injection of the phrenic nerve with local anesthetic causes a temporary paralysis that also encourages the hemidiaphragm to rise. No respiratory compromise due to this practice has been reported. Filling of a residual space with healthy living tissue such as muscle or omentum can also be performed, although this is generally not done during resection because such extreme measures are unlikely to be needed. Last, thoracoplasty can be performed but is rarely used.

Bronchovascular Fistula

Bronchovascular fistula is a rare complication that needs to be considered after bronchoplastic procedures are performed.[122] Fistulas sometimes first appear with a herald bleed, followed by massive hemoptysis. Salvage after a major bleed is rare and the best treatment is to decrease the chance of fistula formation by placing vascularized tissue such as intercostal or extraskeletal muscle, pleura, pericardium, or omentum between the pulmonary artery and the sutured bronchus. If massive hemoptysis does occur, an attempt at placing a double-lumen tube to isolate the nonaffected lung from blood spillage may allow enough time for the chest to be opened and the bleeding controlled. Unfortunately, salvage is rare and the patient dies of suffocation more often than exsanguination.

Postpneumonectomy Syndrome

Postpneumonectomy syndrome is torsion or compression of the trachea, bronchus, esophagus, or pulmonary vasculature caused by mediastinal shift after pneumonectomy. Placement of a tissue expander or a saline breast prosthesis into the post-pneumonectomy space is reported to reverse some of the mediastinal shift and its consequences.[123,124]

Wound Infection and Empyema

Wound infection after thoracotomy is very rare. The wound should be opened to allow adequate drainage. If the patient also has an empyema, tube drainage of the pleural cavity through a separate site can be attempted along with opening of the wound. If the infection goes entirely through, it is better to take the patient back to the operating room for a thorough drainage, irrigation, débridement, and decortication. Strong consideration for leaving the skin open after redo thoracotomy should be given. If the cause of empyema is a bronchopleural fistula, the infection should be cleared, and then definitive treatment of the bronchopleural fistula is undertaken as mentioned earlier.

Post-thoracotomy Pain

Chronic post-thoracotomy pain syndrome remains a devastating and debilitating result after thoracotomy. It is pain that occurs along a thoracotomy scar at least 2 months after surgery, and its incidence is 44% to 67%. Treatment may involve several modalities, including medications, behavioral techniques, and procedures. Combinations of medication include cyclo-oxygenase-2 (COX-2) inhibitors, tricyclic antidepressants, anticonvulsants such as gabapentin, opioids, and Lidoderm patches. Behavioral techniques such as biofeedback, hypnosis, and relaxation techniques may be offered. Procedural treatments include intercostal nerve block, radiofrequency ablation, cryoablation, and transcutaneous electrical nerve stimulation (TENS). Referral to a pain specialty clinic with a team consisting of anesthesiologist, nutritionist, physical therapist, psychiatrist or psychologist, occupational therapist, and pharmacist is recommended for comprehensive care.[125]

Complications after Esophageal Surgery

Many of the complications encountered after thoracotomy or lung resection, particularly the respiratory complications, also occur after esophageal surgery. Atkins and colleagues found that pneumonia was associated with a 20% incidence of death, compared with a 3.1% incidence of death in patients who did not develop pneumonia. Additionally, pneumonia was the cause of 54% of the deaths in their series.[50] Patients are at high risk of aspiration after esophagectomy, especially if they have recurrent laryngeal nerve injury. Aspiration precautions including elevation of the head of the bed at all times, the chin tuck maneuver, eating and drinking only out of bed and sitting straight up, and education by speech pathologists and nutritionists about food choices, mechanics of eating, and concentration during eating are of paramount importance.

Dysphagia

Difficulty swallowing is one of the most frequent complications after any esophageal surgery. At times, it is self-limited and caused by recent surgery. However, persistence of dysphagia after fundoplication, myotomy, or esophageal resection should be investigated. Workup usually includes barium swallow, motility studies, or esophagogastroduodenoscopy, or a combination of these. Anatomic or functional abnormalities such as too tight a fundoplication, slipped fundoplication, recurrent herniation, motility disorder, and ulceration may be found. Treatment depends on the cause of the dysphagia and ranges from simple observation, to dilation, to medical treatment, to need for reoperation.[74,50]

Anastomotic Leak

Anastomotic leak or perforation occurs because of ischemia, distention of conduit and pressure at suture lines, poor nutrition, anastomotic tension, or technical problems.[126] The location and size of the leak determine the treatment. If a neck anastomosis is leaking, the neck wound is opened to allow drainage and healing over time. Stricture may form and require dilation, but that is usually not incapacitating. The patient should generally be kept NPO during that time to reduce the amount of pressure and fluid draining past the hole. Antibiotics are not necessary if the leak is adequately drained. If the leak is more than a quarter of the circumference of the anastomosis, débriding unhealthy tissue and primary reclosure of the anastomosis should be considered.

If the anastomosis is within the chest, a leak may be contained in the space around the conduit, into the pleural cavity, or into the mediastinum. A leak into the pleural cavity should be drained with chest tubes. The patient is made NPO. Intravenous antibiotics are administered unless the patient has no fever or leukocytosis and there is a well-formed drainage tract to the tube. Drainage into the mediastinum can be fatal if it is not evacuated. If the patient is toxic, reoperation for adequate drainage should be performed to prevent mediastinitis and sepsis. If there is adequate healthy tissue after débridement and the patient is not toxic at that time, reanastomosis can be considered. If ischemia or soiling with unhealthy tissue exists, wide débridement with esophageal exclusion may be needed. If a significant amount of the stomach needs to be resected, the hiatus should be closed to prevent herniation.[126] For small persistent anastomotic leaks, both removable polyester/silicone stents and expandable covered metallic stents have been successful.[127,128]

Chylothorax

The incidence of chylothorax is 0.4% to 0.8% after esophagectomy. It usually manifests several days after the operation when tube feedings or oral intake is started. Drainage of moderate to large volumes of milky whitish fluid from the chest tube or with thoracentesis is almost always diagnostic. Analysis of the fluid for lipids with a triglyceride-to-cholesterol ratio of greater than 1 or a triglyceride level greater than 110 g/dL confirms the diagnosis. The thoracic duct may be injured while mobilizing the lower thoracic esophagus, and leakage is usually into the right chest. Conservative measures such as a low-fat or medium-chain triglyceride diet can be tried, but if the drainage does not decrease after several days, full NPO status and total parenteral nutrition should be instituted. Chyle contains abundant proteins, and patients can become nutritionally depleted quickly. Octreotide infusion or subcutaneous administration has been successful in treating chylothorax in case reports.[129,130] Percutaneous embolization of the thoracic duct or cisterna chyli also has good results.[131] Some surgeons prefer not to wait more than 5 days before taking the patient back to the operating room for thoracic duct ligation just above the right hemidiaphragm. This can be done thoracoscopically or with a thoracotomy.[132] Lymphangiography is generally not helpful in localizing the leak, and most radiologists are not trained in this method anymore. Feeding the patient cream or a fat-laden food several hours before surgery can elucidate the leaking portion of the duct. The leaking point is ligated and the duct is also ligated at multiple other points just above the diaphragm. Chest tube output should decrease drastically and the patient can be fed again.

Dumping syndrome occurs because of high osmotic load from the stomach into the small bowel due to lack of antral control after the vagus nerves are divided.[49,77] This can occur approximately 20 minutes or several hours after a meal. Dietary adjustments such as decreasing the intake of foods with simple sugars such as sweets and eating smaller, more frequent meals without a large amount of fluid are helpful in improving symptoms. Fiber intake and acarbose (which interferes with carbohydrate absorption) may help. More severe symptoms can be treated by subcutaneous octreotide.[133,134] Delayed gastric emptying also occurs after esophagectomy because of division of the vagus nerves and decreased stomach motility. Most surgeons perform a drainage procedure at the pylorus to prevent gastric outlet obstruction. At times, dilation of the pylorus or the anastomosis will need to be performed. Medications known to increase gastrointestinal motility, such as metoclopramide and erythromycin, may improve symptoms. Some patients cannot tolerate the extrapyramidal side effects of metoclopramide.

Gas-bloat syndrome occurs after fundoplication. Patients complain of feeling full of gas and being unable to belch for relief. Dietary changes to decrease the amount of gas-producing foods, avoidance of carbonated beverages, and passage of time usually relieve the symptoms of this syndrome. There is some suggestion that a partial fundoplication leads to less gas-bloat syndrome than total fundoplication.[135,136]

Reflux

Gastroesophageal reflux is common after esophagectomy and gastric pull-up. The lower portion of the stomach remains subjected to positive intraperitoneal pressure while negative intrathoracic pressure exerts an influence on the upper portion of the stomach without a lower esophageal sphincter. Patients with a history of Barrett's esophagus or symptoms or findings of esophagitis after gastric pull-up should be on antireflux medication. They need to be counseled to eat and drink in the upright position and remain upright for at least 2 hours after eating. The head of the bed should be elevated 30 degrees, or they should sleep on a foam wedge to avoid nighttime reflux and aspiration. Avoiding damage to the recurrent laryngeal nerves helps to diminish the risk of aspiration when reflux occurs.[133,134]

Stricture

Stricture after esophageal surgery can occur at an anastomosis; at the diaphragmatic hiatus; above, below, or within a fundoplication; at the pylorus; or at the site of previous myotomy. Stricture may be secondary to technical problems, ischemia, leak, ulceration, or reflux, and it may be multifactorial. Most strictures caused by previous esophageal surgery can be treated with either balloon or bougie dilation. Multiple dilations may be necessary in the early period after surgery. With passage of time, the frequency of dilation for each patient decreases until it is no longer necessary. A few patients need repeated dilation on a chronic basis, and some are able to dilate themselves at home after being taught.[126]

Conduit Ischemia

Conduit ischemia can be avoided by assessment of the blood supply before surgery if the patient has had previous gastric or colonic operations. An angiogram of the mesenteric arteries may be desired before the colon is used as a conduit to ensure patency of the marginal artery. Continuous knowledge of the position of the gastroepiploic arteries as the greater curvature dissection is performed prevents inadvertent ligation or damage to the main vascular pedicle used during gastric pull-up. Leaving the right gastric artery intact provides a dual blood supply to ensure adequate blood flow to the stomach as it is transposed into the chest or neck. Careful handling of the gastric tube during passage into the chest or neck and prevention of twisting, torquing, or folding is of paramount importance. The distal tip of the conduit should be pink when positioned and before anastomosis. Bleeding at the gastrostomy site created for stapler insertion or hand-sewn anastomosis and healthy-appearing mucosa should be seen. Conduit ischemia can be difficult to diagnose postoperatively, but symptoms and signs of infection or an inflammatory response without a known source should raise the level of suspicion. Unless diagnosed and treated early, conduit ischemia can lead to further morbidity or mortality. If a significant portion of the conduit is ischemic or the surrounding tissues are unhealthy from inflammation, takedown of the anastomosis, creation of an esophagostomy, and return of the gastric remnant to the peritoneal cavity with closure of the hiatus is recommended.[126]

Recurrent Laryngeal Nerve Damage

Damage to the recurrent laryngeal nerve is more common after transhiatal resection or three-hole resection because of the dissection and retraction in the neck where the recurrent nerves are exposed in the tracheoesophageal groove. Recurrent laryngeal nerve damage not only causes hoarseness but compounds discoordination of swallowing and increased risk of aspiration in patients already at risk for these problems because of the surgical procedure itself. The incidence of this complication can be lowered by careful avoidance of metal retractors deep in the neck wound and visualization of the nerve. If vocal cord paralysis is evident after esophagectomy, assessment for aspiration by modified barium swallow and bedside evaluation by a speech pathologist is necessary before oral intake. If aspiration is present, the patient may need to be kept NPO and nutrition maintained by tube feeding until vocal cord medialization is performed by injection to decrease the risk of aspiration and increase the ability of the patient to make an effective cough.[50,137]

Miscellaneous

Myasthenic crisis is respiratory muscle weakness causing respiratory failure after thymectomy for myasthenia gravis. Positive-pressure mask breathing or ventilation should be used to support the patient through the acute crisis. Mestinon is usually not effective during crisis. If steroids and intravenous immune globulin do not provide enough symptom relief, plasmapheresis may be needed to clear the circulating antibodies.[9,13] Cholinergic crisis results from overtreatment with anticholinesterase medications. The patient may have symptoms related to muscarinic receptor activity (e.g., excessive salivation, sweating, abdominal cramping, urinary urgency, bradycardia). Nicotinic receptor symptoms include fasciculations and muscle weakness. Cholinergic crisis does not respond to neostigmine. Treatment includes respiratory support, atropine, and cessation of anticholinesterase medications.[13]

Cerebrospinal fluid leak is a rare complication seen when tumor is resected near the spine. Assistance of a neurosurgeon is recommended, and primary closure should be done if possible. Coverage with fat or pleura can also be used to help seal the leak. Other treatments involve placing lumbar drains to decrease the amount of cerebrospinal fluid and pressure to allow the leak to seal on its own. The symptoms include leakage of clear fluid and development of intractable headache after resection close to the spine or involving the vertebrae.[138,139]

DISCHARGE PLANNING

Discharge needs should be assessed preoperatively or soon after the surgery. The surgeon can often predict what services will be needed, on the basis of the patient's preoperative health and family support network. The patient and family are made active participants in plans for timely discharge. Team meetings with social workers, nurses, physical therapists, and respiratory therapists about each patient's needs are helpful for planning. Occupational therapists and physical medicine physicians can indicate what level of rehabilitation patients will need after discharge. A list of home-going medications, their purpose, and dosage is reviewed with the patient and the caregivers before discharge, including the changes from preoperative medications. Activity level and home-going exercises should be reviewed, and patients should demonstrate them to the therapist before leaving to ensure they are being done correctly. Driving and lifting are limited for 2 to 3 weeks postoperatively or while on narcotic medications. There is no prohibition for showering or stair climbing.

Outpatient pulmonary rehabilitation programs should be contacted and set up before discharge. The goal is to return the patient to a normal lifestyle as soon as possible. Visiting nurses can be invaluable in helping patients once home, for vital sign check, administration of antibiotics or blood draws, tube care, and wound care. They allow patients to be discharged who need help for only several minutes a day. The follow-up appointment and any laboratory studies or radiology studies that need to be obtained before the appointment should be arranged before the patient's discharge. Appropriate contact phone numbers should be provided should the patient have difficulty after discharge.

REFERENCES

1. Boysen PG. Perioperative management of the thoracotomy patient. *Clin Chest Med* 1993;**14**:321-33.
2. Nici L. Preoperative and postoperative pulmonary rehabilitation in lung cancer patients. *Thorac Surg Clin* 2008;**18**:39-43.
3. Ries AL, Make BJ, Lee SM, et al. The effects of pulmonary rehabilitation in the National Emphysema Treatment Trial. *Chest* 2005;**128**:3799-809.
4. Bartels MN, Kim H, Whiteson JH, Alba AS. Pulmonary rehabilitation in patients undergoing lung volume reduction surgery. *Arch Phys Med Rehabil* 2006;**87**(3 Suppl. 1):s84-8.
5. Karnath B. Smoking cessation. *Am J Med* 2002;**112**:399-405.
6. Vaporciyan AA, Merriman KW, Ece F, Roth JA, Smythe WR, Swisher SG, et al. Incidence of major pulmonary morbidity after pneumonectomy: association with timing of smoking cessation. *Ann Thorac Surg* 2002;**73**:420-6.
7. Camu F, Beckers S. The anesthetic risk of tobacco smoking. *Acta Anaesthesiol Belg* 1991;**42**:45-56.
8. Barrera R, Shi W, Amar D, et al. Smoking and timing of cessation: impact on pulmonary complications after thoracotomy. *Chest* 2005;**127**:1977-83.
9. Krucylak PE, Naunheim KS. Preoperative preparation and anesthetic management of patients with myasthenia gravis. *Semin Thorac Cardiovasc Surg* 1999;**11**:47-53.
10. Eagle KA, Berger PB, Calkins H. ACC/AHA guideline update for perioperative cardiovascular evaluation for non-cardiac surgery: Executive summary. *Circulation* 2002;**105**:1257-67.
11. Jaroszewski DE, Huh J, Chu D, et al. Utility of detailed preoperative cardiac testing and incidence of post-thoracotomy myocardial infarction. *J Thorac Cardiovasc Surg* 2008;**135**:648-55.
12. Marks JB. Perioperative management of diabetes. *Am Fam Physician* 2003;**67**:93-100.
13. Spring PJ, Spies JM. Myasthenia gravis: Options and timing of immunomodulatory treatment. *Biodrugs* 2001;**15**:173-83.
14. Vaporciyan AA, Corea AM, Rice DC, et al. Risk factors associated with atrial fibrillation after noncardiac thoracic surgery: analysis of 2588 patients. *J Thorac Cardiovasc Surg* 2004;**127**:779-86.
15. Cresswell LL, Schuessler RB, Rosenbloom M, Cox JL. Hazards of postoperative atrial arrhythmias. *Ann Thorac Surg* 1993;**56**:539-49.
16. Amar D, Roistacher N, Rusch VW, Leung DHY, Ginsburg I, Zhang H, et al. Effects of diltiazem prophylaxis on the incidence and clinical outcome of atrial arrhythmias after thoracic surgery. *J Thorac Cardiovasc Surg* 2000;**120**:790-8.
17. Dunning J, Treasure T, Versteegh M, et al. Guidelines on the prevention and management of de novo atrial fibrillation after cardiac and thoracic surgery. *Eur J Cardiothorac Surg* 2006;**30**:852-72.
18. Crystal E, Connolly SJ, Sleik K, Ginger TJ, Yusuf S. Interventions on prevention of postoperative atrial fibrillation in patients undergoing heart surgery: a meta-analysis. *Circulation* 2002;**106**:75-80.
19. Asharafian H, Davey P. Is amiodarone an underrecognized cause of acute respiratory failure in the ICU?. *Chest* 2001;**120**:275-82.
20. Attia J, Ray JG, Cook DJ, et al. Deep vein thrombosis and its prevention in critically ill adults. *Arch Intern Med* 2001;**161**:1268-79.
21. Geerts WH, Heit JA, Clagett GP, et al. Prevention of venous thromboembolism. *Chest* 2001;**119**(Suppl. 1):132S-75S.
22. American Society of Health System Pharmacists. ASHP therapeutic guidelines on stress ulcer prophylaxis. *Am J Health-Syst Pharm* 1999;**56**:347-79.
23. Cook DJ. Stress ulcer prophylaxis: Gastrointestinal bleeding and nosocomial pneumonia—Best evidence synthesis. *Scand J Gastroenterol Suppl* 1995;**210**:48-52.
24. Allen ME, Kopp BJ, Erstad BL. Stress ulcer prophylaxis in the postoperative period. *Am J Health-Syst Pharm* 2004;**61**:588-96.
25. Devlin JW, Welage LS, Olsen KM. Proton pump inhibitor formulary considerations in the acutely ill. Part 2: Clinical efficacy, safety and economics. *Ann Pharmacother* 2005;**39**:1844-51.
26. Flannery J, Tucker DA. Pharmacologic prophylaxis and treatment of stress ulcers in critically ill patients. *Crit Care Nurs Clin North Am* 2002;**14**:39-51.
27. Olak J, Jeyasingham K, Forrester-Wood C, et al. Randomized trial of one-dose versus six-dose cefazolin prophylaxis in elective general thoracic surgery. *Ann Thorac Surg* 1991;**51**:956-8.
28. Radu DM, Jaureguy F, Seguin A, et al. Postoperative pneumonia after major pulmonary resections: an unresolved problem in thoracic surgery. *Ann Thorac Surg* 2007;**84**:1669-74.
29. Schussler O, Alifano M, Dermine H, et al. Postoperative pneumonia after major lung resection. *Am J Respir Crit Care* 2006;**173**:1161-9.
30. Website: www.medQIC.org
31. Karger R, Kretschmer V. Modern concepts of autologous haemotherapy. *Transfusion Apheresis Sci* 2004;**32**:185-96.
32. Goodnough LT. Autologous blood donation. *Critical Care* 2004;**8**(Suppl. 2): S49-52.
33. Motoyama S, Okuyama M, Kitamura M, et al. Use of autologous instead of allogeneic blood transfusion during esophagectomy prolongs disease free survival among patients with recurrent esophageal cancer. *J Surg Oncol* 2004;**87**:26-31.

34. Bennett CL, Silver SM, Djulbegovic B, et al. Venous thromboembolism and mortality associated with recombinant erythropoietin and darbepoetin administration for the treatment of cancer related anemia. *JAMA* 2008;**299**:914-24.
35. Bonow RO, Carabello B, de Leon AC, et al. ACC/AHA guidelines for the management of patient with valvular heart disease. *J Am Coll Cardiol* 1998;**32**:1486-582.
36. Campos JH. Lung isolation techniques. *Anesthesiol Clin North Am* 2001;**19**: 455-74.
37. Fernandez-Perez ER, Keegan MT, Brown DR, et al. Intraoperative tidal volume as a risk factor for respiratory failure after pneumonectomy. *Anesthesiology* 2006;**105**:14-8.
38. Kurz A. Thermal care in the perioperative period. *Best Pract Res Clin Anaesthesiol* 2008;**22**:39-62.
39. Faust RJ, Cucchiara RF, Bechtle PS. Patient positioning. In: Miller RD, editor. *Miller's anesthesia*. 6th ed. Philadelphia: Elsevier Churchill and Livingstone; 2005. p. 1151-67.
40. Gomez-Caro A, Roca MJ, Torres J, et al. Successful use of a single chest drain postlobectomy instead of two classical drains: a randomized study. *Eur J Cardiothorac Surg* 2006;**29**:562-6.
41. Veeramachaneni NK, Zoole JB, Decker PA, et al. Lymph node analysis in esophageal resection: American College of Surgeons Oncology Group Z0060 trial. *Ann Thorac Surg* 2008;**86**:418-21.
42. McKenna RJ, Mahtabifard A, Pickens A, et al. Fast tracking after video-assisted thoracoscopic surgery lobectomy, segmentectomy and pneumonectomy. *Ann Thorac Surg* 2007;**84**:1663-8.
43. Slinger PD. Perioperative fluid management for thoracic surgery: the puzzle of postpneumonectomy pulmonary edema. *J Cardiothorac Vasc Anesthesiol* 1995;**9**:442-51.
44. Schierhout G, Roberts I. Fluid resuscitation with colloid or crystalloid solutions in critically ill patients: a systematic review of randomized trials. *BMJ* 1998;**316**:961-4.
45. Hebert PC, Wells G, Blajchman MA, et al. A multicenter, randomized, controlled clinical trial of transfusion requirements in critical care. *N Engl J Med* 1999;**340**:409-17.
46. Hebert PC, Yetisir E, Martin C, et al. Is a low transfusion threshold safe in critically ill patients with cardiovascular diseases?. *Crit Care Med* 2001;**29**: 227-34.
47. Hopkins CC. Antibiotic prophylaxis in clean surgery: peripheral vascular surgery, noncardiovascular thoracic surgery, herniorrhaphy, and mastectomy. *Rev Infect Dis* 1991;**13**(Suppl. 10):S869-73.
48. Headrick JR, Nichols 3rd FC, Miller DL, et al. High-grade esophageal dysplasia: Long-term survival and quality of life after esophagectomy. *Ann Thorac Surg* 2002;**73**:1697-702.
49. McLarty AJ, Deschamps C, Trastek VF, et al. Esophageal resection for cancer of the esophagus: Long term function and quality of life. *Ann Thorac Surg* 1997;**63**:1568-72.
50. Atkins BZ, Shah AS, Hutcheson KA, et al. Reducing hospital morbidity and mortality following esophagectomy. *Ann Thorac Surg* 2004;**78**:1170-6.
51. Burgess FW, Anderson DM, Colonna D, Cavanaugh DG. Thoracic epidural analgesia with bupivacaine and fentanyl for postoperative thoracotomy pain. *J Cardiothorac Vasc Anesth* 1994;**8**:420-4.
52. Moon MR, Luchette FA, Gibson SW, et al. Prospective, randomized comparison of epidural versus parenteral opioid analgesia in thoracic trauma. *Ann Surg* 1999;**229**:684-92.
53. Simpson T, Wahl G, DeTraglia M, et al. The effects of epidural versus parenteral opioid analgesia on postoperative pain and pulmonary function in adults who have undergone thoracic and abdominal surgery: a critique of research. *Heart Lung* 1992;**21**:125-38.
54. Davies RG, Myles PS, Graham JM. A comparison of the analgesic efficacy and side effects of paravertebral vs epidural blockade for thoracotomy: a systematic review and meta-analysis of randomized trials. *Br J Anaesth* 2006;**96**:418-26.
55. Smythe M. Patient-controlled analgesia: a review. *Pharmacotherapy* 1992;**12**:132-43.
56. Michelet P, Guervilly C, Helaine A, et al. Adding ketamine to patient controlled analgesia after thoracic surgery: influence on morphine consumption, respiratory function and nocturnal desaturation. *Br J Anaesth* 2007;**99**:396-403.
57. Wong RHL, Lee TW, Sihoe ADL, et al. Analgesic effect of electroacupuncture in postthoracotomy pain: a prospective randomized trial. *Ann Thorac Surg* 2006;**81**:2031-6.
58. Power I, Bowler GMR, Pugh GC, Chambers WA. Ketorolac as a component of balanced analgesia after thoracotomy. *Br J Anaesthesiol* 1994;**72**:224-6.
59. Singh H, Bossard RF, White PF, Yeatts RW. Effects of ketorolac versus bupivacaine coadministration during patient-controlled hydromorphone epidural analgesia after thoracotomy procedures. *Anesth Analg* 1997;**84**:564-9.
60. McCrory C, Fitzgerald D. Spinal prostaglandin formation and pain perception following thoracotomy: a role for cyclooxygenase-2. *Chest* 2004;**125**:1321-7.
61. D'Andrilli A, Ibrahim M, Ciccone AM, et al. Intrapleural intercostal nerve block associated with mini-thoracotomy improves pain control after major lung resection. *Eur J Cardiothor Surg* 2006;**29**:790-4.
62. Detterbeck FC. Efficacy of methods of intercostal nerve blockade for pain relief after thoracotomy. *Ann Thorac Surg* 2005;**80**:1550-9.
63. Scawn ND, Pennefather SH, Soorae A, et al. Ipsilateral shoulder pain after thoracotomy with epidural analgesia: the influence of phrenic nerve infiltration with lidocaine. *Anesth Analg* 2001;**93**:260-4.
64. Benedetti F, Amanzio M, Casadio C, et al. Control of postoperative pain by transcutaneous electrical nerve stimulation after thoracic operations. *Ann Thorac Surg* 1997;**63**:773-6.
65. Brynitz S, Schroder M. Intraoperative cryolysis of intercostal nerves in thoracic surgery. *Scand J Thor Cardiovasc Surg* 1986;**20**:85-7.
66. Joucken K, Michel L, Schoevaerdts JC, et al. Cryoanalgesia for post-thoracotomy pain relief. *Acta Anaesthesiol Belg* 1987;**38**:179-83.
67. Roxburgh JC, Markland CG, Ross BA, Kerr WF. Role of cryoanalgesia in the control of pain after thoracotomy. *Thorax* 1987;**42**:292-5.
68. McKenna RJ. New approaches to the minimally invasive treatment of lung cancer. *Cancer J* 2005;**11**:73-6.
69. Walker WS, Codispoti M, Soon SY, et al. Long-term outcomes following VATS lobectomy for non-small cell bronchogenic carcinoma. *Eur J Cardiothorac Surg* 2003;**23**:397-402.
70. Sedrakyan A, van der Meulen J, Lewey J, Treasure T. Video assisted thoracic surgery for treatment of pneumothorax and lung resections: systematic review of randomised trials. *BMJ* 2004;**329**:1008-11.
71. Burns HJG. Nutritional support in the perioperative period. *Br Med Bull* 1988;**44**:357-73.
72. Nwiloh J, Freeman H, McCord C. Malnutrition: an important determinant of fatal outcome in surgically treated pulmonary suppurative disease. *J Natl Med Assoc* 1989;**81**:525-9.
73. Wills VL, Hunt DR. Dysphagia after anti-reflux surgery. *Br J Surg* 2001;**88**: 486-99.
74. Johnson DA, Younes Z, Hogan WJ. Endoscopic assessment of hiatal hernia repair. *Gastrointest Endosc* 2000;**52**:650-9.
75. Tanomkiat W, Galassi W. Barium sulfate as contrast medium for evaluation of postoperative anastomotic leaks. *Acta Radiol* 2000;**41**:482-5.
76. Gillinov AM, Heitmiller RF. Strategies to reduce pulmonary complications after transhiatal esophagectomy. *Dis Esophagus* 1998;**11**:43-7.
77. Young MM, Deschamps C, Allen MS, et al. Esophageal reconstruction for benign disease: Self-assessment of functional outcome and quality of life. *Ann Thorac Surg* 2000;**70**:1799-802.
78. Donington JS, Miller DL, Allen MS, et al. Preoperative chemoradiation therapy does not improve early survival after esophagectomy for patients with clinical stage III adenocarcinoma of the esophagus. *Ann Thorac Surg* 2004;**77**:1193-9.
79. Wang JS. Pulmonary function tests in preoperative pulmonary evaluation. *Respir Med* 2004;**98**:598-605.
80. Bonde P, Papachristos I, McCraith A, et al. Sputum retention after lung operation: prospective, randomized trial shows superiority of prophylactic minitracheostomy in high-risk patients. *Ann Thorac Surg* 2002;**74**:196-202.
81. Vermeulen H, Ubbink DT, Goossens A, et al. Systematic review of dressings and topical agents for surgical wounds healing by secondary intention. *Br J Surg* 2005;**92**:665-72.
82. Lambert KV, Hayes P, McCarthy M. Vacuum assisted closure: a review of development and current applications. *Eur J Vasc Endovasc Surg* 2005;**29**: 219-26.
83. Deschamps C, Allen MS, Miller DL, et al. Management of postpneumonectomy empyema and bronchopleural fistula. *Semin Thorac Cardiovasc Surg* 2001;**13**:13-9.
84. Gharagozloo F, Trachiotis G, Wolfe R, et al. Pleural space irrigation and modified Clagett procedure for the treatment of early postpneumonectomy empyema. *J Thorac Cardiovasc Surg* 1998;**116**:943-9.
85. Massera F, Robustellini M, Della Pona C, et al. Predictors of successful closure of open window thoracostomy for postpneumonectomy empyema. *Ann Thorac Surg* 2006;**82**:288-92.
86. Grillo HC, Donahue DM. Post-intubation tracheal stenosis. *Semin Thorac Cardiovasc Surg* 1996;**8**:370-80.
87. Roeckl-Wiedmann I, Bennett M, Kranke P. Systematic review of hyperbaric oxygen in the management of chronic wounds. *Br J Surg* 2005;**92**:24-32.
88. Cerfolio RJ, Pickens A, Bass C, Katholi C. Fast tracking pulmonary resections. *J Thor Cardiovasc Surg* 2001;**122**:318-24.
89. Cerfolio RJ, Tummala RP, Holman WL, et al. A prospective algorithm for the management of air leaks after pulmonary resection. *Ann Thorac Surg* 1998;**66**:1726-31.

90. Marshall MB, Deeb ME, Bleier JIS, et al. Suction versus water seal after pulmonary resection. *Chest* 2002;**121**:831-5.
91. Ferdinand B, Shennib H. Postoperative pneumonia. *Chest Surg Clin North Am* 1998;**8**:529-39.
92. Alam N, Park BJ, Wilton A, et al. Incidence and risk factors for lung injury after lung cancer resection. *Ann Thorac Surg* 2007;**84**:1085-91.
93. Licker M, De Perrot M, Spiliopoulos A, et al. Risk Factors for acute lung injury after thoracic surgery for lung cancer. *Anesth Analg* 2003;**97**:1558-65.
94. Van der Werff YD, Van der Houwen HK, Heijmans PJM, et al. Postpneumonectomy pulmonary edema: a retrospective analysis of incidence and possible risk factors. *Chest* 1997;**111**:1278-84.
95. Cerfolio RJ, Bryant AS, Thurber JS, et al. Intraoperative Solu-Medrol helps prevent postpneumonectomy pulmonary edema. *Ann Thorac Surg* 2003;**76**:1029-35.
96. Allen MS, Darling GE, Pechet TV, et al. Morbidity and mortality of major pulmonary resections in patients with early-stage lung cancer: initial results of the randomized, prospective ACOSOG Z0030 trial. *Ann Thorac Surg* 2006;**81**:1013-9.
97. Alifano M, Boudaya MS, Salvi M, et al. Pneumonectomy after chemotherapy: morbidity, mortality, and long-term outcome. *Ann Thorac Surg* 2008;**85**:1866-73.
98. Mansour Z, Kochetkova EA, Ducrocq X, et al. Induction chemotherapy does not increase the operative risk of pneumonectomy!. *Eur J Cardiothorac Surg* 2007;**31**:181-5.
99. Daly BD, Fernando HC, Ketchedjian A, et al. Pneumonectomy after high-dose radiation and concurrent chemotherapy for nonsmall cell lung cancer. *Ann Thorac Surg* 2006;**82**:227-31.
100. Ruffini E, Parola E, Filosso PL, et al. Frequency and mortality of acute lung injury and acute respiratory distress syndrome after pulmonary resection for bronchogenic carcinoma. *Eur J Cardiothorac Surg* 2001;**20**:30-7.
101. Kutlu CA, Williams EA, Evans TW, et al. Acute lung injury and acute respiratory distress syndrome after pulmonary resection. *Ann Thorac Surg* 2000;**69**:376-80.
102. Algar FJ, Alvarez A, Salvatierra A, et al. Predicting pulmonary complications after pneumonectomy for lung cancer. *Eur J Cardiothorac Surg* 2003;**23**:201-8.
103. Lee H-Y, Lee JM, Kim MS, et al. Low-dose steroid therapy at an early phase of postoperative acute respiratory distress syndrome. *Ann Thorac Surg* 2005;**79**:405-10.
104. Lynch JE, Cheek JM, Chan EY, Zwischenberger JB. Adjuncts to mechanical ventilation in ARDS. *Semin Thorac Cardiovas Surg* 2006;**18**:20-7.
105. Chan KP, Stewart TE, Mehta S. High frequency oscillatory ventilation for adult patients with ARDS. *Chest* 2007;**131**:1907-16.
106. Downar J, Mehta S. Bench to bedside review: high frequency oscillatory ventilation in adults with acute respiratory distress syndrome. *Crit Care* 2006;**10**:240-7.
107. Antman EM, Hand M, Armstrong PW, et al. 2007 focused update of the ACC/AHA 2004 guidelines for the management of patients with ST-elevation myocardial infarction. *J Am Coll Cardiol* 2008;**51**:210-47.
108. Iqbal MB, Westwood MA, Swanton RH. Recent developments in acute coronary syndromes. *Clin Med* 2008;**8**:42-8.
109. Bach RG, Cannon CP, Weintraub MD, et al. The effect of routine early invasive management on outcome for elderly patients with non ST-elevation acute coronary syndromes. *Ann Intern Med* 2004;**141**:186-95.
110. Cummins RO, editor. *ACLS provider manual*. American Heart Association; 2007.
111. Amar D. Postthoracotomy atrial fibrillation. *Curr Opin Anaesth* 2007;**20**:43-7.
112. Andreeti C, Venuta F, Anile M, et al. Pleurodesis with an autologous blood patch to prevent persistent air leaks after lobectomy. *J Thorac Cardiovasc Surg* 2007;**133**:759-62.
113. Droghetti A, Schiavini A, Muriana P, et al. Autologous blood patch in persistent air leaks after pulmonary resection. *J Thorac Cardiovasc Surg* 2006;**132**:556-9.
114. Lang-Lazdunski L, Coonar AS. A prospective study of autologous "blood patch" pleurodesis for persistent air leak after pulmonary resection. *Eur J Cardiothorac Surg* 2004;**26**:897-900.
115. Bayfield MS, Spotnitz WD. Fibrin sealant in thoracic surgery. *Chest Surg Clin North Am* 1996;**6**:567-83.
116. York EL, Lewall DB, Hirji M, et al. Endoscopic diagnosis and treatment of postoperative bronchopleural fistula. *Chest* 1990;**97**:1390-2.
117. Takaoka K, Inoue S, Ohira S. Central bronchopleural fistulas closed by bronchoscopic injection of absolute ethanol. *Chest* 2002;**122**:374-8.
118. Lois M, Noppen M. Bronchopleural fistulas. An overview with special focus on endoscopic management. *Chest* 2005;**128**:3955-65.
119. Ng T, Ryder BA, Maziak DE, Shamji FM. Treatment of postpneumonectomy empyema with debridement followed by continuous antibiotic irrigation. *J Am Coll Surg* 2008;**206**:1178-83.
120. Brunelli A, Refai MA, Muti M, et al. Pleural tent after upper lobectomy: a prospective randomized study. *Ann Thorac Surg* 2000;**69**:1722-4.
121. De Giacomo T, Rendina EA, Venuta F, et al. Pneumoperitoneum for the management of pleural air space problems associated with major pulmonary resections. *Ann Thorac Surg* 2001;**72**:1716-9.
122. Kawahara K, Akamine S, Takahashi T, et al. Management of anastomotic complications after sleeve lobectomy for lung cancer. *Ann Thorac Surg* 1994;**57**:1529-33.
123. Shen KR, Wain JC, Wright CD, et al. Postpneumonectomy syndrome: surgical management and long-term results. *J Thorac Cardiovasc Surg* 2008;**135**:1210-6.
124. Macare van Meurik AFM, Stubenitsky BM, van Swieten HA, et al. Use of tissue expanders in adult postpneumonectomy syndrome. *J Thorac Cardiovasc Surg* 2007;**134**:608-12.
125. Erdek MA, Staats PS. Chronic pain and thoracic surgery. In: Klafta JM, Ferguson MK, editors. *Thoracic surgery clinics: advances in anesthesia and pain management*. Philadelphia: Saunders; 2005. p. 123-30.
126. Cassivi SD. Leaks, strictures and necrosis: a review of anastomotic complications following esophagectomy. *Semin Thorac Cardiovasc Surg* 2004;**16**:124-32.
127. Freeman RK, Ascioti AJ, Wozniak TC. Postoperative esophageal leak management with the Polyflex esophageal stent. *J Thorac Cardiovasc Surg* 2007;**133**:333-8.
128. Kauer WKH, Stein HJ, Dittler HJ, Siewert JR. Stent implantation as a treatment option in patients with thoracic anastomotic leaks after esophagectomy. *Surg Endosc* 2008;**22**:50-3.
129. Kalomenidis I. Octreotide and chylothorax. *Curr Opin Pulm Med* 2006;**12**:264-7.
130. Helin RD, Angeles STV, Bhat R. Octreotide therapy for chylothorax in infants and children: a brief review. *Ped Crit Care Med* 2006;**7**:576-9.
131. Binkert CA, Yucel EK, Davison BD, et al. Percutaneous treatment of high output chylothorax with embolization or needle disruption technique. *J Vasc Interv Radiol* 2005;**16**:1257-61.
132. Fahimi H, Casselman FP, Mariani MA, et al. Current management of postoperative chylothorax. *Ann Thorac Surg* 2001;**71**:448-50.
133. Burrows WM. Gastrointestinal function and related problems after esophagectomy. *Semin Thorac Cardiovasc Surg* 2004;**16**:142-51.
134. Donington JS. Functional conduit disorders after esophagectomy. *Thorac Surg Clin* 2006;**16**:53-62.
135. Chrysos E, Tsiaoussis J, Zoras OJ, et al. Laparoscopic surgery for gastroesophageal reflux disease patients with impaired esophageal peristalsis: total or partial fundoplication?. *J Am Coll Surg* 2003;**197**:8-15.
136. Pessaux P, Arnaud JP, Delattre JF, et al. Laparoscopic antireflux surgery: five-year results and beyond in 1340 patients. *Arch Surg* 2005;**140**:946-51.
137. Lerut TE, van Lanschot JJB. Chronic symptoms after total or subtotal esophagectomy: diagnosis and treatment. *Best Pract Res Clin Gastroenterol* 2004;**18**:901-15.
138. Doss NW, Ambrish M, Ipe J, et al. Epidural blood patch after thoracotomy for treatment of headache caused by surgical tear of dura. *Anesth Analg* 2000;**91**:1372-4.
139. Sganzerla EP, Tisi E, Lucarini C, et al. Acute pneumocephalus: an unusual complication of thoracotomy. *J Neurosurg Sci* 1997;**41**:309-12.

B. Endoscopy

CHAPTER 5

Endoscopic Diagnosis of Thoracic Disease

Benedict J. W. Taylor and Douglas E. Wood

Esophagoscopy
Indications
Pre-Procedure
Flexible Esophagoscopy
Technique
Complications

Rigid Esophagoscopy
Endoscopic Ultrasound
Tracheobronchoscopy
Indications
Endobronchial Ultrasound
Navigational Bronchoscopy

Flexible Bronchoscopy
Technique
Complications
Rigid Bronchoscopy
Technique
Complications

Endoscopy, especially fiberoptic endoscopy, has revolutionized nearly all theaters of medicine in terms of diagnosis and therapeutic intervention.[1] This is particularly true for thoracic surgery, where bronchoscopy and esophagoscopy are essential modalities in the diagnosis, approach, and treatment of tracheal, bronchial, and alimentary tract pathology. As the technology of optics, endoscope instrumentation, and appurtenances such as endoscopic ultrasound and yttrium-aluminum-garnet (YAG) laser have evolved, so have the indications and capabilities of the skilled endoscopist. Although many clinicians may perform endoscopy, thoracic surgeons in particular should be adept and pioneering with these procedures, because new endoscopic technology will continue to enable all aspects of minimally invasive thoracic surgery.

ESOPHAGOSCOPY

In 1868, Kussmaul intubated a sword swallower's stomach via the esophagus with a 13-mm hollow metal tube. This maneuver proved that the oral cavity, esophagus, and stomach could be simultaneously intubated with one rigid instrument. Mikulicz added one crucial aspect to the tube—a distal light to illuminate the esophagus and stomach—and he was able to visualize gastric motility and view probable malignancies. The fiberoptic endoscope was introduced in 1958. This instrument allowed more patient comfort as well as greater therapeutic possibilities in the distal stomach and proximal small intestine. Although the scope itself has not changed greatly, the adjunctive instruments have dramatically changed the way many disease states can be treated.[2]

Indications

For the thoracic surgeon, dysphasia and odynophagia are two of the most common indications for esophageal endoscopy (Box 5-1). Others include reflux, an abnormal esophagogram, trauma, screening, or staging of gastrointestinal (GI) or adjacent masses including tracheoesophageal fistulas. Upper GI bleeding is another very common indication for endoscopy, which has become the first line in management of this clinical scenario.

Dysphagia can arise from a number of pathologic processes. Many causes can be distinguished with a careful history that records the duration and persistence of symptoms and accompanying constitutional symptoms. Endoscopy allows the surgeon to assess the possibility of malignant as opposed to benign causes of dysphagia, thereby guiding therapy.

Reflux is another indication for upper endoscopy. The thoracic surgeon searches for any long-term sequelae associated with chronic gastroesophageal reflux disease (GERD), such as Barrett's esophagus. Esophagoscopy is crucial in the surveillance of known Barrett's esophagus because of the link with the development of adenocarcinoma, although the interval at which these patients should be followed is still unclear.

Upper GI bleeding is another indication for endoscopy, and the procedure is often used therapeutically, as with bleeding esophageal varices, a difficult problem, that can be palliated endoscopically with banding or sclerotherapy.

The most common reason for a thoracic surgeon to perform upper endoscopy is to visualize and biopsy esophageal and proximal stomach masses. Biopsy has a sensitivity of 66% to 96% in esophageal cancers.[3,4] Seven to 10 biopsies are usually taken throughout the area of the lesion, or randomly in the setting of Barrett's esophagitis. For lesions with a tight stricture, the surgeon can use a small-diameter scope, and brushings have been shown to increase the yield of tissue in such cases.[4,5] The role of endoscopic ultrasound in the diagnosis and staging of esophageal disease will be discussed later.

Upper endoscopy can also play a role in the assessment of other mediastinal masses and malignancies that cause esophageal obstructive symptoms. Endoscopy may reveal whether the lesion is causing mass effect or actual erosion through the wall of the esophagus, possibly resulting in a fistula.

Upper endoscopy is also important for investigating trauma—blunt, penetrating, or caustic—and for foreign body

> **Box 5–1**
> **Indications for Upper Endoscopy***
>
> - Persistent nausea and vomiting
> - Upper abdominal pain, heartburn, or acid reflux symptoms (i.e., an acid or burning sensation in the throat or chest)
> - Gastrointestinal (GI) bleeding (vomiting blood or blood found in the stool)
> - Difficulty swallowing; food or liquids get stuck in the esophagus
> - Abnormal or unclear findings on an upper GI radiograph
> - Removal of a foreign body
> - Follow-up on previously found polyps (growths), tumors, or ulcers

According to the American Society for Gastrointestinal Endoscopy. Appropriate use of gastrointestinal endoscopy. Gastrointest Endosc 2000; 52:831-37.

retrieval. The thoracic surgeon is frequently asked to document and manage iatrogenic trauma to the esophagus via instrumentation. Although the esophagogram is the mainstay for the diagnosis of perforation, the usefulness of endoscopy for the diagnosis and documentation of the extent of injury should not be underestimated. When using endoscopy to remove foreign bodies lodged in the esophagus, the surgeon should be alert to the potential for intraesophageal lesions, which may be responsible for the failure of material to pass through.

Corrosive ingestion is another indication for early (within 36 hours) endoscopic inspection,[6] which can help identify transmural involvement and subsequent development of strictures.

Pre-Procedure

Most endoscopies can be performed on an outpatient basis with conscious sedation. Patients should receive nothing by mouth (NPO) after midnight for a morning examination, and those with obstructive symptoms should be placed on a clear liquid diet for 24 to 48 hours before the examination. When the patient arrives, a peripheral intravenous line and electrocardiogram (ECG) leads should be placed. Because the sedatives can cause respiratory depression, ECG and pulse oximetry readings are taken constantly, and blood pressure measurements are obtained frequently during the procedure. Once the monitors are in place, sedation is given to ensure that the patient is comfortable and cooperative. Local anesthesia minimizes the degree of conscious sedation required.

Flexible Esophagoscopy

Technique

The most common position for examination of the outpatient is the left lateral decubitus, with the head flexed. A bite block is placed into the mouth to protect the endoscope from the teeth, and the endoscope is introduced under direct vision. The epiglottis and larynx should be seen and advanced over until the piriform sinuses become apparent. If the vocal cords are visualized, any abnormalities should be documented. Gentle pressure is applied against the upper esophageal sphincter at the cricopharyngeus and the patient is instructed to swallow, which usually results in successful and atraumatic esophageal intubation.

The four normal endoluminal landmarks in the esophagus are as follows: (1) the upper esophageal sphincter at the cricopharyngeus, 15 to 18 cm from the incisors; (2) the aortic arch, usually evident as an indentation on the left anterolateral wall; (3) the left atrium, seen in the distal esophagus as wavelike pulsations of the anterior wall of the esophagus; and (4) the lower esophageal sphincter, which in reality is just a physiologic sphincter, and which can be demonstrated by asking the patient to perform a Valsalva maneuver and noting the pinching off of the lumen. The esophagus is generally easy to assess, and very little air insufflation is required to view its entire course.

Once the gastroesophageal junction has been passed, it is easy to advance into the stomach. The stomach should be insufflated with enough air to flatten out the rugae and allow visualization of the entire mucosal surface. The pylorus is visualized, and the scope can be advanced beyond the sphincter when it is relaxed. The duodenum should be inspected to the third portion. Once this has been performed satisfactorily, the scope should be removed slowly to see any potentially missed pathology. In the stomach, retroflexion of the scope allows the visualization of the body and cardia of the stomach. Insufflated air should be suctioned before leaving the confines of the stomach. During the withdrawal, the scope should be pulled back slowly to more carefully assess the esophagus. Then the endoscope is removed and monitoring of the patient continues.

Complications

Complications are rare after flexible upper endoscopy. Morbidity rates of 0.13% to 0.092% include cardiovascular reactions to premedication, perforation, and bleeding specific to the procedure. Mortality rates are exceedingly rare, quoted at 0.018% to 0.004%.[7,8]

Rigid Esophagoscopy

Rigid esophagoscopy is a rarely used modality, usually reserved for three instances: trauma, removal of impacted food, and removal of foreign bodies. The scope is held in the examiner's right hand while the left hand keeps the mouth open with the left thumb protecting the upper dentition. During the insertion of the scope, the head is initially held forward, in the "sniffing position" used for tracheal intubation; once the cricopharyngeus is passed, the head is extended to eliminate the angle of the mouth and the pharynx. The scope can then be carefully advanced throughout the length of the esophagus and proximal stomach; manipulating the head and cervical spine at the areas of narrowing allows less traumatic passage.

ENDOSCOPIC ULTRASOUND

Endoscopic ultrasound (EUS), for which a small ultrasonic transducer is attached to the end of the endoscope, is a relatively new adjunctive procedure that has expanded the examination of the esophagus and the periesophageal tissues. It is never an initial procedure but is indicated when a previous esophagoscopy has been performed and pathology has been located and evaluated. Indications for esophageal ultrasound range from benign to malignant esophageal disease and include evaluation of periesophageal pathology, usually bronchogenic carcinoma (Box 5-2). The most common indication for EUS

> **Box 5–2**
> **Indications for Endoscopic Ultrasound**
>
> **Esophagus**
> - Staging esophageal cancer
> - Evaluating esophageal submucosal lesions
> - Evaluation of high-grade dysplasia arising in Barrett's esophagus
> - Evaluation of response of esophageal cancer after chemotherapy
> - Differentiating achalasia from pseudoachalasia
> - Evaluation for periesophageal varices
>
> **Mediastinum**
> - Nodal staging of lung cancer
> - Evaluation of selected mediastinal masses
> - Evaluating posterior mediastinal lymphadenopathy

> **Box 5–3**
> **Indications for Flexible Bronchoscopy**
>
> **Diagnostic**
> - Lung cancer
> - Positive sputum cytology
> - Paralyzed vocal cord
> - Localized wheeze
> - Unexplained pleural effusion
> - Hemoptysis
> - Cough
> - Diffuse interstitial infiltrates
> - Immunocompromised state
> - Ventilator-associated pneumonia
> - Endotracheal tube position or patency
> - Atelectasis
> - Tracheoesophageal fistula
> - Acute inhalation injury
> - Bronchography
>
> **Therapeutic**
> - Mucus plug
> - Acute lobar collapse
> - Difficult intubation
> - Foreign body removal
> - Hemoptysis
> - Brachytherapy
> - Laser ablation
> - Electrocautery
> - Stent placement with pulmonary infiltrates
> - Balloon dilation

is the evaluation of esophageal malignancy. The stage of the lesion, as defined by the depth of invasion and nodal involvement, is the best predictor of surgical resection and therefore possible cure.

The normal esophagus has five distinct layers of alternating echogenicity. The first layer, which is the most hyperechoic (white), is the epithelium and lamina propria. The second layer, which is hypoechoic (black), is the muscularis mucosa. The third layer, which is again hyperechoic, is the submucosa. The fourth hypoechoic layer is the muscularis propria. The last layer, the paraesophageal tissue, is thick and hyperechoic. Tumor (T) stage is determined by which layers are invaded. Accumulating data suggest that EUS is the most accurate imaging modality for staging esophageal malignancies. When the EUS results are compared with surgical pathology specimens, EUS demonstrates a preoperative sensitivity of 80% to 92%.[9] The main advantage of EUS over conventional radiology (computed tomography [CT]) is the differentiation of the T stage, especially between the T3 and T4 stages, which may influence the decision to offer the option of surgery to the patient.[10] The accuracy of EUS for staging of regional lymph node metastasis has been in the range of 70% to 80%, which is better than that of CT or magnetic resonance imaging.[10] The regional lymph nodes (N) stage and distant metastasis (M) stage are determined in part by biopsy, which depends on their being seen on examination. Accurate staging is now achieved by five-needle aspiration biopsy, which can be performed on nodal tissue or organ tissues in direct contact with the esophageal wall. After examination of the three different TNM tissues, the patient can be preoperatively staged. EUS is becoming the standard of care in the evaluation of esophageal malignancies.

TRACHEOBRONCHOSCOPY

Gustav Killian, a German laryngologist, is credited with first use of bronchoscopy in 1897. He used a rigid scope to remove a foreign body (bone) from the right main-stem bronchus of a patient. The modern era of flexible bronchoscopy arrived at about the same time as esophagoscopy, once the problem of flexible fiber orientation was solved. Ikeda was the first to report the use of a flexible fiberoptic bronchoscope in a patient.[12] New modalities and techniques such as ultrasound, cautery, fine-needle biopsy, and YAG laser have been coupled with more elegant instrumentation and digital optics to produce the scopes of today. Some of these new modalities have yet to find their particular niche in the modern paradigm.

Tracheobronchoscopy may be performed with a flexible or a rigid instrument, or a combination of the two, depending on the indication and the disease encountered. Flexible bronchoscopy allows the thoracic surgeon not only to diagnose, stage, plan surgical approach, and monitor therapy but also to palliate, temporize, and alleviate a myriad of thoracic pathologies. Rigid bronchoscopy is used less and requires more care, but it is nonetheless indispensible in certain situations. Endobronchial ultrasound (EBUS) is a relatively new modality with growing applications in the diagnosis and staging of primary lung cancer.

Indications

Flexible bronchoscopy can be used for definitive diagnosis of infectious, malignant, and traumatic tracheobronchial diseases (Box 5-3). Pulmonary toilet, endoluminal débridement, endotracheal intubation and extubation, percutaneous tracheostomy placement, and treatment of atelectasis are also elegantly accomplished with the flexible bronchoscope. Perhaps the most important use for the thoracic surgeon, however, is in the staging and assessment of disease before surgery, and in particular, the surgical staging of a primary lung malignancy. After preliminary evaluations with CT and positron emission tomography suggest a resectable lesion, the surgeon surveys the tracheobronchial tree for evidence and extent of endoluminal disease before proceeding with mediastinoscopy and ultimately formal resection. Not only is this evaluation essential from a surgical oncologic perspective but it is also invaluable in terms of defining anatomy and planning resection. If a video-assisted thoracoscopic approach is to be used for resection, the ability to recognize abnormal bronchial anatomy by endoscopy allows resection to be conducted more safely. Furthermore, assessing the cancer's endoluminal involvement can help determine whether lobectomy, sleeve lobectomy, pneumonectomy, or carinal resection should be used.

Direct forceps biopsy, fine-needle aspiration (FNA), endoluminal brush biopsy, and washings are all methods of obtaining tissue that can be performed by flexible bronchoscopy. Mediastinal lymph nodes can be sampled by ultrasound-guided FNA. Although this is inferior, in terms of sensitivity and specificity, to mediastinoscopy as a staging modality, it is often a useful adjunct to cancer staging.

For patients with acute pneumonia in the intensive care setting, flexible bronchoscopy is indispensable for acquiring samples to culture for microbial speciation and antibiotic sensitivities. Routine washings are performed by administering sterile saline though the irrigation port of the bronchoscope, usually in 10-mL volumes. This fluid is then aspirated into a sterile specimen and sent to the laboratory for cytology and culturing. The washing may also be performed by bronchoalveolar lavage (BAL), in which larger volumes of saline are used to reach more terminal bronchioles. The advantage of BAL is that more cellular and noncellular material is retrieved for examination. After the flexible scope is wedged into the fourth or fifth terminal bronchioles, sterile saline is instilled in increments of 50 mL, aiming for a total of 150 to 200 mL, and then aspirated into a specimen trap. The first aspirations contain mostly airway cells, whereas later aspirations can contain alveolar samples. The specimens are handled in the same manner as routine washings, but the absolute cell counts obtained can be useful in the workup of inflammatory, allergic, and autoimmune lung disease. Certain infections, such as atypical tuberculosis, histoplasmosis, and those caused by *Mycobacterium tuberculosis*, *Pneumocystis carinii*, and *Mycoplasma*, are readily diagnosed by BAL.[13]

In intubated patients with copious secretions, endoluminal stents, mucus plugs or clots, and purulent pneumonias, regular bronchoscopy can assist with pulmonary toilet as well as diagnosis. Toilet bronchoscopy is often particularly helpful for patients with impaired mucus clearance, such as active smokers, those with chronic obstructive pulmonary disease or cystic fibrosis, and those who have undergone pulmonary resection or lung transplantation.

Bronchopleural fistula and traumatic tracheobronchial injury are also readily diagnosed by flexible bronchoscopy. Suspicion of either entity should prompt evaluation by endoscopy to definitively and expeditiously rule out such a contingency.

In addition to being used for diagnosis, the flexible bronchoscope is also invaluable for intubation and extubation in precarious airway situations. Small-caliber fiberoptic scopes can be used to define obscure or complex oropharyngeal anatomy, intubate the trachea, and serve as a guide wire over which an endotracheal tube may be securely passed. In these patients, the scope can also withdrawal of the endotracheal tube and then a temporary trial of extubation, providing the ability for a rapid and secure reintubation should the extubation fail.

Percutaneous tracheostomy, the technique of choice for tracheostomy placement in many intensive care units, is considerably safer with the use of flexible bronchoscopy to ensure proper needle, guidewire, dilator, and finally tracheostomy tube placement.

Endobronchial Ultrasound

EBUS uses a small ultrasound probe fitted through a flexible bronchoscope port, and it enhances visualization of the soft tissue of the mediastinum adjacent to the bronchial lumen. Both radial probes, which provide a 360-degree image of the airway and surrounding structures, and convex probes, which provide a 90-degree image, can be used. Soft tissue characteristics of pulmonary nodules, lymph nodes, and tumors can be delineated. This imaging can effectively guide transbronchial FNA to sample pulmonary nodules, tumors, or lymph nodes with greater safety and accuracy. Although primarily used for determining the N staging component of the non–small cell type of lung cancer, EBUS can also help to define the T component if the tumor is adjacent to or approaching the tracheal or bronchial lumen. EBUS allows access to superior and anterior mediastinal lymph nodes and can be combined with EUS access of inferior and posterior mediastinal lymph nodes to allow a more comprehensive sampling of the mediastinum. An advantage of EBUS is that it is a minimally invasive office procedure, but it is not widely available and requires technical training. In terms of pathologic assessment for metastasis, FNA can be performed only with a 22-gauge needle, so comprehensive staging is subject to sampling error. Until convincing randomized trials have compared lymph node sampling by EBUS or EUS with mediastinoscopy for staging non–small cell lung cancer, mediastinoscopy remains the gold standard for N staging of the mediastinum.

Navigational Bronchoscopy

By coupling high-resolution CT imaging with electromagnetic guidance of bronchoscope-delivered biopsy instruments, investigators have sampled more peripheral lung lesions that are inaccessible to conventional methods.[14,15] Lesions that are beyond tertiary bronchioles, and some beyond secondary, are too small to accommodate even small biopsy bronchoscopes. Guiding brushes or biopsy forceps into the distal bronchial tree is assisted somewhat with fluoroscopy, but this is still an almost blind procedure. Real-time, three-dimensional (3D) CT has been coupled to an electromagnetic navigational system (the superDimension bronchus system, superDimension, Ltd., Herzliya, Israel)[14] that can virtually guide the bronchoscopist in sampling peripheral lung lesions. The patient is placed on an electromagnetic board that can define the biopsy probe location in 3D and in real time. The probe's location is then coupled with its anatomic location in a 3D superimposed CT scan map of the patient. The biopsy device is then virtually guided to the sample site. Thus far, only feasibility studies[15] have been performed, which show promise for this new technique as a means to sample peripheral lung lesions heretofore accessible only to surgery or CT-guided biopsy.

Flexible Bronchoscopy

Technique

Most diagnostic bronchoscopy procedures should be performed with an awake patient and with topical anesthesia. When the patient is already intubated or needs general anesthesia for a combined procedure, local anesthesia is not needed. In the outpatient setting, the room should be equipped with monitors for pulse, blood pressure, and continuous pulse oximetry readings.

The size and caliber of the bronchoscope usually depends on the size of the patient and the need for larger working channels if endobronchial intervention is anticipated. The field of vision is generally 80 degrees, and the angle of deflection is usually 160 to 180 degrees. The light source is connected with a flexible cord, and the transmission of light and the resultant resolution are based on the number of flexible fiberoptic bundles. More light, however, results in larger-caliber scopes.

Essential equipment consists of the bronchoscope, a light source, a camera, biopsy tools, suction and irrigation, and a sputum trap. After informed consent has been obtained, the patient is positioned in a seated position so that topical anesthesia (gargled, and spray lidocaine solution) and gentle sedation (intravenous midazolam) can be administered. Either a transnasal or a transoral approach may be used in the awake patient, with the latter being better tolerated. The transnasal approach in the awake patient has the advantage of allowing visualization of the nasal and upper airway.[16] Manipulation of the scope begins with the user holding the handle of the scope in the dominant hand, controlling the shaft with the nondominant hand, and viewing either from an eyepiece or video screen. By manipulating the thumb lever at the scope handle and rotating a taut scope shaft, the tip of the scope can be pointed in all directions. After insertion, the trachea is examined, searching for luminal irregularities. The first landmark is the carina, which should be a sharp bifurcation; any fullness in this area should alert the operator to subcarinal adenopathy or mass involvement of the proximal airway. Orientation is maintained by noting that the membranous trachea is always posterior. The operator then systematically examines all airways to the segmental and subsegmental bronchus level. Digital photography and video are both superb for documenting any disease encountered. This documentation is a useful reference for monitoring disease progression at subsequent procedures or when planning a surgical resection. All pathology should be documented with detailed written descriptions or pictures of the actual findings. Depending on the findings, the surgeon can investigate further with washings, lavage, brushings, and biopsy. Once extracted, the bronchoscope should be irrigated with sterile solution and sent for disinfection.

Complications

In experienced hands, flexible bronchoscopy is very safe. The complication rate reflects the patient's preexisting disease and degree of intervention and therapy. Injudicious suctioning can cause damage to the endobronchial lumen and bleeding, and careless advancement of the scope can disrupt anastomoses and bronchial stump staple lines, dislodge broncholiths or clots, and even cause perforation,[17] all with disastrous consequences. Patients with a history of asthma or bronchospasm should be approached with particular caution, and with appropriate medications at hand. Intubated patients in extremis who manifest refractory hypoxia, elevated airway pressure, or cardiac arrhythmias should undergo bronchoscopy with extreme prejudice only.

Most large series on flexible bronchoscopy cite morbidity rates of 0.05% to 0.1% and a mortality rate of around 0.01%.[18] Morbidity is generally defined as respiratory compromise, symptomatic bradycardia, hypotension, syncope, or arrhythmias. Although manipulation of the instrument may be responsible for some of these manifestations, morbidity is usually related to the administration of and reactivity to the premedication and local anesthesia. Transbronchial FNA, with ultrasound guidance, has a pneumothorax rate of about 5% in most series, and in most cases, this is minor. Significant hemorrhage is also a risk with FNA, because major vessels (e.g., the pulmonary artery) can be inadvertently punctured, but the risk is greatly reduced by Doppler ultrasound.

Rigid Bronchoscopy

Rigid bronchoscopy should be mastered by all thoracic surgeons because it can be life saving in dire situations, and it is a diagnostic and therapeutic intervention that is availed by our specialty alone. Massive hemoptysis, foreign body removal, tracheobronchial obstruction by benign or malignant stricture, airway stenting and dilation, and laser therapy are all best approached with the rigid bronchoscope. This procedure is performed less often than flexible bronchoscopy, because general anesthesia is required, and because it is difficult to become facile with the instrument. However, despite its greater technical difficulty, the rigid scope has several distinct advantages over the flexible scope. First, the rigid scope allows more accurate definition of central airway lesions, and with it the surgeon can palliate these lesions. Second, the rigid scope allows ventilation through its lumen, providing direct control of the airway in the setting of airway disease. Third, the instruments, including suctioning tools, that can be used with the rigid scope are larger and thus more effective than the small instruments developed for use with the flexible scope. Therefore, the rigid scope is more helpful in managing hemoptysis and in foreign body removal.

Massive hemoptysis, defined as 600 mL of blood over 24 hours, mandates urgent rigid bronchoscopy. Once introduced, the airway is controlled. The point of bleeding is then investigated and intervention planned and attempted. Use of a proximal eyepiece allows visualization without compromising ventilation. Rigid bronchoscopy does not obviate the use of the flexible scope; flexible bronchoscopy can be performed through the lumen of the rigid scope to further the examination and possible intervention of the airway disease.

Foreign body extraction is usually technically easier through the rigid scope because of the large caliber of the instrument. Again, airway control is established and the foreign body can be extracted with forceps, or on some occasions with a balloon catheter should the offending mass be lodged in the airway.

Shortcomings of the rigid method include poor visualization of the terminal bronchi, the inability to perform instrumentation and suction with excellent vision, and the need for general anesthesia.

Technique

Elective rigid bronchoscopy is performed on an intubated, paralyzed, and sedated patient. Often, a laryngeal mask airway is used to secure the airway before the intubation. Communication with the anesthesia team concerning the plan and expectations of the procedure is essential to ensuring smooth transitioning between the rigid scope and the endotracheal tube and laryngeal mask airway: adequate sedation and paralysis, and optimal oxygenation via the rigid scope are essential. A shoulder roll is placed under the patient to allow maximal extension of the neck. The rigid scope is introduced with the thumb of the surgeon's nondominant hand braced on the upper incisors and, as when positioning a laryngoscope blade, the scope is advanced around the tongue until the arytenoids and cords are visible. The scope is then delicately insinuated between the cords, a maneuver that is facilitated by the appropriate angle of insertion and by rotating the scope 90 degrees as it is passed between the cords. Once beyond the cords, the scope is rotated back so that its longer lip is placed posteriorly. The side port attachment is then fitted to allow oxygenation via the scope throughout the procedure. At this point, biopsy, foreign body removal, balloon tamponade, YAG laser, and stenting procedures can be executed. A myriad of specialized endobronchial instruments accompany most rigid bronchoscope sets. Should the need arise, modern laparoscopic instruments can be useful for difficult foreign body or biopsy extractions. Passage of the flexible bronchoscope, or videoscope, down the rigid scope provides more magnified viewing of the trachea and bronchi. Measurements for stenting and dilation procedures, as well as for tracheal resection, can be performed accurately with the dual scope configuration. The scope is then withdrawn carefully under direct vision. It is of utmost importance that the scope be stabilized by the operator at all times.

Complications

Although rare, complications of bronchoscopy do occur. Pre-procedure steps include workup of any comorbid cardiac disease or coagulopathy, and careful consideration of the underlying pathology and the possible consequences of bronchoscopic intervention. An essential step to any procedure is the informed consent, which entails educating the patient about the possible complications and the probable effects on the patient.

The risks of rigid bronchoscopy are much more significant than those of flexible bronchoscopy, with the largest series quoting a morbidity of 5.1% and with 1.1% being construed as major.[19] The main reason for the increased risk encountered with rigid bronchoscopy is the greater likelihood that patients selected for this procedure have more complex pathologies and thus require more complex interventional procedures. The increased morbidity also reflects the increased use of the rigid scope for palliative procedures, and the increased risk of subsequent complications.

REFERENCES

1. Fulkerson WJ. Fiberoptic bronchoscopy. *N Engl J Med* 1984;**311**:511-5.
2. Linder TE, Simmen D, Stool SE. The history of endoscopy. *Arch Otolaryngol Head Neck Surg* 1997;**123**:1161-3.
3. Graham D, Schwartz J, Cain G, Gyorkey F. Prospective evaluation of biopsy number in the diagnosis of esophageal and gastric carcinoma. *Gastroenterology* 1982;**82**:228-31.
4. Winawer S, Sherlock P, Belladonna J, et al. Endoscopic brush cytology in esophageal cancer. *JAMA* 1975;**232**:1358.
5. Zargar S, Khuroo M, Jan G, et al. Prospective comparison of the value of brushings before and after biopsy in the endoscopic diagnosis of gastroesophageal malignancy. *Acta Cytol* 1991;**35**:549-52.
6. Ferguson MK, Migliore M, Staszak VM, Little AG. Early evaluation and therapy for caustic esophageal injury. *Am J Surg* 1989;**157**(1):116-20.
7. Enns R, Branch MS. Management of esophageal perforation after therapeutic upper gastrointestinal endoscopy. *Gastrointest Endosc* 1998;**47**(3):318-20.
8. Pasricha PJ, Fleischer DE, Kalloo AN. Endoscopic perforations of the upper digestive tract: A review of their pathogenesis, prevention, and management. *Gastroenterology* 1994;**106**(3):787-802.
9. Botet JF, Lightdale CJ, Zauber AG, et al. Preoperative staging of esophageal cancer: Comparison of endoscopic US and dynamic CT. *Radiology* 1991;**181**(2):419-25.
10. Wu LF, Wang BZ, Feng JL, et al. Preoperative TN staging of esophageal cancer: Comparison of miniprobe ultrasonography, spiral CT and MRI. *World J Gastroenterol* 2003;**9**(2):219-24.
11. Parmar KS, Zwischenberger JB, Reeves AL, Waxman I. Clinical impact of endoscopic ultrasound-guided fine needle aspiration of celiac axis lymph nodes (M1a disease) in esophageal cancer. *Ann Thorac Surg* 2002;**73**(3):916-20.
12. Sackner MA. Bronchofiberoscopy. *Am Rev Respir Dis* 1975;**111**:62-88.
13. Lloveras JJ, Lecuyer I, Dider A. Benefits of bronchoscopy and bronchoalveolar lavage in the diagnosis of pneumonitis is transplant recipients. *Transplant Proc* 1993;**25**:2293.
14. Schwarz Y, Mehta AC, Ernst A, Herth F, Engel A, Besser D, Becker HD. Electromagnetic navigation during flexible bronchoscopy. *Respiration* 2003;**70**:516-22.
15. Schwarz Y, Greif J, Becker H, Ernst A, Mehta A. Real-time electromagnetic navigation bronchoscopy to peripheral lung lesions using overlaid CT images: The first human study. *Chest* April 2006;**129**(4):988-94.
16. Harrell JH. Transnasal approach for fiberoptic bronchoscopy. *Chest* 1978;**73**:704-6.
17. Poe RH, Ortiz C, Israel RH. Sensitivity, specificity, and predictive values of bronchoscopy in neoplasm metastatic to the lung. *Chest* 1985;**88**:84-8.
18. Pue CA, Pacht ER. Complications of fiberoptic bronchoscopy at a university hospital. *Chest* 1995;**107**:430-2.
19. Lukonsky GI, Ovchinnikov AA, Bilal A. Complications of bronchoscopy. *Chest* 1981;**79**:316.

CHAPTER 6
Endoscopic Therapies for Thoracic Diseases

Sébastien Gilbert, Benny Weksler, Hiran C. Fernando, and James D. Luketich

Photodynamic Therapy
   Definition and Mechanism of Action
   Technique
   Contraindications
   Lung Cancer
      Curative Intent
      Palliative Intent
   Barrett's Esophagus and Esophageal Cancer
      Curative Intent
      Palliative Intent
Stents
   Expandable Metal Stents
   Silicone-Based Stents

Technique
   Expandable Metal Stents
   Silicone-Based Stents
Indications
   Benign Airway Strictures
   Malignant Airway Strictures
   Benign Esophageal Strictures
   Malignant Esophageal Strictures
Laser Ablation of Endoluminal Tumors
   Airway
   Esophagus
Brachytherapy
Comparison of Palliative Endoscopic Therapies

Evolving Endoscopic Treatment Modalities for Benign Esophageal Diseases
   Zenker's Diverticulum
      Open Approaches to Zenker's Diverticulum
      Transoral Endoscopic Stapling
   Gastroesophageal Reflux
      Radiofrequency Therapy to the Lower Esophageal Sphincter
      Injection of Biopolymers at the Gastroesophageal Junction
      Endoscopic Plication of the Gastroesophageal Junction

The first recorded bronchoscopic intervention is attributed to Gustav Killian, who in 1897 removed a piece of pork bone from the right main-stem bronchus with an esophagoscope.[1] A few decades later, Chevalier Jackson was instrumental in the advancement of the field of rigid endoscopy of the airway and esophagus.[1] Advancements in endoscopic technology have led to safer and more effective alternatives to surgery in nonoperative candidates. This chapter focuses on endoscopic esophageal and bronchial interventions, such as photodynamic therapy, radiofrequency ablation, stenting, laser ablation, and brachytherapy. Evolving endoscopic procedures for benign esophageal diseases (Zenker's diverticulum and gastroesophageal reflux) are also discussed.

PHOTODYNAMIC THERAPY

Definition and Mechanism of Action

The basic tenant of photodynamic therapy (PDT) is the accumulation in target cells of a photosensitizing substance that is activated by light of a specific spectrum, resulting in selective tissue destruction. Photosensitizers relevant to the thoracic surgeon include purified hematoporphyrin derivatives (porfimer sodium or Photofrin), chlorines (temoporfin or *m*-tetrahydroxyphenyl chlorin [*m*-THPC]), and 5-aminolevulinic acid (5-ALA). The optimal wavelengths of light absorption are 630 nm for porfimer sodium and 5-ALA and 652 nm for *m*-THPC.

Photosensitizers accumulate in all cells of the body. However, after 1 to 4 days, higher concentrations are found within tumor cells and their interstitium. Altered lymphatic drainage, neovascularization, and increased cellular proliferation are some of the mechanisms hypothesized to be responsible for this phenomenon. Laser light delivered directly to cancer cells harboring the photosensitizer triggers a series of events culminating in cell destruction. When cells are bombarded with photons of a wavelength specific to the photosensitizer used, the absorbed energy acts as a catalyst in the formation of highly reactive oxygen species (e.g., superoxide anions, peroxide anions, singlet oxygen). The primary cellular targets of photodamage are cellular membranes, amino acids, and nucleosides.

Technique

The first step in PDT is the administration of the photosensitizer. Porfimer sodium (1.5 to 2.0 mg/kg) and *m*-THPC are injected intravenously; 5-ALA is given orally. Despite an improved side effect profile and increased tumor specificity, 5-ALA has yet to gain widespread clinical acceptance and has limited applications in thoracic surgery.[2,3] At the current oral dosage, 5-ALA PDT produces necrosis only to a depth of 1 mm. Higher 5-ALA doses cannot be used because of severe side effects (e.g., nausea, vomiting, transient elevation of liver enzymes). On the other hand, *m*-THPC is 100 times more photoactive than porfimer sodium and has a shorter elimination half-life; however, it is not yet approved for clinical use in the United States.

PDT is considered effective and is indicated for tumors with a significant endoluminal component. The most commonly used photosensitizer is Photofrin, which has a depth of penetration of approximately 5 mm. It can be given in the outpatient setting, 1 to 4 days before endoscopic light application. Education of the patient is essential to minimize complications related to photosensitivity. All bright light and sunlight exposure must be avoided initially. Patients remain photosensitive for a period of 4 to 8 weeks, after which they can be gradually reexposed to sunlight.

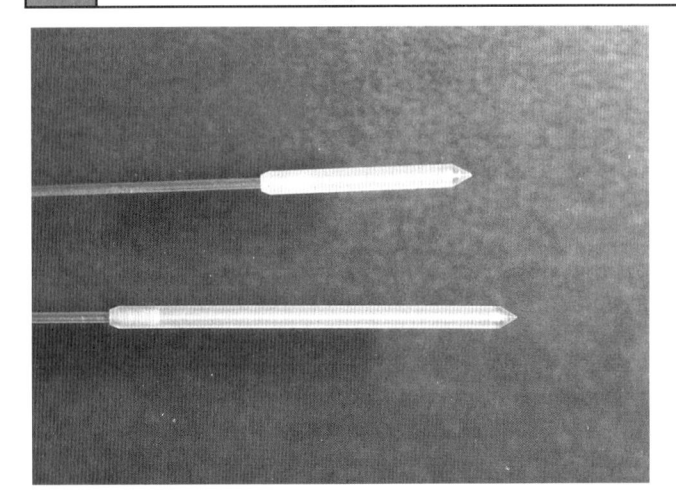

Figure 6–1
PDT diffuser fibers, 2.5 cm and 5 cm.

Our preference has been to use conscious sedation and flexible endoscopy in most cases. A cylindrical diffuser fiber is used to deliver light therapy to the tumor. The sizes used are 1 cm, 2.5 cm, and 5 cm (Fig. 6-1). The diffuser fiber is placed alongside the tumor. If this is not possible because of occlusion of the lumen, the tumor can be impaled with the probe. Multiple light illumination cycles may be needed, depending on the length of the tumor relative to the length of the probe. The diffuser must be positioned to minimize light delivery to normal tissues. Endoscopy is repeated at 48 hours and sometimes a third time after another 48 hours. During the repeated endoscopic procedures, necrotic debris is removed by irrigation and suction. Usually, further light treatments are delivered to the tumor at the time of repeated endoscopy.

In many cases, PDT can be performed in the outpatient setting. However, caution should be exercised in treating the central airways. Perioperative edema and necrotic tissue may temporarily worsen obstruction. We frequently begin the procedure by debulking the tumor with use of a rigid bronchoscope to "core out" the airway. It has been our preference to treat such tumors in the inpatient setting.

Contraindications

Contraindications to PDT are few. Patients suffering from porphyria or those who are allergic to porphyrins cannot receive porfimer sodium. PDT is contraindicated in the presence of an esophagorespiratory fistula or in tumors eroding into a major blood vessel. PDT is not recommended for the treatment of obstruction caused by extraluminal compression.

Lung Cancer

Curative Intent

PDT is approved for the treatment of small proximal endobronchial tumors. These small central tumors are rare, although some centers with active early screening programs, such as sputum cytology or light-induced fluorescence bronchoscopy, may encounter these more frequently.[4] The results of PDT for these small lesions should be compared with the results of surgical resection. The central location of these tumors may necessitate complex airway reconstructions. PDT may be a suitable alternative to resection in patients who are not candidates for surgery. In most cases, these small endobronchial tumors are occult to standard radiologic imaging, such as chest radiography, computed tomography, and positron emission tomography scanning. Assessment of response is difficult and requires bronchoscopic evaluation. It is unclear whether a complete response is the result of tumor eradication or merely reflects the limitations of surveillance techniques. Superficially spreading tumors (<3 cm^2) and small endobronchial tumors (<1 cm^2) are best suited for PDT. Initial complete response can be expected in 65% (<3 cm^2) to 85% (<1 cm^2) of superficial cancers and in 30% (>0.5 cm nodule) to 92% (<0.5 cm nodule) of nodular cancers.[5,6] Long-term response rates (i.e., >1 year) vary between 30% and 80%.[5-9] At 5 years of follow-up, complete response rates of up to 29% to 66% have been reported.[5,7]

In a study of 21 operative candidates treated initially with two courses of PDT, 52% (11 of 21) were free of tumor at 1 year.[7] Curative PDT failed in the remaining 48% (10 of 21), and they were offered surgery; 8 consented. Of the 11 responders, 9 (9 of 21; 43%) did not require surgery (mean follow-up, 68 months), and 2 were operated on for a second primary lung cancer. It is noteworthy that of the patients who eventually underwent resection, 30% were found to have N1 disease, supporting the role of resection, when possible. Our policy has been to reserve PDT for patients with significant comorbid factors or those who refuse pulmonary resection. In this group of patients, PDT is an excellent modality with an expected 1-year survival of 80%.[10] In our initial experience of treating 10 superficial cancers, a complete response was seen in 70% at a follow-up of 30 months.[8] In other prospective series, 80% to 93% of nonsurgical candidates were alive at 5 years of follow-up.[5,11]

Palliative Intent

Resection should continue to be the main therapy for early-stage non–small cell lung cancer. Only a relatively small number of patients will be candidates for PDT with curative intent. A much larger group of patients with advanced lung cancers may benefit from palliative PDT. In this situation, the therapeutic goal should be symptomatic relief and preservation of quality of life and functional status. Most of these patients will complain of dyspnea related to endobronchial obstruction or with hemoptysis.

A cohort of 175 patients with endobronchial non–small cell lung cancer treated with PDT was observed prospectively for a period of 14 years.[11] Most patients had squamous cell carcinoma (89.3%), and treatment by conventional modalities, such as chemotherapy, radiotherapy, laser ablation, and surgery, had failed in 73.1%. The mean number of treatments was 2.8 per patient. Stage had the most significant impact on survival after multivariate analysis. Poor performance status (i.e., Karnofsky performance status < 50) had a negative impact on outcome only in advanced-stage tumors (IIIa-IV). However, patients with a low Karnofsky performance status (<50) secondary to pulmonary symptoms still derived benefit from PDT. Prolonged survival (12 to 37 months) was observed in 66% of stage IIIa-IV patients with poor performance. The median survival for the entire group was 7 months. Of the 44 patients with stage IV disease, 21% survived 12 months or longer.

Our initial experience with palliative PDT involved 44 lung cancer patients with symptoms related to obstruction and hemoptysis.[10] Thirteen patients required a second treatment course at a mean of 2.3 months for recurrent symptoms. There were no fatalities, and 82% of treatments were performed without complications. Hemoptysis was effectively palliated in 90% of treatment courses. Obstruction was successfully palliated in 59% of treatments. Median survival was 2.3 months. PDT is also effective in palliating hemoptysis and dyspnea in patients with endobronchial metastases from nonpulmonary malignant neoplasms.[12] An example of a patient who was treated for a complete lobar obstruction is demonstrated in Figures 6-2 through 6-6.

In a randomized prospective study, PDT was compared with standard laser techniques for inoperable non–small cell lung cancer.[13] The bronchoscopic response rate (PDT, 38.5%; laser, 23.5%) and symptomatic improvement at 1 month were equivalent in each group. PDT provided significantly longer lasting relief (50 days versus 38 days) and improved median survival (265 days versus 95 days) compared with laser resection. However, this finding may be explained in part by the lower proportion of advanced-stage tumors in the PDT group.

In general, PDT is well tolerated with minimal morbidity. In the first 77 treatments that we performed for endobronchial disease, 82% were uneventful. Complications included respiratory failure (7.8%), pleural effusion (1.3%), and sunburn (5.2%). All bright light and sunlight exposure must be avoided initially. Patients remain photosensitive for a period of 4 to 8 weeks, after which they can be gradually reexposed to sunlight.[14,15] Inadvertent direct sunlight exposure has been reported to cause first- and second-degree burns in up to 10% of patients.[35] The restrictions imposed by photosensitivity and their potential impact on quality of life should be considered before treatment. Immediate postprocedure mortality for lung and esophageal PDT (30-day) ranges from 2.6% to 7.1%.[11,13-15]

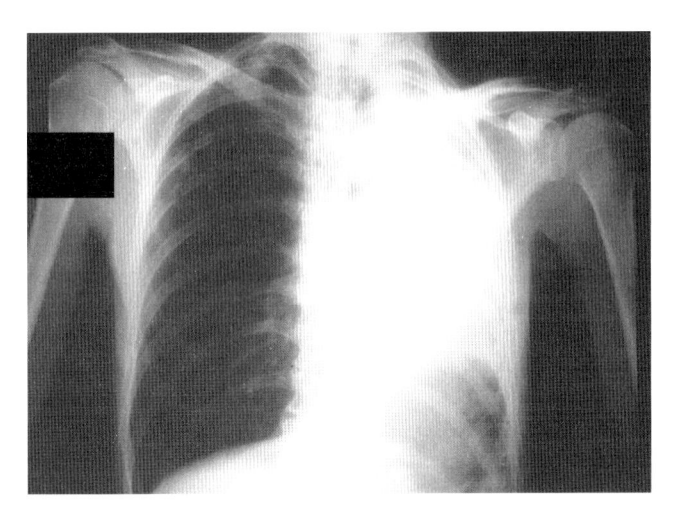

Figure 6–2
Radiographic picture of lung cancer obstructing the left main-stem bronchus before PDT.

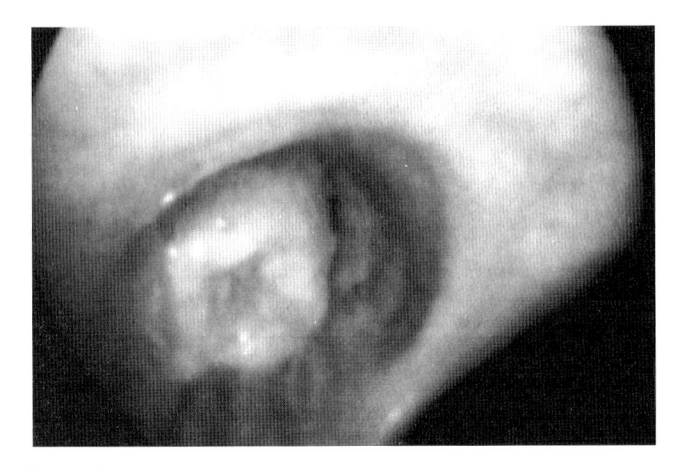

Figure 6–3
Bronchoscopic picture before PDT.

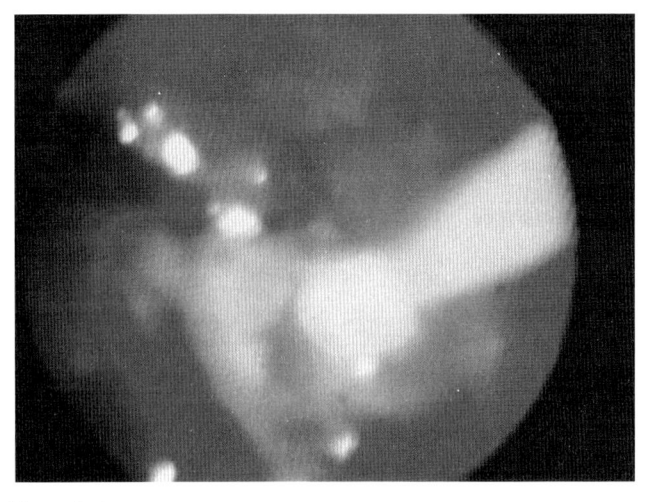

Figure 6–4
Bronchoscopic picture during PDT.

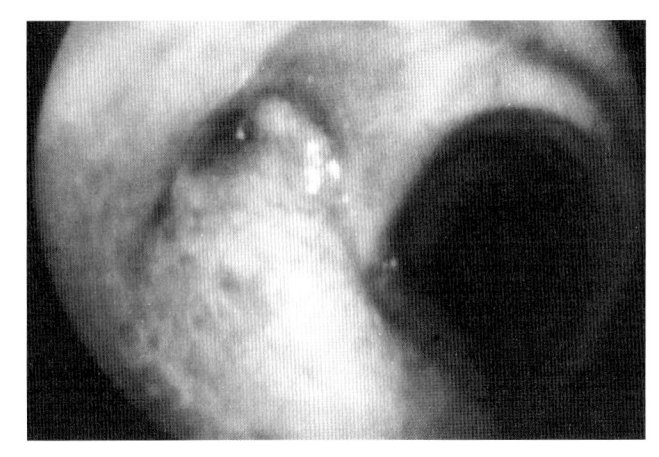

Figure 6–5
Bronchoscopic picture after PDT.

Barrett's Esophagus and Esophageal Cancer

Curative Intent

The management of high-grade dysplasia associated with Barrett's esophagus is controversial. Most surgeons advocate esophagectomy because of the associated risks of occult malignant disease and lymph node metastases.[16] On the other

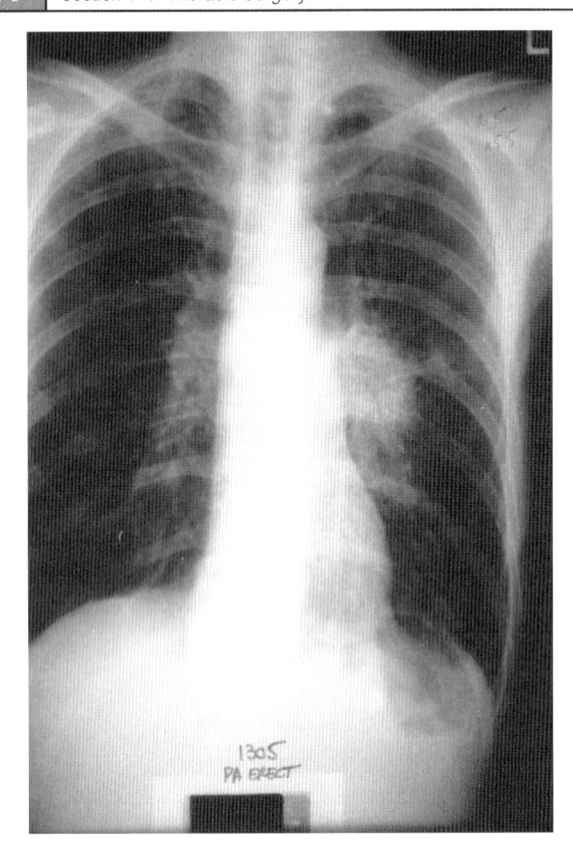

Figure 6–6
Radiographic picture after PDT.

hand, concerns related to the morbidity and mortality of esophagectomy have led some clinicians to advocate alternative approaches, such as surveillance or mucosal ablation.[17] In our experience, we have reported good results with a minimally invasive esophageal resection for patients with Barrett's esophagus and high-grade dysplasia.[18,19] Mucosal ablative methods include laser ablation, argon plasma coagulation, radiofrequency ablation, and PDT.[20-23] All these techniques attempt to eradicate Barrett's epithelium with the hope that it will be replaced by squamous epithelium. Unfortunately, in some instances, islands of columnar epithelium may recur under a normal-appearing squamous epithelial layer.[24] This problem is addressed by other endoscopic techniques, such as endoscopic mucosal resection or endoscopic submucosal dissection, whereby the esophageal mucosa is actually resected piecemeal. An in-depth discussion of endoscopic resection techniques is beyond the scope of this chapter.

PDT is arguably the most established of these ablative techniques. In a large single-institution study, PDT was combined with the neodymium:yttrium-aluminum-garnet (Nd:YAG) laser to treat 73 patients with high-grade dysplasia and 14 with low-grade dysplasia.[25] All patients were observed endoscopically for 12 months. Regression to low-grade dysplasia or no dysplasia was observed in 88% of high-grade dysplasia cases and 93% of low-grade dysplasia cases. Complete eradication of Barrett's epithelium occurred in only 9% of patients after PDT alone. In focusing on the PDT-treated area, a 49% eradication rate was reported. The addition of laser ablation to residual areas of Barrett's epithelium increased the eradication rate to 87%. This group used a transparent centering balloon for PDT delivery, which is no longer available commercially. In a prospective randomized multicenter international trial, omeprazole (20 mg twice daily) was compared with omeprazole plus PDT for the treatment of Barrett's esophagus with high-grade dysplasia.[26] The trial was initially planned for 2 years. However, at the end of 2 years, 65% of the omeprazole-alone group and 59% of the PDT group were enrolled in a long-term follow-up study. At 5 years, the addition of PDT with porfimer sodium to proton pump inhibitor therapy resulted in a 38% increase in Barrett's high-grade dysplasia eradication rate, a 14% decrease in the incidence of invasive carcinoma, and a longer time to progression to cancer. PDT with a centering balloon was the only endoscopic modality used to ablate Barrett's mucosa.

PDT can also be used to treat early-stage esophageal tumors (T1-T2) in patients who refuse or are not candidates for surgical resection. In a group of patients that included mostly T1 tumors (12 of 13), regression to Barrett's esophagus with low-grade dysplasia or without dysplasia was observed in 77% of patients (10 of 13).[25] At our center, PDT with curative intent is reserved for patients with high operative risk. All others undergo minimally invasive esophagectomy.[18] We have reviewed our institutional experience, from 1997 to 2005, using PDT for patients with high-grade dysplasia or superficial esophageal cancer.[27] A total of 50 patients, who either refused or were unfit for surgery, had PDT with curative intent. The majority of patients (70%) had high-grade dysplasia or small (≤T1) tumors. At a median follow-up of 28 months, 32% of patients were alive without recurrence, 30% were alive with recurrent disease, and 38% were deceased from cancer or other causes. The patients with recurrences were re-treated with PDT. There was no procedure-related mortality, and the stricture rate was 42%. Although these results are clearly inferior to esophageal resection, endoscopic ablation appears to be a suitable treatment option for nonsurgical candidates. In another cohort of 28 patients with high-grade dysplasia treated with minimally invasive esophagectomy, 96% remained free of recurrence at 13 months.[18] These results were corroborated by other investigators who have observed excellent long-term survival (100%) after esophagectomy for high-grade dysplasia.[28]

In the treatment of Barrett's esophagus with high-grade dysplasia, PDT is well tolerated with usually transient side effects, such as nausea, regurgitation, constipation, odynophagia, dysphagia, weight loss (average of 6 kg), and noncardiac chest pain.[29,30] Other complications include stricture, tumor growth below the PDT-induced scarring, and Barrett's esophagus and tumor recurrence.[31] In our experience, approximately 30% of patients with high-grade dysplasia undergoing PDT will develop an esophageal stricture.[27] Stricturing is minimized by decreasing the intensity of light therapy compared with doses used for larger tumors.

Another emerging endoscopic treatment modality for patients with Barrett's esophagus is radiofrequency (RF) ablation. The components of the system include a sizing balloon (18 to 34 mm), a 3-cm balloon-based bipolar RF electrode, and a dedicated RF generator. The sizing balloon is used to ensure proper contact between the balloon electrode and the esophageal mucosa. The RF mucosal ablation is achieved by using a power of 300 W to deliver 10 to 12 joules/cm^2. The coagulum is then removed from the esophageal surface by irrigation and suction. The maximum ablation depth is 1 mm, which translates to a depth of injury that is superficial to the muscularis mucosa.[32] The depth of injury is highly reproducible and has been confirmed in the human esophagus. In addition to the balloon electrode, there is an RF ablation device that can be attached to the end of a flexible esophagoscope and used to ablate focal areas of esophageal mucosa. Encouraging results have been published showing complete eradication of Barrett's mucosa and intramucosal carcinoma when RF ablation was used in combination with endoscopic mucosal resection.[33] However, studies involving larger cohorts of patients with longer follow-up time have not yet been published.

Palliative Intent

Stenting of the esophagus is probably the most commonly used modality to palliate dysphagia.[34] However, PDT offers some advantages in certain clinical situations. In addition to relieving obstruction, PDT can control or prevent bleeding from the tumor. It may also prevent the globus sensation associated with stents in the proximal esophagus and the reflux symptoms observed with stents bridging the gastroesophageal junction. PDT is a potential alternative to stenting for endoluminal cancers in both of these locations.

PDT has been compared with laser ablation in a randomized trial. PDT was equivalent to laser ablation for malignant dysphagia and was associated with a lower rate of perforation (PDT, 1%; laser, 7%).[35] We reviewed our experience with PDT in 215 patients suffering from obstructing esophageal cancer.[36] The most common pathologic process was adenocarcinoma (83%). The distal esophagus was involved in 71% of cases. Dysphagia improved in 85% of patients, and bleeding was successfully controlled in 90%. Stenting was subsequently required in 24% of patients. As expected, median survival was poor at 4.9 months; however, effective palliation was provided to these unfortunate patients. In another prospective series of 77 patients for whom conventional therapy had failed or who were deemed unfit for surgery, investigators reported a median survival of 6.3 months after PDT.[14] The only significant predictor of mortality was clinical stage. Photosensitivity appears to be an acceptable tradeoff in these patients. In one study using satisfaction questionnaires, patients reported that the ability to swallow food was more important than the limitations of photosensitivity.[29] In most cases, the potential benefits of PDT far outweigh the risk of complications.

In patients with obstructing aerodigestive tumors, PDT may result in adverse events. Esophageal strictures (4.8% to 5.2%), perforation (0% to 9.1%), and esophagorespiratory fistulas (0% to 5.2%) are among the most serious PDT-related complications.[7,14,37-39] Esophageal perforation and fistula are probably best treated by esophageal stenting. Other factors contributing to the mortality rate and risk of esophageal perforation include the generally poor performance status of this particular group of patients and the fact that some patients with obstructing tumors receive concurrent radiation therapy and chemotherapy.

STENTS

Malignant endoluminal obstruction and extraluminal compression by enlarged lymph nodes or tumor are common indications for stenting of the airway or esophagus. The two major types of stents used in thoracic surgery are expandable metal stents and silicone-based stents.

Expandable Metal Stents

Expandable metal stents are constructed with cobalt alloys (Wallstent, Schneider), stainless steel (Gianturco, Cook), or a nickel-titanium alloy referred to as nitinol (EsophaCoil, Medtronics; Ultraflex, Microvasive). These materials are resistant to corrosion and are biologically inert, even in patients allergic to nickel. The wire stents can be woven (Wallstent), knitted (Ultraflex), or bent into a zigzag (Gianturco) or coil (EsophaCoil) configuration. The stent design influences its retraction properties (i.e., shortening). Retraction percentage is highest with the coil configuration and lowest with the zigzag configuration. The shape memory characteristics of the materials allow the stent to reexpand to its original tubular shape even when it is compressed into a delivery system. The available systems can deploy the stent from the proximal end, the center, or the distal end. Proximal delivery is better suited for proximal strictures, and distal delivery is best for strictures of the gastroesophageal junction. Expandable metal stents can also be partially covered with polyurethane or silicone (e.g., Alimaxx-E, Alveolus; Polyflex, Microvasive; Ultraflex). Covered designs help reduce tumor ingrowth but at the same time have a propensity for migration.[40] The wide range of available diameters and lengths allows expandable metal stents to fit most upper aerodigestive strictures.

Silicone-Based Stents

Silicone-based stents are made of silicone rubber (Silastic, Dow Corning), a ubiquitous component of industrial, household, and medical equipment. Celestin esophageal tubes have fallen out of favor because of the need for an open gastrotomy for anchoring and the higher complication rate in comparison with expandable metal stents.[41]

Flanged (Hood, Hood Laboratories, Pembroke, MA) or studded (Dumon, Bryan Corp., Woburn, MA) cylindrical silicone stents are used in the trachea or bronchi. T-, Y-, and T-Y–shaped silicone stents are also available to treat tracheal and proximal tracheobronchial strictures. If a silicone stent has to be shortened to fit the patient's airway, the manufacturer can provide a customized replacement on request.

Technique

Expandable Metal Stents

The procedure can be performed either under conscious sedation or under general anesthesia. The stricture is identified endoscopically and measured. Esophageal stents are available in a wide range of lengths (60 to 150 mm), but in contrast to airway stents, most have a similar maximal internal diameter (17 to 23 mm). If the opening of the stricture is too small to accept the endoscope, the lumen may require dilation and laser ablation before length can be assessed accurately. Fluoroscopy is then used to mark the location of the stricture on the patient's skin. This is done by use of two radiopaque markers (e.g., small stylets, paper clips) that are aligned with the tip of the endoscope when the endoscope is positioned at the proximal and distal edges of the stricture. Alternatively, some clinicians prefer to inject the submucosa at the proximal and distal ends of the tumor with a radiopaque liquid (Conray). Once the measurement of the tumor length is completed, the proper stent is selected. In general, we use an 18- to 23-mm-diameter stent that is 1 to 2 cm longer than the stricture to avoid crimping and infolding of the ends. A guide wire is passed through the stricture, and the endoscope is withdrawn. Under fluoroscopic control, the delivery system is inserted over the guide wire through the stricture and aligned with the skin or mucosal markers. The stent is deployed and expands within the lumen. Proper positioning and deployment are confirmed fluoroscopically and endoscopically. A postprocedure chest radiograph (in all cases) and barium esophagogram (in esophageal cases) are obtained. Expandable metal stents are popular, as they are easier to insert and do not require expertise in rigid bronchoscopy. Silicone stents are more challenging to place but may be less problematic in the long term. They are preferable for patients with benign strictures.

Silicone-Based Stents

Unless the patient has a tracheal stoma, rigid bronchoscopy is needed to insert a silicone-based stent. A chest tube and the stent are passed over a rigid scope in sequence. The chest tube serves as a pusher to deliver the stent over the rigid scope. For Y-shaped stents, the right main-stem bronchus limb is invaginated and the rigid scope passed through the left main-stem bronchus limb. After it is positioned, the scope is pulled back within the tracheal limb, and biopsy forceps are used to push out the right-sided limb. An alternative technique is to guide the right-sided limb into the right main-stem bronchus by use of a Fogarty catheter while positioning the proximal portion of the stent endoscopically. A complete technical description of rigid endoscopic stent insertion has already been published.[42] Table 6-1 compares some of the features of silicone and metal stents.

Indications

The recommended definitive treatment of benign airway strictures is surgical resection. Stenting is indicated for strictured or malacic airways not amenable to resection or in nonsurgical candidates in whom dilation or laser resection has failed. Stenting may also be used as a bridge to surgery in patients needing time for their general condition to improve. It should be clear that stenting of benign strictures is suboptimal therapy, as 40% of patients will need re-intervention.[43]

Malignant airway strictures, especially those caused by extrinsic tumor compression, can be managed by stenting. In the esophagus, stents are indicated for obstruction or esophagorespiratory fistula associated with malignant disease.

Benign Airway Strictures

Stenting of benign airway strictures should be regarded as second-line therapy, reserved for situations in which surgical resection is not possible. In comparison with the shorter survival expected with malignant strictures, patients with benign strictures live longer and require further intervention over time. For this reason, silicone stents are recommended. Previous experience with silicone stents for benign strictures in nonoperative candidates has been relatively good.[44,45] Of 112 patients with T stents, only 5 (4.5%) required removal for obstructive problems, and 85% were managed successfully for periods of 3 months to more than 5 years.[45] In another case series, 94% of patients with benign strictures had successful palliation of obstruction.[43] Only 3 of 54 silicone stents (5.6%) needed removal or replacement for migration or compression, and the mortality rate was 12.5% at 4 years of follow-up. Other studies involving smaller numbers of patients (6 to 22) reported symptomatic and spirometric improvement after stenting.[46-48] Only one group acknowledged that granulation tissue is a

Table 6–1
Characteristics of Silicone and Expandable Metal Stents

Stent Type	Description	Method of Insertion	Pros	Cons
Silicone based				
Internal	Made of Silastic rubber Straight or Y shaped Studded (Dumon) Flanged (Hood) Silicone mesh with outer polyester coating (Polyflex)	Rigid endoscopy	Resistance to lateral compression Prevents ingrowth Easier to remove	Eliminates mucociliary clearance (airway) Propensity for mucus plugging (airway) Propensity for dislodgment (airway and esophagus)
External	T or T-Y shaped	Rigid bronchoscopy or per tracheal stoma	Maintains tracheal stoma Tracheal port allows suction Prolonged relief of dyspnea in nonoperative candidates Custom-fitted	Cosmesis Regular maintenance (irrigation, suction)
Expandable metal				
Internal, partially or fully covered or noncovered	Nickel-titanium (Ultraflex) Cobalt-steel (Wallstent) Steel (Gianturco) Fully covered (Alimaxx-E, Aero)	Flexible endoscopy	Easy to insert Adapt to irregularly shaped stricture Potentially removable (fully covered)	Weaker expansile force Granulation Allow ingrowth of tumor (noncovered) Nonremovable (noncovered)

common finding (up to 80% of patients), which may lead to removal in 20% of cases.[48]

Our experience supports the use of silicone-based stents over expandable metal stents for benign strictures. In a cohort of 36 patients, re-intervention was necessary in 61% of patients at a mean of 6 months. Nd:YAG lasering was required to ablate granulation in a significantly higher number of patients with metal stents compared with silicone stents. For every five expandable metal stents inserted, one had to be removed for complications. Extirpation of metal stents required thoracotomy in 33% of cases. Despite their relative ease of insertion, expandable metal stents should probably be avoided in nonsurgical candidates with benign airway strictures. A newer silicone-based stent (Polyflex) may be a reasonable temporizing measure. It may be useful in benign strictures associated with inflammation, in which case luminal patency can be maintained while airway remodeling and fibrosis take place. Although the stent is made of silicone, the outside polyester mesh coating may render removal difficult.

Malignant Airway Strictures

Because most patients with malignant airway obstruction usually have a limited survival from the time of stenting, the emphasis should be placed on preserving quality of life more than on the particular type of stent used. Surgeons familiar with silicone stents have achieved relief of dyspnea in 87% to 94% of patients.[43,49] Complications, including migration and occlusion, occurred in 12.5% to 23.1% of stents placed. Mortality was 68.7% at a mean interval of 7.6 months.[49] Polyurethane-covered expandable metal stents can also provide significant improvement in dyspnea and Karnofsky score.[50] However, up to 55.6% of patients experience complications, including stent migration in 22.2%.[50] Although covered stents prevent tumor ingrowth, they have a propensity for dislodgment.

In malignant airway obstruction, stenting is part of a multidisciplinary approach to palliation. In the majority of the studies discussed before, patients received chemotherapy or radiation therapy in addition to stenting. The importance of adjuvant therapy has been highlighted in a prospective trial.[51] In 22 patients with tracheobronchial strictures treated by stenting, 50% eventually had the stent removed after appropriate radiation therapy and chemotherapy regimens.

We recently reviewed 53 cases in which expandable stents were used to treat tracheobronchial obstruction.[52] Concurrent interventions included balloon dilation (29%), Nd:YAG laser (29%), PDT (23%), rigid bronchoscopy with débridement (15%), and brachytherapy (2%). Bronchoscopic patency was achieved in 92% of patients. Radiographic improvement was noted in 46% of patients with lung collapse. Re-intervention was required in 19 patients (36%) for obstruction by mucus plugging or granulation tissue. The median post-stenting survival was relatively short at 41 days.

Benign Esophageal Strictures

In benign esophageal strictures, routine use of stents cannot be recommended in light of a 41% rate of stent-induced restenosis and almost uniform (91%) recurrence of dysphagia.[53,54] In some selected cases when an anastomotic stricture is recalcitrant to repeated endoscopic dilations, insertion of an esophageal stent that is potentially removable (Alimaxx E, Polyflex) may be an acceptable option. It has even been suggested that this approach may be as effective clinically and less costly than repeated endoscopic dilations.[55] We have reported our initial experience with removable esophageal stents (Polyflex) to manage at least 25 patients with benign esophageal strictures, including those associated with an anastomotic leak after esophagectomy.[56] Although dysphagia was significantly improved after stenting, distal migration was a significant problem that occurred in more than two thirds of the patients. Stenting failed to seal anastomotic leaks and malignant tracheoesophageal fistula in 38%. It is hoped that future changes in removable esophageal stent design will address the significant problem of migration.

Malignant Esophageal Strictures

Depending on the referral pattern, up to 80% of malignant esophageal tumors will be inoperable at the time of diagnosis. Endoscopic palliation with laser or stents assumes a preponderant role in providing relief from dysphagia to many of these patients. During the past decade, advances in expandable stent technology have led to smaller, more flexible delivery systems that are easier to manipulate than their silicone counterpart. These attributes often allow successful stent deployment with minimal or no endoscopic dilation, thereby minimizing the risk of perforation.

Both silicone-based and mesh wire stents are susceptible to tumor overgrowth above and below the stent, leading to recurrence of esophageal obstruction. In addition, ingrowth of tumor through noncovered mesh wire interstices can occur. In the absence of an esophagorespiratory fistula, the decision to use a covered stent is influenced by the potential for recurrent obstruction by tumor ingrowth and the likelihood of stent migration. When tumor overgrowth or ingrowth occurs, therapeutic modalities including PDT, laser, and further stenting (i.e., placement of a stent within a stent) may be of additional palliative benefit.[34]

Few studies have compared silicone and metal stents in a prospective randomized fashion.[41,57] In comparable groups of patients, technical success (95% to 100%), improvement in dysphagia (91% to 100%), and the need for re-intervention were similar regardless of stent type. However, the use of silicone stents was associated with a higher rate of complications (43% to 47% for silicone stents versus 0% to 16% for metal stents) and a longer hospital stay (silicone, 6 to 12 days; metal, 4 to 5 days). Even though 30-day mortality was not significantly different (silicone, 29%; metal, 14%), death as a result of stent insertion occurred only in the silicone stent group.[41] Despite a higher purchase price, expandable metal stents were found to be more cost-effective because of shorter hospitalization and lower complication rates.[41]

At the University of Pittsburgh, a review of 100 stented patients demonstrated relief of dysphagia in 85% with a low probability of perforation (0.8%) and no fatalities.[34] Reasons for initial stent failure were inability to resume oral diet, intractable reflux and pain, bulky tumors resulting in inadequate stent expansion, and inadequate stent position. Sixteen stents were placed in patients undergoing neoadjuvant therapy before esophagectomy. Supplemental enteral or intravenous nutrition was not necessary in 88% ($n = 14$) of those patients. At the time of esophagectomy, dissection of the periesophageal planes was more difficult, but no postoperative complications could be directly attributed to preoperative stenting. Patients receiving chemotherapy or radiation therapy at the time of stenting may be prone to perforation or fistulization.[34,58,59] Although this has not been evaluated in controlled trials, alternatives to stenting should be considered in this subgroup of patients. Fully covered esophageal stents may be a better choice in this situation. These stents may be used for temporary relief of dysphagia and can provide the necessary time window for chemotherapy or radiation therapy to take effect. In other large series of patients undergoing stenting (≥100 patients), placement was successful, and improvement of dysphagia was observed in 90% to 100%.[60-64] Patients were stented with a mortality of 0% to 2.5% and a complication rate of 20% to 41%. These findings lend additional support to the use of stents as a relatively safe and effective method of palliation for obstructing esophageal cancer.

LASER ABLATION OF ENDOLUMINAL TUMORS

Various types of lasers are used routinely in medicine. Although carbon dioxide, argon, potassium titanyl phosphate (KTP), and diode lasers are available, the most commonly used laser in thoracic surgery is the neodymium:yttrium-aluminum-garnet (Nd:YAG). The Nd:YAG laser energy can be delivered through a small-caliber fiberoptic conduit, thus making it ideal for use with the flexible bronchoscope or esophagoscope. Adjustments in power level allow either coagulation (low power) or vaporization (high power) of tissue. The maximum depth of penetration of the Nd:YAG laser is approximately 4 mm. Airway and esophageal Nd:YAG laser procedures can be performed safely with sedation alone. During the past 25 years, experience with laser photoresection has led to the emergence of clinical safety guidelines and the characterization of lesions ideally suited to laser therapy. Communication between the surgeon, the anesthesiologist, and the rest of the operating team is essential to minimize risks to the patient and staff during laser procedures. The fractional inspired oxygen (Fio$_2$) should be set to the lowest possible level required to maintain adequate oxygenation and should never exceed 40% because of the risk of airway fire. Experienced centers have published a set of simple rules to increase the safety of lasers in the airway (Table 6-2).[65] These rules, often referred to as the 10 Commandments, are also applicable to the esophagus. Other investigators have contributed an excellent mnemonic to remember favorable lesion characteristics, power and pulse settings, and techniques to optimize the results of airway lasering (Table 6-3).[66] Lesions of the central airways less than 4 cm in length, localized to one wall, and protruding through the lumen (e.g., exophytic, pedunculated) without complete obstruction are ideal for laser ablation.[66]

Airway

Symptomatic relief from cough, dyspnea, hemoptysis, and postobstructive pneumonia and accelerated weaning from mechanical ventilation can be achieved in approximately 80% of patients with malignant airway obstruction.[66] In a series of more than 1800 patients treated with Nd:YAG laser, 93% had improvement in symptoms and quality of life.[67] Even in patients with advanced tumors for whom radiotherapy and chemotherapy have failed, 64% may experience symptomatic

Table 6–2
Adaptation of Dumon's 10 Commandments of Pulmonary Laser Photoresection[65]

1. Know the anatomy. The aortic arch, the pulmonary artery, and the esophagus are danger zones.
2. Have a well-prepared laser team. It includes an anesthetist specialized in conscious sedation and two assistants equipped with emergency response procedures.
3. Any endoluminal growth is amenable to lasering, but purely external compression is a contraindication.
4. Use the rigid bronchoscope with two suction catheters for high-grade obstruction, especially if a malignant neoplasm is involved.
5. Monitor blood gases and cardiac performance. At the least sign of hypoxemia, interrupt treatment long enough to oxygenate the patient, if necessary under closed-circuit conditions.
6. Fire parallel to the wall of the airway. Never aim directly into it.
7. Coagulate at will but avoid using the laser at high-power settings; mechanical resection after laser coagulation is preferable to laser resection alone whenever possible.
8. Control hemorrhage. Even slow bleeding will lead to hypoxemia if it is left unattended.
9. Terminate each procedure with a thorough laser irradiation of the resected area and a tracheobronchial toilet to remove all secretions or debris.
10. Observe and monitor the patient in the recovery room for a reasonable time.

relief after laser ablation.[68] Nd:YAG lasering is successful in controlling hemoptysis in 60% of patients; however, recurrence should be expected within 30 days of treatment.[69] At least 50% of patients can be extubated immediately after laser treatment.[66] There is no difference in response between primary and metastatic airway lesions. Success rate decreases from 90% to 60% in patients with central airway tumors.[70]

The overall complication rate of laser ablation varies between 0% and 2.2%.[66] Serious complications include perforation of vascular structures and endobronchial fire, which usually involves the endotracheal tube, the flexible bronchoscope sheath, or suction catheters. As stated before, fires can be avoided by keeping the Fio$_2$ below 40%, using nonflammable anesthetic agents, and keeping the scope and field as clean as possible. Hemorrhage from the tumor, pneumothorax, and pneumomediastinum are other recognized complications of airway lasering.

Esophagus

Malignant tumors of the esophagus are also amenable to treatment by Nd:YAG laser. Depending on the size of the tumor, several weekly treatments may be necessary to provide significant relief from obstruction. Lasering can also be used to recanalize a tumor in preparation for stenting. The best candidates for laser therapy are patients with small (<5 cm) exophytic tumors located in the middle esophagus, at the site of a previous esophagogastric anastomosis, or above a stent. The incidence of laser-related esophageal

Table 6–3
"Rule of Fours" for Optimal Outcome from Endobronchial Nd:YAG Lasering[66]

Lesion	
Length of lesion	≤4 cm
Duration of collapse	<4 weeks
Initial settings	
Power	40 watts
Pulse duration	0.4 second
Distances	
Endotracheal tube to lesion	>4 cm
Fiber tip to lesion	4 mm
Flexible bronchoscope to tip	4 mm
Technique	
Fio_2	<40%
Number of pulses between cleaning	<40
Procedure time	<4 hours
Total number of treatments	<4
Life expectancy	>4 weeks
Laser team	4 persons

perforation varies between 0% and 6%.[71,72] Recurrence of dysphagia can be expected within 4 to 6 weeks of treatment. The combination of laser ablation with radiotherapy has prolonged the dysphagia-free interval in patients with malignant obstruction.[73]

BRACHYTHERAPY

Brachytherapy can be defined as the placement of interstitial or intracavitary radioactive sources to facilitate the safe delivery of high radiation doses with relative sparing of normal surrounding tissues. High-dose-rate brachytherapy allows the delivery of high doses of radiation to the airway during a short period with minimal effect to surrounding tissue. Typically, bronchoscopy is performed with sedation and local anesthesia. A blind-ended 6-French afterloading catheter is passed through the working channel of a bronchoscope, and dummy seeds are placed within the catheter to confirm its position by fluoroscopy. The catheter is taped securely, and the patient is transferred to the radiation suite. Radiation seeds (iridium Ir 192) are then placed in the afterloading catheter. Typically, a few treatments will be required during a few weeks, each requiring only 10 to 15 minutes of radiation exposure. An advantage of brachytherapy over Nd:YAG laser therapy is the greater depth of penetration (0.5 to 2 cm), making it more suitable for tumors with a predominantly extraluminal component. A disadvantage is that symptomatic improvement will be slower to occur than with PDT or Nd:YAG laser therapy. On longer follow-up, bronchitis with stricturing (9% to 13%) or hemoptysis (7%) may develop as a result of brachytherapy[66,74]; these two complications are more commonly encountered with high radiation doses to the central airways. Symptomatic improvement after brachytherapy occurs in 72% to 94% of cases, depending on the symptom.[66,75] Endobronchial tumor regression may be observed in 54% to 94% of patients.[66] Complete histologic response has been documented in up to 72% of early-stage lung cancers.[76] Finally, there are prospective randomized data suggesting that the combination of brachytherapy and external beam radiation leads to further improvement in symptom-free interval and quality of life.[77]

COMPARISON OF PALLIATIVE ENDOSCOPIC THERAPIES

We have described a number of different approaches to palliate obstruction or bleeding from endoluminal tumors. Because most of these patients have a shortened life expectancy, the goals of therapy should be to improve symptoms and quality of life and to minimize morbidity and hospital stay. No randomized trials are available to compare these modalities. The perception among physicians that palliative treatment modalities are complementary rather than alternative has caused difficulties in patient accrual for randomized trials.[78] Typically, a center will favor one approach over another. It is our opinion that the thoracic surgeon should be familiar with all these modalities, as many clinical scenarios will require the combination of various treatment modalities. An example is given of our approach to palliation of obstructing lung cancer (Fig. 6-7). The relative merits of each treatment modality are summarized in Table 6-4.

EVOLVING ENDOSCOPIC TREATMENT MODALITIES FOR BENIGN ESOPHAGEAL DISEASES

Zenker's Diverticulum

The pharyngoesophageal diverticulum was first described by Ludlow[79] in 1764 but was methodically characterized by Zenker in 1867.[80] Killian elegantly described the anatomic relationship of the diverticulum and Killian's triangle, where it arises.[81] Surgical treatment is indicated to treat symptoms of dysphagia, regurgitation, and aspiration pneumonia. Surgical options include cricopharyngeal myotomy alone, diverticulectomy and myotomy, and diverticulopexy and myotomy. In 1993, Collard first published a small case series of patients treated with the transoral stapling approach.[82] Each technique is briefly reviewed; the transoral technique is described in detail.

Open Approaches to Zenker's Diverticulum

Cricopharyngeal myotomy is an attractive option in the surgical treatment of Zenker's diverticula because the risks of complications are low and the underlying cause of the problem is addressed. Belsey[83] noted that small diverticula disappeared when a myotomy alone was performed. However, when the pouch is large, myotomy alone does not yield satisfactory results.[84] In our opinion, myotomy alone should probably be reserved for the treatment of small (≤2 cm), symptomatic diverticula.

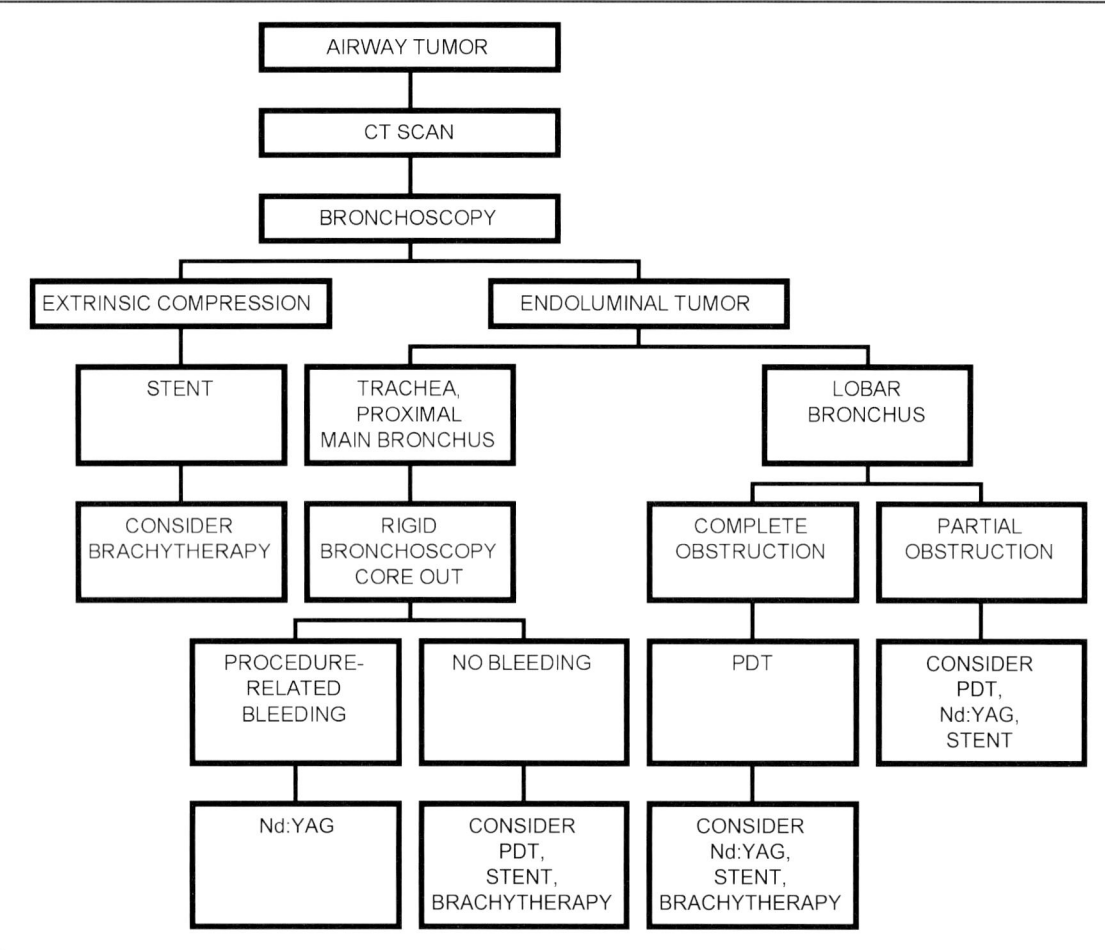

Figure 6–7
Approach to malignant obstruction of the airway.

The combination of a myotomy with a diverticulectomy became popular in the 1960s, and several groups reported lower morbidity and lower recurrence rates when the two procedures were done simultaneously.[84-87] Lerut[86] reported a significant decrease in morbidity from 21% to 11% when a myotomy was performed at the time of diverticulum resection.

Suspension of the diverticulum to the retropharyngeal fascia or to the anterior spinal ligament combined with a myotomy is another acceptable surgical option for the management of symptomatic Zenker's diverticulum. This approach avoids the potential morbidity of a leak at the site of diverticulum resection. Konowitz reported no morbidity in patients undergoing diverticulopexy and myotomy versus 20% morbidity for those undergoing diverticulectomy and myotomy.[88] Additional literature to support the routine use of this technique over diverticulectomy and myotomy is lacking.[84,89,90]

Transoral Endoscopic Stapling

Transoral stapling of the common septum between the diverticulum and the esophagus gained popularity after the first series by Collard, published in 1993.[82] The procedure may result in shorter anesthetic time, decreased hospital stay, and reduced complication rates compared with open procedures. In a recent review of series of transoral stapling published between 1993 and 2002, 94% of 576 attempted staplings were completed successfully, and 96% of the patients had a satisfactory outcome. The incidence of major complications was 3%, and 2.6% of the patients had a perforation or leak.[91]

Patient Positioning

The first step to a successful endoscopic stapling is patient selection. Ideal patient characteristics are ability to fully extend the neck without restriction, low Mallampati classification (I-II), edentulous mouth, and adequate diverticulum size (>2 cm).[92] The procedure is performed under general anesthesia with a single-lumen endotracheal tube. The patient is supine with a small pillow placed for back support and to allow extension of the neck. The surgeon is behind the patient's head.

Endoscopy

All patients should undergo flexible endoscopy, and the esophagus should be carefully inspected for any associated pathologic process (e.g., hiatal hernia, Barrett's esophagus). Care must be taken to find the true esophageal lumen. A guide wire may be left in place during the procedure to mark the location of the true esophageal lumen. After a thorough flexible endoscopy, the Weerda rigid endoscope (Karl Storz, Tuttlingen, Germany) is inserted in the patient's mouth (Fig. 6-8). A 5-mm straight or 30-degree thoracoscope connected to a video camera is used to improve visualization through the rigid endoscope. The blades of the Weerdascope are opened

Table 6-4
Relative Attributes of Endoscopic Therapies for Palliation of Endoluminal Obstruction

	PDT	Stent	Nd:YAG	Brachytherapy
Local anesthesia	Yes	Yes	Yes	Yes
Effective for intraluminal tumor	Yes	Yes	Yes	Yes
Effective for extrinsic compression	No	Yes	No	Yes
Effective for complete obstruction	Yes	No	Occasionally	No
Effective for bleeding	Yes	No	Yes	Yes (not acutely)
Depth of penetration	0.5-1 cm	N/A	N/A	0.5-2 cm
Use in lobar and segmental airways	Yes	No	Yes	Yes
Onset of effect	Rapid	Immediate	Rapid	Slow
Photosensitivity	Yes	No	No	No
Late hemoptysis (non–tumor related)	No	No	No	Yes
Late stricture or dysphagia (non–tumor related)	Yes (if normal tissue treated)	Yes (migration)	No	Yes (radiation bronchitis)

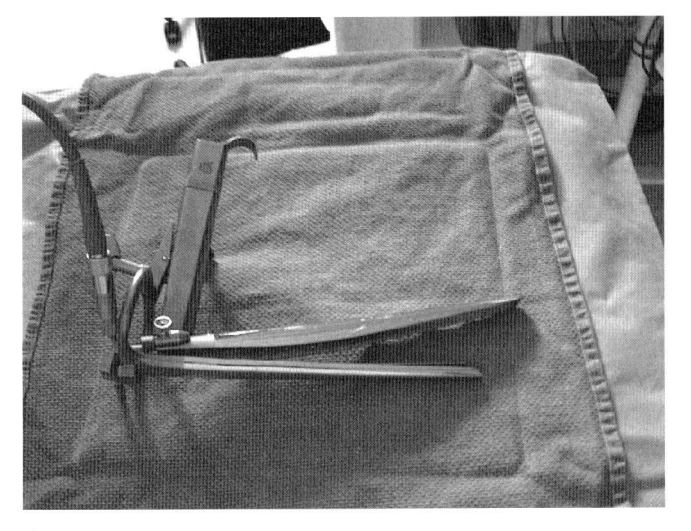

Figure 6-8
The Weerda rigid endoscope. One blade is placed in the esophagus and the other in the diverticulum. *(From Morse CR, Fernando HC, Ferson PF, et al: Preliminary experience by a thoracic service with endoscopic transoral stapling of cervical [Zenker's] diverticulum.)*

gently to demonstrate both the true esophageal lumen and the lumen of the diverticulum. If needed, the diverticulum is cleaned of any residual contents with the help of suction and saline irrigation. The septum between the diverticulum and the true esophageal lumen should be well demonstrated.

Stapling

To facilitate the insertion of the stapling device, a traction suture is placed on the septum, separating the true lumen of the esophagus and the diverticulum, by use of the Endo Stitch device (Fig. 6-9). An Endo GIA 30 is used for stapling. The anvil is modified by shortening its tip, so that the staple line can reach the base of the septum (Fig. 6-10). The stapler is inserted through the rigid endoscope, and the jaws are placed across the septum, in the midline (Fig. 6-11). The suture provides countertraction on the septum.

Results

The two largest series on transoral stapling of Zenker's diverticula come from Italy.[93,94] Peracchia reported his experience with 95 attempted transoral staplings of Zenker's diverticula.[94] Ninety-two patients (97%) had successful stapling. Two patients had limited neck extension, and one patient had a mucosal tear during the procedure. All three patients had an open procedure without complications. The author reported that the three unsuccessful attempts occurred in the early years of the series. Satisfactory outcome was achieved in 94% of the patients, and 5% had recurrence or persistence of the diverticula. Narne described 102 patients,[93] of whom 98 (96%) had successful stapling. A satisfactory outcome was achieved in 96% of patients, with a 4% recurrence rate and no major morbidity.

We recently presented our preliminary results with transoral stapling.[95] Twenty-eight patients had attempted transoral stapling. The procedure was completed in 24 patients (85%). Four patients had conversion to an open procedure because of unfavorable anatomy (two patients), perforation of the diverticula (one patient), and a diverticulum smaller than 2 cm (one patient). There were no significant complications, and the length of stay was 2.2 days. Time to oral intake was 1.38 days, and dysphagia scores improved remarkably after the procedure (2.78 to 1.1).

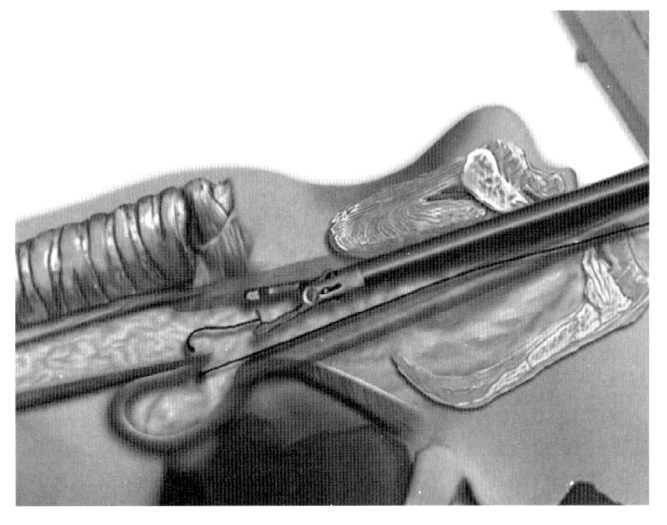

Figure 6–9
Traction stitch placed in the septum with use of 2-0 Ethibond on an Endo Stitch device (U.S. Surgical Corp., Norwalk, CT). This prevents the septum from being "squeezed" out of the stapler jaws. *(From Morse CR, Fernando HC, Ferson PF, et al: Preliminary experience by a thoracic service with endoscopic transoral stapling of cervical [Zenker's] diverticulum.)*

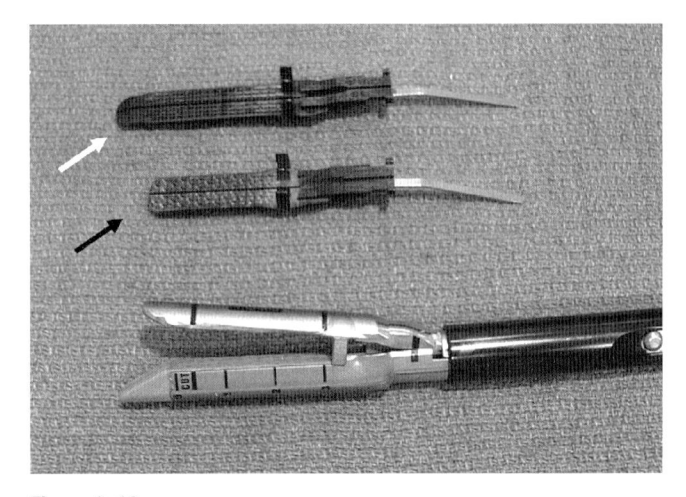

Figure 6–10
The modified Endo GIA 30 stapler (U.S. Surgical Corp., Norwalk, CT). The anvil is modified by shortening the tip to allow the staple to go to the base of the septum. *White arrow*, An unmodified anvil. *Black arrow*, Anvil modified by removal of the tapered end. *(From Morse CR, Fernando HC, Ferson PF, et al: Preliminary experience by a thoracic service with endoscopic transoral stapling of cervical [Zenker's] diverticulum.)*

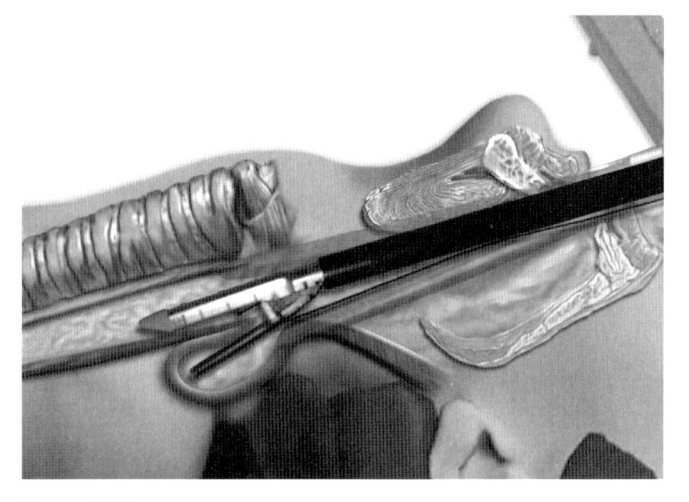

Figure 6–11
Endoscopic transoral stapling of Zenker's diverticulum. *(From Morse CR, Fernando HC, Ferson PF, et al: Preliminary experience by a thoracic service with endoscopic transoral stapling of cervical [Zenker's] diverticulum.)*

Transoral stapling is a safe, rapid, and effective way to treat Zenker's diverticula. Surgeons contemplating the use of this approach should be familiar with rigid esophagoscopy and open surgical management of Zenker's diverticula.

Gastroesophageal Reflux

Gastroesophageal reflux disease (GERD) is defined as the presence of symptoms, such as heartburn or regurgitation, or the presence of esophageal mucosal damage secondary to acid reflux. Up to 44% of the population will experience heartburn at least once a month and 17.8% at least once a week,[96] making GERD the third most common gastrointestinal disorder in the United States. It is responsible for 96,000 hospitalizations a year, at a cost of almost $10 billion.[97] GERD significantly impairs quality of life and may have a worse impact on patients than angina pectoris and congestive heart failure. After initial medical therapy, only 10% to 25% of patients will remain symptom free 6 months after stopping medications; the rest require long-term medical therapy.[98] Up to 20% of GERD patients receiving proton pump inhibitors (PPIs) will experience breakthrough symptoms.[99] The daily dependence on medications, the high associated costs, and the suboptimal symptom control have spurred interest in new, minimally invasive endoscopic approaches to GERD.

Endoscopic procedures for GERD can be classified into three major groups: RF therapy to the lower esophageal sphincter (Stretta, Curon Medical, Fremont, CA), injection of biopolymers at the gastroesophageal junction (Enteryx, Boston Scientific, Natick, MA), and endoscopic plication of the gastroesophageal junction. The first two treatment modalities are mentioned for completeness, as they are no longer commercially available. Endoscopic plicators (e.g., Esophyx, EndoCinch) are currently approved for use in the United States.

Radiofrequency Therapy to the Lower Esophageal Sphincter

Curon Medical, the manufacturer of the Stretta system, stopped making the device after filing for bankruptcy in November 2006. The devices delivered low-power RF energy to the gastroesophageal junction. The procedure involved the delivery of RF energy to the esophageal tissue from 1 cm above the gastroesophageal junction to a level immediately below the squamous-columnar junction. The proposed mechanisms of action for the Stretta procedure include mechanical alteration of the gastroesophageal junction and neural modulation of the lower esophageal sphincter, resulting in decreased relaxation and acid exposure.[100,101]

The short-term results (6 to 12 months) of a prospective study of 118 patients showed significant improvement in DeMeester score, lower esophageal sphincter pressure, heartburn score, GERD health-related quality of life (GERD-HRQL) score, and Short Form 36 (SF-36) questionnaire score.[102] At baseline, 88% of patients required daily PPIs compared with 30% at 12 months. An ad hoc analysis of the results concluded that symptomatic improvement after the Stretta procedure correlated with decreased lower esophageal sphincter acid exposure, linking symptomatic improvement with proximal and distal esophageal acid control.[103]

Corley[104] conducted a blinded, randomized, controlled trial in 64 patients with GERD. At 6 months, treated patients showed a significantly improved heartburn score, GERD-HRQL score, and general quality of life. There was no difference between the groups in daily medication use, median 24-hour pH score, and lower esophageal sphincter pressure or esophageal mucosal erosions. This trial showed that the Stretta procedure was effective in improving symptoms and quality of life but failed to improve acid exposure or healing of mucosal lesions. The authors could not explain the findings. In the largest published study, Wolfsen[105] evaluated GERD symptoms, patients' satisfaction, and medication use in 558 patients treated in 33 centers. Mean follow-up was 8 months, ranging from 2 to 33 months. Satisfaction of patients improved from 23.2% to 86.5%, symptom control improved from 50% to 90%, and 77% of patients reported absent or mild GERD after the Stretta procedure compared with 26.3% at baseline. Subset analysis showed that improvement persisted beyond 1 year after the procedure, and most patients remained off antacid medication.

In summary, the Stretta procedure appears to be effective in controlling GERD symptoms in a selected group of patients. However, questions about the precise mechanism of action and the long-term effects are likely to remain unanswered, given that the device is no longer commercially available.

Injection of Biopolymers at the Gastroesophageal Junction

Enteryx is a biocompatible polymer in the form of a nonviscous liquid that solidifies rapidly when it is injected into tissue, becoming an inert spongy mass. The procedure was usually done under fluoroscopic guidance, and most treatment sessions placed 1-mm blebs circumferentially around the gastroesophageal junction. Enteryx injections can be repeated if symptoms are not fully controlled; however, it is not reversible.[106] The proposed mechanism of action of Enteryx injection to the lower esophageal sphincter is the prevention of lower esophageal sphincter unfolding or relaxation in response to gastric distention. This is supposed to prevent reflux and to improve lower esophageal sphincter tone.[107]

A prospective, multicenter international trial of Enteryx implantation for GERD was conducted, and 12- and 24-month follow-up data are available.[108,109] Results were reported for 85 patients for 12 months and for 144 patients for 24 months. Patients entered the trial if their symptoms were well controlled and symptom scores were normalized with PPIs and returned to abnormal levels after withdrawal of PPIs. At 12 months, 84% of the patients had a reduction in use of PPIs of more than 50%, and 73% of the patients stopped using PPIs completely. This effect was maintained at 24 months; 72% of patients had a reduction in use of PPIs of more than 50%, and 67% had complete cessation of PPIs. GERD-HRQL score improved in 78% of the patients at 12 months and in 80% at 24 months. Median heartburn score improved in 71% at 12 months and 80% at 24 months. Regurgitation score improved in 77% at 12 months and 88% at 24 months. The median score of the physical component of the SF-36 questionnaire improved by 12%, but the mental component did not change significantly. Esophageal manometry was not significantly changed at 12 months. Esophageal acid exposure declined significantly at 12 months. Median supine, upright, and total acid exposure times were decreased by 42%, 28%, and 31%, respectively. Thirty-seven percent of patients had acid exposure normalized 12 months after the procedure. At 12 months, esophagitis was unchanged in 59 patients (55%), decreased in 14 patients (13%), and increased in 34 patients (32%). Of the 34 patients with an increase in esophagitis, 19 had increased by one level and 14 by two levels. One patient had an increase in esophagitis from 0 to III. Adverse effects in the trial were relatively minor, with retrosternal chest pain being the most frequent. One patient presented with a paraesophageal fluid collection, which was treated conservatively. Outside the trial, serious adverse reactions have been reported. One patient died of gastrointestinal bleeding from an aortoesophageal fistula. Enteryx material was found in the patient's aorta at autopsy. Another patient developed severe flank pain and embolization of Enteryx to his aorta and renal arteries.[110] The Food and Drug Administration ordered a recall of the product in 2005. Although the international trial demonstrated good symptomatic relief in patients with GERD controlled with PPIs, 30% worsening in esophagitis and reports of fatalities preclude us from recommending this treatment option.

Endoscopic Plication of the Gastroesophageal Junction

Esophyx

This device, just recently approved by the Food and Drug Administration, tries to restore the angle of His and improve the antireflux mechanism by creating an omega-shaped valve, 3 to 5 cm in length and 200 to 300 degrees in circumference, with use of multiple, full-thickness endoscopic fasteners. The device is essentially an overtube with a channel for the esophagoscope and a flexible section that retroflexes and compresses the tissue at the angle of His.[106] There are scarce clinical data on this device. In a canine model, animals did not show any adverse effects, and the fasteners were effective in creating a stable serosa-to-serosa fusion at 1 year.[111] Animals with a circumferential valve demonstrated a significant and lasting increase in the lower esophageal sphincter pressure compared with animals submitted to a sham procedure. Also, the total and intra-abdominal length of the lower esophageal sphincter was increased compared with baseline and with animals submitted to the sham procedure. Esophageal acid exposure and DeMeester score also decreased significantly. Cadiere[112] published a series of 17 patients treated with the Esophyx device. One year after surgery, GERD-HRQL score improved by 67%, 82% of patients discontinued PPIs, and more than 80% were either satisfied or very satisfied with the procedure. Endoscopy at 1 year revealed that 81% of the valves maintained their tightness, median circumference, and length. Grade A and B esophagitis was observed in 13 patients, and hiatal hernias remained reduced in 8 of 13 patients. There were no significant complications related to the procedure.

EndoCinch

The EndoCinch (Bard Medical, Covington, GA) requires an overtube and two endoscopes, one for the suturing and the other for suction and visualization. The procedure entails plication of a fold of mucosa just below the squamous-columnar junction. Three sutures are placed below the gastroesophageal junction in a circumferential, linear, or helical pattern.[113]

Sham-controlled trials of the EndoCinch have had remarkably different results. Rothstein,[114] in a single-blinded trial, compared 78 patients undergoing the EndoCinch procedure with 81 patients undergoing a sham procedure. At 3 months, more than 50% of patients undergoing the EndoCinch procedure had an improvement in the GERD-HRQL score, as opposed to only 18% in the sham group. Also, patients treated with EndoCinch had a significant improvement in pH acid exposure and a higher rate of discontinuation of PPI therapy (50% versus 24%). There were no significant complications in the treated patients.

In contrast, Montgomery and coworkers[115] randomized 46 patients to the EndoCinch procedure or sham endoscopy. At 12 months, the investigators could not demonstrate differences between groups with regard to GERD-HRQL score, PPI use, acid exposure, or esophageal manometric findings. At 12 months, 33% of the EndoCinch sutures were not visible, leading the investigators to conclude that the detachment of the sutures led to failure of the procedure. Both sham and EndoCinch subjects had significant improvements in GERD symptoms and PPI use after 12 months. The procedure was carried out without major complications. In another sham-controlled trial, Schwartz and colleagues[116] randomized 60 patients to EndoCinch therapy, sham procedure, or observation alone. Heartburn symptoms and the use of PPIs were significantly decreased after EndoCinch compared with sham or control. Quality of life was also significantly improved in treated patients compared with sham patients. Esophageal acid exposure did not significantly differ between the treatment and the sham groups, although both groups experienced a reduction in overall acid exposure after 3 months.

Results of a North American multicenter trial were published in 2005. Eighty-five patients were enrolled and observed for 24 months.[117] Patients had a significant improvement in heartburn symptoms, and 77% reported no or minimal heartburn and no or minimal regurgitation in 2 years. Forty percent of patients reported complete cessation of use of PPIs at 24 months, and the annualized per patient medication costs decreased from $1564 at baseline to $183 at 2 years. Esophageal acid exposure was also significantly decreased at 6 months. One patient experienced severe dysphagia requiring removal of the fundoplication sutures 10 days after the procedure.

NDO Plicator

The NDO plicator (NDO Surgical, Mansfield, MA) was designed to create a full-thickness plication of the gastroesophageal junction by delivery of a suture-based implant. This is accomplished by direct visualization of the gastroesophageal junction in a retroflexed fashion with a pediatric endoscope inserted through a dedicated channel of the plicator device. The plication is done 1.0 to 1.5 cm below the Z line, and either one or two plications are performed. Unfortunately, because of insufficient demand for the device, the company filed for bankruptcy in 2008.

In the North American open-label multicenter trial, 64 patients were treated with one plication by the NDO plicator.[118] At 12 months of follow-up, the GERD-HRQL score improved from 19 to 7 ($P < .0001$). The proportion of patients receiving daily PPI therapy decreased from 93% to 32% at 12 months. At 6 months, there was significant improvement in acid exposure at the distal esophagus, with both the number of episodes and the total acid exposure time showing significant improvement. In a randomized, sham-controlled trial of 159 patients, 56% of plicator patients versus 18.5% of sham patients had an improvement of more than 50% in the GERD-HRQL score at 3 months.[114] Discontinuation of PPI therapy occurred in 50% of the treated patients and 24% of the sham patients at 3 months. Most adverse effects included mild chest and epigastric pain. One patient underwent laparoscopy for persistent epigastric pain and was found to have adhesions between the stomach and the diaphragm. In another study of 33 patients observed for 5 years, there was a significant improvement of the GERD-HRQL score, and 33% had completely discontinued PPI therapy.[119] Adverse effects included sore throat (45%), abdominal pain (41%), chest pain (24%), and transient dysphagia not requiring dilations (21%).

In summary, endoscopic fundoplication is a procedure in evolution that has demonstrated short-term effectiveness in controlling symptoms of GERD. In general, patients with dysphagia, severe esophagitis, Barrett's metaplasia, previous esophageal or gastric surgery, or a type I hiatal hernia larger than 2 cm were excluded from these trials. Most of the trials were also industry sponsored. Overall, it appears that patients with a very small hiatal hernia and a good response to PPIs may be the best candidates for endoluminal therapy. At this time, this treatment modality should probably be reserved for nonsurgical candidates or those who refuse surgery. The role of endoluminal fundoplication in the management of GERD will be further delineated once more complete long-term follow-up data become available.

With technological advancement, these minimally invasive techniques may improve and become even more attractive to patients. It is important for thoracic surgeons to remain aware of further developments and to continue to critically evaluate new therapeutic modalities as they are introduced into clinical practice.

REFERENCES

1. Boyd AD. Chevalier Jackson: the father of American bronchoesophagoscopy. *Ann Thorac Surg* 1994;**57**:502-5.
2. Maier A, Tomaselli F, Matzi V, et al. Photosensitization with hematoporphyrin derivative compared to 5-aminolaevulinic acid for photodynamic therapy of esophageal carcinoma. *Ann Thorac Surg* 2001;**72**:1136-40.
3. Peng Q, Warloe T, Berg K, et al. 5-Aminolevulinic acid–based photodynamic therapy: clinical research and future challenges. *Cancer* 1997;**79**:2282-308.
4. Weigel TL, Kosco PJ, Dacic S, et al. Postoperative fluorescence bronchoscopic surveillance in non–small cell lung cancer patients. *Ann Thorac Surg* 2001;**71**:967-70.
5. Moghissi K, Dixon K, Thorpe JA, et al. Photodynamic therapy (PDT) in early central lung cancer: a treatment option for patients ineligible for surgical resection. *Thorax* 2007;**62**:391-5.
6. Furuse K, Fukuoka M, Kato H, et al. A prospective phase II study on photodynamic therapy with photofrin II for centrally located early-stage lung cancer. The Japan Lung Cancer Photodynamic Therapy Study Group. *J Clin Oncol* 1993;**11**:1852-7.
7. Cortese DA, Edell ES, Kinsey JH. Photodynamic therapy for early stage squamous cell carcinoma of the lung. *Mayo Clin Proc* 1997;**72**:595-602.

8. Weigel TL, Kosco PJ, Christie NA, et al. Photodynamic therapy for early non–small cell lung carcinoma in high-risk patients. *Chest* 2000; **118**:90S.
9. Weigel TL, Kosco PJ, Luketich JD. Photodynamic therapy for endobronchial lesions. In: Pearson FG, editor. *Esophageal surgery*. 2nd ed. New York: Churchill Livingstone; 2002, 901-905.
10. Luketich JD, Fernando HC, Christie NA, et al. Photodynamic therapy in thoracic oncology: a single institution experience (Proceedings Paper). *Proceedings of SPIE* 2001;**4248**:28-33.
11. McCaughan Jr JS, Williams TE. Photodynamic therapy for endobronchial malignant disease: a prospective fourteen-year study. *J Thorac Cardiovasc Surg* 1997;**114**:940-6:discussion 946-947.
12. Litle VR, Christie NA, Fernando HC, et al. Photodynamic therapy for endobronchial metastases from nonbronchogenic primaries. *Ann Thorac Surg* 2003;**76**:370-5:discussion 375.
13. Diaz-Jimenez JP, Martinez-Ballarin JE, Llunell A, et al. Efficacy and safety of photodynamic therapy versus Nd:YAG laser resection in NSCLC with airway obstruction. *Eur Respir J* 1999;**14**:800-5.
14. McCaughan Jr JS, Ellison EC, Guy JT, et al. Photodynamic therapy for esophageal malignancy: a prospective twelve-year study. *Ann Thorac Surg* 1996;**62**:1005-9:discussion 1009-1010.
15. Luketich JD, Christie NA, Buenaventura PO, et al. Endoscopic photodynamic therapy for obstructing esophageal cancer: 77 cases over a 2-year period. *Surg Endosc* 2000;**14**:653-7.
16. Zaninotto G, Parenti AR, Ruol A, et al. Oesophageal resection for high-grade dysplasia in Barrett's oesophagus. *Br J Surg* 2000;**87**:1102-5.
17. Falk GW. Gastroesophageal reflux disease and Barrett's esophagus. *Endoscopy* 2001;**33**:109-18.
18. Fernando HC, Luketich JD, Buenaventura PO, et al. Outcomes of minimally invasive esophagectomy (MIE) for high-grade dysplasia of the esophagus. *Eur J Cardiothorac Surg* 2002;**22**:1-6.
19. Nguyen NT, Schauer P, Luketich JD. Minimally invasive esophagectomy for Barrett's esophagus with high-grade dysplasia. *Surgery* 2000;**127**:284-90.
20. Gossner L, Stolte M, Sroka R, et al. Photodynamic ablation of high-grade dysplasia and early cancer in Barrett's esophagus by means of 5-aminolevulinic acid. *Gastroenterology* 1998;**114**:448-55.
21. May A, Gossner L, Pech O, et al. Local endoscopic therapy for intraepithelial high-grade neoplasia and early adenocarcinoma in Barrett's oesophagus: acute-phase and intermediate results of a new treatment approach. *Eur J Gastroenterol Hepatol* 2002;**14**:1085-91.
22. Sampliner RE, Fennerty B, Garewal HS. Reversal of Barrett's esophagus with acid suppression and multipolar electrocoagulation: preliminary results. *Gastrointest Endosc* 1996;**44**:532-5.
23. Van Laethem JL, Cremer M, Peny MO, et al. Eradication of Barrett's mucosa with argon plasma coagulation and acid suppression: immediate and mid term results. *Gut* 1998;**43**:747-51.
24. Biddlestone LR, Barham CP, Wilkinson SP, et al. The histopathology of treated Barrett's esophagus: squamous reepithelialization after acid suppression and laser and photodynamic therapy. *Am J Surg Pathol* 1998;**22**:239-45.
25. Overholt BF, Panjehpour M, Haydek JM. Photodynamic therapy for Barrett's esophagus: follow-up in 100 patients. *Gastrointest Endosc* 1999;**49**:1-7.
26. Overholt BF, Wang KK, Burdick JS, et al. Five-year efficacy and safety of photodynamic therapy with Photofrin in Barrett's high-grade dysplasia. *Gastrointest Endosc* 2007;**66**:460-8.
27. Keeley SB, Pennathur A, Gooding W, et al. Photodynamic therapy with curative intent for Barrett's esophagus with high grade dysplasia and superficial esophageal cancer. *Ann Surg Oncol* 2007;**14**:2406-10.
28. Romagnoli R, Collard JM, Gutschow C, et al. Outcomes of dysplasia arising in Barrett's esophagus: a dynamic view. *J Am Coll Surg* 2003;**197**:365-71.
29. Hemminger LL, Wolfsen HC. Photodynamic therapy for Barrett's esophagus and high grade dysplasia: results of a patient satisfaction survey. *Gastroenterol Nurs* 2002;**25**:139-41.
30. Overholt BF, Panjehpour M, Ayres M. Photodynamic therapy for Barrett's esophagus: cardiac effects. *Lasers Surg Med* 1997;**21**:317-20.
31. Luketich JD, Wong HY, Buenaventura PO, et al. Photodynamic therapy: results of curative intent for esophageal cancer and Barrett's with high grade dysplasia in high risk patients. Paris, France: International Organization for Statistical Studies on Diseases of Esophagus (OESO), 6th World Congress; 2000.
32. Ganz RA, Utley DS, Stern RA, et al. Complete ablation of esophageal epithelium with a balloon-based bipolar electrode: a phased evaluation in the porcine and in the human esophagus. *Gastrointest Endosc* 2004;**60**:1002-10.
33. Gondrie JJ, Pouw RE, Sondermeijer CM, et al. Effective treatment of early Barrett's neoplasia with stepwise circumferential and focal ablation using the HALO system. *Endoscopy* 2008;**40**:370-9.
34. Christie NA, Buenaventura PO, Fernando HC, et al. Results of expandable metal stents for malignant esophageal obstruction in 100 patients: short-term and long-term follow-up. *Ann Thorac Surg* 2001;**71**:1797-801:discussion 1801-1792.
35. Lightdale CJ, Heier SK, Marcon NE, et al. Photodynamic therapy with portimer sodium versus thermal ablation therapy with Nd:YAG laser for palliation of esophageal cancer: a multicenter randomized trial. *Gastrointest Endosc* 1995;**42**:507-12.
36. Litle VR, Luketich JD, Christie NA, et al. Photodynamic therapy as palliation for esophageal cancer: experience in 215 patients. *Ann Thorac Surg* 2003;**76**:1687-92:discussion 1692-1683.
37. Luketich JD, Westkaemper J, Sommers KE, et al. Bronchoesophagopleural fistula after photodynamic therapy for malignant mesothelioma. *Ann Thorac Surg* 1996;**62**:283-4.
38. Maier A, Anegg U, Fell B, et al. Hyperbaric oxygen and photodynamic therapy in the treatment of advanced carcinoma of the cardia and the esophagus. *Lasers Surg Med* 2000;**26**:308-15.
39. Maier A, Tomaselli F, Gebhard F, et al. Palliation of advanced esophageal carcinoma by photodynamic therapy and irradiation. *Ann Thorac Surg* 2000;**69**:1006-9.
40. Angueira CE, Kadakia SC. Esophageal stents for inoperable esophageal cancer: which to use? *Am J Gastroenterol* 1997;**92**:373-6.
41. Knyrim K, Wagner HJ, Bethge N, et al. A controlled trial of an expansile metal stent for palliation of esophageal obstruction due to inoperable cancer. *N Engl J Med* 1993;**329**:1302-7.
42. Ferson PF, Landreneau RJ, Keenan RL, et al. Interventional bronchoscopy. In: Yim APC, editor. *Minimal access cardiothoracic surgery*. Philadelphia: Saunders; 2000, xxv, 693.
43. Stephens Jr KE, Wood DE. Bronchoscopic management of central airway obstruction. *J Thorac Cardiovasc Surg* 2000;**119**:289-96.
44. Cooper JD, Pearson FG, Patterson GA, et al. Use of silicone stents in the management of airway problems. *Ann Thorac Surg* 1989;**47**:371-8.
45. Gaissert HA, Grillo HC, Mathisen DJ, et al. Temporary and permanent restoration of airway continuity with the tracheal T-tube. *J Thorac Cardiovasc Surg* 1994;**107**:600-6.
46. Ducic Y, Khalafi RS. Use of endoscopically placed expandable nitinol tracheal stents in the treatment of tracheal stenosis. *Laryngoscope* 1999;**109**:1130-3.
47. Gotway MB, Golden JA, LaBerge JM, et al. Benign tracheobronchial stenoses: changes in short-term and long-term pulmonary function testing after expandable metallic stent placement. *J Comput Assist Tomogr* 2002;**26**:564-72.
48. Nashef SA, Dromer C, Velly JF, et al. Expanding wire stents in benign tracheobronchial disease: indications and complications. *Ann Thorac Surg* 1992;**54**:937-40.
49. Sonett JR, Keenan RJ, Ferson PF, et al. Endobronchial management of benign, malignant, and lung transplantation airway stenoses. *Ann Thorac Surg* 1995;**59**:1417-22.
50. Bolliger CT, Heitz M, Hauser R, et al. An airway Wallstent for the treatment of tracheobronchial malignancies. *Thorax* 1996;**51**:1127-9.
51. Witt C, Dinges S, Schmidt B, et al. Temporary tracheobronchial stenting in malignant stenoses. *Eur J Cancer* 1997;**33**:204-8.
52. Litle VR, Fernando HC, Christie NA, et al. Expandable metal stents for malignant tracheobronchial obstruction. *Ann Surg Oncol* 2002;**9**:S82.
53. Morgan R, Adam A. Use of metallic stents and balloons in the esophagus and gastrointestinal tract. *J Vasc Interv Radiol* 2001;**12**:283-97.
54. Sandha GS, Marcon NE. Expandable metal stents for benign esophageal obstruction. *Gastrointest Endosc Clin N Am* 1999;**9**:437-46.
55. Martin RC, Woodall C, Duvall R, et al. The use of self-expanding silicone stents in esophagectomy strictures: less cost and more efficiency. *Ann Thorac Surg* 2008;**86**:436-40.
56. Pennathur A, Chang AC, McGrath KM, et al. Polyflex expandable stents in the treatment of esophageal disease: initial experience. *Ann Thorac Surg* 2008;**85**:1968-72:discussion 1973.
57. Siersema PD, Hop WC, Dees J, et al. Coated self-expanding metal stents versus latex prostheses for esophagogastric cancer with special reference to prior radiation and chemotherapy: a controlled, prospective study. *Gastrointest Endosc* 1998;**47**:113-20.
58. Boulis NM, Armstrong WS, Chandler WF, et al. Epidural abscess: a delayed complication of esophageal stenting for benign stricture. *Ann Thorac Surg* 1999;**68**:568-70.
59. Maier A, Pinter H, Friehs GB, et al. Self-expandable coated stent after intraluminal treatment of esophageal cancer: a risky procedure? *Ann Thorac Surg* 1999;**67**:781-4.
60. Cwikiel W, Tranberg KG, Cwikiel M, et al. Malignant dysphagia: palliation with esophageal stents—long-term results in 100 patients. *Radiology* 1998;**207**:513-8.

61. O'Sullivan GJ, Grundy A. Palliation of malignant dysphagia with expanding metallic stents. *J Vasc Interv Radiol* 1999;**10**:346-51.
62. Raijman I, Siddique I, Ajani J. et al. Palliation of malignant dysphagia and fistulae with coated expandable metal stents: experience with 101 patients. *Gastrointest Endosc* 1998;**48**:172-9.
63. Song HY, Do YS, Han YM, et al. Covered, expandable esophageal metallic stent tubes: experiences in 119 patients. *Radiology* 1994;**193**:689-95.
64. Song HY, Lee DH, Seo TS, et al. Retrievable covered nitinol stents: experiences in 108 patients with malignant esophageal strictures. *J Vasc Interv Radiol* 2002;**13**:285-93.
65. Dumon JF, Reboud E, Garbe L, et al. Treatment of tracheobronchial lesions by laser photoresection. *Chest* 1982;**81**:278-84.
66. Lee P, Kupeli E, Mehta AC. Therapeutic bronchoscopy in lung cancer: laser therapy, electrocautery, brachytherapy, stents, and photodynamic therapy. *Clin Chest Med* 2002;**23**:241-56.
67. Cavaliere S, Venuta F, Foccoli P, et al. Endoscopic treatment of malignant airway obstructions in 2008 patients. *Chest* 1996;**110**:1536-42.
68. Hetzel MR, Nixon C, Edmondstone WM, et al. Laser therapy in 100 tracheobronchial tumours. *Thorax* 1985;**40**:341-5.
69. Jain PR, Dedhia HV, Lapp NL, et al. Nd:YAG laser followed by radiation for treatment of malignant airway lesions. *Lasers Surg Med* 1985;**5**:47-53.
70. Cavaliere S, Foccoli P, Farina PL. Nd:YAG laser bronchoscopy: a five-year experience with 1396 applications in 1000 patients. *Chest* 1988;**94**:15-21.
71. Bisgaard T, Wojdemann M, Heindorff H, et al. Nonsurgical treatment of esophageal perforations after endoscopic palliation in advanced esophageal cancer. *Endoscopy* 1997;**29**:155-9.
72. Casale V, Lapenta R, Gigliozzi A, et al. Endoscopic palliative therapy in neoplastic diseases of the esophagus. *J Exp Clin Cancer Res* 1999;**18**:63-7.
73. Sargeant IR, Tobias JS, Blackman G, et al. Radiotherapy enhances laser palliation of malignant dysphagia: a randomised study. *Gut* 1997;**40**:362-9.
74. Speiser BL, Spratling L. Radiation bronchitis and stenosis secondary to high dose rate endobronchial irradiation. *Int J Radiat Oncol Biol Phys* 1993;**25**:589-97.
75. Mehrishi S, Raoof S, Mehta AC. Therapeutic flexible bronchoscopy. *Chest Surg Clin N Am* 2001;**11**:657-90.
76. Tredaniel J, Hennequin C, Zalcman G, et al. Prolonged survival after high-dose rate endobronchial radiation for malignant airway obstruction. *Chest* 1994;**105**:767-72.
77. Langendijk H, de Jong J, Tjwa M, et al. External irradiation versus external irradiation plus endobronchial brachytherapy in inoperable non–small cell lung cancer: a prospective randomized study. *Radiother Oncol* 2001;**58**:257-68.
78. Moghissi K, Bond MG, Sambrook RJ, et al. Treatment of endotracheal or endobronchial obstruction by non–small cell lung cancer: lack of patients in an MRC randomized trial leaves key questions unanswered. Medical Research Council Lung Cancer Working Party. *Clin Oncol (R Coll Radiol)* 1999;**11**:179-83.
79. Ludlow A. A case of obstructed deglutition from a preternatural bag formed in the pharynx. In: Johnson W, Caldwell T, editors. Medical Observations and inquiries by a society of physicians in London. London: London Medical Society; 1769, 85-101.
80. Zenker FA, von Ziemssen H. Krankheiten des Oesophagus. In: von Ziemssen H, editor. Handbuch des speciellen Pathologie und Therapie. Leipzig: FC Vogel; 1877, 1-87.
81. Killian G. The mouth of the esophagus. *Laryngoscope* 1907;**17**:421-8.
82. Collard JM, Otte JB, Kestens PJ. Endoscopic stapling technique of esophagodiverticulostomy for Zenker's diverticulum. *Ann Thorac Surg* 1993;**56**:573-6.
83. Belsey R. Functional disease of the esophagus. *J Thorac Cardiovasc Surg* 1966;**52**:164-88.
84. Bonafede JP, Lavertu P, Wood BG, et al. Surgical outcome in 87 patients with Zenker's diverticulum. *Laryngoscope* 1997;**107**:720-5.
85. Gutschow CA, Hamoir M, Rombaux P, et al. Management of pharyngoesophageal (Zenker's) diverticulum: which technique? *Ann Thorac Surg* 2002;**74**:1677-82:discussion 1682-1683.
86. Lerut T, van Raemdonck D, Guelinckx P, et al. Zenker's diverticulum: is a myotomy of the cricopharyngeus useful? How long should it be? *Hepatogastroenterology* 1992;**39**:127-31.
87. Orringer MB. Extended cervical esophagomyotomy for cricopharyngeal dysfunction. *J Thorac Cardiovasc Surg* 1980;**80**:669-78.
88. Konowitz PM, Biller HF. Diverticulopexy and cricopharyngeal myotomy: treatment for the high-risk patient with a pharyngoesophageal (Zenker's) diverticulum. *Otolaryngol Head Neck Surg* 1989;**100**:146-53.
89. Duranceau A, Rheault MJ, Jamieson GG. Physiologic response to cricopharyngeal myotomy and diverticulum suspension. *Surgery* 1983;**94**:655-62.
90. Freeland AP, Bates GJ. The surgical treatment of a pharyngeal pouch: inversion or excision? *Ann R Coll Surg Engl* 1987;**69**:57-8.
91. Aly A, Devitt PG, Jamieson GG. Evolution of surgical treatment for pharyngeal pouch. *Br J Surg* 2004;**91**:657-64.
92. Scher RL, Richtsmeier WJ. Long-term experience with endoscopic staple-assisted esophagodiverticulostomy for Zenker's diverticulum. *Laryngoscope* 1998;**108**:200-5.
93. Narne S, Cutrone C, Bonavina L, et al. Endoscopic diverticulotomy for the treatment of Zenker's diverticulum: results in 102 patients with staple-assisted endoscopy. *Ann Otol Rhinol Laryngol* 1999;**108**:810-5.
94. Peracchia A, Bonavina L, Narne S, et al. Minimally invasive surgery for Zenker diverticulum: analysis of results in 95 consecutive patients. *Arch Surg* 1998;**133**:695-700.
95. Morse CR, Fernando HC, Ferson PF, et al. Preliminary experience by a thoracic service with endoscopic transoral stapling of cervical (Zenker's) diverticulum. *J Gastrointest Surg* 2007;**11**:1091-4.
96. Shaheen N, Provenzale D. The epidemiology of gastroesophageal reflux disease. *Am J Med Sci* 2003;**326**:264-73.
97. Sandler RS, Everhart JE, Donowitz M, et al. The burden of selected digestive diseases in the United States. *Gastroenterology* 2002;**122**:1500-11.
98. Dent J, Talley NJ. Overview: initial and long-term management of gastro-oesophageal reflux disease. *Aliment Pharmacol Ther* 2003;**17**(Suppl. 1):53-7.
99. Chiba N, De Gara CJ, Wilkinson JM, et al. Speed of healing and symptom relief in grade II to IV gastroesophageal reflux disease: a meta-analysis. *Gastroenterology* 1997;**112**:1798-810.
100. DiBaise JK, Brand RE, Quigley EM. Endoluminal delivery of radiofrequency energy to the gastroesophageal junction in uncomplicated GERD: efficacy and potential mechanism of action. *Am J Gastroenterol* 2002;**97**:833-42.
101. Tam WC, Schoeman MN, Zhang Q, et al. Delivery of radiofrequency energy to the lower oesophageal sphincter and gastric cardia inhibits transient lower oesophageal sphincter relaxations and gastro-oesophageal reflux in patients with reflux disease. *Gut* 2003;**52**:479-85.
102. Triadafilopoulos G, DiBaise JK, Nostrant TT, et al. The Stretta procedure for the treatment of GERD: 6 and 12 month follow-up of the U.S. open label trial. *Gastrointest Endosc* 2002;**55**:149-56.
103. Triadafilopoulos G. Changes in GERD symptom scores correlate with improvement in esophageal acid exposure after the Stretta procedure. *Surg Endosc* 2004;**18**:1038-44.
104. Corley DA, Katz P, Wo JM, et al. Improvement of gastroesophageal reflux symptoms after radiofrequency energy: a randomized, sham-controlled trial. *Gastroenterology* 2003;**125**:668-76.
105. Wolfsen HC, Richards WO. The Stretta procedure for the treatment of GERD: a registry of 558 patients. J Laparoendosc. *Adv Surg Tech A* 2002;**12**:395-402.
106. Rothstein RI. Endoscopic therapy of gastroesophageal reflux disease: outcomes of the randomized-controlled trials done to date. *J Clin Gastroenterol* 2008;**42**:594-602.
107. Watson TJ, Peters JH. Lower esophageal sphincter injections for the treatment of gastroesophageal reflux disease. *Thorac Surg Clin* 2005;**15**:405-15.
108. Cohen LB, Johnson DA, Ganz RA, et al. Enteryx implantation for GERD: expanded multicenter trial results and interim postapproval follow-up to 24 months. *Gastrointest Endosc* 2005;**61**:650-8.
109. Johnson DA, Ganz R, Aisenberg J, et al. Endoscopic implantation of enteryx for treatment of GERD: 12-month results of a prospective, multicenter trial. *Am J Gastroenterol* 2003;**98**:1921-30.
110. Tintillier M, Chaput A, Kirch L, et al. Esophageal abscess complicating endoscopic treatment of refractory gastroesophageal reflux disease by Enteryx injection: a first case report. *Am J Gastroenterol* 2004;**99**:1856-8.
111. Jobe BA, O'Rourke RW, McMahon BP, et al. Transoral endoscopic fundoplication in the treatment of gastroesophageal reflux disease: the anatomic and physiologic basis for reconstruction of the esophagogastric junction using a novel device. *Ann Surg* 2008;**248**:69-76.
112. Cadiere GB, Rajan A, Germay O, et al. Endoluminal fundoplication by a transoral device for the treatment of GERD: a feasibility study. *Surg Endosc* 2008;**22**:333-42.
113. Haider M, Iqbal A, Filipi CJ. Endoluminal gastroplasty: a new treatment for gastroesophageal reflux disease. *Thorac Surg Clin* 2005;**15**:385-94.
114. Rothstein R, Filipi C, Caca K, et al. Endoscopic full-thickness plication for the treatment of gastroesophageal reflux disease: a randomized, sham-controlled trial. *Gastroenterology* 2006;**131**:704-12.
115. Montgomery M, Hakanson B, Ljungqvist O, et al. Twelve months' follow-up after treatment with the EndoCinch endoscopic technique for gastro-oesophageal reflux disease: a randomized, placebo-controlled study. *Scand J Gastroenterol* 2006;**41**:1382-9.

116. Schwartz MP, Wellink H, Gooszen HG, et al. Endoscopic gastroplication for the treatment of gastro-oesophageal reflux disease: a randomised, sham-controlled trial. *Gut* 2007;**56**:20-8.
117. Chen YK, Raijman I, Ben-Menachem T, et al. Long-term outcomes of endoluminal gastroplication: a U.S. multicenter trial. *Gastrointest Endosc* 2005;**61**:659-67.
118. Pleskow D, Rothstein R, Lo S, et al. Endoscopic full-thickness plication for the treatment of GERD: 12-month follow-up for the North American open-label trial. *Gastrointest Endosc* 2005;**61**:643-9.
119. Pleskow D, Rothstein R, Kozarek R, et al. Endoscopic full-thickness plication for the treatment of GERD: long-term multicenter results. *Surg Endosc* 2007;**21**:439-44.

C. Trauma

CHAPTER 7

Thoracic Trauma

Clinton D. Kemp and Stephen C. Yang

The Primary Survey
Diagnostic Tests
   Chest Radiography
   Ultrasonography
   Echocardiography
   Angiography
Emergency Department Thoracotomy
Blunt Trauma
   Chest Wall
      Rib Fractures
      Flail Chest
      Sternal Fractures
      Clavicular Fractures
      Scapular Fracture

Traumatic Asphyxia
Pulmonary Contusion
Laryngeal Injuries
Tracheobronchial Injuries
Great Vessels
Blunt Cardiac Injuries
Diaphragm
Esophagus
Penetrating Trauma
   Stab Wounds versus Firearm Injuries
   Chest Wall Injury
   Tracheal and Bronchial Penetrating Injuries
   Pulmonary Injuries and Hemothorax
   Cardiac Injuries

Air Embolism and Bullet Embolism
Great Vessels
Diaphragmatic Injuries
Esophageal Injuries
Complications of Thoracic Trauma
   Acute Lung Injury and Respiratory Distress
      Syndrome
   Pneumonia
   Pleural Space Problems
   Bronchopleural Fistula
   Great Vessel Fistula

The earliest recorded reference to thoracic trauma is found in the Edwin Smith Surgical Papyrus written around 3000 BC.[1] In this report of 58 cases, three were related to the chest: a penetrating injury to the cervical esophagus, a stab wound to the sternum, and blunt trauma resulting in rib fractures. During the Trojan war, Homer reported on many thoracic injuries in his *Iliad*, perhaps the most famous of which was that of King Agamemnon, who slayed Odius during the Battle of Troy with a well-placed spear through his chest.[2] At the start of the common era, there are descriptions of fatal thoracic injuries suffered by the ancient Olympians in their often more violent version of the familiar games, as well as those suffered by the Gladiators and depicted by Galen.[3,4] Many of these injuries were the focus of art in the ancient world (Fig. 7-1).[5] More recent was the assassination attempt of President Ronald Reagan by John Hinkley in 1981; a bullet struck the president in his left chest, causing a nonfatal hemothorax (Fig. 7-2).[6,7] In the most recent conflicts in Afghanistan and the Middle East, Operation Enduring Freedom and Operation Iraqi Freedom, respectively, thoracic trauma was responsible for one quarter of on-battlefield deaths and represented up to 20% of all battlefield injuries.[8-10]

Through the eras of Hippocrates and Galen, open packing and local treatment with common ingredients (red meat, honey, lint) was the mainstay of treatment, until the 13th century when wound débridement and closure was advocated.

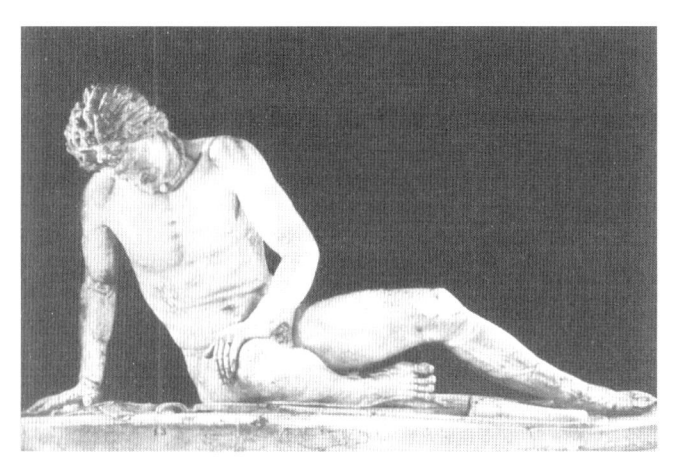

Figure 7–1
The Dying Gaul, from the first or second century BC, the Capitoline Museum of Rome. Note the penetrating trauma to the right hemithorax. *(From Churchill ED. J Hist Med Allied Sci 1971;26[3]:304-5.)*

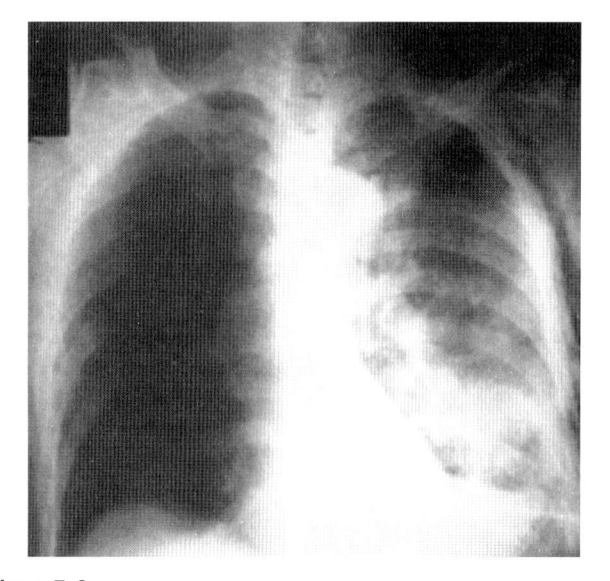

Figure 7–2
Chest radiograph after the assassination attempt on President Ronald Reagan, March 30, 1981. Note the presence of a left-sided chest tube. A bullet fragment is near the left border of the heart. *(From Rockoff SD, Aaron BL. Radiographics 1995;15[2]:407-18.)*

However, wound closure became a topic of great debate, although it was somewhat clarified by Paré in 1514. He advocated immediate closure of wounds without blood (or with only a small amount) in the chest; enlarging of small wounds if better drainage of blood were required; and delaying wound closure until blood drainage had ceased (usually 2 to 4 days).[11] During the next century, various cannulas were developed to irrigate infected wounds and empyemas, which eventually evolved into the closed drainage systems used during World War II.

Also during World War II, thoracotomy became commonplace, not only as the most effective means of draining retained blood and infected debris but also to remove the peel that formed over the lung from the hemothorax. As thoracic surgical principles developed, so too came the advances in endotracheal intubation, mechanical ventilators, and thoracic pain control that became pivotal in the management of most thoracic injuries over the next several decades.

Mortality from chest wounds progressively decreased from a wartime high of 80% to 90% during the Civil War, as reported by Billings,[12] to 4% to 7% in recent civilian experience. Nevertheless, thoracic trauma accounts for 25% of all trauma deaths, representing approximately 160,000 deaths annually.[13] Over 70% of thoracic injuries result from blunt trauma, and most occur in automobile accidents. One in four patients with cardiothoracic trauma regardless of etiology requires hospital admission.

Age of the patient plays an important role in the severity of injuries. In the pediatric patient, where the immature chest wall is elastic and flexible, fractures are rare but intrathoracic injuries are more significant. In the elderly patient, the fragile bony thorax is highly susceptible to even low-impact forces, and offers poor protection for the underlying viscera; mortality is quite high even with minor injuries.

Penetrating injuries are uncommon in age groups at either end of the spectrum, but they are one of the most common causes of death from trauma up to age 40. Low-velocity handguns, seen primarily in the civilian population, transmit very little damage to surrounding tissues. However, much more damage is done and energy conducted along the path of high-velocity missiles, usually associated with the military but now often seen in community violence as well.

THE PRIMARY SURVEY

The standard resuscitation of the trauma patient has been outlined by the American College of Surgeons in the Advanced Trauma Life Support (ATLS) guidelines.[14] When the patient arrives in the trauma bay, a primary survey is rapidly performed. The ABC algorithm is followed so that potentially life-threatening injuries can be recognized before they become lethal: the airway is controlled, then breathing is assessed and assisted with mechanical ventilation if necessary, and third, circulation is supported by establishing reliable, large-bore venous access and initiating fluid resuscitation. Finally, the patient's neurologic disabilities are assessed, and the entire body is exposed to identify any significant deformities or penetrating injuries that might otherwise have been overlooked. The goal of the primary survey is to identify immediate, life-threatening injuries that could account for ventilation or hemodynamic instabilities that, if left uncorrected, could cause the acute demise of the patient.[15]

Table 7-1

Potentially Acutely Lethal Injuries of the Chest and Their Management

Injury	Management
Tension pneumothorax	Tube thoracostomy
Massive intrathoracic hemorrhage	Tube thoracostomy, operative repair
Cardiac tamponade	Pericardiocentesis, operative repair
Deceleration aortic injury	Operative repair
Massive flail chest with pulmonary contusion	Intubation, pain control, fluid restriction
Upper or lower airway obstruction	Intubation, airway, bronchoscopy
Tracheobronchial rupture	Bronchoscopy, operative repair
Diaphragmatic rupture with visceral herniation	Operative repair
Esophageal perforation	Operative repair

Injuries to the thoracic cavity or its contents comprise the majority of this group, and they generally require urgent intervention as a life-saving measure (Table 7-1). These problems should always be kept in mind during the resuscitation of every trauma patient. The mechanism of injury should also influence the index of suspicion for these injuries, as some are more likely to be sequelae of blunt trauma (aortic rupture, diaphragmatic hernia, cardiac tamponade), penetrating trauma (cardiac tamponade, massive intrathoracic hemorrhage), or common to both (pneumothorax).

DIAGNOSTIC TESTS

Approximately a third of all deaths from thoracic trauma occur immediately on or shortly after the patient's arrival at a treatment facility. Diagnostic and emergency management modalities are essential to fully evaluate these injuries and direct care toward the proper therapeutic interventions.[16]

Chest Radiography

For every trauma victim, the chest radiograph is the focal point from which potential life-threatening thoracic problems are suspected. They can be obtained rapidly in the trauma bay with the patient still on the transportation backboard. A systematic review of the film should reveal suspected and unsuspected injures, and the presence of any foreign bodies. Fractures of the bony thorax, including the ribs, clavicles, spine, and scapulas, should be excluded. Fractures of the thoracic cage indicate significant energy transfer to the patient; those of the upper ribs are associated with trauma to the great vessels and those of the clavicle with pulmonary or cardiac contusions. The lung fields should be examined for pneumothorax, hemothorax, or pulmonary contusion. Along the mediastinum, widening, pneumomediastinum, or shifting are highly suspect for aortic transection, tracheobronchial or esophageal injuries, or tension pneumothorax or hemothorax. The soft tissues may reveal subtle subcutaneous air or foreign bodies. Finally, the width of the cardiac silhouette may raise the suspicion of tamponade.

Computerized tomography (CT) is not essential for every patient with chest trauma and should not be performed in the severely hemodynamically unstable patient or in the presence of obvious life-threatening injuries. However, it can be done with rapidity, and it may reveal injuries not seen clearly on plain radiographs: aortic disruption, pneumothorax, pneumomediastinum, hemothorax, or pulmonary contusions. It may be useful to screen all patients with blunt trauma and evaluate unusual or abnormal findings on initial chest radiograph (e.g., diaphragmatic injuries).

CT of the chest has been shown to be more sensitive than plain radiography in detecting thoracic injuries such as pulmonary contusions, hemothorax, and pneumothorax.[17,18] Up to 75% of trauma patients with a normal physical examination and chest radiograph will have an occult injury diagnosed on chest CT, and 5% of these patients will need intervention for their injuries.[19,20] Even when evidence of thoracic trauma is seen on physical examination and plain radiography, the addition of chest CT leads to altered management and therapeutic decisions in up to a third of all patients with thoracic injuries.[18,19] In addition, chest CT can be used to exclude diagnoses made by the less sensitive chest radiograph, which can happen in up to 15% of patients.[19]

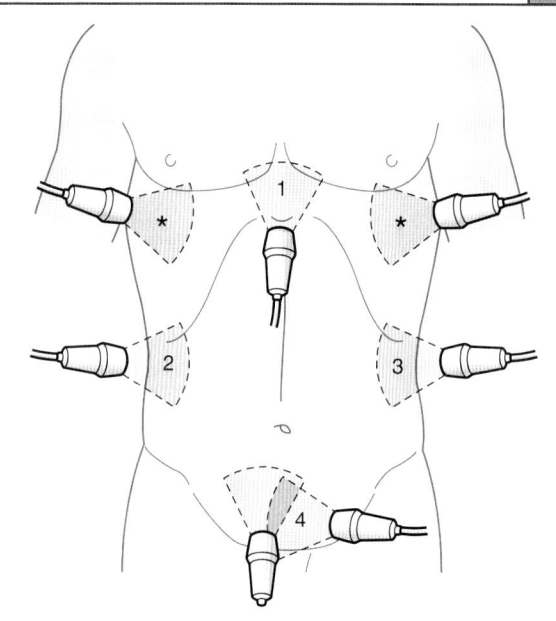

Figure 7-3
The extended focused assessment for the sonographic evaluation of the trauma patient (E-FAST) examination, using four standard viewing ports: right upper quadrant (2), left upper quadrant (3), pelvis (4), subxiphoid (1), and the extended views of the left and right hemithoraces (asterisks). (From Körner M, Krötz MM, Degenhart C, Pfeifer KJ, Reiser MF, Linsenmaier U. Radiographics 2008;28[1]:225-42.)

Ultrasonography

Ultrasonography has now become fairly routine in the early evaluation of the abdomen and pericardium.[21] The focused assessment for the sonographic evaluation of the trauma patient, or FAST examination, four standard viewing ports are used to quickly access for abnormal fluid collection: right upper quadrant, left upper quadrant, pelvis, and subxiphoid. In addition, the extended (E)-FAST, which uses an extension of the right and left upper quadrant views to include the right and left hemithoraces (right and left longitudinal thoracic views), respectively, can aid in the diagnosis of hemothorax or pneumothorax (Fig. 7-3).[22,23] Although not as precise as an ultrasound performed by a board-certified radiologist or cardiologist, this examination is able to detect fluid collections that might influence the need for urgent operative intervention. Of the four views, the subxiphoid view is the most accurate in the hands of surgeons for detecting abnormalities in the trauma setting.[21] It is safe, expeditious, repeatable, and effective even in the hands of surgeons from different specialties[24] and can be useful to identify injuries to the heart, and fluid in the pericardium.

Echocardiography

A major shift in the diagnosis of aortic and great vessel injuries has occurred in recent times.[25] In the 1990s and before, these injuries were diagnosed almost exclusively by aortic angiography or transesophageal echocardiography (TEE). Since the late 1990s, CT angiography (CTA) has become the most prevalent diagnostic modality in this patient population, with only a small percentage of patients undergoing conventional angiography or TEE. In two large trauma-center reviews, CTA was found to be 90% to 95% sensitive and to have a 99% to 100% negative predictive value, making it very useful as a screening modality.[26,27] Meta-analyses of smaller case series from the literature since the late 1980s appear to support these conclusions, with sensitivity and negative predictive values approaching 100%.[26]

Cited reasons for the shift in diagnostic modalities include technical improvements in the quality of CT angiograms with the addition of multirow detector CT techniques to the standard helical CT, the relative ease of performing the test, reliable interpretations of rapidly obtained results, cheaper cost to perform the test, ability to perform real-time three-dimensional (3D) reconstructions, and the ubiquitous nature of CT machines in emergency departments across the nation. CT angiography can be performed at the same time as the common whole-body CT scan that many trauma patients undergo as part of their routine workup. Furthermore, the level of detail achieved with CT aortography far exceeds that from conventional aortography, allowing the radiologist and the surgeon to identify even the most subtle of aortic injuries that may have been missed on conventional aortography. Large case series have identified CT aortography as an appropriate modality for screening, diagnosing, and planning operative repair of aortic injuries.[27]

In addition, results and interpretation of TEE, unlike those of CT angiograms, are extremely user dependent, and the expertise requires an understanding of the anatomic structures and of the sensitivity levels of the machine. TEE may now be reserved for detecting and following small intimal tears not seen on angiography, and for intraoperative imaging before and after a repair.

Angiography

Conventional angiography was once the gold standard in the diagnosis of aortic transection or injuries to the great vessels (Fig. 7-4).[28] In aortic transection, the classic aortographic

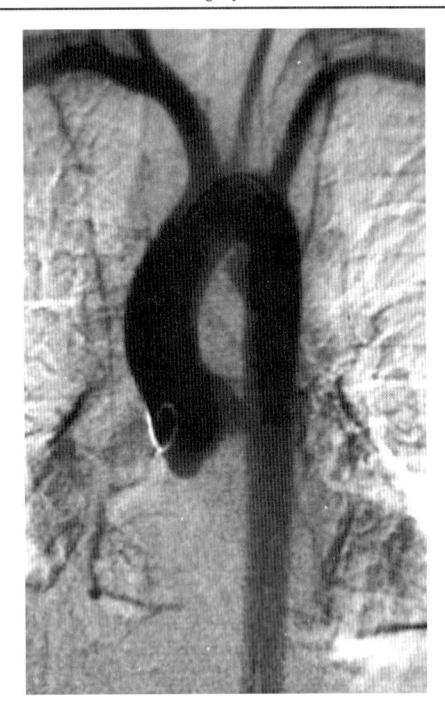

Figure 7-4
Conventional angiogram demonstrating aortic transection injury just distal to the left subclavian artery.

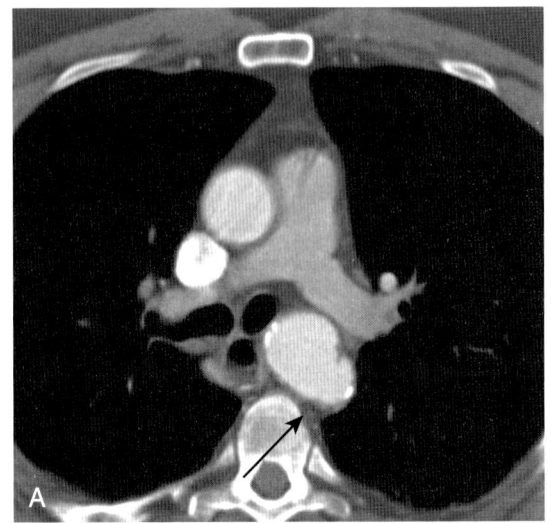

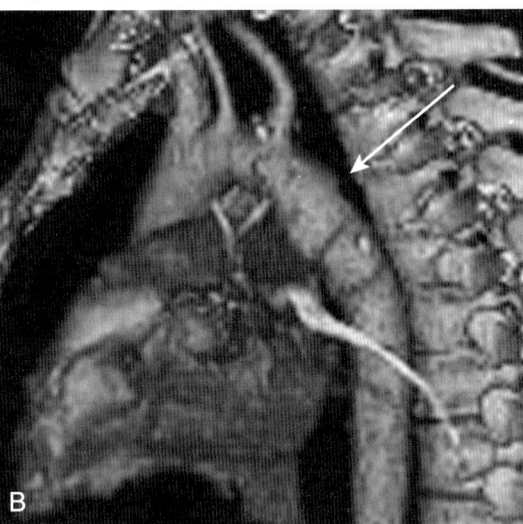

Figure 7-5
Aortic injury with saccular aneurysm *(arrows)* after chest trauma as seen by CT angiogram **(A)** and three-dimensional (3D) reconstruction **(B)**. *(From Steenburg SD, Ravenel JG, Ikonomidis JS, Schonholz C, Reeves S.* Radiology *2008;248[3]:748-62.)*

image displays a pseudoaneurysm near the site of the isthmus. Partial or complete interruption of the aortic contour may be seen when the aortic wall has retracted, or if debris of the wall prolapses into the lumen. Occasionally, a ductus diverticulum, a normal finding at the site of the uninterrupted intimal surface, is seen at the site of the ligamentum arteriosum.[29]

The present role of conventional arteriography is unclear, as many centers now use highly detailed 3D aortic reconstructions alone for diagnosis and operative planning (Fig. 7-5). Others obtain a conventional aortogram if the results of the CT angiogram are equivocal or if the study was technically inadequate. Still others routinely obtain conventional arteriograms to confirm the presence of an aortic injury prior to surgical intervention.[30] When performed, a retrograde femoral arteriogram is the preferred study. Generally agreed on indications for aortography in these patients, by either conventional methods or CT angiography, are listed in Box 7-1.

In fact, use of conventional aortography to further evaluate patients whose CT angiogram has been read as indeterminate is unlikely to aid in a diagnosis of any aortic or other great vessel injuries and thus may no longer be part of the evaluation of these patients.[31] Thus, some have argued that the role of conventional angiography is limited to those centers that do not have adequate multidetector CT scanners with software for 3D reconstruction and an available radiologist for interpretation, for cases where artifact from air or metallic objects precludes adequate imaging, or for cases where angiography is used to direct therapy (e.g., embolization of smaller arteries).[16]

The presence of a mediastinal hematoma is often the first manifestation of an aortic injury seen on CTA.[32] It is important, however, to note the exact location of this hematoma, as hematoma outside of the aortic walls with preservation of the fat plane around the aorta does not represent an aortic injury but rather, usually, damage to surrounding periaortic mediastinal vasculature. If the hematoma extends from a point adjacent to the aortic wall, a true aortic injury can be suspected, and careful examination of the remainder of the thoracic CTA is important. Rarely is active extravasation of contrast material into the mediastinum or thorax seen, as this type of injury is almost always uniformly fatal.

Several radiographic signs on CTA are diagnostic of traumatic aortic injury and should lead to immediate repair without further diagnostic evaluation, especially in the unstable patient. They include any intraluminal thrombi or clear evidence of mural dissection and intimal flap, as well as changes to the diameter or contour of the aorta itself. Delay of definitive repair in these patients may lead to increased mortality in this patient population.

EMERGENCY DEPARTMENT THORACOTOMY

The indications for emergency department (ED) thoracotomy have been widely debated.[33] ED thoracotomy clearly plays a role in the case of penetrating thoracic trauma, particularly

> **Box 7-1**
> **Indications for Angiographic Studies for Potential Thoracic Injuries**
>
> - High-speed deceleration injuries
> - Chest radiographic findings:
>   - Widened mediastinum
>   - Loss of aortic knob shadow
>   - Tracheal or esophageal deviation to the right
>   - Widening of paraspinal stripe and/or apical capping
>   - Downward displacement of left main-stem bronchus
>   - Obliteration of the aortopulmonary window
>   - Fractured first rib, sternum, or scapula
>   - Multiple rib fractures or flail chest
>   - Massive hemothorax
> - Upper extremity hypertension
> - Unexplained hypotension
> - Pulse deficits or asymmetry
> - Systolic murmur

> **Box 7-2**
> **Indications and Contraindications for Emergency Room Thoracotomy**
>
> **Accepted Indications**
> - Unresponsive hypotension (systolic blood pressure [SBP] < 60 mm Hg)
> - Rapid exsanguination from indwelling chest tube (>1500 mL)
> - Traumatic arrest with previously witnessed cardiac activity (before or after hospital admission) after penetrating thoracic injuries
> - Persistent hypotension (SBP < 60 mm Hg) with diagnosed cardiac tamponade, air embolism
>
> **Relative Indications**
> - Traumatic arrest with previously witnessed cardiac activity (before or after hospital admission) after blunt trauma
> - Traumatic arrest without previously witnessed cardiac activity (before or after hospital admission) after penetrating chest injuries
> - Prehospital cardiopulmonary resuscitation: <10 minutes in intubated patient, <5 minutes in nonintubated patient
>
> **Contraindications**
> - Blunt thoracic injuries with no previously witnessed cardiac activity
> - Multiple blunt trauma
> - Severe head injury

Working Group, Ad Hoc Subcommittee on Outcomes, American College of Surgeons-Committee on Trauma: Practice management guidelines for emergency department thoracotomy.[35]

for trauma patients with cardiac tamponade from penetrating chest injuries.[34] There is a very limited role for patients with blunt traumatic injuries, the only accepted indication being the patient who arrives with vital signs and suffers a traumatic arrest in the trauma bay.

Thoracotomy allows relief of cardiac tamponade, the ability to perform open cardiac massage, and control of ongoing intrathoracic hemorrhage. In addition, by applying a cross-clamp to the thoracic aorta, one can limit intra-abdominal bleeding and improve cerebral and coronary perfusion in the setting of exsanguinating hemorrhage. Patients with penetrating cardiac stab wounds and other penetrating cardiac injuries are the most likely to survive resuscitation with ED thoracotomy. The likelihood of patient survival depends on patient downtime, the patient's age and comorbidities, and signs of life on arrival to the ED. General guidelines have been recommended for ED thoracotomies by the American College of Surgeons' Committee on Trauma in the setting of thoracic trauma (Box 7-2).[35]

Although these general guidelines have been debated, most agree that the best results occur in patients with penetrating cardiac trauma and in whom there is a good likelihood for cerebral activity. Even with an experienced team and established protocols, results are still poor. The length of time cardiopulmonary resuscitation (CPR) was performed before the patient reached the hospital has become one of the determinants for whether to perform ED thoracotomy. In one report, there were no survivors from ED thoracotomy when prehospital CPR had been in progress in an intubated patient for more than 10 minutes, or more than 5 minutes in an unintubated patient.[36] Another marker of relatively poor outcome is refractory metabolic acidosis monitored during the initial resuscitation efforts, with a pH of less than 6.8 or severe base deficits restraining the use of ED thoracotomy.

The surgical approach is a left fourth interspace anterolateral thoracotomy. This can be performed with the patient prone or preferably with a few folded blankets placed under the patient's left side to elevate it and allow the incision to be opened more posteriorly if necessary. The incision may also be carried across the sternum into the right chest if necessary to further improve exposure or to evaluate the right side for injury. The pectoralis muscle is divided with a large scalpel, and the intercostal muscles are divided widely using curved mayo scissors. The sternum is transected with an oscillating saw, a Lebsche knife, a Gigli saw, and even (if nothing else is available) a good pair of trauma scissors. The mammary vessels are divided as they are crossed, and ligated once the patient is more stable. The pericardium is opened widely in a craniocaudal direction, staying anterior and avoiding the phrenic nerve. A large pericardiotomy allows easier evacuation of clot, visualization of the heart, and ability to perform more efficient open-heart massage. Cross-clamping the descending aorta requires opening the overlying parietal pleura and then getting around it bluntly using digital dissection. Care should be taken not to avulse any intercostals vessels. At this point, a vascular aortic crossclamp can be placed across it. Aortic crossclamp time should be kept to the minimum (less than 30 minutes) required to resuscitate the patient, to avoid the sequelae of spinal cord ischemia and lactic acidosis caused by distal hypoperfusion. When stable enough, the patient should be taken immediately to the operating room to definitively manage any injuries and to provide a sterile chest washout with antibiotic irrigation and formal closure of the thoracotomy with wide chest tube drainage.

Even with these extraordinary efforts on the part of the ED trauma team, the results from ED thoracotomy are dismal, with overall survival rates of 1.8% to 27.5%.[33] Although the survival rates of patients who undergo ED thoracotomy varies substantially between case series, mechanism of injury is the most important factor affecting mortality, and patients suffering penetrating injuries are more likely to benefit from this procedure, with mean survival rates of 13% (range, 2.7% to 38.9%) compared with a mean of 1% (range, 0% to 12%) for patients who presented with blunt injuries. Even among those who survive their injuries after ED thoracotomy, up to half will have some neurologic deficit, although some authors have reported that over 90% of patients regain neurologic function in their series.

BLUNT TRAUMA

Blunt trauma to the chest in the United States is far more common than penetrating injury. A 2002 report by the National Safety Council reported that of all blunt trauma deaths, 25% resulted from thoracic trauma. The high-speed deceleration and crush injuries involved in automobile accidents have become increasingly prevalent since the 1950s and account for the majority of blunt thoracic trauma. Falls, sports mishaps, assaults, and blast injuries follow. The damage from a powerful blast can be particularly severe, as the blast pressure wave imparts a large amount of kinetic energy to a small area. Blast kinetic energy especially affects gas-containing organs, such as the lung, resulting in pulmonary hemorrhage, hypoxia, and shock. In addition, because of the mechanisms that provide the amount of energy needed to produce significant blunt thoracic trauma, many of these patients will have associated head, abdominal, or extremity injuries along with those of the thorax (as presented here).[37] Nevertheless, even in this multiply injured population, the thoracic injuries are responsible for the majority of mortality.[38]

Chest Wall

Optimal mechanical properties of the chest wall are important determinants for effective functioning of the entire respiratory system. Blunt trauma to the chest wall can disrupt respiratory mechanics and lead to poor pulmonary toilet and significant morbidity. Chest wall trauma alone occurs in only 16% of cases[39] and is more often a marker of more ominous visceral injury in the thoracic cage or below the diaphragm. Because the chest wall provides a protective bony skeleton (ribs, sternum, clavicles, and scapulas) around the vital organs of the chest, the impact of fracturing each of these bones will be considered.

Rib Fractures

Fracture of the ribs is the most common blunt thoracic injury, occurring in an estimated 300,000 people in the United States during 2000, or 39% of patients admitted to major trauma centers.[40,41] Rib fractures are an important indicator of trauma severity. The greater the number of ribs fractured, the higher is the patient's morbidity and mortality, even from nonpulmonary causes, especially if six or more ribs are broken.[42,43] The number of ribs fractured has been significantly correlated with the presence of hemothorax or pneumothorax, with 81% of patients having either condition if two or more ribs were fractured.[44] Fractures of the fourth through the ninth rib are associated with injuries to the lung, bronchus, pleura, and heart, whereas fractures below the ninth rib are indicative of spleen, hepatic, or renal injuries.

The main symptoms include pain, exquisite tenderness, and possibly crepitus. In the initial examination, an upright chest radiograph is performed as a routine part of the trauma series. In the event that special documentation of a crime, such as child abuse, is needed, rib detail films are obtained. Chest radiograph alone fails to diagnose rib fractures in over half of trauma patients with fractures, and the addition of CT to the trauma evaluation improves the sensitivity of the diagnosis of rib fractures.[45] Careless dismissal of a simple rib fracture and underestimating its pathophysiologic potential, especially in the elderly patient, is a common management pitfall. After adjusting for severity of injury, comorbidity, and the presence of multiple rib fractures, elderly patients (≥65 years old) with simple rib fractures still were five times more likely to die than those younger than 65.[46] The first rib fracture has particular significance because of the great force required for it to occur and the likelihood that intrathoracic visceral injury has also taken place. The two most common sites of first rib fractures are at the subclavian sulcus and in the neck of the first rib posteriorly. Subclavian artery or aortic arch angiography (conventional or CTA) is indicated, or both can be done, if the first rib fracture is displaced posteriorly, if the subclavian groove is fractured anteriorly, or if there is widened mediastinum on chest radiograph, an upper extremity pulse deficit, a concomitant brachial plexus injury, or an expanding hematoma.[47]

Although binders, cumbersome rib belts, and taping were advocated in the past, the modern approach to treatment emphasizes relief of pain, prevention of atelectasis, and optimization of pulmonary toilet. The importance of adequate analgesia to proper pulmonary toilet is evident by studies showing decreased mortality among patients with rib fractures who received epidural anesthesia.[43] A prospective case series at a level 1 trauma center found that patients with isolated, simple rib fractures suffered an average of more than 50 days of disability and lost work or usual activity because of pain.[40] Interventions favored for short-term pain relief include epidural analgesia, intercostal rib blocks, intrapleural instillation of anesthesia, and intravenous opiates as well as oral nonsteroidal anti-inflammatory drugs (NSAIDs).[40,48-50] Chronic pain control is invariably required, usually with oral narcotics, NSAIDs, and transdermal patches. Patients must be reminded to practice adequate pulmonary toilet after discharge by using an incentive spirometer, deep breathing, coughing, and ambulation. Patients should be counseled that their pain will probably continue for weeks, and that sustained need for oral analgesics during this time is not uncommon. In addition to chronic pain, other long-term sequelae include chest wall deformities, persistent dyspnea, and neurologic deficits. A relatively uncommon but potential long-term complication of severe blunt trauma is a thoracic lung hernia. Because these entities pose a constant threat of incarceration, pneumothorax, or strangulation, they should be repaired.[51]

Flail Chest

During the primary survey of a patient who has suffered blunt trauma, careful observation for the presence of a flail chest is imperative because of the associated pathophysiologic derangements that accompany this finding.[52] This injury usually occurs with the fracture of four or more ribs at two sites, either unilateral or bilateral, promoting enough instability that the thoracic cage exhibits paradoxical motion locally. This impairs respiratory mechanics and results in hypoventilation, poor pulmonary drainage, and atelectasis. Patients with flail chest are distinct from those with multiple rib fractures as they are at a higher risk of respiratory compromise and often require early intubation.[53] Endotracheal intubation is required in more than two thirds of patients with flail chest and is indicated for a respiratory rate of more than 40 breaths per minute, or a Po_2 of less than 60 mm Hg despite 60% face mask oxygen. Relative indications for intubation include shallow respirations, depressed consciousness, preexisting chronic lung disease, or the presence of associated injuries. In the presence of multiple injuries, intubation of the patient with a flail chest is almost unavoidable, and early controlled intervention often obviates sudden respiratory decompensation and its subsequent morbidity.[53]

A flail chest is invariably caused when the thoracic cage absorbs high kinetic energy, and thus it is an important marker for significant intrathoracic injury in the patient with blunt trauma. It is highly associated with pulmonary contusion, which occurs in about 45% of these patients.[54] Pneumothorax or hemothorax is a common acute sequela, and acute respiratory distress syndrome (ARDS) occurs in as many as a third of these patients and results in mortality rates as high as 33%.[54]

Conservative therapy with emphasis on pain relief with thoracic epidural analgesia is the mainstay of therapy in most centers. In a minority of cases, however, patients require chest wall stabilization (Fig. 7-6).[55,56] These commonly are intubated patients with no possibility of being weaned from the ventilator because of a large unstable flail segment of chest wall.

Sternal Fractures

Isolated fractures of the sternum are seen with increasing frequency in motor vehicle accidents, particularly since the passing of the mandatory seatbelt legislation, because of the rapid deceleration that occurs from this mechanism of injury, especially in vehicles with absent or malfunctioning airbags.[57] Point tenderness, edema, and obvious deformity are occasionally detected on physical examination, but a lateral chest radiograph is diagnostic in the majority of patients.

Morbidity and mortality from isolated sternal fractures is low, and surgical repair is uncommon (<2%). Some have suggested that patients with isolated sternal fractures, a normal echocardiogram, and no elevation of cardiac enzymes in the early hours of injury will have a benign course. They advocate discharging these patients home within 24 hours of arrival in the ED.[58] Still others support selective repair for those with severe deformities or associated chest wall fractures, as this procedure can be performed with low mortality and morbidity and with good outcomes.[59] Surgical management options include metal plates with or without autologous bone grafts.[60,61] Although an isolated sternal fracture carries a favorable prognosis, other life-threatening concomitant injuries occur in up to a third of patients, necessitating careful evaluation and clinical vigilance.

Clavicular Fractures

Because the clavicles are thin and exposed, the mid-clavicular shaft, in particular, is often fractured, and this occurs in three of four patients with clavicular fractures.[62] One of four patients fractures the acromial part of their clavicle. Right and left clavicles tend to be fractured with equal frequencies. Clinical examination reveals tenderness, deformity, crepitus, and occasionally upper extremity neurovascular injury. Routine chest radiographs often demonstrate the diagnosis. Conservative treatment for pain control using closed reduction and figure-eight slings heals 95% of patients. Surgical techniques include placement of steel reconstruction plates and cannulated bone screws. Late sequelae of clavicular fractures include painful nonunions, altered shoulder mechanics, neurogenic thoracic outlet syndrome, vascular abnormalities, and brachial plexus injuries. Contributing factors to nonunion include severe initial trauma, open fracture, marked initial displacement and shortening, soft tissue interposition, primary open reduction and internal fixation, refracture, multiple trauma, and inadequate initial mobilization.[63]

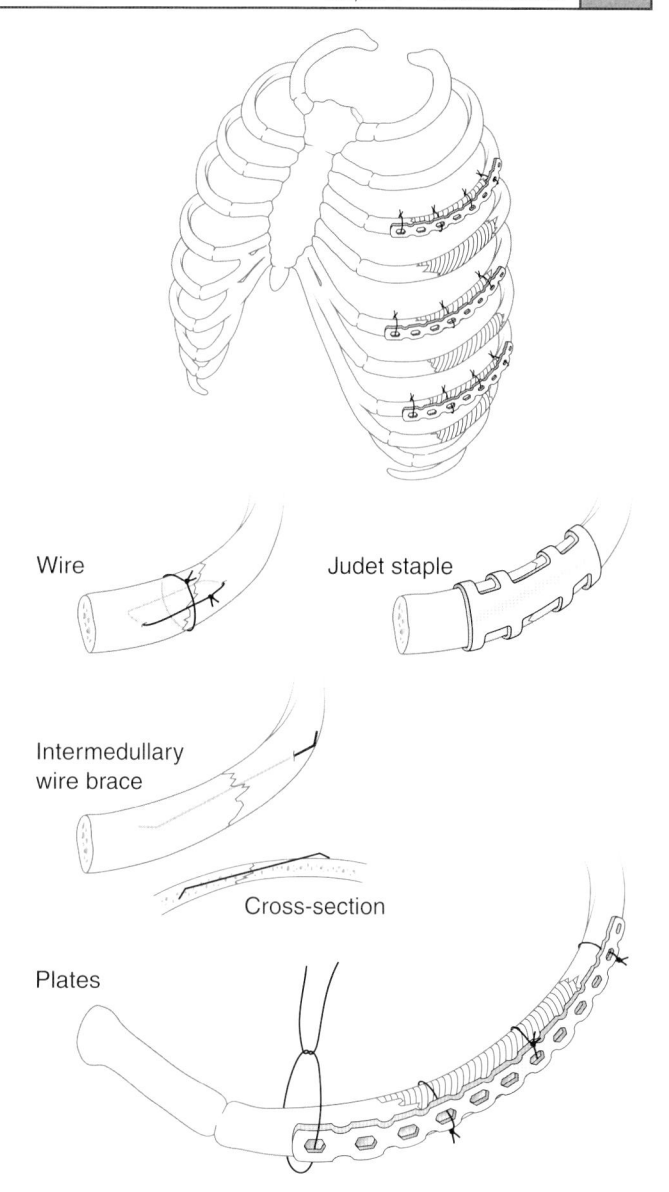

Figure 7–6
Stabilization of flail segments with wire, Judet staple, intermedullary wire brace and periosteal plates. *(From Trunkey DD. Chest wall injuries. In: Blaisdel FW, Trunkey DD, editors. Cervicothoracic trauma. 2nd ed. New York: Thieme Medical; 1994.)*

Scapular Fracture

Because the scapula is thick and well protected, scapular fractures are relatively rare and usually occur only after high-kinetic-energy impacts. In fact, many patients with scapular fractures have other serious injuries to other anatomic sites because of the severe mechanism of energy needed to produce this injury.[64] Still, scapular fractures should always be in the differential diagnosis in any patient who complains of shoulder pain or violent muscular contractions about the shoulder after blunt trauma. Most fractures occur in the neck and body, with glenoid, acromion, and coracoid process injuries being less frequent. As is the case with other thoracic cage trauma caused by severe blunt trauma, associated pulmonary contusions and rib fractures are common. Diagnosis is often difficult on physical examination, occasionally identified by localized tenderness, swelling, and hematoma formation over the fracture site. Scapular fractures are often overlooked on supine chest radiographs, and the three-view trauma series of the shoulder is often necessary to reveal the fracture. Chest CT scans are not recommended.

Immobilization in a sling with pain relief and early range-of-motion exercises is usually all that is needed for recovery of good glenohumeral function. Open surgical reduction is rare. Brachial plexus injuries are often chronic, leading to long-term disability, including loss of shoulder mobility. In these patients, a severely debilitated, insensate extremity may occasionally require amputation.

Traumatic Asphyxia

Traumatic asphyxia is an uncommon clinical syndrome usually occurring after a severe crushing or compression-related injury to the chest. Symptoms and associated physical findings include subconjunctival hemorrhage, cervicofacial cyanosis resulting in a purple-blue discoloration of the neck and face, facial edema, vascular engorgement of the head, mucosal petechiae, and multiple ecchymotic hemorrhages of the face, neck, and upper chest. Cerebral hypoxia resulting from hypoventilation is an ever-present danger that results in varying degrees of cerebral dysfunction. Sore throat, hoarseness, dizziness, numbness, and headaches are common. Pitting lower extremity edema, hemoptysis, hemotympanum, hematuria, rectal bleeding, and transient visual loss may also be evident.[65] The diagnosis is made primarily from the history and physical examination. Chest radiographs are usually normal.

Prompt establishment of the ABCs of trauma management is critical, with special attention to reestablishing oxygenation and perfusion to ensure a successful outcome. Head elevation should be maintained at 30 degrees. If a patient survives the initial insult, the prognosis is excellent. Skin discoloration resolves within 3 weeks, but complete resolution of subconjunctival hemorrhage can take up to 1 month.

Pulmonary Contusion

The lung parenchyma fills a large portion of the chest cavity and lies very close to the bony thorax, making it vulnerable to contusion. In fact, pulmonary contusion is the most common injury in blunt chest trauma.[52] The mechanism of injury usually involves a sudden deceleration injury such as in a motor vehicle accident with the chest hitting the steering wheel, or in a blast injury or a fall from a great height. Although pulmonary contusions are generally associated with concomitant thoracic cage damage and other visceral injuries, they can be isolated and without evidence of rib fracture. Wagner and colleagues have suggested that the pathophysiology of a pulmonary contusion is based on hemorrhage into adjacent alveolar spaces rather than injury to the alveolar capillary wall itself.[66]

Classic symptoms include dyspnea, tachypnea, hemoptysis, cyanosis, and hypotension. Physical examination can demonstrate inspiratory rales, and decreased breath sounds on the affected side. CT is the study of choice and has been found to be more sensitive than radiography in detecting a pulmonary contusion. All patients with a pulmonary contusion should be observed on supplementary oxygen in a hospital setting because of a tendency of their ventilatory status to deteriorate rapidly. By standard ATLS protocol, patients with significant hypoxia (PaO_2 < 65 mm Hg, SaO_2 < 90%) should be intubated and ventilated within 1 hour after injury. If large volumes of fluid are necessary for resuscitation of associated extrathoracic injuries, a pulmonary artery catheter should be placed.

As mentioned, patients with pulmonary contusions are at a high risk of respiratory insufficiency and secondary pneumonia because of the parenchymal damage and large systemic inflammatory response that accompanies this injury. The formation of a pulmonary contusion along with an injury severity score of greater than 65 has been identified as the risk factor that has the greatest contribution to the development of ARDS.[67] The mortality rate from an isolated pulmonary contusion is low, but when combined with other severe injuries, it rises to as high as 50%.[68] Clinical factors predisposing to mortality after a pulmonary contusion include patient age, resuscitation volume, and severity of the pulmonary parenchymal injury as measured by the ratio of PaO_2 to fraction of inspired oxygen (FiO_2) at 24 and 48 hours after the injury.[69]

Laryngeal Injuries

The larynx enjoys a position of relative protection in the neck, shielded laterally by the sternocleidomastoid, posteriorly by the cervical spine, and from the front and above by the mandible. Blunt trauma to the larynx is therefore rare, but its mortality rate reaches as high as 40%, with most patients dying from the injury at the trauma scene.[70] Death is caused primarily by asphyxia from laryngospasm, hemorrhage from an associated major vascular laceration, or laryngeal concussion. Laryngeal trauma is suspected after motor vehicle accidents, hanging attempts, sporting blows such as in karate or soccer, and severe falls.

Signs and symptoms after laryngeal blunt trauma include hoarseness, pain, skin contusions, cervical emphysema, cervical neck crepitance, dysphagia, and upper airway obstruction. Subtle signs of dysphonia including easy fatigue during phonation, marked difficulty with high-pitch and singing voice, and decreased phonation time can also occur. Diagnosis requires a high index of suspicion, because many patients remain asymptomatic at an early stage of injury, and minor symptoms may belie serious abnormalities. Furthermore, patients may be unable to supply critical aspects of the history and physical because of aphonia or intubation. Early diagnosis and appropriate therapy have a significant impact on the patient's condition later, especially in regard to scar formation, ease of breathing, and voice quality.

After securing a patent and stable airway, transnasal flexible laryngoscopy is used for a definitive diagnosis. Because the risk for laryngospasm and sudden airway obstruction is increased in the presence of a laryngeal lesion, preparations for emergency intubation or tracheostomy should be readied before performing endoscopy. Flexible laryngoscopy involves inspection for vocal cord mobility, mucosal edema, hematomas, tears, and arytenoid cartilage luxation. The CT scan is a sensitive diagnostic test for laryngotracheal injury, and it may be indicated despite normal flexible laryngoscopy. The status of the laryngeal skeleton can be determined more precisely via high-resolution CT scanning.

The decision to repair or observe laryngeal trauma is based primarily on the patient's respiratory distress and associated injuries. The presence of laryngeal fractures, air in the soft tissues, and extravasation of contrast material in the neck are helpful in assessing the extent of the injuries before surgical intervention. Immediate initial surgery is aimed at stabilizing the cartilaginous framework of the larynx and repairing the mucosa. Early and low tracheostomy is recommended for patients with endoluminal disruption of the larynx, and immediate surgical exploration with anatomic repair is performed for all laryngeal injuries. Suboptimal results are found in patients with bilateral vocal cord paralysis, displaced cricoid fracture, and arytenoid subluxation.

Tracheobronchial Injuries

Tracheobronchial injuries are uncommon, but they occur usually after high-energy impact and are associated with trauma to other vital organs.[71] According to an extensive review of all published tracheobronchial injuries since 1873, 59% of these injuries were found to be caused by motor vehicle accidents, 76% occurred within 2 cm of the main carina, and 43% were located within 2 cm of the right main bronchus.[72] Three potential mechanisms of blunt tracheobronchial disruption have been identified. The first and most common is a forceful anteroposterior compression of the thoracic cage, the so-called dashboard injury, where an unrestrained automobile occupant hyperextends the neck, striking it on the dashboard or steering wheel and producing a crushing injury of the cervical trachea. The second mechanism is a consequence of high airway pressures, and the third is a rapid deceleration. The typical clinical features include respiratory distress, dyspnea, and air leak. Hoarseness or dysphonia is also common, occurring in up to 45% in some series. Persistence of an undiagnosed air leak is life-threatening and may lead to hypoventilation and, ultimately, respiratory insufficiency. On physical examination, the most common diagnostic signs are subcutaneous emphysema (35% to 85%), pneumothorax (20% to 50%), and hemoptysis (14% to 25%).

The definitive diagnostic study of choice is a flexible bronchoscopy. A careful bronchoscopic examination includes an inspection of the tracheobronchial tree, documenting the site and extent of injury, including a withdrawal of the endotracheal tube in an intubated patient to diagnose proximal tracheal tears. A high level of suspicion is imperative for diagnosis, becausee occasionally patients with tracheobronchial injuries present with normal clinical appearance and negative endoscopic findings. In fact, often the diagnosis of tracheobronchial injury is delayed, and the repair is performed months and even years after the initial injury.[72] In that study, no statistically significant association was found between delay in treatment and successful repair of the injury, with 90% of patients undergoing successful surgical reconstruction more than 1 year after initial injury.

Effective airway management consists of bypassing the lesion with endobronchial intubation to the healthy bronchus using a single- or double-lumen endotracheal tube. Primary surgical repair of the injured airway is often necessary, with the decision to intervene based on the size of the lesion and the respiratory status of the patient. Simple, clean lacerations without much devitalized tissue can be primarily repaired with simple, interrupted 4-0 Vicryl sutures (Ethicon, Cincinnati, OH). More severe injury may even require lobectomy or pneumonectomy. The proximal one half to two thirds of the trachea is best seen via a low cervical collar incision, whereas the distal third of the trachea, the carina, and both the proximal right and left main-stem bronchi should be approached through a right thoracotomy. Prompt diagnosis and treatment generally lead to good functional recovery, but if tracheobronchial injuries remain undetected and untreated, late complications such as bronchial stenosis, recurrent pneumonia, and bronchiectasis can develop.

Great Vessels

The thoracic great vessels consist of the aorta and its major intrathoracic branches, the pulmonary arteries and veins, the venae cavae, and the azygous vein. By far the most lethal injury to any of these is descending aortic injury, which accounts for as many as 40% of fatalities after blunt thoracic trauma, with the majority of deaths at the trauma scene.[73] Most of these deaths result from free intrapleural aortic rupture before surgical repair. The site of injury is usually the medial descending aorta at the ligamentum arteriosum, where shear forces caused by rapid deceleration result in a tear at this point of fixation of the vasculature. Again, a high index of suspicion in a patient who has suffered a high-speed collision is critical, because about half of the patients with contained aortic rupture have no external signs of trauma.[74]

A plain chest film has a 95% negative predictive value for identifying blunt traumatic aortic lesions, so it is an adequate diagnostic screening study.[75] The classic signs on plain chest radiograph (Fig. 7-7) as described by Kirsch and Sloan include a widened mediastinum (>10 cm), loss of aortic knob contour, shift of the endotracheal tube and the trachea to the right, elevation of the left main-stem bronchus, depression of the right main-stem bronchus, shift of the nasogastric tube to the left, apical capping, first rib fracture, acute left-sided hemothorax, and a retrocardiac density. Of these, the finding that most reliably correlates with an aortic tear is loss of aortic knob contour. Spiral-CT scanning with angiography, which has 96.2% sensitivity and 99.8% specificity for blunt traumatic aortic abnormalities, as well as wide availability, has become the preferred confirmatory study in the algorithm of blunt aortic injury for hemodynamically stable trauma patients. Conventional biplane contrast aortography should be considered despite previous negative studies if the clinical suspicion remains high, as it is suggested that 2% of patients with great vessel injuries have this scenario.[76] Those patients with an obviously widened mediastinum on radiograph, along with hypotension and hemothorax, are at high risk for imminent rupture of a contained aortic injury and may

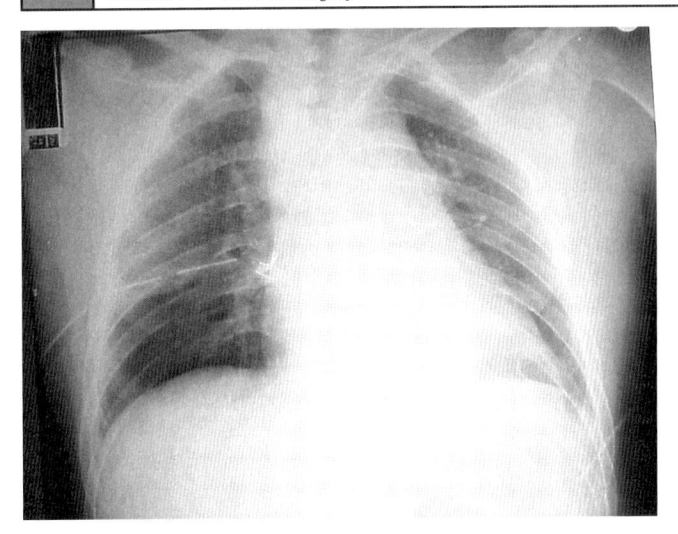

Figure 7-7
Typical chest radiograph with widened mediastinum suggestive of aortic transection from decelerating blunt chest injury.

be taken to the operating room without delaying for further confirmatory studies.[77]

Once a contained, aortic rupture is diagnosed, urgent management is required. Specifically, invasive monitoring and careful blood pressure and heart rate control with intravenous beta-blockade followed by nitroprusside are indicated as a first step. A thorough neurologic examination to document any preoperative deficits is vital. If other life-threatening injuries, such as intra-abdominal bleeding, are detected in the primary or secondary survey, these are repaired first before the thoracic aortic injuries are addressed. If there is little time for preoperative studies, a TEE can even be performed during laparotomy to identify signs of blunt traumatic aortic injury. Since the mid 1990s, the four most dramatic changes in management of these patients have been nonoperative management, delay to definitive treatment, use of endovascular stenting for repair, and the increasing use of left heart bypass via centrifugal pumps in the operating room.[76]

A subset of patients with contained aortic rupture, including those with severe central nervous system injury, extensive burns, hemodynamic instability from other traumatic injuries, respiratory failure, or small intimal defects, are appropriately managed either nonoperatively or with a delayed operation.[78] Mean arterial pressure should be maintained near 60 to 70 mm Hg in a manner similar to that used for patients who have suffered an acute dissection of the descending thoracic aorta.[76] Although the length of time necessary for rigorous antihypertensive therapy is unknown, reports in a small series of patients followed serially by TEE have shown that complete resolution of small (<20 mm) injuries occurs in about 9 days (range, 3 to 19 days).[79]

Since 1991 when the first endovascular stenting of the aorta was performed for an abdominal aortic aneurysm, interest in stent grafting as an alternative to traditional aortic surgery has surged. Preliminary experience is now accumulating from percutaneous positioning of endovascular stent grafts under angiographic guidance for blunt traumatic aortic lesions.[80-83] An analysis of the available data has demonstrated this to be an safe and effective procedure.[83] This procedure has excellent technical success rates, averaging 96.3%, with endo-leak rates of 5.1%, while maintaining low rates of complication, including overall and graft-related mortalities of 7.7% and 2%, respectively, and a 1.1% rate of paraplegia. Similar analyses of open repairs have demonstrated worse outcomes, with mean mortality of 14.7% and a 3.3% rate of paraplegia. In addition, length of hospital stay, transfusion requirement, and need for additional surgical procedures have been shown to be lower among patients who undergo percutaneous stenting compared with open repair of traumatic aortic injuries.[84] As the technology progresses and the grafts and their delivery systems become easier to employ, long-term studies, including randomized, prospective trials evaluating the durability and efficacy of this approach, will be warranted.

The open surgical approach is via a fourth interspace left posterolateral thoracotomy. Proximal and distal control is obtained with care taken to avoid injury of the recurrent laryngeal and vagus nerves as well as the thoracic duct. There has been considerable controversy for more than 2 decades between proponents of the use of "clamp and sew" techniques versus unloading the heart proximally and shunting the blood distally. Traditional arguments against the use of left heart bypass via passive shunts included the need to heparinize a trauma patient with associated injuries and the lack of data showing decreased neurologic injury with passive shunting. Convincing evidence is accumulating, however, demonstrating the benefits of left atrial to femoral shunting via a centrifugal pump. Many of these systems do not require heparin, and there is growing evidence of low rates of paraplegia and mortality.[85-87] Although prolonged clamp times and the increasing complexity of the repair are associated with rising paraplegia rates, another important predictor of paraplegia has been the occurrence of upper body hypotension during surgery. Left atrial to femoral shunting during and immediately after clamping of the aorta allows strict control of upper body blood pressure. In fact, a review of a 30-year experience of blunt traumatic aortic rupture noted the gradual evolution in clinical surgical technique from clamp-and-sew, to passive shunt, to heparin-less partial bypass.[87]

Blunt Cardiac Injuries

For decades, the term *cardiac contusion* has been used to describe a wide clinical spectrum of conditions thought to be associated with blunt injury, ranging from elevation of cardiac enzymes to complex intracardiac defects or rupture. This term should now be omitted entirely because of its inconsistent clinical descriptions, and because it offers little in directing therapy or predicting outcomes.[88] In keeping with the system of assigning trauma scores in the acutely injured patient, a new classification for blunt cardiac injury has been developed and is currently being used at major trauma centers (Table 7-2).[89]

Although blunt cardiac injuries are frequently highlighted in the literature, few patients require management for them. They are usually a result of high-speed motor vehicle accidents, falls from heights, crushing and blast injuries, direct violent assaults. Most motor vehicle–related deaths, however, are related to blunt injuries of the heart and great vessels. Mechanisms of decelerating cardiac trauma include compression by the sternum, impingement between the sternum and vertebral bodies, and increased venous return from crushing lower extremities injuries resulting in rupture of the cardiac chambers from overdistention. Although it was once thought

Table 7-2
Trauma Scores for Blunt Cardiac Injuries

Blunt Cardiac Injury with:	Trauma Score
No electrocardiographic (ECG), physiologic, or anatomic abnormality	1
Minor ECG abnormality	1
Major ECG abnormality	1
Cardiac enzyme elevation	1
Free wall hematoma	2
Septal hematoma	2
Septal defect	2
Valvular insufficiency	4
Free wall rupture	5
Cardiac herniation	5
Coronary artery injury	5

that sternal fractures were associated with a high incidence of blunt cardiac injuries, ironically there has been no proven association between the two. The incidence of these injuries, however, ranges from 10% to 70%, depending on the diagnostic modality and criteria used.

Clinically, there are few signs and symptoms that are specific for blunt cardiac injuries. Sternal or rib abnormalities may not be present. Chest pain is common, usually related to external injuries, and occasionally patients describe angina-type pain not relieved with nitrates. Therefore, the decision of whether a more aggressive workup for cardiac trauma is warranted rests on the mechanism of injury, external chest trauma, and a high index of suspicion. With more significant blunt injuries, hemopericardium is associated with hypotension and elevated central venous pressure. Auscultation may reveal decreased cardiac sounds, or a murmur with septal and valvular defects.

There is no gold standard for making a diagnosis of blunt cardiac injury. Although there is no direct correlation, a diagnosis of blunt cardiac injury should be suspected when a sternal fracture is present. An electrocardiogram (ECG) should be performed on all patients in whom blunt cardiac injury is suspected, but practically all trauma victims eventually get an ECG on admission. New-onset tachyarrhythmias, especially sinus tachycardia, are the most common findings on admission ECG, and this initial ECG is the best indicator of blunt cardiac injury.[90,91] Otherwise, the ECG is unreliable unless ST elevation is present.

Levels of creatine kinase–myocardial bands (CPK-MBs) and troponin have become part of the standard laboratory evaluation tests, but, like the ECG, they are limited by the lack of a precise threshold for the diagnosis of a blunt cardiac injury. However, in the patient with musculoskeletal trauma, the value of a CPK-MB level is questionable. Recently, cardiac troponins I and T were found to be highly sensitive for myocardial injury and useful in the stratification of patients

at risk for complications.[92] However, debate still exists about how the abnormal ECG, echocardiogram, and enzyme levels determine myocardial injury, and how they affect therapy, decision making, and outcomes.[89]

Echocardiography, however, remains the best diagnostic tool for detecting injuries, wall motion abnormalities, effusions, valvular or septal defect, and, particularly, chamber rupture.[93] This should be performed in all patients with an abnormal ECG or who are hemodynamically unstable. An attempt at transthoracic images should be made first, but if they are not optimal or yield limited data, the transesophageal route should be used. Because of their anterior location, the right atrium and ventricle are the most frequently injured chambers, followed by the left atrium and the left ventricle. Mortality from one chamber rupture is 60%, and 100% if two are involved.

Radionucleotide imaging can be helpful in documenting defects and predicting complications, but it may not be practical in the acutely injured patient, and it cannot differentiate new injuries from preexisting chronic disease. Furthermore, in the presence of a normal echocardiogram, it adds little to management decisions or predicting complications. Multigated acquisition scans are recommended, however, if the ECG is abnormal and there is evidence of ventricular failure.[94]

The recommended observation and treatment options depend on a suspicion of blunt cardiac injury, and on there being any associated diagnostic test abnormalities. Because the presence of a sternal fracture does not predict blunt cardiac injury, monitoring is not necessarily indicated. Patients with an abnormal ECG (arrhythmia, ST changes, ischemia, heart block) should be admitted for continuous ECG monitoring for at least 48 hours. However, if the initial ECG and echocardiogram are normal, a prolonged hospital stay with cardiac monitoring is no longer required, and most patients are discharged after 12 hours. Younger patients rarely develop cardiac complications even when there are mild ECG, echocardiogram, and enzyme abnormalities. However, for an older patient with known cardiac disease, hemodynamic instability, multisystem trauma, and ECG changes, and who is facing general anesthesia, appropriate cardiac monitoring is necessary, and placing a pulmonary artery catheter should be considered.

Operative intervention is required in 5% to 10% of patients presenting with nonpenetrating cardiac injuries. Chamber ruptures are usually isolated events and are repaired with simple cardiorrhaphy with a running suture, usually of 4-0 polypropylene; pledgets are required for right and left ventricular repairs. Valvular injuries have been reported in the aortic, mitral, and pulmonary locations. Cardiopulmonary bypass is required for left-sided repairs. Occasionally, valve resuspension or cordae reattachment can be done, but most injuries require valvular replacement. Ventricular septal defects can present either acutely or after several days of progressively worsening congestive heart failure. Operative repair is required for larger defects and for those associated with a left ventricular aneurysm. Pericardial tears with associated cardiac herniation are uncommon and have been described in the left, right, and midline diaphragmatic locations. With small tears and complete herniation, death is almost immediate. Larger tears manifest as intermittent positional hypotension and are usually found at the time of exploration for other injuries. Direct suture closure is required. Patch closure is rarely needed. Finally, arteriovenous fistula or thrombosis is an uncommon complication involving the coronary vessels. The diagnosis is usually made after the appearance of long-term sequelae: left ventricular pseudoaneurysm, cardiac failure, embolism, or arrhythmias. Surgery is directed at the specific complication.

Diaphragm

Since the advent of modern high-speed transportation, injury to or rupture of the diaphragm from blunt truncal trauma is seen with increasing frequency. In North American series, the prevalence of diaphragmatic rupture among blunt trauma victims ranges from 0.8% to 8%. Because of greater awareness, routine use of chest roentgenograms in the initial evaluation of trauma patients, availability of minimally invasive techniques, and improved access to modern trauma care systems, surgeons are increasingly facing the diagnosis and management of diaphragmatic injuries.

Diaphragmatic injuries can be classified according to the mechanism of injury, the side involved, their unilateral or bilateral location, the clinical sequelae after the onset of injury, and the severity of the anatomic disruption. The severity of the disruption has an important practical application in predicting outcome and associated visceral injury, because patients with diaphragmatic injuries are at risk for severe multisystem trauma. Blunt diaphragmatic rupture occurs mainly from high-speed motor vehicle crashes, when the rapid deceleration results in a nonuniform pressure load on the inflexible central tendon. In particular, lateral impact to the torso is three times more likely to rupture the diaphragm than a frontal impact. Because the diaphragm is buffered by the liver on the right, 95% of injuries occur on the left, and bilateral injuries occur in less than 3% of all cases. Compared with the left, patients with right hemidiaphragm ruptures tend to have increased multiorgan involvement, more hypovolemic shock, a lower Glasgow coma scale score, and higher mortality. Bilateral ruptures, including those involving the pericardium, are rare in patients who reach the hospital alive.

Diaphragmatic injury or rupture can also be classified by the time of presentation. After the onset of traumatic diaphragmatic injury, there are three clinical phases: acute, latent, and obstructive. The acute phase begins with the original trauma and ends with the apparent recovery from other injuries, and thus the diaphragm injury may be masked. Most patients (60%) have nonspecific pain in the left upper quadrant, or lower thoracic or shoulder pain. Others have severe acute symptoms of dyspnea, hypotension, or cyanosis as a result of compression of the lung and mediastinal shift from the herniated organs.

In the latent or interval phase, symptoms are variable and nonspecific as the patient compensates for having intrathoracic abdominal contents. The symptoms are suggestive of other disorders such as peptic ulcer disease, gallbladder disorder, partial bowel obstruction, and chronic obstructive pulmonary disease. Symptoms of intermittent bowel obstruction aggravated by eating or lying on the left side are relieved by belching, vomiting, or flatus.

Finally, the obstructive phase may occur at anytime when bowel obstruction occurs after incarceration of herniated viscera, leading to necrosis if diagnosis and treatment are further delayed. In one series, the onset of the obstructive phase ranged from 20 days to 28 years. But 90% usually present with strangulation by 3 years. These patients present with symptoms consistent with slow progressive herniation

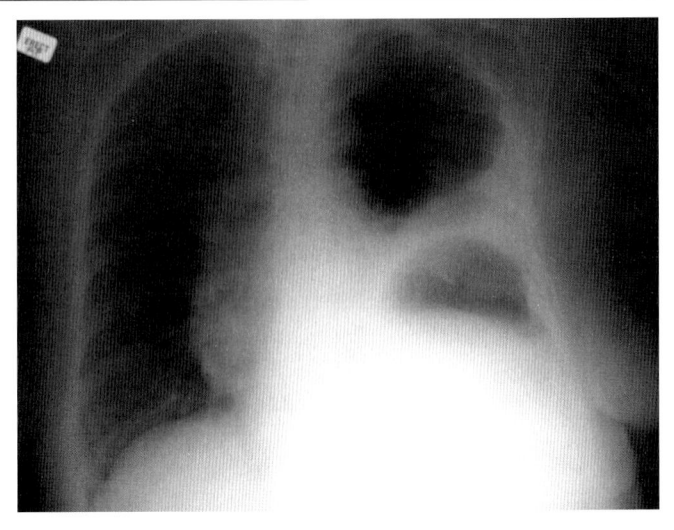

Figure 7–8
Chest radiograph after blunt thoracic trauma suggestive of left diaphragmatic rupture.

of stomach and bowel contents into the chest cavity. These include nausea, vomiting, abdominal pain, and obstipation, finally leading to respiratory distress, shock, obstruction, strangulation, and signs of viscus perforation.

The diagnosis of acute diaphragm injury or rupture is a clinical challenge, especially in patients who do not have obvious indications for emergent exploration. Because diaphragmatic defects do not heal and can eventually lead to a latent visceral herniation, delayed diagnosis can be catastrophic. In a patient who had previous blunt trauma, intermittent bowel obstruction without a previous abdominal incision should raise the possibility of diaphragm disruption. Findings on physical examination, such as paradoxical motion of the left upper abdominal quadrant, decreased intercostal retraction, decreased breath sounds, or shifting of cardiac sounds, should raise suspicion. Diagnosis in the latent phase can also be difficult, particularly with right-sided injuries, because of the vague symptoms. Often, patients do not recall any previous history of trauma, and physical examination may reveal bowel sounds over the chest.

Plain chest films are the initial screening test of choice, but up to 75% are nondiagnostic. Findings suggestive of a diaphragm defect include an indistinct costophrenic angle, elevated or indistinct hemidiaphragm, air–fluid levels in the chest, and abnormal pleural densities (Fig. 7-8). Right diaphragm injuries are rarely detected. CT and ultrasonography are often positive when there is frank visceral protrusion into the chest.

The diagnosis of left-sided ruptures can usually be made if a nasogastric tube passed into the stomach is seen in the hemithorax, or an upper gastrointestinal contrast series reveals a narrowing of the obstructed stomach or bowel segment above the diaphragm (Fig. 7-9). If an aortogram is performed for other reasons, the splenic or gastric vessels may be seen above the diaphragm. Although radionuclide scanning, fluoroscopy, or magnetic resonance imaging has high accuracy in the diagnosis of blunt diaphragmatic rupture, their use in unstable patients with multiple injuries is impractical. Right-sided ruptures may show a total or partial ("mushroom" projection) liver herniation, with or without associated bowel contents.

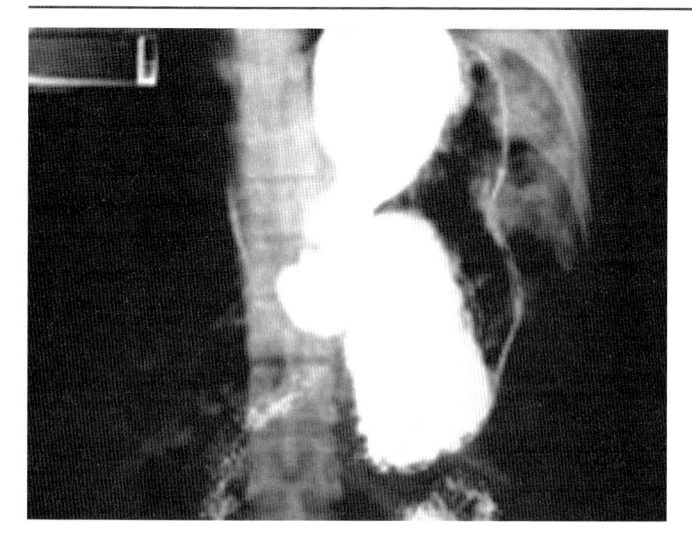

Figure 7–9
Upper gastrointestinal barium study delineating stomach and small bowel contents years after blunt decelerating injury.

Minimally invasive surgery for the evaluation of the diaphragm and other structures can be performed effectively while avoiding the morbidity of an open procedure. Routine laparoscopy is recommended to evaluate occult diaphragmatic injuries in stable patients with a left thoracoabdominal penetrating injury who otherwise have no other indication for an open operation. Among these patients, up to one quarter will have diaphragmatic injuries that were missed during the trauma radiographic workup.[95] These diaphragmatic injuries can be repaired at the time of diagnosis during laparoscopy, and in patients with previous abdominal surgery, a video-assisted thoracic surgical approach may be preferred to evaluate and repair the diaphragm once intra-abdominal injuries have been ruled out.

The surgical approach to repairing acute diaphragmatic injury or rupture depends on the mechanism of injury, the condition of the patient, and the time of presentation. Shock should be corrected, and a nasogastric tube should be in place to decompress the stomach. After immediate life-threatening injuries are addressed, the diaphragm can be thoroughly inspected for defects. Even the smallest of defects should be closed. Laparotomy can be first performed to explore the abdomen for other injuries, but diaphragmatic defects can be repaired from either the abdomen or the chest. When both cavities need to be explored, separate incisions are favored over a continuous one, because morbidity is higher with the latter.

For patients who require emergent laparotomy for suspected intra-abdominal injuries, thorough inspection of both hemidiaphragms is mandatory, regardless of the direction of the blunt impact. Diaphragmatic rupture resulting from blunt trauma should be approached through a laparotomy because of the high incidence of simultaneous intra-abdominal solid-organ injuries. Similarly, for hemodynamically stable patients whose diaphragm injury is confirmed by noninvasive imaging or by laparoscopy, laparotomy should be performed to rule out occult intra-abdominal injuries.

When patients with injuries and hernias present in a delayed fashion, however, a thoracotomy approach is preferred by many. This provides excellent exposure to divide the adhesions between the trapped viscera and the lung parenchyma, but a transabdominal approach may be preferable for left hemidiaphragmatic hernias when segments of small or large bowel may have to be resected and anastomosed. However, a thoracotomy approach should be used for all right-sided diaphragmatic defects, regardless of the timing after initial injury.

The herniated viscera is first carefully reduced and returned to the abdominal cavity. The preferred method of closure of the diaphragmatic defect is by interrupted full-thickness nonabsorbable 0 or no. 1 sutures. Adhesions should be taken down, the lung decorticated, and, if necessary, the diaphragm loosened from the lower rib to take tension off the repair. For the chronic rupture, a splenectomy may need to be performed, followed by enlargement of the defect to facilitate repair. Finally, in the rare case when tissue loss is extensive, closure of the defect can be achieved with fascia lata, biological material such as bovine pericardium, or synthetic material.

Mortality and morbidity in patients with acute diaphragmatic injuries differ considerably from mortality and morbidity in those with a delayed presentation.[96] In the former, multiorgan trauma is usually present, and thus irreversible shock and head injury are most often cited as the causes of early death, with a rate that approaches 40%. With strangulated bowel, the rate goes to 80%. When these injuries are isolated and repaired adequately, complications are rare and usually pulmonary in nature. With the chronic type, sepsis and multisystem organ failure are the usual causes of mortality. In the presence of bowel strangulation and gangrene, a much higher postoperative mortality (66%) and morbidity (80%) are encountered than in those patients with an uncomplicated operative approach.

Esophagus

Blunt and penetrating trauma to the esophagus are both rare because of the relatively protected location of the thoracic esophagus in the posterior mediastinum.[97] Blunt esophageal trauma is much rarer than penetrating injury, and when it occurs, it is usually a result of a direct blow to the cervical region, such as hitting the steering wheel during a decelerating motor vehicle accident or even from padded objects such as boxing gloves. Simultaneous rupture of the esophageal wall and adjacent membranous trachea wall can occur if both are compressed between the sternum and the vertebral body, resulting in fistula formation. It is estimated that a third of all tracheoesophageal fistulas have this etiology, second only to iatrogenic causes. Other blunt force injuries include manual compression during cardiopulmonary resuscitation (an incidence of up to 12% found during autopsy) and the Heimlich maneuver.

A Boerhaave-like rupture injury can occur from increased intraluminal pressure with a closed glottis and increased intra-abdominal pressure. This usually occurs just above the esophagogastric junction, and into the left pleural space where the pleural lining offers less protection. Mortality is high not because of the severity of the injury but rather from the delayed diagnosis and ensuing complications. Other etiologies of barotrauma include blast injuries and introduction of high-pressure gases (e.g., fire extinguisher discharges, eruption of carbonated drinks, and gas ingestions from biting of inner tubes). Finally, localized wall or long-segment necrosis has been described despite its rich blood supply, as the arterial inflow is torn away by the severe blunt trauma.

Blunt esophageal injuries are often difficult to diagnose early, because of multisystem trauma issues and the lack of recognition. Patients may present with signs and symptoms of esophageal leak: subcutaneous air, pneumomediastinum, aspiration (from fistula formation), hypotension, tachycardia, and sepsis in the more advance case. Diagnosis can be made from a contrast swallow study, but in the compromised trauma patient, this usually cannot be performed. A CT scan in some cases may detect small leaks into the neck or mediastinum not seen on contrast esophagography. Esophagoscopy is helpful, and has been reported to have higher sensitivity than contrast studies.[98]

With free perforation or fistula formation, early surgical repair is advocated. Conservative medical therapy (broad-spectrum antibiotics, close observation, parenteral nutritional support) is chosen only in selected patients when the leak is minimal and there are no signs of sepsis. Approaches are dictated by the level of involvement. Cervical incisions usually suffice for the defects in the neck, but exposure with an upper sternal split for the thoracic inlet may be required. A right thoracotomy may be required for the upper third of the thoracic esophagus, whereas the left side is preferred for defects just above the esophagogastric junction. The surgical principles are like those followed for other benign perforations of the esophagus: The edges are trimmed of devitalized tissue and closed in multiple layers. A tissue flap is added to buttress the repair. When a fistula is taken down, the esophageal and tracheal openings are closed primarily, and the suture lines must be separated by a tissue flap to prevent reformation. These flaps include intercostal muscles, strap muscles, mediastinal thymic fat, pericardium, and diaphragm. A tracheostomy has been advocated to help protect the tracheal suture line. Patients whose diagnosis was delayed and who are hemodynamically unstable may require esophageal diversion rather than primary repair.

Extensive necrosis of the esophagus is associated with a much higher mortality rate. When suspected, the diagnosis is made with endoscopy, noting the mucosal ischemic changes. In these circumstances, emergency esophagectomy and proximal diverting esophagostomy is required, with reconstruction of gastrointestinal continuity performed at a later date.

PENETRATING TRAUMA

Stab Wounds versus Firearm Injuries

The evaluation and management of penetrating trauma to the thorax is best broken down by anatomic distribution.[99] This includes the chest wall, the great vessels and other major vascular structures, the trachea and major bronchi, the lung parenchyma, the heart, the esophagus and the diaphragm. Each of these structures can be injured individually or in combination with other intrathoracic or extrathoracic structures. The evaluation of thoracic injury requires a systematic approach founded on anatomy to rapidly identify injury and initiate therapy. The appearance of penetrating injuries to the chest can be subtle or dramatic. Paramount in the management is a rapid assessment and evaluation of the patient's severity of injury. Patients who *appear* stable can deteriorate rapidly and can become acutely moribund through tension pneumothorax, pericardial tamponade, or massive intrathoracic hemorrhage.

Once the initial survey has been performed, the patient's disability should be evaluated, specifically with determination of the location and mechanism of penetrating injury. Puncture wounds can be small and easily missed. The patient must be rolled and completely exposed with close inspection of critical areas such as the axilla. Central wounds and peripheral wounds have different implications. Lower thoracic and upper thoracic wounds suggest potential injuries to neck structures and abdominal structures, respectively, in addition to a thoracic injury. Stab wounds differ from gunshot wounds in their potential depth of penetration and degree of damage to surrounding organs. Knife wounds are limited to the direct track of the blade and impart only the kinetic energy transfer to surrounding tissue that is manually produced. Gunshot wounds, on the other hand, impart kinetic energy to the surrounding tissue produced by the mass and velocity of the bullet (kinetic energy = ½ mass × velocity-squared). In addition to injury along the direct wound path, radial injury is produced by the kinetic energy transferred to the surrounding tissue. Wounds can be classified as low-energy transfer or high-energy transfer.[100] In general, handgun wounds produce low-energy transfer injuries and high-velocity rifles produce high-energy transfer injuries. All of these issues should be rapidly evaluated and considered in the primary survey.

Chest Wall Injury

The chest wall provides a rigid support and protection to the contents of the chest. Injuries that are limited to the chest wall itself rarely require surgical intervention. These injuries include intercostal vascular injuries, which can produce hemothorax as well as injuries to the internal mammary artery. These are usually managed easily with ligation or electrocautery. Blast injuries caused by high velocity missiles usually or shotgun injuries can result in major tissue loss of the chest wall including both soft tissue and the bony thorax. These injuries can be initially covered with adhesive Steri-Drape or a soft Esmark covering with placements of chest tubes inside the thorax to achieve lung inflation and control any air leak. Definitive coverage of the defect using rotational flaps or free flaps of latissimus muscle, pectoralis major, serratus anterior, or omentum can be performed at a later time.

Tracheal and Bronchial Penetrating Injuries

Although penetrating injuries to the trachea and major bronchi are rare, encompassing 1% to 2% of thoracic trauma admissions, the nature of these injuries is quite serious and these patients often present with respiratory distress.[101] Following the principles of ATLS, airway management and control of breathing with endotracheal intubation for adequate ventilation is the first objective in management. The need to establish a surgical airway in more proximal laryngotracheal injuries should be anticipated and performed without hesitation should oral endotracheal intubation prove difficult or impossible. In one series, almost half of these injuries required surgical creation of an airway.[102] Cricothyroidotomy or tracheotomy is unlikely to provide any advantage over endotracheal intubation in more distal tracheal or bronchial injuries. Gunshot wounds are the most common cause of central airway injury, although stab wounds are also possible. Stab wounds that injure the airway are more likely to be in the neck.[103,104]

Signs of airway injury include subcutaneous emphysema, hemoptysis, pneumothorax, and air leak on chest tube insertion. Plain films may reveal pneumothorax, pneumomediastinum, atelectasis in an underinflated lung or lobe, and the fallen lung sign of Kumpe if the lung has collapsed away outward and downward (rather than inward and upward) from the hilum.[105] Adequate ventilation may prove challenging in the setting of a tracheal or hilar injury. Intrapleural injuries produce pneumothorax and should be treated with immediate chest tube insertion. Massive air leak should raise the suspicion of a major bronchial injury, but lack of air leak on chest tube insertion does not rule out the presence of injury. Bronchial edges may be approximated and thus may seal a leak. A clot obstructing the bronchus may prevent air egress from the area of injury. Intubation and bronchoscopy are the first steps in managing a suspected bronchial injury. Extrapleural or mediastinal injury may not manifest as pneumothorax but instead as massive mediastinal air or subcutaneous emphysema.

Flexible bronchoscopy should be performed and the complete tracheobronchial tree examined. If a proximal tracheal injury is suspected, the patient can be intubated over a bronchoscope to fully inspect the airway. Fiberoptic intubation can be performed awake, with sedation and paralysis instituted after the airway has been established. Proximal tracheal injuries are best managed initially with intubation distal to the area of injury and control of the air leak. Injuries to the mainstem bronchi can be more challenging to manage initially. Bronchial blockers or Fogarty catheters are used to occlude the side of the injury and control massive air leak and prevent inadequate ventilation. Double-lumen endotracheal tubes should be used if at all possible for selective ventilation of the uninjured lung. Injuries to the airway can result in significant amounts of blood in the tracheobronchial tree and contribute to problems with ventilation. Aggressive toilet bronchoscopy must be performed, with lavage of the airway until clear.

Surgical management of tracheal or bronchial injuries follows the same principles of tracheobronchial resection and repair used for neoplasms (Fig. 7-10). Proximal tracheal injuries can be managed through a cervical collar incision or an upper sternal split. More distal tracheal injuries are best approached through a right posterolateral incision. Bronchial injuries are best approached through posterolateral thoracotomy to the side of the injury. Proximal left main-stem bronchial injuries and carinal injuries are best managed through a right posterolateral thoracotomy. On initial entry, control of the hilum with isolation of the pulmonary artery and veins is the initial goal. Unsuspected vascular injury may be present, and proximal control of these vessels is critical. We place umbilical tapes and loosely draped tourniquets around the vessels to enable rapid control of bleeding or potential air embolus. The airway is then dissected out and débrided and repaired using interrupted absorbable sutures in the standard manner of sleeve resection or bronchoplasty. A tension-free technique should be used for airway repair. Mobilization of the airway should be adequate to decrease tension but not compromise blood supply. Large defects in the airway may require lung resection, although lung-sparing techniques should be attempted. Injury to a lobar bronchus might be best treated with standard or sleeve lobectomy. Pneumonectomy should be avoided at all costs, given the extremely poor outcomes of patients requiring pneumonectomy for trauma.[106,107] Postoperative care should include aggressive pulmonary toilet and attempts to wean from positive-pressure ventilation as quickly as possible. Aggressive bronchoscopy should be performed to keep the airway clear of secretions and prevent atelectasis. As in all thoracic surgery, early ambulation is critical.

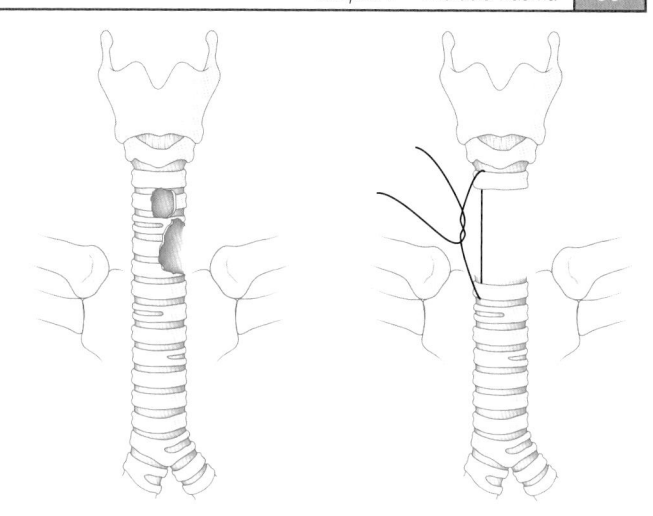

Figure 7–10
Resection and repair after gunshot wound to the cervical trachea. *(From Lee RB. Traumatic injury of the cervicothoracic trachea and bronchi.* Chest Surg Clin N Am *1997;7:300.)*

Pulmonary Injuries and Hemothorax

Pulmonary injuries secondary to penetrating trauma can vary from small pleural or parenchymal lacerations from a stab wound, to massive pulmonary injury secondary to a gunshot wound. The initial evaluation should include, in addition to the ABCs, a routine chest radiograph in the stable patient. Physical examination to detect hemothorax and hemopneumothorax can be unreliable, particularly in a patient who is stable with minimal symptoms. Asymptomatic patients with a normal chest radiograph can be safely observed and discharged after an appropriate time interval.[108] This time interval is a subject of debate, although a serial chest radiograph at 6 hours seems to be a reasonable time period to pick up a delayed hemothorax or pneumothorax. In fact, of all thoracic trauma patients, less than one fifth will have injuries that necessitate placement of a chest tube.[109]

We do not recommend wound exploration and tractotomy of thoracic wounds because of the potential for causing a pneumothorax and contaminating the pleural space. Tube thoracostomy should be performed in all patients with a pneumothorax or findings of pleural fluid after penetrating trauma. We recommend this even if the pneumothorax is small or the fluid appears minimal. Tube thoracostomy allows monitoring of bleeding so that a thoracotomy can be performed if the bleeding becomes significant. In addition, it prevents accumulation of clot that may later prove difficult to drain and require decortication. Patients with minimal chest tube output and no air leak can have the chest tube removed on the first hospital day and can be discharged. Persistent bleeding mandates thoracotomy or thoracoscopy. Massive bleeding on chest tube insertion should be treated with emergent thoracotomy with no attempt to use thoracoscopic techniques.

Most pulmonary lacerations do not require surgery and can be treated by tube thoracostomy. In fact, in a series of 755 penetrating injuries to the chest, more than half of which were gunshot wounds, only 8% required thoracotomy.[110] Drainage of the pleural space with reestablishment of pleural apposition tamponades what is generally low-pressure, venous bleeding and serves to seal an air leak. Even high-velocity war-related injuries usually respond to conservative measures of chest tube drainage, antimicrobial therapy, and wound care.[111] Large air leaks on chest tube insertion should raise the concern for bronchial injury and be followed by prompt bronchoscopy and possible thoracotomy.

If thoracotomy is necessary, the general rule is to spare as much lung as possible and avoid anatomic resection. A posterolateral thoracotomy is performed to gain access to the hilum of the lung. Lung isolation is obtained expeditiously with a double-lumen tube or bronchial blocker. This serves to provide atelectasis to perform a tension-free repair or resection of the lung and to help prevent air embolus. As in all thoracotomies for penetrating thoracic trauma, the hilum and pulmonary vessels are controlled early with umbilical tapes or vessel loops to allow rapid vascular control should an unsuspected central injury be present that was unnoticed. Nonanatomic resections are performed whenever possible. We use stapling devices with a generous margin around the area of injury to resect damaged tissue. Hematomas should be treated with a broad margin and vascular load to the stapler to achieve hemostasis. These staple lines can be oversewn to reinforce the region and support hemostasis if the staple line was not adequate to stop bleeding. Persistent bleeding from deep missile injuries can be opened and exposed by inserting the anvil of the linear stapler into the tract and firing the devise to perform a "tractotomy." If there is extensive tissue loss, anatomic resection of an injured lobe may be necessary. The literature shows that mortality increases with the level of complexity of the procedure.[112] Pneumonectomy is to be avoided and performed only if all other measures to salvage the lung have been exhausted. Anatomic resections require some form of bronchial stump coverage given the contamination of the pleural space and risk for subsequent infection and bronchopleural fistula.

The timing of thoracotomy for thoracic hemorrhage after trauma has been widely discussed. Recommendations have been made for to perform thoracotomy if there is an initial chest tube output of greater than 1500 mL or if the chest tube output is greater than 250 mL per hour for 3 consecutive hours after its placement.[113] Slightly different amounts of chest tube output have been used as guidelines for operative intervention for ongoing bleeding. However, one recent multicenter trial showed that mortality linearly increased as the total amount of chest tube output increased, and the authors used 1500 mL total chest tube output within the first 24 hours after injury as a recommendation to surgically intervene.[112]

Cardiac Injuries

Penetrating injuries to the heart are a significant challenge to manage.[114] They are one of the leading causes of death in urban trauma, accounting for a high rate of prehospital death as well as in-hospital mortality. Most patients who sustain cardiac injuries die before reaching the hospital, and almost two thirds of patients with penetrating cardiac injuries have no vital signs on arrival to the trauma bay. Reported mortality for these injuries varies from one series to another. What is clear is that the mechanism of injury influences survival. In general, these injuries are either stab wounds or gunshot wounds. Penetrating cardiac injuries secondary to blunt trauma that produces fragments of fractured rib or sternum are rare. Gunshot wounds carry higher mortality than knife wounds because stab wounds often seal themselves quickly, and the resulting cardiac tamponade can allow these patients time for definitive management. Ballistic trauma, on the other hand, produces much larger, irregularly contoured wounds that result in hemorrhage without tamponade, as the pericardial sac is no longer intact. The management of patients presenting in extremis or nearly so, with penetrating injury to the heart, consists of airway management with endotracheal intubation, the establishment of intravenous access capable of massive volume resuscitation, and immediate thoracotomy through a left anterolateral approach. This approach allows rapid exposure of the heart and the ability to relieve tamponade from hemorrhage. In addition, it allows the surgeon to perform open heart massage, control cardiac injuries, cross-clamp the descending aorta to preferentially perfuse the brain and coronaries, and allow volume resuscitation in the setting of exsanguination and shock.

The patient's physiologic condition at the time of presentation significantly affects outcome. The clinical features of a patient presenting with a penetrating cardiac injury depend on the degree of pericardial tamponade and the amount of blood loss. Coronary artery injuries are rare but can cause ischemia resulting in hemodynamic instability from myocardial dysfunction. One prospective study of 105 patients with penetrating cardiac injury showed that patients in physiologic collapse on presentation that required emergent ED thoracotomy had a mortality rate of 86%, whereas those who were stable enough to be transported to the operating room for thoracotomy had a 26% mortality rate.[115] The need for aortic cross-clamping was a significant predictor of poor outcome (89% mortality), probably because of the poor physiologic condition of these patients on presentation. Survival from stab wounds (65%) in this study was significantly higher than for gunshot wounds (16%). More recent studies have identified emergency medical services transportation, stab wound (as opposed to gunshot wound), sinus tachycardia, and the presence of vital signs on arrival to the trauma bay as predictors of survival after ED thoracotomy for penetrating cardiac trauma.[116]

All penetrating cardiac injuries have the potential for mortality, and it is not clear that the particular area of the heart that is wounded affects the prognosis. Over a third of all penetrating cardiac trauma results in isolated right ventricular injury, whereas a quarter of patients have isolated left ventricular injury.[73] Thirty percent of patients have multichamber injuries. Ventricular injuries, particularly right ventricular injuries, with their more anterior location, seem to be more common. The left and right atrium, with their smaller size and more protected location, are less commonly injured. Intrapericardial great vessel injuries are also unusual. Although it is not possible to say that one anatomic location of injury portends a worse outcome, it does appear that multichamber and complex cardiac wounds have a worse prognosis than a single-chamber injury.

Although many cardiac injuries are obvious on presentation, as manifested by a hemodynamically unstable patient with a penetrating injury in proximity to the heart, diagnostic evaluation is necessary for other patients who are stable but may harbor occult cardiac injury. These injuries must be identified. Even small knife wounds to the heart are unlikely to seal spontaneously and will eventually result in tamponade. The hole in the pericardium produced by the knife or projectile will frequently seal with clot or pericardial fat. Blood from the heart will accumulate and impinge on the filling of the atrium and ventricle. The incidence of occult injury has been reported to be as high as 20% in asymptomatic patients with penetrating stab wounds to the chest.[117] Workup is indicated in patients with penetrating precordial, right-sided or left-sided chest wounds and those with thoracoabdominal and abdominal wounds. Tachycardia is usually the earliest sign of hypovolemia and impending tamponade. As the pericardium fills with blood, elevated filling pressures are necessary to fill the heart. This results in the clinical findings of distended neck veins and pulsus paradoxus (decrease in systolic pressure with inspiration). These signs can be subtle and difficult to detect in a noisy emergency room or in a hypovolemic patient.

Several modalities can be used to evaluate occult cardiac injuries. Echocardiogram is sensitive for detecting pericardial fluid, and specific signs of tamponade—diastolic collapse of the atrium or ventricle—can be demonstrated by echocardiogram before they become clinically evident. Cardiac ultrasound and echocardiography have been used with good reliability to evaluate penetrating intrapericardial injury.[118] Echocardiography was found to be 97% specific and 90% sensitive in stable patients with precordial wounds.[119]

All patients with penetrating thoracic trauma and echocardiograms positive for free pericardial fluid or that suggest clotted lacerations should be explored surgically. This is based on poor outcomes in patients who are initially managed nonoperatively. One study showed that two out of three patients who were clinically stable, but whose ultrasound suggested clotted laceration, subsequently became unstable, and only one of these patients survived.[120] Patients with echocardiographic evidence of even small amounts of pericardial effusion were found to have major intrapericardial injury at exploration.[121]

CT is another noninvasive modality for evaluating cardiac injury, although it may also fail to pick up subtle injuries or small amounts of pericardial fluid. Although it is not sensitive for small amounts of fluid, it is an excellent means of identifying and localizing intrapericardial or intracardiac foreign bodies such as bullets and gunshot pellets. These should be removed in most circumstances to prevent embolization and infection. Because of the lack of sensitivity of imaging modalities, a high degree of clinical suspicion should be exercised when hemodynamic instability suggests cardiac injury despite a normal echocardiogram, and more invasive measures must be taken. Minimally invasive evaluation has been recommended in selected stable patients using a subxiphoid pericardial window (Fig. 7-11).[117] Pericardial windows have also been performed from laparoscopic and from video-assisted thoracic surgery (VATS) approaches.[122-124]

Management of penetrating injuries to the heart follows standard principles of cardiac surgery. If cardiac injury is suspected and time allows, the patient is transferred to the operating room and a median sternotomy is performed. Otherwise, left anterolateral thoracotomy using a fourth interspace incision, with extension across the sternum to the right chest if necessary, is performed. Minimally invasive procedures are

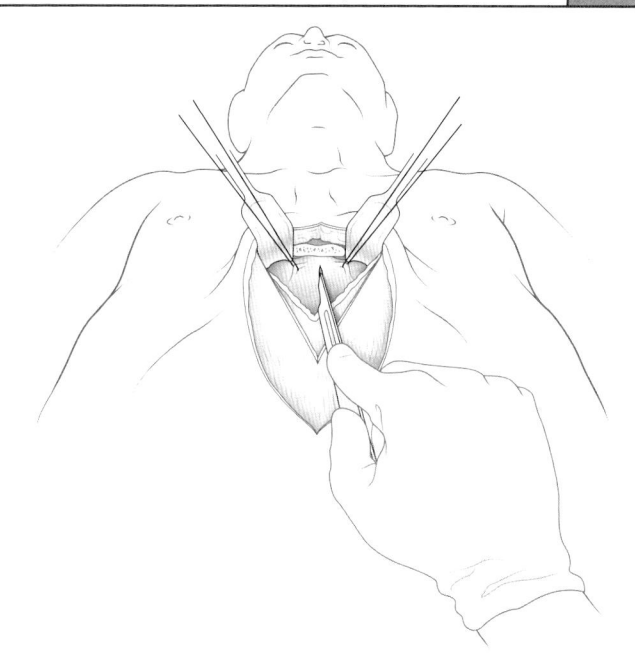

Figure 7-11
Subxiphoid approach for pericardial window. *(From Brown J, Grover FL. Trauma to the heart.* Chest Surg Clinic N Am *1997;**7**:325.)*

not advocated in the setting of hemodynamic compromise and suspected cardiac injury. Unilateral thoracoscopy or laparoscopy is an option in the stable patient when the diagnosis is unclear. Ventricular stab wounds should be repaired using mattress sutures with large, full-thickness bites across the injury. A 2-0 MH needle with Ethibond suture and Teflon pledgets is used to prevent tearing of the myocardium. Bleeding should be controlled using manual pressure or a sponge stick until sutures can be applied. In general, it is not advocated to use of an inflated Foley balloon in a ventricular or atrial defect because of possible interference with the valvular apparatus of the tricuspid or mitral valve, or obstruction of either the right or left ventricular outflow tract. Finally, the use of a Foley catheter increases the likelihood of pulmonary air embolus or stroke.

For atrial injuries, 4-0 Prolene suture with or without pledgets is used, depending on the quality of the atrial tissue and the size of the defect. Autologous pericardium can be used to reconstruct larger defects. Bleeding can be massive and cell-saver technique should be used whenever possible when a perfusionist is available. Coronary injuries present a particularly challenging injury and carry a high mortality because of blood loss and early tamponade, as well as from the resultant myocardial ischemia that can produce hemodynamic instability secondary to myocardial failure. Mattress sutures under the coronary artery, to control bleeding without completely obstructing coronary flow, should be attempted whenever possible (Fig. 7-12).

Left main and anterior descending artery injuries probably produce the most catastrophic outcomes because of the large territory of myocardium that the vessels supply. Hemorrhage from coronary injuries can be temporarily controlled using a peanut to compress the artery both proximal and distal to the injury. Direct repair or coronary bypass on the beating heart is likely to be impractical but might be considered if a cardiac

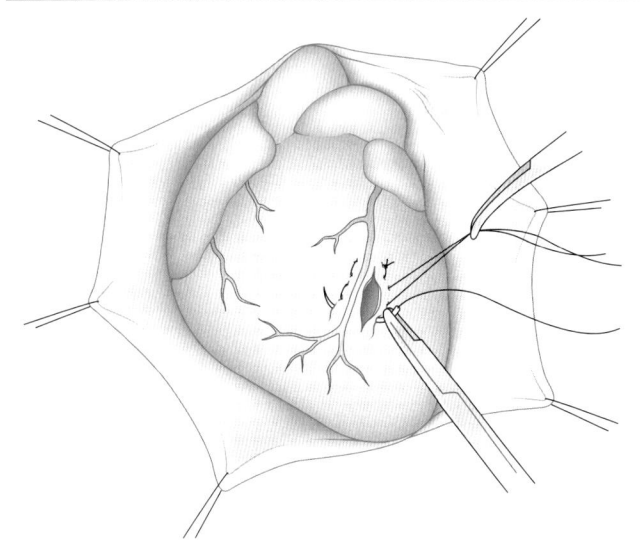

Figure 7–12
Suture repair of ventricular injuries positioned next to the coronary vessels. *(From Blaisdel FW, Trunkey DD, editors. Cervicothoracic trauma. 2nd ed. New York: Thieme Medical; 1994.)*

surgeon with the equipment and experience is available. Ligation or oversewing of a major coronary artery should be undertaken only as a last option. If hemodynamic instability is encountered after ligation, cardiopulmonary bypass should be considered, as well as coronary bypass with standard aortic cross-clamping and saphenous vein grafting distal to the area of ligation.

Intrapericardial great vessel injuries are unusual because of their short segments, but they carry a high mortality. Intrapericardial aortic injuries were uniformly fatal in one series.[125] Lacerations to the intrapericardial aorta can be repaired using basic vascular technique, a side-biting vascular clamp, and oversewing using 3-0 Prolene suture. Temporary inflow occlusion of the inferior vena cava (IVC) and superior vena cava (SVC) can be used to try to minimize hemorrhage while performing the repair. Gunshot injuries producing a significant aortic disruption are usually fatal, but if cardiopulmonary bypass is available, aortic cross-clamping for repair and grafting is optimal.

SVC and IVC injuries are also difficult to control. Lifting or pulling on the heart to expose these injuries usually results in hemodynamic instability in the hypovolemic patient so volume loading is critical. Side-biting vascular clamps can be used to control smaller, tangential injuries but can result in iatrogenic injury if not placed with care on fragile tissue. Shunts such as chest tubes and endotracheal tubes have been recommended to control hemorrhage, but they can be cumbersome and care must be taken not to worsen the original injury. Cardiopulmonary bypass can be used for SVC or IVC drainage and allows more controlled repairs of complex injuries. Cardiopulmonary bypass, while uncommon for use in emergency penetrating injuries to the heart, has been used with success if applied in a timely manner.[126,127] Outcomes for patients with penetrating wounds to the heart show that gunshot wounds have lower survival than stab wounds, and single-chamber injuries have lower survival than multichamber injuries. Patients presenting with lower physiologic status had lower survival than those with higher physiologic status.[125]

Air Embolism and Bullet Embolism

Bullet and other missiles are not routinely removed from the chest if associated injuries are excluded. Foreign body embolism to the heart is rare. This occurs when missiles migrate intravascularly from sites of more peripheral injuries. Diagnosis is made by chest radiograph, CT scan, echocardiogram, or fluoroscopy. The philosophy of management of intracardiac foreign bodies in asymptomatic patients—ranging from removing all intracardiac foreign bodies to expectant management—has been debated. Most surgeons recommend selective management.

The presence of an intracardiac foreign body must first be determined to be embolic and not from direct thoracic injury. Direct injury resulting in a intracardiac foreign body clearly mandates sternotomy to evaluate a penetrating cardiac injury. However, if there is no thoracic injury, intracardiac missiles can be assumed to be embolic. Workup should include chest CT and two-dimensional echocardiogaphy.[128] The CT scan helps localize the foreign body. The echocardiogram confirms its presence and determines the exact location of the embolus in relationship to other cardiac structures and whether there is any valvular dysfunction or septal defect. In addition, echocardiography can help in determining whether the missile is fixed or is mobile. Because of their embolic nature, these missiles are generally on the right side of the heart. If these right-sided missiles appear stable and without tumbling movement on echocardiogram, and if they appear to be lodged in a chamber or ventricular wall, they can be followed expectantly.[129,130] Some authors recommend intervention for larger missiles (greater than 5 mm), irregularly shaped missiles, missiles proximal to an artery, and left-sided intracavitary or partially embedded missiles.[131]

In general, intracardiac embolic missiles should be removed if they are left sided, mobile, large, or symptomatic with valvular incompetence. The use of anticoagulation or prophylactic antibiotics is not recommended for expectant management, but follow-up echocardiograms are recommended at 3 months, 6 months, and 1 year.

Systemic air embolus is a relatively uncommon but frequently unrecognized cause of death in patients with penetrating lung injury. This generally occurs in the setting of a central lung injury. A missile or stab wound creates a fistula from the bronchus to the pulmonary veins, producing an air embolus in patients when placed on positive-pressure ventilation. This may be more likely to occur in the setting of high airway pressures. Cardiovascular collapse occurs when air enters the coronary arteries, causing myocardial ischemia and resulting in ventricular fibrillation or asystole. The hallmark of an air embolism is hemoptysis and bloody, frothy air leak from a lung injury. This can then be confirmed intraoperatively by visualizing air in the coronaries.[132]

If air embolus is suspected, immediate thoracotomy should be performed to the side of the injury. The hilum of the lung should be clamped to prevent further sources of embolus. The patient should be placed head down to prevent cerebral embolus. Removal of a massive air embolus can then be performed using a large-gauge needle and syringe through the left ventricular apex or through the roof of the left atrium as open cardiac massage is performed. Coronary air emboli can also be removed using a syringe and small-gauge needle. Outcomes for massive air embolus are poor with only three of nine patients surviving in the series by Estera and colleagues.[132] Prevention of this problem is paramount and should include lung isolation to prevent positive pressure on an injured lung until repair or resection is performed.[133] Management has also been described using prompt institution of cardiopulmonary bypass to restore circulation while lung resection and cardiac de-airing are performed.[134]

Great Vessels

Over 90% of patients with great vessel injuries present after penetrating thoracic trauma.[135] The thoracic great vessels include the ascending aorta, the aortic arch and descending aorta, the innominate artery and veins, the subclavian artery and veins, the pulmonary artery, and the pulmonary veins. Injuries to the great vessels are challenging to manage. Most patients die before reaching the hospital, and of those who reach the hospital, most require immediate emergency room thoracotomy.[136,137] Workup for major thoracic vascular injuries is frequently limited because of the instability of these patients and the need for immediate thoracotomy. However, a plain chest radiograph may reveal hemothorax, hemopneumothorax, or mediastinal hematoma.

Further workup in the stable patient should include chest CT with intravenous contrast or aortography. This is particularly pertinent in the stable patient with a transmediastinal gunshot wound.[138,139] Given the improved sensitivity of the new generation of CT scanners and the increased speed with which CT can generally be performed, CT angiograms are now replacing angiography as the diagnostic modality for these injuries. In addition, CT allows the identification of other thoracic injuries. Angiography can still be useful as a diagnostic tool in centers without adequate CT scanners or dedicated trauma radiologists, and it is a therapeutic interventional modality to address selective injuries.

The initial management of major vascular thoracic penetrating injuries is prompt thoracotomy and manual tamponade of the injury or control with a vascular clamp. Subclavian injuries can be difficult to tamponade because of their location behind the clavicle. Foley balloon insertion into a neck wound and application of traction to tamponade the bleeding has been recommended until more definitive control can be achieved.[140]

Definitive management of thoracic vascular injuries follows the principles of vascular repair. Aortic injuries are frequently lethal. Rapid exposure of these injuries to establish control is critical so the appropriate choice of incision cannot be overemphasized. Ascending aortic and aortic arch injuries are best approached through a median sternotomy. Manual pressure or control with side-biting vascular clamps (or both) may allow a primary repair. Cross-clamping the ascending aorta is not possible without cardiopulmonary bypass. Repair of complex vascular injuries has been described using cardiopulmonary bypass and deep hypothermic circulatory arrest.[141] Descending thoracic aortic injuries should be approached through a left thoracotomy. The descending aorta can be cross-clamped to achieve proximal and distal control and to perform a primary repair or interposition graft.

Pulmonary artery or vein injuries are best approached through a posterolateral thoracotomy. Proximal control on the pulmonary artery should be achieved as a first step, and a tourniquet placed and cinched down to decrease blood loss and allow better visualization for vascular repair. Similar control can be achieved on the pulmonary veins. Primary repair should be attempted. Pneumonectomy should be avoided if at all possible.

Vena caval and innominate vein injuries are also repaired using standard vascular techniques. The intrapericardial SVC and IVC can be difficult to expose and repair. They can be approached through either a right thoracotomy or a median sternotomy. Ligation of either the SVC or the IVC without shunting is not compatible with survival. Innominate vein injuries are best repaired through a sternotomy. The innominate vein can be ligated if repair is not possible given the existence of adequate collateral venous drainage.

The subclavian vessels are the most frequently injured thoracic great vessels, particularly given their exposure to injury through penetrating neck injury.[137] Surgical exposure for control of bleeding makes these injuries challenging. Recommended approaches for control of these vessels include a clavicular incision, clavicular incision combined with sternotomy (Fig. 7-13), "trapdoor" or upper sternotomy combined with fourth interspace anterior thoracotomy (Fig. 7-14), and a high anterior thoracotomy using a second or third interspace incision (Fig. 7-15). Each of these techniques has its advantages, and the choice of incision should be based on the surgeon's familiarity with the approach and on whether the vascular injury is left- or right-sided, or more proximal or distal. Left-sided subclavian injuries can be difficult to control through a sternotomy. In general, these injuries can be repaired primarily or, if necessary, with an interposition graft of autologous vein or prosthetic graft.[142]

Currently, the role of endovascular stent grafts for great vessel injury (other than aortic) is being addressed.[83] Successful stenting for nontraumatic carotid and subclavian arterial pathologies has been well reported, but its application to traumatic injuries is less so. It has been estimated that well over a third of all nonaortic great vessel injury would be amenable to stent graft placement, but cited reasons for the lack of progress in this area include higher risks of endoleak associated with injuries proximal to arterial origins, and multiple branch points with risk of occlusion and distal ischemia. Limited case series have reported endovascular stenting to be safe and efficacious in selected cases, with up to a 95% success rate at excluding the traumatic lesion, and rates of early graft failure resulting from stenosis or thrombosis and late failure resulting from intimal hyperplasia being in the range of 5% to 10%.[83]

Diaphragmatic Injuries

Diaphragmatic injuries in penetrating trauma can be difficult to diagnose, although once the diagnosis is made, their management is straightforward. Any penetrating injury at the nipple line or below should be considered to have the potential for both abdominal and thoracic injury and traversal of the diaphragm. The dilemmas in management are how to diagnose the injury and how to inspect both the chest and diaphragm for injury. Injuries to the diaphragm may be small, but repair is indicated because of the potential for associated abdominal injuries and the long-term sequelae of chronic diaphragmatic hernia, with the potential for bowel incarceration. Noninvasive methods used to diagnose diaphragmatic injury are chest radiography and chest CT. However, these methods can be unreliable for the diagnosis of diaphragmatic

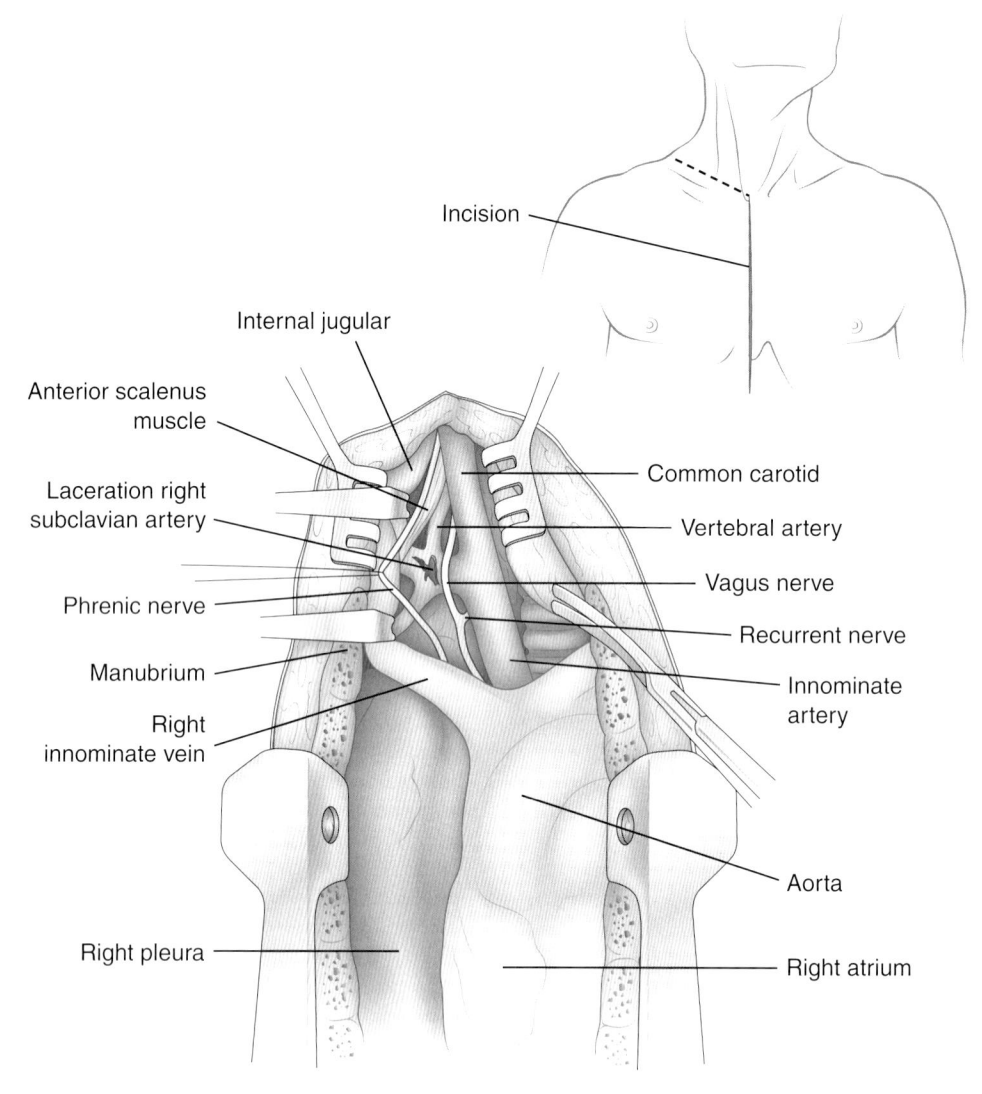

Figure 7-13
Clavicular incision and median sternotomy for exposure and control of the proximal innominate and right subclavian artery. *(From Ravitch MR, Steichen FM, Schlossberg L. Atlas of general thoracic surgery. Philadelphia: WB Saunders; 1988, p. 147.)*

injury, with accuracy rates of only 50%.[143] A more invasive method for diagnosing penetrating diaphragmatic injury, diagnostic peritoneal lavage (DPL), can also miss this injury. Therefore, some have recommended exploratory laparotomy in patients with penetrating wounds inferior to the fourth intercostal space anteriorly, sixth interspace laterally, or eighth interspace posteriorly, because of the contour and insertions of the diaphragm.[144] Laparoscopy and thoracoscopy have been use to improve diagnostic sensitivity in evaluating the diaphragm without resorting to laparotomy. VATS has proven to be a safe and reliable method of evaluating the diaphragm and diagnosing and treating a variety of thoracic trauma. Current recommendations incorporate concepts from these series (Box 7-3).[123,124,145]

Any patient with an indication for thoracotomy or laparotomy should have the diaphragm inspected at the time of surgery. For patients without hard signs for surgery, VATS is a reasonable approach in the setting of an abnormal chest radiograph with an entry wound in the zone of insertion of the diaphragm, as well as in the setting of a high-velocity injury in the proximity of the diaphragm. A high degree of suspicion is needed for diaphragmatic injury. Because the procedure is fast and simple with minimal morbidity, VATS should be used liberally when the diagnosis is uncertain. Repair of the diaphragm can be performed using VATS coupled with standard suturing techniques and a running or interrupted method of repair. The diaphragm can be repaired transabdominally should laparotomy be required. An interrupted repair (of Prolene) rather than a continuous suture of the diaphragm should be used.

In one series of 171 patients with penetrating chest trauma, an algorithm was proposed to identify occult diaphragmatic injury. An initial chest radiograph was obtained, followed by chest tube placement if a pneumothorax or hemothorax was present. In addition, a DPL or abdominal CT was performed to assess abdominal injuries. If the DPL or abdominal CT scan suggested abdominal injury, or if the hemothorax was significant, the patient was taken to the operating room and the diaphragm was evaluated via laparotomy or thoracotomy. In the setting of softer findings that do not mandate thoracotomy

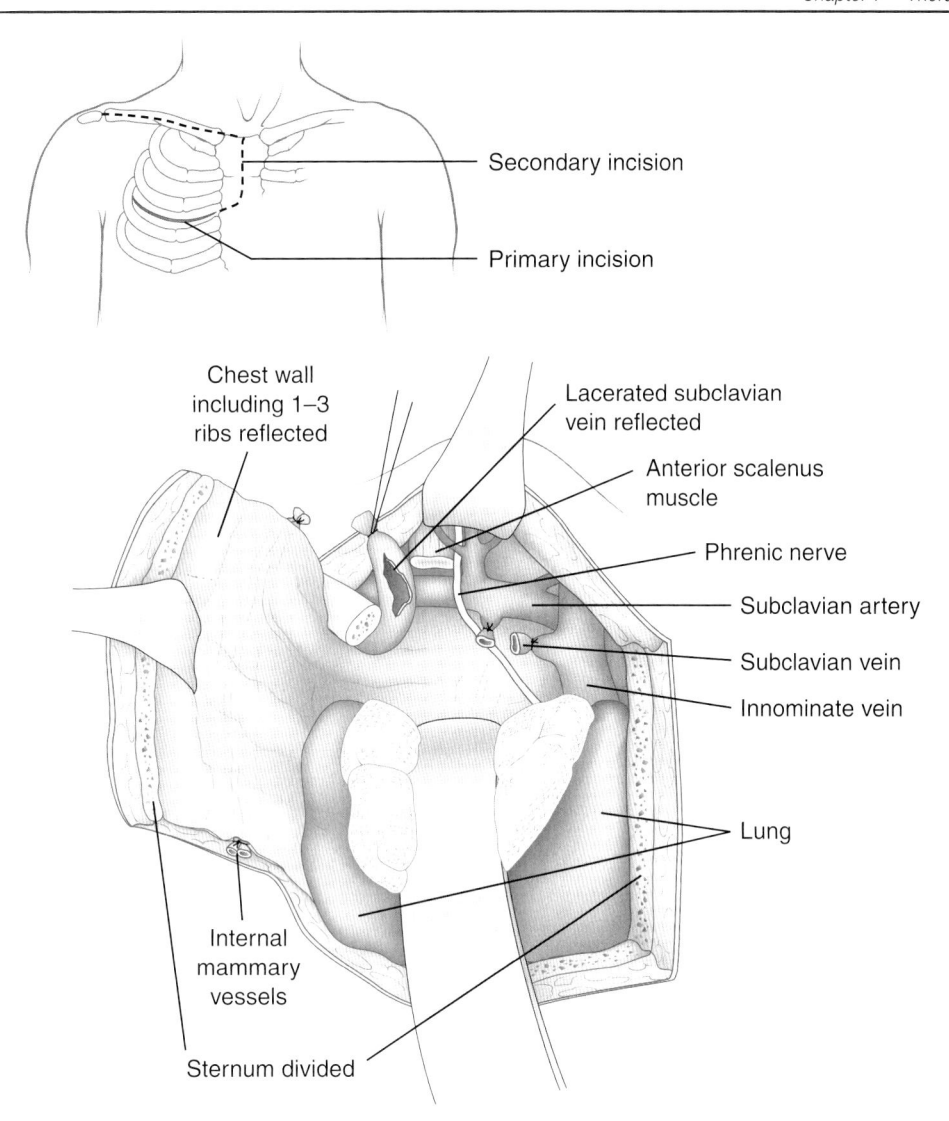

Figure 7–14
"Trapdoor" incision for exposure and control of the distal right subclavian artery injuries, which can be used for the left as well. *(From Ravitch MR, Steichen FM, Schlossberg L.* Atlas of general thoracic surgery. *Philadelphia: WB Saunders; 1988, p. 155.)*

or laparotomy, inspection of the diaphragm using VATS was recommended when two or more of the following findings were present: abnormal chest film, associated abdominal injury, high-velocity injury, injury inferior to the nipple, or a right-sided wound.[146]

Esophageal Injuries

Injuries to the intrathoracic esophagus resulting from penetrating injury are rare. The esophagus is more commonly injured in the neck, where it is most exposed. However, thoracic esophageal injuries carry a high morbidity and mortality for many reasons. Given its central location in the chest, associated injuries are extremely common—98% in one series.[147,148] In addition, these injuries can be missed unless specifically investigated. Finally, repair of the esophagus can be technically difficult and associated with morbid complications. A multicenter study of penetrating esophageal injuries showed that preoperative workup of esophageal injuries resulted in delay in surgery and poorer outcomes.[149] The authors concluded that if selective evaluation and management of injuries were to be performed, this should be done rapidly with the plan of expeditious transfer to the operating room. If this is not possible, they recommend proceeding to prompt surgical exploration.

Investigation for esophageal injuries depends on the stability of the patient. If the patient is stable with a mediastinal or transmediastinal gunshot wound, a CT scan of the chest should be obtained immediately with an intravenous contrast agent and injection of Gastrografin contrast material through a nasogastric tube. This can help delineate associated injuries and the course of the bullet, and it can help in the choice of a surgical approach. If the patient is not stable enough to undergo CT and an emergent operative exploration is necessary, intraoperative flexible bronchoscopy and esophagoscopy should be done first, followed by thoracotomy on the side in which major associated injury is suspected. Thoracotomy should be performed to the left side if the injury is uncertain so as to have access to the descending aorta for cross-clamping should this prove necessary. Lung isolation through a double-lumen tube

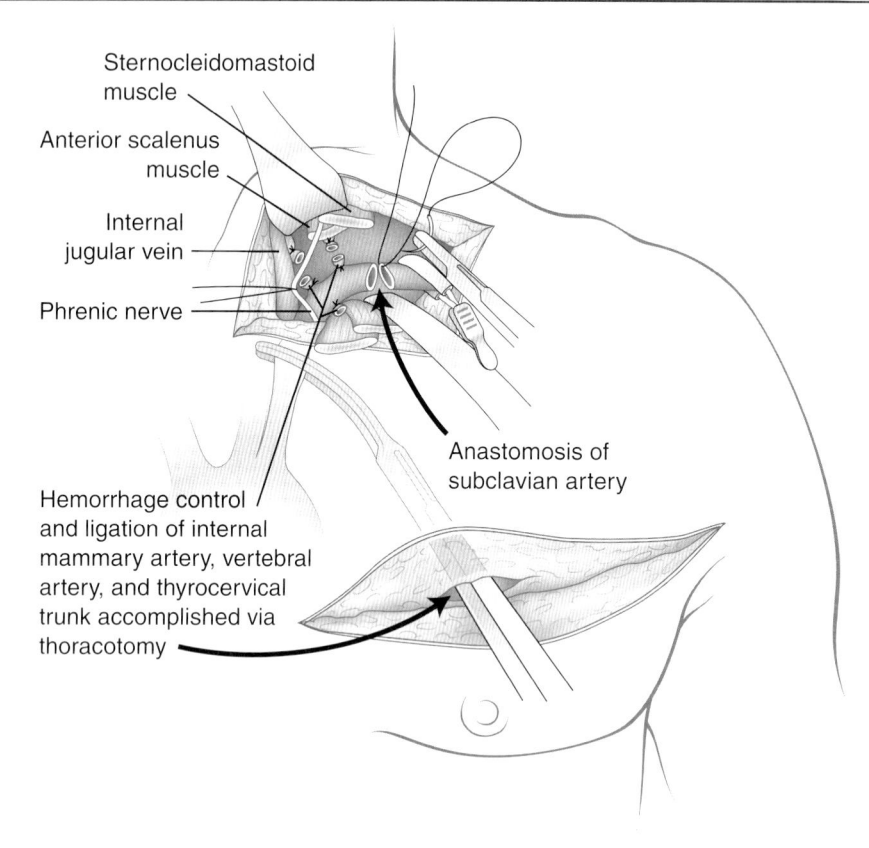

Figure 7–15
Clavicular incision for exposure and control of distal left subclavian artery injuries, and separate upper anterior thoracotomy for proximal control. *(From Ravitch MR, Steichen FM, Schlossberg L.* Atlas of general thoracic surgery. *Philadelphia: WB Saunders; 1988, p. 150.)*

Box 7–3
Role of Video-Assisted Thoracic Surgery in Thoracic Trauma

Indications
- Treatment for ongoing thoracic hemorrhage
- Treatment of retained hemothorax
- Treatment of persistent pneumothorax
- Diagnosis and treatment of diaphragmatic injuries
- Pericardial window for relief of cardiac tamponade
- Management of thoracic duct injuries
- Treatment of post-trauma empyema
- Removal of foreign bodies

Relative Contraindications
- Coagulopathy
- Prior thoracotomy

Absolute Contraindications
- Hemodynamic instability
- Suspected cardiac injury
- Suspected great vessel injury
- Inability to tolerate single-lung ventilation
- Inability to tolerate lateral decubitus position

---

or a bronchial blocker is preferable to provide atelectasis for better visualization and to optimize repair of injuries. Flexible endoscopy for the diagnosis of esophageal trauma has been shown to be an excellent diagnostic tool (100% sensitivity, 96% specificity, and 97% accuracy in one study).[150] Intraoperative insufflation of air through the esophagoscope with the chest filled with saline can help identify a small injury. More proximal injuries are best explored via a right chest through the fifth intercostal space, particularly if associated airway injury is suspected. Bronchoscopy is mandatory to examine both the trachea and the more distal airway for injury. Distal esophageal injuries around the esophagogastric junction are best explored through a sixth-interspace left thoracotomy.

Thoracic esophageal injuries should be repaired using primary closure with wide drainage. Prompt recognition of esophageal injury is critical, and it must be repaired. A missed diagnosis allows mediastinal soilage with ensuing sepsis in a patient who has already undergone one physiologic insult. Nonoperative chest tube drainage alone has no place in the management of penetrating esophageal injuries. One series had a 50% mortality in this setting.[151]

The injured esophagus should be débrided back to clean, viable tissue. Like other esophageal repairs, a two-layer closure is done with attention to a watertight mucosal closure using absorbable suture with an overlying second layer of nonabsorbable suture to close the muscular layer. The repair should be covered with an intercostal muscle flap, or with the fundus of the stomach if the injury is close to the gastroesophageal junction. Multiple chest tubes should be used to ensure complete drainage of the hemithorax and complete reexpansion of the lung to seal the pleura against the closure. In addition to chest tubes, soft, closed suction drains, such as a Jackson-Pratt or Blake drain, should be left close to the area of injury. Therefore, if the repair leaks postoperatively, the chest tubes can be slowly removed and the patient can be eventually discharged from the hospital with the Jackson-Pratt drain still in place controlling the leak until it seals. Gastric and jejunal feeding tubes should be considered and placed operatively either at the time of initial surgery or at a second operation, to provide access for long-term feeding should a postoperative leak preclude oral intake. Esophageal repairs are evaluated for leak with a barium esophagram on postoperative day 7.

COMPLICATIONS OF THORACIC TRAUMA

A complete discussion of complications after thoracic trauma is beyond the scope of this chapter, but the more common problems are listed in Box 7-4. Many complications and their therapies are similar to their counterparts found in nontrauma settings, and the reader is referred to those chapters.

> **Box 7–4**
> **Complications of Thoracic Trauma**
>
> **Pulmonary**
> - Atelectasis
> - Acute respiratory distress syndrome or acute lung injury
> - Pneumonia
> - Infarction
> - Lung abscess
> - Arteriovenous fistula
> - Bronchial stenosis
> - Tracheoesophageal fistula
>
> **Pleural Space**
> - Empyema
> - Bronchopleural fistula
> - Organized hemothorax
> - Chylothorax
> - Fibrothorax
> - Diaphragmatic hernias
>
> **Vascular**
> - Thromboembolism
> - Air embolism
> - Pseudoaneurysm
> - Great vessel fistula
>
> **Chest Wall**
> - Hernias
> - Persistent pain
>
> **Mediastinum**
> - Mediastinitis
> - Pericarditis

However, several issues specific to thoracic injuries are important to note.[152]

Acute Lung Injury and Respiratory Distress Syndrome

Up to 20% of cases of acute respiratory distress syndrome (ARDS) in the United States have thoracic trauma as an etiology. Whether from a direct injury to the lung parenchyma or as a sequela in the critically injured patient, mortality from ARDS remains approximately 50%. Differentiation of ARDS from acute lung injury may be difficult, and they are sometimes included in the same spectrum of diseases. Both reflect the concept of acutely occurring, nonhydrostatic pulmonary edema; infiltrates on the chest radiograph; and hypoxemia—generally worse in ARDS.[153] With alterations in immune competence and production of proinflammatory cytokines, the systemic inflammatory response (SIRS) can develop, which can progress to septic shock and ARDS with a proven infection source.[154] Irrespective of the etiology, the development of ARDS is difficult to predict. Factors that increase the risk of ARDS in these patients are shown in Box 7-5.

Therapy for acute lung injury and ARDS is mainly supportive, directed at correcting the possible underlying etiology that precipitated the pulmonary problem.[155,156] Other therapies include mechanical ventilatory support with or without oscillation, adequate nutritional status, minimization of fluid requirements, and constant rotation of position to redistribute pulmonary edema. Pharmacologic therapy includes inhaled nitric oxide, exogenous or aerosolized surfactant, corticosteroids, and the use of mediator-directed therapy such as nonsteroidal anti-inflammatory drugs and monoclonal antibodies directed against endotoxin. In addition, extracorporeal membrane oxygenation (ECMO) has been used to support these patients. Although most mediators have not shown vast improvement in a prospective fashion, these nonconventional therapies still hold great promise.

Pneumonia

Pneumonia is the most common infectious complication after any multiple trauma, particularly those involving the thorax. The incidence increases with the duration of endotracheal intubation, and it is associated with up to 50% of deaths after

> **Box 7–5**
> **Risk Factors for Acute Respiratory Distress Syndrome (ARDS)**
>
> - Pneumonia or aspiration
> - Pulmonary contusion or penetrating injury
> - Closed head injury
> - Orthopedic injury
> - Sepsis or infection
> - Multiple transfusions
> - Pancreatitis
> - Coagulopathies
> - Inhalation injury
> - Burns

trauma. The etiology of nosocomially acquired pneumonias can be complex and is related to a number of factors: underlying pulmonary conditions, associated injuries, multiple antibiotic therapies, colonization of the upper airway, aspiration at the time of initial injury, impairment of local defenses, and depression of the immune response.

Diagnosis is often difficult, with only half of patients presenting classically with fever, leukocytosis, respiratory distress, and an abnormal chest radiograph. Sputum sampling is essential, however, and in the intubated patient, invasive testing is required, such as transtracheal or bronchoscopic aspiration with bronchoalveolar lavage. Pleural effusions can occur and are seen in 50% of patients with *Haemophilus influenzae* pneumonia.

Broad-spectrum antibiotic therapy is used initially, but the spectrum is narrowed once the offending organism is identified and test results for antibiotic sensitivity are received. Other principles in therapy include good pulmonary care and toilet, and the maintenance of nutritional function. Prophylaxis is paramount and includes effective infection control and prophylactic antibiotic and gastric bleeding measures.

Pleural Space Problems

The incidence of post-trauma empyemas ranges from 2% to 6%, and up to 26% of patients develop pleural space infections after chest tube insertion.[157] The management of these empyemas is the same as for parapneumonic processes, with goals of controlling infection, evacuation of pus, obliteration of the pleural space, and restoration of complete lung reexpansion. However, it is postulated that these empyemas differ from their parapneumonic counterparts in several aspects. Post-trauma empyemas usually have gram-negative organisms in addition to gram-positive organisms, are usually the result of retained hemothorax, often have an effusion that has small volume and is thick, are not in the early or exudative phase, and require open thoracotomy, drainage, and aggressive decortication.[158]

Bronchopleural Fistula

Persistent bronchopleural fistula is a common problem after significant penetrating trauma to the lung parenchyma. Large massive air leaks, identified by loss of 30% to 50% of the tidal volume, are usually caused by main-stem bronchial injuries, and they require immediate surgery. Fistula persisting more than 7 to 10 days is an indication for operative intervention. The use of sclerosing agents has been reported, but failure rates are high. If surgery is performed in the persistent parenchymal fistula, careful dissection and closure is advised because of the friability and fragility of the tissues, sometimes in the presence of ARDS inflammatory changes. The internal parenchymal injury should be exposed, and major bronchioles oversewn. The parenchyma is closed in layers, and the visceral pleural lining oversewn with a running suture to minimize air leaks. If not properly closed in layers, a parenchymal cavity will persist, and it acts as a nidus for a lung abscess. Anatomic resection is rarely needed, and if required, wedge resection usually suffices.

Great Vessel Fistula

Nearly all traumatic arteriovenous fistulas result from penetrating injuries. Although a majority occur in cervico-mediastinal areas, approximately 30% are found in the intrathoracic great vessels.[159] A thrill is heard in only 20% of patients 1 week after the injury, but it is heard in 100% at 2 weeks. At 12 weeks, 85% have some type of significant clinical presentation.

Surgery is recommended once the fistula is documented, usually by angiography. There is no role for fistula "maturation," as venous hypertension can cause bleeding complications during and after the repair. Autogenous vein patch is suggested for peripheral vessels, and prosthetic grafts are reserved for the great vessels, the aorta and main pulmonary artery. Endovascular stenting and embolization have been reported, and selective use of these methods is suggested for smaller vessels.

REFERENCES

1. Breasted J. *The Edwin Smith surgical papyrus*. Vol. 1. Chicago: University of Chicago Press; 1930.
2. Santos GH. Chest trauma during the battle of Troy: ancient warfare and chest trauma. *Ann Thorac Surg* 2000;**69**:1285-7.
3. Menenakos E, Alexakis N, Leandros E, Laskaratos G, Nikiteas N, Bramis J, Fingerhut A. Fatal chest injury with lung evisceration during athletic games in ancient Greece. *World J Surg* 2005;**29**(10):1348-51.
4. Asensio JA, Stewart BM, Murray J, Fox AH, Falabella A, Gomez H, et al. Penetrating cardiac injuries. *Surg Clin North Am.* 1996;**76**(4):685-724.
5. Churchill ED. Chest wounds in ancient sculpture. *J Hist Allied Med Sci* 1971;**26**(3):304-5.
6. Rockoff SD, Aaron BL. The shooting of President Reagan: a radiologic chronology of his medical care. *Radiographics* 1995;**15**(2):407-18.
7. Aaron BL, Rockoff SD. The attempted assassination of President Reagan: medical implications and historical perspective. *JAMA* 1994;**272**(21):1689-93.
8. Brethauer SA, Chao A, Chambers LW, Green DJ, Brown C, Rhee P, Bohman HR. Invasion vs. insurgency: US Navy/Marine Corps forward surgical care during Operation Iraqi Freedom. *Arch Surg* 2008;**143**(6):564-9.
9. Wojcik BE, Humphrey RJ, Fulton LV, Psalmonds LC, Hassell LH. Comparisons of Operation Iraqi Freedom and patient workload generator injury distributions. *Mil Med* 2008;**173**(3):647-52.
10. Rush RM, Stockmaster NR, Stinger HK, Arrington ED, Devine JG, Atteberry L, et al. Supporting the global war on terror: a tale of two campaigns featuring the 250th Forward Surgical Team (Airborne). *Am J Surg* 2005;**189**(5):564-70.
11. Paré, A. *The works of Ambrose Paré*. Translated by Thomas Johnson. London; 1678.
12. Billings, J. *War of the rebellion: medical and surgical history.* 1870, Washington, DC: U.S. Printing Office.
13. LoCicero 3rd J, Mattox KL. Epidemiology of chest trauma. *Surg Clin North Am* 1989;**69**:15.
14. *Advanced Trauma Life Support (ATLS)*. 7th ed. Chicago: American College of Surgeons, Committee on Trauma; 2007.
15. DeArmond D, Carpenter AJ, Calhoun JH. Critical primary survey injuries. *Semin Thorac Cardiovasc Surg* 2008;**20**:6-7.
16. Carpenter A. Diagnostic techniques in thoracic trauma. *Semin Thorac Cardiovac Surg* 2008;**20**:2-5.
17. Trupka A, Waydhas C, Hallfeldt KK, Nast-Kolb D, Pfeifer KJ, Schweiberer L. Value of thoracic computed tomography in the first assessment of severely injured patients with blunt chest trauma: results of a prospective study. *J Trauma* 1997;**43**(3):405-11.
18. Guerrero-López F, Vázquez-Mata G, Alcázar-Romero PP, Fernández-Mondéjar E, Aguayo-Hoyos E, Linde-Valverde CM. Evaluation of the utility of computed tomography in the initial assessment of the critical care patient with chest trauma. *Crit Care Med* 2000;**28**(5):1370-5.
19. Deunk J, Dekker HM, Brink M, van Vugt R, Edwards MJ, van Vugt AB. The value of indicated computed tomography scan of the chest and abdomen in addition to the conventional radiologic work-up for blunt trauma patients. *J Trauma* 2007;**63**(4):757-63.
20. Omert L, Yeaney WW, Protetch J. Efficacy of thoracic computerized tomography in blunt chest trauma. *Am Surg* 2001;**67**(7):660-4.
21. Rozycki GS, Feliciano DV, Schmidt JA, Cushman JG, Sisley AC, Ingram W, Ansley JD. The role of surgeon-performed ultrasound in patients with possible cardiac wounds. *Ann Surg* 1996;**223**:737-46.
22. Körner M, Krötz MM, Degenhart C, Pfeifer KJ, Reiser MF, Linsenmaier U. Current role of emergency US in patients with major trauma. *Radiographics* 2008;**28**(1):225-42.

23. Kirkpatrick AW, Sirois M, Laupland KB, Liu D, Rowan K, Ball CG, et al. Hand-held thoracic sonography for detecting post-traumatic pneumothoraces: the Extended Focused Assessment with Sonography for Trauma (EFAST). *J Trauma* Aug 2004;**57**(2):288-95.
24. Shackford S. Focused ultrasound examination by surgeons: The time is now (editorial). *J Trauma* 1993;**35**:181.
25. Demetriades D, Velmahos GC, Scalea TM, Jurkovich GJ, Karmy-Jones R, Teixeira PG, et al. Diagnosis and treatment of blunt thoracic aortic injuries: changing perspectives. *J Trauma* 2008;**64**(6):1415-8; discussion-1418-9.
26. Mirvis SE. Thoracic vascular injury. *Radiol Clin North Am.* 2006;**44**(2): 181-97:vii.
27. Bruckner BA, DiBardino DJ, Cumbie TC, Trinh C, Blackmon SH, Fisher RG, et al. Critical evaluation of chest computed tomography scans for blunt descending thoracic aortic injury. *Ann Thorac Surg* 2006;**81**(4):1339-46.
28. Pozzato C, Fedriga E, Donatelli F, Gattoni F. Acute posttraumatic rupture of the thoracic aorta: the role of angiography in a 7-year review. *Cardiovasc Intervent Radiol* 1991;**14**:338-41.
29. Morse SS, Glickman MG, Greenwood LH, Denny Jr DF, Strauss EB, Stavens BR, Yoselevitz M. Traumatic Aortic rupture: False-positive aortographic diagnosis due to atypical ductus diverticulum. *Am J Roentgen* 1988;**150**:793-6.
30. Mirvis SE, Shanmuganathan K. Diagnosis of blunt traumatic aortic injury 2007: still a nemesis. *Eur J Radiol* 2007;**64**(1):27-40.
31. Sammer M, Wang E, Blackmore CC, Burdick TR, Hollingworth W. Indeterminate CT angiography in blunt thoracic trauma: is CT angiography enough?. *AJR Am J Roentgenol* 2007;**189**(3):603-8.
32. Steenburg SD, Ravenel JG, Ikonomidis JS, Schonholz C, Reeves S. Acute traumatic aortic injury: imaging evaluation and management. *Radiology* 2008;**248**(3):748-62.
33. Mejia JC, Stewart RM, Cohn SM. Emergency Department Thoracotomy. *Semin Thorac Cardiovasc Surg* 2008;**20**:13-8.
34. Lewis G, Knottenbelt JD. Should emergency room thoracotomy be reserved for cases of cardiac tamponade? *Injury* 1991;**22**:5-6.
35. Working Group. Ad Hoc Subcommittee on Outcomes, American College of Surgeons-Committee on Trauma: Practice management guidelines for emergency department thoracotomy. *J Am Coll Surg* 2001;**193**:303-9.
36. Durham 3rd LA, Richardson RJ, Wall Jr MJ, Pepe PE, Mattox KL. Emergency center thoracotomy: impact of prehospital resuscitation. *J Trauma* 1992;**32**:775-9.
37. Weyant MJ, Fullerton DA. Blunt Thoracic Trauma. *Semin Thorac Cardiovasc Surg* 2008;**20**:26-30.
38. Flores HA, Stewart RM. The multiply injured patient. *Semin Thorac Cardiovasc Surg* 2008;**20**:64-8.
39. Shorr RM, Crittenden M, Indeck M, Hartunian SL, Rodriguez A. Blunt thoracic trauma. Analysis of 515 patients. *Ann Surg* 1987;**206**:200-5.
40. Kerr-Valentic MA, Arthur M, Mullins RJ, Pearson TE, Mayberry JC. Rib fracture pain and disability: can we do better? *J Trauma* 2003;**54**:1058-63.
41. Sirmali M, Türüt H, Topcu S, Gulhan E, Yazici U, Kaya S, Taştepe I. A comprehensive analysis of traumatic rib fractures: morbidity, mortality and management. *Eur J Cardiothorac Surg* 2003;**24**:133-8.
42. Sharma OP, Oswanski MF, Jolly S, Lauer SK, Dressel R, Stombaugh HA. The Perils of Rib Fractures. *Am Surg* 2008;**74**(4):410-4.
43. Flagel BT, Luchette FA, Reed RL, Esposito TJ, Davis KA, Santaniello JM, Gamelli RL. Half a dozen ribs: the breakpoint for mortality. *Surgery* 2005;**138**(4):717-25.
44. Liman ST, Kuzucu A, Tastepe AI, Ulasan GN, Topcu S. Chest injury due to blunt trauma. *J Cardiothorac Surg* 2003;**23**:374-8.
45. Livingston DH, Shogan B, John P, Lavery RF. CT diagnosis of rib fracture and the prediction of acute respiratory failure. *J. Trauma* 2008;**64**(4):905-11.
46. Bergeron E, Lavoie A, Clas D, Moore L, Ratte S, Tetreault S, et al. Elderly trauma patients with rib fractures are at greater risk of death and pneumonia. *J Trauma* 2003;**54**:478.
47. Gupta A, Jamshidi M, Rubin JR. Traumatic first rib fracture: is angiography necessary? A review of 730 cases. *Cardiovasc Surg* 1997;**5**:48-53.
48. Gabram SG, Schwartz RJ, Jacobs LM, Lawrence D, Murphy MA, Morrow JS, et al. Clinical management of blunt trauma patients with unilateral rib fractures: a randomized trial. *World J Surg* 1995;**19**:388-93.
49. Wu CL, Jani ND, Perkins FM, Barquist E. Thoracic epidural analgesia versus intravenous patient-controlled analgesia for the treatment of rib fracture pain after motor vehicle crash. *J Trauma* 1999;**47**:564-7.
50. Haenel JB, Moore FA, Moore EE, Sauaia A, Read RA, Burch JM. Extrapleural bupivacaine for amelioration of multiple rib fracture pain. *J Trauma* 1995;**38**:22-7.
51. Brock MV, Heitmiller RF. Spontaneous anterior thoracic lung hernias. *J Thorac Cardiovasc Surg* 2000;**119**:1046-7.
52. Bastos R, Calhoun JH, Baisden CE. Flail chest and pulmonary contusion. *Semin Thorac Cardiovasc Surg* 2008;**20**:39-45.
53. Velmahos GC, Vassiliu P, Chan LS, Murray JA, Berne TV, Demetriades D. Influence of flail chest on outcome among patients with severe thoracic cage trauma. *Int Surg* 2002;**87**:240-4.
54. Ciraulo DL, Elliott D, Mitchell KA, Rodriguez A. Flail chest as a marker for significant injuries. *J Am Coll Surg* 1994;**178**:466-70.
55. Oyarzun JR, Bush AP, McCormick JR, Bolanowski PJ. Use of 3.5-mm acetabular reconstruction plates for internal fixation of flail chest injuries. *Ann Thorac Surg* 1998;**65**:1471-4.
56. Carbognani P, Cattelani L, Bellini G, Rusca M. A technical proposal for the complex flail chest. *Ann Thorac Surg* 2000;**70**:342-3.
57. Knobloch K, Wagner S, Haasper C, Probst C, Krettek C, Vogt PM, et al. Sternal fractures are frequent following high deceleration velocities in a severe vehicle crash. *Injury* 2008;**39**:36-43.
58. Bar I, Friedman T, Rudis E, Shargal Y, Friedman M, Elami A. Isolated sternal fracture—a benign condition? *Isr Med Assoc J* 2003;**5**:105-6.
59. Richardson JD, Franklin GA, Heffey S, Seligson D. Operative fixation of chest wall fractures: an underused procedure? *Am Surg* 2007;**73**(6):591-6.
60. Kitchens J, Richardson JD. Open fixation of sternal fracture. *Surg Gynecol Obstet* 1993;**177**:423-4.
61. Bertin KC, Rice RS, Doty DB, Jones KW. Repair of transverse sternal nonunions using metal plates and autogenous bone graft. *Ann Thorac Surg* 2002;**73**:1661-2.
62. Nowak J, Mallmin H, Larsson S. The aetiology and epidemiology of clavicular fractures. A prospective study during a two-year period in Uppsala, Sweden. *Injury* 2000;**31**:353-8.
63. Jones GL, McCluskey 3rd GM, Curd DT. Nonunion of the fractured clavicle: evaluation, etiology, and treatment. *South Orthop Assoc* 2000;**9**:43-54.
64. Baldwin KD, Ohman-Strickland P, MehtaHume SE. Scapula Fractures: a marker for concomitant injury? *J. Trauma* 2008;**65**(2):430-5.
65. Yeong EK, Chen MT, Chu SH. Traumatic asphyxia. *Plast Reconstr Surg* 1994;**93**:739-44.
66. Wagner RB, Crawford Jr WO, Schimpf PP, Jamieson PM, Rao KC. Quantitation and pattern of parenchymal lung injury in blunt chest trauma. Diagnostic and therapeutic implications. *J Comput Tomogr* 1988;**12**:270-81.
67. Miller PR, Croce MA, Kilgo PD, Scott J, Fabian TC. Acute respiratory distress syndrome in blunt trauma: identification of independent risk factors. *Am Surg* 2002;**68**:845-50.
68. Nelson L. Ventilatory support of the trauma patient with pulmonary contusion. *Respir Care Clin N Am* 1996;**2**:425-47.
69. Kollmorgen DR, Murray KA, Sullivan JJ, Mone MC, Barton RG. Predictors of mortality in pulmonary contusion. *Am J Surg* 1994;**168**:659-63.
70. Corneille MG, Stewart RM, Cohn SM. Upper airway injury and its management. *Semin Thorac Cardiovasc Surg* 2008;**20**:8-12.
71. Johnson SB. Tracheobronchial injury. *Semin Thorac Cardiovasc Surg* 2008;**20**:52-7.
72. Kiser AC, O'Brien SM, Detterbeck FC. Blunt tracheobronchial injuries: treatment and outcomes. *Ann Thorac Surg* 2001;**71**:2059-65.
73. Navid F, Gleason TG. Great vessel and cardiac trauma diagnostic and management strategies. *Semin Thorac Cardiovasc Surg* 2008;**20**:31-8.
74. Mattox K. Approaches to trauma involving the major vessels of the thorax. *Surg Clin North Am* 1989;**69**:77-91.
75. Wintermark M, Wicky S, Schnyder P. Imaging of acute traumatic injuries of the thoracic aorta. *Eur Radiol* 2002;**12**:431-42.
76. Feliciano D. Trauma to the aorta and major vessels. *Chest Surg Clin N Am* 1997;**7**:305-23.
77. Simon BJ, Leslie C. Factors predicting early in-hospital death in blunt thoracic injury. *J. Trauma* 2001;**51**:906-11.
78. Hirose H, Gill IS, Malangoni MA. Nonoperative management of traumatic aortic injury. *J. Trauma* 2006;**60**:597-601.
79. Kepros J, Angood P, Jaffe CC, Rabinovici R. Aortic intimal injuries from blunt trauma: resolution profile in nonoperative management. *J Trauma* 2002;**52**: 475-8.
80. Dake MD, Miller DC, Semba CP, Mitchell RS, Walker PJ, Liddell RP. Transluminal placement of endovascular stent-grafts for the treatment of descending thoracic aortic aneurysms. *N Engl J Med* 1994;**331**:1729-34.
81. Orford VP, Atkinson NR, Thomson K, Milne PY, Campbell WA, Roberts A, et al. Blunt traumatic aortic transection: the endovascular experience. *Ann Thorac Surg* 2003;**75**:106-11.
82. Kasirajan K, Heffernan D, Langsfield M. Acute thoracic aortic trauma: a comparison of endoluminal stent grafts with open repair and nonoperative management. *Ann Vasc Surg* 2003;**17**:589-95.
83. Hoffer EK. Endovascular intervention in thoracic arterial trauma. *Injury* 2008;**39**:1257-74.
84. Moainie SL, Neschis DG, Gammie JS, Brown JM, Poston RS, Scalea TM, Griffith BP. Endovascular stenting for traumatic aortic injury: an emerging new standard of care. *Ann. Thorac Surg* 2008;**85**(5):1625-9.
85. Forbes AD, Ashbaugh DG. Mechanical circulatory support during repair of thoracic aortic injuries improves morbidity and prevents spinal cord injury. *Arch Surg* 1994;**129**:494-7.

86. Benckart DH, Magovern GJ, Liebler GA, Park SB, Burkholder JA, Maher TD, Magovern GJ. Traumatic aortic transection: repair using left atrial to femoral bypass. *J Card Surg* 1989;**4**:43-9.
87. Cardarelli MG, McLaughlin JS, Downing SW, Brown JM, Attar S, Griffith BP. Management of traumatic aortic rupture: a 30-year experience. *Ann Surg* 2002;**236**:465-9.
88. Mattox KL, Flint LM, Carrico CJ, Grover F, Meredith J, Morris J, et al. Blunt cardiac injury. *J Trauma* 1992;**33**(5):649-50.
89. Adams 3rd JE, Dávila-Román VG, Bessey PQ, Blake DP, Ladenson JH, Jaffe AS. Improved detection of cardiac contusion with cardiac troponin I. *Am Heart J* 1996;**131**:308-12.
90. Foil MB, Mackersie RC, Furst SR, Davis JW, Swanson MS, Hoyt DB, Shackford SR. The asymptomatic patient with suspected myocardial contusion. *Am J Surg* 1990;**160**:638-42.
91. Biffl WL, Moore FA, Moore EE, Sauaia A, Read RA, Burch JM. Cardiac enzymes are irrelevant in the patient with suspected myocardial contusion. *Am J Surg* 1994;**168**:523-7.
92. Sybrandy KC, Cramer MJ, Burgersdijk C. Diagnosing cardiac contusion: old wisdom and new insights. *Heart* 2003;**89**:485-9.
93. Perchinsky MJ, Long WB, Hill JG. Blunt cardiac rupture: The Emanuel Trauma Center experience. *Arch Surg* 1995;**130**:852-7.
94. Keller KD, Shatney CH. Creatine phosphokinase-MB assays in patients with suspected myocardial contusion: Diagnostic test or test of diagnosis? *J Trauma* 1988;**28**:58-63.
95. Murray JA, Demetriades D, Asensio JA, Cornwell E, Velmahos GC, Belzberg H, Berne TV. Occult injuries to the diaphragm: prospective evaluation of laparoscopy in penetrating injuries to the left lower chest. *J Am Coll Surg* 1998;**187**(6):626-30.
96. Reber PU, Schmied B, Seiler CA, Baer HU, Patel AG, Büchler MW. Missed diaphragmatic injuries and their long-term sequelae. *J Trauma* 1998;**44**:183-8.
97. Bryant AS, Cerfolio RJ. Esophageal trauma. *Thorac Surg Clin* 2007;**17**(1):63-72.
98. Bastos RB, Graeber GM. Esophageal injuries. *Chest Surg Clin N Am* 1997;**7**:357-71.
99. Bastos R, Baisden CE, Harker L, Calhoun JH. Penetrating thoracic trauma. *Semin Thorac Cardiovasc Surg* 2008;**20**:19-25.
100. Ryan JM, Rich NM, Dale RF, Morgans BT, Cooper GJ. Biophysics and pathophysiology of penetrating injury. In: *Ballistic trauma: clinical relevance in peace and war*. Oxford University Press; 2007.
101. Karmy-Jones R, Wood DE. Traumatic injury to the trachea and bronchus. *Thorac Surg Clin* 2007;**17**(1):35-46.
102. Grewal H, Rao PM, Mukerji S, Ivatury RR. Management of penetrating laryngotracheal injuries. *Head Neck* 1995;**17**:494-502.
103. Huh J, Milliken JC, Chen JC. Management of tracheobronchial injuries following blunt and penetrating trauma. *Am Surg* 1997;**63**:896-9.
104. Cicala RS, Kudsk KA, Butts A, Nguyen H, Fabian TC. Initial evaluation and management of upper airways in trauma patients. *J Clin Anesth* 1991;**3**:88-90.
105. Kumpe DA, Oh KS, Wyman SM. A characteristic pulmonary finding in unilateral complete bronchial transection. *Am J Roentgenol* 1970;**110**:704-6.
106. Bowling R, Mavroudis C, Richardson JD, Flint LM, Howe WR, Gray LA. Emergency pneumonectomy for penetrating and blunt trauma. *Am Surg* 1985;**51**:136.
107. Karmy-Jones R, Jurkovich GJ, Shatz DV, Brundage S, Wall Jr MJ, Engelhardt S, et al. Management of traumatic lung injury: a Western Trauma Association Multicenter review. *J Trauma* 2001;**51**:1049-53.
108. Brown 3rd PF, Larsen CP, Symbas PN. Management of the asymptomatic patient with a stab wound to the chest. *S Med J* 1991;**84**:591-3.
109. Meyer DM. Hemothorax related to trauma. *Thorac Surg Clin* 2007;**17**:47-55.
110. Inci I, Ozçelik C, Tacyildiz I, Nizam O, Eren N, Ozgen G. Penetrating chest injuries: unusually high incidence of high-velocity gunshot wounds in civilian practice. *World J Surg* 1998;**22**:438-42.
111. Petricevic A, Ilic N, Bacic A, Petricevic M, Vidjak V, Tanfara S. War injuries of the lungs. *Eur J Cardiothorac Surg* 1997;**11**:843-7.
112. Karmy-Jones R, Jurkovich GJ, Nathens AB, Shatz DV, Brundage S, Wall Jr MJ, et al. Timing of urgent thoracotomy for hemorrhage after trauma: a multicenter study. 2001. 136: p. 513–8.
113. Mansour MA, Moore EE, Moore FA, Read RR. Exigent postinjury thoracotomy analysis of blunt vs penetrating trauma. *Surg Gynecol Obstet* 1992;**175**:97-101.
114. Embrey R. Cardiac trauma. *Thorac Surg Clin* 2007;**17**:87-93.
115. Asensio JA, Berne JD, Demetriades D, Chan L, Murray J, Falabella A, et al. One hundred five penetrating cardiac injuries: a 2-year prospective evaluation. *J Trauma* 1998;**44**:1073-82.
116. Molina EJ, Gaughan JP, Kulp H, McClurken JB, Goldberg AJ, Seamon MJ. Outcomes after emergency department thoracotomy for penetrating cardiac injuries: a new perspective. *Interact CardioVasc Thorac Surg* 2008;**7**:845-8.
117. Grewal H, Ivatury RR, Divakar M, Simon RJ, Rohman M. Evaluation of subxiphoid pericardial window used in the detection of occult cardiac injury. *Injury* 1995;**26**(5):305-10.
118. Aaland MO, Bryan 3rd FC, Sherman R. Two-dimensional echocardiogram in hemodynamically stable victims of penetrating precordial trauma. *Am Surg* 1994;**60**(6):412-5.
119. Jimenez E, Martin M, Krukenkamp I, Barrett J. Subxiphoid pericardiotomy versus echocardiography: a prospective evaluation of the diagnosis of occult penetrating cardiac injury. *Surgery* 1999;**108**(108):676-80.
120. Harris DG, Papagiannopoulos KA, Pretorius J, Van Rooyen T, Rossouw GJ. Current evaluation of cardiac stab wounds. *Ann Thorac Surg* 1999;**68**:2119-22.
121. Bolton JW, Bynoe RP, Lazar HL, Almond CH. Two-dimensional echocardiography in the evaluation of penetrating intrapericardial injuries. *Ann Thorac Surg* 1999;**193**(56):506-9.
122. McMahon DJ, Sing RF, Hoff WS, Schwab CW. Laparoscopic transdiaphragmatic diagnostic pericardial window in the hemodynamically stable patient with penetrating chest trauma. *Surg Endosc* 1997;**11**:474-5.
123. Cetindag IB, Neideen T, Hazelrigg SR. Video assisted thoracic surgical applications in thoracic trauma. *Thorac Surg Clin* 2007;**17**:73-9.
124. Reddy VS. Minimally invasive techniques in Thoracic Trauma. *Semin Thorac Cardiovasc Surg* 2008;**20**:72-7.
125. Tyburski JG, Astra L, Wilson RF, Dente C, Steffes C. Factors affecting prognosis with penetrating wounds of the heart. *J Trauma* 2000;**48**(4):587-90.
126. Webb DP, Ramsey JJ, Dignan RJ, Drinkwater Jr DC. Penetrating injury to the heart requiring cardiopulmonary bypass: a case study. *J Extra Corpor Technol* 2001;**33**(4):249-51.
127. Biocina B, Sutlić Z, Husedzinovic I, Rudez I, Ugljen R, Letica D, et al. Penetrating cardiothoracic war wounds. *Eur J Cardiothorac Surg* 1997;**11**(3):399-405.
128. Robison RJ, Brown JW, Caldwell R, Stone KS, King H. Management of asymptomatic intracardiac missiles using echocardiography. *J Trauma* 1988;**28**:1402-3.
129. Symbas PN, Picone AL, Hatcher CR, Vlasis-Hale SE. Cardiac missiles: a review of the literature and personal experience. *Ann Surg* 1990;**211**:639-48.
130. Nagy KK, Massad M, Fildes J, Reyes H. Missile embolization revisited: a rationale for selective management. *Am Surg* 1994;**60**:975-9.
131. Gandhi SK, Marts BC, Mistry BM, Brown JW, Durham RM, Mazuski JE. Selective management of embolized intracardiac missiles. *Ann Thorac Surg* 1996;**62**:290-2.
132. Estera AS, Pass LJ, Platt MR. Systemic arterial air embolism in penetrating lung injury. *Ann Thorac Surg* 1990;**50**:257-61.
133. Ho AM, Lee S, Tay BA, Chung DC. Lung isolation for the prevention of air embolism in penetrating lung trauma. A case report. *Can J Anaesth* 2000;**47**:1256-8.
134. Rawlins R, Momin A, Platts D, El-Gamel A. Traumatic cardiogenic shock due to massive air embolism. A possible role for cardiopulmonary bypass. *Eur J Cardiothorac Surg* 2002;**22**:845-6.
135. Brinkman WT, Szeto WY, Bavaria JE. Overview of great vessel trauma. *Thorac Surg Clin* 2007;**17**:95-108.
136. Demetriades D, Rabinowitz B, Pezikis A, Franklin J, Palexas G. Subclavian vascular injuries. *Br J Surg* 1987;**74**:1001-3.
137. Demetriades D, Asensio JA, Velmahos G, Thal E. Complex problems in penetrating neck trauma. *Surg Clin North Am* 1996;**76**:661-83.
138. Stassen NA, Lukan JK, Spain DA, Miller FB, Carrillo EH, Richardson JD, Battistella FD. Reevaluation of diagnostic procedures for transmediastinal gunshot wounds. *J Trauma* 2002;**53**:635-8.
139. Nagy KK, Roberts RR, Smith RF, Joseph KT, An GC, Bokhari F, Barrett J. Transmediastinal gunshot wounds: are "stable" patients really stable? *World J Surg* 2002;**26**(10):1247-50.
140. Gilroy D, Charalambides LMD. Control of life-threatening hemorrhage from the neck: A new indication for balloon tamponade. *J Trauma* 1992;**23**:557-9.
141. Fulton JO, Brink JG. Complex thoracic vascular injury repair using deep hypothermia and circulatory arrest. *Ann Thorac Surg* 1997;**63**:557-9.
142. Demetriades D. Penetrating injuries to the thoracic great vessels. *J Card Surg* 1997;**12**:173-80.
143. Miller L, Bennett Jr EV, Root HD, Trinkle JK, Grover FL. Management of penetrating and blunt diaphragmatic injury. *J Trauma* 1984;**24**:403-7.
144. Madden MR, Paull DE, Finkelstein JL, Goodwin CW, Marzulli V, Yurt RW, Shires GT. Occult diaphragmatic injury from stab wounds to the lower chest and abdomen. *J Trauma* 1989;**29**:292-7.
145. Uribe RA, Pachon CE, Frame SB, Enderson BL, Escobar F, Garcia GA. A prospective evaluation of thoracoscopy for the diagnosis of penetrating thoracoabdominal trauma. *J Trauma* 1994;**37**:650-4.
146. Freeman RK, Al-Dossari G, Hutcheson KA, Huber L, Jessen ME, Meyer DM, et al. Indications for using video-assisted thoracoscopic surgery to diagnose penetrating chest trauma. *Ann Thorac Surg* 2001;**72**:342-7.
147. Asensio JA, Berne J, Demetriades D, Murray J, Gomez H, Falabella A, et al. Penetrating esophageal injuries: time interval of safety for preoperative evaluation-how long is safe? *J Trauma* 1997;**43**:319-24.

148. Weiman DS, Walker WA, Brosnan KM, Pate JW, Fabian TC. Noniatrogenic esophageal trauma. *Ann Thorac Surg* 1995;**59**:845-50.
149. Asensio JA, Chahwan S, Forno W, MacKersie R, Wall M, Lake J, Trauma J, et al. American Association for the Surgery of Trauma. Penetrating esophageal injuries: multicenter study of the American Association for the Surgery of Trauma. 2001;**50**(2):289-96.
150. Flowers JL, Graham SM, Ugarte MA, Sartor WM, Rodriquez A, Gens DR, et al. Flexible endoscopy for the diagnosis of esophageal trauma. *J Trauma* 1996;**40**(2):261-6.
151. Cohn HE, Hubbard A, Patton G. Management of esophageal injuries. *Ann Thorac Surg* 1989;**48**:309-14.
152. Stewart RM, Corneille MG. Common complications following thoracic trauma: their prevention and treatment. *Semin Thorac Cardiovasc Surg* 2008;**20**:69-71
153. Bernard GR, Artigas A, Brigham KL, Carlet J, Falke K, Hudson L, et al. Report of the American-European Consensus conference on acute respiratory distress syndrome: definitions, mechanisms, relevant outcomes, and clinical trial coordination. Consensus Committee. *Am J Respir Crit Care Med* 1994;**149**:818-24.
154. Bass TL, Miller PK, Campbell DB, Russell GB. Traumatic Adult Respiratory Distress Syndrome. *Chest Surg Clin N Am* 1997;**7**:429-40.
155. Sutyak JP, Wohltman CD, Larson J. Pulmonary Contusions Critical Care management in thoracic trauma. *Thorac Surg Clin* 2007;**17**:11-23.
156. Rico FR, Cheng JD, Gestring ML, Piotrowski ES. Mechanical ventilation strategies in massive chest trauma. *Crit Care Clin* 2007;**23**(2):299-315.
157. Caplan ES, Hoyt NJ, Rodriguez A, Cowley RA. Empyema occurring in the multiply traumatized patient. *J Trauma* 1984;**24**:785-9.
158. Richardson JD, Carrillo E. Thoracic infection after trauma. *Chest Surg Clin N Am* 1997;**7**:401-27.
159. Sebastian MW, Wolfe WG. Traumatic thoracic fistula. *Chest Surg Clin N Am* 1997;**7**:385-400.

D. Trachea

CHAPTER 8

Tracheal Lesions

Todd S. Weiser, Simon K. Ashiku, and Douglas J. Mathisen

Historical Perspective
Anatomy
Tracheal Pathology
   Postintubation Injuries
   Idiopathic Laryngotracheal Stenosis
   Tracheobronchomalacia
   Tracheal Tumors

Clinical Presentation
Radiographic Imaging
Bronchoscopy
Anesthesia
Tracheal Resection
Laryngotracheal Resection
Release Procedures

Repair of Tracheoinnominate
   and Tracheoesophageal Fistulas
Perioperative Management
Results
Complications
Summary

A variety of benign and malignant lesions can develop in the trachea and lead to airway obstruction. The infrequent occurrence of tracheal pathology and its often insidious nature can lead to a delayed diagnosis for patients in whom these conditions exist. Advances in surgical and anesthetic techniques have enabled safe and effective resection with primary reconstruction for many of these lesions. For obstructive lesions whose extent precludes primary tracheal resection and reconstruction, there is still no universally definitive treatment, but several palliative measures exist to provide patients with a satisfactory airway.

This chapter focuses on surgically correctable lesions of the trachea, including those that involve the subglottic larynx. Pathology and treatment of carinal lesions will be discussed in a separate chapter. Historical perspective, along with preoperative assessment, operative strategies, and postoperative care for patients with obstructive pathology of the trachea will be discussed in detail.

HISTORICAL PERSPECTIVE

When the field of tracheal surgery was young, it was widely accepted that only four tracheal rings, or approximately 2 cm, of trachea could be safely resected with immediate reconstruction. It was the work of Dr. Hermes Grillo, considered by most to be the father of modern tracheal surgery, that led to the surgical practices used today. Grillo and colleagues[1-3] systemically investigated the limits of resection of the trachea to permit reconstruction without excessive anastomotic tension. Among other findings, these studies demonstrated that the tracheal blood supply entered in its lateral pedicles, and that safe mobilization of the trachea could be accomplished only with anterior and posterior dissection. Dedo and Fishman[4] described laryngeal release maneuvers to minimize tension on lengthier tracheal resections. These contributions led to the realization that, in select cases, up to 50% of the human trachea could be resected and reconstructed without detrimental tension.

ANATOMY

The trachea averages 11 cm in length from the lower border of the cricoid cartilage to the carinal spur, with an additional 1.5 to 2 cm of subglottic laryngeal airway. The structural support comes from 18 to 22 cartilaginous C-shaped rings, with about two rings per centimeter. The cricoid cartilage is the only complete cartilaginous ring in the normal airway. Most of the trachea lies within the thoracic inlet and the chest. Cervical hyperextension delivers up to half of the trachea into the neck, and flexion devolves most of the trachea into the mediastinum.

The blood supply to the trachea is from many small terminal end arteries. The upper trachea is supplied principally by branches of the inferior thyroid artery, and the lower trachea by branches of the bronchial arteries. These vessels enter the trachea via very fine lateral pedicles that lack collateralization (Fig. 8-1).[5] The pretracheal plane and the plane between the esophagus and the trachea are avascular. The recurrent laryngeal nerves ascend in the tracheoesophageal grooves bilaterally and pass medially to the inferior cornua of the thyroid cartilage to enter the larynx. The nerve on the left is present along the entire length of the trachea, whereas the right recurrent laryngeal nerve is present in the tracheoesophageal groove for only the proximal cervical trachea.

TRACHEAL PATHOLOGY

A wide spectrum of pathology may afflict the trachea, ranging from benign conditions to malignant ones. Most conditions lead to central airway obstruction with subsequent respiratory insufficiency. Others, such as fistulas between the trachea and innominate artery or esophagus, may also occur and be equally deleterious. Direct external trauma, blunt or penetrating, may result in a tear or complete disruption of the trachea at any level. Inhalational burn injuries are usually maximal in the proximal subglottic region and diminish in

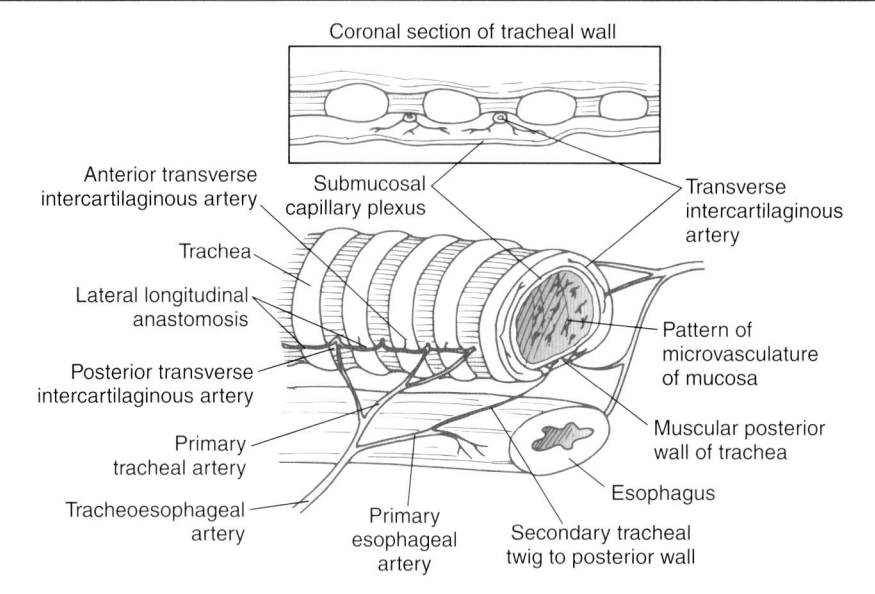

Figure 8–1
Microscopic blood supply of the trachea. Transverse intercartilaginous arteries derived from the lateral longitudinal anastomosis penetrate the soft tissues between the cartilaginous rings to supply a rich vascular network beneath the endotracheal mucosa. *(From Salassa JR, Pearson BW, Payne WS. Ann Thorac Surg 1977;**24**:100-7. Reprinted with permission from the Society of Thoracic Surgeons.)*

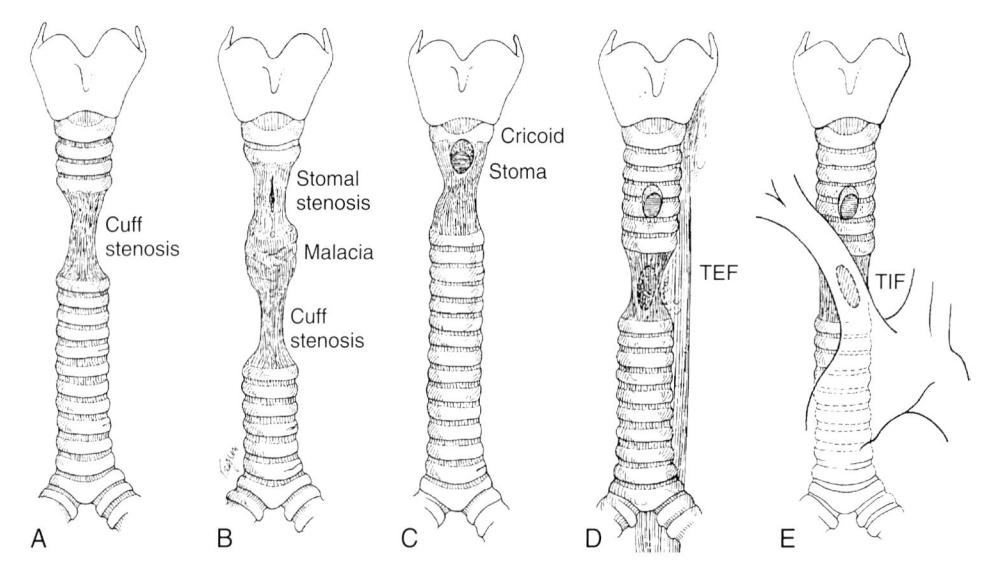

Figure 8–2
Diagrams of principal postintubation tracheal lesions. **A,** Cuff stenosis from the cuff of an endotracheal tube. **B,** Cuff stenosis from the cuff of a tracheostomy tube, usually lower in the trachea than that from an endotracheal tube. Stoma stenosis also occurs at the site of the tracheostomy itself. Malacia may occur either at the level of the cuff or in the segment between the stoma and the cuff stenosis. **C,** Cuff stenosis at the site of a high tracheostomy stoma, which has eroded into the lower margin of the cricoid cartilage. In older patients, this may erode back further into the subglottic larynx, producing a laryngotracheal stenosis. **D,** Tracheoesophageal fistula (TEF) produced by pressure of the cuff against the membranous wall, often abetted by an indwelling, firm, nasogastric tube. **E,** One type of tracheoinnominate fistula (TIF), the result of a high-pressure cuff erosion. The more common type, but also rare, is that seen with a low-placed tracheostomy stoma, which rests against the innominate artery itself. Not shown here are the lesions that occur in the larynx as the result of endotracheal tubes. *(From Grillo HC. Surgical management of postintubation tracheal injuries. J Thorac Cardiovasc Surg 1979;**78**:860.)*

the more distal airway. In most cases, the tracheal rings are not destroyed.[6]

Postintubation Injuries

Iatrogenic injuries resulting from tracheal intubation have long been the most common lesion afflicting the airway. Postintubation injuries include granulomas, strictures, malacia, and tracheoesophageal and tracheoinnominate fistulas (Fig. 8-2).

Postintubation tracheal stenosis represents the most common iatrogenic injury of the trachea. It occurs after intubation and develops principally at the level of the endotracheal tube or tracheostomy tube cuffs. The radial pressure exerted from the cuff causes circumferential pressure necrosis, which results in cicatricial scaring stenosis (Fig. 8-3).[7,8] The route of

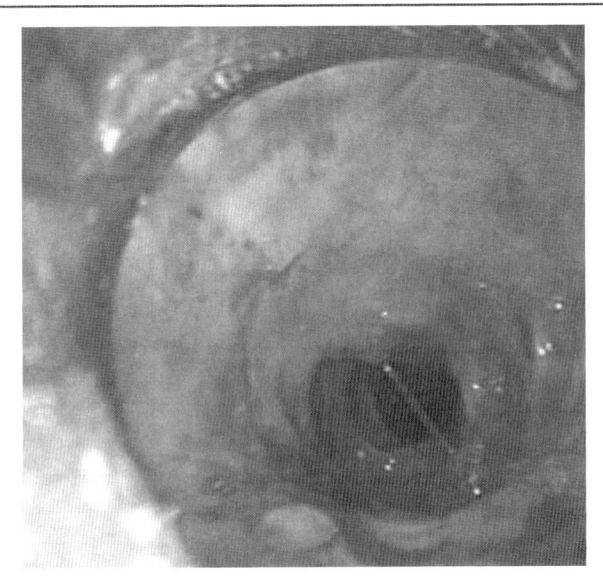

Figure 8–3
Cuff-level stenosis. The stenosis here is circumferential and the remaining lumen round.

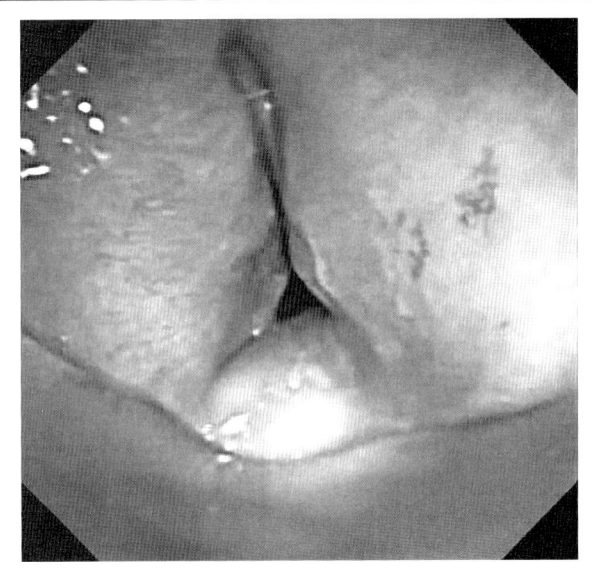

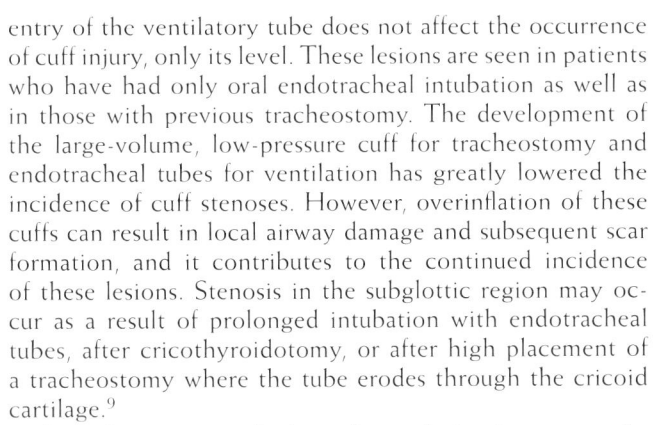

Figure 8–4
Tracheostomy stomal site stenosis. The characteristic A-shaped lumen is evident and results from a primarily anterior and lateral cicatricial process.

entry of the ventilatory tube does not affect the occurrence of cuff injury, only its level. These lesions are seen in patients who have had only oral endotracheal intubation as well as in those with previous tracheostomy. The development of the large-volume, low-pressure cuff for tracheostomy and endotracheal tubes for ventilation has greatly lowered the incidence of cuff stenoses. However, overinflation of these cuffs can result in local airway damage and subsequent scar formation, and it contributes to the continued incidence of these lesions. Stenosis in the subglottic region may occur as a result of prolonged intubation with endotracheal tubes, after cricothyroidotomy, or after high placement of a tracheostomy where the tube erodes through the cricoid cartilage.[9]

Stomal stenosis results from the gradual enlargement of a tracheal stoma and its eventual healing by contraction. This pulls the sides of the defect together, distorting the tracheal lumen to a triangular configuration, with the base of the triangle located posteriorly and consisting of the uninjured membranous wall (Fig. 8-4). The instigating large stoma may result from overzealous excision of anterior tracheal cartilage at the time of the initial tracheostomy, from erosive infection around the margins of the stoma, or, most commonly, from erosion resulting from leverage by equipment attached to the tracheostomy tube during ventilation. The stenotic process may extend into the subglottic larynx if the previous tracheostomy was placed inappropriately high in the trachea.

Prolonged endotracheal intubation combined with a nasogastric tube may lead to a tracheoesophageal fistula (Fig. 8-5). This results from pressure necrosis generated by a ventilating cuff in the trachea and a prolonged feeding tube in the esophagus. Consequently, these fistulas occur in the shared location between the membranous tracheal wall and the anterior wall of the esophagus. Anterior injuries of the trachea may lead to the development of a tracheoinnominate artery fistula. These most often result from direct erosion of the inner elbow of

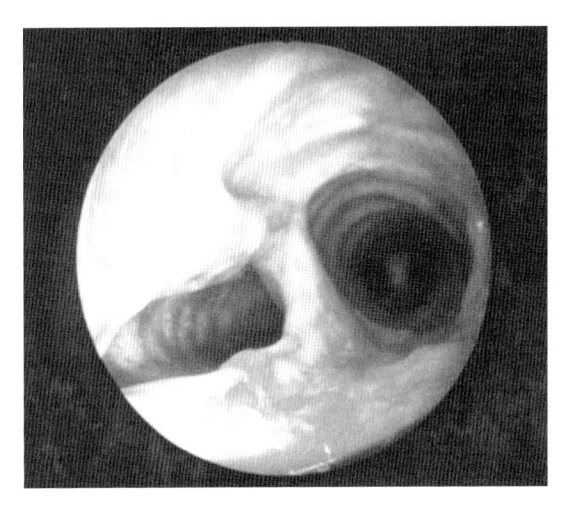

Figure 8–5
Endoscopic view of tracheoesophageal fistula.

the tracheostomy tube in an inferiorly placed stoma, and they may arise either from a tracheostomy tube placed too low in the trachea or from an innominate artery lying high at the sternal notch.

Idiopathic Laryngotracheal Stenosis

Rarely, a patient presents with stenosis of the airway without history of trauma, infection, inhalation injury, or airway intubation. Idiopathic laryngotracheal stenosis is a diagnosis of exclusion, characterized by an inflammatory cicatricial stenosis at the level of the subglottic larynx, cricoid, and upper trachea. An overwhelming majority of these patients are female, and they typically present with signs and symptoms of upper airway obstruction. This process is confined intrinsically to the wall of the airway and the immediately surrounding connective tissue.

It is impossible to predict the future course of the disease. When airway obstruction becomes severe and does not respond for sufficiently long intervals to dilation, surgery may be entertained, with, however, the clear caveat that the disease may progress. Most patients are best treated with definitive laryngotracheal resection and primary reconstruction.[10,11]

Tracheobronchomalacia

Airway malacia may be a consequence of a postintubation injury. However, in patients with chronic obstructive pulmonary disease, malacia may develop in the lower trachea, main bronchi, and sometimes the more distal bronchi, even in the absence of prior intubation.[12] When the patient attempts a deep expiration or a cough, the membranous wall approximates to the anterior, softened cartilaginous wall, causing nearly total obstruction. Subsequently, the posterior membranous wall elongates and becomes redundant. Afflicted patients may present with dyspnea, cough, and secretion retention. It is possible to surgically address the deformity by pulling the ends of the cartilages toward one another posteriorly, restoring a more circular shape to the airway. The redundant membranous wall must be tacked to a posterior splinting material to prevent it from falling forward into the lumen. Various materials have been used for splinting, none with complete success. These have included fascia lata, pericardium, lyophilized bone, polytetrafluoroethylene, and rigid plastic splints. We currently use sheets of polypropylene mesh to plicate the membranous wall as described by Rainer and colleagues.[13]

Tracheal Tumors

Primary tracheal tumors are rare, with an estimated incidence of 2.7 cases per million per year.[14] Approximately two thirds of primary tracheal tumors are either squamous cell carcinomas (SCCs) or adenoid cystic carcinomas (ACCs). These two types occur with equal frequency. The remaining third of the tumors are widely distributed in a heterogeneous group of tumors, both malignant and benign. Secondary tumors that involve the trachea include carcinomas of the larynx, thyroid, lung, and esophagus. Rarely, tumors may metastasize to the submucosa of the trachea or to the mediastinum, with secondary invasion of the trachea.

Squamous cell carcinomas may be either exophytic (Fig. 8-6) or ulcerative. The tumor can metastasize to the regional lymph nodes, and, in its more aggressive and late forms, it invades mediastinal structures. In general, its progress appears to be relatively rapid in comparison with that of adenoid cystic carcinoma. A number of these patients develop synchronous or metachronous second SCC primary cancers of the lung or oropharynx. Squamous cell carcinoma occurs predominantly in men who are cigarette smokers.[15]

ACC often has a very prolonged course of clinical symptoms, sometimes extending for years. After resection, many years may pass before a recurrence is noted. It may extend submucosally over long distances in the airways, and also along perineural tissue. It can spread to regional lymph nodes, although this is less characteristic than in SCC. Although it may invade the thyroid or the muscular coats of the esophagus by contiguity, ACC that has not been surgically interfered

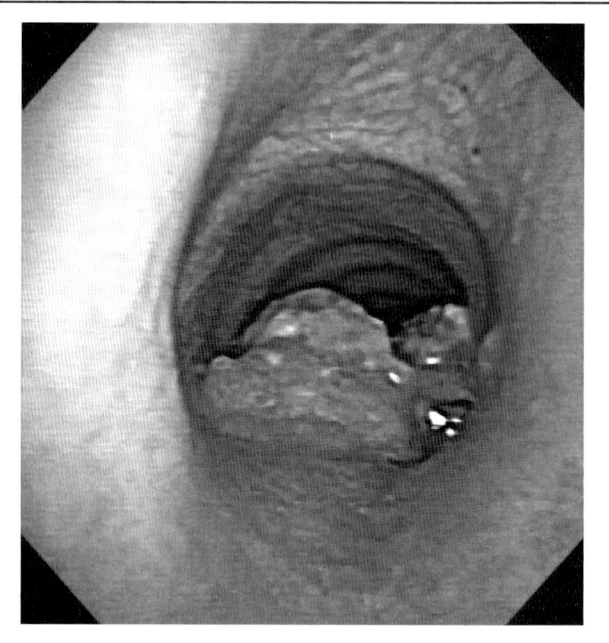

Figure 8–6
An exophytic squamous cell carcinoma of the trachea.

with frequently displaces mediastinal structures before actually invading them. Metastases to the lungs, bone, and other organs can occur. These may grow very slowly over a period of many years and remain asymptomatic until they become quite large. In contrast to patients with tracheal SCC, the male-to-female ratio of ACC is essentially equal, and any smoking history of these patients appears to be incidental.[15]

The third group of primary tracheal tumors is composed of a multitude of tumor types and varying degrees of malignancy, including both epithelial and mesenchymal neoplasms. The list includes pleomorphic adenomas, leiomyomas, chondromas, carcinoid tumors, mucoepidermoid tumors, and sarcomas.

Secondary neoplasms may involve the trachea through direct extension. Thyroid carcinomas typically invade the trachea at the second and third rings, where the thyroid isthmus is adherent to the trachea (Fig. 8-7).[16] More commonly, invasion is seen after thyroidectomy for carcinoma, when the surgeon was aware of shaving off the tumor from the trachea. In such cases, concurrent or early resection of the involved trachea should be considered. Both bronchogenic and esophageal carcinomas can erode into the trachea from local extension.

CLINICAL PRESENTATION

Patients with pathologic lesions of the trachea usually present with signs and symptoms of upper airway obstruction: dyspnea on exertion, wheezing, or stridor. Unfortunately, this presentation is frequently misinterpreted as adult-onset asthma, and it is not uncommon for patients to undergo treatment with corticosteroids before the correct diagnosis is finally made. Any patient who presents with obstructive airway and has a history of tracheal intubation must be considered to have airway stenosis until proven otherwise.

Tumors of the trachea often present insidiously. Their most common signs and symptoms are cough (37%), hemoptysis (41%), and the signs of progressive airway obstruction, including shortness of breath on exertion (54%),

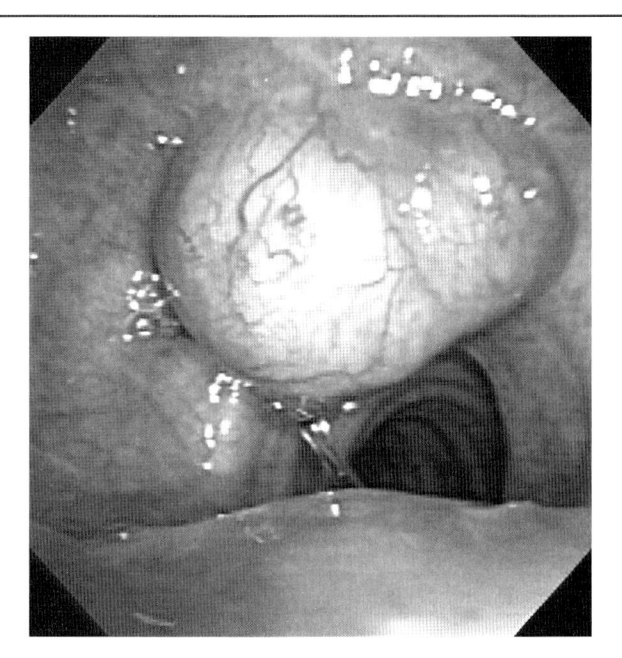

Figure 8–7
Bronchoscopic view of a papillary thyroid carcinoma with tracheal invasion.

wheezing and stridor (35%) and, less commonly, dysphagia or hoarseness (7%).[14] Signs and symptoms may vary with the histology of the tumor. Hemoptysis is prominent in patients with SCC, usually leading to a prompt diagnosis. Patients with ACC more commonly present with wheezing or stridor as the predominant symptom, which often leads to a delay in diagnosis. In one study, the mean duration of symptoms before diagnosis in patients with SCC of the trachea was only 4 months whereas in those with ACC it was 18 months.[17]

A tracheoesophageal fistula frequently presents with an increase in tracheal secretions and the appearance of orally ingested material in the airway. If the patient is on a mechanical ventilator, gastric distension may develop. Tracheoinnominate arterial fistulas may be heralded by a premonitory hemorrhage. In evaluating a patient with bleeding from a tracheostomy tube, it is important to determine whether the source is from erosion of tracheal granulation tissue or mucosal trauma as opposed to the more deleterious arterial fistula.

RADIOGRAPHIC IMAGING

A standard posteroanterior chest radiograph, centered high on the trachea, may reveal some tracheal pathology. Detailed information about the location of the lesion, its longitudinal extent, and the amount of normal trachea available for reconstruction can be demonstrated by computerized axial tomography scans. These are particularly useful in evaluating tracheal tumors, as they characterize extraluminal extension and any mediastinal lymphadenopathy. Recently, the use of high-speed helical computed tomographic scanners to acquire images, combined with powerful three-dimensional-image software, has created impressive two- and three-dimensional airway reconstructions (Fig. 8-8).

BRONCHOSCOPY

Bronchoscopic evaluation is necessary to confirm a diagnosis, design an operative strategy, and ameliorate impending airway obstruction. Measurements taken with a rigid bronchoscope determine the amount of normal trachea that is available, both proximal and distal to the pathology, for reconstruction. Factors such as age, body habitus, prior surgery, and lesion location influence the amount of trachea that can be safely resected. With benign strictures, special attention must be given to assessing the condition of the tracheal mucosa. Indwelling tracheostomy or tracheal T-tubes must be removed and the mucosa assessed. If extensive mucosal inflammation or ulceration exists, definitive repair should be delayed until mucosal healing occurs. This may require a short period of decannulation or a change to a smaller T-tube. Often, patients with idiopathic laryngotracheal stenosis have active inflammation extending into the immediate subglottis. These patients should undergo dilation of their stenosis, and the operation should be delayed until the inflammatory state of the airway mucosa subsides. Patients taking corticosteroids should be weaned from them and should be off for at least a month before an operative repair is undertaken. This is done to minimize the adverse wound-healing effects of these medications.

Expertise with the techniques of interventional bronchoscopy is essential to safely dilate a benign stenosis or "core out" an obstructing airway tumor. This allows evaluation of the distal airway, safe passage of an endotracheal tube, or temporary creation of a patent airway to allow delay in operation. Dilating a narrow, fibrotic stricture is challenging and can result in airway rupture, complete obstruction, or excessive destruction of tracheal mucosa. Progressively larger Jackson dilators passed through a rigid bronchoscope can be used to effectively dilate the stenosis. An assortment of pediatric and adult rigid bronchoscopes can then be used, increasing the sizes and using a gentle corkscrew motion.[18] Balloon dilators placed through the working channel of a flexible bronchoscope permit effective airway dilation.

Obstructing tracheal tumors are managed first by core-out techniques using the rigid bronchoscope, forceps, and suction.[19] Using the tip of the bronchoscope in a corkscrew motion, most tumors can be débrided from the tracheal wall, and forceps can then be used to remove dislodged tumor fragments. If bleeding ensues, the bronchoscope is advanced distal to the lesion and used to tamponade the bleeding. Direct application of epinephrine-soaked pledgets can assist in addressing persistent blood loss.

Patients with critical airway stenosis should be assessed in the operating room where rigid bronchoscopy, biopsy forceps, and instruments required to perform emergent tracheotomy are available. Placement of a tracheostomy tube may be necessary in some patients as the only means to secure an airway. When possible, these should be placed through the stenosis, preserving the uninvolved trachea for future reconstruction.[18]

ANESTHESIA

Anesthesia for bronchoscopy and tracheal surgery, especially when there is a high degree of airway obstruction distally, is best administered by inhalational agents. A slow, patient induction may be necessary if there is a high degree of airway

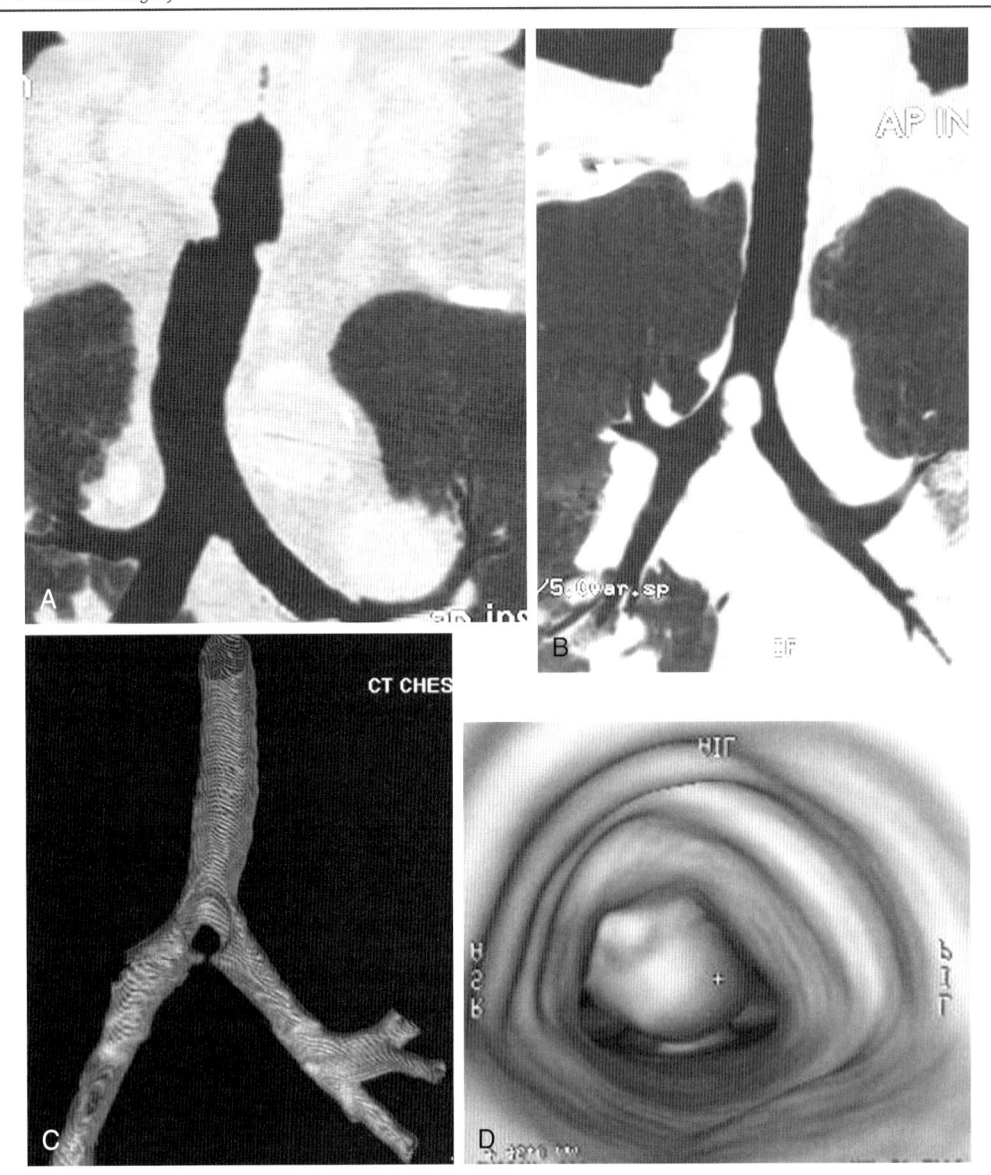

Figure 8-8
A, Reformatted computed tomographic (CT) two-dimensional (2D) image of post-tracheostomy stenosis. **B,** A 2D image of an adenoid cystic carcinoma of the carina. **C,** Three-dimensional (3D) image of a tracheal airway column showing the endobronchial component of the same carinal mass. **D,** The same carinal mass as viewed endobronchially by a 3D image via virtual CT bronchoscopy.

obstruction.[20] This is preferable and safer than the administration of muscle relaxants, which paralyze respiration with a consequent urgent need to establish an airway.

The surgeon should be available with an array of rigid bronchoscopes from pediatric to adult sizes as the induction commences. The residual airway through which the patient is breathing may be as narrow as 2 or 3 mm in diameter. In most cases, tumors are not circumferential. After bronchoscopy, a small endotracheal tube can often be insinuated past a highly obstructive lesion. Although not ideal, an endotracheal tube can be secured above the obstructive pathology.

At the time of tracheal division, the endotracheal tube is pulled back or removed and a sterile, cuffed, and armored endotracheal tube is inserted into the distal airway across the operative field. Sterile connecting tubing is passed to the anesthesiologist to allow ventilation of the patient. This armored tube is removed whenever necessary for suctioning or placement of sutures. Toward the completion of the operation, the original endotracheal tube is advanced into the distal airway and the anastomotic sutures are tied. High-frequency ventilation has been used with equal success intraoperatively, but we have been quite satisfied with the technique described here. High-frequency ventilation is especially useful in certain complex carinal reconstructions.

Anesthesia is maintained with total intravenous anesthesia using short-acting agents such as remifentanil and propofol. This allows immediate extubation at the completion of the procedure and maintains continuous anesthesia during periods when inhalational agents are interrupted by the procedure. Ideally, the patient should be extubated and able to breathe spontaneously at the conclusion of the procedure. Particularly when the trachea has been greatly shortened, it is desirable not to have even a low-pressure cuff lying in contact with the anastomosis. The use of cardiopulmonary bypass is not usually

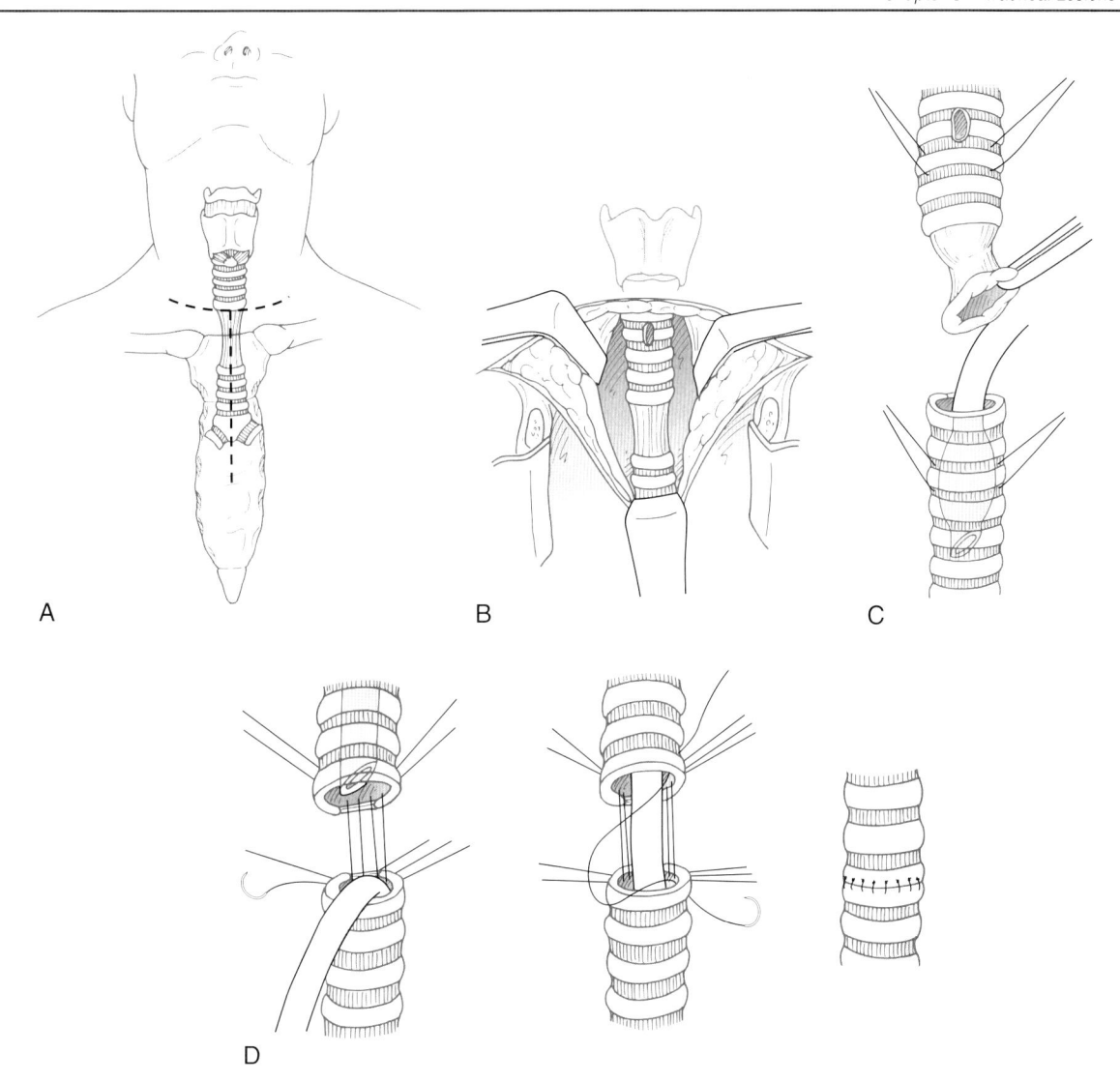

Figure 8–9
Resection of a mid-tracheal airway stenosis. See text for description of **A** to **D**. *(From Grillo HC. Surgery of the trachea: current problems in surgery. Ann Thorac Surg 1970;**7**:3-59. Reprinted with permission from Mosby, Inc.)*

necessary in adult tracheal surgery, even in complex carinal reconstructions. However, it may be requisite in repairing congenital airway lesions in the pediatric population, especially in the presence and correction of cardiac anomalies.[21]

TRACHEAL RESECTION

For uncomplicated resections of the middle and upper trachea, the patient is positioned supine with an inflatable airbag beneath the shoulders and with the neck extended. The inflatable bag facilitates exposure by extending the neck during dissection, and when deflated, it allows cervical flexion just before the anastomotic sutures are tied. The head is supported in a foam ring and the arms are tucked at the sides.

A low collar cervical incision is adequate for most tracheal resections that involve the upper trachea. When the lesion involves the middle to lower trachea, vertical extension with a partial sternal split facilitates exposure (Fig. 8-9A). Dissection is carried through the platysma, and subplatysmal flaps are elevated superiorly to the level of the thyroid cartilage and inferiorly to the level of the sternal notch. The strap muscles are separated in the midline, and a plane of dissection is established very close to the tracheal wall to avoid injury to the recurrent laryngeal nerves (see Fig. 8-9B). The pretracheal plane is dissected to the level of the carina. The investing fascia of the innominate artery and the adjacent mediastinal fat are left intact to guard against postoperative tracheoinnominate fistulization. Retraction on the innominate artery is kept to a minimum to avoid impeding cerebral blood flow.

The area of involved trachea is transilluminated with a flexible bronchoscope through the oral endotracheal tube, allowing the assistant to mark the distal extent of resection. The trachea is sharply dissected circumferentially at the most distal aspect of the lesion, with the dissection plane maintained on the tracheal wall. The oral endotracheal tube is withdrawn into the upper trachea, the trachea is partially divided at the most distal extent of the lesion, and bilateral 2-0 Vicryl traction sutures are placed. These sutures are placed in the mid-lateral aspect of the tracheal wall 1 cm below the anticipated level of transection. Distal tracheal division is completed and circumferential dissection of the residual distal trachea is limited to a centimeter to protect the segmental tracheal blood supply. A cuffed, wire-wound endotracheal tube is promptly passed into the distal tracheal segment and attached to sterile connecting tubing, and cross-table ventilation is instituted (see Fig. 8-9C). The diseased segment of trachea is sharply dissected from the esophagus and amputated at the most proximal extent of the lesion. Proximal 2-0 Vicryl traction sutures are then placed.

The patient's neck is then flexed and the anastomosis tested for tension by crossing the traction sutures. If the limits of flexion and safe dissection have been reached and anastomotic tension exists, then one can proceed with release procedures. When the surgeon is satisfied that the anastomosis will not be under tension, interrupted, 4-0 Vicryl anastomotic sutures are placed so that the knots will be on the outside, beginning posteriorly in the midline and proceeding around either side to the front (see Fig. 8-9D). The sutures are placed 5 to 6 mm from the cut edge of the trachea and 4 mm apart. They should encircle a tracheal ring on either side of the anastomosis to help prevent dehiscence. Frequently, the cross-field endotracheal tube must be withdrawn for short periods to allow accurate placement of the more difficult sutures or for suctioning blood from the distal airway. After placing the anterior sutures, the cross-field endotracheal tube is removed from the distal tracheal segment, and the oral endotracheal tube is advanced carefully beyond the anastomosis.

Before tying down the anastomotic sutures, the inflatable airbag beneath the shoulders is deflated, the 2-0 traction sutures are tied, and any last few degrees of neck flexion that may be required are instituted. The anastomotic sutures are then tied from anterior to posterior—the reverse order to that in which they were placed. The integrity of the suture line is tested under saline immersion with the cuff deflated or placed proximal to the anastomosis. The bilateral sternohyoid muscles are mobilized from their surrounding attachments and sutured to the anterior trachea, above and below the anastomosis, to serve as a vascularized tissue buttress. A closed suction drain is left in the pretracheal space.

A chin-to-chest suture is placed to prevent cervical hyperextension. This suture is tied without slack to prevent neck extension for the first 5 to 7 postoperative days. Patients are extubated in the operating room. When postoperative intubation is thought to be necessary, a small endotracheal tube is left in place, and a stitch is placed at least two rings below the anastomosis to mark the site for possible future tracheostomy. This allows limited dissection and accurate placement in a reoperative field. It is best to wait a few days before placing a tracheostomy to allow skin flaps and other tissue layers to seal before exposing them to airway secretions. This also allows postsurgical airway edema to resolve, possibly obviating the need for a tracheostomy.

For tracheal tumors, the approach is slightly modified. Considerable experience is required to judge whether a tumor can be safely resected with sufficient tissue to provide a clear margin and yet allow successful primary reconstruction of the airway. This can be particularly difficult in patients with adenoid cystic carcinoma, because frozen sections may show microscopic tumor at grossly clear resection margins. The plane of tissue dissection in tumor cases must be kept away from the involved portion of trachea to ensure an adequate radial margin. This endangers the recurrent laryngeal nerves more than during resections for benign disease. If one recurrent laryngeal nerve is involved by tumor, the nerve should be sacrificed. Adjacent paratracheal lymph nodes are resected en bloc with the specimen, but, to minimize devascularization of the airway involved in the tracheal anastomosis, extensive lymph node dissection should not be performed. Postoperative radiation therapy is often recommended in cases of bronchogenic or adenoid cystic carcinoma, unless it is contraindicated by performance status or anastomotic complications.[14]

The transthoracic approach, using a posterolateral thoracotomy through the fourth intercostal space, is used for tumors of the lower trachea and carina and for a few inflammatory lesions. An extra-long, single-lumen endotracheal tube with sufficient diameter is used to intubate the left main-stem bronchus for selective ventilation.

Dissection of the thoracic trachea is carried out in a fashion similar to that for more proximal pathology. In cases of malignancy, effort is made to resect surrounding tissues with the tumor. Eventually, the trachea is dissected circumferentially below the tumor, and sometimes above it, although the upper portion of the dissection may be completed after division of the trachea below. Traction sutures are placed in the midlateral tracheal wall distal to the tumor. If the transection is close to the carina, the sutures are placed in the lateral walls of the right and left main bronchi. Again, anesthesia tubing brought across the field is joined to a flexible armored tube placed in the distal trachea or, preferably, the left main bronchus, to allow collapse of the right lung for better exposure while performing the anastomosis. If this results in significant intrapulmonary shunting, the right pulmonary artery may be gently clamped.

Flexion of the neck, even with the patient in the lateral thoracotomy position, delivers the proximal trachea into the thorax. Dissection anterior to the trachea and both main bronchi will provide additional mobility. These are important maneuvers for obtaining a tension-free anastomosis. In the resection of a malignant tracheal tumor, paratracheal and subcarinal lymph nodes that are not in proximity to the mass should not be radically resected for fear of devascularization of the airway. The technique of anastomosis is similar for that used in the upper trachea.

LARYNGOTRACHEAL RESECTION

When an upper tracheal lesion involves the cricoid cartilage, a laryngotracheal resection will be necessary (Fig. 8-10). The operative procedure must be tailored to address the particular anatomic involvement encountered. The recurrent laryngeal nerves are protected by beveling off the cricoid anteriorly and laterally while preserving the posterior cricoid plate.[22,23] The extent of anterior cricoid resection ranges from complete, with a line of transection through the cricothyroid membrane, to none at all, depending on the extent of involvement. Tracheal resection depends on the distal extent of the lesion (Fig. 8-11A,B). The trachea is appropriately tailored so that the proximal trachea approximates well with the cut edge of the larynx (see Fig. 8-11C,D). Vicryl traction sutures are placed in the mid-lateral position both proximally and distally. Interrupted 4-0 Vicryl sutures are used to fashion the anastomosis. The traction sutures are crossed and tied,

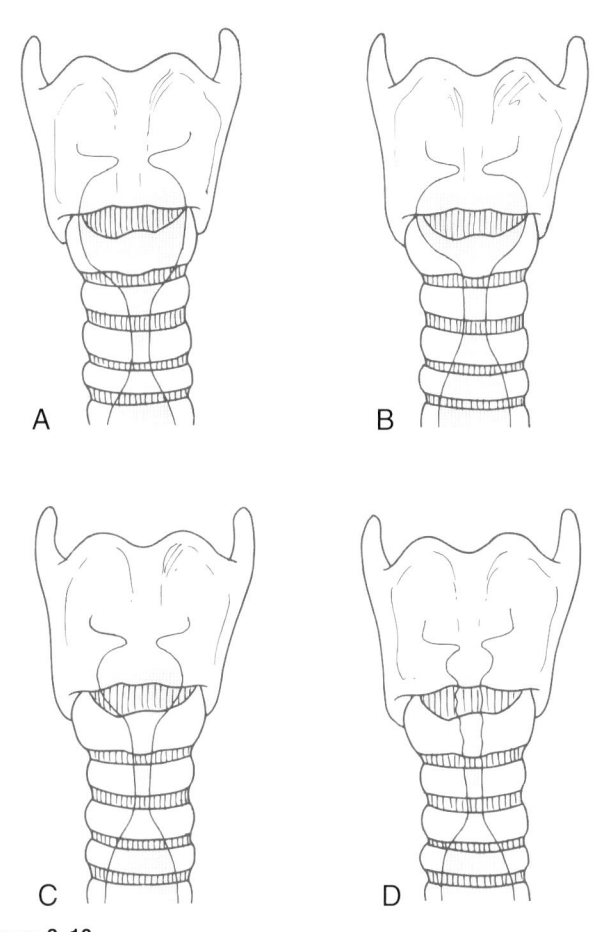

Figure 8-10

Upper airway stenosis. **A,** High tracheal stenosis, easily treated by segmental resection and tracheotracheal anastomosis. **B,** Stenosis that reaches to the lower border of the cricoid cartilage. **C,** Stenosis of the lower subglottic larynx and upper trachea. The extent of the lesion anteriorly is so great that correction requires removal of the anterior portion of the cricoid cartilage. **D,** Stenosis that reaches to the glottis. There is no subglottic space to which an effective anastomosis can be made. *(From Grillo HC. Ann Thorac Surg 1982;**33**:3-18. Reprinted with permission from the Society of Thoracic Surgeons.)*

followed by the individual 4-0 Vicryl anastomotic sutures (see Fig. 8-11E,F).

When the lesion involves the posterior subglottic larynx, a line of mucosal division is performed high on the posterior cricoid plate to excise involved mucosa and submucosa. The posterior cartilage is not resected. Mucosal resection should not extend proximally beyond the superior border of the cricoid plate. A posterior broad-based flap of membranous wall is created and advanced to resurface the posterior cricoid plate (Fig. 8-12). The posterior portion of the anastomosis is made with interrupted 4-0 Vicryl sutures placed only through the full thickness of mucosa and submucosa of the posterior wall of the larynx, and then through the full thickness of the membranous wall of the trachea. They are inverted so that the suture knots lie external to the lumen. Four sutures are placed through the cartilaginous portion of the inferior margin of the cricoid plate and the outer portion of the membranous wall of the trachea below the proximal edge of the flap in order to fix the membranous wall to the inferior edge of the cricoid plate.[22,23]

RELEASE PROCEDURES

Dissection of the pretracheal plane combined with cervical flexion produces sufficient airway mobility to allow tracheal resection and primary reconstruction in most patients. When extensive resections are performed, further mobilization with certain maneuvers may be required to enable a tension-free anastomosis. This has been shown to be necessary in 8.3% of patients undergoing resections for postintubation stenoses and in 15% of patients undergoing resections for tumors.[18] The location of the lesion is an important factor in determining which procedures will be of benefit.

Certain release maneuvers are more effective for achieving additional mobility of the cervical trachea, whereas others are more effective for freeing the intrathoracic trachea. When an upper trachea resection is performed, an additional 1.5 cm of length may be gained by releasing the larynx with a Montgomery suprahyoid release.[24] This is accomplished by dividing the muscles that insert on the superior aspect of the central part of the hyoid bone. The hyoid itself is then divided just medial to its lesser cornua on both sides, and the stylohyoid tendons are divided (Fig. 8-13). Laryngeal release maneuvers may predispose patients to postoperative aspiration, but in time this problem resolves in most patients.

For transthoracic tracheal resections, additional length is best achieved by hilar release.[25] Mobilization of the right hilum should be approached first, along with division of the inferior pulmonary ligament. A U-shaped incision is then made in the pericardium below the inferior pulmonary vein. The pericardium can be incised 360 degrees around the hilum for additional mobility. In this event, the vascular and lymphatic pedicle to the main-stem bronchus is left preserved behind the pericardium. If further mobility is needed, the left hilum may be similarly mobilized (Fig. 8-14). This can be accomplished through a median sternotomy by opening the pericardium, by bilateral thoracotomies, or via an extended clamshell incision. As with most airway surgery, neck flexion is helpful. However, laryngeal release has not been shown to produce meaningful mobility at the level of the carina.[26]

REPAIR OF TRACHEOINNOMINATE AND TRACHEOESOPHAGEAL FISTULAS

Tracheoinnominate fistulas present as either massive airway bleeding or episodic hemoptysis. Significant bleeding from around or through a tracheostomy should be evaluated in the controlled environment of the operating room. The surgeon should be prepared to manage massive airway bleeding before removing the tracheostomy cannula. The patient is then decannulated and a bronchoscopy performed. In the event of massive hemorrhage, control can usually be obtained by finger compression through the stoma, pushing anteriorly against the sternum at the site of bleeding. A small oral endotracheal tube is advanced into the airway beyond the finger and the cuff firmly inflated to ventilate and protect the lungs from aspiration of blood. If the fistula lies beyond reach, hemorrhage may be controlled by placing an inflated endotracheal tube cuff over the bleeding vessel.

Exposure is obtained through a collar incision at the level of the stoma, along with a vertical extension for sternotomy. With finger compression maintaining hemostasis, the vessel is dissected to obtain proximal and distal vascular

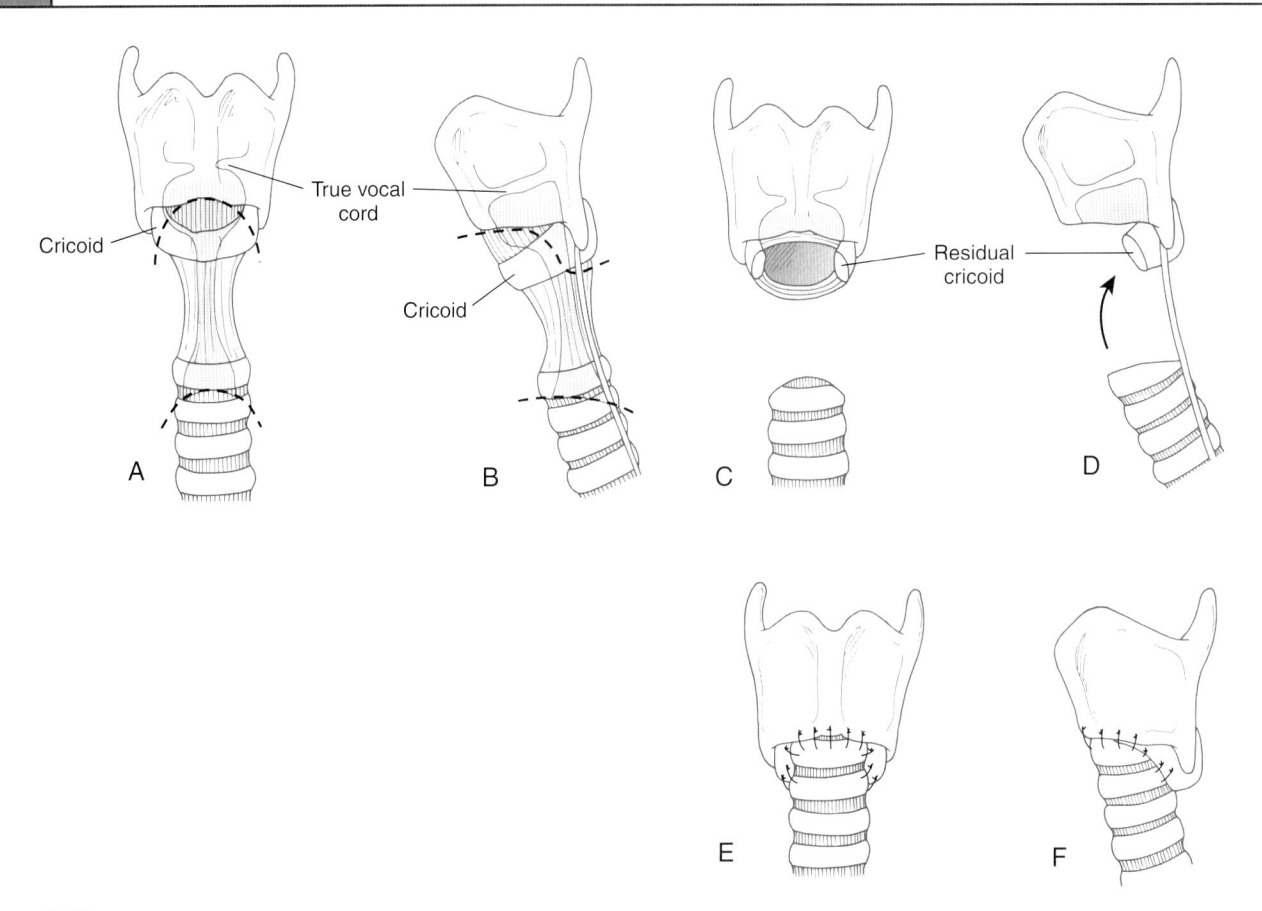

Figure 8–11
Operative repair of anterolateral stenosis of the subglottic larynx and upper trachea. **A,** Anteroposterior view. **B,** Lateral view, showing the extent of disease involvement and the ultimate lines of transection. **C** and **D,** Larynx and trachea after removal of the specimen. Recurrent nerves have been left intact. Mucous membrane of the larynx has been transected sharply at the same level of division as cartilage. Anteroposterior (**E**) and lateral (**F**) views of reconstruction. *(From Grillo HC. Ann Thorac Surg 1982;**33**:3-18. Reprinted with permission from the Society of Thoracic Surgeons.)*

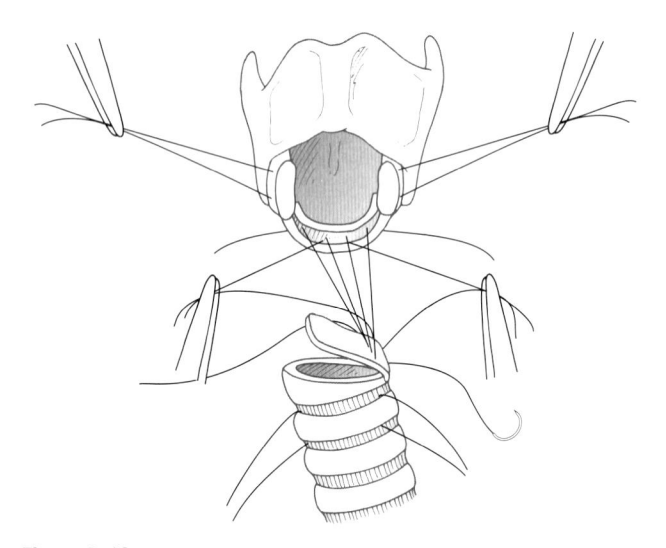

Figure 8–12
Technique of posterior membranous tracheal wall flap with cricoid resurfacing. *(From Grillo HC. Ann Thorac Surg 1982;**33**:3-18. Reprinted with permission from the Society of Thoracic Surgeons.)*

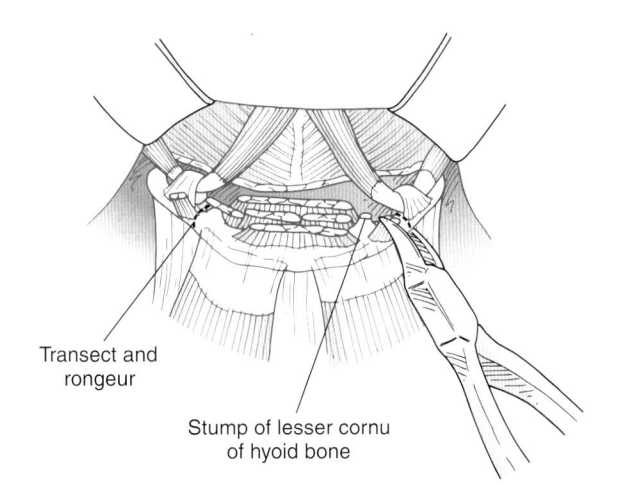

Figure 8–13
The *dotted lines* indicate the point where the hyoid bone is divided, separating its body from the greater horn on each side. *(From Montgomery WW. Arch Otolaryngol 1974;**99**:255-60. Reprinted with permission from the American Medical Association.)*

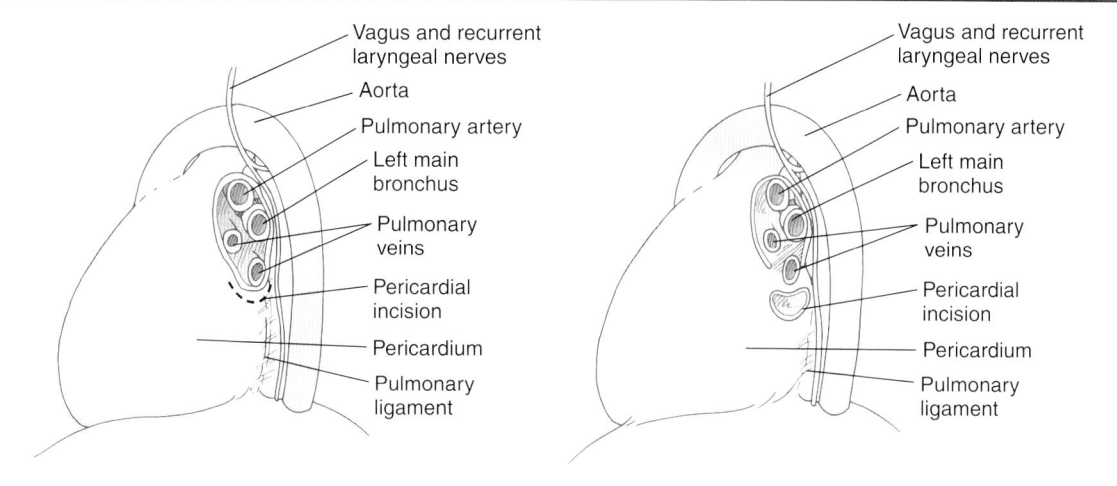

Figure 8–14
The left-sided intrapericardial hilar release technique demonstrates the U-shaped pericardial incision allowing 1 to 2 cm of upward hilar mobility to facilitate the creation of a tension-free anastomosis. *(From Newton JR, Grillo HC, Mathisen DJ. Ann Thorac Surg 1991;**52**:1272-80. Reprinted with permission from the Society of Thoracic Surgeons.)*

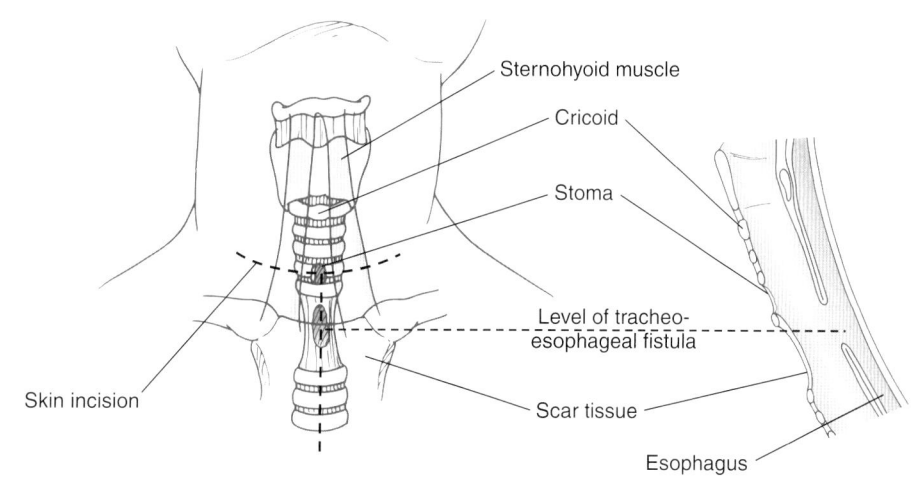

Figure 8–15
Exposure for most tracheoesophageal fistulas is through a low collar incision. Occasionally, a partial upper sternotomy is required for more distal exposure of the trachea. *(From Mathisen DJ, Grillo HC, Wain JC, Hilgenberg AD. Ann Thorac Surg 1991;**52**:759-65. Reprinted with permission from the Society of Thoracic Surgeons.)*

control. The involved segment of artery is resected, and the proximal and distal ends are oversewn. The stumps are covered with surrounding, well-vascularized tissue. Innominate division usually does not result in neurologic sequelae. Depending on the degree of airway destruction, a concomitant tracheal resection may be necessary. A new tracheal stoma is created at a higher level, and a tracheostomy tube long enough to pass beyond the previous stoma is used. Local strap muscle flaps are sutured over the original stoma to hasten its healing.

Acquired, nonmalignant tracheoesophageal fistulas often appear while the patient remains ventilatory dependent. The fistula develops at the level of the cuff and is usually associated with a circumferential tracheal injury.[27] Temporizing measures are taken to allow weaning from the ventilator before repair is undertaken. A tracheostomy tube should be positioned with the occluding cuff located below the fistula to prevent contamination of the tracheobronchial tree. Gastrostomy and jejunostomy tubes should be placed for drainage and feeding, respectively. The esophagus is kept free of tubes, and cuff overinflation is assiduously avoided.

A collar incision is performed that encompasses the stoma (Fig. 8-15). As described previously, the trachea is dissected and divided distal to the fistula. As the posterior wall of the trachea is dissected from inferior to superior, the fistulous connection is isolated circumferentially and detached from the esophagus with a small rim of normal esophageal tissue (Fig. 8-16). After removal of the specimen, the esophagus is closed longitudinally with two layers of 4-0 silk (Fig. 8-17). A strap muscle is used to buttress the esophageal closure and as a flap of vascularized tissue interposed between the esophageal and tracheal suture lines (Fig. 8-18). An end-to-end tracheal anastomosis is then performed. It may be necessary to partially repair the defect in the posterior membranous wall with a vertical suture line to limit the amount of tracheal resection needed to treat a large fistula. Occasionally, there may be only insignificant damage to the trachea; a simple esophageal and tracheal repair with a muscle buttress would then be performed.

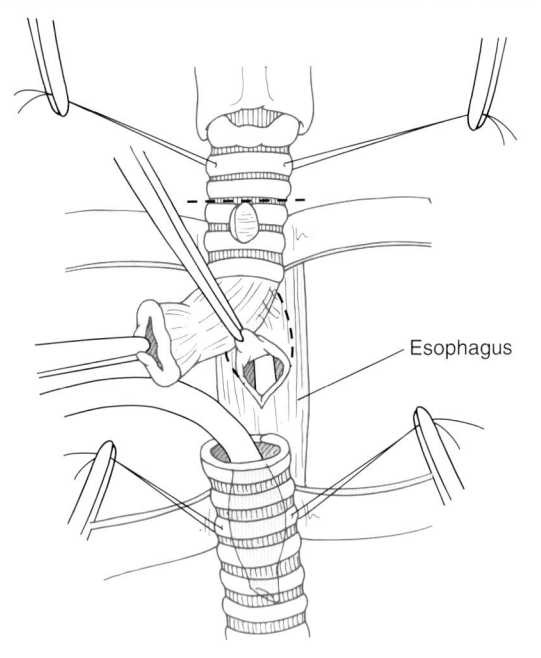

Figure 8–16
Circumferential dissection above and below the fistula is performed in close proximity to the trachea to avoid injury to the recurrent laryngeal nerve. Division of the damaged trachea gives excellent exposure of the esophageal defect. *(From Mathisen DJ, Grillo HC, Wain JC, Hilgenberg AD. Ann Thorac Surg 1991;**52**:759-65. Reprinted with permission from the Society of Thoracic Surgeons.)*

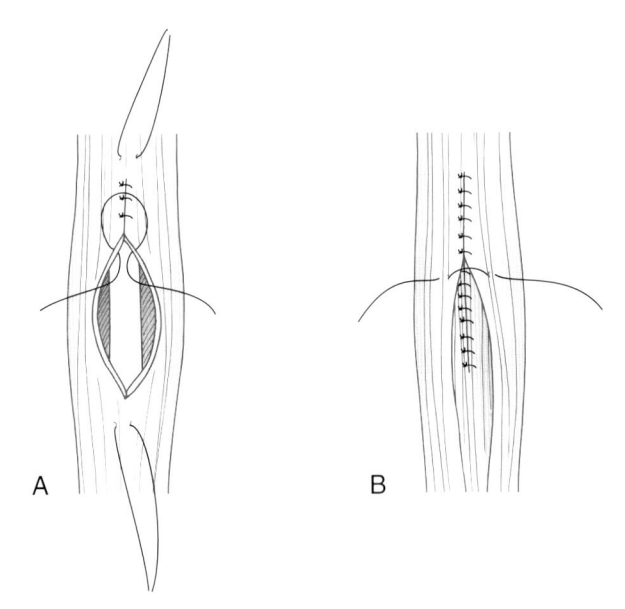

Figure 8–17
The esophageal defect is closed in layers. **A,** The first layer closes the esophageal mucosa. **B,** The esophageal muscle is closed over the first layer. *(From Mathisen DJ, Grillo HC, Wain JC, Hilgenberg AD. Ann Thorac Surg 1991;**52**:759-65. Reprinted with permission from the Society of Thoracic Surgeons.)*

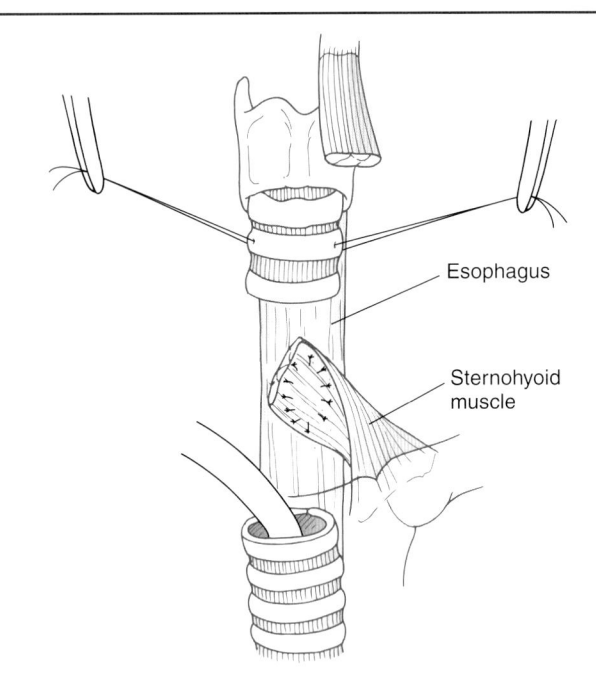

Figure 8–18
A local strap muscle is used to buttress the esophageal closure and separate it from the suture line. *(From Mathisen DJ, Grillo HC, Wain JC, Hilgenberg AD. Ann Thorac Surg 1991;**52**:759-65. Reprinted with permission from the Society of Thoracic Surgeons.)*

PERIOPERATIVE MANAGEMENT

The goals of both intraoperative and postoperative care are the promotion of anastomotic healing and the maintenance of good pulmonary toilet. Ideally, patients are extubated in the operating room. The need for postoperative ventilation is a relative contraindication to tracheal resection. Patients with marginal lung function need careful management during the operation to help avoid the need for postoperative mechanical ventilation. During the procedure, secretions and blood are kept from contaminating the distal tracheobronchial tree, and volume overload is avoided. Rarely, an especially high laryngotracheal resection will cause enough laryngeal edema to necessitate one or two doses of steroids to avoid impending reintubation and tracheostomy. Heliox, with its low viscosity, is sometimes useful in these circumstances, as it can occasionally assist in gaining enough time for the other maneuvers to take effect. The patient is cautioned against unnecessary speech during this period, as it can contribute to the laryngeal edema. Postoperatively, patients are supplied with humidity by face mask to facilitate clearance of secretions. Most patients are able to clear their airway by coughing. Frequently, therapeutic flexible bronchoscopy is performed to suction secretions under direct vision. Cervical flexion is maintained with the chin-to-chest suture for 5 to 7 days, after which the patient is advised not to extend the neck for another week. Before removing the chin-to-chest suture, we routinely examine the anastomosis with a flexible bronchoscope to ensure normal healing. Oral alimentation is begun cautiously in the first few postoperative days.

RESULTS

Postintubation tracheal injuries remain the most common indication for tracheal resection and reconstruction, despite definition of the etiology of these lesions and development of techniques to avoid them. We reported 503 patients who underwent tracheal resection and reconstruction for postintubation lesions.[28] The balloon cuff of an endotracheal or tracheostomy tube accounted for 251 lesions, 178 lesions were at the site of a tracheostomy, and 38 patients had evidence of both lesions. In 36 patients, the exact site was uncertain, often because of prior attempts at treatment including multiple tracheostomies. Of the 503 patients, 441 had lesions that were isolated to the trachea, and 62 had concomitant involvement of the subglottic larynx.

Many patients had undergone prior attempts at surgical treatment before referral. These included resection ($n = 53$), tracheal operations such as wedge resection, splinting, or fissure ($n = 31$), and laryngeal procedures such as stenting, grafting, or fissure ($n = 20$). Sixty had had T-tubes placed, and at least 45 had suffered laser treatment. Eight patients had prior repairs of tracheoesophageal fistulas, three of which had failed.

The initial procedure was carried out through a cervical incision in 350 patients. In 145 patients, a partial upper sternal division through the sternal angle was used, and two more patients required the addition of right anterior thoracotomy to this approach. Six patients underwent repair via a high posterolateral thoracotomy. The amount of trachea resected ranged from 1.0 to 7.5 cm and was most commonly 2 to 4 cm.

Of the 503 initial patients, 324 underwent a trachea-to-trachea anastomosis, and in 117, the reconstruction involved partial resection of the cricoid cartilage with laryngotracheal anastomosis. In the total series of 503 patients, 9.7% underwent laryngeal release procedures. However, only 8% of the 450 patients who had not undergone previous tracheal resection and reconstruction required a laryngeal release, in comparison with 24.5% of the 53 who had prior resection and reconstruction. Many in the former group represent our earlier experience in tracheal surgery. Only one patient required intrapericardial hilar release.

The results have been classified as good, satisfactory, failure, and death. The result is described as good if the patient is functionally able to perform usual activities and if postoperative roentgenograms or bronchoscopic examinations show an anatomically good airway. Patients are placed in the satisfactory category if they can perform normal activities but are stressed on exercise. This is also applied, in the absence of symptoms, to those with abnormalities involving the vocal cords or those with significant airway narrowing evident on either endoscopic or roentgenologic examination. Failure indicated the need for a permanent tracheostomy or T-tube. The average length of follow-up was 3 years. The results were categorized as good in 440 patients, satisfactory in 31 patients, and there were 20 failures and 12 deaths. Failure was treated with tracheostomy ($n = 11$), T-tube ($n = 7$), or dilations ($n = 2$).

In experienced hands, laryngotracheal resection and reconstruction is associated with excellent results and minor complications. The results of single-staged laryngotracheal resection for idiopathic laryngotracheal stenosis were initially reported by Grillo and colleagues[29] and have now been updated to include a series of 73 patients.[30] The majority of these were women (71/73), with a mean age of 46 (range, 13 to 74). Twenty-eight (38%) had undergone a previous laser, dilation, laryngeal, or tracheostomy procedure. After laryngotracheal resection, the majority of patients (67/73) were extubated in the operating room, and 7 required temporary tracheostomies, with only 1 in the last 30 cases. All were successfully decannulated. There was no perioperative mortality. The principal morbidity was alteration in voice quality, which improved with time. Sixty-seven (91%) required no further intervention for idiopathic laryngotracheal stenosis.

Six patients required at least one bronchoscopy for granulation tissue or dilation (or both), and progression of disease was observed in only one patient.

The results from the repair of tracheoesophageal fistulas were reported in a series of 38 patients in whom 41 operations were performed.[27] Simple division and closure of the fistula were done in nine patients. Tracheal resection and reconstruction were combined with esophageal repair in the remainder. The esophageal defect was closed in two layers, and a viable strap muscle was interposed between the airway and esophageal suture lines in all cases. There were four deaths (10.9%); three of these occurred after attempted transthoracic repair of distal tracheoesophageal fistulas. Three patients developed recurrent fistulas and one patient suffered a delayed tracheal stenosis. All were successfully treated with reoperation. Of the 34 survivors, 33 can swallow normally and 32 breathe without the need for a tracheal appliance.

For the oncologic results of primary tumors of the trachea, 208 patients were evaluated in a retrospective multicenter study.[31] Histologic types included 94 squamous cell carcinomas, 4 adenocarcinomas, 65 adenoid cystic carcinomas, and 45 miscellaneous tumors. The procedures performed consisted of 19 laryngotracheal, 165 tracheal, and 24 carinal resections. Operative mortality was 10.5%. As expected, long-term survival was significantly better for ACC than for SCC, with 73% versus 47% at 5 years, and 57% versus 36% at 10 years, respectively.

Gaissert and coworkers[32] published the 40-year cumulative Massachusetts General Hospital experience of treating primary adenoid cystic and squamous cell carcinomas of the trachea. During this time period, 270 patients were evaluated, with histologic distribution equally distributed between ACCs and SCCs. Resection was performed in 191 patients (71%), with an operative mortality of 7.3% (14/191). Importantly, both rates of resection and hospital mortality have improved each decade. As this center's experience has grown, operative mortality has decreased from 21% in the 1960s to 3% in the decade preceding the report.

Resection was not performed in 79 patients, 34 with ACC (25%) and 45 patients with SCC (33%). Contraindications to resection included tumor length (67%) and locoregional extent (24%) in the vast majority of cases, with distant metastases only rarely present (7%). The determination of unresectability was made during operative exploration in 17 of 208 patients (8%). ACC lesions tended to be longer and to be associated with more significant locoregional extension. This explains the more frequent observation of ACC resections having positive microscopic tracheal and radial margins (59%) when compared with SCC (18%).

The overall survival for all patients with primary tracheal carcinoma was 84% at 1 year, 45% at 5 years, and 25% at 10 years. Mean survival was 38 months for resected SCC, 8.8 months for unresectable SCC, 69 months for resected ACC, and 41 months for unresectable ACC. Notably, survival in patients with ACC after incomplete resection was still 14.5% at 15 years. Multivariate analysis identified ACC and complete resection to be associated with 5-year survival, and ACC, complete resection, and age to be associated with 10-year survival. Tumor length, lymph node status, or type of resection did not influence long-term survival.

The presence of tumor at the resection margins of ACC, even by frozen section during operation, has particular importance in airway reconstruction. The surgeon must often compromise complete resection for safety, and the data just cited indicate that a small, though not statistically significant, survival benefit exists in these patients. All these patients now receive postoperative irradiation. Suture line recurrence thus far has been rare, and late recurrence has been related to distant disease. In contrast, irradiation of unresected tumor is all but uniformly characterized by local recurrence in 3 to 5 years despite early good response.

Secondary cancers arising in the thyroid and invading the trachea have also been resected with good results. Of 27 patients undergoing resection and reconstruction of the trachea for thyroid cancer invading the airway, including patients with both simple and complex laryngotracheal reconstructions, 2 died in the postoperative period, 1 had a short segment of tracheal necrosis requiring reoperation, and all others were provided with an adequate airway by their initial operation. Only two patients experienced an airway recurrence.[16] This series was recently updated to include 82 patients treated at the Massachusetts General Hospital.[33] There were no additional operative mortalities in this expanded series. With mean follow-up at greater than 6 years, mean survival was 9.4 years and 10-year survival was 40%.

COMPLICATIONS

Complications after tracheal surgery are similar regardless of the problem for which resection and reconstruction is performed. In 2004, Wright and colleagues[34] presented the most complete analysis of anastomotic complications after tracheal resection. This review of 901 patients identifies relevant risk factors for the development of these problems and further describes their management. Anastomotic complications include granulations at the suture line, stenosis, and tracheal separation.

A significant reduction in suture granuloma formation has been seen since the conversion to absorbable suture material used for the anastomosis. In fact, the use of absorbable Vicryl sutures since 1978 has all but eliminated suture-related granulations. These can be successfully managed with bronchoscopic suture removal and local steroid injection. More extensive processes may require reoperation for resection or placement of a T-tube or tracheostomy.

Several predictors of anastomotic complications were demonstrated: reoperation, diabetes, lengthy (>4 cm) resections, laryngotracheal resections, age less than 17 years, and need for a tracheostomy before operation. The frequency of anastomotic complications was higher in patients undergoing operations for tracheoesophageal fistula than in those with tracheal tumors, postintubation stenoses, and idiopathic laryngotracheal stenoses. Of note, corticosteroid use was not associated with an increased complication rate, probably because of the management strategy used for this group, which is to defer tracheal operations in the presence of high-dose steroids until they can be effectively tapered.

Overall, 81 patients experienced anastomotic complications in this series. Thirty-seven patients had separation of the suture line, another 37 patients developed anastomotic stenosis, and 7 had airway obstruction from granulation tissue formation. Complications were treated with multiple dilations ($n = 2$), temporary tracheostomy ($n = 7$) or tracheal T-tube ($n = 16$), permanent tracheostomy ($n = 14$) or T-tube ($n = 20$), and reoperation ($n = 16$). The mortality of patients who had anastomotic complications was 7.4% (6/81), compared with 0.06% (5/820) in those without anastomotic complications. In this series, no patient has died since 1988. This success can be attributed to the routine use of postoperative bronchoscopy and the early recognition and subsequent definitive management of anastomotic complications.

SUMMARY

Some of the most challenging problems facing thoracic surgeons include benign strictures arising from postintubation stenosis or idiopathic laryngotracheal stenosis, fistulas from the trachea to the esophagus or innominate artery, and primary or secondary tumors of the trachea. Bronchoscopic evaluation is essential to ascertain the diagnosis and in preoperative planning. If critical airway stenosis is suspected, flexible bronchoscopy should be performed only in an operative suite where a rigid bronchoscope is available in case the airway needs to be reestablished. An anesthesia team familiar with the techniques of cross-table ventilation and capable of an interactive team approach is essential.

All patients with tracheal lesions, from benign strictures to malignant tumors, deserve serious consideration for definitive resection. Nonsurgical methods such as dilation, ablation, or stenting are palliative and should be used only as temporizing maneuvers or in poor surgical candidates. Deciding whether a lesion is resectable requires mature surgical judgment. Postoperative radiation should be given to all patients with resected squamous cell or adenoid cystic carcinomas. Patients with thyroid cancer secondarily invading the trachea should be considered for tracheal resection, even with advanced disease, to avoid fatal loss of the airway. With an experienced team, most patients can be successfully treated with a single-stage tracheal resection with low morbidity and mortality and excellent long-term results.

REFERENCES

1. Shaha A, DiMaio T, Money S, Krespi Y, Jaffee BM. Prosthetic reconstruction of the trachea. *Am J Surg* 1988;**156**:306-9.
2. Kim J, Suh SW, Shin JY, Chri YS, Kim H. Replacement of a tracheal defect with a tissue-engineered prosthesis: early results from animal experiments. *J Thorac Cardiovasc Surg* 2004;**128**:124-9.
3. Grillo HC, Dignan EF, Miura T. Extensive resection and reconstruction of mediastinal trachea without prosthesis or graft: An anatomical study in man. *J Thorac Cardiovasc Surg* 1964;**48**:741.
4. Dedo HH, Fishman NH. Laryngeal release and sleeve resection for tracheal stenosis. *Ann Otol Rhinol Laryngol* 1969;**78**:285.
5. Salassa JR, Pearson BW, Payne WS. Gross and microscopical blood supply of the trachea. *Ann Thorac Surg* 1977;**24**:100-107.
6. Gaissert HA, Lofgren RH, Grillo HC. Upper airway compromise after inhalation injury: Complex strictures of larynx and trachea and their management. *Ann Surg* 1993;**218**:672-678.
7. Cooper JD, Grillo HC. The evolution of tracheal injury due to ventilatory assistance through cuffed tubes: A pathologic study. *Ann Surg* 1969;**169**:334-348.
8. Cooper JD, Grillo HC. Experimental production and prevention of injury due to cuffed tracheal tubes. *Surg Gynecol Obstet* 1969;**129**:1235-1241.
9. Whited R-E: A prospective study of laryngotracheal sequelae in long-term intubation. *Laryngoscope* 1984;**94**:367-377.
10. Grillo HC, Mark EJ, Mathisen DJ, Wain JC. Idiopathic laryngotracheal stenosis: The entity and its management. *Ann Thorac Surg* 1993;**56**:80-7.
11. Ashiku SK, Kuzucu A, Grillo HC, Wright CD, Wain JC, Lo B, Mathisen DJ. Idiopathic laryngotracheal stenosis: effective definitive treatment with laryngotracheal resection. *J Thor Cardiovasc Surg* 2004;**127**:99-107.
12. Grillo HC. Surgery of the trachea. In: Keen G, editor. *Operative surgery and management*. 2nd ed. Bristol: Wright; 1987, p. 776-84.

13. Rainer WG, Newby JP, Kelbe DC. Long-term results of tracheal support surgery for emphysema. *Dis Chest* 1968;**53**:765-74.
14. Grillo HC, Mathisen DJ. Primary tracheal tumors: Treatment and results. *Ann Thorac Surg* 1990;**49**:69-77.
15. Gaissert HG, Grillo HC, Shadmehr HB, Wright CD, Gokhale M, Wain JC, Mathisen DJ. Long-term survival after resection of adenoid cystic and squamous cell carcinoma of the trachea and carina. *Ann Thorac Surg* 2004;**78**:1889-96.
16. Grillo HC, Suen HC, Mathisen DJ, Wain JC. Resectional management of thyroid carcinoma invading the airway. *Ann Thorac Surg* 1992;**54**:3-9.
17. Weber AL, Grillo HC. Tracheal tumors: radiological, clinical and pathological evaluation. *Adv Otorhinolaryngol* 1978;**24**:170.
18. Mathisen DJ. Surgery of the trachea. *Curr Probl Surg* 1998;**35**:455-542.
19. Mathisen DJ, Grillo HC. Endoscopic relief of malignant airway obstruction. *Ann Thorac Surg* 1989;**48**:469-475.
20. Wilson RS. Tracheal resection. In Marshall BE, Longnecker DE, Fairley HB, editors: *Anesthesia for thoracic procedures*. Boston: Blackwell Scientific; 1988, p. 415-32.
21. Rutter MJ, Cotton RT, Azizkhan RG, Manning PB. Slide tracheoplasty for the management of complete tracheal rings. *J Pediatr Surg* 2003;**38**:928-34.
22. Grillo HC. Primary reconstruction of airway after resection of subglottic laryngeal and upper tracheal stenosis. *Ann Thorac Surg* 1982;**33**:3-18.
23. Grillo HC, Mathisen DJ, Wain JC. Laryngotracheal resection and reconstruction for subglottic stenosis. *Ann Thorac Surg* 1992;**53**:54-63.
24. Montgomery WW. Suprahyoid release for tracheal anastomosis. *Arch Otolaryngol* 1974;**99**:255-260.
25. Newton JR, Grillo HC, Mathisen DJ. Main bronchial sleeve resection with pulmonary conservation. *Ann Thorac Surg* 1991;**52**:1272-80.
26. Grillo HC. Carinal neoplasia. In: Grillo HC, Austen WG, Wilkins EW, et al, editors. *Current therapy in cardiothoracic surgery*. Ontario, BC: Decker; 1989, p. 134.
27. Mathisen DJ, Grillo HC, Wain JC, Hilgenberg AD. Management of acquired nonmalignant tracheoesophageal fistula. *Ann Thorac Surg* 1991;**52**:759-765.
28. Grillo HC, Donahue DM, Mathisen DJ. Postintubation tracheal stenosis: Treatment and results. *J Thorac Cardiovasc Surg* 1995;**109**:486-493.
29. Grillo HC, Mark EJ, Mathisen DJ, Wain JC. Idiopathic laryngotracheal stenosis and its management. *Ann Thorac Surg* 1993;**56**:80-87.
30. Ashiku SK, Kuzucu A, Grillo HC, Wright CD, Wain JC, Lo B, Mathisen DJ. Idiopathic laryngotracheal stenosis: effective definitive treatment with laryngotracheal resection. *J Thorac Cardiovasc Surg* 2004;**127**:99-107.
31. Regnard JF, Fourquier P, Levasseur P, et al: Results and prognostic factors in resections of primary tracheal tumors: A multicenter retrospective study. *J Thorac Cardiovasc Surg* 1996;**111**:808-814.
32. Gaissert HA, Grillo HC, Shadmehr MB, Wright CD, Gokhale M, Wain JC, Mathisen DJ. Long-term survival after resection of adenoid cystic and squamous cell carcinoma of the trachea and carina. *Ann Thorac Surg* 2004;**78**:1889-96.
33. Gaissert HG, Honings J, Grillo HC, Donahue DM, Wain JC, Wright CD, Mathisen DJ. Segmental laryngotracheal and tracheal resection for invasive thyroid carcinoma. *Ann Thorac Surg* 2007;**83**:1952-9.
34. Wright CD, Grillo HC, Wain JC, Wong DR, Donahue DM, Gaissert HA, Mathisen DJ. Anastomotic complications after tracheal resection: prognostic factors and management. *J Thorac Cardiovasc Surg* 2004;**128**:731-9.

E. Benign Lung Disease

CHAPTER 9

Congenital Lung Diseases

Kemp H. Kernstine, Timothy L. Van Natta, Harold M. Burkhart, and Daniel T. DeArmond

History
Embryology
Tracheal Abnormalities
 Tracheal Agenesis and Atresia
 Congenital Tracheal Stenosis
 Tracheomalacia
Bronchial Branching Abnormalities
 Bronchial Atresia
 Congenital Bronchiectasis
 Tracheobronchomegaly (Mounier-Kuhn Syndrome)
 Laryngotracheoesophageal Cleft
 Tracheobronchial-Esophageal Fistula

Bronchobiliary Fistula
Bronchopulmonary Foregut Malformations
 Sequestrations
 Azygos Lobe
 Horseshoe Lung
 Bronchogenic Cysts
Lung Bud Anomalies
 Pulmonary Agenesis, Aplasia, and Hypoplasia
 Congenital Lobar Emphysema
 Congenital Parenchymal Cysts
 Congenital Cystic Adenomatoid Malformation
 Infantile Pulmonary Emphysema
 Polyalveolar Lobe

Pulmonary Lymphangiectasia
Vascular Abnormalities
 Unilateral Absence of a Main Pulmonary Artery
 Idiopathic, Hyperlucent Lung Syndrome (Swyer-James or Macleod's Syndrome)
 Pulmonary Artery Sling
 Isolated Pulmonary Artery Aneurysm
 Pulmonary Varix
 Pulmonary Arteriovenous Malformations
Conclusion

There are a number of congenital abnormalities involving the pulmonary system. A number of these result in arrested development and stillbirth. Some infants survive delivery only to die shortly thereafter. Neonates with severe anomalies typically display dyspnea and cyanosis at birth. Older children with less critical anomalies may have feeding problems, respiratory infections, developmental delays, or activity limitations. For neonates who are in respiratory distress, speed of diagnosis and early treatment are critical. Intubation may be life-saving. Examination of the naso-oropharynx, neck, and chest along with an emergent radiograph allows rapid diagnosis in most cases. Quality computed tomography (CT) may be necessary to delineate the anomaly. Other important adjuncts that may enhance diagnostic speed and accuracy are echocardiography, magnetic resonance imaging (MRI), and endoscopy.

During the past decade, improvements in prenatal diagnosis[1] have allowed intrauterine repair of some defects.[2] With non–life-sustaining defects such as anencephaly and renal agenesis, parents may opt for pregnancy termination. For potentially correctable lesions, the pregnant mother can be transferred to a tertiary medical center. Advanced supportive and surgical techniques have led to improved survival in these infants.

HISTORY

The first report of a congenital lung defect was by Fontanus in 1639,[3] describing an infant with a lung cyst. In 1777, Huber[4] described an infant with an intralobar sequestration, with blood supply from the thoracic aorta. In the mid-1800s, an extralobar (Rokitansky's lobe) sequestration was reported. The neonatal prevalence of lung infections in the 1900s was so high that it was difficult to formulate concepts of congenital lung disease, and the technology was not sufficiently advanced to correct such defects. In 1917, Gladstone and Cockayne theorized how sequestrations occurred, and in 1925, Koontz reviewed congenital pulmonary cystic diseases. The first surgical correction of a congenital lung anomaly was performed by Rienhoff[5] in 1933, that being local lung cyst excision in a 3-year-old boy.[6] Gross and Lewis[7] performed the first pediatric lobectomy in a child with congenital lobar emphysema. Cystic disease in the right upper and right middle lobes was resected by lobectomy in 1943.[8] In 1946, Gross[9] performed a pneumonectomy in a 3-year-old with cystic lung disease. Potts performed the first neonatal lobectomy in 1949. Lewis later reported the death of a child on whom a lobectomy was being performed for intralobar sequestration, citing exsanguination after lost control of the systemic feeding artery. With development of advanced supportive, anesthetic, vascular, and bypass techniques, the mortality rate for children at high risk for congenital lesions has significantly improved.

EMBRYOLOGY

Lung development occurs both prenatally and postnatally and continues into adulthood. Intrauterine pulmonary development is divided into four phases: embryonic, weeks 1 to 5; pseudoglandular, weeks 5 to 16; canalicular, weeks 16 to 26; and terminal sac, weeks 26 to birth.[10-12]

During the embryonic phase, the foregut begins to develop from the embryonic endoderm beginning on day 9, and the median pharyngeal groove develops from the foregut on day 22. At approximately 4 weeks of gestational age, the respiratory diverticulum, or lung bud, emerges as a 3-mm outpouching from the ventral wall of the embryonic foregut. The respiratory diverticulum at this stage is surrounded by splanchnic mesenchyme that later gives rise to the visceral pleura. Concurrently, the lateral mesoderm grows to form the tracheoesophageal septum, effectively separating the tissues that will become the lung from those that will become the esophagus. The lung bud initially forms the trachea, followed by two bronchial buds that enlarge to form the right and left main bronchi by the start of the fifth week. The individual five lobes become evident during the next few weeks.

In the pseudoglandular stage (weeks 5 to 16), the bronchial tree develops, including the cuboidal and columnar epithelial layers and cartilaginous rings. Repetitive branching of the bronchial tree during this stage gives rise to all the conducting airways. The pulmonary vasculature develops in tandem with the airways; however, the airways and pulmonary arterial branches remain separated by mesenchyme. By the 16th week, the bronchial tree and the pulmonary arteries are fully formed, and the common pulmonary vein drains into the sinoatrial region of the heart.

In the canalicular phase (weeks 16 to 26), respiratory bronchioles divide to form alveolar ducts, and the mesenchymal separation of the airways from pulmonary arterial branches begins to recede, allowing the first appearance of the air-blood barrier. By the 25th week, the pulmonary venous drainage has completely developed.

The terminal sac period (weeks 26 to 40) is marked by continued extension of the air-blood barrier. The primitive alveoli proliferate and become intimately involved with the surrounding capillaries as the mesenchyme separating them thins out. Terminal sac formation from the terminal lung buds occurs in a coordinated interaction between promoter factors, such as fibroblast growth factor 10, and inhibitory factors, such as Sonic hedgehog and transforming growth factor β1.[13,14] Mechanical fluid pressure on the terminal lung bud also appears to play a critical role.[11,15,16] The adult form of alveoli has developed by the 30th to the 36th week, and the airways are nearly fully developed before term. Type II pneumocytes produce surfactant in preparation for delivery.

Lung development continues postnatally with alveolar multiplication that results from progressive septation within the terminal sacs. Septation is driven by transcription factors, growth factors, and extracellular matrix molecules and is closely tied to sprouting angiogenesis (under the influence of vascular endothelial growth factor) followed by the splitting and remodeling of alveolar capillaries. Immediately after birth, alveoli are fairly thick walled and number about 20 million, less than 10% of their eventual number. Acinar development continues to the eighth year of life, but the rate of development diminishes after the second to fourth years. By the end of the eighth year, there are approximately 300 million acini, and after the tenth year of life, alveoli enlarge rather than increase in number. The lung-environmental interface increases from 3 to 4 m^2 at birth to 75 m^2 in adults. From birth to the age of 5 years, airway diameter increases; after the age of 5 years, the proximal airway grows at a faster rate than the more distal airways. The trachea is initially funnel-like but becomes more cylindrical by the age of 4 years. Pulmonary vessel length and diameter rapidly increase until 18 months of age.

Normal airway and vascular development depends on a variety of factors. These include cell-to-cell interactions, local and systemic hormones and growth factors, central and peripheral neural influences, and chest wall effects. The last involve contact influences of the bony and muscular structures. Alterations in normal development may result from defects in any of these factors. Viral infection, hypoxia, starvation, and teratogens also may disrupt normal lung development. In utero airway obstruction may produce a variety of lesions.[17] Eighty-four percent of these patients have additional nonpulmonary anomalies.[18]

Patients with tracheal agenesis may present in utero with maternal polyhydramnios and premature birth. This defect is apparent immediately at birth with respiratory distress, cyanosis, and lack of an audible cry. These infants may be very difficult to ventilate because an endotracheal tube cannot be placed below the level of the vocal cords. Unless there is an esophageal communication allowing ventilation with esophageal intubation, the abnormality is uniformly fatal.

Lung resection in neonates and children is fairly well tolerated. Anatomy is easily defined because there is less mediastinal and hilar fat, adenopathy, and scarring from chronic disease compared with adults. Outcomes after pediatric lung resection are good. Children younger than 5 years develop new alveoli after resection. In those older than 5 to 10 years, the alveoli enlarge, although they no longer increase in number. In an infant pneumonectomy model, lung function returns to normal within 9 to 12 months.[19] Emphysematous changes do occur, as in adults. After lung resection in children in whom the remaining lung is normal, the child appears to grow, develop, and perform normally with maximal exercise.[20,21] The diffusion capacity for carbon monoxide is reduced, and pulmonary artery pressure increases with exercise, but pulmonary vascular resistance is normal after resection.[22]

TRACHEAL ABNORMALITIES

Tracheal Agenesis and Atresia

Payne[23] first described congenital absence of the trachea in 1900. There have been fewer than 100 cases reported.[24] It represents a partial or complete absence of the trachea below the level of the normal larynx. This abnormality is incompatible with life if there is no connection of trachea or bronchi to the esophagus.[25] Floyd and others[26,27] classified three distinct types of tracheal agenesis (Fig. 9-1). In type I, the trachea originates from the esophagus, and the distal trachea, including the carina, is fairly normal; it represents 10% to 13% of the total number of tracheal agenesis cases. In type II, the trachea and carina are fused to the esophagus, and there is no residual trachea; this represents 59% to 62% of the total. In type III, the left and right main-stem bronchi originate from the esophagus, and there is no carina; this represents 22% to 31% of the total. Male incidence predominates in a 2:1 ratio. In 90% of the cases, there are other congenital lesions.[28] Tracheal agenesis may be associated with VACTERL (vertebral, anal, cardiac, tracheal, esophageal, renal, and limb patterns of congenital anomalies)[29] or with complex congenital heart defects as well as with upper extremity defects and duodenal atresia (referred to as TACRD).[30] It is believed that tracheal agenesis is the result of developmental failure of the laryngeal tracheal bud at the third to sixth week of development. The laryngeal tracheal groove fails to develop normally.

Neonates present with severe respiratory distress and the inability to cry. Survival is unlikely, although there are

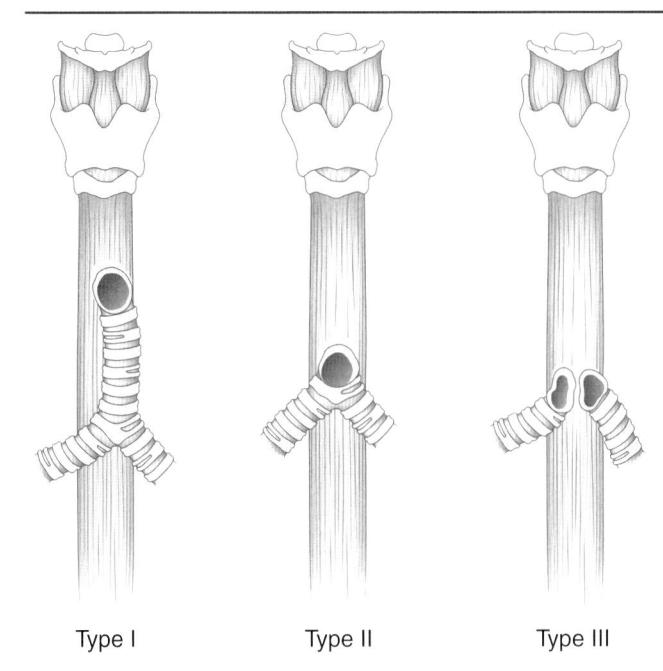

Type I   Type II   Type III

Figure 9–1
Tracheal agenesis classification. There are three types of tracheal agenesis: type I, the trachea originates from the esophagus rather than from the larynx; type II, no trachea is present and the carina originates from the esophagus; and type III, each main-stem bronchus originates from the esophagus. (Modified from Haben CM, Rappaport JM Clarke KD. Tracheal agenesis. J Am Coll Surg 2002;**194**:217-22.)

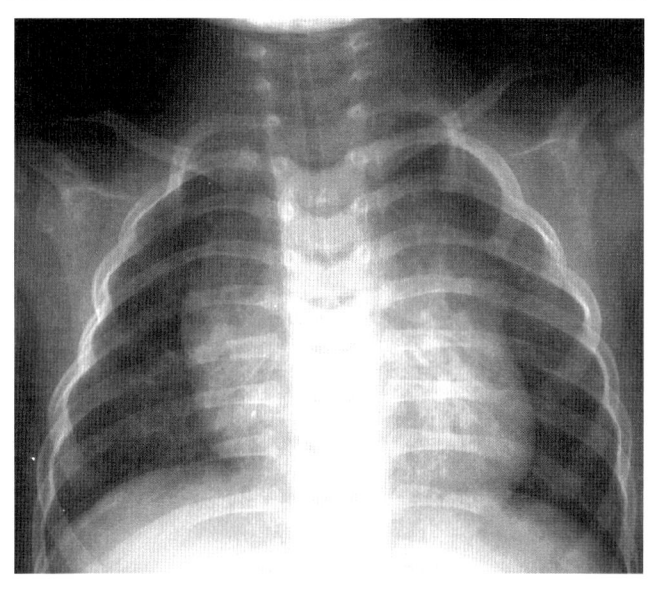

Figure 9–2
Tracheal stenosis (stovepipe trachea) in a 20-month-old boy with stridor since birth. Frontal chest radiograph shows a diffusely narrowed trachea faintly outlined by water-soluble contrast medium. (Courtesy of Simon C. Kao, MD, Iowa City, IA.)

two reported in the literature.[31,32] Those who are successfully managed are endoesophageally intubated,[33] with a nasogastric tube alongside the endotracheal tube for gastric decompression. Urgent bronchoscopy or tracheostomy may assist in diagnosis.[24,34] A survivor is described who had a type II defect and underwent esophageal intubation, gastrostomy, and distal esophageal banding.[31] The patient is reported to have survived to 4 years, undergoing a colonic interposition at 3 years of age. A second patient is described with a type I defect who survived to 6 years of age.[32] Extracorporeal membrane oxygenation (ECMO) may temporize these patients until a more definitive solution can be achieved.[35] If the patients can be stabilized, they should be examined for other life-threatening defects, such as neural and cardiac anomalies, that may require correction. The gastroesophageal continuity can be corrected with colonic interposition or gastric conduit, but there have been no attempts to reconstruct the trachea. Perhaps, for the future, to reconstruct the incompletely developed airway, tracheal allografts[36] or tissue-engineered replacements[37] may be used for long-term success.

Congenital Tracheal Stenosis

Congenital tracheal stenosis (Fig. 9-2) is rare. Cantrell and Guild[38] described three forms of stenosis. Type I is stenosis of the full length of the trachea. Type II is a funnel-shaped stenosis of the upper, lower, or entire trachea. Type III is a segmental stenosis of the lower trachea. This classification assists in identifying patients who are more likely to have associated anomalies and in planning treatment. Stenotic regions have complete cartilaginous rings, the number of which is variable, anywhere from 2 to 18. This rare anomaly is associated with pulmonary vascular sling or vascular ring in 50% of cases.[39] A functional classification system has been proposed to assist in selection of the operative candidate.[40,41]

These patients usually have exertional wheezing or stridor after birth. The type II and type III abnormalities are associated with anomalous location of one more bronchi, most likely a left pulmonary artery sling. All three types are associated with pulmonary agenesis. Symptoms vary according to the degree of stenosis. Patients presenting during the neonatal period or infancy with severe stridor, cyanosis, and recurrent stridor have the highest mortality. Many of these patients have associated congenital malformations and infections. Their prognosis even after surgical correction is variable.[40] Other children presenting at a year of age or soon thereafter have a surgical mortality of 10% to 20%.[42] Some children, late in childhood or early teens, may present for an evaluation for asthma with varying degrees of exertional dyspnea. Typically, these children have a better prognosis. CT, especially multiple detector CT, provides enough detail to assess the tracheobronchial abnormality with a sensitivity of 90%, better than flexible bronchoscopy,[43] and any associated anomalies. Bronchoscopy aids in diagnosis, treatment planning, and evaluation of the surgical repair intraoperatively and postoperatively. Echocardiography is helpful to assess for cardiac and vascular anomalies. Patients should be aggressively treated because they are at high risk for sudden death without surgical correction.[44] Partial tracheal resection is the most frequently performed operation. The neonatal trachea does not tolerate tension as well as in the adult.[45] Up to 50% of the infant trachea can be resected with primary reanastomosis. The repair is much more difficult if more than 50% of the trachea or the carina is involved.

In 1964, the first repair, a primary resection and end-to-end anastomosis, was reported by Cantrell and Guild.[38]

Reconstruction has been performed with pericardium,[46] aortic homograft,[47] costochondral graft,[48] slide tracheoplasty (Fig. 9-3),[49,50] and tracheal autograft.[51] Complete repair of the tracheal stenosis and any vascular ring or sling requires cardiopulmonary bypass and potential circulatory arrest. Backer and coworkers[52] reviewed their 18-year experience in 50 patients, comparing four tracheal stenosis repair techniques: pericardial patch, primary resection, tracheal autograft, and slide tracheoplasty. They concluded that when eight or fewer rings are involved, primary resection is preferable. For stenosis longer than eight rings, an autograft is better. Vascular endothelial growth factor application has the potential of improving the results of tracheal autograft.[53] In contrast, Muraji[54] demonstrated that the slide tracheoplasty technique allowed early extubation and an excellent long-term result in one case. ECMO may be necessary to support the neonate postoperatively.[35,48] Long-term outcome after resection appears to result in normal growth and development.[55] For patients who are considered surgically uncorrectable, palliative maneuvers include balloon dilation and split posterior tracheoplasty,[56,57] stenting, local steroid injection, electroresection, and cryotherapy.[40,41]

Tracheomalacia

In tracheomalacia, weakened cartilage collapses on expiration. With inspiration, there is sufficient suspension of the tracheal wall to maintain patency. The most common pathologic

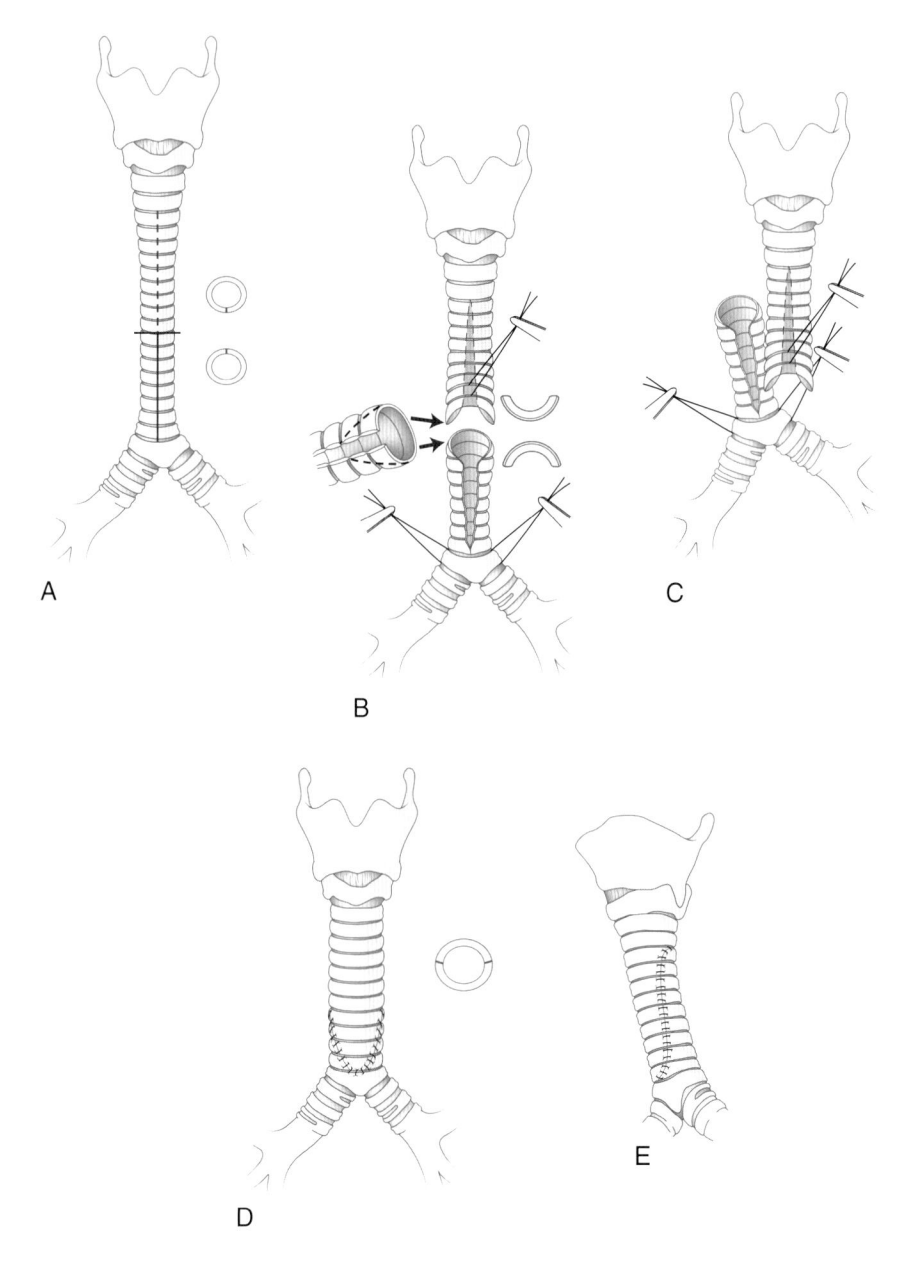

Figure 9–3
Congenital tracheal stenosis. **A,** After identification of the area of stenosis, the midportion of the stenosis is transected, leaving two halves of the trachea disconnected. **B,** A longitudinal tracheal incision is then made in each half, the full length of the stenosis, posterior in the upper half and anterior in the lower half. The corners are trimmed to allow an even, uncrimped anastomosis. **C,** Stay sutures help in retraction and alignment. **D and E,** The anastomosis results in an oblique suture line. The resultant cross-sectional area is quadrupled. *(Modified from the Society of Thoracic Surgeons.* Ann Thorac Surg *1994;**58**:613-21.)*

finding is oval rather than round cartilaginous rings. There is a congenital and an acquired form of tracheomalacia. The congenital form can be diffuse and both proximal and distal, involving the main-stem bronchi. It is associated with tracheoesophageal fistula.[58,59] The more common acquired form results from degeneration of the cartilaginous support, usually by vascular compression such as from a vascular ring or sling, adjacent inflammatory process, tumor, or chest wall deformity (e.g., pectus excavatum).

Tracheomalacia is not usually manifested at birth. It worsens as the child grows, usually after several weeks of life. Coughing, respiratory distress, severe dyspnea, stridor, and cyanosis may occur. Acute apnea, referred to as dying spells, is the most severe presentation. Dyspnea worsens with agitation or respiratory tract infections. These severe symptoms should prompt further investigation.

One fourth of all esophageal atresia patients have tracheomalacia. Tracheoscopy, bronchoscopy, esophagoscopy, and esophagography may be necessary for complete evaluation. CT and MRI provide additional information. The differential includes normal pulsatile collapse, bronchial webs, and tracheal tumors. Many patients suspected of having tracheomalacia may instead have gastroesophageal reflux disease or reflux disease in addition to tracheomalacia. This may warrant either a trial of a proton pump inhibitor and prokinetic agent or a formal evaluation for reflux.[60]

Tracheomalacia improves with age in most cases. "Dying spells," inability to be weaned from the ventilator, and failure to thrive are indications for more aggressive therapy. If tracheomalacia is mild, the infant should be supported and observed because infants usually outgrow their tracheomalacia within the next 2 years. In more severe forms, mortality is as high as 80% with conservative management. Stents have been used with varying success to allow cartilage maturation, usually taking several months.[61,62] Tracheostomy also has been used but is associated with some complications.[63] Aortopexy (Fig. 9-4), by itself or with tracheal resection or stenting, has been performed by a left submammary thoracotomy through the third interspace. The thymus is preserved. After exposure of the ascending aorta, three or four nonabsorbable sutures are placed through the aortic adventitia above and below the innominate artery takeoff. These sutures are attached to the periosteum. Finally, the endotracheal result is visualized by intraoperative bronchoscopy. Eighty percent of the patients are extubated by 4 weeks, and the long-term results are good.[64] The acquired form is treated similarly to the congenital form. Longer segment lesions without vascular compression often require tracheostomy and mechanical ventilation for a time. Bronchomalacia may require both aortopexy and pulmonary artery pexy.[65]

BRONCHIAL BRANCHING ABNORMALITIES

Bronchial branching abnormalities are rarely symptomatic. Accessory bronchi can originate off the trachea or main-stem bronchi and may be attached to rudimentary lung. They are usually incidental findings at autopsy. Cervical diverticula present in utero may regress before birth. There are case reports of bronchi crossing the mediastinum to supply the opposite lung.[66] The most frequent tracheal bronchus is to the right upper lobe. These abnormalities may be isolated or associated with other tracheopulmonary anomalies. They can be associated with wheezing, stridor, pneumonia, bronchiectasis, and hemoptysis. Accessory bronchi and associated abnormal pulmonary tissue should be resected if symptomatic.[67] Chest radiography and high-resolution CT are helpful in defining the anomaly.[68]

The following are anomalies that are more frequently symptomatic, potentially life-threatening, and may be treatable.

Bronchial Atresia

Bronchial atresia, first described by Ramsay in 1953,[69] is the second most common abnormality of the airway after tracheoesophageal fistula. A lobar or segmental bronchus ends blindly in the lung tissue. Lung tissue distal to the bronchial atresia expands and becomes emphysematous as a result of air entering through the pores of Kohn.[70] Beyond the atretic segment but proximal to the hyperinflated lung, the terminal

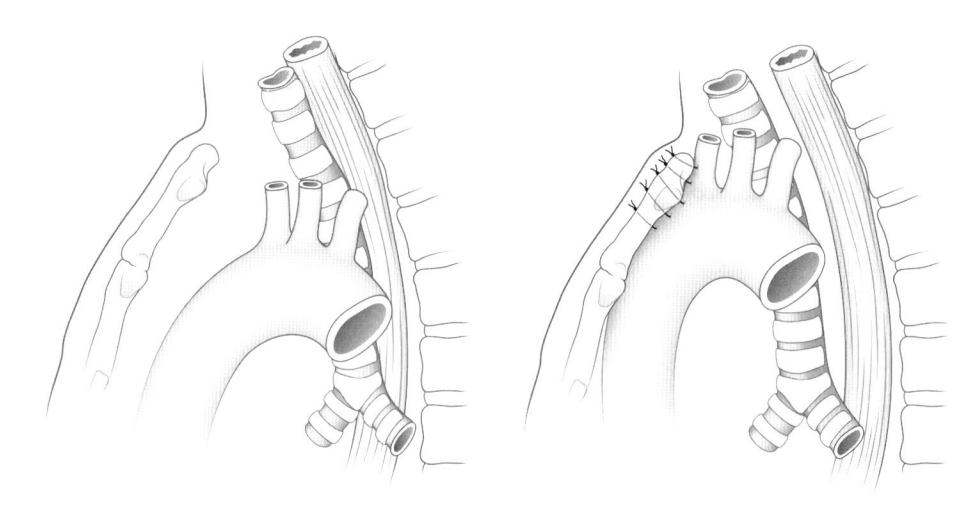

Figure 9–4
Tracheomalacia and aortopexy. In patients with severe tracheomalacia and aortopexy, suturing of the proximal transverse–ascending aorta to the anterior chest wall or sternum may significantly improve the obstructive symptoms. *(Modified from Weber TR, Keller MS, Fiore A. Aortic suspension [aortopexy] for severe tracheomalacia in infants and children. Am J Surg 2002;184:573-77.)*

airway is mucus filled. It is believed that the bronchial bud somehow separates distally from the proximal bronchial bud and continues to develop. Another potential explanation is that there is a vascular insult of the airway in the atretic segment. In either case, the distal airway continues to develop normally.

Infants usually develop respiratory distress 4 or 5 days to several weeks after birth. They may have wheezing, stridor, and repeated pulmonary infections. The most common location is in the left upper lobe, then the left lower lobe, followed by the right upper lobe. A segmental bronchus rather than a lobar bronchus is atretic, most frequently presenting as a lung mass on the first chest radiograph of the newborn. Fetal lung fluid is slowly absorbed, becoming a localized translucency with an opaque circular or oval density at the hilum. Patients rarely mature to adulthood without investigation.

For better assessment of this abnormality, a CT scan should be performed.[71,72] Prenatal diagnosis by ultrasonography has been reported.[73] The differential diagnosis includes acquired bronchial stenosis (which may result from long-term intubation), bronchial adenoma, sequestration, mucoid impaction, vascular compression syndrome, Swyer-James syndrome, and atypical bronchogenic cyst.

Indications for resection in bronchial atresia include a recurrent and possibly serious pulmonary infection, respiratory distress, and increasing size of the translucent lung.[74] Some resect the abnormal tissue to prevent infection. Segmentectomy is possible, but lobectomy is usually required.

Congenital Bronchiectasis

Bronchiectasis is an abnormal dilation of the bronchi or bronchioles. It is believed to be secondary to failure of the mesenchyme to differentiate into cartilage and muscle.[75] It results in a chronic, mildly productive cough with recurrent pneumonia. CT usually achieves the diagnosis,[76] and bronchoscopy typically is unnecessary. Bronchography also is unnecessary, given the detail provided by CT. Treatment and prognosis depend on the number of segments or lobes involved. Patients are provided with humidity, chest physiotherapy, and oxygen as necessary. Therapeutic bronchoscopy is performed for suspected mucoid obstruction or bleeding. Bleeding is initially controlled by embolization, topical epinephrine, or intravenous pitressin. Oral, intravenous, and nebulized antibiotics may be helpful in controlling symptoms.[77] Patients who have localized congenital symptomatic bronchiectasis may require a segmentectomy, lobectomy, or possibly pneumonectomy. The success of surgical intervention is related to the ability to resect all the diseased lung.[78]

Tracheobronchomegaly (Mounier-Kuhn Syndrome)

Tracheobronchomegaly was first described in 1932 by Mounier-Kuhn.[79] It is characterized by excessive dilation of the trachea and main bronchi (Fig. 9-5).[80] This dilation is the result of atrophy of the elastic tissue and smooth muscle of the trachea and main-stem airways.[81] Airway dilation continues to third-order subdivisions. During the course of the disease, mucosal herniations develop between tracheal rings, creating a diverticulosis pattern. Associated conditions include cutis laxa, Ehlers-Danlos syndrome, Marfan

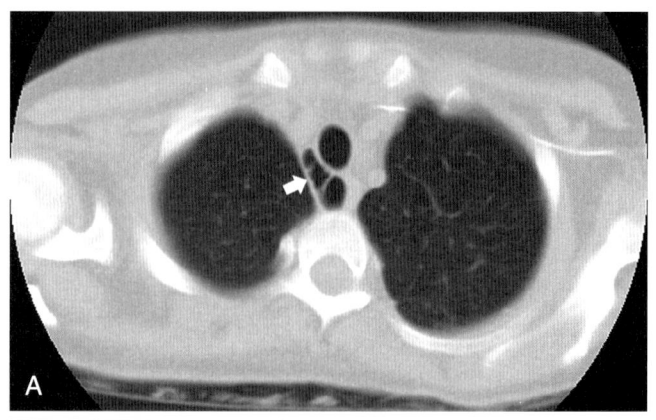

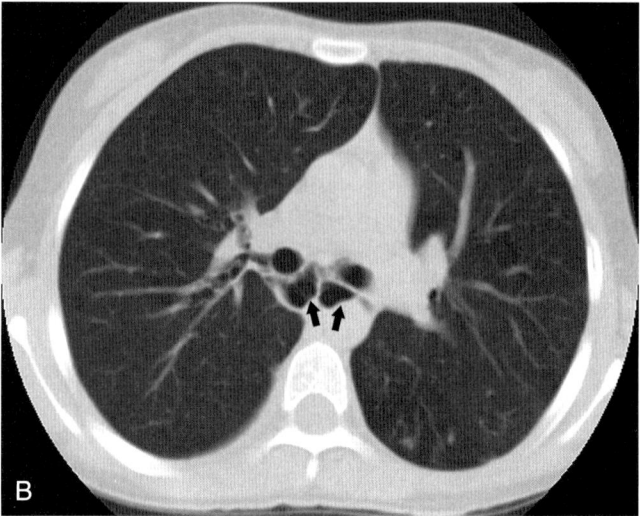

Figure 9-5
Tracheobronchomegaly (Mounier-Kuhn syndrome) in a 13-year-old girl with chronic cough and bronchiectasis. CT scan at the level of the trachea (A) and main-stem bronchi (B) shows air-filled saccules (arrows) around the airway from chronic inflammation destroying the normal elastic properties of the tracheobronchial tree and its smooth muscles. (Courtesy of Simon C. Kao, MD, Iowa City, IA.)

syndrome, Kenny-Caffey syndrome, ataxia-telangiectasia, ankylosing spondylitis, Brachmann–de Lange syndrome, and light chain deposition disease. When an isolated process occurs, there is recessive inheritance.[82] Tracheobronchomegaly also may result from severe pulmonary fibrosis with increased traction on the tracheal wall.[83,84] As these diverticula develop, there is mucus retention with resultant development of bronchiectasis and fibrosis. Patients eventually are unable to clear secretions and succumb to chronic infection and respiratory failure.

The patients are usually men in their third to fourth decades of life. Fifty percent of patients with tracheobronchomegaly have no symptoms until their third decade. They usually have recurrent lower respiratory tract infections. Asymptomatic patients may be identified in that the trachea is three standard deviations larger than normal; for adults, it exceeds 3 cm.[85] Patients with tracheobronchomegaly frequently have recurrent respiratory tract infections and persistent cough. Plain chest radiography demonstrates an enlarged trachea and main-stem airways that may be ectatic. CT more clearly demonstrates changes, and tracheal dimensions for adults[86] and children[87] are helpful in making the diagnosis. Bronchography may be necessary to differentiate it from acquired bronchiectasis. Bronchoscopy generally is unrewarding, with inadequate visualization of the airway lumen as a result of multiple tracheal wall diverticula.

In general, there is no surgical role in the treatment of tracheobronchomegaly. Management of secretions helps minimize the symptoms. Stenting and T-tubes[88,89] may provide significant palliation. Recently, a successful double-lung transplantation with bilateral bronchial stents for tracheobronchomegaly has been reported.[90]

Laryngotracheoesophageal Cleft

Laryngotracheoesophageal cleft is a rare congenital abnormality resulting from failure of the esophagus to separate from the laryngotrachea[91]; infants have a toneless cry and choke with feeding. On an attempt to pass a nasogastric tube, a communication with the airway is seen. A barium study or endoscopy can demonstrate the fistula. One half to more than three fourths of patients survive.[92,93] With late detection, mortality is high. Patients are first treated with a gastrostomy. Then, through a cervical approach, the fistula is divided, the esophagus and larynx are repaired, and a muscle flap is placed between them to reduce likelihood for recurrence. A nasogastric stent is left in place for a time. For large defects, a combined cervical and thoracic approach may be necessary.[94]

Tracheobronchial-Esophageal Fistula

Tracheobronchial-esophageal fistula (TEF) is the most common abnormality of the trachea, occurring in 2.4 per 10,000 births.[95] The most commonly used anatomic classification system for TEF is the one proposed by Gross.[96] type A, esophageal atresia without TEF; type B, esophageal atresia with proximal TEF; type C, atresia with distal TEF; type D, atresia with both proximal and distal TEF; and type E, TEF without esophageal atresia (H-type). Type C is the most common, accounting for 87% of the anomalies, followed by type A (8%), type E (4%), type B (1%), and type D (1%). Associated congenital defects are common[97]; cardiovascular anomalies lead the list, with concomitant occurrence in 35% of TEF cases. In about 20% of cases, TEF occurs as part of the VACTERL constellation of defects.

Patients present with feeding difficulties and excessive salivation. Intermittent cyanosis and tracheobronchial infections are seen as well. Diagnosis of the most common form (type C) is suspected when a large amount of air is seen in the esophagus, stomach, and small bowel. Failure of nasogastric tube passage and its position on plain radiography or contrast fluoroscopy confirm the condition. Cameron Haight is credited with the first successful pediatric TEF repair.[98] Although it was initially accomplished through left thoracotomy, Haight came to prefer right extrapleural thoracotomy for division of the fistula and esophageal anastomosis. Esophageal anastomotic leak is seen in about 15% of cases, but with a functioning chest tube in proximity, 95% of leaks heal spontaneously.[99] Subsequent stricture formation is common, but it generally responds well to dilation. Major, life-threatening leaks occasionally occur. In this situation or in the case of so-called long-gap atresia, wherein esophageal continuity cannot be established despite a variety of elongation techniques, esophageal replacement by colonic interposition or gastric transposition may be necessary. Even in critically ill neonates with a substantial esophageal anastomotic leak, gastric pull-up has been successfully applied as an alternative to temporizing with wide drainage alone.[100] Long-term outcome after surgery for TEF has been the subject of several recent reviews.[101-103]

For ligation of the H-type fistula, a right neck incision is made, allowing avoidance of the thoracic duct. The sternocleidomastoid muscle and carotid sheath contents are retracted laterally. The recurrent laryngeal nerve is identified and protected, and the fistula is divided and oversewn. An interposition muscle flap reduces the likelihood of recurrence. TEF recurrence has been successfully managed with a minimally invasive technique. In one pediatric series, the fistula tracts were de-epithelialized by fulgurating diathermy under endoscopic guidance, with successful track obliteration by way of fibrin glue application.[104] For the lower-lying H-type fistula not accessible through a cervical incision, thoracoscopic ligation has been successful.[105,106]

Not surprisingly, minimally invasive techniques have been increasingly applied not only to management of fistula obliteration but to esophageal reconstruction as well.[107-109] Thoracoscopic repair has been accomplished through an extrapleural approach,[110] and even long-gap esophageal atresia has been amenable to the thoracoscopic approach. The latter consists of initial thoracoscopically mediated esophageal traction followed by staged thoracoscopic creation of the esophageal anastomosis.[111] Nuances of anesthetic and intensive management of neonates undergoing thoracoscopy and laparoscopy are becoming better appreciated.[112,113] Meticulous anesthetic management has allowed successful TEF repair in a neonate with single-ventricle physiology (unpalliated tricuspid atresia).[114]

Preservation of the azygos vein, previously divided with impunity during repairs of esophageal atresia and TEF, has been advanced as desirable. The theory is that postoperative mediastinal edema may be avoided, thereby minimizing esophageal anastomotic complications.[115,116] Clinical significance of this concept awaits further evaluation.

Bronchobiliary Fistula

Bronchobiliary fistula (Fig. 9-6) is a very rare congenital abnormality with perhaps fewer than 50 cases reported.[117] It has generally been reported in infants and children, but a number of cases have been diagnosed in adulthood.[118-120] The fistula track is composed of bronchial and biliary-type tissue from its origin in the airway to the liver. Patients produce green sputum and develop dyspnea and chronic cough. Infants may present with respiratory distress[121]; girls are more commonly affected. The right middle lobe and right main-stem airways are most frequently involved and usually drain to the left hepatic ductal system. Associated anomalies, although not the rule, include esophageal atresia and TEF,[122] biliary atresia,[123] and right-sided diaphragmatic hernia.[117]

Diagnosis is made by bronchoscopy, during which a catheter may be passed into the fistula for administration of contrast material and concomitant radiography.[124] This represents a more modern form of bronchography. Diagnosis also has been achieved with a nuclear biliary scan (^{99m}Tc-HIDA cholescintigraphy)[125,126]; this is useful for postoperative surveillance as well. Finally, MRI for neonatal diagnosis has been

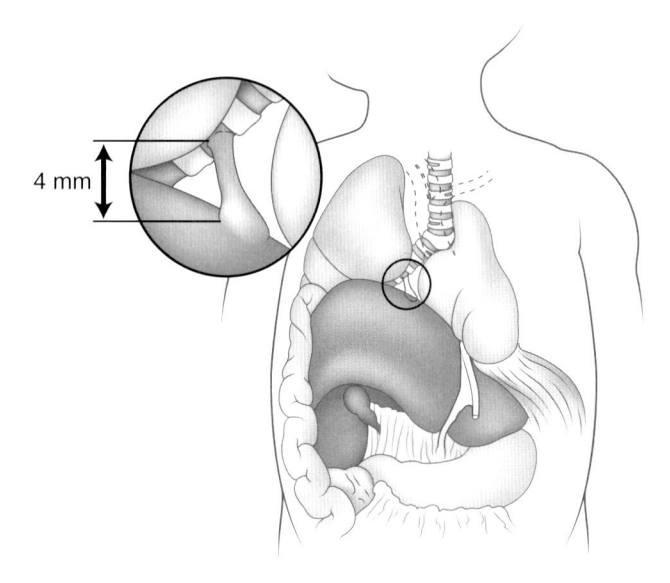

Figure 9–6
Bronchobiliary fistula. In this child with bilious sputum and a congenital diaphragmatic defect, a fistula was found between the right main-stem bronchus and the biliary tree. *(Modified from DiFiore JW, Alexander F. Congenital bronchobiliary fistula in association with right-sided congenital diaphragmatic hernia.* J Pediatr Surg *2002;**37**:1208-09.)*

reported, emphasizing the utility of T1-weighted gradient-echo sequences.[127]

Patients with a confirmed bronchobiliary fistula are treated by ligation and division of the fistula, transecting it as close to the airway as possible. Pulmonary resection has been necessary on occasion.[119] Access is by way of transpleural or extrapleural right thoracotomy. Cholecystography is used selectively to verify biliary drainage into the duodenum.[126] For those with impaired prograde biliary drainage or biliary sepsis, hepatic lobectomy (generally left-sided) or Roux-en-Y hepaticojejunostomy may be necessary.[128]

Bronchopulmonary Foregut Malformations

Bronchopulmonary foregut malformations represent another category of congenital lung diseases. The classification includes sequestrations (intralobar and extralobar), bronchogenic cysts, and other less common entities.

Bronchopulmonary foregut malformations are an abnormal communication between normal lung and esophagus or stomach and represent the second most frequent abnormal communication between the airway and intestinal tract, tracheoesophageal fistula being the most common. Right and left lower lobes are equally and most commonly affected. The fistula rarely involves the gastric fundus or mid-esophagus, almost always tracking to the lower esophagus. It is associated with extralobar sequestrations, more often on the left side. Diagnosis is usually made in the first few months of life up to 18 years of age. The most useful diagnostic test is esophagography. These malformations are associated with other anomalies, such as diaphragmatic hernia and cardiac, gastrointestinal, or vertebral anomalies. Because of chronic infection, lobectomy is usually necessary, and the fistulous communication must be divided and the esophageal defect repaired. If there is no evidence of infection, lung tissue may be preserved.

Sequestrations

Sequestrations are lung defects that have systematic arterial blood supply and abnormal bronchial connections. They are invariably located in the base of the lung, with males more frequently affected than females by a 3:1 ratio. Intralobar sequestrations (Fig. 9-7) are cystic abnormalities within the visceral pleural covering of the lung, whereas extralobar sequestrations (Rokitansky's lobe; Fig. 9-8) are mass lesions that have their own separate visceral covering. Intralobar sequestrations represent 75% of all sequestrations. As a group, intralobar sequestrations receive vascular blood supply from the thoracic aorta in 74% of cases, from the abdominal aorta in 19% of cases, from the intercostals in 3% of cases, and from multiple sources in 20% of cases. The aberrant blood supply most commonly enters the anomalous lung away from the hilum. The venous drainage of sequestrations is usually through pulmonary veins, but it may be through systemic veins. Intralobar sequestration is most frequently found within the posterior segment of the left lower lobe.

Extralobar sequestrations are rounded, smooth, soft masses that usually lie just above the dome of the diaphragm; 90% occur at the base of the left lung. The venous drainage of extralobar sequestrations occurs most frequently through the systemic circulation, to either azygos or hemiazygos systems; only 20% of cases demonstrate venous drainage into the pulmonary veins. On microscopic examination, all lung structures are present in extralobar sequestrations, including alveoli, bronchi, and cartilage.

Intralobar and extralobar sequestrations are both derived from foregut tissue and thus may possess an esophageal fistula. Intralobar sequestrations may present in utero as polyhydramnios or may become symptomatic in adolescents or young adults. Repeated bouts of pulmonary infection and hemoptysis are the most common symptoms. Intralobar sequestration is rarely associated with other congenital anomalies; extralobar sequestration is not uncommonly associated with other anomalies, especially congenital diaphragmatic hernias. Extralobar sequestrations may be found within either the pericardium or the diaphragm or beneath the diaphragm retroperitoneally. Malignant neoplasms have been reported within extralobar sequestrations, and a simultaneous discovery of congenital cystic adenomatoid malformation has been reported, as have other anomalies such as pericardial cysts, esophageal achalasia, and cardiac defects. In the absence of malignant disease, patients with both intralobar and extralobar sequestrations may demonstrate marked serum elevations of the tumor markers CEA and CA19-9.[129]

CT is sensitive and specific for identification of either intralobar or extralobar sequestrations. MRI may be helpful.[130] Bronchography and bronchoscopy are less likely to provide additional information. Barium esophagography may be necessary to demonstrate an esophageal communication. Angiography is seldom necessary, because noninvasive studies generally demonstrate the feeding systemic vessels.

Many lesions are discovered prenatally, and careful follow-up is recommended. If hydropic changes are noted, delivery is indicated.[131,132] In infants, cysts that are large or cause hemodynamic compromise may be temporarily drained by needle aspiration or tube thoracostomy to

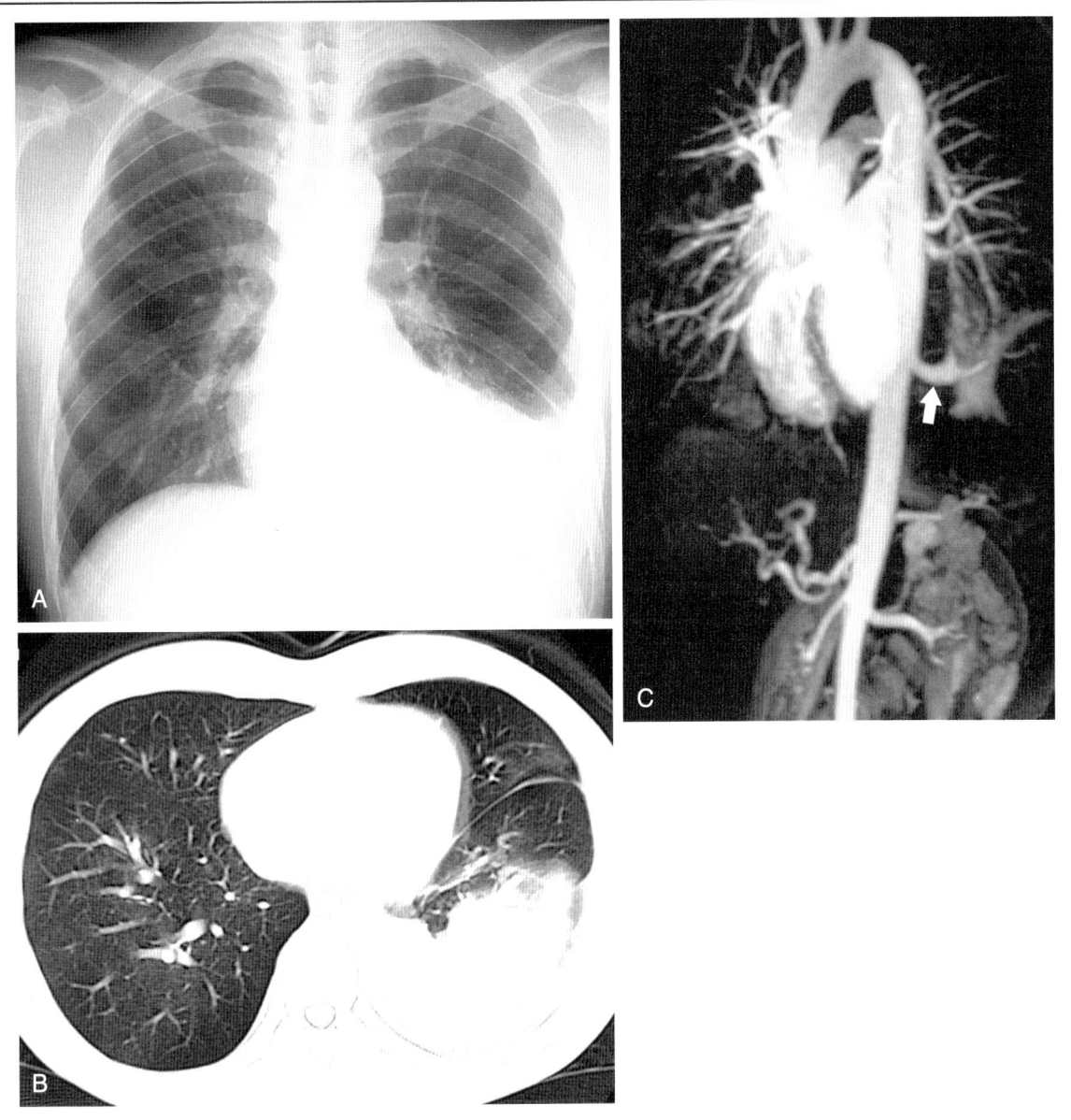

Figure 9–7
Intralobar pulmonary sequestration. **A,** Frontal chest radiograph shows consolidation of the left lower lobe. **B,** CT image of lung base shows opacification of the left posterior lower lobe. **C,** Contrast-enhanced magnetic resonance angiogram shows that a large arterial branch *(arrow)* arising from the low thoracic aorta supplies this region. *(Courtesy of Koji Takahashi, MD, Asahikawa Medical College, Asahikawa, Japan.)*

allow adequate induction of anesthesia. If no infection is involved, the cyst alone, or possibly a segment, may be removed. In most cases, however, lobectomy is required. Early identification of the aberrant arterial blood supply is critical and helps avoid disastrous bleeding. Most of the arteries are less than 1 mm in diameter, but some have been reported to be as large as 2.5 mm. Atherosclerotic changes in the systemic artery may make it difficult to manipulate during surgery. A communication with the gastrointestinal tract should be thoroughly searched for at the time of surgery. Venous drainage also may be aberrant, and it should be ascertained before resection, if possible. Both intralobar and extralobar sequestrations may be amenable to resection by minimally invasive techniques. The outcomes after resection are excellent.[133,134]

Azygos Lobe

An azygos lobe (Fig. 9-9) is present on 0.5% of routine chest radiographs. It is found as an abnormal lobation where the azygos vein creates an additional sulcus separating two portions of the upper lobe, and the azygos vein lies within the substance of the right lung. The term *azygos lobe* is somewhat of a misnomer because this entity does not represent a true anatomic lobe because of the absence of a separate segmental bronchus. Other regions of unusual, separate lobations may be found, particularly in the lingula or in the right and left superior segments. These abnormal lobations are not associated with any other congenital anomaly, nor do they increase the likelihood for any future pathologic or developmental abnormality. They require no treatment.

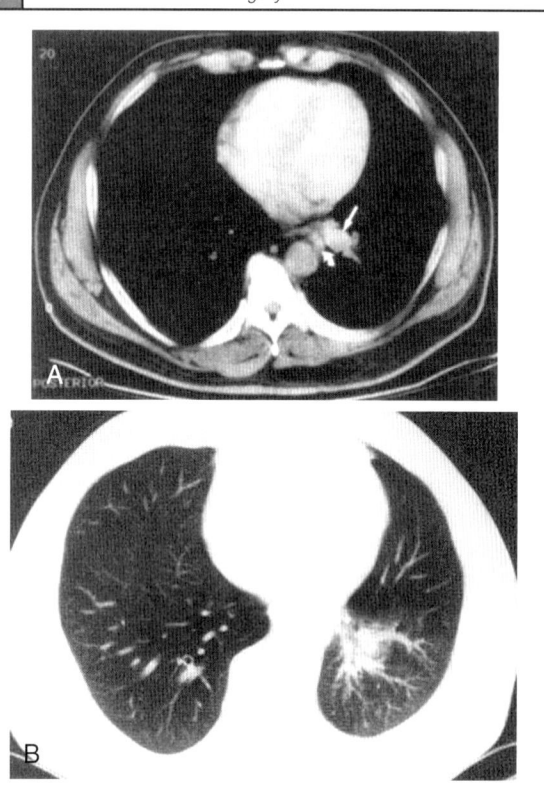

Figure 9–8
Extralobar sequestration. Extralobar sequestration is most frequently found in the lower left chest with its own pleural investment and systemic venous drainage. CT scan is beneficial in better identifying the anatomic details of the defect. *(From Singh SP, Nath H. A 53-year-old man with hemoptysis. Chest 2001;**120**:298-301.)*

Horseshoe Lung

In this rare, recently reviewed pulmonary anomaly,[135] right and left lung bases are fused by common tissue extending through the posterior mediastinum anterior to the aorta but posterior to the heart and esophagus. The clinical relevance lies in its association with recurrent pulmonary infections and pulmonary hypertension. Scimitar syndrome accompanies horseshoe lung in up to 80% of cases.[136] Horseshoe lung also should be suspected in patients with the VACTERL constellation and in patients with other bronchopulmonary foregut anomalies.[135]

Bronchogenic Cysts

Bronchogenic cysts result from abnormal budding from the perimeter of the trachea after it has differentiated from the foregut. They are the most frequent cysts of the mediastinum, accounting for approximately 60% of these lesions. Men are more frequently affected than are women. The usual location of the cysts is along the right paratracheal area, but they may also be attached to the carina, frequently anterior to the esophagus. They may be hilar, attached to a lobar bronchus, and occasionally they are intrapulmonary. They may also be situated below the diaphragm or in the parasternal subcutaneous tissue, skin, or pericardium. The cyst's inner lining is composed of ciliated pseudostratified respiratory epithelium interspersed with goblet cells. Bronchial communication is rare.[137] The cysts are unilocular and usually measure 2 to 10 cm.

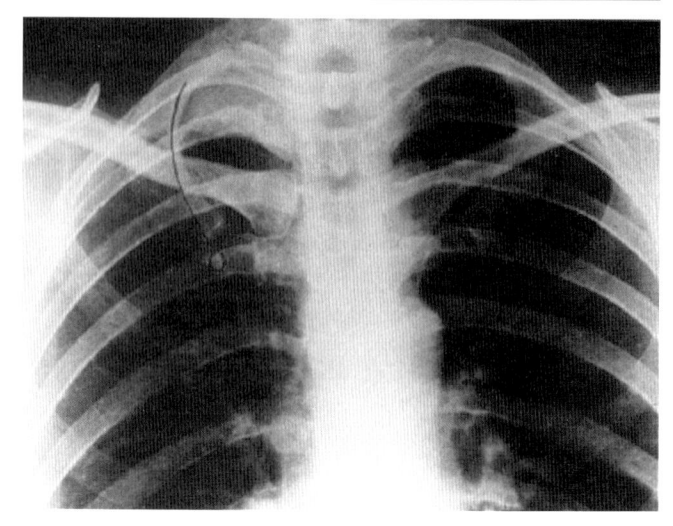

Figure 9–9
Azygos lobe. An additional fissure is found in this chest radiograph. The azygos vein creates a separate division within the right upper lobe.

They may contain normal bronchial elements, including cartilage and smooth muscle, which helps differentiate a bronchogenic cyst from an enteric cyst. Noninfected cysts may contain mucus, blood, or milky material. Symptoms may relate to pulmonary artery compression and possibly paroxysmal atrial fibrillation.[138,139] Bronchogenic cysts most commonly are an incidental finding on chest radiography, usually an air-filled cyst with or without an air-fluid level (Fig. 9-10). Serial radiographs may demonstrate rapid expansion. Intraparenchymal bronchogenic cysts more frequently present with symptoms of infection (90%) compared with mediastinal cysts (36%).[140]

The differential diagnosis of bronchogenic cyst includes lymphadenopathy, pulmonary sequestrations, teratoma, hemangioma, lipoma, hamartoma, neurogenic tumors, foregut and pericardial cysts, and lung abscesses. CT is helpful, and a low Hounsfield unit (<20) is characteristic. MRI may provide additional information. Differentiation of bronchogenic cysts from enteric cysts may be made on the basis of location, as enteric cysts usually present in the posterior mediastinum in close association with the esophagus. Also in the differential diagnosis of bronchogenic cysts, bronchopulmonary foregut malformations are usually multilocular and are more frequently associated with recurrent cough, pneumonia, and hemoptysis. Endoscopic ultrasonography may be beneficial, but endoscopic ultrasonography–directed fine-needle aspiration may be hazardous.[141]

Bronchogenic cysts should be excised completely, if possible, with repair of any associated communication. Needle aspiration alone is likely to result in recurrence. Mediastinoscopic unroofing has been performed and has been diagnostic. Asymptomatic cysts should be removed for diagnosis and to prevent complications associated with the natural history of these cysts, including perforation, hemorrhage, enlargement, infection, and malignant degeneration. In children, the airways are pliable and much more susceptible to life-threatening compression by an enlarging cyst.[142] Malignant degeneration has been reported,[143-145] including an adenocarcinoma in an 8½-year-old girl.[137] Typically, the bronchogenic cyst can be enucleated from the mediastinum.

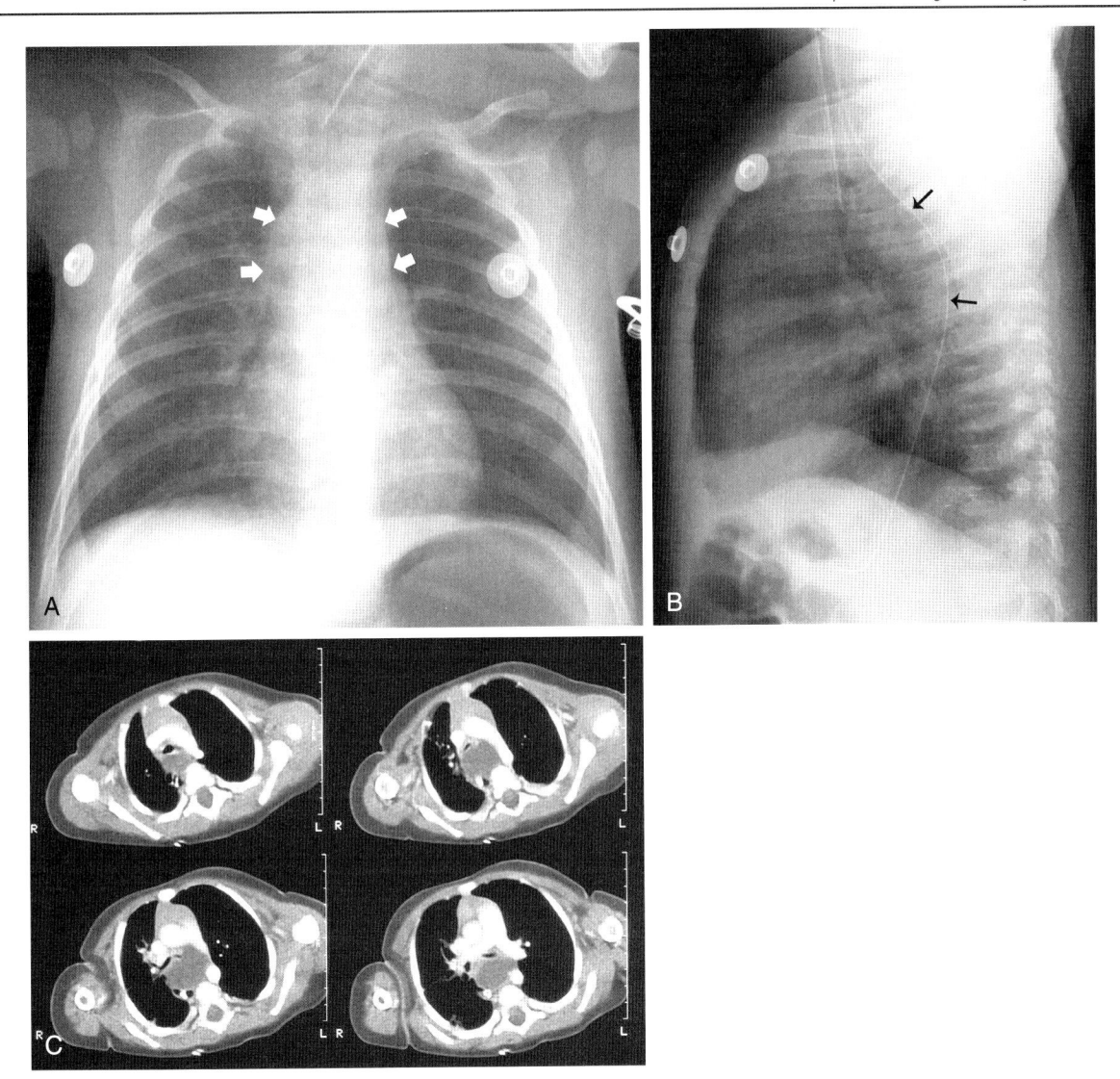

Figure 9–10
Bronchogenic cyst in a 4-month-old boy with cough. Anteroposterior **(A)** and lateral **(B)** chest radiographs show a central mediastinal mass *(arrows)* displacing the esophagus (outlined by nasogastric tube, *arrows*) posteriorly. **C,** Four contiguous axial CT images of the chest show a retrotracheal and subcarinal mass with low-density contents. Excision of the mass and pathologic examination showed bronchogenic cyst. *(Courtesy of Simon C. Kao, MD, Iowa City, IA.)*

If there is a stalk, it is ligated and the bronchial defect repaired. Long-term results are excellent. Video-assisted removal has become increasingly popular,[146] but pericystic adhesions, tracheal or bronchial communications, and the possibility of malignant transformation should be considered indications for thoracotomy.

LUNG BUD ANOMALIES

Pulmonary Agenesis, Aplasia, and Hypoplasia

Pulmonary agenesis is the complete absence of the carina as well as the main-stem bronchus, the lung, and the pulmonary vasculature on the affected side. First described by Morgagni, there are fewer than 20 reported cases. Cardiac anomalies are usually associated when pulmonary agenesis is bilateral. Unilateral cases have cardiac anomalies in 50% and are more frequently associated with right-sided agenesis.[147] The sex distribution is roughly equal. Right and left agenesis is also equally distributed. There is some evidence of a chromosomal abnormality.[148] Left-sided pulmonary agenesis has been reported as part of a syndrome with ipsilateral facial, radial ray, and renal agenesis in a series of three patients.[149] In these three infants, pulmonary artery dilation caused marked bronchial compression. Associated gastroesophageal reflux exacerbated respiratory distress. Other factors associated with impaired intrauterine lung growth include intrathoracic or extrathoracic compression, diminished fetal respiratory movements, and decreased amniotic fluid volume.[150] Abnormal pulmonary development can be detected on fetal ultrasound examination.[151]

When the carina and bronchus are present but the vessels and parenchyma are absent, the defect is referred to as pulmonary aplasia. There is a rudimentary bronchial stump, and the carina appears to be normal. Aplasia may be present in a single lobe or in a combination of lobes. It is most frequently unilobar. The right upper and right middle lobes are the most commonly involved.

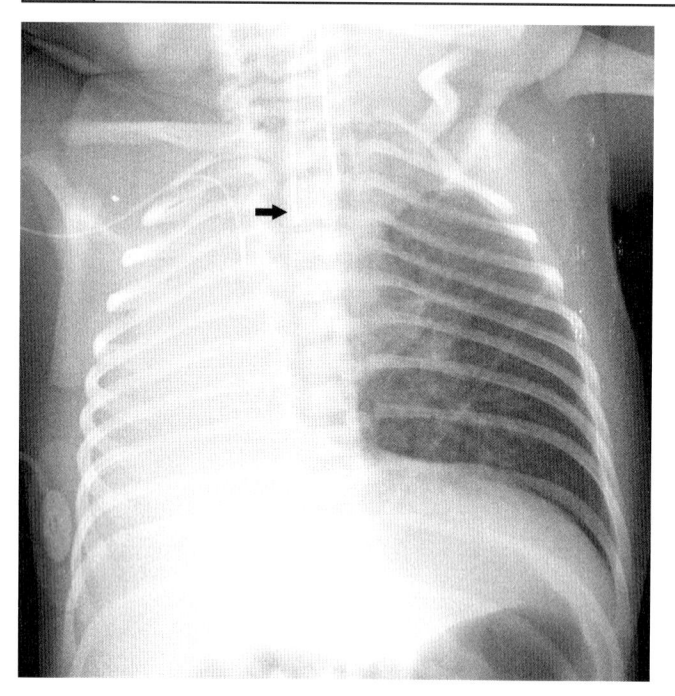

Figure 9-11
Right pulmonary agenesis. Frontal chest radiograph in a newborn with respiratory distress. Note complete opacification of the right hemithorax with mediastinal shift toward the same side. The patient also has esophageal atresia (nasogastric tube lodged in the dilated proximal esophageal pouch, *arrow*) with distal tracheoesophageal fistula (note air in the stomach). *(Courtesy of Simon C. Kao, MD, Iowa City, IA.)*

Agenesis or aplasia may be symptomatic when it is unilateral or even when a single lobe is involved. Patients may have tachypnea, dyspnea, or cyanosis. Older patients may present with wheezing. Boys are more commonly affected than girls are. When congenital cardiac anomalies are present, cyanosis and respiratory distress are generally evident at birth.

Chest radiography shows a shift in the mediastinum toward the area of agenesis or aplasia (Fig. 9-11). Pulmonary angiography shows absence of the ipsilateral pulmonary artery. Bronchoscopy may be helpful to evaluate bronchial stump presence, length, and character in patients with aplasia. CT and esophagography are helpful elements of the evaluation to differentiate agenesis or aplasia from sequestration and atelectasis.

Bilateral agenesis is incompatible with life. Survival periods of up to 6 years in right-sided lesions and up to 16 years in left-sided lesions have been reported.[152] Of those surviving the neonatal period, 30% die within the first year, and 50% succumb within the first 5 years of life.[153]

In pulmonary hypoplasia, the bronchus and the bronchial tissue are poorly formed, and there is a reduced number of alveoli. Lung weight is at least one standard deviation below the mean.[154] Most cases of hypoplasia are the result of another defect that prevents normal lung development, such as a diaphragmatic hernia, chest wall defect, bone dysplasia, or even muscular dystrophy. Primary pulmonary hypoplasia is rare and is frequently associated with Down syndrome.[155] It is often fatal and is the result of hypertrophy of the pulmonary artery smooth muscle and resultant pulmonary artery hypertension. Associated congenital abnormalities also reduce the life expectancy of these patients.

In pulmonary aplasia, removal of the rudimentary stump may be necessary if it is recurrently infected. There is no specific surgical therapy for pulmonary hypoplasia, except to treat the cardiac anomalies or to ameliorate the chest wall anomalies. The severity of the pulmonary artery hypertrophy may result in persistent fetal circulation. At delivery, the affected infant may be hypoxemic, acidotic, and hypercarbic. Such patients are treated with sedation, paralysis, high-frequency ventilation, vasodilators, respiratory alkalosis, and, if necessary, ECMO. Survival has improved with ECMO.[156-158] Another means to treat these patients is with high-frequency oscillatory ventilation.[159] One half of the infants with congenital diaphragmatic hernias require ECMO, and 70% of those patients survive. In patients with a congenital diaphragmatic hernia, it is unnecessary to resect the underdeveloped lung at the time of diaphragmatic repair. There should be no attempt to aggressively inflate the lung. Bilateral lung transplantation has been performed in extreme circumstances.[160] Antenatal surgical therapy has been directed at relief of lung compression, but efficacy is equivocal.[150] Surgical options have recently been reviewed,[161-163] although the absence of large randomized trials precludes robust quantification of risks and benefits of antenatal surgery vis-à-vis postnatal therapy.

Congenital Lobar Emphysema

Congenital lobar emphysema represents 50% of all congenital lung anomalies. It is due to obstruction of a lobar bronchus, usually an upper airway, resulting in overexpansion of alveolar airspaces but lacking parenchymal destruction, in contradistinction to the adult form. The vasculature to the affected lobe is normal.

Expanded lung frequently compresses adjacent lung and in some cases shifts the mediastinum away from the emphysematous lobe. Other descriptive terms include infantile lobar emphysema, congenital segmental bronchomalacia, congenital lobar overinflation, and emphysema of infancy or childhood. A cartilaginous defect obstructs the lobar bronchus in 25% of cases.[164-167] Other potential causes of intrinsic obstruction include mucus plugging and intraluminal granulation tissue. Extrinsic obstruction may result from cardiac or vascular anomalies such as tetralogy of Fallot, pulmonary stenosis, anomalies of pulmonary venous return, adenopathy, mediastinal tumors, and bronchogenic or enteric duplication cysts.[168] In more than one half of the cases, there is no identifiable etiologic factor.[169]

Patients with congenital lobar emphysema are symptomatic at birth. Within several days, they can develop wheezing, dyspnea, or cough.[44] The left upper lobe is most frequently involved, followed by the right upper lobe, then the right middle lobe, and finally the lower lobes.[170] It can present bilaterally. When it does, it is usually the left upper lobe and the right middle lobe that are affected. There is a 3:1 male-to-female ratio of involvement. Of those affected, 80% are symptomatic by 6 months of age. Fourteen percent of patients have an associated cardiac malformation. Rib and thoracic cage abnormalities also are common. If congenital lobar emphysema is symptomatic but left untreated, the mortality is 50% within the first week, and an additional 30% to 40% of patients will die during the next month.

In the newborn with severe respiratory distress, a chest radiograph usually suffices for diagnosis (Fig. 9-12). The of respiratory distress syndrome and long-term mechanical ventilation, and is usually present in the right upper lobe. In acquired childhood emphysema, lung scans demonstrate low flow to the affected lung, in contrast to normal flow in the congenital form.[172] For the congenital form, echocardiography and additional tests (e.g., magnetic resonance angiography) may be required to evaluate for associated cardiac or vascular anomalies. There is no surgical indication for asymptomatic or mildly symptomatic patients. Pulmonary function is likely to remain stable. One half of the patients will normalize during infancy. For patients who are symptomatic, all emphysematous tissue should be resected. Lobectomy is frequently required. Operative mortality is as high as 7% in some series. The greatest risk appears to be at the time of anesthesia induction. Selective intubation has been used to prevent overinflation of the emphysematous lobe, with resulting cardiovascular collapse.[173] High-frequency ventilation also has been employed to prevent mediastinal shift and hemodynamic compromise.[174] Needle aspiration has been performed as necessary.[175] In addition, flexible fiberoptic bronchoscopy has been used in the neonate to decompress an emphysematous lobe.[176] The surgeon should be prepared for immediate thoracotomy soon after induction. Once the chest is open, the emphysematous lobe may spontaneously project out of the chest. Typically, it remains inflated even after the lobe has been removed. The hilar anatomy is usually normal, and the goal should be to resect all of the emphysematous tissue, preserving the adjacent normal lung. Lung function is compromised after resection,[169,177] but the child's development is normal.[178] Long-term follow-up has been reported.[179] In contrast to patients with congenital lobar emphysema, those with acquired lobar emphysema progress to further respiratory difficulties after lung resection.[180] Balloon dilation of the airway stenosis has been used successfully.[181]

Management of coexisting congenital lobar emphysema and congenital heart disease has been described in detail.[182] Presence or absence of pulmonary hypertension is a key factor in the development of an operative strategy. On occasion, the emphysema may be caused by vascular compression of a bronchus, such as in the case of a large ductus arteriosus. The emphysematous changes may resolve after surgical correction of the vascular anomaly.

Congenital Parenchymal Cysts

Congenital parenchymal cysts are rare and may present as a unilocular entity within the parenchyma, most commonly in the left lower lobe. An aberrant systemic artery often supplies the cyst region. Such cysts are lined with mucus-secreting pseudostratified columnar epithelium. The cyst usually communicates with a bronchus. This condition may represent a variant of cystic adenomatoid malformation. It may also result from entrapped lung blood, with subsequent air trapping after the blood has been resorbed. Affected infants present with symptoms ranging from a chronic cough to frank sepsis. Congenital parenchymal cysts are frequently associated with other anomalies. This disease category includes intraparenchymal bronchogenic cysts.[183] There is an association between parenchymal cysts and subtype B Niemann-Pick disease.[184]

Respiratory distress is common within the first few days of life, and the cyst often becomes infected by the first few weeks of age. Air trapping may shift the mediastinum.

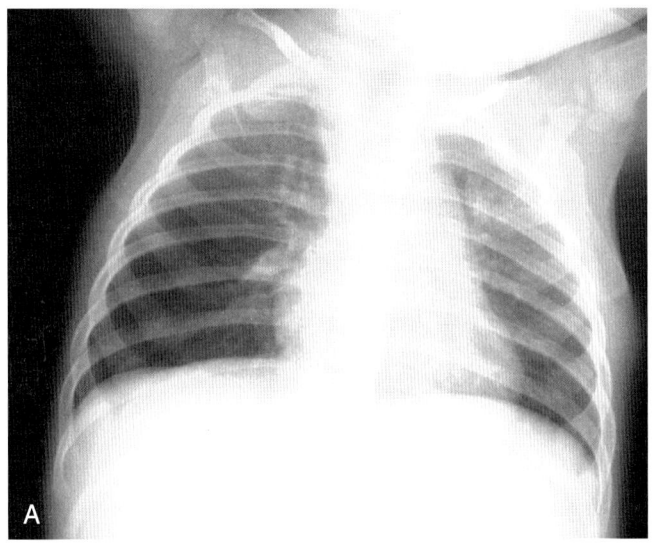

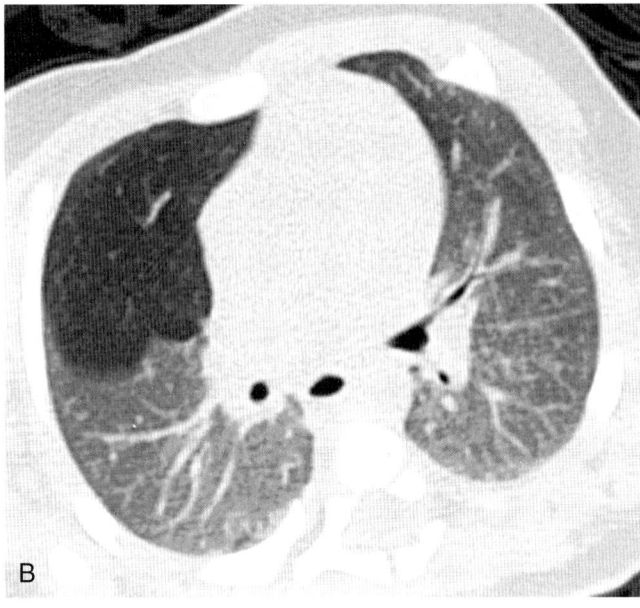

Figure 9–12
Congenital lobar emphysema. **A,** Chest radiograph of a 1-month-old boy shows hyperlucency in the right lower lung field. **B,** CT image of the lungs just below the carinal bifurcation shows right middle lobe emphysema with paucity of blood vessels and decreased attenuation. *(Courtesy of Simon C. Kao, MD, Iowa City, IA.)*

combination of an enlarged, hyperlucent lobe with fairly normal vasculature coupled with compression of adjacent lung tissue and contralateral mediastinal deviation is diagnostic. For mild to moderate symptoms, a CT scan (see Fig. 9-12) may be necessary to rule out mediastinal masses or vascular anomalies. In older children, bronchoscopy can be helpful to assess for mucus plugs or foreign bodies. Bronchography is unlikely to be helpful and is rarely used now. The ventilation-perfusion scan has yielded useful information in some instances.[171] Respiratory distress in the newborn must be differentiated from other lung abnormalities, such as pneumothorax, congenital diaphragmatic hernia, parenchymal lung cysts with a ball-valve mechanism, cystic adenomatoid malformation, and extralobar sequestration. Acquired lobar emphysema is yet a different disease entity, a complication

It may be difficult to differentiate a cyst from an intraparenchymal abscess. The presence of a systemic artery feeding the cyst is diagnostic. Failure of the cyst to completely collapse with tube drainage also is helpful in making the diagnosis. Other anomalies that appear similar include congenital diaphragmatic hernia and postpneumonic staphylococcal pneumatoceles.

Once discovered, congenital parenchymal cysts can be observed unless they become infected, expand, or are otherwise symptomatic. If present for more than a year, they are unlikely to resolve. As noted before, malignant transformation of a pulmonary cyst is a concern.[185] For infected cysts, preliminary antibiotic treatment is followed by resection once sepsis subsides. Lobectomy is usually necessary, although cyst resection can suffice, for example, by right S3 segmentectomy.[183] Pneumonectomy occasionally may be necessary for definitive treatment. Management of congenital parenchymal lung cysts has been grouped with that of congenital cystic adenomatoid malformation, congenital lobar emphysema, and sequestrations to compare and contrast the fine points of each entity.[186] Perioperatively, a combination of one-lung high-frequency ventilation and low-rate intermittent mandatory ventilation has been described for the management of the symptomatic neonatal lung cyst.[187]

Congenital Cystic Adenomatoid Malformation

Congenital cystic adenomatoid malformation (CCAM) was first described in 1949.[188] It is a mass consisting of excessive proliferation of bronchi but without normal alveolar development. Composed of cartilage, smooth muscle, and bronchial glands containing columnar and cuboidal epithelial cells, CCAM represents 25% of all congenital lung anomalies (second only to congenital lobar emphysema). There is normal vascular development, and the affected area communicates with the normal airway. Usually only one lobe is affected, with that lobe generally having a solitary lesion.

The abnormality may be identified in the fetus whose mother develops polyhydramnios by the 23rd week of gestation. Up to one third of those identified in utero resolved before birth.[189-191] For the majority, CCAM presents as neonatal acute respiratory distress with or without associated lung infection. CCAM must be differentiated from congenital diaphragmatic hernia because both entities show multiple air-fluid levels within the affected hemithorax. The initial chest radiograph shows a solid mass. Over time, the fetal fluid is resorbed and the cysts become filled with air (Fig. 9-13). A CT scan may be helpful in achieving a diagnosis. The most commonly associated anomaly is pectus excavatum, and there can be cardiac and pulmonary vessel malformations as well. The Stocker classification assists in treatment planning, categorizing presentations into types I, II, and III.[192] Type I lesions are large, widely spaced, and irregular cystic structures that exceed 1 cm. Affected patients usually reach term but occasionally are stillborn. It is rare to have polyhydramnios or other anomalies associated with a type I lesion. Of these patients, 75% have mediastinal shifting with some associated cyanosis and grunting. The prognosis is generally good. One half of the patients develop pneumonia in infancy and early childhood. In type II CCAM, 40% of cases, the cysts are smaller than 1 cm and have an appearance of dilated bronchioles. The patients are more frequently premature or stillborn.

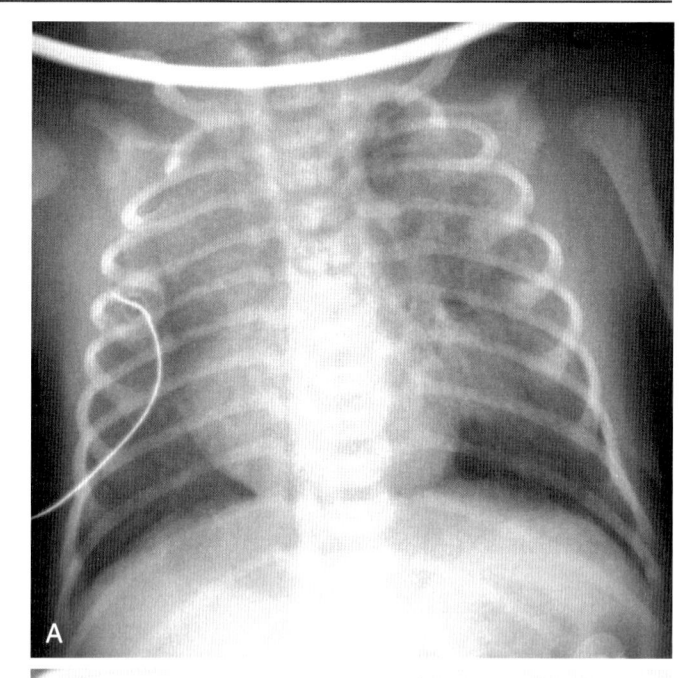

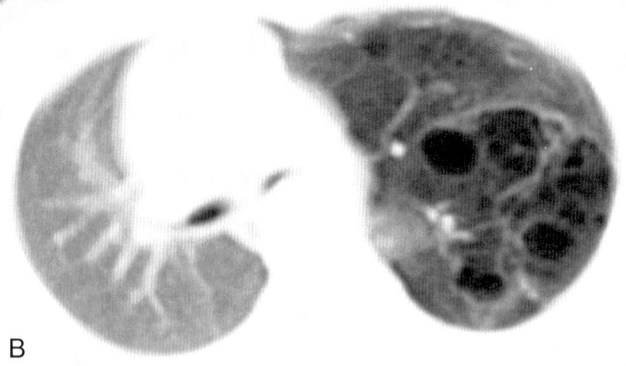

Figure 9–13
Cystic adenomatoid malformation. **A,** Chest radiograph of a newborn with ill-defined lesions in the mid-left lung field. **B,** CT image of the chest shows multicystic lesions in the same region. Excision and histologic examination showed cystic adenomatoid malformation. *(Courtesy of Simon C. Kao, MD, Iowa City, IA.)*

Mediastinal shift is less often seen, and there appears to be more bronchiolar proliferation. Type III lesions are very small cysts, less than 0.5 cm. They represent 10% of all cases. The mass is much firmer, appearing to surround the entire affected lobe, most often the lower lobe. Prognosis is very poor, and patients usually expire within a few hours of birth.

Asymptomatic CCAM patients may be observed for the first 4 to 6 months. Repeated CT at 6 months is performed to assess for CCAM enlargement or malignant degeneration (a consideration but a poorly defined phenomenon in this condition). Delayed intervention allows the child to mature, reducing the operative morbidity. Lesion shrinkage or disappearance, compensatory hypertrophy of normal lung, and unlikely occurrence of later malignant neoplasia all support a conservative approach in asymptomatic patients.[193] Only about 10% of untreated asymptomatic lesions eventually become clinically significant.[194] Any lesion that decreases in size but has not completely regressed should be observed until it has completely resolved. Many authors still favor resection of

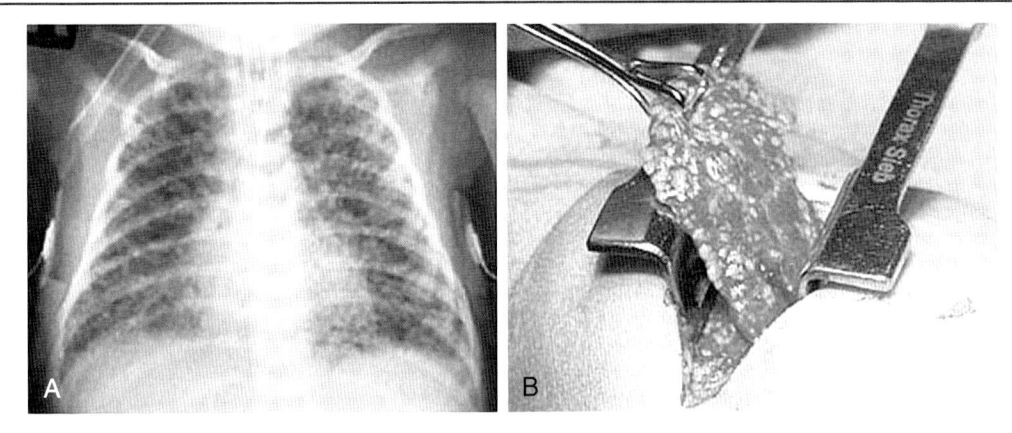

Figure 9–14
Pulmonary lymphangiectasia. The chest radiograph demonstrates the bilateral "soap bubble" appearance of lymphangiectasia. Gross findings at surgery demonstrated the cystic nature of the disease.

cystic lung lesions in asymptomatic neonates, citing persistent risk of infection or malignant transformation.[195,196] Of the total number of primary pulmonary rhabdomyosarcomas and malignant mesenchymomas of lung reported in children, about 50% have antecedent lung cysts.[185] Symptomatic lesions after birth certainly should be resected, and lobectomy has been considered the standard operation. Remaining unaffected lung tissue should be preserved. There is evidence that segmentectomy and wedge resection, when feasible, are just as efficacious as lobectomy, with the obvious advantage of maximizing pulmonary reserve, provided prolonged pulmonary air leaks are avoided.[197] By extension, with ipsilateral multilobar involvement, segmentectomies allow avoidance of pneumonectomy. After *complete* CCAM resection, prognosis is generally excellent.

Antenatal diagnosis suggests the possibility of in utero surgical therapy, but efficacy remains controversial. Successful serial cyst aspiration has been demonstrated in fetal CCAM.[198] However, in one study, only 8 of 20 infants who had a prenatal diagnosis of CCAM were symptomatic in the neonatal period.[199]

Infantile Pulmonary Emphysema

Infantile pulmonary emphysema is uncommon, accounting for about 2% of congenital anomalies. Its morphologic spectrum has been described in detail in a series of 33 cases accessioned to the Armed Forces Institute of Pathology in Washington, DC, during an approximate 30-year period.[200] An entity different from congenital lobar emphysema, it does appear most prominently in the upper lobes and is multilobar in about 20% of cases. Associated anomalies are common. The condition presents as gas surrounding the bronchovascular structures and may evolve to pneumomediastinum or pneumothorax. It occurs in approximately 20% of patients with respiratory distress syndrome and 40% of patients who require positive end-expiratory pressure. Infantile pulmonary emphysema can present as diffuse multicystic abnormalities within all lobes.[201] It must be differentiated from congenital cystic adenomatoid malformation and congenital diaphragmatic hernia. Once the diagnosis is made, less than 2% of patients require surgical resection; most improve with supportive measures alone. Atelectasis, ventilator dependence, and recurrent or persistent infections are indications for surgery. Thoracentesis or thoracostomy is necessary to treat pneumothorax and respiratory embarrassment. Resection of affected tissues with preservation of relatively healthy parenchyma is the objective of surgical intervention.

Polyalveolar Lobe

Polyalveolar lobe is a significant increase in the number of alveoli compared with the bronchi. It was first described in 1970 and was thought to be congenital lobar emphysema.[202] Polyalveolar lobe is differentiated from lobar emphysema in that there is little trapped air and no true emphysematous changes. Radiographic translucency in this condition is the result of a reduction in vasculature to amount of lung, unlike congenital lobar emphysema.[202,203] There appears to be retention of fetal lung liquid in these patients, an occurrence not primarily associated with congenital lobar emphysema.[204] However, polyalveolar lobe may at times give rise to congenital lobar emphysema.[169] There may also be a relationship between polyalveolar lobe and type II congenital cystic adenomatoid malformation[205] and with infantile pulmonary emphysema.[200] In older children, bronchoscopy should be performed to differentiate obstructive emphysema from foreign bodies or bronchial obstructive inflammation. Diagnosis is usually made by high-resolution CT. Resection is performed as necessary for symptomatic patients.

Pulmonary Lymphangiectasia

Pulmonary lymphangiectasia (Fig. 9-14) was first described by Virchow as diffuse cystic lymphatic duct dilation in infancy.[206] There are primary and secondary forms. The primary form involves dilated lymphatic channels within the lung, and the secondary form results from pulmonary venous obstruction. Both forms are symptomatic in neonates, with respiratory distress and cyanosis. One half of these patients have associated cardiac anomalies, usually involving venous return. Their chest radiographs demonstrate a "soap bubble" appearance with ground-glass opacification. CT is more specific in making the diagnosis, but even with current techniques, it may be radiographically difficult to distinguish pulmonary lymphangiectasia from congenital lobar emphysema.[207] Lymphoscintigraphy is a helpful adjunct to CT in distinguishing lymphangiectasia from lobar emphysema.[208] Almost exclusively diagnosed in infants, adult presentation has been seen, with histologic verification after thoracoscopic pulmonary resection.[209]

Lymphatic obstruction may be secondary to venous obstruction. Congenital chylothorax may result. Thus, venous impairment may indirectly produce nonimmune hydrops fetalis, and the concept of a congenital pulmonary lymphangiectasia–congenital chylothorax–hydrops fetalis continuum has been proposed.[208] Patients with pulmonary lymphangiectasia may also have extrapulmonary organ involvement, especially in the alimentary canal and solid organs of the abdomen. Prognosis correlates best with the degree of pulmonary involvement, and outcome is worse when pulmonary involvement is extensive.[210] Prognosis is particularly poor if pulmonary lymphangiectasia is present bilaterally. Survival beyond infancy is unusual, but overall outcome may be better than once believed.[211-213]

To effect survival, immediate postnatal ventilator support and pleural drainage are almost always required. Progress in neonatal intensive care has improved the outlook for these severely ill infants. Surviving patients have a course similar to that of others with major chronic lung disease. Home oxygen therapy, symptomatic treatment of wheezing and cough, and intermittent pleural drainage are generally necessary.[214] Successful pleurodesis employing autologous blood instillation has been reported.[215]

Whereas most cases of pulmonary lymphangiectasia occur sporadically, the condition has been seen in siblings.[216] Candidate gene mutations include vascular endothelial growth factor receptor 3 (VEGFR3) and FOXC2 in families with Milroy and lymphedema-distichiasis syndromes, respectively. According to the same research team, a correlating animal model of fatal chylothorax may be that of α_9-deficient mice. Postmortem examination of one infant who died of pulmonary lymphangiectasis revealed marked upregulation of endothelial nitric oxide synthase in that disorder.[217] From an immunohistochemical standpoint, key antibody markers useful in confirming the diagnosis of lymphangiectasis include CD31, CD34, desmin, smooth muscle actin, and D2-40.[218]

VASCULAR ABNORMALITIES

Unilateral Absence of a Main Pulmonary Artery

Absence of a main pulmonary artery is exceedingly rare and is commonly associated with other cardiac anomalies. The pulmonary vein to the affected lung is normal, but the arterial supply derives from a systemic artery that is usually adjacent to the trachea. Patients develop recurrent respiratory infections and dyspnea in later childhood. Hemoptysis is the most serious complication and may be associated with bronchiectasis. Pulmonary infection warrants surgical resection.

Idiopathic, Hyperlucent Lung Syndrome (Swyer-James or Macleod's Syndrome)

Hyperlucent lung syndrome is defined as a small or normal-sized lung with few pulmonary vessels and associated air trapping. A very rare anomaly with a prevalence of 0.01% in routine chest radiographs,[219] it was first described by Swyer and James[220] and later by Macleod.[221] It is thought to result from chronic childhood lower respiratory tract infections, potentially caused by bronchiolitis obliterans, that lead to pulmonary vascular changes and bronchiectasis.

Patients are usually asymptomatic. A small or normal-sized lobe that is hyperlucent is incidentally discovered by chest radiography. Infants with the condition may have a mildly productive cough or dyspnea. CT and bronchoscopy are helpful in evaluating these patients. Agenesis or hypoplasia of the pulmonary artery can be associated with hyperlucent lung, but air trapping is absent, an important finding in this syndrome. A dynamic inspiratory and expiratory CT scan is performed to assess for trapping. The pulmonary vessels are markedly diminished. Hyperlucent lung usually requires no treatment, although surgical resection as a means of lung volume reduction has been reported.[222]

Pulmonary Artery Sling

Pulmonary artery sling relates to an anomalous origin of the left pulmonary artery. It arises from the right pulmonary artery anteriorly and then passes over the right main-stem bronchus behind the trachea and in front of the esophagus. Prevalence is reported as 59 per million school-age children based on a large two-dimensional echocardiographic study. It may be associated with tracheal stenosis secondary to complete cartilage tracheal rings. Symptoms include respiratory distress, choking, cyanosis, and stridor. The chest radiograph demonstrates hyperinflation. Bronchoscopy should be performed to rule out complete tracheal rings.[223] Esophagography and CT (Fig. 9-15) may help assess the anatomy.

To correct the anomaly, the pulmonary artery is transected through a median sternotomy with the use of extracorporeal circulation. The left pulmonary artery is transected and reanastomosed to the main pulmonary artery anterior to the trachea.[190] If tracheal stenosis is present, it may be treated at the same time. Others have reported an alternative procedure in which the trachea is divided and the left pulmonary artery is moved anterior to the trachea before the trachea repair is performed.[224,225] Backer and Mavroudis[226] reported

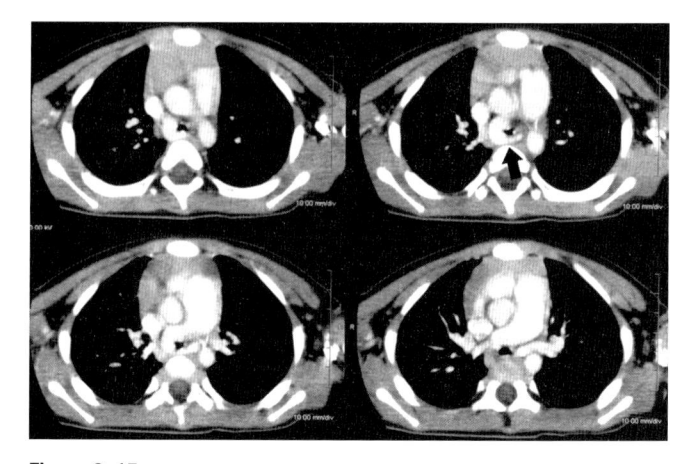

Figure 9–15
Pulmonary sling (aberrant left pulmonary artery). Four contiguous enhanced CT images at the level of the aortopulmonary window show that the left pulmonary artery (arrow) arises from the right pulmonary artery. (Courtesy of Koji Takahashi, MD, Asahikawa Medical College, Asahikawa, Japan.)

no operative mortality in 27 patients who underwent repair of pulmonary artery sling through a median sternotomy.

Isolated Pulmonary Artery Aneurysm

Pulmonary artery aneurysm is a rare vascular anomaly first described in 1947 by Deterling and Clagett.[227] Approximately 40% to 50% of isolated pulmonary artery aneurysms are congenital, and a familial pattern has been described.[228] Sporadic causes include penetrating trauma, prior chest tube placement, and pulmonary artery catheter–related injury. Pulmonary artery aneurysms have also been associated with infection from syphilis, tuberculosis (Rasmussen's aneurysms), or, more frequently, fungus.[229] Isolated aneurysms may also be associated with pulmonary arterial vasculitis in giant cell arteritis or Behçet's syndrome. Behçet's syndrome, which usually presents with oral and genital ulcers and uveitis, is a widespread vasculitis in which 5% of patients have pulmonary artery aneurysms from inflammatory destruction of the pulmonary arterial vasa vasorum. Hughes-Stovin syndrome may represent a subset of Behçet's syndrome without the oral or genital ulcers but with associated peripheral venous thrombosis.

Pulmonary artery aneurysms may occur in a main pulmonary artery or in a lobar or segmental artery and are either fusiform or saccular. Patients with isolated pulmonary artery aneurysms are usually asymptomatic, with lesions only recognized as a mass on chest radiography. Further evaluation is obtained with high-resolution CT, magnetic resonance angiography, or, classically, pulmonary artery angiography. Transesophageal echocardiography may be helpful for assessment of any associated thrombosis.

Rupture of a pulmonary artery aneurysm generally results in overwhelming hemoptysis or hemothorax, and aneurysms that are enlarging or symptomatic should be treated.[230] If the lesions are fairly peripheral, embolization may be performed.[231] In patients who have Behçet's or Hughes-Stovin syndrome, immunosuppressive agents may be helpful in reducing the associated symptoms. Anticoagulation is used cautiously. Resection of the lung, primary resection of the pulmonary artery with reanastomosis, and patch repair have been performed. In the case of vasculitis, there is a 25% recurrence rate[232] that may be mitigated by perioperative medical treatment with steroids and immunosuppressive medications.

Pulmonary Varix

Pulmonary varix is an aneurysmal dilation of a pulmonary vein. It may be seen in any area of the lung, and it is a very rare anomaly; as of 1988, only 71 cases had been reported.[233] It is believed that varying combinations of two processes may be important for the development of a varix: pulmonary venous hypertension and inflammatory changes in the area of the affected pulmonary vein. It has been described with bronchiectasis, tuberculosis, mitral valve disease, and congenital cardiac anomalies. Single lesions are usually asymptomatic; when symptoms are present, they are generally attributable to the associated cardiopulmonary condition. The age range at presentation is between 7 and 82 years, and most symptomatic patients present in their fourth to seventh decades of life.[234] There is an equal gender distribution. Pulmonary varix has been described as a surprise discovery at cervical mediastinoscopy.[235] It may also present with symptoms of cerebral embolism or hemoptysis from spontaneous rupture into a bronchus. In patients who have a varix from mitral valve disease, it is more frequently found in the right lung. When a pulmonary varix is identified incidentally, an evaluation for cardiac disease should ensue. On pulmonary angiography, a Müller maneuver (inspiratory effort against a closed glottis after expiration) increases the size of the varix, whereas a Valsalva maneuver decreases its size. CT or dynamic CT may be helpful. Three anatomic forms are recognized: saccular, tortuous, and confluent. The confluent form designates a dilation of the confluence of veins and is more frequently associated with mitral and left-sided heart disease.[233] Patients with asymptomatic pulmonary varices and without cardiac or infectious disease may be observed with a good prognosis.[236] If a cardiac anomaly is present, it should be repaired, and this will frequently result in regression of the varix.

Pulmonary Arteriovenous Malformations

As the name implies, pulmonary arteriovenous malformations involve a direct connection between branches of a pulmonary artery and vein. They may be acquired lesions from trauma, schistosomiasis, cancer, or actinomycosis and have been associated with the physiologic and hormonal changes of pregnancy. One third of patients have hereditary hemorrhagic telangiectasia (HHT or Osler-Weber-Rendu syndrome). Sixty-five percent of patients with pulmonary arteriovenous malformations have single lesions, of which more than 50% are less than 1 cm in size, and lesions are rarely larger than 5 cm. They are frequently subpleural in location. Patients may present with hemoptysis, chest pain, epistaxis, and palpitations; complications also include cerebral thrombosis, brain abscesses, and pneumothorax. Children are more likely to present with diffuse lesions associated with cyanosis and congestive failure.

The chest radiograph may demonstrate a noncalcified mass, and dynamic CT may be helpful in achieving a diagnosis (Fig. 9-16). Patients with suggestive radiographic findings should be evaluated for recurrent epistaxis, skin lesions, or hematuria (HHT) as well as a family history of similar complaints. HHT is a rare autosomal dominant abnormality that is associated with mucocutaneous and visceral telangiectasias. Between 7% and 15% of patients with HHT have pulmonary arteriovenous malformations; when pulmonary arteriovenous malformations are present, patients have an increased likelihood for complications including hemoptysis, polycythemia, epistaxis, cerebral bleeding, and brain abscesses.[237] Contrast-enhanced transthoracic echocardiography has been helpful in assessing patients with pulmonary arteriovenous malformations, with a sensitivity of 94%.

If the patient has HHT or is symptomatic, if the lesion is large, or if the diagnosis is questionable, surgical resection may be necessary. In the case of HHT, one half of patients left untreated progress to brain abscess and stroke.[238] If the lesion is resected, proximal vessel control is advisable. When telangiectasias are found, only symptomatic or enlarging lesions should be treated. When telangiectasias are present on the lung surface, it is unnecessary to resect them unless they are unusually large.

One other congenital anomaly of note is scimitar syndrome (Fig. 9-17). In this condition, the venous drainage from

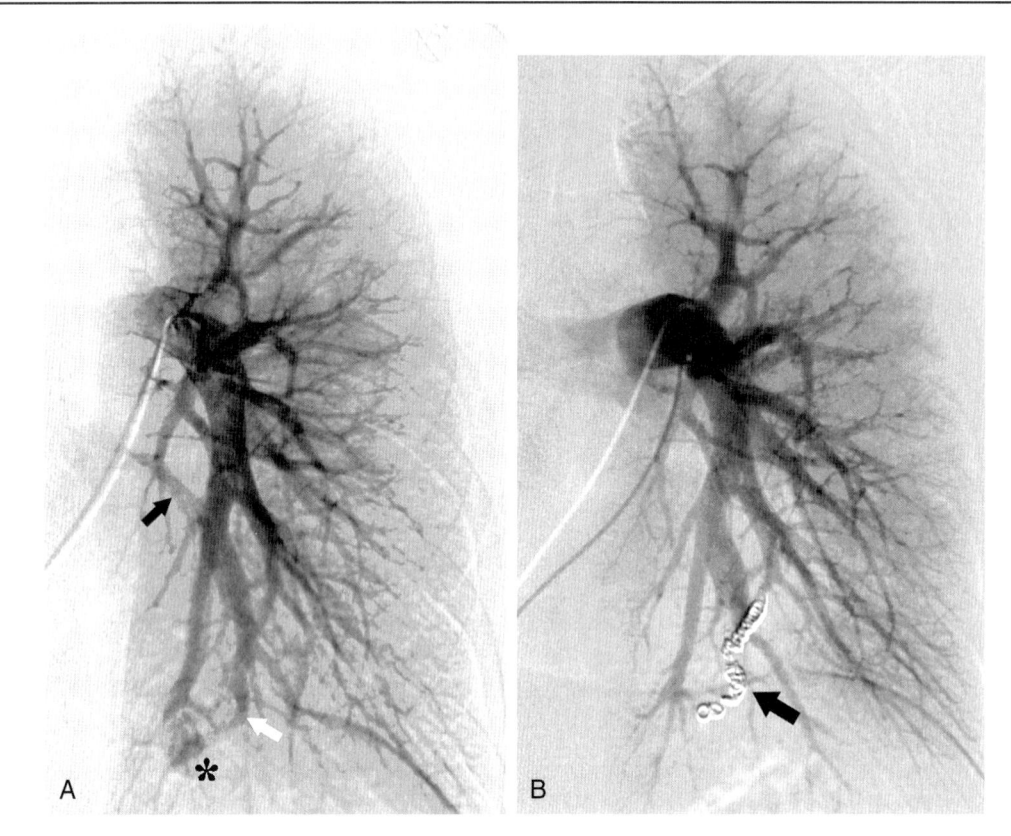

Figure 9–16
Pulmonary arteriovenous malformation. Selective left pulmonary arteriography and coil embolization in a 14-year-old girl. **A,** Left pulmonary arteriogram shows a tangle of vessels *(asterisk)* at left lung base with arterial supply *(white arrow)* from a basal branch of left lower lobe artery and early pulmonary venous opacification *(black arrow)*. **B,** After embolization of coils *(arrow)* by superselective catheterization, the malformation is occluded. *(Courtesy of Simon C. Kao, MD, Iowa City, IA.)*

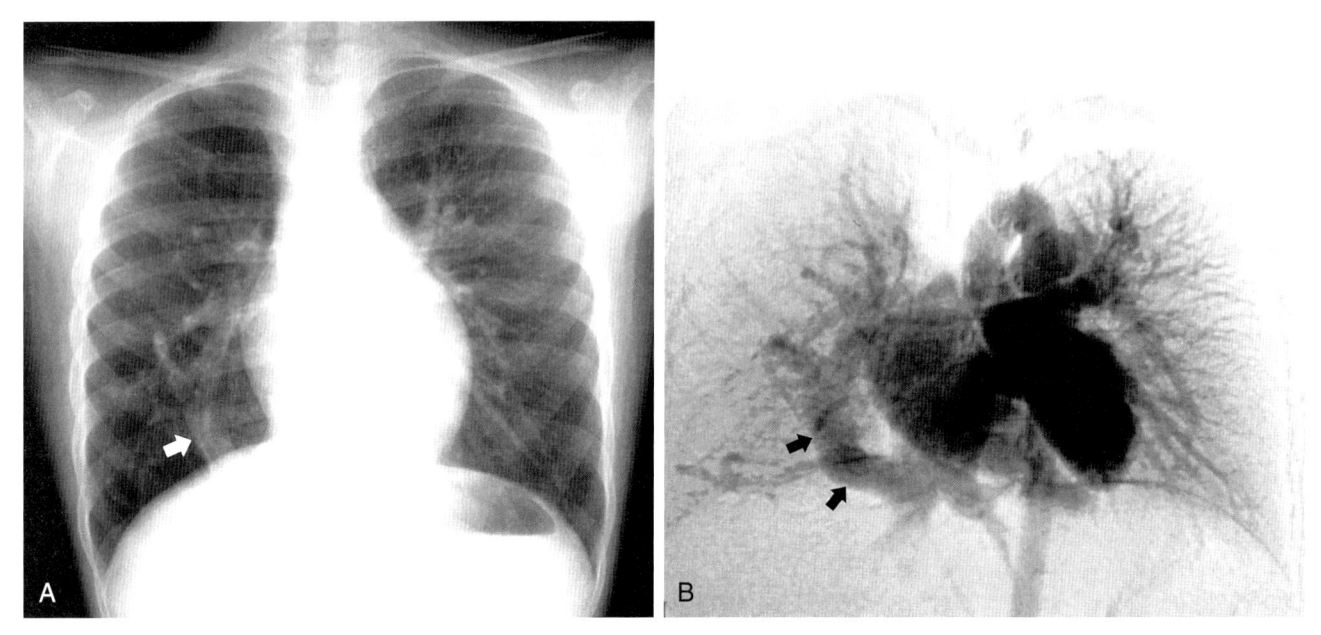

Figure 9–17
Scimitar syndrome. **A,** Frontal chest radiograph shows a curvilinear bandlike shadow *(arrow)* parallel to the right-sided heart border with broadening toward the right hemidiaphragm. **B,** Digital subtraction angiogram shows anomalous right pulmonary venous drainage *(arrows)* to the junction between the hepatic venous confluence and the inferior vena cava. *(Courtesy of Koji Takahashi, MD, Asahikawa Medical College, Asahikawa, Japan.)*

either part of the right lung or the entire right lung enters the inferior vena cava rather than the left atrium. Right lung arterial supply also may be anomalous with associated pulmonary sequestration or pulmonary hypertension. Left-to-right shunting may be so significant, akin to an atrial septal defect, that surgical repair may be necessary. Surgical options have recently been reviewed.[239]

CONCLUSION

This chapter reviews the wide range of congenital lung diseases. Abnormalities may involve the tracheobronchial tree, lung parenchyma, or pulmonary vasculature. Defects may be so severe as to result in stillbirth or profound neonatal respiratory distress. Other manifestations assume a more insidious course. Knowledge of pulmonary embryology and historical contributions relating to these disorders allows a logical diagnostic and therapeutic approach in most instances. Advances in technology, neonatal surgery, and antenatal diagnosis and treatment have led to a markedly improved outlook for patients with congenital lung diseases.

Acknowledgment

We would like to thank Mrs. Leslie James Middlebrooks for her expert assistance in the preparation of this chapter.

REFERENCES

1. Olutoye OO, et al. Prenatal diagnosis and management of congenital lobar emphysema. *J Pediatr Surg* 2000;**35**(5):792-5.
2. Kitano Y, Adzick NS. New developments in fetal lung surgery. *Curr Opin Pulm Med* 1999;**5**(6):383-9.
3. Fontanus N. Responsionum et curationum medicinalium. *Typis Ioannis Ianssonii* 1639.
4. Huber J. Observations aliquot de arteria singulari pulmoni concessa. *Acta Helv* 1777;**9**:85.
5. Rienhoff WFJ. Pneumonectomy; preliminary report of operative technique in 2 successful cases. *Bull Johns Hopkins Hosp* 1933;**53**:390-3.
6. Rienhoff WFJ, Reichert FL, Heuer GJ. Compensatory changes in the remaining lung following total pneumonectomy. *Bull Johns Hopkins Hosp* 1935;**57**:373.
7. Gross RE, Lewis JEJ. Defect of the anterior mediastinum: successful surgical repair. *Surg Gynecol Obstet* 1945;**80**:549.
8. Fisher CC, Tropea FJ, Barley CP. Congenital pulmonary cysts. *J Pediatr Surg* 1943;**23**:219.
9. Gross RE. Congenital cystic lung: successful pneumonectomy in a 3-week-old baby. *Ann Surg* 1946;**123**:229-37.
10. Chinoy MR. Lung growth and development. *Front Biosci* 2003;**8**:d392-415.
11. Galambos C, Demello DE. Regulation of alveologenesis: clinical implications of impaired growth. *Pathology* 2008;**40**(2):124-40.
12. Sadler TW. Respiratory system. In: Sadler TW, editor. *Langman's medical embryology*. Philadelphia: Lippincott Williams & Wilkins; 2004.
13. Bellusci S, et al. Fibroblast growth factor 10 (FGF10) and branching morphogenesis in the embryonic mouse lung. *Development* 1997;**124**(23):4867-78.
14. Lebeche D, Malpel S, Cardoso WV. Fibroblast growth factor interactions in the developing lung. *Mech Dev* 1999;**86**(1-2):125-36.
15. Kitano Y, et al. Tracheal occlusion in the fetal rat: a new experimental model for the study of accelerated lung growth. *J Pediatr Surg* 1998;**33**(12):1741-4.
16. Papadakis K, et al. Fetal lung growth after tracheal ligation is not solely a pressure phenomenon. *J Pediatr Surg* 1997;**32**(2):347-51.
17. Langston C. New concepts in the pathology of congenital lung malformations. *Semin Pediatr Surg* 2003;**12**(1):17-37.
18. Manschot HJ, van den Anker JN, Tibboel D. Tracheal agenesis. *Anaesthesia* 1994;**49**(9):788-90.
19. Longacre JJ, Carter BN, Quill LM. An experimental study of some of the physiological changes following total pneumonectomy. *J Thorac Surg* 1937;**6**:237.
20. Lester CW, Cournand A, Riley RL. Pulmonary function after pneumonectomy in children. *J Thorac Surg* 1942;**11**:529.
21. Peters RM, et al. Respiratory and circulatory studies after pneumonectomy in childhood. *J Thorac Surg* 1950;**20**(3):484-93.
22. Giammona ST, et al. The late cardiopulmonary effects of childhood pneumonectomy. *Pediatrics* 1966;**37**(1):79-88.
23. Payne WA. Congenital absence of the trachea. *Brooklyn Med J* 1900;**14**:568.
24. Lander TA, et al. Tracheal agenesis in newborns. *Laryngoscope* 2004;**114**(9):1633-6.
25. De Jose Maria B, et al. Management of tracheal agenesis. *Paediatr Anaesth* 2000;**10**(4):441-4.
26. Floyd J, Campbell Jr DC, Dominy DE. Agenesis of the trachea. *Am Rev Respir Dis* 1962;**86**:557-60.
27. Koltai PJ, Quiney R. Tracheal agenesis. *Ann Otol Rhinol Laryngol* 1992;**101**(7):560-6.
28. Evans JA, Greenberg CR, Erdile L. Tracheal agenesis revisited: analysis of associated anomalies. *Am J Med Genet* 1999;**82**(5):415-22.
29. Milstein JM, Lau M, Bickers RG. Tracheal agenesis in infants with VATER association. *Am J Dis Child* 1985;**139**(1):77-80.
30. Evans JA, Reggin J, Greenberg C. Tracheal agenesis and associated malformations: a comparison with tracheoesophageal fistula and the VACTERL. association. *Am J Med Genet* 1985;**21**(1):21-38.
31. Hiyama E, et al. Surgical management of tracheal agenesis. *J Thorac Cardiovasc Surg* 1994;**108**(5):830-3.
32. Soh H, et al. Tracheal agenesis in a child who survived for 6 years. *J Pediatr Surg* 1999;**34**(10):1541-3.
33. Josephson GD, Brown-Wagner M, Josephson JS. Agenesis of the trachea. *Clin Pediatr (Phila)* 1995;**34**(1):57-9.
34. Wei JL, Rodeberg D, Thompson DM. Tracheal agenesis with anomalies found in both VACTERL and TACRD associations. *Int J Pediatr Otorhinolaryngol* 2003;**67**(9):1013-7.
35. Kunisaki SM, et al. Extracorporeal membrane oxygenation as a bridge to definitive tracheal reconstruction in neonates. *J Pediatr Surg* 2008;**43**(5):800-4.
36. Jacobs JP, et al. Tracheal allograft reconstruction: the total North American and worldwide pediatric experiences. *Ann Thorac Surg* 1999;**68**(3):1043-51:discussion 1052.
37. Macchiarini P, et al. Clinical transplantation of a tissue-engineered airway. *Lancet* 2008;**372**(9655):2023-30.
38. Cantrell JR, Guild HG. Congenital stenosis of the trachea. *Am J Surg* 1964;**108**:297-305.
39. Loeff DS, et al. Congenital tracheal stenosis: a review of 22 patients from 1965 to 1987. *J Pediatr Surg* 1988;**23**(8):744-8.
40. Anton-Pacheco JL, et al. Management of congenital tracheal stenosis in infancy. *Eur J Cardiothorac Surg* 2006;**29**(6):991-6.
41. Herrera P, et al. The current state of congenital tracheal stenosis. *Pediatr Surg Int* 2007;**23**(11):1033-44.
42. Chiu PP, Kim PC. Prognostic factors in the surgical treatment of congenital tracheal stenosis: a multicenter analysis of the literature. *J Pediatr Surg* 2006;**41**(1):221-5:discussion 221-5.
43. Hoppe H, et al. Grading airway stenosis down to the segmental level using virtual bronchoscopy. *Chest* 2004;**125**(2):704-11.
44. DeLorimer AA. Congenital malformations and neonatal problems of the respiratory tract. In: Welch KJ, Randolph JG, Ravitch MM, editors. *Pediatric surgery*. Chicago: Mosby–Year Book; 1986. p. 631.
45. Grillo HC. Tracheal surgery. *Scand J Thorac Cardiovasc Surg* 1983;**17**(1):67-77.
46. Dykes EH, et al. Reduced tracheal growth after reconstruction with pericardium. *J Pediatr Surg* 1990;**25**(1):25-9.
47. Chahine AA, Tam V, Ricketts RR. Use of the aortic homograft in the reconstruction of complex tracheobronchial tree injuries. *J Pediatr Surg* 1999;**34**(5):891-4.
48. Walker LK, Wetzel RC, Haller Jr JA. Extracorporeal membrane oxygenation for perioperative support during congenital tracheal stenosis repair. *Anesth Analg* 1992;**75**(5):825-9.
49. Grillo HC, et al. Management of congenital tracheal stenosis by means of slide tracheoplasty or resection and reconstruction, with long-term follow-up of growth after slide tracheoplasty. *J Thorac Cardiovasc Surg* 2002;**123**(1):145-52.
50. Hagl S, et al. Modified sliding tracheal plasty using the bridging bronchus for repair of long-segment tracheal stenosis. *Ann Thorac Surg* 2008;**85**(3):1118-20.
51. Backer CL, et al. Repair of congenital tracheal stenosis with a free tracheal autograft. *J Thorac Cardiovasc Surg* 1998;**115**(4):869-74.
52. Backer CL, et al. Tracheal surgery in children: an 18-year review of four techniques. *Eur J Cardiothorac Surg* 2001;**19**(6):777-84.
53. Dodge-Khatami A, et al. Healing of a free tracheal autograft is enhanced by topical vascular endothelial growth factor in an experimental rabbit model. *J Thorac Cardiovasc Surg* 2001;**122**(3):554-61.

54. Muraji T, et al. Slide tracheoplasty: a case report of successful concomitant reconstruction of extensive congenital tracheal stenosis and pulmonary artery sling. *J Pediatr Surg* 1998;**33**(11):1658-9.
55. Harrison MR, et al. Resection of distal tracheal stenosis in a baby with agenesis of the lung. *J Pediatr Surg* 1980;**15**(6):938-43.
56. Brown SB, et al. Tracheobronchial stenosis in infants: successful balloon dilation therapy. *Radiology* 1987;**164**(2):475-8.
57. Messineo A, et al. The balloon posterior tracheal split: a technique for managing tracheal stenosis in the premature infant. *J Pediatr Surg* 1992;**27**(8):1142-4.
58. Rideout DT, et al. The absence of clinically significant tracheomalacia in patients having esophageal atresia without tracheoesophageal fistula. *J Pediatr Surg* 1991;**26**(11):1303-5.
59. Slany E, et al. Tracheal instability in tracheo-esophageal abnormalities. *Z Kinderchir* 1990;**45**(2):78-85.
60. Contencin P, Narcy P. Gastropharyngeal reflux in infants and children. A pharyngeal pH monitoring study. *Arch Otolaryngol Head Neck Surg* 1992;**118**(10):1028-30.
61. Davies MR, Cywes S. The flaccid trachea and tracheoesophageal congenital anomalies. *J Pediatr Surg* 1978;**13**(4):363-7.
62. Filler RM, et al. The use of expandable metallic airway stents for tracheobronchial obstruction in children. *J Pediatr Surg* 1995;**30**(7):1050-5:discussion 1055-6.
63. Greenholz SK, Karrer FM, Lilly JR. Contemporary surgery of tracheomalacia. *J Pediatr Surg* 1986;**21**(6):511-4.
64. Schwartz MZ, Filler RM. Tracheal compression as a cause of apnea following repair of tracheoesophageal fistula: treatment by aortopexy. *J Pediatr Surg* 1980;**15**(6):842-8.
65. Kamata S, et al. Pexis of the great vessels for patients with tracheobronchomalacia in infancy. *J Pediatr Surg* 2000;**35**(3):454-7.
66. Atwell SW. Major anomalies of the tracheobronchial tree: with a list of the minor anomalies. *Dis Chest* 1967;**52**(5):611-5.
67. McLaughlin FJ, et al. Tracheal bronchus: association with respiratory morbidity in childhood. *J Pediatr* 1985;**106**(5):751-5.
68. Sotile SC, Brady MB, Brogdon BG. Accessory cardiac bronchus: demonstration by computed tomography. *J Comput Tomogr* 1988;**12**(2):144-6.
69. Ramsay BH, Byron FX. Mucocele, congenital bronchiectasis, and bronchiogenic cyst. *J Thorac Surg* 1953;**26**(1):21-30.
70. Mori M, et al. Bronchial atresia: report of a case and review of the literature. *Surg Today* 1993;**23**(5):449-54.
71. Jederlinic PJ, et al. Congenital bronchial atresia. A report of 4 cases and a review of the literature. *Medicine (Baltimore)* 1987;**66**(1):73-83.
72. Matsushima H, et al. Congenital bronchial atresia: radiologic findings in nine patients. *J Comput Assist Tomogr* 2002;**26**(5):860-4.
73. Mechoulan A, et al. Is the bronchial atresia prenatal diagnosis possible? *Gynecol Obstet Fertil* 2008;**36**(4):407-12.
74. Haller Jr JA, et al. The natural history of bronchial atresia. Serial observations of a case from birth to operative correction. *J Thorac Cardiovasc Surg* 1980;**79**(6):868-72.
75. Jones VF, et al. Familial congenital bronchiectasis: Williams-Campbell syndrome. *Pediatr Pulmonol* 1993;**16**(4):263-7.
76. Kuhn JP, Brody AS. High-resolution CT of pediatric lung disease. *Radiol Clin North Am* 2002;**40**(1):89-110.
77. Zamir O, et al. Lung resection for bronchiectasis in children. *Z Kinderchir* 1987;**42**(5):282-5.
78. Balkanli K, et al. Surgical management of bronchiectasis: analysis and short-term results in 238 patients. *Eur J Cardiothorac Surg* 2003;**24**(5):699-702.
79. Mounier-Kuhn P. Dilatation de la trachee: constatations radiographiques et bronchoscopiques. *Lyon Med* 1932;**150**:106-9.
80. Woodring JH, Howard 2nd RS, Rehm SR. Congenital tracheobronchomegaly (Mounier-Kuhn syndrome): a report of 10 cases and review of the literature. *J Thorac Imaging* 1991;**6**(2):1-0.
81. Katz I, Levine M, Herman P. Tracheobronchiomegaly. The Mounier-Kuhn syndrome. *Am J Roentgenol Radium Ther Nucl Med* 1962;**88**:1084-94.
82. Johnson FR, Green FA. Tracheobronchomegaly: report of five cases and demonstration of familial occurrence. *Am Rev Respir Dis* 1965;**91**:35-50.
83. Bhutani VK, Ritchie WG, Shaffer TH. Acquired tracheomegaly in very preterm neonates. *Am J Dis Child* 1986;**140**(5):449-52.
84. Woodring JH, et al. Acquired tracheomegaly in adults as a complication of diffuse pulmonary fibrosis. *AJR Am J Roentgenol* 1989;**152**(4):743-7.
85. Blake MA, Chaoui AS, Barish MA. Thoracic case of the day. Thoracic myelolipomatosis. *AJR Am J Roentgenol* 1999;**173**(3):821-823-4.
86. Breatnach E, Abbott GC, Fraser RG. Dimensions of the normal human trachea. *AJR Am J Roentgenol* 1984;**142**(5):903-6.
87. Griscom NT, Wohl ME. Dimensions of the growing trachea related to age and gender. *AJR Am J Roentgenol* 1986;**146**(2):233-7.
88. Gaissert HA, et al. Temporary and permanent restoration of airway continuity with the tracheal T-tube. *J Thorac Cardiovasc Surg* 1994;**107**(2):600-6.
89. Stern Y, Willging JP, Cotton RT. Use of Montgomery T-tube in laryngotracheal reconstruction in children: is it safe? *Ann Otol Rhinol Laryngol* 1998;**107**(12):1006-9.
90. Drain AJ, et al. Double lung transplantation in a patient with tracheobronchomegaly (Mounier-Kuhn syndrome). *J Heart Lung Transplant* 2006;**25**(1):134-6.
91. Chitkara AE, et al. Complete laryngotracheoesophageal cleft: complicated management issues. *Laryngoscope* 2003;**113**(8):1314-20.
92. Hugh-Jones P, Whimster W. The etiology and management of disabling emphysema. *Am Rev Respir Dis* 1978;**117**(2):343-78.
93. Macarthur AM, Fountain SW. Intracavity suction and drainage in the treatment of emphysematous bullae. *Thorax* 1977;**32**(6):668-72.
94. Donahoe PK, Gee PE. Complete laryngotracheoesophageal cleft: management and repair. *J Pediatr Surg* 1984;**19**(2):143-8.
95. Harmon CM, Coran AG. Congenital anomalies of the esophagus. In: O'Neill JAJ, Rowe MI, Grosfeld JL, editors. *Pediatric surgery*. St. Louis: Mosby; 1998.
96. Gross RE. *The Surgery of infancy and childhood*, Philadelphia: W.B. Saunders; 1953.
97. Harmon CM, Coran AG, Grosfeld JL, et al. Congenital anomalies of the esophagus. *Pediatric Surgery*. Philadelphia: Mosby Elsevier; 2006.
98. Haight C, Towsley H. Congenital atresia of the esophagus with tracheoesophageal fistula: extrapleural ligation of the fistula and end-to-end anastomosis of the esophageal segments. *Surg Gynecol Obstet* 1943;**76**:672.
99. Manning PB, et al. Fifty years' experience with esophageal atresia and tracheoesophageal fistula. Beginning with Cameron Haight's first operation in 1935. *Ann Surg* 1986;**204**(4):446-53.
100. Gupta DK, et al. Esophageal replacement in the neonatal period in infants with esophageal atresia and tracheoesophageal fistula. *J Pediatr Surg* 2007;**42**(9):1471-7.
101. Konkin DE, et al. Outcomes in esophageal atresia and tracheoesophageal fistula. *J Pediatr Surg* 2003;**38**(12):1726-9.
102. Kovesi T, Rubin S. Long-term complications of congenital esophageal atresia and/or tracheoesophageal fistula. *Chest* 2004;**126**(3):915-25.
103. Little DC, et al. Long-term analysis of children with esophageal atresia and tracheoesophageal fistula. *J Pediatr Surg* 2003;**38**(6):852-6.
104. Richter GT, et al. Endoscopic management of recurrent tracheoesophageal fistula. *J Pediatr Surg* 2008;**43**(1):238-45.
105. Allal H, et al. Thoracoscopic repair of H-type tracheoesophageal fistula in the newborn: a technical case report. *J Pediatr Surg* 2004;**39**(10):1568-70.
106. Aziz GA, Schier F. Thoracoscopic ligation of a tracheoesophageal H-type fistula in a newborn. *J Pediatr Surg* 2005;**40**:e35-6.
107. Holcomb 3rd GW, et al. Thoracoscopic repair of esophageal atresia and tracheoesophageal fistula: a multi-institutional analysis. *Ann Surg* 2005;**242**(3):422-8:discussion 428-30.
108. Nguyen T, et al. Thoracoscopic repair of esophageal atresia and tracheoesophageal fistula: lessons learned. *J Laparoendosc Adv Surg Tech A* 2006;**16**(2):174-8.
109. Rothenberg SS. Thoracoscopic repair of esophageal atresia and tracheo-esophageal fistula. *Semin Pediatr Surg* 2005;**14**(1):2-7.
110. Tsao K, Lee H. Extrapleural thoracoscopic repair of esophageal atresia with tracheoesophageal fistula. *Pediatr Surg Int* 2005;**21**(4):308-10.
111. van der Zee DC, et al. Thoracoscopic elongation of the esophagus in long gap esophageal atresia. *J Pediatr Surg* 2007;**42**(10):1785-8.
112. Kalfa N, et al. Tolerance of laparoscopy and thoracoscopy in neonates. *Pediatrics* 2005;**116**(6):e785-91.
113. Krosnar S, Baxter A. Thoracoscopic repair of esophageal atresia with tracheoesophageal fistula: anesthetic and intensive care management of a series of eight neonates. *Paediatr Anaesth* 2005;**15**(7):541-6.
114. Mariano ER, et al. Successful thoracoscopic repair of esophageal atresia with tracheoesophageal fistula in a newborn with single ventricle physiology. *Anesth Analg* 2005;**101**(4):1000–102, table of contents.
115. Sharma S, et al. Azygos vein preservation in primary repair of esophageal atresia with tracheoesophageal fistula. *Pediatr Surg Int* 2007;**23**(12):1215-8.
116. Upadhyaya VD, et al. Is ligation of azygos vein necessary in primary repair of tracheoesophageal fistula with esophageal atresia? *Eur J Pediatr Surg* 2007;**17**(4):236-40.
117. DiFiore JW, Alexander F. Congenital bronchobiliary fistula in association with right-sided congenital diaphragmatic hernia. *J Pediatr Surg* 2002;**37**(8):1208-9.
118. Bringas Bollada M, et al. Congenital bronchobiliary fistula diagnosed in adult age. *Med Intensiva* 2006;**30**(9):475-6.
119. de Carvalho CR, et al. Congenital bronchobiliary fistula: first case in an adult. *Thorax* 1988;**43**(10):792-3.
120. Yamaguchi M, et al. Congenital bronchobiliary fistula in adults. *South Med J* 1990;**83**(7):851-2.

121. Chang CC, Giulian BB. Congenital bronchobiliary fistula. *Radiology* 1985;**156**(1):82.
122. Kalayoglu M, Olcay I. Congenital bronchobiliary fistula associated with esophageal atresia and tracheo-esophageal fistula. *J Pediatr Surg* 1976;**11**(3):463-4.
123. Chan YT, et al. Congenital bronchobiliary fistula associated with biliary atresia. *Br J Surg* 1984;**71**(3):240-1.
124. Sane SM, Sieber WK, Girdany BR. Congenital bronchobiliary fistula. *Surgery* 1971;**69**(4):599-608.
125. Aguilar C, et al. Congenital bronchobiliary fistula detected by cholescintigraphy. *Rev Gastroenterol Peru* 2005;**25**(2):216-8.
126. Egrari S, et al. Congenital bronchobiliary fistula: diagnosis and postoperative surveillance with HIDA scan. *J Pediatr Surg* 1996;**31**(6):785-6.
127. Hourigan JS, et al. Congenital bronchobiliary fistula: MRI appearance. *Pediatr Radiol* 2004;**34**(4):348-50.
128. Gauderer MW, Oiticica C, Bishop HC. Congenital bronchobiliary fistula: management of the involved hepatic segment. *J Pediatr Surg* 1993;**28**(3):452-5.
129. Uyama T, et al. CEA and CA 19-9 in benign pulmonary or mediastinal cystic lesions. *J Surg Oncol* 1989;**41**(2):103-8.
130. Cohen MD, et al. Evaluation of pulmonary parenchymal disease by magnetic resonance imaging. *Br J Radiol* 1987;**60**(711):223-30.
131. Becmeur F, et al. Pulmonary sequestrations: prenatal ultrasound diagnosis, treatment, and outcome. *J Pediatr Surg* 1998;**33**(3):492-6.
132. Hubbard AM, Crombleholme TM. Anomalies and malformations affecting the fetal/neonatal chest. *Semin Roentgenol* 1998;**33**(2):117-25.
133. Bailey PV, et al. Congenital bronchopulmonary malformations. Diagnostic and therapeutic considerations. *J Thorac Cardiovasc Surg* 1990;**99**(4):597-602:discussion 602-3.
134. Gustafson RA, et al. Intralobar sequestration. A missed diagnosis. *Ann Thorac Surg* 1989;**47**(6):841-7.
135. Wales PW, et al. Horseshoe lung in association with other foregut anomalies: what is the significance?. *J Pediatr Surg* 2002;**37**(8):1205-7.
136. Takahashi M, et al. Horseshoe lung: demonstration by electron-beam CT. *Br J Radiol* 1997;**70**(837):964-6.
137. Suen HC, et al. Surgical management and radiological characteristics of bronchogenic cysts. *Ann Thorac Surg* 1993;**55**(2):476-81.
138. Volpi A, et al. Left atrial compression by a mediastinal bronchogenic cyst presenting with paroxysmal atrial fibrillation. *Thorax* 1988;**43**(3):216-7.
139. Worsnop CJ, Teichtahl H, Clarke CP. Bronchogenic cyst: a cause of pulmonary artery obstruction and breathlessness. *Ann Thorac Surg* 1993;**55**(5):1254-5.
140. St-Georges R, et al. Clinical spectrum of bronchogenic cysts of the mediastinum and lung in the adult. *Ann Thorac Surg* 1991;**52**(1):6-13.
141. Wildi SM, et al. Diagnosis of benign cysts of the mediastinum: the role and risks of EUS and FNA. *Gastrointest Endosc* 2003;**58**(3):362-8.
142. Haller Jr JA, et al. Surgical management of lung bud anomalies: lobar emphysema, bronchogenic cyst, cystic adenomatoid malformation, and intralobar pulmonary sequestration. *Ann Thorac Surg* 1979;**28**(1):33-43.
143. Bolton JW, Shahian DM. Asymptomatic bronchogenic cysts: what is the best management? *Ann Thorac Surg* 1992;**53**(6):1134-7.
144. Ribet ME, Copin MC, Gosselin B. Bronchogenic cysts of the mediastinum. *J Thorac Cardiovasc Surg* 1995;**109**(5):1003-10.
145. Tanita M, et al. Malignant melanoma arising from cutaneous bronchogenic cyst of the scapular area. *J Am Acad Dermatol* 2002;**46**(2 Suppl Case Reports):S19-21.
146. Hazelrigg SR, et al. Thoracoscopic resection of mediastinal cysts. *Ann Thorac Surg* 1993;**56**(3):659-60.
147. Sbokos CG, McMillan IK. Agenesis of the lung. *Br J Dis Chest* 1977;**71**(3):183-97.
148. Say B, et al. Agenesis of the lung associated with a chromosome abnormality (46, XX,2p+). *J Med Genet* 1980;**17**(6):477-8.
149. Nazir Z, et al. Pulmonary agenesis—vascular airway compression and gastroesophageal reflux influence outcome. *J Pediatr Surg* 2006;**41**(6):1165-9.
150. Greenbough A. Factors adversely affecting lung growth. *Paediatr Respir Rev* 2000;**1**:314-20.
151. Bush A, Hogg J, Chitty LS. Cystic lung lesions—prenatal diagnosis and management. *Prenat Diagn* 2008;**28**(7):604-11.
152. Mardini MK, Nyhan WL. Agenesis of the lung. Report of four patients with unusual anomalies. *Chest* 1985;**87**(4):522-7.
153. Massumi R, Taleghani M, Ellis I. Cardiorespiratory studies in congenital absence of one lung. *J Thorac Cardiovasc Surg* 1966;**51**(4):561-8.
154. Page DV, Stocker JT. Anomalies associated with pulmonary hypoplasia. *Am Rev Respir Dis* 1982;**125**(2):216-21.
155. Cooney TP, Thurlbeck WM. Pulmonary hypoplasia in Down's syndrome. *N Engl J Med* 1982;**307**(19):1170-3.
156. Lally KP, et al. Congenital diaphragmatic hernia. Stabilization and repair on ECMO. *Ann Surg* 1992;**216**(5):569-73.
157. Weber TR, et al. Improved survival in congenital diaphragmatic hernia with evolving therapeutic strategies. *Arch Surg* 1998;**133**(5):498-502:discussion 502-3.
158. West KW, et al. Delayed surgical repair and ECMO improves survival in congenital diaphragmatic hernia. *Ann Surg* 1992;**216**(4):454-60:discussion 460-2.
159. Miguet D, et al. Preoperative stabilization using high-frequency oscillatory ventilation in the management of congenital diaphragmatic hernia. *Crit Care Med* 1994;**22**(Suppl. 9):S77-82.
160. Lee R, et al. Bilateral lung transplantation for pulmonary hypoplasia caused by congenital diaphragmatic hernia. *J Thorac Cardiovasc Surg* 2003;**126**(1):295-7.
161. Azizkhan RG, Crombleholme TM. Congenital cystic lung disease: contemporary antenatal and postnatal management. *Pediatr Surg Int* 2008;**24**(6):643-57.
162. Eber E. Antenatal diagnosis of congenital thoracic malformations: early surgery, late surgery, or no surgery? *Semin Respir Crit Care Med* 2007;**28**(3):355-66.
163. Wilson RD. In utero therapy for fetal thoracic abnormalities. *Prenat Diagn* 2008;**28**(7):619-25.
164. Berlinger NT, Porto DP, Thompson TR. Infantile lobar emphysema. *Ann Otol Rhinol Laryngol* 1987;**96**(1 Pt 1):106-11.
165. Bolande RB, Schneider AF, Boggs JD. Infantile lobar emphysema; an etiological concept. *AMA Arch Pathol* 1956;**61**(4):289-94.
166. Hendren WH. Repair of laryngotracheoesophageal cleft using interposition of a strap muscle. *J Pediatr Surg* 1976;**11**(3):425-9.
167. Lincoln JC, et al. Congenital lobar emphysema. *Ann Surg* 1971;**173**(1):55-62.
168. Scully RE, et al. Case records of the Massachusetts General Hospital. Weekly clinicopathological exercises. Case 20-1997. A 74-year-old man with progressive cough, dyspnea, and pleural thickening. *N Engl J Med* 1997;**336**(26):1895-903.
169. Tapper D, et al. Polyalveolar lobe: anatomic and physiologic parameters and their relationship to congenital lobar emphysema. *J Pediatr Surg* 1980;**15**(6):931-7.
170. Hendren WH, McKee DM. Lobar emphysema of infancy. *J Pediatr Surg* 1966;**1**:24.
171. Markowitz RI, et al. Congenital lobar emphysema. The roles of CT and V/Q scan. *Clin Pediatr (Phila)* 1989;**28**(1):19-23.
172. Cooney DR, Menke JA, Allen JE. "Acquired" lobar emphysema: a complication of respiratory distress in premature infants. *J Pediatr Surg* 1977;**12**(6):897-904.
173. Gupta R, et al. Management of congenital lobar emphysema with endobronchial intubation and controlled ventilation. *Anesth Analg* 1998;**86**(1):71-3.
174. Goto H, et al. High-frequency jet ventilation for resection of congenital lobar emphysema. *Anesth Analg* 1987;**66**(7):684-6.
175. Korngold HW, Baker JM. Non-surgical treatment of unilobar obstructive emphysema of the newborn. *Pediatrics* 1954;**14**(4):296-304.
176. Phillipos EZ, Libsekal K. Flexible bronchoscopy in the management of congenital lobar emphysema in the neonate. *Can Respir J* 1998;**5**(3):219-21.
177. DeMuth GR, Sloan H. Congenital lobar emphysema: long-term effects and sequelae in treated cases. *Surgery* 1966;**59**(4):601-7.
178. Sloan H. Lobar obstructive emphysema in infancy treated by lobectomy. *J Thorac Surg* 1953;**26**(1):1-20.
179. Ozcelik U, et al. Congenital lobar emphysema: evaluation and long-term follow-up of thirty cases at a single center. *Pediatr Pulmonol* 2003;**35**(5):384-91.
180. Azizkhan RG, et al. Acquired lobar emphysema (overinflation): clinical and pathological evaluation of infants requiring lobectomy. *J Pediatr Surg* 1992;**27**(8):1145-51:discussion 1151-2.
181. Jaffe RB. Balloon dilation of congenital and acquired stenosis of the trachea and bronchi. *Radiology* 1997;**203**(2):405-9.
182. Dogan R, et al. Surgical management of infants with congenital lobar emphysema and concomitant congenital heart disease. *Heart Surg Forum* 2004(6):7:E644-9.
183. Tsunezuka Y, et al. Progressive intraparenchymal bronchogenic cyst in a neonate. *Ann Thorac Cardiovasc Surg* 2008;**14**(1):32-4.
184. Baldi BG, et al. Lung cyst: an unusual manifestation of Niemann-Pick disease. *Respirology* 2009;**14**(1):134-6.
185. Domizio P, et al. Malignant mesenchymoma associated with a congenital lung cyst in a child: case report and review of the literature. *Pediatr Pathol* 1990;**10**(5):785-97.
186. Mendeloff EN. Sequestrations, congenital cystic adenomatoid malformations, and congenital lobar emphysema. *Semin Thorac Cardiovasc Surg* 2004;**16**(3):209-14.
187. Randel RC, Mannino FL. One-lung high-frequency ventilation in the management of an acquired neonatal pulmonary cyst. *J Perinatol* 1989;**9**(1):66-8.
188. Ch'In KY, Tang MY. Congenital adenomatoid malformation of one lobe of a lung with general anasarca. *Arch Pathol (Chic)* 1949;**48**(3):221-9.
189. Adzick NS, et al. Fetal lung lesions: management and outcome. *Am J Obstet Gynecol* 1998;**179**(4):884-9.

190. Mashiach R, et al. Antenatal ultrasound diagnosis of congenital cystic adenomatoid malformation of the lung: spontaneous resolution in utero. *J Clin Ultrasound* 1993;**21**(7):453-7.
191. Taguchi T, et al. Antenatal diagnosis and surgical management of congenital cystic adenomatoid malformation of the lung. *Fetal Diagn Ther* 1995;**10**(6):400-7.
192. Stocker JT, Madewell JE, Drake RM. Congenital cystic adenomatoid malformation of the lung. Classification and morphologic spectrum. *Hum Pathol* 1977;**8**(2):155-71.
193. Fitzgerald DA. Congenital cyst adenomatoid malformations: resect some and observe all? *Paediatr Respir Rev* 2007;**8**(1):67-76.
194. Aziz D, et al. Perinatally diagnosed asymptomatic congenital cystic adenomatoid malformation: to resect or not? *J Pediatr Surg* 2004;**39**(3):329-34:discussion 329-34.
195. Adzick NS, Farmer DL, et al. Cysts of the lungs and mediastinum. In: Grosfeld JL, editor. *Pediatric surgery*. Philadelphia: Mosby Elsevier; 2006. p. 956-7.
196. Laberge JM, Bratu I, Flageole H. The management of asymptomatic congenital lung malformations. *Paediatr Respir Rev* 2004;**5**(Suppl A):S305-12.
197. Kim HK, et al. Treatment of congenital cystic adenomatoid malformation: should lobectomy always be performed? *Ann Thorac Surg* 2008;**86**:249-53.
198. Brown MF, et al. Successful prenatal management of hydrops, caused by congenital cystic adenomatoid malformation, using serial aspirations. *J Pediatr Surg* 1995;**30**(7):1098-9.
199. Chow PC, et al. Management and outcome of antenatally diagnosed congenital cystic adenomatoid malformation of the lung. *Hong Kong Med J* 2007;**13**(1):31-9.
200. Mani H, Suarez E, Stocker JT. The morphologic spectrum of infantile lobar emphysema: a study of 33 cases. *Paediatr Respir Rev* 2004;**5**(Suppl A):S313-20.
201. Unger JM, England DM, Bogust GA. Interstitial emphysema in adults: recognition and prognostic implications. *J Thorac Imaging* 1989;**4**(1):86-94.
202. Hislop A, Reid L. New pathological findings in emphysema of childhood. 1. Polyalveolar lobe with emphysema. *Thorax* 1970;**25**(6):682-90.
203. Munnell ER, Lambird PA, Austin RL. Polyalveolar lobe causing lobar emphysema of infancy. *Ann Thorac Surg* 1973;**16**(6):624-8.
204. Cleveland RH, Weber B. Retained fetal lung liquid in congenital lobar emphysema: a possible predictor of polyalveolar lobe. *Pediatr Radiol* 1993;**23**(4):291-5.
205. Wagenvoort CA, Zondervan PE. Polyalveolar lobe and congenital cystic adenomatoid malformation type II: are they related? *Pediatr Pathol* 1991;**11**(2):311-20.
206. Huber A, et al. Congenital pulmonary lymphangiectasia. *Pediatr Pulmonol* 1991;**10**(4):310-3.
207. Chapdelaine J, et al. Unilobar congenital pulmonary lymphangiectasis mimicking congenital lobar emphysema: an underestimated presentation? *J Pediatr Surg* 2004;**39**(5):677-80.
208. Bellini C, et al. Multimodal imaging in the congenital pulmonary lymphangiectasia–congenital chylothorax–hydrops fetalis continuum. *Lymphology* 2004;**37**(1):22-30.
209. Okumura Y, et al. Pulmonary lymphangiectasis in an asymptomatic adult. *Respiration* 2006;**73**(1):114-6.
210. Hirano H, et al. Autopsy case of congenital pulmonary lymphangiectasis. *Pathol Int* 2004;**54**(7):532-6.
211. Barker PM, et al. Primary pulmonary lymphangiectasia in infancy and childhood. *Eur Respir J* 2004;**24**(3):413-9.
212. Dempsey EM, et al. Congenital pulmonary lymphangiectasia presenting as nonimmune fetal hydrops and severe respiratory distress at birth: not uniformly fatal. *Pediatr Pulmonol* 2005;**40**(3):270-4.
213. Ester CR, Barker PM. Pulmonary lymphangiectasis: diagnosis and clinical course. *Paediatr Pulmonol* 2004;**38**:308-13.
214. Bellini C, et al. Congenital pulmonary lymphangiectasia. *Orphanet J Rare Dis* 2006;**1**:43.
215. Akcakus M, et al. Congenital pulmonary lymphangiectasia in a newborn: a response to autologous blood therapy. *Neonatology* 2007;**91**(4):256-9.
216. Stevenson DA, et al. Familial congenital non-immune hydrops, chylothorax, and pulmonary lymphangiectasia. *Am J Med Genet A* 2006;**140**(4):368-72.
217. Hoehn T, et al. Endothelial, inducible and neuronal nitric oxide synthase in congenital pulmonary lymphangiectasis. *Eur Respir J* 2006;**27**(6):1311-5.
218. Rutigliani M, et al. Immunohistochemical studies in a hydroptic fetus with pulmonary lymphangiectasia and trisomy 21. *Lymphology* 2007;**40**(3):114-21.
219. Gaensler EA. Unilateral hyperlucent lung. In: Simon M, Potchen EJ, LeMay M, editors. *Frontiers of pulmonary radiology*. New York: Grune & Stratton; 1969. p. 312-59.
220. Swyer PR, James GC. A case of unilateral pulmonary emphysema. *Thorax* 1953;**8**(2):133-6.
221. Macleod WM. Abnormal transradiancy of one lung. *Thorax* 1954;**9**(2):147-53.
222. Koyama T, et al. Surgically treated Swyer-James syndrome. *Jpn J Thorac Cardiovasc Surg* 2001;**49**(11):671-4.
223. Backer CL, Mavroudis C. Vascular rings and pulmonary artery sling. In: Mavroudis C, Backer CL, editors. *Pediatric cardiac surgery*. Philadelphia: Mosby; 2004.
224. Jonas RA, et al. Pulmonary artery sling: primary repair by tracheal resection in infancy. *J Thorac Cardiovasc Surg* 1989;**97**(4):548-50.
225. van Son JA, et al. Pulmonary artery sling: reimplantation versus antetracheal translocation. *Ann Thorac Surg* 1999;**68**(3):989-94.
226. Backer CL, Mavroudis C, Dunham ME, Holinger LD. Pulmonary artery sling: results with median sternotomy, cardiopulmonary bypass, and reimplantation. *Ann Thorac Surg* 1999;**67**(6):1738-44:discussion 1744-5.
227. Deterling RA, Clagett DT. Aneurysms of the pulmonary artery. *Am Heart J* 1947;**34**:471-98.
228. Aoyagi S, et al. Pulmonary artery aneurysms developed in a family. *J Cardiovasc Surg (Torino)* 2002;**43**(5):661-3.
229. Dransfield MT, Johnson JE. A mycotic pulmonary artery aneurysm presenting as an endobronchial mass. *Chest* 2003;**124**(4):1610-2.
230. Veldtman GR, Dearani JA, Warnes CA. Low pressure giant pulmonary artery aneurysms in the adult: natural history and management strategies. *Heart* 2003;**89**(9):1067-70.
231. Lacombe P, et al. Transcatheter embolization of multiple pulmonary artery aneurysms in Behçet's syndrome. Report of a case. *Acta Radiol Diagn (Stockh)* 1985;**26**(3):251-3.
232. Tuzun H, et al. Surgical therapy of pulmonary arterial aneurysms in Behçet's syndrome. *Ann Thorac Surg* 1996;**61**(2):733-5.
233. Uyama T, et al. Pulmonary varices: a case report and review of the literature. *Jpn J Surg* 1988;**18**(3):359-62.
234. Katagiri S, Itoh T. A case highly suspected of pulmonary varix. *Nippon Kyobu Rinsho* 1977(36):537-40.
235. Arnett Jr JC, Patton RM. Pulmonary varix. *Thorax* 1976;**31**(1):107-12.
236. Hipona FA, Jamshidi A. Observations on the natural history of varicosity of pulmonary veins. *Circulation* 1967;**35**(3):471-5.
237. Dines DE, et al. Pulmonary arteriovenous fistulas. *Mayo Clin Proc* 1974;**49**(7):460-5.
238. Gossage JR, Kanj G. Pulmonary arteriovenous malformations. A state of the art review. *Am J Respir Crit Care Med* 1998;**158**(2):643-61.
239. Brown JW, et al. Surgical management of scimitar syndrome: an alternative approach. *J Thorac Cardiovasc Surg* 2003;**125**(2):238-45.

CHAPTER 10
Benign Lesions of the Lung
Doraid Jarrar, Ayesha S. Bryant, and Robert J. Cerfolio

Definition and Incidence
Evaluation for an Indeterminate Pulmonary Nodule
Hamartoma
Mucous Gland Adenoma
Infectious Granulomatosis
Intrapulmonary Fibrous Tumor

Benign Endobronchial Fibrous Histiocytoma
Granular Cell Tumor
Inflammatory Pseudotumor
Squamous Papilloma
Nodular Amyloid Lesion
Chondroma
Myoepithelioma

Mucinous Cystadenoma
Alveolar Adenoma
Leiomyoma
Clear Cell Tumor (Sugar Tumor)
Primary Pulmonary Thymoma
Conclusion

DEFINITION AND INCIDENCE

Benign lesions of the lung are quite rare. In one of the largest series reported, Martini and colleagues observed that less than 1% of lung lesions resected at the Memorial Sloan-Kettering Cancer Center were benign. A benign lung nodule is difficult to define and classify because some lesions that are called "benign" have malignant properties. However, the best definition of a benign lesion is one in the pulmonary parenchyma that does not metastasize and does not penetrate through surrounding tissue planes. When it is completely resected, a benign tumor should not recur.[1]

Benign lung tumors can be classified pathologically, but a clinically useful classification would combine location (i.e., endobronchial or parenchymal) and information about whether the lesions are single or multiple. Benign lung tumors can also be classified by their presumed origin. Those classifications include unknown (hamartoma, clear cell, teratoma), epithelial (papilloma, polyps), mesodermal (fibroma, lipoma, leiomyoma, chondroma, granular cell tumor, sclerosing hemangioma), and other (myofibroblastic tumor, xanthoma, amyloid, mucosa-associated lymphoid tumor).

The controversy arises because some tumors are often labeled benign (such as pulmonary blastomas) but have the potential to exhibit malignant properties, and thus clear-cut boundaries between malignant and benign often are blurred. Benign tumors of the lung can arise from all of the various cell types that are present in the lung. Box 10-1 lists the most common benign tumors based on their cells of origin.

Most times, benign nodules are resected because of the inability to differentiate them from a malignant process. For this reason, a benign lesion is identified after resection. The typical evaluation of a patient with an indeterminate pulmonary nodule is described next.

EVALUATION FOR AN INDETERMINATE PULMONARY NODULE

The single most important test for a patient who arrives at the office with an indeterminate pulmonary nodule is the review of old chest radiographs and computed tomographic (CT) scans. The radiograph should be interpreted in the context of the patient's medical history. Important factors include a history of a previous solid organ cancer and history of smoking. The physical examination is typically unremarkable, without any cervical lymphadenopathy. If the nodule is new or if the patient did not have a previous chest radiograph, chest computed tomography with contrast enhancement and integrated positron emission tomography–computed tomography (PET/CT) are performed. If the nodule lacks calcification on the chest CT scan, it is indeterminate.[2,3]

Positron emission tomography (FDG-PET) and integrated PET/CT scanning have recently become important adjuncts in the armamentarium of general thoracic surgeons. PET/CT has helped physicians investigate an indeterminate pulmonary nodule that is larger than 5 mm (smaller nodules that are malignant can be missed by PET/CT). If the nodule has glucose avidity and a maximum standard unit value (maxSUV) of 2.5 or greater, it has a significant chance (above 90% in our series) of being malignant.[4] In a study by Bryant and Cerfolio[5] of 585 patients, 496 patients had a malignant nodule, and their median maxSUV was 8.5. Eighty-nine patients had a benign nodule, and the median maxSUV was 4.9 ($P < .001$). They observed that if the maxSUV was between 0 and 2.5, the

---

Box 10-1
Common Benign Tumors of the Lung Based on Cells of origin

Tumors of epithelial origin
- Mucous gland adenoma
- Clara cell adenoma
- Mucous cystadenoma
- Pleomorphic adenoma

Tumors of mesenchymal origin
- Hamartoma
- Inflammatory pseudotumor
- Chondroma
- Fibroma
- Benign endobronchial fibrous histiocytoma

- Leiomyoma
- Lipoma
- Lymphatic lesions

Tumors of miscellaneous origin
- Nodular pulmonary amyloidosis
- Clear cell tumor (sugar tumor)
- Thymoma
- Granular cell tumor
- Teratoma
- Pulmonary paraganglioma

chance that the nodule was malignant was 24%; between 2.6 and 4.0, it was 80%; and for 4.1 or greater, it was 96%. False-negative results occurred from bronchoalveolar carcinoma in 11 patients, carcinoid in 4, and renal cell in 2. False-positives included fungal infections in 16 patients.[5] Similarly, enlarged mediastinal lymph nodes with a maxSUV of greater than 2.5 are likely to be malignant (we have shown that a lymph node with a maxSUV of 5.3 or greater has a 92% chance of being malignant).[6] Patients with lymphadenopathy on CT scans or uptake on PET/CT scans should have mediastinoscopy, endoscopic ultrasound fine-needle aspiration, or endoscopic bronchial ultrasound examination to obtain tissue diagnosis before a thoracotomy. If the CT and FDG-PET scans are equivocal or abnormal, resection is usually best in patients who are good candidates for surgery.

Needle biopsy, by either a transthoracic route or a transbronchial route, rarely changes the management of this type of nodule, especially if there is no lymphadenopathy. Definitive diagnosis is really achieved only by excisional biopsy, which can be performed by a video-assisted approach or an open technique, depending on many variables that are discussed elsewhere in this text.

In this chapter, we discuss the most common benign tumors of the lung (adenomas and hamartomas constitute the largest group of benign lung tumors) and highlight the important clinical factors associated with each one. Each section is organized in the following fashion to help the reader find the pertinent points he or she is looking for: definition, incidence, special history or physical examination findings, unique radiologic characteristics, intraoperative tips for resection if indicated, pathologic characteristics, and special postoperative care or follow-up care including the risk of recurrence. Box 10-2 lists the radiographic characteristics typical of benign lesions.

HAMARTOMA

Hamartomas are the most common benign lung lesions and account for more than 70% of all nonmalignant tumors of the lung.[7] They are mesenchymal tumors with a peak incidence in the sixth decade of life, and approximately 90% are asymptomatic. Men are affected twice as often as women are. Ninety percent of these tumors present as solitary peripheral nodules and account for about 4% of all solitary pulmonary nodules (Fig. 10-1). The 8% to 10% of hamartomas that have presenting symptoms such as cough, hemoptysis, and recurrent pulmonary infections are usually endobronchial lesions. Resection of these is usually needed even when a definitive biopsy has been performed on them and they are proven to be benign because they cause local problems from airway obstruction. These problems include recurrent pneumonia, parapneumonic empyema, hemoptysis, and cough. Laser ablation can be used to help open the airway, but complete resection is preferred.

Cartilage is present in most lesions and is diagnostic of a hamartoma. There are usually nests of cartilage surrounded by cellular fibrotic tissue. Mature fat cells are a frequent

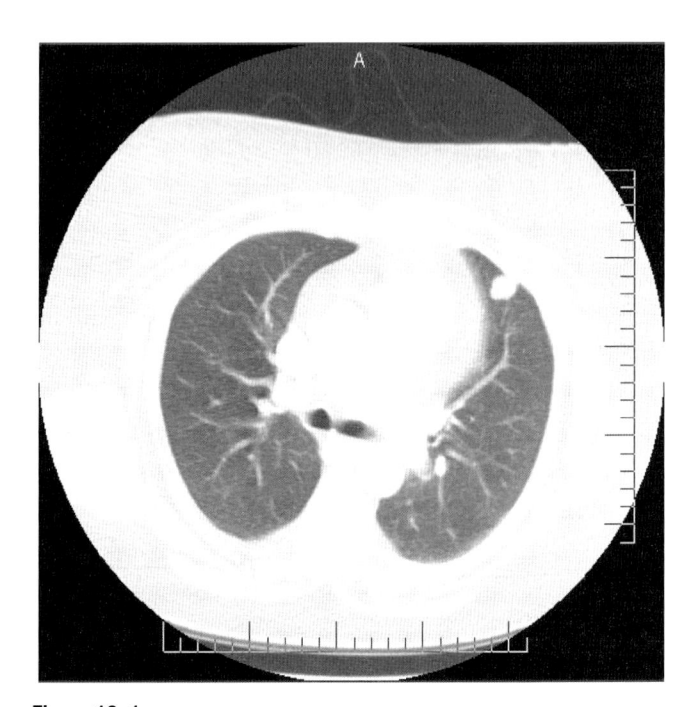

Box 10–2
Radiographic Characteristics of Benign Nodules[31,32]

- Nodular lesions with "tails" toward the hilum include rounded atelectasis (usually has thickening of the associated pleura as well), arteriovenous malformations, and occasional bronchogenic cysts.
- Lesions that are connected to blood vessels include nodular pulmonary infarcts, occasional solitary metastatic lesions, arteriovenous malformations, and bronchopulmonary sequestrations.
- Multiple peripheral triangular or rounded lesions with cavitation and with pulmonary artery branches leading up to them suggest septic embolization.
- In cavitating nodules, wall thickness provides diagnostic information. Thin-walled (<1 mm) cavities are uniformly benign, and 90% of cavitated nodules with wall thickness of 1 to 4 mm are benign. In contrast, cavitated nodules with a wall thickness of more than 16 mm are nearly always malignant.
- Nodules surrounded by a halo may be noted in the setting of angioinvasive aspergillosis, zygomycosis (mucormycosis), lymphoma, bronchioloalveolar carcinoma, coccidioidomycosis, and (rarely) bacterial infections.
- Nodules composed predominantly of ground-glass opacification (nonsolid nodules) can be seen in bronchioloalveolar carcinoma.
- Eighty percent of nodules smaller than 2 cm are benign; 90% of those larger than 3 cm are malignant, yet 40% of malignant nodules are smaller than 2 cm.
- Nodules surrounded by small satellite lesions are benign 90% of the time.
- Nodules with a doubling time of less than 30 days or more than 480 days are usually benign. Bronchioloalveolar carcinoma is an exception to this rule and may have a radiographic doubling time of more than 700 days. Epstein-Barr virus–associated lymphoma or lung cancer in HIV-positive patients may have very fast doubling times.

Figure 10–1
CT scan of the chest showing a chondroid hamartoma measuring 1.4 × 1.7 cm in the inferior lingula of the left lung. The patient was a 49-year-old woman with a normal PET scan. Because her clinical presentation was suggestive of malignant disease, a left upper lobe wedge resection was performed. Ninety percent of hamartomas are located in the periphery, and they account for about 4% of all solitary lung nodules.

component, and their presence on CT scan (low Hounsfield units) is strong evidence for the diagnosis of a hamartoma.[8] Rarely, bone, vessels, bronchioles, and smooth muscle are found. On gross examination, the bosselated appearance is typical for a hamartoma. The usual size is 1 to 3 cm, with the lesion being round and firm. They are easily shelled out from the surrounding lung tissue (Fig. 10-2). As with any indeterminate pulmonary nodule, lung-preserving techniques are best if possible.

On radiographic examination, as shown in Figure 10-3, hamartomas are peripheral lesions that are most often located in the lower lung fields and are well circumscribed. The majority are less than 4 cm in diameter, and calcifications can be appreciated on radiographs in 10% to 30% of cases (Fig. 10-4). Calcifications are described as being "popcorn"-like or diffuse. Hamartomas display a slow growth rate (~3 mm/year) and are rarely multiple. Although it is identifiable in only half of the cases, fat density as identified by CT scan (low Hounsfield units) is strongly suggestive of a benign hamartoma.[9,10] Endobronchial lesions are not identifiable with radiographic examination unless distal parenchymal changes have occurred (e.g., pneumonia or atelectasis).

Although percutaneous transthoracic needle aspiration yields a definitive diagnosis in up to 85% of cases, only a positive and specific result negates the need for excisional biopsy. Depending on the location, lesions might be amenable to resection by video-assisted thoracoscopic surgery (VATS). Endobronchial lesions usually require a sleeve resection with lung preservation if possible. Carbon dioxide or yttrium-aluminum-garnet (YAG) lasers, although effective at opening the airway, are rarely able to completely eradicate the offending lesion because of the lesion's depth of penetration.

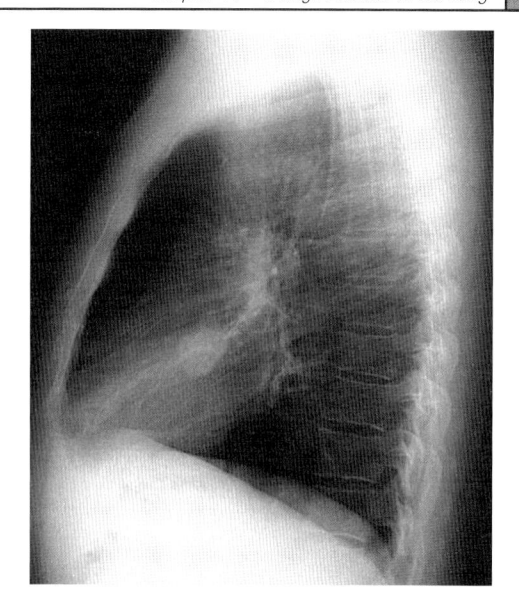

Figure 10–3
Lateral chest radiograph showing a round lesion consistent with a hamartoma.

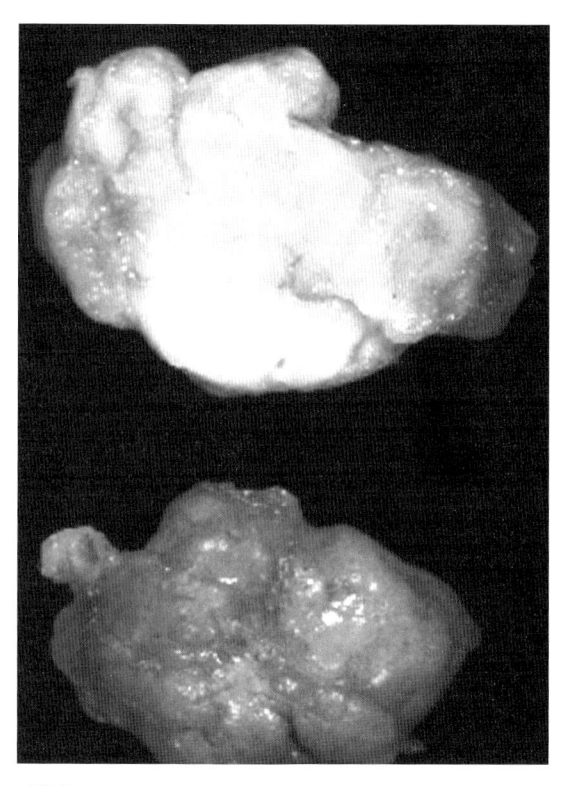

Figure 10–2
Cut surface of a resected hamartoma.

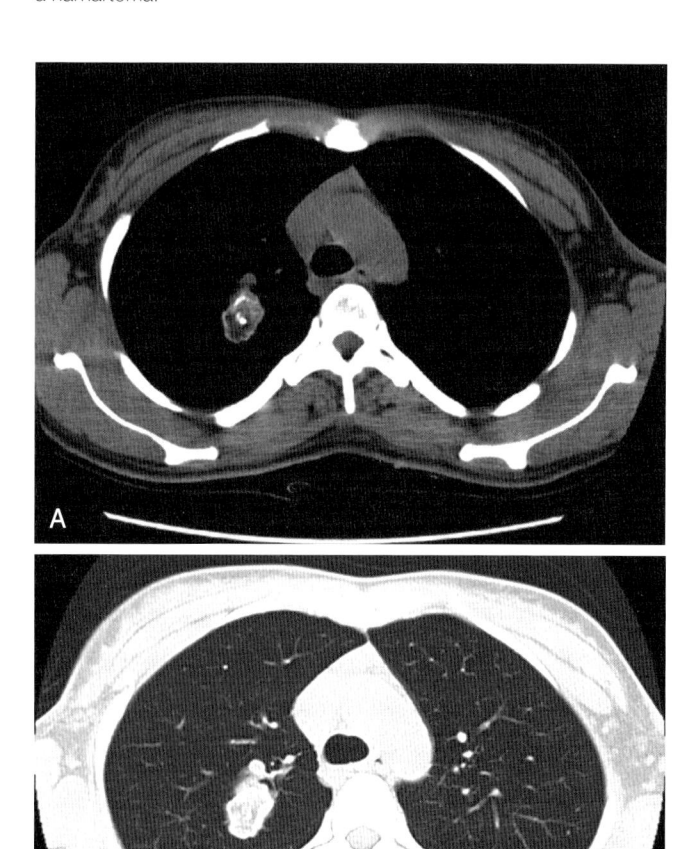

Figure 10–4
Right lung hamartoma. The lesion was resected, and a benign process was confirmed. Lesions are most often located in the lower lung fields and are well circumscribed. The majority are less than 4 cm in diameter, and calcifications can be appreciated on radiographs in 10% to 30% of cases.

Carney's triad is found infrequently and consists of a gastric epithelioid leiomyosarcoma, a functioning extra-adrenal paraganglioma, and a pulmonary hamartoma.[10,11] Most commonly, the gastric lesion is the first cause, followed by the extra-adrenal paraganglioma.

Although hamartomas are benign per se, several cases of malignant transformation arising at the resection site have been reported.[11] However, it appears that these synchronous or metachronous carcinomas are coincidental because the frequency is less than 7%. The etiology of these malignant neoplasms and their relationship to the hamartoma remain unknown.

MUCOUS GLAND ADENOMA

Mucous gland adenoma is a rare, benign tumor arising from the mucous glands of the bronchus. The exact incidence is unknown, and several small series of case reports have been published. To be classified as a mucous gland adenoma, a tumor must contain cystic glands that are superficial to the cartilaginous plate, it must be in the bronchus, and it must contain features of normal bronchial seromucous glands. On histologic examination, numerous small mucus-filled cysts lined by well-differentiated epithelium are observed (Fig. 10-5).[9]

These benign lesions usually present because of hemoptysis, recurrent pneumonia, and persistent cough. The lesion itself does not have distinguishing radiographic features, but the chest radiograph may show obstructive pneumonitis. These tumors are evenly distributed between the left and right lungs, with the major bronchi of the lower lobes being affected more often. They are soft, spherical, polypoid lesions that are usually less than 2 cm in diameter; however, lesions up to 6 cm have been reported.[10] They are noninvasive and well circumscribed. Although the lesions rarely have a stalk, stalks can be completely removed endoscopically by curettage, cryotherapy, or laser ablation. Surgical resection is indicated only if the distal lung tissue is destroyed or chronically infected.

INFECTIOUS GRANULOMATOSIS

Infectious granulomas cause approximately 80% of benign nodules.[11,12] Endemic fungi (e.g., histoplasmosis, coccidioidomycosis) and mycobacteria (either tuberculous or nontuberculous mycobacterial disease) are the most frequently recognized causes of infectious granulomas presenting as a solitary peripheral nodule. When nontuberculous mycobacterial disease presents as a solitary peripheral nodule, the cause of the nodule is typically unrecognized until the lesion is resected as a presumed primary lung cancer. In patients with acquired immunodeficiency syndrome, *Pneumocystis jiroveci* (previously called *Pneumocystis carinii*) infection can present as a solitary peripheral nodule and may cavitate.

INTRAPULMONARY FIBROUS TUMOR

Intrapulmonary fibrous tumors are contiguous with the visceral pleura and are identical to localized fibrous tumors of the pleura. Terms such as intraparenchymal localized fibrous mesotheliomas, intrapulmonary fibrous mesotheliomas, localized fibrous tumor of the pleura, and inverted fibrous tumor of the pleura have been used and are essentially interchangeable. The visceral pleura is the most common location of these tumors, but they also have been found in the retroperitoneum, mediastinum, and parietal surfaces of the intra-abdominal viscera. The tumors are round to oval and contain a smooth cover of visceral pleura (Fig. 10-6). Most lesions are less than 10 cm in diameter, and histologic examinations show spindle cells with oval nuclei, diffuse fine chromatin, and positive staining for vimentin and the surface receptor CD34.[13] In most cases, the tissue of origin is the mesenchymal layer of the visceral pleura. No distinctive radiographic features are known for these lesions, although the radiologist often includes a malignant mesothelioma in the differential diagnosis. The obtuse angle that these tumors make with the chest wall strongly suggests that the tumor is arising from the pleura and not from the lung. Unlike diffuse mesotheliomas, intrapulmonary fibrous tumors are not related to asbestos exposure. Surgical resection is usually performed by VATS, which usually offers complete resection because these lesions are often on a stalk and easy to remove. Resection is curative.

BENIGN ENDOBRONCHIAL FIBROUS HISTIOCYTOMA

A fibrous histiocytoma is a benign lung tumor that is composed of collagen and inflammatory and mesenchymal cells. These are rare endobronchial lesions that occur most often

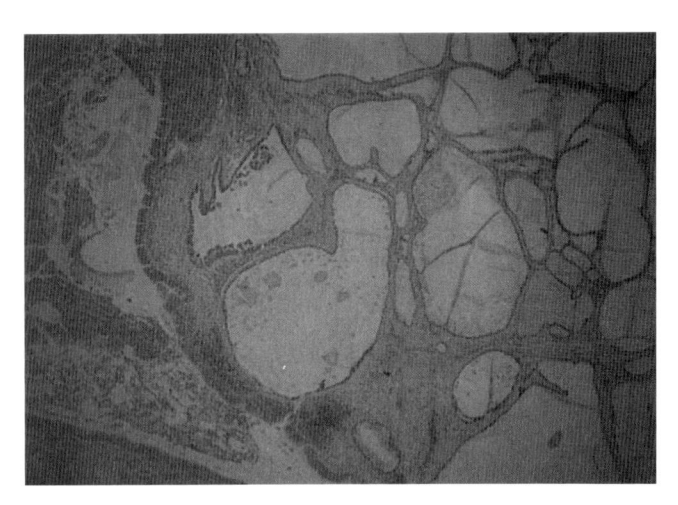

Figure 10–5
Photomicrograph of a mucous gland adenoma.

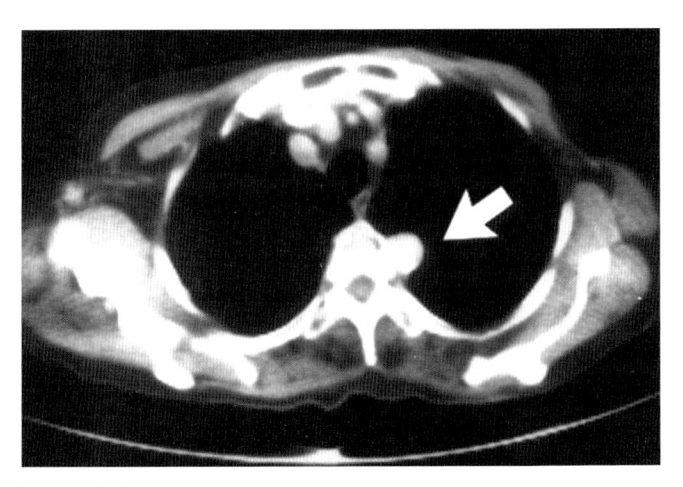

Figure 10–6
The *arrow* shows an intrapulmonary fibrous tumor. Lesions are contiguous with the visceral pleura. Tumors are round to oval and are usually less than 10 cm in diameter.

in either children or young adults. Because they are so rare, their exact incidence is unknown. No specific radiographic findings distinguish these lesions from others. Depending on the location or the extent of bronchial involvement, surgical therapy might entail a lobectomy or sleeve lobectomy. Bueno and coworkers[14] described bronchoplastic resections of five endobronchial fibrous histiocytomas.

GRANULAR CELL TUMOR

Granular cell tumors, also called granular cell myoblastomas, are another type of rare, benign tumor. They initially were thought to derive from skeletal muscle. However, evidence now suggests that these lesions originate from Schwann cells, as Deavers and associates[15] described in 20 cases. In half of the patients, the lesion was an incidental finding. In the other half, symptoms were caused by obstruction, including postobstructive pneumonia and atelectasis. The lesions were solitary in 75% of the cases. Chest radiographs showed lobar infiltrates, coin lesions, and atelectasis. Tumors usually are located in a large bronchus and can protrude into the bronchial lumen, but they also can be found in the pulmonary parenchyma. Tumors usually are circumscribed but not encapsulated and range in size from 0.3 to 5.0 cm. Complete resection is curative, although recurrences have been described.[15] Epstein and Mohsenifar[16] reported the use of neodymium:YAG laser to treat obstructing lesions.

INFLAMMATORY PSEUDOTUMOR

Inflammatory pseudotumors are usually asymptomatic solitary nodules that are found on routine chest radiography or CT scan.[17] However, they can be large or also be primarily of the airway (as shown in Fig. 10-7). Because these tumors go by many other names, such as plasma cell granuloma–histiocytoma complex, plasma cell granuloma, histiocytoma, xanthofibroma, and xanthoma, there is often confusion. Inflammatory pseudotumors usually are well circumscribed, nonencapsulated, firm, white or yellow masses. Two major groups have been identified: fibrohistiocytic and plasma cell granulomas. In both groups, the histologic examinations reveal a mixture of inflammatory cells, including plasma cells, lymphocytes, and macrophages. Some reports have shown that there may be two types of inflammatory pseudotumors.[17] One type is invasive, large, and more difficult to resect as opposed to the other, which is characterized by a small, easily wedged mass without evidence of local tissue invasion. The mechanism for these two types is unclear, although it appears microscopically to depend on the degree of inflammatory cells present. A clinicopathologic series from the Massachusetts General Hospital provided evidence that organizing pneumonia may be the nidus for the formation of inflammatory pseudotumors. Excision of these lesions is usually both diagnostic and curative. In patients with multiple lesions not amenable to excision, radiation therapy and corticosteroid therapy are other options.

These unusual tumors can occur at any age, and there is no predilection for men or women. Although primary lung tumors are infrequent in childhood, plasma cell granuloma is the most common lung lesion in the preadolescent age category. Serial chest radiographs usually show the nodule to be unchanged in size, and it may even shrink without treatment in some patients. Slow growth occurs in less than 10% of cases.[18] On CT scans, these lesions appear as a well-marginated, lobulated mass with some heterogeneous attenuation.

SQUAMOUS PAPILLOMA

Squamous papilloma is a benign epithelial neoplasm formed by squamous epithelium. Papillomas of the endobronchial tree have been classified into two main groups: multiple squamous papillomas and solitary papillomas. Drennan and coworkers[19] also distinguished a third class, inflammatory polyps.

Multiple squamous papillomas are usually seen in children with laryngeal papillomatosis, usually caused by human papillomavirus. Children can become infected during vaginal childbirth because their oropharynges and respiratory systems are exposed during the delivery. Serotypes 16 and 18 may act as promoters in carcinogenesis. On gross examination, the papillomas can be exophytic and have a component outside the bronchial wall and endophytic and obstruct part of the airway. There may be distal bronchiectasis with atelectasis or consolidation of the surrounding lung. Papillomas have a connective tissue stroma that often is heavily infiltrated with lymphocytes and covered completely with cuboidal or squamous epithelium.

Solitary squamous papillomas are rare and affect men, most commonly smokers, in their fifth to seventh decades of life. Productive cough, hemoptysis, wheezing, and dyspnea are common complaints as a result of obstruction by the lesion. On histologic examination, they have a thin central fibrovascular core that is covered by stratified squamous epithelium, and they form multiple papillary fronds. Chest radiography may show a lesion or atelectasis. The papillomas usually are located in segmental or more proximal bronchi. The human papillomavirus is the most common cause of these lesions.

Fibrous polyps are the third group and can be found solitary or in multiple locations. They usually arise from the bronchial mucosa, have a fibrous stalk, and are covered by ciliated columnar epithelium. The stalk usually is composed of loose

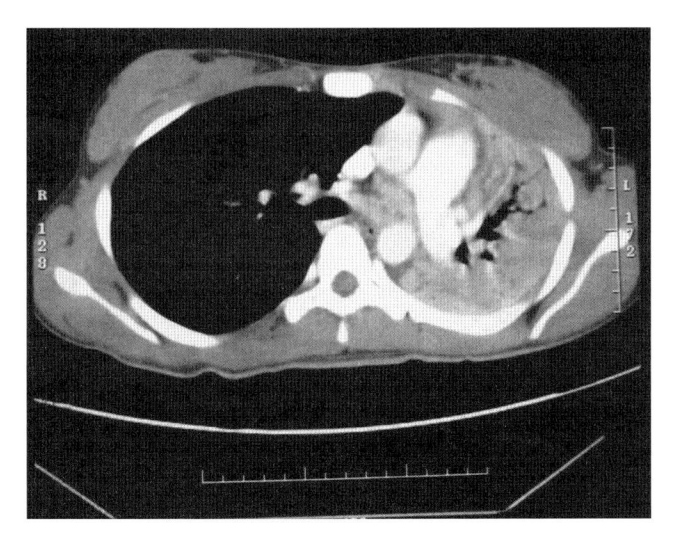

Figure 10–7
Inflammatory pseudotumor of the left main-stem bronchus involving the carina. The patient has been treated successfully in the past with steroids. However, she has recently become afflicted with multiple pneumonias, and radiographic studies suggest that she has obstruction of the main-stem bronchus. The patient did undergo left main-stem bronchial sleeve resection.

connective tissue with an infiltrate of plasma cells, lymphocytes, and eosinophils. These polyps are always benign and may be secondary to chronic inflammatory processes. Photodynamic therapy and laser or endoscopic removal are some of the options available to treat these lesions. Bronchotomy or sleeve resection usually is not needed.

All three of these types of squamous papilloma can be associated with dysplasia, carcinoma in situ, or foci of invasive squamous cell carcinoma. Close surveillance and repeated biopsies are sometimes necessary in observing these patients.

NODULAR AMYLOID LESION

Nodular amyloid lesions represent a focal collection of amyloid deposition in the lung. They are most frequently found in the lower lobes. They are sometimes referred to as amyloidomas. They can occur as either a solitary nodule or multiple nodules. The following three types have been described: tracheobronchial, nodular pulmonary, and diffuse pulmonary. Although nodular amyloid lesions are not associated with primary systemic amyloidosis, multiple myeloma should be ruled out. Patients are usually asymptomatic, and lesions are discovered incidentally on chest radiography. Patients should be followed up long term because of the association with macroglobulinemia and malignant lymphoma. Surgical resection is usually curative.

CHONDROMA

Chondromas are defined as benign cartilaginous tissue that can occur in the lung parenchyma or in the cartilaginous airways. Endobronchial lesions can cause obstructive symptoms, whereas parenchymal tumors are asymptomatic. Histologic examination of chondromas shows benign cartilaginous tissue. Some patients with this unusual lesion may have Carney's triad. This is made up of pulmonary chondroma, multiple gastric smooth muscle tumors, and extra-adrenal paragangliomas.[10] The lesions may contain metaplastic bone, mature cartilage, and myxoid stroma. Single lesions are most commonly resected for diagnosis and have an excellent prognosis. When patients have multiple lesions, a tissue sample, often obtained by a minimally invasive approach with a needle biopsy, usually is sufficient to make the diagnosis.

MYOEPITHELIOMA

Myoepitheliomas are rare, benign tumors arising from myoepithelial cells that lie between the epithelial cells of a gland and the basement membrane. Although these lesions are more commonly found in salivary glands and the breast, rare cases have been reported in the lung parenchyma. Strickler and associates[20] described two patients in whom these lesions were found. Both had a mass on the chest radiograph. Immunostaining for S-100 was positive, which is consistent with the diagnosis of a myoepithelioma. Surgery appears to be curative. Because these lesions are so rare, pathognomonic radiographic and clinical signs have not been described.

MUCINOUS CYSTADENOMA

Mucinous cystadenoma is a unilocular cystic lesion whose fibrous wall is lined by well-differentiated, benign columnar mucinous epithelium.[21] These lesions occur usually in the fifth and sixth decades of life in patients who smoke. However, their exact incidence is unknown. Most patients with this tumor are asymptomatic, and it represents an incidental finding on chest radiography. The lesions usually are located more toward the periphery. Once it is excised, the lesion appears as a unilocular cyst filled with gelatinous material. Sometimes the mucin extravasates into the surrounding lung parenchyma. Because these cysts may harbor adenocarcinoma, they should be completely excised. On microscopic examination, these lesions may look similar to a bronchogenic cyst as well as a bronchoalveolar carcinoma.

ALVEOLAR ADENOMA

Alveolar adenomas are proliferations of alveolar epithelium and septal mesenchyme. These lesions are extremely rare. Yousem and Hochholzer[22] reported one of the largest series with six patients, most of them women. Other smaller reports also have been published.[4] Lesions usually were identified on routine chest radiographs as an indeterminate nodule in the middle lung field. Excision appears to be curative.

LEIOMYOMA

Leiomyomas are benign lesions of the lung that can occur in the trachea, bronchus, or pulmonary parenchyma itself. They account for about 2% of all benign lung lesions. Vera-Roman and coworkers[23] reviewed the literature and found a female-to-male ratio of 1.5:1 (Fig. 10-8). There are no discrete findings on physical examination. Some patients have hemoptysis if it is an endobronchial lesion; in others, the tumor is an incidental finding on chest radiography. It appears that the distribution between tracheobronchial and parenchymal lesions is equal. On histologic examination, smooth muscle differentiation is found. Some of these lesions stain for estrogen and progesterone receptors. They may be dependent on a certain hormonal milieu, and this may explain why some of these lesions occasionally disappear during pregnancy.[24] Surgical treatment consists of excision and is the treatment of choice. Endobronchial lesions sometimes can be treated with laser ablation. Otherwise, sleeve bronchoplasty is needed. Benign metastasizing leiomyomas occur in young women and are associated with leiomyomas of the uterus.[25] Treatment consists of surgery, hormonal manipulation, and chemotherapy. Although labeled a benign condition, these lesions can metastasize and cause death.

Lymphangiomyomatosis is a rare disease primarily found in women of childbearing age and was first described in the medical literature by von Stossel in 1937.[26] It is characterized by progressive proliferation of spindle cells, resembling immature smooth muscle in the lung parenchyma and along lymphatic vessels in the chest and abdomen. The proliferation of spindle cells along the bronchioles leads to air trapping and eventually to the development of thin-walled cysts. Pneumothorax can be a complication when these cysts rupture. The proliferation of spindle cells also can affect the lymphatics and result occasionally in a chylous pleural effusion. Main symptoms stem from either a chylous pleural effusion (up to 80%) or a pneumothorax (30% to 50%). In both cases, dyspnea is the lead symptom.[27]

Radiographic presentation of lymphangiomyomatosis includes reticular, reticulonodular, miliary, and honeycomb

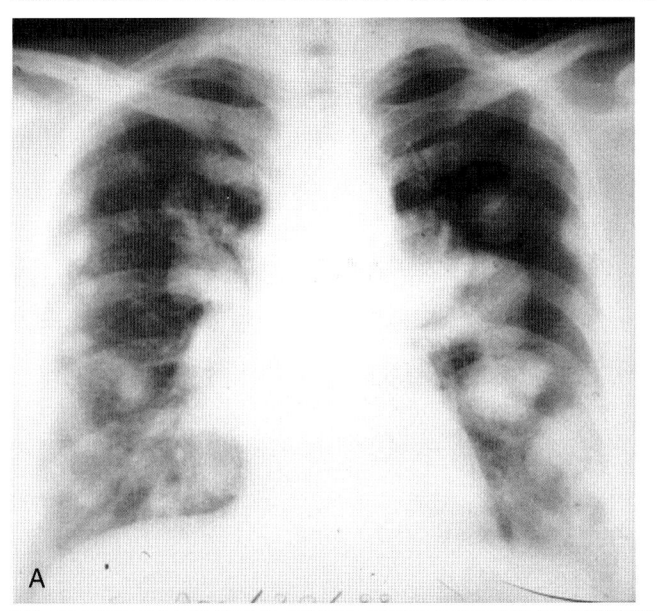

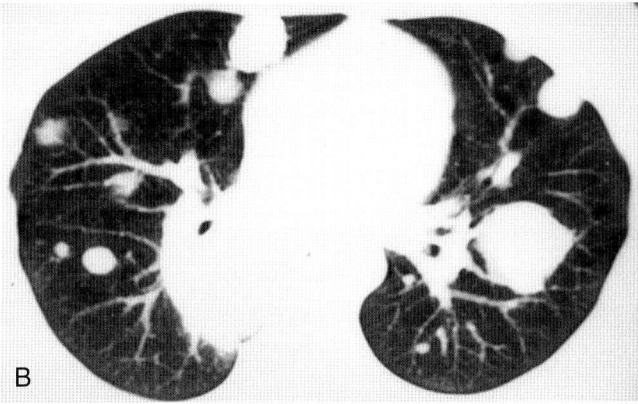

Figure 10–8
Benign metastasizing leiomyoma. These lesions occur in young women and are associated with leiomyomas of the uterus.

patterns on plain radiography. The CT scan usually shows multiple thin-walled lung cysts within normal lung parenchyma. The usual diameter of these cysts is between 0.2 and 5 cm. The disease pattern does not spare any lung zones and is distributed diffusely throughout the lungs. Hilar and mediastinal adenopathy are not uncommon. Diagnostic workup includes plain radiography, chest CT scan, and lung biopsy. Biopsy specimens can be obtained by either thoracoscopy or transbronchial biopsy. Unfortunately, most patients die within 10 years of the onset of symptoms. Although no definitive evidence has linked the disease to the estrogen levels, oophorectomy is an accepted treatment modality. Moreover, for lymphangiomyomatosis patients with severe disease, lung transplantation is an established therapy. The National Institutes of Health currently conducts phase II trials using octreotide in patients with lymphangiomyomatosis to reduce symptoms from chylous effusions or ascites and peripheral lymphedema.

CLEAR CELL TUMOR (SUGAR TUMOR)

Clear cell tumor is a benign lesion of the lung of unknown tissue origin. Recent evidence suggests that it originates from either Clara cells (nonciliated bronchiolar epithelium) or epithelial serous cells. More detailed examination of these tumors showed some neuroendocrine differentiation and positive staining for human melanin black or melanosome-associated protein and S-100. On radiographic examination, the lesions are often peripheral and range in size from 1.5 to 3 cm.[28,29] Excision is curative. The differential diagnosis includes clear cell carcinoma and carcinoid as well as renal cell carcinoma.

PRIMARY PULMONARY THYMOMA

A primary pulmonary thymoma is a tumor that is present in the lung in a patient with a normal mediastinal thymus gland. Pulmonary thymomas are quite rare, and their exact incidence is unknown. They can occur either peripherally or centrally. By definition, the tumor must be within the visceral pleura because ectopic mediastinal thymic tissue can be found in the aortopulmonary window as well as in the aortocaval groove. No distinctive radiologic features are known. Studies have used immunohistochemistry to confirm the diagnosis. Thymic T lymphocytes must be differentiated from lymphoepithelial-like carcinoma of the lung and from primary lymphomas. Surgical resection usually is curative. However, in rare cases, when the tumor is extensive and complete resection is difficult, neoadjuvant therapy with radiation has been described (Fig. 10-9).[30] There are several tumors that are often called benign but that really represent a type of low-grade malignancy.

CONCLUSION

Benign lesions of the lung are extremely rare and often are diagnosed only after complete surgical resection. If a nodule remains indeterminate after a thorough evaluation as described in the preceding sections, resection is best if the patient's risk is acceptable. If surgery is not chosen, careful follow-up is needed to ensure that a malignant neoplasm is not missed. The solitary pulmonary nodule is a common radiologic finding that can require an extensive evaluation to establish a benign or malignant diagnosis. Morphologic evaluation of the size, margins, and contour with conventional imaging techniques alone often is not satisfactory. CT, PET, and PET/CT scans have added to the noninvasive armamentarium available to the general thoracic surgeon. However, careful interpretation of these study results is needed, and no test supplants tissue biopsy or, in some cases, complete excision. A normal finding on needle biopsy does not exclude a malignant process. VATS, which offers minimal morbidity, may afford complete excision as well. Even if the nodule is benign, this procedure offers peace of mind to the patient and obviates the need for repeated, expensive, time-consuming radiologic tests.

Benign lesions of the lung are most commonly a diagnosis of exclusion during the evaluation of an indeterminate pulmonary nodule. Benign lesions can have worrisome clinical presenting symptoms, such as recurrent pneumonia, hemoptysis, and atelectasis. Although they are rare, the general thoracic surgeon should be familiar with the different types of benign lesions to counsel his or her patients and to provide a differential diagnosis. The surgeon must be able to interpret the radiographs and also the disease, which often is equivocal in these lesions.

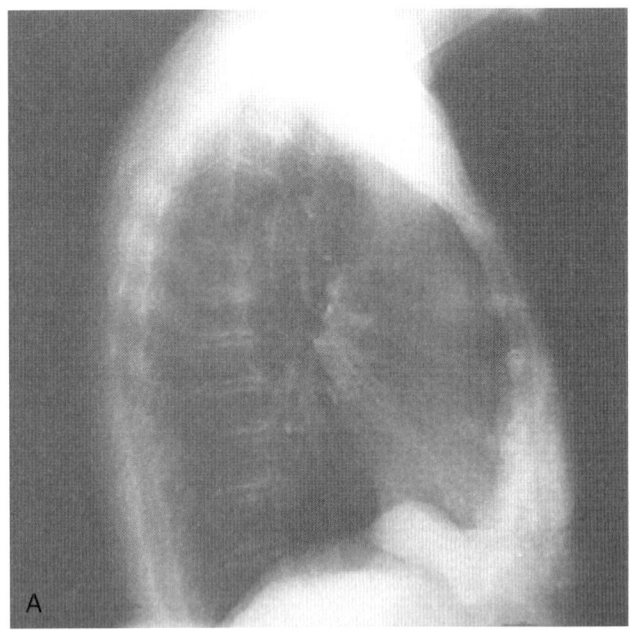

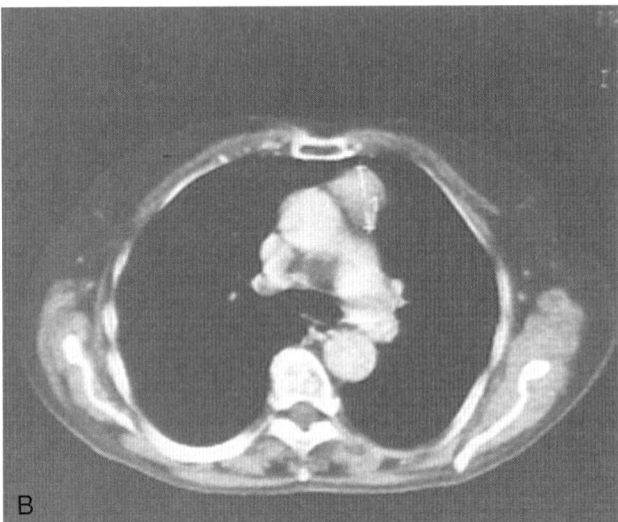

Figure 10–9
Primary pulmonary thymoma. In rare cases, when the tumor is extensive, radiation therapy may be a good alternative.

REFERENCES

1. Scott WJ. Surgical treatment of other bronchial tumors. *Chest Surg Clin N Am* 2003;**13**:111-28.
2. Erasmus JJ, McAdams HP, Connolly JE. Solitary pulmonary nodules: Part II. Evaluation of the indeterminate nodule. *Radiographics* 2000;**20**:59-66.
3. Khouri NF, Meziane MA, Zerhouni EA, et al. The solitary pulmonary nodule. Assessment, diagnosis, and management. *Chest* 1987;**91**:128-33.
4. Wong WL, Campbell H, Saunders M. Positron emission tomography (PET)—evaluation of 'indeterminate pulmonary lesions.' *Clin Oncol (R Coll Radiol)* 2002;**14**:123-8.
5. Bryant AS, Cerfolio RJ. The maximum standardized uptake values on integrated FDG-PET/CT is useful in differentiating benign from malignant pulmonary nodules. *Ann Thorac Surg* 2006;**82**:1016-20.
6. Bryant AS, Cerfolio RJ, Klemm KM, Ojha B. Maximum standard uptake value of mediastinal lymph nodes on integrated FDG-PET/CT predicts pathology in patients with non–small cell lung cancer. *Ann Thorac Surg* 2006 Aug;**82**(2): 417-22.
7. Arrigoni MG, Woolner LB, Bernatz PE, et al. Benign tumors of the lung. A ten-year surgical experience. *J Thorac Cardiovasc Surg* 1970;**60**:589-99.
8. Hamper UM, Khouri NF, Stitik FP, et al. Pulmonary hamartoma: Diagnosis by transthoracic needle-aspiration biopsy. *Radiology* 1985;**155**:15-8.
9. Allen Jr MS, Marsh Jr WL, Geissinger WT. Mucus gland adenoma of the bronchus. *J Thorac Cardiovasc Surg* 1974;**67**:966-8.
10. Dajee A, Dajee H, Hinrichs S, et al. Pulmonary chondroma, extra-adrenal paraganglioma, and gastric leiomyosarcoma: Carney's triad. *J Thorac Cardiovasc Surg* 1982;**84**:377-81.
11. McLaughlin SJ, Dodge EA, Ashworth J, et al. Carney's triad. *Aust N Z J Surg* 1988;**58**:679-81.
12. Altiner M, Paksoy N, Ozturk H. Large cell carcinoma of the lung with unilateral hamartoma. *Pathologica* 1996;**88**:311-2.
13. Chang YL, Lee YC, Wu CT. Thoracic solitary fibrous tumor: Clinical and pathological diversity. *Lung Cancer* 1999;**23**:53-60.
14. Bueno R, Wain JC, Wright CD, et al. Bronchoplasty in the management of low-grade airway neoplasms and benign bronchial stenoses. *Ann Thorac Surg* 1996;**62**:824-8.
15. Deavers M, Guinee D, Koss MN, et al. Granular cell tumors of the lung. Clinicopathologic study of 20 cases. *Am J Surg Pathol* 1995;**19**:627-35.
16. Epstein LJ, Mohsenifar Z. Use of Nd:YAG laser in endobronchial granular cell myoblastoma. *Chest* 1993;**104**:958-60.
17. Cerfolio RJ, Allen MS, Nascimento AG, et al. Inflammatory pseudotumors of the lung. *Ann Thorac Surg* 1999;**67**:933-6.
18. Matsubara O, Tan-Liu NS, Kenney RM, et al. Inflammatory pseudotumors of the lung: Progression from organizing pneumonia to fibrous histiocytoma or to plasma cell granuloma in 32 cases. *Hum Pathol* 1988;**19**:807-14.
19. Drennan J, Douglas A. Solitary papilloma of a bronchus. *J Clin Pathol* 1965;**18**:401.
20. Strickler JG, Hegstrom J, Thomas MJ, et al. Myoepithelioma of the lung. *Arch Pathol Lab Med* 1987;**111**:1082-5.
21. Roux FJ, Lantuejoul S, Brambilla E, et al. Mucinous cystadenoma of the lung. *Cancer* 1995;**76**:1540-4.
22. Yousem SA, Hochholzer L. Alveolar adenoma. *Hum Pathol* 1986;**17**:1066-71.
23. Vera-Roman JM, Sobonya RE, Gomez-Garcia JL, et al. Leiomyoma of the lung. Literature review and case report. *Cancer* 1983;**52**:936-41.
24. Horstmann JP, Pietra GG, Harman JA, et al. Spontaneous regression of pulmonary leiomyomas during pregnancy. *Cancer* 1977;**39**:314-21.
25. Parenti DJ, Morley TF, Giudice JC. Benign metastasizing leiomyoma. A case report and review of the literature. *Respiration* 1992;**59**:347-50.
26. Pacheco-Rodriguez G, Kristof AS, Stevens LA, et al. Filley Lecture. Genetics and gene expression in lymphangioleiomyomatosis. *Chest* 2002;**121**:56S-60S.
27. Hancock E, Osborne J. Lymphangioleiomyomatosis: A review of the literature. *Respir Med* 2002;**96**:1-6.
28. Gaffey MJ, Mills SE, Askin FB, et al. Clear cell tumor of the lung. A clinicopathologic, immunohistochemical, and ultrastructural study of eight cases. *Am J Surg Pathol* 1990;**14**:248-59.
29. Gaffey MJ, Mills SE, Ritter JH. Clear cell tumors of the lower respiratory tract. *Semin Diagn Pathol* 1997;**14**:222-32.
30. Moiseenko V, Craig T, Bezjak A, et al. Dose-volume analysis of lung complications in the radiation treatment of malignant thymoma: A retrospective review. *Radiother Oncol* 2003;**67**:265-74.
31. Henschke CI, Yankelevitz DF, Mirtcheva R, McGuinness G, McCauley D, Miettinen OS. CT screening for lung cancer: frequency and significance of part-solid and nonsolid nodules. *AJR Am J Roentgenol* 2002;**178**:1053-7.
32. Tsubamoto M, Kuriyama K, Kido S, Arisawa J, Kohno N, Johkoh T, et al. Detection of lung cancer on chest radiographs: analysis on the basis of size and extent of ground-glass opacity at thin-section CT. *Radiology* 2002;**224**:139-44.

CHAPTER 11
Interstitial Lung Diseases
Subroto Paul and Yolonda L. Colson

Granulomatous Patterns of Interstitial
  Lung Disease
  Foreign Bodies and Inorganic Dust
  Hypersensitivity Pneumonitis
  Infections
  Sarcoidosis
  Granulomatous Vasculitides: Wegener's
    Granulomatosis and Churg-Strauss
    Syndrome
Eosinophilic Pneumonias
Histiocytosis X
**Alveolitic Patterns of Interstitial Lung
  Disease**
  Drug-Associated Injury
  Goodpasture's Syndrome
  Idiopathic Interstitial Pneumonias
    *Usual Interstitial Pneumonia and Idiopathic
    Pulmonary Fibrosis*
*Desquamative Interstitial Pneumonia
Nonspecific Interstitial Pneumonia
Acute Interstitial Pneumonitis
Respiratory Bronchiolitis–Associated
  Interstitial Lung Disease
Cryptogenic Organizing Pneumonia
Lymphocytic Interstitial Pneumonia*
**Patient Evaluation
Treatment**

Interstitial lung disease (ILD) is a group of more than 200 clinical entities that manifest with chronic, progressive, diffuse inflammation of the pulmonary interstitium. This inflammatory process may result from a primary pulmonary process, or it may be the result of a systemic illness, such as a connective tissue disease. ILD does not include inflammatory responses secondary to known malignant or infectious etiologies, and, for the purposes of this chapter, it will not include adult respiratory distress syndrome. However, these entities may demonstrate very similar clinical and radiographic findings and thus are certainly in the clinical differential diagnosis of immunologic disease of the lung.

The interstitium includes the alveoli, the epithelial and capillary cells within the alveolar wall, the septal tissues, and the connective tissues that surround the vascular, bronchial, and lymphatic structures within the lung parenchyma. An inflammatory response may involve any or all of these structures with varying clinical and radiographic presentations. The pathologic response to the resulting immunologic insult permits a clinically useful, although not strict, categorization of ILD into those entities characterized by alveolitic and diffuse interstitial inflammation and those that result in a predominantly granulomatous pattern of disease (Box 11-1).

Either pathologic response may progress from injury to fibrosis. Thus, all of these entities manifest clinically as progressive dyspnea on exertion, a persistent nonproductive, typically paroxysmal, cough in the setting of radiographic interstitial opacities, or as both. Symptoms are usually chronic, progressing over years. However, presentation may be acute, as in allergic responses seen with hypersensitivity pneumonitis, eosinophilic pneumonia, drug-induced alveolitis, or acute interstitial pneumonia, or subacute, as with sarcoidosis, alveolar hemorrhage syndromes, cryptogenic organizing pneumonia, and some of the connective tissue diseases.

Fatigue and weight loss are common. Wheezing, hemoptysis, or pleuritic chest pain may be present but are relatively rare as presenting symptoms in ILDs. In fact, sudden onset or increased chest pain in the setting of these diseases is more suggestive of spontaneous pneumothorax, particularly in histiocytosis X (pulmonary Langerhans cell histiocytosis), tuberous sclerosis, lymphangiomyomatosis, and neurofibromatosis. Hemoptysis is associated with diffuse alveolar hemorrhage syndromes and the granulomatous vasculitides. Disease manifestation in other organ systems is helpful in the diagnosis of Wegener's granulomatous or Goodpasture's syndrome. Age, sex, past medical, family, and smoking histories, and occupational and environmental exposure all figure prominently in the development of a differential diagnosis for a particular patient. Physical examination usually reveals bibasilar end-inspiratory "Velcro" crackles, but this is less common in the granulomatous diseases. Baseline tachycardia is common. Cyanosis and clubbing can occur with advanced disease.

GRANULOMATOUS PATTERNS OF ILD

Granulomas consist of activated immune cells, typically macrophages, encircling particles that are generally not recognized by the antigen-specific, or adaptive, immune system. The particle

---

**Box 11-1
Categories of Interstitial Lung Disease**

- Granulomatous
- Foreign body/inorganic dust
- Hypersensitivity pneumonitis
- Sarcoidosis
- Granulomatous vasculitides
  - Wegener's granulomatosis
  - Churg-Strauss syndrome
- Eosinophilic pneumonias
- Histiocytosis X
- Alveolitic
- Drug-associated injury
- Goodpasture's syndrome
- Idiopathic interstitial pneumonias

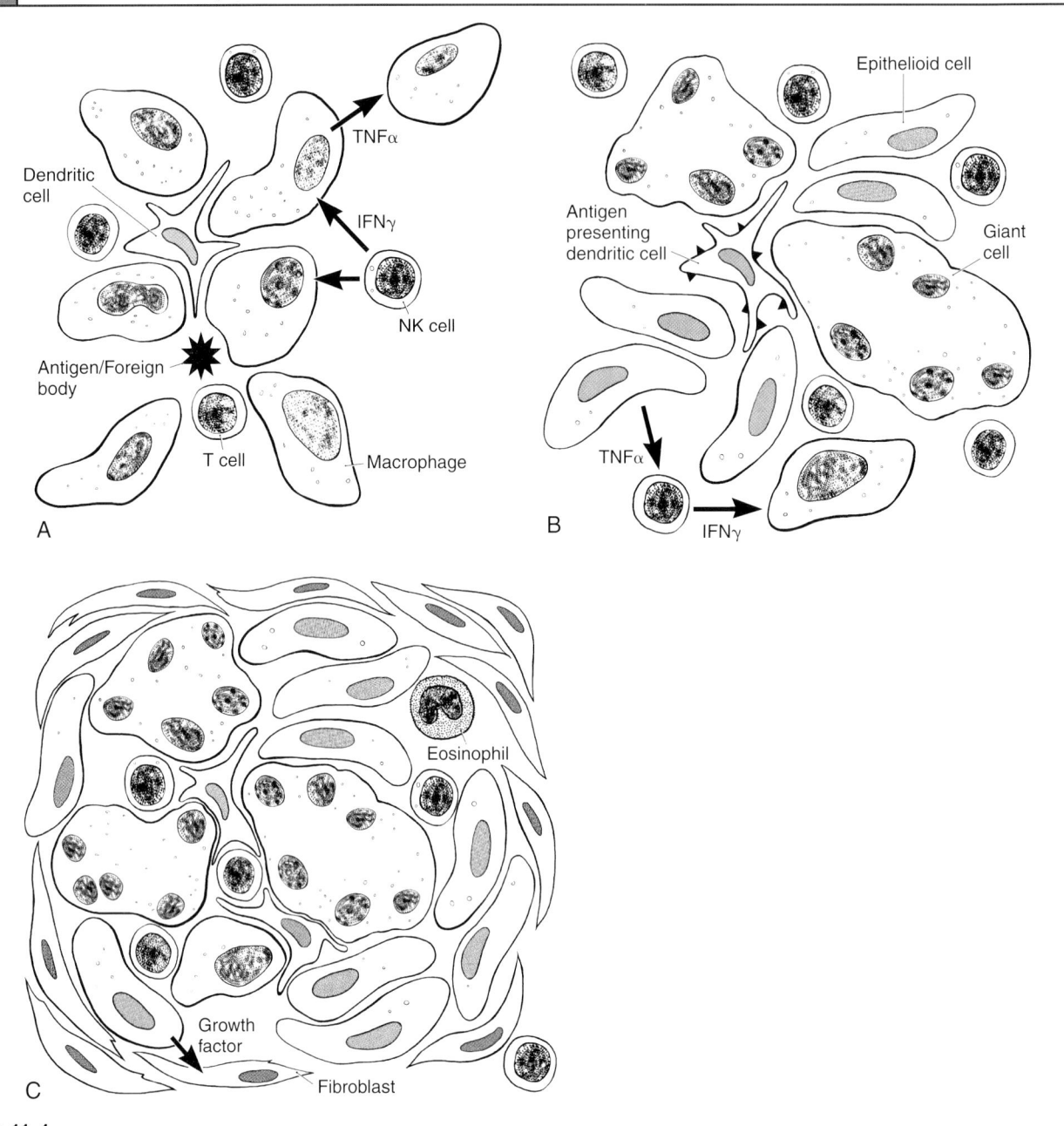

Figure 11–1
Granuloma formation and maturation. **A,** Early accumulation of macrophages around antigen or foreign body. Release of proinflammatory cytokines tumor necrosis factor alpha (TNFα) and interferon-gamma (IFNγ), and chemokines such as macrophage inflammatory protein 1α results in activation of macrophages and recruitment of other immune cells. **B,** Antigen presentation by dendritic cells and macrophages to incoming T cells results in further activation, with development of epithelioid and giant cells. It is at this stage that fibroblasts become activated, resulting in focal areas of fibrosis. **C,** As the granuloma matures, the structure becomes more compact, with giant cells and T cells at the core. The initial helper T cell 1 (T_H1) response leads to the release of T_H2 cytokines as well, with interleukin (IL)-5 recruitment of eosinophils. NK, natural killer.

can be a foreign body or an intrinsic protein antigen that activates the innate immune system. Innate immunity is a non–antigen specific means by which the body provides a first line of defense against foreign pathogens, including inhaled irritants. The innate immune system activates macrophages directly, without any need for prior exposure or antigen processing as is required for an adaptive T- and B-cell-dependent response. Activated macrophages mature to form epithelioid cells around the foreign material and thereby form a granuloma.[1]

However, macrophage activation and granuloma formation are also influenced by specific immune signals generated by other cells of the immune system, including signals triggered in an antigen-specific manner by the foreign particle or protein, as illustrated in Figure 11-1. Fragments of foreign proteins processed by antigen-presenting cells, such as dendritic cells, are displayed on the cell surface in the context of the host major histocompatibility complex (MHC). Through this indirect pathway, antigen-specific CD4+ helper T cells are activated in the context of class II MHC presentation, whereas CD8+ effector T cells traditionally require the class I MHC complex. These activated T cells produce various cytokines that trigger several antigen-specific and nonspecific cellular subsets. For example, the activated T_H1 subsets of $CD4^+$ helper T cells and natural killer (NK) cells produce interferon-gamma (IFN-γ), leading to primarily macrophage activation. On the other hand, the T_H2 subset produces interleukin-4 (IL-4) and interleukin-5 and results in eosinophil production and activation.[1-3] Other T-cell subsets, such as $CD8^+$ effector cells, are also recruited to help clear the protein antigen and thus help regulate the immune system. Once activated, this inflammatory process results in the recruitment of other immune cells, complement, and growth factors to form discrete granulomas, or the process may spread to the alveolar spaces and walls, leading to alveolitic changes (described later). Tumor necrosis factor (TNF), a potent inflammatory cytokine, has been implicated in initiating and driving the inflammatory process in many of these pathologic states. Newer targeted therapies for many inflammatory ILDs involve anti-TNF therapies.[4,5] Granulomatous mechanisms are involved in a variety of pulmonary diseases, yet they all share this fundamental pathophysiologic mechanism. The clinical presentations and findings of these disease entities are described later.

Foreign Bodies and Inorganic Dust

Patients who have inhaled foreign bodies are typically asymptomatic at the time of initial exposure unless the particle is large enough to occlude the tracheobronchial tree. In such cases, as often seen in children, the diagnosis is made by history, confirmed by chest radiography, and, if needed, diagnosed as well as treated via bronchoscopy. However, prolonged exposure to smaller foreign particles, whether organic or inorganic, can lead to a spectrum of pulmonary disease processes. Chronic exposure to metal dusts, such as beryllium, aluminum, and zirconium—foreign particles that cannot be cleared by the mucociliary system or broken down by the pulmonary macrophages—is associated with a marked interstitial granulomatous disease pattern.[6] Continuous exposure to small organic particles in susceptible individuals can also lead to hypersensitivity pneumonitis, with both alveolitic and granulomatous responses. The effect of a one-time massive exposure to inorganic fine particulate matter is less clear. A large subset of the pedestrians and workers exposed to smoke, dust, and particulate matter after the World Trade Center attacks in 2001 presented with a variety of nonspecific respiratory ailments, often with documented nonspecific histologic changes on lung biopsy. However, their long-term outcomes are not yet known.[7,8]

Hypersensitivity Pneumonitis

Hypersensitivity pneumonitis, also known as extrinsic alveolitis, describes a pulmonary disease process characterized by immunologically induced injury of the lung parenchyma with granuloma formation, alveolitis, and an antibody response, as the result of repeated exposure to inhaled protein antigen.[9-11] Numerous antigens have been implicated, from *Aspergillus* and fish meal dust to male rat urine, leading to various interesting, occupation-associated disease names (Table 11-1). Initial exposure to the antigen induces neutrophil and macrophage extravasation to the distal bronchioles and alveoli, thus leading to early alveolitis. Patients may present acutely with cough, fever, and chills several hours after exposure. With continued antigen exposure, patients develop a persistent

Table 11–1
Selected Hypersensitivity Pneumonitis Syndromes

Syndrome	Antigen
Bagassosis	*Actinomycetes* species from sugar cane
Cheese washer's lung	*Penicillium casei* from moldy cheese
Compost lung	*Aspergillus* species from compost
Furrier's lung	Animal fur dust
Hot tub lung	Mold on ceilings
Laboratory worker's lung	Rat urine
Fish meal worker's lung	Fish meal dust
Woodworker's lung	Wood dust

cough with worsening dyspnea secondary to granuloma formation within the pulmonary parenchyma, and progressive interstitial disease.[9,11]

The diagnosis lies in careful history taking, especially when a known occupational exposure is suspected. Chest radiographs have no diagnostic pattern, though may show a reticular nodular pattern consistent with interstitial lung disease. Chest computed tomography (CT) is typically nondiagnostic as well.[10,11] Bronchoalveolar lavage (BAL) may be helpful, showing an increase in $CD4^+$ T cells acutely and $CD8^+$ T cells chronically. However, this narrows the spectrum only marginally, as this is characteristic of nearly all granulomatous disease processes. Serum tests for antibodies to the suspected antigen are often required to make a diagnosis. Lung biopsy, either transbronchially or via video-assisted thoracoscopic surgery (VATS) or open thoracotomy, may be necessary to make a diagnosis in those patients for whom other evidence is lacking. Even this aggressive approach, however, may be nondiagnostic in late stages when the acute granulomatous and alveolitic changes are replaced by interstitial fibrosis.

Treatment consists of removing exposure to the suspected antigen, and steroids for patients with the severe acute form of the disease or with chronic persistent fibrosis.[10-13] Histologic evidence of fibrosis in lung biopsy specimens is correlated with a worse prognosis.[13] Radiologic evidence of fibrosis seen on high-resolution CTs may serve as a surrogate for histologic findings once the diagnosis has been made, and this may correlate with long-term survival and response to therapy.[12]

Infections

Pulmonary infection with *Mycobacterium tuberculosis* is probably the most common cause of granulomatous lung disease worldwide.[2,14] Local as well as disseminated miliary disease leads to granuloma formation in the infected field (Fig. 11-2). Other infectious organisms such as *Aspergillus* and certain helminths can also lead to pulmonary granulomatous disease.[2] Radiologic assessment alone is often inadequate to make a diagnosis, and the clinical context must be taken into account. The clinical pathogenesis, presentation, course, and treatment of pulmonary infections are discussed elsewhere in this book and are not included in this discussion of ILD.

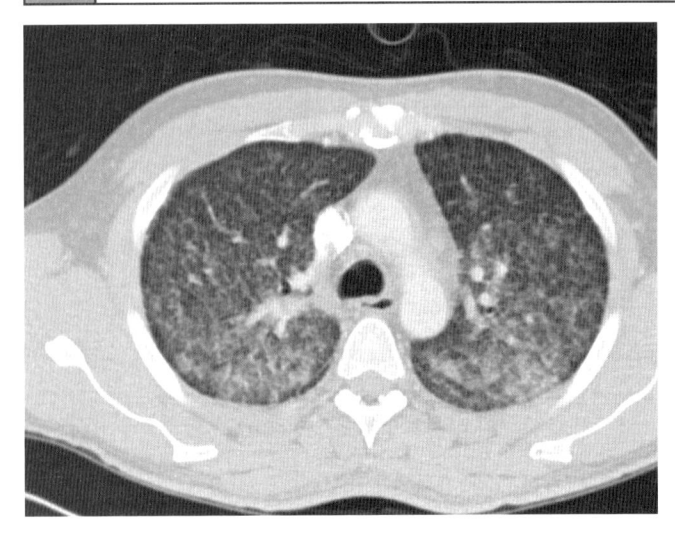

Figure 11-2
Computed tomography of the chest from a patient found to have miliary tuberculosis.

Sarcoidosis

Sarcoidosis is a chronic systemic disorder that, although common, is still poorly understood. Various organ systems of these patients are often affected by granulomatous disease, and some individuals do not manifest pulmonary involvement.[15-17] The incidence of sarcoidosis varies with the population studied. In Western populations, the incidence is estimated to be 10 to 20 per 100,000 population, with a higher rate in women and those of African-American ancestry.[18] Sarcoidosis is uncommon in Asian populations. Although the disease can manifest at any age, most patients present between the ages of 20 and 40.[15,16,19,20]

The etiology of sarcoidosis is unknown. Environmental, infectious, hereditary, and immunologic factors have been postulated, with variable evidence to support each hypothesis.[20] The interstitial granulomatous disease that results from inhalation of metal dusts is pathologically identical to sarcoidosis, suggesting that an unknown environmental exposure may be responsible.[6,21,22] Supporters of an infectious etiology argue that the causative agent must be inhaled, because 80% of affected individuals have pulmonary and mediastinal lymph node involvement. In fact, BAL of individuals with extrapulmonary sarcoid contains inflammatory cells even without evidence of pulmonary disease. The causative agent is suspected by some to be *Mycobacterium tuberculosis* or a nontuberculosis mycobacteria. Genetic analyses of affected tissue by polymerase chain reaction as well as antibody analysis of afflicted individuals have been inconclusive. Other agents implicated have been *Yersinia enterocolitica* and *Borrelia burgdorferi*, but the evidence linking these agents to sarcoidosis is even less well established. There is familial clustering of the disease, and sarcoidosis has been linked to human leukocyte antigens (HLA) A1 and B8 in whites, suggesting that hereditary and genetic factors play an important role in this disease. Non-MHC immunologic factors are probably also involved, as patients with sarcoidosis have numerous abnormalities of the immune system, including altered T-cell ratios, poorly responsive CD4$^+$ T-cell subsets, hyperactive B-cell lines, and altered production of the inflammatory cytokines IFN-γ and RANTES by macrophages.[23-27]

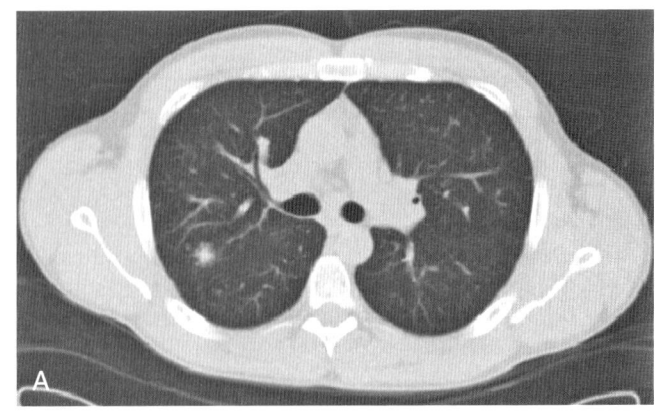

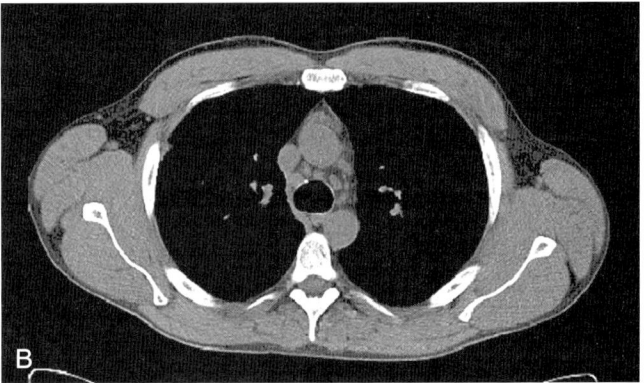

Figure 11-3
Computed tomography of the chest from a patient found to have noncaseating, non-necrotizing granulomata in the mediastinal lymph nodes on cervical mediastinoscopy. These findings are consistent with the diagnosis of sarcoidosis. **A**, Lung window. **B**, Mediastinal window.

Symptoms of sarcoidosis are variable and fluctuate with time. Most patients in whom the disease is identified by routine chest radiography are asymptomatic. Others may present with the acute onset of constitutional symptoms such as fever, chills, fatigue, and weight loss. Afflicted individuals often have an associated connective tissue disorder, such as rheumatoid arthritis, systemic lupus erythematosus, and progressive systemic sclerosis. Pulmonary symptoms commonly include dyspnea and a dry cough.[19] Diagnosis is typically made radiographically, with chest radiographs showing bilateral hilar and mediastinal lymph node enlargement with or without an accompanying reticulonodular pulmonary pattern indicative of interstitial disease. Consolidation and a ground-glass pattern may also be evident, particularly on chest CT (Fig. 11-3). Fibrosis is seen in later stages of the disease. Serum abnormalities may include an increase in levels of angiotensin-converting enzyme (ACE), presumably produced by the activated macrophages in the granulomas. A preponderance of lymphocytes in the BAL suggests an alveolitic process with granulomatous changes. Diagnosis, however, is most often made by mediastinal lymph node biopsy if adenopathy is present.[19,28,29] In rare cases, transbronchial or VATS biopsy may be needed to establish the diagnosis. Histologic findings of affected pulmonary tissue show noncaseating granulomas with high tissue ACE levels.

Treatment consists primarily of steroids in symptomatic patients.[19] Methotrexate and other immunosuppressive agents have also been used for refractory cases. Recent studies have suggested a benefit to tumor necrosis factor inhibitors such as infliximab in patients with poor responses to standard immunosuppressive regimens.[30-32]

Granulomatous Vasculitides: Wegener's Granulomatosis and Churg-Strauss Syndrome

Like sarcoidosis, Wegener's granulomatosis is a systemic disorder characterized by granuloma formation and it may involve multiple organ systems. Wegener's is a rare disease with an incidence of 1 to 3 in 100,000. Affected individuals typically present between the ages of 40 and 60.[33]

In its most extreme form, Wegener's granulomatosis is characterized by necrotizing granulomatous involvement of the pulmonary parenchyma and both pulmonary and renal vasculature.[2,22,33-37] Disease expression is variable and may be limited to the pulmonary system. Numerous etiologies have been suggested, including infectious organisms such as parvovirus B19 and other respiratory agents, inhaled environmental agents such as silica, and genetic factors linked to the HLA alleles DR1, DR2, and DR12. Although all of these possible etiologies are supported by some evidence, no explanation is conclusive. The sera of individuals afflicted with the disease contain antibodies to antineutrophil cytoplasmic antibodies (ANCA). Specifically, 90% of patients with Wegener's granulomatosis have C-ANCA, which chiefly binds to the PR3 plasma serine proteinase in neutrophils, as opposed to P-ANCA, which are antibodies to a perinuclear myeloperoxidase enzyme.[22,34,35] The exact role of C-ANCA in the pathogenesis of Wegener's granulomatosis is unclear and, unfortunately, ANCAs are also found in other disease states, such as systemic lupus erythematosus, in which ILD may develop.[22,34-38]

Individuals with Wegener's granulomatosis may present with fulminant disease, with massive hemoptysis and renal failure secondary to extensive necrotizing granulomatous lesions, or with more subtle findings of fever, malaise, weight loss, and progressive dyspnea, with hemoptysis appearing only as the disease progresses. Neurologic or ocular symptoms may also be present. Diagnosis relies not only on the history but also on laboratory studies such as C-ANCA serologies and other associated systemic abnormalities.[22,34,37] Chest imaging show a reticulonodular pattern consistent with interstitial disease or discrete nodules in only 50% of affected individuals. Central necrosis in these nodules can give the appearance of cavitary lesions (Fig. 11-4). BAL from patients with Wegener's granulomatosis contains neutrophils and eosinophils. Biopsy of pulmonary or renal lesions may be necessary to establish or confirm the diagnosis. Pathology typically shows granulomas with neutrophils, macrophages, and eosinophils. Treatment options vary with the severity of the disease and include steroids and immunosuppressive agents, such as cyclophosphamide.[37] Newer agents currently under active investigation include TNF inhibitors.[4]

Churg-Strauss syndrome is a rare systemic disorder characterized by eosinophilia, vasculitis, and pulmonary parenchymal granuloma formation. Many view this disease as part of a spectrum of disease that includes Wegener's granulomatosis and other connective tissue diseases.[22,35,36] The true incidence is unknown because of the difficulty of establishing a diagnosis, but it is estimated at 1 to 2 per 1 million people, and it affects individuals between the ages of 20 and 50.[22,39] As in

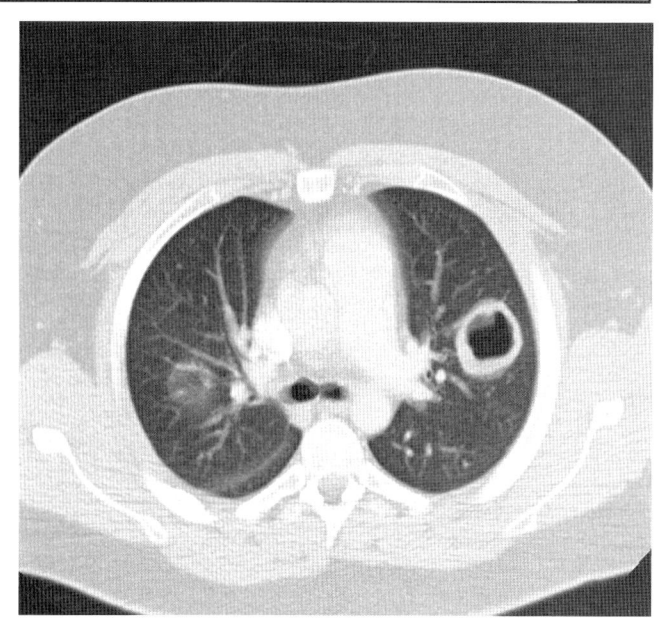

Figure 11–4
Computed tomography of the chest from a young man with Wegener's granulomatosis. Central necrosis in a granulomatous lesion has the appearance of a cavitary lesion. Many other such lesions were present throughout the lung parenchyma.

Wegener's granulomatosis and sarcoidosis, multiple etiologies have been suggested, including pigeon exposure, helminth infection, and cocaine use. Recently, Churg-Strauss syndrome has been associated with the weaning of steroids in asthma patients placed on leukotriene antagonists.[22,36,40,41]

Affected individuals typically have a history of asthma or allergic symptoms and present with fever, cough, and occasionally hemoptysis. Gastrointestinal bleeding or neuropathy may also be present. Diagnosis rests on clinical suspicion and the combination of symptoms, laboratory studies, and pathologic findings. Chest radiographs typically reveal patchy consolidation throughout the lung fields. Levels of immunoglobulin E (IgE) and P-ANCA may be elevated. As expected, the BAL shows large numbers of eosinophils.[28,29] Lung biopsy, usually required for diagnosis, demonstrates vasculitis and parenchymal granulomas with eosinophils. Treatment consists of steroid therapy and other immunosuppressive agents. Anti-TNF therapy has also been investigated.[42] Prognosis for those diagnosed with the syndrome is poor, with a mortality of 50% to 60% at 5 years.[35,36]

Eosinophilic Pneumonias

Eosinophilic pneumonia belongs to a spectrum of pulmonary processes that are distinguished by the accumulation of eosinophils in parenchymal tissue. Eosinophilic pulmonary diseases with known etiologies include those caused by helminth infections, such as *Strongyloides stercoralis* and *Ancylostoma duodenale*, and drug allergies, which cause peripheral blood eosinophilia and can have systemic effects, as well as those conditions associated with the granulomatous vasculitides (discussed earlier) in which the etiology is unclear.[43,44] All of these disease states can have pulmonary involvement. Diagnosis is made by history, blood eosinophil counts, blood serologies, and occasionally lung biopsy.

Idiopathic eosinophilic pneumonias can be divided into simple, acute, and chronic forms. Simple eosinophilic pneumonia, also known as Löeffler's syndrome, is rare and characterized pathologically by interstitial edema with abundant eosinophils. Patients typically present with few or no symptoms. Chest radiographs show patchy parenchymal consolidation, and the diagnosis rests on the demonstration of peripheral blood eosinophilia in patients with a history of asthma or atopy. The disease usually resolves spontaneously, so biopsy or BAL is rarely required to make a diagnosis. Patients with symptoms, even when symptoms are prolonged, may benefit from steroid therapy.[43,44]

Acute eosinophilic pneumonia is a rare disorder that presents as an acute illness with severe respiratory distress that may require ventilatory assistance. The etiology is unclear, but it is thought to be secondary to an eosinophil-mediated immune response to an unknown allergen. Patients present with severe shortness of breath and pleuritic symptoms. Chest radiography show reticular opacities similar to the pattern found with interstitial pulmonary edema. The disease is characterized by a high number of eosinophils, up to 80%, in the BAL. Steroids are the mainstay of treatment, but a high relapse rate is associated with this disease.[43,44]

Chronic eosinophilic pneumonia has a similar histologic and, in most cases, radiographic appearance. Again, diagnosis relies on the demonstration of peripheral blood eosinophilia in patients with a history of asthma or atopy. However, affected patients have chronic symptoms that do not resolve over time, and therefore eosinophilia on BAL, tissue biopsy, or both, are often needed to make the diagnosis.[29,44] Steroid treatment usually results in rapid disease regression.[43,44]

Histiocytosis X

Histiocytosis X, also known as eosinophilic granuloma, pulmonary Langerhans cell histiocytosis, or Langerhans cell granulomatosis, is a rare disorder characterized by the peribronchial accumulation of specialized antigen presenting cells known as Langerhans cells. Letterer-Siwe and Hand-Schüller-Christian diseases are variants typically found in children and may not have pulmonary involvement.[45,46] The adult form, eosinophilic granuloma, is characterized by pulmonary and skeletal system involvement. Although rare, histiocytosis X predominantly occurs in whites and women. Viral infection with Epstein-Barr virus or other members of the herpesvirus family has been suggested as a possible etiology for this disease.[45,46] Recent reports find that the clonal population of cells involved in this disease have short telomeres, much like those in other malignancies.[42] Telomerase activity has also been correlated with the degree of disease expression.[47] Chest radiographs in the early stages of the disease show bilateral nodular opacities. With progression of disease, a reticulonodular pattern is noted. Patients are typically asymptomatic at the time of diagnosis in young adulthood. Diagnosis is commonly made by routine chest radiography. Symptomatic patients present with a dry cough and shortness of breath. BAL can be useful, as Langerhans cell are abundant in the fluid.[28,29,46] Lung biopsy can confirm clinical suspicions in unclear cases, because the demonstration of Langerhans cells infiltrating the pulmonary bronchioles is pathognomonic of this disease. Despite its name, granulomas are not formed in the strict sense, because the chief cellular component in these lesions is Langerhans cells and not macrophages. Long-standing disease leads to interstitial fibrosis. Remission may occur spontaneously and can often be aided with steroid therapy.[48]

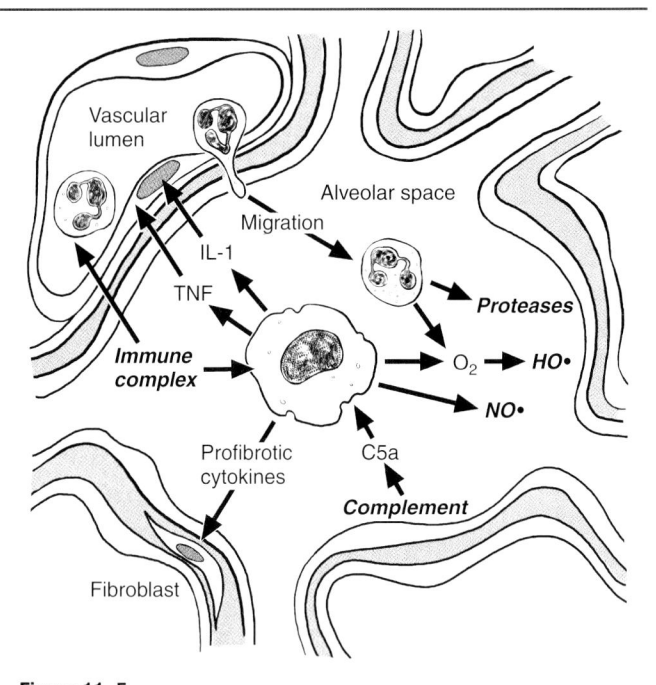

Figure 11–5
Pathogenesis of alveolitic injury. Activation of alveolar macrophages and polymorphonuclear leukocytes by complement, immune complex deposition, and subsequent cytokine/chemokine release trigger a cascade of responses that result in acute lung injury to the surrounding alveolar membrane and interstitium. IL, interleukin; TNF, tumor necrosis factor.

ALVEOLITIC PATTERNS OF ILD

When immunologic injury is primarily directed toward the alveolar epithelial surface, inflammation of the alveolar wall and airspaces results in a histopathologic pattern of alveolitis. Both cellular and humoral components of the immune system are involved in these alveolitic changes in the lung. Alveolitic mechanisms are involved in a variety of pulmonary diseases (see Box 11-1).[49]

Activated macrophages, T cells, and inflammatory cytokines can lead to B-cell activation and antibody production. These antibodies form complexes with the antigen and are deposited within the lung parenchyma, leading to the activation of complement. Although the formation of the membrane attack complex is an attempt to destroy the antigen, injury to the surrounding lung tissue may be significant if this inflammatory reaction is not regulated. A basic diagram of this cascade is illustrated in Figure 11-5.[49]

Chemotactic peptides produced by the complement pathways, such as C5a and C3b, recruit other components of the cellular immune system. Neutrophils and macrophages thus destroy the pathogen and cause further parenchymal destruction. Activated macrophages and other immune cells produce additional cytokines, such as TNF and IL-1, which, together with immune complex deposition and complement activation, lead to direct injury to the lung parenchyma and the surrounding vasculature. Numerous other cytokines and inflammatory modulators, such as prostaglandins, may also play important roles in the pathophysiology of ILDs. If the immune process continues unmitigated, the acute inflammatory response present in the lung parenchyma in the early phase of the disease is replaced by increasing degrees of fibrosis as more and more fibroblasts are recruited into the area of injury to repair the damage. Fibrosis is the final common pathway for both the alveolitic and granulomatous immune responses, making it often impossible to differentiate between these two disease processes in the late stages of ILD. Irreversible scarring and fibrosis of the alveolar–endothelial interface and surrounding parenchyma results in significant impairment in gas exchange and is consistent with end-stage ILD. Current investigational treatments focus on mitigating or abrogating the inflammatory response with targeted therapies directed at many of the cytokines involved in the immune response before the development of fibrosis.

Drug-Associated Injury

Whether directly toxic or immune mediated, drug-associated injury to the lung results in an alveolitic pattern of damage. Chronic concomitant damage often leads to irreversible fibrosis. Numerous drugs have been implicated in pulmonary injury, but only amiodarone and its mechanisms are discussed here. Direct toxic effects can result from radiation, bleomycin, nitrofurantoin, and prolonged exposure to high oxygen concentrations.[50] Injury in these cases is principally the result of free oxygen radical production. Acute changes are predominantly alveolitic, followed by progressive fibrosis as the lungs recover from the initial insult. BAL specimens from patients during the acute phase contain numerous neutrophils or eosinophils.[28,29]

Amiodarone, a potent antiarrhythmic agent, has the ability to induce direct as well as immune-mediated injury. Direct amiodarone toxicity most likely results from the generation of free oxygen radical species. However, the large number of lymphocytes in the BAL, particularly CD8+ T cells, suggests that immune-mediated mechanisms are also involved.[50,51] Pulmonary toxicity has been correlated with patient age and duration of therapy.[52] However, a fulminant form of amiodarone pulmonary toxicity has been described, especially in patients undergoing lung surgery, and is thought to be an idiosyncratic immune response.[51] Chest radiographs in drug-associated ILD demonstrate an interstitial disease pattern. As fibrosis intervenes, the BAL specimen becomes acellular and the chest radiograph shows a more prominent reticulonodular pattern.[28,29] Diagnosis rests on the recognition of prior drug exposure. Lung biopsy, if done in late stages, may show only fibrotic change. Treatment of amiodarone pulmonary toxicity consists of prompt cessation of drug use and management of symptoms.

Goodpasture's Syndrome

Goodpasture's syndrome is characterized by the presence of pulmonary hemorrhage and glomerulonephritis. Its incidence is rare, it predominantly affects males 15 to 25 years in age, and it is linked to the HLA-DR2 MHC allele. Other immunologic and hereditary factors, as well as an association with free-base cocaine use, have been implicated.[53] The pathogenesis of alveolitis, pulmonary hemorrhage, and glomerulonephritis results from the presence of antibodies directed against a collagen protein in the alveolar and glomerular membranes.

Box 11-2
Idiopathic Interstitial Pneumonias

- Usual Interstitial Pneumonia (UIP)/Idiopathic Pulmonary Fibrosis (IPF)
- Desquamative Interstitial Pneumonia (DIP)
- Nonspecific Interstitial Pneumonia (NIP)
- Acute Interstitial Pneumonia (AIP)
- Respiratory Bronchiolitis–Associated Interstitial Lung Disease (RB-ILD)
- Cryptogenic Organizing Pneumonia (COP)
- Lymphocytic Interstitial Pneumonia (LIP)

These antibodies, as a result of complement activation and cell-mediated injury, produce immune complex–mediated injury to both lung and renal parenchyma.[25,54,55]

In most cases, patients present with hemoptysis, and occasionally hematuria. Diagnosis is based on clinical symptoms and the characteristic linear staining of the basement membrane with anti-IgG antibodies present on renal biopsy.[25,55] Chest radiographs demonstrate patchy consolidation secondary to hemorrhage. BAL is nondiagnostic and lung biopsy is rarely needed to make a diagnosis.[28,29] Therapy consists of plasmapheresis to remove the antibodies, and immunosuppressive therapy.

Idiopathic pulmonary hemorrhage is similar to Goodpasture's syndrome in terms of its pulmonary manifestations. However, this disease predominantly affects children younger than 10 years and does not have any renal involvement. Patients present with hemoptysis and weakness secondary to iron deficiency. Radiographic appearance is similar to that in Goodpasture's, but the absence of anti–basement membrane antibodies in lung and renal biopsies differentiates between the two. Prognosis is variable and treatment consists of plasmapheresis and immunosuppressive therapy.[25]

Idiopathic Interstitial Pneumonias

Idiopathic interstitial pneumonias are a spectrum of pulmonary disorders characterized by the infiltration of immune cells into the pulmonary interstitium, and the resultant alveolitic changes. Unabated inflammation leads to fibrosis of the lung parenchyma. Because many terms have been given to the various forms of this disease (Hamman-Rich disease, idiopathic pulmonary fibrosis, usual interstitial pneumonitis, diffuse pulmonary alveolar fibrosis), there has been much confusion in diagnosing this disease entity. A useful subclassification scheme based on pathology has been proposed by Averill Liebow,[55a] and a modification of this scheme is presented in Box 11-2. Many argue that even this classification scheme is arbitrary and that the diseases categorized are merely different manifestations of the same disease.[56-58] Nonetheless, as many of these terms are in clinical use, it is important to have some familiarity with them and the histologic findings (Table 11-2).

Usual Interstitial Pneumonia and Idiopathic Pulmonary Fibrosis

The typical pathologic finding of usual interstitial pneumonia (UIP) is thickened fibrotic alveolar interstitium infiltrated by inflammatory cells, such as lymphocytes and plasma cells.

Table 11–2
Summary of Histologic Findings for Immunologic Lung Diseases

Disease	Histology
Granulomatous	
Foreign body/inorganic dust	Simple granuloma
Hypersensitivity pneumonitis	Granulomas with CD4+/CD8+ T cells; interstitial edema; fibrosis in later stages
Infections	
Tuberculosis	Caseating granulomas
Sarcoidosis	Noncaseating granulomas
Granulomatous vasculitides	
Wegener's granulomatosis	Necrotizing granulomas involving vasculature
Churg-Strauss syndrome	Necrotizing granulomas involving vasculature
Eosinophilic pneumonias	Granulomas with eosinophilic predominance; interstitial edema
Histiocytosis X	Granulomas with Langerhans cells
Alveolitic	
Drug-associated injury	Interstitial edema with inflammatory cells
Goodpasture's syndrome	Linear staining of basement membrane with anti-IgG antibodies typically seen on renal biopsy; interstitial edema with inflammatory cells
Idiopathic interstitial pneumonias	
Usual interstitial pneumonia (UIP)/idiopathic pulmonary fibrosis (IPF)	Interstitial edema and/or fibrosis with inflammatory cells; patchy fibrotic change
Desquamative interstitial pneumonia (DIP)	Interstitial edema with sparse inflammatory cells; mild diffuse fibrotic change
Nonspecific interstitial pneumonia (NIP)	Thickened interstitium with inflammatory cells; some patchy fibrosis
Acute interstitial pneumonia (AIP)	Diffuse alveolar damage with thickened fibrotic interstitium; proliferating fibroblasts
Respiratory bronchiolitis–associated interstitial lung disease (RB-ILD)	Macrophages infiltrating distal bronchioles
Cryptogenic organizing pneumonia (COP)	Chronically inflamed alveoli with granulation tissue in bronchioles and macrophages in alveoli
Lymphocytic interstitial pneumonia (LIP)	Diffuse lymphocytic and plasma cell infiltration; minimal alveolar injury

Histologic analysis in the acute phase of the disease demonstrates alveolitis, with an interstitium overrun with inflammatory cells and areas of patchy fibrotic changes.[56] Patients who demonstrate interstitial lung disease on chest radiography and pathologic evidence of UIP on lung biopsy are given the clinical diagnosis of idiopathic pulmonary fibrosis (IPF) when other causes of interstitial disease (e.g., sarcoidosis, hypersensitivity pneumonitis, histiocytosis X, infection) have been excluded. The pathologic findings of UIP often lead to a diagnosis of IPF in clinical practice.[56,59-63]

IPF occurs with an estimated incidence of 5 to 20 per 100,000 persons, with a slight male predominance.[39,59,64] The etiology of IPF is unknown. Exposure to heavy metal dusts, solvents, and Epstein-Barr and hepatitis C viruses have all been named as possible mediators of the initial lung injury in susceptible individuals, but there has been no definitive proof for any of these theories.[29] Cigarette smoking has been implicated in some case-control studies. IPF has been linked to HLA-B15, HLA-B8, and HLA-B12 loci, and a familial form of IPF has been described, suggesting a hereditary/immunologic component to this disease.[65,66] Further evidence for an immunologic basis is that individuals afflicted with pulmonary disease related to rheumatoid arthritis, systemic lupus erythematosus, and progressive systemic sclerosis have a high incidence of interstitial inflammation and fibrosis that is clinically and pathologically indistinguishable from IPF. Recent studies have implicated matrix metalloproteinases (MMPs) in the pathogenesis of IPF based on microarray analysis and the results of MMP knockout mice. The diagnostic and therapeutic implications of these findings have not yet been determined.[67,68]

Individuals with IPF present with progressive shortness of breath, weight loss, and a nonproductive cough. In 80% of individuals, the chest radiograph reveals linear opacities in a diffuse reticulonodular pattern. The lower lung zones may be preferentially involved. Chest CT can further demonstrate

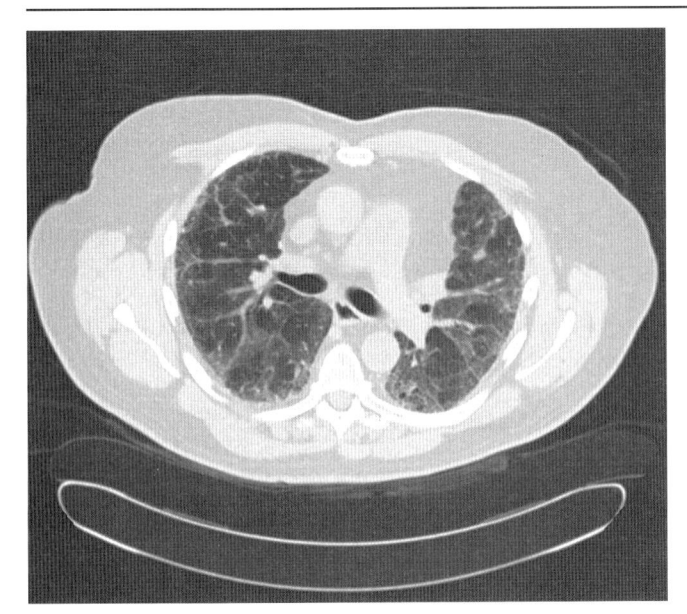

Figure 11–6
Computed tomography of the chest in a patient with idiopathic pulmonary fibrosis. Note the reticular interstitial pattern and honeycombing at the lung bases. The patient subsequently underwent a single-lung transplant.

a reticular pattern, with honeycombing, cysts, and ground-glass opacities (Fig. 11-6).[69,70] Mediastinal lymph node enlargement is common. BAL typically shows large numbers of neutrophils, eosinophils, or lymphocytes.[28,29,59] Patients with high levels of lymphocytes in their BAL fluid have been shown to have a better response to steroid therapy and an improved prognosis in some studies.[71,72] Transbronchial biopsy yields inadequate tissue to make a diagnosis of IPF.[59] The principal role for lung biopsy is to exclude other etiologies of interstitial lung disease, which may alter the therapeutic plan or prognosis.

The mainstay of treatment for IPF is steroids or other immunosuppressive therapies, or both, including methotrexate, penicillamine, colchicine, and cyclosporine. All have variable response rates. Lung transplant is indicated for those patients who deteriorate despite best medical therapy.[73,74] In general, lung transplantation is the procedure of choice for patients with IPF or other end-stage ILDs that fail medical management.[59,75-78] The basic criteria for lung transplantation in this setting are (1) progressive dyspnea/hypoxia despite best medical therapy; (2) a predicted vital capacity of 60% to 70% or less, or a predicted diffusing capacity of 50% to 60% or less; and (3) patient age of 60 or less for double-lung transplant, or 65 for single-lung transplant.[79,80] Diagnosis and treatment of pulmonary fibrosis associated with connective tissue disease is similar to that for IPF.[75-77] However, pulmonary symptoms typically wax and wane with the disease and often respond to treatment of the primary disease.[59] Lung transplantation is indicated in those patients with stable connective tissue disease and progressive pulmonary symptoms refractory to medical therapy.[79] Although the 5-year survival rate is only 50% to 70% after transplantation for IPF, this is a significant improvement over the 28-month median survival reported for medically treated IPF.[80-82]

Desquamative Interstitial Pneumonia

Desquamative interstitial pneumonia (DIP) tends to have a more uniform histologic appearance than UIP or IPF, and the interstitium is only mildly thickened, with a sparse infiltrate of inflammatory cells and mild fibrosis. The incidence of DIP is low, and it affects smokers usually at age 40 to 50.[39,56,59,64,83]

Patients present with dyspnea and fatigue, and the chest radiograph reveals characteristic bilateral ground-glass opacities, which may be linear depending on the degree of fibrosis. Chest CT further highlights these ground-glass abnormalities. BAL specimens typically have fewer inflammatory cells than those from patients with UIP but relative eosinophilia.[28,29,59,83-85] Lung biopsy, as for UIP, may be indicated to exclude other etiologies of ILD. However, the diffuse changes present throughout the lung in DIP may be seen focally in UIP, making it difficult to distinguish UIP from DIP by this means. The presence of eosinophils in the BAL fluid may aid in the diagnosis.[84,85] Patients may respond to steroid therapy, but the disease is typically progressive. Lung transplantation is indicated in end-stage disease.[83]

Nonspecific Interstitial Pneumonia

Lung biopsy specimens from patients with nonspecific interstitial pneumonia (NIP) reveal a mildly thickened interstitium with an infiltrate of inflammatory cells and some fibrosis.[56,58,59,86] The incidence of NIP is rare with no sex predominance, unlike for UIP and IPF. Clinical presentation and radiologic features of the disease are similar to those of UIP and IPF. However, NIP has a much better clinical response to steroid and immunosuppressive therapy and is associated with improved overall survival.[58,59,86]

Acute Interstitial Pneumonitis

Acute interstitial pneumonia (AIP) is rapidly progressive and clinically similar to acute lung injury and acute respiratory distress syndrome (ARDS), with the exception that there is no preceding trauma, sepsis, or known source of injury. The clinical presentation involves rapid onset with progressive dyspnea, respiratory failure, and death usually within a year. Pathologic examination of lung biopsy tissue consists of diffuse alveolar damage with a thickened fibrotic interstitium infiltrated by proliferating fibroblasts.[56,59] In very acute fulminant cases, the fibrosis can be replaced with an exudative interstitial edema similar to that found in diffuse alveolar damage, suggesting that AIP may be a point on the spectrum of disease between IPF and diffuse alveolar damage. Radiologically, AIP is similar to ARDS in that chest radiographs and chest CT demonstrate characteristic bilateral patchy airspace disease and ground-glass opacities. Prognosis for those afflicted with AIP, as for those with ARDS, is poor, with a fatality rate of 70% and most patients dying within 2 weeks of diagnosis.[59,87]

Respiratory Bronchiolitis–Associated Interstitial Lung Disease

Respiratory bronchiolitis-associated interstitial lung disease (RB-ILD) is pathologically distinct in that it is characterized by the infiltration of macrophages surrounding the distal bronchioles.[88] Its incidence is rare, and it chiefly affects men aged 40 to 50. RB-ILD is strongly correlated with a history of recent or current smoking.[59,88,89] Chest radiographs demonstrate a diffuse reticulonodular pattern. BAL samples are characteristic, with abundant macrophages.[28,29] Biopsy is essentially to distinguish the disease from eosinophilic granuloma and histiocytosis X.[88] Treatment consists of steroid therapy and smoking cessation.

Cryptogenic Organizing Pneumonia

Cryptogenic organizing pneumonitis (COP), or idiopathic bronchiolitis obliterans organizing pneumonia (BOOP), is an alveolitic pulmonary disease characterized by chronic inflammation of the alveoli, the production of granulation tissue in the bronchioles and alveoli, and the accumulation of macrophages within the alveoli.[23,88,90-92] The incidence and etiology of COP is unknown, although an association with antibodies to nuclear proteins suggests an immune etiology.[93] Patients with this rare disorder present with weight loss and a nonproductive cough. Chest radiographs often demonstrate bilateral diffuse opacities. Chest CT shows airspace disease with ground-glass opacities, as seen in other peribronchial processes such as RB-ILD and histiocytosis X.[69,70] BAL fluid analysis reveals high levels of immune cells, including lymphocytes, eosinophils, macrophages, and neutrophils. However, the definitive diagnosis is dependent on lung biopsy.[23,88,90-92] Treatment consists of steroid therapy, with a typically rapid response and resolution of the disease. Relapses do occur more often in those who have secondary forms of BOOP from infection, drugs, or connective tissue disease. Relapses are also treated with steroids or other immunosuppressive regimens for longer periods of time.[94]

Lymphocytic Interstitial Pneumonia

Lymphocytic interstitial pneumonia (LIP) is a lymphoproliferative disorder characterized by the infiltration of lymphocytes and plasma cells into the lung parenchyma.[65,95] There is minimal to no alveolar injury. It is included, however, in the differential diagnosis of interstitial lung disease, and a lung biopsy may be required to exclude this disorder in some patients. LIP is a rare disorder predominantly seen in children, immunosuppressed patients, and women between the ages of 40 and 80 years. As with the vast majority of the ILDs discussed here, the etiology is unknown. Afflicted individuals present with the nonspecific symptoms of fever, fatigue, and weight loss. Chest radiography and chest CT illustrate a reticulonodular pattern and sporadic ground-glass opacities. BAL shows a large number of lymphocytes, but lung biopsy is usually required to make the diagnosis in susceptible patient populations.[28,29] Progression to lymphoma has been documented, but initial treatment of LIP consists of steroid therapy.[95,96]

PATIENT EVALUATION

In approaching patients with suspected ILD, a thorough history and physical is critical (Fig. 11-7). The diagnosis may be suggested by a history of environmental or occupational exposure, connective tissue disease, or genetic disease. A similar clinical picture can be seen when intraparenchymal lymphatics are involved by malignant disease, so a history or evidence of malignancy must be sought.[97] Laboratory studies are performed for antibodies that suggest a connective tissue disease, for serum precipitins, or for elevated angiotensin-converting enzyme.

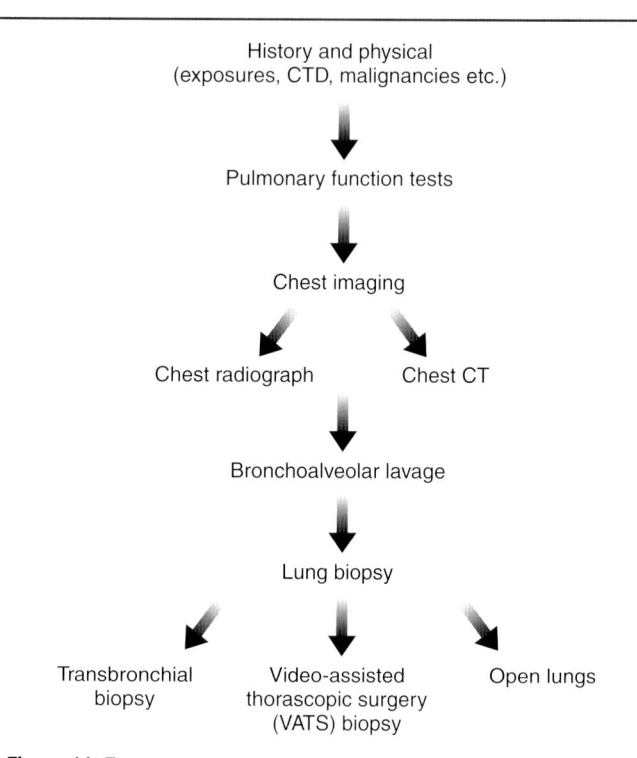

Figure 11–7
Algorithm for the approach to a patient with interstitial lung disease. CTD, connective tissue disease.

Pulmonary function tests are used to measure the extent of pulmonary dysfunction. ILDs are usually characterized by restrictive pulmonary physiology with a reduced total lung capacity, functional residual capacity, and residual volume. The forced expiratory volume in 1 second (FEV_1) and forced vital capacity (FVC) are often decreased as a result of the decrease in total lung capacity. The lung's diffusing capacity for carbon monoxide (DL_{CO}) is impaired because of the reduced compliance of the lung parenchyma and thus reflects the degree of resulting $\dot{V}/\dot{Q}$ mismatch more than the stage of disease. Arterial blood gases may be normal but can reveal hypoxemia as a result of significant $\dot{V}/\dot{Q}$ mismatch, particularly during exercise or sleep. Hypercarbia is usually indicative of end-stage disease. Chest imaging by plain film radiography and chest CT is helpful in separating interstitial disease patterns from consolidative patterns and their associated diseases.[98] Findings on chest radiograph are often nonspecific, with bibasilar reticular markings, and may include nodular opacities, particularly in the upper lung fields in sarcoidosis, hypersensitivity pneumonitis, silicosis, berylliosis, and some of the connective tissue diseases. High-resolution chest CT provides information as to the extent and distribution of disease and is particularly useful in the investigation of early disease, when the chest radiograph may appear normal, and in the evaluation of coexisting adenopathy, malignancy, or emphysema, which have an impact on subsequent treatment. In general, the radiographic appearance may not directly correlate with the histopathologic stage of the disease or the degree of clinical impairment. However, the presence of classic radiographic findings on chest CT may be sufficient for diagnosis and thus obviate the need for tissue diagnosis. Furthermore, evidence of honeycombing and extensive fibrosis is indicative of a poor prognosis.

BAL can be useful in the identification of diseases with a large inflammatory component, such as Wegener's granulomatosis, or in the detection of a particular cellular subset, as seen in eosinophilic pneumonias or histiocytosis X (Langerhans cells), but it is nonspecific in most forms of ILD.[28,29] Therefore, in many cases, lung biopsy by transbronchial, open, or VATS is required to make a definitive diagnosis.[62] Transbronchial biopsy is usually attempted first, particularly if sarcoidosis, Goodpasture's syndrome, or eosinophilic pneumonia is a likely diagnosis, or to rule out lymphangitic carcinomatosis (Fig. 11-8) or an infectious origin. If definitive diagnosis is not possible, surgical biopsy of two distinct disease sites, preferably on two different lobes, is warranted and provides the most effective means of establishing a diagnosis and prognosis. However, some clinicians argue that a single lung biopsy from the lingual or right middle lobe has a diagnostic yield equivalent to two separate biopsies.[99] If adequate-size representative biopsies are obtained early in the disease course before treatment, avoiding areas of honeycombing (which reveals only nonspecific fibrosis), the diagnostic accuracy approaches 90%.[100] Biopsy may not be beneficial if the clinical status or radiographic finding (e.g., extensive honeycombing) suggests that the patient is at high operative risk or that there is little benefit given the extent or prognosis of the disease.

VATS biopsy has proven to be as diagnostically accurate as open lung biopsy through a mini-thoracotomy.[101,102] However, the patient must be able to tolerate single-lung ventilation and to remain in the full lateral decubitus position (Fig. 11-9). Those who are acutely ill or are in a late stage of the disease have decreased pulmonary compliance and decreased DL_{CO} and thus a limited ability to tolerate general anesthesia, particularly with single-lung ventilation. These patients require an open lung biopsy through a mini-thoracotomy. Hence, ideally, lung biopsies should be attempted in patients whose disease stage is early, before diffuse fibrosis has set in,

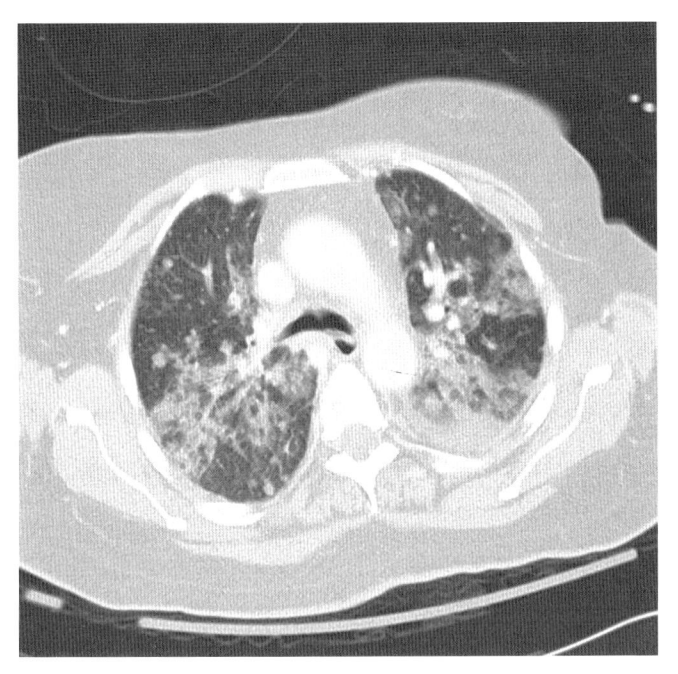

Figure 11–8
Computed tomography of the chest in a patient with a history of breast cancer and rapidly progressive bilateral ground-glass opacities. Lung biopsy revealed metastatic adenocarcinoma. There was a desmoplastic reaction around sites of tumor leading to focal areas of interstitial fibrosis as well.

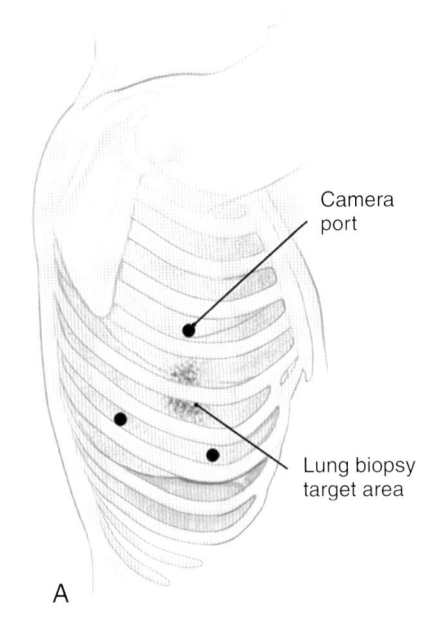

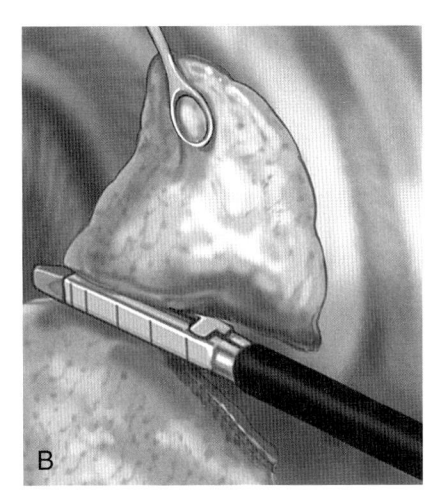

Figure 11–9
Video-assisted thoracoscopic surgery (VATS) lung biopsy. **A,** Patient in full lateral decubitus position after lung isolation. **B,** Lung biopsy performed with endoscopic stapler.

making both diagnosis and intraoperative management increasingly difficult and VATS implausible. Ideal candidates for VATS are ILD patients who are symptomatic but ambulatory with relatively preserved lung function.

TREATMENT

There is currently no known therapy to effectively reverse pulmonary fibrosis once it has occurred. Therefore, treatment of hypoxemia with supplemental oxygen and early intervention to limit injury and prevent progression of the granulomatous or alveolitic process toward fibrosis is the primary goal. Unless a causative agent is identified that can be removed or specifically treated, success is low. Glucocorticoids, usually prednisone at 0.5 to 1.0 mg/kg/day for 4 to 12 weeks, is the cornerstone of medical therapy, and it is recommended for all symptomatic patients diagnosed with idiopathic, interstitial, eosinophilic, or cryptogenic organizing pneumonias; connective tissue disease; sarcoid; or ILDs. A slow taper over several months is attempted if symptoms improve, as a rapid wean can be associated with recurrent disease. Only approximately 20% of patients with IPF respond to steroids, and this failure has led to treatment attempts with cyclophosphamide, azathioprine, methotrexate, and cyclosporine, with variable and inconsistent results. Although recent evidence suggests that IFN-γ may be helpful through its ability to modulate cytokines and the inflammatory response, the only currently available treatment option for the significant number of patients that are medical failures is that of lung transplantation.[57,103]

Diagnosis may not affect treatment, as many of these diseases are treated by steroid or immunosuppressive therapy. It does, however, play a critical role in defining the overall prognosis of these patients and the potential therapeutic options available for treatment. It also allays patient and physician anxiety about diagnostic uncertainty later in the disease course if there is no response to therapy. End-stage therapy consists of lung transplantation. Early diagnosis permits close follow-up and is imperative to ensure evaluation and listing for transplantation in sufficient time to allow survival until a donor organ is available.

REFERENCES

1. Robinson D, Richeldi L, Saltini C, du Bois R. Granulomatous processes. In: Crystal R, West J, Barnes P, editors. *The lung: scientific foundations.* Philadelphia: Lippincott-Raven; 1997. p. 2395-409.
2. Adams DO. The granulomatous inflammatory response: a review. *Am J Pathol* 1976;**84**:164-91.
3. Reynolds HY, Huck JL. Immunologic responses in the lung. *Respiration* 1990;**57**:221-8.
4. Langford CA. Drug insight: anti-tumor necrosis factor therapies for the vasculitic diseases. *Nat Clin Pract Rheumatol* 2008;**4**:364-70.
5. Lee RW, D'Cruz DP. Novel therapies for anti-neutrophil cytoplasmic antibody-associated vasculitis. *Drugs* 2008;**68**:747-70.
6. Maier LA. Clinical approach to chronic beryllium disease and other nonpneumoconiotic interstitial lung diseases. *J Thorac Imaging* 2002;**17**: 273-84.
7. Moline J, Herbert R, Nguyen N. Health consequences of the September 11 World Trade Center attacks: a review. *Cancer Invest* 2006;**24**:294-301.
8. Moscato G, Yacoub MR. World Trade Center disaster: short- and medium-term health outcome. *Monaldi Arch Chest Dis* 2007;**67**:154-8.
9. Bourke SJ, Dalphin JC, Boyd G, McSharry C, Baldwin CI, Calvert JE. Hypersensitivity pneumonitis: current concepts. *Eur Respir J Suppl* 2001;**32**:81s-92.
10. Glazer CS, Rose CS, Lynch DA. Clinical and radiologic manifestations of hypersensitivity pneumonitis. *J Thorac Imaging* 2002;**17**:261-72.
11. Moran JV, Greenberger PA, Patterson R. Long-term evaluation of hypersensitivity pneumonitis: a case study follow-up and literature review. *Allergy Asthma Proc* 2002;**23**:265-70.
12. Hanak V, Golbin JM, Hartman TE, Ryu JH. HRCT findings of parenchymal fibrosis correlate with prognosis in hypersensitivity pneumonitis. *Chest* 2008;**134**: 133-8.
13. Chiodera P. Idiopathic interstitial lung disease: anatomoradiologic pathogenesis. *Rays* 1997;**22**:127-56.
14. Chan ED, Iseman MD. Current medical treatment for tuberculosis. *BMJ* 2002;**325**:1282-6.
15. Gal AA, Koss MN. The pathology of sarcoidosis. *Curr Opin Pulm Med* 2002;**8**:445-51.
16. Hunninghake G, Gadek J, Weinberger S, et al. Comparison of the alveolitis of sarcoidosis and idiopathic pulmonary fibrosis. *Chest* 1979;**75**:266-7.
17. Keogh BA, Hunninghake GW, Line BR, Crystal RG. The alveolitis of pulmonary sarcoidosis: evaluation of natural history and alveolitis-dependent changes in lung function. *Am Rev Respir Dis* 1983;**128**:256-65.
18. Rybicki BA, Major M, Popovich Jr J, Maliarik MJ, Iannuzzi MC. Racial differences in sarcoidosis incidence: a 5-year study in a health maintenance organization. *Am J Epidemiol* 1997;**145**:234-41.
19. Fraser RS, Colman NC, Muller NL, Pare PD. Sarcoidosis. In: Fraser and Pare's, editor. *Diagnosis of diseases of the chest.* Philadelphia: WB Saunders; 1999. p. 1533-83.
20. Rybicki BA, Maliarik MJ, Major M, Popovich Jr J, Iannuzzi MC. Genetics of sarcoidosis. *Clin Chest Med* 1997;**18**:707-17.
21. Costabel U, Teschler H. Biochemical changes in sarcoidosis. *Clin Chest Med* 1997;**18**:827-42.
22. Fraser RS, Colman NC, Muller NL, Pare PD. Vasculitis. In: Fraser and Pare's, editor. *Diagnosis of diseases of the chest.* Philadelphia: WB Saunders; 1999. p. 1489-532.
23. Cordier JF, Loire R, Brune J. Idiopathic bronchiolitis obliterans organizing pneumonia: Definition of characteristic clinical profiles in a series of 16 patients. *Chest* 1989;**96**:999-1004.
24. Conron M, Du Bois RM. Immunological mechanisms in sarcoidosis. *Clin Exp Allergy* 2001;**31**:543-54.
25. Fraser RS, Colman NC, Muller NL, Pare PD. Goodpasture's syndrome and idiopathic pulmonary hemorrhage. In: Fraser and Pare's, editor. *Diagnosis of diseases of the chest.* Philadelphia: WB Saunders; 1999. p. 1757-69.
26. Sharma OP. Sarcoidosis and other autoimmune disorders. *Curr Opin Pulm Med* 2002;**8**:452-6.
27. Hunninghake GW, Crystal RG. Pulmonary sarcoidosis: a disorder mediated by excess helper T-lymphocyte activity at sites of disease activity. *N Engl J Med* 1981;**305**:429-34.
28. Baughman RP, Drent M. Role of bronchoalveolar lavage in interstitial lung disease. *Clin Chest Med* 2001;**22**:331-41.
29. Costabel U, Guzman J. Bronchoalveolar lavage in interstitial lung disease. *Curr Opin Pulm Med* 2001;**7**:255-61.
30. Baughman RP, Costabel U, du Bois RM. Treatment of sarcoidosis. *Clin Chest Med* 2008;**29**:533-48.
31. Judson MA, Baughman RP, Costabel U, et al. Efficacy of infliximab in extrapulmonary sarcoidosis: results from a randomised trial. *Eur Respir J* 2008;**31**:1189-96.
32. Sweiss NJ, Baughman RP. Tumor necrosis factor inhibition in the treatment of refractory sarcoidosis: slaying the dragon?. *J Rheumatol* 2007; **34**:2129-31.
33. Aberle DR, Gamsu G, Lynch D. Thoracic manifestations of Wegener granulomatosis: Diagnosis and course. *Radiology* 1990;**174**:703-9.
34. Falk RJ, Jennette JC. ANCA small-vessel vasculitis.. *J Am Soc Nephrol* 1997;**8**:314-22.
35. Faul JL, Kuschner WG. Wegener's granulomatosis and the Churg-Strauss syndrome. *Clin Rev Allergy Immunol* 2001;**21**:17-26.
36. Jennette JC, Falk RJ. Small-vessel vasculitis. *N Engl J Med* 1997;**337**: 1512-23.
37. Leavitt RY, Fauci AS. Wegener's granulomatosis. *Curr Opin Rheumatol* 1991;**3**:8-14.
38. Sneller MC, Fauci AS. Pathogenesis of vasculitis syndromes. *Med Clin North Am* 1997;**81**:221-42.
39. Coultas DB, Gong Jr H, Grad R, et al. Respiratory diseases in minorities of the United States. *Am J Respir Crit Care Med* 1994;**149**:S93-131.
40. Gross WL. Churg-Strauss syndrome: update on recent developments. *Curr Opin Rheumatol* 2002;**14**:11-4.
41. Stoloff S, Stempel DA. Churg-Strauss syndrome: is there an association with leukotriene modifiers?. *Chest* 2000;**118**:1515-6.

42. Vultaggio A, Matucci A, Parronchi P, et al. Safety and tolerability of infliximab therapy: Suggestions and criticisms based on wide clinical experience. *Int J Immunopathol Pharmacol* 2008;**21**:367-74.
43. Fraser RS, Colman NC, Muller NL, Pare PD. Eosinophilic lung disease. In: Fraser and Pare's, editor. *Diagnosis of diseases of the chest*. Philadelphia: WB Saunders; 1999. p. 1743-56.
44. Pope-Harman AL, Davis WB, Allen ED, Christoforidis AJ, Allen JN. Acute eosinophilic pneumonia: a summary of 15 cases and review of the literature. *Medicine (Baltimore)* 1996;**75**:334-42.
45. Ben-Ezra J, Bailey A, Azumi N, et al. Malignant histiocytosis X: a distinct clinicopathologic entity. *Cancer* 1991;**68**:1050-60.
46. Fraser RS, Colman NC, Muller NL, Pare PD. Langerhans cell histiocytosis. In: Fraser and Pare's, editor. *Diagnosis of diseases of the chest*. Philadelphia: WB Saunders; 1999. p. 1627-40.
47. da Costa CE, Egeler RM, Hoogeboom M, et al. Differences in telomerase expression by the CD1a+ cells in Langerhans cell histiocytosis reflect the diverse clinical presentation of the disease. *J Pathol* 2007;**212**:188-97.
48. Vassallo R, Ryu JH, Schroeder DR, Decker PA, Limper AH. Clinical outcomes of pulmonary Langerhans-cell histiocytosis in adults. *N Engl J Med* 2002;**346**: 484-90.
49. Warren JaW P. Immunoglobulin-and complement-mediated immune injury. In: Crystal R, West J, Barnes P, editors. *The lung: scientific foundations*. Philadelphia: Lippincott-Raven; 1997. p. 2411-9.
50. Martin W. Injury from drugs. In: Crystal R, West J, Barnes P, editors. *The lung: scientific foundations*. Philadelphia: Lippincott-Raven; 1997. p. 2465-73.
51. Van Mieghem W, Coolen L, Malysse I, Lacquet LM, Deneffe GJ, Demedts MG. Amiodarone and the development of ARDS after lung surgery. *Chest* 1994;**105**:1642-5.
52. Ernawati DK, Stafford L, Hughes JD. Amiodarone-induced pulmonary toxicity. *Br J Clin Pharmacol* 2008;**66**:82-7.
53. Garcia-Rostan y Perez GM, Garcia Bragado F, Puras Gil AM. Pulmonary hemorrhage and antiglomerular basement membrane antibody-mediated glomerulonephritis after exposure to smoked cocaine (crack): a case report and review of the literature. *Pathol Int* 1997;**47**:692-7.
54. Ball JA, Young Jr KR. Pulmonary manifestations of Goodpasture's syndrome: antiglomerular basement membrane disease and related disorders. *Clin Chest Med* 1998;**19**:777-91:ix.
55. Bolton WK. Goodpasture's syndrome. *Kidney Int* 1996;**50**:1753-66.
55a. Liebow A. Definition and classification of interstitial pneumonia in human pathology. *Prog Respir Res* 1975;**8**:1-33.
56. Fleming MV, Travis WD. Interstitial lung disease. *Pathology (Phila)* 1996;**4**:1-21.
57. Katzenstein AL, Myers JL. Idiopathic pulmonary fibrosis: clinical relevance of pathologic classification. *Am J Respir Crit Care Med* 1998;**157**:1301-15.
58. Katzenstein AL, Fiorelli RF. Nonspecific interstitial pneumonia/fibrosis: histologic features and clinical significance. *Am J Surg Pathol* 1994;**18**:136-47.
59. Fraser RS, Colman NC, Muller NL, Pare PD. Interstitial pneumonitis and fibrosis. In: Fraser and Pare's, editor. *Diagnosis of diseases of the chest*. Philadelphia: WB Saunders; 1999. p. 1584-626.
60. Hunninghake GW, Zimmerman MB, Schwartz DA, et al. Utility of a lung biopsy for the diagnosis of idiopathic pulmonary fibrosis. *Am J Respir Crit Care Med* 2001;**164**:193-6.
61. Katzenstein AL, Myers JL. Idiopathic pulmonary fibrosis: to biopsy or not to biopsy. *Am J Respir Crit Care Med* 2001;**164**:185-6.
62. Miller JD, Urschel JD, Cox G, et al. A randomized, controlled trial comparing thoracoscopy and limited thoracotomy for lung biopsy in interstitial lung disease. *Ann Thorac Surg* 2000;**70**:1647-50.
63. Ravini M, Ferraro G, Barbieri B, Colombo P, Rizzato G. Changing strategies of lung biopsies in diffuse lung diseases: the impact of video-assisted thoracoscopy. *Eur Respir J* 1998;**11**:99-103.
64. Demedts M, Wells AU, Anto JM, et al. Interstitial lung diseases: an epidemiological overview. *Eur Respir J Suppl* 2001;**32**:2s-16.
65. Bitterman PB, Rennard SI, Keogh BA, Wewers MD, Adelberg S, Crystal RG. Familial idiopathic pulmonary fibrosis: evidence of lung inflammation in unaffected family members. *N Engl J Med* 1986;**314**:1343-7.
66. Fan K, D'Orsogna DE. Diffuse pulmonary interstitial fibrosis: Evidence of humoral antibody mediated pathogenesis. *Chest* 1984;**85**:150-5.
67. Huh JW, Kim DS, Oh YM, et al. Is metalloproteinase-7 specific for idiopathic pulmonary fibrosis?. *Chest* 2008;**133**:1101-6.
68. Hu J, Van den Steen PE, Sang QX, Opdenakker G. Matrix metalloproteinase inhibitors as therapy for inflammatory and vascular diseases. *Nat Rev Drug Discov* 2007;**6**:480-98.
69. Muller NL, Guerry-Force ML, Staples CA, et al. Differential diagnosis of bronchiolitis obliterans with organizing pneumonia and usual interstitial pneumonia: clinical, functional, and radiologic findings. *Radiology* 1987;**162**:151-6.
70. Nagai S, Kitaichi M, Itoh H, Nishimura K, Izumi T, Colby TV. Idiopathic nonspecific interstitial pneumonia/fibrosis: comparison with idiopathic pulmonary fibrosis and BOOP. *Eur Respir J* 1998;**12**:1010-9.
71. King Jr TE, Tooze JA, Schwarz MI, Brown KR, Cherniack RM. Predicting survival in idiopathic pulmonary fibrosis: scoring system and survival model. *Am J Respir Crit Care Med* 2001;**164**:1171-81.
72. King Jr TE, Schwarz MI, Brown K, et al. Idiopathic pulmonary fibrosis: relationship between histopathologic features and mortality. *Am J Respir Crit Care Med* 2001;**164**:1025-32.
73. Mapel DW, Samet JM, Coultas DB. Corticosteroids and the treatment of idiopathic pulmonary fibrosis: Past, present, and future. *Chest* 1996;**110**:1058-67.
74. Rennard SI, Bitterman PB, Ozaki T, Rom WN, Crystal RG. Colchicine suppresses the release of fibroblast growth factors from alveolar macrophages in vitro: the basis of a possible therapeutic approach ot the fibrotic disorders. *Am Rev Respir Dis* 1988;**137**:181-5.
75. Fraser RS, Colman NC, Muller NL, Pare PD. Connective tissue disorders. In: Fraser and Pare's, editor. *Diagnosis of diseases of the chest*. Philadelphia: WB Saunders; 1999. p. 1421-87.
76. Lynch 3rd JP, Hunninghake GW. Pulmonary complications of collagen vascular disease. *Annu Rev Med* 1992;**43**:17-35.
77. Mayberry JP, Primack SL, Muller NL. Thoracic manifestations of systemic autoimmune diseases: radiographic and high-resolution CT findings. *Radiographics* 2000;**20**:1623-35.
78. Sulica R, Teirstein A, Padilla ML. Lung transplantation in interstitial lung disease. *Curr Opin Pulm Med* 2001;**7**:314-22.
79. Maurer JR, Frost AE, Estenne M, Higenbottam T, Glanville AR. International guidelines for the selection of lung transplant candidates. The International Society for Heart and Lung Transplantation, the American Thoracic Society, the American Society of Transplant Physicians, the European Respiratory Society. *Transplantation* 1998;**66**:951-6.
80. Lynch 3rd JP, Saggar R, Weigt SS, Ross DJ, Belperio JA. Overview of lung transplantation and criteria for selection of candidates. *Semin Respir Crit Care Med* 2006;**27**:441-69.
81. Schwartz DA, Helmers RA, Galvin JR, et al. Determinants of survival in idiopathic pulmonary fibrosis. *Am J Respir Crit Care Med* 1994;**149**:450-4.
82. Meltzer EB, Noble PW. Idiopathic pulmonary fibrosis. *Orphanet J Rare Dis* 2008;**3**:8.
83. Carrington CB, Gaensler EA, Coutu RE, FitzGerald MX, Gupta RG. Natural history and treated course of usual and desquamative interstitial pneumonia. *N Engl J Med* 1978;**298**:801-9.
84. Ishiguro T, Takayanagi N, Kurashima K, et al. Desquamative interstitial pneumonia with a remarkable increase in the number of BAL eosinophils. *Intern Med* 2008;**47**:779-84.
85. Kawabata Y, Takemura T, Hebisawa A, et al. Eosinophilia in bronchoalveolar lavage fluid and architectural destruction are features of desquamative interstitial pneumonia. *Histopathology* 2008;**52**:194-202.
86. Katzenstein AL, Myers JL. Nonspecific interstitial pneumonia and the other idiopathic interstitial pneumonias: classification and diagnostic criteria. *Am J Surg Pathol* 2000;**24**:1-3.
87. Swigris JJ, Brown KK. Acute interstitial pneumonia and acute exacerbations of idiopathic pulmonary fibrosis. *Semin Respir Crit Care Med* 2006;**27**:659-67.
88. Guerry-Force ML, Muller NL, Wright JL, et al. A comparison of bronchiolitis obliterans with organizing pneumonia, usual interstitial pneumonia, and small airways disease. *Am Rev Respir Dis* 1987;**135**:705-12.
89. Davies G, Wells AU, du Bois RM. Respiratory bronchiolitis associated with interstitial lung disease and desquamative interstitial pneumonia. *Clin Chest Med* 2004;**25**:717-26:vi.
90. Colby TV. Bronchiolitis: Pathologic considerations. *Am J Clin Pathol* 1998;**109**:101-9.
91. Epler GR, Colby TV, McLoud TC, Carrington CB, Gaensler EA. Bronchiolitis obliterans organizing pneumonia. *N Engl J Med* 1985;**312**:152-8.
92. Izumi T, Kitaichi M, Nishimura K, Nagai S. Bronchiolitis obliterans organizing pneumonia: clinical features and differential diagnosis. *Chest* 1992;**102**:715-9.
93. Chapman JR, Charles PJ, Venables PJ, et al. Definition and clinical relevance of antibodies to nuclear ribonucleoprotein and other nuclear antigens in patients with cryptogenic fibrosing alveolitis. *Am Rev Respir Dis* 1984;**130**:439-43.
94. Basarakodu KR, Aronow WS, Nair CK, et al. Differences in treatment and in outcomes between idiopathic and secondary forms of organizing pneumonia. *Am J Ther* 2007;**14**:422-6.
95. Koss MN, Hochholzer L, Langloss JM, Wehunt WD, Lazarus AA. Lymphoid interstitial pneumonia: clinicopathological and immunopathological findings in 18 cases. *Pathology* 1987;**19**:178-85.

96. Bragg DG, Chor PJ, Murray KA, Kjeldsberg CR. Lymphoproliferative disorders of the lung: histopathology, clinical manifestations, and imaging features. *AJR Am J Roentgenol* 1994;**163**:273-81.
97. Nanki N, Fujita J, Yamaji Y, et al. Nonspecific interstitial pneumonia/fibrosis completely recovered by adding cyclophosphamide to corticosteroids. *Intern Med* 2002;**41**:867-70.
98. Dick JA, Morgan WK, Muir DF, Reger RB, Sargent N. The significance of irregular opacities on the chest roentgenogram. *Chest* 1992;**102**:251-60.
99. Ayed AK. Video-assisted thoracoscopic lung biopsy in the diagnosis of diffuse interstitial lung disease: a prospective study. *J Cardiovasc Surg (Torino)* 2003;**44**:115-8.
100. Green FH. Overview of pulmonary fibrosis. *Chest* 2002;**122**:334S-9.
101. Rena O, Casadio C, Leo F, et al. Videothoracoscopic lung biopsy in the diagnosis of interstitial lung disease. *Eur J Cardiothorac Surg* 1999;**16**:624-7.
102. Kadokura M, Colby TV, Myers JL, et al. Pathologic comparison of video-assisted thoracic surgical lung biopsy with traditional open lung biopsy. *J Thorac Cardiovasc Surg* 1995;**109**:494-8.
103. American Thoracic Society/European Respiratory Society International Multidisciplinary Consensus Classification of the Idiopathic Interstitial Pneumonias. This joint statement of the American Thoracic Society (ATS), and the European Respiratory Society (ERS) was adopted by the ATS board of directors, June 2001 and by the ERS Executive Committee, June 2001. *Am J Respir Crit Care Med* 2002;**165**:277–304.

CHAPTER 12
Infectious Lung Diseases
John D. Mitchell and Marvin Pomerantz

Bacterial Lung Infections
  Community-Acquired Pneumonia
    Clinical Presentation
    Determination of Severity
    Treatment
  Hospital-Acquired (Nosocomial) Pneumonia
    Ventilator-Associated Pneumonia
    Health Care–Associated Pneumonia

Aspiration Pneumonia
Bronchiectasis
Lung Abscess
Mycobacterial Pulmonary Disease
Major Mycotic Lung Infections
  Histoplasmosis
  Coccidioidomycosis
  Blastomycosis

Aspergillosis
  Aspergilloma
  Invasive Aspergillosis
  Allergic Bronchopulmonary Aspergillosis
Cryptococcosis
Mucormycosis

The development of techniques to treat complications of infectious lung disease formed the cornerstone of modern thoracic surgery, dominating the specialty until about 1960. Although advances in critical care, antibiotic therapy, and other alternative treatments have lessened the impact of many lung infections in the practice of today's cardiothoracic surgeon, current evidence suggests that other categories of pulmonary infection are on the rise. There are several reasons for this change: the use of broad-spectrum antimicrobial agents, selecting out resistant organisms; the emergence of new, opportunistic organisms, freshly minted as human pathogens; the widespread application of transplantation techniques, accompanied by the ubiquitous immunosuppression protocols; and more important, the failure of preventive medicine and public hygiene measures to reduce the rate of community-acquired infection. If anything, the infectious challenges facing the cardiothoracic surgeon today are more daunting than they were 40 years ago. In this chapter, we review the more common causes of pulmonary infection and their treatment.

BACTERIAL LUNG INFECTIONS

Community-Acquired Pneumonia

The term *pneumonia* refers to infection of the lower respiratory tract, involving the respiratory bronchioles to the distal alveoli. These illnesses have been subclassified on the basis of the mode and timing of presentation and the existing comorbidities of the affected patient. These distinctions are often useful in considering empiric antibiotic therapy. The terms *typical pneumonia* and *atypical pneumonia*, which refer to the causative organism, are outdated but still occasionally useful in considering this subject. Pneumonias due to so-called atypical organisms (including *Mycoplasma pneumoniae*, *Legionella* species, and *Chlamydia pneumoniae*) can represent up to 40% of cases but are rarely distinguishable from typical bacterial pneumonias at clinical presentation.[1] Thus, the initial therapy chosen should consider both typical and atypical pathogens.

Community-acquired pneumonia (CAP) describes an acute bacterial or viral respiratory infection contracted outside the confines of the hospital or long-term care facility setting.[2,3] It remains a common illness, with an estimated incidence between 5 and 6 million cases, resulting in more than 1 million hospitalizations annually.[4,5] Because CAP is not a reportable illness, these figures probably underestimate the actual magnitude of the problem. The aggregate cost for treatment of these patients approaches $9 billion a year, almost all due to the costs associated with inpatient management.[5] The length of hospitalization has been shown to be the key factor in determining the cost of treatment.[6] Pneumonia remains the sixth leading cause of death in the United States. The mortality rate associated with the development of pneumonia ranges from 1% to 5% for ambulatory patients without comorbidities to close to 40% for those requiring intensive care unit (ICU) admission.[7]

The most common pathogens responsible for CAP are listed in Table 12-1. *Streptococcus pneumoniae* has remained the most commonly identified organism, followed by *Haemophilus influenzae*, *Staphylococcus aureus*, enteric gram-negative bacilli, *Legionella* species, *Mycoplasma pneumoniae*, *Chlamydia pneumoniae*, and respiratory viruses.[3,4,8] In up to 50% of cases, a causative organism is not identified. The likelihood of finding a particular pathogen often depends on the population studied (see Table 12-1) and the diagnostic tests used. For example, sputum culture favors pneumococcus as the most frequently identified organism, whereas *M. pneumoniae* is seen more commonly with serologic testing. A "mixed" infection involving atypical and typical organisms can approach 40%,[9] although it is uncertain whether the atypical organisms, when present, represent an actual coinfection, a preceding infection, or simple colonization. However, empiric antibiotic regimens that cover both typical and atypical organisms have been associated with improved survival and shorter hospitalizations in several large retrospective studies.[10-12]

Certain risk factors may predispose patients to infection with particular organisms. For example, pneumonia due to drug-resistant pneumococcus has been associated with advanced age (>65 years), alcoholism, immune suppressive illness or therapy, recent β-lactam therapy, and other significant comorbidities. Enteric gram-negative infections are seen more frequently in nursing home patients, in those with other significant medical conditions including cardiopulmonary disease, and with recent antibiotic therapy. Pseudomonal infections

Table 12-1
Community-Acquired Pneumonia: Likely Pathogens

Outpatients without Comorbidities*	Outpatients with Comorbidities	Hospitalized Patients without Comorbidities	Hospitalized Patients Requiring ICU Admission
Streptococcus pneumoniae	Streptococcus pneumoniae	Streptococcus pneumoniae	Streptococcus pneumoniae
Mycoplasma pneumoniae	Mycoplasma pneumoniae	Haemophilus influenzae	Legionella spp.
Chlamydia pneumoniae	Chlamydia pneumoniae	Mycoplasma pneumoniae	Haemophilus influenzae
Haemophilus influenzae	Mixed infection†	Chlamydia pneumoniae	Enteric gram-negative bacilli
Respiratory viruses	Haemophilus influenzae	Mixed infection	Staphylococcus aureus
Legionella spp.	Enteric gram-negative bacilli	Enteric gram-negative bacilli	Mycoplasma pneumoniae
Mycobacterium tuberculosis	Respiratory viruses	Aspiration (anaerobes)	Legionella spp.
Endemic fungi	Moraxella catarrhalis	Respiratory viruses	Respiratory viruses
	Legionella spp.	Legionella spp.	Chlamydia pneumoniae
	Aspiration (anaerobes)	Mycobacterium tuberculosis	Mycobacterium tuberculosis
	Mycobacterium tuberculosis	Endemic fungi	Endemic fungi
	Endemic fungi	Pneumocystis carinii	Pseudomonas aeruginosa

*Chronic obstructive pulmonary disease, congestive heart disease, diabetes mellitus.
†Often a polymicrobial infection of typical and atypical organisms.
Modified from Niederman MS, Mandell LA, Anzueto A, et al. Guidelines for the management of adults with community-acquired pneumonia. Diagnosis, assessment of severity, antimicrobial therapy, and prevention.

are more likely to arise in those with structural lung disease, with malnutrition, or in the presence of immune suppressive or broad-spectrum antibiotic therapy.[4] *H. influenzae* infections occur more frequently in smokers than in nonsmokers.

Clinical Presentation

Patients with CAP typically present with cough (90%), dyspnea (66%), sputum production (66%), and pleuritic chest pain (50%). Nonrespiratory symptoms such as malaise, headache, nausea, myalgias, arthralgias, abdominal pain, and mental confusion are seen in 10% to 30% of patients. Elderly patients often have fewer or less severe symptoms than younger patients do. Presenting signs on physical examination include fever (80%), tachypnea, tachycardia, and a generalized toxic state. Crackles on auscultation are common (80%), with indications of consolidation in up to 30% of patients.[13]

Evaluation with chest radiography should be undertaken in all patients who present with symptoms and signs suggestive of pneumonia.[14] Standard posterior-anterior and lateral films classically reveal a segmental (Fig. 12-1) or lobar infiltrate, often with evidence of a parapneumonic effusion. Chest films also will help distinguish pneumonia from other disorders that may present with similar symptoms and can help assess the severity (e.g., multilobar involvement) of the illness. Contributing or causative factors, such as bronchial obstruction, lung abscess, and tuberculosis, can also be seen. The addition of computed tomography may occasionally be helpful in difficult cases, but there are few data to support its routine use in the initial evaluation of patients with CAP.

Routine laboratory studies in ambulatory patients are rarely necessary but may occasionally steer the clinician toward hospital admission in equivocal cases. Laboratory studies in hospitalized patients should include complete blood count, electrolyte values and glucose concentration, renal and liver function tests, and assessment of oxygen saturation. Patients aged 15 to 54 years should undergo testing for human immunodeficiency virus (HIV) infection with informed consent.[14] Tests used to identify an etiologic agent (including blood cultures and sputum Gram stain and culture) should be performed for all patients admitted with pneumonia, although some have questioned the utility of blood cultures in low-risk patients.[15] Viral cultures have not been shown to be useful in the initial evaluation of patients with CAP and should not be routinely performed,[16] although some improvement in the diagnostic yield has been demonstrated with real-time polymerase chain reaction analysis.[17] Every attempt should be made to obtain these culture specimens before initiation of therapy, but not at the expense of unnecessary delays in treatment. Culture data should be correlated with the Gram stain result before narrowing antibiotic therapy. Significant pleural effusions should be tapped and sent for laboratory and culture studies. Routine serologic and cold agglutinin testing is generally not recommended in the initial evaluation of patients with CAP,[3] but it may prove useful in select cases. This recommendation is based on the low failure rate seen with empiric therapy for patients treated in the outpatient setting. A pneumococcal urinary antigen assay recently approved by the Food and Drug Administration may be used to augment the standard diagnostic methods,[18-20] with the advantage of rapid results similar to the Gram stain. Sensitivity and specificity rates of 80% to 90% have been reported. Use of similar technology to detect pneumococcal antigen in sputum has also been reported.[21]

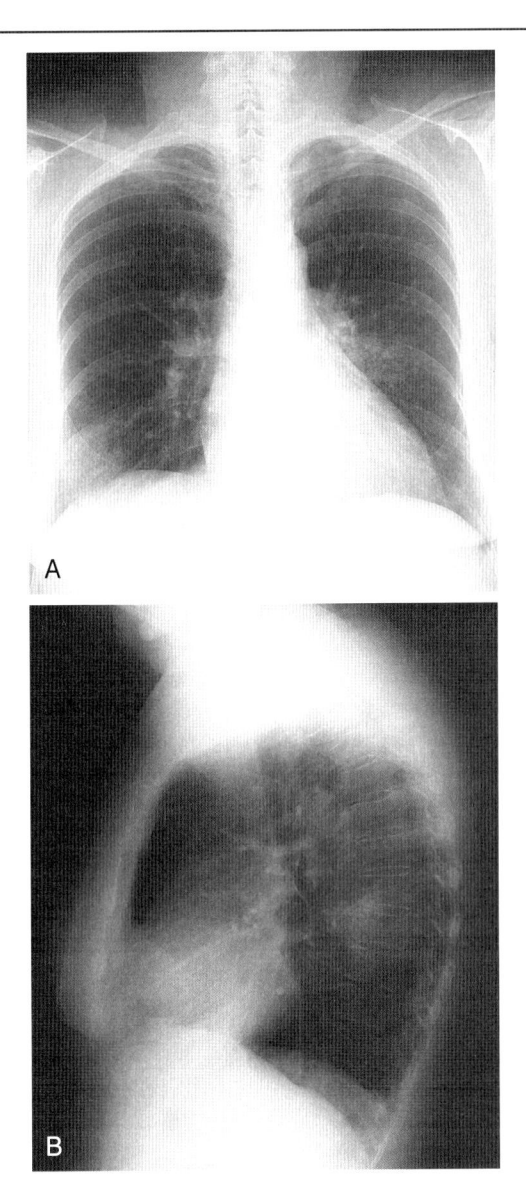

Figure 12–1
Posteroanterior (A) and lateral (B) chest radiographs demonstrating segmental pneumonia involving the superior segment of the left lower lobe.

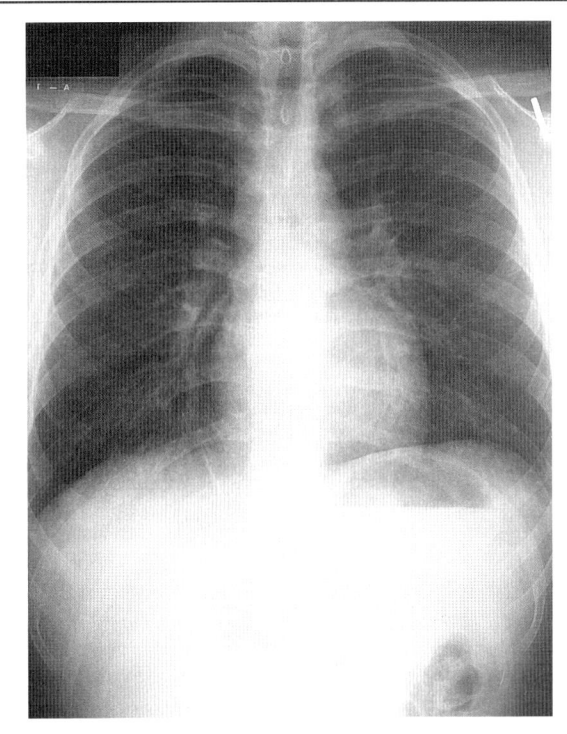

Figure 12–2
Posteroanterior chest radiograph demonstrating a fine interstitial pattern due to *Mycoplasma* pneumonia.

Patients with pneumonia due to *Mycoplasma* species often present with signs and symptoms reminiscent of a mild viral illness, with a more gradual onset and less intense nature. These infections, like other "atypical" infections, occur more frequently in younger patients. Headache, malaise, sore throat, low-grade fever, and rhinorrhea are common. Cough, when it is present, is frequently nonproductive and spasmodic in character. Extrapulmonary manifestations may predominate, with rash, arthralgias, and neurologic abnormalities present. The physical examination of the chest may yield minimal findings, although a wheeze and crackles can sometimes be appreciated. Radiologic findings include nodular or peribronchial infiltrates, an interstitial pattern of disease (Fig. 12-2), and occasional consolidation. Pleural effusions occur frequently. Although the white cell count is often normal, hemolytic anemia can be associated with a positive Coombs test result. Serologic diagnosis may be obtained through measurement of IgM or IgG titer by a complement fixation test.

Pneumonia due to *Legionella* (*Legionella pneumophila*) remains problematic since the initial recognized outbreak of the disease at an American Legion convention in Philadelphia in 1976. The organism is identified in 1% to 5% of patients hospitalized with pneumonia, with considerable variations in detection because of geographic patterns and difficulties in accurate diagnosis. Culture may still be the best way of identifying *Legionella*, along with a urinary antigen assay.[22] However, the urinary antigen assay can remain positive months after the acute infection. Symptoms suggestive of pneumonia predominate (high fever, chills, dyspnea, cough), but extrapulmonary manifestations (gastrointestinal complaints, malaise, myalgias) are not uncommon. Radiographs usually reveal either patchy or diffuse interstitial infiltrates and occasionally consolidation (Fig. 12-3).

Pulmonary infection with *Chlamydia* organisms such as *C. pneumoniae* presents in similar fashion to other atypical pneumonias. Infection with this organism has also been associated with chronic diseases such as atherosclerotic coronary disease. Diagnostic tests used to identify this organism include direct tissue culture (sputum smear and culture are not helpful) and display of a fourfold increase in IgG titer or an IgM titer of 1:16 or higher by a microimmunofluorescence test.

Determination of Severity

One of the key decisions made in the initial evaluation of CAP, beyond establishing a presumptive diagnosis, pertains to the need for inpatient therapy. Many of the patients afflicted with CAP are elderly with significant comorbidities, for whom the progressive pulmonary infection is clearly life-threatening. On the other hand, improper admission for CAP therapy taxes the health-care system billions of dollars

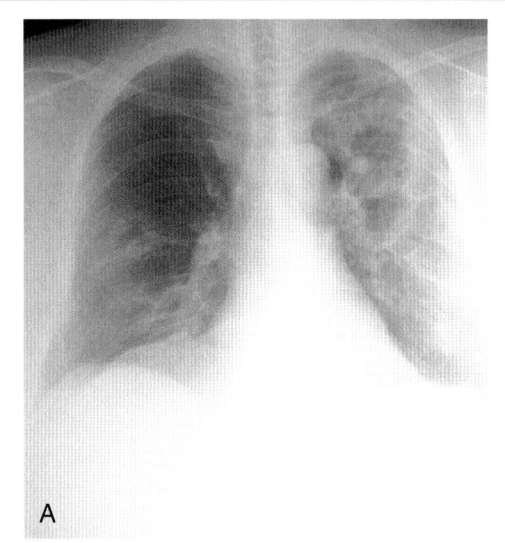

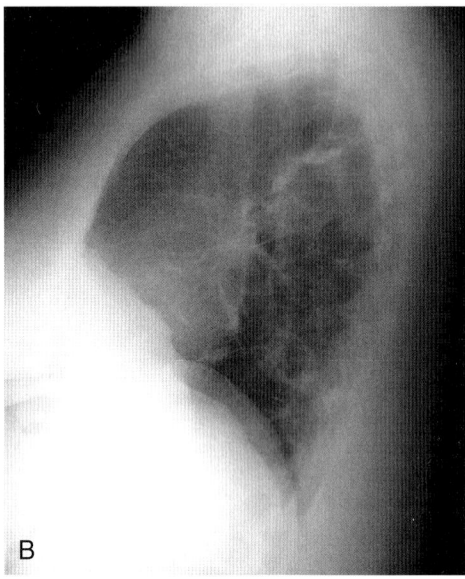

Figure 12–3
Posteroanterior **(A)** and lateral **(B)** chest radiographs demonstrating diffuse infiltrates with cavitation due to *Legionella* infection.

annually, as noted before. In the United States, less than 20% of patients with CAP are admitted for inpatient therapy but account for more than 90% of the costs related to the disease treatment.[5] As a result, various guidelines have been developed to assist clinicians in the assessment of severity of illness at presentation. One such system, the Pneumonia Severity Index (PSI), was validated with data from almost 2300 patients in the Pneumonia Patient Outcomes Research Team (PORT) cohort study.[23] On the basis of clinical parameters obtained at initial presentation, a risk score or class is determined (Fig. 12-4). Patients with a risk class of I to III had a low mortality rate (<1%) and were thought to be at low risk, thus amenable to outpatient management. Patients with a risk class of IV or V had higher mortality rates (9.3 and 27.0, respectfully) and were thought to be appropriate candidates for hospitalization. The value of the PSI has since been confirmed in multiple studies,[24-29] and it is endorsed within the guidelines set forth by the American Thoracic Society/Infectious Diseases Society of America.[3] These guidelines emphasize a multistep process in determining the initial site of treatment based on (1) assessment of factors that compromise the safety of home care, (2) PSI score, and (3) clinical judgment. The PSI has been criticized, though, because of the relative complexity of the assessment required.

In contrast, the British Thoracic Society has adopted an alternative prediction rule for risk stratification in the setting of CAP, termed CURB-65.[30] The CURB-65 uses five prognostic variables: confusion; blood urea nitrogen concentration (>20 mg/dL); respiratory rate (>30 breaths per minute); low blood pressure (systolic, <90 mm Hg; diastolic, <60 mm Hg); and age older than 65 years. Patients with scores of 0 or 1 were thought to be appropriate for outpatient care; those with scores of 2 or 3 should be considered for admission, perhaps to the ICU; and scores of 4 or 5 mandated ICU care. A simplified version of CURB-65, termed CRB-65, drops the blood urea nitrogen measurement and thus is applicable to the outpatient office setting.[31]

The PSI and the CURB-65 have been compared in a variety of studies,[24,32,33] and both have been found to have strengths and weaknesses. The PSI is particularly good at identifying patients with a low risk of mortality but tends to underestimate severity of illness in some populations of patients. Alternatively, the CURB-65 more accurately identifies those patients with severe CAP and at high risk of death. It has been proposed that the two assessment tools may be thought of as complementary rather than competitive tests.[34]

Treatment

The treatment of CAP at initial presentation is outlined in Figure 12-5, as described by the American Thoracic Society/Infectious Diseases Society of America, stratified by the presence or absence of modifying factors, comorbidities, and site of initial treatment.[3] Data from published reports support the use of the guidelines, leading to better outcomes.[10,35-37] The timing of therapy is important, with the first dose of antibiotic given 4 to 8 hours after initial presentation. Prompt administration of therapy has been associated with improved survival.[38] The use of the guidelines facilitates prompt delivery of appropriate therapy. Further, although it is desirable to narrow the spectrum of administered antibiotic agents, this is not possible in up to 50% of cases because of a lack of an identifiable organism. In addition, a significant proportion of cases represent mixed polymicrobial infections. The use of these guidelines employing broad-spectrum therapy allows appropriate treatment in these patients.

Clinical decisions about duration of therapy are poorly supported in the literature. In general, most treatment regimens last 7 to 14 days; the severity of the presenting illness, the response to therapy, and the underlying comorbidities should all be considered in addressing duration of treatment. Most bacterial infections, including those due to *S. pneumoniae*, are treated for 7 to 10 days, provided a good clinical response is seen. *Mycoplasma*, *Chlamydia*, and *Legionella* infections should be treated for 10 to 14 days and perhaps longer if significant comorbidity exists.

Successful response to therapy in a patient with CAP usually follows a predictable course. Stabilization of clinical parameters often occurs by 72 hours, with gradual improvement noted thereafter. The severity of the presenting illness and the underlying disease understandably play a role in the

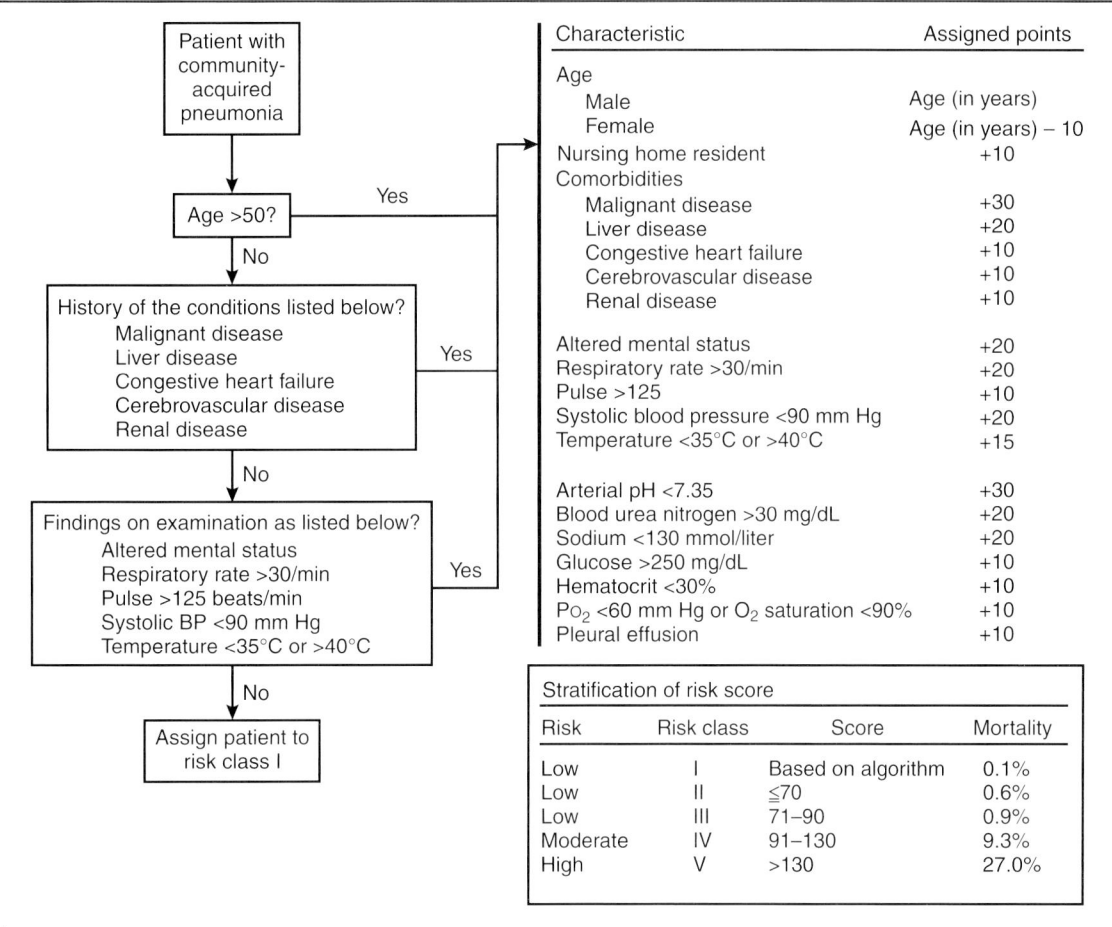

Figure 12–4

The Pneumonia Severity Index. *(Modified from Fine MJ, Auble TE, Yealy DM, et al. A prediction rule to identify low-risk patients with community-acquired pneumonia.)*

Characteristic	Assigned points
Age	
Male	Age (in years)
Female	Age (in years) – 10
Nursing home resident	+10
Comorbidities	
Malignant disease	+30
Liver disease	+20
Congestive heart failure	+10
Cerebrovascular disease	+10
Renal disease	+10
Altered mental status	+20
Respiratory rate >30/min	+20
Pulse >125	+10
Systolic blood pressure <90 mm Hg	+20
Temperature <35°C or >40°C	+15
Arterial pH <7.35	+30
Blood urea nitrogen >30 mg/dL	+20
Sodium <130 mmol/liter	+20
Glucose >250 mg/dL	+10
Hematocrit <30%	+10
P_{O_2} <60 mm Hg or O_2 saturation <90%	+10
Pleural effusion	+10

Stratification of risk score

Risk	Risk class	Score	Mortality
Low	I	Based on algorithm	0.1%
Low	II	≤70	0.6%
Low	III	71–90	0.9%
Moderate	IV	91–130	9.3%
High	V	>130	27.0%

response to therapy. The febrile response and leukocytosis typically resolve by day 4 to 5, with the radiologic findings lagging behind. In fact, the initial radiographic abnormalities may actually worsen before improvement is documented. Only 15% of chest films are clear at discharge, and many take 2 to 3 months to return to normal. With a successful response to treatment, consideration should be given to conversion to oral therapy. The American Thoracic Society describes four criteria that should be met before switching to oral therapy: improvement in cough and dyspnea; afebrile (<100°F) at two consecutive assessments 8 hours apart; resolving leukocytosis; and a functioning gastrointestinal tract with oral intake.[4] Obviously, some leeway may be allowed in these criteria, given the clinical situation. Compliance can be an issue with oral therapy, and drug dosing schedules and side effects should be taken into account in selecting an oral regimen.[39]

Two adjunctive therapies have been recently studied for their effects on outcome in patients with severe CAP. In a retrospective analysis, the administration of activated protein C to a subset of patients in the PROWESS study with CAP was associated with a drop in mortality rates.[40] Further studies, including prospective randomized trials, remain pending. In at least one randomized study, the continuous infusion of corticosteroids in patients with CAP was associated with lower mortality rates, shorter length of ICU stay, and shorter duration of mechanical ventilation.[41] No increase in complications was associated with the use of steroids in this population of patients.

Two serum markers, C-reactive protein and procalcitonin, have been studied to assess response to CAP therapy, to determine outcome, and to guide duration of therapy. Of the two, procalcitonin seems the most promising. Procalcitonin is the precursor to calcitonin and has no hormonal effects. Serum levels of procalcitonin rise in the setting of acute bacterial infections, stimulated by cytokines, microbial toxins, and the cell-mediated immune response. One study determined that higher serum levels of procalcitonin, within 24 hours of admission to the hospital, were associated with higher PSI scores and a greater risk of mortality.[42] Other investigators have found procalcitonin levels useful in predicting outcome and guiding duration of therapy.[43-45]

Clinicians should resist the urge to switch antibiotic therapy within the first 72 hours unless marked clinical deterioration occurs. Failure to respond to initial therapy does occur in up to 10% of patients because of a variety of factors. A drug-resistant or unusual pathogen may be the cause, which may be remedied by further diagnostic tests for the etiologic agent, broadening of the antibiotic therapy, or both. A complication of the initial pneumonia may be present, either local (e.g., lung abscess, empyema) or at a distant site (e.g., meningitis, endocarditis, septic arthritis). Selected imaging such as computed tomography and echocardiography as well as sampling of fluid collections based on these studies and physical examination can often reveal the source of the persistent infection. Finally, several noninfectious illnesses can mimic pneumonia

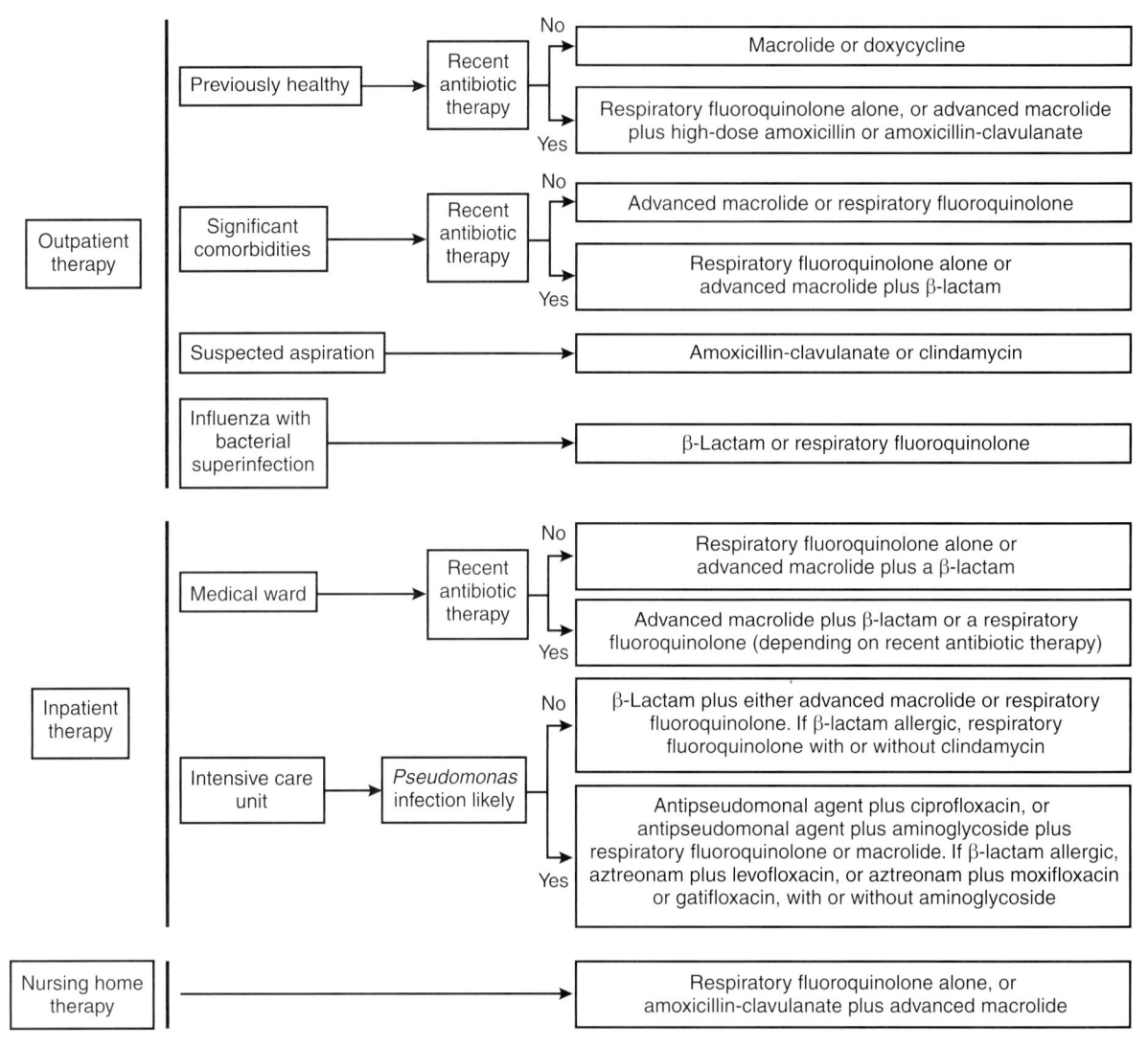

Figure 12–5
Empiric therapy for community-acquired pneumonia. *(Modified from Mandell LA, Wunderink RG, Anzueto A, et al. Infectious Diseases Society of America/American Thoracic Society consensus guidelines on the management of community-acquired pneumonia in adults; and Mandell LA, Bartlett JG, Dowell SF, et al. Update of practice guidelines for the management of community-acquired pneumonia in immunocompetent adults.)*

and should be ruled out. This group of disease states is extensive and includes bronchogenic cancer, lymphoma, and a variety of inflammatory and interstitial lung diseases.

Hospital-Acquired (Nosocomial) Pneumonia

Hospital-acquired pneumonia refers to pulmonary infection after at least 48 to 72 hours of admission to an acute care facility or in intubated patients. The latter situation is termed ventilator-associated pneumonia. Hospital-acquired pneumonia is the second most common nosocomial infection and has the highest mortality,[46-48] with crude mortality rates of 30% previously reported.[49] Risk factors for nosocomial pneumonia have been described and include the extremes of age, chronic lung disease, previous abdominal or thoracic surgery, endotracheal intubation, and duration of mechanical ventilation.[50]

Two factors predispose patients to nosocomial pneumonia: the aerodigestive tract is colonized with bacteria, and the contaminated secretions are aspirated into the lower respiratory system.[51] Several of the preventive strategies described in the following are aimed at interruption of these two processes.

Ventilator-Associated Pneumonia

Ventilator-associated pneumonia is a nosocomial pulmonary infection developing in patients receiving mechanical ventilation. Ventilator-associated pneumonia that occurs early, within 48 to 72 hours after intubation, is typically due to bacteria responsive to antibiotic therapy (e.g., pansensitive *S. aureus*, *H. influenzae*, and *S. pneumoniae*) and frequently results from aspiration complicating the intubation process. In contrast, late-onset ventilator-associated pneumonia is often caused by antibiotic-resistant organisms (e.g., methicillin-resistant *S. aureus*, *Pseudomonas aeruginosa*, *Acinetobacter* and *Enterobacter* species).[52] Risk factors for ventilator-associated pneumonia include the duration of mechanical ventilation, age older than 70 years, H_2 or antacid therapy, chronic lung disease, depressed consciousness, need for reintubation, and gastric aspiration.[46,52-55] The incidence of ventilator-associated pneumonia is significantly higher in surgical ICUs as opposed to medical ICUs, according to the Centers for Disease Control and Prevention.[56]

There is some controversy in the literature about optimal diagnosis of ventilator-associated pneumonia.[57] To date, there seems to be little evidence supporting the use of invasive (bronchoscopic) techniques for diagnosis compared with quantitative tracheobronchial aspirates, with no difference in subsequent mortality, length of hospital stay, or duration of mechanical ventilation.[58-62] Bronchoscopy may be of use in patients who fail to respond to initial therapy.[63] The treatment of ventilator-associated pneumonia consists of general supportive care and the administration of empiric broad-spectrum antibiotics, guided by the severity of the illness.[46,64] The adequacy of initial antibiotic therapy appears to be the most important determinant of outcome.[65,66] Numerous studies have examined preventive measures to limit the development of ventilator-associated pneumonia. Semirecumbent positioning, sucralfate instead of H_2 antagonists for stress ulcer prophylaxis, and selective digestive tract decontamination were found to have the strongest support in the literature.[67]

Health Care–Associated Pneumonia

Health care–associated pneumonia refers to pneumonia that occurs in a nonhospitalized patient with extensive healthcare contacts. Examples of such contacts include outpatient intravenous therapy, hospitalization or treatment at a hospital or dialysis unit within the past 30 days, and residence in a nursing home or other long-term care facility. The recommendations for treatment mirror those suggested for hospital-acquired pneumonia.[46]

Aspiration Pneumonia

Aspiration refers to the inhalation of oropharyngeal or gastric contents into the tracheobronchial tree. This usually results in either a *pneumonitis* caused by a chemical injury from contact with sterile, acidic gastric contents or a *pneumonia* due to inhalation of infected material. Rarely, aspiration can lead to airway obstruction, lung abscess, and other findings. Aspiration pneumonia is a common problem, accounting for 5% to 15% of CAP, and is frequently seen in nursing home residents, those with swallowing disorders, and patients with altered mental states. It is also a recognized complication of general anesthesia, occurring in about 1 in 3000 operations and accounting for 10% to 30% of deaths related to anesthesia.[68]

The acute lung injury or pneumonitis from gastric aspiration, termed Mendelson's syndrome,[69] appears directly related to the acidity and volume of aspirated material. In general, a pH below 2.5 and a volume in excess of 0.3 mL/kg (about 21 mL in a 70-kg adult) are required to initiate lung injury. The injury follows a biphasic pattern; the initial insult is caused by direct damage of the acid on the delicate capillary and alveolar cells, followed several hours later by the rapid accumulation of inflammatory cells and mediators, resulting in a local and systemic inflammatory response. Progression to acute respiratory distress syndrome and multiorgan system failure may ensue. Because the gastric contents are sterile due to the acidity, infection is usually not an initial feature in these cases but may become prominent later in the course of the illness with secondary infection of the damaged lung parenchyma. Efforts to modify the gastric pH may lead to gastric colonization with gram-negative bacteria as well as with other organisms, leading to infection early after the aspiration episode. Treatment is largely supportive in nature. Particularly if the aspiration is witnessed, bronchoscopy is indicated to remove any residual fluid or debris from the airway. The use of corticosteroids in the treatment of aspiration pneumonitis has not been shown to be of benefit. Although it is common practice to initiate antibiotic therapy in these patients, this often overtreats simple pneumonitis, which may resolve with supportive measures only. Further, the use of antibiotics early may encourage the development of resistant organisms. Antibiotic therapy should be considered early in those thought to have gastric colonization and in those patients who do not improve within 48 hours of the inciting event, with evidence of ongoing lung injury, infection, or infiltrate.[70] Empiric coverage with broad-spectrum agents is recommended.

Aspiration pneumonia commonly arises from inhalation of colonized oropharyngeal bacteria, causing the signs, symptoms, and radiographic changes of pneumonia. About half of normal adults aspirate while asleep,[71] and for infection to occur, the normal protective mechanisms must either fail or be overwhelmed by the volume or bacterial burden of the aspirate. In supine patients, the dependent lung segments (posterior aspects of upper lobes, superior segments of lower lobes) are affected most frequently. In upright individuals, the basilar segments, particularly on the right side, are at greatest risk of infection. The aspiration episode in patients developing pneumonia is frequently not observed, and the diagnosis is derived from the clinical picture and characteristic radiographic changes in individuals known to be at risk. Treatment with antimicrobial therapy is appropriate. Use of antibiotics with anaerobic coverage is probably overdone but appropriate in select cases in which severe periodontal disease, alcoholism, and other disorders predominate. In hospitalized patients, coverage of gram-negative bacteria is essential.

Bronchiectasis

Bronchiectasis was first described in 1819 by Laennec. It is defined by the permanent dilation of the bronchi,[72] caused by a recurrent process of transmural infection and inflammation. The disease process is characterized by the pathologic or radiographic appearance of the airways. Cylindrical or tubular bronchiectasis results in dilated, slightly tapered airways; varicose bronchiectasis resembles the chronic venous state of the same name, with areas of dilation and constriction; and in saccular or cystic bronchiectasis, progressive dilation of the airway can end in saclike, cystic structures resembling a cluster of grapes. The cylindrical changes are frequently seen with tuberculosis infections; the saccular or cystic type is more common after obstruction or bacterial infection. Thick, mucoid secretions are often pooled in the dilated airways, causing a chronic inflammatory state involving the airway walls. The lung parenchyma distal to the dilated, ectatic airways is often damaged as well, with fibrosis and emphysematous changes present. The accompanying bronchial arteries and lymph nodes are engorged and hypertrophied as well. The left lower lobe is the area most frequently involved, followed by the lingula and right middle lobe.

Table 12-2
Conditions Causing or Associated with Bronchiectasis

Infection
Bacterial
Mycobacterial
Aspergillus
Viral (including HIV infection)
Congenital conditions
Primary ciliary dyskinesia
α_1-Antitrypsin deficiency
Cystic fibrosis
Tracheobronchomegaly (Mounier-Kuhn syndrome)
Cartilage deficiency (Williams-Campbell syndrome)
Pulmonary sequestration
Marfan syndrome
Immunodeficiency
Hypogammaglobulinemia
Secondary to disease states or therapy
Sequelae of toxic inhalation or aspiration
Chlorine
Foreign body
Rheumatic conditions
Rheumatoid arthritis
Systemic lupus erythematosus
Sjögren's syndrome
Relapsing polychondritis
Inflammatory bowel disease

Modified from Barker AF. Bronchiectasis.

The causes and disease states associated with bronchiectasis are listed in Table 12-2. The common pathway for all these disorders is recurrent, transmural infection of the bronchial wall. Bacterial infections, particularly those involving potentially necrotizing agents such as *S. aureus*, *P. aeruginosa*, *S. pneumoniae*, and various anaerobes, remain important causes of bronchiectasis, particularly when there is a delay in treatment or there are factors present to prevent eradication of the infection. Bronchiectasis in patients with allergic bronchopulmonary aspergillosis is due to an immune reaction to the fungal organism, with production of inflammatory mediators and subsequent direct airway invasion by the fungus. Viral infections can lead to bronchiectatic airways both through direct infection and through a reduction in host defenses. This latter theme is common in the pathophysiologic process of bronchiectasis. Primary ciliary dyskinesia and various immune deficiencies, such as hypogammaglobulinemia, are examples of congenital disorders in which there is impairment in host defense mechanisms. Cystic fibrosis is another important cause of bronchiectasis, with predilection for the upper lobes. On occasion, the appearance of bronchiectasis in middle age will be the presenting symptom in patients with milder forms of cystic fibrosis. Several autoimmune disorders, such as rheumatoid arthritis and inflammatory bowel disease, have been linked to recurrent pulmonary infections and the development of bronchiectasis.

Both focal and diffuse forms of bronchiectasis are seen. The focal variety is often associated with an isolated abnormality causing relative or complete bronchial obstruction. An aspirated foreign body, slow-growing tumor, and broncholith are examples. Rarely, bronchial compression (as seen with middle lobe syndrome) or angulation of the bronchus (after surgical lobectomy) produces obstruction leading to recurrent infection and the development of localized disease. Bronchiectasis due to postinfectious causes is more likely to be localized, whereas disease due to congenital deficiencies is more likely to be diffuse. A study of stable patients with bronchiectasis revealed a 64% incidence of colonization with what were termed potential pathogenic microorganisms. The most frequently isolated potential pathogenic microorganisms were *H. influenzae*, *Pseudomonas* species, and *S. pneumoniae*. Risk factors for colonization by potential pathogenic microorganisms included diagnosis of bronchiectasis before 14 years of age, an FEV_1 of 80% predicted, and the presence of varicose or saccular bronchiectasis.[73]

Patients with bronchiectasis present with recurrent pulmonary infections characterized by dyspnea and an unremitting chronic cough productive of thick, tenacious purulent sputum. Hemoptysis is common and at times can be massive due to erosion into the enlarged bronchial vessels. Patients with bronchiectasis will occasionally describe a nonproductive cough, indicative of upper lobe involvement. Auscultation reveals crackles, wheeze, or rhonchi in the majority of patients.

The radiographic findings in bronchiectasis are understandably important in establishing the diagnosis. Standard radiographs are abnormal in the clear majority of cases, demonstrating focal areas of consolidation, atelectasis, evidence of thickened bronchi (best noted as ring shadows when seen on end), and, in advanced cases, delineation of the dilated, cystic changes in the airway (Fig. 12-6). Computed tomography, particularly with high-resolution images, is more sensitive and specific for the diagnosis of bronchiectasis. Evidence of airway dilation, changes consistent with saccules or varicosities of the airway, and lack of airway tapering toward the periphery are all consistent with bronchiectasis.[74] Upper lobe involvement suggests the diagnosis of cystic fibrosis or allergic bronchopulmonary aspergillosis; middle lobe and lingular disease is more typical of environmental mycobacterial infection, such as *Mycobacterium avium* complex; and lower lobe predominance suggests bacterial involvement.

Therapy for bronchiectasis involves treatment of the underlying disorder, if possible; suppression of the bacterial load through appropriate use of antibiotics; encouragement of proper pulmonary hygiene, including the routine use of bronchodilators, mucolytic agents, and postural drainage; and surgery in select cases. The role of surgery is threefold.

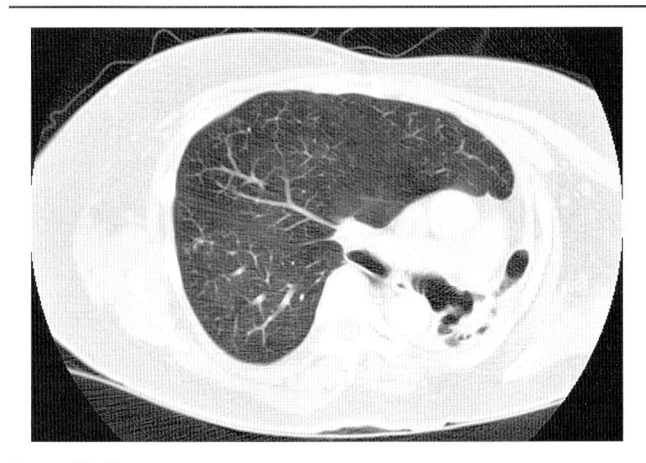

Figure 12–6
Computed tomographic scan demonstrating end-stage bronchiectasis involving the left lung with complete parenchymal destruction.

First, patients with focal areas of disease causing unremitting symptoms and associated with localized lung parenchymal destruction are candidates for resection therapy, usually by a segmentectomy or lobectomy. Second, the rare patient who presents with massive hemoptysis should be considered for surgical therapy if less invasive maneuvers, such as bronchial artery embolization, are unsuccessful. Finally, some patients with end-stage bronchiectasis may be candidates for lung transplantation. As with other patients with end-stage suppurative lung disease, sequential double-lung transplantation is indicated to avoid contamination of the new transplanted lungs.

Lung Abscess

A lung abscess is a circumscribed cavity within the lung parenchyma filled with purulent material and air. The cavity may form as a result of a necrotizing infection or may become secondarily infected. The abscess formation may be singular in nature or multifocal, depending on the etiology. The abscess is arbitrarily termed acute if it is present for 6 weeks or less and chronic if it has been present for a longer time. Further classification comes from the underlying cause, as noted before: a primary lung abscess arises from a necrotizing infection; a secondary lung abscess forms as a result of another pathologic entity.

Table 12-3 lists the causes of lung abscess. The most common cause is inadvertent aspiration of infected oropharyngeal secretions, which can occur in the setting of impaired consciousness, in the presence of poor dental hygiene, and in association with gastroesophageal reflux disease or various dysphagia syndromes (strictures, Zenker's and other diverticula, dysmotility disorders, achalasia, and others). A lung abscess can occur as a sequela of necrotizing lung infections, particularly in the setting of an immunocompromised host. Bronchial obstruction, due to tumor, foreign body, or external compression of the bronchus, can predispose to distal lung infection and subsequent abscess formation. A preexisting cavity within the lung parenchyma, as a result of a cavitating neoplasm, a resolving infarct, or even structural lung disease, can lead to secondary infection and abscess. Direct extension of an adjacent abscess can occur. Finally, hematogenous seeding from another source can produce abscesses within the lung, often multifocal. Recognition of the secondary nature of the abscess can have direct therapeutic implications; for example, an abscess resulting from a foreign body aspiration will likely respond poorly to treatment without removal of the offending item.

The location of lung abscesses is determined by the segmental anatomy of the tracheobronchial tree and the underlying etiology. As aspiration is a major cause, the dependent segments—the posterior segment of the right upper lobe and the superior segments of both lower lobes—tend to be involved frequently. The distribution roughly falls into right upper lobe, 25%; right middle lobe, 10%; right lower lobe, 33%; left upper lobe, 12%; and left lower lobe, 20%.[75]

The bacteriology of lung abscesses frequently falls in line with the underlying cause. Many ambulatory patients with lung abscess have gram-positive bacteria (e.g., alpha- and beta-hemolytic streptococcus, *S. aureus, S. pneumoniae, Streptococcus viridans*) as the source; gram-negative organisms (e.g., *Proteus* spp., *Escherichia coli, P. aeruginosa, Enterobacter,* and *Eikenella*) predominate in nosocomial infections. In lung abscess due to aspiration, mixed flora are often present, and anaerobes play an important part.[76] Aerobic gram-positive cocci and facultative gram-negative bacilli are commonly found, including *S. aureus, Streptococcus pyogenes, Klebsiella pneumoniae,* and *P. aeruginosa.*

Clinically, patients complain of cough, fever, malaise, weight loss, dyspnea, and occasionally pleuritic chest pain. The symptoms are reminiscent of pneumonia and may be insidious in onset. Hemoptysis may rarely be a complicating factor and can vary from blood streaks in the sputum to life-threatening hemorrhage. With cavitation and drainage into the tracheobronchial tree, patients are likely to describe production of large volumes of foul-smelling sputum. The uninvolved lung can become soiled through a spillover effect and produce respiratory failure. If it is large enough, the abscess can exert a mass effect on adjacent structures. Rupture into the pleural space is uncommon but can lead to empyema and fulminant sepsis.

A chest radiograph is likely to show a cavitary space within the lung, accompanied by an air-fluid level (Fig. 12-7). In contrast with a hydropneumothorax, the abscesses are more likely to have equal air-fluid levels on both the posterior-anterior and lateral films.[77] Features of a lung abscess may be difficult to appreciate on plain film examination and can be confused with alternative diagnoses. Computed tomography is helpful in these cases, delineating the exact anatomic features and location of the abscess and its relation to adjacent structures. For example, a cavitary neoplasm may be confused with an abscess. Compared with the thin, smooth walls of the abscess, cavitation secondary to tumor is usually associated with thick, irregular walls, features that do not respond to antibiotic therapy. An interlobar fluid collection or empyema may also be confused with a lung abscess. A lenticular shape, obtuse angle with the chest wall, compression of neighboring bronchovascular structures, and a "split pleura" sign signify the presence of pleural fluid in these cases.[78] In addition to standard laboratory investigation, all patients should undergo bronchoscopy to assess for bronchial obstruction due to tumor or foreign body and possibly to obtain culture specimens. Accurate culture data may be best obtained through percutaneous fine-needle aspiration. In a series reported by Yang and

Table 12-3
Etiology of Lung Abscess

Primary
Aspiration
Impaired consciousness
Severe periodontal disease
Dysphagia syndromes, esophageal reflux
Necrotizing pneumonia
Immunocompromised patient
Secondary
Bronchial obstruction
Neoplasm
Foreign body
Lymphadenopathy
Cavitating lesions
Neoplasm
Pulmonary infarct
Emphysema, bullous disease
Direct extension
Amebiasis (liver)
Subphrenic abscess
Hematogenous dissemination

Modified from Hodder RV, Cameron R, Todd TRJ. Bacterial infections. In: Pearson FG, Deslauriers J, Ginsberg RJ, Hiebert CA, McKneally MF, editors. Thoracic surgery. New York: Churchill Livingstone; 1995; p. 433-69.

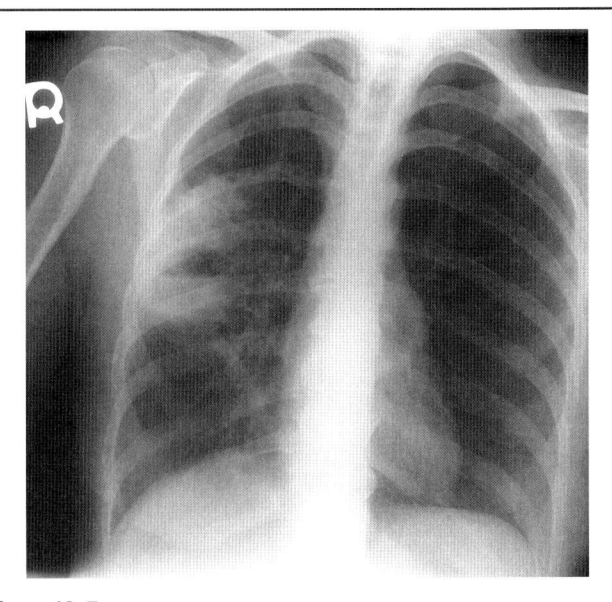

Figure 12–7
Posteroanterior chest radiograph demonstrating a lung abscess with air-fluid level.

colleagues,[79] fine-needle aspiration yielded a 94% success rate in culture of pathogens, compared with 11% from sputum culture and only 3% from lavage. Attempted drainage by bronchoscopic means should be discouraged in most cases because of the risk of flooding the airways with purulent material.

The successful treatment of lung abscess centers around prolonged antimicrobial therapy targeted at the causative organism combined with establishment of adequate drainage. In most cases, the drainage can be accomplished internally, aided by postural techniques and chest physiotherapy. If internal drainage is inadequate, percutaneous drainage may be done, usually with an excellent response (Fig. 12-8). The complications of percutaneous drainage (empyema, pneumothorax, hemothorax) occur in less than 10% of cases, even less so if pleural symphysis is present. The course of antibiotic therapy typically lasts 6 to 8 weeks, with radiographic resolution occurring by 4 to 5 months. Medical therapy for lung abscess is generally successful in 85% to 90% of cases.[80] Indications for surgical intervention include empyema, development of a bronchopleural fistula, significant hemoptysis, persistence of the abscess despite adequate therapy, and suspicion of underlying malignant disease. During surgical procedures for lung abscess, special attention should be paid to protecting the contralateral lung from spillage, usually through the use of a double-lumen tube. Resection of the involved segment of lung is usually performed, although in cases of rupture into the pleural space, simple unroofing of the cavity, decortication, and wide drainage will usually suffice. Some success with endoscopic drainage of lung abscesses has been reported.[81]

MYCOBACTERIAL PULMONARY DISEASE

Mycobacterial pulmonary diseases include infections with *Mycobacterium tuberculosis* and its more virulent forms, multidrug-resistant tuberculosis (MDR-TB) and extensively drug-resistant tuberculosis (XDR-TB).[82] There are other mycobacterial infections caused by organisms that have gone through a series of name changes, including atypical mycobacteria; mycobacterium other than tuberculosis; environmental mycobacteria; and the most commonly used term, nontuberculous mycobacteria.[83] Whereas good epidemiology studies can be found for tuberculosis infections as well as for MDR-TB and XDR-TB, there are poor epidemiology data for these nontuberculous mycobacterial infections. This is probably due to the fact that nontuberculous mycobacterial infections are not transferable from person to person and are not reportable to local or national health authorities.

Annually, there are currently 16,000 new cases of tuberculosis in the United States and 7 to 8 million new cases in the world, with an estimated 2 to 3 million deaths.[84] Unfortunately, the majority of these cases are in countries whose health-care systems are in dire need of help. In India, nearly 500,000 people die of tuberculosis yearly. Fortunately, only 10% to 15% of those exposed to the tuberculosis organism acquire the clinical disease; however, this leaves a large number of individuals who make up a latent source for later activation with tuberculosis if their resistance breaks down because of disease or aging.

The early treatment of tuberculosis gave rise to the sanatoria system. It was thought that rest and fresh air were beneficial in the treatment of tuberculosis. However, it has never

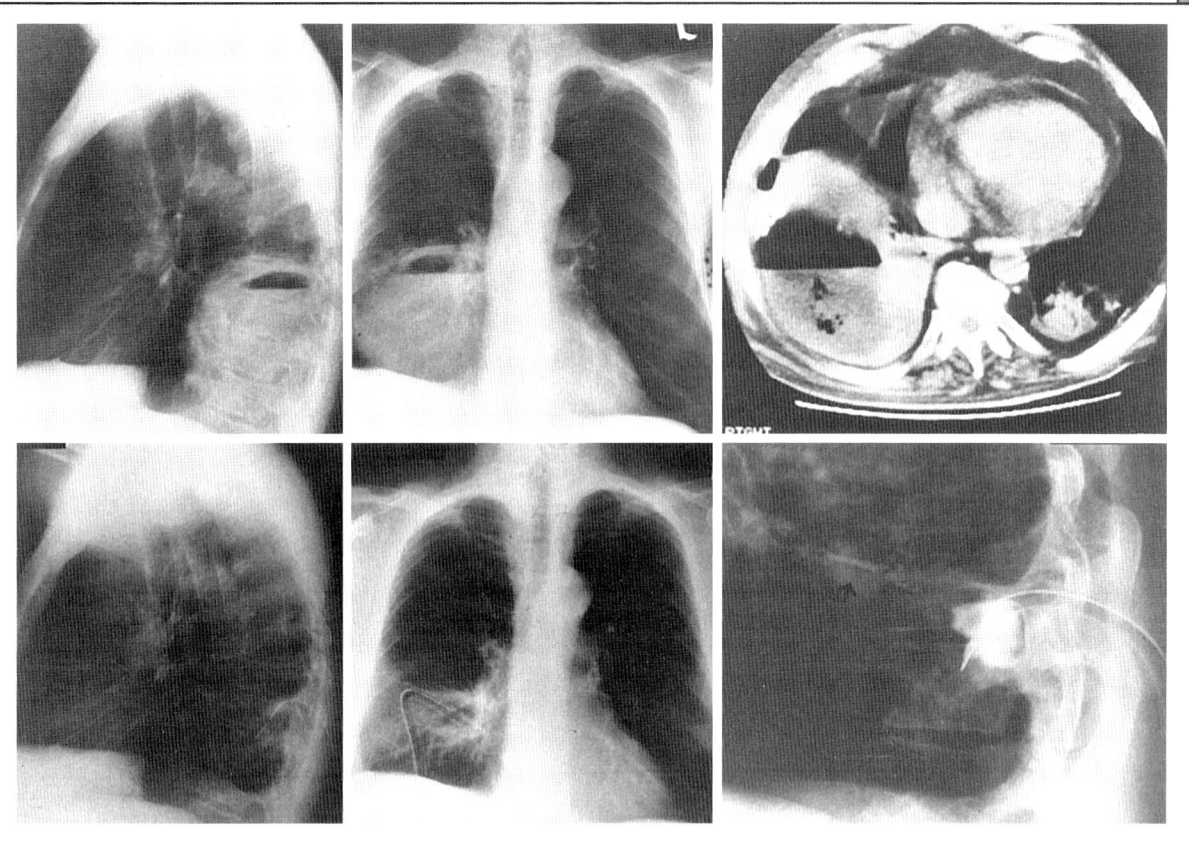

Figure 12–8
Computed tomographic scan and chest radiographs demonstrating a large lung abscess *(upper panels)* with resolution after appropriate percutaneous drainage *(lower panels)*. *(From Pearson FG, Cooper JD, Deslauriers J, et al.* Thoracic surgery, *2nd ed. Philadelphia: Churchill Livingstone; 2002.)*

been well documented that this form of therapy produced any long-term benefit.

Surgery for tuberculosis began with collapse therapy. The tuberculosis organism is an obligate aerobe, and it was reasoned that by preventing oxygen from entering the cavities, this would be beneficial in the treatment of patients with cavitary pulmonary tuberculosis. Various forms of collapse therapy have been used, including thoracoplasty, wax or Lucite ball plombage, phrenic nerve crush or interruption, pneumoperitoneum, and induced pneumothorax. Collapse therapy continued to be the treatment of choice for tuberculosis infections until chemotherapy with streptomycin and p-aminosalicylic acid was introduced in 1945. It was not until the introduction of isoniazid in 1952 that prolonged cures could be obtained with antibiotic therapy.

Resectional surgery gradually replaced collapse therapy as the primary surgical approach to patients with tuberculosis infections having residual destroyed lung or cavitary disease. With the introduction of rifampin in 1966, the need for surgery was markedly reduced and the sanatoria system gradually became extinct. Drug-sensitive tuberculosis in almost all instances can be cured with antibiotic therapy alone. The standard treatment of drug-sensitive tuberculosis is 6 to 9 months of isoniazid and rifampin, with the addition of pyrazinamide and ethambutol during the initial 2 months.[85,86] Patients with drug-sensitive tuberculosis who are treated appropriately are operated on only for complications, such as bronchostenosis, massive hemoptysis (>600 mL in 24 hours), and bronchopleural fistula; to rule out the presence of cancer; and occasionally for decortication of a trapped lung, which occurs by polymicrobial contamination within the pleural cavity in tuberculosis patients who have had a pleural effusion.

Tuberculosis with an organism resistant to both isoniazid and rifampin is classified as MDR-TB. XDR-TB strains are resistant not only to isoniazid and rifampin but also to fluoroquinolones and either aminoglycosides (amikacin, kanamycin) or capreomycin or both.[87,88] The patients with MDR-TB and XDR-TB present a much greater challenge to the treating clinician, and surgery plays a greater role in their management. In addition to the listed indications for surgery, they are also operated on for persistent cavitary disease, destroyed lobe, or destroyed lung with or without culture-positive sputum. In the United States today, patients with MDR-TB make up the largest group of patients operated on for pulmonary infections with tuberculosis.[89] The addition of surgery to the treatment regimen has been shown to be beneficial.[90]

Patients with nontuberculous mycobacterial infection (NTM) present a different challenge. The most common NTM infection is that of the *Mycobacterium avium* complex. This includes both *M. avium* and *Mycobacterium intracellulare*, which are almost indistinguishable from each other on culture. Infections with the so-called rapid growers, such as *Mycobacterium chelonae*, *Mycobacterium abscessus*, and *Mycobacterium fortuitum*, seem to be increasing in the United States, although accurate epidemiologic data are not available. These infections are more difficult to treat because good antibiotic coverage is not available. Some of these rapid grower infections are extremely virulent and may destroy an entire lung

(Figs. 12-9 and 12-10), and surgery offers the only hope to control the process along with continued use of any antibiotics available. Specific types of NTM infection include infection of the middle lobe and lingula of women (Fig. 12-11). This usually occurs in slender women with little or no body fat and is associated frequently with skeletal abnormalities such as scoliosis and pectus excavatum.[91,92] This syndrome has not been found in men, in our experience; however, if it does occur, it is extremely rare.

Preparation for surgery is an important part of the therapeutic approach for patients with mycobacterial infections. The most important aspect of preparation is nutrition. Patients with an albumin concentration below 3.0 g/dL are not operated on. Nutritional supplementation is accomplished either orally or by gastrostomy or jejunostomy feeding tubes to improve the patient's anabolic state before surgery. The best available antibiotic therapy is given for approximately 3 months before surgery. This can be prolonged if bacterial counts are decreasing, and it can be shortened if the sputum becomes negative for acid-fast bacilli. In MDR-TB, only about half the patients have negative sputum before surgery. Routine evaluation, as with other pulmonary surgery, includes pulmonary function tests, ventilation-perfusion scans, and computed tomographic scans.

Surgical principles include leaving enough viable lung tissue to have a functional postoperative patient. Double-lumen tubes or bronchial blockers are used in all operations. All grossly involved lung, which includes cavitary disease and destroyed lung, should be removed; nodular disease remaining in other parts of the lung can be left behind. Fluid administration during surgery is kept to below 1200 mL whenever possible and below 800 mL with pneumonectomies. The use of muscle flaps is controversial. However, it is our opinion that use of muscle flaps to fill space after lobectomies is often helpful. With muscle flaps, we think that the incidence of bronchopleural fistula has been decreased. Muscle flaps are used after pneumonectomy if there is a polymicrobial contamination or positive sputum at the time of surgery.[89] If there is massive contamination, the chest is left open and an omental flap is used. Omental flaps are also used to cover the bronchus in the absence of any muscle due to previous surgery or extreme cachexia. If the chest is left open (Eloesser procedure), it is packed with quarter-strength Dakin's solution with Kerlix gauze and changed on a daily basis for 5 to 6 weeks. When the opening is closed, assuming the intrathoracic chest wall is clean, Clagett's solution is left in the pleural cavity. Pleural tents have been suggested to help eliminate space and to seal air leaks. This is not practical in mycobacterial surgery because most of the dissections over the upper lobe are done in the extrapleural plane. The latissimus dorsi muscle is used whenever there are expected to be significant space problems after lobectomy, and it is also used to cover the bronchus and hilum. If only bronchial support is needed after a pneumonectomy, intercostal muscle can be used. Appropriate antibiotic therapy is continued for 12 to 24 months postoperatively, with some of the injectable antibiotics being stopped before the oral medications are stopped.

Whereas tuberculosis infections can infect normal lung tissue, NTM infections most frequently affect previously diseased lungs and have a much more indolent course than that of tuberculosis or MDR-TB. Lung damage can be due to previous infections such as tuberculosis, bronchiectasis, or chest wall irradiation. Patients with NTM infections often are found to have genetic abnormalities, such as heterozygous cystic fibrosis, α_1-antitrypsin deficiency, or cilia dysfunction. It is also of note that more than 50% of the patients with NTM infections have esophageal dysfunction. These patients often reflux at night, causing contamination and damage to the lungs, making them more susceptible to pulmonary disease.

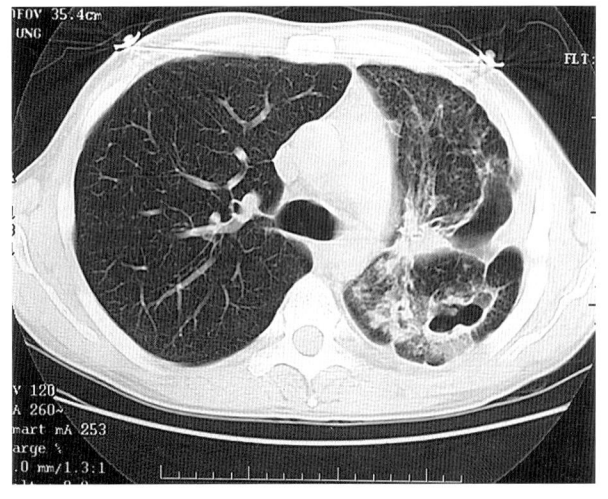

Figure 12–9
Computed tomographic scan showing severe cavitary disease in a patient with *Mycobacterium chelonae* infection.

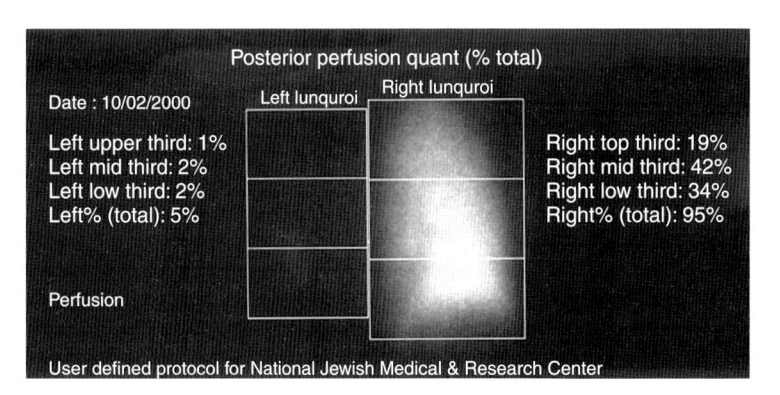

Figure 12–10
Perfusion scan of the same patient depicted in Figure 12-9 demonstrating absence of perfusion to the left lung.

In the United States, there is an abnormally high proportion of patients with NTM disease who are white. In addition, there is an overwhelming majority of patients with NTM infection who are women (relative to men), and the reasons for these two findings are still not clear.

Operative mortality in experienced hands should be less than 3%. The largest study to date involving anatomic lung resection for NTM disease reported a mortality rate of 2.6% in 236 consecutive patients, with no deaths in the second half of the series.[93] Complications after mycobacterial surgery are high, in the 25% to 30% range (but with experience, this can be brought down to less than 15%). Specific complications include a high rate of bronchopleural fistula, most often occurring after right pneumonectomy for NTM infections. Wound infection after *M. chelonae* and *M. abscessus* infections are common, and careful attention to wound closure is necessary. Other complications, such as air leaks, bleeding, and postpneumonectomy pulmonary edema, are similar to those of other thoracic procedures for nonmycobacterial disease.

Results of surgery for tuberculosis or MDR-TB are gratifying; surgery for NTM infections is less successful because of the long duration of indolent disease before surgical intervention. Earlier surgery in these patients should improve the results. Persistence in aggressively treating surgical complications is often necessary to obtain good results and requires dedicated thoracic surgeons experienced in these difficult cases.

With 33% to 40% of the world infected with tuberculosis and with the presence of poverty, this disease will not go away. With the increasing number of NTM infections, at least in the United States, surgery will continue to play a role in the therapy for these patients.

MAJOR MYCOTIC LUNG INFECTIONS

There are at least 100,000 species of fungi, but only 300 or so are associated with pulmonary disease. Fungal infection of the lung results from inhalation of the infectious agent.

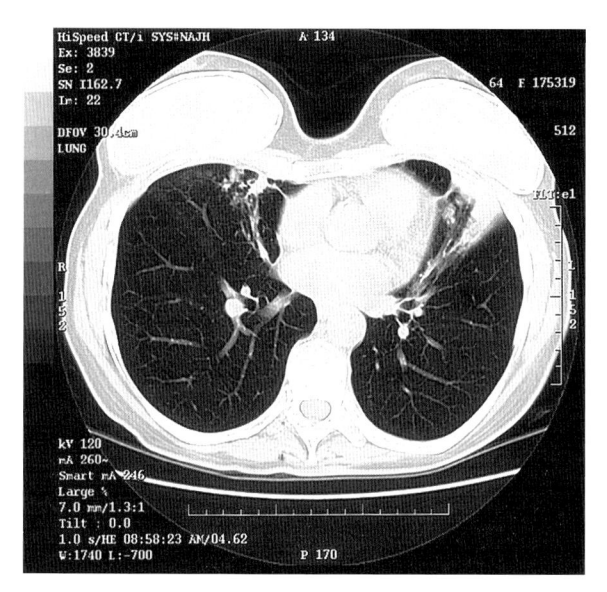

Figure 12-11
Computed tomographic scan of a woman with *M. avium* complex infection of the right middle lobe and lingula.

Colonization or asymptomatic fungal infection is common in the United States; an estimated 30 million are infected with *Histoplasma capsulatum*, and another 10 million with *Coccidioides immitis*. Serious infection is rare but is seen with increasing frequency in immunocompromised populations. The increasingly advanced use of chemotherapy for neoplasms, antibiotics for infections, immunosuppressive therapies for organ transplantation, and corticosteroids for various conditions has increased opportunistic infections by usually harmless saprophytes such as *Aspergillus*, *Candida*, and *Mucor*. Under these conditions, the formerly clear differentiation between so-called pathogenic and nonpathogenic fungi has become blurred.

In addition to detailing the medical conditions that predispose to infection, other areas of the patient's history can yield important clues to the causative agent. The three major fungal infections seen in healthy populations—histoplasmosis, coccidioidomycosis, and blastomycosis—are due to endemic organisms recognized in specific geographic areas of the United States. These organisms are dimorphic; they exist in nature as a mycelium (mold) that bears infectious spores, which later enter the host and develop into a yeast-like phase that is the tissue pathogen. These morphologic differences occur in response to changes in temperature. The spores invade the host through an aerosolized form by the respiratory tract, resulting in a mild or asymptomatic infection. Chronic pulmonary or disseminated infection is uncommon; an intact cell-mediated immune response is critical to prevention of serious illness. The more common opportunistic fungi (*Aspergillus*, *Cryptococcus*, *Mucor*) are ubiquitous and are located in the soil. Proximity to building or construction sites where aerosolization of these organisms can occur has been linked to an increased incidence of aspergillosis, histoplasmosis, coccidioidomycosis, and other infections.[94,95]

Fungal infection of the lung is best established by recovery of the infecting organism by culture, but recognition in smears or tissue sections may be enough for diagnosis. The best two stains for demonstration of fungi in tissue are periodic acid–Schiff and methenamine silver, but no one stain demonstrates all organisms. Specific immunologic changes in the host response may provide a strong indication of the diagnosis and may often lead to therapy before actual isolation of the organism can be achieved.[96] All too often, however, it is not possible to find pathognomonic organisms in the stained specimens, and only a presumptive diagnosis can be made. Cultures of fungi can be made from tissues, sputum, pleural fluid, and other clinical specimens. Induced sputum samples, obtained in the morning and at least six in number, are recommended.[96] Sabouraud's dextrose agar is an excellent general-purpose culture medium. Prompt delivery of the specimens to the laboratory is essential. Because respiratory tract cultures may simply be the result of fungal colonization, the culture isolates from these sites, which are not sterile, may not correspond to infection. However, risk stratification of the host may aid in this matter. One study demonstrated that a culture positive for *Aspergillus* in immunocompromised patients, such as bone marrow transplant recipients, was associated with invasive infection 50% to 70% of the time, whereas a positive culture in cystic fibrosis patients was rarely combined with invasive aspergillosis.[97] Serologic tests for circulating fungal antigens (such as galactomannan in aspergillosis) and circulating antibodies to fungal antigen (histoplasmosis and coccidioidomycosis) can aid in diagnosis. Molecular diagnostic techniques using polymerase chain reaction technology are being developed for *Aspergillus*, *Candida*, and *Cryptococcus*.[98,99]

Histoplasmosis

Histoplasmosis is a fungal infection caused by the dimorphic fungus *Histoplasma capsulatum*, which exists in mycelial form in the soil, its natural habitat, and in yeast form at body temperature. It is endemic in the Mississippi and Ohio River valleys, where the incidence of positive skin reactions to the fungus exceeds 80%.[100] Further, the incidence of skin test reactivity probably underestimates the true incidence because the skin test reaction may revert to negative over time.

The yeast phase of the organism is not contagious, and there is no danger of transmission through direct human contact. It is the microspores from the mycelial phase that act as the transmitted agent, inhaled into the distal airspaces in the lung. The critical inoculum is unknown. Within days, the microspores germinate into yeast spores, attracting neutrophils and macrophages to the site of infection. Neutrophils are largely ineffective against the yeast spores, which are ingested by the macrophages. Infected macrophages transport the spores to other areas in the reticuloendothelial system, producing a subclinical disseminated infection. This process is poorly controlled in those with impaired T-cell immunity. The outcome of infection is determined by the development of a specific cell-mediated immune reaction within about 2 weeks. Granulomas form within the lungs and mediastinal lymph nodes to wall off residual organisms. As the epithelial cell granulomas age, caseating necrosis develops in the central areas and may calcify as the peripheral portions become fibrotic. Within these lesions, *H. capsulatum* organisms are usually found only in the caseous material, seen well with methenamine silver stain. The yeast are often found intracellularly in macrophages.

About half of the cases of acute pulmonary histoplasmosis are asymptomatic. The remaining patients have an influenza-like illness with chills, myalgias, headache, nonproductive cough, dyspnea, and pleuritic chest pain. The disease is self-limited, usually lasting a week or two, but frequently with fatigue lasting for several weeks. On occasion, patients will be troubled by pericarditis or persistent symptoms of arthralgia and erythema nodosum.[101] These symptoms respond well to nonsteroidal anti-inflammatory agents.

Progressive disseminated histoplasmosis develops rarely, usually in those with impaired cell-mediated immunity. The liver, spleen, lymphatic system, bone marrow, and adrenal glands are most frequently involved. Diffuse pulmonary infiltrates may appear and progress rapidly, at times accompanied by shock and disseminated intravascular coagulation.

Chronic cavitary pulmonary histoplasmosis occurs in about 10% of patients with symptomatic histoplasmosis. The majority have chronic obstructive pulmonary disease and other structural defects in the lungs that predispose them to the illness. Clinically, the disease is similar to cavitary tuberculosis, except that the illness is less severe. The radiographic picture mimics that seen in tuberculosis, with fibronodular changes, often involving both pulmonary apices, cavities, and adjacent pulmonary pleural thickening.

Fibrosing mediastinitis represents excessive scarring from prior histoplasmosis. The symptoms are produced by gradual, relentless compression of mediastinal structures, including the superior vena cava, pulmonary vessels, esophagus, and tracheobronchial tree. The calcified nodes may actually erode into the last two structures, presenting as a broncholith with airway obstruction and hemoptysis or with a localized esophageal leak and dysphagia (Fig. 12-12). The progression is fatal in 10% to 20% of cases, and attempts to surgically bypass or to remove the obstructing lesions are difficult and often unrewarding. Antifungal and steroid therapies are of limited use in fibrosing mediastinitis and do not slow the progression of the disease.[102]

Histoplasmomas are the residua of healed primary histoplasmosis and are usually seen as asymptomatic coin lesions on routine chest films. Their significance lies in the fact that the lesions, if uncalcified, may be impossible to differentiate from neoplasm, and surgical excision may be indicated. Computed tomography may reveal central calcification or peripheral calcification, with a "target" appearance indicating a benign diagnosis.

Definitive diagnosis of active histoplasmosis relies on isolation of the fungus in culture. Serologic immunodiffusion tests detect antibodies to *H. capsulatum* in 24 to 48 hours but may also be positive in those with a remote history of the disease. Further, the test result is negative in up to 10% of patients with culture-proven histoplasmosis, usually in immunocompromised patients.

Amphotericin B is the mainstay of significant histoplasmosis infections. The primary, self-limited infection does not require therapy unless progression to severe illness is documented. Treatment is always indicated in the disseminated form of the disease and in immunocompromised populations. Chronic pulmonary histoplasmosis may alternatively be treated with ketoconazole or itraconazole. Surgical intervention in the chronic form of the disease is indicated only if the thick-walled cavities fail to respond to an adequate course of antimicrobial therapy and pulmonary function permits.

Coccidioidomycosis

Coccidioidomycosis is the illness caused by the pathogenic fungus *Coccidioides immitis*. This dimorphic fungus is found in the soil as a mold and in tissues as an endosporulating spherule. Relatively hardy, it can withstand periods of high salinity and drought, but it is intolerant of freezing temperatures. It is endemic in the desert Southwest of the United States, and protection from infection in the endemic area is almost impossible. The infecting structures are termed arthroconidia, which are separated from the mold stalk by wind or other disturbances. The arthroconidia are transported through the air, resulting in inhalation into the distal air sacs of the lung and transformation into spherules. The spherules enlarge in the lung and become packed with endospores, which ultimately rupture, liberating the tiny endospores and perpetuating the invasive process. The severity of the clinical course after inhalation of the endospores is determined mainly by the host's ability to develop cell-mediated immunity against *C. immitis* to control infection. Children exposed are more likely to develop a mild or asymptomatic infection; adults are more likely to have a severe primary infection with dissemination. African Americans are 12 times more likely to develop disseminated disease than whites are; American Indian, Hispanic, and Filipino ethnic groups are also at increased risk.[103] Men are at higher risk than are women.

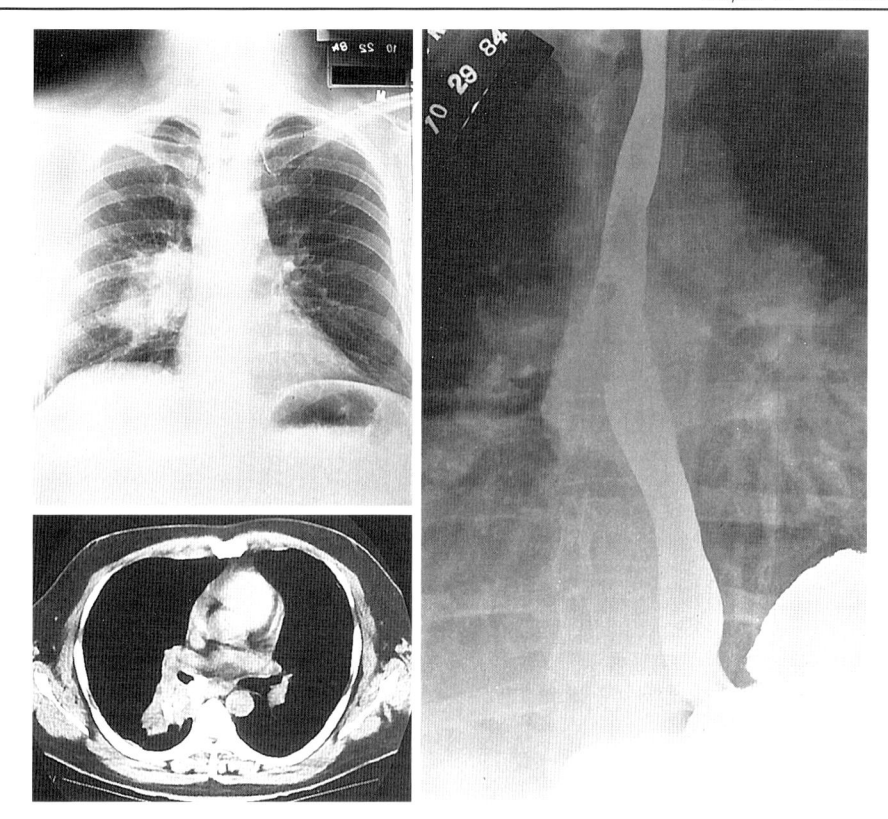

Figure 12–12
Computed tomography, contrast esophagography, and chest radiography demonstrating calcified mediastinal granulomatous disease secondary to histoplasmosis, with erosion into the adjacent esophagus. *(From Pearson FG, Cooper JD, Deslauriers J, et al.* Thoracic surgery, *2nd ed. Philadelphia: Churchill Livingstone; 2002.)*

The most common clinical manifestations of primary pulmonary coccidioidomycosis, termed desert or valley fever, are cough, fever, fatigue, dyspnea, chest pain, and headache. The symptoms develop 1 to 4 weeks after exposure. Approximately 20% of patients will have erythema nodosum or erythema multiforme, indicating an excellent cell-mediated immune response and prognosis. In the majority of cases, the disease is self-limited and remits in a few days. More severe primary infections can be accompanied by high fever, cough, weight loss, and development of pulmonary infiltrates and may take weeks to resolve. If the symptoms persist for more than 6 weeks with concomitant radiologic findings, treatment is usually started.

Patchy infiltrates, which range in size from subsegmental to lobar, are the most common radiographic finding in primary coccidioidomycosis. Infiltrates may be single or multiple. Adenopathy can be present and be so dramatic as to resemble lymphoma. Subsequent necrosis of the infiltrate commonly occurs, resulting in cavitation or coalescence into a granulomatous nodule (Fig. 12-13). The cavities are usually peripheral in location and may rupture into the pleural space, causing a pleural effusion, pneumothorax, bronchopleural fistula, and empyema. Secondary infection of the cavity and hemoptysis may also occur. The nodules that form within the lung parenchyma mimic bronchogenic carcinoma and often require resection to settle the issue.

Disseminated coccidioidomycosis may occur, typically as the result of hematogenous spread. The symptoms are insidious in onset several weeks after the primary infection. Skin and soft tissue lesions, bone and joint lesions, involvement of the genitourinary system, and meningitis may result.

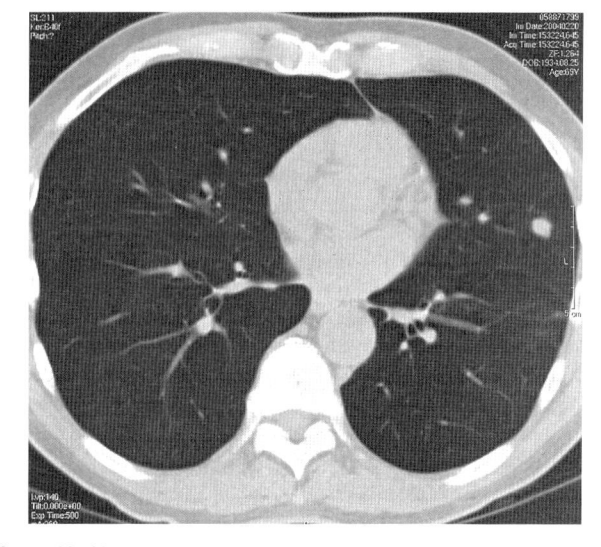

Figure 12–13
Computed tomographic scan demonstrating a granuloma in the lingula due to coccidioidomycosis.

The diagnosis of coccidioidomycosis depends on the identification of *C. immitis* within the body tissues or fluids. Detection by culture may take several weeks. Serum or cerebrospinal fluid may be tested to detect antibodies to *C. immitis*, through an immunodiffusion method. This test result usually becomes positive within 4 weeks after an initial infection and remains positive throughout the clinically active illness.

Some individuals continue to produce detectable antibodies for up to 1 year after recovery. Negative serologic results do not exclude a diagnosis of coccidioidomycosis. A skin test is available that shows a reaction to coccidioidin, prepared from the mycelial phase of the organism. A positive test response is highly correlated with protection and a favorable prognosis. Patients with disseminated disease often lose this measure of cell-mediated immunity, and a persistently negative skin test response at the end of therapy suggests the possibility of relapse.

Most patients with coccidioidomycosis require no therapy. All patients with disseminated disease and those with extensive pulmonary disease should be treated. Amphotericin B is the treatment of choice. Meningeal involvement is treated with intrathecal therapy. Surgical intervention is indicated for resection of old granulomas suggestive of carcinoma and for complications arising from cavitary disease.

Blastomycosis

Blastomycosis is a systemic mycotic infection caused by the dimorphic fungus *Blastomyces dermatitidis*. The fungus is a soil-dwelling organism endemic to the southeastern and central United States, although interestingly it has been cultured from soil only infrequently.[104] This fact as well as the lack of a suitable skin test has made precise definition of the endemic region problematic. The infecting microconidia are inhaled to the level of the alveolus, where the organism converts to its parasitic yeast-like form. The yeast multiplies rapidly, attracting neutrophils and macrophages and later a T cell–mediated immune reaction. An area of pneumonitis forms, with involvement of the regional lymph nodes. As granuloma formation finally occurs, with the organisms walled off, healing begins with "rounding off" of the infiltrate and fibrosis. These produce the late coin lesions suggestive of carcinoma. Late calcification of these lesions is less common than with histoplasmosis or coccidioidomycosis. If delayed hypersensitivity does not develop, the fungus may disseminate throughout the body and involve the skin, bones, meninges, and prostate or adrenal glands, producing disseminated disease. In patients with cell-mediated immune deficiencies, blastomycosis can present as a rapidly progressive infection.[105]

The primary infection site is the lung, although the incidence of asymptomatic infection is difficult to determine. In symptomatic cases, the disease may present acutely with fever, chills, myalgias, arthralgias, and a dry, hacking cough that becomes productive. Hemoptysis and pleuritic pain may occur. Most symptomatic patients recover within 2 to 3 weeks. On occasion, the symptoms will persist, resulting in chronic suppuration and cavitation. Patients who seem to have recovered may develop recurrent infection in areas remote from the primary site.

Radiologic findings are variable. Single or multiple sites of infiltrate or nodularity may occur, often with a lower lobe predilection. Pleural involvement may be seen, including thick, irregular pleura-based lesions.

B. dermatitidis is readily isolated from infected fluid or tissue if proper care is given to the specimen processing. This round, thick-walled, single-budding yeast measuring 8 to 15 μm in diameter may be seen reasonably well with routine hematoxylin and eosin stains, although periodic acid–Schiff and methenamine silver stains usually have many more organisms.

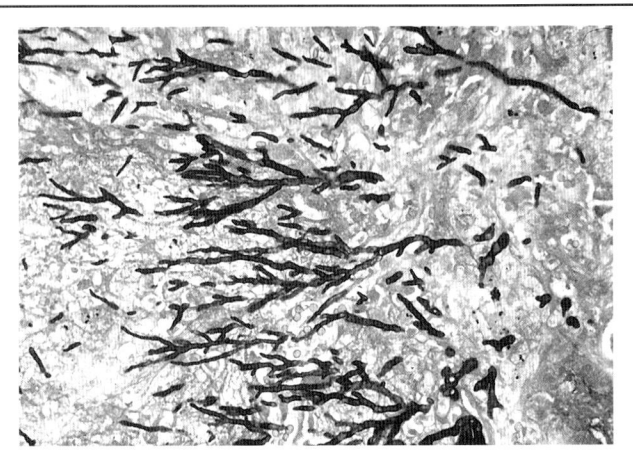

Figure 12–14
Aspergillus fumigatus infection, demonstrating the branching, septate hyphae of the organism. *(From Pearson FG, Cooper JD, Deslauriers J, et al. Thoracic surgery, 2nd ed. Philadelphia: Churchill Livingstone; 2002.)*

Sputum and other fluids should be prepared with a 10% potassium hydroxide solution and examined under a microscope with reduced illumination. A definitive diagnosis may be obtained within an hour. Identification by culture, in contrast, may take weeks. Serodiagnosis of blastomycosis has not been successful to date.

For subclinical disease, treatment may be deferred. In more severe but not life-threatening forms of the illness, itraconazole is used preferentially. Itraconazole may also be used as an adjunct after therapy with amphotericin B in disseminated cases, in those with immune compromise, and in those with mild extrapulmonary disease. For life-threatening and diffuse disease, amphotericin B is the drug of choice. Meningeal involvement also mandates amphotericin B therapy. The role of surgery in blastomycosis is to help with diagnosis and to rule out malignant disease.

Aspergillosis

Aspergillus is a ubiquitous soil-dwelling organism that releases small conidiophores that are easily inhaled (Fig. 12-14). It is inevitable that exposure occurs, and thus the development of active infection depends on other influences. Although more than 200 species of *Aspergillus* are known, only a few are thought to be pathogenic for humans. *Aspergillus fumigatus*, *Aspergillus flavus*, and *Aspergillus niger* are the most common; *A. fumigatus* dominates in human disease. In patients with normal immune function, no chronic or structural lung disease, and no hypersensitivity or allergic concerns, an infection is usually averted. In others, three main types of *Aspergillus* infection may occur, with considerable overlap: noninvasive aspergilloma; invasive aspergillosis; or a hypersensitivity reaction to *Aspergillus*, causing illness. The spectrum of *Aspergillus* infection is detailed in Figure 12-15.

Aspergilloma

Individuals with cavitary lung disease may develop an aspergilloma, a noninvasive infection characterized by a mass of fungal mycelia, inflammatory cells, mucus, and tissue debris, all within a preformed lung cavity (Fig. 12-16). The cavity

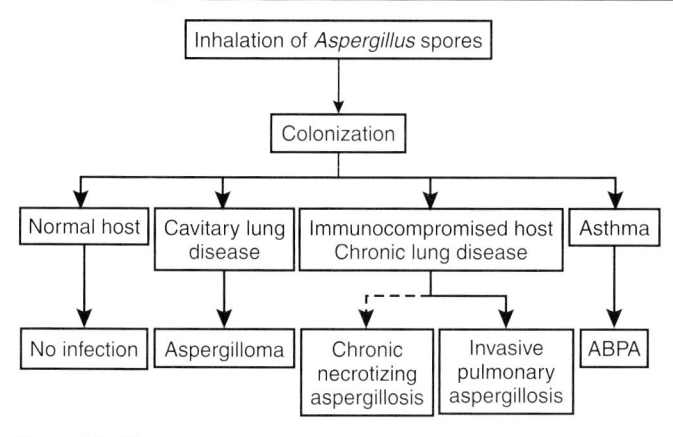

Figure 12–15
The spectrum of *Aspergillus* infection. ABPA, allergic bronchopulmonary aspergillosis.

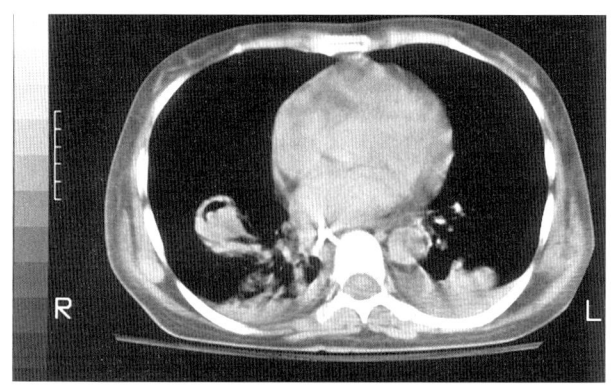

Figure 12–16
Computed tomographic scan demonstrating an aspergilloma involving the right lower lobe.

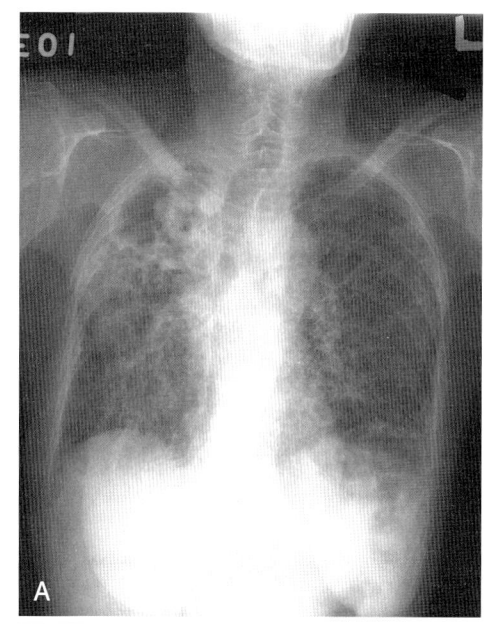

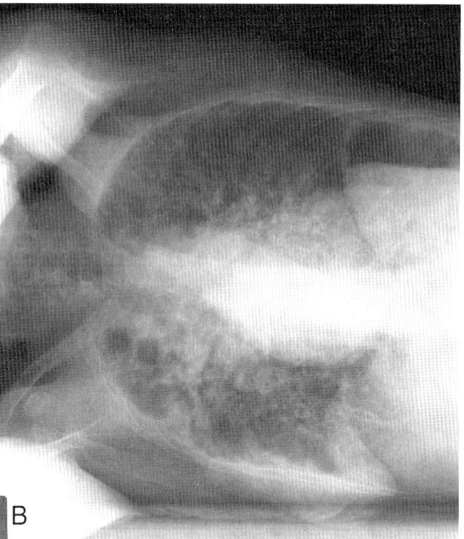

Figure 12–17
Posteroanterior (**A**) and decubitus (**B**) chest radiographs demonstrating an aspergilloma within a right upper lobe cavity. The fungus ball "moves" with change in the patient's position.

classically has been attributed to a prior tubercular infection, although this is obviously not always the case. Other types of fungus may produce a fungal ball, yet *Aspergillus* is by far the most common.[106] The true incidence of aspergilloma is unknown. In a study of 544 patients with a preexisting lung cavity due to tuberculosis, 11% had radiographic evidence of aspergilloma.[107] Most aspergillomas remain asymptomatic, yet some may increase in size or cause hemoptysis requiring intervention. On the other hand, some tend to resolve spontaneously. Invasion and dissemination from an aspergilloma rarely occur. In addition to hemoptysis, which is the most common presenting symptom, chronic cough and weight loss can occur. Rupture of the cavity into the pleural space with subsequent empyema and fistula has been reported.

Radiographic imaging reveals a thick-walled cavity, typically in the upper lobe, with a mass or "fungal ball" within the cavity. Movement of the mass inside the cavity with position change is variable and not a reliable diagnostic test, but it remains an additional interesting finding (Fig. 12-17). Differential diagnoses include cavitating hematoma, neoplasm, abscess, Wegener's granulomatosis, and hydatid cyst. Aspergilloma may coexist with any of these diagnoses. Culture of the sputum may yield *Aspergillus*, but it is frequently negative. Serologic testing will be helpful in the setting of a suggestive radiologic finding.

Systemic antimicrobial agents, including amphotericin B, have limited use in aspergilloma because of poor penetration into the cavity. Asymptomatic mycetomas should be left alone. Surgical resection is indicated if hemoptysis or other symptoms attributable to the lesion occur and adequate pulmonary reserve is present.

Invasive Aspergillosis

Acute invasive *Aspergillus* infection is a rare but dramatic occurrence in immunosuppressed and myelosuppressed patients. Myelosuppression appears to be the greatest risk factor for invasive pulmonary aspergillosis; the incidence is 20 times higher in patients with leukemia than in patients with lymphoma or patients with solid organ transplants.[108] Risk factors for invasive aspergillosis include prolonged neutropenia, corticosteroid therapy, transplantation (highest with lung and bone marrow), hematologic malignant disease, cytotoxic therapy, and AIDS.[109]

The lower respiratory tract is the focus of the invasive infection. As a result, respiratory symptoms predominate, including fever, cough, sputum production, and dyspnea. Pleuritic chest pain (due to pulmonary infarction after vascular invasion) and hemoptysis, in the appropriate clinical setting, should alert the clinician to the possibility of the diagnosis.[110] With vascular invasion, the organism can spread to other organs, particularly the brain but also the heart and intra-abdominal organs.

Radiologic findings can be nonspecific. Rounded densities and peripheral, pleura-based infiltrates are suggestive of infarction. Typical computed tomographic findings include multiple nodules, a halo sign (hemorrhage surrounding a nodule), and the air crescent sign (lucency in the region of the original nodule secondary to necrosis). The presence of *Aspergillus* species in sputum samples could be due to colonization, although studies have shown that positive cultures in patients with leukemia or in those who have undergone bone marrow transplantation have a positive predictive value of 80% to 90%.[111] Bronchoalveolar lavage is helpful in the diagnosis of invasive aspergillosis, particularly in patients with diffuse lung involvement. Transbronchial biopsy adds little to the bronchoalveolar lavage testing except increased risk. Serologic studies are not helpful in this setting. Lung biopsy remains the "gold standard" for diagnosis but should be reserved for equivocal cases.

The mortality for invasive aspergillosis remains high,[112] and empiric therapy should be initiated as early as possible. The treatment of choice remains amphotericin B. Itraconazole and caspofungin are alternatives, and investigation is under way regarding combination therapy.

Allergic Bronchopulmonary Aspergillosis

Allergic bronchopulmonary aspergillosis is a hypersensitivity reaction to *Aspergillus* antigens, particularly *A. fumigatus*. It is typically seen in patients with long-standing asthma or cystic fibrosis. It is believed that IgE- and IgG-mediated reactions play a central role in allergic bronchopulmonary aspergillosis. The diagnosis is usually made on clinical grounds buttressed by radiologic and serologic testing. Patients present with wheezing, fever, and mucus plugging; radiologic studies show pulmonary infiltrates that tend to be in the upper lobe and central in location. Volume loss secondary to mucus impaction may be seen, appearing as bandlike opacities emanating from the hilum with rounded distal margins (Fig. 12-18). Treatment consists of oral corticosteroids to suppress the immunologic response to the *Aspergillus* antigens and the secondary inflammatory reaction. Itraconazole may be added concurrently to the regimen.

Cryptococcosis

Cryptococcus neoformans is an encapsulated yeast that is found worldwide as a soil organism. It is associated with bird (pigeon) droppings, although the birds do not serve as a vector or carrier for the microbe. The portal of entry in humans is the respiratory tract. As a result, pulmonary infection may be the first manifestation of disease, but it is usually variable and

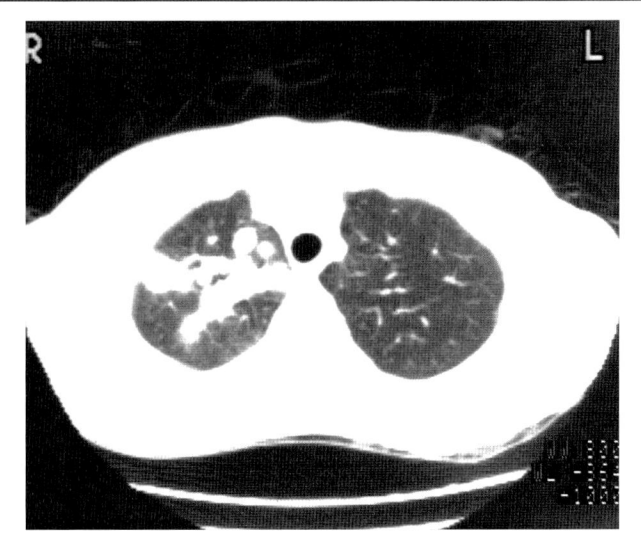

Figure 12–18
Computed tomographic scan demonstrating allergic bronchopulmonary aspergillosis involving the right upper lobe.

nonspecific. Spontaneous remission usually occurs in most patients. In those with suppressed or impaired immune systems, disseminated disease can result. *C. neoformans* has a special predilection for the meninges, and lethal meningitis can occur.

Treatment of cryptococcosis involves amphotericin B and flucytosine. Cryptococcal infections usually come to the attention of the thoracic surgeon after resection of a pulmonary mass that is found to be a chronic granulomatous reaction to a prior *C. neoformans* infection. Central necrosis and cavitation are not commonly seen, as in other major pulmonary mycotic infections. These lesions often involve the lower lobe and are solid. Up to 10% of patients with a resected pulmonary lesion develop cryptococcal meningitis after resection.[113] If incidental resection occurs, sampling of the spinal fluid should be performed. Evidence of extrapulmonary disease or residual pulmonary disease should prompt initiation of therapy.

Mucormycosis

Mucormycosis is a rare fungal infection, commonly fatal, caused by fungi of the subclass Zygomycetes. *Mucor* species are ubiquitous and are found in soil and decaying organic debris. Infection occurs by inhalation of spores and is commonly found in immunocompromised hosts. Risk factors for *Mucor* infection include neutropenia, acidosis, hyperglycemia, corticosteroid therapy, and deferoxamine therapy. This fungus grows best in acidic, hyperglycemic environments, thus accounting for the susceptibility of patients with diabetic ketoacidosis.

Mucor infections may involve several different areas of the body, including rhinocerebral, pulmonary, cutaneous, gastrointestinal, and central nervous system. The rhinocerebral involvement is commonly seen in patients with poorly controlled diabetes, and these patients may also have a pulmonary component. The pulmonary aspect typically presents with bronchopneumonia (Fig. 12-19) and progresses to invade pulmonary vessels, causing infarction. The infection can directly invade the extrapulmonary tissues, including the chest wall and mediastinal structures.

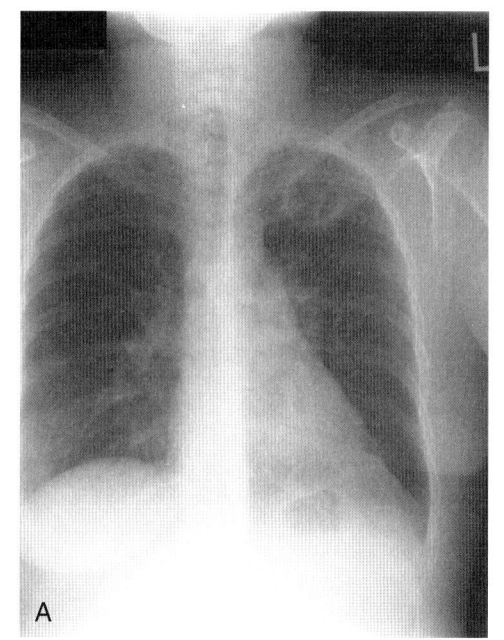

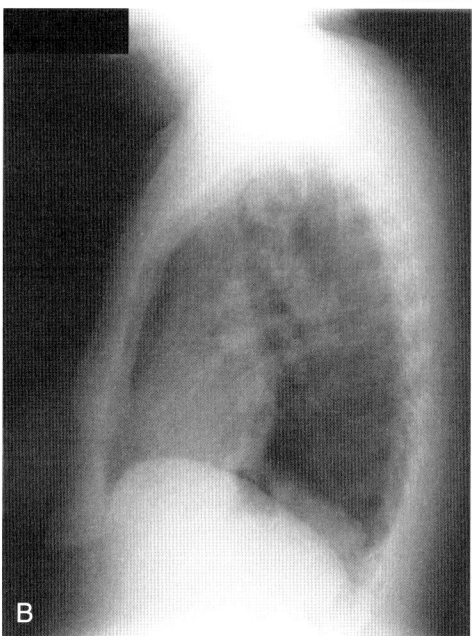

Figure 12–19
Posteroanterior **(A)** and lateral **(B)** chest radiographs demonstrating mucormycosis involving the left upper lobe.

The radiologic findings are variable and contribute little to refining the diagnosis. Culture results are usually negative, but positive results strongly suggest invasive disease. Direct pathologic examination of infected tissue should reveal broad, usually nonseptate hyphae invading the tissue. The side branches are short and at a 90-degree angle.

The overall mortality rate for pulmonary mucormycosis exceeds 50%. Therapy consists of three components: correction of underlying abnormalities, such as the hyperglycemic acidotic state with diabetic ketoacidosis, and reversal of immunosuppression, if possible; early institution of high-dose amphotericin B therapy; and aggressive surgical resection of involved lung and soft tissue, when possible.

REFERENCES

1. Fang GD, Fine M, Orloff J, et al. New and emerging etiologies for community-acquired pneumonia with implications for therapy. A prospective multicenter study of 359 cases. *Medicine* 1990;**69**:307-16.
2. Bartlett JG, Dowell SF, Mandell LA, File Jr TM, Musher DM, Fine MJ. Practice guidelines for the management of community-acquired pneumonia in adults. *Clin Infect Dis* 2000;**31**:347-82.
3. Mandell LA, Wunderink RG, Anzueto A, et al. Infectious Diseases Society of America/American Thoracic Society consensus guidelines on the management of community-acquired pneumonia in adults [see comment]. *Clin Infect Dis* 2007;**44**(Suppl. 2):S27-72.
4. Niederman MS, Mandell LA, Anzueto A, et al. Guidelines for the management of adults with community-acquired pneumonia. Diagnosis, assessment of severity, antimicrobial therapy, and prevention. *Am J Respir Crit Care Med* 2001;**163**:1730-54.
5. Niederman MS, McCombs JS, Unger AN, Kumar A, Popovian R. The cost of treating community-acquired pneumonia. *Clin Ther* 1998;**20**:820-37.
6. Fine MJ, Pratt HM, Obrosky DS, et al. Relation between length of hospital stay and costs of care for patients with community-acquired pneumonia [see comment]. *Am J Med* 2000;**109**:378-85.
7. Fine MJ, Smith MA, Carson CA, et al. Prognosis and outcomes of patients with community-acquired pneumonia. A meta-analysis [see comment]. *JAMA* 1996;**275**:134-41.
8. Bartlett JG, Mundy LM. Community-acquired pneumonia. *N Engl J Med* 1995;**333**:1618-24.
9. Lieberman D, Schlaeffer F, Boldur I, et al. Multiple pathogens in adult patients admitted with community-acquired pneumonia: a one year prospective study of 346 consecutive patients. *Thorax* 1996;**51**:179-84.
10. Gleason PP, Meehan TP, Fine JM, Galusha DH, Fine MJ. Associations between initial antimicrobial therapy and medical outcomes for hospitalized elderly patients with pneumonia. *Arch Intern Med* 1999;**159**:2562-72.
11. Houck PM, MacLehose RF, Niederman MS, Lowery JK. Empiric antibiotic therapy and mortality among medicare pneumonia inpatients in 10 western states. *Chest* 1993;**2001**(119):1420-6:1995, and 1997.
12. Stahl JE, Barza M, DesJardin J, Martin R, Eckman MH. Effect of macrolides as part of initial empiric therapy on length of stay in patients hospitalized with community-acquired pneumonia [see comment]. *Arch Intern Med* 1999;**159**:2576-80.
13. Marrie TJ. Community-acquired pneumonia. *Clin Infect Dis* 1994;**18**:14-5: 501-13; quiz.
14. Mandell LA, Bartlett JG, Dowell SF, et al. Update of practice guidelines for the management of community-acquired pneumonia in immunocompetent adults. *Clin Infect Dis* 2003;**37**:1405-33.
15. Metersky ML, Ma A, Bratzler DW, Houck PM. Predicting bacteremia in patients with community-acquired pneumonia. *Am J Respir Crit Care Med* 2004;**169**:342-7.
16. Bates JH, Campbell GD, Barron AL, et al. Microbial etiology of acute pneumonia in hospitalized patients [see comment]. *Chest* 1992;**101**:1005-12.
17. Oostherheert JJ, van Loon AM, Schuurman R, et al. Impact of rapid detection of viral and atypical bacterial pathogens by real-time polymerase chain reaction for patients with lower respiratory tract infection [see comment]. *Clin Infect Dis* 2005;**41**:1438-44.
18. Andreo F, Dominguez J, Ruiz J, et al. Impact of rapid urine antigen tests to determine the etiology of community-acquired pneumonia in adults. *Resp Med* 2006;**100**:884-91.
19. Briones ML, Blanquer J, Ferrando D, Blasco ML, Gimeno C, Marin J. Assessment of analysis of urinary pneumococcal antigen by immunochromatography for etiologic diagnosis of community-acquired pneumonia in adults. *Clin Vaccine Immunol* 2006;**13**:1092-7.
20. Dominguez J, Gali N, Blanco S, et al. Detection of *Streptococcus pneumoniae* antigen by a rapid immunochromatographic assay in urine samples [see comment]. *Chest* 2001;**119**:243-9.
21. Ehara N, Fukushima K, Kakeya H, et al. A novel method for rapid detection of *Streptococcus pneumoniae* antigen in sputum and its application in adult respiratory tract infections. *J Med Microbiol* 2008;**57**:820-6.
22. Plouffe JF, File Jr TM, Breiman RF, et al. Reevaluation of the definition of Legionnaires' disease: use of the urinary antigen assay. Community Based Pneumonia Incidence Study Group. *Clin Infect Dis* 1995;**20**:1286-91.
23. Fine MJ, Auble TE, Yealy DM, et al. A prediction rule to identify low-risk patients with community-acquired pneumonia [see comment]. *N Engl Med* 1997;**336**:243-50.
24. Aujesky D, Auble TE, Yealy DM, et al. Prospective comparison of three validated prediction rules for prognosis in community-acquired pneumonia. *Am J Med* 2005;**118**:384-92.

25. Aujesky D, Fine MJ. The pneumonia severity index: a decade after the initial derivation and validation. *Clin Infect Dis* 2008;**47**(Suppl. 3):S133-9.
26. American College of Emergency Physicians. Clinical policy for the management and risk stratification of community-acquired pneumonia in adults in the emergency department. *Ann Emerg Med* 2001;**38**:107-13.
27. Halm EA, Teirstein AS. Management of community-acquired pneumonia. *N Engl J Med* 2002;**347**:2039-45.
28. Johnstone J, Eurich DT, Majumdar SR, Jin Y, Marrie TJ. Long-term morbidity and mortality after hospitalization with community-acquired pneumonia: a population-based cohort study. *Medicine* 2008;**87**:329-34.
29. Metlay JP, Fine MJ. Testing strategies in the initial management of patients with community-acquired pneumonia. *Ann Intern Med* 2003;**138**:109-18.
30. Lim WS, van der Eerden MM, Laing R, et al. Defining community acquired pneumonia severity on presentation to hospital: an international derivation and validation study. *Thorax* 2003;**58**:377-82.
31. Bauer TT, Ewig S, Marre R, Suttorp N, Welte T. CRB-65 predicts death from community-acquired pneumonia. *J Intern Med* 2006;**260**:93-101.
32. Buising KL, Thursky KA, Black JF, et al. A prospective comparison of severity scores for identifying patients with severe community acquired pneumonia: reconsidering what is meant by severe pneumonia. *Thorax* 2006;**61**:419-24.
33. Capelastegui A, Espana PP, Quintana JM, et al. Validation of a predictive rule for the management of community-acquired pneumonia. *Eur Respir J* 2006;**27**:151-7.
34. Niederman MS, Feldman C, Richards GA. Combining information from prognostic scoring tools for CAP: an American view on how to get the best of all worlds. *Eur Respir J* 2006;**27**:9-11.
35. Dean NC, Bateman KA, Donnelly SM, Silver MP, Snow GL, Hale D. Improved clinical outcomes with utilization of a community-acquired pneumonia guideline. *Chest* 2006;**130**:794-9.
36. Gleason PP, Kapoor WN, Stone RA, et al. Medical outcomes and antimicrobial costs with the use of the American Thoracic Society guidelines for outpatients with community-acquired pneumonia. *JAMA* 1997;**278**:32-9.
37. Menendez R, Torres A, Zalacain R, et al. Guidelines for the treatment of community-acquired pneumonia: predictors of adherence and outcome. *Am J Respir Crit Care Med* 2005;**172**:757-62.
38. Meehan TP, Fine MJ, Krumholz HM, et al. Quality of care, process, and outcomes in elderly patients with pneumonia [see comment]. *JAMA* 1997;**278**:2080-4.
39. Cockburn J, Gibberd RW, Reid AL, Sanson-Fisher RW. Determinants of non-compliance with short term antibiotic regimens. *Br Med J Clin Research Ed* 1987;**295**:814-8.
40. Laterre P-F, Garber G, Levy H, et al. Severe community-acquired pneumonia as a cause of severe sepsis: data from the PROWESS study [see comment]. *Crit Care Med* 2005;**33**:952-61.
41. Confalonieri M, Urbino R, Potena A, et al. Hydrocortisone infusion for severe community-acquired pneumonia: a preliminary randomized study. *Am J Respir Crit Care Med* 2005;**171**:242-8.
42. Masia M, Gutierrez F, Shum C, et al. Usefulness of procalcitonin levels in community-acquired pneumonia according to the patients outcome research team pneumonia severity index. *Chest* 2005;**128**:2223-9.
43. Boussekey N, Leroy O, Alfandari S, Devos P, Georges H, Guery B. Procalcitonin kinetics in the prognosis of severe community-acquired pneumonia. *Inten Care Med* 2006;**32**:469-72.
44. Boussekey N, Leroy O, Georges H, Devos P. d'Escrivan T, Guery B. Diagnostic and prognostic values of admission procalcitonin levels in community-acquired pneumonia in an intensive care unit. *Infection* 2005;**33**:257-63.
45. Christ-Crain M, Stolz D, Bingisser R, et al. Procalcitonin guidance of antibiotic therapy in community-acquired pneumonia: a randomized trial [see comment]. *Am J Crit Care Med* 2006;**174**:84-93.
46. Guidelines for the management of adults with hospital-acquired. ventilator-associated, and healthcare-associated pneumonia. *Am J Respir Crit Care Med* 2005;**171**:388-416.
47. Craven D, Palladino R, McQuillen D. Healthcare-associated pneumonia in adults: management principles to improve outcomes. *Infect Dis Clin North Am* 2004;**18**:939-62.
48. Mandell LA, Campbell Jr GD. Nosocomial pneumonia guidelines: an international perspective. *Chest* 1998;**113**:188S-93S.
49. Leu H, Kaiser D, Mori M, Woolson R, Wenzel R. Hospital-acquired pneumonia. Attributable mortality and morbidity. *Am J Epidemiol* 1989;**129**:1258-67.
50. Fridkin SK, Welbel SF, Weinstein RA. Magnitude and prevention of nosocomial infections in the intensive care unit. *Infect Dis Clin North Am* 1997;**11**:479-96.
51. Craven DE, Steger KA. Epidemiology of nosocomial pneumonia. New perspectives on an old disease. *Chest* 1995;**108**:1S-6S.
52. Kollef MH. The prevention of ventilator-associated pneumonia. *N Engl J Med* 1999;**340**:627-34.
53. Heyland DK, Cook DJ, Griffith L, Keenan SP, Brun-Buisson C. The attributable morbidity and mortality of ventilator-associated pneumonia in the critically ill patient. The Canadian Critical Trials Group. *Am J Resp Crit Care Med* 1999;**159**:1249-56.
54. Torres A, Aznar R, Gatell JM, et al. Incidence, risk, and prognosis factors of nosocomial pneumonia in mechanically ventilated patients. *Am Rev Respi Dis* 1990;**142**:523-8.
55. Torres A, Carlet J. Ventilator-associated pneumonia. European Task Force on ventilator-associated pneumonia. *Eur Resp J* 2001;**17**:1034-45.
56. Napolitano LM. Hospital-acquired and ventilator-associated pneumonia: what's new in diagnosis and treatment? *Am J Surg* 2003;**186**:4S-14S:discussion 31S-4S.
57. Ewig S, Torres A. Prevention and management of ventilator-associated pneumonia. *Curr Opin Crit Care* 2002;**8**:58-69.
58. Kollef MH. Diagnosis of ventilator-associated pneumonia. *N Engl J Med* 2006;**355**:2691-3.
59. Ruiz M, Torres A, Ewig S, et al. Noninvasive versus invasive microbial investigation in ventilator-associated pneumonia: evaluation of outcome. *Am J Resp Crit Care Med* 2000;**162**:119-25.
60. Shorr AF, Sherner JH, Jackson WL, Kollef MH. Invasive approaches to the diagnosis of ventilator-associated pneumonia: a meta-analysis. *Crit Care Med* 2005;**33**:46-53.
61. Sole Violan J, Fernandez JA, Benitez AB, Cardenosa Cendrero JA, Rodriguez de Castro F. Impact of quantitative invasive diagnostic techniques in the management and outcome of mechanically ventilated patients with suspected pneumonia [see comment]. *Crit Care Med* 2000;**28**:2737-41.
62. The Canadian Critical Care Trials Group. A randomized trial of diagnostic techniques for ventilator-associated pneumonia. *N Engl J Med* 2006;**355**:2619-30.
63. Pereira Gomes JC, Pedreira Jr WL, Araujo EM, et al. Impact of BAL in the management of pneumonia with treatment failure: positivity of BAL culture under antibiotic therapy. *Chest* 2000;**118**:1739-46.
64. Aarts M-AW, Hancock JN, Heyland D, McLeod RS, Marshall JC. Empiric antibiotic therapy for suspected ventilator-associated pneumonia: a systematic review and meta-analysis of randomized trials [see comment]. *Crit Care Med* 2008;**36**:108-17.
65. Kollef MH. Appropriate antibiotic therapy for ventilator-associated pneumonia and sepsis: a necessity, not an issue for debate [comment]. *Inten Care Med* 2003;**29**:147-9.
66. Mehta R, Niederman MS. Adequate empirical therapy minimizes the impact of diagnostic methods in patients with ventilator-associated pneumonia [comment]. *Crit Care Med* 2000;**28**:3092-4.
67. Collard HR, Saint S, Matthay MA. Prevention of ventilator-associated pneumonia: an evidence-based systematic review [see comment]. *Ann Intern Med* 2003;**138**:494-501.
68. Warner MA, Warner ME, Weber JG. Clinical significance of pulmonary aspiration during the perioperative period. *Anesthesiology* 1993;**78**:56-62.
69. Mendelson CL. The aspiration of stomach contents into the lungs during obstetric anesthesia. *Am J Obstet Gynecol* 1946;**52**:191-205.
70. Marik PE. Aspiration pneumonitis and aspiration pneumonia. *N Engl J Med* 2001;**344**:665-71.
71. Gleeson K, Eggli DF, Maxwell SL. Quantitative aspiration during sleep in normal subjects. *Chest* 1997;**111**:1266-72.
72. Reid LM. Reduction in bronchial subdivision in bronchiectasis. *Thorax* 1950;**5**:233-47.
73. Angrill J, Agusti C, de Celis R, et al. Bacterial colonisation in patients with bronchiectasis: microbiological pattern and risk factors. *Thorax* 2002;**57**:15-9.
74. Barker AF. Bronchiectasis. *N Engl J Med* 2002;**346**:1383-93.
75. Hagan JL, Hardy JD. Lung abscess revisited. A survey of 184 cases. *Ann Surg* 1983;**197**:755-62.
76. Bartlett JG. The role of anaerobic bacteria in lung abscess. *Clin Infect Dis* 2005;**40**:923-5.
77. Swensen SJ, Peters SG, LeRoy AJ, Gay PC, Sykes MW, Trastek VF. Radiology in the intensive-care unit. *Mayo Clin Proc* 1991;**66**:396-410.
78. Stark DD, Federle MP, Goodman PC, Podrasky AE, Webb WR. Differentiating lung abscess and empyema: radiography and computed tomography. *AJR Am J Roentgenol* 1983;**141**:163-7.
79. Yang PC, Luh KT, Lee YC, et al. Lung abscesses: US examination and US-guided transthoracic aspiration. *Radiology* 1991;**180**:171-5.
80. Wiedemann HP, Rice TW. Lung abscess and empyema. *Sem thorac Cardiovasc Surg* 1995;**7**:119-28.
81. Herth F, Ernst A, Becker HD. Endoscopic drainage of lung abscesses: technique and outcome. *Chest* 2005;**127**:1378-81.
82. Chan ED, Iseman MD. Multidrug-resistant and extensively drug-resistant tuberculosis: a review. *Curr Opin Infect Dis* 2008;**21**:587-95.

83. Iseman MD, Degroote M. Environmental mycobacterium infections. In: Gorbach SL, Bartlett JG, Blacklow NR, editors. *Infectious Diseases*. 3rd ed Baltimore: Lippincott Williams & Wilkins; 2004. p. 1389-410.
84. Dye C, Scheele S, Dolin P, Pathania V, Raviglione MC. Global burden of tuberculosis: estimated incidence, prevalence, and mortality by country. WHO Global Surveillance and Monitoring Project. *JAMA* 1999;**282**:677-86.
85. American Thoracic Society/Centers for Disease Control and Prevention/Infectious Diseases Society of America. Treatment of tuberculosis. *Am J Respir Crit Care Med* 2003;**167**:603-62.
86. Drugs for tuberculosis. *Treatment Guidelines From the Medical Letter* 2007;**5**:15-22.
87. Grandjean L, Moore DAJ. Tuberculosis in the developing world: recent advances in diagnosis with special consideration of extensively drug-resistant tuberculosis. *Curr Opin Infect Dis* 2008;**21**:454-61.
88. Mitnick CD, Shin SS, Seung KJ, et al. Comprehensive treatment of extensively drug-resistant tuberculosis. *N Engl J Med* 2008;**359**:563-74.
89. Pomerantz BJ, Cleveland JC, Olson HK, Pomerantz M. Pulmonary resection for multi-drug resistant tuberculosis. *J Thorac Cardiovasc Surg* 2001;**121**:448-53.
90. Chan ED, Laurel V, Strand MJ, et al. Treatment and outcome analysis of 205 patients with multidrug-resistant tuberculosis. *Am J Respir Crit Care Med* 2004;**169**:1103-9.
91. Iseman MD, Buschman DL, Ackerson LM. Pectus excavatum and scoliosis. Thoracic anomalies associated with pulmonary disease caused by *Mycobacterium avium* complex. *Am Rev Respir Dis* 1991;**144**:914-6.
92. Pomerantz M, Denton JR, Huitt GA, Brown JM, Powell LA, Iseman MD. Resection of the right middle lobe and lingula for mycobacterial infection. *Ann Thorac Surg* 1996;**62**:990-3.
93. Mitchell JD, Bishop A, Cafaro A, Weyant MJ, Pomerantz M. Anatomic lung resection for nontuberculous mycobacterial disease. *Ann Thorac Surg* 2008;**85**:1887-93.
94. Storch G, Burford JG, George RB, Kaufman L, Ajello L. Acute histoplasmosis. Description of an outbreak in northern Louisiana. *Chest* 1980;**77**:38-42.
95. Werner SB, Pappagianis D, Heindl I, Mickel A. An epidemic of coccidioidomycosis among archeology students in northern California. *N Engl J Med* 1972;**286**:507-12.
96. Seabury JH, Buechner HA, Busey JF. The diagnosis of pulmonary mycoses. Report of the Committee on Fungus Diseases and Subcommittee on Criteria for Clinical Diagnosis, American College of Chest Physicians. *Chest* 1971;**60**:82-8.
97. Perfect JR, Cox GM, Lee JY, et al. The impact of culture isolation of *Aspergillus* species: a hospital-based survey of aspergillosis. *Clin Infect Dis* 2001;**33**:1824-33.
98. Kami M, Fukui T, Ogawa S, et al. Use of real-time PCR on blood samples for diagnosis of invasive aspergillosis. *Clin Infect Dis* 2001;**33**:1504-12.
99. Turin L, Riva F, Galbiati G, Cainelli T. Fast, simple and highly sensitive double-rounded polymerase chain reaction assay to detect medically relevant fungi in dermatological specimens. *Euro J Clin Invest* 2000;**30**:511-8.
100. Edwards LB, Acquaviva FA, Livesay VT, Cross FW, Palmer CE. An atlas of sensitivity to tuberculin, PPD-B, and histoplasmin in the United States. *Am Rev Resp Dis* 1969;**99**(Suppl):1-32.
101. Rosenthal J, Brandt KD, Wheat LJ, Slama TG. Rheumatologic manifestations of histoplasmosis in the recent Indianapolis epidemic. *Arthritis & Rheumatism* 1983;**26**:1065-70.
102. Mathisen DJ, Grillo HC. Clinical manifestation of mediastinal fibrosis and histoplasmosis. *Ann Thorac Surg* 1992;**54**:7-8:1053-7; discussion.
103. Drutz DJ, Catanzaro A. Coccidioidomycosis. Part II. *Am Rev Resp Dis* 1978;**117**:727-71.
104. Davies SF, Sarosi GA. Blastomycosis. In: Sarosi GA, Davies SF, editors. *Fungal Diseases of the Lung*. 2nd ed New York: Raven Press; 1993. p. 51-64.
105. Pappas PG, Threlkeld MG, Bedsole GD, Cleveland KO, Gelfand MS, Dismukes WE. Blastomycosis in immunocompromised patients. *Medicine* 1993;**72**:311-25.
106. Joynson DH. Pulmonary aspergilloma. *Br J Clin Prac* 1977;**31**:207-16:21.
107. Aspergilloma and residual tuberculous cavities—the results of a resurvey. *Tubercle* 1970;**51**:227-45.
108. Burch PA, Karp JE, Merz WG, Kuhlman JE, Fishman EK. Favorable outcome of invasive aspergillosis in patients with acute leukemia. *J Clin Oncol* 1987;**5**:1985-93.
109. Soubani AO, Chandrasekar PH. The clinical spectrum of pulmonary aspergillosis. *Chest* 2002;**121**:1988-99.
110. Albelda SM, Talbot GH, Gerson SL, Miller WT, Cassileth PA. Pulmonary cavitation and massive hemoptysis in invasive pulmonary aspergillosis. Influence of bone marrow recovery in patients with acute leukemia. *Am Rev Resp Dis* 1985;**131**:115-20.
111. Horvath JA, Dummer S. The use of respiratory-tract cultures in the diagnosis of invasive pulmonary aspergillosis. *Am J Med* 1996;**100**:171-8.
112. Meersseman W, Lagrou K, Maertens J, Van Wijngaerden E. Invasive aspergillosis in the intensive care unit. *Clin Infect Dis* 2007;**45**:205-16.
113. Hatcher Jr CR, Sehdeva J, Waters 3rd WC, et al. Primary pulmonary cryptococcosis. *J Thorac Cardiovasc Surg* 1971;**61**:39-49.

CHAPTER 13

Surgery for Emphysema

Bryan F. Meyers, John C. Kucharczuk, and Joel D. Cooper

Selection of Patients for Surgical
  Treatment of Emphysema
Bullectomy
Lung Transplantation
  Techniques

Volume Reduction
  Techniques
Combinations of Lung Transplantation
  and Lung Volume Reduction

Bronchoscopic Treatment of Emphysema
  Endoscopic Placement of One-Way Valves
  Airway Bypass
Summary

The debilitating symptoms of pulmonary emphysema have attracted the interest of surgeons throughout the history of our specialty. Many innovative and creative operations have been devised to treat the dyspnea caused by this disease. Costochondrectomy, phrenic crush, pneumoperitoneum, pleural abrasion, lung denervation, and thoracoplasty all proved to be dead ends in the evolution of surgical treatment for the hyperexpanded and poorly perfused emphysematous lung.[1] Only three surgical procedures have evolved to survive the test of time and to withstand the close scrutiny of the medical community: bullectomy, lung transplantation, and lung volume reduction. Bullectomy has roots dating to the first half of the last century, when external drainage of the giant bulla was attempted to eliminate the space-occupying lesion by collapse rather than by resection. Although vestiges of this conservative approach remain in use for rare high-risk patients, the general approach has evolved to include resection of the bulla with sparing of all functional lung tissue. Lung transplantation was successfully performed in 1963 by Hardy and coworkers,[2] and after a prolonged period of incremental progress, the operation became clinically feasible in the early 1980s as heart-lung transplantation[3] and isolated lung transplantation.[4] Although lung transplantation was initially used as therapy for pulmonary fibrosis and pulmonary hypertension, the indications have evolved such that emphysema is the most common diagnosis leading to transplantation today. Lung volume reduction surgery (LVRS) was first proposed by Brantigan and colleagues[5] in conjunction with lung denervation and was discarded after the initial experience; a mortality of 16% showed the operation to be too risky. Observations about the physiologic behavior of emphysema patients during and after lung transplantation led to the reconsideration of volume reduction by Cooper and associates.[6]

The destruction of pulmonary parenchyma causes a decreased mass of functioning lung tissue and thus decreases the amount of gas exchange that can take place. As the lung tissue is destroyed, it loses elastic recoil and expands in volume. This leads to the typical hyperexpanded chest seen in emphysema patients with flattened diaphragms, widened intercostal spaces, and horizontal ribs. These anatomic changes result in the loss of mechanical advantages exploited in normal breathing and thus lead to increased work of breathing and dyspnea.[7] When the destruction and expansion occur in a nonuniform manner, the most affected lung tissue can expand to crowd the relatively spared lung tissue to impair ventilation of the functioning lung. Finally, there is obstruction in the small airways caused by a combination of reversible bronchospasm and irreversible loss of elastic recoil by adjacent lung parenchyma. The suitability of a given patient for surgical treatment of emphysema depends in part on the relative contributions of lung destruction, lung compression, and small airways obstruction to the overall physiologic impairment of that patient.

SELECTION OF PATIENTS FOR SURGICAL TREATMENT OF EMPHYSEMA

Bullectomy, lung transplantation, and LVRS are invasive procedures with risk of both morbidity and mortality to patients. Therefore, all three procedures are directed only at patients who remain symptomatic despite optimal medical therapy. This optimal medical treatment will include bronchodilators to eliminate any reversible component of airway obstruction. Smoking cessation is an absolute necessity and should be in effect for at least 6 months before surgical therapy is considered. Participation in pulmonary rehabilitation has been shown to relieve subjective dyspnea, to increase functional capabilities, and to improve subjective quality of life.[8,9] All patients considered by the authors for surgical treatment of emphysema are enrolled in a supervised pulmonary rehabilitation program, and their subsequent consideration for surgery is based in part on their compliance and progress with rehabilitation. Finally, because the operations carry an immediate risk of morbidity and mortality, and because none has been shown to reliably increase life expectancy, patients considering an operation must be willing to accept the risks of surgery in exchange for an anticipated relief from dyspnea and an uncertain effect on life expectancy.

BULLECTOMY

Bullectomy is considered whenever a substantial air-filled bulla is detected on a chest radiograph. Most patients considered for surgery are symptomatic with dyspnea, pain, or spontaneous pneumothorax. Other symptoms are rare but include bleeding and infection within the confines of the bulla. The natural history of bullae treated expectantly with observation is one of enlargement causing worsened dyspnea, but the lack of large series of patients treated without surgery makes prediction of the rate of expansion unreliable. Some asymptomatic patients with a single bulla encompassing more than one half the volume of a pleural cavity would be considered surgical candidates, whereas patients with smaller lesions and no symptoms would be more controversial. Factors making surgery less appealing include multiple smaller bullae, advanced emphysema in the nonbullous adjacent lung, and notable comorbidities. The frequency with which bullectomy is performed is low, as demonstrated by a systematic review by Snider,[10] who cited 22 individual reports during a 39-year period that included a total of 476 patients.

The technique of operation is variable and depends on the anatomic details of the bulla as well as the preferred approach of the surgeon. A well-demarcated bulla with a clear pedicle can be excised with a stapler by a muscle-sparing thoracotomy or a video-assisted thoracoscopic approach. Numerous bullae or bullae that merge indistinctly with the comparatively normal adjacent lung will require a large, stapled wedge resection placed to maximize resection of destroyed lung while minimizing resection of spared parenchyma. It is unusual for a formal lobectomy to be necessary, but when a lobe is nearly completely destroyed and the fissures are complete, a lobectomy is an attractive option that might eliminate the possibility of a postoperative air leak and prolonged chest tube drainage. Many surgeons will combine a localized pleurectomy or a pleural tent with the bullectomy to help manage the pleural space and prevent a prolonged chest tube air leak.

The safety of bullectomy in well-selected patients is demonstrated by the 2.3% mortality reported by FitzGerald and colleagues[11] more than 30 years ago. Our modern results are similar, with a single death in 43 operations (2.3%).[12] Because properly selected patients will have an increase in a first second forced expiratory volume (FEV_1) postoperatively, there is a very low rate of respiratory failure and the need for tracheostomy. Parenchymal air leaks are the most frequent single postoperative complication, and they are suitably managed with the surgeon's choice of buttressed stapled lines, pleural tent, pleurectomy, biological glues, or ambulatory Heimlich valves. In our series, 53% of patients experienced chest tube air leaks for more than 7 days.

There are few reports of long-term survival and functional changes after bullectomy, and none of them is a prospective clinical trial. Our clinical series demonstrated a 5-year survival of 91%, with two late deaths attributed to pneumonia and one to pulmonary fibrosis. In general, the freedom from long-term return of dyspnea is proportional to the quality of the remaining lung after bullectomy. All patients with emphysema seem to experience a progressive decline in FEV_1 over time, so patients with nearly normal underlying lung at the time of bullectomy will begin at a higher functional baseline than patients with moderate or severe emphysema in the remaining lung. Our experience demonstrated an improvement in the FEV_1 from 1.2 ± 0.6 L preoperatively to 1.9 ± 0.9 L at 6 months and 1 year postoperatively.[12] The persistence of a measurable airflow obstruction after bullectomy underscores the presence of residual emphysema in the remaining lung, regardless of the normal appearance it may have compared with the destroyed bullous regions.

LUNG TRANSPLANTATION

Pulmonary emphysema was initially thought to be a contraindication for lung transplantation. In the era preceding bilateral lung transplantation, the perceived difficulty of ventilation-perfusion mismatching in the native and newly transplanted lung was thought to be an obstacle worth avoiding. For that reason, early isolated single-lung transplantations were directed at patients with pulmonary fibrosis, in whom the elevated pulmonary vascular resistance and poor compliance of the native lung created a situation in which the transplanted lung was both preferentially perfused and preferentially ventilated. After the initial success with single-lung transplantation for emphysema was reported,[13] and after the development of techniques to allow safe, bilateral lung transplantation,[14,15] the application of lung transplantation for emphysema quickly increased. Management of the recipient of a single lung transplant for emphysema has proved not to be as complicated as feared. The main principles that lead to success are the avoidance of positive end-expiratory pressure and the rapid weaning from mechanical ventilation.

Idiopathic emphysema and α_1-antitrypsin deficiency together have become the most common indications for pulmonary transplantation. These two diagnoses together account for 63% of the adult single-lung transplantations and 32% of the bilateral lung transplantations reported in the 2003 Registry of the International Society for Heart and Lung Transplantation as reported by Trulock and colleagues.[16]

The selection criteria for lung transplantation have been published elsewhere but are chosen to identify patients with sufficient risk of death from lung disease to make the risks of the transplant operation worth bearing. Unfortunately, the survival of emphysema patients has been notably difficult to predict, leading to early listing and an excellent survival rate on the waiting list compared with patients with other diagnoses. Most emphysema patients have deteriorated to a point at which oxygen supplementation is required. In our experience, the mean supplemental oxygen requirement is slightly in excess of 4 L/min. The obstructive physiology in these patients results in FEV_1 of well below 1 L, or approximately 15% of predicted normal values. Progressive elevation in P_{CO_2} has been observed in some patients, however, with several of these individuals undergoing transplantation with the P_{CO_2} in excess of 100 mm Hg.

The advantage of lung transplantation is obvious: a complete replacement of the diseased and nonfunctional lung with a new and healthy donor lung. Initial and long-term function of patients with single or bilateral lung transplantation for emphysema shows a dramatic improvement in pulmonary function and exercise tolerance with elimination of the need for supplementary oxygen. Figure 13-1 demonstrates the magnitude of change in the FEV_1 as a result of single-lung transplantation, bilateral lung transplantation, and LVRS as reported by Gaissert and colleagues.[17] Figure 13-2 shows a similar stratified analysis for exercise tolerance as measured by 6-minute walking distances. It can be seen that although the improvement in both outcome measures is greatest for bilateral lung transplantation and least for LVRS, the absolute differences in exercise tolerance are much less than those seen in pulmonary function.

The disadvantages of lung transplantation are well known but worth reviewing. First, the lack of available donor lungs has created a situation in which the waiting times for transplant recipients in programs such as ours can routinely exceed 2 years. Once lungs become available, the initial morbidity and mortality of lung transplantation are higher than those reported for lung volume reduction, with mortality variously described

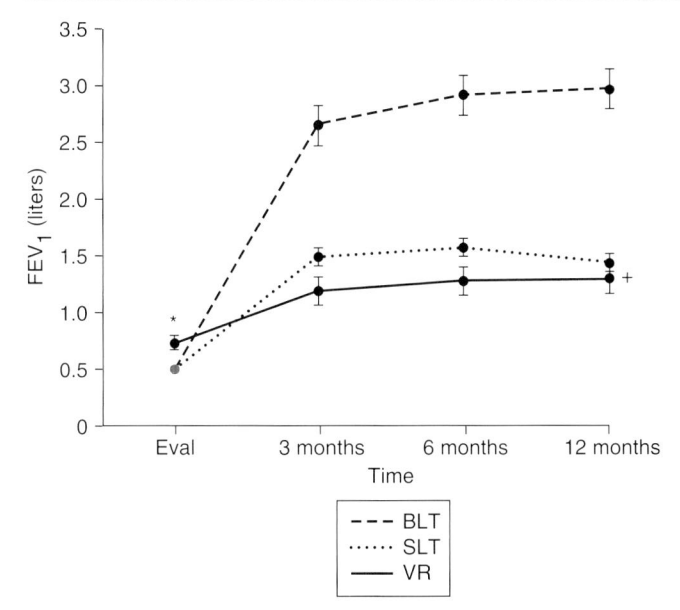

Figure 13-1
Changes observed in first second expired volumes in patients after bilateral lung transplantation (BLT), single-lung transplantation (SLT), and lung volume reduction surgery (VR).

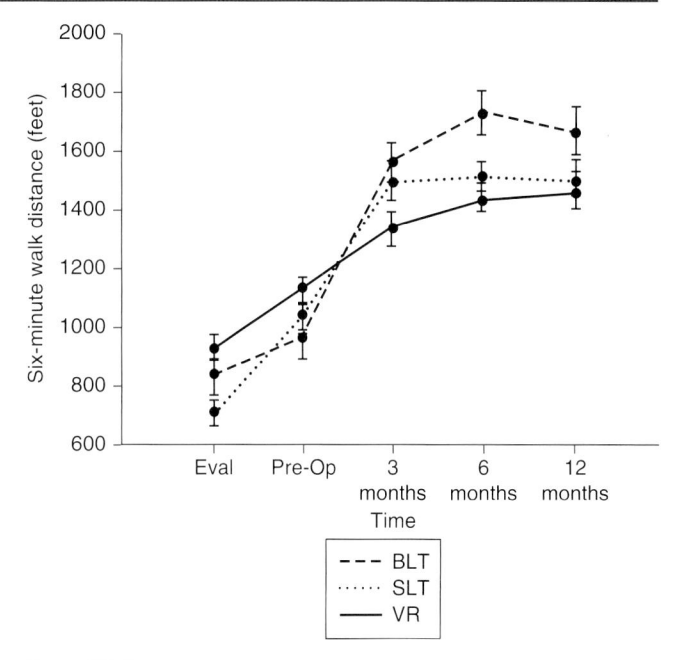

Figure 13-2
Changes observed in 6-minute walk test results after single-lung transplantation (SLT), bilateral lung transplantation (BLT), and lung volume reduction surgery (VR).

as 5% to 15% for the first 30 days and somewhat higher by the end of the first year. For the survivors, the presence of allograft lungs creates the need for lifelong immunosuppression that carries with it higher medical costs to the individual and society as well as increased risk of neoplasm and infection compared with nonimmunosuppressed patients. Finally, the risk for development of chronic allograft dysfunction, or bronchiolitis obliterans syndrome, increases with function of time since transplantation, reaching 50% to 60% by 5 years. The cumulative 5-year survival of our lung transplant experience is 50%, a fact that clearly demonstrates the imperfect solution that transplantation offers to emphysema patients.

A controversial aspect of lung transplantation is the question of whether it conveys a survival benefit to the recipient. There have been no prospective randomized trials in which lung transplantation has been directly compared with medical therapy for treatment of advanced lung disease. As a result, the analysis of this question has been limited to the use of Cox regression analysis, with the transplantation procedure entered into the model as a time-dependent covariable. In essence, the patient's time spent on the waiting list is used as the medical arm of the trial, and the survival after transplantation is used as the surgical arm. One such analysis by Hosenpud and colleagues[18] showed the surprising finding that lung transplantation did not reduce the risk of death compared with the risk faced by remaining on the waiting list. This finding is graphically depicted in Figure 13-3. One explanation for this finding is the stable survival of emphysema patients on the waiting list and the unique situation in the United States that allows listing of patients for transplantation long before they are considered truly ready for such an operation. Other Cox regression models looking at this exact question have shown clear survival benefit for emphysema patients undergoing lung transplantation.[19] More work in this field has been done, but it has been applied to lung transplantation in general and not to emphysema transplant recipients specifically.[20-22]

The choice of bilateral or unilateral transplantation for emphysema patients is controversial. In general, for younger patients, particularly those with α_1-antitrypsin deficiency, we prefer bilateral sequential single-lung transplantation. The bilateral option is also more attractive in larger recipients who might never obtain a sufficiently large single-lung allograft. On the other hand, for smaller recipients, single-lung transplantation offers a suitable option, particularly when an oversized donor lung can be grafted. The earliest reports on the efficacy of lung transplantation for pulmonary emphysema compared the merits and risks of bilateral lung transplantation versus single-lung transplantation for these patients. The authors of these reports demonstrated a higher perioperative risk of the bilateral operation without a demonstrable functional benefit to the bilateral recipients.[23,24] As a result, the single-lung transplantation quickly became the preferred operation for obstructive lung disease.

Our group recently reported a retrospective analysis of outcomes after lung transplantation in patients with chronic obstructive pulmonary disease (COPD).[25] This report included 306 patients, 86 of whom received a single-lung transplant and 220 of whom received a bilateral transplant. In contrast to earlier reports from our institution, the morbidity and mortality were comparable for the two groups, with an overall hospital mortality of 6.2%. There were no differences in hospital stay, intensive care unit stay, or duration of mechanical ventilation. There was, however, a difference in long-term survival; the 5-year survival (Fig. 13-4) of the bilateral transplant recipients was 66.7%, whereas the survival of the single-lung recipients was 44.9%. The International Society for Heart and Lung Transplantation has reported a similar finding, but neither analysis is adjusted for other factors that might bias such a result.[16] There is a likelihood that patients

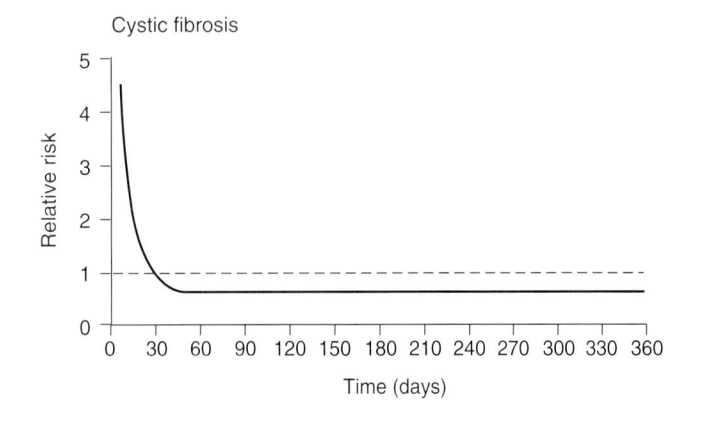

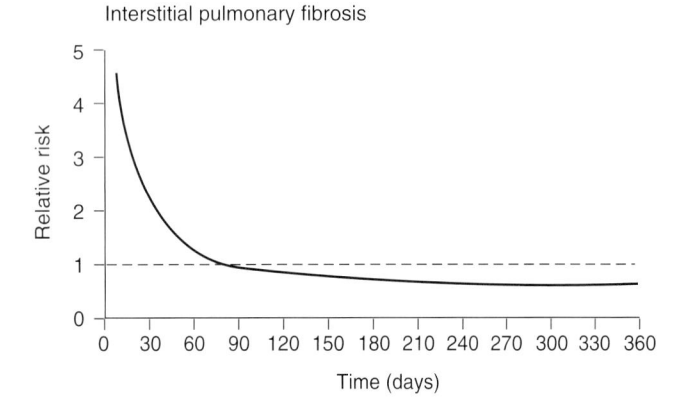

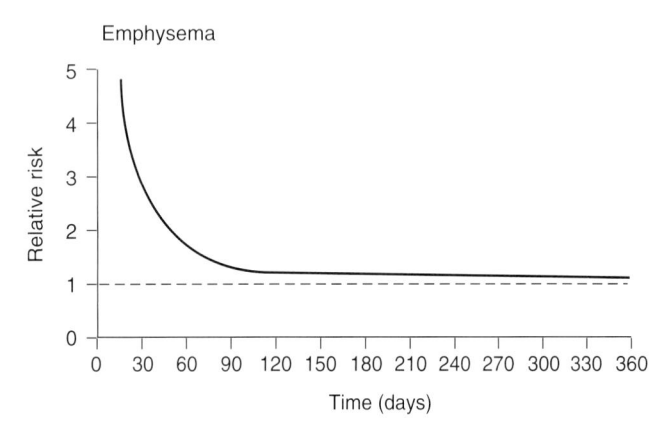

Figure 13–3
Relative risk of death after lung transplantation compared with risk faced by remaining on the waiting list, stratified by underlying diagnosis leading to transplantation.

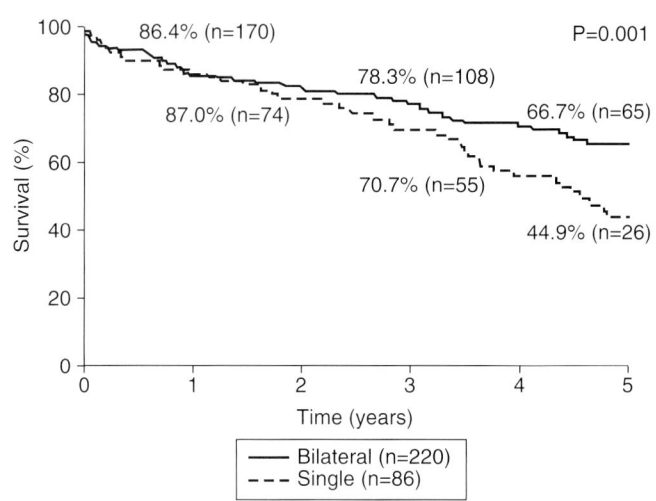

Figure 13–4
Survival curves for bilateral and single-lung transplant recipients at Washington University from 1988 to 2002.

receiving single-lung transplants for emphysema might have a disproportionate share of risk factors, such as advanced recipient age and other comorbidities. Figure 13–4 shows the survival data for all lung transplantations performed by our group. As demonstrated, patients with COPD and α_1-antitrypsin deficiency emphysema make up more than one half of our total recipients. It can also be seen that emphysema patients enjoy a better survival than do all other groups of patients, although the differences are not statistically significant. As a group, these COPD patients experience the best early outcomes after transplantation in most programs; the International Society for Heart and Lung Transplantation database cites a statistically significant 1.65 odds ratio of death in the first year after transplantation for patients with non-COPD diagnoses compared with those with COPD.[16]

Techniques

Our current approach to a bilateral sequential transplantation involves bilateral anterior thoracotomies in the fourth or fifth interspace. The patient is positioned supine with all extremities padded and the arms tucked in at the patient's side. Typically, the fourth intercostal space is entered, and the internal mammary artery is ligated and divided bilaterally. The fourth rib is shingled anteriorly by resecting 1 cm of the costal cartilage at the sternal border. More mobility is obtained by dividing the intercostal muscle from within the pleural space back as far as the posterior axillary line. Should additional access to the thorax become necessary during the conduct of the operation, the sternum is easily divided transversely at the fourth interspace, and the entire chest is clamshelled open. The least functional lung, as determined by preoperative quantitative ventilation and perfusion scans, is resected and replaced first. When numerous adhesions of the visceral and parietal pleura are encountered because of previous pleural sepsis or thoracotomy, care is taken to avoid injury to the lung parenchyma during the first of the two sequential pneumonectomies. Preliminary dissection of both lungs shortens the time that the first implanted lung is exposed to the entire cardiac output and thus lessens the likelihood of reperfusion edema.

The pulmonary arteries and pulmonary veins are dissected beyond their primary bifurcations to preserve the length of the main trunks. The right pulmonary artery is usually transected between firings of a vascular stapling device 1 cm beyond the ligated first branch to the right upper lobe. The left pulmonary artery is kept longer and transected between staple lines beyond the second branch to the left upper lobe. The vein branches are usually not stapled; rather, they are double ligated and divided at their secondary branch points to save length for the future recipient atrial cuff. The arterial and venous dissection and division are accomplished before the bronchial division to avoid prolonged contamination of the operative field by the open distal airway. The bronchus

> **Box 13–1**
> **Indications and Contraindications for Lung Volume Reduction Surgery and Lung Transplantation**
>
> Indications common to both procedures
>   Emphysema with destruction and hyperinflation
>   Marked impairment (FEV_1 <35% predicted)
>   Marked restriction in activities of daily living
>   Failure of maximal medical treatment to correct symptoms
> Contraindications to both procedures
>   Abnormal body weight (<70% or >130% of ideal)
>   Coexisting major medical problems increasing surgical risk
>   Inability or unwillingness to participate in pulmonary rehabilitation
>   Unwillingness to accept the risk of morbidity and mortality of surgery
>   Tobacco use within the past 6 months
>   Recent or current diagnosis of malignant disease
>   Increasing age (>65 years for transplantation, >70 years for volume reduction)
>   Psychological instability, such as depression or anxiety disorder
> Discriminating conditions favoring lung volume reduction surgery
>   Marked thoracic distention
>   Heterogeneous disease with obvious apical target areas
> FEV_1 >20% predicted
>   Age between 60 and 70 years
> Discriminating conditions favoring lung transplantation
>   Diffuse disease without target areas
> FEV_1 <20% predicted
>   Hypercapnia with Pa_{CO_2} >55 mm Hg
>   Pulmonary hypertension
>   Age younger than 60 years
> α_1-Antitrypsin deficiency

is transected between cartilaginous rings, and the posterior bundle of lymphatics and bronchial arteries is exposed to facilitate ligation and subsequent division. The pulmonary artery stump is mobilized centrally, then grasped with a clamp and retracted anteriorly to afford better access to the posterior bronchus. The pulmonary vein stumps are then grasped and retracted anteriorly and laterally to permit circumferential opening of the pericardium. With the pericardium freed, the vein stumps are then retracted and temporarily fixed anteriorly. This provides an excellent view of the bronchus, which is then mobilized well into the mediastinum and divided. Meticulous hemostasis in the mediastinum is achieved at this point, with the knowledge that reaching this portion of the operative field after implantation of the graft lung will be extremely difficult.

Meanwhile, the donor lung is prepared on the back table. The donor bronchus is divided two rings proximal to the upper lobe orifice. Care is taken to minimize dissection of the donor bronchus to preserve collateral flow through the peribronchial nodal tissue. The pulmonary artery and left atrial cuffs are freed from any pericardial attachments that may cause kinking after the anastomosis is completed.

Once the native lung is removed, the atelectatic graft lung is placed into the chest and kept cold with iced saline and slush. We conduct the anastomoses from posterior to anterior in the following sequence: bronchus, artery, and atrium. The first stitch is a running 4-0 PDS that unites the peribronchial tissue and lymphatics of the graft to peribronchial tissue surrounding the recipient bronchus. The back wall of this suture is performed just before the bronchial anastomosis, and the front wall is performed immediately after the bronchus is closed. The next stitches are also 4-0 PDS, and they are placed at the two corners of the bronchial anastomosis at the medial and lateral junction of the membranous and cartilaginous airway. These sutures are tied, and one end is used to join the donor and recipient membranous airways in a continuous suture. The cartilaginous rings of the donor and recipient are joined with interrupted figure-of-eight 4-0 PDS sutures. This process can usually be accomplished with only five such sutures. The anastomosis is finished with the completion of the anterior one half of the peribronchial tissue layer.

The second anastomosis is the pulmonary artery. The pulmonary artery, by now, has already been extensively and circumferentially dissected into the mediastinum. The pulmonary artery is then clamped centrally with a Satinsky clamp, with care taken to avoid including the Swan-Ganz catheter in the jaws of the clamp. The clamp is sewn to the wound edge to immobilize it and to render it less likely to spring open prematurely. The vascular staple line is resected at a location that matches the size of the donor and recipient artery. A larger recipient artery can be divided beyond the first ligated branch to match a smaller donor artery; a smaller recipient artery is divided proximal to the first branch, or through it, to maximize circumference. The donor pulmonary artery is trimmed to an appropriate length, and the anastomosis is created with running 5-0 Prolene suture. This anastomosis must be made with precise, small suture bites to avoid any anastomotic stricture.

The atrial anastomosis is performed last. A Satinsky clamp is placed centrally on the atrium. Placement of this clamp too centrally can reduce venous drainage from the contralateral lung and decrease cardiac output, whereas placement of the clamp too peripherally will compromise the recipient atrial cuff. Once the clamp is placed, an umbilical tape is used to tie the clamp closed to minimize the likelihood of dislodgement during subsequent lateral retraction of the clamp. The ties are then cut off the recipient vein stumps, and the bridge of atrium between vein stumps is divided to create the atrial cuff. The anastomosis is performed with 4-0 Prolene suture, and the last few sutures are left intentionally loose to allow flushing and de-airing of the graft and the recipient atrium. For this maneuver, the lung is partially inflated, and the pulmonary artery clamp is loosened momentarily. The lung is flushed with the atrial clamp still in place to force out the residual pulmonary perfusate solution. The pulmonary artery clamp is then reapplied, and the atrial clamp is opened momentarily to completely de-air the atrium. The atrial sutures are then secured and the clamps removed. All suture lines are then checked for hemostasis as ventilation and perfusion are restored. An identical procedure is then conducted on the opposite side.

VOLUME REDUCTION

The concept of LVRS was first explored by Brantigan many decades ago, but it failed to be widely adopted as a result of a high mortality rate in his reported case series.[5] The idea is conceptually an extension of the bullectomy operation, in which destroyed and functionless lung is resected, and the result is better function of the remaining lung that is relatively spared from emphysematous destruction. In contrast to bullectomy, in which the bulla being resected is truly only an air-filled cavity, the lung tissue resected in LVRS is diseased but does not represent a macroscopic bulla. The advantages of lung volume reduction for suitable candidates are numerous, including the relief of dyspnea and improvement of functional capabilities without the cost and adverse side effects of organ transplantation. There is no built-in waiting time as with transplantation; as soon as candidates can reach the pulmonary rehabilitation exercise goals, they are ready for the procedure. The early and late mortality for lung volume reduction are lower than those seen for transplantation. Because LVRS liberates the patient and the physician from the concern about the distribution of a scarce commodity such as donor lungs, lung volume reduction can be offered with slightly less rigid adherence to selection criteria. For example, a 72-year-old patient who is otherwise an ideal volume reduction candidate would be considered for the procedure, whereas such a patient would be unlikely to be added to a transplant waiting list. Box 13-1 reviews the differences and similarities in the indications and contraindications for lung transplantation and LVRS.

The drawback of volume reduction is that it is dependent on stringent anatomic and pathologic characteristics in the patient's lungs. Early work has shown that the lack of specific target areas and, to a lesser extent, the absence of apical target areas in particular will decrease the likelihood of a good result. Figure 13-5 shows a perfusion scintigram that demonstrates the absence of apical perfusion often seen in ideal candidates for LVRS. Our results have shown a less dramatic and less durable improvement in FEV_1 when LVRS is applied to patients with lower lobe–predominant emphysema.[26]

Many groups have reported preliminary results for LVRS, and these results have consistently shown benefit to the recipient with acceptable mortality and varying morbidity.[17,27-31] The remarkable finding is that these fairly uniform results have been obtained despite the use of a wide array of surgical strategies, including bilateral and unilateral approaches, open and thoracoscopic operations, and buttressed or unbuttressed staplers. The consistent theme among reports of successful lung volume reduction programs has been meticulous selection of patients (Table 13-1), methodical preparation of patients with reduction of risk factors, and attentive postoperative care. Most groups have reported operating on patients with a mean age of 65 years and a preoperative FEV_1 of 600 to 800 mL. The typical postoperative hospitalization is described as 8 to 14 days; somewhat less than one half of the patients are detained because of persistent air leaks from the stapled lung resection. Mortality ranging from 0% to 7% has been described for the initial hospitalization. The expected benefits of the operation vary according to whether a unilateral or bilateral approach has been used, but gains of 20% to 35% in the FEV_1 have been reported for unilateral operations, and gains of 40% to 80% are seen with bilateral operations. Most authors also report substantial gains in exercise tolerance, freedom from oxygen use, freedom from steroid use, and subjective quality of life.

Ciccone and associates,[26] working with us, reported long-term results in 250 bilateral LVRS recipients. After a median follow-up of 4.4 years, the 5-year survival was estimated to be 68%. Of the 250 patients in that report, 18 had gone on to lung transplantation after a median interval of 4.3 years. Five years after surgery, the mean change in FEV_1 was a 7% increase, with 53% of patients demonstrating persistence in benefit over preoperative FEV_1 values. This finding takes on greater importance when one considers the relentless progression in functional impairment seen in the medical arms of the randomized trials described next.

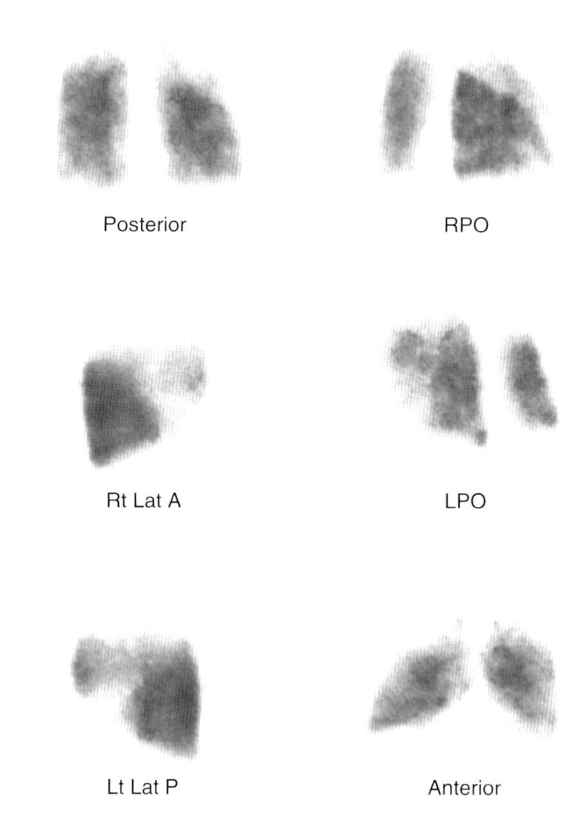

Figure 13–5
Pulmonary perfusion scintigraphy demonstrating typical upper lobe–predominant emphysema that is viewed as the most suitable morphology for lung volume reduction surgery.

After the initial wave of single-institution case series, there has been a handful of reports describing prospective, randomized trials comparing lung reduction surgery with best medical care.[32-37] The results of these trials have been controversial in that they have failed to duplicate the physiologic and functional gains reported in many case series. Furthermore, the mortality and morbidity in the prospective, randomized trials exceeded those seen in most retrospective case series. Part of the discordance between the case series reports and the controlled trials stems from the more liberal selection criteria of the randomized trials compared with individual case series. The inclusion of patients with severe, diffuse emphysema has altered the generalizability of the results by including patients previously thought by many to be contraindicated for the procedure.[33,35,36]

In 2003, the National Emphysema Treatment Trial reported the main results of a 5-year effort. This trial included 1218 patients randomized between LVRS and medical therapy between January 1998 and July 2002.[36] This multicenter trial reported a 90-day surgical mortality of 7.9%, which did

Table 13-1
Selection Criteria for Lung Volume Reduction Surgery

Inclusion Criteria	Exclusion Criteria
General	
Disability despite maximal rehabilitation	Inability to participate in rehabilitation
Cessation of tobacco use >6 months	Continued use of tobacco
Patient's expectation of goals reasonable	Significant comorbidity
	Previous pleurodesis or thoracotomy
	Underweight, overweight
Anatomic-radiographic evaluation	
Marked emphysema	Bronchiectasis
	Minimal radiographic emphysema
Heterogeneously distributed emphysema	Homogeneously distributed emphysema
Target zones of poorly perfused lung	No target zones
Areas with better preserved lung	No preserved lung tissue
Marked thoracic hyperinflation	Chest wall or thoracic cage abnormalities
Physiologic evaluation	
Marked airflow obstruction	Minimal to moderate airflow obstruction
Marked hyperinflation	Minimal to moderate thoracic hyperinflation
Alveolar gas exchange	Markedly disordered alveolar gas exchange
DL_{CO} <50% (steady state)	DL_{CO} <10%
	$Paco_2$ >60 mm Hg
Cardiovascular function	Cardiovascular function
Essentially normal ejection fraction	Mean pulmonary artery pressure >35 mm Hg
	Left ventricular ejection fraction <40%
	Significant coronary artery disease

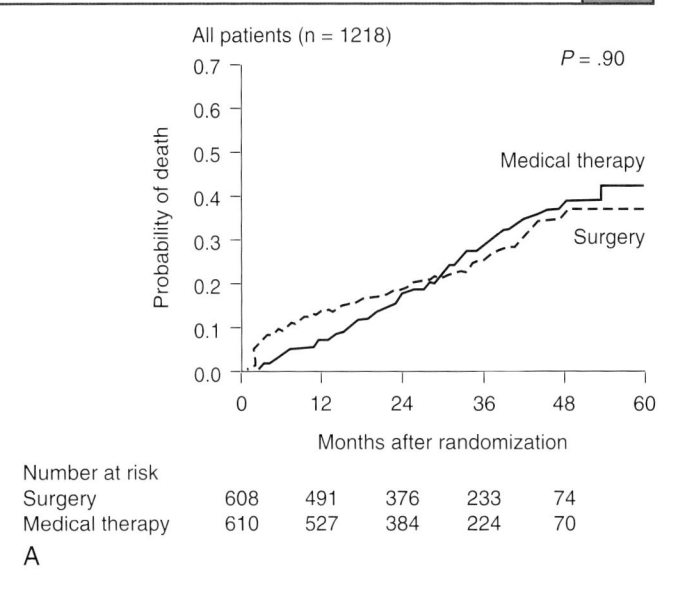

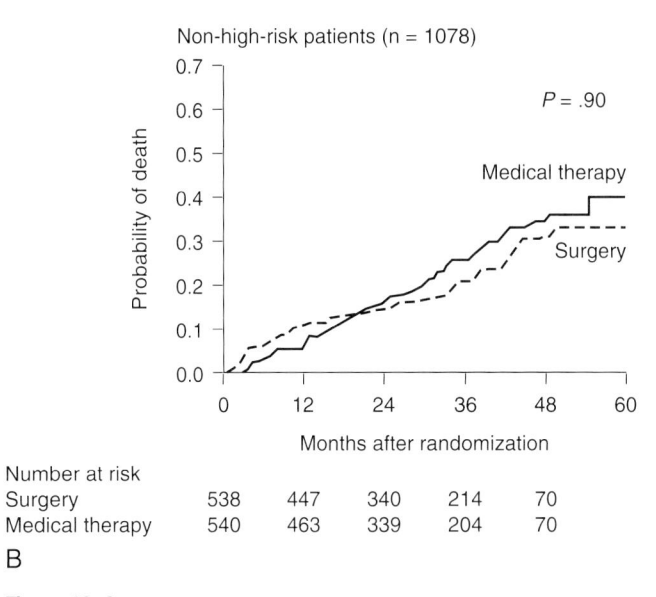

Figure 13-6
National Emphysema Treatment Trial survival curves.

not differ according to surgical approach (sternotomy versus video-assisted thoracoscopic surgery) or specific center. A survival benefit was seen in the surgical arm for patients with upper lobe–predominant emphysema with low baseline exercise capacity, whereas a survival benefit was seen in the medical arm for patients with non–upper lobe–predominant emphysema with high baseline exercise capacity (Fig. 13-6). A previous interim report by the study group identified a subset of patients at high risk for death after surgery, specifically either those with a very low FEV_1 and homogeneous emphysema or those with very low FEV_1 and very low diffusing capacity for carbon monoxide (DL_{CO}).[35] Our group has refrained from offering LVRS to patients with homogenous emphysema from the outset of our experience, but our results in the latter high-risk group are different from those suggested by the National Emphysema Treatment Trial report. Our patients with both FEV_1 and DL_{CO} of less than 20% predicted values experienced a perioperative mortality of 5% and durability of benefit that was not different from that experienced by the rest of the LVRS cohort.[38] The survival curves from that study are shown in Figure 13-7.

Techniques

We continue to favor the median sternotomy approach for bilateral lung volume reduction procedures because of the exposure and flexibility that it provides with a minimum of morbidity. With this exposure, there is no injury to chest wall muscles or to intercostal nerves from the operative approach or even from the chest tubes, which are brought out below the costal arch. Similar results have been obtained with a bilateral video-assisted thoracoscopic surgery approach.

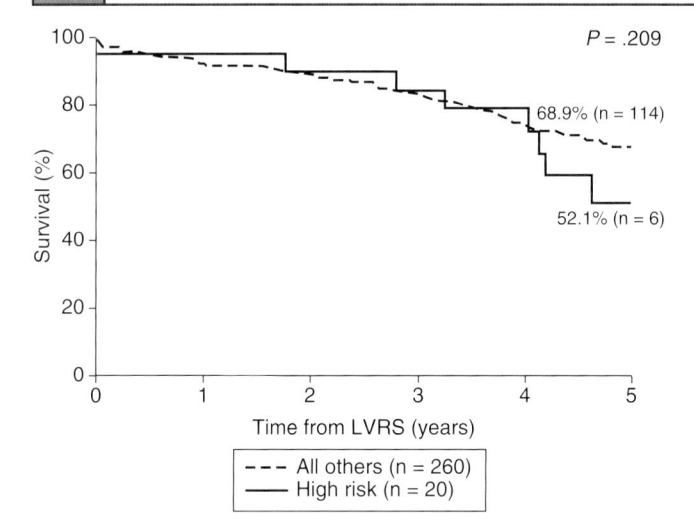

Figure 13–7
Kaplan-Meier survival graph after bilateral LVRS.

Many patients with severe emphysema have a significant element of chronic bronchitis with increased sputum production. After induction of anesthesia, a single-lumen tube is placed and flexible bronchoscopy is carried out to suction secretions and to obtain a specimen for culture and for stat Gram stain. If thick, tenacious secretions are encountered, a mini-tracheostomy may be inserted at the end of the operative procedure to facilitate postoperative pulmonary toilet. After bronchoscopy, the endotracheal tube is replaced with a left-sided double-lumen tube.

Before sternal division, ventilation to both lungs is briefly suspended. A rolled sponge held in a long curved sponge forceps is advanced upward behind the sternum from the subxiphoid position to sweep the pleura away from the retrosternal area on either side. This keeps the mediastinal pleura intact on either side as the sternum is divided. With ventilation suspended, the sternum is divided with a sternal saw. The right mediastinal pleura is incised sharply, with care taken to visualize and to avoid injury to the phrenic nerve near the apex of the chest. Ventilation is maintained to the right lung until just before entrance into the pleural space; this facilitates assessment of the degree of emphysematous damage in various portions of the lung. Demarcation of the fissures, or lack thereof, is also seen best when the lung is inflated. Ventilation to the right lung is then suspended while ventilation to the left lung is continued. Care is taken by the anesthesiologist to avoid overinflation of the left lung, and airway pressures are generally restricted to the range of 15 to 20 cm H_2O pressure. Hypercapnia may well occur, but this is usually well tolerated.

The majority of candidates for this procedure have upper lobe–predominant disease. Several minutes after ventilation is suspended to the right lung, the right middle and lower lobes are usually well deflated and become progressively atelectatic. At that stage, the pulmonary ligament is divided. Dense adhesions are not commonly present but may be a problem if there have been prior episodes of pneumonia. Adhesions are taken down under direct vision, occasionally by an extrapleural dissection if necessary, to avoid injury to the lung.

For upper lobe disease, 70% to 80% of the right upper lobe is excised with multiple applications of a linear stapler buttressed with strips of bovine pericardium. It is often easier to apply the stapler to the deflated lung, and this can rapidly be accomplished by use of the cautery to fenestrate the apex of the right upper lobe. The marked collateral ventilation leads to prompt collapse. A long, straight intestinal clamp can be applied to the lung to create a linear "crush" mark before application of the linear stapler. We initially tailored the upper lobe staple line in the form of an inverted U, but we now go straight across the upper lobe beginning medially just above the hilum and ending just above the upper extent of the oblique fissure. Care should be taken to avoid crossing the fissure as this may damage the lower lobe. Such a practice may also tether the apex of the superior segment to the remaining upper lobe and prevent the superior segment from filling the apex of the chest.

After the first two applications of the linear stapler, it is occasionally awkward to insert the stapler into the chest again for completion of the excision. In this case, an endoscopic stapler, fitted with pericardial strips, can be used to reach deeply into the chest to complete the excision. We prefer to use a single line of excision to remove most of the right upper lobe rather than multiple excisions, remembering that the goal is to reduce volume adequately, not to remove all of the severely diseased lung.

On occasion, the apex of the upper lobe will be densely adherent to the apex of the chest and to the superior mediastinum. In such cases, it may be easier first to transect the upper lobe as described earlier before attempting to dissect the apical and mediastinal adhesions. Once the transection has been accomplished, the specimen can be more easily detached from the chest wall and mediastinum by blunt or sharp dissection, cautery, or even a linear stapler, leaving a small remnant of the lung attached to the mediastinum if necessary to avoid injury to the phrenic nerve.

After upper lobe resection, the chest is filled with warm saline and the lung is gently inflated. Ordinarily, there are no air leaks present at this time. It is not uncommon to find that the reexpanded, remaining lung does not completely fill the apex of the chest. We have explored the use of a pleural tent in this situation but now reserve it for rare instances, in particular when the remaining lung is tethered in the chest by virtue of adhesions to the chest wall or diaphragm. It has not been our practice to do pleurodesis either by abrasion or by talc, even if the patient is not a potential candidate for subsequent lung transplantation.

Two chest tubes are placed in the pleural space and brought out near the midline through small subcostal stab wounds. The posterior tube is brought across the dome of the diaphragm and halfway up the posterior chest. The anterior tube is brought to the apex of the chest near the mediastinum.

Ventilation is shifted from the left lung to the right lung, and the mediastinal pleura is then opened on the left side. Particular care should be taken to visualize the phrenic nerve and to avoid injury to it when the upper portion of the mediastinal pleura is opened; the anatomic location of the left phrenic nerve makes it more vulnerable to injury than the right phrenic nerve. With upper lobe–predominant disease, the goal is to excise the superior subdivision of the left upper lobe, leaving the lingula intact, because this is usually much less diseased. The pulmonary ligament on the left side is divided if possible, but this requires displacement of the heart, and the ligament may be difficult to visualize. In such cases, the ligament is left undivided, although any adhesions between the left lower lobe and the diaphragm are taken down. Unlike the anatomic situation on the right side, the superior segment of the left lower lobe usually reaches easily to the apex of the chest even without division of the pulmonary ligament.

The upper one half to two thirds of the left upper lobe is excised with multiple applications of the linear GIA stapler. This may be facilitated by cautery puncture of the apex of the left upper lobe, allowing it to deflate. The long straight intestinal clamp is often useful in helping to identify and demarcate the proposed line of excision. The line of excision is usually parallel to the oblique fissure separating the upper and lower lobes. As on the right side, care is taken to avoid stapling across the fissure into the superior segment of the left upper lobe.

After left upper lobe excision, the lung is reinflated and inspected for air leaks. Two chest tubes are placed as on the right, one to the base and one to the apex. The mediastinal pleura is closed on either side. Several centimeters are left open inferiorly to allow drainage of any mediastinal fluid collection into the pleural spaces. No mediastinal chest tube is placed.

Because many volume reduction patients are receiving prednisone before the operation, and this might interfere with healing of the sternotomy, we use overlapping figure-of-eight stainless steel wire closure of the sternum for added security. After completion of the operation, the double-lumen tube is removed in the operating room. If a mini-tracheostomy is thought to be necessary on the basis of the initial bronchoscopy, this is placed immediately after removal of the double-lumen tube, generally by a 4-mm-diameter mini-tracheostomy.

COMBINATIONS OF LUNG TRANSPLANTATION AND LUNG VOLUME REDUCTION

There are several permutations in which lung transplantation and lung volume reduction can be combined to optimize treatment of patients with emphysema. These combinations have been reported in anecdotal clusters of patients. The combined approaches can be summarized as follows: volume reduction as a bridge to transplantation, simultaneous single-lung transplantation and unilateral volume reduction to prevent native lung hyperexpansion, early post-transplantation unilateral volume reduction to treat acute native lung hyperexpansion, and late unilateral volume reduction to treat chronic native lung hyperexpansion. Todd and colleagues[39] reported the Toronto experience with simultaneous unilateral volume reduction to prospectively improve overall lung function after single-lung transplantation. They experienced no postoperative problems, and the pulmonary function at 3 months was better than expected on the basis of historic controls receiving a single lung for emphysema.

Yonan and colleagues[40] retrospectively analyzed 27 patients who received 31 single-lung transplants for emphysema. They identified 12 patients who experienced early or late native lung hyperexpansion, and they performed two early lung volume reduction operations to address this problem. Their analysis included an assessment of risk factors, and they concluded that lower pretransplantation FEV_1, higher residual volume, and pulmonary hypertension were all associated with a higher risk for native lung hyperexpansion. They did not perform nor did they advocate volume reduction surgery simultaneously with single-lung transplantation for emphysema.

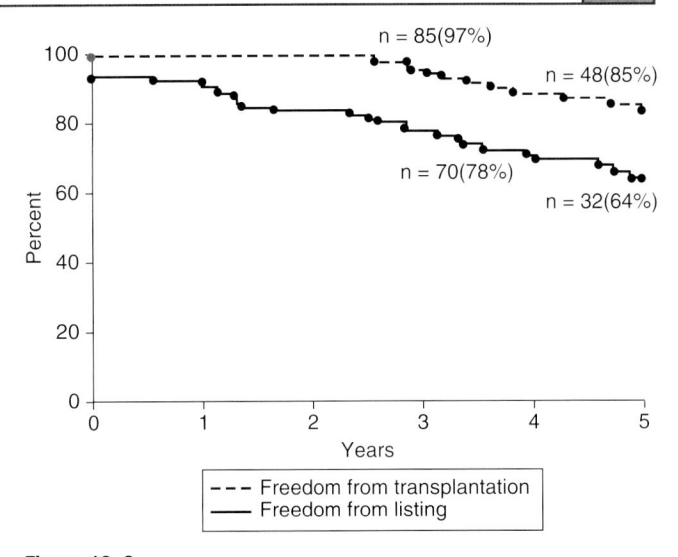

Figure 13–8
Freedom from listing and freedom from transplantation in 99 patients thought to be eligible for either LVRS or transplantation at the time of bilateral LVRS operation.

Volume reduction as a bridge to transplantation is the form of combined procedure that has been most frequently attempted. The concept was introduced to the medical literature by Zenati and colleagues[41] in 1995, when they described two patients who received single-lung transplants 17 months and 4 months after laser ablation of emphysematous bullae. One group has prospectively performed reduction in patients thought to be also eligible for transplantation.[42] This center found 31 patients eligible for both procedures; at the same time, they identified 20 patients who were suitable for LVRS alone and 139 who were thought to be transplantation candidates only. Twenty-four patients had successful LVRS; seven (including one death) were considered LVRS failures. Follow-up was too short at the time of the report to know how frequently late transplantations would be performed. The authors' results with LVRS in patients eligible for transplantation were recently reported.[43] We identified 99 of 200 patients who underwent bilateral LVRS and who were thought to have been eligible for transplantation. With a median follow-up of 5.1 years, 32 of the 99 had been listed for transplantation and 15 had undergone transplantation. The Kaplan-Meier curve depicting freedom from listing and freedom from transplantation is shown in Figure 13-8. The only preoperative or operative factor that was predictive for the subsequent need for transplantation was a lower lobe rather than an upper lobe LVRS procedure. Many of our patients have had LVRS as a functional bridge to transplantation. This has occurred in most cases not as part of an a priori plan to bridge them, as it was a stepwise treatment for crippling dyspnea that was not improved sufficiently either by degree or by duration of effect after lung volume reduction. The concept is attractive on the surface: patients have volume reduction initially and continue to accrue waiting time toward lung transplantation. One potential benefit for the patient successfully completing volume reduction surgery is the possibility that transplantation might be avoided altogether by an excellent response to volume reduction. A second possibility is that transplantation is delayed by several years and the patient is transplanted with a later cohort with the possibility of improved techniques, better immunosuppression, and overall better survival. Finally, because the hazard rate of death after lung transplantation is higher than the hazard rate of death after LVRS, anything that can safely delay entry onto the steeper survival curve seems worth pursuing.

The logic of the potential benefits of LVRS as a bridge to transplantation weakens in the face of some aspects of reality. First, the anatomic and physiologic criteria that require heterogeneous destruction for volume reduction are much more restrictive than the criteria for transplantation, so it is unlikely that a large fraction of emphysema candidates for transplantation could be safely and successfully treated with volume reduction. Also, the dilemma remains as to how to treat a patient near the upper age limit for transplantation. It is quite possible that a patient who is acceptable for both procedures at the age of 62 years might receive volume reduction as a bridge not to transplantation but to ineligibility for future lung transplantation several years later. Our results have confirmed this suspicion: of the 15 patients who have undergone transplantation after bilateral LVRS, only one was older than 60 years at the time of LVRS evaluation. The next oldest was 58 years, and the mean age for the group of LVRS-transplant recipients was 54 years.[43]

The use of LVRS for late native lung hyperexpansion after single-lung transplantation can be described as rare and anecdotal. Kroshus and colleagues[44] described three patients who were treated with unilateral LVRS for native lung hyperinflation and post-transplantation dyspnea that was not attributable to infection or rejection. The patients represented a small fraction of the 66 single-lung transplantations performed at that center for emphysema. The volume reduction operations were performed 12, 17, and 42 months after the initial lung transplantation, and all patients experienced a substantial relief in dyspnea with an improvement in exercise tolerance and an improvement in the appearance of the chest radiograph. A similar report by Le Pimpec-Barthes and associates[45] described successful treatment of symptomatic native lung hyperexpansion by volume reduction of the native side in the form of a right upper lobectomy.

BRONCHOSCOPIC TREATMENT OF EMPHYSEMA

Experience with LVRS has confirmed that reduction of hyperinflation in patients with end-stage emphysema can provide very significant benefit to the patient. On the basis of this principle, several endoscopic approaches to reduce hyperinflation in patients with severe emphysema are being investigated.

Endoscopic Placement of One-Way Valves

One approach has been to develop one-way valves to be placed endoscopically in segmental bronchi leading to markedly destroyed and hyperinflated portions of the lung. It was anticipated that such valves would allow deflation and exit of secretions from the lung, reduce hyperinflation, and even potentially lead to atelectasis and marked volume reduction, thus providing benefits similar to LVRS. A pivotal, randomized clinical trial has recently been completed in the United States, and the initial report indicates that the overall benefits from the procedure, in terms of improved FEV_1, are small. However, a subgroup of patients did show a reduction in hyperinflation and significant functional improvement.

Airway Bypass

Many patients with crippling, end-stage emphysema are not suitable candidates for LVRS because of a homogeneous pattern of destruction. In these patients, there are no "target areas" that could be excised for LVRS or targeted for volume reduction by means of endobronchial valves. Nonetheless, these patients are subject to the same crippling effects of hyperinflation as are other end-stage emphysema patients. With the goal of reducing hyperinflation in these patients, we are developing a procedure, referred to as airway bypass, by which direct communication is provided between segmental bronchi and adjacent lung parenchyma by means of stents placed through the bronchial wall, with one end in the airway and the other in the lung parenchyma. Because of the extensive collateral ventilation in such patients, several such airway bypass stents are capable of deflating an entire lung. This has, in fact, been demonstrated experimentally with use of freshly excised lungs from emphysema patients undergoing lung transplantation.[46] Phase I clinical trials have confirmed the safety and the efficacy of this approach in a small series of patients.[47,48] A pivotal randomized clinical trial of this procedure is now under way in the United States.

SUMMARY

Although bullectomy, LVRS, and lung transplantation are similar in that each represents a surgical procedure aimed at pulmonary emphysema, they are unique in their ideal selection criteria and in their expected outcomes. We favor a meticulous selection process in which all options are considered and the best option is selected for a given patient. Patients referred with a functionless, space-occupying bulla that compresses relatively normal adjacent lung will be offered thoracoscopic or open bullectomy. Patients with ideal circumstances for LVRS—hyperinflation, heterogeneous distribution of disease, FEV_1 greater than 20%, and normal P_{CO_2}—are offered LVRS. Finally, patients with diffuse disease, lower FEV_1, hypercapnia, and associated pulmonary hypertension are directed toward transplantation. LVRS has not been a satisfactory option for patients with α_1-antitrypsin deficiency, and we prefer transplantation in these cases. With strict adherence to these criteria, we find that very few emphysema patients are serious candidates for any surgical procedures. Combinations of lung volume reduction and lung transplantation, either simultaneously or sequentially, are possible but rarely necessary.

Lung transplantation has provided one surgical option for patients with end-stage emphysema and can dramatically improve the quality of life. However, the shortage of organ donors and the need for lifelong immunosuppression make this option suitable for only a small fraction of patients. For patients with upper lobe–predominant emphysematous destruction and marked hyperinflation, LVRS produces significant palliation with a 5-year survival that actually exceeds the 5-year survival after lung transplantation. The success of LVRS has led to the development of multiple endoscopic techniques that may reduce hyperinflation and improve quality of life. This includes the use of one-way endobronchial valves that, in similarity to LVRS, are designed for patients with heterogeneous emphysema and appropriate target zones of hyperinflated lung. In contrast, airway bypass is directed at patients with marked hyperinflation and a homogeneous pattern of severe emphysema. For both endoscopic approaches to LVRS, further experience is required before any firm conclusions can be drawn as to their role and value in the treatment of patients with emphysema.

REFERENCES

1. Cooper JD. The history of surgical procedures for emphysema. *Ann Thorac Surg* 1997;**63**:312-9.
2. Hardy JD, Webb WR, Dalton Jr ML, Walker Jr GR. Lung homotransplantation in man. *JAMA* 1963;**186**(12):1065-74.
3. Reitz BA, Wallwork JL, Hunt SA, et al. Heart-lung transplantation: successful therapy for patients with pulmonary vascular disease. *N Engl J Med* 1982;**306**:557-64.
4. Toronto Lung Transplantation Group. Unilateral lung transplantation for pulmonary fibrosis. *N Engl J Med* 1986;**314**:1140-5.
5. Brantigan OC, Mueller E, Kress MB. A surgical approach to pulmonary emphysema. *Am Rev Respir Dis* 1959;**80**:194-202.
6. Cooper JD, Trulock EP, Triantafillou AN, Patterson GA, Pohl MS, Deloney PA, et al. Bilateral pneumectomy (volume reduction) for chronic obstructive pulmonary disease. *J Thorac Cardiovasc Surg* 1995;**109**(1):106-16.
7. Shrager JB, Kim DK, Hashmi YJ, Lankford EB, Wahl P, Stedman HH, et al. Lung volume reduction surgery restores the normal diaphragmatic length-tension relationship in emphysematous rats. *J Thorac Cardiovasc Surg* 2001;**121**:217-24.
8. Reardon J, Awad E, Normandin E, Vale F, Clark B, ZuWallack RL. The effect of comprehensive outpatient pulmonary rehabilitation on dyspnea. *Chest* 1994;**105**:1046-52.
9. Ries AL, Ellis B, Hawkins RW. Upper extremity exercise training in chronic obstructive pulmonary disease. *Chest* 1988;**93**:688-92.
10. Snider GL. Reduction pneumoplasty for giant bullous emphysema—implications for surgical treatment of non-bullous emphysema. *Chest* 1996;**1996**(109):540-8.
11. FitzGerald MX, Keelan PJ, Gaensler EA. Surgery for bullous emphysema. *Respiration* 1973;**30**:187.
12. Schipper PH, Meyers BF, Battafarano RJ, Guthrie TJ, Patterson GA, Cooper JD. Outcomes following resection of giant emphysematous bullae. *Ann Thorac Surg* 2004;**78**(3):976-82.
13. Mal H, Andreassian B, Pamela F, Duchatelle JP, Rondeau E, Dubois F, et al. Unilateral lung transplantation in end stage pulmonary emphysema. *Am Rev Respir Dis* 1989;**140**:797-802.
14. Pasque MK, Cooper JD, Kaiser LR, Haydock DA, Triantafillou A, Trulock EP. An improved technique for bilateral lung transplantation: rationale and initial clinical experience. *Ann Thorac Surg* 1990;**49**:785-91.
15. Patterson GA, Cooper JD, Goldman B, Weisel RD, Pearson FG, Waters PF, et al. Technique of successful clinical double-lung transplantation. *Ann Thorac Surg* 1988;**45**(6):626-33.
16. Trulock EP, Edwards LB, Taylor DO, Boucek MM, Mohacsi PJ, Keck BM, et al. The Registry of the International Society for Heart and Lung Transplantation: Twentieth Official Adult Lung and Heart-Lung Transplant Report—2003. *J Heart Lung Transplant* 2003;**22**(6):625-35.
17. Gaissert HA, Trulock EP, Cooper JD, Sundaresan RS, Patterson GA. Comparison of early functional results after volume reduction or lung transplantation for chronic obstructive pulmonary disease. *J Thorac Cardiovasc Surg* 1996;**111**:296-307.
18. Hosenpud JD, Bennett LE, Keck BM, Edwards EB, Novick RJ. Effect of diagnosis on survival benefit of lung transplantation for end-stage lung disease. *Lancet* 1998;**351**(9095):24-7.
19. DeMeester J, Smits JM, Persijn GG, Haverich A. Listing for lung transplantation: life expectancy and transplant effect, stratified by type of end-stage lung disease, the Eurotransplant experience. *J Heart Lung Transplant* 2001;**20**(5):518-24.
20. Anyanwu AC, McGuire A, Rogers CA, Murday AJ. An economic evaluation of lung transplantation. *J Thorac Cardiovasc Surg* 2002;**123**(3):411-8:discussion 418-420.
21. Geertsma A, TenVergert EM, et al. Does lung transplantation prolong life? A comparison of survival with and without transplantation. *J Heart Lung Transplant* 1998;**17**:511-6.
22. Ramsey SD, Patrick DL, Albert RK, Larson EB, Wood DE, Raghu G. The cost-effectiveness of lung transplantation: a pilot study. *Chest* 1995;**108**(6):1594-601.
23. Mal H, Sleiman C, Jebrak G, Messian O, Dubois F, Darne C, et al. Functional results of single-lung transplantation for chronic obstructive lung disease. *Am J Respir Crit Care Med* 1994;**149**:1476-81.
24. Patterson GA, Maurer JR, Williams TJ, Cardoso PG, Scavuzzo M, Todd TR. Comparison of outcomes of double and single lung transplantation for obstructive lung disease. *J Thorac Cardiovasc Surg* 1991;**101**:623-32.
25. Cassivi SD, Meyers BF, Battafarano RJ, Guthrie TJ, Trulock EP, Lynch JP, et al. Thirteen-year experience in lung transplantation for emphysema. *Ann Thorac Surg* 2002;**74**(5):1663-9.
26. Ciccone AM, Meyers BF, Guthrie TJ, Davis GE, Yusen RD, Lefrak SS, et al. Long-term outcome of bilateral lung volume reduction in 250 consecutive patients with emphysema. *J Thorac Cardiovasc Surg* 2003;**125**(3):513-25.
27. Argenziano M, Moazami N, Thomashow B, Jellen PA, Gorenstein LA, Rose EA, et al. Extended indications for volume reduction pneumoplasty in advanced emphysema. *Ann Thorac Surg* 1996;**62**:1588-97.
28. Bingisser R, Zollinger A, Hauser M, Bloch KE, Russi EW, Weder W. Bilateral volume reduction surgery for diffuse pulmonary emphysema by video-assisted thoracoscopy. *J Thorac Cardiovasc Surg* 1996;**112**:875-82.
29. Cooper JD, Patterson GA, Sundaresan RS, Trulock EP, Yusen RD, Pohl MS, et al. Results of 150 consecutive bilateral lung volume reduction procedures in patients with severe emphysema. *J Thorac Cardiovasc Surg* 1996;**112**:1319-30.
30. McKenna RJ, Brenner M, Fischel RJ, Gelb AF. Should lung volume reduction for emphysema be unilateral or bilateral?. *J Thorac Cardiovasc Surg* 1996;**112**:1331-9.
31. Naunheim KS, Keller CA, Krucylak PE, Singh A, Ruppel G, Osterloh JF. Unilateral video-assisted thoracic surgical lung reduction. *Ann Thorac Surg* 1996;**61**:1092-8.
32. Criner GJ, Cordova FC, Furukawa S, Kuzma AM, Travaline JM, Leyenson V, et al. Prospective randomized trial comparing bilateral lung volume reduction surgery to pulmonary rehabilitation in severe chronic obstructive pulmonary disease. *Am J Respir Crit Care Med* 1999;**160**(6):2018-27.
33. Geddes D, Davies M, Koyama H, Hansell D, Pastorino U, Pepper J, et al. Effect of lung-volume-reduction surgery in patients with severe emphysema. *N Engl J Med* 2000;**343**:239-45.
34. NETT Research Group. Rationale and design of the National Emphysema Treatment Trial (NETT): a prospective randomized trial of lung volume reduction surgery. *J Thorac Cardiovasc Surg* 1999;**118**:518-28.
35. NETT Research Group. Patients at high risk of death after lung-volume-reduction surgery. *N Engl J Med* 2001;**345**:1075-83.
36. NETT Research Group. A randomized trial comparing lung-volume-reduction surgery with medical therapy for severe emphysema. *N Engl J Med* 2003;**348**(21):2059-73.
37. Pompeo E, Marino M, Nofroni I, Matteucci G, Mineo TC. Reduction pneumoplasty versus respiratory rehabilitation in severe emphysema: a randomized study. *Ann Thorac Surg* 2000;**70**:948-53.
38. Meyers BF, Yusen RD, Guthrie TJ, Patterson GA, Lefrak SS, Davis GE, et al. Results of lung volume reduction surgery in patients meeting a NETT high risk criterion. *J Thorac Cardiovasc Surg* 2004;**127**(3):829-35.
39. Todd TR, Perron J, Winton TL, Keshavjee SH. Simultaneous single-lung transplantation and lung volume reduction. *Ann Thorac Surg* 1997;**63**:1468-70.
40. Yonan NA, el-Gamel A, Egan J, Kakadellis J, Rahman A, Deiraniya AK. Single lung transplantation for emphysema: predictors for native-lung hyperinflation. *J Heart Lung Transplant* 1998;**17**(2):192-201.
41. Zenati M, Keenan RJ, Landreneau RJ, Paradis IL, Ferson PF, Griffith BP. Lung reduction as a bridge to lung transplantation in pulmonary emphysema. *Ann Thorac Surg* 1995;**59**:1581-3.
42. Bavaria JE, Pochettino A, Kotloff RM, Rosengard BR, Wahl PM, Roberts JR, et al. Effect of volume reduction on lung transplant timing and selection for chronic obstructive pulmonary disease. *J Thorac Cardiovasc Surg* 1998;**115**(1):9-18.
43. Meyers BF, Yusen RD, Guthrie TJ, Davis G, Pohl MS, Lefrak SS, et al. Outcome of bilateral lung volume reduction in patients with emphysema potentially eligible for lung transplantation. *J Thorac Cardiovasc Surg* 2001;**122**(1):10-7.
44. Kroshus TJ, Bolman 3rd RM, Kshettry VR. Unilateral volume reduction after single-lung transplantation for emphysema. *Ann Thorac Surg* 1996;**62**:363-8.
45. Le Pimpec-Barthes F, Debrosse D, Cuenod CA, Gandjbakhch I, Riquet M. Late contralateral lobectomy after single-lung transplantation for emphysema. *Ann Thorac Surg* 1996;**61**:231-4.
46. Lausberg HF, Chino K, Patterson GA, Meyers BF, Toeniskotter PD, Cooper JD. Bronchial fenestration improves expiratory flow in emphysematous human lungs. *Ann Thorac Surg* 2003;**75**:393-8.
47. Redina ES, De Giacomo T, Venuta F, Coloni GF, Meyers BF, Patterson GA, et al. Feasibility and safety of the airway bypass procedure for patients with emphysema. *J Thorac Cardiovasc Surg* 2003;**125**:1294-9.
48. Cardosa P, Snell G, Hopkins P, Sybrecht GW, Stamatis G, Ng A, et al. Clinical application of airway bypass with paclitaxel-eluting stents: early results. *J Thorac Cardiovasc Surg* 2007;**134**:974-81.

CHAPTER 14
Lung Transplantation
Varun Puri, Felix G. Fernandez, and G. A. Patterson

Historical Aspects
Selection
  Recipients
  Disease-Specific Guidelines
  Donors
Donor Surgery
  Procurement
    Brain-Dead Donor
    Non-Heart-Beating Donor
  Atrial Cuff and Pulmonary Vein Injuries
  Pulmonary Arteries
  Congenital Bronchial Anomalies
Recipient Surgery
  Anesthesia and Intraoperative Conduct
  Implantation
    Incisions
    Pneumonectomy
    Lung Implantation
    Cardiopulmonary Bypass
Technical Strategies to Overcome Donor Shortage
  Size-Mismatched Lungs
  Living Lobar and Split-Lung Transplantation
  Non-Heart-Beating Donors
  Ex Vivo Reconditioning of Unacceptable Lungs
Postoperative Management
  Ventilation
  Fluid Management
  General Care
Immunosuppression
Infection Prophylaxis
Complications
  Technical Problems
  Primary Graft Dysfunction
  Infectious Complications
    Bacterial
    Viral
    Fungal
  Acute Rejection
  Airway Complications
  Failure of Normal Bronchial Healing
  Anastomotic Stenosis
  Chronic Rejection—Bronchiolitis Obliterans Syndrome
  Post-Transplant Lymphoproliferative Disorder
  Gastrointestinal Complications
Results
Pediatric Lung Transplantation
Summary

The first successful human lung transplantation was performed in 1983, by the Toronto Lung Transplant Group.[1] More than 25 years have passed since this landmark procedure and more than 15,000 lung transplants have been performed. Lung transplantation is now the preferred treatment option for a variety of end-stage pulmonary diseases. Remarkable progress has occurred through refinements in technique and improved understanding of transplant immunology and microbiology. Despite these improvements, donor shortages and chronic lung allograft rejection continue to prevent pulmonary transplantation from reaching its full potential. Attempts made to address these issues include using marginal donors and living-lobar donors, split-lung donor techniques, and non-heart-beating donors.

Chronic rejection of the lung allograft is the major factor limiting long-term survival. Extensive research efforts are underway to find methods to overcome chronic rejection and prolong survival in clinical lung transplantation.

HISTORICAL ASPECTS

In 1947, Vladimir Demikhov performed the first lung transplantation in a dog.[2,3] The animal survived 7 days, dying from complications of bronchial dehiscence. Dr. James D. Hardy and colleagues performed the first human lung transplantation in 1963.[4] Although their patient succumbed after 18 days, their brief success demonstrated the technical feasibility of the operation and stimulated worldwide interest in pulmonary transplantation. Over the next 20 years, approximately 40 lung transplants were attempted, but none achieved long-term success.[5] The only recipient actually discharged from the hospital was a 23-year-old patient of Derom and colleagues,[6] who left the hospital 8 months after transplantation and died a short time later as a result of chronic rejection, sepsis, and bronchial stenosis. Most patients in this era died within 2 weeks of lung transplantation as a result of primary graft failure, sepsis, or rejection. The most frequent cause of death beyond the second week was bronchial anastomotic disruption.

The Toronto Lung Transplant Group's initial attempt at lung transplantation, in 1978, ended with the patient dying after a bronchial dehiscence.[7] Through experimental studies, this group discovered that high-dose perioperative steroid usage contributed significantly to poor bronchial anastomotic healing,[8] and that wrapping an omental pedicle around the bronchus resulted in restoration of blood supply and protection from dehiscence.[9] Recipient selection was also addressed, as most of the early attempts had been in acutely ill, often ventilator-dependent patients. The Toronto group reasoned that end-stage respiratory failure from pulmonary fibrosis would provide the ideal physiologic conditions for single-lung transplantation. The increased resistance to both perfusion and ventilation of the native lung would preferentially direct perfusion and ventilation to the transplanted lung. On November 7, 1983, the first successful isolated lung transplant was performed in a 58-year-old man with pulmonary fibrosis.[1] The use of the omental flap and withholding steroids perioperatively are now mainly of historical interest. In the final analysis, it appears to be the attention to detail that this group practiced that led to long-term success.

Patterson and colleagues used the en bloc double-lung transplant technique to extend the use of lung transplantation to patients with septic lung diseases and emphysema.[10] The en bloc double-lung transplant, however, had several drawbacks: it was technically difficult, it required cardiopulmonary bypass (CPB), tracheal anastomotic ischemic complications were frequent, cardiac denervation occurred, and bleeding into the posterior mediastinum was troublesome because of poor operative exposure. To circumvent these problems, Pasque and colleagues[11] devised the technique of bilateral sequential pulmonary transplantation. A transverse

> **Box 14–1**
> **Recipient Selection Criteria**
>
> - Clinically and physiologically severe disease
> - Medical therapy ineffective or unavailable
> - Substantial limitations in activities of daily living
> - Limited life expectancy
> - Adequate cardiac function without significant coronary disease
> - Ambulatory, with rehabilitation potential
> - Acceptable nutritional status
> - Satisfactory psychosocial profile and emotional support system

> **Box 14–2**
> **Factors That Predict Risk of Death for Patients on the Transplant Waiting List**
>
> - Forced vital capacity
> - Pulmonary artery systolic pressure
> - Oxygen required at rest
> - Age
> - Body mass index
> - Diabetes
> - Functional status
> - Six-minute walk distance
> - Continuous mechanical ventilation
> - Diagnosis
>
> *From Organ Procurement and Transplant Network, available at http://optn.transplant.hrsa.gov/PoliciesandBylaws2/policies/pdfs/policy_9.pdf*

thoracosternotomy provided excellent exposure of the mediastinum and both pleural spaces. Recently, this incision was modified to avoid sternal division, when possible, to eliminate sternal wound complications.

Patients with emphysema were initially felt to be poor candidates for single-lung transplantation, because the overly compliant native lung would be prone to hyperinflation, resulting in mediastinal shift and compression of the transplanted lung. Despite this concern, successful single-lung transplantation for emphysema was reported in 1989 by Mal and colleagues.[12] Pasque and colleagues[13] reported success with single-lung transplantation for patients with pulmonary hypertension. The first applications of living related lobar transplants were reported by Starnes and colleagues.[14]

Split-lung techniques have been developed to allow a large left donor lung to be bipartitioned and the individual lobes transplanted bilaterally.[15] Furthermore, the use of lungs from non-heart-beating donors has moved from the research realm to clinical reality.[16]

SELECTION

Recipients

General selection criteria are listed in Box 14-1 and are summarized by Maurer and colleagues.[17]

Patients with failure of another organ system and patients over the age of 65 are generally not eligible for transplantation. Advanced recipient age is a specific predictor of increased post-transplant mortality.[18] Additionally, a history of malignant disease within the prior 5 years generally precludes pulmonary transplantation. A potential exception is a patient with bilateral bronchoalveolar carcinoma. Etienne and colleagues[19] have reported a single long-term survivor with this therapy, and Zorn and associates[20] have reported a favorable experience in a small number of patients. The patient with a recent extrathoracic malignancy judged to be cured might be considered. Patients with serious psychological dysfunction should not be considered candidates for pulmonary transplantation. Few groups evaluate patients who continue to smoke.

Previous thoracic surgery is not a specific contraindication to pulmonary transplantation, although it may complicate a subsequent transplant procedure. Patients receiving high-dose corticosteroid therapy (≥20 mg prednisone) are not eligible for lung transplantation, as a well-documented negative influence on bronchial healing and susceptibility to postoperative infection has been demonstrated. However, low- or moderate-dose steroid therapy does not result in an increased incidence of bronchial anastomotic complications. Ventilator dependency is not a specific contraindication to transplantation, but it has been identified as a risk factor for increased mortality.[18]

All patients considered for transplantation, except those with primary pulmonary hypertension (PPH) or Eisenmenger's syndrome, participate in a monitored exercise rehabilitation program while awaiting transplantation. Virtually all patients experience an improvement in strength and exercise tolerance without any measurable change in pulmonary function. This improved endurance better enables patients to withstand the rigors of a transplant procedure and subsequent convalescence.

Lung allocation in the United States was previously based on time on the waitlist, regardless of medical urgency or deterioration in medical condition. This system was flawed as it favored recipients well enough to survive on the transplant list, whereas those who might benefit most risked death while waiting. An ideal system of organ allocation balances clinical necessity with ability to recover from a transplant operation. Recently, the United Network for Organ Sharing (UNOS) Thoracic Organ Committee revised the listing algorithm by assigning each patient a lung allocation score (LAS) based on the immediate need for transplant and the probability of post-transplant survival. This led the UNOS, in 2005, to rearrange its waitlist for adult lung transplantation to one based on the LAS score. Details of the new allocation system are found on the official Organ Procurement and Transplantation Network website.[21]

The LAS score is calculated by estimating waitlist urgency, defined as the expected number of days that could be lived without a transplant (Box 14-2), and post-transplantation survival, defined as the expected number of days lived during the first year after transplantation (Box 14-3). The transplant benefit measure is then derived by subtracting the waitlist urgency from the post-transplantation survival to obtain the raw allocation score (calculated in days). This score is normalized to the LAS on a scale of 1 to 100. The highest scores are listed first for transplantation. Factors used to predict risk of death and post-transplantation survival are regularly reviewed by the Thoracic Organ Transplantation Committee and updated as appropriate.

> **Box 14–3**
> **Factors That Predict Survival after Lung Transplantation**
>
> - Forced vital capacity
> - Pulmonary capillary wedge pressure ≥ 20 mm Hg
> - Continuous mechanical ventilation
> - Age
> - Serum creatinine
> - Functional status
> - Diagnosis

From Organ Procurement and Transplant Network, available at http://optn.transplant.hrsa.gov/PoliciesandBylaws2/policies/pdfs/policy_9.pdf

Disease-Specific Guidelines

Obstructive lung disease, notably emphysema and α_1-antitrypsin deficiency, has previously been the most common indication for lung transplantation, accounting for 46% of the adult lung transplantations reported in the 2007 Registry of UNOS and the International Society for Heart and Lung Transplantation (ISHLT).[18]

Before being considered for pulmonary transplantation, patients with obstructive lung disease should have maximization of medical therapy including bronchodilators and oxygen. Consideration should be given to lung volume reduction surgery (LVRS) in ideal patients (with hyperinflation, heterogeneous distribution of disease, forced expiratory volume in 1 second (FEV_1) of more than 20%, and normal PCO_2).[22] We have not found LVRS to be an ideal option in patients with α_1-antitrypsin deficiency, as in general these patients have diffuse disease.[22] Preliminary LVRS does not jeopardize subsequent successful lung transplantation.[23]

We favor a meticulous selection process in which both transplantation and volume reduction are considered, and the best option is selected for each patient. In general, in patients with obstructive lung disease, the FEV_1 should be less than 25% of predicted value, and not reversible, although most patients actually have an FEV_1 of less than 15% of predicted at the time of transplantation. Progressive deterioration as evidenced by hypercarbia ($PaCO_2 \geq 55$ mm Hg), increasing oxygen requirement (resting $PaO_2 < 55$ mm Hg), the development of secondary pulmonary hypertension, rapid decline of FEV_1, or frequent life-threatening infections indicate decreased survival, suggesting the need for transplantation.[17]

Septic lung disease is another common indication for pulmonary transplantation. Cystic fibrosis (CF) is a common inherited disorder resulting in diffuse bronchiectatic destruction of both lungs. Without transplantation, the overwhelming majority of patients die as a result of progressive respiratory failure in the second or third decade of life. As reported in the 2007 ISHLT Registry, CF is now the most common indication for bilateral lung transplantation and the third most common indication for lung transplant in general.[18] The most reliable predictors of life expectancy in CF patients were described by Kerem and associates.[24] An FEV_1 of less than 30% predicted, elevated $PaCO_2$, requirement for supplemental oxygen, frequent admissions to the hospital for control of acute pulmonary infection, and failure to maintain weight are reliable predictors of early mortality in these patients. At this stage of disease, patients with CF usually have a rapidly progressive downhill course. To offset this high waitlist mortality, some of these listed factors have been incorporated into the LAS.

Patients with septic lung disease or those with significant sputum production are evaluated with frequent sputum cultures to assess bacterial sensitivities. Inhaled high-dose aminoglycosides or colistin are frequently used in this population. Patients with multidrug-resistant organisms, especially pan-resistant *Burkholderia cepacia*, are considered at high risk, and many centers consider this a contraindication to transplantation. Early mortality in patients with CF who have *B. cepacia* infection is significantly increased.[25,26] Successful transplantation in these patients often requires the use of multiple combinations of intravenous antibiotics, after in vitro synergy testing to guide antibiotic selection. If no susceptible antibiotic regimen is found on synergy testing, we do not proceed with transplantation.

The diagnoses of pulmonary fibrosis and restrictive lung disease include idiopathic pulmonary fibrosis (IPF), pulmonary fibrosis of other etiologies, sarcoidosis with elevated pulmonary artery pressures, and obliterative bronchiolitis (not retransplant cases). The 2007 ISHLT Registry report indicated that IPF was the second most common indication for single-lung transplantation and the third most common for bilateral lung transplantation.[18] In our experience, candidates for transplantation had classic restrictive findings on spirometry, with a mean forced vital capacity of 1.35 L and an FEV_1 of 1.14 L.[27] All used supplemental oxygen and demonstrated marked impairments in exercise tolerance. Moderate pulmonary hypertension is common in these patients. Patients with pulmonary fibrosis who require a transplant have been observed to have a rapid downhill course. The lung allocation score has been devised to recognize the medical urgency of these patients.

Previously, patients with pulmonary hypertension were considered for lung transplantation early in the course of their disease because of the poor outcome of this disease process. With the use of prostacyclins and other vasodilator therapies, such as endothelin receptor antagonists and phosphodiesterase inhibitors, an improvement in pulmonary artery pressures and relief of symptoms are seen in the majority of patients with primary pulmonary hypertension.[28,29] Transplantation may be delayed as long as these patients remain clinically stable on vasodilatory therapy. For patients with pulmonary hypertension secondary to congenital heart defects or thromboembolic diseases, surgical intervention for the primary diagnosis should be considered. The current indication for transplantation is progressive deterioration despite optimal therapy (e.g., New York Heart Association [NYHA] class III or IV, mean pulmonary artery pressure >50, right atrial pressure >10 mm Hg, cardiac index <2.5 L/min/m², syncopal episodes).[17] We prefer bilateral lung transplantation in this group; if the patient is to undergo single-lung transplantation, we do not use a marginal donor lung, as the bulk of the cardiac output will be through the transplanted lung. Patients with Eisenmenger's syndrome and secondary pulmonary hypertension have not shown an improvement in survival after lung transplantation.[30,31]

Donors

Rapid progress in the field of transplantation has resulted in a shortage of suitable allografts for all organs. This problem is particularly significant for lung transplantation, as only

> **Box 14–4**
> **Ideal Lung Donor Selection Criteria**
>
> - Age < 55 years
> - No history of pulmonary disease
> - Normal serial chest radiograph
> - Adequate gas exchange—PaO_2 > 300 mm Hg; FiO_2, 1.0; positive end-expiratory pressure, 5 cm H_2O
> - Normal bronchoscopic examination
> - Negative serologic screening for hepatitis B and human immunodeficiency virus (HIV)
> - Recipient matching for ABO blood group
> - Size matching

20% of otherwise suitable organ donors have lungs satisfactory for transplantation, according to the criteria listed in Box 14-4. A majority of conditions resulting in brain death (e.g., trauma, spontaneous intracerebral hemorrhage) also lead to significant pulmonary parenchymal pathologic change because of lung contusion, infection, aspiration, or neurogenic pulmonary edema.

Satisfactory gas exchange is essential for donor lungs. This is confirmed by noting a PaO_2 of greater than 300 mm Hg with an inspired oxygen fraction (FiO_2) of 100% and peak end-expiratory pressure (PEEP) of 5 cm H_2O. A PaO_2-to-FiO_2 ratio of 300 or greater provides adequate evidence of satisfactory gas exchange. A donor chest radiograph taken shortly before procurement must reveal clear lung fields. Bronchoscopic assessment at the donor institution often reveals mucopurulent secretions that might contain a variety of microorganisms. This finding is commonly observed and is not a specific contraindication to pulmonary transplantation if the donor is otherwise suitable. Bronchoscopic evidence of aspiration or frank pus in the airway, however, is a definite contraindication to transplantation of that lung.

The donor's medical history is obtained, with particular emphasis on and attention paid to the donor's age, cause of death, timing of death, smoking history, and prior thoracic procedures. Older donor age (greater than 60) is considered a significant risk factor for adverse outcome after pulmonary transplantation, and in general donors younger than 55 are preferred.[32] Although a significant smoking history (≥30 pack-years) in the donor is a concern, it is not an absolute contraindication to the use of otherwise suitable donor lungs. ABO incompatibility between donor and recipient, human immunodeficiency virus positivity, active malignancy (outside the central nervous system), and active hepatitis infection remain absolute contraindications to donor lung procurement. Histocompatibility matching for human leukocyte antigens (HLAs) is not usually performed between donor and recipient before transplantation unless the patient has an elevated panel reactive antibody or known HLA antibodies from prior sensitization.

Size matching between donor and recipient is a significant consideration. An acceptable size match depends on the nature of the recipient's lung disease and the type of transplant anticipated. The most reliable method of size matching predicts donor and recipient lung volumes using standard nomograms based on age, sex, and height, and is used by all pulmonary function laboratories to obtain predicted lung volumes. In patients undergoing single-lung transplantation for obstructive lung disease, we attempt to place allografts with 15% to 20% greater volume than the recipient predicted lung volume. Implantation of a large allograft is easily achieved in a patient with obstructive lung disease because of the enormous size of the recipient pleural space. In patients with pulmonary fibrosis or pulmonary vascular disease, however, the pleural spaces are reduced or normal in size, respectively. It is therefore inadvisable to use excessively oversized lungs in these patients. In patients undergoing bilateral lung replacement, we prefer to match the donor lung volume to the lung volume or anticipated lung dimensions that the recipient would possess in the absence of lung disease. Oversizing a bilateral recipient may produce hemodynamic difficulties on closure of the chest at the termination of the procedure. Donor lungs that are substantially larger than the recipient's chest cavity but are otherwise usable should not preclude transplantation.

Certain circumstances allow relaxation of the typically strict donor selection criteria. A minor degree of pulmonary infiltrate may be accepted in donor lungs being used for a bilateral transplantation. We analyzed 133 consecutive donor lungs and identified 37 with marginal quality, as judged by arterial blood gas analysis and radiographic assessment. The marginal donors provided postoperative function equivalent to those judged excellent.[33]

Novel techniques to optimize donor usage have been introduced. The first is a split-lung technique that bipartitions the left lung of a large cadaveric donor and uses the two lobes to perform a bilateral lobar transplant in the smaller recipient. It requires significant expertise in lung transplantation, but it has been performed successfully with good outcomes at certain institutions.[15,34]

Another technique is the use of non-heart-beating donors.[16] The ability of pulmonary parenchymal cells to continue aerobic cellular metabolism by relying on the oxygen in the alveoli make the lung potentially the ideal organ for transplantation after cessation of circulation—so-called donation after cardiac death. A series from Spain reported excellent early allograft function with no ischemia-reperfusion injury even after 11 hours of total ischemia, and outpatient follow-up to 13 months after transplantation documented adequate lung function and quality of life.[35] More recent follow-up of this experience demonstrates a 3-year survival of 58% in 17 recipients of lungs from non-heart-beating donors.[36] Steen and colleagues from Sweden have advocated extracorporeal perfusion and ex vivo assessment of donor lung function in non-heart-beating donors and have described their initial clinical experience with ex vivo reconditioning of initially unacceptable lungs.[37]

DONOR SURGERY

Procurement

Brain-Dead Donor

Once a candidate is determined to be a suitable donor for lung transplantation on the basis of history, chest radiograph, and arterial blood gas analysis, a flexible bronchoscopy is performed to ensure that there are no copious purulent secretions or signs of aspiration and to thoroughly suction the tracheobronchial tree. A small amount of purulent secretions that clears away with the initial suction does not constitute a contraindication to procurement. Anatomic variations that may complicate implantation are noted. Clear and effective communication between the heart and lung procurement teams should be established. The sites of left and right heart venting, division of the left atrial cuff, and cannulation and division of the main pulmonary artery (PA) should be discussed and agreed on. Also, with multiple procurement teams working simultaneously, we find it useful to establish a small Mayo stand at the head of the table, with selected instruments and sutures that we require.

Via a standard median sternotomy, the pericardium and both pleural spaces are widely opened. A compliance check is performed on the lungs by disconnecting the ventilator at end inspiration. This should result in a prompt deflation of the lungs. The lungs are manually palpated to rule out unsuspected pathology. The pericardium is retracted with heavy silk sutures that are not tied, to allow access to both pleural spaces. At this point, we communicate with the implantation team about the quality of lungs and any concerns before proceeding.

The superior vena cava (SVC) is encircled caudal to the azygous vein with heavy silk suture. Encircling the inferior vena cava (IVC) is optional. The plane between the anterior surface of the right PA and the back of the SVC and the ascending aorta is developed. The aortopulmonary window is dissected, and the aorta is encircled with an umbilical tape; this is useful in the eventual placement of the aortic cross-clamp when the pericardial sac is full of blood. The SVC and the aorta are gently retracted, and the posterior pericardium is incised above the right PA, allowing access to the trachea. The plane around the trachea is developed using finger dissection. Alternatively, the posterior mediastinal dissection, including dissection of the trachea, can be entirely performed after explanting the heart. After completion of the thoracic dissection and ensuring that abdominal organ procurement teams are ready, the donor is systemically heparinized (250 to 300 units/kg). The ascending aorta is cannulated with a routine cardioplegia cannula for cardiac preservation. A U-stitch is placed just proximal to the bifurcation of the main PA, and a Sarns (Sarns, Ann Arbor, MI) 6.5-mm curved metal cannula is placed into the main PA with the cannula tip pointing toward the PA bifurcation (Fig. 14-1).[38]

Using a fine needle, a 500-μg bolus dose of prostaglandin-E_1 is injected directly into the PA. Hypotension should be expected with this maneuver. Next, the SVC is ligated after ensuring that there is no central venous catheter in the lumen and the IVC is divided, thus venting the right heart. The aorta is cross-clamped and cardioplegia initiated. The left atrial appendage is generously incised, venting the left side of the heart (see Fig. 14-1). The pulmonary preservation solution consisting of several liters (50 to 75 mL/kg) of cold (4° C) Perfadex is initiated via the PA cannula. Ice slush is generously used to topically cool the heart and both pleural spaces. Gentle ventilation is continued to prevent atelectasis and homogeneously distribute the perfusate. Clear perfusate exiting the left atriotomy confirms adequate lung flushing. After completion of the cardioplegia and the antegrade pulmonary flush, the cannulae are removed. The IVC is now freed posteriorly and dissected up to the level of the right atrium, ensuring that

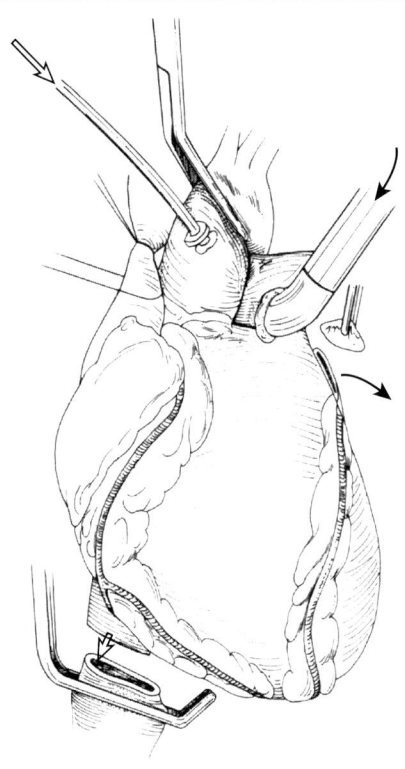

Figure 14-1
Cross-clamping during the procurement operation. The cardioplegia cannula is in place in the ascending aorta, and a perfusion cannula is in the main pulmonary artery. Venting is via the inferior vena cava and the left atrial appendage. *(From Sundaresan S, Trachiotis GD, Aoe M, Patterson GA, Cooper JD. Ann Thorac Surg 1993;**56**:1409-13)*

the right inferior pulmonary vein is not damaged during this maneuver. Division of the left atrium ensues with the cooperation of the heart and lung teams. The heart is retracted toward the right, and an incision is made with a #11-blade scalpel in the left atrium midway between the coronary sinus and the left inferior pulmonary vein. Scissors are then used to extend the opening superiorly and inferiorly while visualizing the orifices of the left superior and inferior pulmonary veins from inside the atrium. The remaining cuff of the left atrium is transected while visualizing the orifice of the right pulmonary veins from within the atrium. An appropriate residual atrial cuff should have a rim of left atrial muscle around each of the pulmonary vein orifices (Fig. 14-2).

The SVC is now transected between ties. This is followed by division of the aorta proximal to the crossclamp and the PA at the site of cannulation. The heart is then passed off the field. Next, we use a Foley catheter to deliver about 250 mL of retrograde pulmonary flush via each of the pulmonary vein orifices, which often delivers residual blood and small clots out of the open PA bifurcation. This retrograde flush may also be performed on the back table at the donor site. Retrograde pulmonary perfusion has been shown to lead to better oxygenation, higher compliance, and a lower extravascular lung water index in transplanted lungs in the experimental setting.[39]

We then proceed with en bloc removal of the mediastinal contents. This technique avoids injury to the membranous trachea, pulmonary arteries, and pulmonary veins, and it

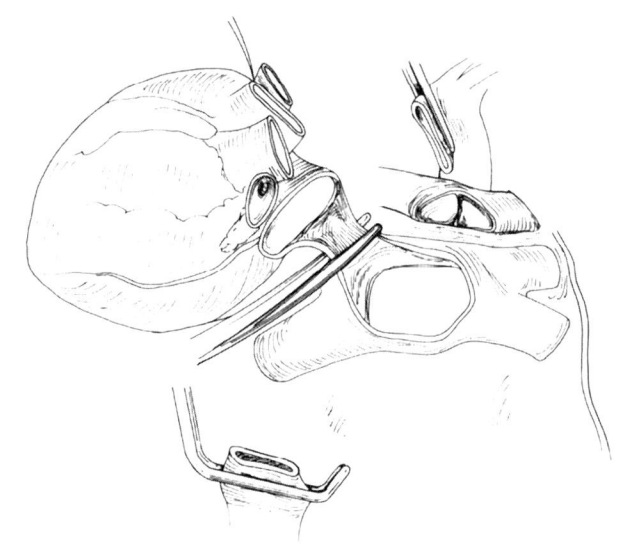

Figure 14–2
The heart is being explanted, leaving a rim of atrium around each pulmonary vein orifice. *(From Sundaresan S, Trachiotis GD, Aoe M, Patterson GA, Cooper JD.* Ann Thorac Surg *1993;**56**:1409-13.)*

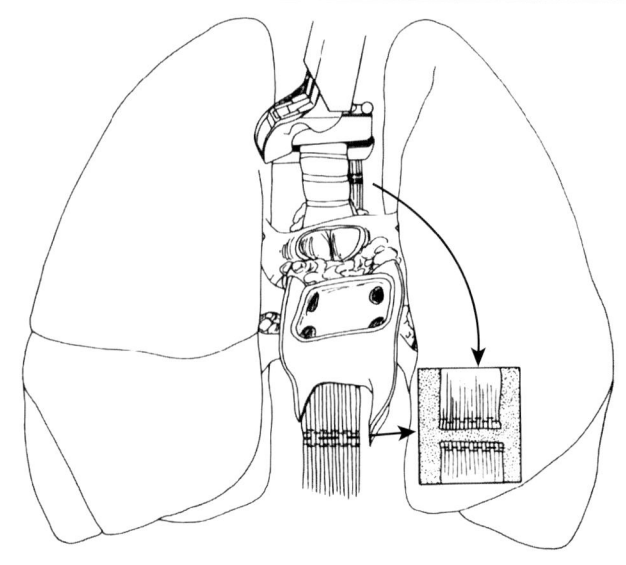

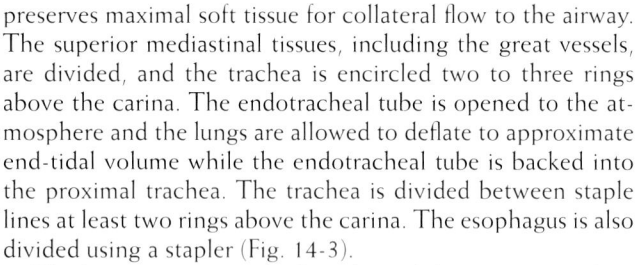

Figure 14–3
Division of the trachea and esophagus prior to double-lung en bloc extraction and after removal of the heart. *Inset,* division of distal donor esophagus. *(From Sundaresan S, Trachiotis GD, Aoe M, Patterson GA, Cooper JD.* Ann Thorac Surg *1993;**56**:1409-13.)*

preserves maximal soft tissue for collateral flow to the airway. The superior mediastinal tissues, including the great vessels, are divided, and the trachea is encircled two to three rings above the carina. The endotracheal tube is opened to the atmosphere and the lungs are allowed to deflate to approximate end-tidal volume while the endotracheal tube is backed into the proximal trachea. The trachea is divided between staple lines at least two rings above the carina. The esophagus is also divided using a stapler (Fig. 14-3).

The lungs are retracted inferiorly, and the superior mediastinal tissue is divided down to the spine. Staying directly on the spine, the posterior mediastinal tissue is divided in a superior-to-inferior direction until the level of the mid-thoracic spine. Now the dissection shifts inferiorly. The pericardium just superior to the diaphragm is divided, and the inferior pulmonary ligaments are divided, avoiding injury to the inferior pulmonary veins and the lung parenchyma. The supradiaphragmatic esophagus is divided with the linear stapler, followed by division of the posterior mediastinal tissue including the aorta. Now the dissection is connected with the superior dissection and the lungs are removed en bloc along with the thoracic esophagus and aorta.

If the lungs are to be used at separate institutions, they are separated on the back table. Otherwise, they are placed in three layers of plastic bags, with cold preservation solution, and transported on ice. Separation of the two lungs is carried out in an ice slush bath. The donor esophagus and aorta are removed and the pericardium is excised. The lungs are separated by division of the posterior pericardium, of the left atrium between the pulmonary veins, of the main PA at the bifurcation, and of the left bronchus close to the carina, in this order. The left bronchus is divided between staples to maintain the inflation of each lung. When the recipient site is reached, if the lungs have been transported en bloc, they are separated as detailed earlier. The right and left pulmonary arteries are dissected back to their first branches. The donor bronchus is divided one ring proximal to the upper lobe orifice while minimizing proximal peribronchial dissection to preserve collateral flow.

Non-Heart-Beating Donor

The mid-term results of the largest single clinical series of non-heart-beating donor lung transplantation have been published,[36] and the technique of donor organ procurement is summarized here. After systemic heparinization, the donor is placed on arteriovenous extracorporeal membrane oxygenation (ECMO) via a femoral approach. A Fogarty catheter is placed in the supradiaphragmatic aorta for better abdominal organ perfusion, and bilateral chest tubes are placed for topical lung cooling with cold Perfadex. De Antonio and colleagues showed that the lung could tolerate a warm ischemia time of 120 minutes and cold preservation time (cooling to harvest) of up to 240 minutes. After obtaining consent, bronchoscopy is performed and the chest is opened. Ventilation is now resumed with 100% FiO_2 and 5 cm of positive end-expiratory pressure (PEEP). The pleural spaces are drained and the pericardium is opened. The aorta is clamped and both venae cavae are ligated. Antegrade lung perfusion is performed with 5 to 6 L of Perfadex, followed by infusion of 300 mL of donor blood through the PA. A blood gas analysis is performed on the left atrial effluent. Retrograde perfusion and the lung procurement are now performed in routine fashion.[36]

Atrial Cuff and Pulmonary Vein Injuries

Injuries most frequently involve the right inferior pulmonary vein and occur during the division of the left atrial cuff or division of the IVC. Pulmonary venous injuries can also occur as a result of excessive dissection of the inferior pulmonary ligament or unnecessary dissection of the atrial cuff within the pericardium. Unidentified, these injuries can lead to troublesome bleeding at reperfusion.

If donor left atrial cuff is inadequate or the superior and inferior veins are completely separated, a reconstructive salvage technique using donor pericardium has been described[40] (Fig. 14-4). It is estimated that up to 2.7% of patients may need atrial cuff reconstruction, and Oto and colleagues have elegantly illustrated their techniques (Fig. 14-5).[41]

Pulmonary Arteries

The right PA is more commonly injured because its course is behind the aorta and the SVC. Because the right PA is substantially longer than the left, injury to this vessel under the aorta often does not require repair, and the artery is simply

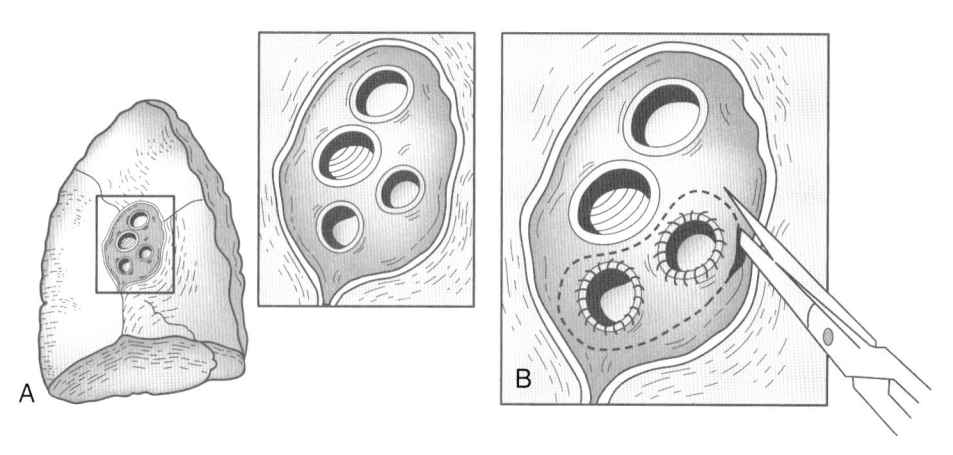

Figure 14–4
Creation of new atrial cuff after suboptimal harvest. **A,** There is complete separation of the superior and inferior pulmonary veins. **B,** Attaching the intima of each vein to the pericardium, then incising pericardium to reconstruct an atrial cuff. *(From Casula RP, Stoica SC, Wallwork J, et al. Ann Thorac Surg 2001;**71**:1373-4, © The Society of Thoracic Surgeons.)*

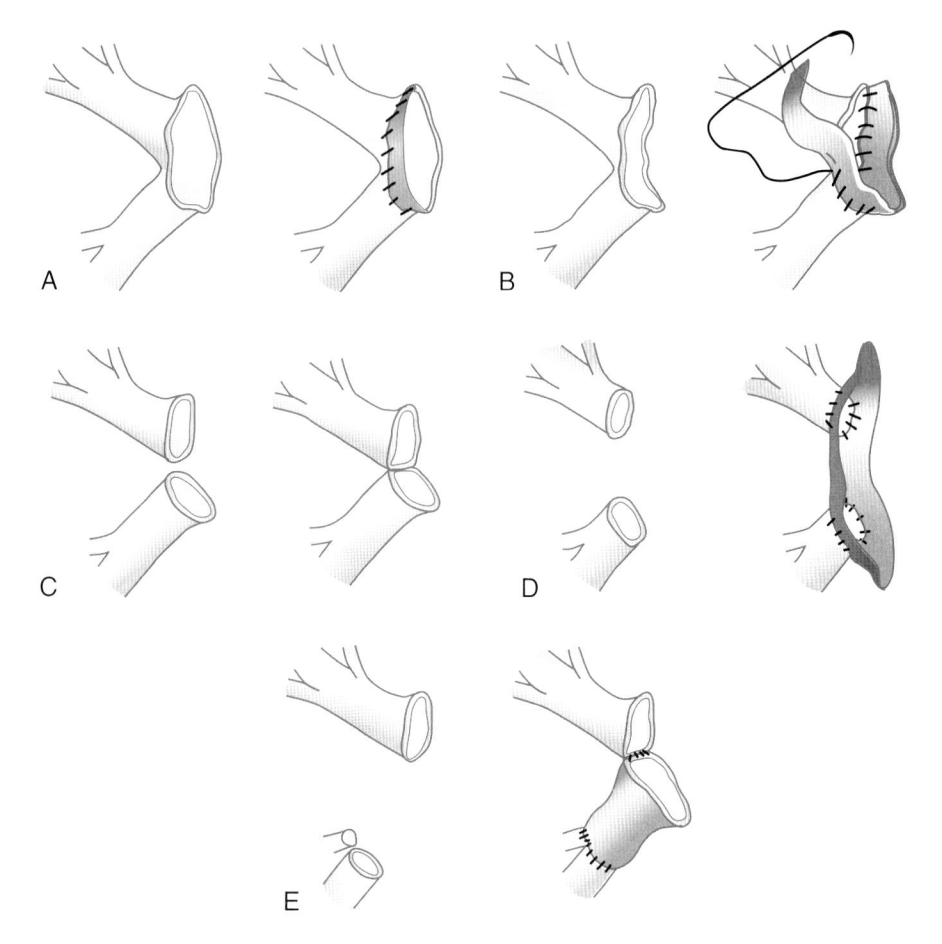

Figure 14–5
Reconstruction for an inadequate left atrial cuff. **A,** Anterior pericardial patch augmentation. **B,** Anterior and posterior pericardial patch augmentation. **C,** Separated but close venous orifices united by suture repair to create oval cross-sectional cuff. **D,** Widely separated veins, cuff reconstruction using pericardium. **E,** Donor pulmonary artery used to reconstruct inferior vein at segmental level. *(From Oto T, Rabinov M, Negri J, et al. Ann Thorac Surg 2006;**81**:1199-204.)*

trimmed distal to the laceration. If repair is required, simple suture or reconstruction using available donor pulmonary artery, azygous vein, or pericardium can be employed.

Congenital Bronchial Anomalies

A tracheal upper lobe bronchus, the most common anomaly, may be a segmental or a lobar bronchus. If the bronchus is determined to be a segmental bronchus, it may be simply oversewn or reimplanted. If the entire upper lobe bronchus arises as an abnormal tracheal bronchus, the options are donor right upper lobectomy, left single-lung transplantation, or incorporation of the bronchus intermedius and the aberrant upper lobe bronchus into a modified anastomosis with the recipient bronchus.[42]

RECIPIENT SURGERY

Anesthesia and Intraoperative Conduct

An experienced anesthesiologist who is well-versed in double-lumen-tube management, bronchoscopy, and the use of transesophageal echocardiography (TEE) is an invaluable part of the transplant team. Our patients undergo placement of an epidural catheter unless systemic heparinization for CPB is anticipated. If the indication for transplantation is septic lung disease, patients undergo therapeutic bronchoscopy and suctioning via a large single-lumen endotracheal tube. Radial and femoral arterial lines, a PA catheter, a TEE probe, and an inframbilical heating blanket are routine. The patient is placed supine with arms tucked. Minimizing intravenous fluids without compromising end-organ perfusion may avoid or reduce postoperative respiratory insufficiency. We use vasopressors as indicated and avoid excessive volume resuscitation.

TEE is useful at various junctures in the operation.[43] In particular, it is useful for TEE, monitoring for acute right ventricular dilation during PA clamping, detecting intracardiac shunts, determining the need for CPB based on classic signs of impending right ventricular decompensation, and assessment of the arterial and venous anastomoses and presence of air in the left atrium. We use epoprostenol or nitric oxide (or both) for acute refractory pulmonary hypertension in the perioperative period. Inhaled nitric oxide is also indicated for poor oxygenation.

Implantation

Incisions

Bilateral anterolateral thoracotomy without sternal division is our preferred incision for bilateral sequential lung transplant.[44] The skin incision follows the inframammary crease at the level of the fourth intercostal space and extends from the lateral sternal edge to the anterior axillary line. The breast tissue is elevated and the pectoralis major muscle is divided. The chest cavity is entered in the fourth interspace. Bilateral internal mammary arteries are ligated and divided. Alternatively, the internal mammary arteries can be preserved if a 1-cm segment of costal cartilage of the fourth rib is resected at the sternal border, allowing upward mobility of the fourth rib when retracted. Further mobility for retraction is obtained by dividing the intercostal muscles from within the pleural space laterally to the paraspinal muscles. We place two chest wall retractors at 90-degree angles to one another (Fig. 14-6). If needed,

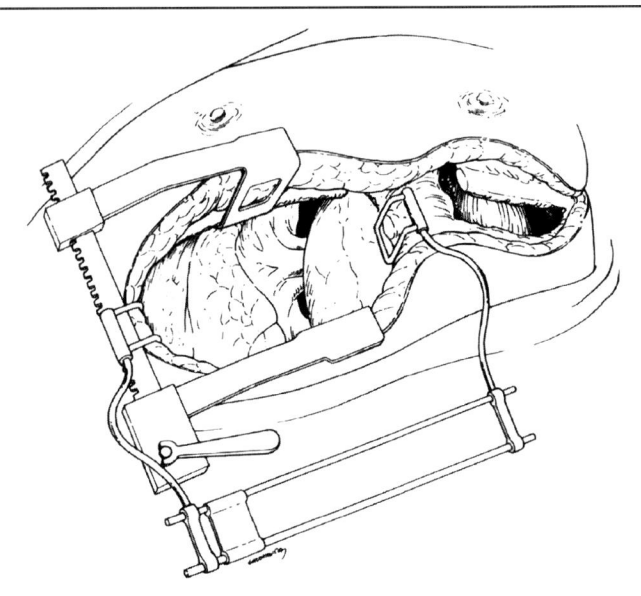

Figure 14–6
Bilateral anterolateral thoracotomy. Two retractors are placed at right angles. *(From Meyers BF, Patterson GA. Technical aspects of adult lung transplantation.* Semin Thorac Cardiovasc Surg *1998;**10**:213-20.)*

a right anterolateral thoracotomy allows adequate exposure of the aorta and right atrium for CPB.

The *clamshell incision* (sternothoracotomy) involves connecting the bilateral anterolateral thoracotomy incisions across the midline by dividing the sternum (Fig. 14-7). This incision provides excellent exposure and requires the division of both mammary arteries. It is used for providing added exposure when a concomitant cardiac procedure is performed, or when cardiomegaly or a relatively small chest cavity makes hilar exposure difficult. The sternum is reapproximated using a heavy-gauge Steinmann pin and two figure-eight #5 sternal wires.

A *median sternotomy* is used if the recipient is undergoing concomitant cardiac surgery, or for women with large breasts that compromise the exposure obtained by anterolateral thoracotomy.

Posterolateral thoracotomy and anterolateral thoracotomy are used when the patient has significant cardiomegaly, which can make exposing the left hilum through an anterolateral thoracotomy difficult. This difficulty can be circumvented by transplanting the left lung via a left posterolateral thoracotomy incision and then repositioning the patient for a right anterolateral thoracotomy to transplant the right lung.

The anterior axillary muscle-sparing thoracotomy incision, which may lead to improved chest wall and shoulder girdle mechanics, was initially described for single-lung transplant in recipients with chronic obstructive pulmonary disease.[45] The small anteroaxillary thoracotomy has been found comparable with the more conventional posterolateral or clamshell incision in terms of operating times and ability to go on central CPB.[46,47]

Pneumonectomy

Before excision of the recipient lungs, the donor lungs should be prepared and ready for implantation, and bilateral hilar dissection and adhesiolysis completed. This allows speedy removal of the second lung, minimizing the amount of time that the

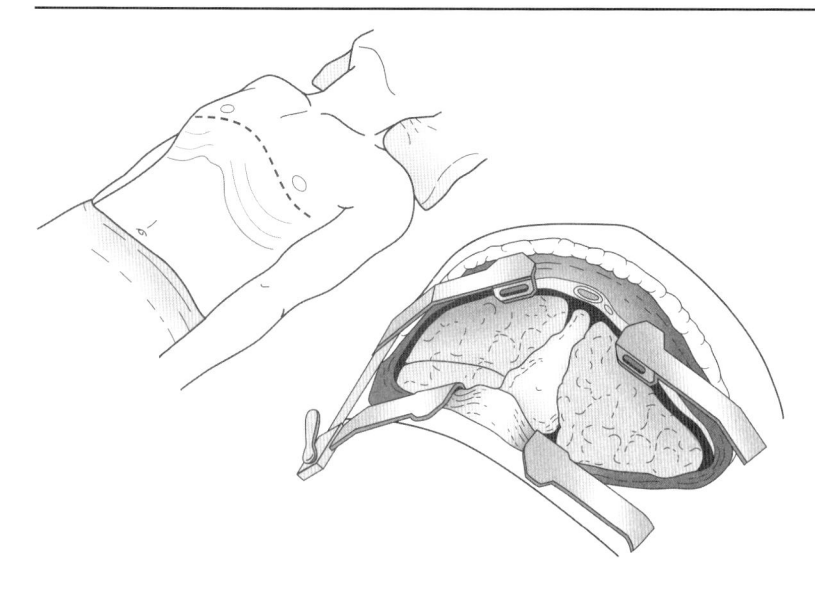

Figure 14-7
The sternum has been divided for a clamshell incision that provides excellent exposure to the thorax. *(From Lau CL, Patterson GA. Technical considerations in lung transplantation. Chest Surg Clin N Am 2003;**13**:463-483.)*

freshly implanted contralateral lung is exposed to the entire cardiac output. The lung with the poorer function, based on a preoperative ventilation perfusion scan, is transplanted first, as the other lung will more likely support single-lung ventilation.

During pneumonectomy, meticulous hemostasis is of prime importance in taking down pleural adhesions, particularly in patients with septic lung disease and prior thoracic procedures. The phrenic, vagus, and recurrent laryngeal nerves must be protected. During hilar dissection, the pulmonary arteries and veins are dissected beyond their first bifurcations to preserve the length of the main trunks. The right PA is transected about 1 cm beyond the truncus anterior branch and the left PA beyond the second branch to the left upper lobe. Vascular staplers are used on the central side of division, and ties are used peripherally. This maneuver downsizes the recipient PA, which may provide a better donor–recipient size match, and the first branch (ligated) of the recipient PA provides an anatomic landmark for orientation during the anastomosis. Next, the pulmonary veins are divided at secondary branch points. The peribronchial tissue is divided, and bronchial artery bleeding is controlled with cautery or ligatures; bronchial arteries are often significantly enlarged in patients with septic lung disease. The bronchus is divided just proximal to the upper lobe origin, and the lung is removed. All posterior mediastinal and posterior chest wall bleeders are controlled, as this is the only opportunity to access this area safely. At implantation, the bronchial anastomosis will be the first step, so we now set up hilar exposure. The pulmonary artery is gently grasped in a clamp, freed centrally, and retracted anteromedially. The superior and inferior pulmonary veins are similarly grasped in clamps, the pericardium around them is widely opened, and the veins are retracted anteriorly. We are now ready for lung implantation.

Lung Implantation

The donor lung is covered with a cold sponge and placed in a bed of ice slush into the thoracic cavity. We start with the bronchial anastomosis. Our preference is an end-to-end

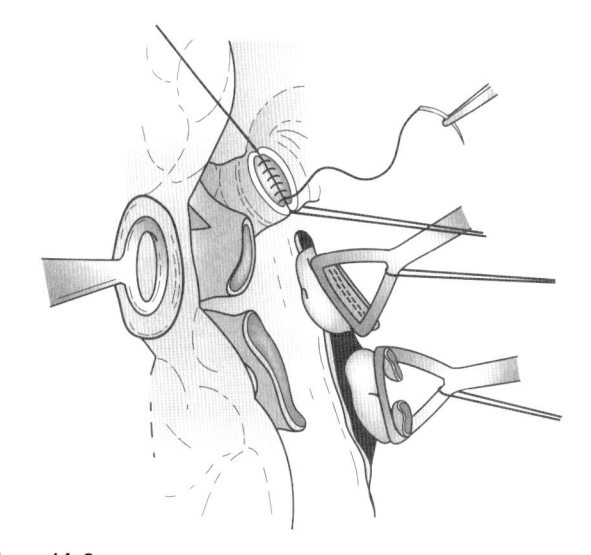

Figure 14-8
Retraction on the pulmonary artery and pulmonary vein stumps provides exposure for the airway anastomosis. The bronchial anastomosis is being performed with 4-0 PDS suture. *(From Meyers BF, Patterson GA. Technical aspects of adult lung transplantation. Semin Thorac Cardiovasc Surg 1998;**10**:213-20.)*

anastomosis using two strands of 4-0 polydioxanone (PDS) in a running stitch. A retraction suture (0 silk) is placed into the anterior aspect of the recipient bronchus to aid exposure. The anastomosis is started on the membranous part in running fashion and carried around over the anterior cartilaginous part with the second suture (Fig. 14-8). In case of significant size mismatch between the bronchi, the membranous portion is completed using a running 4-0 PDS suture, and the cartilaginous part is approximated with simple interrupted 3-0 Vicryl sutures (Fig. 14-9).

The peribronchial tissue on the donor and recipient sides is used to cover the anterior aspect of the anastomosis to offer some protection to the overlying vascular anastomoses in case of bronchial anastomotic breakdown. End-to-end airway

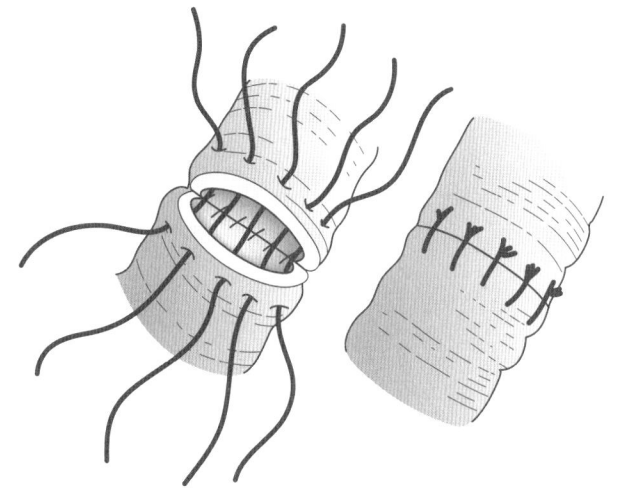

Figure 14–9
The anterior wall of the bronchial anastomosis is performed with interrupted 3-0 Vicryl suture when a significant size mismatch is present. *(From Meyers BF, Patterson GA. Technical aspects of adult lung transplantation. Semin Thorac Cardiovasc Surg 1998;**10**:213-20.)*

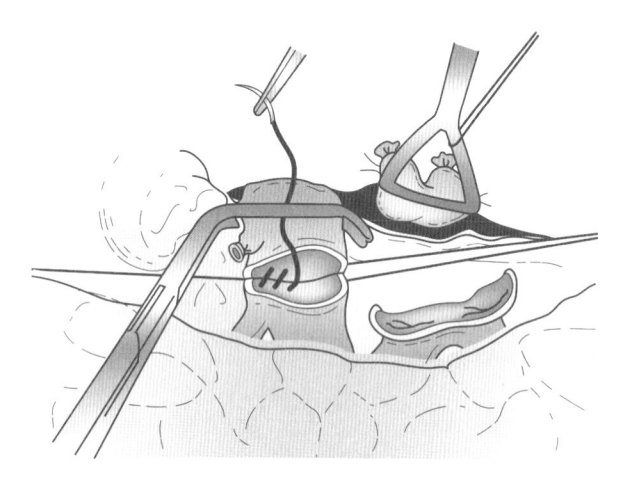

Figure 14–10
The pulmonary artery anastomosis is fashioned using a running 5-0 polypropylene suture. *(From Meyers BF, Patterson GA. Technical aspects of adult lung transplantation. Semin Thorac Cardiovasc Surg 1998;**10**:213-20.)*

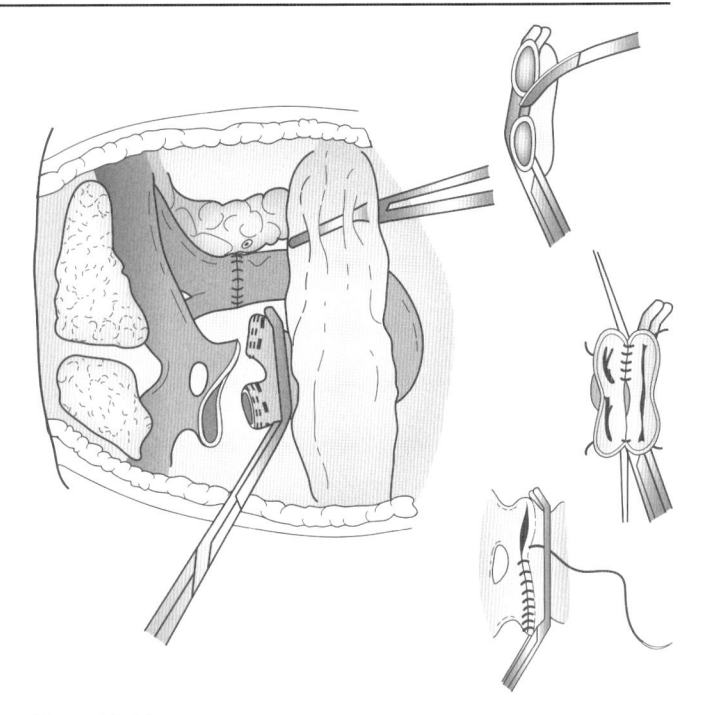

Figure 14–11
A large Satinsky clamp is placed centrally across the left atrium. Both vein stumps are amputated and the bridge between is connected to create a left atriotomy suitable for anastomosis. *(From Patterson GA. Bilateral lung transplant: indications and technique. Semin Thorac Cardiovasc Surg 1992;**4**:95-100.)*

anastomosis has been found to be superior to the telescoped anastomosis technique.[48]

Next, a vascular clamp is placed as proximal as possible on the recipient PA and the staple line resected. The donor and recipient PAs are trimmed to prevent excessive length and possible kinking, and an end-to-end anastomosis is fashioned using a continuous 5-0 polypropylene stitch, using precise small bites to prevent anastomotic stricture (Fig. 14-10).

The vein stumps are then retracted laterally and a Satinsky-type clamp is placed centrally on the recipient's left atrium. The recipient pulmonary venous stumps are amputated and the two openings connected to create the atrial cuff. The anastomosis is fashioned with continuous 4-0 polypropylene suture. Stitches are placed via a mattress technique, which achieves intima-to-intima apposition and excludes potentially thrombogenic atrial muscle (Fig. 14-11).

The last few sutures are left loose, the lung is partially inflated, and the PA clamp is released momentarily. This maneuver flushes out air and perfusate from the lung. The left atrial clamp is then opened to completely de-air the atrium. The atrial suture line is pulled up tight and tied down. All clamps are removed.

If the operation is being performed without CPB, it is important to stabilize the patient after the first lung is implanted. Initial pulmonary hypertension may result from hypercarbia, which is corrected with a period of dual-lung ventilation. Thus the use of CPB for implantation of the second lung can be avoided.

The pleural spaces are usually drained with two #24 Blake drains (Ethicon, Somerville, NJ) in each pleural space, one placed apically and one along the diaphragm. If significant postoperative bleeding is expected, two 28-French conventional chest tubes are preferred over Blake drains. The sternum is typically reapproximated with two figure-of-eight #5 sternal wires. The ribs are reapproximated with heavy interrupted figure-eight monofilament nonabsorbable suture. The chest wall is closed in layers.

A flexible bronchoscopy is performed after exchanging the double-lumen tube for a single-lumen tube, to evaluate the airway anastomoses and remove blood and secretions. The patient is now transported, intubated, to the intensive care unit (ICU).

Cardiopulmonary Bypass

We use CPB selectively in our patients. It is, however, indicated for children, small-statured patients when a double-lumen tube cannot be placed, lobar transplants, concomitant

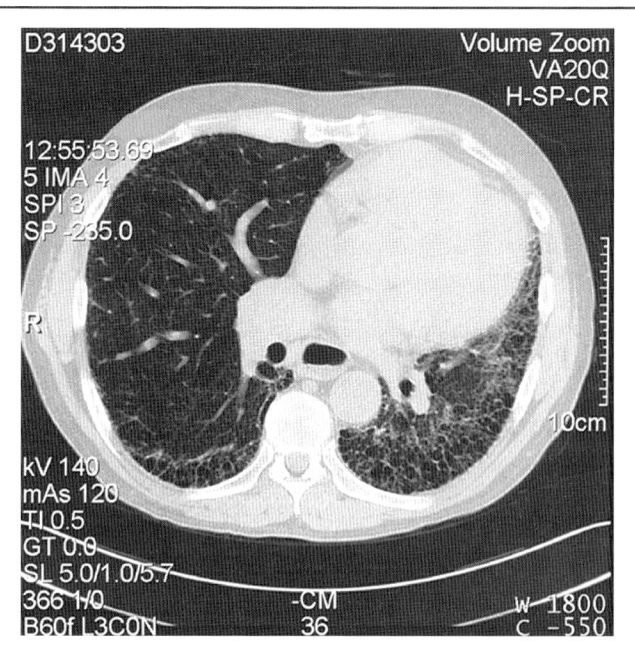

Figure 14–12
Axial CT images from a patient with idiopathic pulmonary fibrosis show a markedly diminished left pleural space with the mediastinum shifted to the left. This mandates the use of cardiopulmonary bypass for adequate exposure.

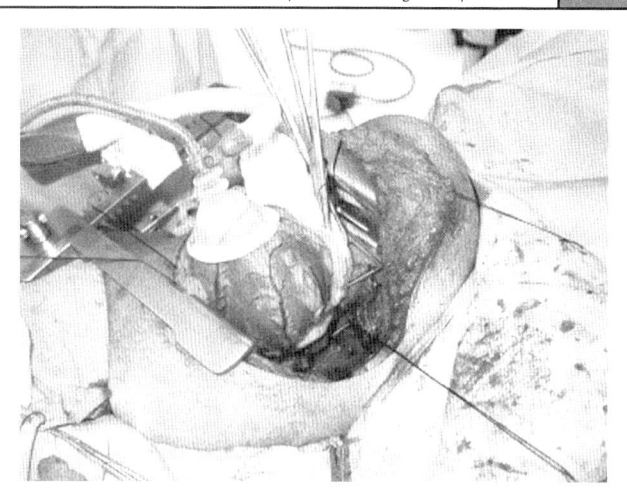

Figure 14–13
An apical suction device is in place, lifting the apex of the heart and improving exposure to the left hilum. *(From Lau CL, Hoganson DM, Meyers BF, Damiano RJ Jr, Patterson GA. Use of an apical heart suction device for exposure in lung transplantation.* Ann Thorac Surg *2006;**81**:1524-5.)*

intracardiac procedures, and most patients with pulmonary hypertension. CPB is also indicated if at any point during the operation the patient develops refractory hypoxemia, hypercarbia, pulmonary hypertension, or hemodynamic instability. Difficult exposure may necessitate CPB, too. This is typically seen in patients with idiopathic pulmonary fibrosis who have a small pleural space with the heart shifted to the left, thus making exposure of the left hilum difficult (Fig. 14-12). A traction suture in the fibrous portion of the diaphragm, brought extracorporeally through a planned chest tube site, can improve exposure. Alternatively, the diaphragm can be depressed using a malleable retractor wedged between the anterior and posterior intercostal spaces in the chest cavity. Inadequate exposure of the left hilum is sometimes the only indication for CPB. We have used the Urchin heart positioning device (Medtronic, Minneapolis, MN) to improve exposure (Fig. 14-13).

When CPB is used electively, we perform most of the dissection prior to systemic heparinization. Standard aortic cannulation is performed, and a two-stage venous cannula is introduced via the right atrial appendage. We avoid the use of pump suckers. After implantation of the first lung, the left atrium is de-aired and the venous clamp removed. This also allows the placement of an atrial clamp for venous anastomosis on the contralateral side.

TECHNICAL STRATEGIES TO OVERCOME DONOR SHORTAGE

Size-Mismatched Lungs

Lungs from otherwise acceptable donors that are larger than the recipient can be safely accepted. We prefer to downsize the lungs by performing a lobectomy on the back table. If the size mismatch is appreciated after implantation, bilateral wedge resection, targeting the lingula and the right middle lobe, is performed using stapling devices.

Living Lobar and Split-Lung Transplantation

Two healthy donors donate one lobe each in this strategy. Donor right lower lobe and left lower lobe are implanted in the recipient on the respective side. In a large series, the operation provided results in the recipient that were comparable with those of conventional transplantation, with no donor mortality but a morbidity rate of 20%.[49]

Pulmonary bipartitioning and lobar transplantation is a technically advanced strategy that Couetil and colleagues have described.[15] Good results have been obtained in experienced programs.[50]

Non-Heart-Beating Donors

The lung is unique among the vital organs because of its tolerance of warm ischemia. In our small initial experience with 11 non-heart-beating-donors, we have had two hospital deaths and two delayed deaths, after a median follow-up of 22 months. The four recipients who died were similar to the seven survivors in the donation-after-cardiac-death group, in age and in preoperative NYHA status, but those who died had longer ischemic time (293 ± 95 minutes versus 232 ± 60 minutes) and higher incidences of nonlocal donors (3 of 4 versus 1 of 7), ECMO requirement (2 of 4 versus 0 of 7), and postoperative renal failure (4 of 4 versus 1 of 7).

Ex Vivo Reconditioning of Unacceptable Lungs

Steen and colleagues used an initially unacceptable lung for transplant after ex vivo reconditioning (Fig. 14-14).[37] In their technique, the lungs are perfused ex vivo with Steen solution, a lung evaluation and preservation solution, and mixed with red blood cells to a hematocrit of 15%. An oxygenator maintains a normal mixed venous blood gas level in the perfusate. The lungs are ventilated and evaluated through analyses of pulmonary vascular resistance, oxygenation capacity, and arterial carbon dioxide pressure minus end-tidal carbon dioxide.

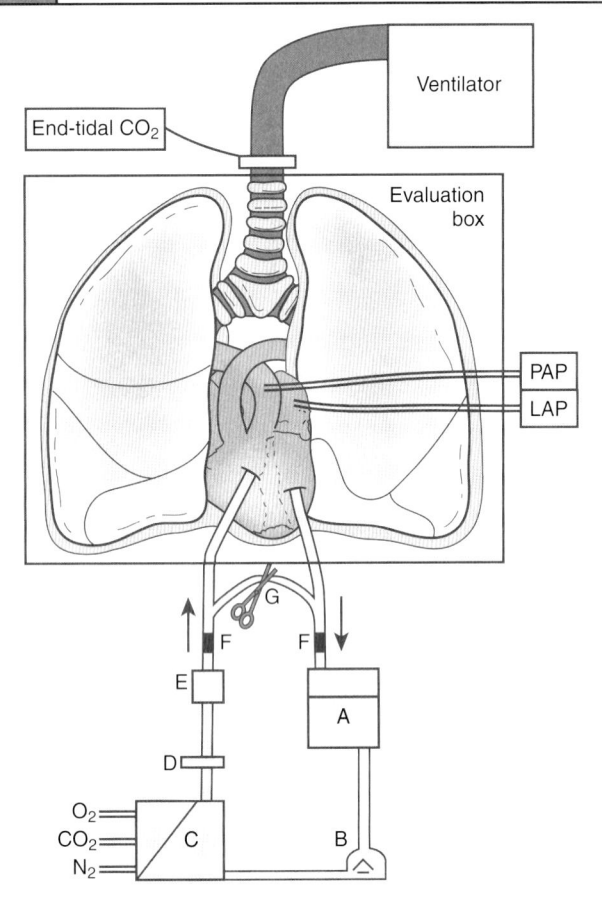

Figure 14–14
Schematic drawing of the ex vivo lung evaluation system. The lungs, placed in the evaluation box, are connected to the perfusion system and a ventilator. End-tidal CO_2, pulmonary arterial pressure (PAP), and left atrial pressure (LAP) are measured. The blood coming out from the left atrium is drained to a reservoir (A), passes a centrifugal pump (B), is deoxygenated in an oxygenator (C) provided with a mixture of gases, passes a flow measurement probe (D) and a leukocyte-arterial filter (E), and is then pumped into the pulmonary artery. F, oxygen, pressure, and temperature sensors; G, shunt to prime the system with Steen solution.

POSTOPERATIVE MANAGEMENT

Ventilation

The patients are transported to the ICU and initially ventilated with standard techniques. The FiO_2 value is adjusted to maintain the PaO_2 greater than 70 mm Hg. Tidal volumes of 7 to 10 mL/kg are usually sufficient, and PEEP of 5 to 7.5 cm H_2O is used in most patients. Frequent arterial blood gas analyses are performed. After an initial period of evaluation, if the patients are hemodynamically stable and have no significant bleeding and if gas exchange is satisfactory, weaning is initiated. Extubation is performed in accordance with standard requirements of gas exchange and respiratory mechanics. Most patients are extubated within 24 to 48 hours of transplantation after standard intermittent mandatory ventilation or pressure support weaning. Before extubation, patients undergo bronchoscopy to ensure adequate clearance of secretions. This standard management is applied in all bilateral lung transplant recipients and single-lung recipients undergoing transplantation for pulmonary fibrosis.

After single-lung transplantation for emphysema or pulmonary vascular disease, patients are managed differently.[51]

Preventing hyperinflation of the native lung and compression of the freshly implanted lung are the main concerns in patients with emphysema. This is accomplished by avoiding the use of PEEP and using lower tidal volumes. If air trapping does occur in the native lung, it leads to high airway pressures, inadequate removal of carbon dioxide, and hypotension from decreased venous return to the heart. This occasionally necessitates volume reduction of the native lung by lobectomy or even pneumonectomy.[52,53]

In single-lung recipients with pulmonary vascular disease, we use a prolonged period (48 to 72 hours) of elective ventilation. The patient is positioned to keep the native lung dependent to maintain inflation and appropriate drainage of the transplanted lung. Tidal volumes are standard, but a higher PEEP of 7.5 to 10 cm H_2O is applied. Should early graft dysfunction, rejection, or infection necessitate a prolonged period of mechanical ventilation, tracheostomy should be performed early in the postoperative course.

Fluid Management

In the early postoperative period, the Swan-Ganz catheter and daily weighings provide objective assessment of fluid status. The patients often return from the operating room with a significant positive fluid balance. Diuretics are used aggressively during the early postoperative period. Occasionally, patients undergoing single-lung transplantation for PPH develop hemodynamic instability if the filling pressures on the right side of the heart are excessively reduced, and these patients may require somewhat higher filling pressures.

General Care

Postoperatively, a quantitative lung perfusion scan to assess for adequate patency and graft flow is usually performed. If a lobar or greater perfusion defect is appreciated, further interrogation for the cause should be undertaken either by catheterization or operative exploration. Vigorous chest physiotherapy, postural drainage, inhalation of bronchodilators, and frequent clearance of pulmonary secretions are required in the postoperative care of these patients. Early and constant involvement of the physical therapy team ensures that transplant recipients are out of bed to chair, ambulatory with assistance, and using the treadmill or exercise bike as soon as possible.

IMMUNOSUPPRESSION

Immunosuppression after solid organ transplantation was revolutionized by the introduction of cyclosporin A in the 1980s. Immunosuppression after lung transplantation has three pillars: induction therapy, maintenance immunosuppression, and treatment for rejection.

Postoperative induction therapy is controversial. Potential benefits include lower rates of acute rejection, protection from nephrotoxicity as a result of the delayed introduction of a calcineurin inhibitor, and a decrease in the occurrence of bronchiolitis obliterans syndrome (BOS). Disadvantages are the higher risk of infectious complications and post-transplantation malignancies. About 40% of patients undergoing lung transplantation receive induction immunosuppression.[18]

The agents used for induction immunosuppression include polyclonal antilymphocyte or antithymocyte preparations, monoclonal OKT3 and interleukin (IL)-2 receptor antagonists. All of the agents used in induction are generally associated with a decrease in the number of episodes of acute rejection, but their true impact on the incidence of BOS or overall survival remains to be determined. Antithymocyte globulin, antilymphocyte globulin, and OKT3 deplete quiescent and activated T lymphocytes, and IL-2 receptor antagonists block activated T lymphocytes and may be associated with a lower risk of infectious complications and possibly post-transplantation lymphoproliferative disease (PTLD).[54,55] Other studies, however, indicate that no single induction agent is superior to another.[56]

For maintenance therapy, lung transplantation programs generally rely on triple-agent therapy, consisting of corticosteroids, a calcineurin inhibitor, and a cell cycle inhibitor. At our center, methylprednisolone (10 to 15 mg/kg IV) is given intraoperatively just before graft perfusion. Most programs use moderate-dose corticosteroid therapy (methylprednisolone, 0.5 to 1 mg/kg/day IV) for several days before initiating an oral dose of prednisone of 0.5 mg/kg/day. About 75% of lung transplant recipients receive a calcineurin inhibitor and a purine synthesis inhibitor at 1 and 5 years after transplantation, respectively.[18]

Cyclosporine and tacrolimus are calcineurin inhibitors that suppress the transcription of IL-2 and inhibit proliferation of T lymphocytes. Azathioprine inhibits de novo purine synthesis and suppresses proliferation of both T and B lymphocytes. Mycophenolate mofetil (MMF) is a prodrug of mycophenolic acid that produces inhibition of de novo purine synthesis. Despite the lack of evidence for the superiority of MMF over azathioprine in lung transplantation, its use now exceeds that of azathioprine in lung transplant recipients.[57,58]

Sirolimus and its derivative everolimus were recently introduced into clinical lung transplantation. These agents block growth factor–driven cell cycle progression and proliferation of lymphocytes and other nonhematopoietic cells such as vascular smooth muscle cells. Initial evidence shows their efficacy in decreasing the incidence of BOS.[59]

INFECTION PROPHYLAXIS

We routinely employ broad-spectrum antibacterial chemotherapy (usually cefepime and vancomycin) for several days after transplantation. Results from donor and recipient airway cultures are used to adjust this empiric regimen. In patients with cystic fibrosis, aerosolized colistin or tobramycin is added, and special emphasis is placed on coverage for *Pseudomonas*.

For the first year after transplantation, we routinely give acyclovir (unless the patient is on ganciclovir or valganciclovir) for herpes simplex prophylaxis. In patients at high risk for cytomegalovirus (CMV) infection (donor⁺–recipient⁻ mismatch), our standard practice is to use 12 weeks of IV ganciclovir (5 mg/kg/day) usually starting 7 to 14 days after transplantation. In other recipients, the ganciclovir is given for shorter courses at the same dosage, but only in the setting of a proved viremia or CMV pneumonitis. For transplant patients, we use CMV-negative or leukocyte-reduced blood products.[60]

We do not routinely use fungal prophylaxis. However, when a heavy growth of yeast is identified after transplantation in donor bronchial culture, prophylactic low-dose fluconazole is used. We have occasionally encountered patients with early postoperative ischemic necrosis of the graft bronchus who have significant growth of *Aspergillus* from the airway. These patients have been treated with itraconazole with good result.

Lifelong *Pneumocystis carinii* prophylaxis is used starting 3 weeks after transplantation. Our current strategy includes Bactrim DS three times per week for life. Alternative agents, such as monthly application of inhaled pentamidine, are administered when there is an allergy to sulfa medications.

As part of the frequent bronchoscopies performed in these patients, we routinely obtain samples from the bronchoalveolar lavage (BAL) for cytology, Gram stain, KOH test, and acid-fast bacilli stain, and immunostains for respiratory viruses, herpes simplex virus, and CMV. Also, bacterial, mycobacterial, fungal, and viral cultures are performed.

It is difficult to distinguish infectious pulmonary problems from rejection in the early post-transplantation lung recipient using radiographic, clinical, and physiologic criteria. This has led to the frequent use of fiberoptic bronchoscopy in these patients. BAL and transbronchial biopsies are performed to look for opportunistic infection and evidence of rejection, respectively. These are routinely performed at 2 to 3 weeks; at 2, 3, 6, and 12 months; and annually thereafter.

COMPLICATIONS

Technical Problems

With increasing experience, the technical aspects of lung transplantation have become more sophisticated and reproducible. However, as with any major operation, technical complications may be seen perioperatively. Perioperative hemorrhage may be related to a large raw surface that is created after explantation from a patient with septic lung disease or who has undergone previous pleurodesis. CPB usually exacerbates this problem. In addition to meticulous attention to stopping all surgically correctible bleeding, we aggressively correct any coagulopathy with blood products and use recombinant factor VII as needed. In this situation, we frequently delay final chest closure until later and proceed to the ICU after approximating the skin and using a transparent sterile dressing. Final chest closure is usually possible within the next 24 to 48 hours. This strategy does not increase wound complications.[61]

A technically unsatisfactory bronchial anastomosis is easily identified in the operating room at postimplantation bronchoscopy. Inadequate anastomotic caliber dictates immediate surgical revision. Pulmonary arterial anastomotic compromise manifests as persistent pulmonary hypertension and unexplained hypoxemia. Intraoperative TEE can also provide a clue to the diagnosis. A nuclear perfusion scan performed immediately postoperatively will demonstrate less than anticipated flow to the affected side. The gold standard for studying the PA anastomosis is contrast angiography, which can additionally look for a gradient across the anastomosis. A gradient of 15 to 20 mm Hg may be found, especially in single-lung recipients, in whom most cardiac output is directed to the transplanted lung, or in bilateral recipients with a high cardiac output. The need for anastomotic revision is dictated by the clinical situation. Significant reduction in flow in the appropriate clinical setting indicates surgical correction, as the donor bronchus depends entirely on pulmonary arterial collateral flow. Pulmonary venous anastomotic compromise can be technical or may be caused by a compressing clot in the setting of significant

Table 14–1

Grading System for Primary Graft Dysfunction

Grade	Pa_{O_2}/Fi_{O_2}	Radiographic Infiltrates
0	>300	Absent
1	>300	Present
2	200-300	Present
3	<200	Present

Fi_{O_2}, fraction of inspired oxygen; Pa_{O_2}, partial pressure of arterial oxygen.
From Christie JD, Carby M, Christie JD, et al. J Heart Lung Transplant 2005;**24**:1454-9.

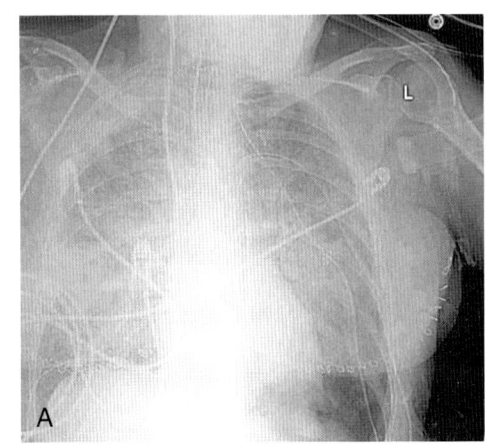

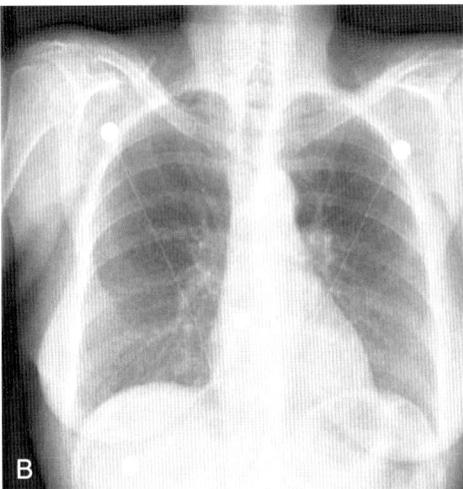

Figure 14–15
A, Chest radiograph showing diffuse consolidation typical of ischemic reperfusion injury. The right lung was implanted first, which explains the increased injury appreciated on this side. **B,** Radiograph of the same patient after complete recovery.

hemorrhage. Similarly, TEE and contrast angiography, with close attention to the venous phase, will identify the problem. Occasionally, surgical exploration is necessary to confirm the diagnosis and conduct appropriate repair.

Primary Graft Dysfunction

Primary graft dysfunction (PGD) develops in up to 25% of lung transplant recipients.[62,63] Mortality from PGD is as high as 30% and it contributes to the majority of patients dying perioperatively. The major diagnostic criteria for PGD are a compromised Pa_{O_2}-to-Fi_{O_2} ratio in the first 48 hours after transplantation, and the presence of panlobar alveolar infiltrates on postoperative chest radiographs (Fig. 14-15). The ISHLT issued a grading system for primary graft dysfunction based on the Pa_{O_2}-to-Fi_{O_2} ratio and findings on chest radiographs (Table 14-1).[64]

Ischemia-reperfusion injury probably accounts for most cases of primary graft dysfunction. Other suspected causes include donor lung pathologic conditions such as aspiration, infection, or contusion. Effects of cold storage can contribute to primary dysfunction by inducing intracellular calcium overload, release of iron from ferritin, reduced production of anticoagulant factors by endothelial cells, and activation of the complement system. Lung-resident macrophages, neutrophils, and T lymphocytes that are recruited to the lung allograft from the recipient on reperfusion are important mediators of ischemia-reperfusion injury. Levels of IL-8, a potent chemoattractant for neutrophils, increase during reperfusion of lung grafts; they correlate with the duration of the ischemic time, and they negatively correlate with early lung function.[65]

Primary graft dysfunction is managed with aggressive cardiopulmonary support in the ICU. Appropriate ventilatory strategies with the use of PEEP, inhaled nitric oxide,[66] and aerosolized prostacyclin[67] are employed. In most patients, primary graft dysfunction resolves over several days of intensive care support, and they obtain satisfactory long-term allograft function.[62]

ECMO support is used if conservative management appears to be unsuccessful. In a review of our experience with 983 lung transplant recipients, 47 required ECMO for PGD during the immediate postoperative phase. ECMO was used in 9.7% of pediatric and 2.8% of adult lung transplant recipients. Only 38% of patients who received ECMO survived to discharge from the hospital.[63] Retransplantation was performed in 11 patients for primary graft dysfunction.

Superior strategies of lung preservation can help prevent PGD. Low-potassium, dextran-containing preservation solutions are routine, and a combination of an antegrade and retrograde pulmonary vascular flush achieves more uniform distribution of flush solution and superior graft cooling.[68,69]

Meticulous attention is paid to avoiding hyperinflation during or after procurement, especially with the majority of organs being transported by airplane. The use of controlled reperfusion in combination with leukocyte depletion has been proposed as a preventive strategy. Lick and colleagues reported a small clinical series using this technique and reported no reperfusion injury.[70] At the time of reperfusion, a modified, leukocyte-filtered perfusate is pumped at a controlled rate (200 mL/min) and pressure (less than 20 mm Hg) for 10 minutes through the transplanted lung. The lung was ventilated with a 50% inspired oxygen concentration during the period.[70] We do not routinely do this.

Primary graft dysfunction probably contributes to chronic rejection. We noted a significant association between PGD and the development of BOS, with the time interval from transplantation to the development of BOS being significantly shorter in patients with PGD.[63]

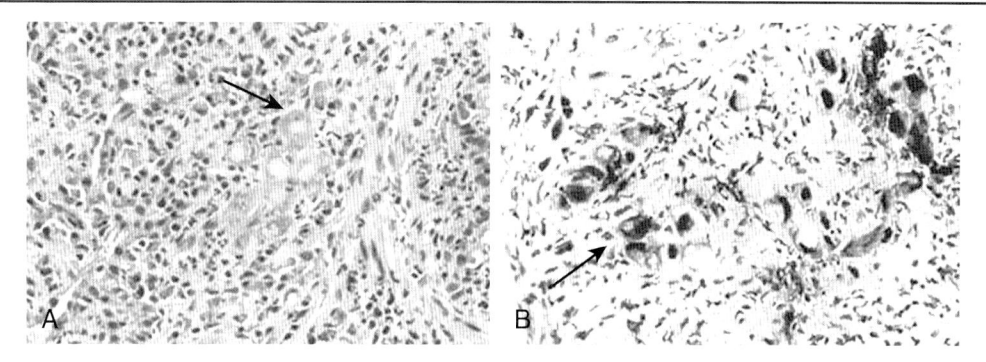

Figure 14–16
A, Transbronchial lung biopsy showing cytomegalovirus (CMV) pneumonitis with demonstration of CMV inclusion bodies *(arrow)* (H&E stain).
B, Demonstration of CMV inclusion bodies by immunoperoxidase staining *(arrow).*

Infectious Complications

Bacterial

Bacterial infections are most common in the early post-transplant period and remain the primary cause of mortality in the early post-transplant period.[71] They may be related to pre-existing colonization of recipient or donor, complications of the transplant operation, nosocomial exposure, or community-acquired infection.[72] Although identification of the organism is important to guide therapy, routine empiric intravenous antibiotic therapy is employed at the initial suspicion. Patients with cystic fibrosis are susceptible to recurrent pulmonary infections from *Pseudomonas* harbored in the airway and upper airway sinuses after transplantation. De Perrot and colleagues reported that *B. cepacia* colonization in patients with CF was associated with poor outcome after transplantation.[73]

Thus, immunosuppressive regimens have been toned down while antimicrobial therapy has been enhanced in this patient population. A recent study outlining the potential transmission of bacterial infections from donor to recipient found the incidence of donor infection to be greater than 50%, which emphasizes the importance of adjusting the antimicrobial regimen according to donor cultures.[74]

Wound infections of thoracotomy, sternotomy, or clamshell incisions are generally caused by conventional bacteria such as staphylococci. Less commonly, *Actinomyces*, *Mycobacterium tuberculosis*, and atypical mycobacterial infections are seen in lung transplant recipients.[72,75]

Lung abscess is occasionally encountered in lung transplantation recipients, and patients with CF are susceptible to multifocal lung abscesses, presumably resulting from inhaled contamination from upper airway or sinus infection. The care of these patients is the same as for any other patient with lung abscess. Appropriate broad-spectrum antibiotic therapy is administered, and bronchoscopy is performed to ensure that no airway obstruction is present.

Viral

Cytomegalovirus disease is the most commonly noted postoperative infectious complication. It occurs in 13% to 75% of transplant patients, depending on definitions of CMV disease and the use of CMV prophylaxis.[60,76] Because the lung can harbor high latent CMV loads, the incidence of CMV infection is higher after lung transplantation than after transplantation of other solid organs. Additionally, CMV may predispose to the development of chronic allograft rejection. CMV induces heightened immunosuppression, so patients are at increased risk for other opportunistic infections and post-transplant lymphoproliferative disease.[77]

The diagnosis of CMV infection at our institution is based on a positive polymerase chain reaction (PCR) test on a blood sample, whereas the presence of cytomegalic cells (CMV inclusion bodies or positive immunoperoxidase stain) in tissue biopsies is considered indicative of CMV disease (Fig. 14-16).

Most programs match seronegative donors with seronegative recipients. The highest incidence of severe CMV infection occurs with donor-negative and recipient-positive transplants. For mismatched recipients, we administer prophylactic therapy for 3 to 6 months. Otherwise, we employ a preemptive treatment approach, where recipients are screened weekly by PCR for CMV in the blood, and treatment is initiated if the PCR test becomes positive. Prophylactic regimens include oral or IV ganciclovir, with or without CMV immunoglobulin (also IV). Valganciclovir, an oral prodrug of ganciclovir with higher bioavailability, has been used as a prophylactic agent.[78] Although CMV infection is uncommon during prophylaxis, the rate of CMV disease increases after cessation of prophylactic therapy, especially with the donor-negative and recipient-positive combination.

Although less common, non-cytomegalovirus viral respiratory tract infections have been reported.[79,80] These include herpesvirus, respiratory syncytial virus, parainfluenza virus, influenza virus, and adenovirus. These infections have also been linked to later development of chronic allograft rejection.[81,82] Treatment includes supportive care and antiviral therapy.

Fungal

Candida albicans is commonly isolated after transplantation. It usually represents colonization,[71] but it may also be invasive.[83] Candidal infections are most commonly associated with airway anastomotic complications.[84,85] These infections may be symptomatic or may be discovered on surveillance bronchoscopy. They can be treated with a combination of systemic and inhaled amphotericin B and fluconazole (some species are resistant).

The most frequent cause of significant fungal infection after transplantation is *Aspergillus*. Invasive infection is the most feared complication; it carries a high mortality, and it is often fatal.[86] More commonly, however, *Aspergillus* growing in

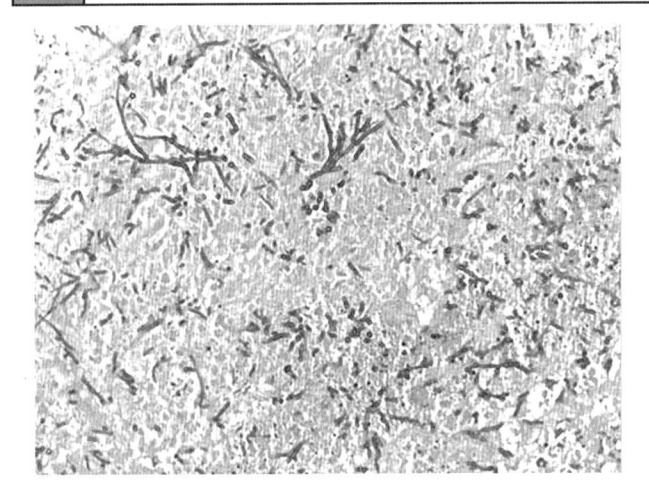

Figure 14–17
Histopathologic examination of a patient with *Aspergillus* infection (H&E stain, ×20).

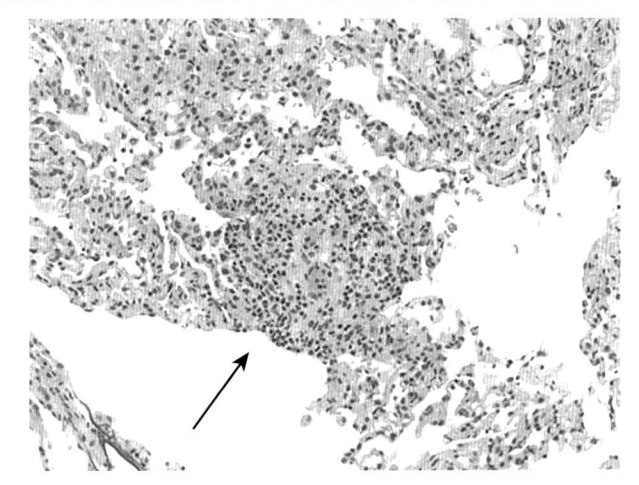

Figure 14–18
Histopathologic examination of acute rejection *(arrow)* (H&E stain, ×20).

sputum or BAL cultures represents colonization (Fig. 14-17). Colonization is a risk factor for invasive disease, but only a fraction of colonized patients develop more serious infections.[72] Prevention of aspergillosis involves infection-control measures such as wearing masks while traversing areas of hospital construction, as well as avoiding gardening, compost, and other outdoor exposures. Once *Aspergillus* has become a resident organism, it is difficult to clear. Postoperative therapy for patients colonized with *Aspergillus* may not be successful in preventing invasive infections.[72]

Aspergillomas found in the recipient explanted lungs have been associated with reduced post-transplant survival.[87] In patients with a single-lung transplant, a potential reservoir of persistent *Aspergillus* is the native lung.[71] These patients should be treated aggressively with the expectation that the *Aspergillus* is not likely to clear from the native lung. In this circumstance, contralateral native lung pneumonectomy may be warranted.

Acute Rejection

Acute rejection is seen more commonly after lung transplantation than after any other solid organ transplant.[88] Although it is an uncommon cause of mortality, its danger lies in its proven association with the development of chronic rejection. The majority of episodes of acute rejection occur early in the postoperative period, and the incidence steadily declines after the first 3 months.[89-91]

Patients with symptomatic episodes of acute rejection present with dyspnea, hypoxemia, low-grade fever, and moderate leukocytosis, which can be difficult to differentiate from early infection. The chest radiograph often shows diffuse-perihilar interstitial infiltrates; however, episodes occurring after the first month may have a normal-appearing chest radiograph.

Episodes of acute rejection may be indicated by a 10% or greater decline in baseline FEV_1 or forced vital capacity. Intensive laboratory investigations are focused on the development of noninvasive techniques by which rejection might be identified. Nuclear scanning may be of some usefulness, as infections are associated with high signals on positron emission tomography, whereas rejection is not.[92]

Cytokines are important mediators in the development of acute rejection, and our group has demonstrated elevated levels of IL-15 as well as granzyme B in the BAL fluid of lung transplant recipients who were undergoing acute rejection.[93]

Bronchoscopic evaluation with transbronchial biopsy is useful in confirming the diagnosis and ruling out infection. A uniform grading system for classification of pulmonary transplant rejection was revised by the ISHLT in 2007.[94] This grading system is based on histologic criteria found on biopsy, with an emphasis on perivascular and interstitial infiltration of mononuclear cells (Fig. 14-18). The previous system, in brief, was as follows: grade A0 (none), grade A1 (minimal), grade A2 (mild), grade A3 (moderate), and grade A4 (severe). The revised (R) categories of small airways inflammation, lymphocytic bronchiolitis, are as follows: grade B0 (none), grade B1R (low grade, 1996, B1 and B2), grade B2R (high grade, 1996, B3 and B4), and BX (ungradeable). Chronic rejection, obliterative bronchiolitis (grade C), is described as present (C1) or absent (C0), without reference to presence of inflammatory activity. Chronic vascular rejection is unchanged as grade D.

Acute rejection is usually treated with IV methylprednisolone, 10 to 15 mg/kg/day for 3 to 5 days. Usually there is dramatic improvement in symptoms and radiographic findings within 8 to 12 hours. Often, this is followed with a steroid taper over 2 to 3 weeks. Baseline immunosuppression is reevaluated with recurrent acute rejection. Two studies have shown a decrease in acute rejection episodes when tacrolimus (FK506; Prograf, Fujisawa) is chosen as the initial calcineurin inhibitor.[95,96]

Other studies have shown a decreased recurrence in acute rejection after switching from cyclosporine to tacrolimus.[97,98] We discontinue cyclosporine and start tacrolimus in patients with severe or recurrent acute rejection episodes. MMF has not been shown to decrease acute rejection episodes compared with azathioprine in lung transplantation,[57,58] but based on its success in other organ transplantations, we often switch to this cell cycle inhibitor when patients have recurrent acute rejection episodes.[99]

We repeat bronchoscopy in 3 to 6 weeks to confirm an appropriate response to therapy. In approximately one third of cases, persistence of acute rejection is detected on follow-up.[100] For refractory acute rejection, a trial of cytolytic therapy is often initiated.[101-103] Other regimens have included aerosolized cyclosporine,[104] alemtuzumab,[105] methotrexate,[106] extracorporeal photopheresis,[107,108] and total lymphoid irradiation.[109]

Airway Complications

Using standard methods of implantation, the donor bronchus is rendered ischemic as the systemic bronchial circulation is interrupted. The donor bronchus thereby relies on collateral pulmonary flow during the first few days after transplantation. Anastomotic complications resulting from airway ischemia include infection, dehiscence, stenosis, and malacia. The reported incidence of these complications is 7% to 14% of patients, although improvements in anastomotic techniques, pulmonary preservation, and care in preserving collateral circulation during harvesting have lessened their occurrence.[110-112]

In a recent review of our experience at Washington University, the rate of airway complications was associated with the time period during which the transplantation was performed. The rate of airway complications during the initial period of the lung transplantation experience at Washington University, from 1988 through 1993, was almost 16%; this decreased to less than 10% during later time periods. Importantly, airway complications did not seem to have an adverse impact on overall survival.[63]

From a technical standpoint, a shortened donor bronchial length (one ring proximal to the upper lobe takeoff) reduces the length of the donor bronchus that is dependent on collateral flow. Peribronchial tissue on the donor bronchus is preserved during preparation of the lung. Telescoping the bronchial anastomosis has not been shown to reduce the rate of airway complications, and we do not use the telescoping technique unless we encounter a significant size mismatch between donor and recipient. Improved techniques of preservation have also resulted in increased bronchial viability after transplantation. Post-transplantation pulmonary parenchymal pathology also compromises collateral flow, rendering the ischemic donor bronchus at increased risk for necrosis and dehiscence. Therefore, pulmonary allograft preservation and adequate postoperative pulmonary blood flow are important. Surprisingly, laboratory evidence points to the beneficial role of steroids in bronchial revascularization and epithelial regeneration.[113,114]

Routine postoperative bronchoscopic surveillance generally provides early evidence that an anastomotic complication is imminent. Computed tomography (CT) is a useful diagnostic tool in the evaluation of documented or suspected donor airway complications. Patients with late airway stenoses present with symptoms of dyspnea, wheeze, or decreased FEV_1. Bronchoscopic assessment confirms the diagnosis.

Failure of Normal Bronchial Healing

Occasionally, patchy areas of superficial necrosis of donor bronchial epithelium are observed. These areas are of no concern and ultimately heal. Minor degrees of bronchial dehiscence are also of little long-term consequence. Membranous wall defects typically heal without airway compromise, whereas cartilaginous defects usually result in some degree of late stricture. Significant dehiscence (greater than 50% of the bronchial circumference) may result in compromise of the airway. This problem should be managed expectantly by laser or mechanical débridement of the area to maintain satisfactory airway patency. A stent can be placed only if the distal main airway remains intact. Occasionally, a significant dehiscence results in direct communication with the pleural space, resulting in pneumothorax and a significant air leak. If the lung remains completely expanded and the pleural space is evacuated, however, the leak will ultimately seal, and the airway may heal without significant stenosis.[115]

Similarly, a dehiscence may communicate directly with the mediastinum, resulting in significant mediastinal emphysema. If the lung remains completely expanded and the pleural space is filled, adequate drainage of the mediastinum can be achieved by placing a drain in close proximity to the anastomotic line by mediastinoscopy. This step will also result in satisfactory healing of the anastomosis, often without stricture.

Surgical revision of the anastomosis is possible only if an adequate length of donor airway is available for resuturing. This procedure is rarely possible, however, if the donor bronchus was cut to an appropriately short length at the time of the initial procedure. Massive dehiscence of the airway with uncontrolled leak or mediastinal contamination has been treated by successful retransplantation.

Necrotic tissue at the bronchial anastomosis is an ideal medium for the growth of saprophytic fungi. These infections can be a significant source of morbidity. In a recent review, Nunley and colleagues found that saprophytic fungal infections involving the bronchial anastomosis occurred in 25% of recipients surviving a minimum of 75 days after transplantation. In 47% of those patients with fungal involvement of the anastomosis, airway complications occurred.[116]

Anastomotic Stenosis

Chronic airway stenoses result from surgical stenosis, granulation tissue, infection, or bronchomalacia, with ischemia as the universal common denominator. Bronchoscopic balloon dilation may be tried as an initial approach, and this may avoid the need for stent placement in these patients.[117] We have used Silastic endobronchial stents for this problem.[118] Daily inhalation of N-acetylcysteine is required, however, to keep the stents patent. Most of these stents have proved to be required only temporarily, as after several months, most patients are able to maintain satisfactory airway patency without a stent. When airways distal to an anastomotic stricture are too small to accept a Silastic stent, or when a Silastic stent will obstruct one bronchus while stenting another, a self-expanding metal stent may be used. However, granulation tissue rapidly overgrows a bare metal mesh stent, sometimes making it impossible to remove. Self-expandable silicone stents have also been used. Treatment of the granulation tissue as a cause of airway stenosis consists of a combination of laser or forceps débridement, dilation, and stenting.[110]

Recurrent airway stenoses have been managed with topical application of mitomycin C,[119] and with high-dose brachytherapy.[120] Finally, if bronchial strictures prove unmanageable by dilation or stent insertion, sleeve resection[121] and retransplantation are available options.[122]

Chronic Rejection—Bronchiolitis Obliterans Syndrome

Chronic rejection of the lung allograft is the major limitation to long-term recipient survival. Five years after transplantation, approximately 50% of recipients have developed chronic rejection,[123] and bronchiolitis obliterans is the histologic hallmark of chronic rejection in the lung allograft (Fig. 14-19). The microscopic picture is characterized by scarring and

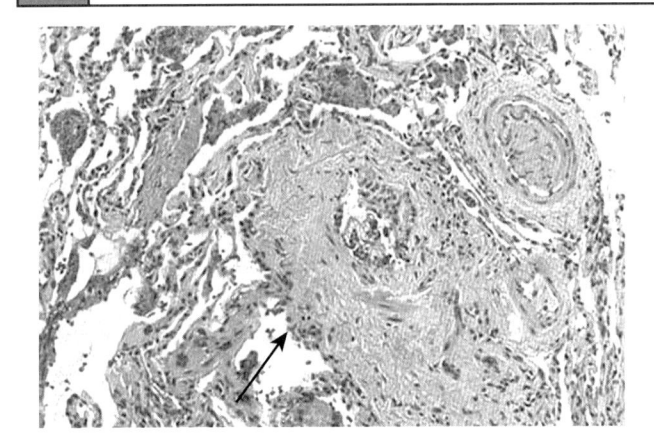

Figure 14–19
Transbronchial lung biopsy showing bronchiolitis obliterans with scarring and fibrosis of the small airways *(arrow)* (H&E stain).

Table 14–2
Criteria* for Bronchiolitis Obliterans Syndrome (BOS)

BOS Score	Degree	Baseline FEV_1(%)
0	None	>90, and FEF_{25-75} > 75%
0-p	Potential	81-90, and/or FEF_{25-75} ≤ 75%
1	Mild	66-80
2	Moderate	51-65
3	Severe	≤50

*Each BOS score has a subcategory noting the histologically documented absence or presence of bronchiolitis obliterans: a indicating "without pathologic evidence of bronchiolitis obliterans," and b indicating "with pathologic evidence of bronchiolitis obliterans."
FEF_{25-75}, forced expiratory flow 25% to 75%; FEV_1, forced expiratory volume in 1 second.
Adapted from Cooper JD, Billingham M, Egan T, et al: J Heart Lung Transplant 1993;**12**:713-6; and Estenne M, Maurer JR, Boehler A, et al: J Heart Lung Transplant 2002;**21**:297-310.

fibrosis of the small airways, with or without an inflammatory component. Because bronchiolitis obliterans is a patchy heterogeneous process, transbronchial biopsy has a sensitivity of only 22% to 73% in the diagnosis of chronic rejection.[124] Because of the difficulty of documenting bronchiolitis obliterans histologically, a clinical deterioration in lung function has been adopted as its surrogate and termed bronchiolitis obliterans syndrome.[125]

The best post-transplant FEV_1 is determined and defined as BOS 0. A decline from this baseline determines the stage of BOS. Importantly, other causes of a decrease in FEV_1 (e.g., infection, acute rejection) must be excluded. Patients cannot receive a diagnosis of BOS until at least 3 months after transplantation. BOS does not require the presence of histologically documented bronchiolitis obliterans. The absence or presence of bronchiolitis obliterans is, however, noted by subcategories "a" and "b," respectively. Table 14-2 shows the currently accepted classification.[126] The FEF_{25-75} is part of the classification and has been shown to be more sensitive than FEV_1 for the detection of early airflow obstruction in bilateral lung transplant recipients,[127] but it has a wide variability with single-lung transplants.

Airway neutrophilia detected on BAL,[127] elevated exhaled nitric oxide fraction,[128] and air trapping on an expiratory CT scan[129] are additional diagnostic tests that indicate BOS. Sharples and colleagues[130] have defined the reported risk factors for BOS as being accepted, potential, or hypothetical based on the available evidence (Box 14-5).

Several recent reports have shown an association between viral respiratory infections and the development of BOS.[81,82] In addition, it has been postulated that chronic aspiration of gastric contents damages the epithelial layer of the lung allograft and contributes to chronic allograft dysfunction.[131] The same group reported that a fundoplication performed early after lung transplantation may reduce the incidence of BOS.

Therapeutic options for established bronchiolitis obliterans are limited, and this condition is generally not reversible. Standard treatment protocols consist of augmenting immunosuppression in an attempt to stabilize the disease process. Regimens such as high-dose corticosteroids, cytolytic therapy, substitution of MMF for azathioprine, and conversion of

Box 14–5
Risk Factors for Bronchiolitis Obliterans or Bronchiolitis Obliterans Syndrome

Definitive Role (Accepted Risk Factors)
- Acute rejection
- Late rejection
- Lymphocytic bronchitis or bronchiolitis
- Late onset

Less Clear Role (Potential Risk Factors)
- Cytomegalovirus
- Other infectious organisms
- Human leukocyte antigen (HLA) matching
- Gastroesophageal reflux disease

Little or No Role (Hypothetical Risk Factors)
- Recipient and donor characteristics

Adapted from Sharples LD, McNeil K, Stewart S, et al. J Heart Lung Transplant 2002;**21**:271-81.

cyclosporine to tacrolimus have on occasion been successful at preserving pulmonary function at a stable level.[132,133] Other therapeutic strategies have included inhaled cyclosporine, inhaled high-dose corticosteroids, and photopheresis. Rapamycin has antiproliferative effects and may also hold some promise in the treatment of BOS. Macrolide antibiotics such as azithromycin and clarithromycin,[134] statins,[135] and IL-2 receptor antagonists[54] may hold promise in altering the outcomes that result from BOS.

Unfortunately, most patients either develop progressive bronchiolitis obliterans or contract a lethal opportunistic infection as a result of the augmented immunosuppression. Retransplantation may be an option in carefully selected patients with BOS. BOS does not appear to occur in an accelerated manner after retransplantation. In the pulmonary retransplant registry, 81% and 56% were free of BOS at 1 and 4 years after retransplantation, respectively.[136]

have reported a 6.8- to 20-fold increased risk of development of PTLD in recipients who were EBV negative before transplantation.[137,144]

When it occurs in the first year after transplantation, PTLD shows a predilection for the thorax and commonly arises in the lung allograft.[137-140] In contrast, when patients present with PTLD after the first year, it is usually extrathoracic, commonly arising in the abdomen and pelvis. In our series, late-occurring abdominal and pelvic PTLD cases were most commonly malignant non-Hodgkin's lymphomas, and despite aggressive therapy, the prognosis was poor. In contrast, patients who presented with early PTLD, unless disseminated at diagnosis, had a favorable prognosis, often responding to simply decreasing immunosuppression.[145]

Treatment of PTLD is based on the stage and progression of disease. Initially, a trial of reduction of immunosuppression is attempted, particularly with disease limited to the allograft. Many also have recommended the simultaneous use of antiviral therapy.[144]

Although chemotherapy (cyclophosphamide, Adriamycin, vincristine, and prednisone [CHOP]) has been used in patients with widespread disease or with progression of disease, treatment-related mortality is considerable. Rituximab, a humanized anti-CD20 monoclonal antibody, is an effective treatment option.[146]

Preventive strategies for children may include matching recipient and donor EBV status, but this is not effective in adults because greater than 90% of the population are EBV positive by the time they are 35 years old. Malouf and colleagues reported that prophylactic use of antiviral therapy may reduce the incidence of PTLD.[147]

Gastrointestinal Complications

Gastrointestinal (GI) complications are frequent in lung transplant recipients, occurring in as many as 50% of patients in some series.[148] Nonsurgical GI complications, including esophagitis, pancreatitis, gastric atony, adynamic colonic ileus, gastroesophageal reflux, peptic ulcer disease, gastritis, GI bleeding, CMV hepatitis, CMV colitis, diverticulitis, cholecystitis, and *Clostridium difficile* colitis or diarrhea, commonly occur in the first month postoperatively, and most patients respond to conservative therapy.

Acute abdominal processes requiring surgical intervention can occur at any point after transplantation and have a reported incidence of 4% to 17% in lung transplant recipients. They include, in decreasing frequency, bowel perforation, appendicitis, cholecystitis, colitis, and pneumatosis intestinalis.[149]

PTLD may present as an acute abdominal process, secondary to intussusception (Fig. 14-21) or bowel perforation. A high index of suspicion is needed for diagnosis, as immunosuppression can mask clinical findings. Emergent operative exploration is associated with significant morbidity and mortality. Elective procedures, however, can be performed safely in this population with acceptable morbidity rates.[150]

RESULTS

Among operative survivors, functional results are excellent. Usually, patients are returned to normal levels of exercise tolerance without oxygen supplementation within 6 to 8 weeks after transplantation. Obstructive pulmonary diseases, such as

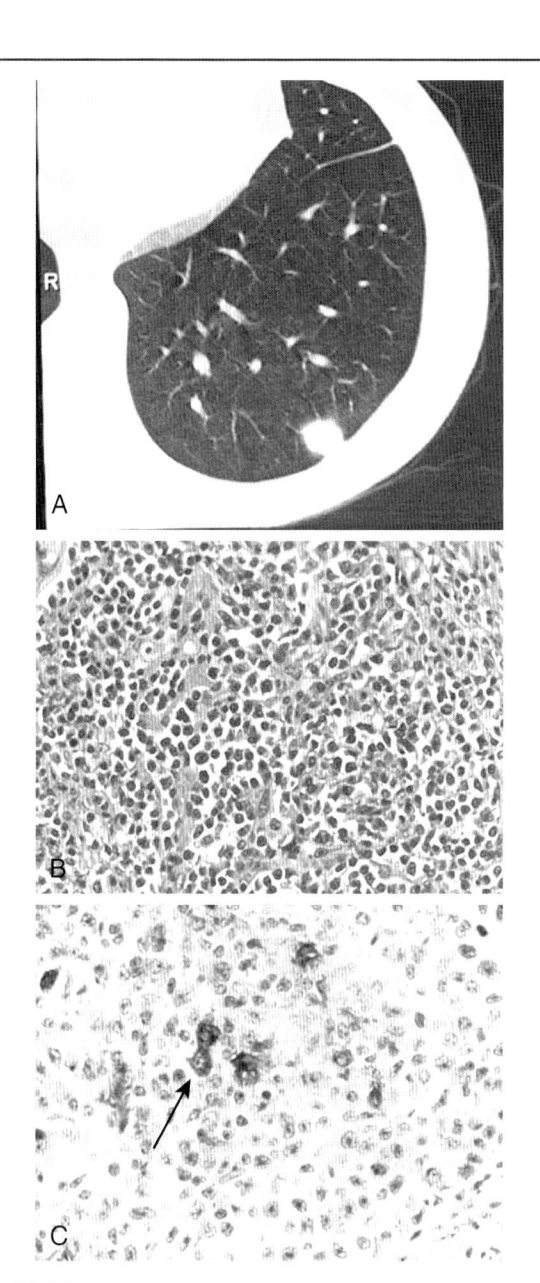

Figure 14–20
A, CT scan of a patient with multiple pulmonary nodules developing several months after bilateral lung transplantation. The patient was found to have post-transplantation lymphoproliferative disease (PTLD). **B,** Histopathologic examination of a post-transplantation lymphoproliferative nodule (H&E stain). **C,** Immunostaining of PTLD nodule positive for Epstein-Barr virus *(arrow)*.

Post-Transplant Lymphoproliferative Disorder

Post-transplant lymphoproliferative disorder is a well-recognized complication after solid-organ and bone marrow transplantation, with an incidence between 4% and 10% after lung transplantation (Fig. 14-20).[137-140] It encompasses a spectrum of disease entities ranging from atypical lymphoid proliferation to malignant non-Hodgkin's lymphoma.[141,142]

Most commonly, the cells are of B-cell origin, and there is an association between PTLD and Epstein-Barr virus (EBV) (see Fig. 14-20).[143] In lung transplant recipients, a strong correlation between negative EBV serology prior to transplantation and the development of PTLD has been reported. Studies chronic obstructive pulmonary disease and α_1-antitrypsin deficiency, are the largest disease-specific experiences in human lung transplantation.[18]

Long-term results of more than 300 patients with emphysema who received transplants at Washington University in St. Louis from 1988 to 2000 have been reported.[151] The overall hospital mortality rate during this 13-year period was 6.2%, but from 1995 to 2000, it was only 3.9%. All patients showed a significant improvement in post-transplantation functional outcomes measured by parameters such as forced vital capacity, FEV_1, and a 6-minute walk test. Overall 5-year survival was 58.6% ± 3.5%, with emphysema patients who received bilateral lung transplants having a significantly better 5-year survival than single-lung transplant recipients. Actuarial survival also improved in the latter period (1995 to 2000) compared with 1988 to 1994. Only single-lung transplantation and use of CPB were found to correlate with poor long-term survival.

A number of centers have reported satisfactory results with the application of bilateral lung transplantations in patients with septic lung disease. Ramirez and colleagues, from Toronto, reported excellent gas exchange, pulmonary function, and exercise capabilities among operative survivors.[152]

The Washington University experience is similar, with overall survival comparable with that of patients with other indications for lung transplantation. Fibrotic lung diseases such as IPF have been the indication for lung transplantation in more than one third of all patients transplanted at our center since revision of the allocation system. The long-term survival appears to be somewhat less than that of patients with other diagnoses at early and later time points (Fig. 14-22). Early mortality is probably affected by the complexity of transplants in fibrotic patients, whereas the late mortality may be affected by the older age of recipients relative to those transplanted for cystic fibrosis, PPH, or α_1-antitrypsin deficiency.[18] Most recent data from the ISHLT Registry, however, now demonstrate an increased survival for bilateral lung transplants in recipients with fibrotic lung disease.[18]

From 1989 to 2001, our program performed 100 transplantations for either PPH or secondary pulmonary hypertension, with 55 adult and 45 pediatric recipients of 51 bilateral-lung, 39 single-lung, and 10 combined heart–lung transplantations.[153] The overall hospital mortality rate in this complicated group of patients was 17%, with a mortality rate of 10.4%

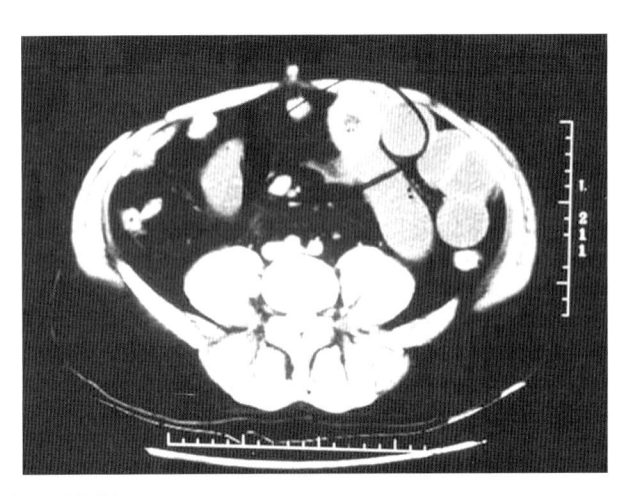

Figure 14–21
CT scan from a patient with small bowel intussusception secondary to post-transplantation lymphoproliferative disease.

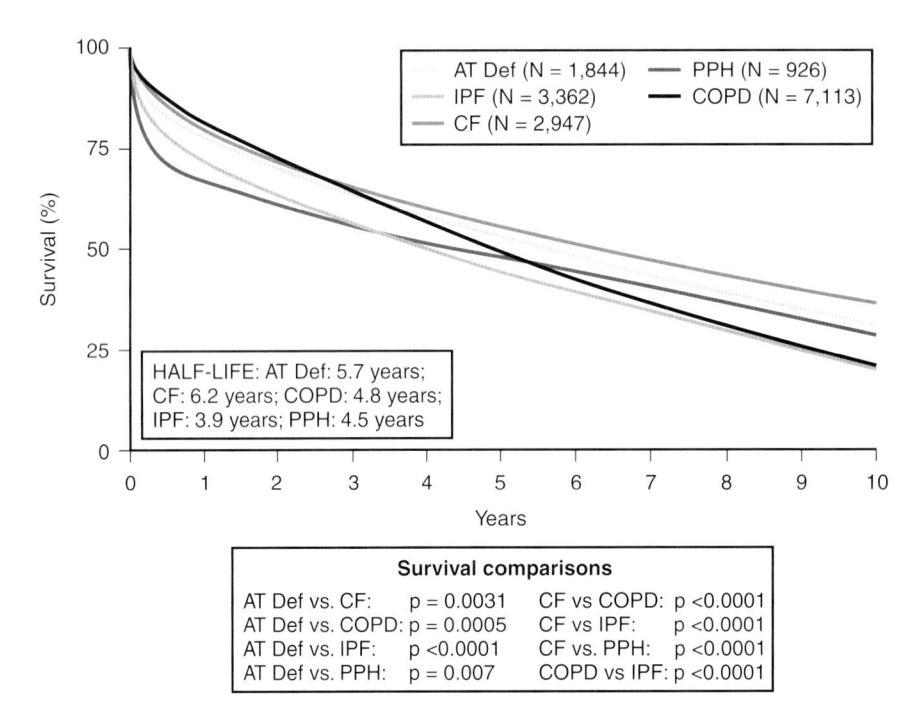

Figure 14–22
Kaplan-Meier survival curves by diagnosis for adult lung transplantations performed between January 1994 and June 2004. AT Def, α_1-antitrypsin deficiency emphysema; CF, cystic fibrosis; COPD, chronic obstructive pulmonary disease; IPF, idiopathic pulmonary fibrosis; PPH, primary pulmonary hypertension. *(From Trulock EP, Christie JD, Edwards LB, et al. Registry of the International Society of Heart and Lung Transplantation: Twenty-fourth Official Adult Lung and Heart-Lung Transplantation Report—2007.* J Heart Lung Transplant 2007;**26**:782-95.)

among those transplanted for PPH and 23.1% among those transplanted for secondary pulmonary hypertension. The morbidity rate was also significantly higher in comparison with patients transplanted for emphysema: almost 25% of patients required reoperation for bleeding, 24% required reintubation, 17% required tracheostomy for prolonged ventilator support, and 16% required ECMO support. Among the surviving patients, there was a significant and sustained improvement in right ventricular function as well as pulmonary artery pressure and resistance. ISHLT Registry data have demonstrated a trend toward improved survival for bilateral versus single-lung transplants in patients with PPH.[18] The standard operation previously offered these patients, combined heart–lung transplantation, has been practiced less frequently due to organ shortages.

PEDIATRIC LUNG TRANSPLANTATION

Lung transplantation was expanded to the pediatric population in a judicious manner in the late 1980s. The number of lung transplantations for recipients younger than 18 years of age was 67 for the year 2004, as reported by the ISHLT.[154] This number has remaided stable over the past decade and represents a small proportion of the total lung transplantation procedures performed. The most common indication for lung transplantation in infants (<1 year) is congenital heart disease, representing 32% of the procedures performed in this age group between 1991 and 2006. Other indications in this age group include PPH, pulmonary vascular disease, and pulmonary alveolar proteinosis. In the group between 1 and 10 years of age, 54% of lung transplantations were performed for cystic fibrosis from 1991 to 2006; other indications include PPH, congenital heart disease, and retransplantations for obliterative bronchiolitis. CF is the predominant indication for lung transplantation in teenagers between 11 and 17 years of age, accounting for about 70% of procedures performed in this age group. The lung allocation system has recently been revised, and currently lungs are allocated to potential recipients younger than 12 years of age on the basis of waiting time on the transplant list. Potential recipients aged 12 to 17 years are prioritized based on their lung allocation score.[155]

Approximately 40% of pediatric lung transplant recipients survive 5 years. Bilateral lung transplant recipients show an improved survival compared with single-lung transplant recipients, but this may be an effect of underlying disease and other recipient factors. The vast majority of pediatric lung transplants are bilateral (89%). As in adults, early mortality after pediatric lung transplantation is secondary to infections and graft failure, and late mortality is attributed mostly to bronchiolitis obliterans, with greater than 50% developing bronchiolitis obliterans by 5 years.[156]

Only 20 to 30 centers are currently performing pediatric lung transplants. Our center began its pediatric lung transplant program in July 1990 and performed its first infant lung transplant in 1993. Now the largest pediatric lung transplant program worldwide, our center has performed 265 pediatric transplants since its inception. Of these, 203 have been bilateral, 39 bilateral lobar (living donor), 14 heart–lung, and 9 single-lung transplants (St. Louis Children's Hospital Lung Transplant Registry; Huddleston, personal communication). The indications for lung transplantation were, in decreasing order, cystic fibrosis (42%), pulmonary vascular disease (21%), bronchiolitis obliterans (10%), pulmonary alveolar proteinosis (6%), pulmonary fibrosis (7%), and other (12%). The average age of recipients at the time of transplantation was 9.5 ± 5.9 years. Actuarial survival at our center was 77% at 1 year, 62% at 3 years, and 55% at 5 years. The most common cause of early mortality was graft failure. Late mortality was most commonly secondary to bronchiolitis obliterans (57%), infection (21%), and post-transplant malignancies (18%).[157]

SUMMARY

Lung transplantation is an effective therapeutic option for selected patients with end-stage pulmonary disease. The use of marginal donors, non-beating-heart donors and ex vivo lung perfusion has been implemented in an attempt to increase the donor pool. Lung preservation and immunosuppression strategies continue to evolve. Extensive research efforts are underway to find methods to overcome chronic rejection and prolong survival in clinical lung transplantation.

REFERENCES

1. Toronto Lung Transplantation Group. Unilateral lung transplantation for pulmonary fibrosis. *N Engl J Med* 1986;**314**:1140-5.
2. Demikhov VP. *Experimental Transplantation of Vital Organs (authorized translation from the Russian by Basil Haigh)*. New York: Consultants Bureau Enterprises; 1962.
3. Konstantinov IE. A mystery of Vladimir P. Demikhov: The 50th anniversary of the first intrathoracic transplantation. *Ann Thorac Surg* 1998;**65**:1171-7.
4. Hardy JD, Webb WR, Dalton ML, et al. Lung homotransplantation in man. *JAMA* 1963;**186**:1065-74.
5. Wildevuur CR, Benfield JR. A review of 23 human lung transplantations by 20 surgeons. *Ann Thorac Surg* 1970;**9**:489-515.
6. Derom F, Barbier F, et al. Ten month survival after lung homotransplantation in man. *J Thorac Cardiovasc Surg* 1971;**61**:835-46.
7. Nelems W. Human lung transplantation. *Chest* 1980;**78**:569-73.
8. Lima O, Cooper JD, Peters WJ, et al. Effects of methylprednisolone and azathioprine on bronchial healing following lung autotransplantation. *J Thorac Cardiovasc Surg* 1981;**82**:211-5.
9. Lima O, Goldberg M, Peters WJ, et al. Bronchial omentopexy in canine lung transplantation. *J Thorac Cardiovasc Surg* 1982;**83**:418-21.
10. Patterson GA, Cooper JD, Goldman B, et al. Technique of successful clinical double-lung transplantation. *Ann Thorac Surg* 1988;**45**:626-33.
11. Pasque MK, Cooper JD, Kaiser LR, et al. An improved technique for bilateral lung transplantation: rationale and initial clinical experience. *Ann Thorac Surg* 1990;**49**:785-91.
12. Mal N, Andreassian B, Pamela F, et al. Unilateral lung transplantation in end-stage pulmonary emphysema. *Am Rev Respir Dis* 1989;**140**:797-802.
13. Pasque MK, Trulock EP, Kaiser LR, et al. Single-lung transplantation for pulmonary hypertension: three month hemodynamic follow-up. *Circulation* 1991;**84**:2275-9.
14. Starnes VA, Lewiston NJ, Luikart H, et al. Current trends in lung transplantation: lobar transplantation and expanded uses of single lungs. *J Thorac Cardiovasc Surg* 1992;**104**:1060-5.
15. Couetil JA, Tolan MJ, Loulmet DF, et al. Pulmonary bipartitioning and lobar transplantation: a new approach to donor organ shortage. *J Thorac Cardiovasc Surg* 1997;**113**:529-37.
16. Steen S, Sjoberg T, Pierre L, et al. Transplantation of lungs from a non-heart-beating donor. *Lancet* 2001;**357**:825-9.
17. Maurer JR, Frost AE, Estenne M, et al. International guidelines for selection of lung transplant candidates. *J Heart Lung Transplant* 1998;**17**:703-9.
18. Trulock EP, Christie JD, et al. Registry of the International Society for Heart and Lung Transplantation: twenty-fourth official adult lung and heart-lung transplantation report-2007. *J Heart Lung Transplant* 2007;**26**:782-95.
19. Etienne B, Bertocchi M, et al. Successful double-lung transplantation for bronchioalveolar carcinoma. *Chest* 1997;**112**:1423-4.
20. Zorn GI, McGiffin DC, et al. Pulmonary transplantation for advanced bronchioloalveolar carcinoma. *J Thorac Cardiovasc Surg* 2003;**125**:45-8.

21. Organ Procurement and Transplantation Network. Available at http://optn.transplant.hrsa.gov/PoliciesandBylaws2/policies/pdfs/policy_9.pdf.
22. Meyers BF, Patterson GA. Lung transplantation versus lung volume reduction as surgical therapy for emphysema. *World J Surg* 2001;**25**:238-43.
23. Meyers BF, Yusen RD, Guthrie TJ, et al. Outcome of bilateral lung volume reduction in patients with emphysema potentially eligible for lung transplantation. *J Thorac Cardiovasc Surg* 2001;**122**:10-7.
24. Kerem E, Reisman J, et al. Prediction of mortality in patients with cystic fibrosis. *N Engl J Med* 1992;**326**:1187-91.
25. Aris RM, Routh JC, LiPuma JJ, et al. Lung transplantation for cystic fibrosis patients with Burkholderia cepacia complex: survival linked to genomovar type. *Am J Respir Crit Care Med* 2001;**164**:2102-6.
26. Chaparro C, Maurer J, Gutierrez C, et al. Infection with Burkholderia cepacia in cystic fibrosis: outcome following lung transplantation. *Am J Respir Crit Care Med* 2001;**163**:43-8.
27. Meyers BF. Single versus bilateral lung transplantation for pulmonary fibrosis: a ten year institutional experience. *J Thorac Cardiovasc Surg* 2000;**120**:99-107.
28. McLaughlin VV, Genthner DE, Panella MM, et al. Reduction in pulmonary vascular resistance with long-term epoprostenol (prostacyclin) therapy in primary pulmonary hypertension. *N Engl J Med* 1998;**338**:273-7.
29. McLaughlin VV, McGoon MD. Pulmonary artery hypertension. *Circulation* 2006;**114**:1417-31.
30. Charman SC, Sharples LD, McNeil KD, et al. Assessment of survival benefit after lung transplantation by patient diagnosis. *J Heart Lung Transplant* 2002;**21**:226-32.
31. De Meester J, Smits JM, Persijn GG, et al. Listing for lung transplantation: life expectancy and transplant effect, stratified by type of end-stage lung disease, the Eurotransplant experience. *J Heart Lung Transplant* 2001;**20**:518-24.
32. Hertz MI, Taylor DO, Trulock EP, et al. The registry of the International Society for Heart and Lung Transplantation: nineteenth official report—2002. *J Heart Lung Transplant* 2002;**21**:950-70.
33. Sundaresan S, Trulock EP, et al. Prevalence and outcome of bronchiolitis obliterans syndrome after lung transplantation. *Ann Thorac Surg* 1995;**60**:1341-7.
34. Barbers RG. Cystic fibrosis: bilateral living lobar versus cadaveric lung transplantation. *Am J Med Sci* 1998;**315**:155-60.
35. Gamez P, Cordoba M, et al. Lung transplantation from out-of-hospital non-heart-beating lung donors: one-year experience and results. *J Heart Lung Transplant* 2005;**24**:1098-102.
36. de Antonio DG, Marcos R, Laporta R, et al. Results of clinical lung transplant from uncontrolled non-heart-beating donors. *J Heart Lung Transplant* 2007;**26**:529-34.
37. Steen S, Ingemansson R, Eriksson L, et al. First human transplantation of a nonacceptable donor lung after reconditioning ex vivo. *Ann Thorac Surg* 2007;**83**:2191-5.
38. Sundaresan S, Trachiotis GD, Aoe M, Patterson GA, Cooper JD. Donor lung procurement: assessment and operative technique. *Ann Thorac Surg* 1993;**56**:1409-13.
39. Kofidis T, Strüber M, Warnecke G, et al. Antegrade versus retrograde perfusion of the donor lung: impact on the early reperfusion phase. *Transplant Int* 2003;**16**:801-5.
40. Casula RP, Stoica SC, Wallwork J, et al. Pulmonary vein augmentation for single lung transplantation. *Ann Thorac Surg* 2001;**71**:1373-4.
41. Oto T, Rabinov M, Negri J, et al. Techniques of reconstruction for inadequate donor left atrial cuff in lung transplantation. *Ann Thorac Surg* 2006;**81**:1199-204.
42. Sekine Y, Fischer S, de Perrot M, et al. Bilateral lung transplantation using a donor with a tracheal right upper lobe bronchus. *Ann Thorac Surg* 2002;**73**:308-10.
43. Serra E, et al. Transesophageal echocardiography during lung transplantation. *Transplant Proc* 2007;**39**:1981-2.
44. Meyers BF, Sundaresan RS, Guthrie T, et al. Bilateral sequential lung transplantation without sternal division eliminates posttransplantation sternal complications. *J Thorac Cardiovasc Surg* 1999;**117**:358-64.
45. Pochettino A, Bavaria JE. Anterior axillary muscle-sparing thoracotomy for lung transplantation. *Ann Thorac Surg* 1997;**64**:1846-8.
46. Toyoda Y. Lung transplantation through minimally invasive approach. *J Heart Lung Transplant* 2008;**27**:S197.
47. Meyer AL, Avsar M, Gottlieb J, et al. Use of cardiopulmonary bypass in patients undergoing minimally invasive bilateral lung transplantation. *J Heart Lung Transplant* 2008;**27**:S198.
48. Aigner C, Jaksch P, Seebacher G, et al. Single running suture—the new standard technique for bronchial anastomoses in lung transplantation. *Eur J Cardiothorac Surg* 2003;**23**:488-93.
49. Barr ML, Schenkel FA, Bowdish ME, et al. Living donor lobar lung transplantation: current status and future directions. *Transplant Proc* 2005;**37**:3983-6.
50. Artemiou O, Birsan T, Taghavi S, et al. Bilateral lobar transplantation with the split lung technique. *J Thorac Cardiovasc Surg* 1999;**118**:369–360.
51. Davis Jr RD, Trulock EP, Manley J, et al. Differences in early results after single lung transplantation. *Ann Thorac Surg* 1994;**58**:1327-35.
52. Kroshus TJ, Kshettry VR, Savik K, et al. Risk factors for the development of bronchiolitis obliterans syndrome after lung transplantation. *J Thorac Cardiovasc Surg* 1997;**114**:195-202.
53. Todd TR, Perron J, Winton TL, et al. Simultaneous single-lung transplantation and lung volume reduction. *Ann Thorac Surg* 1997;**63**:1468-70.
54. Brock MV, Borja MC, Ferber L, et al. Induction therapy in lung transplantation: a prospective, controlled clinical trial comparing OKT3, anti-thymocyte globulin, and daclizumab. *J Heart Lung Transplant* 2001;**20**:1282-90.
55. Burton CM, Andersen CB, et al. The incidence of acute cellular rejection after lung transplantation: a comparative study of anti-thymocyte globulin and daclizumab. *J Heart Lung Transplant* 2006;**25**:638-47.
56. Snell GI, Westall GP. Immunosuppression for lung transplantation: evidence to date. *Drugs* 2007;**67**:1531-9.
57. Corris P, Glanville A, McNeil K, et al. One year analysis of an ongoing international randomized study of mycophenolate mofetil (MMF) vs azathioprine (AZA) in lung transplantation. *J Heart Lung Transplant* 2001;**20**:149-50.
58. Palmer SM, Baz MA, Sanders L, et al. Results of a randomized, prospective, multicenter trial of mycophenolate mofetil versus azathioprine in the prevention of acute lung allograft rejection. *Transplantation* 2001;**71**(12):1772-6.
59. Snell GI, Valentine VG, Vitulo P. Everolimus versus azathioprine in maintenance lung transplant recipients: an international, randomized, double-blind clinical trial. *Am J Transplant* 2006;**6**:169-77.
60. Ettinger NA, Bailey TC, Trulock EP, et al. Cytomegalovirus infection and pneumonitis: impact after isolation lung transplantation. *Am Rev Respir Dis* 1993;**147**:1017-23.
61. Force SD, Miller DL, Pelaez A, et al. Outcomes of delayed chest closure after bilateral lung transplantation. *Ann Thorac Surg* 2006;**81**:2020-4.
62. Haydock DA, Trulock EP, et al. Management of dysfunction in the transplanted lung: experience with 7 clinical cases. *Ann Thorac Surg* 1992;**53**:635-41.
63. Meyers BF, de la Morena M, et al. Primary graft dysfunction and other selected complications of lung transplantation: a single-center experience of 983 patients. *J Thorac Cardiovasc Surg* 2005;**129**:1421-9.
64. Christie JD, Carby M, Christie JD, Carby M, Bag R, Corris P, et al. Report of the ISHLT Working Group on Primary Lung Graft Dysfunction part II: definition. A consensus statement of the International Society for Heart and Lung Transplantation. *J Heart Lung Transplant* 2005;**24**:1454-9.
65. De Perrot M, Sekine Y, et al. Interleukin-8 release during early reperfusion predicts graft function in human lung transplantation. *Am J Respir Crit Care Med* 2002;**165**:211-5.
66. Date H, Triantafillou AN, Trulock EP, et al. Inhaled nitric oxide reduces human lung allograft dysfunction. *J Thorac Cardiovasc Surg* 1996;**111**:913-9.
67. Fiser SM, Cope JT, Kron IL, et al. Aerosolized prostacyclin (epoprostenol) as an alternative to inhaled nitric oxide for patients with reperfusion injury after lung transplantation. *J Thorac Cardiovasc Surg* 2001;**121**:981-2.
68. Chen C, Gallagher RC, Ardery P, et al. Retrograde flush and cold storage for twenty-two to twenty-five hours lung preservation with and without prostaglandin E1. *J Heart Lung Transplant* 1997;**16**:658-66.
69. Venuta F, Rendina EA, Bufi M, et al. Preimplantation retrograde pneumoplegia in clinical lung transplantation. *J Thorac Cardiovasc Surg* 1999;**118**:107-14.
70. Lick SD, Brown Jr PS, Kurusz M, et al. Technique of controlled reperfusion of the transplanted lung in humans. *Ann Thorac Surg* 2000;**69**:910-2.
71. Chaparro C, Kesten S. Infections in lung transplant recipients. *Clin Chest Med* 1997;**18**:339-51.
72. Avery RK. Infections after lung transplantation. *Semin Respir Crit Care Med* 2006;**27**:544-51.
73. de Perrot M, Chaparro C, McRae K, et al. Twenty-year experience of lung transplantation at a single center: influence of recipient diagnosis on long-term survival. *J Thorac Cardiovasc Surg* 2004;**127**:1493-501.
74. Ruiz I, Gavaldà J, Monforte V, et al. Donor-to-host transmission of bacterial and fungal infections in lung transplantation. *Am J Transplant* 2006;**6**:178-82.
75. Bassiri AG, Girgis RE, Theodore S. Actinomyces odontolyticus thoracopulmonary infections: two cases in lung and heart-lung transplant recipients and review of the literature. *Chest* 1996;**109**:1109-11.
76. Gutierrez CA, Chaparro C, Krajden M, et al. Cytomegalovirus viremia in lung transplant recipients receiving ganciclovir and immune globulin. *Chest* 1998;**113**:924-32.
77. Snydman DR. Infections in solid organ transplantation. *Transplant Infect Dis* 1999;**1**:21-8.

78. Humar A, Kumar D, Preiksaitis J, et al. A trial of valganciclovir prophylaxis for cytomegalovirus prevention in lung transplant recipients. *Am J Transplant* 2005;**5**:1462-8.
79. Holt ND, Gould FK, Taylor CE, et al. Incidence and significance of noncytomegalovirus viral respiratory infection after adult lung transplantation. *J Heart Lung Transplant* 1997;**16**:416-9.
80. Chakinala MM, Walter MJ. Community acquired respiratory viral infections after lung transplantation: clinical features and long-term consequences. *Semin Thorac Cardiovasc Surg* 2004;**16**:342-9.
81. Billings JL, Hertz MI, Savik K, et al. Respiratory viruses and chronic rejection in lung transplant recipients. *J Heart Lung Transplant* 2002;**21**:559-66.
82. Khalifah AP, Hachem RR, Chakinala MM, et al. Respiratory viral infections are a distinct risk for bronchiolitis obliterans syndrome and death. *Am J Respir Crit Care Med* 2004;**170**:181-7.
83. Kanj SS, Welty-Wolf K, Madden J, et al. Fungal infections in lung and heart-lung transplant recipients. *Medicine* 1996;**75**:142-56.
84. Hadjiliadis D, Howell DN, Davis RD, et al. Anastomotic infections in lung transplant recipients. *Ann Transplant* 2000;**5**:13-9.
85. Palmer SM, Perfect JR, Howell DN, et al. Candidal anastomotic infection in lung transplant recipients: successful treatment with a combination of systemic and inhaled antifungal agents. *J Heart Lung Transplant* 1998;**17**:1029-33.
86. Cahill BC, Hibbs JR, Savik K, et al. Aspergillus airway colonization and invasive disease after lung transplantation. *Chest* 1997;**112**:1160-4.
87. Hadjiliadis D, Sporn TA, Perfect JR, et al. Outcome of lung transplantation in patients with mycetomas. *Chest* 2002;**121**:128-34.
88. Trulock EP. Lung transplantation. *Am J Respir Crit Care Med* 1997;**155**:789-818.
89. De Hoyos A, Chamberlain D, Schvartzman R, et al. Prospective assessment of a standardized pathologic grading system for acute rejection in lung transplantation. *Chest* 1993;**103**:1813-8.
90. Hopkins PM, Aboyoun CL, Chhajed PN, et al. Prospective analysis of 1,235 transbronchial lung biopsies in lung transplant recipients. *J Heart Lung Transplant* 2002;**21**:1062-7.
91. Trulock EP, Ettinger NA, Brunt EM, et al. The role of transbronchial lung biopsy in the treatment of lung transplant recipients: an analysis of 200 consecutive procedures. *Chest* 1992;**102**:1049-54.
92. Jones HA, Donovan T, Goddard MJ, et al. Use of 18FDG-pet to discriminate between infection and rejection in lung transplant recipients. *Transplantation* 2004;**77**:1462-4.
93. Shi R, Yang J, Jaramillo A, et al. Correlation between interleukin-15 and granzyme B expression and acute lung allograft rejection. *Transpl Immunol* 2004;**12**:103-8.
94. Stewart S, Fishbein MC, Snell GI, et al. Revision of the 1996 working formulation for the standardization of nomenclature in the diagnosis of lung rejection. *J Heart Lung Transplant* 2007;**26**:1229-42.
95. Keenan RJ, Konishi H, Kawai A, et al. Clinical trial of tacrolimus versus cyclosporine in lung transplantation. *Ann Thorac Surg* 1995;**60**:580-4.
96. Treede H, Klepetko W, Reichenspurner H, et al. Tacrolimus versus cyclosporine after lung transplantation: a prospective, open, randomized two-center trial comparing two different immunosuppressive protocols. *J Heart Lung Transplant* 2001;**20**:511-7.
97. Horning NR, Lynch JP, Sundaresan SR, et al. Tacrolimus therapy for persistent or recurrent acute rejection after lung transplantation. *J Heart Lung Transplant* 1998;**17**:761-7.
98. Vitulo P, Oggionni T, Cascina A, et al. Efficacy of tacrolimus rescue therapy in refractory acute rejection after lung transplantation. *J Heart Lung Transplant* 2002;**21**:435-9.
99. Sollinger HW, Group USRTMMS. Mycophenolate mofetil for the prevention of acute rejection in primary cadaveric renal allograft recipients. *Transplantation* 1995;**60**:225-32.
100. Aboyoun CL, Tamm M, Chhajed PN, et al. Diagnostic value of follow-up transbronchial lung biopsy after lung rejection. *Am J Respir Crit Care Med* 2001;**164**:460-3.
101. Barlow CW, Moon MR, Green GR, et al. Rabbit antithymocyte globulin versus OKT3 induction therapy after heart-lung and lung transplantation: effect on survival, rejection, infection, and obliterative bronchiolitis. *Transplant Int* 2001;**14**:234-9.
102. Palmer SM, Miralles AP, Lawrence CM, et al. Rabbit antithymocyte globulin decreases acute rejection after lung transplantation: results of a randomized, prospective study. *Chest* 1999;**116**:127-33.
103. Sheenib H, Massard G, Reynaud M, et al. Efficacy of OKT3 therapy for acute rejection in isolated lung transplantation. *J Heart Lung Transplant* 1994;**13**:514-9.
104. Iacono AT, Smaldone GC, Keenan RJ, et al. Dose-related reversal of acute lung rejection by aerosolized cyclosporine. *Am J Respir Crit Care Med* 1997;**155**:1690-8.
105. Reams BD, Davis RD, Curl J, et al. Treatment of refractory acute rejection in a lung transplant recipient with campath 1H. *Transplantation* 2002;**74**:903-4.
106. Cahill BC, O'Rourke MK, Strasburg KA, et al. Methotrexate for lung transplant recipients with steroid-resistant acute rejection. *J Heart Lung Transplant* 1996;**15**:1130-7.
107. Andreu G, Achkar A, Couetil JP, et al. Extracorporeal photochemotherapy treatment for acute lung rejection episode. *J Heart Lung Transplant* 1995;**14**:793-6.
108. Villanueva J, Bhorade SM, Robinson JA, et al. Extracorporeal photopheresis for the treatment of lung allograft rejection. *Ann Transplant* 2000;**5**:44-7.
109. Valentine VG, Robbins RC, Wehner JH, et al. Total lymphoid irradiation for refractory acute rejection in heart-lung and lung allografts. *Chest* 1996;**109**:1184-9.
110. Chhajed PN, Malouf MA, Tamm M, et al. Interventional bronchoscopy for the management of airway complications following lung transplantation. *Chest* 2001;**120**:1894-9.
111. Griffith BP, Hardesty RL, Armitage JM, et al. A decade of lung transplantation. *Ann Surg* 1993;**218**:310-8.
112. Shennib H, Massard G. Airway complications in lung transplantation. *Ann Thorac Surg* 1994;**57**:506-11.
113. Davreux CJ, Chu NH, Waddell TK, et al. Improved tracheal allograft viability in immunosuppressed rats. *Ann Thorac Surg* 1993;**55**:131-4.
114. Inui K, Schäfers HJ, Aoki M, et al. Bronchial circulation after experimental lung transplantation: the effect of long term administration of prednisolone: *J Thorac Cardiovasc Surg* 1993;**105**:474-9.
115. Patterson GA. Airway complications. *Chest Surg Clin North Am* 1993;**3**:157-66.
116. Nunley DR, Gal AA, Vega JD, et al. Saprophytic fungal infections and complications involving the bronchial anastomosis following human lung transplantation. *Chest* 2002;**122**:1185-91.
117. DeGracia J, Culebras M, Alvarez A, et al. Bronchoscopic balloon dilatation in the management of bronchial stenosis following lung transplantation. *Respir Med* 2007;**101**:27-33.
118. Cooper JD, Pearson FG, Patterson GA, et al. Use of silicone stents in the management of airway problems. *Ann Thorac Surg* 1989;**47**:371-8.
119. Erard AC, Monnier P, Spiliopoulos A, et al. Mitomycin C for control of recurrent bronchial stenosis: a case report. *Chest* 2001;**120**:2103-5.
120. Halkos ME, Godette KD, Lawrence EC, et al. High dose rate brachytherapy in the management of lung transplant airway stenosis. *Ann Thorac Surg* 2003;**76**:381-4.
121. Marulli G, Loy M, Rizzardi G, et al. Surgical treatment of posttransplant bronchial stenoses: case reports. *Transplant Proc.* 2007;**39**(6):1973-5.
122. Novick RJ, Stitt LW, Al-Kattan K, et al. Pulmonary retransplantation: predictors of graft function and survival in 230 patients. *Ann Thorac Surg* 1998;**65**:227-34.
123. Hertz MI, Taylor DO, Trulock EP, et al. The registry of the International Society for Heart and Lung Transplantation: nineteenth official report—2002. *J Heart Lung Transplant* 2002;**21**:950-70.
124. Swanson SJ, Mentzer SJ, Reily JJ. Surveillance transbronchial lung biopsies: implication for survival after lung transplantation. *J Thorac Cardiovasc Surg* 2000;**119**:27-37.
125. Cooper JD, Billingham M, Egan T, et al. A working formulation for the standardization of nomenclature and for clinical staging of chronic dysfunction in lung allografts. *J Heart Lung Transplant* 1993;**12**:713-6.
126. Estenne M, Maurer JR, Boehler A, et al. Bronchiolitis obliterans syndrome 2001: an update of the diagnostic criteria. *J Heart Lung Transplant* 2002;**21**:297-310.
127. Reynaud-Gaubert M, Thomas P, Badier M, et al. Early detection of airway involvement in obliterative bronchiolitis after lung transplantation: functional and bronchoalveolar lavage cell findings. *Am J Resp Care Med* 2000;**161**:1924-9.
128. Gabbay E, Walters EH, Orsida B, et al. Post-lung transplant bronchiolitis obliterans syndrome (BOS) is characterized by increased exhaled nitric oxide levels and epithelial inducible nitric oxide synthase. *Am J Resp Care Med* 2000;**162**:2182-7.
129. Bankier AA, Van Muylem AV, Knoop PC, et al. Bronchiolitis obliterans syndrome in heart-lung transplant recipients: diagnosis with expiratory CT. *Radiology* 2001;**218**:533-9.
130. Sharples LD, McNeil K, Stewart S, et al. Risk factors for bronchiolitis obliterans: a systematic review of recent publications. *J Heart Lung Transplant* 2002;**21**:271-81.
131. Cantu 3rd E, Appel 3rd JZ, Hartwig MG, et al. J. Maxwell Chamberlain Memorial Paper. Early fundoplication prevents chronic allograft dysfunction in patients with gastroesophageal reflux disease. *Ann Thorac Surg* 2004;**78**:1142-51.
132. Ross DJ, Lewis MI, Kramer M, et al. FK 506 'rescue' immunosuppression for obliterative bronchiolitis after lung transplantation. *Chest* 1997;**112**:1175-9.
133. Ross DJ, Waters PF, Levine M, et al. Mycophenolate mofetil versus azathioprine immunosuppressive regimens after lung transplantation: preliminary experience. *J Heart Lung Transplant* 1998;**17**:768-74.

134. O'Hagan AR, Stillwell PC, Arroliga A, et al. Photopheresis in the treatment of refractory bronchiolitis obliterans complicating lung transplantation. *Chest* 1999;**115**:1459-62.
135. Johnson BA, Lacono AT, Zeevi A, et al. Statin use is associated with improved function and survival of lung allografts. *A J Resp Care Med* 2003;**167**:1271-8.
136. Novick RJ, Stitt LW, Al-Kattan K, et al. Pulmonary retransplantation: predictors of graft function and survival in 230 patients. *Ann Thorac Surg* 1998;**65**:227-34.
137. Aris RM, Maia DM, Neuriner IP, et al. Post-transplantation lymphoproliferative disorder in the Epstein-Barr virus-naïve lung transplant recipient. *Am J Respir Crit Care Med* 1996;**154**:1712-7.
138. Armitage JM, Kormos RL, Stuart RS, et al. Posttransplant lymphoproliferative disease in thoracic organ transplant patients: ten years of cyclosporine-based immunosuppression. *J Heart Lung Transplant* 1991;**10**:877-86.
139. Levine SM, Angel L, Anzueto A, et al. A low incidence of posttransplant lymphoproliferative disorder in 109 lung transplant recipients. *Chest* 1999;**116**:1273-7.
140. Paranjothi S, Yusen RD, Kraus MD, et al. Lymphoproliferative disease after lung transplantation: comparison of presentation and outcome of early and late cases. *J Heart Lung Transplant* 2001;**20**:1054-63.
141. Schaar CG, Van Der Pijl JW, Van Hoek B, et al. Successful outcome with a "quintuple approach" of posttransplant lymphoproliferative disorder. *Transplantation* 2001;**71**:47-52.
142. Swedlow SH. Classification of the posttransplant lymphoproliferative disorders: from the past to the present. *Semin Diag Pathol* 1997;**14**:2-7.
143. Montone KT, Litzky LA, Wurster A, et al. Analysis of Epstein-Barr virus associated posttransplantation lymphoproliferative disorder after lung transplantation. *Surgery* 1996;**119**:544-51.
144. Wigle DA, Chaparro C, Humar A, et al. Epstein-Barr virus serology and posttransplant lymphoproliferative disease in lung transplantation. *Transplantation* 2001;**72**:1783-6.
145. Hachem R, Patterson G-A, Trulock EP. Abdominal-pelvic lymphoproliferative disease after lung transplantation. *J Heart Lung Transplant* 2003;**22**:S194.
146. Verschuuren EA, Stevens SJ, van Imhoff GW, et al. Treatment of posttransplant lymphoproliferative disease with rituximab: the remission, the relapse, and the complication. *Transplantation* 2002;**73**:100-4.
147. Malouf MA, Chhajed PN, Hopkins P, et al. Anti-viral prophylaxis reduces the incidence of lymphoproliferative disease in lung transplant recipients. *J Heart Lung Transplant* 2002;**21**:547-54.
148. Lubetkin EI, Lipson DA, Palevsky HI, et al. GI complications after orthotopic lung transplantation. *Am J Gastroenterol* 1996;**91**:2382-90.
149. Hoekstra HJ, Hawkins K, de Boer WJ, et al. Gastrointestinal complications in lung transplant survivors that require surgical intervention. *Br J Surg* 2001;**88**:433-8.
150. Pollard TR, Schwesinger WH, Sako EY, et al. Abdominal operations after lung transplantation. *Arch Surg* 1997;**12**:714-7.
151. Cassivi SD, Meyers BF, Battafarano RJ, et al. Thirteen-year experience in lung transplantation for emphysema. *Ann Thorac Surg* 2002;**74**:1663-9.
152. Ramirez JC, Patterson GA, Winton TL, et al. Bilateral lung transplantation for cystic fibrosis. The Toronto Lung Transplant Group. *J Thorac Cardiovasc Surg* 1992;**103**:287-94.
153. Mendeloff EN, Meyers BF, Sundt TM, et al. Lung transplantation for pulmonary vascular disease. *Ann Thorac Surg* 2002;**73**:209-17.
154. Waltz DA, Boucek MM, Edwards LB, et al. Registry of the International Society for Heart and Lung Transplantation: ninth official pediatric lung and heart-lung transplantation report—2006. *J Heart Lung Transplant* 2006;**25**:904-11.
155. Egan TM, Murray S, Bustami RT, et al. Development of the new lung allocation system in the United States. *Am J Transplant* 2006;**6**:1212-27.
156. Boucek MM, Edwards LB, Keck BM, et al. The registry of the international society for heart and lung transplantation: fifth official pediatric report—2001 to 2002. *J Heart Lung Transplant* 2002;**21**:827-40.
157. Huddleston CB, Bloch JB, Sweet SC, et al. Lung transplantation in children. *Ann Surg* 2002;**236**:270-6.

F. Lung Cancer

CHAPTER 15

Screening for Lung Cancer

Brendon M. Stiles, Jeffrey L. Port, and Nasser K. Altorki

History of Screening for Lung Cancer
Current Lung Cancer Screening Efforts
   Prostate, Lung, Colorectal and Ovarian
     Screening Trial
   National Lung Screening Trial
   Low-Dose Computed Tomography

Novel Technologies with Potential Screening
   Applications
   Sputum Evaluation
   Molecular Detection of Circulating Tumor
     Cells
   Fluorescence Bronchoscopy

The Screening Regimen
Management of the Screen Detected
   Nodule
Summary

Lung cancer is the most common cause of cancer mortality in the United States, resulting in more deaths than breast, prostate, and colon cancer combined.[1] Despite the accepted efficacy of screening for cancers of the breast, prostate, and colon, screening for lung cancer is generally thought to be not beneficial and even potentially harmful. The current recommendations from the National Cancer Institute (NCI) and from the American Cancer Society (ACS) are that no attempt at screening for lung cancer should be performed for patients thought to be at risk for this disease.[2-4] According to the ACS, "Any test for the early detection of lung cancer" is not recommended, and "People with signs or symptoms of lung cancer should consult their physicians."[2] Given the high rates of lung cancer mortality (especially when signs or symptoms become apparent), combined with the lack of an effective screening tool, screening for lung cancer is the subject of active investigation at both the clinical and laboratory levels.

An ideal screening tool would possess adequate sensitivity for detecting a disease, while simultaneously maintaining specificity to reduce the number of false-positive results. In addition, no harm would come to the patient as a result of screening. With regard to sensitivity, the ideal screening test would reduce mortality caused by the screened disease (disease-specific mortality). On the other hand, the false-positive rate would be as low as possible, to ensure that patients without the disease do not undergo unnecessary testing, which might be associated with added morbidity. Finally, the ideal screening test would be painless and would not sequester an unreasonable amount of resources.

The goals of this chapter are to acquaint the reader with (1) the existing published data regarding lung cancer screening, (2) the nature of current clinical investigative efforts for the detection of early disease, (3) management of screen-detected nodules, and (4) studies involving novel screening techniques for this deadly disease.

HISTORY OF SCREENING FOR LUNG CANCER

Interest in screening high-risk patients for lung cancer was sparked when the association between cigarette smoking and lung cancer was first appreciated in the 1950s.[5] Plain chest radiography (CXR) was the first modality used in a mass screening trial to detect lung cancer. The first mass screening project was conducted in London from 1960 to 1964, and although it was not a randomized trial, 55,034 men were assigned to undergo either CXR every 6 months for 3 years (the screened group), or a single CXR at the beginning of the study, followed by a repeat CXR at the end of the 3-year period (the "unscreened" group).[6] At the end of the 3-year period, more lung cancer was detected in the screened group, as a result of the screening protocol, than in the "unscreened" group (132 versus 96 cases). In addition, resectability was enhanced in the screened group. Despite these findings, lung cancer–specific mortality did not differ between the two groups, with 62 patients dying of lung cancer in the screened group and 59 patients in the "unscreened" group.[6]

Interest in lung cancer screening was renewed in the 1970s, when the NCI funded three randomized trials focused on the use of both CXR and sputum cytology.[7-9] At the time, refinements in the technology used for the cytologic assessment of expectorated sputum encouraged the designers of two of these trials (the Johns Hopkins Lung Project and the Memorial Sloan-Kettering Cancer Center [MSKCC] trial) to focus primarily on the effect of the addition of sputum cytology to interval CXRs (Table 15-1).[8,9] In the MSKCC study, patients were randomized to either annual CXR alone or annual CXR plus sputum cytologic assessment every 4 months.[8] Exactly the same number of cancers were detected in both groups. Patients who had sputum cytology in addition to CXR tended to have their tumors detected at an earlier stage than those undergoing CXR alone. However, there was no difference in resectability rates or in lung cancer–specific mortality. This screening protocol was also used in the Johns Hopkins Lung Project randomized trial, with similar results (see Table 15-1).[8,9] No difference in the number of lung cancers or in lung cancer–specific mortality was detected between the two groups.[9]

The design of the Mayo Lung Project was different from that of the MSKCC and Johns Hopkins trials: it focused on the *combined* impact of CXR and sputum cytology in screening for lung cancer (Table 15-2).[7,10,11] In the Mayo trial, considered by many to be the most definitive of the four randomized

Table 15–1

Study Trials* Evaluating the Role of Sputum Cytologic Examination for Lung Cancer Screening

	MSKCC	Johns Hopkins
Years of accrual	1974–1982	1973–1982
Screened arm		
Sample size	4968	5226
Protocol	Annual CXR; sputum cytology every 4 mo	Annual CXR; sputum cytology every 4 mo
Cancers (baseline) (n)	30	39
Cancers (repeat screen) (n)	114	194
Lung cancer mortality†	2.7	3.4
Unscreened arm		
Sample size	5072	5161
Protocol	Annual CXR	Annual CXR
Cancers (baseline) (n)	23	40
Cancers (repeat screen) (n)	121	202
Lung cancer mortality†	2.7	3.8

*The two randomized controlled trials are the Memorial Sloan-Kettering Cancer Center (MSKCC) trial (Melamed MR, Flehinger BJ, Zaman MB, et al. Chest 86:44-53, 1984) and the Johns Hopkins Lung Project (Tockman M. Chest 89:325S-326, 1986).
† Per 1000 person-years.
CXR, chest radiography.

Table 15–2

Trials* Evaluating the Role of CXR Combined with Sputum Cytologic Examination for Lung Cancer Screening

	Mayo	Czechoslovakia
Years of accrual	1971–1983	1976–1980
Screened arm		
Sample size	4618	3172
Protocol	CXR and sputum cytology every 4 mo for 6 yr	CXR and sputum cytology every 6 mo for 3 yr†
Cancers (baseline) (n)	Data not available	Data not available
Cancers (repeat screen) (n)	206	39
Lung cancer mortality‡	3.2	3.6
Unscreened arm		
Sample size	4593	3174
Protocol	Advised for annual CXR and sputum cytology	CXR and sputum cytology initially and after 3 yr†
Cancers (baseline) (n)	Data not available	Data not available
Cancers (repeat screen) (n)	160	27
Lung cancer mortality‡	3.0	2.6

*The two randomized controlled trials are the Mayo Lung Project (Fontana RS, Sanderson DR, Taylor WF, et al. Am Rev Respir Dis 130:561-565, 1984) and the Czech Study on Lung Cancer Screening (Kubik AK, Parkin DM, Zatloukal P. Cancer 89[11 Suppl]:2363-2368, 2000).
†Followed by annual CXR and sputum cytology for an additional 3 years.
‡Per 1000 person-years.

trials, patients were randomized to undergo CXR as well as sputum cytologic assessment every 4 months for 6 years (the screened group), or given the standard Mayo recommendation to undergo both of these examinations annually (the "unscreened" group) without active reminders being sent to the participants.[7] Significantly, in this trial, more than 50% of patients in the "unscreened" group underwent CXR during the study period, whereas 25% of patients in the screened group were not compliant with the screening protocol. After a median follow-up period of 3 years, more lung cancers were detected in the screened group than in the "unscreened" group. Both resectability and the 5-year survival rate were higher for individuals diagnosed with lung cancer in the screened group than in those with detected lung cancer in the control arm. Nevertheless, for the overall study population, there was no difference in lung cancer–specific mortality between the two arms.[7]

In the late 1970s, a screening trial was conducted in Czechoslovakia that was similar to the Mayo Lung Project; it also focused on the combined effects of CXR and sputum cytologic examination for lung cancer screening (see Table 15-2).[7,10,11] In this trial, patients in the screened group underwent CXR and evaluation of sputum cytology every 6 months for 3 years, whereas those in the "unscreened" group had an initial CXR and sputum cytologic examination, both of which were repeated at the end of the 3-year period.[10,11] After the initial screening period, both groups underwent annual CXR and sputum assessment for an additional 3 years. Once again, more lung cancer was diagnosed in the screened group than in the "unscreened" group (39 versus 27 cases). Despite this, no difference was appreciated in lung cancer–specific mortality.[10,11] The interpretation of these four randomized trials continues to be the subject of some controversy. Opponents of lung cancer screening state that although three of these four randomized trials demonstrated that screening may indeed lead to diagnosis of more early-stage lung cancer and improvement in case-specific survival, there was no demonstrable reduction in lung cancer–specific mortality for the whole study population.[12,13]

Overdiagnosis bias has been cited as the most likely reason for this seemingly paradoxical result.[12] Overdiagnosis implies that a significant number of cancers detected by screening are indolent and would not lead to clinical disease in these patients. Indeed, if all screen-detected lung cancers were to grow, spread, and become clinically apparent, it would be expected that the lung cancer incidence rates would be unaffected by screening. If followed long enough, all tumors would become symptomatic and would be detected at equal rates in both screened and unscreened patients. In contrast, if screening led to the diagnosis of lung cancers that were clinically indolent (i.e., overdiagnosis), these tumors would be diagnosed in the screened population but not in the unscreened group, resulting in higher rates of detection but no reduction in mortality in the screened group (as seen in the Mayo Lung Project and the Czechoslovak trials).

Proponents of lung cancer screening criticize the randomized trials using several arguments. First, none of the four randomized trials incorporated a completely unscreened control group, making any positive effects of screening more difficult to detect. Second, two of the trials (the MSKCC and Johns Hopkins trials) evaluated only the effect of sputum cytologic evaluation, as both the experimental and control groups had annual CXRs.[8,9] Standard cytologic examination of expectorated sputum is not currently thought to be a sensitive means of screening for lung cancer. Furthermore, the patients diagnosed with lung cancer in both arms of these two trials had earlier-stage disease and higher resectability and survival rates compared with historical controls of sporadically diagnosed lung cancer patients, implying that annual CXR may be beneficial for lung cancer screening. Third, there was a significant amount of crossover in the Mayo Lung Project, where more than half of the "unscreened" patients had CXRs, and 25% of the screened patients were not compliant with the protocol.[7] Fourth, the Mayo Lung Project was designed to detect a 50% reduction in mortality and was underpowered to detect more subtle differences in mortality (i.e., it had a 19% chance of detecting a 10% decrease in mortality).[14]

In addition to these criticisms, advocates of screening argue that the concept of lung cancer overdiagnosis is erroneous on the basis of the following indirect evidence.[15,16] First, lung cancer is a virulent disease, with nearly 90% of patients diagnosed with lung cancer dying of the disease, making the overdiagnosis hypothesis contrary to the known biological behavior of this disease process.[1] Second, although the undiagnosed autopsy prevalence of some cancers (e.g., prostate) may be very high, this has not been found to be the case for lung cancer.[17] Finally, data from the surgical literature, both prospective and retrospective, suggest that suboptimal treatment or no treatment of early-stage lung cancer is associated with an inferior prognosis when compared with optimally treated patients.[18] Taken together, this information calls the assumption of overdiagnosis into question.

CURRENT LUNG CANCER SCREENING EFFORTS

Prostate, Lung, Colorectal and Ovarian Cancer Screening Trial

The Prostate, Lung, Colorectal and Ovarian (PLCO) trial is a complex, multicenter trial sponsored by the NCI, with a target accrual of 148,000 subjects.[19] Men and women, ages 55 to 74, were randomized to undergo an annual CXR (for 3 years [smokers] or 2 years [nonsmokers]) or routine medical care (unscreened group). Participants will be followed for at least 13 years after randomization to assess health status and cause of death. Accrual to the main phase began in 1994 and was completed in 2001. The PLCO trial has an 89% power to detect a 10% reduction in lung cancer–specific mortality. The results have yet to be reported. Unfortunately, the technology of film-based CXR used in this study has been routinely replaced by digital CXR. Additionally, CXR has already been shown to be inferior to computed tomographic (CT) scans for the detection of nodules, which will certainly lessen the impact of the results of the study.

National Lung Screening Trial

The National Lung Screening Trial (NLST) is an NCI-sponsored randomized controlled trial, previously described by Goldberg.[20] It compares CT to CXR screening in current and former smokers, with baseline studies and then two annual follow-up studies. This trial is powered to detect a 50% reduction in lung cancer mortality within approximately 2 years of follow-up, and a 20% reduction within 6 years of the initial screening. As in the NCI studies performed in the 1970s, the primary endpoint is lung cancer mortality. In addition to the previously discussed limitations of CXR screening, a major concern in regard to the ongoing NLST relates to the number of rounds of screening and the length of follow-up. As is typical in modern screening trials, there are balances between cost concerns in the trial and the various endpoints. Although additional screening rounds would add confidence to the results, they are the most costly aspect of these trials and are therefore limited. In the NLST, there are only two annual repeat rounds, with a median follow-up of about 4 years. It is clear, based on previous studies, that significantly longer follow-up will be necessary before a genuine reduction in mortality can be expected. It thus appears that all of these ongoing studies are subject to critical design issues that might influence interpretation of their results.

Low-Dose Computed Tomography

In the 1990s, increased resolution and data-acquisition speeds of modern CT scanners generated renewed interest in screening for lung cancer. Initial findings from Henschke and colleagues of the Early Lung Cancer Action Project (ELCAP) showed that in a high-risk population, CT was superior to CXR in detection of lung nodules. Notably, 2.7% of those enrolled had lung cancer, the great majority of which were stage I.[21,22] In the initial ELCAP (I-ELCAP) patient population, 27 screen-diagnosed lung cancers were found at baseline screenings, of which 96% were resectable.[21] A subsequent report by the I-ELCAP group addressed overall curability estimated through 10-year survival rates of patients found to have stage I lung cancer by CT screening.[23] The authors reported an estimated 88% 10-year survival rate, markedly higher than survival rates predicted by the current staging system or among those presenting as a result of symptoms. They inferred that because CT screening leads to early detection of lung cancer and because those lung cancers found as a result of CT screening are curable, that CT screening leads to a reduction in lung cancer mortality.

Several other groups have also evaluated CT screening for lung cancer. A recently published review by Black and colleagues identified 12 studies (Table 15-3),[19,24-29] of which two were randomized and the other 10 had no comparator group.[30] Significant variability existed in the study populations and in the definition of a positive finding in each. Nevertheless, the percentage of positive screenings ranged from 5.1% to 51%. From baseline screenings, 1.8% to 18% of positive findings led to a diagnosis of cancer. The majority of the tumors were in stage I (53% to 100%), with a high resectability rate (>78%). Only one of the studies reported 5-year

Table 15–3
Results of Baseline Lung Cancer Screenings with CT Scans

Study, year (ref)	Number screened	Positive screen (%)	Total lung cancer (%)	Lung cancer in screen-positive patients (%)	Percent stage I (for NSCLC) (%)	Percent resectable (for NSCLC) (%)
ELCAP 2001 (21)	1000	23.3	2.7	11.6	88	100
Sone 1998 (24), 2001 (25)	5483	5.1	0.4	7.9	22	100
Garg 2002 (74)	92	33	3.2	10	NR	NR
Tiitola 2002 (75)	602	18.4	0.8	4.5	0	20
Sobue 2002 (26)	1611	11.5	0.8	7.0	77	92
Nawa 2002 (76)	7956	6.8	0.45	6.7	86	NR
Pastorino 2003 (77)	1035	5.9	1.1	18	55	91
Swenson 2002 (27), 2003 (28)	1520	51	1.7	3.3	69	NR
Diederich 2004 (29)	817	43	2.1	4.9	56	100
Gohagan 2004 (19)	1586	20.5	1.9	9.2	53	NR
MacRedmond 2004 (78)	449	24	0.4	1.8	NR	100
Miller 2004 (79)	3598	32	0.61	1.9	NR	NR

NR, not reported; NSCLC, non–small cell lung cancer.

survival: 76% for patients with cancer detected at baseline screening and 65% for patients with cancer detected at annual repeat scanning.[31]

However, the data on CT screening are far from conclusive. In fact, much like the CXR and sputum screening trials, none of the CT trials have yet shown an advantage to survival in screened patient populations versus unscreened populations. This and other shortcomings were highlighted by a recently published multicenter study by Bach and colleagues, which reviewed the findings from CT screening of 3246 high-risk patients.[31] In this study, there was no evidence of a decline in the number of patients with advanced diagnoses or of deaths from lung cancer in the screened groups. Despite this failure to demonstrate a difference in mortality, there was a threefold increase in individuals diagnosed with lung cancer, and a 10-fold increase in patients undergoing lung resection (compared with expected cases). The authors used these data to argue that CT screening is prone to overdiagnosis and thus that the screening may be exposing patients to unnecessary surgery. They concluded that CT screening may not meaningfully reduce the risk of dying from lung cancer.

An important limitation of this study was the relatively short median follow-up time of only 3.9 years. This short period of follow-up may have prevented the detection of any benefit from screening. For most screening studies, any potential benefit is not likely to emerge before at least four to five rounds of screening have been completed. Furthermore, one of the three studies included in the analysis did not require the exclusion of symptomatic individuals. This may have resulted in the inclusion of patients with symptoms of preexisting lung cancer, possibly violating the core concept of screening. Exclusion of symptomatic patients from the analysis may have substantially altered the results.

Novel Technologies with Potential Screening Applications

Sputum Evaluation

The examination of expectorated sputum using standard cytologic techniques is generally regarded as insensitive in screening for lung cancer, based on the results of the MSKCC and Johns Hopkins Lung Projects, which randomized subjects to either annual CXR alone, or CXR plus sputum cytologic evaluation every 4 months (see Table 15-1).[8,9] Both trials demonstrated that the examination of expectorated sputum did not enhance the ability to detect lung cancer.

To improve the sensitivity of sputum analysis as a screening tool, more sophisticated assays using sputum cells are being investigated. In a retrospective analysis of archived sputum specimens containing moderately atypical cells from the Johns Hopkins Lung Project, 64% of specimens possessing positive immunostaining for a nuclear ribonucleoprotein, hnRNP A2/B1, were from patients who eventually developed lung cancer, whereas 88% with negative staining did not develop cancer.[32] Further prospective investigation in a population of Chinese tin miners as well as a population of North American patients with a history of resected, stage I non–small cell lung cancer have echoed the retrospective data, with the sensitivity and specificity of hnRNP A2/B1 immunostaining reported as 77% and 82%, respectively, for the detection of second primary lung cancer, and 82% and 65% for the detection of new primary lung cancer.[33,34] Whether these data will be reproducible and applicable to lung cancer screening remains to be determined.

Other sputum-based investigational approaches to lung cancer early detection, and potentially screening, include the use of the polymerase chain reaction (PCR) to detect mutations in expectorated bronchial epithelial cells, and the detection of malignancy-associated changes. Although PCR is a very sensitive assay (it detects one mutated cell in more than 100,000 normal cells), and mutations in genes including *KRAS* and p53 have indeed been detected in the sputum of patients with lung cancer using PCR,[35] the usefulness of this technique is unclear because these mutations are also found in the sputum of smokers without cancer, and many different mutations can exist for a particular gene (e.g., p53).[36,37]

The presence of malignant cells is thought to induce changes in the chromatin pattern in neighboring, nontransformed cells. These subtle, subvisual changes in DNA are termed malignancy-associated changes (MACs), and they can be quantified using computer-assisted imaging technology.[38-40] In a retrospective analysis using archived sputum specimens from the Mayo Lung Project, MACs were present in 74% of the specimens from patients who went on to develop cancer.[41] One advantage of this technology is that a positive result is not dependent on the presence of malignant cells in the sputum, which may serve to offset some of the inefficiencies of the sputum induction process. The clinical application of image cytometry is the subject of ongoing investigation, including its combined role with low-dose CT in detecting early lung cancer.

It has become increasingly evident that abnormal methylation of the promoter region of a variety of specific genes may be responsible for the inhibition of gene expression seen in multiple tumor types (e.g., tumor suppressor genes).[42] Such epigenetic changes have also been shown to occur in lung cancers and can be demonstrated in the sputum of lung cancer patients.[42-45] Specifically, a recent study has demonstrated aberrant methylation of the p16 and O^6-methylguanine DNA methyltransferase (*MGMT*) genes in 100% of squamous cell cancers and their corresponding sputum specimens.[43] Another study demonstrated aberrant methylation of the p16, *MGMT*, *DAPK*, and other genes in sputum specimens of patients with cancer.[46] Abnormal methylation of the promoter region of a variety of specific genes may be responsible for the inhibition of gene expression and the subsequent development of cancer. Belinsky and colleagues reported that the risk of lung cancer increases with the number of hypermethylated genes.[46] However, as seen in the detection of mutations (genetic changes), false-positive results were relatively common, with aberrant methylation being demonstrable in nearly one out of four long-term smokers without cancer,[43] implying that this method may be more useful for identifying high-risk patients than for identifying definite cancer cases.

Regardless of the technology used, when evaluating sputum for the presence of malignant cells, the quality of the sputum specimen remains a source of some of the insensitivity associated with these techniques. As an example, in the study evaluating hnRNP A2/B1 immunostaining for the detection of a second primary lung cancer by the Lung Cancer Early Detection Working Group, approximately 25% of sputum samples were unsatisfactory for analysis.[33] As a result of this problem, recent investigations have also focused on the development of technology that will enhance the quality of these specimens. Potential advances include the high-frequency chest wall oscillation vest[47] and the use of inhaled uridine 5′-triphosphate (UTP), a compound that stimulates salt and water transport and cilia beat frequency in airway epithelium.[48]

Molecular Detection of Circulating Tumor Cells

In addition to the analysis of sputum, molecular diagnostic techniques are beginning to be evaluated for the detection of circulating tumor cells in the bloodstream in patients with lung cancer. The use of methylation-specific PCR has revolutionized the detection of circulating, epigenetic alterations (aberrant promoter methylation).[42] Numerous genes have now been found to be abnormally methylated in both small cell and non–small cell lung cancer specimens, including p16, *DAP-K*, *GSTP1*, *MGMT*, adenomatous polyposis coli (APC), and the retinoic acid receptor-beta.[42,49-51] Significantly, identical aberrant methylation is often found in the serum of patients from whom these tumor specimens are obtained, but not in the serum of patients whose tumors had unmethylated DNA, or in serum from normal subjects.

Other detectable alterations in the blood of patients with lung cancer (mainly small cell) include microsatellite alterations and levels of prepro-gastrin-releasing peptide mRNA, the latter being detected using reverse transcriptase PCR.[52,53] Whether these findings as well as changes in promoter methylation will play a role in screening patients for lung cancer remains to be determined.

Fluorescence Bronchoscopy

Conventional white-light bronchoscopy has an overall sensitivity of only approximately 40% for the detection of preinvasive lung cancer (carcinoma in situ).[54] Fluorescence bronchoscopy relies on the difference in autofluorescence spectra between normal and malignant airway epithelia. Using the He-Cad laser (442 nm), normal epithelium fluoresces green, whereas malignant tissue fluoresces brown to red. In a recent review of the published literature regarding the use of fluorescence bronchoscopy for the detection of preinvasive lesions, Lam and colleagues found that the addition of fluorescence bronchoscopy to conventional white-light bronchoscopy improved the detection rate from 40% to 80%.[54] Importantly, autofluorescence bronchoscopy may also detect lung cancers that are not visible on CT. In a recent screening study by McWilliams and colleagues, one quarter of detected cancers were CT occult and seen only with autofluorescence bronchoscopy.[55] Future work regarding fluorescence bronchoscopy will entail the design and evaluation of thinner bronchoscopes, as the major limitation of this modality is related to the size of the instrument.

THE SCREENING REGIMEN

Our current screening regimen begins with a low-dose helical CT scan and an a priori definition of what constitutes a positive or negative reading. In its first iteration, ELCAP defined a positive result on baseline as finding one to six noncalcified nodules.[21] If no nodules, only calcified nodules, or more than six nodules were identified, the result was negative and the person was referred to the first annual repeat screening.

On the annual repeat scan, a positive result is defined as the presence of any growing noncalcified nodule, including newly identified nodules.[22] If the initial test is positive, a well-defined diagnostic algorithm is followed until a diagnosis of cancer is established. If the CT result is negative or the diagnostic algorithm does not lead to a diagnosis of malignancy, the person is referred to the next routinely scheduled screening round.

As technology improved and more knowledge was gained about performing the algorithm, the definition of a positive result was updated, as was the choice of additional tests. Helical CT scanning has rapidly advanced since the initiation of the I-ELCAP project. Using modern multislice scanners, images from a slice less than 1 mm thick can be obtained in a single breath hold. Because resolution markedly improves with thinner slices, it is not surprising that many more nodules are being detected. Most of these nodules, however, are less than 5.0 mm in diameter. The current I-ELCAP definition of a positive result on baseline is as follows: one or more noncalcified solid or part-solid nodules 5.0 mm or larger, or a nonsolid nodule 8.0 mm or larger (from www.ielcap.org). Using this updated definition, the percentage of positive results on the baseline low-dose screening is reduced to less than 15% without any increase in the false-negative rate. The definition of positive results on annual repeat screening has remained unchanged. Positive results continue to occur in less than 6% of these screening studies.

Notably, there have also been changes in the diagnostic workup. These include changes in time intervals for follow-up scans, the use of biopsy as a possible alternative without documenting growth (only when the nodule is ≤15 mm at baseline), the use of antibiotics, and the use of positron emission tomography (PET) or CT scans. As technological innovations continue, the definition of positive results for baseline and annual repeat screening and the algorithm of diagnostic workup will need to be further updated.

MANAGEMENT OF THE SCREEN-DETECTED NODULE

No matter how the current debate on screening unfolds or how the technology evolves, thoracic surgeons will continue to have to evaluate individuals with either screen-detected or incidentally discovered small pulmonary nodules. The management of these patients presents several challenges, such as the relationship between nodule size and the likelihood of malignancy. The overwhelming majority of nodules found by screening or on incidental studies are not cancer. A large proportion of these nodules are less than 5 mm on the baseline round of screening and therefore do not actually constitute a positive result. Even for larger nodules, it is important to reassure patients that a positive CT scan does not mean that they have cancer. In the I-ELCAP data, 11.6% of patients with positive baseline CT scans were found to have cancer.[22]

Several factors influence the probability of cancer in a pulmonary nodule. Of these factors, nodule size is the most critical. In the initial ELCAP publication, the rate of malignant disease was 1% in nodules less than or equal to 5 mm, 24% in nodules 6 to 10 mm, 33% in nodules 11 to 20 mm, and 80% in those greater than 20 mm.[21] Change in size is also an important factor to consider, because nodules that demonstrate growth are considered to be active. Time to follow-up CT scanning is in part dependent on the initial size of the nodule (as documentation of growth in small nodules is more challenging) and on whether the nodules were initially detected on the baseline or a repeat round. The time to follow-up is typically shorter on the repeat round, because cancers found on repeat screening are typically faster growing. Sophisticated three-dimensional software packages are available to more accurately assess doubling times.

Several factors other than size play a role in the probability of malignancy. Patients with numerous small nodules (>6) are generally thought to be at low risk for malignancy and more likely to have inflammatory lung disease. The consistency of the nodule also has an impact on the probability of cancer. According to data from the initial ELCAP group, part-solid nodules have a higher rate of malignancy (63%) than nonsolid nodules (18%), and solid nodules have the lowest malignancy rate (7%).[56] Patients with part-solid or nonsolid nodules predominantly had bronchioloalveolar carcinoma or adenocarcinoma with bronchioloalveolar features. Other factors to consider are patient age, smoking history, occupational history, and endemic rates of granulomatous disease.

Our algorithm for radiographic follow-up is generally guided by the I-ELCAP protocol (www.ielcap.org). For nodules less than 5 mm in diameter or for nonsolid nodules less than 8 mm found on baseline CT, we recommend repeat CT in 1 year. For nodules 5 to 15 mm in diameter (8 to 15 mm for nonsolid nodules), we obtain a repeat CT scan in 3 months to assess for growth or resolution. For nodules found on annual repeat screening, those less than 3 mm in diameter should have another CT in 6 months, and those greater than 3 mm and less than 5 mm should have CT follow-up within 3 months. For those larger than 5 mm, a course of antibiotics and a repeat in 1 month is an additional option. In the I-ELCAP patient population, an initial 7- to 10-day course of antibiotics resulted in partial or complete resolution of 29% of nodules on baseline screening and 74% of nodules on repeat screening.[57] In all instances, nodule growth should prompt careful consideration of a biopsy or closer follow-up. PET scans may be another diagnostic option for screen-detected nodules, particularly for patients with nodules greater than 1 cm in diameter. Veronesi and colleagues reported the sensitivity and specificity of PET for screen-detected lung nodules to be 89% and 93%, respectively.[58] Median nodule size was 14 mm for their cohort of patients. Even for nodules less than 10 mm, sensitivity and specificity were 83% and 100%, respectively. As part of their diagnostic strategy, the authors suggested lowering the positive maximal standard uptake value cutoff for smaller nodules to 1.5.

Once the possibility of cancer exists, it is imperative to establish an accurate tissue diagnosis. When a nodule is deemed to be suspect for malignancy, either based on baseline characteristics, positive PET scan findings, or the demonstration of growth, we typically proceed to fine needle aspiration (FNA), even for nodules less than 10 mm in size. FNA performed at high-volume centers can be extremely accurate, with a sensitivity of 82% and a diagnostic accuracy of 88%, although the yield decreases with nodules less than 8 mm.[59] FNA produces four possible outcomes: malignant, specific benign, nonspecific benign, and nondiagnostic. For malignant and specific benign nodules, the treatment course is typically obvious. However, those patients with nonspecific benign and nondiagnostic results require further workup. A review of 74 cases of FNA with either nonspecific benign or nondiagnostic findings demonstrated an eventual malignancy rate of almost

18%.[60] Such nonspecific diagnoses may include atypical cells or inflammation. We typically repeat CT scans at short intervals (within 3 months), with or without a course of antibiotics, and gradually increase the interval to the subsequent scan so that nodule stability can be ascertained. Volumetric analysis with serial CT scans can also be performed to assess nodule growth over time and to infer malignancy. Unfortunately, such techniques are not universally available, are costly, and potentially delay treatment in patients in whom there may be significant concern for malignancy. Further growth necessitates repeat FNA or surgical biopsy, depending on clinical suspicion and surgical risk.

In institutions where CT-guided FNA is not routinely performed, there should be a higher reliance on more invasive diagnostic techniques for suspicious nodules, such as bronchoscopic biopsy or surgical biopsy, either by open thoracotomy or via video-assisted thoracoscopic surgery (VATS). Bronchoscopic biopsy is an option for establishing tissue diagnosis, although the yield for flexible bronchoscopy has historically been low, especially in small peripheral nodules. Newer techniques including endobronchial ultrasound and electromagnetic navigation have been reported to increase the diagnostic yield of transbronchial biopsy to upward of 60%, even for small peripheral lesions.[61,62]

When surgical biopsy is necessary, VATS is thought to decrease postoperative morbidity when compared with open thoracotomy, but it is occasionally accompanied by difficulty of palpating and visualizing the small lesions that are often found on screening studies. Several techniques are available to localize and excise small pulmonary nodules using a minimally invasive approach.[63-68] Preoperative marking with methylene blue, wire hooks, and metallic coils have all been described. Reported complications are rare but include marker dislodgement, pneumothorax, intrapulmonary hemorrhage, and air embolism. Recently, Sortini and colleagues and other investigators have reported good results with ultrasound localization,[69] although this method is strongly operator dependent. Other groups have described a VATS radiotracer localization technique, with a success rate of 92% for nodules with a median size of 8 mm.[70] The technique can be applied to all pleural surfaces including interlobar regions with complete fissures, and it enables rapid and predictable intraoperative localization. The procedure uses readily available technical components with minimal additional cost. Regardless of the method used to localize small nodules, VATS resection is typically performed with low morbidity, short hospital stays, and excellent diagnostic accuracy.

Summary

Lung cancer continues to be a deadly disease, curable only in its early stages. Over the past 5 decades, attempts have been made to screen high-risk patients for lung cancer, with the goal of detecting tumors in these earlier, curable stages and thus reducing disease-specific mortality. Four reports of randomized, controlled trials of lung cancer screening currently exist, none of which has shown a reduction in lung cancer–specific mortality in the screened groups. As a result, it is currently not recommended that physicians perform screening for this disease. The interpretation of these four trials, however, has been the subject of several criticisms, and many clinicians question this conclusion in favor of screening.

Current clinical investigation has focused on the role of low-dose CT in screening for lung cancer, with multiple studies demonstrating that this modality is more sensitive than CXR for detecting early lung cancer. Despite this enhanced sensitivity, high numbers of false-positive scans have raised issues including cost-effectiveness and overdiagnosis of indolent disease, leading many to challenge the advocates of this strategy. This controversy underscores the need for large, randomized, controlled trials of low-dose CT in this capacity. The endpoints of these trials should be critically examined. It should be noted that no randomized control study has ever demonstrated a reduction in lung cancer mortality as a result of smoking cessation.[71-73] In fact, one such study, the Multiple Risk Factor Intervention Trial, indicated that lung cancer mortality was 15% higher in the group of patients who quit smoking, after several years of follow-up.[68] When viewed only through the mortality prism, this would suggest that continuing to smoke cigarettes prevents deaths from lung cancer. Certainly, we do not hold this to be true. This anomaly illustrates the deficiencies of mortality endpoints in screened patient populations. Other endpoints such as cure rate and resectability are perhaps more appropriate and should be closely examined when reviewing the data that has accumulated with regard to screening for lung cancer. Finally, novel technologies are currently being developed in the laboratory that may possess usefulness in the detection of preclinical lung cancer. These include assays for molecular alterations in sputum and peripheral blood, and novel imaging techniques including fluorescence bronchoscopy and computer-assisted imaging of expectorated sputum cells. Whether any of these new technologies will play a role in the future of lung cancer screening remains to be determined.

REFERENCES

1. Greenlee RT, Murray T, Bolden S, Wingo PA. Cancer statistics. *CA Cancer J Clin* 2000;**50**:7-33.
2. American Cancer Society. Report on the cancer-related health checkup: cancer of the lung. *CA Cancer J Clin* 1980;**30**:199-207.
3. National Cancer Institute website, Screening for lung cancer (PDQ): www.nci.nih.gov/cancerinfo/pdq/screening/lung/HealthProfessional#Section_15.
4. Smith RA, von Eschenbach AC, Wender R, et al. American Cancer Society guidelines for the early detection of cancer: update of early detection guidelines for prostate, colorectal, and endometrial cancers. Also: update 2001: testing for early lung cancer detection. *CA Cancer J Clin* 2001;**51**:38-75.
5. Doll R, Hill AB. Smoking and carcinoma of the lung: preliminary report. *BMJ* 1950;**2**:739-48.
6. Brett GZ. The value of lung cancer detection by six-monthly chest radiographs. *Thorax* 1968;**23**:414-20.
7. Fontana RS, Sanderson DR, Taylor WF, et al. Early lung cancer detection: results of the initial (prevalence) radiologic and cytologic screening in the Mayo Clinic study. *Am Rev Respir Dis* 1984;**130**:561-5.
8. Melamed MR, Flehinger BJ, Zaman MB, et al. Screening for early lung cancer: results of the Memorial Sloan-Kettering study in New York. *Chest* 1984;**86**:44-53.
9. Tockman M. Survival and mortality from lung cancer in a screened population: the Johns Hopkins study. *Chest* 1986;**89**:325s-326.
10. Kubik AK, Parkin DM, Zatloukal P. Czech Study on Lung Cancer Screening: post-trial follow-up of lung cancer deaths up to year 15 since enrollment. *Cancer* 2000;**89**(11 Suppl):2363-8.
11. Kubik A, Polak J. Lung cancer detection: results of a randomized prospective study in Czechoslovakia. *Cancer* 1986;**57**:2427-37.
12. Bach PB, Kelley MJ, Tate RC, et al. Screening for lung cancer: a review of the current literature. *Chest* 2003;**123**(1 Suppl):72S-82.
13. Eddy DM. Screening for lung cancer. *Ann Intern Med* 1989;**111**:232-7.
14. Fontana RS, Sanderson DR, Woolner LB, et al. Screening for lung cancer: a critique of the Mayo Lung Project. *Cancer* 1991;**67**(4 Suppl):1155-64.
15. Strauss GM, Gleason RE, Sugarbaker DJ. Screening for lung cancer: another look, a different view. *Chest* 1997;**111**:754-68.

16. Yankelevitz DF, Kostis WJ, Henschke CI, et al. Overdiagnosis in chest radiographic screening for lung carcinoma: frequency. *Cancer* 2003;**97**:1271-5.
17. McFarlane MJ, Feinstein AR, Wells CK. Clinical features of lung cancers discovered as a postmortem "surprise. *Chest* 1986;**90**:520-3.
18. Sugarbaker DJ, Strauss GM. Extent of surgery and survival in early lung carcinoma: implications for overdiagnosis in stage IA nonsmall cell lung carcinoma. *Cancer* 2000;**89**(11 Suppl):2432-7.
19. Gohagan JK, Prorok PC, Hayes RB, et al. The Prostate, Lung, Colorectal and Ovarian (PLCO) Cancer Screening Trial of the National Cancer Institute: history, organization, and status. *Control Clin Trials* 2000;**21**(6 Suppl):251S-72.
20. Goldberg KB. *NCI Lung Cancer Screening Trial. Cancer Letter*. Washington, DC: National Cancer Institute; 2002.
21. Henschke CI, McCauley DI, Yankelevitz DF, et al. Early Lung Cancer Action Project: overall design and findings from baseline screening. *Lancet* 1999;**354**:99-105.
22. Henschke CI, Naidich D, Yankelevitz DF, et al. Early Lung Cancer Action Project: initial findings on repeat screening. *Cancer* 2001;**92**:153-9.
23. International Early Lung Cancer Action Program Investigators, Henschke CI, Yankelevitz DF, Libby DM, et al. Survival of patients with stage I lung cancer detected on CT screening. *N Engl J Med* 2006;**355**:1763-71.
24. Sone S, Takashima S, Li F, et al. Mass screening for lung cancer with mobile spiral computed tomography scanner. *Lancet* 1998;**351**:1242-5.
25. Sone S, Li F, Yang Z-G, et al. Results of three-year mass screening programme for lung cancer using mobile low-dose spiral computed tomography scanner. *Br J Cancer* 2001;**84**:25-32.
26. Sobue T, Moriyama N, Kaneko M, et al. Screening for lung cancer with low-dose helical computed tomography: anti-Lung Cancer Association Project. *J Clin Oncol* 2002;**20**:911-20.
27. Swensen SJ, Jett JR, Sloan JA, et al. Screening for lung cancer with low-dose spiral computed tomography. *Am J Respir Crit Care Med* 2002;**165**:508-13.
28. Swensen SJ, Jett JR, Hartman TE, et al. Lung cancer screening with CT: Mayo Clinic experience. *Radiology* 2003;**226**:756-61.
29. Diederich S, Wormanns D, Semik M, et al. Screening for early lung cancer with low-dose spiral CT: prevalence in 817 asymptomatic smokers. *Radiology* 2002;**222**:773-81.
30. Black C, de Verteuil R, Walker S, et al. Population screening for lung cancer using computed tomography, is there evidence of clinical effectiveness? A systematic review of the literature. *Thorax* 2007;**62**:131-8.
31. Bach PB, Jett JR, Pastorino U, et al. Computed tomography screening and lung cancer outcomes. *JAMA* 2007;**297**:953.
32. Tockman MS, Gupta PK, Myers JD, et al. Sensitive and specific monoclonal antibody recognition of human lung cancer antigen on preserved sputum cells: a new approach to early lung cancer detection. *J Clin Oncol* 1988;**6**:1685-93.
33. Tockman MS, Erozan YS, Gupta P, et al. The early detection of second primary lung cancers by sputum immunostaining. LCEWDG Investigators. Lung Cancer Early Detection Group. *Chest* 1994;**106**(6 Suppl):385S-90.
34. Tockman MS, Mulshine JL, Piantadosi S, et al. Prospective detection of preclinical lung cancer: results from two studies of heterogeneous nuclear ribonucleoprotein A2/B1 overexpression. *Clin Cancer Res* 1997;**3**(12 Pt 1):2237-46.
35. Mao L, Hruban RH, Boyle JO, et al. Detection of oncogene mutations in sputum precedes diagnosis of lung cancer. *Cancer Res* 1994;**54**:1634-7.
36. Hollstein M, Rice K, Greenblatt MS, et al. Database of p53 gene somatic mutations in human tumors and cell lines. *Nucleic Acids Res* 1994;**22**:3551-5.
37. Wistuba II, Lam S, Behrens C, et al. Molecular damage in the bronchial epithelium of current and former smokers. *J Natl Cancer Inst* 1997;**89**:1366-73.
38. Hu YC, Sidransky D, Ahrendt SA. Molecular detection approaches for smoking associated tumors. *Oncogene* 2002;**21**:7289-97.
39. Ikeda N, MacAulay C, Lam S, et al. Malignancy associated changes in bronchial epithelial cells and clinical application as a biomarker. *Lung Cancer* 1998;**19**:161-6.
40. McWilliams A, MacAulay C, Gazdar AF, et al. Innovative molecular and imaging approaches for the detection of lung cancer and its precursor lesions. *Oncogene* 2002;**21**:6949-59.
41. Payne PW, Sebo TJ, Doudkine A, et al. Sputum screening by quantitative microscopy: a reexamination of a portion of the National Cancer Institute Cooperative Early Lung Cancer Study. *Mayo Clin Proc* 1997;**72**:697-704.
42. Plass C. Cancer epigenomics. *Hum Mol Genet* 2002;**11**:2479-88.
43. Palmisano WA, Divine KK, Saccomanno G, et al. Predicting lung cancer by detecting aberrant promoter methylation in sputum. *Cancer Res* 2000;**60**:5954-8.
44. Wang YC, Lu YP, Tseng RC, et al. Inactivation of hMLH1 and hMSH2 by promoter methylation in primary non-small cell lung tumors and matched sputum samples. *J Clin Invest* 2003;**111**:887-95.
45. Zochbauer-Muller S, Minna JD, Gazdar AF. Aberrant DNA methylation in lung cancer: biological and clinical implications. *Oncologist* 2002;**7**:451-7.
46. Belinsky SA, Liechty KC, Gentry FD, et al. Promoter hypermethylation of multiple genes in sputum precedes lung cancer incidence in a high-risk cohort. *Cancer Res* 2006;**66**:3338.
47. Fink JB, Mahlmeister MJ. High-frequency oscillation of the airway and chest wall. *Respir Care* 2002;**47**:797-807.
48. Johnson FL, Donohue JF, Shaffer CL. Improved sputum expectoration following a single dose of INS316 in patients with chronic bronchitis. *Chest* 2002;**122**:2021-9.
49. Bearzatto A, Conte D, Frattini M, et al. p16(INK4A) Hypermethylation detected by fluorescent methylation-specific PCR in plasmas from non-small cell lung cancer. *Clin Cancer Res* 2002;**8**:3782-7.
50. Esteller M, Sanchez-Cespedes M, Rosell R, et al. Detection of aberrant promoter hypermethylation of tumor suppressor genes in serum DNA from non-small cell lung cancer patients. *Cancer Res* 1999;**59**:67-70.
51. Oshita F, Sekiyama A, Suzuki R, et al. Detection of occult tumor cells in peripheral blood from patients with small cell lung cancer by promoter methylation and silencing of the retinoic acid receptor-beta. *Oncol Rep* 2003;**10**:105-8.
52. Chen XQ, Stroun M, Magnenat JL, et al. Microsatellite alterations in plasma DNA of small cell lung cancer patients. *Nat Med* 1996;**2**:1033-5.
53. Saito T, Kobayashi M, Harada R, et al. Sensitive detection of small cell lung carcinoma cells by reverse transcriptase-polymerase chain reaction for prepro-gastrin-releasing peptide mRNA. *Cancer* 2003;**97**:2504-11.
54. Lam S, MacAulay C, leRiche JC, et al. Detection and localization of early lung cancer by fluorescence bronchoscopy. *Cancer* 2000;**89**:2468-73.
55. McWilliams AM, Mayo JR, Ahn MI, et al. Lung cancer screening using multi-slice thin-section computed tomography and autofluorescence bronchoscopy. *J Thorac Oncol* 2006;**1**:61.
56. Henschke CI, Yankelevitz DF, Mirtcheva R, et al. CT screening for lung cancer: frequency and significance of part-solid and nonsolid nodules. *Am J Roentgenol* 2002;**178**:1053.
57. Libby DM, Smith JP, Altorki NK, et al. Managing the small pulmonary nodule discovered by CT. *Chest* 2004;**125**:1522.
58. Veronesi G, Bellomi M, Veronesi U, et al. Role of positron emission tomography scanning in the management of lung nodules detected at baseline computed tomography screening. *Ann Thorac Surg* 2007;**84**:959.
59. Wallace MJ, Krishnamurthy S, Broemeling LD, et al. CT-guided percutaneous fine-needle aspiration biopsy of small (≤1-cm) pulmonary lesions. *Radiology* 2002;**225**:823.
60. Savage C, Walser EM, Schnadig V, et al. Transthoracic image-guided biopsy of lung nodules: when is benign really benign? *J Vasc Interv Radiol* 2004;**15**:161.
61. Kurimoto N, Miyazawa T, Okimasa S, et al. Endobronchial ultrasonography using a guide sheath increases the ability to diagnose peripheral pulmonary lesions endoscopically. *Chest* 2004;**126**:959.
62. Gildea TR, Mazzone PJ, Karnak D, et al. Electromagnetic navigation diagnostic bronchoscopy: a prospective study. *Am J Respir Crit Care Med* 2006;**174**:982.
63. Santambrogio R, Montorsi M, Bianchi P, et al. Intraoperative ultrasound during thoracoscopic procedures for solitary pulmonary nodules. *Ann Thorac Surg* 1999;**68**:218.
64. Chella A, Lucchi M, Ambrogi MC, et al. A pilot study of the role of Tc-99m radionuclide in localization of pulmonary nodular lesions for thoracoscopic resection. *Eur J Cardiothorac Surg* 2000;**18**:17.
65. Partik BL, Leung AN, Müller MR, et al. Using a dedicated lung-marker system for localization of pulmonary nodules before thoracoscopic surgery. *AJR Am J Roentgenol* 2003;**180**:805.
66. Powell TI, Jangra D, Clifton JC, et al. Peripheral lung nodules: fluoroscopically guided video-assisted thoracoscopic resection after computed tomography-guided localization using platinum microcoils. *Ann Surg* 2004;**240**:481.
67. Torre M, Ferraroli GM, Vanzulli A, Fieschi S. A new safe and stable spiral wire needle for thoracoscopic resection of lung nodules. *Chest* 2004;**125**:2289.
68. Eichfeld U, Dietrich A, Ott R, Kloeppel R. Video-assisted thoracoscopic surgery for pulmonary nodules after computed tomographic-guided marking with a spiral wire. *Ann Thorac Surg* 2005;**79**:313.
69. Sortini A, Carrella G, Sortini D, Pozza E. Single pulmonary nodules: localization with intrathoracoscopic ultrasound: a prospective study. *Eur J Cardiothorac Surg* 2002;**22**:440.
70. Stiles BM, Altes TA, Jones DR, et al. Clinical experience with radiotracer-guided thoracoscopic biopsy of small, indeterminate lung nodules. *Ann Thorac Surg* 2006;**82**:1191.
71. Anthonisen NR, Connett JE, Kiley JP, et al. Effects of smoking intervention and the use of an inhaled anticholinergic bronchodilator on the rate of decline of FEV1: the Lung Health Study. *JAMA* 1994;**272**:1497.
72. Rose G, Hamilton PJ, Colwell L, Shipley MJ. A randomized controlled trial of anti-smoking advice: 10 year results. *J Epidemiol Community Health* 1982;**36**:102.
73. Shaten BJ, Kuller LH, Kjelsberg MO, et al. Lung cancer mortality after 16 years in MRFIT participants in intervention and usual-care groups: Multiple Risk Factor Intervention Trial. *Ann Epidemiol* 1997;**7**:125.

74. Garg K, Keith RL, Byers T, et al. Randomized contolled trial with low-dose spiral CT for lung cancer screening: feasibility study and preliminary results. *Radiology* 2002;**225**:506-10.
75. Tiitola M, Kivisaari L, Huuskonen MS, et al. Computed tomography screening for lung cancer in asbestos-exposed workers. *Lung Cancer* 2002;**35**:17-22.
76. Nawa T, Nakagawa T, Kusano S, et al. Lung cancer screening using low-dose spiral CT: results of baseline and 1-year follow-up studies. *Chest* 2002;**122**:15-20.
77. Pastorino U, Bellomi M, Landoni C, et al. Early lung-cancer detection with spiral CT and positron emission tomography in heavy smokers: 2-year results. *Lancet* 2003;**362**:593-7.
78. MacRedmond R, Logan PM, Lee M, et al. Screening for Lung cancer using low dose CT scanning. *Thorax* 2004;**59**:237-41.
79. Miller A, Markowitz S, Mankowitz A, et al. Lung cancer screening using low-dose high resolution CT scanning in a high-risk workforce: 3500 nuclear fuel workers in three US states. *Chest* 2004;**125**:152S-3S.

CHAPTER 16

Lung Cancer Workup and Staging

Bernard J. Park and Valerie W. Rusch

The Staging System
Diagnosis and Staging
  History and Physical Examination
Noninvasive Modalities
  Chest Radiography
  Sputum Cytology
  High-Resolution Computed Tomography
  Positron Emission Tomography

Bone Scan
Magnetic Resonance Imaging
Invasive Modalities
  Bronchoscopy
  Endobronchial Ultrasound
  Autofluorescence Bronchoscopy
  Percutaneous Transthoracic
    Needle Biopsy

Cervical Mediastinoscopy
Left Anterior Mediastinotomy and Extended
  Cervical Mediastinoscopy
Scalene Node Biopsy
Video-Assisted Thoracic Surgery
Thoracotomy
Metastatic Workup
Summary

It was estimated that in 2008 there were approximately 215,020 new cases of lung cancer in the United States,[1] and with 161,840 deaths projected for 2008, lung cancer remains the leading cause of cancer-related deaths in both men and women. Of newly diagnosed cases, approximately 80% will be non–small cell lung cancer (NSCLC), and of these, 80% will involve disseminated or locally advanced disease. Unfortunately, only 20% will be in potentially surgically curable patients with early stage disease, where complete resection yields a 5-year survival rate approaching 70%.[2]

Thorough workup and staging of the lung cancer patient are critical for a number of reasons. First, determining a patient's clinical TNM (tumor, node, metastasis) stage allows appropriate therapeutic decisions to be made on the basis of the specific stage of disease. This is particularly important for locally advanced disease in which multimodality therapy (induction or adjuvant) is now the standard of care, as well as for metastatic disease when unnecessary surgery should be avoided. Second, accurate staging allows the clinician to give the patient valuable prognostic information. Third, staging allows evaluation of new therapeutic interventions, and comparison of results of treatments between studies and institutions.

There are differences and controversies regarding the extent of workup and staging that should be performed, as well as about the appropriate modalities employed. Newer modalities, such as positron emission tomography (PET) and endobronchial ultrasound (EBUS), and their roles in the characterization of lung cancer will be reviewed.

THE STAGING SYSTEM

Staging is a process through which the extent of lung cancer in a patient is measured by a combination of techniques that includes history, physical examination, imaging studies, and invasive procedures where appropriate. Before initiation of treatment, a clinical stage (cTNM) is generated. If surgical resection occurs, the operative findings and pathologic features determine the final pathologic stage (pTNM).

In 1974, the American Joint Committee for Cancer (AJCC) Staging developed a lung cancer staging system based on TNM descriptors.[3] Naruke and coauthors[4] devised the original lymph node mapping schema that placed nodes into stations on the basis of clearly defined anatomic boundaries. Used to define the N (nodal) descriptors, it was modified for North America by the American Thoracic Society[5] and by Mountain and Dresler.[6] The current form of the map is seen in Figure 16-1. In 1986, the AJCC, Union Internationale Contre le Cancer (UICC), and representatives from Japan and Germany proposed an International Staging System (ISS) for lung cancer that grouped patients with similar survival outcomes using anatomic and morphologic criteria.[7] This system was originally applied to a database of over 3000 patients from the M. D. Anderson Cancer Center and the Lung Cancer Study Group and verified significant survival differences between stages. The applicability of the ISS was subsequently confirmed by studies from Naruke and colleagues[8] and Watanabe and coworkers.[9] The version of the ISS adopted in 1997 attempted to further minimize heterogeneity within stages and refine prognostic groupings after reviewing the survival data of 5319 patients.[10] The significant changes included dividing stages I and II into A and B subsets and incorporating T3N0M0 tumors into stage IIB. In addition, satellite nodules in the same lobe of the lung as the primary lesion were designated as T4 disease, whereas all other ipsilateral synchronous lesions were designated as M1. The current sixth edition of TNM Classification of Malignant Tumours introduced in 2002 made no alterations to the previous edition with respect to lung cancer.[11]

In 1996, the International Association for the Study of Lung Cancer (IASLC) initiated an international staging project to form the basis of the seventh edition of the TNM staging system.[12] The goals of the project were to validate the individual T, N, and M descriptors using a larger database made up of medical and surgical patients from a wide geographic distribution.[13] Data on 100,869 patients, including 67,725 cases of NSCLC, were submitted to the database, and several changes were proposed.[14] The existing N descriptors were validated

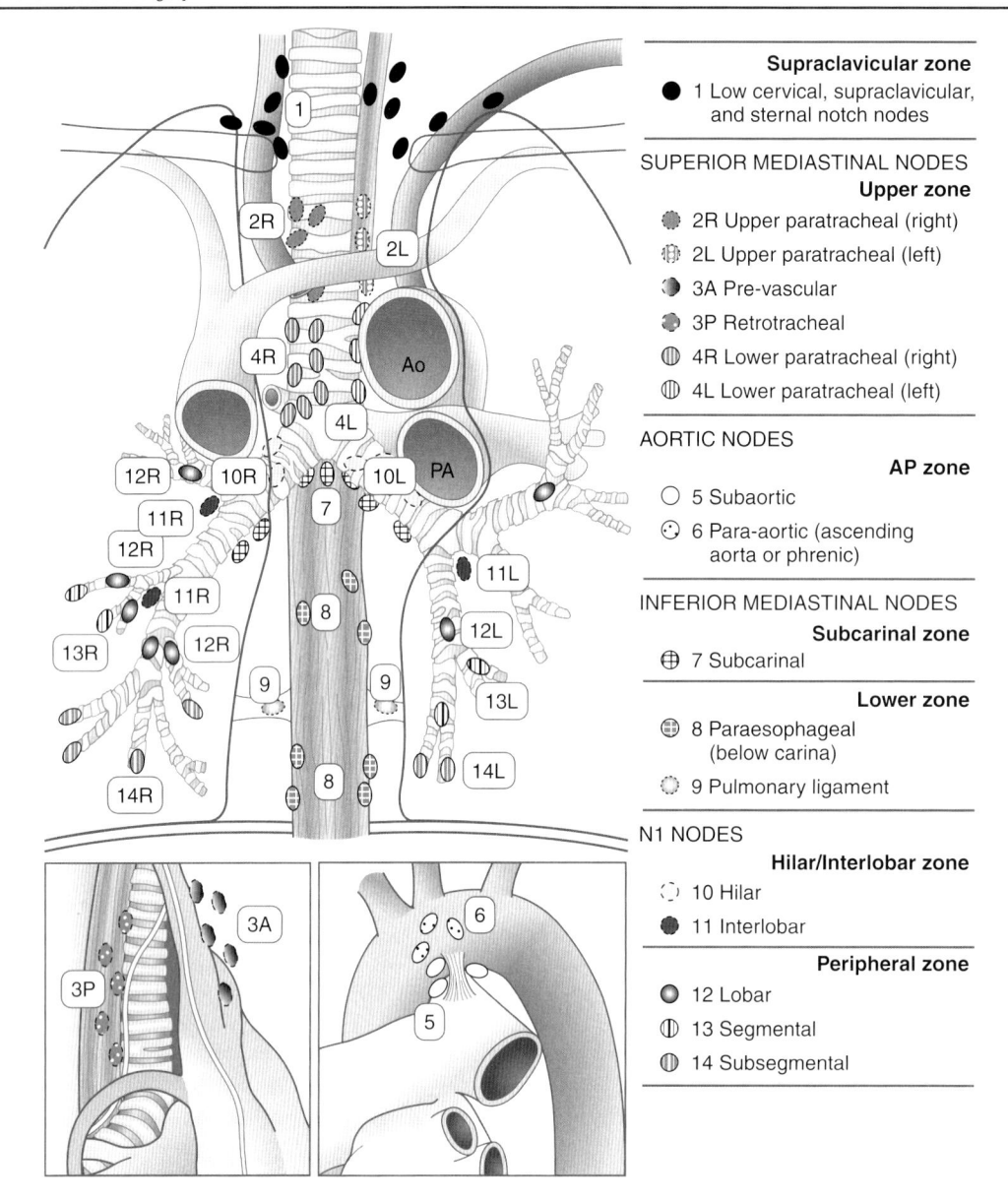

Figure 16–1
Regional lymph node stations for the staging of non–small cell lung cancer. Ao, aorta; PA, pulmonary artery. *(From Rusch VW, Asamura H, Watanabe H, Giroux DJ, Rami-Porta R, Goldstraw P. The IASLC Lung Cancer Staging Project: a proposal for a new international lymph node map in the forthcoming seventh edition of the TNM Classification for Lung Cancer.* J Thorac Oncol 2009;**4**:568.)

and not changed.[15] For the T descriptors, suggestions were made to make additional size cutoffs to the T1 and T2 tumors and to designate tumors greater than 7 cm in greatest dimension as T3, recognizing the poor prognostic significance of increasing size of the primary tumor (Table 16-1).[16] Furthermore, additional tumor nodules in the same lobe as the primary are proposed to be T3, whereas other nodules in the ipsilateral lobes become T4. It was recommended that the M descriptor be divided into M1a (for pleural metastases, malignant effusion, or contralateral pulmonary disease) and M1b (for extrathoracic metastases).[17] After incorporating the suggested changes into the data and reanalyzing the TNM subsets, new stage groupings were identified that yield even distributions between stages, particularly between stages IIA and IIB (Table 16-2).

DIAGNOSIS AND STAGING

Diagnosis and clinical staging take place concurrently, beginning with the initial history and physical examination. A variety of noninvasive and invasive tests are available to evaluate a patient suspected of having lung cancer, and often a single study serves the dual purpose of securing a diagnosis and staging the patient. If a patient's treatment is nonsurgical or involves multimodality therapy, obtaining a tissue diagnosis prior to treatment is mandatory. If it appears that the patient's clinical stage will be most appropriately managed by surgical resection alone, tissue confirmation of malignancy can be secured either preoperatively or at the time of exploration, depending on the preference of the operating surgeon.

Table 16–1
Proposed Definitions for T, N, and M Descriptors

T (Primary Tumor)	
TX	Primary tumor cannot be assessed, or tumor proven by the presence of malignant cells in sputum or bronchial washings but not visualized by imaging or bronchoscopy
T0	No evidence of primary tumor
Tis	Carcinoma in situ
T1	Tumor ≤ 3 cm in greatest dimension, surrounded by lung or visceral pleura, without bronchoscopic evidence of invasion more proximal than the lobar bronchus (i.e., not in the main bronchus)*
T1a	Tumor ≤ 2 cm in greatest dimension
T1b	Tumor > 2 cm but ≤ 3 cm in greatest dimension

T2	Tumor > 3 cm but ≤ 7 cm or tumor with any of the following features (T2 tumors with these features are classified T2a if ≤ 5 cm)
	    Involves main bronchus, ≥ 2 cm distal to the carina
	    Invades visceral pleura
	    Associated with atelectasis or obstructive pneumonitis that extends to the hilar region but does not involve the entire lung

T2a	Tumor > 3 cm but ≤ 5 cm in greatest dimension
T2b	Tumor > 5 cm but ≤ 7 cm in greatest dimension
T3	Tumor > 7 cm or one that directly invades any of the following: chest wall (including superior sulcus tumors), diaphragm, phrenic nerve, mediastinal pleura, parietal pericardium; or tumor in the main bronchus < 2 cm distal to the carina* but without involvement of the carina; or associated atelectasis or obstructive pneumonitis of the entire lung or separate tumor nodule(s) in the same lobe
T4	Tumor of any size that invades any of the following: mediastinum, heart, great vessels, trachea, recurrent laryngeal nerve, esophagus, vertebral body, carina; separate tumor nodule(s) in a different ipsilateral lobe
N (Regional Lymph Nodes)	
NX	Regional lymph nodes cannot be assessed
N0	No regional lymph node metastasis
N1	Metastasis in ipsilateral peribronchial and/or ipsilateral hilar lymph nodes and intrapulmonary nodes, including involvement by direct extension
N2	Metastasis in ipsilateral mediastinal and/or subcarinal lymph node(s)
N3	Metastasis in contralateral mediastinal, contralateral hilar, ipsilateral or contralateral scalene, or supraclavicular lymph node(s)
M (Distant Metastasis)	
MX	Distant metastasis cannot be assessed
M0	No distant metastasis
M1	Distant metastasis
M1a	Separate tumor nodule(s) in a contralateral lobe; tumor with pleural nodules or malignant pleural (or pericardial) effusion†
M1b	Distant metastasis (extrathoracic mets)

*The uncommon superficial spreading tumor of any size with its invasive component limited to the bronchial wall, which may extend proximally to the main bronchus, is also classified as T1.
†Most pleural (and pericardial) effusions with lung cancer are due to tumor. In a few patients, however, multiple cytopathologic examinations of pleural (pericardial) fluid are negative for tumor, and the fluid is nonbloody and is not an exudate. Where these elements and clinical judgment dictate that the effusion is not related to the tumor, the effusion should be excluded as a staging element and the patient should be classified as T1, T2, T3, or T4.
From Goldstraw P, Crowley J, Chansky K, Giroux DJ, Groome PA, Rami-Porta R, et al. The IASLC Lung Cancer Staging Project: proposals for the revision of the TNM stage groupings in the forthcoming (seventh) edition of the TNM classification of malignant tumours. J Thorac Oncol 2007;2(8):709.

History and Physical Examination

Patients often present for evaluation with a number of studies already performed. However, for several reasons, the history and physical examination remain the most important initial steps in evaluating patients who are suspected of having lung cancer. A detailed history focusing on risk factors such as duration of cigarette smoking, exposure to asbestos and other industrial hazards, a prior history of lung cancer, and the presence of symptoms allow the clinician to assess the probability of the diagnosis of lung cancer. Bach and associates showed that the duration of tobacco smoking, more so than the amount of daily usage, increases an individual's

Table 16-2
Descriptors, Proposed T and M Categories, and Proposed Stage Groupings

Sixth Edition T/M Descriptor	Proposed T/M	N0	N1	N2	N3
T1 (≤ 2 cm)	T1a	IA	IIA	IIIA	IIIB
T1 (>2–3 cm)	T1b	IA	IIA	IIIA	IIIB
T2 (≤ 5 cm)	T2a	IB	**IIA**	IIIA	IIIB
T2 (> 5–7 cm)	T2b	**IIA**	IIB	IIIA	IIIB
T2 (> 7 cm)	T3	**IIB**	**IIIA**	IIIA	IIIB
T3 invasion		IIB	IIIA	IIIA	IIIB
T4 (same-lobe nodules)		**IIB**	**IIIA**	**IIIA**	IIIB
T4 (extension)	T4	**IIIA**	**IIIA**	IIIB	IIIb
M1 (ipsilateral lung)		**IIIA**	**IIIA**	**IIIB**	IIIB
T4 (pleural effusion)	M1a	**IV**	**IV**	**IV**	**IV**
M1 (contralateral lung)		IV	IV	IV	IV
M1 (distant)	M1b	IV	IV	IV	IV

Cells in bold indicate a change from the sixth edition for a particular TNM category.
From Goldstraw P, Crowley J, Chansky K, Giroux DJ, Groome PA, Rami-Porta R, et al. The IASLC Lung Cancer Staging Project: proposals for the revision of the TNM stage groupings in the forthcoming (seventh) edition of the TNM classification of malignant tumours. J Thorac Oncol 2007;2(8):709.

risk of developing lung cancer.[18] Similarly, the risk associated with asbestos increases with the intensity and length of exposure, and together, tobacco use and asbestos exposure have a multiplicative effect. Certain symptoms, such as bone pain, hoarseness, weight loss, and neurologic changes, can indicate the presence of metastatic disease and mandate further investigation.

A thorough physical examination is also critical. It provides an estimate of a patient's overall health status, which has significant implications for the types of treatments available to that individual. Certain physical findings, such as ptosis, miosis, and anhidrosis in patients with Horner's syndrome, or the presence of clubbing, can support the suspicion of lung cancer. Furthermore, the physical examination can often demonstrate advanced disease even before any radiographic or other studies are performed. For example, palpation of the supraclavicular fossae can reveal lymph node metastases, and auscultation of the lung fields can detect the presence of a malignant pleural effusion.

NONINVASIVE MODALITIES

Chest Radiography

The standard posteroanterior and lateral chest radiographs are the most common initial study in which a suspected lung cancer is identified. Lesions are detected on a chest radiograph performed for symptoms or for unrelated reasons, such as part of a routine health assessment or preoperative clearance. Most lesions are not visible until they are at least 7 to 10 mm in diameter,[19] at which time they contain roughly 1 billion cells, representing 30 doublings.[20] A high-quality chest radiograph can impart a large amount of information and should be reviewed carefully. It localizes the site of suspect lesions (central or peripheral) and the local extent and effects of disease, showing areas of atelectasis, consolidation, or proximity to the pleural surface. The presence of a pleural effusion indicative of a T4 tumor can be seen, as well as elevation of the hemidiaphragm in the event of phrenic nerve involvement. Advanced disease may be identified in the case of rib destruction from bone metastases or synchronous lesions in the pulmonary parenchyma. Hilar and mediastinal lymph node metastasis is more difficult to identify, unless there is substantial enlargement.

Sputum Cytology

Cytologic analysis of sputum for malignant cells is a simple diagnostic technique, although it is being used less often in North America than in the past because bronchoscopy and percutaneous needle biopsy are used more now, and because of the decrease in the proportion of squamous cell cancers. Samples obtained may be induced by saline nebulization or collected as a 3-day pool of sputum produced from spontaneous coughing in the morning. Induced specimens should be immediately fixed and stained. Pooled samples are preserved in Saccomanno's solution (50% ethanol and 2% polyethylene glycol), or 70% ethanol until fixation and staining can be performed. Schreiber and McCrory[21] performed a meta-analysis of the published data on the diagnostic accuracy of sputum cytology in lung cancer. Most studies included a variety of indications for testing with only a few evaluating the sensitivity and specificity of sputum cytology in patients suspected of having lung cancer. Based on 16 published studies of at least 50 patients each, the overall sensitivity is 66% (range, 42% to 97%) and the overall specificity is 99% (range, 68% to 100%). The false-positive and false-negative rates are 9% and 6%, respectively. When sputum cytology is used for patients suspected of having lung cancer on clinical grounds, the diagnostic yield is higher, with a sensitivity of 87% and a specificity of 90%, as demonstrated by Jay and colleagues.[22]

A number of authors have shown that the sensitivity of sputum cytology for detecting lung cancer depends on the number of specimens collected per patient. Pilotti and coworkers,[23] Liang,[24] and Böcking and coworkers[25] confirmed that the optimal diagnostic sensitivity requires three specimens per patient. Other factors that influence the diagnostic sensitivity of sputum cytology include tumor location, size, and histologic type. Schreiber and McCrory[21] reviewed 17 studies that compared the sensitivity of sputum cytology in central versus peripheral lung lesions. Meta-analysis showed that the overall sensitivity was 71% for central lesions and 49% for peripheral lesions. The most likely explanation is that central tumors have a higher likelihood of shedding tumor cells into expectorated sputum because of their proximal bronchial location. Kato and associates[26] found that large tumors (greater than 3 cm), tumors associated with atelectasis or consolidation, and lower lobe location had higher diagnostic yields. In their study, the lowest sensitivity (20%) for sputum cytology occurred with peripheral tumors less than 3 cm in diameter. Histology of the tumor generally has less influence on the diagnostic accuracy of sputum cytology than the other

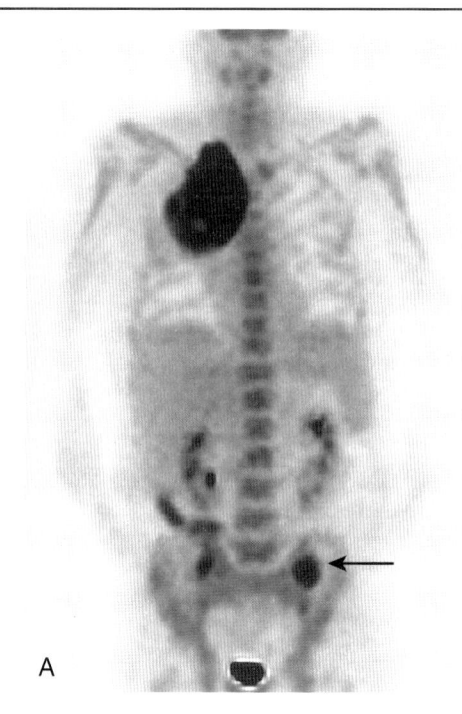

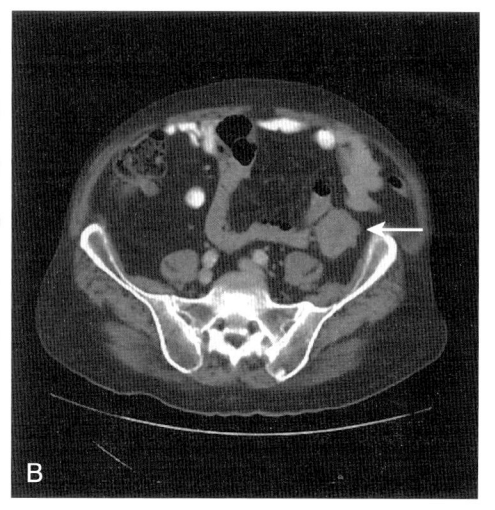

Figure 16-2
Positron emission tomography–computed tomography (PET-CT) showing a right superior sulcus tumor (**A**) and the presence of an asymptomatic retroperitoneal metastasis (**B**).

factors mentioned. Squamous carcinomas are, however, more frequently diagnosed by sputum analysis than adenocarcinomas or large cell carcinomas. This is probably related to the fact that squamous tumors are more commonly central in location.

High-Resolution Computed Tomography

Once a suspect lesion is detected on a chest radiograph or a low-dose computed tomography (CT) scan, the standard next step in the evaluation is a high-resolution CT of the chest and upper abdomen. This will yield information about the features and local extent of a potential lung cancer, giving precise size measurements and demonstrating signs of malignancy within a given lesion (spiculation, ground-glass opacification, lack of calcification). Evidence of invasion of contiguous structures, such as chest wall or mediastinal structures, can be assessed. This is especially critical when planning operative intervention, although unresectable involvement of surrounding structures may require surgical exploration for verification.

CT also provides details about the remaining lung parenchyma and pleural spaces. Satellite or additional nodules, bullous or emphysematous changes, pleural thickening, masses, or effusion may be identified. Typically, the chest CT for a suspected lung cancer includes the upper abdomen, specifically the liver and adrenal glands. Although most asymptomatic, incidental lesions in the upper abdomen are benign (adrenal adenoma, hepatic cysts), unsuspected metastases are identified in a small percentage of patients.

In addition to providing information about the primary tumor and the possibility of distant metastases, CT of the chest allows assessment of mediastinal lymph nodes. If not contraindicated, intravenous contrast is useful in distinguishing nodes from vascular structures. The most widely used criterion to define metastatic involvement is a short-axis diameter of 1 cm or greater. Although it is the most effective radiographic method of measuring lymph node enlargement, CT alone is inadequate to reliably predict metastatic nodal disease. In a prospective study of 143 patients with bronchogenic carcinoma in which CT findings were correlated with surgical pathologic staging, McLoud and coauthors[27] reported that the sensitivity of CT in predicting mediastinal nodal status was 64%, with a specificity of 62%. Toloza and colleagues[28,29] reported results of a meta-analysis of 20 studies with 3438 evaluable patients that showed an overall sensitivity of 57% and specificity of 82%. Therefore, staging of the mediastinum and subsequent therapeutic decisions should not be based solely on the results of the CT in most cases.

Positron Emission Tomography

Whole-body PET is a physiologic imaging technique based on the detection of positrons emitted by low-atomic-weight isotopes (carbon, fluorine, oxygen, nitrogen). Fluorodeoxyglucose (FDG) labeled with radioactive fluoride (^{18}F) is a D-glucose analog that is phosphorylated after cellular uptake and accumulates intracellularly, rather than being metabolized. Because lung cancer cells have an increased rate of glycolysis and overexpress the glucose transporter, there is preferential accumulation and visualization of FDG in the primary tumor and in potentially metastatic sites (Fig. 16-2).[30] The criterion for an abnormal PET scan is either a standardized uptake value (SUV) of greater than 2.5 or uptake in the lesion that is greater than the background activity of the mediastinum. Currently, the lower limit of resolution of PET is approximately 1.0 to 1.2 cm. In addition, certain non-neoplastic processes (such as inflammatory conditions and infections) can produce false-positive PET findings. Despite these limitations, PET has become an invaluable tool in lung cancer staging.

Several recent studies have shown that PET is superior to CT in staging the mediastinum in lung cancer patients. Pieterman and colleagues[31] prospectively compared standard staging approaches to PET for detection of mediastinal lymph node and distant metastases in 102 patients with resectable NSCLC who underwent histologic staging of the mediastinum. The sensitivity and specificity of PET for detection of mediastinal nodal metastases were 91% and 86%, respectively, compared with a sensitivity of 75% and a specificity of 66% for CT. Similarly, meta-analysis of 18 studies by Toloza and coworkers[28,29] demonstrated an overall sensitivity of 84% and specificity of 89%. Pieterman and associates[31] also showed that combining CT and PET resulted in the highest diagnostic accuracy, with a sensitivity of 94% and a specificity of 86%, supporting the use of both modalities for staging of the mediastinum.

Another significant result in the study by Pieterman and coauthors[31] was the observation that PET resulted in a stage different from the one arrived at by the standard methods in 62 of 102 patients, correctly indicating a lower stage in 20 patients and higher-stage disease in 42 patients. More importantly, PET was effective in identifying occult metastatic disease. In 11 patients (11%), PET demonstrated distant metastatic disease that was not detected by the usual staging tests. The sites of metastasis included bone, liver, and adrenal gland.

Within the past 10 years, integrated PET-CT scanners have replaced dedicated PET alone because of improved diagnostic accuracy and anatomic localization of disease.[32] Lardinois and colleagues[33] compared the diagnostic accuracy of integrated PET-CT with CT alone, PET alone, and visually correlated PET and CT in 50 patients with proved or suspected NSCLC. In 40 patients who underwent histologic confirmation, tumor staging was significantly more accurate with integrated PET-CT than with CT alone ($P = .001$), PET alone ($P < .001$), or visual correlation of PET and CT ($P = .013$). In 37 patients with histologic confirmation of nodal status, integrated PET-CT was more accurate in assessing the mediastinum than PET alone ($P = .013$). Moreover, unsuspected extrathoracic metastases were discovered in 16% (8 of 49 patients). Similarly, Cerfolio and coauthors compared PET with and without integrated CT in 129 patients with biopsy-proved or suspected NSCLC who subsequently underwent surgical staging.[34] PET-CT was a significantly better predictor of stages I and II disease and demonstrated superior accuracy for both T status (70% versus 47%, $P = .001$) and N status (78% versus 56%, $P = .008$) compared with PET alone. Moreover, PET-CT was more sensitive and more specific and had a higher positive predictive value for the status of N1 and N2 disease ($P < .05$). As in prior studies, PET-CT identified 19 (14.7%) patients with M1 disease.

With respect to the evaluation for the presence of bone metastases, PET-CT has proved to be more accurate than a bone scan, with a similar sensitivity and a higher specificity.[35-37] In the largest study comparing PET with bone scan, Song and colleagues retrospectively analyzed 1000 newly diagnosed patients, 105 of whom were eventually diagnosed with bone metastases and underwent PET-CT and bone scan.[37] PET-CT was more accurate (98.3% versus 95.1%, $P < .001$), sensitive (94.3% versus 78.1%, $P = .001$) and specific (98.8% versus 97.4%, $P = .006$) than bone scan. PET-CT also showed a lower incidence of false positives (1.2% versus 2.9%) and false-negative results (5.7% versus 21.9%) compared with a bone scan. Agreement between PET-CT and bone scan findings was good, with a calculated $\varkappa = 0.732$. Based on its clear advantages in noninvasive intrathoracic staging, and particularly in the identification of occult extrathoracic disease, PET-CT should be a routine part of pretreatment staging.

Bone Scan

Although PET-CT has essentially replaced it for evaluation of potential skeletal metastases, when utilized in the setting of a positive clinical assessment (e.g., bone pain or tenderness), a technetium-99m methylene diphosphate (^{99m}Tc MDP) whole-body bone scan is relatively sensitive, but not specific. In their meta-analysis of seven studies and 633 patients, Toloza and colleagues[28,29] showed that bone scans have an overall sensitivity of 87% and specificity of 67%. False-positive abnormalities are more common when scans are done in asymptomatic patients and can be the result of degenerative or traumatic skeletal injury. Follow-up imaging with magnetic resonance imaging (MRI) may or may not aid in establishing a definitive diagnosis. False-negative results, although uncommon, do occur, and in one series 6% of patients with an initially negative bone scan developed confirmed skeletal metastases within 1 year.[38]

Magnetic Resonance Imaging

MRI of the chest for the evaluation and characterization of pulmonary lesions and the mediastinum offers few advantages over CT in the diagnosis or staging of lung cancer. Heelan and coworkers[39] evaluated both CT and MRI in otherwise operable patients with NSCLC and found that MRI was no more accurate than CT in identifying hilar or mediastinal lymph node metastases and actually had a higher false-positive rate. In some situations, however, MRI can be useful. When tumors are adjacent to the vertebral body or spinal canal, MRI provides superior visualization of the spinal canal and can more accurately detect subtle changes in the marrow suggestive of invasion. In addition, MRI can more accurately delineate a superior sulcus tumor's relationship to major vessels and the brachial plexus at the thoracic outlet.

INVASIVE MODALITIES

Bronchoscopy

Rigid or flexible bronchoscopy with conventional white light allows visualization of the tracheobronchial tree and is a standard part of evaluating patients with known or suspected lung cancer. It serves several critical purposes: diagnosis, staging, assessment of resectability, and visualization of the remaining bronchial tree. Flexible video-assisted bronchoscopy has become a widely used technique, replacing rigid bronchoscopy for all but a few special circumstances. Flexible bronchoscopy is generally performed as an outpatient procedure on a spontaneously breathing patient through the nasal or oral route, following topical anesthesia and sedation. The tracheobronchial tree up to the second or third subsegmental bronchi is easily visualized. The options available to secure a diagnosis include direct biopsy, brushing, saline lavage for cytology, and transbronchial needle aspiration (TBNA) with or without fluoroscopic guidance. Employing more than one

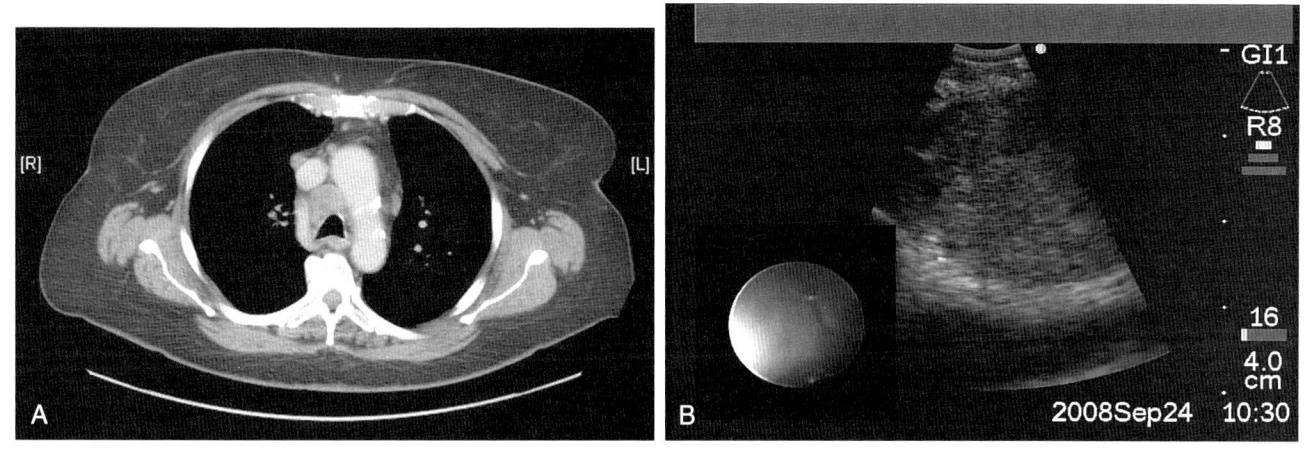

Figure 16–3
A, CT scan of the chest revealing enlarged right paratracheal lymph node. **B,** Endobronchial ultrasound (EBUS)–guided transbronchial needle aspirate of an enlarged right paratracheal lymph node.

technique (e.g., biopsy, brushing, and cytologic lavage) generally improves the diagnostic yield.

When bronchoscopy reveals an endobronchial tumor, biopsy is best accomplished with either a forceps or brush biopsy, with sensitivities in the range of 80% to 100%.[40,41] Positive endobronchial findings are more common with squamous and small cell cancers because of their central location. In contrast, a normal bronchoscopic examination is usually seen with peripheral lesions, and the diagnostic sensitivity of bronchoscopy varies widely from 37% to 98%, depending on the size and location of the target lesion. Increasing size and presence of a bronchus sign (a bronchus leading to or contained in a lesion on CT) portend a higher diagnostic yield.[41] The use of fluoroscopy to guide a transbronchial biopsy or TBNA and lavage can improve diagnostic accuracy up to 80%.[42]

TBNA can also be used when there is bronchial distortion (thickening or blunting of the carina, extrinsic compression) secondary to the lesion or metastatic lymph nodes. Popularized by Wang and Terry, TBNA employs a 20- to 22-gauge, rigid needle through the channel of the fiberoptic bronchoscope to puncture the airway in the area of interest.[43] It is a safe and inexpensive procedure with an overall sensitivity of 50% and a specificity of 96%.[40,41] As previously mentioned, diagnostic yield is enhanced by the use of fluoroscopy, as well as the use of rapid, on-site cytopathology. A positive result, especially from a mediastinal lymph node station, can obviate further surgical staging, although a negative result should still be confirmed surgically. Limitations include a sensitivity of only 30% for small (<2 cm), peripheral lesions, and inaccessibility of certain lymph node stations, including anterior, aortopulmonary, paraesophageal, and pulmonary ligament nodes.

Endobronchial Ultrasound

In an effort to improve on the diagnostic accuracy of TBNA, EBUS was developed and commercially introduced in the early 1990s.[44] The original probe was radial, and radial EBUS guidance was shown to improve the yield of TBNA in the lymph node staging of lung cancer.[45,46] More recently, a new ultrasonic endoscope with a built-in linear-array, convex probe at the tip was developed by the Olympus Corporation (Tokyo) to enable real-time EBUS-guided TBNA. This EBUS is integrated with a convex transducer at 7.5 MHz at the tip of a flexible bronchoscope (XBF-UC260F-OL8, Olympus), whose angle of view is 90 degrees and direction of view is 30 degrees forward oblique. The ultrasound scans parallel to the insertion direction of the scope, and images are obtained by directly contacting the probe, with or without a saline-filled balloon at the tip. The ultrasound image is processed by a dedicated scanner (EU-C2000) that allows for image freezing, size measurement, and Doppler mode. A special 22-gauge needle is passed under direct visualization through the instrument channel to biopsy the target lesion through the bronchial wall (Fig. 16-3). The procedure can be done under monitored anesthesia care or general anesthesia. Indications for EBUS-TBNA include diagnosis of lung and mediastinal tumors and assessment of mediastinal and hilar lymph nodes. Accessible nodal stations include levels 2, 3, 4, 7, 10, and 11. Subaortic, paraesophageal, peribronchial, segmental, and subsegmental nodes are general not approachable.

Several retrospective studies have demonstrated excellent accuracy of EBUS-TBNA for mediastinal and hilar nodal staging in NSCLC.[47-49] In one of the earliest and largest series of patients, Yasufuku and colleagues[48] successfully performed EBUS-TBNA in 105 patients with proved or suspected lung cancer and suspect adenopathy by CT criteria alone. They sampled 163 lymph nodes and reported an overall diagnostic accuracy rate of 96.3%, with a sensitivity of 94.6% and a specificity of 100%. Of note, patients who proved to have benign disease were excluded from analysis, and not all patients had confirmatory surgical biopsy of the nodal stations biopsied by EBUS. No studies to date have compared results of EBUS-TBNA with those of cervical mediastinoscopy. Despite the lack of studies with histologic confirmation of all nodal stations sampled by EBUS, this new technology is clearly emerging as a potential alternative to more invasive mediastinal and hilar staging.

Autofluorescence Bronchoscopy

Detection and treatment of subtle dysplastic or early invasive neoplastic lesions whose presence is suggested by positive sputum cytology remain a challenge. In one study,

Woolner[50] reported that only 29% of the carcinoma in situ detected by sputum cytology could be localized by conventional bronchoscopy. Additional studies have shown that roughly one third of patients with positive sputum cytology, but radiographically occult lung cancers, require more than one bronchoscopy for localization.[51,52] In an effort to improve identification of superficial bronchial mucosal malignancy, Hung and associates[53] were able to demonstrate that normal and malignant bronchial mucosa have different autofluorescence intensities under blue light (wavelength, 442 nm). This led to the development of the LIFE (light imaging fluorescence endoscope) Lung system (Xillix Technologies, Richmond, BC, Canada). Whereas normal bronchial mucosa appears green, premalignant and malignant tissue appears brown-red.[54] Subsequent prospective trials comparing white-light bronchoscopy alone with white-light bronchoscopy plus LIFE have shown enhanced sensitivity in detection of intraepithelial neoplasms and invasive carcinoma.[54-57] Lam and coauthors[57] reported the results of a multicenter North American trial of 173 patients that showed the relative sensitivity of white-light bronchoscopy plus LIFE versus white-light bronchoscopy alone to be 6.3 for intraepithelial lesions, and 2.71 if invasive cancers were included. The role of LIFE was in preoperative screening for synchronous squamous carcinomas, but follow-up for recurrence or second primary tumors, and for monitoring intraepithelial dysplasia in some chemoprevention trials, it is not currently in widespread use.

Percutaneous Transthoracic Needle Biopsy

Percutaneous transthoracic needle biopsy is a well-established procedure used in confirming a tissue diagnosis of lung cancer in patients who are not surgical candidates because of advanced disease or medical contraindications. However, with the identification of increasing numbers of noncalcified pulmonary nodules by low-dose CT, transthoracic needle biopsy is becoming a critical tool in the detection of early stage lung cancer. Although both fluoroscopic and CT guidance are employed, CT is the preferred modality for several reasons. CT allows planning precise trajectories that avoid aerated lung, blood vessels, bullae, and vital cardiovascular structures in the mediastinum. Smaller lesions can be biopsied, and CT can enable differentiation between necrotic and viable areas in a larger tumor, improving diagnostic yield.[58] The most common complications of the procedure are pneumothorax and mild hemoptysis. Although the reported incidence of pneumothorax varies greatly, the rate of postprocedure pneumothoraces requiring intervention ranges from 1.6% to 17%.[59,60] The most important risk factor is underlying chronic obstructive pulmonary disease (COPD).[61] Hemoptysis occurs in 5% to 10% of cases and is usually self-limited. Massive hemoptysis is extremely rare with the use of 20-gauge or smaller needles.[62,63] Relative contraindications to transthoracic biopsy, therefore, are the presence of severe COPD, a bleeding disorder, contralateral pneumonectomy, and severe pulmonary hypertension. When successful, the results of percutaneous transthoracic biopsy are positive in patients with lung cancer in roughly 90% of cases, with a low false-positive rate of less than 2%.[64] However, false-negative results can be frequent, so all results should be considered indeterminate unless a specific benign diagnosis is made.

Cervical Mediastinoscopy

Accurate assessment is paramount as mediastinal lymph node involvement by metastatic carcinoma strongly influences treatment decisions. Cervical mediastinoscopy is the most accurate pre-thoracotomy method of staging the mediastinum in bronchogenic carcinoma. Described by Carlens in 1959, mediastinoscopy employs a rigid, lighted scope placed in the avascular, pretracheal space to access the superior mediastinum.[65] Its efficacy is well established, with a pooled procedural sensitivity of 81% and a specificity of 100% in a recent meta-analysis of 5687 patients.[29] Moreover, a negative mediastinoscopy predicts a high rate of complete resection at thoracotomy. Luke and colleagues[66] demonstrated that of 590 patients with a negative mediastinoscopy, 93% had complete tumor resection. Cervical mediastinoscopy is an outpatient procedure that is extremely safe. In a review of 2137 patients, Hammoud and coworkers[67] reported overall morbidity and mortality rates of 0.6% and 0.05%, respectively.

The indications for mediastinoscopy are often debated, and routine mediastinoscopy is controversial. Most thoracic surgeons would agree that mediastinoscopy should be performed for the following: (1) lymph node enlargement greater than 1 cm in the short axis on CT, (2) hypermetabolic uptake on PET, and (3) possible enrollment into induction therapy protocols. Relative indications include the presence of T2 or T3 tumor, adenocarcinoma, or large cell carcinoma.[68] Those who support the practice of routine mediastinoscopy emphasize its low complication rate and accuracy, the high rate of complete resection after a negative mediastinoscopy, the relatively low sensitivity of CT, the prevalence of nodal disease even in T1 tumors (Table 16-3), and the ability to select patients who might benefit from induction therapy.

Left Anterior Mediastinotomy and Extended Cervical Mediastinoscopy

One limitation of mediastinoscopy can be in the setting of a left upper lobe cancer, in which aortopulmonary window and para-aortic lymph nodes (levels 5 and 6) may need to be sampled. In this situation, there are two options for surgical staging. Most commonly, level-5 and level-6 mediastinal lymph nodes can be accessed from a left anterior or parasternal approach, as described by McNeill and Chamberlain.[69] A transverse incision is placed over the second rib, and the costal cartilage is removed. The retrosternal extrapleural space is entered by blunt dissection and the para-aortic space is explored. Modifications of the procedure include preservation of the internal mammary vessels, use of the mediastinoscope for better visualization, and preservation of the cartilaginous rib. In three reported series totaling 194 patients with left upper lobe cancers who underwent a Chamberlain procedure, 38% (73 of 194) had positive biopsy results, and resectability in those patients with a negative anterior mediastinotomy was 95%.[70] As with cervical mediastinoscopy, morbidity and mortality in previously reported series are low—8% and 0%, respectively.

A second, less commonly employed surgical approach to the anterior mediastinum in left upper lobe cancers is extended mediastinoscopy, as described by Ginsberg and associates.[71] After a pathologically negative standard cervical mediastinoscopy, the mediastinoscope is withdrawn, and blunt digital

Table 16-3
Prevalence of Nodal Metastases in Clinical T1 Non–Small Cell Lung Cancer

Author (ref)	Patients (N)	Node + (%)	N1 (%)	N2 (%)	Skip N (%)
Ishida et al. (87)	221	28	9	19	28
Naruke (88)	714	33	18	15	30
Asamura et al. (89)	337	26	10	16	25
Oda et al. (90)	524	22	8	14	51
Graham et al. (91)	86	29	19	10	34

dissection is used to create a window between the innominate and left carotid arteries posterior to the innominate vein. The mediastinoscope is reinserted and advanced along the anterolateral surface of the aortic arch into the node-containing fat pad. Extended mediastinoscopy should be avoided in patients with a dilated or calcified aortic arch or previous sternotomy. Because of the nature of the dissection and the emergence of other minimally invasive alternatives to accessing the aortopulmonary window, such as EUS and video-assisted thoracic surgery (VATS), extended mediastinoscopy is not widely performed.

Scalene Node Biopsy

Scalene node biopsy is used to assess suspect nodes in the supraclavicular fossa, identified by either palpation or imaging (specifically, PET). It has also been shown to be valuable to rule out N3 disease in patients with proven N2 disease. In the event that there are grossly palpable nodes in the supraclavicular fossa, a fine-needle aspiration (FNA) in the office is often sufficient. Should an FNA be nondiagnostic, or if metastatic disease is suspected on imaging alone, a formal excision of the fat pad may be performed. A 3- to 4-cm incision is placed over the insertion of the sternocleidomastoid muscle parallel to the clavicle. Dissection is performed between the clavicular and sternal heads, exposing the scalene fat pad on top of the scalenus anterior muscle. Care must be taken to preserve the phrenic nerve lying posterior on the scalenus anterior muscle. Alternatively, Lee and Ginsberg[72] reported a technique whereby scalene node biopsy can be done during a positive cervical mediastinoscopy employing a single incision. They showed that 15.4% of patients (6 of 39) with positive N2 disease had positive scalene nodes as well, indicating N3 disease.

Video-Assisted Thoracic Surgery

Video-assisted thoracic surgery, with a thoracoscope and enhanced video optics and instrumentation, provides another valuable tool for the diagnosis and staging of NSCLC. It requires general anesthesia and a patient who can tolerate single-lung ventilation. With the patient in a standard lateral decubitus position, the thoracoscope and endoscopic instruments are inserted through two or more operating ports placed via small incisions through the intercostal space. With this technique, the entire hemithorax can be explored, including the hilum, mediastinum, visceral and parietal pleural surfaces, and chest wall. The principal use of VATS has been to perform the excisional biopsy of peripheral lung nodules for the diagnosis of primary lung cancer or to rule out synchronous or metastatic disease.[73,74] However, VATS is less effective for lesions located in the posterior paravertebral space or situated deep in the lung parenchyma. It can be used to evaluate mediastinal lymph nodes in patients with lung cancer. In particular, VATS can be used to sample nodes inaccessible by cervical mediastinoscopy (anterior, aortopulmonary, para-aortic) or anterior mediastinotomy (hilar, inferior pulmonary ligament).[75,76] Several studies have shown that the sensitivity and accuracy of VATS approach 100% for diagnosis and staging of lung cancer, with minimal morbidity and mortality.

Thoracotomy

When other diagnostic and staging modalities have failed, thoracotomy is indicated for accurate diagnosis, staging, and subsequent curative treatment of potential lung cancers. With the myriad of accurate, less invasive diagnostic methods available, more than 95% of tumors can be characterized without thoracotomy. Exploratory thoracotomy, however, still allows the most thorough assessment of the primary lesion, the pleural space, and the ipsilateral mediastinal lymph nodes. The tumor is typically biopsied by Tru-Cut needle, and the local extent and status of the mediastinal lymph nodes are assessed while the pathologists analyze the specimen by frozen section.

METASTATIC WORKUP

Approximately 40% of patients with newly diagnosed lung cancer are found to have extrathoracic metastases. Identifying these patients is critical to avoid unnecessary thoracotomy and delaying appropriate systemic therapy. Currently, the standard multiorgan imaging techniques used to rule out the most common metastases in patients with NSCLC (adrenal, liver, brain, bone) are CT of the chest and upper abdomen, CT or MRI of the brain with contrast, and whole-body PET-CT.

Who should undergo evaluation for distant metastatic disease? There are precious few prospective randomized trials of extrathoracic imaging for NSCLC. It is well accepted that patients who have certain symptoms, abnormal physical findings, or laboratory abnormalities are at increased risk of having metastatic disease. Silvestri and coauthors showed in a large meta-analysis that a positive clinical evaluation was

Table 16-4
Clinical Evaluation for Metastatic Disease

Clinical Evaluation	Finding
Symptoms	Constitutional: weight loss > 5% of body weight, malaise Musculoskeletal: focal skeletal pain Neurologic: headache, seizure, mental status or personality changes
Physical signs	Focal neurologic deficit Supraclavicular lymphadenopathy Hoarseness Superior vena cava syndrome Bony tenderness Skin or soft tissue mass Hepatomegaly
Laboratory tests	Anemia Elevated liver function tests Hypercalcemia

associated with a roughly 50% rate of abnormal scans.[77] These results underscore how critical the findings of the initial history, physical examination, and laboratory tests are in guiding subsequent workup. Patients with a positive clinical evaluation (Table 16-4) should undergo multiorgan scanning.

What about asymptomatic patients? Routine multiorgan imaging in patients without symptoms or signs is controversial. Several studies have shown that routine preoperative scanning in asymptomatic patients is associated with a low percentage (3% to 10%) of positive results, with silent metastases found in 2.7% to 15%.[78,79] In their meta-analysis, Silvestri and colleagues[77] calculated the probability that a scan will be negative if the clinical evaluation is negative (i.e, the negative predictive value of the clinical evaluation). For CT of the abdomen or brain, and for bone scan, the negative predictive values were 94%, 95%, and 89%, respectively. The only prospective, randomized trial that compared routine multiorgan scanning with chest CT and mediastinoscopy in asymptomatic patients with clinically operable lung cancer showed no statistically significant difference in the rate of unnecessary thoracotomy, postoperative recurrence, or overall survival.[80] Despite this, more recent data have shown whole-body PET and PET-CT to be invaluable in disclosing non–central nervous system metastatic disease in up to 10% to 20% of cases missed by standard methods.[31,81-83] On this basis, PET-CT should be considered a standard staging modality in all cases of biopsy-proved or suspected lung cancer, and it obviates the need for bone scan as well.

In addition, some authors have reported that more locally advanced lesions (T3 or N2) have a higher rate of asymptomatic distant metastases.[84,85] Others have shown that adenocarcinomas have a higher rate of asymptomatic cerebral metastases than squamous carcinomas.[79,86]

Based on the available information, we believe that all patients with established or suspected lung cancer should undergo high-resolution, contrast CT of the chest and whole-body PET-CT. Additional appropriate multiorgan scanning should be considered for (1) any patient with a positive clinical evaluation (symptoms, signs, blood work), (2) patients with locally advanced disease (stage IIIA) being considered for multi-modality therapy, and (3) patients with earlier-stage disease (stages I, II) who are marginal operative candidates.

Summary

Lung cancer remains a challenging and deadly disease. Proper diagnosis and staging are critical for determining the best treatment strategy for each individual patient. The most important components of the workup are the initial history and the physical examination. Numerous noninvasive and invasive techniques can be employed to establish an accurate and valid clinical estimate of tumor stage.

REFERENCES

1. Jemal A, Siegel R, Ward E, et al. Cancer statistics, 2008. *CA Cancer J Clin* 2008;**58**:71-96.
2. Nesbitt JC, Putnam JB, Walsh GL, et al. Survival in early-stage non-small cell lung cancer. *Ann Thorac Surg* 1995;**60**:466-72.
3. Mountain CF, Carr DT, Anderson WA. A system for the clinical staging of lung cancer. *AJR Am J Roentgenol Radium Ther Nucl Med* 1974;**120**:130-8.
4. Naruke T, Suemasu K, Ishikawa S. Lymph node mapping and curability at various levels of metastasis in resected lung cancer. *J Thorac Cardiovasc Surg* 1978;**76**:832-9.
5. American Thoracic Society. Medical section of the American Lung Association. Clinical staging of primary lung cancer. *Am Rev Respir Dis* 1983;**127**:659-64.
6. Mountain CF, Dresler CM. Regional lymph node classification for lung cancer staging. *Chest* 1997;**111**:1718-23.
7. Mountain CF. A new international staging system for lung cancer. *Chest* 1986;**89**:225-33.
8. Naruke T, Goya T, Tsuchya R, et al. Prognosis and survival in resected lung cancer based on the new international staging system. *J Thorac Cardiovasc Surg* 1988;**96**:440-7.
9. Watanabe Y, Shimizu J, Oda M, et al. Proposals regarding some deficiencies in the new international staging system for non-small cell lung cancer. *Jpn J Clin Oncol* 1991;**21**:160-8.
10. Mountain CF. Revisions in the international system for staging lung cancer. *Chest* 1997;**111**:1710-7.
11. Sobin L, Wittekind Ch, editors. TNM Classification of Malignant Tumors. Sixth Edition New York: Wiley-Liss; 2002. p. 99-103.
12. Goldstraw P, Crowley JJ. on behalf of the IASLC International Staging Project The International Association for the Study of Lung Cancer International Staging Project on Lung Cancer. *J Thorac Oncol* 2006;**1**:281-6.
13. Groome PA, Bolejack V, Crowley J, et al. on behalf of the International Staging Committee, Cancer Research and Biostatistics, Observers to the Committee and Participating Institutions. The IASLC Lung Cancer Staging Project: Validation of the Proposals for Revision of the T, N, and M Descriptors and Consequent Stage Groupings in the Forthcoming (Seventh) Edition of the TNM Classification of Malignant Tumours. *J Thorac Oncol* 2007;**2**:694-705.
14. Goldstraw P, Crowley J, Chansky K, et al. on behalf of the International Association for the Study of Lung Cancer International Staging Committee and Participating Institutions. The IASLC Lung Cancer Staging Project: Proposals for the Revision of the TNM stage groupings in the forthcoming (seventh) Edition of the TNM classification of malignant tumours. *J Thorac Oncol* 2007;**2**:706-14.
15. Rusch VW, Crowley J, Giroux DJ, et al. on behalf of the International Staging Committee, Cancer Research and Biostatistics, Observers to the Committee, and Participating Institutions. The IASLC Lung Cancer Staging Project: proposals for the revision of the N descriptors in the forthcoming seventh edition of the TNM classification for lung cancer. *J Thorac Oncol* 2007;**2**:603-12.
16. Rami-Porta R, Ball D, Crowley J, et al. on behalf of the International Staging Committee, Cancer Research and Biostatistics, Observers to the Committee, and Participating Institutions. The IASLC Lung Cancer Staging Project: Proposals for the revision of the T descriptors in the forthcoming (seventh) edition of the TNM classification for lung cancer. *J Thorac Oncol* 2007;**2**:593-602.
17. Postmus PE, Brambilla E, Chansky K, et al. on behalf of the International Staging Committee, Cancer Research and Biostatistics, Observers to the Committee, and Participating Institutions. The IASLC Lung Cancer Staging Project: Proposals for revision of the M descriptors in the forthcoming (seventh) edition of the TNM classification of lung cancer. *J Thorac Oncol* 2007;**2**:686-93.
18. Bach PB, Kattan MW, Thornquist MD, et al. Variations in lung cancer risk among smokers. *J Natl Cancer Inst* 2003;**95**:470-8.

19. Rigler LG. The earliest roentgenographic signs of carcinoma of the lung. *JAMA* 1966;**195**:655-7.
20. Geddes DM. The natural history of lung cancer: A review board on rates of tumor growth. *Br J Dis Chest* 1979;**73**:1-7.
21. Schreiber G, McCrory DC. Performance characteristics of different modalities for diagnosis of suspected lung cancer. Summary of published evidence. *Chest* 2003;**123**:115S-28S.
22. Jay SJ, Wehr K, Nicholson DP, et al. Diagnostic sensitivity and specificity of pulmonary cytology: Comparison of techniques used in conjunction with flexible fiberoptic bronchoscopy. *Acta Cytol* 1980;**24**:304-12.
23. Pilotti S, Rilke F, Gribaudi G, et al. Sputum cytology for the diagnosis of carcinoma of the lung. *Acta Cytol* 1982;**26**:649-54.
24. Liang XM. Accuracy of cytologic diagnosis and cytotyping of sputum in primary lung cancer: Analysis of 161 cases. *J Surg Oncol* 1989;**40**:107-11.
25. Böcking A, Biesterfeld S, Chatelain R, et al. Diagnosis of bronchial carcinoma on sections of paraffin-embedded sputum: Sensitivity and specificity of an alternative to routine cytology. *Acta Cytol* 1992;**36**:37-47.
26. Kato H, Konako C, Ono J, et al. *Cytology of the lung: Techniques and interpretation*. Tokyo: Igaku-Shoin; 1983.
27. McLoud TC, Bourgouin PM, Greenberg RW, et al. Bronchogenic carcinoma: Analysis of staging in the mediastinum with CT by correlative lymph node mapping and sampling. *Radiology* 1992;**182**:319-23.
28. Toloza EM, Harpole L, McCrory DC. Noninvasive staging of non-small cell lung cancer. A review of the current evidence. *Chest* 2003;**123**:137S-46S.
29. Toloza EM, Harpole L, Detterbeck F, et al. Invasive staging of non-small cell lung cancer. A review of the current evidence. *Chest* 2003;**123**:157S-66S.
30. Brown RS, Leung JY, Kison PV, et al. Glucose transporters and FDG uptake in untreated primary human non-small cell lung cancer. *J Nucl Med* 1999;**40**:556-65.
31. Pieterman RM, van Putten JWG, Meuzelaar JJ, et al. Preoperative staging of non-small-cell lung cancer with positron-emission tomography. *N Engl J Med* 2000;**343**:254-61.
32. Beyer T, Townsend DW, Brun T, et al. A combined PET/CT scanner for clinical oncology. *J Nucl Med* 2000;**41**:1369-79.
33. Lardinois D, Weder W, Hany TF, et al. Staging of non-small-cell lung cancer with integrated positron-emission tomography and computed tomography. *N Engl J Med* 2003;**348**:2500-7.
34. Cerfolio RJ, Buddhiwardhani O, Bryant AS, et al. The Accuracy of integrated PET-CT compared with dedicated PET alone for the staging of patients with nonsmall cell lung cancer. *Ann Thorac Surg* 2004;**78**:1017-23.
35. Bury T, Barreto A, Daenen F, et al. Fluorine-18 deoxyglucose positron emission tomography for the detection of bonemetastases in patients with non-small cell lung cancer. *Eur J Nucl Med* 1998;**25**:1244-7.
36. Gayed I, Vu T, Johnson M, et al. Comparison of bone and 2-deoxy-2-[18F]fluoro-D-glucose positron emission tomography in the evaluation of bony metastases in lung cancer. *Mol Imaging Biol* 2003;**5**:26-31.
37. Song JW, Oh YM, Shim TS, Kim WS, Ryu JS, Choi CM. Efficacy comparison between 18F-FDG PET/CT and bone scintigraphy in detecting bony metastases of non-small-cell lung cancer. *Lung Cancer* 2009:doi:10.1016/j.lungcan.2008.12.004.
38. Michel F, Soler M, Imhof E, et al. Initial staging of non-small cell lung cancer: Value of routine radioisotope bone scanning. *Thorax* 1991;**46**:469-73.
39. Heelan RT, Martini N, Westcott JW, et al. Carcinomatous involvement of the hilum and mediastinum: Computed tomographic and magnetic resonance evaluation. *Radiology* 1985;**156**:111-5.
40. Gasparini S. Bronchoscopic biopsy techniques in the diagnosis and staging of lung cancer. *Monaldi Arch Chest Dis* 1997;**52**:392-8.
41. Shure D. Fiberoptic bronchoscopy-diagnostic applications. *Clin Chest Med* 1987;**8**:1-3.
42. Schenk DA, Bryan CL, Bower JH, et al. Transbronchial needle aspiration in the diagnosis of bronchogenic carcinoma. *Chest* 1987;**92**:83-5.
43. Wang KP, Terry PB. Transbronchial needle aspiration in the diagnosis and staging of bronchogenic carcinoma. *Am Rev Respir Dis* 1983;**127**:344-7.
44. Hurter T, Hanrath P. Endobronchial sonography: feasibility and preliminary results. *Thorax* 1992;**47**:565-7.
45. Herth F, Becker HD, Ernst A. Ultrasound-guided transbronchial needle aspiration: an experience in 242 patients. *Chest* 2003;**123**:604-7.
46. Herth F, Becker HD, Ernst A. Conventional vs endobronchial ultrasound-guided transbronchial needle aspiration: a randomized trial. *Chest* 2004;**125**:322-5.
47. Yasufuku K, Chiyo M, Sekine Y, et al. Real-time endobronchial ultrasound guided transbronchial needle aspiration of mediastinal and hilar lymph nodes. *Chest* 2004;**126**:122-8.
48. Yasufuku K, Chiyo M, Koh E, et al. Endobronchial ultrasound guided transbronchial needle aspiration for staging of lung cancer. *Lung Cancer* 2005;**50**:347-54.
49. Krasnik M, Vilman P, Larsen SS, et al. Preliminary experience with a new method of endoscopic transbronchial real time ultrasound guided biopsy for diagnosis of mediastinal and hilar lesions. *Thorax* 2003;**58**:1083-6.
50. Woolner LB. Pathology of cancer detected cytologically. In: *Atlas of early lung cancer*. National Cancer Institute, National Institutes of Health, U.S. Department of Health and Human Services. Tokyo: Igaku-Shoin; 1983, p. 107-213.
51. Bechtel JJ, Kelly WR, Petty TL, et al. Outcome of 51 patients with roentgenographically occult lung cancer detected by sputum cytologic testing: A community hospital program. *Arch Intern Med* 1994;**154**:975-80.
52. Cortese DA, Pairolero PC, Bergstralh EJ, et al. Roentgenographically occult lung cancer: A 10-year experience. *J Thorac Cardiovasc Surg* 1983;**86**:373-80.
53. Hung J, Lam S, LeRiche JC, et al. Autofluorescence of normal and malignant bronchial tissue. *Laser Surg Med* 1991;**11**:99-105.
54. Kennedy TC, Lam S, Hirsch FR. Review of recent advances in fluorescence bronchoscopy in early localization of central airway lung cancer. *Oncologist* 2001;**6**:257-62.
55. Hirsch FR, Prindiville SA, Miller YE, et al. Fluorescence versus white-light bronchoscopy for detection of preneoplastic lesions: a randomized study. *J Natl Cancer Inst* 2001;**93**:1385-91.
56. Lam S, Kennedy TC, Unger M, et al. Localization of bronchial intraepithelial neoplastic lesions by fluorescence bronchoscopy. *Cancer* 1998;**113**:696-702.
57. Lam S, MacAulay C, LeRiche JC, et al. Detection and localization of early lung cancer by fluorescence bronchoscopy. *Cancer* 2000;**89**:2468-73.
58. Pinstein ML, Scott RL, Salazar J. Avoidance of negative percutaneous lung biopsy using contrast-enhanced CT. *AJR Am J Roentgenol* 1983;**140**:265-7.
59. Moore EH, Shepard JO, McLoud TC, et al. Positional precautions in needle aspiration lung biopsy. *Radiology* 1990;**175**:733-5.
60. Permutt LM, Johnson WW, Dunnick NR. Percutaneous transthoracic needle aspiration: A review. *AJR Am J Roentgenol* 1989;**152**:451-5.
61. Fish GD, Stanley JH, Miller KS, et al. Post-biopsy pneumothorax: Estimating the risk by chest radiography and pulmonary function tests. *AJR Am J Roentgenol* 1988;**150**:71-4.
62. Moore EH. Technical aspects of needle aspiration lung biopsy: A personal perspective. *Radiology* 1998;**208**:303-18.
63. Wescott JL. Percutaneous transthoracic needle biopsy. *Radiology* 1988;**169**:593-601.
64. Charig MJ, Stutley JE, Padley SPG, et al. The value of negative needle biopsy in suspected operable lung cancer. *Clin Radiol* 1991;**44**:147-9.
65. Carlens EJ. Mediastinoscopy: A method for inspection and tissue biopsy in the superior mediastinum. *Dis Chest* 1959;**36**:343-52.
66. Luke WP, Pearson FG, Todd TPU, et al. Prospective evaluation of mediastinoscopy for assessment of carcinoma of the lung. *J Thorac Cardiovasc Surg* 1986;**91**:53-6.
67. Hammoud ZT, Anderson RC, Meyers BF, et al. The current role of mediastinoscopy in the evaluation of thoracic disease. *J Thorac Cardiovasc Surg* 1999;**118**:894-9.
68. Vallieres E, Waters PF. Incidence of mediastinal node involvement in clinical T1 bronchogenic carcinomas. *Can J Surg* 1987;**30**:341-2.
69. McNeill T, Chamberlain J. Diagnostic anterior mediastinotomy. *Ann Thorac Surg* 1966;**2**:532-9.
70. Olak J. Parasternal mediastinotomy (Chamberlain procedure). *Chest Surg Clin North Am* 1993;**6**:31-9.
71. Ginsberg RJ, Rice TW, Goldberg M, et al. Extended cervical mediastinoscopy: A single staging procedure for bronchogenic carcinoma of the left upper lobe. *J Thorac Cardiovasc Surg* 1987;**94**:673-8.
72. Lee JD, Ginsberg RJ. Lung cancer staging: The value of ipsilateral scalene lymph node biopsy performed at mediastinoscopy. *Ann Thorac Surg* 1996;**62**:338-41.
73. Hazelrigg SR, Nunchuck SK, LoCicero III J, et al. Video-assisted thoracic surgery study group data. *Ann Thorac Surg* 1993;**56**:1039-44:69.
74. Nomori H, Horio H, Fuyuno G, et al. Lung adenocarcinomas diagnosed by open lung or thoracoscopic biopsy. *Chest* 1998;**114**:40-4.
75. Landreneau RJ, Hazelrigg SR, Mack MJ, et al. Thoracoscopic mediastinal lymph node sampling: Useful for mediastinal lymph node stations inaccessible by cervical mediastinoscopy. *J Thorac Cardiovasc Surg* 1993;**106**:554-8.
76. Rendina EA, Venura F, DeGiaconio T, et al. Comparative merits of thoracoscopy, mediastinoscopy, and mediastinotomy for mediastinal biopsy. *Ann Thorac Surg* 1994;**57**:992-5.
77. Silvestri GA, Littenberg B, Colice GL. The clinical evaluation for detecting metastatic lung cancer: A meta-analysis. *Am J Respir Crit Care Med* 1995;**152**:225-30.
78. Quinn DL, Ostrow LB, Porter DK, et al. Staging of non-small cell bronchogenic carcinoma: Relationship of the clinical evaluation to organ scans. *Chest* 1986;**89**:270-5.
79. Salvatierra A, Baamonde C, Llamas JM, et al. Extrathoracic staging of bronchogenic carcinoma. *Chest* 1990;**97**:1052-8.

80. The Canadian Lung Oncology Group. Investigating extrathoracic metastatic disease in patients with apparently operable lung cancer. *Ann Thorac Surg* 2001;**71**:425-34.
81. MacManus MP, Hicks RJ, Matthews JP, et al. High rate of unsuspected distant metastases by PET in apparent stage III non-small-cell lung cancer: Implications for radical radiation therapy. *Int J Radiat Oncol Biol Phys* 2001;**50**:287-93.
82. Saunders CAB, Dussek JE, O'Doherty MJ, et al. Evaluation of fluorine-18-deoxyglucose whole body positron emission tomography imaging in the staging of lung cancer. *Ann Thorac Surg* 1999;**67**:790-7.
83. Weder W, Schmid RA, Bruchhaus H, et al. Detection of extrathoracic metastases by positron emission tomography in lung cancer. *Ann Thorac Surg* 1998;**66**:886-93.
84. Grant D, Edwards K, Goldstraw P. Computed tomography of the brain, chest, and abdomen in the preoperative assessment of non-small cell lung cancer. *Thorax* 1988;**43**:883-6.
85. Silvestri GA, Lenz JE, Harper SN, et al. The relationship of clinical findings to CT scan evidence of adrenal gland metastases in the staging of bronchogenic carcinoma. *Chest* 1992;**102**:1748-51.
86. Tarver RD, Richmond BD, Klatte EC. Cerebral metastases from lung carcinoma: Neurological and CT correlation work in progress. *Radiology* 1984;**153**:689-92.
87. Ishida Y, Yano T, Maeda K, et al. Strategy for lymphadenectomy in lung cancer three centimeters or less in diameter. *Ann Thorac Surg* 1990;**50**:708-13.
88. Naruke T. Significance of lymph node metastases in lung cancer. *Semin Thorac Cardiovasc Surg* 1993;**5**:210-8.
89. Asamura H, Nakayaa H, Kondo H, et al. Lymph node involvement, recurrence, and prognosis in resected, small peripheral non-small-cell lung carcinomas: are these carcinomas candidates for video-assisted lobectomy? *J Thorac Cardiovasc Surg* 1996;**111**:1125-34.
90. Oda M, Watanabe Y, Shimizu J, et al. Extent of mediastinal node metastasis in clinical stage I non-small-cell lung cancer: the role of systematic nodal dissection. *Lung Cancer* 1998;**22**:23-30.
91. Graham AN, Chan KJ, Pastorino U, et al. Systematic nodal dissection in the intrathoracic staging of patients non-small cell lung cancer. *J Thorac Cardiovasc Surg* 1999;**117**:246-51.

CHAPTER 17
Lung Cancer: Surgical Treatment
Masaki Anraku and Shaf Keshavjee

Historical Note
Pulmonary Surgical Operations: Indications and Technique
  Lobectomy
    Positioning and Incisions
    Mobilization and Hilar Dissection
    Management of Vessels
    Management of Bronchus
    Placement of Chest Tubes
  Pneumonectomy
    Incision
    Hilar Dissection
  Management of Bronchus
  Management of the Postpneumonectomy Space
  Sublobar Resection (Segmentectomy and Wedge Resection)
    Surgical Principles
  Mediastinal Lymph Node Dissection
    Rationale
    Techniques
Surgical Treatment of Non–Small Cell Lung Cancer

T Category: T1 and T2
  Sublobar Resection versus Lobectomy for Node-Negative, Small-Size NSCLC
T Category: T3
  Tumors Invading the Chest Wall
  Superior Sulcus Tumors
  Tumors in Proximity to the Carina
  Tumors Invading the Mediastinum or Diaphragm
  Additional Nodules in the Primary Lobe
T Category: T4
  Heart and Great Vessels
  Carina and Trachea
  Ipsilateral Pulmonary Metastasis in Nonprimary Lobe(s)
  Vertebral Body
  Esophagus
N Category: N0 and N1
N Category: N2
  N2 Found on Pretreatment Staging
  N2 Found at Thoracotomy
N Category: N3
M Category: M1a

  Additional Nodule(s) in the Contralateral Lung
  Malignant Pleural Effusion
M Category: M1b
  Adrenal Gland
  Brain
Special Considerations
Mediastinal Lymph Node Dissection versus Systematic Sampling
  Operative Morbidity
  Staging Accuracy
  Local Control and Long-Term Survival
Multifocal Bronchioloalveolar Carcinoma
  Treatment Strategy and Outcome
Surgical Treatment of Small Cell Lung Cancer
  Rationale for Surgery
  Improved Local Control
  Mixed-Histology Tumors
  Surgery as Salvage Therapy
  Ongoing Randomized Trials
Summary

This chapter provides an overview of the surgical treatment for lung cancer. The indications for surgery, types and extent of lung resection, and mediastinal lymphadenectomy are reviewed, with an emphasis on recent published evidence and the new international tumor-node-metastasis (TNM) staging system (seventh edition, 2009). Minimally invasive lung resection (see Chapter 18), tracheal lesions (see Chapter 8), tumor invading the chest wall (see Chapter 20), and multimodality approaches (see Chapter 19) are specifically covered separately.

Lung cancer remains the leading cause of cancer death worldwide, with an estimated 160,390 deaths and 213,380 new cases in the United States in 2007.[1] Complete surgical resection is the treatment of choice for patients with early-stage (stages I and II) and selected locally advanced (stage III) non–small cell lung cancer (NSCLC). There are also several situations where surgery may have a role to play: NSCLC with isolated adrenal metastasis, isolated brain metastasis, or highly selected small cell lung cancer (SCLC). Adjuvant chemotherapy has been established as a modality to improve survival in selected resectable NSCLC on the basis of published clinical studies including phase III randomized trials.[2] Neoadjuvant therapy (induction chemotherapy or chemoradiotherapy) improves outcome in patients with N2 disease or resectable, locally advanced NSCLC.[3]

HISTORICAL NOTE

The first lobectomy for lung cancer was described by Davies[4] in 1912; the patient died 8 days after resection, with empyema. As water-sealed drainage system and anesthetic techniques advanced, surgical resection for lung cancer became prevalent. In 1933, Graham and Singer[5] reported the first successful one-stage pneumonectomy. Since then, the standard operation for lung cancer became pneumonectomy with the technique of individual hilar ligation of the pulmonary vessels and suturing of the bronchus. Around the same time, Churchill and coworkers[6] described their experience of lobectomies with hilar dissections. The technique of segmentectomy for lung cancer was described by Overholt and Langer.[7] As refinements progressed, more advanced techniques were developed, including sleeve resection by Price-Thomas[8] in 1947, carinal resection by Mathey and colleagues[9] and Thompson,[10] and Pancoast tumor resection by Chardak and MacCallun.[11] Grillo and colleagues[12] reported on carinal resection with airway reconstruction in 1963. In 1973, Jensik and colleagues[13] reported a large series of segmental resections as intentional curative procedures for the treatment of bronchogenic carcinoma. Since the early 1990s, as the system of video endoscopy and endoscopic instruments have evolved, video-assisted thoracoscopic surgery (VATS) for major pulmonary resection has continued to develop worldwide.[14]

PULMONARY SURGICAL OPERATIONS: INDICATIONS AND TECHNIQUE

Lobectomy

Lobectomy with complete en bloc tumor removal remains the standard surgical procedure in patients with resectable NSCLC. Resections less extensive than lobectomy (i.e., segmentectomy and wedge resection) are chosen in patients with limited pulmonary reserve, or recently, in those with small peripheral tumors without nodal disease for curative intent. The indications for curative-intent sublobar resection are discussed later. On occasion, sleeve lobectomy is required when the tumor protrudes into the main-stem bronchus. A concern with sleeve lobectomy is that it might be an inferior oncologic resection compared with pneumonectomy; however, sleeve lobectomy has proved to be superior to pneumonectomy with regard to long-term outcome, with lower morbidity and mortality.[15,16]

Positioning and Incisions

The patient is placed into the lateral decubitus position. Entry into the pleural space via a posterolateral incision is the standard that provides an excellent exposure to the hilum of the lung. The anterior serratus muscle can be mobilized and spared whenever possible. The intercostal muscle, in most cases the fifth intercostal, is cut along the rib both anteriorly and posteriorly to obtain wider rib-spreading. Anterior, lateral, or axillary thoracotomies are other alternatives. Occasionally, a hemi-clamshell incision or median sternotomy is selected for extended resection of apical tumors because either provides excellent exposure of the thoracic inlet, superior pulmonary veins, and main pulmonary arteries.

Mobilization and Hilar Dissection

After the pleural cavity is entered, careful inspection of the pleural space is performed. Any pleural fluid is sampled for cytology and culture. All lobes of the lung are then palpated to assess the extent of the disease, to identify unexpected pleural or parenchymal lesions, and to confirm resectability. The inferior pulmonary ligament is incised up to the inferior pulmonary vein, and the mediastinal pleura of the hilum is incised circumferentially to totally mobilize the lung. Care must be taken to prevent injury to the phrenic nerve by electrocautery when the anterior hilum is opened. The posterior views of right and left pulmonary hila are shown in Figure 17-1.

The hilar vascular structures (the main pulmonary artery and the superior and inferior pulmonary veins) are identified and dissected. The fissures between the lobes are often not completely open, so dissection is required to reach the interlobar structures. The incomplete fissures usually necessitate a combination of sharp and blunt dissection. Care must be taken to avoid violation of the tumor if an extension of the tumor from one lobe to another is seen. The interlobar views of right and left lungs are shown in Figure 17-2.

Management of Vessels

Once the interlobar pulmonary artery is identified, the segmental arteries are exposed to the appropriate plane by dissecting down onto the pulmonary arterial vascular plane. The fissures can be divided with electrocautery or with a mechanical stapler (e.g., Auto Suture GIA [Tyco Healthcare, Hampshire, UK]), depending on the amount of parenchymal tissue to be transected. For division of pulmonary arteries, some surgeons prefer transfixing ligatures (especially for larger vessels), and others apply simple nonabsorbable ligatures. The mechanical stapler can be also used to divide large vessels. It is

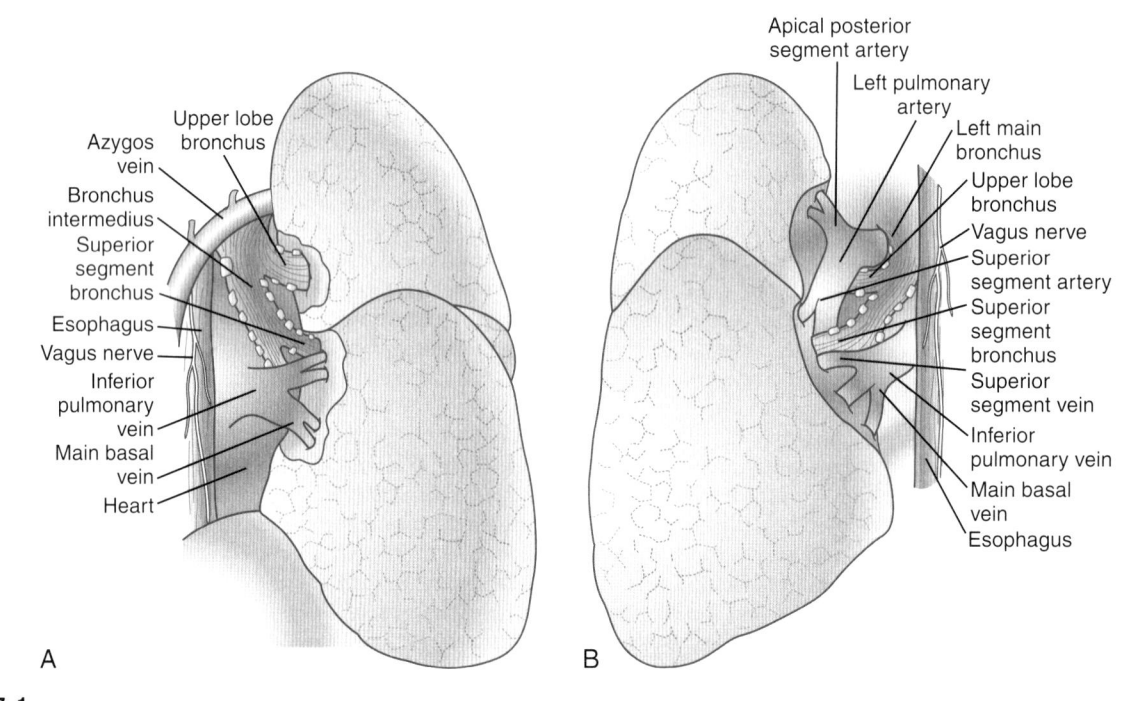

Figure 17–1
Posterior views of the right (**A**) and left (**B**) pulmonary hila. The mediastinal pleura is opened and the lung retracted anteriorly. *(Illustrations by Dennis Wei.)*

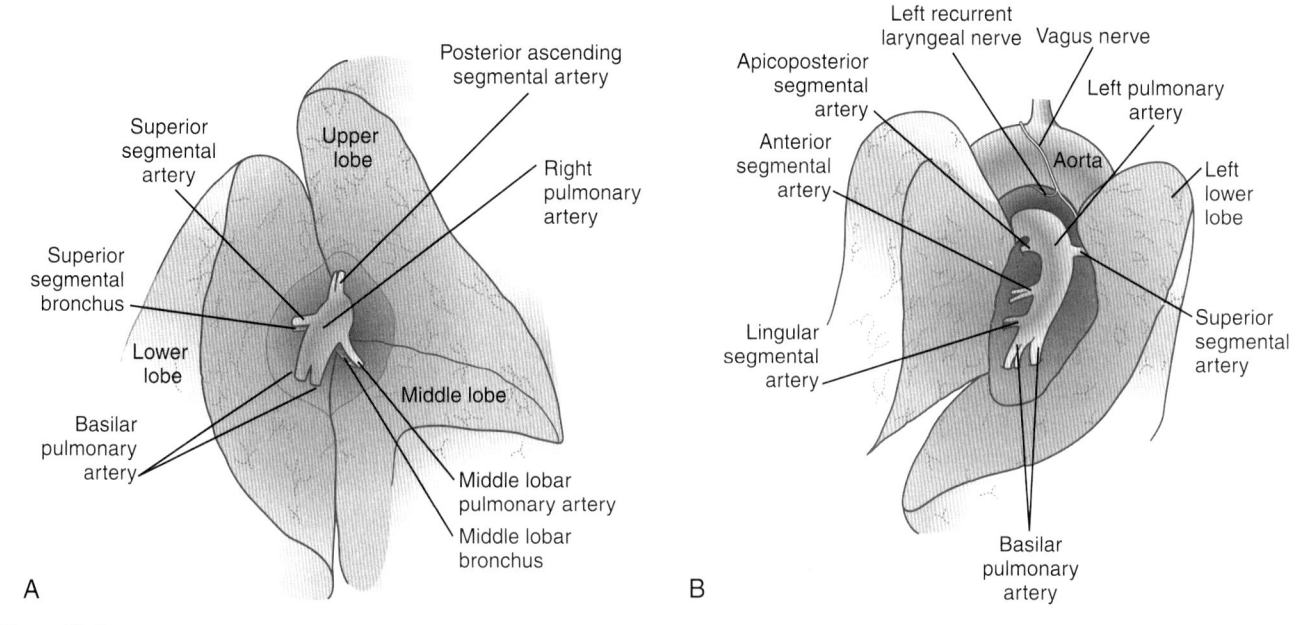

Figure 17-2
The interlobar views of the right (A) and left (B) lungs. The fissures are incised and pulmonary artery branches are exposed. *(Illustrations by Dennis Wei.)*

preferable to isolate and tape the main pulmonary artery and pulmonary veins for control before starting vessel dissections in the following cases: (1) tumor invasion to the main trunk of the pulmonary artery, (2) tumor involving the roots of segmental arterial branches, or (3) significant inflammatory scarring or adhesions encountered around the pulmonary arteries. Using this technique, the main pulmonary artery and veins can be easily clamped for control if an arterial injury occurs.

The order of division of the vasculature is flexible; however, it is safe to divide pulmonary artery branches, then veins, followed by bronchus, in most cases. Some prefer to divide veins first to avoid possible tumor cell dissemination into the blood circulation during the manipulation of the lung, but it has not been proven that this maneuver affects long-term outcome. The disadvantage of dividing the pulmonary vein before arterial division is that the diseased lobe may become congested with retained blood, making the surgery difficult. It is often advantageous to first divide the structure whose absence allows better exposure of the remaining structures. For example, the bronchus can be divided first to obtain better exposure and dissection of the pulmonary arterial branches if needed.

Management of Bronchus

After obtaining the proposed bronchial margin by clearing of peribronchial lymph nodes of the diseased lobe, bronchial closure is performed with a bronchial stapler. Excessive devascularization of the bronchial stump should be avoided to prevent bronchopleural fistula (BPF). Although closure can be performed by hand-suturing techniques, the stapling technique is faster and equally safe. Before firing the bronchial stapler, the anesthesiologist is asked to inflate the operative lung to confirm no impingement of the main bronchus or other remaining bronchi. Frozen-section pathologic examination of the bronchial margins should be obtained if there is any concern of tumor invasion. For poor-risk patients or those who received induction chemoradiotherapy, the bronchial stump should be covered with pericardial fat pad, pericardium, pleura, or intercostal muscle to minimize the chances of a postoperative BPF. In cases of sleeve lobectomy, cancer-free margins on both proximal and distal bronchial ends should be confirmed by frozen section. For the bronchial anastomosis, two traction stitches on both bronchial ends are placed. Interrupted sutures of 4-0 monofilament absorbable sutures on the cartilaginous portion and a running monofilament absorbable suture on the membranous portion are performed without any tension on the bronchial anastomosis.

Placement of Chest Tubes

Chest tubes are placed for evacuation of residual fluid and air to reexpand the residual lung. Another purpose of tube placement is for monitoring of postoperative bleeding. Although there are no standardized rules in terms of the tube size and number, we usually place an apical chest tube and an angled basilar chest tube above the diaphragm (28 French).

Pneumonectomy

As anatomic lobectomy has become the standard form of curative resection for bronchogenic carcinoma, pneumonectomy has become less prevalent. Pneumonectomy is reserved for central lesions, traditionally, but even in patients with tumor invasion of the main-stem bronchus or bronchus intermedius, sleeve lobectomy is the procedure of choice, with acceptable morbidity, mortality, and long-term survival.[17] After careful assessment and patient selection, pneumonectomy is used for patients with centrally located NSCLC that cannot be completely resected using bronchoplastic procedures.

Incision

Posterolateral thoracotomy via the fifth intercostal space is the standard approach, as it provides excellent access to both the anterior and the posterior hila. On entering the pleural cavity, a careful assessment is performed to identify the extent of tumor. This includes bronchoscopic assessment at the time of surgery. The decision to perform pneumonectomy is usually made preoperatively on the basis of the tumor location and the cardiopulmonary reserve; however, occasionally, it is not possible to make a decision before the intraoperative assessment. A lesser resection such as sleeve lobectomy with or without pulmonary arterioplasty should always be considered as long as a complete en bloc tumor resection can be achieved.

Hilar Dissection

Once the need for pneumonectomy is confirmed, the hilum is dissected to identify the main pulmonary artery and the superior and inferior pulmonary veins. After retracting the lung anterosuperiorly, the inferior pulmonary ligament is divided up to the level of the inferior pulmonary vein. The inferior pulmonary vein is exposed and isolated by dissecting surrounding connective tissues. On the right side, a plane between the main pulmonary artery and the superior pulmonary vein should be developed for dissection. On the left side, the superior pulmonary vein resides anterior to the left main bronchus, so a plane for dissection should be found between these structures. The division of the superior and inferior pulmonary veins can be performed by double ligation or stapling. When the tumor involves the pericardial reflection, the pericardium is opened for more proximal vessel isolation, and a vascular clamp is applied across the atrium for division of the pulmonary vein. After division of the vein, the stump is closed with a double-layer nonabsorbable suture.

When the tumor is in close proximity to the proximal pulmonary artery, and thus it is not possible to obtain a sufficient margin to apply a stapler, the pericardium should be opened to obtain additional length for division (Fig. 17-3). On the right side, mobilization of the superior vena cava is often required to encircle the proximal right main pulmonary artery. On the left side, division of the ligamentum arteriosum produces additional length for division of the left main pulmonary artery proximally. During this maneuver, special attention should be paid to avoiding injury to the left recurrent laryngeal nerve, if the nerve is not involved by the tumor. Dissecting proximally after opening the pericardium at its reflection, one can divide the left pulmonary artery at its origin. It is important not to impinge on the right pulmonary artery when applying traction to staple the left main pulmonary artery.

Management of Bronchus

The division of the main-stem bronchus should be performed as proximally as possible (3 to 5 mm from the carina) to avoid creating an unnecessarily long bronchial stump. On the right side, the carina and the anticipated point of bronchial division is often visualized easily. The division of the left main-stem bronchus requires some traction on the bronchus, because the carina is poorly visualized from the left side. Peribronchial tissues and lymph nodes around the bronchus are cleared to better expose the bronchus, but an excessive devascularization should be avoided to preclude poor healing that could lead to postoperative BPF. In patients who received induction radiotherapy, the stump of the right main bronchus should be covered by a pericardial fat pad, mediastinal pleura, pericardium, intercostal muscle flap, or even omentum. Although it is generally desirable to protect the right main bronchial stump, it is not always necessary on the left side because the left main stump retracts into mediastinal tissues after division. Darling and colleagues[18] reported the rates of BPF around 13% on the right side and 5% on the left side, with 8% overall.

Management of the Postpneumonectomy Space

The goal of management of the postpneumonectomy space is to normalize (i.e., reposition) mediastinum to the midline. To accomplish this, some leave a small chest tube to evacuate

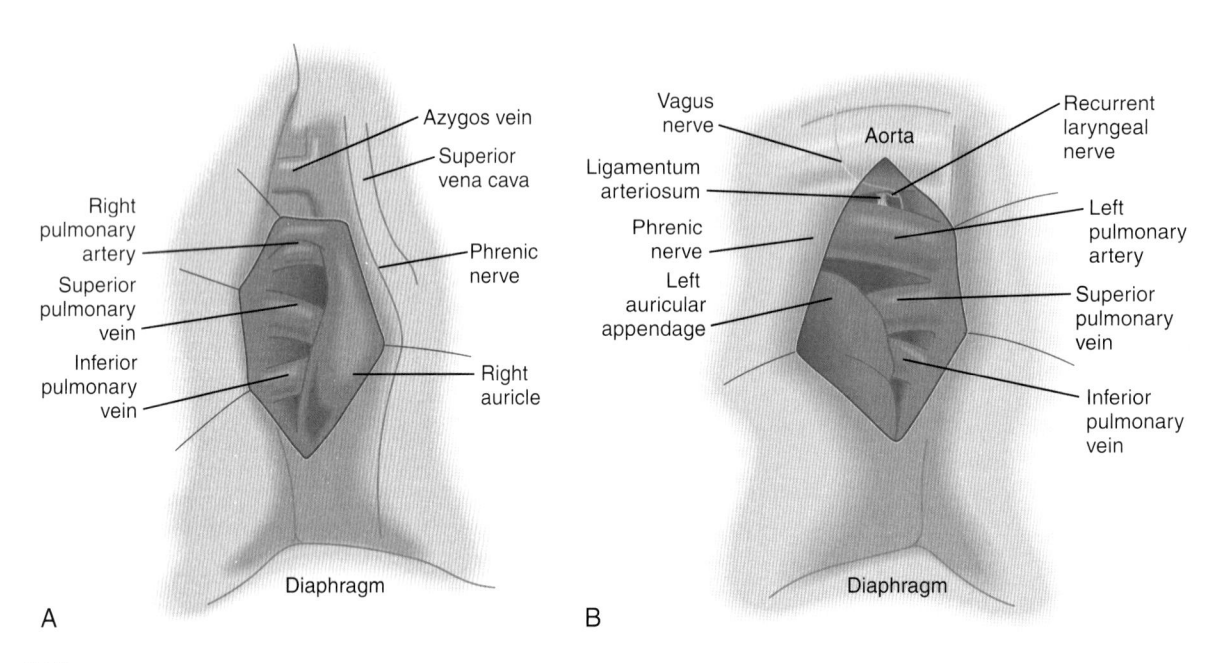

Figure 17-3
The anterior intrapericardial views of the right (**A**) and the left (**B**). *(Illustrations by Dennis Wei.)*

a measured quantity of air immediately after surgery in the operating room, and then remove the tube, whereas others leave a chest tube with balanced pneumonectomy drainage systems (e.g., Pleur-Evac [Genzyme, Cambridge, MA] balanced pneumonectomy drainage system) to avoid mediastinal shift while maintaining normal pressures. Alternatively, a chest tube can be left clamped and intermittently unclamped briefly to reposition the mediastinum. In any case, negative pressure to the chest tube must not be applied, as it may cause a significant mediastinal shift to the operative side.

Sublobar Resection (Segmentectomy and Wedge Resection)

Sublobar resection was originally developed for the surgical management of infectious lung diseases such as tuberculosis and bronchiectasis, in which bilateral or multisegmental disease is frequently seen. For the treatment of NSCLC, this has generally been the option for patients with poor pulmonary function who may not tolerate anatomic lobectomy, because limited resections have demonstrated a higher local recurrence rate and worse long-term outcome than anatomic lobectomy.[19] However, recent evidence suggests that sublobar resection, especially anatomic segmentectomy, may in fact be the surgical procedure of choice, not only for patients with poor cardiopulmonary reserve but also for those with early stage NSCLC at low risk.[20] In general, anatomic segmentectomy is preferred over simple wedge resection to clear the lymphatics draining the tumor bed. Generous wedge resection with cancer-free margins may be acceptable for small, peripheral, "nonsolid" bronchioloalveolar carcinoma.[21] Sampling or formal dissection of hilar and mediastinal lymph nodes with intraoperative frozen-section pathology should be performed to confirm any nodal disease. If proven to be positive for nodal disease intraoperatively, the surgical resection should be converted to anatomic lobectomy whenever possible.

Surgical Principles

The landmark of a diseased segment used to guide resection is its bronchus. Thus identification of the bronchus of the diseased segment is a key step. Therefore, the division of segmental structures tends to begin with the segmental arterial branch, because this often allows good exposure of the segmental bronchus, which runs along with the segmental artery. The segmental vein is best divided last, after identification of the intersegmental plane. Intersegmental veins, the venous drainage of adjacent segments, are usually preserved. The separation at the intersegmental lung parenchymal plane is performed with differential lung deflation and inflation. First, the segmental bronchus of the diseased segment is clamped in a deflated state. Then the lung is inflated, and the demarcation line can be identified because the diseased segment remains airless while other parts of the lung are expanded. Alternatively, the lung is expanded first, followed by clamping the bronchus of the diseased segment, then the lung is deflated to demarcate the diseased segment that remains expanded. Manual monofilament absorbable interrupted suturing (4-0 polydioxanone [PDS] or Maxon) is usually used for the bronchial closure. Stapling may be performed if sufficient length of the diseased segmental bronchus is available. In this case, care must be taken to avoid compromising adjacent segmental bronchi. Blunt or sharp dissection of the intersegmental plane is traditionally performed by scissors, a sponge on a stick, or the surgeon's fingers. Small bridging veins or bronchi are individually clipped or ligated for division. Stapling the intersegmental plane is also applicable and desirable, and this is achievable if the resection is extended into an adjacent segment to achieve an adequate margin from the tumor. Any air leaks from the dissecting plane are controlled by nonabsorbable suturing. Various types of segmentectomy are shown in Figure 17-4.

The use of wedge resection as a surgical procedure for primary lung cancer should be strictly limited to small, peripheral, early-stage NSCLC. Although wedge resection is often accomplished by VATS, it is often difficult to assess the interlobar lymph nodes. Whenever there is any doubt about the resection margins, the procedure should be converted to anatomic segmentectomy.

Mediastinal Lymph Node Dissection

Rationale

Recent advances in mediastinal staging with computed tomography (CT), positron emission tomography (PET), and endoscopic ultrasound bronchoscopy with real-time guided fine-needle aspiration (EBUS-FNA) have improved diagnostic accuracy.[22,23] However, there is no doubt that intraoperative mediastinal lymph node staging remains the gold standard, and it is an integral part of the surgical treatment of lung cancer to determine accurate nodal (N) status, which is a significant outcome predictor.[24] Generally, *lymph node sampling* indicates the removal of macroscopically abnormal lymph nodes. When biopsies are performed from all lymph node stations, it is said to be *systematic sampling*. If systematic removal of all the mediastinal tissue containing lymph nodes within anatomic landmarks is performed, it is referred to as *complete lymph node dissection*. Bilateral mediastinal and cervical lymph node clearance is referred to as *extended lymph node dissection*.[25] It has been a subject of controversy as to whether complete lymph node dissection is superior to systematic sampling in diagnostic accuracy and long-term survival. These issues are discussed later. The classification and graphic representation of lymph node levels for lung cancer staging by the American Joint Committee on Cancer (AJCC) and the Union Internationale Contre le Cancer (UICC)[26] are shown in Figure 17-5.

Techniques

Mediastinal lymph node dissection is almost always accompanied by lung resection for lung cancer, so the procedure is most frequently performed via a posterolateral thoracotomy. It can also be achieved via median sternotomy, anterior thoracotomy, or, more recently, VATS incisions. Although the surgical procedure and extent of mediastinal lymph node dissection may vary from surgeon to surgeon, dissection of stations 2R, 4R, 7, 8, 9, and 10R for the right side and stations 5, 6, 7, 8, 9, and 10L on the left side is generally accepted. On the right side, the superior mediastinum bordered by the superior vena cava anteriorly, the trachea posteriorly, the innominate artery superiorly, and the azygos vein inferiorly, is dissected for lymphadenectomy. After incision of the mediastinal pleura, the mediastinal fat pad is dissected from the posterior aspect of the superior vena cava and the anterolateral surface of the trachea. One or two small draining veins are frequently seen

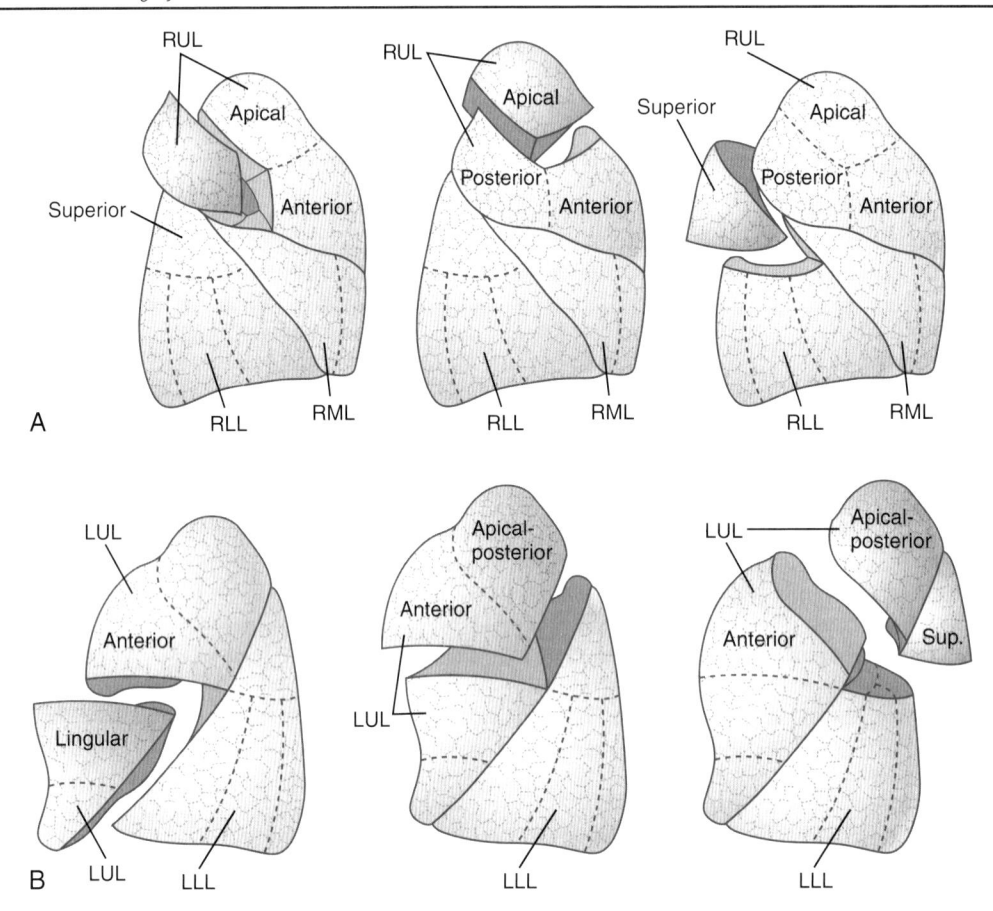

Figure 17-4
Segmental resections of the lung. **A,** Right lung. Upper lobe: posterior and apical segmentectomies. Lower lobe: superior segmentectomy. **B,** Left lung. Upper lobe: lingual and superior division segmentectomies. Combined segmentectomies of apical-posterior (upper lobe) and superior (Sup.) segments (lower lobe). LLL, left lower lobe; LUL, left upper lobe; RLL, right lower lobe; RML, right middle lobe; RUL, right upper lobe. *(From Jensik RJ, Faber LP, Milloy FJ, Monson DO. J Thorac Cardiovasc Surg 1973;**66**:563–72.)*

from the mediastinal fat pad into the superior vena cava, and they are ligated or simply clipped. Right station 2 (2R) nodes are located between the cephalic border of the aortic arch and the cephalic border of the right innominate artery. Right station 4 (4R) nodes are found between the cephalic border of the aortic arch and the origin of the right upper lobe bronchus. Lymph nodes at station 3 posterior (3p) are dissected between the esophagus and the membranous portion of the trachea, and at station 3 anterior (3a) are taken anterior to the superior vena cava (anterior to the right phrenic nerve) where necessary. Right station 10 (10R) nodes are dissected along the anterior border of the right bronchus distal to the pleural reflection.

To expose the subcarinal lymph nodes (7), the lung is retracted anteriorly. After incision of the mediastinal pleura along with the anterior border of the esophagus, the subcarinal fat pad is dissected from the medial border of the right main bronchus laterally, the anterior aspect of the esophagus posteriorly, and the pericardium anteriorly. The attachments between the main bronchus and the fatty tissues containing subcarinal nodes are freed. The bronchial arterial branches running into the fat tissues are clipped before division to avoid unnecessary bleeding. The inferior pulmonary ligament nodes (9) are easy to dissect, and the paraesophageal nodes (8) are taken if they are present. On the left side, aortopulmonary (5 and 6) and subcarinal (7) nodes are dissected. For the upper mediastinal node dissection, the mediastinal pleura is incised just above the left main pulmonary artery, all the way up to the cephalic border of the aortic arch, midway between the phrenic nerve and the vagus nerve. Para-aortic (6) nodes are dissected from the phrenic nerve posteriorly and the ligamentum arteriosum anteriorly, and subaortic (5) nodes are removed posterior to the ligamentum arteriosum. During dissection, small arteries or veins should be controlled by ligation or clipping to avoid any thermal injury of the phrenic, vagus, and recurrent laryngeal nerves by electrocautery. Subcarinal (7) nodes can be removed in the same way as on the right side.

SURGICAL TREATMENT OF NON–SMALL CELL LUNG CANCER

Surgical resection is generally considered in patients with stage I or II NSCLC. Those with locally advanced stage IIIA or IIIB NSCLC are usually treated with chemotherapy and radiotherapy. However, stages IIIA and IIIB represent heterogeneous groups of patients, and select patients will benefit from surgical resection.

The decision regarding surgical intervention is made on the basis of several variables, including the extent of disease (both T and N factors), age, cardiopulmonary reserve, performance status, and comorbid risk factors. Induction or adjuvant (postsurgical) chemotherapy with or without radiotherapy is offered

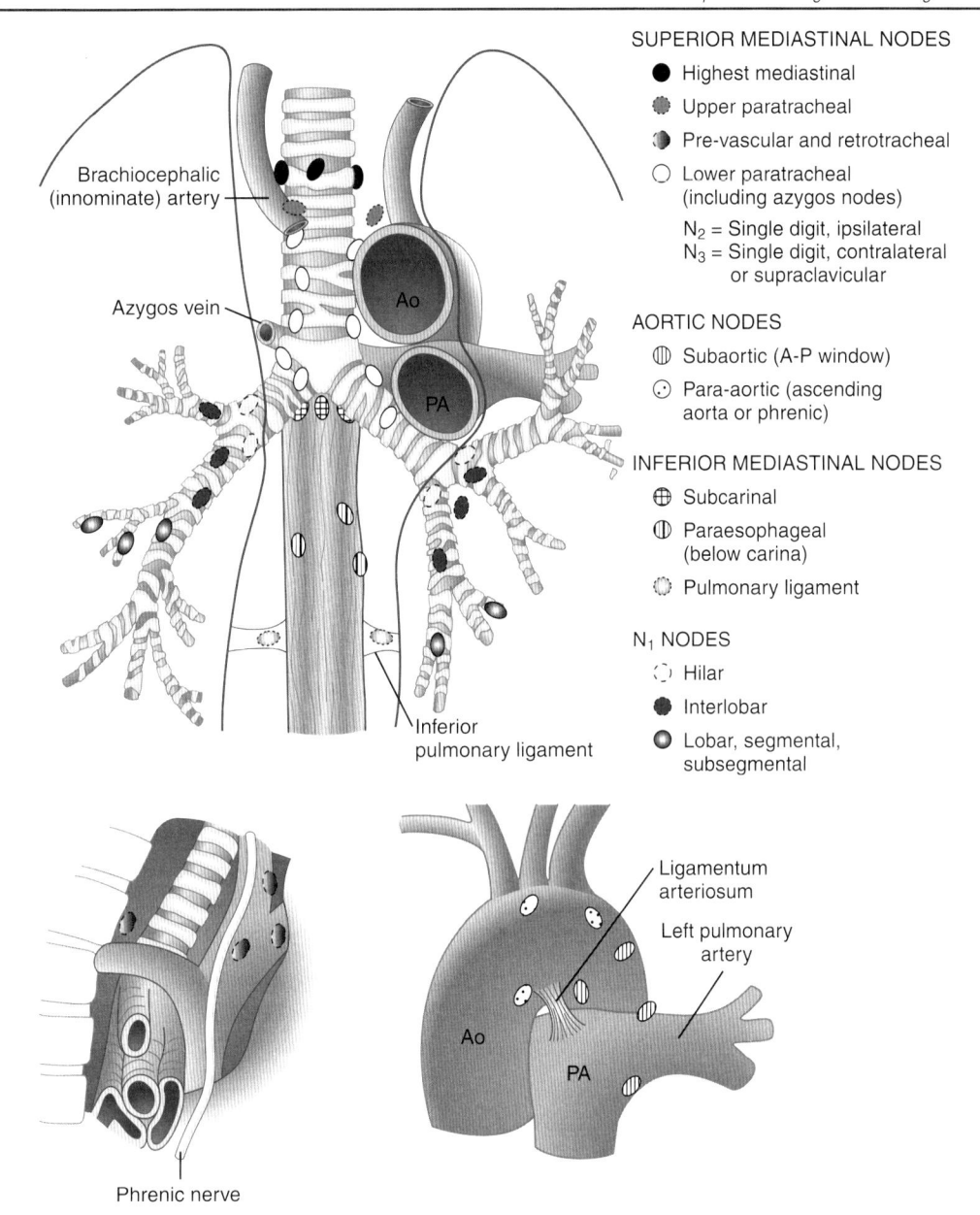

Figure 17–5
Regional lymph node stations for lung cancer staging by the American Thoracic Society and the North American Lung Cancer Study Group. Ao, aorta; PA, pulmonary artery. *(From Mountain CF, Dresler CM.* Chest *1997;**111**:1718–23.)*

to surgical candidates with locally advanced NSCLC. Recently, adjuvant or neoadjuvant chemotherapy has been also offered to patients with early-stage resectable NSCLC in clinical trial settings, and the combined approach appears to prolong survival.

The International Association for the Study of Lung Cancer (IASLC) staging committee recently published proposals for the revision of the TNM classification scheduled for 2009.[27] The proposed definitions of TNM descriptors are shown in Table 17-1. Specific surgical issues related to each stage (T, N, and M) are discussed here.

T Category: T1 and T2

T1 and T2 tumors will be subcategorized in the next edition of the TNM staging according to the proposals by the IASLC Lung Cancer Staging Project.[28] The proposed changes in the T classification in the T1 and T2 categories are as follows: (1) T1 will be T1a if the tumor is 2 cm or less, and T1b if the tumor is greater than 2 cm but not greater than 3 cm; (2) T2 tumors are greater than 3 cm, and they will be T2a if equal to or less than 5 cm, and T2b if greater than 5 cm and equal to or less than 7 cm. Tumors greater than 7 cm will be moved into the T3 category (see Table 17-1).

For the T1 and T2 categories, the surgical procedure of choice is essentially the same if patients are medically fit and have good cardiopulmonary reserve; anatomic lobectomy is the preferred mode of resection. However, recent refinements of prognostication suggest that sublobar resection (segmentectomy or wide wedge resection) can be performed on patients with small, peripheral, early-stage NSCLC without jeopardizing the clinical outcome. Additional multicenter trials comparing lobectomy with lesser resections are under way. On another front, a growing body of

Table 17-1

Proposed Definitions for T, N, and M Descriptors by the International Association for the Study of Lung Cancer (IASLC)

T (Primary Tumor)		T (Primary Tumor)	
TX	Primary tumor cannot be assessed, or tumor proven by the presence of malignant cells in sputum or bronchial washings but not visualized by imaging or bronchoscopy	T4	Tumor of any size that invades any of the following: mediastinum, heart, great vessels, trachea, recurrent laryngeal nerve, esophagus, vertebral body, carina; separate tumor nodule(s) in a different ipsilateral lobe
T0	No evidence of primary tumor	**N (Regional Lymph Nodes)**	
Tis	Carcinoma in situ	NX	Regional lymph nodes cannot be assessed
T1	Tumor ≤ 3 cm in greatest dimension, surrounded by lung or pleura, without bronchoscopic evidence of invasion more proximal than the lobar bronchus (i.e., not in the main bronchus)*	N0	No regional lymph node metastasis
		N1	Metastasis in ipsilateral peribronchial and/or ipsilateral hilar lymph nodes and intrapulmonary nodes, including involvement by direct extension
T1a	Tumor ≤ 2 cm in greatest dimension	N2	Metastasis in ipsilateral mediastinal and/or subcarinal lymph node(s)
T1b	Tumor > 2 cm but ≤ 3 cm in greatest dimension	N3	Metastasis in contralateral mediastinal, contralateral hilar, ipsilateral or contralateral scalene, or supraclavicular lymph node(s)
T2	Tumor > 3 cm but ≤ 7 cm or tumor with any of the following features (T2 tumors with these features are classified T2a if ≤ 5 cm)	**M (Distant Metastasis)**	
T2a	Involves main bronchus, ≥2 cm distal to the carina	MX	Distant metastasis cannot be assessed
T2b	Invades visceral pleura	M0	No distant metastasis
	Associated with atelectasis or obstructive pneumonitis that extends to the hilar region but does not involve the entire lung	M1	Distant metastasis
	Tumor > 3 cm but ≤ 5 cm in greatest dimension	M1a	Separate tumor nodule(s) in a contralateral lobe; tumor with pleural nodules or malignant pleural (or pericardial) effusion†
	Tumor > 5 cm but ≤ 7 cm in greatest dimension	M1b	Distant metastasis
T3	Tumor > 7 cm or one that directly invades any of the following: chest wall (including superior sulcus tumors), diaphragm, phrenic nerve, mediastinal pleura, parietal pericardium; or tumor in the main bronchus < 2 cm distal to the carina* but without involvement of the carina; or associated atelectasis or obstructive pneumonitis of the entire lung or separate tumor nodule(s) in the same lobe		

*The uncommon superficial spreading tumor of any size with its invasive component limited to the bronchial wall, which may extend proximally to the main bronchus, is also classified as T1.
†Most pleural (and pericardial) effusions with lung cancer are due to tumor. In a few patients, however, multiple cytopathologic examinations of pleural (pericardial) fluid are negative for tumor, and the fluid is nonbloody and is not an exudate. Where these elements and clinical judgment dictate that the effusion is not related to the tumor, the effusion should be excluded as a staging element and the patient should be classified as T1, T2, T3, or T4.
(Adapted from Goldstraw P, Crowley J, Chansky K, et al. J Thorac Oncol 2000;2:706–14.)

evidence suggests that surgical resection alone is not adequate for the treatment of large-sized NSCLC without any nodal disease.[2]

Sublobar Resection versus Lobectomy for Node-Negative, Small-Size NSCLC

Historically, Jensik and coworkers[13] reported their 15-year experience of segmental resections of peripheral lung cancer as a curative-intent procedure in 1973. The 5-year survival rate of 69 patients who underwent curative resections by segmentectomy was 56%. Of these, six (9%) developed local recurrence in the primary lobe. The authors concluded that segmentectomy can be a valid procedure for selected, peripherally located lung cancer. In the early 1980s, the Lung Cancer Study Group (LCSG) performed a multicenter randomized clinical trial of lobectomy versus a lesser resection by wedge or segmentectomy in T1N0 NSCLC in patients presenting with small peripheral tumors, and the report suggested a threefold increase in the incidence of local recurrence in patients treated by resections smaller than lobectomy.[19] Therefore, the authors recommended that the use of sublobar resection should be limited to poor-risk patients with compromised pulmonary function.

However, more recent evidence suggests that radical, curative-intent sublobar resection can be offered for clinical T1N0 NSCLC even in good-risk patients. The survival outcome and locoregional recurrence rates of anatomic segmentectomy in comparison with lobectomy are summarized in Table 17-2.[19,29-32] Although most of the evidence is from retrospective studies comparing the outcome of segmentectomy with that of lobectomy, several key factors have been identified to obtain optimal results by anatomic segmentectomy. The factors include (1) surgical margins, (2) tumor size, and (3) lymph node assessment.

It is clear that positive surgical margins must be avoided to achieve complete resection; however, it remains unresolved as to what is the optimal adequate surgical margin (i.e., the distance from the tumor to the cut margin) for localized tumors in the setting of segmentectomy. Sawabata and colleagues[33] conducted a prospective study to define optimal surgical margins in

Table 17-2
Long-Term Outcome and Local Recurrence Rate of Sublobar Resection in Comparison to Lobectomy in Patients with Early-Stage Non–Small Cell Lung Cancer

Author (Year)	N (Sublobar/Lobectomy)	Stage	Sublobar Resection versus Lobectomy	
			Local Recurrence (%)	5-Year Survival (%)
Ginsberg et al. (1995)	125/122	cT1N0	6.3 vs 2.1*	83 vs 89
Koike et al. (2003)	74/159	cT1N0	2.7 vs 1.3	89 vs 90
Fernando et al. (2005)	124/167	pT1N0	17.5 vs 10.0 (tumor size < 2 cm)	56 vs 85 months (MS)
			4.4 vs 3.5 (tumor size, 2-3 cm)	45 vs 70 months* (MS)
Okada et al. (2006)	305/262	cT1N0	4.9 vs 6.9	90 vs 90
Okumura et al. (2007)	55/187	pT1N0†	NS	83 vs 81

*Statistically significant.
†Large cell carcinoma excluded.
c, clinical; MS, median survival; NS, not stated; p. pathologic.

excision of NSCLC. In the study, the surgical margins were microscopically 100% negative for malignancy when the margin distance was greater than 20 mm, or when the resected tumors had a margin distance greater than the maximum tumor diameter (a margin-to-tumor size ratio > 1). Schuchert and coworkers[34] reported that the local recurrence rate was significantly higher in patients with a margin-to-tumor ratio less than 1, than in those with the ratio greater than 1 (25% versus 6.2%). In the study, the mean surgical margin in patients with local recurrence was 12.8 mm, and that in those without local recurrence was 18.6 mm. Therefore, lobectomy or extended segmentectomy should be performed when an adequate surgical margin (preferably 2 cm) cannot be obtained, especially if tumors are located centrally. Intraoperative pathologic assessment of surgical margins should generally be performed to confirm the margins.

Tumor size is also an important factor when segmental resection is considered. A large tumor size is associated with increased risk of local recurrence and distant metastasis. Fernando and colleagues reported that there was no difference in survival between sublobar resection and lobar resection groups when the tumor size was smaller than 2 cm in pathologic T1N0 NSCLC, whereas the median survival was significantly better in the lobar resection group when tumor size was greater than 2 cm (68.7 versus 50.6 months).[30] Okada and colleagues[35] reported the 5-year cancer-specific survivals of patients with pathologic stage I disease with tumors of 2 cm or less and 2.1 to 3 cm in diameter were similar: 92.4% and 87.4% after lobectomy, and 96.7% and 84.6% after segmentectomy, respectively. On the other hand, in patients with a tumor greater than 3 cm in diameter, survivals were significantly worse in the segmentectomy group than in the lobectomy group (62.9% versus 81.3%). Bando and colleagues[36] reported a higher locoregional recurrence rate of segmentectomy in patients with tumors 2.1 to 3 cm than in those with tumors 2 cm or smaller. In the report by Schuchert and associates,[34] recurrence was observed more frequently in stage IB patients than stage IA patients. Jones and coworkers[37] reported no locoregional recurrence in 43 patients with pathologic T1N0 NSCLC who underwent segmentectomy. El-Sherif and colleagues[38] recently reviewed their experience of sublobar resection versus lobectomy and demonstrated that the disease-free survival rate of sublobar resection was equivalent to that of lobectomy in patients with stage IA NSCLC, but in those with stage IB NSCLC, survival was worse in the sublobar resection group. Several recent series have also reported comparable long-term outcomes of segmentectomy and lobectomy in small (tumor size, <2 cm) T1N0 NSCLC.[29,31,39] Based on the current evidence, patients with early-stage small NSCLC (preferably 2 cm or less in size) may undergo anatomic segmentectomy if negative nodal disease is confirmed.

Intraoperative lymph node assessment is an integral part of sublobar resection. Miller and colleagues[40] evaluated the frequency of lymph node metastasis in patients who underwent resection of NSCLC 1 cm or less. The tumors were located in the periphery in 89 patients, centrally in three, and endobronchially in eight. Of these, seven (7%) had lymph node metastasis (N1 = 5 and N2 = 2). In the prospective nonrandomized trial of sublobar resection reported by Okada and colleagues,[31] of 305 patients with clinical T1 (tumor size, <2 cm) N0 NSCLC who were assigned to undergo sublobar resection, 20 (7%) were found to have lymph node metastasis (N1 = 11 and N2 = 9) intraoperatively, so the procedure was converted to lobectomy. Therefore, even for tumors smaller than 1 cm, intraoperative hilar and mediastinal lymph node sampling or dissection is recommended whenever sublobar resection is performed.

Wedge resection has appeared to be suboptimal for the surgical treatment of lung cancer except for localized, small-size pure bronchioloalveolar carcinoma because of a higher local recurrence rate. Landreneau and associates[41] documented high local recurrence rates in patients with T1N0 NSCLC who underwent wedge resection (wedge versus lobectomy: 24% versus 9%). Sienel and coworkers[42] analyzed local recurrence rates in patients with pathologic T1N0 NSCLC who underwent either segmentectomy or wedge resection. Segmentectomies were followed by systematic lymph node dissection, and wedge resections by lymph node sampling. The local recurrence rate was significantly higher in the wedge resection group than in the segmentectomy group (55% versus 16%), and the difference of recurrence rates was significant even in patients with tumors 2 cm or less (40% versus 11%). The observed higher locoregional recurrence rates may be partly explained by an inadequate lymph node assessment, because sampling of interlobar lymph nodes or segmental hilar nodes is often impractical or impossible, resulting in the missing of positive nodes and false downstaging. Wedge resection may also leave draining lymphatic vessels containing cancer cells behind in the residual diseased segment, thus increasing the risk of local recurrence. Therefore, anatomic segmentectomy, but not wedge resection, is recommended for patients with early-stage small NSCLC when sublobar resection is considered. If anatomic segmentectomy might not be tolerated because of poor cardiopulmonary reserve, wedge resection combined with radiotherapy or brachytherapy could be an alternative approach to reduce the risk of local recurrence.[30,43]

Although the topic of adjuvant therapy is not in the scope of this chapter, recent evidence suggests that patients with early-stage, resectable NSCLC (including N1 disease) appear to benefit from adjuvant or neoadjuvant therapy.[2,44-47] This topic is discussed in Chapter 19.

T Category: T3

The T3 category includes (1) tumors greater than 7 cm; (2) additional nodules in the primary lobe; (3) tumors of any size invading the chest wall, diaphragm, mediastinal pleura, or parietal pericardium; (4) tumors in the main-stem bronchus less than 2 cm from the carina without invading the carina; and (5) tumor-associated atelectasis or obstructive pneumonitis of the entire lung (see Table 17-1). Some of these subsets are discussed with respect to their specific surgical considerations later.

Tumors Invading the Chest Wall

Technical details and the outcome of this subset are reviewed in Chapter 20. NSCLC invading the chest wall is usually peripheral in location, so mediastinal lymph nodes are less likely to be involved. The degree of chest wall involvement with tumor varies from the parietal pleura to the muscles and ribs of the chest wall. Those with NSCLC involving the chest wall, but without mediastinal node disease, are good candidates for surgical treatment whenever medically fit. Postoperative mortality has continued to be reduced, in recent reports ranging between 0% to 6.3%.[48-54] In general, factors affecting long-term survival include (1) completeness of resection,[48,50,54] (2) extent of invasion of the chest wall,[49,50,54] and (3) nodal status.[48,50,51,53,54] In patients with incomplete resection (macroscopic or microscopic disease) or unresectable tumors, the 5-year survival was essentially zero.[48,54] It is a matter of controversy as to whether en bloc (full-thickness chest wall) resection is necessary for all depths of tumors invading the chest wall, but some authors advocate a full-thickness resection to achieve complete tumor clearance.[50,51,53] The roles of chemotherapy and radiotherapy for this group of patients are still uncertain and clearly require further investigation.[53]

Superior Sulcus Tumors

Superior sulcus tumors (Pancoast tumors) are a unique subset of carcinomas of the lung, invading the thoracic inlet. Because of the close proximity to thoracic inlet structures, the tumors often invade adjacent tissues early, with symptomatic consequences. In case of tumor invasion to the posterior compartment of the thoracic inlet, involvement of the lower brachial plexus, particularly the T1 nerve root, is common. Shoulder and arm pain radiating to the inner aspect of the upper arm (T1) or the ulnar distribution in the fourth and fifth fingers of the hand (C8), or both, are commonly seen in these cases. Extension to the stellate ganglion with a consequent Horner's syndrome, or extension to the ribs or vertebrae is also observed. Tumors invading the anterior compartment of the thoracic inlet may involve the subclavian vessels.

Advances in surgical techniques and combined-modality approaches recently led to the conduct of two prospective multicenter phase II clinical trials, where induction chemoradiotherapy was performed followed by surgical resection in patients with superior sulcus NSCLC.[55,56] The North American Intergroup trial (Southwest Oncology Group 9416, INT 0160) report by Rusch and colleagues[55] suggested that both T3N0-1 and T4N0-1 tumors benefit from preoperative chemoradiation with high response rates by pathologic examination (61% with complete pathologic response or minimal microscopic tumor) and high complete resection rates (76% overall, and 94% of patients who underwent thoracotomy). The median survival was 33 months for all patients, and 94 months for the patients who achieved an R0 resection. Kunitoh and coworkers[56] reported mature results of induction chemoradiotherapy followed by surgical resection in patients with T3 ($n = 56$) or T4 ($n = 20$) NSCLC (Japan Clinical Oncology Group Trial, JCOG 9806). Of these, 57 patients (76%) underwent surgical resection and, again, a high R0 resection rate (68% overall, and 90% of patients who received surgical resection) was achieved. The overall 5-year survival rate was 56%. In both studies, the pattern of cancer recurrence was predominantly distant, and the brain is the leading organ of relapse. In the INT 0160 trial, 19 of 57 patients (41%) who developed recurrence had brain metastasis only, and 5 of 39 patients (13%) did so in the JCOG 9806 trial.

Tumors in Proximity to the Carina

A tumor extending to within 2 cm of the carina is said to be a T3 tumor, and patients with this subset of tumors benefit from surgical resection in published series. Since the introduction of lung-sparing techniques by Price-Thomas[8] in 1947, sleeve lobectomy has been adopted by many thoracic surgeons,[57] and it is now the standard of procedure for NSCLC extending into the large airway whenever appropriate. The techniques can be applied to not only tumors in proximity to the carina, but also those located at the origin of a lobar bronchus, those with positive margin after standard lobectomy, and those that are N1 disease and can be completely resected. Pneumonectomy or sleeve pneumonectomy should be strictly considered for lesions that cannot be completely removed by a lung-sparing procedure because of the higher postoperative morbidity and mortality. Deslauriers and colleagues[16] reported a lower operative mortality in the sleeve lobectomy group compared with the pneumonectomy group (1.6% versus 5.3%). The authors reported the 5-year survival rates of 52% in the sleeve lobectomy group and 31% in the pneumonectomy group. The 5-year survival rates in the sleeve lobectomy group by nodal involvement were 63% in N0, 48% in N1, and 8% in N2. Although no series specifically reported on results of surgical resection of T3 tumors defined by proximity to the carina, negative mediastinal node disease and complete resection are keys for improved survival.[16,58]

When a tumor involves not only the main-stem bronchus but also the proximal pulmonary artery, vascular sleeve resection is combined for complete resection. In the report by Yildizeli and coworkers[58] of 218 patients with sleeve lobectomy, 28 patients (13%) underwent vascular sleeve resection and most of them (20/28) were associated with left upper lobectomy. A meta-analysis reported by Ma and associates[17] suggested that sleeve lobectomy with or without vascular reconstruction can be performed without increasing mortality or morbidity compared with pneumonectomy, and it offers better survival than pneumonectomy.

Tumors Invading the Mediastinum or Diaphragm

The outcome in patients with mediastinal pleural involvement is generally poor because of frequent mediastinal node involvement. Riquet and colleagues[59] documented that 25 out of 68 patients (36%) with mediastinal pleural invasion who underwent surgical resection had N2 disease. The 5-year survival rate was reported as 31% in the study. Pitz and associates[60] documented a 5-year survival rate of 25% in patients with complete resection.

NSCLC invading the diaphragm is a rare condition and infrequently diagnosed preoperatively. Yokoi and coworkers[61] noted only one third of these patients (17/63 patients) had a diagnosis of diaphragmatic invasion before surgery, and Riquet and colleagues[62] reported only three out of 68 patients (4%) had the diagnosis preoperatively. Prognostic factors reported in this subset were nodal disease, completeness of resection, and the depth of diaphragmatic invasion. In the series of Yokoi and coworkers, 5-year survival rates by nodal disease were 28% (N0) versus 18% (N1/2), and those by the depth of diaphragmatic invasion were 33% (parietal pleura) versus 14% (diaphragmatic muscle or deeper). Rocco and colleagues[63] reported the 5-year survival rate of 27% in patients with N0 disease and diaphragmatic invasion. The relatively poor prognosis of mediastinal or diaphragmatic involvement even in patients with N0 disease after complete resection can be explained by the extensive lymphatic and venous drainage,[59,62] so adjuvant or neoadjuvant therapy should probably be offered for these subsets of patients.

Additional Nodules in the Primary Lobe

It is recognized that patients with pulmonary metastasis in a primary lobe have better survival than those with contralateral pulmonary metastasis or with other metastatic disease. In addition, it is often not possible to determine whether a satellite nodule seen on a CT scan is a metastatic lesion or an inflammatory lesion preoperatively, so satellite lesions in a primary lobe still warrant surgical resection. In recent surgical series, the 5-year survival rates in patients with pathologically proven pulmonary metastasis in a primary lobe have been reported to be from 45% to 57%.[64-67] The node status is a significant prognostic factor in this subset of patients who underwent complete surgical resection, but whether the number of satellite lesions is a prognostic factor has yet to be clarified.

T Category: T4

The T4 category includes tumors directly invading important mediastinal structures such as heart, esophagus, great vessels, trachea, vertebral body, or carina (see Table 17-1). Tumors with a malignant pleural effusion will be reclassified into M1 category, because the prognosis of this subset of patients is comparable with that of those with metastatic disease. The median survival of patients with malignant pleural dissemination is only 8 months, and the 5-year survival rate is 2%.[28] On the other hand, M1 based on additional nodules in the ipsilateral lung (different lobe) will be reclassified as T4.

Generally, T4 tumors are deemed unresectable; however, curative surgical resection can be performed in highly selected patients with surgery alone or with a combined multimodality approach including chemotherapy or radiotherapy, or both. Patients with T4 tumors with mediastinal node disease (N2) are generally excluded from being surgical candidates, because their prognosis is in general not improved. Therefore, every effort should be made to exclude N2 disease if surgical resection is considered.

Heart and Great Vessels

Patients with T4 tumors by virtue of invasion to the heart are rarely candidates for surgical treatment. On occasion, central tumors extending around the inferior pulmonary vein and the left atrium may be amenable to complete surgical resection.[68] The tumor resection can be achieved by clamping the left atrium and then suturing the defect, or by removing tumors with the patient on cardiopulmonary bypass, if indicated (e.g., for cardiac chamber invasion with main pulmonary artery involvement).[68,69] Tsuchiya and coworkers[70] reported a 5-year survival after left atrium resection of 22% in 44 patients with NSCLC.

Surgical resection of NSCLC involving great vessels, including the aorta, the main pulmonary artery, and the superior vena cava (SVC), can be performed either primarily or as a part of multimodality treatment. In patients with tumors invading the thoracic aorta or the subclavian artery, the surgical procedure varies from intra-adventitial dissection or direct lateral clamping and suturing with or without a patch, to replacement of a portion of artery with a prosthetic graft.[71,72] These aggressive surgical resections are further justified when tumors extend into the arterial wall, because they carry a risk of sudden rupture or embolism. Several reports of SVC resections for NSCLC have depicted survival rates according to the degree of primary tumor or nodal involvement. In general, a poor prognosis is seen in patients with mediastinal node disease (5-year survival, 52% in N0-1 versus 21% in N2),[73] those with SVC invasion by metastatic lymph nodes (5-year survival, 36% in SVC tumor invasion versus 6.6% in SVC lymph nodal invasion),[74] or those with pneumonectomy (hazard ratio = 2.9 compared with lobectomy).[75] Induction treatment should be considered, because it may allow less pulmonary resection (i.e., lobectomy or sleeve lobectomy) by reducing tumor burden, and it may also decrease the distant failure rate.[75,76]

Carina and Trachea

Carinal resection has been performed for patients with NSCLC invading the carina or extending to the lower part of the trachea since the 1950s as a potentially curative treatment.[77] As a result of improvements in surgical techniques, perioperative management, and patient selection, the surgery-related hospital mortality continues to decrease. In the past decade, acceptable mortality rates in patients who underwent carinal pneumonectomy have been reported from several experienced institutions, ranging from 4% to 15%.[78-82]

As a part of mediastinal staging, some prefer to perform mediastinoscopy at the time of planned thoracotomy to avoid the development of scar tissue along the trachea, to help in reducing anastomotic tension by allowing good tracheal mobilization.[78,80] Others perform mediastinoscopy preoperatively for possible induction chemoradiotherapy if pathologic N2 disease is confirmed.[79,81] A rigid bronchoscopy is frequently used to better assess the involved tracheobronchial tree, to determine resectability, and to plan airway reconstruction.

Various tracheobronchial anastomoses after carinal resection have been described by Mitchell and associates,[83] who reviewed the surgical experience at Massachusetts General Hospital. The techniques are described in Chapter 8. A right carinal pneumonectomy is generally performed via right posterolateral thoracotomy, or occasionally bilateral thoracotomy, or sometimes median sternotomy is performed for bilateral reconstruction of the tracheobronchial tree. The approach for a left carinal pneumonectomy varies: median sternotomy, clamshell incision, left thoracotomy, or bilateral thoracotomies is used.

Mediastinal lymph node involvement is a strong prognostic factor.[78-82] Whether adjuvant or neoadjuvant, or chemotherapy or chemoradiotherapy, should be used for those with N2 disease in this subset is still under debate. Recent series of carinal resection are summarized in Table 17-3.

Ipsilateral Pulmonary Metastasis in Nonprimary Lobes

A recent report of a surgical series by Nagai and colleagues[84] demonstrated 5-year survival rates of patients with nonprimary lobe lung metastases of 42.1% (p-N0, $n = 38$), 7.9% (p-N1, $n = 19$), and 10.0% (p-N2, $n = 52$). In the study, around 60% of these patients received R0 (complete) resection, and 11% of cases received pneumonectomy. Significant survival differences were detected between node-negative (N0) and node-positive (N1 or N2) groups. Because the stage of the mediastinal node disease is a key prognostic factor, careful preoperative mediastinal investigation is necessary if surgical resection is to be considered in this subset of patients.

Vertebral Body

Patients with vertebral body involvement historically have been deemed unresectable; however, advances in surgical techniques, postoperative care, and induction chemoradiotherapy allow aggressive complete resection with an acceptable mortality for patients with vertebral body invasion.[85,86] Several groups have reported outcomes of vertebral body resection (either total or hemi) in patients with NSCLC invading the spine. Grunenwald and associates[85] reported a 53% 2-year survival rate in 19 patients treated with vertebral body resection. Gandhi and coworkers[87] primarily performed surgery followed by radiotherapy in this subset and achieved a 2-year survival rate of 54%. Fadel and colleagues[88] documented a 3-year survival rate of 39%. The Toronto Group[89] reported a 3-year survival rate of 58% in patients ($n = 23$) with T4 (vertebral body) N0 disease who underwent surgery including multiple total vertebrectomy (Fig. 17-6A). In the study, all the patients received preoperative chemotherapy or chemoradiotherapy, and 45% of them achieved complete response to the neoadjuvant therapy by pathologic examination. R0 resection rate was high: 19 out of 23 patients (83%) achieved complete resection. The outcome in patients who demonstrated pathologic complete response or near complete response (viable cells < 1% in the resected specimen) was excellent, whereas the outcome in those who did not was poor (3-year survival, 93% versus 20%; see Fig. 17-6B). Because the high rates of both R0 resection and pathologic complete response were associated with better survival, a multimodality treatment approach with induction chemoradiotherapy should be strongly considered in carefully selected patients. Recent series of vertebral body resection are summarized in Table 17-4.

Esophagus

NSCLC invading the esophagus is rarely amenable to complete resection and the outcomes have been disappointing, so the presence of frank invasion to the esophagus is considered unresectable. Pitz and associates[90] reported that only three out of 12 patients (25%) achieved complete resection in this subset of patients.

Table 17-3
Recent Series of Carinal Resection in Non–Small Cell Lung Cancer

Author (Year)	N (Number of N2/3)	Mortality(%)	Overall	5-Year Survival(%)	
				N0/1	N2/3
Mitchell et al. (2001)	60 (11)	15	42	51 (N0), 32 (N1)	12
Regnard et al. (2005)	65 (23)	7.7	26.5	38	5.3
de Perrot et al. (2006)	100 (27)	7.6	44	53	15
Macchiarini et al. (2006)	50 (18)	4	51	NS*	NS
Roviaro et al. (2006)	53 (NS)	7.5	33	NS	NS

NS, not stated.
*Nodal status was a significant prognostic factor in multivariate analysis.

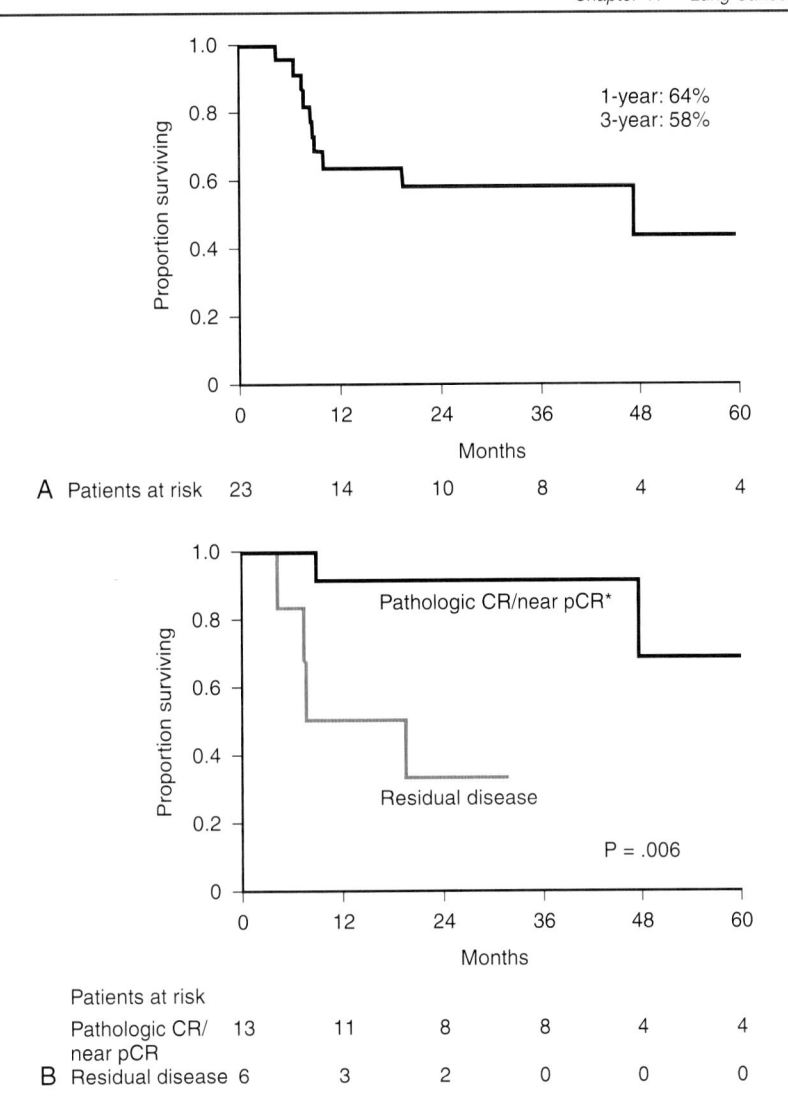

Figure 17-6
Survival after induction chemoradiotherapy followed by radical vertebrectomy for patients with non–small cell lung cancer invading the spine. **A,** Overall survival (n = 23). **B,** Survival according to the pathologic complete response (pCR) in the resected specimen in patients with R0 resection (pCR, n = 10; near pCR*, n = 3; pathologic residual disease, n = 6). *Viable tumor cells less than 1% in a resected tumor. *(From Anraku M, Waddell TK, de Perrot M, et al.* J Thorac Cardiovasc Surg *2009;**137**:441-7.)*

N Category: N0 and N1

Decision making in the treatment of patients with stage I/II (N0 or N1) NSCLC is relatively straightforward, as surgical resection (in most cases, lobectomy) is the mainstay of therapy if patients have good cardiopulmonary reserve. However, there is a growing body of evidence on types of surgical resection and combined neoadjuvant and adjuvant therapy in the management of stage I/II disease.

In patients with clinical N0-1 disease, the type of pulmonary resection is dependent on T category and intraoperative assessment of nodal disease. As described (see Sublobar Resection versus Lobectomy, earlier), lesser resection such as segmentectomy would be an option for small-size peripheral NSCLC (T1 disease) if no nodal disease is confirmed intraoperatively. Therefore, intraoperative interlobar or hilar nodal assessment (or both) is critical in decision making for sublobar resection. VATS has been widely accepted for resection in this category. On the other hand, for patients with N0 NSCLC with local tumor invasion (T3 disease), an extended en bloc resection such as pneumonectomy, sleeve resection, chest wall resection, or other procedures can be performed to obtain cancer-free margins. Mediastinal lymph node sampling is essential for accurate cancer staging. The controversy as to whether complete mediastinal lymph node dissection is included is discussed later in this chapter.

Cisplatin-based adjuvant chemotherapy has been shown to improve survival in patients with N1 and even in pathologic N0 disease, with completely resected, T1b or higher NSCLC based on recent phase III randomized clinical trials.[44,45,47] Various combinations of chemotherapeutic agents, new non-platinum agents including molecular targeted drugs, or techniques of tumor molecular profiling are under investigation in efforts to further improve outcomes in patients with NSCLC.

N Category: N2

The option of offering surgery to patients with N2 disease (ipsilateral mediastinal or subcarinal node involvement) has been long debated. N2 disease comprises heterogeneous groups of patients, from those with micrometastatic

Table 17-4
Recent Surgical Series of Vertebrectomy in Non–Small Cell Lung Cancer

Author (Year)	All Patients (N)	Vertebrectomy (n of Patients)			Treatment Protocol (n)	R0 Resection (%)	Survival (%)
		Total	Hemi*	Multilevel† (%)			
Gandhi et al. (1999)	17	7	10	3 (18)	S alone (1), R → S (1)	65	54 (2-year)
					S → R (6), C+R → S (3)		
					S → C+R (6)		
Grunenwald et al. (2002)	19	4	15	3 (16)	S (8), R → S (2)	79	53 (2-year)
					C → S (5), C+R → S (4)		
Fadel et al. (2002)	17‡	1	16	1 (6)	S → R (9), C → S → R (7)	77	39 (3-year)
					C+R → S → R (1)		
Anraku et al. (2009)	23	6	17	4 (17)	C+R → S (22), C → S (1)	83	58 (3-year)

*Partial vertebrectomy and transverse process resection included.
†Number of cases with two or more total vertebrectomies.
‡All had direct tumor spread into the intervertebral foramina without spinal canal or vertebral body invasion.
C, chemotherapy; NS, not stated; R, radiotherapy; S, surgery.
From Anraku M, Waddell TK, de Perrot M, et al. J Thorac Cardiovasc Surg 2009;137:441–7.

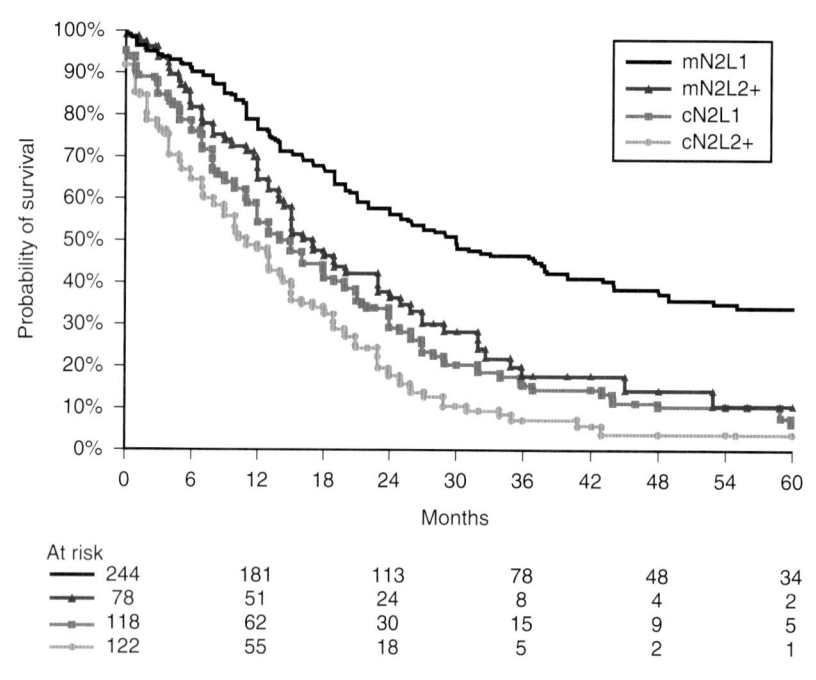

Figure 17-7
Survival of patients with N2 disease treated with primary surgery according to N2 status and number of levels involved. cN2, N2 disease proven by CT (lymph node > 1 cm in short-axis diameter) or mediastinoscopy before surgical resection; mN2, N2 disease not proven before surgery (all lymph nodes < 1 cm in short-axis diameter by CT or negative mediastinoscopy); L1, a single lymph node level involved; L2+, multiple lymph node levels involved. (From Andre F, Grunenwald D, Pignon JP, et al. J Clin Oncol 2000;**18**:2981–9.)

mediastinal node involvement found intraoperatively (on frozen section) or postoperatively (on final pathologic examination) to those with bulky mediastinal node involvement recognized by the pretreatment staging workup. In a study by Andre and coworkers,[91] patients with N2 disease proven before surgery (either by CT or mediastinoscopy) had significantly worse survival than those who did not have a diagnosis of N2 disease before surgery (Fig. 17-7). Patients with N2 disease are subjected to a combined treatment strategy including chemotherapy, radiotherapy, and surgery, but it remains controversial as to which of these treatment modalities should be included or in what sequence (i.e., before or after surgery). Furthermore, it has been under substantial debate as to which patients with N2 disease should be offered surgical resection at all.

In the context of decision making in the treatment of N2 disease, there are two distinct scenarios according to when the nodal disease is definitely confirmed: (1) N2 disease confirmed by the pretreatment staging workup, and (2) N2 disease found at thoracotomy or at postsurgical pathologic examination (unexpected N2 disease).

N2 Found on Pretreatment Staging

Patients with multistation, bulky (involved lymph nodes >2 cm in short-axis diameter measured by CT scan), histologically or cytologically proven N2 disease are generally treated with nonsurgical modalities (i.e., chemotherapy or chemoradiotherapy), because complete resection would not be expected. On the other hand, those with nonbulky, multistation or single-station N2 disease found at staging, but without any sign of distant metastasis, are still potential candidates for curative surgical resection. In such cases, the use of neoadjuvant (induction) should be considered based on several randomized phase III clinical trials[92-94] and recent phase II studies.[3,95,96] Theoretical advantages of neoadjuvant treatment include (1) downsizing of the primary and nodal disease that may facilitate complete clearance of the nodal disease, (2) decreased chance of surgical seeding of tumor cells, (3) in vivo chemosensitivity or radiosensitivity checking of the tumor, and (4) better patient compliance with the treatment.[97] The Toronto group[3] recently reported an improved overall median survival of 40 months in patients with biopsy-proven N2 NSCLC treated with induction chemoradiation followed by surgery (Fig. 17-8A), and in this patient population, pathologic response to induction treatment was also prognostic (see Fig. 17-8B). However, the decision to proceed with surgical resection requires careful assessment after induction treatment including restaging, performance status, and pulmonary function tests. Especially for poor-risk patients who respond to induction chemotherapy, definitive radiotherapy is an option for treatment, as a recent randomized clinical trial conducted by the European Organisation for Research and Treatment of Cancer (EORTC) Lung Cancer Group demonstrated comparable outcomes in the radiotherapy arm and the surgery arm.[98]

Mediastinal restaging and assessment after neoadjuvant treatment is of great importance, because residual N2 disease after chemotherapy appears to be an unfavorable prognostic factor, and surgical resection for these patients remains controversial.[95,99] Although clinical restaging with chest CT is suboptimal for predicting pathologic response of metastatic lymph nodes to induction chemotherapy, integrated PET and CT,[100,101] and endobronchial ultrasound with transbronchial needle aspiration (EBUS-TBNA)[102] have been used and may be promising in this context. In a prospective study by Cerfolio and colleagues[101] in patients with biopsy-proven N2 disease treated with induction chemoradiotherapy, PET plus CT was more accurate than CT alone for restaging. In their study, a greater than 50% decrease in the maximum standardized uptake value (SUV_{max}) in the metastatic lymph nodes was highly suggestive of pathologic clearance of cancer. Repeat mediastinoscopy after induction chemotherapy has been reported as useful with high sensitivity by Stamatis and colleagues[103] and others.[104] However, because it is an invasive procedure and known to be technically demanding, it is not regularly performed in clinical practice.

Bueno and coworkers[105] stressed the importance of residual disease after induction chemotherapy. In their study, it was found that patients down-staged to pN0 had a 5-year survival of 35.8%, whereas those who did not achieve down-staging

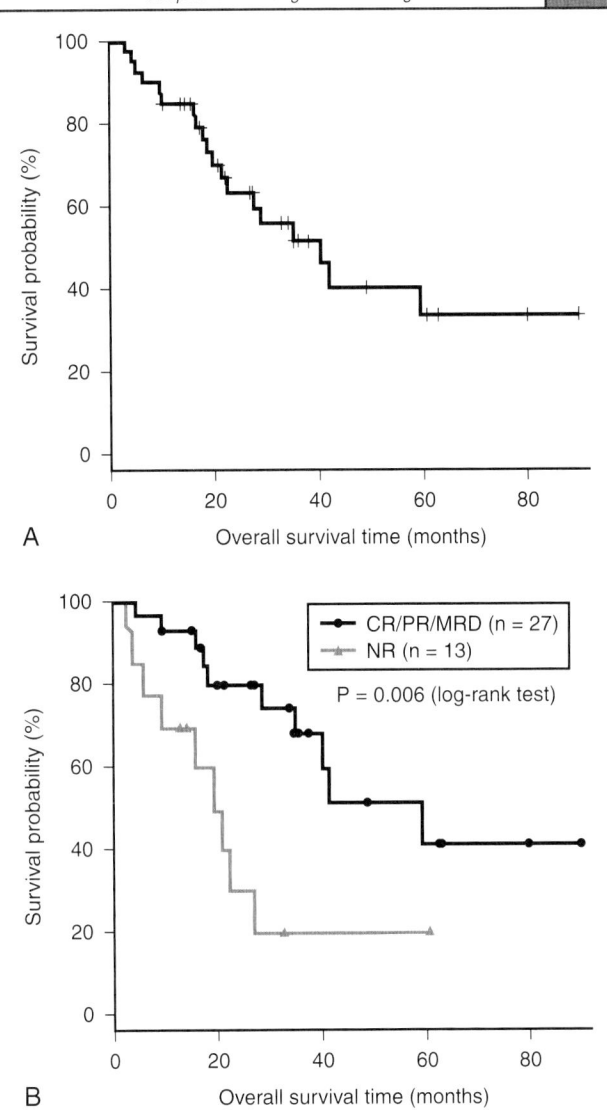

Figure 17–8
Survival after induction chemoradiotherapy followed by surgical resection in patients with N2 non–small cell lung cancer. **A,** Overall survival. **B,** Survival by pathologic response. CR, complete pathologic response; PR, partial pathologic response; MRD, minimal residual disease, defined as less than 10% viable tumor cells; NR, no response. *(From Uy KL, Darling G, Xu W, et al. J Thorac Cardiovasc Surg 2007;**134**:188–93.)*

demonstrated a disappointing 9% 5-year survival. In a phase II study of induction chemotherapy followed by surgery in patients with mediastinoscopy-proven N2 disease, reported by Garrido and coworkers,[96] the 5-year survival was 17.6% in patients with residual pN1-3 disease (Fig. 17-9). In their study, patients down-staged to pN0 had significantly better survival (5-year survival, 51.6%) than those with pN1-3 disease. However, persistent minor mediastinal disease after induction chemotherapy may not always exclude surgical resection; in other words, some of those may be cured by surgical clearance of residual mediastinal disease. Dooms and colleagues[106] tried to select this subset of patients by means of serial [^{18}F]fluoro-2-deoxyglucose (FDG) PET scans taken before and after induction therapy. The authors demonstrated significantly better survival in patients with persistent minor mediastinal disease and a more than 60% decrease in the SUV_{max} than in patients with persistent minor disease but with a less than 60% decrease in SUV_{max}.

N2 Found at Thoracotomy

The optimal management in patients with N2 disease found at thoracotomy (unsuspected N2 disease) is controversial. Treatment options include aborting lung resection followed by induction therapy and possibly followed by surgical resection, or proceeding with lung resection followed by adjuvant therapy. The rationale for the former decision is based on the favorable outcome of induction therapy followed by surgery obtained from published evidence including randomized clinical trials.[107] In this era of VATS lung resection, however, it is reasonable to stop lung resection for induction therapy if N2 disease is discovered at the time of a VATS lobectomy, in which case the morbidity of the incision is small. On the other hand, with open thoracotomy, one may favor the latter option because the patient has already been exposed to the risks of general anesthetic and thoracotomy. In addition, one might presume that patients who underwent thoracotomy (even without lung resection) may not be as compliant as those who undergo induction therapy before surgery. Cerfolio and colleagues[108] reported a 5-year survival of 35% in patients who have completely resected unsuspected N2 disease after PET plus CT and thin-slice CT assessments (most likely reflecting minimal disease N2 status).

Controlling distant relapse is critical in patients with resected N2 NSCLC, because presence of N2 disease is known to be an indicator for high risk of metastatic relapse. Albain and coworkers[99] reported cancer relapse patterns in patients with N2 disease who underwent induction chemoradiotherapy followed by surgical resection. Of 65 relapses in the study, 11% were only locoregional and 61% were only distant. Pisters and Le Chevalier[109] summarized similar relapse rates in operable stage IIIA (N2) NSCLC (Table 17-5).

On this background, the use of adjuvant chemotherapy or radiotherapy has been extensively studied in resected N2 NSCLC, and adjuvant cisplatin-based chemotherapy appears to be beneficial, as proven by two recent randomized clinical trials. The Adjuvant Navelbine International Trialist Association (ANITA) trial demonstrated a reduced risk for death (Hazard Ratio, 0.69), with prolonged survival in patients who received adjuvant chemotherapy with or without radiotherapy compared with those without adjuvant therapy after complete surgical resection (Table 17-6).[45] A hazard ratio of 0.79 was reported in

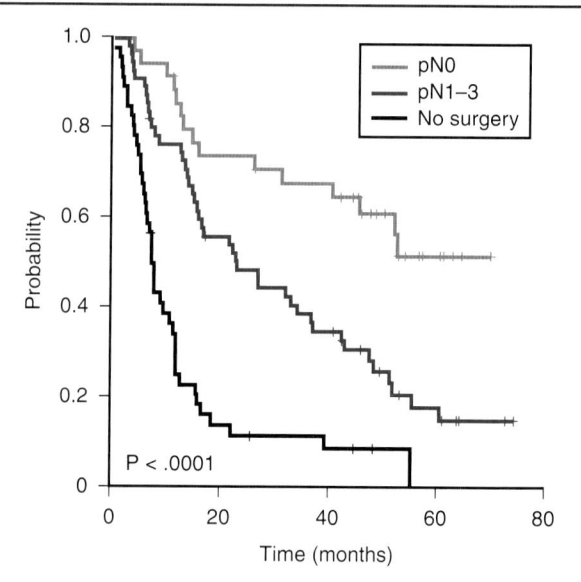

Figure 17-9
Median survival according to pathologic down-staging in patients with mediastinoscopy-proof N2 with induction chemotherapy followed by surgery. (From Garrido P, Gonzalez-Larriba JL, Insa A, et al. J Clin Oncol 2007;25:4736–42.)

Table 17-5

Expected Outcome after Surgical Resection in Operable Non–Small Cell Lung Cancer

Surgical Stage		5-Year Survival (%)	Relapse (%)	
			Local	Distant
IA	T1N0	67	10	15
IB	T2N0	57	10	30
IIA	T1N1	55	—	—
IIB	T2N1	39	12	40
	T3N0	38		
IIIA	T3N1	25	15	60
	T1-3N2	23		

Modified from Pisters KM, Le Chevalier T. J Clin Oncol 2005;23:3270–8.

Table 17-6

Overall Survival Estimates for Resected Patients* with N2 Non–Small Cell Lung Cancer with or without Cisplatin-Based Adjuvant Chemotherapy

	Survival (%)			
	Chemotherapy		Control	
Survival Interval	Radiotherapy	No Radiotherapy	Radiotherapy	No Radiotherapy
1-year	98	71	74	57
2-year	77	49	48	35
5-year	47	34	21	17

*N = 224.
Modified from Douillard JY, Rosell R, De Lena M, et al. Lancet Oncol 2006;7:719–27.

the International Adjuvant Lung Cancer Trial (IALT), in favor of adjuvant chemotherapy compared with observation alone.[47]

Postoperative mediastinal radiotherapy for patients with resected NSCLC has not been proven to be effective in a past meta-analysis.[110] However, a more recent meta-analysis using the Surveillance, Epidemiology, and End Results (SEER) database of postoperative radiotherapy demonstrated prolonged survival in patients with stage IIIA (N2) disease.[111] Results from the ANITA trial (nonrandomized subanalysis) also showed a benefit with postoperative radiation (see Table 17-6). An ongoing randomized trial of three-dimensional conformal postoperative radiotherapy versus no radiotherapy in patients resected for N2 NSCLC (Lung Adjuvant Radiotherapy Trial [Lung ART]) may give us a more definitive answer to the question of whether modern radiotherapy should be a part of combined treatment in patients resected for N2.

N Category: N3

Contralateral mediastinal lymph node metastases are considered a contraindication for surgery because long-term outcome with surgery has been dismal. The Southwest Oncology Group[99] reported a 0% 3-year survival rate of patients with N3 NSCLC who underwent induction chemotherapy and radiotherapy followed by surgery. Because N3 lymph nodes are outside the surgical field and considered to be extensive lymphatic spread of cancer, complete surgical resection cannot be achieved. Therefore, we believe that patients with N3 disease should be treated nonsurgically.

M Category: M1a

M1a includes separate tumor nodules in a contralateral lobe, tumor with pleural nodules, and tumor with malignant pleural effusion.

Additional Nodules in the Contralateral Lung

Additional nodules in the *contralateral lung* are designated as M1a (previously M1), whereas those in the *primary lobe* are designated as T3, and those in the *ipsilateral lung (different lobe)* as T4, according to the proposal from the IASLC Staging Project to the seventh edition of the TMN Classification for Lung Cancer.[27] Based on the IASLC data, the median survival of patients with M1a disease was 10 months, with a 5-year survival rate of 3%,[112] which was significantly worse than that of same-lobe nodules or ipsilateral lung nodules (5-year survival, 28% and 21%, respectively). The median survivals of this subset of patients in the IASLC database and the SEER database were 6 and 7 months, respectively. Therefore, additional nodules in the contralateral lung generally preclude surgery, although surgery may be offered for the primary NSCLC if the contralateral pulmonary lesions are questionable and mediastinal staging is negative. FDG PET has appeared to be sensitive for detecting malignant metastatic disease,[113] but pathologic confirmation should be made by a percutaneous transthoracic needle biopsy or an excisional biopsy of those identified by PET, especially in the case of a solitary lesion.[114]

When tumors represent double primaries (synchronous primaries) without mediastinal disease, the optimal treatment is two-staged lobectomy for contralateral tumors if the patient's lung function permits. When the cardiopulmonary reserve is limited, a lobectomy could be performed for the more advanced tumor and a limited resection (segmentectomy or wedge resection) for the contralateral tumor. Limited resection is in general reserved for smaller tumors or squamous carcinomas, as they are less likely to spread via the local lymphatic system, although this concept needs further study. Alternatively, bilateral segmentectomies can be considered for patients with very limited pulmonary function.

A subtype of adenocarcinoma of the lung, bronchioloalveolar carcinoma (BAC), is characterized as being multicentric and is frequently identified in its early stage with the advent of high-resolution CT. BAC can also exist with other cell types of NSCLC. The management of multifocal BACs or BAC with other non–small cell types is discussed later (see Multifocal Bronchioloalveolar Carcinoma).

Malignant Pleural Effusion

A histologically documented malignant pleural effusion is a contraindication for surgery because it is not amenable to complete resection. However, Ichinose and coworkers[115] reported a 5-year survival rate of 23% in surgical patients with a minimal amount of malignant pleural effusions (average, 37 mL) found at thoracotomy. Long-term survivals (>5 years) have also been reported by Yokoi and colleagues[116] in highly selected patients with carcinomatous pleuritis without N2 disease who underwent extrapleural pneumonectomy.

M Category: M1b

Category M1b includes all distant metastasis outside the lung. The vast majority of lung cancer patients with distant metastasis are not curable by surgical treatment and surgery is therefore precluded. However, there is some evidence for a potential role for surgical resection in patients with NSCLC who have an isolated distant metastasis in adrenal gland or brain.

Adrenal Gland

A solitary adrenal metastasis in patients with otherwise operable NSCLC is a rare condition (incidence, 1.6%), because adrenal metastases are usually accompanied by other metastatic disease.[117] Based on reported series of adrenalectomy for isolated adrenal metastases in NSCLC, complete surgical resection of both the primary tumor and adrenal metastasis may improve survival in selected cases. Mercier and associates[118] reported a 5-year survival rate of 23% in 23 patients with NSCLC who underwent complete resection of an adrenal metastasis after surgical treatment of lung cancer. In the study, six patients presented with an adrenal metastasis found on the preoperative workup, and the remaining 17 patients were found to have an isolated adrenal metastasis during follow-up after lung resection. The complete adrenalectomy necessitated combined kidney ($n = 2$), inferior vena cava ($n = 1$), or liver ($n = 1$) resection. In the case series by Pfannschmidt and coworkers,[119] the median survival after adrenalectomy was 12.6 months ($n = 11$). Tanvetyanon and colleagues[120] analyzed the pooled data from 114 cases in 10 publications describing outcomes of adrenalectomy in NSCLC. The authors concluded that the time between diagnosis of primary lung cancer and the discovery of adrenal metastasis (disease-free interval [DFI]) was prognostic. Patients with a DFI of 6 months or less demonstrated significantly shorter median survival than those with a DFI greater than 6 months (12 versus 31 months).

The impact of adjuvant chemotherapy or radiation to the adrenal bed on long-term outcome remains undefined because of the scarcity of this population subset; however, the treatment strategy should be refined further, as this subset may be detected more frequently as a result of improvements in diagnostics including CT, magnetic resonance imaging, and PET.[121]

Brain

NSCLC is known for its propensity to metastasize to the brain, and the form of dissemination is often multiple. It has been reported that 30% to 50% of patients with NSCLC are found to develop brain metastasis during the course of their disease.[122] A solitary brain metastasis from lung cancer can be categorized into three subsets: (1) a synchronous primary lung cancer with a single brain metastasis, (2) a solitary brain metastasis found after successful treatment of the primary tumors, and (3) a single brain metastasis from an uncontrolled primary lung cancer. Here we will discuss only the first presentation of the brain metastases, because thoracic surgical oncologists may encounter such cases and be involved in the decision-making process. Thoracic surgeons should be aware, as they advise new surgical colleagues, that resection of a solitary brain metastasis in a patient with completely resected NSCLC does carry a potential cure rate.

In a retrospective report from the Mayo Clinic by Billing and coworkers,[123] 28 out of 220 patients underwent surgical treatment of brain metastases from NSCLC. These patients were treated with surgical resection of synchronous brain metastases and the primary lung cancer. In this series, all craniotomies were performed before the primary lung cancer resections, with a median time between craniotomy and thoracotomy of 14 days. The most responsible factor influencing survival after surgery was the presence of thoracic lymph node metastases. The overall 5-year survival rate was 21.4%, but no patient with lymph node metastases (N1 and N2) survived longer than 3 years.

The use of whole-brain radiation (WBR) alone or WBR combined with surgical resection for a solitary brain metastasis was reported by Rodrigus and associates.[124] In this retrospective study, 32 patients with a solitary brain metastasis undergoing metastasectomy had a significantly better 1-year survival rate than 89 patients with a solitary brain lesion but without surgery (58% versus 14%). All the patients with a solitary brain metastasis received WBR with a dosage of 20 to 45 Gy.

The advent of stereotactic radiosurgery (SRS) has offered another treatment option for patients with a solitary brain metastasis. Hu and coworkers[122] reported on outcomes of NSCLC patients with a solitary brain metastasis treated with either SRS or neurosurgery, in conjunction with chemotherapy or radiotherapy, or both, for the lung primary site. The median survivals for patients who had received treatment for their primary cancers and those who had not were 15.5 and 5.9 months, respectively. In addition, the survival times were thoracic stage–dependent: median survivals by thoracic stage (I, II, and III) were 25.6, 9.5, and 9.9 months, respectively.

The optimal treatment for the primary site and a metastatic site of newly diagnosed NSCLC with a solitary brain metastasis is still under debate because of the lack of randomized trials. However, based on the reported series, patients with thoracic stage I NSCLC with a solitary brain metastasis appear to benefit from aggressive treatment including surgical resection of the primary site. Surgical resection or SRS, with or without WBR to a solitary brain lesion, is the treatment of choice, although randomized trials are required to determine the impact of these modalities on local control and survival.

SPECIAL CONSIDERATIONS

Mediastinal Lymph Node Dissection versus Systematic Sampling

Tumor staging is critical for predicting prognosis, for comparing clinical studies, and, most importantly, for planning therapy in lung cancer. To obtain more accurate mediastinal lymph node staging, intraoperative lymph node examination is necessary in early-stage (I and II) or selected stage III resectable disease. However, current practice varies from simple visual inspection of the mediastinum to radical mediastinal lymph node dissection (MLND) without having solid consensus among thoracic surgeons. In fact, it was reported that nodes were sampled at any mediastinal level during surgery in only 42% of patients with lung cancer in the United States.[125] The points of current debate with regard to surgical mediastinal staging, in particular, in comparing MLND with systematic sampling (SS) include safety, staging accuracy, and local control and long-term survival.

Operative Morbidity

The argument against MLND is that it might be associated with higher morbidity than SS. It can be assumed that chylothorax, phrenic or recurrent laryngeal nerve injury, increased lymphatic drainage/bleeding, or decreased host defense may occur because of resection of whole lymphatic drainage pathways and lymphatic tissues along with the local blood supply. However, recent reports, including a randomized clinical trial, demonstrated that MLND does not increase operative morbidity.[126-128] Allen and colleagues[128] reported a large multi-institutional randomized trial (the American College of Surgeons Oncology Group trial, ACOSOG Z0030), in which patients with lung cancer were randomized to either lymph node sampling ($n = 498$) or lymph node dissection ($n = 525$). Operative mortality was 2.0% for the sampling group and 0.76% for the dissection group. Morbidity including minor complications was 38% in each group. Specifically, there were no statistical differences in the rates of chylothoraces, postoperative hemorrhage, recurrent nerve injuries, or bronchopleural fistulas. No statistical difference was observed in the duration of chest tube drainage (sampling versus dissection, 4 versus 5 days), median total chest tube drainage (1.34 versus 1.46 L), or the length of hospitalization (6 days in both groups).

Staging Accuracy

One of the critical questions needing to be answered is whether SS is as accurate as MLND in surgical mediastinal staging. If mediastinal lymph node assessment is not adequately performed, the true N stage remains unrecognized, which may result in false down-staging. In the ACOSOG Z0030 trial, all patients first received lymph node sampling with frozen section examination. When all required lymph nodes biopsied were negative for malignancy on frozen section, then those patients were randomized to either sampling only with no further dissection or to complete MLND. Positive mediastinal nodes were found in 20 patients (3.8%) who had negative sampling and were randomized to MLND. Therefore, these patients would have unrecognized N2 disease without the dissection.

In the nonrandomized trial reported by Keller and colleagues,[126] SS was as efficacious as MLND in accurate nodal staging, with rates of detected N2 disease of 60% in the SS group (n = 112/187) and 59% in the MLND group (n = 110/186). However, MLND detected significantly more levels of N2 disease (multiple N2 levels: 30% in MLND versus 12% in SS) in the study. The result is comparable to prospective randomized trials reported by Izbicki and associates (17.4% in SS versus 57.2% in MLND),[129] and by Wu and colleagues (28% in SS versus 48% in MLND).[130]

One might ask whether complete MLND is always necessary for patients with early-stage, small-size NSCLC, as such cases are frequently and increasingly identified today. In a prospective randomized trial for patients with clinical T1N0 NSCLC less than 2 cm in diameter (n = 115) by Sugi and coworkers,[131] the authors concluded that SS is adequate, as there were no statistical differences in N2 detection rates (13% in both groups) or in survival between groups.

A unique multicenter cross-sectional study was performed by Massard and associates[132] to answer the question of whether MLND elevates diagnostic accuracy. The authors performed lymph node sampling first, followed by complete MLND in each patient enrolled in the study (N = 208). The sampled nodes and the nodes from MLND were examined separately, so each case served as its own control. Of 60 patients with pathologic N2 disease, lymph node sampling identified only 31 patients (52%) as having N2 disease. Furthermore, multilevel N2 disease was detected by sampling in 10 out of 25 patients (40%). The authors concluded that lymph node sampling is inadequate in determining accurate N stage.

Local Control and Long-Term Survival

A postulated argument is that MLND contributes not only to improved staging but also to tumor control and long-term prognosis; however, the therapeutic efficacy of MLND remains under debate. If SS fails to identify positive mediastinal nodes, it may result in an increased risk of local recurrence in comparison with MLND. On the other hand, it might be hypothesized that MLND may help in clearing occult micrometastatic cells in the mediastinal lymph nodes that are not identified by conventional histopathologic methods,[133] and thus may increase the rate of complete resection. The latter hypothesis is supported by the fact that local tumor recurrence is significantly higher in patients with pathologic stage I or pathologic N0-1 disease who underwent SS than in those who underwent MLND (45% versus 13%, and 46% versus 13%, respectively).[127]

A few prospective randomized studies have examined these issues. A study by Izbicki and colleagues[134] demonstrated that MLND appeared to prolong the relapse-free interval compared with SS in patients with pathologic N1-2 disease; however, there was no significant difference in survival. Sugi and associates[131] conducted a prospective randomized study of SS and MLND in patients with clinically diagnosed peripheral NSCLC less than 2 cm in diameter. The patients were assigned to a lobectomy with SS (n = 56) or a lobectomy with MLND (n = 59). In the study, no significant differences were found in recurrence rate or survival between the groups. On the other hand, a more recent prospective randomized trial conducted by Wu and coworkers[130] demonstrated a survival benefit of MLND over SS (median survival, 59 versus 34 months) with a reduced local recurrence rate (2.9% versus 4.8%). The difference in survival was prominent in stage I (5-year survival, 82.2% versus 57.5%) and stage IIIA (27.0% versus 6.2%). Recent evidence from the literature relating to the potential benefit of MLND on both local control and long-term outcome are summarized in Table 17-7.

The large (more than 1000 cases), prospective, randomized multicenter trial of MLND versus SS during pulmonary resection in patients with clinically resectable NSCLC is currently underway (ACOSOG Z0030).[128] Whether there is a favorable impact of MLND on long-term outcome awaits the result of this trial.

Multifocal Bronchioloalveolar Carcinoma

Bronchioloalveolar carcinoma is a subtype of adenocarcinoma with distinct pathologic, radiographic, and clinical features. BAC may have two entities—focal and diffuse forms—with similar histologic features.[135] The incidence of focal BAC is rising, representing 4% of all NSCLCs over the past 2 decades in the United States.[136] Focal BAC is discussed here because it is often amenable to surgical treatment with good outcome.

Pathologically, BAC originates from Clara cells or type II pneumocytes, and it grows along alveolar walls without stromal invasion.[137] It frequently presents as a part of an adenocarcinoma with mixed subtypes, characterized by a mixture of a noninvasive BAC component and invasive subtypes.[138] BAC is also known for its multifocal nature, including bilateral lung involvement, although the etiology of the multifocality is under debate.[139]

One radiographic appearance of BAC, known as ground-glass opacity (GGO), is characterized as a localized, mild-to-moderate increase in density on a CT scan without obscuring preexisting bronchovascular structures. A focal GGO can contain solid parts in the lesion that often represent invasive components. High-resolution CT is useful for correlating the radiographic appearance of GGO with pathologic features, including mediastinal node involvement.[140,141]

Treatment Strategy and Outcome

In small (<2 cm) peripheral BAC, stromal invasion is associated with lymph node metastasis and worse outcome after surgical resection; on the other hand, noninvasive BAC demonstrated no lymph node involvement and an excellent 5-year survival rate (100%).[142] Given its multifocal process and better outcome compared with other non–small cell types, attempts have been made with complete surgical resection for multifocal BAC, or for BAC with other non–small cell types. Roberts and colleagues[143] reported a 5-year survival rate of 64% after complete surgical resection in patients

Table 17–7

Impact of Mediastinal Lymph Node Dissection (MLND) or Systematic Sampling (SS) on Local Recurrence and Long-Term Outcome in Patients with Resectable Non–Small Cell Lung Cancer

Author (Year)	Study Design (N of Patients)	Clinical Stage	MLND vs SS Local Recurrence (%)	MLND vs SS Disease-Free Median Survival (mo, but % when 5-yr)
Izbicki (1998)	Randomized (169)	I-III	28.9 vs 34.4 (NS)	48 vs 24 (NS)
Sugi (1998)	Randomized (115)	I	10 vs 13 (NS)*	81.4% vs 83.9% (overall 5-yr, NS)
Keller (2000)	Nonrandomized (373)	II, IIIA	52 vs 58 (NS)*	57.5% vs 29.2†
Wu (2002)	Randomized (471)	I-IIIA	2.9 vs 4.8	59 vs 34†
				p-St. I, 82.2% vs 57.5%† (5-yr)
				p-St. II, 50.4% vs 34.1% (5-yr, NS)
				p-St. IIIA, 27.0% vs 6.2%† (5-yr)
Lardinois (2005)	Nonrandomized (100)	I, II	p-St. I, 13 vs 45†	p-St. I, 60.2 vs 44.8†
			p-St. II, 17 vs 55 (NS)	p-N0, 52.8 vs 44.8†
			p-St. IIIA, 23 vs 10 (NS)	All, 46.2 vs 41.1 (NS)

NS, not significant; p-St., pathologic stage.
*Statistically significant.
†Distant recurrence included.

with multifocal BAC (unilateral, n = 9; and bilateral, n = 5). Nakata and coworkers[144] reported a 3-year survival rate of 92% in patients with multiple primary adenocarcinoma treated with combinations of lobectomy and sublobar resections. Mun and colleagues[145] also reported clinicopathologic results of thoracoscopic resections for patients with small, peripheral, multifocal BAC (105 BAC lesions in 27 patients). In the study, the authors performed lobectomies or lesser resections (segmentectomy or wedge resection) with or without lymph node dissection. All lesions demonstrated GGO with no solid components (pure GGO) on the preoperative CT scan. The 5-year disease-free survivals were excellent—70% overall, 65% in lobectomy, and 75% in lesser resection cases. There was no local recurrence observed; however, interestingly, de novo BAC lesions developed in 26% of the patients after the surgical treatment.

Based on a limited number of published case series of BAC, sublobar resection may be offered for solitary, small, peripheral BAC with no sign of invasive growth (radiographically pure GGO), although standard lobectomy should be performed for those with invasive growth features radiographically. Complete surgical resection appears to be a promising option for multifocal BAC if mediastinal nodes are not involved.

SURGICAL TREATMENT OF SMALL CELL LUNG CANCER

Small cell lung cancer (SCLC) represents 15% of all lung cancer in the North America[146] and is characterized by rapid growth and early dissemination. Only approximately 30% of the patients with SCLC present with limited disease (LD). LD-SCLC is treated with curative intent with chemoradiotherapy with median survival of 23 months and a 5-year survival rate of 12% to 17%, whereas extensive-disease SCLC is treated primarily with chemotherapy with a median survival of approximately 7 to 12 months, and the proportion surviving 5 years is only 2%.[146]

The treatment for patients with lung cancer including SCLC was primarily surgery before 1970, but surgery was largely discouraged after a report from the Medical Research Council in the United Kingdom.[147] This trial showed a small but significant difference in the survival rate—a 4-year survival of 3% in the surgery arm versus 7% in the radiotherapy arm. Because all patients who survived 5 years were treated in the radiotherapy arm, this became the standard form of treatment for LD-SCLC. The role of surgery as initial treatment was reevaluated after introduction of the TNM staging system. Shields and colleagues[148] reported the experience of the Veterans Administration Surgical Oncology Group (VASOG) and concluded that surgical resection is indicated in patients with T1N0 SCLC. Around the same time, the reduction of local recurrence of LD-SCLC by surgical resection was emphasized by the Toronto group.[149] These findings revived interest in the role of surgery in the treatment of early-stage SCLC. Furthermore, the role of adjuvant chemotherapy after surgical resection was investigated by several groups,[150-152] which enhanced the benefit on improved survival. In 1983, the Lung Cancer Study Group initiated a prospective randomized trial in which patients treated with induction chemotherapy were randomized to undergo surgical resection or to receive radiotherapy.[153] Although several criticisms can be made, this is the only prospective randomized trial for LD-SCLC comparing surgery with radiotherapy to date. Median survival was 15.4 months in the surgery arm (n = 70) and 18.6 months in the radiation arm (n = 76). The authors concluded that surgical resection did not contribute to either prolonged survival or local control. Conclusions are limited by the fact that in the surgical arm only 77% (n = 54) of patients underwent complete resection. Also, neither platinum-based chemotherapy nor concurrent chemoradiotherapy was used, and the modern preoperative neoadjuvant therapy might be more potent. Finally, patients with peripheral nodules, assumed to be T1N0, who might be the best candidates for surgery, were specifically excluded in this study.

Rationale for Surgery

Evolving from a number of case-series reports and prospective phase II trials, the role of surgery in LD-SCLC has been shaped by several rationales: (1) small peripheral lesions without any nodal involvement can occasionally be misdiagnosed as SCLC when they are in fact typical or atypical carcinoid tumors, (2) surgical resection for LD-SCLC (T1N0, T2N0) may improve local control compared with chemoradiotherapy, (3) mixed-histology tumors (a SCLC tumor with an NSCLC component) may not be completely eradicated by chemoradiotherapy because the NSCLC component is less sensitive to chemotherapy, (4) salvage surgery for chemoresistant localized SCLC or local relapse after an initial response to chemotherapy or chemoradiotherapy may be more effective than current second-line chemotherapy. A final indication for surgery is a second primary tumor with NSCLC histology after cure of initial SCLC. Although only a small percentage of patients with SCLC survive longer than 2 years, the occurrence of a second primary NSCLC is becoming more common with current advances in the treatment of SCLC. It is worth noting that any new tumor arising longer than 2 years after initial treatment for SCLC is in fact more likely to be of non–small cell histology. Patients without mediastinal node metastases can be treated with surgery. However, survival is reduced in patients with a stage I second NSCLC who underwent wedge resection compared with patients with primary stage I NSCLC receiving wedge resection (median survival, 24.5 versus 58.4 months).[154]

Improved Local Control

Although the mainstay of the current treatment for LD-SCLC is chemotherapy with or without radiotherapy, even the current active chemoradiotherapy protocols have demonstrated local failure rates of 36% and 52%.[155] The first site of recurrence in patients with LD-SCLC who achieve complete remission is the primary tumor site, followed by hilar or mediastinal lymph nodes.[156] In an autopsy series, only 31% of patients who underwent surgery had residual primary tumor, whereas 92% of patients with LD-SCLC who had negative mediastinoscopy but were treated without surgery had residual disease at the primary site. Shepherd and colleagues[149] reported on the Toronto experience, with a combined treatment program including surgical resection, and demonstrated local relapse in only two of 35 patients. A recent report from a German group has demonstrated 100% local or locoregional control after complete surgical resection following induction chemoradiotherapy for LD-SCLC, with a 5-year survival rate of 63%.[157] There are no available data from randomized control trials comparing modern chemoradiotherapy protocols with chemoradiotherapy with surgery; however, the impact of surgical resection on local control seems to be evident. In this context, surgical treatment for SCLC appearing as a solitary pulmonary nodule without nodal involvement would be a justifiable strategy. Particularly if the diagnosis is uncertain or in question, surgery can be an initial step in the management of T1-2 N0 SCLC. In a recent Japanese trial, the 5-year survival rates in patients with clinical stage IA (T1N0) and IB (T2N0) postoperatively proven SCLC who underwent complete resection followed by chemotherapy were an encouraging 73% and 67%, respectively.[158]

Mixed-Histology Tumors

According to the World Health Organization classification of lung carcinoma (1999), the variants of SCLC admixed with various other histologic types are defined as combined small cell carcinoma. Recent surgical series of neuroendocrine lung tumors revealed that 26.6% of resected SCLC fell into this category.[159] In studies of induction chemotherapy followed by adjuvant surgery for pathologically confirmed SCLC, an NSCLC component was found in the resected specimen in 11% to 15% of cases.[153,160] The high percentage of combined SCLC in surgical reports is partially because combined SCLC tends to be in the periphery rather than in the hilum and thus surgical resection may be more feasible. In addition, because of the large amount of tissue available in surgical cases (i.e., the entire tumor), the chance of finding other components may increase. Another possible reason is that, since the NSCLC component is less sensitive to chemotherapy than the SCLC component, residual tumors, which are more likely to be surgically treated, may be more likely to contain an NSCLC component. Therefore, it is reasonable to offer surgical resection to improve local control if a histologic diagnosis of mixed SCLC without nodal involvement is obtained. It must be part of a combined modality approach, because surgery alone is not adequate for the SCLC component. An NSCLC component may be responsible for local relapse or the poor response to chemoradiotherapy, so surgery may be offered as salvage treatment as discussed next.

Surgery as a Salvage Treatment

Because the treatment of relapsed or unresponsive LD-SCLC with second-line chemotherapy is generally unsatisfactory, salvage surgery for these cases offers another treatment option. The Toronto group has identified a small but curable subset of patients who benefit from salvage surgery.[161] In this prospective study, the authors offered surgery for patients with residual disease after chemotherapy or radiotherapy (or both), or with local failure after the initial response to chemotherapy. After resection, 10 of 28 patients were found to have a mixed histology or pure-NSCLC tumor, although 25 of 28 patients were thought to have a pure-SCLC tumor preoperatively. The 10 patients with mixed histology or pure-NSCLC tumor achieved a median survival of more than 2 years. In contrast, patients with pure-SCLC tumors rarely survived more than 2 years. Therefore, patients with mixed histology in their residual or nonresponsive tumor without nodal disease may be good candidates for salvage surgery. In this view, it is worth considering a second biopsy to reevaluate the cell type.

Ongoing Randomized Trials

On the basis of promising results from several phase II trials,[158,162] prospective randomized trials for LD-SCLC with platinum-based induction chemotherapy combined with

Table 17–8
Ongoing Randomized Trials of Multimodality Treatment Program Including Surgery for Limited-Disease Small Cell Lung Cancer

Trial	Regimen	Study design
Essen Thoracic Oncology Group	Cisplatin, etoposide	Arm A: CT × 3 + CT/Hf-RT (45 Gy; twice daily) → surgery
		Arm B: CT × 3 + CT/Hf-RT (45 Gy; twice daily) → boost CT/RT
West Japan Thoracic Oncology Group	Cisplatin, etoposide	Arm A: CT × 3 + CT/Hf-RT (45 Gy; twice daily) + PCI* + surgery
		Arm B: CT × 2/Hf-RT (45 Gy; twice daily) + CT × 2 + PCI*
German multicenter randomized trial	Carboplatin, etoposide, paclitaxel	Arm A: CT × 5 + surgery ± RT (50 Gy; once daily) + PCI
		Arm B: CT × 5 + RT (50 Gy; once daily) + PCI

*PCI is planned only for patients with complete remission after induction chemoradiotherapy.
CT, chemotherapy; Hf-RT, hyperfractionated radiotherapy; PCI, prophylactic cranial irradiation.
From Anraku M, Waddell TK. Surgery for small-cell lung cancer. Semin Thorac Cardiovasc Surg 2006;18:211–6.

concurrent hyperfractionated accelerated radiotherapy, followed by either surgery, chemotherapy, or chemoradiotherapy, are now under investigation (Table 17-8). In the Essen Thoracic Oncology Group trial, based on historically dismal results of surgical treatment for pathologic node-positive disease, only patients with N0 status confirmed by repeat mediastinoscopy after induction chemoradiotherapy proceed to surgery. In the West Japan Thoracic Oncology Group trial, patients who have no response to induction chemoradiotherapy are specifically excluded from the surgery arm. Also, because of the pattern of failure after combined-modality treatment including surgery, prophylactic cranial irradiation is given to reduce the risk of recurrence in the brain either before or after surgery in these trials. The trials may give more solid answers as to the question of whether surgery has any role in the treatment of not only early-stage SCLC (IB-IIB) but also more locally advanced SCLC (i.e., IIIA disease).

In summary, surgery is indeed a viable option for the treatment of LD-SCLC. How best to integrate it into multimodality treatment programs and how to improve patient selection for surgery are key considerations for further refinement of the treatment strategy in these patients.

Summary

Surgical resection in patients with NSCLC continues to be the mainstay of curative treatment, and the techniques continue to evolve. On one hand, VATS allows thoracic surgeons to perform minimally invasive surgery on early-stage tumors while not violating key oncologic principles. On the other hand, improvements in surgical techniques, intraoperative management, and postoperative care allow more radical resections of tumor invading other organs. Neoadjuvant, adjuvant, or both therapies should be considered in the treatment for most patients with resectable NSCLC (excluding stage IA) if medically fit. Accurate tumor staging continues to be the key to determining optimal treatment strategy.

REFERENCES

1. Jemal A, Siegel R, Ward E, et al. Cancer statistics. *CA Cancer J Clin* 2007;**57**:43-66:2007.
2. Pisters KM, Evans WK, Azzoli CG, et al. Cancer Care Ontario and American Society of Clinical Oncology adjuvant chemotherapy and adjuvant radiation therapy for stages I-IIIA resectable non small-cell lung cancer guideline. *J Clin Oncol* 2007;**25**:5506-18.
3. Uy KL, Darling G, Xu W, et al. Improved results of induction chemoradiation before surgical intervention for selected patients with stage IIIA-N2 non-small cell lung cancer. *J Thorac Cardiovasc Surg* 2007;**134**:188-93.
4. Davies HM: Recent advances in the surgery of the lung and pleura. Br J Surg 1:**228**, 1913-1914.
5. Graham EA, Singer JJ. Successful removal of the entire lung for carcinoma of the bronchus. *JAMA* 1933;**101**:1371.
6. Churchill ED, Sweet RH, Sutter L, Scannel JG. The surgical management of carcinoma of the lung: a study of cases treated at the Massachusetts General Hospital from 1930-1950. *J Thorac Cardiovasc Surg* 1950;**20**:349.
7. Overholt RH, Langer L. *The technique of pulmonary resection.* Springfield, MO: Charles C Thomas; 1951.
8. Price-Thomas C. Conservative resection of the bronchial tree. *J R Coll Surg Edinb* 1956;**1**:169.
9. Mathey J, Binet JP, Galey JJ, et al. Tracheal and tracheobronchial resections: technique and results in 20 cases. *J Thorac Cardiovasc Surg* 1966;**51**:1.
10. Thompson DT. Tracheal resection with left lung anastomosis following right pneumonectomy. *Thorax* 1966;**21**:560.
11. Chardak WM, MacCallun JD. Pancoast tumor (5 yr survival without recurrence or metastases following radical resection and postoperative irradiation). *J Thorac Surg* 1956;**31**:535.
12. Grillo HC, Bendixen HH, Gephart T. Resection of the carina and lower trachea. *Ann Surg* 1963;**158**:889-93.
13. Jensik RJ, Faber LP, Milloy FJ, Monson DO. Segmental resection for lung cancer. a fifteen year experience. *J Thorac Cardiovasc Surg* 1973;**66**:563.
14. Yim AP. VATS major pulmonary resection revisited-controversies, techniques, and results. *Ann Thorac Surg* 2002;**74**:615-23.
15. Ferguson MK, Lehman AG. Sleeve lobectomy or pneumonectomy: optimal management strategy using decision analysis techniques. *Ann Thorac Surg* 2003;**76**:1782-8.
16. Deslauriers J, Gregoire J, Jacques LF, et al. Sleeve lobectomy versus pneumonectomy for lung cancer: a comparative analysis of survival and sites or recurrences. *Ann Thorac Surg* 2004;**77**:1152-6:discussion 1156.
17. Ma Z, Dong A, Fan J, et al. Does sleeve lobectomy concomitant with or without pulmonary artery reconstruction (double sleeve) have favorable results for non-small cell lung cancer compared with pneumonectomy? A meta-analysis. *Eur J Cardiothorac Surg* 2007;**32**:20-8.
18. Darling GE, Abdurahman A, Yi QL, et al. Risk of a right pneumonectomy: role of bronchopleural fistula. *Ann Thorac Surg* 2005;**79**:433-7.
19. Ginsberg RJ, Rubinstein LV. Randomized trial of lobectomy versus limited resection for T1 N0 non-small cell lung cancer. Lung Cancer Study Group. *Ann Thorac Surg* 1995;**60**:615-22:discussion 622-3.
20. Okada M. Radical sublobar resection for lung cancer. *Gen Thorac Cardiovasc Surg* 2008;**56**:151-7.
21. Asamura H. Minimally invasive approach to early, peripheral adenocarcinoma with ground-glass opacity appearance. *Ann Thorac Surg* 2008;**85**:S701-4.
22. Lardinois D, Weder W, Hany TF, et al. Staging of non-small-cell lung cancer with integrated positron-emission tomography and computed tomography. *N Engl J Med* 2003;**348**:2500-7.
23. Yasufuku K, Chiyo M, Koh E, et al. Endobronchial ultrasound guided transbronchial needle aspiration for staging of lung cancer. *Lung Cancer* 2005;**50**:347-54.
24. Scott WJ, Howington J, Feigenberg S, et al. Treatment of non-small cell lung cancer stage I and stage II: ACCP evidence-based clinical practice guidelines. *Chest* 2007;**132**:234S-42S:2nd edition.
25. Lardinois D, De Leyn P, Van Schil P, et al. ESTS guidelines for intraoperative lymph node staging in non-small cell lung cancer. *Eur J Cardiothorac Surg* 2006;**30**:787-92.
26. Mountain CF, Dresler CM. Regional lymph node classification for lung cancer staging. *Chest* 1997;**111**:1718-23.
27. Goldstraw P, Crowley J, Chansky K, et al. The IASLC Lung Cancer Staging Project: proposals for the revision of the TNM stage groupings in the forthcoming (seventh) edition of the TNM Classification of malignant tumours. *J Thorac Oncol* 2007;**2**:706-14.

28. Rami-Porta R, Ball D, Crowley J, et al. The IASLC Lung Cancer Staging Project: proposals for the revision of the T descriptors in the forthcoming (seventh) edition of the TNM classification for lung cancer. *J Thorac Oncol* 2007;**2**:593-602.
29. Koike T, Yamato Y, Yoshiya K, et al. Intentional limited pulmonary resection for peripheral T1 N0 M0 small-sized lung cancer. *J Thorac Cardiovasc Surg* 2003;**125**:924-8.
30. Fernando HC, Santos RS, Benfield JR, et al. Lobar and sublobar resection with and without brachytherapy for small stage IA non-small cell lung cancer. *J Thorac Cardiovasc Surg* 2005;**129**:261-7.
31. Okada M, Koike T, Higashiyama M, et al. Radical sublobar resection for small-sized non-small cell lung cancer: a multicenter study. *J Thorac Cardiovasc Surg* 2006;**132**:769-75.
32. Okumura M, Goto M, Ideguchi K, et al. Factors associated with outcome of segmentectomy for non-small cell lung cancer: long-term follow-up study at a single institution in Japan. *Lung Cancer* 2007;**58**:231-7.
33. Sawabata N, Ohta M, Matsumura A, et al. Optimal distance of malignant negative margin in excision of nonsmall cell lung cancer: a multicenter prospective study. *Ann Thorac Surg* 2004;**77**:415-20.
34. Schuchert MJ, Pettiford BL, Keeley S, et al. Anatomic segmentectomy in the treatment of stage I non-small cell lung cancer. *Ann Thorac Surg* 2007;**84**:926-32:discussion 932-3.
35. Okada M, Nishio W, Sakamoto T, et al. Effect of tumor size on prognosis in patients with non-small cell lung cancer: the role of segmentectomy as a type of lesser resection. *J Thorac Cardiovasc Surg* 2005;**129**:87-93.
36. Bando T, Miyahara R, Sakai H, et al. A follow-up report on a new method of segmental resection for small-sized early lung cancer. *Lung Cancer* 2009;**63**:58-62.
37. Jones DR, Stiles BM, Denlinger CE, et al. Pulmonary segmentectomy: results and complications. *Ann Thorac Surg* 2003;**76**:343-8:discussion 348-9.
38. El-Sherif A, Gooding WE, Santos R, et al. Outcomes of sublobar resection versus lobectomy for stage I non-small cell lung cancer: a 13-year analysis. *Ann Thorac Surg* 2006;**82**:408-15:discussion 415-6.
39. Kondo D, Yamada K, Kitayama Y, et al. Peripheral lung adenocarcinomas: 10 mm or less in diameter. *Ann Thorac Surg* 2003;**76**:350-5.
40. Miller DL, Rowland CM, Deschamps C, et al. Surgical treatment of non-small cell lung cancer 1 cm or less in diameter. *Ann Thorac Surg* 2002;**73**:1545-50:discussion 1550-1.
41. Landreneau RJ, Sugarbaker DJ, Mack MJ, et al. Wedge resection versus lobectomy for stage I (T1 N0 M0) non-small-cell lung cancer. *J Thorac Cardiovasc Surg* 1997;**113**:691-8:discussion 698-700.
42. Sienel W, Dango S, Kirschbaum A, et al. Sublobar resections in stage IA non-small cell lung cancer: segmentectomies result in significantly better cancer-related survival than wedge resections. *Eur J Cardiothorac Surg* 2008;**33**:728-34.
43. McKenna Jr RJ, Mahtabifard A, Yap J, et al. Wedge resection and brachytherapy for lung cancer in patients with poor pulmonary function. *Ann Thorac Surg* 2008;**85**:S733-6.
44. Winton T, Livingston R, Johnson D, et al. Vinorelbine plus cisplatin vs. observation in resected non-small-cell lung cancer. *N Engl J Med* 2005;**352**:2589-97.
45. Douillard JY, Rosell R, De Lena M, et al. Adjuvant vinorelbine plus cisplatin versus observation in patients with completely resected stage IB-IIIA non-small-cell lung cancer (Adjuvant Navelbine International Trialist Association [ANITA]): a randomised controlled trial. *Lancet Oncol* 2006;**7**:719-27.
46. Kato H, Ichinose Y, Ohta M, et al. A randomized trial of adjuvant chemotherapy with uracil-tegafur for adenocarcinoma of the lung. *N Engl J Med* 2004;**350**:1713-21.
47. Arriagada R, Bergman B, Dunant A, et al. Cisplatin-based adjuvant chemotherapy in patients with completely resected non-small-cell lung cancer. *N Engl J Med* 2004;**350**:351-60.
48. Downey RJ, Martini N, Rusch VW, et al. Extent of chest wall invasion and survival in patients with lung cancer. *Ann Thorac Surg* 1999;**68**:188-93.
49. Chapelier A, Fadel E, Macchiarini P, et al. Factors affecting long-term survival after en-bloc resection of lung cancer invading the chest wall. *Eur J Cardiothorac Surg* 2000;**18**:513-8.
50. Facciolo F, Cardillo G, Lopergolo M, et al. Chest wall invasion in non-small cell lung carcinoma: a rationale for en bloc resection. *J Thorac Cardiovasc Surg* 2001;**121**:649-56.
51. Burkhart HM, Allen MS, Nichols 3rd FC, et al. Results of en bloc resection for bronchogenic carcinoma with chest wall invasion. *J Thorac Cardiovasc Surg* 2002;**123**:670-5.
52. Roviaro G, Varoli F, Grignani F, et al. Non-small cell lung cancer with chest wall invasion: evolution of surgical treatment and prognosis in the last 3 decades. *Chest* 2003;**123**:1341-7.
53. Doddoli C, D'Journo B, Le Pimpec-Barthes F, et al. Lung cancer invading the chest wall: a plea for en-bloc resection but the need for new treatment strategies. *Ann Thorac Surg* 2005;**80**:2032-40.
54. Voltolini L, Rapicetta C, Luzzi L, et al. Lung cancer with chest wall involvement: predictive factors of long-term survival after surgical resection. *Lung Cancer* 2006;**52**:359-64.
55. Rusch VW, Giroux DJ, Kraut MJ, et al. Induction chemoradiation and surgical resection for superior sulcus non-small-cell lung carcinomas: long-term results of Southwest Oncology Group Trial 9416 (Intergroup Trial 0160). *J Clin Oncol* 2007;**25**:313-8.
56. Kunitoh H, Kato H, Tsuboi M, et al. Phase II trial of preoperative chemoradiotherapy followed by surgical resection in patients with superior sulcus non-small-cell lung cancers: report of Japan Clinical Oncology Group trial 9806. *J Clin Oncol* 2008;**26**:644-9.
57. Jensik RJ, Faber LP, Kittle CF, et al. Survival in patients undergoing tracheal sleeve pneumonectomy for bronchogenic carcinoma. *J Thorac Cardiovasc Surg* 1982;**84**:489-96.
58. Yildizeli B, Fadel E, Mussot S, et al. Morbidity, mortality, and long-term survival after sleeve lobectomy for non-small cell lung cancer. *Eur J Cardiothorac Surg* 2007;**31**:95-102.
59. Riquet M, Lang-Lazdunski L, Le PB, et al. Characteristics and prognosis of resected T3 non-small cell lung cancer. *Ann Thorac Surg* 2002;**73**:253-8.
60. Pitz CC, Brutel de la Riviere A, Elbers HR, et al. Results of resection of T3 non-small cell lung cancer invading the mediastinum or main bronchus. *Ann Thorac Surg* 1996;**62**:1016-20.
61. Yokoi K, Tsuchiya R, Mori T, et al. Results of surgical treatment of lung cancer involving the diaphragm. *J Thorac Cardiovasc Surg* 2000;**120**:799-805.
62. Riquet M, Porte H, Chapelier A, et al. Resection of lung cancer invading the diaphragm. *J Thorac Cardiovasc Surg* 2000;**120**:417-8.
63. Rocco G, Rendina EA, Meroni A, et al. Prognostic factors after surgical treatment of lung cancer invading the diaphragm. *Ann Thorac Surg* 1999;**68**:2065-8.
64. Battafarano RJ, Meyers BF, Guthrie TJ, et al. Surgical resection of multifocal non-small cell lung cancer is associated with prolonged survival. *Ann Thorac Surg* 2002;**74**:988-93:discussion 993-4.
65. Bryant AS, Pereira SJ, Miller DL, et al. Satellite pulmonary nodule in the same lobe (T4N0) should not be staged as IIIB non-small cell lung cancer. *Ann Thorac Surg* 2006;**82**:1808-13:discussion 1813-4.
66. Rao J, Sayeed RA, Tomaszek S, et al. Prognostic factors in resected satellite-nodule T4 non-small cell lung cancer. *Ann Thorac Surg* 2007;**84**:934-8:discussion 939.
67. Port JL, Korst RJ, Lee PC, et al. Surgical resection for multifocal (T4) non-small cell lung cancer: is the T4 designation valid?. *Ann Thorac Surg* 2007;**83**:397-400.
68. Park BJ, Bacchetta M, Bains MS, et al. Surgical management of thoracic malignancies invading the heart or great vessels. *Ann Thorac Surg* 2004;**78**:1024-30.
69. de Perrot M, Fadel E, Mussot S, et al. Resection of locally advanced (T4) non-small cell lung cancer with cardiopulmonary bypass. *Ann Thorac Surg* 2005;**79**:1691-6:discussion 1697.
70. Tsuchiya R, Asamura H, Kondo H, et al. Extended resection of the left atrium, great vessels, or both for lung cancer. *Ann Thorac Surg* 1994;**57**:960-5.
71. Klepetko W, Wisser W, Birsan T, et al. T4 lung tumors with infiltration of the thoracic aorta: is an operation reasonable?. *Ann Thorac Surg* 1999;**67**:340-4.
72. Grunenwald DH. Surgery for advanced stage lung cancer. *Semin Surg Oncol* 2000;**18**:137-42.
73. Spaggiari L, Leo F, Veronesi G, et al. Superior vena cava resection for lung and mediastinal malignancies: a single-center experience with 70 cases. *Ann Thorac Surg* 2007;**83**:223-9:discussion 229-30.
74. Suzuki K, Asamura H, Watanabe S, et al. Combined resection of superior vena cava for lung carcinoma: prognostic significance of patterns of superior vena cava invasion. *Ann Thorac Surg* 2004;**78**:1184-9:discussion 1184-9.
75. Spaggiari L, Magdeleinat P, Kondo H, et al. Results of superior vena cava resection for lung cancer. Analysis of prognostic factors. *Lung Cancer* 2004;**44**:339-46.
76. Shargall Y, de Perrot M, Keshavjee S, et al. 15 years single center experience with surgical resection of the superior vena cava for non-small cell lung cancer. *Lung Cancer* 2004;**45**:357-63.
77. Grillo HC. Development of tracheal surgery: a historical review. Part 1: Techniques of tracheal surgery. *Ann Thorac Surg* 2003;**75**:610-9.
78. Mitchell JD, Mathisen DJ, Wright CD, et al. Resection for bronchogenic carcinoma involving the carina: long-term results and effect of nodal status on outcome. *J Thorac Cardiovasc Surg* 2001;**121**:465-71.
79. Regnard JF, Perrotin C, Giovannetti R, et al. Resection for tumors with carinal involvement: technical aspects, results, and prognostic factors. *Ann Thorac Surg* 2005;**80**:1841-6.

80. de Perrot M, Fadel E, Mercier O, et al. Long-term results after carinal resection for carcinoma: does the benefit warrant the risk?. *J Thorac Cardiovasc Surg* 2006;**131**:81-9.
81. Macchiarini P, Altmayer M, Go T, et al. Technical innovations of carinal resection for nonsmall-cell lung cancer. *Ann Thorac Surg* 1997;**82**:2006:1989-97; discussion.
82. Roviaro G, Vergani C, Maciocco M, et al. Tracheal sleeve pneumonectomy: long-term outcome. *Lung Cancer* 2006;**52**:105-10.
83. Mitchell JD, Mathisen DJ, Wright CD, et al. Clinical experience with carinal resection. *J Thorac Cardiovasc Surg* 1999;**117**:39-52:discussion 52-3.
84. Nagai K, Sohara Y, Tsuchiya R, et al. Prognosis of resected non-small cell lung cancer patients with intrapulmonary metastases. *J Thorac Oncol* 2007;**2**:282-6.
85. Grunenwald DH, Mazel C, Girard P, et al. Radical en bloc resection for lung cancer invading the spine. *J Thorac Cardiovasc Surg* 2002;**123**:271-79.
86. Mazel C, Hoffmann E, Antonietti P, et al. Posterior cervicothoracic instrumentation in spine tumors. *Spine* 2004;**29**:1246-53.
87. Gandhi S, Walsh GL, Komaki R, et al. A multidisciplinary surgical approach to superior sulcus tumors with vertebral invasion. *Ann Thorac Surg* 1999;**68**:1778-84:discussion 1784-5.
88. Fadel E, Missenard G, Chapelier A, et al. En bloc resection of non-small cell lung cancer invading the thoracic inlet and intervertebral foramina. *J Thorac Cardiovasc Surg* 2002;**123**:676-85.
89. Anraku M, Waddell TK, de Perrot M, et al. Induction chemoradiotherapy facilitates radical resection of T4 non-small cell lung cancer invading the spine. *J Thorac Cardiovasc Surg* 2009;**137**:441-7.
90. Pitz CC, Brutel de la Riviere A, van Swieten HA, et al. Results of surgical treatment of T4 non-small cell lung cancer. *Eur J Cardiothorac Surg* 2003;**24**:1013-8.
91. Andre F, Grunenwald D, Pignon JP, et al. Survival of patients with resected N2 non-small-cell lung cancer: evidence for a subclassification and implications. *J Clin Oncol* 2000;**18**:2981-9.
92. Roth JA, Fossella F, Komaki R, et al. A randomized trial comparing perioperative chemotherapy and surgery with surgery alone in resectable stage IIIA non-small-cell lung cancer. *J Natl Cancer Inst* 1994;**86**:673-80.
93. Rosell R, Gomez-Codina J, Camps C, et al. Preresectional chemotherapy in stage IIIA non-small-cell lung cancer: a 7-year assessment of a randomized controlled trial. *Lung Cancer* 1999;**26**:7-14.
94. Depierre A, Milleron B, Moro-Sibilot D, et al. Preoperative chemotherapy followed by surgery compared with primary surgery in resectable stage I (except T1N0), II, and IIIa non-small-cell lung cancer. *J Clin Oncol* 2002;**20**:247-53.
95. Lorent N, De Leyn P, Lievens Y, et al. Long-term survival of surgically staged IIIA-N2 non-small-cell lung cancer treated with surgical combined modality approach: analysis of a 7-year prospective experience. *Ann Oncol* 2004;**15**:1645-53.
96. Garrido P, Gonzalez-Larriba JL, Insa A, et al. Long-term survival associated with complete resection after induction chemotherapy in stage IIIA (N2) and IIIB (T4N0-1) non small-cell lung cancer patients: the Spanish Lung Cancer Group Trial 9901. *J Clin Oncol* 2007;**25**:4736-42.
97. Robinson LA, Ruckdeschel JC, Wagner Jr H, et al. Treatment of non-small cell lung cancer-stage IIIA: ACCP evidence-based clinical practice guidelines. *Chest* 2007;**132**:243S-65S:2nd edition.
98. van Meerbeeck JP, Kramer GW, Van Schil PE, et al. Randomized controlled trial of resection versus radiotherapy after induction chemotherapy in stage IIIA-N2 non-small-cell lung cancer. *J Natl Cancer Inst* 2007;**99**:442-50.
99. Albain KS, Rusch VW, Crowley JJ, et al. Concurrent cisplatin/etoposide plus chest radiotherapy followed by surgery for stages IIIA (N2) and IIIB non-small-cell lung cancer: mature results of Southwest Oncology Group phase II study 8805. *J Clin Oncol* 1995;**13**:1880-92.
100. De Leyn P, Stroobants S, De Wever W, et al. Prospective comparative study of integrated positron emission tomography-computed tomography scan compared with remediastinoscopy in the assessment of residual mediastinal lymph node disease after induction chemotherapy for mediastinoscopy-proven stage IIIA-N2 Non-small-cell lung cancer: a Leuven Lung Cancer Group Study. *J Clin Oncol* 2006;**24**:3333-9.
101. Cerfolio RJ, Bryant AS, Ojha B. Restaging patients with N2 (stage IIIa) non-small cell lung cancer after neoadjuvant chemoradiotherapy: a prospective study. *J Thorac Cardiovasc Surg* 2006;**131**:1229-35.
102. Herth FJ, Annema JT, Eberhardt R, et al. Endobronchial ultrasound with transbronchial needle aspiration for restaging the mediastinum in lung cancer. *J Clin Oncol* 2008;**26**:3346-50.
103. Stamatis G, Fechner S, Hillejan L, et al. Repeat mediastinoscopy as a restaging procedure. *Pneumologie* 2005;**59**:862-6.
104. Marra A, Hillejan L, Fechner S, et al. Remediastinoscopy in restaging of lung cancer after induction therapy. *J Thorac Cardiovasc Surg* 2008;**135**:843-9.
105. Bueno R, Richards WG, Swanson SJ, et al. Nodal stage after induction therapy for stage IIIA lung cancer determines patient survival. *Ann Thorac Surg* 2000;**70**:1826-31.
106. Dooms C, Verbeken E, Stroobants S, et al. Prognostic stratification of stage IIIA-N2 non-small-cell lung cancer after induction chemotherapy: a model based on the combination of morphometric-pathologic response in mediastinal nodes and primary tumor response on serial 18-fluoro-2-deoxy-glucose positron emission tomography. *J Clin Oncol* 2008;**26**:1128-34.
107. Farray D, Mirkovic N, Albain KS. Multimodality therapy for stage III non-small-cell lung cancer. *J Clin Oncol* 2005;**23**:3257-69.
108. Cerfolio RJ, Bryant AS. Survival of patients with unsuspected N2 (stage IIIA) nonsmall-cell lung cancer. *Ann Thorac Surg* 2008;**86**:362-6:discussion 366-7.
109. Pisters KM, Le Chevalier T. Adjuvant chemotherapy in completely resected non-small-cell lung cancer. *J Clin Oncol* 2005;**23**:3270-8.
110. Burdett S, Stewart L. Postoperative radiotherapy in non-small-cell lung cancer: update of an individual patient data meta-analysis. *Lung Cancer* 2005;**47**:81-3.
111. Lally BE, Zelterman D, Colasanto JM, et al. Postoperative radiotherapy for stage II or III non-small-cell lung cancer using the surveillance, epidemiology, and end results database. *J Clin Oncol* 2006;**24**:2998-3006.
112. Postmus PE, Brambilla E, Chansky K, et al. The IASLC Lung Cancer Staging Project: proposals for revision of the M descriptors in the forthcoming (seventh) edition of the TNM classification of lung cancer. *J Thorac Oncol* 2007;**2**:686-93.
113. Fletcher JW, Kymes SM, Gould M, et al. A comparison of the diagnostic accuracy of 18F-FDG PET and CT in the characterization of solitary pulmonary nodules. *J Nucl Med* 2008;**49**:179-85.
114. Reed CE, Harpole DH, Posther KE, et al. Results of the American College of Surgeons Oncology Group Z0050 trial: the utility of positron emission tomography in staging potentially operable non-small-cell lung cancer. *J Thorac Cardiovasc Surg* 2003;**126**:1943-51.
115. Ichinose Y, Tsuchiya R, Koike T, et al. Prognosis of resected non-small cell lung cancer patients with carcinomatous pleuritis of minimal disease. *Lung Cancer* 2001;**32**:55-60.
116. Yokoi K, Matsuguma H, Anraku M. Extrapleural pneumonectomy for lung cancer with carcinomatous pleuritis. *J Thorac Cardiovasc Surg* 2002;**123**:184-5.
117. Ettinghausen SE, Burt ME. Prospective evaluation of unilateral adrenal masses in patients with operable non-small-cell lung cancer. *J Clin Oncol* 1991;**9**:1462-6.
118. Mercier O, Fadel E, de Perrot M, et al. Surgical treatment of solitary adrenal metastasis from non-small cell lung cancer. *J Thorac Cardiovasc Surg* 2005;**130**:136-40.
119. Pfannschmidt J, Schlolaut B, Muley T, et al. Adrenalectomy for solitary adrenal metastases from non-small cell lung cancer. *Lung Cancer* 2005;**49**:203-7.
120. Tanvetyanon T, Robinson LA, Schell MJ, et al. Outcomes of adrenalectomy for isolated synchronous versus metachronous adrenal metastases in non-small-cell lung cancer: a systematic review and pooled analysis. *J Clin Oncol* 2008;**26**:1142-7.
121. Kumar R, Xiu Y, Yu JQ, et al. 18F-FDG PET in evaluation of adrenal lesions in patients with lung cancer. *J Nucl Med* 2004;**45**:2058-62.
122. Hu C, Chang EL, Hassenbusch 3rd SJ, et al. Non small cell lung cancer presenting with synchronous solitary brain metastasis. *Cancer* 2006;**106**:1998-2004.
123. Billing PS, Miller DL, Allen MS, et al. Surgical treatment of primary lung cancer with synchronous brain metastases. *J Thorac Cardiovasc Surg* 2001;**122**:548-53.
124. Rodrigus P, de Brouwer P, Raaymakers E. Brain metastases and non-small cell lung cancer. Prognostic factors and correlation with survival after irradiation. *Lung Cancer* 2001;**32**:129-36.
125. Little AG, Rusch VW, Bonner JA, et al. Patterns of surgical care of lung cancer patients. *Ann Thorac Surg* 2005;**80**:2056:2051-6; discussion.
126. Keller SM, Adak S, Wagner H, et al. Mediastinal lymph node dissection improves survival in patients with stages II and IIIa non-small cell lung cancer. Eastern Cooperative Oncology Group. *Ann Thorac Surg* 2000;**70**:358-65:discussion 365-6.
127. Lardinois D, Suter H, Hakki H, et al. Morbidity, survival, and site of recurrence after mediastinal lymph-node dissection versus systematic sampling after complete resection for non-small cell lung cancer. *Ann Thorac Surg* 2005;**80**:268-74:discussion 274-5.
128. Allen MS, Darling GE, Pechet TT, et al. Morbidity and mortality of major pulmonary resections in patients with early-stage lung cancer: initial results of the randomized, prospective ACOSOG Z0030 trial. *Ann Thorac Surg* 2006;**81**:1013-9:discussion 1019-20.
129. Izbicki JR, Passlick B, Karg O, et al. Impact of radical systematic mediastinal lymphadenectomy on tumor staging in lung cancer. *Ann Thorac Surg* 1995;**59**:209-14.
130. Wu Y, Huang ZF, Wang SY, et al. A randomized trial of systematic nodal dissection in resectable non-small cell lung cancer. *Lung Cancer* 2002;**36**:1-6.

131. Sugi K, Nawata K, Fujita N, et al. Systematic lymph node dissection for clinically diagnosed peripheral non-small-cell lung cancer less than 2 cm in diameter. *World J Surg* 1998;**22**:290-4:discussion 294-5.
132. Massard G, Ducrocq X, Kochetkova EA, et al. Sampling or node dissection for intraoperative staging of lung cancer: a multicentric cross-sectional study. *Eur J Cardiothorac Surg* 2006;**30**:164-7.
133. Osaki T, Oyama T, Gu CD, et al. Prognostic impact of micrometastatic tumor cells in the lymph nodes and bone marrow of patients with completely resected stage I non-small-cell lung cancer. *J Clin Oncol* 2002;**20**:2930-6.
134. Izbicki JR, Passlick B, Pantel K, et al. Effectiveness of radical systematic mediastinal lymphadenectomy in patients with resectable non-small cell lung cancer: results of a prospective randomized trial. *Ann Surg* 1998;**227**:138-44.
135. Jang HJ, Lee KS, Kwon OJ, et al. Bronchioloalveolar carcinoma: focal area of ground-glass attenuation at thin-section CT as an early sign. *Radiology* 1996;**199**:485-8.
136. Read WL, Page NC, Tierney RM, et al. The epidemiology of bronchioloalveolar carcinoma over the past two decades: analysis of the SEER database. *Lung Cancer* 2004;**45**:137-42.
137. Travis WD, Colby TV, Corrin B, et al. *Histological typing of lung and pleural tumors.* In: Wechsler AS, editor. World Health Organization Histologic Typing of Lung Tumors. 3rd Ed Berlin: Springer; 1999. p. 25-47.
138. Terasaki H, Niki T, Matsuno Y, et al. Lung adenocarcinoma with mixed bronchioloalveolar and invasive components: clinicopathological features, subclassification by extent of invasive foci, and immunohistochemical characterization. *Am J Surg Pathol* 2003;**27**:937-51.
139. Holst VA, Finkelstein S, Yousem SA. Bronchioloalveolar adenocarcinoma of lung: monoclonal origin for multifocal disease. *Am J Surg Pathol* 1998;**22**:1343-50.
140. Matsuguma H, Yokoi K, Anraku M, et al. Proportion of ground-glass opacity on high-resolution computed tomography in clinical T1 N0 M0 adenocarcinoma of the lung: a predictor of lymph node metastasis. *J Thorac Cardiovasc Surg* 2002;**124**:278-84.
141. Okada M, Nishio W, Sakamoto T, et al. Correlation between computed tomographic findings, bronchioloalveolar carcinoma component, and biologic behavior of small-sized lung adenocarcinomas. *J Thorac Cardiovasc Surg* 2004;**127**:857-61.
142. Sakurai H, Maeshima A, Watanabe S, et al. Grade of stromal invasion in small adenocarcinoma of the lung: histopathological minimal invasion and prognosis. *Am J Surg Pathol* 2004;**28**:198-206.
143. Roberts PF, Straznicka M, Lara PN, et al. Resection of multifocal non-small cell lung cancer when the bronchioloalveolar subtype is involved. *J Thorac Cardiovasc Surg* 2003;**126**:1597-602.
144. Nakata M, Sawada S, Yamashita M, et al. Surgical treatments for multiple primary adenocarcinoma of the lung. *Ann Thorac Surg* 2004;**78**:1194-9.
145. Mun M, Kohno T. Efficacy of thoracoscopic resection for multifocal bronchioloalveolar carcinoma showing pure ground-glass opacities of 20 mm or less in diameter. *J Thorac Cardiovasc Surg* 2007;**134**:877-82.
146. Jackman DM, Johnson BE. Small-cell lung cancer. *Lancet* 2005;**366**:1385-96.
147. Fox W, Scadding JG. Medical Research Council comparative trial of surgery and radiotherapy for primary treatment of small-celled or oat-celled carcinoma of bronchus. Ten-year follow-up. *Lancet* 1973;**2**:63-5.
148. Shields TW, Higgins Jr GA, Matthews MJ, et al. Surgical resection in the management of small cell carcinoma of the lung. *J Thorac Cardiovasc Surg* 1982;**84**:481-8.
149. Shepherd FA, Ginsberg RJ, Evans WK, et al. Reduction in local recurrence and improved survival in surgically treated patients with small cell lung cancer. *J Thorac Cardiovasc Surg* 1983;**86**:498-506.
150. Meyer JA, Comis RL, Ginsberg SJ, et al. The prospect of disease control by surgery combined with chemotherapy in stage I and stage II small cell carcinoma of the lung. *Ann Thorac Surg* 1983;**36**:37-41.
151. Friess GG, McCracken JD, Troxell ML, et al. Effect of initial resection of small-cell carcinoma of the lung: a review of Southwest Oncology Group Study 7628. *J Clin Oncol* 1985;**3**:964-8.
152. Shepherd FA, Evans WK, Feld R, et al. Adjuvant chemotherapy following surgical resection for small-cell carcinoma of the lung. *J Clin Oncol* 1988;**6**:832-8.
153. Lad T, Piantadosi S, Thomas P, et al. A prospective randomized trial to determine the benefit of surgical resection of residual disease following response of small cell lung cancer to combination chemotherapy. *Chest* 1994;**106**:320S-.
154. Smythe WR, Estrera AL, Swisher SG, et al. Surgical resection of non-small cell carcinoma after treatment for small cell carcinoma. *Ann Thorac Surg* 2001;**71**:962-6.
155. Turrisi 3rd AT, Kim K, Blum R, et al. Twice-daily compared with once-daily thoracic radiotherapy in limited small-cell lung cancer treated concurrently with cisplatin and etoposide. *N Engl J Med* 1999;**340**:265-71.
156. Elliott JA, Osterlind K, Hirsch FR, et al. Metastatic patterns in small-cell lung cancer: correlation of autopsy findings with clinical parameters in 537 patients. *J Clin Oncol* 1987;**5**:246-54.
157. Eberhardt W, Stamatis G, Stuschke M, et al. Prognostically orientated multimodality treatment including surgery for selected patients of small-cell lung cancer patients stages IB to IIIB: long-term results of a phase II trial. *Br J Cancer* 1999;**81**:1206-12.
158. Tsuchiya R, Suzuki K, Ichinose Y, et al. Phase II trial of postoperative adjuvant cisplatin and etoposide in patients with completely resected stage I-IIIa small cell lung cancer: the Japan Clinical Oncology Lung Cancer Study Group Trial (JCOG9101). *J Thorac Cardiovasc Surg* 2005;**129**:977-83.
159. Asamura H, Kameya T, Matsuno Y, et al. Neuroendocrine neoplasms of the lung: a prognostic spectrum. *J Clin Oncol* 2006;**24**:70-6.
160. Shepherd FA, Ginsberg RJ, Feld R, et al. Surgical treatment for limited small-cell lung cancer. The University of Toronto Lung Oncology Group experience. *J Thorac Cardiovasc Surg* 1991;**101**:385-93.
161. Shepherd FA, Ginsberg R, Patterson GA, et al. Is there ever a role for salvage operations in limited small-cell lung cancer? *J Thorac Cardiovasc Surg* 1991;**101**:196-200.
162. Eberhardt W, Korfee S. New approaches for small-cell lung cancer: local treatments. *Cancer Control* 2003;**10**:289-96.

CHAPTER 18

Lung Cancer: Minimally Invasive Approaches

Mark Onaitis and Thomas A. D'Amico

Definition	Right Upper Lobectomy	Postoperative Pulmonary Function
History	Right Middle Lobectomy	Systemic Inflammatory Effects
Indications	Lower Lobectomy (Right or Left)	Oncologic Effectiveness
Contraindications	Segmentectomy	Cost-Effectiveness
Strategy for Thoracoscopic Lobectomy	Wedge Resection	Overall Complications
Technical Considerations	Results	Summary
Left Upper Lobectomy	Postoperative Pain	

The surgical approach in the management of patients with lung cancer continues to evolve and improve. Conventional surgical approaches (including standard posterolateral thoracotomy, muscle-sparing thoracotomy, trans-sternal thoracotomy, and median sternotomy) remain viable options for the majority of patients with resectable lung cancer. However, minimally invasive procedures have been used in selected patients with early-stage lung cancer to minimize operative morbidity without sacrificing oncologic efficacy.

DEFINITION

Minimally invasive procedures, using operative telescopes and video technology, are referred to synonymously as thoracoscopic procedures or video-assisted thoracic surgery (VATS). For clarity, the terms *VATS* and *thoracoscopic* refer to totally thoracoscopic approaches, where visualization depends on video monitors, and rib spreading is avoided. A hybrid procedure, which employs rib spreading and direct visualization in addition to thoracoscopy, may be referred to as video-assisted thoracotomy.

Thoracoscopy has been widely used diagnostically in the management of patients with lung cancer; thoracoscopic wedge resection to confirm malignancy prior to thoracotomy for anatomic resection is commonly performed. In addition, thoracoscopic therapeutic procedures, including pleurodesis for malignant pleural effusion and pericardial window for pericardial effusions, are also frequently performed. The application of thoracoscopic anatomic resections is no longer new and is increasingly used internationally.

Thoracoscopic lobectomy is defined as the anatomic resection of an entire lobe of the lung, using a videoscope and an access incision, without the use of a mechanical retractor and without rib spreading.[1-4] The anatomic resection includes individual dissection and stapling of the involved pulmonary vein, pulmonary artery, and bronchus and appropriate management of the mediastinal lymph nodes, as would be performed with thoracotomy. In selected patients, thoracoscopic anatomic segmentectomy may be performed, adhering to the same oncologic principles that guide resection at thoracotomy.

Some surgeons have advocated simultaneous stapling of hilar structures with video assistance and the avoidance of rib spreading.[5,6] Such an approach has been termed video-assisted simultaneously stapled lobectomy. Although this technique has been used successfully in selected patients, the reference to thoracoscopic lobectomy is limited to anatomic resection with individual vessel ligation. VATS wedge resection describes nonanatomic thoracoscopic resection of a lesion, which is considered useful for diagnostic procedures.

To be considered a viable alternative to conventional lobectomy, thoracoscopic lobectomy must be applied with the same oncologic principles: individual vessel ligation, complete anatomic resection with negative margins, complete hilar lymph node dissection, and appropriate management of the mediastinal lymph nodes. Theoretical advantages to minimally invasive resection include reduced surgical trauma, decreased postoperative pain, shorter chest tube duration, shorter length of stay, preserved pulmonary function, and superior cosmetic result when compared with lobectomy via open thoracotomy.[7-9]

HISTORY

The history of minimally invasive thoracic surgery began in 1910 when Jacobeus used a cystoscope to lyse adhesions in order to collapse the lung to treat tuberculosis.[10] This technique was widely applied in the early part of the century but was largely abandoned after streptomycin was introduced in 1945. However, with the emergence of laparoscopic cholecystectomy, minimally invasive approaches were applied more widely. The first descriptions of VATS to perform anatomic lobectomy were published in 1993 by Kirby and Rice[1] and Walker and colleagues.[2] The first randomized trial of VATS lobectomy versus the conventional open approach was presented in 1994 and demonstrated no significant benefits for VATS.[11] With more widespread application of technology and refinements in technique, other groups have published series of VATS lobectomy (Table 18-1).

Table 18-1
Recent Series of Thoracoscopic Lobectomy

Author (ref)	N	Conversion rate(%)	Method	LN dissection	Mortality (%)	Stage I survival (actuarial/actual)(%)
Lewis et al. (6)	200	0	SSL	Dissection	0	92 (3 yr) (actuarial)
Solaini et al. (9)	125	10.4	IHD	Sampling	0	90 (3 yr) (actuarial)
Brown (59)	105	7.6	IHD	Sampling	0	NA
Kaseda et al. (25)	128	11.7	IHD	Dissection	0.8	94 (4 yr) (actuarial)
Rovairo et al. (60)	171	19.9	IHD	Sampling	0	91 (1 yr) (actuarial)
Walker (61)	150	11.8	IHD	Sampling	2	81 (5 yr)
Yim et al. (12)	214	0	IHD	Sampling	0.5	NA
McKenna et al. (14)	1100	2.5	IHD	Sampling/Dissection	0.8	80 (5 yr) (actuarial)
Onaitis et al. (15)	500	1.6	IHD	Dissection	1.0	80 (5 yr) (actuarial)
Swanson et al. (CALGB) (18)	127	13.5	IHD	Sampling/Dissection	2.7	78 (3 yr) (actuarial)
Nicastri et al. (54)	153	9.2	IHD	Dissection	0.7	75 (3 yr) (actuarial)
Sawada et al. (26)	198	2.5	IHD	Dissection	0	89 (5 yr) (actual)

IHD, individual hilar dissection; LN, lymph node; NA, not assessed; SSL, simultaneously stapled lobectomy.

INDICATIONS

In general, the indications for thoracoscopic lobectomy are similar to those for lobectomy using the open approach.[12-15] Thus, the procedure is applied to patients with known or suspected lung cancer (clinical stage I) if the disease appears amenable to complete resection by lobectomy. Preoperative staging and patient selection for thoracoscopic lobectomy should be conducted as for conventional thoracotomy.[16]

Tumor size may preclude the option of thoracoscopic lobectomy in some patients, as some large specimens may not be amenable to removal without rib spreading; however, no absolute size criteria are used. Although it is controversial, some have also argued that the thoracoscopic approach may allow recruitment and resection of some patients considered medically inoperable, who could not undergo conventional thoracotomy.[17,18] A recent report demonstrates improved tolerance of thoracoscopic lobectomy as compared with thoracotomy lobectomy in patients older than 70.[19] The minimal physiologic requirements for resection have not been agreed on; however, the selection of patients for thoracoscopic lobectomy must take into account that conversion to thoracotomy may be necessary.

CONTRAINDICATIONS

Absolute contraindications to thoracoscopic lobectomy include the inability to achieve complete resection with lobectomy, T3 (chest wall) or T4 tumors, active N2 or N3 disease, and inability to achieve single-lung ventilation.[14,15,18] Relative contraindications include tumors visualized in the lobar orifice at bronchoscopy (although successful thoracoscopic sleeve resection has been reported[20]), the presence of complex, calcified benign hilar lymphadenopathy that would complicate vascular dissection, and prior thoracic irradiation. Prior thoracic surgery; T3 tumors that involve the pericardium, mediastinal pleura, or diaphragm; incomplete or absent fissures; and benign noncalcified mediastinal adenopathy should not be considered contraindications.[15,17,18,21] Increasing experience has allowed successful thoracoscopic lobectomy after induction therapy, including for patients with stage IIIA (N2) disease.[22] Finally, chest wall involvement would obviate thoracoscopic resection for most patients, but successful en bloc resection via VATS has been reported.[23]

STRATEGY FOR THORACOSCOPIC LOBECTOMY

After bronchoscopy and mediastinoscopy (when indicated), single-lung anesthesia is established using a dual-lumen endotracheal tube or bronchial blocker. The patient is positioned in a full lateral decubitus position with slight flexion of the table at the level of the hip, which provides splaying of the ribs to improve thoracoscopic access and exposure. Care must be taken to secure and pad the patient so that the risk of neurologic injury is minimized. Once the patient is positioned, the anesthesiologist should reconfirm the desired position of the endotracheal tube. Before sterile preparation and draping, the chest is marked for the placement of thoracoscopic incisions.

Port placement is a matter of surgeon preference. Most surgeons use three or four incisions, although lobectomy can usually be accomplished using only two incisions.[15] Using this strategy, the first incision, a 10-mm port access used predominantly for the thoracoscope, is placed in the seventh or eighth intercostal space in the midaxillary line. The location of this incision is chosen so that it does not compete with the anterior incision, yet it still provides anterior and superior visualization of the hilum. A port is used for placement of the telescope, but ports are not used for the other incisions. Before making the second incision, evidence that the patient is unresectable, such as parietal pleural involvement, should be sought.

The second incision, an anterior access incision (4.5 to 6.0 cm) for dissection and specimen retrieval, is placed in the fifth or sixth intercostal space, just inferior to the breast. The location of this incision, where the intercostal spaces are the widest, is chosen to provide access for hilar dissection and is usually not dependent on whether the planned procedure is an upper or lower lobectomy. Additional incisions may be used, either in the axilla or posteriorly, to improve visualization or to provide retraction.

Instrumentation for thoracoscopic lobectomy is critical to successful completion of the procedure. The thoracoscope should be a 30-degree angled scope to optimize the ability to achieve panoramic visualization during dissection and to minimize competition with the operative instruments. Alternatively, a 45-degree angled scope or a flexible scope may be used. A spectrum of surgical instruments may be used for dissection, including conventional instruments and dedicated thoracoscopic or laparoscopic instruments. It is especially beneficial to use curved instruments for retraction during dissection, as they minimize the tendency for instruments to compete or collide with each other. Thoracoscopic (linear) mechanical staplers, such as the EndoGIA (Covidien, Norwalk, CT), are employed for control of the vessels (2.0- or 2.5-mm staples), bronchus (3.5- or 4.8-mm staples), and fissure.

After placing the second incision, the surgeon performs thoracoscopic exploration, which includes confirming the location of the tumor, excluding the presence of pleural metastases, and dividing the pulmonary ligament. If a malignant diagnosis has not been achieved preoperatively, thoracoscopic wedge resection is performed using an automatic stapling device, and the specimen is removed in a protective bag. After frozen section confirms a malignant diagnosis, thoracoscopic lobectomy may be completed. Mediastinal lymph node dissection may be performed at this point or may be deferred until the lobectomy is completed.

The approach to the staging of mediastinal lymph nodes is controversial. Many advocate systematic sampling of mediastinal lymph nodes because of concerns about the adequacy and safety of formal dissection.[24] Others accomplish mediastinal lymph node dissection by complete resection of the mediastinal nodes thoracoscopically, including levels 2, 4, 7, 8, and 9 on the right and levels 5, 6, 7, 8, and 9 on the left.[15,25,26] A minimum of three mediastinal stations should be assessed.[16]

Hilar dissection is carried out through the access incision, to achieve visualization and mobilization of the hilar structures. For any anatomic thoracoscopic lobectomy, hilar dissection is begun with mobilization of the pulmonary vein. For upper lobectomy, the lung is reflected posteriorly and inferiorly to facilitate dissection. For lower lobectomy, the lung is retracted superiorly. Moving the thoracoscope to the anterior incision may improve visualization of the superior hilum and may facilitate placement of the linear stapler for

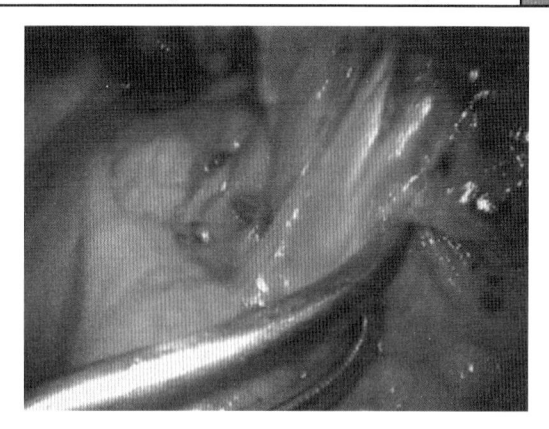

Figure 18–1
Left superior pulmonary vein, encircled with a curved clamp. (See color version in the online edition through Expert Consult.)

upper lobectomy, if it is introduced through the midaxillary port.

The risk of intraoperative hemorrhage is minimized with careful hilar dissection, which is facilitated with the visual clarity and magnification available with the video thoracoscope. Unexpected bleeding from a major branch of the pulmonary artery or pulmonary vein may occur, however. In most cases, the source of the bleeding is easily identifiable and tamponade is possible, allowing conversion to thoracotomy. To minimize the risk of vascular injury, surgeons have employed a variety of techniques to isolate the pulmonary arterial and venous branches, including ligatures to retract the vessels, and catheters to guide the stapling devices. These techniques may be helpful in difficult cases but are not required for the majority of patients.

All lobectomy specimens are removed using a protective specimen bag, to prevent implantation of tumor cells in the incision. The lobectomy specimen and hilum are each inspected to ascertain that anatomic lobectomy has been performed. After retrieval, the hemithorax is irrigated with warm saline and the bronchial stump is inspected. If an air leak is encountered, repeat stapling or endoscopic suturing may be performed.[27]

TECHNICAL CONSIDERATIONS

Left Upper Lobectomy

With the thoracoscope in the midaxillary incision, the horizontal and oblique fissures are inspected and the presence of the tumor in the left upper lobe is confirmed. The lung is retracted posteriorly, and the superior pulmonary vein is identified and mobilized. The left superior pulmonary vein is then encircled using a curved clamp; dissection behind the superior pulmonary vein allows identification of the pulmonary artery (Fig. 18-1). The stapling device is then applied (Fig. 18-2) and the superior pulmonary vein is divided, exposing the pulmonary artery. The pulmonary artery is mobilized, focusing on the apical and anterior branches (Fig. 18-3), which may then be stapled and divided. The left upper lobe bronchus is now visualized and may be stapled and divided (Fig. 18-4). Subsequently, the branches of the posterior and lingular arteries are stapled (Fig. 18-5). Finally, the fissures are completed and the specimen is retrieved.

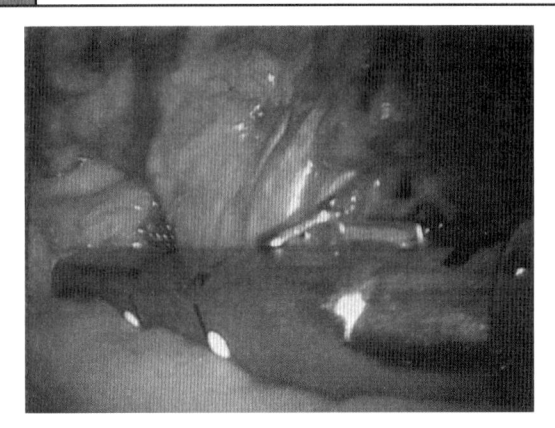

Figure 18–2
Left superior pulmonary vein, just prior to division with stapler. (See color version in the online edition through Expert Consult.)

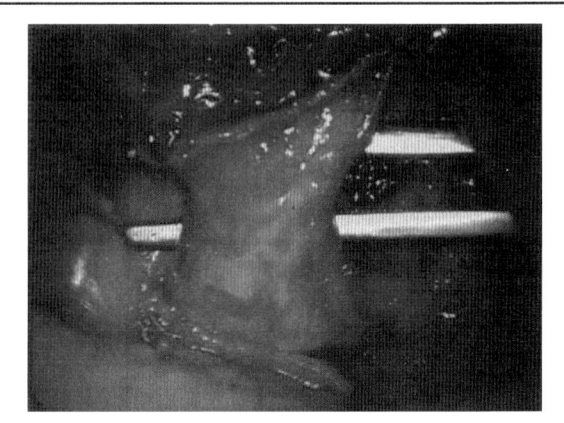

Figure 18–4
Left upper lobe bronchus, encircled with a curved clamp. (See color version in the online edition through Expert Consult.)

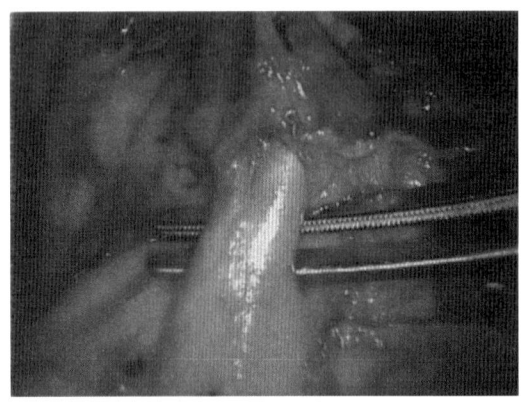

Figure 18–3
Apical anterior branches of the left pulmonary artery. (See color version in the online edition through Expert Consult.)

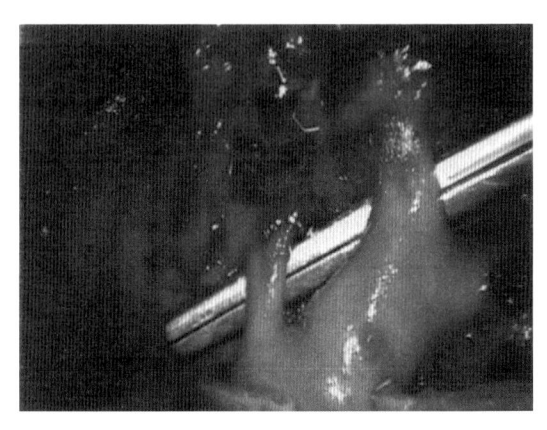

Figure 18–5
Posterior and lingular branches of the left pulmonary artery. (See color version in the online edition through Expert Consult.)

Right Upper Lobectomy

Right upper lobectomy is slightly more difficult than left upper lobectomy because both the horizontal and oblique fissures must be managed. With the thoracoscope in the midaxillary incision, the horizontal and oblique fissures are inspected and the presence of the tumor in the right upper lobe is confirmed. The right lung is retracted posteriorly, and the superior pulmonary vein is identified and mobilized, to identify the division between the middle lobe and upper lobe venous branches. The upper lobe branches are encircled using a curved clamp; dissection behind the superior pulmonary vein allows identification of the pulmonary artery. The stapling device is then applied and the vein is divided, exposing the pulmonary artery. The pulmonary artery is mobilized, and the apical anterior trunk (truncus anterior) may then be stapled and divided. The right bronchus is now exposed, and the upper lobe bronchus may be stapled and divided. Subsequently, the posterior ascending arterial branch is stapled. Finally, the fissures are completed and the specimen is retrieved.

Right Middle Lobectomy

With the thoracoscope in the midaxillary incision, the horizontal and oblique fissures are inspected and the presence of the tumor in the middle lobe is confirmed. The lung is retracted posteriorly, and the superior pulmonary vein is identified and mobilized, to identify the division between the middle lobe and upper lobe venous branches. The middle lobe vein is encircled and stapled, exposing the middle lobe bronchus and artery. Retraction of the middle lobe laterally and posteriorly optimizes exposure of the bronchus. At this point, the bronchus is encircled and stapled, further exposing the middle lobe artery. The middle lobe artery is then stapled and divided as well, allowing completion of the fissures.

Lower Lobectomy (Right or Left)

The strategy for lower lobectomy is similar on the right and left sides. With the thoracoscope in the midaxillary incision, the presence of the tumor in the lower lobe is confirmed. The lung is retracted anteriorly, and the pleura is incised between the lung and the esophagus. The lung is then retracted laterally and superiorly to incise the pleura overlying the inferior pulmonary vein, which can then be encircled and stapled after ascertaining that the superior segment branch is included in the dissection. Further superior retraction of the lower lobe improves exposure of the bronchus, at the bifurcation of the lower lobe bronchus and the middle lobe bronchus (right lung) or lingular bronchus (left lung). The lower lobe bronchus is then encircled and stapled, exposing the lower lobe arterial trunk, which is then stapled and divided. Finally, the fissure is completed and the specimen retrieved.

Segmentectomy

Thoracoscopic segmentectomy is an option for anatomic resection in patients with poor lung function or synchronous primary tumors. In addition, small, peripheral primary tumors (particularly with bronchoalveolar histology) may be candidates. These resections may be successfully completed thoracoscopically.[28,29]

Wedge Resection

Lobectomy is considered the procedure of choice in most patients with early stage lung cancer, as it is associated with a lower rate of local recurrence and higher overall survival compared with wedge resection.[30] However, in patients with small peripheral tumors who will not tolerate anatomic resection, wedge resection followed by radiotherapy is an option.[31-33] VATS wedge resection of small (<3 cm) peripheral nodules is usually carried out using endoscopic stapling devices to transect lung parenchyma. Larger and more centrally located nodules are more challenging. A neodymium:yttrium-aluminum-garnet (Nd:YAG) laser[34] and a monopolar floating ball device[27] are two methods that have been reported to achieve precise tumor resection without unnecessary sacrifice of lung parenchyma.

RESULTS

The safety and efficacy of thoracoscopic lobectomy for patients with early-stage lung cancer have been established. Although there are no prospective, randomized series that compare thoracoscopic lobectomy with conventional approaches, a sufficient number of series have been published, both single-institution and multi-institution experiences, to conclude that thoracoscopic lobectomy is a reasonable strategy for patients with clinical stage I lung cancer.

As Figure 18-1 demonstrates, excellent 5-year survival is possible with minimally invasive approaches. The first study detailing actual, rather than actuarial, 5-year survival in thoracoscopic lobectomy patients reveals an excellent 89% rate.[26] This single-institution figure will have to be repeated at other centers. The Cancer and Leukemia Group B (CALGB) reported on the results of a prospective, multi-institutional registry series of 127 patients who underwent thoracoscopic lobectomy.[18] In this series, the mortality was 2.7%, the operative time was 130 min, and the median length of stay was 3 days. Numerous other series have been published and are summarized in Table 18-1. In summary, thoracoscopic lobectomy has been demonstrated to be equivalent in terms of safety and oncologic efficacy, as measured by complete resection rate, operative time, extent of lymph node dissection, operative mortality, and short-term survival, when compared with published results for thoracotomy and lobectomy.[35]

Morbidity and mortality associated with thoracoscopic resection are comparable with or lower than expected for conventional thoracotomy and resection (see Table 18-1). The mortality reported in several recent series ranges from 0% to 4%. Conversion rates range from 0% to 20% and appear to decrease with experience over time. Persistent air leak, defined as lasting greater than 7 days, is the most common major complication but may be expected to decrease with experience and the use of endoscopic suturing.[27,36] Wound recurrence due to tumor implantation was first described in 1996,[37] but its risk can be minimized by use of specimen bags and copious irrigation. Perhaps the most feared major complication is hemorrhage into a closed chest, but careful hilar dissection has led to only rare cases.

Postoperative Pain

Post-thoracotomy pain is related to rib spreading, which is obviated by the totally thoracoscopic approach. Many groups have analyzed acute pain after VATS. Although Kirby's randomized trial of VATS versus muscle-sparing lobectomy revealed no difference in postoperative pain, many of the VATS patients had undergone rib spreading during the operation.[11] This study also did not differentiate between acute and more chronic pain. Nomori and colleagues compared a group of age- and sex-matched patients who underwent thoracoscopic lobectomy ($n = 33$) or limited anterior thoracotomy ($n = 33$).[38] The patients who underwent thoracoscopic lobectomy experienced less pain between postoperative day (POD) 1 and POD 7 ($P < .05$-$.001$) and had lower analgesic requirements up to POD 7 ($P < .001$).

Demmy and colleagues reported on their results in a series of patients who underwent either thoracoscopic lobectomy or conventional thoracotomy.[17] In this series, the percentage of patients reporting severe pain was 6% after thoracoscopic lobectomy and 65% after thoracotomy. Moreover, the percentage of patients reporting minimal or no pain was 63% after thoracoscopic lobectomy and 6% after thoracotomy. Other studies analyzing acute pain have concluded that VATS results in either less pain[8,39-41] or a lower analgesia requirement[42,43] in the early postoperative period.

Chronic discomfort is also an important issue in postoperative recovery. Although more difficult to measure than acute pain, chronic pain and shoulder dysfunction have been studied. Stammberger and colleagues, in addressing long-term quality of life following VATS, reported that 53% of 173 patients undergoing VATS had insignificant pain 2 weeks after the operation. At 6 months, 75% had no complaints, and only 4% had mild or moderate discomfort at 2 years.[44] Landreneau's group questioned patients about shoulder dysfunction and concluded that although dysfunction is the same between VATS and conventional groups at 3 weeks, it lasted significantly longer in the conventional group.[39] This group's next examination of these issues revealed a significantly lower proportion of patients experiencing pain and shoulder dysfunction within the first year after operation.[45]

Postoperative Pulmonary Function

Many have theorized that smaller incisions and absence of rib spreading may improve lung function in the postoperative period, and several studies have reported pulmonary function test (PFT) data after thoracoscopic resection. Two studies examined postoperative PaO_2 after both VATS and muscle-sparing thoracotomy and found that VATS patients had better oxygenation during the first postoperative week.[41,46] Others have revealed improvements in early postoperative forced expiratory volume in 1 second (FEV_1) and forced vital capacity, in the first weeks and months after VATS.[8,39,47] These differences probably disappear over time, because Nakata and coworkers revealed no PFT differences at follow-up of longer than 1 year.[46]

Systemic Inflammatory Effects

Minimally invasive procedures appear to produce less of a systemic insult than more conventional, invasive procedures.[7,8,48-50] Many groups have studied inflammatory mediators after VATS and open resection and have found lower levels of C-reactive protein and interleukins (IL) in those having undergone VATS.[7,8,48] Yim and colleagues analyzed the cytokine responses in a series of 36 matched patients who underwent thoracoscopic lobectomy or conventional thoracotomy and lobectomy.[7] Analgesic requirement was significantly lower in the patients who underwent VATS lobectomy. In addition, the levels of IL-6 and IL-8 were lower in the VATS group than in the group that underwent thoracotomy. A recent study from the same group compared cytokine levels after thoracoscopic lobectomy ($n = 20$) and thoracotomy lobectomy ($n = 22$) and demonstrated higher circulating levels of insulin-like growth factor binding protein 3 (IGFBP-3) and lower circulating levels of matrix metalloproteinase-9 (MMP-9) and tissue inhibitor of metalloproteinase-1 (TIMP-1) in the thoracoscopy group.[50] Leaver and coworkers examined immunosuppression due to systemic effects of surgery and found higher numbers of CD4 lymphocytes and natural killer cells and less suppression of lymphocyte oxidation in the VATS group.[48] Whether these trends toward more effective immune function after VATS resection lead to faster recovery or toward better oncologic outcomes will be important endpoints of future studies.

Oncologic Effectiveness

The ultimate acceptance of thoracoscopic lobectomy will be dependent on its oncologic effectiveness as compared with conventional lobectomy. Although there has been no prospective, randomized trial with sufficient power to assess differences between the operations, the studies performed are sufficient for limited analysis. First, no differences were seen in number of lymph nodes obtained either by dissection or sampling between conventional and VATS lobectomy.[17,43,51] Second, data from existing series reveal survival rates for patients with stage I disease that were at least as good as those published in the literature for conventional thoracotomy (see Table 18-1). Some groups have documented improved survival when VATS was used.[6,25,27] Reasons for the possible differences are unclear, but it has been postulated that preservation of immune function and less systemic release of inflammatory cytokines may contribute.[52] Final resolution of these issues awaits a rigorously controlled, prospective, randomized trial.

In addition, the benefit of adjuvant treatment for resected stage II lung cancer necessitates attempts to maximize planned chemotherapy doses postoperatively. Thoracoscopic lobectomy, with its lower morbidity rates, allows a high proportion of patients to receive all intended doses.[53,54]

Cost-Effectiveness

The assessment of cost-effectiveness is controversial because of the difficulty in identifying and including all costs. Clearly, VATS can be associated with high costs of consumables and with longer operative times in inexperienced hands. However, numerous disposable instruments that are essential to the performance of thoracoscopic lobectomy, such as linear endoscopic staplers, are also employed by many in performing either conventional thoracotomy or limited thoracotomy. Nakajima and colleagues recently published a study from Japan demonstrating that hospital charges were actually lower for the VATS approach.[55] One important variable in the assessment of cost-effectiveness is length of hospital stay. In a recent series of thoracoscopic lobectomy, the median length of stay was only 3 days.[15] As experience increases with thoracoscopic lobectomy, the operative time will become comparable with that of conventional approaches. In fact, the mean operative time in the CALGB multi-institutional study was only 130 minutes.[18]

Overall Complications

The observation that thoracoscopic lobectomy may have a lower complication profile has recently been supported in studies analyzing outcomes of series including patients undergoing thoracoscopic lobectomy and patients undergoing open lobectomy. In one study, 122 patients undergoing thoracoscopic lobectomy and 122 patients undergoing thoracotomy were compared.[56] Overall, the incidence of postoperative complications was lower in the thoracoscopic group (17.2% versus 27.9%, $P = .046$); however, these patients were matched for age and sex only, and there was no significant difference in the incidence of any of the specific complications reported. Whitson and colleagues analyzed the outcomes of 147 (unmatched) patients who underwent lobectomy, including 88 by thoracotomy and 59 by thoracoscopy.[57] Thoracoscopic lobectomy was associated with a lower incidence of pneumonia but with no difference in other complications, including blood loss, atrial fibrillation, or number of ventilator days.

In another study, the outcomes of patients undergoing either thoracoscopic lobectomy ($n = 300$) or open lobectomy ($n = 283$) were analyzed using a prospective outcomes database.[58] In the entire cohort of 583 patients, thoracoscopic lobectomy was associated with a lower incidence of atrial fibrillation, pneumonia, sepsis, renal failure, overall complications, and death. A propensity-matching method was then used to create two groups with similar baseline characteristics based on 15 preoperative variables, comparing 153 patients who underwent thoracotomy and 153 patients who underwent thoracoscopic lobectomy. The overall complication rate was lower in patients who underwent thoracoscopic lobectomy: 110/153 patients (72%) who underwent thoracoscopic lobectomy had no complications, in comparison with only 89/153 patients (58%) who underwent lobectomy by thoracotomy. In addition, thoracoscopic lobectomy was associated with a lower incidence of atrial fibrillation (13% versus 22%). A second propensity analysis was performed based on stage, comparing 151 patients with stage I disease with 151 patients with disease later than stage I. In this analysis, thoracoscopic lobectomy was associated with lower postoperative mortality; lower incidence of atrial fibrillation, atelectasis, pneumonia, transfusion, and renal failure; and shorter chest tube duration and length of stay. This study demonstrates that thoracoscopic lobectomy is associated with fewer overall complications than lobectomy by thoracotomy, using propensity-matched populations based on preoperative variables and on stage.

Summary

Minimally invasive approaches to lung cancer treatment have been demonstrated to be safe and effective for patients with early-stage lung cancer. Thoracoscopic lobectomy is designed to achieve the same oncologic result as conventional lobectomy: complete hilar dissection and individual vessel control. The recognized advantages of thoracoscopic anatomic resection include less short-term postoperative pain, shorter hospital stay, and preserved pulmonary function. Although there are no prospective randomized studies comparing the thoracoscopic approach with conventional thoracotomy, there are no data from published series to suggest any difference in oncologic efficacy.

REFERENCES

1. Kirby TJ, Rice TW. Thoracoscopic lobectomy. *Ann Thorac Surg* 1993;**56**:784-6.
2. Walker WS, Carnochan FM, Pugh GC. Thoracoscopic pulmonary lobectomy: early operative experience and preliminary clinical results. *J Thorac Cardiovasc Surg* 1993;**106**:1111-7.
3. McKenna RJ. Thoracic lobectomy with mediastinal sampling in 80-year-old patients. *Chest* 1994;**106**:1902-4.
4. Mason DP, Swanson SJ. Lung cancer: diagnosis and treatment. In: Demmy TL, editor. *Video-Assisted Thoracic Surgery (VATS)*. Georgetown, TX: Landis Bioscience; 2001. p. 71-98.
5. Lewis RJ, Caccavale RJ. Video-assisted thoracic surgical non-rib spreading simultaneously stapled lobectomy (VATS(n)SSL). *Semin Thorac Cardiovasc Surg* 1998;**10**:332-9.
6. Lewis RJ, Caccavale RJ, Bocage JP, Widmann MD. Video-assisted thoracic surgical non-rib spreading simultaneously stapled lobectomy: a more patient-friendly oncologic resection. *Chest* 1999;**116**:1119-24.
7. Yim APC, Wan S, Lee TW, Arifi AA. VATS lobectomy reduced cytokine responses compared with conventional surgery. *Ann Thorac Surg* 2000;**70**:243-7.
8. Nagahiro I, Andou A, Aoe M, et al. Pulmonary function, postoperative pain, and serum cytokine level after lobectomy: a comparison of VATS and conventional procedure. *Ann Thorac Surg* 2001;**72**:362-5.
9. Solaini L, Prusciano F, Bagioni P, et al. Video-assisted thoracic surgery major pulmonary resections: present experience. *Eur J Cardiothorac Surg* 2001;**20**:437-42.
10. Jacobeus HC. Ueber die Moglichkeit die Zystoskopie bei untersuchung Seroser Hohlungen Anzuwenden. *Munchen Med Wochenschur* 1910;**57**:2090-2.
11. Kirby TJ, Mack MJ, Landreneau RJ, Rice TW. Lobectomy: video-assisted thoracic surgery versus muscle-sparing thoracotomy: a randomized trial. *J Thorac Cardiovasc Surg* 1995;**109**:997.
12. Yim APC, Izzat MB, Liu HP, Ma CC. Thoracoscopic major lung resections: an Asian perspective. *Semin Thorac Cardiovasc Surg* 1998;**10**:326-31.
13. Daniels LJ, Balderson SS, Onaitis MW, D'Amico TA. Thoracoscopic lobectomy: a safe and effective strategy for patients with stage I lung cancer. *Ann Thorac Surg* 2002;**74**:860-4.
14. McKenna Jr RJ, Houck W, Fuller CB. Video-assisted thoracic surgery lobectomy: experience with 1,100 cases. *Ann Thorac Surg* 2006;**81**:421-5:discussion 425-426.
15. Onaitis MW, Petersen RP, Balderson SS, et al. Thoracoscopic lobectomy is a safe and versatile procedure: experience with 500 consecutive patients. *Ann Surg* 2006;**244**:420-5.
16. Ettinger DS, Bepler G, Bueno R, et al. Non-small cell lung cancer clinical practice guidelines in oncology. *J Natl Compr Canc Netw* 2006;**4**:548-82.
17. Demmy TL, Curtis JJ. Minimally invasive lobectomy directed toward frail and high-risk patients: a case control study. *Ann Thorac Surg* 1999;**68**:194-200.
18. Swanson SJ, Herndon 2nd JE, D'Amico TA, et al. Video-assisted thoracic surgery lobectomy: report of CALGB 39802: a prospective, multi-institution feasibility study. *J Clin Oncol* 2007;**25**(31):4993-7.
19. Cattaneo SM, Park BJ, Wilton AS, et al. Use of video-assisted thoracic surgery for lobectomy in the elderly results in fewer complications. *Ann Thorac Surg* 2008;**85**:231-5:discussion 235-236.
20. Mahtabifard A, Fuller CB, McKenna Jr RJ. Video-assisted thoracic surgery sleeve lobectomy: a case series. *Ann Thorac Surg* 2008;**85**:S729-732.
21. Yim APC, Liu HP, Hazelrigg SR, et al. Thoracoscopic operations on reoperated chests. *Ann Thorac Surg* 1998;**65**:328.
22. Petersen RP, Pham D, Toloza EM, et al. Thoracoscopic lobectomy: a safe and effective strategy for patients receiving induction therapy for non-small cell lung cancer. *Ann Thorac Surg* 2006;**82**:214-8:discussion 219.
23. Widmann MD, Caccavale RJ, Bocage JP, Lewis RJ. Video-assisted thoracic surgery resection of chest wall en bloc for lung carcinoma. *Ann Thorac Surg* 2000;**70**:2138.
24. Naruke T, Tsuchiya R, Kondo H, et al. Lymph node sampling in lung cancer: how should it be done? *Eur J Cardiothorac Surg* 1999;**16**:S17-24.
25. Kaseda S, Aoki T, Hangai N. Video-assisted thoracic surgery (VATS) lobectomy: the Japanese experience. *Semin Thorac Cardiovasc Surg* 1998;**10**:300-4.
26. Sawada S, Komori E, Yamashita M. Very long-term outcomes of video-assisted thoracoscopic surgery for lung cancer. *Surg Endosc* 2008;**22**:2407-11.
27. Yim APC. VATS major pulmonary resection revisited: controversies, techniques, and results. *Ann Thorac Surg* 2002;**74**:615-23.
28. Atkins BZ, Harpole Jr DH, Mangum JH, et al. Pulmonary segmentectomy by thoracotomy or thoracoscopy: reduced hospital length of stay with a minimally-invasive approach. *Ann Thorac Surg* 2007;**84**:1107-12:discussion 1112-1113.
29. D'Amico TA. Thoracoscopic segmentectomy: technical considerations and outcomes. *Ann Thorac Surg* 2008;**85**:S716-718.
30. Ginsberg RJ, Rubinstein LV. Lung Cancer Study Group randomized trial of lobectomy versus resection for T1 non-small cell lung cancer. *Ann Thorac Surg* 1995;**60**:615.
31. Asamura H, Nakayama H, Kondo H, et al. Lymph node involvement, recurrence, and prognosis in resected small, peripheral non-small cell lung carcinomas: are these carcinomas candidates for video-assisted lobectomy?. *J Thorac Cardiovasc Surg* 1996;**111**:1125-34.
32. Shennib H, Kohman L, et al. a multicenter phase II prospective study of video-assisted wedge resection followed by radiotherapy for T1N0 NSCLC in high-risk patients: preliminary analysis of technical outcome. Toronto: American Association of Thoracic Surgery; 2000, CALGB 9335.
33. Swanson SJ, Bueno R, et al. Subcentimeter non-small cell lung cancer: early detection and resection is warranted. 80th American Association of Thoracic Surgery; Toronto, 2000.
34. Landreneau RJ, Keenan RJ, Hazelrigg SR, et al. VATS wedge resection of the lung using the neodymium: yttrium-aluminum garnet laser. *Ann Thorac Surg* 1993;**56**:758.
35. Allen MS, Darling GE, Pechet TT, et al. Morbidity and mortality of major pulmonary resections in patients with early-stage lung cancer: initial results of the randomized, prospective ACOSOG Z0030 trial. *Ann Thorac Surg* 2006;**81**:1013-9:discussion 1019-1020.
36. Yim APC, Liu HP. Complications and failures from video-assisted thoracic surgery: experience from two centers in Asia. *Ann Thorac Surg* 1996;**61**:538.
37. Downey RJ, McCormack P, LoCicero 3rd J. Dissemination of malignant tumors after video-assisted thoracic surgery: a report of twenty-one cases. *J Thorac Cardiovasc Surg* 1996;**111**:954.
38. Nomori H, Horio H, Naruke T, Suemasu K. What is the advantage of a thoracoscopic lobectomy over a limited thoracotomy procedure for lung cancer surgery?. *Ann Thorac Surg* 2001;**72**:879-84.
39. Landreneau RJ, Hazelrigg SR, Mack MJ, et al. Postoperative pain-related morbidity: video-assisted thoracic surgery versus thoracotomy. *Ann Thorac Surg* 1993;**56**:1285-9.
40. Giudicelli R, Thomas P, Lonjon T, et al. Video-assisted minithoracotomy versus muscle-sparing thoracotomy for performing lobectomy. *Ann Thorac Surg* 1994;**58**:712-8.
41. Tschernko EM, Hofer S, Bieglmayer C, et al. Early postoperative stress: video-assisted wedge resection/lobectomy vs conventional axillary thoracotomy. *Chest* 1996;**109**:1636-42.
42. Walker WS, Pugh GC, Craig SR, Carnochan FM. Continued experience with thoracoscopic major pulmonary resection. *Int Surg* 1996;**81**:255-8.
43. Ohbuchi T, Morikawa T, Takeuchi E, Kato H. Lobectomy: video-assisted thoracic surgery versus posterolateral thoracotomy. *Jpn J Thorac Cardiovasc Surg* 1998;**46**:519-22.
44. Stammberger U, Steinacher C, Hillinger S, et al. Early and long-term complaints following video-assisted thoracoscopic surgery: evaluation in 173 patients. *Eur J Cardiothorac Surg* 2000;**18**:7-11.
45. Landreneau RJ, Mack MJ, Hazelrigg SR, et al. Prevalence of chronic pain after pulmonary resection by thoracotomy or video-assisted thoracic surgery. *J Thorac Cardiovasc Surg* 1994;**107**:1079-86.
46. Nakata M, Saeki H, Yokoyama N, et al. Pulmonary function after lobectomy: video-assisted thoracic surgery versus thoracotomy. *Ann Thorac Surg* 2000;**70**:938-41.
47. Kaseda S, Aoki T, Hangai N, Shimizu K. Better pulmonary function and prognosis with video-assisted thoracic surgery than with thoracotomy. *Ann Thorac Surg* 2000;**70**:1644-6.

48. Leaver HA, Craig SR, Yap PL, Walker WS. Lymphocyte responses following open and minimally invasive thoracic surgery. *Eur J Clin Invest* 2000;**30**:320-8.
49. Sugi K, Kaneda Y, Esato K. Video-assisted thoracoscopic lobectomy reduces cytokine production more than conventional open thoracotomy. *Jpn J Thorac Cardiovasc Surg* 2000;**48**:161-5.
50. Ng CS, Wan S, Hui CW, et al. Video-assisted thoracic surgery lobectomy for lung cancer is associated with less immunochemokine disturbances than thoracotomy. *Eur J Cardiothorac Surg* 2007;**31**:83-7.
51. Iwasaki A, Shirakusa T, Kawahara K, et al. Is video-assisted thoracoscopic surgery suitable for resection of primary lung cancer? *Thorac Cardiovasc Surg* 1997;**45**:13-5.
52. Yim APC, et al. Video-assisted pulmonary resections. In: Pearson FG, Cooper JD, Deslauriers J, editors. *Thoracic surgery*. Philadelphia: Churchill Livingstone; 2002. p. 1073-84.
53. Petersen RP, Pham D, Burfeind WR, et al. Thoracoscopic lobectomy facilitates the delivery of chemotherapy after resection for lung cancer. *Ann Thorac Surg* 2007;**83**:1245-9:discussion 1250.
54. Nicastri DG, Wisnivesky JP, Litle VR, et al. Thoracoscopic lobectomy: report on safety, discharge independence, pain, and chemotherapy tolerance. *J Thorac Cardiovasc Surg* 2008;**135**:642-7.
55. Nakajima J, Takamoto S, Kohno T, Ohtsuka T. Costs of video-assisted thoracoscopic surgery versus open resection for patients with lung carcinoma. *Cancer* 2000;**89**:2497-501.
56. Park BJ, Zhang H, Rusch VW, Amar D. Video-assisted thoracic surgery does not reduce the incidence of postoperative atrial fibrillation after pulmonary lobectomy. *J Thorac Cardiovasc Surg* 2007;**133**:775-9.
57. Whitson BA, Andrade RS, Boettcher A, et al. Video-assisted thoracoscopic surgery is more favorable than thoracotomy for resection of clinical stage I non-small cell lung cancer. *Ann Thorac Surg* 2007;**83**:1965-70.
58. Villamizar NR, Darrabie MD, et al. Thoracoscopic lobectomy is associated with lower morbidity compared to thoracotomy. J Thorac Cardiovasc Surg in press; 2009.
59. Brown WT. Video-assisted thoracic surgery: the Miami experience. *Semin Thorac Cardiovasc Surg* 1998;**10**:305-12.
60. Roviaro G, Varoli F, Vergani C, Maciocco M. Video-assisted thoracoscopic surgery (VATS) major pulmonary resections: the Italian experience. *Semin Thorac Cardiovasc Surg* 1998;**10**:313-20.
61. Walker WS. Video-assisted thoracic surgery: the Edinburgh experience. *Semin Thorac Cardiovasc Surg* 1998;**10**:291-9.

CHAPTER 19
Lung Cancer: Multimodal Therapy

Sudish C. Murthy, David P. Mason, and Thomas W. Rice

Adjuvant Therapy
   Adjuvant Chemotherapy
   Adjuvant Radiotherapy
Induction Therapy

Induction Chemotherapy for Early-Stage
   Non–Small Cell Lung Cancer
Induction Therapy for Stage IIIA/B
   Non–Small Cell Lung Cancer

Induction Chemotherapy
Induction Chemoradiotherapy
Special Circumstance: Superior Sulcus Tumors
Recommendations

Though long regarded as the best chance for cure, surgery alone has shortcomings in the management of non–small cell lung cancer (NSCLC). Even in the most favorable of circumstances (stage I), failure of therapy is anticipated in 20% to 40% of patients.[1-3] Moreover, because most patients do not have localized disease at the time of the initial diagnosis, surgical resection is offered to only a minority of all patients with NSCLC.

Considerable effort has been directed toward developing preoperative (induction or neoadjuvant) and postoperative (adjuvant) strategies to improve long-term outcome after surgery and to increase the total number of resectable patients. These strategies employ chemotherapy and radiation used either singly, sequentially, or concurrently.

Predicting which patients will not be cured by resection permits identification of appropriate candidates for multimodality therapy. To this end, locoregional lymph node involvement is a powerful predictor of cancer recurrence and should be thoroughly investigated during treatment planning.[4] Tumor histology and size also affect cancer-related and overall survival of resected patients.[5-7] Moreover, numerous genetic markers are being discovered that may aid outcome prognostication, and when combined with current imaging modalities (e.g., positron emission tomography), outcome prediction may be further refined.[8-10] Recent reports have proposed systems using histologic and molecular criteria to stratify predicted survival of resected patients.[11-13]

In developing strategies for combined therapies, patterns of failure must be considered. Locoregional recurrence after resection of stage I cancers is rare, but it is more common when regional lymph nodes are involved. However, because patients seldom die from local recurrence, the impact of improving local control with adjuvant radiotherapy may not translate to a survival advantage. Even in the presence of local lymph node involvement, resected patients with stage II cancers are still twice as likely to fail systemically as locally,[14] suggesting that adjuvant systemic therapy (chemotherapy) might be more useful than adjuvant local therapy (radiotherapy) and, if effective, may ultimately result in a survival advantage.

ADJUVANT THERAPY

Despite enthusiasm for multimodality treatment of NSCLC, and after more than 35 years of promising clinical trials, it has only recently become apparent that there is a clear and consistent benefit of adjuvant therapy for resected lung cancer. The delay may have been partly because chemotherapy and radiation protocols changed frequently, resulting in large numbers of studies that were difficult to compare. Few studies have been designed to critically examine treatment effects on specific NSCLC stages; most studies tend to group stages I through III in their treatment arms. This shortcoming has been compounded by a lack of accurate pathologic staging in most trials. Moreover, promising results generated at high-volume academic centers may not be easily reproduced at less specialized smaller institutions.[15,16]

Adjuvant Chemotherapy

Early randomized trials of adjuvant chemotherapy focused on the use of nitrogen mustard,[17,18] cyclophosphamide,[17,19] and a combination of lomustine and hydroxyurea.[20] Cumulatively, these trials demonstrated that treated patients had more postoperative complications without any survival benefit than did untreated patients. In fact, patients treated with postoperative cyclophosphamide experienced a poorer long-term survival than did untreated patients.[19] This was independently confirmed by meta-analysis.[20] Findings from these early studies have been largely invalidated because histologic type and pathologic stage were not considered during trial design. Moreover, chemotherapeutic agents used in these early trials have since been demonstrated to be ineffective, if not detrimental, for patients with NSCLC.

As several studies began documenting the efficacy of platinum-based agents for advanced (stage IV) NSCLC, platinum-based adjuvant in combination chemotherapy regimens became the preferred choice for resected patients. Initial enthusiasm was generated when the Lung Cancer Study Group trial 772,[21] a randomized study, suggested a disease-free and overall survival benefit in the treatment arm. Although the survival advantage was not considered statistically significant, sufficient optimism was generated to continue investigations of these types of chemotherapeutic protocols. Early subsequent trials, however, proved to be far less promising, although sufficient flaws were identified in the design or conduct of each to rationalize their failure.

A randomized study of cyclophosphamide, Adriamycin, and cisplatin adjuvant therapy for resected stage I to II NSCLC[22] did not demonstrate treatment efficacy. This trial suffered from the inability to deliver the prescribed chemotherapeutic regimen (four cycles) over the prescribed time. Fewer than 30% of patients in the treatment arm actually received chemotherapy as intended. Other randomized studies have been similarly plagued by incomplete delivery of prescribed postoperative therapies,[23,24] which partly contributes to the negative findings of these trials. Additionally, the dose of cisplatin (40 to 60 mg/m^2/cycle) was lower than that currently recommended (80 to 120 mg/m^2/cycle).[25]

Although all of these early platinum trials were considered statistically negative, subtle survival differences were noted between control and treated patients in essentially every study. Not surprisingly, a 1995 meta-analysis of several randomized adjuvant platinum-based trials demonstrated a 13% reduction in the risk of death ($P = .08$) for treated patients.[26] This rekindled interest in this adjuvant strategy and spawned multiple modern trials. Platinum dosage was adjusted so that patients were scheduled to receive 300 to 400 mg/m^2 (total dose). Adjuvant radiation therapy was left to the discretion of participating centers. Two studies demonstrated trends favoring survival benefit in treated patients, although neither was considered to be a positive trial.[27,28] The International Adjuvant Lung Cancer Trial,[29] however, demonstrated a clear survival benefit of adjuvant platinum-based chemotherapy. This study included resected stage I to III patients and found a survival advantage, 5% percent benefit after 5 years ($P = .003$), favoring the adjuvant chemotherapy arm versus surgery alone. This survival advantage is similar in magnitude to that achieved by adjuvant chemotherapy for resected breast and colon cancers.[30,31]

The Lung Adjuvant Cisplatin Evaluation (LACE) pooled data from the five largest randomized trials completed since 2004 and reanalyzed this collective.[32] This study amassed information from more than 4500 patients who were previously randomized to treatment and concluded that postoperative cisplatin-based chemotherapy significantly improves survival in patients with NSCLC. Because the index trials feeding LACE were heterogeneous with regard to stage (I to III), subgroup analysis of the pooled data allowed some insight into the differential effect of adjuvant therapy on specific stages of resected cancer. From LACE, there is little doubt that resected stage II and III patients will enjoy a meaningful survival advantage from adjuvant chemotherapy—at least 5% for overall survival and 6% for disease-free survival.[32] Patients with resected stage IB disease, however, have a much less obvious benefit, although the trend is toward some advantage. The confidence intervals of the hazard ratio are wide and quite similar to those of the final analysis of the Cancer and Leukemia Group B (CALGB) 9633, a trial of adjuvant carboplatin and paclitaxel for resected stage IB patients only.[33] An important finding of CALGB 9633 was that patients with primary tumors larger than 4 cm do, in fact, benefit from adjuvant chemotherapy.[33]

Adjuvant Radiotherapy

Studies of the efficacy of adjuvant radiotherapy are confounded by many of the same factors that have plagued and continue to plague chemotherapy trials. Many randomized adjuvant radiotherapy studies are composed of patients from all stages of resected NSCLC. Consequently, the expected negligible (or deleterious) effects on patients with early-stage cancer may obscure small beneficial effects for patients with more advanced disease. Also, because the field of radiation oncology has evolved so quickly, many early randomized studies became obsolete before their data had matured. Moreover, most of the early randomized trials were underpowered to demonstrate small but relevant differences in outcome. Consequently, it is not surprising that, although many feasibility and retrospective studies have yielded promising results, no randomized data yet exist to suggest a survival benefit of postoperative radiotherapy.

Currently, there is no justification to include adjuvant radiotherapy in the management of resected stages I and II NSCLC. Three randomized trials,[34-36] as well as meta-analyses of trials (postoperative radiotherapy [PORT] studies),[37,38] document a deleterious effect (a survival disadvantage) of adjuvant radiotherapy for early-stage NSCLC. Reasons for this include poor radiotherapy planning,[36] larger fraction size,[34] greater total radiation dosage,[34-36] outdated equipment, and poor quality control.[39]

Although there was optimism that hilar lymph node (N1)-positive patients (stage II) would provide a good substrate for adjuvant radiotherapy, this appears not to be the case. From subgroup analysis of several randomized trials,[37,38,40,41] radiotherapy has no significant effect on either local control or overall survival for these patients.

Finally, there are insufficient randomized data to defend the use of adjuvant radiotherapy for resected stage III (N2/N3) disease. Even though improved local control has been reported,[40-42] it has not translated into a meaningful survival benefit. The strongest argument to support adjuvant radiotherapy for resected stage III NSCLC comes from a nonrandomized, single-institution, retrospective study.[17,43] These investigators found that postoperative radiotherapy was the strongest independent predictor of survival for resected N2-positive disease. This study, however, has been widely criticized,[39] and PORT meta-analyses consistently do not demonstrate clear efficacy for adjuvant radiotherapy for stage III disease.[37,38] Yet, controversy still remains over radiotherapy used in this setting, as one recent trial of adjuvant chemotherapy demonstrated the best survival when patients received thoracic radiation after their chemotherapy for resected stage III disease.[44]

INDUCTION THERAPY

Induction or neoadjuvant therapy is any systemic or regional cytoreductive treatment (e.g., chemotherapy, radiotherapy, chemoradiotherapy) administered before definitive locoregional therapy (e.g., surgery). Aggressive surgical (mediastinoscopy or video-assisted thoracoscopic surgery [VATS]) or interventional (transbronchial needle aspiration or endoscopic ultrasound-guided fine-needle aspiration) staging is imperative to ensure that induction therapy protocols are applied to homogeneous patient populations. Some patients may be rendered inoperable because of grade 3 or 4 induction therapy toxicities, and this must be considered and discussed with patients during treatment planning.

Use of chemotherapy in the induction setting has several potential advantages. First, there is earlier treatment of micrometastatic systemic disease. Because distant recurrence is the most common mode of failure, early eradication of systemic disease might translate into a survival advantage, and chemotherapy is most efficacious when the tumor burden is small.[45] Also, drug delivery and cytotoxic effects may be enhanced as a result of preservation of tumor blood supply. Perhaps most importantly, however, a higher percentage of patients will probably receive their intended dose of chemotherapy when drugs are delivered preoperatively.[46]

Induction radiotherapy in combination with chemotherapy has been and continues to be investigated vigorously. Two large phase III trials comparing only induction radiotherapy (40 to 50 Gy) were reported several decades ago.[47,48] Both demonstrated inferior survival rates for radiated patients. Since then, limited data have emerged to suggest a role for radiotherapy alone as an induction modality. Consequently, discussions of induction radiotherapy are primarily in the context of chemoradiotherapy protocols.

Induction therapies are not without concerns. Subsequent resections are generally more technically challenging and may result in lung-sparing operations becoming less feasible. Morbidity and mortality rates for surgery after induction therapy may be greater,[27,49] and for an early-stage cancer, given the expected relatively good survival, the risks may well exceed any benefits. Despite these concerns, several groups are pursuing rigorous induction strategies and demonstrating reasonable safety profiles.[50,51]

Induction Chemotherapy for Early-Stage Non–Small Cell Lung Cancer

Observations from other solid tumor treatment trials suggest that chemotherapy response rates improve as similar drug regimens are applied to earlier stages of disease.[52] The feasibility of induction chemotherapy for early-stage lung cancer was demonstrated in 2000 by the Bimodality Lung Oncology Team study.[46] This phase II trial examined the response, toxicity, resectability rate, surgical morbidity, and intermediate survival for patients treated preoperatively with carboplatin and paclitaxel. Two preoperative cycles were administered and three postoperative cycles planned for patients undergoing complete resections. After induction therapy, 56% of patients had a major objective response; 86% of patients underwent complete resection. Impressively, 96% of patients received the intended preoperative chemotherapy, and 46% received the planned postoperative courses. Treated patients appeared to have standard postoperative recoveries.

A more recent randomized trial suggests a benefit of induction chemotherapy for stages I and II NSCLC.[27] The induction regimen consisted of two cycles of mitomycin, ifosfamide, and cisplatin. Two additional cycles were given postoperatively for responding patients. The patient population was heterogeneous, with some stage IIIA patients included in the study. Nonetheless, despite a slightly higher mortality rate for chemotherapy-treated patients, disease-free survival was longer than for untreated patients with stage I or II cancers.

Induction Therapy for Stage IIIA/B Non–Small Cell Lung Cancer

Induction Chemotherapy

In 1982, Pearson and colleagues reported on the dismal outcome of surgery alone for stage IIIA (N2 lymph node–positive) patients.[53] They noted a 9% 5-year survival rate for gross mediastinal lymph node involvement and a 24% survival rate for patients with microscopically positive nodes. Even for occult, single-station N2 disease, the best reported survival rate is less than 30% after 5 years.[54] Local recurrence seldom contributed to mortality, because the vast majority of these patients die of metastatic disease. Consequently, induction chemotherapy as the systemic component of multimodality treatment for patients with locally advanced NSCLC has been investigated.

By the mid 1990s, the recognized standard of care for resectable stage IIIA (N2-positive) NSCLC was changed by the near-simultaneous reports of two small randomized trials designed to study the efficacy of induction chemotherapy followed by resection. Until this time, most had considered combined definitive chemoradiotherapy as the standard of care. Collectively, these two reports represented data acquired from only 120 patients. Rosell and associates[55] compared surgery alone with three cycles of induction chemotherapy (platinum based) followed by surgery. All patients in the study were scheduled to receive postoperative thoracic irradiation. A second, more chemotherapy-intensive trial consisted of three cycles of a cisplatin regimen given as induction with three additional cycles planned postoperatively for responding patients.[56] In this trial, radiotherapy was reserved for unresectable or incompletely resected patients. Entry into either trial required pathologic confirmation of mediastinal lymph node involvement (N2 disease) by mediastinoscopy, or T3 disease.

Although neither study was without shortcomings, surprisingly both trials were stopped early because interim analyses demonstrated a significant advantage favoring patients given induction chemotherapy. Mature, actual (not actuarial) survival updates have been published, with an average of 7 years of follow-up.[57,58] These reports document a durable and statistically significant survival benefit of induction chemotherapy with surgery versus surgery alone, and they translate into a 20% better 5-year survival rate.

Induction Chemoradiotherapy

Radiotherapy in sequence after chemotherapy (with or without surgery) has long been used to consolidate the local component of therapy for stage III NSCLC.[59-61] Concurrent chemoradiotherapy has several theoretical advantages over the sequential strategy. Contemporary drugs active in NSCLC (e.g., cisplatin, paclitaxel) are radiation sensitizers and allow a synergistic tumoricidal effect when given concurrently with ionizing radiation. Although combined therapy is clearly more toxic,[62] several investigators have found the subsequent operative mortality and morbidity to be similar to induction chemotherapy alone, if appropriate perioperative safeguards and patient selection are optimized.[49,63] A hypothetical advantage of concurrent chemoradiation induction therapy is reduction in tumor bulk, which might permit unresectable lesions to be removed with negative margins, or, potentially, for lesser resections to be performed (lobectomy as opposed to pneumonectomy). Finally, delivery of ionizing radiation when tumor vascularity has not yet been disrupted by surgical dissection may enhance response.

Since 1990, the standard of care for patients with unresectable stage IIIA disease (bulky N2 involvement), and for most patients with stage IIIB NSCLC, has been concurrent chemoradiotherapy.[64] Based on encouraging observations with regard to clinical response rates but a disappointing rate of local failure, investigations were conducted to explore addition of surgery to provide "more definitive" local control.[65] The Southwest Oncology Group (SWOG) conducted the most widely reported, multi-institutional feasibility trial of this strategy, SWOG 8805. The treatment protocol consisted of two cycles of induction chemotherapy (cisplatin and etoposide) and 45 Gy of concurrent radiotherapy for patients with stage IIIA or IIIB NSCLC.[66] Of the 126 patients enrolled, 60% had stage IIIA disease and 40% were stage IIIB. Fifty-three percent of the stage IIIB patients had N3 lymph node involvement. There was a 6% operative mortality rate even though nearly one third of the operations required pneumonectomy.[67] This compared favorably with contemporary surgical series without induction therapies,[68,69] and it underscored the possibility of safely performing resection after combined neoadjuvant therapy.[66] This notion has since been reaffirmed by more recent studies.[50,51]

Stage IIIB disease with N3 lymph node involvement is generally considered inoperable because of an inability to obtain a complete resection and a near-universal pattern of systemic failure after aggressive local therapy. Growing experience with surgery after induction chemoradiation has allowed certain centers to offer resection to selected stage IIIB patients. In SWOG 8805, patients with stage IIIA and IIIB disease had equivalent clinical and pathologic responses and, surprisingly, similar survival rates.[66] These investigators, as well as others,[70-73] noted that only patients who had sterilization of their mediastinal disease after induction treatment benefited from treatment. For patients experiencing complete pathologic responses (i.e., no viable tumor found in the resected specimen), a 40% to 55% 5-year survival rate is expected.[63,73] Because of this, more recent therapeutic regimens have attempted to improve the preoperative sterilization rate by increasing the dosage of radiation in the induction chemoradiation treatment to above 5900 cGy.[50,51]

A single-institution experience using hyperfractionated radiotherapy with concurrent induction chemotherapy (cisplatin and paclitaxel) has identified an intermediate prognostic group.[74,75] Patients with stage IIIA/B disease who were treated with this regimen were equally likely to benefit whether they had N2 or N3 disease before treatment. Patients downstaged from N3 to N2, or those IIIA patients with residual N2 disease at surgery, still had a median survival rate of 27 months and a 31% 5-year survival rate.[63]

A few recent randomized studies of induction chemotherapy and chemoradiotherapy for stage IIIA NSCLC question the usefulness of surgery as part of any treatment algorithm. In the much older SWOG 8805 study, 21% of resected patients had a complete pathologic response with sterilization of primary lesion and regional lymph nodes (i.e., primary T0N0). An additional 37% of patients had only microscopic residual cancer.[66] Such observations led some investigators to speculate whether resection actually contributed to survival at all or merely provided prognostic information of response to therapy. To address the usefulness of surgery in patients with stage III NSCLC, the National Cancer Institute sponsored a multi-institutional phase III trial (INT 0139), in which 429 patients received two cycles of cisplatin and etoposide with concurrent thoracic radiotherapy (45 Gy), followed by either resection or additional chemoradiation therapy. Resected patients were scheduled for two postoperative cycles of chemotherapy, whereas patients randomized to the no-surgery arm were to receive uninterrupted radiation up to 61 Gy with two additional cycles of chemotherapy. Although there were more early deaths in the surgical arm (14 versus 3), disease-free survival rates were superior when resection was a component of treatment (log-rank, $P = .02$). The 3-year survival rate in the operated group was 29% compared with only 19% in the chemoradiation-alone cohort.[76] The outcomes update, however, did not demonstrate a clear survival advantage for the whole group, although subgroup analysis showed a benefit favoring induction chemoradiation therapy followed by surgery when a lobectomy (not pneumonectomy) was performed.[77]

Still more recently, another randomized trial of induction chemotherapy followed by either resection or definitive radiotherapy demonstrated equivalence of the two treatment arms.[78] The 5-year overall survival rates were 15.7% and 14% for surgery and radiotherapy, respectively. The authors were left to conclude that, because of the lower side-effect profile and lower treatment-related mortality, radiotherapy, and not surgical resection, should be considered the preferred locoregional treatment for these patients.

Current investigative efforts to enhance survival in patients with stage III disease are focused on novel induction chemotherapy drug combinations, different dosage schedules and intensities, altered radiation fractionation schemes, and the use of biological response modifiers targeting inflammation, angiogenesis, tissue invasion, cellular proliferation, apoptosis, and metastasis.[79-81]

Surgery remains central in the accurate staging of these patients and enhances survival for some patients with stage IIIA or IIIB NSCLC. Unfortunately, no patient or tumor characteristics can predict response to induction therapy. Moreover, clinical, noninvasive, and radiographic assessments of response have been disappointing.[61] Semiquantitative positron emission tomography (PET)[82] and some minimally invasive techniques (e.g., endoscopic ultrasound-guided fine-needle aspiration,[83] VATS,[84] repeat mediastinoscopy[85-87]) may permit identification of patients most likely to benefit from resection after induction therapies. Nonresponders might be best served by alternative or experimental therapies.

For these reasons, the optimal treatment of patients with stage III NSCLC continues to remains undefined. The role of surgery is still unclear and the impact of improved postinduction staging unknown. There is little doubt that pneumonectomy after induction chemoradiotherapy should be avoided.

Special Circumstance: Superior Sulcus Tumors

Patients with superior sulcus (Pancoast) tumors represent a unique group who serve as attractive candidates for induction protocols. The biological behavior of some of these tumors seems different from that of other NSCLC in that extensive local disease can occur without the obligate systemic disease that accompanies other T3 tumors.[88] Nonetheless, presence of regional lymph node involvement still remains a powerful negative predictor of survival after Pancoast tumor resection. In approximately one third of Pancoast tumor resections, complete resection is not obtained.[89] This is significant because an incomplete resection does not benefit the patient.[90-93]

Long-term survival after resection of a superior sulcus tumor was first observed only after the addition of adjuvant radiation therapy.[94] Subsequently, an induction radiation therapy strategy was developed that dramatically improved survival over historical controls.[95,96] Despite these advances, complete resection for node-negative T3 tumors was possible in less than two thirds of patients. Unlike standard stage II/III disease, locoregional disease was the most common form of recurrence.[97]

The feasibility of induction chemoradiation therapy for patients with superior sulcus tumors was evaluated in a 2001 multi-institutional trial.[98] The study population included patients who had N2/N3 node-negative disease with T3 or T4 tumors and adequate cardiopulmonary fitness to tolerate resection. Patients were given two cycles of cisplatin and etoposide with concurrent radiation (45 Gy). The radiation field included the primary tumor and ipsilateral supraclavicular fossa, but it excluded the hilum or mediastinum. Surgery was performed 3 to 5 weeks after the end of the induction therapy. Two cycles of "boost" (adjuvant) chemotherapy were scheduled after recovery from surgery.

The induction therapy was completed as planned in 92% of patients. The related mortality rate was 3%. Of the enrolled patients, 75% underwent surgery. Of these, 92% underwent complete resection. The 2-year survival for completely resected patients was a surprising 70%. Updated mature results of this phase II trial demonstrated a 44% 5-year survival for the entire cohort and a 12% local relapse rate versus 40% for historical controls.[99,100]

RECOMMENDATIONS

The extent of NSCLC at initial diagnosis, as defined by American Joint Committee on Cancer staging, is currently the only reliable predictor of survival. It is therefore essential to exhaust all reasonable efforts to obtain accurate staging information before consideration of adjuvant or induction therapies. Multimodality therapy planning should then be used in a stage-dependent manner.

Staging protocols must include a thorough search for distant metastatic disease, as well as providing accurate information regarding locoregional lymph node involvement. We currently favor using PET as part of the metastatic survey, and we prefer mediastinoscopy for evaluation of mediastinal lymph nodes, although endoscopic and endobronchial staging modalities are becoming increasingly more refined and accurate. Our institutional experience with PET to stage the mediastinum has not measured up to that reported elsewhere[101,102] and has not replaced mediastinoscopy for this purpose in our practice.

There is little doubt that adjuvant chemotherapy has a role in the management of resected stage II/III NSCLC and should be considered the standard of care at this time. Chemotherapy should revolve around a platinum-based regimen, and it is becoming increasingly apparent that patients benefit most when the intended dose of chemotherapy is delivered.

There is still active debate regarding the use of adjuvant chemotherapy for stage IB disease. Ongoing trials should help clarify this issue, although on the basis of current data, it is reasonable to consider adjuvant chemotherapy for patients with larger IB tumors who demonstrate good performance status.

Patients with stage IIIA/B NSCLC do poorly with surgery alone. After numerous studies and much debate, the optimal use of induction chemoradiation therapy still remains largely unresolved, although recent randomized trials do not favor the inclusion of surgical resection, particularly pneumonectomy, in the treatment algorithm.

REFERENCES

1. Green FL, Page DL, Fleming ID. *Cancer staging manual.* New York: Springer-Verlag; 2002. p. 167-77.
2. Martini N, Bains MS, Burt ME, et al. Incidence of local recurrence and second primary tumors in resected stage I lung cancer. *J Thorac Cardiovasc Surg* 1995;**109**(1):120-9.
3. Mountain CF. Prognostic implications of the International Staging System for Lung Cancer. *Semin Oncol* 1988;**15**(3):236-45.
4. Mountain CF. Revisions in the International System for Staging Lung Cancer. *Chest* 1997;**111**(6):1710-7.
5. Mountain CF, Lukeman JM, Hammar SP, et al. Lung cancer classification: the relationship of disease extent and cell type to survival in a clinical trials population. *J Surg Oncol* 1987;**35**(3):147-56.
6. Ou SH, Zell JA, Ziogas A, Anton-Culver H. Prognostic factors for survival of stage I nonsmall cell lung cancer patients: a population-based analysis of 19,702 stage I patients in the California Cancer Registry from 1989 to 2003. *Cancer* 2007 Oct 1;**110**(7):1532-41.
7. Ost D, Goldberg J, Rolnitzky L, Rom WN. Survival after surgery in stage IA and IB non-small cell lung cancer. *Am J Respir Crit Care Med* 2008;**177**(5):516-23:Mar 1.
8. Lau CL, D'Amico TA. Clinical and molecular prognostic factors and models for non-small cell lung cancer. In: Pass HI, Mitchell JB, Johnson DH, editors. *Lung cancer: principles and practice.* Philadelphia: Lippincott Williams & Wilkins; 2000. p. 602-11.
9. Taylor MD, Smith PW, Brix WK, Wick MR, et al. Fluorodeoxyglucose positron emission tomography and tumor marker expression in non-small cell lung cancer. *J Thorac Cardiovasc Surg* 2009;**137**(1):43-8.
10. Vesselle H, Salskov A, Turcotte E, Wiens L, et al. Relationship between non-small cell lung cancer FDG uptake at PET, tumor histology, and Ki-67 proliferation index. *J Thorac Oncol* 2008(9):971-8:Sep;3.
11. D'Amico TA, Massey M, Herndon 2nd JE, et al. A biologic risk model for stage I lung cancer: immunohistochemical analysis of 408 patients with the use of ten molecular markers. *J Thorac Cardiovasc Surg* 1999;**117**(4):736-43.
12. Kwiatkowski DJ, Harpole Jr DH, Godleski J, et al. Molecular pathologic substaging in 244 stage I non-small-cell lung cancer patients: clinical implications. *J Clin Oncol* 1998;**16**(7):2468-77.
13. Zhu ZH, Sun BY, Ma Y, Shao JY, et al. Three Immunomarker Support Vector Machines-Based Prognostic Classifiers for Stage IB Non-Small-Cell Lung Cancer. *J Clin Oncol* 2009:Feb 2.
14. Ginsberg RJ, Vokes EE, Raben A. Non-small cell lung cancer. In: Devita VTJ, Hellman S, Rosenberg SA, editors. *Cancer principles and practice of oncology.* Philadelphia: Lippincott-Raven; 1997. p. 858-911.
15. Bach PB, Cramer LD, Schrag D, Downey RJ, et al. The influence of hospital volume on survival after resection for lung cancer. *N Engl J Med* 2001;**345**(3):181-8:Jul 19.
16. Sioris T, Sihvo E, Sankila R, Salo J. Effect of surgical volume and hospital type on outcome in non-small cell lung cancer surgery: a Finnish population-based study. *Lung Cancer* 2008;**59**(1):119-25.
17. Higgins GA, Shields TW. Experience of the Veterans Administration Surgical Adjuvant Group. In: Muggia F, Rozencwieg M, editors. Lung Cancer: Progress in Therapeutic Research. New York: Raven Press; 1979. p. 433.
18. Slack NH. Bronchogenic carcinoma: Nitrogen mustard as a surgical adjuvant and factors influencing survival. University surgical adjuvant lung project. *Cancer* 1970;**25**(5):987-1002.
19. Brunner KW, Marthaler T, Muller W. Effects of long-term adjuvant chemotherapy with cyclophosphamide (NSC-26271) for radically resected bronchogenic carcinoma. *Cancer Chemother Rep* 1973;**4**(2):125-32.

20. Shields TW, Higgins Jr GA, Humphrey EW, et al. Prolonged intermittent adjuvant chemotherapy with CCNU and hydroxyurea after resection of carcinoma of the lung. *Cancer* 1982;**50**(9):1713-21.
21. Holmes EC, Gail M. Surgical adjuvant therapy for stage II and stage III adenocarcinoma and large-cell undifferentiated carcinoma. *J Clin Oncol* 1986;**4**(5):710-5.
22. Feld R, Rubinstein L, Thomas PA. Adjuvant chemotherapy with cyclophosphamide, doxorubicin, and cisplatin in patients with completely resected stage I non-small-cell lung cancer. The Lung Cancer Study Group. *J Natl Cancer Inst* 1993;**85**(4):299-306.
23. Ohta M, Tsuchiya R, Shimoyama M, et al. Adjuvant chemotherapy for completely resected stage III non-small-cell lung cancer. Results of a randomized prospective study. The Japan Clinical Oncology Group. *J Thorac Cardiovasc Surg* 1993;**106**(4):703-8.
24. Pisters KM, Kris MG, Gralla RJ, et al. Randomized trial comparing postoperative chemotherapy with vindesine and cisplatin plus thoracic irradiation with irradiation alone in stage III (N2) non-small cell lung cancer. *J Surg Oncol* 1994;**56**(4):236-41.
25. Rapp E, Pater JL, Willan A, et al. Chemotherapy can prolong survival in patients with advanced non-small-cell lung cancer: report of a Canadian multicenter randomized trial. *J Clin Oncol* 1988;**6**(4):633-41.
26. Carbone DP, Minna JD. Chemotherapy in non-small cell lung cancer: a meta-analysis using updated data on individual patients from 52 randomised clinical trials. Non-small Cell Lung Cancer Collaborative Group. *Br J Med* 1995;**311**(7010):889-90.
27. Depierre A, Milleron B, Moro-Sibilot D, et al. Preoperative chemotherapy followed by surgery compared with primary surgery in resectable stage I (except T1N0), II, and IIIa non-small-cell lung cancer. *J Clin Oncol* 2002;**20**(1):247-53.
28. Scagliotti GV, Fossati R, Torri V, et al. Randomized study of adjuvant chemotherapy for completely resected stage I, II, or IIIA non-small-cell lung cancer. *J Natl Cancer Inst* 2003;**95**(19):1453-61.
29. Arriagada R, Bergman B, Dunant A, et al. Cisplatin-based adjuvant chemotherapy in patients with completely resected non-small-cell lung cancer. *N Engl J Med* 2004;**350**(4):351-60.
30. Early Breast Cancer Trialists Collaborative Group. Systemic treatment of early breast cancer by hormonal, cytotoxic, immune therapy: 133 randomised trials involving 31,000 recurrences and 24,000 deaths among 75,000 women. *Lancet* 1992;**339**:1-5.
31. International Multicentre Pooled Analysis of Colon Cancer Trials (IMPACT) Investigators. Efficacy of adjuvant fluorouracil and folinic acid in colon cancer. *Lancet* 1995;**345**:939-44.
32. Pignon JP, Tribodet H, Scagliotti GV, Douillard JY, et al. Lung adjuvant cisplatin evaluation: a pooled analysis by the LACE Collaborative Group. *J Clin Oncol* 2008;**26**(21):3552-9.
33. Strauss GM, Herndon 2nd JE, Maddaus MA, Johnstone DW, et al. Adjuvant paclitaxel plus carboplatin compared with observation in stage IB non-small-cell lung cancer: CALGB 9633 with the Cancer and Leukemia Group B, Radiation Therapy Oncology Group, and North Central Cancer Treatment Group Study Groups. *J Clin Oncol* 2008;**26**(31):5043-51:Nov 1.
34. Bonner JA. The role of postoperative radiotherapy for patients with completely resected non-small cell lung carcinoma: seeking to optimize local control and survival while minimizing toxicity. *Cancer* 1999;**86**(2):195-6.
35. Lafitte JJ, Ribet ME, Prevost BM, et al. Postresection irradiation for T2 N0 M0 non-small cell carcinoma: a prospective, randomized study. *Ann Thorac Surg* 1996;**62**(3):830-4.
36. Van Houtte P, Rocmans P, Smets P, et al. Postoperative radiation therapy in lung cancer: a controlled trial after resection of curative design. *Int J Radiat Oncol Biol Phys* 1980;**6**(8):983-6.
37. PORT Meta-analysis Trialists Group. Postoperative radiotherapy in non-small-cell lung cancer: systematic review and meta-analysis of individual patient data from nine randomised controlled trials. *Lancet* 1998;**352**(9124):257-63.
38. PORT Meta-analysis Trialists Group. Postoperative radiotherapy for non-small cell lung cancer. *Cochrane Database Syst Rev* 2005 Apr 18(2):CD002142.
39. Sawyer TE, Bonner JA. Postoperative irradiation in non-small cell lung cancer. In: Pass HI, Mitchell JB, Johnson DH, editors. *Lung Cancer: principles and practice*. Philadelphia: Lippincott Williams & Wilkins; 2000. p. 778-97.
40. Effects of postoperative mediastinal radiation on completely resected stage II and stage III. epidermoid cancer of the lung. The Lung Cancer Study Group. *N Engl J Med* 1986;**315**(22):1377-81.
41. Stephens RJ, Girling DJ, Bleehen NM, et al. The role of post-operative radiotherapy in non-small cell lung cancer: a multicentre randomised trial in patients with pathologically staged T1-2, N1-2, M0 disease. Medical Research Council Lung Cancer Working Party. *Br J Cancer* 1996;**74**(4):632-9.
42. Muggia FM, Rozencweig M. *Lung Cancer: Progressive Therapeutic Research*. New York: Raven Press; 1979, p. 443.
43. Miller DL, McManus KG, Allen MS, et al. Results of surgical resection in patients with N2 non-small cell lung cancer. *Ann Thorac Surg* 1994;**57**(5):1100-1:1095-1000; discussion.
44. Douillard JY, Rosell R, De Lena M, Carpagnano F, et al. Adjuvant vinorelbine plus cisplatin versus observation in patients with completely resected stage IB-IIIA non-small-cell lung cancer (Adjuvant Navelbine International Trialist Association [ANITA]): a randomised controlled trial. *Lancet Oncol* 2006 Sep;**7**(9):719-27.
45. Goldie JH, Coldman AJ. A mathematic model for relating the drug sensitivity of tumors to their spontaneous mutation rate. *Goldie Cancer Treat Rep* 1979;**63**(11-12):1727-33.
46. Pisters KM, Ginsberg RJ, Giroux DJ, et al. Induction chemotherapy before surgery for early-stage lung cancer: a novel approach. Bimodality Lung Oncology Team. *J Thorac Cardiovasc Surg* 2000;**119**(3):429-39.
47. Shields TW, Higgins Jr GA, Lawton R, et al. Preoperative x-ray therapy as an adjuvant in the treatment of bronchogenic carcinoma. *J Thorac Cardiovasc Surg* 1970;**59**(1):49-61.
48. Warram J. Preoperative irradiation of cancer of the lung: final report of a therapeutic trial. A collaborative study. *Cancer* 1975;**36**(3):914-25.
49. Roberts JR, Eustis C, Devore R, et al. Induction chemotherapy increases perioperative complications in patients undergoing resection for non-small cell lung cancer. *Ann Thorac Surg* 2001;**72**(3):885-8.
50. Daly BD, Fernando HC, Ketchedjian A, Dipetrillo TA, et al. Pneumonectomy after high-dose radiation and concurrent chemotherapy for nonsmall cell lung cancer. *Ann Thorac Surg* 2006 Jul;**82**(1):227-31.
51. Sonett JR, Suntharalingam M, Edelman MJ, Patel AB, et al. Pulmonary resection after curative intent radiotherapy (>59 Gy) and concurrent chemotherapy in non-small-cell lung cancer. *Ann Thorac Surg* 2004;**78**(4):1200-5:discussion 1206.
52. Song S, Wientjes MG, Gan Y, et al. Fibroblast growth factors: an epigenetic mechanism of broad spectrum resistance to anticancer drugs. *Proc Natl Acad Sci U S A* 2000;**97**(15):8658-63.
53. Pearson FG, DeLarue NC, Ilves R, et al. Significance of positive superior mediastinal nodes identified at mediastinoscopy in patients with resectable cancer of the lung. *J Thorac Cardiovasc Surg* 1982;**83**(1):1-1.
54. Martini N, Flehinger BJ, Zaman MB, et al. Results of resection in non-oat cell carcinoma of the lung with mediastinal lymph node metastases. *Ann Surg* 1983;**198**(3):386-97.
55. Rosell R, Gomez-Godina J, Camps C, et al. A randomized trial comparing preoperative chemotherapy plus surgery with surgery alone in patients with non-small cell lung cancer. *N Engl J Med* 1994;**330**(3):153-8.
56. Roth JA, Fossella F, Komaki R, et al. A randomized trial comparing perioperative chemotherapy and surgery with surgery alone in resectable stage IIIA non-small-cell lung cancer. *J Natl Cancer Inst* 1994;**86**(9):673-80.
57. Rosell R, Gomez-Codina J, Camps C, et al. Preresectional chemotherapy in stage IIIA non-small-cell lung cancer: a 7-year assessment of a randomized controlled trial. *Lung Cancer* 1999;**26**(1):7-14.
58. Roth JA, Atkinson EN, Fossella F, et al. Long-term follow-up of patients enrolled in a randomized trial comparing perioperative chemotherapy and surgery with surgery alone in resectable stage IIIA non-small-cell lung cancer. *Lung Cancer* 1998;**21**(1):1-6.
59. Dillman RO, Seagren SL, Propert KJ, et al. A randomized trial of induction chemotherapy plus high-dose radiation versus radiation alone in stage III non-small-cell lung cancer. *N Engl J Med* 1990;**323**(14):940-5.
60. Le Chevalier T, Arriagada R, Quoix E, et al. Radiotherapy alone versus combined chemotherapy and radiotherapy in nonresectable non-small-cell lung cancer: first analysis of a randomized trial in 353 patients. *J Natl Cancer Inst* 1991;**83**(6):417-23.
61. Sugarbaker DJ, Herndon J, Kohman LJ, et al. Results of cancer and leukemia group B protocol 8935. A multiinstitutional phase II trimodality trial for stage IIIA (N2) non-small-cell lung cancer. Cancer and Leukemia Group B Thoracic Surgery Group. *J Thorac Cardiovasc Surg* 1995;**109**(3):473-83:discussion 483-485.
62. Fowler WC, Langer CJ, Curran Jr WJ, et al. Postoperative complications after combined neoadjuvant treatment of lung cancer. *Ann Thorac Surg* 1993;**55**(4):986-9.
63. DeCamp MM, Rice TW, Adelstein DJ, et al. Value of accelerated multimodality therapy in stage IIIA and IIIB non-small cell lung cancer. *J Thorac Cardiovasc Surg* 2003;**126**(1):17-27.
64. Schaake-Koning C, van den Bogaert W, Dalesio O, et al. Effects of concomitant cisplatin and radiotherapy on inoperable non-small-cell lung cancer. *N Engl J Med* 1992;**326**(8):524-30.
65. Albain KS. Induction therapy followed by definitive local control for stage III non-small-cell lung cancer. A review, with a focus on recent trimodality trials. *Chest* 1993;**103**(Suppl. 1):43S-50S.

66. Albain KS, Rusch VW, Crowley JJ, et al. Concurrent cisplatin/etoposide plus chest radiotherapy followed by surgery for stages IIIA (N2) and IIIB non-small-cell lung cancer: mature results of Southwest Oncology Group phase II study 8805. *J Clin Oncol* 1995;**13**(8):1880-92.
67. Rusch VW, Albain KS, Crowley JJ, et al. Surgical resection of stage IIIA and stage IIIB non-small-cell lung cancer after concurrent induction chemoradiotherapy. a Southwest Oncology Group trial. *J Thorac Cardiovasc Surg* 1993;**105**(1):97-104;discussion 104-106.
68. Ginsberg RJ, Hill LD, Eagan RT, et al. Modern thirty-day operative mortality for surgical resections in lung cancer. *J Thorac Cardiovasc Surg* 1983;**86**(5):654-8.
69. Harpole Jr DH, DeCamp Jr MM, Daley J, et al. Prognostic models of thirty-day mortality and morbidity after major pulmonary resection. *J Thorac Cardiovasc Surg* 1999;**117**(5):969-79.
70. Andre F, Grunewald D, Le Chevalier T. Persistence of viable tumor cells after radiation and chemotherapy for stage IIIB non-small cell lung cancer: an early marker of treatment failure. *J Thorac Cardiovasc Surg* 2001;**121**(2):403.
71. Choi NC, Carey RW, Daly W, et al. Potential impact on survival of improved tumor downstaging and resection rate by preoperative twice-daily radiation and concurrent chemotherapy in stage IIIA non-small-cell lung cancer. *J Clin Oncol* 1997;**15**(2):712-22.
72. Eberhardt W, Wilke H, Stamatis G, et al. Preoperative chemotherapy followed by concurrent chemoradiation therapy based on hyperfractionated accelerated radiotherapy and definitive surgery in locally advanced non-small-cell lung cancer: mature results of a phase II trial. *J Clin Oncol* 1998;**16**(2):622-34.
73. Grunenwald DH, Andre F, Le Pechoux C, et al. Benefit of surgery after chemoradiotherapy in stage IIIB (T4 and/or N3) non-small cell lung cancer. *J Thorac Cardiovasc Surg* 2001;**122**(4):796-802.1
74. Thames Jr HD, Peters LJ, Withers HR, et al. Accelerated fractionation vs hyperfractionation: rationales for several treatments per day. *Int J Radiat Oncol Biol Phys* 1983;**9**(2):127-38.
75. Withers HR. Biologic basis for altered fractionation schemes. *Cancer* 1985;**55**(Suppl. 9):2086-95.
76. Albain KS, Scott CB, Rusch VR, et al. Phase III comparison of concurrent chemotherapy plus radiotherapy (CT/RT) and CT/RT followed by surgical resection for stage IIIA (pN2) non-small cell lung cancer (NSCLC): initial results from intergroup trial 0139 (RTOG93-09). *Proc Am Soc Clin Onc* 2003;**22**:621.
77. Albain KS, Swann RS, Rusch VR, Turrisi AT, et al. Phase III study of concurrent chemotherapy and radiotherapy (CT/RT) vs CT/RT followed by surgical resection for stage IIIA(pN2) non-small cell lung cancer (NSCLC): outcomes update of North American Intergroup 0139 (RTOG 9309). *J Clin Oncol* 2005;**23**:16S:(June 1 Supplement):7014.
78. van Meerbeeck JP, Kramer GW, Van Schil PE, Legrand C, et al. Randomized controlled trial of resection versus radiotherapy after induction chemotherapy in stage IIIA-N2 non-small-cell lung cancer. *J Natl Cancer Inst* 2007 Mar 21;**99**(6):442-50.
79. Ciardiello F, Caputo R, Bianco R, et al. Inhibition of growth factor production and angiogenesis in human cancer cells by ZD1839 (Iressa), a selective epidermal growth factor receptor tyrosine kinase inhibitor. *Clin Cancer Res* 2001;**7**(5):1459-65.
80. Huang SM, Harari PM. Epidermal growth factor receptor inhibition in cancer therapy: biology, rationale and preliminary clinical results. *Invest New Drugs* 1999;**17**(3):259-69.
81. Woodburn JR. The epidermal growth factor receptor and its inhibition in cancer therapy. *Pharmacol Ther* 1999;**82**(2-3):241-50.
82. Akhurst T, Downey RJ, Ginsberg MS, et al. An initial experience with FDG-PET in the imaging of residual disease after induction therapy for lung cancer. *Ann Thorac Surg* 2002;**73**(1):259-64;discussion 264-266.
83. Wallace MB, Silvestri GA, Sahai AV, et al. Endoscopic ultrasound-guided fine needle aspiration for staging patients with carcinoma of the lung. *Ann Thorac Surg* 2001;**72**(6):1861-7.
84. Mentzer SJ, Swanson SJ, DeCamp MM, et al. Mediastinoscopy, thoracoscopy, and video-assisted thoracic surgery in the diagnosis and staging of lung cancer. *Chest* 1997;**112**(Suppl. 4):239S-241.
85. Mateu-Navarro M, Rami-Porta R, Bastus-Piulats R, et al. Remediastinoscopy after induction chemotherapy in non-small cell lung cancer. *Ann Thorac Surg* 2000;**70**(2):391-5.
86. Rami-Porta R. Restaging after induction therapy for non-small cell lung cancer. *Ann Thorac Cardiovasc Surg* 2002;**8**(6):325-7.
87. Van Schil P, van der Schoot J, Poniewierski J, et al. Remediastinoscopy after neoadjuvant therapy for non-small cell lung cancer. *Lung Cancer* 2002;**37**(3):281-5.
88. Detterbeck FC. Changes in the treatment of Pancoast tumors. *Ann Thorac Surg* 2003;**75**(6):1990-7.
89. Detterbeck F. *Diagnosis and treatment of lung cancer: an evidence-based guide for the practicing clinician.* Philadelphia: WB Saunders; 2001, p. 233-43.
90. Detterbeck FC. Pancoast (superior sulcus) tumors. *Ann Thorac Surg* 1997;**63**(6):1810-8.
91. Ginsberg RJ, Martini N, Zaman M, et al. Influence of surgical resection and brachytherapy in the management of superior sulcus tumor. *Ann Thorac Surg* 1994;**57**(6):1440-55.
92. Muscolino G, Valente M, Andreani S. Pancoast tumours: clinical assessment and long-term results of combined radiosurgical treatment. *Thorax* 1997;**52**(3):284-6.
93. Niwa H, Masaoka A, Yamakawa Y, et al. Surgical therapy for apical invasive lung cancer: different approaches according to tumor location. *Lung Cancer* 1993;**10**(1-2):63-71.
94. Chardack WM, Maccallum JD. Pancoast tumor: Five-year survival without recurrence or metastases following radical resection and postoperative irradiation. *J Thorac Surg* 1956;**31**(5):535-42.
95. Paulson DL. Carcinomas in the superior pulmonary sulcus. *J Thorac Cardiovasc Surg* 1975;**70**(6):1095-104.
96. Paulson DL. Carcinomas in the superior sulcus. *J Thorac Cardiovasc Surg* 1975;**70**(6):1095-104.
97. Rusch VW, Parekh KR, Leon L, et al. Factors determining outcome after surgical resection of T3 and T4 lung cancers of the superior sulcus. *J Thorac Cardiovasc Surg* 2000;**119**(6):1147-53.
98. Rusch VW, Giroux DJ, Kraut MJ, et al. Induction chemoradiation and surgical resection for non-small cell lung carcinomas of the superior sulcus: initial results of Southwest Oncology Group Trial 9416 (Intergroup Trial 0160). *J Thorac Cardiovasc Surg* 2001;**121**(3):472-83.
99. Rusch VW, Giroux DJ, Kraut MJ, Crowley J, et al. Induction chemoradiation and surgical resection for superior sulcus non-small-cell lung carcinomas: long-term results of Southwest Oncology Group Trial 9416 (Intergroup Trial 0160). *J Clin Oncol* 2007;**25**(3):313-8;Jan 20.
100. Rusch VW, Giroux D, Kraut MJ, Crowley J. Induction chemoradiotherapy and surgical resection for non-small cell lung carcinomas of the superior sulcus: prediction and impact of pathologic complete response. *Lung Cancer* 2003;**41**(2):S78.
101. Gonzalez-Stawinski GV, Lemaire A, Merchant F, et al. A comparative analysis of positron emission tomography and mediastinoscopy in staging non-small cell lung cancer. *J Thorac Cardiovasc Surg* 2003;**126**(6):1900-5.
102. Reed CE, Harpole DH, Posther KE, et al. Results of the American College of Surgeons Oncology Group Z0050 trial: the utility of positron emission tomography in staging potentially operable non-small cell lung cancer. *J Thorac Cardiovasc Surg* 2003;**126**(6):1943-51.

CHAPTER 20

Lung Cancer: Surgical Strategies for Tumors Invading the Chest Wall

Matthew A. Steliga, Michaela Straznicka, and Garrett L. Walsh

Historical Note
Demographics and Symptoms
Diagnosis
Staging
Treatment

Preoperative Assessment
Operative Techniques
Reconstruction
Postoperative Care
Complications

Pathology
Results
Summary

Lung cancer continues to be the leading cause of cancer-related deaths in both men and women. More than 75% of non–small cell lung cancer (NSCLC) is advanced in stage at presentation, with extensive locoregional disease or distant metastasis. The majority of resectable lung cancers are confined to the pulmonary parenchyma, but 5% to 8% extend beyond the lungs and invade the pleura, soft tissues, or osseous structures of the chest wall.[1,2] Chest wall invasion for surgical staging (T3) is defined as any tumor involvement into or beyond the parietal pleura. Pathologists can further describe these tumors by their depth of chest wall invasion, but this is infrequently reported in this subset of T3 patients.

HISTORICAL NOTE

Historically, chest wall invasion by a tumor of any histology was considered unresectable. Early surgical experience demonstrated that the surgical violation of the parietal pleura resulted in a sucking chest wound with immediate pulmonary collapse, often leading to the rapid demise of the patient. Dr. M. Michellau presented to the Institute of France in Paris in March of 1818 with a fungating mass protruding from his left chest wall. Dr. Richerand proposed a resection of the involved rib and pleura, an unprecedented operation at that time. On March 31, 1818, Dr. Richerand resected the left sixth and seventh ribs of Dr. Michellau, but acute respiratory distress occurred unexpectedly as the chest cavity was entered. The patient was saved by covering the aperture with a linen cloth plastered with cerate. Despite a rocky postoperative course, Dr. Michellau survived and returned home 27 days postoperatively. The pathology of the lesion is not known, but a primary rib malignancy is suspected.[3]

In the summer of 1883, a brilliant young surgeon, H. M. Block, in what was then called Danzig, East Prussia (now Gdansk, Poland) carried out the first planned pulmonary resection. Dr. Block had performed successful open chest surgery on experimental animals and was eager to apply his experience to humans.[4] He chose a young female relative with a diagnosis of bilateral pulmonary tuberculosis and performed a thoracotomy to resect her diseased lung. Although the details of the operation are not known, we do know that it had a tragic end.

A few days later, the short, brilliant career of Dr. Block ended with a self-inflicted gunshot wound to the head.[5]

Murphy[6] described his experiments and clinical experiences with open pneumothorax during his address to the American Medical Association in 1898. Parham,[7] in 1899, was the first in the United States to report resection of a bony chest wall tumor involving three ribs. A controlled pneumothorax with soft tissue coverage was created. This patient survived, but many who followed did not.

The difficulties of operating with an opened pleural space in a spontaneously breathing patient were all too apparent to the surgeons of those times. Working without adequate control of the airway and without ventilator support was difficult, and the patient quickly deteriorated once the chest was open. Many ideas were investigated to overcome these deficiencies and problems with anesthesia techniques.

Major surgical and anesthesia advances were introduced in 1904 at the German Surgical Congress in Berlin. Two techniques designed to surmount the open chest problem were proposed. Ferdinand Sauerbruch,[8] from the surgical clinic of von Mickulykz at the University of Breslau, introduced his method of *unterdruck* (low-pressure) ventilation. Lung expansion was maintained after thoracotomy by keeping an experimental animal's body inside a negative-pressure chamber (at −15 cm H_2O) while the head remained outside the chamber with the anesthesiologist. Brauer[9] described the benefits of *uberdruck* (high pressure) anesthesia, in which the lung was kept expanded by placing the patient's head in a glass positive-pressure chamber.

Surprisingly, the *unterdruck* method was initially the preferred technique. Sauerbruch and von Mickulykz built a negative-pressure operating room large enough to accommodate an entire surgical team, in which successful thoracic operations were carried out. These rooms continued to be built by Sauerbruch in Munich as late as 1918, making this approach the favored method in Germany through the 1930s. Sauerbruch's ideas and methods so dominated his associates' and contemporaries' ideas that little progress in other anesthetic techniques issued from Germany during this era.

Major progress, however, had already begun and would continue in France, England, and the United States during roughly the same period. The use of positive-pressure ventilation of the lungs was slowly being developed. Reliable delivery of positive pressure to the lungs was possible only by direct intubation of the trachea, and, at that time, a tracheotomy was the only technique for tracheal intubation. Most surgeons were unwilling to perform a tracheotomy simply to deliver an anesthetic under positive pressure. The first systematic use of intubation through the mouth using bellows to inflate the lung was by the Frenchman DePaul, who intubated and resuscitated neonates in the mid 1800s. Other French surgeons, Tuffier, Quenu, and Doyen, and Milton in Egypt, also used positive pressure during thoracotomies in the last few years of the 19th century.

In the late 1800s, two physicians from New York, Joseph O'Dwyer and George Fell, described intubation techniques and positive-pressure ventilation. Dr. O'Dwyer developed a practical method of endotracheal intubation for the treatment of diphtheria, which was applied in thousands of cases and resulted in a gratifying decrease in the mortality rate of that dreaded disease.[10,11] Dr. Fell used a crude device to maintain ventilation in patients suffering from drug overdoses.[12] In New Orleans, Parham and Matas used the combined Fell-O'Dwyer apparatus in 1898 to administer positive-pressure surgical anesthesia.[13]

The use of positive-pressure ventilation identified the need for cuffed endotracheal tubes for the reliable delivery of anesthesia to the lungs. Eisenmenger first described a cuffed endotracheal tube in 1893. Placement of such tubes was facilitated by Kirstein,[14] who introduced direct laryngoscopy in 1895 for safe, reliable placement of endotracheal tubes in the trachea. In 1907, Chevalier Jackson improved the laryngoscope and produced the instrument that is still in use today and bears his name.[15] A practical endotracheal tube design for general use was introduced by Guedel in 1928,[16] and its use became widespread starting in the 1930s. In 1938, the first operative use of ventilators was made with the Freckner Spiropulsator, developed in Sweden. In 1942, Griffith, in Montreal, Canada, introduced curare to facilitate intraoperative controlled ventilation.[17]

With these international advances in intubation techniques and airway management, positive-pressure anesthesia slowly became a clinical reality during the last few years of the 19th century and the first few decades of the 20th century. As a direct result, surgeons became increasingly willing to transgress the parietal pleura to address the complex pathologies of the thoracic cavity. From 1904 to 1929, surgeons began to specialize and to perform a series of pulmonary resections, and by 1929, thoracic surgery had become an established specialty. Most early lung resections and thoracoplasties were performed because of infections. Surgical morbidity and mortality rates were horrifying at first, and only the bravest patients and the most resilient surgeons chose to continue to work in the field. Sepsis was the predominant cause of death and was correlated mainly with an open pleural cavity.

In 1947, Coleman[18] reported long-term survival after en bloc excision of the chest wall with pulmonary resection. Concurrently, significant strides in chest wall reconstructive techniques were occurring through the use of fascia lata grafts, autogenous rib grafts, large cutaneous flaps, and latissimus dorsi muscle flaps, as described by Campbell in 1950[19] and Grillo and colleagues in 1966.[20] In the past 40 years, we have witnessed further refinements in surgical procedures, the use of prophylactic antibiotics, improved anesthesia delivery and monitoring, and the implementation and use of critical care units for postoperative ventilation. Today, these advances permit the safe and effective resection of locally advanced lung cancer with extensive chest wall involvement on a routine basis.

Pancoast tumors comprise a distinct surgical entity and are discussed separately (see Chapter 21).

DEMOGRAPHICS AND SYMPTOMS

Patients with lung cancer are usually 50 to 70 years old. Lung cancer is rarely seen in patients younger than 30 years, although with the ongoing epidemic of children and young teenage smokers, advanced lung cancer can be seen even in younger age groups (Fig. 20-1). Lung cancer with chest wall invasion most typically presents in patients in their

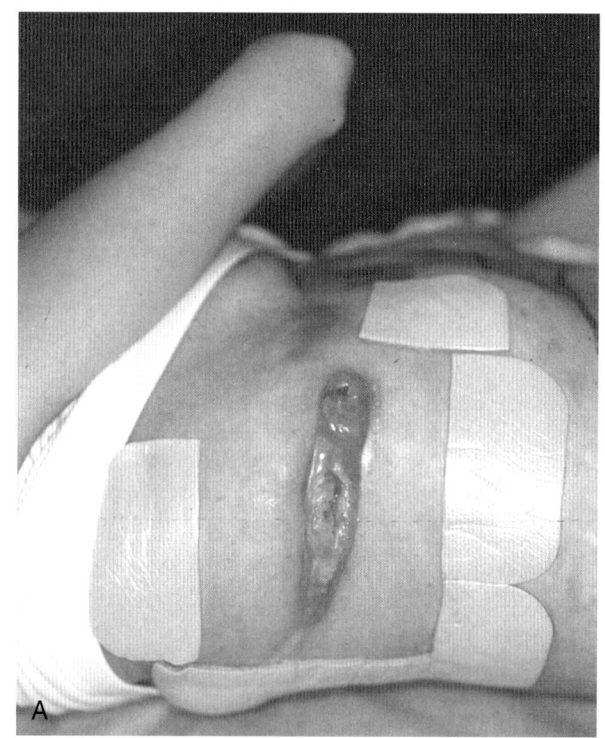

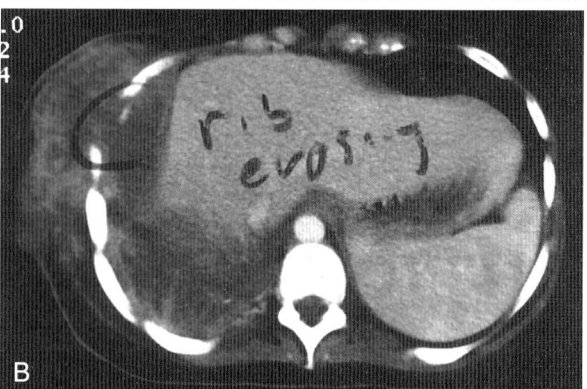

Figure 20–1
A, This 25-year-old woman presented to our institution with a nonhealing thoracotomy incision and a draining wound after an attempted decortication for what was initially believed to be a postpneumonic empyema. **B,** CT scan demonstrates a large right lower lobe adenocarcinoma of the lung with direct invasion of the chest wall as the cause for the nonhealing wound.

7th decade, with a median age of 64 to 66 years (range, 38 to 93 years).[21-23] Overall, lung cancer incidence and mortality continue to be disproportionately higher in men than in women, although the gap is narrowing. Lung cancer with chest wall invasion has an overwhelming predominance in men; women represent only 10% to 30% of patients in several recent studies.[2,21-23] A current or previous smoking history is elicited in approximately two thirds of patients, with an average 50-pack-year history per patient.[2,21]

The lung parenchyma has no sensory nerve fibers, which accounts for the often late clinical appearance of most bronchogenic tumors. The majority of patients have presenting symptoms related to compression, invasion, or obstruction of the lung parenchyma or airways, or invasion of the chest wall or mediastinal structures. Metastasis to distant organs, including neurologic symptoms and bone pain, unfortunately are common.

Patients whose lung cancer has invaded the chest wall have similar presenting symptoms, including chest pain (40% to 60%), cough (14%), recurrent lower respiratory tract infection (10% to 25%), weight loss (10% to 18%), hemoptysis (12%), and dyspnea (11%). However, as many as 25% of patients can be asymptomatic (Table 20-1).[2,21,22]

The right lung has a slight predominance for the location of lung cancers, both in general and for those with chest wall invasion.[2] Okada and coworkers described a marked predilection for the upper lobes in their series of lung cancers that invade the chest wall, although not all series confirm this finding.[23] Lung cancers in general have a slight predilection for upper lobes rather than lower lobes, which theoretically may be related to the relative increase in ventilation (and associated carcinogens) to the upper portions of the lungs.

Squamous cell carcinoma is the classic smoking-related tumor, and for many years it was the most common histology. In recent years, however, adenocarcinoma has overtaken squamous cell carcinoma as the most common lung cancer worldwide. Several series of patients with lung cancer invading the chest wall have demonstrated that squamous cell carcinoma remains the most common, followed closely by adenocarcinoma; large cell carcinoma and adenosquamous carcinoma comprise fewer of these tumors.[2,22,23] Average tumor diameter in these patients, by computed tomography (CT) measurements, was 6.5 cm; tumors ranged from 2 to 18 cm in maximum diameter.[2]

DIAGNOSIS

Chest roentgenography is useful for the identification of parenchymal lesions, although it has poor specificity and sensitivity for detecting chest wall involvement. Rib destruction is a reliable indicator of chest wall invasion, but it is identified on routine chest radiographs in only a fraction of cases. Tissue diagnosis of malignancy in these T3 lesions is usually obtained by transthoracic needle aspiration by interventional radiologists.

Peripheral lung lesions with the suggestion of chest wall involvement may require additional radiographic testing to confirm invasion. These radiographic techniques include CT scans, nuclear medicine (scintigraphic) bone scans, magnetic resonance imaging (MRI), and positron emission tomography (PET) scans. Although gross tumor involvement of the chest wall is easily diagnosed with these radiographic modalities, confirmation of isolated parietal or mediastinal pleural invasion is more difficult and often unreliable.[24-27]

The use of CT scans has greatly increased the precision of tumor localization, has allowed accurate evaluation of contiguous organ involvement, has improved assessment of lymph nodes, and has improved the identification of pulmonary metastasis. A CT scan is excellent for assessing rib destruction and intercostal muscle tumor extension, but it is relatively inaccurate for invasion limited to the parietal or mediastinal pleura.[24,25,27] Helical three-dimensional reconstruction has been shown to be superior to standard two-dimensional images, but the latter technology is universally used.[28] Shirakawa and associates[29] identified patients who had parietal pleural invasion by using inspiratory and expiratory CT scans. They demonstrated that a respiratory phase shift of greater than one half of a vertebral body height in middle and lower lobe tumors reliably predicted the absence of parietal pleural invasion. The accuracy and negative predictive value were 90% and 86%, respectively, in tumors located in the lower and middle lobes. For upper lobe tumors, however, the respiratory phase shift did not correlate with operative findings regardless of whether invasion was present. This discrepancy results from the minimal normal respiratory phase shift of these lung fields when the patients were studied in the supine position.

MRI has the advantages of multiplanar reconstruction and high differential signal intensity, which are invaluable for determining vascular invasion and spinal involvement. Conventional MRI, unfortunately, is just as limited as CT for evaluation of parietal and mediastinal pleural invasion. Kodalli and associates[26] used breath-hold inspiration and expiration MRI to assess parietal pleural invasion. Pleural invasion was excluded when tumor displacement exceeded 5 mm in reference to chest wall structures or relevant mediastinal structures (e.g., the aortic arch). This study identified 100% sensitivity and specificity for pleural invasion of tumors located in the middle lobe and basilar segments of the lower lobes. Studies of upper lobe tumors and those located in the apical segments of the lower lobes demonstrated a positive predictive value of only 40% but a negative predictive value of 100%. The superiority of MRI to CT lies in its ability to assess lung and diaphragm movement in a coronal plane. Insufficient respiratory motion is evident by a less-than-1-cm movement of the

Table 20–1
Presenting Symptoms in Patients with Lung Cancer with Chest Wall Invasion

Presenting Symptom	Occurrence(%)
Chest wall pain	40-60
Recurrent lower respiratory tract infection	10-25
Weight loss	10-18
Hemoptysis	12
Dyspnea	11
Cough	11
Asymptomatic	25

diaphragm on coronal images, and necessary scans could be repeated by asking the patient to take a deeper breath.

In a recent report, ultrasonography (US) was compared with CT for detection of chest wall involvement. In this series, 90 patients with suspected chest wall involvement were evaluated preoperatively with CT and US. Their ultrasound criteria for determining chest wall invasion were any two of the following: (1) tumor ingrowth seen into the chest wall, (2) interruption of the pleural reflection, (3) invasion of the ribs, and (4) impairment of movement with respiration. Using these criteria, US was deemed more sensitive than CT (89% versus 42%) with similar specificity (95% versus 100%).[30] Perhaps the real-time imaging of ultrasound during respiration leads to more accurate imaging data.

More invasive methods have been used for detection of parietal pleural invasion, including the use of expiratory dynamic CT after the introduction of a diagnostic pneumothorax.[31,32] Lack of invasion was diagnosed on the basis of an air space between the mass and adjacent structures. Sensitivity was 100% in both studies for chest wall invasion, although sensitivity dropped to 76% in cases of mediastinal invasion. Specificity for tumor involvement was 80% in the study by Watanabe and colleagues.[31] Benign pleural adhesions caused false-positive results in both of these studies. Complications were reported as mild and included chest pain, shortness of breath, and subcutaneous emphysema.

Despite these results from a variety of imaging techniques, we do not use these special imaging studies. We feel that these tests are not warranted because they may subject high-risk patients to a pneumothorax and ultimately are unlikely to alter the planned operative procedure. In some cases, reviewing the CT scans obtained during transthoracic needle biopsy reveals minimal pneumothoraces, incidentally obtained as a result of biopsy. Often, these images show clear separation from the chest wall (Fig. 20-2).

For most patients, preoperative assessment of chest wall involvement is not critical, as it does not often alter resectability or treatment strategy. However, for the marginal patient, who may be borderline for toleration of lung resection, identifying significant chest wall invasion, and thus the necessity for combined pulmonary and chest wall resection, may lead the clinician to pursue definitive nonoperative treatment with chemoradiotherapy. Often, regardless of imaging studies, the final assessment of chest wall involvement can be made only by direct palpation at the time of surgery.

STAGING

Accurate staging of NSCLC is critical for effective clinical management. Standard preoperative evaluation includes a complete history and physical examination, laboratory tests (including complete blood cell counts, serum electrolytes, glucose, calcium, phosphorous, and liver function tests), electrocardiogram (ECG), chest radiograph, and CT scans of the chest and upper abdomen to include the adrenal glands. Combined CT-PET scans have become routine in our staging workup of patients with lung cancer. MRI of the brain is performed whenever a patient has neurologic symptoms or when a lesion is locally advanced or nodal disease is suspected.

Surgical-pathologic staging is performed according to the International Staging System for Lung Cancer, using information about the primary tumor (T), nodal status (N), and distant metastasis (M).[33] T status denotes characteristics of the primary tumor, including size, location, and local aggressiveness. Chest wall involvement increases the T status to T3. *Chest wall involvement*, however, includes a wide pathologic spectrum, from invasion of the parietal pleura only, to full-thickness chest wall replacement by tumor. Other characteristics that denote T3 status include invasion of the diaphragm, mediastinal pleura, or parietal pericardium, or a tumor in a main-stem bronchus 2 cm or less from the carina but not involving the carina. Full-thickness invasion into the mediastinum, including the heart, great vessels, trachea, or vertebral bodies, denotes a T4 classification. Pancoast tumors by definition are at least T3 because of the chest wall invasion. Further invasion with involvement of the subclavian artery or vein or the brachial plexus is not specifically described in the staging system, although we consider them T4 because of their poorer prognosis. Satellite lesions located in the involved lobe also denote T4 classification, but they will be considered T3 under

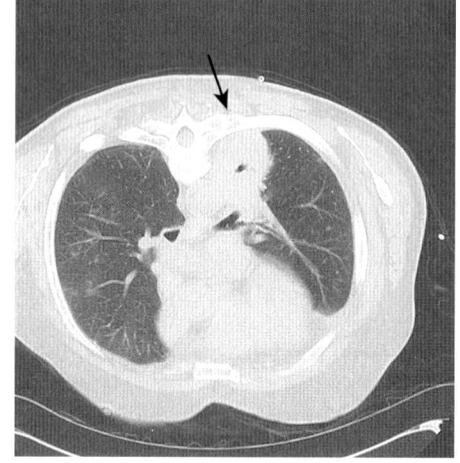

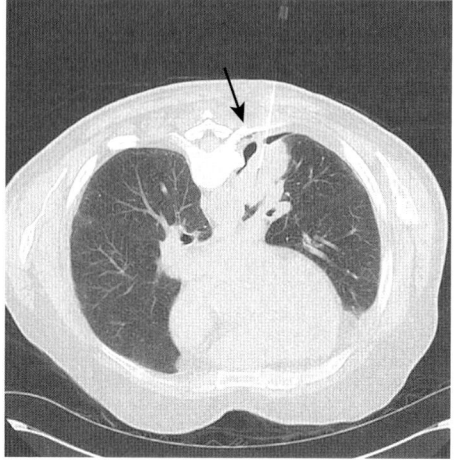

Figure 20–2
CT of the chest reveals a lung mass abutting the posterior rib (*arrow* in left image). By reviewing the images obtained during transthoracic needle biopsy, the mass can be seen moving away from the chest wall with a minimal focal area of pneumothorax (*arrow* in right image). Other images revealed complete separation from the chest wall. Note: The patient is prone in these scans for obtaining the biopsy.

the International Association for the Study of Lung Cancer (IASLC) proposed changes to the staging system.[34] Most T4 tumors are not considered suitable for surgical resection, although those patients in whom an R0 resection (microscopically negative margins) is possible may be treated surgically.

Nodal status (N) is the second feature of the International Staging System. Ipsilateral hilar node involvement is classified as N1 disease and is not considered a contraindication for resection. Ipsilateral adenopathy of the mediastinum increases the nodal status to N2. The most effective treatment modality for these patients is controversial and is best managed with a multidisciplinary board. Chemotherapy and radiation is the primary management of patients with N2 disease. Surgical resection may be an option for those not responding to induction therapy. Spread of tumor to the contralateral mediastinal, scalene, or supraclavicular nodal basins denotes N3 status, and these patients are not considered surgical candidates.

Patients without evidence of distant metastatic disease are considered to have M0 disease and may be candidates for surgical resection if T and N status are acceptable. Distant metastatic disease is noted as M1 and is almost always considered inoperable. Systemic treatment in the form of chemotherapy is currently the treatment of choice, often in combination with radiation therapy for local control.

In 1997, an important change was made to the TNM staging system regarding tumors with chest wall involvement. NSCLC defined as T3N0M0 was classified as stage IIIA by the prior system described by Mountain in 1986.[35] Survival data of patients with these tumors revealed that their clinical course with surgery alone was more favorable than that of other patients with stage IIIA disease (i.e., those with hilar or mediastinal lymph node involvement: T3N1, T3N2, T1N2, or T2N2). Subsequently, T3N0M0 tumors were down-staged to stage IIB with this revision.

Changes on the horizon for the TNM staging system are proposed but have not been implemented at this time.[34] The proposed changes are included in the upcoming 17th edition of the IASLC staging manual. Same-lobe satellite lesions will be down-staged from T4 to T3, and there are new size criteria for the different T groupings. However, the proposed changes will not alter the management or staging of tumors with chest wall invasion, which will still be classified as T3. The staging of T3N0 will still be considered stage IIB, and T3N1 or T3N2 will still be considered stage IIIA.

Because the survival rate of lung cancer patients with chest wall involvement and nodal disease is significantly worse than that of patients with chest involvement alone, the clinical challenge for surgeons is to identify nodal involvement by imaging or by minimally invasive biopsy techniques before subjecting patients to extensive chest wall resections. The importance of correct pretreatment staging cannot be overemphasized. Hilar and mediastinal nodes can be assessed before surgery with CT, MRI, and PET scans. Integrated CT-PET scans measure metabolic activity of tissues and can detect disease in otherwise normal-size-appearing nodal tissue, but accuracy for sub-centimeter nodules is reduced.

Despite advances in imaging techniques, mediastinoscopy still remains the most sensitive and specific test for evaluating the mediastinal nodes and should be considered before any major chest wall resection. Another option for staging the mediastinum is endobronchial ultrasound (EBUS)-guided fine-needle aspiration. EBUS involves the use of a specially designed bronchoscope with an ultrasound transducer at the tip allowing real-time image guided biopsy of nodes adjacent to the airway, and it can access some nodes at levels 10, 11, and 12.[36,37] Sensitivity and specificity of EBUS have been reported to be higher than those of CT or PET and comparable with those of mediastinoscopy, and it is less invasive.[38] Because of the anatomic location, the preoperative assessment of N1 disease is more problematic via mediastinoscopy, but these nodes are easily reached with EBUS. Patients with T3N1 disease should still be considered for en bloc resections, and they have a better survival rate than those with N2 disease.

Although it is unlikely that peripheral lung tumors involving the chest wall extend into the airway, it is our practice to perform bronchoscopy immediately before resection to identify any unsuspected endobronchial disease and to assess the airway anatomy. Navigational bronchoscopy can access peripheral tumors out of the range of standard bronchoscopy to obtain tissue for diagnosis[39]; although this is not commonplace today, it may have a more widespread role for biopsying peripheral tumors in the future.

Extrathoracic metastases are found in up to 50% of patients with newly diagnosed lung cancer.[40] Patients with symptoms suggestive of central nervous system involvement are evaluated with an MRI scan of the brain. Symptoms or laboratory findings suggestive of disseminated malignancy, such as weight loss, bone pain, or elevated alkaline phosphatase, are evaluated with bone scintigraphy scans.

Bone scintigraphy scans are used to detect occult bony metastases and confirm bony lesions in symptomatic patients. The vertebral column is the most commonly affected region for bone metastases. MRI is accepted as the most accurate imaging modality in detecting bone metastases in the vertebral column, and focal imaging can be guided by bone scan abnormalities or symptoms.[41-43] Suspect uptake in bones other than the vertebral column also requires further investigation, although MRI scans become less useful. False positives are seen in the bony thorax when a history of rib fractures or trauma is noted. False negatives can be appreciated when bone scans are correlated with PET scans. Positive lesions on PET scans, which are not seen on bone scans, may represent soft tissue metastasis.[44] Durski and associates[44] recommend that all patients be staged with a PET scan, and that bone scans should be performed only if symptomatically indicated when PET scans are negative. In their series, the use of bone scans in addition to PET scans did not change the clinical stage of any of their patients, although it allowed more precise localization of skeletal abnormalities.

PET scans using [F^{18}]fluorodeoxyglucose (FDG) are routinely used in addition to CT scans for both initial diagnosis and staging of NSCLC. One study suggests that obtaining both a PET and a CT scan is more cost-effective than performing a CT scan alone for staging.[45] The reported sensitivity and specificity of PET for thoracic lymph node involvement are 70% to 100% and 81% to 100%, respectively. CT has a sensitivity and specificity of 25% to 81% and 56% to 94%, respectively.[46-50] The American College of Surgeons Oncology Group trial ACOSOG Z0050 evaluated the usefulness of PET for staging NSCLC. The results support staging all NSCLC patients with PET to reduce the rate of nontherapeutic thoracotomy, but they recommend confirming PET-positive mediastinal nodes with mediastinoscopy. In addition, their recommendations include using PET to guide tissue biopsy in the cases of suspected single-site distant metastases.[51] Integrated PET-CT was compared with PET alone in a prospective blinded trial in which the same radiologist read an integrated scan, and at a later date was asked to read the PET images only. Integrated PET-CT was shown to be more accurate at predicting T and N status of patients, and better at determining stage I and stage II disease.[52] Integrated PET-CT scans have become standard for preoperative evaluation of all our patients with NSCLC.

TREATMENT

Patients with confirmed N2 disease who are devoid of distant metastatic disease are offered a treatment protocol with induction chemotherapy. Surgery is offered to those patients whose tumors show an objective response to chemotherapy and whose disease can be completely resected.[22] Progression of disease while on chemotherapy is generally regarded as a contraindication to surgery, as is evidence of N3 disease. Preoperative radiation therapy has not been shown to increase survival in several studies, but it has demonstrated an increased operative mortality.[1,22,53] Preoperative radiation therapy therefore is not used at our institution.

Patients with evidence of metastatic spread should not be considered surgical candidates except in extraordinary circumstances. These circumstances may include isolated brain metastases that can be resected before lung resection.

PREOPERATIVE ASSESSMENT

The most important risk factors for perioperative complications for patients who are undergoing resection of lung tumors are cardiovascular and pulmonary disease, metabolic disorders (e.g., diabetes), and malnutrition. A complete preoperative assessment therefore includes physiologic testing for cardiac and pulmonary reserve, optimal management of diabetes, and nutritional support when needed. Spirometry, arterial blood gases, alveolocapillary carbon monoxide diffusion capacity (DL_{CO}), and xenon ventilation scans determine pulmonary reserve and predict postoperative function. Cardiac evaluation, including ECG, echocardiography, stress testing, and even cardiac catheterization, may be required to identify correctable disease in high-risk patients. Nutritional assessment includes aggressive diabetic control, optimization of protein stores, and possible enteral or parenteral feeds for severely malnourished patients. Serial measurements of prealbumin levels may be used as a guide to nutritional improvement.

Most surgeons try to leave a patient with at least 33% of predicted forced expiratory volume in 1 second (FEV_1) postoperatively. Spirometry, xenon scanning, and exercise oxygen testing are helpful in identifying patients who are truly medically inoperable on the basis of these pulmonary function criteria. There are no studies, however, that can accurately predict the increased postoperative pulmonary compromise of patients with T3 lesions who require chest wall resections. It is often difficult to predict preoperatively the extent of required rib resection and the requirement for chest wall stabilization and reconstruction. Often, a surgeon ends up removing more chest wall than anticipated. Phrenic nerve or diaphragmatic involvement may lead to further impaired respiratory physiology. The overall effect on chest wall mechanics and respiratory physiology must be taken into account when evaluating the medical condition of the patient and the extent of pulmonary resection. Occasionally, in patients with marginal lung function, a nonanatomic or subsegmental resection of the lung may be required if the chest wall component of the operation is extensive.

OPERATIVE TECHNIQUES

Good communication and cooperation with our anesthesia colleagues are crucial to the success of these operations. Several anesthesia techniques have dramatically improved our intraoperative course and our patients' postoperative recovery. The placement of epidural catheters before the institution of general anesthesia is encouraged for all of our patients. A double-lumen endotracheal tube greatly facilitates visualization during the surgery.

In the great majority of patients, the tumor can be approached via a posterolateral thoracotomy. For tumors that involve the chest wall and the apex of the chest (either superior sulcus tumors proper or large upper lobe tumors with chest wall and neck extensions), an initial anterior neck approach to dissect the subclavian vessels and the brachial plexus may be beneficial before addressing the posterior chest wall component (Fig. 20-3). Depending on the tumor location, the incision may be tailored more posteriorly and extended superiorly between the scapula and spinous processes. Review of the radiographic studies and palpation of the interspaces should identify an intercostal space at least one rib space below the inferior margin of the tumor for entry into the chest cavity. On entry into the hemithorax, careful digital examination of the lung and chest wall is performed to determine tumor attachment and assess chest wall fixation. The chest cavity is examined closely for pleural dissemination or metastatic deposits at other sites. Great care should be taken to prevent disruption of thin adhesions of the tumor to the parietal pleura that may be involved with tumor.

When tumor invasion into the chest wall is radiographically evident before surgery, an en bloc chest wall resection should be carried out with at least one uninvolved rib and intercostal muscle above and below the mass.[54] An en bloc resection is defined as removal of lung parenchyma in continuity with a portion of the adjacent parietal pleura and chest wall soft tissues. The overlying integument is generally left intact, although complete extension of tumors through the skin can be seen (Fig. 20-4).

On rare occasions when the tumor is large, its bulk can impede safe exposure of hilar structures. In this situation, several firings of a stapler through normal, uninvolved pulmonary parenchyma can permit the initial removal of the tumor and chest wall, with safer dissection of the delicate hilar vessels without the risk of torsion and traction created by the weight of the tumor and attached chest wall. An en bloc resection is preferred whenever it is feasible.

It is more difficult to determine the extent of malignant pleural involvement when the adhesions are thin and filmy between the tumor and the chest wall. The tumor may be somewhat mobile on palpation. A surgeon must resist the temptation to simply lyse these adhesions. An extrapleural dissection must be initiated away from the site of attachment. If the plane is not easily identified at any time during the extrapleural dissection, then the extrapleural dissection must be immediately halted and a full-thickness chest wall resection performed. If the extrapleural dissection appears to proceed easily, frozen section analysis of the parietal pleura is recommended.[2] If the tumor transgresses the parietal pleura on frozen section,

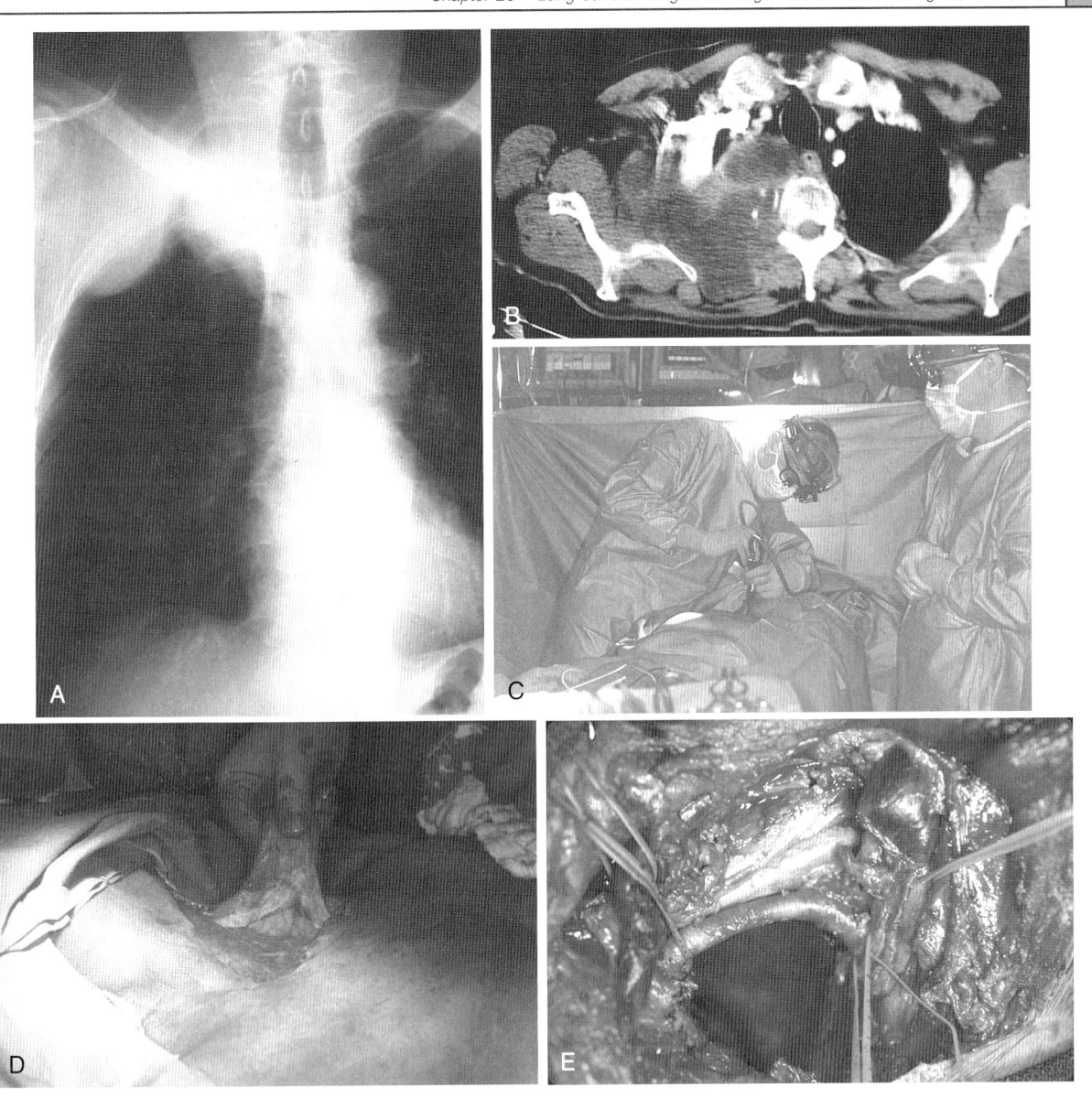

Figure 20–3
A, Chest radiograph demonstrating a large right upper lobe apical tumor, which was diagnosed a sarcomatoid carcinoma by transthoracic needle biopsy. **B,** CT scan demonstrates the full-thickness chest wall involvement with tumor extension into the posterior chest wall musculature. **C,** A mediastinoscopy is performed routinely to rule out N2 or N3 nodal involvement before proceeding with the extensive lung and chest wall resection. **D,** An initial supraclavicular neck dissection is performed to dissect the subclavian vessels and brachial plexus. This is the initial hockey-stick skin incision along the anterior border of the sternocleidomastoid muscle and along the clavicle. **E,** A close-up of the resection of the first and second ribs from the anterior approach with resection of the subclavian vein and preservation of the subclavian artery and brachial plexus, as shown.

then additional resection of the chest wall is required. When performing an extrapleural dissection, marking the extent of the extrapleural dissection with metal clips on the chest wall can leave a permanent radiographic landmark as to the prior extent of attachment and guide adjuvant radiotherapy if final pathologic margins do come back as positive.

Circumferential margins of 2 cm are generally regarded as adequate, although some surgeons advocate a larger margin of 4 cm on the rib resection.[2,55] In these studies, the mean number of ribs resected was three, with a range of one to five.[2,21] The oncologic resection should never be compromised by a less-than-complete resection.

Several circumstances deserve additional mention. Special attention needs to be paid to tumors extending into the intervertebral foramen without intraspinal extension. Disarticulation of the ribs is performed through the costotransverse joints with ligation of the nerve roots as they exit the spinal column.[56] Tumors that extend into the vertebral column may require a laminectomy to expose the epidural tumor and involved nerve root. The tumor is dissected free from the dura, and the nerve roots are identified and transected. When the tumor invades the vertebral bodies themselves, a partial resection of the vertebral body may be performed without the need for instrumentation. Resection should be carried out to grossly uninvolved bone and can include complete vertebrectomy with spinal reconstruction (Fig. 20-5). Further discussion regarding vertebral resection and reconstruction is beyond the scope of this chapter.

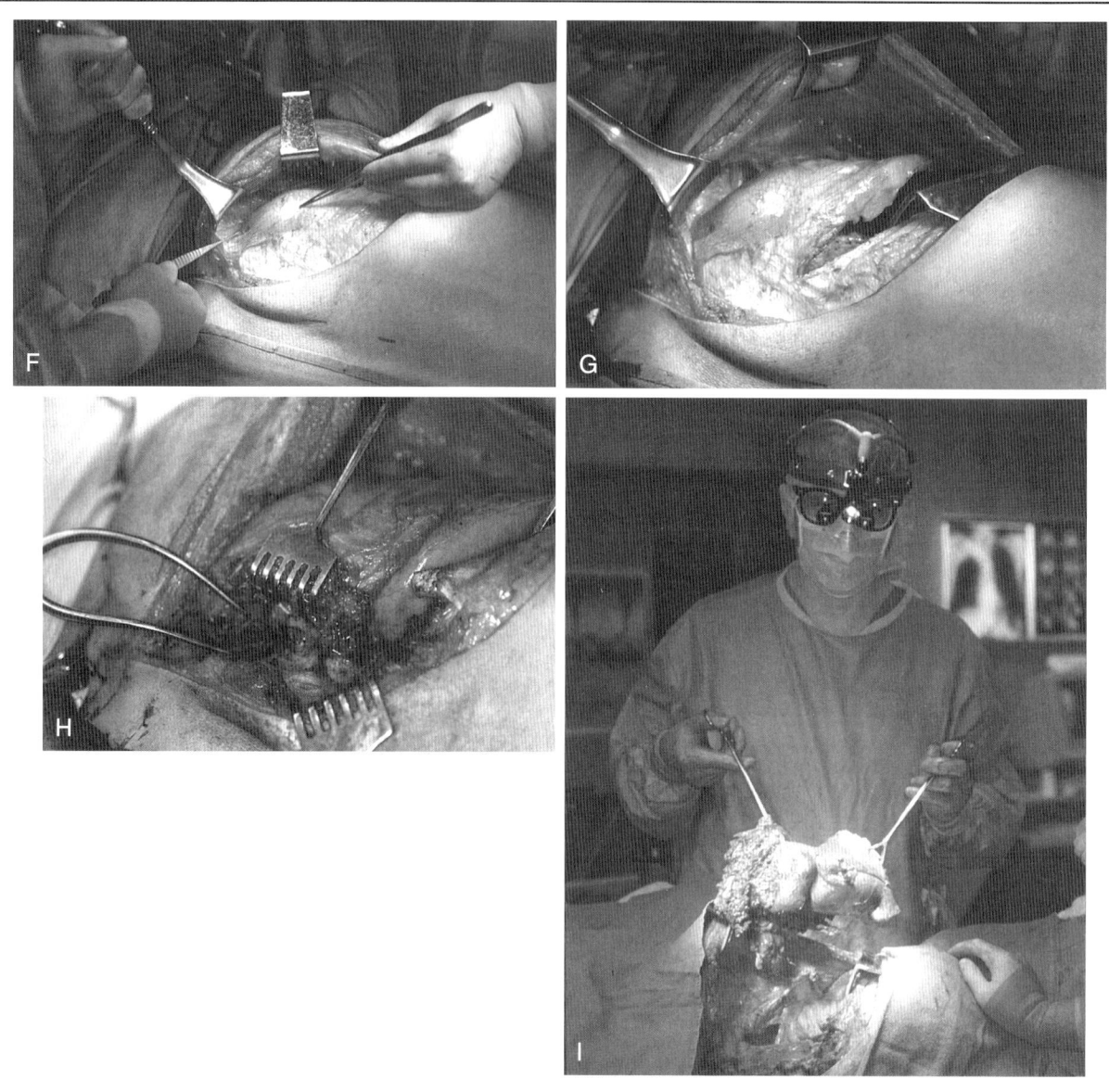

Figure 20–3, cont'd
F, The patient is repositioned. The initial dissection is through a posterolateral thoracotomy with elevation of the scapula after division of the latissimus dorsi muscle and reflection of the serratus anterior muscle. The tumor bulge into the interspaces of the chest wall can be appreciated. There is no gross tumor involvement of the external surface of the chest wall, however. **G,** An interspace is entered caudal to the inferior extent of the tumor involvement. **H,** The posterior elevation of the paraspinous muscles and disarticulation of the posterior ribs from the transverse processes and vertebral bodies. **I,** Complete en bloc removal of the chest wall (ribs one to five) and the right upper lobe. (See color versions of **C, D, F,** and **I** in the online edition through Expert Consult.)

Anterior tumors that invade into the sternum are resected en bloc with the involved portion of the sternum and attached ribs. An adequate resection may necessitate a complete sternectomy. Reconstruction with a rigid prosthesis to prevent flail is usually required after a complete sternectomy. If the resection is limited to either the manubrium or less than one third of the sternum, reconstruction is often unnecessary.[57]

The resected portion of the chest wall remains attached to the lung and is allowed to drop into the hemithorax, where pulmonary resection is then carried out in the usual manner. The extent of pulmonary resection is determined by the amount of parenchymal involvement, as well as by the pulmonary reserve of the patient. A crucial determinant for long-term survival is the ability to achieve a complete (R0) resection.[1] The survival rate of patients who undergo incomplete resection (R1) is comparable with that of patients who have not had a resection at all.[1] Most frequently, lobectomy is sufficient to achieve an R0 resection.

Burkhart and associates,[21] in 95 operations for bronchogenic carcinoma with chest wall involvement, performed a lobectomy in 80% of patients in their series, pneumonectomy in 13%, bi-lobectomy in 4%, and sublobar resection in 3%. Okada and associates,[23] in their series of 132 patients, favored a more lung-preserving approach, with 49% undergoing lobectomy, 15% segmentectomy, 13% sleeve lobectomy, 10% pneumonectomy, 8% lobectomy with partial resection, and 5% sleeve bi-lobectomy or sleeve pneumonectomy. In both series, a complete mediastinal and hilar lymph node dissection was performed in each patient. In all cases, the operating surgeon confirmed the clinical impression of an R0 resection. In our practice, we agree with the general recommendation to perform a complete mediastinal and hilar nodal dissection in these patients.

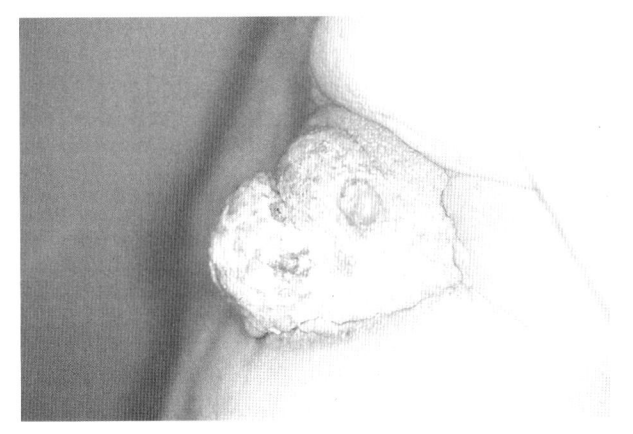

Figure 20–4
A fungating tumor in the left anterior chest wall in a 75-year-old man. It originated from a bronchogenic carcinoma of the lingula with transmural invasion of the chest wall and skin.

RECONSTRUCTION

Reconstruction of the chest wall defect is controversial. Some surgeons do not routinely reconstruct chest wall defects in any patients, and they report minimal morbidity. Facciolo and associates[2] performed 104 thoracotomies with full-thickness chest wall resection without prosthetic reconstruction of the costal elements in any patient. Chest wall defects were closed with scapula repositioning or chest wall muscle transfers. Exact details regarding location and complexity of the defects were not described, although the results were excellent.

In general, all full-thickness skeletal defects that have the potential for paradox should be considered for reconstruction. Both the size and location of the chest wall resection should guide the decision for reconstruction. When the defect is small, approximately 5 cm or less, the skeletal component can be ignored and the defect closed with overlying soft issues only. Posterior defects up to 10 cm in diameter may not require reconstruction because the overlying scapula provides support. Exceptions include midthoracic posterior defects that allow the scapular tip to become entrapped in the bony thorax during full range of motion of the arm. In these cases, either the chest wall can be reconstructed or the scapular tip can be amputated.

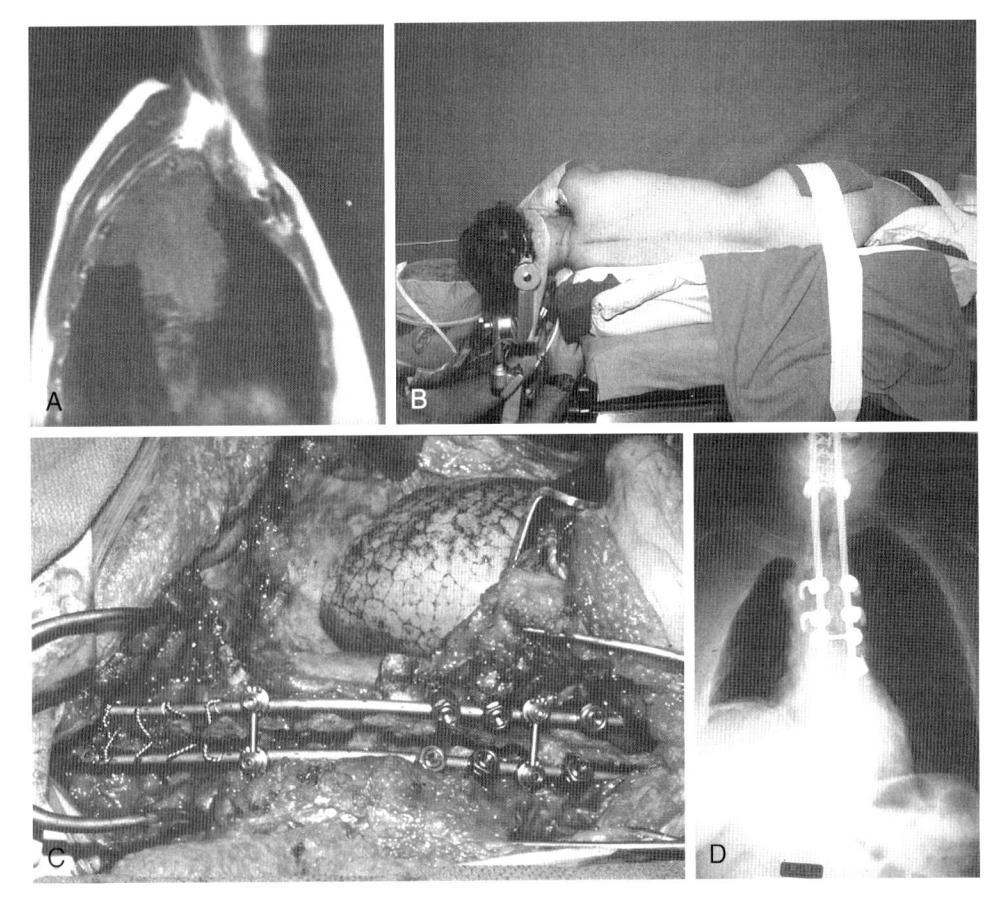

Figure 20–5
A, Lateral chest radiograph demonstrating a large right upper lobe lung cancer with involvement of the chest wall and T1 through T3 vertebral bodies. **B,** Operative positioning of the patient with the head in cervical tongs to immobilize it and to maintain the alignment of the cervical and thoracic spines. The patient is additionally secured on a beanbag and taped with padding appropriate to the anterior superior iliac spine. **C,** Intraoperative photograph showing the resected chest wall, right upper lobe, and multilevel vertebral body resection, with reconstruction with posterior rods and anterior stabilization. **D,** Posteroanterior chest radiograph demonstrating postoperative instrumentation. (See color version of **B** in the online edition through Expert Consult.)

Many complex chest wall chest defects require not only skeletal stabilization, but also skin and soft-tissue coverage to protect the reconstruction. Indications for reconstruction include the need for structural stability, cosmesis for anterior and lateral chest wall defects, obliteration of dead space, and a need to restore the chest wall integrity (by recruitment of healthy soft tissue from nonanatomic areas).

Reconstruction can be performed using autogenous tissues, such as fascia lata grafts or muscle transpositions, or various prosthetic materials, including mesh, metals, or soft-tissue patches. The use of autogenous tissue is favored when the wound to be closed is contaminated. Grossly contaminated wounds may need to remain open for a period of time for aggressive local wound care before attempted closure, sometimes at the expense of prolonged mechanical ventilation.

The most commonly used autogenous grafts are locally advanced muscle flaps. Although transposition of the latissimus dorsi muscle for chest wall coverage was described in 1896 by Tansini, it was Jurkiewicz and associates who reintroduced the musculocutaneous concept in 1977 and created a surge of interest in muscle and musculocutaneous flap reconstruction of the thoracic cavity.[58] The use of muscle flaps should be anticipated before surgery, and the operation conducted to protect the muscle of choice and its vascular pedicle at all times (Fig. 20-6).

The most widely used local muscle flaps are the latissimus dorsi, pectoralis major, rectus abdominis, serratus anterior, trapezius, and deltoid muscles. The latissimus dorsi muscle has excellent versatility because of its large size and wide arc of motion, allowing it to reach both the anterior and the posterior thorax. The pectoralis major muscle also displays great versatility, with significant limitations seen only when posterior thoracic coverage is needed. In those cases, it can be used as a free flap. Less frequently, the transverse rectus abdominis musculocutaneous (TRAM) flap is used. It is used almost exclusively for anterior defects and is rotated about its vascular pedicle.

When muscle flaps are not available or cannot be used, a variety of prosthetic materials are available. In fact, because of the availability and easy handling of synthetic materials, many surgeons prefer to use synthetic grafts for reconstruction even if muscle flaps are available. The choice of prosthetic material can vary, but the type of material used often depends on the surgeon's preference. LeRoux and Shama have set forth the ideal characteristics of a prosthetic material: rigidity to abolish paradoxical chest motion, inertness to permit ingrowth of fibrous tissues and decrease the likelihood of infection, malleability so that it can be fashioned to the appropriate shape at the time of the operation, and radiolucency to allow follow-up of the underlying problem.[59]

Additional desirable features include hypoallergenicity, lack of proven carcinogenicity, the ability to withstand sterilization, the ability to not be modified by bodily fluids, and adequate strength. Although no substance to date perfectly fulfills all of these criteria, various synthetic and alloplastic materials can be used with satisfactory results.

Polypropylene mesh (PM) (Marlex, Cranston, RI) with or without methylmethacrylate sandwich, polytetrafluoroethylene (PTFE) mesh, and Vicryl mesh are examples of materials that have been used in different situations. PTFE is made in a variety of thickness sizes; a 2-mm thickness is required for chest wall reconstruction to tolerate the tension generated during closure. Some surgeons consider PTFE to be easier to handle than PM because it lends itself to a slight stretch, can be sutured with fewer wrinkles and surface irregularities, and may create a watertight seal of the pleural space.[57] However, Deschamps and associates[60] compared PM mesh with PTFE and observed no significant differences in outcomes or complications.

Polypropylene mesh with methylmethacrylate (PPMM) sandwich provides the most rigidity and perhaps the best cosmetic result, at the price of greater difficulty of implantation. When the chest wall resection is extensive and the possibility of paradoxical movement of the reconstruction is suspected, this level of rigidity is desired. A few key points need to be kept in mind when working with this unyielding material. After the specimen in removed, the patient is returned to a neutral position by unflexing the operating table if initially flexed on positioning. An imprint of the defect is made to determine the size of the reconstruction, and the mesh is tailored to leave approximately 2 to 3 cm of extra material circumferentially with which to secure the patch to the remaining chest wall. A thin layer of methylmethacrylate is applied directly to the mesh, leaving 2 to 3 cm of mesh circumferentially overlapping the chest wall and free of cement. The layer of cement should not extend completely to the edges of the ribs, but leave a gap of at least 1 cm. If the cement is allowed to extend to the rib edges, respiratory motion and movement of the torso can lead to undesirable and often painful clicking as the unyielding solid prosthesis moves against the bony elements of the chest wall. A second layer of mesh, of identical size, is quickly applied to the cement, thereby creating the sandwich. The cement generates a significant amount of heat as it hardens, so care must be taken to avoid contact with unprotected tissue. When the reconstruction is of the lateral chest wall, it is important to re-create the curvature of the thorax. This may be accomplished by allowing the sandwich to harden on a malleable retractor that has been shaped appropriately, or by allowing the sandwich to harden on the patient's (protected) iliac crest.

Regardless of the material used, the patch is secured taut with heavy interrupted nonabsorbable sutures either through or around the remaining ribs. If the spine constitutes the posterior border of the defect, the sutures may be placed through drill holes in the transverse processes. The patch is then covered with adequate healthy soft tissue. Intrathoracic chest tubes are tunneled a distance from the reconstruction and positioned to avoid direct contact with the synthetic material. Subcutaneous closed suction drains should be used when extensive flaps have been raised and a large potential dead space has been created.

The simplest and most practical method of coverage is local tissue advancement. This is particularly important in patients who have received high doses of radiation; the local tissues may have impaired healing potential, and in many cases rotation of a pedicled muscle flap from a nonirradiated area may be advantageous. Sometimes the local muscle flaps are unavailable because the muscles have been extirpated or the vascular pedicle has been destroyed by surgical ablation or irradiation. In those cases, free tissue transfer of flaps using microvascular reconstruction can be performed with excellent results.[61] Often, these complex cases require the close interaction of the thoracic surgical team with our plastic surgeon colleagues. Available grafts can include contralateral latissimus

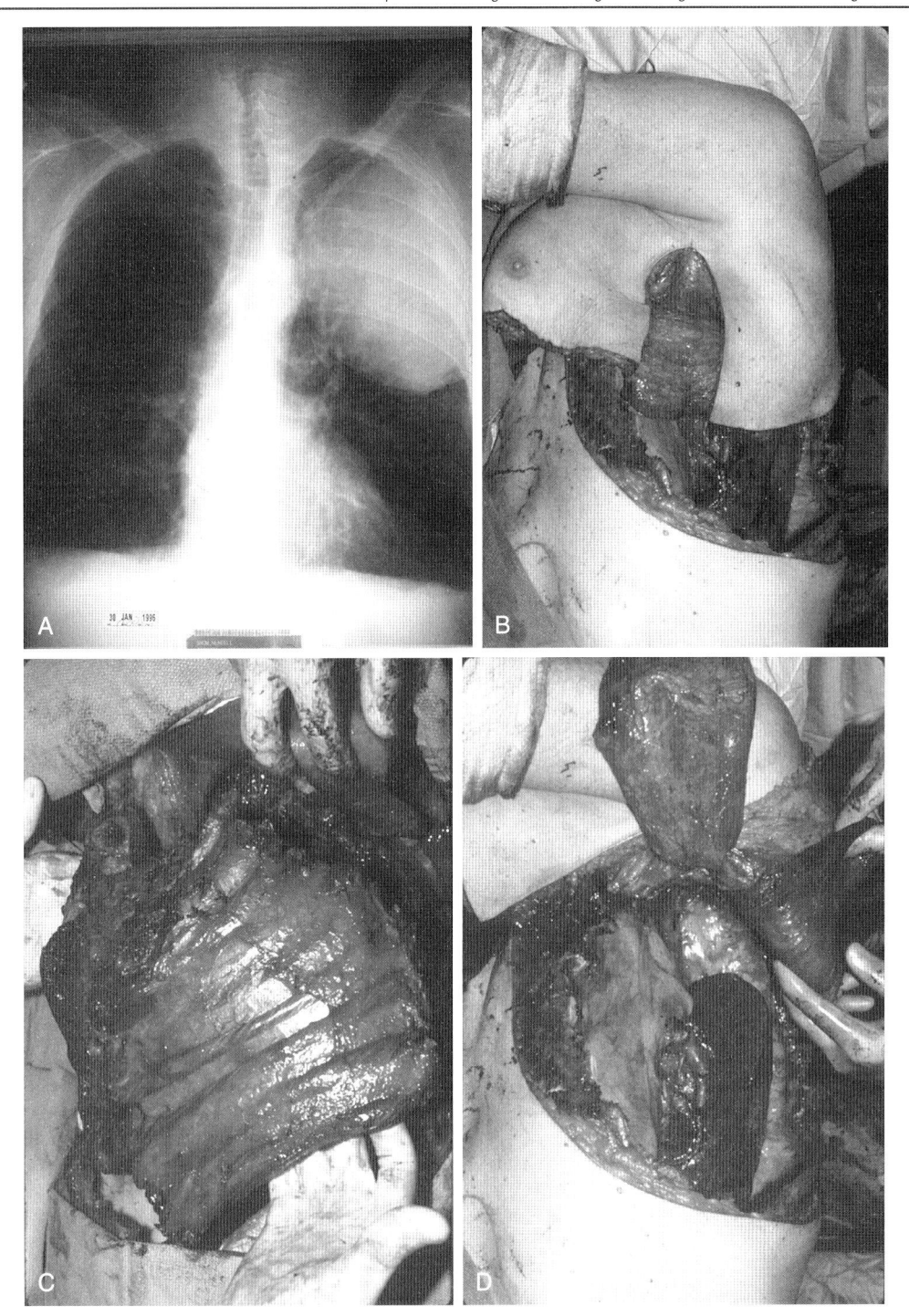

Figure 20–6
A, Posteroanterior chest radiograph demonstrating a large squamous cell carcinoma of the left upper lobe involving ribs one through seven. Mediastinoscopy was negative. **B,** Lateral operative positioning with the entailed skin incision raised for muscle flaps. **C,** Operative photo demonstrating extensive chest wall resection of seven ribs with en bloc left upper lobe attached. **D,** Resulting surgical chest wall defect with previously mobilized muscle flaps (latissimus, serratus, and pectoralis) that are used to cover the prosthetic chest wall reconstruction. (See color version in the online edition through Expert Consult.)

dorsi and serratus anterior muscles, as well as both ipsilateral and contralateral TRAM flaps.[61] The omentum is an excellent salvage flap that can be used when the pedicled muscle flap fails. Suction drains are frequently used to eliminate dead space, or when there are large raw surfaces over the prosthetic reconstruction. Drains are usually removed when the daily output is less than 25 mL/day from each drain.

Lung tumors that involve the chest wall are exceedingly rare in children, but children present a unique challenge to the thoracic surgeon when reconstruction is necessary. Depending on the age of the child, growth of the chest wall continues, thereby limiting the ability to use prosthetic materials for reconstruction. As the child outgrows the reconstruction, the mesh may cut through its anchors and re-create the defect.

If a more solid reconstruction is used, permanent mesh can act as a tether, eventually leading to contracture and deformity. Tuggle and colleagues[62] have reported successful chest wall reconstruction using bioabsorbable copolymer plates in four children. This material has been used for cranial and facial reconstruction in the pediatric population. They cite benefits that include excellent tensile strength and the ability to be molded and resorbed, which would leave residual firm fibrous tissue but theoretically not limit growth. Their report in this limited series indicates follow-up (only 2 years) without instability or growth limitation at that point.[62] Ideally, reconstruction should be performed with rotational muscle flaps whose nerve supplies are carefully preserved, to allow for growth and a dynamic contribution to chest wall development.[63]

POSTOPERATIVE CARE

Postoperative care should be tailored to each individual patient. A patient with good preoperative pulmonary function who had a limited resection and reconstruction should be extubated in the operating room at the conclusion of the surgery and allowed to convalesce on a telemetry ward. A frailer patient with an extensive resection and reconstruction may require intubation for 24 to 48 hours in the intensive care unit, with meticulous respiratory hygiene. For all patients, we prefer to continue epidural analgesia until the chest tubes are removed, or up to 7 days after surgery (whichever comes first). Aggressive pulmonary hygiene, including early ambulation, incentive spirometry, and bronchodilators, is essential and is attended by a full-time respiratory therapy staff on the wards. All patients remain on telemetry monitors throughout their hospital stay. The use of antibiotics postoperatively is usually limited to 24 hours of a broad-spectrum cephalosporin. Chest tubes are removed when air leaks have been sealed and when drainage is less than 100 mL per 8-hour shift. Additional postoperative care is similar to that of other thoracotomy patients.

COMPLICATIONS

Complications specific to chest wall resection and reconstruction include wound seroma formation, wound infection involving the prosthesis, and respiratory mechanical changes subsequent to prosthetic placement.[60-64] Small seromas are best managed with observation, because the majority resolve with time. Large or symptomatic seromas can be repeatedly aspirated under strict sterile conditions with little risk of contamination. Surgical obliteration is infrequently necessary and is reserved for recalcitrant seromas.[60]

Wound infections that occur with synthetic grafts usually require removal of the prosthesis and replacement with either autogenous reconstruction or open wound care with delayed closure. Prolonged air leaks from violated visceral pleural surfaces or fissures can allow respiratory bacteria to infect the overlying prosthesis. Every attempt must be made to seal or oversew any raw lung surfaces and decrease the remaining free space in the hemithorax before placement of the prosthetic material. In all pulmonary resections, including the upper lobes, the inferior pulmonary ligament should be divided to permit sufficient mobility of the remaining lung in the hemithorax. Chest tubes should be placed in the hemithorax, minimizing their direct contact with the mesh. Polypropylene mesh is preferable to PTFE when significant air leaks are present. The smooth surface of PTFE often makes it more difficult for a lung prosthesis apposition to occur and can result in a localized bronchopleural fistula that declares itself months later. Polypropylene mesh permits more vigorous adhesions, leading to rapid ingrowth of the lung, and is better suited for the "contaminated" environment of an air leak.

The development of a bronchopleural fistula after pneumonectomy is an extremely morbid complication to treat, and in cases with chest wall resection and synthetic reconstruction, the treatment options are limited and complex. The majority of patients require removal of the prosthesis and prolonged open wound care. Patients who survive the initial sepsis and demonstrate signs of wound healing may be considered for complex reconstructions, which may include muscle flaps, omental flaps, and even thoracoplasty. Frequently, these complicated cases are best handled using a multispecialty approach, with the aid of talented plastic surgeons familiar in reconstructive techniques.

Delayed wound infections can occur as a result of seroma aspiration or hematogenous seeding from distant infection. In these cases, careful inspection of the prosthesis in the operating room is required. The majority of early prosthesis infections require removal of the prosthesis, followed by local wound care. When infections appear months after the primary surgery, removal of the prosthesis without replacement is often well tolerated without pulmonary compromise. After several months, sufficient fibrous tissue has developed to support the chest wall mechanics. Delayed wound infections may have had adequate time for incorporation of the prosthesis by granulation tissue, especially in the case of polypropylene, making prosthesis removal difficult and even unnecessary. Deschamps and associates[60] allowed those prostheses that were well incorporated by granulation tissue to remain in situ, using aggressive wound débridement and frequent dressing changes. They were able to salvage about one half of these infected reconstructions without removal of the prosthesis, and without development of delayed wound infections or draining sinus tracts.

Rarely, complications occur that are related to mechanical failure of the prosthesis, with patch dehiscence resulting in lung herniation, or flail physiology. We encountered one case in which a particularly active teenage patient fractured his PPMM prosthesis in a fall, resulting in uncomfortable clicking and instability. This necessitated replacement (Fig. 20-7).

Postoperative respiratory mechanical changes are often difficult to measure, and they vary with the type of prosthesis used. The loss of viscoelasticity and inhomogeneity result from the replacement of a dynamic chest wall with a rigid structure that prevents chest wall mobility. Animal studies suggest that PTFE is preferable to PPMM because it allows the chest wall to remain dynamic during the respiratory cycle.[64] Lardinois and associates[65] studied patients preoperatively and 6 months postoperatively and found no significant deterioration of FEV_1, and they noted concordant chest wall to prosthesis movements in the majority of patients.

Cerebrospinal fluid (CSF) leaks can occur when the dura is violated during dissection in the intervertebral foramina or during partial or complete vertebrectomies. The nerve roots should be ligated distal to the emergence of the external

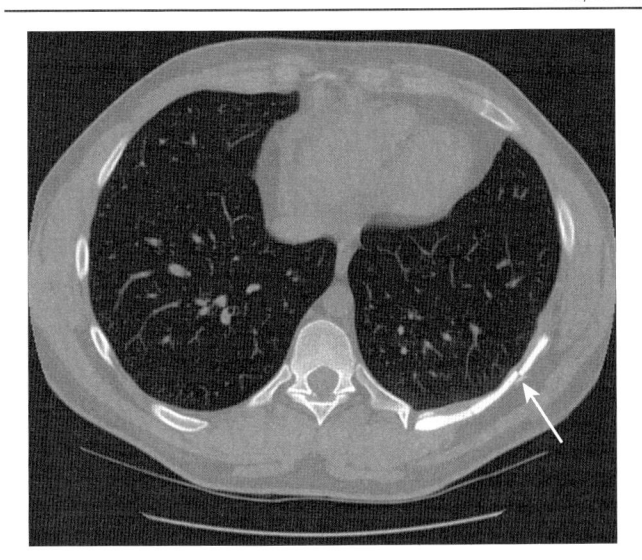

Figure 20-7
An active young patient fractured his polypropylene-methylmethacrylate chest prosthesis *(arrow)*. The instability and clicking were uncomfortable, necessitating reoperation.

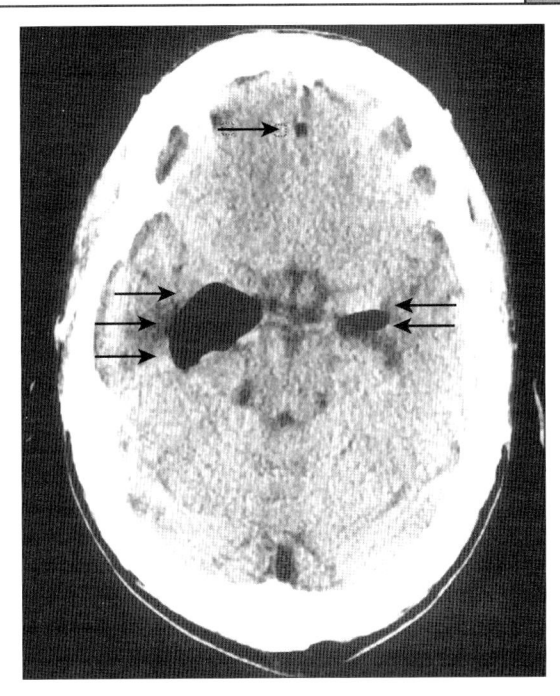

Figure 20-8
CT scan of the brain demonstrating the pathognomonic finding of air in the ventricular system of the brain *(arrows)* secondary to a bronchopleural-subarachnoid fistula from a combined chest wall, lung, and vertebral body resection.

sheath covering the cord. Potential spinal fluid leaks should be carefully evaluated during the initial operation. If a small dural tear has occurred during the resection, it needs to be repaired with fine monofilament sutures and covered with an autogenous tissue transfer using intercostal muscle, diaphragm, or pleura. Negative intrathoracic pressure coupled with positive pressure created in the CSF can lead to a chronic CSF leak. Initial treatment includes a lumbar drain and patient immobility in a supine position to minimize the CSF pressure. Supine bed rest of a post-thoracotomy patient can be associated with significant pulmonary complications.

Caution with hemostasis around the vertebral foramina is of paramount importance. Excessive use of monopolar electrocautery in this region could lead to transmitted cautery current, resulting in nerve or even spinal injury; judicious use of bipolar cautery is warranted. Aggressive packing of oxycellulose to control hemorrhage at an intervertebral foramen has led to a report of paraplegia caused by swelling of the oxycellulose. Fortunately this was reversible with immediate reoperation, removal of the oxycellulose and coverage with fibrin glue, and a pericardial fat pad.[66]

Patients who have required extensive combined lung and chest wall resections that extend to the vertebral bodies and dural sac can have fascinating delayed complications. For example, a patient in whom a small dural rent was identified and repaired during the resection of a tumor involving the vertebrae required a chest tube for 10 days for a prolonged air leak that occurred during the dissection of the interlobar fissure. The patient had no problems after the removal of the chest tubes and discharge from the hospital. Several months later, he had mental status changes and a seizure that was thought, on clinical grounds, to probably represent metastatic disease to the brain. A CT scan demonstrated a significant amount of air in the brain (Fig. 20-8), which originated from a small bronchopleural subarachnoid fistula. This required a re-do thoracotomy with interposition of a pedicled omental flap between the lung and the dural sac to close the small communication. Within 48 hours, the patient's neurologic status normalized.

PATHOLOGY

A complete resection (R0) is defined as pathologic evidence of disease-free (negative) tissue margins on final pathology and an assessment by the surgeon that all grossly detectable disease, including nodal disease, has been removed. Patients who had complete gross resection at thoracotomy but were found to have positive margins on final microscopic pathologic review are classified as having undergone an incomplete (R1) resection. Gross residual disease after an attempted resection is classified as an R2 resection, including residual nodal disease that could not be removed.

Depth of chest wall invasion can be grouped into three levels on the basis of the final pathologic examination: parietal pleura only; parietal pleura and soft tissues; and parietal pleura, soft tissues, and bone. Complete pathologic stage (TNM) is based on microscopic examination of the primary mass, all surrounding margins, and nodes.

The evaluation of the world literature pertaining to chest wall resections in patients with lung cancer is often complicated because surgical practices vary. Some surgeons proceed directly to en bloc full-thickness chest wall resections rather than attempting to strip the parietal pleura by extrapleural maneuvers. In Facciolo and associates' series of 104 patients who underwent full-thickness, en bloc resections of lung with attached chest wall, the pathologic depth of invasion was limited to parietal pleura in only 27%, parietal pleura and soft tissues in 35%, and parietal pleura, soft tissue, and bone in 38%.[2] All margins were microscopically negative on final pathologic review. All lymph nodes were negative in 80% (N0), 5% had positive hilar or lobar nodes (N1), and 15% had positive mediastinal (N2) nodes.

Chapelier and associates[67] also exclusively performed full-thickness resection of any tumors found by the naked eye to be invading at least the parietal pleura. A total of 100 patients were treated by this method. Pathologic evaluation revealed parietal pleural invasion in 29% of cases, parietal pleura and intercostal muscle invasion in 47% of cases, and osseous invasion in 24% of cases. Microscopically negative margins were attained in all but one patient. Nodal status was 65% N0, 28% N1, and 7% N2.

Burkhart and associates[21] reviewed their experience with 95 resections in patients with bronchogenic carcinoma with invasion of the chest wall, all treated with full-thickness chest wall resection. Depth of invasion extended into the parietal pleura only in 31% of patients, into the parietal pleura and soft tissues in 45% of patients, and into the osseous structures in 24% of patients. Seventeen percent of patients had pathologically involved N1 nodes, and 15% had pathologically involved N2 nodes. A presumed R0 resection was obtained in all cases.

Downey and associates[1] reported on 334 patients who underwent thoracic exploration for T3 tumors involving the chest wall at Memorial Sloan-Kettering Hospital. Intraoperative results included 175 patients who achieved an R0 resection, 94 who achieved an R1 or R2 resection, and 65 who underwent exploration only. Of the 175 patients who did attain an R0 resection, 80 (46%) underwent an extrapleural resection based on intraoperative surgeon judgment of the level of invasion. All 80 had evidence of parietal invasion only. The remaining 95 patients underwent full-thickness chest wall resection, and 19% had parietal pleural invasion, 25% had parietal pleural and soft tissue invasion, and 56% had invasion involving the osseous structures.

Magdeleinat and associates[22] attempted an extrapleural resection in all patients whose parietal pleura could be easily removed. Intraoperative frozen sections were obtained when any doubt existed about negative margins. Tumors fixed to the deeper structures were removed with the associated full-thickness chest wall. A total of 201 patients were studied, of whom 89 (44%) had tumor invasion limited to the parietal pleura. Ten of these patients underwent a full-thickness chest wall resection because the surgeon suspected deeper invasion intraoperatively. Only one patient who underwent an extrapleural resection had an underestimation of invasion, with microscopic residual identified at final pathology. Thirty-four patients (17%) did not achieve an R0 resection, most often because of residual tumor at the lateral edges of the resection. Nodal disease was absent in 58% (N0), lobar or hilar nodal disease was seen in 26% (N1), and mediastinal nodal disease was seen in 13% (N2). Three percent of patients had T4 disease.

Pathologic staging with standard histopathologic evaluation has been augmented with the use of immunohistochemical (IHC) stains to detect micrometastatic disease in lymph nodes and at resection margins. Mineo and colleagues analyzed nodes and margins of their en bloc lung and chest wall resections ($N = 47$) with IHC stains and found that greater than 10% of patients had only margins positive on IHC, which strongly correlated with local failure, and 12% had only nodal micrometastases seen with IHC staining, which correlated with distant relapse.[68] None of their patients who were IHC positive in the lymph nodes or margins lived to the 4-year follow-up, whereas those who were node negative and margin negative by IHC had a 73% 5-year survival. This appears to be a strong prognostic factor, but whether IHC detection of disease can lead to improved delivery of adjuvant therapy and subsequent survival advantage remains to be seen.

RESULTS

Operative mortality is defined as mortality within 30 days of surgery or within the same hospitalization. Improvements in preoperative screening, anesthesia techniques, and postoperative care have decreased the incidence of postoperative mortality in many studies. Long-term results are affected most importantly by complete resection to microscopically negative margins and by absence of N2 nodal involvement.[69] The extent (number of ribs) of chest wall resection is not a determinant for 5-year survival as long as an R0 resection is accomplished. These results are validated by several studies.

Overall complications and mortality in patients with combined pulmonary and chest wall resection are greater than of pulmonary resection alone. This is not only because of the added potential complications unique to chest wall resection but also because of the increased surgical insult and physiologic impairment from chest wall resection. A review by Martin-Ucar and colleagues[70] from Leicester of their experience with lung and chest wall resection in 41 patients indicated increased 60-day mortality in those with any of the following: significant weight loss (BMI < 18.5), advanced age (>75 years old), and decreased preoperative FEV_1 (<70% of predicted), with a 47% 60-day mortality for patients with one or more of the aforementioned risks, and 0% mortality for their patients who did not have any of the three factors.

Weyant and colleagues[71] reported on 262 chest wall reconstructions (141 were pulmonary resections with chest wall resection). In their series, the greatest predictor of postoperative respiratory complications was the size of the chest wall resection; they advocated rigid repair with PPMM sandwich for physiologic stability of the chest wall. They caution against performing pneumonectomy with chest wall resection; in their series, four of nine patients who underwent pneumonectomy with chest wall resection died postoperatively.

Facciolo and associates[2] reported no operative mortality and a rate of major complications of 20%, which included atrial fibrillation, bleeding, prolonged air leak, and empyema. Forty percent of patients received postoperative radiation therapy, and all patients with N2 disease received postoperative chemotherapy. The overall 5-year survival rate was 61%, with a median survival period of 74 months. Statistically worse 5-year survival rates were noted in patients with N2 disease when compared with patients with N0 disease (18% versus 67%). Depth of invasion also affected survival rates, with a 79% survival rate at 5 years for pleural involvement only, compared with a 56% survival rate for pleural, soft-tissue, and bone involvement. An impressive 90% 5-year survival rate was noted in the subset of patients with N0 disease whose tumors were limited to the parietal pleural invasion only. The addition of postoperative radiation therapy dramatically increased 5-year estimated survival rates from 47% to 74%, although the criteria for administering postoperative radiation are not clearly defined.

Chapelier and associates[67] had different results. The operative mortality rate was 4%, and postoperative complications were noted in 16% of patients. The median survival period was 18 months, the 2-year survival rate was 41%, and the 5-year survival rate was 18%. Significantly worse 5-year survival rates were noted in patients with N2 disease when compared with those with N0 or N1 disease (0% versus 22% versus 9%, respectively). Invasion limited to the pleura only was an independent factor favoring long-term survival when compared with deeper invasion ($P = .02$). The long-term survival for patients with well-differentiated tumors was significantly better than that for those with poorly differentiated tumors ($P = .005$). Postoperative radiation therapy or adjuvant chemotherapy did not improve survival in this study.

Burkhart and associates[21] summarized the Mayo Clinic experience, with somewhat higher mortality and morbidity rates. The operative mortality rate was 6.3%, and the complication rate was 45%. The overall 5-year actuarial survival rate was 39%, with best survival rates noted in patients with stage IIB disease (T3N0M0) (44%), and worse rates for patients with stage IIIA (26%). Interestingly, women in their study had a significantly improved 5-year survival rate over that of men (53% versus 39%, respectively), and women without evidence of nodal disease had the best survival rate (61% 5-year survival). Survival rates in all groups were affected by depth of invasion; tumors that invaded the parietal pleura only resulted in a 5-year survival rate of 50%, compared with 35% in patients with tumor invasion into the soft tissues, and 31% in patients with osseous involvement. Although these results did not reach statistical significance, the trend is suggestive of results seen at other institutions. Of their patients, 10% received neoadjuvant chemotherapy or radiation therapy, or both, with a disappointing increase in operative mortality rates noted in those patients who received radiation. No improvement in survival rates was seen in pretreated patients.

Volotini and colleagues[72] retrospectively analyzed outcomes of their lung resections with chest wall involvement in 68 patients. A multivariate analysis revealed that survival was affected by nodal status, complete resection, and depth of chest wall invasion. Their node negative patients had a 42% 5-year survival, but those who were node positive (N1 or N2) had 17% survival at 5 years. Those with tumors involving the parietal pleura had significantly better 5-year survival rates than those with deeper invasion (43% versus 9%). They had three patients with positive margins; none lived to 1 year.

Matsuoka and colleagues[73] reported similar conclusions with their experience of lung resections involving the chest wall. They also found poorer 5-year survival for N2 positive patients compared with node negative patients (6% versus 44%), and poorer survival for those with incomplete resections (14% compared with 34% for complete resections). They, however, did not find depth of chest wall invasion to correlate with outcome.

Doddoli and colleagues[74] in France reported their series of 309 patients from three institutions. In their experience, lung resection involving the chest wall was associated with an 8% operative mortality rate and a 33% complication rate. They reported a 5-year survival of 40% for patients with stage IIB (T3N0) disease, but only 12% for patients with stage IIIA (T3N1-2). In their population of patients with stage IIB (T3N0) disease, en-bloc resection afforded better 5-year survival (60%) than extrapleural resection (39%). The impact of R1 or R2 resection could not be determined, because their series only included those with R0 resection.

The Memorial Sloan-Kettering experience, as summarized by Downey and associates,[1] is comparable with other reports. The operative mortality rate, including all patients who underwent surgery, was 3%. Patients who left the operating room with either R1 or R2 disease had a dismal 5-year survival rate of 4%, which was comparable with those patients who underwent exploration without resection (0%). Patients who received R0 resection had an overall 5-year survival rate of 32%. Further analysis in the R0 group demonstrated a survival advantage in node-free patients: a 5-year survival rate in patients with T3N0 of 49%, with T3N1 of 27%, and with T3N2 of 15% ($P < .0003$). After either complete extrapleural or en bloc resection, there was no significant difference in survival rates between histologic groups, nor was there any difference in survival rates, by univariate analysis, based on pathologic demonstration of depth of tumor invasion in the chest wall. Overall, there was no observed significant difference in survival rates after a complete extrapleural resection compared with a complete en bloc resection. However, further subgroup analysis demonstrated that patients with N0 disease had a prolonged survival period when receiving an extrapleural resection as opposed to an en bloc resection (65 months versus 21 months, respectively, $P < .01$). This conflicts with the aforementioned series by Doddoli and coworkers, where stage IIB patients had better survival with en bloc resection.[74] They also noted no survival advantage to radiation therapy given preoperatively, intraoperatively, or postoperatively.

Magdeleinat and associates[22] documented a 7% operative mortality rate and a 36% complication rate. Predictably, perioperative complications were more frequent in older patients and in patients with limited pulmonary reserve. Actuarial 5- and 10-year survival rates for the entire population were 21% and 13%, respectively. After complete and incomplete resection, 5-year survival rates were 24% and 13%, respectively. The highest survival rate was noted again in the subgroup of patients without nodal involvement. The authors noted an increased 5-year survival rate in patients whose tumor did not extend beyond the parietal pleura (37%) as compared with those whose tumor did extend past the parietal pleura into the chest wall proper (15%). Of note, in patients with disease limited to the pleura, the type of resection (extrapleural or chest wall) did not affect survival rates (37% and 31%, respectively).

Elia and colleagues[75] from Italy reported similar outcomes in their 110 patients: a 0% mortality rate and 28% complication rate. Again, nodal status was strongly correlated with 5-year survival (47% for N0 versus 0% for N1 or N2). They also analyzed survival of their N0 patients by type of resection and found no difference in survival for extrapleural versus en bloc resection. The survival of R1 resections was not reported, and breakdown of survival by depth of chest wall involvement was not analyzed. Comparison of outcomes between the various studies can be seen in Table 20-2.

Summary

In summary, bronchogenic lung cancer with invasion into the chest wall is seen in less than 10% of patients with resectable disease. Although chest wall invasion denotes a T3 tumor classification, it does not preclude resectability. Extensive preoperative staging is required because metastatic disease is a contraindication for surgical treatment. Patients diagnosed

Table 20–2
Results of Surgical Resection of Lung Cancer with Chest Wall Invasion

Lead Author (Date)	Mortality (%)	Major Morbidity (%)	5-Year Survival Overall (%)	5-Year Survival with N0 (%)	5-Year Survival with N2 (%)	5-Year Survival: Pleural Invasion Only (%)	5-Year Survival: Invasion Beyond Pleura (%)	5-Year Survival: R1 or R2 Resection (%)
Burkhart (2002)	6	45	39	44	26	30	31	N/A
Chapelier (2000)	4	16	18	22	0	N/A	N/A	N/A
Doddoli (2005)	8	33	31	40	8	45	N/A	N/A
Downey (1999)	6	N/A	32	49	15	33	34	4
Elia (2001)	0	28	35	47	0	N/A	N/A	N/A
Facciolo (2001)	0	19	61	67	18	79	54	N/A
Magdeleinat (2001)	7	36	24	25	21	37	15	13
Matsuoka (2004)	N/A	N/A	30	44	6	33	36	14
Volotini (2006)	4	N/A	32	42	17 (N1 or N2)	43	9	0

N/A, not available.

with N2 disease should not be considered candidates for primary surgical treatment. When they are available, these patients should be considered for protocol treatments that may include induction chemotherapy followed by surgery if an appropriate response is seen.

The operative approach may include an extrapleural resection only, when tumor invasion is limited to the parietal pleura, or it may include a more extensive en bloc resection when deeper soft-tissue and bony chest wall invasion demonstrated. The most important predictors of long-term patient survival are the achievement of an R0 resection and nodal status. Reconstruction is generally required for anterior and lateral defects when a flail segment is created, and for large posterior defects that may cause a trapped scapula. Reconstruction options are numerous, including autogenous tissue flaps, rotational muscle flaps, and a variety of prosthetic materials. The choice of reconstruction is based on each individual patient and the clinical situation, surgeon preference, and the availability of specialized plastic surgical assistance.

Long-term results are encouraging in those patients who, after final pathologic review, are found to have N0 disease (stage IIB). The role of postoperative adjuvant treatment in patients with incidental N1 or N2 (IIIA) disease is not defined.

REFERENCES

1. Downey RJ, Martini N, Rusch VW, et al. Extent of chest wall invasion and survival in patients with lung cancer. Ann Thorac Surg 1999;**68**:188-93.
2. Facciolo F, Cardillo G, Lopergolo M, et al. Chest wall invasion in non-small cell lung carcinoma: a rationale for en bloc resection. J Thorac Cardiovasc Surg 2001;**121**:649-56.
3. Richerand A, Deschamps JFP, Percy P-F, et al. Account of a resection of the ribs and the pleura. Read before the Royal Academy of Sciences of the Institute of France, April 27, 1818. Translated by Thomas Wilson. Philadelphia, printer for the translator by Thomas Town, 1818.
4. Block HM. Experimentelles zur Lungenresection. Deutche Med Wochenschrift 1881;**7**:634-6.
5. Walton GL. Letter from Berlin. Resection of the lung as proposed by Dr. Block. Boston Med Surg J 1883;**108**:262.
6. Murphy JB. Surgery of the lung. JAMA 1898;**31**:165.
7. Parham FW. Thoracic resection for tumors growing from the bony wall of the chest. Trans South Surg Gynecol Assoc 1898;**11**:223-363.
8. Sauerbruch F. Uber die Auschaltung der schadlichen Wirkung des Pneumothorax bei intrathorakelen Operationen. Zentralbl Chir 1904;**31**:146-9.
9. Brauer L. Die Ausschaltung der Pneumothoraxfolgen met Hilfe des Uberdruckverfahrens. Mitteilungen aus den Grenzgebieten der Medizin und Chirurgie 1904:398-486.
10. Northrop WP, O'Dwyer J. His methods of work on intubation: the measure of his success; the interest of both to young graduates. Med Rec 1904;**65**:561.
11. O'Dwyer J. Fifty cases of croup in private practice treated by intubation of the larynx, with a description of the method and of the dangers incident thereto. Med Rec 1887;**32**:557.
12. Fell GW. Forced respiration. JAMA 1891;**16**:325.
13. O'Dwyer J. Chronic stenosis of the larynx treated by a new method with report of a case. Med Rec 1886;**29**:641.
14. Kirstein A. Autoskopie des larynx und der trachea (laryngoscopia directa, euthyskopie, besichtigung ohne Spiegel. Arch Laryngol Rhinol 1895;**3**:156-64.
15. Scott J. Oral endotracheal intubation. In: Dailey RH, Simon B, Young GP, editors. The airway: emergency management.. St Louis: Mosby; 1993. p. 73-91.
16. Guedel AE. A new intratracheal catheter. Curr Res Anes Anal 1928;**7**:238-9.
17. Griffith HR, Johnson GE. The use of curare in general anesthesia. Anesthesiology 1942;**3**:418-20.
18. Coleman FP. Primary carcinoma of the lung, with invasion of the ribs: pneumonectomy and simultaneous en bloc resection of chest wall. Ann Surg 1947;**126**:168.
19. Campbell DA. Reconstruction of anterior thoracic wall. J Thorac Cardiovasc Surg 1950;**19**:456-61.
20. Grillo HC, Greenberg JJ, Wilkins Jr EW. Resection of bronchogenic carcinoma involving thoracic wall. J Thorac Cardiovasc Surg 1966;**51**:417-21.
21. Burkhart HM, Allen MS, Nichols III FC, et al. Results of en bloc resection for bronchogenic carcinoma with chest wall invasion. J Thorac Cardiovasc Surg 2002;**123**:670-5.
22. Magdeleinat P, Alifano M, Benbrahem C, et al. Surgical treatment of lung cancer invading the chest wall: results and prognostic factors. Ann Thorac Surg 2001;**71**:1094-9.

23. Okada M, Tsubota N, Yoshimura M, et al. How should interlobar pleural invasion be classified? Prognosis of resected T3 non-small cell lung cancer. *Ann Thorac Surg* 1999;**68**:2049-52.
24. Glazer HS, Duncanmeyer J, Aronberg DJ, et al. Pleural and chest wall invasion in bronchogenic-carcinoma: CT evaluation. *Radiology* 1985;**157**:191-4.
25. Glazer HS, Kaiser LR, Anderson DJ, et al. Indeterminate mediastinal invasion in bronchogenic-carcinoma: CT evaluation. *Radiology* 1989;**173**:37-42.
26. Kodalli N, Erzen C, Yuksel M. Evaluation of parietal pleural invasion of lung cancers with breathhold inspiration and expiration MRI. *Clin Imaging* 1999;**23**:227-35.
27. Pennes DR, Glazer GM, Wimbish KJ, et al. Chest wall invasion by lung-cancer: limitations of CT evaluation. *Am J Roentgenol* 1985;**144**:507-11.
28. Kuriyama K, Tateishi R, Kumatani T, et al. Pleural invasion by peripheral bronchogenic-carcinoma: assessment with 3-dimensional helical CT. *Radiology* 1994;**191**:365-9.
29. Shirakawa T, Fukuda K, Miyamoto Y, et al. Parietal pleural invasion of lung masses: evaluation with CT performed during deep inspiration and expiration. *Radiology* 1994;**192**:809-11.
30. Bandi V, Lunn W, Ernst A, Eberhardt R, Hoffman H, Herth FJF. Ultrasound vs. CT in detecting chest wall invasion by tumor. *Chest* 2008;**133**:881-6.
31. Watanabe A, Shimokata K, Saka H, et al. Chest CT combined with artificial pneumothorax: value in determining origin and extent of tumor. *Am J Roentgenol* 1991;**156**:707-10.
32. Yokoi K, Mori K, Miyazawa N, et al. Tumor invasion of the chest wall and mediastinum in lung-cancer: evaluation with pneumothorax CT. *Radiology* 1991;**181**:147-52.
33. Mountain CF. Revisions in the international system for staging lung cancer. *Chest* 1997;**111**:1710-7.
34. Rami-Porta R, Ball D, Crowley G, et al. The IASLC lung cancer staging project: proposals for the revision of the T Descriptors in the forthcoming (seventh) edition of the TNM classification for lung cancer. *J Thorac Oncol* 2007;**2**:593-602.
35. Mountain CF. A new international staging system for lung cancer. *Chest* 1986;**89**(4S):225S-33S.
36. Yasufuku K, Chiyo M, Koh E, et al. Endobronchial ultrasound guided transbronchial needle aspiration for staging of lung cancer. *Lung Cancer* 2005;**50**:347-54.
37. Herth FJF, Eberhardt R, Vilmann P, Krasnik M, Ernst A. Real-time endobronchial ultrasound guided transbronchial needle aspiration for sampling mediastinal lymph nodes. *Thorax* 2006;**62**:795-8.
38. Yasufuku K, Nakajima T, Motoori K, et al. Comparison of endobronchial ultrasound, positron emission tomography, and CT for lymph node staging of lung cancer. *Chest* 2006;**130**:710-8.
39. Schwartz M, Grief J, Becker HD, et al. Real-time electromagnetic navigational bronchoscopy to peripheral lung lesions using overlaid CT images. *Chest* 2006;**129**:988-94.
40. Jemal A, Thomas A, Murray T, et al. Cancer statistics. *Cancer J Clin* 2002;**52**:23-47:2002.
41. Frank JA, Ling A, Patronas NJ, et al. Detection of malignant bone tumors: MR imaging vs.scintigraphy. *Am J Roentgenol* 1990;**155**:1043-8.
42. Hauboldreuter BG, Duewell S, Schilcher BR, et al. The value of bone scintigraphy, bone marrow scintigraphy and fast spin-echo magnetic resonance imaging in staging of patients with malignant solid tumors: A prospective study. *Eur J Nucl Med* 1993;**20**:1063-9.
43. Smoker WRK, Godersky JC, Knutzon RK, et al. The role of MR imaging in evaluating metastatic spinal disease. *Am J Roentgenol* 1987;**149**:1241-8.
44. Durski JM, Srinivas S, Segall G. Comparison of FDG-PET and bone scans for detecting skeletal metastases in patients with non-small cell lung cancer. *Clinical Positron Imaging* 2000;**3**:97-105.
45. Gambhir SS, Hoh CK, Phelps ME, et al. Decision tree sensitivity analysis for cost-effectiveness of FDG-PET in the staging and management of non-small-cell lung carcinoma. *J Nucl Med* 1996;**37**:1428-36.
46. Albes JM, Lietzenmayer R, Schott U, et al. Improvement of non-small-cell lung cancer staging by means of positron emission tomography. *J Thorac Cardiovasc Surg* 1999;**47**:42-7.
47. Chin R, Ward R, Keyes JW, et al. Mediastinal staging of non-small-cell lung cancer with positron emission tomography. *Am J Respir Crit Care Med* 1995;**152**:2090-6.
48. Gupta NC, Graeber GM, Rogers JS, et al. Comparative efficacy of positron emission tomography with FDG and computed tomographic scanning in preoperative staging of non-small cell lung cancer. *Ann Surg* 1999;**229**:286-91.
49. Marom EM, McAdams HP, Erasmus JJ, et al. Staging non-small cell lung cancer with whole-body PET. *Radiology* 1999;**212**:803-9.
50. Steinert HC, Hauser M, Allemann F, et al. Non-small cell lung cancer: nodal staging with FDG PET versus CT with correlative lymph node mapping and sampling. *Radiology* 1997;**202**:441-6.
51. Reed CE, Harpole DH, Posther KE, et al. Results of the American College of Surgeons Oncology Group Z0050 Trial: the utility of positron emission tomography in staging potentially operable non-small cell lung cancer. *J Thorac Cardiovasc Surg* 2003;**126**(6):1943-51.
52. Cerfolio RJ, Ojha B, Bryant AS, Raghuveer V, Mountz JM, Bartolucci AA. The accuracy of integrated PET-CT compared with dedicated PET alone for the staging of patients with nonsmall cell lung cancer. *Ann Thorac Surg* 2004;**78**:1017-23.
53. Albertucci M, DeMeester TR, Rothberg M, et al. Surgery and the management of peripheral lung tumors adherent to the parietal pleura. *J Thorac Cardiovasc Surg* 1992;**103**:8-13.
54. Ravitch MM, Steichen FM. Pulmonary resections. In: Ravitch MM, Steichen FM, editors: atlas of general thoracic surgery. Philadelphia: WB Saunders; 1988. p. 189-292.
55. Grillo HC. Technical considerations in stage III disease: Pleural and chest wall involvement. In: Delarue NC, Eschapasse H, editors. International trends in general thoracic surgery. 1st ed. Philadelphia: WB Saunders; 1985. p. 134-8.
56. York JE, Walsh GL, Lang FF, et al. *Combined chest wall resection with vertebrectomy and spinal reconstruction for the treatment of Pancoast tumors. J Neurosurg* 1999;**91**:74-80.
57. Nesbitt JC, Wind GG. *Thoracic surgical oncology exposures and techniques.* Philadelphia: Lippincott Williams & Wilkins; 2003.
58. Brown R, Fleming W, Jurkiewicz M. *An island flap of the pectoralis major muscle. Br J Plast Surg* 1977;**30**:161-5.
59. Le Roux BT, Shama DM. Resection of tumors of the chest wall. *Curr Probl Surg* 1983;**20**:345-86.
60. Deschamps C, Tirnaksiz BM, Darbandi R, et al. Early and long-term results of prosthetic chest wall reconstruction. *J Thorac Cardiovasc Surg* 1999;**117**:588-91.
61. Netscher DT, Valkov PL. Reconstruction of oncologic torso defects: emphasis on microvascular reconstruction. *Semin Surg Oncol* 2000;**19**:255-63.
62. Tuggle DW, Mantor PC, Foley DS, Markley MM, Puffinbarger N. Using a bioabsorbable copolymer plate for chest wall reconstruction. *J Pediatr Surg* 2004;**39**:626-8.
63. Hosalkar H, Thatte MR, Yagnik MG. Chest-wall reconstruction in spondylocostal dysostosis: rare use of a latissimus dorsi flap. *Plast Reconstr Surg* 2002;**110**:537-40.
64. Macedo-Neto AV, Santos LV, Menezes SL, et al. Respiratory mechanics after prosthetic reconstruction of the chest wall in normal rats. *Chest* 1998;**113**:1667-72.
65. Lardinois D, Müller M, Furrer M, et al. Functional assessment of chest wall integrity after methylmethacrylate reconstruction. *Ann Thorac Surg* 2000;**69**:919-23.
66. Shimizu K, Otani Y, Ibe T, et al. Successful treatment of subarachnoid-pleural fistula using pericardial fat pad and fibbrin glue after chest wall resection for lung cancer. *Jpn J Thorac Cardiovasc Surg* 2005;**53**:93-6.
67. Chapelier A, Fadel E, Macchiarini P, et al. Factors affecting long-term survival after en-bloc resection of lung cancer invading the chest wall. *Eur J Cardiothorac Surg* 2000;**18**:513-8.
68. Mineo TC, Ambrogi V, Pompeo E, Baldi A. Immunohistochemistry-detected microscopic tumor spread after en-bloc resection for T3-chest wall lung cancer. *Eur J Cardiothorac Surg* 2007;**31**:1120-4.
69. Incarbone M, Pastorino U. Surgical treatment of chest wall tumors. *World J Surg* 2001;**25**:218-30.
70. Martin-Ucar AE, Nicum R, Oey I, et al. En-bloc chest wall and lung resection for non-small cell lung cancer: predictors of 60-day non-cancer related mortality. *Eur J Cardiothor Surg* 2003;**23**:859-64.
71. Weyant MJ, Bains MS, Venkatraman E, et al. Results of chest wall resection and reconstruction with and without rigid prosthesis. *Ann Thorac Surg* 2006;**81**:279-85.
72. Volotini L, Rapicetta C, Luzzi L, et al. Lung cancer with chest wall involvement: predictive factors of long-term survival after surgical resection. *Lung Cancer* 2006;**52**:359-64.
73. Matsuoka H, Nishio W, Okada M, et al. Resection of chest wall invasion in patients with non-small cell lung cancer. *Eur J Cardiothor Surg* 2004;**26**:1200-4.
74. Doddoli C, D'Journo B, Le Pimpec-Barthes F, et al. Lung cancer invading the chest wall: a plea for en-bloc resection but the need for new treatment strategies. *Ann Thorac Surg* 2005;**80**:2032-40.
75. Elia S, Griffo S, Gentile M, et al. Surgical treatment of lung cancer invading chest wall: a retrospective analysis of 110 patients. *Eur J Cardiothor Surg* 2001;**20**:356-60.

CHAPTER 21
Anterior Approach to Superior Sulcus Lesions
Philippe G. Dartevelle, Sacha Mussot, and Chuong D. Hoang

Presentation
Preoperative Studies

Treatment
Anterior Transcervical Technique

Surgical Morbidity and Mortality
Results and Prognosis

Henry K. Pancoast, a radiologist at the University of Pennsylvania, described a patient afflicted with a carcinoma of uncertain histologic origin occupying the extreme apex of the chest, associated with shoulder and arm pain, atrophy of the hand muscles, and Horner's syndrome.[1] This clinical entity has become known as Pancoast's syndrome. Unknown to Pancoast, Tobias had already characterized the anatomic and clinical aspects of this lesion, correctly recognizing that the tumor was a peripheral lung cancer. Anatomically, the pulmonary sulcus refers to the costovertebral gutter extending from the first rib to the diaphragm. The superior pulmonary sulcus lies at the uppermost extent of this recess, as reviewed by Teixeira.[2] Generally, it is understood that non–small cell lung carcinomas of this region are termed Pancoast tumors, and we refer to this association throughout. However, the term *superior sulcus lesion* encompasses other, more diverse etiologies, both benign and malignant. Furthermore, this definition has been expanded to include patients who do not have evidence of brachial plexus or stellate ganglion involvement. Chest wall involvement in this region might be restricted to involvement of the parietal pleura or could extend deeper to the upper ribs, vertebral bodies, or subclavian vessels according to Detterbeck.[3] Invasion of the chest wall at or lower than the level of the second rib, or of the visceral pleura only, does not meet the criteria for a superior sulcus lesion. Additionally, Macchiarini and colleagues[4] reported that a wide variety of superior sulcus lesions can result in Pancoast's syndrome (Box 21-1); thus, a histologic diagnosis is required when the syndrome is encountered.

PRESENTATION

Superior sulcus lesions of non–small cell histology account for less than 5% of all bronchial carcinomas, as reported by Ginsberg and associates.[5] These tumors may arise from either upper lobe and tend to invade parietal pleura, endothoracic fascia, subclavian vessels, brachial plexus, vertebral bodies, or the first rib. However, their clinical features are influenced by their location.

Tumors located anterior to the anterior scalene muscle may invade the platysma and sternocleidomastoid muscles, the external and anterior jugular veins, the inferior belly of the omohyoid muscle, the subclavian and internal jugular veins including major branches, and the scalene fat pad (Fig. 21-1). They invade the first intercostal nerve and the first rib more frequently than the phrenic nerve or superior vena cava. Patients usually complain of pain distributed to the upper anterior chest wall.

Tumors located between the anterior and middle scalene muscles may invade the anterior scalene muscle (phrenic nerve lying on its anterior aspect); the subclavian artery including primary branches, except the posterior scapular artery; and the trunks of the brachial plexus and middle scalene muscle (Fig. 21-2). These tumors manifest with signs and symptoms related to the compression or infiltration of the middle and lower trunks of the brachial plexus (e.g., pain and paresthesia radiating to the shoulder and upper limb).

Tumors lying posterior to the middle scalene muscles are usually located in the costovertebral groove and invade the nerve roots of T1, the posterior aspect of the subclavian and vertebral arteries, the paravertebral sympathetic chain, the inferior cervical (stellate) ganglion, and the prevertebral muscles. Some of these posterior tumors can invade transverse processes (Fig. 21-3) or extend to the vertebral bodies (only those abutting the costovertebral angle or extending into the intraspinal foramen without intraspinal extension may be resected).

Because of the peripheral location of these lesions, pulmonary symptoms, such as cough, hemoptysis, and dyspnea, are uncommon in the initial stages of the disease. Abnormal sensation and pain in the axilla and medial aspect of the upper arm in the distribution of the intercostobrachial (T2) nerve are more frequently observed in the early stage of the disease process. With further tumor growth, patients may present with overt Pancoast's syndrome.

PREOPERATIVE STUDIES

Any patient presenting with signs and symptoms that suggest the involvement of the thoracic inlet should undergo a detailed preoperative evaluation to establish the diagnosis of bronchial carcinoma and to assess for operability. These patients usually present with small apical tumors that are hidden behind the clavicle and the first rib on routine chest radiographs. The diagnosis is established by history and physical examination,

Box 21-1
Causes of Pancoast's Syndrome

Neoplasms
- Primary bronchogenic carcinomas
- Other primary thoracic neoplasms: adenoid cystic carcinomas
- Hemangiopericytoma
- Mesothelioma
- Metastatic neoplasms: carcinoma of the larynx, cervix, urinary bladder, and thyroid gland
- Hematologic neoplasms: plasmacytoma, lymphoid granulomatosis, lymphoma

Infectious processes
- Bacterial: staphylococcal and pseudomonal pneumonia, thoracic actinomycosis
- Fungal: aspergillosis, allescheriasis, cryptococcosis
- Tuberculosis
- Parasitic: echinococcosis (hydatid cyst)

Adapted from Arcasoy SM, Jett JR. Superior pulmonary sulcus tumors and Pancoast's syndrome. N Engl J Med 1997;337:1370.

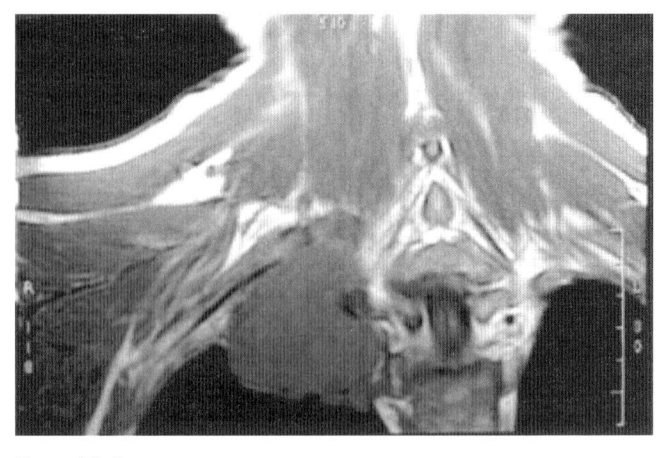

Figure 21-2
MR image showing a left superior sulcus bronchial carcinoma invading the middle thoracic inlet, including the subclavian artery.

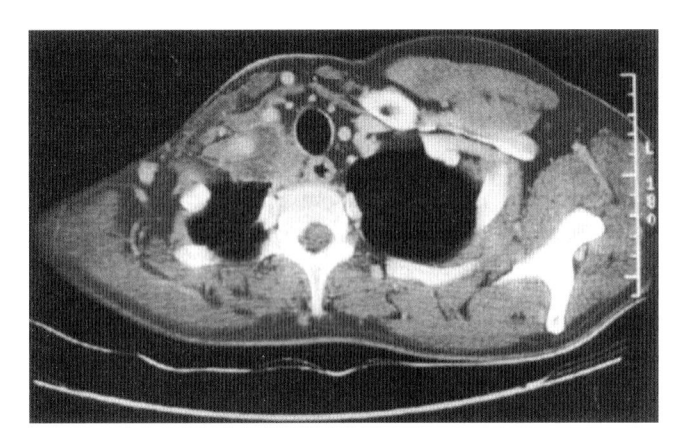

Figure 21-1
CT scan showing a right superior sulcus bronchial carcinoma invading the anterior thoracic inlet, including the subclavian vein.

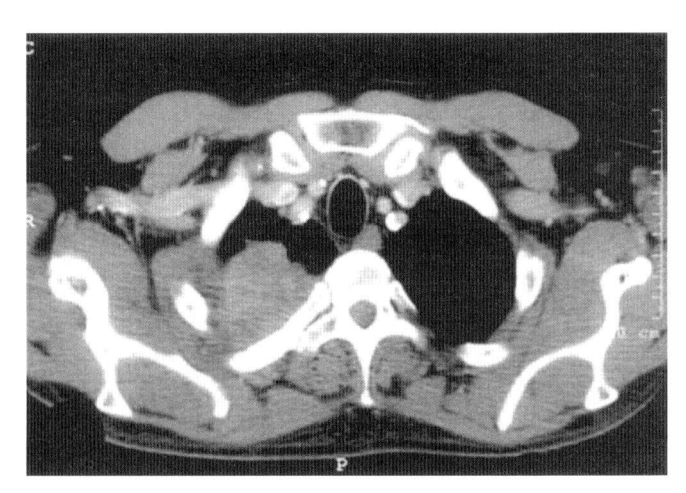

Figure 21-3
CT scan showing a right superior sulcus bronchial carcinoma invading the posterior arch and the transverse process of the first rib and abutting the costovertebral angle.

biochemical profile, chest radiographs, bronchoscopy with sputum cytology, fine-needle transthoracic or transcutaneous biopsy, and computed tomography of the chest. A tissue diagnosis via video-assisted thoracoscopy may be indicated when other investigations are negative and to eliminate the possibility of pleural metastatic disease. If there is evidence of mediastinal adenopathy on computed tomographic scanning, mediastinoscopy is mandatory because patients with clinical N2 disease are not operative candidates.

Neurologic examination, magnetic resonance imaging (MRI), or electromyography may delineate the tumor's extension to the brachial plexus, phrenic nerve, or epidural space. Vascular invasion is evaluated by venous angiography, subclavian arteriography, Doppler ultrasonography (cerebrovascular disorders may contraindicate resection of the vertebral artery), or MRI (Fig. 21-4). Additional MRI is mandatory if the workup suggests tumor encroachment into the intervertebral foramina, to rule out invasion of the extradural space (Fig. 21-5).

The initial evaluation also includes routine cardiopulmonary function tests and investigative procedures (e.g., positron emission tomography) to identify the presence of any metastatic disease. Extrathoracic metastases are rare.

TREATMENT

Tumors of the superior sulcus are deemed universally and rapidly fatal lesions. For many years, it was believed that these tumors were not amenable to surgery, until Chardack and MacCallum[6] successfully performed a lobectomy and chest wall excision followed by radiation therapy. Five years later, Shaw and colleagues[7] approached superior sulcus tumors with preoperative radiation therapy (30 to 45 Gy in 4 weeks, including the primary tumor, mediastinum, and supraclavicular region) followed by surgical resection. This radiosurgical approach shortly became the standard treatment, yielding better disease control and survival than other treatments. More recently, Ginsberg and colleagues[5] provided evidence that en bloc resection of the tumor combined with external radiation (preoperative,

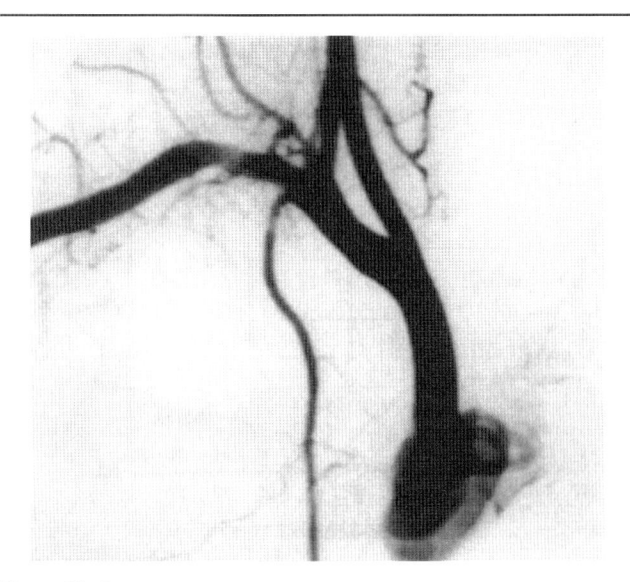

Figure 21–4
Angiography illustrating a massive tumoral invasion of the intrascalenic left subclavian artery.

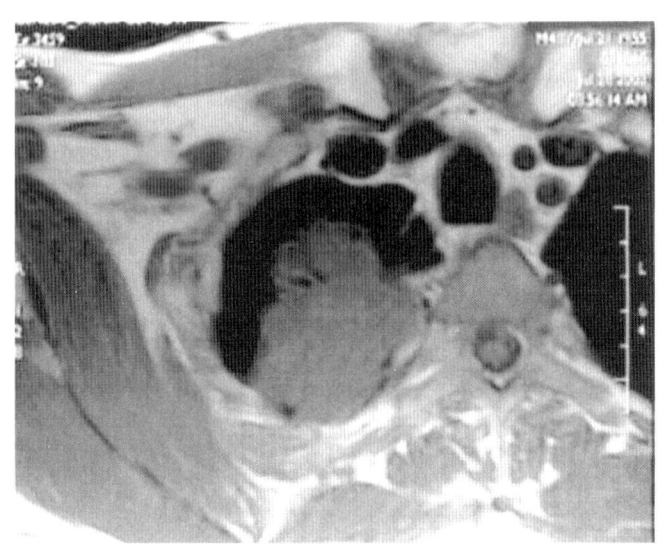

Figure 21–5
MR image that rules out invasion of the intervertebral foramina by the tumor.

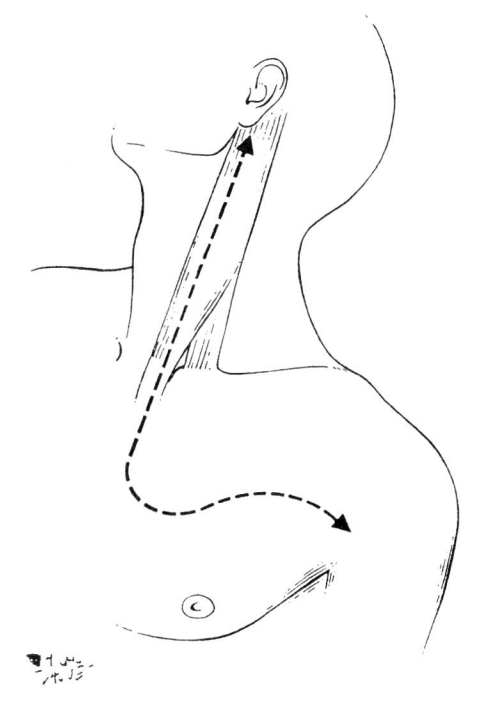

Figure 21–6
Anterior transcervical approach. (As described in Dartevelle PG, Chapelier AR, Macchiarini P, et al. Anterior transcervical-thoracic approach for radical resection of lung tumors invading the thoracic inlet. J Thorac Cardiovasc Surg 1993;**105**:1025.).

postoperative, or both) must be considered the standard therapeutic approach for superior sulcus tumors. The goal of resection is the complete removal of the upper lobe in continuity with the invaded ribs, transverse processes, subclavian vessels, T1 nerve root, upper dorsal sympathetic chain, and prevertebral muscles.

In 1999, we reviewed various surgical approaches for treating superior sulcus lesions.[8] In general, superior sulcus lesions not invading the thoracic inlet are completely resectable through the classic posterior approach of Shaw and colleagues.[7] However, the posterior approach does not allow direct, safe visualization, manipulation, or complete oncologic clearance of all anatomic structures of the thoracic inlet. Superior sulcus lesions extending to the thoracic inlet should be resected by an anterior transcervical approach according to our previous description.[9]

This operation has been increasingly accepted as a standard approach for all benign and malignant lesions of the thoracic inlet. Additionally, this approach facilitates exposure of the anterolateral aspects of the upper thoracic vertebrae. Contraindications to this approach include extrathoracic metastasis, invasion of the brachial plexus above the T1 nerve root, invasion of the vertebral canal or sheath of the medulla, massive invasion of the scalene muscles or extrathoracic muscles, mediastinal lymph node involvement, and advanced cardiopulmonary disease.

ANTERIOR TRANSCERVICAL TECHNIQUE

One-lung anesthesia with measurements of urine output and body temperature are necessary. An arterial line opposite to the primary lesion, and at least two venous lines for volume expansion should be used. The patient is supine with the neck hyperextended and the head turned away from the involved side. A bolster behind the shoulder elevates the operative field. The skin preparation extends from the mastoid downward to the xiphoid process and from the midaxillary line laterally to the contralateral midclavicular line medially. An L-shaped cervicotomy incision is made, including a vertical pre-sternocleidomastoid incision carried horizontally below the clavicle up to the deltopectoral groove (Fig. 21-6). To increase the exposure, the interception between the vertical and horizontal branches of the L-shaped incision is lowered to the level of the second or third intercostal space, depending on tumor extent. The incision is then deepened with cautery. The sternal attachment of the sternocleidomastoid muscle is divided. The cleidomastoid muscle, along with the upper digitations of the ipsilateral pectoralis major muscle, is scraped from the clavicle. A myocutaneous flap is then folded

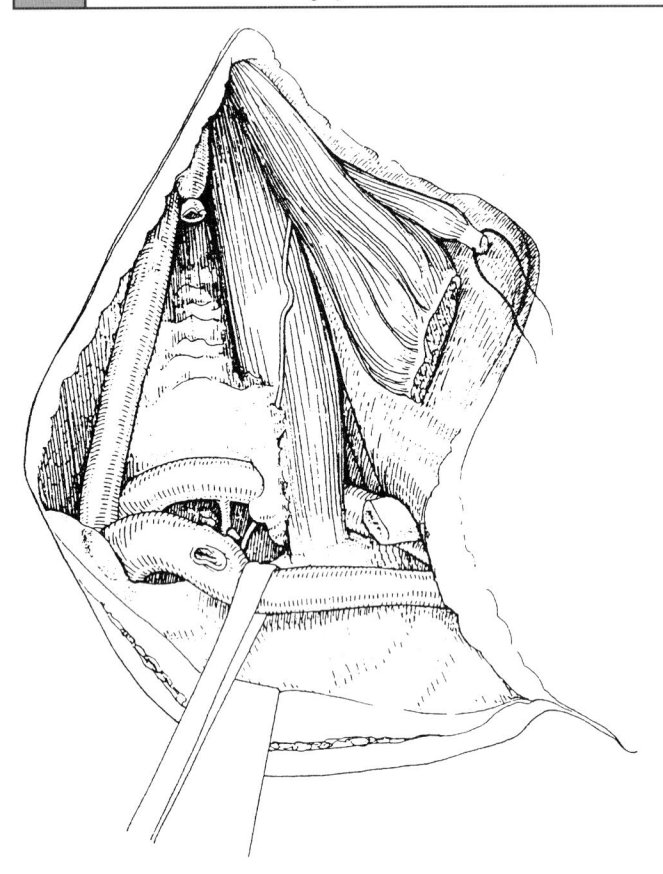

Figure 21–7
Illustration of the resected scalene fat pad and the internal half of the clavicle after division of the sternal head of the sternocleidomastoid and the inferior belly of the omohyoid muscles. The exposure, dissection, and division of the external and internal jugular vein greatly facilitates the exposure of the subclavian vein and permits assessment of tumor resectability. *(Adapted from Dartevelle PG, Chapelier AR, Macchiarini P, et al. Anterior transcervical-thoracic approach for radical resection of lung tumors invading the thoracic inlet. J Thorac Cardiovasc Surg 1993;**105**:1025.)*

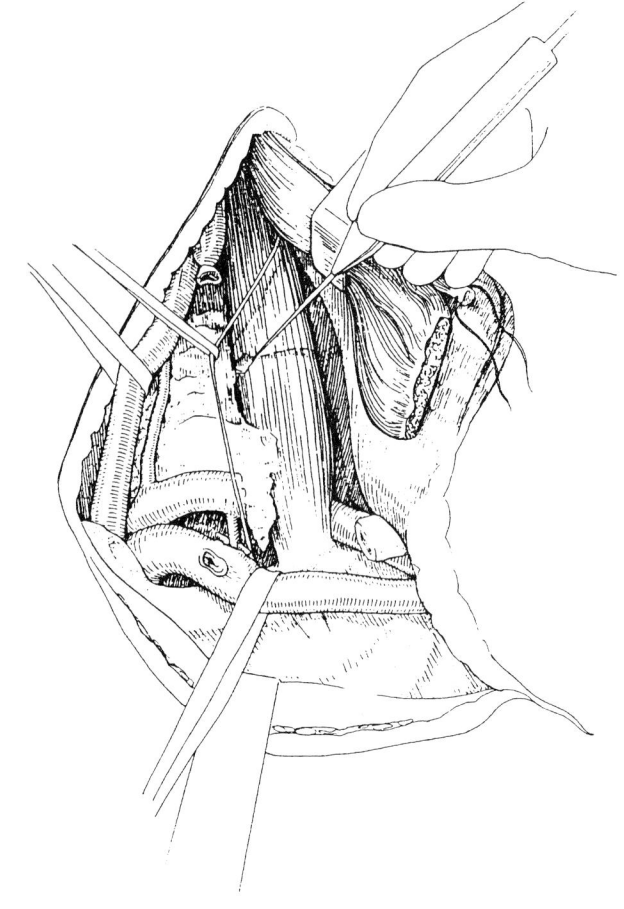

Figure 21–8
The subclavian artery is exposed after division of the insertion of the anterior scalenus muscle on the first rib. The phrenic nerve is protected and preserved. *(Adapted from Dartevelle PG, Chapelier AR, Macchiarini P, et al. Anterior transcervical-thoracic approach for radical resection of lung tumors invading the thoracic inlet. J Thorac Cardiovasc Surg 1993;**105**:1025.)*

back, providing full exposure of the neck and cervicothoracic junction.

Once the inferior belly of the omohyoid muscle is divided, the scalene fat pad is dissected and sent for pathologic examination to exclude scalene lymph node metastasis. Inspection of the ipsilateral superior mediastinum after division of the sternothyroid and sternohyoid muscles is made by the surgeon's finger along the tracheoesophageal groove. Tumor extension to the thoracic inlet is carefully assessed next. We recommend resection of the medial half of the clavicle only if the tumor is deemed resectable. The jugular veins are dissected first, so that branches to the subclavian vein can eventually be divided. On the left side, ligation of the thoracic duct is usually required. Division of the distal part of the internal, external, and anterior jugular veins facilitates visualization of the venous confluence at the origin of the innominate vein. The internal jugular vein can be ligated to increase exposure of the subclavian vein (Fig. 21-7). If the subclavian vein is involved, it can be easily resected after proximal and distal control has been achieved. Direct extension of the tumor to the innominate vein does not preclude resection. Next, the anterior scalene muscle is divided with cautery either at its insertion on the scalene tubercle of the first rib or in a tumor-free margin (Fig. 21-8). If the tumor has invaded the upper part of this muscle, it needs to be divided at its insertions on the anterior tubercles of the transverse processes of C3 to C6. Before dealing with the anterior scalene muscle, the status of the phrenic nerve is carefully assessed because its unnecessary division has a deleterious influence on postoperative respiratory function. It should be preserved whenever possible.

The subclavian artery is dissected (Fig. 21-9). To improve mobilization, branches are divided. The vertebral artery is resected only if invaded and if no significant extracranial occlusive disease was detected on preoperative Doppler ultrasound. If the tumor rests against the subclavian artery wall, the artery can be freed following a subadventitial plane. If there is invasion of the arterial wall, resection is necessary to obtain tumor-free margins. After proximal and distal control is obtained, the artery is divided on either side of the tumor (Fig. 21-10). Revascularization is performed using either polytetrafluoroethylene graft (6 or 8 mm) or, more often, an end-to-end primary anastomosis after freeing the carotid and subclavian arteries. During these maneuvers, the pleural space is usually opened by dividing Sibson's fascia.

The middle scalene muscle is divided above its insertion on the first rib or higher, as dictated by tumor extent. This may require division of its insertions on the posterior tubercles of the transverse processes of vertebrae C2 to C7, especially

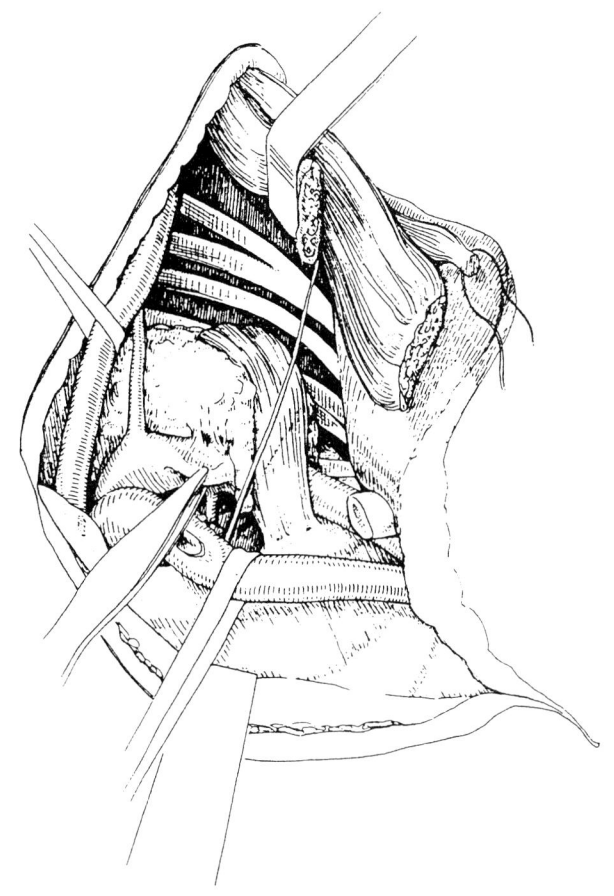

Figure 21–9
Retraction of the anterior scalenus muscles allows identification of the interscalenic trunks of the brachial plexus. The subclavian artery can be gently freed from the tumor by dividing all collateral branches (the vertebral artery is generally preserved if not invaded). *(Adapted from Dartevelle PG, Chapelier AR, Macchiarini P, et al. Anterior transcervical-thoracic approach for radical resection of lung tumors invading the thoracic inlet. J Thorac Cardiovasc Surg 1993;**105**:1025.)*

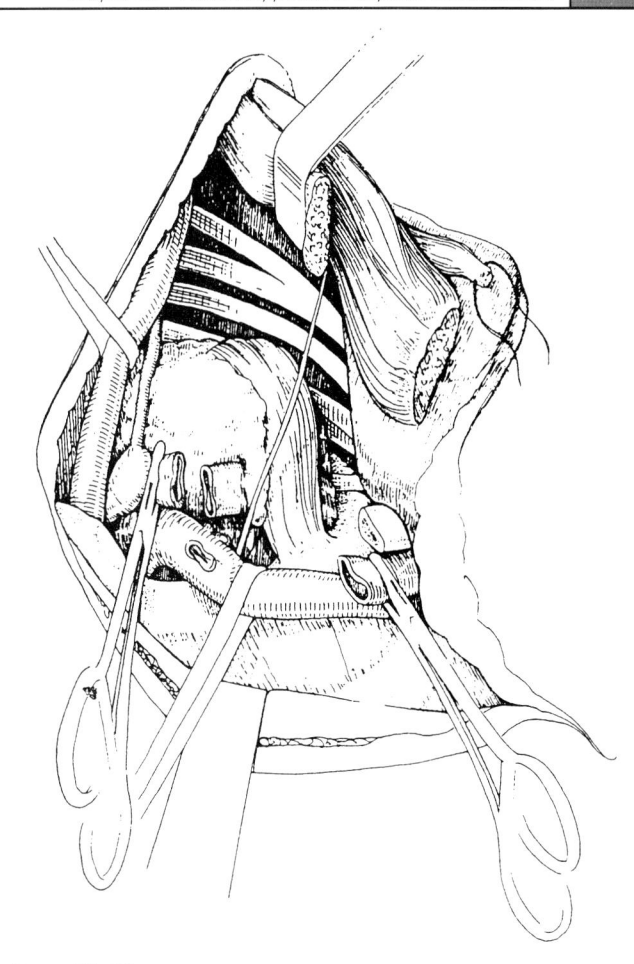

Figure 21–10
If involved by the tumor, the subclavian artery can be divided after its proximal and distal control. *(Adapted from Dartevelle PG, Chapelier AR, Macchiarini P, et al. Anterior transcervical-thoracic approach for radical resection of lung tumors invading the thoracic inlet. J Thorac Cardiovasc Surg 1993;**105**:1025.)*

for apical tumors invading the middle compartment of the thoracic inlet. The nerve roots of C8 and T1 are easily identified and dissected free from outside to inside, up to where they join to form the lower trunk of the brachial plexus. Thereafter, the ipsilateral prevertebral muscles are resected, along with the paravertebral sympathetic chain and stellate ganglion, from the anterior surface of the vertebral bodies of C7 and T1 (Fig. 21-11). This permits oncologic clearance of the major lymphatic vessel draining the thoracic inlet and the visualization of the intervertebral foramina. The T1 nerve root is usually divided proximally beyond visible tumor, just lateral to the T1 intervertebral foramen. Although tumor involvement of the brachial plexus may be high, neurolysis is usually achieved without division of the nerve roots above T1 (Fig. 21-12). Lateral and long thoracic nerves should be preserved to avoid winged scapula.

The chest wall resection is completed before the upper lobectomy (Fig. 21-13). The anterolateral arch of the first rib is divided at the costochondral junction. The second rib is divided at the middle arch. The third rib is scraped on the superior border toward the costovertebral angle. The specimen is progressively freed. The divided ribs are disarticulated from the transverse processes of the first two or three thoracic vertebrae. An upper lobectomy can be accomplished through this cavity, although it is technically more demanding. The additional posterior thoracotomy, as in our original description,[9] is usually not required. The cervical incision is closed in two layers after the sternal insertion of the sternocleidomastoid muscle is sutured. Conventional tube drainage of the ipsilateral chest cavity is carried out.

There is increasing concern about the functional and aesthetic benefit of preserving the clavicle. We believe that the indications for preserving and reconstructing the clavicle are limited to the combined resection of the serratus anterior muscle and the long thoracic nerve, because this causes the scapula to rotate and draw forward. This entity (scapula alata), combined with the resection of the internal half of the clavicle, pushes the shoulder anteriorly and medially, leading to severe cosmetic, functional discomfort. If this circumstance is anticipated, we recommend an oblique section of the manubrium that fully preserves the sternoclavicular articulation, its intra-articular disc, and the costoclavicular ligaments, rather than the simple sternoclavicular disarticulation. Clavicular osteosynthesis can be accomplished by placing metallic wires across the lateral clavicular edges and across the divided manubrium.

We developed a technique for resecting superior sulcus tumors extending into the intervertebral foramen without intraspinal extension[10] (Fig. 21-14). The underlying principle

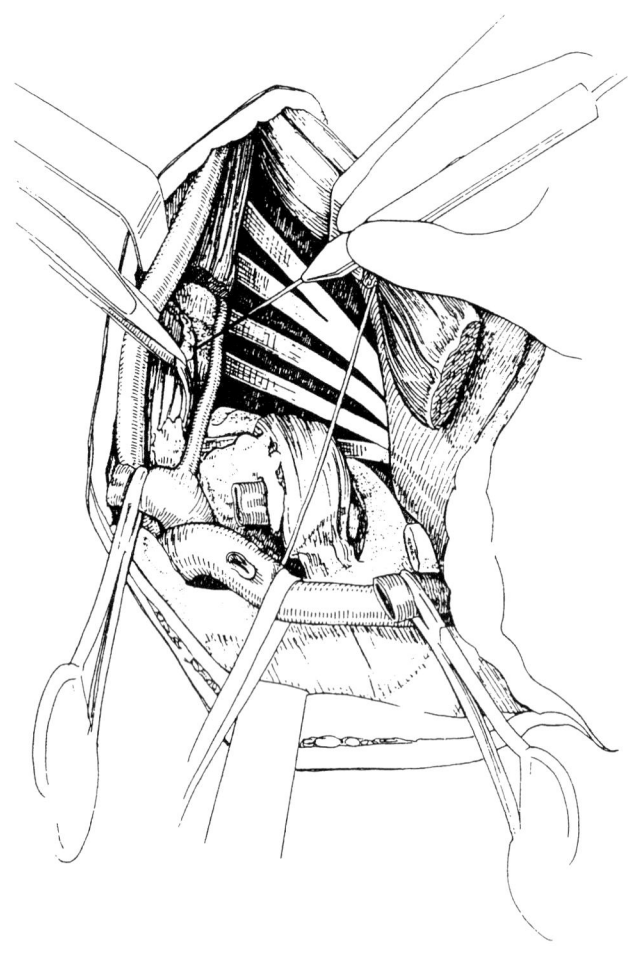

Figure 21–11
The prevertebral muscles are extensively detached from the vertebral bodies, and both the stellate ganglion and dorsal sympathetic chain are isolated and finally released, using raspatories, from all surrounding attachments. *(Adapted from Dartevelle PG, Chapelier AR, Macchiarini P, et al. Anterior transcervical-thoracic approach for radical resection of lung tumors invading the thoracic inlet. J Thorac Cardiovasc Surg 1993;**105**:1025.)*

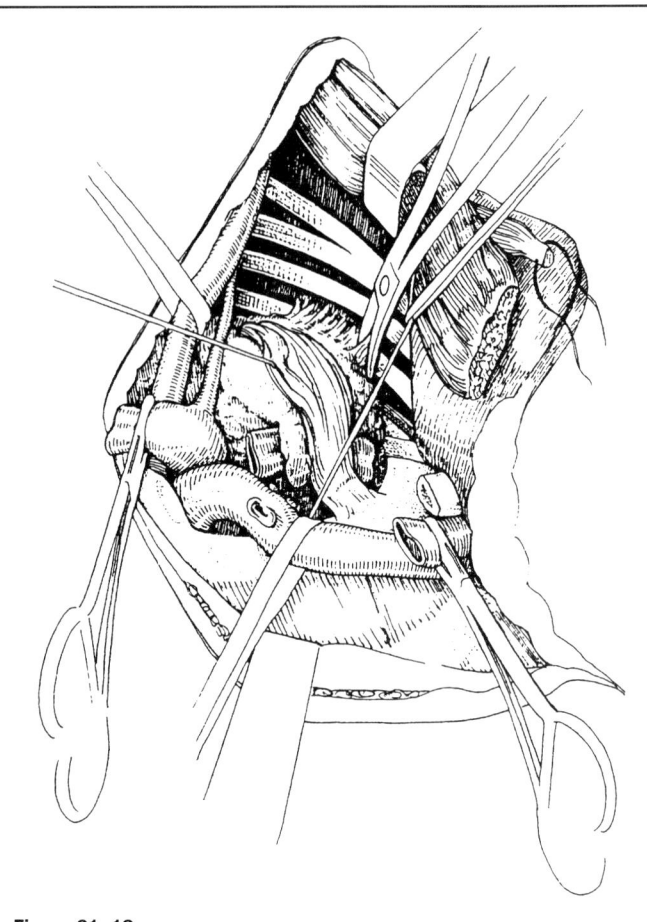

Figure 21–12
Tumoral involvement of the brachial plexus requires an inside-out neurolysis if the upper trunks are involved, or a resection of T1 if the lower trunk or nerve roots are involved. *(Adapted from Dartevelle PG, Chapelier AR, Macchiarini P, et al. Anterior transcervical-thoracic approach for radical resection of lung tumors invading the thoracic inlet. J Thorac Cardiovasc Surg 1993;**105**:1025.)*

is the use of a combined anterior transcervical and posterior midline approach, allowing resection of the intervertebral foramen and division of the nerve roots inside the spinal canal. The procedure starts with a transcervical approach; resectability is assessed. All tumor-involved areas are resected with tumor-free margins, as described. Next, the patient is placed in a ventral position, and a median vertical incision is extended from spinal processes C7 to T4.

After a unilateral laminectomy on three levels, the nerve roots are divided inside the spinal canal at their emergence from the external sheath covering the spinal cord. The specimen is resected en bloc, with the lung, ribs, and vessels through the posterior incision (Fig. 21-15) after division of the ipsilateral hemivertebral bodies. On the side of the tumor, spinal fixation is performed from the pedicle above to the pedicle below the resected hemivertebrae. On the contralateral side, a screw is placed in each pedicle (Fig. 21-16). However, if an anterior spinal artery is discovered to be penetrating the spinal canal through an invaded intervertebral foramen, surgery is contraindicated. Tumors involving transverse processes should be resected with the anterior approach. The maneuver is similar to that used with the posterior approach but from the front to the back, with a finger placed behind the transverse process of T1 and T2 to direct the chisel correctly (Fig. 21-17).

SURGICAL MORBIDITY AND MORTALITY

Surgical complications are numerous and vary in severity. Spinal fluid leakage occurs secondary to injury to the spinal cord sheath. The risks of air embolism into the subarachnoid space, ventricles, central canal of the brain, and spinal cord space justify reoperation, during which a cerebral ventricular-venous shunt may be required.

Horner's syndrome occurs after injury to the stellate ganglion. The clinical consequences are usually well tolerated. Various nerve deficits can occur as well. Although division of the T1 nerve root does not induce significant muscular palsy in the nerve distribution, resection of the lower trunk of the brachial plexus may result in atrophic paralysis of the forearm and small muscles of the hand, with paralysis of the cervical sympathetic system (Klumpke-Déjérine syndrome). This scenario should be discussed with the patient preoperatively. Relief of the preoperative pain and potential cancer cure are worth the nerve sacrifice, however, and adaptation is usually reasonable.

Hemothorax may result from the extensive pleural adhesions encountered during resection, the chest wall resection,

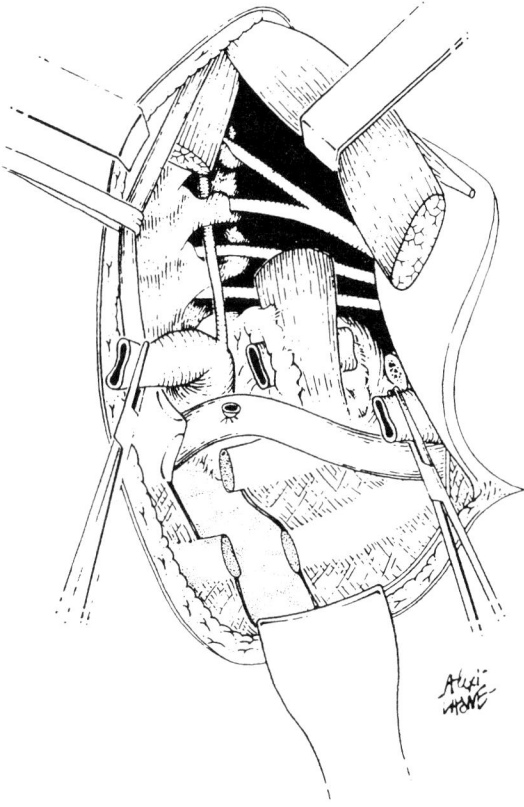

Figure 21-13
Once structures above the thoracic inlet are freed from the tumor, the first two ribs might be separated anteriorly at its chondrocostal junction and resected posteriorly in tumor-free margins. The third rib is scribed on its superior border toward the costovertebral angle and retracted inferiorly. *(Adapted from Dartevelle PG, Chapelier AR, Macchiarini P, et al. Anterior transcervical-thoracic approach for radical resection of lung tumors invading the thoracic inlet. J Thorac Cardiovasc Surg 1993;**105**:1025.)*

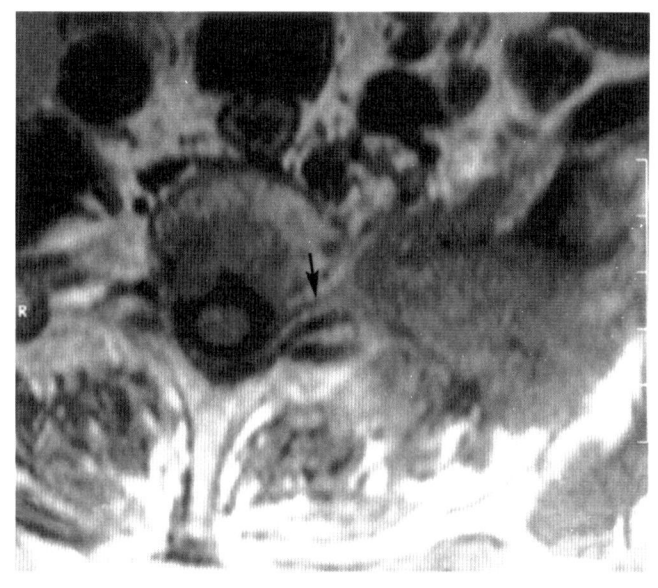

Figure 21-14
MR image of a right superior sulcus bronchial carcinoma extending into the intervertebral foramen without intraspinal extension.

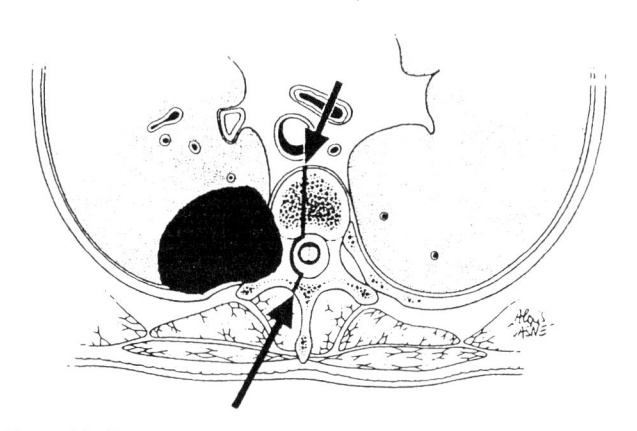

Figure 21-15
Right-sided apical tumor involving the costo-transverse space, intervertebral foramen, and part of the ipsilateral vertebral body. This tumor is first approached anteriorly as described in the text, and then the operation is completed through a hemivertebrectomy performed via the posterior midline approach. *Arrows* show the line of vertebral resection. *(Adapted from Dartevelle PG, Chapelier AR, Macchiarini P, et al. Anterior transcervical-thoracic approach for radical resection of lung tumors invading the thoracic inlet. J Thorac Cardiovasc Surg 1993;**105**:1025.)*

or the blood spillage from veins around the intervertebral foramina. Chylothorax should be prevented intraoperatively by extensive ligation of the cervical and intrathoracic lymphatic vessels after meticulous dissection. Whenever this occurs, continued chest tube drainage, lung expansion, or reoperation may be necessary.

Patients having a combined transcervical and midline approach are more likely than others to develop postoperative atelectasis and perfusion-ventilation mismatch. This is due to chest wall dyskinesia and phrenic nerve resection or even temporary paresis from the dissection. Thus, they are unable to breathe spontaneously in the early postoperative course.

The postoperative course is characterized by atelectasis because of the extended chest wall resection, with or without phrenic nerve sacrifice. Treatment involves measures to achieve complete lung expansion by ensuring the following: ventilation (mechanical support as necessary); chest tube function; prevention of retained secretions by mobilization, coughing, chest physiotherapy, and airway suctioning (even a temporary tracheostomy); optimal analgesia; and incentive spirometry.

Fluid overload should be avoided and diuretics used judiciously to avoid adult respiratory distress syndrome. Chest tubes remain in place until all air leaks have stopped and there is complete lung expansion. Fluid drainage should be minimal. Incomplete lung expansion with persistent intrapleural air space should be ignored because the space will ultimately be filled with serous fluid.

Resection of the subclavian vein should be accompanied by elevation of the ipsilateral forearm to facilitate venous drainage and generation of a collateral venous pathway (within 1 to 2 months). The radial pulse should be followed closely to control the patency of the revascularized subclavian artery; after a preoperative loading dose of intravenous heparin, anticoagulant treatment should be switched to oral doses for a 6-month postoperative period only.

RESULTS AND PROGNOSIS

The overall 5-year survival rates after combined radiosurgical (posterior approach) treatment of superior sulcus tumors caused by bronchial carcinoma range from 18% to 56%

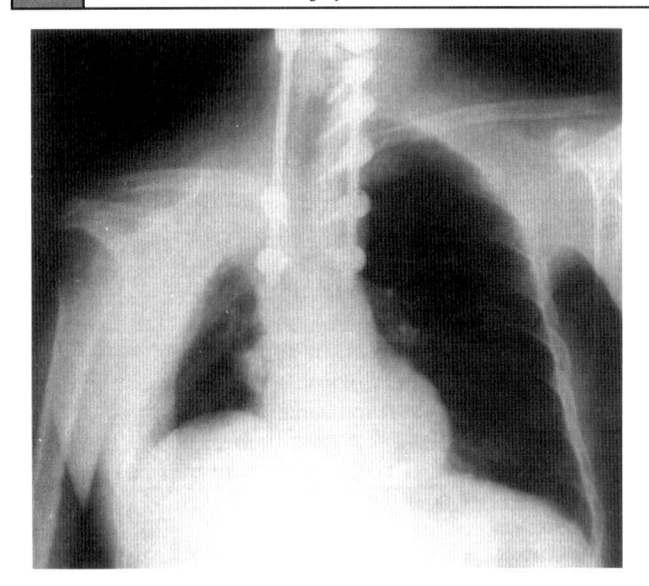

Figure 21–16
Chest radiograph showing bilateral spinal fixation with metal rods interposed. *(From Dartevelle PG. Extended operations for lung cancer. Ann Thorac Surg 1997;**63**:12, with permission.)*

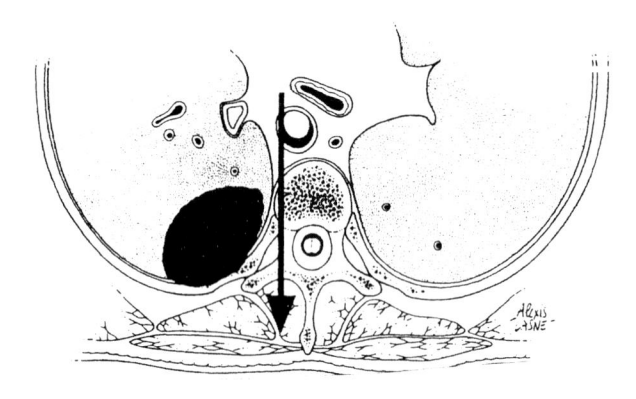

Figure 21–17
Right-sided apical tumor involving the posterior arch of the rib only and resected from the anterior cervical approach by a vertical en bloc resection of part of the lateral vertebral body, the costo-transverse space, and transverse process. *Arrow* shows the line of vertebral resection. *(Adapted from Dartevelle PG, Chapelier AR, Macchiarini P, et al. Anterior transcervical-thoracic approach for radical resection of lung tumors invading the thoracic inlet. J Thorac Cardiovasc Surg 1993;**105**:1025.)*

(Table 21-1). The best prognosis is found in patients without nodal involvement who have had a complete resection, as noted by Arcasoy and Jett[11] and Ginsberg and colleagues.[5] We reported a complete resection rate of 100% with no postoperative mortality or major complications.[12] The 5-year and median survival rates were approximately 35% and 18 months, respectively. The local recurrence rate was less than 1.8% using our approach. Fadel and coworkers reported 17 en bloc resections of non–small cell lung cancers invading the thoracic inlet and intervertebral foramina, with 5-year and median survival rates of 20% and 27 months, respectively.[13] Among the adverse prognostic factors, the nodal status is the only predictor of disease-free survival (Box 21-2). Recently, we reviewed our current experience with superior sulcus tumors in 126 patients.[14] Complete resection was achieved in 90% of cases, resulting in a median survival time of 28 months and

Table 21–1
Results of Surgical Treatment for Superior Sulcus Tumors

Author (year)	Cases (N)	5-Year survival (%)	Mortality (%)
Paulson DL (1985)[15]	79	35	3
Anderson et al (1986)[16]	28	34	7
Devine et al (1986)[17]	40	10	8
Miller et al (1987)[18]	36	31	NS
Wright et al (1987)[19]	21	27	—
Shahian et al (1987)[20]	18	56	—
McKneally et al (1987)[21]	25	51	NS
Komaki et al (1990)[22]	25	40	NS
Sartori et al (1992)[23]	42	25	2.3
Maggi et al (1994)[24]	60	17.4	5
Ginsberg et al (1994)[5]	100	26	4
Okubo et al (1995)[25]	18	38.5	5.6
Dartevelle P (1998)[26]	70	34	—
Totals	562	33±12*	3.5±3*

Adapted from Dartevelle P, Macchiarini P. Optimal management of tumors in the superior sulcus. In: Franco KL, Putman Jr J, editors. Advanced therapy in thoracic surgery. Hamilton, Ont: BC Decker; 1998, with permission.
NS, not stated.
*Values are percent ± standard deviation.

Box 21–2
Factors Influencing Survival and Disease-Free Survival* of Patients with Superior Sulcus Tumor†

Adverse prognostic factors
- Female sex
- Positive bronchoscopy
- Abnormal serum carcinoembryonic antigen (CEA)
- Full-blown Pancoast-Tobias syndrome
- Positive lymph nodes (N1-3)

Factors without prognostic influence
- Side and site of the tumor
- Type of surgery (wedge versus lobectomy)
- Subclavian vessel invasion (absent versus present)
- Invasion of the intervertebral foramen

Adapted from Macchiarini P, Dartevelle P: Extended resections for lung cancer. In Roth JA, Hong WK, Cox JD, editors. Lung cancer. 2nd ed. Cambridge, MA: Blackwell Scientific; 1998, with permission.
*By multivariate analysis, only the nodal status adversely affected disease-free survival.
†The superior sulcus tumors had invaded the thoracic inlet, and they were completely resected through the anterior approach.

a 5-year survival of 39.3%. There was one death during the study period. By multivariate analysis, incomplete resection and subclavian artery involvement adversely affected survival ($P = .01$, each). Overall, our results suggest that radical surgery for superior sulcus tumors may be performed in experienced centers with low mortality and favorable survival rates.

REFERENCES

1. Pancoast HK. Superior pulmonary sulcus tumor. *JAMA* 1932;**99**:1391.
2. Teixeira JP. Concerning the Pancoast tumor: what is the superior pulmonary sulcus?. *Ann Thorac Surg* 1983;**35**:577.
3. Detterbeck FC. Changes in the treatment of Pancoast tumors. *Ann Thorac Surg* 1990;**75**:2003.
4. Macchiarini P, Dartevelle P, Chapelier A, et al. Technique for resecting primary and metastatic nonbronchial carcinomas of the thoracic outlet. *Ann Thorac Surg* 1993;**55**:611-8.
5. Ginsberg RJ, Martini N, Zaman M, et al. Influence of surgical resection and brachytherapy in the management of superior sulcus tumor. *Ann Thorac Surg* 1994;**57**:1440-5.
6. Chardack WM, MacCallum JD. Pancoast syndrome due to bronchogenic carcinoma: Successful surgical removal and postoperative irradiation: a case report. *J Thorac Surg* 1953;**54**:831.
7. Shaw RR, Paulson DL, Kee JLJ. Treatment of the superior sulcus tumor by irradiation followed by resection. *Ann Surg* 1961;**154**:29.
8. Dartevelle PG, Macchiarini P. Surgical management of superior sulcus tumors. *Oncologist* 1999;**4**:398-407.
9. Dartevelle PG, Chapelier AR, Macchiarini P, et al. Anterior transcervical-thoracic approach for radical resection of lung tumors invading the thoracic inlet. *J Thorac Cardiovasc Surg* 1993;**105**:1025-34.
10. Dartevelle PG. Extended operations for lung cancer. *Ann Thorac Surg* 1997;**63**:12.
11. Arcasoy SM, Jett JR. Superior pulmonary sulcus tumors and Pancoast's syndrome. *N Engl J Med* 1997;**337**:1370.
12. Macchiarini P, Dartevelle PG. Extended resections for lung cancer. In: Roth JA, Hong WK, Cox JD, editors. *Lung cancer.* 2nd ed Cambridge, UK: Blackwell Scientific; 1998. pp 135-62.
13. Fadel E, Missenard G, Chapelier A, et al. En bloc resection of non-small cell lung cancer invading the thoracic inlet and intervertebral foramina. *J Thorac Cardiovasc Surg* 2002;**123**:676-85.
14. Yildizeli B, Dartevelle PG, Fadel E, et al. Results of primary surgery with T4 non-small cell lung cancer over a 25-year period in a single center: the benefit is worth the risk. *Ann Thorac Surg* 2008;**86**:1065-75.
15. Paulson DL. The "superior sulcus lesion. In: Delarue N, Eschapasse H, editors. *International trends in general thoracic surgery.* Vol. 1: *Lung canc* Philadelphia: WB Saunders; 1985. p. 121-31.
16. Anderson TM, Moy PM, Holmes EC. Factors affecting survival in superior sulcus tumors. *J Clin Oncol* 1986;**4**:1598-603.
17. Devine JW, Mendenhall WM, Million RR, Carmichael MJ. Carcinoma of the superior pulmonary sulcus treated with surgery and/or radiation therapy. *Cancer* 1986;**57**:941-3.
18. Miller JI, Mansour KA, Hatcher CR. Carcinoma of the superior pulmonary sulcus. *Ann Thorac Surg* 1979;**28**:44-7.
19. Wright CD, Moncure AC, Shepard JOA, et al. Superior sulcus lung tumors. *J Thorac Cardiovasc Surg* 1987;**94**:69-74.
20. Shahian DM, Wildford BN, Ellis Jr FH. Pancoast tumors:improved survival with preoperative and postoperative radiotherapy. *Ann Thorac Surg* 1987;**43**:32-8.
21. McKneally M, Discussion of Shahian DM, Neptune WB, Ellis FH. Pancoast tumors: improved survival with preoperative and postoperative radiotherapy. *Ann Thorac Surg* 1987;**43**:32-8.
22. Komaki E, Mountain CF, Holbert JM, et al. Superior sulcus tumors:treatment selection and results for 85 patients without metastasis (M0) at presentation. *Int J Radiat Oncol Biol Phys* 1990;**19**:31-6.
23. Sartori F, Rea F, Calabro F, et al. Carcinoma of the superior sulcus. Results of irradiation and radical resection. *J Thorac Cardiovasc Surg* 1990;**104**:679-83.
24. Maggi G, Casadio C, Pischedda F, et al. Combined radiosurgical treatment of Pancoast tumors. *Ann Thorac Surg* 1994;**57**:198-202.
25. Okubo K, Wada H, Fukuse T, et al. Treatment of Pancoast tumors. Combined irradiation and radical resection. *Thorac Cardiovasc Surg* 1995;**43**:284-6.
26. Dartevelle P, Macchiarini P. Optimal management of tumors in the superior sulcus. In: France KL, Putnam Jr J, editors. *Advanced therapy in thoracic surgery.* Hamilton, Ontario: BC Decker; 1998. pp 106-15.

G. Other Lung Malignancy

CHAPTER 22
Other Primary Tumors of the Lung

Alykhan S. Nagji and David R. Jones

- **Bronchopulmonary Carcinoid Tumors**
  - Pathology
  - Genetics and Biochemistry
  - Clinical Presentation
  - Diagnosis
    - *Imaging*
    - *Bronchoscopy*
    - *Tumor Markers*
  - Staging
  - Management and Treatment
    - *Surgery*
    - *Endobronchial Management*
    - *Radiation and Chemotherapy*
  - Prognosis
- **Carcinoid Tumorlets**
  - Pathology and Diagnosis

- Management, Treatment, and Prognosis
- **Primary Pulmonary Salivary Gland–Type Neoplasms**
  - Pathology
  - Diagnosis
  - Management and Treatment
    - *Surgery*
    - *Endobronchial Treatment Strategies*
    - *Adjuvant Treatment*
  - Prognosis
- **Primary Pulmonary Sarcomas**
  - *Primary Pulmonary Leiomyosarcoma*
  - *Primary Pulmonary Synovial Sarcoma*
  - *Primary Pulmonary Epithelioid Hemangioendothelioma*
  - *Primary Pulmonary Angiosarcoma*

- **Primary Solitary Pulmonary Plasmacytoma**
  - Diagnosis
  - Treatment and Prognosis
- **Primary Pulmonary Lymphoma**
  - Pathology
  - Diagnosis
  - Management and Treatment
  - Prognosis
- **Primary Pulmonary Melanoma**
  - Pathology
  - Diagnosis
  - Treatment
- **Primary Pulmonary Carcinosarcoma**
  - Diagnosis
  - Treatment and Prognosis

On occasion, the thoracic surgeon must diagnose and treat an unusual primary lung cancer, and, although the clinical presentation of these uncommon tumors is often similar to that of the more common tumors, treatment may be quite different. The goal of this chapter is to provide an understanding of some of the features and treatment strategies for these unusual tumors.

CARCINOID TUMORS

Approximately 25% of carcinoid tumors are bronchopulmonary (BP).[1] The Surveillance, Epidemiology, and End Results (SEER) database shows that BP carcinoid tumors represent approximately 1.2% of primary lung malignancies.[2] The current BP neuroendocrine tumor classification is based on 2004 World Health Organization (WHO) guidelines and describes four histologic subtypes of BP neuroendocrine tumors: typical carcinoid tumor (low grade), atypical carcinoid tumor (intermediate grade), large-cell neuroendocrine carcinoma (high grade), and small cell lung carcinoma (high grade).[3]

BP carcinoid tumors occur almost equally in men and women; however, in patients less than 50 years of age, they are observed nearly twice as often in women.[4] Modlin and colleagues conducted a 5-decade meta-analysis of carcinoid tumors, which demonstrated that BP carcinoid tumors were more common in whites (black-to-white ratio, 0.45), Asians (Asians-to-non-Asians ratio, 0.52), and non-Hispanics (Hispanics-to-non-Hispanics ratio, 0.23).[1]

Unlike high-grade BP neuroendocrine tumors (large cell and small cell), typical and atypical BP carcinoid tumors rarely occur in combination with other adenocarcinomas; however, their risk of occurring synchronously with breast or prostate cancer is slightly elevated.[5,6]

Pathology

The WHO histologic classification of BP neuroendocrine tumors is based on specific morphologic features: organoid or trabecular growth pattern, palisading of the tumor cells around the periphery of tumor nests, and the formation of rosette structures. Although the WHO places these four subtypes under the general heading of BP neuroendocrine tumors, histopathologic and immunochemical studies support the idea that BP carcinoid tumors are distinct from those of the more malignant and higher-grade neuroendocrine tumors.[7]

The majority of BP carcinoid tumors are typical and tend to be centrally located.[8] Davila and coworkers reported that 75% of BP carcinoid tumors arise in the lobar bronchi, 10% in the main-stem bronchi, and 15% peripherally.[9] Bronchoscopic evaluation of typical carcinoid tumors demonstrates sessile, red-brown to bluish tan endobronchial masses with variable vascularity and a smooth surface. On gross pathologic examination, typical carcinoid tumors appear as a white or gray cut surface with minimal evidence of hemorrhage or necrosis.[10] The WHO diagnostic criteria for typical carcinoid tumors include a 0.5-cm or larger tumor with carcinoid morphology, with fewer than two mitoses per 2 mm^2, and without necrosis (Fig. 22-1A and Table 22-1).[11]

In contrast, atypical carcinoid tumors tend to be located peripherally in the lungs.[8] On gross pathologic examination, they appear white-gray on section but can be tan, pink to yellow brown, or red.[12] The WHO diagnostic criteria for atypical carcinoid tumors include a tumor with carcinoid morphology with two to 10 mitoses per 2 mm^2, with or without necrosis (see Fig. 22-1B and Table 22-1).[11]

Genetics and Biochemistry

Leotlela and colleagues report development of BP neuroendocrine tumors as a result of loss of heterozygosity in multiple chromosomes, including 3p, 11q13 (*MEN1* gene), 13q13 (the retinoblastoma *[RB]* gene), and 17p13 (*p53* gene).[13] Loss of heterozygosity at chromosome 3p is the most frequent change in BP neuroendocrine tumors and has been observed in 40% of typical carcinoid tumors and 73% of atypical carcinoid tumors.[14]

BP carcinoid tumors are known to occur, although rarely, as components of familial endocrine cancer syndromes—namely, multiple endocrine neoplasia I (MEN-1). Inactivation of the *MEN1* gene by mutation is seen in approximately 47% of typical carcinoid tumors and 70% of atypical carcinoid tumors.[15-17] A study of 129 patients with MEN-1 found that six individuals (5%) had been diagnosed with BP carcinoid tumors on initial diagnosis.[18] A review of the chest computed tomography (CT) scans of 32 of these patients showed that 12 patients had pulmonary nodules that were suspected to be BP carcinoid tumor, and four of these were histologically confirmed as BP carcinoid tumor. Therefore, it is recommended that patients with a diagnosis of MEN-1 be screened for BP carcinoid tumors with chest CT scanning every 3 years beginning at 20 years of age.[18,19]

The *p53* gene is important for maintaining genomic stability in addition to numerous other functions. Loss of heterozygosity or abnormal expression of the *p53* locus has been detected in 4% of typical carcinoid tumors and 29% of atypical carcinoid tumors.[20,21] Kobayashi and coworkers evaluated the frequency of p53 protein expression in BP neuroendocrine tumors and found that typical carcinoid tumors demonstrated 0% expression, whereas atypical carcinoid tumors have 20% expression.[22]

E-cadherin and β-catenins, transmembrane glycoproteins involved in cell–cell adhesion, are expressed in BP carcinoid tumors at levels of 50% and 37%, respectively, which is a lower level than their expression in high-grade BP neuroendocrine tumors.[23] A decrease in expression of E-cadherin and β-catenin also correlates with lymph node metastases,

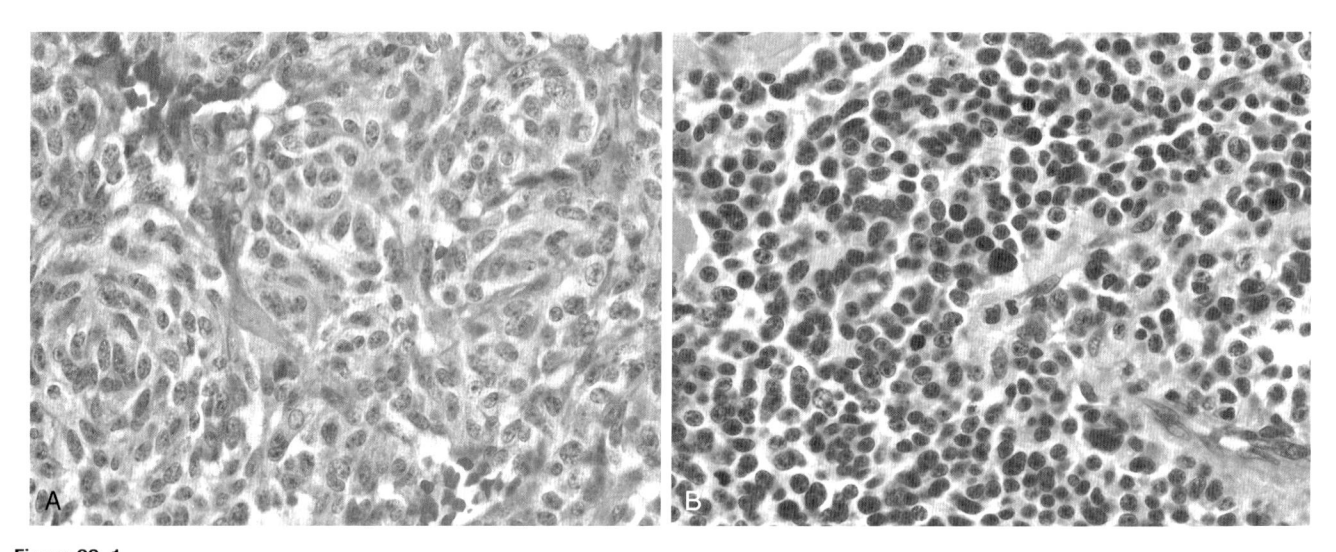

Figure 22–1
A, Typical carcinoid tumor (hematoxylin & eosin). **B,** Atypical carcinoid tumor (H&E).

Table 22–1
WHO Diagnostic Criteria for Bronchopulmonary Carcinoid Tumors

	Location	Nodal Metastases	Gross Pathologic Examination	WHO Criteria
Typical carcinoid tumor	Central	Rare	White or gray, with minimal evidence of necrosis or hemorrhage	<2 mitoses per 2 mm^2 Size > 0.5 cm Lack of necrosis
Atypical carcinoid tumor	Peripheral	Frequent	White-gray; on section, tan, pink, red, or yellow-brown	2-10 mitoses per 2 mm^2 Size > 0.5 cm Necrosis

suggesting that an abnormal E-cadherin or β-catenin expression pattern is an independent predictor of atypical carcinoid tumor progression.[24]

Clinical Presentation

Because of the high proportion of centrally located BP carcinoid tumors,[9] most patients are symptomatic at presentation. The most common symptoms are cough, hemoptysis, and pneumonia, representing the consequences of endoluminal obstruction secondary to the tumor. Symptoms may be present for many years before diagnosis, and, almost entirely, they reflect the anatomic location of the lesion as opposed to the secreted bioactive products.[25] Interestingly, a population-based study in Denmark observed that 24% of typical carcinoid tumors and 7% of atypical carcinoid tumors were discovered on autopsy.[25]

Carcinoid syndrome (diarrhea, flushing, wheezing, and heart disease) as a presentation of BP carcinoid tumors is rare (1% to 3%) and is associated with liver metastases. The incidence of liver metastases is very rare (typical carcinoid tumor, 2%; atypical carcinoid tumor, 5%).[26,27]

Cushing syndrome (ectopic production and secretion of adrenocorticotropic hormone [ACTH]) can occur in 2% of patients with BP carcinoid tumors; however, less than 1% of those with Cushing syndrome have a BP carcinoid tumor.[28] Aniszewski and colleagues studied 106 patients with ectopic production of ACTH and found that BP carcinoid tumors (25%) were the most frequent cause, followed by islet cell tumors (16%) and small cell lung cancer (11%).[29]

Other rare endocrinopathies that afflict patients with BP carcinoid tumors include acromegaly (increased production and secretion of growth hormone), hypercalcemia, and hypoglycemia.[30,31]

Diagnosis

Imaging

Chest radiographs are nonspecific for BP carcinoid tumors. Those tumors that do appear are often isolated, well-defined hilar or perihilar masses. Suspect lesions should be examined further with chest CT (Fig. 22-2). The usual CT appearance of a typical carcinoid tumor is that of a well-defined, spherical to ovoid mass that exerts a mass effect or obstruction of airways. They are often vascular and more often centrally located. In contrast, atypical carcinoid tumors are usually located peripherally and 30% have calcifications (Fig. 22-3).[8]

A majority of BP neuroendocrine tumors express (80%) somatostatin receptors, predominantly subtype 2.[32] Somatostatin receptor scintigraphy uses radiolabeled somatostatin analogs (indium-111–labeled octreotide and ^{111}In-lanreotide) to locate BP neuroendocrine tumors.[33] This imaging modality is rarely used, however, in the diagnosis or workup of BP carcinoid tumors.

Positron emission tomography (PET) detects uptake of radiolabeled biological fluorodeoxyglucose labeled with radioactive fluoride (^{18}F) (FDG) by neoplastic cells. FDG-PET has shown false-negative results with solitary BP carcinoid tumors, as they are usually hypometabolic on FDG-PET[34]; however, a more recent retrospective study by Marom and coworkers examined 192 T1 lung cancers, six of which were BP carcinoid tumors, and five of the six were detected using FDG-PET.[35] Chong and colleagues reviewed seven FDG-PET scans of two typical carcinoid tumors and five atypical

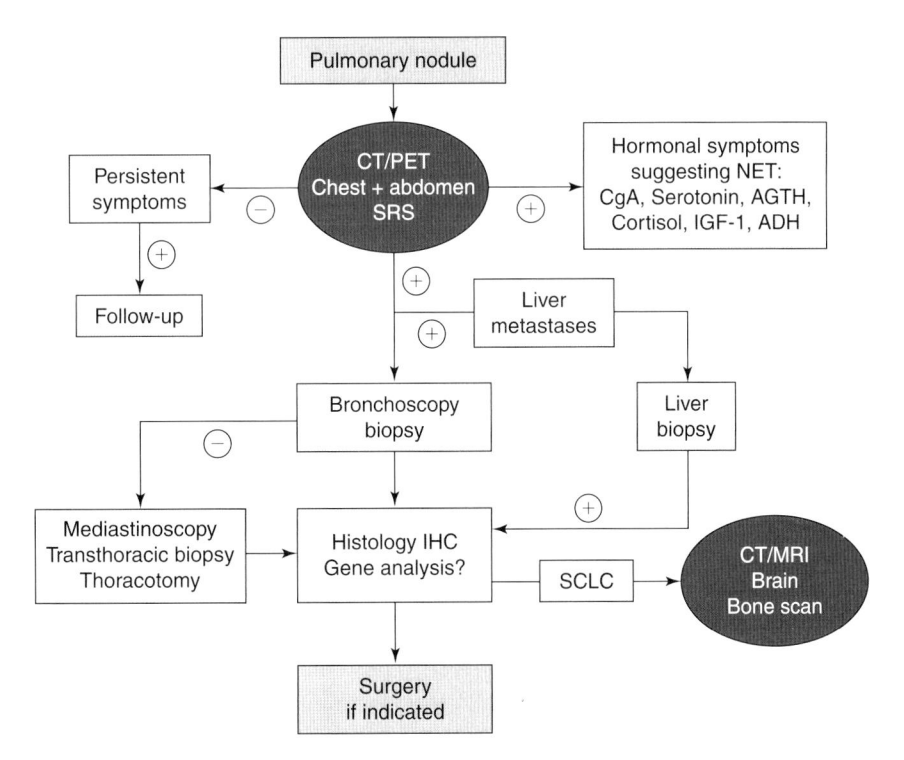

Figure 22–2
Algorithm for diagnosis of bronchopulmonary carcinoid tumors. ADH, antidiuretic hormone; AGTH, adrenoglomerulotropic hormone; CgA, chromogranin A; IGF, insulin-like growth factor; IHC, immunohistochemistry; NET, neuroendocrine tumor; SCLC, small cell lung cancer; SRS, somatostatin receptor scintigraphy. *(From Gustafsson BI, Kidd M, Chan A, Malfertheiner MV, Modlin IM.* Cancer 2008;**113**:5-21.)

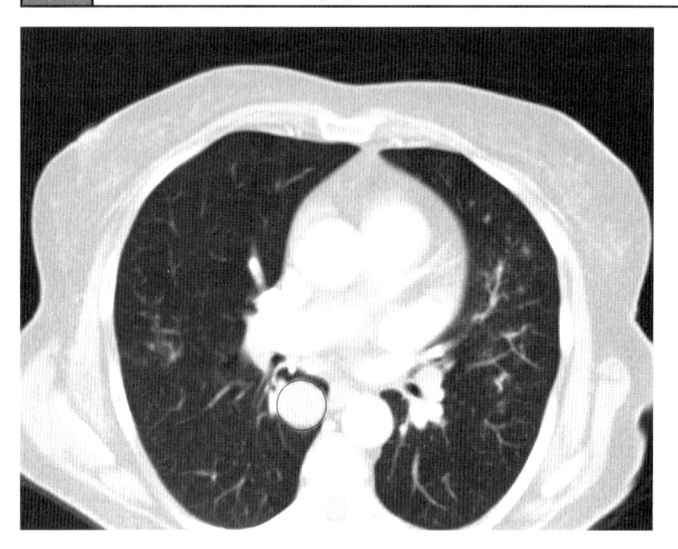

Figure 22-3
Chest CT of a right-sided typical carcinoid tumor.

carcinoid tumors for the maximal standardized uptake value (SUV). The two typical carcinoid tumors had an SUV range of 3.2 to 3.4, with both specimens exhibiting less than mediastinal uptake. Three of the five atypical carcinoid tumors had higher than mediastinal uptake (4.0 to 7.1). One of the five atypical carcinoid tumors had a maximal SUV of 1.7, with an ipsilateral hilar lymph node measuring 11.2 SUV.[36] Given the propensity for false-negatives in FDG-PET scans, a lesion that is suspected of being a carcinoid tumor on CT should be resected if the patient is operable.

Bronchoscopy

Rivera and coworkers reviewed nearly 3800 patients with central, endobronchial lesions and found the overall sensitivity of flexible fiberoptic bronchoscopy for detecting lesions was 88%.[37] Because the majority (75%) of BP carcinoid tumors are centrally located, they are amenable to bronchoscopic evaluation. Even with direct visualization of BP carcinoid tumors, it is difficult to distinguish typical from atypical carcinoid tumor with the small biopsy typically obtained by flexible bronchoscopy. As 5% to 20% of typical carcinoid tumors and 30% to 70% of atypical carcinoid tumors metastasize, lymph nodes should be assessed to adequately stage the BP carcinoid tumor.[12]

In the past, a feared complication of flexible bronchoscopy was major hemorrhage; however, this is now rare. In a review of 587 biopsies by flexible and rigid bronchoscopy, significant hemorrhage occurred in 15 patients (2.6%), with only four (0.7%) requiring emergency intervention for massive uncontrollable hemorrhage.[38] To reduce the risk of hemorrhage, an epinephrine solution can be administered through the bronchoscope before the biopsy. In the event of significant bleeding that is difficult to control, a neodymium:yttrium-aluminum-garnet (Nd:YAG) laser is helpful.[39] In summary, it is safe to bronchoscopically biopsy a suspected carcinoid tumor.

Peripheral BP carcinoid lesions can be evaluated by CT-guided percutaneous transthoracic needle biopsy, video-assisted thoracic surgery (VATS), or thoracotomy.

Tumor Markers

Serotonin and urinary 5-hydroxyindoleacetic acid are well-known markers of hormonally active carcinoid tumors; however, they are not specific for BP carcinoid tumors. Chromogranin A elevation in plasma is a relatively (75%) sensitive marker of BP carcinoid tumors.[40] Care must be taken in patients with renal impairment or atrophic gastritis, and during proton-pump inhibitor therapy, as these conditions cause elevations in chromogranin A and thus false-positive results. In clinical practice, there is no evidence that measurement of tumor marker levels adds value or alters patient management, so they are not routinely performed.

Staging

The TNM classification for lung cancer remains the most useful staging classification for BP carcinoid tumors. Fink and colleagues[26] analyzed nearly 142 cases of BP carcinoid tumors (128 typical and 14 atypical) and found that 87% of typical carcinoid tumors were without lymph node metastases, 10% demonstrated N1 disease (ipsilateral hilar lymph node involvement), and 3% demonstrated N2 disease (ipsilateral mediastinal lymph node involvement). None were found to exhibit N3 disease. Two (1.5%) patients with typical carcinoid tumor presented with distant metastases. Of the atypical carcinoid tumors, 43% were N0, 29% demonstrated N1 disease, 14% demonstrated N2 disease, and 14% exhibited N3 disease. Three patients (14%) with atypical carcinoid tumor presented with distant metastases.[26]

More recently, an Italian study retrospectively analyzed 252 patients (174 typical and 78 atypical) over a 38-year period and found 96% of patients with typical carcinoid tumors presented without nodal metastases, 3.4% with N1 disease, and 0.6% with N2 disease. In contrast, only 72% of patients with atypical carcinoid tumors presented without nodal metastases, 17% with N1 disease, and 11% with N2 disease. Thus, typical carcinoid tumors rarely have nodal disease, whereas atypical carcinoid tumors commonly have either N1 or N2 disease, again highlighting the different profiles of these two tumors.

Management and Treatment

Surgery

Complete surgical resection with preservation of normal lung tissue remains the only curative treatment of BP carcinoid tumors (Fig. 22-4).[7] Centrally located typical carcinoid tumors should be resected using lung- and parenchyma-sparing resections such as a sleeve resection, or an anatomic segmentectomy.[27,41] Surgical treatment of typical carcinoid tumors does not require a wide margin of resection, as local recurrence is rare.[42] Ferguson and coworkers in a multicenter retrospective study found that a wide nonanatomic wedge resection or segmentectomy was justified in the case of peripheral typical carcinoid tumors because of the low likelihood of local recurrence.[43]

Although most agree that a nonanatomic resection, when possible, is acceptable in the management of typical carcinoid tumors, the surgical approach for atypical carcinoid tumors is typically a lobectomy or, rarely, a pneumonectomy. Because of the greater propensity of atypical carcinoid tumors to metastasize to lymph nodes, a more extensive and aggressive

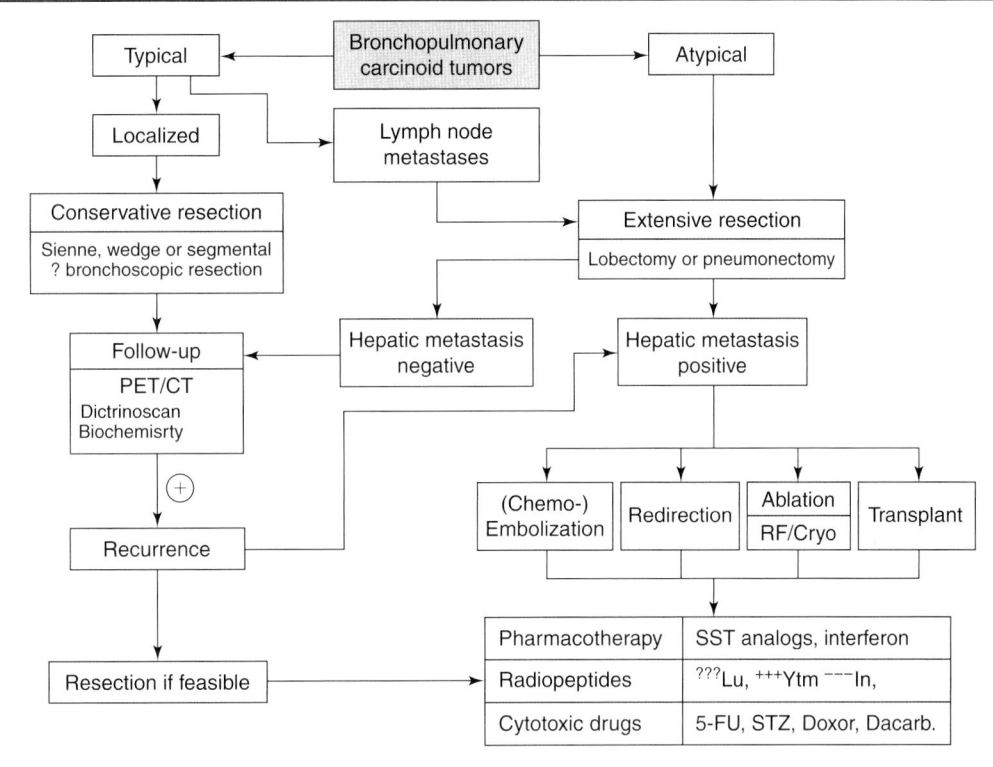

Figure 22–4
Algorithm for treatment of bronchopulmonary carcinoid tumors. FU, fluorouracil; RF, radiofrequency; SST, somatostatin; STZ, streptozocin. Dacarb., dacarbazine; Doxor, doxorubicin; Lu, lutetium; Ytm, yttriium; In, indium. *(From Gustafsson BI, Kidd M, Chan A, Malfertheiner MV, Modlin IM. Cancer 2008;**113**:5-21.)*

resection (lobectomy, bi-lobectomy, and pneumonectomy) and nodal dissection is recommended.[9,44,45]

Surgical resection of BP carcinoid tumors should be combined with ipsilateral mediastinal lymph node dissection or sampling.[42] Lymph node dissection is justified by the possibility of lymph node metastasis, which has an incidence of 4% to 13% in typical carcinoid tumors and 28% to 67% in atypical carcinoid tumors.[26,27,42,46]

Endobronchial Management

Bertoletti and colleagues recently conducted a study of 18 patients (all with typical carcinoid tumor, strict endoluminal disease, and no evidence of lymph node invasion) treated with flexible bronchoscopy and cryotherapy. Patients were followed for 55 months, and there was one recurrence in 7 years, with no long-term complications.[47] Although these results are encouraging, endobronchial resection should be reserved for patients who are not amenable to surgical intervention.

Radiation and Chemotherapy

BP carcinoid tumors respond poorly to radiotherapy, so this is generally used only when surgical resection is impractical, or as an adjunct when resection is incomplete.[7]

There is no role for adjuvant chemotherapy after resection of a typical carcinoid tumor regardless of the lymph node status. In patients with atypical carcinoid tumors, the recommendations for adjuvant doublet, platinum-based chemotherapy are largely based on similar indications for other non–small cell lung cancer histologies and the presence of N1 or N2 disease. No clinical trials have specifically addressed the role of chemotherapy, or the agent or dosing regimen, for atypical carcinoid tumors.

Prognosis

With an increase in the number of chest imaging studies as well as the enhanced quality of the imaging techniques, there has been an increase in the reported incidence of BP carcinoid tumors. Despite what could be perceived as earlier detection of all carcinoid tumors, a review of the SEER database demonstrates that there is a decrease in the 5-year survival rate of all patients with carcinoid tumors (including atypical ones) over the past 30 years.[2] Reasons for this observation are unclear; it may be related to an increase in the incidence of atypical carcinoid tumor histology.

Patients with typical carcinoid tumors have better prognoses than those with atypical carcinoid tumors. This difference is primarily explained by the differences in tumor biology between the two (Table 22-2). Recent studies have shown that the 5- and 10-year survival rates for patients with typical carcinoid tumors are 89% to 99% and 82% to 93%, respectively, whereas the 5- and 10-year survival rates for patients with atypical carcinoid tumors are 70% to 77% and 52% to 64%, respectively.[26,27,42,46]

The prognostic significance of lymph node involvement has been addressed by many studies in the past decade (see Table 22-2). Cardillo and coworkers and Garcia-Yuste and colleagues have demonstrated a significant 5-year survival difference for patients with node-positive atypical carcinoid tumors disease (59% and 60%, respectively) when compared with node-negative disease (100% and 83%, respectively).

Table 22–2
Comparison of Typical and Atypical Bronchopulmonary (BP) Carcinoid Tumors

Author, Year (ref)	BP Carcinoid Tumor	Patients (N)	N0	N1	N2	5-yr Survival (%)	10-yr Survival (%)	5-yr Survival (Node Negative) (%)	10-yr Survival (Node Negative) (%)	5-yr Survival (Node Positive) (%)	10-yr Survival (Node Positive) (%)
Fink et al., 2001 (26)	Typical	128	111	13	4	89	82	n/a	n/a	n/a	n/a
	Atypical	12	6	4	2	75	56				
Filosso et al., 2002 (27)	Typical	75	69	2	4	97	93	92	87	85	52
	Atypical	38	24	7	7	77	52				
Cardillo et al., 2004 (46)	Typical	121	107	14	0	99	n/a	100	n/a	90	n/a
	Atypical	42	15	18	9	70	n/a	100	n/a	59	n/a
Garcia-Yuste et al., 2007 (48)	Typical	569	517	32	20	97	92	97	92	100	66
	Atypical	92	59	14	19	78	67	83	70	60	60
Rea et al., 2007 (42)	Typical	174	167	6	1	n/a	93	n/a	87	n/a	50
	Atypical	78	56	13	9	n/a	64				
Totals	Typical	1067	971	67	29	89-99	82-93	—	—	—	—
	Atypical	262	160	56	46	70-77	52-67	—	—	—	—

n/a, not available.

For typical carcinoid tumors, the presence or absence of nodal disease does not correlate with survival.[46,48] Both Filosso and associates and Rea and coworkers have found there to be significantly better 10-year survival in patients diagnosed with BP carcinoid tumors and N0 disease regardless of histology (87% and 87%, respectively) when compared with those with N1 and N2 disease (52% and 50%, respectively).[26,42]

CARCINOID TUMORLETS

Gustafsson and colleagues discussed diffuse idiopathic pulmonary neuroendocrine cell hyperplasia (DIPNECH), a rare preneoplastic condition involving proliferation of pulmonary neuroendocrine cells and neuroepithelial bodies. When this proliferation extends beyond the basement membrane, the group of cells is identified as a tumorlet. A BP tumorlet is a nodular proliferation of neuroendocrine cells that constitutes a nodule less than 5 mm, and those that proliferate to greater than 5 mm are classified as BP carcinoid tumors.[7] DIPNECH can be both an adaptive response, as seen in persons living at high altitudes, and a reactive response to lung injury, as seen in patients with obliterative bronchiolitis,[49] chronic cough,[50] and interstitial lung disease.[51]

Carcinoid tumorlets and carcinoid tumors have long been associated, but a definitive relationship has not been established. Studies have demonstrated the presence of tumorlets in normal lungs or in association with carcinoid tumors.[52,53] There have also been case reports of isolated peribronchial[54] and hilar[55] lymph node metastases that point to the possible neoplastic potential[7] of carcinoid tumorlets. In each of these circumstances, the lymph nodes appeared grossly normal but were found to have microscopic metastases on pathologic examination.

Pathology and Diagnosis

Carcinoid tumorlets develop from Kulchitsky cells, which are hyperplastic neuroendocrine cells in the bronchial and bronchiolar mucosa. It has been suggested that these cells secrete neuropeptides that can elicit peribronchiolar reaction leading to fibrotic lung disease.[49,56]

The majority of pulmonary carcinoid tumorlets are often asymptomatic, even if multiple tumorlets are present. Pulmonary symptoms, dysfunction, and radiologic abnormalities have been attributed to multiple tumorlets.[57]

Aubry and coworkers[57] retrospectively reviewed 28 patients (26 were women) and their imaging. Patients were grouped according to results of imaging studies: multiple nodules (17), solitary nodule/opacity (seven), and obstructive lung disease (four). Those with multiple nodules were most likely to present with cough (59%) and dyspnea (47%); however, 41% of the patients had no presenting symptoms. Nearly one half of the patients (47%) with multiple nodules were nonsmokers, but 59% had test findings of obstructive pulmonary function. Thirteen patients with multiple nodules had both a carcinoid tumor and tumorlet, and four had only tumorlets. Three patients (11%) with a dominant carcinoid tumor had lymph node metastases.[57]

Management, Treatment, and Prognosis

There is no consensus on the management of carcinoid tumorlets. If a carcinoid tumorlet is discovered on pathologic examination, further surgical resection is not advocated. When carcinoid tumorlets are associated with BP carcinoid tumors, the appropriate management and treatment are dictated by the histology and stage of the BP carcinoid tumor. Clinical surveillance may be indicated for patients with carcinoid tumorlets, because they can (but rarely) progress to a true carcinoid tumor.

The risk of developing clinically significant neuroendocrine lung neoplasms is low for patients with neuroendocrine cell hyperplasia.[57] Neuroendocrine cell hyperplasia has been suggested to be a preneoplastic lesion, as it had been associated with tumorlets and peripheral carcinoid tumors.[58]

Most patients have persistent and stable disease without the need for adjuvant therapy. Progressive disease, although uncommon, is demonstrated by metastases in patients with a dominant carcinoid tumor or progressive diffuse disease with underlying obstructive airway disease.[57]

PRIMARY PULMONARY SALIVARY GLAND–TYPE NEOPLASMS

Primary salivary gland–type lung tumors are rare intrathoracic malignancies and account for 0.2% of all lung tumors.[59] These tumors include adenoid cystic carcinomas (ACC), mucoepidermoid carcinomas (MEC), and mixed tumors (ACC and MEC).[60] ACC, MEC, and mixed tumors are nearly indistinguishable from other salivary gland tumors. It has been postulated that these tumors arise from the submucosal glands of the tracheobronchial tree.[60,61]

Molina and colleagues[62] performed a retrospective review of 62 patients with primary salivary-type lung cancer and found that ACC was diagnosed in 64.5% of patients, MEC was diagnosed in 32.3% of patients, and mixed tumor was diagnosed in 3.2% of patients. These results are consistent with tose of previous series, although MEC is usually considered the most frequent form of primary salivary gland–type lung tumor contained in the lung parenchyma. Patients diagnosed with ACC were older than those with MEC (54 years versus 40 years, $P = .02$). A history of smoking or current smoking is more associated with ACC than with MEC.[62]

Pathology

MEC tumors are defined by the presence of mucous cells mixed with epidermoid, clear, and "intermediate" cell types. Brandwein and coworkers developed a three-stage grading system (low to high grade).[63] ACC tumors exhibit myoepithelial cells with various degrees of ductal-type cells and are recognized on the basis of their predominant architectural pattern: tubular (grade 1), cribriform (grade 2), or solid (grade 3). Tumors that had a greater than 30% solid growth pattern are classified as solid (Table 22-3).[62]

Diagnosis

The majority of salivary gland tumors are endobronchial lesions that arise centrally in large airways, although primary peripheral ACC of the lung has rarely been reported.[60,64] Symptoms are typically related to the sequelae of either endoluminal obstruction or extraluminal compression as a result of the central tumor location.

Table 22-3
Primary Pulmonary Salivary Gland–Type Neoplasms

Tumor Type	Location	Pathology	Sputum Cytology	Treatment
Adenoid cystic carcinoma (ACC)	Trachea, bronchi, lung	Myoepithelial cells, ductal-type cells	Negative	Surgery, radiation therapy
Mucoepidermoid carcinoma (MCC)	Bronchi	Mucous cells, epidermoid cells, clear-type cells, "intermediate" cells	Negative	Surgery
Mixed tumors (ACC and MCC)	Trachea, bronchi	Mix of ACC and MEC	Negative	Surgery

Molina and colleagues retrospectively reviewed 49 patients with MEC and 115 patients with ACC and found the most common symptoms to be cough, dyspnea, hemoptysis, wheezing, and fever. Dyspnea (60% versus 35%) and wheezing (42.5% versus 30%) were more common in patients with ACC than in those with MEC.[62]

Chest radiographs usually appear normal unless the tumor obstructs the airway, so chest CT scans are recommended to obtain more detail about the intraluminal and extraluminal extents of both ACC and MEC.[65]

Because of the predominance of centrally located primary salivary gland–type lung tumors, flexible bronchoscopy is the primary invasive diagnostic modality.

Management and Treatment

Surgery

Complete surgical resection with preservation of normal lung tissue is the only curative treatment for ACCs and MECs. Given the propensity of ACCs to have submucosal and perineural spread, intraoperative frozen sections must be used to confirm negative margins.[66] Transmucosal bronchoscopic biopsies conducted intraoperatively can help direct operative planning. Because of the tendency of ACC to extend longitudinally in a perineural manner, a microscopically positive surgical margin may be acceptable if further resection would jeopardize a successful tracheobronchial anastomosis.[67]

A recent retrospective analysis of 62 of patients with primary salivary gland–type lung tumors, 43 (71.7%) of whom underwent surgical resection, found that the most common procedures performed were lobectomy (44%), tracheal resection (26%), and pneumonectomy (19%). Interestingly, patients with MEC (95%) underwent surgical resection more often than patients with ACC (60%).[62]

Endobronchial Treatment Strategies

Brutinel and coworkers[68] compiled a 2-year experience with endobronchial Nd:YAG laser therapy to relieve endobronchial obstruction. Of the 116 patients in the study, eight had ACC. When these patients were treated with laser therapy for palliation, they remained asymptomatic for longer than those with more common forms of lung cancer.[68] Endobronchial laser therapy should precede radiation therapy if possible, because edema from radiation therapy may temporarily exacerbate the airway obstruction.[69,70] Endobronchial brachytherapy can be used to extend the palliative treatment of ACC.[71]

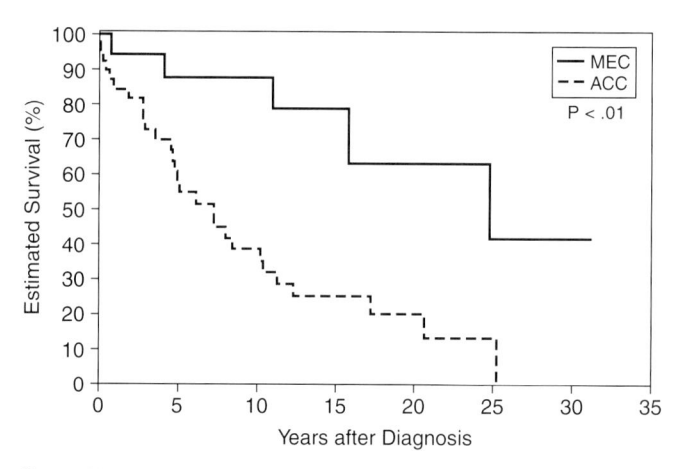

Figure 22-5
Kaplan-Meier curves comparing adenoid cystic carcinomas (ACC) and mucoepidermoid carcinomas (MEC). (From Molina JR, Aubry MC, Lewis JE, et al. Cancer 2007;**110**: 2253-2259.)

Adjuvant Treatment

ACCs are relatively radiosensitive; the role of radiation therapy for MEC is more controversial. The likelihood of a complete response for ACC correlates significantly with a dose of 60 Gy or more.[72] Molina and colleagues treated 14 patients with adjuvant radiation therapy, some for positive resection margins at the time of surgery and some for palliation.[62] It is generally recommended to offer adjuvant radiation to centrally located ACC lesions, regardless of whether it is an R0, R1, or R2 resection.

Hotte and coworkers[73] conducted a phase II consortium study to assess the antitumor activity of imatinib (Gleevac) in ACC, as these tumors are known to express a high level of c-kit. Imatinib inhibits autophosphorylation of the *bcr-abl*, platelet-derived growth factor receptor beta, and c-*kit* tyrosine kinases. Of the 16 patients enrolled in the study, 15 had an assessable response. Nine patients had stable disease and six had progressive disease after two cycles. Therefore, there is no role for routine administration of imatinib to patients with ACC.[73]

Prognosis

Patients with primary salivary-type lung tumors have significantly better outcomes than those with non–small cell lung cancers, as the former are considered low-grade malignancies. Patients with ACC had significantly poorer 5- and 10-year survival rates than patients with MEC (55% and 39% compared with 88% and 88%, respectively) (Fig. 22-5).[62]

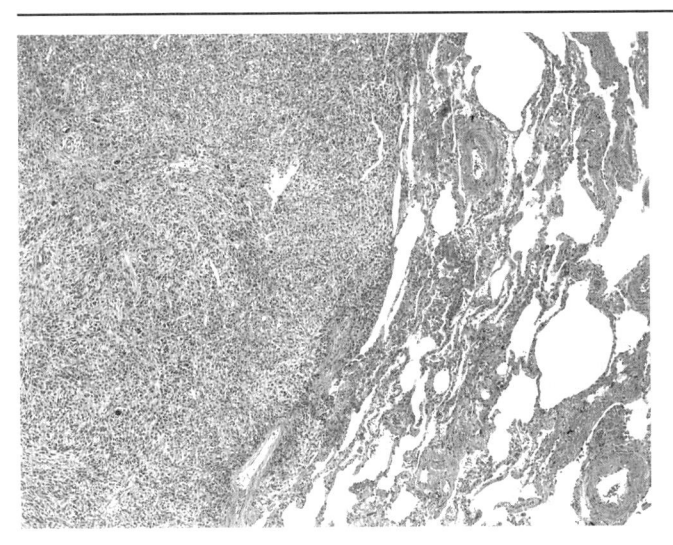

Figure 22-6
Leiomyosarcoma (hematoxylin & eosin).

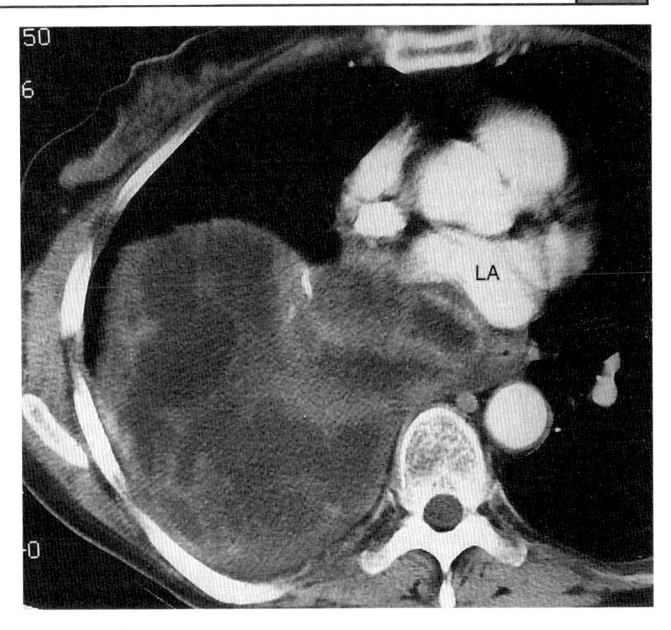

Figure 22-7
Chest CT scan of primary pulmonary leiomyosarcoma. LA, left atrium. *(From Gladish GW, Sabloff BM, Munden RF, Truong MT, Erasmus JJ, Chasen MH.* Radiographics 2002;**22**: 621-637.)

Tumor grade is both a prognostic marker and a factor in determining adjuvant therapy for MEC.[74] Yousem and colleagues reported a 95% survival rate for low-grade MEC tumors, and they found that nearly 25% of patients with high-grade MEC tumors experienced recurrences.[74] The rate of nodal metastasis is related to tumor grade, with 2% of low-grade and 15% of high-grade MEC tumors metastasizing to regional lymph nodes, respectively.[61] It has been suggested that patients with grade 1 MEC undergo surgery alone, whereas those with grade 2 and 3 tumors should receive surgery followed by adjuvant therapy.[67]

PRIMARY PULMONARY SARCOMAS

Primary pulmonary sarcomas are rare neoplasms, making up only 1% of lung carcinomas. They must be distinguished from the more common sarcomas metastatic to the lung, primary pulmonary sarcomatoid carcinomas, and diffuse malignant mesotheliomas involving the lung.[75,76] Diagnosis requires a tissue biopsy, along with confirmation that the patient does not have a history of cancer or a current remote neoplasm consistent with a sarcoma of another primary site.

In 2004, the WHO reclassified primary pulmonary sarcomas. Tumors previously thought to be primary sarcomas are now classified into other neoplastic groups. For example, pulmonary blastomas, rhabdomyosarcomas, osteosarcomas, and chondrosarcomas are all now designated as primary pulmonary sarcomatoid carcinomas.[75] With advances in molecular pathology diagnostics and histopathologic technology, lesions once thought to be primary pulmonary sarcomas, such as hemangiopericytoma, are now rarely described in the literature.[77] The primary pulmonary sarcomas described in the following paragraphs retain their classification and occur as such in the literature.

Primary Pulmonary Leiomyosarcoma

Primary pulmonary leiomyosarcomas can be subdivided into those that are primarily in the pulmonary artery (10%) and those that arise from the bronchus (20%) and pulmonary parenchyma (70%).[78] Gross pathology studies reveal well-circumscribed, grayish white, firm, and rubbery lesions. Those lesions considered high grade demonstrated areas of hemorrhage and necrosis. Histologically, Moran and coworkers separated the lesions from low to intermediate to high grade (Fig. 22-6).[79] Radiologically, pulmonary leiomyosarcomas manifest as well-marginated smooth or lobular homogeneous nodules or large necrotic masses (Fig. 22-7).[80]

Because of the rarity of primary pulmonary leiomyosarcomas, there is little consensus on treatment. The most commonly accepted therapy is surgical excision, as is performed for other pulmonary sarcomas.[81] There is a lack of evidence for radiation and chemotherapy in the treatment of primary pulmonary leiomyosarcomas; however, doxorubicin and ifosfamide are considered the most effective agents for soft tissue sarcomas.[82]

A study reviewing 18 patients with primary leiomyosarcomas of the lung found a mean age of 50 (5 to 76 years). A majority of the patients were asymptomatic on presentation, and the neoplasms were incidentally discovered. The review indicated that those patients with high-grade lesions had significantly poorer prognosis, with 89% (eight of nine) of patients dead within 2 years of diagnosis.[79]

Primary Pulmonary Synovial Sarcoma

Primary pulmonary synovial sarcoma comprises 0.5% of all lung malignancies. Tumors may derive from the lung parenchyma, the bronchial tree, or the pulmonary arteries.[83] The 2004 WHO classification defines primary pulmonary synovial sarcomas as being mesenchymal spindle cell tumors.

On gross pathologic examination, the tumors are soft, tan masses, with foci of necrosis, hemorrhage, and cystic change. Histologically, these tumors are indistinguishable from those of monophasic synovial sarcomas of the soft tissues; however, many groups, including Begueret and colleagues,[84] found that a characteristic t(X;18) chromosomal translocation helps diagnostically confirm pulmonary synovial sarcomas in greater than 90% of cases. Additionally, Jiang and coworkers demonstrated the presence of two embryonic tumor markers, epithelial membrane antigen and vimentin, that help differentiate primary pulmonary synovial sarcomas from other lesions.[83]

In a study of 75 patients with primary pulmonary synovial sarcomas with no characteristic symptoms on presentation, the majority of patients were asymptomatic. The most common presenting symptoms, if any were present, were cough (21%), chest pain (20%), and hemoptysis (20%). The median age at diagnosis was 40 years, and there was no significant sex preponderance.[85,86] Most pulmonary tumors are peripheral, with occasional endobronchial lesions.[84,87] Metastatic synovial sarcoma to the lungs is more common than its primary counterpart; therefore, metastatic disease must be ruled out before therapy is begun. The standardized therapy for patients with primary pulmonary synovial sarcoma is surgical resection and adjuvant radiation or chemotherapy, depending on the findings at the time of surgery. Synovial sarcoma is chemosensitive to doxorubicin and ifosfamide with an overall response rate of 24%.[88] Tumors tend to recur locally with extension into the chest wall, pericardium, paraspinal soft tissue, diaphragm, and abdomen.[75] The overall prognosis for patients with primary pulmonary synovial sarcoma is poor, with an overall 5-year survival rate of 50%.[89] Risk factors that predict a poorer prognosis for patients with primary pulmonary synovial sarcoma are age greater than 20 years, tumor size greater than 5 cm, incomplete resection, and large number of mitotic figures.[83]

Primary Pulmonary Epithelioid Hemangioendothelioma

Pulmonary epithelioid hemangioendothelioma, previously called intravascular bronchioloalveolar tumor, is a primary pulmonary sarcoma that is considered a low- to intermediate-grade vascular tumor. It affects young patients and is more common in women.[90]

On gross examination, the tumor is gray-white or gray-tan. The cut surface has a cartilaginous consistency with occasional calcification. Histologically, the tumor has a distinctive appearance, with short cords and nests of epithelioid cells associated with a myxohyaline matrix.[75]

Preoperative diagnosis is difficult, as most diagnoses are made from pathologic evaluation of surgical biopsies. Immunohistochemistry shows diffuse cytoplasmic staining of the malignant cells with factor VIII-related antigen, confirming lineage of tumor cells.[90] Fifty percent of patients present with clinical symptoms similar to those of other lung neoplasms (cough, dyspnea, chest pain). Imaging often demonstrates the presence of multiple bilateral nodules, with occasional calcification.[91-94]

Because primary pulmonary epithelioid hemangioendothelioma is rare, data related to a standard treatment strategy are limited. In patients with a unilateral nodule, a wedge resection offers a survival benefit similar to that of anatomic resection.[90] Lymph node sampling or dissection is typically done, but the prognostic value is unknown because of the small number of patients who demonstrate lymph node metastases.[95] Patients with bilateral nodules have undergone a variety of treatments, such as interferon-alpha-2a,[96] azathioprine,[97] multiple wedge resections,[98] or just follow-up. Bagan and colleagues endorse evaluation for lung transplantation in patients with vascular aggressiveness because of a life expectancy of less than 1 year.[90]

Prognosis is, in part, dependent on the site of metastases; however, unlike in other lung cancers, simultaneous lesions in the lung and the liver do not necessarily mean metastases. Epithelioid hemangioendothelioma may also be found as a second concurrent primary in the liver. This is important in the transplant community because surgeons who manage transplantation for hepatic hemangioendothelioma do not consider a focal lesion in the lung as a metastasis.[99] Bagan and coworkers indicate that the current staging system for lung cancer does not predict outcome for primary pulmonary epithelioid hemangioendothelioma, and they advocate the use of clinical and radiologic disease to guide prognosis.[90] Prognosis in patients with primary pulmonary epithelioid hemangioendothelioma can be sorted into two groups: asymptomatic patients with nodules, who have a median survival of 180 months, and patients with symptoms of vascular endothelial cell proliferation (alveolar hemorrhage, hemoptysis, hemorrhagic pleural effusion), who have a significantly worse survival.[90]

Primary Pulmonary Angiosarcoma

Malignant vascular tumors are highly uncommon, with angiosarcomas constituting less than 1% of all sarcomas.[100] Pulmonary angiosarcomas are usually the consequence of metastases from the skin or subcutaneous tissue, breast, liver, or heart. Primary pulmonary angiosarcoma is characterized by an insidious growth pattern, with the tumor showing extensive local invasion and hematogenous metastases at the time of presentation.[101] Demographically, angiosarcomas typically arise in middle-aged adults. These tumors have been associated with radiation therapy and with exposure to vinyl chloride and arsenic.[102]

Pathologically, these lesions can mimic carcinomas and exhibit cytokeratin positivity.[103] Some patients present with bilateral infiltrates that mask pulmonary hemorrhage. The most common clinical presentation is that of hemoptysis.[103] Radiologically, these lesions usually present as multiple bilateral nodules.[104]

Surgery remains the mainstay treatment for primary pulmonary angiosarcomas. Angiosarcomas are radiosensitive. Some studies have shown promising results with intratumoral injection of recombinant interleukin-2, and, if high enough dosages are given, regression of pulmonary metastasis has been demonstrated.[105] Additionally, paclitaxel, which exerts antiangiogenic and apoptotic effects, has been shown to be effective against angiosarcoma.[106] Prognosis of patients with angiosarcomas is quite poor: most patients die within months of initial presentation.[100]

PRIMARY SOLITARY PULMONARY PLASMACYTOMA

Extramedullary plasmacytomas are uncommon neoplasms of plasma cell origin. Most of these tumors arise in the head and neck region, and in very rare occasions they may arise in the lung as a solitary nodule or less commonly as a lobar consolidation or diffuse pulmonary infiltrates.[107] Joseph and colleagues evaluated 19 cases of primary pulmonary plasmacytoma and found both men and women were affected equally and that the median age at diagnosis was 42 years.[108]

Diagnosis

Patients are either asymptomatic on presentation or have nonspecific pulmonary symptoms of cough, wheeze, or shortness of breath.[107] Diagnosis of primary pulmonary plasmacytoma is difficult. The clinician should undertake the workup of a lung nodule or mass. Most commonly, the diagnosis is made after excision of the tumor and proper histopathologic examination.

Treatment and Prognosis

Treatment for primary pulmonary plasmacytoma is usually resection alone or a combination of surgery with chemotherapy or radiotherapy. A review of 19 patients with primary pulmonary plasmacytomas showed that the patients underwent surgery alone (11), radiation therapy (3), surgery with radiation (3), or surgery with chemotherapy (2), and only one patient had a local recurrence 9 years after excision.[108] A solitary pulmonary plasmacytoma has been reported to develop into multiple myeloma over time.[109,110] Therefore, once the diagnosis is made, a complete evaluation should be done to exclude systemic disease. After resection, patients should be monitored closely with serum and urine electrophoresis, skeletal bone survey, and bone marrow examination.[107]

PRIMARY PULMONARY LYMPHOMA

Primary pulmonary lymphomas are uncommon, representing less than 1% of lung cancers,[111] less than 1% of malignant lymphomas,[112] and only 3.6% of extranodal lymphomas.[113] The peak incidence of primary pulmonary lymphomas is in the 6th and 7th decades of life with no sex predominance.[114] Immunosuppression has been shown to be a risk factor for the development of lymphoma.[115]

Pathology

All mucosa-associated lymphoid tissue (MALT) lymphomas are of B-cell origin, often with plasmacytoid differentiation. Most MALT lymphomas are low grade, but transition to higher grade can occur in a minority of cases.[116]

Diagnosis

Graham and coworkers[116] reported a series of 18 patients with primary pulmonary lymphoma. The most common pulmonary symptoms on presentation were cough (50%), dyspnea (39%), and chest pain (17%). Additionally, these patients suffered from the systemic symptoms of fatigue (11%) and weight loss (6%). Four patients (22%) were asymptomatic on presentation.[116]

Management and Treatment

Once diagnosed, the primary pulmonary lymphoma must be appropriately staged to rule out extrathoracic disease. This includes further imaging, possible bone marrow biopsy, and laboratory tests (lactate dehydrogenase and beta-2-microglobulin).[117,118]

Management for an isolated primary pulmonary MALT lymphoma diagnosed by CT-guided biopsy is observation only, reserving treatment for possible future progression of disease based on symptoms and radiographic progression. When the diagnosis was established after a wedge resection or lobectomy, with negative margins and no evidence of high-grade transformation or disease elsewhere, a complete resection is considered definitive and no further therapy is required. If there is residual disease, disease in the contralateral chest, high-grade lymphoma, or extrathoracic disease, then chemotherapy, and rarely radiation, should be considered.[116]

Prognosis

Cordier and colleagues reported a 94% 5-year survival for low-grade primary pulmonary lymphoma, and a median survival of 3 years for high-grade disease.[119] Ferraro and coworkers reported a 68% 5-year survival for primary pulmonary MALT lymphoma.[120]

PRIMARY PULMONARY MELANOMA

Primary pulmonary melanomas are among the rarest of primary lung tumors, and only approximately 20 cases have been reported in the English language literature.[121] Because of their scarcity, the clinical presentation, natural history, treatment, and prognosis are not well defined.

Pathology

It has been proposed that three histologic criteria may help differentiate primary pulmonary melanoma from metastatic disease. These criteria are nesting of malignant cells beneath the bronchial epithelium, invasion of the bronchial epithelium in an area without epithelial ulceration, and demonstration of melanoma beneath the aforementioned changes.[122]

Attempts have been made to classify primary pulmonary melanomas. It would seem that to have a primary pulmonary melanoma, there must be a melanin-containing precursor cell. However, melanin-containing cells have not been demonstrated in the normal tracheobronchial tree.[121] It has been postulated that because the trachea shares an embryologic origin with the pharynx and esophagus, both of which are known to give rise to primary melanomas, the primary pulmonary melanoma may be a consequence of residual melanoblasts.[121]

Diagnosis

In a literature review of 20 cases, Ost and colleagues[121] found that the common presenting symptoms of primary pulmonary melanoma to be cough (50%), hemoptysis (40%), and postobstructive pneumonia (25%). Of note, 30% of patients were asymptomatic and the lesion was found incidentally on chest radiographs. Constitutional symptoms of weight loss, night sweats, or fever were present in 25% of patients.[121]

In addition to the pathologic criteria for the identification of primary pulmonary melanomas, a complete evaluation of the patient must be conducted to exclude any other primary source. Jensen and coworkers proposed criteria for clinical diagnosis of primary pulmonary melanoma as follows: pigmented skin tumors were not previously removed and melanomas in other organs were not demonstrable at the time of surgical resection, these is no history of excised ocular tumors, and the tumor must be solitary with morphologic features compatible with a primary tumor.[123]

Treatment

If a pulmonary melanoma is encountered and it is determined to be a primary lesion after a thorough examination, the appropriate treatment is an anatomic resection (usually a lobectomy) and lymph node dissection.[121]

PRIMARY PULMONARY CARCINOSARCOMA

Primary pulmonary carcinosarcomas were once considered primary pulmonary sarcomas, but because of their varied histologic makeup, they now have a designation of their own. Carcinosarcomas contain a mixture of carcinomatous and sarcomatous components[124] and generally affect older adults.[125,126]

Diagnosis

Cytokeratin and vimentin antibodies can be used to readily distinguish between carcinomatous and sarcomatous tumor formation.[124] Carcinosarcomas are rarely diagnosed preoperatively, although there have been reports of diagnosis by sputum cytology[127] and transthoracic needle biopsy.[128]

Treatment and Prognosis

Complete surgical resection with clear margins is the most commonly accepted treatment for primary pulmonary carcinosarcomas. Huwer and colleagues advocated chemotherapy and radiation, the standard treatment modalities for soft tissue sarcoma therapy, for those with primary pulmonary carcinosarcoma, because the prognosis depends on the sarcoma component of the tumor.[124]

The prognosis of primary pulmonary carcinosarcomas is poor because of their propensity to metastasize to distant sites and their high rate of local recurrence.[129,130] Petrov and coworkers reported a 5-year survival of 49% with a mean survival of 37 months.[131]

REFERENCES

1. Modlin IM, Lye KD, Kidd M. A 5-decade analysis of 13,715 carcinoid tumors. Cancer 2003;**97**:934-59.
2. Institute TUNC: Surveillance Epidemiology and End Results (SEER) data base, 1973-2004. http://seercancergov/2007, 2007.
3. Beasley MB, Brambilla E, Travis WD. The 2004 World Health Organization classification of lung tumors. Semin Roentgenol 2005;**40**:90-7.
4. Quaedvlieg PF, Visser O, Lamers CB, Janssen-Heijen ML, Taal BG. Epidemiology and survival in patients with carcinoid disease in The Netherlands. An epidemiological study with 2391 patients. Ann Oncol 2001;**12**:1295-300.
5. Cote ML, Wenzlaff AS, Philip PA, Schwartz AG. Secondary cancers after a lung carcinoid primary: a population-based analysis. Lung Cancer 2006;**52**:273-9.
6. Fernandez FG, Battafarano RJ. Large-cell neuroendocrine carcinoma of the lung. Cancer Control 2006;**13**:270-5.
7. Gustafsson BI, Kidd M, Chan A, Malfertheiner MV, Modlin IM. Bronchopulmonary neuroendocrine tumors. Cancer 2008;**113**:5-21.
8. Marty-Ane CH, Costes V, Pujol JL, Alauzen M, Baldet P, Mary H. Carcinoid tumors of the lung: do atypical features require aggressive management? Ann Thorac Surg 1995;**59**:78-83.
9. Davila DG, Dunn WF, Tazelaar HD, Pairolero PC. Bronchial carcinoid tumors. Mayo Clin Proc 1993;**68**:795-803.
10. Huang Q, Muzitansky A, Mark EJ. Pulmonary neuroendocrine carcinomas. A review of 234 cases and a statistical analysis of 50 cases treated at one institution using a simple clinicopathologic classification. Arch Pathol Lab Med 2002;**126**:545-53.
11. Travis WD, Rush W, Flieder DB, et al. Survival analysis of 200 pulmonary neuroendocrine tumors with clarification of criteria for atypical carcinoid and its separation from typical carcinoid. Am J Surg Pathol 1998;**22**:934-44.
12. Beasley MB, Thunnissen FB, Brambilla E, et al. Pulmonary atypical carcinoid: predictors of survival in 106 cases. Hum Pathol 2000;**31**:1255-65.
13. Leotlela PD, Jauch A, Holtgreve-Grez H, Thakker RV. Genetics of neuroendocrine and carcinoid tumours. Endocr Relat Cancer 2003;**10**:437-50.
14. Onuki N, Wistuba II, Travis WD, et al. Genetic changes in the spectrum of neuroendocrine lung tumors. Cancer 1999;**85**:600-7.
15. Zhao J, de Krijger RR, Meier D, et al. Genomic alterations in well-differentiated gastrointestinal and bronchial neuroendocrine tumors (carcinoids): marked differences indicating diversity in molecular pathogenesis. Am J Pathol 2000;**157**:1431-8.
16. Debelenko LV, Brambilla E, Agarwal SK, et al. Identification of MEN1 gene mutations in sporadic carcinoid tumors of the lung. Hum Mol Genet 1997;**6**:2285-90.
17. Walch AK, Zitzelsberger HF, Aubele MM, et al. Typical and atypical carcinoid tumors of the lung are characterized by 11q deletions as detected by comparative genomic hybridization. Am J Pathol 1998;**153**:1089-98.
18. Sachithanandan N, Harle RA, Burgess JR. Bronchopulmonary carcinoid in multiple endocrine neoplasia type 1. Cancer 2005;**103**:509-15.
19. Schussheim DH, Skarulis MC, Agarwal SK, et al. Multiple endocrine neoplasia type 1: new clinical and basic findings. Trends Endocrinol Metab 2001;**12**:173-8.
20. Lohmann DR, Fesseler B, Putz B, et al. Infrequent mutations of the p53 gene in pulmonary carcinoid tumors. Cancer Res 1993;**53**:5797-801.
21. Sugio K, Osaki T, Oyama T, et al. Genetic alteration in carcinoid tumors of the lung. Ann Thorac Cardiovasc Surg 2003;**9**:149-54.
22. Kobayashi Y, Tokuchi Y, Hashimoto T, et al. Molecular markers for reinforcement of histological subclassification of neuroendocrine lung tumors. Cancer Sci 2004;**95**:334-41.
23. Takeichi M. Cadherin cell adhesion receptors as a morphogenetic regulator. Science 1991;**251**:1451-5.
24. Pelosi G, Scarpa A, Puppa G, et al. Alteration of the E-cadherin/beta-catenin cell adhesion system is common in pulmonary neuroendocrine tumors and is an independent predictor of lymph node metastasis in atypical carcinoids. Cancer 2005;**103**:1154-64.
25. Skuladottir H, Hirsch FR, Hansen HH, Olsen JH. Pulmonary neuroendocrine tumors: incidence and prognosis of histological subtypes. A population-based study in Denmark. Lung Cancer 2002;**37**:127-35.
26. Fink G, Krelbaum T, Yellin A, et al. Pulmonary carcinoid: presentation, diagnosis, and outcome in 142 cases in Israel and review of 640 cases from the literature. Chest 2001;**119**:1647-51.
27. Filosso PL, Rena O, Donati G, et al. Bronchial carcinoid tumors: surgical management and long-term outcome. J Thorac Cardiovasc Surg 2002;**123**:303-9.
28. Limper AH, Carpenter PC, Scheithauer B, Staats BA. The Cushing syndrome induced by bronchial carcinoid tumors. Ann Intern Med 1992;**117**:209-14.
29. Aniszewski JP, Young Jr WF, Thompson GB, Grant CS, van Heerden JA. Cushing syndrome due to ectopic adrenocorticotropic hormone secretion. World J Surg 2001;**25**:934-40.
30. Zatelli MC, Maffei P, Piccin D, et al. Somatostatin analogs in vitro effects in a growth hormone-releasing hormone-secreting bronchial carcinoid. J Clin Endocrinol Metab 2005;**90**:2104-9.
31. Shames JM, Dhurandhar NR, Blackard WG. Insulin-secreting bronchial carcinoid tumor with widespread metastases. Am J Med 1968;**44**:632-7.
32. Bruns C, Weckbecker G, Raulf F, et al. Molecular pharmacology of somatostatin-receptor subtypes. Ann N Y Acad Sci 1994;**733**:138-46.
33. Granberg D, Sundin A, Janson ET, Oberg K, Skogseid B, Westlin JE. Octreoscan in patients with bronchial carcinoid tumours. Clin Endocrinol (Oxf) 2003;**59**:793-9.
34. Taal BG, Hoefnagel CA, Valdes Olmos RA, Boot H, Beijnen JH: Palliative effect of metaiodobenzylguanidine in metastatic carcinoid tumors. J Clin Oncol 1996;**14**:1829-38.
35. Marom EM, Sarvis S, Herndon 2nd JE, Patz Jr EF. T1 lung cancers: sensitivity of diagnosis with fluorodeoxyglucose PET. Radiology 2002;**223**:453-9.
36. Chong S, Lee KS, Kim BT, et al. Integrated PET/CT of pulmonary neuroendocrine tumors: diagnostic and prognostic implications. AJR Am J Roentgenol 2007;**188**:1223-31.
37. Rivera MP, Detterbeck F, Mehta AC. Diagnosis of lung cancer: the guidelines. Chest 2003;**123**:129S-36S.

38. Dusmet ME, McKneally MF. Pulmonary and thymic carcinoid tumors. *World J Surg* 1996;**20**:189-95.
39. Hage R, de la Riviere AB, Seldenrijk CA, van den Bosch JM. Update in pulmonary carcinoid tumors: a review article. *Ann Surg Oncol* 2003;**10**:697-704.
40. Seregni E, Ferrari L, Bajetta E, Martinetti A, Bombardieri E. Clinical significance of blood chromogranin A measurement in neuroendocrine tumours. *Ann Oncol* 2001;**12**(Suppl. 2):S69-72.
41. Cooper WA, Thourani VH, Gal AA, Lee RB, Mansour KA, Miller JI. The surgical spectrum of pulmonary neuroendocrine neoplasms. *Chest* 2001;**119**:14-8.
42. Rea F, Rizzardi G, Zuin A, et al. Outcome and surgical strategy in bronchial carcinoid tumors: single institution experience with 252 patients. *Eur J Cardiothorac Surg* 2007;**31**:186-91.
43. Ferguson MK, Landreneau RJ, Hazelrigg SR, et al. Long-term outcome after resection for bronchial carcinoid tumors. *Eur J Cardiothorac Surg* 2000;**18**:156-61.
44. McCaughan BC, Martini N, Bains MS. Bronchial carcinoids. Review of 124 cases. *J Thorac Cardiovasc Surg* 1985;**89**:8-17.
45. Mezzetti M, Raveglia F, Panigalli T, et al. Assessment of outcomes in typical and atypical carcinoids according to latest WHO classification. *Ann Thorac Surg* 2003;**76**:1838-42.
46. Cardillo G, Sera F, Di Martino M, et al. Bronchial carcinoid tumors: nodal status and long-term survival after resection. *Ann Thorac Surg* 2004;**77**:1781-5.
47. Bertoletti L, Elleuch R, Kaczmarek D, Jean-Francois R, Vergnon JM. Bronchoscopic cryotherapy treatment of isolated endoluminal typical carcinoid tumor. *Chest* 2006;**130**:1405-11.
48. Garcia-Yuste M, Matilla JM, Cueto A, et al. Typical and atypical carcinoid tumours: analysis of the experience of the Spanish Multi-centric Study of Neuroendocrine Tumours of the Lung. *Eur J Cardiothorac Surg* 2007;**31**:192-7.
49. Aguayo SM, Miller YE, Waldron Jr JA, et al. Brief report: idiopathic diffuse hyperplasia of pulmonary neuroendocrine cells and airways disease. *N Engl J Med* 1992;**327**:1285-8.
50. Carmichael MG, Zacher LL. The demonstration of pulmonary neuroendocrine cell hyperplasia with tumorlets in a patient with chronic cough and a history of multiple medical problems. *Mil Med* 2005;**170**:439-41.
51. Armas OA, White DA, Erlandson RA, Rosai J. Diffuse idiopathic pulmonary neuroendocrine cell proliferation presenting as interstitial lung disease. *Am J Surg Pathol* 1995;**19**:963-70.
52. Bonikos DS, Archibald R, Bensch KG. On the origin of the so-called tumorlets of the lung. *Hum Pathol* 1976;**7**:461-9.
53. Felton 2nd WL, Liebow AA, Lindskog GE. Peripheral and multiple bronchial adenomas. *Cancer* 1953;**6**:555-67.
54. D'Agati VD, Perzin KH. Carcinoid tumorlets of the lung with metastasis to a peribronchial lymph node. Report of a case and review of the literature. *Cancer* 1985;**55**:2472-6.
55. Hausman DH, Weimann RB. Pulmonary tumorlet with hilar lymph node metastasis. Report of a case. *Cancer* 1967;**20**:1515-9.
56. Bennett GL, Chew FS. Pulmonary carcinoid tumorlets. *AJR Am J Roentgenol* 1994;**162**:568.
57. Aubry MC, Thomas Jr CF, Jett JR, Swensen SJ, Myers JL. Significance of multiple carcinoid tumors and tumorlets in surgical lung specimens: analysis of 28 patients. *Chest* 2007;**131**:1635-43.
58. Gosney JR. Diffuse idiopathic pulmonary neuroendocrine cell hyperplasia as a precursor to pulmonary neuroendocrine tumors. *Chest* 2004;**125**:108S.
59. Heitmiller RF, Mathisen DJ, Ferry JA, Mark EJ, Grillo HC. Mucoepidermoid lung tumors. *Ann Thorac Surg* 1989;**47**:394-9.
60. Moran CA. Primary salivary gland-type tumors of the lung. *Semin Diagn Pathol* 1995;**12**:106-22.
61. Turnbull AD, Huvos AG, Goodner JT, Foote Jr FW. Mucoepidermoid tumors of bronchial glands. *Cancer* 1971;**28**:539-44.
62. Molina JR, Aubry MC, Lewis JE, et al. Primary salivary gland-type lung cancer: spectrum of clinical presentation, histopathologic and prognostic factors. *Cancer* 2007;**110**:2253-9.
63. Brandwein MS, Ivanov K, Wallace DI, et al. Mucoepidermoid carcinoma: a clinicopathological study of 80 patients with special reference to histological grading. *Am J Surg Pathol* 2001;**25**:835-45.
64. Yokouchi H, Otsuka Y, Otoguro Y, et al. Primary peripheral adenoid cystic carcinoma of the lung and literature comparison of features. *Intern Med* 2007;**46**:1799-803.
65. Spizarny DL, Shepard JA, McLoud TC, Grillo HC, Dedrick CG. CT of adenoid cystic carcinoma of the trachea. *AJR Am J Roentgenol* 1986;**146**:1129-32.
66. Pearson FG, Todd TR, Cooper JD. Experience with primary neoplasms of the trachea and carina. *J Thorac Cardiovasc Surg* 1984;**88**:511-8.
67. Conlan AA, Payne WS, Woolner LB, Sanderson DR. Adenoid cystic carcinoma (cylindroma) and mucoepidermoid carcinoma of the bronchus. Factors affecting survival. *J Thorac Cardiovasc Surg* 1978;**76**:369-77.
68. Brutinel WM, Cortese DA, McDougall JC, Gillio RG, Bergstralh EJ. A two-year experience with the neodymium-YAG laser in endobronchial obstruction. *Chest* 1987;**91**:159-65.
69. Munsch C, Westaby S, Sturridge M. Urgent treatment for nonresectable, asphyxiating tracheal cylindroma. *Ann Thorac Surg* 1987;**43**:663-4.
70. Personne C, Colchen A, Leroy M, Vourc'h G, Toty L. Indications and technique for endoscopic laser resections in bronchology. A critical analysis based upon 2,284 resections. *J Thorac Cardiovasc Surg* 1986;**91**:710-5.
71. Chin HW, DeMeester T, Chin RY, Boman B. Endobronchial adenoid cystic carcinoma. *Chest* 1991;**100**:1464-5.
72. Fields JN, Rigaud G, Emami BN. Primary tumors of the trachea. Results of radiation therapy. *Cancer* 1989;**63**:2429-33.
73. Hotte SJ, Winquist EW, Lamont E, et al. Imatinib mesylate in patients with adenoid cystic cancers of the salivary glands expressing c-kit: a Princess Margaret Hospital phase II consortium study. *J Clin Oncol* 2005;**23**:585-90.
74. Yousem SA, Hochholzer L. Mucoepidermoid tumors of the lung. *Cancer* 1987;**60**:1346-52.
75. Litzky LA. Pulmonary sarcomatous tumors. *Arch Pathol Lab Med* 2008;**132**:1104-17.
76. Gebauer C. Primary pulmonary sarcomas: etiology, clinical assessment and prognosis with a comparison to pulmonary carcinomas—a review of 41 cases and 394 other cases of the literature. *Jpn J Surg* 1982;**12**:148-59.
77. Gengler C, Guillou L. Solitary fibrous tumour and haemangiopericytoma: evolution of a concept. *Histopathology* 2006;**48**:63-74.
78. Ohta H, Komibuchi T, Nishiyama H, Shizuki K, Miyaki Y. 99mTc(V)-DMSA and 99mTc-MDP uptake and no 67Ga-citrate uptake in a case of primary pulmonary leiomyosarcoma. *Ann Nucl Med* 1992;**6**:191-3.
79. Moran CA, Suster S, Abbondanzo SL, Koss MN. Primary leiomyosarcomas of the lung: a clinicopathologic and immunohistochemical study of 18 cases. *Mod Pathol* 1997;**10**:121-8.
80. Fitoz S, Atasoy C, Kizilkaya E, Basekim C, Karsli F. Radiologic findings in primary pulmonary leiomyosarcoma. *J Thorac Imaging* 2000;**15**:151-2.
81. Janssen JP, Mulder JJ, Wagenaar SS, Elbers HR, van den Bosch JM. Primary sarcoma of the lung: a clinical study with long-term follow-up. *Ann Thorac Surg* 1994;**58**:1151-5.
82. Kasper B, Gil T, D'Hondt V, Gebhart M, Awada A. Novel treatment strategies for soft tissue sarcoma. *Crit Rev Oncol Hematol* 2007;**62**:9-15.
83. Jiang J, Zhou J, Ding W. Primary pulmonary synovial sarcoma, a rare primary lung neoplasm: two case reports and review of the current literature. *Respirology* 2008;**13**:748-50.
84. Begueret H, Galateau-Salle F, Guillou L, et al. Primary intrathoracic synovial sarcoma: a clinicopathologic study of 40 t(X;18)-positive cases from the French Sarcoma Group and the Mesopath Group. *Am J Surg Pathol* 2005;**29**:339-46.
85. Zeren H, Moran CA, Suster S, Fishback NF, Koss MN. Primary pulmonary sarcomas with features of monophasic synovial sarcoma: a clinicopathological, immunohistochemical, and ultrastructural study of 25 cases. *Hum Pathol* 1995;**26**:474-80.
86. Hartel PH, Fanburg-Smith JC, Frazier AA, et al. Primary pulmonary and mediastinal synovial sarcoma: a clinicopathologic study of 60 cases and comparison with five prior series. *Mod Pathol* 2007;**20**:760-9.
87. Essary LR, Vargas SO, Fletcher CD. Primary pleuropulmonary synovial sarcoma: reappraisal of a recently described anatomic subset. *Cancer* 2002;**94**:459-69.
88. Spillane AJ, A'Hern R, Judson IR, Fisher C, Thomas JM. Synovial sarcoma: a clinicopathologic, staging, and prognostic assessment. *J Clin Oncol* 2000;**18**:3794-803.
89. Skytting B, Meis-Kindblom JM, Larsson O, et al. Synovial sarcoma: identification of favorable and unfavorable histologic types: a Scandinavian sarcoma group study of 104 cases. *Acta Orthop Scand* 1999;**70**:543-54.
90. Bagan P, Hassan M, Le Pimpec Barthes F, et al. Prognostic factors and surgical indications of pulmonary epithelioid hemangioendothelioma: a review of the literature. *Ann Thorac Surg* 2006;**82**:2010-3.
91. Eggleston JC. The intravascular bronchioloalveolar tumor and the sclerosing hemangioma of the lung: misnomers of pulmonary neoplasia. *Semin Diagn Pathol* 1985;**2**:270-80.
92. Dail DH, Liebow AA, Gmelich JT, et al. Intravascular, bronchiolar, and alveolar tumor of the lung (IVBAT). An analysis of twenty cases of a peculiar sclerosing endothelial tumor. *Cancer* 1983;**51**:452-64.
93. Weiss SW, Ishak KG, Dail DH, Sweet DE, Enzinger FM. Epithelioid hemangioendothelioma and related lesions. *Semin Diagn Pathol* 1986;**3**:259-87.
94. Ross GJ, Violi L, Friedman AC, Edmonds PR, Unger E. Intravascular bronchioloalveolar tumor: CT and pathologic correlation. *J Comput Assist Tomogr* 1989;**13**:240-3.
95. Cronin P, Arenberg D. Pulmonary epithelioid hemangioendothelioma: an unusual case and a review of the literature. *Chest* 2004;**125**:789-93.

96. Erasmus JJ, McAdams HP, Carraway MS. A 63-year-old woman with weight loss and multiple lung nodules. *Chest* 1997;**111**:236-8.
97. Ledson MJ, Convery R, Carty A, Evans CC. Epithelioid haemangioendothelioma. *Thorax* 1999;**54**:560-1.
98. Kantelip B, Champiat B, Mignot P, Fonck Y, Molina C. [Intravascular bronchioloalveolar tumor or I.V.B.A.T. Apropos of a case and review of the literature]. *Rev Pneumol Clin* 1985;**41**:273-82.
99. Madariaga JR, Marino IR, Karavias DD, et al. Long-term results after liver transplantation for primary hepatic epithelioid hemangioendothelioma. *Ann Surg Oncol* 1995;**2**:483-7.
100. Kojima K, Okamoto I, Ushijima S, et al. Successful treatment of primary pulmonary angiosarcoma. *Chest* 2003;**124**:2397-400.
101. Patel AM, Ryu JH. Angiosarcoma in the lung. *Chest* 1993;**103**:1531-5.
102. Gladish GW, Sabloff BM, Munden RF, Truong MT, Erasmus JJ, Chasen MH. Primary thoracic sarcomas. *Radiographics* 2002;**22**:621-37.
103. Sheppard MN, Hansell DM, Du Bois RM, Nicholson AG. Primary epithelioid angiosarcoma of the lung presenting as pulmonary hemorrhage. *Hum Pathol* 1997;**28**:383-5.
104. Suster S. Primary sarcomas of the lung. *Semin Diagn Pathol* 1995;**12**:140-57.
105. Masuzawa M, Mochida N, Amano T, et al. Evaluation of recombinant interleukin-2 immunotherapy for human hemangiosarcoma in a SCID mice model (WB-SCID). *J Dermatol Sci* 2001;**27**:88-94.
106. Fata F, O'Reilly E, Ilson D, et al. Paclitaxel in the treatment of patients with angiosarcoma of the scalp or face. *Cancer* 1999;**86**:2034-7.
107. Edelstein E, Gal AA, Mann KP, Miller Jr JI, Mansour KA. Primary solitary endobronchial plasmacytoma. *Ann Thorac Surg* 2004;**78**:1448-9.
108. Joseph G, Pandit M, Korfhage L. Primary pulmonary plasmacytoma. *Cancer* 1993;**71**:721-4.
109. Hagl S, Jakob H, Sebening C, et al. External stabilization of long-segment tracheobronchomalacia guided by intraoperative bronchoscopy. *Ann Thorac Surg* 1997;**64**:1412-20:discussion 1421.
110. Wadsworth SJ, Juniper MC, Benson MK, Gleeson FV. Fatal complication of an expandable metallic bronchial stent. *Br J Radiol* 1999;**72**:706-8.
111. Miller DL, Allen MS. Rare pulmonary neoplasms. *Mayo Clin Proc* 1993;**68**:492-8.
112. Rosenberg SA, Diamond HD, Jaslowitz B, Craver LF. Lymphosarcoma: a review of 1269 cases. *Medicine (Baltimore)* 1961;**40**:31-84.
113. Freeman C, Berg JW, Cutler SJ. Occurrence and prognosis of extranodal lymphomas. *Cancer* 1972;**29**:252-60.
114. Li G, Hansmann ML, Zwingers T, Lennert K. Primary lymphomas of the lung: morphological, immunohistochemical and clinical features. *Histopathology* 1990;**16**:519-31.
115. Rabkin CS, Yellin F. Cancer incidence in a population with a high prevalence of infection with human immunodeficiency virus type 1. *J Natl Cancer Inst* 1994;**86**:1711-6.
116. Graham BB, Mathisen DJ, Mark EJ, Takvorian RW. Primary pulmonary lymphoma. *Ann Thorac Surg* 2005;**80**:1248-53.
117. Thieblemont C, de la Fouchardiere A, Coiffier B. Nongastric mucosa-associated lymphoid tissue lymphomas. *Clin Lymphoma* 2003;**3**:212-24.
118. Kahl BS. Update: gastric MALT lymphoma. *Curr Opin Oncol* 2003;**15**:347-52.
119. Cordier JF, Chailleux E, Lauque D, et al. Primary pulmonary lymphomas. A clinical study of 70 cases in nonimmunocompromised patients. *Chest* 1993;**103**:201-8.
120. Ferraro P, Trastek VF, Adlakha H, Deschamps C, Allen MS, Pairolero PC. Primary non-Hodgkin's lymphoma of the lung. *Ann Thorac Surg* 2000;**69**:993-7.
121. Ost D, Joseph C, Sogoloff H, Menezes G. Primary pulmonary melanoma: case report and literature review. *Mayo Clin Proc* 1999;**74**:62-6.
122. Allen Jr MS, Drash EC. Primary melanoma of the lung. *Cancer* 1968;**21**:154-9.
123. Jensen OA, Egedorf J. Primary malignant melanoma of the lung. *Scand J Respir Dis* 1967;**48**:127-35.
124. Huwer H, Kalweit G, Straub U, Feindt P, Volkmer I, Gams E. Pulmonary carcinosarcoma: diagnostic problems and determinants of the prognosis. *Eur J Cardiothorac Surg* 1996;**10**:403-7.
125. Grahmann PR, Swoboda L, Bonnet R, Riede UN, Hasse J. Carcinosarcomas of the lung. Three case reports and literature review. *Thorac Cardiovasc Surg* 1993;**41**:312-7.
126. Heremans A, Verbeken E, Deneffe G, Demedts M. Carcinosarcoma of the lung. Report of two cases and review of the literature. *Acta Clin Belg* 1989;**44**:110-5.
127. Ishizuka T, Yoshitake J, Yamada T, et al. Diagnosis of a case of pulmonary carcinosarcoma by detection of rhabdomyosarcoma cells in sputum. *Acta Cytol* 1988;**32**:658-62.
128. Cabarcos A, Gomez Dorronsoro M. Lobo Beristain JL: Pulmonary carcinosarcoma: a case study and review of the literature. *Br J Dis Chest* 1985;**79**:83-94.
129. Summermann E, Huwer H, Seitz G. Carcinosarcoma of the lung, a tumour which has a poor prognosis and is extremely rarely diagnosed preoperatively. *Thorac Cardiovasc Surg* 1990;**38**:247-50.
130. Ishida T, Tateishi M, Kaneko S, et al. Carcinosarcoma and spindle cell carcinoma of the lung. Clinicopathologic and immunohistochemical studies. *J Thorac Cardiovasc Surg* 1990;**100**:844-52.
131. Petrov DB, Vlassov VI, Kalaydjiev GT, et al. Primary pulmonary sarcomas and carcinosarcomas: postoperative results and comparative survival analysis. *Eur J Cardiothorac Surg* 2003;**23**:461-6.

CHAPTER 23
Secondary Lung Tumors
Scott Cowan, Melissa Culligan, and Joseph Friedberg

History of Metastasectomy
Pathophysiology of Pulmonary Metastases
   Do Metastases Metastasize?
   Does Lung Cancer Metastasize to Lung?
Evaluation of the Patient with Secondary Pulmonary Tumors
   Symptoms and Presentation
   Radiographic Evaluation
   Tissue Diagnosis

Indications for Surgery
Surgical Approach
Lymph Node Dissection
Results of Pulmonary Metastasectomy
Metastases to the Lung
   Soft Tissue Sarcomas
   Osteosarcoma (Osteogenic Sarcoma)
   Large Bowel Cancer
   Breast Carcinoma

   Head and Neck Carcinoma
   Renal Cell Carcinoma
   Germ Cell Tumors
   Gynecologic Tumors
   Melanoma
   Endocrine Tumors
Alternative Treatment Options
Palliative Therapy
Conclusions

After the liver, the lung is the second most common site for metastatic involvement in neoplastic disease when all tissues and organs are considered, and 20% to 54% of patients with cancer will have pulmonary metastases at some point in the natural history of their disease (Boxes 23-1 and 23-2). In the absence of extrathoracic metastases (i.e., in about 25% of patients with disseminated disease), complete resection is associated with increased survival, regardless of histology. With appropriate patient selection, life expectancy is often improved with pulmonary metastasectomy. Cures are reported with either resection alone or in combination with chemotherapy.[1,2] Even in the context of unresectability, surgical forms of palliation may serve to improve quality of life. For other patients (e.g., those with nonseminomatous germ cell tumors), surgery may have a more diagnostic role, such as defining residual disease that is potentially amenable to salvage forms of therapy.

HISTORY OF METASTASECTOMY

During the 19th century, there were sporadic reports of lung resections for metastatic tumors in the European literature. The first of these reports was in 1855, by the French surgeon Sédillot, who removed a chest wall tumor and excised disease extending into the lung.[3] The first case of a true pulmonary metastasectomy was described by Weinlechner in 1882 in a patient with a rib sarcoma, who was found to have two incidental pulmonary metastases at the time of the sarcoma resection.[4] Kronlein reported the first long-term survivor after pulmonary metastasectomy in a patient with recurrent chest wall sarcoma and a metastatic lung nodule. The patient went on to survive 7 years, eventually succumbing to recurrent pulmonary disease.[5-7]

The first, and perhaps most famous, report of a planned pulmonary metastasectomy in the United States was performed in 1933 by Barney and Churchill.[1] Soon after resection of a renal cell carcinoma, they noted that the patient's pulmonary nodule, seen on a chest radiograph preoperatively and presumed to be tuberculosis, had doubled in size. The lesion, now thought to represent metastatic disease, was treated with radiation therapy. They noted a poor response and elected to resect the nodule. The patient went on to live 23 years, eventually dying of coronary artery disease with no evidence of tumor recurrence at autopsy. Despite the early discovery that survival could be improved by resection of metastatic disease, it was not for another 40 years that metastasectomy was performed as a separate procedure by Divis in Europe.[8] This was followed soon after by similar reports in the American literature by Torek and Tudor Edwards in the early 20th century.[9,10]

These early reports, and others like them, paved the way toward general acceptance of pulmonary metastasectomy. Although initial indications for surgery were reserved for those with a solitary metastasis, with time and experience more aggressive metastasectomies were performed. In 1947, Alexander and Haight described the first case series of 24 patients who underwent pulmonary metastasectomy.[11] In this series, they described a woman, in her 20s, with a spindle cell neurogenic sarcoma. She initially underwent a right lower lobectomy for metastatic disease in 1939. She had a recurrence in 1940 for which she underwent a left upper lobectomy. This article was the first to define criteria for resection of pulmonary metastases, including control of the primary tumor, absence of extrathoracic disease, and sufficient pulmonary reserve. Today, the indications for resection of secondary pulmonary malignancies have been broadened to include not only patients with recurrent disease but also those with multiple metastases, bilateral lesions, and essentially all histologies.[12]

The largest effort aimed at evaluating patients undergoing pulmonary metastasectomy was undertaken by the International Registry of Lung Metastases (IRLM). Established in 1991, the IRLM accrued 5206 patients in North America and Europe. This landmark report demonstrated that complete resection, short disease-free interval, and single lesions were favorable measurements for long-term survival. This and other studies have helped to develop current criteria for performing pulmonary metastasectomies and to define anticipated survival after resection.[13,14,66]

PATHOPHYSIOLOGY OF PULMONARY METASTASES

In 1889, the British surgeon Stephen Paget observed that metastatic disease followed a nonrandom pattern. Using autopsy records of patients with a variety of primary tumors,

> **Box 23–1**
> **Primaries Most Commonly Metastatic to the Lung***
>
> - Breast
> - Colon
> - Kidney
> - Uterus
> - Prostate
> - Oropharyngeal carcinoma

*Most common because of greater prevalence.

> **Box 23–2**
> **Tumors with the Highest Predilection for Pulmonary Metastasis**
>
> - Choriocarcinoma
> - Osteosarcoma
> - Testicular tumors
> - Melanoma
> - Ewing's sarcoma
> - Kaposi's sarcoma

he hypothesized that factors in certain tumors have an affinity for certain factors in target organs. Theories have subsequently evolved that attempt to explain the propensity for metastases to spread to specific organs. The "cascade spread" theory hypothesizes that a single organ represents the first site of spread, followed by systemic dissemination.[15] This metastatic cascade is considered to be a complex series of events culminating in the generation of metastases. The initial phase of the cascade involves tumor growth via neovascularization, which is stimulated by growth factors secreted by the tumor cells and local host cells. The invasive phase of tumor growth involves the local production and activation of proteolytic enzymes (matrix metalloproteinases, collagenases, serine proteinases, cysteine proteinases) derived from both the host and tumor tissue. These enzymes serve to decrease cell adhesiveness, stimulate cell migration, and enhance chemotaxis and subsequent tumor cell detachment.

Metastasis is most likely initiated after cell detachment from the primary tumor mass. Typically, epithelial cells undergo anoikis (apoptosis) because of the loss of cell–cell interactions once they are separated from parent tissue. Metastatic cells are thought to resist anoikis by forming cell–cell attachments with other tumor cells or host cells and through the overexpression of proteins that inhibit anoikis.

Movement from the extracellular space into a vascular compartment is termed *intravasation*. Cancer cells have been shown to degrade basement membranes via local release of extracellular matrix-degrading proteins (matrix metalloproteinases), facilitating migration into the lymphatic and circulatory system. Once in the circulatory system, tumor cells must avoid recognition and destruction by the host immune system. Only 0.1% of tumors cells in circulation go on to generate metastases.[16] Mechanisms that cancer cells use to survive include human leukocyte antigen (HLA) class I downregulation (mediator of immune cell recognition) and loss of immunogenic antigens. Cancer cells also downregulate the immune system via the production of immunosuppressive cytokines. Some evidence suggests that clots form around tumor cells that protect these cells from immunologic and physiologic stresses in the bloodstream.[17]

Tumor cells bind to pulmonary vasculature which, via a platelet-induced reaction, stimulates endothelial cell retraction.[18] The lung is thought to play a role as the primary capillary filter for drainage of most organs, and its rich capillary network provides an ideal environment for deposition. Movement of tumor cells from the circulatory system into the interstitium is called *extravasation*. Basement membrane disruption is thought to occur in a manner similar to intravasation.

Once extravasated, tumors may remain quiescent or proliferate. Proliferation and local invasion requires neovascularization, which is induced via a shift toward the intracellular and extracellular production of pro-angiogenic factors. Epidermal growth factor (EGF), platelet-derived growth factor (PDGF), and transforming growth factor α (TGF-α) foster tumor cell proliferation in the new environment. On the other hand, the host organ produces inhibitors, such as TGF-β, mammastatin, and amphiregulin, to prevent metastatic implantations.[19] These compounds are under investigation to assess their ability to control metastatic disease.

Do Metastases Metastasize?

It is thought that metastases need to follow the same steps as the primary tumor to metastasize: angiogenesis, intravasation, arrest, and extravasation. In 1975, Hoover and Ketcham demonstrated, experimentally, that metastases do have the ability to metastasize.[20] In their experiment, the primary tumor in mice was amputated after pulmonary metastasis developed. These mice were then placed into parabiosis with normal syngeneic partners. Metastases were demonstrated in the non–tumor-bearing partners, supporting the theory that metastases can re-metastasize. In addition, both autopsy and experimental data have defined the concept of metastases from metastatic disease.[21] On the other hand, Sugarbaker and colleagues took pieces of healthy lungs and transplanted them into mice that had established pulmonary metastases. Their results demonstrated no evidence of secondary tumor development, this leading to the conclusion that metastases do not metastasize.[22]

Whether metastases metastasize is still poorly understood and remains a challenge for medical oncologists and surgeons alike as they struggle to determine the best treatment and the proper timing of that treatment for patients with pulmonary metastases.[23]

Does Lung Cancer Metastasize to Lung?

Lung cancer can metastasize via lymphatic channels to the ipsilateral lung and, as suggested by some autopsy series, less commonly to the contralateral lung. These are patients with one primary lung cancer and intrapulmonary metastases. According to the proposed seventh revision of the lung cancer staging system of the International Association for the Study of Lung Cancer (IASLC), ipsilateral nodules in the same lobe as the primary tumor will be considered T4 and ipsilateral nodules in a different lobe from the primary tumor will be considered M1.[24] It is difficult, however, to determine if these patients have synchronous lesions or a primary lung cancer with intrapulmonary metastases. Ichinose and coworkers have used DNA flow cytometry to evaluate these lesions.[25,26] Using this technique, lesions are determined to be synchronous if they demonstrate completely different DNA ploidy. If both tumors show diploidy, or when at least one DNA index of abnormal clones between two aneuploidy tumors is the same or almost identical, they are considered metastatic. In addition, loss of heterozygosity and p53 mutational status have been used to distinguish multicentric lung cancers from intrapulmonary metastases.[27,28] Using these criteria, it appears that lung cancer can metastasize to lung, albeit less commonly than synchronous tumors. These molecular genetic techniques will continue to be used to determine whether two lung lesions are synchronous primary lung tumors or a single primary lung tumor with metastases.

EVALUATION OF THE PATIENT WITH SECONDARY PULMONARY TUMORS

Symptoms and Presentation

Approximately 75% to 90% of patients with secondary pulmonary malignancies are asymptomatic and, therefore, their disease is most commonly discovered incidentally on routine or follow-up radiologic examinations.[29,30] The usual lack of symptoms may, in part, be secondary to the common, nonobstructing peripheral location of pulmonary metastases. The asymptomatic nature of pulmonary metastases emphasizes the importance of obtaining lung imaging studies in the follow-up of cancer patients.

Symptoms, when they do occur, typically result from a delayed diagnosis with endobronchial or pleural involvement, large bulky disease, or central tumors. Patients may present with cough and hemoptysis suggesting an endobronchial lesion and thus warranting bronchoscopic examination. Endobronchial metastatic lesions are extremely rare, less than 2%, in patients who die of solid tumors, with breast, kidney, pancreas, colon, and melanoma as the most common sources.[31] Another presenting symptom may be dyspnea, which is usually secondary to airway obstruction, a pleural effusion, parenchymal replacement by multiple metastatic lesions, or lymphatic spread. Finally, chest pain, wheezing, or pneumothorax may occur, but these are unusual presenting symptoms.

During physical examination, wheezing may be heard, which is a sign of airway obstruction. Occasionally, a pericardial rub is heard, representing pericardial involvement. Pleural and pericardial involvement are usually the result of ovarian, breast, or lung adenocarcinomas. Thymomas are notorious for their pleural involvement when they metastasize.[32] In addition, decreased breath sounds and egophony may be appreciated when an obstructing lesion is present with associated lobar or segmental atelectasis, which could be seen on a chest radiograph as postobstructive pneumonia.

Radiographic Evaluation

Most pulmonary metastases are detected by chest radiography (Fig. 23-1) or computed tomography (CT) (Fig. 23-2) during routine follow-up for the primary cancer. Radiologic testing is used to define the extent of the disease and to

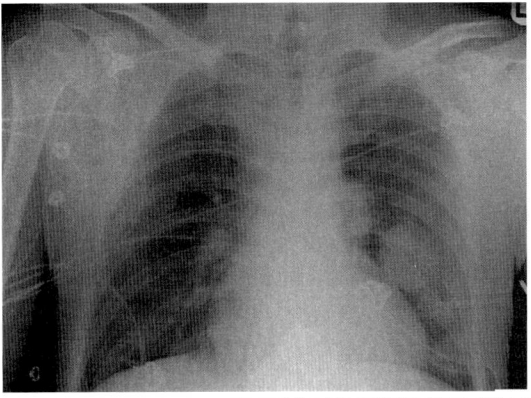

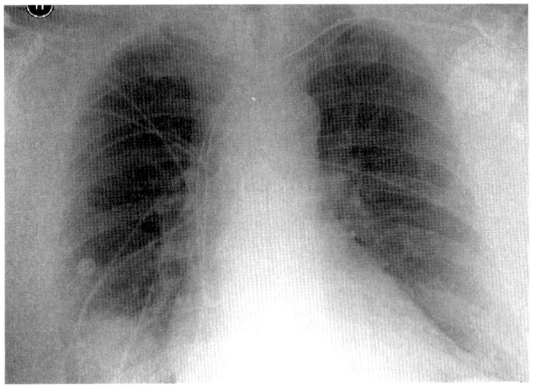

Figure 23–1
Pulmonary metastases as detected by chest radiography.

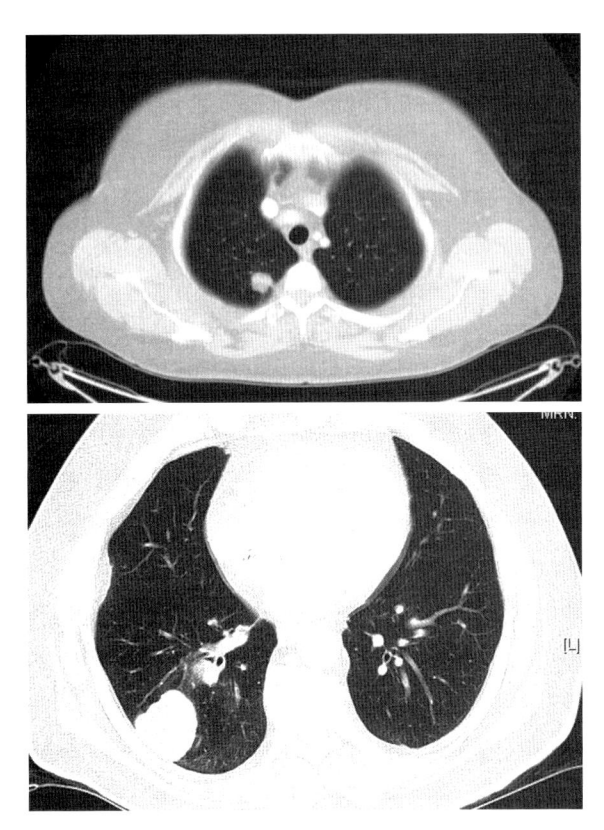

Figure 23–2
Pulmonary metastases as detected by chest CT.

determine whether an individual is a candidate for pulmonary metastasectomy. A search for extrathoracic disease may involve imaging the original primary disease site as well as looking for distant disease. A new pulmonary nodule in a patient with a prior malignancy should be considered cancer until proven otherwise.

A standard chest radiograph is often obtained as a screening test in patients with prior malignancies, and it provides a baseline for future studies. The sensitivity of plain radiography is low in comparison to that of CT. The resolution of a routine chest radiograph is approximately 9 mm, whereas that of a CT scan is 1 to 2 mm. CT is the gold standard imaging modality for evaluating the lungs and characterizing metastatic lesions. Lung metastases tend to be small, usually less than 1 cm, and they appear as multiple lesions in 75% of cases. The majority, nearly 75%, of secondary malignancies appear with multiple lung nodules. Distinguishing between a metastatic lesion and a new lung primary carcinoma can be difficult. Most metastatic lesions to the lung are found on the lung periphery, and they have a predilection for the basilar lung fields, probably because of increased blood flow to this region when the patient is in an upright position.[33,34]

CT characteristics of metastatic lesions include spherical shape with well-circumscribed, smooth borders. Lesions with irregular or spiculated borders with associated linear densities are more commonly associated with primary lung cancers, although this is not a universal finding.[33] Calcifications in lung nodules are rarely seen in metastatic pulmonary disease. Metastases that may have associated calcifications include osteosarcomas, chondrosarcomas, and breast and ovarian primaries. Cavitation can occur in both benign and malignant lesions. Benign etiologies include lung abscesses, aspergillosis, and tuberculosis. Malignant nodules that cavitate include squamous cell carcinomas (primary lung or metastatic carcinomas), sarcomas, and testicular tumors.

Although CT is useful for identifying and characterizing pulmonary metastases, it has been shown to underestimate the number of lesions compared with thoracotomy. In 1996, McCormack and colleagues prospectively performed video-assisted thoracoscopic surgery (VATS) resections based on CT findings, followed by thoracotomies with lung palpation, and found additional lesions in 14 of 18 patients.[35] Parsons and coworkers confirmed that helical CT missed metastases in 47% of cases.[36] Other studies have shown that, at least for patients who underwent metastasectomy for colorectal cancer, there is no statistically significant difference in survival between the open and the thoracoscopic approaches.[37] Furthermore, as CT scanning technology evolves, the detection of nodules as small as 1 mm can be achieved, further narrowing the disparity between CT scanning and manual palpation.[38] At this point, the data support thoracotomy and manual palpation as being the more sensitive method for detecting nodules. However, the choice between thoracotomy and VATS involves many factors and should be individualized for every patient.

Positron emission tomography (PET) has proved to be beneficial when considering patients for metastasectomy. In a series of patients with melanoma, [^{18}F]fluorodeoxyglucose (FDG)-PET had a sensitivity of 92%, a specificity of 88%, and accuracy of 91%.[39] PET is helpful in assessing extent of disease, including the primary disease site as well as thoracic and extrathoracic potential sites of metastases, but it is limited by false-negative results in patients with sub-centimeter pulmonary metastases.

The mediastinum should be evaluated carefully, because metastatic disease involves the mediastinum 2% to 3% of the time.[31,40] Head and neck tumors, testicular tumors, renal cell carcinomas, breast carcinomas, and melanomas have been known to appear with mediastinal disease.

Tissue Diagnosis

Obtaining tissue diagnosis prior to thoracotomy may be advantageous during the workup of a patient with a pulmonary nodule. In a patient with a history of cancer, a solitary pulmonary nodule may be benign or malignant. If malignant, the lesion may represent a primary lung cancer or metastatic disease. Under normal circumstances, the standard of care for a primary lung cancer is a formal anatomic resection, whereas metastatic disease may be removed by simple wedge resection. Consequently, this diagnosis has significant implications for the patient's therapeutic options. Furthermore, some patients may not be surgical candidates but still require a tissue diagnosis for appropriate nonsurgical management.

Sputum cytology is generally not indicated, as it is often nondiagnostic because of the peripheral location of most pulmonary metastases.[41] Bronchoscopic examination and diagnosis of pulmonary metastases is useful in the case of endobronchial or centrally located lesions. Fine-needle aspiration (FNA) is another option for obtaining a tissue diagnosis. It is associated with a risk of pneumothorax, in some series as high as 27%.[42] In addition, the sensitivity of this procedure may be relatively low (80%). Equivocal or "negative" results do not establish a diagnosis of benign disease. Generally, this procedure is thought to yield useful information only when it establishes a diagnosis of cancer.[43] When a nonsurgical therapy is indicated for a suspected histologic diagnosis, or when a patient is not a surgical candidate, FNA represents an excellent diagnostic option. Success of this procedure depends not only on the skill of the operator but also on the diagnostic prowess of the interpreting cytologist. The emerging field of bronchoscopic biopsies using electromagnetic navigation has demonstrated promising results and has potential to fall into the preferred armamentarium of clinicians attempting to establish a diagnosis for lung nodules.[44] The role of this technology in the care of patients with pulmonary metastatic disease has not yet been established.

For excisional biopsy, VATS has a sensitivity and specificity approaching 100%.[45-47] It is a more significant procedure than FNA and requires general anesthesia with selective lung ventilation. It is indicated when FNA has failed to or is unlikely to establish a diagnosis, or when more information or tissue is required for treatment purposes. Also, under appropriate circumstances, it may be therapeutic as well as diagnostic, as the nodules can be completely excised.

Occasionally, there is a role for thoracoscopic FNA, such as in cases of multiple lesions not amenable to complete surgical resection when treatment hinges on a tissue diagnosis and all less-invasive diagnostic modalities have proved fruitless or are deemed less safe than a VATS approach.[48]

INDICATIONS FOR SURGERY

Reasons to perform surgery for secondary pulmonary malignancy include curative resection, tissue diagnosis, or evaluation of residual disease after chemotherapy (see Germ Cell

Table 23-1

Most Common Site of Metastasis, and Percentage with Isolated Disease

Histology	Most Common Site of Metastasis (%)	Second Most Common Site of Metastasis	Those with Isolated Pulmonary Metastases (% of All Patients)
Breast carcinoma	Lung[138] (59-65)		22[107]
Colorectal	Liver[139]	Lung[139]	2-4[2]
Germ cell tumors	Lung[140]		
Head and neck squamous cell carcinoma	Lung (75)[72]		
Melanoma	Lung[129],*,† (18-36)		5[129]
Osteosarcoma	Lung (85)[90]		
Renal cell carcinoma	Lung[108]		4[108]
Soft tissue sarcoma	Lung[141] (80-90)		20[83]
All histologies	Liver	Lung[142]	15-20[143,144]

*Secondary to skin, subcutaneous, lymph nodes.
†In clinical series; however, 70% to 87% in autopsy series.

Tumors, later). Before proceeding with resection, a number of questions should be considered in the preoperative assessment of the patient.

Does the pulmonary nodule represent one site of multiorgan spread, thereby contraindicating resection? Pulmonary metastases are common in the advanced stages of cancer, with as many as one third of patients presenting with secondary nodules. Of these patients, however, the majority of pulmonary nodules (75% to 85%) are a manifestation of widespread disease. Consequently, only 15% to 25% of patients have lesions confined to the lung and are appropriate candidates for curative resection (Table 23-1). Preoperative evaluation, therefore, should exclude extrathoracic disease.

When pleural or pericardial effusions are present, thoracentesis or pericardiocentesis should be performed to rule out malignancy. Positive cytology contraindicates resection. Cytology may be falsely negative, however, in up to 40% to 60% of cases.[49,50] Consequently, a negative cytology returned in the context of a high index of suspicion for malignancy warrants pericardial or pleural biopsy, or both. A VATS approach can be used to access the pleural space, and it offers a minimally invasive transthoracic approach to the pericardium. It also affords the option of visualizing and palpating the lung as well as biopsying the mediastinal lymph nodes. Bronchoscopy should always be performed before thoracoscopy or thoracotomy, to rule out endobronchial lesions.

Is a nonsurgical therapeutic option available? Although surgical resection of secondary pulmonary malignancies may give patients a significant survival advantage, nonsurgical management may be more appropriate for certain histology. For example, in the context of nonseminomatous germ cell tumors, great success has been obtained with chemotherapy alone, with cure rates approaching 90% (see Germ Cell Tumors, later). In addition, high-dose multidrug chemotherapy and bone marrow rescue is the primary form of treatment offered to patients for disseminated pulmonary involvement secondary to breast carcinoma, although this is an area of some controversy (see Breast Carcinoma, later).

Will the patient tolerate the procedure? Risk factors associated with metastatic disease (e.g., smoking and advanced age) require that patients being considered for surgical resection receive a thorough medical assessment with particular attention to their pulmonary and cardiac status. Stress testing, echocardiograms, arterial blood gases, pulmonary function testing, and ventilation-perfusion scans may be necessary to assess a patient's tolerance for a proposed resection or their ability to undergo single-lung ventilation. Also, previously administered chemotherapeutic agents such as bleomycin or mitomycin may result in additional compromise of pulmonary function, and doxorubicin may be associated with cardiac impairment. The thoracic surgeon expecting to perform a metastasectomy must always be prepared to perform a formal lobectomy should the pathology reveal a primary lung cancer, or should wedge resection result in incomplete resection. Thus, performing the preoperative assessment with an eye toward a potential lobectomy is prudent.

Are the lesions resectable? Unresectability is defined as noncontiguous involvement beyond the visceral pleural envelope.[29] This is best determined at operation. Preoperatively, imaging modalities can only provide an estimate of resectability. In addition, thoracoscopy can sometimes be useful to assess for disseminated disease or bulky tumors that involve major structures and preclude complete resection, or to access a pleural or pericardial effusion that cannot be reached percutaneously. If the pericardium or pleura is involved with neoplastic disease from direct extension of an underlying parenchymal lesion, but there is no associated effusion, they should be resected en bloc with the specimen. Direct metastases to the pleura or pericardium in a discontinuous manner (i.e., disseminated spread) and malignant pleural or pericardial effusions are generally contraindications for resection.

Box 23-3
Selection Criteria* for Metastasectomy

- Local control of the primary tumor or ability to completely resect the primary with synchronous presentations[20]
- Radiologic findings consistent with metastatic disease
- Absence of extrathoracic metastases (i.e., metastasis is confined to the lung)
- Ability to perform a complete resection of the metastases
- No significant comorbidity that would preclude surgery
- No alternative therapy that is superior to surgery

*Approximately a third of patients with metastatic disease meet these criteria.

Is the primary tumor controlled? Efficacy of pulmonary metastasectomy depends on, among other factors, the ability to control the primary neoplasm. The primary neoplasm, therefore, should generally be addressed before resection of the pulmonary metastases. Therefore, thorough preoperative testing should be performed to rule out other possible metastatic sites or local recurrence of the primary tumor prior to pulmonary metastasectomy (Box 23-3).

Alexander and Haight, in the 1940s, were the first to describe specific selection criteria for consideration of pulmonary metastasectomy. They realized that the benefits of surgical resection depended on primary tumor control, absence of extrathoracic spread, and adequate patient selection. Approximately a third of patients meet these selection criteria and can appropriately undergo metastatic resection.

SURGICAL APPROACH

Surgery for pulmonary metastases is based on the principle of performing a complete resection while preserving as much lung tissue as possible in case metastasectomies are required in the future.[51] The specific location of the tumor in the lung plays a role in determining the resection volume necessary to remove all disease. Wedge resection of the lung to include a negative resection margin is the standard therapy. Deeply located lesions or central lesions may require an anatomic resection—segmentectomy, lobectomy, or, rarely, pneumonectomy.

Bronchoscopy is performed routinely at the time of resection to exclude endobronchial involvement. Epidural analgesia has become the gold standard in thoracic surgery for managing postoperative pain and facilitating postoperative secretion clearance in the metastasectomy patient. Single-lung isolation using a double-lumen endotracheal tube or a bronchial blocker allows the surgeon to perform a thorough manual inspection of the superficial and deep parenchyma of the deflated lung. A reticulating stapler that cuts and staples simultaneously is useful for removing palpable nodules while sparing lung tissue. A 1-cm or greater margin is thought to be adequate when excising metastases to the lung.

The choice of incision should reflect the extent of disease, the goal of complete resection, and the patient's ability to undergo the procedure. The surgical options for metastasectomy include minimally invasive VATS and the traditional open procedure. VATS procedures typically involve three-port access to the pleural space, ipsilateral lung collapse via a double-lumen tube with digital palpation of the lung, and nodule localization through the nearest trocar site. Central lesions may be difficult to palpate through the trocar incision, which may justify an open procedure for their removal. Lin and colleagues reported on 99 potentially curative resections of metastases using a VATS approach and demonstrated long-term survival comparable to historic results with an open approach.[52] Landreneau and coworkers observed less pain and a shorter hospital stay after VATS resection of colorectal metastases to the lungs.[53] Critics of the VATS approach say that the loss of bimanual tactile ability results in a higher rate of missed metastases.

Open approaches include standard thoracotomy, bilateral simultaneous or staged thoracotomy, a clamshell and hemi-clamshell incision, and median sternotomy. Standard thoracotomy can be performed as the definitive procedure in patients with unilateral disease or as a staged procedure, with a contralateral thoracotomy performed approximately 6 weeks later in patients with bilateral disease. Muscle-sparing thoracotomy is frequently performed to preserve mechanical function postoperatively. Bilateral submammary incisions including a transverse sternotomy (a clamshell incision) is useful for accessing both thoracic cavities for metastasectomy. A hemi-clamshell incision, consisting of a unilateral anterior thoracotomy with a partial or complete sternotomy, has been described. Each of these incisions may at times be the correct approach, but, generally, each of them tends to be more morbid and painful than VATS or a median sternotomy.

Median sternotomy, preferred by some surgeons, provides access to both thoracic cavities, but it provides limited exposure to lesions in the left lower lobe and large posterior central lesions. Some surgeons may find that central lesions necessitating lobectomy are more easily excised via a thoracotomy. Patients with a history of radiation therapy, obesity, chronic obstructive pulmonary disease, diabetes, and steroid use may be at higher risk for sternal complications after median sternotomy. Morbidity and mortality rates for lung metastasectomy by conventional means range between 0% and 31.6% and between 0% and 7.6%, respectively.[54]

The metastasectomy itself usually consists of a wedge resection. This is facilitated by the tendency of metastatic disease to be found at the periphery of the lung, and it is easily performed with lung clamps and a pulmonary stapling device. Excision with electrocautery or laser may also be performed under select circumstances.[55-58] Posterior areas of the lung may be better assessed by filling the hemithorax with saline to float the lung anteriorly. Alternatively, posterior packs may be used. Only rarely are metastases found in regional lymph nodes, so formal nodal dissection is generally not indicated.[29] Although in primary lung cancer, lobectomy has been shown to give higher survival rates than wedge resections, no such difference has been found with metastasectomy.[59] Resection with a 1- to 2-cm margin of uninvolved tissue has proved to be adequate in this setting. Lobectomy is indicated if a lesser procedure would result in an incomplete resection or is not technically possible. This is most commonly the case with large, centrally located lesions or lesions in such close proximity to bronchovascular structures that an anatomic resection is required to avoid leaving fatally compromised lung tissue behind. Chest wall resection of contiguous lesions not associated with other disease, or even pneumonectomy, has been shown to improve survival when used in the appropriate setting.[3,60,61]

When considering a unilateral procedure for the treatment of presumed (on the basis of preoperative imaging) unilateral pulmonary metastases, the question is whether this approach will miss undiagnosed contralateral disease and whether this would be detrimental to the patient. One study tried to answer this question by looking at sternotomy versus unilateral thoracotomy in patients with metastases that appeared unilateral in preoperative imaging studies.[62] Unilateral thoracotomy was used, and the contralateral lung was not assessed. One might expect residual disease in the unevaluated thorax, resulting in a worse prognosis for this group. In fact, no difference in long-term survival was found. Furthermore, repeat resection of recurrences have been shown to improve survival, thus making the argument that any missed subclinical disease could be resected subsequently.[62,63] These results have been corroborated by Younes and colleagues.[64] In this study, patients undergoing unilateral thoracotomy for unilateral disease ($n = 179$) and patients undergoing bilateral thoracotomies for bilateral disease ($n = 88$) were investigated. The two groups of patients with confirmed bilateral metastases (synchronous or metachronous) were compared. Patients who experienced recurrence in the contralateral lung within 3, 6, or 12 months had overall 5-year survival rates of 24%, 30%, and 37%, respectively. When patients with recurrence in the contralateral lung were compared with patients with bilateral metastases on admission, there was no significant difference in overall survival. The only two predictors of contralateral recurrence were histology and the number of pathologically proven metastases. The authors concluded that bilateral exploration of unilateral lung metastases is not warranted in all cases.[64]

A newer technique involves placement of a substernal handport used in conjunction with thoracoscopy. After thoracoscopy is performed, an epigastric incision is made, the linea alba is divided, and the xyphoid is usually excised. The substernal space is then entered by blunt dissection, and both pleural spaces are accessed, allowing manual lung palpation.[65] Detterbeck and colleagues reported that this technique allowed adequate resection in 67% of patients; conversion to an open procedure was necessary in 33% of patients for anatomic and technical reasons.

LYMPH NODE DISSECTION

The role of systematic lymph node dissection performed during pulmonary resections for metastases is being defined. In the literature, the reported incidence of mediastinal nodal metastases ranges from 5% to 28.6%.[66,67] Most studies do not include nodal data because a lymph node dissection was not routinely performed as part of the operation. Putnam and coworkers demonstrated a very low incidence of lymph node metastases in patients with sarcomatous pulmonary metastases.[77]

There is evidence that the presence of nonsarcomatous lymph node metastases at the time of metastasectomy has an adverse effect on survival.[67] Omitting lymphadenectomy from the metastasectomy may incorrectly classify patients as being free of disease. Furthermore, lymph node involvement may influence the ensuing postoperative treatment plan. The feasibility of VATS nodal dissection has been established.[69] Certainly the need to perform a nodal dissection should not be the sole criterion for choosing an open over a VATS approach.

Finally, if involvement of the paratracheal lymph nodes is suspected, a mediastinoscopy should be performed. This minimally invasive outpatient procedure can save a patient from a metastasectomy that is unlikely to be of benefit.

RESULTS OF PULMONARY METASTASECTOMY

Approximately two thirds of patients experience recurrence after metastasectomy, so close follow-up is required.[70] Pastorino and colleagues[78] observed a higher probability of recurrence for sarcomas and melanomas (64%) than for epithelial (46%) or germ cell (26%) tumors.

A second or third metastasectomy has been shown to yield reasonably good survival if the primary tumor is controlled and all lesions are resectable. In the National Cancer Institute series reported by Temeck and colleagues,[78a] 70 of 152 patients required more than one operative procedure for removal of metastases. There was still a 50% long-term survival in patients whose tumors were felt to have been completely resected at the time of the second operation. Kandioler and colleagues observed a 5-year survival rate of 48% after repeated metastasectomy in 35 patients who underwent 82 metastasectomies. A significant survival advantage was seen among patients with long disease-free intervals.

Pulmonary metastasectomy in appropriately selected patients has been shown to improve survival. When all histologies are considered, the 5-year survival rate for patients undergoing resection of secondary pulmonary malignancy is 25% to 40% (Table 23-2). Many series have evaluated potential prognostic indicators to more clearly define the patients who are most likely to benefit from metastasectomy.

Table 23-2

Five-Year Survival Rates of Various Histologic Metastatic Resections

Histology	5-Yr Survival Rate without Metastasectomy (%)	5-Yr Survival Rate with Metastasectomy (%)
All histologies	—	25-40[77,145]
Breast cancer	11[107]	35-50[109,146,147]
Colorectal cancer	<5[54]	40-45[99,148]
Germ cell tumors	—	68[77]
Head and neck squamous cell carcinoma	—	29-60[77]
Melanoma	3-4[128,129]	21-36[77,128,129]
Osteosarcoma	0-17[90,149]	20-40[75,77,150,151]
Renal cell carcinoma	—	13-54[152]
Soft tissue sarcomas	—	20-40[77,79]
Urinary tract cancer	—	25-43[152]

Table 23-3
Prognostic Factors in Metastasectomy

Absolute	Equivocal
Complete resectability	Tumor doubling time
	Disease-free survival
	Number of nodules
	Histology
	Nodal status

Table 23-4
Prognostic Staging System

Prognostic Stage	# of Prognostic Indicators*	5-Yr Survival Rate (%)
Stage I	None	61
Stage II	Two	34
Stage III	Three	24
Stage IV	Unresectable	14

*The three possible indicators are resectability, disease-free interval greater than 36 months, and solitary (as opposed to multiple) metastases.
From Pastorino U, McCormack PM, Ginsberg RJ. Chest Surg Clin N Am 1998;8:197-202.

For example, short *tumor doubling time* is frequently a sign of an aggressive lesion, and it has been proposed that patients with these tumors, therefore, might not derive a survival benefit from resection. The results seen in these studies, however, are equivocal.[71-74] Moreover, the practical application of such a measurement is difficult. Disease-free interval has also been studied in an attempt to predict outcomes. Longer disease-free intervals, however, have not been consistently associated with a better prognosis.[74-77] It might seem that a finding of an increased number of nodules on preoperative testing would be associated with a poor prognosis, but in general, patients with multiple nodules do more poorly then those with a solitary nodule. However, there is great variability.[66,74,77,78] Also, it is not clear whether there is a number of nodules above which resection is unwarranted. As many as 20 to 30 metastasectomies have been performed at one operation with good results.[79] In addition, the number of nodules estimated with preoperative testing is often inaccurate. Thus, multiplicity may be more appropriately used to assist in the assessment of tumor resectability. None of these criteria for predicting positive outcome from metastasectomy has been universally established. Most studies have proposed that complete resectability is the only universal determinant of prognosis across histologies (Table 23-3).[78]

Many of the aforementioned studies attempting to evaluate prognostic determinants in pulmonary metastasectomy have been faulted because they lack sufficient statistical power to demonstrate clinical significance. One group, however, reported 5206 cases of pulmonary metastases from various sites from the 18 medical centers of the International Registry of Lung Metastases.[66] In this retrospective review, three indicators were shown to have prognostic significance regardless of primary histology: resectability, a disease-free interval of greater than 36 months, and solitary versus multiple metastasis. As a result, the authors proposed a four-group staging system based on the number of prognostic indicators present in a given patient (Table 23-4). Although staging systems such as this may better define the patients most likely to benefit from metastasectomy, survival rates after surgery, even with poor prognostic indicators, may be better than after any other treatment. Consequently, some feel that metastasectomy should be offered to appropriate patients regardless of these factors, with the possible exception of inability to perform complete resection.[66]

In addition to the aforementioned factors equivocally associated with prognosis, other factors have been shown to clearly not affect outcome. These factors include unilateral (as opposed to bilateral) disease, age, sex, and wedge resection versus formal lobectomy (Box 23-4).

Box 23-4
Factors Not Affecting Prognosis in Patients with Metastasectomy

- Age
- Sex
- Unilateral versus bilateral disease
- Wedge resection versus formal lobectomy

From Pass HI, Donington JS. Metastatic cancer of the lung. In: De Vita V, Hellman S, Rosenberg SA, editors. Principles and practice of oncology. Philadelphia: JB Lippincott; 1997, p. 2436-551; and Putnam JB, Roth JA, Wesley MN, et al. J Thorac Cardiovasc Surg 1984;87:260-8.

After complete pulmonary resection of metastatic disease, recurrence is the most common cause of death. Despite this, repeat resections have contributed to prolonged survival for a number of histologies.[63,77,80,81] The most studied of these is soft tissue sarcoma. For example, in a study by the National Cancer Institute in which patients underwent re-resection for soft tissue sarcomas, no difference in the actuarial 5-year survival was found in those undergoing one, two, and even three resections for recurrence.[80] To appropriately choose patients for repeat resection, it is important to use preoperative selection criteria that are similar to those used for the initial resection. This ensures the absence of disseminated disease and the ability of a given patient to tolerate the proposed procedure. Once patients have been screened, therefore, resection of recurrent disease will be offered to approximately 70%, if no extrathoracic dissemination is present and if the lesion is amenable to resection.

METASTASES TO THE LUNG
Soft Tissue Sarcomas

Soft tissue sarcomas are a group of nonossifying malignant neoplasms derived from mesenchymal connective tissue. In a 1997 report from the International Pulmonary Metastases Registry, soft tissue sarcomas were the most common type of pulmonary metastases resected, and they accounted for 42% of all patients undergoing metastasectomy.[82] Unfortunately, only 50% of patients with lung metastases from sarcoma are operative candidates, and of those, 80% undergo complete resection. It is from that 80% that the 5-year survival rates of

20% to 40% are obtained.[83] Soft tissue sarcomas typically respond poorly to systemic chemotherapy, making surgery the only potentially curative treatment option.

Patients with extremity soft tissue sarcomas tend to develop pulmonary metastases more frequently than those with sarcomas at other sites.[84] Gadd and coworkers analyzed histopathologic findings of soft tissue extremity sarcomas and their relationship to pulmonary metastases.[83] The probability of pulmonary metastases developing from a soft tissue sarcoma is influenced by histopathologic findings including grade, size, and location of the primary tumor. Patients with spindle cell sarcoma had the highest incidence of pulmonary metastases, whereas those with liposarcomas had the lowest incidence.

Regardless of histology, primary and repeat metastasectomy has been associated with improved long-term survival. A study from Memorial Sloan-Kettering focusing on 719 patients with sarcoma who had pulmonary metastases showed a 3-year survival rate of 46% for patients undergoing resection, compared with 17% for those treated nonsurgically.[85] Significant prognostic variables include completeness of resection, disease-free interval, tumor doubling time greater than 40 days, number of nodules (four or fewer), grade, tumor histology, radicality of resection, and age.[71,85-87]

Pulmonary re-recurrence after complete resection of metastatic soft tissue sarcomas has been reported to occur in 45% to 83% of patients, and the lungs represent the main reason for ultimate treatment failure in up to 80% of patients.[88] Five-year survival rates of 36% after re-resection of soft tissue sarcomas have been reported.[89] Patients whose metastases cannot be completely resected, those with large metastases, and those with high-grade primary tumor pathology tend to have worse outcomes.[89]

Osteosarcoma (Osteogenic Sarcoma)

Like soft tissue sarcomas, osteosarcoma has a strong predilection for metastasis to the lung. In addition, the lesions themselves are frequently multiple and often recur despite resection. Consequently pulmonary involvement is responsible for most deaths in patients with this disease. Approximately 10% to 20% of patients have distant metastases on initial evaluation and, as with other histologies, CT of the chest is the imaging modality of choice for detection.

Before the introduction of chemotherapy, the overall survival from osteogenic sarcoma was only 10% to 20%.[75,90] In the early 1970s, however, the use of chemotherapy, especially high-dose methotrexate, substantially improved outcomes.[91] Later, with the introduction of multimodality therapy, chemotherapy (doxorubicin, high-dose cyclophosphamide, and cisplatin) combined with resection improved 5-year survival rates to 32% to 40%.[47,66,92] In some cases, treatment resulted in cure. As a consequence of these improved results early in the history of metastasectomy, a more aggressive approach toward resection of pulmonary metastases developed. Furthermore, simultaneous resection of the primary osteosarcoma and lung metastasectomy after neoadjuvant chemotherapy has been associated with improved outcomes.[24]

Despite the survival advantage imparted by surgical resection in osteogenic carcinoma, tumor recurs in 50% of patients within 1 year. Eventually, 85% of these patients relapse with recurrent pulmonary disease, despite adequate removal of the primary tumor and no earlier evidence of gross secondary disease. Resection of these recurrences is indicated, as numerous studies have demonstrated improved survival.[27,93] If the patient is not a surgical candidate, radiotherapy may be an option.[94] In addition, brachytherapy has been used successfully in patients with metastatic endobronchial lesions.[81]

No prognostic factors, except complete resection, have consistently been associated with improved survival after metastasectomy.[66] A number of studies have looked at the aforementioned characteristics (age, sex, location, doubling time, disease-free survival, number of nodules, resectability) but found that few consistent conclusions could be drawn. Most studies do correlate a worse outcome with an increased number of nodules.[66,95] All studies conclude that complete surgical resection is indicated, and when resectability was studied, incomplete resection was always associated with a worse outcome.[66,78,96,97] In addition, the location of the primary lesion has been associated with worse prognosis in the case of pelvic and vertebral tumors.[98]

Her-2/neu expression has also been associated with increased risk for pulmonary metastases.[66] These findings suggest that these patients may benefit from additional biological therapy. Phase I/II gene therapy trials using an adenovirus vector containing a murine osteocalcin promoter for the treatment of refractory osteosarcomas metastatic to the lung are under way.[78]

Large Bowel Cancer

Among all patients with colorectal cancer, about 20% have metastases at the time of diagnosis. After resection of the primary cancer, approximately 10% of patients develop lung metastases and only 2% are suitable for resection.[99,100] Surgical resection is still commonly considered the treatment of choice for local control of pulmonary metastases from colorectal cancer according to the National Comprehensive Cancer Network's 2007 *Clinical Practice Guidelines in Oncology*. Pulmonary resection of colorectal carcinoma results in long-term survival in selected patients, with 5-year survival rates ranging from 27% to 61%. Prognostic factors found to be significant in patients with pulmonary metastases from large bowel cancers include primary tumor stage and completeness of the resection.[100,101] Other prognostic factors may include number of pulmonary metastases, pre-thoracotomy carcinoembryonic antigen (CEA) serum level, and presence of lymph node metastases.[99,101-104]

The liver is the most common intra-abdominal site of metastases in patients with colorectal cancer. Successful resections of liver metastases have been reported, with resulting 5-year survival rates of 25% to 35%. Because chemotherapy for metastatic disease results in a median survival of only 16 to 20 months, an aggressive approach to synchronous and metachronous colorectal metastases to the lung and liver is recommended. Barlow and colleagues observed a median survival of 44 months after liver and lung resection.[105] Long-term results are influenced by the disease-free interval and the completeness of the resection.[106]

Breast Carcinoma

Breast cancer accounts for 30,000 deaths each year and is currently the second most common cause of cancer deaths in women in the United States, behind lung cancer. Pulmonary involvement in breast cancer is most commonly associated with widespread disease, which contraindicates resection in the majority of patients. A thorough search for extrathoracic disease is warranted before considering metastasectomy. In a series of 5143 patients with breast cancer, Staren and coworkers reported lung metastases in 284 patients, and only 1% of these had metastatic disease confined to the lung.[107] They observed a significant 5-year survival advantage for patients who underwent metastasectomy (36% versus 11%). Factors conferring a more favorable prognosis include estrogen and progesterone receptor (ER/PR) status and a complete resection.[98,108,109]

A solitary pulmonary nodule in a patient with prior breast cancer has a 50% chance of being a new lung primary or a benign nodule. Resection of the nodule with histologic comparison to the patient's breast primary and an analysis of immunohistochemical markers distinct for breast cancer help to identify the tumor cell origin. Differentiating breast cancer metastases from primary lung cancer is important because lung cancers are best treated with an anatomic lobectomy, whereas wedge resection is an adequate treatment for metastatic breast cancer. Currently, metastasectomy is recommended in a select group of patients with metastatic breast cancer.

Head and Neck Carcinoma

Head and neck carcinomas most commonly spread through local lymphatics. The lung is among the more common sites of distant spread, followed by bone and liver. Patients with head and neck cancer and a history of frequent tobacco use are at risk for other foregut malignancies. A solitary nodule in a patient with a history of head and neck cancer has a greater chance of being a lung primary and should be treated as such. Five-year survival rates after metastasectomy for head and neck cancers range from 29% to 59%.[110]

Renal Cell Carcinoma

The lung is a frequent site of renal cell metastases, with prevalence rates as high as 72% to 76% in autopsy studies.[111,112] Since the first resection of a renal cell carcinoma by Barney and Churchill in 1939,[113] a number of studies have been published demonstrating the beneficial effect of resecting renal cell cancer metastases to the lung. Han and colleagues reported that patients with evidence of disease in multiple organs fare significantly worse than those with metastatic disease limited to the lungs.[114] Patients with a solitary renal metastases fare best, with a 5-year survival of up to 54%.[115] Assouad and colleagues[115a] observed that 5-year survival was significantly affected by the size of the largest metastasis and by mediastinal lymph node involvement. Synchronous metastases, greater than six metastases, absence of regional and mediastinal nodes, and resectability have been identified as being important prognostic factors.[108,116] Results of long-term follow-up studies support an aggressive surgical approach in patients with renal carcinoma metastases to the lungs.[117]

Germ Cell Tumors

Germ cell tumors account for only 1% of all cancers, but they are the most common malignancy in male patients between the ages of 15 and 35 years. The majority of germ cell tumors are highly responsive to chemotherapy and have an excellent prognosis even in patients with metastatic disease. The majority of patients with metastatic testicular tumors demonstrate a complete clinical remission after treatment with chemotherapy. Surgical intervention for pulmonary metastases from germ cell tumors is primarily reserved for evaluation of a residual mass after chemotherapy.

In patients with a residual mass after chemotherapy, it is difficult to differentiate necrosis from a mature teratoma or persistent tumor. Cagini and coworkers reported on a series of 144 patients who underwent resection of a residual mass after chemotherapy for metastatic germ cell tumors.[118] Viable malignant elements were found in 44 patients, and 63 patients were found to have a differentiated teratoma. An overall 5-year survival rate of 77% was observed, with a worse rate (51%) in patients with malignant teratomatous elements. Resection of a residual mass is advocated in these patients to determine the need for further chemotherapy.

Gynecologic Tumors

The lung represents the most common organ involved in uterine cancer spread, with isolated pulmonary metastases observed in approximately 6% of patients.[119] Pulmonary metastasectomy for uterine cancers is associated with a 5-year survival rate of 53%.[120] Anderson and colleagues observed improved median survival in patients undergoing pulmonary metastasectomy for adenocarcinomas (46 months) compared with leiomyosarcomas (25 months).[119] Completeness of resection, longer disease-free interval, and three or fewer metastases have been associated with an improved survival rate in this patient population.[119,121] Additionally, ER/PR status of pulmonary metastases is significant, as patients with positive ER/PR receptors have an 80% response rate and average survival rates of up to 33 months.[122]

Isolated lung metastases occur in approximately 1.5% to 6% of patients with cervical cancer.[123,124] Five-year survival rates range from 0% to 52% for cervical cancers metastatic to the lung treated by pulmonary resection.[120] Hormonal therapy has shown no benefit thus far in the treatment of cervical metastases, and ER/PR receptors are not typically measured.

The majority of patients with ovarian cancer metastatic to the lung present with malignant effusions.[125] Disease confined to the lung amenable to metastasectomy is exceedingly rare.

Melanoma

Patients with metastatic melanoma often present with widely disseminated disease, and isolated pulmonary metastases are rare. The lungs are the second most common site of metastases in patients with melanoma, with a prevalence of between 12% and 36%.[126,127] The annual probability of developing pulmonary metastases increases progressively from 10% at 5 years to 17% at 15 years.

An aggressive surgical approach to pulmonary metastatic disease from melanoma is warranted as long as a complete metastasectomy can be performed. Evidence for this is based in part on studies from Harpole and colleagues and Tafra and coworkers, who reported 5-year survival rates of 20% and 27%, respectively, in patients undergoing pulmonary metastasectomy, versus 4% and 3%, respectively, in patients treated medically.[128,129]

If a complete resection cannot be performed, little or no benefit is provided in terms of prolonging patient survival. Additional factors influencing survival include prolonged disease-free interval, prior chemotherapy, the presence of no more than two pulmonary nodules, and negative lymph nodes.[129]

Endocrine Tumors

The lungs represent an uncommon site of metastases for malignant endocrine tumors. A select group of patients with slow-growing endocrine tumors, including carcinoids, well-differentiated thyroid cancers, and parathyroid cancers, may benefit from resection of their metastases. In a retrospective review, Khan and coworkers reported shorter survival in patients with positive mediastinal lymph nodes at the time of resection and a shorter disease-free interval.[130] Occasionally, metastases may be resected to alleviate symptoms of hormone production.[131,132]

ALTERNATIVE TREATMENT OPTIONS

Radiofrequency ablation (RFA) is a thermal energy delivery system that applies an alternating current through a needle electrode into a tissue. The result of energy delivery is coagulative necrosis and tissue destruction in the vicinity of the probe. Lung parenchyma is thought to be a good place to use RFA because pulmonary tissue surrounding solid tumors acts as a thermal insulator, allowing energy to focus on the area of the solid tumor.[133-135] Lesions can be approached percutaneously with CT guidance or by mini-thoracotomies in the operating suite.

Inclusion criteria for RFA include lesions no larger than 5 cm in diameter, inoperable non–small cell lung cancer, and no more than four secondary lesions in both lungs. The feasibility of RFA depends on factors including the presence of an "access window" and proximity to hilar structures. Complications of RFA include pneumothorax, pleural effusion, hyperpyrexia, infection, and hemorrhage. Yasui and colleagues achieved local control of disease in 90% of cases at 7 months after treating 96 metastases and three primary tumors. Lagana and coworkers achieved immediate total ablation for almost 90% of patients (16 of 18 lesions), with a recurrence rate of 13.3%.

Isolated lung perfusion, first reported by Creech and associates in 1958, is an alternative method of chemotherapy delivery that allows administration of high local doses while reducing the incidence of systemic toxicities.[136] Phase I trials have been completed that examine safety aspects of different chemotherapeutic agents.[137] The technique provides a novel means for examining the efficacy of other agents, both biologic and chemotherapeutic, on metastatic disease. More studies are needed to define the role of lung perfusion in metastatic disease. Researchers at Roswell Park Cancer Institute are working on minimally invasive techniques for isolated lung perfusion.

PALLIATIVE THERAPY

Palliative therapies include laser ablation of airway lesions, tracheobronchial photodynamic therapy (PDT), radiation (external beam, cyber knife, localized), and airway stenting. Hemoptysis resulting from pulmonary metastases is usually controlled with either external beam radiation, laser ablation, or PDT. The neodymium:yttrium-aluminum garnet laser provides effective coagulation and tumor necrosis, and it is helpful in the removal of endobronchial tumors causing obstruction. It can be used effectively via a flexible or rigid endoscope. PDT has been shown to prolong airway patency and can be used as the primary treatment modality or in conjunction with the laser. Finally, airway stenting is frequently used either alone or in conjunction with other palliative therapies to improve patient quality of life.

CONCLUSIONS

Currently, metastasectomy is the treatment of choice in select patients with metastatic disease to the lungs. Selection guidelines now available are useful in determining which patients benefit from metastasectomy. The role of pulmonary metastasectomy may change as more effective systemic chemotherapy treatment regimens become available. Controlled clinical trials are needed to clarify this issue.

REFERENCES

1. Barney JD. Twelve-year cure following nephrectomy for adenocarcinoma and lobectomy for solitary metastasis. *J Urol* 1944;**52**:406-7.
2. Burt M. In: Fishman AP, editor. Pulmonary disease. Philadelphia: JB Lippincott; 1998, p. 1851-60.
3. Koong HN, Pastorino U, Ginsberg RJ. Is there a role for pneumonectomy in pulmonary metastases? International Registry of Lung Metastases. *Ann Thorac Surg* 1999;**68**(6):2039-43.
4. Weinlechner JW. Zur Kasuistic der Tumoren an der Brustwand und deren Behandlung (Resektion der Rippen, Eroffnung der Brusthohle, partielle Entfernung der Lunge). *Wein Med Wochenschr* 1882;**32**(589-591):624-8.
5. Attinger B, Jaggi F, Haag M, et al. The first successful lung resection. *Schweiz Rundsch Med Prax* 1993;**82**:435-40.
6. Kronlein RU. Ueber Lungenchirurgie. *Berl Klin Wochnschr* 1884;**21**:129-32.
7. Naef AP. *The story of thoracic surgery: milestones and pioneers*. Toronto: Hogrefe and Huber; 1990.
8. Divis G. Ein Beitrag Zur Operativen Lungeschwulste. *Acta Chir Scand* 1927;**62**:329-41.
9. Edwards AT. Malignant disease of the lung. *J Thorac Surg* 1934;**4**:107-24.
10. Torek F. Removal of metastatic carcinoma of the lung and mediastinum. *Arch Surg* 1930;**21**:1416-24.
11. Alexander J, Haight C. Pulmonary resection for solitary metastatic sarcomas and carcinomas. *Surg Gynecol Obstet* 1947;**85**:129-46.
12. Martini N, McCormack PM. Evolution of the surgical management of pulmonary metastases. *Chest Surg Clin North Am* 1998;**8**:13-27.
13. Treasure T. Pulmonary metastasectomy for colorectal cancer: weak evidence and no randomized trials. *Eur J Cardiothor Surg* 2008;**33**:300-2.
14. Treasure T. Surgical resection of pulmonary metastases. *Eur J Cardiothor Surg* 2007;**32**:351-5.
15. Viadana E, Bross IDJ, Pickren JW. Cascade spread of blood-borne metastases in solid and nonsolid cancers in humans. In: Weiss L, Gilbert HA, editors. *Pulmonary metastasis*. Boston: GK Hall; 1978, p. 142-67.
16. Liotta LA, Saidel MG, Kleinerman J. The significance of hematogenous tumor cell clumps in the metastatic process. *Cancer Res* 1976;**36**:889-94.
17. Im JH, Fu W, Wang H, Bhatia SK, Hammer DA, Kowalska MA, Muschel RJ. Coagulation facilitates tumor cell spreading in the pulmonary vasculature during early metastatic colony formation. *Cancer Res* 2004;**64**:8613-9.
18. Honn KV, Tang DG, Grossi IM, et al. Enhanced endothelial cell retraction mediated by 12(S)-HETE: a proposed mechanism for the role of platelets in tumor cell metastasis. *Exp Cell Res* 1994;**210**:1-9.
19. Liotta LA. Cancer metastasis and angiogenesis: an imbalance of positive and negative regulation. *Cell* 1991;**64**:327-36.
20. Hoover Jr HC, Ketcham AS. Metastasis of metastases. *Am J Surg* 1975;**130**(4):405-11.
21. Pass HI, Temeck BA. Biology of metastatic disease. *Chest Surg Clin North Am* 1998;**8**:1-1.

22. Sugarbaker EV, Cohen AM, Ketcham AS. Do metastases metastasize? *Ann Surg* 1971;**174**(2):161-6.
23. Tait CR, Dodwell D, Horgan K. Do metastases metastasize? *J Pathology* 2004;**203**:515-8.
24. Ramii-Porta R, Ball D, et al. The IASLC Lung Cancer Staging Project: proposals for the revision of the T descriptors in the forthcoming (seventh) edition of the TNM classification for lung cancer. *J Thor Oncology* 2007;**2**(7):593-602.
25. Ichinose Y, Hara N, Ohta M, et al. DNA ploidy patterns of tumors diagnosed as metachronous or recurrent lung cancers. *Ann Thor Surg* 1991;**52**(3):469-73.
26. Ichinose Y, Hara N, Ohta M. Synchronous lung cancers defined by deoxyribonucleic acid flow cytometry. *J Thorac Cardiovasc Surg* 1991;**102**(3):418-24.
27. Kandioler D, Kromer E, Tuchler H, End A, Muller MR, Wolner E, Eckersberger F. Long-term results after repeated surgical removal of pulmonary metastases. *Ann Thor Surg* 1998;**65**:909-12.
28. Matsuzoe D, Hideshima T, Ohshima K, et al. Discrimination of double primary lung cancer from intrapulmonary metastases by p53 gene mutation. Br J Cancer 1999; **79**(9-10):1549-52.
29. Pass HI, Donington JS. Metastatic cancer of the lung. In: De Vita V, Hellman S, Rosenberg SA, editors. *Principles and practice of oncology*. Philadelphia: JB Lippincott; 1997, p. 2436-551.
30. Toomes H, Delphendahl A, Manke H, et al. The coin lesion of the lung. *Cancer* 1983;**51**:534-9.
31. Snyder BJ, Pugatch RD. Imaging characteristics of metastatic disease to the chest. *Chest Surg Clin North Am* 1998;**8**(1):29-48.
32. Graeber GM, Tamin W. Current status of the diagnosis and treatment of thymoma. *Sem Thorac Cardiovasc Surg* 2000;**12**(4):268-77.
33. Crow J, Slavin G, Kreel L. Pulmonary metastases: A pathologic and radiologic study. *Cancer* 1981;**47**:2595-601.
34. Khan A, Herman PG, Vorwerk P, Stevens P, Rojas KA, Graver M. Solitary pulmonary nodules: comparison of classification with standard, thin-section, and reference phantom CT. *Radiology* 1991;**179**:477-81.
35. McCormack PM, Bains MS, Begg CB, et al. Role of video-assisted thoracic surgery in the treatment of pulmonary metastases: results of a prospective trial. *Ann Thor Surg* 2004;**78**:1910-8.
36. Parsons AM, Ennis EK, Yankaskas BC, Parker LA, Hyslop WB, Detterbeck FC. Helical computed tomography inaccuracy in the detection of pulmonary metastases: can it be improved? *Ann Thor Surg* 2007;**84**:1830-7.
37. Nakajima J, Murakawa T, Fukami T, Takamoto T. Is thoracoscopic surgery justified to treat pulmonary metastasis from colorectal cancer? *Interactive Cardiovascular and Thoracic Surgery* 2008;**7**(2):212-7.
38. Kang MC, Kang CH, Lee HJ, Goo JM, Kim YT, Kim JH. Accuracy of 16-channel multi-detector row chest computed tomography with thin sections in the detection of metastatic pulmonary nodules. *Eur J Cardiothorac Surg* 2008;**33**(3):473-9.
39. Harris MT, Berlangieri SU, Cebon JS, Davis ID, Scott AM. Impact of 2-deoxy-2[F-18]fluoro-D-glucose positron emission tomography on the management of patients with advanced melanoma. *Mol Imaging Biol* 2005;**7**: 304-8.
40. Gross BH, Glazer GM, Brookstein FL. Multiple pulmonary nodules detected by computed tomography, diagnostic implications. *J Comput Assist Tomogr* 1985;**9**:880-5.
41. Vincent RG, Choksi LB, Takita H. Surgical resection of solitary pulmonary metastasis. In: Weiss L, Gilbert HA, editors. *Pulmonary metastasis*. Boston: GK Hall; 1978, p. 232-42.
42. Crosby JH, Kager B, Hoeg K. Transthoracic fine needle aspiration. *Cancer* 1985;**56**:2504-7.
43. McCormack PM. Surgical resection of pulmonary metastases. *Semin Surg Oncol* 1990;**6**:297-302.
44. Eberhardt R, Anantham D, Herth F, Feller-Kopman D, Ernst A. Electromagnetic navigation diagnostic bronchoscopy in peripheral lung lesions.[see comment]. *Chest* 2007;**131**(6):1800-5.
45. DeCamp Jr MM, Jaklitsch MT, Mentzer SJ, Harpole Jr D, Sugarbaker DJ. The safety and versatility of video-thoracoscopy: A prospective analysis of 895 consecutive cases. *J Am Coll Surg* 1995;**181**:165-7.
46. Mack MJ, Hazelrigg SR, Landreneau RJ, Acuff TE. Thoracoscopy for the diagnosis of the indeterminate solitary pulmonary nodule. *Ann Thor Surg* 1993;**56**:830-2.
47. Mitruka S, Landreneau RJ, Mack MJ, Fetterman LS, Gammie J, Bartley S, et al. Diagnosing the indeterminate pulmonary nodule: percutaneous biopsy versus thoracoscopy. *Surgery* 1995;**118**:676-84.
48. Sterman DH, Sztejman E, Rodriguez E, Friedberg JS. Diagnosis and staging of "other bronchial tumors." *Chest Surg Clin North Am* 2003;**13**(1):79-94.
49. Emad A, Rezaian GR. Closed percutaneous pleural brushing: a new method for the diagnosis of malignant pleural effusions. *Respir Med* 1998;**92**:659-63.

50. Prakash UB, Reiman HM. Comparison of needle biopsy with cytologic analysis for the evaluation of pleural effusion: analysis of 414 cases. *Mayo Clin Proc* 1985;**60**:158-64.
51. Downey R. Surgical treatment of pulmonary metastases. *Surg Oncol Clin North Am* 1999;**8**(2):341-54.
52. Lin JC, Wiechmann RJ, Szwerc MF, et al. Diagnostic and therapeutic video-assisted thoracic surgery resection of pulmonary metastases. *Surgery* 1999;**126**:636-41:discussion 641-2.
53. Landreneau RJ, De Giacomo T, Mack MJ, et al. Therapeutic video-assisted thoracoscopic surgical resection of colorectal pulmonary metastases. *Eur J Cardiothor Surg* 2000;**18**:671-6:discussion 676-7.
54. Ponn RB, Fernieni A, D'Agostino RS, et al. Comparison of late pulmonary function after posterolateral thoracotomy and muscle-sparing thoracotomy. *Ann Thor Surg* 1992;**53**:675-9.
55. Alsabeh R, Wilson CS, Ahn CW, et al. Expression of bcl-2 by breast cancer: a possible diagnostic application. *Mod Pathol* 1996;**9**:439-44.
56. Branscheid D, Krysa S, Wollkopf G, et al. Does Nd-YAG laser extend the indications for resection of pulmonary metastases? *Eur J Cardiothorac Surg* 1992;**6**:590-7.
57. Kodama K, Doi O, Higashiyama M, et al. Surgical management of lung metastases. Usefulness of resection with the neodymium:yttrium-aluminum-garnet laser with median sternotomy. *J Thorac Cardiovasc Surg* 1991;**101**: 901-8.
58. Rolle A, Pereszlenyi A, Koch R, Richard M, Baier B. Is surgery for multiple lung metastases reasonable? A total of 328 consecutive patients with metastasectomies with a new 1318-nm Nd:YAG laser. *J Thorac Cardiovasc Surg* 2006;**131**(6):1236-42.
59. Ginsberg RJ, Rubinstein LV. Randomized trial of lobectomy versus limited resection for T1N0 non-small cell lung cancer. *Ann Thorac Surg* 1995;**60**: 615-22.
60. Hendricks JM, van Putte B, Romijn S. Pneumonectomy for lung metastases: report of ten cases. *Thor Cardiov Surg* 2003;**51**(1):38-41.
61. Spaggiari L, Grunenwald DH, Girard P, et al. Pneumonectomy for lung metastases: indications, risks and outcomes. *Ann Thoracic Surg* 1998;**66**(6):1930-3.
62. Roth JA, Pass HI, Wesley MN, et al. Comparison of median sternotomy and thoracotomy for resection of pulmonary metastases in patients with adult soft tissue sarcoma. *Ann Thorac Surg* 1986;**42**:134-8.
63. Saltzman DA, Snyder CL, Ferrell KL, et al. Aggressive metastasectomy for pulmonic sarcomatous metastases: A follow-up study. *Am J Surg* 1993;**17**: 543-7.
64. Younes RN, Gross JL, Deheinzelin D. Surgical resection of unilateral lung metastases: is bilateral thoracotomy necessary? *World J Surg* 2002;**26**(9): 1112-6.
65. Detterbeck FC, Egan TM. Thoracoscopy using a substernal handport or palpation. *Ann Thor Surg* 2004;**78**:1031-6.
66. Pastorino U, Buyse M, Friedel G, et al. Long-term results of lung metastasectomy: Prognostic analysis on 5206 cases. *J Thorac Cardiovasc Surg* 1997;**113**:37-49.
67. Ercan S, Nichols FC, Trastek VF, Deschamps C, Allen MS, Miller DT, et al. Prognostic significance of lymph node metastases found during pulmonary metastasectomy for extrapulmonary carcinoma. *Ann Thor Surg* 2004;**77**: 1786-91.
68. Putnam JB. Secondary tumors of the lung. In: Shields TW, LoCicero J, Ponn RB, editors. *General thoracic surgery*. 5th ed. Philadelphia: Lippincott Williams and Wilkins; 2000, p. 1555-76.
69. Watanabe A, Koyanagi T, Ohsawa H, et al. Systematic node dissection by VATS is not inferior to that through an open thoracotomy: a comparative clinicopathologic retrospective study. *Surgery* 2005;**138**:510-7.
70. Sadoff JD, Detterbeck FC. Pulmonary metastases from extrapulmonary cancer. In: Detterbeck FC, Rivera MP, Socinski MA, Rosenman JG, editors. *Diagnosis and treatment of lung cancer: an evidence based guide for the practicing clinician*. Philadelphia: WB Saunders; 2004, p. 450-64.
71. Casson AG, Putnam JB, Natarajan G, Johnston DA, Mountain C, McMurtrey M, Roth JA. Five year survival after pulmonary metastasectomy for adult soft tissue sarcoma. *Cancer* 1992;**69**(3):662-8.
72. D'Amico TA, Sabiston DC. Surgical management of pulmonary metastases. In: Sabiston DC, Spencer FC, editors. *Surgery of the chest*. Philadelphia: WB Saunders; 1995. p. 669-75.
73. Joseph WL, Morton DL, Adkins PC. Prognostic significance of tumor doubling time in evaluating operability in pulmonary metastatic disease. *J Thorac Cardiovasc Surg* 1971;**61**:23-32.
74. Putnam JB, Roth JA, Wesley MN, et al. Survival following aggressive resection of pulmonary metastases from soft tissue sarcomas. *J Thorac Cardiovasc Surg* 1984;**87**:260-7.

75. Beattie Jr EJ, Matini N, Rosen G. The management of pulmonary metastases in children with osteogenic sarcoma with surgical resection combined with chemotherapy. *Cancer* 1975;**35**:618-21.
76. Meyer WH, Schell MJ, Kumar AP, et al. Thoracotomy for pulmonary metastatic osteosarcoma: an analysis of prognostic indicators of survival. *Cancer* 1987;**59**:374-9.
77. Putnam Jr JB, Roth JA, Wesley MN, et al. Survival following aggressive resection of pulmonary metastases from osteogenic sarcoma: analysis of prognostic factors. *Ann Thor Surg* 1983;**36**:516-23.
78. Pastorino U, McCormack PM, Ginsberg RJ. A new staging proposal for pulmonary metastases: the results of analysis of 5206 cases of resected pulmonary metastases. *Chest Surg Clin N Am* 1998;**8**:197-202.
78a. Temeck B, Wexler LH, Stemberg S. Metastasectomy for sarcomatous Pediatric histologies: results and prognostic factors. *Ann Thor Surg* 1995;**59**:1385-90.
79. Martini N, McCormack PM, Bains MS, et al. Surgery for solitary and multiple pulmonary metastases. *N Y State J Med* 1978;**78**:1711-3.
80. Rizzoni WE, Pass HI, Wesley MN, et al. Resection of recurrent pulmonary metastases in patients with soft-tissue sarcomas. *Arch Surg* 1986;**121**:1248-52.
81. Roth JA, Putnam Jr JB, Wesley MN, Rosenberg SA. Differing determinants of prognosis following resection of pulmonary metastases from osteogenic and soft tissue sarcoma patients. *Cancer* 1985;**55**:1361-6.
82. International Registry of Lung Metastases. Long-term results of lung metastasectomy. *J Thorac Cardiovasc Surg* 1997;**113**:37-49.
83. Gadd MA, Casper ES, Woodruff JM, et al. Development and treatment of pulmonary metastases in adult patients with extremity soft tissue sarcoma. *Ann Surg* 1993;**218**:705-12.
84. Vezeridis MP, Moore R, Karakousis CP. Metastatic patterns in soft tissue sarcomas. *Arch Surg* 1983;**118**:915-8.
85. Billingsley KG, Burt ME, Jara E, Ginsberg RJ, Woodruff JM, Leung DHY, Brennan MF. Pulmonary metastases from soft tissue sarcomas: analysis of patterns of disease and postmetastasis survival. *Ann Surg* 1999;**229**(5):602-12.
86. Abecasis N, Cortez F, Bettencourt A, Costa CS, Orvalho F. Mendez de Almeida JM: Surgical treatment of lung metastases: prognostic factors for long-term survival. *J Surg Oncol* 1999;**72**:193-8.
87. van Geel AN, Pastorino U, Jauch KW, Judson IR, Coevorden FV, Buesa JM, et al. Surgical treatment of lung metastases: the European Organization for Research and Treatment of Cancer—Soft Tissue and Bone Sarcoma Group study of 255 patients. *Cancer* 1996;**77**:675-82.
88. Marcove R, Mike V, Hajek JV, Levin AG, Hutter RVP. Osteogenic sarcoma under the age of 21: a review of 145 cases. *J Bone Joint Surg* 1970;**52**:411-8.
89. Weiser MR, Downey RJ, Leung DH, Brennan MF. Repeat resection of pulmonary metastases in patients with soft-tissue sarcoma. *J Am Coll Surg* 2000;**191**:184-91.
90. La Quaglia MP. Osteosarcoma: Specific tumor management and results. *Chest Surg Clin North Am* 1998;**8**:77-95.
91. Rosen G, Suwansirikul S, Kwon C, et al. High-dose methotrexate with citrovorum factor rescue and Adriamycin in childhood osteogenic sarcoma. *Cancer* 1974;**33**:1151-63.
92. Skinner KA, Eilber FR, Holmes EC, et al. Surgical treatment and chemotherapy for pulmonary metastases from osteosarcoma. *Arch Surg* 1992;**127**:1065-71.
93. Antunes M, Bernardo J, Salete M, Prieto D, et al. Excision of pulmonary metastases of osteogenic sarcoma of the limbs. *Eur J Thor Cardiovasc Surg* 1999;**15**:592-6.
94. Gossost D, Radu C, Girard P, et al. Resection of pulmonary metastases from sarcoma: can some patients benefit from a less invasive approach. *Ann Thorac Surg* 2009;**87**:238-44.
95. Belli L, Scholl S, Livartowski A, et al. Resection of pulmonary metastases in osteosarcoma. A retrospective analysis of 44 patients. *Cancer* 1989;**63**:2546-50.
96. Goorin AM, Delorey MJ, Lack E, et al. Prognostic significance of complete surgical resection of pulmonary metastases in patients with osteogenic sarcoma: analysis of 32 patients. *J Clin Oncol* 1984;**2**:425-31.
97. Meyers PA, Heller G, Healey JH, et al. Osteogenic sarcoma with clinically detectable metastasis at initial presentation. *J Clin Oncol* 1993;**11**:449-53.
98. Friedel G, Hurtgen M, Penzenstadler M, et al. Resection of pulmonary metastases from renal cell carcinoma. *Anticancer Res* 1999;**19**(2C):1593-6.
99. McCormack P, Burt ME, Bains MS, Martini N, Rush W, Ginsberg RJ. Lung resection for colorectal cancer. *Arch Surg* 1992;**127**:1403-6.
100. Lee WS, Yun SH, Chun HK, Lee WY, Yun HR, Kim J. Pulmonary resection for metastases from colorectal cancer: prognostic factors and survival. *Inter J Colorect Dis* 2007;**22**:699-704.
101. Melloni G, Doglioni C, Bandiera A, et al. Prognostic factors and analysis of microsatellite instability in resected pulmonary metastases from colorectal carcinoma. *Ann Thorac Surg* 2006;**81**:2008-13.
102. Baron O, Amini M, Duveau D, Despins P, Sagan CA, Michaud JL. Surgical resection of pulmonary metastases from colorectal cancer. Five-years survival and main prognostic factors. *Eur J Cardiothorac Surg* 1996;**10**:347-51.
103. Pfannschmidt J, Dienemann H, Hoffman H. Surgical resection of pulmonary metastases from colorectal cancer: a systematic review of published series. *Ann Thor Surg* 2007;**84**:324-38.
104. Pfannschmidt J, Muley T, Hoffman H, Dienemann H. Prognostic factors and survival after complete resection of pulmonary metastases from colorectal cancer: experience in 167 patients. *J Thorac Cardiovasc Surg* 2007;**126**:732-9.
105. Barlow AD, Nakas A, Pattenden C, Martin-Ucar AE, Dennison AR, Berry DP, et al. Surgical treatment of combined hepatic and pulmonary colorectal metastases. *Eur J Surg Oncol* 2008;**35**(3):1-6.
106. Imdahl A, Fischer E, Tenckhof C, Hasse J, Hopt UT, Stoelben E. Resection of combined or sequential lung and liver metastases of colorectal cancer: indication for everyone? *Zentralbl Chir* 2005;**130**(6):539-43.
107. Staren ED, Salerno C, Rongione A, Witt TW, Faber LP. Pulmonary resection for metastatic breast cancer. *Arch Surg* 1992;**127**:1282-4.
108. Hofmann HS, Neef H, Krohe K, Andreev P, Solber RE. Prognostic factors and survival after pulmonary resection of metastatic renal cell carcinoma. *Eur Urol* 2005;**48**:77-82.
109. Lanza LA, Natarajan G, Roth JA, et al. Long-term survival after resection of pulmonary metastases from carcinoma of the breast. *Ann Thor Surg* 1992;**54**:244-8.
110. Wedman J, Balm AJ, Hart AA, et al. Value of resection of pulmonary metastases in head and neck cancer patients. *Head Neck* 1998;**18**(4):311-6.
111. Saito H. Distant metastases of renal cell carcinoma: a single institution study. *Cancer* 1981;**48**:1487-91.
112. Weiss L, Harlos JP, Torhorst J, et al. Metastatic patterns of renal cell carcinomas: an analysis of 687 necropsies. *J Cancer Res Clin Oncol* 1988;**114**:605-12.
113. Barney JD, Churchill EJ. Adenocarcinoma of the kidney with metastasis to the lung: cured by nephrectomy and lobectomy. *J Urol* 1961;**42**:269.
114. Han KR, Pantuck AJ, Bui MH, Shvarts O, Freitas DG, Zisman A, et al. Number of metastatic sites rather than location dictates overall survival of patients with node-negative metastatic renal cell carcinoma. *Urology* 2003;**61**:314-9.
115. Kavolius J, Mastorakos D, Pavlovich C, et al. Resection of metastatic renal cell carcinoma. *J Clin Oncol* 1998;**16**:2261-6.
115a. Assouad J, Petkova B, Beuva P, et al. Lung metastasis surgery: pathologic findings and prognostic factors. *Ann Ther Surg* 2007;**84**:1114-20.
116. Lam JS, Shvarts O, Leppert JT, et al. Renal cell carcinoma 2005: new frontiers in staging, prognostication and targeted molecular therapy. *J Urol* 2005;**173**:1853-62.
117. Piltz S, Meimarakis G, Wichmann MW, Hatz R, Schildberg FW, Fuerst H. Long-term results after pulmonary resection of renal cell carcinoma metastases. *Ann Thor Surg* 2002;**73**(4):1082-7.
118. Cagini L, Nicholson AG, Horwich A, Goldstraw P, Pastorino U. Thoracic metastasectomy for germ cell tumours: long term survival and prognostic factors. *Ann Oncol* 1998;**9**(11):1185-91.
119. Anderson TM, McMahon JJ, Nwogu CE, Pombo MW, Urschel JD, Driscoll DL, Lele SB. Pulmonary resection in metastatic uterine and cervical malignancies. *Gynecol Oncol* 2001;**83**:472-6.
120. Mountain CF, McMurtrey MJ, Hermes KE. Surgery for pulmonary metastases: a 20-year experience. *Ann Thor Surg* 1984;**38**:323-30.
121. Fuller AF, Scannell JG, Wilkins EW. Pulmonary resection for metastases from gynecologic cancers: Massachusetts General Hospital experience, 1943-1982. *Gynecol Oncol* 1985;**22**:174-80.
122. Byers LJ, Fowler JM, Twiggs LB, Abeloff MD, Armitage JO, Lichter AS, Niederhuber JE, editors. *Clinical oncology*, 2nd ed. Philadelphia: Churchill Livingstonce; 2000, p. 1987-2015.
123. Barte JF, Soong SJ, Hatch KD, Orr JW, Shingleton HM. Diagnosis and treatment of pulmonary metastases from cervical carcinoma. *Gynecol Oncol* 1990;**38**(3):347-51.
124. Carlson V, Delclos L, Fletcher G. Distant metastases in squamous cell carcinoma of the uterine cervix. *Radiology* 1967;**88**:961-6.
125. Kerr VE, Cadman E. Pulmonary metastases in ovarian cancer: Analysis of 357 patients. *Cancer* 1985;**56**:1209-13.
126. O'Day SJ, Gammon G, Boasberg PD, et al. Advantages of concurrent biochemotherapy modified by decrescendo interleukin-2, granulocyte colony-stimulating factor, and tamoxifen for patients with metastatic melanoma. *J Clin Oncol* 1999;**17**(9):2752-61.
127. Pfannenberg C, Aschoff P, Schanz S, et al. Prospective comparison of 18-fluorodeoxyglucose positron emission tomography and whole-body magnetic resonance imaging in staging of advanced malignant melanoma. *Eur J Cancer* 2007;**43**(3):557-64.
128. Tafra L, Dale PS, Wanek LA, Ramming KP, Morton DL. Resection and adjuvant immunotherapy for melanoma metastatic to the lung and thorax. *J Thorac Cardiovasc Surg* 1995;**110**:119-24.

129. Harpole Jr DH, Johnson CM, Wolfe WG, George SL, Seigler HF. Analysis of 945 cases of pulmonary metastatic melanoma. *J Thorac Cardiovasc Surg* 1997;**103**:743-50.
130. Khan JH, McElhinney DB, Rahman SB, George TI, Clark OH, Merrick SH. Pulmonary metastases of endocrine origin: the role of surgery. *Chest* 1998;**114**(2):526-34.
131. Flye MW, Brennan MR. Surgical resection of metastatic parathyroid carcinoma. *Ann Surg* 1981;**193**:425-35.
132. Jensen JC, Pass HI, Sindelar WF, et al. Recurrent or metastatic disease in select patients with adrenocortical carcinoma. *Arch Surg* 1991;**126**:457-61.
133. Dupuy DE, Zagoria RJ, Akerley W, Mayo-Smith WW, Kavanagh PV, Safran H. Percutaneous radiofrequency ablation of tumors of the lung. *Am J Roentgenol* 2000;**174**(1):57-9.
134. Gadaleta C, Mattioli V, Colucci G, Cramarossa A, Lo Russo V, Cannello E, et al. Radiofrequency ablation of 40 lung neoplasms: preliminary results. *Am J Roentgenol* 2004;**183**:361-8.
135. Lee JM, Jin GY, Goldberg SN, Lee YC, Chung GH, Han YM, et al. Percutaneous radiofrequency ablation for inoperable non–small cell lung cancer and metastasis: Preliminary report. *Radiology* 2004;**230**:125-34.
136. Creech O, Krementz ET, Ryan RF, Winblad JN. Chemotherapy of cancer. *Ann Surg* 1958;**148**:616-32.
137. Burt ME, Liu D, Abolhoda A, et al. Isolated lung perfusion for patients with unresectable metastases from sarcoma: a phase I trial. *Ann Thor Surg* 2000;**69**:1542-9.
138. Warren S, Witman E. Studies on tumor metastases: The distribution of metastases in cancer of the breast. *Surg Gynecol Obstet* 1937;**57**:1018.
139. Cohen AL, Minsky BD, Schilsky RL. In: DeVita VT, Hellman S, Rosenberg SA, editors. *Cancer: principles and practice of oncology*. Philadelphia: JB Lippincott; 1993. p. 929-77.
140. Lee M, Hendrickson FR. Analysis of patterns of recurrence in nonseminomatous testicular tumor. *Radiology* 1978;**127**:775.
141. Pass HI, Dwyer A, Makuch R, et al. Detection of pulmonary metastases in patients with osteogenic and soft-tissue sarcomas: The superiority of CT scan compared to conventional linear tomograms using dynamic analysis. *J Clin Oncol* 1985;**3**:1261-5.
142. Willis RA. *The spread of tumors in the human body*. London: Butterworths; 1973, p. 167-74.
143. Farrell JJ. Pulmonary metastasis: A pathologic, clinical, roentgenologic study based on 78 cases seen at necropsy. *Radiology* 1935;**24**:444.
144. Gilbert HA, Kagan AR. In: Weiss L, editor. Fundamental aspects of metastasis. Amsterdam: North Holland; 1976. p. 315.
145. McCormack PM, Bains MS, Beatti JR, et al. Pulmonary resection for metastatic disease. *Chest* 1978;**73**:163-6.
146. Friedel G, Linder A, Toomes H. The significance of prognostic factors for the resection of pulmonary metastases of breast cancer. *Thorac Cardiovasc Surg* 1994;**42**:71-5.
147. McDonald ML, Deschamp C, Ilstrup DM, et al. Pulmonary resection for metastatic breast cancer. *Ann Thorac Surg* 1994;**58**:1599-602.
148. Regnard JF, Grunenwald D, Spaggiar L, et al. Surgical treatment of hepatic and pulmonary metastases from colorectal cancers. *Ann Thorac Surg* 1998;**66**:214-9.
149. Coley BL. *Neoplasms of bone and related conditions: etiology, pathogenesis, diagnosis and treatment*. New York: Hoeber 1960.
150. Di Lorenzo M. Collin PP: Pulmonary metastases in children: Results of surgical treatment. *J Pediatr Surg* 1988;**23**:762-5.
151. Mogulkoc N, Goker E, Atasever A, et al. Endobronchial metastases from osteosarcoma of bone: Treatment with intraluminal radiotherapy. *Chest* 1999;**116**(6):1811-4.
152. Pogrebniak HW, Haas G, Linehan M, et al. Renal cell carcinoma: resection of solitary and multiple metastases. *Ann Thor Surg* 1988;**52**:197-203.

H. Chest Wall

CHAPTER 24
Congenital Chest Wall Deformities
Robert C. Shamberger

Pectus Excavatum
  Etiology and Incidence
  Symptoms
  Pathophysiology
    Pulmonary Function Studies
    Cardiovascular Studies
    Echocardiographic Studies of Mitral Valve Prolapse
  Surgical Repair
    Minimally Invasive Repair of Pectus Excavatum

Open Surgical Repair of Pectus Excavatum
Pectus Carinatum
  Etiology
  Surgical Repair
    Surgical Technique
    Operative Results
Poland's Syndrome
  Surgical Repair
Sternal Defects
  Cleft Sternum
    Surgical Repair

Ectopia Cordis
  Etiology
  Thoracic Ectopia Cordis
  Thoracoabdominal Ectopia Cordis (Cantrell's Pentalogy)
Thoracic Deformities in Diffuse Skeletal Disorders
  Asphyxiating Thoracic Dystrophy (Jeune's Disease)
  Spondylothoracic Dysplasia (Jarcho-Levin Syndrome)

A great variety of congenital abnormalities of the chest wall occur. Their physiologic implications are also quite varied and span the spectrum from the rare entities of ectopia cordis and asphyxiating thoracic dystrophy, which are often lethal, to the much more common pectus excavatum and pectus carinatum with their limited physiologic impact. In this chapter, anterior thoracic deformities will be considered in five categories: pectus excavatum, pectus carinatum, Poland's syndrome, sternal defects including ectopia cordis, and miscellaneous conditions including asphyxiating thoracic dystrophy (Jeune's syndrome).

PECTUS EXCAVATUM

Pectus excavatum is the most frequent anterior chest wall deformity. The central depression of the chest is produced by posterior angulation of the sternum and the costal cartilages. The first and second costal cartilages and the manubrium are usually in a normal position (Fig. 24-1), but the lower costal cartilages, which insert into the sternum, and the body of the sternum are depressed. The most anterior segment of the ossified portion of the ribs may also be curved posteriorly in older adolescents and adults. The extent of sternal and cartilaginous deformity is quite variable. Numerous methods of grading these deformities have been proposed by Hümmer and Willital,[1] von der Oelsnitz,[2] Welch,[3] Haller and associates,[4] and others, but none has been universally accepted. Asymmetry of the depression is often present. The right side is frequently more depressed than the left, and the sternum may be rotated as well. A system to quantify the asymmetry based on computed tomography (CT) of the chest has been reported.[5] The majority of affected children (86%) with pectus excavatum are identified at birth or within the first year of life (Fig. 24-2). They have a characteristic physique—a broad thin chest, dorsal lordosis, "hook shoulder" deformity, costal flaring, and poor posture. The deformity rarely resolves with increasing age, and it may worsen during the period of rapid growth in adolescence. Waters and associates identified scoliosis in 26% of 508 patients with pectus excavatum,[6] so all patients with pectus deformities should be evaluated clinically for scoliosis. Asymmetric pectus excavatum with a deep right gutter and sternal rotation is often accompanied by scoliosis. Congenital heart disease was identified in 1.5% of infants and children undergoing chest wall correction at the Children's Hospital in Boston (Table 24-1).[7] The frequency of chest wall deformities among all patients with congenital heart disease evaluated at this institution was only 0.17%.

Asthma may be identified in association with pectus excavatum and carinatum. However, in a review of 694 consecutive cases, 35 patients with asthma were identified (5.2%), a frequency comparable to that of asthma in the general pediatric population.[8]

Etiology and Incidence

Ravitch reported that pectus excavatum may occur as frequently as 1 in 300 to 400 live births and that it is rare in blacks.[9] It occurs more frequently in boys than girls, by an almost 4:1 ratio. Although the sternal depression appears to be caused by overgrowth of costal cartilages, the etiology of pectus deformities is unknown. Lester attributed its development to an abnormality of the diaphragm that tethered the sternum posteriorly.[10] This theory was supported by the occurrence of pectus excavatum in children after repair of agenesis of the diaphragm and the frequent association of pectus excavatum and congenital diaphragmatic hernia.[11,12] Histopathologic changes in the costal cartilages similar to those seen in scoliosis, aseptic osteonecrosis, and inflammatory

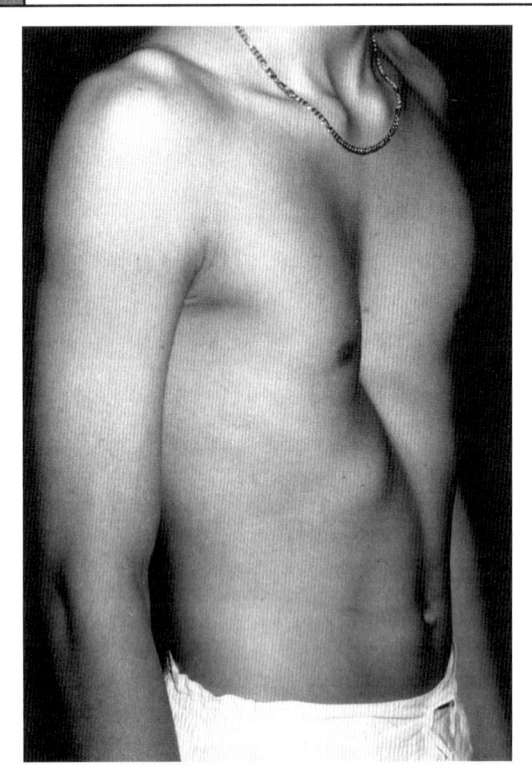

Figure 24–1
A 16½-year-old boy with a symmetric pectus excavatum deformity. Note that the depression extends to the sternal notch.

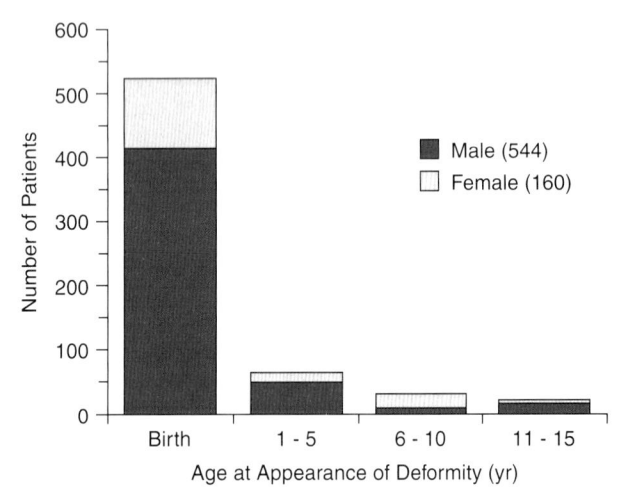

Figure 24–2
Age at appearance of pectus excavatum deformity in 704 infants and children. Note the large proportion identified at birth or within the first year of life, and the predominance of males with this deformity. *(From Shamberger RC, Welch KJ. J Pediatr Surg 1988;**23**:615, with permission.)*

Table 24–1
Congenital Heart Disease Associated with Pectus Excavatum and Carinatum

Congenital Heart Disease	Number of Cases
Aortic ring	1
Aortic regurgitation	1
Atrial septal defect primum	2
Atrial septal defect secundum	3
Complete atrioventricular canal	3
Dextrocardia	3
Ebstein's malformation	1
Idiopathic hypertrophic subaortic stenosis	2
Patent ductus arteriosus	1
Pulmonic stenosis	1
Total anomalous pulmonary venous return	1
Transposition of great arteries	6
Tetralogy of Fallot	3
Tricuspid atresia	1
Truncus arteriosus	1
Ventricular septal defect	6

*From Shamberger RC, Welch KJ, Castaneda AR, Keane JF, Fyler DC. Anterior chest wall deformities and congenital heart disease. J Thorac Cardiovasc Surg 1988;**96**:427-32, with permission.*

processes are reported, but the etiology of these findings and their significance are unknown.[13]

A family history of chest wall deformity in 37% of 704 patients suggests a genetic predisposition to pectus excavatum.[14] Three of four siblings were affected in one family. Analysis of 34 families with more than one family member with pectus excavatum has shown a variable pattern of inheritance that appears to be multifactorial.[15]

A high incidence of chest wall deformities occurs in children with Marfan syndrome, and these deformities are often severe and usually accompanied by scoliosis.[16] Pectus excavatum is also commonly seen in individuals with the abdominal musculature deficiency syndrome (prune-belly syndrome).[17] Pectus excavatum also occurs in association with other myopathies and chromosomal defects such as Turner's syndrome. A summary of the associated musculoskeletal abnormalities is shown in Table 24-2.

Symptoms

Pectus excavatum is well tolerated in infancy and childhood. The anterior depression in an infant with a flexible chest may be accentuated by upper airway obstruction as from tonsillar and adenoidal hypertrophy, but this obstruction does not produce the pectus deformity. Older children may complain of pain in the area of the deformed cartilages or of precordial pain after sustained exercise. Symptomatic limitations to sustained exercise may also appear in these children and teenagers and limit their participation in athletic activities. Palpitations, presumably resulting from transient atrial arrhythmias, are occasionally reported. These patients may have mitral valve prolapse.

Table 24-2
Musculoskeletal Abnormalities Identified in 130 of 704 Cases of Pectus Excavatum

Musculoskeletal Abnormality	Number of Cases
Scoliosis	107
Kyphosis	4
Myopathy	3
Marfan syndrome	2
Pierre Robin syndrome	2
Prune-belly syndrome	2
Neurofibromatosis	3
Cerebral palsy	4
Tuberous sclerosis	1
Congenital diaphragmatic hernia	2

From Shamberger RC, Welch KJ. J Pediatr Surg 1988;23:615, with permission.

Pathophysiology

The cardiopulmonary implications of the pectus excavatum deformity have been debated for many decades. Although some authors feel this deformity has a limited physiologic effect, many patients report increased stamina after surgical repair. These findings date back to the first surgical repair performed by Sauerbruch in 1913.[18] The patient was an 18-year-old man who developed dyspnea and palpitations with very limited exercise. Three years after his operation, he could work 12 to 14 hours a day without tiring and without palpitations. Anecdotal reports during the next 3 decades repeated this observation. Investigators have sought to identify the physiologic abnormality or combination of abnormalities that could explain this symptomatic improvement after surgery. Early physiologic measurements of cardiac and pulmonary function were crude and did not yield convincing evidence of a cardiopulmonary deficit. In many early studies, the results fell within the broad range of normal values, if often at the lower limit.[7] A recent analysis of a large multi-institutional cohort of 408 patients with pectus excavatum found that the median values for forced vital capacity (FVC) and forced expiratory volume in 1 second (FEV_1) were 13% below predicted values, and the forced expiratory flow, midexpiratory phase ($FEF_{25\%-75\%}$) median was 20% below the predicted value.[19]

A systolic ejection murmur is frequently present in individuals with pectus excavatum, and it is magnified by a short interval of exercise. This murmur is attributed to the close proximity of the sternum and the pulmonary artery, which results in transmission of a flow murmur.

Electrocardiographic abnormalities are common and result from the abnormal configuration of the chest wall, which produces displacement of the heart into the left thoracic cavity.[20] Patients with a history of palpitations should have a 24-hour electrocardiogram to document the presence or absence of arrhythmias, as well as an echocardiogram to evaluate for mitral valve prolapse. Resolution of these supraventricular arrhythmias has been anecdotally reported after correction of a pectus excavatum deformity.

Many authors attribute the symptomatic improvement in exercise tolerance after surgery to improvement in pulmonary function. This has been difficult to prove, however, because of the wide range of pulmonary function that exists from individual to individual and its dependence on physical training and body habitus. Several of the key studies will be reviewed.

Pulmonary Function Studies

As early as 1951, Brown and Cook performed pulmonary evaluations on patients before and after surgical repair.[21] They demonstrated that although vital capacity (VC) was normal, the maximum breathing capacity was diminished (50% or more) in 9 of 11 cases, and it increased an average of 31% after surgical repair. Weg and associates in 1967 evaluated 25 Air Force recruits with pectus excavatum and compared them with 50 unselected basic trainees.[22] Although the lung compartments of both groups were equal, as were the vital capacities, the maximal voluntary ventilation was significantly lower in those with pectus excavatum than in the control population. Castile and coworkers in 1982 evaluated seven patients with pectus excavatum, five of whom were symptomatic with exercise.[23] The mean total lung capacity of the group was 79% of predicted. Flow volume configurations were normal, excluding airway obstruction as a cause of the symptoms. Workload tests demonstrated normal response to exercise in the deadspace-to-tidal-volume ratio and in alveolar-to-arterial oxygen difference. The measured oxygen uptake, however, increasingly exceeded predicted values as workload approached maximum in the four "symptomatic" patients with pectus excavatum. This pattern of oxygen consumption was different from that in normal subjects and in the three asymptomatic patients with pectus excavatum, in whom a linear response was seen. The mean oxygen uptake in the symptomatic patients at maximal effort exceeded the predicted values by 25.4%. The three asymptomatic patients, on the other hand, demonstrated normal linear oxygen uptake during exercise. Increased oxygen uptake suggests increased work of breathing in these symptomatic individuals despite the normal or mildly reduced VCs. Increases in tidal volume with exercise were uniformly depressed in those with pectus excavatum.

Cahill and coworkers in 1984 performed preoperative and postoperative studies in five children and adolescents with pectus carinatum and in 14 with pectus excavatum.[24] No abnormalities were demonstrated in the pectus carinatum group. The low normal vital capacities in excavatum patients were unchanged by operation, but a small improvement in the total lung capacity and a significant improvement in the maximal voluntary ventilation were seen. Exercise tolerance improved in those with pectus excavatum after operation, as determined both by total exercise time and maximal oxygen consumption. In addition, at any given workload, those with pectus excavatum demonstrated a lower heart rate, stable oxygen consumption, and higher minute ventilation after repair. Mead and associates in 1985 studied rib cage mobility by assessing intra-abdominal pressure.[25] Normal abdominal pressure tracings in pectus excavatum suggested normal rib cage mobility.

Blickman and colleagues in 1985 assessed pulmonary function in 17 children with pectus excavatum by xenon perfusion and ventilation scintigraphy before and after surgery.[26] Ventilation studies were abnormal in 12 children before surgery and improved in seven after repair. Perfusion scans were abnormal in 10 children before surgery and improved after operation in six children. The ventilation-perfusion ratios were abnormal in 10 of the 17 children preoperatively and normalized after repair in six children.

Derveaux and associates in 1989 evaluated 88 patients with pectus excavatum and carinatum by pulmonary function tests before and 1 to 20 years after repair (mean, 8 years).[27] The surgical technique used a fairly extensive chest wall dissection. Preoperative studies were within the normal range (>80% of predicted) except in patients who had both scoliosis and pectus excavatum. The postoperative values for FEV_1 and VC expressed as percent of expected were decreased in all groups, although the absolute values at follow-up may have been greater than at preoperative evaluation. Improved chest wall configuration was confirmed by radiologic evaluation, so the relative deterioration in pulmonary function was not the result of recurrence of the pectus deformity. An inverse relationship was found between preoperative and postoperative function. Those with less than 75% of predicted function had improved function after surgery, but function was worse after repair if the preoperative values were greater than 75% of predicted. Almost identical results were found in a study by Morshuis and coworkers in 1994.[28] They evaluated 152 patients before and a mean of 8 years after surgery for pectus excavatum. These results of pulmonary evaluation were in contrast to the subjective symptomatic improvement reported by the patients and their improved chest wall configuration. The decline in pulmonary function in the postoperative studies was attributed to the operation, because the preoperative pulmonary defect appeared to be stable regardless of the age at initial repair. Both studies were marred by the obvious lack of an age- and severity-matched control group without surgery.

Derveaux and colleagues in 1988 evaluated transpulmonary and transdiaphragmatic pressures at total lung capacity in 17 individuals with pectus excavatum.[29] Preoperative and long-term follow-up evaluations were performed a mean of 12 years apart. Reduced transpulmonary and transdiaphragmatic pressures demonstrated that the increased restrictive defect was produced by extrapulmonary rather than pulmonary factors, suggesting that surgery produced increased rigidity of the chest wall.

Wynn and others in 1990 assessed 12 children with pectus excavatum by pulmonary function tests and exercise testing.[30] Eight children had repair and were evaluated preoperatively and postoperatively. Four children had two sets of evaluations but no operation. A decline in total lung capacity was identified in the repaired children compared with stable values in the control group. Cardiac output and stroke volume increased appropriately with exercise before and after operation in both groups, and the operation was believed to have produced no physiologically significant effect on the response to exercise.

Kaguraoka and associates in 1992 evaluated pulmonary function in 138 individuals before and after repair of pectus excavatum.[31] A decrease in VC occurred during the first 2 months after surgery, with recovery to preoperative levels by 1 year after operation. At 42 months, the values were maintained at baseline, despite a significant improvement in the chest wall configuration. Tanaka and coworkers in 1993 found similar results in individuals who had the more extensive sternal turnover technique; in fact, they demonstrated a more significant and long-term decrease in VC.[32] Morshuis and coworkers in 1994 evaluated 35 patients who had had pectus excavatum repaired as teenagers or young adults; ages were 17.9 ± 5.6 years.[33] Preoperative evaluations were performed and repeated 1 year after surgery. Preoperative total lung capacity (86.0% ± 14.4% of predicted) and VC (79.7% ± 16.2%) were significantly decreased from predicted values and decreased further after surgery (−9.2% ± 9.2% and −6.6% ± 10.7%, respectively). The efficiency of breathing at maximal exercise improved significantly after operation. Exercise was limited by ventilation in 43% of the patients before repair. A tendency toward improvement occurred after operation. However, the group with no ventilatory limitation initially demonstrated one after operation, with a significant increase in oxygen consumption.

Quigley and colleagues in 1996 evaluated 36 adolescents with pectus excavatum and 10 age-matched healthy controls at baseline and then an average of 8 months after surgery for 15 patients and 9 months for controls.[34] Adolescents with pectus excavatum had a decrease in VC compared with controls, although the mean values remained in the normal range. The mean total lung capacity was also normal. There was no difference in workload performance between patients with pectus excavatum and the controls, with both groups achieving a similar duration and level of exercise. No significant change in pulmonary function tests was seen at follow-up in either group. The duration of exercise and the level of work increased significantly in those who had surgery but not in the controls. The absence of adverse effects on pulmonary function after surgery was attributed to a less extensive surgical procedure than was used in the studies reported by Derveaux[29] and Morshuis[28,33] and their colleagues. Two series reported the effects on pulmonary function of the minimally invasive repair of pectus excavatum (MIRPE) described by Nuss.[35,36] In these series, there were limited or no preoperative abnormalities and mild or no significant change after repair. Similar results were reported in a prospective study of 145 patients having a MIRPE.[37] There was no improvement in static values 6 months after removal of the struts.

In composite, these studies of pulmonary function over the last 4 decades failed to document consistent improvement in pulmonary function resulting from surgical repair. In fact, some studies have demonstrated deterioration in pulmonary function at long-term evaluation, which was attributed to increased chest wall rigidity after repair. A meta-analysis of 12 of these studies revealed no statistically significant change in pulmonary function.[38] Despite this finding, workload studies have shown improvement in exercise tolerance after repair, suggesting a cardiac basis for this enhanced performance.[24,39]

Cardiovascular Studies

Posterior displacement of the sternum can produce a deformity of the heart, particularly indentation of the right ventricle. Displacement of the heart to the left, often with a sternal "imprint" on the anterior wall of the right ventricle, was demonstrated angiographically by Garusi and D'Éttorre in 1964,[40] and Howard[41] demonstrated its resolution after surgical repair. Elevated right heart pressures have been reported by some authors, as have pressure curves similar to those seen in constrictive pericarditis.

In 1962, Bevegård studied 16 individuals with pectus excavatum by right heart catheterization and exercise testing.[42] The physical work capacity in pectus excavatum at a given heart rate was significantly lower in the sitting than in the supine position. Those with 20% or greater decline in physical work capacity from the supine to the sitting position had shorter sternovertebral distances than those with less decrease in their physical work capacity. The measured stroke volume at rest decreased from supine to sitting positions by a mean of 40.3%, similar to that in normal subjects. In the supine position, stroke volume increased with exercise by 13.2%. In the sitting position, the increase in stroke volume from rest to exercise was 18.5% for the pectus excavatum group, significantly lower ($P < .001$) than the 51% increase seen in normal subjects. Thus, in the pectus excavatum group, an increased cardiac output could be achieved primarily by increased heart rate because only limited enhancement of the stroke volume could occur. Intracardiac pressures measured at rest and with exercise were normal in all patients despite this apparent limitation of ventricular volume.

Gattiker and Bühlmann in 1967 confirmed this limitation of the stroke volume in a study of 19 patients.[43] In the upright position at a heart rate of 170 beats per minute, the physical work capacity was lower than in the supine position (mean 18% decrease) because of the decrease in stroke volume. Beiser and associates in 1972 performed cardiac catheterization in six adolescents and young adults with moderate degrees of pectus excavatum.[44] Normal pressure and cardiac index were obtained at rest in the supine position. The cardiac index during moderate exercise was normal, but the response to upright exercise was below that predicted in two patients and at the lower limit of normal in three patients. The cardiac index was 6.8 ± 0.8 L/min/m^2 compared with 8.9 ± 0.3 L/min/m^2 in a group of 16 normal controls ($P < .01$). The difference in cardiac performance again appeared to be produced primarily by a smaller stroke volume in the group with pectus excavatum in an upright position. Stroke volume was 31% lower and cardiac output 28% lower during upright as compared with supine exercise. Postoperative studies were performed in three individuals, and two of them achieved a higher level of exercise tolerance after surgery. The cardiac index increased an average of 38%. Because heart rate at maximal exercise was not higher after repair, an enhanced stroke-volume response was responsible for this increase.

Peterson and associates in 1985 performed radionuclide angiography and exercise studies in 13 children with pectus excavatum.[45] Ten of 13 were able to reach the target heart rate before surgical repair, four without symptoms. After operation, all but one child reached the target heart rate during the exercise protocol, and nine of 13 reached the target without becoming symptomatic. The left and right ventricular end-diastolic volumes were consistently increased after repair at rest, and the mean stroke volume was increased 19% after repair. These findings substantiated the ventricular volume changes previously demonstrated by cardiac catheterization, although an increase in the cardiac index was not demonstrated. Recent echocardiographic studies by Kowalewski and associates of 42 patients before and 6 months after surgery revealed statistically significant changes in the right ventricular volume indices after surgery.[46] There was no correlation seen, however, between the pectus index and the changes in the right ventricular volume indices.

Malek and coauthors in 2003 performed maximal exercise testing and pulmonary function tests on 21 individuals with pectus excavatum, 18 of whom routinely did aerobic exercise.[39] Their maximal oxygen uptake and oxygen pulse were both significantly lower than expected, and these limitations were attributed to cardiovascular and not ventilatory factors, and they resulted in an abnormally low threshold for lactate accumulation. Of note, patients with a Haller index of greater than 4.0 were eight times more likely to have reduced aerobic capacity than those with a lower severity index.

Results of cardiac function have more recently been assessed in patients having the MIRPE procedure.[36] In 11 patients, an increase was demonstrated in the stroke volume measured echocardiographically 3 months after repair, to which subjective improvement in exercise tolerance was attributed.

A meta-analysis was performed of eight studies (representing 169 patients) that reported quantitative data on the cardiovascular function of patients before and after repair.[47] The analysis suggested that surgical repair did not significantly improve cardiovascular function.

Additional studies are needed to further define the relationship between pectus excavatum and cardiopulmonary function. Recent dynamic or exercise studies have been most promising in this area. Methods to more effectively evaluate preoperative cardiopulmonary function are needed to identify which children may achieve symptomatic and physiologic improvement from surgical repair.

Echocardiographic Studies of Mitral Valve Prolapse

Bon Tempo, Salomon, and Schutte and their associates reported mitral valve prolapse in patients with narrow anterior-posterior chest diameters, anterior chest wall deformities, and scoliosis.[48-50] Prospective echocardiographic studies of adults with pectus excavatum demonstrated mitral valve prolapse in six of 33 patients (18%) studied by Udoshi and associates[51] and in 11 of 17 patients (65%) of Saint-Mezard and colleagues.[52] Anterior compression of the heart by the depressed sternum may deform the mitral annulus or the ventricular chamber and produce mitral valve prolapse in these patients. We performed a preoperative echocardiographic evaluation of children and adolescents with pectus excavatum and identified 23 with mitral valve prolapse.[53] Postoperative studies did not demonstrate mitral valve prolapse in 10 (43%) of these children, suggesting its resolution after correction of the chest wall deformity.

Coln and coauthors performed echocardiography on patients during exercise (123 preoperatively and 107 postoperatively).[54] They demonstrated chamber compression in 117 (95%) before surgery and in none of the patients after repair. They also found in patients with chamber compression resolution of mitral valve prolapse (16 of 23) and mitral valve regurgitation (28 of 29) after repair, as I had previously demonstrated. Symptoms related to exertion, reported in 106 (86%) of the patients, resolved remarkably in all, which was attributed to the cardiac effects of repair.

Surgical Repair

The first surgical corrections of pectus excavatum were reported by Meyer[55] in 1911 and Sauerbruch in 1920,[18] and Ochsner and DeBakey[56] summarized the early experience with various techniques. In 1949, Ravitch reported a technique that included excision of all deformed costal cartilages with the perichondrium, division of the xiphoid from the sternum, division of the intercostal bundles from the sternum, and a transverse sternal osteotomy securing the sternum anteriorly in an overcorrected position.[57] Kirschner wire fixation was used in the first two patients, and silk suture fixation in later patients.

Baronofsky (1957) and Welch (1958) subsequently reported a technique for the correction of pectus excavatum that emphasized total preservation of the perichondrial sheaths as well as attachment of the upper sheaths and intercostal bundles to the sternum.[58,59] Anterior fixation of the sternum was achieved with silk sutures. Haller and associates later developed a technique that they labeled as *tripod fixation*.[60] Subperichondrial resection of the abnormal cartilages is performed, followed by a posterior sternal osteotomy. The most cephalad normal cartilages are then divided obliquely in a posterolateral direction. When the sternum is elevated, the sternal ends of the cartilage rest on the costal ends, providing further anterior support of the sternum. Support of the sternum by metallic struts after mobilization of the costal cartilages has been promoted by several authors. Rehbein and Wernicke developed struts that could be placed into the marrow cavity of the ribs at the costochondral junction.[61] An arch was then formed by the struts anterior to the sternum, and the sternum was secured to this arch. Paltia and associates placed a transverse strut through the caudal end of the sternum, firmly fixing its location.[62] The two ends of the strut are supported by the ribs laterally. Adkins and Blades,[63] and Jensen and associates[63a] used retrosternal elevation by a metallic strut. Willital employed a similar retrosternal strut after creating multiple chondrotomies in the costal cartilages to provide flexibility.[64] Recent innovations in these methods include bioabsorbable struts, or use of Marlex mesh or a Dacron vascular graft as a strut, but there is no evidence that these methods are preferable to traditional methods with metallic struts.[65] Robicsek and Fokin described a large series of chest wall deformities.[66] For patients with pectus excavatum, the sternum is mobilized more extensively with this technique than with others, except for the sternal turnover. The sternum is divided from the intercostal muscles and perichondrial sheaths from its tip to the upper extent of the deformity. It is then supported in an anterior position by a hammock of Marlex mesh, which is sewn to the ends of the ribs on each side. The advantages of this extensive mobilization and permanent implantation of the mesh are not clear. No randomized studies have compared the recurrence or complication rates between suture or strut fixation techniques. Von der Oelsnitz[2] and Hecker and coworkers,[13] using suture fixation, reported satisfactory repairs in 90% to 95% in their large series.

The *sternal turnover* was first proposed by Judet and Judet[67] in 1954 and Jung[68] in 1956 in the French literature. The sternum is mobilized and the costal cartilages are divided, allowing the sternum to be rotated 180 degrees. Wada and colleagues[69] in 1970 reported a very large series from Japan using this technique, which is essentially a free graft of sternum. It is a radical approach and has been associated with major complications if infection occurs. Modifications of this technique by Taguchi and associates in 1975 have involved either preservation of the internal mammary vessels by wide dissection or reimplantation of the internal mammary artery.[70] These modifications were developed because of the reported incidence of osteonecrosis and fistula formation, which occurred in up to 46% of patients older than 15 years.

Allen and Douglas implanted Silastic molds into the subcutaneous space to fill the depression in pectus excavatum.[71] Although this approach may improve the external contour of the chest, extrusion of the molds has occurred, and this method does nothing to increase the volume of the thoracic cavity or relieve compression on the heart. Recently, other authors have reported favorable cosmetic results in adults, with no pulmonary restrictions but with a significant frequency of seroma and hematoma formation.[72,73] Schier and coworkers[73] described the use of a suction device placed over the chest in children and adults with pectus excavatum, and early results were encouraging, but the durability of the correction was not established. Haecker and Mayr[74] described a similar device. Although improvement was seen, only 14.7% of the patients had the sternum lifted to a "normal" position after 12 months of therapy.

Minimally Invasive Repair of Pectus Excavatum

A method of elevation of the sternum with a retrosternal bar without resection or division of the costal cartilages was first reported by Nuss and associates in 1998.[75] He repaired 42 patients younger than 15 years (median age, 5 years) by placing a convex steel bar under the sternum and anterior to the heart through small bilateral thoracic incisions. A long clamp was passed blindly behind the sternum and out an opening in the contralateral chest (Fig. 24-3A). A tape was then drawn across the chest in the clamp and used to pull the bar through the pleural cavity and anterior to the pericardium. The bar was initially placed with the concave side anteriorly and then it was rotated once it was in position (see Fig. 24-3B). The bar was left in position for 2 years before removal, when presumed permanent remodeling of the cartilages had occurred. Although in the initial report Nuss warned that the "upper limits of age for this procedure require further evaluation," the technique has been widely used in older patients, and Hebra and colleagues reported the use of this technique in adults.[76]

In 2002, the results by Nuss and his associates using this technique in 303 patients were reported by Croitoru and coworkers.[77] This included a group of children who were older than in the initial report (range, 21 months to 29 years; median age, 12.4 years). Two bars were required in 12.5% of the patients. Routine use of thoracoscopy to avoid cardiac injury was instituted in 1998 and routinely used thereafter. Lateral stabilizers were placed in 69.4% of the cases and were wired to the bar in 65.4% of cases. It is now recommended that the bars be left in the chest for 3 years. Epidural analgesic was administered for 2 to 4 days, and the median length of stay was 5 days, with a range of 3 to 10 days. The frequency of early complications was low. They included pneumothorax requiring aspiration, 1.0%; pericarditis, 2.3%, with only 0.3% requiring drainage; pneumonia, 0.7%; hemothorax, 0.3%; transient extremity paralysis, 0.3%; superficial wound infection, 2.3%; and bar infection requiring eventual removal of the bar, 0.7%.

Late complications in this series included bar displacement requiring repositioning in 8.6%, which included a high proportion (greater than 50%) of patients in whom a stabilizer was not used, or in patients where the stabilizer was not wired to the bar. When both modifications were employed, displacement occurred in only 5% of the patients. An unexpected occurrence of allergy to the metal bar was

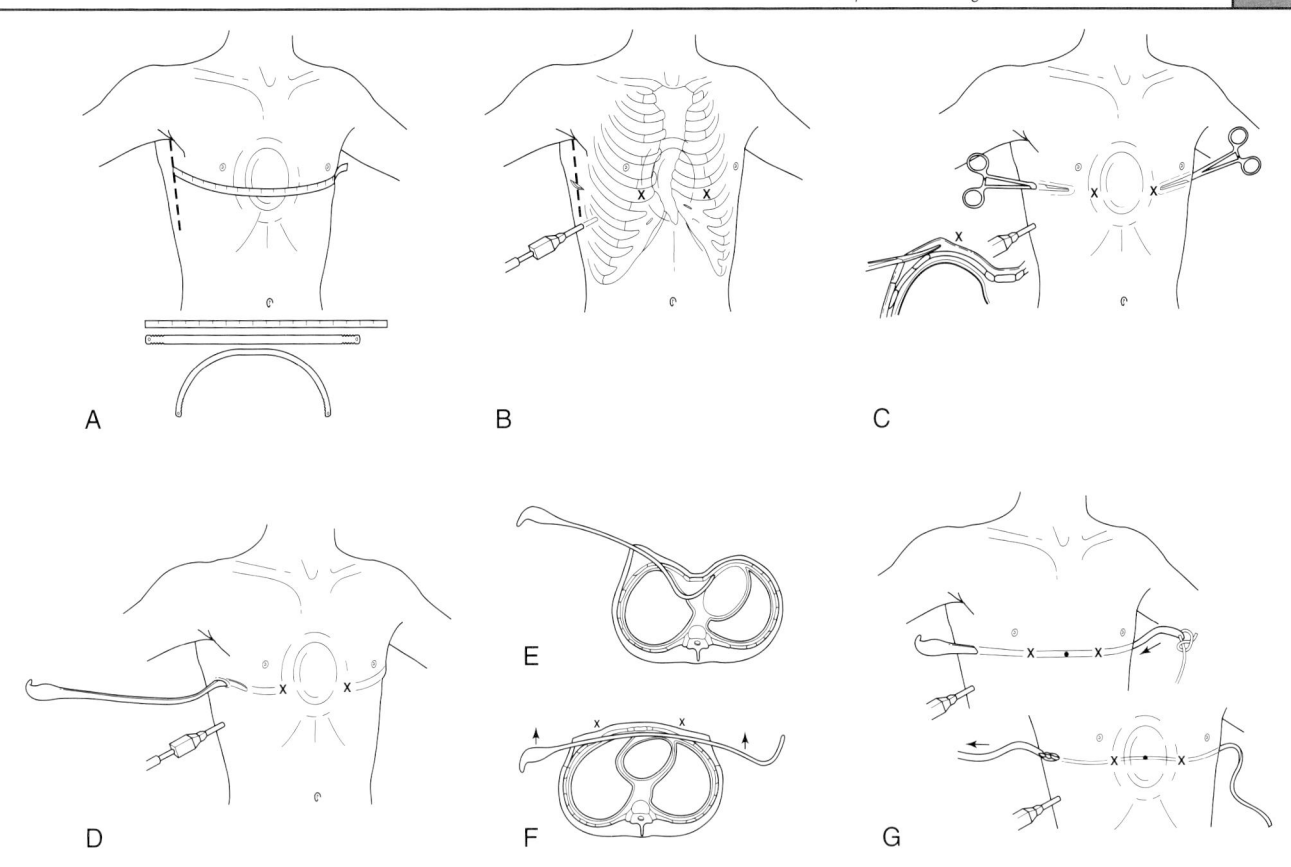

Figure 24–3
A, The length of the pectus bar is determined by measuring the distance from the right midaxillary line to the left midaxillary line and subtracting 2 cm or 1 inch, because the bar takes a shorter course than the tape measure. The measurement is done over the area of the deepest depression that is still part of the sternum. The bar is bent to the desired convex configuration, making note that the center of the bar should be flat for 2 to 4 cm to allow greater stability. **B,** A thoracoscope is inserted into the right chest two intercostal spaces below the planned bar placement to check that the internal anatomy corresponds with the external markings and to look for unexpected pathology. If all is well, the lateral thoracic incisions are made in the region of the midaxillary line, and subcutaneous tunnels are created to the greatest apex of the pectus deformity (X). The X's represent the entrance and exit sites of the bar from the chest. They are in the intercostal space that is in the same horizontal place as the deepest depression and care should be taken that they are placed medial to the greatest apex of the chest. **C,** Skin tunnels are created above the muscle starting from each of the lateral thoracic incisions and going to the top of the pectus ridge on each side. The tunnels should be created so that the entry and exit sites of the bar from inside the chest are medial to the top of the pectus ridge on each side. With the thoracoscope in place, a tonsil clamp is inserted into the subcutaneous tunnel on the right, and a blunt thoracostomy is created at the X, taking care not to injure the intercostal vessels, lung, or pericardium. **D,** Under continued thoracoscopic visualization, a Lorenz (W. Lorenz Surgical, Jacksonville, FL) introducer is inserted into the chest through the right tunnel and thoracostomy site at the top of the pectus ridge. With great care and thoracoscopic guidance, the pleura and pericardium are dissected off the undersurface of the sternum, creating a substernal tunnel. The introducer is slowly advanced across the mediastinum and brought out through the corresponding intercostal space on the left and advanced out of the incision on the contralateral side. Again, this exit site is medial to the top of the pectus ridge. **E,** A 30-degree scope facilitates visualization during the substernal dissection, and care is taken to keep the point of the dissector underneath the sternum at all times to push the heart out of the way of the dissection plane. During the dissection, the ECG monitor should be turned to maximum volume to listen for any ectopy or arrhythmias. **F,** The introducer is pushed out of the thorax through the previously marked intercostal space (X) on the left and advanced out through the corresponding tunnel and incision. When the introducer is fully in place, the sternum is elevated by lifting the introducer on each side, thus correcting the pectus excavatum. The sternum is lifted out of its depressed position with the introducer, numerous times. This is facilitated by pressing down on the lower chest wall while lifting the introducer. **G,** Once the sternal depression has been corrected, umbilical tape is attached to the introducer, and the introducer is slowly withdrawn from the chest cavity with the umbilical tape attached.

encountered in 1% of the patients, who presented with rashes in the area of the bar. This required conversion to bars composed of other alloys. Late hemothorax occurred in two patients, one secondary to undefined trauma. The occurrence of a mild overcorrection in the deformity was seen in 3.6%, and a pectus carinatum deformity developed in 1.3%, all of whom had either Marfan syndrome or Ehlers-Danlos syndrome. The reported outcome of children in this large series was excellent appearance in 84.5%, good in 14.8%, and failed in only one patient. However, the bars had been removed from only 23.4% of the patients at the time of the report.

A more recent summary by Shin and associates reported a series of 863 consecutive patients and showed a 1.5% incidence of infectious complications.[78] This included six bar infections, four cases of cellulitis, and three stitch abscesses. Antibiotics and surgical drainage resolved the infection in three of the bar infections, but removal of the bar was required in three, one 3 months after surgery, and two 18 months after surgery. *Staphylococcus aureus* was involved in 83% of the cases. This degree of success in preserving the struts despite infectious complications was mirrored by the experience in two subsequent reports.[79,80]

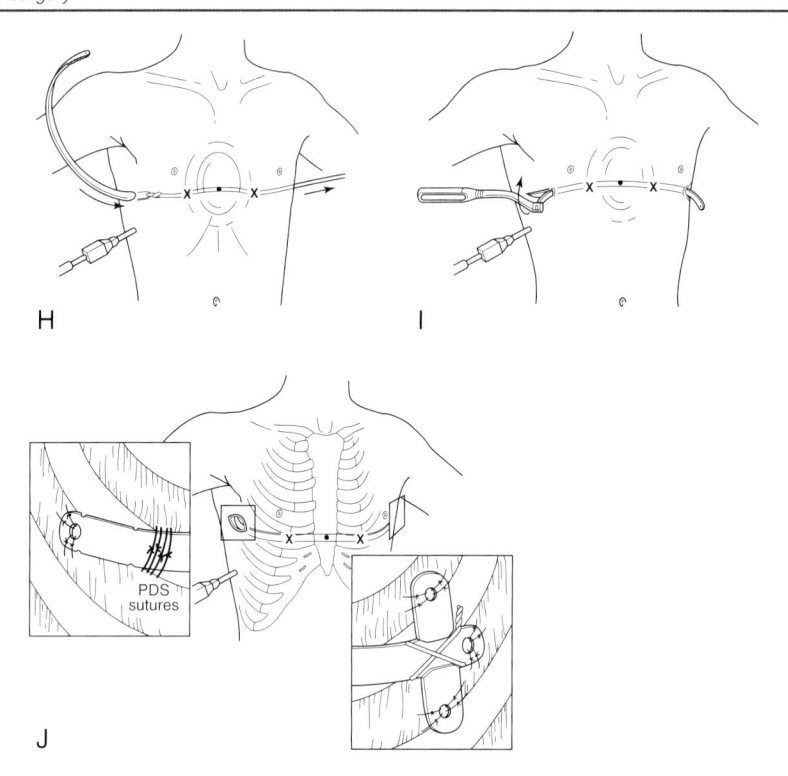

Figure 24–3, cont'd
H, The pectus bar that was previously bent into a convex shape is then attached to the umbilical tape and slowly guided through the right subcutaneous tunnel under thoracoscopic visualization, and then through the substernal tunnel, with its convexity facing posteriorly until it emerges on the contralateral side. **I,** The pectus bar is positioned inside the chest with its convexity facing posteriorly and an equal amount of bar protruding on each side. Using the specially designed Lorenz bar flippers, the bar is rotated 180 degrees, giving instant correction to the pectus deformity. The sides of the bar should be resting comfortably against the musculature and should not be too tight or too loose. If the bar does not fit snugly on each side because of pressure on the middle, the bar can be re-flipped and molded as necessary while still in place in the chest. **J,** The bar is stabilized by attaching a stabilizer to the left end of the bar and wiring the bar and stabilizer together with #3 surgical steel wire. The stabilizer and bar are also secured by placing numerous interrupted absorbable sutures through the holes in the bar and adjacent fascia. An additional stabilizing technique involves a laparoscopic auto-suture needle to place multiple 0 PDS or Vicryl sutures around the bar and underlying ribs under thoracoscopic guidance. *(From Shamberger RC, Nuss D, Goretsky MJ. Surgical treatment of chest wall deformities. In: Spitz L, Coran AG, editors. Operative pediatric surgery, 6th edition. London: Hodder Arnold, 2006, with permission.)*

Allergy to the retrosternal bars was also identified in 2.2% of the patients having MIRPE by Nuss and his group.[81] The majority (63%) presented with rash and erythema, 32% had pleural effusions, and 15% were diagnosed on preoperative screening. It is critical to distinguish between allergic and infectious complications. The importance of placing the bars and stabilizers in a subcutaneous and not a submuscular position, to avoid extra-osseous bone formation around the strut and increased blood loss at the time of removal, has been demonstrated.[82]

Hebra and associates reported the results of a survey of members of the American Pediatric Surgery Association who had employed the minimally invasive (Nuss) technique.[83] Thirty institutions contributed 251 cases, although it should be noted that 42% were performed by one surgeon. The complications reported were similar to those of Nuss and his associates, but the frequency was higher, presumably because the procedures were performed by more individuals less familiar with the operation. Displacement of the bar occurred in 9.2% of cases and pneumothorax requiring tube thoracostomy in 4.8%. Less frequently encountered complications included thoracic outlet syndrome, pericarditis, blood loss requiring a transfusion, cardiac injury, persistent cardiac arrhythmias, and erosion of the sternum by the bar. Many of the surgeons had adopted the use of thoracoscopy to improve the safety of passing the clamp anterior to the heart. Other surgeons elevate the sternum with a bone hook during passage of the clamp to open the retrosternal space anterior to the heart.

Engum and coauthors reported their series of 21 patients with a mean age of 8.2 years.[84] Their patients had an average hospital stay of 4.9 days, which was comparable with the open repair. Complications encountered in their series were similar to the experience of others and included rotation of the bar, production of a marked pectus carinatum deformity, progressive chest wall asymmetry, and chronic persistent pain requiring removal of the bar in one case.

Molik and colleagues later enlarged this single-institution review and in a retrospective analysis compared 68 patients with standard surgical repair with 35 patients with a Nuss repair.[85] The Nuss procedure required less time (3.3 hours) than the open technique (4.7 hours), but it had a higher complication rate (43%) than the open method (20%). Four patients with the standard operation (6%) and eight with the Nuss technique (29%) required reoperation. Length of stay was comparable between the open (4.8 days) and Nuss (4.0 days) techniques. The Nuss patients had a higher frequency of epidural analgesics postoperatively and an increased duration of patient-controlled analgesia after surgery.

Fonkalsrud and associates reported a similar retrospective comparison of the two techniques, each used at one institution.[86] During a 5-year interval, 68 patients had the minimally invasive procedure and 139 had the open technique. There was a higher incidence of reoperations and hospitalizations in the Nuss group, but it was noted that 90% of the complications of this method occurred in the first 25 cases, again clearly demonstrating the role of experience in determining the frequency of surgical complications. It was difficult to determine in this study whether the differences noted in the use of epidural catheters and intravenous narcotics were attributable to truly different patient requirements or was a manifestation of institutional bias for analgesic techniques. There was a shorter mean hospitalization noted for the open procedure (2.9 days) than for the minimal-access procedure (6.5 days), and a similar difference between mean time before return to work or school (12 versus 18 days). These authors concluded that "long-term follow-up also will be required to assure both health professionals and the public that this is the procedure of choice for patients with pectus excavatum."

The occurrence of "overcorrection" of the deformity or production of a true carinate deformity was first reported by Croitoru and associates and was associated with underlying connective tissue disorders (Marfan syndrome and Ehlers-Danlos syndrome).[77] However, it was reported by Hebra to have occurred in an otherwise healthy 13-year-old boy 1 year after Nuss repair.[87] What factors predispose some patients to this complication is not understood.

Other rare complications for the MIRPE include exsanguinating hemorrhage during removal of the strut, resulting from laceration of a pulmonary vessel, and bilateral sternoclavicular dislocation; cardiac tamponade and shock produced by erosion of the aorta by a strut that had rotated 90 degrees; and a near-fatal hemorrhage from erosion of the internal mammary vessel by a bar that had rotated 45 degrees.[88-90]

A prospective multi-institutional study of patients undergoing repair of pectus excavatum has been completed. It is hoped that this study will better define the physiologic effects of repair. Early reports from this study suggest that the pain and complications from the MIRPE and open procedures are similar and that repair can be accomplished with limited risks to the patients.[91]

Children should be followed after repair by any technique until they reach full stature. Only by so doing can each surgeon assess the ultimate results of the surgical technique. Regrettably, recurrence can occur until full stature is achieved.

Open Surgical Repair of Pectus Excavatum

The open surgical technique for correction of pectus excavatum is depicted in Figure 24-4. In girls, particular attention is taken to place the incision in the projected inframammary crease, thus avoiding the complications of breast deformity and development described by Hougaard and Arendrup.[92] Skin flaps are mobilized by electrocautery to the angle of Louis superiorly and a shorter distance to the xiphoid inferiorly. Pectoral muscle flaps are elevated off the sternum and costal cartilages, preserving the entire pectoralis major and portions of the pectoralis minor and serratus anterior muscles in the flap (see Fig. 24-4A). Ellis and associates described elevating the skin and muscle together in a single flap, which is a reasonable but not widely adopted alternative method.[93]

Perioperative antibiotics are used, giving one dose of cefazolin immediately before operation and three postoperative doses. The Hemovac drain (Snyder Laboratories, New Philadelphia, OH) is removed when the drainage is less than 15 mL in an 8-hour period. All patients are warned to avoid aspirin and nonsteroidal anti-inflammatory agent–containing compounds for 2 weeks before surgery.

I currently use the retrosternal bar (Baxter Healthcare, Deerfield, IL) for internal fixation to secure the sternum firmly in an anterior position and to avoid the need to skeletonize the sternum to achieve adequate mobility for suture fixation. Although correction of pectus excavatum is technically most easily performed in a young child, I have become increasingly concerned about long-term recurrence in these children, as well as about impairment in the growth of the chest wall. I delay surgery until the children are well into their pubertal growth. At this age, the chest has less remaining growth and opportunity for recurrence of the pectus excavatum (Fig. 24-5). Fonkalsrud and coworkers recommend delay of surgery until at least 10 years of age because of recurrence most frequently seen during pubertal growth.[86] In contrast, Backer and associates have found no correlation between the age at repair and frequency of recurrence.[94,95]

Complications are few and relatively unimportant, except for major recurrence, which occurred in 17 of 704 patients in a series from Children's Hospital in Boston (Table 24-3).[14] Pneumothorax occurred in 2% of the patients and required only observation or aspiration. Tube thoracostomy was required in only four patients in the entire series and in no patients during the last 2 decades of the report. Wound infection is rare with use of perioperative antibiotic coverage.

The most distressing complication after surgical correction of pectus excavatum is major recurrence of the deformity. It is difficult to predict which patients will have a major recurrence, but it appears to occur with increased frequency in children who have poor muscular development and an asthenic or "marfanoid" habitus. All children with Marfan syndrome should be repaired with strut fixation because of the high risk of recurrence reported without strut fixation. Scherer and associates reported a low recurrence rate (one of eight cases) using a retrosternal strut.[16]

Although recurrences appear symmetrical, many are in fact right-sided, with a deep right parasternal gutter and sternal obliquity. The third, fourth, and fifth rib ends migrate medially, with apparent foreshortening of the costal cartilages. Correction of recurrent pectus excavatum is generally a formidable task. Sanger and associates reported their experience in secondary correction.[96] They resected the regenerated fibrocartilage plate, repeated the sternal osteotomy, and closed the pectoral muscles behind the sternum. Ten patients had an early good result. In the Children's Hospital Boston experience, 12 children and adolescents underwent secondary repair. Resection of the segments of the third to fifth costal cartilages was necessary to correct the deformity. After clearing the tip of the sternum, resection of the left fibrocartilage plate to the level of the third or second perichondrial sheath allowed the sternum to be brought forward and rotated into an acceptable position. Ten of 12 repeat operations were accomplished without pleural entry. Follow-up of patients with secondary correction ranged from 10 to 17 years. Eight had an acceptable thoracic contour; two had a broad shallow depression; and two had frank recurrence. I recommend use of

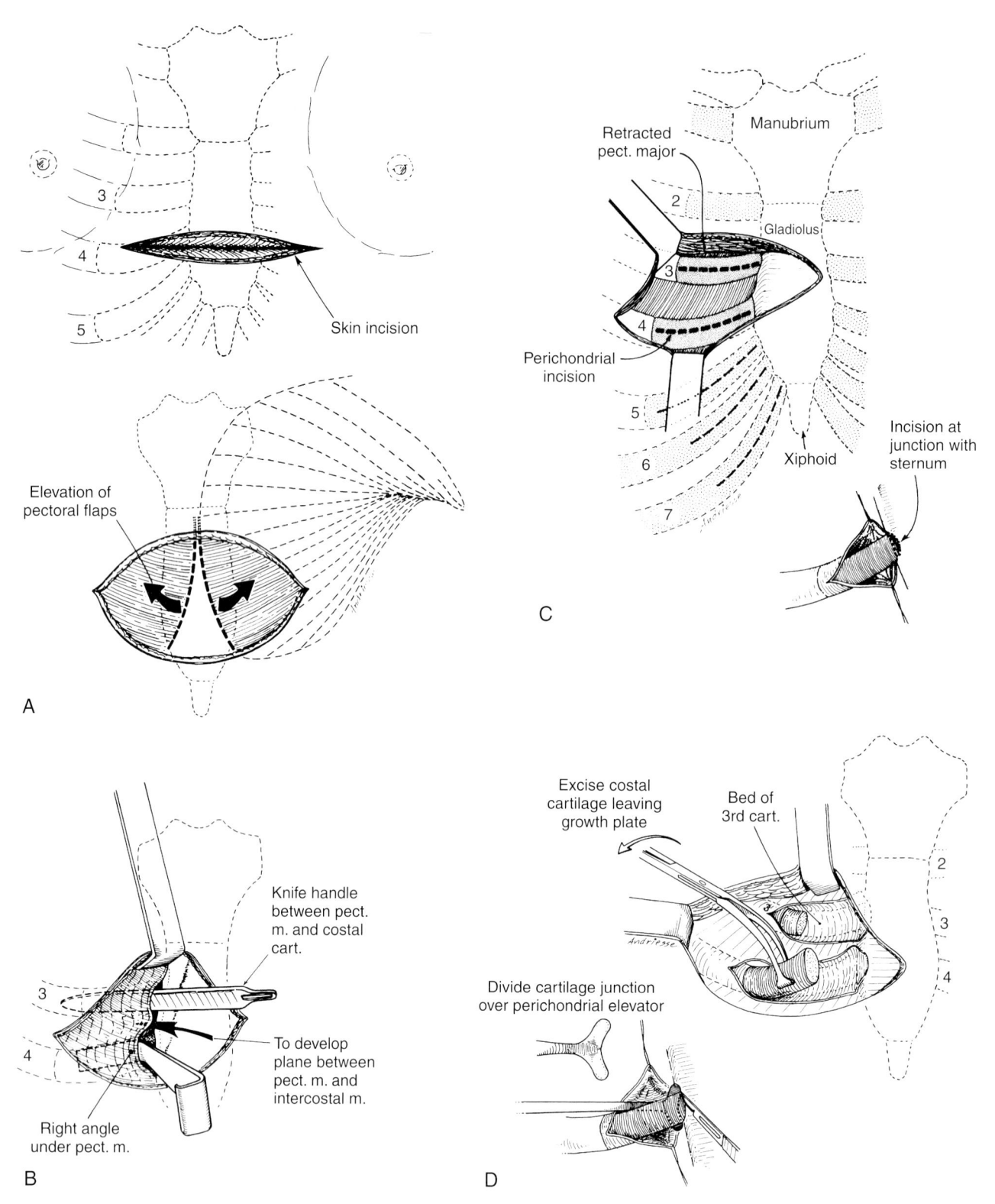

Figure 24–4

Open surgical technique for repair of pectus excavatum. **A,** A transverse incision is placed below and well within the nipple lines and, in females, at the site of the future inframammary crease. The pectoralis major muscle is elevated from the sternum along with portions of the pectoralis minor and serratus anterior bundles. **B,** The correct plane of dissection of the pectoral muscle flap is defined by passing an empty knife handle directly anterior to a costal cartilage after the medial aspect of the muscle is elevated with electrocautery. The knife handle is then replaced with a right-angle retractor, which is pulled anteriorly. The process is then repeated anterior to an adjoining costal cartilage. Anterior distraction of the muscles during the dissection facilitates identification of the avascular areolar plane and avoids entry into the intercostal muscle bundles. Muscle elevation is extended bilaterally to the costochondral junctions of the third to fifth ribs and a comparable distance for ribs six and seven. **C,** Subperichondrial resection of the costal cartilages is achieved by incising the perichondrium anteriorly. It is then dissected away from the costal cartilages in the bloodless plane between perichondrium and costal cartilage. Cutting back the perichondrium 90 degrees in each direction at its junction with the sternum *(inset)* facilitates visualization of the back wall of the costal cartilage. **D,** The cartilages are divided at their junction with the sternum with a knife having a Welch perichondrial elevator and held posteriorly to elevate the cartilage and protect the mediastinum *(inset)*. The divided cartilage can then be held with an Allis clamp and elevated. The costochondral junction is preserved with a segment of costal cartilage on the osseous ribs by incising the cartilage with a scalpel. Costal cartilages three through seven are generally resected, but occasionally the second costal cartilages must be removed if posterior displacement or funneling of the sternum extends to this level, as may be seen in older patients (see Fig. 24–1). Segments of the sixth and seventh costal cartilages are resected to the point where they flatten to join the costal arch. Familiarity with the cross-sectional shape of the medial ends of the costal cartilages facilitates their dissection. The second and third cartilages are broad and flat, the fourth and fifth are circular, and the sixth and seventh are narrow and deep.

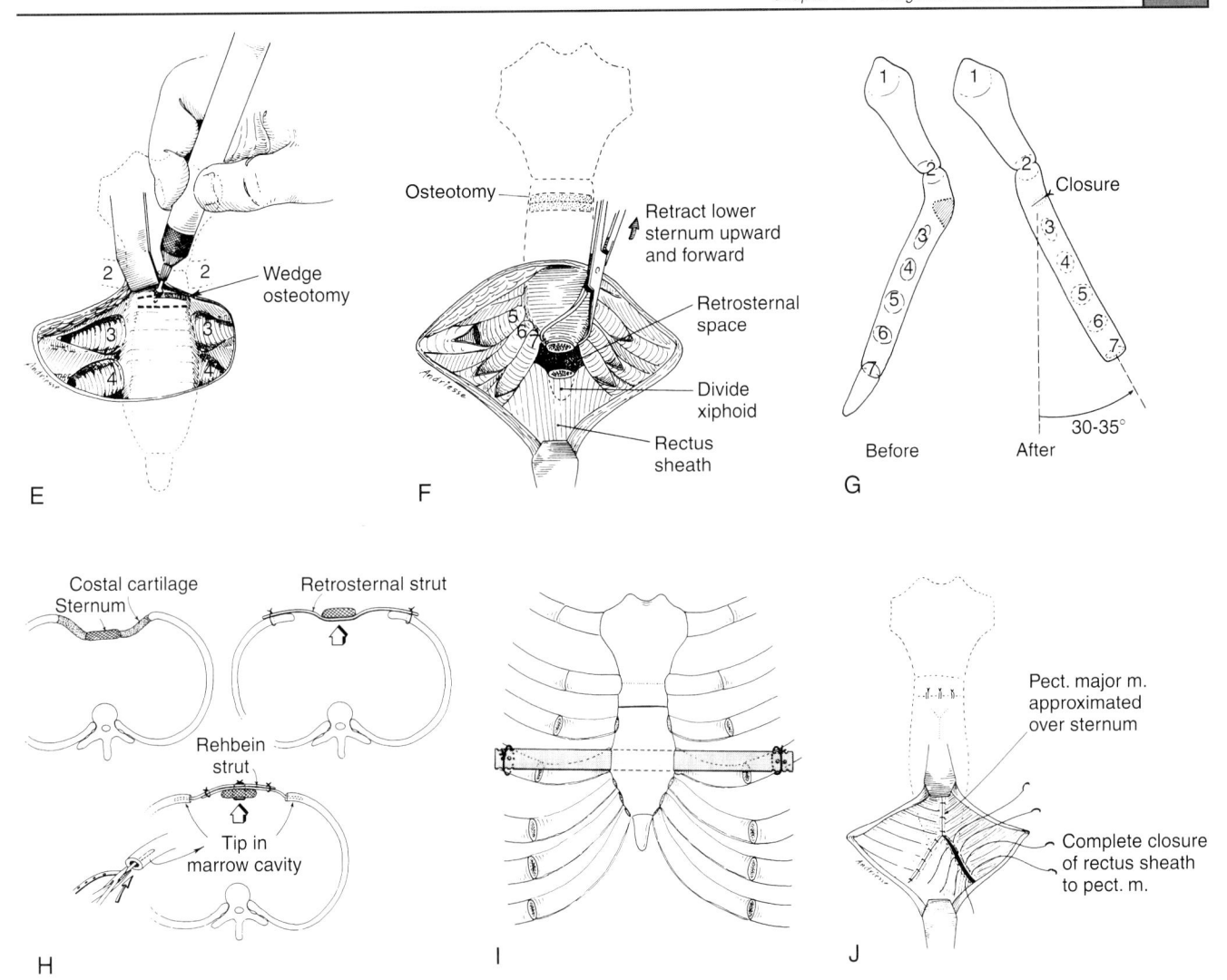

Figure 24–4, cont'd

E, The sternal osteotomy is created above the level of the last deformed cartilage and the posterior angulation of the sternum—generally the third cartilage but occasionally the second. Two transverse sternal osteotomies are created through the anterior cortex with a Hall air drill (Zimmer USA, Warsaw, IN) 3 to 5 mm apart. **F,** The base of the sternum and the rectus muscle flap are elevated with two towel clips, and the posterior plate of the sternum is fractured. The xiphoid can be divided from the sternum with electrocautery, allowing entry into the retrosternal space. This step is not necessary with the use of a retrosternal strut unless the xiphoid is protruding anteriorly when the sternum is in its corrected position. Preservation of the attachment of the perichondrial sheaths and xiphoid avoids an unsightly depression that can occur below the sternum. **G,** Correction of the abnormal position of the sternum is achieved by creation of a wedge-shaped osteotomy, which is then closed with elevation by the strut, bringing the sternum anteriorly into a slightly overcorrected position. **H,** Demonstration of the use of retrosternal and Rehbein struts. Rehbein struts are inserted into the marrow cavity *(insert)* of the third or fourth rib, and the struts are then joined medially to create an arch anterior to the sternum. The sternum is sewn to the arch to secure it in its new anterior position. The retrosternal strut is placed behind the sternum and is secured to the rib ends laterally to prevent migration. **I,** Anterior depiction of the retrosternal strut. The perichondrial sheath to either the third or fourth rib is divided from its junction with the sternum, and the retrosternal space is bluntly dissected to allow passage of the strut behind the sternum. It is secured with two pericostal sutures laterally to prevent migration. The wound is then flooded with warm saline and cefazolin solution to remove clots and to inspect for a pleural entry. A single-limb medial Hemovac drain (Snyder Laboratories, New Philadelphia, OH) is brought through the inferior skin flap to the left of the sternum and placed in a parasternal position to the level of the highest resected costal cartilage. **J,** The pectoral muscle flaps are secured to the midline of the sternum, advancing the flaps inferiorly to obtain coverage of the entire sternum. The rectus muscle is then joined to the pectoral muscle flaps, closing the mediastinum. *(A-G and J from Shamberger RC, Welch KJ. J Pediatr Surg 1988;23:615, with permission. D and F adapted from original figures. H and I from Shamberger RC. Chest wall deformities. In: Shields TW, Locicero III J, Ponn RB. General thoracic surgery, 5th edition. Philadelphia: Lippincott Williams & Wilkins; 2000, p. 535-61.)*

strut fixation on all patients with secondary repair, because cartilage regeneration will be slower and less adequate than that after primary operation. Successful repair of recurrent pectus excavatum has also been reported using the MIRPE technique.[97,98]

In 1990, Martinez and associates first described a deficiency in thoracic growth in children after repair of pectus excavatum during the preschool years.[99] Subsequently, in 1996, Haller and colleagues reported three boys who presented in their teens with apparent limited growth of the ribs after resection

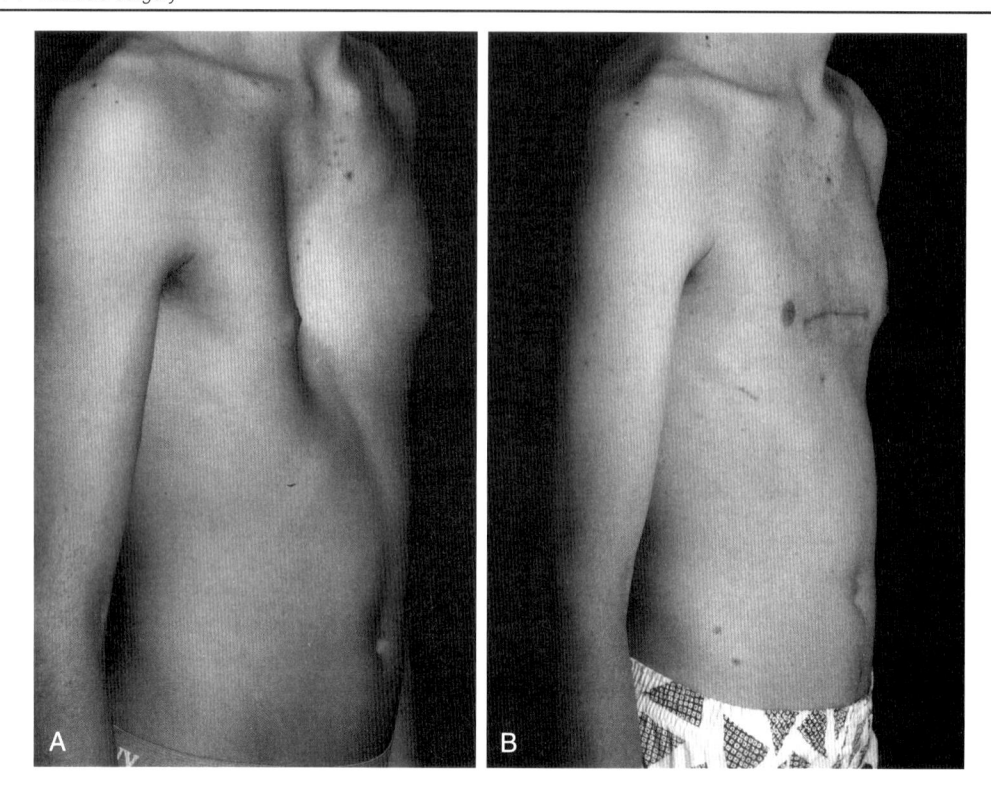

Figure 24–5
A, Preoperative photographs of a 14-year-old boy with pectus excavatum. **B,** Postoperative photograph 7 months after repair using a retrosternal strut.

of the costal cartilages at an early age.[100] This produced a bandlike narrowing of the mid chest, which was labeled acquired Jeune's disease by the authors (Fig. 24-6). In some cases, the first and second ribs in which the costal cartilages had not been resected had relative overgrowth, producing anterior protrusion of the upper sternum (see Fig. 24-6C). Haller's group attributed this to injury of the costochondral junctions during surgical repair.[100] As these junctions are the longitudinal growth centers for the ribs, early operation resulted in decreased growth of the ribs and of the sternum because of injury to the growth centers or vascular supply.

Martinez and associates demonstrated experimentally in 6-week-old rabbits that resection of the costal cartilages produced a marked impairment in chest growth, particularly the anterior-posterior diameter, during a 5.5-month period of observation.[99] Less severe impairment occurred if only the medial three fourths of the costal cartilage was resected, preserving the growth centers at the costochondral junction. This impairment was attributed to fibrosis and scarring in the perichondrial sheaths. Perichondrial sheaths, bone, or other prosthetic tissues that cannot grow also should not be joined posterior to the sternum because they will form a bandlike stricture across the chest. This complication of delayed thoracic growth was described primarily in children repaired in early childhood and can be avoided by delaying surgery until the children are older. Preservation of the costochondral junction by leaving a segment of the cartilage on the osseous portion of the rib may partially minimize growth impairment.

Weber and Kurkchubasche described a method of improving the severe pulmonary impairment encountered in one

Table 24–3
Complications of Pectus Excavatum Repair: 70 Cases in 704 Patients

Complication	Number of Cases
Pneumothorax*	11
Wound infection	5
Wound hematoma	3
Wound dehiscence	5
Pneumonia	3
Seroma	1
Hemoptysis	1
Hemopericardium	1
Major recurrence	17
Mild recurrence	23

*Four patients required chest tube placement.
From Shamberger RC, Welch KJ. J Pediatr Surg 1988;**23**:615, with permission.

patient with "acquired Jeune's syndrome."[101] A sternotomy was performed and wedged open permanently with rib struts. The pleura was opened bilaterally, along with subperichondral resection of six ribs. Pulmonary function was improved after the procedure in this patient. A subsequent report involving

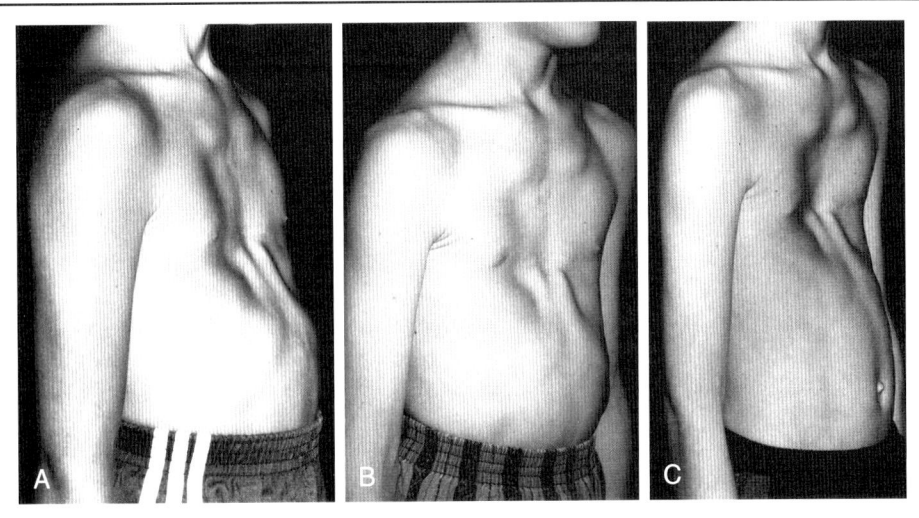

Figure 24-6
Sequence of photographs demonstrating deterioration in the quality of a repair that can occur with time. This boy had an initial excellent result from a Welch repair with suture fixation of the sternum at age 4 years 3 months. The follow-up photographs at 7 years 6 months (**A**), 9 years 3 months (**B**), and 12 years 9 months (**C**) demonstrate progressive depression of the sternum and costal cartilages and relative "overgrowth" of the upper chest.

10 patients further substantiates the efficacy of this technique to improve pulmonary function in eight of the 10 cases.[102] Patients are followed after surgery to full growth: age 16 for girls and 19 for boys. Use of clinical and Moiré photography for initial evaluation and follow-up studies leads to improved clinical assessment of results and obviates the need for multiple radiographic examinations.[103]

PECTUS CARINATUM

Pectus carinatum, an anterior protrusion of the sternum or chest wall, is much less frequent than pectus excavatum and comprises 16.7% of all chest wall deformities in the Children's Hospital Boston experience. The anterior protrusion occurs in a spectrum of configurations often divided into four categories (Table 24-4).[104] The most frequent form, termed *chondrogladiolar* by Brodkin,[105] consists of anterior protrusion of the body of the sternum with protrusion of the lower costal cartilages. It is described as appearing as if a giant hand had pinched the chest from the front, forcing the sternum and medial portion of the costal cartilages forward and the lateral costal cartilages and ribs inward (Fig. 24-7).[106] Asymmetric deformities with anterior displacement of the costal cartilages on one side and normal cartilages on the contralateral side are less common (Fig. 24-8). Mixed lesions have a carinate deformity on one side and a depression or excavatum deformity on the contralateral side, often with sternal rotation. Some authors classify these as a variant of the excavatum deformities. The least frequent deformity is the *chondromanubrial* or "pouter pigeon" deformity, with protrusion of the upper chest involving the manubrium and second and third costal cartilages and with relative depression of the body of the sternum (Fig. 24-9).

Etiology

The etiology of pectus carinatum is no better understood than that of pectus excavatum. It appears as an overgrowth of the costal cartilages, with forward buckling of the cartilages

Table 24-4
Frequency of Pectus Carinatum Deformities

Deformity	Number of Cases
Chondrogladiolar	
Symmetric	89
Asymmetric	49
Mixed carinatum and excavatum	14
Chondromanubrial	3
Total	155

From Shamberger RC, Welch KJ. J Pediatr Surg 1987;22:48-53.

and anterior displacement of the sternum. Again, the clear-cut increased family incidence suggests a genetic basis. In our review of 152 patients, 26% had a family history of chest wall deformity and 12% of scoliosis.[104] It is much more frequent in boys than in girls, with a 3:1 ratio. Scoliosis and other deformities of the spine are the most common associated musculoskeletal anomalies (Table 24-5).[104]

Pectus carinatum is rarely present at birth, and in almost half of the patients, the deformity was not identified until after the 11th birthday (Fig. 24-10). The deformity often progresses during early childhood, particularly in the period of rapid growth at puberty. The chondromanubrial deformity, in contrast with the chondrogladiolar form, is often noted at birth and is associated with a truncated, comma-shaped sternum with absent sternal segmentation or premature obliteration of the sternal sutures (Fig. 24-11). Currarino and Silverman described its association with an increased risk of congenital heart disease.[107] Lees and Caldicott reviewed 1915

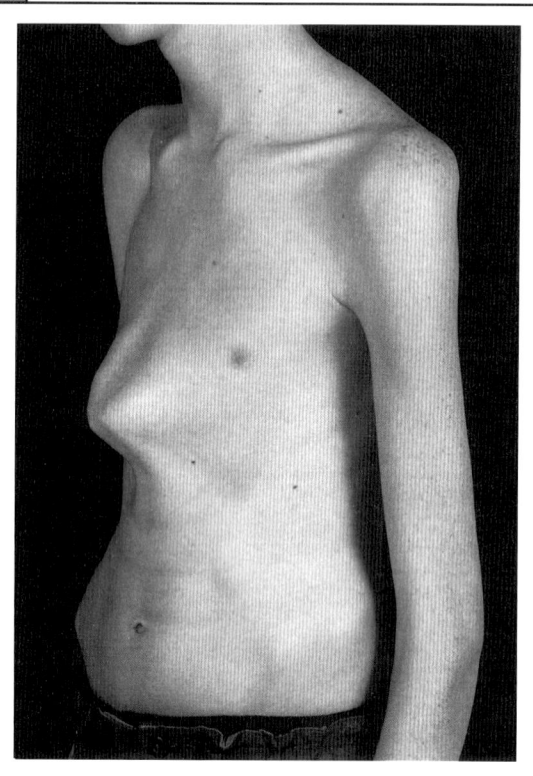

Figure 24–7
Symmetric chondrogladiolar pectus carinatum in a 11½-year-old boy.

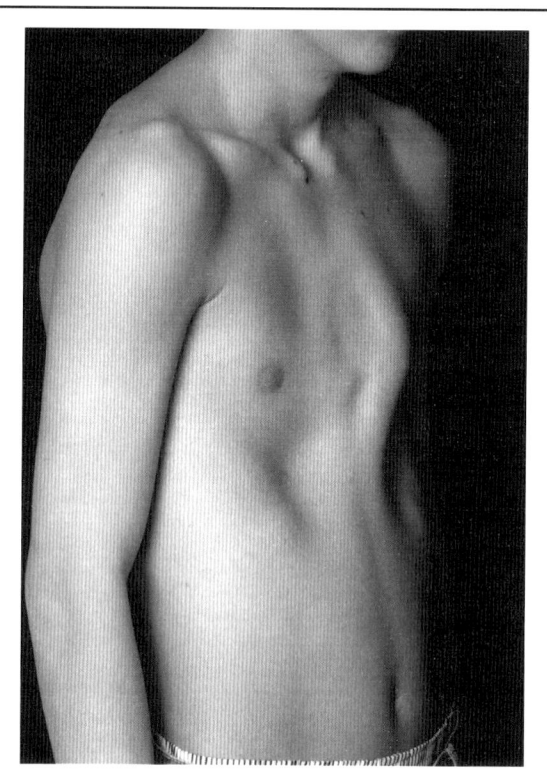

Figure 24–8
A 15-year-old boy with marked asymmetric pectus carinatum. The protrusion of the costal cartilages is limited to the left side of his chest.

thoracic radiographs and identified 135 children with sternal fusion anomalies.[108] Of these children, 18% had documented congenital heart disease.

Surgical Repair

Correction of carinate deformities has had a colorful history, beginning in 1952 with the first repair by Ravitch of an upper chondromanubrial deformity.[109] He resected multiple costal cartilages and performed a double sternal osteotomy. In 1953, Lester reported two methods of repair for a lower chondrogladiolar deformity.[110] The first approach, resection of the anterior portion of the sternum, was abandoned because of excessive blood loss and unsatisfactory results. The second method, subperiosteal resection of the entire sternum, was a no less radical technique. Chin[111] and later Brodkin[112] (1958), in a technique called the xiphosternopexy, advanced the transected xiphoid and the attached rectus muscles to a higher site on the sternum. This produced posterior displacement of the sternum in younger patients with a flexible chest wall. Howard combined this method with subperichondrial resection of the costal cartilages and a sternal osteotomy.[106] Ravitch reported repair of the chondrogladiolar deformity by resection of costal cartilage in a one- or two-stage procedure, with placement of "reefing" sutures to shorten and posteriorly displace the perichondrium.[113] A sternal osteotomy was used in one of three cases. Robicsek and associates described repair by subperichondrial resection of costal cartilages, transverse sternal osteotomy, and resection of the protruding lower portion of the sternum.[114] The xiphoid and rectus muscles were reattached to the new lower margin of the sternum, pulling it posteriorly. In 1973, Welch and Vos reported an approach to these deformities that I continue to use today.[115] Recent attempts at treating children with pectus carinatum by orthotic bracing have been reported, and success has been achieved in younger children.[116-120] Compliance in using the brace is the rate-limiting factor for success in older patients. However, significant to complete correction has been reported in up to 75% of patients. The asymmetric lesions appear the most difficult to correct.

Surgical Technique

The placement of the skin incision, mobilization of the pectoral muscle flaps, and subperichondrial resection of the involved costal cartilage are identical to the method described for pectus excavatum. Management of the sternum is shown in Figure 24-12 for the various deformities. In the chondromanubrial deformity, the costal cartilages must be resected from the second cartilage inferiorly.[121] A single-limb medium Hemovac drain is brought through the inferior skin flap, as for excavatum patients, with the suction ports in a parasternal position to the level of the highest resected costal cartilage. The pectoralis muscle flaps and skin flaps are closed. Perioperative antibiotics are used as in pectus excavatum.

Operative Results

Results are overwhelmingly successful in these patients. In our review of 152 cases, postoperative recovery was generally uneventful.[104] Blood transfusions are rarely required, and none has been given in the last 10 years of the report. There is a 3.9%

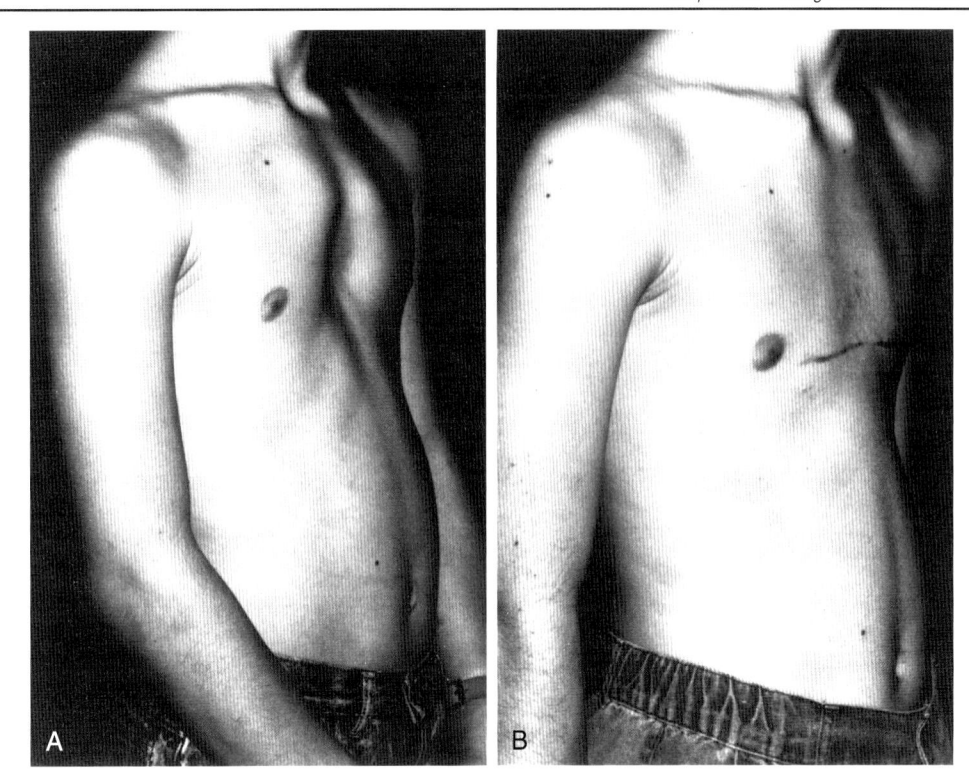

Figure 24–9
A, A 15-year-old boy with the chondromanubrial deformity. Note the posterior depression of the lower sternum, accentuated by the anterior bowing of the second and third costal cartilages. **B,** After repair, the sternal contour is improved and costal cartilages are re-formed in a more appropriate fashion.

complication rate (Table 24-6). Only three patients have required revision, each having additional lower costal cartilages resected for persistent unilateral malformation of the costal arch.

POLAND'S SYNDROME

In 1841, while Poland was a medical student, he described congenital absence of the pectoralis major and minor muscles associated with syndactyly.[122] Despite a prior report of this entity by Froriep in 1839,[123] the eponym *Poland's syndrome* has been used since 1962, when Clarkson first applied it to a group of similar patients.[124] Subsequent reports have described other components of the syndrome, including absence of ribs, chest wall depression, and abnormalities of the breasts. Each component of the syndrome occurs with variable severity. The extent of thoracic involvement may range from hypoplasia of the sternal head of the pectoralis major and minor muscles with normal underlying ribs, to complete absence of the anterior portions of the second to fifth ribs and costal cartilages (Figs. 24-13 and 24-14). Breast involvement is frequent and ranges from mild hypoplasia to complete absence of the breast (amastia) and nipple (athelia) (see Fig. 24-13C).[125] Minimal subcutaneous fat and an absence of axillary hair are additional components of the syndrome. Hand deformities may include hypoplasia of the fingers (brachydactyly) and fused fingers (syndactyly), primarily involving the central three digits. The most severe expression of the anomaly, mitten or claw deformity (ectromelia), is rare.[124,126] An extensive classification of the associated hand anomalies has been developed.[127] Poland's syndrome may also occur in combination with Sprengel's

Table 24–5

Musculoskeletal Abnormalities Identified in 30 of 152 Cases of Pectus Carinatum

Musculoskeletal Abnormality	Number of Cases
Scoliosis	23
Neurofibromatosis	2
Morquio's disease	2
Vertebral anomalies	1
Hyperlordosis	1
Kyphosis	1

From Shamberger RC, Welch KJ. J Pediatr Surg 1987;**22**:48, with permission.

deformity, in which there is decreased size, elevation, and winging of the scapula.

Poland's syndrome is present at birth and has an estimated incidence of 1 in 30,000 to 32,000.[128,129] Abnormalities of the breast can be defined at birth by absence of the underlying breast bud and by the hypoplastic nipple, which is often superiorly displaced. The etiology of Poland's syndrome is unknown. Bouvet and associates[130] proposed hypoplasia of the ipsilateral subclavian artery as the origin of this malformation, but, as noted by David,[131] decreased blood flow to the extremity may be the result of decreased muscle mass

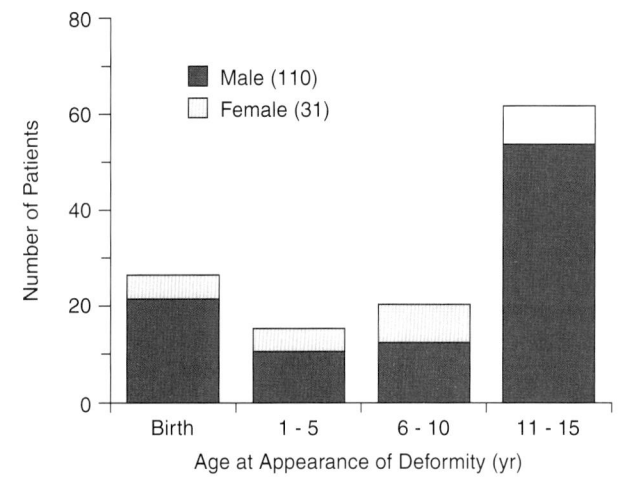

Figure 24-10
Age at appearance of pectus carinatum deformity in 141 infants and children. Note the appearance of protrusion in almost one half of the children at puberty. (From Shamberger RC, Welch KJ. J Pediatr Surg 1987;**22**:48-53, with permission.)

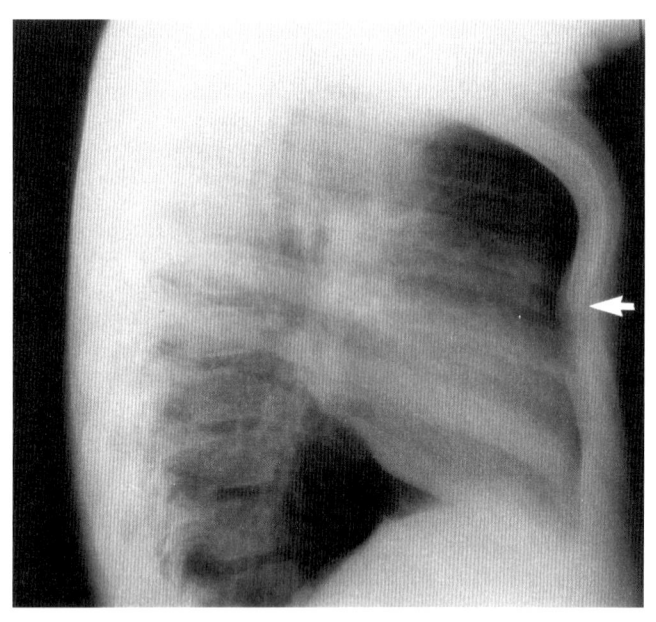

Figure 24-11
Lateral chest radiograph of a boy with chondromanubrial pectus carinatum. The short, comma-shaped sternum lacking segmentation is apparent. *Arrow* is at the tip of the truncated sternum. (From Shamberger RC, Welch KJ. J Pediatr Surg 1988;**23**:319-22, with permission.)

of the hypoplastic limb rather than its cause. Although some forms of syndactyly are autosomal dominant traits, a similar pattern has not been demonstrated in patients with Poland's syndrome, which is generally sporadic. Multiple cases within a family are rare, and its appearance in one of two identical twins was described.[132-135] Poland's syndrome is associated with a second rare syndrome, the Möbius syndrome: bilateral or unilateral facial palsy and abducens oculi palsy. Nineteen such cases have been identified, but a unifying etiology is lacking. Familial occurrence of these two syndromes was reported.[136,137] An unusual association between Poland's syndrome and childhood leukemia has also been reported.[138,139]

The experience with Poland's syndrome at Children's Hospital Boston from 1970 to 1987 included 41 children and adolescents, of whom 21 were boys.[140] The lesion was right-sided in 23 patients, left-sided in 17 patients, and bilateral in one patient. Hand anomalies were noted in 23 (56%) and breast anomalies in 25 (61%). In 10 children, the underlying thoracic abnormality required reconstruction, and in three children, rib or cartilage grafts were needed for complete repair.

Surgical Repair

Assessment of the extent of involvement of the various musculoskeletal components is critical for optimal thoracic reconstruction. If the deformity is limited to the sternal component of the pectoralis major and minor muscles without underlying chest wall deformity, there is little functional deficit and repair is unnecessary, except to facilitate breast augmentation in girls (see Fig. 24-14). If the underlying costal cartilages are depressed or absent, repair must be considered to minimize the concavity, to eliminate the paradoxical motion of the chest wall if ribs are absent, and in girls to provide an optimal base for breast reconstruction. Ravitch reported correction of posteriorly displaced costal cartilages by unilateral resection of the cartilages; a wedge osteotomy of the sternum allowing rotation of the sternum; and fixation with Rehbein struts and Steinmann pins.[109] I have achieved suitable repair in most cases with bilateral costal cartilage resection and an oblique osteotomy, which corrects both the sternal rotation and the posterior displacement, as in patients with mixed pectus carinatum and excavatum deformity (Fig. 24-15). The sternum is then displaced anteriorly and is supported with a retrosternal strut, which allows correction of the posteriorly displaced costal cartilages. An unappreciated carinate deformity is often present on the contralateral side, which accentuates the ipsilateral concavity (see Fig. 24-14B).

Absence of the medial portion of the ribs can be managed with split rib grafts taken from the contralateral side. These must be secured to the sternum medially and to the "dagger point" ends of the hypoplastic ribs laterally. The grafts can be covered with a prosthetic mesh if needed for further support. In these cases, little tissue is present between the endothoracic fascia and the fascial remnants of the pectoral muscles. Soft tissue coverage of the area can be augmented with transfer of a latissimus dorsi muscle flap. This is particularly helpful in girls, who will require breast augmentation.[140a,141-143] Flap rotation is seldom, if ever, required in boys and has the disadvantage of adding a second posterior thoracic scar and decreasing the strength of the latissimus dorsi muscle.

STERNAL DEFECTS

Sternal defects are rare compared with pectus excavatum and carinatum, yet they have received a great deal of attention in the medical literature because of their dramatic presentation and often fatal outcome. Deformities resulting from failure of ventral fusion of the sternum can be divided into four groups: cleft sternum, thoracic ectopia cordis, thoracoabdominal ectopia cordis, and cervical ectopia cordis. The heart is in a normal position in cleft sternum, but it is displaced in the other

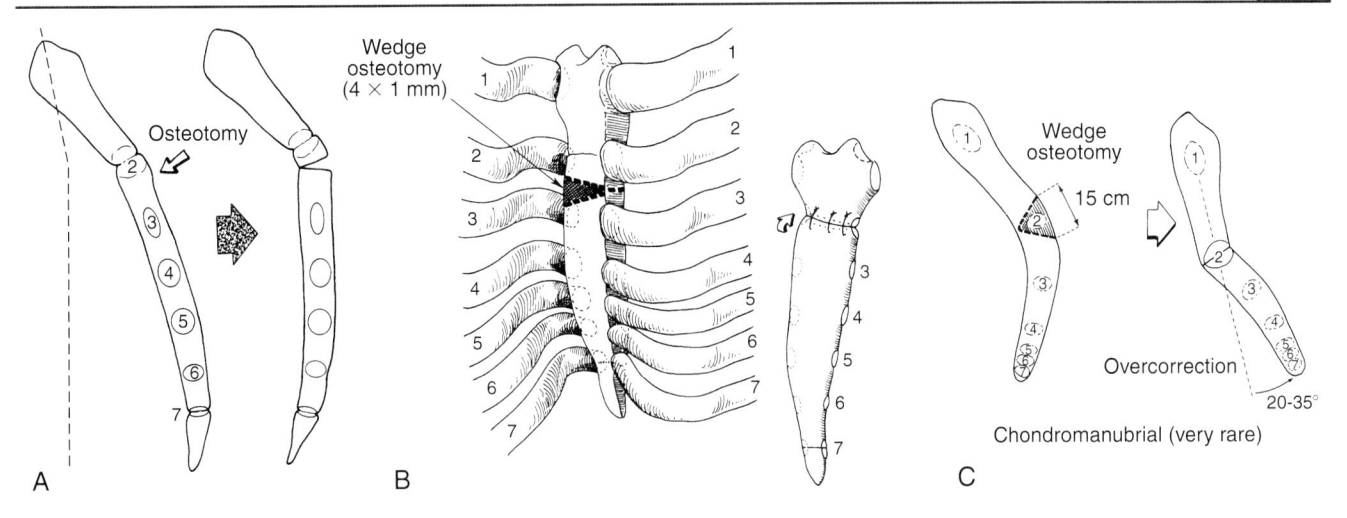

Figure 24–12
A, A single or double osteotomy after resection of the costal cartilages allows posterior displacement of the sternum to an orthotopic position.
B, The mixed pectus deformity is corrected by full and symmetric resection of the third to seventh costal cartilages, followed by transverse offset (0- to 10-degree wedge-shaped sternal osteotomy). Closure of this defect achieves both anterior displacement and rotation of the sternum.
C, The chondromanubrial type of deformity is depicted, with a broad, wedge-shaped sternal osteotomy placed through the anterior cortex of the obliterated sternomanubrial junction. Closure of the osteotomy after fracture of the posterior cortex achieves a posterior displacement of the superior portion of the sternum, which is secured only by its attachment to the first rib. The lower portion of the sternum is overcorrected 20 to 35 degrees and is secured in position by strut or suture fixation. (***A*** and ***B*** *from Shamberger RC, Welch KJ. J Pediatr Surg 1987;**22**:48-53, with permission;* ***C*** *from Shamberger RC, Welch KJ. J Pediatr Surg 1988;**23**:319-22, with permission.)*

Table 24-6
Complications of Pectus Carinatum Repair: 7 Cases in 152 Patients

Complication	Number of Cases
Pneumothorax*	4
Atelectasis	1
Wound infection	1
Local tissue necrosis	1

Two patients required chest tube placement.

three entities. In thoracic ectopia cordis, the heart protrudes anteriorly and there are no tissues covering the heart. In cervical ectopia cordis, the protrusion is even more pronounced, and the heart is often fused with the head. In thoracoabdominal ectopia cordis, the heart is covered but often displaced into the abdomen through a defect in the diaphragm.

Cleft Sternum

An infant with cleft sternum has a complete or partial separation of the sternum but a normally positioned intrathoracic heart. This deformity results from failure of fusion of the sternal bars, which should occur about the 8th week of gestation. In all such cases, despite the sternal separation, normal skin coverage is present, with an intact pericardium and a normal diaphragm. Abdominal wall defects such as omphalocele do not occur in these children. The condition causes few functional problems. A dramatic increase in the protrusion of the deformity occurs with crying or Valsalva's maneuver. The sternal defects described in 109 cases are summarized in Table 24-7.[144] The cleft involves primarily the upper sternum, whereas patients with thoracic or thoracoabdominal ectopia cordis have clefts primarily of the lower sternum.

The second distinction between cleft sternum and the other sternal defects is that children with cleft sternum rarely have intrinsic congenital heart disease. An unexplained association does exist, however, between cleft sternum and cervicofacial hemangiomas, which were reported in 14 cases since the first description of this association by Fischer in 1879.[145]

Surgical Repair

Maier and Bortone accomplished the first primary repair of cleft sternum in 1949 in a 6-week-old infant.[146] The flexibility of the newborn chest allows approximation of the sternal bars without producing cardiac compression (Fig. 24-16). A summary of the reported repairs for cleft sternum in 69 cases is shown in Table 24-8.

Sabiston reported reconstruction of cleft sternum using multiple oblique chondrotomies.[147] The chondrotomies increase the chest wall dimensions and flexibility. The technique is useful in older infants and children with a less flexible chest and a wide defect. Meissner described a variation of the repair, in which the cartilages are divided laterally and swung medially to cover the defect.[148] Autologous grafts of costal cartilage, split ribs, and segments of the costal arch have been used since Burton first repaired this defect with a portion of the costal arch.[149] Repairs with prosthetic material are far less satisfactory because of the risks of infection and the inability of these tissues to grow with the child. Most authors now recommend treatment of cleft sternum in the newborn period, when simple direct closure is possible without the use of prosthetic materials or grafts.

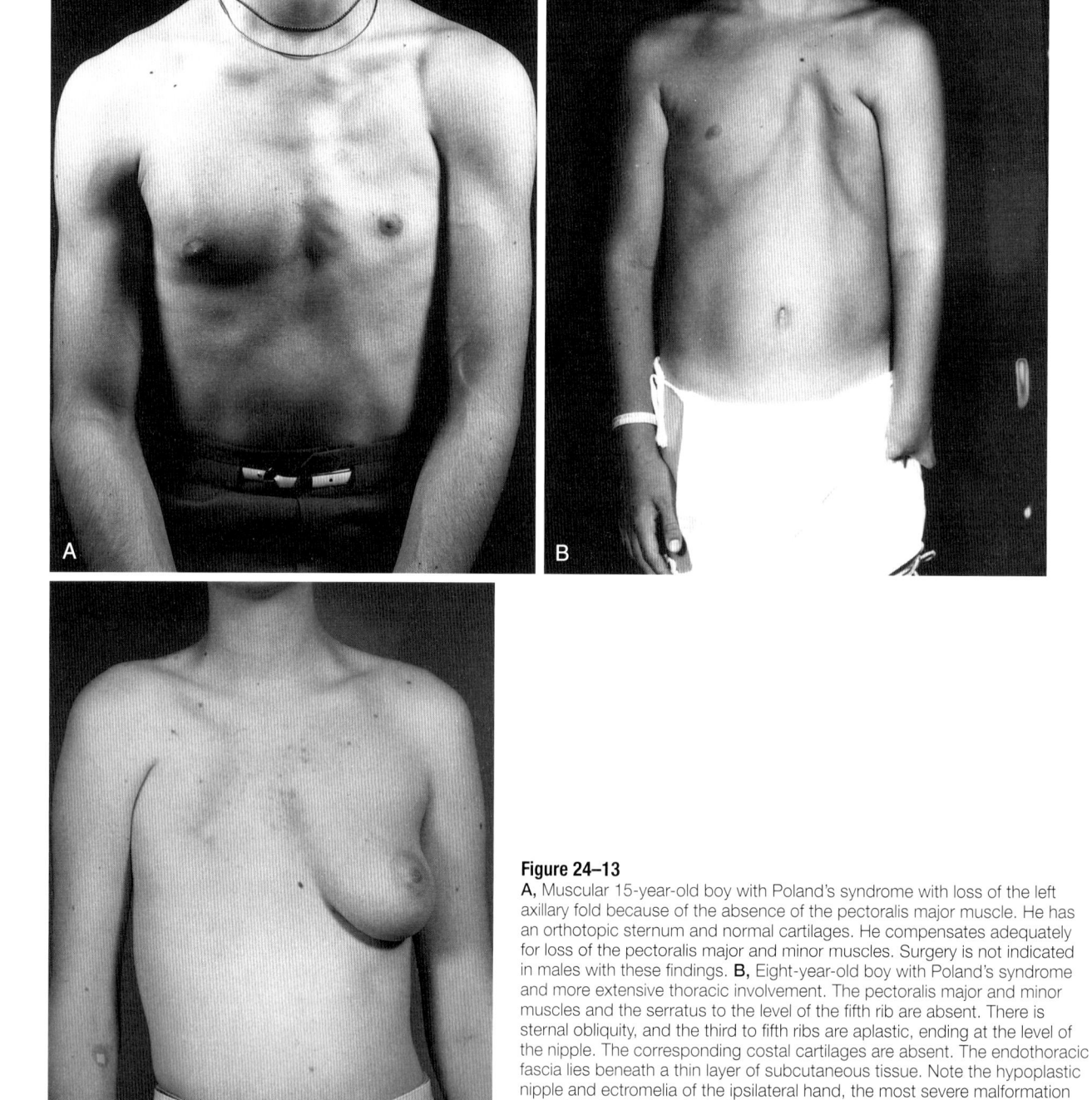

Figure 24-13
A, Muscular 15-year-old boy with Poland's syndrome with loss of the left axillary fold because of the absence of the pectoralis major muscle. He has an orthotopic sternum and normal cartilages. He compensates adequately for loss of the pectoralis major and minor muscles. Surgery is not indicated in males with these findings. **B,** Eight-year-old boy with Poland's syndrome and more extensive thoracic involvement. The pectoralis major and minor muscles and the serratus to the level of the fifth rib are absent. There is sternal obliquity, and the third to fifth ribs are aplastic, ending at the level of the nipple. The corresponding costal cartilages are absent. The endothoracic fascia lies beneath a thin layer of subcutaneous tissue. Note the hypoplastic nipple and ectromelia of the ipsilateral hand, the most severe malformation of the hand associated with Poland's syndrome. **C,** A 14-year-old girl with Poland's syndrome. Note the high position of the right nipple, amastia, sternal rotation, and depressed right chest. The anterior second to fourth ribs and cartilages were missing. Breast augmentation will be required after the contralateral breast achieves full growth.

Ectopia Cordis

Although treatment of isolated cleft sternum is routinely successful, surgical repair of ectopia cordis, particularly thoracic ectopia cordis, has a high mortality. The lethal factor in thoracic ectopia cordis and cervical ectopia cordis is the extrathoracic location of the heart, which makes tissue coverage difficult. In thoracoabdominal ectopia cordis (the Cantrell pentalogy), the major impediment to survival is the high incidence of intrinsic congenital heart disease.[150]

Etiology

The etiology of thoracic ectopia cordis and thoracoabdominal ectopia cordis is much debated. Some consider these anomalies to be the result of disruption of the amnion and possibly disruption of the chorionic layer or yolk sac as well.[151-154] This disruption occurs during the 3rd or 4th week of gestation at a time when cardiac chamber formation is occurring rapidly. This timing may account for the high incidence of abnormal cardiac development. Von Praagh (personal communication, 1987) has the intriguing notion, based on embryology studies by Patten[155] and Bremer,[156] that acute hyperflexion of the craniocervical segment of the embryo pins the heart down in the extrathoracic position with the submental cardiac apex. The abnormal fetal configuration produced by oligohydramnios may persist to delivery and oppose traction by the gubernaculum cordis, which normally pulls the cardiac apex into caudal alignment. Chromosome abnormalities have been reported.[157-159]

Thoracic Ectopia Cordis

Thoracic ectopia cordis is one of the most dramatic occurrences in the delivery room (Fig. 24-17). The naked beating heart is external to the thorax. Clearly visible are the atrial appendages, coronary vasculature, and cephalic orientation of the cardiac apex. The gubernaculum cordis initially extends to the supraumbilical raphe. Thoracic ectopia cordis was first reported by Stensen[160] in 1671 and the report later translated by Willius.[161] Stensen identified the four components of the tetralogy of Fallot in this patient with thoracic ectopia cordis (such is the fate of eponyms). Cardiac anomalies are unusually frequent in thoracic ectopia cordis. Table 24-9 lists the associated cardiac anomalies reported up to 1990. Only four of 75 cases had no intrinsic cardiac anomalies.

Infants with thoracic ectopia cordis are severely deficient in the midline somatic tissues that normally cover the heart. Many attempts at primary closure fail because of the inability to mobilize adequate tissues for coverage. An abdominal defect is often present as well. Recent CT evaluation by Haynor and associates also shows reduced intrathoracic volume in these infants.[162] Most allegedly successful repairs have been not of true thoracic ectopia cordis but, rather, of thoracoabdominal ectopia cordis. Cutler and Wilens first attempted repair in 1925 by skin flap coverage, but they failed because of cessation of cardiac function, presumably from compression of the heart.[163] Only three survivors of more than 29 attempts have been recorded (Table 24-10).

The first successful repair of ectopia cordis was achieved by Koop in 1975 and was reported by Saxena.[164] An infant with a normal heart had skin flap coverage at 5 hours of age, with inferior mobilization of the anterior attachments of the diaphragm. The sternal bars were 2 inches apart and could not be approximated primarily without cardiac compression and compromise. When the infant was 7 months old, an acrylic resin of Dacron and Marlex mesh was inserted to close the sternal cleft, followed by primary skin closure. Necrosis of the skin flaps complicated the postoperative course with infection of the prosthetic material, which was later removed. This child survives to age 20 years and is reported to be entirely well.

Successful closure in two other infants is reported. Dobell and associates achieved closure in two stages.[165] Skin flap coverage was provided for the newborn. Rib strut grafts were placed over the sternal defect at 19 months of age and covered

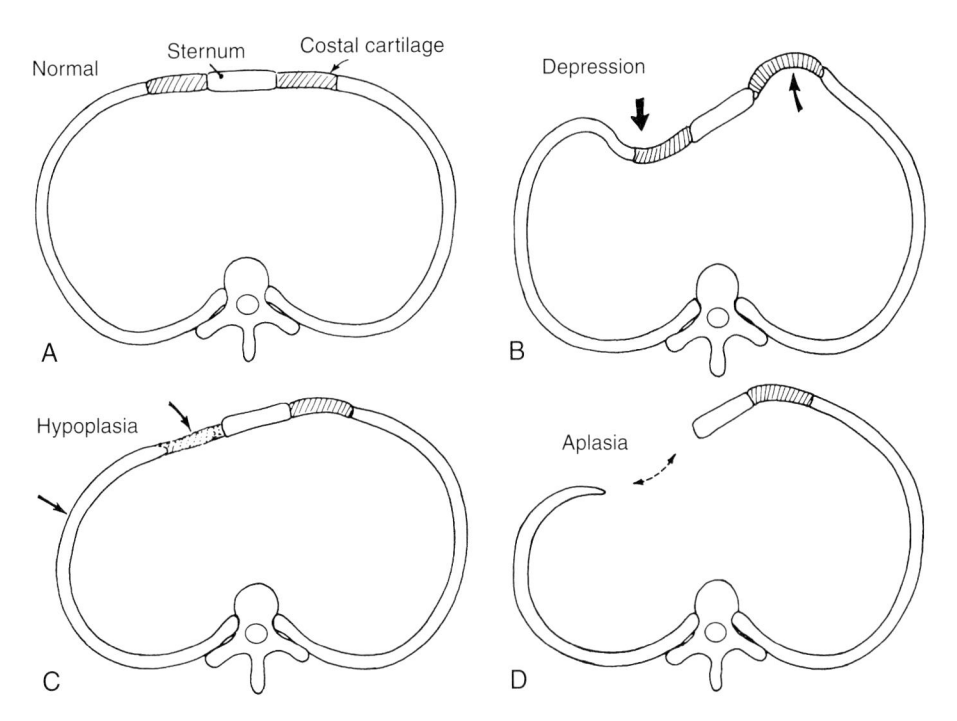

Figure 24–14
The spectrum of thoracic abnormality seen in Poland's syndrome. **A,** Most frequently, an entirely normal thorax is present, and only pectoral muscles are absent. **B,** Depression of the involved side of the chest wall, with rotation and often depression of the sternum. A carinate protrusion of the contralateral side is frequently present. **C,** Hypoplasia of ribs on the involved side but without significant depression may be seen. It usually does not require surgical correction. **D,** Aplasia of one or more ribs is usually associated with depression of adjacent ribs on the involved side and rotation of the sternum. *(From Shamberger RC, Welch KJ, Upton J III. J Pediatr Surg 1989;**24**:760-5, with permission.)*

Figure 24–15
Poland's syndrome. **A,** A transverse incision is placed below the nipple lines and, in females, in the inframammary crease. **B,** Schematic depiction of the deformity, with rotation of the sternum, depression of the cartilages of the involved side, and carinate protrusion of the contralateral side. **C,** In patients with aplasia of the ribs, the endothoracic fascia is encountered directly below the attenuated subcutaneous tissue and pectoral fascia. The pectoral muscle flap is elevated on the contralateral side and the pectoral fascia, if present, on the involved side. Subperichondrial resection of the costal cartilages is then carried out, as shown by the *bold dashed lines*. Rarely, this must be carried to the level of the second costal cartilages. **D,** A transverse, offset, wedge-shaped sternal osteotomy is created below the second costal cartilage. Elevation of the sternum with a retrosternal strut corrects both the posterior displacement and the rotation of the sternum. **E,** In patients with rib aplasia, split rib grafts are harvested from the contralateral fifth or sixth rib and then secured medially with wire sutures into previously created sternal notches and with wire to the native ribs laterally. Ribs are split as shown along their short axis to maintain maximal mechanical strength. *(From Shamberger RC, Welch KJ, Upton J III. J Pediatr Surg 1989;**24**:760-5, with permission.)*

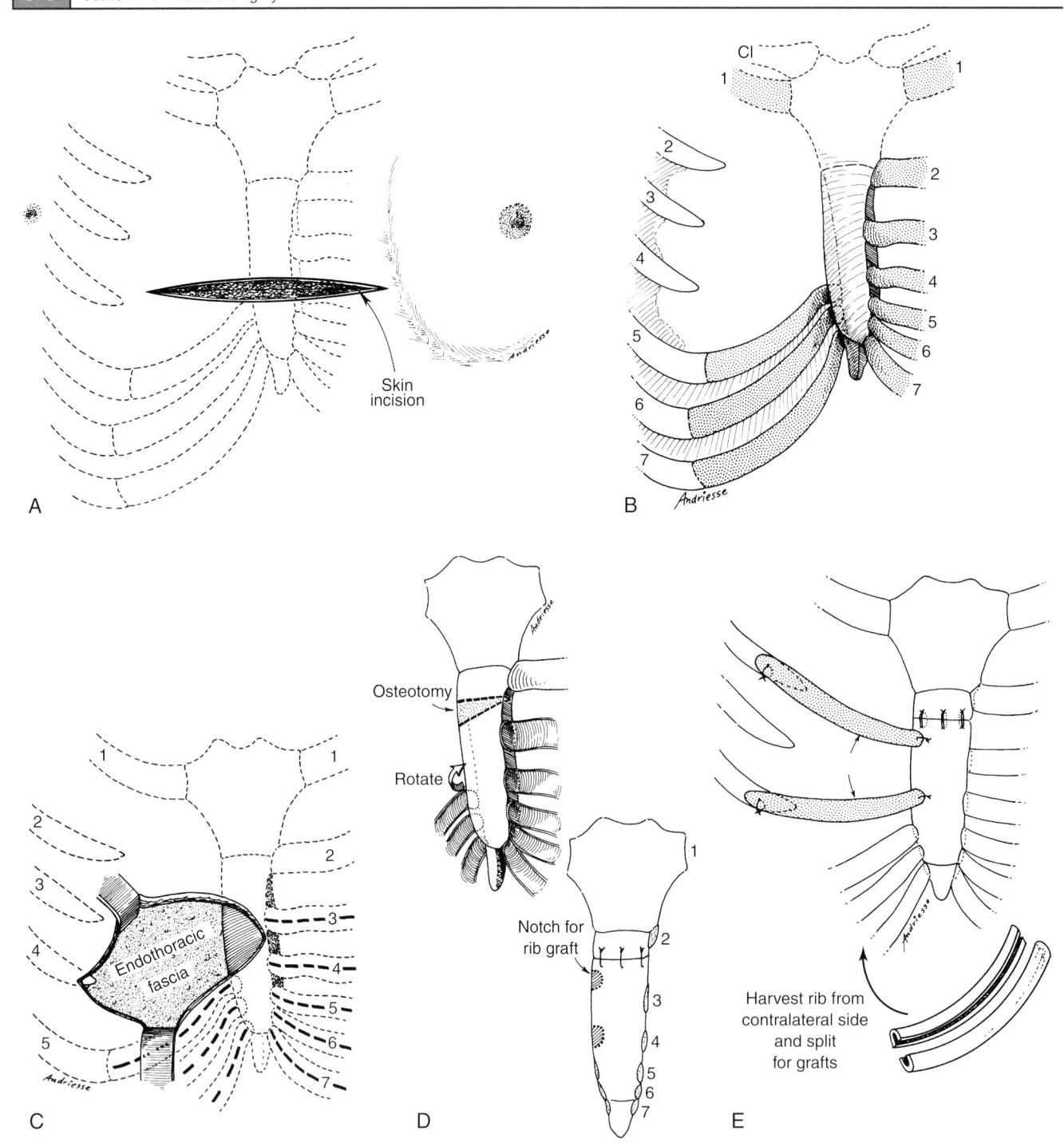

Table 24–7
Sternal Defects Reported in 109 Cases of Cleft Sternum

Sternal Defect	Number of Cases
Upper cleft	46
Upper cleft to xiphoid	33
Complete cleft	23
Lower defect with manubrium or mid-segment intact	5
Central defect with manubrium and xiphoid intact	2
Skin ulceration noted in only three of 109 cases	3

From Shamberger RC, Welch KJ. Pediatr Surg Int 1990;5:156-64, with permission.

with pectoral muscle flaps. The pericardium was divided from its anterior attachments to the chest wall, allowing the heart to fall back partially into the thoracic cavity. Only Amato and colleagues achieved complete coverage of the heart in one stage.[166] The unifying theme of successfully managed cases is mobilization of adequate soft tissue to cover the heart in its extrathoracic location and avoiding attempts to return the heart to an orthotopic location. Of note, in the successful cases, intrinsic cardiac lesions and associated abdominal defects were absent. These are the characteristics that most distinguish the successes from the failures, rather than any differences in surgical techniques. Coverage of the heart with autologous tissues, whether by flap rotation or bipedicle flaps, generally produces excessive compression on the heart, which limits cardiac output either by kinking outflow vessels or impeding cardiac filling. In most instances, attempts are abandoned in the operating room because of severe impairment of cardiac function. In patients who are repaired with autologous tissue grafts (bone or cartilage) or synthetic materials, infection

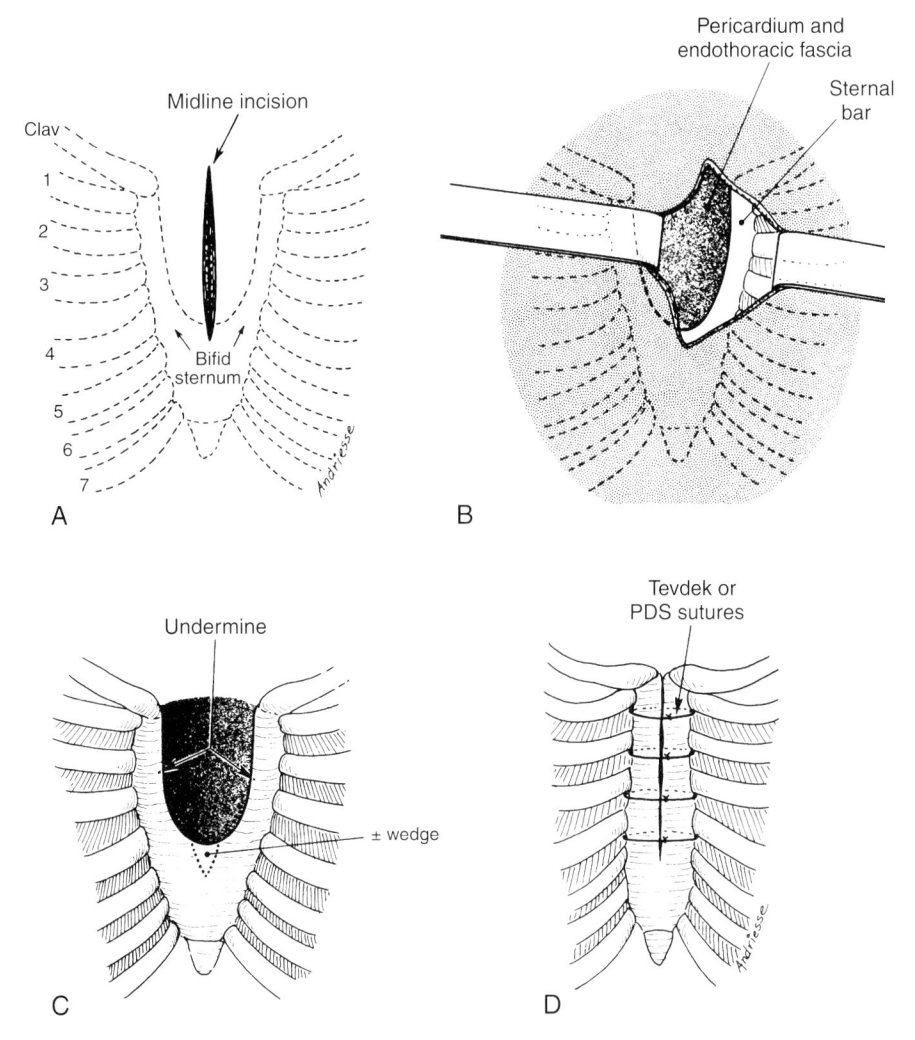

Figure 24–16
Repair of cleft sternum. **A,** Repair of bifid sternum is best performed through a longitudinal incision extending the length of the defect. **B,** Directly beneath the subcutaneous tissues, the sternal bars are encountered, with pectoral muscles present lateral to the bars. **C,** The endothoracic fascia is mobilized off the sternal bars posteriorly with blunt dissection to allow safe placement of the sutures. Approximation of the sternal bars may be facilitated by excising a wedge of cartilage inferiorly. **D,** Closure of the defect is achieved with 2-0 Tevdek or PDS (Ethicon, Somerville, NJ) sutures. (From Shamberger RC, Welch KJ. Pediatr Surg Int 1990;5:156-64, with permission.)

Table 24–8
Methods of Repair of Cleft Sternum in 69 Cases

Method of Repair	Number of Cases
Primary approximation and repair	25
Primary repair with sliding chondrotomies (Sabiston)	19
Primary repair with rotating chondrotomies (Meissner)	3
Primary repair with other chondrotomy	4
Bone or cartilage graft	8
Prosthetic mesh graft	4
Sternocleidomastoid muscle transposition	3
Transposition of local soft tissues	2
Skin closure with excision of ulcer	1

From Shamberger RC, Welch KJ. Pediatr Surg Int 1990;**5**:156-64, with permission.

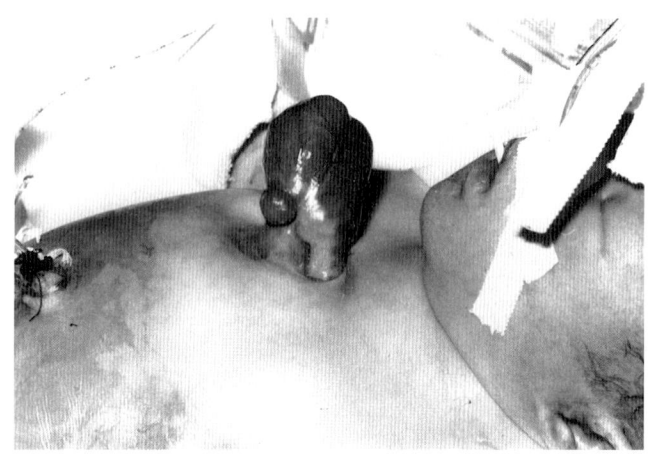

Figure 24–17
An infant with thoracic ectopia cordis with no abdominal wall defect. The cardiac apex is cephalad. Any movement of the heart results in bradycardia and arrest. The patient had complex tetralogy of Fallot.

Table 24–9
Intrinsic Cardiac Lesions Reported: 75 Cases of Thoracic Ectopia Cordis

Cardiac Lesion	Number of Cases
Tetralogy of Fallot	16
Pulmonary artery stenosis	6
Transposition of great arteries and pulmonary artery stenosis or atresia	8
Patent ductus arteriosus (PDA)	2
Tricuspid and pulmonary atresia	3
Ventricular septal defect (VSD) and atrial septal defect (ASD)	6
VSD	5
ASD and PDA	4
ASD	1
Truncus arteriosus	3
Coarctation, ASD, and PDA	1
Coarctation	1
Aortic hypoplasia	1
Double-outlet left ventricle	2
Double-outlet right ventricle	2
Aortic stenosis, ASD, and PDA	1
Single atrium, single ventricle	3
Double atrium, single ventricle	3
Cor triatriatum	1
Aberrant right subclavian artery	1
Bilateral superior vena cava*	1
Normal	4

*Also present in association with many of the listed anomalies.
From Shamberger RC, Welch KJ. Pediatr Surg Int 1990;**5**:156-64, with permission.

and extrusion of the graft invariably occur. Ultimate success with this lesion will be achieved only by accomplishing tissue coverage of the heart that avoids posterior displacement into an already limited thoracic space. This will require use of tissues from sites distant from the chest wall or engineered tissue materials. Severe intracardiac defects associated with thoracic ectopia cordis in most cases also limit survival. The only recent advancement in management of this lesion has been early ultrasonographic diagnosis, including definition of the intracardiac lesion and termination of the pregnancy, if acceptable to the parents.[167,168]

Abdominal wall defects are also frequent in these patients, including an upper abdominal omphalocele or diastasis recti and, rarely, eventration of the abdominal viscera (Fig. 24-18). Associated abdominal wall defects are summarized in Table 24-11. The presence of abdominal defects should not, however, lead to classification of these lesions as thoracoabdominal ectopia cordis. This term should be reserved for those infants in whom the heart is covered at birth.

Thoracoabdominal Ectopia Cordis (Cantrell's Pentalogy)

In thoracoabdominal ectopia cordis, the heart is covered by an omphalocele-like membrane or thin skin, which is often pigmented. The sternum is generally cleft inferiorly, and the heart lacks the severe anterior rotation present in thoracic ectopia cordis. An early report of this lesion by Wilson[168a] in 1798 clearly defined the associated somatic defects of the abdominal wall, diaphragm, and pericardium (Fig. 24-19), as well as

Table 24-10
Reported Survivors of Thoracic Ectopia Cordis and Method of Repair

Author (ref)	Year	Lesion	Method of Sternal Closure
Koop (Saxena, 164)	1975	None	Skin flap closure at 5 hr. Acrylic resin applied to sternal cleft at 7 months.
Dobell et al. (165)	1982	None	Perinatal skin closure in one stage. Second-stage repair with skin grafts.
Amato et al. (166)	1988	None	Skin flaps mobilized, diaphragm moved inferiorly, Gore-Tex* membrane used to close defect with skin flaps over it. Child survived, but died of aspiration at 11 months of age.

*Gore-Tex: WL Gore, Flagstaff, AZ.
From Shamberger RC, Welch KJ. Pediatr Surg Int 1990;5:156-64, with permission.

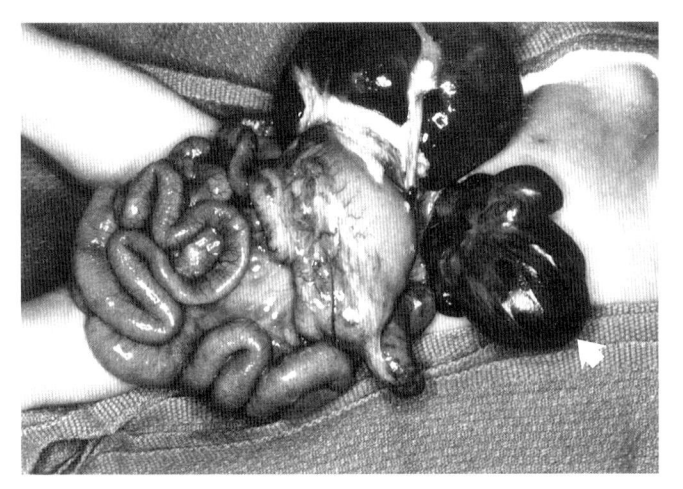

Figure 24-18
Infant with thoracic ectopia cordis (arrow) and eventration of the abdominal viscera. (From Shamberger RC, Welch KJ. Pediatr Surg Int 1990;**5**:156-64, with permission.)

Table 24-11
Abdominal Wall Defects Reported in 75 Cases of Thoracic Ectopia Cordis

Abdominal Wall Defect	Number of Cases
Omphalocele	36
Diastasis recti (or ventral hernia)*	6
Eventration	4

*Often covered by thin, pigmented dermis.
From Shamberger RC, Welch KJ. Pediatr Surg Int 1990;**5**:156-64, with permission.

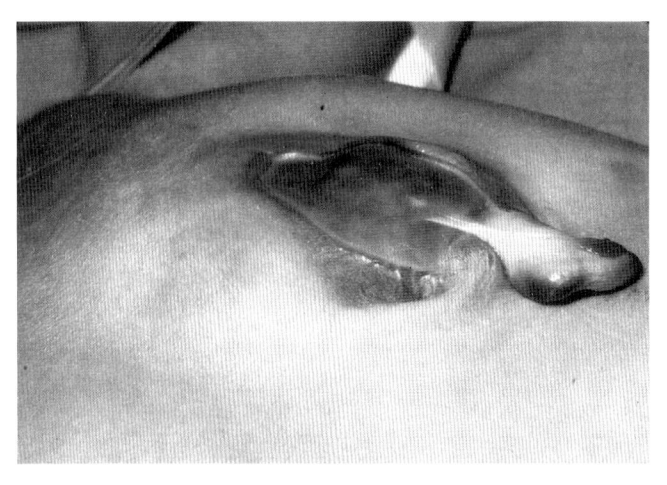

Figure 24-19
Male newborn with thoracoabdominal ectopia cordis. The head is to the left. Note the epigastric omphalocele extending superior to the umbilicus. The cardiac apex was visible below the costal arch just at the superior aspect of the omphalocele.

the intrinsic cardiac anomalies. This entity was subsequently reviewed by Major[169] in 1953 and Cantrell and associates[150] in 1958. It is now frequently called Cantrell's pentalogy, although it was described long before Cantrell's relatively recent review. The five essential features of thoracoabdominal ectopia cordis are a cleft lower sternum, a half moon–shaped anterior diaphragmatic defect resulting from lack of development of the septum transversum, absence of the parietal pericardium at the diaphragmatic defect, omphalocele (Table 24-12), and, in most patients, an intrinsic cardiac anomaly (Table 24-13; see Fig. 24-19). A left ventricular diverticulum occurs with surprising frequency in this anomaly. In many cases, the diverticulum protrudes through the diaphragmatic and pericardial defects into the abdominal cavity.

Successful repair and long-term survival are more frequent in thoracoabdominal ectopia cordis than in thoracic ectopia cordis. Arndt attempted the first repair in 1896, but return of the heart to the thoracic cavity resulted in death.[170] Wieting performed the first successful surgical repair in 1912.[171] He achieved primary closure of the diaphragm and abdominal wall fascia but ignored the ventricular diverticulum. Initial surgical intervention must address the skin defects overlying the heart and abdominal cavity. Primary excision of the omphalocele with skin closure avoids infection and mediastinitis, although several cases have been successfully managed by local application of topical astringents, thus allowing

Table 24-12
Abdominal Wall Defects Reported in Patients with Thoracoabdominal Ectopia Cordis

Abdominal Wall Defect	Number of Cases
Omphalocele	64
Diastasis recti (or ventral hernia)	40
Diaphragmatic defect	71
Pericardial defect	46

From Shamberger RC, Welch KJ. Pediatr Surg Int 1990;**5**:156-64, with permission.

Table 24-13
Intrinsic Cardiac Lesions Reported in Patients with Thoracoabdominal Ectopia Cordis

Cardiac Lesion	Number of Cases
Tetralogy of Fallot	13
Tetralogy of Fallot and diverticulum of left ventricle	1
Diverticulum of left ventricle	16
Diverticulum of left ventricle and VSD	9
Diverticulum of left ventricle, pulmonary stenosis, and VSD	1
Diverticulum of left ventricle and ASD	1
Diverticulum of left ventricle, ASD, and VSD	1
Diverticulum of left ventricle, VSD, and mitral stenosis	1
Diverticulum left ventricle, hypoplastic left ventricle, and VSD	1
VSD	8
VSD and ASD	2
VSD and single atrium	1
ASD	3
ASD, VSD, and total anomalous pulmonary venous connection	1
Truncus arteriosus	5
Single atrium and single ventricle	5
Pulmonary atresia and single ventricle	2
Pulmonary atresia, VSD, and PDA	1
Pulmonary stenosis and VSD	3
Tricuspid atresia	4
Double-outlet left ventricle	2
Double-outlet right ventricle	2
Transposition of the great arteries, mitral atresia, and pulmonary artery hypoplasia	1
Transposition of the great arteries and pulmonary artery stenosis	2
Transposition great arteries and VSD	1
Aortic stenosis, ASD, and VSD	1
Bilateral superior vena cava	1
Normal	5

*Also present in association with many of the listed anomalies.
ASD, atrial septal defect; PDA, patent ductus arteriosus; VSD, ventricular septal defect.
From Shamberger RC, Welch KJ. Pediatr Surg Int 1990;**5**:156-64, with permission.

secondary epithelialization to occur. Several early cases, such as in that of Cullerier in 1806, document the long-term viability of individuals with thoracoabdominal ectopia cordis with intact skin coverage despite the abnormal location and coverage of the heart.[172]

Advances in cardiac surgery now allow correction of the intrinsic cardiac lesions, which were previously fatal. An aggressive approach to repair in infants with thoracoabdominal ectopia cordis is appropriate. Repair of the abdominal wall defect or diastasis has been achieved by primary closure or prosthetic mesh (Table 24-14). Primary closure of the thoracoabdominal defect may be difficult to achieve because of the wide separation of the rectus muscles and their superior attachment to the costal arches. Complete repair of the intracardiac defect is best performed before placement of prosthetic mesh overlying the heart. Repair of the abdomen and chest wall is important, primarily for mechanical protection of the heart and abdominal viscera. Early diagnosis by prenatal ultrasound has not altered the surgical approach or overall mortality of this lesion. Three cases in the Children's Hospital Boston series had severe pulmonary hypoplasia, which was lethal in two; this was a previously unreported association.[144]

THORACIC DEFORMITIES IN DIFFUSE SKELETAL DISORDERS

Asphyxiating Thoracic Dystrophy (Jeune's Disease)

In 1954, Jeune and colleagues described a newborn with a narrow rigid chest and multiple cartilage anomalies.[173] The patient died of respiratory insufficiency early in the perinatal period. Subsequent authors have further characterized this form of osteochondrodystrophy, which has variable degrees of skeletal involvement. It is inherited in an autosomal recessive pattern and is not associated with chromosomal abnormalities. Its most prominent feature is a narrow, bell-shaped thorax and protuberant abdomen. The thorax is narrow in both the transverse and sagittal axes and has little respiratory motion because of the horizontal direction of the ribs (Fig. 24-20). The ribs are short and wide, and the splayed costochondral junctions barely reach the anterior axillary line. The costal cartilage is abundant and irregular, like a rachitic rosary. Microscopic examination of the costochondral junction demonstrates disordered and poorly progressing endochondral ossification, resulting in decreased rib length.

Table 24–14
Reported Methods of Repair of Thoracoabdominal Ectopia Cordis

Method of Repair	Number of Cases
Primary closure of diaphragm and abdominal wall defect	8
Primary closure of skin only and excision of omphalocele	7
Primary closure of diaphragm	4
Primary closure of abdominal wall defect	2
Coverage of abdominal defect with Silastic pouch and secondary epithelialization	3
Resection of lower ribs and sternum to increase room in chest with inferior attachment of diaphragm and primary skin coverage	1
Staged repair with initial skin closure with secondary prosthetic mesh closure of the abdominal and thoracic defect	1
Staged repair with initial skin closure with secondary closure of abdominal wall and diaphragm	1

From Shamberger RC, Welch KJ. Pediatr Surg Int 1990;**5**:156-64, with permission.

Skeletal abnormalities associated with this syndrome include short stubby extremities with relatively short and wide bones. The clavicles are in a fixed and elevated position, and the pelvis is small and hypoplastic, with square iliac bones.

The syndrome has a variable extent of pulmonary impairment. Although the initial reported cases resulted in neonatal deaths, subsequent reports by Kozlowski and Masel and others have documented that infants can survive for longer intervals of time with this syndrome.[174] The pathology findings in autopsy cases reveal a range of abnormal pulmonary development. In most cases, the bronchial development is normal and there are fewer alveolar divisions, as described by Williams and associates.[175]

Spondylothoracic Dysplasia (Jarcho-Levin Syndrome)

Spondylothoracic dysplasia is an autosomal recessive deformity with multiple vertebral and rib malformations, described by Jarcho and Levin in 1938.[176] Infants and children with this syndrome have multiple alternating hemivertebrae in most, if not all, of the thoracic and lumbar spine. The vertebral ossification centers rarely cross the midline, although bone formation is normal. Multiple posterior fusions of the ribs and remarkable shortening of the thoracic spine result in a crablike appearance of the ribs on the chest radiograph (Fig. 24-21).

The thoracic deformity is secondary to the spine anomaly, which results in close posterior approximation of the origin of the ribs. Although most infants with the entity succumb before 15 months of age, as reviewed by Roberts and colleagues,

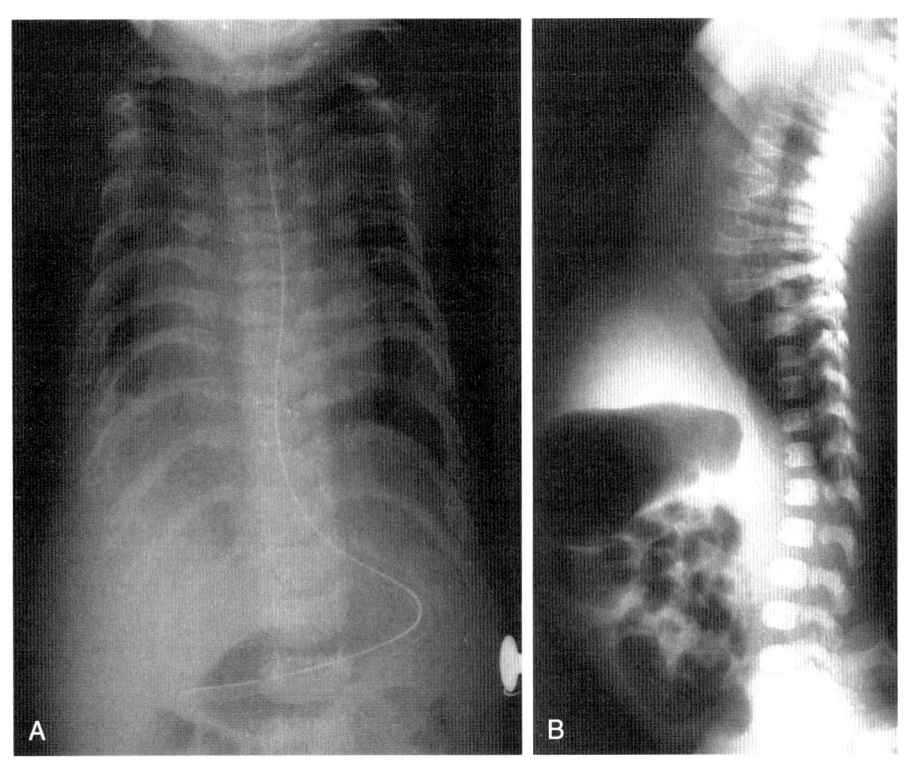

Figure 24–20
Jeune's disease (asphyxiating thoracic dystrophy). **A**, Anteroposterior radiograph shows short horizontal ribs and narrow chest. **B**, Lateral radiograph demonstrates that the short ribs end at the midaxillary line. Abnormal flaring at the costochondral junctions is also present. The patient died of progressive respiratory insufficiency at 1 month of age. There was no surgical intervention. Postmortem examination revealed alveolar hypoplasia.

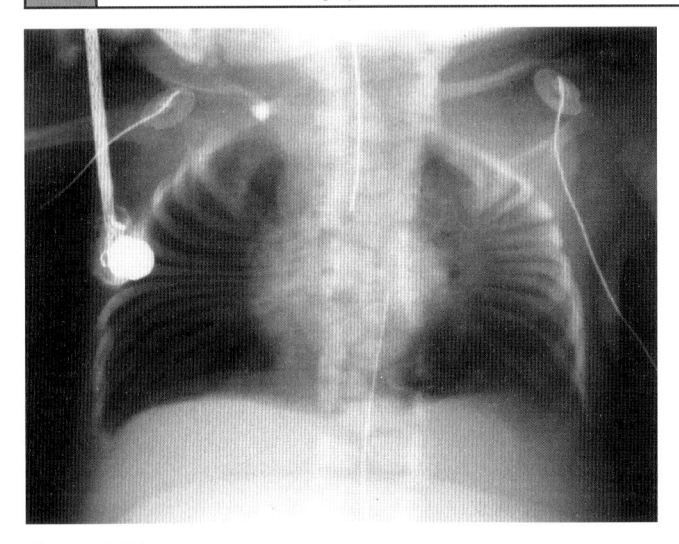

Figure 24–21
Chest radiograph of an infant with spondylothoracic dysplasia. Severe abnormality of the spine is apparent, with multiple alternating hemivertebrae producing a crablike configuration of the ribs.

no surgical efforts have been proposed or attempted.[177] One third of patients with this syndrome have associated malformations, including congenital heart disease and renal anomalies. Heilbronner and Renshaw have reported its occurrence primarily in Puerto Rican families (15 of 18 cases).[178]

REFERENCES

1. Hümmer H, Willital GH. Morphologic findings of chest deformities in children corresponding to the Willital-Hummer classification. *J Pediatr Surg* 1984;**19**:562-6.
2. von der Oelsnitz G. Anomalies of the chest (author's translation). *Z Kinderchir* 1981;**33**:229-36.
3. Welch KJ. Chest wall deformities. In: Holder TH, Ashcraft K, editors. *Pediatric surgery*. Philadelphia: WB Saunders; 1980. p. 162-82.
4. Haller JJ, Kramer S, Lietman S. Use of CT scans in selection of patients for pectus excavatum surgery: a preliminary report. *J Pediatr Surg* 1987;**22**:904-6.
5. Lawson M, Barnes-Eley M, Burke B, et al. Reliability of a standardized protocol to calculate cross-sectional chest area and severity indices to evaluate pectus excavatum. *J Pediatr Surg* 2006;**41**:1219-25.
6. Waters P, Welch K, Micheli L, et al. Scoliosis in children with pectus excavatum and pectus carinatum. *J Pediatr Orthop* 1989;**9**:551-6.
7. Shamberger R, Welch K. Cardiopulmonary function in pectus excavatum. *Surg Gynecol Obstet* 1988;**166**:383-91.
8. Shamberger R, Welch K. Chest wall deformities. In: Ashcraft KW, Holder TM, editors. *Pediatric surgery*. 2nd ed Philadelphia: WB Saunders; 1993. p. 146-62.
9. Ravitch M. *Congenital deformities of the chest wall and their operative correction*. Philadelphia: WB Saunders; 1977.
10. Lester C. The etiology and pathogenesis of funnel chest, pigeon chest, and related deformities of the anterior chest wall. *J Thorac Surg* 1957;**34**:1-0.
11. Greig J, Azmy A. Thoracic cage deformity: a late complication following repair of an agenesis of diaphragm. *J Pediatr Surg* 1990;**25**:1234-5.
12. Vanamo K, Peltonen J, Rintala R, et al. Chest wall and spinal deformities in adults with congenital diaphragmatic defects. *J Pediatr Surg* 1996;**31**:851-4.
13. Hecker W, Procher G, Dietz H. Results of operative correction of pigeon and funnel chest following a modified procedure of Ravitch and Haller (author's translation). *Z Kinderchir* 1981;**34**:220-7.
14. Shamberger R, Welch K. Surgical repair of pectus excavatum. *J Pediatr Surg* 1988;**23**:615-22.
15. Creswick H, Stacey M, Kelly RJ, et al. Family study of the inheritance of pectus excavatum. *J Pediatr Surg* 2006;**41**:1699-703.
16. Scherer L, Arn P, Dressel D, et al. Surgical management of children and young adults with Marfan syndrome and pectus excavatum. *J Pediatr Surg* 1988;**23**:1169-72.
17. Welch K, Kraney G. Abdominal musculature deficiency syndrome prune belly. *J Urol* 1974;**111**:693-700.
18. Sauerbruch F. *Die Chirurgie der Brustorgane*. Berlin: Springer; 1920.
19. Lawson M, Mellins R, Tabangin M. Impact of pectus excavatum on pulmonary function before and after repair with the Nuss procedure. *J Pediatr Surg* 2005;**40**:174-80.
20. Schaub V, Wegmann T. Elektrokardiographische veranderungen bei trichterbrust. *Cardiologia* 1954;**24**:39-46.
21. Brown A, Cook O. Cardio-respiratory studies in pre and postoperative funnel chest. *Dis Chest* 1951;**20**:378-91.
22. Weg J, Krumholz R, Harkleroad L. Pulmonary dysfunction in pectus excavatum. *Am Rev Respir Dis* 1967;**96**:936-45.
23. Castile R, Staats B, Westbrook P. Symptomatic pectus deformities of the chest. *A Rev Respir Dis* 1982;**126**:564-8.
24. Cahill J, Lees G, Robertson H. A summary of preoperative and postoperative cardiorespiratory performance in patients undergoing pectus excavatum and carinatum repair. *J Pediatr Surg* 1984;**19**:430-3.
25. Mead J, Sly P, Le Souef P, Hibbert M, Phelan P. Rib cage mobility in pectus excavatum. *Am Rev Respir Dis* 1985;**132**:1223-8.
26. Blickman J, Rosen PR, Welch KJ, Papanicolaou N, Treves ST. Pectus excavatum in children. *Radiology* 1985;**156**:781-2.
27. Derveaux L, Clarysse I, Ivanoff I, et al. Preoperative and postoperative abnormalities in chest x-ray indices and in lung function in pectus deformities. *Chest* 1989;**95**:850-6.
28. Morshuis W, Folgering H, Barentsz J, et al. Pulmonary function before surgery for pectus excavatum and at long-term follow-up. *Chest* 1994;**105**:1646-52.
29. Derveaux L, Ivanoff I, Rochette F, Demedts M. Mechanism of pulmonary function changes after surgical correction for funnel chest. *Eur Respir J* 1988;**1**:823-5.
30. Wynn S, Driscoll D, Ostrom N, et al. Exercise cardiorespiratory function in adolescents with pectus excavatum. *J Thorac Cardiovasc Surg* 1990;**99**:41-7.
31. Kaguraoka H, Ohnuki T, Itaoka T, et al. Degree of severity of pectus excavatum and pulmonary function in preoperative and postoperative periods. *J Thorac Cardiovasc Surg* 1991;**104**:1483-8.
32. Tanaka F, Kitano M, Shindo T, Huang CL, Nagasawa M, Tatsumi A. Postoperative lung function in patients with funnel chest. *Nippon Kyobu Geka Gakkai Zasshi* 1993;**41**:2161-5.
33. Morshius W, Folgering H, Barentsz J, et al. Exercise cardiorespiratory function before and one year after operation for pectus excavatum. *J Thorac Cardiovasc Surg* 1994;**107**:1403-9.
34. Quigley P, Haller JJ, Jelus K, et al. Cardiorespiratory function before and after corrective surgery in pectus excavatum. *J Pediatr* 1996;**128**:638-43.
35. Borowitz D, Cerny F, Zallen G. Pulmonary function and exercise response in patients with pectus excavatum after Nuss repair. *J Pediatr Surg* 2003;**38**:544-7.
36. Sigalet D, Montgomery M, Harder J. Cardiopulmonary effects of closed repair of pectus excavatum. *J Pediatr Surg* 2003;**38**:380-5.
37. Aronson D, Bosgraaf R, Merz E, et al. Lung function after minimal invasive pectus excavatum repair (Nuss procedure). *World J Surg* 1007;**31**:1518-22.
38. Malek M, Berger D, Marelich W, et al. Pulmonary function following surgical repair of pectus excavatum: a meta-analysis. *Eur J Cardiothorac surg* 2006;**30**:637-43.
39. Malek M, Fonkalsrud E, Cooper C. Ventilatory and cardiovascular responses to exercise in patients with pectus excavatum. *Chest* 2003;**124**:870-82.
40. Garusi G. D'Éttorre A. Angiocardiographic patterns in funnel-chest. *Cardiologia* 1964;**45**:313-30.
41. Howard R. Funnel chest: its effect on cardiac function. *Arch Dis Child* 1959;**32**:5-7.
42. Bevegård S. Postural circulatory changes at rest and during exercise in patients with pectus excavatum. *Acta Med Scan* 1962;**171**:695-713.
43. Gattiker H, Bühlmann A. Cardiopulmonary function and exercise tolerance in supine and sitting position in patients with pectus excavatum. *Helv Med Acta* 1966;**33**:122-38.
44. Beiser G, Epstein S, Stampfer M, et al. Impairment of cardiac function in patients with pectus excavatum, with improvement after operative correction. *N Engl J Med* 1972;**287**:267-72.
45. Peterson R, Young Jr W, Godwin J, et al. Noninvasive assessment of exercise cardiac function before and after pectus excavatum repair. *J Thorac Cardiovasc Surg* 1985;**90**:251-60.
46. Kowalewski J, Brocki M, Dryjanski T, et al. Pectus excavatum: increase of right ventricular systolic, diastolic, and stroke volumes after surgical repair. *J Thorac Cardiovasc Surg* 1999;**118**:92-3:Discussion.
47. Malek M, Berger D, Housh T, et al. Cardiovascular function following surgical repair of pectus excavatum: A metaanalysis. *Chest* 2006;**130**:506-16.
48. Bon Tempo C, Ronan Jr J, de Leon Jr A, et al. Radiographic appearance of the thorac in systolic click-late systolic murmur syndrome. *Am J Cardiol* 1975;**31**:27-31.
49. Salomon J, Shah P, Heinle R. Thoracic skeletal abnormalities in idiopathic mitral valve prolapse. *Am J Cardiol* 1975;**36**:32-6.

50. Schutte J, Gaffney F, Blend L, et al. Distinctive anthropometric characteristics of women with mitral vale prolapse. *Am J Med* 1981;**71**:533-8.
51. Udoshi M, Shah A, Fisher V, et al. Incidence of mitral valve prolapse in subjects with thoracic skeletal abnormalities—a prospective study. *Am Heart J* 1979;**97**:303-11.
52. Saint-Mezard G, Duret J, Chanudet X, et al. Mitral vale prolapse and pectus excavatum. Fortuitous association or syndrome? *Presse Med* 1986;**15**:439.
53. Shamberger RC, Welch KJ, Sanders SP. Mitral valve prolapse associated with pectus excavatum. *J Pediatr* 1987;**111**(3):404-7.
54. Coln E, Carrasco J, Coln D. Demonstrating relief of cardiac compression with the Nuss minimally invasive repair for pectus excavatum. *J Pediatr Surg* 2006;**41**:683-6.
55. Meyer L. Zur Chirurgischen behandlung der angeborenen trichterbrust. *Verh Berliner Med Gesellschaft* 1911;**42**:364-73.
56. Ochsner A, DeBakey M. Chone-chondrosternon: report of a case and review of the literature. *J Thorac Surg* 1939;**8**:469-511.
57. Ravitch M. The operative treatment of pectus excavatum. *Ann Surg* 1949;**129**:429-44.
58. Baronofsky I. Technique for the correction of pectus excavatum. *Surgery* 1957;**42**:884-90.
59. Welch K. Satisfactory surgical correction of pectus excavatum deformity in childhood: a limited opportunity. *J Thorac Surg* 1980;**36**:697-713.
60. Haller JJ, Peters G, Mazur D, et al. Pectus excavatum: a 20 year surgical experience. *J Thorac Cardiovasc Surg* 1970;**60**:375-83.
61. Rehbein F. The operative treatment of the funnel chest. *Arch Dis Child* 1957;**32**:5-8.
62. Paltia V. Operative technique in funnel chest: experience in 81 cases. *Acta Chir Scan* 1958;**116**:90-8.
63. Adkins P, Blades B. A stainless steel strut for correction of pectus excavatum. *Surg Gynecol Obstet* 1961;**113**:111-3.
63a. Jensen NK, Schmidt WR, Garamella JJ, Lynch MF. Pectus excavatum and carinatum: the how, when, and why of surgical correction. *J Pediatr Surg* 1970;**5**:4-13.
64. Willital G. Indication and operative technique in chest deformities. *Z Kinderchir* 1981;**33**:244-52.
65. Lansman S, Serlo W, Linna O, et al. Treatment of pectus excavatum with bioabsorbable polylactide plates: preliminary results. *J Pediatr Surg* 2002;**37**:1281-6.
66. Robicsek F, Fokin A. Surgical correction of pectus excavatum and carinatum. *J Thorac Cardiovasc Surg (Torino)* 1999;**40**:725-31.
67. Judet J, Judet R. Thorax en entonnoir. Un procede operatoire. *Rev Orthop* 1954;**40**:248-57.
68. Jung A. Le traitement du thorax en entoinnoir par le "retournement pedicule" de la cuvette sterno-chondrale. *Mem Acad Cir* 1956;**82**:242-9.
69. Wada J, Ikeda K, Ishida T, et al. Results of 271 funnel chest operations. *Ann Thorac Surg* 1970;**10**:526-32.
70. Taguchi K, Mochizuki T, Nakagaki N, et al. A new plastic operation for pectus excavatum: sternal turnover surgical procedure with preserved internal mammary vessels. *Chest* 1975;**67**:606-8.
71. Allen R, Douglas M. Cosmetic improvement of thoracic wall defects using a rapid setting Silastic mold: a special technique. *J Pediatr Surg* 1979;**14**:745-9.
72. Wechselberger G, Ohlbauer M, Haslinger J, Schoeller T. Silicone implant correction of pectus excavatum. *Ann Plast Surg* 2001;**47**:489-93.
73. Schier F, Bahr M, Klobe E. The vacuum chest wall lifter: an innovative, nonsurgical addition to the management of pectus excavatum. *J Pediatr Surg* 2005;**40**:496-500.
74. Haecker F, Mayr J. The vacuum bell for treatment of pectus excavatum: an alternative to surgical correction? *Eur J Cardiothorac surg* 2006;**29**:557-61.
75. Nuss D, Kelly RJ, Croitoru D, et al. A 10-year review of a minimally invasive technique for the correction of pectus excavatum. *J Pediatr Surg* 2998;**33**:545-52.
76. Hebra A, Jacobs J, Feliz A, et al. Minimally invasive repair of pectus excavatum in adult patients. *American Surgeon* 2006;**72**:837-42.
77. Croitoru D, Kelly RJ, Goretsky J, et al. Experience and modification update for the minimally invasive Nuss technique for pectus excavatum repair in 303 patients. *J Pediatr Surg* 2002;**37**:437-45.
78. Shin S, Goretsky J, Kelly RJ, et al. Infectious complications after the Nuss repair in a series of 863 patients. *J Pediatr Sug* 2007;**42**:87-92.
79. Van Renterghem K, von Bismarck S, Bax N, et al. Should an infected Nuss bar be removed? *J Pediatr Surg* 2005;**40**:670-3.
80. Calkins C, Shew S, Sharp R, et al. Management of postoperative infections after the minimally invasive pectus excavatum repair. *J Pediatr Surg* 2005;**40**:1004-8.
81. Rushing GD, Goretsky MJ, Gustin T, Morales M, Kelly Jr RE, Nuss D. When it is not an infection: metal allergy after the Nuss procedure for repair of pectus excavatum. *J Pediatr Surg* 2007;**42**:93-7.
82. Ostlie D, Marosky J, Spilde T, et al. Evaluation of pectus bar position and osseous bone formation. *J Pediatr Surg* 2003;**38**(June):953-6.
83. Hebra A, Swoveland B, Egbert M, et al. Outcome analysis of minimally invasive repair of pectus excavatum: review of 251 cases. *J Pediatr Surg* 2000;**35**:252-7.
84. Engum S, Rescorla F, West K, et al. Is the grass greener? Early results of Nuss procedure. *J Pediatr Surg* 2000;**35**(2):51-246:discussion 257–8.
85. Molik K, Egum S, Rescorla F, et al. Pectus excavatum repair: experience with standard and minimal invasive techniques. *J Pediatr Surg* 2001;**36**:324-8.
86. Fonkalsrud E, Beanes S, Hebra A, et al. Comparison of minimally invasive and modified Ravitch pectus excavatum repair. *J Pediatr Surg* 2002;**37**:413-7.
87. Hebra A. Pectus carinatum as a sequela of minimally invasive pectus excavatum repair. *Pediatr Endosurg & Innovative Techniques* 2002;**6**:41-4.
88. Leonhardt J, Kulber J, Feiter J, et al. Complications of the minimally invasive repair of pectus excavatum. *J Pediatr Surg* 2005;**40**:E7-9.
89. Hoel T, Rein K, Svennevig J. A life-threatening complication of the Nuss-procedure for pectus excavatum. *Ann Thorac Surg* 2004;**81**:370-2.
90. Barsness K, Bruny J, Janik J, Partrick D. Delayed near-fatal hemorrhage after Nuss bar displacement. *J Pediatr Surg* 2005;**40**:E5-6.
91. Kelly RJ, Shamberger R, Mellins R, et al. Prospective multicenter study of surgical correction of pectus excavatum: design, perioperative complications, pain, and baseline pulmonary function facilitated by internet-based data collection. *J Am Coll Surg* 2007;**205**:205-16.
92. Hougaard K, Arendrup H. Deformities of the female breasts after surgery for funnel chest. *Scan J Thorac Cardiovasc Surg* 1983;**17**:171-4.
93. Ellis D, Snyder C, Mann C. The "re-do" chest wall deformity correction. *J Pediatr Surg* 1997;**32**:1267-71.
94. Humphreys GH 2nd, Jaretzki A 3rd. Pectus excavatum: late results with and without operation. *J Thorac Cardiovasc Surg* 1980;**80**:686-95.
95. Backer OG, Brunner S, Larsen V. The surgical treatment of funnel chest: initial and follow-up results. *Acta Chir Scand* 1961;**121**:253-61.
96. Sanger P, Robicsek F, Daaugherty H. The repair of recurrent pectus excavatum. *J Thorac Cardiovasc Surg* 1968;**56**:141-3.
97. Miller K, Ostlie D, Wade K, et al. Minimally invasive bar repair for "redo" correction of pectus excavatum. *J Pediatr Surg* 2002;**37**:1090-2.
98. Croitoru D, Kelly RJ, Goretsky J, et al. The minimally invasive Nuss technique for recurrent or failed pectus excavatum repair in 50 patients. *J Pediatr Surg* 2005;**40**:181-7.
99. Martinez D, Juame J, Stein T. The effect of costal cartilage resection on chest wall development. *Pediatr Surg Int* 1990;**5**:170-3.
100. Haller JA Jr, Columbani P, Humphries C, et al. Chest wall constriction after too extensive and too early operations for pectus excavatum. *Ann Thorac Surg* 1996;**61**:1618-24.
101. Weber T, Kurkchubasche A. Operative management of asphyxiating thoracic dystrophy after pectus repair. *J Pediatr Surg* 1998;**33**:262-5.
102. Weber T. Further experience with the operative management of asphyxiating thoracic dystrophy after pectus repair. *J Pediatr Surg* 2005;**40**:170-3.
103. Shochat S, Csongradi J, Hartman G, et al. Moire photopography in the evaluation of anterior chest wall deformities. *J Pediatr Surg* 1981;**16**:353-7.
104. Shamberger RC, Welch KJ. Surgical correction of pectus carinatum. *J Pediatr Surg* 1987;**22**:48-53.
105. Brodkin H. Congenital chondrosternal prominence (pigeon breast): a new interpretation. *Pediatrics* 1949;**3**:286-95.
106. Howard R. Pigeon chest (protrusion deformity of the sternum). *Med J Aust* 1958;**45**:664-6.
107. Currarino G, Silverman F. Premature obliteration of the sternal sutures and pigeon-breast deformity. *Radiology* 1958;**70**:532-40.
108. Lees R, Caldicott J. Sternal anomalies and congenital heart disease. *Am J Roentgenol Radium Ther Nucl Med* 1975;**124**:423-7.
109. Ravitch M. Unusual sternal deformity with cardiac symptoms: operative correction. *J Thorac Surg* 1952;**23**:138-44.
110. Lester C. Pigeon breast (pectus carinatum) and other protrusion deformities of the chest of developmental origin. *Ann Surg* 1953;**137**:482-9.
111. Chin E. Surgery of funnel chest and congenital sternal prominence. *Br J Surg* 1957;**44**:360-76.
112. Brodkin H. Pigeon breast: congenital chondrosternal prominence. *Arch Surg* 1958;**77**:261-70.
113. Ravitch M. The operative correction of pectus carinatum (pigeon breast). *Ann Surg* 1960;**151**:705-14.
114. Robicsek F, Sargar P, Taylor F, et al. The surgical treatment of chondrosternal prominence (pectus carinatum). *J Thorac Cardiovasc Surg* 1963;**45**:691-701.
115. Welch K, Vos A. Surgical correction of pectus carinatum (pigeon breast). *J Pediatr Surg* 1973;**8**:659-67.
116. Haje S, Bowen J. Preliminary results of orthotic treatment of pectus deformities in children and adolescents. *J Pediatr Orthop* 1992;**12**:795-800.

117. Mielke C, Winter R. Pectus carinatum successfully treated with bracing. A case report. *Int Orthop* 1993;**17**:350-2.
118. Egan J, DuBois J, Morphy M, et al. Compressive orthotics in the treatment of asymmetric pectus carinatum: A preliminary report with an objective radiographic marker. *J Pediatr Surg* 2000;**35**:1183-6.
119. Frey A, Garcia V, Brown R, et al. Nonoperative management of pectus carinatum. *J Pediatr Surg* 2006;**41**:40-5.
120. Banever G, Konefal Jr S, Gettens K, Moriarty K. Nonoperative correction of pectus carinatum with orthotic bracing. *J Laparoendoscop & advanced surgical techniques* 2006;**16**:164-7.
121. Shamberger R, Welch K. Surgical correction of chondromanubrial deformity (Currarino Silverman syndrome). *J Pediatr Surg* 1988;**23**:319-22.
122. Poland A. *Deficiency of the pectoralis muscles* 1841;**6**:191-3.
123. Froriep R. Beobachtung eines Falles von Mangel der Brustdruse. *Notizen aus dem Gebiete der Naturund Heilkunde* 1839;**10**:9-14.
124. Clarkson P. Poland's syndactyly. *Guy's Hosp Rep* 1962;**111**:335-46.
125. Mestak J, Zadorozna M, Cakrtova M. Breast reconstruction in women with Poland's syndrome. *Acta Chir Plasticae* 1991;**33**:137-44.
126. Walker R, Meijer R, Aranda D. Syndactylism with deformity of the pectoralis muscle—Poland's syndrome. *J Pediatr Surg* 1969;**4**:569-72.
127. Al-Qattan M. Classification of hand anomalies in Poland's syndrome. *Br J Plast Surg* 2001;**54**:132-6.
128. Freire-Maia N, Chautard E, Opitz J, et al. The Poland Syndrome—Clinical and genealogical data, dermatoglyphic analysis, and incidence. *Hum Hered* 1973;**23**:97-104.
129. McGillivray B, Lowry R. Poland syndrome in British Columbia: incidence and reproductive experience affected persons. *Am J Med Genet* 1977;**1**:65-74.
130. Bouvet J, Lerque D, Bermetieres F, Gros J. Vascular origin of Poland syndrome? A comparative radiographic study of the vascularization of the arms in either patients. *Eur J Pediatr* 1978;**128**:17-26.
131. David T. Vascular origin of Poland syndrome?. *Eur J Pediatr* 1979;**130**:299-301.
132. Sujansky E, Riccardi V, Matthew A. The familial occurrence of Poland syndrome. *Birth Defects* 1977;**13**:117-32.
133. David T. Familial Poland anomaly. *J Med Genet* 1982;**19**:293-6.
134. Cobben J. Poland anomaly in mother and daughter. *Am J Med Genet* 1989;**33**:519-21.
135. Stevens D, Fink B, Prevel C. Poland's syndrome in one identical twin. *J Pediatr Orthop* 2000;**20**:392-5.
136. Larrandaburu M, Schuler L, Ehlers J, et al. The occurrence of Poland and Poland-Moebius syndromes in the same family: further evidence of their genetic component. *Clin Dysmorpho* 1999;**8**:93-9.
137. Rojas MA, Garcia-Cruz D, Garcia A, et al. Poland-Moebius syndrome in a boy and Poland syndrome in his mother. *Clin Genet* 1991;**40**:225-8.
138. Fontaine G, Ovlaque S. Le syndrome de Poland-Mobius. *Arch Fr Pediatr* 1984;**41**:351-2.
139. Boaz D, Mace J, Gotlin R. Poland's syndrome and leukemia. *Lancet* 1971;**1**:349-50.
140. Shamberger R, Welch K, Upton J III. Surgical treatment of thoracic deformity in Poland's syndrome. *J Pediatr Surg* 1989;**24**:760-5.
140a. Ravitch MM. Atypical deformities of the chest wall—absence and deformities of the ribs and costal cartilage. *Surgery* 1966;**59**:438-39.
141. Ohmori K, Takada H. Correction of Poland's pectoralis major muscle anomaly with latissimus dorsi musculocutaneous flaps. *Okast Reconstr Surg* 1980;**65**:400.
142. Haller JA Jr, Colombani P, Miller D, et al. Early reconstruction of Poland's syndrome using autologous rib grafts combined with latissimus muscle flap. *J Pediatr Surg* 1984;**19**:423-9.
143. Gatti J. Poland's deformity reconstruction with a customized, extrasoft silicone prosthesis. *Ann Plast Surg* 1997;**39**:122-30.
144. Shamberger R, Welch K. Sternal defects. *Pediatr Surg Int* 1990;**5**:156-64.
145. Fischer H. Fissurea sterno congenita mit partieller Bauchspalte. *Dtsch Z Chir* 1879;**12**:367.
146. Maier H, Bortone F. Complete failure of sternal fusion with herniation of pericardium. *J Thorac Surg* 1949;**18**:851-9.
147. Sabiston DC Jr. The surgical management of congenital bifid sternum with partial ectopia cordis. *J Thorac Surg* 1958;**35**:118-22.
148. Meissner F. Fissura sterni congenita. *Zentralbl Chir* 1964;**89**:1832-9.
149. Burton J. Method of correction of ectopia cordis. *Arch Surg* 1947;**77**:79-84.
150. Cantrell J, Haller JJ, Ravitch M. A syndrome of congenital defects involving the abdominal wall, sternum, diaphragm, pericardium, and heart. *Surg Gynecol Obstet* 1958;**107**:602-14.
151. Higginbottom M, Jones K, Hall V, et al. The amniotic band disruption complex: timing of amniotic rupture and variable spectra of consequent defects. *J Pediatr Surg* 1979;**95**:544-9.
152. Opitz J, et al. Editorial comment following paper by Hersh, et al and Kapland et al on sternal cleft. *Am J Med Genet* 1985;**21**:201-2.
153. Hersh J, Wadterfill D, Rutledge J, et al. Sternal malformation/vascular dysplasia association. *Am J Med Genet* 1985;**21**:177-86.
154. Kaplan L, Matsuoka R, Gilbert E, et al. Ectopia cordis and cleft sternum: evidence for mechanical teratogenesis following rupture of the chorion or yolk sac. *Am J Med Genet* 1985;**21**:187-99.
155. Patten B. *Human embryology*. Philadelphia: Blakiston; 1946.
156. Bremer L. *Textbook of embryology*. Philadelphia: WB Saunders; 1936.
157. Say B, Wilsey C. Chromosome aberration in ectopia cordis. *Am Heart J* 1978;**95**:274-5.
158. King C. Ectopia cordis and chromosomal errors. *Pediatrics* 1980;**66**:328.
159. Stoll SC, Vivier M, Renaud R. A supraumbilical midline raphe with sternal cleft in a 47, XXX woman. *Am J Med Genet* 1987;**27**:229-31.
160. Stensen N. An unusually early description of the so-called tetralogy of Fallot. *Acta Medica et Philosophica Hafnienca* 1671;**1**(202):1671-2.
161. Willius F. An unusually early description of the so-called tetralogy of Fallot. *Proc Staff Meeting Mayo Clin* 1948;**23**:316-20.
162. Haynor D, Shuman W, Brewer D, et al. Imaging of fetal ectopia cordis: roles of sonography and computed tomography. *J Ultrasound Med* 1984;**3**:25-7.
163. Cutler G, Wilens G. Ectopia cordis: report of a case. *Am J Dis Child* 1925;**30**:76-81.
164. Saxena N. Ectopia cordis child surviving: prosthesis fails. *Pediatr News* 1976;**10**:3.
165. Dobell A, Williams H, Long R. Staged repair of ectopia cordis. *J Pediatr Surg* 1982;**17**:353-8.
166. Amato J, Cotroneo J, Gladiere R. *Repair of complete ectopia cordis (film)*. Chicago: Presented at American College of Surgeons Clinical Congress; 1988, October 23, p. 23-28.
167. Kragt H, Aarnoudse J, Meyboom E, et al. Case report: Prenatal ultrasonic diagnosis and management of ectopia cordis. *Eur J Obstet Gynecol Reprod Biol* 1985;**20**:177-80.
168. Mercer L, Petres R, Smeltzer J. Ultrasound diagnosis of ectopia cordis. *Obstet Gynecol* 1983;**61**:523-5.
168a. Wilson J. A description of a very unusual formation of the human heart. *Philos Tran R Soc London*. 1798;**2**:346-56.
169. Major J. Thoracoabdominal ectopia cordis. *J Thorac Surg* 1953;**26**:309-17.
170. Arndt C. Nabelschnurbruch mit Herzhernie: Operation durch laparotomie mit todlichem Ausgang. *Centralbl Gynakol* 1896;**20**:632-3.
171. Wieting. Eine operative behandelte Herzmissbildung. *Dtsch Z Chir* 1912;**114**:293-5.
172. Cullerier M. Observation sue un deplacement remarquable du coeur; par M. Deschamps, medecin a laval. *J General Med Chir Pharmacie* 1806;**26**:275.
173. Jeune M, Caroon R, Beraud C, et al. Polychondrodystrophie avec blocage thoracique d'évolution fatale. *Pediatrie* 1954;**9**:390-2.
174. Kozlowski K, Masel J. Asphyxiating thoracic dystrophy without respiratory disease: report of two cases of the latent form. *Pediatr Radiol* 1976;**5**:30-5.
175. Williams A, Vauterg G, Reid L. Lung structure in asphyxiating thoracic dystrophy. *Arch Pathol Lab Med* 1984;**108**:658-61.
176. Jarcho S, Levin P. Hereditary malformation of the vertebral bodies. *Bull Johns Hopkins Hospital* 1938;**62**:216-62.
177. Roberts AP, Conner AN, Tolmie JL, Connor JM. Spondylothoracic and spondylocostal dysostosis: hereditary forms of spinal deformity. *J Bone Joint Surg Br* 1988;**70**(1):123-6.
178. Heilbronner D, Renshaw T. Spondylothoracic dysplasia. *J Bone Joint Surg* 1984;**66A**:302-3.

CHAPTER 25
Chest Wall Tumors
Mark S. Allen

Clinical Presentation
Surgical Management
   Chest Wall Reconstruction
      History
      Indications
   Methods of Reconstruction

Soft Tissue Coverage
Benign Chest Wall Tumors
   Osteochondroma
   Chondroma
   Desmoid
Malignant Chest Wall Tumors

Malignant Fibrous Histiocytoma
Chondrosarcoma
Rhabdomyosarcoma
Clinical Experience
   Summary

Tumors of the chest wall encompass a variety of bone and soft tissue disorders.[1-3] Primary and metastatic neoplasms of both the bony skeleton and the soft tissues as well as primary neoplasms that invade the thorax from adjacent structures, such as the breast, lung, pleura, and mediastinum, are included; benign, nonmalignant conditions of the chest wall, such as infections, cysts, and fibromatosis, are also included (Box 25-1). Almost all of these tumors have been irradiated as the treatment of choice or have been irradiated in combination with chest wall resection.[4] It is also not uncommon to have patients present with a postradiation necrotic chest wall neoplasm. The thoracic surgeon is frequently asked to establish a diagnosis for most of these patients, to treat some for cure, and to manage a few for necrotic, foul-smelling chest wall ulcers. All of these entities represent a diagnostic and therapeutic challenge. In many patients, surgical extirpation is often the only remaining method of treatment, and this may be compromised by an incorrect diagnosis or an inability to reconstruct large chest wall defects. From a practical standpoint, however, chest wall resection is most frequently used to treat primary chest wall neoplasms.[1-3,5]

Because primary chest wall neoplasms are uncommon, relatively few series historically have been reported. Moreover, most early reports included only patients with bone tumors.[6-8] When bone tumors are combined with primary soft tissue tumors, however, the soft tissues become a major source of chest wall neoplasms and today account for nearly half of all tumors.

The incidence of malignancy in primary chest wall neoplasms varies and ranges from 50% to 80%. The higher malignancy rates occur in soft tissue tumors. Consequently, when bone and soft tissue tumors are combined, malignant fibrous histiocytomas (fibrosarcomas), chondrosarcomas, and rhabdomyosarcomas are the most common primary malignant neoplasms, and cartilaginous tumors (osteochondroma and chondroma) and desmoid tumors are the most common primary benign tumors.[2,5]

The type and incidence of chest wall tumors in the pediatric population are somewhat difficult to determine; primitive neuroectodermal tumors, Ewing's rhabdomyosarcoma, and neuroblastoma dominate the malignant cell types, and chondroma, hamartomas, and desmoid tumors are the frequent types of benign tumors. Chest wall masses are more likely to be malignant in children.[9,10]

Box 25-1
Primary Chest Wall Neoplasms

Malignant
   Malignant fibrous histiocytoma
   Chondrosarcoma
   Rhabdomyosarcoma
   Myeloma
   Ewing's sarcoma
   Liposarcoma
   Neurofibrosarcoma
   Osteogenic sarcoma
   Hemangiosarcoma
   Leiomyosarcoma
   Lymphoma

Benign
   Osteochondroma
   Chondroma
   Desmoid
   Lipoma
   Fibroma
   Neurilemoma

CLINICAL PRESENTATION

Chest wall tumors generally present as slowly enlarging, asymptomatic masses. With continued growth, pain invariably occurs. Initially, the pain is often generalized, and the patient is frequently treated for a neuritis or a musculoskeletal complaint. Nearly all malignant neoplasms eventually become painful, compared with only two thirds of benign tumors. In some patients with rib tumors, a mass may not be apparent on physical examination but is detected on conventional chest radiography.

Evaluation of patients with suspected chest wall tumors should include a careful history, physical examination, and laboratory examination followed by conventional radiographs of the involved area. Previous chest radiographs are important to determine the rate of growth. In general, magnetic resonance imaging is the preferred method of imaging chest wall tumors. Magnetic resonance imaging not only distinguishes the tumor from nerves and blood vessels but also allows visualization in different planes, such as coronal and sagittal planes. However, magnetic resonance imaging does not accurately assess pulmonary nodules or the extent of calcification within the lung. Thus, if the lung parenchyma needs evaluation for metastatic disease, computed tomography is preferable. Positron emission tomography may be useful to rule out metastases but not to differentiate benign or malignant tumors.

SURGICAL MANAGEMENT

Chest wall neoplasms that are clinically suspected of being primary tumors require tissue diagnosis. A tumor thought to be a metastasis from a known primary neoplasm elsewhere can be accurately diagnosed by incisional or needle biopsy. However, if a primary chest wall neoplasm (either benign or malignant) is suspected, excisional biopsy rather than incisional or needle biopsy should be done because the last two limited biopsies tend to underdiagnose certain low-grade malignant neoplasms (e.g., chondrosarcoma as being benign). Consequently, wide resection is invariably not done, and the opportunity for cure is denied. Also, the location of the excisional biopsy should not interfere with subsequent treatment. An improperly placed biopsy site, extensive soft tissue dissection, and wound infection can all complicate subsequent treatment by delaying definitive resection, radiation therapy, or chemotherapy. If frozen tissue diagnosis of a primary chest wall tumor cannot be established at the time of excisional biopsy, the chest wound should be closed, most often without skeletal reconstruction, because the chest wall defect is usually small. If the neoplasm is later determined to be benign, no further surgical therapy is required. If, however, malignancy is diagnosed, wide resection is then required, which must also include en bloc resection of the entire biopsy site (skin, subcutaneous tissue, and muscle) because of potential tumor contamination of the overlying muscle, subcutaneous tissue, and skin.

Wide resection of a primary malignant chest wall neoplasm is now recognized as being essential to successful management. However, the extent of resection should not be compromised because of an inability to close large chest wall defects.[1-3,5] Opinions differ with regard to what constitutes wide resection. In a report from the Mayo Clinic that analyzed the effect of the extent of resection on long-term survival in patients with primary malignant chest wall neoplasm,[11] 56% of patients with a margin of resection of 4.0 cm or more remained free from cancer at 5 years compared with only 29% of patients with a margin of 2.0 cm (Fig. 25-1). For many surgeons, a resection margin of 2.0 cm is considered to be adequate. Although this margin may be adequate for chest wall metastases and benign tumors, a 2.0-cm margin for resection is *inadequate* for malignant neoplasms. Moreover, more aggressive malignant tumors, such as osteogenic sarcoma and malignant fibrous histiocytoma, have the potential to spread within the marrow cavity or along tissue planes such as the periosteum or parietal pleura. Consequently, all primary malignant neoplasms that are initially diagnosed by excisional biopsy should be resected further to include at least a 4.0-cm margin

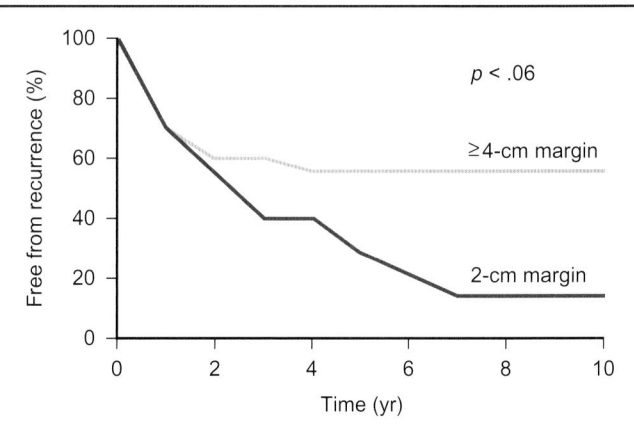

Figure 25–1
Percentage of patients with malignant chest wall tumors free from recurrent tumor by extent of resection margin. Zero time on abscissa represents day of chest wall resection. *(From King RM, Pairolero PC, Trastek VF, et al. Primary chest wall tumors: factors affecting survival. Reprinted with permission of The Society of Thoracic Surgeons.)*

of normal tissue on all sides. High-grade malignant neoplasms should also have the entire involved bone resected. For neoplasms of the rib, this includes removal of the entire involved rib, removal of the corresponding anterior costal arch if the tumor is located anteriorly, and partial resection of several ribs above and below the neoplasm. For tumors of the sternum and manubrium, resection of the entire involved bone and corresponding costal arches bilaterally is indicated.[12] Any attached structures, such as lung, thymus, pericardium, or chest wall muscles, should also be excised. Radiofrequency thermoablation has been described for treatment of a mesenchymal hamartoma of the chest wall in an infant, but its efficacy is unknown.[13]

The role of resection for chest wall metastases and recurrent breast cancer is controversial. Nonetheless, most thoracic surgeons would agree that tumor ulceration is an indication for excision. For these patients, wound hygiene is crucial, and surgical excision is frequently the only treatment option available. The goal in treating patients with necrotic tumors should be a healed wound after local excision. Although the length of survival is not increased after resection, the quality of life is certainly improved.

The ability to close large chest wall defects is of prime importance in the surgical treatment of chest wall neoplasms. The critical question of whether the reconstructed thorax will support respiration and protect the underlying organs must be answered in considering both the extent of resection and the method of reconstruction. Adequate resection and dependable reconstruction are the mandatory ingredients for successful treatment. These two important items are accomplished most safely by the joint efforts of a thoracic surgeon and a plastic surgeon.

Chest Wall Reconstruction

Indications for chest wall resection include primary or metastatic chest wall neoplasms, tumors contiguous from breast or lung, radiation necrosis, congenital defects, and trauma or infectious processes from osteomyelitis or median sternotomy or lateral thoracotomy wounds.[14,15] Improvements in preoperative imaging, intraoperative anesthetic management, techniques available for reconstruction, and postoperative care allow almost any pathologic process to be successfully managed by chest wall resection and reconstruction. The tenets of chest wall resection and reconstruction are (1) to remove all devitalized tissue; (2) to restore rigidity to the chest wall if the defect is large, to prevent a flail chest; and (3) to cover with healthy soft tissue to seal the pleural space; to protect underlying organs, and to prevent infection. Because successful management of chest wall lesions often requires input from multiple different specialties, these types of problems are best cared for by a team of physicians including plastic surgeons, pulmonologists, and anesthesiologists as well as the thoracic surgeon.

History

Holden reported the first successful partial sternectomy in 1878, and in 1898, Parham reported resection of the chest wall in continuity with a pulmonary tumor.[16] Reconstruction was particularly difficult in these early efforts because of the problems involved in sealing the pleural cavity. With the advent of endotracheal intubation, the difficulties of pneumothorax during chest wall resection were mitigated. Closed-chest drainage, positive-pressure ventilation, and antibiotics further enhanced the success rate of chest wall resection and reconstruction. The 1940s and the war injuries seen in World War II advanced the management of an infected pleural space and ventilation mechanics and brought advances in soft tissue coverage. Watson and James[17] described the use of fascia lata grafts to close chest wall defects. The use of rib grafts to reinforce the anterior chest wall after sternectomy was discussed by Bisgard and Swenson.[18] The advent of musculocutaneous flaps to cover defects in the chest wall is a major advance in the reconstruction of chest wall defects. The latissimus dorsi musculocutaneous flap was initially described by Tansini[19] in 1906 for coverage of the chest wall after a radical mastectomy. The musculocutaneous flap was again described in the late 1930s and by Campbell in 1950 but, for unknown reasons, was not noticed until 20 years later. The idea of a musculocutaneous flap was then repopularized by Blades and Paul,[20] Converse and associates,[21] and Myre and Kirklin.[22] In the field of thoracic surgery, Jurkiewicz expanded the idea of using muscle flaps to reconstruct the chest wall. Through him and the residents he trained, these techniques are now commonly in use.

There have recently been numerous reports of the use of chest wall musculature to reconstruct the chest wall.[23,24] Almost all the thoracic muscles, including the latissimus dorsi, pectoralis major and minor, serratus anterior, rectus abdominis, and external obliques, are now used. Tissue expanders have been added to facilitate transfer of the muscle, and free microvascular transfer has been described to cover chest wall defects. Currently, it is almost always possible to cover aggressive resections with autologous tissue by modern techniques.

For stabilization of the resected bony chest wall, either autologous tissue or synthetic materials have been described. The use of transposed ribs or diced cartilage is of historic interest and is rare today. Fascia lata for reconstruction of chest wall deformities was first described in 1947 by Watson and James.[17] Donor cryopreserved rib allografts have been described.[25] Synthetic materials are the most commonly used objects today. Marlex, as a material to reconstruct the chest wall, was first described in 1960 by Graham and colleagues.[26] Similar meshes were developed with Prolene and Vicryl. More recently, Gore-Tex patches have been constructed for this purpose.

Indications

Malignant neoplasms—primary, metastatic, or those with contiguous invasion of the chest wall—are the primary indication for a chest wall resection. It has been shown that lung cancer that invades the chest wall is best treated by resection of the bony chest wall in continuity with pulmonary resection. Similar although much less common is breast cancer that invades the chest wall directly from the breast tissue. This is uncommon today because most breast cancer is found when it is small. Primary tumors of the chest wall also dictate a full-thickness resection and often require reconstruction of the bone and soft tissues. Infection necessitates a chest wall resection, usually when an infected median sternotomy has not healed properly after an initial attempt to close it. Resection of all devitalized tissue with open packing and serial débridement is often necessary to obtain a closed, healed wound. Radiation therapy can cause serious problems in the chest wall. Although this problem is less common today because of more accurate portals and improved knowledge of the dangers of radiation therapy, it is still seen all too commonly. A fungating, painful, infected, or bleeding mass on the chest wall that results from radiation therapy can be resected with a great improvement of quality. Traumatic lesions are another reason to resect and reconstruct the chest wall but are not as common. Finally, congenital defects exist that require chest wall reconstruction.

Reasons for resection of the chest wall vary among different series. The four main reasons are shown in Box 25-2. In a large series by Arnold and Pairolero,[27] chest wall tumor was the indication in 275 patients, infected median sternotomy in 142, radiation necrosis in 119, and a combination of these reasons in the remaining 121 patients (Table 25-1). In Cohen's series of 113 patients, the indications for resection were infection (mostly infected median sternotomies) in 76, radiation necrosis in 23, tumor in 12, and trauma in 2 patients.[28] Finally, in another large series by Mansour and coworkers,[14] the indications were malignancy in 171, infection in 31, radiation necrosis in 29, and other reasons in 29 patients. The actual distribution is largely determined by the practice patterns of each reporting physician.

When a portion of the bony chest wall is removed, reconstruction is not always necessary. Restoration of chest wall stability minimizes paradoxical movement and ensures adequate ventilatory mechanics. If the defect is less than 5 cm in diameter, it is unlikely that it will cause much physiologic impairment of ventilation. Thus, whether to reconstruct becomes a question of cosmetic outcome. If the defect is located anteriorly and the patient is thin or is going to lose a great deal of weight, most defects should be reconstructed to avoid a noticeable deformity of the chest wall. Conversely, if the defect is small and located posteriorly or if it will be covered by the scapula, reconstruction is not necessary. However, when the defect is at or near the tip of the scapula, it should be reconstructed to prevent the tip of the scapula from catching on the edge of the chest wall and causing an uncomfortable sensation for the patient. Resection of the upper thoracic ribs, as occurs when a Pancoast tumor is resected, does not require reconstruction of the bony chest wall because the scapula will cover the defect.

In general, it is not necessary to replace the sternum with prosthetic material after removal. It has been shown that reconstruction of the sternum with rigid material does not improve the mechanics of breathing or pulmonary function.[29-31] However, the defect should be covered with muscle and skin to obtain a closed wound.

Methods of Reconstruction

Once the resection of all devitalized or malignant tissue has been accomplished, the chest wall must be closed to provide for adequate respiratory mechanics, to protect the underlying organs and vessels, and to obtain an acceptable cosmetic outcome. If the defect is small, as mentioned previously, the bony chest wall does not need reconstruction, and the soft tissue can be closed primarily. With larger resections, the bony chest wall and the soft tissues will need some more creative techniques for a closed wound to be obtained.

For reconstruction of the bony chest wall, some type of firm tissue needs to be placed. This usually means synthetic material; however, Murakawa and colleagues[32] described using fascia lata in eight patients who had a chest wall resection. All had a good outcome, and they claimed that harvesting of the graft was easy because it did not require repositioning and was markedly cheaper than use of synthetic material. They did acknowledge the disadvantage of having to make another incision to harvest the graft.

The choice of the specific type of synthetic tissue to use is confusing and is usually based on the surgeon's preference. A 2-mm-thick expanded polytetrafluoroethylene (PTFE) or Gore-Tex (W. L. Gore & Associates, Inc., Flagstaff, AZ) patch is the preferred material despite the high cost. Advantages are its impermeability to water and air, strength, and ease of use. It is sutured into place by large (#0) polypropylene sutures. Use of the thinner 1-mm patch is not recommended in chest wall reconstruction because it does not hold sutures as well as the thicker patch does. Because the patch is fairly rigid in all directions, it is easier to place tightly into the chest wall defect than are other synthetic materials that are knitted (Figs. 25-2 and 25-3). The PTFE patch has a characteristic appearance on follow-up computed chest tomography (Fig. 25-4).

Synthetic mesh made of polypropylene, either single knitted (Marlex by Davol and Bard, Cranston, RI) or double-stitch knitted (Prolene by Ethicon, Inc., Somerville, NJ), is an excellent material for reconstruction. The material is not impermeable to water and air, which is of some concern for chest wall reconstructions. It is less expensive than PTFE and has been shown to yield results just as good as those with PTFE.[33,34]

These meshes can also be combined with methylmethacrylate to form a rigid prosthesis for the chest wall. This is rarely necessary, as shown by Arnold and Pairolero.[27] They used this rigid material only once in 500 reconstructions, and it had to be removed 2 months later for infection. The material must be used with care because when it is mixed, the reaction is exothermic and the heat given off may damage lung or surrounding tissues. It can be useful for reconstruction of a huge defect when a curved prosthesis is needed. With a piece of lead plate formed to the correct shape, a Marlex methylmethacrylate sandwich can be formed over the lead template.

Box 25–2
Etiology of Chest Wall Defects[16]

Neoplasm
    Primary chest wall
        Chondrosarcoma
        Osteosarcoma
        Solitary plasmacytoma
        Ewing's tumor
        Desmoid tumor
    Contiguous lung cancer
    Contiguous breast cancer
    Metastatic chest wall
        Breast
        Kidney
        Colon
        Thyroid
        Sarcoma
Infection
    Median sternotomy wound
    Lateral thoracotomy wound
    Osteomyelitis
Radiation necrosis
Trauma

Table 25–1
Indications for Chest Wall Resection: Selected Series

Series	Malignancy	Infection	Radiation Necrosis	Other	Total
Arnold and Pairolero[27]	275	142	119	536	1072
Mansour et al[14]	171	31	29	29	260
Cohen and Ramasastry[28]	12	76	23	2	113
Weyant et al[34]	242	4	7	9	262
Total (%)	700	253	178	576	1707

Chapter 25 Chest Wall Tumors   383

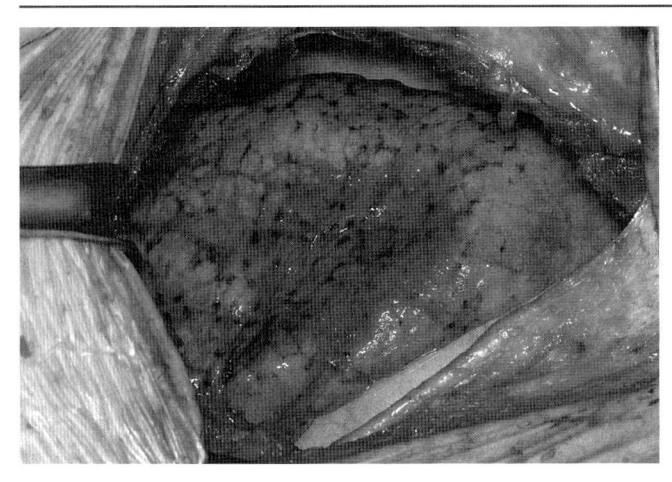

Figure 25-2
Defect in left chest wall after resection of a metastatic tumor.

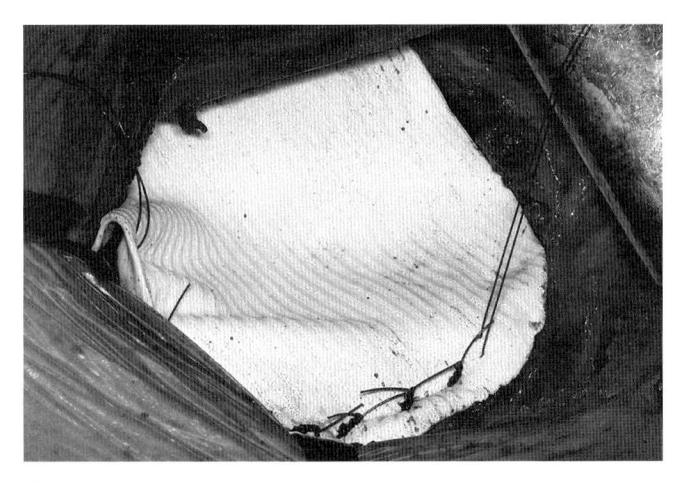

Figure 25-3
Gore-Tex patch being placed to reconstruct the bony chest wall.

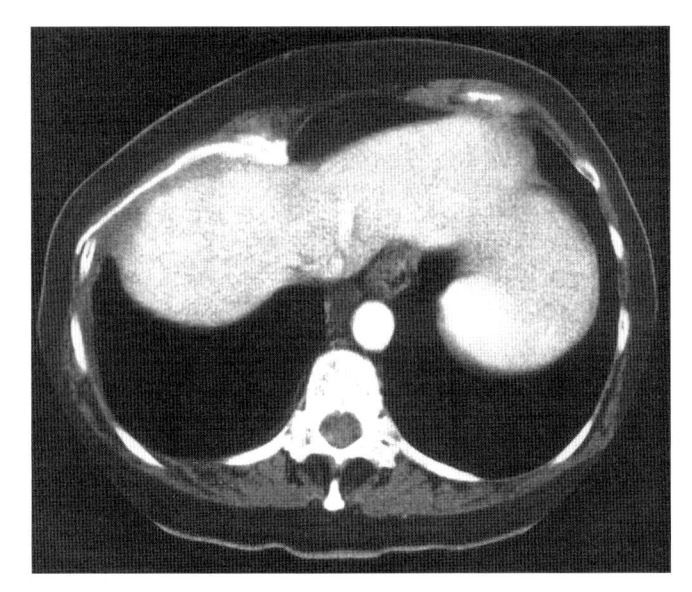

Figure 25-4
Postoperative chest computed tomographic scan of a patient who has had a 2-mm Gore-Tex patch placed in the right lower anterior chest wall.

Once this mixture has cooled, it can be sutured into the defect in the chest wall by passing large sutures through the Marlex that is at the perimeter of the prosthesis. Infection of a rigid prosthesis remains a problem. The constant motion of the chest wall tends to loosen the material unless it is secured very carefully. In one series, three of the nine prostheses had to be removed for infection even though all were placed in clean incisions.[35] It was thought that methylmethacrylate led to more chest wall pain and respiratory problems than other synthetic materials did.

Whatever prosthetic material is chosen, it should be securely attached to the chest wall. The suture material should be nonabsorbable polypropylene, usually #0 or #1. The sutures can be passed around the rib for a secure closure and should be placed interruptedly so that if one fails, the patch does not fail. The patch should be placed on the outside edge of the bony chest wall for the best cosmetic result. If the diaphragm is involved in the resection, it can be attached to the patch in a similar manner. The patch should be under tension after it is sewn in place; therefore, if a patient is in a flexed lateral decubitus position, the flex in the operation room should be removed before the patch is placed.

Seromas will often occur after a synthetic material is used to reconstruct the chest wall. It is unclear whether placement of a drain at the time of surgery to prevent the formation of a seroma is a good idea. The drain will certainly decrease the incidence of seromas but may increase the incidence of infection, a far more serious problem. Postoperative seromas can be managed by observation with a gentle pressure dressing or, if the seroma is large, aspiration under strict aseptic conditions. Aspiration may have to be performed several times until the problem resolves. Infection of a prosthetic patch is a grave problem and usually means that the patch must be removed. A fibrin layer has usually formed under the patch, so the risk of creating an open pneumothorax is low if the patch has been in place for sufficient time, usually a week or two. If the patch is made of Gore-Tex, it is relatively easy to slip the patch out, place drains in the space, and allow the incision to heal by secondary intention. Marlex is much more difficult to remove because of the ingrowth of fibrous tissue.

Soft Tissue Coverage

Once the bony chest wall has been stabilized, the incision is closed. This is best accomplished by primary closure with local tissue. Unfortunately, this is often not possible because much of the overlying skin and muscle required resection. In this situation, myocutaneous flaps have become an invaluable resource to cover the prosthetic material and to provide closure. A variety of different myocutaneous flaps are available; the choice of which one to use depends on the location of the defect and what is available.[36]

For anterior central chest wall defects, the pectoralis major is an excellent choice. In Arnold's series, this muscle was used in 355 patients.[27] It is mobilized with preservation of the thoracoacromial neurovascular leash and can easily reach the midline (Fig. 25-5). Mobilization in this fashion permits another median sternotomy to be done in the future without dividing the blood supply of the flaps.

Another extremely versatile myocutaneous flap is based on the latissimus dorsi muscle (see Fig. 25-5). This flap covers anterior or anterior lateral defects quite well. It is transposed

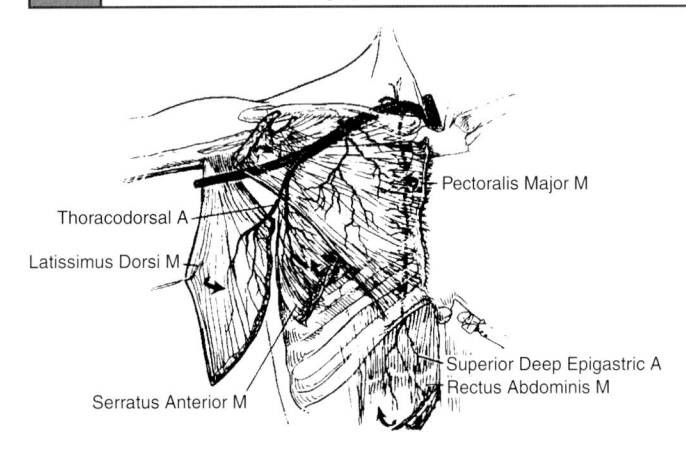

Figure 25–5
Diagram demonstrating the dominant blood supply to the chest wall muscles. *(From Black SB, Mendez-Eastman SK. Repair and care of chest wall defects.* Plast Surg Nurs *2001;**21**:13-21. Originally from Shaw, Aston, Zide, 1990).*

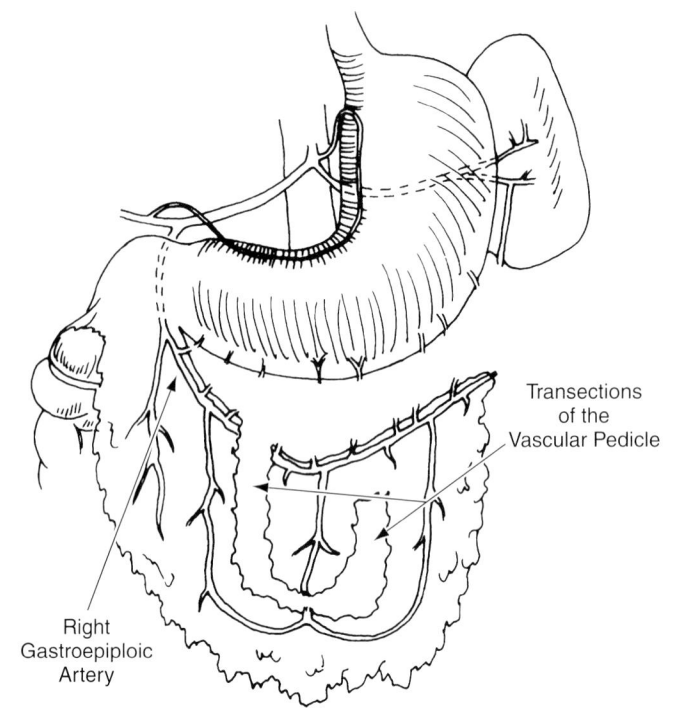

Figure 25–6
Diagram demonstrating the blood supply of the omentum and the divisions necessary to harvest the omentum based on the right gastroepiploic artery and the omental arcade. *(From Graeber GM. Chest wall resection and reconstruction.* Semin Thorac Cardiovasc Surg *1999;**11**:251-63.)*

on the dominant thoracodorsal neurovascular leash and can retain its function when the nerve is left intact. It is an extremely reliable source of tissue coverage.

The serratus anterior muscle is rarely used for chest wall defects but can be rotated into the chest cavity to cover defects in the airway (see Fig. 25-5).

For lower anterior chest wall defects, the rectus abdominis can be used for coverage. The muscle can be harvested with its overlying skin as a transverse rectus abdominis myocutaneous flap, known as the TRAM flap. This will provide excellent coverage for the lower chest wall. The muscle depends on the blood supply from the superior epigastric artery, so if the ipsilateral mammary artery has been taken, this flap is not the first choice.

The external oblique can also be used to cover lower anterior chest wall defects. It is not commonly used. It can reliably cover up only to the inferior mammary crease.

The omentum can also be used to provide viable tissue on a damaged chest wall. It is not thick enough to cover prosthetic material, but it can be used when the bony chest is intact and the skin and subcutaneous tissue have been lost as a result of radiation damage or infection. It requires a laparotomy for harvest. Laparoscopic harvesting has been described, but most patients with a chest wall defect do not tolerate the pneumoperitoneum required for a laparoscopic approach. It is usually based on the right gastroepiploic arcade, and if the omental arc is divided, the tissue can reach almost anywhere on the chest wall (Fig. 25-6). The omentum is most useful for coverage of the chest wall after radiation damage. In the large series by Arnold, omentum was of little use for treatment of an infected median sternotomy.[27]

BENIGN CHEST WALL TUMORS

Osteochondroma

Osteochondroma, the most common benign bone neoplasm, constitutes nearly 50% of all benign rib tumors. The incidence, however, may actually be higher because most patients are asymptomatic and the tumors are often not removed. Men are affected three times more frequently than women are. The neoplasm begins in childhood and continues to grow until skeletal maturity is reached. The onset of pain in a previously asymptomatic tumor may indicate malignant degeneration.

Osteochondromas arise from the metaphyseal region of the rib and present as a stalked bony protuberance with a cartilaginous cap. A rim of calcification may be present at the periphery of the tumor, and stippled calcification is often found within the tumor. On microscopic examination, bone proliferation occurs to varying degrees, and the thickness of the cartilaginous cap also varies.

All osteochondromas occurring in children after puberty or in adults should be resected. Asymptomatic osteochondromas may occur before puberty, but if pain or increase in size occurs, the tumor should be resected.

Chondroma

Chondromas constitute 15% of all benign neoplasms of the rib cage. Most occur anteriorly at the costochondral junction. Both sexes are affected equally, and the tumor can occur at any age. These neoplasms usually present as a slowly enlarging mass that may be nontender or slightly painful. On radiographic examination, chondroma is an expansile lesion causing thinning of the cortex. The differentiation between a chondroma and a chondrosarcoma is impossible on clinical and radiographic examination. In gross appearance, chondroma is as a lobulated mass. On microscopic examination, the tumor is characterized by lobules of hyaline cartilage. The microscopic differentiation between a chondroma and a low-grade chondrosarcoma can be extremely difficult. All chondromas must be considered malignant and should be treated by wide excision. Although this extent of resection may seem extensive for what may turn out to be a benign tumor, modern reconstructive techniques make the risk negligible, and long-term results are excellent.

Desmoid

Desmoid tumor deserves special consideration.[37] Forty percent of all desmoids occur in the shoulder and chest wall. Encapsulation of the brachial plexus and the vessels of the arm and neck is common. The tumor often extends into the pleural cavity, markedly displacing mediastinal structures. Initially, the tumor presents as a poorly circumscribed mass with little or no pain. Paresthesias, hyperesthesia, and motor weakness occur later, after neural encasement. Veins or arteries are rarely occluded. Desmoid occurs most commonly between puberty and 40 years of age and is rarely observed in infants or the very old. Men and women are affected equally.

On gross examination, the tumor originates in muscle and fascia and frequently extends along tissue planes. On microscopic examination, a monotonous pattern of elongated spindle-shaped cells infiltrating the surrounding tissue is invariably seen. Most pathologists consider desmoid to be a form of benign fibromatosis.[38,39] Because these tumors can invade adjacent structures and have been reported to have malignant degeneration, other pathologists consider desmoid to be a low-grade fibrosarcoma.[40,41] Whatever the cause, the tumor tends to be recurrent if it is inadequately excised and should be treated with wide resection. Encapsulation of thoracic outlet structures presents a special problem in management. Enucleation of the tumor from these structures followed by radiation therapy is the current practice.

MALIGNANT CHEST WALL TUMORS

Malignant Fibrous Histiocytoma

Malignant fibrous histiocytoma is the most common primary chest wall neoplasm that the thoracic surgeon is asked to evaluate.[5,11] The tumor characteristically occurs in late adult life, with the majority of cases occurring between the ages of 50 and 70 years. These neoplasms are rare in childhood, and approximately two thirds occur in men. Malignant fibrous histiocytoma often presents as a painless, slowly enlarging mass. Pregnancy, however, may accelerate the growth rate, resulting in pain. Fever and leukocytosis with neutropenia or eosinophilia are occasionally present.[42] Excellent circumstantial evidence suggests that some chest wall malignant fibrous histiocytomas are radiation induced.[42]

On gross examination, malignant fibrous histiocytoma tends to be lobulated and to spread for considerable distances along fascial planes or between muscle fibers, which accounts for its high recurrence rate after resection. The neoplasm is unresponsive to both irradiation and chemotherapy and should be treated by wide resection. Five-year survival is approximately 38%.

Chondrosarcoma

Chondrosarcoma accounts for 30% of all primary malignant bone tumors. It occurs most frequently in the anterior chest wall, with 75% arising in either the costochondral arches or the sternum. The tumor most commonly occurs in the third and fourth decades of life and is relatively uncommon in persons younger than 20 years. Chondrosarcoma is more frequent in men. Nearly all patients present with a slowly enlarging mass, which has usually been painful for many months. Differentiation from chondroma may be extremely difficult. From a practical standpoint, all tumors arising in the costal cartilages should be considered to be malignant and should be treated by wide resection.

The cause of chondrosarcoma is unknown. Although malignant degeneration of benign cartilaginous tumors—secondary chondrosarcoma—has been reported, most chondrosarcomas arise de novo. An association has been suggested between trauma and chondrosarcoma.[39] In the Mayo Clinic series, 12.5% of patients had sustained severe crushing injury to the ipsilateral chest wall.[43]

Definitive diagnosis of chondrosarcoma can only be made pathologically. Histologic confirmation may be difficult, however, because most tumors are well differentiated. This well-differentiated tendency frequently results in a misdiagnosis of chondroma and subsequent undertreatment, leading to local recurrences. For this reason, excisional biopsy rather than incisional or needle biopsy of all chest wall masses suspected of being chondrosarcoma is indicated.

Chest wall chondrosarcoma typically grows slowly and recurs locally. If it is left untreated, metastases occur late. Prompt, complete control of the primary neoplasm is the main determinant of survival; the objective of the first operation should be resection wide enough to prevent local recurrence. This involves resection of a 4-cm margin of normal tissue on all sides. Wide resection results in cure in nearly all patients.[43,44]

Rhabdomyosarcoma

This is the second most common chest wall soft tissue malignant neoplasm and occurs most frequently in children and young adults. These tumors are rare after the age of 45 years, and men are affected only slightly more than women are. Rhabdomyosarcomas present as a rapidly enlarging mass that is usually deep seated and is intimately associated with striated muscle tissue. In general, the tumor is neither painful nor tender, despite evidence of rapid growth. Both grossly and microscopically, it has few neoplastic characteristics. As with most rapidly growing tumors, the overall appearance reflects the degree of cellularity and the extent of secondary changes such as hemorrhage and necrosis.

Modern therapy has profoundly altered the clinical course of this disease. Wide resection followed by irradiation and multidrug chemotherapy has resulted in 5-year survivals of 70%. Inadequately treated, the tumor rapidly recurs both locally and metastatically.

CLINICAL EXPERIENCE

Since the early 1980s, more than 500 chest wall resections for primary neoplasms were performed at the Mayo Clinic by one team of surgeons.[1,3,5,45] Nearly two thirds of these neoplasms were malignant. Malignant fibrous histiocytoma and chondrosarcoma were the most common malignant neoplasms, and desmoid tumor was the most common benign tumor. The age of patients ranged from 11 to 85 years, with a median of 45.2 years. An average of 3.9 ribs were resected. Total or partial sternectomies were performed in 23 patients. Skeletal defects were closed with prosthetic material in 67 patients and with autogenous ribs in 5 patients. Eighty-eight patients underwent 126 muscle transpositions including 48 pectoralis major, 35 latissimus dorsi, 16 serratus anterior, 3 external oblique, 2 rectus abdominis, 2 trapezius, and 20 other. The omentum was transposed in 14 patients. Median hospitalization was 8.5 days. There were no 30-day operative deaths. Patients were generally extubated during the evening of the operation or on the following morning. Three patients required tracheostomy. Most other patients had only minor changes in pulmonary function.[46]

Long-term survival of patients with primary chest wall malignant neoplasm is dependent on cell type and the extent of chest wall resection.[47,48] In the Mayo Clinic series, overall 5-year survival was 57%.[11] Wide resection for chondrosarcoma resulted in a 5-year survival of 96% compared with only 70% for patients who had local excision (Fig. 25-7).[46] Five-year overall survival for patients with either chondrosarcoma or rhabdomyosarcoma was 70% in contrast to only 38% for patients with malignant fibrous histiocytoma (Fig. 25-8).[11] Recurrent neoplasm, however, was an ominous sign; only 17% of patients in whom recurrence developed survived 5 years.

Summary

Resection and reconstruction of chest wall lesions can be a challenging endeavor. However, by approaching the problems of each patient with a careful, well-thought plan, the results should be excellent in the majority of patients. Use of expertise of a variety of other specialties, including plastic surgeons, anesthesiologists, and pulmonary medicine specialists, will greatly facilitate successful results.

The key to successful treatment of primary chest wall neoplasms remains early diagnosis and aggressive surgical resection. This procedure can generally be performed in one operation with minimal respiratory insufficiency and with low operative mortality. In combination with current methods of reconstruction, potential cure is likely for most patients with primary chest wall neoplasms.

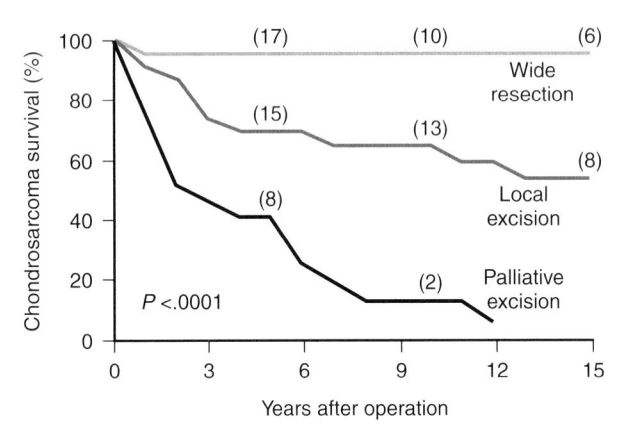

Figure 25–7
Survival of patients with chest wall chondrosarcoma by extent of operation. Zero time on abscissa represents day of chest wall resection. *(From McAfee MK, Pairolero PC, Bergstralh EJ, et al. Chondrosarcoma of the chest wall: factors affecting survival. Reprinted with permission of The Society of Thoracic Surgeons.)*

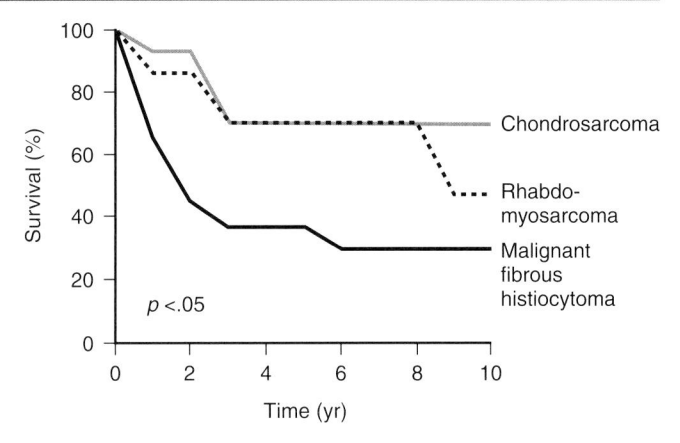

Figure 25–8
Survival for patients with chondrosarcoma and rhabdomyosarcoma compared with malignant fibrous histiocytoma. Zero time on abscissa represents day of chest wall resection. *(From King RM, Pairolero PC, Trastek VF, et al. Primary chest wall tumors: factors affecting survival. Reprinted with permission of The Society of Thoracic Surgeons.)*

REFERENCES

1. Arnold PG, Pairolero PC. Chest wall reconstruction: Experience with 100 consecutive patients. *Ann Surg* 1984;**199**:725.
2. Arnold PG, Pairolero PC. Chest wall reconstruction: An account of 500 consecutive patients. *Plast Reconstr Surg* 1996;**98**:804.
3. Pairolero PC, Arnold PG. Thoracic wall defects: Surgical management of 205 consecutive patients. *Mayo Clin Proc* 1986;**61**:557-63.
4. Arnold PG, Pairolero PC. Surgical management of the radiated chest wall. *Plast Reconstr Surg* 1986;**77**:605-12.
5. Pairolero PC, Arnold PG. Chest wall tumors: Experience with 100 consecutive patients. *J Thorac Cardiovasc Surg* 1985;**90**:367-72.
6. Groff DB, Adkins PC. Chest wall tumors. *Ann Thorac Surg* 1967;**4**:260.
7. Pascuzzi CA, Dahlin DC, Clagett OT. Primary tumors of the ribs and sternum. *Surg Gynecol Obstet* 1957;**104**:390.
8. Stelzer P, Gay Jr WA. Tumors of the chest wall. *Surg Clin North Am* 1980;**60**:779.
9. La Quaglia MP. Chest wall tumors in childhood and adolescence. *Semin Pediatr Surg* 2008;**17**:173-80.
10. van den Berg H, van Rijn RR, Merks JHM. Management of tumors of the chest wall in childhood: A review. *J Pediatr Hematol Oncol* 2008;**30**:214-21.
11. King RM, Pairolero PC, Trastek VF, et al. Primary chest wall tumors: Factors affecting survival. *Ann Thorac Surg* 1986;**41**:597-601.
12. Chapelier AR, Missana M-C, Couturaud B, Fadel E, Fabre D, Mussot S, et al. Sternal resection and reconstruction for primary malignant tumors. *Ann Thorac Surg* 2004;**77**:1001-7.
13. Bertocchini A, Falappa P, Accinni A, Devito R, Inserra A. Radiofrequency thermoablation in chest wall mesenchymal hamartoma of an infant. *Ann Thorac Surg* 2007;**84**:2091-3.
14. Mansour KA, Thourani VH, Losken A, Reeves JG, Miller Jr JI, Carlson GW, Jones GE. Chest wall resections and reconstruction: A 25-year experience. *Ann Thorac Surg* 2002;**73**:1720-6.
15. Thomas-de-Montpreville V, Chapelier A, Fadel E, Mussot S, Dulmet E, Dartevelle P. Chest wall resection for invasive lung carcinoma, soft tissue sarcoma, and other types of malignancy. Pathologic aspects in a series of 107 patients. *Ann Diagn Pathol* 2004;**8**:198-206.
16. Sabanathan S, Shah R, Mearns AJ, Richardson J. Chest wall resection and reconstruction. *Br J Hosp Med* 1997;**57**:255-9.
17. Watson WL, James AG. Fascia lata grafts for chest wall defects. *J Thorac Surg* 1947;**16**:399-406.
18. Bisgard JD, Swenson Jr SA. Tumors of the sternum: Report of a case with special operative technique. *Arch Surg* 1948;**56**:570.
19. Tansini I. Sopra il mio nuovo processo di amputazione della mammella. *Gazz Med Ital Torino* 1906;**57**:141.
20. Blades B, Paul JS. Chest wall tumors. *Ann Surg* 1950;**131**:976.
21. Converse JM, Campbell RM, Watson WL. Repair of large radiation ulcers situated over the heart and the brain. *Ann Surg* 1951;**133**:95.

22. Myre TT, Kirklin JW. Resection of tumors of the sternum. *Ann Surg* 1956;**144**:1023.
23. Novoa N, Benito P, Jimenez MF, de Juan A, Aranda JL, Varela G. Reconstruction of chest wall defects after resection of large neoplasms: ten-year experience. *Interact Cardiovasc Thorac Surg* 2005;**4**:250-5.
24. Skoracki RJ, Chang DW. Reconstruction of the chest wall and thorax. *J Surg Oncol* 2006;**94**:455-65.
25. Aranda JL, Varela G, Benito P, de Juan A. Donor cryopreserved rib allografts for chest wall reconstruction. *Interact Cardiovasc Thorac Surg* 2008;**7**:858-60.
26. Graham J, Usher FC, Perry JL, Barkley HT. Marlex mesh as a prosthesis in the repair of thoracic wall defects. *Ann Surg* 1960;**151**:469-79.
27. Arnold PG, Pairolero PC. Chest-wall reconstruction: An account of 500 consecutive patients. *Plast Reconstr Surg* 1996;**98**:804-10.
28. Cohen M, Ramasastry SS. Reconstruction of complex chest wall defects. *Am J Surg* 1996;**172**:35-40.
29. Daigeler A, Druecke D, Hakimi M, Duchna HW, Goertz O, Homann HH, et al. Reconstruction of the thoracic wall—long-term follow-up including pulmonary function tests. *Langenbecks Arch Surg* 2009;**394**:705-15.
30. McCormack PM. Use of prosthetic materials in chest-wall reconstruction: Assets and liabilities. *Surg Clin North Am* 1989;**69**:965-76.
31. Meadows III JA, Statts BA, Pairolero PC. Effect of resection of the sternum and manubrium in conjunction with muscle transposition on pulmonary function. *Mayo Clin Proc* 1985;**60**:604.
32. Murakawa T, Nakajima J, Maeda K, Tanaka M, Takamoto S. Reappraisal of fascia lata grafts for the reconstruction of chest wall defects. *Asia Cardiovasc Thorac Ann* 2002;**10**:285-6.
33. Deschamps C, Tirnaksiz BM, Darbandi R, Trastek VF, Allen MS, Miller DL, et al. Early and long-term results of prosthetic chest wall reconstruction. *J Thorac Cardiovasc Surg* 1999;**117**:588-92.
34. Weyant MJ, Bains MS, Venkatraman E, Downey FJ, Park BJ, Flores RM, et al. Results of chest wall resection and reconstruction with and without rigid prosthesis. *Ann Thorac Surg* 2006;**81**:279-85.
35. Gayer G, Yellin A, Rozenman Y. Reconstruction of the sternum and chest wall with methyl methacrylate: CT and MRI appearance. *Eur Radiol* 1998;**8**:239-43.
36. Chang RR, Mehrara BJ, Hu Q-Y, Disa JJ, Cordeiro PG. Reconstruction of complex oncologic chest wall defects. A 10-year experience. *Ann Plast Surg* 2004;**52**:471-9.
37. Abbas AE, Deschamps C, Cassivi SD, Nichols III FC, Allen MS, Schleck CD, Pairolero PC. Chest wall desmoid tumors: Results of surgical intervention. *Ann Thorac Surg* 2004;**78**:1219-23.
38. Goellner JR, Soule EH. Desmoid tumors: An ultrastructural study of eight cases. *Hum Pathol* 1980;**11**:43.
39. Hayry P, Reitamo JJ, Totterman S, et al. The desmoid tumor. II. Analysis of factors possibly contributing to the etiology and growth behavior. *Am J Clin Pathol* 1982;**77**:674.
40. Hajdu SI. *Pathology of Soft Tissue Tumors*. Philadelphia: Lea & Febiger; 1979, p. 122.
41. Soule EG, Scanlon PW. Fibrosarcoma arising in an extraabdominal desmoid tumor: Report of a case. *Mayo Clin Proc* 1962;**37**:443.
42. Weiss SW, Enzinger FM. Malignant fibrous histiocytoma: An analysis of 200 cases. *Cancer* 1978;**41**:2250.
43. McAfee MK, Pairolero PC, Bergstralh EJ, et al. Chondrosarcoma of the chest wall: Factors affecting survival. *Ann Thorac Surg* 1985;**40**:535.
44. Arnold PG, Pairolero PC. Chondrosarcoma of the manubrium. Resection and reconstruction with pectoralis major muscle. *Mayo Clin Proc* 1978;**53**:54-7.
45. Arnold PG, Pairolero PC, Waldorf JC. The serratus anterior muscle: Intrathoracic and extrathoracic utilization. *Plast Reconstr Surg* 1984;**73**:240-8.
46. Meadows III JA, Staats BA, Pairolero PC, et al. Effect of resection of the sternum and manubrium in conjunction with muscle transposition on pulmonary function. *Mayo Clin Proc* 1985;**60**:604-9.
47. Fong Y-C, Pairolero PC, Sim FH, Cha SS, Blanchard CL, Scully SP. Chondrosarcoma of the chest wall. A retrospective clinical analysis. *Clin Orthop* 2004;**427**:184-9.
48. Gross JL, Younes RN, Haddad FJ, Deheinzelin D, Pinto CAL, Costa MLV. Soft-tissue sarcomas of the chest wall: Prognostic factors. *Chest* 2005;**127**:902-8.

CHAPTER 26
Thoracic Outlet Syndrome and Dorsal Sympathectomy
Harold C. Urschel, Jr. and Amit N. Patel

Historical Aspects
Surgical Anatomy
Functional Anatomy
Compression Factors
Symptoms and Signs
Diagnosis
  Clinical Maneuvers
  Radiographic Findings
  Nerve Conduction Velocity and
    Electromyography
  Method of Measuring Conduction
    Velocities
  Equipment
  Technique
  Calculation of Velocities

Normal Ulnar Nerve Conduction Velocities
Grading of Compression
Angiography
Differential Diagnosis
Therapy
  Technique of Transaxillary Resection of the
    First Rib
Effort Thrombosis: Paget-Schroetter
  Syndrome
Dorsal Sympathectomy and Thoracic Outlet
  Syndrome Management with VATS
  Pathophysiology
  Complications
    Horner's Syndrome
    Postsympathetic Neuralgia

Recurrent Symptoms
Surgical Approaches for Dorsal
  Sympathectomy
Variations of Dorsal Sympathectomy
Technique
  Transaxillary Approach with a Transthoracic
    Sympathectomy
  Transaxillary First Rib Resection
    for Thoracic Outlet Syndrome
    with Retraction of the Pleura and
    Sympathectomy
Results
Reoperation for Recurrent Thoracic Outlet
  Syndrome
Summary

Thoracic outlet syndrome, a term coined by Rob and Standover,[1] refers to compression of the subclavian vessels and brachial plexus at the superior aperture of the chest. It was previously designated, according to presumed etiologies, as scalenus anticus, costoclavicular, hyperabduction, cervical rib, and first thoracic rib syndromes. The various syndromes are similar, and the compression mechanism is often difficult to identify. Most compressive factors operate against the first rib (Fig. 26-1).[2,3]

HISTORICAL ASPECTS

Until 1927, the cervical rib was commonly thought to be the cause of symptoms of this syndrome. Galen and Vesalius first described the presence of a cervical rib.[4] Hunauld, who published an article in 1742, is credited by Keen[5] as being the first to describe the importance of the cervical rib in causing symptoms. In 1818, Cooper treated symptoms of cervical rib with some success,[6] and in 1861, Coote[7] did the first cervical rib removal. Halsted[8] stimulated interest in dilation of the subclavian artery distal to cervical ribs, and Law[9] reported the role of adventitious ligaments in the cervical rib syndrome. In 1927, Adson and Coffey[6] suggested the role of the scalenus anticus muscle in cervical rib syndrome. Naffziger and Grant[10] and Ochsner and associates[11] popularized sectioning of the scalenus anticus muscle. Falconer and Weddell[12] and Brintnall and colleagues[13] incriminated the costoclavicular membrane in the production of neurovascular compression. In 1945, Wright[14] described the hyperabduction syndrome with compression in the costoclavicular area by the tendon of the pectoralis minor. Rosati and Lord[15] added claviculectomy to anterior exploration, scalenotomy, cervical rib resection (when one was present), and sectioning of the pectoralis minor and subclavian muscles and of the costoclavicular membrane. The role of the first rib in causing symptoms of neurovascular compression was recognized by Bramwell[16] in 1903. Murphy[17] is credited with the first resection of the first rib. Brickner,[18] Brickner and Milch,[19] and Telford and coworkers[20,21] suggested that the first rib was the culprit. Clagett[2] emphasized the first rib and its resection through the posterior thoracoplasty approach to relieve neurovascular compression. In 1962, Falconer and Li[22] reported the anterior approach for first rib resection, whereas Roos[23] introduced the transaxillary route for first rib resection and extirpation. Caldwell and colleagues[24] introduced the method of measuring motor conduction velocities across the thoracic outlet in diagnosing thoracic outlet syndrome. Urschel and Razzuk[25] popularized reoperation for recurrent thoracic outlet syndrome.

SURGICAL ANATOMY

At the superior aperture of the thorax, the subclavian vessels and the brachial plexus traverse the cervicoaxillary canal to reach the upper extremity. The cervicoaxillary canal is divided by the first rib into two sections: the proximal one, composed of the scalene triangle and the costoclavicular space, and the distal one, composed of the axilla. The proximal division is the more critical for neurovascular compression. It is bounded superiorly by the clavicle, inferiorly by the first rib, anteromedially by the costoclavicular ligament, and posterolaterally by the scalenus medius muscle and the long thoracic nerve. The scalenus anticus muscle, which inserts on the scalene tubercle of the first rib, divides the costoclavicular space into two compartments: the anteromedial one containing the subclavian vein and the posterolateral one containing the subclavian artery and the brachial plexus (Fig. 26-2). The latter

```
                    Scalenus anticus and medius muscles              Cervical rib
                    Pectoralis minor muscle and                       First rib anomalies
                    costocoracoid ligament
                                                                      Long transverse process
                    Costoclavicular membrane        Compression       Clavicle abnormalities
                    Subclavius muscle

                                                   First rib

                         Vascular                                           Nerve

              Subclavian vein    Subclavian artery       Sympathetic        Peripheral
                                                  Pain
                                            Color and
                                         temperature change
                                              Ischemia
                                           Trophic change

                   Edema         Loss of pulse         Raynaud's              Pain
              Venous distention   Claudication        phenomenon          Paresthesias
           Paget-Schroetter syndrome Thrombosis                          Motor weakness
```

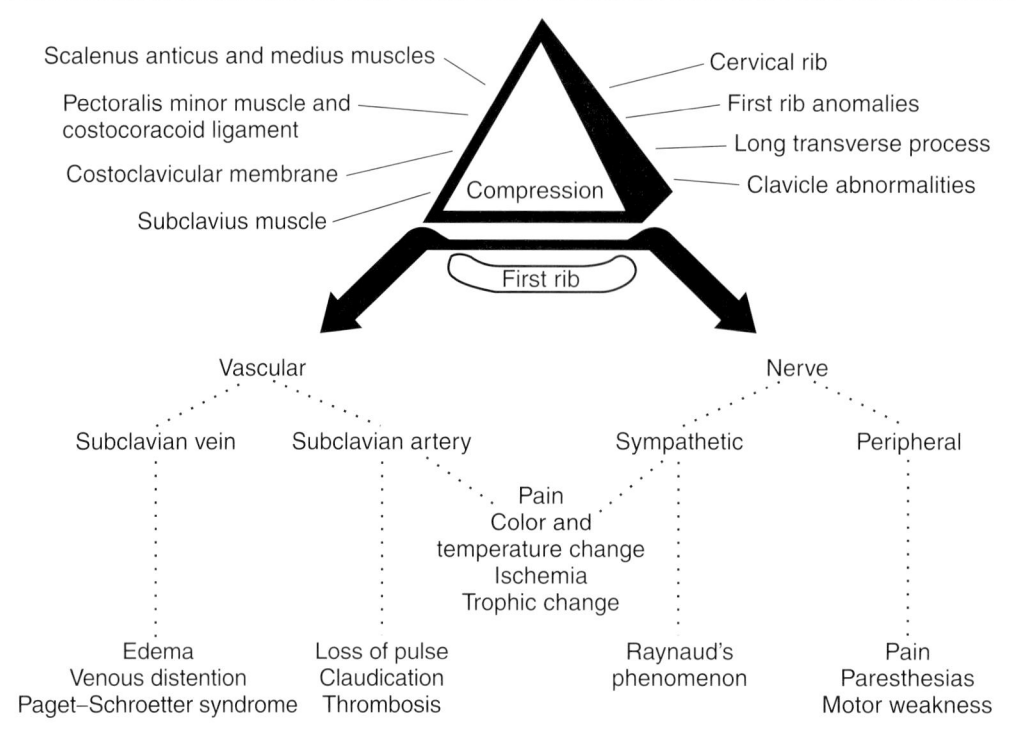

Figure 26–1
Diagram of the relationships of muscle, ligament, and bone abnormalities in the thoracic outlet that may compress neurovascular structures against the first rib.

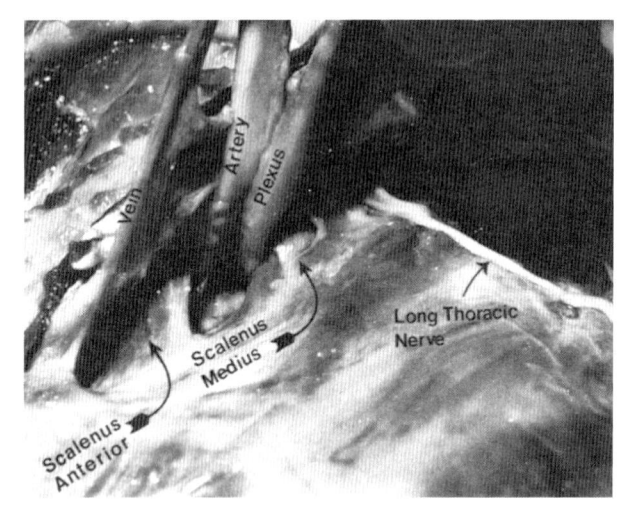

Figure 26–2
Anatomic dissection from the transaxillary approach, showing the relationship of the neurovascular bundle, the scalenus anterior muscle, and the long thoracic nerve along the posterior border of the scalenus medius muscle.

compartment, which is bounded by the scalenus anticus anteriorly, the scalenus medius posteriorly, and the first rib inferiorly, is called the scalene triangle.

FUNCTIONAL ANATOMY

The cervicoaxillary canal, particularly its proximal segment, the costoclavicular area, normally has ample space for passage of the neurovascular bundle without compression. Narrowing of this space occurs during functional maneuvers. It narrows during abduction of the arm because the clavicle rotates backward toward the first rib and the insertion of the scalenus anticus muscle. In hyperabduction, the neurovascular bundle is pulled around the pectoralis minor tendon, the coracoid process, and the head of the humerus. During this maneuver, the coracoid process tilts downward and thus exaggerates the tension on the bundle. The sternoclavicular joint, which ordinarily forms an angle of 15 to 20 degrees, forms a smaller angle when the outer end of the clavicle descends (as in drooping of the shoulders in poor posture), and narrowing of the costoclavicular space may occur.[15] Normally, during inspiration, the scalenus anticus muscle raises the first rib and thus narrows the costoclavicular space. This muscle may cause an abnormal lift of the first rib, as in cases of severe emphysema or excessive muscular development, which is seen in young adults.

The scalene triangle, which normally occurs between the scalenus anticus anteriorly, the scalenus medius posteriorly, and the first rib inferiorly, permits the passage of the subclavian artery and the brachial plexus, which are in direct contact with the first rib. The space of the triangle is 1.2 cm at its base and approximately 6.7 cm in height (Fig. 26-3). There is a close-fitting relationship between the neurovascular bundle and this triangular space. Anatomic variations may narrow the superior angle of the triangle, cause impingement on the upper components of the brachial plexus, and produce the upper type of scalenus anticus syndrome that involves the trunk containing elements of C5 and C6. If the base of the triangle is raised, compression of the subclavian artery and the trunk containing components of C7, C8, and T1 results in the lower type of scalenus anticus syndrome. Both types have been described by Swank and Simeone.[26]

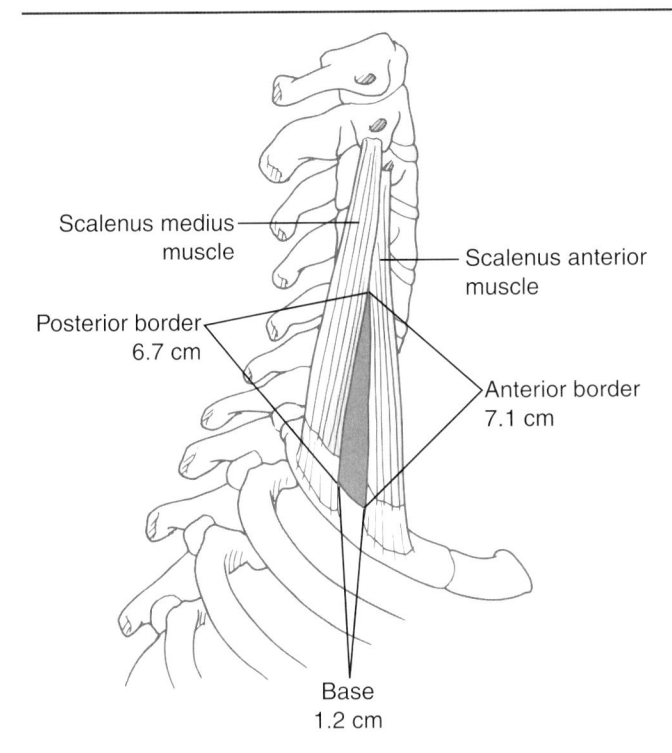

Figure 26-3
The scalene (anterior) triangle, with its measurements and the narrow interval through which the neurovascular bundle passes. *(From Rosati LM, Lord JV. Neurovascular compression syndromes of the shoulder girdle. New York: Grune & Stratton; 1961.)*

> **Box 26-1**
> **Causes of Neurovascular Compression Syndromes**
>
> **Anatomic**
> - Potential sites of neurovascular compression
>   - Interscalene triangle
>   - Costoclavicular space
>   - Subcoracoid area
>
> **Congenital**
> - Cervical rib and its fascial remnants
> - Rudimentary first thoracic rib
> - Scalene muscles
>   - Anterior
>   - Middle
>   - Minimus
> - Adventitious fibrous bands
> - Bifid clavicle or first rib
> - Exostosis of first thoracic rib
> - Enlarged transverse process of C7
> - Omohyoid muscle
> - Anomalous course of transverse cervical artery
> - Abnormal lateral insertion of costoclavicular ligament
> - Flat clavicle
>
> **Traumatic**
> - Fracture of clavicle
> - Dislocation of head of humerus
> - Crushing injury to upper thorax
> - Sudden, unaccustomed muscular efforts involving shoulder girdle muscles
> - Cervical spondylosis and injuries to cervical spine
>
> **Atherosclerosis**

COMPRESSION FACTORS

Many factors may cause compression of the neurovascular bundle at the thoracic outlet, but the basic factor is deranged anatomy, to which congenital, traumatic, and, occasionally, atherosclerotic factors may contribute (Box 26-1).[15] Bony abnormalities are present in approximately 30% of patients, either as cervical rib, bifid first rib, and fusion of first and second ribs; clavicular deformities; or previous thoracoplasties.[3] These abnormalities can be visualized on the plain posteroanterior chest film, but special radiographic views of the lower cervical spine may be required in some cases of cervical ribs.

SYMPTOMS AND SIGNS

The symptoms of thoracic outlet syndrome depend on whether the nerves or blood vessels, or both, are compressed in the cervicoaxillary canal. Neurogenic manifestations are observed more frequently than vascular ones. Symptoms consist of pain and paresthesias, which are present in approximately 95% of cases, and motor weakness and occasionally atrophy of hypothenar and interosseous muscles, which is the ulnar type of atrophy, in approximately 10%. The symptoms occur most commonly in areas supplied by the ulnar nerve, which include the medial aspects of the arm and hand, the fifth finger, and the lateral aspects of the fourth finger. The onset of pain is usually insidious and commonly involves the neck, shoulder, arm, and hand. The pain and paresthesias may be precipitated by strenuous physical exercise or sustained physical effort with the arm in abduction and the neck in hyperextension. Symptoms may be initiated by sleeping with the arms abducted and the hands clasped behind the neck. In other cases, trauma to the upper extremities or the cervical spine is a precipitating factor. Physical examination may be noncontributory. When present, objective physical findings usually consist of hypesthesia along the medial aspects of the forearm and hand. Atrophy, when evident, is usually described in the hypothenar and interosseous muscles with clawing of the fourth and fifth fingers. In the upper type of thoracic outlet syndrome, in which components of C5 and C6 are involved in compression, pain is usually in the deltoid area and the lateral aspects of the arm. The presence of this pain should induce action to exclude a herniated cervical disc.[15] Entrapment of C7 and C8 components that contribute to the median nerve produces symptoms in the index finger and sometimes the middle finger. Components of C5, C6, C7, C8, and T1 can occur at the thoracic outlet by a cervical rib and produce symptoms of various degrees in the distribution of these nerves (Fig. 26-4).

In some patients, the pain is atypical, involving the anterior chest wall or parascapular area, and is termed pseudoangina because it simulates angina pectoris. These patients may have normal coronary arteriograms and ulnar nerve conduction velocities decreased to values of 48 m/sec and less, which

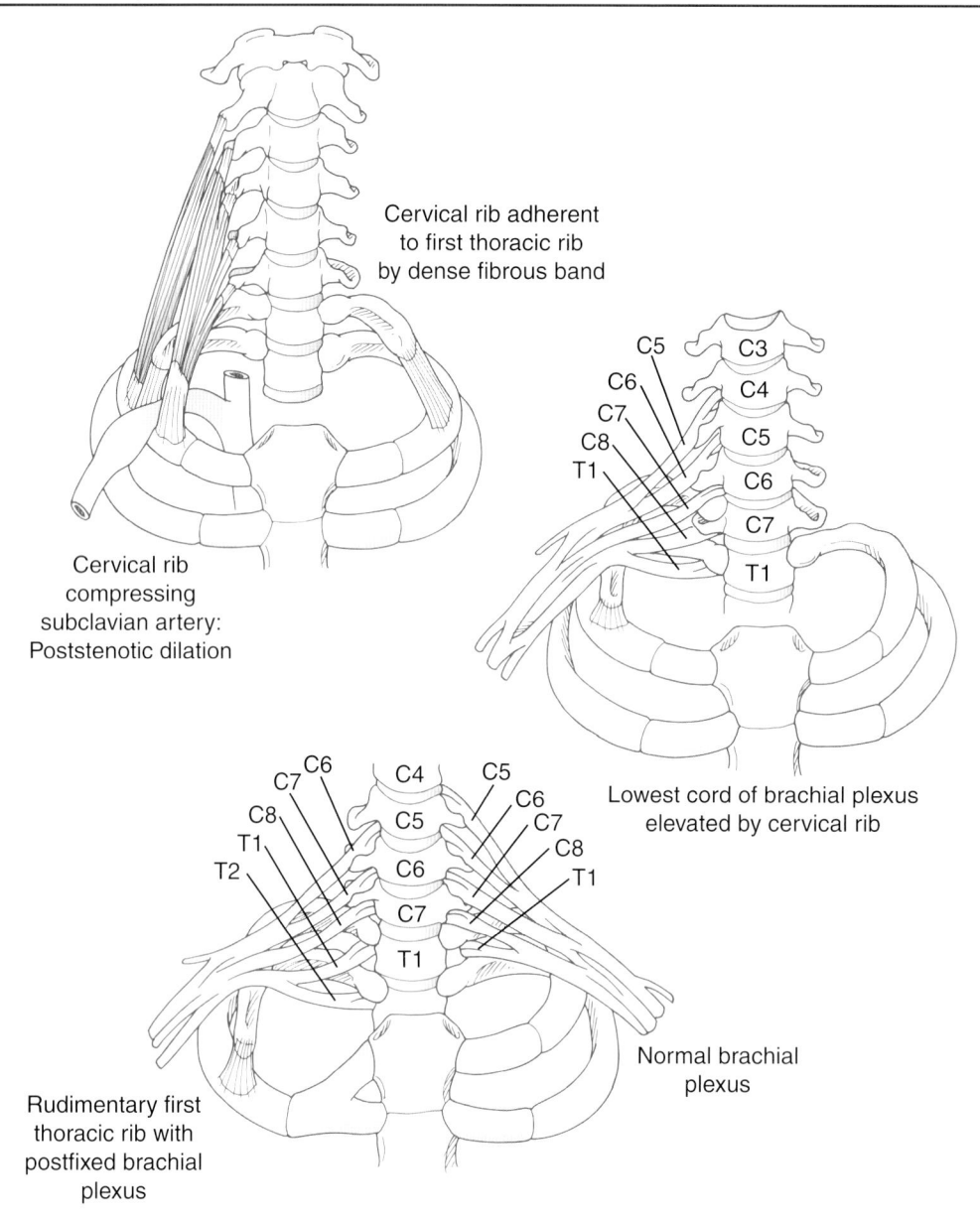

Figure 26–4
Compression caused by congenital rib abnormalities. *(Reprinted from www.netterimages.com © elsevier Inc. All rights reserved.)*

strongly suggests the diagnosis of thoracic outlet syndrome. The shoulder, arm, and hand symptoms that usually provide the clue for the diagnosis of thoracic outlet syndrome may initially be absent or minimal compared with the severity of the chest pain. The diagnosis of thoracic outlet syndrome is frequently overlooked; many of these patients are committed to becoming "cardiac cripples" without an appropriate diagnosis, or they develop severe psychological depression when told that their coronary arteries are normal and that they have no significant cause for their pain.[27]

Symptoms of arterial compression include coldness, weakness, easy fatigability of the arm and hand, and pain that is usually diffuse.[28,29] Raynaud's phenomenon is noted in approximately 7.5% of patients with thoracic outlet syndrome.[28] Unlike Raynaud's disease, which is usually bilateral and symmetrical and elicited by cold or emotion, Raynaud's phenomenon in neurovascular compression is usually unilateral and is more likely to be precipitated by hyperabduction of the involved arm, turning of the head, or carrying of heavy objects. Sensitivity to cold may also be present. Symptoms include sudden onset of cold and blanching of one or more fingers, followed slowly by cyanosis and persistent rubor. Vascular symptoms in neurovascular compression may be precursors of permanent arterial thrombosis.[15] Arterial occlusion, usually of the subclavian artery, when present, is manifested by persistent coldness, cyanosis or pallor of the fingers, and in some instances, ulceration or gangrene. Palpation in the parascapular area may reveal prominent pulsation, which indicates poststenotic dilation or aneurysm of the subclavian artery (Fig. 26-5).[30]

Less frequently, the symptoms are those of venous obstruction or occlusion, commonly recognized as effort thrombosis,

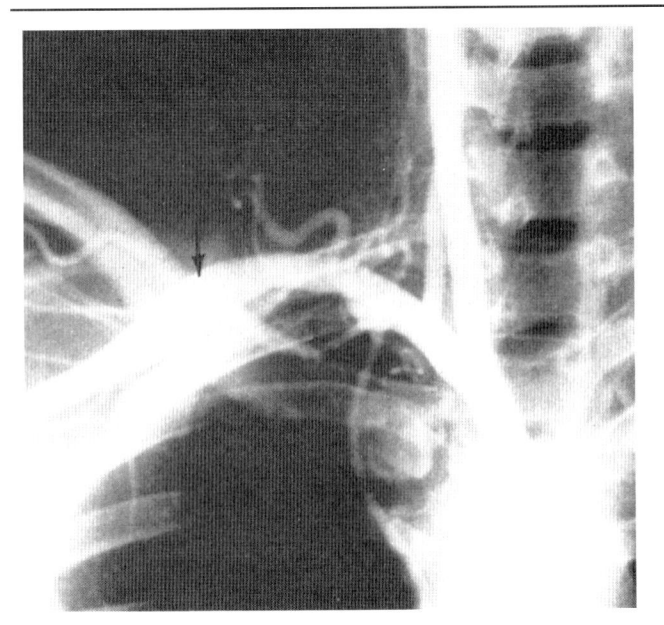

Figure 26–5
Arteriogram showing poststenotic dilation *(arrow)* of the right subclavian artery secondary to thoracic outlet compression.

or Paget-Schroetter syndrome. The condition characteristically results in edema, discoloration of the arm, distention of the superficial veins of the limb and shoulder, and some degree of aches and pains. In some patients, the condition is observed on waking; in others, it follows sustained efforts with the arm in abduction. Sudden backward and downward bracing of the shoulders or heavy lifting or strenuous physical activity involving the arm may constrict the vein and initiate venospasm, with or without subsequent thrombosis. On examination, in cases of definite venous thrombosis, there is usually moderate tenderness over the axillary vein, and a cordlike structure may be felt that corresponds to the course of the vein. The acute symptoms may subside in a few weeks or days as the collateral circulation develops. Recurrence follows with inadequacy of the collateral circulation.[31]

Objective physical findings are more common in patients with primarily vascular rather than neural compression. Loss or diminution of radial pulse and reproduction of symptoms can be elicited by the three classic clinical maneuvers: the Adson's or scalene test,[32] the costoclavicular test, and the hyperabduction test.[33]

DIAGNOSIS

The diagnosis of thoracic outlet syndrome includes history, physical and neurologic examinations, films of the chest and cervical spine, electromyogram, and ulnar nerve conduction velocity (UNCV). In some cases with atypical manifestations, other diagnostic procedures such as cervical myelography, peripheral[30] or coronary arteriography, or phlebography[34] should be considered. A detailed history and physical and neurologic examinations can often result in a tentative diagnosis of neurovascular compression. This diagnosis is strengthened when one or more of the classic clinical maneuvers is positive and is confirmed by the finding of decreased UNCV.[35]

Clinical Maneuvers

The clinical evaluation is best based on the physical findings of loss or decrease of radial pulses and reproduction of symptoms that can be elicited by the following three classic maneuvers[15,33]:

- Adson or scalene test[32] (Fig. 26-6). This maneuver tightens the anterior and middle scalene muscles and thus decreases the interspace and magnifies any preexisting compression of the subclavian artery and brachial plexus. The patient is instructed to take and hold a deep breath, extend the neck fully, and turn the head toward the side. Obliteration or decrease of the radial pulse suggests compression.
- Costoclavicular test (military position) (Fig. 26-7). The shoulders are drawn downward and backward. This maneuver narrows the costoclavicular space by approximating the clavicle to the first rib and thus tends to compress the neurovascular bundle. Changes in the radial pulse with production of symptoms indicate compression.
- Hyperabduction test (Fig. 26-8). When the arm is hyperabducted to 180 degrees, the components of the neurovascular bundle are pulled around the pectoralis minor tendon, the coracoid process, and the head of the humerus. If the radial pulse is decreased, compression should be suspected.

Radiographic Findings

Films of the chest and cervical spine are helpful in revealing bony abnormalities, particularly cervical ribs (Fig. 26-9) and bony degenerative changes. If osteophytic changes and intervertebral space narrowing are present on plain cervical films, a cervical computed tomography (CT) scan should be obtained to rule out bony encroachment and narrowing of the spinal canal and the intervertebral foramina.

Nerve Conduction Velocity and Electromyography

This test is widely used in differential diagnosis of the causes of arm pain, tingling, and numbness with or without motor weakness of the hand. Such symptoms may result from compression at various sites: in the spine; at the thoracic outlet; around the elbow, where it causes tardy ulnar nerve palsy; or on the flexor aspects of the wrist, where it produces carpal tunnel syndrome. For diagnosis and localization of the site of compression, cathodal stimulation is applied at various points along the course of the nerve. Motor conduction velocities of the ulnar, median, radial, and musculocutaneous nerves can be measured reliably.[36] Caldwell and colleagues[24] have improved the technique of measuring UNCV for evaluation of patients with thoracic outlet compression. Conduction velocities over proximal and distal segments of the ulnar nerve are determined by recording the action potentials generated in the hypothenar or first dorsal interosseous muscles. The points of stimulation are the supraclavicular fossa, middle upper arm, below the elbow, and at the wrist (Fig. 26-10).[29]

Method of Measuring Conduction Velocities

Equipment

Electromyographic examination of each upper extremity and determination of the conduction velocities are done with the Meditron 201 AD or 312 or the TECA-3 electromyograph;

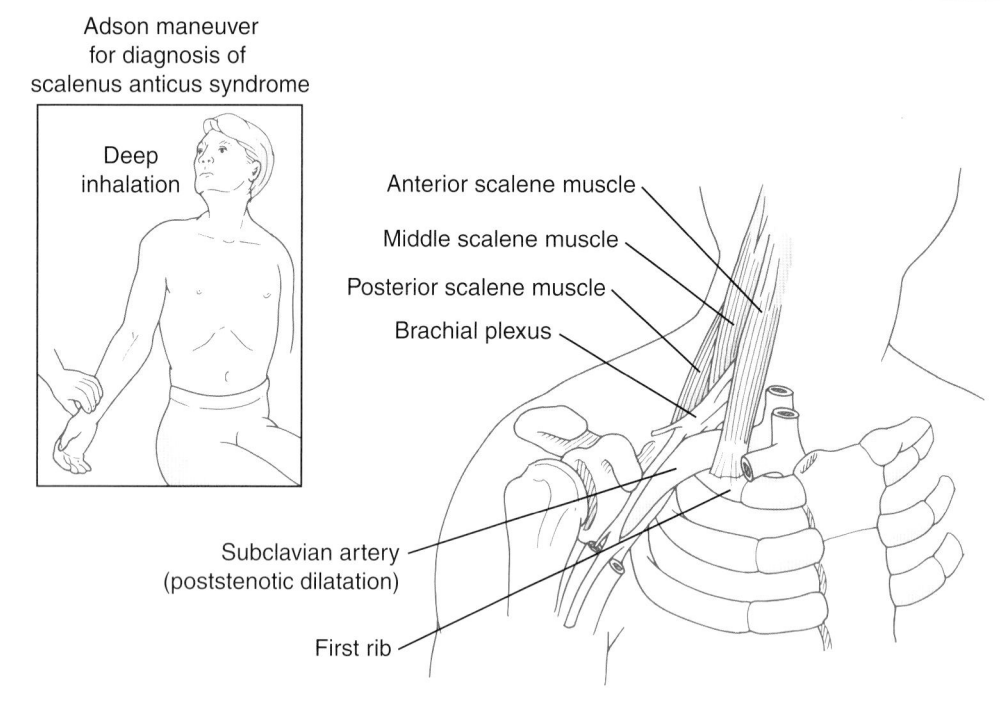

Figure 26–6
Adson's maneuver. Relationship of the scalene triangle to the neurovascular bundle. *(Reprinted from www.netterimages.com @ elsevier inc. All rights reserved.)*

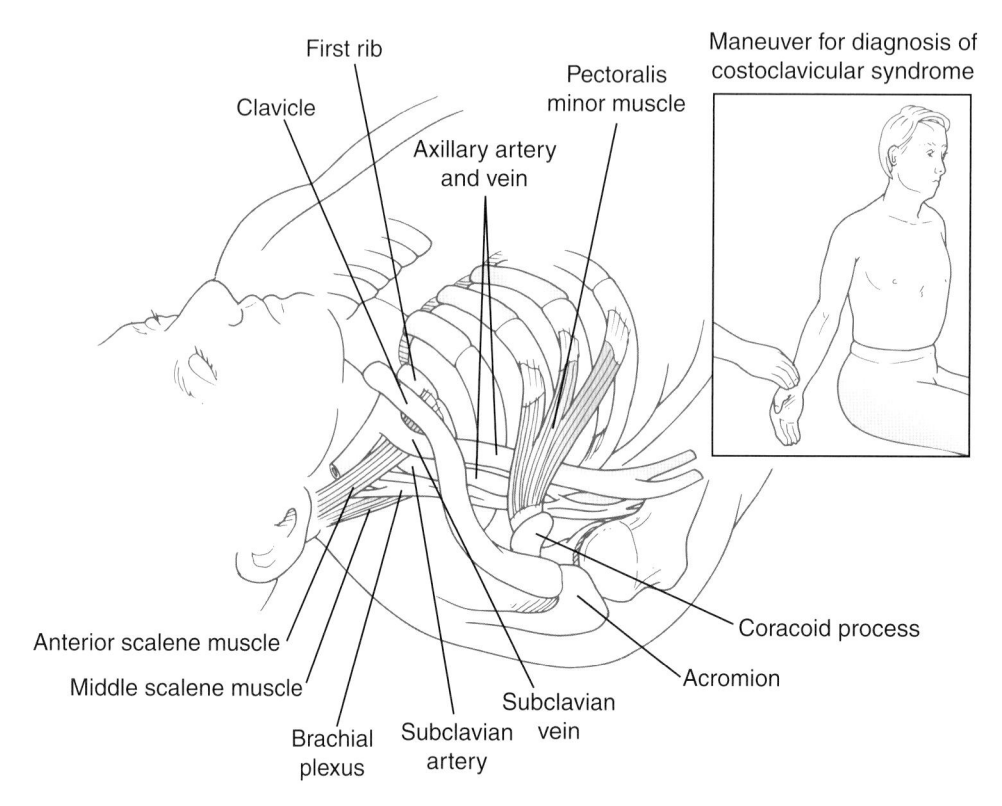

Figure 26–7
Costoclavicular maneuver (military position). Relationship of the costoclavicular space to the neurovascular bundle. *(Reprinted from www.netterimages.com @ elsevier inc. All rights reserved.)*

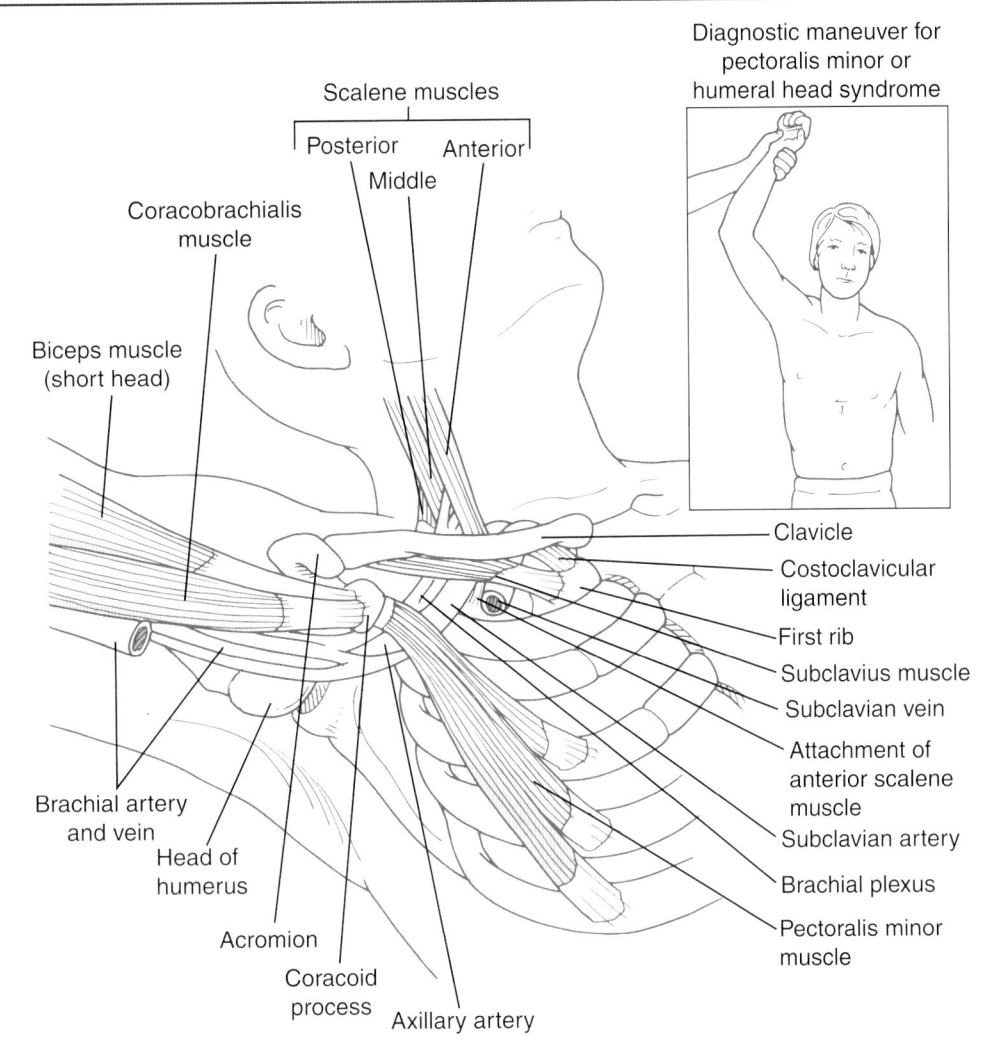

Figure 26–8
Hyperabduction maneuver. Relationship of the neurovascular bundle to the pectoralis minor tendon, the coracoid process, and the humeral head (pulley effect). *(Reprinted from www.netterimages.com © elsevier inc. All rights reserved.)*

coaxial cable with three needles or surface electrodes are used to record muscle potentials, which appear on the fluorescent screen (Fig. 26-11).

Technique

The conduction velocity is determined by the Krusen-Caldwell technique.[24] The patient is placed on the examination table with the arm fully extended at the elbow and in about 20 degrees of abduction at the shoulder to facilitate stimulation over the course of the ulnar nerve. The ulnar nerve is stimulated at the four points by a special stimulation unit (Fig. 26-12) that imparts an electrical stimulus with strength of 350 V with the patient's load, which is approximately equal to 300 V with the patient's load with a skin resistance of 5000 Ω. Supramaximal stimulation is used at all points to obtain maximal response. The duration of the stimulation is 0.2 msec, except for muscular individuals, for whom it is 0.5 msec. Time of stimulation, conduction delay, and muscle response appear on the TECA screen; time markers occur each millisecond on the sweep.

The latency period to stimulation from the four points of stimulation to the recording electrode is obtained from the TECA digital recorder or calculated from the tracing on the screen.

Calculation of Velocities

After the latencies, which are expressed in milliseconds, are obtained, the distance in millimeters between two adjacent sites of stimulation is measured with steel tape. The velocities, which are expressed in meters per second, are calculated by subtracting the distal latency from the proximal latency and dividing the distance between two points of stimulation by the latency difference (Fig. 26-13) according to the following formula:

Velocity (m/sec) = distance between adjacent stimulation points (mm) ÷ difference in latency between adjacent stimulation points (msec)

Normal Ulnar Nerve Conduction Velocities

The normal values of the UNCVs according to the Krusen-Caldwell technique[24] are 72 m/sec or greater across the outlet, 55 m/sec or greater around the elbow, and 59 m/sec or

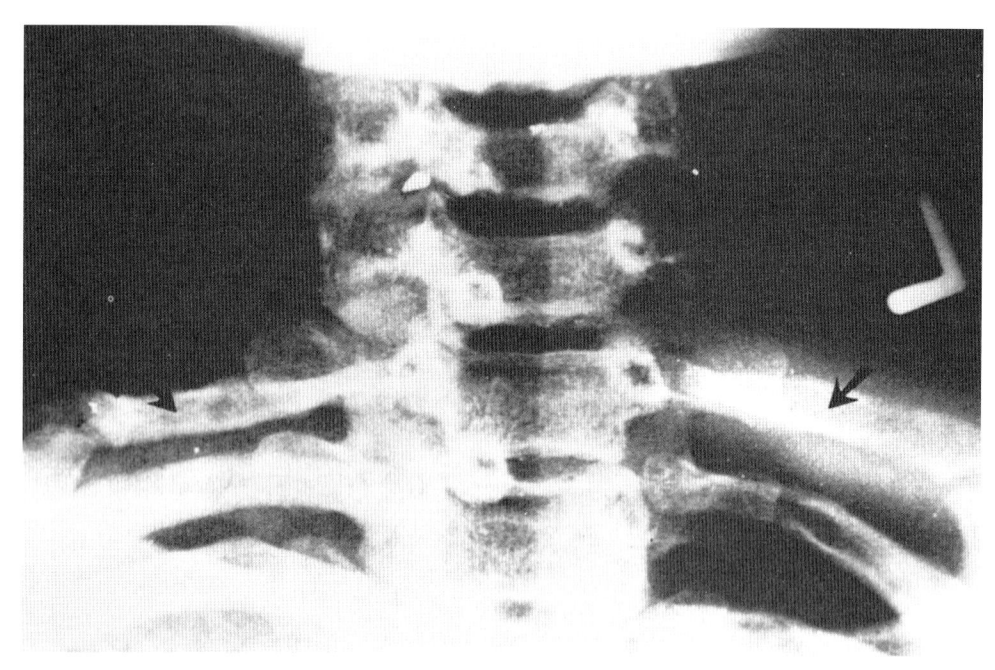

Figure 26–9
Radiographic film showing bilateral cervical ribs *(arrows)*.

greater in the forearm. Wrist delay is 2.5 to 3.5 msec. Decreased velocity in a segment or increased delay at the wrist indicates compression, injury, neuropathy, or neurologic disorders. Decreased velocity across the outlet is consistent with thoracic outlet syndrome. Decreased velocity around the elbow signifies ulnar nerve entrapment or neuropathy. Increased delay at the wrist is encountered in carpal tunnel syndrome.

Grading of Compression

The clinical picture of thoracic outlet syndrome correlates fairly well with the conduction velocity across the outlet. Any value less than 70 m/sec indicates neurovascular compression. The severity is graded according to decrease of velocity across the thoracic outlet: compression is called slight when the velocity is 66 to 69 m/sec, mild when the velocity is 60 to 65 m/sec, moderate when the velocity is 55 to 59 m/sec, and severe when the velocity is 54 m/sec and less.

Angiography

Simple clinical observations usually suffice to determine the degree of vascular impairment in the upper extremity. Peripheral angiography[30,37] is indicated in some cases, as in the presence of a paraclavicular pulsating mass, the absence of radial pulse, or the presence of supraclavicular or infraclavicular bruits. Retrograde or antegrade arteriograms of the subclavian and brachial arteries to demonstrate or localize the pathology should be obtained. In cases of venous stenosis or obstruction, as in Paget-Schroetter syndrome, phlebograms are used to determine the extent of thrombosis and the status of the collateral circulation (Fig. 26-14).

DIFFERENTIAL DIAGNOSIS

The thoracic outlet syndrome should be differentiated from various neurologic, vascular, cardiac, pulmonary, and esophageal conditions (Box 26-2).[3,15,35,38]

Neurologic causes of pain in the shoulder and arm are more difficult to recognize and may arise from involvement of the nervous system in the spine, the brachial plexus, or the peripheral nerves. A common neurologic cause of pain in the upper extremities is a herniated cervical intervertebral disc. The herniation almost invariably occurs at the interspace between the fifth and the sixth or the sixth and the seventh cervical vertebrae and produces characteristic symptoms. Onset of pain and stiffness of the neck is manifested with varying frequency. The pain radiates along the medial border of the scapula into the shoulder, occasionally into the anterior chest wall, and down the lateral aspect of the arm, at times into the fingers. Numbness and paresthesias in the fingers may be present. The segmental distribution of pain is a prominent feature. A herniated disc between the C5 and the C6 vertebrae, which compresses the C6 nerve root, causes pain or numbness primarily in the thumb and to a lesser extent in the index finger. The biceps muscle and the radial wrist extensor are weak, and the reflex of the biceps muscle is reduced or abolished. A herniated disc between the C6 and the C7 vertebrae, which compresses the C7 nerve root, produces pain or numbness in the index finger and weakness of index finger flexion and ulnar wrist extension; the triceps muscle is weak and its reflex is reduced or abolished. Any of these herniated discs may cause numbness along the ulnar border of the arm and hand due to spasm of the scalenus anticus muscle. Rarely, pain and paresthesias in the ulnar distribution may be related to herniation between the C7 and the T1 vertebrae, which causes compression of the C8 nerve root. Compression of the latter

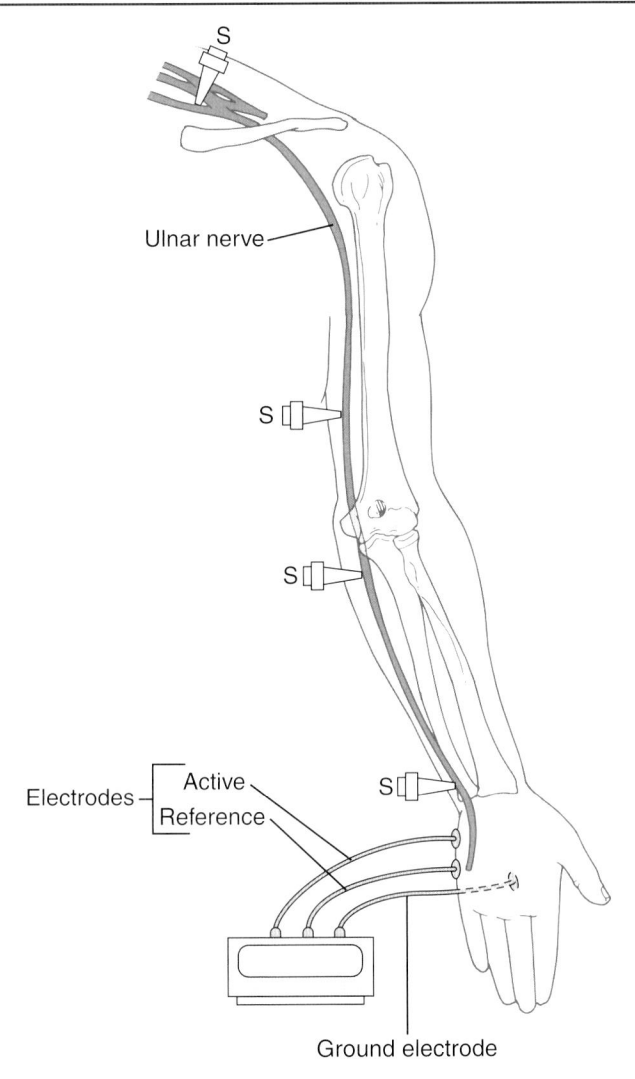

Figure 26-10
The four ulnar nerve stimulation points: in the supraclavicular fossa (Erb's point over the trunks of the plexus), above the elbow, below the elbow, and at the wrist.

nerve root produces weakness of intrinsic hand muscles.[15,39] Although rupture of the fifth and sixth discs produces hypesthesia in this area, only rupture of the seventh disc produces pain down the medial aspect of the arm.[15]

The diagnosis of a ruptured cervical disc is based primarily on the history and physical findings; lateral films of the cervical spine reveal loss or reversal of cervical curvature with the apex of the reversal of curvature at the level of the disc involved. Electromyography can localize the site and extent of the nerve root irritation. When a herniated disc is suspected, cervical myelography should be done to confirm the diagnosis.[15,39]

Another condition that causes upper extremity pain is cervical spondylosis, a degenerative disease of the intervertebral disc and the adjacent vertebral margin that causes spur formation and the production of ridges into the spinal canal or intervertebral foramina. Radiographic films and a CT scan of the cervical spine and electromyography help in making the diagnosis of this condition (Fig. 26-15).

Several arterial and venous conditions can be confused with thoracic outlet syndrome (see Box 26-2); the differentiation can often be made clinically.[15]

In atypical patients who present with chest pain alone, it is important to suspect the thoracic outlet syndrome in addition to angina pectoris. Exercise stress testing and coronary angiography may exclude coronary artery disease when there is a high index of suspicion of angina pectoris.[27,33]

THERAPY

Patients with neurogenic thoracic outlet syndrome should be given physiotherapy when the diagnosis is made. Proper physiotherapy includes heat massages, active neck exercises, stretching of the scalenus muscles, strengthening of the upper trapezius muscle, and posture instruction. Because sagging of the shoulder girdle, which is common among middle-aged people, is a major cause in this syndrome, many patients with less severe cases are improved by strengthening the shoulder girdle and by improving posture.[39]

Most patients with thoracic outlet syndrome who have UNCVs of more than 60 m/sec improve with conservative management. If the conduction velocity is below that level, most patients, despite physiotherapy, may remain symptomatic, and surgical resection of the first rib and correction of other bony abnormalities may be needed to provide relief of symptoms.[28,29,40]

If symptoms of neurovascular compression continue after physiotherapy, and the conduction velocity shows slight or no improvement or regression, surgical resection of the first rib and cervical rib, when present, should be considered.[28,29,40] Clagett[2] popularized the high posterior thoracoplasty approach for first rib resection, Falconer and Li[22] emphasized the anterior approach, and Roos[23] introduced the transaxillary route.

The transaxillary route is an expedient approach for complete removal of the first rib with decompression of the seventh and eighth cervical and first thoracic nerve roots and the lower trunks of the brachial plexus. First rib resection can be performed without the need for major muscle division, as in the posterior approach[2]; the need for retraction of the brachial plexus, as in the anterior supraclavicular approach[22]; and the difficulty of removing the posterior segment of the rib, as in the infraclavicular approach. In addition, first rib resection shortens the postoperative disability and provides better cosmetic results than the anterior and posterior approaches, particularly because 80% of patients are female.[28,29,35,41]

Technique of Transaxillary Resection of the First Rib

The patient is placed in the lateral position with the involved extremity abducted to 90 degrees by traction straps wrapped around the forearm and attached to an overhead pulley. An appropriate weight, usually 2 lb, is used to maintain this position without undue traction (Fig. 26-16).[3,33] Two arm holders are employed to hold the arm at 90 degrees from the body and prevent further hyperabduction.

A transverse incision is made in the axilla below the hairline between the pectoralis major and the latissimus dorsi muscles and deepened to the external thoracic fascia (Fig. 26-17). Care should be taken to prevent injury to the intercostobrachial cutaneous nerve, which passes from the chest wall to the subcutaneous tissue in the center of the operative field.

The dissection is extended cephalad along the external thoracic fascia up to the first rib. With gentle dissection, the

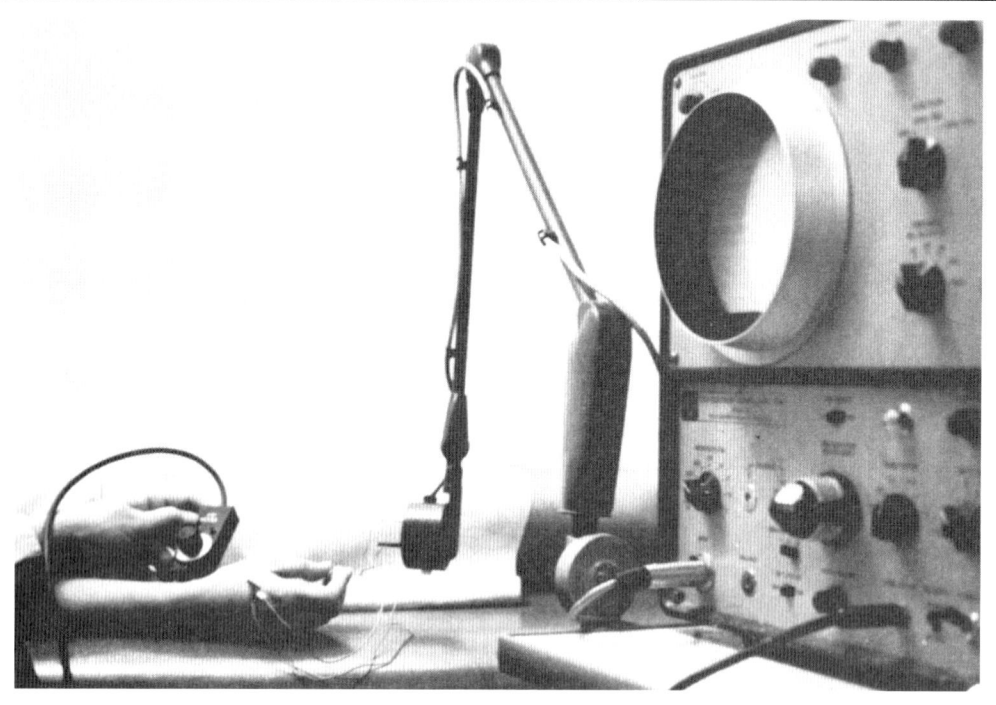

Figure 26–11
TECA-3 electromyograph using a coaxial cable and three needles to record generated action potentials.

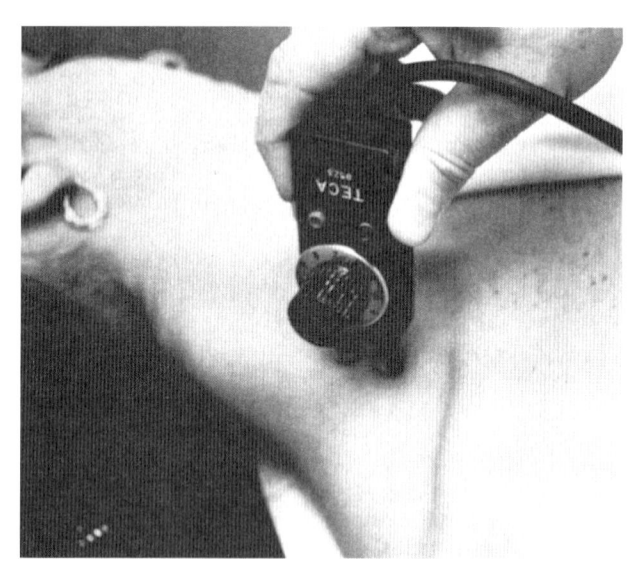

Figure 26–12
A stimulating electrode positioned over the cords of the brachial plexus at Erb's point in the supraclavicular fossa posterior to the sternocleidomastoid muscle, which is the stimulation site of the brachial plexus across the outlet.

neurovascular bundle and its relationship to the first rib and both scalenus muscles are clearly outlined, which helps avoid injury to its components (Fig. 26-18). The insertion of the scalenus anticus muscle is identified, skeletized, and divided (Fig. 26-19). The first rib is dissected subperiosteally with a periosteal elevator and separated carefully from the underlying pleura to avoid pneumothorax. A segment of the middle portion of the rib is resected, followed by subperiosteal dissection and resection of the anterior portion of the rib at the costochondral junction. After the costoclavicular ligament is cut, the posterior segment of the rib is similarly dissected subperiosteally and resected in fragments, including the articulation with the transverse process, the neck, and the head. The scalenus medius muscle should not be cut from its insertion on the second rib but rather stripped with a periosteal elevator to avoid injury to the long thoracic nerve that lies on its posterior margin. The neck and head of the first rib are removed completely with a long, special Urschel double-action pituitary and Urschel Lexel rongeurs. The eighth cervical and first thoracic nerve roots can be visualized at this point. If a cervical rib is present, its anterior portion, which usually articulates with the first rib, should be resected when the middle portion of the first rib is removed. The remaining segment of the cervical rib should be removed after removal of the posterior segments of the first rib. The wound is drained, and only the subcutaneous tissues and skin require closure, because no large muscles have been divided. The patient is encouraged to use the arm for self-care but to avoid heavy lifting until at least 3 months after operation. Cervical muscle stretching should be started at the end of the 1st week, and gentle exercising of the arm can be started at the end of the 3rd week after operation.

It is preferable to remove the first rib entirely, including the head and neck, to avoid future irritation of the plexus, because a residual portion, particularly if long, will cause recurrence of symptoms.

EFFORT THROMBOSIS: PAGET-SCHROETTER SYNDROME

Effort thrombosis of the axillary-subclavian vein (Paget-Schroetter syndrome) is generally secondary to unusual or excessive use of the arm in addition to the presence of one or more compressive elements in the thoracic outlet.[34,42]

Calculation of UNCV

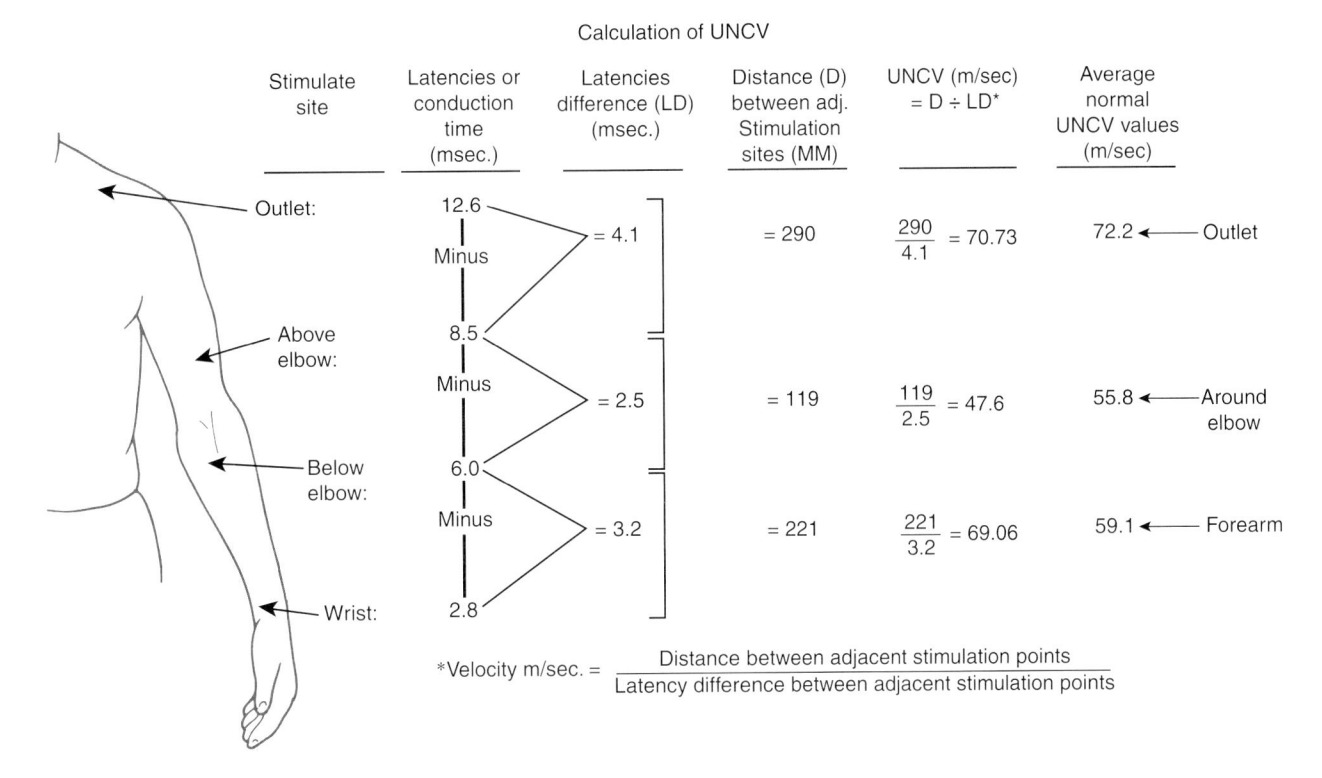

Stimulate site	Latencies or conduction time (msec.)	Latencies difference (LD) (msec.)	Distance (D) between adj. Stimulation sites (MM)	UNCV (m/sec) = D ÷ LD*	Average normal UNCV values (m/sec)
Outlet:	12.6	= 4.1	= 290	$\frac{290}{4.1}$ = 70.73	72.2 ← Outlet
Above elbow:	8.5	= 2.5	= 119	$\frac{119}{2.5}$ = 47.6	55.8 ← Around elbow
Below elbow:	6.0	= 3.2	= 221	$\frac{221}{3.2}$ = 69.06	59.1 ← Forearm
Wrist:	2.8				

*Velocity m/sec. = $\frac{\text{Distance between adjacent stimulation points}}{\text{Latency difference between adjacent stimulation points}}$

Figure 26–13
The sites of stimulation and the formula for calculating ulnar nerve conduction velocity (UNCV).

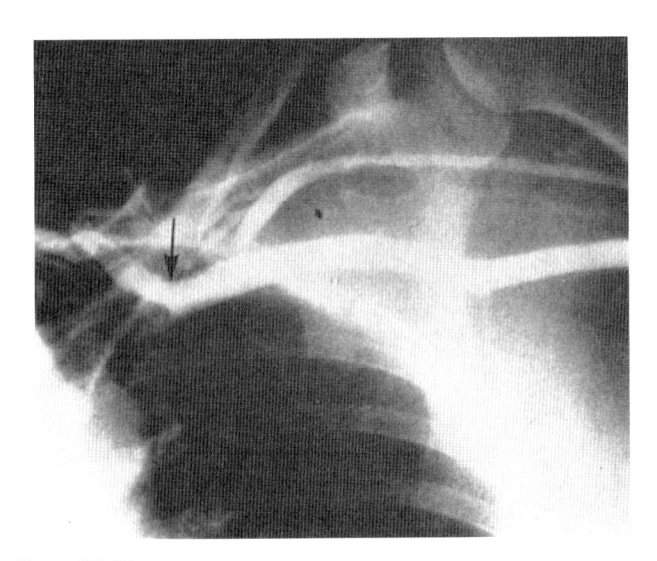

Figure 26–14
Phlebogram showing total occlusion (arrow) with minimal collateral circulation of the left subclavian vein resulting from thoracic outlet compression. At operation, no thrombus was present in the vein, and obstruction was relieved by removing the first rib.

Historically, Paget[43] in 1875 in London and Von Schroetter[44] in 1884 in Vienna described this syndrome of thrombosis of the axillary-subclavian vein, which bears their names. The word *effort*[45] was added to thrombosis because of the frequent association with exertion producing either direct or indirect compression of the vein. The thrombosis is caused by trauma[46] or is associated with unusual occupations requiring repetitive muscular activity, as has been observed in professional athletes, Linotype operators, painters, and beauticians. Cold and traumatic factors, such as carrying skis over the shoulder, tend to increase the proclivity for thrombosis.[47] Elements of increased thrombogenicity also increase the incidence of the problem and exacerbate its symptoms on a long-term basis.

In Paget-Schroetter syndrome, which is always secondary to thoracic outlet syndrome, the costoclavicular ligament congenitally inserts into the first rib much farther laterally than normal in all cases we have seen (Fig. 26-20 is normal; Fig. 26-21 is abnormal). Subsequent hypertrophy of the scalenus anticus muscle (e.g., in weightlifters), which is lateral to the axillary-subclavian vein, produces severe external compression of the vein. This established the abnormal anatomic structure which may produce vein occlusion—the Paget-Schroetter syndrome.[48]

Adams and colleagues[34,49] reported long-term results in patients treated conservatively with elevation and warfarin sodium (Coumadin). There was a 12% incidence of pulmonary embolism. Development of occasional venous distention occurred in 18%, and late residual arm symptoms of swelling, pain, and superficial thrombophlebitis were noted in 68% of patients (deep venous thrombosis with postphlebitic syndrome). Phlegmasia cerulea dolens was present in one patient.

For many years, therapy included elevation of the arm and use of anticoagulants, with subsequent return to work. If symptoms recurred, the patient was considered for a first rib resection, with or without thrombectomy,[49] as well as resection of the scalenus anterior muscle and removal of any other compressive element in the thoracic outlet, such as the cervical rib or abnormal bands.[50-52]

> **Box 26–2**
> **Differential Diagnoses of Thoracic Outlet Syndrome Nerve Compression**
>
> **Cervical Spine**
> - Ruptured intervertebral disc
> - Degenerative disease
> - Osteoarthritis
>
> **Tumors**
> - Spinal cord tumors
> - Brachial plexus superior pulmonary sulcus tumors
>
> **Peripheral Nerve**
> - Postural palsy
> - Peripheral nerves entrapment neuropathy
> - Carpal tunnel—median nerve
> - Ulnar nerve—elbow
> - Radial nerve
> - Suprascapular nerve
> - Medical neuropathies
>
> **Vascular Phenomena**
> - Arterial arteriosclerosis-aneurysm occlusive
> - Thromboangiitis obliterans
> - Embolism
> - Vasculitis, collagen disease, panniculitis
> - Venous thrombophlebitis
> - Mediastinal venous obstruction
> - Raynaud's disease
> - Reflex vasomotor dystrophy
> - Causalgia
>
> **Other Diseases**
> - Angina pectoris
> - Esophageal spasm

Increased availability of thrombolytic agents,[53-55] combined with prompt surgical decompression of the neurovascular compressive elements in the thoracic outlet,[56] reduced morbidity and the necessity for thrombectomy and substantially improved clinical results, including the ability to return to work.[38]

One advantage of urokinase over streptokinase is the direct action of urokinase on the thrombosis distal to the catheter, producing a local thrombolytic effect.[57-59] Streptokinase produces a systemic effect involving potential complications. Heparin is given postoperatively until the catheter is removed. Another advantage is that the need for thrombectomy decreases after use of the thrombolytic agent followed by aggressive surgical intervention because some of the long-term disability is related to morbidity from thrombectomy as well as recurrent thrombosis.[60-62]

The natural history of Paget-Schroetter syndrome suggests moderate morbidity[63-65] with conservative treatment alone. Bypass with vein or other conduits[66-68] has a limited application in this low-pressure system. Causes other than thoracic outlet syndrome must be treated individually[69,70] using the basic principles mentioned. Intermittent obstruction of the subclavian vein[71] can lead to thrombosis, and decompression should be employed prophylactically.[67,68] Over 600 patients with Paget-Schroetter syndrome have now undergone operations. By far the best results are seen when the clot is lysed less than 6 weeks after the axillary-subclavian vein is occluded, and then the first rib is promptly removed and neurovascular decompression is provided. This gives uniformly good results. If the time of treatment is greater than 6 weeks from the time of the initial thrombosis, the results are less good, but the same procedure should be performed to obtain optimal results.[35,72,73]

After successful thrombolysis, there often appears to be a stenosis in the vein on venography. Therefore, interventional radiologists or cardiologists sometimes dilate this vein, suspecting an "internal" problem rather seeing it as the result of external compression. Because the stenosis immediately closes down after balloon dilation, they may insert intravascular stents. These have all failed in our experience[72,92] and in the experiences of others.[74]

DORSAL SYMPATHECTOMY AND THORACIC OUTLET SYNDROME MANAGEMENT WITH VATS

Dorsal sympathectomy and the management of thoracic outlet syndrome are significantly improved with video assistance through magnification and an improved light system. Video-assisted thoracic surgery (VATS) offers better visualization of anatomic structures in a "deep hole," with an additional bonus of excellent visualization for other members of the team, which is particularly helpful for surgical residents. In addition, for sympathectomy alone, it offers less pain to the patient and a shorter hospitalization.

Video assistance is employed in two techniques. One involves the sympathectomy through three ports, with the standard VATS. The second technique involves a transaxillary incision with removal of the first rib using video-assistance magnification and light; the surgeon operates either directly or secondarily while visualizing the image on the television screen. This last technique was popularized by Martinez.[75]

Major indications for dorsal sympathectomy include hyperhidrosis, Raynaud's phenomenon and Raynaud's disease, causalgia, reflex sympathetic dystrophy (RSD), and vascular insufficiency of the upper extremity. Except for hyperhidrosis, all of these indications require the usual diagnostic techniques, including cervical sympathetic block to assess whether the symptoms are relieved by temporary blockade of the sympathetic ganglia. When Raynaud's phenomenon of a minor to moderate degree is associated with thoracic outlet syndrome, the simple removal of the first rib with any cervical rib, in addition to stripping the axillary-subclavian artery (neurectomy), will relieve most symptoms after the initial operation.[28]

It is rarely necessary to perform a sympathectomy unless Raynaud's is a very severe type, in which case a dorsal sympathectomy is carried out with first rib resection. In contrast, with recurrent thoracic outlet syndrome and causalgia, it has been found that the dorsal sympathectomy should be performed with the initial reoperation procedure.[27,76]

Chapter 26 Thoracic Outlet Syndrome and Dorsal Sympathectomy   401

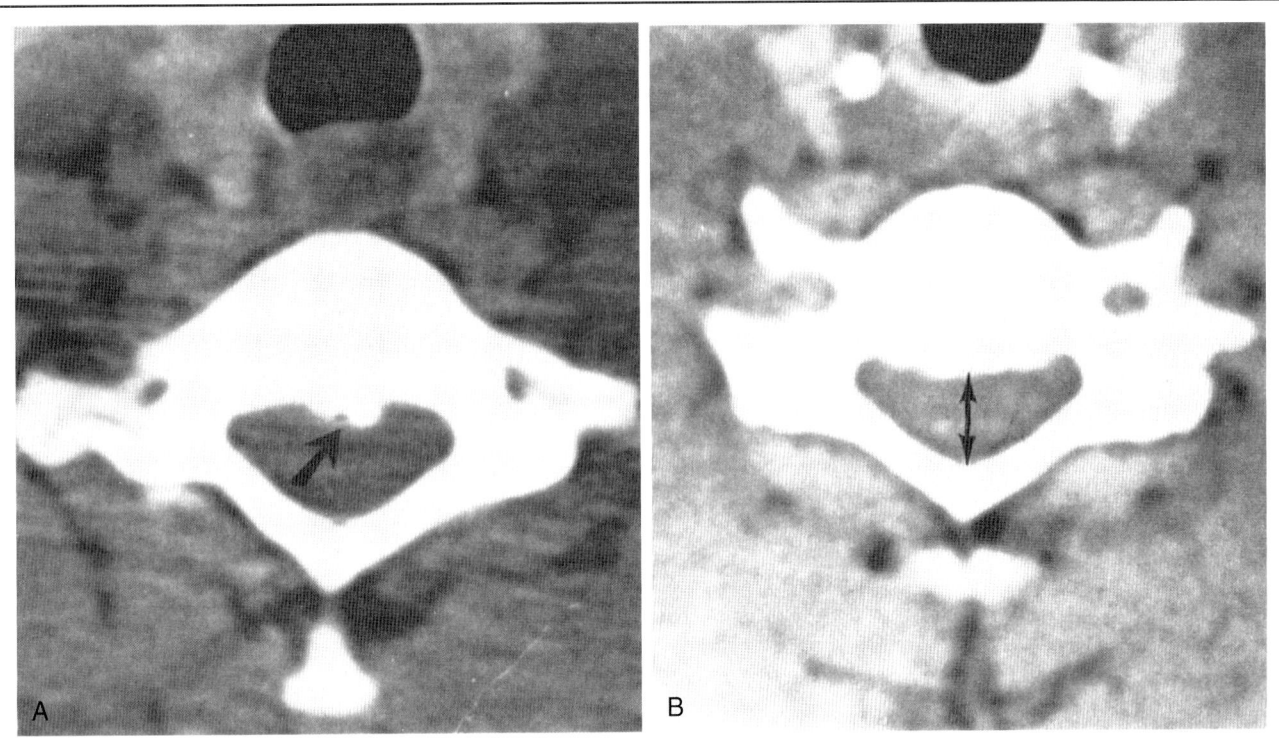

Figure 26–15
CT scan showing osteophytic ingrowth in the spinal canal (**A**) and narrowing of the anteroposterior diameter of the spinal canal (**B**) in a patient with the typical clinical picture of thoracic outlet syndrome.

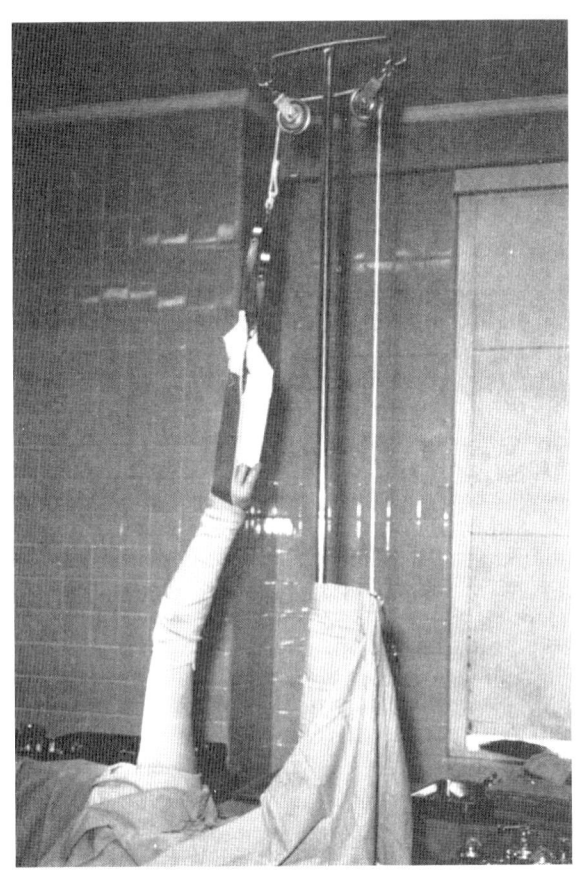

Figure 26–16
The arm is abducted to 90 degrees by traction straps on the forearm and is attached to an overhead pulley.

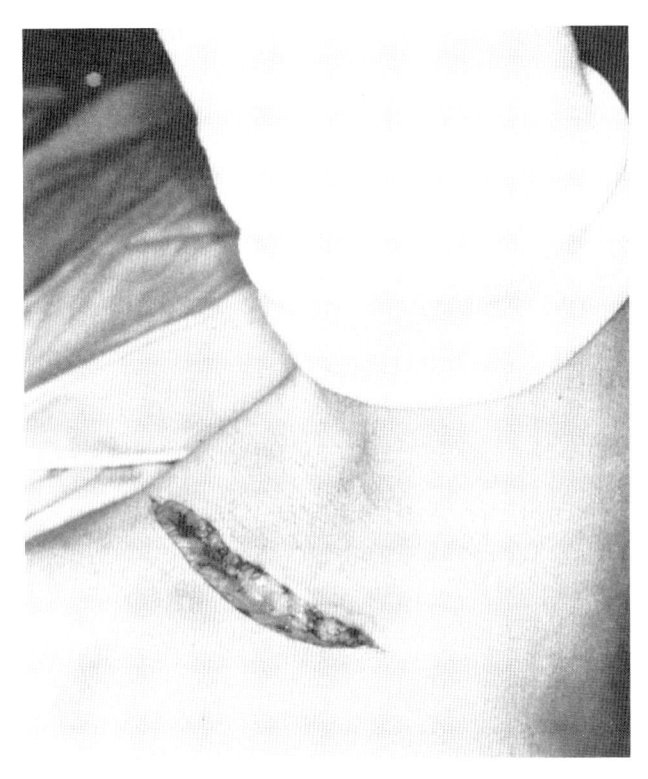

Figure 26–17
A transverse incision is made in the axilla below the hairline between the pectoralis major and the latissimus dorsi muscles and is extended to the chest wall.

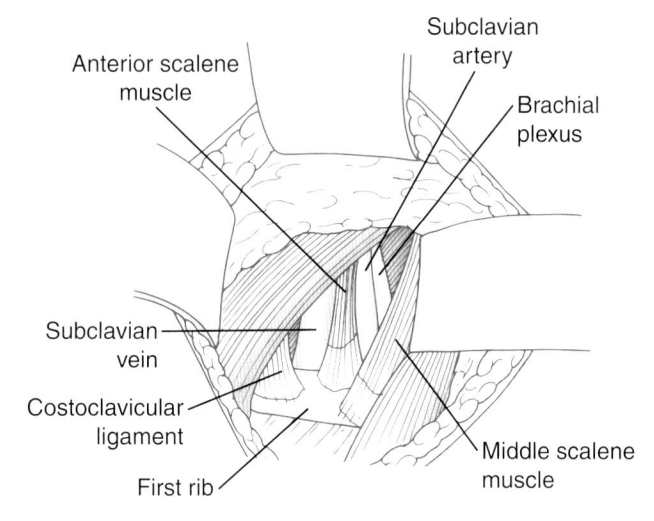

Figure 26–18
Schematic drawing showing the relationship of the neurovascular bundle to the scalene muscles, first rib, costoclavicular ligament, and subclavius muscle.

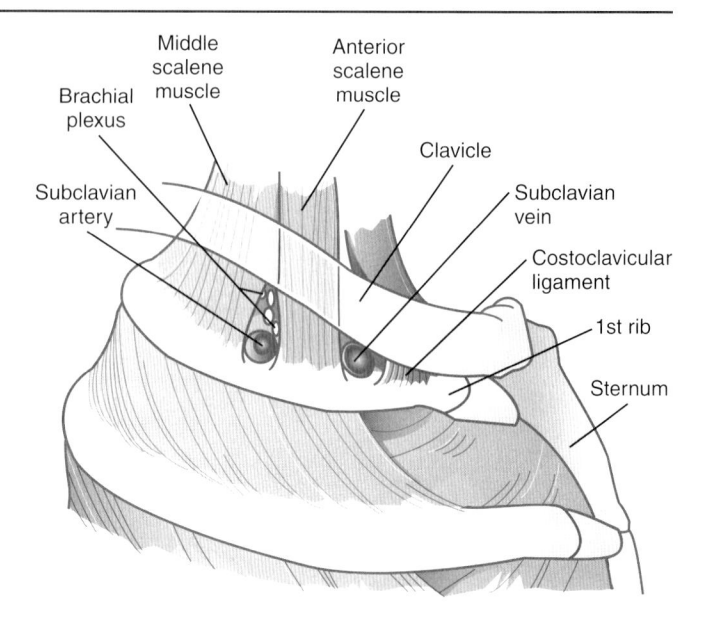

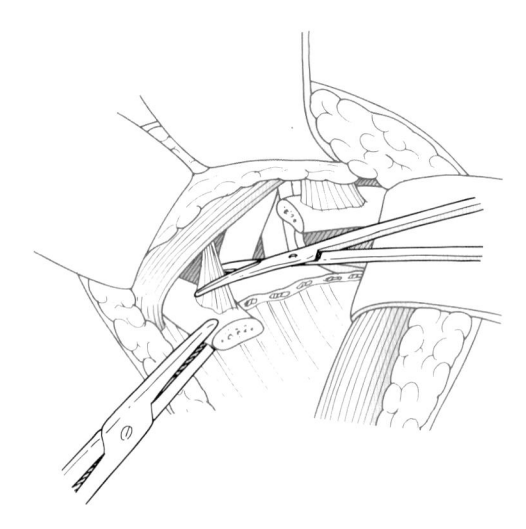

Figure 26–19
Schematic drawing showing division of the insertion of the scalenus anterior muscle on the first rib and removal of a segment of the midportion of the first rib.

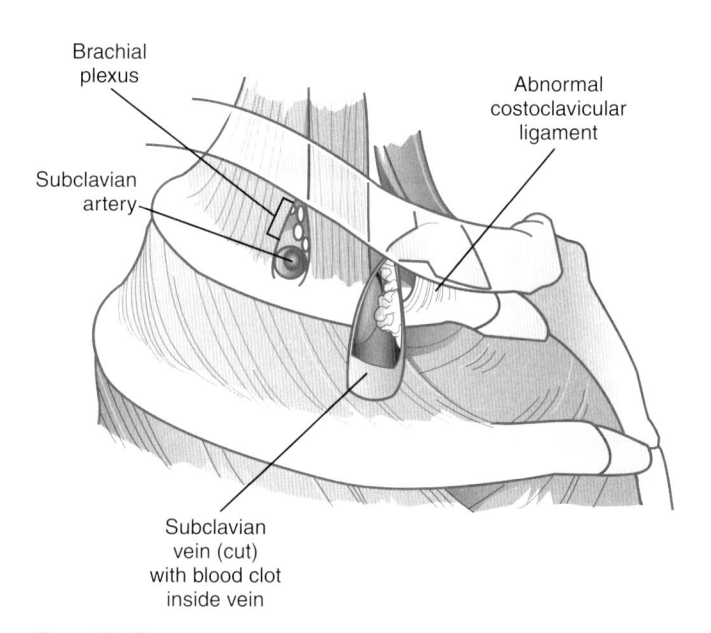

Figure 26–20
The cross-sectional view of the neurovascular structures traversing the thoracic outlet, with the clavicle above and the first rib below.

Figure 26–21
The costoclavicular ligament inserts much farther laterally on the first rib, causing vein occlusion.

Pathophysiology

The principal physiologic effect expected of sympathectomy is the release of vasomotor control and hyperactive tone of the arterioles and smaller arteries that have a muscular element in the vessel wall. Circulation to the skin, peripheral extremity, and bone receives major improvement, but the effect on skeletal muscle of the arm is minimal. The other known function is the control of cutaneous sweating, which is profuse and undesirable. Sympathectomy eliminates perspiration in that quadrant of the body but increases it elsewhere. RSD is associated with pain, neurasthenia, and cutaneous atrophy (Sudeck-Leriche) and post-traumatic limb. These patients also benefit from a sympathectomy if a diagnostic block is effective. Sympathectomy is not recommended for patients with diabetic neuropathy. Nor should it be performed in any of the vascular vasospastic syndromes until after conservative management, including cessation of tobacco products and institution of β-blockers, peripheral vasodilators, and calcium channel blockers, has been tried.[77]

Preganglionic sympathetic nerves derived from the spinal cord do not follow a corresponding relationship to the accompanying somatic nerves. The cervical ganglia of C1 to C4 are fused into a superior cervical ganglion, C5 and C6 into the middle cervical ganglion, and C7 and C8 into the inferior ganglion, which combines with the ganglion from T1 to the larger stellate ganglion. Cervical ganglionectomy is not used for denervation of the upper extremity, because the preganglionic sympathetic outflow from the spinal cord to the arm is usually from T2 through T9, mostly from T2 through T4. In about 10% of cases, T1 preganglionic fibers also supply the upper extremity. For removal of preganglionic fibers to the upper extremity in most patients, removal of paravertebral ganglia T2 and T3 with the interconnecting chain is sufficient. Postganglionic fibers from these two segments often join and branches then follow the nerves of the brachial plexus. The joined T2 and T3 fibers that bypass the stellate ganglion are known as the nerve of Kuntz.[78] For all of the remaining patients who have a T1 connection through the stellate ganglion to obtain adequate sympathetic denervation, the lower third of the stellate ganglion should also be removed, as recommended by Palumbo.[79,80]

Patients with RSD or sympathetic maintained pain syndrome (SMPS) must complain of pain outside a peripheral nerve distribution.[81] Although the injury itself may have been minor, the pain appears out of proportion to the injury. We have seen two types of RSD or SMPS; one involves the hand or even a greater majority of the upper extremity and a second is localized to one or more digits. In no instance can the patient's pain be completely accounted for by an injury to a specific nerve, although injury to a specific nerve may cause the more diffuse symptoms. The patient also demonstrates diminished hand function. Several patients have been referred with a diagnosis of SMPS, and, on examination, it is quite apparent that although they may complain of diffuse pain, the hand functions normally with a full range of movement, and motor power is demonstrated. These patients, of course, do not have SMPS. The patient must also demonstrate some joint stiffness. The skin and soft tissue trophic changes demonstrate varying amounts of vasomotor instability, depending on the stage of SMPS.

According to Mackinnon and Dellon,[81] there are early, intermediate, and late stages of SMPS. In the early stages, vasomotor instability is noted, with very dramatic sympathetic overactivity apparent in the hand or digit involved. Instability, with symptoms varying between redness and warmth and cyanosis and sweating, is noted in this early stage. Edema is also a classic finding in the early stage. In the intermediate stage of SMPS, pain is a less dramatic component and is usually elicited by attempts to move the joints. At rest, the patient may be quite comfortable. The edema and vasomotor changes have settled by this time, and the hand has the appearance of a "burned out" dystrophic hand, with marked stiffness and atrophy of the soft tissue noted. The normal wrinkles on the dorsum of the hand are no longer apparent. The fingertips may have a tapered appearance. The nail growth is usually more exaggerated than in the normal hand, and the hand is often cool and pale. The intermediate stage extends over a number of months. During the late stage, all the superimposed problems of disuse atrophy may take effect. During this stage, problems with the elbow and shoulder are very common, even though the initial SMPS involved only the hand or one or more digits. The degree of pain experienced during the late phase is variable and is often the result of disuse and stiffness. SMPS can affect other areas of the body and has been observed in the foot, face, and penis.

Complications

Horner's Syndrome

If the fibers of C7 and C8 (the upper part of the stellate ganglion) are removed, Horner's syndrome results. This involves miosis, enophthalmos, drooping of the eyelid (ptosis), and flushing of that side of the face, with loss of sweating in that area.[82]

Postsympathectomy Neuralgia

The complication of postsympathectomy neuralgia is less common in the upper extremities than in the lower extremities. The pain usually occurs in the shoulder and upper arm on the lateral aspect. Clinical history usually substantiates this diagnosis if the symptoms occur within the first 3 months. The confirmation may be obtained by a test involving skin resistance and sudomotor activity detection. Tests reveal increased sympathetic activity and suggest a rebound phenomenon from the nonsympathectomized adjacent dermatomes. Rebound may be a regeneration of nerve fibers or an increased response of peripheral nerves to catecholamines. Symptoms are usually resolved in 3 to 6 weeks with conservative management. Phenytoin sodium (Dilantin), carbamazepine (Tegretol), and calcium channel blockers are all used in the medical management of these symptoms.[83]

Recurrent Symptoms

Occasionally, after an excellent sympathectomy, with a warm hand and good circulation, recurrent symptoms occur as early as 3 months. These may be secondary to the regeneration or sprouting and rehooking of nerves, or to failure to strip the sympathetic nerves from the artery and the transfer of sympathetic tone through these nerves. Therefore, stripping of the axillary-subclavian artery of its local sympathetic nerves is performed in each case at the initial operation.[84] Also, during the initial procedure, cauterization of the bed of the sympathectomy area produces sympathetic effects that usually last at least 3 years.

Surgical Approaches for Dorsal Sympathectomy

Historically, the anterior cervical approach has been used, with the division of the scalenus-anticus muscle as the approach to the cervical sympathetic chain.[44] The stellate ganglion lies on the transverse process of C6, and this approach is used primarily by both neurosurgeons and vascular surgeons. For hypertension, Smithwick[85] and Urschel and Razzuk[86] popularized the posterior approach using a longitudinal parasternal incision with the patient in the prone position. A small piece of both the first and the second rib is removed and the sympathetic chain is identified in the usual position. This approach has the advantage of allowing bilateral procedures at the same time without changing the patient's surgical position.

The most common approach is the transaxillary transthoracic approach, which is performed through the second or third interspace with the transverse sub-hairline incision.[79,80,87,88] This is more painful than the other approaches, but with VATS, it can be performed with minimal discomfort. The approach most frequently employed when the patient also has thoracic outlet syndrome is the transaxillary approach, with resection of the first rib, retraction of the pleura caudad, and a dorsal sympathectomy.[28,40] This combined procedure causes minimal pain and low morbidity. Video assistance is used frequently for this approach as well.

Variations of Dorsal Sympathectomy

Standard sympathectomy involves removal of the sympathetic chain with thoracic ganglia 1, 2, and 3. This involves removing the lower third of the stellate ganglion[28] with the second and third ganglia and the interconnecting sympathetic chain. This is the standard approach for hyperhidrosis, Raynaud's phenomenon, causalgia, and RSD. It is advantageous that Horner's syndrome does not occur after removal of C8 or the upper two thirds of the stellate ganglia. Complete dorsal sympathectomy includes the removal of C8 with the total stellate ganglion including 1, 2, and 3 and the cervical chain in between. This procedure is primarily for patients with Raynaud's disease and actual ulceration of the fingers, as well as recurrent problems from the other indications. Newer evidence suggests that removal of only the T2 and T3 ganglia, avoiding the stellate ganglia altogether, offers adequate sympathectomy for the standard indications of hyperhidrosis, Raynaud's phenomenon, causalgia, and RSD. This is yet to be proved in our experience, because careful attention to anatomy virtually eliminates the possibility of Horner's syndrome; thus, there is no advantage in leaving T1 if it presents potential problems.

Technique

Two approaches are employed. The first is the transaxillary approach with a transthoracic sympathectomy.[89] This involves leaving the first rib, collapsing the lung, and performing the sympathectomy with video-assisted technique.[90] The second is a transaxillary removal of the first rib and the retraction of the pleura with a dorsal sympathectomy, which was used in most patients.

Transaxillary Approach with a Transthoracic Sympathectomy

The patient is placed in the lateral thoracotomy position with an axillary roll under the downside arm. The upper arm is suspended at 90 degrees from the chest wall over a pulley system with a 1-lb weight.[88] An arm holder is used to ensure that no hyperabduction or hyperextension of the shoulder occurs and that relaxation occurs every 3 minutes. Three ports are used between the second and the fourth interspaces. The camera should be placed either anteriorly or in the midaxillary port. A double-lumen endobrachial tube is used, and the upside lung is collapsed, ventilating only the downside lung.[91] This shunts blood through the downside lung selectively, and excellent oxygenation usually results.

The lung is retracted and the sympathectomy performed. The mediastinal pleurae are cut open and the sympathetic chain is identified on the vertebral body near the neck of the ribs. Nerve hooks are employed to elevate the dorsal sympathetic chain, and the nerve connections, including the gray and white rami, are clipped before cutting or cauterization. The stellate ganglion is divided at the junction of the lower third, where it looks like a cat's claw. The lower third is cut, but it is not photoablated or cauterized, because Horner's syndrome may result from either heat or light injury in the adjacent C8 ganglion. The lower ganglia can be cauterized, photoablated with the laser, or cut. Hemostasis is achieved with the cautery. The pleurae are left open and the chest tube is placed through one of the ports for drainage. There is a curvature of the sympathetic chain, so in many cases the stellate ganglion lies transversely, rather than vertically, on the transverse process of the vertebral body. Special knowledge of the anatomy is important, especially the location of the thoracic duct, which can simulate the sympathetic chain and be injured if not appropriately identified.

Transaxillary First Rib Resection for Thoracic Outlet Syndrome with Retraction of the Pleura and Sympathectomy

This technique differs slightly from the usual VATS in that an actual incision is made transversely below the axillary hairline and the technique for rib resection is carried out.

A right-angle breast retractor with a light is employed, and a Dever retractor is placed on the other side of the incision. The video camera is a standard thoracoscope, a Wolf scope, or an Olympus flexible operating esophagogastroscope.

The pleurae are retracted inferiorly using a sponge stick, and the sympathetic chain is identified on the transverse process of the vertebral bodies. It is vertical between the T2 and T3 ganglia. However, T1, the lower part of the stellate ganglion, angles anteriorly and lies in almost a transverse position. Clips are placed on all the communicating rami of the sympathetic chain. T2 and T3 ganglia are resected. The stellate ganglion is divided at the junction of its lower third and T1 is removed. This division is carried out with a sharp knife. Cauterization or laser photoablation is not employed in the stellate ganglion. Cautery is used after the removal of the sympathetic chain to prevent sprouting. Hemostasis is secured. A large, round Jackson-Pratt drain is placed, and methylprednisolone acetate (Depo-Medrol) is injected over the nerve roots and plexus that have undergone neurolysis. The camera is removed and the wound closed in the usual manner.

Results

In 926 patients, sympathectomy alone or in conjunction with first rib removal for thoracic outlet syndrome has been successful.[94] In only six patients has sympathetic activity recurred in less than 6 months. All of these were initially treated conservatively. Three of the six required repeat sympathectomy. Postsympathectomy neuralgia occurred in only two of the 926 patients. Both of these were managed successfully in a conservative manner. Among the patients in whom Horner's syndrome was not created deliberately, four patients developed the syndrome. All resolved spontaneously in several months. Forty-two cases of Raynaud's phenomenon were successfully treated with first rib resection alone or with periarterial neurectomy without initial sympathectomy.[35,92]

REOPERATION FOR RECURRENT THORACIC OUTLET SYNDROME

Extirpation of the first rib relieves symptoms in patients with thoracic outlet syndrome not relieved by physiotherapy. Of the surgically treated patients, 10% develop various degrees of shoulder, arm, and hand pain and paresthesias that are usually mild and short-lasting and that respond well to a brief course of physiotherapy and muscle relaxants. In a few patients (1.6%), symptoms persist, become progressively more severe, and often involve a wider area of distribution because of entrapment of the immediate trunk in addition to the lower trunk and C8 and T1 nerve roots. Symptoms may recur 1 month to 7 years after rib resection; in most patients, they recur within the first 3 months. Symptoms consist of an aching or burning type of pain, often associated with paresthesias, involving the neck, shoulder, parascapular area, anterior chest wall, arm, and hand. Vascular lesions are uncommon and consist of causalgia minor and an occasional injury of the subclavian artery with subsequent false aneurysm formation caused by the sharp edge of a remaining posterior stump of an incompletely resected first rib (Fig. 26-22). Recurrence is diagnosed on the basis of history, physical examination, and decreased nerve conduction velocity across the outlet. Diagnostic evaluation should also include thorough neurologic evaluation, chest and cervical spine films (Fig. 26-23), cervical myelography, subclavian artery angiography, and magnetic resonance imaging of cervical spine and brachial plexus,[93] when indicated.

Two groups of patients who require reoperation can be identified. Pseudorecurrence occurred in patients who did not have relief of symptoms after the initial operation. These patients can be separated etiologically as those in whom the second rib was mistakenly resected instead of the first; the first rib was resected, leaving a cervical rib; a cervical rib was resected, leaving an abnormal first rib; or a second rib was resected, leaving a rudimentary first rib. True recurrence occurred in patients whose symptoms were relieved after the first operation but who retained a significant segment of the first rib or who had complete resection of the first rib but showed excessive scar formation around the brachial plexus.

Physiotherapy should be given to all patients with symptoms of neurovascular compression after first rib resection. If the symptoms persist and the conduction velocity remains below normal, reoperation is indicated.

Reoperation for thoracic outlet syndrome is performed with the posterior thoracoplasty approach to provide better exposure of the nerve roots and brachial plexus, which reduces the danger of injury to these structures and provides adequate exposure of the subclavian artery and vein. This incision also provides a wider field for resection of any bony abnormalities or fibrous bands and allows extensive neurolysis of the nerve roots and brachial plexus, which is not always possible with the limited exposure of the transaxillary approach. The anterior or supraclavicular approach is inadequate for reoperation.

The basic elements of reoperation include resection of persistent or recurrent bony remnants of a cervical first rib, neurolysis of the brachial plexus and nerve roots, and dorsal sympathectomy. Sympathectomy removes T1, T2, and T3 thoracic ganglia. Care is taken to avoid damage to the C8 ganglion (upper aspect of the stellate ganglion), which produces Horner's syndrome. The reoperation provides relief of major and minor causalgia and alleviates the paresthesias in the supraclavicular and infraclavicular areas. The incidence of "postsympathetic" syndrome has been negligible in this group of patients. A nerve stimulator is used to differentiate scar from nerve root to avoid damage with reoperations in these patients.

The technique of the operation includes a high thoracoplasty incision that extends from 3 cm above the angle of the scapula, halfway between the angle of the scapula and the spinous processes, and caudad 5 cm from the angle of the scapula. The trapezius and rhomboid muscles are split the length of the incision. The scapula is retracted from the chest wall by making a subperiosteal incision over the fourth rib. The posterior superior serratus muscle is divided and the sacrospinalis muscle retracted medially. The first rib remnant and cervical rib remnant, if present, are located and removed subperiosteally. After the rib remnants (Fig. 26-24) have been resected,

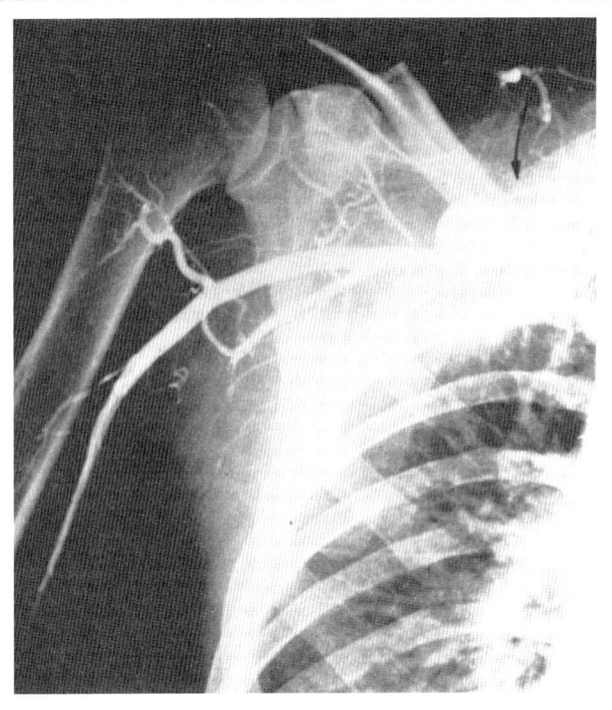

Figure 26–22
Arteriogram showing a false aneurysm of the right subclavian artery caused by the pointed end of a posterior stump *(arrow)* of an incompletely resected first rib.

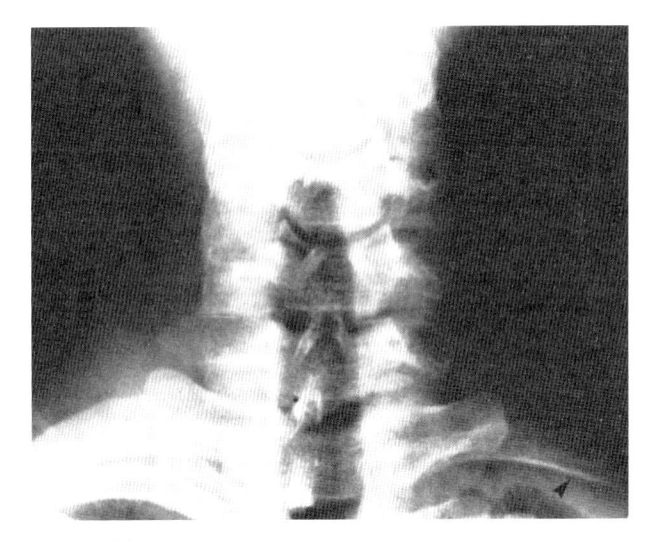

Figure 26–23
Cervical film showing a posterior remnant *(arrowhead at lower right)* of an incompletely resected first rib in a patient who developed recurrent thoracic outlet syndrome.

the regenerated periosteum is removed (Fig. 26-25). In our experience, most regenerated ribs occur from the end of an unresected rib segment rather than from periosteum, although the latter is possible. For a reduction in the incidence of bony regeneration, it is important in the initial operation to remove the first rib totally in all patients with primarily nerve compression and pain.

If there is excessive scar after removal of a bony rib remnant, it may be prudent to do the sympathectomy initially. A 1-inch segment of the second rib is resected posteriorly to locate the

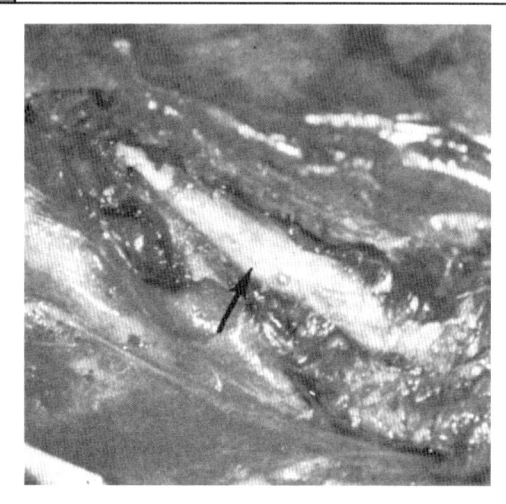

Figure 26–24
A long posterior remnant *(arrow)* of an incompletely resected first rib in a patient with recurrent thoracic outlet syndrome.

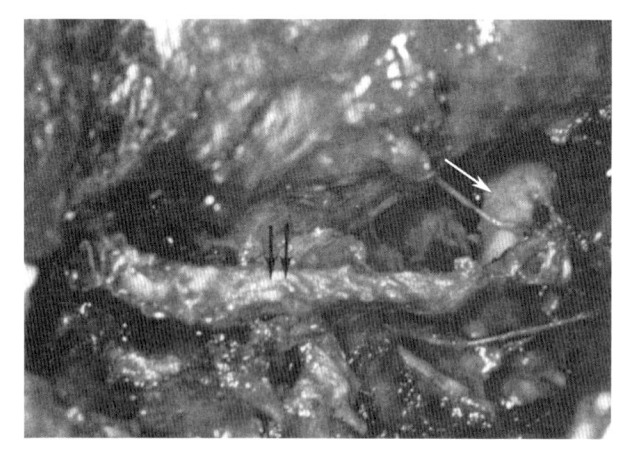

Figure 26–25
Fibrocalcific band *(two black arrows)* of regenerated periosteum in continuity with a posterior remnant *(white arrow)* of the first rib in a patient with recurrent thoracic outlet syndrome.

sympathetic ganglion. In that way, the first thoracic nerve may be easier to locate below rather than through the scar.

Neurolysis of the nerve root and brachial plexus is done with a nerve stimulator and is carried down to but not into the nerve sheath. Neurolysis is extended peripherally over the brachial plexus as far as any scarring persists. Excessive neurolysis is not indicated, and opening of the nerve sheath produces more scarring than it relieves. For scarring to be minimized, the initial operation for thoracic outlet syndrome should include complete extirpation of the first rib, avoidance of hematomas with adequate drainage either by catheter or by opening the pleura, and avoidance of infection.

The subclavian artery and vein are released if symptoms mediate. The scalenus medius muscle is débrided. The dorsal sympathectomy is completed by extrapleural dissection. Meticulous hemostasis is effected, and a large, round Jackson-Pratt catheter drain is placed in the area of, but not touching, the brachial plexus and is brought out through the subscapular space via a stab wound into the axilla. Sepraseal (hyaluronidase) and methylprednisolone acetate (Depo-Medrol; 80 mg) are left in the area of the brachial plexus, but the patient is not given systemic steroids unless keloid formation has occurred. The wound is closed in layers with interrupted heavy Vicryl and Neurolon sutures to provide adequate strength. Range-of-motion exercises are performed to prevent shoulder limitation, but overactivity is avoided to minimize excessive scar formation.

When the problem is vascular and involves false or mycotic aneurysms, special techniques are used for reoperation. A bypass graft is interposed from the innominate or carotid artery proximally, through a separate tunnel distally, to the brachial artery. The graft is usually performed with the saphenous vein, although other conduits may be used. The arteries supplying and leaving the infected aneurysm are ligated. Subsequently, the aneurysm is resected by a transaxillary approach with no fear of bleeding or ischemia of the arm.

Special instruments have been devised to provide adequate resection through the transaxillary or posterior route. They include a modified strengthened pituitary rongeur and a modified Leksell double-action rongeur for removal of the first rib without danger to the nerve root.

The sympathectomy relieves chest wall pain that resembles angina pectoris, esophageal disease, or even a tumor in the lung by denervating the deep fibers that accompany the arteries and bone.

The results of reoperation are good if an accurate diagnosis is made and the proper procedure is used.[28] More than 1200 patients have been followed for 6 months to 15 years. All patients improved initially after reoperation, and in 79%, the improvement was maintained for more than 5 years. In 14% of the patients, symptoms were managed with physiotherapy; 7% required a second reoperation, in every case because of re-scarring. There were no deaths, and only two patients had infections that required drainage.[94]

SUMMARY

Thoracic outlet syndrome is recognized in approximately 8% of the population. Its manifestations may be neurologic or vascular, or both, depending on the component of the neurovascular bundle predominantly compressed. The diagnosis is suspected from the clinical picture and is usually substantiated by determination of the UNCV. Treatment is initially conservative, but persistence of significant symptoms, which occurs in approximately 5% of patients with diagnosed thoracic outlet syndrome, is an indication for first rib resection. Primary resection is performed preferably through the transaxillary approach. Symptoms of various degrees recur after first rib resection in approximately 10% of patients. Most patients improve with physiotherapy, and only 1.6% require reoperation. Reoperation for recurrent symptoms is performed through a high posterior thoracoplasty incision.[76,94]

Acknowledgments

The contributions of Mrs. Rachel Montano and Mrs. Brenda Knee have been of immeasurable value. We are grateful for their excellent assistance in organizing, preparing, and transcribing this chapter.

REFERENCES

1. Rob CG, Standover A. Arterial occlusion complicating thoracic outlet compression syndrome. *Br Med J* 1958;**2**:709.
2. Clagett OT. Presidential address: research and prosearch. *J Thorac Cardiovasc Surg* 1962;**44**:153.
3. Urschel Jr HC, Cooper JC. *Atlas of Thoracic Surgery*. New York City/London: Churchill Livingstone; 1995.
4. Borchardt M. Symptomatologie und therapie der Halsrippen. *Berl Klin Wochenschr* 1901;**38**:1265.
5. Keen WW. The symptomatology, diagnosis and surgical treatment of cervical ribs. *Am J Sci* 1907;**133**:173.
6. Adson AW, Coffey JR. Cervical rib: A method of anterior approach for relief of symptoms by division of the scalenus anticus. *Ann Surg* 1927;**85**:839.
7. Coote H. Pressure on the axillary vessels and nerve by an exostosis from a cervical rib; Interference with the circulation of the arm; removal of the rib and exostosis; recovery. *Med Times Gaz* 1861;**2**:108.
8. Halsted WS. An experimental study of circumscribed dilation of an artery immediately distal to a partially occluding band, and its bearing on the dilation of the subclavian artery observed in certain cases of cervical rib. *J Exp Med* 1916;**24**:271.
9. Law AA. Adventitious ligaments simulating cervical ribs. *Ann Surg* 1920;**72**:497.
10. Naffziger HC, Grant WT. Neuritis of the brachial plexus-Mechanical in origin: the scalenus syndrome. *Surg Gynecol Obstet* 1938;**67**:722.
11. Ochsner A, Gage M, DeBakey M. Scalenus anticus (Naffziger) syndrome. *Am J Surg* 1935;**28**:699.
12. Falconer MA, Weddell G. Costoclavicular compression of the subclavian artery and vein: relation to scalenus syndrome. *Lancet* 1943;**2**:539.
13. Brintnall ES, Hyndman OR, VanAllen WM. Costoclavicular compression associated with cervical rib. *Ann Surg* 1956;**144**:921.
14. Wright IS. The neurovascular syndrome produced by hyperabduction of the arm. *Am Heart J* 1945;**29**:1.
15. Rosati LM, Lord JW. *Neurovascular compression syndromes of the shoulder girdle*. Modem Surgical Monographs. New York: Grune & Stratton; 1961.
16. Bramwell E. Lesion of the first dorsal nerve root. *Rev Neurol Psychiatr* 1903;**1**:236.
17. Murphy T. Brachial neuritis caused by pressure of first rib. *Aust Med J* 1910;**15**:582.
18. Brickner WM. Brachial plexus pressure by the normal first rib. *Ann Surg* 1927;**85**:858.
19. Brickner WM, Milch H. First dorsal vertebra simulating cervical rib by maldevelopment or by pressure symptoms. *Surg Gynecol Obstet* 1925;**40**:38.
20. Telford ED, Mottershead S. Pressure of the cervicobrachial junction. *J Bone Joint Surg Am* 1948;**30**:249.
21. Telford ED, Stopford JSB. The vascular complications of the cervical rib. *Br J Surg* 1937;**18**:559.
22. Falconer MA, Li FWP. Resection of the first rib in costoclavicular compression of the brachial plexus. *Lancet* 1962;**11**:59.
23. Roos DB. Transaxillary approach for first rib resection to relieve thoracic outlet syndrome. *Ann Surg* 1966;**163**:354.
24. Caldwell JW, Crane CR, Krusen EM. Nerve conduction studies in the diagnosis of the thoracic outlet syndrome. *South Med J* 1971;**64**:210.
25. Urschel Jr HC, Patel AN. *Thoracic Outlet Syndromes. Mastery of Cardiothoracic Surgery*. 2nd ed. Philadelphia: Lippincott-Raven; 2007.
26. Swank WL, Simeone FA. The scalenus anticus syndrome. *Arch Neurol Psychiatr* 1944;**51**:432.
27. Urschel Jr HC, Razzuk MA, Albers JE, Paulson DL. Reoperation for recurrent thoracic outlet syndrome. *Ann Thorac Surg* 1976;**21**:19.
28. Urschel Jr HC, Paulson DL, McNamara JJ. Thoracic outlet syndrome. *Ann Thorac Surg* 1968;**6**:1.
29. Urschel Jr HC, Razzuk MA. Current concepts: management of the thoracic outlet syndrome. *N Engl J Med* 1972;**286**:1140.
30. Rosenberg JC. Arteriography demonstrations of compression syndromes of the thoracic outlet. *South Med J* 1966;**59**:400.
31. Lord JW, Urschel HC. Total claviculectomy. *Surg Rounds* 1988;**11**:17.
32. Adson AW. Cervical ribs: symptoms and differential diagnosis for section of the scalenus anticus muscle. *J Int Coll Surg* 1951;**16**:546.
33. Urschel Jr HC, Razzuk MA. Thoracic outlet syndrome. *Surg Ann* 1973;**5**:229.
34. Adams JT, DeWeese JA. Effort thrombosis of the axillary and subclavian veins. J Trauma 11:923, 1971. Adams JT, DeWeese JA, Mahoney EB, Rob CG: Intermittent subclavian vein obstruction without thrombosis. *Surgery* 63:147, 1968.
35. Urschel Jr HC, Kourlis Jr H. Thoracic Outlet Syndrome: a 50-year experience at Baylor University Medical Center. *Bayl Univ Med Cent Proc* 2007;**20**:125-35.
36. Jebsen RH. Motor conduction velocities in the median and ulnar nerves. *Arch Phys Med* 1967;**48**:185.
37. Lang ER. Roentgenographic diagnosis of the neurovascular compression syndromes. *Radiology* 1962;**79**:58.
38. Urschel Jr HC, Razzuk MA. Improved management of the Paget-Schroetter syndrome secondary to thoracic outlet compression. *Ann Thorac Surg* 1991;**52**:1217.
39. Krusen EM. Cervical pain syndromes. *Arch Phys Med* 1968;**49**:376.
40. Urschel Jr HC, Razzuk MA, Hyland JW, et al. Thoracic outlet syndrome masquerading as coronary artery disease. *Ann Thorac Surg* 1973;**16**:239.
41. Urschel Jr HC, Razzuk MA, Wood RE, Paulson DL. Objective diagnosis (ulnar nerve conduction velocity) and current therapy of the thoracic outlet syndrome. *Ann Thorac Surg* 1971;**12**:608.
42. Johnston RW. Neurovascular conditions involving the upper extremity. In: Rutherford RB, editor. *Vascular Surgery*. 3rd ed. Philadelphia: W.B. Saunders; 1989. p. 801-98.
43. Paget J. *Clinical Lectures and Essays*. London: Longmans Green; 1875.
44. Von Schroetter L. Erkrankungen der Gefossl. In: Nathnogel AK, editor. *Handbuch der Pathologie und Therapie*. Wein: Holder; 1884.
45. Aziz R, Straenley CJ, Whelan TJ. Effort-related axillasubclavian vein thrombosis. *Am J Surg* 1986;**152**:57.
46. Cikrit DF, Dalsing MC, Bryant BJ, et al. An experience with upper-extremity vascular trauma. *Am J Surg* 1990;**160**:229.
47. Daskalakis E, Bouhoutsos J. Subclavian and axillary vein compression of musculoskeletal origin. *Br J Surg* 1980;**67**:573.
48. Urschel HC Jr: Anatomy of the Thoracic Outlet. Thorac Surg Clin 17:4:511–520. Editors: Mark K. Ferguson, MD & Jean Deslauriers, MD, FRCS (C). November 2007.
49. DeWeese JA, Adams JT, Gaiser DI. Subclavian venous thrombectomy. *Circulation* 1970;**16**(Suppl. 2J):158.
50. Inahara T. Surgical treatment of "effort" thrombosis of the axillary and subclavian veins. *Am J Surg* 1968;**34**:479.
51. Prescott SM, Tlkoff G. Deep venous thrombosis of the upper extremity: a reappraisal. *Circulation* 1979;**59**:350.
52. Roos DB. Thoracic outlet nerve compression. In: Rutherford RB, editor. *Vascular Surgery*. 3rd ed. Philadelphia: W.B. Saunders; 1989. p. 858-75.
53. Rubenstein N, Greger WP. Successful streptokinase therapy for catheter-induced subclavian vein thrombosis. *Arch Intern Med* 1980;**140**:1370.
54. Sundqvist SB, Hedner U, Rullenberg RHE, et al. Deep venous thrombosis of the arm: a study of coagulation and fibrinolysis. *Br Med J* 1981;**283**:265.
55. Zimmerman R, Marl H, Harenberg J, et al. Urokinase therapy of subclavian axillary vein thrombosis. *Klin Wochenschr* 1981;**59**:851.
56. Taylor LN, McAllister WR, Dennis DL, et al. Thrombolytic therapy followed by first rib resection for spontaneous subclavian vein thrombosis. *Am J Surg* 1985;**149**:644.
57. Becker GJ, Holden RW, Robe FE, et al. Local thrombolytic therapy for subclavian and axillary vein thrombosis. *Radiology* 1983;**149**:419.
58. Drury EM, Trout HH, Giordono JM, et al. Lytic therapy in the treatment of axillary and subclavian vein thrombosis. *J Vasc Surg* 1984;**2**:821.
59. Eisenbud DE, Brener BJ, Shoenfeld R, et al. Treatment of acute vascular occlusions with intra-arterial urokinase. *Am J Surg* 1990;**160**:160.
60. Campbell CB, Chandler JG, Tegtmeyer CJ. Axillary, subclavian and brachiocephalic vein obstruction. *Surgery* 1977;**82**:816.
61. Drapanas T, Curran WL. Thrombectomy in the treatment of "effort" thrombosis of the axillary and subclavian veins. *J Trauma* 1966;**6**:107.
62. Painter TD, Rarpf M. Deep venous thrombosis of the upper extremity: 5 years' experience at a university hospital. *Angiology* 1984;**35**:743.
63. Coon WW, Willis PW. Thrombosis of axillary subclavian veins. *Arch Surg* 1966;**94**:657.
64. Gloviczki P, Razmier RJ, Hollier LH. Axillary-subclavian venous occlusion: the morbidity of a nonlethal disease. *J Vasc Surg* 1986;**4**:333.
65. Tilney ML, Griffiths HJ, Edwards EA. Natural history of major venous thrombosis of the upper extremity. *Arch Surg* 1970;**101**:792.
66. Hansen B, Feins RS, Detmar DE. Simple extra-anatomic jugular vein bypass for subclavian vein thrombosis. *J Vasc Surg* 1985;**2**:291.
67. Hashmonai M, Schramek A, Farbstein J. Cephalic vein cross-over bypass for subclavian vein thrombosis: a case report. *Surgery* 1976;**80**:563.
68. Jacobson JH, Haimov M. Venous revascularization of the arm: report of three cases. *Surgery* 1977;**81**:599.
69. Loring WE. Venous thrombosis in the upper extremities as a complication of myocardial failure. *Am J Med* 1952;**12**:397.
70. Stoney WS, Addlestone RB, Alford Jr WC, et al. The incidence of venous thrombosis following long-term transvenous pacing. *Ann Thorac Surg* 1976;**22**:166.
71. McLaughlin CW, Popma AM. Intermittent obstruction of the subclavian vein. *JAMA* 1960;**113**:1939.

72. Urschel Jr HC, Patel AN. Surgery remains the most effective treatment for paget-schroetter syndrome: 50 years' experience. *Ann Thor Surg* July 2008;**86**:254-60.
73. Urschel Jr HC, Razzuk MA. Paget-Schroetter syndrome: what is the best management? *Ann Thorac Surg* 2000;**69**(2):1693.
74. Sharafuddin MD, Melhem J. Endovascular management of venous thrombotic diseases of the upper torso and extremities. *J Vasc Radiol* 2002;**13**:975.
75. Martinez NS. Posterior first rib resection for total thoracic outlet syndrome decompression. *Contemp Surg* 1979;**15**:13.
76. Urschel Jr HC, Razzuk MA. The failed operation for thoracic outlet syndrome: the difficulty of diagnosis and management. *Ann Thorac Surg* 1986;**42**:523.
77. Cooley DA, Wukasch DC. *Techniques in Vascular Surgery*. Philadelphia: W.B. Saunders; 1979, p. 211-12.
78. Kuntz A. Distribution of the sympathetic rami to the brachial plexus. *Arch Surg* 1927;**15**:871.
79. Palumbo LT. Upper dorsal sympathectomy without Horner's syndrome. *Arch Surg* 1955;**71**:743.
80. Palumbo LT. Anterior transthoracic approach for upper extremity thoracic sympathectomy. *Arch Surg* 1956;**72**:659.
81. Mackinnon SE, Dellon AL. *Surgery of the Peripheral Nerve*. New York: Thieme Medical; 1988, p. 210-14.
82. Galbraith NF, Urschel Jr HC, Wood RE, et al. Fracture of first rib associated with laceration of subclavian artery: report of a case and review of literature. *J Thorac Cardiovasc Surg* 1973;**65**:649.
83. Litwin MS. Postsympathectomy neuralgia. *Arch Surg* 1962;**84**:591.
84. Urschel Jr HC. Dorsal sympathectomy and management of thoracic outlet syndrome with VATS. *Ann Thorac Surg* 1993;**56**:717.
85. Smithwick RH. Modified dorsal sympathectomy for vascular spasm (Raynaud's disease) of the upper extremity. *Ann Surg* 1936;**104**:339.
86. Urschel Jr HC, Razzuk MA. Posterior thoracic sympathectomy. In: Malt RA, editor. *Surgical Techniques Illustrated: A Comparative Atlas*. Philadelphia: W.B. Saunders; 1985. p. 612-5.
87. Atkins HJB. Peraxillary approach to the stellate and upper thoracic sympathetic ganglia. *Lancet* 1949;**2**:1152.
88. Atkins HJB. Sympathectomy by the axillary approach. *Lancet* 1954;**1**:538.
89. Ravitch MM, Steichen FM. *Atlas of General Thoracic Surgery*. Philadelphia: W.B. Saunders; 1988, p. 101-9.
90. Urschel Jr HC. Video-assisted sympathectomy and thoracic outlet syndrome. *Chest Surg Clin North Am* 1993;**3**:299.
91. Wood RE, Campbell DC, Razzuk MA, et al. Surgical advantages of selective unilateral ventilation. *Ann Thorac Surg* 1972;**14**:2.
92. Urschel HC Jr, Patel AN: Paget-Schroetter syndrome therapy: failure of intravenous stents. Ann Thorac Surg 75:1693–1696, 2003. (Presented at STSA Meeting, Miami, FL; Nov. 8, 2002.)
93. Rapoport S, Blair DN, McCarthy SM, et al. Brachial plexus: correlation of MR imaging and CT pathologic findings. *Radiology* 1988;**167**:161.
94. Urschel Jr HC, Razzuk MA. Neurovascular decompression in the thoracic outlet: changing management over 50 years. *Ann Thorac Surg* 1998; **228**:609.

I. Pleura

CHAPTER 27

Spontaneous Pneumothorax

Karl G. Reyes and David P. Mason

Epidemiology
Etiology
Clinical Presentation
Imaging
Management

Observation
Aspiration
Tube Thoracostomy
Pleurodesis
Surgery

Special Considerations
Secondary Spontaneous Pneumothorax
Catamenial Pneumothorax

The term *pneumothorax* was first coined by Jean Marc Gaspard Itard[1] in 1803, when he called attention to five cases in which free air was found in the thorax after trauma. Derived from the Greek words *pneuma* (air) and *thorakos* (breastplate or chest), it is an apt description for the accumulation of air in the pleural space that leads to partial or total collapse of the affected lung. The clinical features of pneumothorax were first described in 1819 by René Laennec,[2] who postulated the relationship to preexisting blebs and unprovoked rupture and, hence, the term *spontaneous pneumothorax*. This pathophysiologic mechanism was confirmed by Kjærgaard[3] in later decades. Today, the classification of pneumothoraces is based on clinical presentation and underlying lung disease. Multiple management strategies range from simple evacuation of air from the pleural space to potential prevention of future pneumothoraces.

EPIDEMIOLOGY

Spontaneous pneumothorax (SP) may be termed either a primary or secondary event, dependent on underlying lung disease. Primary spontaneous pneumothorax (PSP) typically occurs in young patients with localized blebs but otherwise normal lungs. Secondary spontaneous pneumothorax (SSP) occurs in patients with marked structural lung disease and directly contributes to SP. Approximately 20,000 new cases of PSP are diagnosed annually in the United States,[4] with an estimated economic impact of $130 million per year due to lost wages. The annual estimated incidence of PSP is between 7.4 and 18 cases per 100,000 population among men and 1.2 and 6 cases per 100,000 population among women.[4] Patients prone to PSP are usually tall and thin and between 10 and 30 years of age.[5] A significant factor is cigarette smoking, which can increase the risk of PSP by a factor as high as 20.[6]

SSP develops as a complication of underlying lung disease, most commonly chronic obstructive pulmonary disease (COPD).[7] The annual incidence of SSP is approximately 6.3 cases per 100,000 population among men and 2 cases per 100,000 population among women.[4] The peak incidence occurs between the ages of 60 and 65 years.[5]

ETIOLOGY

PSP manifests without forewarning signs or symptoms and is most likely due to rupture of a subpleural bleb. This premise is based on cumulative results of patients undergoing computed tomography (CT), which demonstrated subpleural blebs in as many as 80%.[8,9] Surgical experience confirmed the presence of bullae in more than 75% of patients who underwent video-assisted thoracoscopic surgery and thoracotomy.[10-12] After the first episode of PSP, recurrence varies, ranging from 16% to 54%. Most studies indicate an average of 30%.[13,14] Most recurrences develop between 6 months and 2 years after the initial episode.[13] Men who are tall and with a smoking history are at the greatest risk of recurrence. Counseling for smoking cessation should be strongly encouraged.[13] After the second episode of PSP, the likelihood of recurrence increases markedly and can reach as high as 83%.[7,14]

CLINICAL PRESENTATION

PSP typically manifests with sudden pleuritic chest pain and dyspnea.[6,15] Classic findings on physical examination include diminished breath sounds, hyperresonance, and fremitus; however, patients with small pneumothoraces may have normal findings on physical examination. Most patients with PSP are stable. This is primarily due to their young age and otherwise normal lung function. Patients with SSP are more likely to present with respiratory distress, a result of respiratory compromise caused by SP superimposed on preexisting lung disease.[12] Whereas tension SP is unusual, indicators include tachycardia, cyanosis, and hypotension.

IMAGING

Chest radiography is the most common diagnostic tool for SP. A thin pleural line can be identified that has been displaced from the chest wall. A small SP may be difficult to identify on plain radiography; an expiratory view may prove more beneficial in determining the presence of SP. Frequently, attempts are made to measure the size of the SP as a percentage of the hemithorax it occupies, although this method is typically inaccurate.[16,17] On occasion, a giant bulla can mimic a pneumothorax. Subtle lines demarcate a bulla, which tends to be surrounded by thickened visceral pleura. In addition, a pleural line can frequently be seen with lung markings visible beyond the suspected bulla (double wall sign).[18,19]

CT is seldom required for routine diagnosis of SP, but it can help differentiate between SP and a giant bulla.[17] Controversy exists about the significance of routine chest CT to evaluate for subpleural blebs. Proponents contend that identification of large or multiple subpleural blebs on CT is an indication for early surgical intervention to prevent recurrence.[11,20,21] Opponents of this principle argue that management should not be influenced by these findings alone.[22,23]

MANAGEMENT

Algorithms for the management of SP range from established management protocols to operative intervention. Selected therapies depend on a number of variables: SP size, stability of the patient, symptom complex, initial SP onset or recurrent episode, and presence or absence of structural lung disease.[17,24] The principal procedure is evacuation of air from the pleural space (spontaneous resolution versus instrumentation). Additional procedures targeted to prevent future SP episodes should also be considered.

Observation

Small pneumothoraces are those that are less than 3 cm in distance between the apical parietal pleura and the thoracic cupula, with no lateral component. Asymptomatic patients should be managed expectantly[24-26] by close monitoring, physical examination, continuous pulse oximetry, and repeated chest radiography within 6 hours. Our practice is to monitor patients in the hospital for a minimum of 24 hours. Even though some patients with stable radiographic features may be discharged from the hospital with follow-up within 12 to 24 hours,[24] the potential for catastrophic consequences from a missed tension pneumothorax is a great risk.[27] Small pneumothoraces usually resolve without intervention, but recurrence is possible. If chest radiography reveals that the SP is enlarging, immediate intervention is crucial.

Aspiration

Aspiration allows evacuation of pleural air and complete reexpansion of the lung. This technique can be applied even for larger pneumothoraces if the patient is stable. We prefer the Seldinger technique,[28,29] which uses a small, single-lumen central line placed over the superior rib edge in the second interspace in the midclavicular line. A three-way stopcock and large syringe are used to aspirate until resistance is felt, usually signifying full lung expansion. Chest radiography is then performed to confirm the findings, and the catheter is removed.[25,26,30-34] Commercially prepared kits with one-way valves (Heimlich valve)[7] allow air to exit but prevent air entry. These valves can be left in place until full lung expansion is achieved. For more rapid resolution, however, it is our preference to perform tube thoracostomy with a small chest tube. Complications of aspiration, although rare, may include bleeding and possible lung injury. Reported success is higher in resolving PSP (66% to 83%) than for SSP (37%).[25,33] SP that does not respond successfully to aspiration requires tube thoracostomy.

Tube Thoracostomy

Tube thoracostomy is recommended for patients with large or symptomatic SP and for most patients with SSPs. Patients presenting with a tension pneumothorax should be treated without hesitation, even before chest radiography. Tube placement is through the fifth intercostal space in the midaxillary line. Apical placement speeds resolution, and a subcutaneous track prevents "sucking air" during removal. A small chest tube can be difficult to direct to the apex of the chest, so a 28 French is preferable. The chest tube is left in place between 24 and 48 hours. Our practice is to place the chest tube on water seal once lung expansion is confirmed. If an air leak persists and nonoperative management is preferred, a Heimlich valve can be placed. The patient can then be discharged for outpatient management. The efficacy of suction is debated, but there is no evidence that it speeds the resolution of SP. If it is used, it should be used judiciously.[35] Tube thoracostomy successfully resolves PSP in approximately 90% of patients for the first occurrence, 50% for the first recurrence, and 15% after a second recurrence.[36] For this reason, tube thoracostomy is recommended only for definitive management of PSP for the first event.

Pleurodesis

After tube thoracostomy, chemical pleurodesis may help prevent SP recurrence. Sclerosing agents are instilled to create pleural symphysis. The most commonly used agents are sterile talc slurry and doxycycline solution. Because adult respiratory distress syndrome may be triggered by high doses of talc, use should be limited to 5 g.[37,38] In theory, talc has the potential to induce malignant transformation after decades of use, but thus far, this has not been demonstrated in humans.[39] Nonetheless, our agent of preference is doxycycline to sclerose benign pleural processes. A total of 500 mg of doxycycline combined with lidocaine is infused through the chest tube, and the patient's position is shifted from side to side to distribute the sclerosant. Suction is then placed for 48 hours. Recurrence of SP in patients treated with bedside pleurodesis is high, ranging from 8% to 40%.[38,40,41] In our institution, this treatment is reserved for patients who are not considered good operative candidates, most commonly patients with SSP.

Surgery

Surgical indications for PSP are recurrence, large or persistent air leaks, and incomplete lung expansion after tube thoracostomy. Other surgical indications include patients with a history of bilateral SP and those in occupations that would place them at high risk if a pnemothorax recurred, such as commercial pilots and professional scuba divers.[17,24,35,36] Although some thoracic surgeons do recommend surgery in patients with a first-time PSP if bullae are detected on CT scan,[20] we think that this strategy is highly aggressive, unnecessary, and unproven and do not incorporate this practice into our treatment strategies.

Video-assisted thoracoscopic surgery (VATS) is the surgical procedure of choice for SP, replacing the previous procedure,

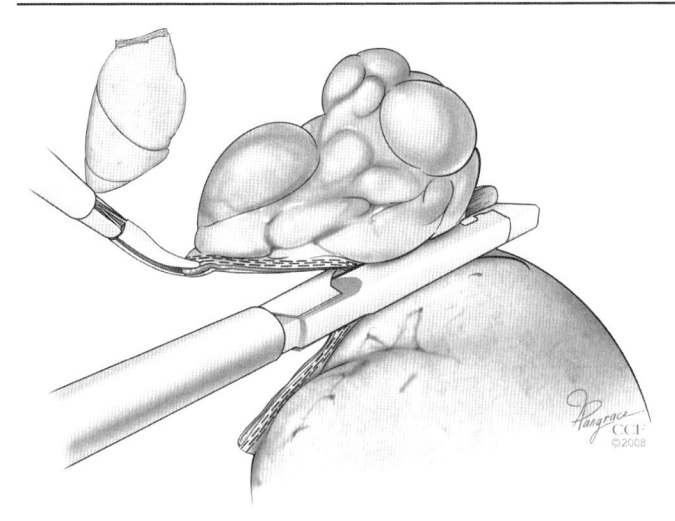

Figure 27–1
Video-assisted technique of apical bleb resection. (*Reprinted with permission of the Cleveland Clinic Center for Medical Art Photography. © 2008.*)

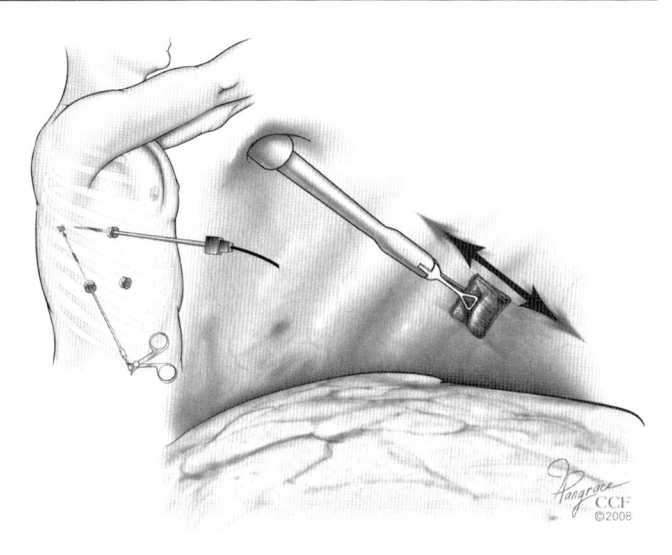

Figure 27–2
Video-assisted mechanical pleurodesis with use of an electrocautery scratch pad. (*Reprinted with permission of the Cleveland Clinic Center for Medical Art Photography. © 2008.*)

axillary thoracotomy.[42,43] The goals of surgery are resection of the offending bulla, complete lung expansion, and pleurodesis to prevent recurrence. A standard three-port VATS technique is used with lung isolation through a double-lumen endotracheal tube. The entire lung is carefully inspected, with particular attention to the apex and superior segments, as these are typical bullae locations. Saline flooding of the hemithorax during gentle lung inflation can help locate a ruptured bleb. Some surgeons resect the apex of the lung even if no bleb is located, although our practice is to perform lung resection only when a bleb is identified (Fig. 27-1). Buttressed staple lines are not necessary with otherwise normal lung parenchyma.

Intraoperative pleurodesis should be performed in addition to blebectomy. Mechanical pleurodesis is our most common method and is performed with use of a Bovie scratch pad with aggressive abrasion of the parietal pleura (Fig. 27-2). Some surgeons instill chemical sclerosing agents, such as talc, at the time of surgery with good results and minimal impairment of pulmonary function over time.[44,45] Another effective method of obtaining pleural symphysis is parietal pleurectomy, by either VATS or open techniques. Results are similar to those of mechanical abrasion.[46,47] One should make every effort to control air leak before leaving the operating room. Apical chest tube placement is crucial to full lung expansion. Postoperatively, we prefer 48 hours of suction before removal. VATS successfully resolves SP and prevents recurrence in more than 90% of patients.[48] Whereas some studies show that recurrence of SP is slightly higher with VATS compared with thoracotomy, this small increment does not justify the discomfort and lost work days in this generally young population.[49] Thoracotomy is reserved for VATS failures and complex giant bleb resections not amenable to VATS.

SPECIAL CONSIDERATIONS

Secondary Spontaneous Pneumothorax

Clinical presentation of SSP is similar to that of PSP; however, dyspnea and respiratory compromise are often more profound, given the presence of underlying lung disease, even with small pneumothoraces. In this setting, intervention should be performed quickly with tube thoracostomy. Major causes of SSP are COPD with bleb rupture followed by *Pneumocystis* infection in patients with HIV infection, asthma, cystic fibrosis, necrotizing pneumonia, and tuberculosis. Less common causes are idiopathic pulmonary fibrosis, Langerhans cell histiocytosis, lung cancer, lymphangioleiomyomatosis, sarcoidosis, and catamenial pneumothorax.[12] SP in patients with COPD portends poor long-term prognosis.[50] Management strategies must be tailored to the individual patient. Operative risk in a markedly compromised patient must be weighed against the potential morbidity and prolonged hospital course that can accompany nonoperative intervention. We have found Heimlich valves particularly valuable in managing patients with prolonged air leak as they allow easy ambulation and outpatient management.

Catamenial Pneumothorax

Catamenial pneumothorax is a rare form of SP usually occurring within 72 hours of menstruation. The typical patient is between 30 and 40 years of age, although age may range substantially. Theories are unproven but suggest that catamenial pneumothorax is caused by congenital diaphragmatic fenestrations that allow passage of air through the peritoneum to the pleura or pathologic intrathoracic endometrial implants that cause perforation of the visceral pleura.[51,52] Right-sided catamenial pneumothorax is more common, but the reasons for this are unclear. When catamenial pneumothorax recurs despite intervention, treatment can be challenging. Hormonal manipulation with gonadotropin-releasing hormone agonists has been recommended; however, side effects can be unpleasant, and it should be combined with surgery for optimal results.[52] Our approach is to inspect the diaphragm for fenestrations thoracoscopically. If they are identified, fenestrations should be closed. This should be combined with mechanical pleurodesis or pleurectomy. Hormonal manipulation for one or two menstrual cycles can be considered while awaiting complete pleural symphysis.[52]

REFERENCES

1. Myers JA. Simple spontaneous pneumothorax. *Dis Chest* 1954;**26**:420-41.
2. Driscoll PJ, Aronstam EM. Experiences in the management of recurrent spontaneous pneumothorax. *J Thorac Cardiovasc Surg* 1961;**42**:174-8.
3. Kjærgaard H, Anderson H. *Spontaneous pneumothorax in the apparently healthy.* Copenhagen: Levin & Munksgaard; 1932, 159.
4. Melton LJ 3rd, Hepper NG, Offord KP. Incidence of spontaneous pneumothorax in Olmsted County, Minnesota: 1950 to 1974. *Am Rev Respir Dis* 1979;**120**:1379-82.
5. Primrose WR. Spontaneous pneumothorax: a retrospective review of aetiology, pathogenesis and management. *Scott Med J* 1984;**29**:15-20.
6. Bense L, Eklund G, Wiman LG. Smoking and the increased risk of contracting spontaneous pneumothorax. *Chest* 1987;**92**:1009-12.
7. Baumann MH, Strange C. Treatment of spontaneous pneumothorax: a more aggressive approach? *Chest* 1997;**112**:789-804.
8. Lesur O, Delorme N, Fromaget JM, Bernadac P, Polu JM. Computed tomography in the etiologic assessment of idiopathic spontaneous pneumothorax. *Chest* 1990;**98**:341-7.
9. Mitlehner W, Friedrich M, Dissmann W. Value of computer tomography in the detection of bullae and blebs in patients with primary spontaneous pneumothorax. *Respiration* 1992;**59**:221-7.
10. Donahue DM, Wright CD, Viale G, Mathisen DJ. Resection of pulmonary blebs and pleurodesis for spontaneous pneumothorax. *Chest* 1993;**104**:1767-9.
11. Inderbitzi RG, Leiser A, Furrer M, Althaus U. Three years' experience in video-assisted thoracic surgery (VATS) for spontaneous pneumothorax. *J Thorac Cardiovasc Surg* 1994;**107**:1410-5.
12. Sahn SA, Heffner JE. Spontaneous pneumothorax. *N Engl J Med* 2000;**342**:868-74.
13. Lippert HL, Lund O, Blegvad S, Larsen HV. Independent risk factors for cumulative recurrence rate after first spontaneous pneumothorax. *Eur Respir J* 1991;**4**:324-31.
14. Light RW. *Pleural diseases.* 5th ed. Philadelphia: Lippincott Williams & Wilkins; 2007, xiii.
15. Seremetis MG. The management of spontaneous pneumothorax. *Chest* 1970;**57**:65-8.
16. Engdahl O, Toft T, Boe J. Chest radiograph—a poor method for determining the size of a pneumothorax. *Chest* 1993;**103**:26-9.
17. Henry M, Arnold T, Harvey J. BTS guidelines for the management of spontaneous pneumothorax. *Thorax* 2003:58:Suppl. 2:ii39-52.
18. Waitches GM, Stern EJ, Dubinsky TJ. Usefulness of the double-wall sign in detecting pneumothorax in patients with giant bullous emphysema. *AJR Am J Roentgenol* 2000;**174**:1765-8.
19. Waseem M, Jones J, Brutus S, et al. Giant bulla mimicking pneumothorax. *J Emerg Med* 2005;**29**:155-8.
20. Sawada S, Watanabe Y, Moriyama S. Video-assisted thoracoscopic surgery for primary spontaneous pneumothorax: evaluation of indications and long-term outcome compared with conservative treatment and open thoracotomy. *Chest* 2005;**127**:2226-30.
21. Schramel FM, Postmus PE, Vanderschueren RG. Current aspects of spontaneous pneumothorax. *Eur Respir J* 1997;**10**:1372-9.
22. Cole Jr FH, Cole FH, Khandekar A, et al. Video-assisted thoracic surgery: primary therapy for spontaneous pneumothorax? *Ann Thorac Surg* 1995;**60**:931-933; discussion:934-5.
23. Massard G, Thomas P, Wihlm JM. Minimally invasive management for first and recurrent pneumothorax. *Ann Thorac Surg* 1998;**66**:592-9.
24. Baumann MH, Strange C, Heffner JE, et al. Management of spontaneous pneumothorax: an American College of Chest Physicians Delphi consensus statement. *Chest* 2001;**119**:590-602.
25. Bevelaqua FA, Aranda C. Management of spontaneous pneumothorax with small lumen catheter manual aspiration. *Chest* 1982;**81**:693-4.
26. Light RW. Management of spontaneous pneumothorax. *Am Rev Respir Dis* 1993;**148**:245-8.
27. O'Rourke JP, Yee ES. Civilian spontaneous pneumothorax. Treatment options and long-term results. *Chest* 1989;**96**:1302-6.
28. Ayed AK, Chandrasekaran C, Sukumar M. Aspiration versus tube drainage in primary spontaneous pneumothorax: a randomised study. *Eur Respir J* 2006;**27**:477-82.
29. Noppen M, Alexander P, Driesen P, Slabbynck H, Verstraeten A. Manual aspiration versus chest tube drainage in first episodes of primary spontaneous pneumothorax: a multicenter, prospective, randomized pilot study. *Am J Respir Crit Care Med* 2002;**165**:1240-4.
30. Andrivet P, Djedaini K, Teboul JL, Brochard L, Dreyfuss D. Spontaneous pneumothorax. Comparison of thoracic drainage vs immediate or delayed needle aspiration. *Chest* 1995;**108**:335-9.
31. Archer GJ, Hamilton AA, Upadhyay R, Finlay M, Grace PM. Results of simple aspiration of pneumothoraces. *Br J Dis Chest* 1985;**79**:177-82.
32. Delius RE, Obeid FN, Horst HM, et al. Catheter aspiration for simple pneumothorax. Experience with 114 patients. *Arch Surg* 1989;**124**:833-6.
33. Hamilton AA, Archer GJ. Treatment of pneumothorax by simple aspiration. *Thorax* 1983;**38**:934-6.
34. Vallee P, Sullivan M, Richardson H, Bivins B, Tomlanovich M. Sequential treatment of a simple pneumothorax. *Ann Emerg Med* 1988;**17**:936-42.
35. So SY, Yu DY. Catheter drainage of spontaneous pneumothorax: suction or no suction, early or late removal? *Thorax* 1982;**37**:46-8.
36. Jain SK, Al-Kattan KM, Hamdy MG. Spontaneous pneumothorax: determinants of surgical intervention. *J Cardiovasc Surg (Torino)* 1998;**39**:107-11.
37. Kennedy L, Rusch VW, Strange C, Ginsberg RJ, Sahn SA. Pleurodesis using talc slurry. *Chest* 1994;**106**:342-6.
38. Kennedy L, Sahn SA. Talc pleurodesis for the treatment of pneumothorax and pleural effusion. *Chest* 1994;**106**:1215-22.
39. NTP Toxicology and Carcinogenesis Studies of Talc (CAS No. 14807-96-6) (Non-Asbestiform) in F344/N Rats and B6C3F1 Mice (Inhalation Studies). *Natl Toxicol Program Tech Rep Ser* 1993;**421**:1-287.
40. Heffner JE, Standerfer RJ, Torstveit J, Unruh L. Clinical efficacy of doxycycline for pleurodesis. *Chest* 1994;**105**:1743-7.
41. Kitamura S, Sugiyama Y, Izumi T, Hayashi R, Kosaka K. Intrapleural doxycycline for control of malignant pleural effusion. *Curr Ther Res Clin Exp* 1981;**30**:515-21.
42. Murray KD, Matheny RG, Howanitz EP, Myerowitz PD. A limited axillary thoracotomy as primary treatment for recurrent spontaneous pneumothorax. *Chest* 1993;**103**:137-42.
43. Simansky DA, Yellin A. Pleural abrasion via axillary thoracotomy in the era of video assisted thoracic surgery. *Thorax* 1994;**49**:922-3.
44. Cardillo G, Carleo F, Giunti R, et al. Videothoracoscopic talc poudrage in primary spontaneous pneumothorax: a single-institution experience in 861 cases. *J Thorac Cardiovasc Surg* 2006;**131**:322-8.
45. Lange P, Mortensen J, Groth S. Lung function 22-35 years after treatment of idiopathic spontaneous pneumothorax with talc poudrage or simple drainage. *Thorax* 1988;**43**:559-61.
46. Nathan DP, Taylor NE, Low DW, Raymond D, Shrager JB. Thoracoscopic total parietal pleurectomy for primary spontaneous pneumothorax. *Ann Thorac Surg* 2008;**85**:1825-7.
47. Nkere UU, Kumar RR, Fountain SW, Townsend ER. Surgical management of spontaneous pneumothorax. *Thorac Cardiovasc Surg* 1994;**42**:45-50.
48. Ng CS, Lee TW, Wan S, Yim AP. Video assisted thoracic surgery in the management of spontaneous pneumothorax: the current status. *Postgrad Med J* 2006;**82**:179-85.
49. Barker A, Maratos EC, Edmonds L, Lim E. Recurrence rates of video-assisted thoracoscopic versus open surgery in the prevention of recurrent pneumothoraces: a systematic review of randomised and non-randomised trials. *Lancet* 2007;**370**:329-35.
50. Videm V, Pillgram-Larsen J, Ellingsen O, Andersen G, Ovrum E. Spontaneous pneumothorax in chronic obstructive pulmonary disease: complications, treatment and recurrences. *Eur J Respir Dis* 1987;**71**:365-71.
51. Alifano M, Roth T, Broet SC, et al. Catamenial pneumothorax: a prospective study. *Chest* 2003;**124**:1004-8.
52. Peikert T, Gillespie DJ, Cassivi SD. Catamenial pneumothorax. *Mayo Clin Proc* 2005;**80**:677-80.

CHAPTER 28

Empyema

Daniel L. Miller

Historical Notes
Stages of Progression
Complications
   Parapneumonic Effusions
Pathogenesis
   Bacteriology
Diagnosis
Management

Acute Empyema
   Drainage
   Antibiotics
   Intrapleural Enzymes and Talc
   Supportive Measures
Chronic Empyema
   Rib Resection Drainage and Open Thoracic Window

Space Sterilization
Space-Filling Procedures
Bronchopleural Fistula
   Clinical Presentation and Diagnosis
   Management
Conclusions

An empyema is a collection of pus in a natural body cavity. One of the most common varieties of empyema is empyema thoracis, which can be localized (i.e., encapsulated) or can involve the entire pleural space.[1] Empyema thoracis is defined as a purulent pleural effusion. Although this infection usually originates from the lung, it may enter through the chest wall, from below the diaphragm, or from the mediastinum. Complications from elective thoracic surgery or from post-traumatic hemithoraces are other possible causes. Most empyemas are, however, parapneumonic, and they occur when the host is overwhelmed by the number and virulence of the organisms in the inoculum. Whereas the normal pleural space is resistant to infection, the abnormal space, such as one containing air, blood, or other fluids, is highly susceptible to empyema formation. The therapy for empyema depends on the pathogenesis of the pleural infection. In this chapter, some of the most controversial issues concerning pathogenesis, diagnosis, and management of postpneumonic empyemas are addressed. The problems associated with post-traumatic or postoperative empyemas are covered extensively in other chapters.

HISTORICAL NOTES

Empyema of the pleural cavity was recognized approximately 2400 years ago, when Hippocrates made the distinction between empyema and hydrothorax.[2] Hippocrates diagnosed an empyema on the basis of its clinical presentation. Fever was constant, but mild during the day and increased at night. The patient's cough was nonproductive, the eyes were hollow, and the cheeks showed red spots. When the patient was shaken by the shoulders, splash succussion sounds could be heard from the thorax, depending on the presence and amount of air and fluid. In his book on chest auscultation, Laennec translated Hippocrates' description that distinguished hydrothorax from empyema: "When applying the ear on the ribs, during a certain time you hear a noise like boiling wine gar, which suggests that the chest contains water and no pus."[3] Sometimes, the noises were not heard, depending on the quantity and physical characteristics of the intrathoracic liquid.

Hippocrates is also credited with the first drainage operation for empyema by using cautery or trephination of a rib. As reported by Paget, Hippocrates opened the chest where the pain and swelling were most evident.[4] He packed the wound with a strip of linen cloth, which was changed every day. He observed that this packing allowed fluid to escape around the strip but prevented air from entering the space. Daily irrigations with "warm wine and oil" cleaned the lung surfaces, and when the empyema had healed, metal rods were used to close the wound. He clearly understood the natural history of undrained empyemas when he wrote in a treatise on pleurisy and peripneumonia, "Patients with pleurisy who, from the beginning, have sputum of different colors or consistencies die on the third or the fifth day, or they become suppurative by the eleventh day."[5] Hippocrates also wrote, "When empyemas are opened by the cautery or by the knife, and the pus flows pale and white, the patient survives, but if it is mixed with blood, muddy, and foul smelling, he will die."

In the 19th century, aspiration of acute pleural effusions was introduced. Wyman and his colleague Bowditch are credited with establishing this procedure.[6,7] Wyman described the first therapeutic thoracentesis in a letter addressed to Sir William Osler: "With Dr. Homans' advice and assistance, the chest was punctured with an exploring trocar and cannula between the sixth and seventh ribs about six inches from the spine, and twenty ounces of straw colored serum drawn off slowly with great relief of the symptoms." Needles used for pleural aspiration, cannulas, devices preventing the entry of air, and suctioning systems were developed during the 19th century.[8]

Thoracentesis was modified with a closed-tube thoracostomy, according to descriptions by Playfair[9] and Hewitt,[10] who performed drainage with a trocar and then placed a rubber tube through the cannula into the pleural space. The rubber drain was connected to a glass tube that went through a cork into a bottle with a sealing level of antiseptic solution. It acted like a unidirectional valve, allowing the liquid to leave the thoracic cavity but keeping air from entering the space. The sealing level could be adjusted depending on the type and amount of fluid being drained. This system constituted a true siphon drainage system that also allowed pleural irrigation. In 1891, von Bulau popularized the underwater drainage system throughout Europe. His name is still associated with this "no suction" method of pleural drainage.[11]

Eloesser flap

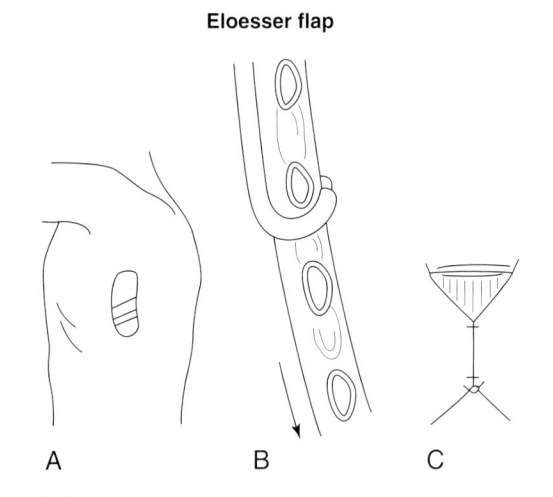

Figure 28–1
The original Eloesser flap.

The consequences of open pneumothorax and the importance of closed-tube drainage were not truly appreciated until a clear understanding of the pathogenesis of pleural infection was provided by Graham and Bell.[12] Prior to their report, acute empyemas were managed by rib resection and open drainage; unfortunately, mortality rates averaged 30%. Death frequently occurred within 30 minutes of the procedure and was attributed to the open pneumothorax and mediastinal instability rather than to the empyema itself. Soon after Graham and Bell recommended closed rather than open drainage to treat early empyemas, the mortality rates decreased to 5% to 10%.[13,14] The principles of empyema management as described by Graham and Bell included (1) careful avoidance of open pneumothorax during the acute stage, (2) prevention of chronicity by rapid sterilization and obliteration of the space, and (3) careful attention to the patient's nutritional status.

Open drainage is indicated only when fibrotic changes have occurred within the space. In 1935, Leo Eloesser described a tissue flap for the treatment of pleural tuberculosis. This flap was constructed as a one-way valve (Fig. 28-1), allowing the exit of pus but preventing the entry of air.[15]

As thoracic surgery evolved rapidly during the end of the 19th century, procedures such as thoracoplasty[16,17] and decortication[18,19] were introduced. These procedures described the obliteration of space either by collapsing the chest wall over the lung or by attempting to reexpand the lung itself. The results were not always good, but in 1901, Fowler stated that decortication was applicable to all patients with nontuberculous empyemas who could tolerate the procedure.[20] He even said that "decortication could be used instead of Estlander's thoracoplasty operation in most cases and should replace the Schede's thoracoplasty altogether." In 1923, Eggers reported on 146 patients who underwent decortication, and he described in full details the procedure as it is still used today.[21]

At the end of the 20th century, another modality was introduced for the diagnosis and treatment of empyema—video-assisted thoracic surgery (VATS), or thoracoscopy. Wakabashi first used thoracoscopy for the drainage of an empyema.[22] Today, VATS is the modality of choice for the diagnosis and treatment of early empyema.[23]

With the onset of the antibiotic era, the incidence of pneumococcal and streptococcal empyemas fell sharply, and the mortality rate also declined dramatically. Subsequently, the increasing significance of anaerobic infection and the development of new generations of drug-resistant organisms have led to a new spectrum of problems. In addition, the number of patients with acquired immunodeficiency syndrome (AIDS) has increased, as has the number of patients receiving chemotherapy, and this has somewhat modified the natural history of empyema, because patients are no longer able to produce the inflammatory reaction that is fundamental to localizing the empyema and obliterating the space.[24]

STAGES OF PROGRESSION

The American Thoracic Society in 1962 divided the formation of an empyema into three distinct stages indicative of disease progression in the pleural space. Progression through these stages usually occurs over a 3- to 6-week period. During the exudative phase (stage I), the pleural membranes swell considerably and discharge a thin exudative fluid. Fibrin is deposited over all pleural surfaces and, despite early angioblastic and fibroblastic proliferation that extends outward from the pleura, the peel is not thickened enough to prevent complete lung reexpansion once the space is emptied. During the fibrinopurulent phase (stage II), fibrin is heavily deposited over all pleural surfaces—more over the parietal pleura than over the visceral pleura. The pleural fluid is turbid or frankly purulent and has a large number of polymorphonuclear white cells. At this stage, the pleura is still relatively intact, and the lung, although less mobile, can be reexpanded. Loculations form during this stage. Usually within 3 to 4 weeks, organization (stage III) begins, with massive ingrowth of fibroblasts and formation of collagen fibers over both parietal and visceral surfaces. The pus is very thick, and the lung, which is now virtually functionless, is imprisoned within a thick fibrous peel. The lung can no longer expand without being decorticated. Finally, arterioles infiltrate the peel within 6 weeks. In a 10-year retrospective analysis of 101 patients with empyema, Renner and colleagues found that 17 patients had stage I empyema, eight were in the purulent stage, and 76 (75%) had an organized empyema.[25] (For management purposes, two stages are recognized: an acute process [stages I and II] and a chronic process phase [stage III].)

COMPLICATIONS

Complications can occur at any time during the formation of an empyema, but they are more likely to develop during the chronic stage of the disease process. One of the most common but often unrecognized complications is increased fibrosis and scar tissue in the lung, which produce pulmonary fibrosis. Scar tissue can also penetrate the parietal pleura and reach the intercostal spaces, which become narrowed and contracted, giving the chest wall the appearance of a carapace.[1] This penetration can to lead severe pleuritic pain with ensuing shortness of breath. In extreme cases, the shape of the ribs is altered, and on cross section, they appear triangular. In other instances, calcifications may develop in the fibrous tissue, and bone may be formed. *Empyema necessitatis* is characterized by the dissection of pus through the soft tissues of the chest wall and eventually through the skin. Similarly, the sudden appearance of purulent sputum signals the development of a bronchopleural fistula with spontaneous drainage of pus into

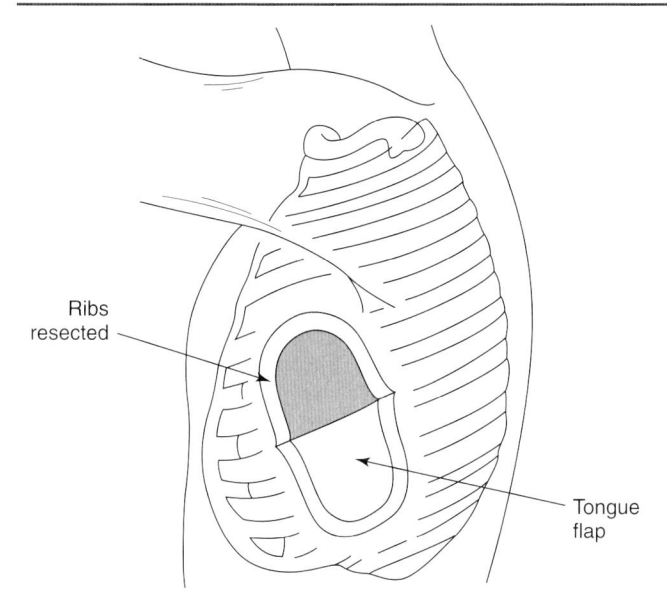

Figure 28-2
Incision, with tongue flap reflected and proposed ribs resected.

the bronchial tree (Fig. 28-2). In a series of 77 patients with bronchopleural fistula studied by Hankins and colleagues, spontaneous fistulas (n = 28) were secondary to tuberculosis in 23 patients and to bacterial pneumonia or lung abscess in five.[26] Unusual complications include rib or spine osteomyelitis, pericarditis, mediastinal abscesses, or transdiaphragmatic drainage of the empyema into the peritoneal cavity.

Parapneumonic Effusions

Patients with bacterial pneumonia may have an associated pleural effusion, which is called a parapneumonic or postpneumonic effusion. Uncomplicated effusions are nonpurulent, are negative by Gram stain and by culture, and do not loculate in the pleural space. They resolve spontaneously with antibiotic treatment of the underlying pneumonia.[27] Complicated effusions are either empyemas or loculated parapneumonic effusions that require surgical drainage for adequate resolution. According to Light and colleagues, the pH of the pleural fluid as well as its lactate dehydrogenase (LDH) and glucose levels appear to be useful to differentiate uncomplicated from complicated parapneumonic effusions.[28]

PATHOGENESIS

Most empyemas are the result of bacterial suppuration in organs that are contiguous with the pleural surface. Among these, the lungs are the most common source. In such cases, empyema occurs by direct bacterial spread across the visceral pleura or by free intrapleural rupture of microscopic and peripherally located lung abscesses. In a classic description of putrid empyemas, Maier and Grace showed that most were associated with bronchiectasis, pulmonary abscess, and suppurative pneumonia.[29] In most series, empyemas are secondary to bronchopulmonary infections in 50% to 60% of cases and nearly all of the so-called primary empyemas result from subclinical pneumonic processes.[20,30,31]

In 1971, Vianna showed that several patients with postpneumonic empyemas had various underlying conditions, such as alcoholism or chronic pulmonary disease.[32] Inactive pulmonary tuberculosis, diabetes mellitus, long-term steroid therapy, and various malignancies are other common predisposing conditions. Substance abusers and immunosuppressed individuals, such as patients with AIDS, are also at risk for bacterial and aspiration pneumonia and other pulmonary infections.[33] These may lead to parenchymal destruction with subsequent contamination of the pleural space, which results in either simple empyema or complex infections including bronchopleural fistula.

Other potential sources of contamination should be sought when the cause of empyema is unclear. Rupture of the esophagus, for example, nearly always results in empyema formation. Rare causes of contamination, including infection in the deep posterior region of the neck and, less frequently, infections in the chest wall or thoracic spine. Although subphrenic abscesses can occasionally contaminate the pleural space through direct transdiaphragmatic erosion, most effusions associated with these abscesses are sterile exudates known as sympathetic effusions. LeRoux showed that lymph drainage from subphrenic spaces can travel cephalad through the diaphragm, and this is the likely route of transferal of subphrenic infections to the pleural space.[34] He also noted that silent paracolic abscesses can occasionally erode through the diaphragm and infect the pleural space.

Virtually all post-traumatic empyemas are associated with penetration of the chest wall or the presence of a hemothorax. In a large series of trauma patients seen between 1972 and 1996, Mandal and Thadepalli reported a 1.6% incidence of empyema formation.[35] In penetrating thoracic injuries, empyema formation is usually the result of organic foreign bodies being carried into the pleural space.[36] In an interesting study, Ogilvie showed that the nature of the missile (e.g., shell splinters, bullets, or bayonets) played little part in determining the rate of infection in empyemas secondary to penetrating injuries.[37]

After blunt thoracic injury, hemothoraces become secondarily infected via contamination through the chest tube or from an infection in the adjacent lung. In 1977, Arom and colleagues made a distinction between post-traumatic empyemas and infected organizing hemothoraces (clotted hemothoraces) in which masses of blood clot became secondarily infected.[38] Ogilvie showed that air in the pleural space that is associated with blood is more likely to get infected than is a pneumothorax or a hemothorax alone.[37] In an experimental model for empyema thoracis, Mavroudis and colleagues showed that a concomitant hemothorax increased the incidence of empyema and early death after *Staphylococcus* was inoculated into the pleural space.[39] In rarer cases, traumatic empyemas follow blunt esophageal rupture, acute diaphragmatic hernia with bowel strangulation or necrosis, or aspiration of a foreign body with perforation of the lung.[40] Direct inoculation of the pleural space can occur as a result of minor thoracic interventions, such as thoracentesis, thoracic biopsies, or chest tube drainage when sterile technique is not followed.

Postoperative empyemas are seen almost exclusively after operations in which the esophageal or bronchial lumina have been entered. The incidence of this complication is in the range of 2% to 4% after pulmonary resection. In recent years, prophylactic use of antibiotics during the postoperative period and improved surgical technique have played a significant role in lowering the incidence of these events. There is limited evidence that hematogenous infection of the pleural space can occur from a distant infection site (classically, osteomyelitis) without an intermediate lung infection, which then contaminates the pleural space. In Sherman and colleagues' series, only four cases represented true metastatic hematogenous seeding of the pleural space.[31]

Bacteriology

In the pre-antibiotic era, the predominant organisms recovered from empyemas were pneumococci and *Streptococcus pneumoniae*.[41,42] In summarizing a total of 3000 empyemas reported from 1934 to 1939, Ehler noted that pneumococci were found in 64% of cases, *Streptococcus pyogens* in 9%, and *Staphylococcus aureus* in 7%.[43] He concluded that other organisms were found rarely and should be considered curiosities. The incidence of empyema was greater (80%) with streptococcal pneumonia than with other types of pneumonia because of greater lung destruction associated with the causative organism. In those cases, myriads of tiny lung abscesses occurred along the lymphatic channels and discharged the infecting organisms into the effusion in great quantities; this converted the effusion into an empyema in a matter of hours.[44]

The introduction and increasing use of antibiotics was accompanied not only by a marked reduction in the incidence and mortality rates of empyemas but also by a change in the spectrum of causative organisms. In a study on the changing etiology of acute bacterial empyema, Finland and Barnes showed that although the incidence of streptococcal pneumonia generally declined from 1950 to 1953, it still continued to occur in community-acquired empyemas.[45] The incidence of *S. aureus*–related empyemas increased, and it became the most frequently found organism in empyemas in 1955. It declined to its original levels after 1965, but gram-negative rods increased in importance.

The predominant isolates in recent years have been *S. aureus* (29% to 69% of culture-positive cases) and enteric gram-negative bacilli (29% to 60% of culture-positive cases).[46] In a report by Vianna, 41 patients with bacterial pneumonia complicated by empyema were studied, and *S. aureus* was the most common causative organism isolated (34%).[32] Gram-negative bacteria were isolated in 64% of empyemas that complicated some other underlying disease, probably as a result of previous antibiotic therapy. The incidence of *S. aureus*–induced empyema has also increased in children. From 1955 to 1958, it was the causative organism in 92% of cases in children younger than 2 years, as reported by Ravitch and Fein.[47] In countries where the introduction of new antibiotics and new administration techniques was delayed, the changes in the bacteriology of empyemas were seen at a later date.

The recovery rates of anaerobes isolated from empyemas vary from 19% to 76%.[46,48] These microorganisms are normal inhabitants of the mouth, intestine, and female genital tract. They reach the lung by aspiration from the mouth or bacteremic spread from the intestines or areas of pelvic suppuration. In a series reported by Sullivan and colleagues, 226 culture-proven empyemas were analyzed, and anaerobes were isolated from 44 patients.[48] More than 50 anaerobic bacteria were identified, but the most common was *Streptococcus*.

In the series by Bartlett and colleagues, 76% of patients with empyemas had anaerobes either alone (35%) or in combination with aerobic agents.[46] In most cases, the flora were complex, with an average of three different species of bacteria per case. According to these authors, the paucity of anaerobic isolates in most reports of empyema is related to the inadequacy of methods to preserve oxygen-sensitive forms during transfer to the laboratory and the lack of adequate anaerobic culture technique.

Often, a culture of empyema fluid does not establish a microbiologic diagnosis. In the series by LeRoux, a causative organism could not be isolated in 80% of patients.[34] In other series, the percentage of negative cultures varied from 25% to 60%.[49,50] In general, negative cultures result from inadequate culture techniques or very effective antibiotics that can penetrate the empyema and prevent bacterial growth. When empyema necessitatis occurs, the pathogens recovered do not necessarily represent the microorganism responsible for the disease, because the skin fistula may be contaminated with skin flora or hospital pathogens.[49]

DIAGNOSIS

The diagnosis of an empyema is made on clinical grounds, by the presence of leukocytosis, by characteristic findings on chest radiographs, and by the recovery of purulent fluid from the pleural space. In several cases, however, the real problem is to distinguish between a noninfected parapneumonic pleural effusion and a true empyema, or to correlate radiographic findings and fluid analysis with the stage of empyema. An empyema should be suspected in patients with acute respiratory illnesses with associated pleural effusion. Typical symptoms, such as pleuritic pain, high fever, cough, tachypnea, tachycardia, toxicity, or local tenderness, are often present. Other symptoms include generalized malaise, anorexia, and weight loss. These symptoms can occur very acutely or develop insidiously over a period of a few days or even weeks. Physical examination nearly always shows diminished mobility of the involved hemithorax, decreased breath sounds, and dullness to percussion.

In the series by Varkey and colleagues of 72 cases of empyema, the most common initial manifestations were dyspnea (82%), fever (81%), cough (70%), and chest pain (67%).[51] In addition, a major underlying disease was present in 45 patients. Because the symptoms are related to the cause and stage of empyema, the amount of pus in the pleural space, the status of the host defense mechanisms, and the virulence of the microorganisms involved, patient experience may vary from a few symptoms to several, with severe toxicity. Symptoms may also vary with the cause of the empyema. Patients with parapneumonic empyemas, for example, often present with cough and purulent sputum, whereas the symptoms of patients with empyemas secondary to subphrenic abscesses may be exclusively abdominal complaints. On the basis of the clinical history, Maier and Grace divided cases of putrid anaerobic empyemas into two groups.[29] In the first, expectoration of foul sputum indicated the presence of a pulmonary anaerobic process or of an anaerobic empyema with an associated bronchopleural fistula. In the second group, the foul sputum was absent, and the symptoms suggested ordinary pneumonia. Most patients with an empyema have leukocytosis with a shift of the cell count to the left.

Chest radiographs show a pleural effusion with or without underlying pneumonia or lung abscess. On lateral radiographs, the empyemas are nearly always posterior and lateral, and most extend to the diaphragm. The classic image is that of a posteriorly located, inverted D-shaped density ("pregnant lady" sign) as seen in a lateral chest film. Decubitus views are useful to determine if the collection is free flowing in the pleural space (stage I) or if it is loculated (stage II). Because it is often difficult to differentiate between lung consolidation and pleural fluid, computed tomographic (CT) scanning is used to ascertain the underlying pulmonary pathologic condition. It is also useful to stage the empyema as determined by the presence of loculations, thickness of the pleura, and presence or absence of a trapped lung. As reported by Stark and colleagues, visualization of thickened and separated pleural surfaces, compression of the parenchyma, and pleural thickening are specific CT signs of empyema.[52] In 1991, Hanna and colleagues described the "split pleura sign," which is indicative of the presence of pleural fluid between the thickened visceral and parietal pleurae.[53]

Ultrasonography may be used to document the presence of fluid or to distinguish between pleural fluid, pleural thickening, and parenchymal consolidation. It is also useful for guided needle aspiration of pleural fluid, especially when the position of the diaphragm cannot be documented with certainty on standard radiographs, and for entering loculated areas. As described by Moran[54] and Orringer,[55] an empyemagram can be done by injecting contrast material at the time of the initial thoracentesis and then obtaining posteroanterior and lateral chest films and decubitus views. Although this technique has seldom been used since the advent of CT, it may provide information about the extent of the empyema cavity and the presence or absence of loculations in the space. After the presence of pleural fluid has been confirmed, diagnostic thoracentesis should be done, and the aspirate should be sent for cytologic study, biochemical analysis, Gram stain, aerobic and anaerobic studies, and antibiotic sensitivity tests.

Orringer showed that the gross appearance and odor of pleural fluid are among the most significant items of information obtainable by thoracentesis.[55] Thin fluid, even with positive bacteriologic findings, may respond to selective antibiotic therapy and therapeutic thoracentesis; thick pus requires formal surgical drainage. Anaerobic pus is usually foul; aerobic pus has no offensive odor. Several authors have shown that recovery of anaerobes requires careful technique. Varkey and colleagues noted that the variability in the reported incidence of anaerobic empyemas may be caused by differences in the methods of transportation and processing of the pleural fluid specimens.[51] Pleural fluid should be sent for viral, tuberculosis, and fungal cultures in addition to the standard bacteriologic examinations.

The relevance of pleural fluid analysis in empyema diagnosis is controversial, especially with regard to its biochemistry. Several authors[56-58] believe that pleural effusions with low fluid pH (<7.0), low glucose concentration (<50 mg/dL), and high LDH level (>1000 IU/L) should be drained because these parameters indicate a complicated effusion or impending empyema. These changes can be detected before organisms are found on Gram stain or culture, and they usually occur concomitantly. In uncomplicated effusions, the pH is greater than 7.3, the glucose level is higher than 60 mg/dL, and the LDH level is less than 1000 IU/L; these do not need to be drained. If the patient has free-flowing, nonpurulent fluid with borderline biochemical parameters, Sahn and Light recommend appropriate antibiotic therapy and repeated thoracentesis 12 hours later.[59] If the pleural fluid values are stable or improving, continued antibiotic therapy is warranted, but if there is worsening of these values, chest tube or VATS drainage is generally necessary for resolution. In a series by Potts and colleagues, three categories of parapneumonic effusions were characterized.[60] The pH was greater than 7.3 in all 10 benign effusions, and spontaneous resolution occurred in each case. All 10 empyemas and the four loculated effusions had pH levels that were less than 7.3.

Physiologically, these biochemical changes are explained by an increased leukocytic activity and acid production in the pleural fluid. Based on all these diagnostic parameters, Van Way III and colleagues proposed a method of regrouping patients with empyemas by diagnostic class.[61] Patients with class I empyemas ($n = 12$) were treated with short-duration chest tubes, and there were no deaths. Patients with class II empyemas ($n = 28$) were treated with chest tubes, and there were two deaths (7%). There were 40 patients with class III empyemas, and most required some form of surgical intervention.

Despite the usefulness of all of these tests, the proper clinical staging of parapneumonic effusions remains difficult. How does one distinguish a simple inflammatory reaction (likely to respond to antibiotics and drainage) from early organization? How does one differentiate between the very acute stage in which pleural fluid is thin and the purulent stage in which fibrin is deposited over pleural surfaces? Values of pleural fluid chemistry, such as pH less than 7.2, correlate with loculated effusions but not necessarily with the presence of frank empyema.[62] In experienced hands, CT and ultrasonography provide significant information by detecting loculations and thickness of the fibrinous deposits encasing the lung.[63] Currently, VATS has been incorporated earlier to help determine stage and appropriate treatment. During the investigation of patients with empyema, it is also important to look for the causative process. Sullivan and colleagues, for example, showed that decayed teeth, retained food, or advanced periodontal disease were present in 17 of 24 patients with anaerobic empyemas of pulmonary origin.[48] Bronchoscopy should be performed to rule out foreign bodies or endobronchial tumors, especially if the patient requires surgery.

MANAGEMENT

As emphasized by Cohen and colleagues, empyema management depends on its cause, its clinical stage, the state of the underlying lung, the presence or absence of a bronchopleural fistula, and the patient's clinical and nutritional status.[64]

Acute Empyema

In acute empyemas, antibiotics are used to control the infection, and intercostal tube drainage is both simple and effective to drain and obliterate the space. Repeated thoracentesis, in conjunction with antibiotic therapy, may be indicated when the fluid is thin and the toxicity is well controlled. According to Moran, antibiotics and thoracentesis can be curative in a large proportion of parapneumonic effusions if the mode of therapy is instituted early enough.[54] On the other hand, Personne suggests that performing thoracentesis alone is usually a mistake, because the chances of complete success are minimal.[65] It often leads to the formation of multiloculated pockets, which eventually become difficult to drain. Ferguson[66] noted that "although simple drainage and antibiotic therapy remain the norm, an enlarging group of patients, particularly those with complicated or postoperative empyemas, will require aggressive surgical intervention," such as VATS. Early recognition of these patients and institution of surgical intervention, as primary therapy rather than as a last resort, is likely to result in improved survival and shortened hospital stay. Open drainage plays no role in the therapy of acute empyemas.

Drainage

Surgical removal of pus by proper pleural space drainage remains the gold standard of empyema management. This procedure not only evacuates the pus but also allows the apposition of pleural surfaces, which eventually leads to obliteration of the space and resolution of the infection. The timing of the surgical drainage and the choice of a drainage procedure must be tailored to the individual patient.[54]

Pleural drainage can be accomplished by closed-tube thoracostomy, by pigtail catheter, by VATS, or by open thoracotomy. The technique of intercostal tube drainage is simple and well described in every textbook of thoracic surgery. When inserting a chest tube without proper visualization of the space, the surgeon must be careful not to penetrate the diaphragm, which is often retracted upward. The chest tube (28 to 36 French) is connected to an active suction system, usually with a negative pressure of 20 cm H_2O. If the lung expands well, the chest tube is left under suction drainage for 5 to 7 days, or until the space is permanently obliterated. This is likely to have occurred when the daily amount of drainage is low (<100 mL/day), when there are no up-and-down movements of fluid in the tubing, or when no pneumothorax develops if the tube is opened to atmospheric pressure. At this point, the tube can simply be removed or closed drainage can be changed to open drainage by cutting the tube close to the chest wall. The tube is then shortened at the rate of about 1 inch per week or until granulation tissue and fibrosis lead to its spontaneous expulsion from the pleural space.

When the lung expands well with tube drainage and there is no persistent empyema cavity, intrapleural irrigation of antibiotics does not appear to provide additional advantages.[67-69] Intrapleural irrigations were required in 96 of 236 patients (44%) with empyema reported by Blasco and colleagues.[70] In these individuals, initial drainage was inadequate either because fibrin clots occluded the chest tube or because persistent loculations and adhesions prevented adequate lung reexpansion. Several patients (n = 36) required more than one chest tube for these irrigations. In that series, the overall mortality was low (2%), and only 20 patients had permanent radiologic sequelae.

Another option for closed pleural space drainage is to use small-base pigtail catheters positioned with ultrasound or CT guidance. This technique is less traumatic, but often these patients need several CT scans and replacement of blocked or misplaced catheters. Lee and colleagues[71] and Crouch and colleagues[72] have reported success rates ranging from 70% to 90%, but this was for very early disease. Pigtail catheters should not be used when thick pus is found, because it is likely to clog these small-bore tubes. The use of pigtail catheters is usually reserved for patients who are not surgical candidates because of significant comorbidities or other contraindications to surgery. A team approach is needed among pulmonologist, intervention radiologist, and thoracic surgeons to expedite the treatment of empyemas to improve overall success and to decrease associated morbidity, hospital stay, and cost to patients.

In 1991, Wakabayashi reported on expanded applications of therapeutic VATS.[22] In his series, 20 patients underwent thoracoscopic débridement of chronic empyema; the lungs reexpanded in 18, in whom the duration of empyema had been less than 2 months, and failed to reexpand in two patients who had had empyema for 4 and 7 months. Since then, several authors have used this technique as a primary method to drain acute empyemas.[63,73-76] Following ultrasound or CT delineation of the location and size of the collection, VATS techniques are used to evacuate the pus, disrupt the loculations containing fibrin clots and membranes, remove the fibrinous membranes, reexpand the lung, perform biopsies of the lung or pleura if necessary, and position the chest tubes in the most dependent portion of the space. Because it is minimally invasive, VATS is also an ideal procedure for most critically ill patients, who are at high surgical risk not only because of their illness but also because of a prior debilitating condition or immunosuppressed status. Deslauriers feels that VATS débridement of fibrinopurulent empyemas represents one of the best indications for therapeutic VATS techniques.[77] In 1996, Angelillo Mackinlay and colleagues reported 64 cases of fibrinopurulent empyemas treated by formal thoracotomy (n = 33) or thoracoscopy (n = 31).[75] The mortality was similar in both groups (3%), but VATS techniques had substantial advantages over thoracotomy in terms of resolution of the disease, hospital stay, and cosmetic outcome. In 1999, Cassina and colleagues presented a prospective, selected single-institution series of 45 patients with pleural empyema who underwent operation.[63] In 37 patients (82%), VATS débridement was successful, and there were no complications during the procedure. At follow-up, 35 of the patients (95%) treated by VATS showed normal values on pulmonary function tests. A summary of the world's literature on thoracoscopic treatment of empyema is shown in Table 28-1.[63,73,75,76,78-80] Overall, these techniques are safe and efficient for stage I and II empyemas but inefficient for organized disease.[81]

Before the advent of VATS techniques, several authors[33,61,65,82] proposed early open thoracotomy to drain acute empyemas that could not be adequately evacuated by tube thoracostomy because of multiple loculations or inaccessible purulent collections.[39] This procedure was incorrectly called "early decortication" by these authors.[35,83,84] Under general anesthesia, a small incision is made over the cavity, and a short segment of rib is resected. The empyema is then completely evacuated and, through a separate incision, a large-bore chest tube is secured in the most dependent portion of the space. In Fishman and Ellertson's series, six of eight immunosuppressed patients survived early decortication and were discharged 3 to 6 weeks after the operation.[83]

Morin and colleagues also reported excellent results with early thoracotomy in 23 patients with posteriorly located, D-shaped densities seen on lateral chest radiograph.[82] Miller[84] and Pothula and Krellenstein[85] also advocate early aggressive surgical approach when the standard chest tube does not relieve the loculated fluid, because the surgical risk is low and

Table 28-1
Thoracoscopic Treatment of Empyema

Primary Author (ref)	Patients	Stage	Success (%)	Complications (%)	Mortality (%)
Angelillo Mackinlay (75)	31	2	90	16	19
Landreneau (73)	76	2 & 3	83	3	0
Striffeler (76)	67	2	72	4	6
Cassina (63)	45	2 & 3	82	11	0
Luh (78)	210	2 & 3	86	25	3
Wurnig (79)	130	2 & 3	97	9	0
Solaini (80)	80	2	97	11	0

the expected outcome is good in more than 95% of patients. Of 52 patients reported by Pothula and Krellenstein, there were no operative deaths, and good results were obtained in 50 of 52.[85] In substance-abuse patients, exploration thoracotomy is recommended within 24 to 48 hours if the patient has toxic manifestations despite drainage or if there is evidence of parenchymal destruction, multiple loculations, or trapped lung.[33]

Antibiotics

Several factors, such as the pathogen involved, the stage of the empyema, and the immune status of the host, determine the response to antibiotics. Concentrations of antibiotics in the infected pleural space must be high enough to neutralize the pathogens, a feature possible during the exudative phase of disease but less likely during the fibrinopurulent or organization stages.[49] Initially, and while awaiting the results of antibiotic susceptibility, a semisynthetic penicillin, such as methicillin, or clindamycin should be given if the empyema has been acquired in the community or if the Gram staining reveals clusters of gram-positive cocci that are compatible with *S. aureus*.[49] In patients with anaerobic, gram-negative empyema, penicillin is the antibiotic of choice; clindamycin can also be used. It is generally agreed that antibiotics should be continued for 2 to 4 weeks.

Intrapleural Enzymes and Talc

During the transitional stage of empyema progression, fibrin is deposited in the pleural space, and fibrin strands develop between visceral and parietal pleura, forming loculi and preventing lung reexpansion despite well-placed chest tubes. During that period, the use of intrapleural fibrinolytic enzymes has been described as a method to break up these strands and to improve drainage. The use of intrapleural streptokinase for the therapy of acute empyemas was first described by Tillett and Sherry in 1949.[86] However, allergy and bleeding complications, probably related to impure preparations and prolonged dwelling times, prevented adoption of this technique.[87] In 1977, Bergh and colleagues showed that streptokinase at the dose of 250,000 U diluted in 100 mL of physiologic saline solution stimulates the liquefaction of fibrin clots and, in some cases, facilitates the subsequent drainage of the pleural space.[88] In 1994, Robinson and colleagues presented a series of 13 consecutive patients with fibrinopurulent empyemas who had incomplete drainage.[89] Streptokinase (250,000 U in 100 mL of 0.9% saline solution) or urokinase (100,000 U in 100 mL of 0.9% saline solution) was instilled daily into the chest tube, and the tube was clamped for 6 to 12 hours, followed by suction. This regimen was completely successful in 10 of 13 patients (77%), with resolution of the empyema, eventual withdrawal of the chest tubes, and no recurrence. In 1997, Davies and colleagues reported the benefits of this technique in a randomized, controlled trial.[90] Twenty-four patients with infected community-acquired parapneumonic effusions were studied, and all had either frankly purulent pleural fluid or the presence of gram-positive organisms. These patients were treated by drainage and either intrapleural saline flushes or intrapleural streptokinase (250,000 IU in 20 mL of saline) with a 2-hour dwelling time daily for 3 days. The streptokinase group drained more fluid and showed greater improvement on chest radiograph at discharge. Surgery was required in three control patients but none in the streptokinase group. Another randomized trial of empyema therapy by Wait and colleagues compared pleural drainage and fibrinolytic therapy with VATS with regard to efficacy and duration of hospitalization.[91] In patients with loculated, complex, fibrinopurulent, parapneumonic empyema, this study showed that a primary treatment strategy of VATS was associated with a higher efficacy, shorter hospital duration, and lower cost. Unfortunately, streptokinase is not available for clinical use in the United States.

Urokinase, an enzyme isolated from human urine and acting through activation of plasminogen, can also be used for the lysis of loculated pleural effusions.[92,93] In a prospective, double-blind study, Bouros and colleagues concluded that urokinase could be the thrombolytic of choice given the potential of dangerous allergic reaction to streptokinase and the relatively small cost of urokinase.[94] In a series by Lopez-Rivero and colleagues, 22 patients with empyema were treated by intrapleural instillation of urokinase (200,000 IU) three times a day.[95] Depending on the clinical and radiologic response, this treatment was continued for 48 hours, sometimes with lower dosage. After an average dose of 900,000 IU, 95% of the empyemas were completely drained, and only one patient had to undergo surgery because of treatment failure.

The use of talc has also been described by Weissberg and Kaufman.[96] They reported on five patients with fibrinopurulent empyema who did not respond to conventional therapy and in whom intrapleurally insufflated talc powder led to pleurodesis. Although no side effects were observed, this technique should clearly be restricted to a few selected patients. Currently, talc is not recommended in patients with culture-proven or suspected infected pleural space.

Supportive Measures

Supportive measures, including proper respiratory care with therapy of associated respiratory infection and obstructive pulmonary disease and maintenance of nutrition by enteral feedings, are essential for the successful management of early empyemas. Active chest physiotherapy is particularly important to promote lung reexpansion and prevent chest wall contraction. Because nearly 50% to 60% of patients have a major associated medical illness, it is imperative that this condition is diagnosed and appropriately managed.

Chronic Empyema

Usual causes of chronicity include a delay in diagnosis, inadequate antibiotic therapy, improper drainage during the acute phase, continuing reinfection (such as that which occurs with a bronchopleural fistula or lung abscess), presence of a foreign body, or presence of a specific infection (such as tuberculosis or a fungal infection). Chronicity is diagnosed by persistent or increasing fever and chest pain, thick pleural fluid, unresolving radiologic findings, and incomplete reexpansion of the lung after closed drainage.[24] When the empyema has reached this stage, simpler forms of therapy, such as rib resection, open drainage, or window thoracostomy, may be useful initially, but they are, as a rule, ineffective for definitive space obliteration. Decortication of the lung, space filling by muscle flaps, space collapse (thoracoplasty or pneumoperitoneum), and space sterilization are alternative therapeutic options that should be considered before a final decision is made. It is most important to weigh all options before a decision is reached so that nonreversible procedures are not performed.

Rib Resection Drainage and Open Thoracic Window

The first therapeutic priority is to provide adequate drainage of the empyema. In poor-risk patients, this can be done either by inserting a large drainage tube or by creating an open thoracic window. Lemmer and colleagues noted that early rib resection, especially for postoperative empyemas and for empyemas that have occurred in immunosuppressed patients, was likely to result in fewer therapeutic failures.[97] In their series, control of the empyema was obtained in 10 of 11 patients treated by this method. Rib resection drainage is a relatively minor procedure, but it should be done only when sufficient adhesions have formed between the visceral and parietal pleura. When the pleural fluid produces 75% of sediment, the empyema can be considered to be in a chronic stage, and rib resection with open thoracic window can be safely performed. It is primarily indicated for debilitated, poor-risk patients and for patients with small residual spaces that are expected to obliterate early.[98] Rib resection is usually performed under general anesthesia. It requires the resection of a short segment of rib over the most dependent part of the cavity, the opening and de-loculation of the space, and the insertion of a large multifenestrated tube into the cavity. If the visceral pleura is thin and "stretchable," space may eventually be obliterated through lung reexpansion, contraction of the space, and filling by granulation tissue. With this technique, the recovery period is long, and frequent dressing and tube changes are usually needed. In Conlan and colleagues' series, 50 patients with chronic empyema without bronchopleural fistula were treated with rib resection, closed-tube drainage, and twice-daily instillation of 2% taurolidine solution into the empyema space through the drainage tube.[99] Forty-one patients underwent further therapy, which consisted of drain removal, decortication, or open-window thoracostomy.

A more permanent form of drainage can be established by the creation of an open-window thoracostomy. This was first described by Samuel Robinson from the Mayo Clinic in 1916 in a patient with nontuberculous empyema.[100] This technique of open-window thoracostomy is usually credited to Dr. Leo Eloesser (the Eloesser flap bears his name), who described it in 1935 as a drainage procedure for acute tuberculous empyemas.[15] This open thoracic window is particularly useful when long-term drainage may be required.[101] The advantages of the technique are that the cavity can be easily irrigated and cleaned, and the dressings can be changed daily on an outpatient basis. Given time, some of these windows close spontaneously, either by filling of the space with granulation tissue or by complete reepithelialization from the skin flaps. Free skin grafts can also be used to stimulate faster closure. In most cases, however, the space is too large for spontaneous closure to occur. In these cases, the window may have to be left open permanently, or it may be closed at a later stage with a pedicle muscle interposition flap. More recently, Thourani and colleagues from my institution reported a series of patients who underwent a modified Eloesser flap procedure for chronic empyema.[102] The flap differed from the original flap in that it was an based on an "inverted" U-shaped flap of skin and subcutaneous tissue (Figs. 28-3 through 28-7). This modification was originally described by Symbas and colleagues from Emory University in 1971.[103]

Space Sterilization

Sterilization of chronic persistent empyema cavities was originally described as a therapeutic option for parapneumonic empyema spaces. According to Virkkula and colleagues,[101] Heuer in 1929 first described space sterilization techniques when he discussed the therapy of 24 patients with chronic empyemas, some of which were of tuberculous origin.[104] He used drainage and sterilization of the empyema cavities with antiseptic chemicals. In a number of the patients, he tried, in addition to space sterilization, operative maneuvers that involved the parietal pleura.

One of the most important contributions to the therapy of chronic empyema was made by Clagett and Geraci in 1963, when they reported a technique of sterilization for the treatment of postpneumonectomy empyemas.[105] This technique has been effective in 50% to 70% of patients who do not have an associated bronchopleural fistula.[106,107] More recently, an updated series from Dr. Clagett's former institution (the Mayo Clinic) reported on 84 patients who underwent a Clagett procedure consisting of open pleural drainage, serial operative

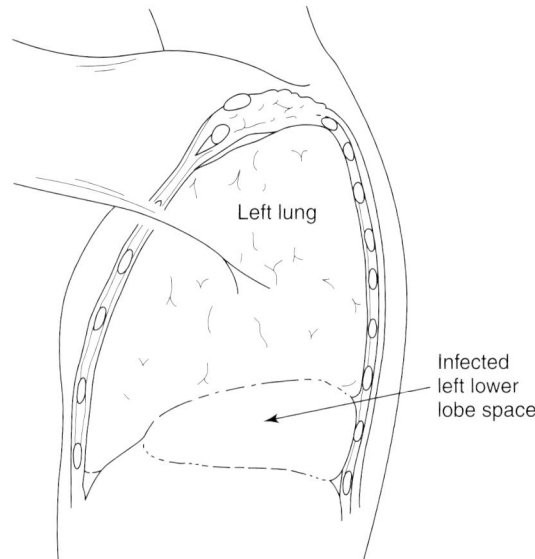

Figure 28–3
Left chronic empyema.

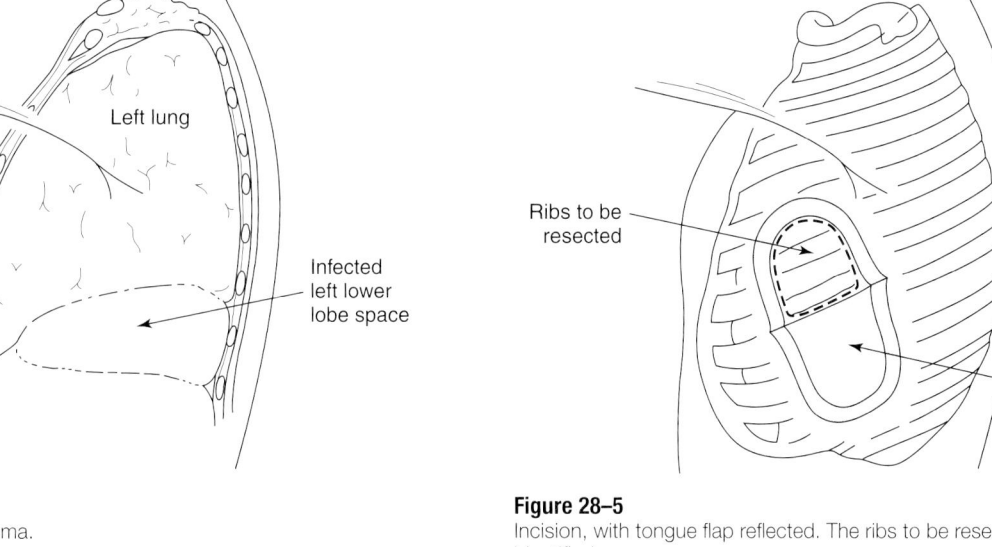

Figure 28–5
Incision, with tongue flap reflected. The ribs to be resected are identified.

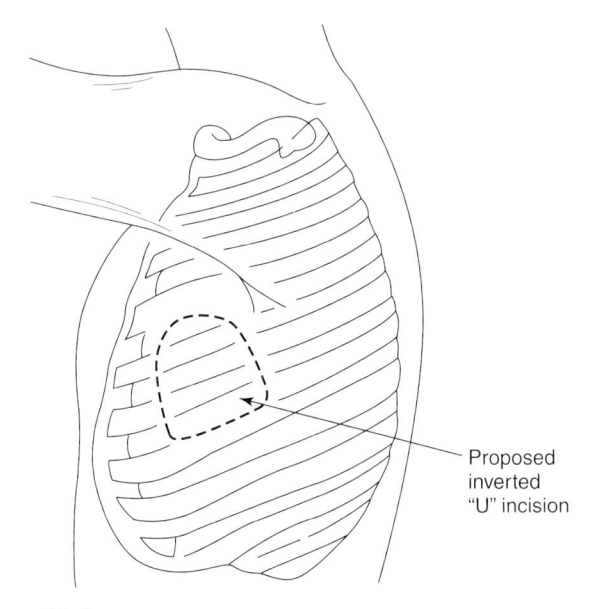

Figure 28–4
Proposed incision for modified Eloesser flap. The proposed inverted U incision is in the left side of the chest.

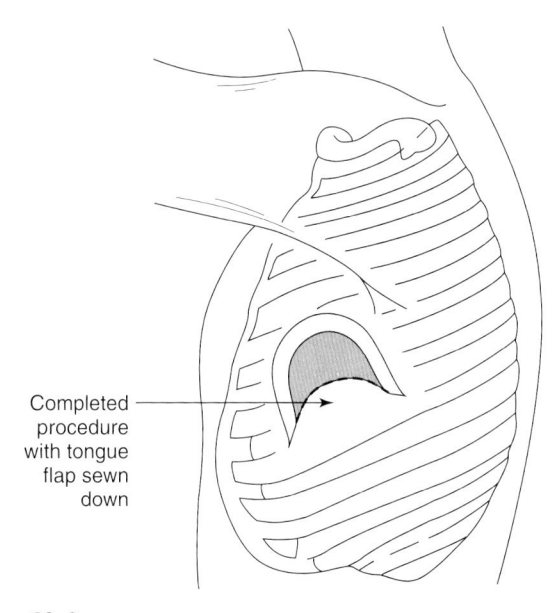

Figure 28–6
Completed modified Eloesser flap with tongue flap sewn to the base of the empyema cavity.

débridements, and eventual chest closure after filling the pleural cavity with a débridement antibiotic solution containing gentamicin, neomycin, and polymyxin B.[108] Modification of the procedure was performed if a bronchopleural fistula (BPF) was present. The bronchial stump would be isolated in the mediastinum and reclosed at the carina with interrupted polypropylene suture. The reclosed stump is reinforced with an intrathoracic transposition of extrathoracic skeletal muscle, usually the serratus anterior muscle if available. In the Mayo series, a BPF was present in 55 patients (65%) and was successfully closed in all of them.[108] Overall, 81% of patients had a healed chest cavity without evidence of recurrent infection at a median follow-up of 1.5 years. The BPF remained closed in all patients. An intrathoracic muscle transposition flap is essential for successful and persistent closure of a postpneumonectomy BPF, as previously described by Pairolero and colleagues.[109] Patients less than 65 years of age, and an interval between pneumonectomy and empyema of greater than 15 weeks, were independent predictors of long-term survival.

Space sterilization techniques can also be used in patients who have empyemas but no previous pneumonectomy.[110,111] In Weissberg's series,[111] open-window thoracostomy was created in 12 patients with empyema and sepsis after conventional therapy with antibiotics and drainage had failed. Complete obliteration of the empyema cavity by granulation tissue occurred in 11 of 12 patients within 1 to 8 months;

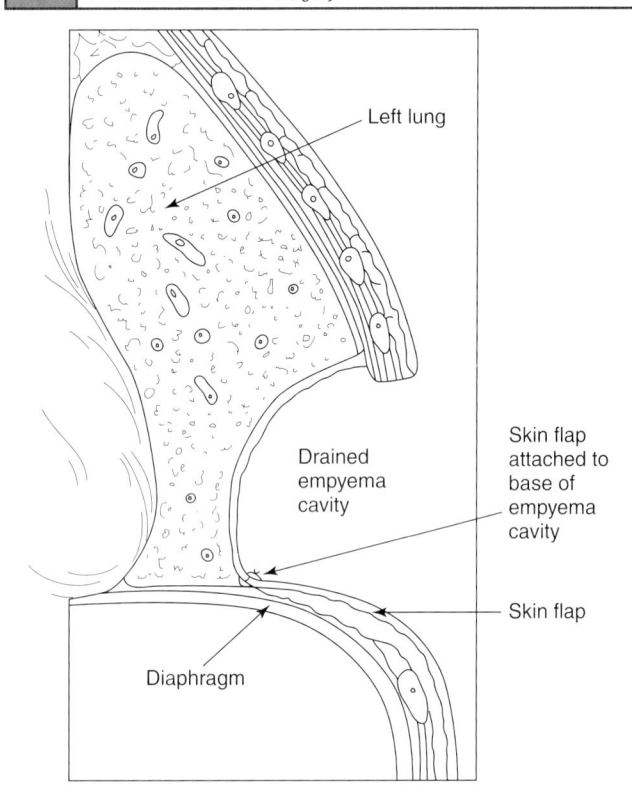

Figure 28–7
Cross-sectional view of the drained empyema cavity and the completed modified Eloesser flap, with tongue flap sewn to the base of the empyema cavity.

the time variation depended on the size of the space. Smolle-Jutner and colleagues also showed that open-window thoracostomy is worthwhile because of its potential for rapid and low-risk control of severe, life-threatening, septic conditions in desperate cases of pleural empyema.[112]

Space-Filling Procedures

Decortication and Empyemectomy

Decortication is defined as the removal of a constricting peel over the lung, and empyemectomy is the complete excision of the empyema space and of its contents without entering it. In empyemectomy, both visceral and parietal peels are excised together, avoiding contamination of either the thoracotomy incision or the free pleural space. Although decortication is the procedure most commonly used, both operations are performed to encourage lung reexpansion in the hope of filling the space.

In general, decortication is seldom required because most patients with parapneumonic empyemas are treated before the disease process reaches the chronic organizing stage. In Blasco and colleagues' series, only eight of 236 patients (3%) required decortication.[70] Personne also emphasized that decortication should be reserved for patients with obvious treatment failures.[65] The timing of decortication in relationship to the diagnosis of chronic empyema remains somewhat controversial. Many authors believe that it is best to wait 3 or more months after diagnosis to achieve maximal functional respiratory recovery.[36,65,82] Others recommend decortication at an earlier stage when the peel of the empyema is not excessively adherent to the lung and therefore may be removed without important blood losses or parenchymal tears.[113] In addition, when decortication is performed before significant ingrowth of fibrous tissue into the lung has occurred, the visceral pleura does not need to be removed, so the likelihood of lung injuries is minimized.

The success rates of decortication depend on an intact visceral pleura, a lung that is expandable, and, most important, a space that can be completely obliterated by pulmonary reexpansion. In a series of 94 patients reported by Sensenig and colleagues, the results of decortication for chronic, nontuberculous empyema were as follows: good, 79; passable, 9; and poor 2.[114] Four patients died; all were older than 45 years. In another report of 25 patients with chronic empyemas, Martella and Santos showed that decortication should be the preferred treatment of chronic postpneumonic empyemas because it was the only procedure that permitted complete débridement of the space and full reexpansion of the affected lung.[115]

To eradicate any potential source of chronic infection completely, it is occasionally necessary to resect a segment of lobe of the lung adjacent to the empyema. In a few cases when the lung is completely destroyed, total pleuropneumonectomy may be necessary. Several authors have also noted that significant functional improvement cannot be achieved after decortication in patients with significant underlying lung disease.[116-118]

Muscle Transposition

Since first reported by Abrashanoff[119] in 1911 and Robinson[120] in 1915 and 1916, transposing muscle flaps on pedicles has been used extensively for the therapy of residual infected pleural spaces, whether closed or in the form of open-window thoracostomies.[100,101,109,121-129] The indications for muscle transposition include obliteration of persistent pleural spaces and reinforcement of the bronchial stump after closure of an associated bronchopleural fistula.[123] Viable tissue in the cavity is essential for successful surgery. The muscle selection should be based not only on its availability but also on the location, size, and shape of the empyema space. The blood supply, innervation, and bulk of the muscle must be preserved, and it must fill the entire space, because empyema is likely to recur if a residual space is left. No attempt to close small bronchopleural fistulas (<2 mm) should be made; however, large fistulas must be débrided and closed. The space should always be drained during the first 10 to 12 postoperative days.

Thoracoplasty

The concept of resecting ribs to decrease the size of the thorax and collapse infected spaces was first described by Estlander in 1879 and Schede in 1890.[16,17] In 1937, Alexander redefined some of these principles.[130] He proposed a posterior extramusculoperiosteal approach through which residual spaces could be collapsed in most cases. During the last 30 years of the 20th century, collapse therapy lost much of its popularity because it is considered by many to be a mutilating and poorly tolerated operation. Two studies have shown, however, that extrapleural thoracoplasty is an excellent therapeutic option for selected patients. In the Hopkins and colleagues series of 30 patients, the operative mortality was 10%, and permanent space closure was obtained in 82% of the survivors.[131] Gregoire and colleagues showed that in a series of 17 patients who underwent one-stage thoracoplasty for therapy of postpneumonectomy empyemas, there were no operative deaths, and immediate control of the empyema was obtained in 15 patients (88%).[132]

In 1989, Nakaoka and colleagues presented the cases of 22 patients with chronic empyema thoracis who underwent decortication.[133] In 11 patients, decortication alone did not achieve sufficient lung reexpansion, and the parietal wall was collapsed, without rib resection, to contact the surface of the decorticated lung. All 11 patients had a one-stage cure, and in all, pulmonary function was well preserved. In another series, Laisaar and Ilves described the use of partial thoracoplasty with omental transplant as a method to treat postpneumonectomy empyemas.[134] In five patients, there were no recurrences of the empyema, and the authors emphasized that the procedure was a one-stage operation without open-window thoracostomy.

BRONCHOPLEURAL FISTULA

Bronchopleural fistulas aggravate the course of empyemas and present a major therapeutic challenge. The presence of a bronchopleural fistula indicates persistent contamination of the pleural space, difficulties in reexpansion of the lung, and possible aspiration in the remaining lung. For many patients with empyema, the presence or absence of a fistula makes the difference between recovery, chronicity, or death. Bronchopleural fistulas most commonly occur after pulmonary resection, but the incidence is low. In the series of Malave and colleagues, 1307 resections were performed, and 35 patients (2.7%) developed a bronchopleural fistulas.[135] In another study by Vester and colleagues, the overall incidence of postresection fistulas was 1.6% (35 of 2243 resections), and approximately two thirds of the patients with postoperative fistulas had undergone preoperative radiotherapy, chemotherapy, or both.[136] Postoperative bronchopleural fistulas can be either at the bronchial or at the peripheral level (alveolar peripheral air leak). Pertinent etiologic factors include endobronchial tuberculosis or infection, contamination of the pleural space during the procedure, devascularization of the bronchus, previous radiation treatment, long bronchial stump, poor surgical technique, or concomitant illnesses.

Patients are considered to have a spontaneous fistula if no previous pulmonary resection has been performed.[26] These usually occur in association with tuberculosis, bacterial pneumonia, or lung abscesses. They also occur with spontaneous pneumothoraces, especially those secondary to chronic obstructive lung disease or to AIDS. In a series by Crawford and colleagues, 44 patients with AIDS were treated for spontaneous pneumothorax, and in 14 of them, a bronchopleural fistula that persisted for more than 10 days developed.[137]

Clinical Presentation and Diagnosis

The most common presenting symptoms of postoperative bronchopleural fistulas are the coughing up of serosanguineous fluid or pus, fever, malaise, and general symptoms of toxicity. On chest radiograph, a previously small space may be enlarging, or a newly formed air–fluid level may be noted. Other radiologic signs include lowering or sudden disappearance of a pleural effusion or a mediastinal shift toward the contralateral side.

At least a two–intercostal space drop is considered enough to suggest a bronchopleural fistula. The diagnosis is usually made by bronchoscopy or by observing persistent air leak through the chest tube. Occasionally, late-occurring fistulas and empyemas are overlooked until they drain spontaneously through the skin of the chest wall (empyema necessitatis), and they may be misdiagnosed as a cancer recurrence.

Management

The management of postresection fistulas depends on why the bronchial stump or lung tissue failed to hold the sutures.[138] Primary failures result from poor closure technique, persistent pathologic changes in the bronchus, or impaired healing, such as that seen in patients who have undergone radiotherapy. In these cases, the therapy may be conservative, with suction drainage of the pleural cavity and possible use of fibrin sealants applied through the rigid bronchoscope[139] or through the flexible fiberoptic bronchoscope.[140-142] In some cases, reclosure of the bronchus, reamputation of the stump, additional sealing of the pulmonary sutures, or additional resection may be advisable.[138]

Secondary failures occur in empyemas in which the bronchial stump reopens because of local pressure by the purulent collection.[138] In this situation, drainage should be done initially followed by definitive management, which consists of bronchial reclosure, muscle flap, or thoracoplasty. These patients are usually very ill, and definitive therapy should be delayed until the empyema has become chronic and the patient's overall medical condition has improved. Puskas and colleagues showed that direct surgical repair of chronic bronchopleural fistulas may be achieved in most patients by suture closure and aggressive transposition of vascularized pedicle flaps.[143]

CONCLUSIONS

Empyema thoracis has been a major medical concern throughout recorded medical history. During the 20th century, and particularly over the past 2 decades, management has been influenced by the identification of a spectrum of new and more virulent pathogens and by the increasing incidence of immunologically compromised hosts. New antibacteriologic agents have contributed to major advances in the therapy of these infectious problems. In many centers, early decortication by thoracoscopic techniques is performed to reexpand the lung and prevent the more serious complications associated with chronicity.

The overall mortality rate associated with empyemas continues to decline. Most deaths occur in elderly patients or from conditions that predispose patients to the empyema, rather than from the empyema itself. Other important factors include the cause of the empyema, the bacteria involved, the correct use of antibiotics, and the immunologic status of the host.

REFERENCES

1. Le Roux BT, Mohlala ML, Odell JA, Whitton ID. Suppurative disease of the lung and pleural space. Part 1: Empyema thoracis and lung abscess. *Curr Probl Surg* 1986;23:1-89.
2. Chadwick J, Mann WN. *The medical works of Hippocrates*. Springfield, IL: Charles C Thomas; 1950.
3. Lain-Entralgo P. *Clásicos de le medicina: Laenec*. Madrid: CSIC, Instituto Arnaldo de Vilanova; 1954.
4. Paget S, Empyema. In: Paget S, editor. The surgery of the chest. New York: EB Treat; 1897. p. 204-29.

5. Major RH. *Classic descriptions of disease.* London: Ballière Tindall and Cox; 1945.
6. Atwater EC. Morrill Wyman and the aspiration of acute pleural effusion, 1850 [letter]. *N Engl Bull Hist Med* 1972;**36**:235.
7. Bowditch HI. On pleuritic effusions and the necessity of paracentesis for their removal. *Am J Med Sci* 1852;**22**:320.
8. Hurt R. The diagnosis and treatment of empyemas. In: Hurt R, editor. The history of cardiothoracic surgery, New York: Parthenon; 1996.
9. Playfair GE. Case of empyema treated by aspiration and subsequently by drainage: recovery. *Br Med J* 1875;**1**:45.
10. Hewitt LF. Thoracentesis: the place of continuous aspiration. *Br Med J* 1876;**1**:317.
11. Von Bulau G. Fur die Heber Drainage bei Behandlung der Empyema. *Z Klin Med* 1891;**18**:31.
12. Graham EA, Bell RD. Open pneumothorax: Its relation to the treatment of acute empyema. *Am J Med Sci* 1918;**156**:939.
13. Graham EA. *Some fundamental considerations in the treatment of empyema thoracis.* St. Louis: CV Mosby; 1925.
14. Peters RM. Empyema thoracis: historical perspective. *Ann Thorac Surg* 1989;**48**:306.
15. Eloesser L. An operation for tuberculous empyema. *Surg Gynecol Obstet* 1935;**60**:1096.
16. Estlander JA. Résection des côtes dans l'empyème chronique. *Rev Med Chir (Paris)* 1879;**3**:156.
17. Schede M. Die Behandlung der Empyema. *Verh Dtsch Ges Imm Med* 1890;**9**:41.
18. Delorme E. Nouveau traitement des empyèmes chroniques. *Gaz Hôp* 1894;**67**:94.
19. Fowler GR. *A history of thoracic surgery (quoted by R. Meade).* Springfield, IL: Charles C Thomas; 1961.
20. Yeh TJ, Hall DP, Ellison RG. Empyema thoracis: A review of 110 cases. *Am Rev Respir Dis* 1963;**88**:785.
21. Eggers C. Radical operation for chronic empyema. *Ann Surg* 1923;**77**:327.
22. Wakabayashi A. Expanded applications of diagnostic and therapeutic thoracoscopy. *J Thorac Cardiovasc Surg* 1991;**102**:721.
23. Gossot D, Stern JB, Galetta D, et al. Thoracoscopic management of postpneumonectomy empyema. *Ann Thorac Surg* 2004;**78**:273.
24. Delarue NC. Empyema: Principles of management: an old problem revisited. In: Deslauriers Lacquet LK, editor. International trends in general thoracic surgery. St. Louis: Mosby–Year Book; 1990, Vol 6.
25. Renner H, Gabor S, Pinter H, et al. Is aggressive surgery in pleural empyema justified? *Eur J Cardiothorac Surg* 1998;**14**:117.
26. Hankins JR, Miller JE, Alter S, et al. Bronchopleural fistula: thirteen-year experience with 77 cases. *J Thorac Cardiovasc Surg* 1978;**76**:755.
27. Potts DE, Taryle DA, Sahn SA. The glucose-pH relationship in parapneumonic effusions. *Arch Intern Med* 1978;**138**:1378.
28. Light RW, Girard WM, Jenkinson SG, George RB. Parapneumonic effusions. *Am J Med* 1980;**69**:507.
29. Maier AC, Grace EJ. Putrid empyema. *Surg Gynecol Obstet* 1942;**74**:69.
30. Ali L, Unruh H. Management of empyema thoracis. *Ann Thorac Surg* 1990;**50**:355.
31. Sherman MM, Subramanian V, Berger RL. Management of thoracic empyema. *Am J Surg* 1977;**133**:474.
32. Vianna NJ. Nontuberculous bacterial empyema in patients with and without underlying disease. *JAMA* 1971;**215**:69.
33. Hoover EL, Hsu HK, Ross MJ, et al. The surgical management of empyema thoracis in substance abuse patients: A 5-year experience. *Ann Thorac Surg* 1988;**46**:563.
34. LeRoux BT. Empyema thoracis. *Br J Surg* 1965;**52**:89.
35. Mandal AK, Thadepalli H. Treatment of spontaneous bacterial empyema thoracis. *J Thorac Cardiovasc Surg* 1987;**94**:414.
36. Thurer RJ, Palatinos GM. Surgical aspects of the pleural space. *Semin Respir Med* 1987;**9**:98.
37. Ogilvie AG. Final results in traumatic haemothorax: A report of 230 cases. *Thorax* 1950;**5**:116.
38. Arom KK, Grover FL, Richardson JD, Trinkle JK. Posttraumatic empyema. *Ann Thorac Surg* 1977;**23**:254.
39. Mavroudis C, Ganzel BL, Katzmark S, Polk HC. Effect of hemothorax on experimental empyema thoracis in the guinea pig. *J Thorac Cardiovasc Surg* 1985;**89**:42.
40. Baethge BA, Eggerstedt JM, Olash FA. Group F streptococcal empyema from aspiration of a grass inflorescence. *Ann Thorac Surg* 1990;**49**:319.
41. Brown B, Ory EM, Meads M, et al. Penicillin treatment of empyema: Report of 24 cases and review of the literature. *Ann Intern Med* 1956;**24**:343.
42. Keefer CS, Rantz LA, Rammelkamp CH. Hemolytic streptococcal pneumonia and empyema: study of 55 cases with special reference to treatment. *Ann Intern Med* 1941;**14**:1533.
43. Ehler AN. Non-tuberculous thoracic empyema: a collective review of the literature from 1934 to 1939. *Int Abstr Surg* 1941;**72**:17.
44. Thomas DF, Glass JL, Vaisch BF. Management of streptococcal pneumonia. *Ann Thorac Surg* 1966;**2**:658.
45. Finland M, Barnes MW. Changing ecology of acute bacterial empyema occurrence and mortality at Boston City Hospital during 12 selected years from 1935 to 1972. *J Infect Dis* 1978;**137**:274.
46. Bartlett JG, Thadepalli H, Gorbach SL, Finegold SM. Bacteriology of empyema. *Lancet* 1974;**1**:338.
47. Ravitch M, Fein R. The changing picture of pneumonia and empyema in infants and children: A review of the experience at the Harriet Lane Home from 1934 through 1958. *JAMA* 1961;**175**:1039.
48. Sullivan KM, O'Toole RD, Fisher RH, Sullivan KN. Anaerobic empyema thoracis: the role of anaerobes in 226 cases of culture proven empyemas. *Arch Intern Med* 1973;**131**:521.
49. Bergeron MG. The changing bacterial spectrum and antibiotic choice in thoracic surgery: Surgical management of pleural diseases. In: Deslauriers J, Lacquet LK, editors. International trends in general thoracic surgery. St. Louis: Mosby–Year Book; 1990, Vol 6. p. 197-207.
50. Paris F, Blasco E, Tarazona V et al: El empyema pleural como complicacion de la bronchopneumopathia aguda. Proceedings II Symposium Internatiónal sobre antibioticos. Beecham, Valencia, 1970.
51. Varkey B, Rose HD, Kesavan-Kurry CP, Politis J. Empyema thoracis during a ten-year period: Analysis of 72 cases and comparison to a previous study (1952 to 1967). *Arch Intern Med* 1981;**141**:1771.
52. Stark DD, Federle MP, Goodman PC, et al. Differentiating lung abscess and empyema: radiography and computed tomography. *AJR Am J Roentgenol* 1983;**141**:163.
53. Hanna JW, Read JC, Choplin RH. Pleural infections: a clinical radiological review. *J Thorac Imaging* 1991;**6**:68-79.
54. Moran JF. Surgical management of pleural space infections. *Semin Respir Infect* 1988;**3**:383.
55. Orringer MB. Thoracic empyema: Back to basics. *Chest* 1988;**93**:901.
56. Houston MC. Pleural fluid pH: Diagnostic, therapeutic and prognostic value. *Am J Surg* 1987;**154**:333.
57. Light RW. Parapneumonic effusion and empyema. *Clin Chest Med* 1985;**6**:55.
58. Light RW. Parapneumonic effusions and empyema. *Semin Respir Med* 1987;**9**:37.
59. Sahn SA, Light RW. The sun should never set on a parapneumonic effusion. *Chest* 1989;**95**:945.
60. Potts DE, Levin DC, Sahn SA. Pleural fluid pH in parapneumonic effusions. *Chest* 1976;**70**:328.
61. Narrod III C, Narrod J, Hopeman A. The role of early limited thoracotomy in the treatment of empyema. *J Thorac Cardiovasc Surg* 1988;**96**:436.
62. Himelman RB, Callen PW. The prognostic value of loculations in parapneumonic pleural effusion. *Chest* 1986;**90**:852.
63. Cassina PC, Hauser M, Hillejan L, et al. Video-assisted thoracoscopy in the treatment of pleural empyema: stage-based management and outcome. *J Thorac Cardiovasc Surg* 1999;**117**:234.
64. Cohen RG, DeMeester TR, Lafontaine E. The pleura. In: Sabiston DC, Spencer FC, editors. Surgery of the chest. 6th ed. Philadelphia: WB Saunders; 1995.
65. Personne C. Role of early thoracotomy in the treatment of empyema. In: Deslauriers J, Lacquet LK, editors. International trends in general thoracic surgery. St. Louis: Mosby–Year Book; 1990, Vol 6.
66. Ferguson MK. The healing hand. *Chest* 1990;**97**:4.
67. Luizy J, Mathey J, Le Brigand H, Galey JJ. Technique d'irrigation pleurale sous depression continue dans le traitement des pyothorax. *Rev Tuberc Pneumol* 1966;**30**:393.
68. Dieter RA, Pifarré R, Neville WE, et al. Empyema treated with neomycin irrigation and closed-chest drainage. *J Thorac Cardiovasc Surg* 1970;**59**:496.
69. Rosenfeldt FL, McGibney D, Braimbridge MV, Watson DA. Comparison between irrigation and conventional treatment for empyema and pneumonectomy space infections. *Thorax* 1981;**36**:272.
70. Blasco E, Paris F, Padilla J. Acute postpneumonic empyema treated by intercostal tube drainage with suction and pleural washing but without rib resection. In: Deslauriers J, Lacquet LK, editors. International trends in general thoracic surgery. St. Louis: Mosby–Year Book; 1990, Vol 6.
71. Lee KS, Im JG, Kim YH, Hwang SH, Bae WK, Lee BH. Treatment of thoracic multiloculated empyemas with intra-cavity urokinase: a prospective study. *Radiology* 1991;**179**:771.
72. Crouch JD, Keagy BA, Delany DJ. Pigtail" catheter drainage in thoracic surgery. *Am Rev Respir Dis* 1987;**136**:174.
73. Landreneau RJ, Keenan RJ, Hazelrigg SR, et al. Thoracoscopy for empyema and hemothorax. *Chest* 1995;**109**:18.
74. Lawrence DR, Obri SK, Moxon RE, et al. Thoracoscopic débridement of empyema thoracis. *Ann Thorac Surg* 1997;**64**:1448.

75. Angelillo Mackinlay TA, Lyons GA, Chimondeguy DJ, Piedras MA, Angaramo G, Emery J. VATS debridement versus thoracotomy in the treatment of loculated postpneumonia empyema. *Ann Thorac Surg* 1996;**61**:1626-30.
76. Striffeler H, Gugger M, Imhof V. Video-assisted thoracoscopic surgery for fibrino-purulent empyema in 67 patients. *Ann Thorac Surg* 1998;**65**:319.
77. Deslauriers J, Invited commentary to Cassina PC, et al. Video-assisted thoracoscopy in the treatment of pleural empyema: Stage-based management and outcome. *J Thorac Cardiovasc Surg* 1999;**117**:238.
78. Luh SP, Chou MC, Wang LS, et al. Video-assisted thoracoscopic surgery in the treatment of complicated parapneumonic effusions or empyemas: outcome of 234 patients. *Chest* 2005;**127**:1427.
79. Wurnig PN, Wittmer V, Pridun NS, et al. Video-assisted thoracic surgery for pleural empyema. *Ann Thorac Surg* 2006;**81**:309.
80. Solaini L, Prusciano F, Bagioni P. Video-assisted thoracic surgery in the treatment of pleural empyema. *Surg Endosc* 2007;**21**:280.
81. Silen ML, Naunheim KS. Thoracoscopic approach to the management of empyema thoracis: indications and results. *Chest Surg Clin North Am* 1996;**6**:491.
82. Morin JE, Munro DD, MacLean LD. Early thoracotomy for empyema. *J Thorac Cardiovasc Surg* 1972;**64**:530.
83. Fishman NH, Ellertson DG. Early pleural decortication for thoracic empyema in immunosuppressed patients. *J Thorac Cardiovas Surg* 1977;**74**:537.
84. Miller JI. Empyema thoracis. *Ann Thorac Surg* 1990;**50**:343.
85. Pothula V, Krellenstein DJ. Early aggressive surgical management of parapneumonic empyemas. *Chest* 1994;**105**:832.
86. Tillett WS, Sherry S. The effect in patients of streptococcal fibrinolysin (streptokinase) and streptococcal desoxyribonuclease on fibrinous, purulent and sanguineous pleural exudations. *J Clin Invest* 1949;**28**:173.
87. Muers MF. Streptokinase for empyema. *Lancet* 1997;**349**:1491.
88. Bergh NP, Ekroth R, Larsson S, Nagy P. Intrapleural streptokinase in the treatment of haemothorax and empyema. *Scand J Thorac Cardiovasc Surg* 1977;**11**:265.
89. Robinson LA, Moulton AL, Fleming WH, et al. Intrapleural fibrinolytic treatment of multiloculated thoracic empyemas. *Ann Thorac Surg* 1994;**57**:803.
90. Davies RJO, Traill ZC, Gleeson FV. Randomized controlled trial of intrapleural streptokinase in community acquired pleural infection. *Thorax* 1997;**52**:416.
91. Wait MA, Sharma S, Hohn J, Dal Nogare A. A randomized trial of empyema therapy. *Chest* 1997;**111**:1548.
92. Moulton JS, Moore PT, Mencini RA. Treatment of loculated pleural effusions with transcatheter intracavity urokinase. *AJR Am J Roentgenol* 1989;**153**:941.
93. Pollack JS, Passik CS. Intrapleural urokinase in the treatment of loculated pleural effusions. *Chest* 1994;**105**:868.
94. Bouros D, Schiza S, Patsourakis G, et al. Intrapleural streptokinase versus urokinase in the treatment of complicated parapneumonic effusions: a prospective double-blind study. *Am J Respir Crit Care Med* 1997;**155**:291.
95. Lopez-Rivero L, Lopez-Pujol J, Quevedo S, et al. Urokinase in the management of loculated intrapleural effusion. Abstracts from the 2nd European Conference on General Thoracic Surgery. In: E.S.T.S. Gotti G, Elias S, Paldini P, editors. Universita degli Studi di Siena. Siena, Italy: Cattedra de Chirugia Toracia; 1994.
96. Weissberg D, Kaufman M. The use of talc for pleurodesis in the treatment of resistant empyema. *Ann Thorac Surg* 1986;**41**:143.
97. Lemmer JH, Botham MJ, Orringer MB. Modern management of adult thoracic empyema. *J Thorac Cardiovasc Surg* 1985;**90**:849.
98. Samson PE. Empyema thoracis: essentials of present-day management. *Ann Thorac Surg* 1971;**11**:210.
99. Conlan AA, Abramor E, Delikaris O, Hurwitz SS. Taurolidine instillation as therapy for empyema thoracis. *S Afr Med J* 1983;**64**:653.
100. Robinson S. The treatment of chronic non-tuberculous empyema. *Surg Gynecol Obstet* 1916;**22**:557.
101. Virkkula L, Eerola S. Treatment of postpneumonectomy empyema and large fistula. *Les Bronches* 1973;**23**:230.
102. Thourani VH, Lancaster RT, Mansour KA, et al. Twenty-six years of experience with the modified Eloesser flap. *Ann Thorac Surg* 2003;**76**:401.
103. Symbas PN, Nugent JT, Abbott OA, et al. Nontuberculous pleural empyema in adults. *Ann Thorac Surg* 1971;**12**:69.
104. Heuer GA. Observations on the treatment of chronic empyema. *Ann Surg* 1929;**72**:80.
105. Claggett OT, Geraci JE. A procedure for the management of postpneumonectomy empyema. *J Thorac Cardiovasc Surg* 1963;**45**:141.
106. Goldstraw P. Treatment of the post-pneumonectomy empyema: the case for fenestration. *Thorax* 1979;**34**:740.
107. Stafford EG, Claggett OT. Post-pneumonectomy empyema: neomycin instillations and definitive closure. *J Thorac Cardiovasc Surg* 1972;**63**:771.
108. Zaheer S, Allen MS, Cassivi SD, et al. Postpneumonectomy empyema: results after the Clagett procedure. *Ann Thorac Surg* 2006;**82**:279.
109. Pairolero PC, Arnold PHG, Piehler JM. Intrathoracic transposition of extrathoracic skeletal muscle. *J Thorac Cardiovasc Surg* 1983;**86**:809.
110. Bayes AJ, Wilson JAS, Chiu RCJ, et al. Claggett open-window thoracostomy in patients with empyema who had and had not undergone pneumonectomy. *Can J Surg* 1987;**30**:329.
111. Weissberg D. Empyema and bronchopleural fistula: Experience with open-window thoracostomy. *Chest* 1982;**82**:447.
112. Smolle-Juttner E, Beuster W, Pinter H, et al. Open-window thoracoscopy in pleural empyema. *Eur J Cardiothorac Surg* 1992;**6**:635.
113. Moir R, Telander RL. Complications of lower respiratory tract infection, empyema complicating pneumonia, pneumatoceles, and respiratory embarrassment. In: Fallis JC, Piller RM, Lemoine G, editors. Current topics in general thoracic surgery. New York: Elsevier; 1991, Vol 1.
114. Sensenig DM, Rossi NP, Ehrenhaft JL. Decortication for chronic non-tuberculous empyema. *Surg Gynecol Obstet* 1963;**1117**:443.
115. Martella AT, Santos GH. Decortication for chronic postpneumonic empyema. *J Am Coll Surg* 1995;**180**:573.
116. Carroll LD, McClement J, Himmelsteen A, et al. Pulmonary function following decortication. *Am Rev Tuberc* 1951;**63**:231.
117. Morton JR, Boushy SF, Guin GA. Physiological evaluation of results of pulmonary decortication. *Ann Thorac Surg* 1970;**9**:321.
118. Patton WE, Warson TR, Gaensler EA. Pulmonary function before and at intervals after surgical decortication of the lung. *Surg Gynecol Obstet* 1952;**95**:477.
119. Abrashanoff A. Plastishe methode zur Schliesslung von Fistel-gangrenn welch von immeran organen Komman. *Zentralbi Chir* 1911;**38**:186.
120. Robinson S. The treatment of chronic non-tuberculous empyema (Collected Papers). *Mayo Clin* 1915;**7**:618.
121. Baena-Montilla P, Tarasona V. Bronchopleural fistula: management with muscle transposition. In: Grillo H, Eschapasse H, editors. *International trends in general thoracic surgery*, Vol 2. Philadelphia: WB Saunders; 1987.
122. Borro JM, Tarazona V, Paris F. Management of postpneumonectomy empyema of the pleural space. In: Peters RM, Toledo J, editors. Current topics in general thoracic surgery: an international series. New York: Elsevier; 1991, Vol 2.
123. Deschamps C, Trastek VF, Arnold PG, Pairolero PC. Surgical approach to chronic Empyema: decortication and muscle transposition. In: Deslauriers J, Lacquet LK, editors. International trends in general thoracic surgery. St. Louis: Mosby–Year Book; 1990, Vol 6.
124. Garcia-Yuste M, Ramos G, Duque JL, et al. Open-window thoracostomy and thoracomyoplasty to manage chronic pleural empyema. *Am Thorac Surg* 1998;**65**:818.
125. Miller JI, Mansour KA, Nahai F, et al. Single-stage complete muscle flap closure of the post-pneumonectomy empyema space: a new method and possible solution to a disturbing complication. *Ann Thorac Surg* 1984;**38**:227.
126. Pairolero PC, Arnold PHG. Bronchopleural fistula: treatment by transposition of pectoralis major. *J Thorac Cardiovasc Surg* 1980;**79**:142.
127. Miller JI. Management of post-pneumonectomy empyema of the pleural space. In: Peters RM, Toledo J, editors. Current topics in general thoracic surgery: an international series. New York: Elsevier; 1991.
128. Tarazona V, Paris F, Chamorro JJ, et al. Comblement des poches résiduelles aprè pneumonectomie par transposition complète du grand dorsal, du grand dentale et du grand pectoral: a propos de quatre malades. *Ann Chir Thorac Cardiovasc* 1981;**35**:681.
129. Uri SU, Nahai F. Intrathoracic muscle transposition: surgical anatomy and techniques of harvest. *Chest Surg Clin North Am* 1996;**6**:501.
130. Alexander J. *The collapse therapy of pulmonary tuberculosis*. Springfield, IL: Charles C Thomas; 1937.
131. Hopkins RA, Ungerleider RM, Staub EN, Young WG. The modern use of thoracoplasty. *Ann Thorac Surg* 1985;**40**:181.
132. Gregoire R, Deslauriers J, Beaulieu M, Piraux M. Thoracoplasty: Its forgotten role in the management of non-tuberculous post-pneumonectomy empyema. *Can J Surg* 1987;**30**:343.
133. Nakaoka K, Nakalara K, Iioka S, et al. Postoperative preservation of pulmonary function in patients with chronic empyema thoracis: a one-stage operation. *Ann Thorac Surg* 1989;**47**:848.
134. Laisaar T, Ilves A. Omentoplasty together with partial thoracoplasty: a one-stage operation for postpneumonectomy pleural empyema. *Ann Chir Gynaecol* 1997;**86**:319.
135. Malave G, Foster ED, Wilson JA, Munro DD. Bronchopleural fistula: present day study of an old problem. *Ann Thorac Surg* 1971;**11**:1.
136. Vester SR, Faber LP, Kittle F, et al. Bronchopleural fistula after stapled closure of bronchus. *Ann Thorac Surg* 1991;**52**:1253.
137. Crawford BK, Galloway AC, Boyd AD, Spencer FC. Treatment of AIDS-related bronchopleural fistula by pleurectomy. *Ann Thorac Surg* 1992;**54**:212.
138. Perelman ME, Rymko LP. Management of empyemas: the problems of associated bronchopleural fistulas. In: Deslauriers J, Lacquet LK, editors. *International trends in general thoracic surgery*, Vol 6. St. Louis: Mosby–Year Book; 1990.

139. Onotera RT, Unruh HW. Closure of post-pneumonectomy bronchopleural fistula with fibrin sealant (Tisseel). *Thorax* 1988;**43**:1015.
140. Jensen C, Sharna P. Use of fibrin glue in thoracic surgery. *Ann Thorac Surg* 1985;**39**:521.
141. Glover W, Chavis TV, Daniel TM, et al. Fibrin glue application through the flexible fiberoptique bronchoscope: closure of bronchopleural fistulas. *J Thorac Cardiovasc Surg* 1987;**93**:470.
142. York JEL, Lewall DB, Hidi M, et al. Endoscopic diagnosis and treatment of postoperative bronchopleural fistula. *Chest* 1990;**197**:1390.
143. Puskas JD, Mathisen DJ, Grillo HC, et al. Treatment strategies for bronchopleural fistula. *J Thorac Cardiovasc Surg* 1995;**109**:989.

CHAPTER 29
Chylothorax
Gaetano Rocco

Classification and Etiology
Anatomic Considerations
Pathophysiology
Symptoms and Diagnosis
Treatment
Chylothorax after Pulmonary Resection
Chylothorax after Esophagectomy

Chylothorax is the collection of an excessive amount of chyle in the pleural space. The continued loss of chyle—which can amount to 2 to 3 L/day after a thoracic duct injury[1]—leads to significant depletion of fats (up to 70% of dietary intake), proteins, and T lymphocytes.[2] As a consequence, marked disturbances in the immunologic and nutritional profile occur in these patients, along with a mass effect created by dislocation of intrathoracic structures by the enlarging fluid collection. Indeed, the flow rate of chyle within the thoracic duct can be as high as 110 mL/hr.[1] If left untreated, chylothorax may yield an overall mortality rate of 50%.[3]

CLASSIFICATION AND ETIOLOGY

The term *traumatic* is often used to include both iatrogenic and postinjury chylothoraces,[2] which usually represent the most common causes of significant chyle accumulation in the chest. Neoplastic etiology can account for up to 20% of chylothoraces.[2] In a recent report from the Mayo Clinic, the etiology was surgery or trauma in 50% of the patients, medical conditions in 44%, and unknown in 6%.[4] This unusual distribution compared with the commonly reported series[5] was explained by the high volume of surgical cases being performed each year at that institution.

In the pediatric group, congenital chylothorax appears early after birth, possibly because of a combination of thoracic duct malformation and sudden elevation of venous pressure.[6] Neonatal chylothorax has been reported in conjunction with several syndromes, such as Noonan's syndrome and Down syndrome.[2,6] In addition, the incidence of chylothorax after cardiothoracic procedures in children is reported to be as high as 3.8%.[7] The detection of a pleural effusion in this age group should immediately arouse suspicion of chylothorax.[6] Tuberculosis with significant mediastinal adenopathy may still be responsible for "spontaneous" bilateral chylothoraces in children because of the obstruction to centripetal flow.[8]

Excessive chyle collection in the pleural space may occur in association with benign and malignant tumors. Reportedly, almost 50% of patients with chylothorax have cancer. Of these, 70% have lymphoma.[5] Conversely, chylothorax was reported in 10% of the patients with lymphangioleiomyomatosis (LAM) treated at the Mayo Clinic over a 24-year period.[9]

Intraoperative injuries may ensue from surgical procedures conducted in the proximity of the thoracic duct anatomic course.[2,10,11] Even minor maneuvers, such as raising a pleural flap over the thoracic aorta or dividing the inferior pulmonary ligament, can cause this complication.[12] In 1999, the Mayo Clinic reported that after 11,315 general thoracic surgical procedures, 47 patients (0.42%) had postoperative chylothorax.[1]

Chylothorax has been reported to complicate the postoperative course in 1% of patients who underwent esophagectomy,[13] requiring surgical reexploration in almost 90% of those cases.[3] Although it occurred in less than 1% of patients subjected to pulmonary resection, only 38% of those underwent reoperation for final treatment.[1] A detailed list of possible causes of chylothorax was reported by De Meester[14] in the 4th edition of this book, and it was recently modified by Nair.[2]

ANATOMIC CONSIDERATIONS

A certain variability in the distribution of the thoracic duct and its tributaries is not uncommon. At some point in embryogenesis, the thoracic duct is a bilateral structure,[15] and it can be double or triple in up to 40% of the population.[15] A single thoracic duct is found in about 65% of individuals. Chylothorax can result from leak of lymph from major collectors—the most sizable being the thoracic duct—or from multiple lymphatic channels that make up a network of tributaries consistently demonstrated by several anatomic studies.[11]

The centripetal flow toward the left subclavian vein is regulated by three factors[16]: (1) the *vis a tergo* created by the continuous enteral absorption of chyle constituents, which pushes the chyle from the cisterna chyli to the left subclavian vein, (2) the aspiration effect given by the negative effect of the intrathoracic pressure facilitating the cephalad flow, and (3) lymphatic vessel contractions, generated by smooth musculature to empty the duct into the subclavian vein.

PATHOPHYSIOLOGY

A chylothorax can result from a chyle leak (by direct injury or obstruction of the major lymphatic vessel) or from generalized transdiaphragmatic flow from chylous ascites.[9] The distinction between idiopathic (sometimes called spontaneous) and secondary causes of chylothorax depends on the presence of an identified etiology. Secondary causes include neoplastic and inflammatory conditions, as chylothorax may result from obstruction to centripetal flow or from increased flow rate with extreme dilation of lymphatic vessels. As a consequence, lymphatic vessels are thought to preserve—at the beginning—their structural integrity at the expense of increased permeability into the pleural space.[2,9] Constrictive pericarditis, superior vena cava obstruction, and mediastinal fibrosis resulting from cancer treatment can generate chylothorax according to this pathophysiologic model.[5] Thus, patients with liver cirrhosis can develop spontaneous chylothorax because of a twofold or threefold increase in diameter of the thoracic duct from an unusual backflow and pressure.[17]

Another factor implied in the onset of chylothorax is valve competency in the lymphatic vessels, as demonstrated by the rarity of such complication after pulmonary resection and extensive mediastinal nodal dissection. Valve insufficiency–induced backflow from the thoracic duct into the areas of nodal dissection and injury of the lymphatic network may explain the chylous effusion[11] after pulmonary resections with concurrent nodal dissection.

Clinically, chylothorax resulting from pleural carcinomatosis or from tubercular involvement may have a gradual onset and development. This can be explained by progressive lung trapping caused when the visceral pleura are thickened by the persistent chemical irritation of chyle components.[12] In time, fibrotic visceral pleura may impose a restrictive physiology on the affected lung by significantly reducing its compliance. This scenario is more often the case with the so-called pseudochylothorax (see later).

Induced or secondary causes of chylothorax include traumatic and iatrogenic causes, which have in common the interruption of the vessel by direct injury, inadvertent division, or blunt trauma to the thoracic duct or its tributaries. Rupture of the thoracic duct may also occur after sudden hyperextension of the spine (e.g., seat belt injury),[18] with vertebral fractures or dislocation, or after protracted and vigorous vomiting or coughing.[6]

SYMPTOMS AND DIAGNOSIS

Biochemically, chyle is usually characterized by a content of triglycerides in the pleural fluid greater than the content detected in the plasma (>110 mg/dL[1]), a cholesterol-to-triglycerides ratio of less than 1, and the presence of chylomicrons.[2,6,19-21] A detailed description of the chemical components of chyle is available in the surgical literature.[1,6]

The differential diagnosis for chylothorax includes pseudochylothorax, which refers to chronic effusions that resemble chylothorax but do not have its biochemical composition.[2] The pleural effusions seen in patients with tuberculosis and rheumatoid arthritis, for example, may be sterile and yellowish or milky in color and have high cholesterol levels.

It is interesting that chyle does not contain fibrinogen, which could seal a small leak.[3] Chyle is bacteriostatic and can be a chemical irritant for the pleural surfaces,[12] although this finding is disputed.[2,16] In addition, chylothorax can affect the bioavailability of drugs such as amiodarone, digoxin, and cyclosporine.[2]

The acute onset of a significant chyle leak may be characterized by dyspnea and cough associated with a sense of pressure in the chest.[2] Hemodynamic disturbance is also common with high-flow chylous fistulas.[2] Conversely, severe malnourishment and cachexia may result from persistent chylothorax.[2] Symptoms related to chyle accumulation were described in a recent report from the Mayo Clinic.[4] During a 21-year observation period, 203 patients developed chylothorax (male-to-female ratio, 1.21; median age, 54 years). Of these patients, 57% presented with dyspnea whereas 37% were asymptomatic. More than 7 weeks elapsed from symptom development to diagnosis.[4]

A milky pleural effusion accumulating at a rate of greater than 400 to 700 mL per day is suggestive of chylothorax.[12] An empty pleural space after pneumonectomy may accommodate a greater chyle flow.[12] The administration of a high-fat meal 3 hours before surgery, with or without dye, or the subcutaneous injection of dye 1 hour before surgical exploration can facilitate the identification of the site of leakage when the decision to surgically ligate the duct is made.[12]

Some authors rely on the findings of pedal lymphography to define further management.[17,22] Indeed, the discontinuation of chyle leak after lymphography is a distinct therapeutic possibility[17] because of the sclerosing effect of the iodine contrast medium. Controversies exist about whether to proceed to lymphography only in candidates for surgical reexploration or to proceed routinely in all patients who develop chylothorax after pulmonary resection.[23] However, the adoption of a rigorous management protocol including lymphography has been reported to minimize the need for reoperation, which seems to argue for the latter option.[22]

Nevertheless, the lymphographic finding of a leak from small tributaries may predict the success of conservative management.[17]

TREATMENT

The three approaches to treatment are (1) conservative (nonsurgical), (2) surgical, aimed at identifying and isolating the lymphatic duct causing the leak so as to close it, and (3) surgical, aimed at obliterating the space that would otherwise become filled by chyle (Table 29-1). Conservative management is the mainstay of treatment of children who develop postoperative chylothorax after cardiothoracic interventions.[7] Conservative treatment includes parenteral nutrition (nothing by mouth) and a medium-chain triglyceride diet.[12]

In adults, it has been suggested that the detection of chylothorax greater than 1 L/day after 1 week or between 0.1 and 1 L/day of chyle loss during the first 2 weeks[17] is evidence of failure of conservative management. Others[12] suggest surgical intervention if the leak is greater than 1 L/day for 5 days, if the chylothorax does not subside after 2 weeks, or when there is severe nutritional or metabolic imbalance. Advocates of early surgical intervention after esophagectomy support the idea of re-intervention if the leak is consistently greater than 2 L/day during 2 consecutive days.[3] An interesting perspective for chylothorax treatment has been outlined by Cope, who suggested percutaneously injecting a sclerosing agent into the cisterna chyli.[24]

Surgical intervention or re-intervention can be performed via an open or a video-assisted thoracic surgery (VATS)/robotic approach.[25] The increasing use of minimally invasive techniques to achieve control of the thoracic duct may change the balance between conservative and operative approaches. The therapeutic possibilities center on identification of the leak, closure of the fistula, and obliteration of the pleural space, especially if the chylothorax complicates an esophagectomy. On principle, the side of the identified leak should be preferentially approached and surgically treated.[3] In the event of a bilateral chylothorax, the right side should be preferentially

Table 29–1
Therapeutic Modalities in the Management of Chylothorax

Nonsurgical (ref)	Operative: Open or VATS/robotic (ref)
Chest drain only (5)	Fibrin glue plugging (3, 12)
Medium-chain triglycerides diet and total parenteral nutrition (12)	Mass ligation (1, 12)
Somatostatin (12)	Thoracoscopic clipping (3, 12)
Octreotide (12)	Ultrasonic coagulation (3)
Etilefrine (12)	Pledget suturing (3)
Postoperative radiation, up to 20 Gy (2, 12)	Pleurovenous or peritoneal shunting (12, 20, 28)
Nitric oxide (12)	Decortication or pleurectomy (3)
Tetracycline/doxycycline pleurodesis (12, 20)	VATS talc pleurodesis (12)
Povidone pleurodesis (29)	
OK-432 interferon or interleukins (20)	
Bleomycin (20)	
Embolization during lymphangiography (27)	
Positive-pressure ventilation (20)	

VATS, video-assisted thoracoscopic surgery.

entered to ligate the supradiaphragmatic thoracic duct. If the duct cannot be isolated, mass ligation of the fibrotic area around the duct should be performed.[12] Treatment options suggested in the literature are listed in Table 29-1.

Chylothorax after Pulmonary Resection

Although a well-expanded residual lung after lobectomy and a postpneumonectomy chylothorax share similar etiologies and pathophysiologies, a conservative approach is usually preferred for the former.[21] In postpneumonectomy chylothorax, a sudden accumulation of chyle in the empty hemithorax can cause a contralateral shift of the mediastinum, with attendant cardiorespiratory functional impairment. This rare clinical scenario, reported in almost half of the pneumonectomy patients who developed chylothorax,[26] mandates a more aggressive protocol to ensure early ligation of the thoracic duct—within 3 to 5 days of onset if the chyle loss is greater than 400 mL after an observation period lasting two consecutive 8-hour shifts.[21]

Reportedly, chylothorax occurs more frequently on the right side, possibly as a result of the more radical mediastinal nodal dissection after resection for bronchial carcinoma.[17]

Chylothorax after Esophagectomy

Patients undergoing esophagectomy are often older, with significant cardiorespiratory comorbidities and malnourishment.[13] In addition, multiple operative fields are necessary to complete the esophageal resection and to restore gastrointestinal continuity. VATS has reduced the impact of this operation on patients' overall condition. In a series of 1787 patients operated on during an 18-year period, 26% underwent a transhiatal esophagectomy because of substantial cardiorespiratory comorbidities.[13] However, no significant difference in the prevalence of chylothorax was noted between transthoracic and transhiatal approaches.[13] In a Mayo Clinic series, the incidence of this complication after esophagectomy was reported to be 2.9%.[1] Recently, investigators renowned for their long-standing experience with transhiatal esophagectomy (reaching almost 2000 such patients) reported an incidence of chylothorax of 1.5%, favorably comparing with the 2% to 4% range reported in the literature.[21]

Early reoperation with mass ligation of the thoracic duct is advocated to limit the immunologic and nutritional imbalances that can heavily affect the postoperative course of these patients.[13] The mortality rates for reoperation reach 16%, compared with more than 80% after conservative treatment,[3] suggesting that the early surgery option to control chylothorax is preferable. The prophylactic ligation of the immediately supradiaphragmatic azygos vein along with the thoracic duct at the time of resection may be a maneuver that could reduce the incidence of chylothorax after esophagectomy.[2,13]

REFERENCES

1. Cerfolio RJ, Allen MS, Deschamps C, et al. Postoperative chylothorax. *J Thorac Cardiovasc Surg* 1996;**112**:1361-6.
2. Nair SK, Petko M, Hayward MP. Aetiology and management of chylothorax in adults. *Eur J Cardiothorac Surg* 2007;**32**:362-9.
3. Cerfolio RJ. Chylothorax after esophagogastrectomy. *Thorac Surg Clin* 2006;**16**:49-52.
4. Doerr CH, Allen MS, Nichols 3rd FC, et al. Etiology of chylothorax in 203 patients. *Mayo Clin Proc* 2005;**80**:867-70.
5. Jimenez CA, Mhatre AD, Martinez CH, et al. Use of an indwelling pleural catheter for the management of recurrent chylothorax in patients with cancer. *Chest* 2007;**132**:1584-90.
6. Malthaner RA, Inculet RI, et al. The thoracic duct and chylothorax. In: Pearson FG, Deslauries J, Ginsberg RJ, editors. *Thoracic surgery*. 2nd ed. Churchill Livingstone; 2005. p. 1128-240.
7. Chan EH, Russell JL, Williams WG, et al. Postoperative chylothorax after carsdiothoracic surgery in children. *Ann Thorac Surg* 2005;**80**:1864-70.
8. Grobbelaar M, Andronikou S, Goussard P, et al. Chylothorax as a complication of pulmonary tuberculosis in children. *Pediatr Radiol* 2008;**38**:224-6.
9. Ryu JH, Doerr CH, Fisher SD, et al. Chylothorax in lymphangioleiomyomatosis. *Chest* 2003;**123**:623-7.
10. Le Pimpec-Barthes F, D'Attellis N, Assouad J, et al. Chylous leak after cervical mediastinoscopy. *J Thorac Cardiovasc Surg* 2003;**126**:1199-200.
11. Riquet M, Le Pimpec-Barthes F, Souilamas R, Hidden G. Thoracic duct tributaries from intrathoracic organs. *Ann Thorac Surg* 2002;**73**:892-8.
12. Platis IE, Nwogu CE. Chylothorax. *Thorac Surg Clin* 2006;**16**:209-14.
13. Merigliano S, Molena D, Ruol A, et al. Chylothorax complicating esophagectomy for cancer: a plea for early thoracic duct ligation. *J Thorac Cardiovasc Surg* 2000;**119**:453-7.
14. De Meester TR. The pleura. In: Sabinston DC, Spencer EC, editors. *Surgery of the chest*, 4th ed. Philadelphia: WB Saunders; 1983.
15. Sersar SI. Chylothorax revisited. *Eur J Cardiothorac Surg* 2008;**33**:1159.
16. Miller JI. Anatomy of the thoracic duct and chylothorax. In: Shields TW, editor. *General thoracic surgery*. Philadelphia: Lippincott Williams and Wilkins; 1999. p. 747-56.
17. Le Pimpec-Barthes F, D'Attellis N, Dujon A, et al. Chylothorax complicating pulmonary resection. *Ann Thorac Surg* 2002;**73**:1714-9.
18. Agrawal V, Doelken P, Sahn SA. Seat belt-induced chylothorax: a cause of idiopathic chylothorax? *Chest* 2007;**132**:690-2.
19. Agrawal V, Doelken P, Sahn SA. Pleural fluid analysis in chylous pleural effusion. *Chest* 2008;**133**:1436-41.
20. Cortina RM, Johnstone DW. Benign pleural diseases. Chylothorax. In: Sabinston DC, Spencer EC, editors. *Surgery of the chest*, 7th ed. Philadelphia: WB Saunders; 2005. p. 443-45.

21. Ammori JB, Pickens A, Chang AC, et al. Tension chylothorax. *Ann Thorac Surg* 2006;**82**:729-30.
22. Boffa DJ, Sands MJ, Rice TW, et al. A critical evaluation of a percutaneous diagnostic and treatment strategy for chylothorax after thoracic surgery. *Eur J Cardiothorac Surg* 2008;**33**:435-9.
23. Vallieres E, Shamji FM, Todd JR. Postpneumonectomy chylothorax. *Ann Thorac Surg* 1993;**55**:1006-8.
24. Cope C. Diagnosis and treatment of postoperative chyle leakage via percutaneous transabdominal catheterization of the cisterna chyli: a preliminary study. *J Vasc Interv Radiol* 1998;**9**:727-34.
25. Thompson KJ, Kernstine KH, Grannis FW, et al. Treatment of chylothorax by robotic thoracic duct ligation. *Ann Thorac Surg* 2008;**85**:334-6.
26. Sarsam MA, Rahman AN, Deiraniya AK. Postpneumonectomy chylothorax. *Ann Thorac Surg* 1994;**57**:689-90.
27. Hoffer EK, Bloch RD, Mulligan RS, et al. Treatment of chylothorax: percutaneous catheterization and embolization of the thoracic duct. *AJR Am J Roentgenol* 2001;**176**:1040-2.
28. Gupta D, Ross K, Piacentino V, et al. Use of LeVeen pleuroperitoneal shunt for refractory high-volume chylothorax. *Ann Thorac Surg* 2004;**78**:e9-12.
29. Rizzardi G, Loy M, Marulli G, et al. Persistent chylothorax in lymphangioleiomyomatosis treated by intrapleural instillation of povidone. *Eur J Cardiothorac Surg* 2008; **34**: 214-5.

CHAPTER 30
Malignant Pleural and Pericardial Effusions
Sai Yendamuri, Chukwumere Nwogu, and Todd L. Demmy

Malignant Pleural Effusions
  Etiology
  Demographics
  Evaluation
    Historical and Physical Findings
    Imaging
    Diagnostic Procedures

Treatment
  Drainage-Based Methods of Malignant Effusion Control
  Sclerosis-Based Pleural Effusion Management
  Radiopharmaceutical Interventions
  Mechanical Abrasion or Laser

  Pleurectomy
  Prognosis and Future Trends
Malignant Pericardial Effusions
  Mechanism
  Evaluation
  Treatment

MALIGNANT PLEURAL EFFUSIONS

Pleural effusions are common clinical problems, occurring in more than 1 million patients each year.[1] In some settings, up to 22% of these effusions are caused by malignant disease, and more than 100,000 malignant effusions require treatment annually.[2] Affected patients with advanced neoplastic disease experience considerable morbidity as a result of these pleural fluid collections.

Etiology

Pleural effusion results from a derangement in the normal physiology such that there is increased production of pleural fluid or a change in its composition with or without a reduction in the absorption of the fluid. It can result from primary or secondary tumors of the pleura, with seeding of the intrapleural space and lymphatic obstruction. Free-floating tumor cells block absorption of fluid and produce vasoactive substances that in turn increase the production and block the absorption of intrapleural protein and fluid.

Demographics

In adults, 95% of neoplastic pleural effusions arise from a metastatic source, with lung and breast carcinoma accounting for 75% of all cases.[3] Other common causes are lymphoma, gastric cancer, and ovarian cancer. About half of patients with breast cancer develop a pleural effusion within their lifetime, compared with one fourth of patients with lung cancer and one third of patients with lymphoma.

Most pediatric effusions, on the other hand, are benign. If malignant, lymphomas or leukemias account for half, with the remainder a mix of tumors such as neuroblastoma, Wilms' tumor, and germ cell neoplasms.[4]

Adenocarcinomas whose primary is unknown constitute a distinct entity in patients in whom the source of the pleural malignancy is never found. They are associated with exposure to environmental tobacco smoke.[5]

Evaluation
Historical and Physical Findings

Patients with malignant pleural effusions are typically symptomatic and complain of dyspnea, cough, or chest pain. The discomfort is often independent of respiration and is aggravated by activity. With invasive pleural metastases, the affected nerve roots may radiate pain. As with pericardial effusions, rapid fluid accumulation amplifies the symptoms. For at least 10% of patients, the dyspnea is multifactorial and does not improve after drainage. Physical findings indicating pleural effusion are decreased tactile fremitus and dullness to percussion on examination of the posterior chest, accompanied by decreased breath sounds. As the effusion increases in size, there may be hyperresonance on percussion immediately above the fluid level because of compression and overdistention of the lung. Bronchial breath sounds may be prominent. As effusions become massive, tracheal deviations from mediastinal shifts are detectable. Malignant pleural effusions rarely cause hemodynamic compromise from tension hydrothorax.

Imaging

Early chest radiographic evidence of pleural effusion is costodiaphragmatic sulcus blunting caused by as little as 125 to 250 mL of fluid, depending on the quality of the film (Fig. 30-1). Occasionally, a spurlike shadow projects into the fissure. Massive effusions are uncommon, but when they occur they are likely to be malignant. In patients in whom the finding is uncertain, a decubitus film might show shifting of the fluid. Effusions wider than 10 mm by decubitus film are often successfully tapped.[6]

There are specific computed tomography (CT) criteria for pleural effusions. In general, loculation, pleural thickening, pleural nodules, and extrapleural fat of increased density are present only in exudative effusions. Multiple pleural nodules and nodular pleural thickening are generally limited to effusions of malignant etiology (Fig. 30-2). Pleural thickening greater than 1 cm is also a reliable criterion.[7] Magnetic resonance imaging (MRI) has limited use,

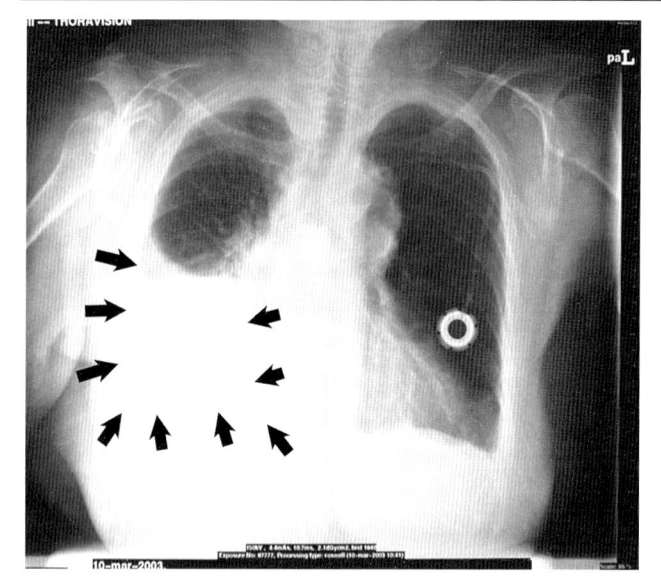

Figure 30–1
Chest roentgenogram showing large right pleural effusion (outlined by *arrows*).

but it may be slightly more useful for certain pleural tumors such as lipoma, and it also can be helpful in determining the extent of invasion for mesothelioma.[8] Thoracic ultrasound shows the optimal site for diagnostic thoracentesis of a small pleural effusion. It also helps select ideal entry points for thoracoscopes or pleural biopsy instruments by avoiding adhesions.[9]

Positron emission tomography (PET)-CT scans may detect early pleural metastases before other imaging tests. If nuclear imaging reveals pleural activity and pleural fluid is scant, diagnostic thoracoscopy is necessary to exclude pleural disease if this staging is relevant. Limited data suggest a high degree of diagnostic accuracy in differentiating benign from malignant pleural effusions.[10] Figure 30-3 is an image of a PET scan demonstrating a malignant pleural effusion.

Diagnostic Procedures

Thoracentesis

The diagnosis of pleural effusion is confirmed by thoracentesis. Withdrawing only a small portion of pleural fluid is indicated occasionally when full lung reexpansion is unlikely, or as a prelude to a definitive drainage procedure. It is usually preferable to attempt drainage of as much pleural fluid as possible (Fig. 30-4).

Several commercial kits facilitate drainage by allowing insertion of soft catheters with side holes to completely evacuate the fluid. The catheters can be readjusted during drainage if the lung temporarily occludes the holes. Needles with retractable blunt obturators (e.g., a Turkel needle) also prevent lung injury during pleural entry. Physical examination can guide a pleural tap. On the other hand, in more complex situations, ultrasound or other imaging can optimize needle or chest tube placement for effusion drainage (Fig. 30-5). This is particularly useful for a small effusion or pleural disease of long duration complicated by lung consolidation or pleural loculation. Marking of the area of "deepest" fluid is useful, but it is important to perform the thoracentesis with the patient

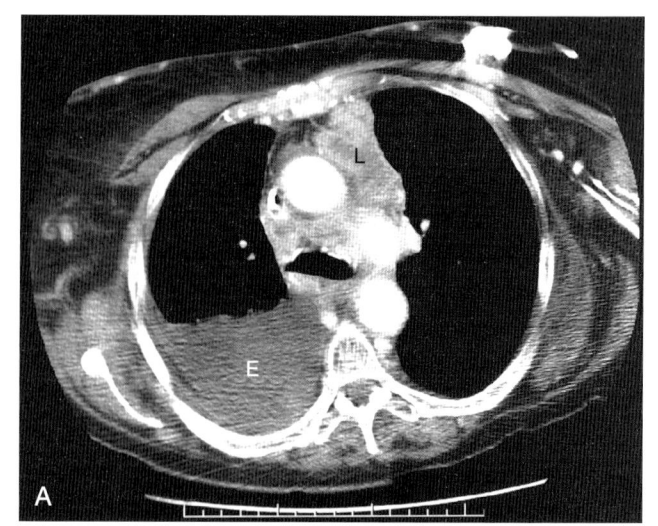

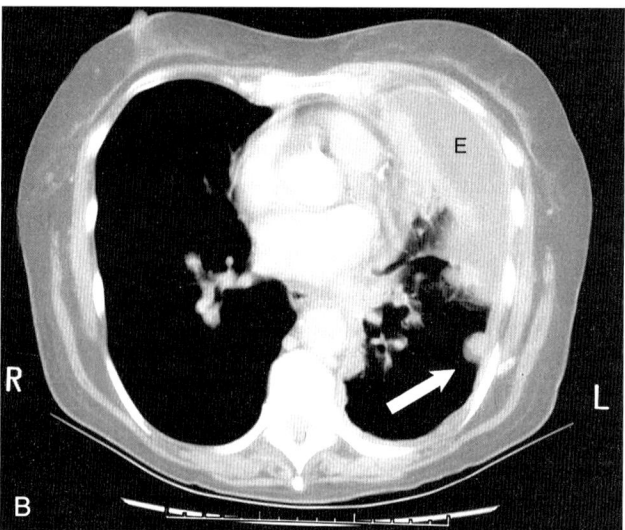

Figure 30–2
A, CT images of a malignant pleural effusion. **B,** Chest CT from a patient with breast carcinoma, with recurrent basilar left pleural effusion after partially successful chemical sclerosis. The image shows partial pleurodesis, pleural thickening, and a pleural nodule *(arrow)* at the level of the mid thorax. E, effusion; L, prevascular lymphadenopathy.

in the same position as during the imaging. Attempts to completely aspirate chronic effusions should be undertaken carefully. High vacuum applied to the pleural space, by either syringe aspiration or vacuum bottle, is sufficient to rupture alveoli and cause a complicated hydropneumothorax.

Standard Chemistry and Cell Counts

Practically all malignant pleural effusions are exudates. Laboratory criteria to establish exudative effusions are based on absolute values or on ratios to systemic parameters. One of the most useful sets of criteria to classify effusions as exudative was described by Light, as follows[1,11]:

- Ratio of pleural fluid to serum total protein, greater than 0.5
- Ratio of pleural fluid to serum lactate dehydrogenase (LDH), greater than 0.6

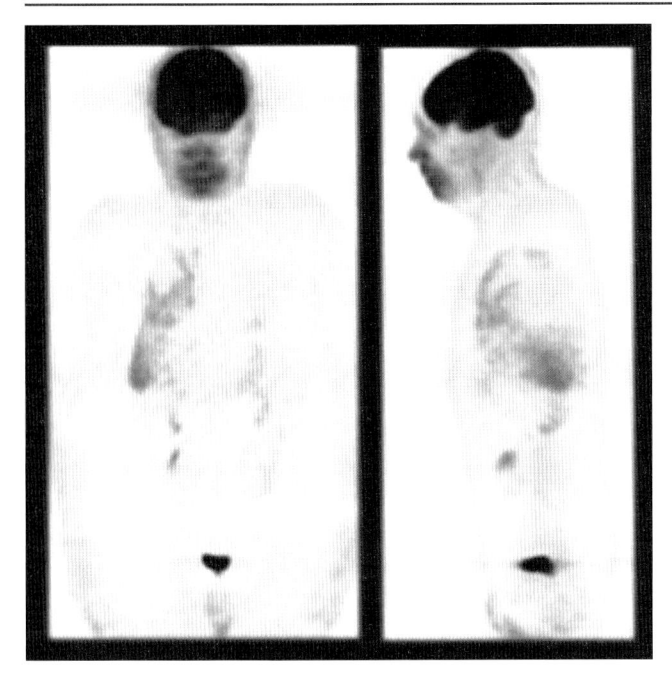

Figure 30-3
PET scan demonstrating uptake on the side of the chest with the malignant pleural effusion.

- Value of LDH in pleural fluid, greater than 200 U/L, or greater than two thirds of the laboratory's upper limit of normal for serum

Low glucose (<60 mg/dL) and pH (<7.20) levels are common in malignant pleural effusions.[12] This is attributed to glucose use and acid production by the malignant cells, leukocytes within the pleural fluid, and increased pleural membrane metabolism. Investigators have also implicated abnormal pleural membrane transport of glucose, carbon dioxide, or hydrogen ion.[13] Pleural fluid amylase is elevated in about 10% of patients with malignant pleural effusions even without pancreas gland disease.[14] In fact, the most common cause of an amylase-rich pleural effusion is neoplasm.[15] The cell count can also indicate malignancy. For some investigators, bloody fluid is the strongest positive predictor of malignant effusion. Fluid viscosity has also been studied as a diagnostic test.[16]

Immunocytochemistry and Special Chemistry
Many investigators focused their explorations on staining patterns of cells obtained from pleural fluid to confirm malignancy and, if present, to correctly classify its origin. Unfortunately, markers are not yet sufficiently sensitive and specific, but they generally show twice the positivity of cytology alone (80% versus 40%).[17] These tests are usually used after standard cytologic screening and also are combined with cytogenetic and other miscellaneous tests to establish a diagnosis. A more complete list is displayed in Table 30-1.

Some of these markers, such as p53, predict a worse prognosis for malignant effusions that are p53 negative.[18] Another marker, Ki-67, is associated with a worse prognosis when its labeling index is low.[19]

Vascular endothelial growth factor (VEGF) has been found to be a useful discriminator for malignant effusions.[20] Other special chemistry values (Table 30-2) are occasionally useful to categorize malignancy. The sensitivities and specificities vary by specific cell type.

Cytogenetics

DNA testing by flow cytometry or chromosome analysis predicts the likelihood of malignancy. The evidence of a marker chromosome, aneuploidy, or a hyperdiploid state suggests malignancy. Aneuploid samples (by flow cytometry) yield predictive values as high as 96%.[21] No aneuploidy was found in benign reactive effusions in one series.[22] Telomerase activity occurs in 92% of malignant effusions and in only 6% of benign effusions (with a specificity of 94.2%).[23]

Pleural Cytology and Biopsy

Cytologic evaluations with standard staining (Papanicolaou smears) can sometimes confirm malignant pleural effusions. In very unusual cases (0.5%), the results are falsely positive.[24] In cytologic specimen reviews, lung adenocarcinoma is the most frequent diagnosis. Breast cancer effusion specimens have a higher cytology diagnostic yield (about 78%) than lung or other tissue primaries.[25] The sensitivity of cytologic evaluation of pleural fluid is frequently greater than that of undirected pleural biopsy.

When standard pleural effusion cytology is nondiagnostic, pleural needle biopsy occasionally provides some additional useful diagnostic information (48% in one series).[26] However, whether pleural biopsy adds much beyond fluid cytologic evaluation in cases of suspected malignancy is controversial. In another series, only 7% of patients had a diagnosis made by pleural biopsy when the cytology result was negative.[27] For difficult cases, cytology combined with needle biopsy results are inferior to those obtained by video-assisted thoracic surgery (VATS) (41% versus 97%).[28] In several series, a typical yield of undirected pleural needle biopsy of 50% to 60% was far inferior to the yield of biopsies obtained by VATS. A directed VATS approach in these cases achieves greater than 90% success.[29] With idiopathic effusions (20% in some series), uncertainty is reduced to 4% by using thoracoscopy. The complication rate from thoracoscopic biopsy is low, with mortality rates less than 1% and complication rates less than 10%.[30] Figure 30-6 shows thoracoscopic images that confirmed pleural malignancy.

A technique variation that might shift results of "blind" biopsy toward those of directed biopsy is the use of a pleural brush to increase the cytologic yield. In one series, this technique was positive in 90% of the cases, as opposed to 67% with the routine cytologic aspirate and 58% with biopsy.[31] Thoracotomy to perform pleural biopsy is unusual given the successful directed methods such as VATS.

When patients remain without a definitive diagnosis after VATS or thoracotomy, about one third demonstrate a cause (typically lymphoma or mesothelioma) months to years later.[32] For patients with massive malignant effusions of uncertain etiology, fiberoptic bronchoscopy may establish lung cancer. When effusions are mild to moderate and without associated symptoms, the chance of finding a neoplasm is not great enough to warrant bronchoscopy.

In summary, clinical information, conventional cytology results, immunocytochemistry, flow cytometry, and special

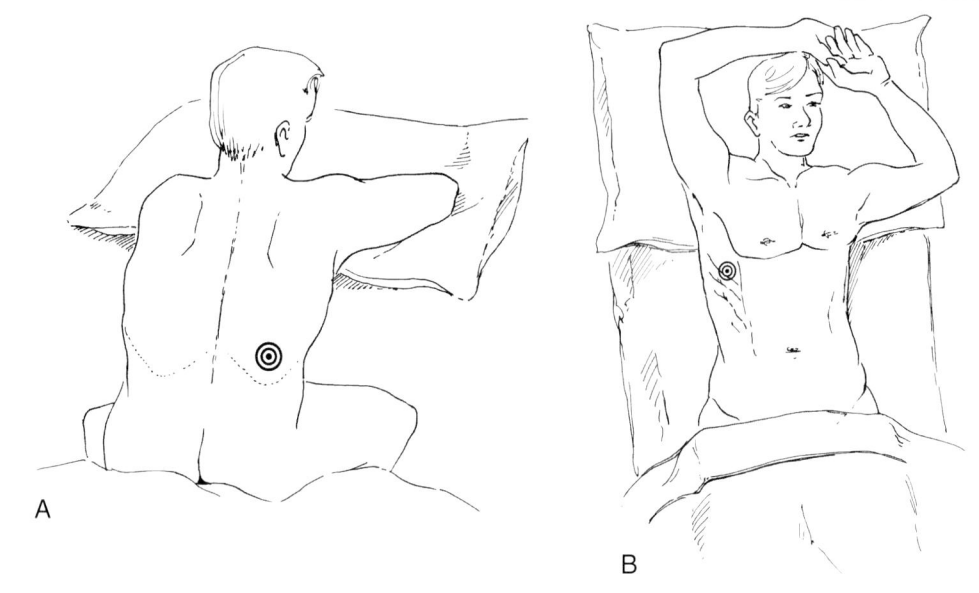

Figure 30–4
A, Common patient position for insertion of a thoracentesis needle or catheter. Posterior approach allows access to the most dependent (posterior pleural) sulcus to allow maximal drainage of nonloculated fluid. **B,** Lateral patient positioning for thoracentesis or chest tube placement is also useful for effusions with large lateral collections of fluid. The patient's arm is abducted and flexed over his head to facilitate access to the lateral chest.

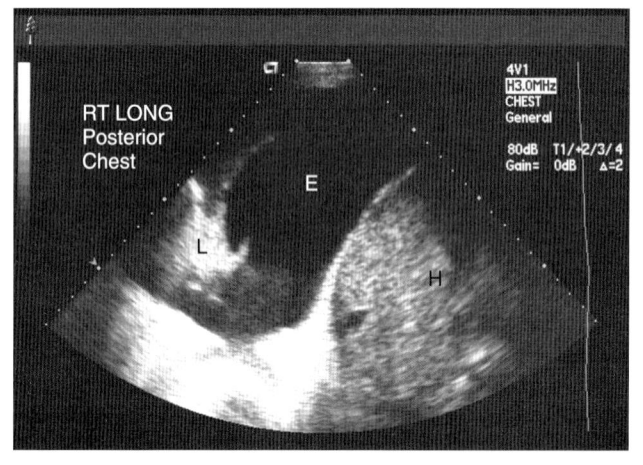

Figure 30–5
Ultrasound of right lateral chest to facilitate safe pleural access. E, effusion; H, hepatic lobe; L, lung.

chemistry test results must all be integrated to yield the most accurate diagnosis.

Treatment

The optimal treatment for malignant pleural effusion is controversial. Multiple technologies control malignant pleural effusions successfully. The best selection for a patient is guided by factors including the individual's frailty and the prognosis of the primary malignancy. The need for additional pleural tissue or directed biopsy as well as concomitant diagnostic or therapeutic procedures requiring general anesthesia also guide the choice and timing of pleural interventions.

The anatomic state of the affected thorax is important. For example, a pleural effusion of relatively rapid onset typically yields full expansion of the lung and pleural coaptation after the effusion is evacuated. On the other hand, malignant disease of long duration can prevent full lung expansion because of visceral pleural restriction, endobronchial obstruction, parenchymal fibrosis, or replacement by tumor. To help with planning, good diagnostic imaging is important.

Treatment options can be classified into those that rely on drainage alone and those that also obliterate the pleural space. As there is an inflammatory response associated with most pleural effusions, persistent and complete pleural drainage may also achieve pleural fusion. Evidence shows cytokine activation from repetitive pleural draining that supports this view.[33] Although pleural malignancy traditionally means surgical incurability, some investigational multidisciplinary methods include operations, for selected cases, that are designed to improve the chance for cure.[34]

A chest radiograph after pleurodesis commonly shows multiloculated fluid collections suggestive of empyema. This finding probably represents regions of rapid pleural adhesion formation with intervening accumulations of inflammatory fluid. This is probably an acceptable variation of treatment effect rather than a nonuniform distribution of sclerosing agent.

This imaging appearance generally resolves by 1 to 3 weeks. However, to avoid this phenomenon, some physicians wait for effusion drainage rates to decrease before instilling pleurodesis agents. It is not clear whether this practice is necessary. Long delays before pleurodesis may simply reduce the thoracic cavity area to which the instilled agent is exposed when significant pleural adhesions have already occurred in regions remote to the drainage catheter. Occasionally, significant pleural thickening or even fibrothoraxes occur as long-term sequelae of pleurodesis. The use of thoracic ultrasound (see Fig. 30-5) can guide the optimal drainage site for small pleural effusions or the optimal point of entry of a thoracoscope to avoid adhesions.

Table 30–1
Immunocytochemistry Markers

Authors (ref)	Test	Benign mesothelial	MM	General CA	Adeno CA	Other CA	Other type
Cascinu et al (17)	AFP	—	—	—	—	++	Hepatocellular
Mason et al (80)	Alcian blue	0	—	+	—	—	—
Betta et al (81)	B 72.3	—	0	++	+++	—	—
Cascinu et al (17)	B-19	—	—	—	—	++	Prostate
Loy et al (82)	BCA-225	0	—	++	—	—	—
Stoop et al (83)	BER-EP4	0	0	++/+++	+++	—	—
Cascinu et al (17)	CA 15.3	—	—	—	—	+++	Breast
Cascinu et al (17)	CA 19.9	—	—	—	—	+++	Gastric
Ko et al (84)	Calretinin	+++	+++	0	0	—	—
Berner et al (85)	CD44 s	+++	—	- - -	—	—	—
Berner et al (85)	CD44 v 3-10	0	—	+	—	—	—
Ko et al (84) Shi et al (86)	CEA	0	—	+++	++	+++	Colorectal
Davidson et al (87)	Desmin	++/+++	0	0	—	—	—
Kitazume et al (88)	E-cadherin	0	+++	++	—	—	—
Stoop et al (83)	EMA	- -	+++	+++	—	—	—
Burstein et al (89)	GLUT1	- -	—	+++	—	—	—
Mason et al (80)	Keratin	0	+++	+	+++	—	—
Saleh et al (90)	Ki67	0	—	++	—	—	—
Bailey et al (91)	Leu M1	—	—	—	++	—	—
Cascinu et al (17)	MCA	—	—	—	—	++	Breast
Stoop et al (83)	MCA-b-12	- -	—	+++	—	—	—
Morgan et al (92)	MOC31	0	—	—	+++	—	—
Ko et al (84)	Mucicarmine	—	—	—	+	—	—
Cibas et al (93)	Mucin	0	—	—	+	—	—
Davidson et al (87)	N-cadherin	++	+++	+	—	—	—
Mayall et al (94)	p53	0	—	+	—	—	—
Rosen-Levin et al (95)	UEA	0	—	+	—	—	—
Giarnieri et al (96)	TIMP-2	—	—	—	++	—	—
Mocanu et al (97)	Vimentin	—	—	+	—	—	—
Mocanu et al (97)	CKMNF 116	—	—	+	—	—	—

Scale: +++, >90%; ++, 60% to 90%; +, 30% to 59%; - -, 10% to 29%; 0, <10%; —, not studied.
Adeno CA, specific diagnosis of adenocarcinoma; AFP, α-fetoprotein; CKMNF, cytokeratin; EMA, epithelial membrane antigen; general CA, nonspecific diagnosis of cancer; GLUT1, glucose transport protein 1; MM, malignant mesothelioma; other CA, specific diagnosis of certain histologic type; TIMP, tissue inhibitor of metalloproteinase; UEA, Ulex europaeus agglutinin.

Table 30-2
Sensitivity and Specificity of Various Pleural Fluid Assays in the Detection of Malignancy

Authors (ref)	Assay	Sensitivity (%)	Specificity (%)
Alatas et al (98)	Ca 19-9	36	83
Alatas et al (98)	Ca 15.3	80–95	93
Alatas et al (98)	CEA	52	77
Alatas et al (98)	CYFRA 21-1	91	90
Okamoto et al (99)	MUC-1 >0.126	64	95.7
Okamoto et al (99)	MUC-5AC >0.028	72	98
Imecik et al (100)	Sialic acid >0.075	68	77
Lee et al (101)	Sialyl EA	64	95
Odeh et al (102)	TNF ratio	84	90
Alatas et al (98)	TSA	80	67
Gu et al (103)	CYFRA 21-1	47	92
Li et al (104)	MN/CA9	89	91
Roncella et al (105)	Mammaglobin by RT-PCR	82	75

CEA, carcinoembryonic antigen; CYFRA, cytokeratin fragment; RT-PCR, reverse transcriptase–polymerase chain reaction; sialyl EA, sialyl embryonic antigen; TNF, tumor necrosis factor; TSA, total sialic acid.

Drainage-Based Methods of Malignant Effusion Control

Serial thoracenteses appropriately control malignant pleural effusions for some patients. This option is not effective for durable effusion control but provides temporary symptomatic relief in patients with extremely poor prognoses. Thoracentesis is also ideal when an alternative therapy could cause a major reduction in the patient's effusion. For example, a lymphoma-related effusion may resolve with chemotherapy.

Occasionally, thoracentesis creates a hydropneumothorax because of poor compliance or entrapment of the ipsilateral lung. If the pneumothorax and dyspnea symptoms remain stable and noncompelling, tube thoracostomy should be avoided, because pleural coaptation and effective ventilation from that lung are unlikely. Fluid will replace the airspace over time.

Small Catheter Drainage

Implantation of a long-term pleural catheter or percutaneous medium-durability pleural catheter placement for continuous or intermittent drainage is better than serial percutaneous aspirations.[35] The former methods have the advantage of obtaining nearly complete removal of the pleural fluid in the same way that a tube thoracostomy evacuates the pleural space. Needle aspiration rarely evacuates the fluid completely and rarely maintains the lung expansion long enough for a spontaneous pleurodesis to occur. Even without introduction of any pleural sclerosing agents, pleurodesis occurs simply by maintaining pleural apposition, in a select group of patients, probably from the underlying inflammation and invasive effects of the neoplasms.[36]

Using a small silicone catheter (Fig. 30-7) with a valve that allows drainage only when connected to a closed system, similar success at 30 days has been achieved in prospective randomized clinical trials compared with traditional pleurodesis methods.

This research was replicated with the Tenckhoff catheter, the pigtail catheter, and the Pleuracan device (Braun, Helsungen, Germany).[37-39] All controlled dyspnea in greater than 90% of the cases. Intermittent pleural drainage is an attractive option for patients in whom pleurodesis is less likely to occur because of the inability of the visceral pleura to touch the parietal pleura. As a consequence, this method is often used to complement sclerosis options at various centers.

Pleuroperitoneal Shunting

Another way to drain pleural fluid is to pump it into the peritoneal cavity using a device similar to that crafted to drain ascites into the venous system. This generally requires the patient to pump the shunt chamber (Fig. 30-8) at least 20 times four times a day, and perhaps more because of the need to overcome the negative intrapleural pressure.[40]

More than 80% of patients reported excellent results with this method, and it avoided the need for an appliance to traverse the skin. Unfortunately with this technology, at least 10% to 20% of patients occlude their shunt, possibly requiring revision; furthermore, determination of shunt obstruction may be difficult.[41] Otherwise, this shunt appears to have survival rates similar to talc pleurodesis. Also, there is generally no evidence that peritoneal deposits result from this pleuroperitoneal shunting technology. The decision to use the shunt can be made during thoracoscopy when pleural coaptation seems unlikely, and it is relatively easy to place the shunt while the patient is under general anesthesia.

Sclerosis-Based Pleural Effusion Management

Generally, accelerating the process of pleurodesis (which might not occur by prolonged drainage alone) is done by accessing the pleural space, draining the majority of fluid, and then inserting a substance that increases the inflammatory response and thus causes intense adhesions within the pleural envelope. There is controversy regarding how pleural fluid characteristics affect the success of pleurodesis and the prognosis of the patient. For example, investigators have shown that a low pleural-fluid glucose level (<60 mg/dL), low pH (<7.2), low performance status (Karnofsky, <70), massive effusion, and high pleural LDH levels (>600 U/L) are associated with a higher rate of failure of pleurodesis efforts. These values also predict positive pleural fluid cytology and a poor overall prognosis.[42] However, other investigators have contradicted this finding, particularly with respect to pleural effusion pH.[43] Experimental evidence supports the concept that the inflammatory effect needed by some sclerosant agents is inhibited by steroid use, thereby decreasing the effectiveness of the pleurodesis.[44]

Rolling the patient into different positions after instilling the desired sclerosant is another common practice. This is unnecessary in patients with normal pleural spaces in whom aqueous sclerosing agents were used. Rapid intrapleural dispersion occurs in just one position, as demonstrated by radiopharmaceutical

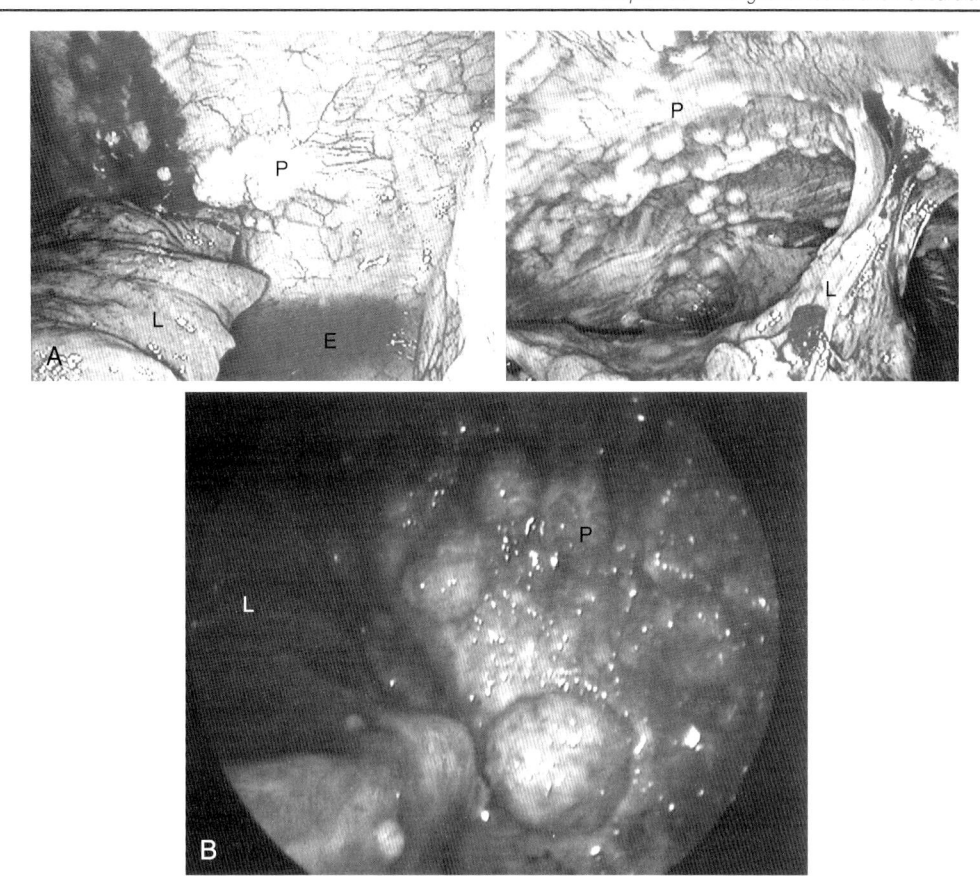

Figure 30–6
A, Lung carcinoma. Parietal and visceral pleural implants with residual effusion are displayed. B, Malignant mesothelioma with the "grape cluster" pattern characteristic of pleural tumors. E, residual effusion; L, lung; P, parietal pleura.

labeling and nuclear medicine imaging.[45] However, when the pleural space is loculated or there is lack of full lung expansion, rolling may be useful. Sclerosing agents that are particulate, such as talc slurry, might achieve more uniform distribution with rolling, but this has been disproved in one small prospective trial.[46] There also appear to be variations in the practice of pleurodesis, with some surgeons more likely to use an agent such as talc and other physicians using bleomycin or cycline-based drugs.

Another controversy is whether the pleural effusion drainage rate should be tapered before instilling a sclerosing agent. This may be unnecessary. Investigators have shown that daily drainage of pleural fluid is much less useful than achieving full pleural fluid evacuation and lung reexpansion on chest roentgenogram.[47] Pleurodesis appears to have only a minor adverse effect on respiratory function, although the studies on this are limited.[48] Finally, whereas sclerosis of the pleural cavity is generally practiced on inpatients, there have been successful outpatient pleurodesis programs.

When pleurodesis is performed as an inpatient procedure, a chest tube is generally inserted. Chest tube size can vary quite significantly, ranging from 20 to 36 French depending on local institution or operator preference. Also, there appears to be considerable variation in sedation practices, with occasional episodes of high discomfort and anxiety during the insertion of chest tubes. Generally, patients with dyspnea from malignant effusions are not decompensated enough to require emergent placement without analgesic preparation. It is appropriate to establish a protocol to standardize intravenous sedative and analgesic use to supplement the generous use of local anesthetics during placement of a chest catheter.

The trend has been toward the use of smaller catheters, both for drainage and for the pleurodesis of malignant pleural effusions. In a prospective randomized study, a 12-Fr catheter was comparable to a standard large bore tube.[49] This has been reproduced in other studies of both inpatient and outpatient pleurodeses using the pigtail, Cystofix (Braun), Elecath (Electro-Catheter, Rahway, NJ), and PleurX (Denver Biomedical, Golden, CO) catheters and talc, doxycycline, or similar traditional sclerosing agents.[50-53]

Techniques of Sclerosis

Chemical Sclerosis: Talc

Talc was first used to create pleural adhesions for tuberculosis management in 1935, and about 25 years later it started to become popular for controlling malignant effusions. Generally, there are two ways to administer talc into the pleural space. One is as an insufflated powder (talc poudrage) and the other is by instillation of a particulate slurry, with the talc in a liquid vehicle. The amount of talc needed depends somewhat on the route of delivery and its preparation method. A fine powder from an aerosol gives a broader distribution with less mass (Fig. 30-9). Nevertheless, reported successful talc pleurodeses generally used between 2 and 8 g, with 5 g being the most common amount used in multicenter trials.

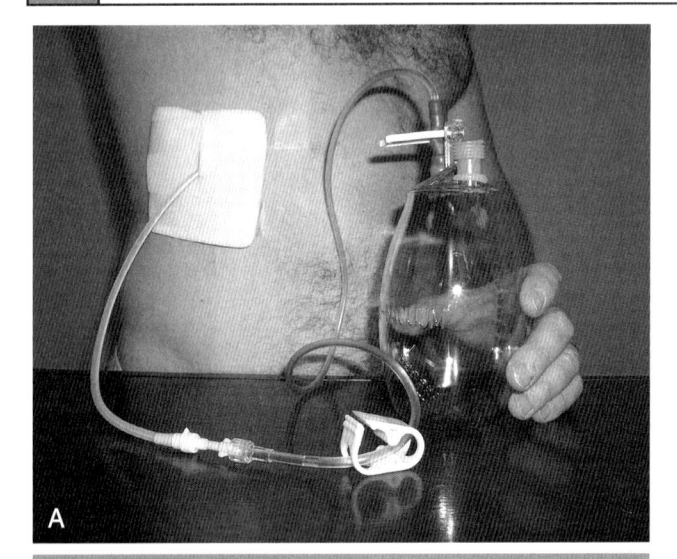

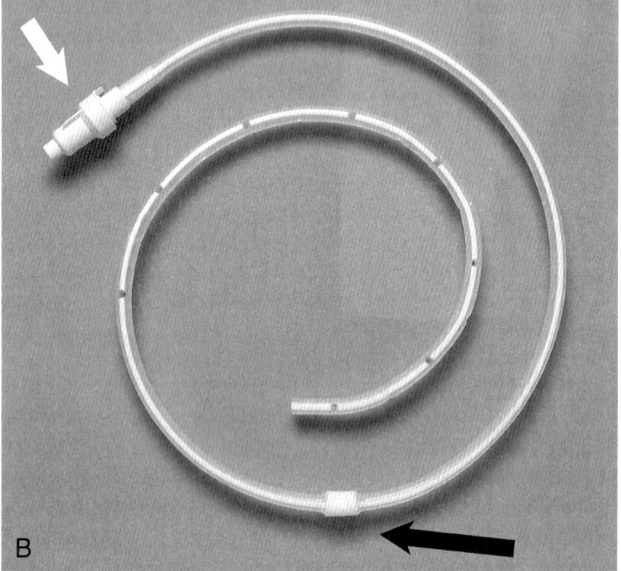

Figure 30–7
PleurX catheter. **A,** Patient connects the PleurX catheter to a bottle for self-drainage. **B,** Close-up of the catheter. Note the one-way valve mechanism *(white arrow)* and Velcro cuff to provide tissue ingrowth *(black arrow).*

Talc is often prepared preferentially in the hospital pharmacy rather than purchasing it from expensive vendors. In fact, the cost compares favorably to that of most other non-talc agents. The use of purified but not sterilized talc may be acceptable because a tremendous inflammatory response kills contaminating bacteria. Nevertheless, the standard, preferred practice is to use talc sterilized by prolonged baking at 132° C, ethylene oxide (talc in cellophane pouches), or gamma radiation.

Although the use of talc for malignant pleural effusions has become widespread and is considered a safe clinical practice, some patients sustain an inflammatory response severe enough to cause respiratory insufficiency. Such responses have prompted experts to question its use. Clinical outcomes and laboratory testing show that talc administered intrapleurally is distributed systemically. The extent to which this might adversely affect somewhat frail patients who receive it is unclear. Some investigators have suggested that the patient should be observed as an inpatient for up to 72 hours after its use. Talc causes mesothelial denuding and an exudative neutrophilic pleural effusion similar to what occurs with the tetracycline class of sclerosis agents. For some tumors, such as mesothelioma, talc may also induce apoptosis. On the other hand, if there is evidence of increased fibrinolytic activity, talc sclerosis may be less effective.

Table 30-3 lists good to excellent results of talc and other sclerosing agents in noncomparative studies. Hospital stays ranged from 3.3 to 4.4 days.[54,55] Associated mortality ranges from 0% to 16%, and morbidity ranges between 4% and 14%, with respiratory complications being most frequent.

When talc is tested in comparison trials (Table 30-4), the results are not as favorable, but they are still equal or superior to other common pleurodesis methods. Most of these investigations had good risk profiles, with complication rates less than 20% and mortality attributed to the talc in less than 5% of cases. Are the differences in results dependent on the patient population or, perhaps, the method or composition of the talcum powder used? Particle size might affect dissemination. At least 20% of the patients who receive talc pleurodesis have a transient interstitial haziness on the chest roentgenogram, possibly from endothelial damage and capillary leak syndrome. Talc slurry was thought to be the more risky delivery route because there seemed to be more anecdotal reports of respiratory distress associated with this method. Some investigators feel that intraoperative talc leads to shorter hospital stays. A prospective study has not shown a significant difference between talc poudrage administered in the operating room and a bedside talc slurry, based on a 30-day prevention of an effusion.[56]

Chemical Sclerosis: Cycline Drugs and Bleomycin
Multiple doses of chemical sclerosants have been studied, but a single dose is probably sufficient. A dose of tetracycline at 20 mg/kg was found to be effective as a single-dose regimen.[57] Now doxycycline is available to be used instead of tetracycline. A dose of doxycycline is typically 500 mg in 100 to 200 mL of 0.9% saline. Despite interest in using cycline-based drugs intraoperatively, there is no advantage to this over bedside use. Results of noncomparison studies with tetracycline and bleomycin are presented in Table 30-3.

In general, bleomycin shows results that are equivalent to or just less than that of talc pleurodesis. Pleural effusions from breast tumors may respond better than those of other tumors to this drug. Many times these drugs work better in the pleural cavity than in other spaces such as the peritoneal cavity.

Pain and transient fever occurred in 5% of patients after intrapleural instillation in a multicenter trial.[58] In other studies, the fever occurred in as many as 60% of patients. It is unclear why there is so much variation in the reporting of these side effects.

Reports of pleural sclerosis need to be compared on the basis of how long the treatment effects are followed. One investigation found 70% long-term success with combined bleomycin and tetracycline. Although a favorable early result was found with either agent, after 4 months the single-sclerosant success fell to 25% to 35%.[59]

Other Sclerosing Compounds
Other compounds that have been used include three doses of *Corynebacterium parvum* (7 mg in 20 mL saline). Good results (76% to 100% success) were obtained, but this preparation is

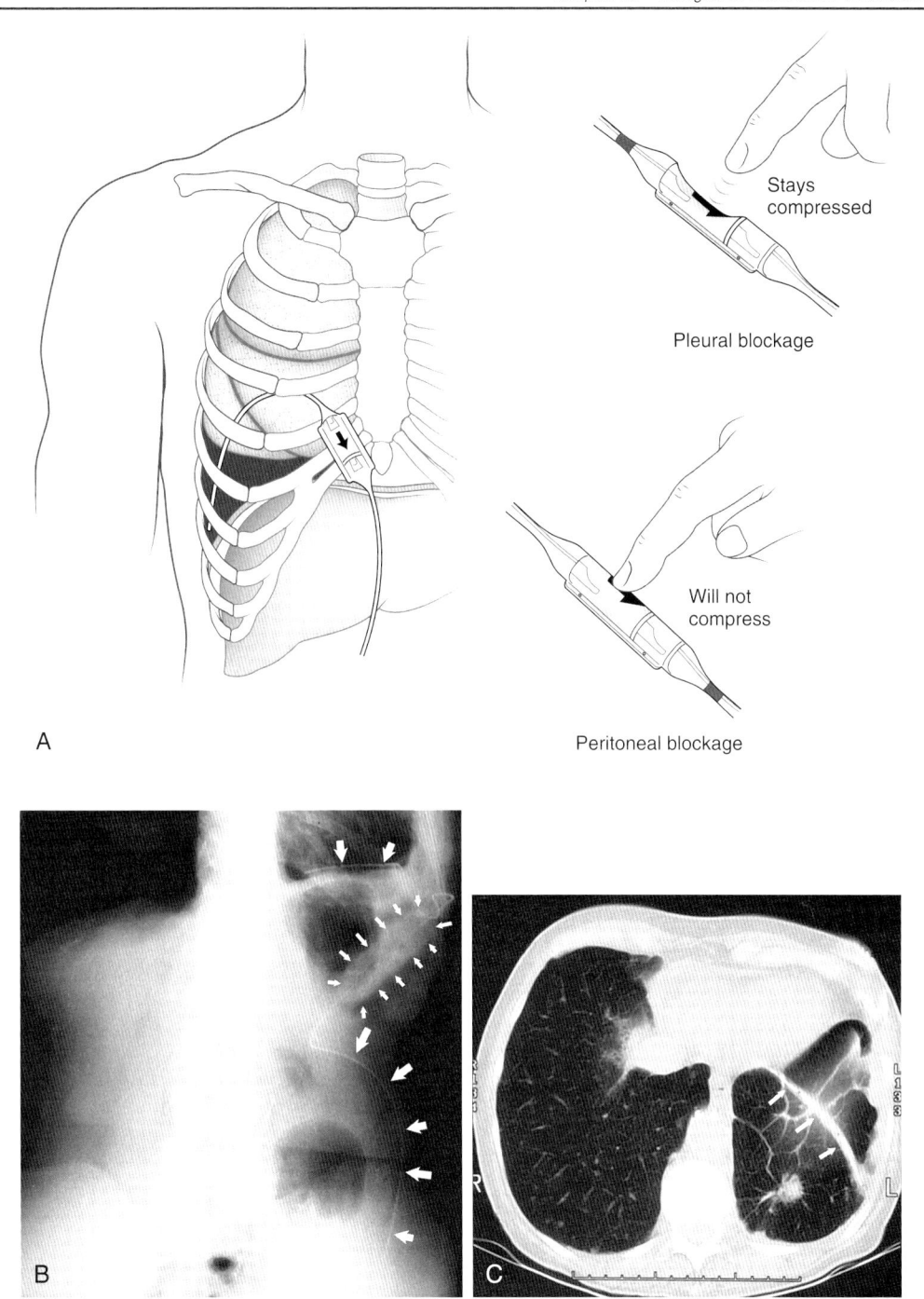

Figure 30–8
Pleuroperitoneal shunt. **A,** Diagram of shunt position and demonstration of proximal and distal obstruction. **B,** Roentgenogram of lower chest and upper abdomen, showing left pleuroperitoneal shunt *(arrows)* with chamber placed at costal margin for patient self-pumping. **C,** CT image showing the catheter *(arrows)* in the left lower pleural space. This image was obtained 3 months after shunt placement in the patient whose left lower lung loculated pleural breast carcinoma effusion as depicted in Figure 30-2B. *(**A,** reprinted with permission from Ponn RB, Blancaflor J, D'Agostino RS, Kiernan ME, Toole AL, Stern H. Pleuroperitoneal shunting for intractable pleural effusions. Ann Thorac Surg 1991;**51**:605-09.)*

no longer available. Intrapleural interferon-β (5 to 20 million units in a maximum of three administrations) can be used alone, but the remission rate is only 30%. However, when interferon-β is cycled with immunotherapy such as interleukin-2 and interferon-α, the response rate is 56% to 70%.[60] Tumor necrosis factor therapy yielded an 87% recurrence-free rate at 4 weeks with a dose of 0.15 to 1.01 mg per patient. These patients have flulike symptoms including fevers, chills, and fatigue.[61]

Radiopharmaceutical Interventions

Radioactive compounds used in the 1960s to control malignant pleural effusions have seen renewed interest. The most commonly used is an intracavitary colloidal suspension of chromic phosphate (as phosphorus 32) because of its safer emission and faster decay than elements such as gold. Results of these therapies in uncontrolled trials have success rates

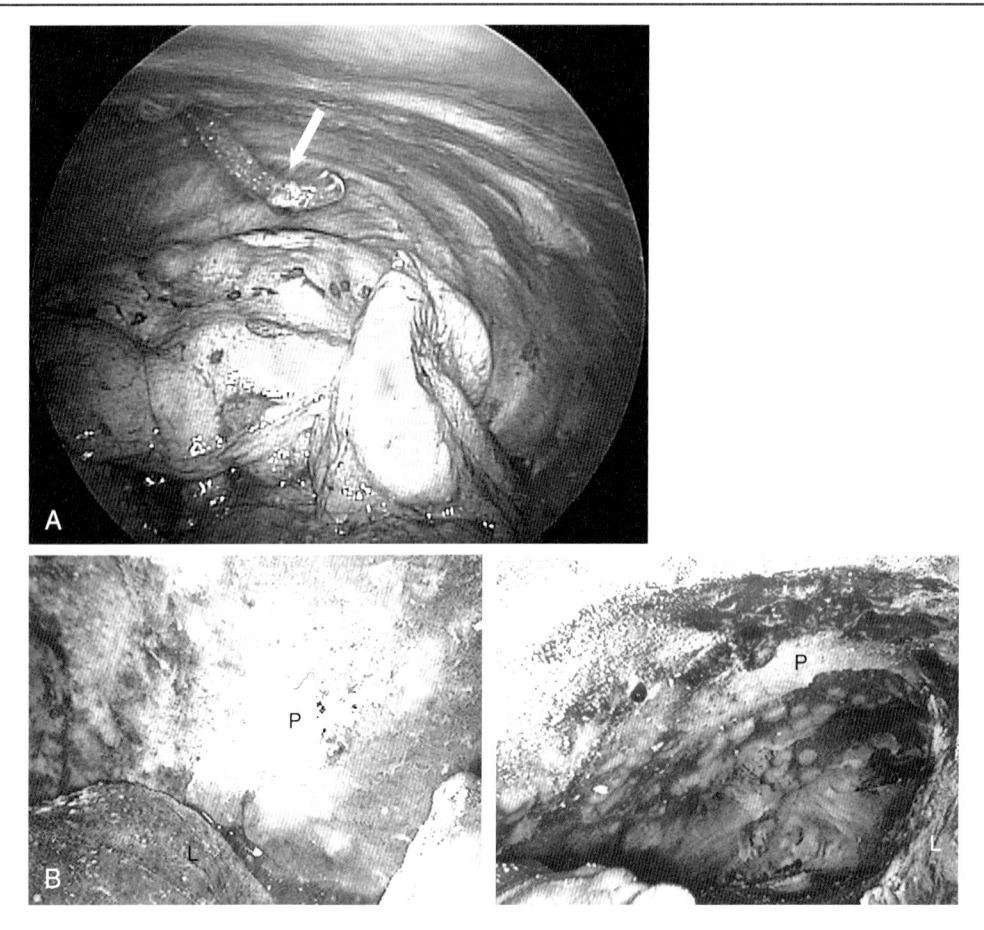

Figure 30-9
A, Thoracoscopic image of left chest before insufflation of talc. Angled tip on insufflation catheter *(arrow)* facilitates directing talc to desired areas.
B, Thoracoscopic image of left chest after insufflation of talc (see same patient, Fig. 30-6A). L, lung; P, parietal pleura.

of 75%.[62] Generally, a dose of 6 to 12 mCi of ^{32}P is used, which has a half-life of 14 days. A therapeutic thoracentesis (maximal drainage) is performed using a temporary thoracentesis catheter. The catheter remains in place until the ^{32}P is instilled. It is then flushed and withdrawn. The patient may then be discharged if there are no complications.

Mechanical Abrasion or Laser

Limited data exist regarding the use of mechanical pleural abrasion, which is effective for other types of pleural disease such as pneumothorax. Experimental data suggest that the mechanical abrasions are no better than the addition of sclerosing agents such as talc. Similarly, laser treatments that cause superficial pleural destruction are probably not as effective in controlling effusions. Both are inhibited by their erratic effects in poorly healing neoplastic tissue.

Pleurectomy

The poor prognosis of patients with malignant pleural effusions limits enthusiasm for aggressive surgical options because the anticipated recovery times for such operations are long. However, the less invasive therapies previously noted are used when thoracoscopy is needed to achieve a directed diagnosis of the pleural pathology. The use of thoracotomy and pleurectomy is accepted more for patients with malignant mesothelioma in whom early mortality from distant metastases is less certain. The mortality rate for pleurectomy of malignant effusions is at least 12%. Patients were considered for pleurectomy if they failed traditional drainage and sclerosing agents, had trapped lung, or were found to have malignant pleural effusion or pleural carcinomatosis at the time of thoracotomy. Nevertheless, these indications are now unusual outside a clinical trial. To reduce the concern regarding thoracotomy morbidity, there is interest in VATS pleurectomy (Fig. 30-10), which results in a shorter hospital stay and good effusion control. In a series of VATS pleurectomy patients,[63] there was 0% mortality with a mean hospital stay of 5 days. Six of 19 patients died within 12 months, and of the remaining 13 patients, two developed recurrent effusions.

Prognosis and Future Trends

The prognoses of patients with malignant effusions vary between clinical settings because of population variations in primary cell types and regional preferences in therapies used to control effusions. A survival rate of less than 50% at 6 months and 6% at 2 years after diagnosis of malignant pleural effusion is typical. Also, in these series, patients treated only with serial thoracenteses rather than with more aggressive therapies had a particularly short survival time (13.9 weeks).

Table 30-3
Results of Nonrandomized Trials of Common Sclerosant Agents

Authors (ref)	Patients (N)	Success(%)
Talc poudrage		
Daniel et al (106)	40	90
Aelony et al (107)	42	82
Ohri et al (108)	44	96
Danby et al (55)	24	88
Sanchez-Armengol et al (109)	125	87
Talc slurry		
Kennedy et al (110)	58	81
Weissberg et al (111)	34	100
Bleomycin		
Paladine et al (112)	38	63
Bitran et al (113)	20	85
Patz et al (114)	19	79
Cyclines		
Gravelyn et al (115)	25	59
Robinson et al (116)	21	88
Pulsiripunya et al (117)	31	100
Iodopovidone		
Olivares-Torres et al (118)	52	96
Vincristine		
Vidyasagar et al (119)	15	80

Most investigators defined 100% success as complete or near complete control of pleural effusion at 30 days after pleurodesis based on both symptom control and repeat chest imaging. One month was a common interval for assessing this endpoint, but some investigators used longer follow-up. Studies also differed on whether early deaths were considered failures.

A longer interval between the initial diagnosis of cancer and the malignant effusion favors survival.

Breast cancer effusions are associated with a more favorable survival rate, particularly when they are estrogen receptor positive and when the cells show a morula clustering pattern on cytology. The presence of large clusters of malignant cells on smears also indicates a favorable prognosis in other cancers. Unfavorable tumor surface receptors adversely affects prognosis (see Immunocytochemistry and Special Chemistry, earlier).

Like the treatment modality, patient performance status is an important factor in determining optimal therapy. A Karnovsky score of 70 or greater is preferred before using more aggressive surgical approaches, such as thoracoscopy, that require general anesthesia. This yields a survival rate that makes the morbidity risk tenable.

Occasionally, trivial malignant effusions are discovered with minimal nearby carcinomatous pleuritis at the time of thoracotomy. If there is only a small primary tumor with little other regional disease, it may be reasonable to perform a formal resection if the patient has good pulmonary function. Although it is controversial, the logic for this follows from the finding that occult pleural metastases treated by pleural washings may have prolonged survival times or cure. Accordingly, for patients with minimal pleural carcinomatosis and N0 tumors, there is interest in performing ablative therapy of the pleura to improve cancer control and possibly effect a cure. One of these treatments has been the use of pleurectomy and intracavitary photodynamic therapy, which has been used for mesothelioma but may also be useful for primary lung cancer. A phase II trial on carefully selected patients demonstrated a 6-month local control rate of 73% and a median survival of 21.7 months.[64]

Hyperthermic chemotherapy and hypotonic chemotherapy are other investigational methods of effusion control. Thrombolytic agents may disrupt loculations for more effective pleurodesis or pleural ablation therapy. Transfer of lymphokine-activated killer cells improved tumor lysis in the pleural space, and intrapleural interleukin-2 induced a 37% complete response in a multi-institutional study, possibly by restoring the immunocompetence of effusion-associated lymphocytes.[65] Cytokine therapy, particularly the use of VEGF receptor blocker, can control some pleural effusions. In related research, indomethacin blocks prostanoid-related endothelial cell permeability associated with adenocarcinomas. Intrapleural steroids, however, do not slow effusion reaccumulation. Finally, intrapleural chemotherapy can control effusions without pleurodesis, per se. Mixed results have occurred with agents such as cisplatin and cytarabine, and doxorubicin. One of the trials by the Lung Cancer Study Group showed a combined complete and partial response at 3 weeks of 49%.[66] More commonly, systemic chemotherapy is administered; recent drugs used for this include gemcitabine and vinorelbine or combinations with cisplatin, ifosfamide, and irinotecan. Zoledronic acid and hypotonic cisplatin therapy have also been proposed.[67,68] Gene therapy is yet another strategy being explored.[69] Fusing of a sclerosing agent with a chemotherapy agent is another novel approach. A bioadhesion compound linked to Adriamycin achieved a 100% response rate in 14 patients in a preliminary report.[70] Similarly, microspheres can deliver chemotherapy intrapleurally at high local concentrations with low systemic exposures.

Diverse managements are offered for patients with malignant pleural effusions. Optimally, the treatment selected conforms to the patient's anticipated survival based on histologic diagnosis, molecular markers, extent of metastatic disease, and other comorbidities. There is some promising research but the overall prognoses for these patients are limited, and therapy should focus on improving quality of life. Accordingly, less invasive, outpatient, small catheter–based methods are replacing inpatient therapies such as the traditional chest tube with talc slurry. A randomized multicenter trial (Cancer and Leukemia Group B, 30102) was designed to compare chest tube talc slurry (inpatient) with intermittent small-catheter drainage (outpatient); however, accrual was limited because potential subjects wanted to choose the hospital or ambulatory setting. Because malignant pleural effusions are a common problem with considerable morbidity, further study is

Table 30-4
Results of Randomized Trials of Common Sclerosant Agents

Authors (ref)	Patients (N)	Talc slurry (% success)	Talc poudrage (% success)	Bleomycin (% success)	Tetracycline (% success)	Other agent in study (% success)
Dresler et al (56)	469*	70	79	—	—	—
Noppen et al (120)	26	79	—	75	—	—
Fentiman et al (121)	33	92	—	—	48	—
Hartman et al (122)	134	—	97	64	33	—
Diacon et al (123)	36	—	87	59	—	—
Martinez-Moragon et al (124)	62	—	—	64	52	—
Ruckdeschel et al (125)	115*	—	—	64	33	—
Emad et al (59)	60	—	—	25	35	Bleomycin + Tetracycline (70)
Patz et al (126)	106	—	—	72	—	Doxycycline (79)
Ostrowski et al (127)	38	—	—	74	—	*Corynebacterium parvum* (43)
Hillerdal et al (128)	32	—	—	13	—	*Corynebacterium parvum* (65)
Koldsland et al (129)	40	—	—	50	—	Mepacrine (80)
Loutsidis et al (130)	40	—	—	—	80	Methenamine (60)
Yoshida et al (131)	102	—	—	69	—	OK-432 (76) Cisplatin +etoposide (71)
Sartori et al (132)	160	—	—	85	—	Interferon alpha-2b (62)
Paschoalini Mda et al (133)	49	84	—	—	—	Silver nitrate (96)
Bayly et al (134)	18	—	—	—	83	Quinacrine (90)

Most investigators defined 100% success as complete or near complete control of pleural effusion at 30 days after pleurodesis based on symptom control and repeat chest imaging.
*Multicenter trial.

necessary to help determine the optimal therapy for patients so afflicted.

MALIGNANT PERICARDIAL EFFUSIONS

Pericardial effusion is the most common cardiac problem in malignant disease and is reported in 1.5% to 21% of cancer cases.[71] Moreover, nonmalignant conditions also cause pericardial effusions in cancer patients. Examples of these conditions are infection, uremia, congestive heart failure, hypothyroidism, and autoimmune disorders. Radiation, drug-induced pericarditis, and idiopathic pericarditis are also known etiologies.

The most common malignancies to involve the pericardium are metastatic lung cancer, breast cancer, leukemia, lymphoma, and melanoma. Less commonly, secondary involvement by esophageal, gastric, colonic, oral, nasopharyngeal, prostate, and ovarian carcinoma may be seen. Primary tumors of the pericardium are rare and include mesothelioma, fibrosarcoma, angiosarcoma, and malignant teratoma.

Mechanism

Tumors spread to the pericardium by direct extension or by hematogenous or lymphatic spread. Mediastinal lymph node metastases subsequently spread to the pericardium by retrograde movement through lymphatic vessels draining that space. Increased visceral pericardial fluid production may result from direct involvement of the serosal surface by tumor. When tumor obstructs flow, lymphatic and venous hydrostatic pressure increase, which also drives pericardial fluid accumulation. The hemodynamic consequences of a pericardial effusion depend on its rate of accumulation and the pericardial compliance. Thus, large effusions may cause no symptoms if they accumulate slowly in compliant pericardia.

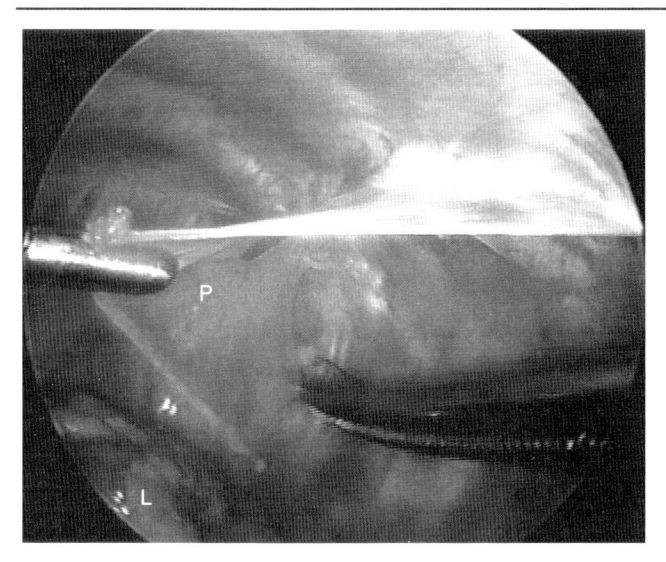

Figure 30–10
Video-assisted thoracic surgery (VATS) image of parietal pleurectomy. L, lung; P, parietal pleural peel.

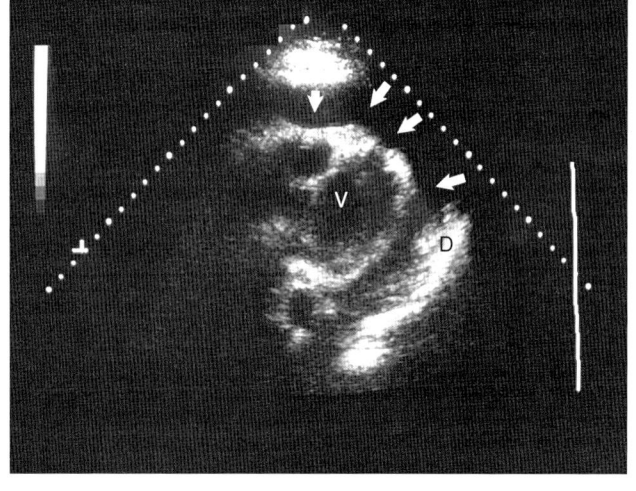

Figure 30–11
Echocardiogram shows a large pericardial effusion (arrows). D, diaphragmatic pericardium; V, ventricle.

Evaluation

Frequent symptoms of pericardial effusion are dyspnea, cough, and chest pain. Physical examination findings are tachycardia, pulsus paradoxus, diminished heart sounds, elevated jugular venous pressure, hypotension, and pulsus alternans. Pericardial tamponade is more likely after rapid accumulations of fluid and may be the initial clinical presentation of malignant pericardial disease.

The chest radiograph often shows an enlarged cardiac silhouette, mediastinal widening, or hilar densities. A normal plain radiograph does not exclude pericardial effusion. Electrocardiographic effusion criteria are sinus tachycardia, nonspecific ST segment or T wave changes, low-voltage tracings, and electrical alternans.

Echocardiography is very sensitive in detecting the presence of fluid and has become the most useful diagnostic tool for pericardial effusions (Fig. 30-11). Right atrial or right ventricular compression with decreased left ventricular dimension and failure of the inferior vena cava to collapse on deep inspiration suggests hemodynamic compromise. The echocardiogram also safely guides pericardiocentesis and drainage catheter placement. Cytologic examination of the pericardial fluid may then be performed. The rate of positive cytologic results reported in published series ranges from 57% to 100% among patients with malignancy.[72] Both CT and MRI provide excellent anatomic detail of the pericardial space but do not yield physiologic or functional information (Fig. 30-12).

Treatment

Various therapeutic interventions are used, alone or in combination, for patients with malignant pericardial effusions. One of the main objectives is obliteration of any potential pericardial space by fusion of the epicardium and pericardium. Patient performance status, medical comorbidities, malignant disease stage, prognosis, and response to other cancer treatments influence selections of these options.

Pericardiocentesis provides immediate decompression of the pericardial space and is usually performed with

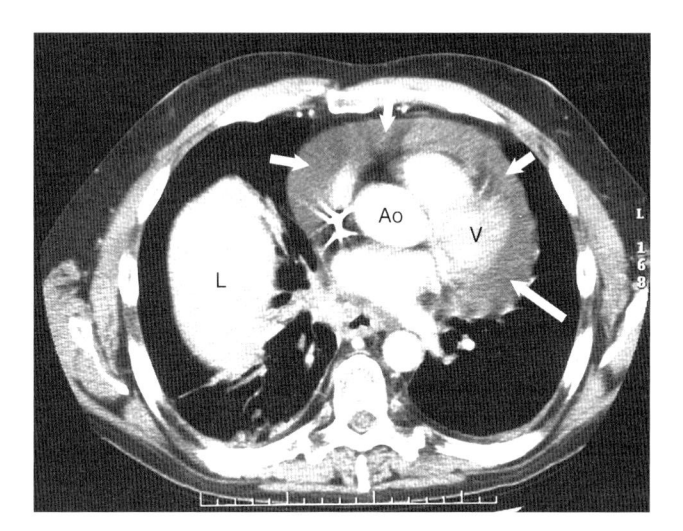

Figure 30–12
CT scan shows moderately large pericardial effusion (arrows). Ao, aortic root; L, liver dome (left); V, atrioventricular junction with adjacent pulmonary outflow tract.

echocardiographic guidance. Hemodynamic impairment is thereby relieved but can recur quickly. Recurrence rates as high as 25% have been reported.[73] Thus, this procedure is seldom durable enough except for terminal patients with brief anticipated survival.

A pericardial catheter left in place at the time of pericardiocentesis allows drainage of additional fluid with or without administration of a sclerosing agent. Numerous investigators induced pericardial sclerosis to avoid pericardial effusion recurrences and described their small series. Some of the agents administered were thiotepa, tetracyclines, OK-432 (an immunomodulator), bleomycin, aclarubicin, mitomycin C, 5-fluorouracil, and radiocolloids such as ^{32}P and gold 154 (^{154}Au). Doxycycline may produce intense pain and, like bleomycin, may produce a febrile response in a significant number of patients. Thiotepa does not cause pain and rarely evokes a fever.

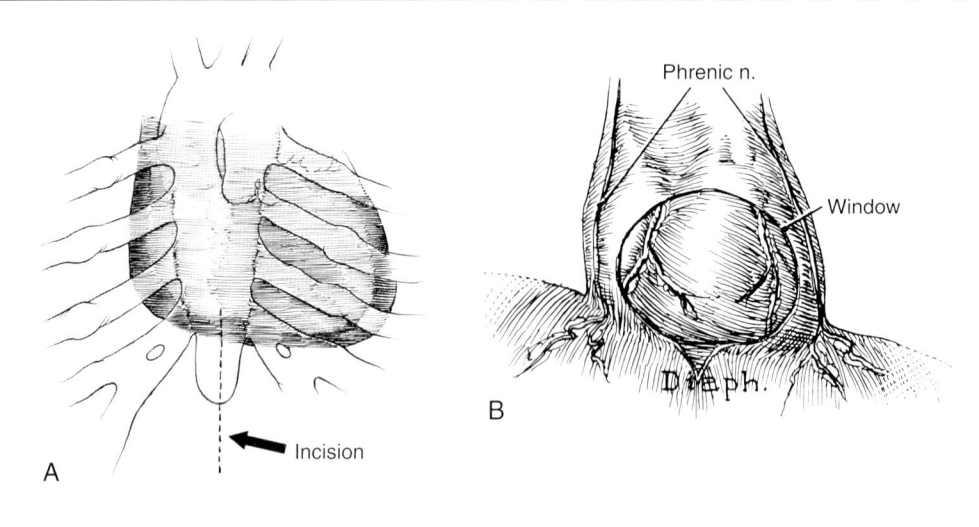

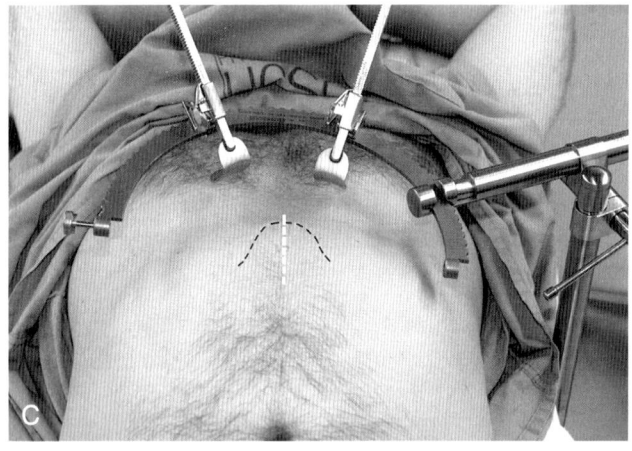

Figure 30–13
A, Relation of pericardial effusion to planned subxiphoid incision (arrow). **B,** Large pericardial window has been resected. Exposure can be facilitated by partial excision of the subxiphoid cartilage. Drainage may be facilitated by placement of a drainage tube, opening of the pleural spaces, or a preperitoneal space, depending on the surgeon's preference. **C,** Exposure can also be facilitated by a self-retaining retractor system that lifts the costal margin and sternum anteriorly to expose the superior pericardium. The model is positioned under partial ring of the Bookwalter retractor system with small blades that provide this traction. *Black dashed line* shows the costal margin and the *white dashed line* overlies the xiphoid process, denoting the planned incision. *(**A** and **B** reprinted with permission from Ravitch M, Steichen F: Atlas of general thoracic surgery. Philadelphia: WB Saunders, 1988, p 175.)*

It is inexpensive and is the sclerosant of choice at some centers because of these advantages. Intrapericardial sclerosis has an overall success rate of greater than 80%.[73] A few centers use intrapericardial radiocolloids, but their popularity is limited, in part because of logistic problems related to their administration. Intrapericardial interferon has also been used.[74] It reportedly enhances cell-mediated cytotoxicity and has an antiproliferative effect. Colchicine has been described to have an inhibitory effect on leukocyte chemotaxis, and it decreases the production of interleukin-1 by monocytes.[75] These effects have been exploited in the use of colchicine in the treatment of refractory malignant pericardial effusion. The minimally invasive nature of these catheter-based interventions is attractive, and they reduce the recurrence rate after simple pericardiocentesis to an acceptable level. When less invasive options fail, surgical treatment can still be offered to appropriate candidates.

Of the surgical options, subxiphoid pericardial window creation has been used most extensively (Fig. 30-13). It can be performed using local or general anesthesia, it has low complication rates, and it does not require single-lung ventilation, as some thoracoscopic methods do. Success rates over 90% have been reported.[73] Much of the pericardial fluid drainage occurs in the space posterior to the ascending aorta through abundant carinal lymphatic systems. A relatively small tumor burden in that space (which is not visible to surgeons performing subxiphoid pericardial windows) may create an effusion. This accounts for some pericardial window specimens that do not show malignancy by pathologic review.

Thoracotomy may be used either to create a pleuropericardial window or to perform pericardiectomy. The latter has been claimed to have the greatest durability of all the surgical procedures. However, it does require general anesthesia and optimal single-lung ventilation, and it has relatively high morbidity and mortality rates.

Thoracoscopic approaches aim to provide the same quality of pericardial drainage without the morbidity of a thoracotomy.[76] This has been well tolerated in very ill patients but still requires single-lung ventilation and general anesthesia. When both pleural and pericardial effusions are present, a thoracoscopic approach should be favored (Fig. 30-14). This permits treatment

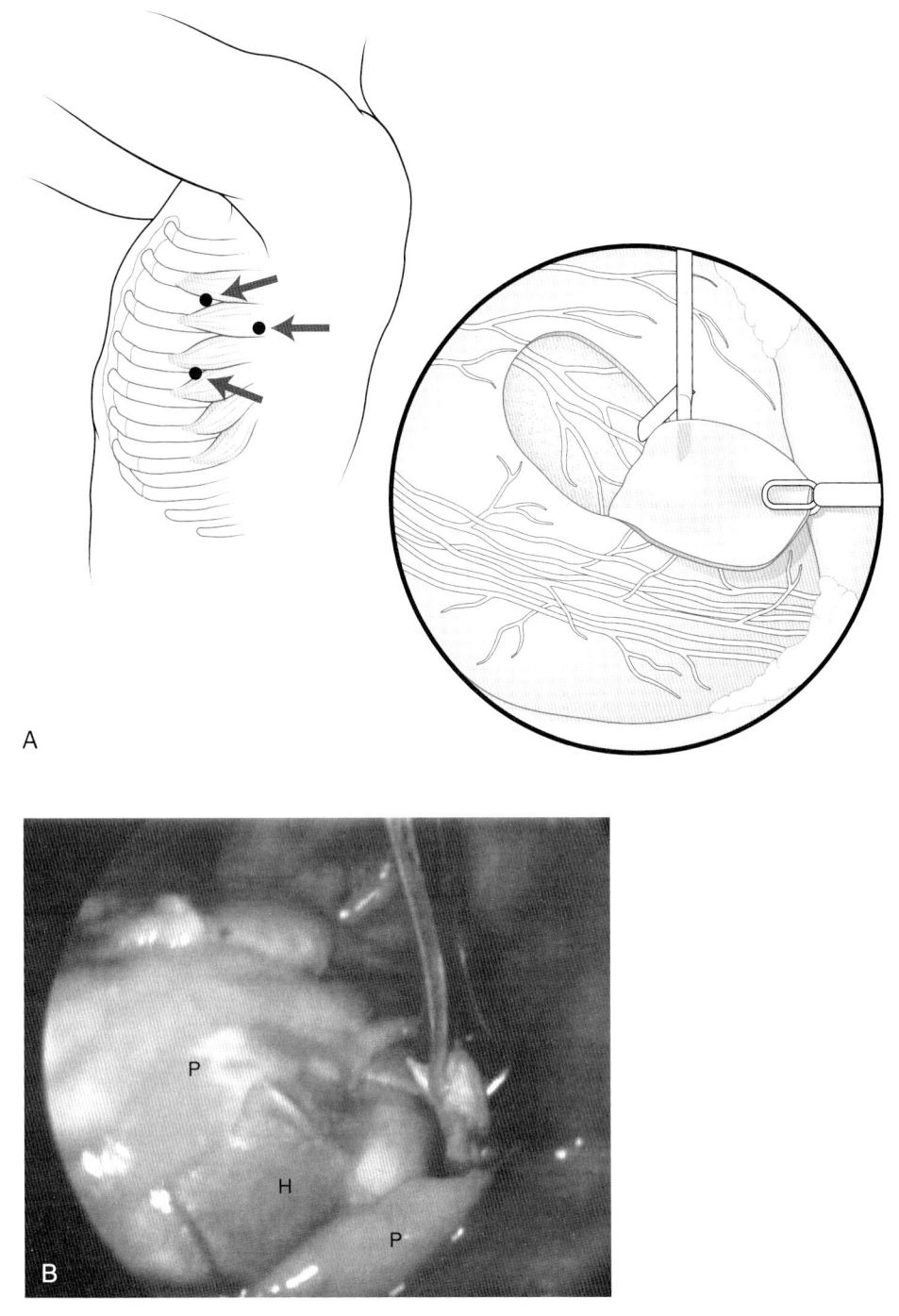

Figure 30–14
A, Trocar positions in preparation for creation of a thoracoscopic pericardial window. The patient is in the decubitus position. The camera trocar site lies most posteriorly, and the remaining two sites are used for manipulating instruments. B, Thoracoscopic image of left thoracoscopic pericardial window (left chest). H, heart; P, pericardium. (A *from Inderbitzi R, Furrer M, Leupi F. Pericardial biopsy and fenestration. Eur Heart J 1993;**14**:135-137.*)

of both spaces. Also, excellent visualization of the thoracic cavity permits directed biopsies in undiagnosed cases.

Creation of a pericardial window by percutaneous balloon has been reported.[77] Complications included pleural effusions requiring drainage, transient fever, and small pneumothoraces. This was performed with patients under local anesthesia and usually permitted prompt hospital discharge.

The Denver pleuroperitoneal shunt has also been used to drain pericardial effusions into the peritoneal space.[78] This requires only local anesthesia and a short hospital stay. The patients need to compress the pumping chamber of the device several times daily. Possible shortcomings of this drainage method include lack of patient cooperation and shunt thrombosis.

Passive pericardioperitoneal shunting can be accomplished using a video-assisted technique.[79] This essentially involves a laparoscopic approach that creates a generous transdiaphragmatic pericardial window without an external drain.

Chemotherapy and radiation therapy can be quite effective in patients with neoplasms that are sensitive to these modalities. They can be used in conjunction with direct pericardial interventions.

The choice of procedure depends on the patient. No modality is clearly superior to others, but the degree of invasiveness, the morbidity, and the cost vary widely. The clinical focus should be placed on providing rapid and durable relief from the effusion with the least possible morbidity.

REFERENCES

1. Light RW. Pleural diseases. *Dis Mon* 1992;**38**:261-331.
2. Lynch Jr TJ. Management of malignant pleural effusions. *Chest* 1993; **103**(4 Suppl):385S-389.
3. Fiocco M, Krasna MJ. The management of malignant pleural and pericardial effusions. *Hematol Oncol Clin North Am* 1997;**11**:253-65.
4. Hallman JR, Geisinger KR. Cytology of fluids from pleural, peritoneal and pericardial cavities in children: a comprehensive survey. *Acta Cytol* 1994;**38**:209-17.
5. Ang P, Tan EH, Leong SS, et al. Primary intrathoracic malignant effusion: a descriptive study. *Chest* 2001;**120**:50-4.
6. Light RW. Pleural effusions. *Med Clin North Am* 1977;**61**:1339-52.
7. Traill ZC, Davies RJ, Gleeson FV. Thoracic computed tomography in patients with suspected malignant pleural effusions. *Clin Radiol* 2001;**56**:193-6.
8. McLoud TC. CT and MR in pleural disease. *Clin Chest Med* 1998;**19**:261-76.
9. Macha HN, Reichle G, von Zwehl D, et al. The role of ultrasound assisted thoracoscopy in the diagnosis of pleural disease: clinical experience in 687 cases. *Eur J Cardiothorac Surg* 1993;**7**:19-22.
10. Toaff JS, Metser U, Gottfried M, et al. Differentiation between malignant and benign pleural effusion in patients with extra-pleural primary malignancies: assessment with positron emission tomography-computed tomography. *Invest Radiol* 2005;**40**:204-9.
11. Roth BJ, O'Meara TF, Cragun WH. The serum-effusion albumin gradient in the evaluation of pleural effusions. *Chest* 1990;**98**:546-9.
12. Rodriguez-Panadero F, Lopez MJ. Low glucose and pH levels in malignant pleural effusions: diagnostic significance and prognostic value in respect to pleurodesis. *Am Rev Respir Dis* 1989;**139**:663-7.
13. Good Jr JT, Taryle DA, Sahn SA. The pathogenesis of low glucose, low pH malignant effusions. *Am Rev Respir Dis* 1985;**131**:737-41.
14. Light RW, Murray JF, Nadel JA. Tumors of the pleura. Textbook of respiratory medicine. Philadelphia: WB Saunders; 1988. p. 1770-80.
15. Villena V, Pérez V, Pozo F, et al. Amylase levels in pleural effusions: a consecutive unselected series of 841 patients. *Chest* 2002;**121**:470-4.
16. Chang LC, Hua CC, Liu YC, et al. Pleural fluid viscosity may help identifying malignant pleural effusions. *Respirology* 2008;**13**:341-5.
17. Cascinu S, Del Ferro E, Barbanti I, et al. Tumor markers in the diagnosis of malignant serous effusions. *Am J Clin Oncol* 1997;**20**:247-50.
18. Lai CL, Tsai CM, Tsai TT, et al. Presence of serum anti-p53 antibodies is associated with pleural effusion and poor prognosis in lung cancer patients. *Clin Cancer Res* 1998;**4**:3025-30.
19. Shiba M, Kakizawa K, Kohno H, et al. Prognostic implication of Ki-67 immunostaining in treating subclinical pleural cancer found at thoracotomy in lung cancer patients. *Ann Thorac Surg* 2001;**71**:1765-71.
20. Momi H, Matsuyama W, Inoue K, et al. Vascular endothelial growth factor and proinflammatory cytokines in pleural effusions. *Respir Med* 2002;**96**:817-22.
21. Motherby H, Friedrichs N, Kube M, et al. Immunocytochemistry and DNA-image cytometry in diagnostic effusion cytology: II. Diagnostic accuracy in equivocal smears. *Anal Cell Pathol* 1999;**19**:59-66.
22. Motherby H, Kube M, Friedrichs N, et al. Immunocytochemistry and DNA-image cytometry in diagnostic effusion cytology: I. Prevalence of markers in tumour cell positive and negative smears. *Anal Cell Pathol* 1999;**19**:7-20.
23. Yang CT, Lee MH, Lan RS, Chen JK. Telomerase activity in pleural effusions: diagnostic significance. *J Clin Oncol* 1998;**16**:567-73.
24. Irani DR, Underwood RD, Johnson EH, Greenberg SD. Malignant pleural effusions: a clinical cytopathologic study. *Arch Intern Med* 1987;**147**:1133-6.
25. Sears D, Hajdu SI. The cytologic diagnosis of malignant neoplasms in pleural and peritoneal effusions. *Acta Cytol* 1987;**31**:85-97.
26. Von Hoff DD, LiVolsi V. Diagnostic reliability of needle biopsy of the parietal pleura: a review of 272 biopsies. *Am J Clin Pathol* 1975;**64**:200-3.
27. Prakash UB, Reiman HM. Comparison of needle biopsy with cytologic analysis for the evaluation of pleural effusion: analysis of 414 cases. *Mayo Clin Proc* 1985;**60**:158-64.
28. Boutin C, Rey F. Thoracoscopy in pleural malignant mesothelioma: a prospective study of 188 consecutive patients. Part 1: Diagnosis. *Cancer* 1993;**72**:389-93.
29. Page RD, Jeffrey RR, Donnelly RJ. Thoracoscopy: a review of 121 consecutive surgical procedures. *Ann Thorac Surg* 1989;**48**:66-8.
30. Allen MS, Deschamps C, Jones DM, et al. Video-assisted thoracic surgical procedures: the Mayo experience. *Mayo Clin Proc* 1996;**71**:351-9.
31. Emad A, Rezaian GR. Closed percutaneous pleural brushing: a new method for diagnosis of malignant pleural effusions. *Respir Med* 1998;**92**:659-63.
32. Ryan CJ, Rodgers RF, Unni KK, Hepper NG. The outcome of patients with pleural effusion of indeterminate cause at thoracotomy. *Mayo Clin Proc* 1981;**56**:145-9.
33. Chung CL, Chen YC, Chang SC. Effect of repeated thoracenteses on fluid characteristics, cytokines, and fibrinolytic activity in malignant pleural effusion. *Chest* 2003;**123**:1188-95.
34. Friedberg JS, Mick R, Stevenson JP, et al. Phase II trial of pleural photodynamic therapy and surgery for patients with non-small-cell lung cancer with pleural spread. *J Clin Oncol* 2004;**22**:2192-2201. Available from www.asco.org/asco/publications/abstract_print_view/0, 1148,_12-002326-00_18-002001-00_19-001303-00_29-00A,00. html.
35. Ohm C, Park D, Vogen M, et al. Use of an indwelling pleural catheter compared with thoracoscopic talc pleurodesis in the management of malignant pleural effusions. *Am Surg* 2003;**69**:198-202.
36. Putnam Jr JB, Light RW, Rodriguez RM, et al. A randomized comparison of indwelling pleural catheter and doxycycline pleurodesis in the management of malignant pleural effusions. *Cancer* 1999;**86**:1992-9.
37. Robinson RD, Fullerton DA, Albert JD, et al. Use of pleural Tenckhoff catheter to palliate malignant pleural effusion. *Ann Thorac Surg* 1994;**57**:286-8.
38. Sahin U, Unlü M, Akkaya A, Ornek Z. The value of small-bore catheter thoracostomy in the treatment of malignant pleural effusions. *Respiration* 2001;**68**:501-5.
39. Chen YM, Shih JF, Yang KY, et al. Usefulness of pig-tail catheter for palliative drainage of malignant pleural effusions in cancer patients. *Support Care Cancer* 2000;**8**:423-6.
40. Cimochowski GE, Joyner LR, Fardin R, et al. Pleuroperitoneal shunting for recalcitrant pleural effusions. *J Thorac Cardiovasc Surg* 1986;**92**:866-70.
41. Tzeng E, Ferguson MK. Predicting failure following shunting of pleural effusions. *Chest* 1990;**98**:890-3.
42. Sahn SA, Good Jr JT. Pleural fluid pH in malignant effusions: diagnostic, prognostic, and therapeutic implications. *Ann Intern Med* 1988;**108**:345-9.
43. Heffner JE, Nietert PJ, Barbieri C. Pleural fluid pH as a predictor of pleurodesis failure: analysis of primary data. *Chest* 2000;**117**:87-95.
44. Girardi LN, Ginsberg RJ, Burt ME. Pericardiocentesis and intrapericardial sclerosis: Effective therapy for malignant pericardial effusions. *Ann Thorac Surg* 1997;**64**:1422-7.
45. Lorch DG, Gordon L, Wooten S, et al. Effect of patient positioning on distribution of tetracycline in the pleural space during pleurodesis. *Chest* 1988;**93**:527-9.
46. Mager HJ, Maesen B, Verzijlbergen F, Schramel F. Distribution of talc suspension during treatment of malignant pleural effusion with talc pleurodesis. *Lung Cancer* 2002;**36**:77-81.
47. Villanueva AG, Gray Jr AW, Shahian DM, et al. Efficacy of short term versus long term tube thoracostomy drainage before tetracycline pleurodesis in the treatment of malignant pleural effusions. *Thorax* 1994;**49**:23-5.
48. Ukale V, Bone D, Hillerdal G, et al. The impact of pleurodesis in malignant effusion on respiratory function. *Respir Med* 1999;**93**:898-902.
49. Parulekar W, Di Primio G, Matzinger F, et al. Use of small-bore vs large-bore chest tubes for treatment of malignant pleural effusions. *Chest* 2001;**120**:19-25.
50. Clementsen P, Evald T, Grode G, et al. Treatment of malignant pleural effusion: pleurodesis using a small percutaneous catheter—A prospective randomized study. *Respir Med* 1998;**92**:593-6.
51. Hsu WH, Chiang CD, Chen CY, et al. Ultrasound-guided small-bore Elecath tube insertion for the rapid sclerotherapy of malignant pleural effusion. *Jpn J Clin Oncol* 1998;**28**:187-91.
52. Parker LA, Charnock GC, Delany DJ. Small bore catheter drainage and sclerotherapy for malignant pleural effusions. *Cancer* 1989;**64**:1218-21.
53. Saffran L, Ost DE, Fein AM, Schiff MJ. Outpatient pleurodesis of malignant pleural effusions using a small-bore pigtail catheter. *Chest* 2000;**118**:417-21.
54. Aelony Y. Thoracoscopic talc poudrage: comparison with tetracycline and use in Hodgkin's disease. *Chest* 1992;**102**:1922-4.
55. Danby CA, Adebonojo SA, Moritz DM. Video-assisted talc pleurodesis for malignant pleural effusions utilizing local anesthesia and I.V. sedation. *Chest* 1998;**113**:739-42.
56. Dresler CM, Herndon J, Daniels T, et al. Cancer and Leukemia Group B (CALGB) 9334: a phase III, intergroup study of sclerosis of malignant pleural effusion by talc. *Proc Am Soc Clin Oncol* 2000:p 2455.
57. Landvater L, Hix WR, Mills M, et al. Malignant pleural effusion treated by tetracycline sclerotherapy: a comparison of single vs repeated instillation. *Chest* 1988;**93**:1196-8.

58. Ostrowski MJ, Halsall GM. Intracavitary bleomycin in the management of malignant effusions: a multicenter study. *Cancer Treat Rep* 1982;**66**:1903-7.
59. Emad A, Rezaian GR. Treatment of malignant pleural effusions with a combination of bleomycin and tetracycline: a comparison of bleomycin or tetracycline alone versus a combination of bleomycin and tetracycline. *Cancer* 1996;**78**:2498-501.
60. Goldman CA, Skinnider LF, Maksymiuk AW. Interferon instillation for malignant pleural effusions. *Ann Oncol* 1993;**4**:141-5.
61. Rauthe G, Sistermanns J. Recombinant tumour necrosis factor in the local therapy of malignant pleural effusion. *Eur J Cancer* 1997;**33**:226-31.
62. Izbicki R, Weyhing 3rd BT, Baker L, et al. Pleural effusion in cancer patients: a prospective randomized study of pleural drainage with the addition of radioactive phosphorous to the pleural space vs. pleural drainage alone. *Cancer* 1975;**36**:1511-8.
63. Waller DA, Morritt GN, Forty J. Video-assisted thoracoscopic pleurectomy in the management of malignant pleural effusion. *Chest* 1995;**107**:1454-6.
64. Friedberg JS, Mick R, Stevenson JP, et al. Phase II trial of pleural photodynamic therapy and surgery for patients with non–small-cell lung cancer with pleural spread. *J Clin Oncol* 2004;**22**:2192-201.
65. Yasumoto K, Ogura T. Intrapleural application of recombinant interleukin-2 in patients with malignant pleurisy due to lung cancer: a multi-institutional cooperative study. *Biotherapy* 1991;**3**:345-9.
66. Rusch VW, Figlin R, Godwin D, Piantadosi S. Intrapleural cisplatin and cytarabine in the management of malignant pleural effusions: a Lung Cancer Study Group trial. *J Clin Oncol* 1991;**9**:313-9.
67. Stathopoulos GT, Moschos C, Loutrari H, et al. Zoledronic acid is effective against experimental malignant pleural effusion. *Am J Respir Crit Care Med* 2008;**178**:50-9.
68. Seto T, Ushijima S, Yamamoto H, et al. Intrapleural hypotonic cisplatin treatment for malignant pleural effusion in 80 patients with non-small-cell lung cancer: a multi-institutional phase II trial. *Br J Cancer* 2006;**95**:717-21.
69. Sterman DH, Recio A, Carroll RG, et al. A phase I clinical trial of single-dose intrapleural IFN-beta gene transfer for malignant pleural mesothelioma and metastatic pleural effusions: high rate of antitumor immune responses. *Clin Cancer Res* 2007;**13**(15 Pt 1):4456-66.
70. Sugitachi A, Takatsuka Y, Kido T, et al. Bio-adhesio-chemo (BAC) therapy for patients with malignant pleural effusion. *Am J Clin Oncol* 1989;**12**:156-61.
71. Kralstein J, Frishman WH. Malignant pericardial diseases: diagnosis and treatment. *Cardiol Clin* 1987;**5**:583-9.
72. Maher EA, Shepherd FA, Todd TJ. Pericardial sclerosis as the primary management of malignant pericardial effusion and cardiac tamponade. *J Thorac Cardiovasc Surg* 1996;**112**:637-43.
73. Vaitkus PT, Herrmann HC, LeWinter MM. Treatment of malignant pericardial effusion. *JAMA* 1994;**272**:59-64.
74. Wilkins 3rd HE, Cacioppo J, Connolly MM, et al. Intrapericardial interferon in the management of malignant pericardial effusion. *Chest* 1998;**114**:330-1.
75. Austin EH, Flye MW. The treatment of recurrent malignant pleural effusion. *Ann Thorac Surg* 1979;**28**:190-203.
76. Liu HP, Chang CH, Lin PJ, et al. Thoracoscopic management of effusive pericardial disease: indications and technique. *Ann Thorac Surg* 1994;**58**:1695-7.
77. Wang HJ, Hsu KL, Chiang FT, et al. Technical and prognostic outcomes of double-balloon pericardiotomy for large malignancy-related pericardial effusions. *Chest* 2002;**122**:893-9.
78. Wang N, Feikes JR, Mogensen T, et al. Pericardioperitoneal shunt: an alternative treatment for malignant pericardial effusion. *Ann Thorac Surg* 1994;**57**:289-92.
79. Molnar TF, Biki B, Horvath OP. Pericardioperitoneal shunt: further development of the procedure using VATS technique. *Ann Thorac Surg* 2002;**74**:593-5.
80. Mason MR, Bedrossian CW, Fahey CA. Value of immunocytochemistry in the study of malignant effusions. *Diagn Cytopathol* 1987;**3**:215-21.
81. Betta PG, Pavesi M, Pastormerlo M, et al. Use of monoclonal antibody B72.3 as a marker of metastatic carcinoma cells in neoplastic effusions. *Pathologica* 1991;**83**:99-104.
82. Loy TS, Diaz-Arias AA, Bickel JT. Value of BCA-225 in the cytologic diagnosis of malignant effusions: an immunocytochemical study of 197 cases. *Mod Pathol* 1990;**3**:294-7.
83. Stoop JA, Hendriks JG, Berends D. Identification of malignant cells in serous effusions using a panel of monoclonal antibodies Ber-EP4, MCA-b-12 and EMA. *Cytopathology* 1992;**3**:297-302.
84. Ko EC, Jhala NC, Shultz JJ, Chhieng DC. Use of a panel of markers in the differential diagnosis of adenocarcinoma and reactive mesothelial cells in fluid cytology. *Am J Clin Pathol* 2001;**116**:709-15.
85. Berner HS, Davidson B, Berner A, et al. Differential expression of CD44s and CD44v3-10 in adenocarcinoma cells and reactive mesothelial cells in effusions. *Virchows Arch* 2000;**436**:330-5.
86. Shi HZ, Liang QL, Jiang J, et al. Diagnostic value of carcinoembryonic antigen in malignant pleural effusion: a meta-analysis. *Respirology* 2008;**13**:518-27.
87. Davidson B, Nielsen S, Christensen J, et al. The role of desmin and N-cadherin in effusion cytology: a comparative study using established markers of mesothelial and epithelial cells. *Am J Surg Pathol* 2001;**25**:1405-12.
88. Kitazume H, Kitamura K, Mukai K, et al. Cytologic differential diagnosis among reactive mesothelial cells, malignant mesothelioma, and adenocarcinoma: utility of combined E-cadherin and calretinin immunostaining. *Cancer* 2000;**90**:55-60.
89. Burstein DE, Reder I, Weiser K, et al. GLUT1 glucose transporter: a highly sensitive marker of malignancy in body cavity effusions. *Mod Pathol* 1998;**11**:392-6.
90. Saleh H, Bober P, Tabaczka P. Value of Ki67 immunostain in identification of malignancy in serous effusions. *Diagn Cytopathol* 1999;**20**:24-8.
91. Bailey ME, Brown RW, Mody DR, et al. Ber-EP4 for differentiating adenocarcinoma from reactive and neoplastic mesothelial cells in serous effusions: comparison with carcinoembryonic antigen, B72.3 and Leu-M1. *Acta Cytol* 1996;**40**:1212-6.
92. Morgan RL, De Young BR, McGaughy VR, et al. MOC-31 aids in the differentiation between adenocarcinoma and reactive mesothelial cells. *Cancer* 1999;**87**:390-4.
93. Cibas ES, Corson JM, Pinkus GS. The distinction of adenocarcinoma from malignant mesothelioma in cell blocks of effusions: the role of routine mucin histochemistry and immunohistochemical assessment of carcinoembryonic antigen, keratin proteins, epithelial membrane antigen, and milk fat globule–derived antigen. *Hum Pathol* 1987;**18**:67-74.
94. Mayall F, Heryet A, Manga D, Kriegeskotten A. p53 immunostaining is a highly specific and moderately sensitive marker of malignancy in serous fluid cytology. *Cytopathology* 1997;**8**:9-12.
95. Rosen-Levin E, Patil JR, Watson CW, Jagirdar J. Distinguishing benign from malignant pleural effusions by lectin immunocytochemistry. *Acta Cytol* 1989;**33**:499-504.
96. Giarnieri E, Alderisio M, Mancini R, et al. Tissue inhibitor of metalloproteinase 2 (TIMP-2) expression in adenocarcinoma pleural effusions. *Oncol Rep* 2008;**19**:483-7.
97. Mocanu L, Cimpean AM, Raica M. Expression of cytokeratin MNF116 and vimentin in pleural serous effusions. *Rom J Morphol Embryol* 2007;**48**:291-4.
98. Alatas F, Alata O, Metinta M, et al. Diagnostic value of CEA, CA 15-3, CA 19-9, CYFRA 21-1, NSE and TSA assay in pleural effusions. *Lung Cancer* 2001;**31**:9-16.
99. Okamoto I, Morisaki T, Sasaki J, et al. Molecular detection of cancer cells by competitive reverse transcription-polymerase chain reaction analysis of specific CD44 variant RNAs. *J Natl Cancer Inst* 1998;**90**:307-15.
100. Imecik O, Ozer F. Diagnostic value of sialic acid in malignant pleural effusions. *Chest* 1992;**102**:1819-22.
101. Lee YC, Chern JH, Lai SL, Perng RP. Sialyl stage-specific embryonic antigen-1: a useful marker for differentiating the etiology of pleural effusion. *Chest* 1998;**114**:1542-5.
102. Odeh M, Sabo E, Srugo I, Oliven A. Tumour necrosis factor alpha in the diagnostic assessment of pleural effusion. *Q J Med* 2000;**93**:819-24.
103. Gu P, Huang G, Chen Y, et al. Diagnostic utility of pleural fluid carcinoembryonic antigen and CYFRA 21-1 in patients with pleural effusion: a systematic review and meta-analysis. *J Clin Lab Anal* 2007;**21**:398-405.
104. Li G, Passebosc-Faure K, Feng G, et al. MN/CA9: a potential gene marker for detection of malignant cells in effusions. *Biomarkers* 2007;**12**:214-20.
105. Roncella S, Ferro P, Bacigalupo B, et al. Assessment of RT-PCR detection of human mammaglobin for the diagnosis of breast cancer derived pleural effusions. *Diagn Mol Pathol* 2008;**17**:28-33.
106. Daniel TM, Tribble CG, Rodgers BM. Thoracoscopy and talc poudrage for pneumothoraces and effusions. *Ann Thorac Surg* 1990;**50**:186-9.
107. Aelony Y, King R, Boutin C. Thoracoscopic talc poudrage pleurodesis for chronic recurrent pleural effusions. *Ann Intern Med* 1991;**115**:778-82.
108. Ohri SK, Oswal SK, Townsend ER, Fountain SW. Early and late outcome after diagnostic thoracoscopy and talc pleurodesis. *Ann Thorac Surg* 1992;**53**:1038-41.
109. Sanchez-Armengol A, Rodriguez-Panadero F. Survival and talc pleurodesis in metastatic pleural carcinoma, revisited: report of 125 cases. *Chest* 1993;**104**:1482-5.
110. Kennedy L, Harley RA, Sahn SA, Strange C. Talc slurry pleurodesis: pleural fluid and histologic analysis. *Chest* 1995;**107**:1707-12.
111. Weissberg D, Ben Zeev I. Talc pleurodesis: experience with 360 patients. *J Thorac Cardiovasc Surg* 1993;**106**:689-95.
112. Paladine W, Cunningham TJ, Sponzo R, et al. Intracavitary bleomycin in the management of malignant effusions. *Cancer* 1976;**38**:1903-8.
113. Bitran JD, Brown C, Desser RK, et al. Intracavitary bleomycin for the control of malignant effusions. *J Surg Oncol* 1981;**16**:273-7.

114. Patz Jr EF, McAdams HP, Goodman PC, et al. Ambulatory sclerotherapy for malignant pleural effusions. *Radiology* 1996;**199**:133-5.
115. Gravelyn TR, Michelson MK, Gross BH, Sitrin RG. Tetracycline pleurodesis for malignant pleural effusions: a 10-year retrospective study. *Cancer* 1987;**59**:1973-7.
116. Robinson LA, Fleming WH, Galbraith TA. Intrapleural doxycycline control of malignant pleural effusions. *Ann Thorac Surg* 1993;**55**:1115-21.
117. Pulsiripunya C, Youngchaiyud P, Pushpakom R, et al. The efficacy of doxycycline as a pleural sclerosing agent in malignant pleural effusion: a prospective study. *Respirology* 1996;**1**:69-72.
118. Olivares-Torres CA, Laniado-Laborín R, Chávez-García C, et al. Iodopovidone pleurodesis for recurrent pleural effusions. *Chest* 2002;**122**:581-3.
119. Vidyasagar MS, Ramanujam AS, Fernandes DJ, et al. Vincristine (Vinca-alkaloid) as a sclerosing agent for malignant pleural effusions. *Acta Oncol* 1999;**38**:1017-20.
120. Noppen M, Degreve J, Mignolet M, Vincken W. A prospective, randomised study comparing the efficacy of talc slurry and bleomycin in the treatment of malignant pleural effusions. *Acta Clin Belg* 1997;**52**:258-62.
121. Fentiman IS, Rubens RD, Hayward JL. A comparison of intracavitary talc and tetracycline for the control of pleural effusions secondary to breast cancer. *Eur J Cancer Clin Oncol* 1986;**22**:1079-81.
122. Hartman DL, Gaither JM, Kesler KA, et al. Comparison of insufflated talc under thoracoscopic guidance with standard tetracycline and bleomycin pleurodesis for control of malignant pleural effusions. *J Thorac Cardiovasc Surg* 1993;**105**:743-7.
123. Diacon AH, Wyser C, Bolliger CT, et al. Prospective randomized comparison of thoracoscopic talc poudrage under local anesthesia versus bleomycin instillation for pleurodesis in malignant pleural effusions. *Am J Respir Crit Care Med* 2000;**162**(4 Pt 1):1445-9.
124. Martinez-Moragon E, Aparicio J, Rogado MC, et al. Pleurodesis in malignant pleural effusions: a randomized study of tetracycline versus bleomycin. *Eur Respir J* 1997;**10**:2380-3.
125. Ruckdeschel JC, Moores D, Lee JY, et al. Intrapleural therapy for malignant pleural effusions: a randomized comparison of bleomycin and tetracycline. *Chest* 1991;**100**:1528-35.
126. Patz Jr EF, McAdams HP, Erasmus JJ, et al. Sclerotherapy for malignant pleural effusions: a prospective randomized trial of bleomycin vs doxycycline with small-bore catheter drainage. *Chest* 1998;**113**:1305-11.
127. Ostrowski MJ, Priestman TJ, Houston RF, Martin WM. A randomized trial of intracavitary bleomycin and *Corynebacterium parvum* in the control of malignant pleural effusions. *Radiother Oncol* 1989;**14**:19-26.
128. Hillerdal G, Kiviloog J, Nöu E, Steinholtz L. *Corynebacterium parvum* in malignant pleural effusion. A randomized prospective study. *Eur J Respir Dis* 1986;**69**:204-6.
129. Koldsland S, Svennevig JL, Lehne G, Johnson E. Chemical pleurodesis in malignant pleural effusions: a randomised prospective study of mepacrine versus bleomycin. *Thorax* 1993;**48**:790-3.
130. Loutsidis A, Bellenis I, Argiriou M, Exarchos N. Tetracycline compared with mechlorethamine in the treatment of malignant pleural effusions: a randomized trial. *Respir Med* 1994;**88**:523-6.
131. Yoshida K, Sugiura T, Takifuji N, et al. Randomized phase II trial of three intrapleural therapy regimens for the management of malignant pleural effusion in previously untreated non–small cell lung cancer: JCOG 9515. *Lung Cancer* 2007;**58**:362-8.
132. Sartori S, Tassinari D, Ceccotti P, et al. Prospective randomized trial of intrapleural bleomycin versus interferon alfa-2b via ultrasound-guided small-bore chest tube in the palliative treatment of malignant pleural effusions. *J Clin Oncol* 2004;**22**:1228-33.
133. Paschoalini Mda S, Vargas FS, Marchi E, et al. Prospective randomized trial of silver nitrate vs talc slurry in pleurodesis for symptomatic malignant pleural effusions. *Chest* 2005;**128**:684-9.
134. Bayly TC, Kisner DL, Sybert A, et al. Tetracycline and quinacrine in the control of malignant pleural effusions: a randomized trial. *Cancer* 1978;**41**:1188-92.

CHAPTER 31
Pleural Tumors
Ciaran McNamee, Christopher T. Ducko, and David J. Sugarbaker

Pleural Embryology and Anatomy
Asbestos-Associated Pleural Pathology
  Biologic Capabilities of Asbestos Fibers
  Epidemiology of Mesothelioma
  Population Exposure
  Pathogenesis of Asbestos Fibers
    Mesothelial Cell Neoplastic Changes Attributed to Asbestos Exposure
    Tumor Suppressor Genes in Mesothelioma

Viral Activation of Mesothelioma Cells
Apoptotic Processes
Clinical Aspects of Pleural Tumors
  Inflammatory Pleural Reactions
  Pulmonary Tumors That May Resemble Pleural Tumors
  Benign Pleural Tumors
    Benign Pleural Tumors That May Remain Benign

    Pleural Tumors with Low Malignant Potential
    Primary Malignant Pleural Tumors That May Look Like Benign Tumors
  Malignant Pleural Tumors
    Metastatic Malignant Tumors
    Diffuse Malignant Pleural Mesothelioma
    Multimodality Therapy
    Innovative Adjunctive Therapies

PLEURAL EMBRYOLOGY AND ANATOMY

The pleura is a thin continuous membrane that separates during embryologic development into two layers as the developing lung buds encroach on the pleural cavity. The component of the pleural membrane that envelopes the lung is called the visceral pleura, which then continues as a contiguous serosal layer, called the parietal pleura, to cover the chest wall, the mediastinum, and the diaphragm. These layers fuse at the hilum, creating the pleural space. The pleural space contains a small quantity of glycoprotein-rich fluid that allows the opposing pleural surfaces to glide over each other during respiration. These pleural membranes are derived from the mesoderm during embryogenesis; the separation by the ingrowth of the lung bud permits the parietal pleura to fuse with the ectoderm to form the somatopleure, and the visceral pleura to fuse with the endoderm to form the splanchnopleure. Thus, all three germ layers are represented in the histiogenesis of the pleurae, which explains the later de-differentiation of pleural tumors into both epithelial and mesenchymal elements.

The blood supply of the parietal pleura emanates from systemic sources: intercostal arteries, subclavian artery, internal thoracic artery, and phrenic arteries. The visceral pleura derives its arterial blood supply from the bronchial arterial circulation and from the lung parenchyma. The lymphatic drainage for the parietal pleura follows the arterial blood supply and drains to systemic sources. The visceral pleura drains into the pulmonary parenchyma. There are naturally occurring pores or stomata in the caudal aspect of the parietal and mediastinal pleurae that transfer particulate matter into lymphatic channels for drainage. Most of the fluid that accumulates in the pleural space is derived from the lung and is absorbed by the parietal pleura. The visceral pleura is devoid of somatic innervation, whereas the parietal pleura has a rich network of somatic, sympathetic, and parasympathetic neural innervation.

The pleural membrane is thin and translucent. It is composed of five separate layers: (1) the mesothelial layer (flattened mesothelial cells joined by tight junctions), (2) a thin submesothelial connective tissue layer, (3) a superficial elastic tissue layer, (4) a loose subpleural connective tissue layer in which run lymphatics, nerves, arteries, and veins, and (5) a fibroelastic layer that is adherent to the underlying structures (lung, mediastinum, diaphragm, chest wall). The mesothelial cell features long slender microvilli that extend into the pleural space and are believed to release hyaluronic acid into the pleural fluid.[1]

The pleural response to injury is characterized by edema and exudation of protein and neutrophils. This response is known as an exudative pleural reaction. It is orchestrated by the release of inflammatory mediators (cytokines, chemokines, oxidants, and proteases) from mesothelial cells, which also have phagocytic capabilities. Lesser inflammatory conditions can be resolved by the absorption of inflammatory products by mesothelial cells aided by the lymphatic evacuation of fluid and particles. Severe or persistent damage encourages a submesothelial fibroblastic response and the formation of dense adhesions.

The pleural reaction can occur in response to an infectious or a noninfectious injury, usually acquired through the respiratory system. Infectious organisms are associated with empyema. However, the visceral pleura responds to autoimmune diseases, drug reactions, radiation, or pneumoconiosis by creating cytokines (transforming growth factor beta [TGFβ] and tumor necrosis factor alpha [TNFα]), which in turn lead to the formation of a fibrin matrix. Asbestos, silica, and coal dust all are associated with the development of circumferential plaques of dense hyaline fibrosis on the parietal pleural surface that typically involve the diaphragm and chest wall.

ASBESTOS-ASSOCIATED PLEURAL PATHOLOGY
Biologic Capabilities of Asbestos Fibers

Asbestos is divided into two main types based on fiber length and other physical properties that may account for its biopersistence in humans. The fibers of the first type are short and serpentine. Chrysotile (or white asbestos) is the predominant member. The second type, known as amphibole asbestos, has long, thin, straight fibers. It has several subtypes, including crocidolite, actinolyte, tremolite, anthophyllite, and amosite.[2] Approximately 95% of the asbestos currently used worldwide is chrysotile. The remaining 5% is amosite and crocidolite, although these groups of fibers are commonly mixed together.[3]

Two conflicting theories have been advanced to explain the oncogenic potential of asbestos fibers based on their physical properties of dimension, shape, and length. The amphibole hypothesis proposes that amphibole fibers owe their durability and their biopersistence in the lung to their long length. Proponents of this hypothesis believe that the short serpentine chrysotile fibers are broken down and cleared too quickly to provoke cancer.[4] The Stanton theory postulates that amphibole asbestos is carcinogenic because the long fibers are able to penetrate deeper into the pleura, where they come in contact with and incite mesothelial cell proliferation.[5] Whatever the cause, it appears that chrysotile fibers are cleared from the body by macrophages much more quickly than amphibole fibers, which can remain in the lung for many years after exposure, accounting for their high degree of biopersistence.

There is evidence that the biopersistence of asbestos fibers is associated with malignancy in animals[6,7] and in humans.[8] Although consensus has not been reached on the precise carcinogenic potential of the different fiber types, or the level or length of exposure needed for the malignant transformation to mesothelioma, an expert panel (level 4 evidence) has recently published an opinion on this matter. The consensus decision of this panel suggests that the longer, biopersistent fibers associated with amphibole asbestos (particularly, crocidolite) have greater carcinogenic potential than the short fibers of the serpentine asbestos.[9]

Epidemiology of Mesothelioma

The causal association between asbestos exposure and the later development of pleural tumors is strong. However, the lack of a clinically recognizable, premalignant, noninvasive form of malignant mesothelioma, coupled with the difficulty of obtaining invasive biopsy material, has hampered the identification of the agent or agents responsible for initiating or promoting the development of pleural tumors in vivo. Thus, much of current knowledge is empirically derived from three sources: epidemiologic data, in vitro investigation of asbestos and mesothelial cell lines, and retrograde assumptions made from mesothelioma chromosome studies.

Malignant mesothelioma was first identified as a discrete diagnosis in 1870.[10] The name was coined in the 1930s.[11] Suspicion of an association between asbestos exposure and mesothelioma development was initially documented in the medical literature between 1920 and 1950.[12-14] Despite the numerous case reports, it was not until 1960 that Wagner and colleagues reported a series of cases that demonstrated a strong association between mesothelioma and occupational exposure to asbestos in asbestos miners in South Africa.[10] A clear link between asbestos exposure and pleural tumor development was documented in the United States by Selikoff and colleagues in the 1960s and 1970s.[15,16] Further evidence of this association followed, with multiple case-control series from 1965 to 1975. These reports were summarized in an epidemiologic review of mesothelioma by Britton.[17] In this review, the most notable risk of mesothelioma was associated with occupational exposure to asbestos, primarily in shipyards where crocidolite asbestos was used in naval insulation materials. Other defined exposure groups with varied relative risks of mesothelioma development included workers who installed insulation and workers in the asbestos product manufacturing industry or in heating and construction industries.[17] After Wagner's publication, further worldwide case series comparing amphibole and chrysotile fiber exposures from 1980 to 1999 confirmed the association of asbestos exposure (particularly amphibole fibers) and mesothelioma. Even chrysotile miners were identified to be at high risk for mesothelioma, although contamination of the chrysotile asbestos by amphibole fibers (particularly tremolite) has been questioned in these miners as the true cause.[17,18]

Based on the suspicion of an association between asbestos and cancer development, industrial regulation began to occur. As early as 1932, the United Kingdom issued the first antiasbestos regulation, entitled "Asbestos Industry Regulation 1931." Crocidolite asbestos was not banned in the United Kingdom, however, until 1970. By 1980, most western European countries had followed suit. The United States Environmental Protection Agency listed asbestos as a hazardous air pollutant in 1971. By 1972, exposure limits for asbestos had been published, and by 1979 asbestos use was curtailed. Asbestos control or regulation in many other world regions has yet to be achieved.

The latency period (20 to 50 years) between exposure to asbestos and mesothelioma development is substantial.[19] Although the epidemiologic data linking asbestos exposure to mesothelioma are clear, the lifetime risk of mesothelioma development in workers exposed to asbestos ranges from 4.5% to 10.0%.[20-23] Thus, the lack of a strong, direct, quantifiable association between asbestos exposure and pleural tumor development impedes the prediction of individual disease development, and future predictions are relevant only in broad demographic terms.

Western populations were exposed to asbestos as an environmental hazard when it was used in an uncontrolled fashion in the shipbuilding and construction industries between 1940 and 1970. Despite worldwide attention by environmental regulatory bodies, the latency of the disease suggests that the peak incidence of the disease in Europe, North America, and Australia may be in the next 10 to 15 years.[24,25] Prediction risks for mesothelioma development suggest that the disease will continue to increase in Europe, to peak in 2020, and thereafter to rapidly decline, as the workforce exposure should affect only the population born before 1950 (assuming the commencement of work at age 20, when asbestos regulations were initiated).[17,24] The prediction for a mesothelioma peak in the United States is 2004; Australia, 2015; and Japan, 2025. However, these assumptions do not include many unanticipated factors such as the attack on the World Trade Center in 2001, where an estimated 10 million New Yorkers were exposed to asbestos dust.[26,27]

Population Exposure

Individuals with asbestos disease can be divided into four groups based on the degree of exposure to asbestos: direct occupational exposure, secondary occupational exposure, passive occupational exposure, and nonoccupational exposure.

The first group comprises individuals with direct exposure either through work or by direct inadvertent exposure to asbestos fibers. An example of this exposure group is the miners of asbestos in Wittenoom, Australia. These miners were exposed at work, but because asbestos was used in lieu of grass to cover the schoolyards and playgrounds, their children also received direct exposure.[25]

The secondary exposure group represents persons whose exposure could be termed as occasional, such as plumbers, carpenters, navy personnel, and installers of asbestos as insulation.

The third group represents those who are passively exposed through other family members who work directly with asbestos and carry the fibers home on their clothing. This group includes persons in close contact with the first two groups (e.g., wives of asbestos workers).[28]

A small number of individuals have mesothelioma but no history of occupational exposure to asbestos. Some may have contacted asbestos fibers in their natural habitat,[29] or they may have a genetic predisposition.[30,31] It has been postulated that simian virus 40 (SV40) plays a synergistic role with asbestos in the development of mesothelioma, either as a clastogenic transformer (an inducer of chromosomal damage) or as a cytologic protector, which permits chromosomally damaged cells to survive and propagate rather than die (apoptosis).[32,33] SV40 was identified as a contaminant in polio vaccines from 1950 to 1963, and the extent of its role in mesothelioma development is still both very controversial and undetermined.

Finally, 2% to 5% of mesothelioma cases arise in a pediatric population, which suggests a genetic rather than an environmental cause of mesothelioma in these individuals.[34]

Pathogenesis of Asbestos Fibers

Benign asbestos-related pleural disease is thought to manifest as either discrete parietal pleural plaques or as diffuse disease involving visceral pleural hyperplasia and fibrosis.[35] The mechanism whereby asbestos fibers reach the parietal pleura to evoke pleural plaque formation is unknown. However, as described earlier, it is suspected that the inability of pulmonary macrophages to phagocytose these particles is a result of their length, and that the fibers burrow through the lung and eventually come into contact with the mesothelial cells in the pleural membranes. Several theories have been proposed to explain how the fibers pass from the visceral to the parietal mesothelial cells. There are several putative causes. The fibers may protrude through the visceral pleura, abrading and irritating the parietal pleural surface. The fibers may migrate across the pleura from the visceral to the parietal surface, or they may disseminate via lymphatic drainage to the parietal mesothelial cells.[27,35]

The effect of asbestos on mesothelial cells is complex, multifactorial, and difficult to explain. It has been shown, for example, that human mesothelial cells often die in vitro after contact with, or phagocytosis of, asbestos fibers.[36,37] A possible explanation is that asbestos fibers may induce the proliferation of cellular cytokines that have cytoprotective effects and that allow asbestos-transformed mesothelial cells to survive and proliferate. TNFα expression has been shown to increase after mesothelial cells and macrophages are been exposed to asbestos, and this factor may enable the asbestos-damaged cells to survive.[38] Fiber persistence may lead to chronic inflammation with increased cycles of cell growth that might induce cellular mitotic changes. These changes may gradually cause the mesothelial cells to acquire genetic and epigenetic changes that lead to neoplasia. Even without directly interfering with the DNA machinery of the cell, these fibers may secondarily select for cells with oncologic potential.

In addition to inducing cellular proliferation, asbestos fibers have other cytologic and clastogenic properties that could lead to neoplasia. Incorporation of asbestos fibers into the mesothelial cell, for example, produces oxygen free radicals,[39,40] cytokines, chemokines, and growth factors such as epidermal growth factor (EGF) and TGFα.[41-43] These elements can promote the proliferation of mesothelial cells, rendering them more susceptible to DNA and genetic damage.[44] Asbestos induces phosphorylation of mitogen-activated protein (MAP) kinases and of the extracellular signal–regulated kinases (ERKs) 1 and 2 with increased downstream expression of tumor proto-oncogenes.[43]

Asbestos fibers also have clastogenic properties—that is, they may act directly on the chromosomes.[45] They may sever or disrupt the mitotic spindle of cells, causing chromosomal abnormalities such as aneuploidy to occur.[46] Finally, they may induce epigenetic tumor suppressor silencing via promoter DNA CpG methylation, which permits tumorigenic cells to enter the cell cycle instead of halting them at the G_1/S interphase of mitosis.[47]

Mesothelial Cell Neoplastic Changes Attributed to Asbestos Exposure

Retrograde analysis of molecular biologic changes in the malignant mesothelial cell has revealed several different areas of molecular variance from normal mesothelial cellular mechanics. These variations are thought to lead to neoplasia.

Chromosomal Abnormalities in Mesothelioma

Karyotypic alterations result from somatic mutations; however, gene deletions, gene silencing, and RNA editing are also common chromosomal aberrations in malignant mesothelioma. DNA sequencing techniques and comparative genomic hybridization permit discrimination between clonal proliferations of tumor cells.[48,49] These techniques may also help in the histologic identification and sorting of mesothelioma subtypes. They may aid by distinguishing mesothelioma from similar-appearing tumors such as adenocarcinoma.[50] Whole-transcriptome, deep sequencing of single mesothelioma tumors has revealed unique individual tumor profiles of chromosomal and mRNA expression.[51]

These chromosomal changes in malignant mesothelioma often are multiple, leading to clonal proliferations that show individual variation (losses are more common than gains).[50] In mesothelioma, a common deletion occurs at the 9p21 locus. This occurs at a frequency of 70% in mesothelioma cell lines and in up to 22% of primary tumor specimens.[52,53] This locus encodes two inhibitors of the cyclin-dependent kinases (CDKs)—namely, p16^{INK4a} (CDKN2A) and P15^{INK4b} (CDKN2B), which prevent the phosphorylation of retinoblastoma (Rb) protein. The Rb protein modulates cell entrance into the S phase from G_1 of the cell cycle. Phosphorylation of this protein, which is prevented by CDK inhibitors, allows uncontrolled cellular entry into S phase. The 9p21 gene also codes for p14^{ARF}, which acts as a regulator for an important tumor suppressor oncogene, *p53*. This gene encodes tumor protein p53, which responds to diverse cellular stresses such as hypoxia, DNA damage, and oncogene activation, to regulate target genes that induce cell cycle arrest, apoptosis, senescence, DNA repair, or changes in metabolism. P53 protein is expressed at a low level in normal cells and at a high level in a variety of transformed cell lines, where it is believed to contribute to transformation and malignancy. P53 is a DNA-binding protein containing transcription activation, DNA-binding, and oligomerization domains. It is postulated to bind to a p53-binding site and activate expression of downstream genes that inhibit growth and invasion, and thus function as a tumor suppressor by initiating the transcription of genes leading to downstream effects on cell cycle arrest in G_0 and apoptosis. A downstream target of p53 is p21, a multifunctional CDK inhibitor. Loss of p21 expression is associated with decreased patient survival.[54] Also, there is a frequent loss of chromosome 22 in malignant mesothelioma.[55] The tumor suppressor gene *NF2* is located on this chromosome.

Tumor Suppressor Genes in Mesothelioma

Tumor Suppressor Genes and CDK Inhibitor Loss

Ironically, malignant mesothelial cells lack mutation of the two most common genetic mutations found in most cancers—namely, tumor suppressor genes *p53* and *pRb*.[56] The tumor suppressor gene *p53* is important for cell cycle arrest, as it prevents propagation of DNA-damaged cells or genetically unstable cells. It acts by stimulating the expression of p21 which, in turn, acts as a CDK inhibitor. In an equivalent manner, the retinoblastoma gene *(Rb)*, as noted earlier, also halts chromosomal synthesis and therefore tumor proliferation.

However, the chromosomal aberrations of malignant mesothelioma cells ultimately adversely affect these two tumor suppressor genes by upstream regulation of their gene products. Mutational deletion of the 9p21 locus in mesothelioma cells affects p14^{ARF}, an upstream regulator of p53. Deletional interruptions of this gene inactivate TP53-MDM2, which is extremely important for intrinsic cellular control of chromosomally damaged cells. Inactivation of this pathway by decreasing p21 gene products allows CDK to phosphorylate Rb protein, which then allows damaged cells to enter the S phase of the cell cycle.[57] Viral transduction of p14^{ARF} into mesothelioma cells in culture leads to increased production of p53 and p21, resulting in an increase in dephosphorylated Rb and G_1 arrest and an inhibition of mesothelioma cell growth.[58]

In an equivalent manner, the loss of p16^{INK4a} leads to loss of CDK 4 and 6, leading to phosphorylation of Rb gene by the lack of CDK inhibition.[57] Deletion of p16/CDKN2A has been reported in greater than 70% of mesothelioma cells.[50,59] As seen with p53, mesothelioma cells transfected with adenovirus expressing p16^{INK4a} demonstrate decreased phosphorylation of Rb,[60] leading to cell cycle arrest, cell death, and tumor regression.

Merlin and RAS-ERK Pathway

Changes in chromosome 22 may lead to altered expression of NF2, or somatic mutational changes may lead to NF2 alterations, which occur in approximately 50% of patients with mesothelioma.[61] NF2 encodes for a protein named merlin (alternatively called schwannomin). This protein is important in the connection between the plasma membrane and the cytoskeleton of the cell and may act as a tumor suppressor gene by inhibiting the RAS-ERK pathway and inducing cyclin D1 expression. Inhibition or abrogation of NF2 function and its downstream product merlin may lead to a lack of contact-dependent growth arrest,[62-64] leading to tumor proliferation at the expense of neighboring normal cells.

Oncogene Activation in Mesothelioma

The transcription factors AP-1 and β-catenin are often upregulated in malignant mesothelioma; AP-1 is upregulated by Fra-1 which is a member of the Fos family of transcription factors. Fra-1 expression is increased in malignant mesothelioma cells, in response to asbestos or EGF and reduced with inhibitors of ERK. Mesothelioma cells transfected with either an ERK inhibitor or a dominant negative fra-1 reverse their transformed phenotype.[65]

The transcription factor β-catenin is controlled by Wnt signaling, so that the presence of Wnt inhibits phosphorylation of adenomatous polyposis coli (APC) and axin, allowing persistence of β-catenin. Increased presence of β-catenin leads to nuclear binding of T-cell factor/lymphoid-enhancer factor (Tcf/Lef) proteins with downstream activation of transcription factors. Mesothelioma cells have been shown to have altered APC expression,[66] and they may express upstream negative inhibitors of the Wnt pathway (Wnt inhibitory factor [WIF-1] and secreted frizzled-related protein [sFRP]).[67,68] Extracellular signaling, through the overexpression of membrane disheveled proteins with downstream activation of β-catenin, may play an important role in malignant mesothelioma.[57]

Epigenetic Maneuvers

Promoter methylation has been shown to be effective in inactivating WIF-1 and sFRP.[69,70] Hypermethylation of DNA is a common epigenetic method of inhibition of tumor suppressor gene function.[71,72] In the context of asbestos exposure, however, there may be a dose-dependent increased induction of methylation as a result of asbestos fibers.[47] The precise mechanism for hypermethylation of this phenotypically important pathway is still not established. It may also be directly attributable to the clastogenic properties of asbestos fibers, or alternatively to repeated inflammatory insults of asbestos-generating reactive oxygen species, which may lead to increased mitotic stimulation and promoter methylation. Acquired generations of accrued genetic and epigenetic chromosomal changes leading to malignancy may thus be induced.[47]

Growth Factors in Mesothelioma

Platelet-derived growth factor (PDGF) chains A and B increase in response to asbestos exposure; they have been implicated in the development and progression of malignant mesothelioma.[50,73] Asbestos also induces autophosphorylation of EGF receptor (EGFR). This may result in the activation of the MAP kinase cascade and ERK1 and ERK2 kinases, leading to expression of proto-oncogenes that encode members of the fos-jun and activator protein 1 families.[43] Hepatocyte growth factor (HGF) can promote cell growth and migration mediated via downstream AKT and ERK pathways by binding to its receptor c-met. Circulating levels of this growth factor are elevated in mesothelioma patients, so inhibition of HGF receptor c-met may be a therapeutic option.[74] EGFR (member of the erbB family of tyrosine kinase receptors) is overexpressed in malignant mesothelioma in association with angiogenesis and proliferation.[75] There are multiple ligands which can bind to and activate this receptor, leading to intracellular tyrosine kinase autophosphorylation and signaling pathways of cell proliferation, differentiation, and immortality. The two most important ligands are EGFR and TGFα, both of which are increased by mesothelial asbestos exposure. Inhibition of EGFR and VEGF pathways by tyrosine kinase inhibitors[76] and inhibitors to VEGF production or VEGF receptors[77] will decrease or inhibit mesothelioma cell growth. VEGF production is increased by SV40 infection of mesothelioma cells.[78] Inhibitors of VEGF[79,80] and EGFR pathways[76] in mesothelioma patients are currently used in clinical studies.

Viral Activation of Mesothelioma Cells

SV40 is a double-stranded circular polyomavirus that contaminated polio vaccines in the United States, Canada, Europe, Asia, and Africa between 1955 and 1963. This virus has the potential, based on molecular, pathologic, and clinical evidence, to cause cancer.[81] It has two major chromosomal regions, one of which harbors latent oncogenic potential. The early region encodes for SV40Tag (large tumor antigen), SV40tag (small tumor antigen), and 17 KT; the late region encodes for structural proteins of the virus.

It has been postulated that SV40 infection may increase the cellular production of growth factors, such as VEGF[82] and HGF, through autocrine and paracrine mechanisms.[78] It may also protect cells from apoptosis by the ectopic production of telomerase, which prevents chromosomal shortening with successive cell divison.[83]

SV40Tag can bind to and inactivate the tumor suppressor genes $p53$ and Rb, unleashing uncontrolled tumor growth. Small tumor antigen (SV40tag) may inhibit PP2A, leading to dephosphorylation of members of the MAPK family and deactivation of Wnt and ERK, which may lead to increased cellular transcription.[84]

Despite the powerful putative oncologic attributes of SV40 virus, however, there is much debate in the literature as to the role of SV40 in cellular transformation; the oncologic potential of SV40 is very controversial and current opinion discounts its oncologic potential.[85,86] The counter-argument to the role of SV40 in inducing neoplasia in mesothelial cells is supported by the lack of viral particles identified within mesothelioma cells.[87] Further support for this counter-argument is empirically derived from the knowledge that $p14^{ARF}$ and $p16^{INK4a}$ cause mesothelioma mutational changes, with upstream deactivation of $p53$ and Rb, thus rendering SV40 inactivation of these tumor suppressor genes redundant and therefore obsolete.

Apoptotic Processes

Extracellular ligands of the caspase pathway, such as TNF, TNF-related apoptosis-inducing ligand (TRAIL), and Fas ligand, induce programmed cell death in normal cells. Intracellular mediators of apoptosis, including telomerase (see Viral Activation of Mesothelioma Cells, earlier) and proteins from the bcl-2 family, which may have proapoptotic and antiapoptotic properties, are increased in mesothelioma patients. Protein expression from this family may have a diagnostic and prognostic role in clinical medicine.[75,88] Proapoptotic Bcl-2 proteins induce apoptosis by increasing mitochondrial membrane permeability, in turn leading to caspase pathway activation. Antiapoptotic Bcl-xl expression is increased in mesothelioma. This can also be targeted by inhibitors of antisense oligonucleotides[89] or viral vector transfection of mesothelioma cells.[90]

CLINICAL ASPECTS OF PLEURAL TUMORS

Pleural tumors are recognized by the characteristic radiographic appearance of a thickened pleural layer that contains fluid, solid tumor, or a combination of both. Patients may present with or without symptoms of chest pain or dyspnea consequent to lung restriction or compression. Rarely, pleural tumors are associated with other symptoms, such as hypoglycemia or hypertrophic pulmonary osteoarthropathy. Radiographic evidence of pleural thickening in either symptomatic or asymptomatic patients is often the stimulus to initiate clinical studies to confirm the benign or malignant nature of the pathology or to redress, if possible, the underlying lung compression.

It is often difficult to distinguish benign from malignant pleural reactions (Box 31-1). As with other benign pleural conditions, the mesothelial cell also may release mediators such as cytokines, chemokines, oxidants, and proteases. These mediators may induce an exudative pleural reaction that gives rise to a proliferative hyperplasia of the mesothelial and submesothelial layers.[1,35] This reaction can resemble a malignant process. Thus, pleural thickening can be attributable to multiple causes, ranging from benign inflammation to malignancy, as summarized in Box 31-2.

Inflammatory Pleural Reactions

The pleura reacts to pleural injury either by development of a reactive mesothelial hyperplasia or organizing pleuritis (as opposed to atypical mesothelial hyperplasia, described later) or by the formation of nodular pleural plaques. Plaques are acellular deposits on the parietal pleura that often calcify. They are usually associated with asbestos exposure.[91,92] These benign lesions are often multiple and occur bilaterally. Their

---

Box 31-1
Benign Causes of Pleural Hyperplasia

- Pleural infections
- Radiation
- Surgery
- Trauma
- Intracavitary treatments (chemotherapy or sclerosing agents)
- Collagen vascular diseases
- Systemic immune diseases (systemic lupus erythematosus, rheumatoid arthritis, Sjögren's syndrome, Wegener's granulomatosis)
- Subpleural pulmonary abnormalities (infarction, infection, neoplasia)
- Pneumothorax
- Drug reactions (nitrofurantoin, bromocriptine, methysergide, procarbazine)
- Pancreatitis, uremia
- Pneumoconiosis (asbestosis)

Modified from Cagle PT, Churg A. *Arch Pathol Lab Med* 2005;**129**:1421-7 [95]; and King J, Thatcher N, Pickering C, Hasleton P. *Histopathology* 2006;**49**:561-8.[96]

> **Box 31-2**
> **Causes of Pleural Masses**
>
> - Inflammatory pleural reactions
>   - Reactive mesothelial hyperplasia or organizing pleuritis versus atypical mesothelial hyperplasia
>   - Nodular pleural plaques
> - Pulmonary tumors that may resemble pleural tumors
>   - Inflammatory pseudotumor of the lung
> - Benign pleural tumors
>   - Solitary fibrous tumor
>   - Lipomas and lipoblastomas
>   - Adenomatous tumors
>   - Calcifying fibrous tumors
>   - Mesothelial cysts
>   - Multicystic mesothelioma
>   - Schwannoma
> - Pleural tumors with low malignant potential
>   - Desmoid tumors
>   - Well-differentiated papillary mesothelioma
>   - Pleural thymoma
> - Primary malignant pleural tumors that may look like benign tumors
>   - Malignant solitary fibrous tumor
>   - Pleuropulmonary blastoma
>   - Localized malignant mesothelioma
>   - Vascular sarcoma
>   - Liposarcoma
>   - Pleuropulmonary synovial sarcoma
>   - Askin tumor or primitive neuroectodermal tumor (PNET)
>   - Desmoplastic small round cell tumor
> - Malignant pleural tumors
>   - Metastatic malignancies to the pleura
>   - Malignant mesothelioma

presence raises the possibility of mesothelioma or lung cancer, either on presentation or in the future.

Pulmonary Tumors That May Resemble Pleural Tumors

Inflammatory pseudotumor of the lung is a rare pulmonary tumor in adults, but it is the most common primary pulmonary tumor in children.[93] These tumors may be associated with a pleural thickening that responds to steroid therapy.[94]

The specific histologic features of a *benign reactive mesothelial hyperplasia* that mimics malignancy include high cellularity, cytologic mitoses, necrosis, papillary excrescences, and entrapment of mesothelial cells in organizing pleuritis. Immunohistochemistry may be of limited help in differentiating benign from malignant pleural pathology. Its primary value may be in the demonstration of invasion by immunostaining of invasive cells. Invasion is a key marker for malignancy and must be differentiated pathologically from entrapment, pseudo-invasion, or sequestration.[95,96]

Indeterminate lesions may occur on pleural biopsy. These are revealed by a proliferation of atypical mesothelial cells, either in a monolayer or piled up with cellular accumulations. These lesions may demonstrate increased cytologic atypia without evidence of true invasion; they may remain benign or degenerate into malignancy.[95,97]

Benign Pleural Tumors

Benign pleural tumors comprise less than 5% of all pleural tumors. Far more commonly, they represent either metastatic cancer or a diffuse malignant pleural mesothelioma. These malignant tumors share common properties with benign pleural tumors, which can make it difficult to establish the diagnosis, particularly with small biopsies of minimal amounts of tissue. The common properties of benign and malignant pleural tumors are that both originate from or metastasize to mesothelial or submesothelial surfaces, both may recur after surgical removal, and both are difficult to identify with limited tissue biopsy material because of patterns of heterogeneous cellularity.[98]

However, it is important to be able to distinguish a benign from a malignant pleural tumor, because the benign form confers excellent survival potential. Some benign tumors may recur after complete resection and they may still be treated surgically with curative intent.

A radiograph of a patient with benign tumors of the pleura reveals a thickened parietal layer with underlying lung compression. Occasionally, these tumors have the appearance of lung invasion (particularly if they are visceral pleura based), as in the inverted fibroma form of solitary fibrous tumors. These pleural abnormalities are identified by a variable thickening of either the visceral or parietal pleura. This imposes a diagnostic dilemma because of the many possible etiologies for pleural masses in the differential diagnosis. Furthermore, fine-needle aspirates of these abnormalities are often unreliable for confirming a diagnosis as a benign pleural tumor.[96,99-101]

From a clinical perspective, primary pleural tumors span a pathologic spectrum ranging from benign tumors, to benign tumors with some malignant features, to frankly malignant tumors. The most common pleural tumor (solitary fibrous tumor of the pleura) can occur in either a benign or a malignant form; and they may also recur in either a benign or a malignant form.[98,102]

Benign Pleural Tumors That May Remain Benign

Solitary Fibrous Tumors

The solitary fibrous tumor is the most common benign pleural tumor, and it is rare (by 2002, only 800 cases had been reported).[98] (In contrast, 3000 new cases of diffuse mesothelioma are diagnosed yearly in the United States.[103]) This tumor arises from the submesothelial layer of the mesothelioma and it is usually solitary, although it may occur in multiple sites.[104,105] It is associated with hypertrophic pulmonary osteoarthropathy in up to 22% of cases, and with severe hypoglycemia in 3% to 4% of cases.[106] The latter syndrome (Doege-Potter syndrome) is attributable to tumor-derived growth factor (insulin-like growth factor II).[107]

These tumors are often (>80%) attached to the visceral pleura, and they are often pedunculated (80%). In the remaining 20% of cases, they originate from the parietal pleura on the diaphragmatic or mediastinal surface, and parietal-based tumors are more likely to be sessile than pedunculated.[105]

Pedunculated tumors have a 2% recurrence rate, whereas sessile tumors have an 8% recurrence rate.[98]

Because the solitary fibrous tumor is often pedunculated, it is amenable to resection by video assisted thoracic surgery (VATS). However, resection should be complete and without tumor disruption to prevent tumor recurrence from either incomplete resection or microscopic seeding of the resected bed. It is important to remove not only the tumor but also the stalk with a 1-cm base of underlying lung. If the tumor is too large for VATS surgery, a thoracotomy may be required.[98,100] Tumors originating from the parietal pleura require at least a partial pleurectomy with the tumor resection. Occasionally, chest wall resection along with tumor removal is required if there is concern about recurrence or invasion from possible malignant transformation.

Sessile lesions larger than 5 cm should probably be removed by thoracotomy to prevent recurrences.[100] These tumors may appear to invade the lung if visceral growth (inverted fibroma) is seen, so lung resection may be required. Peritumoral adhesions, in which microscopic tumor deposits may hide, are common (60%), so a wide resection is needed. This can include lung, diaphragm, chest wall, and pericardium with frozen section determination that all margins are free of tumor at resection.[100] Recurrent tumors may be multifocal and may undergo malignant transformation.[102] Histologic characteristics do not always predict the potential for recurrence, necessitating long-term follow-up.

Lipomas and Lipoblastomas

Chest wall lipoma is a common incidental finding, occurring in 0.1% of all computed tomography (CT) scans of the chest.[108] Lipoblastoma is a tumor of embryonic white fat that typically occurs in infancy or early childhood.[109] Both lipomas and lipoblastomas are benign and are best treated by surgical excision of the involved area.

Adenomatoid Tumors

Adenomatoid tumors are very rare incidental findings appearing as solitary circumscribed lesions on either the parietal or visceral pleura. They are usually identified at the time of pulmonary resection for unrelated pathology. They occur more commonly in other sites (most commonly the genital tract) and resection is performed to exclude other malignant pleural tumors.[110]

Calcifying Fibrous Tumors

Calcifying fibrous tumors are rare and are characterized by dense collagenous tissue with psammoma bodies containing dystrophic calcifications. They commonly occur in subcutaneous tissue or in deep soft tissue, but rarely in the pleura (there have been nine reports of this tumor since the initial report in 1996). They can occur as solitary tumors or in multiple sites; calcifications are typically not seen on plain chest films but are seen on a CT scan.[111-118]

Simple Mesothelial Cysts

The pleura is an uncommon site for the development of a mesothelial cyst, which is thought to arise from persistence of the ventral pericardial recess after embryonic development. These lesions often occur in the anterior right cardiophrenic angle. The cysts that retain a connection to the pericardium are called pleuropericardial cysts, and if the neck to the pericardium is pinched off they are classified as mesothelial cysts. They can be treated with surveillance unless symptoms develop, and then they can be treated by either aspiration or excision by VATS.[119,120]

Multicystic Mesothelial Cysts

Multicystic inclusion cysts (multicystic mesothelioma or multilocular inclusion cysts) appear as multilocular fluid-filled cysts spread along the serosal surface of the pleura. There are extremely rare abnormalities occurring in asymptomatic individuals, and their removal to exclude other pathologies can be accomplished by VATS surgery.[121]

Schwannoma

Schwannomas are peripheral nerve sheath tumors that may occur spontaneously or after radiotherapy.[122] They may arise in paraspinal intrathoracic locations and may mimic loculated fibrous deposits or localized pleural tumors. The key to the removal of this tumor is to exclude the possibility of spinal extension to prevent paraplegia from compressive spinal cord hematoma formation caused by bleeding into the peritumoral area.

Pleural Tumors with Low Malignant Potential

Well-Differentiated Papillary Mesothelioma

Well-differentiated papillary mesothelioma typically occurs with a diffuse nodular growth over the mesothelial surface, although there is only superficial invasion without deep invasion except in recurrent or long-standing lesions. Diagnosing this lesion is difficult because it looks similar to invasive mesothelioma (diffuse malignant mesothelioma) on small biopsy specimens. These lesions have an indolent course in the absence of invasive features, and in most instances they do not shorten life expectancy.[123]

Desmoid Tumors

Desmoid tumors, which usually arise from facial or musculoaponeurotic structures, commonly arise from the chest wall with visceral invasion, although pleural desmoid tumors have been documented.[124,125] They may be associated with aggressive fibromatosis via the APC tumor suppressor gene or the β-catenin oncogene acting through the main intracellular effector pathway of the Wingless/Wnt signaling pathway.[126,127]

The treatment of these tumors requires complete resection with negative margins,[124,125,128] although recurrence may occur even with negative margins.[125] However, surgical resection of recurrences has excellent potential for long-term cure.[128]

Pleural Thymoma

Pleural thymomas may arise from the pleura and can appear in either a localized or diffuse form. They probably arise from ectopic thymic tissue in the pleura, although this occurrence is rare (only 15 cases reported by 2002).[129] The localized form can be surgically removed for cure; the diffuse form may require radiotherapy.[123,130]

Primary Malignant Pleural Tumors That May Look Like Benign Tumors

Malignant Solitary Fibrous Tumor

Patients with this tumor, which arises from mesenchymal cells in the submesothelial layer with malignant degeneration, are more likely to present with larger, symptomatic, sessile tumors than their benign pedunculated counterparts.[98,99,131] Visceral-based tumors are less likely to be malignant,[132] and they are more often pedunculated than the parietal-based tumors.[98,100] Malignancy is also more often associated with CT heterogeneity of these tumors, pleural effusions, chest wall invasion, and positivity with positron emission tomography (PET).[99,100] CT-guided aspiration to determine malignancy is notoriously inaccurate,[99,100] possibly because the tumor heterogeneity results in sampling error.

After tumor removal, malignancy is determined on the basis of cellularity and high mitotic counts, nuclear pleomorphism, presence of areas of tumor necrosis, and stromal or vascular invasion. Malignancy occurs in approximately 37% of case series of solitary fibrous tumors (range, 7% to 60%).[100] Recurrence is usually local and strongly associated with malignancy. It occurs with the following frequencies: benign pedunculated, 2%; benign sessile, 8%; malignant pedunculated, 14%; malignant sessile, 63%.[98]

Benign tumors may also recur as malignant tumors,[102,133] indicating the need for long-term follow-up. All tumors and recurrences are best treated with aggressive surgical resection or extended resection if necessary.[98,100] The value of adjuvant therapy for malignant tumors is debated.[98,100,131]

Pleuropulmonary Blastoma

Pleuropulmonary blastoma (PPB) arises from either the lung or the visceral pleural lining and affects children less than 6 years of age. This tumor is unique in its progression from a cystic stage (type I, multilocular cystic tumors), to a more aggressive stage (type II, mixed cystic and solid tumors), and finally to the most aggressive stage (type III, solid tumor). Age correlates with the type of PBB: younger patients (median age, 9 months) tend to have type I, whereas older patients (median age, 42 months) tend to have type III.[134] There is strong evidence for sequential progression of tumor from type I to type II to type III, and recurrences after surgical removal of type I tumors always arise as type II or III tumors, with a low salvage rate.[135] The survival rate after successful resection of type I tumors is 85% to 90%, but it drops to 60% for type II and 45% for type III tumors.[134,136] Important treatment points concerning this tumor are a thorough histologic review of any multiloculated pediatric lung cyst, continued CT surveillance of these patients, and consideration of adjuvant chemotherapy for resected type I tumors.[136]

Localized Malignant Mesothelioma

Localized malignant mesothelioma is a rare tumor: by 2007, only 46 cases had been reported in the English literature.[137] By all histologic, immunohistochemical, and ultrastructural criteria, these tumors are similar to diffuse malignant mesothelioma.[138] Their diagnosis depends on the following factors: (1) radiologic, surgical, or pathologic evidence of a localized serosal or subserosal tumor mass without evidence of diffuse serosal spread, and (2) a microscopic pattern identical to that of diffuse malignant mesothelioma.[139] The small number of case series in the literature do not show it to have a strong association with asbestos exposure.[137] Recurrence after surgical resection may occur either locally or with distant metastases, although only rarely does diffuse pleural spread occur with recurrence, and, in contradistinction to diffuse malignant mesothelioma, many cases are cured by surgical excision.[137,138]

Vascular Sarcoma

The two types of pleural vascular sarcomas are epithelioid hemangioendothelioma and angiosarcoma, and the former has a lesser histologic grade. Both may demonstrate smooth to nodular pleural thickening resembling diffuse malignant mesothelioma. Differentiating these vascular sarcomas from mesothelioma can be done by immunostaining for vascular markers (CD34, CD31, factor VIII).[123,138] Both types are very aggressive, and the outcome is often poor despite aggressive treatment.[140]

Liposarcoma

Liposarcomas are rare (15 cases in the English literature to 2007). They are thought to be derived from residual nests of primitive mesenchymal cells in the pleural cavity. Surgical resection with consideration of postoperative chemotherapy is recommended for these tumors.[123,141]

Pleuropulmonary Synovial Sarcoma

Pleuropulmonary synovial sarcoma is a distinct histologic subtype of sarcoma that is identified as a mesenchymal spindle cell tumor with a specific chromosomal translocation of t(X;18)(p11.2;q11.2). The name is a misnomer, as these tumors have no relationship to synovial tissue. They are thought to derive from totipotential mesenchymal cells with epithelial differentiation. The majority of these tumors are large and pleural based with heterogeneous areas of necrosis or hemorrhage; it is important to differentiate these rare primary pleural tumors from the more frequently seen metastatic synovial sarcoma to the lungs.[142] Only a few anecdotal reports appear in the literature with respect to the treatment of this tumor. All include surgical resection and adjuvant therapy. Chemotherapy or radiotherapy may be added to the treatment regimen, based on soft tissue synovial sarcoma experiences and poor anecdotal results with this tumor in thoracic locations.[142,143]

Askin Tumor or Primitive Neuroectodermal Tumor (PNET)

The Askin tumor, or primitive neuroectodermal tumor (PNET), is a soft tissue tumor that appears either as a single lesion or as multiple pleural nodules in children and young adults. It is classified as a member of the Ewing's sarcoma family because the chromosomal aberration t(11;22)(q24;q12) is peculiar to both tumors. However, PNET originates from soft tissue, whereas Ewing's sarcoma is a tumor of bone. Extrapolated data from a single-center report of treatment of PNET[144] or the combined results of both tumors[145] suggest consideration of neoadjuvant chemotherapy, surgical resection, and adjuvant chemoradiotherapy.

Desmoplastic Small Round Cell Tumor

The desmoplastic small round cell tumor is a rare aggressive malignancy of adolescents and young men; fewer than 10 thoracic cases have been described.[95,146,147] These tumors may remain localized, but more commonly they involve the pleura diffusely. They have a unique expression of epithelial, muscle, and neural markers, with a characteristic fusion protein as a result of gene fusion transcript between the Ewing's sarcoma gene on chromosome 22 and the Wilms' tumor gene on chromosome 11, t(11;22)(p13;q22).[123,138] The prognosis is poor, as it is in patients with abdominal presentations of this tumor.

Malignant Pleural Tumors

Metastatic Malignant Tumors

Metastatic tumors to the pleura are common (>150,000 new cases per year in the United States); the tumor of origin in 75% of cases is lung, breast, or lymphoma, with minor contributions from ovary and stomach. In 5% to 10% of cases, the primary is unknown.[148,149] Patients with metastatic pleural tumors often present with symptoms from a pleural effusion because of lymphatic obstruction of pleural fluid or because of increased capillary permeability in response to tumor invasion, either by direct local tumor extension or by tumors (ovary, breast) with a predilection for serosal invasion by a hematogenous route.[150] Examples of secondary pleural effusions (paramalignant effusions) caused by tumor-associated effusions without direct neoplastic involvement of serosal surfaces are chylothoraces, proximal bronchus obstruction with postobstructive atelectasis, and effusions resulting from cancer cachexia.[149] Metastatic tumors to serosal surfaces resulting in effusions develop site-based cellular differences between effusion tumor cells and cells from the primary or other metastatic sites. Such differences include upregulation of matrix metalloprotein (MMP)-2, and other adhesion molecules (cadherins, integrins), reduced reliance on ERK-driven pathways or chemokines for proliferation, and apoptosis resistance despite increased death receptor expression and in accordance with increased inhibitors of apoptosis proteins.[150]

Determination of malignancy by cytologic examination of pleural effusions ranges from 62% to 90% of patients with malignant pleural effusions; increased test sensitivity can be achieved by repeated thoracocenteses, electro-chemiluminescence immunoassay, genetic analysis by microsatellite analysis, DNA methylation, determination of aneuploidy, and immunocytochemistry by a variety of techniques.[151] Gene expression tests such as EGFR mutation and receptor analysis can be useful both for tumor differentiation and for response to treatment.[152] Malignant pleural effusions can be managed by a variety of techniques with a goal of creating a pleural symphysis. Such techniques range from a variety of catheter drainage procedures with the option of several different sclerosing agents, to pleuroperitoneal shunting or a surgical pleurectomy and decortication.[148,149,151,153,154]

Restraint with respect to aggressive surgical strategies is appropriate, because, apart from breast cancer, the median survival from malignant pleural effusions is less than 6 months.[155] Massive effusions fare worse than lesser effusions.[156]

Diffuse Malignant Pleural Mesothelioma

Diffuse malignant pleural mesothelioma (MPM) is the most common primary pleural tumor, but it occurs less commonly than distant malignancy with metastatic involvement of the pleural surfaces.[151,154] An aggressive tumor, MPM arises from the mesothelial cells of the pleura. Although it can spread systemically, it grows preferentially over serosal surfaces, penetrating the interlobar fissure and eventually encasing the lung. The disease can occur at any site where mesothelial cells de-differentiate from mesenchymal cells, including the peritoneum, pericardium, tunica vaginalis of the testes, and ovary. The pleura, however, is the most common site of involvement of MPM. In the United States, there are approximately 2000 to 3000 new cases each year. Annual mortality rates in Britain and the rest of the world are projected to continue to rise into the next decade, peaking in 2020.[24,157]

Mesothelioma has several histologic subtypes (Fig. 31-1). Epithelial mesothelioma is the most prevalent type, followed by mixed/biphasic, sarcomatous, and, rarely, desmoplastic types.[158] In a large study of 1517 cases, the epithelial cell type was found in 61.5% of the specimens, followed by the biphasic type in 22%, and the sarcomatous type in 16.4%.[159] Unusual histologic subtypes of mesothelioma include tubular, capillary, solid, large or giant cell, small cell, clear-cell, signet cell, glandular, microcystic, myxoid, and adenoid cystic.[160]

Clinical Presentation

In early-stage disease, the symptoms are often subtle and the disease may be identified only because of a serendipitous finding on a chest radiograph performed for other complaints. The most common presenting symptom associated with mesothelioma is dyspnea (80%) caused by restrictive compression of the affected lung. Cough (69%) and weight loss (40%) may also occur; fatigue and weakness are generally later symptoms.[161] Mesothelioma is usually not associated with pleuritic chest pain,[162] which may suggest chest wall invasion. If invasion is confined to a localized area of the chest wall, this may still permit surgical resection. If diffuse, it may indicate nonresectable disease.

Physical examination may reveal a spectrum of signs from minimal disease to an absence of breath sounds suggestive of a unilateral pleural reaction in the involved hemithorax.

The chest radiographs typically reveal a large pleural opacity; this may also be associated with evidence of pleural-based masses (identified as nodular or irregular pleural thickening).[163] In advanced cases, mediastinal compression or intercostal narrowing can be seen on the chest radiograph; rib erosion or periosteal reaction is indicative of chest wall invasion. The chest CT scan is more accurate than plain films for identifying the extent of disease, the potential for lung compression or invasion of local structures, and metastatic spread to the mediastinal nodes. Magnetic resonance imaging (MRI) is generally superior to CT for evaluating diaphragmatic or mediastinal invasion. However, neither mode is 100% accurate, and operative exploration may be required to determine resectability.

Recently, PET-CT imaging has been shown to increase the accuracy of MPM staging,[164] and to indicate extrathoracic

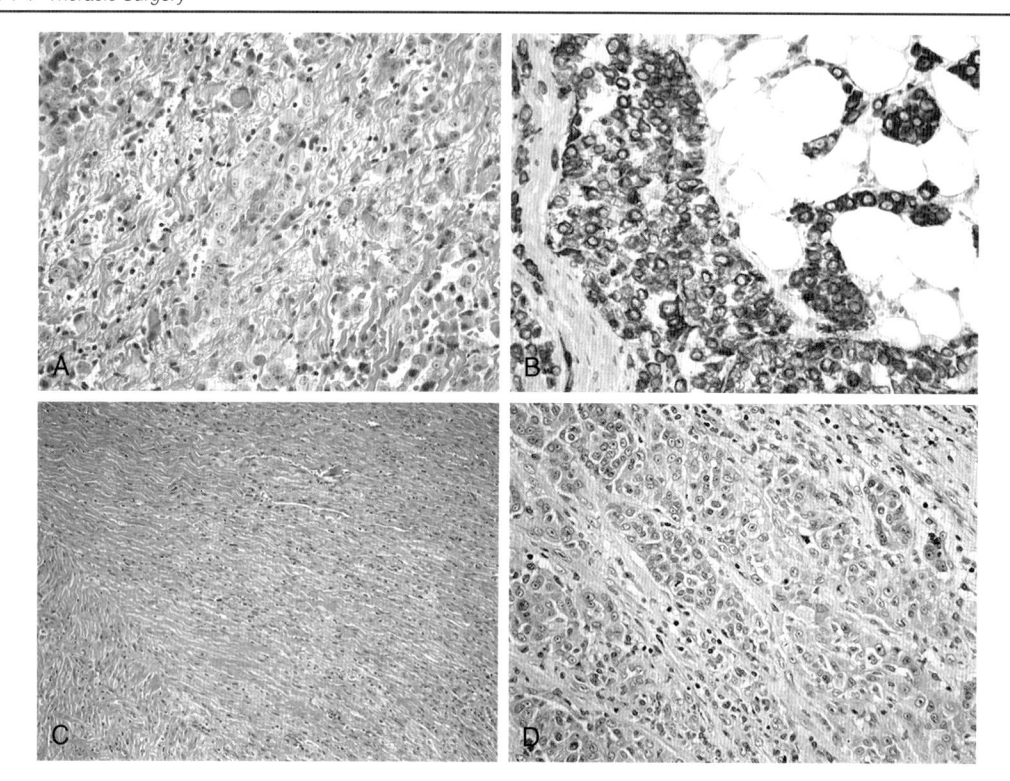

Figure 31–1
The pathologic classification of mesothelioma reveals three histologic patterns. Diffuse malignant mesothelioma is categorized as epithelioid, sarcomatoid, or biphasic (mixed) epithelioid mesothelioma. **A,** Epithelioid subtype (hematoxylin & eosin, ×4000). In this typical photomicrograph of epithelioid mesothelioma, the cells are arranged in a tubular pattern. **B,** Immunostaining pattern of malignant mesothelioma, epithelioid subtype. Note the more solid pattern of cells highlighted with cytokeratin immunostaining (AE1/AE3, ×400). The photomicrograph also demonstrates invasion of tumor cells into the chest wall adipose tissue. **C,** Sarcomatoid subtype (H&E, ×400). Spindle-shaped cells are arranged in sheets or fascicles that form nonspecific architectural patterns resembling those seen in the various sarcomas. **D,** The biphasic or mixed subtype is characterized by the presence of both epithelioid and sarcomatoid components (H&E, ×400). *(Courtesy of Lucian Chirieac, MD, Brigham and Women's Hospital, Boston.)*

occult disease. PET-CT scans are 91% sensitive and 100% specific in differentiating benign from malignant pleural disease.[165]

Histologic identification of the pleural abnormality is required to determine the malignant nature of the pleural mass, as well as to identify the tumor type and subtype. Often, thoracentesis is the initial step for both symptomatic relief of a pleural effusion and diagnosis. However, the cytologic yield from this type of sample is relatively poor, only 62%.[166] The yield from pleural needle biopsy is somewhat better, at 86%.[167] VATS has been shown to be an effective method of enhancing the diagnosis of MPM, and it provides specimens from selected biopsy areas of parietal, visceral, and diaphragmatic pleura.[168] Extensive sampling is often still needed, but collection in this fashion is diagnostic in 98% of patients.

The visual manifestations of mesothelioma as seen either at open thoracotomy or by VATS can be described as localized mass lesions (rarest form), pleural studding and small plaques (discontinuous), pleural masses with variable confluence, and lung encasement with tumor invasion of chest wall and lung.[139,169]

Tissue samples that are removed for histologic evaluation must be carefully evaluated to differentiate between benign proliferative mesothelial processes and malignant mesothelioma. It is also difficult to determine differences between epithelial mesothelioma, sarcomatoid mesothelioma, and sarcoma. Definite stromal invasion is the most reliable indicator of malignancy in both epithelial and spindle cell neoplasms.[170]

Densely packed mesothelial cells in the pleural space are consistent with a benign disease process, but if they are found in the stroma, it is more suggestive of malignant mesothelioma. The three histologic subtypes of malignant mesothelioma are classified according to the relative proportions of epithelial and spindle cells. These include epithelial, sarcomatoid (spindle), and mixed (see Fig. 30-1). The epithelial subtype accounts for over 50% of tumors and needs to be carefully differentiated from adenocarcinoma.[171,172] Electron microscopy may aid in this differentiation. The basement membrane underlying adenocarcinoma cells has a more complete structure than that which underlies mesothelioma cells.[173] Mucopolysaccharide stains (i.e., periodic acid–Schiff, Mayer's mucicarmine) are strongly positive in adenocarcinomas and usually absent in mesotheliomas. The presence of hyaluronic acid strongly supports the diagnosis of mesothelioma. Epithelial mesotheliomas are further characterized not only by their architectural pattern, including tubular, tubulopapillary, papillary, solid, or microcystic types, but also on the basis of their cytologic features, including small cell, large cell, deciduoid, or clear cell types.[174] The sarcomatoid subtype accounts for 15% to 20% of tumors and must be distinguished from sarcomas.[175,176]

Although no single immunohistochemical marker is sufficiently sensitive and specific to differentiate mesothelioma from adenocarcinoma, sarcoma, or reactive mesothelial hyperplasia, a panel of markers is currently used to aid in this distinction.[177] The antibody calretinin demonstrates good specificity for mesothelial cells, whereas carcinoembryonic antigen (CEA) is highly specific for adenocarcinoma.[178] Low-molecular-weight cytokeratin is a general marker of mesothelioma, whereas the high-molecular-weight cytokeratins favor epithelial mesothelioma in particular.[179] Thyroid transcription factor-1 (TTF-1) and E-cadherin stains also help differentiate mesothelioma from adenocarcinoma, as mesothelioma specimens are negative for TTF-1 and adenocarcinomas are positive for E-cadherin.[180] These two markers serve as the frontline immunohistochemical staining for mesothelioma, which can be followed by a secondary panel of antibodies including BerEP4, Leu M1, calretinin, cytokeratin 5/6, and N-cadherin, if necessary. Bueno's group has investigated the role of a technique involving microarray RNA profiling to help distinguish between mesothelioma and adenocarcinoma.[181] This work uses gene product ratios and is a novel approach to diagnosing MPM, with an accuracy of between 95% and 99%.

After histologic confirmation of mesothelioma, the staging of this disease becomes central to determining the best therapy for a particular patient. Staging is equally important in assessing the effectiveness of a new therapy; and it helps to ensure that proper comparisons are made between treatment groups. When study results are reported or compared, it is important to distinguish between clinical and pathologic staging. Unfortunately, there is lack of consensus for a single mesothelioma staging system, and several different staging systems are in use today. These include the Butchart staging system,[182] the TNM staging system set forth by the Union Internationale Contre le Cancer (UICC),[183] the International Mesothelioma Interest Group (IMIG) staging system based on TNM status,[184] and the Brigham and Women's Hospital/Dana-Farber Cancer Institute staging system.[185]

Butchart's classification system for MPM described in 1976 was the first to be introduced and is quite simple, but it fails to provide any prognostic information, as anything beyond stage I is considered unresectable.[182]

The UICC staging system, described in 1990, was based on the TNM cancer staging system used for non–small cell lung cancer (NSCLC).[183] Because of the nature of mesothelioma tumor growth in the pleural space, the T variable as it is described in terms of NSCLC is not always applicable in patients with mesothelioma. Furthermore, although the N nodal description is the same as for NSCLC, in mesothelioma it is often difficult to evaluate nodal stations when the pleural space is completely filled with tumor or effusion. Owing to the short overall survival in mesothelioma, patients often do not live long enough for metastatic disease (M) to be found. Once again, this staging system falls short clinically because it fails to correlate with patient survival and prognosis.

In 1994, another staging system was proposed by the IMIG (Box 31-3). This classification system attempts to account for the unique features of mesothelioma while using the accepted T and N status indicators. In this system, T1a tumors involve the ipsilateral parietal pleura with or without diaphragmatic involvement, and T1b tumors involve the visceral pleura. T2 disease invades the lung parenchyma, so that lung resection would be necessary for complete removal of tumor. These tumors are associated with a pleural effusion. T3 tumors are locally advanced but are still amenable to resection in that there is involvement of endothoracic fascia, mediastinal fat, localized chest wall, or pericardium. T4 disease is technically unresectable and involves invasion of tumor into the chest wall, through the diaphragm into the peritoneum, or into the contralateral pleura, mediastinal organs, spine, internal pericardial surface, or myocardium. Staging of nodal involvement in the IMIG system is similar to NSCLC staging. Stages Ia and Ib correlate with T1aN0 and T1bN0, respectively. Stage II includes T2N0 tumors. Stage III is any T3 or any N1 or N2, and stage IV involves any T4, N3, or M1 disease.

The Brigham and Women's Hospital/Dana-Farber Cancer Institute staging system is simpler than a TNM-based system (Table 31-1) and offers better prognostic value for patients treated with different modalities. Stage I disease is resectable without lymph node involvement. Stage II tumors are also confined to the pleural envelope, but they include positive lymph node (N0 or N1) involvement. Stage III disease is unresectable, with locally aggressive tumors invading the mediastinum, diaphragm, or chest wall with or without extrathoracic or contralateral (N2 or N3) lymph node involvement. Stage IV tumors are associated with extrathoracic metastases. This system stratifies patients according to survival and accounts for resectability, tumor histology, and nodal status. The validity of this staging system has been confirmed in an analysis of a series of 120 patients.[186]

Prognosis

Malignant pleural mesothelioma is a rare but highly aggressive tumor of the pleura that has defied a standard approach to treatment. Without treatment, the median survival ranges from 4 to 12 months.[187-189] Recommended treatment strategies are based on the same principles applied to other solid tumors and include chemotherapy, radiation, surgery, and combinations thereof. Assessment of response to treatment can be measured according to certain criteria.[190] However, mesothelioma tumors have a unique growth pattern with a preference for serosal spreading, which makes the application of conventional response criteria sometimes difficult.[191] A modification of these criteria for tumor response correlates with survival and lung function, and can be used to measure outcome in mesothelioma treatments.[192] In addition to tumor stage, several independent prognostic variables are important and have been defined in two scoring systems.[193,194] These include age, performance status, and histologic subtype. Less important variables include chest pain, dyspnea, presence of pleural effusion, asbestos exposure, weight loss, anemia, leukocytosis, thrombocytosis (platelet count > 400,000/μL), and elevated lactate dehydrogenase (>500 IU/L). The prognostic value of these scoring systems was confirmed in a retrospective review of an independent cohort of patients.[195] Tumors with epithelial histology carry a better prognosis.[196]

Treatment

To date, there are no evidence-based consensus guidelines on the management of MPM. Because of its rare incidence, there are no randomized controlled trials that compare different surgical approaches with one another or that compare surgery to alternative treatments. The cumulative evidence in the literature lies in retrospective case series reports and prospective noncontrolled studies. These data are further confounded by the changing classification and staging systems for mesothelioma.

Box 31-3
International Mesothelioma Interest Group (IMIG) Staging System

T Primary Tumor and Extent

T1
- a Tumor limited to ipsilateral parietal pleura, including mediastinal and diaphragmatic pleura: no involvement of the visceral pleura
- b Tumor involving the ipsilateral parietal pleura, including mediastinal and diaphragmatic pleura; scattered foci or tumor also involving the visceral pleura

T2 Tumor involving each of the ipsilateral pleural surfaces (parietal, mediastinal, diaphragmatic pleura; scattered foci or tumor also involving the visceral pleura)
- Involvement of diaphragmatic muscle
- Confluent visceral pleura (including the fissures) or extension of tumor from visceral pleura into the underlying pulmonary parenchyma

T3 Locally advanced but potentially resectable tumor; tumor involving all of the ipsilateral pleural surfaces (parietal, mediastinal, diaphragmatic, and visceral pleura) with at least one of the following features:
- Involvement of the endothoracic fascia
- Extension into mediastinal fat
- Solitary, complete resectable focus or tumor extending into the soft tissues of the chest wall
- Nontransmural involvement of the pericardium

T4 Locally advanced, technically nonresectable tumor; tumor involving all of the ipsilateral pleural surfaces (parietal, mediastinal, diaphragmatic, and visceral pleura) with at least one of the following features:
- Diffuse extension or multifocal mass of tumor in the chest wall, with or without associated rib destruction
- Direct transdiaphragmatic extension of the tumor to the peritoneum
- Direct extension of tumor to the contralateral pleura
- Direct extension of tumor to one or more mediastinal organs
- Direct extension of tumor into the spine
- Tumor extending through the internal surface of the pericardium without or without a pericardial effusion or tumor involving the myocardium

N Lymph Nodes
- Nx Regional lymph nodes cannot be assessed
- N0 No regional lymph node metastases
- N1 Metastases in ipsilateral bronchopulmonary or hilar lymph nodes
- N2 Metastases in the subcarinal or the ipsilateral mediastinal lymph nodes, including the ipsilateral internal mammary nodes
- N3 Metastases in contralateral mediastinal, contralateral internal mammary, ipsilateral, or contralateral supraclavicular scalene lymph nodes

M Metastases
- Mx Presence of distant metastases cannot be assessed.
- M0 No (known) metastasis
- M1 Distant metastasis present

Stage Grouping

I
- a T1aN0M0
- b T1bN0M0

II T2N0M0

III Any T3M0, any N1M0, any N2M0

IV Any T4, any N3, any M1

Radiation Therapy

Mesothelioma cells have a modest sensitivity to radiation, less sensitive than small cell lung cancer but more than NSCLC.[197] Effective treatment with an intact lung is largely limited by the collateral damage associated with the vital organs in the necessary radiation field.[198] It is difficult to assess the value of radiation therapy, as no large study has compared radiation therapy to no treatment at all. In a small series of 23 patients reported by Ball and coworkers, those patients who received less than 40 Gy did not have effective palliation, whereas those receiving higher dosages were better palliated.[199]

Radiation therapy has been shown to be effective in the prevention of local recurrence after thoracentesis or thoracoscopic biopsy.[200] However, radiation is usually ineffective in controlling disease after partial surgical resections. Dosages must be limited to 20 Gy because of toxicity to the remaining lung. When a patient can undergo extrapleural pneumonectomy (EPP), adjuvant radiation can help reduce local recurrence,

Table 31-1
Brigham Women's Hospital Revised Staging System

I	Disease confined to the capsule of the parietal pleura: ipsilateral pleura, lung, pericardium, diaphragm, or chest wall disease limited to previous biopsy sites
II	All stage I with positive intrathoracic (N0, N1) lymph nodes
III	Local extension of disease into chest wall, mediastinum, or heart, or through diaphragm or peritoneum, with or without extrathoracic or contralateral (N2,3) lymph node involvement
IV	Distant metastatic disease

Box 31-4
Eligibility Criteria for Extrapleural Pneumonectomy

- Karnofsky performance, >70
- Renal function: creatinine, <2
- Liver function: AST, <80 IU/L; total bilirubin, <1.9 mg/dL; PT, <15 sec
- Pulmonary function: postoperative FEV_1, > 0.8 L, as calculated from PFTs and quantitative $\dot{V}/\dot{Q}$ scans
- Cardiac function: normal electrocardiogram and echocardiogram (EF, >45%)
- Extent of disease: limited to ipsilateral hemithorax, with no transdiaphragmatic, transpericardial, or extensive chest wall involvement

AST, aspartate aminotransferase; EF, ejection fraction; FEV_1, forced expiratory volume in 1 sec; PFT, pulmonary function tests; PT, prothrombin time; $\dot{V}/\dot{Q}$, lung ventilation/perfusion quotient.

which arises in the ipsilateral hemithorax in more than 60% of cases. In one nonrandomized study, which did not reach statistical significance, 31% of patients treated with radiation after EPP had local recurrence, as opposed to 45% of patients not treated with adjuvant radiation.[200] Those patients with negative margins did not show any decrease in local recurrence after postoperative radiation, whereas postoperative radiation was found to possibly benefit those with positive resection margins. External beam radiation therapy, previously based on chest radiographs, has evolved to include intensity-modulated regimens based on three-dimensional field planning.[201] With careful intraoperative marking by the surgeon and postoperative planning by the radiation oncologist, intensity-modulated radiation beams maximize targeting of the tumor bed and avoid toxicity to surrounding vital structures.[202]

Chemotherapy

Mesothelioma is relatively chemoresistant, with response rates to single agents less than 20% and no effect on overall survival. The antimetabolites, anthracyclines, and platinum compounds seem to be the most active in mesothelioma. Methotrexate showed a 37% response rate in a phase II trial of 63 patients.[203] However, toxicity was seen in 58% of patients. Detorubicin showed a greater response than doxorubicin in 35 patients, where a response rate of 26% was found.[204] Cisplatin was demonstrated to have a 14% response rate in a Southwest Oncology Group study.[205] At a higher dosing schedule, a 36% response rate was seen.[206] However, there were significant side effects, and these prompted discontinuation in 34% because of toxicity. Carboplatin showed a similar response rate of 11% and is somewhat better tolerated than cisplatin.[204] Vinorelbine also has single-agent activity against mesothelioma, with a low incidence of serious side effects.[207] Partial response with 50% reduction in tumor thickness was seen in 24% of patients, whereas 55% had stable disease (neither 25% increase nor 50% decrease in tumor thickness). Gemcitabine has limited activity when used alone.[208] Pemetrexed has shown some encouraging results in single-agent therapy in 64 patients, where 14% experienced a partial response.[209]

Response rates are increased for combination therapies compared with single-agent treatments.[210] Therefore, single-agent treatment has given way to combination regimens. The results reported by Vogelzang and colleagues showed superior survival time, time to progression, and response rates for patients treated with pemetrexed plus cisplatin versus cisplatin alone.[211] This was a randomized, multicenter, phase III trial in 456 patients. Epithelial histology dominated in over two thirds of the patients, and stage III or IV disease was seen in 78% of cases. Median survival time was 12.1 months in the combined group versus 9.3 months for cisplatin alone, with response rates of 41.3% versus 16.7%, respectively. This combination is now generally accepted as the standard treatment for mesothelioma patients,[212] and further investigations into second-line chemotherapy regimens have begun.[213]

Surgery

Patients must be suitable surgical candidates for thoracotomy before being considered for pleurectomy/decortication (P/D) or EPP. Age and functional status are the first markers to assess. There is no upper age limit; however, caution is required for patients older than 70 or with a Karnofsky performance status of less than 70. Cardiopulmonary function is closely studied: a preoperative forced expiratory volume in 1 second (FEV_1) of less than 2 L, or a predicted postoperative FEV_1 of less than 0.8 L requires more intensive pulmonary investigation. A marginal preoperative FEV_1 warrants a quantitative radionuclide perfusion scan to predict the postoperative pulmonary capacity.[214] Echocardiography provides valuable information, with its ability to assess cardiac function, wall motion abnormalities, valvular disease, and particularly pulmonary artery pressure. If required for further assessment, right heart catheterization may be performed. Left and right ventricular function must be preserved (>45%). Pulmonary hypertension (>45 mm Hg) is a contraindication to EPP.

CT and MRI are used to define the anatomic extent of the tumor and mediastinal or chest wall invasion, and to rule out abdominal extension of disease. CT-PET scanning and cervical mediastinoscopy provide additional staging for extrathoracic disease and lymph node involvement. Metastatic mediastinal node disease confirmed at mediastinoscopy is treated with neoadjuvant chemotherapy in an attempt to downstage the tumor, followed by restaging. The primary goal of surgery is to remove all gross visible tumor (macroscopic complete resection). The eligibility criteria for EPP are listed in Box 31-4.[17,32,82,182,215-219] Patients who do not meet these criteria may still be candidates for pleurectomy.

Extrapleural pneumonectomy. With routine hemodynamic monitoring, an epidural and a double-lumen endotracheal tube in position, a posterolateral thoracotomy is made. The incision begins midway between the posterior scapula and the spine, and extends under the scapular tip along the course of the sixth rib to the costochondral junction.[220] The latissimus and serratus muscles are divided. In general, any prior thoracoscopy port sites or incisions are excised and incorporated into the thoracotomy incision when feasible. The sixth rib is carefully identified and removed from just anterior to the paraspinal ligament posteriorly to the costochondral junction anteriorly. This sets up the start of the extrapleural dissection plane, which is established next. The fused pleura is dissected away from the chest wall until there is room to insert a retractor. Then, the dissection proceeds in an organized manner, packing off any dissected planes to tamponade bleeding during mobilization elsewhere. Blunt dissection using a sponge stick or a finger complements sharp dissection with scissors. Careful attention is given to the subclavian vessels superiorly; the contralateral pleural space and internal thoracic vessels medially; and the azygos vein, superior vena cava, and esophagus (right side) and aorta, intercostal arteries, and esophagus (left side) posteriorly. Continuous reorientation helps avoid inadvertent injury, as does palpation of a properly positioned nasogastric tube.

At this point, a determination is made as to the resectability of the tumor. Once this has been confirmed, the diaphragm is dissected at the anterior border with the chest wall and pericardium. The diaphragm is avulsed from the chest wall by careful manual traction, as opposed to sharp dissection, which can actually lead to more bleeding. Care must be taken to ensure removal of all gross tumor, but it is necessary to leave a rim of the diaphragmatic crus intact for later patch reconstruction. The peritoneum is left intact if at all possible. Next, the pericardium is opened caudally. It is incised anteromedially toward the phrenic nerve and the hilar vessels. The pulmonary veins are divided intrapericardially. The pulmonary artery is taken in similar fashion on the right, but extrapericardially on the left. Each vascular division is done using the endoleader technique and the endoscopic stapling device. Posteriorly, the pericardium is opened at the level of the esophagus on the right and the aorta on the left. The subcarinal lymph nodes are then removed and the bronchus is divided last using a heavy-wire stapler. The ability to visualize this bronchoscopically during the dissection aids in achieving the proper bronchus length. A short, nearly flush bronchial stump reduces the possibility of stump syndrome from airway secretions and helps minimize stump breakdown.

Once the specimen has been removed, additional lymph node stations are sampled and the bronchial stump is leak tested. At this point, a chemical wash is performed, followed by intracavitary heated chemotherapy if not contraindicated. Next, the omentum is mobilized for use as a bronchial stump buttress. Alternatively, this can be covered with a pericardial fat pad buttress. Next, the diaphragm and pericardium are reconstructed using 2- and 1-mm expanded polytetrafluoroethylene (e-PTFE) patches, respectively (Gore-Tex Micro-Mesh; WL Gore, Flagstaff, AZ) (Fig. 31-2). A series of nine stitches is used to secure the patch circumferentially from the posterior paraspinous ligament around to the sixth costal cartilage anteriorly. Gore-Tex buttons or bumpers are used to keep the sutures from pulling through the chest wall (Fig. 31-3). The dynamic two-piece diaphragm patch is then sewn to the base of the pericardium from the anterior costophrenic angle posteriorly toward the esophagus and inferior vena cava (right) or aorta and crus (left) (Fig. 31-4). The impermeable nature of the patch prevents peritoneal fluid from freely crossing into the pleural space postoperatively.

The pericardial patch is fenestrated and sewn in place posteriorly first. It is then secured to the diaphragmatic patch inferiorly and the residual pericardium anteriorly and

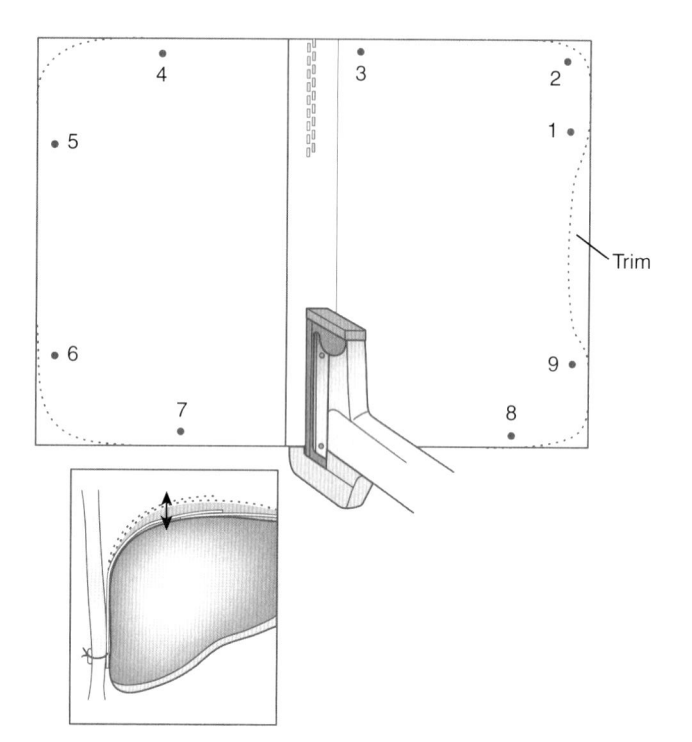

Figure 31–2
Creation of the diaphragmatic patch. Two 2-mm impermeable Gore-Tex patches (Gore-Tex Dual Mesh; WL Gore, Flagstaff, AZ) are overlapped, stapled together, and trimmed to create a dynamic patch with reduced tension along its edges. Nine holes are made along the periphery of the patch to receive interrupted 0 Gore-Tex sutures.

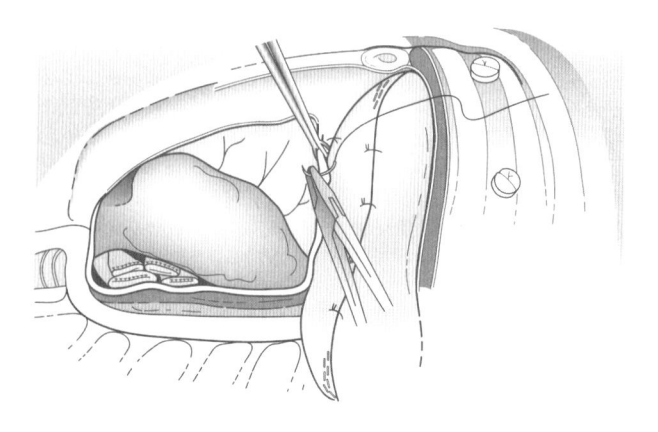

Figure 31–3
Diaphragmatic reconstruction. The sutures on the patch are pulled through the chest wall with an awl and securely tied, from the paraspinous ligament posteriorly to the sixth rib anteriorly. Polytetrafluorethylene (PTFE) buttons or bumpers are placed to prevent the sutures from pulling through the chest wall.

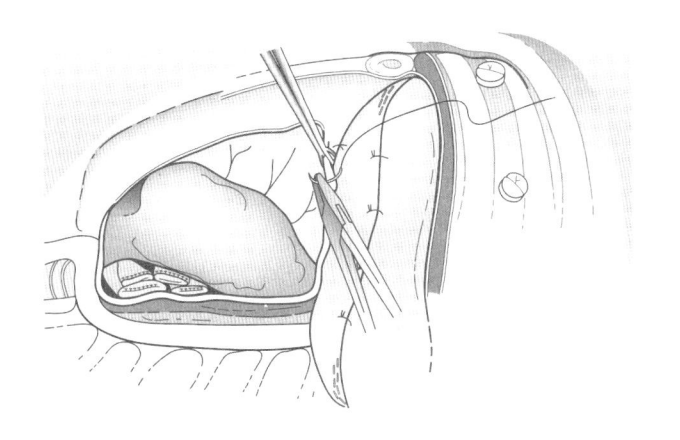

Figure 31–4
Completion of patch reconstruction. The posterior or mediastinal edge of the diaphragmatic patch is sutured to the inferior cut edge of the pericardium. Care is taken to avoid constriction of the inferior vena cava (right side), slitting the patch if necessary, and to avoid intra-abdominal herniation (left side) with healthy bites along the crus and posterior chest wall.

Figure 31–5
The pericardial patch is secured to the posterior, anterior, and superior cut edges of the pericardium. Inferiorly, it is sutured to the diaphragmatic patch itself. Depending on patient size, it may be necessary to splice in an additional patch to avoid cardiac or caval constriction. Displacement of the heart into the pneumonectomy space after closure needs to be taken into account when sizing the pericardial patch during implantation. The pericardial patch should be fenestrated before reconstruction to reduce the chance of pericardial tamponade from fluid accumulation behind the patch.

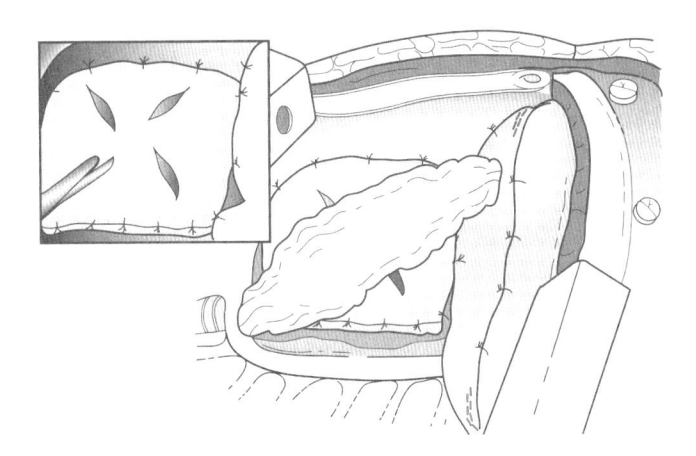

Figure 31–6
A portion of omentum can be mobilized and carefully pulled through the patch to serve as a buttress on the bronchial stump to help prevent bronchopleural fistula.

superiorly (Fig. 31-5). It should not be made too tight, as this may constrict filling of the heart, causing a tamponade effect. This is more important on the right side, given the potential for the heart to turn about the axis of the cavae and herniate. In fact, the left-sided pericardium does not always have to be patched. Once the patches have been placed, an elliptical opening is made in the diaphragmatic patch, and the omentum is pulled through this aperture (Fig. 31-6). It is secured to the bronchus, primarily, with additional bites taken along the surrounding tissues to minimize direct tension. The diaphragmatic patch can be reefed up between the two pieces that make up the dynamic patch, with care not to make the neodiaphragm too tight. Additional bites are taken to secure this patch with the chest wall and diaphragmatic crura posterolaterally. Thorough hemostasis is achieved with an argon beam coagulator. The thoracotomy is closed in standard fashion with care to make it watertight. A 12-French red rubber catheter is left in place for use in balancing the mediastinum intraoperatively. In men, 1000 mL is removed initially after a right EPP (750 mL from the left), whereas in women, 750 mL is taken from the right chest (500 mL from the left side). Additional air is removed in the postoperative setting as needed based on the chest radiograph, with the intention of removing the catheter altogether by the 3rd day.

Pleurectomy. Pleurectomy is a palliative debulking procedure that is combined with decortication for patients with mesothelioma whose pulmonary function or physiologic status contraindicates pneumonectomy. The incision and initial dissection are identical to that described for an EPP. Once the parietal pleura has been dissected free, the tumor itself is incised down to the visceral pleura for an internal pleurectomy. Bleeding can be controlled with an argon beam coagulator or hilar clamping, if needed. It is important to remove as much tumor tissue as possible, especially that extending into the fissures, for a macroscopic complete resection.[221] On the right side, reconstruction of the diaphragm is not always needed, because the liver is there and the lung is left in place.

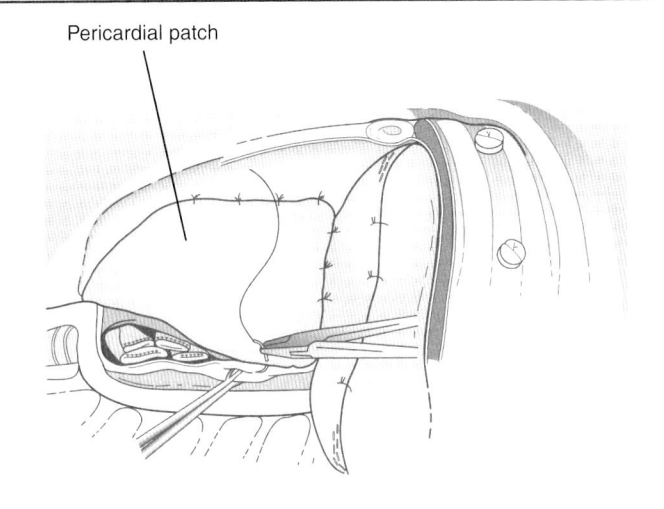

Postoperative Management

Key points in successful recovery of patients in the postoperative setting include pain management, careful fluid balance, and early vigilance for, and diagnosis of, common postoperative complications. These include deep venous thrombosis, pulmonary embolism, vocal cord paralysis, chylothorax, empyema, bronchopleural fistula, and mediastinal shift.[222] Pain is controlled with a thoracic epidural and a patient-controlled analgesia (PCA) pump when needed. Proper pain control and vigorous ambulation (after an initial 48-hour period of mediastinal equilibration for pneumonectomy patients) are critical to preventing contralateral lung atelectasis.

Patients are given a nasogastric tube and nothing by mouth for the first 48 hours. Diet and activity are then advanced as tolerated. There is a low threshold for evaluating the vocal cords in any patient with a voice change or signs of aspiration, as aspiration can have devastating consequences in this patient population. Fluid restriction and liberal use of diuretics help achieve proper fluid balance: pulmonary edema is a dreaded complication of pneumonectomy. Perioperative beta-blockade is administered for prophylaxis of atrial fibrillation. Aggressive screening and prophylaxis for deep venous thrombosis is carried out in every patient.

Operative Results

Several large studies of pleurectomy for mesothelioma have been reported. A series from Memorial Sloan-Kettering listed a mortality rate of 1.8%, complication rate of 25%, and 1-year survival of 49% in 64 patients.[223] In Germany, Achatzy and colleagues reviewed 245 partial and complete pleurectomy cases and showed a 30-day mortality of 8.5% with a median survival of 9.2 months.[224] In 1991, Brancatisano and associates described a series of 45 pleurectomy patients with a mortality rate of 2.2%, morbidity rate of 16%, and median survival of 16 months.[225] Allen and coworkers reported a series of 56 patients with a perioperative mortality of 5.4%, morbidity of 26.8%, and 1-year survival of 30%.[226] More recently, Richards and colleagues reported a retrospective analysis of patients under a protocol for a combined regimen of cytoreduction surgery (pleurectomy or EPP) plus intraoperative intracavitary chemotherapeutic lavage with hyperthermic cisplatin.[221] In a subgroup of patients undergoing pleurectomy at two different dosages of hyperthermic drug delivery—low dosage (50 to 150 mg/m^2) versus high dosage (175 to 250 mg/m^2)—the study found that the subset of patients receiving high-dose chemotherapy demonstrated an apparent survival benefit warranting further investigation. The EPP arm of this phase I study was published in 2009 and reported overall median survival of 17 months (resected 20 months; unresected 10 months). Median survivals for patients receiving the higher cisplatin dose was 26 months and for patients receiving the lower dose, median survival was 16 months (P=.35).[274]

Extrapleural pneumonectomy carries a higher mortality than pleurectomy in most series. The perioperative mortality in Butchart's original series was 30%, which was comparable to that of contemporary studies in the 1970s.[182] Since then, experience from high-volume centers has shown a significant reduction in mortality from EPP to rates of less than 10%. DaValle and colleagues[227] published a mortality rate of 9%, and Rusch and coworkers[228] reported a rate of 6%. Recently, Sugarbaker's group reported a perioperative mortality of 3.4% and morbidity of 25%.[188]

Multimodality Therapy

Early efforts to treat malignant pleural mesothelioma with single therapies failed to have a significant impact on patient survival (Box 31-5). As a result of these failures, a multimodality strategy evolved. The multidisciplinary approach for surgical candidates includes P/D or EPP, external beam radiation to the hemithorax, and systemic combined chemotherapy. Treatment plans involving two modalities, such as chemotherapy and surgery, radiation and surgery, or chemotherapy and

---

Box 31–5
Therapeutic Options for Malignant Pleural Mesothelioma

Single-Modality Therapy
- Debulking surgery (pleurectomy/decortication or extrapleural pneumonectomy)
- Radiation (external beam, brachytherapy)
- Chemotherapy (single- or double-agent approach: doxorubicin, cyclophosphamide, cisplatinum; gemcitabine, pemetrexed (see ref. 265), and cisplatin)

Multimodality Therapy
- Surgery and adjuvant radiation
- Surgery and adjuvant chemotherapy
- Surgery and adjuvant chemoradiotherapy

Innovative Therapies under Investigation
- Intracavitary lavage with hyperthermic chemotherapy
- Photodynamic therapy
- Gene therapy
- Angiogenesis
- Immunogenic therapy

---

radiation, have shown some improvement over single-modality treatment in nonrandomized studies. Chemotherapy or radiation without surgery has had very limited success.[229] Surgery, either as P/D or EPP, combined with chemotherapy or radiation has been found to show some improvement in survival when compared with historical controls. Rusch and colleagues from Memorial Sloan-Kettering reported a series of 105 patients with malignant pleural mesothelioma who underwent P/D combined with intraoperative brachytherapy plus adjuvant external beam radiation.[183] Median survival was 12.5 months, with local relapse the most common treatment failure. In another study from the same institution, 28 mesothelioma patients underwent P/D, this time in conjunction with intrapleural and adjuvant systemic chemotherapy.[230] Overall survival was 68% at 1 year and 40% at 2 years, with locoregional disease the most common relapse.

A seminal article in 1980 by Antman and associates advocated a multimodality approach to malignant mesothelioma after a retrospective review suggested an advantage to aggressive intervention.[231] Antman initiated a prospective multimodality protocol that included EPP followed by adjuvant chemoradiation. In 1991, Sugarbaker reported his first case series of 31 patients who underwent EPP in a trimodality setting. The mortality rate was low (6%), and this study identified trends toward improved survival in the subset of patients with negative histologic margins.[232] During this period, other centers produced case series with improved mortality rates after EPP.[189,227]

A prospective trial by Rusch and coworkers noted a longer progression-free survival with EPP but showed no difference in survival when compared with patients who underwent less radical procedures or nonsurgical treatment.[228] Allen and colleagues published a retrospective case series of patients who underwent either pleurectomy or EPP with adjuvant chemotherapy or radiation therapy.[226] There was a trend toward higher median survival in those who underwent EPP, but it was not statistically significant. Sugarbaker's group described a substantial reduction in operative mortality (4.6%), and in 1993, the Brigham and Women's Hospital/Dana-Farber Cancer Institute combined cancer treatment program identified a subset of patients with epithelial histology and node-negative status that exhibited improved survival.[233,234] The next update in the Brigham series reported a median survival of 21 months in 120 patients.[186] Based on the Brigham staging system, median survival was 22 months for stage I, 17 months for stage II, and 11 months for stage III disease. These data were subsequently updated in 183 patients using the revised Brigham staging system, where N2 disease was reclassified as stage III (instead of stage II) disease, beyond the pleural envelope.[185] This reclassification was in response to a multivariate analysis that showed that the most important predictor of poor outcome after EPP in a trimodal setting was histologic subtype (nonepithelial), positive N2 nodal disease, and positive resection margins.

During this time, the IMIG consortium led by Rusch developed another staging system (see Box 31-3).[184] TNM staging designates the majority of patients as stage III, which has the effect of coalescing patients with different tumor characteristics and obscuring survival benefits associated with such prognostic markers. Nonetheless, the TNM staging system continues to be more widely used. Rusch published a prospective noncontrolled study of a cohort of mesothelioma patients treated with either EPP or pleurectomy followed by adjuvant treatment. Tumor stage had a significant impact on overall survival when considered across all stage groups: stage I had a median survival of 30 months, stage II 19 months, stage III 10 months, and stage IV 8 months. Although there was no significant difference in survival based on type of surgical resection, it should be noted that pleurectomy was performed in patients with minimal visceral pleural tumor, whereas those with more locally advanced tumors underwent EPP.[184] It is important to recognize such a selection bias in operative planning when interpreting results.

As there is much controversy as to the importance of type of surgical resection (P/D versus EPP), the issue is likely to remain unresolved in the absence of randomized controlled trials comparing the two approaches. A recent case series by Stewart and colleagues supports the benefit of EPP over P/D by demonstrating a longer progression-free survival and longer time to local disease progression with EPP.[235] Studies of patterns of failure after multimodality therapy have implicated locoregional recurrence as the most common site of treatment failure. Baldini and colleagues revealed that 25 of 46 patients (54%) developed documented recurrences, with a median time to recurrence of 19 months. The ipsilateral hemithorax was the most common site of recurrence (35%), followed by the abdomen (26%), contralateral hemithorax (17%), and distant disease (8%).[236] This study clearly indicates the locally aggressive nature of malignant mesothelioma and suggests that more effective methods to prevent locoregional recurrence are needed after macroscopic complete resection of this tumor.

Innovative Adjunctive Therapies

Intraoperative Heated Chemotherapy

Intracavitary chemotherapy has been studied in patients with abdominal malignancies as a means of improving locoregional control.[237,238] With intracavitary administration, the chemotherapy agent enters the tumor cells directly by diffusion, thereby minimizing the toxicity associated with systemic delivery. The depth of penetration for chemotherapy agents is only several centimeters deep from surface application[239]; however, this may be sufficient for locoregional control if microscopic control is needed after gross tumor removal. It is important to achieve a macroscopic complete resection before the administration of intracavitary chemotherapy to ensure complete exposure of the chemotherapeutic agent to all surfaces that may harbor cancer cells.[221] The optimal timing for chemotherapy lavage is in the operating room immediately after tumor resection and before the development of adhesions. This allows maximal drug exposure to occur before tumor cells become entrapped in fibrinous exudates and loculated adhesion pockets. In addition, the best time for drug delivery is immediately after resection, when the volume of residual tumor cells is small enough to be penetrated by the chemotherapy drug.

Systemic absorption of intrapleural chemotherapy will occur, with peak plasma levels occurring within 1 hour of intrapleural administration of cisplatin; however, there is a local advantage with respect to pleural to plasma levels using this drug delivery system.[240] Intraoperative caution is needed with respect to crystalloid infusion to prevent postpneumonectomy pulmonary edema, and there is also significant concern about renal toxicity because of potential systemic absorption of cisplatin. Adjunctive methods to mitigate the potential for renal toxicity include the intraoperative administration of thiosulfate and amifostine as cytoprotective agents in combination with intravenous hydration postoperatively.

Hyperthermia has been shown to increase cell permeability, alter cellular metabolism, and improve membrane transport of drugs.[241] A synergistic effect of hyperthermia and cisplatin has been demonstrated (Table 31-2).[242,243] Initial studies with this approach after EPP suggested that median survival could be increased to 18 months,[244] and, in selected patients, long-term control could be achieved.[245] Tilleman et al has recently reported a series of 121 patients treated with heated intraoperative chemotherapy after EPP.[274] In this series, in the group of patients who completed the protocol, there was a mortality of 1.1% and a postoperative morbidity of 48.9%, with significant renal toxicity of 9.8%. The overall median survival of the treatment cohort was 13.1 months, with a cancer-specific survival of 16.9 months. However, in patients with epithelial histology and early stage disease (Brigham and Women's Hospital stage I or II), there was an improved cancer-specific median survival of 21.4 months and 22 months, respectively.[246]

Because of the potential for local recurrence in the hemithorax as well as for regional relapse in the abdomen, the practice of bicavitary intraoperative heated chemotherapy is now used in conjunction with EPP or P/D as part of a multimodality treatment approach in patients with mesothelioma.

Antiangiogenic Therapy

Angiogenesis plays a central role in tumor growth and therefore lends itself as a target in the treatment of cancer patients. The three antiangiogenesis inhibitors currently under trial include thalidomide, SU5416, and bevacizumab. Thalidomide is one of the few orally available antiangiogenic agents. It has shown promise in prolonging disease stabilization with a relatively mild toxicity profile.[247] Studies involving the other

Table 31-2
Hyperthermic Intracavitary Chemotherapy Studies

Study	Patients (N)	Surgery (# Patients)	Intracavitary Chemotherapy	Overall Median Survival (mo)	Cytoprotection	Renal Toxicity (# Patients)
Rusch et al., 1994 (266)	27	P/D	Cisplatin (100-75 mg/m^2) Mitomycin C (8 mg/m^2)	18.3	IV hydration	(2)
Rice et al., 1994 (267)	19	P/D (9) EPP (10)	Cisplatin (100 mg/m^2) Mitomycin C (8 mg/m^2)	13	IV hydration	None
Lee et al., 1995 (268)	15	P/D	Cisplatin (100 mg/m^2) Cytosine arabinoside (1200 mg)	11.5	IV hydration	(1) grade III
Sauter et al., 1995 (269)	13	P/D	Cisplatin (100 mg/m^2) Cytosine arabinoside (1200 mg)	9	IV hydration	(1) grade IV
Colleoni et al., 1996 (270)	20	P/D	Cisplatin (100 mg/m^2) Cytarabine (1000 mg/m^2)	11.5	IV hydration	(2) grade III/IV
Yellin et al., 2001 (245)	7	EPP (4) P/D (1) Thor (2)	Cisplatin (150 mg or 200 mg)	NR	IV hydration	None
Monneuse et al., 2003 (244)	16	P/D	MMC (max, 60 mg), +/- cisplatin (max, 80 mg)	18	IV hydration	None
van Ruth et al., 2003 (271)	20	P/D (12) EPP (8)	Cisplatin 80 mg/m^2 Doxorubicin (20-35 mg/m^2)	11	IV hydration	None
Chang and Sugarbaker, 2004 (272)	50	EPP	Dosage-escalation study. MTD cisplatin 250 mg/m^2	NR	IV sodium thiosulfate concomitant with lavage	NR
Richards et al., 2006 (221)	44	P/D	Cisplatin (MTD 225 mg/m^2)	Survival benefit for high dosage range (18 mo versus 6 mo)	IV sodium thiosulfate after lavage (16 g/m^2 for 6 hr)	(1) grade IV, 2 grade III, 4 grade II
Zellos et al., 2009 (273)	29	EPP	Cisplatin (225 mg/m^2)*	20	IV amifostine (910 mg/m^2) after EPP/before lavage	(8) grade III/IV (reversible in all but 1)
Tilleman et al., 2008 (274)	92	EPP	Cisplatin (225 mg/m^2)	13.1	IV sodium thiosulfate after lavage with and without amifostine (910 mg/m^2) before lavage	(9) grade III/IV (1 not attributable to cisplatin)

*Renal toxicity not related to cisplatin dose; MTD could not be established.
EPP, extrapleural pneumonectomy; MTD, maximum tolerated dose; P/D, pleurectomy/decortication; Thor, thoracotomy (exploration and thoracotomy only followed by intracavitary chemotherapy was performed in 2 patients).
Reproduced with permission from Mujoomdar A, Sugarbaker D: Sem Thorac Cardiovasc Surg 2009;20:298-304.

two drugs involve the vascular endothelial growth factor (VEGF) and endpoints include time to progression of disease and tumor response rate. SU5416 is an inhibitor of the VEGF-1 receptor flk-1 and is being studied by the National Cancer Institute, and bevacizumab is a recombinant anti-VEGF monoclonal antibody under investigation at M. D. Anderson Cancer Center, the University of Chicago, and the University of Pennsylvania.[248]

Photodynamic Therapy

Photodynamic therapy (PDT) is a two-step process that involves first the administration of a photosensitizing agent, such as Photofrin or Foscan. Tumor cells preferentially take up these compounds. The second step involves exposing the affected tumor tissue to light at a certain wavelength. This light catalyzes a cellular reaction in which free radicals are produced and ischemic necrosis occurs. These events lead to damage from direct cytotoxic effects on cellular membranes and from vascular occlusion. Because the depth of tissue penetration of the light is limited, PDT is well suited for use as an intraoperative adjunct after surgical debulking.

Applications of this therapy in mesothelioma patients have been ongoing at a few centers.[249-251] Takita and his group studied Photofrin in 40 patients from 1991 to 1996.[251] Patients underwent pleurectomy or extrapleural pneumonectomy for removal of all gross disease or were debulked to a depth of less than 0.5 cm, followed by intraoperative PDT. Median survival for patients in stages I and II was 36 months and 10 months for patients in stage III and IV. Because of its better profile in terms of increased oxygen singlet production and decreased duration of skin photosensitivity, the photosensitizer Foscan was studied in 26 patients undergoing P/D or EPP in a phase I trial from 1997 to 2001.[249] Median progression-free survival and overall survival were each 12.4 months. These preliminary results will probably lead to a phase II trial.

Immunotherapy

Several studies suggest that mesothelioma cells are susceptible to destruction by immunologic means.[253] Boutin described the activity of intrapleural recombinant gamma-interferon against malignant mesothelioma in 1991.[254] His group has also made use of an implantable access system for prolonged administration of the immunotherapy agents directly into the affected hemithorax, reducing the toxicity and allowing treatment on an outpatient basis.[255] A recent prospective multicenter study of 89 patients with early-stage disease showed an overall response rate of 20%, and the treatment was well tolerated.[256] The exact mechanism of action is not clear, but it may relate to a gamma interferon–mediated inhibitory effect on interleukin-6 (IL-6) production, which may abrogate the systemic manifestations associated with mesothelioma cells.[257]

Other work has been done using the cytokine interleukin-2, which is known to stimulate proliferation of T cells, natural killer cells, and lymphokine activated killer cells. Repeated intrapleural instillation of IL-2 was given twice weekly for 4 weeks during a phase II trial in 31 patients, 22 of whom were in stage I.[258] Pleural fluid collections were effectively treated in 90% of patients, and median overall survival was 15 months. In another study, treatment with IL-2 yielded an overall response rate of 47% in a phase I trial and 55% in phase II testing.[259] Monti demonstrated the in situ activation of CD8+ cells and macrophages after the administration of gamma-interferon.[260] Despite the theoretical considerations, a phase II trial using an infusion of activated macrophages and gamma-interferon did not show an improvement in antitumoral activity.[261]

Gene Therapy

Gene transfer techniques can be used to alter cells to enhance immunogenicity. This can be done in several ways, including by transfection and expression of genes for various cytokines and costimulatory molecules.[262] In a murine model of mesothelioma, flank tumors were treated with adenovirus-encoding beta-interferon.[263] Tumors treated before debulking increased long-term tumor-free survival and resulted in twofold to sixfold smaller foci of implanted tumor cells at 2 weeks postoperatively. It was postulated that elimination of residual tumor cells occurred because of an amplification of the cytotoxic T-lymphocyte antitumor response mediated by adenovirus-encoding beta-interferon.

Recently, a small study of 21 patients with mesothelioma used high-dose therapy with a vector that encoded the herpes simplex virus thymidine kinase.[264] A spectrum of clinical responses was observed, including in two patients followed for 6 years after gene transfer therapy. It is thought that in the future, augmenting the immune effects of gene transfers may lead to increased numbers of therapeutic responses.

Acknowledgments

The authors wish to thank Bill Richards, PhD, and Ann S. Adams, Medical Editor, for contributions made to this chapter.

REFERENCES

1. English JC, Leslie KO. Pathology of the pleura. *Clin Chest Med* 2006;**27**:157-80.
2. Craighead JE, Mossman BT, Bradley BJ. Comparative studies on the cytotoxicity of amphibole and serpentine asbestos. *Environ Health Perspect* 1980;**34**:37-46.
3. Mancuso TF. Relative risk of mesothelioma among railroad machinists exposed to chrysotile. *Am J Ind Med* 1988;**13**:639-57.
4. Nicholson WJ. The carcinogenicity of chrysotile asbestos: a review. *Ind Health* 2001;**39**:57-64.
5. Stanton MF, Wrench C. Mechanisms of mesothelioma induction with asbestos and fibrous glass. *J Natl Cancer Inst* 1972;**48**:797-821.
6. Miller BG, Searl A, Davis JM, Donaldson K, Cullen RT, Bolton RE, et al. Influence of fibre length, dissolution and biopersistence on the production of mesothelioma in the rat peritoneal cavity. *Ann Occup Hyg* 1999;**43**:155-66.
7. Miller BG, Jones AD, Searl A, Buchanan D, Cullen RT, Soutar CA, et al. Influence of characteristics of inhaled fibres on development of tumours in the rat lung. *Ann Occup Hyg* 1999;**43**:167-79.
8. McDonald JC, Armstrong BG, Edwards CW, Gibbs AR, Lloyd HM, Pooley FD, et al. Case-referent survey of young adults with mesothelioma: I. Lung fibre analyses. *Ann Occup Hyg* 2001;**45**:513-8.
9. Report on the expert panel on health effects of asbestos and synthetic vitreous fibers: the influence of fiber length. Prepared for Agency for Toxic Substances and Disease Registry Division of Health Assessment and Consultation, Atlanta, GA; 2003. Available at www.atsdr.cdc.gov/HAC/asbestospanel/finalpart1.pdf. Accessed 4/12/09.
10. Wagner JC, Sleggs CA, Marchand P. Diffuse pleural mesothelioma and asbestos exposure in the North Western Cape Province. *Br J Ind Med* 1960;**17**:260-71.
11. Stout A. Localized pleural mesothelioma: investigation of its characteristics and histogenesis by the method of tissue culture. *Arch Pathol* 1942;**34**:951-64.
12. Cooke W. Fibrosis of the lungs due to the inhalation of asbestos dust. *BMJ* 1924;**2**:147.
13. Lynch K, Smith W. Pulmonary asbestosis III: Carcinoma of lung in asbestos-silicosis. *Am J Cancer* 1935;**24**:56-64.
14. Lynch K, Smith W. Pulmonary asbestosis: a report of bronchial carcinoma and epithelial metaplasia. *Am J Cancer* 1939;**36**:567-73.
15. Selikoff I, Churg J, Hammond E. Asbestos exposure and neoplasia. *JAMA* 1964;**188**:22-6.
16. Selikoff I. Cancer risk of asbestos exposure. In: Hiatt R, Winston J, editors. *Origins of human cancer.* New York: Cold Spring Harbor; 1977. p. 1765-84.
17. Britton M. The epidemiology of mesothelioma. *Semin Oncol* 2002;**29**:18-25.
18. Kukreja J, Jaklitsch MT, Wiener DC, Sugarbaker DJ, Burgers S, Baas P. Malignant pleural mesothelioma: overview of the North American and European experience. *Thorac Surg Clin* 2004;**14**:435-45.
19. McDonald JC. Health implications of environmental exposure to asbestos. *Environ Health Perspect* 1985;**62**:319-28.
20. Pass HI, Lott D, Lonardo F, Harbut M, Liu Z, Tang N, et al. Asbestos exposure, pleural mesothelioma, and serum osteopontin levels. *N Engl J Med* 2005;**353**:1564-73.
21. Rizzo P, Bocchetta M, Powers A, Foddis R, Stekala E, Pass HI, Carbone M. SV40 and the pathogenesis of mesothelioma. *Semin Cancer Biol* 2001;**11**:63-71.
22. Roggli VL, Sharma A, Butnor KJ, Sporn T, Vollmer RT. Malignant mesothelioma and occupational exposure to asbestos: a clinicopathological correlation of 1445 cases. *Ultrastruct Pathol* 2002;**26**:55-65.
23. Powers A, Carbone M. The role of environmental carcinogens, viruses and genetic predisposition in the pathogenesis of mesothelioma. *Cancer Biol Ther* 2002;**1**:348-53.

24. Peto J, Decarli A, La Vecchia C, Levi F, Negri E. The European mesothelioma epidemic. *Br J Cancer* 1999;**79**:666-72.
25. Leigh J, Robinson B. The history of mesothelioma in Australia 1945-2001. In: Robinson BWS, Chahinian PA, editors. *Mesothelioma*. London: Martin Dunitz; 2002. p. 55-110.
26. Robinson BW, Lake RA. Advances in malignant mesothelioma. *N Engl J Med* 2005;**353**:1591-603.
27. Ismail-Khan R, Robinson LA, Williams Jr CC, Garrett CR, Bepler G, Simon GR. Malignant pleural mesothelioma: a comprehensive review. *Cancer Control* 2006;**13**:255-63.
28. Ferrante D, Bertolotti M, Todesco A, Mirabelli D, Terracini B, Magnani C. Cancer mortality and incidence of mesothelioma in a cohort of wives of asbestos workers in Casale Monferrato, Italy. *Environ Health Perspect* 2007;**115**:1401-5.
29. Baris YI, Artvinli M, Sahin AA. Environmental mesothelioma in Turkey. *Ann N Y Acad Sci* 1979;**330**:423-32.
30. Roushdy-Hammady I, Siegel J, Emri S, Testa JR, Carbone M. Genetic-susceptibility factor and malignant mesothelioma in the Cappadocian region of Turkey. *Lancet* 2001;**357**:444-5.
31. Das PB, Fletcher AG, Deodhare SG. Mesothelioma in an agricultural community of India: a clinicopathological study. *Aust N Z J Surg* 1976; **46**:218-26.
32. Carbone M, Kratzke RA, Testa JR. The pathogenesis of mesothelioma. *Semin Oncol* 2002;**29**:2-17.
33. Cristaudo A, Foddis R, Vivaldi A, Buselli R, Gattini V, Guglielmi G, et al. SV40 enhances the risk of malignant mesothelioma among people exposed to asbestos: a molecular epidemiologic case-control study. *Cancer Res* 2005;**65**:3049-52.
34. Fraire AE, Cooper S, Greenberg SD, Buffler P, Langston C. Mesothelioma of childhood. *Cancer* 1988;**62**:838-47.
35. Jantz MA, Antony VB. Pleural fibrosis. *Clin Chest Med* 2006;**27**:181-91.
36. Bocchetta M, Di Resta I, Powers A, Fresco R, Tosolini A, Testa JR, et al. Human mesothelial cells are unusually susceptible to simian virus 40-mediated transformation and asbestos cocarcinogenicity. *Proc Natl Acad Sci U S A* 2000;**97**:10214-9.
37. Adamson IY, Bakowska J, Bowden DH. Mesothelial cell proliferation after instillation of long or short asbestos fibers into mouse lung. *Am J Pathol* 1993;**142**:1209-16.
38. Yang H, Bocchetta M, Kroczynska B, Elmishad AG, Chen Y, Liu Z, et al. TNF-alpha inhibits asbestos-induced cytotoxicity via a NF-kappaB-dependent pathway, a possible mechanism for asbestos-induced oncogenesis. *Proc Natl Acad Sci U S A* 2006;**103**:10397-402.
39. Gulumian M, van Wyk JA. Hydroxyl radical production in the presence of fibres by a Fenton-type reaction. *Chem Biol Interact* 1987;**62**:89-97.
40. Kamp DW, Israbian VA, Preusen SE, Zhang CX, Weitzman SA. Asbestos causes DNA strand breaks in cultured pulmonary epithelial cells: role of iron-catalyzed free radicals. *Am J Physiol* 1995;**268**:L471-80.
41. Adamson IY, Bakowska J. KGF and HGF are growth factors for mesothelial cells in pleural lavage fluid after intratracheal asbestos. *Exp Lung Res* 2001;**27**:605-16.
42. Walker C, Everitt J, Ferriola PC, Stewart W, Mangum J, Bermudez E. Autocrine growth stimulation by transforming growth factor alpha in asbestos-transformed rat mesothelial cells. *Cancer Res* 1995;**55**:530-6.
43. Zanella CL, Posada J, Tritton TR, Mossman BT. Asbestos causes stimulation of the extracellular signal-regulated kinase 1 mitogen-activated protein kinase cascade after phosphorylation of the epidermal growth factor receptor. *Cancer Res* 1996;**56**:5334-8.
44. Xu A, Huang X, Lien YC, Bao L, Yu Z, Hei TK. Genotoxic mechanisms of asbestos fibers: role of extranuclear targets. *Chem Res Toxicol* 2007;**20**:724-33.
45. Jaurand MC. Mechanisms of fiber-induced genotoxicity. *Environ Health Perspect* 1997;**105**(Suppl. 5):1073-84.
46. Ault JG, Cole RW, Jensen CG, Jensen LC, Bachert LA, Rieder CL. Behavior of crocidolite asbestos during mitosis in living vertebrate lung epithelial cells. *Cancer Res* 1995;**55**:792-8.
47. Christensen BC, Godleski JJ, Marsit CJ, Houseman EA, Lopez-Fagundo CY, Longacker JL, et al. Asbestos exposure predicts cell cycle control gene promoter methylation in pleural mesothelioma. *Carcinogenesis* 2008;**29**:1555-9.
48. Haber DA, Settleman J. Cancer: drivers and passengers. *Nature* 2007;**446**:145-6.
49. Greenman C, Stephens P, Smith R, Dalgliesh GL, Hunter C, Bignell G, et al. Patterns of somatic mutation in human cancer genomes. *Nature* 2007;**446**:153-8.
50. Musti M, Kettunen E, Dragonieri S, Lindholm P, Cavone D, Serio G, Knuutila S. Cytogenetic and molecular genetic changes in malignant mesothelioma. *Cancer Genet Cytogenet* 2006;**170**:9-15.
51. Sugarbaker DJ, Richards WG, Gordon GJ, Dong L, De Rienzo A, Maulik G, et al. Transcriptome sequencing of malignant pleural mesothelioma tumors. *Proc Natl Acad Sci U S A* 2008;**105**:3521-6.
52. Cheng JQ, Jhanwar SC, Klein WM, Bell DW, Lee WC, Altomare DA, et al. p16 alterations and deletion mapping of 9p21-p22 in malignant mesothelioma. *Cancer Res* 1994;**54**:5547-51.
53. Hirao T, Bueno R, Chen CJ, Gordon GJ, Heilig E, Kelsey KT. Alterations of the p16(INK4) locus in human malignant mesothelial tumors. *Carcinogenesis* 2002;**23**:1127-30.
54. Baldi A, Groeger AM, Esposito V, Cassandro R, Tonini G, Battista T, et al. Expression of p21 in SV40 large T antigen positive human pleural mesothelioma: relationship with survival. *Thorax* 2002;**57**:353-6.
55. Flejter WL, Li FP, Antman KH, Testa JR. Recurring loss involving chromosomes 1, 3, and 22 in malignant mesothelioma: possible sites of tumor suppressor genes. *Genes Chromosomes Cancer* 1989(1):148-54.
56. Mor O, Yaron P, Huszar M, Yellin A, Jakobovitz O, Brok-Simoni F, et al. Absence of p53 mutations in malignant mesotheliomas. *Am J Respir Cell Mol Biol* 1997;**16**:9-13.
57. Lee AY, Raz DJ, He B, Jablons DM. Update on the molecular biology of malignant mesothelioma. *Cancer* 2007;**109**:1454-61.
58. Yang CT, You L, Yeh CC, Chang JW, Zhang F, McCormick F, Jablons DM. Adenovirus-mediated p14(ARF) gene transfer in human mesothelioma cells. *J Natl Cancer Inst* 2000;**92**:636-41.
59. Illei PB, Rusch VW, Zakowski MF, Ladanyi M. Homozygous deletion of CDKN2A and codeletion of the methylthioadenosine phosphorylase gene in the majority of pleural mesotheliomas. *Clin Cancer Res* 2003;**9**:2108-13.
60. Frizelle SP, Grim J, Zhou J, Gupta P, Curiel DT, Geradts J, Kratzke RA. Re-expression of p16INK4a in mesothelioma cells results in cell cycle arrest, cell death, tumor suppression and tumor regression. *Oncogene* 1998;**16**:3087-95.
61. Schipper H, Papp T, Johnen G, Pemsel H, Bastrop R, Muller KM, et al. Mutational analysis of the nf2 tumour suppressor gene in three subtypes of primary human malignant mesotheliomas. *Int J Oncol* 2003;**22**:1009-17.
62. Xiao GH, Gallagher R, Shetler J, Skele K, Altomare DA, Pestell RG, et al. The NF2 tumor suppressor gene product, merlin, inhibits cell proliferation and cell cycle progression by repressing cyclin D1 expression. *Mol Cell Biol* 2005;**25**:2384-94.
63. Jung JR, Kim H, Jeun SS, Lee JY, Koh EJ, Ji C. The Phosphorylation status of merlin is important for regulating the Ras-ERK pathway. *Mol Cells* 2005;**20**:196-200.
64. Lallemand D, Curto M, Saotome I, Giovannini M, McClatchey AI. NF2 deficiency promotes tumorigenesis and metastasis by destabilizing adherens junctions. *Genes Dev* 2003;**17**:1090-100.
65. Ramos-Nino ME, Timblin CR, Mossman BT. Mesothelial cell transformation requires increased AP-1 binding activity and ERK-dependent Fra-1 expression. *Cancer Res* 2002;**62**:6065-9.
66. Abutaily AS, Collins JE, Roche WR. Cadherins, catenins and APC in pleural malignant mesothelioma. *J Pathol* 2003;**201**:355-62.
67. Lee AY, He B, You L, Xu Z, Mazieres J, Reguart N, et al. Dickkopf-1 antagonizes Wnt signaling independent of beta-catenin in human mesothelioma. *Biochem Biophys Res Commun* 2004;**323**:1246-50.
68. Lee AY, He B, You L, Dadfarmay S, Xu Z, Mazieres J, et al. Expression of the secreted frizzled-related protein gene family is downregulated in human mesothelioma. *Oncogene* 2004;**23**:6672-6.
69. Batra S, Shi Y, Kuchenbecker KM, He B, Reguart N, Mikami I, et al. Wnt inhibitory factor-1, a Wnt antagonist, is silenced by promoter hypermethylation in malignant pleural mesothelioma. *Biochem Biophys Res Commun* 2006;**342**:1228-32.
70. He B, Lee AY, Dadfarmay S, You L, Xu Z, Reguart N, et al. Secreted frizzled-related protein 4 is silenced by hypermethylation and induces apoptosis in beta-catenin-deficient human mesothelioma cells. *Cancer Res* 2005;**65**:743-8.
71. Toyooka S, Carbone M, Toyooka KO, Bocchetta M, Shivapurkar N, Minna JD, Gazdar AF. Progressive aberrant methylation of the RASSF1A gene in simian virus 40 infected human mesothelial cells. *Oncogene* 2002;**21**:4340-4.
72. Baylin SB, Ohm JE. Epigenetic gene silencing in cancer: a mechanism for early oncogenic pathway addiction? *Nat Rev Cancer* 2006;**6**:107-16.
73. Versnel MA, Hagemeijer A, Bouts MJ, van der Kwast TH, Hoogsteden HC. Expression of c-sis (PDGF B-chain) and PDGF A-chain genes in ten human malignant mesothelioma cell lines derived from primary and metastatic tumors. *Oncogene* 1988;**2**:601-5.
74. Jagadeeswaran R, Ma PC, Seiwert TY, Jagadeeswaran S, Zumba O, Nallasura V, et al. Functional analysis of c-Met/hepatocyte growth factor pathway in malignant pleural mesothelioma. *Cancer Res* 2006;**66**:352-61.
75. Whitson BA, Kratzke RA. Molecular pathways in malignant pleural mesothelioma. *Cancer Lett* 2006;**239**:183-9.

76. Govindan R, Kratzke RA, Herndon 2nd JE, Niehans GA, Vollmer R, Watson D, et al. Gefitinib in patients with malignant mesothelioma: a phase II study by the Cancer and Leukemia Group B. *Clin Cancer Res* 2005;**11**:2300-4.
77. Masood R, Kundra A, Zhu S, Xia G, Scalia P, Smith DL, Gill PS. Malignant mesothelioma growth inhibition by agents that target the VEGF and VEGF-C autocrine loops. *Int J Cancer* 2003;**104**:603-10.
78. Cacciotti P, Libener R, Betta P, Martini F, Porta C, Procopio A, et al. SV40 replication in human mesothelial cells induces HGF/Met receptor activation: a model for viral-related carcinogenesis of human malignant mesothelioma. *Proc Natl Acad Sci U S A* 2001;**98**:12032-7.
79. Kindler HL. Moving beyond chemotherapy: novel cytostatic agents for malignant mesothelioma. *Lung Cancer* 2004;**45**(Suppl. 1):S125-7.
80. Catalano A, Gianni W, Procopio A. Experimental therapy of malignant mesothelioma: new perspectives from anti-angiogenic treatments. *Crit Rev Oncol Hematol* 2004;**50**:101-9.
81. Vilchez RA, Kozinetz CA, Arrington AS, Madden CR, Butel JS. Simian virus 40 in human cancers. *Am J Med* 2003;**114**:675-84.
82. Cacciotti P, Strizzi L, Vianale G, Iaccheri L, Libener R, Porta C, et al. The presence of simian-virus 40 sequences in mesothelioma and mesothelial cells is associated with high levels of vascular endothelial growth factor. *Am J Respir Cell Mol Biol* 2002;**26**:189-93.
83. Foddis R, De Rienzo A, Broccoli D, Bocchetta M, Stekala E, Rizzo P, et al. SV40 infection induces telomerase activity in human mesothelial cells. *Oncogene* 2002;**21**:1434-42.
84. Barbanti-Brodano G, Sabbioni S, Martini F, Negrini M, Corallini A, Tognon M. Simian virus 40 infection in humans and association with human diseases: results and hypotheses. *Virology* 2004;**318**:1-9.
85. Shah K. SV40 and human cancer: a review of recent data. *Int J Cancer* 2007;**15**:215-23.
86. Engels E. Does simian virus 40 cause non-Hodgkin lymphoma? A review of the laboratory and epidemiological evidence. *Cancer Invest* 2005;**23**:529-36.
87. Manfredi JJ, Dong J, Liu WJ, Resnick-Silverman L, Qiao R, Chahinian P, et al. Evidence against a role for SV40 in human mesothelioma. *Cancer Res* 2005;**65**:2602-9.
88. Soini Y, Kinnula V, Kaarteenaho-Wiik R, Kurttila E, Linnainmaa K, Paakko P. Apoptosis and expression of apoptosis regulating proteins bcl-2, mcl-1, bcl-X, and bax in malignant mesothelioma. *Clin Cancer Res* 1999;**5**:3508-15.
89. Smythe WR, Mohuiddin I, Ozveran M, Cao XX. Antisense therapy for malignant mesothelioma with oligonucleotides targeting the bcl-xl gene product. *J Thorac Cardiovasc Surg* 2002;**123**:1191-8.
90. Pataer A, Smythe WR, Yu R, Fang B, McDonnell T, Roth JA, Swisher SG. Adenovirus-mediated Bak gene transfer induces apoptosis in mesothelioma cell lines. *J Thorac Cardiovasc Surg* 2001;**121**:61-7.
91. Mollo F, Andrion A, Colombo A, Segnan N, Pira E. Pleural plaques and risk of cancer in Turin, northwestern Italy. An autopsy study. *Cancer* 1984;**54**:1418-22.
92. Chapman SJ, Cookson WO, Musk AW, Lee YC. Benign asbestos pleural diseases. *Curr Opin Pulm Med* 2003;**9**:266-71.
93. Bahadori M, Liebow AA. Plasma cell granulomas of the lung. *Cancer* 1973;**31**:191-208.
94. Ishioka S, Maeda A, Yamasaki M, Yamakido M. Inflammatory pseudotumor of the lung with pleural thickening treated with corticosteroids. *Chest* 2000;**117**:923.
95. Cagle PT, Churg A. Differential diagnosis of benign and malignant mesothelial proliferations on pleural biopsies. *Arch Pathol Lab Med* 2005;**129**:1421-7.
96. King J, Thatcher N, Pickering C, Hasleton P. Sensitivity and specificity of immunohistochemical antibodies used to distinguish between benign and malignant pleural disease: a systematic review of published reports. *Histopathology* 2006;**49**:561-8.
97. Scurry J, Duggan MA. Malignant mesothelioma eight years after a diagnosis of atypical mesothelial hyperplasia. *J Clin Pathol* 1999;**52**:535-7.
98. de Perrot M, Fischer S, Brundler MA, Sekine Y, Keshavjee S. Solitary fibrous tumors of the pleura. *Ann Thorac Surg* 2002;**74**:285-93.
99. Kohler M, Clarenbach CF, Kestenholz P, Kurrer M, Steinert HC, Russi EW, Weder W. Diagnosis, treatment and long-term outcome of solitary fibrous tumours of the pleura. *Eur J Cardiothorac Surg* 2007;**32**:403-8.
100. Magdeleinat P, Alifano M, Petino A, Le Rochais JP, Dulmet E, Galateau F, et al. Solitary fibrous tumors of the pleura: clinical characteristics, surgical treatment and outcome. *Eur J Cardiothorac Surg* 2002;**21**:1087-93.
101. Moran CA, Suster S, Koss MN. The spectrum of histologic growth patterns in benign and malignant fibrous tumors of the pleura. *Semin Diagn Pathol* 1992;**9**:169-80.
102. Krishnadas R, Froeschle PO, Berrisford RG. Recurrence and malignant transformation in solitary fibrous tumour of the pleura. *Thorac Cardiovasc Surg* 2006;**54**:65-7.
103. Zellos L, Sugarbaker DJ. Current surgical management of malignant pleural mesothelioma. *Curr Oncol Rep* 2002;**4**:354-60.
104. Tastepe I, Alper A, Ozaydin HE, Memis L, Cetin G. A case of multiple synchronous localized fibrous tumor of the pleura. *Eur J Cardiothorac Surg* 2000;**18**:491-4.
105. Cardillo G, Facciolo F, Cavazzana AO, Capece G, Gasparri R, Martelli M. Localized (solitary) fibrous tumors of the pleura: an analysis of 55 patients. *Ann Thorac Surg* 2000;**70**:1808-12.
106. Robinson LA. Solitary fibrous tumor of the pleura. *Cancer Control* 2006;**13**:264-9.
107. Hirai A, Nakanishi R. Solitary fibrous tumor of the pleura with hypoglycemia associated with serum insulin-like growth factor II. *J Thorac Cardiovasc Surg* 2006;**132**:713-4.
108. Buirski G, Goddard P, The CT. diagnosis of pleural lipoma. *Bristol Med Chir J* 1986;**101**:43.
109. Kwak JY, Ha DH, Kim YA, Shim JY. Lipoblastoma of the parietal pleura in a 7-month-old infant. *J Comput Assist Tomogr* 1999;**23**:952-4.
110. Kaplan MA, Tazelaar HD, Hayashi T, Schroer KR, Travis WD. Adenomatoid tumors of the pleura. *Am J Surg Pathol* 1996;**20**:1219-23.
111. Jang KS, Oh YH, Han HX, Chon SH, Chung WS, Park CK, Paik SS. Calcifying fibrous pseudotumor of the pleura. *Ann Thorac Surg* 2004;**78**:e87-8.
112. Soyer T, Ciftci AO, Gucer S, Orhan D, Senocak ME. Calcifying fibrous pseudotumor of lung: a previously unreported entity. *J Pediatr Surg* 2004;**39**:1729-30.
113. Ammar A, El Hammami S, Horchani H, Sellami N, Kilani T. Calcifying fibrous pseudotumor of the pleura: a rare location. *Ann Thorac Surg* 2003;**76**:2081-2.
114. Cavassa A, Gelli M, Agostini L, Sgarbi G, De Marco L, Gardini G. Calcified pseudotumor of the pleura: a description of a case. *Pathologica* 2002;**94**:201-5.
115. Hainaut P, Lesage V, Weynand B, Coche E, Noirhomme P. Calcifying fibrous pseudotumor (CFPT): a patient presenting with multiple pleural lesions. *Acta Clin Belg* 1999;**54**:162-4.
116. Jeong HS, Lee GK, Sung R, Ahn JH, Song HG. Calcifying fibrous pseudotumor of mediastinum: a case report. *J Korean Med Sci* 1997;**12**:58-62.
117. Pinkard NB, Wilson RW, Lawless N, Dodd LG, McAdams HP, Koss MN, Travis WD. Calcifying fibrous pseudotumor of pleura. A report of three cases of a newly described entity involving the pleura. *Am J Clin Pathol* 1996;**105**:189-94.
118. Mito K, Kashima K, Daa T, Kondoh Y, Miura T, Kawahara K, et al. Multiple calcifying fibrous tumors of the pleura. *Virchows Arch* 2005;**446**:78-81.
119. Walker MJ, Sieber SC, Boorboor S. Migrating pleural mesothelial cyst. *Ann Thorac Surg* 2004;**77**:701-2.
120. Mouroux J, Venissac N, Leo F, Guillot F, Padovani B, Hofman P. Usual and unusual locations of intrathoracic mesothelial cysts. Is endoscopic resection always possible? *Eur J Cardiothorac Surg* 2003;**24**:684-8.
121. Sasaki H, Yano M, Kiriyama M, Kaji M, Fukai I, Yamakawa Y, et al. Multicystic mesothelial cyst of the mediastinum: report of a case. *Surg Today* 2003;**33**:199-201.
122. Morbidini-Gaffney S, Alpert TE, Hatoum GF, Sagerman RH. Benign pleural schwannoma secondary to radiotherapy for Hodgkin disease. *Am J Clin Oncol* 2005;**28**:640-1.
123. Granville L, Laga AC, Allen TC, Dishop M, Roggli VL, Churg A, et al. Review and update of uncommon primary pleural tumors: a practical approach to diagnosis. *Arch Pathol Lab Med* 2005;**129**:1428-43.
124. Wilson RW, Gallateau-Salle F, Moran CA. Desmoid tumors of the pleura: a clinicopathologic mimic of localized fibrous tumor. *Mod Pathol* 1999;**12**:9-14.
125. Abbas AE, Deschamps C, Cassivi SD, Nichols 3rd FC, Allen MS, Schleck CD, Pairolero PC. Chest-wall desmoid tumors: results of surgical intervention. *Ann Thorac Surg* 2004;**78**:1219-23; discussion 1223.
126. Latchford A, Volikos E, Johnson V, Rogers P, Suraweera N, Tomlinson I, et al. APC mutations in FAP-associated desmoid tumours are non-random but not 'just right'. *Hum Mol Genet* 2007;**16**:78-82.
127. Lips DJ, Barker N, Clevers H, Hennipman A. The role of APC and beta-catenin in the aetiology of aggressive fibromatosis (desmoid tumors). *Eur J Surg Oncol* 2008.
128. Allen PJ, Shriver CD. Desmoid tumors of the chest wall. *Semin Thorac Cardiovasc Surg* 1999;**11**:264-9.
129. Attanoos RL, Galateau-Salle F, Gibbs AR, Muller S, Ghandour F, Dojcinov SD. Primary thymic epithelial tumours of the pleura mimicking malignant mesothelioma. *Histopathology* 2002;**41**:42-9.
130. Sugiura H, Morikawa T, Ito K, Ono K, Okushiba S, Satoshi K, Katoh H. Long-term results of surgical treatment for invasive thymoma. *Anticancer Res* 1999;**19**:1433-7.
131. Sung SH, Chang JW, Kim J, Lee KS, Han J, Park SI. Solitary fibrous tumors of the pleura: surgical outcome and clinical course. *Ann Thorac Surg* 2005;**79**:303-7.
132. Carretta A, Bandiera A, Melloni G, Ciriaco P, Arrigoni G, Rizzo N, et al. Solitary fibrous tumors of the pleura: immunohistochemical analysis and evaluation of prognostic factors after surgical treatment. *J Surg Oncol* 2006;**94**:40-4.
133. Odom SR, Genua JC, Podesta A, Rubin HP. Recurrence of a solitary fibrous tumor of the pleura: a case report. *Conn Med* 2004;**68**:367-70.

134. Hill DA, Jarzembowski JA, Priest JR, Williams G, Schoettler P, Dehner LP. Type I pleuropulmonary blastoma: pathology and biology study of 51 cases from the international pleuropulmonary blastoma registry. *Am J Surg Pathol* 2008;**32**:282-95.
135. Priest JR, Watterson J, Strong L, Huff V, Woods WG, Byrd RL, et al. Pleuropulmonary blastoma: a marker for familial disease. *J Pediatr* 1996;**128**:220-4.
136. Priest JR, Hill DA, Williams GM, Moertel CL, Messinger Y, Finkelstein MJ, Dehner LP. Type I pleuropulmonary blastoma: a report from the International Pleuropulmonary Blastoma Registry. *J Clin Oncol* 2006;**24**:4492-8.
137. Takahashi H, Harada M, Maehara S, Kato H. Localized malignant mesothelioma of the pleura. *Ann Thorac Cardiovasc Surg* 2007;**13**:262-6.
138. Guinee DG, Allen TC. Primary pleural neoplasia: entities other than diffuse malignant mesothelioma. *Arch Pathol Lab Med* 2008;**132**:1149-70.
139. Allen TC, Cagle PT, Churg AM, Colby TV, Gibbs AR, Hammar SP, et al. Localized malignant mesothelioma. *Am J Surg Pathol* 2005;**29**:866-73.
140. Zhang PJ, Livolsi VA, Brooks JJ. Malignant epithelioid vascular tumors of the pleura: report of a series and literature review. *Hum Pathol* 2000;**31**:29-34.
141. Peng C, Zhao X, Dong X, Jiang X. Liposarcoma of the pleural cavity: a case report. *J Thorac Cardiovasc Surg* 2007;**133**:1108-9.
142. Frazier AA, Franks TJ, Pugatch RD, Galvin JR. From the archives of the AFIP: pleuropulmonary synovial sarcoma. *Radiographics* 2006;**26**:923-40.
143. Galetta D, Pelosi G, Leo F, Solli P, Veronesi G, Borri A, et al. Primary thoracic synovial sarcoma: factors affecting long-term survival. *J Thorac Cardiovasc Surg* 2007;**134**:808-9.
144. Veronesi G, Spaggiari L, De Pas T, Solli PG, De Braud F, Catalano GP, et al. Preoperative chemotherapy is essential for conservative surgery of Askin tumors. *J Thorac Cardiovasc Surg* 2003;**125**:428-9.
145. Smorenburg CH, van Groeningen CJ, Meijer OW, Visser M, Boven E. Ewing's sarcoma and primitive neuroectodermal tumour in adults: single-centre experience in The Netherlands. *Neth J Med* 2007;**65**:132-6.
146. Parkash V, Gerald WL, Parma A, Miettinen M, Rosai J. Desmoplastic small round cell tumor of the pleura. *Am J Surg Pathol* 1995;**19**:659-65.
147. Ostoros G, Orosz Z, Kovacs G, Soltesz I. Desmoplastic small round cell tumour of the pleura: a case report with unusual follow-up. *Lung Cancer* 2002;**36**:333-6.
148. Khaleeq G, Musani AI. Emerging paradigms in the management of malignant pleural effusions. *Respir Med* 2008;**102**:939-48.
149. Neragi-Miandoab S. Malignant pleural effusion, current and evolving approaches for its diagnosis and management. *Lung Cancer* 2006;**54**:1-9.
150. Davidson B. Biological characteristics of cancers involving the serosal cavities. *Crit Rev Oncog* 2007;**13**:189-227.
151. Heffner JE. Diagnosis and management of malignant pleural effusions. *Respirology* 2008;**13**:5-20.
152. Hung MS, Lin CK, Leu SW, Wu MY, Tsai YH, Yang CT. Epidermal growth factor receptor mutations in cells from non-small cell lung cancer malignant pleural effusions. *Chang Gung Med J* 2006;**29**:373-9.
153. Haas AR, Sterman DH, Musani AI. Malignant pleural effusions: management options with consideration of coding, billing, and a decision approach. *Chest* 2007;**132**:1036-41.
154. Spector M, Pollak JS. Management of malignant pleural effusions. *Semin Respir Crit Care Med* 2008;**29**:405-13.
155. Marel M, Stastny B, Melinova L, Svandova E, Light RW. Diagnosis of pleural effusions. Experience with clinical studies, 1986 to 1990. *Chest* 1995;**107**:1598-603.
156. Jimenez D, Diaz G, Gil D, Cicero A, Perez-Rodriguez E, Sueiro A, Light RW. Etiology and prognostic significance of massive pleural effusions. *Respir Med* 2005;**99**:1183-7.
157. Peto J, Hodgson JT, Matthews FE, Jones JR. Continuing increase in mesothelioma mortality in Britain. *Lancet* 1995;**345**:535-9.
158. Boutin C. Malignant pleural mesothelioma. *Eur Respir J* 1981;**12**:972-81.
159. Suzuki Y. Pathology of human malignant mesothelioma: preliminary analysis of 1,517 mesothelioma cases. *Ind Health* 2001;**39**:183-5.
160. Corson JM. Pathology of diffuse malignant pleural mesothelioma. *Semin Thorac Cardiovasc Surg* 1997;**9**:347-55.
161. Maggi G, Casadio C, Cianci R, Rena O, Ruffini E. Trimodality management of malignant pleural mesothelioma. *Eur J Cardiothorac Surg* 2001;**19**:346-50.
162. Dimitrov N, McMahon S. Presentation, diagnostic methods, staging, and natural history of malignant mesothelioma. In: Antman K, Aisnee J, editors. Asbestos-related malignancy. Orlando: Grune & Stratton; 1986;225-38.
163. Viallat J, Boutin C. [Malignant pleural effusions: recourse to early use of talc.]. *Rev Med Interne* 1998;**19**:811-8.
164. Erasmus JJ, Truong MT, Smythe WR, Munden RF, Marom EM, Rice DC. Asbestos-related malignancy: Integrated computed tomography-positron emission tomography in patients with potentially resectable malignant pleural mesothelioma: staging implications. *J Thorac Cardiovasc Surg* 2005;**129**:1364-70.
165. Jaklitsch MT, Grondin SC, Sugarbaker DJ. Treatment of malignant mesothelioma. *World J Surg* 2001;**25**:210-7.
166. Whitaker D, Shilkin KB. Diagnosis of pleural malignant mesothelioma in life: a practical approach. *J Pathol* 1984;**143**:147-75.
167. Adams RF, Gleeson FV. Percutaneous image-guided cutting-needle biopsy of the pleura in the presence of a suspected malignant effusion. *Radiology* 2001;**219**:510-4.
168. Boutin C, Rey F. Thoracoscopy in pleural malignant mesothelioma: a prospective study of 188 consecutive patients. Part 1: Diagnosis. *Cancer* 1993;**72**:389-93.
169. Crotty T. Localized malignant mesothelioma. A clinical pathologic and flow cytometric study. *Am J Surg Pathol* 1994;**18**:357-63.
170. Churg A, Colby TV, Cagle P, Corson J, Gibbs AR, Gilks B, et al. The separation of benign and malignant mesothelial proliferations. *Am J Surg Pathol* 2000;**24**:1183-200.
171. Law MR, Hodson ME, Heard BE. Malignant mesothelioma of the pleura: relation between histological type and clinical behaviour. *Thorax* 1982;**37**:810-5.
172. Thurlbeck S, Miller R. The respiratory system, disease of the pleura. In: Rubin E, editor. *Pathology*. Philadelphia: Lippincott; 1998. p. 615-9.
173. Dewar A, Valente M, Ring NP, Corrin B. Pleural mesothelioma of epithelial type and pulmonary adenocarcinoma: an ultrastructural and cytochemical comparison. *J Pathol* 1987;**152**:309-16.
174. Attanoos RL, Gibbs AR. Pathology of malignant mesothelioma. *Histopathology* 1997;**30**:403-18.
175. Battifora H, McCaughey WTE. *Tumors of the Serosal Membranes*. Washington, DC: Armed Forces Institute of Pathology; 1995:**9**-14. Atlas of Tumor Pathology, 3rd series, fascicle 15.
176. Henderson B, editor. Pathology and diagnosis of mesothelioma. New York: Hemisphere; 1982, p. 183-222.
177. Roberts F, McCall AE, Burnett RA. Malignant mesothelioma: a comparison of biopsy and postmortem material by light microscopy and immunohistochemistry. *J Clin Pathol* 2001;**54**:766-70.
178. Leers MP, Aarts MM, Theunissen PH. E-cadherin and calretinin: a useful combination of immunochemical markers for differentiation between mesothelioma and metastatic adenocarcinoma. *Histopathology* 1998;**32**:209-16.
179. Battifora H. *The pleura*. New York: Raven Press; 1989, pp. 828-55.
180. Abutaily A, Addis B, Roche W. Immunohistochemistry in the distinction between malignant mesothelioma and pulmonary adenocarcinoma: a critical evaluation of new antibodies. *J Clin Pathol* 2002;**55**:662-8.
181. Gordon GJ, Jensen RV, Hsiao LL, Gullans SR, Blumenstock JE, Ramaswamy S, et al. Translation of microarray data into clinically relevant cancer diagnostic tests using gene expression ratios in lung cancer and mesothelioma. *Cancer Res* 2002;**62**:4963-7.
182. Butchart EG, Ashcroft T, Barnsley WC, Holden MP. Pleuropneumonectomy in the management of diffuse malignant mesothelioma of the pleura. Experience with 29 patients. *Thorax* 1976;**31**:15-24.
183. Rusch VW, Ginsberg R. *new concepts in the staging of mesothelioma*. Invited comment to Chapter 26. St. Louis: C.V. Mosby; 1990, p 336-43.
184. Rusch VW. A proposed new international TNM staging system for malignant pleural mesothelioma. From the International Mesothelioma Interest Group. *Chest* 1995;**108**:1122-8.
185. Sugarbaker DJ, Flores RM, Jaklitsch MT, Richards WG, Strauss GM, Corson JM, et al. Resection margins, extrapleural nodal status, and cell type determine postoperative long-term survival in trimodality therapy of malignant pleural mesothelioma: results in 183 patients. *J Thorac Cardiovasc Surg* 1999;**117**:54-63:discussion 63-5.
186. Sugarbaker DJ, Garcia JP, Richards WG, Harpole Jr DH, Healy-Baldini E, DeCamp Jr MM, et al. Extrapleural pneumonectomy in the multimodality therapy of malignant pleural mesothelioma. Results in 120 consecutive patients. *Ann Surg* 1996;**224**:288-94:discussion 294-6.
187. Chahinian P, Ambinder R, Mandel E. Evaluation of 63 patients with diffuse malignant mesothelioma. *Proc Am Soc Clin Oncol* 1980;**21**:360A.
188. Law MR, Hodson ME, Turner-Warwick M. Malignant mesothelioma of the pleura: clinical aspects and symptomatic treatment. *Eur J Respir Dis* 1984;**65**:162-8.
189. Ruffie P, Feld R, Minkin S, Cormier Y, Boutan-Laroze A, Ginsberg R, et al. Diffuse malignant mesothelioma of the pleura in Ontario and Quebec: a retrospective study of 332 patients. *J Clin Oncol* 1989;**7**:1157-68.
190. Therasse P, Arbuck SG, Eisenhauer EA, Wanders J, Kaplan RS, Rubinstein L, et al. New guidelines to evaluate the response to treatment in solid tumors. European Organization for Research and Treatment of Cancer, National Cancer Institute of the United States, National Cancer Institute of Canada. *J Natl Cancer Inst* 2000;**92**:205-16.
191. van Kalveren R, Aerts J, de Bruin H, et al. Inadequacy of the RECIST criteria for the evaluation of response in patients (pts) with malignant pleural mesothelioma (MPM). *Proc Am Soc Clin Oncol* 2002;**21**:310A.

192. Byrne MJ, Nowak AK. Modified RECIST criteria for assessment of response in malignant pleural mesothelioma. *Ann Oncol* 2004;**15**:257-60.
193. Herndon JE, Green MR, Chahinian AP, Corson JM, Suzuki Y, Vogelzang NJ. Factors predictive of survival among 337 patients with mesothelioma treated between 1984 and 1994 by the Cancer and Leukemia Group B. *Chest* 1998;**113**:723-31.
194. Curran D, Sahmoud T, Therasse P, van Meerbeeck J, Postmus PE, Giaccone G. Prognostic factors in patients with pleural mesothelioma: the European Organization for Research and Treatment of Cancer experience. *J Clin Oncol* 1998;**16**:145-52.
195. Edwards JG, Abrams KR, Leverment JN, Spyt TJ, Waller DA, O'Byrne KJ. Prognostic factors for malignant mesothelioma in 142 patients: validation of CALGB and EORTC prognostic scoring systems. *Thorax* 2000;**55**:731-5.
196. Merritt N, Blewett CJ, Miller JD, Bennett WF, Young JE, Urschel JD. Survival after conservative (palliative) management of pleural malignant mesothelioma. *J Surg Oncol* 2001;**78**:171-4.
197. Carmichael J, Degraff WG, Gamson J, Russo D, Gazdar AF, Levitt ML, et al. Radiation sensitivity of human lung cancer cell lines. *Eur J Cancer Clin Oncol* 1989;**25**:527-34.
198. Gordon Jr W, Antman KH, Greenberger JS, Weichselbaum RR, Chaffey JT. Radiation therapy in the management of patients with mesothelioma. *Int J Radiat Oncol Biol Phys* 1982;**8**:19-25.
199. Ball DL, Cruickshank DG. The treatment of malignant mesothelioma of the pleura: review of a 5-year experience, with special reference to radiotherapy. *Am J Clin Oncol* 1990;**13**:4-9.
200. Boutin C, Rey F, Viallat JR. Prevention of malignant seeding after invasive diagnostic procedures in patients with pleural mesothelioma. A randomized trial of local radiotherapy. *Chest* 1995;**108**:754-8.
201. Tobler M, Watson G, Leavitt DD. Intensity-modulated photon arc therapy for treatment of pleural mesothelioma. *Med Dosim* 2002;**27**:255-9.
202. Forster KM, Smythe WR, Starkschall G, Liao Z, Takanaka T, Kelly JF, et al. Intensity-modulated radiotherapy following extrapleural pneumonectomy for the treatment of malignant mesothelioma: clinical implementation. *Int J Radiat Oncol Biol Phys* 2003;**55**:606-16.
203. Solheim OP, Saeter G, Finnanger AM, Stenwig AE. High-dose methotrexate in the treatment of malignant mesothelioma of the pleura. A phase II study. *Br J Cancer* 1992;**65**:956-60.
204. Baas P. Chemotherapy for malignant mesothelioma: from doxorubicin to vinorelbine. *Semin Oncol* 2002;**29**:62-9.
205. Zidar BL, Green S, Pierce HI, Roach RW, Balcerzak SP, Militello L. A phase II evaluation of cisplatin in unresectable diffuse malignant mesothelioma: a Southwest Oncology Group Study. *Invest New Drugs* 1988;**6**:223-6.
206. Planting AS, Schellens JH, Goey SH, van der Burg ME, de Boer-Dennert M, Stoter G, Verweij J. Weekly high-dose cisplatin in malignant pleural mesothelioma. *Ann Oncol* 1994;**5**:373-4.
207. Steele JP, Shamash J, Evans MT, Gower NH, Tischkowitz MD, Rudd RM. Phase II study of vinorelbine in patients with malignant pleural mesothelioma. *J Clin Oncol* 2000;**18**:3912-7.
208. Kindler HL, van Meerbeeck JP. The role of gemcitabine in the treatment of malignant mesothelioma. *Semin Oncol* 2002;**29**:70-6.
209. Scagliotti GV, Shin DM, Kindler HL, Vasconcelles MJ, Keppler U, Manegold C, et al. Phase II study of pemetrexed with and without folic acid and vitamin B12 as front-line therapy in malignant pleural mesothelioma. *J Clin Oncol* 2003;**21**:1556-61.
210. Berghmans T, Paesmans M, Lalami Y, Louviaux I, Luce S, Mascaux C, et al. Activity of chemotherapy and immunotherapy on malignant mesothelioma: a systematic review of the literature with meta-analysis. *Lung Cancer* 2002;**38**:111-21.
211. Vogelzang NJ, Rusthoven JJ, Symanowski J, Denham C, Kaukel E, Ruffie P, et al. Phase III study of pemetrexed in combination with cisplatin versus cisplatin alone in patients with malignant pleural mesothelioma. *J Clin Oncol* 2003;**21**:2636-44.
212. Green J, Dundar Y, Dodd S, Dickson R, Walley T. Pemetrexed disodium in combination with cisplatin versus other cytotoxic agents or supportive care for the treatment of malignant pleural mesothelioma. *Cochrane Database Syst Rev* 2007;**1**:CD005574.
213. Janne PA. Chemotherapy for malignant pleural mesothelioma. *Clin Lung Cancer* 2003;**5**:98-106.
214. Sterman DH, Kaiser LR, Albelda SM. Advances in the treatment of malignant pleural mesothelioma. *Chest* 1999;**116**:504-20.
215. Carbone M, Pass HI, Rizzo P, Marinetti M, Di Muzio M, Mew DJ, et al. Simian virus 40-like DNA sequences in human pleural mesothelioma. *Oncogene* 1994;**9**:1781-90.
216. Brenner J, Sordillo PP, Magill GB, Golbey RB. Malignant mesothelioma of the pleura: review of 123 patients. *Cancer* 1982;**49**:2431-5.
217. Bussolino F, Di Renzo MF, Ziche M, Bocchietto E, Olivero M, Naldini L, et al. Hepatocyte growth factor is a potent angiogenic factor which stimulates endothelial cell motility and growth. *J Cell Biol* 1992;**119**:629-41.
218. Byrne MJ, Davidson JA, Musk AW, Dewar J, van Hazel G, Buck M, et al. Cisplatin and gemcitabine treatment for malignant mesothelioma: a phase II study. *J Clin Oncol* 1999;**17**:25-30.
219. Carbone M, Rizzo P, Grimley PM, Procopio A, Mew DJ, Shridhar V, et al. Simian virus-40 large-T antigen binds p53 in human mesotheliomas. *Nat Med* 1997;**3**:908-12.
220. Zellos L, Jaklitsch MT, Bueno R, Sugarbaker DJ. Treatment of malignant mesothelioma: Extrapleural pneumonectomy with intraoperative chemotherapy. *Op Tech Thorac Cardiovasc Surg* 2006;**11**:45-56.
221. Richards WG, Zellos L, Bueno R, Jaklitsch MT, Janne PA, Chirieac LR, et al. Phase I to II study of pleurectomy/decortication and intraoperative intracavitary hyperthermic cisplatin lavage for mesothelioma. *J Clin Oncol* 2006;**24**:1561-7.
222. Sugarbaker DJ, Jaklitsch MT, Bueno R, Richards W, Lukanich J, Mentzer SJ, et al. Prevention, early detection, and management of complications after 328 consecutive extrapleural pneumonectomies. *J Thorac Cardiovasc Surg* 2004;**128**:138-46.
223. McCormack PM, Nagasaki F, Hilaris BS, Martini N. Surgical treatment of pleural mesothelioma. *J Thorac Cardiovasc Surg* 1982;**84**:834-42.
224. Achatzy R, Beba W, Ritschler R, Worn H, Wahlers B, Macha HN, Morgan JA. The diagnosis, therapy and prognosis of diffuse malignant mesothelioma. *Eur J Cardiothorac Surg* 1989;**3**:445-7, discussion 448.
225. Brancatisano RP, Joseph MG, McCaughan BC. Pleurectomy for mesothelioma. *Med J Aust* 1991;**154**:455-7.
226. Allen KB, Faber LP, Warren WH. Malignant pleural mesothelioma. Extrapleural pneumonectomy and pleurectomy. *Chest Surg Clin N Am* 1994;**4**:113-26.
227. DaValle MJ, Faber LP, Kittle CF, Jensik RJ. Extrapleural pneumonectomy for diffuse, malignant mesothelioma. *Ann Thorac Surg* 1986;**42**:612-8.
228. Rusch VW, Piantadosi S, Holmes EC. The role of extrapleural pneumonectomy in malignant mesothelioma. A Lung Cancer Study Group trial. *J Thorac Cardiovasc Surg* 1991;**102**:1-9.
229. Linden CJ, Mercke C, Albrechtsson U, Johansson L, Ewers SB. Effect of hemithorax irradiation alone or combined with doxorubicin and cyclophosphamide in 47 pleural mesotheliomas: a nonrandomized phase II study. *Eur Respir J* 1996;**9**:2565-72.
230. Rusch VW, Rosenzweig K, Venkatraman E, Leon L, Raben A, Harrison L, et al. A phase II trial of surgical resection and adjuvant high-dose hemithoracic radiation for malignant pleural mesothelioma. *J Thorac Cardiovasc Surg* 2001;**122**:788-95.
231. Antman KH, Blum RH, Greenberger JS, Flowerdew G, Skarin AT, Canellos GP. Multimodality therapy for malignant mesothelioma based on a study of natural history. *Am J Med* 1980;**68**:356-62.
232. Sugarbaker DJ, Heher EC, Lee TH, Couper G, Mentzer S, Corson JM, et al. Extrapleural pneumonectomy, chemotherapy, and radiotherapy in the treatment of diffuse malignant pleural mesothelioma. *J Thorac Cardiovasc Surg* 1991;**102**:10-4; discussion 14-5.
233. Sugarbaker DJ, Mentzer SJ, Strauss G. Extrapleural pneumonectomy in the treatment of malignant pleural mesothelioma. *Ann Thorac Surg* 1992;**54**:941-6.
234. Sugarbaker DJ, Strauss GM, Lynch TJ, Richards W, Mentzer SJ, Lee TH, et al. Node status has prognostic significance in the multimodality therapy of diffuse, malignant mesothelioma. *J Clin Oncol* 1993;**11**:1172-8.
235. Stewart DJ, Martin-Ucar A, Pilling JE, Edwards JG, O'Byrne KJ, Waller DA. The effect of extent of local resection on patterns of disease progression in malignant pleural mesothelioma. *Ann Thorac Surg* 2004;**78**:245-52.
236. Baldini EH, Recht A, Strauss GM, et al. Patterns of failure after trimodality therapy for malignant pleural mesothelioma. *Ann Thorac Surg* 1997;**63**:334-8.
237. Grant DC, Seltzer SE, Antman KH, Finberg HJ, Koster K. Computed tomography of malignant pleural mesothelioma. *J Comput Assist Tomogr* 1983;**7**:626-32.
238. Sugarbaker PH, Jablonski KA. Prognostic features of 51 colorectal and 130 appendiceal cancer patients with peritoneal carcinomatosis treated by cytoreductive surgery and intraperitoneal chemotherapy. *Ann Surg* 1995;**221**:124-32.
239. Averbach A, Sugarbaker P. Methodological considerations in treatment using intraperitoneal chemotherapy. In: Sugarbaker PH, editor. *Peritoneal carcinomatosis: diagnosis and treatment*. Boston: Kluwer Academic; 1996. p. 289-309.
240. Rusch VW, Niedzwiecki D, Tao Y, Menendez-Botet C, Dnistrian A, Kelsen D, et al. Intrapleural cisplatin and mitomycin for malignant mesothelioma following pleurectomy: pharmacokinetic studies. *J Clin Oncol* 1992;**10**:1001-6.
241. Ausmus PL, Wilke AV, Frazier DL. Effects of hyperthermia on blood flow and cis-diamminedichloroplatinum(II) pharmacokinetics in murine mammary adenocarcinomas. *Cancer Res* 1992;**52**:4965-8.

242. Giovanella BC, Stehlin JS, Yim SO. Correlation of the thermosensitivity of cells to their malignant potential. *Ann N Y Acad Sci* 1980;**335**:206-14.
243. Azzarelli A. Intra-arterial infusion and perfusion chemotherapy for soft tissue sarcomas of the extremities. *Cancer Treat Res* 1986;**29**:103-29.
244. Monneuse O, Beaujard AC, Guibert B, Gilly FN, Mulsant P, Carry PY, et al. Long-term results of intrathoracic chemohyperthermia (ITCH) for the treatment of pleural malignancies. *Br J Cancer* 2003;**88**:1839-43.
245. Yellin A, Simansky DA, Paley M, Refaely Y. Hyperthermic pleural perfusion with cisplatin: early clinical experience. *Cancer* 2001;**92**:2197-203.
246. Mujoomdar A, Sugarbaker D. Hyperthermic chemoperfusion for the treatment of malignant pleural mesothelioma. *Sem Thorac Cardiovasc Surg* 2009:298-304.
247. Baas P, Boogerd W, Dalesio O, Haringhuizen A, Custers F, van Zandwijk N. Thalidomide in patients with malignant pleural mesothelioma. *Lung Cancer* 2005;**48**:291-6.
248. Nowack A, Lake RA, Kindler HL. New approaches for mesothelioma: Biologics, vaccines, gene therapy, and other novel agents. *Semin Oncol* 2002;**29**:82-96.
249. Friedberg JS, Mick R, Stevenson J, Metz J, Zhu T, Buyske J, et al. A phase I study of Foscan-mediated photodynamic therapy and surgery in patients with mesothelioma. *Ann Thorac Surg* 2003;**75**:952-9.
250. Ris HB. Photodynamic therapy as an adjunct to surgery for malignant pleural mesothelioma. *Lung Cancer* 2005;**49**(Suppl. 1):S65-8.
251. Moskal TL, Dougherty TJ, Urschel JD, Antkowiak JG, Regal AM, Driscoll DL, Takita H. Operation and photodynamic therapy for pleural mesothelioma: 6-year follow-up. *Ann Thorac Surg* 1998;**66**:1128-33.
252. Pass HI, Temeck BK, Kranda K, Thomas G, Russo A, Smith P, et al. Phase III randomized trial of surgery with or without intraoperative photodynamic therapy and postoperative immunochemotherapy for malignant pleural mesothelioma. *Ann Surg Oncol* 1997;**4**:628-33.
253. Upham JW, Garlepp MJ, Musk AW, Robinson BW. Malignant mesothelioma: new insights into tumour biology and immunology as a basis for new treatment approaches. *Thorax* 1995;**50**:887-93.
254. Boutin C, Viallat JR, Van Zandwijk N, Douillard JT, Paillard JC, Guerin JC, et al. Activity of intrapleural recombinant gamma-interferon in malignant mesothelioma. *Cancer* 1991;**67**:2033-7.
255. Driesen P, Boutin C, Viallat JR, Astoul PH, Vialette JP, Pasquier J. Implantable access system for prolonged intrapleural immunotherapy. *Eur Respir J* 1994;**7**:1889-92.
256. Boutin C, Nussbaum E, Monnet I, Bignon J, Vanderschueren R, Guerin JC, et al. Intrapleural treatment with recombinant gamma-interferon in early stage malignant pleural mesothelioma. *Cancer* 1994;**74**:2460-7.
257. Antoniou KM, Ferdoutsis E, Bouros D. Interferons and their application in the diseases of the lung. *Chest* 2003;**123**:209-16.
258. Castagneto B, Zai S, Mutti L, Lazzaro A, Ridolfi R, Piccolini E, et al. Palliative and therapeutic activity of IL-2 immunotherapy in unresectable malignant pleural mesothelioma with pleural effusion: Results of a phase II study on 31 consecutive patients. *Lung Cancer* 2001;**31**:303-10.
259. Bard M, Ruffie P. Malignant mesothelioma. Medical oncology: standards, new trends, trials: the French experience. *Lung Cancer* 2004;**45**(Suppl. 1):S129-31.
260. Monti G, Jaurand MC, Monnet I, Chretien P, Saint-Etienne L, Zeng L, et al. Intrapleural production of interleukin 6 during mesothelioma and its modulation by gamma-interferon treatment. *Cancer Res* 1994;**54**:4419-23.
261. Monnet I, Breau JL, Moro D, Lena H, Eymard JC, Menard O, et al. Intrapleural infusion of activated macrophages and gamma-interferon in malignant pleural mesothelioma: a phase II study. *Chest* 2002;**121**:1921-7.
262. Culver KW, Blaese RM. Gene therapy for cancer. *Trends Genet* 1994;**10**:174-8.
263. Kruklitis RJ, Singhal S, Delong P, Kapoor V, Sterman DH, Kaiser LR, Albelda SM. Immuno-gene therapy with interferon-beta before surgical debulking delays recurrence and improves survival in a murine model of malignant mesothelioma. *J Thorac Cardiovasc Surg* 2004;**127**:123-30.
264. Sterman DH, Recio A, Vachani A, Sun J, Cheung L, DeLong P, et al. Long-term follow-up of patients with malignant pleural mesothelioma receiving high-dose adenovirus herpes simplex thymidine kinase/ganciclovir suicide gene therapy. *Clin Cancer Res* 2005;**11**:7444-53.
265. Vogelzang NJ. Standard therapy for the treatment of malignant pleural mesothelioma. *Lung Cancer* 2005;**50**(Suppl. 1):S23-4.
266. Rusch V, Saltz L, Venkatraman E, Ginsberg R, McCormack P, Burt M, et al. A phase II trial of pleurectomy/decortication followed by intrapleural and systemic chemotherapy for malignant pleural mesothelioma. *J Clin Oncol* 1994;**12**:1156-63.
267. Rice TW, Adelstein DJ, Kirby TJ, Saltarelli MG, Murthy SR, Van Kirk MA, et al. Aggressive multimodality therapy for malignant pleural mesothelioma. *Ann Thorac Surg* 1994;**58**:24-9.
268. Lee JD, Perez S, Wang HJ, Figlin RA, Holmes EC. Intrapleural chemotherapy for patients with incompletely resected malignant mesothelioma: the UCLA experience. *J Surg Oncol* 1995;**60**:262-7.
269. Sauter ER, Langer C, Coia LR, Goldberg M, Keller SM. Optimal management of malignant mesothelioma after subtotal pleurectomy: revisiting the role of intrapleural chemotherapy and postoperative radiation. *J Surg Oncol* 1995;**60**:100-5.
270. Colleoni M, Sartori F, Calabro F, Nelli P, Vicario G, Sgarbossa G, et al. Surgery followed by intracavitary plus systemic chemotherapy in malignant pleural mesothelioma. *Tumori* 1996;**82**:53-6.
271. van Ruth S, Baas P, Haas RL, Rutgers EJ, Verwaal VJ, Zoetmulder FA. Cytoreductive surgery combined with intraoperative hyperthermic intrathoracic chemotherapy for stage I malignant pleural mesothelioma. *Ann Surg Oncol* 2003;**10**:176-82.
272. Chang MY, Sugarbaker DJ. Extrapleural pneumonectomy for diffuse malignant pleural mesothelioma: techniques and complications. *Thorac Surg Clin* 2004;**14**:523-30.
273. Zellos L, Richards WG, Capalbo L, Jaklitsch MT, Chirieac LR, Johnson BE, et al. A phase I study of extrapleural pneumonectomy and intracavitary intraoperative hyperthermic cisplatin with amifostine cytoprotection for malignant pleural mesothelioma. *J Thorac Cardiovasc Surg* 2009;**137**:453-8.
274. Tilleman TR, Richards GW, Zellos L, et al. Extrapleural pneumonectomy followed by intracavitary intraoperative hyperthermic cisplatin with pharmacologic cytoprotection for treatment of malignant pleural mesothelioma: a phase II prospective study. *J Thorac Cardiovasc Surg* 2009;**138**:405-11.

J. Diaphragm

CHAPTER 32

Surgery of the Diaphragm: A Deductive Approach

Daniel C. Wiener, Jonathan Daniel, and Michael T. Jaklitsch

Embryology
Structure and Function
Pleural and Peritoneal Attachments
Arterial and Venous Anatomy
Lymphatics
Diaphragmatic Innervation
Diaphragmatic Incisions
Traumatic Diaphragmatic Injury
Diaphragmatic Elevation
Diaphragmatic Hernias
Diaphragmatic Pacing
Oncology of the Diaphragm
Diaphragmatic Resection and Repair with Prosthetic Patch
Summary

And on a day we meet to walk the line
And set the wall between us once again.
We keep the wall between us as we go....
He only says, "Good fences make good neighbors."
 — Robert Frost, "Mending Wall"

The muscular diaphragm acts as a boundary between the positive-pressure abdominal cavity and the negative-pressure thoracic cavity. Perhaps because it is a boundary structure, or perhaps because the horizontal diaphragm is poorly visualized on a plain chest radiograph and computed tomography (CT) scan, discussion of the surgical approach to the diaphragm is neglected in many surgical textbooks.

In our opinion, there is some misinformation about the surgical treatment of the diaphragm in the current literature. This misinformation seems to reflect a lack of understanding of the basic anatomy and physiology of the diaphragm. Although diaphragmatic disease is infrequent, exposure to the diaphragm is commonplace because it is visualized during every thoracic surgical procedure and most intra-abdominal operations. Therefore, the basic principles advocated by this chapter can be verified or denied by the curious reader in the operating room.

Two fundamental principles can be applied to all surgical approaches to the diaphragm: (1) the muscles contract in a radial manner like the spokes of a wheel; and (2) the balance of positive pressure pushing up from the abdomen and negative pressure within the thorax created by the elastic recoil of the lung during quiet expiration displaces the central tendon into the chest, whereas contraction of the diaphragmatic muscle pulls the tendon back toward the costal margin and elevates the lower ribs, enlarging the volume of the thorax. We hope to apply these two fundamental principles in an understanding of the physiology and pathophysiology of the diaphragm. Furthermore, we believe that these two principles will allow the reader to use new technologies and to develop better operations to treat diaphragmatic disease.

EMBRYOLOGY

In utero, the diaphragm forms from the septum transversum and pleuroperitoneal folds.[1] The septum transversum is an unpaired ventral membrane that separates the pericardium from the remainder of the thorax and creates the central trileaflet of the diaphragmatic tendon (Fig. 32-1).[2] One of the trileaflet tendons lies within the right hemithorax, one within the left hemithorax, and the third beneath the pericardium. The dorsolateral portions of the diaphragm start with the formation of pleuroperitoneal folds. The mesothelium of the pleura binds to the mesothelium of the peritoneum in a membrane only two cell layers deep. Myotomes from C3, C4, and C5 then migrate from the lateral border toward the center of each hemithorax within the interspace between these two mesothelial layers in the 7th week of life. The outer rim of muscle of the diaphragm is from myotomes that carry nerve innervation from T7 through T12.[2] The intestines return to the abdomen from the yolk sac in the 10th week of life and will be displaced into the chest if the diaphragm has not successfully formed (a congenital diaphragmatic hernia).

STRUCTURE AND FUNCTION

This simplified embryologic description provides several fundamental concepts of diaphragm function and pathology. Muscle contraction is in a radial manner along the lines of migration of the myotomes. Thus, fiber shortening is along the lines of a wheel spoke, between the central tendon and the circumferential rib cage. Furthermore, any congenital loss of muscle or tendon may present as a hernia within the diaphragm.

In the adult, each hemidiaphragm resembles the surface of an upside-down fairway wooden golf club. The fan-shaped tendon is like the flat metal sole plate, and the circumferential muscle curves away into the sulcus like the curved wooden club head. The muscle fascicles of the crus coalesce and attach to the lumbar spine, just as the wooden club curves down to attach to the metal shaft.

There are three natural openings within the diaphragm (Fig. 32-2). The aortic opening is the most posterior of the three and is formed from fibers composing the right and left diaphragmatic crura.[3] This tunnel is actually behind the diaphragm, not within it, and contains the aorta, azygos vein, and thoracic duct. The esophageal hiatus is slightly more ventral from the aortic hiatus and consists of fibers passing between the aorta and the esophagus toward the right crus and fibers converging on the pericardial tendon. The opening of the inferior vena cava lies within the confluence of the tendons of the right hemithorax and the tendon beneath the pericardium.

The fan-shaped muscle of the diaphragm arises from the internal circumference of the thorax, with attachments to the sternum, the lower six or seven ribs, and the vertebral bodies of the lumbar vertebrae. Posteriorly, the muscle fibers originate from the aponeurotic arch of the ligamentum arcuatum externum, which overrides the psoas and quadratus lumborum muscle. Laterally, the fibers of the diaphragm interdigitate with slips from the transversalis muscle of the abdomen as they originate from the ribs.[3] The right crus is larger and longer than the left and arises from the bodies of the upper three or four lumbar vertebrae. The left crus arises from the upper two lumbar vertebral bodies.

During inspiration, the first rib is elevated and fixed by the scalene muscles of the neck. The external intercostal muscles raise, in turn, each of the lower ribs. Raising these ribs, like a bucket handle that is attached to the sternum and vertebral column, enlarges the thorax and creates the negative pressure that ventilates the lung.[3]

The diaphragm is the major muscle of inspiration.[4] In the resting state, the central tendon is displaced cephalad into the thorax by the positive intra-abdominal pressure. During contraction, the radial muscle fibers pull the tendon down toward the abdominal cavity like a drumhead. This further augments the negative intrathoracic pressure and further increases the positive pressure in the abdomen.

The diaphragmatic crura contribute to the magnitude of displacement of the central tendon. In fact, if there were only circumferential attachments to the rib cage, the diaphragm would be limited in its ability to displace the lower ribs and to enlarge the thoracic cavity. The thicker fascicles of the crura, which lie at a 45- to 90-degree angle to the plane of the fan, pull on the anchoring lumbar spine like a lever and thus fix the central tendon in place. In descending, the fan of the diaphragm displaces the intra-abdominal viscera, which do not yield completely because they are bolstered by the anterior abdominal wall. The central tendon becomes a fixed point from which the radial muscles of the fan contract and are thus able to elevate the lower ribs. Even though the points of muscle attachment to the lumbar spine are more caudal than the attachments to the rib cage, the domed tendon acts as a fulcrum cephalad to the attachments to the rib cage. In fact, contraction of the diaphragm can raise the lower ribs only if the intra-abdominal viscera are in situ and not if the organs have been removed.[3] Injuries to the crura have a more disproportionate effect on the respiratory function of the ipsilateral diaphragm than a similar injury to the peripheral muscle.

A forced inspiration descends the central tendon one or two rib interspaces. Under normal respiration, each hemidiaphragm provides between 15% and 25% of respiratory muscle function, with each side of the combined intercostals providing the remaining percentage.[5,6] Under strained respiration, however, the diaphragm can increase its workload to provide up to 80% of the work of breathing.

PLEURAL AND PERITONEAL ATTACHMENTS

The pleura is tightly adherent to the top surface of the diaphragmatic central tendon and most of the musculature. It is impossible to separate the pleura from the central tendon of each hemidiaphragm. As the pleura curves off the chest wall and folds back on itself on the surface of the diaphragm, there is a circumferential diaphragmatic recess of approximately 1 cm that does not contain pleura.[7] This recess of uncovered diaphragm is used to good advantage during an extrapleural

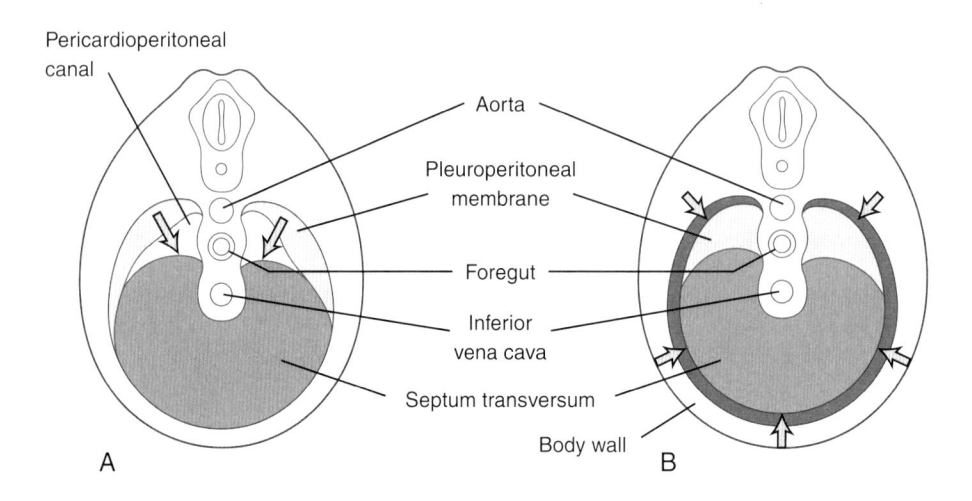

Figure 32–1
Transverse schematic of developing embryo during weeks 5 to 7. Bilateral pleuroperitoneal folds extend anteriorly to reach the posterior edge of the septum transversum, thus forming the posterior portions of the diaphragm. The septum transversum develops into the majority of the central tendon. *(From Larsen W. Human embryology. 2nd ed. New York: Churchill Livingstone; 1997.)*

dissection when the surgeon wraps his or her fingers into this recess and pulls downward, thus exposing the diaphragmatic musculature for division (Fig. 32-3).

The peritoneum is less adherent to the undersurface of the diaphragm and can be bluntly mobilized off the diaphragm during extraperitoneal approaches to the abdominal aorta. The plane of dissection lies between the inferior phrenic artery and vein on the muscle side and the peritoneal membrane. The peritoneum separates from the central tendon of the right diaphragm to form the falciform ligament and produces an area directly under the central tendon that does not have peritoneal covering. This is known as the bare area.

ARTERIAL AND VENOUS ANATOMY

The superior phrenic arteries are located on the thoracic surface of the diaphragm. They are small branches from the lower thoracic aorta and traverse the posterior diaphragm over the top portion of each crus close to the mediastinum.[3] They terminate in small anastomoses with the musculophrenic and pericardiophrenic arteries, which are both branches from the internal mammary artery. These two arteries also supply blood to the phrenic nerve and the pericardial fat pad.[8]

The inferior phrenic arteries lie on the undersurface of the crus and the dome of the diaphragm (Fig. 32-4). They are small paired vessels with frequent anatomic variations. They can originate separately or as a common trunk from the aorta above the celiac artery or from the celiac artery itself. Alternatively, a common trunk arising from either the aorta or the celiac artery gives rise to these two arteries. On occasion, one vessel originates from the aorta and the other emerges from one of the renal arteries. Diverging near the crura, the inferior phrenic arteries then course obliquely superior and lateral along the inferior surface of the diaphragm. The left inferior phrenic artery passes posterior to the esophagus and then runs anteriorly along the lateral side of the esophageal hiatus. The right inferior phrenic artery passes behind the inferior vena cava.[3]

Close to the posterior aspect of the central tendon, both the left and right inferior phrenic arteries divide into a medial and a lateral branch. The medial branch extends anteriorly, close to the mediastinum. Branches of this vessel traverse the muscular portion of the diaphragm to anastomose with the musculophrenic and pericardiophrenic arteries. The lateral

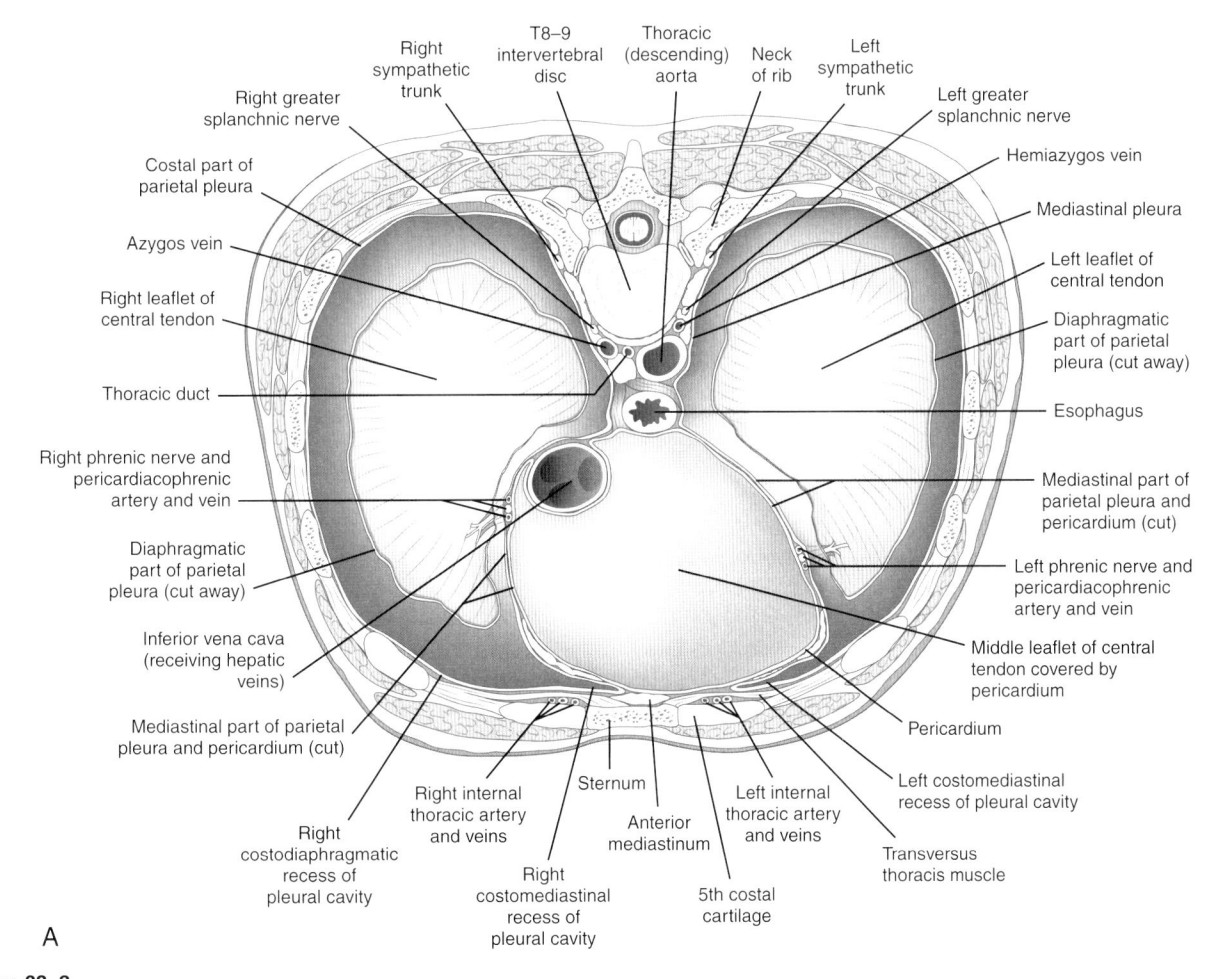

Figure 32–2
Superior (**A**) and inferior (**B**) views of the diaphragm, including phrenic nerve anatomy. The intradiaphragmatic course of the phrenic nerves is often difficult to visualize at the time of surgery. Familiarity with the nerve's path as it traverses the muscle is helpful in deciding where to make diaphragmatic incisions.

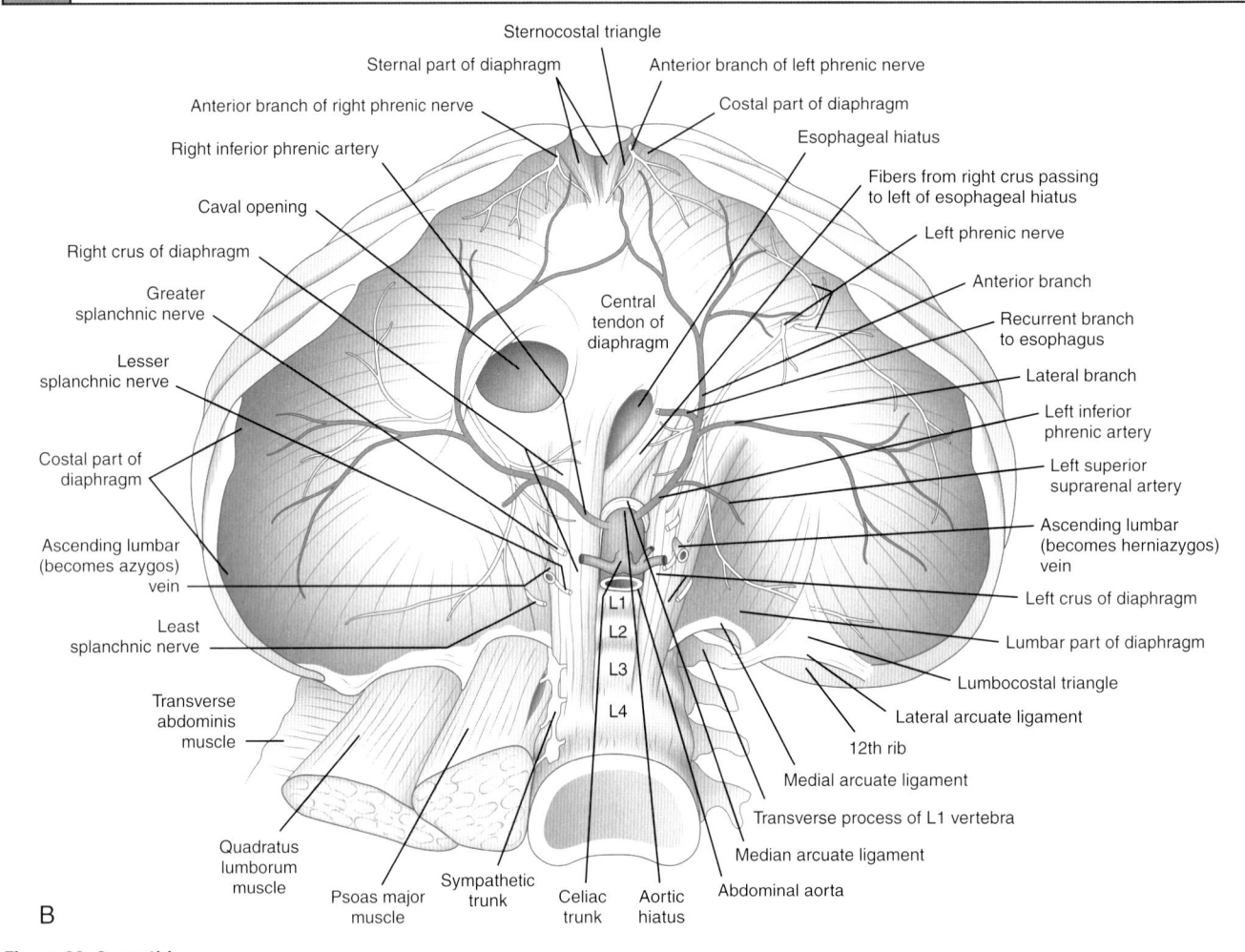

Figure 32–2, cont'd

branch of the inferior phrenic artery courses laterally and forms anastomoses with the lower intercostal arteries. The left inferior phrenic artery provides a minor contribution to the blood supply of the lower esophagus. Both the right and left inferior phrenic arteries have branches to the ipsilateral suprarenal gland. These branches are called the right and left superior suprarenal arteries.[3]

In general, the venous anatomy in this region parallels that of the arteries. The superior phrenic veins are small and drain anteriorly to the internal mammary vein. The much larger inferior phrenic veins parallel the course of the inferior phrenic arteries. The right vein empties directly into the inferior vena cava. The left vein usually has two branches, one of which drains into the left renal or suprarenal vein; the other passes anterior to the esophageal hiatus and empties into the inferior vena cava.[3]

LYMPHATICS

The lymphatics of the diaphragm drain toward the internal mammary chain anteriorly and the thoracic duct posteriorly. Smaller lateral lymphatic branches follow the course of the intercostal vessels along the lateral and posterior margins of the chest wall.[3] Although these vessels are rarely seen in the nonpathologic state, engorged vessels are frequently seen on both the upper and lower surfaces of the diaphragm in patients who have congenital heart disease with elevated central venous pressures and in primary pathologic conditions of the lymphatics, such as cavernous lymphangioma.

DIAPHRAGMATIC INNERVATION

The phrenic nerve originates from the C3, C4, and C5 nerve roots and then enters the chest anterior to the subclavian artery. On the left side, the nerve lies medial to the internal mammary artery 64% of the time; on the right side, it lies medial to the internal mammary artery only 46% of the time.[9] Thus, the left nerve is more susceptible to injury during mobilization of the left internal mammary artery through a median sternotomy incision.

The majority of diaphragmatic muscle originates from cervical myotomes innervated by fibers from the spinal nerve roots at cervical levels C3, C4, and C5. These fibers join and form the phrenic nerve, which elongates as the septum transversum migrates caudally. There is, however, an outer rim of diaphragmatic muscle that originates from migrating mesenchymal cells of the nearby body wall innervated by spinal nerves from thoracic levels T7-12. In addition, there is a contribution from mesenchyme associated with the foregut at levels L1-3 that coalesces to form the right and left crura.[2,3]

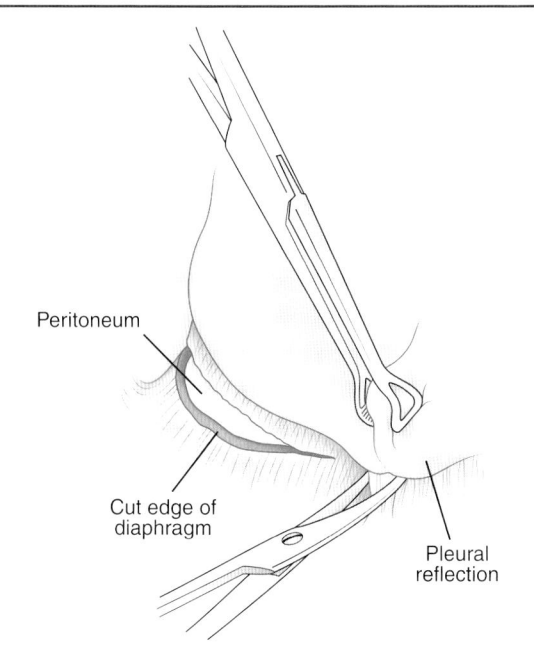

Figure 32–3
The parietal pleura folds off the rib cage and onto the diaphragm but does not extend into the deep recess of the diaphragmatic sulcus. A bare area of diaphragmatic muscle can be exposed with traction on the parietal pleura.

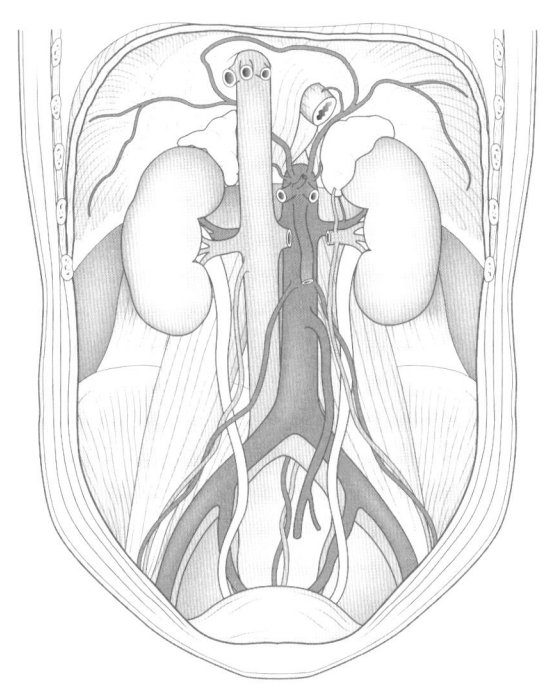

Figure 32–4
Arterial anatomy of the inferior diaphragmatic surface.

Despite the contributions from the thoracic and spinal nerve roots, the majority of the diaphragm is innervated by the phrenic nerve. Although the origin of the phrenic nerve and its proximal course through the mediastinum are well known, the distal extent of the nerve as it branches into the diaphragm proper is less well described. In 1956, Merendino and colleagues[10] published the most descriptive and often-cited reference regarding this intradiaphragmatic portion of the phrenic nerve. Their anatomic findings and frequently adapted schematized drawings are based on electrical stimulation studies and gross dissection in dogs as well as on intraoperative dissection of approximately 40 human diaphragms.

The phrenic nerve usually divides at the level of the diaphragm or just above it. The right phrenic nerve enters the diaphragm just lateral to the inferior vena cava within the central tendon. The left phrenic nerve enters lateral to the left border of the heart just anterior to the central tendon within the muscle itself. The intradiaphragmatic course of the phrenic nerve can be predicted, even when it is not directly seen, by knowing the distribution of the four main motor divisions. The phrenic nerve first splits into an anterior and a posterior trunk (see Fig. 32-2B). The anterior trunk subsequently divides into a sternal and an anterolateral branch near the anteromedial border of the central tendon. The posterior trunk likewise divides into a crural and a posterolateral branch along the posteromedial border of the central tendon. The sternal and crural branches are short and continue to run in an anteromedial and posteromedial direction, respectively. The anterolateral and posterolateral branches are much longer and run close to the muscular fiber insertions into the central tendon. These two branches innervate the majority of the diaphragm. Their anatomic relation to one another is often described as a pair of handcuffs or manacles. These branches are often within the muscle layers and are not readily visible.

DIAPHRAGMATIC INCISIONS

There are a variety of suitable locations for diaphragmatic incisions that one can deduce from knowledge of diaphragmatic anatomy and function. Certain areas of the diaphragm can be incised safely without causing significant damage or loss of function. Other regions are likely to result in bleeding, structural weakness, or diaphragmatic hemiparesis if they are incised or cauterized inappropriately.

Diaphragmatic incisions can be divided into three groups: circumferential, central tendon, and radial. Circumferential incisions in the periphery result in little loss of function. These circumferential incisions, however, must be at least 5 cm lateral to the edge of the central tendon to avoid the posterolateral and anterolateral branches of the phrenic nerve. These incisions can be difficult to correctly realign after a long operation. Placement of surgical clips on each side of the muscular incision can greatly facilitate the correct spatial orientation on closing (Fig. 32-5).

Incisions in the central tendon, as far centrally as within 2 cm of the entrance of the phrenic nerve, do not interrupt any major branch of the nerve itself. This type of incision can provide excellent visualization of the abdomen from the thorax, and vice versa. These incisions are easy to open and to close.

A transverse radial incision made from the midaxillary line centrally is relatively safe because it courses between the distal aspects of the anterolateral and posterolateral branches of the phrenic nerve (i.e., through the opening of the handcuffs). Radial incisions from the costal margin extending all the way to the esophageal hiatus, however, may result in segmental diaphragmatic paralysis if the incision transects the crural or posterolateral branches of the phrenic nerve.

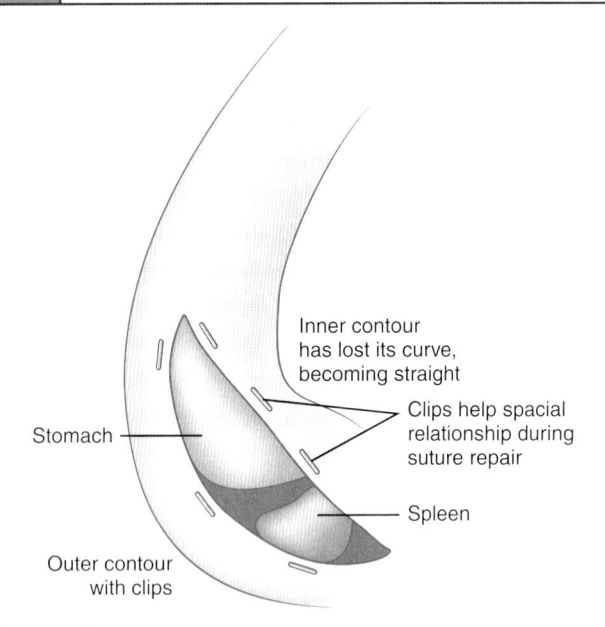

Figure 32–5
Curvilinear diaphragmatic incision between strategically placed surgical clips. Diaphragmatic incisions disrupt the radial tension and distort the muscular anatomy. Placement of surgical clips before incision facilitates closure with proper realignment of the diaphragmatic musculature.

TRAUMATIC DIAPHRAGMATIC INJURY

Both blunt and penetrating trauma can injure the diaphragm. Penetrating injuries to the lower thorax and upper abdomen place the diaphragm at risk of injury. The nipples, marking the most cephalad displacement of the central tendon, and the base of the 12th rib, marking the most caudal attachment of the muscle, are important landmarks that identify a potential diaphragmatic injury from penetrating trauma. Any missile traversing this area or knife wound within this zone may create a diaphragmatic laceration.

Blunt trauma that dramatically increases the intra-abdominal pressure may cause a central tendon rupture of the diaphragm. A common mechanism for rupture is seen in patients involved in high-speed motor collisions who are wearing seat belts. Imminent awareness of an approaching accident can cause inspiration with tensing of abdominal muscles and contraction of the diaphragm. This increases intra-abdominal pressure and in combination with additional force from the seat belt at impact can result in rupture of the diaphragm at the dome or central attachments. Diaphragmatic rupture occurs in 0.8% to 1.6% of patients arriving at the emergency department with blunt trauma.[11] Because the liver protects the right hemidiaphragm from this mechanism of injury, most diaphragmatic ruptures from blunt trauma are recognized on the left side.

An abnormal diaphragm contour on plain chest radiograph or CT scan after a traumatic injury should raise the possibility of diaphragmatic injury. These findings may be easier to appreciate if a radiopaque nasogastric tube is in place at the time of imaging. Nonetheless, radiographic findings may still be as subtle as blurring of the costophrenic angle. Because of this subtlety, delayed diagnoses are not uncommon. Review of the literature suggests that the diagnosis is missed in as many as 66% in some series.[12] This may be in part related to traditional CT imaging, which has yielded poor detection of diaphragmatic injury; however, reports of new helical CT scanners show increasing sensitivity as high as 84%.[13] If clinical suspicion is high, minimally invasive techniques with laparoscopy or thoracoscopy have improved detection of occult diaphragmatic laceration, especially in penetrating left thoracoabdominal injuries.

Diaphragmatic injuries that are diagnosed promptly should be explored from the abdomen with either laparotomy or laparoscopy because of the frequent association of other abdominal organ injury (liver, spleen, stomach, kidney). During insufflation, the surgeon must be prepared to place an emergent chest tube in the event that a tension pneumothorax arises from communication through the diaphragmatic hole. In those cases with a significant delay in diagnosis, injuries generally should be explored from the thorax, with either thoracotomy or thoracoscopy, because the herniated abdominal structure is frequently adherent to the ipsilateral lung.

Diaphragmatic injuries need to be repaired when they are recognized. Repair corrects or prevents complications, such as respiratory compromise or herniation of abdominal viscera with the associated risk of incarceration and strangulation. If no other indication for surgical exploration is present and the diagnosis of diaphragmatic rupture remains in question, exploratory thoracoscopy is a simple and effective diagnostic procedure. Small tears can be sutured with thoracoscopic techniques after reduction of abdominal contents displaced across the defect. Thoracoscopic exploration and repair require general anesthesia with single-lung ventilation. Timing therefore depends on underlying pulmonary and neurologic function.

Lateral avulsions of the diaphragm may require reattachment to a rib at a higher level. Diaphragmatic lacerations can be closed with nonabsorbable heavy suture, with care taken to prevent injury to the main phrenic nerve branches. If the defect is large and unable to be repaired primarily, a prosthetic mesh is a good option. In the presence of heavy contamination during damage control surgery, use of an absorbable or biological substitute is preferable to prevent continued retraction of the defect and pleural contamination. At reoperation, provided there is no remaining soilage, the mesh can be exchanged for a permanent prosthetic.

DIAPHRAGMATIC ELEVATION

The two most common causes of diaphragmatic elevation are congenital eventration of the diaphragm and phrenic nerve palsy (Fig. 32-6A).

Congenital eventration of the diaphragm is a spectrum of disorders that share the underlying cause of impaired fetal myotome migration.[14] Mild cases may lack only the central tendon, whereas severe cases may lack the central tendon as well as the entire muscular diaphragm. The area of congenitally missing muscle tissue is usually closed with a fused single membrane of pleura and peritoneum. This membrane is generally displaced within the ipsilateral hemithorax because of the absence of muscle.

Phrenic nerve paralysis in the child can be due to a viral palsy, an iatrogenic injury (typically after pediatric thoracic surgery), or a traction injury to the phrenic nerve at the base

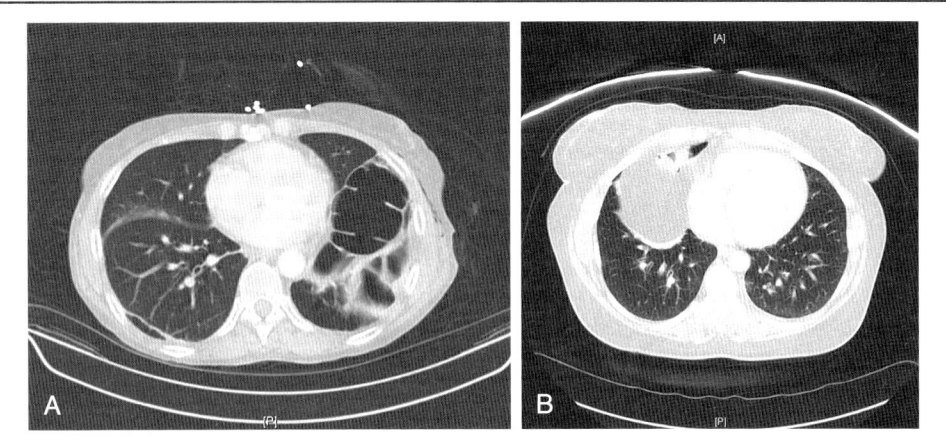

Figure 32–6
A, CT scan of left diaphragmatic elevation. Note the lung tissue at the anterior and posterior thorax. **B,** CT scan of Morgagn's hernia. Note the lack of lung tissue at the extreme hemithorax.

of the neck after a forceps delivery. In addition, there can be congenital absence of the phrenic nerve.

Diaphragmatic elevation is poorly tolerated in neonates. The flaccid diaphragm itself compresses the lower lobe of the ipsilateral lung. In addition, if there is a large displacement of abdominal components into the negative-pressure thorax, this bulk mechanically shifts the mediastinum with compression of the contralateral lung. Thus, there is atelectasis of the ipsilateral lower lobe, compression of the left atrium and impediment to pulmonary venous blood flow, and contralateral lung compression with additional atelectasis.[15] The end result may be complete pulmonary failure requiring intubation. Mechanical ventilation reinflates the atelectatic lungs and balances the mobile mediastinum. The ipsilateral diaphragm is shifted into the abdomen.

Surgical intervention is nearly mandatory in symptomatic infants with eventration; but in the adult population, the indications for surgery are less clear. In children, plication is readily successful in achieving weaning from ventilation. In adults, however, this is not the case. In addition, regarding nonventilated patients, the condition is better tolerated in adults, and in general only patients with progressive symptoms should be offered surgery. Causes of eventration in adults are usually related to phrenic nerve involvement through spinal cord disease, cervical trauma, infiltration of the nerve by tumors or lymph nodes, and iatrogenic injury. In certain conditions, conservative management will eventually lead to recovery of function; however, in the remaining patients, plication remains a low-risk procedure that continues to be underused. A study of patients who underwent unilateral plication by video-assisted thoracoscopic surgery (VATS) documented substantial increases in spirometry readings at 6 months after the procedure.[16] The mechanism for improvement in these patients is due to increased tension of the diaphragmatic barrier between the thorax and abdomen. This allows patients to generate a more negative intrapleural pressure than is possible with a floppy, paralytic diaphragm.

A variety of techniques have been described in the literature for plication of the diaphragm. Severe forms of congenital eventration of the diaphragm with only a pleuroperitoneal membrane will require patching.[14] A rim of rudimentary diaphragmatic tissue can generally be found around the lateral contour of the chest with enough substance to hold sutures to anchor the patch. Along the medial side, the patch can be stitched to the pericardium and the anterior thoracic spinal ligaments.

The easiest technique of plication is to place imbricating stitches within the central tendon of the diaphragm.[17,18] If the sutures extend far enough from the edge of the diaphragmatic tendon, they can produce substantial caudal displacement of the tendon toward the abdominal cavity and allow expansion of the ipsilateral lower lobe as well as balancing of the mediastinum (Fig. 32-7).[19] A number of variants of the central tendon repair exist and are performed by thoracoscopic, laparoscopic, or hybrid techniques. With improved videoscopic equipment and experience, the trend toward less invasive procedures will continue and may encourage more physicians to refer their patients for surgery. Mouroux and colleagues[20] described a series of 12 patients who underwent thoracoscopically assisted plication with a utility 5-cm incision. A Duval grasper is used to invaginate the apex of the eventration caudad, creating a fold that is closed in two layers. A VATS reproduction of the traditional pleating or "accordion" repair was performed by Freeman and colleagues[16] in 22 patients with use of an Endo Stitch (Ethicon Endo-Surgery, Cincinnati, OH) device to create six to eight parallel U stitches for patients with unilateral diaphragm paralysis. Improvement in pulmonary function and quality of life was seen along with a shortened hospital stay compared with patients who underwent thoracotomy. A total thoracoscopic technique with three ports has been described by Kim and associates[21] and uses the additional adjuncts of carbon dioxide insufflation and steep reverse Trendelenburg position to push the diaphragm down and to increase the effective working space. Laparoscopic plication with four working trocars has been performed by Huttl and colleagues.[22] Retention sutures are placed on the dome of the diaphragm and then used for traction. This allows creation of an intra-abdominal fold for plication with 12 to 15 U-type sutures. Finally, to counter the difficulty in placing adequate sutures through minimal access techniques, Moon and coworkers[23] reported grasping and rolling of the redundant diaphragm followed by placement of noncutting linear endoscopic staplers underneath for creation of folds that are left in situ.

Because of the rarity of diaphragmatic surgery for eventration and the multitude of presentations, a true randomized

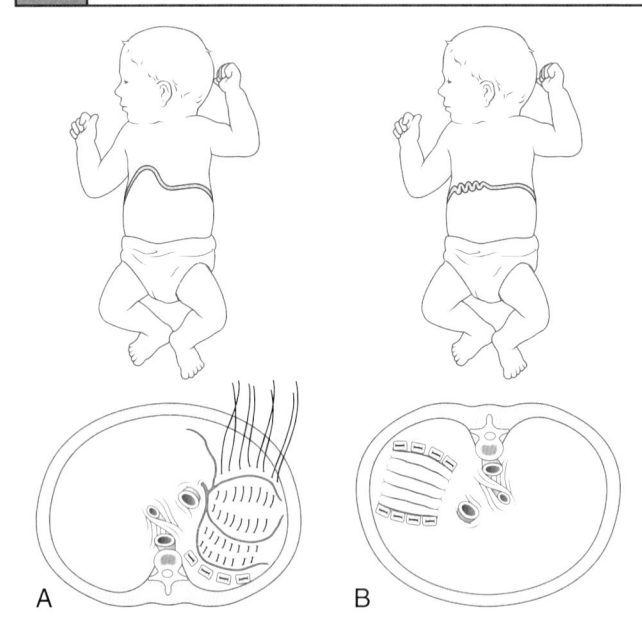

Figure 32–7
Diaphragmatic plication by pleating of the central tendon. Sutures extend beyond the junction of the central tendon with the muscle and should not directly strike the branches of the phrenic nerve. Unfortunately, the phrenic branches lie within the muscle and frequently cannot be visualized.

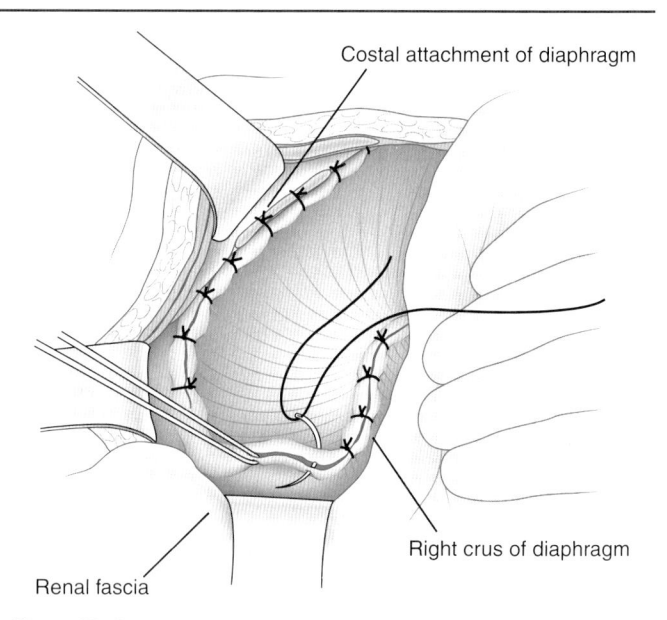

Figure 32–8
Original description of a radial plication technique by David State in 1949. A generous subcostal incision was used, and the muscle was sewn circumferentially to the lateral chest wall and crus to make the tendon taught.

study to compare these methods is difficult, and at present, most surgeons will continue to practice the procedure with which they are most familiar. The drawback of the previous techniques, however, is that the majority of the pleats will fold the noncompliant central tendon. The compliant muscular remnant can be expected to stretch with time. It has been our experience that the central tendon pleating technique is associated with re-elevation of the diaphragm to the level of the hilum within several years. Long-term follow-up of this technique has included reports of recurrent diaphragmatic elevation requiring additional intervention in as many as 19% of treated patients.[24] Furthermore, the phrenic vessels and branches of the nerve travel near the insertion of the muscle into the edge of the tendon and cannot be visualized from the thoracic surface of the diaphragm. Yet, to adequately displace the central tendon, these stitches need to extend into the muscle area, and this places the branches of the nerve at risk of injury. For these reasons, our preference is the radial plication method, which we believe more closely approximates the natural physiology of the diaphragm.

David State first described a subcostal radial plication technique for congenital eventration of the diaphragm in 1949.[25] The original description of this technique included a generous incision across the right upper quadrant of the abdomen and placement of radial sutures along the muscular portion of the diaphragm, pulling it toward the lateral chest wall (Fig. 32-8). A transthoracic radial plication has also been described.[19,26]

John Foker at the University of Minnesota has used a transthoracic radial plication technique since 1976 to treat 35 children with elevation of the diaphragm.[27] The repairs were performed with interrupted horizontal mattress pledgeted sutures, imbricating the muscular portion of the diaphragm in a radial manner toward the chest wall through a posterolateral thoracotomy (Fig. 32-9). The plication sutures extended in an unbroken band from the xiphoid area to the vertebral body. No sutures were placed along the mediastinal pleura. The goal was to produce a taut diaphragm that appeared as a straight-angled line from mediastinum to chest wall on the anteroposterior view of the chest radiograph. We believe that this produces a plication that mimics the contraction of the fan-shaped muscle while minimizing injury to the branches of the nerve or vessels.

In this series, 31 of the 36 operations (86%) led to extubation within 3 days, even though 15 patients had been ventilator dependent before plication.[27] There were no deaths within 30 days, and no morbidity was directly attributed to plication. Only one patient (3%) suffered a recurrence requiring repeated plication. Twenty-six of these patients survived long term (median, 12 years at time of analysis), and 18 of these patients were reevaluated with diaphragmatic ultrasound examination in 1996. Some degree of function had returned to 14 (78%) of the diaphragms.

We have extended this technique to a thoracoscopic approach in adults with elevated hemidiaphragms with some success (Fig. 32-10). Currently, we use a three-port technique, with an anterior and posterior port at the sixth and eighth intercostal space, respectively. The third port is subcostal and is used to pass an O-ring clamp through the abdominal cavity to grasp the undersurface of the central tendon of the diaphragm. This allows the vigorous caudal displacement of the muscle to see the muscular imbrications for plication. The posterior thoracic port is then used to plicate the anterior and lateral borders of the muscle; the anterior thoracic port is used to plicate the lateral and posterior borders.

DIAPHRAGMATIC HERNIAS

Several types of hernias involve the diaphragm, including hernias of the foramen of Morgagni, hernias of the foramen of Bochdalek, and central tendon and paraesophageal hernias.

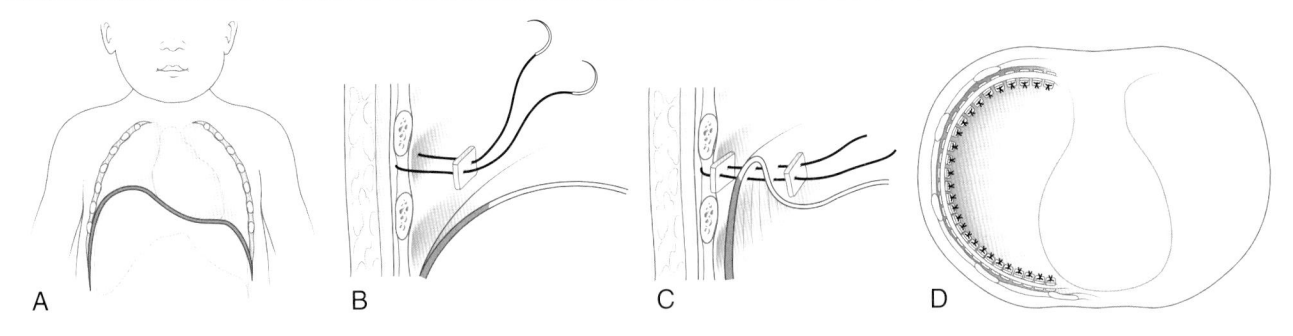

Figure 32–9
Radial plication of the diaphragm with interrupted double-pledgeted sutures extending from the xiphoid to the vertebral spine. Each suture pleats the flaccid muscle to the lateral chest wall.

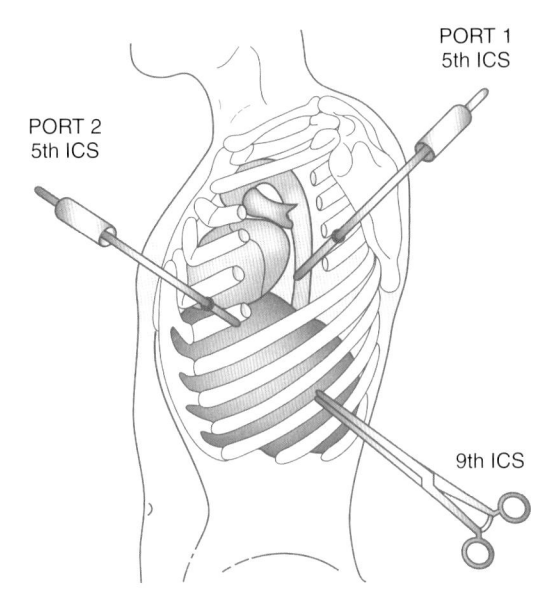

Figure 32–10
Thoracoscopic port placement for radial plication in an adult. (From Mouroux J, Padovani B, Poirer NC, et al. Technique for the repair of diaphragmatic eventration. *Ann Thorac Surg* 1996; 62: 905.)

The foramen of Morgagni is a potential space that lies in the parasternal area where the internal mammary vessels pass from the thoracic cavity into the upper abdominal cavity. Slips of diaphragmatic muscle insert medially onto the back of the xiphisternum and laterally to the costal margin (see Fig. 32-2B). This produces a small triangular gap of muscle tissue around the mammary vessels.

In the presence of increased intra-abdominal pressure, omentum, small intestine, or colon can pass through this defect into the anterior mediastinum. Dull pain along the right subcostal area is the most common presenting symptom. Others are found incidentally on radiographic imaging for unrelated reasons. Foramen of Morgagni hernias are more common in women, in obese individuals, and on the right side because the left side is partially occluded by the pericardial sac. These hernias appear as a density in the parasternal area. CT scans of the chest are helpful in distinguishing these hernias from the pericardial fat pad or a pericardial cyst (see Fig. 32-6B).[28]

Foramen of Morgagni hernias are frequently repaired from an abdominal approach. Both laparoscopic and thoracoscopic repairs have been described.[29,30] A small rim of the internal transthoracic muscle is frequently found behind the sternum and is sutured to the diaphragm to close the hernia. We perform this closure with interrupted mattress sutures using a heavy nonabsorbable suture. Alternatively, the posterior rectus sheath or a rib can be used to help close the hernia. Rarely, the hernia cannot be closed without tension, and a patch is used.

Foramen of Bochdalek hernias can occur in adults. These are rare disorders that either are found incidentally on radiographs for other reasons or are recognized after organ incarceration or volvulus.[31] Most of these hernias are small and are repaired primarily. This can be performed with minimally invasive techniques. Larger defects may require a patch.

A congenital hernia can occur in each of the three central tendons of the trileaflet diaphragm. These can be confused radiographically with tumors lying over the dome of the diaphragm. When the hernia occurs in the central trileaflet, it is frequently associated with a congenital absence of the inferior pericardial sac. This can lead to the phenomenon of abdominal contents within the pericardial sac. Repair of these hernias is straightforward because of the laxity of the central tendon. Primary repair is frequently possible. Very large defects may require patching.

The most frequent diaphragmatic hernia is the paraesophageal hernia. The most commonly used descriptive classification system defines four types of hiatal hernias. A sliding or type I hiatal hernia accounts for as many as 95% of paraesophageal hernias and involves the circumferential weakening of the phrenoesophageal ligament with symmetric displacement of the proximal stomach into the thoracic cavity. This is frequently associated with a shortened esophagus. Most type I hernias are asymptomatic, discovered incidentally on radiographic studies or endoscopy. When symptoms occur, they are primarily related to the associated loss of lower esophageal sphincter tone and gastroesophageal reflux. The likelihood of these symptoms increases in proportion to the size of the hernia.[32]

A paraesophageal or type II hiatal hernia involves a focal weakening of the phrenoesophageal ligament. These hernias tend to occur either anterior or lateral to the esophagus. The gastric cardia remains within the abdomen, and the lower esophageal sphincter remains at the level of the diaphragm. A portion of the gastric fundus, however, rolls through the defect into the chest and produces extrinsic compression of the lower esophagus.

A mixed or type III hiatal hernia has both a sliding and a rolling component. The lower esophageal sphincter has been displaced up into the thorax because of a shortened esophagus. A portion of the gastric fundus then rolls through the enlarged hiatal hernia, producing extrinsic compression of the distal esophagus as well. We agree with Pearson and colleagues[33] that a type II hernia with the gastroesophageal junction below the diaphragm is rarely seen, and type I and type III with the gastroesophageal junction displaced into the thorax are far more common.

Type IV hernias are associated with a large enough defect in the phrenoesophageal membrane to allow other organs, such as the colon, spleen, and small intestine, to enter the hernia sac and the chest cavity. Unrepaired type I, II, or III hiatal hernias can progress, resulting in a large defect between the crura of the diaphragm. As the hernia enlarges, the stomach has a tendency to migrate into the thoracic cavity. The positive pressure in the abdomen and the negative thoracic pressure can lead to the herniation of the greater curvature of the stomach into the right side of the chest and twisting of the stomach on itself. This gastric volvulus produces a gastric outlet obstruction. If air or gastric juices distend the proximal stomach above the gastric outlet, the intraluminal pressure can exceed the perfusion pressure of the organ. This leads to ulceration, bleeding, and the potential for gastric rupture. Recognition of a gastric volvulus or displacement of intra-abdominal organs into the chest is an indication for urgent surgical repair. Because of this potential life-threatening complication, most surgeons recommend repair of these hernias even in the asymptomatic patient.

The initial step in operative repair of a hiatal hernia is to clearly delineate the muscular limits of the hiatal defect. Some experienced surgeons advocate a transthoracic approach for long-standing hernias to facilitate lysis of inflammatory adhesions under direct vision but at the cost of more postoperative pain. More recently, laparoscopic approaches have proved somewhat superior in this goal of identifying the limits of hiatal hernia. This is due to the cephalad displacement of the diaphragmatic muscle during insufflation of carbon dioxide into the abdomen, making the two crura of the diaphragm taut. This tautness and extra space between the stomach and the diaphragmatic muscle greatly facilitate the dissection.

The fat between the proximal stomach and the diaphragmatic muscle needs to be removed. Dividing the muscular fibers of the left diaphragmatic crus in a straight lateral manner can enlarge tight hiatal rings. This will not divide the branches of the phrenic nerve that lie far anteriorly, nor the phrenic vein, which lies medially. The left inferior phrenic artery may be divided without causing ischemia because anastomosing vessels continue to perfuse the area. The enlargement of the tight hiatal ring can greatly facilitate the reduction of a large bulky hernia. Alternatively, a red rubber catheter can be passed across the neck of the hiatal hernia and air insufflated within the sac to facilitate reduction of the hernia contents. This breaks the natural vacuum that occurs in trying to reduce the abdominal contents through the hiatal neck.

The diaphragmatic defect needs to be closed as part of the surgical repair of the hiatal hernia. In fact, it is the pathologic process of the diaphragm that has contributed to the disease of gastroesophageal reflux by disrupting the lower esophageal sphincter. Closure of the dilated esophageal diaphragmatic hiatus is frequently performed by placement of sutures reapproximating the right and left crura of the diaphragm. In large hiatal hernias, this defect can be sizable. If the fibers of the diaphragmatic crura have been thinned, we frequently use pledgeted nonabsorbable sutures to reapproximate the right and left muscle bundles. The tenant of all hernia repairs is to prevent tension at closure, and some defects may require patch or mesh reinforcement. Two randomized studies comparing mesh versus primary crural closure are available. Frantzides and colleagues[34] randomized 36 patients to closure with or without a polytetrafluoroethylene (PTFE) mesh onlay. At 3-year follow-up, 22% in the primary group had hernia recurrence compared with 0% in the mesh group. Another study with 50 patients used polypropylene rather than PTFE. The simple cruroplasty cohort had a 26% recurrence rate compared with 8% in the mesh group.[35]

A late complication of the use of prosthetic mesh for this indication has been mesh migration and esophageal or gastric erosion, often ending in sepsis and need for esophageal exclusion. Biological mesh options now exist that decrease the risk of this complication. The use of porcine small intestine submucosa has been described for closure of large hiatal defects.[36] This is now our preferred approach to reinforcement of the crura associated with giant paraesophageal hernias. A radial incision leading to a keyhole slit is made in the mesh to accommodate the esophagus, and the mesh incision is then closed with endoscopic placement of sutures. The material allows a remodeling of the hiatus and is eventually incorporated with the neighboring tissue so that a permanent material is not left in place.

The postoperative complication rate after laparoscopic antireflux surgery is approximately 8%. Between 3% and 6% of all patients undergoing antireflux surgery require reoperation for recurrent, persistent, or new symptoms secondary to complications of the initial repair.[37] In one published series of 627 patients, 7% of the entire group had demonstrable anatomic failure, most of which were due to intrathoracic migration of the wrap with or without disruption of the fundoplication.[38] A number of factors has been attributed to this problem, including inadequate closure of the crura, lack of appreciation of a shortened esophagus, and physiologic factors that increase intra-abdominal pressure, such as valsalva, coughing, or retching in the postoperative period.

We believe that one of the most common errors in the surgical repair of hiatal hernias is not recognizing that an esophagus has shortened. If the esophagus is not of adequate length to allow the fundoplication to reside within the abdomen without undue pressure, the fundoplication will likely herniate into the thorax within a few years. We have a low threshold for extending the length of the esophagus with a Collis gastroplasty to ensure that the fundoplication will lie beneath the diaphragmatic hiatus without tension.

A rare but devastating complication of fundoplication herniation into the chest from an unrecognized shortened esophagus is a gastropericardial fistula[39] (Fig. 32-11). This rare condition has an associated mortality rate of more than 50% and is most often seen in patients with prior gastroesophageal surgery. Most likely, these fistulas originate at the site of gastric ulcerations. Approximately 3% to 5% of open Nissen fundoplication procedures are complicated by gastric ulceration. In most cases, the ulcerations occur high on the lesser curvature of the stomach, in proximity to the fundoplication, and are seen most often in patients with recurrent hiatal hernias. Fistulas from the stomach to the aorta, diaphragm, pericardium, right ventricle, and bronchus have been reported as late complications from open Nissen fundoplication.[39]

Repair of a gastropericardial fistula involves the removal of a circle of pericardium (see Fig. 32-11) and the fistulous entry into the stomach. The muscle of the diaphragm can then be used as a pedicled muscle flap to lie between the exposed heart and the staple line along the lesser curve of the stomach. In our experience, we have used pledgeted sutures to close the muscles of the crura and secure the wrap beneath the diaphragm.[39]

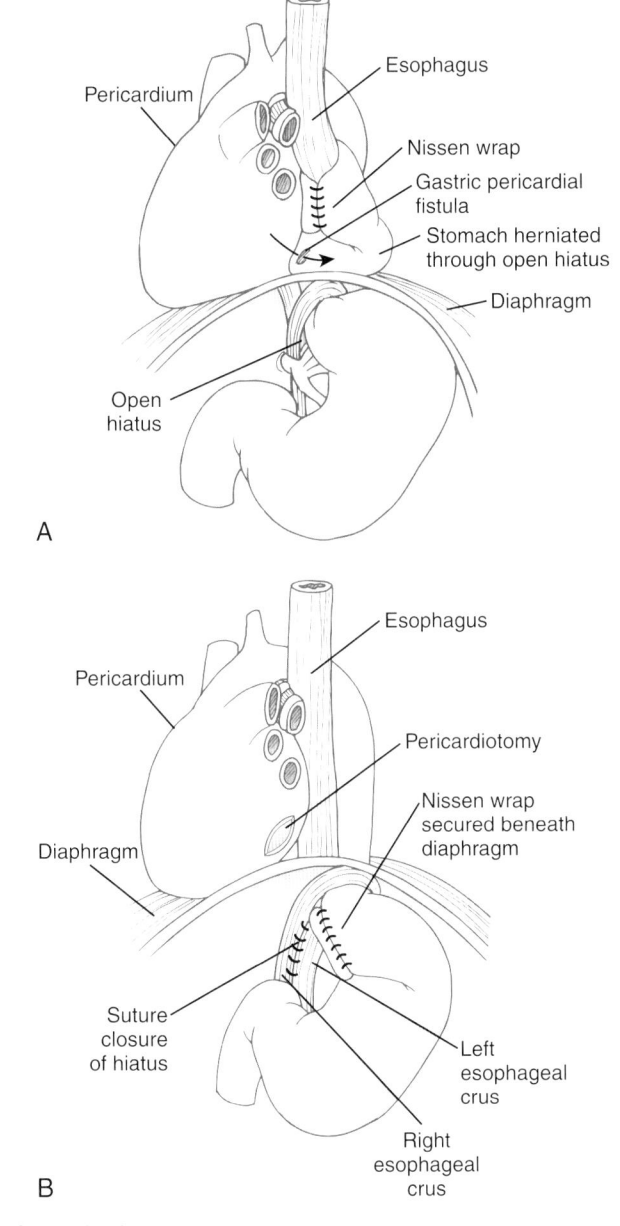

Figure 32-11
A, Gastropericardial fistula is a devastating complication of a fundoplication herniating into the chest from failure to close the diaphragmatic crura. The fistula is typically along the lesser curve of the stomach distal to the fundoplication. B, We repaired this fistula by using the diaphragm as a muscle flap to place between the heart and the stomach. (From Murthy S, Looney J, Jaklitsch MT. Gastropericardial fistula after laparoscopic surgery for reflux disease. *N Eng J Med*: 2002; **346**: 328-32.)

DIAPHRAGMATIC PACING

Diaphragmatic pacing may have a role to play for patients with compromised pulmonary function and diaphragmatic paralysis. The technology was first used clinically in 1967, and more than 700 patients with chronic hypoventilation have been treated in this manner, some for as much as 18 years.[40] Expertise in this technique, however, is limited to a few centers. Technical details of long-term continuous pacing were mostly worked out by William Glenn of Yale. He and his colleagues rapidly moved from a successful animal model in 1964[41] to treatment of a patient with central hypoventilation in 1967.[42] Excellent detailed reviews of this subject have been published by Glenn and Koda[40] and Elefteriades and Quin,[43] also from Yale.

Diaphragmatic pacing has largely been supplanted by noninvasive methods of ventilatory support, including bi-level positive airway pressure and continuous positive airway pressure, particularly in the setting of temporary respiratory compromise or comorbid disease, such as chronic obstructive pulmonary disease. A select subset of patients, however, may be helped by this diaphragmatic pacing. The ideal patient for this technique has central nervous system or upper motor neuron disease and an intact phrenic nerve and diaphragm.[43] The major experience with phrenic nerve pacing has come from quadriplegic patients and central alveolar hypoventilation patients. Patients with spinal cord injury above C3 are especially good candidates because the whole phrenic nerve is denervated from upper motor neurons but intact within the chest. Because pacing will not produce normal excursion of an atrophied diaphragmatic muscle, it is recommended that the pacemaker be placed soon after the neurologic insult.

The major therapeutic objective of diaphragmatic pacing is oxygenation rather than the elimination of carbon dioxide. Expiratory flow must be adequate, thus limiting the use of pacing in severe chronic obstructive pulmonary disease or other conditions that have significantly altered the shape of the chest wall or diaphragm.[43] Sufficient diaphragmatic strength, nearly normal function of the distal phrenic nerve, and satisfactory excursion of the thoracic skeleton must be demonstrated.

The topic of phrenic nerve pacing is frequently discussed in the setting of phrenic nerve palsy. The inherent lack of electrical conductivity of skeletal muscle, unlike the heart, does not allow uniform contraction of the muscle by multiple surface electrodes. An intact lower motor neuron (i.e., phrenic nerves) is thus required to deliver the electrical impulse by neurotransmitters throughout the muscle for coordinated contraction. Because axonal damage precludes conduction of electrical impulses to the neuromuscular junction, direct phrenic nerve injury is not amenable to pacing. These patients may be better treated with direct intervention (i.e., primary phrenic nerve repair or nerve transplantation with an intercostal or recurrent laryngeal nerve) or supportive measures (i.e., diaphragmatic plication, nocturnal bi-level positive airway pressure, or tracheostomy).[43]

The best placement of the phrenic nerve pacemaker with current technology is within the upper thorax by an anterolateral thoracotomy through the third intercostal space. This allows placement of the electrode around the main phrenic trunk below the entry of the accessory nerve from the C5 nerve root, which frequently joins the phrenic nerve within the upper thorax.[44] It is important to avoid handling of the nerve as injury would prevent accurate pacing. The site of implantation of the electrode is above the azygos vein and superior vena cava on the right (Fig. 32-12). In the left side of the chest, the preferred site is between the aortic arch and the pulmonary artery.[45] The wire attached to the electrode is then tunneled to the receiver in the chest wall. Although the nerve trunk is easily found in the neck, the phrenic nerve is missing the C5 accessory nerve at this level in 76% of patients.[46] Furthermore, placement of the electrode over the superior vena cava avoids direct conduction of the electrical signal to the atrium, which can occur lower in the thorax. Electrodes can now be placed thoracoscopically.[43] Implantation through the cervical approach has largely been abandoned because of its inability to bring the pacing electrode in proximity to the C5 branch of the phrenic nerve.

The phrenic nerve should be tested transcutaneously for patients with a central nervous system cause of hypoventilation to verify intact nerve and muscle function. This test was described by Shaw and colleagues in 1975.[47] An indifferent electrode is placed on the skin of the neck, and a pacing electrode delivering 5 to 10 mA for 1 msec is placed at the lateral border of the sternocleidomastoid muscle. A forceful contraction of the diaphragm signifies normal or nearly normal diaphragmatic function. Forceful diaphragmatic movement can be observed by physical examination. Quantification of diaphragmatic excursion can be made by fluoroscopy or ultrasonography. An excursion of at least 5 cm should be seen for pacing intervention to be considered.[43]

The initial diaphragmatic pacemaker consisted of a monopolar electrode attached to an antenna and a radiofrequency generator. A bipolar electrode would be used if the patient also has a cardiac pacemaker. To overcome the lack of natural electrical conductivity of the skeletal muscle of the diaphragm, a train of pulse currents with increasing amplitude is delivered by the pacemaker to stimulate all axons within the nerve.[43] One consequence of the pulse train to induce uniform muscle contraction is that every fascicle is stimulated to contract. Because 24% of the fascicles are fast-twitch, fatigue-prone type IIB fibers,[48] full-time pacing can occur only after a period of muscle conditioning. Part-time pacing in quadriplegic patients does not start for 14 days to avoid pleural effusion.[43] Pacing starts at 15 minutes per hour and changes every 7 to 14 days. Conditioning thus takes 3 to 6 months. A permanent tracheostomy is recommended for all patients on full-time, continuous phrenic nerve pacing.[43]

Three pacing systems are currently available: the Avery model (Avery Laboratories, Glen Cove, NY), the Atrotech OY (Tampere, Finland), and the MedImplant (Vienna, Austria). All models have a two-part system with an extracorporeal radiofrequency generator and implantable receiver–nerve electrode. Further technological improvements may make diaphragmatic pacing a more generalizable technique for patients with long-term but ultimately reversible dysfunction, such as viral palsies and iatrogenic injuries. The largest reported series of diaphragmatic implantation pacers observed 165 patients; 68% were paced for less than 5 years, 20% for 5 to 10 years, and 10% for 10 to 15 years.[49]

Onders and colleagues[50] have developed a separate diaphragm pacing system that can be implanted through a laparoscopic technique. For this form of pacing to be effective, an intact phrenic nerve is still required to recruit muscle contraction by conduction pathways. After laparoscopic ports are placed, the initial step is to map the diaphragm with a specially developed probe to see which point causes the greatest diaphragmatic excursion. Once this point is identified, electrodes are placed on each side and retested. The lead wires are then tunneled to exit from the chest wall. Limited studies have shown results comparable to those of standard phrenic nerve pacing.[51] Potential advantages compared with currently available phrenic nerve pacing include less expensive equipment and the ability to implant electrodes in both diaphragms without the need for repositioning or single-lung ventilation that is required during VATS procedures. Current experimentation with natural orifice transluminal endoscopic surgery may further decrease the invasiveness of this procedure and make temporary pacing in the intensive care unit a more realistic possibility.[52]

At present, the impact on improved quality of life for patients is the reason for continued research into the science of diaphragmatic pacing. Besides the obvious benefit of freedom from mechanical ventilation, pacing can also lead to improved speech patterns, conversion from tracheostomy to stoma devices, and return of olfactory sensation.[45]

In summary, diaphragmatic pacing is useful for carefully selected patients with intact phrenic nerve and diaphragmatic muscle function but impaired upper motor neurons. Results of unilateral pacing are not beneficial because the phrenic nerve is usually not functional. The potential exists for a large group of patients with lower motor neuron disease (i.e., temporary or permanent phrenic nerve injury) to benefit once further advances in technology can produce smooth, coordinated muscle contraction of the diaphragm with direct muscle stimulation.

ONCOLOGY OF THE DIAPHRAGM

Primary tumors of the diaphragm are rare, and the literature is notable for scattered case reports only. Benign tumors include variants of fibrous tumors and lipomas, neurogenic

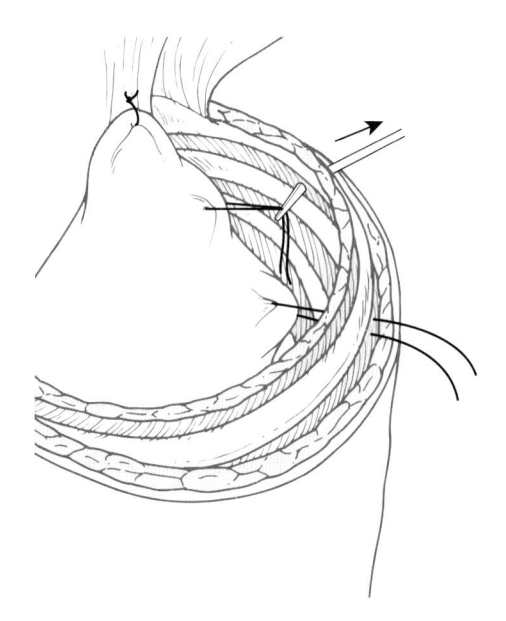

Figure 32–12
Diaphragmatic resection for extrapleural pneumonectomy necessitates patch closure. A sterile leatherworking awl is used to pass anchoring sutures through the chest wall to re-create radial lines of tension. These sutures are secured along the outside of the rib cage with use of angiocaths through the holes of sterile buttons.

tumors, and cysts. These tumors generally present as incidental findings on imaging studies, and the majority of patients are asymptomatic. Surgical resection with primary closure or reconstruction is the standard treatment. Primary malignant tumors may arise from muscles, tendon, or mesothelial elements on either side of the diaphragm. Most of these lesions are sarcomatous in origin and are locally aggressive and best treated with complete diaphragmatic resection. The benefits of chemotherapy are limited. Because recurrence is usually local, various methods of irradiation delivered preoperatively or postoperatively have been used. We have also used intraoperative placement of brachytherapy seeds after resection of primary or secondary tumors of the diaphragm.

Invasion of the diaphragm from tumors on either side of the "fence" can occur. In the abdomen, this is most commonly seen with large retroperitoneal sarcomas, hepatocellular carcinoma, or upper gastrointestinal tumors including direct extension into the hiatus by gastroesophageal junction adenocarcinomas.

Mesothelioma and chest wall sarcomas are thoracic malignant neoplasms that may involve the diaphragm and are discussed elsewhere in greater detail. Invasion of the diaphragm by primary lower lobe lung adenosquamous cancers is considered T3 disease, and these patients are often not considered for surgery on the basis of preoperative imaging because a corresponding pleural effusion is present that up-stages the disease to T4. Others are given chemotherapy first to determine responders who will most benefit from surgery. Between 0.17% and 0.4% of patients are found to have diaphragm disease at explorative thoracotomy.[53,54] Because of the rarity of this occurrence, limited data have been published about this topic. Weksler and associates[55] were the first to address this population of patients, describing eight patients between 1974 and 1995 who underwent exploratory thoracotomy for non–small cell lung cancer. All patients underwent en bloc resection with an overall survival of 52.8 weeks.

To improve on the limited data from the previous series, two multicentric retrospective studies have been done. Riquet and colleagues[55] reviewed 68 patients from 17 centers who underwent thoracotomy with resection of non–small cell lung cancer invading the diaphragm and found a 67% rate of lymph node involvement. This was thought to be due to the extensive lymphatic drainage of the diaphragm. Sixty-three patients in a study from the Lung Cancer Surgical Study Group of Japan were identified from 31 institutions. Complete resection was performed in 55 patients (87.3%), and the 5-year survival in these patients was 22.6%.[53] The depth of diaphragm involvement was noted to affect prognosis; patients with shallow invasion of the diaphragm had a 33% 5-year survival versus 14.3% in those with deep muscular or peritoneal invasion. The overall survival of these patients after complete resection compared with T3 lung cancers with chest wall involvement was significantly less.

DIAPHRAGMATIC RESECTION AND REPAIR WITH PROSTHETIC PATCH

Partial diaphragmatic resections are necessary to remove tumors that have invaded a portion of the diaphragm. The redundancy of the muscle frequently allows primary repair for small to modest resections. Larger defects are easily repaired with a mesh or impermeable graft sutured to the remnant of muscle. We use mesh for patients with lung tissue remaining in the ipsilateral hemithorax and impermeable grafts for patients who have had a pneumonectomy to prevent fluid shifts between the thorax and abdomen.

Complete diaphragmatic resection may be required for large tumors invading the diaphragm, such as lung cancer of the lower lobe or sarcomas of the chest. We have gained our extensive experience with complete diaphragmatic resection as part of an extrapleural pneumonectomy for mesothelioma.[7]

An extrapleural pneumonectomy is the complete removal of the pleural envelope and all its contents, including the ipsilateral lung, lateral pericardium, and underlying diaphragm. Because the pleura cannot be separated from the central tendon of the diaphragm, the diaphragm must be resected if the pleural envelope is to be kept intact during removal.

Diaphragmatic resection begins with traction of the pleura away from the chest wall deep into the diaphragmatic sulcus. This exposes the bare area of the lateral diaphragm where the pleura folds off the rib cage and back onto the upper surface of the diaphragm (Fig. 32-13).[7] The division of these lateral radial bands of the fan-shaped portion of the diaphragm is started at the most anterior portion of the chest close to the pericardium. The fingers of the surgeon bluntly dissect the peritoneum from beneath the muscle, then pull the fibers taut to facilitate visualization to divide the muscle with cautery. It is not unusual for the posterolateral portion of the diaphragm to be beyond the direct vision of the surgeon. Fibers in this area can be bluntly avulsed with minimal risk of bleeding. Once the ligamentum arcuatum externum (external arcuate ligament) is reached in the paravertebral sulcus, the perinephric fat of Gerota's fascia not the peritoneum, is directly beneath the fan-shaped muscle. This part of the dissection quickly progresses to the lateral margin of the crus. The diaphragm can then be separated from the peritoneum up toward the lateral border of the pericardium. Defects in the peritoneum are closed as they are recognized.

An extrapleural pneumonectomy requires the removal of the lateral portion of the pericardium because the mediastinal pleura cannot be removed from that structure. The pericardium

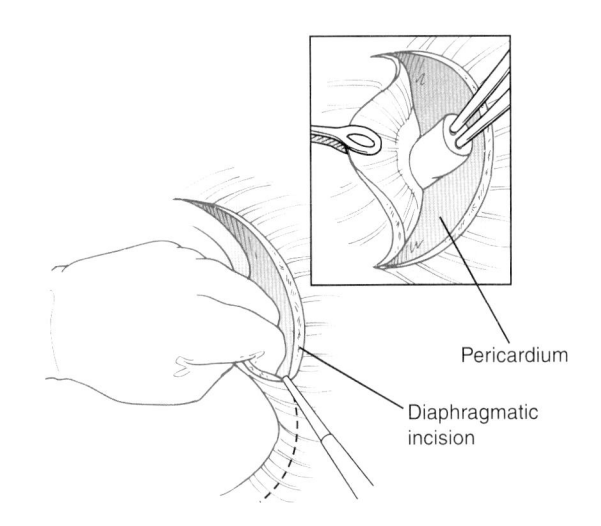

Figure 32–13
Circumferential incision of the right hemidiaphragm exposing the underlying peritoneum. Pericardial and crural attachments remain after division of the fan-shaped muscle.

is opened anteriorly. The phrenic nerve is divided cephalad to the pulmonary artery. The trileaflet of the diaphragmatic tendon is divided along the line demarcating the central tendon of the ipsilateral muscle from the tendon lying beneath the pericardium. This cut is made medial to the insertion of the phrenic nerve into the anterior muscle. This medial cut is extended along the fused portion of diaphragmatic tendon and pericardium to the inferior vena cava on the right or the esophageal hiatus on the left.

At this point, the only attachment of the diaphragm remaining is the crus. Blunt dissection of the pleura of the deep diaphragmatic sulcus needs to be completed before division of the crus to prevent buttonholing of the inferior extent of the posterolateral pleura. The superior phrenic arteries are surgically inconsequential and rarely identified. The inferior phrenic vessels, however, lie on the deep surface of the crus and are easily seen and ligated. These vessels may bifurcate low over the crus, and a second branch may therefore be found after ligation of a branch thought to be the main trunk. The left inferior phrenic vein usually has two branches, one of which drains into the left renal or suprarenal vein and another that passes anterior to the esophageal hiatus and empties into the inferior vena cava. The right inferior phrenic vein empties directly into the inferior vena cava and therefore requires careful dissection and ligation. Vigorous lateral traction can avulse this vessel from the inferior vena cava, close to the insertion of the hepatic veins. Once these vessels have been divided, the crus is easily divided. This completes the diaphragmatic resection.

The postpneumonectomy space fills with fluid. To prevent fluid shifts between the thorax and abdomen, we use a 2-mm impermeable Gore-Tex prosthetic patch to reconstruct the resected diaphragm. This patch prevents herniation of abdominal contents into the chest, holds the abdominal viscera out of the thoracic irradiation field, and bolsters the contralateral diaphragm by fixing the medial edge of the fan into place. This then facilitates the function of the opposite diaphragm by allowing its central tendon to become the anchor point for the lateral fan fascicles. Without patching of the ipsilateral diaphragmatic defect, the contralateral muscle function is compromised.

After the patch has been cut to the shape of the removed diaphragm, the medial edge is sewn to the pericardial tendon with a soft nonabsorbable stitch. We prefer 0 Ethibond for this suture. This suture line runs from the free edge of the divided anterior fan muscles, along the pericardial edge, to either the inferior vena cava or esophageal hiatus. A reliable lateral anchorage system has been devised, requiring a sterilized leatherworking awl (Fig. 32-14). Loops of suture material that have been passed through the lateral edge of the patch are then brought through the chest wall with the awl. The sutures are then passed through a small postage stamp–sized patch of the same material as well as a sterile plastic button, with the assistance of two angiocaths. The loop of suture is then tied down to itself onto the button, resulting in excellent lateral displacement of the patch.

The posterior mediastinum between the thoracic spine and the inferior vena cava or esophagus is the area where patch ruptures occur, with abdominal contents herniating into the chest. This is due to a lack of strong mediastinal tissue available to anchor the patch. Our group of surgeons have developed the following three potential solutions: (1) a suture anchoring the patch to the anterior spinal ligament, (2) a tongue of

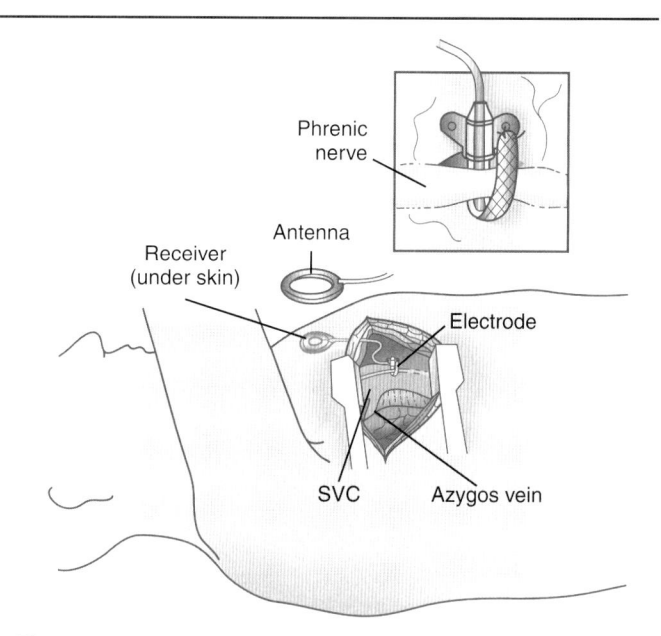

Figure 32–14
Placement of phrenic nerve pacing lead to an intra-lateral thoracotomy. SVC, superior vena cava. (From Kaanan S, Ducko. CT. Diaphragmatic pacing. In: *Harrison's Principles of Internal Medicine*, 17th ed. Online update, 2008. http://www.accessmedicine.com.)

extra patch material folded inferiorly along the lumbar spine in simulation of the diaphragmatic crus, and (3) a composite of two patches of 2-mm Gore-Tex stapled together in the middle with a thoracoabdominal stapler to create a dynamic patch at the center with less tension at the lateral suture lines. The first technique uses the dense spinous ligament to anchor the posterior mediastinal portion of the patch and decreases the free defect between the anterior suture line at the inferior vena cava and the thoracic spine to a few centimeters. The second technique allows the medial portion of the patch to be partially displaced into the chest but prevents visceral herniation unless the entire tongue becomes displaced into the chest. The last technique allows the prosthetic patch to "give" without rupture if the patient experiences abdominal distention.

SUMMARY

The diaphragm serves several functions as a result of its unique anatomic location. It is the major muscle of respiration, by creating the intrathoracic vacuum and moving the lower ribs. It is a barrier between the positive-pressure abdomen and the negative-pressure thorax. It is important in the function of the lower esophageal sphincter.

Surgical approaches to the diaphragm are easily learned and depend on an understanding of the anatomy and physiology of the muscle, nerve, and blood vessels. A variety of incisions are possible once the locations of the nerve and vessel branches have been learned. These structures frequently lie within the muscle itself and are not seen on the surface of the structure. Therefore, the concept of a handcuff around the junction of the central tendon to the muscle is helpful.

Diaphragmatic repair and patching are helpful in traumatic injuries, congenital absence of a part of the diaphragm, and diaphragmatic hernias. Diaphragmatic pacing is not useful in phrenic nerve palsies because an intact lower motor neuron is required for the current level of technology to function. Plication of the diaphragm for these cases is useful. We prefer a radial plication technique that mimics the radial contraction of the fan-shaped muscle to that of a central tendon pleat.

Repair of gastroesophageal reflux depends on the construction of a new lower esophageal sphincter. A major contributor of the pathologic process, however, is a diaphragmatic hernia between the crura: a hiatal hernia. Therefore, we believe that tightening of the crus around the repair and lengthening of a shortened esophagus are important steps to keep the repair within the abdomen and to prevent complications such as gastropericardial fistula.

The entire hemidiaphragm can be resected. Small resections can be repaired primarily, but large resections should be patched to assist the function of the contralateral muscle. The choice between permeable and impermeable patches depends on the remaining presence of ipsilateral lung. The principles of the patch repair include a tight apposition to the medial remnant of the diaphragm and then radial lateral displacement of anchoring sutures.

Although the diaphragm acts as a boundary between the thorax and abdomen, it should not serve as a boundary between the realm of thoracic surgeons and gastrointestinal surgeons. The diaphragm makes a good fence, but neighbors on both sides of that fence should know its anatomy, physiology, and surgical principles of resection and repair.

REFERENCES

1. Schumpelick V, Steinau G, Schluper I, et al. Surgical embryology and anatomy of the diaphragm with surgical applications. *Surg Clin North Am* 2000;**80**(1): 213-39, xi.
2. Larsen W. *Human embryology*. 2nd ed. New York: Churchill Livingstone; 1997. 136-137.
3. Gray H. Anatomy, descriptive and surgical. In: Pick T, Howden R, editors. *Revised American, from the 15th English ed.* New York: Bounty Books; 1977. p. 1257.
4. Epstein S. An overview of respiratory muscle function. *Clin Chest Med* 1994;**15**:619-39.
5. Bergofsky E. Relative contributions of the rib cage and the diaphragm to ventilation in man. *J Appl Physiol* 1964;**19**:698-706.
6. Wade O. Movements of the thoracic cage and diaphragm in respiration. *J Physiol* 1954;**124**:193-212.
7. Sugarbaker D, Mentzer S, Strauss G. Extrapleural pneumonectomy in the treatment of malignant pleural mesothelioma. *Ann Thorac Surg* 1992;**54**:941-6.
8. Anderson T, Miller J. Surgical technique and application of pericardial fat pad and pericardiophrenic grafts. *Ann Thorac Surg* 1995;**59**:1590-1.
9. Owens W, Gladstone D, Heylings D. Surgical anatomy of the phrenic nerve and internal mammary artery. *Ann Thorac Surg* 1994;**58**:843-4.
10. Merendino KA, Johnson RA, Skinner HH, et al. The intradiaphragmatic distribution of the phrenic nerve with particular reference to the placement of diaphragmatic incisions and controlled segmental paralysis. *Surgery* 1956;**39**:189-98.
11. Reber PU, Schmied B, Seiler CA, et al. Missed diaphragmatic injuries and their long term sequelae. *J Trauma* 1998;**44**(1):183-8.
12. Shah R, Sabanthan S, Mearns AJ, et al. Traumatic rupture of diaphragm. *Ann Thorac Surg* 1995;**60**:1444-9.
13. Larici AR, Gotway MB, Litt HI, et al. Helical CT with sagittal and coronal reconstructions: accuracy for detection of diaphragmatic injury. *Am J Roentgenol* 2002 Aug;**179**(2):451-7.
14. Beck W, Motsay D. Eventration of the diaphragm. *Arch Surg* 1952;**65**:557-63.
15. Marcos J, Grover F, Trinkle J. Paralyzed diaphragm—effect of plication on respiratory mechanics. *J Surg Res* 1974;**16**:523-6.
16. Freeman RK, Wozniak TC, Fitzgerald EB. Functional and physiologic results of video-assisted thoracoscopic diaphragm plication in adult patients with unilateral diaphragm paralysis. *Ann Thorac Surg* 2006;**81**(5):1855-7.
17. Garbaccio C, Gyepes M, Fonkalsrud E. Malfunction of the intact diaphragm in infants and children. *Arch Surg* 1972;**105**:57-61.
18. Schwartz M, Filler R. Plication of the diaphragm for symptomatic phrenic nerve paralysis. *J Pediatr Surg* 1978;**13**(3):259-63.
19. Shoemaker R, Palmer G, Brown JW, et al. Aggressive treatment of acquired phrenic nerve paralysis in infants and small children. *Ann Thorac Surg* 1981;**32**(3):251-9.
20. Mouroux J, Padovani B, Poirer NC, et al. Technique for the repair of diaphragmatic eventration. *Ann Thorac Surg* 62: 905, 1996.
21. Kim DH, Hwang JJ, Kim KD. Thoracoscopic diaphragmatic plication using three 5 mm ports. *Int J Cardiovasc and Thorac Surg* 2007;**6**:280-2.
22. Huttl TP, Wichmann MW, Reichart B, et al. Laparoscopic diaphragmatic plication. *Surg Endosc* 2004;**18**:547-51.
23. Moon SW, Young-Pil W, Yong-Whan K, et al. Thoracoscopic plication of diaphragmatic eventration using endostaplers. *Ann Thorac Surg* 2000; **70**:299-300.
24. Smith C, Sade RM, Crawford FA, et al. Diaphragmatic paralysis and eventration in infants. *J Thorac Cardiovasc Surg* 1986;**91**:490-7.
25. State D. The surgical correction of congenital eventration of the diaphragm in infancy. *Surgery* 1949;**25**:461-8.
26. Sethi G, Reed W. Diaphragmatic malfunction in neonates and infants: Diagnosis and treatment. *J Thorac Cardiovasc Surg* 1971;**62**(1):138-43.
27. Jaklitsch M, et al: Twenty year experience with peripheral radial plication of the diaphragm. Presented at 33rd Annual Meeting of the Society of Thoracic Surgeons, San Diego, 1997.
28. Naunheim K. Adult presentation of unusual diaphragmatic hernias. *Chest Surg Clin N Am* 1998;**8**(2):359-69.
29. Huntington T. Laparoscopic transabdominal preperitoneal repair of a hernia of foramen of Morgagni. *J Laparoendosc Surg* 1996;**6**:131-3.
30. Hussong R, Landrenau R, Cole F. Diagnosis and repair of a Morgagni hernia with video-assisted thoracic surgery. *Ann Thorac Surg* 1997;**63**:1474-5.
31. Karanikas ID, Dendrinos SS, Liakakos TD, et al. Complications of congenital posterolateral diaphragmatic hernia in adults. *J Cardiovasc Surg (Torino)* 1994;**35**:555-8.
32. Patti MG, Goldberg HI, Arcerito M, et al. Hiatal hernia size affects lower esophageal sphincter function, esophageal acid exposure, and the degree of mucosal injury. *Am J Surg* 1996;**171**:182-6.
33. Pearson FG, Cooper JD, Ilves R, et al. Massive hiatal hernia with incarceration: a report of 53 cases. *Ann Thorac Surg* 1983;**35**(1):45-51.
34. Frantzides CT, Richards CG, Carlson MA. Laparoscopic repair of large hiatal hernia with polytetrafluoroethylene. *Surg Endosc* 1999;**13**:906-8.
35. Granderath FA, Schweiger UM, Kamolz T, et al. Laparoscopic Nissen fundoplication with prosthetic hiatal closure reduces postoperative intrathoracic wrap herniation: preliminary results of a prospective randomized functional and clinical study. *Arch Surg* 2005;**140**:40-8.
36. Zilberstein B, Eshkenazy R, Pajecki D, et al. Laparoscopic mesh repair antireflux surgery for treatment of large hiatal hernia. *Dis Esophagus* 2005;**18**:166-9.
37. Soper N, Dunnegan D. Anatomic fuxdoplication failure after laparoscopic surgery. *Ann Surg* 1999;**229**:669-76.
38. Steir HJ, Feussner H, Siewert JR. *Am J Surg* 1996;**171**:36-9.
39. Murthy S, Looney D, Jaklitsch MT. Gastropericardeal fistula after laparoscopic surgery for reflux disease. *N Engl J Med* 2002;**346**:328-32.
40. Glenn W, Koda H. Pacing the diaphragm in chronic ventilatory insufficiency. In: Shields TW, editor. *Thoracic surgery*. Philadelphia: Lea & Febiger; 1989. p. 595-610.
41. Glenn WW, Hageman JH, Mauro A, et al. Electrical stimulation of excitable tissue by radio-frequency transmission. *Ann Surg* 1964;**160**:338-50.
42. Judson J, Glenn W. Radiofrequency electrophrenic respiration: long-term application to a patient with primary hypoventilation. *JAMA* 1968;**203**:1033-7.
43. Elefteriades J, Quin J. Diaphragm pacing. *Chest Surg Clin N Am* 1998;**8**(2):331-57.
44. Glenn W, Sairenji H. Diaphragm pacing in the treatment of chronic ventilatory insufficiency. In: Roussos C, Macklem P, editors. *The thorax*. New York: Marcel Dekker; 1985. p. 1407-49.
45. Kanaan S, Ducko CT. Diaphragmatic pacing. In: *Harrison's principles of internal medicine*. 17th edi. Online Update. 2008. http://www.accessMedicine.com
46. Kelley W. Phrenic nerve paralysis: Special consideration of the accessory phrenic nerve. *J Thorac Cardiovasc Surg* 1950;**19**:923-8.
47. Shaw R, Glenn W, Holcomb W. Phrenic nerve conduction studies in patients with diaphragm pacing. *Surg Forum* 1975;**26**:195-7.
48. Lieberman D, Faulkner JA, Craig Jr AB, et al. Performance and histochemical composition of guinea pig and human diaphragm. *J Appl Physiol* 1973;**34**:233-7.
49. Glenn WW, et al. Fundamental consideration in pacing of the diaphragm for chronic ventilatory insufficiency: a multi-center study. *Pacing Clin Electrophysiol* 1988;**11**:2121-7.
50. Onders RP, DiMarco AF, Ignagni AR, et al. Mapping the phrenic nerve motor point: The key to a successful laparoscopic diaphragm pacing system in the first human series. *Surgery* 2004;**136**:819-26.
51. DiMarco AF, Onders RP, Ignagni A, et al. Phrenic nerve pacing via intramuscular diaphragm electrodes in tetraplegic subjects. *Chest* 2005;**127**:671-8.

52. Onders RP, McGee MF, Marks J, et al. Diaphragm pacing with natural orifice transluminal endoscopic surgery: potential for difficult-to-wean intensive care unit patients. *Surg Endosc* 2007;**21**:475-9.
53. Yokoi K, Tsuchiya R, Mori T, et al. Results of surgical treatment of lung cancer involving the diaphragm. *J Thorac Cardiovasc Surg* 2000;**120**:799-805.
54. Weksler B, Bains M, Burt M, et al. Resection of lung cancer invading the diaphragm. *J Thorac Cardiovasc Surg* 1997;**114**:500-1.
55. Riquet M, Porte H, Chapelier A, et al. Resection of lung cancer invading the diaphragm. *J Thorac Cardiovasc Surg* 2000;**120**:417-8.

CHAPTER 33
Congenital Diaphragmatic Hernia
Dario O. Fauza and Jay M. Wilson

History
Epidemiology
Embryology of the Diaphragm
Pathology
  Etiology
  Pathogenesis
  Pathologic Anatomy
    Gross Findings
    Microscopy
  Pathophysiology
Clinical Manifestations
Diagnosis
Associated Anomalies
Prognostic Factors
Treatment
  Preoperative Care
    Pulmonary Vasodilators
    Nitric Oxide
    Surfactant
    Alternative Forms of Mechanical Ventilation
    Extracorporeal Membrane Oxygenation
  Surgery
  Postoperative Care
  Late-Presentation Congenital Diaphragmatic Hernia
Results
Long-Term Follow-Up
  Diaphragmatic Hernia Recurrence
Future Perspectives
Other Diaphragmatic Anomalies
  Diaphragmatic Eventration
  Morgagni Hernia
  Hiatal Hernia
  Pericardial Hernia
  Diaphragmatic Agenesis
  Diaphragmatic Duplication
  Cribriform Diaphragm

Various congenital diaphragmatic anomalies include one or more defects that allow herniation of abdominal contents into the chest. However, the term *congenital diaphragmatic hernia* (CDH), also referred to as Bochdalek's hernia, refers specifically to congenital defects located on the posterolateral aspect of the diaphragm. Despite the term *hernia*, there is a true hernia sac in only approximately 15% of the cases.

HISTORY

The first known written description of a diaphragmatic herniation was made by Ambroise Parè in 1579.[1] However, the two cases described by Parè were caused by trauma. In his 1679 *Sepulchretum*, Teophile Bonet attributed the first description of a congenital case to Lazare Rivere, at the beginning of the 17th century, even though it was from the autopsy of an adult.[2] The first report of a CDH in a newborn was made by George Macaulay, in 1754, also as an autopsy finding, in an infant who died from respiratory failure a little over 1 hour after birth.[3]

In 1761, Giambattista Morgagni, then a pupil of Valsalva, wrote a review of diaphragmatic herniations and credited Stehenius with the first observation that CDH was associated with pulmonary hypoplasia.[4] In the review, Morgagni described the first case of a parasternal hernia, henceforth termed Morgagni hernia, in an elderly man. In 1848, Vincent Alexander Bochdalek reported two cases, and he described the location of the diaphragmatic defect as being in the posterolateral aspect of the muscle—hence the origins of the terms *Bochdalek hernia* and *Bochdalek foramen*.[5] Although widely employed, these terms are actually improper, as the mechanisms and exact location proposed by Bochdalek—namely, rupture of the lumbocostal triangle—are inaccurate.[6-8]

The link between CDH and deviations of the embryonic development of the pleuroperitoneal membrane only started to be established from the studies by Broman, in 1902 and 1905.[9,10] Nevertheless, although this anatomic location for the diaphragmatic defect is universally accepted, it is not yet known where the primary disorder that leads to CDH takes place.

The first successful repair of a CDH was performed by Aue in a 9-year-old boy in 1901, but it ws published only in 1920.[11] The first publication of a successful CDH repair was by Heidenhain, in 1905, and he reported a procedure, also in a 9-year-old boy, that took place in 1902.[12] In 1940, the first survival of a neonate, who underwent CDH repair on the second day of life, was reported by Ladd and Gross.[13] Gross was also the first to report on a good outcome after repair before the first 24 hours of life, in 1946.[14]

In 1977, German and coworkers reported the first child with CDH to survive after being placed on extracorporeal membrane oxygenation (ECMO).[15] Since the mid 1980s, ECMO has played a major role in maximizing the survival rates of neonates with CDH.[16-18]

In 1989, Harrison and associates presented the first series of patients with CDH treated by open prenatal repair of the diaphragmatic defect in humans, leading to live births but no midterm survival.[19] Survival after this procedure was reported by this same group in 1992, but only in 28.6% of the operated fetuses.[20]

In the early 1990s, Wung and colleagues introduced the concept of avoiding hyperventilation and minimizing barotrauma.[21,22] This led to marked reduction in iatrogenic insult to the lungs, which was very common with the old, aggressive ventilation strategies, and the consequent improvement in survival has been significant.[16,23-25]

The first successful lung transplantation for the treatment of CDH was performed in a newborn in 1992, by the groups of Shochat and Starnes.[26,27] Also in 1992, Wilson first showed, in an ovine model of CDH, that fetal lung growth could be significantly accelerated after occlusion of the fetal trachea, leading to reversal of the pulmonary hypoplasia associated with experimental CDH.[28] In 1994, Harrison's group applied this maneuver successfully in a human fetus with CDH.[29] Nonetheless, the results of fetal tracheal occlusion, whether performed as an open or a video-fetoscopic procedure, remain worse than those of postnatal care, at least at the referral centers in North America.[30-32] Still, fetal tracheal occlusion continues to be offered systematically at a few European centers, and (anecdotally) elsewhere, although its current indications, if any, remain to be clearly defined.[33,34]

In 1994, the Congenital Diaphragmatic Hernia Registry was created as a meta-institutional organization dedicated to the exchange and analysis of data related to this disease, as well as to the design and implementation of multicenter prospective trials. This initiative, molded after the pediatric oncology groups first established in the 1980s, has had a major beneficial impact on CDH survival and on management guidelines.[35]

In 1995, we demonstrated experimentally that lung growth could be accelerated after birth, through continuous intrapulmonary distention with a perfluorocarbon.[36,37] The first series of patients that received this treatment, under ECMO support, was presented in 2000.[38] A multicenter prospective trial of this principle has proven difficult to pursue because of regulatory and logistical hurdles, yet it remains an anticipated perspective. Also in 2000, the use of a tissue-engineered construct for the repair of the diaphragmatic defect was first proposed in an animal model.[39] Further experimental developments have validated engineered diaphragmatic repair, and a clinical trial is expected in the foreseeable future, pending regulatory clearance.[40-43]

In general, efforts are now aimed at defining the patients who would benefit from lung growth acceleration (whether prenatal or postnatal), enhancing diaphragmatic repair through tissue engineering, and minimizing morbidity of the increasing number of long-term survivors.

EPIDEMIOLOGY

The prevalence of CDH has been reported as being between 1:1200 and 1:12,000 births.[44-56] The main reason for such disparity is probably the so-called hidden mortality of CDH, which means that many babies die before reaching a referral center and thus are not included in the statistics.[57] The better-controlled studies show CDH as occurring in 1:2107 to 1:3163 births.[44,47,49,50,52,54] One of the largest series, by Torfs and colleagues, involving over 718,000 births and stillbirths in California, revealed that CDH occurred in 1:3163 births and in 1:3340 live births.[54] Among the major congenital anomalies, CDH is one of the most common, accounting for approximately 8% of the cases.[58]

There are no clear racial differences in the prevalence of CDH.[52,54] The study by Torfs and coworkers showed a higher prevalence in rural rather than urban areas, but this has not yet been confirmed by other series.[54] The prevalence of prematurity and weight deviations in neonates with CDH is no different from that in the general population.[54] Although isolated CDH is a little more common in boys than in girls (1.5:1), sex distribution is equal in CDH associated with other congenital anomalies and in the whole CDH population.[54,59]

There is limited controversy as to the risk of CDH recurrence in families. In the vast majority of cases, CDH is sporadic, with no genetic component described and with the risk for further offspring being practically equal to that in the general population.[44,47] At the same time, many families with more than one child with CDH, usually siblings, have been identified.[49,54,58,60-66] Less frequently, relatives other than siblings present with this anomaly.[61,67,68] The epidemiologic profile of familial cases of CDH differs little from that of the total of cases: it is slightly more common in males (approximately 2:1),[60,63,67,69] and the data are conflicting as to other variables.[62,68] The occurrence of familial CDH follows a pattern suggestive of multifactorial inheritance as the most likely mode of transmission, with recurrence estimated between 1.3% and 2%.[54,58,62,65] The possibility that a genomic imprinting phenomenon takes place has also been proposed.[66] A recent extensive review of a single-hospital-based malformation surveillance program (the largest to date of consecutively collected cases of CDH) showed low precurrence among siblings.[70]

EMBRYOLOGY OF THE DIAPHRAGM

The development of the diaphragm from the mesoderm is complex and not yet fully understood. It results from the fusion of four embryonic components: two odd ones—the transverse septum and the mediastinum (also known as the dorsal mesentery of the esophagus)—and two paired structures—both sides of the body wall musculature and both pleuroperitoneal membranes (Fig. 33-1).[9]

The diaphragm begins to develop during the 3rd and 4th weeks of gestation, with the appearance of the first component of the diaphragm, the transverse septum (see Fig. 33-1). At this point, the transverse septum is an incomplete mesenchymal divider, related cranially to the pericardial cavity and caudally to the midgut. Dorsally, the transverse septum blends with the mediastinum. On each side of the mediastinum there are the pleural canals, which connect the pericardial and peritoneal cavities. The subsequent development of the diaphragm depends on the closure of these dorsal pleural canals, which will give rise to the pleural cavities.

During the 4th week, the pulmonary buds, which are developing inside the mediastinum, begin to protrude into the pleural canals. At this stage, the pleural canals are very small and the pericardial cavity is very large. Crests formed on both extremities of the pleural canals will separate the future pleural cavities from the pericardial cavity, cranially, and from the peritoneal cavity, caudally. The cranial crest

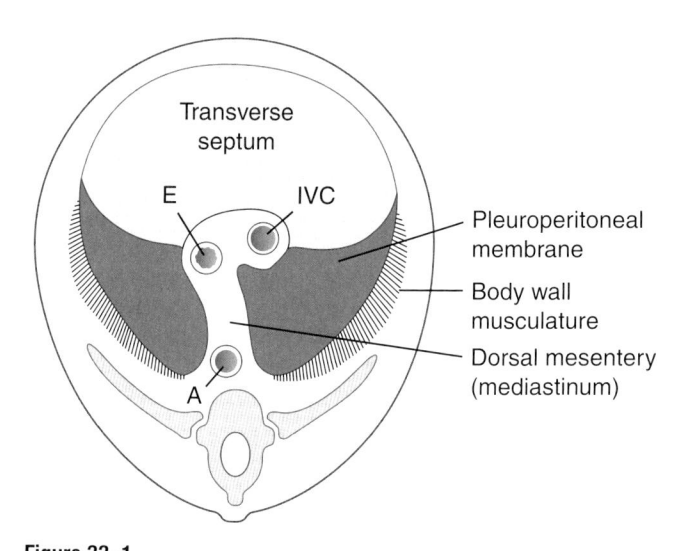

Figure 33–1
The four embryonic components of the diaphragm. A, aorta; E, esophagus; IVC, inferior vena cava.

will give rise to the pleuropericardial membrane and the caudal crest will form the pleuroperitoneal membrane (see Fig. 33-1).

The enlargement of what are now the pleural cavities leads to a progressive narrowing of the opening between them and the pericardial cavity, as well as to the development of the pleuropericardial membrane. In like manner, there is progressive narrowing of the pleuroperitoneal canals and the development of the pleuroperitoneal membranes.[6,7] The definitive closure of the pleuroperitoneal canals, now small, will occur during the 8th week of gestation.[6]

After closure of the pleuroperitoneal canals, the pleural cavities continue to expand, in parallel to lung growth. Cranially, they spread out beyond the limits of the pericardial space. Caudally, they extend into the body wall.[6] During this process, which takes place from the 9th to the 12th week, the mesoderm in the posterior thoracic wall appears to be carved out by the caudal borders of the expanding pleural cavities, so that its inner portion will become part of the diaphragm. At the same time, a similar process happens at another, more lateral and anterior portion of both the thoracic and the abdominal walls. As a consequence, part of the diaphragmatic muscle originates from the musculature of the thoracic and the abdominal walls.[6,71]

Despite the almost universal acceptance of this explanation for the development of the diaphragmatic muscle, there is some controversy related to the role of the phrenic nerve in that process. In accordance with the principle that muscles in general retain their original segmental innervation, certain authors believe that myoblasts derived from the caudal portion of the infrahyoid mesoderm migrate, together with the phrenic nerve, from the third and fourth cervical somites, toward the diaphragm, so that this would be the origin of the diaphragmatic muscle.[72,73] However, the phenomenon of myoblasts migrating together with the phrenic nerve has not yet been proven; it is but a partially accepted theory. The fact that the tendinous center of the diaphragm is a fibrous structure completely devoid of muscle fibers speaks against this theory.[7] In any event, even if myoblasts from the superior cervical myotomes do follow the phrenic nerve, at least part of the diaphragmatic innervation should be later transferred to muscular portions derived from the thoracic and abdominal walls.

Deviations from the normal development of each one of the various components of the diaphragm bring about different variants of diaphragmatic anomalies. Table 33-1 shows the diverse embryonic origins of the diaphragm and their relationship to different diaphragmatic defects.

PATHOLOGY

Etiology

The etiology of CDH is unknown. In a few rare syndromes in which a diaphragmatic defect is present, there is a well-defined genetic cause, such as in trisomies of chromosomes 13 and 18. On the other hand, a recent single-institution review showed that 17% of all cases of CDH (both isolated and in association with other congenital anomalies) had a recognizable genetic etiology.[70] In addition, there was no concordance for CDH among five monozygotic twin pairs. These findings, in conjunction with previous reports of de novo dominant mutations in CDH patients, suggest that new mutations may be an important mechanism in the etiology of this disease. The twin data also point to the possibility that epigenetic abnormalities contribute to its development. Different strategies to reveal eventual CDH-critical chromosome loci and candidate genes in humans are now being actively pursued.[74]

Experimental CDH can be produced in diverse animal species through different interventions, other than surgical creation of the defect, including exposure to diet deficient in either vitamin A,[75,76] zinc,[77] or cadmium[78]; administration of either thalidomie,[79] antirat rabbit serum,[80] 2,4-dichlorophenyl-p-nitrophenyl ether (nitrofen, a herbicide),[81-83] or polybromate biphenyls[84,85]; and genetic manipulations, such as FOG-2, COUP-TFII, and GATA-4 mutations.[86-88] However, a conclusive relationship between these experimental models and clinical or epidemiologic data in humans has not been shown.

Pathogenesis

The pathogenesis of CDH is also unknown. Normally, before the return of the bowel from the umbilical cord to the abdominal cavity, which occurs during the 10th week of gestation, it is necessary for the pleuroperitoneal canal and the lumbocostal triangle to firmly close, which happens between the 8th and 10th weeks. If such closure does not take place, the bowel will pass through the pleuroperitoneal canal, sometimes also through the lumbocostal triangle, and will invade the chest, resulting in a "herniation" without a hernia sac. If there is only a membranous closure, the same phenomenon will happen, albeit with a hernia sac that may, or may not, rupture sometime later. In any case, although it is well established that the diaphragmatic defect is at the level the pleuroperitoneal canal,[6,7,9,10] the sequence of events that culminates in disturbances of its closure remain to be determined.

Table 33–1
Embryologic Origins of the Diaphragm and Corresponding Diaphragmatic Defects

Embryonic Structure	Time (wk)	Portion Formed	Diaphragmatic Defect
Transverse septum	3 and 4	Central tendon	Pericardial hernia (ventral defect)
Pleuroperitoneal membranes	7 and 8	Primitive diaphragm	Bochdalek hernia (posterolateral defect)
Mediastinum (dorsal mesentery)	—	Median portion and crura	—
Body wall	9 to 12	Muscle periphery (ventral-lateral and dorsal)	Morgagni hernia (parasternal defect) and eventration

The prevailing theory as to CDH development has been that the incomplete closure of the pleuroperitoneal canal was a primarily diaphragmatic defect and that the abdominal viscera herniated to the thorax impeded normal lung development and resulted in the pulmonary hypoplasia and hypertension observed almost universally in association with CDH. This perception was widely confirmed by animal models in which a diaphragmatic defect was surgically produced in fetuses of different species,[89-91] or in which the diaphragmatic herniation was mimicked by an inflatable prosthesis placed in the pleural cavity.[92] All these models resulted in lung hypoplasia and pulmonary hypertension at birth.

Nonetheless, the foremost notion today is that the primary defect is not in the diaphragm but in the lung buds, and that the diaphragmatic defect would actually be secondary to a primary pulmonary hypoplasia. Such pulmonary hypoplasia, in turn, could be intensified even more by the presence of abdominal viscera herniated into the chest. Starting at the 4th week of gestation, the growth of the pulmonary buds and of the pleural cavities result in a progressive narrowing of the pleuroperitoneal canals and in the formation of the pleuroperitoneal membranes.[6,7] The development of the diaphragm, more specifically of the pleuroperitoneal membranes, is intimately related to lung development itself. Researchers that have worked with the experimental model of CDH induced by nitrofen have shown that, in that model, the pulmonary hypoplasia precedes the diaphragmatic defect.[82,83,93,94] These findings are in accordance with the fact that nitrofen exposure can lead to pulmonary hypoplasia independently of the existence of CDH.[95-97] Iritani has concluded that the lung buds, which are primarily hypoplastic because of exposure to nitrofen, cause hypoplasia of the posthepatic mesenchymal plate, which in turn develops in intimate association with the lung buds.[82] The hypoplasia of this mesenchymal plate, which is one of the precursor portions of the primitive diaphragm, would then give rise to the diaphragmatic defect and, consequently, to the CDH.[82] Moreover, it is thought that the morphogenesis and differentiation of the pulmonary respiratory epithelium is intimately dependent on the kind of extracellular matrix synthesized by the mesenchyme.[83,98,99] Kluth and colleagues have shown that lungs of embryos exposed to nitrofen display an abnormal expression of factors normally found in the extracellular mesenchymal matrix, with a delayed pattern of epithelial differentiation.[99] Iritani speculates further that the reason that CDH is more common on the left in humans is that lung bud development tends to be slower on the left than on the right[82,100,101] and, also, the fusion of the pleuroperitoneal membranes happens later on the left side than on the right.[89] Independent of the possibility of a primary pulmonary hypoplasia in the nitrofen model, Alles and coworkers have shown that there is also cell death in the mesoderm of some cervical somites that are precursors of the diaphragm, suggesting a concomitant primary disorder of diaphragmatic development. Consequently, the mechanism behind the emergence of CDH in this model is still to be clarified.[102] Knockout models, such as FOG-2 −/− mice, are further evidence of a primary pulmonary hypoplasia associated with CDH.[86]

A so-called smooth muscle hypothesis, pointing to abnormalities in airway smooth muscle development as central to the pathogenesis of CD, has been proposed but not yet fully validated,[103] and other, less accepted theories for the pathogenesis of CDH exist.[73,104-106] Whatever the location and nature of the primary defect may be, the presence of a diaphragmatic defect per se usually leads to herniation of abdominal viscera to the chest, which, in turn, at least contributes to worsen the pulmonary hypoplasia.[89-91] The sooner the herniation occurs in gestation and the larger the herniation content, the more intense the pulmonary hypoplasia tends to be.

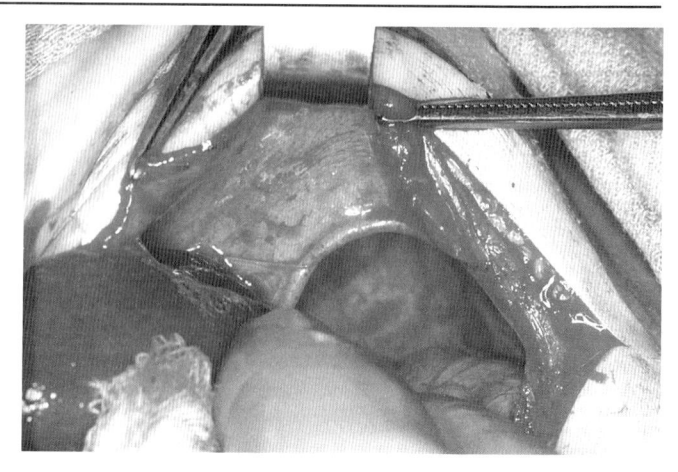

Figure 33–2
Typical intraoperative finding, through a left subcostal laparotomy, in a neonate with congenital diaphragmatic hernia. Note the defect on the posterolateral aspect of the left diaphragm.

Pathologic Anatomy

Gross Findings

The diaphragmatic defect, or Bochdalek foramen, is located in the posterolateral aspect of the diaphragm and involves at least the area that would have originated from the pleuroperitoneal membrane and, many times, also the area immediately posterior to it—the lumbocostal triangle (Fig. 33-2). The size of the defect is highly variable, from less than 1 cm in diameter to an almost complete absence of the hemidiaphragm, extending beyond the dome, practically to the midline, preserving merely a small anterolateral band of muscle. There is no fibrosis or any evidence of inflammation at the level of the diaphragmatic opening. The left side is affected in approximately 80% to 90% of the cases, the right side in 10% to 20%, and bilateral cases are rare, occurring in approximately 1% of the patients.[17,107]

In most cases, the pleura and the peritoneum are in continuity over the borders of the diaphragmatic defect, which may render the identification of the residual posterior muscle band difficult. In only approximately 15% of the patients is there a hernia sac. The size of the diaphragmatic opening does not necessarily relate to the volume of the herniation.

Because of the herniation to the chest, the mediastinum is usually deviated to the contralateral side of the hernia (Fig. 33-3). Both lungs, but particularly the one ipsilateral to the defect, are smaller than normal in both volume and weight (Fig. 33-4).[108-110] Pulmonary lobulation is ordinarily normal but may be compromised in a few cases.[108,111] On the other hand, the shape of the pulmonary lobes is commonly distorted.[108,111] The pulmonary ligament is almost always absent on the side of the hernia.[108] The number of airway generations and their dimensions are reduced, especially in the ipsilateral

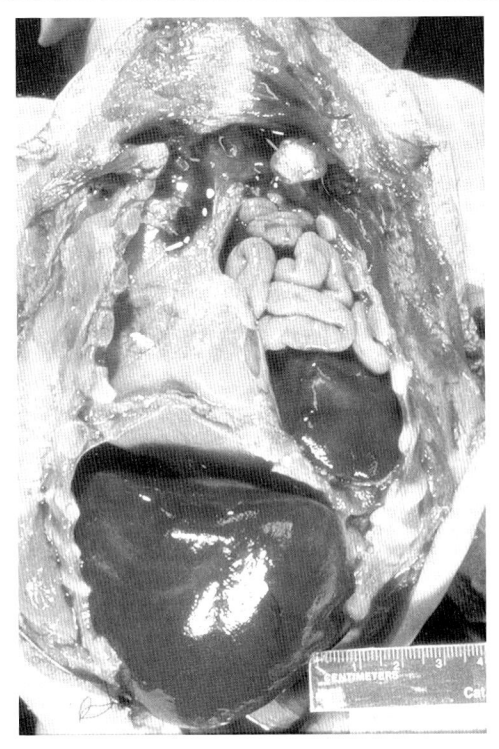

Figure 33–3
Typical gross autopsy finding from a neonate with congenital diaphragmatic hernia. Note the abdominal organs herniated to the left hemithorax through the posterolateral defect on the ipsilateral diaphragm, and the mediastinal deviation to the right. There is no hernia sac.

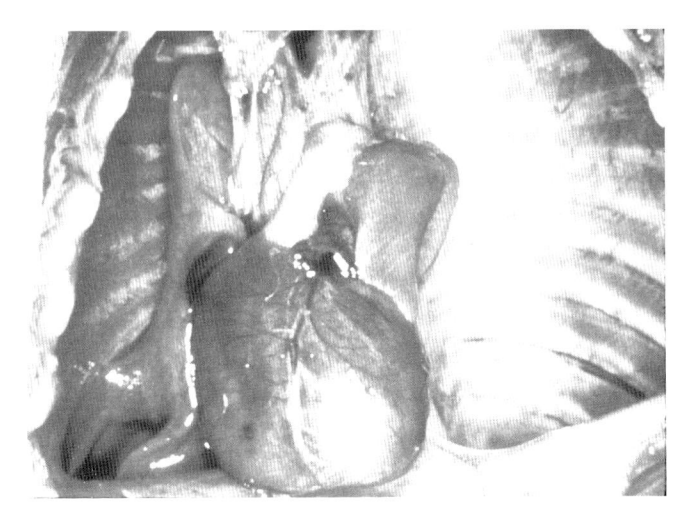

Figure 33–4
Thoracic cavity in the neonate shown on Figure 33-3, after removal of the abdominal organs herniated to the left hemithorax. Note the reduced size of the lungs, especially on the left.

side of the defect.[108,111] The pulmonary arteries, as well as the number and dimensions of their branches, are smaller than normal, in proportion to the reduced size of the lungs, and also particularly on the side of the hernia.[108]

The herniation of abdominal contents to the thorax and the pulmonary hypoplasia may both lead to the appearance of many other abnormalities. Therefore, such abnormalities are not considered other anomalies associated with CDH but actually integral components of the CDH syndrome.[112] The most frequent of such abnormalities are persistent ductus arteriosus, persistent foramen ovale, and intestinal malrotation.[112] Less frequently, the following abnormalities can also be a direct consequence of CDH: gastric volvulus, abnormally sized chest cavity, accessory spleen or congenital splenic fibrosis in left CDH, abnormal hepatic lobulation or hepatopulmonary fusion in right CDH, and hypoplasia or fibrosis of the lobe of the liver ipsilateral to the hernia.[112-114] Also, the volume of the abdominal cavity is frequently reduced.

Microscopy

Except for the defect itself, the diaphragm does not exhibit any other deformity. A local decrease of the density of branches of the phrenic and intercostal nerves has been described by some[73] but not yet confirmed by others and is considered of limited value.[102]

The impact of CDH on the lungs vary in an ample spectrum. The lung ipsilateral to the hernia is impaired the most, but both lungs are affected. In a given patient, the effects of the hernia are not uniform on the different portions of each lung.

The airway branching order is abnormal, with a reduced number of generations of lower bronchi and bronchioli, often with complete absence of the latter, so that bronchi may end directly in alveoli.[108,110,111] Given that normal airway branching is complete by 16 weeks of gestation,[100,115] the reduction in airway generations observed both grossly and microscopically is further evidence of the fact that CDH and pulmonary hypoplasia start before this time, more specifically between the 10th and 12th weeks. On the other hand, the development of airway cartilage itself does not seem to be affected, so the proportion of cartilage-bearing airways to the total number of airways is normal.[108,111] However, the number of bronchi containing mucous glands is diminished.[111]

The total alveolar number is reduced, both in absolute terms and in relation to total lung volume.[108,110,111] However, the number of alveoli per acinus may be either reduced or normal, suggesting that the reduction in total alveolar number is mostly a consequence of the lower number of terminal bronchioli.[108,110] The alveoli are also smaller than normal.[108] The fate of type II pneumocytes is not yet completely clear. Many studies uncover evidence that the surfactant system is depressed, but it is not absolutely clear whether this has to do with a reduction in the density of type II pneumocytes.[116-122]

In parallel to the lower number of airway generations, the absolute number of arterial branches is reduced,[108] yet the density of intra-acinar arteries may be normal.[110] The arterial diameters are reduced.[108,110] There is hypertrophy of the arterial muscle layer at all levels, as well as extension of such muscle layers into more distal branches, which normally would not bear any muscle.[108,110,123,124] There seems to be a direct relationship between pulmonary hypoplasia and arterial muscularization, so that the more hypoplastic the lung, the more intense is the abnormally augmented muscularization.[123]

Pathophysiology

The cardinal aspects of CDH pathophysiology are pulmonary hypertension with persistence of a fetal circulatory pattern, along with a reduction in both pulmonary tidal volume and compliance. The intensity of such manifestations varies a great deal, going from almost nonexistent to incompatible with life, depending mostly on the severity of the anatomic abnormalities of a given patient. According to some, a deficiency of the surfactant system is also part of CDH pathophysiology.[116-119] However, this notion has been increasingly challenged by more recent data.[122,125,126]

In children, total peripheral airway cross-sectional area is proportionally larger than in adults, so the reduction in airway generation present in CDH usually does not lead to significant increases in airway resistance.[127] The difficulty in ventilating children with CDH stems mostly from the lower pulmonary compliance and lower tidal volumes. The pressure–volume curves of these hypoplastic lungs are abnormal, so that, at a given pressure, lung volume is lower than normal.[128] Microscopic analyses under insufflation show that, although certain airspaces may open at 15 to 20 cm H_2O, many are still closed at 30 to 35 cm H_2O.[129] Thus, higher inspiratory pressures are transferred only to the alveoli that are open, leading to alveolar rupture and a tendency to develop pneumothorax.[130] It is not yet clear whether the decreased pulmonary compliance is a result of a quantitative or qualitative (or both) depression of the surfactant system, or is a result a relative increase in the total amount of collagen in the lungs.[116-118,131] The lower tidal volumes are a direct consequence of the reductions in both lung volume and total alveolar number.[108-111] All these ventilatory abnormalities are the main reasons for the tendency of infants with CDH to retain CO_2.[130]

Contrary to what happens with the airways, the peripheral vessels (lower arteries, arterioles, and capillaries) account for most of the pulmonary vascular resistance (PVR). Therefore, as a result of the reduction in the total number of arterial branches and their lower than normal diameters, the total arterial cross-sectional area is diminished and the PVR is usually significantly increased in CDH.[132,133] Further contributing factors to the increased PVR are the hypermuscularization of the arteries and amplified arterial reactivity. Because of the latter, certain physiologic stimuli such as alveolar hypoxia, hypoxemia, hypercapnia, acidosis, cyanosis, hypothermia, and any "disturbances," such as certain inflammatory mediators and simple manipulations of the patient, may trigger intense pulmonary vasoconstriction and marked increase in PVR.[134,135] Other than the possibility of a role played by the muscular hypertrophy present in pulmonary arteries and arterioles, the reason these vessels tend to overreact to stimuli is not yet known. Recent data suggest that the pulmonary vasculature's ability to synthesize nitric oxide is depressed in patients with CDH and thus may be part of the mechanism.[136] The possibility of an imbalance involving prostanoids, which are vasoactive agents that include prostaglandins, playing a role has been suggested.[133,137-139] A potential role for other endogenous vasoactive agents, such as endothelins, in the increase in PVR has proved debatable.[133,140,141]

This increase in PVR leads to pulmonary hypertension, which is almost universally observed in neonates with CDH.[129,133,142] Pulmonary hypertension leads to a decrease in total blood flow to the lungs, an increase in end-diastolic pressure in the right ventricle, and a tendency for persistence of a fetal circulatory pattern, with right-to-left shunt through the ductus arterious and foramen ovale.[129,134] The decrease in total pulmonary blood flow and the right-to-left shunt lead to hypoxemia, hypercapnia, and acidosis, which, in turn, are stimuli to pulmonary vasoconstriction, which worsens the pulmonary hypertension, with consequent intensification of the fetal circulatory pattern and so forth, establishing a vicious circle difficult to break. Not infrequently, patients may be satisfactorily oxygenated and fairly stable, until a random stimulus, or nothing immediately discernible, triggers the vicious circle of fetal circulation. This period of temporary stability that precedes the emergence or worsening of pulmonary hypertension has been coined *honeymoon*. It was described for the first time by Collins and colleagues in the mid 1970s and remains a frequent observation in neonates with CDH.[133,143] The mechanisms responsible for the end of the honeymoon have been elusive until the past few years, when mounting evidence points to it being a cardiac event—more specifically, variable degrees of right heart failure.[144] Patients who present soon after birth with persistent hypoxemia, without ever going through a honeymoon period, usually have severe pulmonary hypoplasia and serious abnormalities of the pulmonary vasculature.[124]

In the fetus, the oxygenated blood that comes from the placenta returns to the right heart through the umbilical vein and crosses either the foramen ovale or the ductus arteriosus toward the aorta, so that only approximately 7% of the cardiac output goes through the lungs.[145] Therefore, the hemodynamic disturbances associated with pulmonary hypertension almost never manifest in utero. After birth, however, the hemodynamic status tends to deteriorate, often with overload and potential failure of the right side of the heart. Thus, cardiac failure is typically part of the pathophysiology of CDH,[144,146,147] and survival depends, to a great extent, on the ability of the myocardium to withstand the overload imposed by the pulmonary vasculature.[129,144,146] The deviation of the mediastinum by the herniated content may lead to a decrease in the venous return to the heart, possibly contributing to further worsening of the patient's hemodynamic status.

It has been suggested that neonates with CDH may have adrenal insufficiency, with an inadequate response to stress.[148] At the same time, there is preliminary experimental evidence pointing to the possibility that lower than normal glucocorticoid levels may contribute to the abnormal lung development and maturation found in patients with CDH.[149] The true meaning of these findings in CDH pathophysiology remains to be better defined. Indeed, at least as far as receptors are concerned, hypoplastic lungs of fetuses and newborns with CDH seem to be as responsive to glucocorticoids, thyroid hormone, and retinoic acid (all relevant to normal pulmonary development) as the lungs of normal children.[150]

Of the different aspects of the pathophysiology of CDH, it is the pulmonary hypertension that is most responsible for mortality in the neonatal period. Because otherwise healthy neonates who undergo total pneumonectomy are often able to maintain good oxygenation and ventilation, without clinically relevant pulmonary hypertension, the lack of pulmonary parenchyma alone cannot explain all the manifestations commonly observed in infants with CDH.[151] Rarely in CDH is the bilateral lung impairment intense enough to cause a neonate to have less than half of the normal total alveolar surface area. Consequently, it would appear that, more often than not, the pulmonary vasculature abnormalities are clinically much more relevant than the lack of alveoli (pulmonary hypoplasia).

CLINICAL MANIFESTATIONS

Ninety percent of the patients with CDH are symptomatic within the first 24 hours of life.[152] However, this disease may first manifest at any age and, more rarely, go unnoticed until very late in life or even never be diagnosed.[153-155]

When a child is symptomatic within the first 24 hours of life, the main clinical manifestation is respiratory distress. The earlier the onset of signs and symptoms, the more severe the pulmonary disease. Newborns who are symptomatic in the first 6 hours after birth are considered at high risk and account for 88% of the cases.[152] Tachypnea associated with sternal, subcostal, and supraclavicular retraction is common. Cyanosis and pallor are also frequent. Apgar scores tend to be low. If untreated, the dyspnea tends to worsen with time, for three reasons: the progressive distention of the intrathoracic bowel by gas, which is accelerated by aerophagy, common in children in respiratory distress; the gradual increase of the volume herniated to the chest, which is a result of the negative pressure exerted during respiration; and the escalating hypoxemia, hypercapnia, and acidosis, resulting from the vicious circle generated by persistent pulmonary hypertension. The abdomen is often scaphoid because of the migration of abdominal viscera to the chest. However, because of possible bowel distention inside the abdominal cavity, the abdomen may assume a normal appearance with time. The chest may be asymmetrical, larger on the side of the hernia, especially after the bowel fills with gas. The heart sounds are commonly dislocated to the contralateral side of the hernia. Sometimes the same happens with the trachea. In the ipsilateral hemithorax, the respiratory sounds may be diminished or absent altogether, and bowel sounds may be present. There may be hemodynamic instability, with a tendency to arterial hypotension, because of a decreased venous return to the heart resulting from the mediastinal deviation or because of right heart failure due to pulmonary hypertension. Occasionally, mediastinal deviation can also lead to superior vena cava syndrome.[156] If untreated, a symptomatic newborn usually expires in a few minutes or hours.

Rarely in the neonatal period, there may be manifestations stemming from perforations or strangulation, or both, of a hollow viscus, gastric, or midgut volvulus, or rupture of a herniated spleen, such as gastrointestinal (GI) obstructions, empyema, hemothorax, fever, arterial hypotension, coagulopathy, anemia, or hypovolemic shock. Anecdotal associations between CDH and septicemia with group B streptococci in premature babies have also been described.[157]

When CDH first manifests after the neonatal period, partial or complete GI obstructions are more common than respiratory distress, which, if present at all, tends to be mild. Unlike in the neonates, the spectrum of manifestations of late-presentation CDH is quite broad, including, in addition to GI obstruction and respiratory distress, sudden death, growth retardation, perforations or strangulations of intrathoracic hollow viscera (which may lead to sepsis, empyema, pneumothorax, and hemothorax), rupture of a herniated spleen (with hemothorax, anemia, and possibly hypovolemic shock), airway infections or recurrent pneumonias, urinary tract obstruction due to herniation of the ureter, chest pain, abdominal pain, vomiting, diarrhea, anorexia, acute abdomen, intrathoracic appendicitis, and other rare presentations.[153,154]

In bilateral CDH, both sides may not manifest at the same time, and staggered presentation has been described.[158]

DIAGNOSIS

The majority of cases are diagnosed before birth, during routine prenatal ultrasound.[159] The relative proportion of cases diagnosed in utero is constantly climbing, because of the increasing application of prenatal ultrasound screening and improvements in ultrasound technology and resolution. Fetal ultrasonography should always be performed whenever there is polyhydramnios, as CDH is one of its causes, apparently because of a reduction in the volume of amniotic fluid swallowed by the fetus, probably as a consequence of the GI obstruction caused by the hernia. A few authors also recommend careful ultrasonographic examination whenever an amniocentesis shows abnormally low levels of lecithin and sphingomyelin, because of the possibility of an association between CDH and a deficiency in the surfactant system.[118,119] Such an association, however, has been increasingly less accepted.[121,122,125,126] CDH can be diagnosed by prenatal ultrasound from the 11th week of gestation until term; previously negative examinations may become positive at any time during the pregnancy.[159,160] False-negative and false-positive examinations may occur; fetal ultrasonography is precise in approximately 90% of cases.[134,161] Not infrequently, the herniated content identified by prenatal ultrasound moves in and out of the chest, as if the hernia were a dynamic process.[162] A case of CDH diagnosed in the second trimester of pregnancy that seemed to have resolved spontaneously during the third trimester, with delivery of a normal infant, has been reported.[163] There may be inaccuracies as to the side of the hernia when it is unilateral, and sometimes a bilateral CDH may be diagnosed as unilateral.[162] The differential diagnoses of CDH identified by prenatal ultrasound include congenital cystic adenomatoid malformation of the lung (CCAM), diaphragmatic eventration, Morgagni hernia, hiatal hernia, pentalogy of Cantrell, primary diaphragmatic agenesis, pericardial hernia, pulmonary sequestration, lung cysts, diaphragmatic duplication, leiomyosarcoma of the lung, mediastinal teratoma, esophageal atresia with tracheoesophageal fistula, primary pulmonary agenesis, primary pulmonary hypoplasia, and intrathoracic duplications of the GI tract.[134,164] Color Doppler, three-dimensional ultrasonography, and magnetic resonance imaging (MRI) may all facilitate the prenatal diagnosis of CDH.[165,166] In extremely rare, selected cases, if in doubt, more invasive examinations might be considered, such as amniography, computerized tomography (CT), or ultrasonography with concomitant intrathoracic or intra-abdominal injection of saline as a contrast.[162,167] But as MRI becomes more accessible, these more invasive examinations will become of historical interest only. At most referral centers, the prenatal diagnosis of CDH automatically leads to an amniocentesis to determine the fetal karyotype. Should certain chromosomal abnormalities be detected, pregnancy termination may be considered.

After birth, a plain chest radiograph is almost always enough to confirm the diagnosis. The typical image is that of bowel loops seen in the lung field(s), with deviation of the mediastinum to the contralateral side of the hernia, and decrease or absence of gas in the abdomen (Fig. 33-5). When

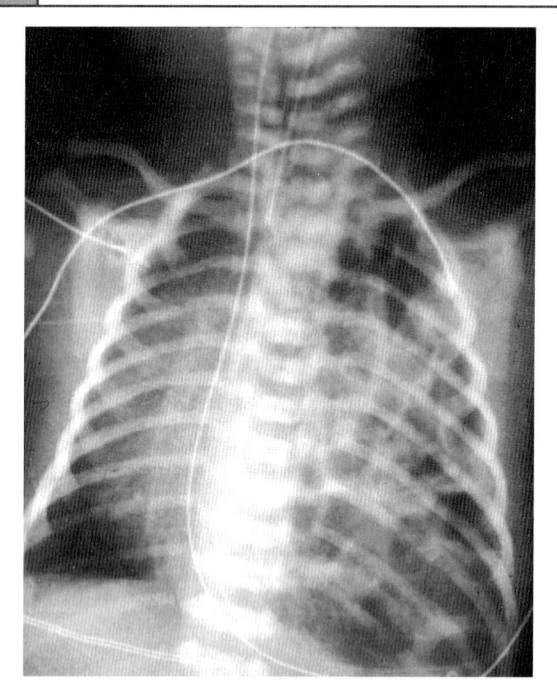

Figure 33–5
Typical aspect of plain radiograph from a neonate with a left congenital diaphragmatic hernia. Note the presence of bowel loops in the left hemithorax, the mediastinal deviation to the right, and the gastric tube in the chest.

the radiograph is obtained before the GI tract could be filled with gas, or if the intestines are not herniated (which is more common in right hernias), there may be confusion in the diagnosis. The introduction of a radiopaque gastric tube often helps, in case the stomach is herniated (see Fig. 33-5). Should any uncertainty persist, which is highly uncommon, the diagnosis can be confirmed through a radiograph performed after infusion of contrast through the gastric tube. Even less frequently, an ultrasound may be of help. More rarely, a CT, MRI, or contrast enema may have a role.

The differential diagnoses of CDH after birth include diaphragmatic eventration, pneumonia, CCAM, lung cysts, pneumothorax, pleural collections, Morgagni hernia, hiatal hernia, primary agenesis of the diaphragm, primary pulmonary agenesis, primary pulmonary hypoplasia, pericardial hernia, pulmonary sequestration, cardiac tumors, and duplication of the diaphragm. Despite all these possibilities, the diagnosis of CDH after birth tends to be relatively easy.

For late-presentation CDH, the diagnosis is usually made through a simple chest radiograph as well. Also in these cases, a gastric tube may be of help during the interpretation of the radiograph. Many times, there is previous history of a normal chest radiograph.[168] The possibility of late-presentation CDH should always be considered, to avoid delay or confusion with either pneumonia, pneumatoceles, CCAM, pneumothorax, pleural collections, diaphragmatic eventration, lung cysts, lung nodules, or pulmonary sequestrations. Because late-presentation CDH is relatively rare, the need for other imaging in addition to the chest radiograph is somewhat more common. Such imaging may include an upper GI series (often with the patient in Trendelenburg position), ultrasound, CT, MRI, fluoroscopy, and, more rarely, a contrast enema. CDH may be diagnosed as an incidental imaging finding in an asymptomatic patient.[169]

ASSOCIATED ANOMALIES

Children bearing any major congenital anomaly are known to carry a much higher risk of having another anomaly than the general population, and neonates with CDH are no exception. The incidence of other anomalies associated with CDH in the literature varies from "rare" to as much as 60%.[54,56,112,170,171] Explanations for this disparity include other anomalies directly linked to CDH and considered integral components of the so-called CDH syndrome, as mentioned earlier; stillbirths or patients who die before reaching a referral center; and variabilities in diagnostic routines, autopsy rates, patient populations in terms of the proportion of high-risk neonates included in the analysis, and regional prevalences of certain congenital anomalies. Studies have identified many different associated anomalies, in all body systems, usually with a predominance of cardiac malformations.

In a detailed review of 166 high-risk neonates (i.e., symptomatic within the first 6 hours of life), we noticed that approximately 40% of the children had one or more congenital anomalies associated with CDH.[112] This index was obtained even after exclusion of all the other anomalies that are part of the CDH syndrome. Cardiac anomalies were by far the most common, found in 63% of the patients who had an associated anomaly, followed by anomalies in the genitourinary tract (23%), GI tract (17%), central nervous system (CNS) (14%), muscles and skeleton (10%), chromosomes (10%), lungs (5%), and others (5%); in many children, there were more than one associated anomaly (Table 33-2).[112] Our results were comparable to those from another large series.[54,171]

The high proportion of cardiac anomalies associated with CDH in many series deserves special attention. In our review, for example, they were more frequent than all other anomalies put together (see Table 33-2).[112] Among the cardiac anomalies, heart hypoplasia was the most common.[112] This finding is in accordance with many observations pointing to the fact that the cardiac hypoplasia associated with CDH, especially that of the cardiac chambers ipsilateral to the hernia, occurs, like the pulmonary hypoplasia itself, at least in part because of compression of the heart by the herniated content and, perhaps, should also be considered part of the CDH syndrome, as it probably plays a role in the cardiac failure often manifested clinically.[112,172-174] The presence of an associated cardiac anomaly may lead to significant further reduction of the postductal P_{O_2} when compared with isolated CDH.[112] In fact, in neonates with an excessively low postductal P_{O_2}, a potential associated cardiac anomaly should be searched for very carefully.

The side of the hernia has recently been linked to differences in the frequency and pattern of associated malformations.[175] This interesting first observation needs further validation. Patients with late-presentation CDH also seem to have a higher prevalence of other anomalies than the general population. However, the related series published thus far are too small for definitive conclusions. For example, in a review of 26 patients, spanning 20 years, Berman and coworkers found one or more associated anomalies in 31% of them.[176]

Table 33–2
Associated Anomalies Indentified in 166 High-Risk Patients with Congenital Diaphragmatic Hernia*

Anomaly	Patients (N)	Anomaly	Patients (N)
Cardiac		Microcephaly	1
Heart hypoplasia	13	Myelomeningocele	1
Atrial septal defect	10	Open spine	1
Ventricular septal defect	9	Vascular malformation of cord	1
Hypoplasia of aortic isthmus	3	**Gastrointestinal**	
Aortic coarctation	3	Meckel's diverticulum	6
Persistent left superior vena cava	3	Absent gallbladder	1
Ebstein's anomaly	2	Absent vermiform appendix	1
Parachute mitral valve	2	Accessory pancreas	1
"Abnormal" mitral valve	1	Annular pancreas	1
"Abnormal" tricuspid valve	1	Duodenal atresia	1
Absent left pericardium	1	Ectopic liver	1
Absent right pulmonary artery	1	Ectopic pancreas	1
Bicommissural aortic valve	1	Esophageal atresia with transesophageal fistula	1
Bifid apex of the heart	1	Imperforate anus	1
Common atrioventricular canal	1	Neuroenteric cyst	1
Cor triatriatum	1	Phrygian cap deformity of gallbladder	1
Double outlet of right ventricle	1	**Musculoskeletal**	
Double coronary ostia	1	Hemivertebrae	2
Scimitar syndrome	1	Absent rib	1
Single coronary artery	1	"Abnormal" rib	1
Genitourinary		Accessory rib	1
Undescended testes	6	Hip dislocation	1
Bicornuate uterus	2	"Limb dystrophy"	1
Hydronephrosis	2	Polydactyly	1
Horseshoe kidneys	1	Sacral dysgenesis	1
Hypospadias	1	Scoliosis	1
Renal dysplasia	1	**Chromosomal**	
Single kidney	1	Trisomy 18	2
Ureteropelvic junction obstruction	1	"Abnormal" chromosome 14 centromere	1
Vaginal or uterine atresia	1	Balanced 12/15 translocation	1
Central Nervous System		Chromosome 7Q deletion	1
Hydrocephalus	4	Chromosome 12P	1
Rachischisis	2	Mosaic trisomy	1
Circle of Willis anomaly	1	Tetraploidy 21	1

(Continued)

Table 33-2

Associated Anomalies Indentified in 166 High-Risk Patients with Congenital Diaphragmatic Hernia*—cont'd

Anomaly	Patients (N)	Anomaly	Patients (N)
Trisomy 13	1	**Other**	
Pulmonary		Inguinal hernia	2
Pulmonary sequestration	2	Omphalocele	2
Pulmonary lymphangiectasia	1	Cleft lip or palate	1
Trifurcated trachea	1	Conotruncal facies	1
		Torticollis	1

*Excluding pulmonary hypoplasia, persistent ductus arteriosus, persistent foramen ovale, intestinal malrotation, gastric volvulus, size abnormalities of the chest wall, accessory spleen or congenital splenic fibrosis in left congenital diaphragmatic hernia (CDH), abnormalities of liver lobulation in right CDH, and hypoplasia or fibrosis of the liver lobe ipsilateral to the hernia.
Reproduced with permission from Fauza DO, Wilson JM. J Pediatr Surg 1994;29:1113-7.

PROGNOSTIC FACTORS

The search for reliable prognostic markers has been an essential aspect of the study of CDH for many years. Because of the very broad pathology spectrum related to CDH, such markers are critical for any meaningful comparisons among different therapeutic strategies, as well as for the identification of cases incompatible with life, in which further efforts would not be justified.

Certain clinical variables are known to be associated with different survival rates. Ever since the study by Young, in 1969, there is a well-established inverse relationship between age at the beginning of symptoms and mortality rates.[55,177] Neonates symptomatic within the first 6 hours of life are considered high risk, as they have the lowest survival rates.[55] There is no difference in mortality between the sexes in isolated CDH, but higher mortality rates have been reported in females than in males, when CDH is associated with other anomalies.[54] Some studies have shown that the lower the gestational age at birth, or the lower the birth weight, the lower is the survival rate.[55,178] Lower Apgar scores, particularly in the 5th minute, are also linked to higher mortality.[55] Contrary to what a few studies have suggested, the side of the hernia has not had any prognostic impact in the larger series.[55] At the same time, the size of the defect is well established as a determining factor in survival.[24,55] It is not yet known whether the presence of a hernia sac is of any prognostic significance. The variable with the highest impact on CDH survival rates is the presence of other associated congenital anomalies. The prognosis for neonates with associated anomalies, especially cardiac, is worse than that of infants with isolated CDH.[55,112,179,180]

Since the beginning of the 1970s, countless studies have tried to correlate mortality with blood gas values or ventilation parameters, either independently or mutually integrated in often intricate equations. Examples include pH values; "best" P_{CO_2} or "best" P_{O_2}, either postductal or preductal; alveolar–arterial O_2 gradient; mean airway pressure; respiratory rate; pulmonary compliance; dead space; and tidal volume.[181-186] In the past, perhaps the most popular of these markers was the best postductal P_{O_2} obtained during maximal mechanical ventilation, either prior to surgical repair of the hernia or prior to placing the patient on ECMO. Children with values higher than 100 mm Hg were labeled "responsive" and had a better prognosis, and vice versa.[184,185] Other parameters also used until recently were the so-called Bohn criteria, which related P_{CO_2} with the ventilation index (VI = respiratory rate × mean airway pressure); for example, a P_{CO_2} greater than 40 mm Hg with a VI of 1000 or greater would suggest high mortality.[182,184,185] Some authors have proposed that preductal blood gases are more predictive of the degree of pulmonary hypoplasia than postductal blood gases, as the latter are more influenced by the intensity of pulmonary hypertension and right-to-left shunt; a preductal P_{O_2} of less than 100 mm Hg and a preductal P_{CO_2} of greater than 60 mm Hg would be related to very high mortality.[183,187] As a result of the now universal acceptance of the principle of gentle ventilation, permissive hypercapnia, and minimization of iatrogenic injury related to mechanical ventilation, even preductal blood gases have had increasingly limited prognostic value, and at the same time, postductal gases such as best P_{O_2} during maximal ventilation have been practically abandoned.

Imaging criteria as severity predictors have also been extensively studied. One example is the value of prenatal ultrasonography. Until the early 1990s, a positive prenatal ultrasound was considered a marker of bad prognosis, particularly if the hernia was diagnosed before 25 weeks of gestation.[188,189] Lately, probably as a result of the widespread use of fetal ultrasound during routine prenatal care, the improvements in ultrasound technology, and the novel therapeutic strategies for CDH, it is quite clear that the prenatal diagnosis of an isolated CDH is, by itself, of no prognostic value, regardless of the gestational age at which it is made.[159,179] In the event that other associated anomalies, especially cardiac, are diagnosed prenatally in addition to the diaphragmatic hernia, the prognosis is still comparable to that of a diagnosis made after birth.[112] Several specific findings on fetal ultrasound have been proposed as bad prognostic markers, such as polyhydramnios, herniation of the liver or the stomach into the chest, underdevelopment of the left side of the heart, disproportionate cardiac ventricles, high ratio of the herniated area to the cardiac area, low ratio of the lung area to the total thoracic area, depression or absence of fetal breathing movements, severe mediastinal deviation, reduction of liquid flow through the nose and oropharynx during fetal breathing movements, and disturbances of blood flow modulation through the ductus arteriosus.[160,188-191] The merit of all these markers, however, is highly controversial and of very limited acceptance. Somewhat recently, the value of liver herniation, as well as of the so-called lung-to-head ratio (LHR), which measures the relative proportion between the areas of the lung and the head at predetermined locations, has been emphasized by a few groups.[192,193] For example, fetuses with liver in the chest and an LHR of less than 1 would have a particularly bad prognosis. Although debate continues over the value of the presence of the liver in the chest, the same cannot be said of the LHR, which has been shown to be significantly inconsistent, especially across different institutions.[152,194] Three-dimensional measurements of fetal lung volume via MRI are being increasingly refined and adopted as a more reliable imaging-based prognostic marker, including at our institution.[165,195]

Similarly, some studies suggest that certain postnatal imaging findings, either independently or in combination, can also be linked to poor outcome. On plain chest radiograph, examples of such findings include presence of the stomach in the chest, ipsilateral or contralateral pneumothorax, presence of interstitial emphysema, and a low ratio of aerated ipsilateral lung area over that of the contralateral lung.[196-198] On echocardiogram, examples are decreased left ventricular mass, disproportionate dimensions between both pulmonary arteries, and a disproportionately large pulmonary artery trunk in relation to the aorta.[199,200] Finally, on pulmonary arteriogram, examples are reduced dimensions of both pulmonary arteries, reduced size of the ipsilateral lung, and severe peripheral compromise.[184] Yet, as with prenatal imaging, the predictive value of these proposed postnatal findings is questionable, to say the least, and very few institutions adopt any of them at this time.

Only the following variables have been clearly validated by well-controlled, extensive multicenter data as being of predictive value in CDH: age at the onset of symptoms, birth weight, 5-minute Apgar score, defect size, and the presence of an associated cardiac anomaly.[24,55] The meaning of all other suggested prognostic markers is debatable and of limited acceptance.[201] The impact of various prognostic markers seems to differ depending on the side of the hernia.[202] One of the most common shortcomings of the studies involving prognostic markers is that most of them are reviews from a single institution. Hence, the data are unavoidably linked to the unique patient population and peculiar therapeutic strategies of each service, which are aspects known to still be highly variable from one center to another in CDH. On the other hand, even if well-controlled multicenter trials were performed, the fact that the treatment of CDH is constantly evolving could lessen the significance of their results. The introduction of ECMO and of the principle of gentle ventilation are clear examples of the vulnerability of data of this kind, as these therapies rendered the conclusions obtained prior to their availability nearly useless, even in a given institution.

TREATMENT

Except for the rare cases of strangulation of the herniated content, CDH is not a surgical emergency. Rather, CDH is a physiologic emergency. In fact, not infrequently, mechanical aspects of respiration tend to deteriorate after the repair of the hernia.[203,204] Indeed, not only is emergency surgery unnecessary and often deleterious, but also a period of preoperative stabilization is known to improve outcome.[22,205] The child should not go to the operating room while unstable. The time needed for stabilization may vary from less than 12 hours to several days. A few authors even suggest that waiting until well beyond stabilization has been reached is beneficial.[22] In certain premature neonates at higher surgical risk, one may wait weeks, or even more than a month, before proceeding to the repair.[152]

The therapeutic strategy in children with CDH and other associated anomalies must be individualized for the patient. Usually, the hernia is repaired before the other anomalies. However, when CDH is associated with cardiac anomalies, such strategy may lead to unacceptably high mortality.[112,152] Unless the cardiac defect is very mild, the current tendency is to repair the heart before the diaphragm, or, occasionally, both during the same intervention. However, guidelines for the different scenarios are still being defined.

One of the benefits of the prenatal diagnosis of CDH is that delivery can be planned at a tertiary referral center. The initial results of postnatal resuscitation are known to be maximized when the presence of CDH is detected before birth.[159] At our institution and others, high-risk outborn infants have a significantly lower survival rate than inborn neonates. Unless there is any obstetrical contraindication, vaginal delivery is preferred over cesarean section.

Preoperative Care

The neonate should be intubated in the delivery room. Ventilation by mask before intubation should be avoided because of the risk for distention of hollow viscera in the chest. A gastric tube should be introduced and kept under mild continuous suction, to minimize such distention and to drain air that may have been swallowed. Central venous access is established, usually through the umbilical vein (occasionally, however, particularly in patients with right-sided CDH, there may be significant distortions of the liver anatomy because of the herniation, which may impede the use of this vein). One of the umbilical arteries is catheterized for blood pressure and postductal blood gas monitoring. Preductal blood gases are obtained through access to the right radial artery, or to one of the superficial temporal arteries. Transcutaneous pulse oximetry monitors and, if available, transcutaneous P_{O_2} and P_{CO_2} monitors are placed both on preductal and postductal territories. Monitors for body temperature and respiratory rate should also be positioned. At least in the high-risk cases, a Foley catheter is introduced. The volumes of intravenous infusions should be carefully controlled to minimize the chances of a pulmonary edema developing. Prophylactic antibiotics covering both gram-positive and gram-negative bacteria are commonly administered. Whenever possible, inotropic agents should be avoided, as these drugs usually increase not only cardiac output but also peripheral vascular resistance, both of which may, together with the ever-present pulmonary hypertension, lead to excessive cardiac overload not always tolerated, especially when there is some degree of cardiac hypoplasia.[112,173] When the use of these drugs is inescapable, many prefer dobutamine, amrinone, or epinephrine to dopamine or norepinephrine, because the former drugs may produce pulmonary vasodilation at low dosages.[134] One should limit any manipulation or interaction with the infant to a minimum because of the great volatility of the pulmonary vasculature.

Every neonate with CDH should undergo an echocardiogram with Doppler, given the relatively common occurrence and prognostic impact of both right heart failure and associated cardiac anomalies. Should any functional or structural cardiac disease be identified, its treatment must be carefully coordinated with that of the hernia. Not infrequently, a pediatric cardiologist is a member of the multidisciplinary team caring for these patients. Certain variables, such as prenatal diagnosis prior to the 25th week of gestation, low Apgar scores, and "excessively low" postductal PO_2, have been shown to be risk factors for the presence of other associated anomalies.[112] Should these variables be present, further examinations such as genitourinary tract and head ultrasounds, as well as a karyotype (if this was not already done during pregnancy) should be strongly considered, in addition to the echocardiogram.[112]

Until the early 1990s, neonates were typically sedated, paralyzed, and hyperventilated, and they also received systemic alkalinization with sodium bicarbonate or tromethamine to minimize pulmonary hypertension. Ventilation parameters used to be controlled by postductal blood gases. This strategy, which unfortunately is still practiced by many centers today, is clearly associated with unacceptably high risks for iatrogenic lung injury. Pulmonary hypoplasia and, in particular, pulmonary hypertension are both expected to lead to low PO_2 and high PCO_2, especially in postductal gases. Attempts to normalize postductal blood gas values often lead to marked increases in ventilator parameters—namely, respiratory rate (RR), inspired O_2 fraction (FiO_2), peak inspiratory pressure (PIP), positive end-expiratory pressure (PEEP), and mean airway pressure (MAP), which, in turn, commonly lead to hyperdistention of the lungs and severe barotrauma, not to mention the toxicity of high FiO_2 levels. A survey involving clinical and autopsy data from 68 children with CDH treated in this fashion showed a tremendously high frequency and severity of iatrogenic insult to the pulmonary parenchyma.[174] In that study, 91% of the patients had evidence of diffuse alveolar damage with development of hyaline membrane, more obvious in the ipsilateral lung. Moreover, 65% of the children developed pneumothorax, 51% had pulmonary hemorrhage, and 6% already had variable degrees of interstitial fibrosis.[174] Other studies also showed alveolar ruptures, damage to the alveolar basal membrane, alveolar hemorrhage, and edema, all of which contributed to atelectasis, a decline in lung compliance, and even further deterioration of gas exchange.[16,122] In addition to barotrauma, to which CDH neonates are particularly vulnerable,[129] pulmonary hyperdistention leads to even further increases of the already elevated pulmonary vascular resistance, thus worsening the effects associated with pulmonary hypertension.[206,207] Systemic alkalinization with sodium bicarbonate may lead to increases in PCO_2 and to both volume and sodium overloads. Tromethamine may be useful at times in the short term, but relatively large volumes of this drug are usually necessary, which tends to result in both generalized and pulmonary edema.

It is very clear that a completely different strategy, first proposed by Wung and colleagues, should be offered to high-risk neonates with CDH.[21,22] It is based on the following guidelines: minimal sedation; no muscle paralysis; respiration merely assisted by the mechanical ventilator, if possible through pressure support under flow synchronization, or, if this is not available, then through simple or synchronized intermittent mandatory volume; permissive hypercapnia with no hyperventilation; and no systemic alkalinization. Patient monitoring is mostly through preductal gases. Ventilator parameters are left at the minimum necessary to maintain a preductal arterial O_2 saturation (SaO_2) of 90% or greater, whatever the postductal values may be, with tolerance to high PCO_2 levels. In general, the ventilator parameters are left at a base RR of 40 breaths or fewer per minute, and the PIP and PEEP no higher than 30 and 5 cm H_2O, respectively, and the FiO_2 should be the lowest possible to prevent severe preductal hypoxemia. That is to say, unless there is metabolic acidosis, suggesting excessively low O_2 delivery, one should tolerate low postductal PO_2 and SaO_2, as long as there is an adequate amount of oxygen in the preductal blood that is going to the brain and to the heart. As long as the pH is at "acceptable" levels, one should tolerate hypercapnia. The main goal of this therapeutic strategy is the prevention of barotrauma, probably the most common cause of death whenever the old, conventional hyperventilation strategy is employed.[16,22,187] Despite the known benefits of sedation in patients with CDH, which raises the excitability threshold of the pulmonary vasculature,[208] in this "new" strategy, one must use sedation with great caution, so that a child can effectively activate the mechanical ventilator, preferably in pressure support under flow synchronization. A child who is able to control both the RR and the airflow from the respirator can contribute more to the minute volume without compromising the functional residual capacity. This therapeutic strategy also avoids the side effects of systemic alkalinization.

As discussed earlier, the lungs of newborns with CDH are particularly vulnerable to barotrauma, so the occurrence of pneumothorax is relatively common. Except on very rare, select occasions, a pneumothorax should not be drained if it is ipsilateral to the hernia prior to surgical repair, because of the risk of iatrogenic injury to the herniated content.

Pulmonary Vasodilators

Regardless of the ventilation strategy, many vasodilators administered systemically have been used in an attempt to control the pulmonary hypertension. Examples of these agents are tolazoline, nitroglycerin, nitroprusside, acetylcholine, prostaglandin E_1, prostaglandin D_2, prostacyclin, isoprenaline, and nifedipine. Despite the theoretical appeal of these drugs, they are not selective enough to the pulmonary vasculature and usually lead to a drop in both total peripheral vascular resistance and systemic arterial pressure. Therefore, their effects on the pressure gradient through the ductus arteriosus is either minimal or nonexistent, so that the tendency to right-to-left shunt is unchanged. Furthermore, they may lead to vasodilation of poorly ventilated areas of the lungs, which may even worsen the intrapulmonary right-to-left shunt. The drop in systemic arterial pressure, on the other hand, may lead to the administration of volume or inotropic agents (or both), both of which should be avoided. Bos and coworkers reported a reduction of both the alveolar–arterial O_2 gradient and the oxygenation index (OI = MAP × FiO_2/PO_2) after administration of prostacyclin in high-risk CDH patients, but this had no impact on survival.[209] The use of prostacyclin is also associated with an increase in bleeding time, which is clearly undesirable in surgical patients.[209,210]

Inhalational prostacyclin has been investigated experimentally but has found no clinical applicability yet.[211,212] The response to prostaglandin D_2 is variable, and systemic hypotension is a common side effect.[133,209,212] The most popular of these vasodilators was, perhaps, tolazoline, an α-adrenergic receptor blocking agent with a mild inotropic and chronotropic effect on the myocardium. This drug also lowers the levels of thromboxane B_2, which is possibly a mediator of pulmonary hypertension in CDH and which also has histamine-like effects.[134,213] Children who respond to tolazoline usually do so within 4 hours after an initial bolus of 1 to 2 mg/kg, which may be noticed by an increase in the postductal Po_2. This bolus is commonly followed by a continuous infusion of 1 mg/kg/hr. The infusion of vasodilators directly into the pulmonary artery has been shown not to have any advantage over their systemic or peripheral administration.[214] Tolazoline side effects may be severe and include systemic arterial hypotension, upper GI hemorrhage, thrombocytopenia, hyponatremia, and skin rubor.[134,213] If there is upper GI hemorrhage, one should give priority to antacids and gastric lavage, as tolazoline may inhibit the effects of cimetidine.[215] Tolazoline, as well as these other vasodilators, may occasionally contribute to the stabilization of the patient, sometimes lengthening the honeymoon period. However, more often than not, this is not the case and, even when there is some improvement in oxygenation, no beneficial impact on survival has been demonstrated.[22,205,209] Indeed, most referral centers no longer use systemically administered pulmonary vasodilators.

More recently, sildenafil has been proposed as beneficial in the management of pulmonary hypertension associated with CDH.[216-218] Although the initial reports are arguably encouraging, its therapeutic value remains to be defined.

Nitric Oxide

The most potent selective pulmonary vasodilator known is nitric oxide (NO) administered by the endotracheal route. NO is a natural mediator of smooth muscle relaxation in general, but it acts only locally because of its extremely short half-life. It is responsible for the biological activity of the so-called endothelium-derived relaxing factor.[219] When given as part of the inspired air, NO crosses the alveolar-capillary membrane by diffusion and stimulates the cyclic guanosine 3′,5′-monophosphate (cyclic GMP) in the smooth muscle of the pulmonary arterioles, inducing vasodilation. Its effects are limited to the pulmonary vasculature because it quickly combines with hemoglobin and is deactivated.

At first, there was great enthusiasm about the use of NO for the treatment of CDH, but clinical experience has been disappointing. Occasionally, NO does help in stabilizing the patient, but even when there is an initially satisfactory response, there may be tachyphylaxis, and improvements in outcome related to its use remain to be demonstrated.[152,220,221] In fact, studies involving term neonates with respiratory failure of different causes have shown that inhalation NO improves oxygenation and lowers the need for ECMO in all diagnoses except CDH.[222] The underlying reason why CDH neonates are often unresponsive to NO is unknown. There has been some evidence that, if combined with the administration of surfactant or with liquid ventilation, NO may improve oxygenation and lower the pulmonary vascular resistance of children with CDH.[122,223] At most referral centers, the role of NO in CDH remains confined to the management of right cardiac failure, when present.

Surfactant

Because of the possibility of a deficiency in the surfactant system in children with CDH, endotracheal instillation of exogenous surfactant has been studied as a therapeutic adjunct for many years. The results obtained thus far, however, do not justify its widespread application, except when prematurity itself is the indication for its use.[125,126]

Prenatal administration of corticosteroids is known to induce, or at least increase, the production of endogenous surfactant.[224] Although the precise mechanisms behind this phenomenon have yet to be elucidated, studies exploring this response in the treatment of CDH have been proposed.[224]

Alternative Forms of Mechanical Ventilation

Alternative forms of mechanical ventilation have also been employed for CDH. One example is high-frequency oscillatory ventilation (HFOV), which mobilizes volumes smaller than the anatomic dead space, at frequencies of up to 40 Hz. Gas exchange seems to occur not from the delivery of gas under positive pressure, as in conventional mechanical ventilation, but through a diffusion process. Compared with conventional ventilation, it is thought that HFOV minimizes barotrauma and facilitates gas exchange, especially CO_2 elimination, in select circumstances. This form of ventilation, either isolated or combined with NO, has been tested in many institutions for the support of CDH patients, usually with less than satisfactory results.[152,225] Like NO, HFOV seems to be an option only in selected cases and still needs to be better defined. When analyzed as a whole, the experience with HFOV in CDH has been disappointing.[122] However, Bohn proposed that, as long as HFOV is not used for lung recruitment, but with mean airway pressures no higher than 14 to 16 cm H_2O and peak-to-peak airway pressures limited to 35 to 45 cm H_2O, it can lead to improved survival, especially if used early, rather than in a rescue mode.[226] Other authors have also seen the value of HFOV in CDH, within specific guidelines.[180]

Intratracheal pulmonary ventilation, a form of ventilation that promotes active expiration, which drastically lowers dead space, thus enhancing CO_2 elimination and minimizing barotrauma, has been used in a handful of CDH cases, with very promising preliminary results.[227] Regrettably, broader, definitive studies have been stalled by regulatory constraints and conflicting patent interests.

Liquid ventilation with a perfluorocarbon (PFC) has also been examined for some time. PFCs are bio-inert, nonabsorbable by the alveolar-capillary membrane, and may carry large amounts of both O_2 (in particular) and CO_2. Also, they display low surface tension levels, thus acting as truly artificial surfactants. Hybrid liquid ventilation (i.e., with a PFC and a gas) is known to increase pulmonary compliance and to improve gas exchange, especially oxygenation.[228] The improved oxygenation, in turn, optimizes redistribution of pulmonary blood flow, hence alleviating the pulmonary hypertension.[228] Liquid ventilation, either isolated or in combination with NO, has been applied in a few CDH cases, with encouraging results.[228,229] However, its impact on outcome and role in the treatment of CDH, if any, is yet to be established.[122,230]

Extracorporeal Membrane Oxygenation

Since the mid 1980s, extracorporeal life support has left the realm of experimental therapy and has become part of the standard therapeutic options for patients with CDH. Several early studies showed that the introduction of ECMO resulted in a significant increase in survival of these patients.[16,205,231-233] The significance of these studies, however, was limited by the relatively small number of patients and by the fact that each involved a single institution. A multicenter review by the Congenital Diaphragmatic Hernia Registry, involving 632 patients from 65 centers, showed that ECMO improved survival from 53% to 77% in children with high mortality markers and comparable prognoses.[122] That same study also showed a direct relationship between the severity of the cases and the beneficial impact of ECMO on outcome.

During extracorporeal support, there is not enough time for the lungs to grow to the point of reversing the pulmonary hypoplasia. However, ECMO acts as a bridge, lessening, if not eliminating, the component of pulmonary vascular hyperreactivity, allowing maximal pulmonary remodeling, with an increase in compliance of the pulmonary arteries and arterioles, which normally takes place after birth,[110,124] as well as reducing barotrauma to a minimum. There is still some debate regarding the best moment to place the patient on ECMO in relation to the time of surgical repair of the hernia.[17] There were no differences in survival between preoperative and postoperative commencement of ECMO.[234,235] The current trend at most referral centers, however, is to use ECMO during preoperative stabilization, with repair of the hernia done either after ECMO decannulation or while still under bypass.[16,236,237] Despite the need for anticoagulation during ECMO, it has been shown that certain pharmacologic precautions and technical principles allow safe surgical intervention during bypass, with a minimal risk of hemorrhagic complications.[16,237-239] Occasionally, a patient may be stable without the need for ECMO in the preoperative period, and then deteriorate either during or soon after the operation and need to go on bypass.

A few authors have proposed criteria for the contraindication of both ECMO and surgical repair, which would supposedly be linked to pulmonary disease incompatible with life.[22,109,183,187,205] Given the many reports by other groups showing survival of patients who had met such criteria,[16,232,234,240] not to mention the controversies related to the prognostic markers of CDH in general,[201] we offer ECMO and surgery to every patient, unless the presence of other associated anomalies is deemed incompatible with life.[112]

The specific criteria for placing a patient on ECMO are equally debatable. Because many controversies surround prognostic markers in CDH, it is no surprise that the many proposed indications for ECMO in this disease have not been widely accepted. Usually, the indications for ECMO in other diseases do not apply to CDH, mainly because the mechanical ventilation parameters used in other diagnoses prior to ECMO being considered would be unacceptably toxic to the lungs of children with CDH, who are particularly vulnerable to iatrogenic injury.[241] In most centers, ECMO is considered when the patient with CDH cannot be adequately maintained without the use of "toxic" ventilator parameters. The definition of *toxic* parameters varies from one institution to another. As mentioned, in general we do not allow the PIP and PEEP to be higher than 30 and 5 cm H_2O, respectively; it should be possible to gradually lower the FiO_2 to 60% or less in no more than 72 hours, and the base RR on the ventilator should not exceed 40 breaths per minute, although a much higher RR is tolerated when the child is under flow synchronization on the ventilator. The ventilation parameters are controlled mostly by preductal blood gases. When the patient cannot be maintained under these guidelines, the use of HFOV or NO may be considered in selected cases. However, most of the time, extracorporeal bypass is indicated right away. A potential benefit in placing infants with severe pulmonary hypoplasia on bypass already in the delivery room is currently being evaluated at select referral centers. Whenever possible, venovenous ECMO is preferred over the venoarterial mode.[16,235] When ECMO is initiated preoperatively, we perform the repair with the patient on bypass.

Surgery

If the patient is on ECMO, we begin a continuous infusion of aminocaproic acid (AMICAR), an inhibitor of fibrinolysis, approximately 2 hours before the operation, concomitantly with reductions of the activated clotting time (ACT).[237,239] Patients on HFOV or NO administration (or both) need not be discontinued during the procedure, but these can be useful in selected cases. If neither ECMO, HFOV, nor NO is being used, the best form of intraoperative ventilation is at low pressures and high respiratory rates, with a dedicated infant or pediatric ventilator. Conventional anesthesia ventilators are excessively compliant and have too much dead space, hence are not suitable for these children.

In addition to general inhalation anesthesia, we recommend the routine introduction of a catheter for continuous epidural anesthesia, which allows early withdrawal of curare in the postoperative period, and maintenance of abdominal wall relaxation.[16] All these effects, in turn, facilitate early postoperative resumption of flow synchronization, as well as minimizing volume retention, commonly associated with the continued use of curare. Nitrous oxide should not be used, as it tends to cause bowel distention, which may hinder hernia reduction and abdominal closure.

The patient is positioned supine and slightly tilted to the side contralateral to the hernia by a small support placed under the ipsilateral thoracoabdominal transition. An abdominal access is preferred over a thoracic one, usually through a subcostal laparotomy.[17] After careful reduction of the herniated content, the ipsilateral lung should always be inspected. Should it not be visible, the presence of a hernia sac, which is not always easily identifiable, must be investigated. If present, the hernia sac should be separated from the diaphragm and at least partially resected. Very often, the posterior aspect of the residual diaphragm must be detached from the posterior abdominal wall, after opening the peritoneum and the pleura, which usually cover that area.

Whenever possible, a primary repair of the hernia is performed, with nonabsorbable sutures (Fig. 33-6). However, one should not force a primary repair under tension, because of the following potentially harmful consequences: the diaphragm will become flat and tense, minimizing, if not eliminating, its functionality; there will be an excessive enlargement of the thoracic cavity, which may lead to alveolar hyperextension in the ipsilateral lung and consequent worsening of the pulmonary hypertension and barotrauma; the tension exerted on the diaphragm may be transmitted to the rib cage, resulting in chest wall deformities; and, finally, there will be further

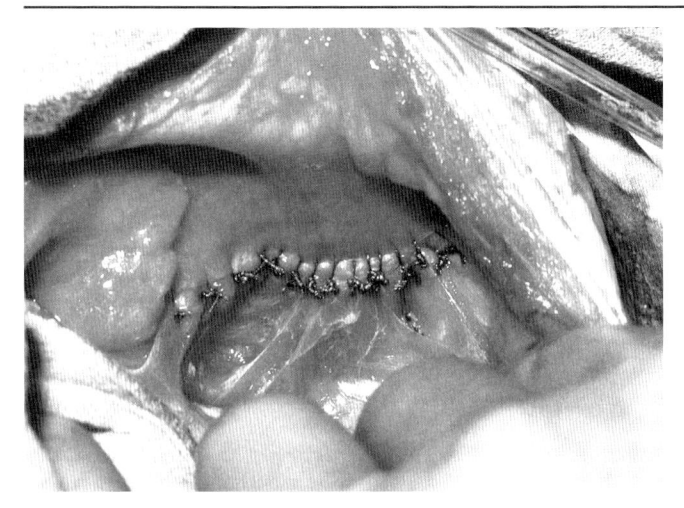

Figure 33-6
Primary repair of a diaphragmatic defect in a newborn with congenital diaphragmatic hernia.

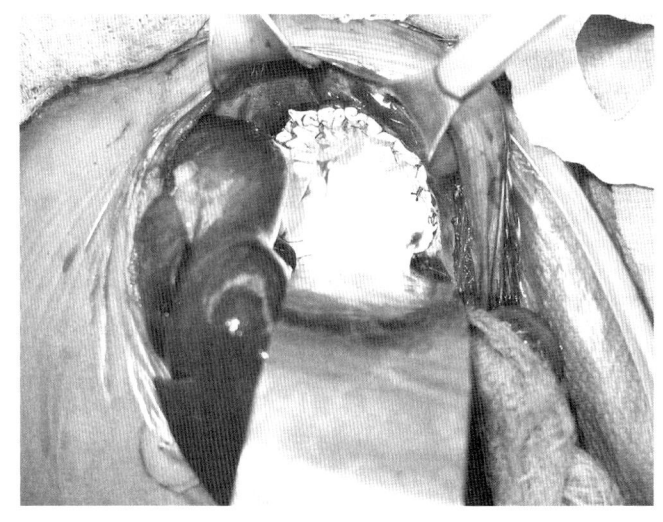

Figure 33-7
Prosthetic repair of a diaphragmatic defect with expanded Teflon, in a newborn with congenital diaphragmatic hernia.

decrease of the abdominal cavity volume, hampering closure of the laparotomy.[242] In a review by the Congenital Diaphragmatic Hernia Registry, 51% of the patients had to receive a patch of some kind to have the diaphragm closed.[17] In case a tension-free primary repair is not possible, several alternative techniques have been proposed, including abdominal or thoracic muscle flaps, free fascia lata grafts, and a myriad of prostheses, such as lyophilized dura mater, silicone, Dacron, polypropylene (Marlex), polytetrafluoroethylene (PTFE, or Teflon), and others.[17,205,243-248] Regardless of the technique used, care should be taken not to leave the diaphragm too flat, but with a slight to moderate-sized dome, so that the same problems associated with primary closure under tension may be avoided.[242] If the dome is too pronounced, local paradoxical respiration may ensue. We do not favor muscle flaps because of the residual defects left in the abdominal or thoracic walls, as well as the increased risk for local hemorrhage, particularly if ECMO is or may be employed. At most U.S. centers, pediatric surgeons prefer the use of a prosthesis made of expanded Teflon (Fig. 33-7). At least part of the reasons for this preference derive from a study showing improved Teflon incorporation by the host and a better motility pattern of this prosthesis in the short term, when compared with silicone prostheses and muscle flaps.[249] A number of acellular biological prostheses, including acellular human dermis and small intestinal submucosa (SIS), have also been studied experimentally, with conflicting results.[250-253] SIS has already been used clinically, with disappointing results (unpublished data). When the posterior residual diaphragm is not large enough for proper suturing, one option is to pass the suture around the subjacent rib, after gentle anterior traction of the rib with a clamp to avoid injury to its neurovascular bundle.

Soon before completion of the diaphragmatic closure, a multiperforated tube is placed into the pleural cavity, exteriorized through the chest, and typically just placed under water seal. Continuous suction through the chest is usually avoided, to circumvent the possibility of pulmonary overdistention, which is highly detrimental in CDH. Many authors even recommend that a chest tube not be placed at all.[22,254] In a review by the Congenital Diaphragmatic Hernia Registry, 24% of the patients did not receive a chest tube.[17]

We prefer to correct the intestinal malrotation, almost always present. However, most centers do not perform this maneuver.[17] In most institutions, including ours, an appendectomy is not routinely done, to minimize morbidity.[17] Given the reduced abdominal volume, difficulty closing the abdominal wall is not uncommon. Should there be excessive intra-abdominal tension after abdominal wall closure, a syndrome of compression of the inferior vena cava may develop, along with a decrease in thoracic expansibility and tidal volume. To prevent this, repeated digital distention of the abdominal wall and evacuation of intestinal gas may be of help. Some have suggested a routine gastrostomy as an additional means to decompress the stomach, facilitate abdominal closure, and minimize postoperative respiratory complications, but there has been no evidence-based support for this idea.[236,255] When tension-free closure of the abdominal wall is not possible, the use of an abdominal silo should be considered, followed by postoperative serial reductions and definitive primary closure.[22,205,256] Another option is simply to close the skin, leaving the proper, definitive closure for a later date.[237] The need for either of these maneuvers, however, should be extremely rare.

In children on ECMO, a few technical precautions should be taken to prevent excessive bleeding: the skin should be opened with needle-tip electrocautery; when primary diaphragmatic closure is unlikely, the posterior residual diaphragm should not be dissected if it is adhered to the posterior abdominal wall, but the stitches should be passed around the subjacent rib, as described earlier; finally, fibrin glue should be applied to the diaphragmatic suture line and other raw surfaces.[237] We do not leave a drain in the abdomen. If the abdominal wall cannot be closed primarily and a silo is implanted, serial reductions should commence only after the child comes off bypass.

Thoracoscopic and laparoscopic repairs of CDH have been increasingly employed.[257-259] During thoracoscopy, reduction of the hernia can be facilitated by the mild positive intrathoracic pressure often applied intraoperatively. These procedures have also proved viable in the presence of associated cardiac anomalies, as well as for the placement of prosthetic patches. The precise indications, the pros and cons of the so-called minimally invasive repair of CDH, are yet to be fully clarified. A possible beneficial role for intratracheal pulmonary ventilation during the procedure in severe cases has been proposed in an animal model.[260]

Postoperative Care

If the patient was not on ECMO during surgery, mild ventilatory support under flow synchronization, as described earlier, should resume as soon as possible—if necessary, with pharmacologic reversal of the muscle paralysis if it had to be used. This transition can be tremendously facilitated if the child was placed under continuous epidural anesthesia intraoperatively.[16] The principles guiding mechanical ventilation described for the preoperative period also apply to the postoperative period. The same is true for the criteria to go on ECMO.

Although some children improve after repair of the hernia, there is frequently (at least temporary) deterioration of the respiratory mechanics in the immediate postoperative period.[203,261] This phenomenon is thought to result from anatomic distortions on the diaphragm and thoracic cavity, hyperinflation of both lungs, and an increase of the intra-abdominal pressure.[261] Under these circumstances, the ventilator parameters may need to be temporarily "increased," sometimes to the point that alternative modes of ventilation and even ECMO may have to be used. Occasionally, children who had been on bypass preoperatively and were decannulated before the operation may need to go back on ECMO (this is another reason we prefer to perform the repair on bypass).

Another potential complicating factor is the administration of intravenous fluids, which must be controlled very carefully. Along with the common risk of hypovolemia, related to surgical trauma and bleeding, neonates with CDH, more so than newborns with other surgical diseases, initially behave as if there is inappropriate secretion of antidiuretic hormone, and they may tend to retain excessive amounts of water.[256] The explanation for this phenomenon is not yet clear. If this predisposition is not recognized early, patients can be easily overloaded with fluids, with harmful consequences to their respiratory and cardiac status.

Sometimes, intra-abdominal pressure may rise significantly in the immediate postoperative period. Signs of inferior vena cava syndrome should be watched for, as it may lead to a decrease in the venous return to the heart, impairment of renal blood flow, and a reduction in tidal volume. Should there be any evidence of renal insufficiency or major worsening of the respiratory or cardiac status, muscle paralysis should be considered, as it may lower the intra-abdominal pressure. In the more severe cases, it may be necessary to take the child back to the operating room for placement of an abdominal silo.

Whenever used, the chest tube is not continuously aspirated but only placed under a passive water seal to avoid pulmonary hyperdistention, which may occur on both lungs, caused by the large empty residual space in the ipsilateral pleural cavity.[22,261] The chest tube should be removed only after the patient is extubated, usually after liquid drainage ceases. Not infrequently, liquid drainage lasts for a long time, until the lung can occupy the whole pleural space. In these circumstances, one may consider removing the chest tube while it is still draining fluid and tolerating a temporary pleural collection.

Children on ECMO should continue to receive AMICAR, in parallel to the maintenance of ACT levels lower than usual for bypass.[237] When AMICAR is not used, or the technical precautions described here are not duly followed, the incidence and severity of hemorrhagic complications tend to be high.[205,262] Should there be bleeding, surgical dressings must be regularly weighed and the losses through the chest tube and abdominal drain (if present) must be quantified. In our service, either blood loss equal to or higher than 20% of a patient's total blood content in 8 hours or less, or progressive abdominal distention, is a criterion for surgical reexploration. Frequently, one cannot find specific areas of bleeding during reoperation, but a diffuse oozing is seen throughout the operative field. In these cases, more aggressive pharmacologic management related to AMICAR and ACT levels must be pondered. In addition to these potential surgical complications related to ECMO, the common risks associated with extracorporeal bypass itself are, clearly, also a possibility.

More rarely, GI obstruction resulting from adhesions, gastric volvulus, or midgut volvulus may occur even in the immediate postoperative period.[263] Other rare complications are chylothorax and chylous ascites.[264-266] In the very few cases reported to date, the causes for these chylous collections were not clearly determined. Their treatment should be based on parenteral nutrition, feedings with middle-chain triglycerides, and, if necessary, occasional needle drainages.[264-266]

Late-Presentation Congenital Diaphragmatic Hernia

Regardless of its initial clinical presentation, even when found incidentally, late-presentation CDH should be repaired as soon as possible, because of the risks of incarceration and strangulation of the herniated content, and even sudden death.[267-269] A laparotomy is still the preferred access, although a thoracotomy may be considered much more frequently than in neonates, whenever the presence of firm adhesions in the herniated content into the chest is suspected. Often, one cannot determine preoperatively whether a laparotomy or a thoracotomy would be the best access, and personal, somewhat subjective preferences may play a role in the decision process. Minimally invasive access can be justified in selected cases.

RESULTS

Even at referral centers with all known therapeutic options for treatment of CDH available, there may be a sizeable variability of the survival rates associated with this disease, for several reasons. On one hand, patient population profiles may vary with regard to the proportion of high-risk neonates from one institution to another. Also, patients may die before reaching a center and thus not be included in the final numbers—the hidden mortality originally described by Harrison.[270] At the same time, a few authors deliberately exclude children considered to have pulmonary hypoplasia incompatible with life, often based on arguable criteria, which artificially improve survival rates.[183,187] The same is true for the inclusion of children bearing other congenital anomalies associated with CDH.[112,179] In addition, there are still major differences among institutions related to therapeutic protocols and strategies. Such heterogeneities, combined with the different sizes of the review series and the constant evolution of the treatment options for CDH, may limit the interpretation of the results.

Bearing in mind these limitations, the latest meaningful reviews have shown that overall survival for patients with isolated CDH at many referral centers has been close to 90%, a sharp increase from the depressing figures of less than 20 years ago, when ECMO was not widely available and aggressive hyperventilation was still the norm.[24,35,122,187] At our institution, over 80% of the patients are diagnosed prenatally. As a consequence, their delivery can be planned, usually at one of two sister institutions linked to our hospital. The few cases diagnosed only after birth in our referral base are rapidly transferred to us, consequently our hidden mortality is practically zero and our patient population is large and illustrative. In accordance with the data from other referral centers, our survival rates for high-risk neonates (about 90% of our cases) had varied between approximately 85% and 90% for isolated CDH and had been approximately 70% when all cases, including those with other associated anomalies, were considered.[16,122,271] These numbers were intimately related to the application of the principle of gentle ventilation and permissive hypercapnia, as well to the liberal and early indication for ECMO. In the past 3 years, our overall survival has surpassed 90%, by adding careful attention to the right side of the heart to our management principles.[272]

In patients not at high risk (i.e., when an isolated CDH becomes symptomatic after 6 hours of life), survival is close to 100%.[122,187]

LONG-TERM FOLLOW-UP

At the same time that CDH survival rates have almost skyrocketed lately, perhaps predictably so, morbidity rates have worsened. High-risk children, who would otherwise have died not long ago, now survive, often with multiple problems, in various systems, and need to be followed by a dedicated, multidisciplinary team.[266,271,273-276] Although this seems to be somewhat more evident in patients who had to go on ECMO, it is currently a universal trend that also applies to those who did not need bypass.[266,271,275,276] In many series, including ours, there is a direct relationship between the need for prosthetic diaphragmatic repair and the incidence and severity of late complications.[271,273,275,276]

One of the most common problems in CDH survivors is gastroesophageal reflux (GER).[205,236,266,271,273,274,276,277] In our experience, virtually every child has some manifestation of GER, but only about 20% of them need to undergo a fundoplication.[276] It has been suggested that, in addition to GER, esophageal motility is often abnormal, not infrequently with concurrent esophageal dilation, hindering management of the GER itself.[277,278] In our series, over half of the children stayed below the 25th percentile for weight during the first year of life, despite a higher than normal caloric intake.[276] Up to two thirds of the children may need a gastric tube or gastrostomy to be fed adequately, usually because of oral feeding difficulties.[266,273,277] Prolonged endotracheal intubation is predictive for severe oral aversion, which was found in one quarter of our patients during the first year of life.[276] Most of these GI and nutritional complications tend improve with age.[276]

Bronchopulmonary dysplasia, or "chronic lung disease," is present in a third to two thirds of the patients.[273,279] The need for continuous oxygen delivery through a nasal catheter after hospital discharge is not uncommon (16% of the cases, in our experience), in some patients for more than 2 years.[152,266,273,275] Volume restrictions, usually through diet based on hyperosmolar formula, may help minimize pulmonary complications.[266] Diuretics, sometimes in association with bronchodilators or steroids (or both), may also be useful.[273,275] In our patients, prophylaxis against respiratory syncytial virus has been proposed as a means to decrease both the incidence and severity of acute respiratory failure related to this disease.[275]

Although the alveoli continue to multiply during the first 8 years of life,[115,280] their total numbers do not reach normal values in patients with CDH.[108,110,111,281] Emphysematous changes may occasionally be seen on plain chest radiographs, especially in the more caudal portions of the lungs.[282] Radioisotopic pulmonary scans usually show reductions on both ventilation and perfusion, which are also typically disproportionate to each other.[275,282] Interestingly, despite all these initial disturbances, pulmonary function seems to normalize in the long term.[127,283,284] Pulmonary artery pressure, estimated by Doppler echocardiogram, tends to normalize with time in most children. However, deaths from right cardiac failure have been reported at as late as 18 months of age.[205]

Different factors, including hypoxemia, ventilation strategy, and ECMO, may affect the neurodevelopmental outcome. In general, the overall incidence of neurologic complications in patients who received ECMO for CDH is comparable to that found in infants who went on bypass because of other diseases.[285,286] There is some controversy, however, about purely cognitive development. Although a few authors have found cognition problems to be more frequent in children with CDH than in those who went on ECMO for other reasons, others have not confirmed such findings.[271,285,286] In most cases, such impairment is mild or moderate.[266,271,273,285,286] Children with continued need for oxygen therapy or with failure to thrive are more susceptible to neurodevelopmental complications. Otherwise, neurodevelopmental delays tend to disappear, or at least improve, with age.[266,271]

Hearing deficits and need for hearing aids have been noticed in up to one fifth of the children, for reasons yet to be completely clarified.[266,271,273,274] Putative causes include prolonged alkalosis, the use of aminoglycoside antibiotics, and the administration of high doses of furosemide.[266] ECMO is also a risk factor.[287] Every child with CDH, particularly those with speech delays, must undergo screening audiometry and brainstem auditory-evoked response testing periodically, as hearing deficits may have a delayed onset.[266,271]

Chest wall development may be affected both by the disease itself and by its treatment. The volume of the ipsilateral thoracic cavity may be reduced, apparently as a consequence of the reduced size of the lungs.[288] Overall, up to one third of the children have some degree of chest wall deformity, more commonly pectus excavatum and thoracic scoliosis (the latter is a risk factor for hernia recurrence in children who receive a diaphragmatic prosthesis).[266,271] In general, chest wall deformities associated with CDH are mild and rarely need surgical repair.[266,271]

Several other complications have been reported in different systems. Intestinal obstruction is the most frequent reason for reoperation in our experience, occurring in just under 20% of the cases.[266] Its most common cause is adhesions, followed by midgut volvulus and gastric volvulus.[266,271,273] Other ailments also reported in association with CDH, albeit much less frequently, include vesicoureteral reflux, cholelithiasis, asymptomatic renal calculi, chylothorax, hypertrophic pyloric stenosis, retinal vasculopathy without functional visual deficit, and chronic superior vena cava syndrome (the latter two complications were probably related to ECMO).[266,271,273]

Diaphragmatic Hernia Recurrence

Overall postoperative recurrence rates have been reported to be between 6% and 80%.[205,236,266,285,289] Hernia recurrence is more common within the first 18 months of life, but it can happen at any age.[289] The vast majority of the cases occur in children in whom a prosthetic patch was used for repair of the hernia, with a little over half of them progressing with a recurrence in the larger or longer series.[236,266,285,289] Diaphragmatic repair with a prosthesis has also been associated with higher rates of infection, adhesions, and both thoracic and spinal column deformities, when compared with primary repair.[273,290,291] The main mechanism behind hernia recurrence is believed to be related to normal growth, which is supposed to lead to traction and eventual detachment of the prosthesis, usually at its posteromedial aspect.[236] The most common clinical manifestations of hernia recurrence are intestinal obstruction and respiratory distress, in that order.[271,289] Asymptomatic recurrences are not uncommon,[266,289] nor are multiple recurrences.[289] Diagnosis is usually made through a plain chest radiograph. However, sometimes a contrast GI radiograph is necessary. Occasionally, depending on the herniated content, ultrasound, CT, or, more rarely, a contrast enema, may be of help. Hernia recurrence should be surgically repaired, because of the risk for incarceration or strangulation. In selected cases of short-term small and stable recurrences, reoperation may be postponed, depending on the overall condition of the patient.[292] Because hernia recurrence is frequently asymptomatic at first, a plain chest radiograph should be performed at least once a year postoperatively in every patient who underwent prosthetic repair.[266]

FUTURE PERSPECTIVES

Since the mid 1990s, much progress has been made on the treatment of CDH. Survival rates consistently hovering around 90% are now commonplace at major referral centers. At the same time, one could say that a formerly fatal illness has been turned into a chronic disease, as morbidity rates have increased in parallel to survival. The challenges ahead relate to both minimizing morbidity and rescuing the cases with extreme pulmonary hypoplasia, which remains the leading cause of death in patients with this disease. These challenges have been the stimuli for some of the most fertile research efforts in pediatric surgery lately. Summarized accounts of some of these efforts will follow, along with a few brief historical notes.

Despite a few anecdotal successes, the results of the actual repair of the hernia in the fetus were very disappointing.[19,20] One of the reasons for the bad results was the fact that reduction of the hernia increased intra-abdominal pressure, hampering umbilical blood flow, and also frequently leading to kinking of the umbilical vein and of the ductus venosus.[20,293] More than 10 years ago, Wilson and colleagues showed that a complete occlusion of the fetal trachea drastically accelerated fetal lung growth, reversing both the pulmonary hypoplasia and its associated pulmonary vascular abnormalities in experimental CDH, resulting in marked improvements of lung function at birth[28,294,295] (Fig. 33-8). This led almost immediately to clinical trials in which fetal tracheal occlusion was accomplished first through open surgery, then video-fetoscopically.[31,32,296-298] The tracheal occlusion device is typically removed at birth before occluding the umbilical cord, during a so-called ex utero, intrapartum (EXIT) procedure. Once again, despite a few, mostly isolated successes, results have been significantly worse than those of postnatal care, mostly because of postoperative preterm labor, dislodgment of the tracheal occlusion device, erratic secretion of the pulmonary liquid by the fetus, and pulmonary dysfunction in a few patients in whom there was reversal of the lung hypoplasia (the cause of which remains to be determined).[30-32,297] Even so, recent experimental developments may contribute to the refinement and optimization of fetal tracheal occlusion in the future.[299-301]

The acceleration of pulmonary growth observed after fetal tracheal occlusion depends on sustained intrapulmonary distention by retained lung liquid, which is actively secreted by the alveolar-capillary membrane.[28,294,295] One result of this finding was our demonstration that lung growth can also be accelerated after birth by continuous intrapulmonary distention with a liquid medium, namely PFC, which is bio-inert and nonabsorbable by the alveolar-capillary membrane.[36] This phenomenon cannot be reproduced in the lungs of adults.[37] Thus, apparently, liquid-based pulmonary distention simply accelerates normal growth and cannot induce hyperplasia in mature, developed lungs. Long-term studies in animal models have revealed no deleterious effects of PFC-based lung distention.[302] The first series of neonates who underwent pulmonary distention with PFC under extracorporeal support was presented in 2000, with encouraging results (Fig. 33-9).[38] A larger, multicenter study

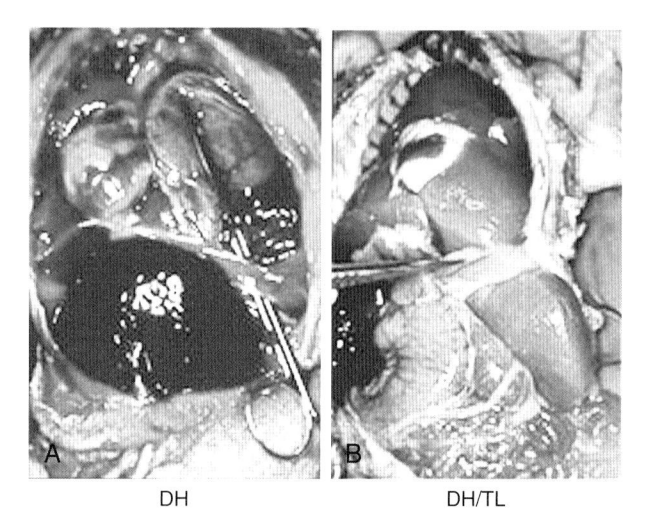

Figure 33–8
(A) Gross necropsy finding in a newborn lamb with experimental congenital diaphragmatic hernia (CDH). The scissors are placed through a defect on the left diaphragm. Abdominal viscera are present in the left hemithorax. The lungs are small and not visible. **(B)** Gross necropsy finding in a newborn lamb with experimental CDH and complete tracheal occlusion. The forceps are holding the left diaphragm. Both lungs are markedly enlarged. The left lung has completely reduced the herniated abdominal viscera and has grown into the abdomen, through the diaphragmatic defect. DH, diaphragmatic hernia; TL, tracheal ligation. *(Reproduced with permission from DiFiore JW, Fauza DO, Slavin R, Peters CA, Fackler JC, Wilson JM. J Pediatr Surg 1994;29:248-57.)*

with longer distention times than those allowed by the U.S. Food and Drug Administration (FDA) in the first series is now being pursued.

The concept of lung transplantation in CDH involves the notion that the transplanted lung (or lobe) should maintain the patient only until the native lung contralateral to the hernia develops enough to allow resection of the graft, so that immunosuppression is no longer necessary. Successful conventional lung transplantations have been performed in very few patients with CDH.[26,27] Survival after living-donor, reduced-lung transplantations has been achieved as well, albeit only experimentally.[303] Chronic donor shortage and the many difficulties yet to be overcome in reduced-lung transplantation to newborns render these options of limited, if any, value, at least for the foreseeable future.

Diaphragmatic reconstruction with an autologous engineered construct was first proposed in 2000 and has since continued to develop experimentally as a viable and potentially improved alternative for diaphragmatic replacement in the neonatal period.[39,40] Diaphragmatic repair with an autologous tendon engineered from mesenchymal cells isolated from the amniotic fluid has been shown to lead to improved mechanical and functional outcomes when compared with an equivalent acellular bioprosthetic repair, given a suitable scaffold environment.[40] Cell manufacturing for engineered diaphragmatic replacement has recently proved viable under FDA-mandated guidelines.[42,43] Translation of these findings into clinical practice is expected in the not-too-distant future, pending the generation of additional animal safety data.

Fundamental knowledge and basic aspects of the management of CDH should also continue to improve. A better understanding of the pathogenesis and pathophysiology of this disease are expected. A large, detailed multicenter study sponsored by the National Institutes of Health aimed at uncovering genetic aspects of CDH is under way.[74,304] The notion of prenatal gene therapy for CDH has started to be explored experimentally in rodent models.[305] The recent addition of computer simulation models, including cell-based simulation, could shed additional light on the pathogenesis of CDH.[306,307] The search for prognostic markers will continue—for example, through ever-improving imaging methods such as three-dimensional anatomic measurements via MRI. The role of adjunct therapies and alternative ventilation methods should be better defined.

The role of the Congenital Diaphragmatic Hernia Registry is as important as any of the initiatives just mentioned. Like its pediatric oncology counterparts, this organization, now embracing several tens of centers, has had major impact on both the understanding and treatment of this disease, and its influence should continue to flourish.

OTHER DIAPHRAGMATIC ANOMALIES

In addition to conventional CDH, many other congenital diaphragmatic anomalies have been described. An overview of their location and frequency at different ages can be seen in Figure 33-10.[151] CDH is, by far, the most common diaphragmatic anomaly of the neonatal period. Hiatal hernia seldom manifests prior to adulthood. In the following paragraphs, only the general aspects of these other diaphragmatic anomalies are briefly discussed.

Diaphragmatic Eventration

Eventration is a term used to describe an abnormal elevation of the diaphragm. It can be congenital or acquired. Acquired cases, also known as diaphragmatic paralysis or paresis, usually

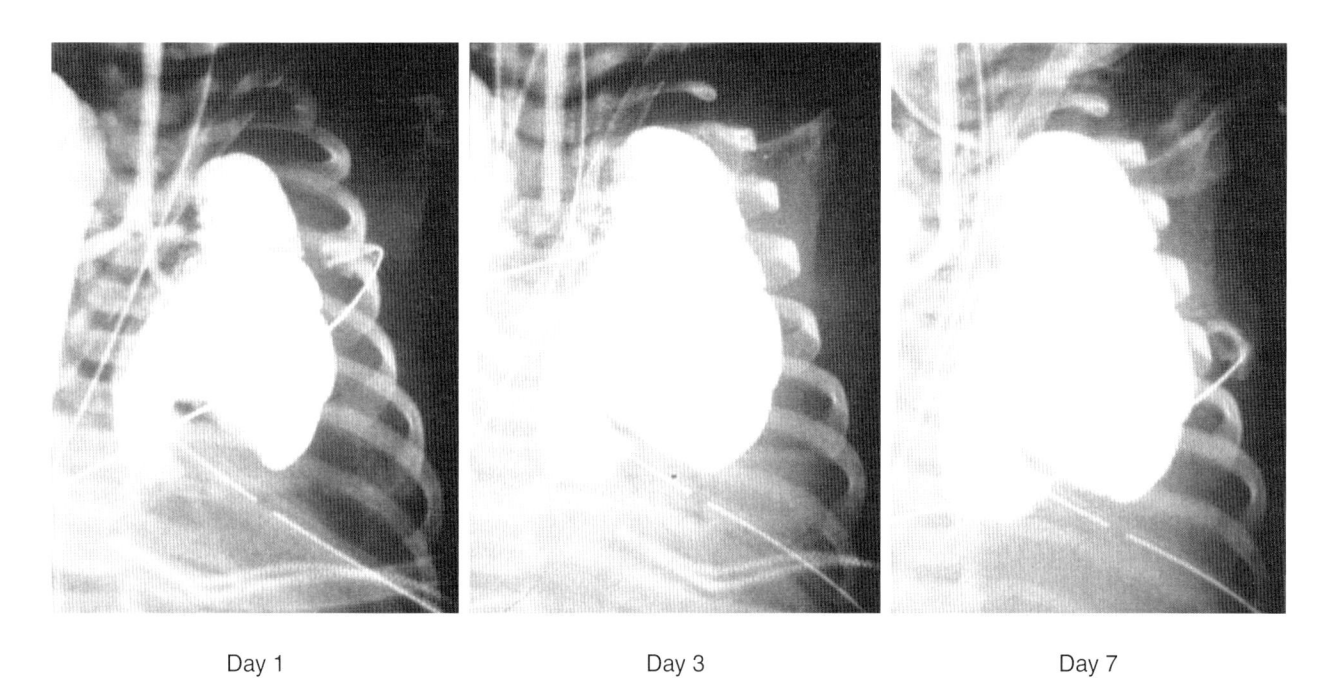

Figure 33–9
Plain chest radiographs from a neonate with congenital diaphragmatic hernia, showing the progress of the ipsilateral lung during intrapulmonary distention with a perfluorocarbon (radiopaque) for 7 days. Notice its obvious increase in size, which did not happen in the contralateral lung. *(Reproduced with permission from Fauza DO, Hirschl R, Wilson JM. J Pediatr Surg 2001;36:1237-40.)*

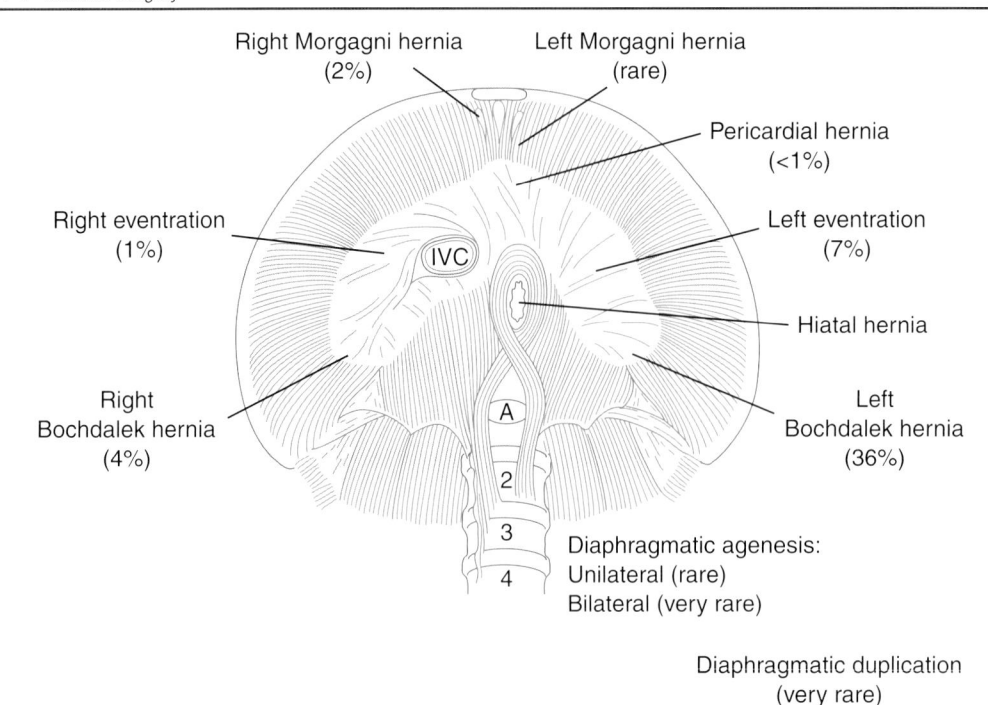

Figure 33-10
Overall relative incidence and location of different diaphragmatic anomalies at all ages, including children and adults. Bochdalek hernia is, by far, the most common in infants. Hiatal hernia rarely manifests before adulthood. IVC, inferior vena cava.

result from damage to the phrenic nerve, which in turn may be caused by traumatic delivery, thoracic surgery, tumors, inflammation, or CNS conditions such as poliomyelitis and Werdnig-Hoffmann disease.[308-310] In congenital cases, the phrenic nerve is almost always normal. Often, it is difficult to differentiate a congenital case from one caused by obstetric trauma. Acquired eventration should be suspected whenever there is a history of complications at delivery or concomitant signs of injury to the brachial plexus.

In congenital eventration, either the whole diaphragm may be affected, or only part of it—usually its dome, which is not a meeting point of embryonic components. Indeed, it is thought that diaphragmatic eventration represents a failure of muscularization of the diaphragm, not a failed fusion of all its embryonic components. Its cause is unknown. It can be present on either side but is more frequent on the left. Bilateral cases have been reported.[311] Diaphragmatic thickness and its muscle fiber density vary within a broad spectrum in the eventrated area, going from normal, with practically all fibers present, to very thin, without any fibers. The eventrated portion of the diaphragm does not function. In certain cases, the differentiation between it and CDH containing a hernia sac is purely arbitrary. As in CDH, there may be associated pulmonary hypoplasia, intestinal malrotation, and other anomalies in various systems.[312-314]

Clinical manifestations also vary within an ample spectrum that, to a certain extent, is analogous to that of CDH. However, presentation after the neonatal period is much more common, and symptoms are usually much less exuberant than in CDH. In older children, (often recurrent) pneumonia may be the first manifestation. GI symptoms, usually obstructive in nature, and failure to thrive are not uncommon. In cases linked to Werdnig-Hoffmann disease, respiratory distress resulting from the eventration may the initial manifestation of disease.[309] The patient may also be completely asymptomatic. The diagnosis is typically made through a plain chest radiograph, although sometimes it may have to be confirmed through an ultrasonography or a fluoroscopy, both of which may also be helpful in eventually differentiating it from CDH. In the latter two examinations, one should be able to notice paradoxical respiration in the affected area, as long as the patient is not being artificially ventilated.

Symptomatic patients should undergo surgical repair. In asymptomatic patients, surgery is recommended when there is a large eventration or pulmonary function tests are abnormal, as lung growth may be compromised if the eventration is not treated. In a few patients with an asymptomatic acquired eventration, there may be variable degrees of recovery of the diaphragmatic function with time and spontaneous reversal of the eventration, so that conservative treatment may be initially justified, but not for long.

At surgery, plication of the diaphragm with nonabsorbable sutures is usually preferred, but, in selected patients, partial resection followed by overlapped reconstruction of the residual diaphragm may be the best option (simple end-to-end suturing commonly leads to recurrence). In right eventrations, most authors prefer to perform the repair through a thoracotomy. For left eventrations, there is some controversy as to whether a thoracotomy or a laparotomy would be the most suitable access. We favor the thoracic access, mostly because it allows visualization of the branches of the phrenic nerve, which thus can be preserved during diaphragmatic plication. This is particularly relevant in view of the fact that, after plication, there may be at least partial recovery of diaphragmatic function.[315] When a thoracotomy is used, regardless of the side, usually the 7th intercostal space is the one to be opened. An abdominal access may be preferred in certain bilateral cases. Over the past few years, thoracoscopic repair has been increasingly favored by many centers.[316] The minimally invasive approach may well become the method of choice for many patients.

Morgagni Hernia

Also known as retrosternal or parasternal hernia, the Morgagni diaphragmatic hernia occurs through the parasternal spaces, also called Morgagni foramina, or Larrey clefts, which are small, triangular portions of the diaphragm on each side of the inferior limit of the sternum that form as a result of the union between the transverse septum and the thoracic wall. This hernia can occur on either side but is more common on the right. Bilateral cases have been reported.[317,318] If a hernia sac is present, the superior epigastric artery normally stays lateral to it. This hernia is more frequent in adults and in older children. In childhood, it occurs in a ratio of approximately 1:20 to the occurrence of classic CDH.[318-320] Predisposing factors include obesity and a history of trauma. Morgagni hernia is usually asymptomatic. Only occasionally does it lead to mild symptoms such as respiratory discomfort, vague GI manifestations, or epigastric tenderness. In children, it tends to be symptomatic more often than in adults.[318] Most of the time, this hernia is diagnosed as an incidental finding of a chest roentgenogram. A lateral radiograph is usually more helpful than an anteroposterior image, sometimes after a barium swallow, or, more rarely, after contrast enema. Occasionally, ultrasound or CT can be valuable to confirm the diagnosis as well.[318]

Incarceration of the herniated content is rare. Open repair is frequently performed through a supraumbilical, usually subcostal, laparotomy. After hernia reduction and resection of the hernia sac (if present), the diaphragm is sutured to the posterior sheath of the rectus abdominis muscle. A prosthesis is rarely necessary for diaphragmatic repair. Also here, the laparoscopic approach has been increasingly favored.[321-323]

Various other anomalies can be associated with Morgagni hernia, more frequently cardiac.[318,320] Intestinal malrotation is somewhat common.[318] A Morgagni hernia may be part of the pentalogy of Cantrell, if associated with defects of the inferior aspect of the sternum, of the supraumbilical abdominal wall, and of the pericardium (all of which lead to cardiac ectopia), in addition to a cardiac anomaly.[324] In these cases, the surgeon usually tries to suture the diaphragm to the sternum and may need to use a prosthesis more frequently than in isolated hernias.

Hiatal Hernia

Hernias through the esophageal hiatus can be divided into four main types: sliding esophageal hernia, the most common, in which the esophagus moves freely through the hiatus, so that the esophagogastric junction may be either in the chest or in the abdomen at different times; paraesophageal hernia, in which the esophagogastric junction remains below the diaphragm and the stomach rolls up into the chest parallel to the esophagus; combined hernia, in which the two previous types coexist; and the controversial congenital short esophagus.

Hiatal hernia may manifest as early as the neonatal period, but most cases first appear in adulthood. Vomiting is the most common manifestation, but patients are often asymptomatic. The diagnosis is usually made through a contrast upper GI series. An upper GI endoscopy is frequently part of the diagnostic evaluation as well. Surgical treatment is the norm, particularly because of the risks of incarceration and strangulation. Either through a laparoscopy or a laparotomy, the hernia is reduced, the diameter of the esophageal hiatus is normalized, and a gastroesophageal fundoplication is performed. The treatment of choice for certain cases of short esophagus remains a subject of much debate. Hiatal hernia is discussed in more detail in chapter 36.

Pericardial Hernia

Pericardial hernia, also known as hernia of the central diaphragmatic tendon, is the rarest and least understood of the diaphragmatic defects that may lead to a hernia. In this defect, there is a communication between the peritoneal and pericardial cavities, with or without herniation.[325] In general, there is no hernia sac.[325-327] It has been identified from soon after birth up to late adulthood, but most cases are diagnosed in neonates.[327-329] It is thought that the primary defect affects the transverse septum directly.[151] The data are not sufficient for typical clinical manifestations to be described; it can be asymptomatic and only incidentally suspected on a plain chest radiograph.[328,329] Surgical repair through the abdomen is recommended.[328]

Diaphragmatic Agenesis

Diaphragmatic agenesis is customarily confused with CDH in which the diaphragmatic defect is particularly large, especially if the residual posterior diaphragm is not dissected from the abdominal wall. True diaphragmatic agenesis is rare. It is usually unilateral, more common on the left, and very rarely bilateral.[330-332] It is generally identified in the neonatal period, but cases uncovered only in adulthood have been described.[333,334] It can be associated with multiple other anomalies, especially if bilateral.[331,335] Clinical manifestations, diagnosis, and treatment are analogous to those of CDH, except that a prosthesis is always necessary for diaphragmatic closure.[334] Survival data are unreliable, as in many studies, its differentiation from classic CDH is not clear. In general, it is thought that the prognosis for diaphragmatic agenesis is worse than that for classic CDH, given the dimensions of the diaphragmatic defect.

Diaphragmatic Duplication

Diaphragmatic duplication, be it partial or complete, is exceedingly rare.[336,337] It consists of a fibromuscular membrane that separates the affected hemithorax in two cavities and represents a duplication of the pleuroperitoneal membrane. In most cases, the accessory diaphragm is not innervated by the phrenic nerve. The accessory diaphragm may be eminently muscular and the orthotopic diaphragm fibrous, or vice versa.[338,339] The accessory diaphragm may be located in the chest in such a way that the ipsilateral lung is divided into two compartments; it may also be associated with anomalous airways or pulmonary vessels, as well as with partial pulmonary agenesis.[339-342] Clinically, it may cause respiratory distress in the neonatal period, recurring airway infections during childhood, and chronic pulmonary inflamation in adulthood, occasionally with bronchiectasis.[336,341] Apparently, it can also be asymptomatic.[340,343] Because, when present, symptoms are nonspecific, the diagnosis is commonly confirmed only intraoperatively. In the rare cases in which a diaphragmatic duplication was resected, an improvement of respiratory symptoms resulted. At least one case of association between (right-sided) CDH and diaphragmatic duplication in a neonate has been reported.[344]

Cribriform Diaphragm

A case of an incidental intraoperative finding of a cribriform aspect of the right diaphragm, with several portions of the liver protruding to the chest through the many diaphragmatic defects, has been described in an elderly patient.[345] It is not yet possible to know whether this is another diaphragmatic anomaly, with a distinct embryonic pathogenesis, or an extremely rare variant of CDH, or even simply an acquired diaphragmatic defect.

REFERENCES

1. Paræo A. *Opera chirurgica*. Frankfurt; 1610;**230**.
2. Bonetus T. Suffocatione De, Observatio XLI. Suffocatio excitata a tenuium intestorum vulnus diaphramatis, in thoracem ingrestu. In: *Sepulchretum sive anatomia practica et cadareribus morbo denatus*. Geneva; 1679.
3. Macaulay G. An account of viscera herniation. *Phil Trans Roy Coll Phys* 1754;**6**:25-35.
4. Morgagni GB. The seats and causes of disease investigated by anatomy. In: Alexander BT, editor. London: Miller & Caldwell; 1769. p. 205-6.
5. Bochdalek VA. Einige Betrachtungen uber die Entstehung des angelborenen Zwerchfellbruches. Als Bietrag zur pathologischen. Anatomie der Hernien. *Vjsch Prakt Heik* 1848;**19**:89-97.
6. Bremer JL. The diaphragm and diaphragmatic hernia. *Arch Pathol* 1943;**36**:539-49.
7. Wells LJ. Development of the human diaphragm and pleural sacs. *Contrib Embryol Carnegie Inst Wash* 1954;**35**:109.
8. White JJ, Suzuki H. Hernia through the foramen of Bochdalek: a misnomer. *J Pediatr Surg* 1972;**7**:60-1.
9. Broman I. Uber die Entwicklung des Zwerchfells beim Menschen. *Verh Anat Ges* 1902;**16**:9-17.
10. Broman I. Ueber die Entwicklung und Bedeutung der Mesenterien und der Körperhöhlen bei den Wirbeltieren. *Ergeb Anat Entw* 1905;**15**:332-409.
11. Aue O. Uber angeborene Zwerchfellhernien. *Deutsch Z Chir* 1920;**160**:14.
12. Heidenhain L. Gesichte eines Falles von chronisher Incarceration des Mageus in einer angeborenen Zwerchfellhernie welcher durcher Laparotomie geheilt wurde, mitansheissenden Bermerkungen uber die Moglichkeit, das Kardiacarcinom der Speiserihre zu reseciren. *Deutsch Z Chir* 1905;**76**:394-407.
13. Ladd WE, Gross RE. Congenital diaphragmatic hernia. *N Engl J Med* 1940;**233**:917-25.
14. Gross RE. Congenital hernia of the diaphragm. *Am J Dis Child* 1946;**71**:579-92.
15. German JC, Gazzaniga AB, Amlie R, et al. Management of pulmonary insufficiency in diaphragmatic hernia using extracorporeal circulation with a membrane oxygenator (ECMO). *J Pediatr Surg* 1977;**12**:905-12.
16. Wilson JM, Lund DP, Lillehei CW, et al. Congenital diaphragmatic hernia—a tale of two cities: the Boston experience. *J Pediatr Surg* 1997;**32**:401-5.
17. Clark RH, Hardin Jr WD, Hirschl RB, et al. Current surgical management of congenital diaphragmatic hernia: a report from the Congenital Diaphragmatic Hernia Study Group. *J Pediatr Surg* 1998;**33**:1004-9.
18. Harting MT, Lally KP. Surgical management of neonates with congenital diaphragmatic hernia. *Semin Pediatr Surg* 2007;**16**:109-14.
19. Harrison MR, Langer JC, Adzick NS, et al. Correction of congenital diaphragmatic hernia in utero, V. Initial clinical experience. *J Pediatr Surg* 1990;**25**:56-7:47-55; discussion.
20. Harrison MR, Adzick NS, Flake AW, et al. Correction of congenital diaphragmatic hernia in utero: VI. Hard-earned lessons. *J Pediatr Surg* 1993;**28**:1411-7, discussion 1417-8.
21. Wung JT, James LS, Kilchevsky E, et al. Management of infants with severe respiratory failure and persistence of the fetal circulation, without hyperventilation. *Pediatrics* 1985;**76**:488-94.
22. Wung JT, Sahni R, Moffitt ST, et al. Congenital diaphragmatic hernia: survival treated with very delayed surgery, spontaneous respiration, and no chest tube. *J Pediatr Surg* 1995;**30**:406-9.
23. Kays DW, Langham Jr MR, Ledbetter DJ, et al. Detrimental effects of standard medical therapy in congenital diaphragmatic hernia. *Ann Surg* 1999;**230**:340-8, discussion; 348-51.
24. Lally KP, Lally PA, Lasky RE, et al. Defect size determines survival in infants with congenital diaphragmatic hernia. *Pediatrics* 2007;**120**:e651-7.
25. Lally KP, Engle W. Postdischarge follow-up of infants with congenital diaphragmatic hernia. *Pediatrics* 2008;**121**:627-32.
26. Van Meurs KP, Rhine WD, Benitz WE, et al. Lobar lung transplantation as a treatment for congenital diaphragmatic hernia. *J Pediatr Surg* 1994;**29**:1557-60.
27. Shochat SJ: Personal communication, 1995.
28. Wilson JM, DiFiore JW, Peters CA. Experimental fetal tracheal ligation prevents the pulmonary hypoplasia associated with fetal nephrectomy: possible application for congenital diaphragmatic hernia. *J Pediatr Surg* 1993;**28**:1439-40:1433-9; discussion.
29. Adzick NS: Personal communication, 1994.
30. Flake AW, Crombleholme TM, Johnson MP, et al. Treatment of severe congenital diaphragmatic hernia by fetal tracheal occlusion: clinical experience with fifteen cases. *Am J Obstet Gynecol* 2000;**183**:1059-66.
31. Harrison MR, Albanese CT, Hawgood SB, et al. Fetoscopic temporary tracheal occlusion by means of detachable balloon for congenital diaphragmatic hernia. *Am J Obstet Gynecol* 2001;**185**:730-3.
32. Harrison MR, Keller RL, Hawgood SB, et al. A randomized trial of fetal endoscopic tracheal occlusion for severe fetal congenital diaphragmatic hernia. *N Engl J Med* 2003;**349**:1916-24.
33. Done E, Gucciardo L, Van Mieghem T, et al. Prenatal diagnosis, prediction of outcome and in utero therapy of isolated congenital diaphragmatic hernia. *Prenat Diagn* 2008;**28**:581-91.
34. Deprest JA, Flemmer AW, Gratacos E, et al. Antenatal prediction of lung volume and in-utero treatment by fetal endoscopic tracheal occlusion in severe isolated congenital diaphragmatic hernia. *Semin Fetal Neonatal Med* 2008.
35. Tsao K, Lally KP. The Congenital Diaphragmatic Hernia Study Group: a voluntary international registry. *Semin Pediatr Surg* 2008;**17**:90-7.
36. Fauza DO, DiFiore JW, Hines MH, et al. Continuous intrapulmonary distention with perfluorocarbon accelerates postnatal lung growth: possible application for congenital diaphragmatic hernia. *Surg Forum* 1995;**46**:666-9.
37. Nobuhara KK, Fauza DO, DiFiore JW, et al. Continuous intrapulmonary distension with perfluorocarbon accelerates neonatal (but not adult) lung growth. *J Pediatr Surg* 1998;**33**:292-8.
38. Fauza DO, Hirschl RB, Wilson JM. Continuous intrapulmonary distention with perfluorocarbon accelerates lung growth in infants with congenital diaphragmatic hernia: initial experience. *J Pediatr Surg* 2001;**36**:1237-40.
39. Fauza DO, Marler JJ, Koka R, et al. Fetal tissue engineering: diaphragmatic replacement. *J Pediatr Surg* 2001;**36**:146-51.
40. Fuchs JR, Kaviani A, Oh JT, et al. Diaphragmatic reconstruction with autologous tendon engineered from mesenchymal amniocytes. *J Pediatr Surg* 2004;**39**:834-8:834-8; discussion.
41. Kunisaki SM, Fuchs JR, Kaviani A, et al. Diaphragmatic repair through fetal tissue engineering: a comparison between mesenchymal amniocyte- and myoblast-based constructs. *J Pediatr Surg* 2006;**41**:34-9:34-9; discussion.
42. Kunisaki SM, Armant M, Kao GS, et al. Tissue engineering from human mesenchymal amniocytes: a prelude to clinical trials. *J Pediatr Surg* 2007;**42**:974-9, discussion; 979-80.
43. Steigman SA, Armant M, Bayer-Zwirello L, et al. Preclinical regulatory validation of a 3-stage amniotic mesenchymal stem cell manufacturing protocol. *J Pediatr Surg* 2008;**43**:1164-9.
44. Butler N, Claireaux AE. Congenital diaphragmatic hernia as a cause of perinatal mortality. *Lancet* 1962;**1**:659-63.
45. Ravitch MM, Barton BA. The need for pediatric surgeons as determined by the volume of work and the mode of delivery of surgical care. *Surgery* 1974;**76**:754-63.
46. Touloukian RJ, Cole D. A state-wide survey of index pediatric surgical conditions. *J Pediatr Surg* 1975;**10**:725-32.
47. David TJ, Illingworth CA. Diaphragmatic hernia in the south-west of England. *J Med Genet* 1976;**13**:253-62.
48. Harrison MR, de Lorimier AA. Congenital diaphragmatic hernia. *Surg Clin North Am* 1981;**61**:1023-35.
49. Czeizel A, Kovacs M. A family study of congenital diaphragmatic defects. *Am J Med Genet* 1985;**21**:105-17.

50. Leck I, Record RG, McKeown T, et al. The incidence of malformations in Birmingham, England, 1950-1959. *Teratology* 1968;**1**:263-80.
51. Puri P, Gorman WA. Natural history of congenital diaphragmatic hernia: Implications for management. *Pediatr Surg Int* 1987;**2**:327-30.
52. Sarda P, Devaux P, Lefort G, et al. Epidemiology of diaphragmatic hernia in Languedoc-Roussillon. *Genet Couns* 1991;**2**:77-81.
53. Wenstrom KD, Weiner CP, Hanson JW. A five-year statewide experience with congenital diaphragmatic hernia. *Am J Obstet Gynecol* 1991;**165**:838-42.
54. Torfs CP, Curry CJ, Bateson TF, et al. A population-based study of congenital diaphragmatic hernia. *Teratology* 1992;**46**:555-65.
55. Estimating disease severity of congenital diaphragmatic hernia in the first 5 minutes of life. The Congenital Diaphragmatic Hernia Study Group. *J Pediatr Surg* 2001;**36**:141-5.
56. Yang W, Carmichael SL, Harris JA, et al. Epidemiologic characteristics of congenital diaphragmatic hernia among 2.5 million California births, 1989-1997. *Birth Defects Res A Clin Mol Teratol* 2006;**76**:170-4.
57. Stauffer UG, Rickham PP. Congenital diaphragmatic hernia and eventration of the diaphragm. In: Rickham PP, Lister J, Irvings JM, editors. *Neonatal surgery* London: Butterworth; 1978. p. 163.
58. Narayan H, De Chazal R, Barrow M, et al. Familial congenital diaphragmatic hernia: prenatal diagnosis, management, and outcome. *Prenat Diagn* 1993;**13**:893-901.
59. Boychuk RB, Nelson JC, Yates KA. Congenital diaphragmatic hernia (an 8-year experience in Hawaii). *Hawaii Med J* 1983;**42**:400-2.
60. Welch RG, Cooke RT. Congenital diaphragmatic hernia. *Lancet* 1962;**1**:975.
61. Lilly JR, Paul M, Rosser SB. Anterior diaphragmatic hernia: familial presentation. *Birth Defects Orig Artic Ser* 1974;**10**:257-8.
62. Wolff G. Familial congenital diaphragmatic defect: review and conclusions. *Hum Genet* 1980;**54**:1-5.
63. Mishalany H, Gordo J. Congenital diaphragmatic hernia in monozygotic twins. *J Pediatr Surg* 1986;**21**:372-4.
64. Carmi R, Meizner I, Katz M. Familial congenital diaphragmatic defect and associated midline anomalies: further evidence for an X-linked midline gene? *Am J Med Genet* 1990;**36**:313-5.
65. Frey P, Glanzmann R, Nars P, et al. Familial congenital diaphragmatic defect: transmission from father to daughter. *J Pediatr Surg* 1991;**26**:1396-8.
66. Austin-Ward ED, Taucher SC. Familial congenital diaphragmatic hernia: is an imprinting mechanism involved? *J Med Genet* 1999;**36**:578-9.
67. Turpin R, Petit P, Chigot P, et al. Hernie diaphragmatique congénitale de type embryonnaire (fente pleuro-péritonéale gauche). Coincidence chez deux cousins germains de cette malformation isolée. *Ann Pédiatr* 1959;**35**:272-9.
68. Norio R, Kaariainen H, Rapola J, et al. Familial congenital diaphragmatic defects: aspects of etiology, prenatal diagnosis. treatment. *Am J Med Genet* 1984;**17**:471-83.
69. Mäkelä V. Hernia diaphragmatica congenita spuria. *Finska Läk Sällsk Handl* 1916;**58**:1107-27.
70. Pober BR, Lin A, Russell M, et al. Infants with Bochdalek diaphragmatic hernia: sibling precurrence and monozygotic twin discordance in a hospital-based malformation surveillance program. *Am J Med Genet A* 2005;**138A**:81-8.
71. Moore KL. *The developing human.* 4th ed. Philadelphia: WB Saunders; 1988.
72. Lewis WH. The development of the muscular system. In: Keibel F, Mall FP, editors. *Manual of human embryology.* Philadelphia: J.B. Lippincott; 1910.
73. Dussault J, Godlewski G, Pignodel C. Pathogenesis of congenital diaphragmatic hernia of the newborn infant: apropos of 2 cases. *Bull Assoc Anat (Nancy)* 1981;**65**:77-81.
74. Kantarci S, Donahoe PK. Congenital diaphragmatic hernia (CDH) etiology as revealed by pathway genetics. *Am J Med Genet C Semin Med Genet* 2007;**145C**:217-26.
75. Andersen DH. Incidence of congenital diaphragmatic hernia in the young of rats bred on a diet deficient in vitamin A. *Am J Dis Child* 1941;**62**:888.
76. Warkany J, Roth CB. Congenital malformations induced in rats by maternal vitamin A deficiency. II. Effect of varying the preparatory diet upon the yield of abnormal young. *J Nutr* 1948;**35**:1-2.
77. Hurley LS. Teratogenic aspects of manganese, zinc, and copper nutrition. *Physiol Rev* 1981;**61**:249-95.
78. Barr M. Jr. The teratogenicity of cadmium chloride in two stocks of Wistar rats. *Teratology* 1973;**7**:237-42.
79. Drobeck HP, Coulston F, Cornelius D. Effects of thalidomide on fetal development in rabbits and on establishment of pregnancy in monkeys. *Toxicol Appl Pharmacol* 1965;**7**:165-78.
80. Brent RL. Antibodies and malformations. In: Tuchmann-Duplessis H, editor. *Malformations congénitales des mammiféres.* Paris: Masson City; 1971. p. 187-222.
81. Ambrose AM, Larson PS, Borzelleca JF, et al. Toxicologic studies on 2,4-dichlorophenyl-p-nitrophenyl ether. *Toxicol Appl Pharmacol* 1971;**19**:263-75.
82. Iritani I. Experimental study on embryogenesis of congenital diaphragmatic hernia. *Anat Embryol* 1984;**169**:133-9.
83. Kluth D, Tenbrinck R, von Ekesparre M, et al. The natural history of congenital diaphragmatic hernia and pulmonary hypoplasia in the embryo. *J Pediatr Surg* 1993;**28**:462-3:456-62; discussion.
84. Beaudoin AR. Teratogenicity of polybrominated biphenyls in rats. *Environ Res* 1977;**14**:81-6.
85. Sutherland MF, Parkinson MM, Hallett P. Teratogenicity of three substituted 4-biphenyls in the rat as a result of the chemical breakdown and possible metabolism of a thromboxane A2-receptor blocker. *Teratology* 1989;**39**:537-45.
86. Ackerman KG, Herron BJ, Vargas SO, et al. Fog2 is required for normal diaphragm and lung development in mice and humans. *PLoS Genet* 2005;**1**:58-65.
87. You LR, Takamoto N, Yu CT, et al. Mouse lacking COUP-TFII as an animal model of Bochdalek-type congenital diaphragmatic hernia. *Proc Natl Acad Sci U S A* 2005;**102**:16351-6.
88. Jay PY, Bielinska M, Erlich JM, et al. Impaired mesenchymal cell function in Gata4 mutant mice leads to diaphragmatic hernias and primary lung defects. *Dev Biol* 2007;**301**:602-14.
89. deLorimier AA. Tierney OF, and Parker HR: Hypoplastic lungs in fetal lambs with surgically produced congenital diaphragmatic hernia. *Surgery* 1967;**62**:12-7.
90. Kent GM, Olley PM, Creighton RE, et al. Hemodynamic and pulmonary changes following surgical creation of a diaphragmatic hernia in fetal lambs. *Surgery* 1972;**72**:427-33.
91. Fauza DO, Tannuri U, Ayoub AA, et al. Surgically produced congenital diaphragmatic hernia in fetal rabbits. *J Pediatr Surg* 1994;**29**:882-6.
92. Harrison MR, Jester JA, Ross NA. Correction of congenital diaphragmatic hernia in utero. I. The model: intrathoracic balloon produces fatal pulmonary hypoplasia. *Surgery* 1980;**88**:174-82.
93. Nakao Y, Iritani I, Kishimoto H. Experimental model of congenital diaphragmatic hernia induced chemically. *Teratology* 1981;**24**:11A.
94. Molenaar JC, Bos AP, Hazebroek FW, et al. Congenital diaphragmatic hernia, what defect? *J Pediatr Surg* 1991;**26**:248-54.
95. Kimbrough RD, Gaines TB, Linder RE. 2,4-Dichlorophenyl-p-nitrophenyl ether (TOK): effects on the lung maturation of rat fetus. *Arch Environ Health* 1974;**28**:316-20.
96. Gray Jr LE, Kavlock RJ, Chernoff N, et al. Prenatal exposure to the herbicide 2,4-dichlorophenyl-p-nitrophenyl ether destroys the rodent Harderian gland. *Science* 1982;**215**:293-4.
97. Ueki R, Nakao Y, Nishida T, et al. Lung hypoplasia in developing mice and rats induced by maternal exposure to nitrofen. *Cong Anom* 1990;**30**:133-43.
98. Taderera JV. Control of lung differentiation in vitro. *Dev Biol* 1967;**16**:489-512.
99. Kluth D, Keijzer R, Hertl M, et al. Embryology of congenital diaphragmatic hernia. *Semin Pediatr Surg* 1996;**5**:224-33.
100. Bucher U, Reid L. Development of the intrasegmental bronchial tree: the pattern of branching and development of cartilage at various stages of intrauterine life. *Thorax* 1961;**16**:207-18.
101. Skandalakis JE, Gray SW, Symbas P. The trachea and the lungs. In: Skandalakis JE, Gray SW, editors. *Embryology for surgeons.* Baltimore: Williams & Wilkins; 1994. p. 415.
102. Alles AJ, Losty PD, Donahoe PK, et al. Embryonic cell death patterns associated with nitrofen-induced congenital diaphragmatic hernia. *J Pediatr Surg* 1995;**30**:359-60:353-8; discussion.
103. Jesudason EC. Small lungs and suspect smooth muscle: congenital diaphragmatic hernia and the smooth muscle hypothesis. *J Pediatr Surg* 2006;**41**:431-5.
104. Heine H. Zur Entwicklungsgeschichte angeborener Zwerchfellhernien bei Saugetieren. *Anat Anaz* 1973;**133**:382-93.
105. Holder RM, Ashcraft KW, et al. Congenital diaphragmatic hernia. In: Ravitch MM, Welch KJ, Benson CD, editors. *Pediatric surgery.* Chicago: Year–Book Medical Publishers; 1979. p. 432-45.
106. Gattone VHd and Morse DE. A scanning electron microscopic study on the pathogenesis of the posterolateral diaphragmatic hernia. *J Submicrosc Cytol* 1982;**14**:483-90.
107. Zamir O, Eyal F, Lernau OZ, et al. Bilateral congenital posterolateral diaphragmatic hernia. *Am J Perinatol* 1986;**3**:56-7.
108. Kitagawa M, Hislop A, Boyden EA, et al. Lung hypoplasia in congenital diaphragmatic hernia. A quantitative study of airway, artery, and alveolar development. *Br J Surg* 1971;**58**:342-6.
109. Bohn D, Tamura M, Perrin D, et al. Ventilatory predictors of pulmonary hypoplasia in congenital diaphragmatic hernia, confirmed by morphologic assessment. *J Pediatr* 1987;**111**:423-31.
110. Beals DA, Schloo BL, Vacanti JP, et al. Pulmonary growth and remodeling in infants with high-risk congenital diaphragmatic hernia. *J Pediatr Surg* 1992;**27**:997-1001, discussion 1001-2.

111. Areechon W, Reid L. Hypoplasia of the lung with congenital diaphragmatic hernia. *Br Med J* 1963;**1**:230-3.
112. Fauza DO, Wilson JM. Congenital diaphragmatic hernia and associated anomalies: their incidence, identification, and impact on prognosis. *J Pediatr Surg* 1994;**29**:1113-7.
113. Kovarik JL, Jensen NK. Congenital aplasia of the right hepatic lobe with right-sided diaphragmatic hernia and intestinal malrotation. *Int Surg* 1969;**51**:499-503.
114. Robertson DJ, Harmon CM, Goldberg S. Right congenital diaphragmatic hernia associated with fusion of the liver and the lung. *J Pediatr Surg* 2006;**41**:e9-10.
115. Reid LM. Lung growth in health and disease. *Br J Dis Chest* 1984;**78**:113-34.
116. Blackburn WR, Logsdon P, Alexander JA. Congenital diaphragmatic hernia: studies of lung composition and structure. *Am Rev Respir Dis* 1977;**115S**:275.
117. Wigglesworth JS, Desai R, Guerrini P. Fetal lung hypoplasia: biochemical and structural variations and their possible significance. *Arch Dis Child* 1981;**56**:606-15.
118. Hisanaga S, Shimokawa H, Kashiwabara Y, et al. Unexpectedly low lecithin/sphingomyelin ratio associated with fetal diaphragmatic hernia. *Am J Obstet Gynecol* 1984;**149**:905-6.
119. Asabe K, Tsuji K, Handa N, et al. Immunohistochemical distribution of surfactant apoprotein-A in congenital diaphragmatic hernia. *J Pediatr Surg* 1997;**32**:667-72.
120. Gandy G, Bradbrooke JG, Naidoo BT, et al. Comparison of methods for evaluating surface properties of lung in perinatal period. *Arch Dis Child* 1968;**43**:8-16.
121. Sullivan KM, Hawgood S, Flake AW, et al. Amniotic fluid phospholipid analysis in the fetus with congenital diaphragmatic hernia. *J Pediatr Surg* 1994;**29**:1023-4;1020-3; discussion.
122. Muratore CS, Wilson JM. Congenital diaphragmatic hernia: where are we and where do we go from here? *Semin Perinatol* 2000;**24**:418-28.
123. Naeye RL, Shochat SJ, Whitman V, et al. Unsuspected pulmonary vascular abnormalities associated with diaphragmatic hernia. *Pediatrics* 1976;**58**:902-6.
124. Geggel RL, Murphy JD, Langleben D, et al. Congenital diaphragmatic hernia: arterial structural changes and persistent pulmonary hypertension after surgical repair. *J Pediatr Surg* 1985;**107**:457-64.
125. Boucherat O, Benachi A, Chailley-Heu B, et al. Surfactant maturation is not delayed in human fetuses with diaphragmatic hernia. *PLoS Med* 2007:4:e237.
126. Engle WA. Surfactant-replacement therapy for respiratory distress in the preterm and term neonate. *Pediatrics* 2008;**121**:419-32.
127. Wohl ME, Griscom NT, Strieder DJ, et al. The lung following repair of congenital diaphragmatic hernia. *J Pediatr* 1977;**90**:405-14.
128. Starrett RW, de Lorimier AA. Congenital diaphragmatic hernia in lambs: hemodynamic and ventilatory changes with breathing. *J Pediatr Surg* 1975;**10**:575-82.
129. Dibbins AW. Congenital diaphragmatic hernia: hypoplastic lung and pulmonary vasoconstriction. *Clin Perinatol* 1978;**5**:93-104.
130. Dibbins AW, Wiener ES. Mortality from neonatal diaphragmatic hernia. *J Pediatr Surg* 1974;**9**:653-62.
131. Hassett MJ, Glick PL, Karamanoukian HL, et al. Pathophysiology of congenital diaphragmatic hernia. XVI: Elevated pulmonary collagen in the lamb model of congenital diaphragmatic hernia. *J Pediatr Surg* 1995;**30**:1191-4.
132. Levin DL. Congenital diaphragmatic hernia: a persistent problem. *J Pediatr* 1987;**111**:390-2.
133. Nobuhara KK, Wilson JM. Pathophysiology of congenital diaphragmatic hernia. *Semin Pediatr Surg* 1996;**5**:234-42.
134. Weinstein S, Stolar CJ. Newborn surgical emergencies. Congenital diaphragmatic hernia and extracorporeal membrane oxygenation. *Pediatr Clin North Am* 1993;**40**:1315-33.
135. Shochat SJ. Pulmonary vascular pathology in congenital diaphragmatic hernias. *Pediatr Surg Int* 1987;**2**:331-5.
136. Shehata SM, Sharma HS, Mooi WJ, et al. Pulmonary hypertension in human newborns with congenital diaphragmatic hernia is associated with decreased vascular expression of nitric-oxide synthase. *Cell Biochem Biophys* 2006;**44**:147-55.
137. Ford WD, James MJ, Walsh JA. Congenital diaphragmatic hernia: association between pulmonary vascular resistance and plasma thromboxane concentrations. *Arch Dis Child* 1984;**59**:143-6.
138. Stolar CJ, Dillon PW, Stalcup SA. Extracorporeal membrane oxygenation and congenital diaphragmatic hernia: modification of the pulmonary vasoactive profile. *J Pediatr Surg* 1985;**20**:681-3.
139. Inamura N, Kubota A, Nakajima T, et al. A proposal of new therapeutic strategy for antenatally diagnosed congenital diaphragmatic hernia. *J Pediatr Surg* 2005;**40**:1315-9.
140. Kobayashi H, Puri P. Plasma endothelin levels in congenital diaphragmatic hernia. *J Pediatr Surg* 1994;**29**:1258-61.
141. Cloutier M, Seaborn T, Piedboeuf B, et al. Effect of temporary tracheal occlusion on the endothelin system in experimental cases of diaphragmatic hernia. *Exp Lung Res* 2005;**31**:391-404.
142. Haller Jr JA, Signer RD, Golladay ES, et al. Pulmonary and ductal hemodynamics in studies of simulated diaphragmatic hernia of fetal and newborn lambs. *J Pediatr Surg* 1976;**11**:675-80.
143. Collins DL, Pomerance JJ, Travis KW, et al. A new approach to congenital posterolateral diaphragmatic hernia. *J Pediatr Surg* 1977;**12**:149-56.
144. Mohseni-Bod H, Bohn D. Pulmonary hypertension in congenital diaphragmatic hernia. *Semin Pediatr Surg* 2007;**16**:126-33.
145. Fox WW, Duara S. Persistent pulmonary hypertension in the neonate: diagnosis and management. *J Pediatr* 1983;**103**:505-14.
146. Dibbins AW. Neonatal diaphragmatic hernia: a physiologic challenge. *Am J Surg* 1976;**131**:408-10.
147. Hill AC, Adzick NS, Stevens MB, et al. Fetal lamb pulmonary hypoplasia: pulmonary vascular and myocardial abnormalities. *Ann Thorac Surg* 1994;**57**:946-51.
148. Pittinger TP, Sawin RS. Adrenocortical insufficiency in infants with congenital diaphragmatic hernia: a pilot study. *J Pediatr Surg* 2000;**35**:225-6;223-5; discussion.
149. Muglia LJ, Bae DS, Brown TT, et al. Proliferation and differentiation defects during lung development in corticotropin-releasing hormone-deficient mice. *Am J Respir Cell Mol Biol* 1999;**20**:181-8.
150. Rajatapiti P, Keijzer R, Blommaart PE, et al. Spatial and temporal expression of glucocorticoid, retinoid, and thyroid hormone receptors is not altered in lungs of congenital diaphragmatic hernia. *Pediatr Res* 2006;**60**:693-8.
151. Skandalakis JE, Gray SW, Ricketts RR. The diaphragm. In: Skandalakis JE, Gray SW, editors. *Embryology for surgeons*. Baltimore: Williams & Wilkins; 1994. p. 502.
152. Unpublished data from the Department of Surgery, Children's Hospital, Boston; 2001.
153. Osebold WR, Soper RT. Congenital posterolateral diaphragmatic hernia past infancy. *Am J Surg* 1976;**131**:748-54.
154. Amirav I, Kramer SS, Schramm CM. Radiological cases of the month. Delayed presentation of congenital diaphragmatic hernia. *Arch Pediatr Adolesc Med* 1994;**148**:203-4.
155. Folkman J. Personal communication, 1995.
156. Giacoia GP. Right-sided diaphragmatic hernia associated with superior vena cava syndrome. *Am J Perinatol* 1994;**11**:129-31.
157. Falcao MC, Carvalho MF, Tannuri U, et al. (Early-onset neonatal sepsis and late-appearing diaphragmatic hernia) (in Process Citation). *Rev Hosp Clin Fac Med Sao Paulo* 1998;**53**:152-5.
158. Barker DP, Hussain S, Frank JD, et al. Bilateral congenital diaphragmatic hernia—delayed presentation of the contralateral defect [letter]. *Arch Dis Child* 1993;**69**:543-4.
159. Wilson JM, Fauza DO, Lund DP, et al. Antenatal diagnosis of isolated congenital diaphragmatic hernia is not an indicator of outcome. *J Pediatr Surg* 1994;**29**:815-9.
160. Kamata S, Hasegawa T, Ishikawa S, et al. Prenatal diagnosis of congenital diaphragmatic hernia and perinatal care: assessment of lung hypoplasia. *Early Hum Dev* 1992;**29**:375-9.
161. Sherer DM, Abramowicz JS, D'Angio C, et al. Hepatic interlobar fissure sonographically mimicking the diaphragm in a fetus with right congenital diaphragmatic hernia. *Am J Perinatol* 1993;**10**:319-22.
162. Adzick NS, Harrison MR, Glick PL, et al. Diaphragmatic hernia in the fetus: prenatal diagnosis and outcome in 94 cases. *J Pediatr Surg* 1985;**20**:357-61.
163. Sherer DM, Woods Jr JR. Second trimester sonographic diagnosis of fetal congenital diaphragmatic hernia, with spontaneous resolution during the third trimester, resulting in a normal infant at delivery. *J Clin Ultrasound* 1991;**19**:298-302.
164. Kelly DR, Grant EG, Zeman RK, et al. In utero diagnosis of congenital diaphragmatic hernia by CT amniography. *J Comput Assist Tomogr* 1986;**10**:500-2.
165. Duncan KR. Fetal and placental volumetric and functional analysis using echo-planar imaging. *Top Magn Reson Imaging* 2001;**12**:52-66.
166. Luks FI, Carr SR, Ponte B, et al. Preoperative planning with magnetic resonance imaging and computerized volume rendering in twin-to-twin transfusion syndrome. *Am J Obstet Gynecol* 2001;**185**:216-9.
167. Haeusler MC, Ryan G, Robson SC, et al. The use of saline solution as a contrast medium in suspected diaphragmatic hernia and renal agenesis. *Am J Obstet Gynecol* 1993;**168**:1486-92.
168. Berman L, Stringer DA, Ein S, et al. Childhood diaphragmatic hernias presenting after the neonatal period. *Clin Radiol* 1988;**39**:237-44.
169. Movsowitz HD, Jacobs LE, Movsowitz C, et al. Transesophageal echocardiographic evaluation of a transthoracic echocardiographic pitfall: a diaphragmatic hernia mimicking a left atrial mass. *J Am Soc Echocardiogr* 1993;**6**:104-6.
170. Puri P, Gorman F. Lethal nonpulmonary anomalies associated with congenital diaphragmatic hernia: implications for early intrauterine surgery. *J Pediatr Surg* 1984;**19**:29-32.

171. Stoll C, Alembik Y, Dott B, et al. Associated malformations in cases with congenital diaphragmatic hernia. *Genet Couns* 2008;**19**:331-9.
172. Greenwood RD, Rosenthal A, Nadas AS. Cardiovascular abnormalities associated with congenital diaphragmatic hernia. *Pediatrics* 1976;**57**:92-7.
173. Karamanoukian HL, Glick PL, Wilcox DT, et al. Pathophysiology of congenital diaphragmatic hernia. XI: Anatomic and biochemical characterization of the heart in the fetal lamb CDH model. *J Pediatr Surg* 1995;**30**:925-8, discussion 929.
174. Sakurai Y, Azarow K, Cutz E, et al. Pulmonary barotrauma in congenital diaphragmatic hernia: a clinicopathological correlation. *J Pediatr Surg* 1999;**34**:1813-7.
175. Slavotinek AM, Warmerdam B, Lin AE, et al. Population-based analysis of left- and right-sided diaphragmatic hernias demonstrates different frequencies of selected additional anomalies. *Am J Med Genet A* 2007;**143A**:3127-36.
176. Berman L, Stringer D, Ein SH, et al. The late-presenting pediatric Bochdalek hernia: a 20-year review. *J Pediatr Surg* 1988;**23**:735-9.
177. Young D. Diaphragmatic hernia in infancy. In: Wilkinson AW, editor. Recent advances in paediatric surgery London: Churchill; 1969. p. 142-51.
178. Walker LK. Use of extracorporeal membrane oxygenation for preoperative stabilization of congenital diaphragmatic hernia. *Crit Care Med* 1993;**21**:S379-80.
179. Steinhorn RH, Kriesmer PJ, Green TP, et al. Congenital diaphragmatic hernia in Minnesota. Impact of antenatal diagnosis on survival. *Arch Pediatr Adolesc Med* 1994;**148**:626-31.
180. Migliazza L, Bellan C, Alberti D, et al. Retrospective study of 111 cases of congenital diaphragmatic hernia treated with early high-frequency oscillatory ventilation and presurgical stabilization. *J Pediatr Surg* 2007;**42**:1526-32.
181. Boix-Ochoa J, Peguero G, Seijo G, et al. Acid-base balance and blood gases in prognosis and therapy of congenital diaphragmatic hernia. *J Pediatr Surg* 1974;**9**:49-57.
182. Bohn D. Ventilatory and blood gas parameters in predicting survival in congenital diaphragmatic hernia. *Pediatr Surg Int* 1987;**2**:336-40.
183. Stolar C, Dillon P, Reyes C. Selective use of extracorporeal membrane oxygenation in the management of congenital diaphragmatic hernia. *J Pediatr Surg* 1988;**23**:207-11.
184. O'Rourke PP, Vacanti JP, Crone RK, et al. Use of the postductal PaO2 as a predictor of pulmonary vascular hypoplasia in infants with congenital diaphragmatic hernia. *J Pediatr Surg* 1988;**23**:904-7.
185. Wilson JM, Lund DP, Lillehei CW, et al. Congenital diaphragmatic hernia: predictors of severity in the ECMO era. *J Pediatr Surg* 1991;**26**:1033-4:1028-33; discussion.
186. Arnold JH, Bower LK, Thompson JE. Respiratory deadspace measurements in neonates with congenital diaphragmatic hernia. *Crit Care Med* 1995;**23**:371-5.
187. Boloker J, Bateman DA, Wung JT, et al. Congenital diaphragmatic hernia in 120 infants treated consecutively with permissive hypercapnia/spontaneous respiration/elective repair. *J Pediatr Surg* 2002;**37**:357-66.
188. Nakayama DK, Harrison MR, Chinn DH, et al. Prenatal diagnosis and natural history of the fetus with a congenital diaphragmatic hernia: initial clinical experience. *J Pediatr Surg* 1985;**20**:118-24.
189. Adzick NS, Vacanti JP, Lillehei CW, et al. Fetal diaphragmatic hernia: ultrasound diagnosis and clinical outcome in 38 cases. *J Pediatr Surg* 1989;**24**:654-7, discussion 657-8.
190. Hasegawa T, Kamata S, Imura K, et al. Use of lung-thorax transverse area ratio in the antenatal evaluation of lung hypoplasia in congenital diaphragmatic hernia. *J Clin Ultrasound* 1990;**18**:705-9.
191. Fox HE, Badalian SS. Ultrasound prediction of fetal pulmonary hypoplasia in pregnancies complicated by oligohydramnios and in cases of congenital diaphragmatic hernia: a review. *Am J Perinatol* 1994;**11**:104-8.
192. Harrison MR, Adzick NS, Bullard KM, et al. Correction of congenital diaphragmatic hernia in utero VII: a prospective trial. *J Pediatr Surg* 1997;**32**:1637-42.
193. Harrison MR, Mychaliska GB, Albanese CT, et al. Correction of congenital diaphragmatic hernia in utero IX: fetuses with poor prognosis (liver herniation and low lung-to-head ratio) can be saved by fetoscopic temporary tracheal occlusion. *J Pediatr Surg* 1998;**33**:1017-22, discussion 1022-3.
194. Arkovitz MS, Russo M, Devine P, et al. Fetal lung-head ratio is not related to outcome for antenatal diagnosed congenital diaphragmatic hernia. *J Pediatr Surg* 2007;**42**:107-10, discussion 110-1.
195. Barnewolt CE, Kunisaki SM, Fauza DO, et al. Percent predicted lung volumes as measured on fetal magnetic resonance imaging: a useful biometric parameter for risk stratification in congenital diaphragmatic hernia. *J Pediatr Surg* 2007;**42**:193-7.
196. Srouji MN, Buck B, Downes JJ. Congenital diaphragmatic hernia: deleterious effects of pulmonary interstitial emphysema and tension extrapulmonary air. *J Pediatr Surg* 1981;**16**:45-54.
197. Touloukian RJ, Markowitz RI. A preoperative x-ray scoring system for risk assessment of newborns with congenital diaphragmatic hernia. *J Pediatr Surg* 1984;**19**:252-7.
198. Burge DM, Atwell JD, Freeman NV. Could the stomach site help predict outcome in babies with left sided congenital diaphragmatic hernia diagnosed antenatally? *J Pediatr Surg* 1989;**24**:567-9.
199. Hasegawa S, Kohno S, Sugiyama T, et al. Usefulness of echocardiographic measurement of bilateral pulmonary artery dimensions in congenital diaphragmatic hernia. *J Pediatr Surg* 1994;**29**:622-4.
200. Callahan PF, Short BL, Rais-Bahrami K, et al. Pulmonary artery size is larger in nonsurvivors with congenital diaphragmatic hernia. In: 10th Annual Children's National Medical Center ECMO Symposium. Keystone, CO: EUA; 1994.
201. O'Rourke PP. Congenital diaphragmatic hernia: are there reliable clinical predictors? *Crit Care Med* 1993;**21**:S380-1.
202. Fisher JC, Jefferson RA, Arkovitz MS, et al. Redefining outcomes in right congenital diaphragmatic hernia. *J Pediatr Surg* 2008;**43**:373-9.
203. Nakayama DK, Motoyama EK, Tagge EM. Effect of preoperative stabilization on respiratory system compliance and outcome in newborn infants with congenital diaphragmatic hernia. *J Pediatr* 1991;**118**:793-9.
204. Cartlidge PH, Mann NP, Kapila L. Preoperative stabilisation in congenital diaphragmatic hernia. *Arch Dis Child* 1986;**61**:1226-8.
205. West KW, Bengston K, Rescorla FJ, et al. Delayed surgical repair and ECMO improves survival in congenital diaphragmatic hernia. *Ann Surg* 1992;**216**:454-60, discussion 460-2.
206. Levine G, Goetzman B, Milstein J, et al. Influence of airway state on hemodynamics of the pulmonary circulation in newborn lambs. *Pediatr Res* 1992;**31**:314A.
207. Mansell AL, McAteer AL, Pipkin AC. Maturation of interdependence between extra-alveolar arteries and lung parenchyma in piglets. *Circ Res* 1992;**71**:701-10.
208. Vacanti JP, Crone RK, Murphy JD, et al. The pulmonary hemodynamic response to perioperative anesthesia in the treatment of high-risk infants with congenital diaphragmatic hernia. *J Pediatr Surg* 1984;**19**:672-9.
209. Bos AP, Tibboel D, Koot VC, et al. Persistent pulmonary hypertension in high-risk congenital diaphragmatic hernia patients: incidence and vasodilator therapy. *J Pediatr Surg* 1993;**28**:1463-5.
210. Bloss RS, Aranda JV, Beardmore HE. Congenital diaphragmatic hernia: pathophysiology and pharmacologic support. *Surgery* 1981;**89**:518-24.
211. Walmrath D, Schneider T, Pilch J, et al. Aerosolised prostacyclin in adult respiratory distress syndrome. *Lancet* 1993;**342**:961-2.
212. Bindl L, Fahnenstich H, Peukert U. Aerosolised prostacyclin for pulmonary hypertension in neonates. *Arch Dis Child Fetal Neonatal Ed* 1994;**71**:F214-6.
213. Caplan MS, MacGregor SN. Perinatal management of congenital diaphragmatic hernia and anterior abdominal wall defects. *Clin Perinatol* 1989;**16**:917-38.
214. Wiener ES. Congenital posterolateral diaphragmatic hernia: new dimensions in management. *Surgery* 1982;**92**:670-81.
215. Ahlquist RP, Huggins RA, Woodbury RA. The pharmacology of benzyl-imidazoline (Priscoline). *J Pharmacol Exp Ther* 1947;**89**:271-4.
216. Noori S, Friedlich P, Wong P, et al. Cardiovascular effects of sildenafil in neonates and infants with congenital diaphragmatic hernia and pulmonary hypertension. *Neonatology* 2007;**91**:92-100.
217. Rocha GM, Bianchi RF, Severo M, et al. Congenital diaphragmatic hernia. The post-neonatal period. Part II. *Eur J Pediatr Surg* 2008;**18**:307-12.
218. Rocha GM, Bianchi RF, Severo M, et al. Congenital diaphragmatic hernia—the neonatal period (part I). *Eur J Pediatr Surg* 2008;**18**:219-23.
219. Palmer RM, Ferrige AG, Moncada S. Nitric oxide release accounts for the biological activity of endothelium-derived relaxing factor. *Nature* 1987;**327**:524-6.
220. Leveque C, Hamza J, Berg AE, et al. Successful repair of a severe left congenital diaphragmatic hernia during continuous inhalation of nitric oxide. *Anesthesiology* 1994;**80**:1171-5.
221. Shah N, Jacob T, Exler R, et al. Inhaled nitric oxide in congenital diaphragmatic hernia. *J Pediatr Surg* 1994;**29**:1010-4, discussion 1014-5.
222. Finer NN, Barrington KJ. Nitric oxide therapy for the newborn infant. *Semin Perinatol* 2000;**24**:59-65.
223. Karamanoukian HL, Glick PL, Wilcox DT, et al. Pathophysiology of congenital diaphragmatic hernia. VIII: Inhaled nitric oxide requires exogenous surfactant therapy in the lamb model of congenital diaphragmatic hernia. *J Pediatr Surg* 1995;**30**:1-4.
224. Finer NN, Tierney A, Etches PC, et al. Congenital diaphragmatic hernia: developing a protocolized approach. *J Pediatr Surg* 1998;**33**:1331-7.
225. Kinsella JP, Truog WE, Walsh WF, et al. Randomized, multicenter trial of inhaled nitric oxide and high-frequency oscillatory ventilation in severe, persistent pulmonary hypertension of the newborn. *J Pediatr* 1997;**131**:55-62.
226. Bohn D. Congenital diaphragmatic hernia. *Am J Respir Crit Care Med* 2002;**166**:911-5.
227. Wilson JM, Thompson JR, Schnitzer JJ, et al. Intratracheal pulmonary ventilation and congenital diaphragmatic hernia: a report of two cases. *J Pediatr Surg* 1993;**28**:484-7.

228. Wilcox DT, Glick PL, Karamanoukian HL, et al. Partial liquid ventilation and nitric oxide in congenital diaphragmatic hernia. *J Pediatr Surg* 1997;**32**:1211-5.
229. Pranikoff T, Gauger PG, Hirschl RB. Partial liquid ventilation in newborn patients with congenital diaphragmatic hernia. *J Pediatr Surg* 1996;**31**:613-8.
230. Greenspan JS, Fox WW, Rubenstein SD, et al. Partial liquid ventilation in critically ill infants receiving extracorporeal life support. Philadelphia Liquid Ventilation Consortium. *Pediatrics* 1997;**99**:E2.
231. Bartlett RH, Gazzaniga AB, Toomasian J, et al. Extracorporeal membrane oxygenation (ECMO) in neonatal respiratory failure. 100 cases (published erratum appears in Ann Surg 1987;205(1):11A). *Ann Surg* 1986;**204**:236-45.
232. Stolar CJ, Snedecor SM, Bartlett RH. Extracorporeal membrane oxygenation and neonatal respiratory failure: experience from the extracorporeal life support organization. *J Pediatr Surg* 1991;**26**:563-71.
233. Steimle CN, Meric F, Hirschl RB, et al. Effect of extracorporeal life support on survival when applied to all patients with congenital diaphragmatic hernia. *J Pediatr Surg* 1994;**29**:997-1001.
234. Wilson JM, Lund DP, Lillehei CW, et al. Delayed repair and preoperative ECMO does not improve survival in high risk congenital diaphragmatic hernia. *J Pediatr Surg* 1992;**27**:368-72, discussion 373-5.
235. Rais-Bahrami K, Short BL. The current status of neonatal extracorporeal membrane oxygenation. *Semin Perinatol* 2000;**24**:406-17.
236. Lally KP, Paranka MS, Roden J, et al. Congenital diaphragmatic hernia. Stabilization and repair on ECMO. *Ann Surg* 1992;**216**:569-73.
237. Wilson JM, Bower LK, Lund DP. Evolution of the technique of congenital diaphragmatic hernia repair on ECMO. *J Pediatr Surg* 1994;**29**:1109-12.
238. Wilson JM, Bower LK, Fackler JC, et al. Aminocaproic acid decreases the incidence of intracranial hemorrhage and other hemorrhagic complications of ECMO. *J Pediatr Surg* 1993;**28**:536-40, discussion 540-1.
239. Downard CD, Betit P, Chang RW, et al. Impact of AMICAR on hemorrhagic complications of ECMO: a ten-year review. *J Pediatr Surg* 2003;**38**:1212-6.
240. Clark RH, Yoder BA, Sell MS. Prospective, randomized comparison of high-frequency oscillation and conventional ventilation in candidates for extracorporeal membrane oxygenation [see comments]. *J Pediatr* 1994;**124**:447-54.
241. v.d. Staak FH, Thiesbrummel A, de Haan AF, et al. Do we use the right entry criteria for extracorporeal membrane oxygenation in congenital diaphragmatic hernia? *J Pediatr Surg* 1993;**28**:1003-5.
242. Bax NM, Collins DL. The advantages of reconstruction of the dome of the diaphragm in congenital posterolateral diaphragmatic defects. *J Pediatr Surg* 1984;**19**:484-7.
243. Benjamin HB. Agenesis of the left diaphragm. *J Thorac Cardiovasc Surg* 1963;**46**:265-70.
244. Simpson JS, Gossage JD. Use of abdominal wall muscle flap in repair of large congenital diaphragmatic hernia. *J Pediatr Surg* 1971;**6**:42-4.
245. Lister J. Recent advances in the surgery of the diaphragm in the newborn. *Prog Pediatr Surg* 1971;**2**:29-39.
246. Bray RJ. Congenital diaphragmatic hernia. *Anaesthesia* 1979;**34**:567-77.
247. Bianchi A, Doig CM, Cohen SJ. The reverse latissimus dorsi flap for congenital diaphragmatic hernia repair. *J Pediatr Surg* 1983;**18**:560-3.
248. Koot VC, Bergmeijer JH, Bos AP, et al. Incidence and management of gastroesophageal reflux after repair of congenital diaphragmatic hernia. *J Pediatr Surg* 1993;**28**:48-52.
249. Newman BM, Jewett TC, Lewis A, et al. Prosthetic materials and muscle flaps in the repair of extensive diaphragmatic defects: an experimental study. *J Pediatr Surg* 1985;**20**:362-7.
250. Lally KP, Cheu HW, Vazquez WD. Prosthetic diaphragm reconstruction in the growing animal. *J Pediatr Surg* 1993;**28**:45-7.
251. Koot VC, Bergmeijer JH, Molenaar JC. Lyophylized dura patch repair of congenital diaphragmatic hernia: occurrence of relapses. *J Pediatr Surg* 1993;**28**:667-8.
252. Ramadwar RH, Carachi R, Young DG. Collagen-coated Vicryl mesh is not a suitable material for repair of diaphragmatic defects. *J Pediatr Surg* 1997;**32**:1708-10.
253. Dalla Vecchia L, Engum S, Kogon B, et al. Evaluation of small intestine submucosa and acellular dermis as diaphragmatic prostheses. *J Pediatr Surg* 1999;**34**:167-71.
254. Yazbeck S, Cloutier R, Laberge JM. La hernie diaphragmatique congénitale: les résultas changent-ils vraiment? *Chir Pediatr* 1986;**27**:37-40.
255. Mishalany HG, Nakada K, Woolley MM. Congenital diaphragmatic hernias: eleven years' experience. *Arch Surg* 1979;**114**:1118-23.
256. Schnitzer JJ, Kikiros CS, Short BL, et al. Experience with abdominal wall closure for patients with congenital diaphragmatic hernia repaired on ECMO. *J Pediatr Surg* 1995;**30**:19-22.
257. van der Zee DC, Bax NM. Laparoscopic repair of congenital diaphragmatic hernia in a 6-month-old child. *Surg Endosc* 1995;**9**:1001-3.
258. Becmeur F, Reinberg O, Dimitriu C, et al. Thoracoscopic repair of congenital diaphragmatic hernia in children. *Semin Pediatr Surg* 2007;**16**:238-44.
259. Shah SR, Wishnew J, Barsness K, et al. Minimally invasive congenital diaphragmatic hernia repair: a 7-year review of one institution's experience. *Surg Endosc* 2008.
260. Fuchs JR, Kaviani A, Watson K, et al. Intratracheal pulmonary ventilation improves gas exchange during laparoscopy in a pediatric lung injury model. *J Pediatr Surg* 2005;**40**:22-5.
261. Sakai H, Tamura M, Hosokawa Y, et al. Effect of surgical repair on respiratory mechanics in congenital diaphragmatic hernia. *J Pediatr* 1987;**111**:432-8.
262. Vazquez WD, Cheu HW. Hemorrhagic complications and repair of congenital diaphragmatic hernias: does timing of the repair make a difference? Data from the Extracorporeal Life Support Organization. *J Pediatr Surg* 1994;**29**:1005-6:1002-5; discussion.
263. Welch KJ. The thoracic parietes. In: Welch KJ, editors. Complications of pediatric surgery. Philadelphia: W.B. Saunders; 1982. p. 170-81.
264. Wiener ES, Owens L, Salzberg AM. Chylothorax after Bochadalek herniorrhaphy in a neonate. Treatment with intravenous hyperalimentation. *J Thorac Cardiovasc Surg* 1973;**65**:200-6.
265. Tilmont P, Alessandri JL, Duthoit G, et al. Epanchement chyleaux apres cure chirurgicale d'une hernie diaphragmatique chez 2 nouveau-nés. *Arch Fr Pediatr* 1993;**50**:783-6.
266. Lund DP, Mitchell J, Kharasch V, et al. Congenital diaphragmatic hernia: the hidden morbidity. *J Pediatr Surg* 1994;**29**:258-62, discussion 262-4.
267. Nunez R, Rubio JL, Pimentel J, et al. Congenital diaphragmatic hernia and intrathoracic intestinal volvulus. *Eur J Pediatr Surg* 1993;**3**:293-5.
268. Chui PP, Tan CT. Sudden death due to incarcerated Bochdalek hernia in an adult. *Ann Acad Med Singapore* 1993;**22**:57-60.
269. Phillpott JW, Cumming WA. Torsion of the spleen: an unusual presentation of congenital diaphragmatic hernia. *Pediatr Radiol* 1994;**24**:150-1.
270. Harrison MR, Bjordal RI, Langmark F, et al. Congenital diaphragmatic hernia: the hidden mortality. *J Pediatr Surg* 1978;**13**:227-30.
271. Nobuhara KK, Lund DP, Mitchell J, et al. Long-term outlook for survivors of congenital diaphragmatic hernia. *Clin Perinatol* 1996;**23**:873-87.
272. Downard CD, Jaksic T, Garza JJ, et al. Analysis of an improved survival rate for congenital diaphragmatic hernia. *J Pediatr Surg* 2003;**38**:729-32.
273. D'Agostino JA, Bernbaum JC, Gerdes M, et al. Outcome for infants with congenital diaphragmatic hernia requiring extracorporeal membrane oxygenation: the first year. *J Pediatr Surg* 1995;**30**:10-5.
274. Stolar CJ. What do survivors of congenital diaphragmatic hernia look like when they grow up? *Semin Pediatr Surg* 1996;**5**:275-9.
275. Muratore CS, Kharasch V, Lund DP, et al. Pulmonary morbidity in 100 survivors of congenital diaphragmatic hernia monitored in a multidisciplinary clinic. *J Pediatr Surg* 2001;**36**:133-40.
276. Muratore CS, Utter S, Jaksic T, et al. Nutritional morbidity in survivors of congenital diaphragmatic hernia. *J Pediatr Surg* 2001;**36**:1171-6.
277. Stolar CJ, Levy JP, Dillon PW, et al. Anatomic and functional abnormalities of the esophagus in infants surviving congenital diaphragmatic hernia. *Am J Surg* 1990;**159**:204-7.
278. Taylor GA, Short BL. Esophageal dilatation and reflux in neonates on extracorporeal membrane oxygenation after diaphragmatic hernia repair (letter). *AJR Am J Roentgenol* 1988;**151**:1055.
279. Bos AP, Hussain SM, Hazebroek FW, et al. Radiographic evidence of bronchopulmonary dysplasia in high-risk congenital diaphragmatic hernia survivors. *Pediatr Pulmonol* 1993;**15**:231-4.
280. Dunnill MS. Quantitative methods in the study of pulmonary pathology. *Thorax* 1962;**17**:320-8.
281. Hislop A, Reid L. Persistent hypoplasia of the lung after repair of congenital diaphragmatic hernia. *Thorax* 1976;**31**:450-5.
282. Jeandot R, Lambert B, Brendel AJ, et al. Lung ventilation and perfusion scintigraphy in the follow up of repaired congenital diaphragmatic hernia. *Eur J Nucl Med* 1989;**15**:591-6.
283. Reid IS. Hutcherson RJ: Long-term follow-up of patients with congenital diaphragmatic hernia. *J Pediatr Surg* 1976;**11**:939-42.
284. Butler MW, Stolar CJ, Altman RP. Contemporary management of congenital diaphragmatic hernia. *World J Surg* 1993;**17**:350-5.
285. Van Meurs KP, Robbins ST, Reed VL, et al. Congenital diaphragmatic hernia: long-term outcome in neonates treated with extracorporeal membrane oxygenation. *J Pediatr* 1993;**122**:893-9.
286. Stolar CJ, Crisafi MA, Driscoll YT. Neurocognitive outcome for neonates treated with extracorporeal membrane oxygenation: are infants with congenital diaphragmatic hernia different? *J Pediatr Surg* 1995;**30**:366-71, discussion 371-2.
287. ECMO Registry Report, Extracorporeal Life Support Organization, 2001.

288. Moessinger AC, Harding R, Adamson TM, et al. Role of lung fluid volume in growth and maturation of the fetal sheep lung. *J Clin Invest* 1990;**86**:1270-7.
289. Moss RL, Chen CM, Harrison MR. Prosthetic patch durability in congenital diaphragmatic hernia: a long-term follow-up study. *J Pediatr Surg* 2001;**36**:152-4.
290. Cullen ML. Congenital diaphragmatic hernia: operative considerations. *Semin Pediatr Surg* 1996;**5**:243-8.
291. Greenholz SK. Congenital diaphragmatic hernia: an overview. *Semin Pediatr Surg* 1996;**5**:216-23.
292. Cohen D, Reid IS. *Recurrent diaphragmatic hernia. J Pediatr Surg* 1981;**16**:42-4.
293. MacGillivray TE, Jennings RW, Rudolph AM, et al. Vascular changes with in utero correction of diaphragmatic hernia. *J Pediatr Surg* 1994;**29**:992-6.
294. DiFiore JW, Fauza DO, Slavin R, Peters CA, Fackler JC, Wilson JM. Experimental fetal tracheal ligation reverses the structural and physiological effects of pulmonary hypoplasia in congenital diaphragmatic hernia. *J Pediatr Surg* 1994;**29**:248-56, discussion 256-7.
295. DiFiore JW, Fauza DO, Slavin R, et al. Experimental fetal tracheal ligation and congenital diaphragmatic hernia: a pulmonary vascular morphometric analysis (see comments). *J Pediatr Surg* 1995;**30**:917-23, discussion 923-4.
296. Bealer JF, Skarsgard ED, Hedrick MH, et al. The 'PLUG' odyssey: adventures in experimental fetal tracheal occlusion. *J Pediatr Surg* 1995;**30**:361-4, discussion 364-5.
297. Harrison MR, Adzick NS, Flake AW, et al. Correction of congenital diaphragmatic hernia in utero VIII: Response of the hypoplastic lung to tracheal occlusion. *J Pediatr Surg* 1996;**31**:1339-48.
298. Papadakis K, Luks FI, Deprest JA, et al. Single-port tracheoscopic surgery in the fetal lamb. *J Pediatr Surg* 1998;**33**:918-20.
299. Dzakovic A, Kaviani A, Jennings RW, et al. Positive intrapulmonary oncotic pressure enhances short-term lung growth acceleration after fetal tracheal occlusion. *J Pediatr Surg* 2002;**37**:1007-10:1007-10; discussion.
300. Chang R, Komura M, Andreoli S, et al. Rapidly polymerizing hydrogel prevents balloon dislodgment in a model of fetal tracheal occlusion. *J Pediatr Surg* 2004:in press.
301. Chang R, Komura M, Andreoli S, et al. Hyperoncotic enhancement of pulmonary growth after fetal tracheal occlusion: a comparison between dextran and albumin. *J Pediatr Surg* 2004;**39**:324-8:324-8; discussion.
302. Nobuhara KK, Ferretti ML, Siddiqui AM, et al. Long-term effect of perfluorocarbon distension on the lung. *J Pediatr Surg* 1998;**33** 1024-8, discussion 1028-9.
303. Crombleholme TM, Adzick NS, Hardy K, et al. Pulmonary lobar transplantation in neonatal swine: a model for treatment of congenital diaphragmatic hernia. *J Pediatr Surg* 1990;**25**:11-8.
304. Clugston RD, Zhang W, Greer JJ. Gene expression in the developing diaphragm: significance for congenital diaphragmatic hernia. *Am J Physiol Lung Cell Mol Physiol* 2008;**294**:L665-75.
305. Larson JE, Cohen JC. Improvement of pulmonary hypoplasia associated with congenital diaphragmatic hernia by in utero CFTR gene therapy. *Am J Physiol Lung Cell Mol Physiol* 2006;**291**:L4-10.
306. Martinez L, Gonzalez-Reyes S, Hernandez F, et al. (Aplication of a 3D reconstruction model for the analysis of nitrofen induced intrathoracic malformations.) *Cir Pediatr* 2005;**18**:165-9.
307. Fisher JC, Bodenstein L. Computer simulation analysis of normal and abnormal development of the mammalian diaphragm. *Theor Biol Med Model* 2006;**3**:9.
308. Christensen P. Eventration of the diaphragm. *Thorax* 1959;**14**:311-9.
309. Mellins RB, Hays AP, Gold AP, et al. Respiratory distress as the initial manifestation of Werdnig-Hoffmann disease. *Pediatrics* 1974;**53**:33-40.
310. Abad P, Lloret J, Martinez Ibanez V, et al. (Diaphragmatic paralysis: pathology at the reach of the pediatric surgeon.) *Cir Pediatr* 2001;**14**:21-4.
311. McNamara JJ, Eraklis AJ, Gross RE. Congenital posterolateral diaphragmatic hernia in the newborn. *J Thorac Cardiovasc Surg* 1968;**55**:55-9.
312. Reed JA, Borden DL. Eventration of the diaphragm. *Arch Surg* 1935;**31**:30-64.
313. Laxdal OE, McDougal H, Mellin GW. Congenital eventration of the diaphragm. *N Engl J Med* 1954;**205**:401-8.
314. Irving IM, Booker PD. Congenital diaphragmatic hernia and eventration of the diaphragm. In: Lister J, Irving IM, editors. *Neonatal surgery*. London: Butterworths; 1990. p. 199-200.
315. Anderson KD. Congenital diaphragmatic hernia. In: Welch KJ, Randolph JG, Ravitch MM, editors. *Pediatric surgery*. Chicago: Year–Book Medical Publishers; 1986. p. 599.
316. Hines MH. Video-assisted diaphragm plication in children. *Ann Thorac Surg* 2003;**76**:234-6.
317. Fitchett CW, Tavarez V. Bilateral congenital diaphragmatic herniation: case report. *Surgery* 1965;**57**:305-8.
318. Nawaz A, Matta H, Jacobsz A, et al. Congenital Morgagni's hernia in infants and children. *Int Surg* 2000;**85**:158-62.
319. Carter REB, Waterston DJ, Aberdeen E. Hernia and eventration of the diaphragm in childhood. *Lancet* 1962;**1**:656-9.
320. Pokorny WJ, McGill CW, Harberg FJ. Morgagni hernias during infancy: presentation and associated anomalies. *J Pediatr Surg* 1984;**19**:394-7.
321. Georgacopulo P, Franchella A, Mandrioli G, et al. Morgagni-Larrey hernia correction by laparoscopic surgery. *Eur J Pediatr Surg* 1997;**7**:241-2.
322. Becmeur F, Chevalier-Kauffmann I, Frey G, et al. (Laparoscopic treatment of a diaphragmatic hernia through the foramen of Morgagni in children. A case report and review of eleven cases reported in the adult literature.) *Ann Chir* 1998;**52**:1060-3.
323. Lima M, Domini M, Libri M, et al. Laparoscopic repair of Morgagni-Larrey hernia in a child. *J Pediatr Surg* 2000;**35**:1266-8.
324. Cantrell JR, Haller JA, Ravitch MM. A syndrome of congenital defects involving the abdominal wall, sternum, diaphragm, pericardium and heart. *Surg Gynecol Obstet* 1958;**197**:602-14.
325. Casey AE, Hidden EH. Nondevelopment of septum transversum, with congenital absence of anterocentral portion of the diaphragm and the suspensory ligament of the liver and presence of an elongated ductus venosus and a pericardioperitoneal foramen. *Arch Pathol* 1944;**38**:370-4.
326. Keith A. Diaphragmatic herniae. *Br Med J* 1910;**2**:1297.
327. Wilson AK, Rumel WR, Ross OL. Peritoneopericardial diaphragmatic hernia: report of a case in a newborn infant, successfully corrected by surgical operation with recovery of patient. *AJR Am J Roentgenol* 1947;**57**:42-9.
328. Rogers JF, Lane WZ, Gibbs R. Herniation through the diaphragm into the pericardium. *Conn Med J* 1958;**22**:653-6.
329. Wetzel H. Parasternale Zwerchfellhernie mit Verlagerung des Colon in den Herzbeutel. *Fortschr Rontgenstr* 1963;**98**:501-3.
330. Sagal Z. Absence of left diaphragm associated with inverted thoracic stomach. *AJR Am J Roentgenol* 1933;**30**:206-14.
331. Coca MA, Landin F. Malformations congénitales multiples avec absence presque complète de diaphragme. *Semin Hop Paris* 1957;**33**:3839.
332. Hatzitheofilou C, Conlan AA, Nicolaou N. Agenesis of the diaphragm. A case report. *S Afr Med J* 1982;**62**:999-1001.
333. Jenkinson EL. Absence of half of the diaphragm (thoracic stomach; diaphragmatic hernia). *AJR Am J Roentgenol* 1931;**26**:899-903.
334. Shaffer JO. Prosthesis for agenesis of the diaphragm. *JAMA* 1964;**188**:1000-2.
335. Kajii T, Oikawa K, Itakura K, et al. A probable 17-18 trisomy syndrome with phocomelia, exomphalos, and agenesis of hemidiaphragm. *Arch Dis Child* 1964;**39**:519-22.
336. Wille L, Holthusen W, Willich E. Accessory diaphragm. Report of 6 cases and a review of the literature. *Pediatr Radiol* 1975;**4**:14-20.
337. Krzyzaniak R, Gray SW. Accessory septum transversum. The first case report. *Am Surg* 1986;**52**:278-81.
338. Sappington Jr TB, Daniel Jr RA. Accessory diaphragm: a case report. *Am Surg* 1951;**21**:212-6.
339. Hashida Y, Sherman FE. Accessory diaphragm associated with neonatal respiratory distress. *J Pediatr* 1961;**59**:529-32.
340. Allen L. Transpleural muscles. *J Thorac Surg* 1950;**19**:290-1.
341. Drake EH, Lynch JP. Bronchiectasis associated with anomaly of the right pulmonary vein and right diaphragm: report of a case. *J Thorac Surg* 1950;**19**:433.
342. Sullivan HJ. Supernumerary diaphragm with agenesis of upper lobe. *J Thorac Surg* 1957;**34**:544-7.
343. Nigogosyan G, Ozarda H. Accessory diaphragm: a case report. *AJR Am J Roentgenol* 1961;**83**:309-11.
344. Ildstad ST, Stevenson RJ, Tollerud DJ, et al. High apical insertion of the right diaphragm in an infant with right- sided Bochdalek diaphragmatic hernia. *J Pediatr Surg* 1990;**25**:553-5.
345. Appelquist E, Hoier-Madsen K. Cribriform diaphragm: a variant of congenital diaphragmatic herniation. A case report. *Scand J Thorac Cardiovasc Surg* 1986;**20**:185-7.

K. Esophagus—Benign Disease

CHAPTER 34
Esophageal Anatomy and Function
John C. Lipham and Tom R. DeMeester

Embryology and Anatomy
  Cervical Esophagus
  Thoracic Esophagus
  Abdominal Esophagus
  Blood Supply, Lymphatics, and Innervation
Physiology
  The Swallowing Mechanism

Lower Esophageal Sphincter
  Causes and Consequences of the Failure of the Gastroesophageal Barrier
Evaluation of Esophageal Function
  Radiographic Evaluation
  Endoscopic Examination
  Esophageal Manometry

Lower Esophageal Sphincter
Lower Esophageal Sphincter Relaxation
Esophageal Body Motility
Upper Esophageal Sphincter
High-Resolution Manometry
Ambulatory 24-Hour pH Monitoring

The esophagus is a muscular tube that starts as the continuation of the pharynx and ends as the cardia of the stomach. Knowledge of the anatomy of the esophagus and its relationship with other organs and structures is essential for the surgeon to evaluate the location of lesions seen by endoscopy, barium swallow study, or computed tomography; to interpret esophageal function studies; and to safely expose the esophagus during surgery (Fig. 34-1). Similarly, a knowledge of foregut embryology is key to the understanding of the pathogenesis of congenital malformations of the esophagus.

EMBRYOLOGY AND ANATOMY

The embryonic esophagus forms when paired longitudinal grooves appear on each side of the laryngotracheal diverticulum. These grooves subsequently grow medially and fuse to form the tracheoesophageal septum. This septum divides the foregut into the ventral laryngotracheal tube and the dorsal esophagus. Incomplete fusion of the two lateral grooves was formerly thought to be the major factor in the pathogenesis of congenital tracheoesophageal fistula, but the anomaly is now attributed to abnormal growth and differentiation of the lung buds. The esophagus is initially short, but it rapidly elongates; the relative final length is attained by the seventh week of gestation.[1] This is followed by endodermal proliferation, which nearly obliterates the esophageal lumen. Subsequent recanalization occurs by the development of large vacuoles that coalesce. The adult position of the vagal nerves on the lower third of the esophagus results from the unequal growth of the greater and lesser curvature of the stomach, so the left vagus rotates anteriorly and the right vagus posteriorly.

The cricopharyngeal sphincter and the most proximal 1 to 2 cm of the cervical esophagus are primarily striated muscle. The striated muscle is derived from the caudal branchial arches and innervated by the vagus nerve and its recurrent laryngeal branches. The cricopharyngeal sphincter is made up primarily of the cricopharyngeus muscle, but it is also aided by the inferior pharyngeal constrictors and the circular muscles of the upper esophagus. Studies have indicated that the transition from predominantly striated to predominantly smooth muscle occurs in the proximal 4 to 5 cm of the esophagus and that only 1 cm of the proximal esophagus below the cricopharyngeal sphincter is entirely striated muscle.[2] In contrast with the proximal portion of the cervical esophagus, the thoracic and abdominal esophagus and the lower esophageal sphincter

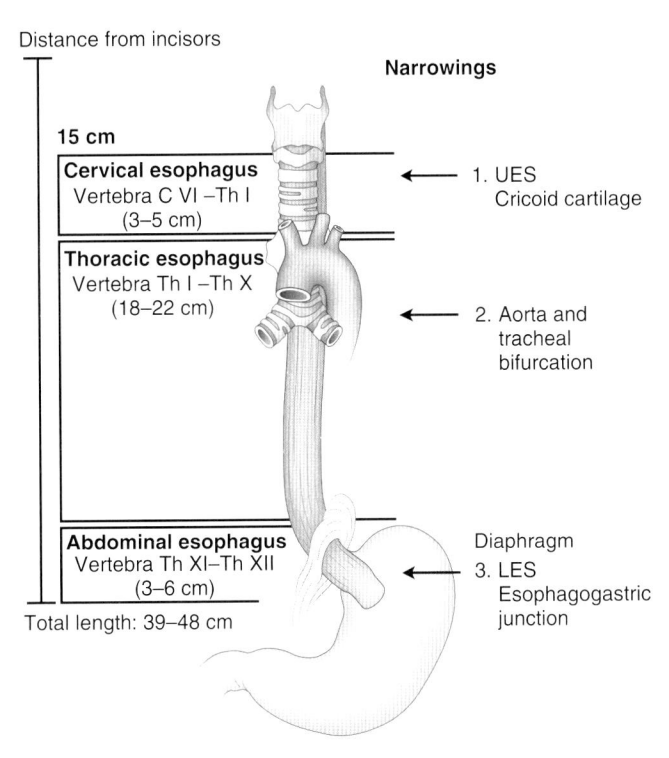

Figure 34-1
Classic division of the esophagus and relationships to the cervical and thoracic vertebrae as radiologic landmarks. The approximate lengths and narrowings (arrows) of the esophagus are shown. UES, upper esophageal sphincter; LES, lower esophageal sphincter.

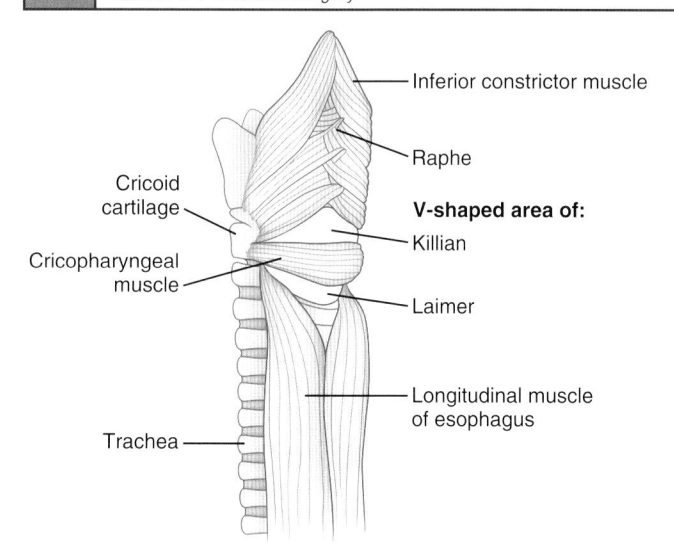

Figure 34-2
Muscular architecture of the pharyngoesophageal junction, which is the region of the upper esophageal sphincter. The triangular areas of the sparse muscle cover are shown in the scheme. Zenker's diverticulum arises from Killian's triangle. *(Modified from Liebermann-Meffert D. Anatomy, embryology, and histology. In: Pearson FG, Deslauriers J, Ginsberg RJ, et al, editors. Esophageal surgery. New York: Churchill Livingstone; 1995. p. 1-25.)*

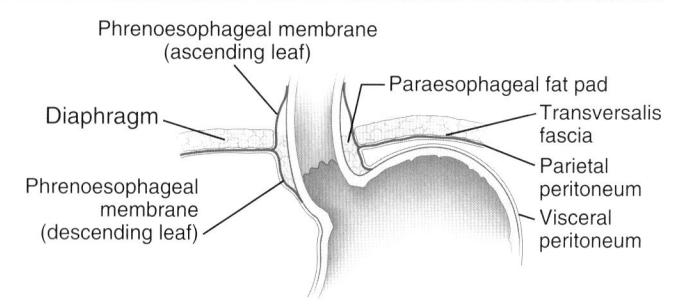

Figure 34-3
Attachments of the phrenoesophageal membrane.

(LES) consist entirely of smooth muscle and are composed of an inner circular and outer longitudinal layer. Throughout the length of the esophagus, there is no serosa overlying the muscle layers. The smooth muscle of the lower esophagus arises from the splanchnic mesenchyme and is supplied by nerves of the esophageal plexus derived from neural crest cells.[1]

Cervical Esophagus

The cervical portion of the esophagus is about 5 cm long. It starts below the cricopharyngeus muscle and appears as a continuation of the inferior constrictor muscle of the pharynx. A space between the right and left inferior constrictor muscles posteriorly just above the cricopharyngeus muscle is called killian triangle and is the site where a Zenker's diverticulum develops (Fig. 34-2). The beginning of the cervical esophagus is marked by the level of C6, and the end by the lower border of T1. The cervical esophagus curves slightly to the left as it descends. Anteriorly, it abuts the trachea and larynx and can be dissected off both organs. Posteriorly, the cervical esophagus lies on the vertebral bodies in a prevertebral or retroesophageal space. This space continues with a retropharyngeal space superiorly and is continuous with the posterior mediastinum. Laterally, the omohyoid muscle crosses the cervical esophagus obliquely, and it is usually divided to expose this portion of the esophagus. The carotid sheaths lie laterally, and the lobes of the thyroid and the strap muscles lie anteriorly. The recurrent laryngeal nerves lie in the grooves between the esophagus and the trachea. The right recurrent nerve runs a more lateral and oblique course to reach the groove and is more prone to anatomic variation. The surgical approach to the cervical esophagus may be from either side of the neck through an incision along the medial border of the sternocleidomastoid muscle. The left-sided approach is preferred to avoid injury to the right recurrent nerve.

Thoracic Esophagus

The thoracic portion of the esophagus is approximately 20 cm long (see Fig. 34-1) and starts at the thoracic inlet. In the upper portion of the thorax, it is closely related to the posterior wall of the trachea. This close relationship is responsible for the early spread of cancer of the upper esophagus into the trachea, and it may limit the surgeon's ability to resect such a tumor. Above the level of the tracheal bifurcation, the esophagus courses to the right of the aortic arch and the descending aorta and then moves to the left, passing behind the tracheal bifurcation and the left main bronchus.

In the lower portion of the thorax, the esophagus again deviates to the left and anteriorly to pass through the diaphragmatic hiatus. The lower thoracic esophagus is buttressed only by mediastinal pleura on the left, making this portion the weakest and the most common site of perforation in Boerhaave's syndrome. The azygos vein is closely related to the esophagus as it arches from its paraspinal position over the right main bronchus to enter the superior vena cava. The thoracic duct ascends behind and to the right of the distal thoracic esophagus; but at the level of T5, it passes posterior to the aorta and ascends on the left side of the esophagus, which is posterior and medial to the left subclavian artery.

Abdominal Esophagus

The abdominal portion of the esophagus is approximately 2 cm long and includes the abdominal portion of the LES. It begins as the esophagus passes through the diaphragmatic hiatus and is surrounded by the phrenoesophageal membrane, a fibroelastic ligament that arises from the subdiaphragmatic fascia as a continuation of the transversalis fascia lining the abdomen (Fig. 34-3). The upper leaf of the membrane attaches in a circumferential fashion around the esophagus about 1 to 2 cm above the level of the hiatus. The lower limit of the phrenoesophageal membrane blends with the serosa of the stomach, and its end is marked anteriorly by a prominent fat pad, which corresponds approximately with the gastroesophageal junction. The LES is a zone of high pressure 3 to 4 cm long at the lower end of the esophagus[3] and does not correspond to any macroscopic anatomic change except for a slight thickening of the esophageal muscular wall. Its function is derived from the microscopic architecture of the muscle fibers. The esophageal hiatus is surrounded by the right and left crura, which together form a sling of skeletal muscle around the esophagus that originates from tendinous bands attached to the anterolateral surface of the first lumbar vertebra (Fig. 34-4).

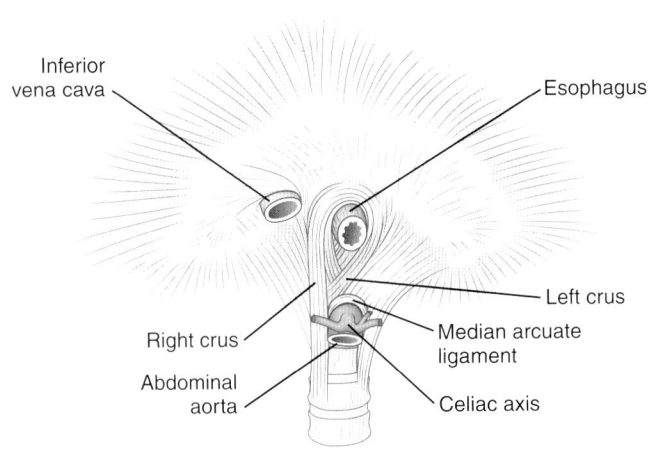

Figure 34–4
Diaphragm and esophageal hiatus viewed from the abdomen.

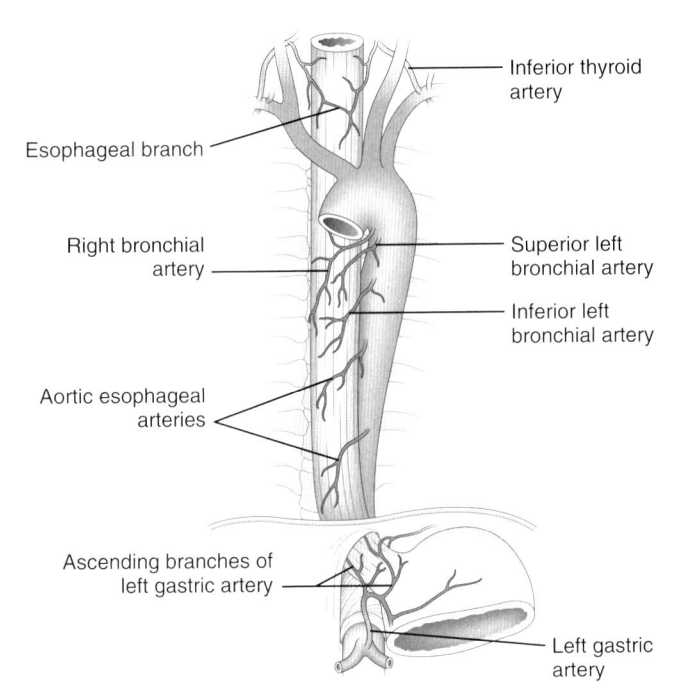

Figure 34–5
Arterial blood supply of the esophagus. *(Modified from Rothberg M, DeMeester TR. Surgical anatomy of the esophagus. In: Shields TW, editor. General thoracic surgery, 3rd ed. Philadelphia: Lea & Febiger; 1989. p. 84.)*

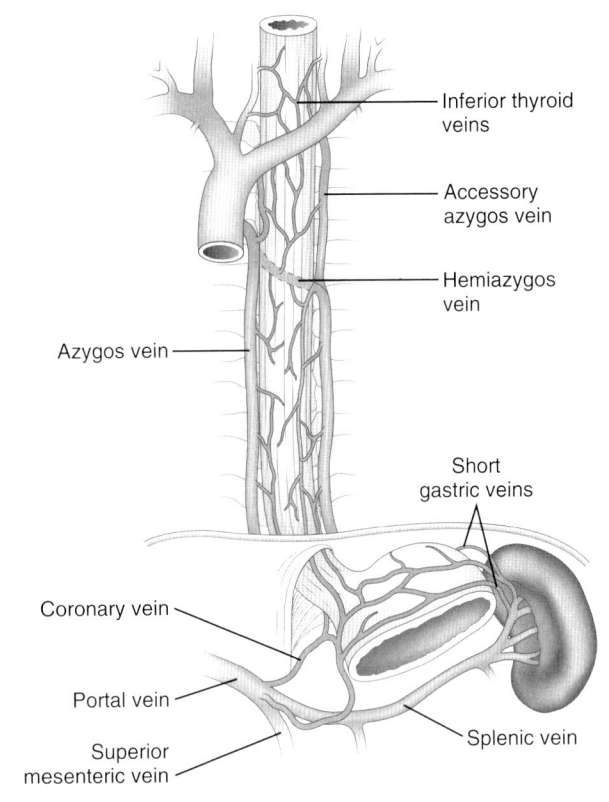

Figure 34–6
Venous drainage of the esophagus. *(Modified from Rothberg M, DeMeester TR. Surgical anatomy of the esophagus. In: Shields TW, editor. General thoracic surgery, 3rd ed. Philadelphia: Lea & Febiger; 1989. p. 85.)*

The relative contribution of the right and left crura to this sling is variable. Posterior to the esophagus, the crura are united by a tendinous arch—the median arcuate ligament—that lies just anterior to the aorta.

Blood Supply, Lymphatics, and Innervation

The cervical portion of the esophagus receives its main blood supply from the inferior thyroid artery. The thoracic portion receives blood from the bronchial and esophageal arteries. Seventy-five percent of individuals have one right-sided and two left-sided bronchial arteries, and usually two esophageal branches arise directly from the aorta. The blood supply of the abdominal portion of the esophagus comes from the ascending branch of the left gastric artery and from the right and left inferior phrenic arteries (Fig. 34-5). After the vessels have entered the muscular wall of the esophagus, branching occurs at right angles to provide an extensive longitudinal vascular plexus. The rich blood supply provided by this vascular plexus allows mobilization of the esophagus from the stomach to the aortic arch without causing ischemic injury.[4]

The capillaries of the esophagus drain into a submucosal and periesophageal venous plexus, from which the esophageal veins originate. In the cervical region, the esophageal veins empty into the inferior thyroid vein; in the thoracic region, they empty into the bronchial, azygos, or hemiazygos veins; and in the abdominal region, they empty into the coronary vein (Fig. 34-6).

The lymphatic channels are located almost exclusively below the muscularis mucosa in the submucosa of the esophagus. They are so dense and interconnected that they constitute a plexus (Fig. 34-7) with more lymph vessels than blood capillaries. Lymph flow in the submucosal plexus runs in a longitudinal direction, and after the injection of a contrast medium, the longitudinal spread is six times that of the transverse spread. In the upper two thirds of the esophagus, the lymphatic flow is mostly cephalad; in the lower third, it is mostly caudad. In the thoracic portion of the esophagus, the submucosal lymph plexus extends over a long distance in a longitudinal direction before penetrating the muscle layer to enter lymph vessels in the adventitia. As a consequence of this nonsegmental lymph drainage, the lymphatic spread of tumor cells can extend for a considerable distance superiorly and inferiorly within the submucosal lymphatics before the cells pass through lymphatic channels in the muscularis and

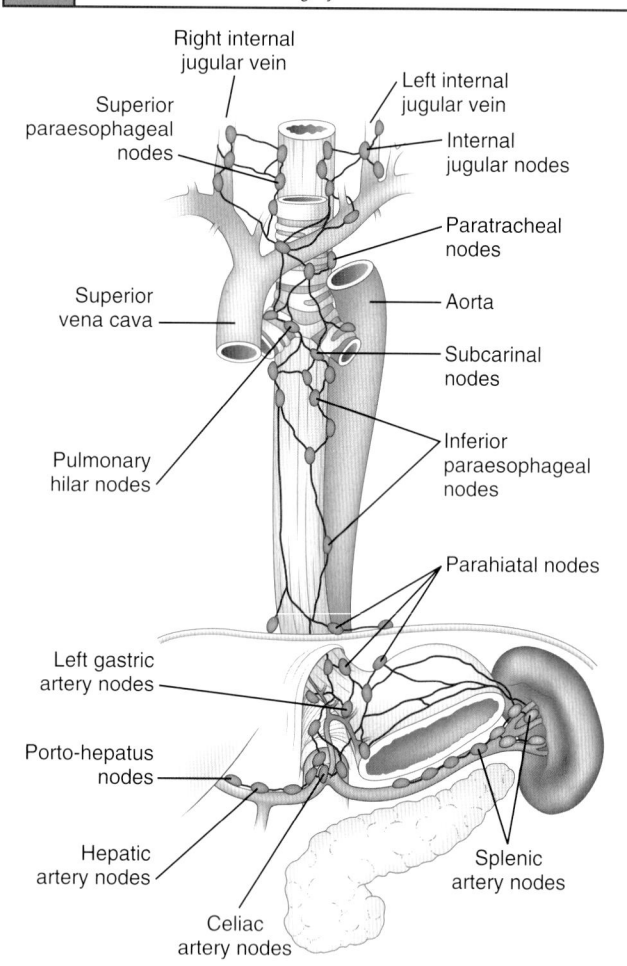

Figure 34–7
Lymphatic drainage of the esophagus. (From DeMeester TR, Barlow AP. Surgery and current management for cancer of the esophagus and cardia: Part 1. Curr Probl Surg 1988;**25**:498.)

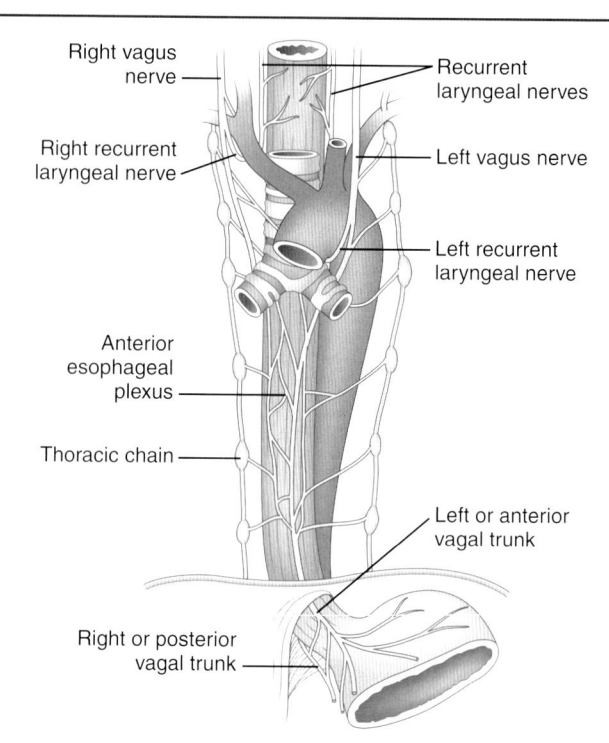

Figure 34–8
Innervation of the esophagus. (Modified from Rothberg M, DeMeester TR. Surgical anatomy of the esophagus. In: Shields TW, editor. General thoracic surgery, 3rd ed. Philadelphia: Lea & Febiger; 1989. p. 85.)

on into the regional lymph nodes. By contrast, the cervical esophagus has a more segmental lymph drainage into the regional lymph nodes, and as a result, tumors in this portion of the esophagus have less submucosal extension.

Lymph from the cervical esophagus drains into the paratracheal and deep cervical lymph nodes, whereas lymph from the upper thoracic esophagus flows mainly into the paratracheal lymph nodes. The lymph from the lower thoracic esophagus drains into the subcarinal and inferior pulmonary nodes. Lymph from the distal thoracic and abdominal portion of the esophagus drains into the parahiatal and left gastric nodes.[1]

The parasympathetic innervation of the pharynx and esophagus is provided mainly by cranial nerve X or the vagal nerve. The constrictor muscles of the pharynx receive branches from the pharyngeal plexus, which is located on the posterior lateral surface of the middle constrictor muscle and is formed by pharyngeal branches of the vagus nerve, with a small contribution from cranial nerves IX and XI. The cricopharyngeal sphincter and the cervical portion of the esophagus receive branches from both the right and left recurrent laryngeal nerves (Fig. 34-8). Damage to these recurrent nerves interferes not only with the movement of the vocal cords but also with the function of the cricopharyngeal sphincter and the motility of the cervical esophagus and predisposes the patient to pulmonary aspiration on swallowing. The upper thoracic esophagus receives innervation from the left recurrent laryngeal nerve and both vagal nerves. The esophageal plexus, which is formed by the branches of the right and left vagal nerves and thoracic sympathetic chain, lies on the anterior and posterior walls of the esophagus and innervates the lower thoracic portion.[5] The branches of the plexus coalesce into the left (anterior) and right (posterior) vagal trunks.

Afferent visceral sensory fibers from the esophagus end without synapse in the first four segments of the thoracic spinal cord by a combination of sympathetic and vagal pathways. These pathways are also occupied by afferent visceral sensory fibers from the heart, which explains the similarity of symptoms in esophageal and cardiac diseases.

PHYSIOLOGY

To comprehend the mechanics of alimentation, it is useful to visualize the gullet as a series of pumps and valves. In the pharyngeal segment, the tongue and pharyngeal muscle function as pumps, whereas the soft palate, the epiglottis, and the cricopharyngeus serve as the valves that regulate flow. In the esophageal segment, the esophageal body functions as the pump to propel the food bolus, whereas the LES serves as a one-way valve to allow transport into the stomach and to prevent the flow of gastric contents back into the esophagus.

The Swallowing Mechanism

Swallowing can be started at will, or it can be reflexively elicited by the stimulation of the anterior and posterior tonsillar pillars or the posterior lateral walls of the hypopharynx. The

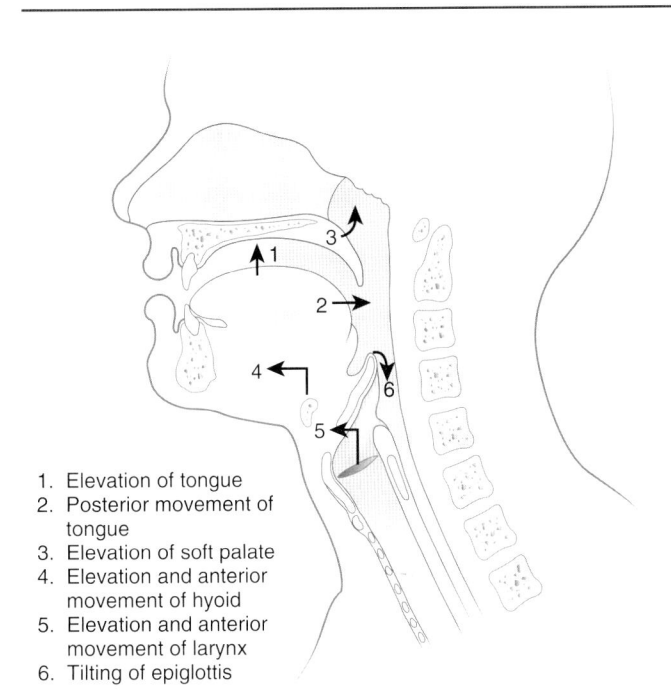

1. Elevation of tongue
2. Posterior movement of tongue
3. Elevation of soft palate
4. Elevation and anterior movement of hyoid
5. Elevation and anterior movement of larynx
6. Tilting of epiglottis

Figure 34-9
Sequence of events during the oropharyngeal phase of swallowing. *(From DeMeester TR, Stein HJ, Fuchs KH. Physiologic diagnostic studies. In: Zuidema GD, Orringer MB, editors. Shackelford's surgery of the alimentary tract, 3rd ed, vol 1. Philadelphia: WB Saunders; 1991. p. 95.)*

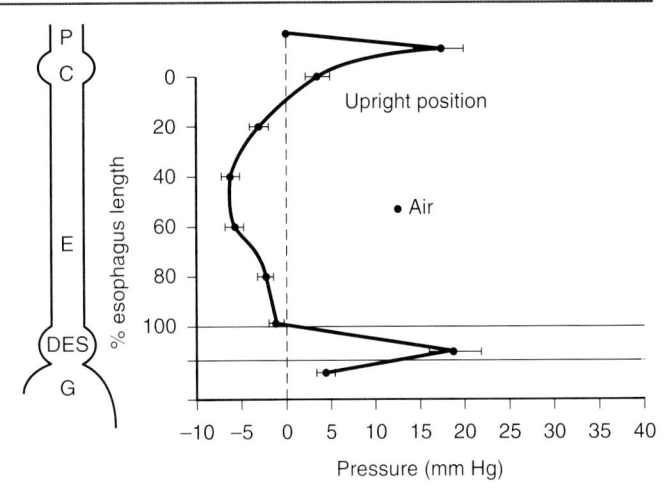

Figure 34-10
Resting pressure profile of the foregut showing the pressure differential between the atmospheric pharyngeal pressure (P) and the less-than-atmospheric midesophageal pressure (E) and the greater-than-atmospheric intragastric pressure (G), with the interposed high-pressure zones of the cricopharyngeus (C) and the distal esophageal sphincter (DES). The necessity for relaxation of the cricopharyngeus and DES pressure to move a bolus into the stomach is apparent. Esophageal work occurs when a bolus is pushed from the midesophageal area with a pressure that is less than atmospheric (E) and into the stomach, which has a pressure that is greater than atmospheric (G). *(From Waters PF, DeMeester TR. Foregut motor disorders and their surgical management. Med Clin North Am 1981;**65**:1237.)*

afferent sensory nerves of the pharynx are the glossopharyngeal nerves and the superior laryngeal branches of the vagal nerves. Once it is aroused by stimuli entering through these nerves, the swallowing center in the medulla coordinates the complete act of swallowing by discharging impulses through cranial nerves V, VII, X, XI, and XII and the motor neurons of C1 through C3. Discharges through these nerves always occur in a specific pattern and last for approximately 0.5 second. Little is known about the swallowing center except that it can trigger swallowing after a variety of different inputs. Once it is triggered, the swallow response is always a rigidly ordered pattern of outflow neurogenic impulses.

The act of alimentation requires the passage of food and drink from the mouth into the stomach. Food is taken into the mouth in a variety of bite sizes, after which it is broken up by the teeth, mixed with saliva, and lubricated. When food is ready for swallowing, the tongue, acting as a pump, moves the bolus into the posterior oropharynx and forces it into the hypopharynx (Fig. 34-9). Concomitantly with the posterior movement of the tongue, the soft palate is elevated, thereby closing the passage between the oropharynx and nasopharynx. With the initiation of the swallow, the hyoid moves superiorly and anteriorly, thereby elevating the larynx and enlarging the retropharyngeal space. At the same time, the epiglottis covers the laryngeal inlet to prevent aspiration.

During swallowing, the pressure in the hypopharynx rises abruptly to 60 mm Hg as a result of the backward movement of the tongue and contraction of the posterior pharyngeal constrictors. A sizable pressure difference develops between the hypopharyngeal pressure and the subatmospheric midesophageal or intrathoracic pressure (Fig. 34-10). This pressure gradient speeds the movement of food from the hypopharynx into the esophagus when the cricopharyngeus or upper esophageal sphincter (UES) relaxes. The bolus is both propelled by the peristaltic contraction of the posterior pharyngeal constrictors and sucked into the thoracic esophagus by this pressure gradient.

Critical to receiving the bolus is the compliance of the cervical esophageal muscle and the timing and degree of relaxation of the UES. Abnormalities of compliance and UES opening result in pharyngeal dysphagia. During the transfer of the bolus from the mouth into the esophagus, the UES is mechanically pulled open. Elevation of the larynx by muscles attached to the hyoid bone pulls the UES open at the time muscle relaxation of the UES occurs. This is an active relaxation caused by a reduction in the tone of the tonic cricopharyngeus muscle, and it is dependent on a neurologically mediated reflex. This is an all-or-nothing event; partial relaxation does not normally occur. The UES closes within 0.5 second of the initiation of the swallow, with a postrelaxation contraction pressure that is approximately twice the resting pressure of 30 mm Hg. The postrelaxation contraction continues down the esophagus as a peristaltic wave (Fig. 34-11). The high closing pressure and the initiation of the peristaltic wave prevent reflux of the bolus from the esophagus into the pharynx. After completion of the swallow, the pressure of the UES returns to its normal resting pressure.

The pharyngeal activity in swallowing initiates the esophageal phase of swallowing. Because of the helical arrangement of its circular muscles, the body of the esophagus functions as a worm-drive propulsive pump, and it is responsible for transmitting a bolus of food into the stomach. With the act of swallowing, the longitudinal muscle of the esophageal body shortens, thus enlarging the lumen to accept the bolus (this is called the "on response"), after which the circular smooth muscle contraction forms the peristaltic wave (the "off response"). During the esophageal phase of swallowing, the bolus is moved into the stomach over a gradient of 12 mm Hg (i.e., from a negative intrathoracic pressure environment of −6 mm Hg to a positive intra-abdominal pressure environment of +6 mm Hg). Effective and coordinated smooth muscle function in the lower two thirds of the esophageal body is important to allow this movement to occur.

The peristaltic wave generates an occlusive pressure that varies from 30 to 120 mm Hg. The wave rises to a peak in 1 second, remains at the peak for about 0.5 second, and then subsides in about 1.5 seconds. The whole course of the rise and fall of an occlusive contraction may occupy one point in the esophagus for 3 to 5 seconds.[6,7] The peak of the primary peristaltic contraction moves down the esophagus at a rate of 2 to 4 cm per second and reaches the distal esophagus about 9 seconds after swallowing starts. A consecutive swallow in 20 seconds produces a similar primary peristaltic wave; however, if the swallow occurs sooner, the esophagus is inhibited and unresponsive.

To be effective, peristaltic contractions must be of sufficient amplitude to occlude the esophageal lumen and sufficiently organized in a peristaltic waveform to propel a bolus aborally. Low-amplitude contractions that do not occlude the lumen merely indent a semisolid bolus rather than propel it, and simultaneous contractions throughout the body of the esophagus result in splitting the bolus or even propelling it orally. Clinically, defects in peristalsis occur in three broad categories, depending on which major feature is the most impaired. First, there is a neural abnormality that results in the defective organization of the peristaltic wave; this is recognized by the presence of simultaneous contractions with a loss of the peristaltic sequence and results in typical primary motility disorders (e.g., diffuse esophageal spasm). The second category defect is evident when there is a reduction of the amplitude of the contraction but the peristaltic sequence remains; this is usually due to muscle damage and the formation of fibrous tissue within the muscle. Examples include end-stage gastroesophageal reflux disease and connective tissue disorders such as scleroderma. The third category defect results from altered anatomy of the esophageal body. A loss in the efficiency of the peristaltic sequence can result when the esophagus is not anchored distally, as occurs with a large sliding hiatal hernia; this will look like an accordion esophagus on barium swallow study, with ineffective clearance of barium from the esophagus.

Lower Esophageal Sphincter

The LES represents the barrier that confines the gastric juice to the stomach and protects the acid-sensitive squamous esophageal mucosa from injury by refluxed gastric juice. As is true for any valve, failure of the LES can occur in two completely opposite ways, which lead to two distinct clinical disease entities. Regardless of the type of LES failure, the secondary effects are produced proximally in the esophagus. Failure of the LES to relax or to open appropriately leads to the inability of the esophagus to propel food into the stomach, esophageal distention, and the condition known as achalasia. On the other hand, failure of the LES to remain closed leads to an increased exposure of the squamous epithelium to gastric juice and the condition known as gastroesophageal reflux disease (GERD).

The LES has no anatomic landmarks, but its presence can be identified by a rise in pressure over gastric baseline pressure when a pressure transducer is pulled from the stomach into the esophagus. This high-pressure zone is normally present except in two situations: (1) after a swallow, when it is momentarily dissipated or relaxes to allow passage of food into the stomach; and (2) during a belch, when it allows gas to be vented from a distended fundus. The common denominator for virtually all episodes of gastroesophageal reflux is the loss of this normal high-pressure zone or barrier. When the barrier is absent, resistance to the flow of gastric juice from an environment of higher pressure (the stomach) to an environment of lower pressure (the esophagus) is lost. In early GERD, this is usually caused by a transient loss of the barrier. In advanced GERD, there is usually a permanent loss of the barrier.[8]

There are three characteristics of the LES or high-pressure zone that maintain its function as a barrier to intragastric and

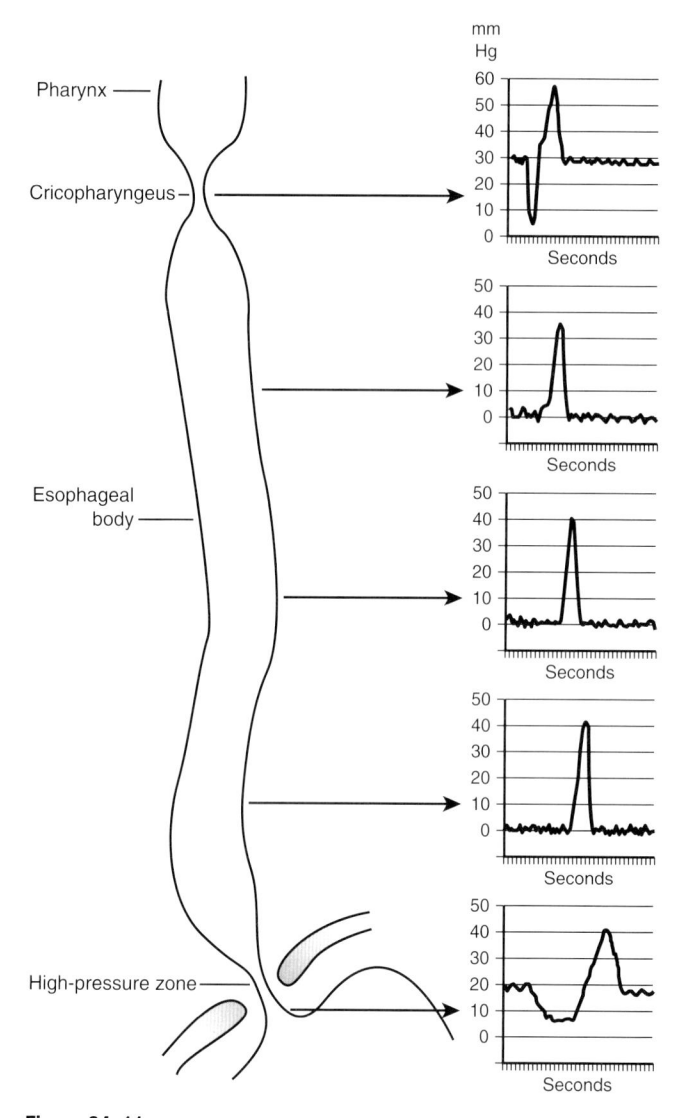

Figure 34–11
Intraluminal esophageal pressures in response to swallowing. *(From Waters PF, DeMeester TR. Foregut motor disorders and their surgical management.* Med Clin North Am 1981;**65**:1237.)

intra-abdominal pressure challenges. Two of these characteristics—the overall length and pressure of the LES—work together and depend on each other to provide resistance to the flow of gastric juice from the stomach into the esophagus.[9] The shorter the overall length, the higher the pressure must be for the LES to maintain sufficient resistance to remain competent (Fig. 34-12). Consequently, the effect of a normal LES pressure can be nullified by a short overall LES length, and the effect of a normal overall LES length can be nullified by a low LES pressure. For practical purposes, the pressure of the LES is measured at a single point, but in actuality, pressure is applied over the entire length of the LES; this allows the computer formation of a three-dimensional image of the LES or barrier (Fig. 34-13). The volume of this image reflects the resistance of the LES to the flow of fluid through it, which is called the *sphincter pressure vector volume*. A calculated volume below that of the fifth percentile of normal resting subjects indicates a permanently defective LES.[10] A fundamental principle for surgeons to understand is that the length of the barrier or LES is critical to its function. Shortening of LES length occurs naturally with gastric filling as the terminal esophagus is "taken up" by the expanding fundus (Fig. 34-14)[11]; this is similar to the shortening of the neck of a balloon as it is inflated. With excessive gastric distention (e.g., with overeating), the length of the LES shortens to a critical point at which it gives way, the pressure drops precipitously, and reflux occurs (Fig. 34-15).[12] If the length of the LES is permanently shortened, then further shortening caused by the normal gastric distention with normal-volume meals results in postprandial reflux. In this situation, competency of the barrier is an ever-constant

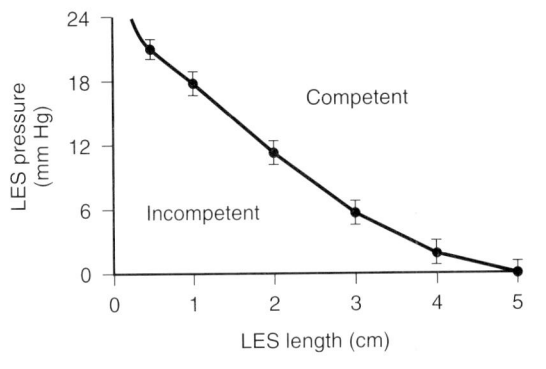

Figure 34–12
The relationship of the LES pressure (measured at the respiratory inversion point) and overall LES length with the resistance to the flow of fluid through the barrier. Note that the shorter the overall length of the high-pressure zone, the higher the pressures must be to maintain sufficient resistance to remain competent. Competent, no flow; incompetent, flow of varied volumes.

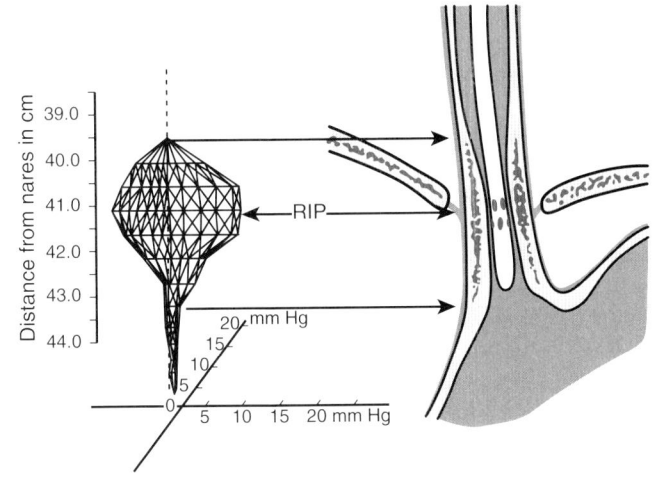

Figure 34–13
A graphic illustration of how a three-dimensional computerized image of the LES can be constructed by measuring the pressure of the high-pressure zone in four quadrants at 0.5-cm intervals over the entire length of the zone. RIP, respiratory inversion point. *(From Stein HJ, DeMeester TR, Naspetti R, et al. Three-dimensional imaging of the lower esophageal sphincter in gastroesophageal reflux disease. Ann Surg 1991;* **214** *: 374-84.)*

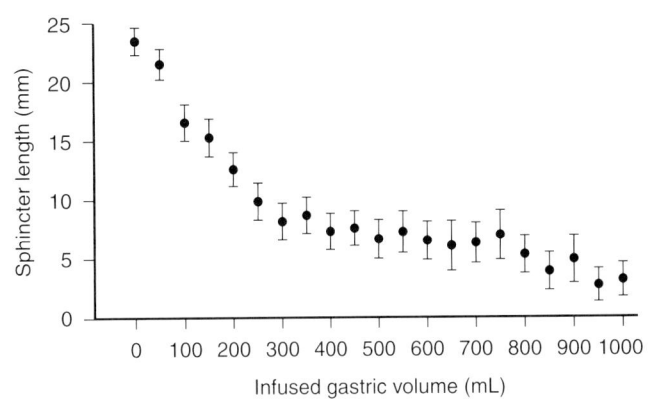

Figure 34–14
The relationship between overall sphincter length and gastric distention with increasing volumes of water. *(From Mason RJ, Lund RJ, DeMeester TR, et al. Nissen fundoplication prevents shortening of the sphincter during gastric distention. Arch Surg 1997;* **132** *: 719-26.)*

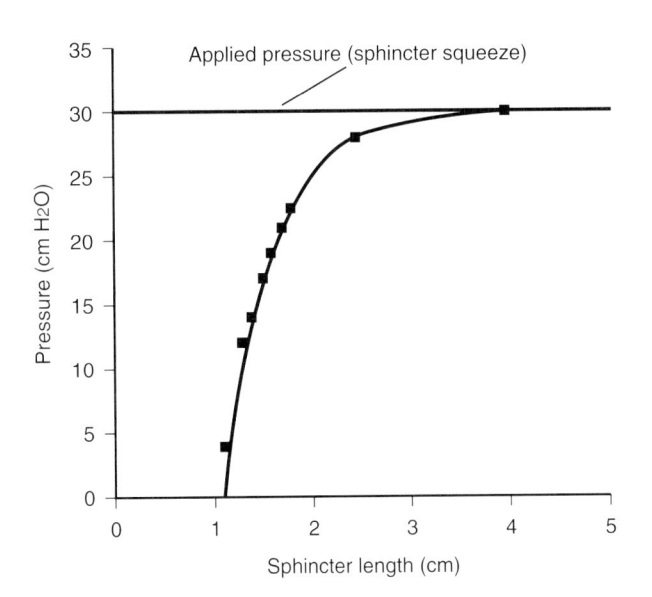

Figure 34–15
The relationship between resting LES pressure measured by manometry and LES length when applied pressure or "sphincter squeeze" is kept constant. Analysis was made with a model of the LES high-pressure zone. Note that as the LES length decreases, the pressure recorded within the LES decreases only slightly until a length of 2 cm is reached, when LES pressure drops precipitously and its competency is lost. *(From Pettersson GB, Bombeck CT, Nyhus LM. The lower esophageal sphincter: mechanisms of opening and closure. Surgery 1980;* **88** *: 307-14.)*

clinical problem. The observation that gastric distention results in shortening of the LES down to a critical length so that the pressure dissipates, the lumen opens, and reflux occurs provides a mechanical explanation for transient LES relaxations without invoking a neuromuscular reflex. If only the LES pressure and not its length is measured (e.g., with a Dent sleeve), the event appears as a spontaneous relaxation of LES pressure.[13] In reality, it is the progressive shortening of the LES rather than the transient LES relaxations that results in the loss of LES pressure.

Variations in the anatomy of the cardia, from a normal acute angle of His to an abnormal dome architecture of a sliding hiatal hernia, influence the ease with which the sphincter is shortened by gastric distention. A hernia can result from the pulsion force of abdominal pressure on the esophageal hiatus or from the traction produced by inflammatory fibrosis of the esophageal body. The resulting alteration in the geometry of the cardia places the sphincter at a mechanical disadvantage in maintaining its length with progressive degrees of gastric distention. Greater gastric distention is necessary to open the barrier in patients with an intact angle of His than in those with a hiatal hernia.[14] The reason is that the dome or funnel shape of a hiatal hernia allows the wall tension forces that pull open the barrier with gastric distention to be more effectively applied to the gastroesophageal junction,[15] and it accounts for the common association of a hiatal hernia with GERD. Kahrilas and colleagues[16] demonstrated this mechanical disadvantage by studying the effect of intragastric air infusion on the number of transient LES relaxations or "shortenings" per hour. Patients with hiatal hernias had significantly more transient LES relaxations per hour than did control subjects without hernias. The reduction in length became significant 20 to 30 minutes after the beginning of air infusion and occurred in a distal to cephalad direction before a loss of LES pressure was observed.

The third characteristic of the LES high-pressure zone is its position. A portion of the overall length of the high-pressure zone is normally exposed to the positive intra-abdominal pressure environment and is commonly referred to as the abdominal length of the LES.[17] During periods of increased intra-abdominal pressure, the resistance of the LES would easily be overcome if its position were such that abdominal pressure is unable to be applied equally to the LES and the stomach.[18-20] Think of sucking on a soft soda straw immersed in a bottle of liquid; the positive hydrostatic pressure of the fluid and the negative pressure inside the straw from sucking cause the straw to collapse instead of allowing the liquid to flow up the straw in the direction of the negative pressure. If the LES is positioned so that the abdominal length is inadequate, it cannot collapse in response to applied positive intra-abdominal pressure. On the other hand, intragastric pressure would be augmented by the applied positive intra-abdominal pressure, and the sphincter pressure would be easily overcome; the negative intrathoracic pressure will encourage reflux to occur. More than 1 cm of the LES needs to be exposed to the abdominal pressure environment for it to respond effectively to changes in intra-abdominal pressure.[13]

If, in the fasting state, the LES has an abnormally low pressure, a short overall length, or a minimal length exposure to the abdominal pressure environment, the result is a permanent loss of resistance with unhampered reflux of gastric contents into the esophagus; this is known as a permanently defective barrier or LES. The most common consequence of a permanently defective LES is increased esophageal exposure to gastric juice, which results in inflammatory injury to the mucosa and the muscularis propria of the esophageal body, thereby causing a reduced contraction amplitude of the esophageal body and interrupted or dropped peristaltic sequences. If the reflux is not brought under control, the progressive loss of effective esophageal clearance results in an ever-increasing esophageal exposure to gastric juice, with further organ injury (Fig. 34-16).[21,22]

Causes and Consequences of the Failure of the Gastroesophageal Barrier

Early GERD is initiated by increased transient losses of the barrier as a result of gastric overdistention from excessive air and food ingestion.[8,23] The tension vectors produced by gastric wall distention pull on the gastroesophageal junction, which results in the terminal esophagus being "taken up" into the stretched fundus, thereby reducing the length of the LES. With overeating, a critical length is reached (usually about 1 to 2 cm) at which the sphincter gives way; its pressure drops precipitously, and reflux occurs (see Fig. 34-14). If the swallowed air is vented, gastric distention is reduced, the length of the LES is restored, and competency returns until subsequent distention again shortens it and further reflux occurs. Aerophagia is common in patients with GERD because they swallow their saliva more frequently to neutralize the acidic gastric juice that is refluxed into the esophagus.[24] Together, the actions of overeating and air swallowing result in the common complaint of postprandial bloating, repetitive belching, and heartburn in patients with early GERD. The high prevalence of the disease in the Western world is thought to be a result of the eating habits of Western society.[25] Gastric distention from overeating, along with delayed gastric emptying

PROGRESSION OF GERD

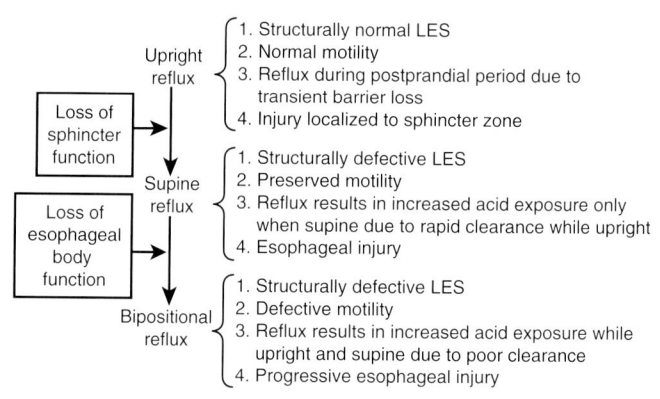

Upright reflux:
1. Structurally normal LES
2. Normal motility
3. Reflux during postprandial period due to transient barrier loss
4. Injury localized to sphincter zone

Loss of sphincter function → Supine reflux:
1. Structurally defective LES
2. Preserved motility
3. Reflux results in increased acid exposure only when supine due to rapid clearance while upright
4. Esophageal injury

Loss of esophageal body function → Bipositional reflux:
1. Structurally defective LES
2. Defective motility
3. Reflux results in increased acid exposure while upright and supine due to poor clearance
4. Progressive esophageal injury

Figure 34–16
Schema of the progression of gastroesophageal reflux disease. Initially, esophageal acid exposure occurs only after meals and when the patient is in the upright, awake position, as a result of the transient losses of the barrier. With inflammatory injury to the LES, the barrier becomes permanently defective, and an increase in the esophageal acid exposure occurs with the patient in the supine position, whereas gravity and the esophageal body effectively clear the refluxed acid during the day when the patient is upright. Inflammatory injury to the esophageal body from supine acid exposure results in the loss of esophageal body clearance function and increased esophageal acid exposure during the day and night; this is known as bipositional reflux.

resulting from the increased ingestion of fatty foods, leads to prolonged periods of postprandial gastric distention with shortening of the LES and repetitive transient loss of the barrier. A Nissen fundoplication prevents the shortening of the barrier with progressive degrees of gastric distention by diverting the forces produced by gastric wall tension that pull on the gastroesophageal junction.[12]

In advanced GERD, permanent loss of sphincter length occurs from inflammatory injury that extends from the mucosa into the muscular layers of the LES. Fletcher and colleagues[26] showed that in the fasting state, there is a persistent region of high acidity in the area of the gastroesophageal junction and that this region of acidity migrates 2 cm proximally after meals. This migration occurs from distention of the stomach with eating and pulling apart of the distal high-pressure zone or LES, thus allowing the area of high acidity to move proximal to the squamocolumnar junction. This proximal movement exposes the distal esophageal squamous mucosa to acid and results in the formation of cardiac mucosa. Cardiac mucosa is an acquired mucosa and results from inflammatory injury to the squamous mucosa in the terminal esophagus.[27] The inflammatory process extends into the muscular layer of the LES, thereby resulting in muscle cell injury with permanent shortening of the high-pressure zone or LES and a concomitant reduction in the amplitude of the high-pressure zone or barrier pressure.[27-29] A defective barrier is recognized when the length or pressure of the LES measured during the fasting state is below the 2.5 percentile of normal.[30] For clinicians, the finding of a permanently defective LES has several implications. First, symptoms in patients with a defective LES can be difficult to control, and mucosal damage may be difficult to control with medical therapy.[31] Surgery is usually required to achieve consistent long-term symptom relief in these patients and to interrupt the natural history of the disease. It has been shown repeatedly that a laparoscopic Nissen fundoplication can restore the length and pressure of the LES to normal.[32] Second, a permanently defective LES is commonly associated with reduced contractility and abnormal wave progression of the esophageal body[33]; this makes the clearance of reflux acid difficult and leads to excessive esophageal exposure to acid. Third, a permanently defective LES and the loss of effective esophageal clearance lead to increased esophageal exposure to gastric juice with mucosal injury and the potential for Barrett's metaplasia, repetitive regurgitation, aspiration, and pulmonary fibrosis.

EVALUATION OF ESOPHAGEAL FUNCTION

A thorough understanding of the patient's underlying anatomic and functional deficits is fundamental to the successful treatment of esophageal disease. The diagnostic tests that are employed to evaluate the esophagus are those used to visualize structural abnormalities, to detect functional abnormalities, and to measure esophageal exposure to gastric juice.

Radiographic Evaluation

Radiographic assessment of the anatomy and function of the esophagus and stomach is one of the more important aspects of the esophageal evaluation, provided the surgeon has a working knowledge of esophageal physiology. The first diagnostic test in patients with suspected esophageal disease should be a barium swallow that includes a full assessment of the stomach and the duodenum.[34] Videotaping of the study greatly aids in the evaluation by providing the surgeon with a real-time visualization of bolus transport and the size and reducibility of the hiatal hernia. The study also provides anatomic information, such as the presence of obstructing lesions and structural abnormalities of the foregut.

The pharynx and the UES are evaluated in the upright position, with the performance of an assessment of the relative timing and coordination of the events of pharyngeal transit.[35] This includes oropharyngeal bolus transport, pharyngeal contraction, opening of the pharyngoesophageal segment, and degree of airway protection during swallowing. It readily identifies a diverticulum, stasis of the contrast medium in the valleculae, cricopharyngeal bar, or narrowing of the pharyngoesophageal segment.[36] These are anatomic manifestations of neuromuscular disease and result from the loss of muscle compliance from the deinnervation of the skeletal muscle of the pharynx and the cervical esophagus.[37]

The assessment of peristalsis on video esophagography often adds to or complements the information obtained by esophageal manometry. Esophageal motility is optimally assessed by observing several individual swallows of barium with the patient in both the upright and supine positions; the study can be performed with both liquid and solid bolus material. During normal swallowing, a primary peristaltic wave is generated that completely strips the bolus out of the esophagus and into the stomach. Residual material rarely stimulates a secondary peristaltic wave; rather, an additional pharyngeal swallow is usually required.

Normal subjects in the prone position can clear at least three of five 10-mL liquid barium boluses with one swallow and have only one episode of proximal escape or distal retention of a barium bolus with the five swallows. Normal subjects can clear a solid barium bolus with four or fewer swallows in the upright position. Motility disorders with disorganized or simultaneous esophageal contraction give a segmented appearance to the barium column. This can often give a beading or corkscrew appearance to the barium within the esophagus. In patients with dysphagia, the use of a barium-impregnated marshmallow, piece of bread, or hamburger can identify an esophageal transport disturbance that is not evident on the liquid barium study.

A hiatal hernia is present in a high percentage of patients with gastroesophageal reflux.[38] These are best demonstrated with the patient in the prone position; the increased intra-abdominal pressure produced in this position promotes displacement of the hernia above the diaphragm. The hiatal hernia is an important component of the underlying pathophysiology of reflux. A large (>5 cm) or irreducible hiatal hernia suggests a shortening of the esophagus, and a paraesophageal hernia can explain the complaint of dysphagia. Reflux is not easily seen on video esophagography, and only rarely in patients with classic symptoms of GERD does the radiologist observe spontaneous reflux (i.e., unprovoked retrograde flow of barium from the stomach into the esophagus). When spontaneous reflux is seen by the radiologist, it is a dependable sign of GERD; however, failure to observe reflux does not indicate the absence of disease.

A full-column technique with distention of the esophageal wall can discern extrinsic compression of the esophagus, and a fully distended esophagogastric region is necessary to identify narrowing from a ring, stricture, or obstructing lesion. Mucosal relief or double-contrast films can be obtained to enhance the detection of small neoplasms, esophagitis, and varices. Assessment of the stomach and duodenum during the barium study is helpful for the evaluation of the patient with esophageal symptoms. A gastric or duodenal ulcer, a neoplasm, or poor gastroduodenal transit can mimic many of the symptoms that are suggestive of an esophageal disorder.

Endoscopic Examination

Endoscopic evaluation of the esophagus in practice is the physical examination of the foregut. It is a critical part of the assessment of a patient with esophageal disease and is indicated even if the video esophagogram is normal. A barium study obtained before esophagoscopy is helpful to the endoscopist by directing attention to locations of subtle change and alerting the examiner to such potential danger spots as a cervical vertebral osteophyte, an esophageal diverticulum, a deeply penetrating ulcer, or a carcinoma. Regardless of the radiologist's interpretation of an abnormal finding, each structural abnormality of the esophagus should be examined visually with an endoscope.

During every examination, the locations of the diaphragmatic crura, gastroesophageal junction, and squamocolumnar junction are measured. The crura are usually evident, and their location can be confirmed by having the patient sniff. The squamocolumnar junction is the location at which the velvet and darker rose-colored columnar epithelium changes to the lighter squamous epithelium. The anatomic gastroesophageal junction is the location at which the gastric rugal folds meet the tubular esophagus; it is often at or just below the squamocolumnar junction. Particular effort should be exerted to detect esophagitis and Barrett's columnar epithelium–lined esophagus when GERD is suspected. Barrett's esophagus is a condition in which the tubular esophagus is lined with columnar epithelium as opposed to the normal squamous epithelium. On histologic examination, it appears as columnar mucosa with goblet cells and is called intestinal metaplasia.[39-41] It is suspected at endoscopy when there is difficulty with visualization of the squamocolumnar junction at its normal location and by the appearance of a redder, more luxuriant mucosa than is normally seen in the lower esophagus; its presence is confirmed by biopsy. Multiple biopsy specimens should be taken in a cephalad direction to determine the length of the metaplastic mucosa. Barrett's esophagus is susceptible to ulceration, bleeding, stricture formation, and malignant degeneration.[42] The earliest histologic sign of malignant degeneration is high-grade dysplasia or intramucosal adenocarcinoma.[43] These dysplastic changes have a patchy distribution, so a minimum of four biopsy specimens every 2 cm should be taken from the Barrett's mucosa–lined portion of the esophagus.

Abnormalities of the cardia or gastroesophageal junction can be visualized by retroflexion of the endoscope. Hill and colleagues[44] have graded the appearance of the gastroesophageal valve from I to IV according to the degree of unfolding or deterioration of the normal architecture (Fig. 34-17).

A hiatal hernia is confirmed by finding a pouch lined with gastric rugal folds lying 2 cm or more above the margins of the diaphragmatic crura. A prominent sliding hiatal hernia is frequently associated with GERD. When a hernia is observed, particular care is taken to exclude a gastric ulcer or gastritis within the herniated stomach.

As the endoscope is removed, the esophagus is again examined, and biopsy samples are taken. The location of the cricopharyngeus is identified, and the larynx and vocal cords are visualized. Acid reflux may result in inflammation of the larynx. Vocal cord movement should also be recorded, both as a reference for subsequent surgery and as an assessment of the patient's ability to protect the airway.

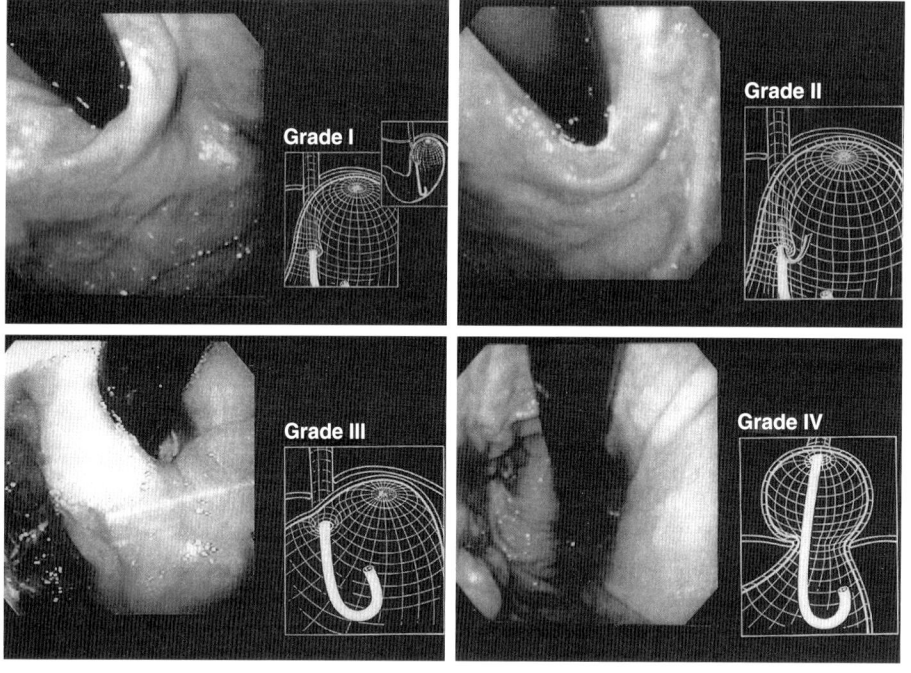

Figure 34–17
Endoscopic Hill grading of the gastroesophageal valve.

Esophageal Manometry

Fundamental to the evaluation of a patient with benign esophageal disease is the assessment of esophageal contractility and sphincter function. Stationary esophageal manometry is performed by passing a catheter containing pressure sensor ports (usually spaced 5 cm apart) into the esophagus to measure contraction pressures and waveform in the esophageal body and the sphincters' resting pressure and response to swallowing. Manometry is indicated whenever an abnormality of the esophagus is suggested by the symptoms of dysphagia, odynophagia, chest pain, heartburn, and regurgitation.[45] It is particularly necessary to confirm the diagnosis of specific primary esophageal motility disorders, such as achalasia, diffuse esophageal spasm, nutcracker esophagus, and hypertensive LES.[46] It can also identify ineffective esophageal motility abnormalities that result from GERD and systemic disease, such as scleroderma, dermatomyositis, polymyositis, or mixed connective tissue disease. In patients with symptomatic GERD, esophageal manometry can identify a mechanically defective LES and evaluate the adequacy of the esophageal body contraction amplitudes and waveform.

Esophageal manometry is performed by insertion of a lubricated manometric catheter through the nostril and into the esophagus (Fig. 34-18). The catheter is advanced until all recording ports are in the stomach. A complete manometric study assesses the characteristics of the LES, the degree of LES relaxation, the esophageal body contraction amplitude and waveform, and the UES function.

Lower Esophageal Sphincter

As the catheter is slowly withdrawn in 1-cm increments, the high-pressure zone of the LES is reached by the uppermost pressure port. The lower (distal) border of the LES is the point at which the resting pressure rises above the gastric baseline; the upper border is the point at which sphincter pressure reaches the esophageal baseline. The respiratory inversion point is identified when the positive excursions that occur with breathing in the abdominal environment change to negative deflections in the thoracic environment. The respiratory inversion point is the functional division between the abdomen and thorax. The resting pressure of the LES is the pressure above gastric baseline measured during mid-respiration at the respiratory inversion point. The overall length of the sphincter is the distance from the distal border to the proximal border. The abdominal length is the distance from the distal border to the respiratory inversion point and represents the portion of the LES that is subject to fluctuations in intra-abdominal pressure (Fig. 34-19). The measurements for each of these components from each transducer are expressed as an average. A mechanically defective sphincter is identified by one or more of the following characteristics: (1) an average LES pressure of less than 6 mm Hg, (2) an average abdominal length of less than 1 cm, and (3) an average overall length of less than 2 cm. As compared with normal volunteers, these values are below the 2.5 percentile. A defect in one or even two components of the LES may be compensated by good esophageal body function, but when all three components are defective, excessive esophageal acid exposure is inevitable.[47]

Lower Esophageal Sphincter Relaxation

The catheter is positioned with four pressure ports at the same level in the LES, one port in the stomach, and at least one in the esophageal body. A series of swallows are obtained by giving the patient 5-mL boluses of water. The LES pressure normally drops to gastric baseline immediately after the swallow, before the oncoming peristaltic wave reaches the lower esophagus.

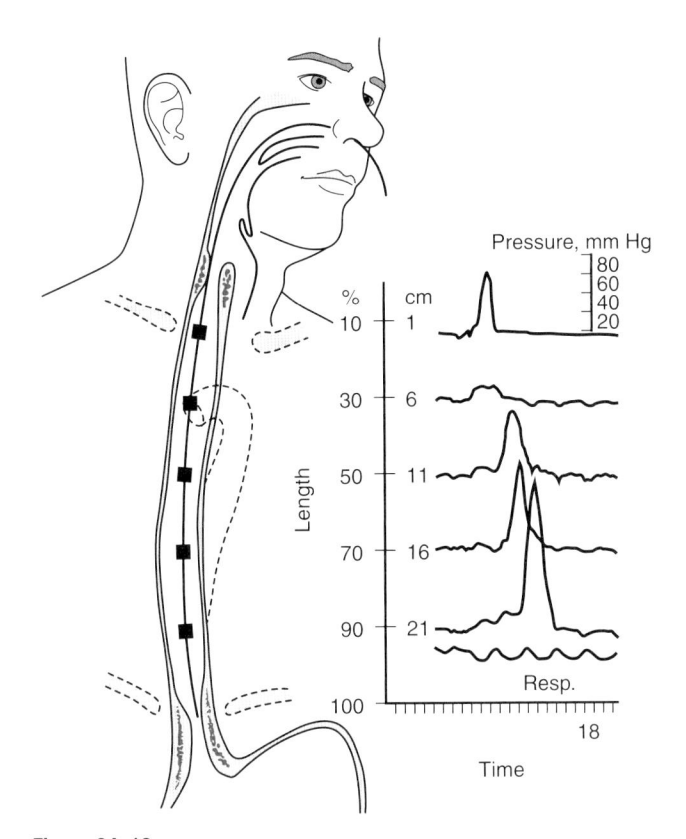

Figure 34-18
Illustration of the position of the five-channel esophageal motility catheter during the esophageal body portion of the study.

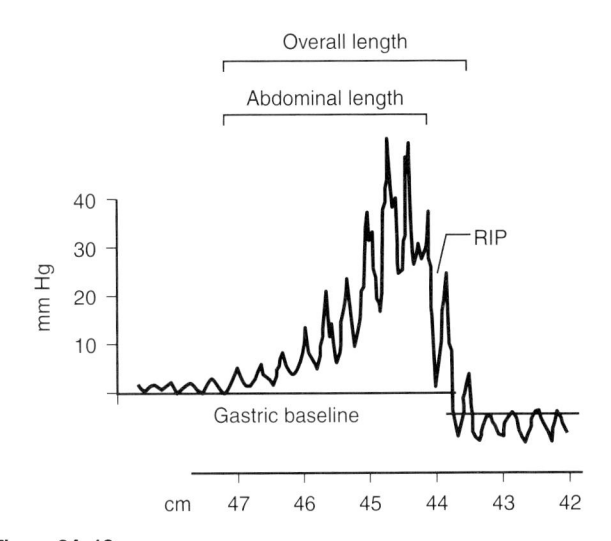

Figure 34-19
Manometric tracing as a transducer is pulled across the lower esophageal sphincter, showing pressure, overall length, and abdominal length. RIP, respiratory inversion point.

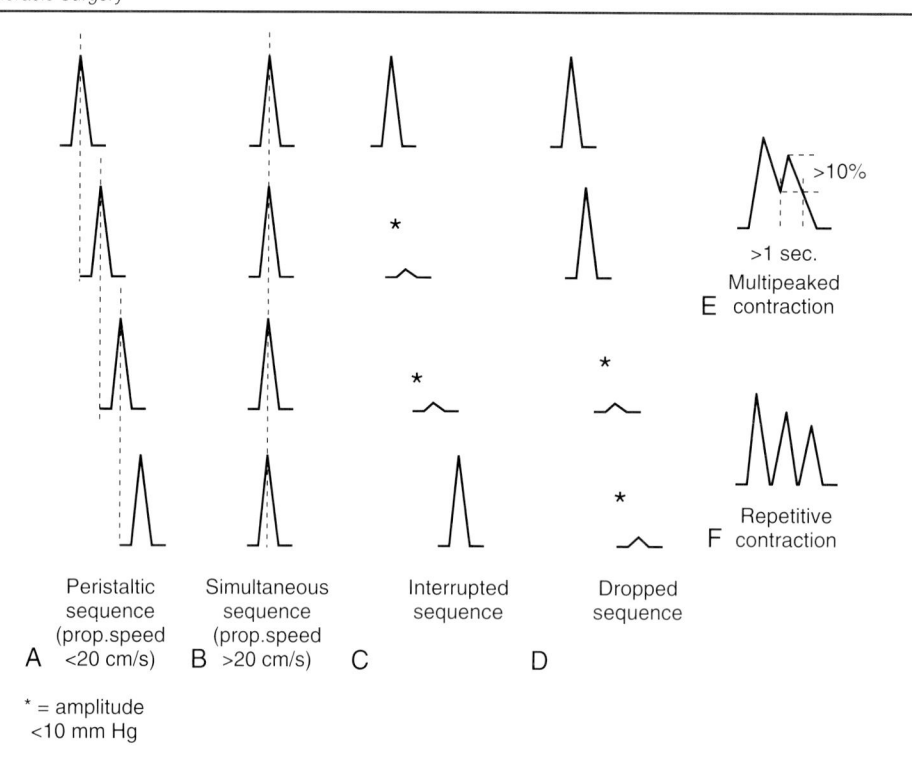

Figure 34–20
Classification of esophageal contraction waves on stationary manometry. **A,** A complete peristaltic sequence is a series of detectable contractions at each esophageal level, with a progression speed of less than 20 cm/s. **B,** A simultaneous sequence is a series of detectable contractions at each esophageal level, with a progression speed of more than 20 cm/s. **C,** An interrupted sequence is a series of detectable contractions in which an initial contraction is followed by no detectable contractions (<10 mm Hg), with a normal contraction subsequently reappearing. **D,** A dropped sequence is a series of detectable contractions in which an initial contraction is followed by no detectable contractions (<10 mm Hg). The morphology of the contractions is classified as normal, multipeaked, or repetitive. The difference between multipeaked **(E)** and repetitive **(F)** contractions is that in the latter, the pressure between two consecutive peaks returns to baseline. prop., propagation.

Esophageal Body Motility

To evaluate the esophageal body, the catheter is positioned so that the pressure-sensing ports span the length of the esophagus, and the peristaltic response to 10 swallows of 5 mL of water is measured. The features of individual contractions are the amplitude, duration, slope, and morphology (i.e., single, double, or triple peaked). Transmission of waves from one level to the next is assessed by the speed of wave propagation and by noting any interruption (Fig. 34-20). Most commercially available manometric systems automatically measure these features and compare the results with those of normal subjects (Figs. 34-21 and 34-22).

Upper Esophageal Sphincter

The position, length, and resting pressure of the UES and its relaxation with swallowing are assessed with a technique similar to that used for the LES. The key features to be assessed are the adequacy of pharyngeal contraction and the timing and extent of UES relaxation. An indirect measure of UES stiffness or loss of compliance is the intrabolus pressure, which appears as a pressure rise or shoulder on the upstroke of the pharyngeal contraction (Figs. 34-23 and 34-24).

High-Resolution Manometry

High-resolution manometry is an advancement in the technology used to assess esophageal contractility and sphincter function. It represents an improvement in methodology that leads to a more detailed data collection and simpler data interpretation. The concept behind this technology is that by vastly increasing the number of sensors and reducing the space between the sensors, it can provide representation of the entire pressure profile along the esophagus from the pharynx to the proximal stomach without the need to reposition or to pull back the catheter as in conventional manometry.

The most commonly used high-resolution system is a solid-state manometric assembly with 36 circumferential sensors spaced at 1-cm intervals (Sierra Scientific Instruments, Inc., Los Angeles, CA). This system uses a proprietary pressure transduction technology (TactArray). These transducers detect the pressure over a length of 25 mm in each of 12 radially dispersed sectors. The recorded pressure at each sector is then averaged, making each of the 36 sensors a circumferential pressure detector with the extended frequency response characteristic of solid-state manometric systems and free of the hydrostatic influence characteristic of water-perfused systems. The increased number of circumferential pressure sensors results in a vastly greater amount of data and detail.

Interpretation of the data has also been simplified by a sophisticated topographic plotting algorithm that converts the normal waveform data into a three-dimensional topographic display. Sphincter characteristics and esophageal motor function are represented by isocontour manometric plots, potentially eliminating the need for the tedious analysis of the increased waveform data that are generated by the 36 sensors. High-resolution manometry is a major evolution over conventional manometry and should help researchers and

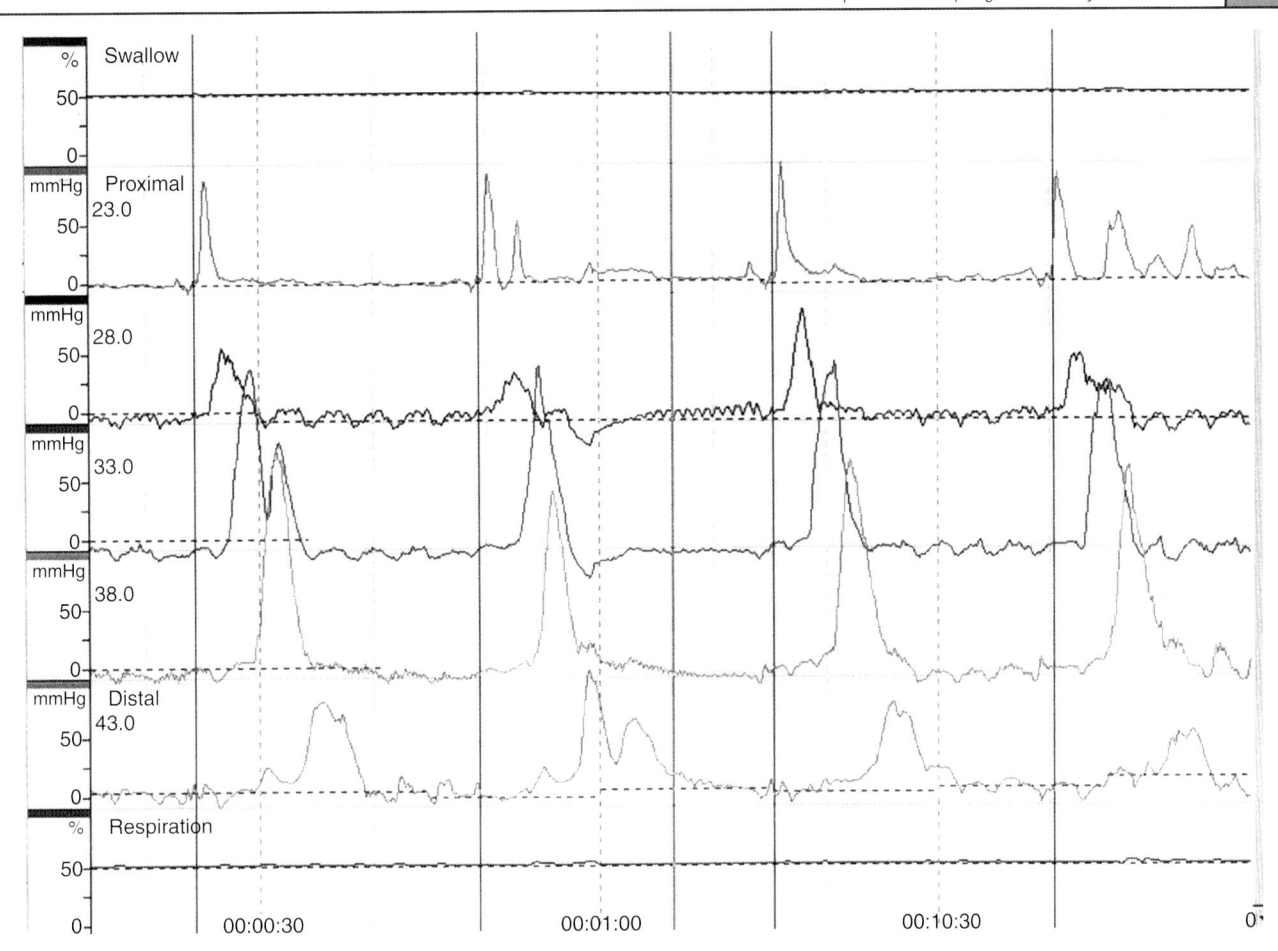

Figure 34–21
Illustration of progressive peristaltic contraction sequences in response to wet swallows.

clinicians assess esophageal motor function in a more simplified and detailed manner.

Ambulatory 24-Hour pH Monitoring

The development of 24-hour pH monitoring was a major advance in the unraveling of the pathophysiology of GERD. All previous tests had relied on the identification of reflux by a provocative maneuver, which had little relevance to the patient's daily activities. The 24-hour pH monitoring made it possible to determine if the time of esophageal exposure to gastric juice in a patient during a 24-hour period was greater than what was found in normal subjects.

The 24-hour pH monitoring is considered by many to be the gold standard for the diagnosis of GERD because it has the highest sensitivity and specificity of all tests currently available. It is indicated in any patient with symptoms suggestive of GERD, unless the symptoms are trivial or permanently abolished by a short course of acid-suppression therapy. The need for continued acid suppression should stimulate objective study. A 24-hour pH monitoring study is especially important in patients who are being considered for antireflux surgery. Atypical presentations of GERD are also a common indication; they include such symptoms as noncardiac chest pain (i.e., pain despite a normal cardiac evaluation) and respiratory symptoms such as shortness of breath, cough, nocturnal wheezing, and chronic hoarseness. In such patients, 24-hour pH monitoring allows confirmation of the diagnosis of GERD and can relate the occurrence of the symptoms to an episode of reflux.[48]

To perform the test, a small pH electrode is passed transnasally into the esophagus and placed 5 cm above the upper border of the LES, a position that has been previously determined by manometry. Different probes are available, but bipolar glass electrodes are preferred for their greater reliability[49] and their elimination of the need for an external reference electrode. The electrode is connected to an external portable digital storage device that is strapped to the patient's side, and pH values are continuously recorded at 6-second intervals for 24 hours (i.e., a complete circadian cycle). Precalibration and postcalibration of the system to pH levels of 1 and 7 is important to exclude electrode drift. The patient is instructed to carry out normal daily activities but to avoid strenuous exertion. He or she is asked to remain in the upright position while awake during the day, lying down supine only at night while sleeping, and to ingest two meals at the usual time. The diet is standardized only by its absence of food and beverages with a pH value of less than 5.0 and greater than 6.0. The patient notes in a diary the times of meals, retiring for sleep, and rising the following morning as well as the presence and duration of any symptoms. Figure 34-25 shows typical 24-hour pH tracings from a healthy subject and from a patient

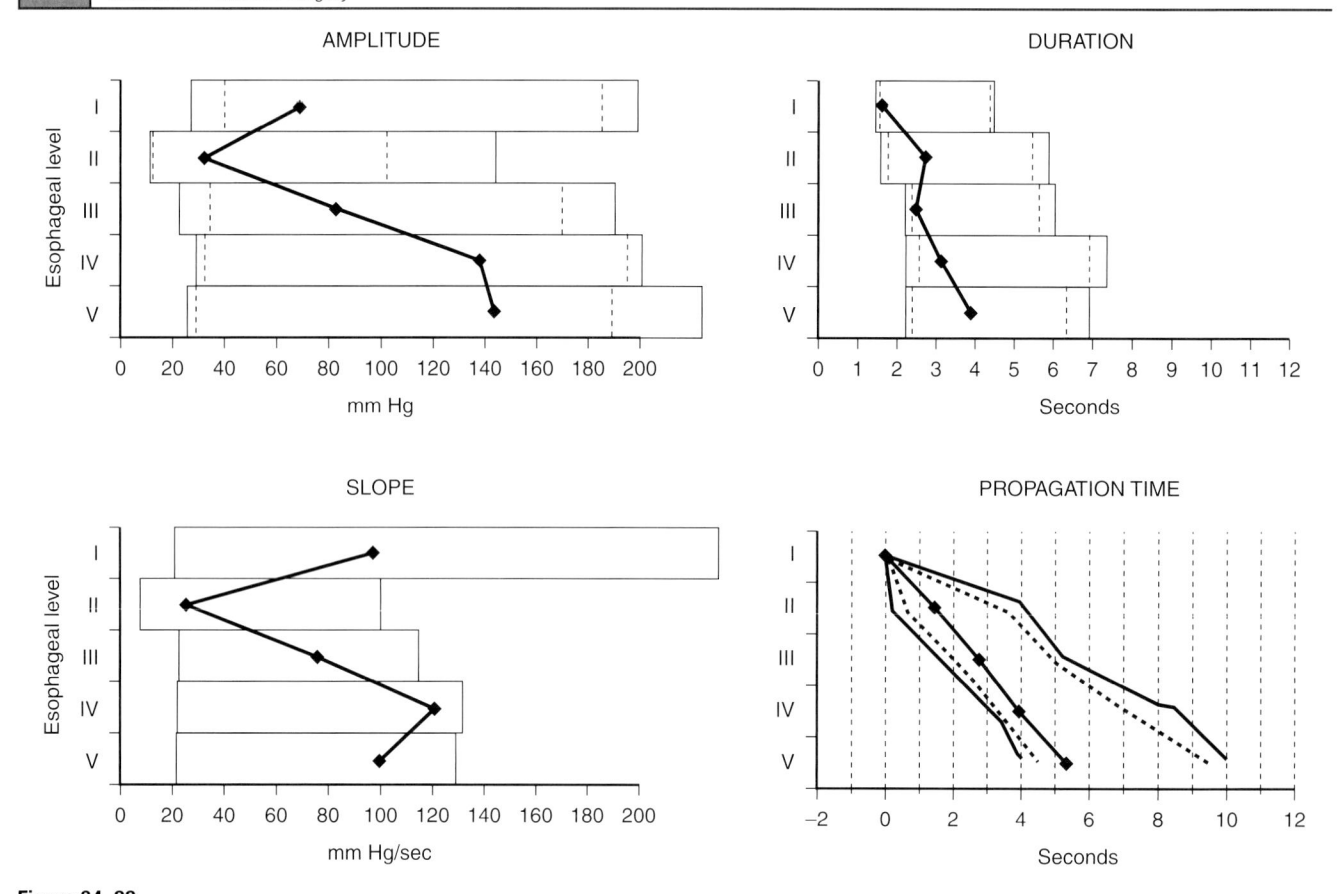

Figure 34–22
Computerized printout of an esophageal body motility study. Median patient values are related to the normal range obtained from healthy volunteers. The 2.5th and 97.5th percentiles are shown by solid lines; the 5th and 95th percentiles are shown by dotted lines.

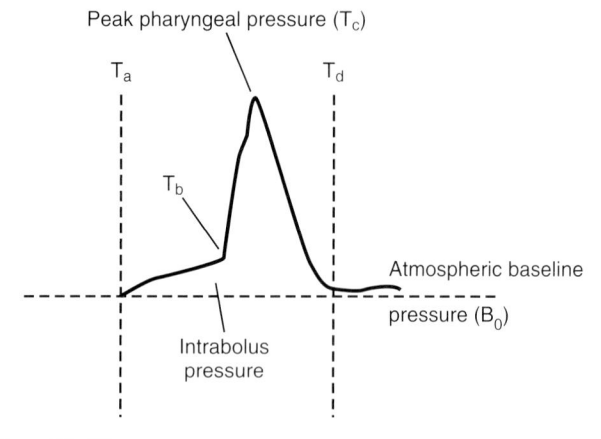

Figure 34–23
Diagram of a typical pharyngeal pressure tracing. T_a, arrival of the bolus head; T_b, the bolus tail; T_c, peak pressure of the pharyngeal stripping wave; T_d, completion of the pharyngeal pressure wave; B_0, baseline atmospheric pressure.

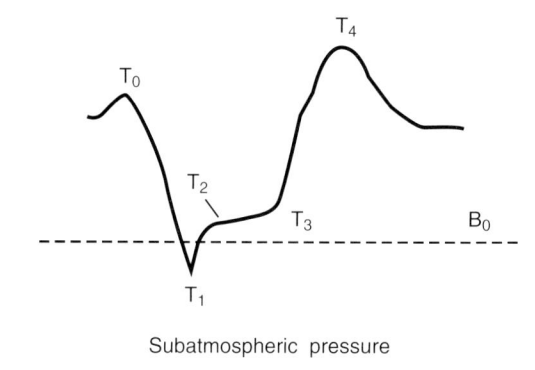

Figure 34–24
Diagram of a typical UES pressure and its relaxation on swallowing. T_0, pressure at beginning of the swallow; T_1, complete opening of the sphincter (with complete opening, pressure is subatmospheric); T_2, transition from subatmospheric to a supra-atmospheric pressure as the head of the bolus flows into the sphincter; T_3, pressure at the bolus tail ahead of the pharyngeal stripping wave; T_4, peak pressure after luminal closure by the pharyngeal stripping wave; B_0, baseline atmospheric pressure.

with GERD. Medications such as H_2 blockers and prokinetics should be discontinued for 48 hours before the testing begins. Proton pump inhibitors (e.g., omeprazole) should be stopped for 2 weeks before pH monitoring because of their long-lasting action.

It is important to emphasize that 24-hour esophageal pH monitoring should not be considered a test for reflux; rather, it is a measurement of the esophageal exposure to gastric juice. The measurement is expressed as the percentage of time that the esophageal pH was below 4 during the 24-hour period. Just measuring the percentage of time that the pH is less than 4, although concise, does not reflect how the exposure has occurred; for example, it may have occurred in a few long or several short reflux episodes. Consequently, two other

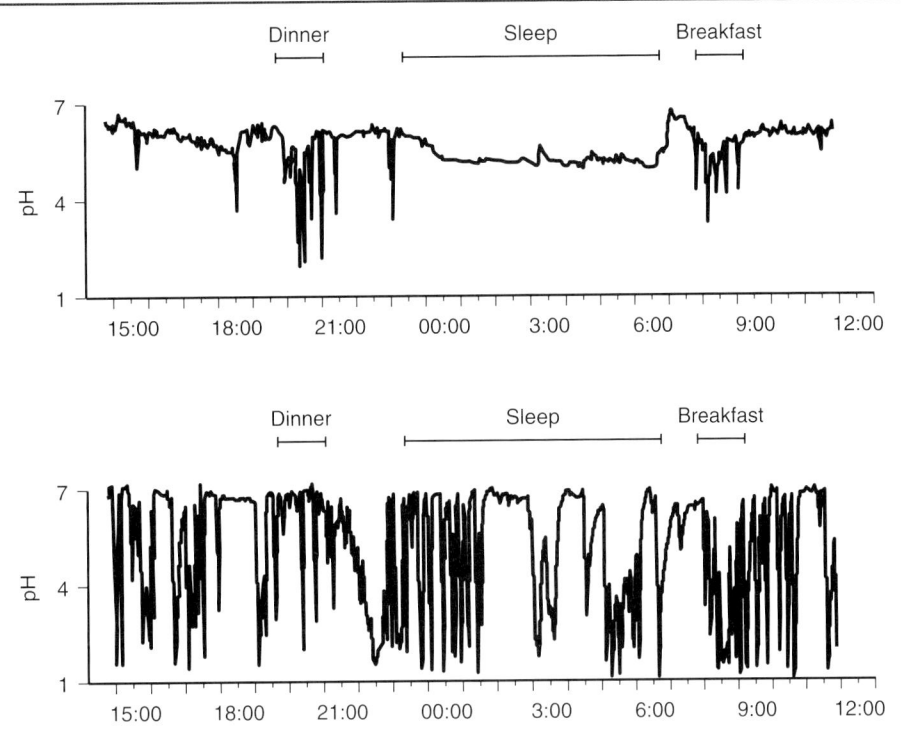

Figure 34–25
Tracings of 24-hour pH monitoring of the distal esophagus in a healthy subject *(top)* and in a patient with GERD *(bottom)*. Physiologic reflux occurs in the normal subject, mainly in the upright position after meals. The patient's record shows an increased number of reflux episodes in both the upright and supine positions, some of them with prolonged clearing time.

Table 34–1
Normal Values for Ambulatory Esophageal pH Monitoring in 50 Healthy Volunteers

	Mean	Standard Deviation	Median	Minimum	Maximum	95th Percentile
Percentage of total time with pH < 4	1.5	1.4	1.2	0	6.0	4.5
Percentage of upright time with pH < 4	2.2	2.3	1.6	0	9.3	8.4
Percentage of supine time with pH < 4	0.6	1.0	0.1	0	4.0	3.5
Number of episodes	19.00	12.8	16.0	2.0	56.0	46.9
Number of episodes > 5 minutes	0.8	1.2	0	0	5.0	3.5
Longest episode (minutes)	6.7	7.9	4.0	0	46.0	19.8
Composite score	6.0	4.4	5.0	0.4	18.0	14.7

assessments are necessary: (1) the frequency of the reflux episodes and (2) their duration. For this reason, esophageal exposure to gastric juice is best assessed by the following measurements[28]:

- the cumulative time that the esophageal pH is below 4 expressed as the percentage of the total, upright, and supine monitored times;
- the frequency of reflux episodes, when the pH drops below 4, expressed as the number of episodes per 24 hours;
- the number of episodes during which the pH remained below 4 for longer than 5 minutes per 24 hours; and
- the time in minutes of the longest recorded reflux episode, the longest time the pH consistently remained below 4.

Normal values for these six components of the 24-hour record were derived from 50 asymptomatic control subjects. The upper limits of normal were established at the 95th percentile.[50] If the values of symptomatic patients are outside of the 95th percentile of normal subjects, they are considered to be abnormal for the component measured. There is a uniformity of normal values for these six components as reported by centers throughout the world. The normal values for the six components obtained from 50 healthy volunteers are shown in Table 34-1. A composite scoring system has been derived that integrates the different components of the pH record into a single measurement of esophageal acid exposure. This composite score is calculated from the six parameters with use of their standard deviations as weighing factors.[51]

In patients with symptoms of chronic cough, hoarseness, or pulmonary aspiration, placement of an additional pH electrode in the proximal part of the esophagus or pharynx can be helpful.[52] If the accumulated acid sequence is greater than 1% in the proximal esophagus or the number of reflux episodes is more than 24 (particularly if there is a temporal relationship between the reflux episodes and the onset of the symptoms), reflux can be documented and assumed to be the cause of the patient's respiratory symptoms.[53]

Advances in technology have made pH testing more comfortable for the patient. The development of a catheter-free miniaturized pH electrode has revolutionized the way that standard 24-hour pH testing is performed. The Bravo system (Medtronic, Minneapolis, MN) allows the transnasal or transoral deployment of a small capsule attached to the esophageal mucosa that is capable of transmitting pH data by radiotelemetry to a pager-sized receiver, thus eliminating the need for an unpleasant catheter. It may also provide a more accurate physiologic picture by allowing patients to perform their normal daily activities without the social and behavioral restrictions imposed by the catheter. The Bravo capsule also has the ability to record for prolonged periods, 48 to 96 hours, which may increase the accuracy of pH testing in the diagnosis of GERD.[54-56]

Additional testing may be necessary if the standard methods of assessing esophageal function fail to yield conclusive results. The 24-hour esophageal bile probe can be useful for detecting bilirubin during a 24-hour period in those patients who reflux a preponderance of duodenal contents. Ambulatory 24-hour esophageal manometry can give a much more comprehensive picture of esophageal function during a patient's normal daily activity, especially during meals. In normal subjects, the esophagus becomes progressively more organized from the supine position to the upright position to the meal period; this feature is reflected in the higher prevalence of effective peristaltic waves during meals. Loss of this improved organization of esophageal activity during meals is a subtle sign of a motility disorder. Additional information may also be gained by multichannel intraluminal esophageal impedance measurement. This type of measurement determines the resistance to the flow of current through a given medium (impedance). The impedance to current changes as the composition of the medium in which the current is traveling changes (i.e., air, liquids, or solids). The application of this technology provides a better insight into esophageal bolus transport. Coupled with a pH probe, it can also differentiate acid reflux from nonacid reflux. Last, the assessment of gastric function can be important in many patients with esophageal symptoms. Disorders of gastric emptying frequently can contribute to or be confused with esophageal disease, especially GERD.

These technological advances in esophageal diagnostics—and others yet to come—will undoubtedly provide a better understanding of esophageal physiology and function and ultimately lead to the improved treatment of esophageal disorders.

REFERENCES

1. Liebermann-Meffert D, Duranceau A. Embryology, anatomy and physiology of the esophagus. In: Orringer MB, Zuidema GD, editors. *Shackelford's surgery of the alimentary tract. The esophagus.* 3rd ed. Philadelphia: Saunders; 1991. p. 3-9.
2. Meyer GW, Austin RM, Brady CE, Castell DO. Muscle anatomy of the human esophagus. *J Clin Gastroenterol* 1986;**8**:131-7.
3. Gray SW, Rowe Jr JS, Skandalakis JE. Surgical anatomy of the gastroesophageal junction. *Am Surg* 1979;**45**:575-87.
4. Liebermann-Meffert D, Luescher U, Neff U, et al. Esophagectomy without thoracotomy: is there a risk of intramediastinal bleeding? A study on blood supply of the esophagus. *Ann Surg* 1987;**206**:184-92.
5. Liebermann-Meffert D, Walbrun B, Hiebert CA, Siewert JR. Recurrent and superior laryngeal nerves: a new look with implications for the esophageal surgeon. *Ann Thorac Surg* 1999;**67**:217-23.
6. Pouderoux P, Lin S, Kahrilis PJ. Timing, propagation, coordination, and effect of esophageal shortening during peristalsis. *Gastroenterology* 1997;**112**:1147-54.
7. Pouderoux P, Shi G, Tatum RP, et al. Esophageal solid bolus transport: studies using concurrent videofluoroscopy and manometry. *Am J Gastroenterol* 1999;**94**:1457-63.
8. DeMeester TR, Peters JH, Bremner CG, Chandrasoma P. Biology of gastroesophageal reflux disease: pathophysiology relating to medical and surgical treatment. *Annu Rev Med* 1999;**50**:469-506.
9. Bonavina L, Evander A, DeMeester TR, et al. Length of the distal esophageal sphincter and competency of the cardia. *Am J Surg* 1986;**151**:24-34.
10. Stein HJ, DeMeester TR, Naspetti R, et al. Three-dimensional imaging of the lower esophageal sphincter in gastroesophageal reflux disease. *Ann Surg* 1991;**214**:374-84.
11. Mason RJ, Lund RJ, DeMeester TR, et al. Nissen fundoplication prevents shortening of the sphincter during gastric distention. *Arch Surg* 1997;**132**:719-26.
12. Pettersson GB, Bombeck CT, Nyhus LM. The lower esophageal sphincter: mechanisms of opening and closure. *Surgery* 1980;**88**:307-14.
13. Dent J. A new technique for continuous sphincter pressure measurement. *Gastroenterology* 1976;**71**:263-7.
14. Ismail T, Bancewicz J, Barlow J. Yield pressure, anatomy of the cardia and gastroesophageal reflux. *Br J Surg* 1995;**82**:943-7.
15. Marchand P. The gastro-oesophageal "sphincter" and the mechanism of regurgitation. *Br J Surg* 1955;**42**:504-13.
16. Kahrilas PJ, Shi G, Manka M, Joehl RJ. Increased frequency of transient lower esophageal sphincter relaxation induced by gastric distention in reflux patients with hiatal hernia. *Gastroenterology* 2000;**118**:688-95.
17. DeMeester TR, Wernly JA, Bryant GH, et al. Clinical and in vitro analysis of gastroesophageal competence: a study of the principles of antireflux surgery. *Am J Surg* 1979;**137**:39-46.
18. Johnson LF, Lin YC, Hong SK. Gastroesophageal dynamics during immersion in water to the neck. *J Appl Physiol* 1975;**38**:449-54.
19. O'Sullivan GC, DeMeester TR, Joelsson BE, et al. The interaction of the lower esophageal sphincter pressure and length of sphincter in the abdomen as determinants of gastroesophageal competence. *Am Surg* 1982;**143**:40-7.
20. Pellegrini CA, DeMeester TR, Skinner DB. Response of the distal esophageal sphincter to respiratory and positional maneuvers in humans. *Surg Forum* 1976;**27**:380-2.
21. Stein HJ, Barlow AP, DeMeester TR, Hinder RA. Complications of gastroesophageal reflux disease: role of the lower esophageal sphincter, esophageal acid and acid/alkaline exposure, and duodenogastric reflux. *Ann Surg* 1992;**216**:35-43.
22. Zaninotto G, DeMeester TR, Bremner CG, et al. Esophageal function in patients with reflux-induced strictures and its relevance to surgical treatment. *Ann Thorac Surg* 1995;**47**:362-70.
23. Barham CP, Gotley DC, Mills A, Alderson D. Precipitating causes of acid reflux episodes in ambulant patients with gastro-oesophageal reflux disease. *Gut* 1995;**36**:505-10.
24. Bremner RM, Hoeft SF, Costantini M, et al. Pharyngeal swallowing: the major factor in clearance of esophageal reflux episodes. *Ann Surg* 1993;**218**:364-70.
25. Iwakiri K, Kobayashi M, Kotoyari M, et al. Relationship between postprandial esophageal acid exposure and meal volume and fat content. *Dig Dis Sci* 1996;**41**:926-30.
26. Fletcher J, Wirz A, Young J, et al. Unbuffered highly acidic gastric juice exists at the gastroesophageal junction after a meal. *Gastroenterology* 2001;**121**:775-83.
27. Öberg S, Peters JH, DeMeester TR, et al. Inflammation and specialized intestinal metaplasia of cardiac mucosa is a manifestation of early gastroesophageal reflux disease. *Ann Surg* 1997;**226**:522-32.
28. DeMeester TR, Wang CI, Wernly JA, et al. Technique, indications and clinical use of 24-hour esophageal pH monitoring. *J Thorac Cardiovasc Surg* 1980;**79**:656-70.
29. Theisen J, Oberg S, Peters JH, et al. Gastro-esophageal reflux disease confined to the sphincter. *Dis Esophagus* 2001;**14**:235-8.
30. DeMeester TR, Ireland AP. Gastric pathology as an initiator and potentiator of gastroesophageal reflux disease. *Dis Esophagus* 1997;**10**:1-8.
31. Kuster E, Ros E, Toledo-Pimentel V, et al. Predictive factors of the long term outcome in gastro-oesophageal reflux disease: six year follow up of 107 patients. *Gut* 1994;**35**:8-14.

32. Peters JH, DeMeester TR, Crookes P, et al. The treatment of gastroesophageal reflux disease with laparoscopic Nissen fundoplication. *Ann Surg* 1998;**228**:40-50.
33. Singh P, Adamopoulos A, Taylor RH, Colin-Jones DG. Oesophageal motor function before and after healing of oesophagitis. *Gut* 1992;**33**:1590-6.
34. Dodds WJ. Current concepts of esophageal motor function: clinical implications for radiology. *AJR Am J Roentgenol* 1977;**128**:549-61.
35. Ekberg Walgreen L. Dysfunction of pharyngeal swallowing: a cineradiographic investigation in 854 dysphagial patients. *Acta Radiol Diagn* 1985;**26**:389-95.
36. Seaman WB. Roentgenology of pharyngeal disorders. In: Margulis AR, Burhenne JH, editors. *Alimentary tract roentgenology*. 2nd ed. St. Louis: Mosby; 1973, vol. I. p. 305-36.
37. Donner MW. Swallowing mechanism and neuromuscular disorders. *Semin Roentgenol* 1974;**9**:273-82.
38. Schwizer W, Hinder RA, DeMeester TR. Does delayed gastric emptying contribute to gastroesophageal reflux disease? *Am J Surg* 1989;**157**:74-81.
39. Chandrasoma P. Norman Barrett: so close, yet 50 years away from the truth. *J Gastrointest Surg* 1999;**3**:7-14.
40. Salo JA, Kivilaakso EO, Kiviluoto TA, et al. Cytokeratin profile suggests metaplastic epithelial transformation in Barrett's oesophagus. *Ann Med* 1996;**28**:305-9.
41. Sawney RA, Shields HM, Allan CH, et al. Morphological characterization of the squamocolumnar junction of the esophagus in patients with and without Barrett's epithelium. *Dig Dis Sci* 1996;**41**:1088-98.
42. Hameeteman W, Tytgat GNJ, Houthoff HJ, et al. Barrett's esophagus: development of dysplasia and adenocarcinoma. *Gastroenterology* 1989;**96**:1249-56.
43. Zhuang Z, Vortmeyer AO, Mark EJ, et al. Barrett's esophagus: metaplastic cells with loss of heterozygosity at the APC gene locus are clonal precursors to invasive adenocarcinoma. *Cancer Res* 1996;**56**:1961-4.
44. Hill LD, Kozarek RA, Kraemer SJ, et al. The gastroesophageal flap valve: in vitro and in vivo observations. *Gastrointest Endosc* 1996;**44**:541-7.
45. Castell DO, Richter JE, Dalton CB, editors. *Esophageal motility testing*. New York: Elsevier; 1987.
46. Benjamin SB, Richter JE, Cordova CM, Knuff TE, Castell DO. Prospective manometric evaluation with pharmacologic provocation of patients with suspected esophageal motility dysfunction. *Gastroenterology* 1983;**84**:893-901.
47. Zaninotto G, DeMeester TR, Schwizer W, et al. The lower esophageal sphincter in health and disease. *Am J Surg* 1988;**155**:104-11.
48. Miller FA. Utilization of inlying pH-probe for evaluation of acid peptic diathesis. *Arch Surg* 1964;**89**:199-203.
49. Johnson LF, DeMeester TRP. Development of the 24-hour intraesophageal pH monitoring composite scoring system. *J Clin Gastroenterol* 1986;**8**(Suppl. 1): 52-8.
50. McLaughlan G, Rawlings JM, Lucas ML, et al. Electrodes for 24-hour pH monitoring: a comparative study. *Gut* 1987;**28**:935-9.
51. Johnson LF, DeMeester TR. Twenty-four-hour pH monitoring of the distal esophagus: a quantitative measure of gastroesophageal reflux. *Am J Gastroenterol* 1974;**62**:325-32.
52. DeMeester TR. Prolonged oesophageal pH monitoring. In: Read NW, editor. *Gastrointestinal motility: which test?* Petersfield, England: Wrightson Biomedical; 1989. p. 41.
53. Ayazi S, Hagen JA, Hindoyan AH, et al. Dual probe pH monitoring: improved definition of normal proximal acid exposure. *Gastroenterology* 2008;**134**(4): Suppl. 1:A-598.
54. Scarpulla G, Camilleri S, Galante P, Manganaro M, Fox M. The impact of prolonged pH measurements on the diagnosis of gastroesophageal reflux disease: 4-day wireless pH studies. *Am J Gastroenterol* 2007;**102**:2642-7.
55. Tseng D, Rizvi A, Fennerty MB, et al. Forty-eight-hour pH monitoring increases sensitivity in detecting abnormal esophageal acid exposure. *J Gastrointest Surg* 2005;**9**:1043-52.
56. Ayazi S, Lipham JC, Portale G, Peyre CG, Streets CG, Leers JM, et al. Bravo catheter-free pH monitoring: normal values, concordance, optimal diagnostic thresholds and accuracy. *Clin Gastroenterol Hepatology* 2009; doi:10.1016/ j.cgh.2008.08.020.

CHAPTER 35

Surgery for Congenital Lesions of the Esophagus

Kurt Newman, David Spurlock, and Alfred Chahine

Embryology
Esophageal Atresia
  Historical Aspects
  Epidemiology
  Anatomy
  Presentation
  Workup
  Initial Management
  Operative Principles

Complications and Long-term Effects
Esophageal Duplications
  Anatomy and Embryology
  Incidence
  Presentation
  Diagnosis
  Treatment
Congenital Esophageal Stenosis
  Anatomy

Presentation
Diagnosis
Treatment
Laryngotracheoesophageal Cleft
  Anatomy
  Presentation
  Diagnosis
  Treatment

EMBRYOLOGY

At about the 18th or 19th day of fetal life, the notochord, the anlage of the vertebral column, starts to form, first in close association with endodermal cells, then separating from them. The foregut develops from the endodermal cells as they are separating from the notochord. At about 3 weeks of embryonic development, the tracheal primordium appears as a ventral diverticulum in the cephalad portion of the foregut. During the next few weeks, growth and elongation of the diverticulum and the foregut along the tracheoesophageal groove contribute to the separation of the esophagus and the trachea, which is complete by about 5 to 6 weeks of fetal life. During the seventh and eighth weeks, the esophageal epithelium proliferates and fills the lumen almost completely. Vacuoles appear in the lumen and eventually coalesce to recanalize it by the tenth week.[1]

The major anomalies of the esophagus are a result of some aberration in this orderly development. Failure of separation of the trachea and esophagus may result in esophageal atresia (EA) with or without a tracheoesophageal fistula (TEF) and laryngotracheoesophageal clefts. Tracheobronchial elements including cartilage can be left behind in the distal esophagus, causing congenital esophageal stenosis. Failure of recanalization of the esophageal lumen may contribute to the pathogenesis of EA and esophageal webs. Intramural esophageal duplication cysts may result from failure of the esophageal vacuoles to completely coalesce and disappear. Aberrations in the orderly separation of endodermal cells and the notochord may explain the formation of duplication cysts in the posterior mediastinum and vertebral defects associated with EA.

A doxorubicin (Adriamycin)–induced murine model of EA has been described.[2] With use of this model, investigators are studying the role that patterning genes and proteins like Sonic hedgehog (*Shh*) might play in the morphogenesis of EA.[3,4] In the same rat model as well as in neonates with EA/TEF, Spilde and coworkers have studied the molecular expression of foregut patterning genes to shed a light on the origin of TEF. The distal esophagus seems to arise as a diverticulum of the trachea, which elongates and joins the stomach, rather than from the foregut itself.[2,5,6] They speculate that this might explain the well-known poor motility of the reconstructed esophagus in patients with TEF.

ESOPHAGEAL ATRESIA

Historical Aspects

The historical background relevant to EA is thoroughly reviewed by Harmon and Coran.[7] Durston in 1670 and Gibson in 1697 described the first cases of EA. It took about 250 years before the first reported cases of survivors by Leven and Ladd independently in 1939. Both were able to achieve success by performing a series of operations including gastrostomy, ligation of the fistula, marsupialization of the upper pouch, and final reconstruction with an antethoracic skin tube. The early attempts at primary repair were all unsuccessful. It was not until 1941 that Haight reported the first survivor of a primary repair. In the decade that followed, it became evident that the mortality was very high in infants of lower birth weights, in those with severe associated anomalies, and in those critically ill from aspiration pneumonia.[8-10] There followed a shift toward staging of the operation for sick infants, with a gastrostomy followed by division of the TEF and the esophageal reconstruction performed as a third stage.[8-10] In 1962, Waterston proposed a classification based on birth weight, presence of pneumonia, and associated anomalies.[9] The 1970s and 1980s witnessed major advances in respiratory, neonatal, anesthetic, and surgical care as well as the introduction of more effective antibiotics. These advances included endotracheal intubation, which made it easier to prevent aspiration from the esophageal pouch and to deal with its sequelae. As a result, multiple groups started to recommend either direct primary anastomosis (anastomosis shortly after birth) or delayed primary anastomosis (anastomosis delayed for the treatment of other life-threatening anomalies or stabilization of the patient) regardless of the patient's weight but based on physiologic criteria.[11-19] The end of the 20th century ushered in the

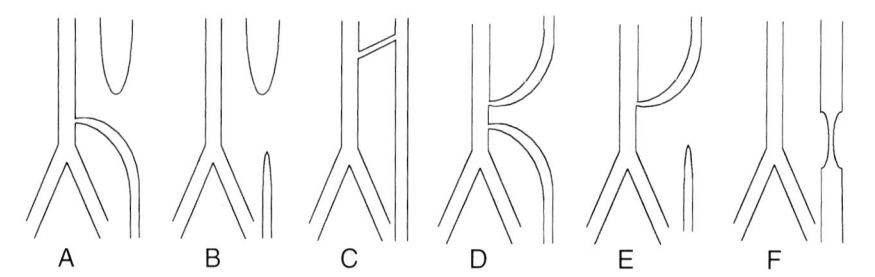

Figure 35–1
Classification of types of esophageal anomalies. **A,** EA with distal TEF. **B,** EA without TEF. **C,** TEF without EA (H-type fistula). **D,** EA with proximal and distal TEF. **E,** EA with proximal TEF. **F,** Esophageal stenosis. EA, esophageal atresia; TEF, tracheoesophageal fistula.

application of thoracoscopy to the repair of EA/TEF and other congenital anomalies of the esophagus.[20-27]

Epidemiology

The average rate of EA is reported to be about 2.4 per 10,000 births.[28] No significant sex predilection is described. Other congenital anomalies occur in patients with EA frequently, ranging from 30% to 76%.[29-33] This might be due to the fact that the malformation in EA occurs early in the first trimester when there is active organogenesis. As a result, the developmental cause of EA/TEF might also affect other organ systems at the same time. The number of associated anomalies occurring in each patient increases with decreasing birth weight.[29,34,35] With the improvement in anesthetic, respiratory, and neonatal techniques during the last few decades, the associated anomalies are now the major contributor to mortality in patients with EA.[31] The most common associated anomaly is congenital heart disease, present in some form in about a fifth of the patients.[29,33-37] About 20% of patients have some combination of the constellation of anomalies referred to as VATER or VACTERL association: vertebral, anorectal, cardiac, tracheoesophageal, renal or radial, and limb anomalies.[36,37]

Infants born with EA often have low birth weight and are premature.[35,38] In one study, 90% of the patients with EA were below the 50th percentile for gestational age, and 40% were below the 10th percentile or small for gestational age.[39] The growth retardation might be secondary to decreased absorption of the amniotic fluid protein or a mechanical factor.[39] Severe intrauterine growth retardation increases the mortality rate of the neonate who is small for gestational age by 5 to 20 times that of neonates who are appropriate for gestational age.[40]

Anatomy

There are five types of EA with or without TEF. Different classification schemes have numbered them differently, so it is preferred to describe the actual anomaly rather than assign it a number or a letter (Fig. 35-1): EA with distal TEF, EA without TEF, EA with proximal TEF, EA with proximal and distal fistula, and isolated TEF (H-type TEF). The distribution of the different types in large series has been relatively uniform across different decades and countries, with the most common being EA with distal TEF (Table 35-1).[11,29,41-43] The fistula is usually small and most of the time arises from the midline of the membranous portion of the trachea just above the bifurcation, but there are significant variations.

Table 35–1
Distribution of Types of Esophageal Atresia

Type of Anomaly	Number	Percentage
EA with distal TEF	1024	87.1
EA	82	7.0
H-type TEF	37	3.1
EA with proximal TEF	11	0.9
EA with double TEF	22	1.9

EA, esophageal atresia; TEF, tracheoesophageal fistula.
Compiled from references 11, 29, 41-43.

Presentation

A significant number of cases of EA are now suspected on prenatal ultrasonography; polyhydramnios, absent or small stomach bubble, and visualization of an esophageal pouch in the neck are the most prominent features.[44,45] Suspecting the diagnosis prenatally is invaluable in preparing the family. Prenatal counseling with a pediatric surgeon and a neonatologist and planning for appropriate delivery arrangements are extremely helpful. Postnatally, EA is diagnosed in most patients in the first few hours after birth. Choking with feeding, regurgitation of saliva and feeds, and respiratory distress from aspiration of saliva or gastric contents through the TEF are the most common signs and symptoms. Inability to pass a feeding tube confirms the diagnosis.

Isolated TEF (H-type TEF) may not be diagnosed until later in life. Recurrent episodes of aspiration pneumonia and choking and coughing with feedings should raise the suspicion. Contrast esophagography and rigid bronchoscopy are complementary in making the diagnosis.[46]

Patients with isolated EA often have a scaphoid abdomen because of the absence of gas in the intestines. If EA is suspected, one should always look for other physical signs of the VATER association: anorectal malformations, limb anomalies, and vertebral defects (Fig. 35-2).

Workup

A chest radiograph showing a curved catheter in the proximal esophageal pouch is often all that is required to make the diagnosis (Fig. 35-3). In patients with isolated EA, the radiograph reveals absence of intestinal air (Fig. 35-4). If there is

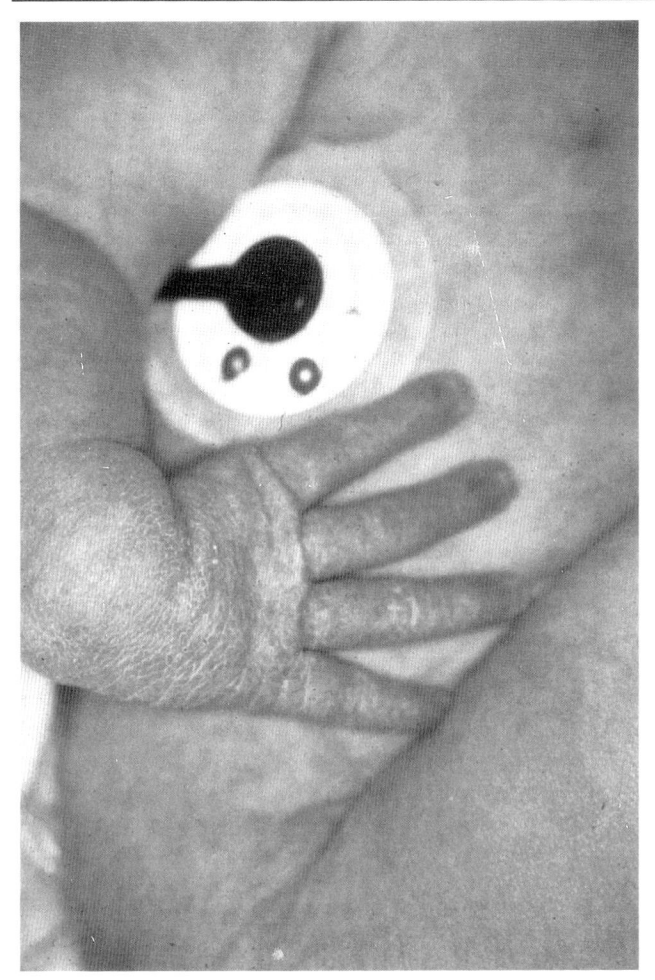

Figure 35–2
Radial aplasia, one component of the VATER association. *(Courtesy of Dr. R. Ricketts, Emory University Medical Center.)*

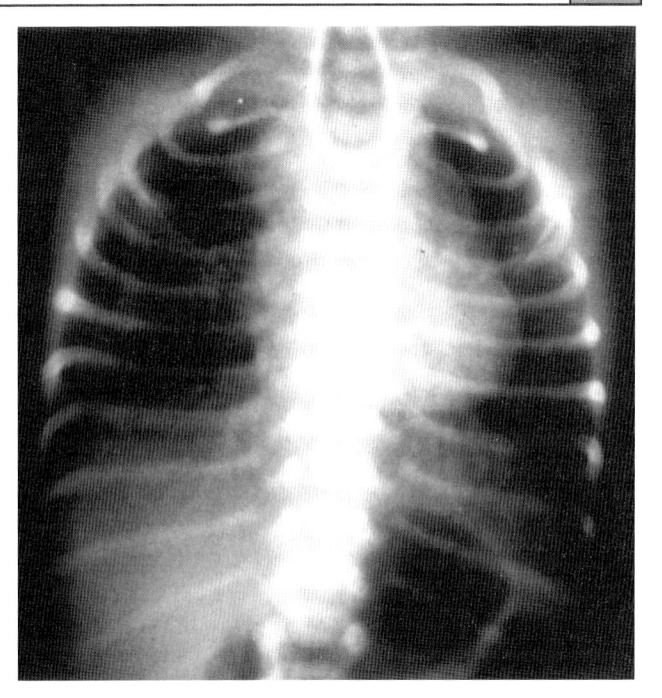

Figure 35–3
Chest radiograph of a patient with esophageal atresia and tracheoesophageal fistula. Note the catheter curved in the upper pouch and the presence of air in the intestinal tract. *(Courtesy of Dr. R. Ricketts, Emory University Medical Center.)*

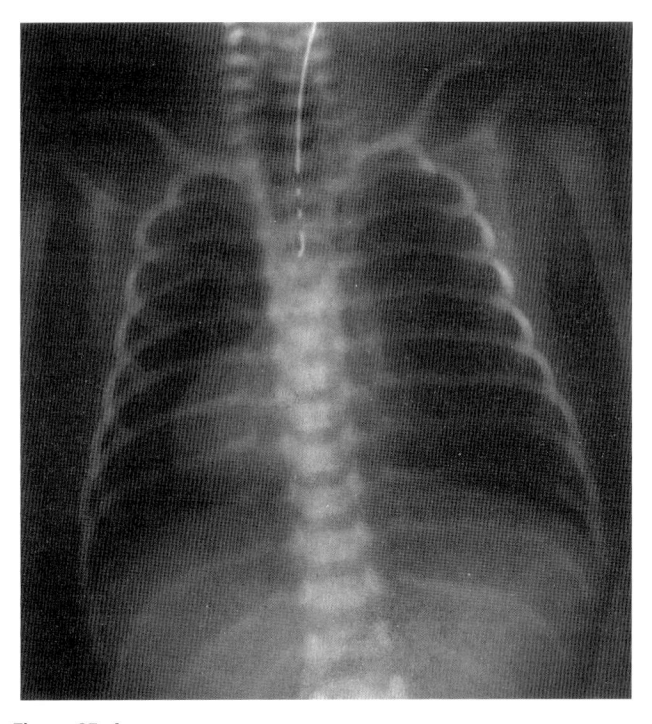

Figure 35–4
Chest radiograph of a patient with isolated esophageal atresia. Note the absence of air in the intestinal tract. *(Courtesy of Dr. C. Leftridge, Georgetown University Medical Center.)*

still doubt, a small amount of air injected into the pouch accentuates it on a plain radiograph and confirms EA (Fig. 35-5). The use of barium to look for an upper pouch fistula should be discouraged because it may potentially lead to aspiration. Upper pouch fistulas are rare and are usually found at the time of repair by either bronchoscopy or a careful dissection of the proximal pouch. Esophagography performed through a catheter being pulled up along the esophagus while the patient is prone is invaluable in making the diagnosis of H-type fistula (Fig. 35-6).

An echocardiogram, renal ultrasound examination, and vertebral films should be obtained to rule out major cardiac, renal, and vertebral anomalies as part of the VATER association. The echocardiogram is also helpful in determining the location of the aortic arch and of any aberrant central vessels, which might alter the surgical approach.

Initial Management

Patients born with EA are at risk for aspiration of saliva or gastric contents into the tracheobronchial tree. A Replogle-type soft sump suction catheter with the holes all close to the tip should be placed in the upper pouch and put on continuous suction. In the presence of a TEF, the patient should be placed in the reverse Trendelenburg position with the head up to minimize reflux of gastric contents into the trachea. Having the patient prone might also help in keeping the gastroesophageal junction at a less dependent position and decrease gastric reflux. With isolated EA, the Trendelenburg position facilitates the passive drainage of the hypopharynx and complements the active suction of the catheter. Even with a drainage catheter in place, frequent suctioning of the hypopharynx helps decrease the risk of aspiration. If there is any evidence of aspiration pneumonitis on a radiograph, broad-spectrum antibiotics should be started.

Positive-pressure ventilation should be avoided in a patient with a TEF if at all possible to minimize shunting through the TEF and abdominal distention. Because the majority of the fistulas are located just proximal to the carina, the tip of the tube should be kept high in the trachea to prevent the tip of the tube from getting lodged in the TEF. The TEF is sometimes significant enough that adequate ventilation cannot be maintained, especially in the face of respiratory distress syndrome of the premature with its attendant high intraparenchymal pressures. In that case, emergent ligation of the TEF might be warranted.[47] A more difficult way to control the TEF emergently is obliteration of the TEF with a Fogarty balloon introduced by bronchoscopy.[48] A hazardous situation can occur when a patient with significant steal through a TEF also has a very high intestinal obstruction, such as duodenal atresia. The massive gastric distention exacerbates the respiratory compromise and could lead to perforation of the stomach. Emergent gastric decompression has to be performed, sometimes at the bedside with a needle.

The timing of repair of EA is of particular interest. The key issues affecting the timing include severity of the infant's condition, associated abnormalities, and birth weight. The Spitz classification acknowledges low birth weight (<1500 g) and major congenital heart disease as two major risk factors associated with EA.[49] This system stratifies patients into groups. Survival was estimated at 97% for group I (weight >1500 g with no major congenital cardiac defect), 59% for group II (birth weight <1500 g or major congenital cardiac defect), and 22% for group III (birth weight <1500 g and major congenital cardiac defect). In 2006, Lopez and colleagues[50] examined the same risk factors in 188 neonates and found survival results comparable to those of Spitz, thus validating the Spitz classification.

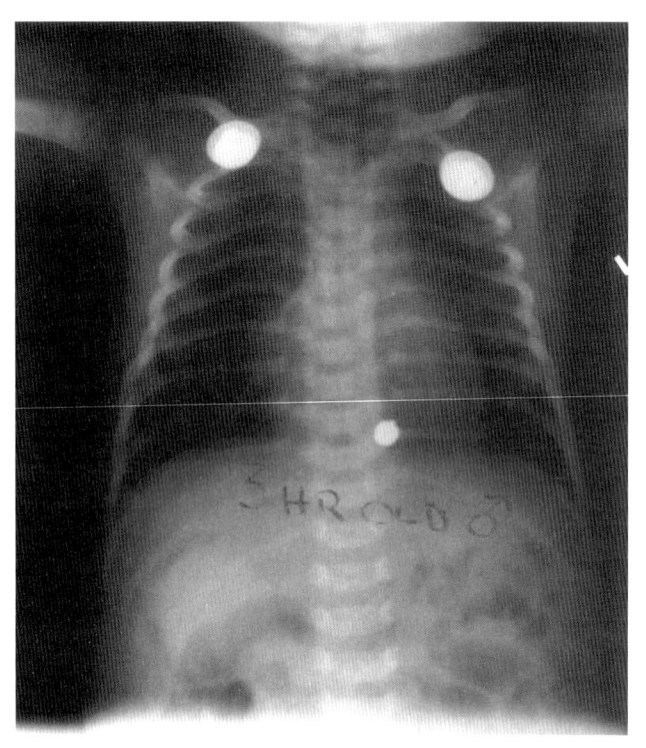

Figure 35–5
Air-contrast esophagogram in patient with esophageal atresia showing the distended proximal pouch. *(Courtesy of Dr. C. Leftridge, Georgetown University Medical Center.)*

Operative Principles

Rigid bronchoscopy is helpful at the beginning of the procedure to identify the exact location of the TEF, to recognize rare variants like double fistulas or H-type fistula and laryngotracheoesophageal clefts, to identify tracheomalacia, and to help in placement of the endotracheal tube to avoid dislodgement into the TEF (Fig. 35-7).[51-53]

Primary repair of EA with division of the TEF and end-to-end anastomosis is the ideal goal (Fig. 35-8). The standard approach is a right posterolateral thoracotomy. If the patient has a right-sided aortic arch, it might be easier to approach the esophagus from the left thorax. Having the patient tilted forward in the nearly prone position facilitates access to the posterior mediastinum. To minimize some of the complications reported with thoracotomy in neonates, namely, winged scapula and scoliosis, an axillary skin crease thoracotomy has been reported by Bianchi[54] and used with good results.[55] Traditionally, an extrapleural approach has been advocated to decrease the risk of empyema if an esophageal leak occurs. With the introduction of more powerful antibiotics in the 1970s and 1980s, the importance of a retropleural approach with the potential increase in operative time has been questioned.[41,56]

The posterior mediastinum is exposed by dividing the parietal pleura. The azygos vein is divided to allow access to the TEF, which is usually behind it. The fistula is circumferentially

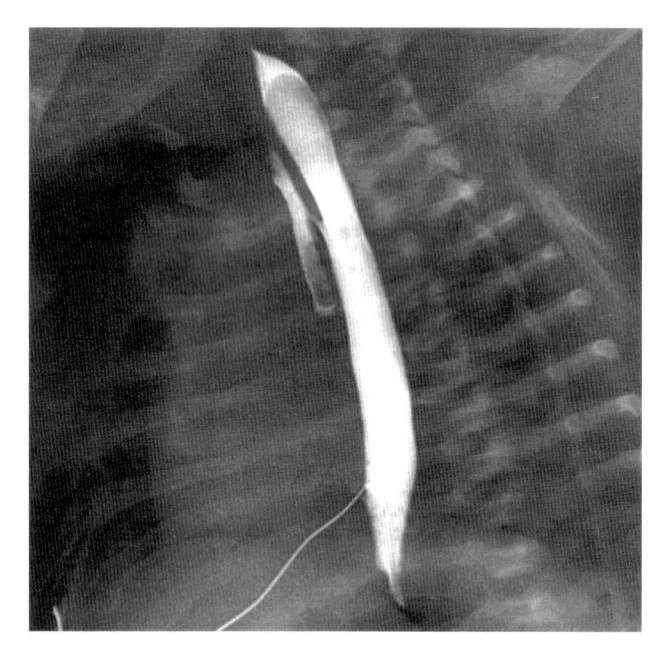

Figure 35–6
Contrast esophagogram showing an isolated tracheoesophageal fistula (H-type) with contrast material delineating the trachea. *(Courtesy of Dr. C. Leftridge, Georgetown University Medical Center.)*

controlled and occluded. The fistula is divided, leaving about 1 mm of esophageal tissue on the tracheal side to avoid narrowing of the tracheal lumen. Leaving more than a minimal amount of esophageal rim might create a pouch, which could accumulate secretions and cause repeated aspirations. The tracheal defect is closed in an airtight manner, usually with an absorbable monofilament suture.

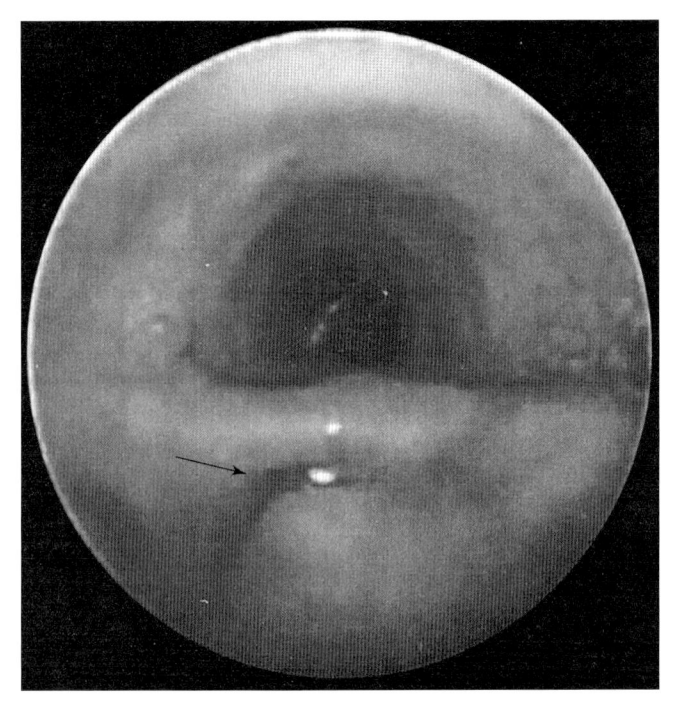

Figure 35–7
Bronchoscopic appearance of a tracheoesophageal fistula in the membranous portion of the trachea proximal to the carina.

Gentle pressure by the anesthesiologist on the pouch catheter helps identify the upper pouch, which is usually high in the thoracic inlet. A transmural suture placed through the fistula and incorporating the catheter makes the manipulation of the upper esophagus less traumatic. The upper pouch and the trachea are intimately juxtaposed, often sharing a common wall. The dissection between the esophageal pouch and the trachea is delicate. Extreme caution should be applied to avoid injury to both vagus and recurrent laryngeal nerves. The pouch is mobilized as high as possible to minimize the tension of the anastomosis. The blood supply of the upper esophagus is intramural, allowing minimal ischemia even after extensive mobilization. In contradistinction, the lower esophagus is supplied by segmental branches from the aorta; therefore, its mobilization should be minimized to prevent ischemia. The ends of the esophagus are trimmed, and an end-to-end anastomosis is built in a single-layer fashion with a fine monofilament absorbable suture. The knots are tied extraluminally if possible. It is crucial to identify the mucosa of both the upper and lower esophagus and to incorporate it in the sutures. If there is significant tension, it is helpful to leave the sutures untied and to approximate all at the same time as the knots are tied to take some of the tension off. The esophageal and tracheal suture lines must be separated to avoid fistula formation. This is usually accomplished by the interposition of a pleural flap, but a pericardial flap is sometimes required. The routine use of gastrostomy and transanastomotic feeding tubes remains controversial.[7] Before the anastomosis is constructed, congenital esophageal stenosis needs to be ruled out by passing a tube through the distal esophagus into the stomach.[57] At the completion of the procedure, a small chest tube is placed and secured to the endothoracic fascia away from the anastomosis. At about 5 or 7 days postoperatively, a contrast study is obtained to assess the anastomosis. The disparity in size between the distended proximal pouch and the small distal esophagus gives the appearance of a narrowing,

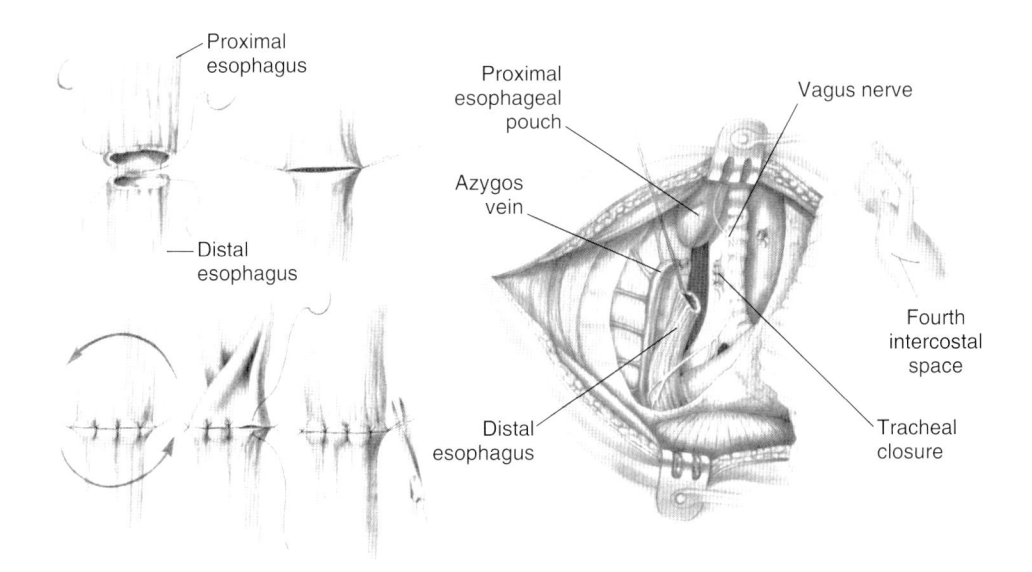

Figure 35–8
Construction of the anastomosis in a patient with esophageal atresia and tracheoesophageal fistula. End sutures are placed to draw the ends of the esophageal segments together. A single row of simple sutures completes the front-presenting portions of the anastomosis, with the knots tied on the outside. One of the corner sutures is passed behind the esophagus, which is then rotated 180 degrees. The anastomosis is completed with simple sutures in the presenting posterior surface, which has been rotated into view. It is essential that the sutures are full thickness because the mucosa has a tendency to retract.

but usually prompt emptying of contrast material attests to the wide patency of the anastomosis (Fig. 35-9A). With time, the size discrepancy becomes less pronounced (Fig. 35-9B). If there is no leak, the chest tube is removed and feedings are started. Because of the frequent occurrence of gastroesophageal reflux and the deleterious effects acid can have on a fresh anastomosis, serious consideration should be given to keeping the patient on acid suppressive and promotility drugs until the anastomosis is well healed.

Repair of EA in patients with significant gaps between the two ends of the esophagus can be challenging. The magnitude of the challenge is reflected in the number of innovative techniques described to save the native esophagus. Rehbein proposed approximating the two ends as much as possible and waiting for a fistula to develop around the sutures, then dilating that fistula.[58] Staging of the operation with initial ligation of the TEF and delayed primary anastomosis has been advocated.[59] The growth of the esophagus can be spontaneous or active with serial bougienage of the upper pouch. Delayed primary anastomosis is certainly a safe and effective strategy in patients with very low birth weight, in whom the tissues are friable, or in patients who are unstable.[13,35] Livaditis described performing a circular myotomy on the upper esophagus to gain length.[19] This has been used with good results by multiple groups.[60-62] Delayed ballooning and diverticulum formation are two described long-term complications of circular myotomy.[63,64] A second circular myotomy can be added through a cervical incision if more length is still needed. Kimura advocates elongation of the esophagus by a series of cervical esophagostomies with gradual elongation.[65] Foker proposed the application of tension on the two ends through sutures brought out of the skin and tightened sequentially.[66] Elongation of the distal esophagus by a Collis-Nissen fundoplication at the time of repair of EA has been described.[67] Schärli advocates division of the lesser curvature of the stomach to elongate it and partial gastric transfer to gain as much as 6 cm in length in the treatment of long gap atresia and pure EA.[68] Tubularization of the upper pouch after creation of a U-shaped flap is an attractive technique described by Bar-Maor and associates.[69]

The repair of pure EA without a TEF is even more challenging. The distal esophagus is usually very short and the gap significant. All of the preceding techniques can be tried in this situation. Most series report the most success with either

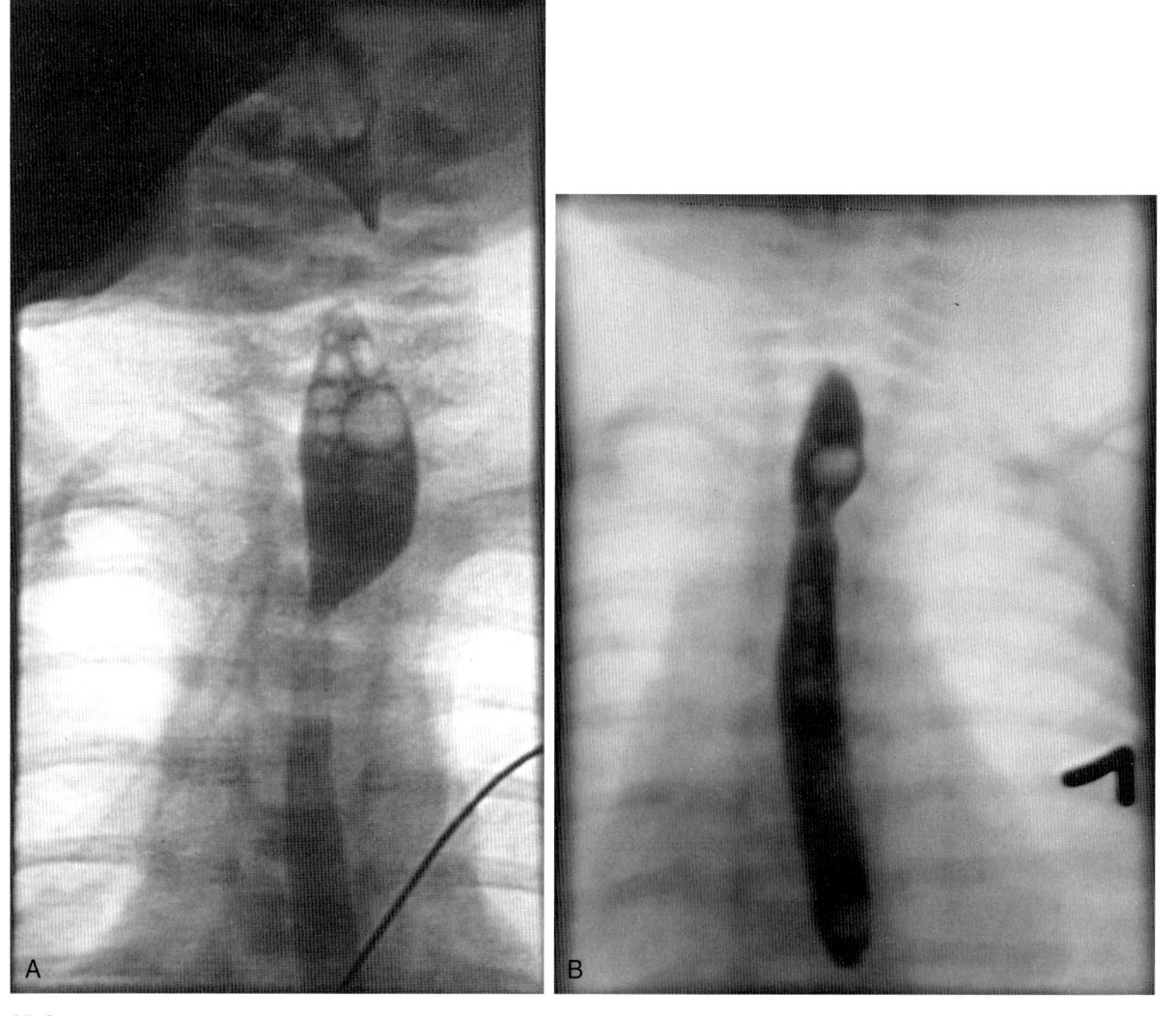

Figure 35–9
A, Postoperative esophagogram at 1 week revealing a patent anastomosis and a size discrepancy between the proximal and distal esophagus.
B, Esophagogram at 2 months postoperatively showing a decrease in the size discrepancy.

delayed primary anastomosis or esophageal replacement.[70] Colonic interposition, jejunal interposition, creation of a gastric tube, and gastric transposition are well-established techniques for esophageal replacement in children.[71-73]

The approach to an H-type fistula is usually through a right cervical incision because the majority of them are in the neck. Direct division of the fistula and repair of the esophagus and tracheal components are the goals (Fig. 35-10). Placement of a wire through the fistula by bronchoscopy and its retrieval from the mouth assist in the identification of the fistula and offer the opportunity to apply cephalad traction on the fistula to bring it up from the thorax if it is more distal than usual.[74]

In 1999, Lobe and Rothenberg performed the first thoracoscopic repair of isolated EA.[21] Since then, multiple groups have reported the successful thoracoscopic repair of EA with TEF (Fig. 34-11).[24,25,75] This method of repair has become more widely practiced. In 2005, Holcomb and colleagues[76] performed a multi-institutional retrospective review of 104 newborns with EA/TEF. Their results demonstrated advantages such as superior visualization of the anatomy within the thoracic cage and decreased musculoskeletal deformities (i.e., winged scapula, thoracic wall asymmetry, serratus anterior muscle atrophy, thoracic scoliosis). In comparison to open repair, operative time was slightly shorter at approximately 2 hours, and time on the ventilator was slightly longer at 3.5 days. Time at discharge (18 days) was comparable with the two techniques. However, this is a phase I study and does not answer the question of whether thoracoscopic technique is superior to the open approach.

Several other papers have been published on thoracoscopic treatment of EA.[77,78] However, none directly compares outcomes between thoracoscopic and open approaches.

This remains a point of interest and potential area of further research.

Complications and Long-term Effects

Complications of EA repair can be thought of as short term (leak, stricture) and long term (tracheomalacia, gastroesophageal reflux, nutrition, recurrent fistula, foreign body impaction).

Most large series report the rate of anastomotic leak to be between 15% and 20%.[36,41,79] Most leaks are small and can be managed nonoperatively with broad-spectrum antibiotics and thoracic drainage. Very rarely, suture repair or cervical diversion is required for a major leak.

The rate of esophageal stricture after repair is variable, ranging from 4% to about 50%.[36,41,79] The wide range probably reflects the variability in the criteria for defining the stenosis (whether it requires dilatations, the number of dilatations, and the need for resection). Singh and Shun[80] have proposed to spatulate the distal esophagus, creating a wider anastomosis, as a way to decrease the rate of stricture formation. Symptoms include choking, apnea, near-death spells, and food impaction. Most strictures are adequately treated with dilatations. Strictures that are refractory to dilatations should prompt a diligent search for and control of gastroesophageal reflux, often with a fundoplication. Recalcitrant strictures can also be secondary to the occurrence of ectopic tissues, tumors, or tracheobronchial remnants near the anastomosis.[57,81,82] The standard approach to refractory strictures has been a resection and reanastomosis. The application of interventional radiologic techniques has allowed the recanalization of impassable strictures that could not be dilated.[83,84]

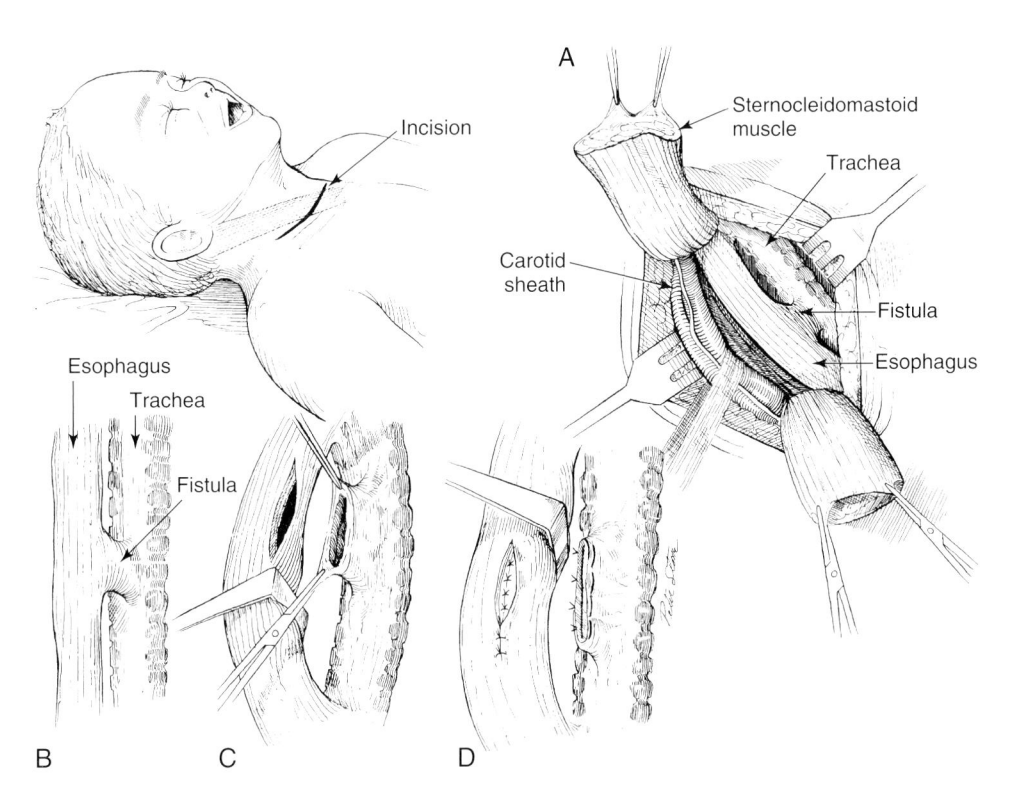

Figure 35–10
Repair of H-type fistula. An incision is made in the neck. The sternocleidomastoid is retracted or severed. The fistula is divided flush with the esophagus to ensure closure of the trachea without narrowing of the lumen.

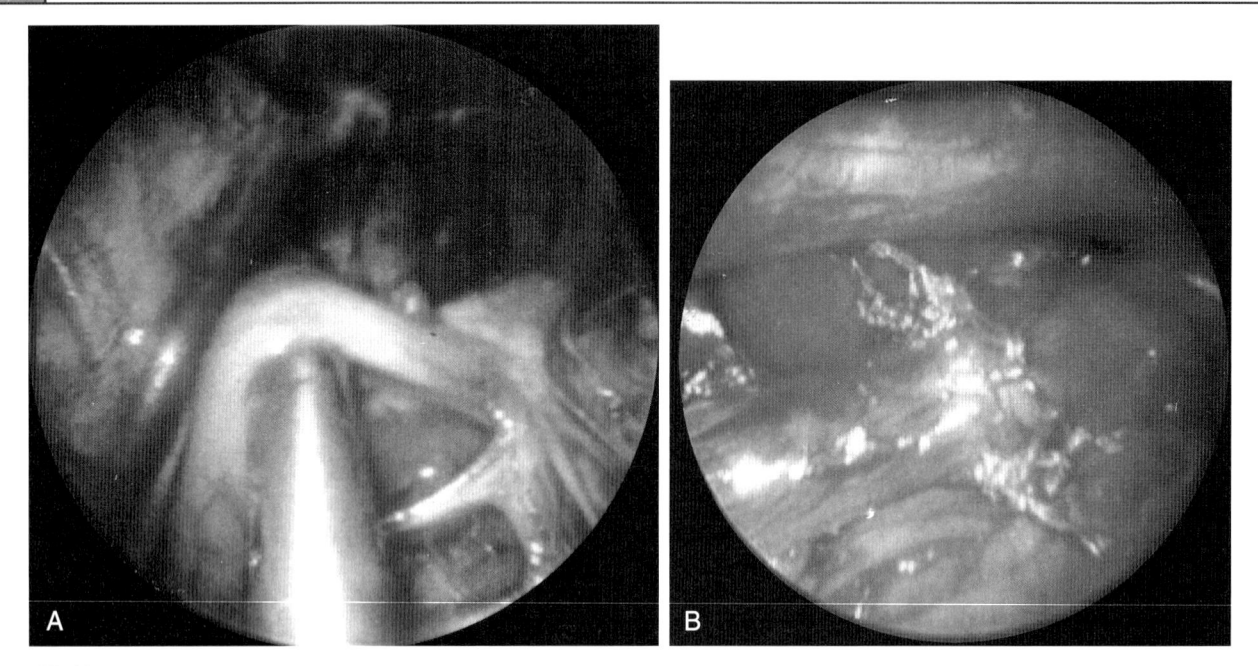

Figure 35–11
A, Thoracoscopic mobilization of the tracheoesophageal fistula. **B,** Thoracoscopic view of completed esophageal anastomosis. *(Courtesy of Dr. C. Albanese, Stanford University Medical Center.)*

Gastroesophageal reflux is a major concern in patients with EA, occurring in as many as 54% of patients.[36,79] It is a significant contributor to the rate of occurrence of leaks and strictures as well as to respiratory complications including aspiration pneumonia and cyanotic, near-death spells.[79] The majority of patients with significant gastroesophageal reflux eventually require a fundoplication to control their symptoms. The short-term morbidity of fundoplication in patients with EA is higher than in the general population, perhaps because of the dysmotility of the distal esophagus. A partial fundoplication, like the Toupet 270-degree wrap, could be considered in patients with severe dysmotility or small stomachs.

TEF recurs in as many as 10% of the patients after EA repair.[36,41,79,85] Symptoms include coughing, gagging, cyanotic and apneic spells, and recurrent respiratory infections. The diagnosis is difficult to make and relies heavily on contrast studies. Most will require repeated resection, but a few reports of bronchoscopic obliteration with fibrin glue, laser, or tissue adhesives have been published.[86-90]

Tracheomalacia is common in patients with EA and is thought to be secondary to the prolonged compression of the developing trachea by the enlarged esophageal pouch. Patients with EA and severe tracheomalacia often have a characteristic barking cough. Severe symptoms include stridor, choking, apnea, and near-death spells. The diagnosis is confirmed by bronchoscopy performed while the patient is spontaneously breathing and more recently by cine computed tomography and magnetic resonance imaging.[91,92] Symptomatic patients usually benefit from aortosternopexy. Sutures are placed in the adventitia of the aorta and fixed anteriorly to the sternum, therefore suspending the trachea and increasing its diameter. The improvement in diameter is monitored bronchoscopically (Fig. 34-12). This can be accomplished through a left thoracotomy or an anterior thoracotomy and more recently thoracoscopically.[91-93]

Andrassy and coworkers[94] have studied the long-term nutritional status of patients with EA. They found that even though the patients suffered from malnutrition in the first few years after repair, they seem to "catch up" in the later years, especially after the age of 13 years.

Foreign body impaction in the esophagus after EA repair occurs in at least 13% of patients.[95] Esophagoscopy is often needed to clear the esophagus, to evaluate for a stricture, and potentially to dilate the esophagus. No specific predisposing factors were identified, but the incidence of food impaction decreases after 5 years of age.

Several studies have discussed quality of life in adults who have undergone EA repair. In 2005, Deurloo and colleagues[96] investigated these quality of life issues in 97 patients 16 years and older who had undergone EA repair. A questionnaire was sent that included questions from the Gastrointestinal Quality of Life Index, the Illness Cognition Questionnaire, and three open-ended questions. The results to the open-ended questions included 8% who responded in the affirmative to a question asking if there were things that the patient would like to do but could not because of the EA repair. Limitations mentioned included inability to play certain sports, inability to lift heavy objects, and dysphagia. Thirty-three percent of participants thought that there were negative consequences of EA. Gastrointestinal symptoms were the most common responses. Fourteen percent of patients stated that they have positive experiences of EA in their daily life; 50% of these responders stated they were grateful to be alive.

In 2008, Deurloo and colleagues[97] investigated gastroesophageal reflux, esophageal function, and quality of life in 25 patients older than 18 years after EA repair. Manometry, pH measurement, and the patient's subjective feeling of dysphagia or heartburn were used to evaluate esophageal function. The study found that 70% of patients met manometric criteria for "ineffective esophageal motility." In this study, 20% of patients showed minor or pathologic reflux based on pH measurements.

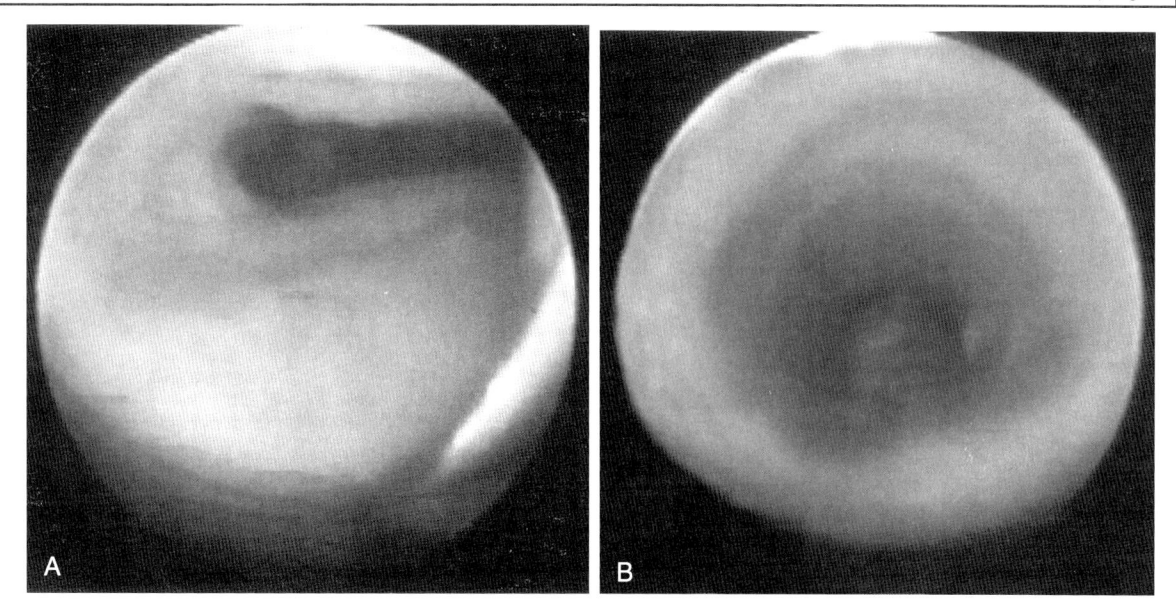

Figure 35–12
A, Bronchoscopic appearance of tracheomalacia in a patient with esophageal atresia with tracheoesophageal fistula. Note that the anterior and posterior walls of the trachea are almost touching. **B,** Bronchoscopic appearance of the same patient after aortosternopexy. The anterior wall is now stented open by the suspension of the aorta. *(Courtesy of Dr. D. Powell, Children's National Medical Center.)*

Interestingly, when these symptoms are compared with their effect on quality of life, dysphagia had a negative effect on quality of life but gastroesophageal reflux did not.

ESOPHAGEAL DUPLICATIONS

Anatomy and Embryology

The nomenclature of esophageal duplications is confusing. They have been referred to as enterogenous cysts, esophageal duplication cysts, neuroenteric cysts, and gastrocytomas, among others. In addition, there has been some confusion with bronchogenic cysts when these occur in the mediastinum between the esophagus and the trachea. Because the foregut and the notochord originate in direct continuity with each other and because both trachea and esophagus arise from the primitive foregut, it is helpful to view all these cysts as part of a continuum of foregut duplication cysts.[98] The duplications can be lined by alimentary or tracheobronchial mucosa, regardless of where they are located. About 50% of the cysts will contain ectopic gastric mucosa. They can be located in the posterior mediastinum or between the trachea and the esophagus. Cysts located in the posterior mediastinum are often associated with vertebral defects. Intramural duplications probably originate from a failure of vacuolization of the esophageal lumen.[1]

Most esophageal duplications do not communicate with the lumen, but they can be tubular, with one or more openings into the lumen. They can be localized to the chest or extend into the abdomen with extensive thoracoabdominal components. The majority are located in the distal esophagus, but they can occur anywhere along the length of the esophagus.[99,100]

Incidence

Esophageal duplications are rare, with an incidence of 1 in 8200.[99] Only 10% to 22% of alimentary duplications are esophageal.[100]

Presentation

About a third of patients with esophageal duplications are asymptomatic. Symptomatic patients present with a variety of respiratory and intestinal symptoms: dyspnea, wheezing, recurrent infections and pneumonias, dysphagia, anorexia, and bleeding if they have ectopic gastric mucosa.[98] If the cyst has a fistula to the spinal canal, meningitis can be the presenting symptom.

Diagnosis

Plain chest radiographs often show a mediastinal mass. These are also helpful in detecting any associated vertebral anomalies. A computed tomographic scan will delineate the mass further and allow an exact anatomic localization. If there are any vertebral anomalies, magnetic resonance imaging is helpful to rule out intraspinal disease. Contrast esophagography can show extrinsic or intrinsic compression.

Treatment

Complete resection is the preferred method of treatment, traditionally through a thoracotomy. Marsupialization and simple aspiration have a high recurrence rate. If the cyst shares a common wall with either the tracheobronchial tree or the esophagus, part of the wall can be left behind, but the mucosa has to be stripped to prevent recurrence. Intramural cysts are enucleated without violating the esophageal lumen. A bougie inserted into the esophagus might make the dissection easier. Posterior mediastinal cysts are usually easily excised unless they have an intraspinal component. Cysts located between the esophagus and the trachea can be challenging to remove because of the close association with the trachea. Long tubular thoracoabdominal duplications might require a combined thoracoabdominal approach.

Thoracoscopy and minimal access techniques have been used to resect a significant number of these cysts.[20,22,23,26,101]

As these techniques gain more acceptance and popularity, undoubtedly more and more of these lesions will be treated thoracoscopically.

CONGENITAL ESOPHAGEAL STENOSIS

Congenital esophageal stenosis is a rare anomaly.

Anatomy

Three types of congenital esophageal stenosis have been described: fibromuscular, membranous, and those secondary to tracheobronchial remnants. The last two are usually refractory to dilatations and require surgical relief. These lesions can coexist with EA and should be ruled out at the time of EA repair by insertion of a catheter into the distal esophagus.[57]

Presentation

Patients with congenital esophageal stenosis usually present with progressive feeding intolerance and regurgitation. The symptoms often are not manifested until the patient starts solid foods.

Diagnosis

An esophagogram is frequently diagnostic, showing the tapered narrowing in the distal esophagus similar to achalasia. Endoscopic ultrasonography has been employed to differentiate stenosis secondary to tracheobronchial remnants from that associated with fibromuscular hyperplasia.[102,103]

Treatment

Stenosis due to tracheobronchial remnants and intraluminal membranes does not respond to dilatation and requires resection with end-to-end anastomosis. One of the complications is esophageal shortening and gastroesophageal reflux. Nihoul-Fékété and colleagues[104] have recommended the addition of a Nissen fundoplication to the management of distal esophageal stenosis to prevent this complication. The combined Collis gastroplasty and Nissen fundoplication has been proposed to prevent both the shortening and the reflux.[105]

LARYNGOTRACHEOESOPHAGEAL CLEFT

Laryngotracheoesophageal cleft is a rare anomaly arising from the failure of orderly separation of the trachea and esophagus.

Anatomy

There are four subtypes of laryngotracheoesophageal cleft[106]:

Type I: cleft present to, but not below, the vocal cords
Type II: cleft extends into, but not through, the posterior cricoid cartilage
Type III: cleft extends through the cricoid cartilage
Type IV: cleft extends to the trachea

Presentation

There is a wide spectrum of presenting symptoms. Patients with types I to III can have subtle symptoms: chronic cough, wheezing, and repeated chest infections. Patients with type IV often have severe symptoms similar to those of patients with TEF: choking with feeding, severe aspiration pneumonia, and respiratory distress.

Diagnosis

Rigid bronchoscopy and esophagoscopy are essential in making the diagnosis. Other associated anomalies including TEF, gastroesophageal reflux disease, congenital heart disease, and cleft lip and palate should be sought.

Treatment

Observation of asymptomatic patients with type I clefts is often warranted. If they are symptomatic, repair can be performed endoscopically or open. Types II to IV clefts need to be repaired. The lateral pharyngotomy approach has been abandoned because of the high risk of recurrent laryngeal nerve injury and poor access to longer defects. The standard method is a transtracheal approach splitting the airway and trachea in the midline to expose the laryngotracheoesophageal cleft, which is then repaired. Long type IV clefts can be challenging to repair and might require cardiopulmonary bypass or extracorporeal membrane oxygenation. A multidisciplinary collaboration among pediatric surgeons, otorhinolaryngologists, and cardiac surgeons is often required.

If gastroesophageal reflux disease is significant, aggressive therapy with fundoplication enhances the chances of success of laryngotracheoesophageal cleft repair.

REFERENCES

1. Skandalakis JE, Gray SW, Ricketts R. The esophagus. In: Skandalakis JE, Gray SW, editors. *Embryology for surgeons.* Baltimore: Williams & Wilkins; 1994, 65-112.
2. Diez-Pardo JA, et al. A new rodent experimental model of esophageal atresia and tracheoesophageal fistula: preliminary report. *J Pediatr Surg* 1996;**31**(4):498-502.
3. Ioannides AS, et al. Role of *Sonic hedgehog* in the development of the trachea and oesophagus. *J Pediatr Surg* 2003;**38**(1):29-36.
4. Ioannides AS, et al. Dorsoventral patterning in oesophageal atresia with tracheo-oesophageal fistula: evidence from a new mouse model. *J Pediatr Surg* 2002;**37**(2):185-91.
5. Spilde TL, et al. Complete discontinuity of the distal fistula tract from the developing gut: direct histologic evidence for the mechanism of tracheoesophageal fistula formation. *Anat Rec* 2002;**267**(3):220-4.
6. Spilde TL, et al. Thyroid transcription factor-1 expression in the human neonatal tracheoesophageal fistula. *J Pediatr Surg* 2002;**37**(7):1065-7.
7. Harmon CM, Coran AG. Congenital anomalies of the esophagus. In: O'Neill JA, editor. *Pediatric surgery.* St. Louis: Mosby; 1998. p 941–967.
8. Koop CE, Hamilton JP. Atresia of the esophagus: increased survival with staged procedures in the poor-risk infant. *Ann Surg* 1965;**162**(3):389-401.
9. Waterston DJ, Bonham Carter RE, Aberdeen E. Oesophageal atresia: tracheo-oesophageal fistula. A study of survival in 218 infants. *Lancet* 1962;**1**:819-22.
10. Holder TM, McDonald VG, Woolley MM. The premature or critically ill infant with esophageal atresia: increased success with a staged approach. *J. Thorac Cardiovasc Surg* 1962;**44**(3):344-58.
11. Myers NA. Oesophageal atresia: the epitome of modern surgery. *Ann R Coll Surg Engl* 1974;**54**(6):277-87.
12. Abrahamson J, Shandling B. Esophageal atresia in the underweight baby: a challenge. *J Pediatr Surg* 1972;**7**(5):608-13.
13. Rickham PP. Infants with esophageal atresia weighing under 3 pounds. *J Pediatr Surg* 1981;**16**(4 Suppl. 1):595-8.
14. Pohlson EC, Schaller RT, Tapper D. Improved survival with primary anastomosis in the low birth weight neonate with esophageal atresia and tracheoesophageal fistula. *J Pediatr Surg* 1988;**23**(5):418-21.
15. Koop CE, Schnaufer L, Broennie AM. Esophageal atresia and tracheoesophageal fistula: supportive measures that affect survival. *Pediatrics* 1974;**54**(5):558-64.

16. Ito T, Sugito T, Nagaya M. Delayed primary anastomosis in poor-risk patients with esophageal atresia associated with tracheoesophageal fistula. *J Pediatr Surg* 1984;**19**(3):243-7.
17. Randolph JG, Newman KD, Anderson KD. Current results in repair of esophageal atresia with tracheoesophageal fistula using physiologic status as a guide to therapy. *Ann Surg* 1989;**209**(5):526-30:discussion 530-1.
18. Hays DM, Snyder WH. Results of conventional operative procedures for esophageal atresia in premature infants. *Am J Surg* 1963;**106**:19-23.
19. Livaditis A, Eklof O. Esophageal atresia with tracheoesophageal fistula: results of primary anastomosis in premature infants. *Z Kinderchir* 1973;**12**(1):32-9.
20. Rothenberg SS. Thoracoscopy in infants and children. *Semin Pediatr Surg* 1994;**3**(4):277-82.
21. Lobe TE, et al. Thoracoscopic repair of esophageal atresia in an infant: a surgical first. *Pediatr Endosurg Innov Tech* 1999;**3**:141-8.
22. Koizumi K, et al. Thoracoscopic enucleation of a submucosal bronchogenic cyst of the esophagus: report of two cases. *Surg Today* 1998;**28**(4):446-50.
23. Merry C, Spurbeck WE, Lobe TE. Resection of foregut-derived duplications by minimal-access surgery. *Pediatr Surg Int* 1999;**15**(3-4):224-6.
24. Rothenberg SS. Thoracoscopic repair of a tracheoesophageal fistula in a newborn infant. *Pediatr Endosurg Innov Tech* 2000;**4**(4):289-94.
25. Rothenberg SS. Thoracoscopic repair of tracheoesophageal fistula in newborns. *J Pediatr Surg* 2002;**37**(6):869-72.
26. Watson DI, Britten-Jones R. Thoracoscopic excision of bronchogenic cyst of the esophagus. *Surg Endosc* 1995;**9**(7):824-5.
27. Bax KM, van Der Zee DC. Feasibility of thoracoscopic repair of esophageal atresia with distal fistula. *J Pediatr Surg* 2002;**37**(2):192-6.
28. Harris J, Kallen B, Robert E. Descriptive epidemiology of alimentary tract atresia. *Teratology* 1995;**52**:15-29.
29. German JC, Mahour GH, Woolley MM. Esophageal atresia and associated anomalies. *J Pediatr Surg* 1976;**11**(3):299-306.
30. Cozzi F, Wilkinson AW. Low birthweight babies with oesophageal atresia or tracheo-oesophageal fistula. *Arch Dis Child* 1975;**50**(10):791-5.
31. Ein SH, et al. Esophageal atresia with distal tracheoesophageal fistula: associated anomalies and prognosis in the 1980s. *J Pediatr Surg* 1989;**24**(10):1055-9.
32. Depaepe A, Dolk H, Lechat MF. The epidemiology of tracheo-oesophageal fistula and oesophageal atresia in Europe. EUROCAT Working Group. *Arch Dis Child* 1993;**68**(6):743-8.
33. van Heurn LW, et al. Anomalies associated with oesophageal atresia in Asians and Europeans. *Pediatr Surg Int* 2002;**18**(4):241-3.
34. Saing H, Mya GH, Cheng W. The involvement of two or more systems and the severity of associated anomalies significantly influence mortality in esophageal atresia. *J Pediatr Surg* 1998;**33**(11):1596-8.
35. Chahine AA, Ricketts RR. Esophageal atresia in infants with very low birth weight. *Semin Pediatr Surg* 2000;**9**(2):73-8.
36. Manning PB, et al. Fifty years' experience with esophageal atresia and tracheoesophageal fistula. Beginning with Cameron Haight's first operation in 1935. *Ann Surg* 1986;**204**(4):446-53.
37. Driver CP, et al. Phenotypic presentation and outcome of esophageal atresia in the era of the Spitz classification. *J Pediatr Surg* 2001;**36**(9):1419-21.
38. Robert E, et al. An international collaborative study of the epidemiology of esophageal atresia or stenosis. *Reprod Toxicol* 1993;**7**(5):405-21.
39. Jolleys A. An examination of the birthweights of babies with some abnormalities of the alimentary tract. *J Pediatr Surg* 1981;**16**(2):160-3.
40. Anderson MS, Hay Jr WW. Intrauterine growth restriction and the small-for-gestational-age infant. In: Avery GB, Fletcher MA, MacDonald MG, editors. *Neonatology: pathophysiology and management of the newborn*. Philadelphia: Lippincott Williams & Wilkins; 1999. p 411-445.
41. Louhimo I, Lindahl H. Esophageal atresia: primary results of 500 consecutively treated patients. *J Pediatr Surg* 1983;**18**(3):217-29.
42. Spitz L, Kiely E, Brereton RJ. Esophageal atresia: five year experience with 148 cases. *J Pediatr Surg* 1987;**22**(2):103-8.
43. Holder TM, et al. Care of infants with esophageal atresia, tracheoesophageal fistula, and associated anomalies. *J Thorac Cardiovasc Surg* 1987;**94**(6):828-35.
44. Haeusler MC, et al. Prenatal ultrasonographic detection of gastrointestinal obstruction: results from 18 European congenital anomaly registries. *Prenat Diagn* 2002;**22**(7):616-23.
45. Shulman A, et al. Prenatal identification of esophageal atresia: the role of ultrasonography for evaluation of functional anatomy. *Prenat Diagn* 2002;**22**(8):669-74.
46. Benjamin B, Pham T. Diagnosis of H-type tracheoesophageal fistula. *J Pediatr Surg* 1991;**26**(6):667-71.
47. Templeton Jr JM, et al. Management of esophageal atresia and tracheoesophageal fistula in the neonate with severe respiratory distress syndrome. *J Pediatr Surg* 1985;**20**(4):394-7.
48. Filston HC. The Fogarty balloon catheter as an aid to management of the infant with esophageal atresia and tracheoesophageal fistula complicated by severe RDS or pneumonia. *J Pediatr Surg* 1982;**17**:149.
49. Spitz L, et al. Oesophageal atresia: at-risk groups for the 1990s. *J Pediatr Surg* 1994;**29**(6):723-5.
50. Lopez PJ, et al. Oesophageal atresia: improved outcome in high-risk groups? *J Pediatr Surg* 2006;**41**(2):331-4.
51. Filston HC, Rankin JS, Grimm JK. Esophageal atresia. Prognostic factors and contribution of preoperative telescopic endoscopy. *Ann Surg* 1984;**199**(5):532-7.
52. Garcia NM, Thompson JW, Shaul DB. Definitive localization of isolated tracheoesophageal fistula using bronchoscopy and esophagoscopy for guide wire placement. *J Pediatr Surg* 1998;**33**(11):1645-7.
53. Pigna A, et al. Bronchoscopy in newborns with esophageal atresia. *Pediatr Med Chir* 2002;**24**(4):297-301.
54. Bianchi A, et al. Aesthetics and lateral thoracotomy in the neonate. *J Pediatr Surg* 1998;**33**(12):1798-800.
55. Kalman A, Verebely T. The use of axillary skin crease incision for thoracotomies of neonates and children. *Eur J Pediatr Surg* 2002;**12**(4):226-9.
56. Schaarschmidt K, et al. Delayed primary reconstruction of an esophageal atresia with distal esophagotracheal fistula in an infant weighing less than 500 g. *J Pediatr Surg* 1992;**27**(12):1529-31.
57. Vasudevan SA, et al. Management of congenital esophageal stenosis. *J Pediatr Surg* 2002;**37**(7):1024-6.
58. Rehbein F, Schweder N. Reconstruction of the esophagus without colon transplantation in cases of atresia. *J Pediatr Surg* 1971;**6**(6):746-52.
59. Puri P, et al. Delayed primary anastomosis for esophageal atresia: 18 months' to 11 years' follow-up. *J Pediatr Surg* 1992;**27**(8):1127-30.
60. Lindahl H, Louhimo I. Livaditis myotomy in long-gap esophageal atresia. *J Pediatr Surg* 1987;**22**(2):109-12.
61. Ricketts RR, Luck SR, Raffensperger JG. Circular esophagomyotomy for primary repair of long-gap esophageal atresia. *J Pediatr Surg* 1981;**16**(3):365-9.
62. Slim MS. Circular myotomy of the esophagus: clinical application in esophageal atresia. *Ann Thorac Surg* 1977;**23**:62-6.
63. Janik JS, et al. Long-term follow-up circular myotomy for esophageal atresia. *J Pediatr Surg* 1980;**15**(6):835-41.
64. Otte JB, et al. Diverticulum formation after circular myotomy for esophageal atresia. *J Pediatr Surg* 1984;**19**(1):68-71.
65. Kimura K, et al. Multistaged extrathoracic esophageal elongation procedure for long gap esophageal atresia: Experience with 12 patients. *J Pediatr Surg* 2001;**36**(11):1725-7.
66. Foker JE, et al. Development of a true primary repair for the full spectrum of esophageal atresia. *Ann Surg* 1997;**226**(4):533-41:discussion 541-3.
67. Kawahara H, et al. Collis-Nissen procedure in patients with esophageal atresia: long-term evaluation. *World J Surg* 2002;**26**(10):1222-7.
68. Schärli AF. Esophageal reconstruction in very long atresias by elongation of the lesser curvature. *Pediatr Surg Int* 1992;**7**:101-5.
69. Bar-Maor JA, Shoshany G, Sweed Y. Wide gap esophageal atresia: a new method to elongate the upper pouch. *J Pediatr Surg* 1989;**24**(9):882-3.
70. Ein SH, Shandling B, Heiss K. Pure esophageal atresia: outlook in the 1990s. *J Pediatr Surg* 1993;**28**(9):1147-50.
71. Spitz L. Esophageal atresia: past, present, and future. *J Pediatr Surg* 1996;**31**(1):19-25.
72. Pedersen JC, Klein RL, Andrews DA. Gastric tube as the primary procedure for pure esophageal atresia. *J Pediatr Surg* 1996;**31**(9):1233-5.
73. Spitz L. Gastric transposition for esophageal substitution in children. *J Pediatr Surg* 1992;**27**(2):252-9.
74. Ko BA, et al. Simplified access for division of the low cervical/high thoracic H-type tracheoesophageal fistula. *J Pediatr Surg* 2000;**35**(11):1621-2.
75. Lovvorn HN, et al. Update on thoracoscopic repair of esophageal atresia with and without tracheoesophageal fistula. *Pediatr Endosurg Innov Tech* 2001;**5**(2):135-9.
76. Holcomb 3rd GW, et al. Thoracoscopic repair of esophageal atresia and tracheoesophageal fistula: a multi-institutional analysis. *Ann Surg* 2005;**242**(3):422-8:discussion 428-30.
77. Lima M, et al. Thoracoscopic treatment of oesophageal atresia. *Pediatr Med Chir* 2007;**29**(5):262-6.
78. Nguyen T, et al. Thoracoscopic repair of esophageal atresia and tracheoesophageal fistula: lessons learned. *J Laparoendosc Adv Surg Tech A* 2006;**16**(2):174-8.
79. Leenderste-Verloop K, et al. Postoperative morbidity in patients with esophageal atresia. *Pediatr Surg Int* 1987;**2**:2-5.
80. Singh SJ, Shun A. A new technique of anastomosis to avoid stricture formation in oesophageal atresia. *Pediatr Surg Int* 2001;**17**(7):575-7.
81. De La Hunt MN, Jackson CR, Wright C. Heterotopic gastric mucosa in the upper esophagus after repair of atresia. *J Pediatr Surg* 2002;**37**(5):E14.

82. Lee H, et al. Leiomyoma at the site of esophageal atresia repair. *J Pediatr Surg* 2001;**36**(12):1832-3.
83. Gilchrist BF, et al. The application of vascular technology to esophageal and airway strictures. *J Pediatr Surg* 2002;**37**(1):47-9.
84. Chahine AA, et al. Recanalization of an esophageal atresia anastomosis by an interventional radiologic technique. *Pediatr Endosurg Innov Tech* 2003;**7**(1):71-7.
85. Ein SH, et al. Recurrent tracheoesophageal fistulas: a seventeen-year review. *J Pediatr Surg* 1983;**18**(4):436-41.
86. Bhatnagar V, et al. Endoscopic treatment of tracheoesophageal fistula using electrocautery and the Nd:YAG laser. *J Pediatr Surg* 1999;**34**(3):464-7.
87. Lopes MF, et al. Endoscopic obliteration of a recurrent tracheoesophageal fistula with enbucrilate and polidocanol in a child. *Surg Endosc* 2003;**17**(4):657.
88. Hoelzer DJ, Luft JD. Successful long-term endoscopic closure of a recurrent tracheoesophageal fistula with fibrin glue in a child. *Int J Pediatr Otorhinolaryngol* 1999;**48**(3):259-63.
89. Gutierrez C, et al. Recurrent tracheoesophageal fistula treated with fibrin glue. *J Pediatr Surg* 1994;**29**(12):1567-9.
90. Brands W, Joppich I, Lochbuhler H. Use of highly concentrated human fibrinogen in paediatric surgery—a new therapeutic principle. *Z Kinderchir* 1982;**35**(4):159-62.
91. Weber TR, Keller MS, Fiore A. Aortic suspension (aortopexy) for severe tracheomalacia in infants and children. *Am J Surg* 2002;**184**(6):573-7:discussion 577.
92. Kimura K, et al. Aortosternopexy for tracheomalacia following repair of esophageal atresia: evaluation by cine-CT and technical refinement. *J Pediatr Surg* 1990;**25**(7):769-72.
93. Schaarschmidt K, et al. A technique for thoracoscopic aortopericardiosternopexy. *Surg Endosc* 2002;**16**(11):1639.
94. Andrassy RJ, et al. Long-term nutritional assessment of patients with esophageal atresia and/or tracheoesophageal fistula. *J Pediatr Surg* 1983;**18**(4):431-5.
95. Zigman A, Yazbeck S. Esophageal foreign body obstruction after esophageal atresia repair. *J Pediatr Surg* 2002;**37**(5):776-8.
96. Deurloo JA, et al. Quality of life in adult survivors of correction of esophageal atresia. *Arch Surg* 2005;**140**(10):976-80.
97. Deurloo JA, et al. Adults with corrected oesophageal atresia: is oesophageal function associated with complaints and/or quality of life? *Pediatr Surg Int* 2008;**24**(5):537-41.
98. Nobuhara KK, et al. Bronchogenic cysts and esophageal duplications: common origins and treatment. *J Pediatr Surg* 1997;**32**(10):1408-13.
99. Arbona JL, Fazzi JG, Mayoral J. Congenital esophageal cysts: case report and review of literature. *Am J Gastroenterol* 1984;**79**(3):177-82.
100. Fowler CL. Esophageal duplications. In: *Operative pediatric surgery*, Ziegler MM, Azizkhan RG, Weber T, editors. New York: McGraw-Hill; 2003. p 355–365.
101. Lewis RJ, Caccavale RJ, Sisler GE. Imaged thoracoscopic surgery: a new thoracic technique for resection of mediastinal cysts. *Ann Thorac Surg* 1992;**53**(2):318-20.
102. Usui N, et al. Usefulness of endoscopic ultrasonography in the diagnosis of congenital esophageal stenosis. *J Pediatr Surg* 2002;**37**(12):1744-6.
103. Kouchi K, et al. Endosonographic evaluation in two children with esophageal stenosis. *J Pediatr Surg* 2002;**37**(6):934-6.
104. Nihoul-Fékété C, et al. Congenital esophageal stenosis: a review of 20 cases. *Pediatr Surg Int* 1987;**2**:86-92.
105. Chahine AA, Campbell AB, Hoffman MA. Management of congenital distal esophageal stenosis with combined Collis gastroplasty–Nissen fundoplication. *Pediatr Surg Int* 1995;**10**:23-5.
106. Rutter MJ, Azizkhan RG, Cotton RT. Posterior laryngeal cleft. In: Ziegler MM, Azizkhan RG, Weber T, editors. *Operative pediatric surgery*. New York: McGraw-Hill; 2003, 313–320.

CHAPTER 36
Surgical Treatment of Benign Esophageal Diseases
Thomas W. Rice, Steven S. Shay, and Sudish C. Murthy

The Esophagus and Its Surroundings
  Esophageal Wall
  Regional Anatomy
Esophageal Function
Evaluation of the Esophagus
  History and Physical Examination
  Investigations
    Barium Esophagram
    Esophagoscopy
    Esophageal Manometry
    Ambulatory Conventional and Wireless pH
      Monitoring
    Impedance-pH Monitoring for Nonacid
      Reflux
  Endoscopic Esophageal Ultrasound

Other Investigations
  Bilitech 2000
  Impedance-Manometry
Benign Esophageal Diseases and Their
  Treatment
  Hiatal Hernia
  Gastroesophageal Reflux Disease
  Motility Disorders
    Achalasia
    Hypermotility Disorders
    Hypomotility Disorders
    Secondary Esophageal Motility Disorders
  Diverticula
    Zenker's Diverticulum
    Midthoracic Diverticula

Epiphrenic Diverticula
Benign Esophageal Tumors and Cysts
  Tumors of the Mucosa
  Tumors of the Submucosa
  Tumors of the Muscularis Propria
  Esophageal Cysts
Esophageal Injuries
  Strictures
  Corrosive Injuries
  Perforations
  Esophageal Foreign Bodies
Conclusions

It is preferable to bring your own esophagus to dinner.
                                   Lucius D. Hill, MD

The esophagus actively transports solids and liquids from the pharynx to the stomach. It has no digestive, absorptive, metabolic, or endocrine functions. A muscular tube subtended by two sphincters performs this rudimentary transfer task. Despite simplicity in esophageal function and form, surgical treatment of benign esophageal disorders is challenging. Few options are available to repair damaged sphincters; disorders of the esophageal body are rarely amenable to surgical correction. Often, progressive disease and failed surgical therapy result in a nonrepairable esophagus. The only treatment option is resection and replacement. Successful surgical therapy requires a sound understanding of esophageal anatomy, physiology, investigative techniques, and disease processes.

THE ESOPHAGUS AND ITS SURROUNDINGS

Esophageal Wall

The esophagus is lined with stratified, nonkeratinizing squamous epithelium (Fig. 36-1), isolated from the remainder of the esophageal wall by a basement membrane. Immediately beneath the basement membrane is the lamina propria, a thin layer of loose connective tissue with a complex of collagen and elastic fibers. It contains a network of endothelium-lined channels, both capillaries and lymphatics. The muscularis mucosae supports the lamina propria and is composed of a longitudinal layer of smooth muscle. This continuous muscle layer pleats the inner layers of the esophagus into a series of folds that disappear with distension. The epithelium, lamina propria, and muscularis mucosae comprise the esophageal mucosa.

The submucosa is composed of connective tissue that contains a network of blood vessels and lymphatics. Elastic fibers and collagen combine to make this the strongest esophageal layer. Submucosal glands are mixed types, producing a combination of serous and mucous secretions. These submucosal glands are unique to the esophagus and allow differentiation of the esophagus from the stomach in instances of glandular epithelial metaplasia. Ducts from these glands pierce the mucosa to drain into the esophageal lumen.

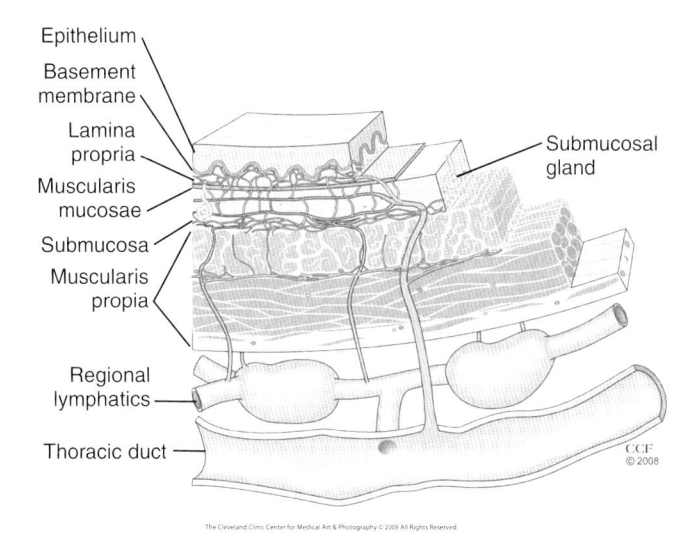

Figure 36–1
Esophageal wall and its unique lymphatic drainage. *(The Cleveland Clinic Center for Medical Art and Photography. © 2009. All rights reserved.)*

The muscularis propria is the muscular sleeve that provides the propulsive force necessary for swallowing. There are two layers of muscle: an inner circular layer and an outer longitudinal layer. The proximal 4% to 5% of the esophagus is composed completely of striated muscle and the distal 54% to 62% completely of smooth muscle.[1] Smooth muscle first appears in the anterior circular layer. The transition from striated to smooth muscle in the circular muscle layer is gradual, and the 50% point is approximately 5 cm from the cricopharyngeus muscle.

The cricopharyngeus (upper esophageal sphincter [UES]) is a continuous transverse band of muscle originating from the cricoid cartilage (Fig. 36-2). Superiorly, the muscle of the cricopharyngeus blends with the inferior pharyngeal constrictor muscle. A posterior defect, Killian's triangle, is an inverted fan–shaped weakness in the inferior constrictor at the superior border of the cricopharyngeus. Inferiorly, the cricopharyngeus merges with the inner, circular layer of the muscularis propria. The longitudinal muscle layer of the muscularis propria originates from the lateral aspect of the cricoesophageal tendon. Posteriorly, these anterior and lateral components converge to meet at the midline. Thus, the proximal 1 to 2 cm of the posterior cervical esophagus is composed only of inner circular muscle, creating a potential for a mirror-image triangular area of weakness called Laimer's triangle.

Contraction of the longitudinal muscle fibers of the esophageal body produces esophageal shortening. The inner circular muscle is arranged in incomplete rings producing a helical pattern. Muscle layers are equal and uniform in thickness until the distal 3 to 4 cm of the esophagus. Here, the inner circular layer thickens and divides into incomplete horizontal muscular clasps on the lesser curve aspect of the distal esophagus, and oblique fibers on the greater curve aspect. These become gastric sling fibers (see Fig. 36-2). Although no complete circular bands exist at the lower esophageal sphincter (LES), it is this area of rearranged circular fibers that corresponds to the high-pressure zone of the LES.

The esophagus lies in a bed of fat, neurovascular, and connective tissue and elastic fibers termed the adventitia. This layer of loose connective tissue surrounding the esophagus contains lymphatics and regional lymph nodes, blood vessels, and nerves. Unlike the stomach, small bowel, and colon, it has no serosa, except in its short abdominal segment.

Lymphatics begin as blind endothelium-lined saccules in the lamina propria just below the epithelium and basement membrane. Recent immunohistochemical study of the esophageal wall using lymphatic endothelial marker D2-40 has provided new insight into the lymphatic anatomy of the esophageal wall (see Fig. 36-1).[2] There is a dense longitudinal plexus of lymphatic vessels in the lamina propria. Rare perforating lymphatics have been found draining into a sparse circumferential lymphatic network in the outer margin of the submucosa. Perforating lymphatics from the submucosal plexus, usually running with an artery and vein, penetrate the inner circular layer of the muscularis propria. Here, they drain into a circumferential intramuscular plexus that accompanies the artery, vein, and nerves of this space. Afferent lymphatics usually accompanied by an artery and a vein drain the intramuscular plexus into the lymphatic channels in the adventitia. No direct connection from the lamina propria network and the thoracic duct has been identified.[2] Existence of direct routes from mural lymphatics to the thoracic duct, without a relay through regional lymphatics and lymph nodes, has been documented by many authors; however, the exact patterns and occurrence of these pathways are highly variable.[3-5]

The arterial supply of the esophagus is parasitic. It is derived from blood vessels supplying other organs in the neck, chest, and abdomen. Generally, these vessels divide at a distance from the esophagus and send small segmental branches to that segment of the esophagus. Esophageal blood supply has three principal sources. The superior and inferior thyroid arteries supply the cervical esophagus. The proximal and middle thoracic esophagus receives blood from branches of the bronchial arteries. The only dedicated esophageal arteries are one or two branches that arise from the anterior aspect of the aorta below the tracheal carina. In a third of autopsy specimens, no esophageal artery could be identified.[6] These esophageal arteries directly supply the lower thoracic esophagus. The lower thoracic esophagus and abdominal esophagus receive arterial branches from the left gastric and, occasionally, the splenic arteries. The combination of a segmented arterial supply derived from multiple sources and a rich intramural vascular plexus ensures an excellent esophageal blood flow and permits extensive esophageal mobilization without esophageal arterial insufficiency or ischemia. Because esophageal arteries branch from larger arteries some distance from the esophagus, stripping of the esophagus from its bed during transhiatal (blunt) esophagectomy is possible without direct ligation of the esophageal arterial supply. Arterial spasm provides adequate hemostasis; thus, significant bleeding does not complicate this procedure.

Subepithelial esophageal venules drain into a substantial submucosal venous plexus that extends the length of the

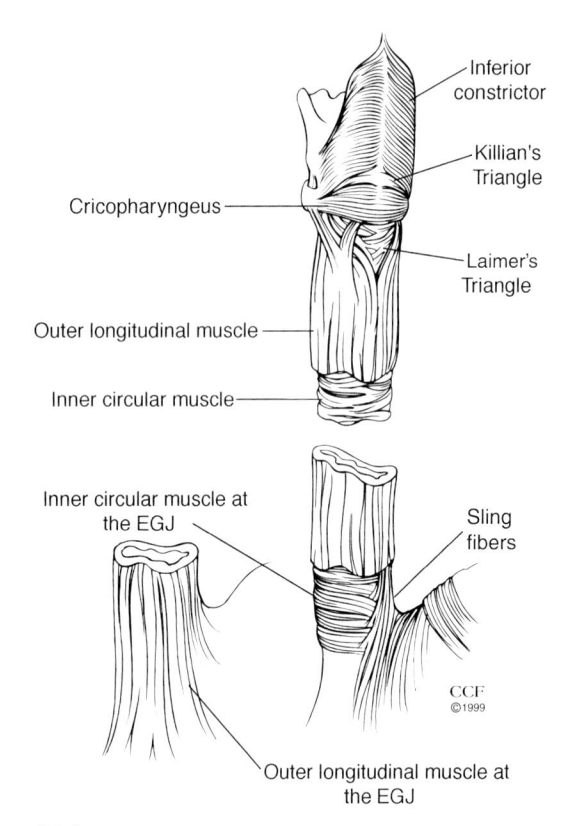

Figure 36–2
Esophageal musculature. EGJ, esophagogastric junction.

esophagus.[7] There are venous connections between the lower thoracic and abdominal esophagus and the portal venous system. Venules then pierce the muscularis propria to drain into veins on the surface of the esophagus. Regional drainage is directed to the inferior thyroid and brachiocephalic veins in the neck, the azygos and hemiazygos veins in the chest, and the left gastric and splenic veins in the abdomen.

Both parasympathetic and sympathetic nerves innervate the esophagus. Branches of the vagus nerve supply parasympathetic fibers that are motor to the muscle coat and secretomotor to the submucosal glands. The cervical and thoracic sympathetic chain and the celiac plexus provide sympathetic fibers that promote contraction of sphincters and relaxation of the esophageal body muscle, increase peristaltic and glandular activity, and cause vasoconstriction. These fibers enter the esophageal wall with the blood supply and form fibers and ganglia within it. The myenteric (Auerbach's) plexus is positioned between the longitudinal and circular layers of the muscularis propria, and it controls these muscles. The submucosal (Meissner's) plexus controls the muscularis mucosae and submucosal glands.

Regional Anatomy

The esophagus spans the lower neck, thoracic cavity, and upper abdomen (Fig. 36-3). The anatomy of the esophagus is best divided into fifths: cervical, upper thoracic, middle thoracic, lower thoracic, and abdominal esophagus. The anterior wall of the cervical esophagus is in intimate contact with the posterior membranous trachea. The recurrent laryngeal nerves course anteriorly and laterally in the tracheoesophageal groove. The carotid sheaths bind the cervical esophagus laterally. The posterior wall of the cervical esophagus lies on the vertebral bodies.

The thoracic esophagus occupies the posterior mediastinum and passes anteriorly to the vertebral bodies. The upper thoracic esophagus lies posteriorly to the trachea and is bound laterally by the mediastinal pleura. In its lower left aspect, it is sandwiched between the azygos vein on the right and the aortic arch on the left. The middle thoracic esophagus lies behind the pulmonary hilum and between the azygos vein and descending aorta. The lower thoracic esophagus has the same lateral and posterior boundaries, but it lies behind the pericardium. The thoracic duct is situated between the azygos vein and the descending thoracic aorta, and posteriorly and to the right of the lower and midthoracic esophagus. At approximately the level of the fourth thoracic vertebra, it crosses the midline to become a left-sided structure.

The abdominal esophagus is cradled in the muscular esophageal hiatus. The inferior vena cava is on the right posterolateral aspect, the abdominal aorta on the left posterolateral aspect. Superiorly, the left lateral segment of the liver overlies the esophagus and the esophagogastric junction.

ESOPHAGEAL FUNCTION

Swallowing has three phases: oral, pharyngeal, and esophageal. The action of swallowing is voluntarily initiated and is followed by a cascade of involuntary muscle activities that propels the swallowed bolus aborally. The esophageal phase of swallowing commences with the relaxation of the UES during the initiation of pharyngeal contraction. Food is pushed by pharyngeal contraction, and its transit is facilitated by negative intrathoracic pressure. Duration of UES relaxation is between 0.5 and 1 second. After passage of the bolus, the UES contracts, reaching twice resting pressure. The primary peristaltic wave is a progressive contraction activated by

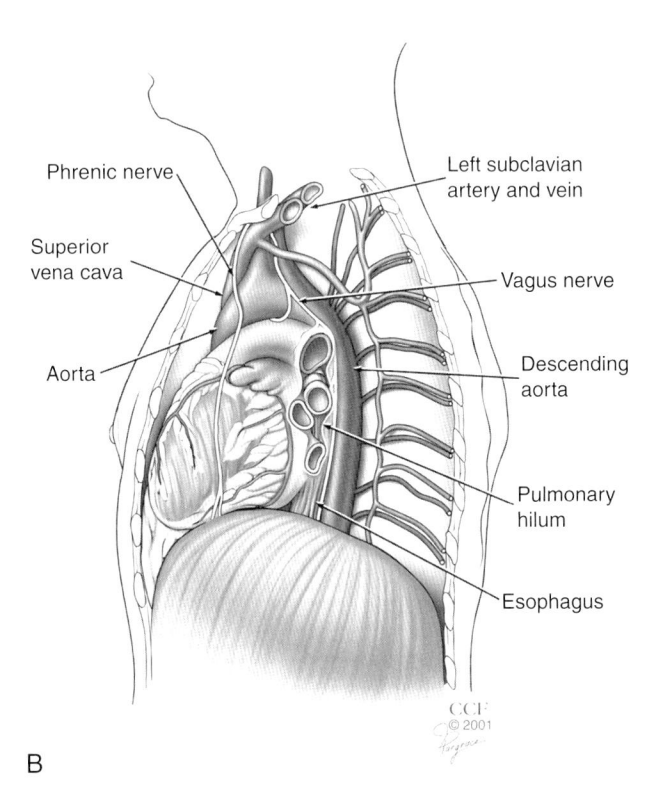

Figure 36–3
Regional anatomy. **A**, Right mediastinal view. **B**, Left mediastinal view.

voluntary swallowing. With an antegrade peristaltic contraction speed of 2 to 7 cm/sec, a wave carries the bolus into the stomach. The strength of the primary peristaltic contraction increases with propagation along the esophagus. In more than 90% of wet swallows, a primary wave normally follows. If impaction occurs, esophageal distension produces closure of the UES, and a secondary peristaltic wave begins at the site of obstruction and passes distally. Tertiary contractions are nonperistaltic contractions occurring spontaneously between swallows, and they are ineffective in antegrade bolus transit.

Resting pressure of the LES exceeds intragastric pressure and prevents reflux of gastric contents into the distal esophagus. Within 2 seconds of pharyngeal contraction, the LES relaxes to near intragastric pressure for 7 to 10 seconds. The LES then contracts to greater than resting pressure for 8 to 12 seconds before return to resting pressure.

EVALUATION OF THE ESOPHAGUS

History and Physical Examination

The symptoms most commonly associated with esophageal diseases are heartburn, regurgitation, dysphagia, and odynophagia. Other symptoms that may be associated with esophageal disease are sore throat, hoarseness, cough, bad taste, globus, hiccup, aspiration, wheezing, chest pain, nausea, vomiting, choking, hematemesis, and melena. Symptom composition depends on the esophageal disorder and is discussed in various sections of this chapter. Physical examination of the esophagus is indirect and focuses on head and neck, thoracic, and abdominal findings.

Box 36-1 lists systemic diseases with esophageal manifestations. Some are discussed later in this chapter. These potential underlying disorders should be considered while obtaining the patient's history and performing the physical examination.

Investigations

Patients with suspected esophageal disease will typically undergo barium esophagram or esophagoscopy, or both, in their initial diagnostic testing.

Barium Esophagram

A three-phase study assessing mucosa, contour, and function of the esophagus is optimal.[8] First, the mucosa is examined in the double-contrast phase, in which the patient, in the upright position, ingests high-density barium and CO_2 tablets (Fig. 36-4). Next, esophageal function is assessed with the patient in the right anterior oblique (RAO) position and ingesting low-density barium in single swallows at 20- to 30-second intervals (Fig. 36-5). The examination is videotaped. The value of attempting to elicit reflux in this phase is questionable, because 20% of normal individuals have radiologic reflux.[9] Barium tablets, or barium-coated marshmallows or solids, may demonstrate abnormalities not visualized by liquid barium studies. The final phase, the full-column technique, is performed with the patient in a semiprone RAO position and with low-density barium. Multiple quick swallows produce a column of barium that fully distends the esophagus. This optimizes imaging of the distal esophagus and can demonstrate small hiatal hernias, subtle strictures, or distal rings (Fig. 36-6). The esophagus is allowed to empty, and the remaining barium coating the esophageal wall provides a mucosal relief study, now rarely performed.

A timed barium esophagogram is a simple test of esophageal emptying (Fig. 36-7). After ingestion of a premeasured amount of barium, usually 250 mL, spot films are taken at 1-, 2- and 5-minute intervals and, if necessary, at 10 minutes and 20 minutes after barium ingestion. This allows simple quantification of esophageal emptying and is useful for evaluating motility disorders and to follow therapy.[10,11]

Esophagoscopy

Esophagoscopy is used to visually assess mucosal and structural esophageal abnormalities. Biopsies of epithelial abnormalities such as esophagitis, mucosal nodules, columnar

---

Box 36–1
Systemic Diseases of the Esophagus

Connective tissue disorders
　Scleroderma
　Systemic lupus erythematosus
　Polymyositis
　Dermatomyositis
　Mixed connective tissue disorder
　Raynaud's disease
Allergic diseases
　Eosinophilic esophagitis
Metabolic diseases
　Amyloidosis
　Diabetes mellitus
　Hypothyroidism
　Hyperthyroidism
Dermatologic diseases
　Epidermolysis bullosa
　Pemphigus vulgaris
　Pemphigoid
　Erythema multiforme
　Lichen planus
　Behçet's disease
Infectious diseases
　Histoplasmosis
　Tuberculosis
　Actinomycosis
　In the immunocompromised host:
　　Fungal: *Candida* species
　　Viral: herpes simplex, cytomegalovirus
　　Mycobacterial
　　Bacterial: *Streptococcus viridans*, *Staphylococcus*, bacilli, *Treponema pallidum*
　　Protozoal
Miscellaneous disorders
　Sarcoidosis
　Crohn's disease

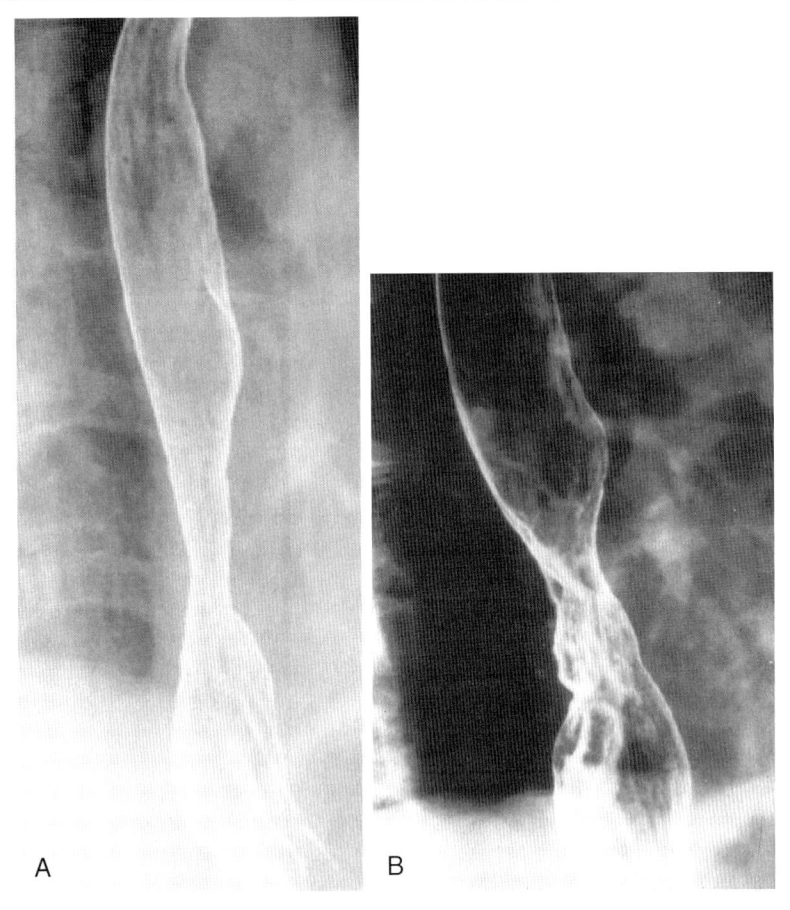

Figure 36–4
Barium esophagram: mucosa. Double-contrast phase of the barium esophagram provides mucosal definition. **A,** Patient with a hiatal hernia and peptic stricture; no significant ulceration is seen. **B,** Patient with a columnar cell–lined esophagus, distal peptic stricture, ulcers, and nodules.

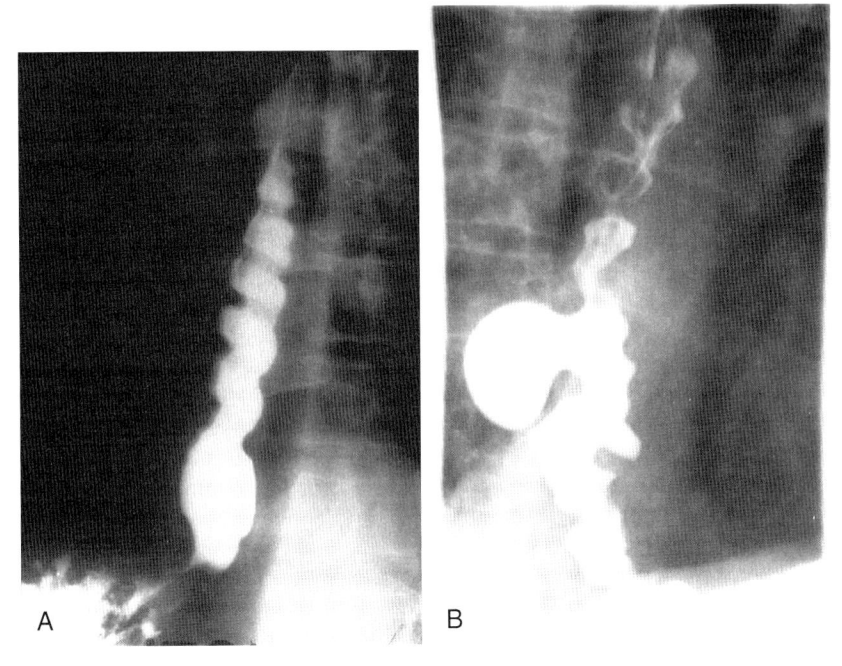

Figure 36–5
Barium esophagram: function. Single swallows every 20 to 30 seconds with the patient in the right anterior oblique semiprone position assesses esophageal function. **A,** Patient with diffuse esophageal spasm (cork-screw esophagus). **B,** Patient with abnormal motility and a midthoracic diverticulum.

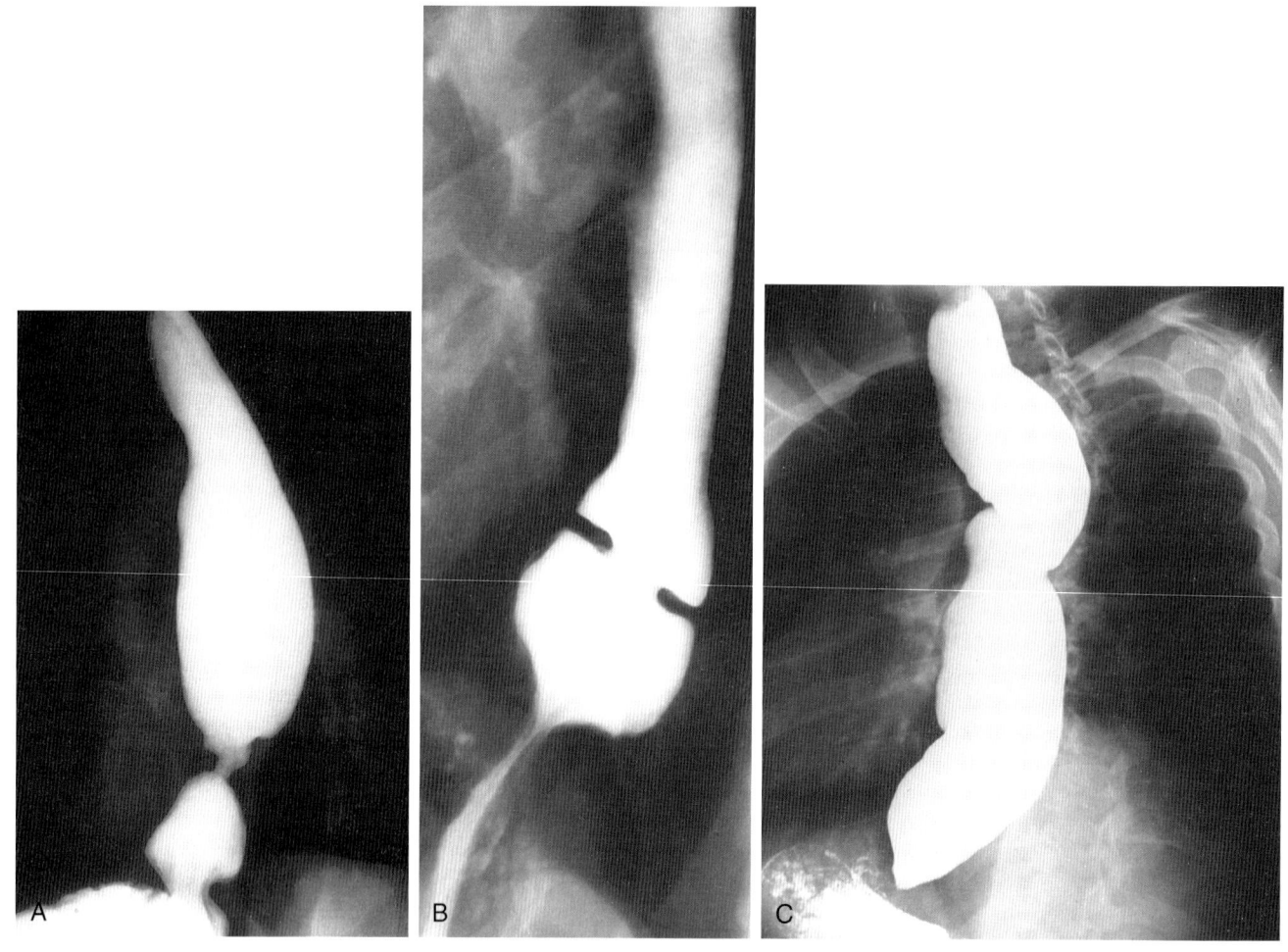

Figure 36–6
Barium esophagram: contour. The full-column phase of the barium esophagram fills and fully distends the esophagus, providing an opportunity to examine the esophageal contour. **A,** Patient with an obstructed esophagus due to a peptic stricture and associated nonreducible hiatal hernia. **B,** Patient with a Schatzki's ring. **C,** Patient with achalasia.

cell–lined segments, and strictures are an integral part of flexible fiberoptic esophagoscopy. However, the biopsies are limited to the mucosa. Indirect evidence of deeper mural abnormalities or extraesophageal lesions may be appreciated by extrinsic compression or displacement of the overlying epithelium.

Esophageal Manometry

Esophageal manometry is most commonly performed in patients with esophageal dysphagia, in patients with chest pain after excluding cardiac disease, and prior to antireflux surgery. Water-perfused fine capillary tubes or solid-state microtransducers with three to eight pressure sensors at variable distances apart have traditionally been used. However, a catheter has been developed with 36 solid-state pressure sensors 1 cm apart that offers high-resolution manometry (HRM) from the pharynx to the proximal stomach (Manoscan, Sierra Scientific, Los Angeles). It makes accurate catheter placement easier and markedly shortens procedure length by eliminating the LES pull-through. A disadvantage is its higher cost. In addition, it has not been demonstrated that the new observations with HRM translate to better outcomes.

LES resting pressure and length, but most importantly completeness of LES relaxation, are measured (Table 36-1). HRM allows more accurate measurement of LES relaxation than traditional manometry by compensating for the LES movement with swallows. Esophageal body parameters to assess are antegrade esophageal peristalsis, contraction amplitude, and duration. HRM allows generation of a spatiotemporal plot, where segments of the peristaltic wave-front can be separately analyzed (Fig. 36-8).[12] Direct comparison with traditional manometry shows that HRM is more accurate at predicting abnormal barium bolus transport, especially with mild or moderate esophageal dysmotility.[13] Reclassification of esophageal motility disorders based on HRM has been suggested,[12,14] but further reports, including outcome studies, are needed to confirm validity. UES measurements have not been found to be clinically useful.

Ambulatory Conventional and Wireless pH Monitoring

Ambulatory pH monitoring detects and quantifies acid gastroesophageal reflux. Because this test is typically performed without acid-suppression medication, proton pump inhibitors should be discontinued for 1 week, histamine 2 (H_2) blockers

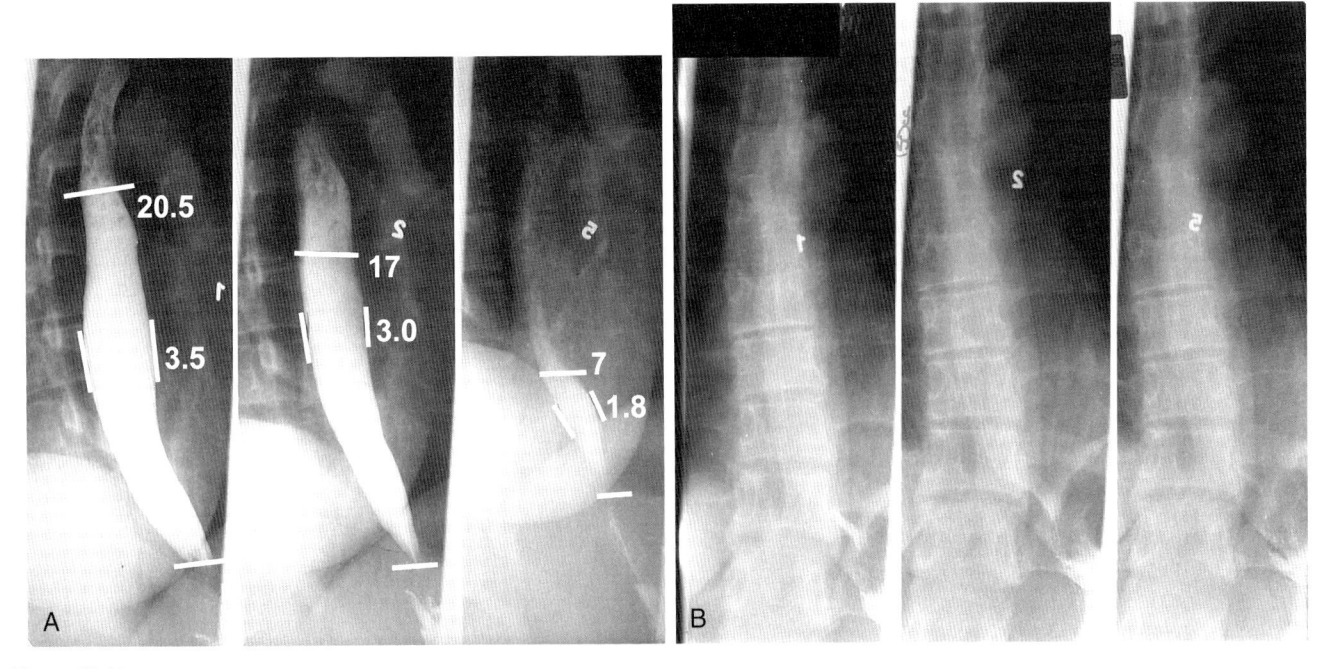

Figure 36–7
Timed-barium esophagram. **A,** Before Heller's myotomy, this patient was able to ingest only 70 of the 250 mL of barium requested. Height (barium-coated saliva not included) and width of the column are measured at 1, 2, and 5 minutes after ingestion. Note markedly delayed esophageal emptying and incomplete emptying at 5 minutes. **B,** After Heller's myotomy, ingestion of 70 mL of barium resulted in trace barium in the esophagus at 1 and 2 minutes and clearance by 5 minutes.

Table 36–1
Normal Values for Traditional Esophageal Manometry at Cleveland Clinic

	Normal*	High	Low
Lower esophageal sphincter pressure (mm Hg)	24 ± 10	>45	<10
Contraction amplitude† (mm Hg)	99 ± 40	>180	<30
Contraction duration† (sec)	3.9 ± 0.9	>7	<1.3

*Mean ± standard deviation.
†Mean of measurements at 3 cm and 8 cm above the LES.
From Richter JE, Wu WC, Johns DN, et al. Dig Dis Sci 1987;32(6):583-92.[190]

for 24 hours, and antacids for 8 hours. Transnasal monitoring is done for 24 hours with the thin pH catheter placed 5 cm above the LES, located by manometry. Patients are instructed to have a "typical day" regarding activity and eating. Because symptom correlation is an important component of this test, the patient presses a symptom button when a symptom is felt.

A pH below 4 has arbitrarily been chosen to define an acid reflux episode. The normal parameters for 24-hour pH monitoring, based on this reference, have been defined (Table 36-2). Total acid exposure time, expressed as a percentage of study time, is the best discriminator between normal and abnormal.[15,16] Composite scores, such as the DeMeester score and the frequency-duration index, are no better than simple measured parameters in identifying abnormal reflux. The symptom index relates symptoms to reflux events and is calculated by dividing symptom episodes with reflux by the total number of symptom episodes multiplied by 100%; 50% is the optimum threshold.[17]

Wireless pH monitoring is a recent technological advance. The Bravo delivery system "pins" a 6 × 5.5 × 25-mm capsule to the esophagus 6 cm above the squamocolumnar junction, identified by endoscopy. Manometry is not required. Improved patient tolerance allows increased activities and improved food intake; moreover, monitoring is traditionally extended to 48 hours (Fig. 36-9).[18] A 2008 American Gastroenterological Association Institute position paper states that wireless pH monitoring has superior sensitivity for detecting pathologic acid reflux.[19] Drawbacks are cost, occasional premature detachment, and severe pain requiring endoscopic removal in less than 2% of cases. Like nasal pH monitoring, it is unable to detect nonacid reflux.

Impedance-pH Monitoring for Nonacid Reflux

When an ionic fluid bolus traverses an electrode pair, impedance to current flow decreases. Impedance pairs placed on a pH catheter at multiple sites can detect retrograde fluid flow throughout the esophagus as acid reflux if the pH is less than 4, or nonacid reflux if pH is greater than 4.[20] An expert panel concluded that impedance-pH monitoring when the patient is *off* proton pump inhibitor (PPI) therapy is the best test to detect all reflux episodes in a patient[21] and thus is the best test for symptom association in patients with gastroesophageal reflux disease (GERD). However, it has limitations: a nasal catheter is necessary, and inaccuracies in current software require manual data correction of the study.

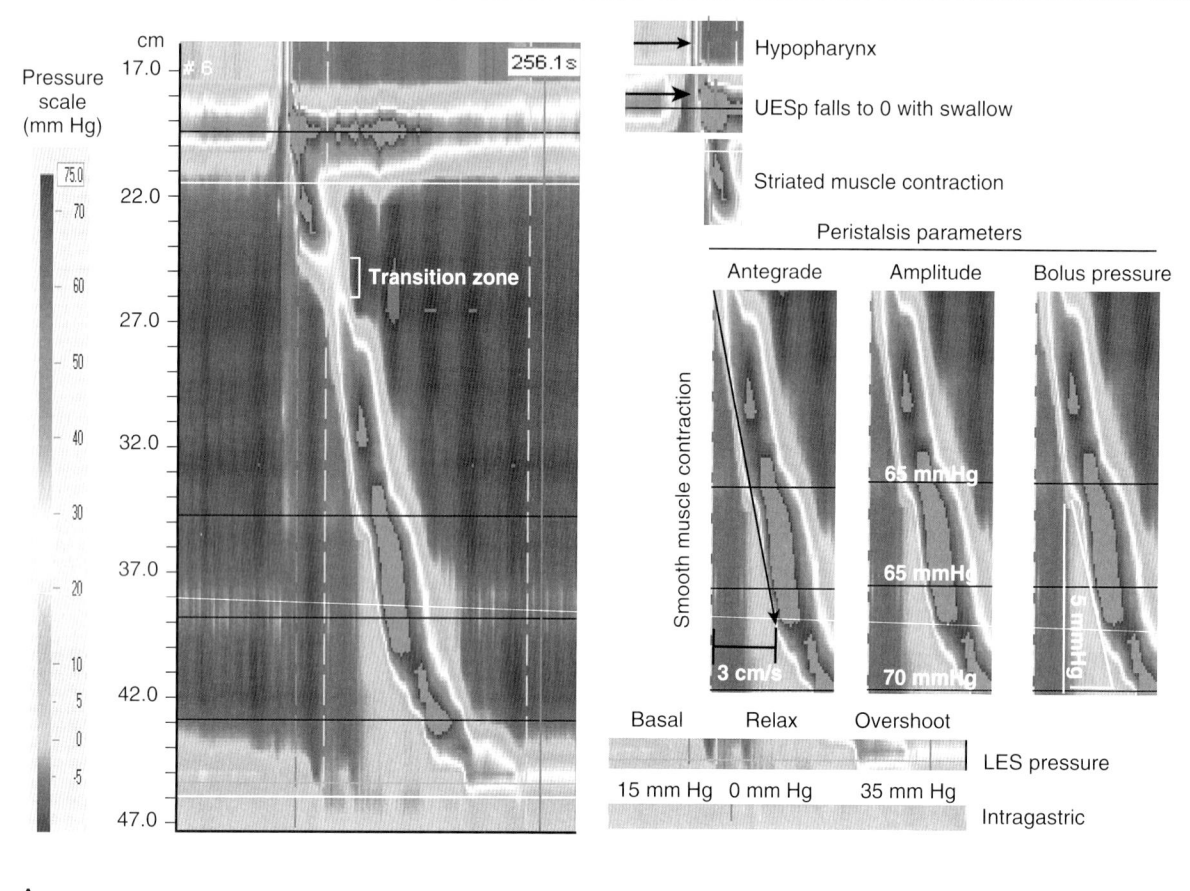

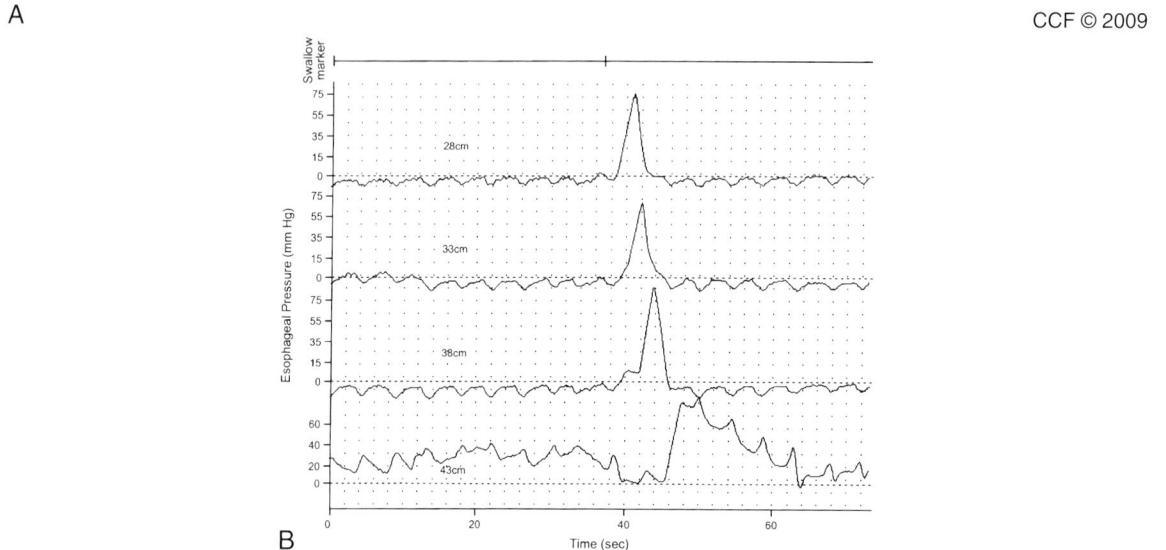

Figure 36–8

A, High-resolution manometry (HRM) tracing derived from 36 pressure sites 1 cm apart. HRM tracing on the left is divided into anatomic segments from pharynx to stomach on the right. Pharynx is from 16 to 18 cm, and pharyngeal contraction *(black arrow)* occurs as the upper esophageal sphincter (UES) (18 to 20 cm) relaxes, after a 5-mL swallow, and the UESp (UES pressure) falls from 50 to 0 mm Hg. Striated muscle contraction wave begins as the UES recovers, and it advances from 21 to 24 cm, where a transition zone (24 to 26 cm) of lower pressure occurs. Smooth muscle peristaltic contraction wave extends from 26 to 44 cm, is antegrade (3 cm/sec [normal, <8]), and normal in amplitude (50 to 75 mm Hg [normal, <180]), duration, and intrabolus pressure. The lower esophageal sphincter (LES) extends from 44 to 47 cm, relaxes, just after a swallow occurs, from 15 mm Hg to near 0, and then overshoots to 30 mm Hg. **B,** Traditional esophageal manometry, with four sites 5 cm apart, shows antegrade contraction waves at 5, 10, and 15 cm above the LES, and normal LES relaxation.

Table 36–2
Normal Distal Values for 24-Hour pH Monitoring

Parameter	Johnson[191] 95th percentile	Richter[192] 95th percentile	Jamieson[193] Mean	Percentile
Total time (%)	4.45	5.78	4.5	95
Upright time (%)	8.42	8.15	7.1	93
Supine time (%)	3.45	3.45	1.5	86
No. of episodes	47	46	56	98
No. of episodes >5 min.	3	4	3	94
Longest episode (min)	19.8	18.5	12	84
Composite score	14.7	—	16.7	96

From Adhami T, Richter JE. Twenty-four hour pH monitoring in the assessment of esophageal function. Semin Thorac Cardiovasc Surg 2001;13(3):241-54.[194]

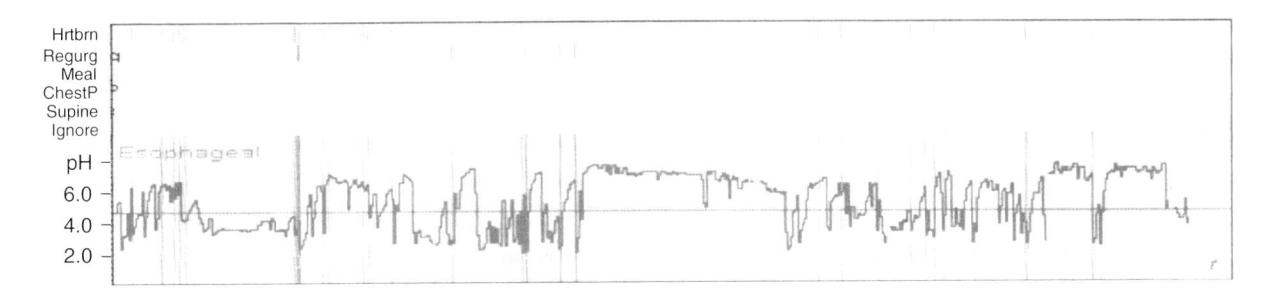

Reflux table - Acid reflux analysis - Day 1

	Total	(Normal)	Upright	(Normal)	Supine	(Normal)
Fraction time pH<4 ((%))	33.0	5.5	20.9	8.2	38.8	3.0
Number of refluxes	104		49		55	
Number of long refluxes(>5 (min))	14		3		11	
Duration of longest reflux (min)	111		39		111	
Time pH <4 ((min))	474		98		375	

Reflux table - Acid reflux analysis - Day 2

	Total	(Normal)	Upright	(Normal)	Supine	(Normal)
Fraction time pH <4 ((%))	141	5.5	18.6	82	7.3	3.0
Number of refluxes	100		87		13	
Number of long refluxes(>5 (min))	8		6		2	
Duration of longest reflux (min)	29		29		8	
Time pH <4 ((min))	178		140		37	

Symptom index
SI table - Total

	Total	(Abnormal)
HrtBrn	57.1	>50%
ChestP	50.0	
Regurg	100.0	
Cough	n/a	

Figure 36–9
Example of 48-hour Bravo pH monitoring in a symptomatic patient with suspected gastroesophageal reflux disease. Severe (day 1) and moderate (day 2) bipositional acid exposure is present, as well as positive symptom index (>50%) for heartburn and regurgitation.

Impedance-pH monitoring when the patient is *on* PPI therapy has been used when suspected esophageal or extraesophageal GERD symptoms (or both) persist despite PPIs (Fig. 36-10). Small case series in patients with a positive symptom index have shown good results after fundoplication.[22] However, we believe that long-term controlled studies, performed in centers with experience in impedance-pH monitoring, are needed to identify the role of such monitoring when only symptom association and nonacid reflux are found.

Endoscopic Esophageal Ultrasound

Endoscopic ultrasound (EUS) provides definition of the esophageal wall and periesophageal tissue not possible by routine fiberoptic esophagoscopy. It is indispensable in evaluating abnormalities of the esophageal wall and in diagnosing nonmucosal esophageal tumors. Ultrasound endoscopes scan the wall with ultrasound waves from 7.5- and 12-MHz. The probes, which can be passed through the biopsy channel of

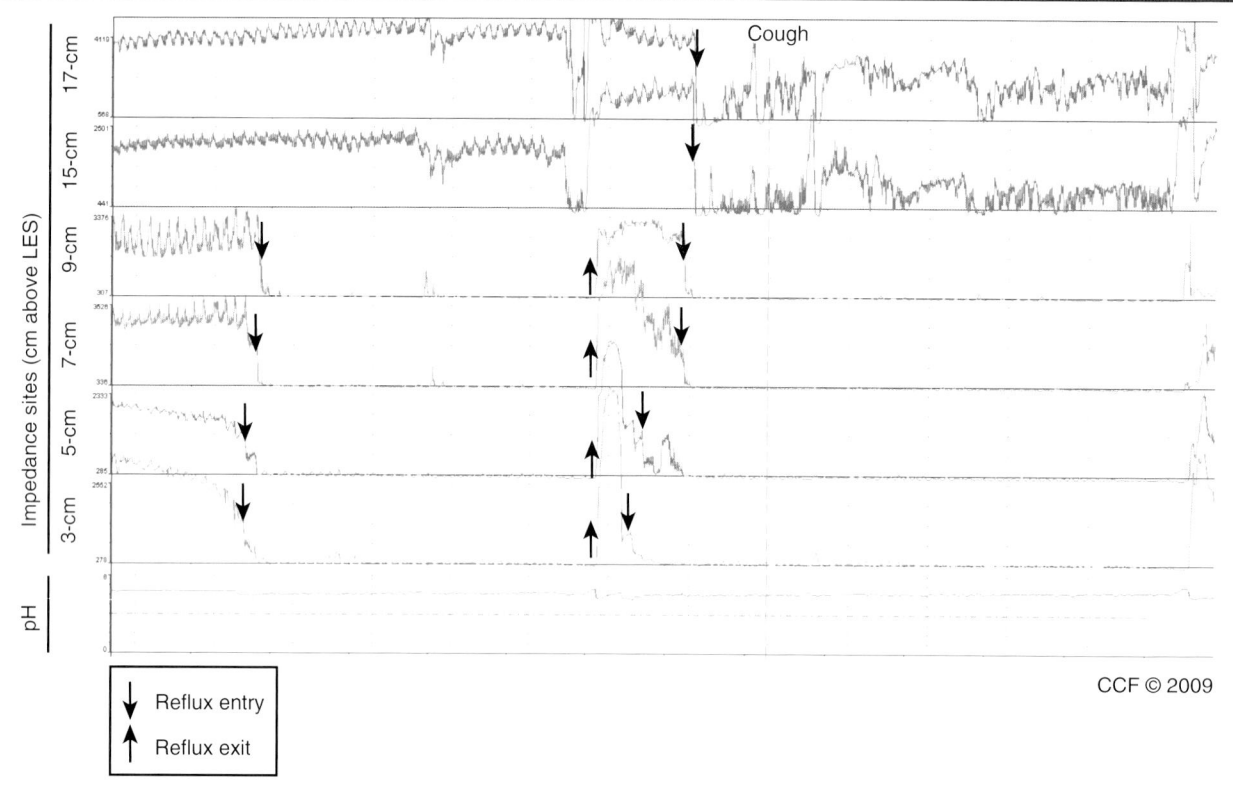

Figure 36–10
Simultaneous impedance and pH monitoring shows two nonacid liquid reflux episodes in a patient receiving acid suppression. The first episode shows retrograde liquid reflux to 9 cm above the lower esophageal sphincter (LES) *(down arrows)*, and subsequent clearance after 2 minutes at all sites *(up arrows)*. The second episode shows retrograde liquid reflux to the most proximal site, and cough occurs 40 seconds later.

flexible endoscopes, can be used to evaluate esophageal strictures that prevent passage of standard ultrasound equipment. The esophagus and periesophageal tissues are seen as five alternating layers of different echogenicities (Fig. 36-11). This examination also images periesophageal structures, including regional lymph nodes. Both the layer of origin and the ultrasound characteristics of a mass are critical for diagnosing benign esophageal tumors. Periesophageal masses and regional lymph nodes can also be studied. EUS-directed fine-needle aspiration (FNA) provides cytologic and pathologic assessment of esophageal tumors, periesophageal masses, and regional lymph nodes.

Other Investigations

Bilitec 2000

The Bilitec 2000 fiberoptic spectrophotometer detects the presence of bilirubin, the principal component of bile, by absorption of the band of light (450 nm) characteristic for bilirubin.[23] Because impedance-pH monitoring can detect nonacid reflux, the role of Bilitec in GERD is limited. Moreover, it is not widely available. However, measuring duodenogastroesophageal reflux may be useful in the patient with previous esophagogastric surgery and with suspected symptoms from bile reflux.

Impedance-Manometry

In impedance-manometry, multiple impedance electrode pairs on a manometry catheter allow transport of a swallowed bolus to be assessed as it traverses the esophagus (Fig. 36-12). Bolus transit can be compared with simultaneous esophageal peristalsis and contraction amplitude.[24] Among 350 patients studied at a single center, all those who had achalasia and scleroderma had abnormal bolus transit, and 95% or more of those who had normal manometry, nutcracker esophagus, and LES dysfunction (high or low) had normal bolus transit. However, only 50% of patients with esophageal spasm and ineffective esophageal motility had normal bolus transit.[25] Impedance-manometry may define different treatment strategies for patient subpopulations. For example, patients with abnormal rather than normal bolus transit may develop dysphagia after antireflux surgery, or patients with esophageal spasm and with poor as opposed to normal bolus transit may respond better to approaches improving esophageal emptying. Clinical studies with outcome data will assess if impedance-manometry improves patient management in these and other situations.

BENIGN ESOPHAGEAL DISEASES AND THEIR TREATMENT

Hiatal Hernia

Herniation of abdominal contents through the esophageal hiatus is a common occurrence. With provocative maneuvers that increase intra-abdominal pressure, 55% of patients undergoing barium esophagram were found to have herniation of the stomach into the chest.[26] Symptoms are secondary to reflux, incarceration or strangulation of herniated organs, or compression of thoracic structures. There are four types of hiatal hernia, each with its own symptom presentation. Type I, or sliding hiatal hernia, is the most common (Fig. 36-13, and

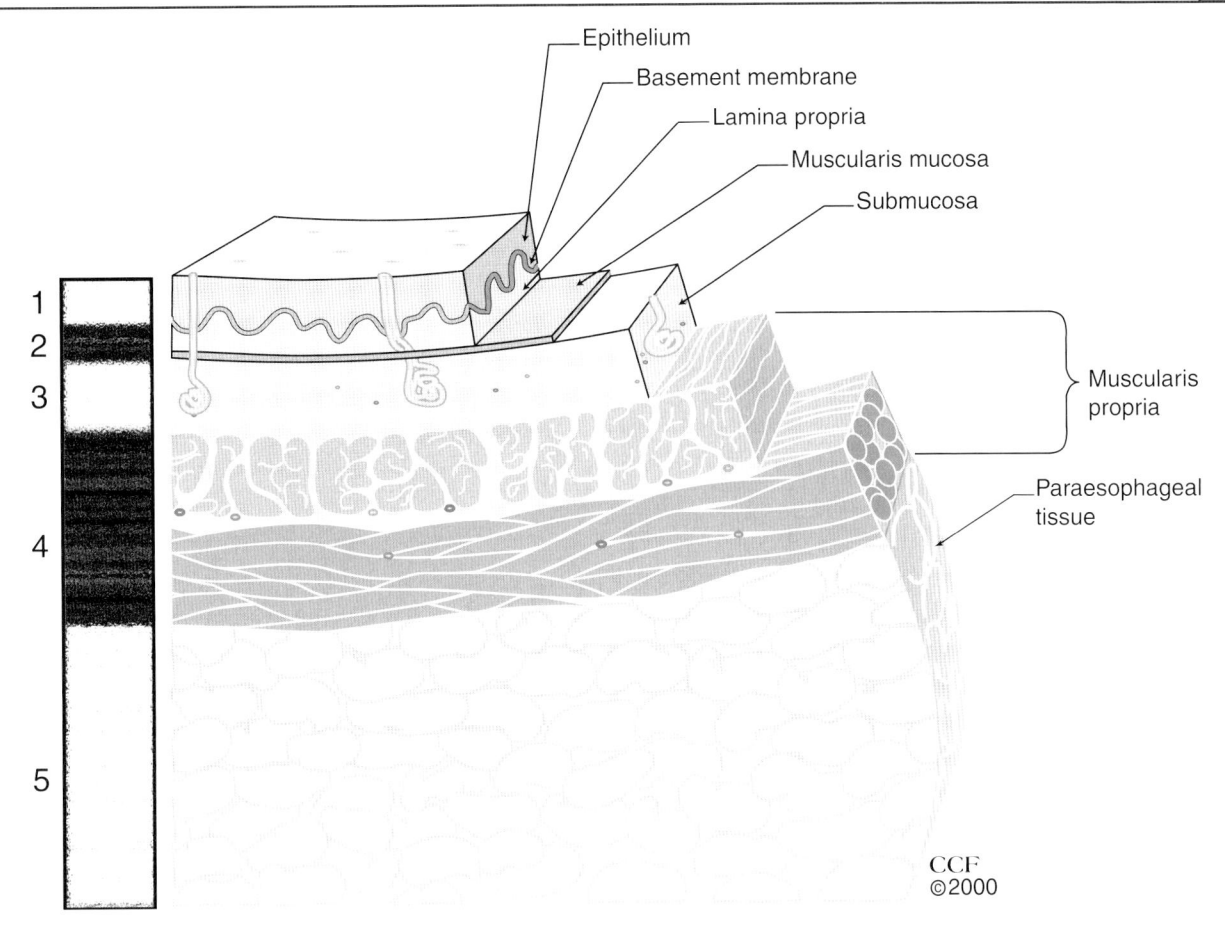

Figure 36–11
Esophageal wall is visualized as five alternating layers of differing echogenicity by esophageal ultrasound (EUS). The first (inner) layer is hyperechoic (white) and represents the superficial mucosa (epithelium and lamina propria). The second layer is hypoechoic (black) and represents the deep mucosa (muscularis mucosae). The third layer is hyperechoic and represents the submucosa. The fourth layer is hypoechoic and represents the muscularis propria. The fifth layer is hyperechoic and represents the paraesophageal tissue. The thickness of the layers as indicated by ultrasound does not equal the actual thickness of the anatomic layers.

see Fig. 36-6A). Herniation of the esophagogastric junction into the posterior mediastinum occurs because of thinning and elongation of the phrenoesophageal ligament. There is no potential for incarceration. The majority of patients with type I hiatal hernias are asymptomatic. If symptoms occur, they are related to GERD. Type II, or rolling, hiatal hernias are uncommon (Fig. 36-14). They result from a defect in or isolated weakness of the phrenoesophageal ligament, allowing a portion of the stomach to herniate through the hiatus while the esophagogastric junction remains anchored in the abdomen. Symptoms of gastric obstruction, strangulation, anemia, and, less commonly, shortness of breath and arrhythmia result from gastric herniation through the hiatus and presence of the stomach in the chest. Type III, or mixed, hiatal hernias are the second most common type (Fig. 36-15). Patients may present with reflux or with symptoms of type II hernias, or with both. As type III hernias increase in size, there may be organoaxial volvulus with the potential for strangulation. In many patients, these hernias may be a progression of type I hernias.[27] Type IV hiatal hernias contain the stomach and other abdominal contents such as colon, spleen, small bowel, and pancreas (Fig. 36-16). The term *paraesophageal hernia* is sometimes used to describe any type II, III, or IV hiatal hernia.

Symptomatic hiatal hernias should be repaired. Repair of asymptomatic types II and III hernias is controversial. The potential for strangulation and gastric necrosis has been advocated as the prime reason to repair paraesophageal hernias in all patients, particularly because 50% mortality was initially reported when this complication occurred.[28] However, strangulation is an uncommon occurrence without antecedent symptoms; therefore, this is an overestimate, and careful follow-up of asymptomatic patients is a viable alternative to repair in all patients.

Repair follows the principles of surgical management of GERD. Addition of a fundoplication is controversial, but it is definitely indicated if symptomatic GERD is present. Laparoscopic repairs have been reported to have an earlier and increased rate of failure.[29] A meta-analysis showed this rate to be 25%, at variable follow-up periods.[30] This high incidence of recurrence has prompted the use of a variety of mesh reinforcement of laparoscopic hiatal reconstruction. Although mesh has been reported to decrease recurrence at 6 months,[31] the clinical significance of this finding[32] and long-term durability[33] are in question. In most patients, addition of a gastrostomy or gastropexy is not required. Compared with patients with GERD, patients with type III hiatal hernias are older and have more comorbidities. Adjusting for these factors demonstrates that patients with type III hernias are more likely to have pulmonary, thromboembolic, and bleeding complications in their postoperative course than those with type I hiatal hernias.[34]

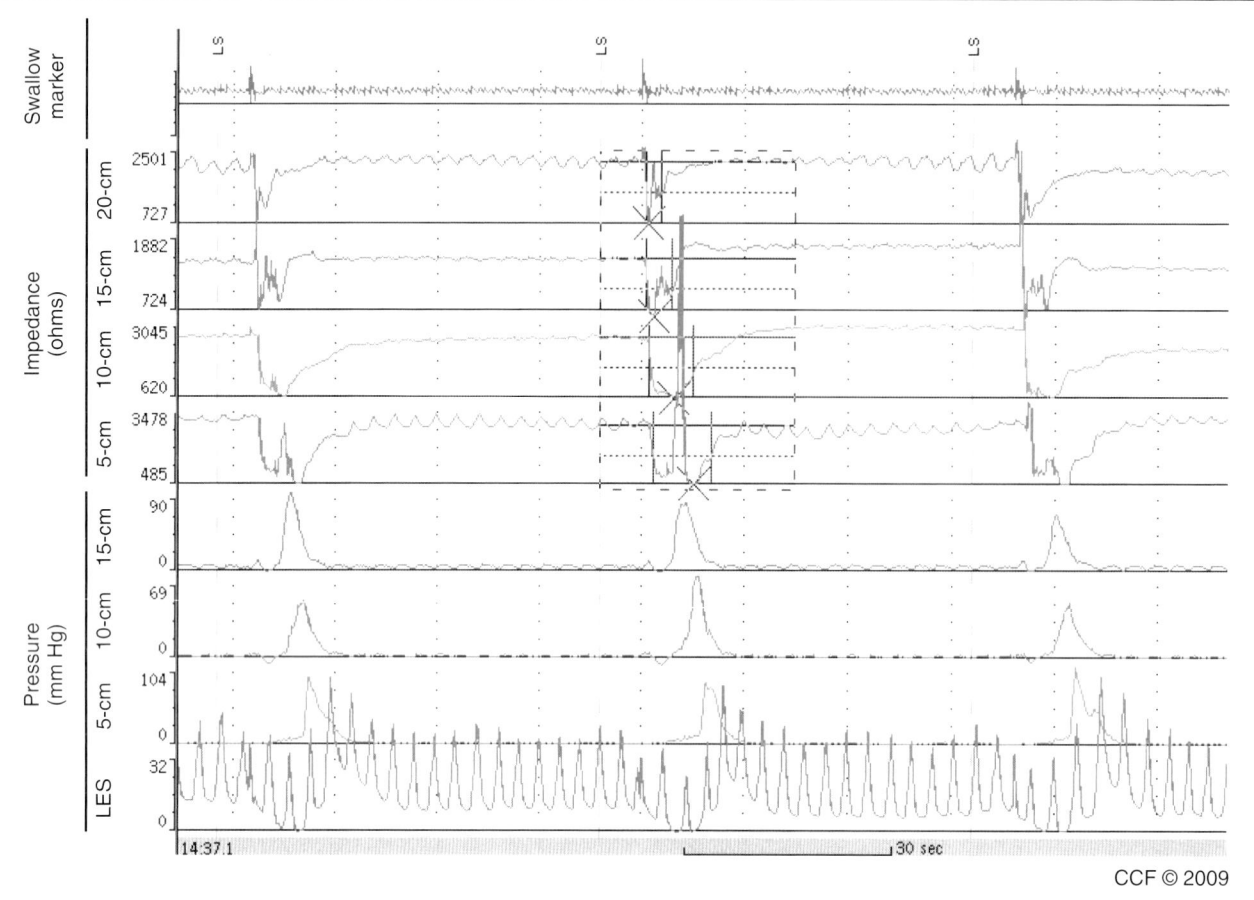

Figure 36–12
Simultaneous impedance and manometry showing normal bolus transit after each of three 5-mL saline swallows. Bolus entry occurs at each of four impedance sites as impedance decreases (see first vertical line in second swallow). Antegrade decrease in impedance in the four sites shows normal bolus advance through the esophagus. After bolus persistence with a low impedance value, a rise in impedance toward baseline occurs at each site from bolus clearing (see second vertical line in second swallow) due to simultaneous esophageal contraction at the same level. Antegrade increase in the four impedance sites shows normal bolus clearing from the esophagus. Normal lower esophageal sphincter relaxation and overshoot is seen.

Gastroesophageal Reflux Disease

GERD was defined at the recent Montreal consensus conference as "a condition which develops when the reflux of stomach contents causes troublesome symptoms and/or complications."[35] Typical symptoms of GERD are heartburn, regurgitation, and dysphagia. Extra-esophageal (or atypical) symptoms or disorders having an established association with GERD are cough, laryngitis, and asthma. Other atypical symptoms or disorders (pulmonary fibrosis, pharyngitis, otitis media, and sinusitis) are often linked to reflux and are proposed associations, but data are insufficient to establish causation.[35] It is important that abdominal pain, gas, and bloating not be misinterpreted as GERD symptoms.

Complicated GERD includes reflux esophagitis, esophageal stricture, and Barrett's esophagus. The mucosal response to acid may produce intestinal metaplasia (Barrett's esophagus), and damage to the submucosa and muscularis propria can result in a short esophagus (see Figs. 36-4 and 36-6A). Two feared complications of GERD are peptic stricture and the development of high-grade dysplasia or intramucosal cancer in Barrett's esophagus.

The LES and diaphragmatic hiatal mechanism are the major components of the reflux barrier.[36,37] A hiatal hernia is seen in 50% to 90% of GERD patients.[38-41] However, reflux events are most commonly caused by transient LES relaxations, although reflux over a low basal LES is also important.[42] Poor acid clearance from peristaltic dysfunction and delayed gastric emptying contribute to prolonged acid exposure in some patients.

The mainstay of therapy for patients with GERD is medical management. PPIs can heal esophagitis in more than 90% of patients; randomized studies do not demonstrate a superiority of surgery over medical therapy.[43-45] Atypical symptoms or disorders respond less predictably to PPIs, especially in the absence of typical symptoms. Controlled trials of PPIs showing benefit in patients with laryngitis or asthma have been predominantly in those having concomitant typical symptoms. However, a recent controlled trial in patients with chronic posterior laryngitis symptoms and endoscopic findings, but no typical GERD symptoms, found no benefit with esomeprazole.[46]

Surgical management of uncomplicated GERD should be considered in patients who are PPI intolerant and who have typical GERD symptoms responsive to PPI, and persistent typical GERD symptoms despite PPI, especially volume regurgitation.[47] The following preoperative GERD evaluation is suggested. First, endoscopy should be performed to assess for presence of esophagitis, Barrett's mucosa, stricture, hiatal hernia,

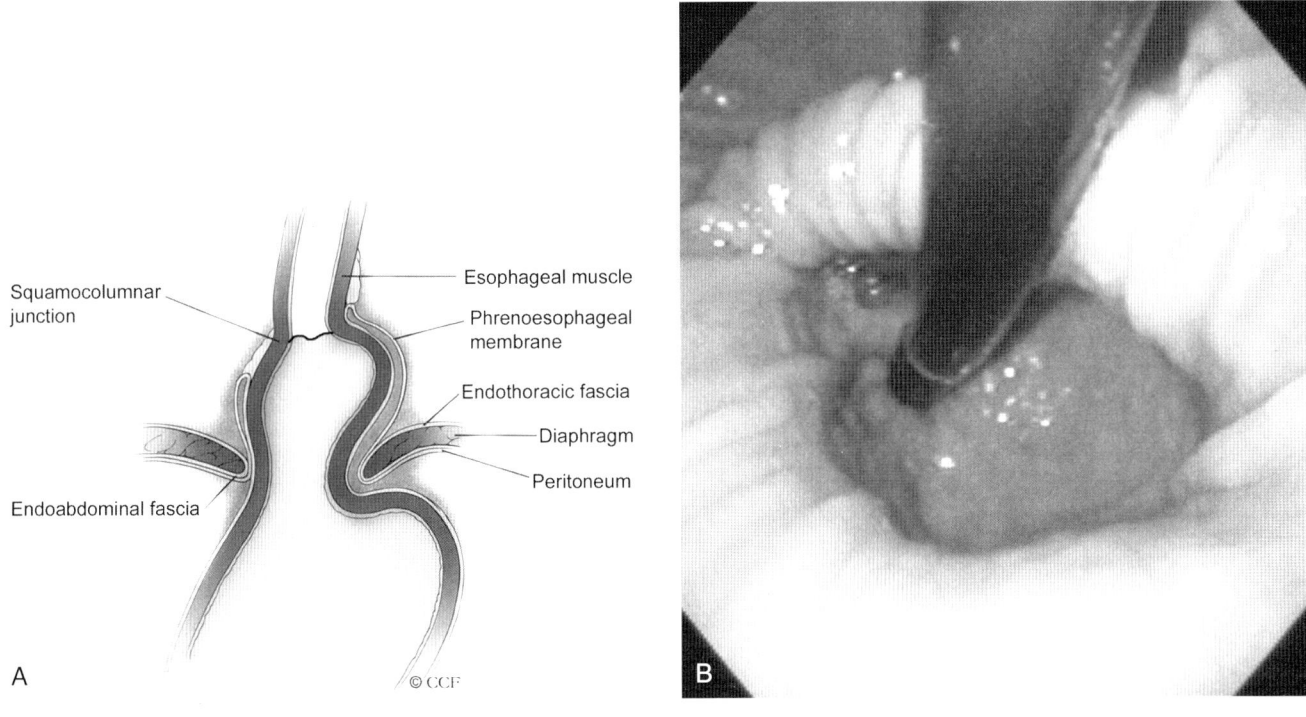

Figure 36-13
Type I hiatal hernia. **A,** Drawing. **B,** Retroflexed view from the intra-abdominal stomach at esophagoscopy. Diaphragmatic impression and intrathoracic stomach can be seen.

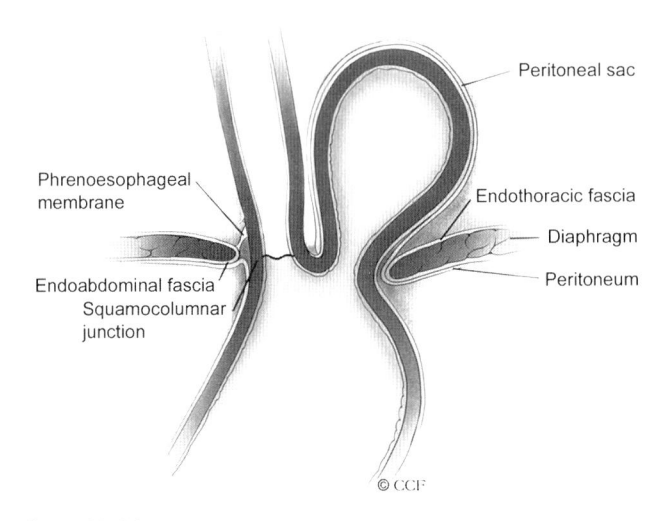

Figure 36-14
Type II hiatal hernia.

and alternative upper gastrointestinal diagnoses such as ulcer disease. Second, manometry should be performed to locate and measure LES, to exclude another diagnosis such as esophageal spasm, and to assess peristalsis. Third, a barium esophagram should be performed to assess the anatomy of the esophagus and esophagogastric junction, mucosal changes, and esophageal function. Fourth, ambulatory pH monitoring off therapy should be performed to confirm excessive acid exposure. The presence of typical symptoms that respond to PPI therapy, and of abnormal acid exposure as determined by pH monitoring, are reliable predictors of successful surgical treatment of GERD.[48,49] In patients with suspected gastric drainage abnormalities, a nuclear medicine gastric emptying study is required.

Surgical management is less likely to be effective in patients with persistent atypical symptoms or disorders in the absence of typical GERD symptoms. Thus, antireflux surgery primarily for atypical symptoms or disorders should be reserved for patients with concomitant typical GERD symptoms, and in whom causality of reflux for the atypical symptom or disorder has been established to the greatest degree possible during the preoperative evaluation just described. Although small case series have shown good results for antireflux surgery in patients with persistent cough on PPIs and reflux by impedance-pH monitoring,[50] long-term controlled studies are needed to validate this approach.

Complicated GERD is first managed with aggressive medical therapy; however, peptic esophageal stricture and chronic Barrett's ulcer may require surgery. The columnar cell–lined esophagus is not in itself an indication for surgery. It is debatable that surgery can reverse the changes of columnar lining. Partial reversal, although interesting, is not a compelling argument for surgical correction of GERD.[51] Effective reflux control may reduce the incidence of malignant degeneration in the columnar cell–lined esophagus. However, failure of antireflux repairs is frequently seen in patients with adenocarcinoma of the esophagus. Patients with a columnar cell–lined esophagus have the most disordered physiology, largest hernias, and most disrupted hiatal mechanisms.[52] Therefore, either prevention of or halting malignant degeneration in a columnar-lined esophagus is not an indication for surgery. If a patient with a columnar cell–lined esophagus has antireflux surgery, the need for endoscopic surveillance is not eliminated. Thus, the patient with a columnar cell–lined esophagus has the same indications for surgery as the patient with a squamous cell–lined esophagus.

The principles of antireflux surgery are restoration of the intra-abdominal length of esophagus, reconstruction of

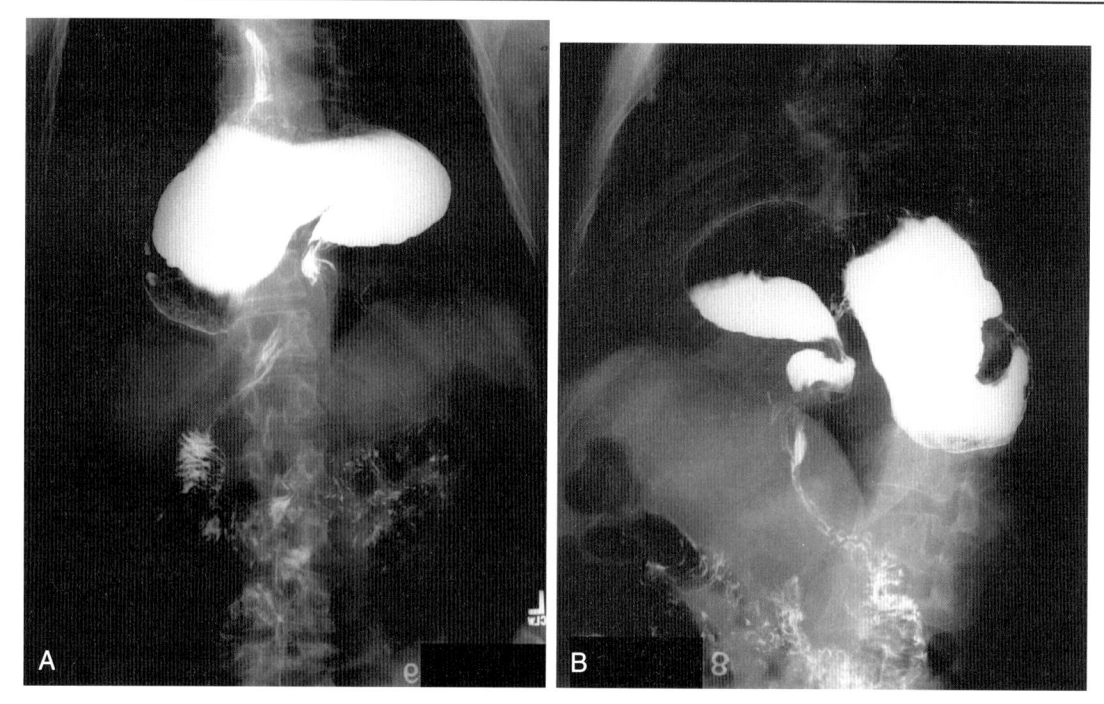

Figure 36–15
Barium esophagram demonstrates a type III hiatal hernia with organoaxial rotation. **A,** Posteroanterior view. **B,** Lateral view.

the esophageal hiatus, and reinforcement of the LES.[53] These can be accomplished by a number of approaches and techniques. Possible approaches, in descending order of morbidity, are thoracoabdominal, thoracotomy, laparotomy, and laparoscopy. Facility with all of these approaches is necessary.

Restoration of the intra-abdominal esophagus requires reducing the hiatal hernia and mobilizing the esophagus. This portion of the operation necessitates recognition of the short esophagus.[54] Failure to lengthen the short esophagus by extensive esophageal mobilization to the aortic arch or by addition of a Collis gastroplasty will result in a repair under tension and early failure. The short esophagus should be suspected by history of a stricture or previous dilation or findings of a long segment of columnar cell–lined esophagus, a large type I hiatal hernia (>4 cm), a type III hiatal hernia, or failure of the hernia to reduce below the diaphragm on upright barium esophagram.

The importance of reconstruction of the hiatus cannot be underestimated. It plays a role in reflux prevention equal to that of the LES.[55] The recent addition of mesh reinforcement of the hiatal closure ignores the past history of antireflux surgery and the dynamic nature of this structure. Complete mobilization of the hiatal crura and careful removal of the hernia sac will allow primary suture reconstruction of the hiatus. Failure to reconstruct the hiatus is a common cause of failure of laparoscopic antireflux surgery.[56] The principal reason for reherniation after an otherwise adequate repair is tension on the repair, either because the short esophagus was ignored or because it was not recognized, and not an unbuttressed reconstruction of the hiatus.

The final step in the surgical correction of GERD is reinforcing the LES by constructing a fundoplication, which may be either total or partial. The Nissen fundoplication, a 360-degree total fundoplication, completely encircles the esophagus. Partial fundoplication is typically 270 degrees and is either anteriorly placed (Belsey Mark IV repair), or posteriorly placed (Toupet repair). Theoretically, the tradeoff is between better reflux control with a total fundoplication and less dysphagia with a partial fundoplication. Some surgeons tailor the fundoplication to suit the peristaltic activity of the esophageal body.[57] High-resolution manometry should allow a more precise cutoff at which the severity of peristaltic dysfunction requires partial fundoplication. Until then, we consider total fundoplication to be appropriate for all except the patient with an aperistaltic esophagus.[15,58-61] The use of a partial fundoplication for complicated GERD is associated with an increased incidence of failed repair.[62] Dysphagia after surgery for GERD is usually transient with a properly constructed fundoplication. Prolonged dysphagia is indicative of a malformed fundoplication, either long, tight, or twisted. Return of normal esophageal motility with resolution of GERD after fundoplication is hypothetically possible. It is more likely that the amplitude of the peristaltic wave will increase than that failure of propagation will be corrected. Therefore, any fundoplication should be constructed under the assumption that the peristaltic abnormalities will not improve. Finally, the potential for postprandial symptoms of gas bloat and early satiety must be mentioned to any patient being considered for fundoplication.

An often ignored but essential part of the physical examination is measuring and recording weight and height and calculating body mass index (BMI). Overweight (BMI, 25 to 29) and obese (BMI, 30 to 34) GERD patients should be counseled on weight loss and encouraged to reach their ideal weight before elective surgery. Because obesity and GERD are interrelated,[63,64] successful and sustained weight loss may eliminate the need for surgery. Although there is disagreement about the impact of obesity on the outcome of antireflux surgery,[65-70] the health benefits of weight loss in severely (BMI,

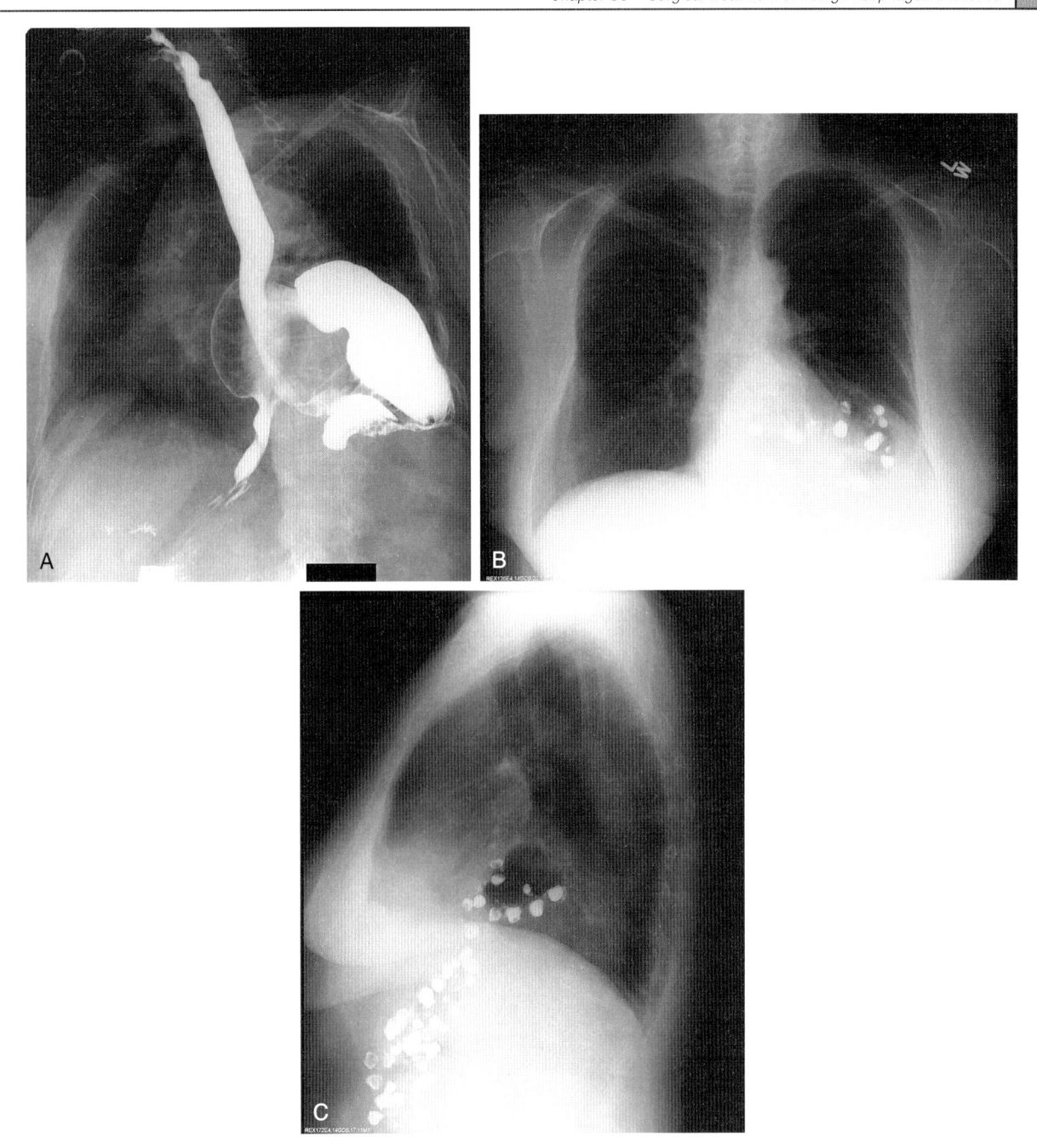

Figure 36-16
Barium esophagram **(A)** demonstrates a type III hiatal hernia with organoaxial rotation. Three days later, barium is seen in the colonic diverticulum on preoperative chest radiograph, posteroanterior view **(B)** and lateral view **(C)**. Therefore, this is a type IV hiatal hernia.

35 to 39) and morbidly (BMI, ≥40) obese patients with GERD should make weight loss surgery the operation of choice in these patients.

Antireflux operations are not infinitely durable. It is important that all patients are instructed to avoid activities that excessively increase intra-abdominal pressure and to maintain their ideal weight.[71] Unrealistic patient expectations and widespread application of laparoscopic fundoplication without careful patient selection in low-volume centers by inexperienced surgical teams have produced poor results and have had a negative impact on this operative approach.[72-74]

Motility Disorders

Achalasia

Achalasia is a degenerative esophageal disease culminating in aperistalsis of the esophageal body and abnormal relaxation of the LES. The underlying cause of this T cell–mediated destruction and eventual fibrous replacement of the esophageal myenteric neural plexus is unknown.[75-77] Patients complain of progressive dysphagia, regurgitation, and weight loss. Chest pain affects a minority of patients, and it may persist when other symptoms improve after successful therapy. Recurrent respiratory infection, aspiration pneumonia, and lung abscess may be initial presentations and herald advanced disease. Most patients seek medical attention only after significant and irreversible damage to the esophageal myenteric neural plexus has occurred.

Barium esophagogram and esophagoscopy are usually the first diagnostic tests because the usual symptoms are dysphagia and regurgitation. Classic findings at esophagram are esophageal dilation, aperistalsis, impaired esophageal emptying, and symmetric tapering at the esophagogastric junction (bird's beak or ace of spades appearance) (see Fig. 36-6C). Timed barium esophagogram allows quantification of esophageal obstruction and emptying (see Fig. 36-7). Esophagoscopy usually shows some degree of retention (occasionally only saliva) and a "tight" esophagogastric junction. When achalasia is suspected, it is essential to exclude pseudoachalasia (esophageal obstruction secondary to malignancy), which may be clinically indistinguishable from primary achalasia.

Manometry confirms achalasia suggested by symptoms and other studies mentioned earlier. Achalasia is defined by incomplete or failed relaxation of the LES and aperistalsis of the esophageal body. Because resting LES pressure is normal in 40% of patients, elevated LES pressure is not required for diagnosis.[78,79] High-resolution manometry has recently identified three subtypes of achalasia with different treatment responses (Fig. 36-17): minimal esophageal pressurization (type I, classic), esophageal pressure greater than 30 mm Hg throughout the entire esophagus (type II), and 30% or more swallows being followed by a spastic contraction (type III). Type II achalasia has been reported to be a predictor of very good outcome after treatment, whereas type III and pretreatment esophageal dilation were predictive of poorer outcomes.[80]

Goals of therapy are symptom relief, improving esophageal emptying by barium radiographs,[81] and preventing megaesophagus. Achalasia patients require follow-up by their gastroenterologist or surgeon every 1 to 2 years to accomplish this. Variable emptying in patients with achalasia is possible,[82] but repeated studies in the long-term follow-up are valuable.

Treatment of achalasia is palliative and directed at reducing LES pressure and improving esophageal emptying. Calcium channel blockers and long-acting nitrates relax smooth muscle and provide transient, but incomplete, relief of symptoms. Unpleasant side effects may limit their use.

Endoscopic injection of botulinum toxin has been used to treat achalasia. Palliation is temporary, lasting a mean of 6 months, with recurrent symptoms in more than 50% of patients.[83] Resistance to repeat injections is thought to result from antibody production against botulinum toxin. Use of botulinum toxin may complicate future surgery because it causes inflammation and fibrosis in the plane between the submucosa and the muscularis propria.[84-86] This therapy is reserved for patients who cannot tolerate more aggressive forms of treatment.

Pneumatic dilation and surgical myotomy are the two most effective treatment modalities for achalasia. Pneumatic dilation with the modern Rigiflex balloon dilator is successful in controlling symptoms in most patients. Graded dilation is performed to the desired result with 3.0 cm, 3.5 cm if necessary, and 4.0 cm if necessary, and response rates are 74%, 86%, and 90%, respectively.[87] A recent summary of 22 studies with 1212 patients treated with Rigiflex balloon dilation reported a 2.0% perforation rate and 78% good or excellent results at 3-year follow-up. More than a third of patients will have symptom recurrence during a 4-year period, but they may respond to repeat dilation.[88]

Open modified Heller myotomy performed transabdominally or transthoracically has been successful in treatment of achalasia. Two prospective studies have been reported comparing pneumatic dilation to myotomy.[89,90] After 4.8 years of follow-up, laparotomy and myotomy provided symptom control in 95% of patients, whereas pneumatic dilation with the Mosher system provided symptom control in 65%.[89]

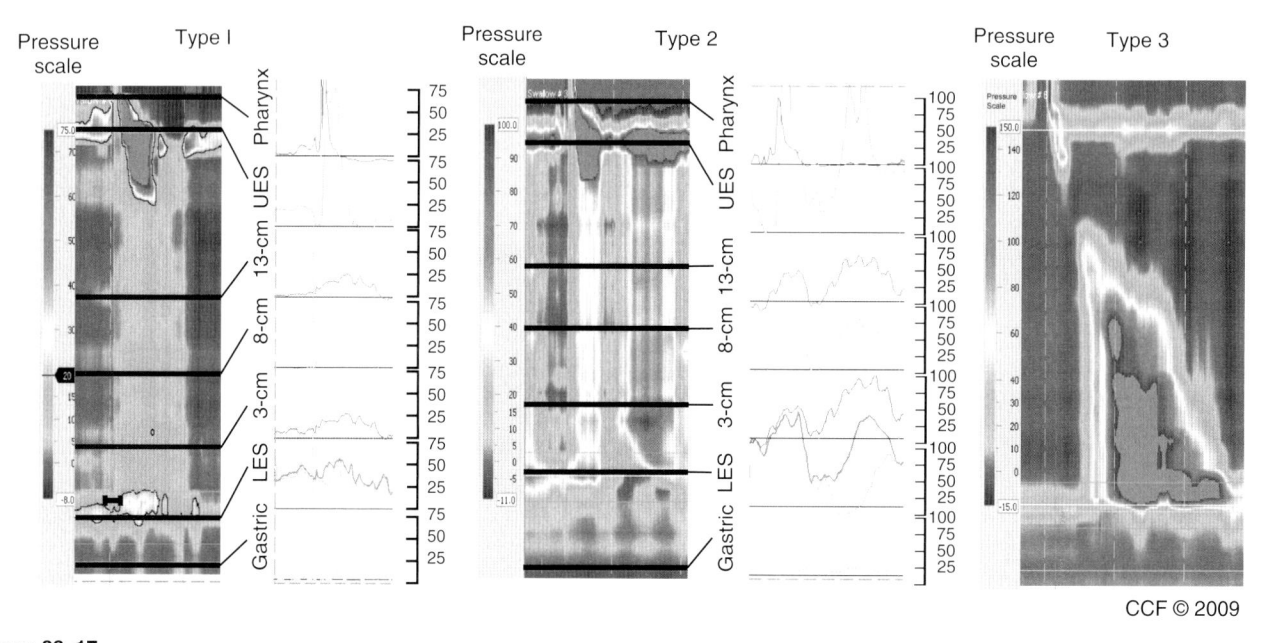

Figure 36–17
Three achalasia subtypes. *Type 1* has no contraction identified in the smooth muscle portion of the esophagus. Lower esophageal sphincter pressure (LESp) is > 30 mm Hg, and LES relaxation is never to < 20 mm Hg (normal, <15). *Type 2* has esophageal pressurization > 40 mm Hg extending from upper esophageal sphincter (UES) to LES, that is simultaneous and repetitive. *Type 3* has a prolonged, simultaneous, high-amplitude contraction characteristic of "vigorous achalasia." The contraction does not extend from UES to LES as in type 2.

In a small randomized study of 40 patients, no difference was observed between modalities, except that myotomy was associated with a lower LES pressure and less reflux.[90]

Development of laparoscopic Heller myotomy has resulted in more patients being referred for surgery and fewer for pneumatic dilation.[91] Laparoscopic Heller myotomy results in a shorter hospital stay.[92] Improved outcome is associated with increased surgical volume. With short follow-up (mean, 1 year), good to excellent symptom control is seen in 94% of patients, but 11% report reflux.[87] A recent review of 33 published studies of laparoscopic Heller myotomy reported that 85% of 1812 patients had a good to excellent response at a mean follow-up of 32 months, and 17% reported GERD as a postoperative complication.[88] Preoperative pneumatic dilation has been reported to increase the risk of intraoperative esophageal perforation during laparoscopic Heller myotomy.[93]

Regardless of surgical approach, the extent of myotomy is critical to good long-term outcome. A 3-cm extension of the myotomy onto the stomach is superior to a lesser myotomy for symptomatic and physiologic effects.[94] Controversy continues regarding the need for fundoplication added to myotomy. A fundoplication has been reported to be less essential when a thoracotomy is used. This finding most likely reflects a lesser myotomy. However, with the adoption of longer extensions of the myotomy onto the stomach, it is prudent to add a partial fundoplication to reduce reflux. The addition of a partial fundoplication has been demonstrated to reduce reflux[95] without impairing esophageal emptying.[96]

Failure to reduce LES pressure may produce a dilated sigmoid esophagus, which may require esophagectomy.[97-101]

Hypermotility Disorders

Diffuse esophageal spasm (DES) is a disorder of unknown etiology. Patients typically present with dysphagia and chest pain, often after an extensive but negative cardiac evaluation. Barium esophagram classically demonstrates a normal upper esophagus with a corkscrew pattern in the smooth muscle (distal two-thirds) portion (see Fig. 36-5A). Diagnosis is made by esophageal manometry. Simultaneous contractions of normal or increased amplitude occurring after more than 20% of swallows is required for diagnosis, as is presence of normal peristaltic contractions. Other findings that may be present are repetitive or prolonged contractions.[102] Standard manometry has found that LES function is usually normal, but both abnormal relaxation and hypertensive resting pressure have been reported. Because high-resolution manometry compensates for LES movement, more DES patients with poor LES relaxation may be identified, which will have an impact on treatment. Moreover, high-resolution manometry has demonstrated that apparently simultaneous contractions by traditional manometry are not true spasm; as a result, DES was rare in this large study population.[12]

Because DES is poorly understood and there are probably subgroups, multiple therapies have been tried with variable success. Medical therapy includes calcium channel blockers and nitrates and, recently, sildenafil in small series.[103] Endoscopic therapy with botulinum toxin injection into the LES and esophageal muscle has successfully controlled symptoms in selected patients. Pneumatic dilation has been used for the subgroup of DES patients with poor relaxation of the LES.

Future studies are necessary to assess the efficacy of tailoring therapy for different DES subgroups.

An excellent review emphasizes the need for careful selection of patients for DES surgery, and that surgery is rarely indicated.[104] For patients with severe DES refractory to medical therapy, a long myotomy extending from the aortic arch to the proximal stomach has been reported to provide good to excellent symptom control in 70%,[105] and to provide excellent medium-term control of dysphagia and chest pain. However, 10% of patients have been reported to experience postoperative reflux.[106]

Nutcracker esophagus is characterized by high-amplitude contractions of the distal esophagus, but esophageal peristalsis is normal. It is common and has been found in up to 48% of patients with noncardiac chest pain undergoing esophageal manometry, and in 10% with dysphagia (Fig. 36-18).[107] Treatment is medical. GERD is often present, and these patients should be treated with a PPI. Calcium channel blockers have not been found to be consistently effective. Trazodone and imipramine have been found to improve chest pain in some patients.[103] Surgery should be avoided.

Hypomotility Disorders

Hypocontractile motility abnormalities occur in some patients and have been lumped together as ineffective esophageal motility (IEM). IEM is associated with GERD, especially erosive esophagitis.[108] Unfortunately, therapeutic options to restore contractility are limited. Impedance-manometry can assess which patients with IEM have abnormal bolus transport,[109] and high-resolution manometry can assess the entire peristaltic wave-front rather than just three to four pressure sites, as with standard manometry. The role for these new methods in IEM is promising. Perhaps they will identify which patients with hypocontractility, but not total aperistalsis, should have partial fundoplication.

Secondary Esophageal Motility Disorders

Scleroderma, or progressive systemic sclerosis, is a systemic disease that commonly results in esophageal dysfunction. Fibrosis, collagen deposition, and patchy smooth muscle atrophy are histologic hallmarks of esophageal involvement. Skeletal muscle is unaffected. Destruction of esophageal smooth muscle results in diminished peristalsis of the lower esophagus and a hypotensive LES (see Fig. 36-18). Reflux and dysphagia are common complaints. Therapy includes aggressive acid suppression with potent PPIs and dilation of strictures. Surgery should be avoided if possible, especially if aperistalsis is present. When surgery is performed, it usually requires esophageal lengthening (Collis gastroplasty) and a partial fundoplication.[110] For extensive, unrepairable esophageal damage, resection may be required.

Neurologic and muscular disorders such as stroke, amyotrophic lateral sclerosis, and muscular dystrophies may be accompanied by esophageal dysfunction. Esophageal involvement is also seen in patients with diabetes or alcoholic neuropathy.

Diverticula

A diverticulum is an outpouching that protrudes from the gastrointestinal wall. True diverticula contain all layers of the gastrointestinal wall and are uncommon in the esophagus.

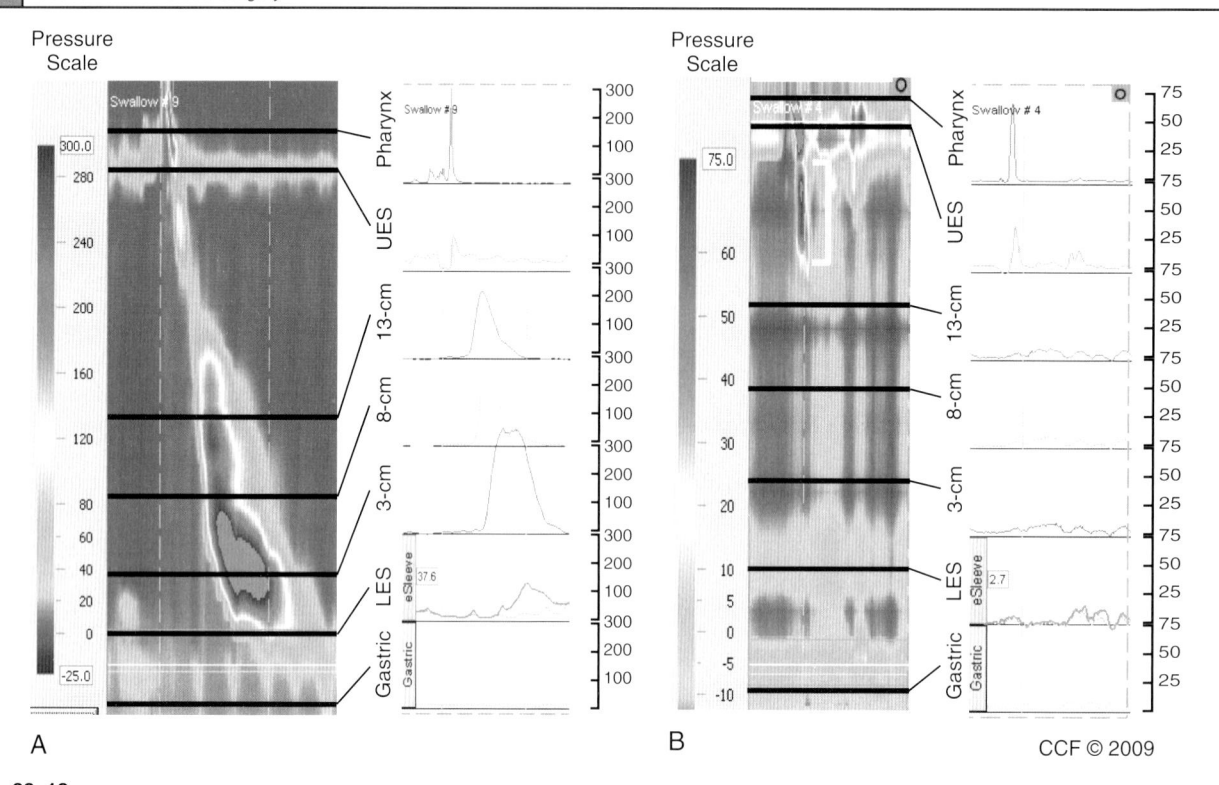

Figure 36–18
High-resolution and traditional manometry. **A,** In a patient with nutcracker esophagus, esophageal contraction amplitude is greater than 200 mm Hg (normal, <180 mm Hg) in the distal half of the esophagus. Esophageal peristalsis is normal. **B,** In a patient with scleroderma, there is a complete absence of smooth muscle contraction in the distal 75% of the esophagus. However, there is preserved striated muscle contraction in proximal 25% of esophagus *(white bracket)*. Lower esophageal sphincter (LES) pressure is less than 5 mm Hg. UES, upper esophageal sphincter.

Most esophageal diverticula consist of mucosa, submucosa, and strands of muscle fibers and are, therefore, false diverticula. The mechanisms by which diverticula develop are not completely understood. However, diverticula are termed pulsion, traction, or congenital, according to the *suspected* mechanism of formation. A pulsion diverticulum usually occurs at or proximal to an esophageal sphincter or proximal to areas of prolonged or increased pressure. They are assumed to result from excessive outward pressure on the gastrointestinal wall. Generally, these are false diverticula. Traction diverticula result from forces arising outside the gastrointestinal wall and are usually true diverticula. They are far less common and are found adjacent to regions of periesophageal inflammation, such as chronic lymphadenitis.

Diverticula of the esophagus are most commonly acquired. Pulsion diverticula can be located anywhere along the esophagus. Traction and congenital diverticula are rare. There are three common anatomic sites of focal diverticula. Proximally, they occur in the hypopharyngeal or pharyngoesophageal region. Mid-esophageal diverticula are seen near the tracheal carina. Distal or epiphrenic diverticula appear within a few centimeters of the gastroesophageal junction.

Zenker's Diverticulum

Zenker's diverticulum, the most common esophageal diverticulum, occurs above the cricopharyngeus at Killian's triangle. Typically, it is located opposite the C6 or C7 vertebral body (Fig. 36-19). Cook and colleagues demonstrated incomplete UES opening in patients with Zenker's diverticula.[111] Over

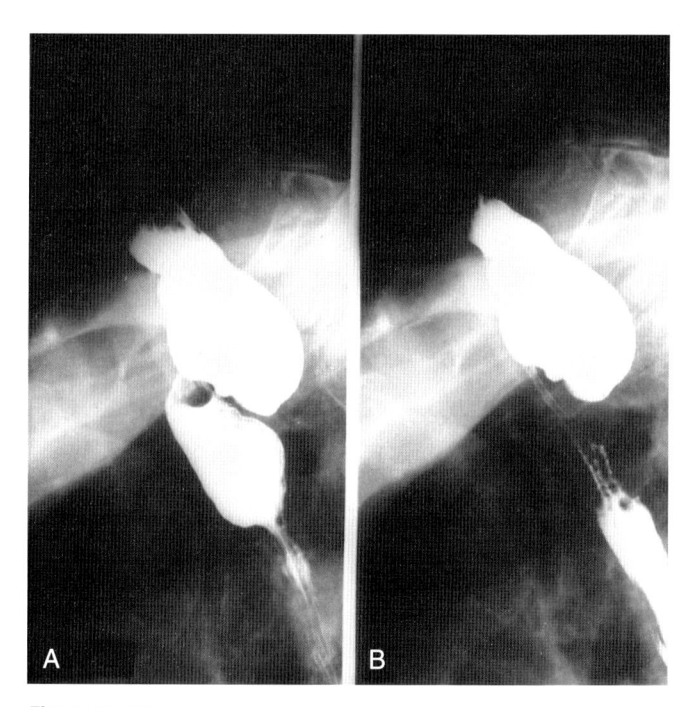

Figure 36–19
Zenker's diverticulum. Lateral view during barium esophagram shows a large diverticulum **(A)** that does not clear with repeated swallowing **(B)**.

time, a permanent narrow-mouthed outpouching of the posterior pharynx and esophagus develops and enlarges inferiorly. As a result, saliva and ingested foodstuffs pool dependently in the sac and cannot empty easily into the esophagus.

Early on, patients may complain of a vague sensation or sticking in their throat, intermittent cough, excessive salivation, and intermittent solid food dysphagia. These minor symptoms may be dismissed as globus hystericus. As the sac enlarges, symptoms worsen as dysphagia becomes more frequent. This usually occurs in patients who are older than 50 years. Gurgling sounds during swallowing, regurgitation of undigested food ingested, halitosis, voice change, retrosternal pain, and respiratory problems may be accompanying symptoms. To aid swallowing, patients perform unusual maneuvers such as throat clearing, coughing, or placing manual pressure on the neck. In rare cases, the diverticulum can become large enough to obstruct the esophagus. A neck mass may be observed in these patients. The most serious complication associated with a Zenker's diverticulum is aspiration, which can lead to pneumonia or lung abscess. Perforation, hemorrhage, or carcinoma may complicate Zenker's diverticula.

A Zenker's diverticulum is best identified and evaluated by barium esophagram, which can also evaluate the esophagus, as described earlier. Endoscopy is not required in all cases, but it is indicated when the esophagram is abnormal or when concomitant esophageal or gastric symptoms exist. Experience is necessary to safely navigate past large diverticula. Manometric testing of the cricopharyngeal area is not clinically useful. Esophageal manometry is performed when symptoms or esophagram findings warrant it, and it usually requires endoscopic placement.

Treatment goals of Zenker's diverticula are to increase UES compliance and reduce resting pressure in the cricopharyngeus. This can be accomplished endoscopically by creating an esophago-diverticulostomy with an endoscopic stapler.[112] Medium-term results with this technique are excellent.[113] Large diverticula and redundant mucosa are reported as risk factors for failure of endoscopic transoral stapling.[114] An open surgical myotomy is adequate treatment for small diverticula. For large diverticula, a myotomy with suspension or excision of the diverticulum is indicated.[115] Both of these procedures provide similar outcomes with the same incidence of complications.[116,117]

Midthoracic Diverticula

Midthoracic diverticula usually develop within 4 to 5 cm of the tracheal carina. Until recently, these diverticula were commonly caused by traction secondary to mediastinal fibrosis or chronic lymphadenopathy from pulmonary tuberculosis or histoplasmosis. Many patients with these diverticula are found to have abnormal peristaltic waves from achalasia, DES, or other nonspecific esophageal motor disorders (see Fig. 36-5B).[118,119]

Patients with mid-esophageal diverticula may be asymptomatic; however, a history of dysphagia, retrosternal pain, regurgitation, belching, epigastric pain, heartburn, and weight loss may be elicited. Although attributed to the diverticulum, these symptoms may be the result of the associated motor disorder. Complications are unusual, but spontaneous rupture, hemorrhage, aspiration, esophagobronchial fistula, and carcinoma have been reported.

Most patients with mid-thoracic diverticula require no treatment. Borrie and Wilson reported that although 80% of patients had a proven motility disorder, only 20% required surgery.[120] Diverticulectomy with esophageal myotomy is the preferred treatment for mid-thoracic diverticula associated with esophageal motility disorders. Right thoracotomy provides excellent exposure of the esophagus and airway at the tracheal bifurcation. Placing a bougie in the esophagus avoids compromise of the esophageal lumen and helps guide diverticulectomy. The mural defect should be repaired in two layers: the mucosal and submucosal layers closed with a continuous absorbable suture or staples and the muscularis propria reapproximated with interrupted absorbable sutures. The esophageal repair may be buttressed with pleura, pleuropericardial fat pad, or omentum. A myotomy can be carried out on the esophageal wall opposite the diverticulectomy. Diverticulopexy with suspension of the diverticulum superiorly from the prevertebral fascia,[121] a myotomy alone,[122] and diverticulectomy alone[123] have been successfully applied in treating mid-thoracic esophageal diverticula. Treatment of true traction diverticulum, secondary to periesophageal inflammation, is often in the setting of an esophagobronchial fistula. Excision of the diverticulum, repair of the esophagus, removal of inflammatory nodes, closure of the airway fistula, and interposition of muscle are required.

Epiphrenic Diverticula

Epiphrenic diverticula occur in the distal third of the esophagus, and the distal margin of the diverticulum is less than 4 cm from the gastroesophageal junction. There is usually an associated esophageal motor disorder or hiatal hernia.[124] Epiphrenic diverticula are occasionally asymptomatic, but most patients present with dysphagia, regurgitation, vomiting, chest and epigastric pain, anorexia, weight loss, cough, halitosis, or noisy swallowing. There is no apparent relationship between symptoms and the size of the diverticulum.

Barium esophagogram best identifies epiphrenic diverticula and often characterizes the underlying motility disorder (Fig. 36-20). Many patients show bizarre, nonpropulsive tertiary contractions during examination. In addition to fixed, wide-mouthed diverticula, transient outpouchings can occur proximally in segments where peristalsis is absent. Timed barium esophagogram may be used in any patient in whom an emptying disorder is suspected, particularly in achalasia (see Fig. 36-7). Esophagoscopy generally yields little information about diverticula, but it may rule out malignancy and assess associated esophageal problems. Esophageal motility is essential before surgery. Esophagoscopy may be required to pass the manometry catheter past the diverticulum into the stomach.

Most authors agree that a diverticulectomy alone may result in a recurrence and advocate adding a myotomy.[125-127] Addition of an antireflux procedure to diverticulectomy and myotomy is controversial. However, if added, a partial (nonobstructing) wrap, such as a Belsey, Toupet, or Dor fundoplication, may minimize postoperative dysphagia.

Benign Esophageal Tumors and Cysts

Benign esophageal tumors are uncommon and represent less than 1% of esophageal neoplasms. EUS is essential in the diagnosis. Thus, classification by layer of origin in the esophageal

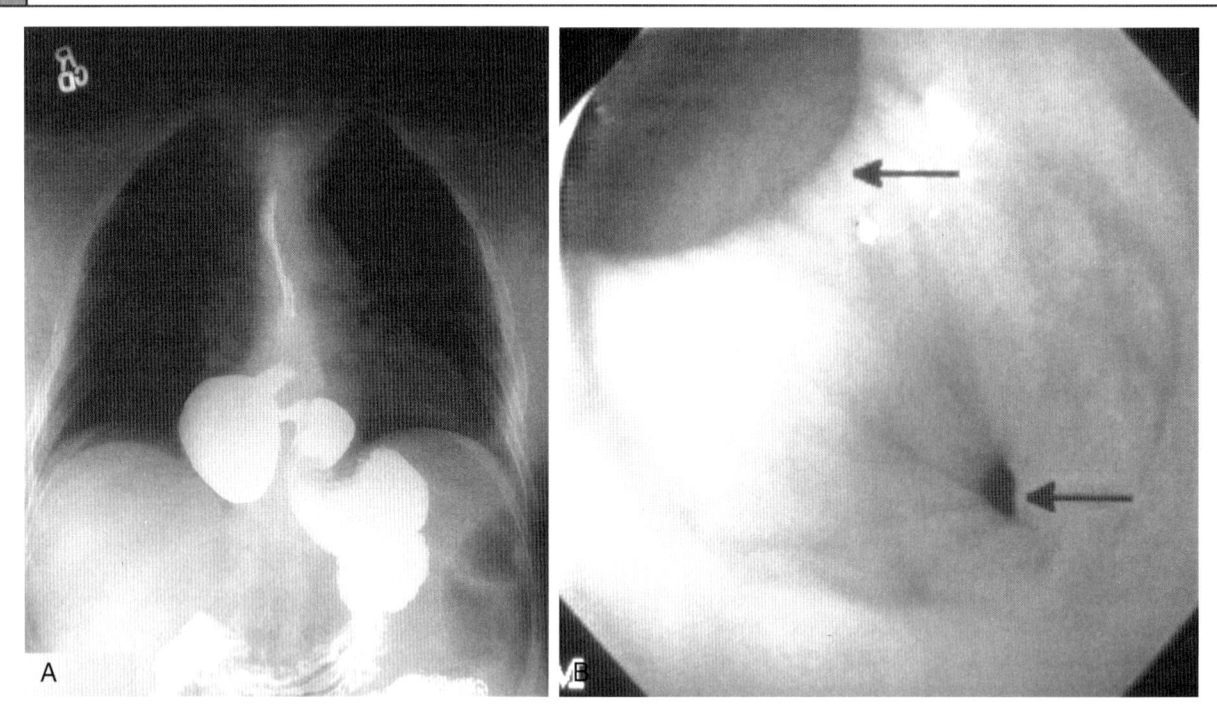

Figure 36–20
Epiphrenic diverticulum. **A,** Barium esophagram shows a large diverticulum. **B,** At esophagoscopy, the wide-mouthed diverticulum *(upper arrow)* and deviated distal esophageal lumen *(lower arrow)* are seen. Preferential filling of the diverticulum with swallowing can be appreciated from this examination.

Box 36–2
Classification of Benign Esophageal Tumors

Mucosa (First and Second Esophageal Ultrasound [EUS] Layers)
  Squamous papilloma
  Fibrovascular polyp
  Retention cyst

Submucosa (Third EUS Layer)
  Lipoma
  Fibroma
  Neurofibroma
  Granular cell tumor
  Hemangiomas
  Salivary gland–type tumor

Muscularis Propria (Fourth EUS Layer)
  Leiomyoma
  Duplication cyst

Periesophageal Tissue (Fifth EUS Layer)
  Foregut cyst

---

wall is the most clinically useful categorization of benign esophageal tumors (Box 36-2).

Tumors of the Mucosa

Squamous papillomas are small (<1 cm), solitary, sessile projections in the distal esophagus and are usually found incidentally.[128] Histologic evaluation shows vascularized projections of the lamina propria covered by hyperplastic squamous epithelium. Biopsy differentiates squamous papillomas from small superficial squamous cell carcinomas. Because progression to malignancy is rare, asymptomatic patients require no follow-up. Symptomatic papillomas or those with atypical histologic features require excision, usually endoscopic. Although their cause is unknown, associations with human papilloma virus and GERD have been reported.[129]

Fibrovascular polyps are collections of fibrous, vascular, and adipose tissue lined by normal squamous epithelium. These polyps, which usually arise in the cervical esophagus and extend into the esophageal lumen, may reach into the stomach. Most patients complain of dysphagia and respiratory symptoms.[130] Regurgitation into the hypopharynx with subsequent aspiration and asphyxia is possible. These lesions can be detected by either barium esophagogram or esophagoscopy (Fig. 36-21). Because fibrovascular polyps fill the esophageal lumen and have a composition similar to that of the mucosa, diagnosis by esophagoscopy or EUS may be difficult or impossible.[131] Most polyps are surgically treated, although some have been removed endoscopically. Recurrence after resection is rare.

Tumors of the Submucosa

At esophagoscopy, lipomas are noted as a bulging of the overlying esophageal mucosa. They have a pale yellow appearance and a soft or pillow-like texture when probed endoscopically. Esophagoscopic biopsies demonstrate only normal squamous epithelium because forceps rarely penetrate the submucosa. EUS demonstrates a hyperechoic homogeneous lesion that originates in and is confined to the submucosal layer. If asymptomatic, only observation is required.

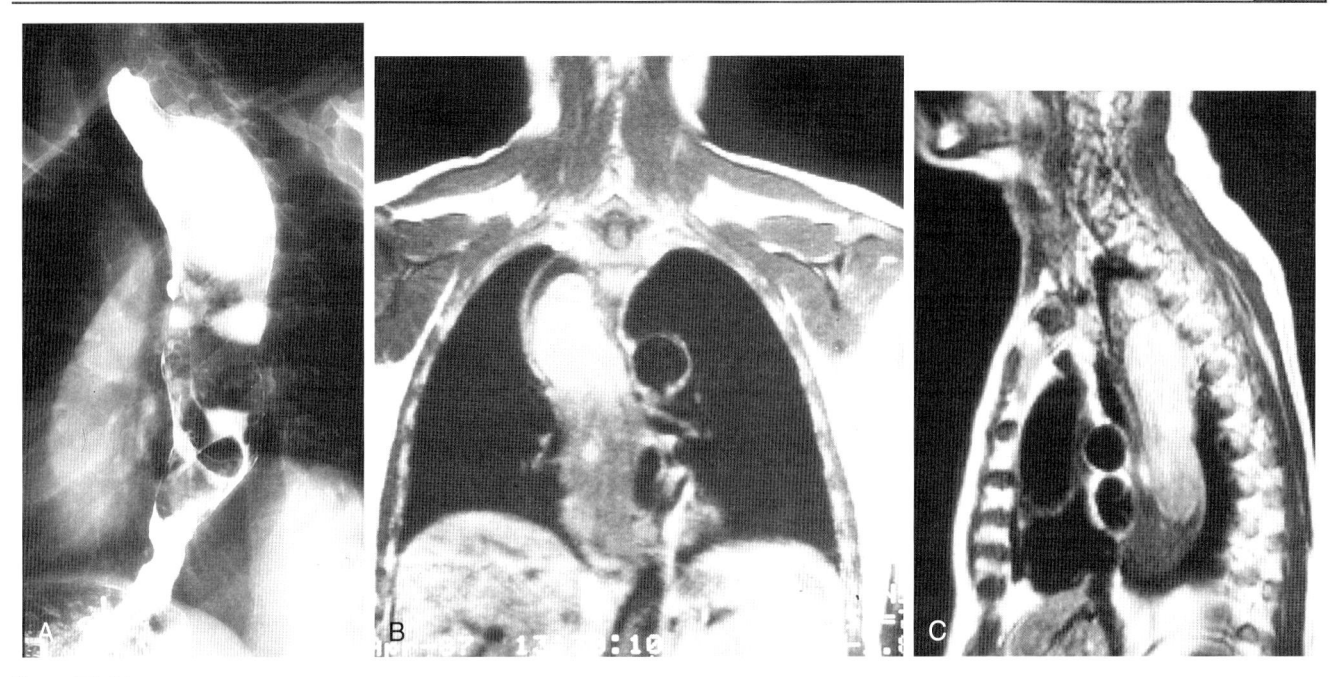

Figure 36–21
Fibrovascular polyp. **A,** Large polypoid filling defect of the intrathoracic esophagus. **B** and **C,** Magnetic resonance images show a large, soft tissue mass filling the esophagus.

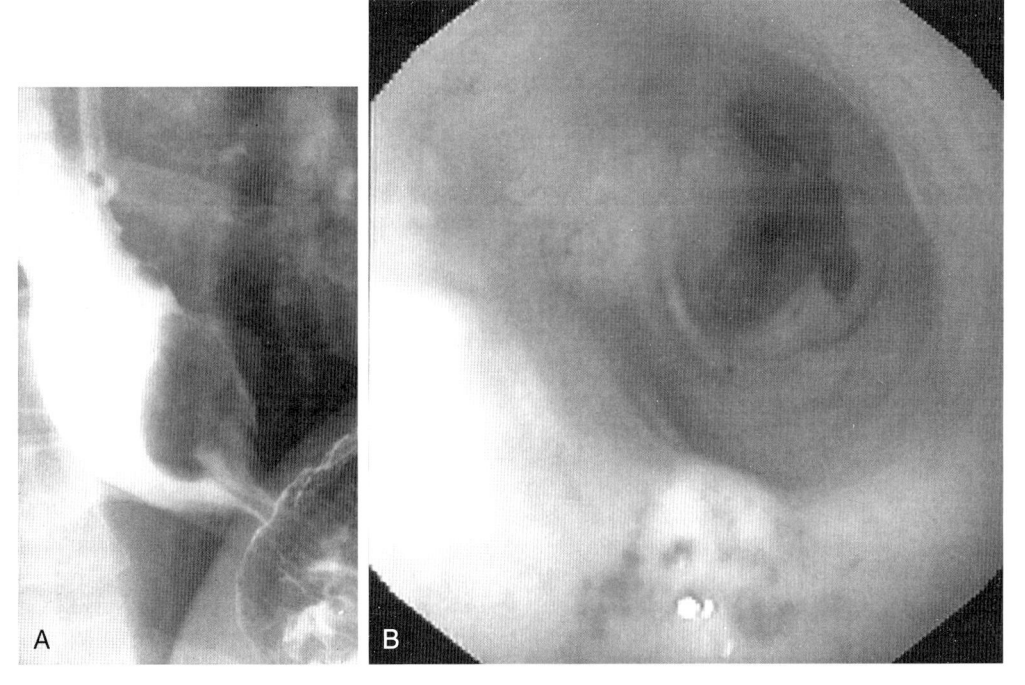

Figure 36–22
Granular cell tumor. **A,** In a patient with dysphagia and acid reflux symptoms, barium esophagram shows a polypoid filling defect in the distal esophagus. **B,** Esophagoscopy of another patient with a granular cell tumor shows a tumor that is extra-epithelial. Biopsy of this tumor was diagnostic for granular cell tumor.

Fibromas and neurofibromas are rare. At endoscopy, unlike lipomas, they are firm "to the touch." These lesions, which arise from the submucosa, are less hyperechoic by EUS than lipomas. Symptomatic submucosal tumors have been enucleated with minimally invasive techniques.[132]

Granular cell tumors are of neural origin and arise from Schwann cells. The majority of patients with granular cell tumors are asymptomatic and rarely require surgery.[133] At endoscopy, these lesions are yellow, firm nodules, which can be diagnosed by routine endoscopic biopsies (Fig. 36-22). On EUS, granular cell tumors arise from the submucosa and are hyperechoic, but less so than lipomas.[134] Nests of cells with pyknotic nuclei, abundant granular cytoplasm, absence of mitotic figures, and strong S-100 protein expression

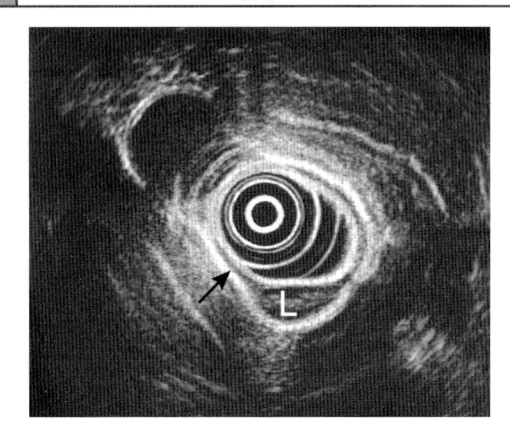

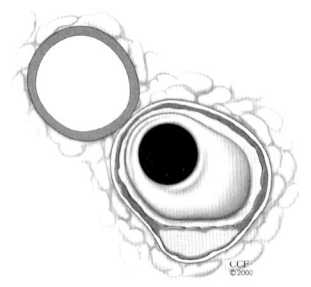

Figure 36–23
An esophageal leiomyoma (L). *Above:* Esophageal ultrasound (EUS) of this most common benign tumor demonstrates a hypoechoic, homogeneous, well-demarcated tumor with no associated lymphadenopathy. EUS balloon overdistention blends the first three ultrasound layers into one hyperechoic layer. Tumor arises from and is confined to the fourth ultrasound layer *(arrow). Below:* A benign leiomyoma arises from and is confined to the muscularis propria.

characterize these tumors. Malignant variants have been reported.[133,134]

Hemangiomas can present with dysphagia and bleeding. Most are found in the lower esophagus, where they may be mistaken for esophageal varices. EUS examination reveals a hypoechoic mass with sharp margins arising from the second or third EUS layer.[135,136] Treatment options include observation, simple excision, fulgarization, or radiotherapy.[137] Salivary gland–type tumors have been rarely reported in the esophagus and probably arise from submucosal esophageal glands.

Tumors of the Muscularis Propria

Leiomyomas are benign, smooth muscle tumors of the muscularis propria. They are the most common benign esophageal tumor and account for more than 70% of these neoplasms. Most arise from the inner circular muscle layer of the distal and mid-thoracic esophagus. They have no sex preponderance, and they typically occur in younger patients (20 to 50 years old) than esophageal cancer. Although frequently asymptomatic and discovered incidentally, leiomyomas can cause dysphagia, pain, or bleeding. In addition, distal esophageal leiomyomas are often associated with symptoms of GERD. Barium esophagogram demonstrates smooth-contoured filling defects. At esophagoscopy and EUS, a normal overlying mucosa is seen over a hypoechoic tumor arising from the fourth ultrasound layer (Fig. 36-23). Atypical EUS findings are a tumor 4 cm or larger, irregular margins, mixed internal echo characteristics and associated regional lymphadenopathy. Definitive diagnosis is difficult to obtain, because endoscopic biopsies do not reach the muscularis propria, and EUS-directed FNA does not provide enough information to differentiate leiomyomas from leiomyosarcomas.

Symptomatic neoplasms should be resected. For asymptomatic tumors with typical EUS features, expectant therapy and EUS observation are indicated. Leiomyosarcomas are exceedingly rare,[138] and malignant transformation of benign leiomyomas has been infrequently reported.[139] Gastrointestinal stromal tumors (GIST) rarely occur in the esophagus and must be differentiated from leiomyomas. These tumors, which originate from the gastrointestinal pacemaker cells of Cajal, stain positively for tyrosine kinase and should be excised by esophagectomy.[140]

Esophageal Cysts

Esophageal cysts are the second most common benign esophageal tumor, accounting for 20% of these lesions. The minority are acquired epithelial cysts, arising in the lamina propria.[141] Submucosal glandular inflammation is the suspected cause. The majority of esophageal cysts are congenital foregut cysts.[142] They are lined with squamous, respiratory, or columnar epithelium and may contain smooth muscle, cartilage, or fat. An esophageal duplication is a type of foregut cyst; it is lined with squamous epithelium, and its submucosal and muscularis elements interdigitate with the muscularis propria of the esophagus. Duplication cysts may be associated with vertebral and spinal cord abnormalities. Many patients with foregut cysts present in the first year of life with life-threatening respiratory compromise resulting from mass effect. EUS can clearly define the intramural or extra-esophageal nature of these tumors and further determine their anechoic, cystic nature (Fig. 36-24).[143-146] Regardless, removal of all discovered cysts is suggested because most become symptomatic by adulthood.[147] In addition, transesophageal drainage has also been reported, but drainage of the cyst without destroying its lining often results in recurrence.[148]

Esophageal Injuries

Strictures

A variety of benign congenital and acquired disorders as well as malignant lesions can result in esophageal stricture. Congenital esophageal strictures, although rare, occur in the distal esophagus. They may result from the same developmental abnormalities that produce tracheoesophageal fistula or esophageal atresia.[149] Acquired esophageal strictures can be either benign or malignant (Box 36-3). Although most benign strictures result from chronic injury and resultant fibrous repair, they can occur after a single injury. Malignant strictures are usually primary esophageal adenocarcinomas or squamous cell carcinomas. Local invasion of a bronchogenic carcinoma or secondary involvement from breast, lung, or renal primary sites can produce a malignant stricture.

The patient typically does not perceive difficulty swallowing until the esophageal lumen is half its normal diameter. Because the obstruction is structural, dysphagia associated with esophageal stricture is unremitting and reproducible. Dysphagia from strictures can often be distinguished from other causes by history. Dysphagia in esophageal motility disorders

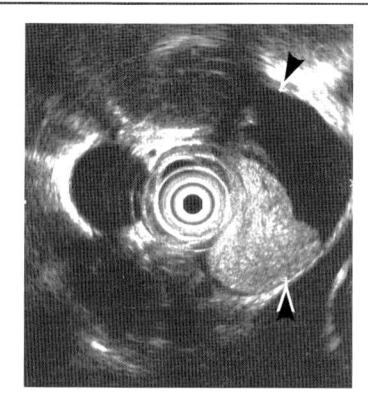

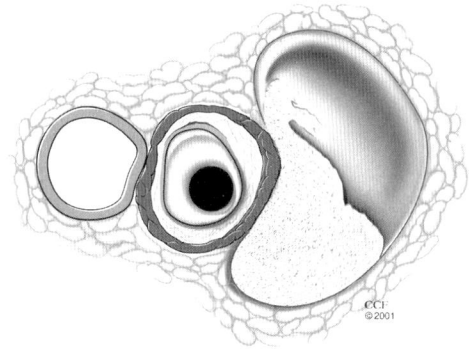

Figure 36-24
Foregut cyst. *Above:* Esophageal ultrasound (EUS) demonstrates a mass *(arrowheads)* adjacent to the trachea and esophagus. The cyst has two components, one hyperechoic *(white)*, representing proteinaceous material, and one hypoechoic *(black)*, representing fluid. *Below:* Foregut cyst in close proximity to esophagus and trachea.

> **Box 36-3**
> **Causes of Esophageal Strictures**
>
> **Benign**
>   Congenital
>   Esophageal atresia
>   Tracheoesophageal fistula
>   Web
>   Acquired
>   Peptic
>   Gastroesophageal reflux
>   Scleroderma
>   Schatzki's ring
>   Caustic ingestion
>   Drug induced
>   Anticholinergic medications
>   Aspirin
>   Clinitest
>   Fosamax
>   Nonsteroidal anti-inflammatory
>   Quinidine
>   Potassium supplements
>   Tetracycline
>   Vitamin C
>   Eosinophilic esophagitis
>   Iatrogenic
>   Variceal ligation/injection
>   Postoperative (anastomotic)
>   Radiation
>   Instrumentation
>   Nasogastric tube
>   Infections
>   Fungal: moniliasis
>   Bacterial: syphilis
>   Mycobacterial: tuberculosis
>   Granulomatous
>   Crohn's disease
>   Dermatosis
>   Epidermolysis bullosa dystrophica
>   Pemphigoid
>   Behçet's disease
> **Malignant**
>   Primary
>   Secondary

is typically intermittent, with both liquids and solids. Chest pain is often present. Oropharyngeal dysphagia is suggested by choking, aspiration, drooling, or nasal regurgitation, in addition to a sense of solid bolus retention in the neck, resulting in repeated swallowing.

Barium esophagram is usually the first test in evaluation of dysphagia and suspected esophageal stricture. Subtle strictures may be found with a barium tablet (13 mm). Once the stricture anatomy is defined, esophagoscopy is crucial to characterize, biopsy, and dilate the stricture. EUS is an important diagnostic adjunct after successful dilation in strictures with submucosal or extrinsic features at esophagoscopy or esophagram.

A treatment algorithm for esophageal stricture is given in Figure 36-25. For benign dilatable strictures, the inciting agent must be identified and removed and the stricture treated by dilation as necessary. Simple benign strictures can usually be treated with bougie or through-the-scope balloon dilators. More complex strictures typically need wire guided dilation, which is best done with fluoroscopy. Longer, more complex, and tight strictures are typically from corrosive ingestion, radiation, nasogastric tubes, eosinophilic esophagitis, or congenital esophageal stenosis. These are particularly challenging to dilate. Frequent dilation may be necessary, and stricture injection with steroids should be considered.[150] Recent encouraging reports of self-expanding plastic esophageal stents suggest that they play a role as a nonpermanent dilator.[151] Nondilatable benign strictures and resectable malignant strictures are treated by excision and reconstruction. Inoperable malignant strictures are palliated.

Peptic esophageal stricture is a late complication of severe, poorly controlled GERD. Fortunately, peptic stricture is much less common since the widespread use of PPIs.[152] Although initial damage is confined to the epithelium, with continued exposure to refluxed gastric contents, the injury progresses to involve the submucosa, the esophageal musculature, and, eventually, periesophageal tissue. The components of this

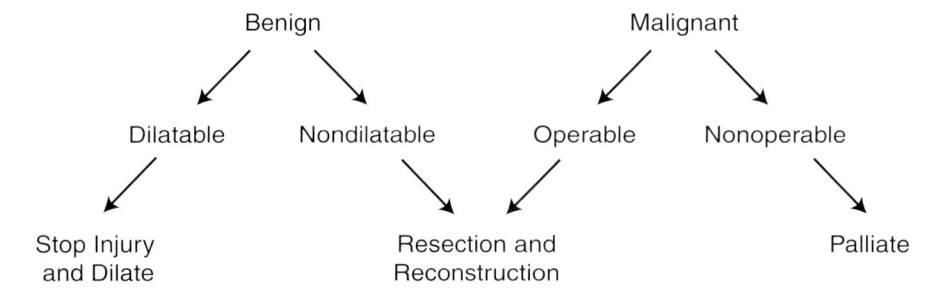

```
                    Benign                              Malignant
                   /      \                            /         \
             Dilatable   Nondilatable              Operable    Nonoperable
                /              \                   /                \
         Stop Injury        Resection and                          Palliate
         and Dilate         Reconstruction
```

Figure 36–25
Treatment algorithm for esophageal strictures.

injury are spasm, inflammation, and fibrosis. Eventually, the injury–repair cycle ends in cicatricial fibrosis and obstructive physiology of the distal esophagus. Most patients with peptic strictures present with dysphagia. It is less common for a patient to develop a symptomatic stricture during the treatment and follow-up of GERD. Although patients often do not have a prior diagnosis of GERD, more than 75% have symptoms of reflux.[153]

Most peptic strictures are located in the distal esophagus, usually above a hiatal hernia (see Figs. 36-5 and 36-6A). They are smooth, tapered areas of concentric narrowing. Occasionally, asymmetric peptic scarring produces an eccentric stricture mimicking carcinoma. Symptomatic peptic strictures are usually 1 to 4 cm in length and 2 to 15 mm in diameter. They may be difficult to dilate, and they often recur, although aggressive PPI therapy makes this uncommon. Most peptic strictures occur at the squamocolumnar junction. Occurrence of the stricture well above the esophagogastric junction is suggestive of Barrett's mucosa, which has been reported in 44% of patients with peptic esophageal strictures.[154]

Surgery should be considered for young patients who would require lifelong medication and for those who cannot tolerate medication. Early surgical correction provides better long-term results than late intervention, because the esophageal injury is more likely to be reversible.

Scleroderma should be suspected in patients with refractory and complicated GERD. The disease affects the smooth muscle of the esophagus and results in an incompetent LES and poor motility of the esophageal body. Massive reflux and insufficient esophageal clearance causes severe GERD and peptic complications that are difficult to treat. The mainstay of treatment is acid suppression and repeated dilation. Antireflux surgery should be avoided if possible because of poor or absent peristalsis. If required, an esophageal lengthening procedure and partial fundoplication are indicated. Total fundoplication may worsen the dysphagia because inadequate peristalsis and poor clearance may not overcome a reconstructed LES. Peptic damage may be so severe that it requires resecting the amotile strictured esophagus.

Schatzki's ring occurs precisely at the squamocolumnar junction (see Fig. 36-6B). These ringlike narrowings involve the mucosa and submucosa. They are thin, web-like constrictions, usually associated with hiatal hernia, and are best seen radiographically. These rings may be missed at esophagoscopy because of incomplete distension of the esophagus. Schatzki's rings, thought to be reflux related, are amenable to dilation.

Patients with pill-induced esophageal injury generally have no previous esophageal disease history. The initial injury is an ulcer, and patients typically present with chest pain and odynophagia.[155,156] Then, painless dysphagia heralds the onset of a pill-induced stricture. Many patients recall the initial episode of pill lodging, typically a rushed ingestion done without caution, often without liquids and in a recumbent position. Pill injury is more common in women than in men.

Common locations of pill injury are in the cervical esophagus and the thoracic esophagus at the aortic arch, but other areas of anatomic or pathologic narrowing may trap a pill. Most medications produce superficial injuries that usually heal spontaneously. However, quinidine, potassium chloride, and Fosamax can produce severe esophagitis, and transmural injury may occur, leading to scarring and a stricture requiring dilation.

Rarely, an esophageal stricture can be caused by a nasogastric tube in place for days to weeks. Patients develop symptoms weeks to months after tube removal. The mechanism of injury is unknown but is postulated to be trauma from tube insertion, chronic irritation by the tube, uncontrolled gastroesophageal reflux from an indwelling tube stenting the LES open, or impaired esophageal clearance secondary to the tube. Typically, barium esophagram demonstrates a long stricture with extensive ulceration in the mid and distal esophagus (Fig. 36-26). Initially, the strictures are smooth, tapered concentric narrowings that mimic peptic strictures. Progression can be rapid, with increased stricture length and severity resembling caustic strictures. Treatment includes dilation, avoidance of esophageal intubation, and aggressive antireflux medication.

Eosinophilic esophagitis (EE) has been recognized recently as a cause of esophageal symptoms, especially dysphagia and strictures.[157] Diagnosis is made by mucosal biopsy when at least 15 eosinophils per high-power field are present. Endoscopic findings suggesting EE are multiple rings, linear furrowing, and a narrow-caliber esophagus with normal mucosa. In retrospect, many patients previously diagnosed with "ringed esophagus" or "congenital esophageal stenosis" in fact had EE. It is believed to be of allergic origin, as some patients have an allergic history, and allergy testing is suggested.

Treatment of EE is in evolution. Swallowed steroids (Fluticasone) are recommended. Elimination diets, which have been particularly beneficial in children, are suggested for selected adult patients with EE. Immune therapies are being evaluated and offer promise. For persistent dysphagia, PPI and dilation are indicated. Esophageal dilation has drawbacks, including frequent tears and occasional perforation in advanced cases. When a long tight stricture is present, multiple dilation sessions may be necessary, and a goal diameter of 14 to 15 mm is suggested.[158]

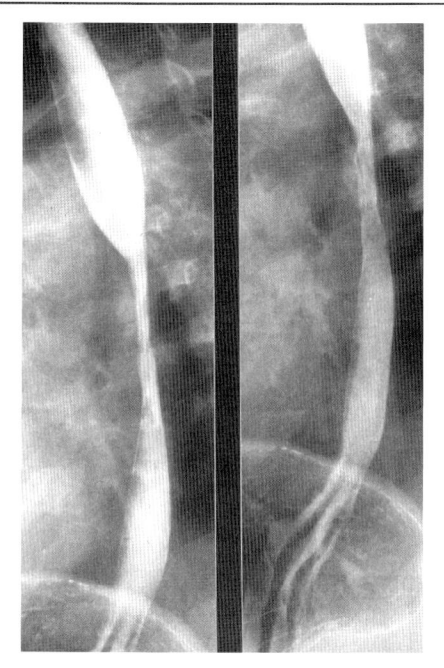

Figure 36–26
Nasogastric tube stricture. This patient had a prolonged stay in the intensive care unit and a protracted period of nasogastric tube drainage. A barium esophagram 1 month after discharge demonstrates a long, smooth, benign-appearing stricture of the midthoracic esophagus.

Radiation strictures can occur as early as 3 to 8 months after radiation dosages between 30 and 60 Gy.[159,160] They are smooth, concentric, and tapered, and they lie in the radiation portals. Low-dose radiotherapy and concurrent doxorubicin administration can also produce esophageal strictures. Other esophageal complications attributed to these therapies include esophagotracheal and esophagobronchial fistulae.

Anastomotic strictures complicate as many as a third of reconstructions after esophagectomy. Factors that produce these strictures include anastomotic tension, ischemia, infection, and radiation. Strictures are more common after anastomotic leaks, local infection, and adjuvant radiotherapy. Treatment is usually repeated dilation. Recurrent carcinoma may be difficult to detect by esophagoscopy and may require endoscopic ultrasound.[161,162]

Corrosive Injuries

Corrosive injuries of the esophagus are caused by the ingestion of strong acid or alkali. There is a bimodal distribution of age and etiology. In children less than 5 years of age, ingestion is usually accidental—the result of an inquisitive toddler ingesting improperly stored corrosive agents. The first swallow of the noxious substance usually stops further ingestion and injury. In adults, ingestion of large volumes of caustic agents is usually a suicide attempt.

Early Management

Obtaining a history of the estimated amount and nature of the ingested agent is critical to directing treatment.[163] Bleach and phosphate detergents are irritants that rarely produce significant injury. Ingestion of strong acid produces coagulation necrosis, which may limit the depth of injury. However, rapid passage and pooling in the stomach can promote gastric injury.[164] Ingesting viscous alkali produces liquefaction necrosis and increased depth of injury. Historically, most alkali agents were solids, generally restricting injuries to the mouth, oropharynx, hypopharynx, esophagus, and trachea. Significant solid corrosive ingestion may produce oral pain, drooling, excessive salivation, inability or refusal to swallow or drink, hoarseness, aphonia, dyspnea, stridor, and ulceration of the mouth, pharynx, or larynx. Currently, the availability of liquid alkali has altered the pattern of injury. These agents pass rapidly through the upper gastrointestinal tract, producing severe injury to the esophagus at physiologic points of narrowing (cricopharyngeus, upper thoracic esophagus at the tracheal bifurcation, and the distal thoracic esophagus) as well as the stomach and adjacent intra-abdominal organs. Significant liquid caustic ingestion typically produces dysphagia, odynophagia, chest and abdominal pain, and signs of mediastinitis or peritonitis.

Patients should be admitted to the hospital and given orders not to receive anything by mouth. Because the injury is immediate, dilution or induction of emesis is not helpful. In fact, regurgitation of the alkali may worsen the injury by repeat exposure of the injured area to the agent. Fluid resuscitation and broad-spectrum antibiotic therapy is essential. Early administration of corticosteroids does not limit the depth of injury or reduce the incidence of late strictures.[165,166] Intubation or tracheostomy and ventilation may be urgently required if there is significant laryngotracheal injury. Rapid evaluation of the upper gastrointestinal tract with flexible fiberoptic esophagogastroduodenoscopy is important to identify location and extent of injury. This is facilitated by the smallest esophagoscope available with limited use of insufflation. Grading of caustic injury is similar to that of cutaneous burns.[167] First-degree injuries exhibit only mucosal edema and hyperemia. Second-degree injuries demonstrate blisters with vesicle and pseudomembrane formation. Third-degree injuries produce deep ulcers with eschar formation.

Patients with first-degree injuries require no specific treatment; the incidence of stricture is low. Patients with second- and third-degree burns are at increased risk of early mortality and late complications. The esophagus should be allowed to reepithelialize; early dilation may increase stricture formation and risk for perforation.[168] Frequent clinical assessment is necessary to detect and treat necrosis of the esophagus or stomach. Resection of the involved organ or organs with delayed reconstruction is recommended for transmural necrosis with mediastinitis or peritonitis. Tracheoesophageal fistula complicating caustic injury should be managed with esophageal resection and exclusion and tracheostomy.[169] Reconstruction is delayed for several months. Patients without acute complications should be placed on a bland liquid or mechanical soft diet and prophylactic acid-suppression medication.

Ingestion of small alkali disc batteries presents a particular threat to small children. Severe esophageal injury may result within hours of ingestion, as a result of current generation, seepage of extremely corrosive contents from damaged cases, and pressure necrosis. Careful endoscopic removal is aimed at preserving the integrity of the battery case.[170] Passage of batteries through the stomach or lower gastrointestinal tract is uneventful.

Late Management

Dilation of caustic strictures should begin a few weeks after injury if the patient is symptomatic or a stricture is demonstrated radiographically. Although retrograde dilation has been proposed as the safest dilation technique, it requires gastrostomy. Prograde guided bougienage or balloon dilation has been successful. Short strictures not responding to initial dilation may benefit from local steroid injection followed by repeat dilation.[171] Axial shortening of the esophagus results in hiatal hernia and GERD and may worsen the original corrosive injury. Need for excessive dilation and inability to dilate to a sufficient diameter are indications for resection and reconstruction. Colonic interposition used to be preferred for replacement after resection of corrosive esophageal injuries, but stomach, if not injured by the ingestion, is now the organ of choice.[172] Lye ingestion places patients at 1000 times the cancer risk of the general population.[173,174]

Perforation

Perforation of the esophagus results in chemical and infectious mediastinitis, which is lethal unless treated early and effectively. Iatrogenic injury is the most common cause of perforation.[172] The incidence of this complication is less than 0.05% during diagnostic endoscopy, but it increases with the complexity of the procedure and the underlying esophageal pathology. A perforation rate up to 17% has been documented after dilation of caustic strictures.[175,176] The esophagus may be injured not only by instrumentation but during any procedure performed in the vicinity of the esophagus. Trauma and spontaneous (barogenic) rupture are the next most common causes of perforation. The esophagus is normal in about 50% of perforations. Pathologic changes in the remaining cases include benign strictures in 25% of patients, diverticula in 15%, carcinoma in 10%, and achalasia in 5%.[172,177]

A high index of suspicion is important for early recognition of injury. Symptoms of spontaneous rupture are often nonspecific and include acute chest and abdominal pain, odynophagia, dyspnea, and fever. A catastrophic presentation with acute sepsis may be seen. Any patient reporting symptoms after instrumentation of the esophagus should be considered to have a perforation until proved otherwise. Pleural effusion, pneumothorax, pneumomediastinum, and subcutaneous emphysema are nonspecific chest radiograph findings. However, chest radiographs are diagnostic in only 15% of patients and may be normal in 10%.[178] Clinical diagnosis of esophageal perforation is confirmed by esophagram (Fig. 36-27). This is first performed with Gastrografin aqueous contrast material and, if that is negative, repeated with barium. Up to 22% of perforations are missed if only aqueous contrast is used.[179] Computed tomographic scanning with ingestion of oral contrast has replaced barium esophagram in many institutions.

Some injuries may be contained within the wall of the esophagus. When the laceration is limited to the esophageal wall or when contrast material drains freely into the esophagus without distal esophageal obstruction, patients without fever or elevated white cell count can be followed by observation.[180,181] However, if a transmural injury with mediastinal soilage is identified, definitive surgical management is required after fluid resuscitation and administration of intravenous antibiotics. The principles of treatment are débridement of infected or necrotic tissue, closure of the perforation, treatment of underlying esophageal pathology (if present), and drainage of the mediastinum. A myotomy at the site of perforation allows the full extent of damage to the mucosa to be recognized and repaired. Reinforcement of the repair decreases mortality and fistula formation.[182] Delayed recognition of a perforation makes successful primary repair less likely. Therapy should be directed toward defunctioning, débridement, drainage, and resection.[183-185] Surgical drainage without repair is possible for most cervical perforations. Descending mediastinitis requires prompt treatment of the mediastinal component of a cervical perforation and may necessitate addition of a right thoracotomy to the cervical incision.[186] Palliation of perforated esophageal carcinoma has been successful with self-expanding, covered metallic stents.[187] One third of patients experience dysphagia after repair of esophageal perforations and require either dilation or further surgery.[188] The best results are seen in patients with achalasia and other motor disorders who undergo a myotomy during perforation repair. In patients with strictures or diffuse esophageal disease, esophagectomy may produce the best long-term results.

Esophageal Foreign Bodies

The majority of ingested foreign bodies are seen in toddlers.[189] In younger adults, ingested foreign bodies are usually associated with drug or alcohol use or psychiatric illness. In older adults, with either dentures or esophageal pathology, a food bolus may serve as the impacted foreign body. The site of impaction is invariably at a physiologic or pathologic area of narrowing. Plain film and contrast radiography are diagnostic for the majority of patients. Most small blunt objects pass into the distal gastrointestinal tract without difficulty. Blunt impacted foreign bodies may be removed with a flexible esophagoscope and balloon catheters or baskets. Sharp or pointed objects, if the sharp edge is directed aborally, may be removed with flexible esophagoscopy; little damage is incurred from the sharp trailing edge. However, if the leading edge is sharp,

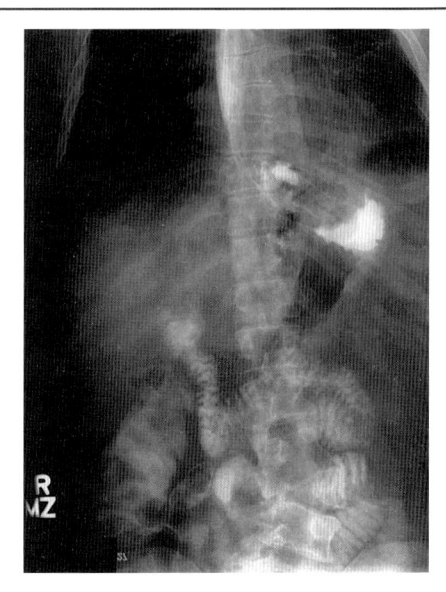

Figure 36–27
Perforation. The patient has just undergone unguided esophageal dilation of a distal esophageal stricture, and barium esophagram shows extravasation of barium into the mediastinum.

rigid esophagoscopy with retraction of the sharp edge into the barrel of the rigid esophagoscope may be necessary. Surgical removal is rarely required for impacted foreign objects or those complicated by lacerations and mediastinitis.

CONCLUSIONS

The understanding of esophageal anatomy, function, and physiology is essential to correctly diagnose and successfully treat benign esophageal diseases. Esophageal conditions amenable to surgery are uncommon except hiatal hernia and GERD. Restoration of esophageal function and the ability to swallow are essential. It is imperative that the first operation be successful, or the patient is started down the path of multiple reoperations that will ultimately end in esophagectomy for benign disease.

REFERENCES

1. Meyer GW, Austin RM, Brady 3rd CE, Castell DO. Muscle anatomy of the human esophagus. *J Clin Gastroenterol* 1986;**8**(2):131-4.
2. Yajin S, Murkami G, Takeuchi H, Hasagawa T, Kitano H. The normal configuration and interindividual differences in intramural lymphatic vessels of the esophagus. *J Thorac Cardiovasc Sur* 2009;**137**:1406-14.
3. Kuge K, Murakami G, Mizobuchi S, Hata Y, Aikou T, Sasaguri S. Submucosal territory of the direct lymphatic drainage system to the thoracic duct in the human esophagus. *J Thorac Cardiovasc Surg* 2003;**125**(6):1343–9.
4. Murakami G, Sato I, Shimada K, Dong C, Kato Y, Imazeki T. Direct lymphatic drainage from the esophagus into the thoracic duct. *Surg Radiol Anat* 1994;**16**(4):399-407.
5. Riquet M, Saab M, Le Pimpec Barthes F, Hidden G. Lymphatic drainage of the esophagus in the adult. *Surg Radiol Anat* 1993;**15**(3):209-11.
6. Liebermann-Meffert DM, Luescher U, Neff U, Rüedi TP, Allgöwer M. Esophagectomy without thoracotomy: is there a risk of intramediastinal bleeding? A study on blood supply of the esophagus. *Ann Surg* 1987;**206**(2):184-92.
7. Butler H. The veins of the oesophagus. *Thorax* 1951;**6**(3):276-96.
8. Baker ME, Einstein DM, Herts BR, Remer EM, Motta-Ramirez GA, Ehrenwald E, et al. Gastroesophageal reflux disease: integrating the barium esophagram before and after antireflux surgery. *Radiology* 2007;**243**(2):329-39.
9. Ott DJ, Gelfand DW, Wu WC. Reflux esophagitis: radiographic and endoscopic correlation. *Radiology* 1979;**130**(3):583-8.
10. de Oliveira JM, Birgisson S, Doinoff C, Einstein D, Herts B, Davros W, et al. Timed barium swallow: a simple technique for evaluating esophageal emptying in patients with achalasia. *AJR Am J Roentgenol* 1997;**169**(2):473-9.
11. Kostic SV, Rice TW, Baker ME, Decamp MM, Murthy SC, Rybicki LA, et al. Timed barium esophagogram: a simple physiologic assessment for achalasia. *J Thorac Cardiovasc Surg* 2000;**120**(5):935-43.
12. Pandolfino JE, Ghosh SK, Rice J, Clarke JO, Kwiatek MA, Kahrilas PJ. Classifying esophageal motility by pressure topography characteristics: a study of 400 patients and 75 controls. *Am J Gastroenterol* 2008;**103**(1):27-37.
13. Fox M, Hebbard G, Janiak P, Brasseur JG, Ghosh S, Thumshirn M, et al. High-resolution manometry predicts the success of oesophageal bolus transport and identifies clinically important abnormalities not detected by conventional manometry. *Neurogastroenterol Motil* 2004;**16**(5):533-42.
14. Fox MR, Bredenoord AJ. Oesophageal high-resolution manometry: moving from research into clinical practice. *Gut* 2008;**57**(3):405-23.
15. Manifold DK, Anggiansah A, Marshall RE, Owen WJ. Oesophageal dysmotility is not associated with poor outcome after laparoscopic Nissen fundoplication. *Br J Surg* 1999;**86**(7):969.
16. Wiener GJ, Morgan TM, Copper JB, Wu WC, Castell DO, Sinclair JW, Richter JE. Ambulatory 24-hour esophageal pH monitoring. Reproducibility and variability of pH parameters. *Dig Dis Sci* 1988;**33**(9):1127-33.
17. Singh S, Richter JE, Bradley LA, Haile JM. The symptom index. Differential usefulness in suspected acid-related complaints of heartburn and chest pain. *Dig Dis Sci* 1993;**38**(8):1402-8.
18. Pandolfino JE, Richter JE, Ours T, Guardino JM, Chapman J, Kahrilas PJ. Ambulatory esophageal pH monitoring using a wireless system. *Am J Gastroenterol* 2003;**98**(4):740-9.
19. Kahrilas PJ, Shaheen NJ, Vaezi MF, Hiltz SW, Black E, Modlin IM, et al. American Gastroenterological Association Medical Position Statement on the management of gastroesophageal reflux disease. *Gastroenterology* 2008;**135**(4):1383-91, 1391 e1-5.
20. Shay S, Tutuian R, Sifrim D, Vela M, Wise J, Balaji N, et al. Twenty-four hour ambulatory simultaneous impedance and pH monitoring: a multicenter report of normal values from 60 healthy volunteers. *Am J Gastroenterol* 2004;**99**(6):1037-43.
21. Sifrim D, Castell D, Dent J, Kahrilas PJ. Gastro-oesophageal reflux monitoring: review and consensus report on detection and definitions of acid, non-acid, and gas reflux. *Gut* 2004;**53**(7):1024-31.
22. Mainie I, Tutuian R, Shay S, Vela M, Zhang X, Sifrim D, Castell DO. Acid and non-acid reflux in patients with persistent symptoms despite acid suppressive therapy: a multicentre study using combined ambulatory impedance-pH monitoring. *Gut* 2006;**55**(10):1398-402.
23. Vaezi MF, Shay SS. New techniques in measuring nonacidic esophageal reflux. *Semin Thorac Cardiovasc Surg* 2001;**13**(3):255-64.
24. Bredenoord AJ, Tutuian R, Smout AJ, Castell DO. Technology review: esophageal impedance monitoring. *Am J Gastroenterol* 2007;**102**(1):187-94.
25. Tutuian R, Castell DO. Combined multichannel intraluminal impedance and manometry clarifies esophageal function abnormalities: study in 350 patients. *Am J Gastroenterol* 2004;**99**(6):1011-9.
26. Stilson WL, Sanders I, Gardiner GA, Gorman HC, Lodge DF. Hiatal hernia and gastroesophageal reflux. A clinicoradiological analysis of more than 1,000 cases. *Radiology* 1969;**93**(6):1323-7.
27. Maziak DE, Todd TR, Pearson FG. Massive hiatus hernia: evaluation and surgical management. *J Thorac Cardiovasc Surg* 1998;**115**(1):53-60:discussion 61-2.
28. Hill LD. Incarcerated paraesophageal hernia. A surgical emergency. *Am J Surg* 1973;**126**(2):286-91.
29. Hashemi M, Peters JH, DeMeester TR, Huprich JE, Quek M, Hagen JA, et al. Laparoscopic repair of large type III hiatal hernia: objective followup reveals high recurrence rate. *J Am Coll Surg* 2000;**190**(5):553-60:discussion 560-1.
30. Rathore MA, Andrabi SI, Bhatti MI, Najfi SM, McMurray A. Metaanalysis of recurrence after laparoscopic repair of paraesophageal hernia. *Jsls* 2007;**11**(4):456-60.
31. Oelschlager BK, Pellegrini CA, Hunter J, Soper N, Brunt M, Sheppard B, et al. Biologic prosthesis reduces recurrence after laparoscopic paraesophageal hernia repair: a multicenter, prospective, randomized trial. *Ann Surg* 2006;**244**(4):481-90.
32. Rice TW, Blackstone EH. Does a biologic prosthesis really reduce recurrence after laparoscopic paraesophageal hernia repair? *Ann Surg* 2007;**246**(6):1116-7, author reply 1117-8.
33. Fumagalli U, Bona S, Caputo M, Elmore U, Battafarano F, Pestalozza A, Rosati R. Are Surgisis biomeshes effective in reducing recurrences after laparoscopic repair of large hiatal hernias? *Surg Laparosc Endosc Percutan Tech* 2008;**18**(5):433-6.
34. Gupta A, Chang D, Steele KE, Schweitzer MA, Lyn-Sue J, Lidor AO. Looking beyond age and co-morbidities as predictors of outcomes in paraesophageal hernia repair. *J Gastrointest Surg* 2008.
35. Vakil N, van Zanten SV, Kahrilas P, Dent J, Jones R. Global Consensus Group. The Montreal definition and classification of gastroesophageal reflux disease: a global evidence-based consensus. *Am J Gastroenterol* 2006;**101**(8):1900-20, quiz 1943.
36. Mittal RK, Balaban DH. The esophagogastric junction. *N Engl J Med* 1997;**336**(13):924-32.
37. Kahrilas PJ, Lin S, Chen J, Manka M. The effect of hiatus hernia on gastro-oesophageal junction pressure. *Gut* 1999;**44**(4):476-82.
38. Berstad A, Weberg R, Frøyshov Larsen I, Hoel B, Hauer-Jensen M. Relationship of hiatus hernia to reflux oesophagitis. A prospective study of coincidence, using endoscopy. *Scand J Gastroenterol* 1986;**21**(1):55-8.
39. Kaul B, Petersen H, Myrvold HE, Grette K, Røysland P, Halvorsen T. Hiatus hernia in gastroesophageal reflux disease. *Scand J Gastroenterol* 1986;**21**(1):31-4.
40. Ott DJ, Gelfand DW, Chen YM, Wu WC, Munitz HA. Predictive relationship of hiatal hernia to reflux esophagitis. *Gastrointest Radiol* 1985;**10**(4):317-20.
41. Sontag SJ, Schnell TG, Miller TQ, Nemchausky B, Serlovsky R, O'Connell S, et al. The importance of hiatal hernia in reflux esophagitis compared with lower esophageal sphincter pressure or smoking. *J Clin Gastroenterol* 1991;**13**(6):628-43.
42. Holloway RH, Dent J. Pathophysiology of gastroesophageal reflux. Lower esophageal sphincter dysfunction in gastroesophageal reflux disease. *Gastroenterol Clin North Am* 1990;**19**(3):517-35.
43. Spechler SJ, Lee E, Ahnen D, Goyal RK, Hirano I, Ramirez F, et al. Long-term outcome of medical and surgical therapies for gastroesophageal reflux disease: follow-up of a randomized controlled trial. *JAMA* 2001;**285**(18):2331-8.
44. Lundell L, Miettinen P, Myrvold HE, Pedersen SA, Liedman B, Hatlebakk JG, et al. Continued (5-year) followup of a randomized clinical study comparing antireflux surgery and omeprazole in gastroesophageal reflux disease. *J Am Coll Surg* 2001;**192**(2):172-9, discussion 179-81.
45. Mehta S, Bennett J, Mahon D, Rhodes M. Prospective trial of laparoscopic Nissen fundoplication versus proton pump inhibitor therapy for gastroesophageal reflux disease: Seven-year follow-up. *J Gastrointest Surg* 2006;**10**(9):1312-6, discussion 1316-7.

46. Vaezi MF, Richter JE, Stasney CR, Spiegel JR, Iannuzzi RA, Crawley JA, et al. Treatment of chronic posterior laryngitis with esomeprazole. *Laryngoscope* 2006;**116**(2):254-60.
47. Kahrilas PJ, Shaheen NJ, Vaezi MF. American Gastroenterological Association Institute technical review on the management of gastroesophageal reflux disease. *Gastroenterology* 2008;**135**(4):1392-413, 1413 e1-5.
48. Campos GM, Peters JH, DeMeester TR, Oberg S, Crookes PF, Tan S, et al. Multivariate analysis of factors predicting outcome after laparoscopic Nissen fundoplication. *J Gastrointest Surg* 1999;**3**(3):292-300.
49. So JB, Zeitels SM, Rattner DW. Outcomes of atypical symptoms attributed to gastroesophageal reflux treated by laparoscopic fundoplication. *Surgery* 1998;**124**(1):28-32.
50. Tutuian R, Mainie I, Agrawal A, Adams D, Castell DO. Nonacid reflux in patients with chronic cough on acid-suppressive therapy. *Chest* 2006;**130**(2):386-91.
51. Gurski RR, Peters JH, Hagen JA, DeMeester SR, Bremner CG, Chandrasoma PT, DeMeester TR. Barrett's esophagus can and does regress after antireflux surgery: a study of prevalence and predictive features. *J Am Coll Surg* 2003;**196**(5):706-12, discussion 712-3.
52. Cameron AJ. Barrett's esophagus: prevalence and size of hiatal hernia. *Am J Gastroenterol* 1999;**94**(8):2054-9.
53. Rice TW, Blackstone EH. Surgical management of gastroesophageal reflux disease. *Gastroenterol Clin North Am* 2008;**37**(4):901-19.
54. Gastal OL, Hagen JA, Peters JH, Campos GM, Hashemi M, Theisen J, et al. Short esophagus: analysis of predictors and clinical implications. *Arch Surg* 1999;**134**(6):633-6, discussion 637-8.
55. Pandolfino JE, Kim H, Ghosh SK, Clarke JO, Zhang Q, Kahrilas PJ. High-resolution manometry of the EGJ: an analysis of crural diaphragm function in GERD. *Am J Gastroenterol* 2007;**102**(5):1056-63.
56. Hunter JG, Smith CD, Branum GD, Waring JP, Trus TL, Cornwell M, Galloway K. Laparoscopic fundoplication failures: patterns of failure and response to fundoplication revision. *Ann Surg* 1999;**230**(4):595-604, discussion 604-6.
57. Wetscher GJ, Glaser K, Wieschemeyer T, Gadenstaetter M, Prommegger R, Profanter C. Tailored antireflux surgery for gastroesophageal reflux disease: effectiveness and risk of postoperative dysphagia. *World J Surg* 1997;**21**(6):605-10.
58. Heider TR, Behrns KE, Koruda MJ, Shaheen NJ, Lucktong TA, Bradshaw B, Farrell TM. Complete fundoplication is not associated with increased dysphagia in patients with abnormal esophageal motility. *J Gastrointest Surg* 2001;**5**(1):36-41.
59. Bessell JR, Finch R, Gotley DC, Smithers BM, Nathanson L, Menzies B. Chronic dysphagia following laparoscopic fundoplication. *Br J Surg* 2000;**87**(10):1341-5.
60. Tew S, Jamieson GG, Holloway RH, Ferguson S, Tew P. A prospective study of the effect of fundoplication on primary and secondary peristalsis in the esophagus. *Dis Esophagus* 1997;**10**(4):247-52.
61. Rydberg L, Ruth M, Abrahamsson H, Lundell L. Tailoring antireflux surgery: A randomized clinical trial. *World J Surg* 1999;**23**(6):612-8.
62. Horvath KD, Jobe BA, Herron DM, Swanstrom LL. Laparoscopic Toupet fundoplication is an inadequate procedure for patients with severe reflux disease. *J Gastrointest Surg* 1999;**3**(6):583-91.
63. de Vries DR, van Herwaarden MA, Smout AJ, Samsom M. Gastroesophageal pressure gradients in gastroesophageal reflux disease: relations with hiatal hernia, body mass index, and esophageal acid exposure. *Am J Gastroenterol* 2008;**103**(6):1349-54.
64. Pandolfino JE. The relationship between obesity and GERD: "big or overblown"? *Am J Gastroenterol* 2008;**103**(6):1355-7.
65. Morgenthal CB, Lin E, Shane MD, Hunter JG, Smith CD. Who will fail laparoscopic Nissen fundoplication? Preoperative prediction of long-term outcomes. *Surg Endosc* 2007;**21**(11):1978-84.
66. Fraser J, Watson DI, O'Boyle CJ, Jamieson GG. Obesity and its effect on outcome of laparoscopic Nissen fundoplication. *Dis Esophagus* 2001;**14**(1):50-3.
67. Patterson EJ, Davis DG, Khajanchee Y, Swanström LL. Comparison of objective outcomes following laparoscopic Nissen fundoplication versus laparoscopic gastric bypass in the morbidly obese with heartburn. *Surg Endosc* 2003;**17**(10):1561-5.
68. Anvari M, Bamehriz F. Outcome of laparoscopic Nissen fundoplication in patients with body mass index >or=35. *Surg Endosc* 2006;**20**(2):230-4.
69. Winslow ER, Frisella MM, Soper NJ, Klingensmith ME. Obesity does not adversely affect the outcome of laparoscopic antireflux surgery (LARS). *Surg Endosc* 2003;**17**(12):2003-11.
70. Perez AR, Moncure AC, Rattner DW. Obesity adversely affects the outcome of antireflux operations. *Surg Endosc* 2001;**15**(9):986-9.
71. Soper NJ, Dunnegan D. Anatomic fundoplication failure after laparoscopic antireflux surgery. *Ann Surg* 1999;**229**(5):669-76, discussion 676-7.
72. Hogan WJ, Shaker R. Life after antireflux surgery. *Am J Med* 2000;**108**(Suppl. 4a):181S-91S.
73. Richter JE. Let the patient beware: the evolving truth about laparoscopic antireflux surgery. *Am J Med* 2003;**114**(1):71-3.
74. Vakil N, Shaw M, Kirby R. Clinical effectiveness of laparoscopic fundoplication in a U.S. community. *Am J Med* 2003;**114**(1):1-5.
75. Goldblum JR, Whyte RI, Orringer MB, Appelman HD. Achalasia. A morphologic study of 42 resected specimens. *Am J Surg Pathol* 1994;**18**(4):327-37.
76. Goldblum JR, Rice TW, Richter JE. Histopathologic features in esophagomyotomy specimens from patients with achalasia. *Gastroenterology* 1996;**111**(3):648-54.
77. Clark SB, Rice TW, Tubbs RR, Richter JE, Goldblum JR. The nature of the myenteric infiltrate in achalasia: an immunohistochemical analysis. *Am J Surg Pathol* 2000;**24**(8):1153-8.
78. Sifrim D, Janssens J, Vantrappen G. Failing deglutitive inhibition in primary esophageal motility disorders. *Gastroenterology* 1994;**106**(4):875-82.
79. Goldenberg SP, Burrell M, Fette GG, Vos C, Traube M. Classic and vigorous achalasia: a comparison of manometric, radiographic, and clinical findings. *Gastroenterology* 1991;**101**(3):743-8.
80. Pandolfino JE, Kwiatek MA, Nealis T, Bulsiewicz W, Post J, Kahrilas PJ. Achalasia: a new clinically relevant classification by high-resolution manometry. *Gastroenterology* 2008;**135**(5):1526-33.
81. Vaezi MF, Baker ME, Richter JE. Assessment of esophageal emptying post-pneumatic dilation: use of the timed barium esophagram. *Am J Gastroenterol* 1999;**94**(7):1802-7.
82. Kostic S, Andersson M, Hellström M, Lönroth H, Lundell L. Timed barium esophagogram in the assessment of patients with achalasia: reproducibility and observer variation. *Dis Esophagus* 2005;**18**(2):96-103.
83. Tsui JK. Botulinum toxin as a therapeutic agent. *Pharmacol Ther* 1996;**72**(1):13-24.
84. Bonavina L, Incarbone R, Antoniazzi L, Reitano M, Peracchia A. Previous endoscopic treatment does not affect complication rate and outcome of laparoscopic Heller myotomy and anterior fundoplication for oesophageal achalasia. *Ital J Gastroenterol Hepatol* 1999;**31**(9):827-30.
85. Horgan S, Hudda K, Eubanks T, McAllister J, Pellegrini CA. Does botulinum toxin injection make esophagomyotomy a more difficult operation? *Surg Endosc* 1999;**13**(6):576-9.
86. Ferguson MK, Reeder LB, Olak J. Results of myotomy and partial fundoplication after pneumatic dilation for achalasia. *Ann Thorac Surg* 1996;**62**(2):327-30.
87. Vaezi MF, Richter JE. Current therapies for achalasia: comparison and efficacy. *J Clin Gastroenterol* 1998;**27**(1):21-35.
88. Richter JE. A young man with a new diagnosis of achalasia. *Clin Gastroenterol Hepatol* 2008;**6**(8):859-63.
89. Csendes A, Braghetto I, Henríquez A, Cortés C. Late results of a prospective randomised study comparing forceful dilatation and oesophagomyotomy in patients with achalasia. *Gut* 1989;**30**(3):299-304.
90. Felix VN, Cecconello I, Zilberstein B, Moraes-Filho JP, Pinotti HW, Carvalho E. Achalasia: a prospective study comparing the results of dilatation and myotomy. *Hepatogastroenterology* 1998;**45**(19):97-108.
91. Patti MG, Fisichella PM, Perretta S, Galvani C, Gorodner MV, Robinson T, Way LW. Impact of minimally invasive surgery on the treatment of esophageal achalasia: a decade of change. *J Am Coll Surg* 2003;**196**(5):698-703, discussion 703-5.
92. Wang YR, Dempsey DT, Friedenberg FK, Richter JE. Trends of Heller myotomy hospitalizations for achalasia in the United States, 1993-2005: effect of surgery volume on perioperative outcomes. *Am J Gastroenterol* 2008;**103**(10):2454-64.
93. Morino M, Rebecchi F, Festa V, Garrone C. Preoperative pneumatic dilatation represents a risk factor for laparoscopic Heller myotomy. *Surg Endosc* 1997;**11**(4):359-61.
94. Oelschlager BK, Chang L, Pellegrini CA. Improved outcome after extended gastric myotomy for achalasia. *Arch Surg* 2003;**138**(5):490-5, discussion 495-7.
95. Richards WO, Torquati A, Holzman MD, Khaitan L, Byrne D, Lutfi R, Sharp KW. Heller myotomy versus Heller myotomy with Dor fundoplication for achalasia: a prospective randomized double-blind clinical trial. *Ann Surg* 2004;**240**(3):405-12, discussion 412-5.
96. Rice TW, McKelvey AA, Richter JE, Baker ME, Vaezi MF, Feng J, et al. A physiologic clinical study of achalasia: should Dor fundoplication be added to Heller myotomy? *J Thorac Cardiovasc Surg* 2005;**130**(6):1593-600.
97. Orringer MB, Stirling MC. Esophageal resection for achalasia: indications and results. *Ann Thorac Surg* 1989;**47**(3):340-5.
98. Pinotti HW, Cecconello I, da Rocha JM, Zilberstein B. Resection for achalasia of the esophagus. *Hepatogastroenterology* 1991;**38**(6):470-3.
99. Peters JH, Kauer WK, Crookes PF, Ireland AP, Bremner CG, DeMeester TR. Esophageal resection with colon interposition for end-stage achalasia. *Arch Surg* 1995;**130**(6):632-6, discussion 636-7.
100. Miller DL, Allen MS, Trastek VF, Deschamps C, Pairolero PC. Esophageal resection for recurrent achalasia. *Ann Thorac Surg* 1995;**60**(4):922-5, discussion 925-6.

101. Banbury MK, Rice TW, Goldblum JR, Clark SB, Baker ME, Richter JE, et al. Esophagectomy with gastric reconstruction for achalasia. *J Thorac Cardiovasc Surg* 1999;**117**(6):1077-84.
102. Spechler SJ, Castell DO. Classification of oesophageal motility abnormalities. *Gut* 2001;**49**(1):145-51.
103. Lacy BE, Weiser K. Esophageal motility disorders: medical therapy. *J Clin Gastroenterol* 2008;**42**(5):652-8.
104. Almansa C, Hinder RA, Smith CD, Achem SR. A comprehensive appraisal of the surgical treatment of diffuse esophageal spasm. *J Gastrointest Surg* 2008;**12**(6):1133-45.
105. Ellis Jr FH, Crozier RE, Shea JA. Long esophagomyotomy for diffuse esophageal spasm and related disorders. In: Siewert Jr HA, editor. *Diseases of the esophagus*. New York: Springer-Verlag; 1988. p. 913-7.
106. Leconte M, Douard R, Gaudric M, Dumontier I, Chaussade S, Dousset B. Functional results after extended myotomy for diffuse oesophageal spasm. *Br J Surg* 2007;**94**(9):1113-8.
107. Katz PO, Dalton CB, Richter JE, Wu WC, Castell DO. Esophageal testing of patients with noncardiac chest pain or dysphagia. Results of three years' experience with 1161 patients. *Ann Intern Med* 1987;**106**(4):593-7.
108. Hong SJ, Ko BM, Jung IS, Ryu CB, Moon JH, Cho JY, et al. Relevance of ineffective esophageal motility and hyperactive acid sensitization in patients with gastroesophageal reflux. *J Gastroenterol Hepatol* 2007;**22**(10):1662-5.
109. Blonski W, Hila A, Jain V, Freeman J, Vela M, Castell DO. Impedance manometry with viscous test solution increases detection of esophageal function defects compared to liquid swallows. *Scand J Gastroenterol* 2007;**42**(8):917-22.
110. Orringer MB. Surgical management of scleroderma reflux esophagitis. *Surg Clin North Am* 1983;**63**(4):859-67.
111. Cook IJ, Gabb M, Panagopoulos V, Jamieson GG, Dodds WJ, Dent J, Shearman DJ. Pharyngeal (Zenker's) diverticulum is a disorder of upper esophageal sphincter opening. *Gastroenterology* 1992;**103**(4):1229-35.
112. Collard JM, Otte JB, Kestens PJ. Endoscopic stapling technique of esophagodiverticulostomy for Zenker's diverticulum. *Ann Thorac Surg* 1993;**56**(3):573-6.
113. Peracchia A, Bonavina L, Narne S, Segalin A, Antoniazzi L, Marotta G. Minimally invasive surgery for Zenker diverticulum: analysis of results in 95 consecutive patients. *Arch Surg* 1998;**133**(7):695-700.
114. Visosky AM, Parke RB, Donovan DT. Endoscopic management of Zenker's diverticulum: factors predictive of success or failure. *Ann Otol Rhinol Laryngol* 2008;**117**(7):531-7.
115. Lerut T, van Raemdonck D, Guelinckx P, Dom R, Geboes K. Zenker's diverticulum: is a myotomy of the cricopharyngeus useful? How long should it be? *Hepatogastroenterology* 1992;**39**(2):127-31.
116. Laccourreye O, Ménard M, Cauchois R, Huart J, Jouffre V, Brasnu D, Laccourreye H. Esophageal diverticulum: diverticulopexy versus diverticulectomy. *Laryngoscope* 1994;**104**(7):889-92.
117. Bonafede JP, Lavertu P, Wood BG, Eliachar I. Surgical outcome in 87 patients with Zenker's diverticulum. *Laryngoscope* 1997;**107**(6):720-5.
118. Kaye MD. Oesophageal motor dysfunction in patients with diverticula of the mid-thoracic oesophagus. *Thorax* 1974;**29**(6):666-72.
119. Schima W, Schober E, Stacher G, Franz P, Uranitsch K, Pokieser P, et al. Association of midoesophageal diverticula with oesophageal motor disorders. Videofluoroscopy and manometry. *Acta Radiol* 1997;**38**(1):108-14.
120. Borrie J, Wilson RL. Oesophageal diverticula: principles of management and appraisal of classification. *Thorax* 1980;**35**(10):759-67.
121. Evander A, Little AG, Ferguson MK, Skinner DB. Diverticula of the mid- and lower esophagus: pathogenesis and surgical management. *World J Surg* 1986;**10**(5):820-8.
122. Fekete F, Vonns C. Surgical management of esophageal thoracic diverticula. *Hepatogastroenterology* 1992;**39**(2):97-9.
123. Fegiz G, Paolini A, De Marchi C, Tosato F. Surgical management of esophageal diverticula. *World J Surg* 1984;**8**(5):757-65.
124. Rice TW, Goldblum JR, Yearsley MM, Shay SS, Reznik SI, Murthy SC, et al. Myenteric plexus abnormalities associated with epiphrenic diverticula. *Eur J Cardiothorac Surg* 2009;**35**(1):22-7.
125. Benacci JC, Deschamps C, Trastek VF, Allen MS, Daly RC, Pairolero PC. Epiphrenic diverticulum: results of surgical treatment. *Ann Thorac Surg* 1993;**55**(5):1109-13, discussion 1114.
126. Feussner H, Kauer W, Siewert JR. The surgical management of motility disorders. *Dysphagia* 1993;**8**(2):135-45.
127. Reznik SI, Rice TW, Murthy SC, Mason DP, Apperson-Hansen C, Blackstone EH. Assessment of a pathophysiology-directed treatment for symptomatic epiphrenic diverticulum. *Dis Esophagus* 2007;**20**(4):320-7.
128. Quitadamo M, Benson J. Squamous papilloma of the esophagus: a case report and review of the literature. *Am J Gastroenterol* 1988;**83**(2):194-201.
129. Politoske EJ. Squamous papilloma of the esophagus associated with the human papillomavirus. *Gastroenterology* 1992;**102**(2):668-73.
130. Levine MS, Buck JL, Pantongrag-Brown L, Buetow PC, Hallman JR, Sobin LH. Fibrovascular polyps of the esophagus: clinical, radiographic, and pathologic findings in 16 patients. *AJR Am J Roentgenol* 1996;**166**(4):781-7.
131. Schuhmacher C, Becker K, Dittler HJ, Höfler H, Siewert JR, Stein HJ. Fibrovascular esophageal polyp as a diagnostic challenge. *Dis Esophagus* 2000;**13**(4):324-7.
132. Salo JA, Kiviluoto T, Heikkilä L, Perhoniemi V, Lamminen A, Kivilaakso E. Enucleation of an intramural lipoma of the oesophagus by videothoracoscopy. *Ann Chir Gynaecol* 1993;**82**(1):66-9.
133. Goldblum JR, Rice TW, Zuccaro G, Richter JE. Granular cell tumors of the esophagus: a clinical and pathologic study of 13 cases. *Ann Thorac Surg* 1996;**62**(3):860-5.
134. Palazzo L, Landi B, Cellier C, Roseau G, Chaussade S, Couturier D, Barbier J. Endosonographic features of esophageal granular cell tumors. *Endoscopy* 1997;**29**(9):850-3.
135. Araki K, Ohno S, Egashira A, Saeki H, Kawaguchi H, Ikeda Y, et al. Esophageal hemangioma: a case report and review of the literature. *Hepatogastroenterology* 1999;**46**(30):3148-54.
136. Maluf-Filho F, Sakai P, Amico EC, Pinotti HW. Giant cavernous hemangioma of the esophagus: endoscopic and echo-endoscopic appearance. *Endoscopy* 1999;**31**(4):S32.
137. Govoni AF. Hemangiomas of the esophagus. *Gastrointest Radiol* 1982;**7**(2):113-7.
138. Perch SJ, Soffen EM, Whittington R, Brooks JJ. Esophageal sarcomas. *J Surg Oncol* 1991;**48**(3):194-8.
139. Seremetis MG, De Guzman VC, Lyons WS, Peabody Jr JW. Leiomyoma of the esophagus. A report of 19 surgical cases. *Ann Thorac Surg* 1973;**16**(3):308-16.
140. Blum MG, Bilimoria KY, Wayne JD, de Hoyos AL, Talamonti MS, Adley B. Surgical considerations for the management and resection of esophageal gastrointestinal stromal tumors. *Ann Thorac Surg* 2007;**84**(5):1717-23.
141. Hover AR, Brady 3rd CE, Williams JR, Stewart DL, Christian C. Multiple retention cysts of the lower esophagus. *J Clin Gastroenterol* 1982;**4**(3):209-12.
142. Nobuhara KK, Gorski YC, La Quaglia MP, Shamberger RC. Bronchogenic cysts and esophageal duplications: common origins and treatment. *J Pediatr Surg* 1997;**32**(10):1408-13.
143. Bhutani MS, Hoffman BJ, Reed C. Endosonographic diagnosis of an esophageal duplication cyst. *Endoscopy* 1996;**28**(4):396-7.
144. Faigel DO, Burke A, Ginsberg GG, Stotland BR, Kadish SL, Kochman ML. The role of endoscopic ultrasound in the evaluation and management of foregut duplications. *Gastrointest Endosc* 1997;**45**(1):99-103.
145. Massari M, De Simone M, Cioffi U, Rosso L, Chiarelli M, Gabrielli F. Endoscopic ultrasonography in the evaluation of leiomyoma and extramucosal cysts of the esophagus. *Hepatogastroenterology* 1998;**45**(22):938-43.
146. Lim LL, Ho KY, Goh PM. Preoperative diagnosis of a paraesophageal bronchogenic cyst using endosonography. *Ann Thorac Surg* 2002;**73**(2):633-5.
147. St-Georges R, Deslauriers J, Duranceau A, Vaillancourt R, Deschamps C, Beauchamp G, et al. Clinical spectrum of bronchogenic cysts of the mediastinum and lung in the adult. *Ann Thorac Surg* 1991;**52**(1):6-13.
148. Kuhlman JE, Fishman EK, Wang KP, Siegelman SS. Esophageal duplication cyst: CT and transesophageal needle aspiration. *AJR Am J Roentgenol* 1985;**145**(3):531-2.
149. Spitz L. Congenital esophageal stenosis distal to associated esophageal atresia. *J Pediatr Surg* 1973;**8**(6):973-4.
150. Kochhar R, Ray JD, Sriram PV, Kumar S, Singh K. Intralesional steroids augment the effects of endoscopic dilation in corrosive esophageal strictures. *Gastrointest Endosc* 1999;**49**(4 Pt 1):509-13.
151. Ragunath K. Refractory benign esophageal strictures: extending the role of expandable stents. *Am J Gastroenterol* 2008;**103**(12):2995-6.
152. Ruigómez A, García Rodríguez LA, Wallander MA, Johansson S, Eklund S. Esophageal stricture: incidence, treatment patterns, and recurrence rate. *Am J Gastroenterol* 2006;**101**(12):2685-92.
153. Watson A. Reflux stricture of the oesophagus. *Br J Surg* 1987;**74**(6):443-8.
154. Spechler SJ, Sperber H, Doos WG, Schimmel EM. The prevalence of Barrett's esophagus in patients with chronic peptic esophageal strictures. *Dig Dis Sci* 1983;**28**(9):769-74.
155. McCord GS, Clouse RE. Pill-induced esophageal strictures: clinical features and risk factors for development. *Am J Med* 1990;**88**(5):512-8.
156. Kikendall JW. Pill-induced esophageal injury. *Gastroenterol Clin North Am* 1991;**20**(4):835-46.
157. Furuta GT, Liacouras CA, Collins MH, Gupta SK, Justinich C, Putnam PE, et al. Eosinophilic esophagitis in children and adults: a systematic review and consensus recommendations for diagnosis and treatment. *Gastroenterology* 2007;**133**(4):1342-63.
158. Bohm M, Richter JE. Treatment of eosinophilic esophagitis: overview, current limitations, and future direction. *Am J Gastroenterol* 2008;**103**(10):2635-44, quiz 2645.

159. Chowhan NM. Injurious effects of radiation on the esophagus. *Am J Gastroenterol* 1990;**85**(2):115-20.
160. Ng TM, Spencer GM, Sargeant IR, Thorpe SM, Bown SG. Management of strictures after radiotherapy for esophageal cancer. *Gastrointest Endosc* 1996;**43**(6):584-90.
161. Lightdale CJ, Botet JF, Kelsen DP, Turnbull AD, Brennan MF. Diagnosis of recurrent upper gastrointestinal cancer at the surgical anastomosis by endoscopic ultrasound. *Gastrointest Endosc* 1989;**35**(5):407-12.
162. Catalano MF, Sivak Jr MV, Rice TW, Van Dam J. Postoperative screening for anastomotic recurrence of esophageal carcinoma by endoscopic ultrasonography. *Gastrointest Endosc* 1995;**42**(6):540-4.
163. Goldman LP, Weigert JM. Corrosive substance ingestion: a review. *Am J Gastroenterol* 1984;**79**(2):85-90.
164. Maull KI, Scher LA, Greenfield LJ. Surgical implications of acid ingestion. *Surg Gynecol Obstet* 1979;**148**(6):895-8.
165. Anderson KD, Rouse TM, Randolph JG. A controlled trial of corticosteroids in children with corrosive injury of the esophagus. *N Engl J Med* 1990;**323**(10):637-40.
166. Howell JM, Dalsey WC, Hartsell FW, Butzin CA. Steroids for the treatment of corrosive esophageal injury: a statistical analysis of past studies. *Am J Emerg Med* 1992;**10**(5):421-5.
167. Zargar SA, Kochhar R, Mehta S, Mehta SK. The role of fiberoptic endoscopy in the management of corrosive ingestion and modified endoscopic classification of burns. *Gastrointest Endosc* 1991;**37**(2):165-9.
168. Knox WG, Scott JR, Zintel HA, Guthrie R, McCabe RE. Bouginage and steroids used singly or in combination in experimental corrosive esophagitis. *Ann Surg* 1967;**166**(6):930-41.
169. Burrington JD, Raffensperger JG. Surgical management of tracheoesophageal fistula complicating caustic ingestion. *Surgery* 1978;**84**(3):329-34.
170. Litovitz T, Schmitz BF. Ingestion of cylindrical and button batteries: an analysis of 2382 cases. *Pediatrics* 1992;**89**(4 Pt 2):747-57.
171. Gandhi RP, Cooper A, Barlow BA. Successful management of esophageal strictures without resection or replacement. *J Pediatr Surg* 1989;**24**(8):745-9, discussion 749-50.
172. Jones 2nd WG, Ginsberg RJ. Esophageal perforation: a continuing challenge. *Ann Thorac Surg* 1992;**53**(3):534-43.
173. Appelqvist P, Salmo M. Lye corrosion carcinoma of the esophagus: a review of 63 cases. *Cancer* 1980;**45**(10):2655-8.
174. Isolauri J, Markkula H. Lye ingestion and carcinoma of the esophagus. *Acta Chir Scand* 1989;**155**(4-5):269-71.
175. Quine MA, Bell GD, McCloy RF, Matthews HR. Prospective audit of perforation rates following upper gastrointestinal endoscopy in two regions of England. *Br J Surg* 1995;**82**(4):530-3.
176. Karnak I, Tanyel FC, Büyükpamukçu N, Hiçsönmez A. Esophageal perforations encountered during the dilation of caustic esophageal strictures. *J Cardiovasc Surg (Torino)* 1998;**39**(3):373-7.
177. Bladergroen MR, Lowe JE, Postlethwait RW. Diagnosis and recommended management of esophageal perforation and rupture. *Ann Thorac Surg* 1986;**42**(3):235-9.
178. Goldstein LA, Thompson WR. Esophageal perforations: a 15 year experience. *Am J Surg* 1982;**143**(4):495-503.
179. Buecker A, Wein BB, Neuerburg JM, Guenther RW. Esophageal perforation: comparison of use of aqueous and barium-containing contrast media. *Radiology* 1997;**202**(3):683-6.
180. Cameron JL, Kieffer RF, Hendrix TR, Mehigan DG, Baker RR. Selective nonoperative management of contained intrathoracic esophageal disruptions. *Ann Thorac Surg* 1979;**27**(5):404-8.
181. Altorjay A, Kiss J, Vörös A, Bohák A. Nonoperative management of esophageal perforations. Is it justified? *Ann Surg* 1997;**225**(4):415-21.
182. Gouge TH, Depan HJ, Spencer FC. Experience with the Grillo pleural wrap procedure in 18 patients with perforation of the thoracic esophagus. *Ann Surg* 1989;**209**(5):612-7, discussion 617-9.
183. Bufkin BL, Miller Jr JI, Mansour KA. Esophageal perforation: emphasis on management. *Ann Thorac Surg* 1996;**61**(5):1447-51, discussion 1451-2.
184. Wang N, Razzouk AJ, Safavi A, Gan K, Van Arsdell GS, Burton PM, et al. Delayed primary repair of intrathoracic esophageal perforation: is it safe? *J Thorac Cardiovasc Surg* 1996;**111**(1):114-21, discussion 121-2.
185. Altorjay A, Kiss J, Vörös A, Sziránýi E. The role of esophagectomy in the management of esophageal perforations. *Ann Thorac Surg* 1998;**65**(5):1433-6.
186. Kiernan PD, Hernandez A, Byrne WD, Bloom R, Dicicco B, Hetrick V, et al. Descending cervical mediastinitis. *Ann Thorac Surg* 1998;**65**(5):1483-8.
187. Watkinson A, Ellul J, Entwisle K, Farrugia M, Mason R, Adam A. Plastic-covered metallic endoprostheses in the management of oesophageal perforation in patients with oesophageal carcinoma. *Clin Radiol* 1995;**50**(5):304-9.
188. Iannettoni MD, Vlessis AA, Whyte RI, Orringer MB. Functional outcome after surgical treatment of esophageal perforation. *Ann Thorac Surg* 1997;**64**(6):1606-9, discussion 1609-10.
189. Webb WA. Management of foreign bodies of the upper gastrointestinal tract. *Gastroenterology* 1988;**94**(1):204-16.
190. Richter JE, Wu WC, Johns DN, Blackwell JN, Nelson 3rd JL, Castell JA, Castell DO. Esophageal manometry in 95 healthy adult volunteers. Variability of pressures with age and frequency of "abnormal" contractions. *Dig Dis Sci* 1987;**32**(6):583-92.
191. Johnson LF, Demeester TR. Twenty-four-hour pH monitoring of the distal esophagus. A quantitative measure of gastroesophageal reflux. *Am J Gastroenterol* 1974;**62**(4):325-32.
192. Richter JE, Bradley LA, DeMeester TR, Wu WC. Normal 24-hr ambulatory esophageal pH values. Influence of study center, pH electrode, age, and gender. *Dig Dis Sci* 1992;**37**(6):849-56.
193. Jamieson JR, Stein HJ, DeMeester TR, Bonavina L, Schwizer W, Hinder RA, Albertucci M. Ambulatory 24-h esophageal pH monitoring: normal values, optimal thresholds, specificity, sensitivity, and reproducibility. *Am J Gastroenterol* 1992;**87**(9):1102-11.
194. Adhami T, Richter JE. Twenty-four hour pH monitoring in the assessment of esophageal function. *Semin Thorac Cardiovasc Surg* 2001;**13**:241-54.

L. Esophagus—Cancer

CHAPTER 37
Staging Techniques for Carcinoma of the Esophagus

Virginia R. Litle

- Esophageal Cancer TNM Staging
- Staging by Endoscopic Ultrasonography
  - Endoscopic Ultrasonography and Neoadjuvant Therapy
  - Metastatic Disease
- Computed Tomography
- Positron Emission Tomography
  - Initial Staging
- PET/CT
  - Initial Staging
  - Interval Staging
  - Restaging
- Surgical Staging
- Additional Metastatic Tests: Brain Scan
- Future Direction: Molecular Staging
  - Summary

In the United States in 2008, there were 16,470 estimated new cases of esophagus cancer diagnosed and 14,280 estimated deaths.[1] Worldwide, the overall survival from esophageal cancer remains dismal at less than 10% at 5 years[2] because fewer than half of the patients will be eligible for potentially curative resection at the time of presentation. The incidence of esophageal adenocarcinoma continues to increase in the United States, with a more than 20% increase per year in white men in particular but also a significant rise in African-American men and white women.[3]

Although the prognosis of patients with esophageal adenocarcinoma remains poor, there have been improvements in the staging modalities available to enhance the appropriate selection of treatment for patients. In addition, significant advances have been made in less invasive therapeutic modalities, from endoscopic resection of intramucosal cancers to minimally invasive approaches for esophagogastrectomy. Improvements in early detection of the disease, selection of appropriate treatment for patients, and surgical approaches may eventually translate into improved overall survival rates. Currently we see 3-year survival rates for patients with stage I esophageal adenocarcinoma reported from 65%[4-6] to at least 80% at 5 years for carefully staged patients.[7,8] Historically, however, esophagectomy has been associated with mortality rates exceeding 20%[9]; thus, oncologists have been reluctant to refer patients for potentially curative surgical resection. With modernization of approaches and improved perioperative care, the surgical mortality rates after esophagectomy have improved to less than 4% in the past decade.[5,6,8] Esophagectomy, however, should be considered a potentially curative option and not a palliative modality, considering the negative impact on quality of life after potentially palliative resection.[10] More palliative options are now currently available in the form of stents and laser therapy,[11] and resection may be reserved for the significantly bleeding or perforated tumor. Accurate staging is also important to determine the best mode of palliation for patients with stage IV disease. The information gained may allow a realistic discussion with the family. For example, does a patient benefit from a feeding tube if the disease is stage IV?

In addition to early detection of this disease, identification of early-stage disease with accurate staging tests should allow optimal selection of surgical candidates. Routine noninvasive preoperative staging modalities available at most institutions should include endoscopic ultrasonography (EUS), and positron emission tomography–computed tomography (PET/CT). Previously, only CT scans, bone scans, and brain magnetic resonance imaging (MRI) scans were available for diagnosis of distant disease, or patients would undergo potentially morbid surgical exploration only for their cancer to be deemed unresectable. Patients with early-stage disease benefit from surgical resection, whereas patients in an advanced stage may benefit from palliative options to improve quality of life. Patients assigned to an intermediate stage can benefit from neoadjuvant therapy followed by restaging and surgical resection with curative intent. Although clinical trials of neoadjuvant chemotherapy or chemoradiation have generally not shown a consistent survival benefit,[12-15] a few individual studies and a meta-analysis have shown some benefit.[16-19] It is increasingly becoming the standard of care to offer neoadjuvant chemotherapy or chemoradiation to patients with clinical stage T3 or N1 esophagus cancer.[17,20-22] The earlier studies did not have PET or PET/CT available to help with restaging, and this absence may have contributed to esophagectomies in patients with metastatic disease. In addition, because neoadjuvant treatment is still considered controversial, accurate staging is important to determine which patients may be eligible for clinical trials, to assess response to treatment with PET and CT scans, and then to determine which patients should be offered potentially curative esophagectomy.

In spite of technological and diagnostic advances, however, most patients currently do not go through a standardized multimodality staging program. In addition, many investigators reporting accuracy rates for these tests do not have actual pathologic confirmation of the stage. This is particularly true with the more recent staging modality of PET/CT. Some of the modalities simply are not available everywhere, but even when they are available, many new esophageal cancer patients do not undergo a standardized staging routine before receiving operative or nonoperative therapy. This chapter outlines what is available now for staging of thoracic esophageal cancer.

ESOPHAGEAL CANCER TNM STAGING

The current staging system for esophageal cancer follows the American Joint Committee on Cancer TNM system of T for tumor, N for regional nodal status, and M for presence or absence of distant metastases (Table 37-1).[23] The TNM staging system is in the process of being revised. Several changes may include subdividing T1 to include T1a for intramucosal cancers and T1b for submucosal lesions. This T stage modification is based on the incidence of lymph node involvement and subsequent survival differences for tumors of increasing depth. In addition, as has been done for pathologic staging of other malignant neoplasms,[24-26] there will also likely be a subdivision of the nodal stage based on number of lymph nodes involved with metastases. Again, this change is based on several studies from different esophageal groups in the United States that have found significant survival differences based on absolute number of positive lymph nodes,[27-31] absolute number of negative lymph nodes,[32] and ratio of positive to negative lymph nodes.[31,30,33]

STAGING BY ENDOSCOPIC ULTRASONOGRAPHY

Endoscopic ultrasound staging of esophageal cancers was first advanced in the literature by Lightdale[34] in 1992. In the next decade, the modality became a standard part of staging of esophageal cancer in newly diagnosed patients.[35] Before EUS, CT was the primary modality available to decide whether to proceed with an esophagectomy for an otherwise medically fit patient presenting with esophagus cancer, although MRI and bone scans were sometimes indicated by clinical presentation. Now EUS is available to help determine locoregional stage of esophagus cancer as well as distant disease by providing cytology of liver, adrenal, or celiac lymph nodes metastases.

With increased utility of preoperative chemoradiation, especially after the Walsh study,[36] EUS helped determine the locoregional stage of the cancer so that neoadjuvant treatment could potentially be offered to those with locally advanced disease. Although clinical signs and symptoms can determine T stage with a fair degree of accuracy, with substernal chest pain, dysphagia, and weight loss all being highly suggestive of T3 or T4 disease,[37] symptoms alone are probably not enough to determine surgical resectability. In addition, EUS has improved on CT evaluation of distant metastatic disease by providing fine-needle aspiration (FNA) and cytologic confirmation of hepatic or celiac lymph node metastases with accuracy rates of 90%.[38,39]

Conventional EUS is carried out with conscious sedation by use of the 360-degree radial mechanical echoendoscope with a 7.5-MHz ultrasound probe. Conventional EUS is the best approach to assess depth of primary tumor into the esophageal wall (Fig. 37-1). For EUS-guided FNA of suspicious lymph nodes, a curved linear array echoendoscope is used with a 22- or 25-gauge needle. A 7.5-MHz or lower frequency endoscope is better than the high-frequency one for assessment of regional lymph nodes because of the greater depth of visualization. Endoscopic criteria for potentially malignant lymph nodes include at least two of the following characteristics: round, discrete, hypoechoic, and a dimension of more than 1 cm.[40,41] EUS imaging of nodes alone is not specific enough, but FNA of the suspicious nodes can result in a specificity rate of up to 95%.[42]

Table 37-1

Current TNM Classification of Esophageal Cancer

T	Primary tumor	N	Regional nodes
X	Tumor cannot be assessed	X	Regional nodes cannot be assessed
0	No primary tumor	0	No regional nodes
is	High-grade dysplasia (in situ)	1	Regional nodes involved
1	Tumor invades the lamina propria or submucosa		
2	Tumor invades muscularis propria	**M**	**Distant metastases**
3	Tumor invades adventitia	X	Metastases cannot be assessed
4	Tumor invades adjacent structures	1a	Upper thoracic tumor metastatic to cervical nodes Lower thoracic tumor metastatic to celiac nodes
		1b	Upper thoracic tumor metastatic to other distant sites Midthoracic tumor metastatic to nonregional nodes and/or distant sites Lower thoracic tumor metastatic to other distant sites

Stage Group	T	N	M
0	Tis	N0	M0
I	T1	N0	M0
IIA	T2	N0	M0
	T3	N0	M0
IIB	T1	N1	M0
	T2	N1	M0
III	T3	N1	M0
	T4	Any N	M0
IV	Any T	Any N	M1
IVA	Any T	Any N	M1a
IVB	Any T	Any N	M1b

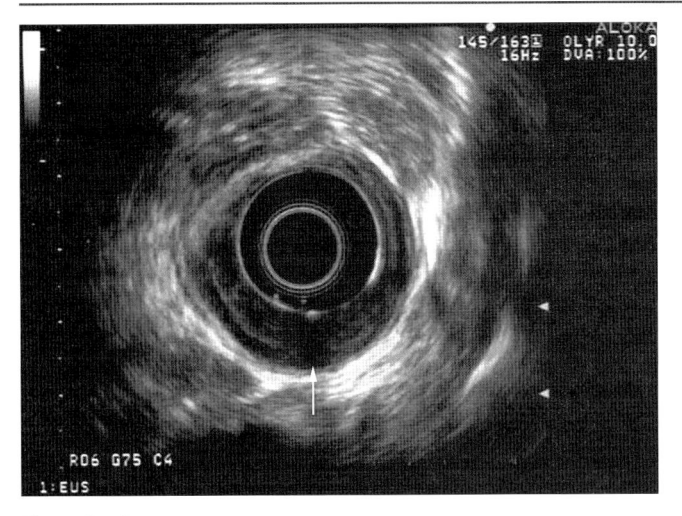

Figure 37-1
Endoscopic ultrasound picture of T2 tumor (arrow) invading the muscularis propria.

Table 37-2
Accuracy of Endoscopic Ultrasound Staging in Various Series with Pathologic Stage Available

Author (year)	Neoadjuvant Treatment (n)	pT Stage (%)	pN Stage (%)
Barbour et al[43] (2007)	No (209)	61	75
Davies et al[44] (2006)	No (94)	78	70
Larghi et al[45] (2005) with miniprobe (15-20 MHz)	No	85	NA
Cen et al[40] (2008)	No (87)	NA	81
Vickers and Alderson[48] (1998)	No (50)	92	86
Flamen et al[47] (2000)	No (42)	64	NA
Zhang et al[55] (2005)	No (34) / Yes (39)	79 / 51	74 / 54
Zuccaro et al[41] (1999)	Yes (59)	37	38
Isenberg et al[54] (1998)	Yes (23)	43	NA

NA, not available; p, pathologic.

EUS remains the most accurate modality for determination of T stage, with accuracy rates ranging from 64% to 80% for the low-frequency probe[38,43,44] and up to 85% to 92% for the high-frequency probe.[38,40,45] Accuracy can be calculated only when patients have undergone histologic confirmation of the tumor and nodal status. The accuracy of EUS for staging of T and N stage in the most recent series of patients since the mid-1990s is summarized in Table 37-2. As summarized, EUS staging is indicated before initiation of chemotherapy or radiation therapy. The accuracy rates as confirmed by pathologic staging decrease by 25% to 50% for both T and N stages when it is done after induction therapy. EUS is more accurate for T3 and T4 stages[38,44] (80% to 90%) than for T1 and T2 stages (74%).[44] In a large series of more than 200 patients with pathologic confirmation of the tumor and nodal stages, most EUS staging errors were understaging of T0 and T1 and overstaging of T2.[46] EUS accurately staged T3 and T4 lesions in 85% of cases.[43] In another series of 47 patients undergoing surgical resection for adenocarcinoma or squamous cell carcinoma, EUS overstaged T stage in 19% of the patients and understaged it in 17%.[47]

In studies with pathologic confirmation, the accuracy rates for N stage range from 70% to 86%.[38,40,43,44,48] Before FNA-guided biopsy of lymph nodes by EUS was applied, the false-negative rate of EUS for nodal stage exceeded 33%.[47,49]

Although EUS has added much to the clinical staging and management of esophageal cancer patients, it still is limited by malignant stenoses preventing staging of the primary tumor. In these cases, however, tumor obstruction almost always represents T3 or T4Nx.[48] In addition, the probability of a T3 or T4 tumor being N1 exceeds 80%.[50]

With the continued expansion of endoscopic therapy for early esophageal cancers, accurate staging of T1 adenocarcinoma with EUS will be important to determine which patients may be offered endoscopic therapy with potential cure and which patients should undergo esophagectomy. From experienced EUS groups, the accuracy of staging of an intramucosal (T1a) cancer was 82% to 94%.[38,40,51] A T1b cancer has about a 20% likelihood of lymph node metastases versus the intramucosal lesion, which is less than 5%; thus, the EUS T stage may help in deciding between endoscopic and surgical resection.[52] EUS before endoscopic resection of T1 tumors remains controversial, and resection may be diagnostic.

For the patient initially presenting with a localized cancer, conventional EUS with a 7.5- to 12-MHz radial ultrasound probe is good for initial assessment of tumor infiltration and to look for suspicious lymph nodes (hypoechoic, >1 cm). The examination should include a full evaluation of the liver and lymph nodes in the perigastric, subhepatic, and celiac stations. If a suspicious node is identified, a curvilinear echoendoscope allows FNA of the suspicious node.

Endoscopic Ultrasonography and Neoadjuvant Therapy

Although EUS is feasible in 70% of patients after neoadjuvant chemoradiation,[53] its accuracy rate with current neoadjuvant modalities drops below 50%.[41,54] It overstages the tumor depth and nodal status in more than 49% and more than 38%, respectively.[55] The accuracy for T stage after chemoradiation at current radiation doses of 45 Gy ranges from 37% to 43%.[41,54] Radiation fibrosis causes overstaging or understaging of T stage about 40% of the time.[53,56] T stage by EUS after chemotherapy may be accurate only when the tumors do not respond to the chemotherapy.[41] EUS essentially is not recommended after neoadjuvant chemotherapy or chemoradiation because of the low accuracy rate[54] secondary to the postinflammatory changes,[41,57] although post-chemoradiation CT or endoscopy alone is not as good as EUS in assessing treatment response.[58]

Metastatic Disease

EUS is also helpful in confirming metastases to celiac lymph nodes, which assigns the patient to stage IV cancer.[42,59,60] Celiac lymph nodes could be evaluated in 95% of 62 patients in Reed's series from 1999, and in this group, EUS sensitivity was 72% and specificity 97%.[59] The presence of celiac lymph node metastases as detected by EUS has also been associated with a worse survival for all T stages. In another study from the Medical University of South Carolina, the authors concluded that the 5-year survival rate of patients without celiac nodal involvement by EUS was three times better than that of patients with celiac lymph node involvement (39.8 versus 13.8 months).[60] EUS can also be helpful in evaluating and allowing biopsy of liver metastases.[61] In a study of 132 patients, EUS-FNA of noncystic liver lesions confirmed liver metastases in 20% of the cases, and EUS was superior to CT in quantifying liver metastases, especially in cases in which the metastases were too small to be characterized by CT scan.[61]

COMPUTED TOMOGRAPHY

Accuracy rates of CT scanning for assessment of depth of esophageal and gastroesophageal junction cancers are notoriously poor: 33% for T2, 0% for T3, and 50% for T4 for an overall rate of 15%. CT tends to understage depth of penetration,[62] although the overall accuracy of CT for T stage was 59% in more recent series.[38,49,62,63] CT is used to identify distant metastases and suspicious regional nodes more than tumor depth. Historically, nodal staging by CT averaged 50% for node-positive patients,[62] whereas the combination of EUS and CT for detection of regional nodal involvement accurately was 82% in a series of 42 patients undergoing surgical resection.[50] The sensitivity of CT staging of celiac lymph nodes was only 8% in slightly older series, although the specificity was 100%,[59] but it was only 64% accurate for diagnosis of stage IV disease by solid organ metastases or distant lymph node metastases in 74 Belgian patients.[47]

Before the advent of CT scanning for staging of esophagus cancer, other noninvasive tests including linear tomography and bone scans accurately staged esophagus cancer in less than 30% of cases.[64] Routine CT scanning has improved the detection of distant metastases, but it generally has been replaced by the more sensitive PET/CT. CT scanning may still have a role in evaluating chemoradiation response, however. Some groups have suggested that a reduction in maximal cross-sectional area of the tumor on CT scanning may be helpful in assessing chemoradiation response preoperatively.[38,54] Similarly, earlier studies suggested that preoperative CT width of the cancer may be a prognostic factor,[58] even without neoadjuvant downstaging.[65] New interest is developing in this staging of tumor measurements on radiographic measurements, with assessment of treatment response based on tumor length.[66]

POSITRON EMISSION TOMOGRAPHY

Most of the EUS data were published and quoted before PET/CT. Just as EUS contributes to the preoperative evaluation and management of the new esophagus cancer patient, PET/CT adds additional biological information about the primary tumor as well as important staging information. The standardized uptake value (SUV) may potentially play an important role in triage of patients for therapy both before any treatment and as it has begun as an indicator of pathologic response to neoadjuvant treatment.

Initial Staging

PET scans initially and currently use ^{18}F-2-fluoro-2-deoxy-D-glucose ([^{18}F]FDG) as the tracer for glucose metabolism. [^{18}F]FDG is taken up into the cell and phosphorylated but cannot be metabolized as glucose 6-phosphate and instead is trapped within cells using high rates of glucose. Patients must fast for 4 to 6 hours before the PET scan so that they are normoglycemic at the time of the study. Forty to 60 minutes after intravenous injection of 10 to 15 mCi of FDG, the scan is obtained with the patient supine. The minimum lesion size that can be detected by PET scan alone is 5 mm,[67] although with PET/CT, we may see improvements in the resolution as lesion size and intensity influence detectability. PET is very sensitive at detection of primary tumor, with the primary tumor being hypermetabolic in more than 95% of cases.[47,68,69] One of the big advantages of PET scanning over CT is the three-dimensional imaging with PET. This modality also is more likely than CT to identify second primary tumors.[68] PET is not typically used to diagnose esophageal cancer, however, but instead is used to evaluate regional nodal disease and distant metastases. Lymph node status is the most important prognostic predictor for patients with potentially resectable disease,[70] and clinical staging of lymph nodes currently may lead to induction therapy. Thus, optimal clinical staging of lymph nodes is an important part of esophageal cancer workup. From many series, sensitivity and specificity of PET are 51% and 84% for detection of regional nodal disease and 67% and 97% for metastatic disease.[67] PET/CT improved the accuracy of PET alone for identification of malignant lymph nodes in a series of 39 patients because CT improved the localization of the PET tracer.[71] In this particular study, small lymph nodes (6 to 11 mm) that were negative on PET were detected with PET/CT. PET findings for detection or elimination of metastatic disease have been shown to change management of the patient in about 20% of cases staged by CT initially.[67]

There is currently growing enthusiasm for use of PET and SUV data to give prognostic information as well as response to neoadjuvant therapy. Although it is controversial whether T stage correlates with PET SUV, with Flamen and coworkers[47] finding no relationship between primary tumor SUV and pathologic T stage or extent of nodal metastases, Cerfolio and Bryant[72] did find a significant correlation between T stage and N stage with increasing SUV. In general, PET is not considered a useful determinant of T stage.[67] In the PET study by Downey and associates[73] of patients receiving neoadjuvant treatment, pretreatment SUV, however, did not correlate with survival in 39 esophagectomy patients.

The first studies demonstrating that PET would be useful for staging of esophagus cancer came from Flanagan and colleagues at Washington University. This group found that in 29 patients who underwent curative surgery (19 with adenocarcinoma), PET scan accurately detected regional nodal disease in 76% of the patients and distant metastases in 93% of the patients. PET identified regional nodal involvement twice as often as CT did in 21 patients undergoing esophagectomy for adenocarcinoma or squamous cell carcinoma and improved detection of metastatic disease by 80% (45% by CT and 82% by PET and CT).⁶⁸ For detection of stage IV disease in patients with esophageal adenocarcinoma or squamous cell carcinoma, PET alone had sensitivity, specificity, and accuracy rates of 74%, 90%, and 82% compared with rates of 41%, 83%, and 64% for CT scan, respectively.⁴⁷ Small (<1 cm) hepatic metastases were missed by both PET and CT scans in one patient, and in a second, a pancreatic metastasis was missed.⁷⁴ The authors concluded that PET changed clinical management in 17% of 36 patients with adenocarcinoma or squamous cell carcinoma.⁷⁴ False-positive results on PET scanning of esophagus cancer patients can result from granulomatous disease, reactive hyperplasia, or local extension of tumor misinterpreted as regional nodal involvement.⁴⁷,⁷⁴ False-negative regional lymph node involvement can result from occult micrometastatic disease in normal-sized nodes and in nodes adjacent to the primary tumor, where the PET uptake of the primary tumor obscures the nodal uptake. False-negative findings of stage IV disease by PET can result from peritoneal metastases, small (<1 cm) or superficial hepatic metastases, and presumably small lung lesions.⁴⁷

Results of the American College of Surgeons Oncology Group Z0060 trial of PET staging in esophagus cancer were published in 2007.⁷⁵ This is the only intergroup trial that has looked at PET scans in esophageal cancer to determine whether PET can improve on an acceptable 5% rate of metastasis detection and hence prevent unnecessary surgery for esophageal cancer patients with metastatic disease. All patients underwent a CT scan of the abdomen and chest first; if that was normal, they had a PET scan to look for stage IV disease. Although tissue confirmation of PET-positive suspicious lesions was part of the study algorithm, not all patients were able to undergo confirmatory biopsies of PET-positive areas. Indeed, two patients who did undergo procedures sustained complications after biopsy or after an adrenalectomy for a false-positive PET result. Of the 145 patients who had a PET scan negative for metastases and who underwent potentially surgical resection, 5.6% developed recurrent cancer (location not otherwise specified) within 6 months of surgery. The group concluded that confirmed metastatic disease was detected in 4.8% of patients otherwise potentially eligible for curative surgery after body CT staging and as-needed brain or bone imaging and that tissue confirmation is important for avoiding the 3.7% false-positive rate resulting from PET scanning of these patients. In the PET study of 39 patients undergoing induction treatment, PET identified distant metastatic disease in 15% of patients, with tissue confirmation or support by another imaging modality.⁷³

PET/CT

Initial Staging

With the advent of PET/CT in 2000,⁴⁷,⁷⁶,⁷⁷ this modality has become increasingly used at most major institutions. The PET/CT study is carried out in a fashion similar to PET, with the patient fasting for at least 4 hours before the scan to standardize glucose metabolism. The patient receives FDG, followed by the CT scan; then, within 45 to 60 minutes of injection of the radiotracer, the PET images are obtained. The PET and CT images are fused, and both PET and PET/CT images are analyzed. Figure 37-2 shows PET/CT images of the primary tumor, hilar regional nodal involvement, and metastatic disease to the T8 vertebra. PET/CT has been

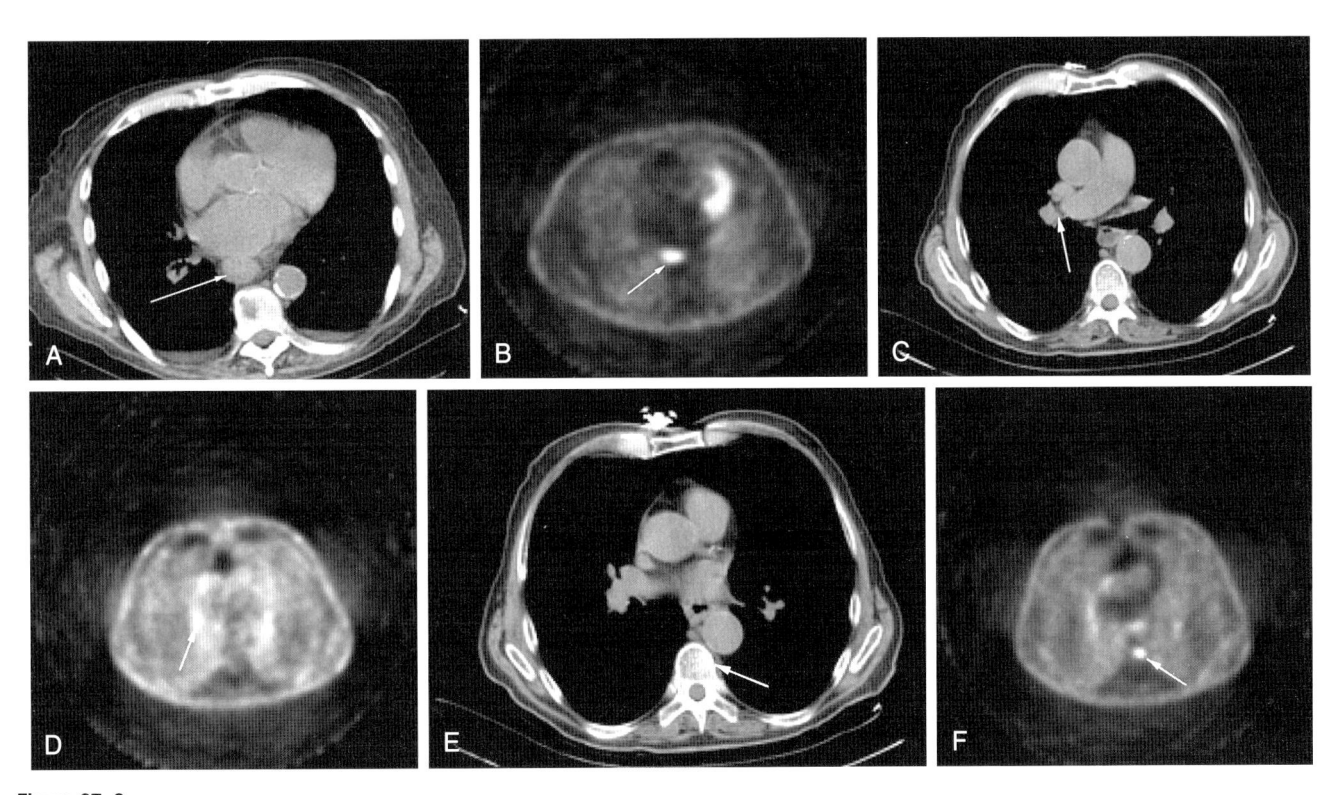

Figure 37-2
PET/CT scans of three patients with esophageal cancer: **A, B,** localized disease; **C, D,** locally advanced to the left hilum; and **E, F,** metastatic disease to the T8 vertebra.

shown to increase the accuracy of lymph node staging in esophageal adenocarcinoma from 78% with PET alone to 83% with fused PET/CT.[71] The authors in this study also increased the staging accuracy to 95% when they included the diameter of the primary tumor.

In a diagnostic imaging study from the M. D. Anderson Cancer Center, PET/CT was used to detect distant metastases in 22% of esophageal cancer patients undergoing initial staging.[78] The most common sites of metastases were liver (10%), bone (9%), lung (9%), adrenal glands (2%), and peritoneum (1.4%). In addition, "atypical" metastases were found in the skeletal muscle, brain, and thyroid in 0.3% to 1.7% of the patients. One patient (0.5%) was also found to have a synchronous colon cancer after colonoscopy for focal uptake by PET/CT. Although some authors have suggested that it is not ethically possible to always confirm histologically metastatic disease,[67] the counterargument is that it is ethically right to proceed with a biopsy if possible and if potentially curative options are available.

Patients who respond to chemotherapy or chemoradiation therapy have a better prognosis after surgical resection,[13,15,20,36,79,80] and some groups have found that only the complete responders had survival benefit.[81] Complete pathologic response ranges from 17% to 22%.[69,82] For patients undergoing neoadjuvant treatment, what is the role of interval staging (e.g., obtaining a PET/CT scan after two cycles of induction chemotherapy)? As seen before, EUS is inaccurate at restaging because of radiation fibrosis and inflammation. PET scanning, however, provides a functional or metabolic picture of the tumor, not an anatomic one.

What is the role of a PET scan in assessing response to the neoadjuvant treatment? In patients with proximal esophageal squamous cell carcinoma, a 52% response by PET after chemoradiation therapy correlated with nearly complete pathologic response, with a positive predictive value of 72%, and PET responders had more than double the survival rate of nonresponders.[80] The interval PET or PET/CT scan is done after two cycles of chemotherapy[82] and selects out the responders and the nonresponders. The restaging scan is done after completion of neoadjuvant treatment to identify metastatic disease.

Interval Staging

In some centers, a PET or PET/CT scan is obtained after two cycles of chemotherapy to differentiate the nonresponders from the responders. The nonresponders could then be spared subsequent chemotherapy that is not working and then could be offered "salvage" therapy, including different chemotherapy, chemoradiation, or surgery[67]; the responders could complete the neoadjuvant treatment, stage could be reassigned, and surgical resection could be considered. There is increasing evidence supporting this approach for patients undergoing neoadjuvant treatment. Indeed, in the MUNICON trial for esophageal adenocarcinomas, interval metabolic response evaluation determined whether patients continued with chemotherapy or underwent surgical resection.[67] What is the ideal timing for the interval PET/CT? At the M. D. Anderson Cancer Center, the findings of Bruzzi and coworkers[82] were at a median interval of 83 days between baseline PET/CT scan and repeated scan after one or two cycles of chemotherapy.

Restaging

A metabolic response by PET or PET/CT scan is increasingly being shown to correlate with histologic response to induction therapy with a sensitivity of 89%.[83,84] In one study of 37 patients with gastroesophageal junction adenocarcinomas (98% clinical stage T3Nx, 2% T4Nx), those with a significant decrease in SUV also were able to undergo complete surgical resection.[83] In addition, a significant decrease from maximum SUV on repeated PET images after induction therapy predicts a lower likelihood of disease recurrence[83] and improved disease-free and overall survival.[69,73,83-85] The optimal timing of the repeated PET/CT scan after neoadjuvant chemotherapy or chemoradiation therapy is typically 3 to 4 weeks after completion of treatment (Fig. 37-3). Metastatic disease is identified in 8% to 17% in post-treatment PET/CT.[69,82,86] Additional distant metastases can be found intraoperatively, in spite of a normal PET/CT scan, however, in an additional 2% to 6% of patients.[69,82] In one series, 29% of patients had pathologic N1 nodes despite a normal PET/CT scan before esophagectomy.[82]

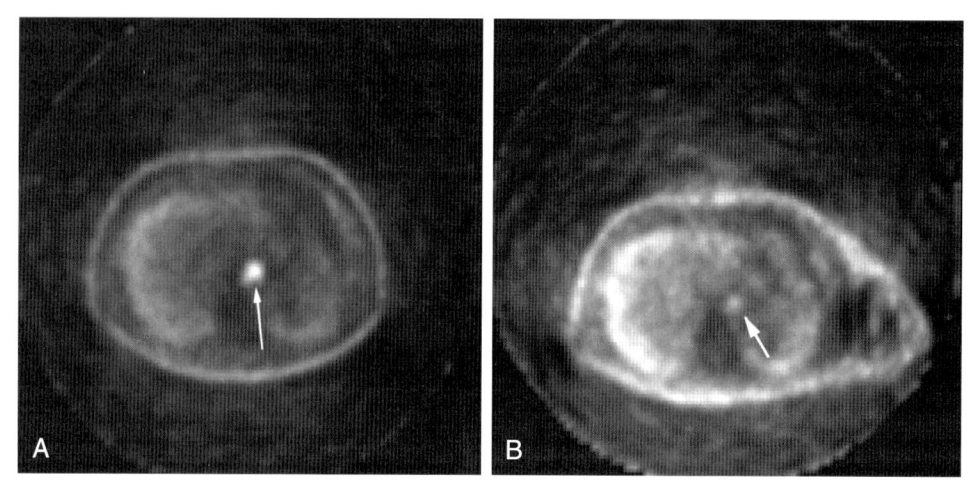

Figure 37-3
Complete metabolic response to induction chemoradiation on PET/CT images before therapy **(A)** and 3 weeks after completion of therapy **(B)** in a patient with a gastroesophageal junction adenocarcinoma.

An interesting aspect of restaging with PET and now PET/CT scans is the potential prognostic information from the decrease in SUV, as suggested initially by Downey and colleagues,[73] who stratified 17 patients after induction therapy into those with a greater or less than 60% change in SUV before and after chemoradiation. Of the eight surgically resected patients who had greater than 60% decrease in SUV peri-treatment, 67% were disease free at 2 years postoperatively. The 2-year overall survival rate difference was 89% versus 63% for the two groups with the 60% SUV cutoff. Other studies support use of a relative decrease in SUV as a predictor of histologic response to induction chemotherapy, and the sensitivity was 86% for identification of responders in the study of Roedl and coworkers.[66] The correlation of change in primary tumor SUV and histologic response to chemoradiation is controversial, though.[69,82] In a set of 55 patients who underwent esophagectomy, PET/CT had only a 39% positive predictive value for differentiation of patients with a pathologic response.[82] In another study, the positive predictive value of PET for determination of a pathologic complete response was only 50%.[69] The optimal cutoff point of what is considered significant is not known. Some groups use greater than 35% for a sensitivity and specificity of 75% and greater than 45% decrease in SUV for a specificity of 86%,[83] whereas greater than 60% was used to predict improved survival.

Finally, the Massachusetts General Hospital group concluded that in their 47 patients with esophageal or gastroesophageal junction cancers, decrease in tumor length as assessed by PET/CT was a better predictor of treatment response than was change in SUV.[66] We can conclude that the literature does not yet support use of PET or PET/CT scanning to determine treatment response and to triage patients for potentially curative or morbid resection.

The standard interval for the restaging PET/CT after completion of neoadjuvant chemotherapy or chemoradiation therapy is about 21 to 40 days.[69,82] At most institutions, it is not yet standard to forego an esophagectomy in patients without a significant decrease in SUV of the primary tumor; it is controversial.[82] Although it is not the standard to repeat EUS, the M. D. Anderson group gave it a positive predictive value of 88% for evaluation of tumor response to neoadjuvant therapy.[82] They have also found that adding PET/CT to postinduction repeated endoscopy significantly improved the ability to detect residual tumor compared with repeated endoscopy alone.[87] This was suggested in 1998, for esophagus cancer, in a study of 48 patients in Japan, where patients with an SUV of more than 7.0 had a poor prognosis, with earlier recurrence within 2 years of surgery.[88]

SURGICAL STAGING

What is the role of surgical staging for the patient with newly diagnosed esophageal cancer? That question has been examined by a few groups and then the feasibility evaluated in a multicenter trial led by Krasna.[89] Minimally invasive surgical staging is superior to EUS staging alone for assessment of N status,[90] but whether it is cost-effective is debatable. Early results of surgical staging for esophageal cancer entered the literature in 1995, when Krasna and associates reported the CALGB pilot study findings of staging by video-assisted thoracoscopic surgery (VATS).[91,92] The three institutions involved concluded that VATS staging of disease in patients with thoracic esophageal cancer was feasible in 95% of patients enrolled and that 88% of the patients undergoing esophagectomy with confirmatory pathologic stage were correctly assigned to stage. Bonavina and Luketich then separately reported the use of laparoscopy.[90,93] In the Italian study, 50 patients with distal esophageal adenocarcinoma or squamous cell carcinoma underwent CT, EUS, and laparoscopy. The investigators concluded that laparoscopy was safe and quick (mean time, 20 minutes) and changed the therapeutic approach in 10% of patients.[93] Luketich and coworkers[90] at the same time published results of minimally invasive staging of 26 patients with esophageal adenocarcinoma (92%) or squamous cell carcinoma and compared laparoscopic/right VATS staging with EUS staging. They concluded that surgical staging improved the accuracy of lymph node staging by 16%.

Krasna led the CALGB 9380 prospective trial, looking at the feasibility of surgical staging with laparoscopy and right VATS, and found that the approach was feasible and that the number of positive lymph nodes doubled compared with those detected by less invasive staging modalities.[89] An unanswered question, as it was not an endpoint of the study, is the cost-effectiveness of surgical staging. In addition, since the study's completion, PET/CT and enhanced EUS techniques have improved the accuracy of clinical staging modalities. In reality, most groups do not perform routine surgical staging. VATS does not appear to increase the identification of metastatic disease, whereas laparoscopy may be used judiciously for patients with suspected celiac nodal or liver metastases.

ADDITIONAL METASTATIC TESTS: BRAIN SCAN

Brain metastases from esophageal cancer are rare. Brain metastases are detected at initial diagnosis of esophagus cancer in 1.7% to 5% of patients in large series of patients with adenocarcinoma or squamous cell carcinoma.[94-96] Brain metastasis in a recent series of 27 patients with esophageal cancer (82% adenocarcinoma) was associated with a median survival of 3.8 months.[96] After potentially curative esophagectomy, intracranial metastases occur in an estimated 2% of patients in multiple series.[96] Esophageal metastases are typically to liver, lung, bone, and less commonly adrenal gland and kidney. In a series of 27 patients (1.7% of all esophagus cancer patients) with esophageal brain metastases during an 8-year period, only one presented with the brain metastasis as the index sign of his esophagus cancer.[96] Of 916 patients presenting for whole-brain irradiation for brain metastases, only 6% originated from the gastrointestinal malignant neoplasms and none from the esophagus.[97] In a high-volume esophageal cancer center, however, 28% of patients presenting for stereotactic radiosurgery for gastrointestinal tract brain metastases had esophageal primaries.[98] Most reports of patients developing brain metastases identify stage IV disease after potentially curative resection.[99-101] In one Japanese study of 803 patients treated for brain metastases, 2% originated from primary esophageal cancer (52% squamous cell carcinoma).[100] The authors recommended whole-brain irradiation to improve median survival from 18 to 66 months in patients who underwent metastasectomy or stereotactic radiosurgery.[100] Other Japanese groups have found the brain as the sole site of recurrent disease in 2% of patients and a median survival of 17 months after craniotomy and resection.[99,102]

Currently, the indications for a brain scan, either CT or MRI, for a patient initially presenting with esophagus cancer are similar to those for patients with other solid tumors, which are new-onset headaches and neurologic complaints including ataxia or paresthesias. As routine CT scanning of the brain was not cost-effective at the University of Michigan, the authors did note that risk factors for brain metastases included large locally and regionally advanced primary cancers.[94]

What about restage scanning after neoadjuvant treatment and before potential resection? There is evidence from the Cleveland Clinic that there is a higher occurrence of brain metastases in esophageal cancer patients treated with neoadjuvant or adjuvant chemotherapy and that the adjuvant treatment itself may facilitate development of brain metastases.[96] The significance of this concept is that we may not yet know the role of routine brain MRI or CT in patients treated with neoadjuvant therapy before esophagectomy. It seems the incidence is still too low and that the same guidelines of neuropathy and headache should dictate evaluation for brain metastases.

FUTURE DIRECTION: MOLECULAR STAGING

Potti and colleagues[103] recently introduced a genomic strategy to identify subsets of lung cancer patients who may have a worse prognosis and thus may benefit from adjuvant chemotherapy. Subsequently, molecular signatures with microarrays and quantitative reverse transcriptase–polymerase chain reaction have been reported by several other groups for prognostication of lung cancer patients.[104,105] Molecular profiling of esophageal cancers is nascent, but some early prognostic predictors of survival include distinct microRNA profiles[106] and gene expression variants of cyclin D1 gene expression.[107] Given the 30% to 40% response rate of esophageal cancers to induction chemotherapy, molecular analysis of esophageal tumors would allow targeted smart induction therapy. Pretreatment gene expression profiles to predict response to chemoradiation therapy have been shown to be significant in several studies in both squamous cell carcinoma and esophageal adenocarcinoma,[108-110] and there is increasing evidence that gene expression profiling of tumors may help predict an individual patient's response to chemotherapy.[111] Microarray analysis of gene expression profiles also should help identify targeted therapy tailored to an individual patient's tumor.[112,113] Although pathologic response to chemoradiation has been associated with molecular subtypes of endoscopic biopsy specimens in preliminary studies,[109] the significant genes and proteins have not been validated through prospective studies. We can begin, however, to envision a future staging system of genomic profiling of esophageal cancers wherein the easily accessible endoscopic biopsy specimen of esophageal cancer would allow molecular staging. Expression profiling of primary tumors thus would assist therapeutic stratification of patients to endoscopic resectional therapy, targeted induction therapy, minimally invasive esophagectomy, en bloc esophagectomy, palliative therapy, perhaps chemoradiation therapy, or no therapy.

Summary

Esophageal adenocarcinoma is on the rise in the United States, and treatment and staging modalities are evolving to translate into a much-needed improvement in survival rates. Appropriate staging of the newly diagnosed esophageal cancer can only result in the least and most invasive therapies being offered only to patients who may potentially benefit. The staging algorithm outlined in Figure 37-4 applies to most patients presenting with thoracic esophageal cancer under the current TNM staging system. As we obtain longer follow-up

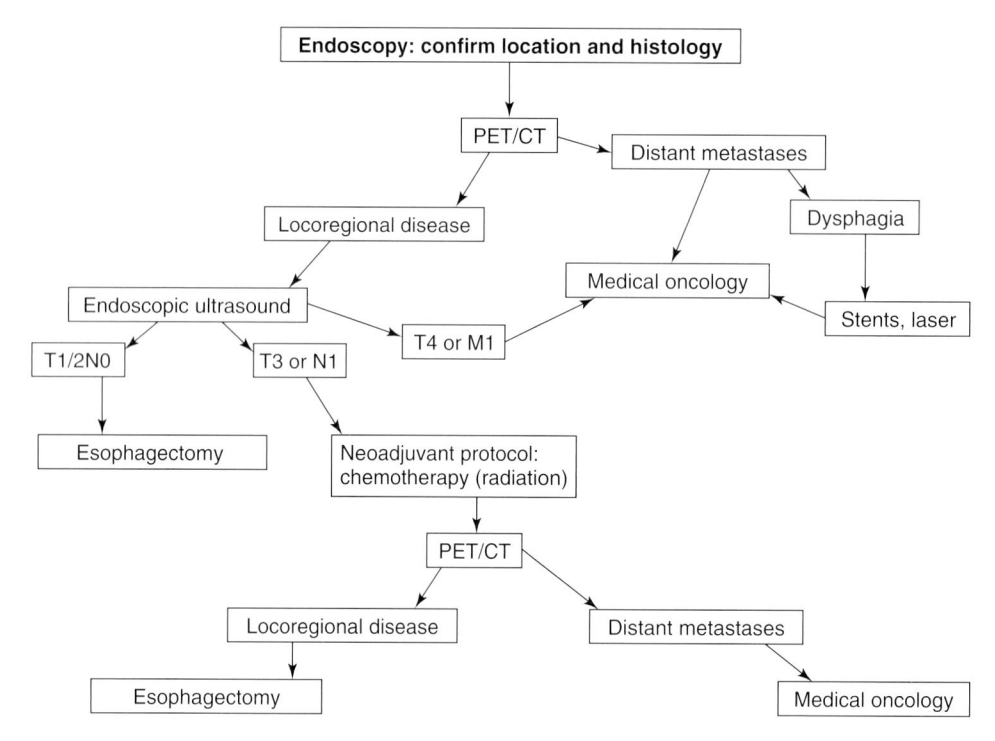

Figure 37–4
An algorithm for staging of thoracic esophageal cancer. Metastatic disease must always be confirmed by evaluating the tissue in question pathologically.

after endoscopic resection for treatment and staging of superficial tumors, this modality may be incorporated into the algorithm.

The next modification of the TNM staging system will likely include the subdivisions of T1 tumors and the number of lymph nodes resected or involved with metastases. Molecular staging of tumors, however, is still not ready for inclusion in a revised staging system. Complete but appropriate staging of esophageal cancer and ideally discussion of the results at a multidisciplinary team meeting can improve selection of patients for esophagectomy and may improve patient outcomes.[44]

REFERENCES

1. Jemal A, Siegel R, Ward E, Hao Y, Xu J, Murray T, et al. Cancer statistics. *CA Cancer J Clin* 2008;**58**(2):71-96:2008 Mar-Apr.
2. Parkin DM, Bray F, Ferlay J, Pisani P. Global cancer statistics. *CA Cancer J Clin* 2002;**55**(2):74-108:2005 Mar-Apr.
3. Bollschweiler E, Wolfgarten E, Gutschow C, Holscher AH. Demographic variations in the rising incidence of esophageal adenocarcinoma in white males. *Cancer* 2001 Aug 1;**92**(3):549-55.
4. Swanson SJ, Batirel HF, Bueno R, Jaklitsch MT, Lukanich JM, Allred E, et al. Transthoracic esophagectomy with radical mediastinal and abdominal lymph node dissection and cervical esophagogastrostomy for esophageal carcinoma. *Ann Thorac Surg* 2001 Dec;**72**(6):1924-5:1918-24; discussion.
5. Orringer MB, Marshall B, Chang AC, Lee J, Pickens A, Lau CL. Two thousand transhiatal esophagectomies: Changing trends, lessons learned. *Ann Surg* 2007 Sep;**246**(3):372-4:363-72; discussion.
6. Luketich JD, Alvelo-Rivera M, Buenaventura PO, Christie NA, McCaughan JS, Litle VR, et al. Minimally invasive esophagectomy: Outcomes in 222 patients. *Ann Surg* 2003 Oct;**238**(4):494-5:486,94; discussion.
7. Portale G, Hagen JA, Peters JH, Chan LS, DeMeester SR, Gandamihardja TA, et al. Modern 5-year survival of resectable esophageal adenocarcinoma: Single institution experience with 263 patients. *J Am Coll Surg* 2006 Apr;**202**(4):596-8:588-96; discussion.
8. Low DE, Kunz S, Schembre D, Otero H, Malpass T, Hsi A, et al. Esophagectomy—it's not just about mortality anymore: Standardized perioperative clinical pathways improve outcomes in patients with esophageal cancer. *J Gastrointest Surg* 2007 Nov;**11**(11):1395-402:discussion 1402.
9. Dimick JB, Cowan Jr JA, Ailawadi G, Wainess RM, Upchurch Jr GR. National variation in operative mortality rates for esophageal resection and the need for quality improvement. *Arch Surg* 2003 Dec;**138**(12):1305-9.
10. Blazeby JM, Farndon JR, Donovan J, Alderson D. A prospective longitudinal study examining the quality of life of patients with esophageal cancer. *Cancer* 2000 Apr 15;**88**(8):1781-7.
11. Blazeby JM, Alderson D, Farndon JR. Quality of life in patients with oesophageal cancer. *Recent Results Cancer Res.* 2000;**155**:193-204.
12. Kelsen DP, Ginsberg R, Pajak TF, Sheahan DG, Gunderson L, Mortimer J, et al. Chemotherapy followed by surgery compared with surgery alone for localized esophageal cancer. *N Engl J Med* 1998;**339**(27):1979-84:Dec 31.
13. Law S, Fok M, Chow S, Chu KM, Wong J. Preoperative chemotherapy versus surgical therapy alone for squamous cell carcinoma of the esophagus: A prospective randomized trial. *J Thorac Cardiovasc Surg* 1997 Aug;**114**(2):210-7.
14. Urba SG, Orringer MB, Turrisi A, Iannettoni M, Forastiere A, Strawderman M. Randomized trial of preoperative chemoradiation versus surgery alone in patients with locoregional esophageal carcinoma. *J Clin Oncol* 2001;**19**(2):305-13:Jan 15.
15. Berger AC, Farma J, Scott WJ, Freedman G, Weiner L, Cheng JD, et al. Complete response to neoadjuvant chemoradiotherapy in esophageal carcinoma is associated with significantly improved survival. *J Clin Oncol* 2005 Jul 1;**23**(19):4330-7.
16. Medical Research Council Oesophageal Cancer Working Group. Surgical resection with or without preoperative chemotherapy in oesophageal cancer: A randomised controlled trial. *Lancet* 2002;**359**(9319):1727-33:May 18.
17. Pennathur A, Luketich JD, Landreneau RJ, Ward J, Christie NA, Gibson MK, et al. Long-term results of a phase II trial of neoadjuvant chemotherapy followed by esophagectomy for locally advanced esophageal neoplasm. *Ann Thorac Surg* 2008 Jun;**85**(6):1936-7:1930-6; discussion.
18. Luu TD, Gaur P, Force SD, Staley CA, Mansour KA, Miller Jr JI, et al. Neoadjuvant chemoradiation versus chemotherapy for patients undergoing esophagectomy for esophageal cancer. *Ann Thorac Surg* 2008 Apr;**85**(4):1223-4:1217-23; discussion.
19. Urschel JD, Vasan H. A meta-analysis of randomized controlled trials that compared neoadjuvant chemoradiation and surgery to surgery alone for resectable esophageal cancer. *Am J Surg* 2003;**185**(6):538-43:Jun.
20. Donington JS, Miller DL, Allen MS, Deschamps C, Nichols 3rd FC, Pairolero PC. Tumor response to induction chemoradiation: Influence on survival after esophagectomy. *Eur J Cardiothorac Surg* 2003 Oct;**24**(4):636-7:631-6; discussion.
21. Ku GY, Ilson DH. Multimodality therapy for the curative treatment of cancer of the esophagus and gastroesophageal junction. *Expert Rev Anticancer Ther* 2008 Dec;**8**(12):1953-64.
22. Ku GY, Ilson DH. Preoperative therapy in esophageal cancer. *Clin Adv Hematol Oncol* 2008 May;**6**(5):371-9.
23. Greene F, Page D, Fleming I, Fritz A, Balch C, Haller D, editors. American joint committee on cancer: Manual for staging of cancer. 6th ed. New York: Springer-Verlag; 2002.
24. Lee HY, Choi HJ, Park KJ, Shin JS, Kwon HC, Roh MS, et al. Prognostic significance of metastatic lymph node ratio in node-positive colon carcinoma. *Ann Surg Oncol* 2007 May;**14**(5):1712-7.
25. Rodriguez Santiago JM, Munoz E, Marti M, Quintana S, Veloso E, Marco C. Metastatic lymph node ratio as a prognostic factor in gastric cancer. *Eur J Surg Oncol* 2005 Feb;**31**(1):59-66.
26. Nitti D, Marchet A, Olivieri M, Ambrosi A, Mencarelli R, Belluco C, et al. Ratio between metastatic and examined lymph nodes is an independent prognostic factor after D2 resection for gastric cancer: Analysis of a large European monoinstitutional experience. *Ann Surg Oncol* 2003 Nov;**10**(9):1077-85.
27. Bollschweiler E, Baldus SE, Schroder W, Schneider PM, Holscher AH. Staging of esophageal carcinoma: Length of tumor and number of involved regional lymph nodes. Are these independent prognostic factors?. *J Surg Oncol* 2006 Oct 1;**94**(5):355-63.
28. Rice TW, Blackstone EH, Rybicki LA, Adelstein DJ, Murthy SC, DeCamp MM, et al. Refining esophageal cancer staging. *J Thorac Cardiovasc Surg* 2003 May;**125**(5):1103-13.
29. Greenstein AJ, Litle VR, Swanson SJ, Divino CM, Packer S, Wisnivesky JP. Prognostic significance of the number of lymph node metastases in esophageal cancer. *J Am Coll Surg* 2008 Feb;**206**(2):239-46.
30. Eloubeidi MA, Desmond R, Arguedas MR, Reed CE, Wilcox CM. Prognostic factors for the survival of patients with esophageal carcinoma in the U.S. The importance of tumor length and lymph node status. *Cancer* 2002 Oct 1;**95**(7):1434-43.
31. Kunisaki C, Akiyama H, Nomura M, Matsuda G, Otsuka Y, Ono HA, et al. Developing an appropriate staging system for esophageal carcinoma. *J Am Coll Surg* 2005 Dec;**201**(6):884-90.
32. Greenstein AJ, Litle VR, Swanson SJ, Divino CM, Packer S, Wisnivesky JP. Effect of the number of lymph nodes sampled on postoperative survival of lymph node–negative esophageal cancer. *Cancer* 2008 Mar 15;**112**(6):1239-46.
33. van Sandick JW, van Lanschot JJ, ten Kate FJ, Tijssen JG, Obertop H. Indicators of prognosis after transhiatal esophageal resection without thoracotomy for cancer. *J Am Coll Surg* 2002 Jan;**194**(1):28-36.
34. Lightdale CJ. Endoscopic ultrasonography in the diagnosis, staging and follow-up of esophageal and gastric cancer. *Endoscopy* 1992 May;**1**(24 Suppl):297-303.
35. Melzer E, Avidan B, Heyman Z, Bar-Meir S. Accuracy of endoscopic ultrasonography for preoperative staging of esophageal malignancy. *Isr J Med Sci* 1995;**31**(2-3):119-21:Feb-Mar.
36. Walsh TN, Noonan N, Hollywood D, Kelly A, Keeling N, Hennessy TP. A comparison of multimodal therapy and surgery for esophageal adenocarcinoma. *N Engl J Med* 1996;**335**(7):462-7:Aug 15.
37. Heidemann J, Schilling MK, Schmassmann A, Maurer CA, Buchler MW. Accuracy of endoscopic ultrasonography in preoperative staging of esophageal carcinoma. *Dig Surg* 2000;**17**(3):219-24.
38. Lightdale CJ, Kulkarni KG. Role of endoscopic ultrasonography in the staging and follow-up of esophageal cancer. *J Clin Oncol* 2005 Jul 10;**23**(20):4483-9.
39. Chang KJ, Katz KD, Durbin TE, Erickson RA, Butler JA, Lin F, et al. Endoscopic ultrasound-guided fine-needle aspiration. *Gastrointest Endosc* 1994 Nov-Dec;**40**(6):694-9.
40. Cen P, Hofstetter WL, Lee JH, Ross WA, Wu TT, Swisher SG, et al. Value of endoscopic ultrasound staging in conjunction with the evaluation of lymphovascular invasion in identifying low-risk esophageal carcinoma. *Cancer* 2008 Feb 1;**112**(3):503-10.
41. Zuccaro Jr G, Rice TW, Goldblum J, Medendorp SV, Becker M, Pimentel R, et al. Endoscopic ultrasound cannot determine suitability for esophagectomy after aggressive chemoradiotherapy for esophageal cancer. *Am J Gastroenterol* 1999 Apr;**94**(4):906-12.
42. Giovannini M, Monges G, Seitz JF, Moutardier V, Bernardini D, Thomas P, et al. Distant lymph node metastases in esophageal cancer: Impact of endoscopic ultrasound-guided biopsy. *Endoscopy* 1999 Sep;**31**(7):536-40.

43. Barbour AP, Rizk NP, Gerdes H, Bains MS, Rusch VW, Brennan MF, et al. Endoscopic ultrasound predicts outcomes for patients with adenocarcinoma of the gastroesophageal junction. *J Am Coll Surg* 2007 Oct;**205**(4):593-601.
44. Davies AR, Deans DA, Penman I, Plevris JN, Fletcher J, Wall L, et al. The multidisciplinary team meeting improves staging accuracy and treatment selection for gastro-esophageal cancer. *Dis Esophagus* 2006;**19**(6):496-503.
45. Larghi A, Lightdale CJ, Memeo L, Bhagat G, Okpara N, Rotterdam H. EUS followed by EMR for staging of high-grade dysplasia and early cancer in Barrett's esophagus. *Gastrointest Endosc* 2005 Jul;**62**(1):16-23.
46. Heidemann J, Schilling MK, Schmassmann A, Maurer CA, Buchler MW. Accuracy of endoscopic ultrasonography in preoperative staging of esophageal carcinoma. *Dig Surg* 2000;**17**(3):219-24.
47. Flamen P, Lerut A, Van Cutsem E, De Wever W, Peeters M, Stroobants S, et al. Utility of positron emission tomography for the staging of patients with potentially operable esophageal carcinoma. *J Clin Oncol* 2000 Sep 15;**18**(18):3202-10.
48. Vickers J, Alderson D. Oesophageal cancer staging using endoscopic ultrasonography. *Br J Surg* 1998 Jul;**85**(7):994-8.
49. Botet JF, Lightdale CJ, Zauber AG, Gerdes H, Urmacher C, Brennan MF. Preoperative staging of esophageal cancer: Comparison of endoscopic US and dynamic CT. *Radiology* 1991 Nov;**181**(2):419-25.
50. Peters JH, Hoeft SF, Heimbucher J, Bremner RM, DeMeester TR, Bremner CG, et al. Selection of patients for curative or palliative resection of esophageal cancer based on preoperative endoscopic ultrasonography. *Arch Surg* 1994 May;**129**(5):534-9.
51. Murata Y, Suzuki S, Ohta M, Mitsunaga A, Hayashi K, Yoshida K, et al. Small ultrasonic probes for determination of the depth of superficial esophageal cancer. *Gastrointest Endosc* 1996 Jul;**44**(1):23-8.
52. Rice TW, Zuccaro Jr G, Adelstein DJ, Rybicki LA, Blackstone EH, Goldblum JR. Esophageal carcinoma: Depth of tumor invasion is predictive of regional lymph node status. *Ann Thorac Surg* 1998 Mar;**65**(3):787-92.
53. Laterza E, de Manzoni G, Guglielmi A, Rodella L, Tedesco P, Cordiano C. Endoscopic ultrasonography in the staging of esophageal carcinoma after preoperative radiotherapy and chemotherapy. *Ann Thorac Surg* 1999 May;**67**(5):1466-9.
54. Isenberg G, Chak A, Canto MI, Levitan N, Clayman J, Pollack BJ, et al. Endoscopic ultrasound in restaging of esophageal cancer after neoadjuvant chemoradiation. *Gastrointest Endosc* 1998 Aug;**48**(2):158-63.
55. Zhang X, Watson DI, Lally C, Bessell JR. Endoscopic ultrasound for preoperative staging of esophageal carcinoma. *Surg Endosc* 2005 Dec;**19**(12):1618-21.
56. Isenberg G, Chak A, Canto MI, Levitan N, Clayman J, Pollack BJ, et al. Endoscopic ultrasound in restaging of esophageal cancer after neoadjuvant chemoradiation. *Gastrointest Endosc* 1998 Aug;**48**(2):158-63.
57. Beseth BD, Bedford R, Isacoff WH, Holmes EC, Cameron RB. Endoscopic ultrasound does not accurately assess pathologic stage of esophageal cancer after neoadjuvant chemoradiotherapy. *Am Surg* 2000 Sep;**66**(9):827-31.
58. Giovannini M, Seitz JF, Thomas P, Hannoun-Levy JM, Perrier H, Resbeut M, et al. Endoscopic ultrasonography for assessment of the response to combined radiation therapy and chemotherapy in patients with esophageal cancer. *Endoscopy* 1997 Jan;**29**(1):4-9.
59. Reed CE, Mishra G, Sahai AV, Hoffman BJ, Hawes RH. Esophageal cancer staging: Improved accuracy by endoscopic ultrasound of celiac lymph nodes. *Ann Thorac Surg* 1999 Feb;**67**(2):319-21:discussion 322.
60. Eloubeidi MA, Wallace MB, Hoffman BJ, Leveen MB, Van Velse A, Hawes RH, et al. Predictors of survival for esophageal cancer patients with and without celiac axis lymphadenopathy: Impact of staging endosonography. *Ann Thorac Surg* 2001 Jul;**72**(1):219-20:212,9; discussion.
61. Singh P, Mukhopadhyay P, Bhatt B, Patel T, Kiss A, Gupta R, et al. Endoscopic ultrasound versus CT scan for detection of the metastases to the liver: Results of a prospective comparative study. *J Clin Gastroenterol* 2009 Apr;**43**(4):367-73.
62. Greenberg J, Durkin M, Van Drunen M, Aranha GV. Computed tomography or endoscopic ultrasonography in preoperative staging of gastric and esophageal tumors. *Surgery* 1994 Oct;**116**(4):701-2:696-701; discussion.
63. Kelly S, Harris KM, Berry E, Hutton J, Roderick P, Cullingworth J, et al. A systematic review of the staging performance of endoscopic ultrasound in gastro-oesophageal carcinoma. *Gut* 2001 Oct;**49**(4):534-9.
64. Inculet RI, Keller SM, Dwyer A, Roth JA. Evaluation of noninvasive tests for the preoperative staging of carcinoma of the esophagus: A prospective study. *Ann Thorac Surg* 1985 Dec;**40**(6):561-5.
65. Lefor AT, Merino MM, Steinberg SM, Dwyer A, Roth JA, Flanagan M, et al. Computerized tomographic prediction of extraluminal spread and prognostic implications of lesion width in esophageal carcinoma. *Cancer* 1988;**62**(7):1287-92:Oct 1.
66. Roedl JB, Harisinghani MG, Colen RR, Fischman AJ, Blake MA, Mathisen DJ, et al. Assessment of treatment response and recurrence in esophageal carcinoma based on tumor length and standardized uptake value on positron emission tomography–computed tomography. *Ann Thorac Surg* 2008 Oct;**86**(4):1131-8.
67. Ott K, Weber W, Siewert JR. The importance of PET in the diagnosis and response evaluation of esophageal cancer. *Dis Esophagus* 2006;**19**(6):433-42.
68. Block MI, Patterson GA, Sundaresan RS, Bailey MS, Flanagan FL, Dehdashti F, et al. Improvement in staging of esophageal cancer with the addition of positron emission tomography. *Ann Thorac Surg* 1997 Sep;**64**(3):776-7:770-6; discussion.
69. Flamen P, Van Cutsem E, Lerut A, Cambier JP, Haustermans K, Bormans G, et al. Positron emission tomography for assessment of the response to induction radiochemotherapy in locally advanced oesophageal cancer. *Ann Oncol* 2002 Mar;**13**(3):361-8.
70. Hagen JA, DeMeester SR, Peters JH, Chandrasoma P, DeMeester TR. Curative resection for esophageal adenocarcinoma: Analysis of 100 en bloc esophagectomies. *Ann Surg* 2001 Oct;**234**(4):520-30:530-1; discussion.
71. Roedl JB, Blake MA, Holalkere NS, Mueller PR, Colen RR, Harisinghani MG. Lymph node staging in esophageal adenocarcinoma with PET-CT based on a visual analysis and based on metabolic parameters. *Abdom Imaging* 2008:Oct 1 [Epub ahead of print]..
72. Cerfolio RJ, Bryant AS. Maximum standardized uptake values on positron emission tomography of esophageal cancer predicts stage, tumor biology, and survival. *Ann Thorac Surg* 2006 Aug;**82**(2):394-5:391-4; discussion.
73. Downey RJ, Akhurst T, Ilson D, Ginsberg R, Bains MS, Gonen M, et al. Whole body ^{18}FDG-PET and the response of esophageal cancer to induction therapy: Results of a prospective trial. *J Clin Oncol* 2003;**21**(3):428-32:Feb 1.
74. Flanagan FL, Dehdashti F, Siegel BA, Trask DD, Sundaresan SR, Patterson GA, et al. Staging of esophageal cancer with ^{18}F-fluorodeoxyglucose positron emission tomography. *AJR Am J Roentgenol* 1997;**168**(2):417-24:Feb.
75. Meyers BF, Downey RJ, Decker PA, Keenan RJ, Siegel BA, Cerfolio RJ, et al. The utility of positron emission tomography in staging of potentially operable carcinoma of the thoracic esophagus: Results of the American College of Surgeons Oncology Group Z0060 trial. *J Thorac Cardiovasc Surg* 2007;**133**(3):738-45:Mar.
76. Beyer T, Townsend DW, Brun T, Kinahan PE, Charron M, Roddy R, et al. A combined PET/CT scanner for clinical oncology. *J Nucl Med* 2000 Aug;**41**(8):1369-79.
77. Charron M, Beyer T, Bohnen NN, Kinahan PE, Dachille M, Jerin J, et al. Image analysis in patients with cancer studied with a combined PET and CT scanner. *Clin Nucl Med* 2000 Nov;**25**(11):905-10.
78. Bruzzi JF, Munden RF, Truong MT, Marom EM, Sabloff BS, Gladish GW, et al. PET/CT of esophageal cancer: Its role in clinical management. *Radiographics* 2007 Nov-Dec;**27**(6):1635-52.
79. Chirieac LR, Swisher SG, Ajani JA, Komaki RR, Correa AM, Morris JS, et al. Posttherapy pathologic stage predicts survival in patients with esophageal carcinoma receiving preoperative chemoradiation. *Cancer* 2005 Apr 1;**103**(7):1347-55.
80. Brucher BL, Weber W, Bauer M, Fink U, Avril N, Stein HJ, et al. Neoadjuvant therapy of esophageal squamous cell carcinoma: Response evaluation by positron emission tomography. *Ann Surg* 2001 Mar;**233**(3):300-9.
81. Ancona E, Ruol A, Santi S, Merigliano S, Sileni VC, Koussis H, et al. Only pathologic complete response to neoadjuvant chemotherapy improves significantly the long term survival of patients with resectable esophageal squamous cell carcinoma: Final report of a randomized, controlled trial of preoperative chemotherapy versus surgery alone. *Cancer* 2001 Jun 1; **91**(11):2165-74.
82. Bruzzi JF, Swisher SG, Truong MT, Munden RF, Hofstetter WL, Macapinlac HA, et al. Detection of interval distant metastases: Clinical utility of integrated CT-PET imaging in patients with esophageal carcinoma after neoadjuvant therapy. *Cancer* 2007 Jan 1;**109**(1):125-34.
83. Weber WA, Ott K, Becker K, Dittler HJ, Helmberger H, Avril NE, et al. Prediction of response to preoperative chemotherapy in adenocarcinomas of the esophagogastric junction by metabolic imaging. *J Clin Oncol* 2001 Jun 15; **19**(12):3058-65.
84. Ott K, Weber WA, Lordick F, Becker K, Busch R, Herrmann K, et al. Metabolic imaging predicts response, survival, and recurrence in adenocarcinomas of the esophagogastric junction. *J Clin Oncol* 2006 Oct 10;**24**(29):4692-8.
85. Lerut T, Flamen P. Role of FDG-PET scan in staging of cancer of the esophagus and gastroesophageal junction. *Minerva Chir* 2002 Dec;**57**(6):837-45.
86. Cerfolio RJ, Bryant AS, Ohja B, Bartolucci AA, Eloubeidi MA. The accuracy of endoscopic ultrasonography with fine-needle aspiration, integrated positron emission tomography with computed tomography, and computed tomography in restaging patients with esophageal cancer after neoadjuvant chemoradiotherapy. *J Thorac Cardiovasc Surg* 2005 Jun;**129**(6):1232-41.
87. Erasmus JJ, Munden RF, Truong MT, Ho JJ, Hofstetter WL, Macapinlac HA, et al. Preoperative chemo-radiation–induced ulceration in patients with esophageal cancer: A confounding factor in tumor response assessment in integrated computed tomographic–positron emission tomographic imaging. *J Thorac Oncol* 2006 Jun;**1**(5):478-86.

88. Fukunaga T, Okazumi S, Koide Y, Isono K, Imazeki K. Evaluation of esophageal cancers using fluorine-18-fluorodeoxyglucose PET. *J Nucl Med* 1998 Jun;**39**(6):1002-7.
89. Krasna MJ, Reed CE, Nedzwiecki D, Hollis DR, Luketich JD, DeCamp MM, et al. CALGB 9380: A prospective trial of the feasibility of thoracoscopy/laparoscopy in staging esophageal cancer. *Ann Thorac Surg* 2001 Apr;**71**(4):1073-9.
90. Luketich JD, Schauer P, Landreneau R, Nguyen N, Urso K, Ferson P, et al. Minimally invasive surgical staging is superior to endoscopic ultrasound in detecting lymph node metastases in esophageal cancer. *J Thorac Cardiovasc Surg* 1997 Nov;**114**(5):821-3:817-21; discussion.
91. Krasna MJ, Reed CE, Jaklitsch MT, Cushing D, Sugarbaker DJ. Thoracoscopic staging of esophageal cancer: A prospective, multiinstitutional trial. Cancer and Leukemia Group B Thoracic Surgeons. *Ann Thorac Surg* 1995 Nov;**60**(5):1337-40.
92. Sugarbaker DJ, Jaklitsch MT, Liptay MJ. Thoracoscopic staging and surgical therapy for esophageal cancer. *Chest* 1995 Jun;**107**(6 Suppl):218S-23S.
93. Bonavina L, Incarbone R, Lattuada E, Segalin A, Cesana B, Peracchia A. Preoperative laparoscopy in management of patients with carcinoma of the esophagus and of the esophagogastric junction. *J Surg Oncol* 1997 Jul;**65**(3):171-4.
94. Gabrielsen TO, Eldevik OP, Orringer MB, Marshall BL. Esophageal carcinoma metastatic to the brain: Clinical value and cost-effectiveness of routine enhanced head CT before esophagectomy. *AJNR Am J Neuroradiol* 1995 Oct;**16**(9):1915-21.
95. Mandard AM, Chasle J, Marnay J, Villedieu B, Bianco C, Roussel A, et al. Autopsy findings in 111 cases of esophageal cancer. *Cancer* 1981 Jul 15;**48**(2):329-35.
96. Weinberg JS, Suki D, Hanbali F, Cohen ZR, Lenzi R, Sawaya R. Metastasis of esophageal carcinoma to the brain. *Cancer* 2003 Nov 1;**98**(9):1925-33.
97. Bartelt S, Momm F, Weissenberger C, Lutterbach J. Patients with brain metastases from gastrointestinal tract cancer treated with whole brain radiation therapy: Prognostic factors and survival. *World J Gastroenterol* 2004 Nov 15;**10**(22):3345-8.
98. Hasegawa T, Kondziolka D, Flickinger JC, Lunsford LD. Stereotactic radiosurgery for brain metastases from gastrointestinal tract cancer. *Surg Neurol* 2003 Dec;**60**(6):514-5:506-14; discussion.
99. Kawabata R, Doki Y, Ishikawa O, Nakagawa H, Takachi K, Miyashiro I, et al. Frequent brain metastasis after chemotherapy and surgery for advanced esophageal cancers. *Hepatogastroenterology* 2007 Jun;**54**(76):1043-8.
100. Yoshida S. Brain metastasis in patients with esophageal carcinoma. *Surg Neurol* 2007 Mar;**67**(3):288-90.
101. Rice TW, Khuntia D, Rybicki LA, Adelstein DJ, Vogelbaum MA, Mason DP, et al. Brain metastases from esophageal cancer: A phenomenon of adjuvant therapy? *Ann Thorac Surg* 2006 Dec;**82**(6):2042-9:e1-2 2049.
102. Ogawa K, Toita T, Sueyama H, Fuwa N, Kakinohana Y, Kamata M, et al. Brain metastases from esophageal carcinoma: Natural history, prognostic factors, and outcome. *Cancer* 2002 Feb 1;**94**(3):759-64.
103. Potti A, Mukherjee S, Petersen R, Dressman HK, Bild A, Koontz J, et al. A genomic strategy to refine prognosis in early-stage non-small-cell lung cancer. *N Engl J Med* 2006 Aug 10;**355**(6):570-80.
104. Chen HY, Yu SL, Chen CH, Chang GC, Chen CY, Yuan A, et al. A five-gene signature and clinical outcome in non-small-cell lung cancer. *N Engl J Med* 2007 Jan 4;**356**(1):11-20.
105. Guo NL, Wan YW, Tosun K, Lin H, Msiska Z, Flynn DC, et al. Confirmation of gene expression–based prediction of survival in non–small cell lung cancer. *Clin Cancer Res.* 2008 Dec 15;**14**(24):8213-20.
106. Guo Y, Chen Z, Zhang L, Zhou F, Shi S, Feng X, et al. Distinctive microRNA profiles relating to patient survival in esophageal squamous cell carcinoma. *Cancer Res.* 2008 Jan 1;**68**(1):26-33.
107. Gupta VK, Feber A, Xi L, Pennathur A, Wu M, Luketich JD, et al. Association between CCND1 G/A870 polymorphism, allele-specific amplification, cyclin D1 expression, and survival in esophageal and lung carcinoma. *Clin Cancer Res.* 2008 Dec 1;**14**(23):7804-12.
108. Duong C, Greenawalt DM, Kowalczyk A, Ciavarella ML, Raskutti G, Murray WK, et al. Pretreatment gene expression profiles can be used to predict response to neoadjuvant chemoradiotherapy in esophageal cancer. *Ann Surg Oncol* 2007 Dec;**14**(12):3602-9.
119. Luthra R, Wu TT, Luthra MG, Izzo J, Lopez-Alvarez E, Zhang L, et al. Gene expression profiling of localized esophageal carcinomas: Association with pathologic response to preoperative chemoradiation. *J Clin Oncol* 2006 Jan 10;**24**(2):259-67.
110. Izzo JG, Malhotra U, Wu TT, Ensor J, Luthra R, Lee JH, et al. Association of activated transcription factor nuclear factor κB with chemoradiation resistance and poor outcome in esophageal carcinoma. *J Clin Oncol* 2006 Feb 10;**24**(5):748-54.
111. Kihara C, Tsunoda T, Tanaka T, Yamana H, Furukawa Y, Ono K, et al. Prediction of sensitivity of esophageal tumors to adjuvant chemotherapy by cDNA microarray analysis of gene-expression profiles. *Cancer Res* 2001 Sep 1;**61**(17):6474-9.
112. Watts GS, Tran NL, Berens ME, Bhattacharyya AK, Nelson MA, Montgomery EA, et al. Identification of Fn14/TWEAK receptor as a potential therapeutic target in esophageal adenocarcinoma. *Int J Cancer* 2007 Nov 15;**121**(10):2132-9.
113. Kashyap MK, Marimuthu A, Kishore CJ, Peri S, Keerthikumar S, Prasad TS, et al. Genomewide mRNA profiling of esophageal squamous cell carcinoma for identification of cancer biomarkers. *Cancer Biol Ther* 2009 Jan 1;**8**(1).

CHAPTER 38

Esophageal Resection and Replacement

Cynthia S. Chin, Philip A. Linden, and Scott J. Swanson

History of Esophageal Resection
Techniques of Esophageal Resection
  Modified McKeown or Tri-incisional
    Technique
    Indications
    Contraindications
    Preparation
    Technique
  Ivor Lewis Esophagectomy
    Indications
    Contraindications
    Technique
  Transhiatal Esophagectomy
    Indications
    Contraindications
    Preparation
    Technique
  Trials Comparing Transhiatal
    with Transthoracic Resection

Minimally Invasive Esophagectomy
  Tri-incisional
  Ivor Lewis
  Transhiatal
  Results
Left Thoracoabdominal Approach
  Indications
  Contraindications
  Technique
En Bloc Resection
  Technique
  Results
Three-Field Lymph Node Dissection
  *Prognostic Significance of Number
    of Lymph Nodes Resected*
Techniques of Alternative Conduits: Colon
  and Jejunum
  Colon
  Left Colon

  Right Colon
  Jejunum
Considerations in Esophageal Resection
  Perioperative Mortality
  Early Perioperative Complications
    Anastomotic Leak
    Respiratory Complications
    Recurrent Laryngeal Nerve Injury
    Bleeding
    Chyle Leak
    Cardiovascular Morbidity
  Late Perioperative Complications
    Anastomotic Stricture
    Postresection Reflux
    Impaired Conduit Emptying
  Local Recurrence
  Long-term (5-Year) Survival
  Summary

The incidence of esophageal carcinoma, particularly adenocarcinoma, has risen in the Western Hemisphere. The American Cancer Society "Cancer Statistics, 2008" reports that the 5-year survival rate for all patients with esophageal cancer is 15.6%. Patients treated with an esophagectomy have a 5-year survival rate close to 35%.[1]

HISTORY OF ESOPHAGEAL RESECTION

The first esophageal resection was performed more than 125 years ago, yet it remains one of the most formidable operations, carrying the highest morbidity of any commonly performed resection. The perioperative mortality has decreased from 40% to less than 3% in selected academic centers, largely because of advances in surgical and anesthetic technique, intensive care, and management of complications. The rate of morbidity for this surgery has not decreased as dramatically as the rate for mortality. With average mortality rates at 10% and complication rates exceeding 50%, careful selection of patients, thoughtful surgical planning, meticulous technique, and timely management of complications are essential to ensure good outcome for the patient. The esophageal surgeon must be familiar with the anatomy of the neck, chest, and abdomen and be skilled in surgery of the entire alimentary tract to provide complete care of the patient requiring esophageal resection. Only with this knowledge can the surgeon fit the operation to the patient, not the patient into the operation. These issues are detailed in this chapter.

Ivor Lewis, writing in 1946, is credited with popularizing transthoracic resection of the esophagus. He initially performed the operation in two stages, first mobilizing the stomach through a laparotomy and second, several days later, resecting the esophagus and performing an intrathoracic anastomosis through a right thoracotomy. Lewis showed a sophisticated understanding of the challenges involved in esophageal surgery when he stated that "the oesophagus is a difficult surgical field for three reasons: its inaccessibility; its lack of a serous coat, and its enclosure in structures where infection is especially dangerous and rapid."[2] The Ivor Lewis and transhiatal approaches are the most commonly employed techniques of esophageal resection used today. In 1962, McKeown described a three-stage esophagectomy, with the addition of a cervical incision and anastomosis to allow better margins for proximal tumors.[3] It is now called the three-hole or tri-incisional esophagectomy.

Open esophagectomy has up to 60% reported morbidity.[4,5] For this reason, several approaches have been supplemented with thoracoscopic or laparoscopic modifications. Since Cuschieri first introduced the concept of a minimally invasive approach to esophagectomy in 1992,[6] there have been numerous descriptions in the literature.[7-11]

TECHNIQUES OF ESOPHAGEAL RESECTION

Modified McKeown or Tri-incisional Technique

Indications

The tri-incisional esophagectomy (modified McKeown) is a versatile technique that can be employed for tumors at any level and for a variety of benign and malignant conditions.

It combines the advantages of the Ivor Lewis approach with those of a transhiatal technique. These include complete lymph node dissection in the chest, direct visualization of the intrathoracic dissection, avoidance of an intrathoracic anastomosis, maximal margins, and diminution of chances for postoperative gastroesophageal reflux disease. It is especially useful for tumors of the mid and upper esophagus and for tumors arising in a long Barrett's segment where nearly total excision of the esophagus is required.

Contraindications

Fusion of the right pleural space or inability to support ventilation with the left lung would make an approach through a right thoracotomy difficult. Relative contraindications include small gastric conduits secondary to tumor or limited vascular supply. Patients with tumor extending onto the stomach require more gastric resection than do those with tumor isolated to the esophagus. These patients are most suited for an Ivor Lewis or a jejunal reconstruction if there is not enough stomach.

Preparation

A detailed history and physical examination are necessary to evaluate for coexistent comorbid disease. Computed tomography and positron emission tomography of the chest and abdomen should be performed to evaluate for metastatic disease, anatomic abnormalities, and location of the tumor adjacent to vital structures. Pulmonary function tests should be obtained. Poor forced expiratory volume in 1 second (FEV_1) is not a contraindication to a muscle-sparing limited thoracotomy, although increased risk of pulmonary complications may be expected. Computed tomography and positron emission tomography of the head are useful in ruling out metastatic disease. Preoperative bowel preparation is generally done in the rare and unfortunate instance in which there needs to be a change in conduit.

Technique

Esophagogastroduodenoscopy is performed to identify the location of the tumor and to rule out disease of the stomach or duodenum. Retroflexion of the esophagogastroduodenoscopy is important for proper evaluation of the gastroesophageal junction. The carina is at the level of 25 cm from the incisor on esophagogastroduodenoscopy. Tumors in this area should be carefully evaluated by bronchoscopy for tumor invasion of the trachea. A double-lumen tube is placed, and the patient is positioned in a left lateral decubitus position. A right posterolateral thoracotomy incision is made wide enough to insert the surgeon's hand (approximately 10 cm). A portion of the latissimus is divided; the serratus is spared (Fig. 38-1). Division of the intercostal muscle from the vertebral bodies posteriorly to the mammary vessels anteriorly usually provides enough working space without division of a rib. The chest is entered through the fifth or sixth interspace, depending on the location of the tumor.

The lung is retracted anteriorly, and the inferior pulmonary ligament is divided by use of cautery. In a region away from the tumor and away from any scarring, the pleura overlying the esophagus is incised anteriorly and posteriorly and the

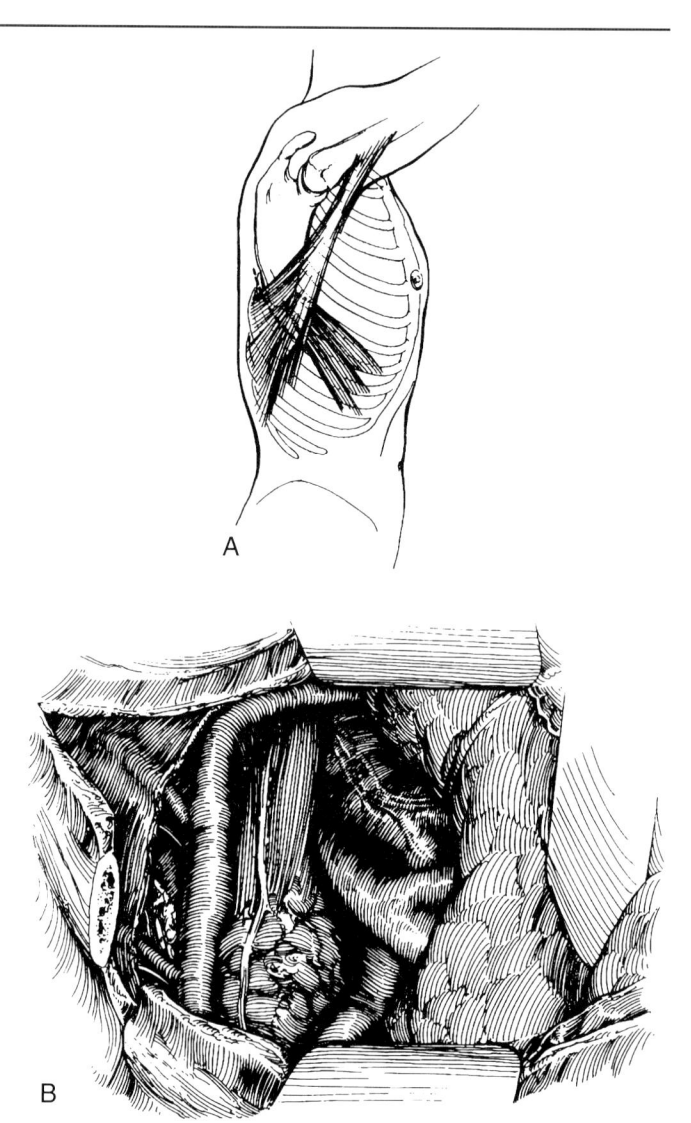

Figure 38-1
A limited right posterolateral thoracotomy is performed, dividing the latissimus. *(From Swanson S, Grondin S, Sugarbaker D. Total esophagectomy: the Brigham and Women's Hospital approach. Oper Tech Thorac Cardiovasc Surg 1999;4:197-209.)*

esophagus is surrounded with a Penrose drain. With traction on the Penrose drain, the esophagus is retracted both anteriorly and posteriorly and is dissected by electrocautery, including all adjacent lymph node tissue. Arterial branches supplying the esophagus from the aorta are clipped before being divided. Any cautery performed in the region of the carina must be at low settings to avoid thermal injury to the trachea. The azygos vein is typically divided. At the level of the azygos vein, the vagus nerves are identified on the esophagus and divided between clips. Division of the vagal nerve is important because an intact vagus nerve can lead to a traction injury of the recurrent laryngeal nerve. Further cranial dissection proceeds with the vagus nerves away from the esophagus to avoid recurrent nerve injury. Blunt dissection is useful high in the right chest (Fig. 38-2). Most dissection should be in the posterior plane to avoid injury to the recurrent laryngeal nerve, which is in the groove between the esophagus and trachea. A knotted Penrose drain is placed around the cervical esophagus and

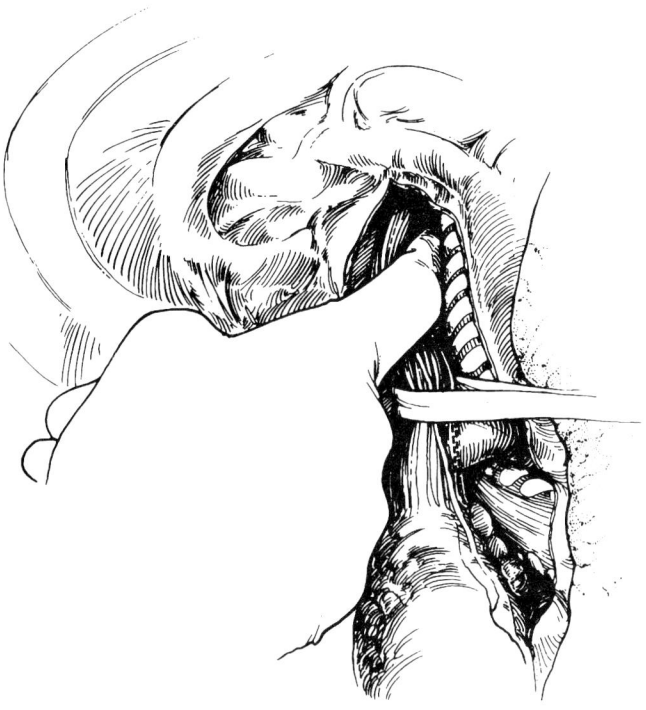

Figure 38–2
Blunt finger dissection close to the esophagus is used to free the esophagus up into the neck. *(From Sugarbaker D, DeCamp M, Liptay M. Surgical procedures to resect and replace the esophagus. In: Zinner M, Schwartz S, Ellis H, et al, editors.* Maingot's abdominal operations. *Stanford, CT: Appleton & Lange; 1997. p. 885-910.)*

Figure 38–3
A knotted Penrose drain is placed into the left side of the neck for later retrieval during the cervical dissection. This helps ensure isolation of the esophagus without injury to the recurrent nerves. *(From Sugarbaker D, DeCamp M, Liptay M. Surgical procedures to resect and replace the esophagus. In: Zinner M, Schwartz S, Ellis H, et al, editors.* Maingot's abdominal operations. *Stanford, CT: Appleton & Lange; 1997. p. 885-910.)*

pushed into the posterior neck for retrieval during the cervical portion of the case (Fig. 38-3). This Penrose drain, positioned inside the vagus nerves relative to the esophagus, permits isolation of the cervical esophagus without traction on the recurrent nerve. A sponge is packed high in the chest to assist in hemostasis and is removed before closure. The lower portion of the esophagus is encircled with a second Penrose drain and the remaining distal esophagus is dissected, including in the specimen all tissue lateral to the pericardium and medial to the aorta and spine.

If the tumor is near the gastroesophageal junction, a 2-cm rim of diaphragm is resected with the esophagus (Fig. 38-4). The Penrose drain is knotted and left in the abdomen for retrieval during the abdominal portion of the operation. Mass ligature of the thoracic duct at the level of the hiatus is performed by encircling all tissue between the aorta and spine with a 0 silk suture. The chest is inspected for hemostasis, the sponge previously placed is removed, and a 28 French straight chest tube is inserted through a separate stab incision and directed to the apex of the chest. The ribs are approximated with interrupted #2 Vicryl sutures. The latissimus is closed with running 0 Vicryl suture. The subdermal fascia is closed with a running 2-0 Vicryl suture. The skin is closed with staples or suture. The patient is repositioned in the supine position and is reintubated with a single-lumen tube. A transverse roll is placed under the scapula, and the head is turned 45 degrees to the right. An upper midline laparotomy is performed from the umbilicus to the junction of the costal margin and the left side of the xiphoid; the xiphoid is occasionally resected for better visualization. The abdomen is

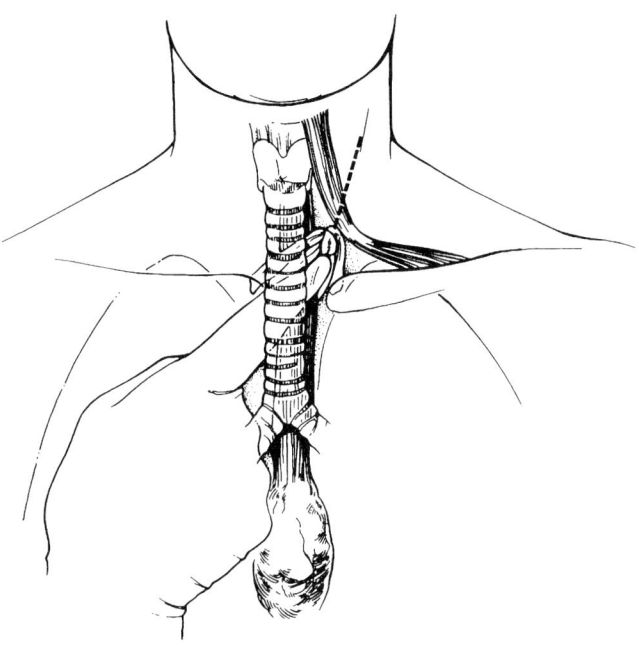

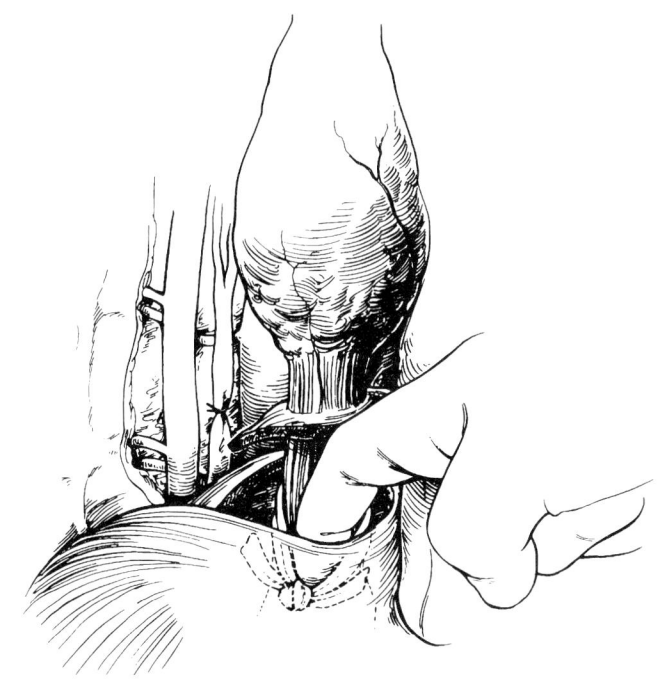

Figure 38–4
A rim of diaphragm is incorporated into the specimen for all gastroesophageal junction tumors. A knotted Penrose drain is placed into the abdomen to aid dissection of the esophagus at the gastroesophageal junction during the abdominal phase of the operation. *(From Sugarbaker D, DeCamp M, Liptay M. Surgical procedures to resect and replace the esophagus. In: Zinner M, Schwartz S, Ellis H, et al, editors.* Maingot's abdominal operations. *Stanford, CT: Appleton & Lange; 1997. p. 885-910.)*

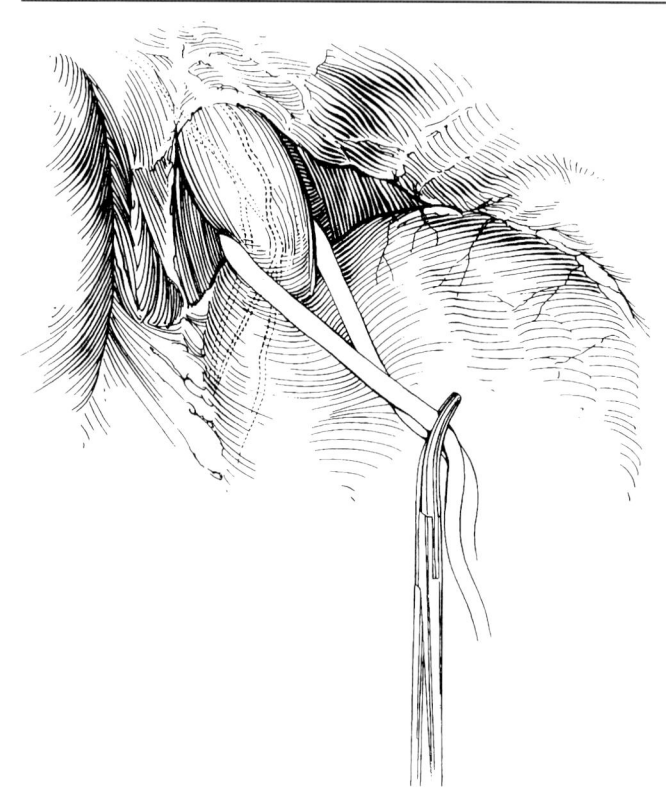

Figure 38–5
The phrenoesophageal ligament is divided fully after retrieval of the Penrose drain. *(From Swanson S, Grondin S, Sugarbaker D. Total esophagectomy: The Brigham and Women's Hospital approach.* Oper Tech Thorac Cardiovasc Surg *1999;4:197-209.)*

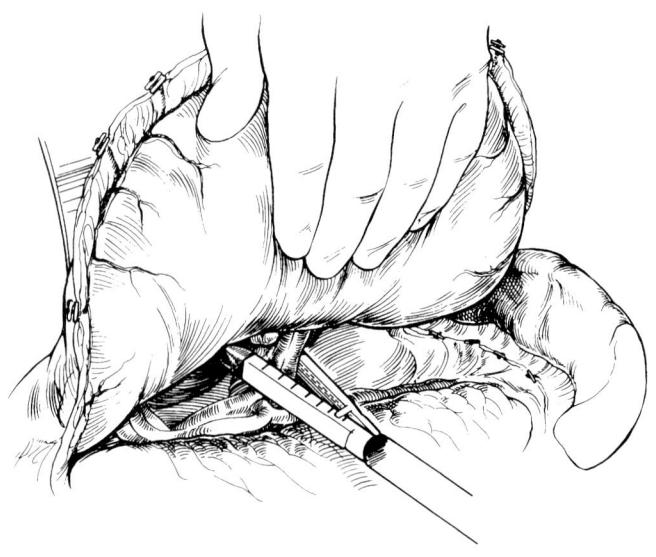

Figure 38–6
After complete mobilization of the greater curvature of the stomach and division of the gastrohepatic ligament, the left gastric vessels are identified. An endoscopic vascular stapler is used to divide these vessels, with care taken not to impinge on the celiac axis. *(From Sugarbaker D, DeCamp M, Liptay M. Surgical procedures to resect and replace the esophagus. In: Zinner M, Schwartz S, Ellis H, et al, editors.* Maingot's abdominal operations. *Stanford, CT: Appleton & Lange; 1997. p. 885-910.)*

explored for metastatic disease, which includes inspection of the liver, omentum, and peritoneal surfaces. The left lobe of the liver is mobilized by dividing the triangular ligament. Close to the triangular ligament are large diaphragmatic veins that should be avoided during this dissection. The Penrose drain surrounding the gastroesophageal junction is grasped, and the remaining phrenoesophageal ligament is divided (Fig. 38-5). The gastroepiploic pulse is palpated. At a point 2 cm away from the gastroepiploic artery on the greater curvature of the stomach, the lesser sac is entered. Dissection along the greater curvature of the stomach toward the spleen proceeds with division of vascular branches by use of double clips, silk ties, or the harmonic scalpel. Short gastric vessels are taken in identical fashion. Displacement of the spleen anteriorly by placement of lap pads behind the spleen may aid in dissection of the short gastric vessels. Once the short gastric arteries are divided, additional dissection toward the pylorus is performed. The gastroduodenal artery travels behind the pylorus before branching into the right gastric epiploic and superior pancreaticoduodenal arteries. The duodenum is mobilized from its retroperitoneum connections by a Kocher maneuver. The duodenum is adequately mobilized when the pylorus can reach the esophageal hiatus.

The stomach is then lifted anteriorly, and any adhesions between the stomach and pancreas are divided with electrocautery. The left gastric artery is identified and skeletonized, sweeping lymph node tissue onto the specimen. With a 30-mm vascular stapler, the base of the left gastric artery is clamped. A continued strong pulse in the gastroepiploic artery is confirmed, and the left gastric artery is divided (Fig. 38-6). The gastrohepatic ligament is divided by a combination of cautery and the stapler. Either a pyloromyotomy or pyloroplasty may be performed. If a pyloroplasty is performed, it should be a single layer with interrupted 3-0 silk sutures, carefully incorporating mucosa and muscular wall.

Attention is then turned to the neck, and a 6-cm incision is made from the sternal notch along the anterior border of the sternocleidomastoid muscle. The platysma is divided, and dissection proceeds between the carotid sheath laterally and the strap muscles medially. The omohyoid muscle may be divided. The knot of the Penrose drain should be palpable on the spine. The Penrose drain is grasped, and the esophagus is gently mobilized. The nasogastric tube is partially withdrawn, and the cervical esophagus is divided with a 75-mm linear stapler (Fig. 38-7). A #2 silk suture ligature is fastened to the distal end of the divided esophagus, and the specimen is drawn into the abdomen with the attached silk suture. The cervical end of the silk suture is fastened to a clamp.

A gastric tube is fashioned by resecting the gastroesophageal junction and the lesser curve of the stomach with a series of 75-mm-thick tissue staples (Fig. 38-8). A narrow gastric tube aids in gastric emptying. A diameter of less than 6 cm, however, can compromise venous and arterial blood supply. The line of division ends at a point on the lesser curve near the crow's-feet of veins. At this point along the lesser curve, the right gastric artery and associated tissue can be divided to maximize conduit length.

With the specimen removed, a final check for hemostasis is made in the bed of the stomach and spleen. Before the conduit is pulled into the neck, the esophageal hiatus should be dilated to four fingers. The gastric conduit may be pulled to the neck in relatively atraumatic fashion by the use of an endoscopic camera bag attached to a Foley catheter. The heavy silk

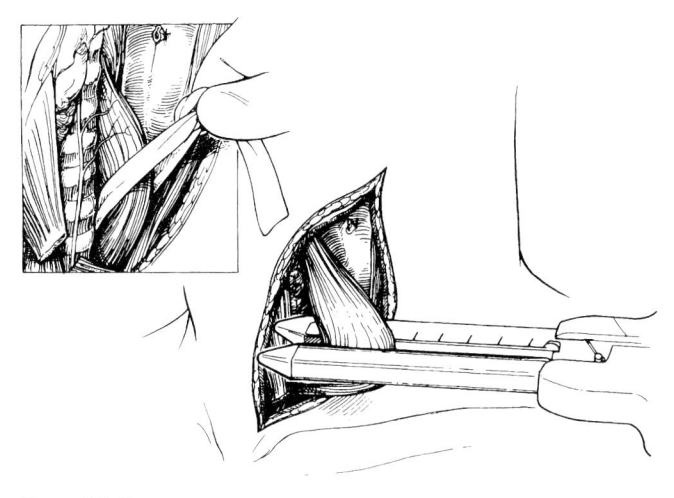

Figure 38–7
Retrieval of the Penrose drain placed around the esophagus inside the recurrent nerves during chest dissection. This aids in the prevention of recurrent nerve injury. The esophagus is divided after removal of the nasogastric tube. *(From Sugarbaker D, DeCamp M, Liptay M. Surgical procedures to resect and replace the esophagus. In: Zinner M, Schwartz S, Ellis H, et al, editors.* Maingot's abdominal operations. *Stanford, CT: Appleton & Lange; 1997. p. 885-910.)*

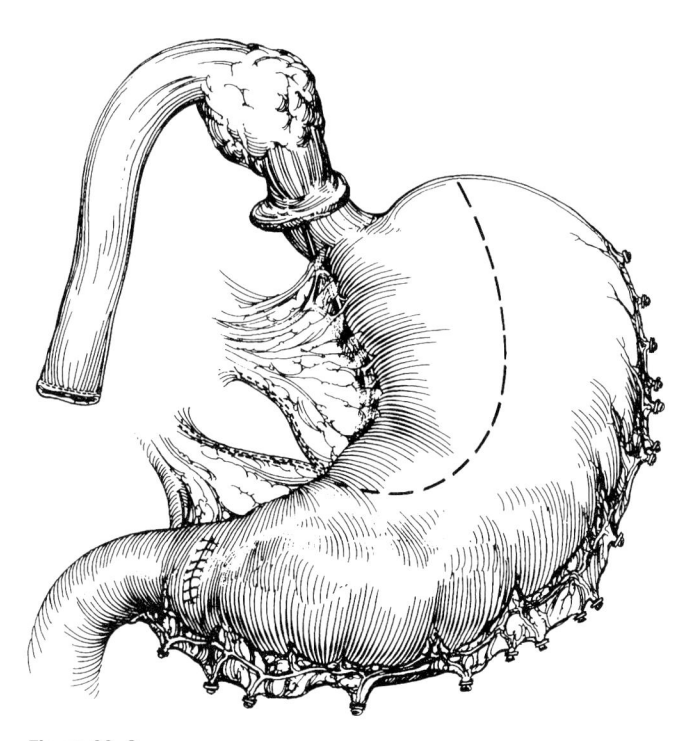

Figure 38–8
The gastric tube is created after complete dissection of the stomach and after the cervical esophagus is divided and brought into the abdomen. The gastric tube should be kept at least 5 cm in diameter. This also allows longer margins for gastroesophageal junction tumors. A pyloroplasty has been performed. *(From Swanson S, Grondin S, Sugarbaker D. Total esophagectomy: The Brigham and Women's Hospital approach.* Oper Tech Thorac Cardiovasc Surg *1999;4:197-209.)*

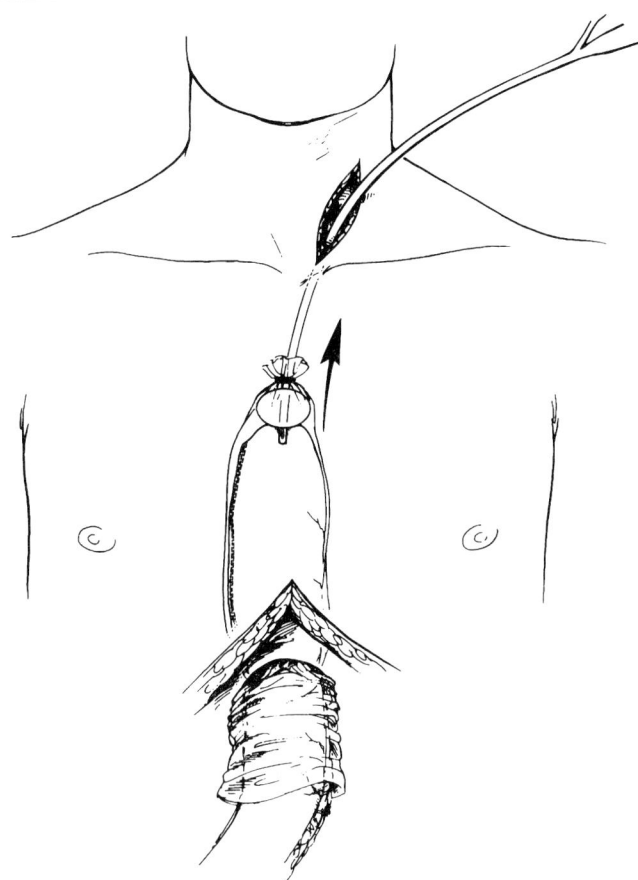

Figure 38–9
An endoscopic camera bag is used as an atraumatic means of drawing the conduit into the neck for anastomosis. Suction is applied to the Foley catheter as it is pulled into the neck. *(From Sugarbaker D, DeCamp M, Liptay M. Surgical procedures to resect and replace the esophagus. In: Zinner M, Schwartz S, Ellis H, et al, editors.* Maingot's abdominal operations. *Stanford, CT: Appleton & Lange; 1997. p. 885-910.)*

tie that traverses the mediastinum from the neck is tied to the valved end of a 30-cm^3 three-way Foley urinary catheter. The endoscopic bag is secured to the Foley balloon. The conduit is placed in the bag, and the valved end is drawn into the neck (Fig. 38-9). The assistant must guide the conduit through the hiatus and up the lower mediastinum, ensuring that there is no torsion. The bag is cut away from the conduit in the neck, and the conduit is grasped with a Babcock instrument. The pylorus should sit at the hiatus. A side-to-side, functional end-to-end stapled anastomosis may be performed. The anastomosis is created with a 75-mm linear stapler followed by a 30-mm endoscopic stapler. Alternatively, the neck anastomosis can be hand sewn with interrupted circumferential full-thickness 3-0 silk sutures (Fig. 38-10). The nasogastric tube is advanced across the anastomosis and positioned just proximal to the pylorus before closure of the remaining anastomotic defect (Fig. 38-11). A drain is placed along the spine posterior to the anastomosis, and the platysma is run closed with 2-0 Vicryl sutures. The skin is closed with staples. A feeding tube is inserted in the jejunum at a point 40 cm distal to the ligament of Treitz. The abdominal fascia is closed with a running #2 monofilament suture, and the skin is closed with staples.

Ivor Lewis Esophagectomy

Indications

The indications are similar to those for a tri-incisional approach.

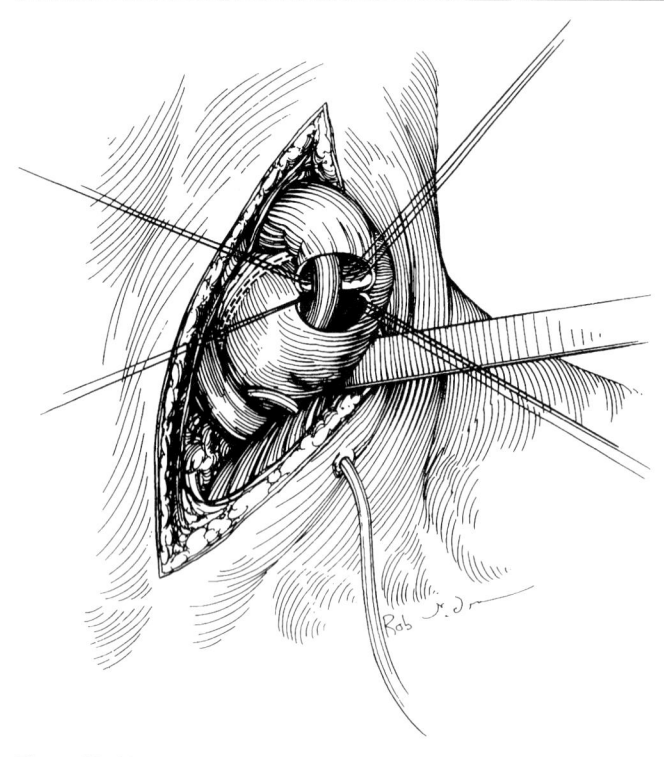

Figure 38-10
The cervical anastomosis may be hand sewn with interrupted silk sutures over a nasogastric tube. *(From Swanson S, Grondin S, Sugarbaker D. Total esophagectomy: The Brigham and Women's Hospital approach. Oper Tech Thorac Cardiovasc Surg 1999;4: 197-209.)*

Contraindications

Tumors located in the upper third of the thoracic esophagus, above the carina, are better approached with resection of the cervical esophagus and anastomosis in the neck to ensure adequate margins. Long-segment Barrett's esophagus with extension into the cervical esophagus is also a contraindication to an anastomosis in the right chest. A fused pleural space or severely compromised lung function should lead to reconsideration of a thoracotomy.

Technique

The patient is positioned supine. Preoperative bronchoscopy and esophagogastroduodenoscopy are performed. An upper midline incision is made extending from the umbilicus to the xiphoid. The abdominal portion of the operation is identical to that described for a tri-incisional esophagectomy, with complete mobilization of the stomach, kocherization of the duodenum, pyloroplasty, construction of the gastric tube, and placement of a J-tube. The conduit is advanced into the chest as far as possible before the abdomen is closed. After placement of a double-lumen endotracheal tube, the patient is repositioned in the left lateral decubitus position, and a standard right posterolateral thoracotomy is performed. Entry into the chest is through the fourth or fifth interspace. The azygos vein is divided and the intrathoracic esophagus is dissected, including all adjacent areolar and lymphatic tissue. A margin of at least 5 cm and ideally 10 cm is desirable, and thus the anastomosis is usually performed high in the right chest. The esophagus is dissected free to a point only several centimeters above the proposed line of transection to preserve blood supply to the anastomosis. The esophagus is divided and the stomach is pulled up, and the gastric conduit is fashioned with a GIA stapler. A variety of techniques may be used to perform the anastomosis, including single-layer hand sewn, double-layer hand sewn, end-to-end stapled, and side-to-side functional end-to-end stapled.

With all techniques, wrapping of the anastomosis with omentum and passage of the nasogastric tube before completion of the final portion of the anastomosis are advised. A stapled anastomosis may be performed in a side-to-side, functional end-to-end manner with creation of the anastomosis by a GIA 75-mm or sequential 30-mm endoscopic stapler and closure of the defect with a TA 30-mm or 60-mm stapler. A similar technique involves lining up the gastric conduit and esophagus in a linear fashion and stapling the back wall of the anastomosis with a linear stapler or endostapler and sewing the front wall by either a one- or two-layer technique. This type of approach is used in the neck as described by Orringer. The anastomosis can also be performed with an EEA stapler, although anastomoses created with EEA staplers smaller than 33 mm carry a significant risk of stricture.[12] With the EEA stapler, passage of the nasogastric tube is, of course, performed after completion of the anastomosis.

If a hand-sewn anastomosis is to be performed, the proximal esophagus is divided with a knife after clamping the esophagus proximally with a noncrushing bowel clamp. A single-layer anastomosis is performed with interrupted 3-0 silk stitches with full-thickness bites of the mucosa and muscularis and careful approximation of tissues. Knots on the posterior row may be tied inside the lumen (Fig. 38-12).[13] A double-layer anastomosis was described by Churchill and Sweet in 1942.[14,15] At a point at least 2 cm beyond the staple line, a 2-cm-diameter area of gastric serosa is scored. Underlying vessels are ligated with interrupted silk sutures. The posterior layer of the anastomosis is created with interrupted 3-0 silk stitches. An inner, full-thickness layer is performed with a fine 4-0 absorbable suture, either catgut or Monocryl, by a running Connell stitch to invert the mucosa. Before completion of the inner layer, the nasogastric tube is passed to the hiatus. An anterior outer layer is then performed with interrupted 3-0 silk. Omentum is used to wrap the anastomosis. The distal portion of the stomach is reduced into the abdomen to avoid excess redundancy of the stomach in the chest, which might impair conduit emptying. Stitches are placed anchoring the conduit to the diaphragmatic hiatus. Some use additional stitches anchoring the intrathoracic conduit to the pleura, although the effectiveness of these stitches is debated.

Transhiatal Esophagectomy

Indications

Some believe that transhiatal esophagectomy is ideally suited for benign esophageal disease and possibly Barrett's esophagus with high-grade dysplasia, for which complete lymphadenectomy may not be necessary. Other factors, such as poor pulmonary function (FEV_1 <800 mL or <35% predicted) and pleural symphysis, would favor a technique that avoids a thoracotomy.

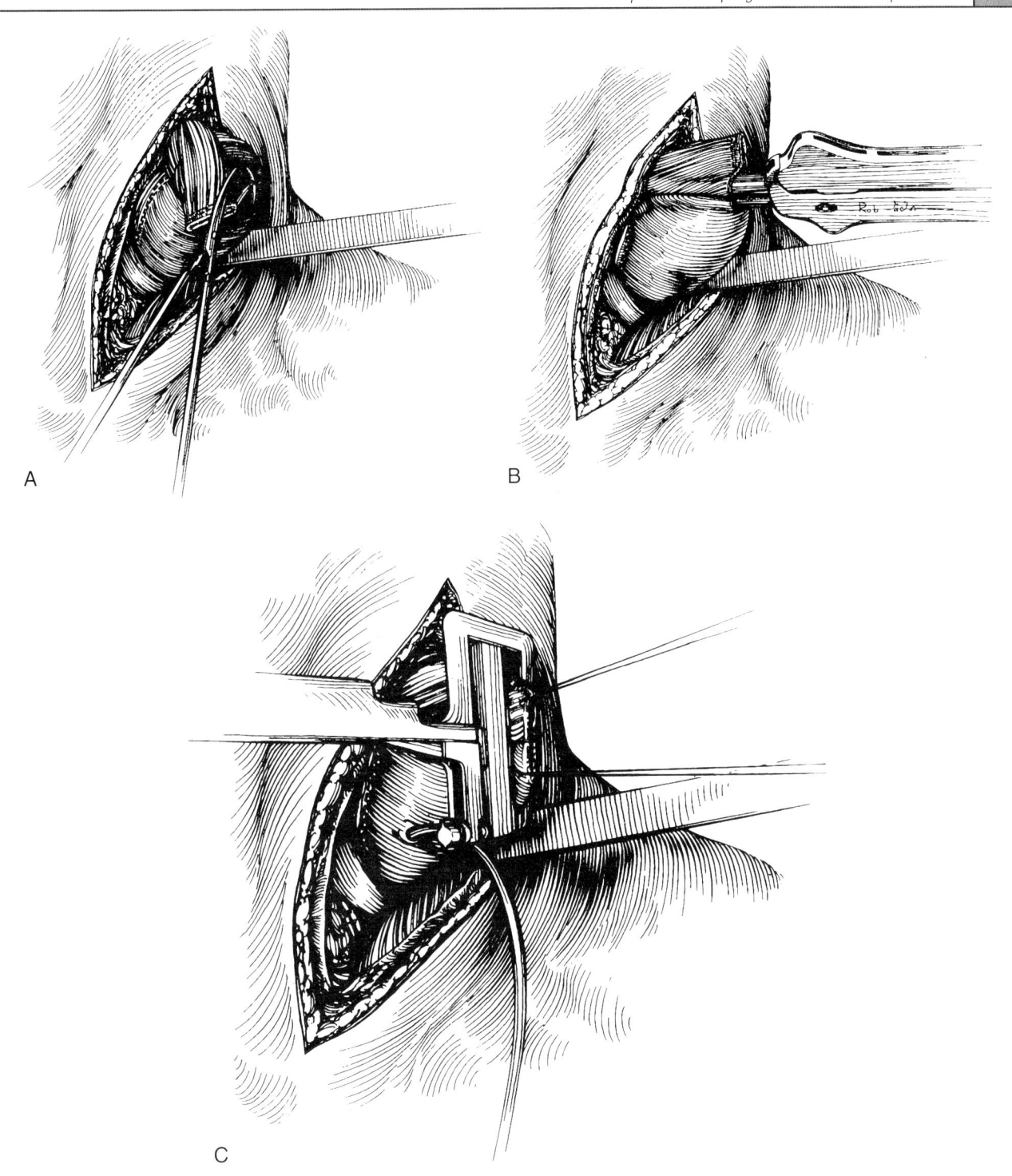

Figure 38–11

A, A corner of the proximal esophageal staple line is trimmed, and an enterotomy is made in the proximal gastric conduit away from the staple line. **B,** A GIA stapler is used to create the back wall of the cervical anastomosis. Additional length may be obtained with an additional fire of an endoscopic 30-mm stapler. **C,** The anterior wall of the anastomosis is closed with a TA stapler. In this illustration, a gastric drainage tube exits through the neck. These tubes can be used in place of a nasogastric tube and are more comfortable for the patient. *(From Swanson S, Grondin S, Sugarbaker D. Total esophagectomy: The Brigham and Women's Hospital approach.* Oper Tech Thorac Cardiovasc Surg 1999;4:197-209.)

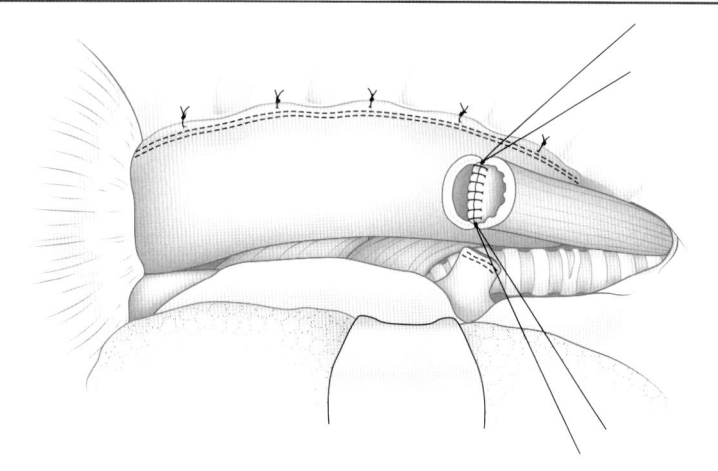

Figure 38–12
The Ivor Lewis anastomosis is performed at the level of the azygos vein, in two layers, after creation of a circular enterotomy in the proximal conduit. The edges of the conduit are shown here tacked to the pleura, although it is debatable whether this effectively reduces tension on the anastomosis. *(Modified from Sugarbaker D, DeCamp M, Liptay M. Surgical procedures to resect and replace the esophagus. In: Zinner M, Schwartz S, Ellis H, et al, editors.* Maingot's abdominal operations. *Stanford, CT: Appleton & Lange; 1997. p. 885-910.)*

Contraindications

Bulky tumors of the midthoracic esophagus are difficult to visualize from the transhiatal approach, and injury to adjacent structures may occur. Scarring after neoadjuvant treatment of esophageal tumors may also make the transhiatal approach difficult. The need to perform a complete lymphadenectomy is a contraindication to this approach.

The presence of severe coronary or valvular disease makes the episodic drops in blood pressure associated with blunt dissection behind the heart especially treacherous. A transthoracic approach may be preferable in these instances.

Preparation

The preparation is identical to preparation for a tri-incisional esophagectomy.

Technique

Bronchoscopy and esophagogastroduodenoscopy are performed as previously described. The abdominal portion of the procedure is performed as described in the previous section. An upper hand retractor aids in raising the xiphoid and sternum for visualization of the mediastinum. The esophagophrenic attachments are divided with cautery, the gastroesophageal junction is separated from the crura, and the distal esophagus is encircled with a Penrose drain. The hiatus is dilated to allow entry of the surgeon's hand. Various hand-held malleable retractors may be used in dissection of the mediastinum through the hiatus. With the use of the Penrose drain to retract the lower esophagus, the lower esophagus is dissected through the hiatus. Arterial branches supplying the lower esophagus from the aorta are clipped under direct vision. With the fingertips against the esophagus, the esophagus is dissected off the vertebral plane bluntly into the upper chest. The palmar aspect of the fingertips is kept directly against the esophagus. Arteries supplying the esophagus branch approximately 1 cm away from the esophagus, and dissection close to the esophagus disrupts only the smaller arterial branches directly entering the esophagus. Close dissection of the esophagus also avoids injury to adjacent structures. A cervical incision is made along the lower border of the left sternocleidomastoid muscle. Dissection proceeds as described in the previous section with the exception that the esophagus must be identified and encircled from the neck. An approach from the left side of the neck aids in avoiding injury to the right recurrent laryngeal nerve, which is farther from the esophagus than the left recurrent nerve at this level. Dissection is kept immediately on the esophagus to avoid recurrent nerve injury. Metal retractors should not be placed near the tracheoesophageal groove. A Penrose drain is placed around the cervical esophagus.

Dissection caudally is performed with two fingers against the esophagus in the posterior plane. Depending on the length of the surgeon's fingers and the width of the abdominal surgeon's hand, it should be possible for the two hands to contact directly. There always remains a thin plane of tissue that must be torn for the two hands to touch. Alternatively, a sponge stick can be advanced posteriorly from the neck to touch the dissecting hand from the abdomen (Fig. 38-13). Dissection then proceeds in a similar fashion on the anterior surface of the esophagus. Extreme care must be taken in the region of the trachea and especially the carina to avoid injury to the membranous trachea. (At this point in the operation, any difficulty in dissecting the esophagus from the trachea or any concern of adhesion to or invasion of the trachea should result in repositioning of the patient in the left lateral decubitus position, and a right thoracotomy should be performed for direct visualization and dissection.) The fingers from above and below should meet in the region of the carina (Fig. 38-14).

As much dissection as possible should be performed under direct vision from the neck and from the abdomen. Portions of the lateral dissection near the lower aspect of the trachea often cannot be visualized, and lateral dissection must be performed bluntly. The surgeon's right hand is advanced from the abdomen high up in the chest to the point where circumferential dissection has been completed from the neck. The first and second fingers surround the esophagus, and with a raking motion, the lateral attachments are avulsed as the hand

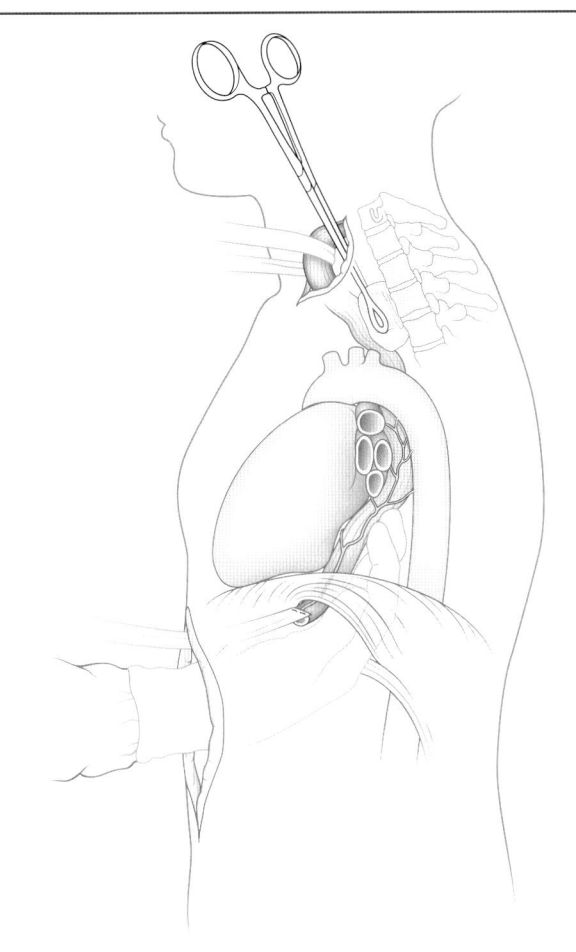

Figure 38-13
Posterior dissection is performed with the fingertips adjacent to the esophagus. Dissection from the cranial aspect may be performed with a sponge stick if the surgeon's upper hand cannot reach the lower hand. *(Modified from Orringer MB, Sloan H. Esophagectomy without thoracotomy.* J Thorac Cardiovasc Surg *1978;76:643-54.)*

is drawn back into the abdomen. Care must be taken near the region of the azygos vein (Fig. 38-15). After complete mobilization of the esophagus, it is divided in the neck, and the specimen is brought out into the abdomen. The mediastinum is packed for hemostasis. Before the gastric tube is drawn up into the neck, the mediastinal packing is removed and both pleural spaces are inspected for integrity. Entry into the pleural space is managed by chest tube placement before removal of the drapes.

Trials Comparing Transhiatal with Transthoracic Resection

Numerous nonrandomized, retrospective trials have been performed in an attempt to define differences in either perioperative complication rate or long-term survival between the transhiatal and transthoracic approaches (Table 38-1).[16-18] Most of these were limited by small study size and selection bias. A large meta-analysis review was performed by Rindani and coworkers[19] in 1999. Forty-four trials published in the English literature between 1986 and 1996 consisting of 5483 patients undergoing either Ivor Lewis or transhiatal esophagectomy were reviewed. The overall incidence of pneumonia was 25%, and it was not appreciably different between the two techniques. The incidence of bleeding and cardiac complications was also not different. The most significant differences were seen in the anastomotic leak rate (16% transhiatal versus 10% Ivor Lewis), stricture (28% transhiatal versus 16% Ivor Lewis), and recurrent nerve injury (11% transhiatal versus 5% Ivor Lewis). Perioperative mortality was higher in the Ivor Lewis population (9.5%) than in the transhiatal population (6.3%). Overall long-term (5-year) survival was similar in the two groups, 25%. Hulscher and colleagues[20] also performed a meta-analysis of trials between 1990 and 1999 published in English language journals. Fifty publications were identified, some randomized, some comparing transthoracic with transhiatal approaches, and some evaluating only one technique. Overall, cardiac complications (20% versus 7%), anastomotic leakage (14% versus 7%), and vocal cord paralysis (10% versus 4%) were higher in the transhiatal versus the transthoracic groups. Pulmonary complications (19% versus 13%), in-hospital mortality (9% versus 6%), and operative time (5.6 versus 4.0 hours) were higher in the transthoracic versus the transhiatal group. Overall 5-year survival was similar among all the studies and patients evaluated (23% for transthoracic resections and 21.7% for transhiatal resections). These reviews are of historical and factual interest only, and little can be concluded about the relative merits of each technique in matched populations.

Orringer and colleagues[21] reviewed their 30-year experience with transhiatal esophagectomies in 2007 patients. The patients were divided into two groups: group I, those operated on between 1976 and 1998; and group II, those operated on from 1998 to 2006. Postoperative mediastinal bleeding requiring reoperation occurred in less than 1%. The incidence of recurrent laryngeal nerve injury was significantly lower in group II (2%) compared with group I (7%; $P < .0001$). They believed that this decrease in injury was secondary to an increase in operative volume. Chylothorax was seen in 1%. The incidence of respiratory complications that required a hospital stay beyond 10 days was 2%. They also reported that the routine use of side-to-side stapled cervical esophagogastric anastomosis after 1997 has led to a notable decrease in leak rate and need for postoperative dilation. The overall hospital mortality was 3%. The hospital mortality fell with increased volume (group I, 4%; group II, 1%). It is clear that the high volume at this center has produced impressive results with regard to transhiatal esophagectomy.

Wolff and associates[22] retrospectively reviewed all esophagectomies at the Mayo Clinic between 1994 and 2004. Of the 517 esophagectomies performed, the type of surgery was as follows: transhiatal (68), Ivor Lewis (392), and extended Ivor Lewis (57). The mean lymph nodes retrieved for the Ivor Lewis and extended Ivor Lewis were 18.7 and 17.4, respectively. This was not statistically different. The transhiatal patients had a mean of 8.99 lymph nodes in the specimen. They found that the combined Ivor Lewis group and the transhiatal group were significantly different, showing on average 9.5 lymph nodes in the surgical specimen ($P < .001$). The importance of the number of lymph nodes harvested at the time of surgery is discussed in a later section.

Orringer and associates[23] reviewed outcomes after transhiatal and transthoracic surgery using the Surveillance, Epidemiology, and End Results (SEER) cancer registry. They identified patients between 1992 and 2002 undergoing esophagectomy.

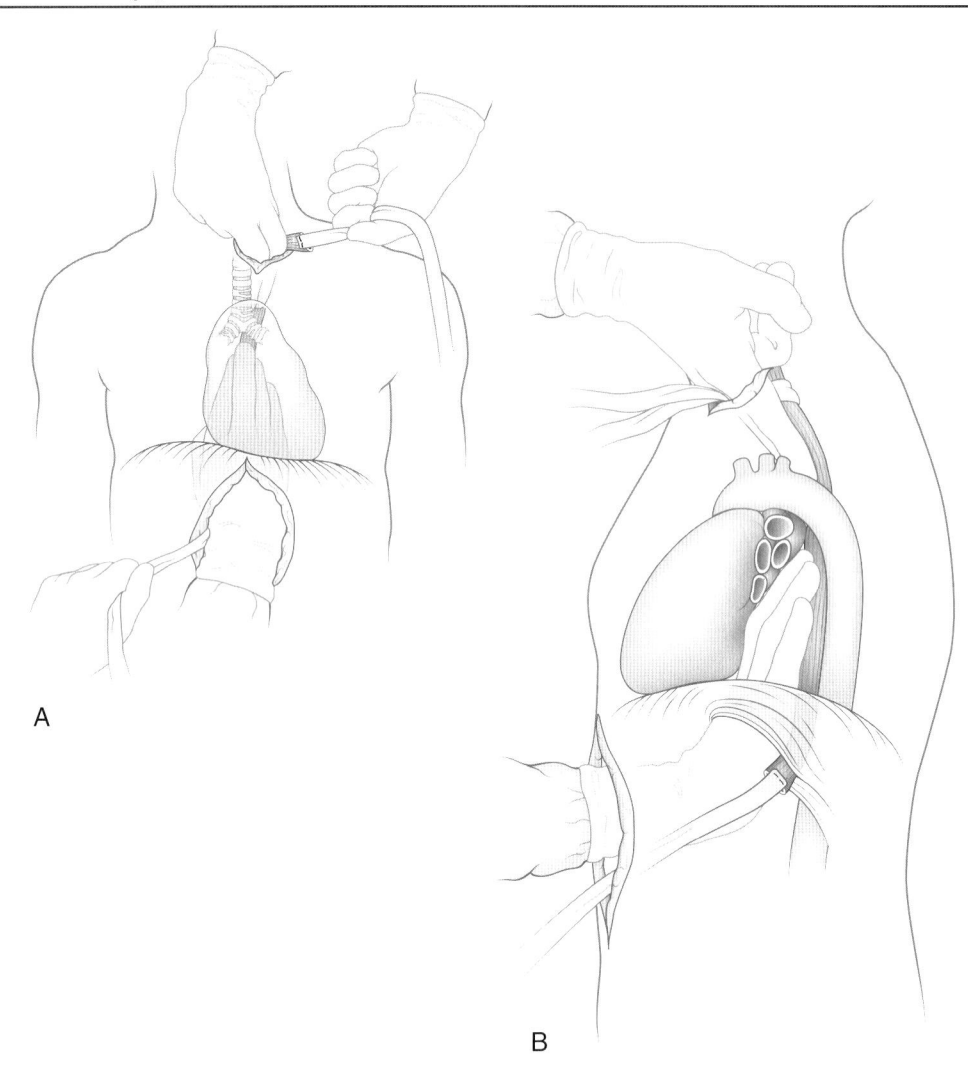

Figure 38–14
Blunt dissection of the esophagus off of the trachea is performed with the fingertips immediately against the esophagus. The fingertips are united. The fingertips from above should be able to reach near the carina, as they do during cervical mediastinoscopy. *(Modified from Orringer MB. Transhiatal esophagectomy without thoracotomy. In: Cohn LH, editor. Modern techniques in surgery. New York: Futura Publishing; 1983.)*

Of the 868 patients studied, 643 had a transthoracic approach and 225 underwent a transhiatal esophagectomy. They concluded that patients undergoing a transhiatal esophagectomy had a lower operative mortality rate than did those undergoing transthoracic operations (6.7% versus 13.1%; $P = .009$). The need for anastomotic dilation was higher in the transhiatal group (43.1%) compared with the transthoracic patients (34.5%; $P = .02$). The 5-year survival was significantly higher in the transhiatal group; however, this benefit over the transthoracic group was diminished after adjustments were made for patient and hospital or provider characteristics, such as volume performed at the center and involvement of trainees.

Three randomized, prospective trials comparing transhiatal resection with transthoracic resection demonstrated that either technique may be performed safely in skilled hands, and no clear differences have been shown between the two techniques. This is in large part due to an inadequate number of patients enrolled in the trials. Extrapolating from their retrospective meta-analysis, Rindani and colleagues[19] estimated that 2360 patients would have to be randomized for a significant difference to be shown in perioperative mortality, and 6400 patients would be needed for a difference to be shown in long-term survival. Clearly, this is beyond the capacity of any prospective esophagectomy trial.

The first randomized, prospective trial was published in 1993 by Goldminc and coworkers.[24] They randomized 67 patients younger than 70 years with squamous cell cancer of the esophagus to Ivor Lewis esophagectomy or transhiatal esophagectomy. Operative time was longer (6 versus 4 hours) in the transthoracic group. There was no difference in incidence of pneumonia (20%), anastomotic leak, recurrent nerve injury, bleeding, perioperative mortality, or length of hospitalization. At a mean follow-up of 3 years, survival was not statistically different between the two groups. For those patients with nodal disease, however, none of the transhiatal patients was alive at 18 months, whereas 30% of the transthoracic patients were alive at 18 months.

Wong and colleagues reported a prospective, randomized series of 39 patients with lower third esophageal cancers treated with either an Ivor Lewis resection or a transhiatal

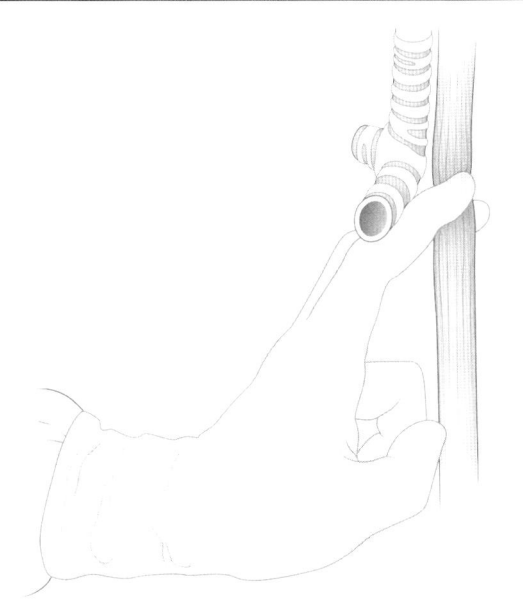

Figure 38–15
After dissection of the anterior and posterior planes, the lateral stalks can be torn between the first and second fingers in a "raking" motion. *(Modified from Orringer MB. Transhiatal esophagectomy without thoracotomy. In: Cohn LH, editor.* Modern techniques in surgery. *New York: Futura Publishing; 1983.)*

Table 38–1

Comparison of Transthoracic and Transhiatal Approaches to Esophagectomy: Perioperative Complications

Complication	Transthoracic	Transhiatal
Blood loss (mL)	1001	728
Operative time (hours)	5.6	4.0
Cardiac complications (%)	6.6	19.5
Pulmonary complications (%)	18.7	12.7
Anastomotic leak (%)	7.2	13.6
Vocal cord paralysis (%)	3.5	9.5
Chyle leak (%)	2.4	1.4
In-hospital mortality (%)	9.2	5.7

Modified from Hulscher J, Tijssen J, Lanschot J. Transthoracic versus transhiatal resection for carcinoma of the esophagus: a meta-analysis. Cumulative review of all English literature publications (searched via MEDLINE) between 1990 and 1999 comparing transhiatal with transthoracic esophageal resection.

resection.[25] Patients undergoing neoadjuvant therapy or those with an FEV_1 below 70% were excluded from the study. There were no perioperative (30-day) deaths in either group, although the in-hospital mortality was 15% for the transhiatal group and 0% for the transthoracic group (not significantly different). Intraoperative hypotension occurred in 60% of transhiatal patients but in only 5% of transthoracic patients. There was no difference in blood loss, pneumonia, or recurrent nerve injury. Operating time was longer for the transthoracic group. The mean proximal margin was 3 cm longer in the transhiatal group. No significant difference was seen in tumor recurrence or survival. This group recently published their 5-year results from this study.[26] After a complete 5-year follow-up, they concluded that overall survival was not significantly different between the two groups. They did report a trend toward improved survival in the extended transthoracic group over the transhiatal group in the patients with a type I esophageal cancer.

More recently, a randomized study was completed in the Netherlands comparing transhiatal resection with extended transthoracic en bloc resection for distal adenocarcinomas of the esophagus or cardia[27]; 106 patients had a transhiatal resection, and 114 patients had a transthoracic resection. The median follow-up was 4.7 years. In-hospital mortality was 2% to 4% in each group. Respiratory complications including atelectasis and pneumonia were higher in the transthoracic group (57% versus 27%), as was the incidence of chyle leak (10% versus 2%). The high incidence of respiratory complications in the transthoracic group (57%) should be questioned, as it is much higher than that quoted in many prior transthoracic resection series.[19] Although statistical significance was not reached, there was a trend toward improved survival at 5 years in the transthoracic group (39% versus 29%).

Minimally Invasive Esophagectomy

Cuschieri is credited with first applying minimally invasive techniques to an esophagectomy. Since his initial description of subtotal endoscopic esophagectomy using thoracoscopic techniques for mobilization of the esophagus, there have been numerous descriptions with varying degrees of endoscopic involvement. The three most widely performed open procedures for esophageal resection—tri-incisional, Ivor Lewis, and transhiatal esophagectomy—have endoscopic counterparts. These are discussed.

Minimally Invasive Tri-incisional Esophagectomy

Minimally invasive techniques can be used to perform a modified McKeown esophagectomy. All or part of the procedure may be replaced with thoracoscopic or laparoscopic dissection.

Indications

There are no finite indications for minimally invasive esophagectomy. There are relative indications advocated by those who specialize in this surgery. These reported benefits of minimally invasive esophagectomy are discussed in a later section.

Contraindications

Fusion of the right pleural space or inability to maintain isolated lung ventilation is a contraindication to the approach. Unlike its open counterpart, video-assisted thoracoscopic esophagectomy requires nearly perfect lung isolation to allow adequate room to thoracoscopically maneuver within the thoracic cavity. On occasion, continuous positive airway pressure to the right lung will aid in achieving adequate ventilation and oxygenation with minimal effect on exposure. Relative contraindications with respect to minimally invasive surgery are the same as those in the open sections. As with any endoscopically assisted surgery, the surgeon's comfort is a strong determining factor in use of this technology. Those not trained in minimally invasive surgery should consider performing this highly technical surgery with a surgeon who is facile with this procedure.

Technique

Video-Assisted Thoracoscopic Mobilization of the Thoracic Esophagus

Video-assisted thoracoscopic esophageal mobilization utilizes four thoracoscopic incisions. After the patient is prepared and draped in the left lateral decubitus position, a 1-cm incision is made in the eighth intercostal space at the posterior axillary line. Ideally, the camera needs to be as posterior as possible for optimal visualization. However, this port will be used for the chest tube, and any position farther posterior will result in an ineffective chest tube because the patient will be lying on it.

With the thoracoscope, the right hemithorax is examined for pleural disease that may prohibit further surgery. Three access incisions are placed next, with two of the ports in line with the tip of the scapula, at the level of the sixth and ninth intercostal spaces. The final access incision will be in the fourth intercostal space in line with the camera. This is used mainly for lung retraction and suctioning of the operative field.

The majority of authors use a port only for the camera. Standard open instruments, such as a ring forceps, are passed through the other incisions without a port. Some surgeons prefer laparoscopic instruments, so they use 5-mm and 10-mm ports to allow easy passage of these surgical tools.

Some surgeons place a stitch in the central tendon of the diaphragm and bring it out through a separate intercostal space to retract the diaphragm. The authors place an endoscopic Kittner (Ethicon, Somerville, NJ) alongside the camera to provide gentle caudal retraction on the diaphragm.

Through the posterior ports, the surgeon uses an ultrasonic scalpel, the harmonic scalpel (Ethicon, Somerville NJ), to divide the inferior pulmonary ligament. The posterior mediastinal pleura is opened, and the lymph nodes are swept off the pericardium toward the esophagus. This dissection is carried to the azygos vein. The pleura above the azygos vein is opened close to the esophagus. An endovascular stapler is used to ligate the azygos vein. Once this is achieved, the pleura on the posterior aspect of the esophagus is opened at an area away from the tumor and carina. Once circumferentially around the esophagus, a Penrose drain is placed. The Penrose drain is stapled together with an endovascular stapling device. This Penrose drain can be used as a handle to hold the esophagus during dissection. The vagus is divided just above the azygos vein to prevent traction injury to the recurrent laryngeal nerve. The thoracic esophagus is circumferentially dissected for its entire length. The diaphragmatic hiatus is not opened in the chest to allow adequate pneumoperitoneum during the laparoscopic portion. After adequate mobilization, the Penrose drain is placed into the apex of the thoracic cavity to allow retrieval from the neck. A complete thoracic lymphadenectomy is an important aspect of this component of the operation and should be performed routinely. The chest tube is placed, and all thoracic incisions are closed. The patient is turned supine, and the double-lumen endotracheal tube is changed to a single-lumen tube. The patient is prepared and draped for laparoscopic surgery.

Laparoscopic Mobilization of the Gastric Conduit, Pyloroplasty, and Formation of a Jejunostomy Tube

Four 5-mm ports and one 10-mm port are placed as they would be in preparation for a laparoscopic Nissen fundoplication. The liver retractor is used to retract the left lobe of the liver so the underlying esophageal hiatus is visualized. The assistant standing to the patient's left will maintain the camera and provide countertraction for the surgeon. The harmonic scalpel is used to open the gastrocolic ligament. Great care is taken to maintain a 2-cm distance from the gastroepiploic arcade. The short gastric arteries can be divided with the harmonic scalpel. The gastric hepatic ligament is opened to allow access to the right crus of the diaphragm. The lymph nodes along the celiac and left gastric are swept toward the stomach. The left gastric artery is ligated. A gastric tube is created by dividing the stomach starting at the distal lesser curve with use of a 3.5- or 4.8-mm endovascular stapler. The conduit is formed with several firings of the endovascular stapler until this area on the lesser curve is connected with the cardia-fundus of the greater curvature. Once achieved, the proximal gastric tube is attached to the gastric remnant with several Endo Stitch sutures (U.S. Surgical Corp., Norwalk, CT).

A pyloroplasty is done by use of the harmonic scalpel to open the pylorus in a longitudinal fashion and placement of interrupted Endo Stitch sutures to close the opening in a transverse manner.[28]

Before a neck dissection is performed, a jejunostomy is created. The ligament of Treitz is identified by elevating the transverse colon. A place on the jejunum, approximately 40 cm from the ligament of Treitz, is attached to the anterior abdominal wall with the Endo Stitch. A needle catheter kit (Compat Biosystems, Minneapolis, MN) is placed percutaneously into the jejunal loop. The Seldinger technique is used to guide a catheter into the jejunum. The placement is visually confirmed by injecting air into the catheter and watching for jejunal distention.

Finally, a neck incision and dissection are performed as described earlier. The esophagus is pulled out of the neck while an assistant laparoscopically guides the conduit through the hiatus, ensuring proper alignment. The specimen is sent for pathologic examination, and the anastomosis is performed as previously described.

Of interest, Fabian and coworkers[29] published a report of 21 patients who had a thoracoscopic mobilization of the esophagus in the prone position. The authors thought the prone position for thoracoscopic esophageal mobilization to be equivalent to lateral decubitus position with respect to blood loss, number of lymph nodes dissected, and complications. The operative time, however, was significantly reduced in the group of prone patients.

Minimally Invasive Ivor Lewis Esophagectomy

Indications, contraindications, and preparation for this procedure are identical to those for open surgery. After esophagogastroduodenoscopy and bronchoscopy, the patient is prepared and draped in the supine position. The laparoscopic portion of this surgery, including jejunostomy tube formation and pyloroplasty, is almost identical to that for minimally invasive tri-incisional surgery.

After gastric conduit formation and completion of the laparoscopic surgery, a double-lumen endotracheal tube is placed. The patient is prepared and draped in the lateral decubitus position. The thoracoscopic incisions are identical to those described in the minimally invasive tri-incisional section with one exception. The posterior eighth intercostal access incision is 3 to 4 cm to allow placement of a laparoscopic wound protector.[30] A combination of the wound protector and lubrication allows easy introduction of the EEA stapler through this port. The esophagus is mobilized to a few centimeters above the azygos vein. The gastroesophageal junction and conduit are then delivered through the hiatus. The proximal esophagus is divided above the azygos vein, and the specimen is brought out the protected port. The anvil of the EEA stapler is secured in the proximal esophagus with an Endo Stitch. The EEA stapler is then maneuvered into the proximal gastric conduit. An end-to-side (esophagus to stomach) circular anastomosis is formed. A linear stapler is used to close the gastric conduit. Chest tubes and standard closure are performed.

Minimally Invasive Transhiatal Esophagectomy

Laparoscopic transhiatal surgery has been described by various centers.[31-33] The procedure has the same preparation and positioning as a transhiatal esophagectomy. Laparoscopic instruments are used for mediastinal dissection, thus avoiding the blind, blunt dissection done in open transhiatal surgery. The esophagogastric anastomosis is made in the left neck. Limited visualization of the middle and upper third of the mediastinum and incomplete mediastinal lymphadenectomy are the main criticisms of this surgery. A mediastinoscope placed in the superior mediastinum has been employed to help address this concern.[34]

Results of Minimally Invasive Esophagectomy

Regardless of surgical approach and the use of minimally invasive techniques, esophageal surgery for malignant disease must adhere to certain principles. The procedure must ensure safe and complete resection of the tumor with adequate margins and provide restoration of gastrointestinal continuity. The literature contains numerous descriptions and outcome data of minimally invasive esophagectomy. However, the publications at present are almost entirely composed of case series.

Luketich and associates[35] at the University of Pittsburgh Medical Center published their results of 222 consecutive minimally invasive esophagectomies performed between 1996 and 2002. The median age was 66.5 years. The indications for surgery were carcinoma (78%) and high-grade dysplasia (21.2%). Of the patients with invasive esophageal cancer, 31 were assigned to stage I, 71 to stage II, and 81 to stage III. Neoadjuvant chemotherapy was given to 78 patients (35.1%) and radiation therapy to 36 patients (16.2%). Fifty-five patients had previous abdominal surgery. A pyloromyotomy was performed in 28 patients and a pyloroplasty in 136 patients. The authors abandoned the pyloroplasty mid series when they made a narrower gastric conduit (4 cm). The leak rate increased, and the pyloroplasty was reinstituted as part of a minimally invasive esophagectomy. A laparoscopic jejunostomy tube was placed in 202 patients. The authors completed a minimally invasive esophagectomy in 206 patients (92.8%). Twelve patients required a thoracotomy, and four patients needed a laparotomy to complete the esophagectomy. Patients were given oral intake by postoperative day 4. Median intensive care stay was 1 day (range, 1 to 30 days), with an average hospital stay of 7 days (range, 3 to 75 days). The mean follow-up was 19 months (range, 1 to 68 months). Dysphagia scores were assigned during follow-up. The mean Health-Related Quality of Life score was 4.6, which represented a normal score. Significant reflux (score of >15) was reported by 4% of the patients. The 30-day operative mortality was 1.4% (three patients). The first death was related to development of pneumonia. The second and third deaths were secondary to a myocardial infarct and pericardial tamponade, respectively. The minor and major complications were 23.9% and 32%, respectively. The most common complications in this series were atrial fibrillation (11.7%) and pleural effusions requiring a chest tube (6.3%). Interestingly, patients with 6-cm conduits had an anastomotic leak rate of 6.1%, and patients with a smaller conduit had a significantly increased leak rate (27.6%; $P < .001$). The authors compared their results with those published in a prospective U.S. Department of Veterans Affairs (VA) database of 1777 patients undergoing esophagectomy.[36] Luketich and associates considered that their 1.3% mortality rate compared well with the results of the VA study, which reported a 10% perioperative mortality rate. The incidence of complications in the VA database was reported at 50%, with the most frequent complications being pneumonia (21%), respiratory failure (16%), and prolonged ventilatory support (22%). Of the 222 studied cases of minimally invasive esophagectomy, pneumonia was reported in 7.6% and acute respiratory distress syndrome in 5%. It was thought that this suggested an advantage for minimally invasive esophagectomy.

This large series also compared its results with the single-institution report by Swanson and coworkers.[13] In their series of 250 patients undergoing a modified McKeown esophagectomy, the reported 3-year survivals for their patients assigned to stages I, IIa, IIb, and III were 65%, 41%, 45%, and 17%. Luketich and associates noted similar survival rates. The higher percentage of induction therapy might be the reason for increased mortality (3.9%) and length of stay (13 days) in the open series compared with that reported by the minimally invasive esophagectomy group.

Berrisford and colleagues[11] found that the operating time for a total minimally invasive esophagectomy decreased significantly ($P < .001$) as experience with the procedure increased.

One study evaluated minimally invasive esophagectomy in 41 elderly patients (range, 75 to 89 years).[37] In this cohort of patients, the mean intensive care unit time was 1 day, and the median hospital stay was 7 days. Major morbidity was reported as 19%, and there was no perioperative mortality.

There are a handful of case-controlled studies. Nguyen and colleagues[38] reported on a direct comparison of open and minimally invasive esophagectomy. There was a trend toward shorter operating times, less blood loss, and lower intensive care and hospital stays for this group. However, it has been noted that the minimally invasive group had less advanced stage cancers and the technique was performed by one surgeon, whereas the open cases were performed by one of four surgeons. Law and coworkers[39] compared 22 patients who underwent thoracoscopic esophageal mobilization with

63 open esophagectomy patients. Blood loss was significantly lower in the thoracoscopic group; however, there was no significant difference in morbidity or mortality. Laparoscopically assisted transhiatal surgery in 17 patients was compared with open transhiatal esophagectomy in 14 patients.[40] This published series also reported shorter operative times and decreased blood loss in the minimally invasive group. In a series of 166 patients, 47 minimally invasive esophagectomy patients were compared with 60 open transthoracic patients and 59 open transhiatal patients.[5] A lower mortality and reduced morbidity were noted in the minimally invasive esophagectomy group.

The largest series to date comparing minimally invasive surgery with open surgery is that published by Smithers and associates.[41] This group compared open (114) with thoracoscopically assisted (309) and total minimally invasive (23) esophagectomy. Decreased blood loss in the thoracoscopically assisted (400 mL) and minimally invasive (300 mL) esophagectomy was noted compared with the open (600 mL). Open surgery had shorter operative times (300 minutes) compared with total minimally invasive esophagectomy (330 minutes) but longer times compared with thoracoscopically assisted surgery (285 minutes). Minimally invasive esophagectomy patients had the shortest reported hospital stay (11 days), followed by thoracoscopically assisted patients (13 days) and the open patients (14 days). Stage for stage, there was no difference in overall median or 3-year survival among the three groups.

Finally, Gemmill and McCulloch[42] performed a systematic review of minimally invasive surgery for gastric and esophageal surgery spanning 1997 to 2007. Of the 46 articles that met criteria, 23 pertained to esophageal surgery. Most studies reviewed from that period were case series. There were no randomized, controlled studies of minimally invasive esophagectomy published during that time. There were 1398 patients in the combined papers. A completely endoscopic surgery was performed in 405 patients; 103 patients had laparoscopic mobilization and a thoracotomy; 561 patients had the reverse, thoracoscopic mobilization and laparotomy. The 30-day in-hospital mortality was 2.3%, and the morbidity was 46.2%. The anastomotic leak was 7.7%. Respiratory complications at a rate of 13.2% were reported in 1268 patients. Mean operating room time reported for 981 patients was 281 minutes. One group noted that the operating time for a total minimally invasive esophagectomy decreased significantly ($P < .001$) as experience with the procedure increased.[11] Hospital stay was 2 to 195 days, with a mean of 11 days. The average number of lymph nodes retrieved in 607 patients was 17.6. Interestingly, length of stay and overall morbidity rates were not different from their open counterparts. Clearly, these results have several inherent weaknesses. A randomized, controlled trial in this field would be helpful in understanding any benefit that minimally invasive surgery may have over an open esophagectomy. Long-term follow-up of these patients also needs to be reported to assess whether smaller-access surgery provides equal oncologic outcomes.

Left Thoracoabdominal Approach

Indications

The indications for a left thoracoabdominal approach are limited. A distal esophageal tumor beyond 30 to 35 cm in a patient with compromised physiologic status may be a suitable candidate, although some would argue that a transhiatal approach is preferable.

Contraindications

The presence of tumor at or above 30 cm makes an approach from the left chest much more difficult, as the anastomosis must be placed above the aortic arch or in the neck. A distal esophageal peptic stricture is considered by many to be a contraindication to limited distal esophagectomy as gastroesophageal reflux is often a severe problem after distal esophagectomy and placement of the anastomosis low in the chest.

Technique

The left thoracoabdominal approach can be performed in a variety of ways. Isolation with a double-lumen tube is necessary in all of the approaches. In the supine position, an upper midline laparotomy can be extended across the costal margin into the left chest through the seventh interspace and the diaphragm taken down in circumferential fashion. This position is least versatile and is generally used only when extension into the chest is unanticipated, as with proximal extension of certain tumors of the gastric cardia. Conversely, the patient may be placed in the full lateral position, and a complete esophagectomy may be performed through a thoracic incision. Abdominal dissection can be performed, although with some difficulty, through an enlarged hiatus or through a circumferential peripheral incision in the diaphragm (Fig. 38-16).

The most versatile thoracoabdominal approach involves placement of the patient in the right lateral decubitus position with the abdomen rolled back 45 degrees. The abdomen is readily accessible for extension of the distal aspect of the thoracotomy across the costal margin and across the rectus muscle. The neck is prepared in the field if extension to the cervical esophagus is a possibility. An incision is made from a point behind the tip of the scapula along the seventh interspace across the costal margin to the middle of the abdomen. The inferior pulmonary ligament is divided by cautery. The esophagus is encircled with a Penrose drain at a point away from the tumor where there is minimal scarring. Complete dissection of the esophagus and all surrounding lymphatic and connective tissue is performed up, including all tissue in between the aorta and the pericardium in the specimen. Dissection proceeds cranially posterior to the left pulmonary veins. Cranial dissection should be performed only to a point approximately 3 cm above the proposed line of transection to preserve blood supply to the anastomosis.

At the diaphragmatic hiatus, a 2-cm rim of diaphragm is included with the specimen. Although it is at times possible to continue dissection of the short gastric vessels and gastrohepatic ligament through the hiatus, exposure is improved by taking the diaphragm down circumferentially at a point 2 to 3 cm away from its insertion on the chest wall. Dissection proceeds from the gastroesophageal junction along the greater curvature, dividing all short gastric vessels. Dissection of the remainder of the gastric conduit is performed as detailed in the section on tri-incisional esophagectomy. Complete dissection of the stomach may not be required if

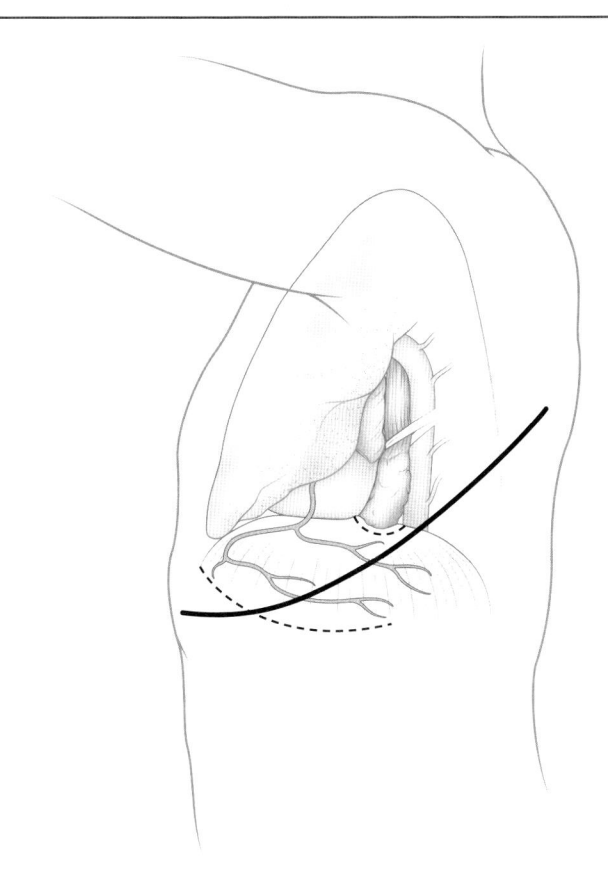

Figure 38-16
The left thoracoabdominal approach. The abdomen can be entered through incisions in the diaphragm as delineated by the *dotted lines*. Alternatively, the incision can be taken across the costal margin onto the abdomen and the diaphragm taken down circumferentially from the costal margin incision. *(Modified from Sugarbaker D, DeCamp M, Liptay M. Surgical procedures to resect and replace the esophagus. In: Zinner M, Schwartz S, Ellis H, et al, editors.* Maingot's abdominal operations. *Stanford, CT: Appleton & Lange; 1997. p. 885-910.)*

only a very limited portion of distal esophagus is resected. Minimizing dissection at the expense of an entirely tension-free anastomosis, however, is unwise. Kocherization of the duodenum and either pyloroplasty or pyloromyotomy are performed. The conduit is lifted into the chest. The anastomosis can be hand sewn in either a single layer or double layer. It may also be performed with a large (33-mm) EEA stapler or as a side-to-side, functional end-to-end anastomosis. A nasogastric tube is positioned before completion of the anastomosis. The conduit should be tacked to the diaphragm and may also be tacked to the adjacent pleura. Buttressing of the anastomosis with available omentum is recommended. The diaphragmatic rim is reattached to the chest wall with interrupted horizontal mattress 0 silk stitches. The costal margin is reattached with a single figure-of-eight wire or heavy Prolene stitch. The abdominal fascia is closed in layers. Before closure of the thoracotomy, a soft drain may be inserted dependently near the anastomosis, and an apical chest tube should be placed, each through separate stab incisions. The thoracotomy incision is closed with #2 Vicryl paracostal sutures, a 0 Vicryl latissimus layer, a 2-0 subdermal layer, and a 3-0 subcuticular stitch.

En Bloc Resection

The long-term survival rate after esophagectomy for esophageal cancer remains approximately 20% despite recent advances in surgical technique, instrumentation, and perioperative care. A large percentage of esophageal cancers manifest with invasion through the esophageal wall (T3) or nodal involvement (N1 or N2). Because radial margins are difficult to assess grossly and even microscopically, it is difficult to ensure complete removal of all invasive and nodal disease. To ensure complete margins and removal of all adjacent nodal tissue, several surgeons have advocated en bloc resection of the esophagus, including all adjacent tissues in the resected specimen. DeMeester and Skinner recommend en bloc esophagectomy for all patients in whom the cardiopulmonary morbidity is not prohibitive.[43,44] In one of these studies, an FEV_1 of less than 1.5 L was considered prohibitive. In their nonrandomized series, long-term survival was significantly better in the en bloc resection group versus the conventional approach.

Technique

Although an en bloc resection may be performed through either the left or right side of the chest, only very distal esophageal tumors may be resected with ease and with adequate margins through a left thoracotomy. Because of the high incidence of postoperative reflux esophagitis, an approach through a right thoracotomy is advised. Entry into the chest is through the right sixth interspace. Two parallel incisions are made in the pleura. An incision is made anteriorly, entering the pericardium, and posteriorly, behind the azygos vein. Intercostal veins draining into the azygos are ligated individually, and the thoracic duct and azygos vein are included in the specimen. Some surgeons do not resect the azygos vein. The left pleura bordering the specimen is harvested and included in the specimen. This plane of dissection is continued cranially to the carina. Above the carina, the margins are limited by the proximity of the trachea anteriorly and the spine posteriorly.

At the hiatus, a 2-cm rim of diaphragm is included with the specimen. In the abdomen, the lesser curvature of the stomach and all nodal tissue along the left gastric artery are taken. All tissue posterior to the stomach and superior to the border of the pancreas is removed. Nodes along the celiac axis, splenic artery, and superior mesenteric artery are dissected. The gastric tube is then pulled up to the neck for esophageal replacement. DeMeester and his group routinely resect the proximal two thirds of stomach, the greater omentum, and the spleen and its associated nodes. They replace the esophagus with isoperistaltic colon.

Results

Retrospective trials comparing en bloc resection with conventional resection have been associated with heavy selection and staging bias. Patients with poor cardiopulmonary reserve are typically excluded from en bloc resection. Moreover, in conventional resection, the disease is commonly understaged as a limited nodal dissection is performed. Both factors would favor stage per stage improved survival in the en bloc group. In Skinner's series of 128 patients, 78 underwent en bloc resection and the remainder underwent a simpler resection, most through the transthoracic route. Perioperative mortality was similar at 4% to 5% in each group. The incidence of pneumonia, leak, and recurrent nerve injury was similar. Four-year survival in patients assigned to stage III was 37% after en bloc resection and 0% after transhiatal resection. Survival was also better in patients with early-stage disease after en bloc resection compared with non–en bloc resection. In DeMeester's series, 69 patients with gastroesophageal junction tumors were studied. Patients in good health with resectable disease underwent en bloc resection, whereas those in poor health or with apparently unresectable disease underwent a transhiatal resection. Five-year survival was significantly better in the en bloc resection group (41%) compared with the transhiatal group (14%). The complication rate was not mentioned in this study.

Three-Field Lymph Node Dissection

Three-field lymph node dissection is a term applied to the addition of a cervical nodal dissection to the traditional thoracic and abdominal nodal dissections that are performed during esophagectomy for cancer. Ten percent to 30% of patients with lower esophageal cancers have cancers that spread to cervical nodal areas, and the same is true of celiac nodes in patients with cervical esophageal cancers.[45-47] Proponents of this technique argue that cervical nodes should be considered resectable even in lower esophageal cancers and should routinely be resected with the specimen.

The abdominal and thoracic phases of the operation are nearly identical to those performed during a tri-incisional en bloc resection of the esophagus. Attention is paid to dissection of the recurrent nerve lymph node chain in the thorax. The neck is incised bilaterally with a U-shaped incision. The sternocleidomastoid muscles are divided. The deep cervical nodes deep and lateral to the jugular vein are dissected, dissection of the recurrent nerve nodes in the neck is continued, and the supraclavicular nodes are also removed.

In experienced hands, the incidence of recurrent nerve injury is no higher than with any other esophagectomy requiring a cervical incision. Altorki and Skinner[46] described a recurrent nerve injury rate of 6%. In their series, there was only one perioperative death from their only case of pneumonia. Although the benefit of three-field lymph node dissections is not clear, several older studies suggested an improved survival.[48,49] More recently, a Japanese study by Ando and coworkers[47] and a U.S. study by Altorki and coworkers[50] have shown 5-year survival rates in the range of 40% to 50% after en bloc esophagectomy with three-field lymph node dissection. The study of Ando and coworkers was limited to patients with squamous carcinoma; the U.S. study included patients with adenocarcinoma and squamous cell carcinoma. Perioperative mortality was 5% to 8% in both studies. There was a 20% to 25% pulmonary complication rate in each study. The recurrent nerve injury rate was 9% in the study of Altorki and coworkers; it was not mentioned in the study by Ando and coworkers. In these selected studies, the perioperative morbidity is comparable to that in other studies, although perioperative mortality in the Ando study is higher than the quoted rate of 3% to 4% from several large academic studies of esophagectomy without en bloc or three-field dissections.[13,51] Long-term survival is impressive, although it is not clear if selection factors or differences in tumor biology between the Japanese and U.S. populations might account for some of the difference.

Prognostic Significance of Number of Lymph Nodes Resected

Rizk and colleagues[52] reported the prognostic significance of the number of involved lymph nodes in patients with esophageal cancer. This retrospective review examined the records of 336 patients operated on between January 1996 and September 2003. The patients studied received surgery as their only treatment. Recursive partitioning analysis using lymph nodes as a variable in addition to T, N, and M status showed that the presence of more than four positive lymph nodes was the most important prognostic factor. This group also reported that the likelihood of finding positive N1 nodes increased when more than 18 nodes were present in the specimen. They concluded that when the appropriate number of lymph nodes is obtained, depth of invasion of the tumor is not a prognostic indicator because survival assessment will be based on lymph node involvement. Since this landmark article, several articles have been published confirming that the number of lymph nodes removed has prognostic significance.

Greenstein and associates[53] evaluated 972 patients in the SEER cancer registry treated with an esophagectomy for esophageal malignant disease diagnosed between 1988 and 2003. Interestingly, on multivariate regression controlling for age, race or ethnicity, sex, histology, tumor status, and postoperative radiotherapy, patients with pathologic node-negative disease in 18 lymph nodes or more were found to have a higher disease-specific survival.

Another group also using the SEER database reported that the number of lymph nodes removed is an independent predictor of survival after an esophagectomy for malignant disease.[54] Of the 2303 patients studied, 1700 patients had an esophagectomy with a thoracotomy and 603 patients had an esophagectomy without a thoracotomy. The Cox regression analysis showed that the number of lymph nodes removed was an independent factor for survival. They concluded that it was necessary to have 23 to 29 lymph nodes in the specimen to provide optimal survival.

Altorki and coworkers[55] retrospectively reviewed their single-institution experience with 264 patients with esophageal cancer treated with esophagectomy between 1988 and 2006. They also concluded that increased nodal resection is an independent factor that favorably influences survival.

Techniques of Alternative Conduits: Colon and Jejunum

Colon

Indications

The stomach is the preferred conduit for esophageal replacement. It has several advantages over the colon, including a reliable blood supply that is usually free of atherosclerotic disease, a low intraluminal bacterial burden, and the need for only a single anastomosis. In those instances when stomach is not available, usually because of previous abdominal or gastric surgery or involvement of the stomach with tumor, the colon becomes the preferred conduit. The left colon differs from the right in that its lumen is smaller and more closely approximates that of the esophagus. Its usable length is usually greater than that of the right colon. The vascular anatomy on the left is more consistent than on the right; however, involvement by atherosclerotic disease of the inferior mesenteric artery is more common than in any other mesenteric vessel.

In general, isoperistaltic orientation is preferred and can be achieved without tension.

Contraindications

Intrinsic disease of the colon by neoplasia, stricture, or extensive diverticulosis precludes its use as an esophageal replacement. In addition, prior abdominal surgery that may have interrupted either the arterial blood supply or venous drainage of the colon may render a segment of the colon unusable. The inferior mesenteric vein drains into the splenic vein, and prior severe pancreatitis or other causes of splenic vein thrombosis may render the left colon unusable as a conduit because of inferior mesenteric vein thrombosis.

Preparation

The patient should be screened for cardiopulmonary disease as for esophagectomy with gastric reconstruction. In addition, preoperative mesenteric angiography should be performed for any patient older than 40 years or otherwise with risk factors for atherosclerotic disease. A barium enema study or colonoscopy should be performed to rule out a coexistent neoplasia or extensive diverticular disease. Mechanical and antibiotic bowel preparation is administered.

Left Colon

As stated previously, the left colon has several advantages over the right, including a longer length, a less-vascular anatomic variation, and a caliber more similar to that of the esophagus. A midline laparotomy is performed, and the abdomen is explored. The peritoneal attachments of the left colon to the retroperitoneum are divided along the white line of Toldt. The length of the conduit that is needed should be estimated by passing an umbilical tape from the proposed proximal line of transection of the esophagus through the proposed route of placement of the conduit to the point of proposed anastomosis to the stomach. The umbilical tape can then be used to measure an appropriate length of colon.

The vessels supplying the left colon are visualized by transillumination. The middle colic artery should be test clamped with a noncrushing bulldog clamp. A palpable pulse should still be present in the marginal artery. If there is any question, a Doppler probe may be used, or the bulldog clamp should be left in place and the conduit inspected for adequate perfusion. Only after it is determined that the conduit is of satisfactory quality should the esophagectomy be completed. The left colon should then be prepared. The omentum is separated from the left colon and splenic flexure that is to be used as a conduit. The middle colic artery is divided, and the mesentery is divided near its root, away from the marginal artery of Drummond (Fig. 38-17). The colon is reanastomosed, and the mesenteric defect is closed.

Either the proximal or distal anastomosis may be done first; however, we believe that construction of the proximal anastomosis first allows better determination of conduit length and ensures that the conduit will sit properly in the neck. The proximal end of the conduit may be drawn up into the neck by use of an atraumatic method, such as an endoscopic camera bag (see tri-incisional technique). The posterior mediastinal (in situ) route is preferred as this is the shortest route

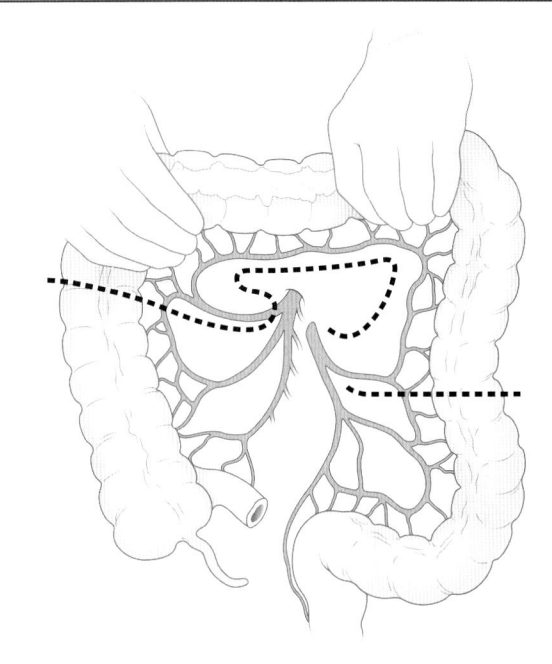

Figure 38–17
The mesentery of the mobilized colon is transilluminated, revealing the mesenteric vessels. The *dotted lines* are the lines of division for a conduit based on the left colic artery. *(Modified from Sugarbaker D, DeCamp M, Liptay M. Surgical procedures to resect and replace the esophagus. In: Zinner M, Schwartz S, Ellis H, et al, editors. Maingot's abdominal operations. Stanford, CT: Appleton & Lange; 1997. p. 885-910.)*

between the stomach and esophagus (Fig. 38-18). If the posterior mediastinal route is unavailable because of prior infection or scarring, as occurs with a prior gastric conduit leak, the substernal or transpleural route is an option. These routes, however, result in more conduit angulation and may impair emptying. Routine resection of the manubrium or a portion of the manubrium is necessary to prevent obstruction and to allow adequate space for the colon if the substernal route is used. Excess length is taken out of the conduit. If there is significant excess length, the proximal end may be trimmed as needed. The proximal anastomosis is typically constructed with a single- or two-layer hand-sewn anastomosis of the end of the esophagus to the side of the antimesenteric taenia. A stapled technique may also be used as detailed in the section on tri-incisional esophagectomy. The anastomosis should be constructed over a nasogastric tube with its tip positioned in the center of the stomach. The conduit should be monitored for arterial insufficiency or venous engorgement. The gastrocolic anastomosis is performed with a large EEA stapler or in a side-to-side functional end-to-end stapled manner. Before closure, the conduit should be sutured to the crus to prevent migration of the colon into the chest or herniation of abdominal viscera into the chest.

Right Colon

A variety of conditions may make the left colon unusable as a conduit. These include extensive diverticular disease, stricture secondary to ischemia or prior diverticular infection, atherosclerotic occlusion of the inferior mesenteric artery, and splenic vein thrombosis with thrombosis of the inferior

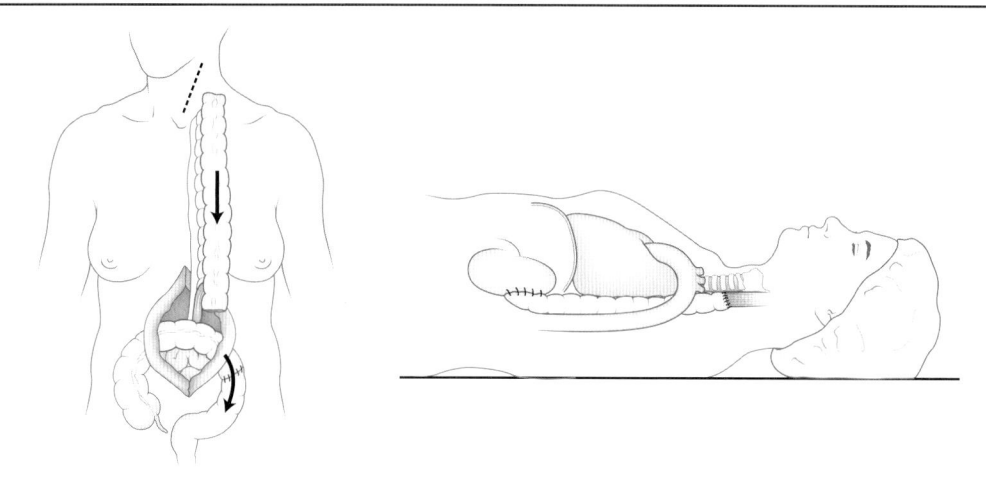

Figure 38–18
The posterior mediastinal (in situ) route is the shortest route between the stomach and esophagus. *(Modified from Sugarbaker D, DeCamp M, Liptay M. Surgical procedures to resect and replace the esophagus. In: Zinner M, Schwartz S, Ellis H, et al, editors.* Maingot's abdominal operations. *Stanford, CT: Appleton & Lange; 1997. p. 885-910.)*

mesenteric vein. The right colon is an acceptable conduit and will readily reach the esophagus in the neck.

The right colon is inspected for any disease, and its retroperitoneal attachments are lysed. The mesentery of the right colon may be transilluminated, showing the ileocolic, right colic, marginal, and middle colic arteries. Soft clamps are placed on the ileocolic and right colic arteries, and the right colon is inspected for adequate perfusion through the marginal artery. The right colon is then harvested, leaving the marginal artery intact. An appendectomy is performed. Whether the ileocecal valve and short segment of ileum should be included in the conduit for esophageal anastomosis is controversial. The ileum does provide a better size match for anastomosis with the esophagus, and in theory, the ileocecal valve should guard against reflux in the neck. Opponents argue that despite the size mismatch, a hand-sewn anastomosis of the end of the esophagus to the side of the colon is easy, reflux esophagitis is rare high in the neck, and the ileocecal valve may contribute to anterograde obstruction.

Appropriate lengths of right colon are divided with a GIA 75-mm stapler, and the colocolonic anastomosis is performed. From the surgeon's perspective, the right colon conduit is rotated counterclockwise, and the proximal end is drawn up into the neck in atraumatic fashion. The proximal anastomosis is created most easily by a single-layer end of esophagus to the side of the colon along a taenia. Excess length is brought out into the abdomen, and the conduit is tacked to the hiatus. At this point, excess length in the distal conduit can be managed by excising colon at the end of the vascular conduit. The cologastric anastomosis is usually constructed with either EEA staplers or a side-to-side stapled technique. The colon may be brought into the anterior aspect or posterior aspect of the stomach.

Jejunum

Indications

Jejunum may be used to replace a portion of the esophagus as a free graft, pedicled graft, or Roux-en-Y replacement.[56,57] Replacement of the esophagus with jejunum is indicated when the stomach is not available because of prior surgery or intrinsic disease. When limited distal esophagectomy is planned, jejunum or colon is preferred to stomach as these two conduits are more resistant to the effects of gastroesophageal reflux. Replacement of a distal esophageal peptic stricture should be performed with colon or jejunum in preference to stomach. Interposition of an isoperistaltic segment of intestine is preferable to gastric pull-up, which has a very high incidence of recurrent severe reflux. Free jejunal graft is indicated in limited reconstruction of the cervical esophagus. Roux-en-Y jejunal replacement may be used to replace the stomach and distal esophagus after total gastrectomy including distal esophagectomy.

Contraindications

Intrinsic disease of the small bowel, whether it is due to inflammatory bowel disease or previous surgery, may prevent its use as a conduit. In general, total esophageal replacement cannot be accomplished with jejunum alone as the length is insufficient to reach the neck.

Preparation

Although mechanical bowel preparation is not necessary for jejunal interposition, it is advisable so that colon is available if the jejunum is found to be unacceptable as a conduit or if the blood supply to the jejunum is damaged during harvest, rendering it unusable as a conduit. Antibiotics (a cephalosporin and an anaerobic antibiotic) should be administered preoperatively.

Roux-en-Y Replacement

Roux-en-Y replacement (Fig. 38-19) may be used for reconstruction after total gastrectomy and distal esophageal resection as indicated in proximal gastric tumors or for esophageal resection into the upper chest. On occasion, a Roux-en-Y replacement may reach the neck, but this is variable, and unlike the stomach, it will not reliably reach the cervical esophagus.

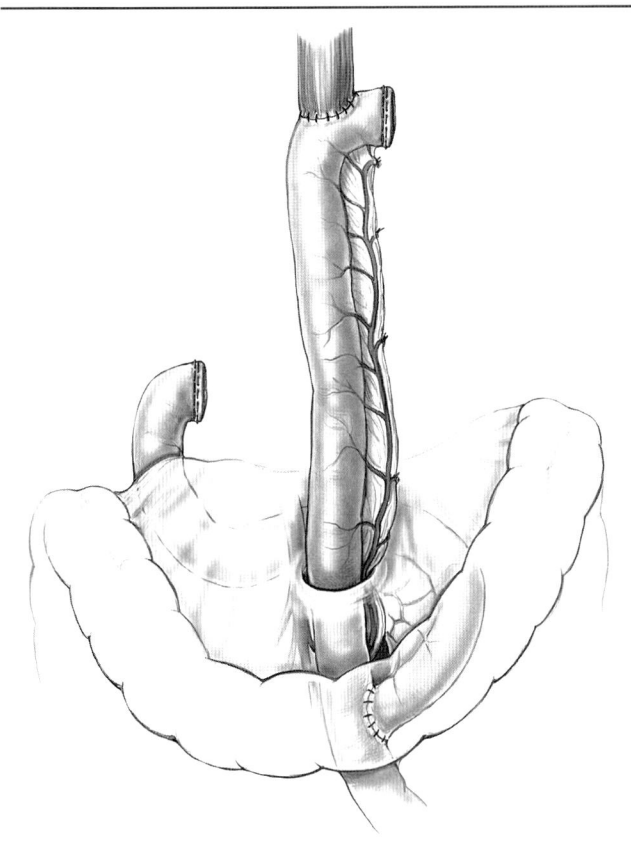

Figure 38-19
Roux-en-Y replacement with jejunum is useful for reconstruction after esophagectomy with gastrectomy, as with proximal gastric tumors.

When it is used after total gastrectomy, jejunum is divided approximately 20 to 30 cm beyond the ligament of Treitz. The jejunum is elevated outside the abdomen, and the vascular arcade is transilluminated. The proposed point of division is identified, and the line of division of the mesentery is also identified along with the proposed division of several vessels of the mesentery, which will allow movement of the jejunum up into the chest. The proposed feeder vessel is identified and preserved. The serosal surface of the mesentery is scored, and the vessels to be transected are clamped with a soft bulldog clamp. The conduit is observed for several minutes for evidence of ischemia or congestion. By this technique, 60 cm of jejunal conduit can be mobilized. A hole in the transverse mesocolon is made to the left of the middle colic vessels large enough for the jejunum and its mesentery to pass through. For replacement after total gastrectomy, the proximal anastomosis is to the very distal esophagus in the upper abdomen. If distal esophagectomy is also performed as for a malignant lesion of the cardia extending to the gastroesophageal junction, the abdominal incision must be brought across the costal margin into the left sixth or seventh interspace. If, after division of the esophagus and mobilization of the Roux-en-Y limb into the lower chest, additional length of jejunum is needed, the next vessel in the mesenteric arcade is test clamped and then divided.

The esophagojejunal anastomosis can be performed by stapled or hand-sewn techniques. The stapled anastomosis is most easily performed with an EEA stapler. Ideally, a size 33-mm EEA stapler should be used to protect against the development of strictures. The distal esophagus may be gently dilated with a lubricated dilator. A full-thickness 2-0 Prolene suture is used to create a pursestring in the distal esophagus. The shaft of the EEA stapler can be introduced through the stapled end of the proximal jejunum. Care must be taken not to occlude the ongoing lumen of the jejunum with the stapler. Two full-thickness anastomotic doughnuts should be verified. After removal of the EEA stapler, the jejunal end can be closed with a TA 60-mm stapler. A hand-sewn anastomosis in two layers may also be performed. The outer layer is seromuscular on the jejunum to muscular esophagus with 3-0 silk, and the inner layer is full thickness with interrupted 3-0 or 4-0 chromic gut.

The jejunum should be tacked to the hiatus at several points with interrupted silk sutures. This prevents herniation of abdominal contents into the chest and limits tension on the esophagojejunal anastomosis. Likewise, the defect in the colonic mesentery should be closed to prevent an internal hernia. The distal anastomosis can be hand sewn or performed by a side-to-side functional end-to-end stapled technique.

Pedicled Jejunal Interposition

A left thoracoabdominal incision is used with a left seventh interspace incision extended across the costal margin and across the rectus muscle. As with the harvest of a Roux-en-Y loop, the jejunum is transilluminated, and an appropriate length of jejunum is selected from a point 20 cm distal to the ligament of Treitz. A single large vessel is used as a feeding vessel for the conduit. The jejunum is transected proximally and distally with a GIA stapler, and the mesentery is divided down each side to the origin of the vessel. The remaining jejunum is reconnected by a side-to-side functional end-to-end stapled technique. The pedicled jejunum is tunneled through the mesocolon and brought into the left chest. The proximal anastomosis is constructed like the Roux-en-Y esophagojejunal anastomosis. The jejunogastric anastomosis may be hand sewn in two layers or stapled with an EEA stapler (Fig. 38-20).

Free Jejunal Interposition

Free jejunal graft may reach portions of the upper esophagus that pedicled grafts may not. It is not clear whether the use of a short jejunal interposition is preferable to total esophageal replacement with a normal gastric conduit. The use of jejunum does carry a lower incidence of gastroesophageal reflux; however, the increased risk of life-threatening graft ischemia and necrosis is significant. Moreover, two anastomoses are required, increasing the risk of anastomotic leak.

As with the pedicled jejunal graft, a short segment of jejunum is chosen for harvest. A left cervical incision is made, and the esophagus and carotid and jugular vessels are isolated. Soon after division of the jejunal vessels with a scalpel, the artery and vein are flushed with heparinized saline. The proximal hand-sewn anastomosis is constructed first, an operating microscope and fine 9-0 or 10-0 suture are used to anastomose the jejunal vessels to the carotid and jugular vessels, and the distal anastomosis is then constructed (Fig. 38-21). The graft is covered with a meshed split-thickness skin graft to monitor graft viability in the postoperative period.

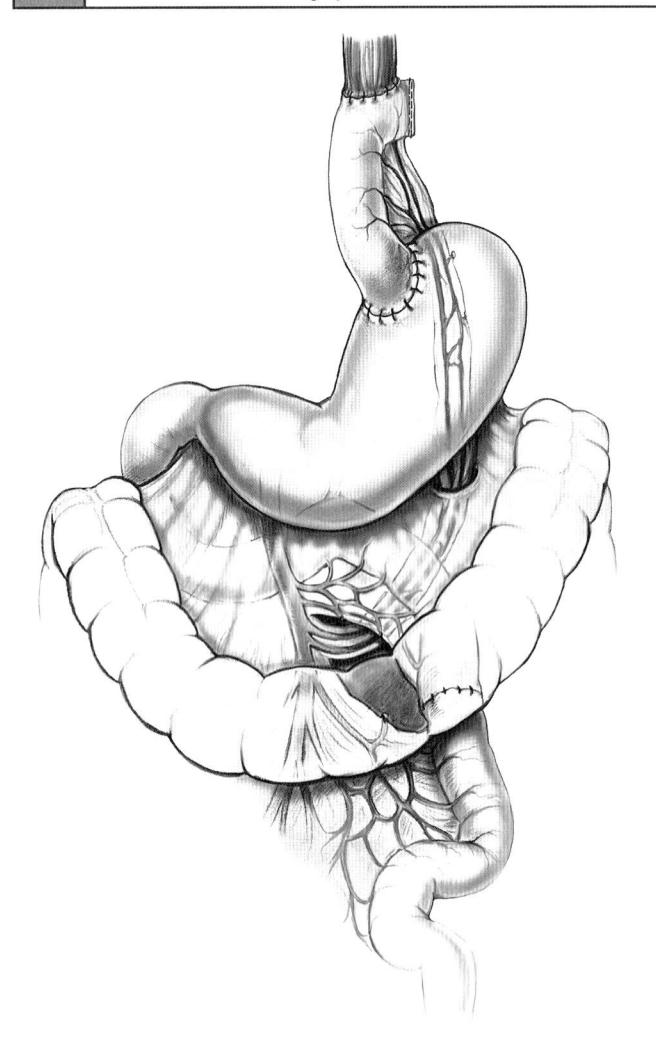

Figure 38–20
Pedicled jejunum is ideally suited for distal esophageal replacement. An appropriate length of jejunum is harvested beginning 20 cm beyond the ligament of Treitz.

CONSIDERATIONS IN ESOPHAGEAL RESECTION

Perioperative Mortality

Historically, esophagectomy has been associated with the highest perioperative mortality of any commonly performed resection. The combination of a long operation traversing three body compartments in an elderly, potentially malnourished individual with the potential for overwhelming mediastinal sepsis has produced perioperative mortality rates that were initially quoted at 15% to 40%.[58,59] Reports published after 1980 showed improvement in the mortality rates to approximately 15%, with a large meta-analysis of papers published between 1986 and 1996 showing mortality rates averaging 6% to 10%.[19,60] Several large academic centers have published large series with mortality rates ranging from 3% to 4%.[13,51,61]

A relationship with hospital volume and outcome has been long described. This particular relationship has been reported for esophagectomy as far back as the late 1970s.[62] Chang and Birkmeyer[63] reviewed this topic for *Thoracic Surgery Clinics*. They noted 11 of 12 studies publishing statistically significant volume-outcome relationships pertaining to esophagectomy. One of the authors had used the Medicare database to produce the largest study to date evaluating mortality and esophagectomy.[64] His analysis showed that 6337 patients underwent an esophagectomy at 1575 hospitals. Low-volume hospitals were defined as those with fewer than two operations per year. Higher-volume hospitals performed more than 19 such operations per year. The in-hospital mortality of the high-volume center was considerably lower (8.1%) than that of the low-volume hospital (23.1%). A second report from this same group examined surgeon volume and outcomes.[65] Using the Medicare database from 1998 to 1999, they reported that surgical outcome with regard to operative mortality was inversely related to surgeon volume. They found the surgeon volume and hospital volume to be independent factors in outcomes. A low-volume surgeon at a high-volume center has higher mortality rates than does a high-volume surgeon at a high-volume center. The application of this information to policy and certification of hospitals and surgeons for this highly technical operation is beyond the scope of this chapter.

Several studies have identified age as a risk factor for increased morbidity and mortality after an esophagectomy. It has recently been observed in an analysis of the Nationwide Inpatient Sample database that there is a 19.9% perioperative mortality in octogenarians after esophagectomy. This is significantly different from the 8.8% perioperative mortality after similar surgery in patients 65 to 69 years old ($P < .0001$).[66] It is clear that advances in surgical technique, anesthesia, and intensive care have markedly improved the safety of esophagectomy during the past several decades. In older series, the greatest contributor to perioperative mortality was intrathoracic sepsis caused by either an anastomotic or a conduit leak. The mortality rate from a clinically overt intrathoracic leak may be greater than 50%.[67] Aggressive, early management of an intrathoracic esophageal leak is essential in limiting its possible fatal effects.

In the more recent, larger series published with mortality rates below 5%, the most common cause of perioperative death is not conduit leak; rather, it is pulmonary in etiology: respiratory insufficiency, pneumonia, or pulmonary embolus.[13,51,61] The combination of a low incidence of leak with early, aggressive management has made the intrathoracic enteric leak less of a factor in perioperative mortality.

Early Perioperative Complications

Anastomotic Leak

The incidence of intrathoracic leak after Ivor Lewis esophagectomy is typically 5% to 10%.[15,19] The incidence of leak after a cervical anastomosis is higher, generally in the 10% to 15% range.[19,51] Older studies have quoted cervical leak rates at 25% to 26%, whereas a recent large study described a leak rate of 8%.[13,59,68] A retrospective evaluation of anastomotic leaks revealed that albumin level below 3 g/dL, positive margins, and cervical anastomosis were risk factors for anastomotic leak after esophagectomy.[68] Several factors are believed to be responsible for the increased incidence of leak in the cervical position. The increase in length needed may cause increased tension on the anastomosis. Blood supply to the anastomosis may be compromised as it is farther away from the origin of the gastroepiploic artery, and arterial inflow and venous drainage may be compromised by a tight thoracic inlet.

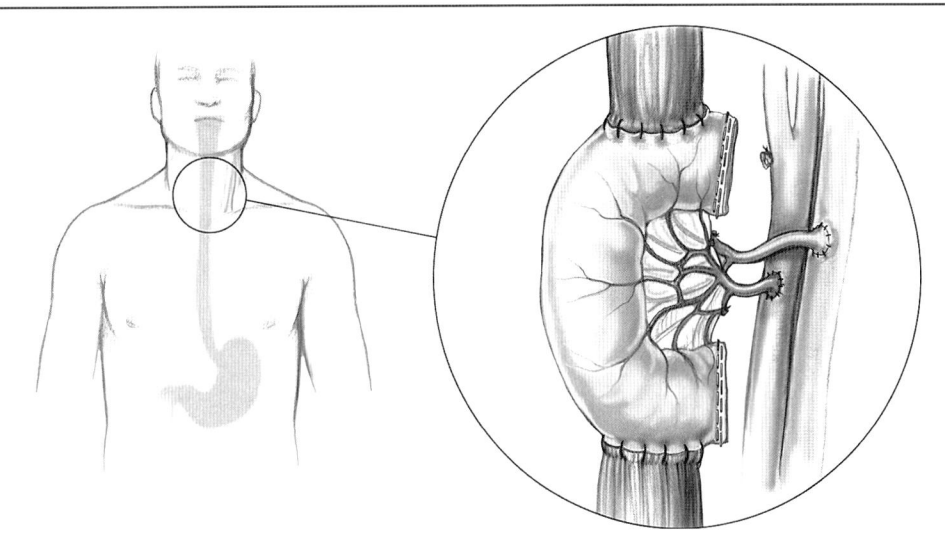

Figure 38-21
Free jejunal interposition may be used where pedicled graft will not reach, such as in the proximal esophagus. The arterial and venous supplies are anastomosed to the carotid and jugular vessels under the operating microscope. A split-thickness skin graft covers the graft to allow inspection of graft viability in the perioperative period.

In a randomized trial of hand-sewn versus stapled anastomosis in 102 patients undergoing Ivor Lewis esophagectomy, no significant difference was seen in the incidence of leaks between the two groups. The incidence of leak was 5% after a single hand-sewn monofilament anastomosis and 2% after stapled anastomosis.[69]

The Mayo Clinic published its retrospective review of stapled versus hand-sewn esophagogastric anastomosis.[70] Hand-sewn esophagogastric anastomosis was performed at the Mayo Clinic only until 2002, when stapling devices were used to resume gastrointestinal continuity. Around this time, 280 patients who underwent an esophagectomy by the transhiatal, transthoracic, or tri-incisional approach were evaluated. It was found that the method of stapling of the anastomosis was safe and associated with a lower leak rate and need for dilation compared with the hand-sewn group. Clearly, the incidence of leak after hand-sewn anastomosis is more operator dependent than with stapled anastomosis, and the reproducibility of the stapled anastomosis is its main advantage.

An intrathoracic leak is a life-threatening event that usually requires immediate operative intervention. Although the mortality rate from this complication has been lowered at large centers during the last few decades, the cost in intensive care unit and hospital stay and delayed recovery remains high. The intervention required may range from repair and drainage of a limited leak, to placement of a T-tube, to complete diversion by split fistula and reduction of viable gastric conduit into the abdomen. The more critically ill the patient is as a result of the leak, the more aggressive and definitive the treatment required. In rare instances (a clinically silent, small contained leak draining back into the conduit not near vital structures such as the trachea or aorta), such a leak may be treated conservatively with antibiotics and maintenance of strict NPO status.

Historically, a thoracic leak is associated with a higher mortality than a cervical anastomotic leak is. With adequate drainage, some authors are questioning this belief.[71,72] As stent technology has developed, there have been reports of its use for control of an anastomotic leak.[73-76] Siewert and co-workers inserted a self-expanding covered metal stent at the site of intrathoracic leak in 10 patients. Radiologic methods confirmed closure of anastomotic leak in all but one patient. In this patient the stent was adjusted, and closure of the leak was confirmed. Stent migration requiring new stents and adjustment occurred in four patients. The authors found that in all but one patient, complete leak closure was achieved. Two patients died of reasons not related to stent placement, but further details were missing from the report. Stent technology continues to develop new indications for its use; however, indications for control of an anastomotic leak have not been confirmed by large randomized trials.

Leak after a cervical anastomosis, although more frequent, is uncommonly a life-threatening event. Older series have described mortality from a cervical leak as high as 20%, although recent series have described mortality rates that are much lower.[13,67] Cervical anastomotic leak occurs, in general, later than intrathoracic leaks do, with many diagnosed only on routine postoperative barium swallow study or on commencement of oral feeds after a normal barium swallow study.[77] Patients with cervical leaks may present with low-grade fevers, localized redness, or wound discharge. Treatment usually entails limited opening of the neck incision and placement of a wick. Larger leaks resulting from anastomotic necrosis may be treated with a Silastic stent or T-tube. Leaks into the chest after cervical anastomosis, due to either retraction of the anastomosis into the chest or dependent drainage of enteric contents into the chest, must be treated in the same manner as any intrathoracic leak. The main long-term sequela of a cervical anastomotic leak without signs of systemic sepsis is an increased incidence of delayed stricture formation.

Respiratory Complications

Pneumonia, atelectasis, and respiratory failure, in the modern era, are probably the most serious complications after esophagectomy when one takes into account their relatively high incidence and potentially life-threatening consequences. The incidence of pneumonia after esophagectomy ranges from 2% to 47%.[27,51] Respiratory failure after esophagectomy occurs in 4% of patients.[19] The assumption that avoidance of thoracotomy results in fewer pulmonary complications than with a transthoracic esophagectomy has not conclusively been supported by the literature. In the randomized trial of Goldminc and associates[24] comparing transhiatal with Ivor Lewis esophagectomy, the incidence of pneumonia was 20% for both groups. In the randomized trial of Chu and coworkers[25] comparing transhiatal with Ivor Lewis esophagectomy in 39 patients, the incidence of pneumonia was 10% after transhiatal and 0% after Ivor Lewis resection (no significant difference). A recent European randomized trial comparing transhiatal with en bloc tri-incisional esophagectomy did show a difference in the rate of pulmonary complications (pneumonia or lobar atelectasis) in the tri-incisional (57%) versus the transhiatal group (27%).[27] The unusually high incidence of pulmonary complications in both groups of this series should be questioned. Typically, rates of pulmonary complications are in the 20% range.[20] Previous series involving en bloc resections have described pneumonia rates of 5%.[43]

A muscle-sparing, limited thoracotomy, epidural anesthesia, and early ambulation are essential in limiting post-thoracotomy respiratory complications. Multivariate analysis has shown that age and decreased FEV_1 were predictive of postoperative respiratory failure.[78] Age, preoperative chemoradiation, and decreased FEV_1 have also been identified as risk factors for respiratory compromise after an esophagectomy.[79]

As discussed in the earlier section on minimally invasive esophagectomy, many proponents of smaller-access surgery have reported fewer pulmonary complications with this approach to an esophagectomy.

Recurrent Laryngeal Nerve Injury

The incidence of recurrent nerve injury and vocal cord dysfunction after esophagectomy is higher with a cervical anastomosis than with an intrathoracic anastomosis. Malfunction of a single vocal cord, although seemingly a minor complication resulting in hoarseness, can lead to a series of life-threatening complications if it is not recognized early and treated. The lack of vocal cord apposition makes an effective cough and clearance of pulmonary secretions difficult. This is exacerbated by the loss of airway protection during swallowing and repeated episodes of overt aspiration or microaspiration.

As expected, the incidence of recurrent nerve injury is higher with a cervical anastomosis (11%) than with an intrathoracic anastomosis (5%).[19] In the right thorax, the recurrent nerve may be injured by traction on the vagus nerves or by cautery near the nerve as it recurs around the subclavian artery. In addition, a neck dissection may result in direct injury to the recurrent nerves as the esophagus is dissected away from the tracheoesophageal groove. In the neck, dissection must be performed immediately against the esophagus, with care taken to recognize and to avoid the recurrent nerve. Dissection close to the recurrent nerves does not necessarily place them at risk; one series of three-field lymph node dissection with direct dissection of all lymph nodes adjacent to both recurrent nerves resulted in a recurrent nerve injury rate of only 6%.[46]

Early recognition and treatment of a recurrent nerve injury (in itself a non–life-threatening condition unless both cords are simultaneously injured) are essential in preventing the potentially lethal complications of aspiration and pneumonia. Any patient who presents with hoarseness and an ineffective cough after esophagectomy should undergo fiberoptic laryngoscopy. Unilateral paralyzed vocal cords should be medialized by either injection or prosthesis implantation. Early intervention can lead to a low incidence of pulmonary complications.[13]

Bleeding

The incidence of bleeding after esophagectomy is approximately 5% and does not vary according to the techniques used.[19] In a meta-analysis, average blood loss was slightly higher for the transthoracic approach, averaging 1000 mL, than for the transhiatal approach, averaging 728 mL.[20] Anticoagulants and antiplatelet agents should be stopped in advance of esophagectomy. Low-dose subcutaneous heparin does not increase the incidence of bleeding after esophagectomy. Direct arterial branches from the aorta to the esophagus usually found in the lower thorax should be clipped, not simply cauterized. Larger arteries supplying the esophagus branch into a fine plexus of arterioles at a point 1 to 2 cm away from the esophagus. If blunt dissection of the esophagus is used, it should be kept immediately adjacent to the esophagus with disruption of only the smaller arterioles.

Chyle Leak

The thoracic duct drains the cisterna chyli in the abdomen beginning at the L2 level. It enters the chest through the aortic hiatus and ascends through the right chest behind the esophagus along the vertebral bodies between the azygos vein and the aorta. On occasion, more than one channel exists in the lower chest at the level of the hiatus. At approximately the T6 level, it crosses to the left side behind the aorta and ascends along the left side of the esophagus posterior to the left subclavian artery. Above the clavicle, the duct descends behind the carotid sheath and anterior to the anterior scalene muscle and phrenic nerve to empty into the junction of the left internal jugular and subclavian vein. The duct can be injured at any point along dissection of the esophagus. The incidence of chyle leak after esophagectomy ranges from 2% to 10%.[19,27] The incidence is higher after transthoracic resection, probably as a result of an extended radial dissection of the esophagus and associated nodal tissue. Prophylactic mass ligation of the duct at the hiatus may help decrease the incidence of postoperative leak. If chest tube output is 1000 mL/day or more 48 hours after esophagectomy, chylothorax should be suspected. Diagnosis can be difficult as the classic milky appearance of chyle is apparent only in a fed patient. Gram stain will exclude polymorphonuclear cells. Fluid should be sent for determination of triglyceride level, cholesterol level, and cell count. A triglyceride level of greater than 1 mmol/L is highly suggestive of a chyle leak, as is a lymphocyte count of greater than 90%. A cholesterol to triglyceride ratio of less than 1 and confirmation of chylomicrons on electrophoresis have also been suggested to be diagnostic of a chyle leak. Perhaps the best and simplest test is feeding cream at 30 mL/hr through the

J-tube for 3 to 4 hours, watching for a change from serous pleural fluid to a milky fluid.

There is no role for conservative management of a high-output chyle leak after esophagectomy. Continued loss of lymphocytes, protein, fats, and fluid at a rate of 1 L/day or more in a malnourished patient healing from a major operation invites disaster. Once the diagnosis is confirmed, or even if the diagnosis is highly suspected, the patient should be brought back to the operating room for ligation of the duct at the level of the hiatus. Cream should be instilled through the J-tube for several hours before reoperation. The approach to ligation of the duct should be through a right thoracotomy or thoracoscopy. The exact site of injury can often be located after the patient has been given cream enterally. It may be repaired with pledgeted 4-0 or 5-0 monofilament sutures. If there is any doubt about the integrity of the repair, the duct should be mass ligated at the level of the hiatus. The pleura is incised, and a 0 silk mass ligature is used to encompass all tissue between the azygos vein and aorta along the spine. A pledgeted suture should be used if tissue integrity is poor. A careful search to confirm cessation of the leak should be performed before closure.

Noninvasive methods for closure of thoracic duct leaks have been proposed. The thoracic duct can be cannulated percutaneously by puncture into the cisterna chyli and embolized with coils or fibrin glue. In a trial of 42 patients (9 of whom were postesophagectomy patients), the thoracic duct could be embolized in 26 patients, and 16 of these were cured.[80] This technology is in evolution and at this point should be reserved for complex patients for whom surgical repair has failed or for patients who are not candidates for surgical repair.

Cardiovascular Morbidity

Perioperative arrhythmias after esophagectomies have a reported incidence of 20% to 60%.[81-86] The development of new-onset perioperative atrial fibrillation has been linked to anastomotic leaks and pulmonary complications.[83] Although arrhythmias can be treated effectively with calcium channel blockers and beta-blockers,[87] patients given prophylactic digoxin did not have a reduced incidence of cardiac arrhythmias.[82]

The incidence of myocardial infarction after esophageal resection is 1% to 2%.[81,85,86] Currently, a double-blinded, randomized trial is under way in 182 centers in 21 countries to evaluate the benefit of perioperative beta-blockage in patients undergoing noncardiac thoracic surgery. The study has entered 6400 patients and is set to accrue 10,000 patients.[88]

Late Perioperative Complications

Anastomotic Stricture

Although anastomotic stricture is never life-threatening, it is not uncommon and, if severe, negates the primary benefit of intestinal continuity after esophageal replacement. A large retrospective meta-analysis concluded that the incidence of symptomatic stricture is somewhat higher after anastomosis in the cervical position (28%) than after Ivor Lewis resection (16%).[19] This is in part due to the higher incidence of leak after cervical anastomosis. In an examination of risk factors of benign stricture after transhiatal esophagectomy, the use of a stapled anastomosis, an anastomotic leak, and the presence of cardiac disease were the only risk factors identified for the development of stricture.[89] Earlier studies had identified intraoperative blood loss and poor vascularization of the gastric conduit as risk factors.[90,91] From these studies, it is apparent that three factors influence the development of postoperative stricture: infection, ischemia, and mechanical issues.

Anastomotic leak is a well-known risk factor for the development of a delayed stricture. Curiously, Honkoop and associates[89] found no difference in the incidence of delayed stricture between clinically overt leaks and those detected by swallow only. Preemptive bougienage dilation (7 to 10 days after operation) has been advocated by some to prevent the development of stricture after cervical leak.[92] Ischemia is one of the major contributors to anastomotic leak, and it is difficult to determine what effect this alone has on the development of postoperative stricture. All efforts to avoid ischemia (adequate blood supply, systemic oxygen delivery, avoidance of congestion) should certainly be made to prevent both leak and stricture. It is also evident that mechanical factors influence the development of stricture. Law and colleagues[69] performed a randomized trial of hand-sewn versus EEA-stapled Ivor Lewis anastomosis. The incidence of stricture after the hand-sewn anastomosis was 9%, whereas that after stapled anastomosis was 40%. Strictures were not seen with the 33-mm EEA stapler but had a 12.5% incidence with the 29-mm stapler and a 43% incidence when a 25-mm stapler was used. Not every esophagus will allow a 33-mm stapler, but it should be used whenever possible. Otherwise, a hand-sewn anastomosis or a different stapling technique should be considered. A retrospective study performed at the University of Texas M. D. Anderson Cancer Center indicated that side-to-side stapled esophagogastric anastomosis represented a trend in which this technique had lower associated postoperative dysphagia and need for stricture dilation compared with its hand-sewn counterparts.[93]

Postoperative stricture is usually managed by repeated bougie dilation. In Honkoop's study, three dilations, on average, were needed to achieve normal swallowing. Perforation occurred in 2 of 519 episodes of dilation. Both of these perforations resulted in death of the patient. In the study by Law and colleagues, 53% were treated by one dilation, 20% by two, 12% by three, and 8% by four. No patient in either study was treated by reoperation.

Martin and coworkers[94] reported that a majority of postesophagectomy patients will have some degree of dysphagia. Some have advocated early dilation of the anastomosis and conduit in patients with dysphagia even if there is no anatomic reason for the dysphagia.[95]

Barthel and colleagues[96] advocate the use of a silicone stent as an alternative to serial dilations. They evaluated eight patients who had persistent anastomotic strictures after a transhiatal esophagectomy. They placed 13 stents in eight patients with strictures between 20 and 23 cm from the incisors. All strictures were less than 2 cm and had a predilation luminal diameter of 2 to 5 mm. The authors concluded that stent placement significantly prolonged the interval between endoscopic interventions that are necessary for management of strictures. However, their data did not show permanent resolution of the stricture after the stent was removed.

Postresection Reflux

Reflux of duodenal contents into the conduit occurs to some degree after esophagectomy in virtually all patients. It is not clear that preservation of the integrity of the pylorus protects against bile reflux. In fact, a study by Romagnoli and colleagues[97] involving 24-hour bile monitoring of the denervated gastric conduit in 16 patients showed elevated concentrations of bile in the stomach irrespective of the presence or absence of a drainage procedure.

The incidence of severe postoperative reflux requiring intervention after distal esophagectomy with esophagogastric anastomosis low in the chest approaches 20%.[98] For this reason, when esophageal replacement is contemplated for a distal peptic stricture, colon or jejunal interposition should be employed. These conduits, in the isoperistaltic position, are more resistant to the effects of gastric reflux and provide active peristalsis that allows clearance of bile.

Impaired Conduit Emptying

Several factors have been implicated in delayed conduit emptying after esophagectomy; these include truncal vagotomy, absence of pyloric drainage procedure, swelling at the pyloroplasty site, kinking of redundant conduit in the lower chest, and conduit that is too wide and patulous. Some of these variables are difficult to assess, whereas others have been carefully studied. After truncal vagotomy for ulcer disease, there is a 25% incidence of impaired gastric emptying.[99] Whether this applies to transposed stomach after esophagectomy is not clear. One study showed that delayed emptying after esophagectomy with gastric replacement was less in those undergoing pyloroplasty (the time of emptying of radiolabeled water was 378 minutes with no pyloroplasty versus 161 minutes in patients undergoing pyloroplasty).[100] Other studies showed no objective difference in gastric conduit emptying.[101] In any event, there is often poor correlation between gastric emptying tests and symptoms.

Fok and associates[102] conducted a prospective randomized trial of pyloroplasty versus no pyloroplasty in 200 patients undergoing Ivor Lewis esophagectomy with gastric reconstruction. There were no complications from the pyloroplasty procedure. Of the 100 patients who had no drainage procedure, 13 patients had symptoms of delayed gastric emptying. Two of these patients died as a result of aspiration pneumonia, one required reoperation, and three others had prolonged symptoms. The daily postoperative nasogastric drainage was not significantly different between the two groups. Gastric emptying measured at 6 months was 6 minutes in the pyloroplasty group and 24 minutes in the patients without pyloroplasty. The patients without pyloroplasty also had more symptoms attributable to impaired gastric emptying at 6 months than the pyloroplasty patients did. The authors strongly advocate a routine pyloric drainage procedure. The same group conducted a randomized trial of pyloroplasty to pyloromyotomy and found both to be effective and safe procedures.[103] Six months after the procedure, gastric emptying was twice as fast in the pyloroplasty groups versus the pyloromyotomy group; however, the incidence of symptoms appeared to be no different.

Kim and associates[104] reported on balloon dilation in 21 patients who had delayed gastric emptying after an esophagectomy. Gastric emptying before and after dilation was measured by radioisotope imaging. Single dilation was performed in 19 patients. Two patients required a second dilation. Gastric emptying improved after dilation in 67% of the patients; seven patients were greatly improved and six patients were slightly improved, whereas six patients showed no improvement. There were no complications. This is clearly a small case report, and larger studies need to be performed to observe any benefit from balloon dilation.

The width of the gastric conduit is also believed to influence the rate of emptying. The gastric tube should be kept narrow, with the width not significantly exceeding that of the antrum. A retrospective study examined the relationship between conduit emptying and size and found that patients with a narrow gastric tube had a far lower incidence of symptoms attributable to delayed gastric emptying (3%) than did patients with whole stomach (38%) or distal two-thirds stomach (14%) conduits.[105] A conduit that is too narrow, however, may become ischemic from a compromised arterial inflow and venous congestion. In the authors' opinion, conduit diameter should not be less than 5 cm. Proper length of the gastric conduit is also important as excess conduit can fold over into the right chest and has been associated with impaired emptying.

Local Recurrence

Factors involved in local recurrence include resection margins and clearance of adjacent nodal disease. Tam and coworkers[106] found a correlation between the incidence of local recurrence and the lateral spread of tumor outside the esophageal wall (T3) but no correlation with tumor differentiation or lymph node metastasis. As discussed earlier, the importance of complete clearance of nodal tissue is debated among proponents of complete lymphadenectomy (by transthoracic or en bloc dissection) and proponents of simple transhiatal dissection.

The issue of recurrence with an incomplete linear margin is better understood. The palpable intraoperative in situ resection margin will be larger than the contracted gross postresection margin, which in turn is longer than the final fixed margin. Siu and colleagues[107] estimated that margins after removal of the esophagus were only about 50% of the in situ margin. Descriptions of margin length must take this factor into account. Tam and coworkers[106] examined the in situ resection margins of 100 patients with squamous cell carcinoma of the esophagus. When the in situ margin was less than 5 cm, there was a 20% incidence of anastomotic recurrence; between 5 and 10 cm, there was an 8% chance; and when the margin was greater than 10 cm, there were no anastomotic recurrences. Wong[12] further pointed out that it is difficult to obtain a 10-cm margin, as the length of the average esophageal tumor is 6 cm. Assuming the average esophagus is 25 cm in length, only distal esophageal tumors can, on average, be resected with a 10-cm margin if the larynx is to be conserved. Another author suggested that an adequate distal margin after resection of adenocarcinoma of the gastroesophageal junction should be 6 cm.[108]

Long-term (5-Year) Survival

Long-term survival remains an elusive goal for the medical and surgical oncologist caring for a patient with esophageal cancer. Despite advances in perioperative care that have reduced the perioperative mortality rate to 7% and below, 5-year survival has not changed appreciably during the past 2 decades. The 5-year survival described by Cunha-Melo and associates between 1953 and 1978 (18%) is similar to that described in the meta-analysis by Hulscher and coworkers[27] between 1990 and 1999 (22%). It remains to be seen whether the introduction of neoadjuvant treatment for advanced esophageal cancers (invading through the esophageal wall or with positive nodes) will change the overall survival of patients with esophageal cancer. Three randomized trials employing neoadjuvant chemoradiation before esophagectomy have been performed. A trial randomizing 100 esophageal cancer patients to preoperative chemoradiation followed by transhiatal esophagectomy versus transhiatal esophagectomy alone showed that survival in the neoadjuvant group was 30% at 3 years versus 16% in the surgery-alone group; the difference was not statistically significant.[109] A European study randomizing 282 patients with squamous cell cancer to neoadjuvant chemoradiation followed by en bloc transthoracic esophagectomy and to esophagectomy alone found no difference in 5-year survival.[110] Walsh and coworkers[111] randomized 113 patients with adenocarcinoma to surgery alone versus chemoradiation followed by surgery. Five-year survival was approximately 50% in the neoadjuvant group and unusually poor in the surgery-alone group (8%); the difference was statistically significant. Larger trials have been attempted; however, they have encountered difficulty in enrolling patients in a randomized fashion, and the true benefit of neoadjuvant chemoradiation may never be measured.

A few isolated series in selected centers employing radical en bloc dissection of the esophagus with three-field lymph node dissection have described 5-year survival rates in the 40% to 50% range.[47,50] These results are discussed in the sections on en bloc resection and three-field lymph node dissection.

Summary

The reduction in perioperative mortality of esophagectomy from more than 40% during the past 50 years to as low as 3% as described in several large academic centers is attributable to improvements in selection of patients, operative technique, and intensive care and early recognition and aggressive management of perioperative complications. Minimizing complications and optimizing chances of cure require that the skilled esophageal surgeon be familiar with the anatomy of the neck, chest, and abdomen and well trained in and ready to use a variety of routes of esophageal resection and methods of reconstruction. As minimally invasive esophagectomy has become more prominent, numerous institutions have reported their experience, suggesting an advantage to a minimally invasive esophagectomy over an open surgery. However, randomized, controlled trials need to be performed to affirm these claims.

REFERENCES

1. Jemal A, Siegel R, Ward E, et al. Cancer statistics 2008. *CA Cancer J Clin* 2008;**58**:71-96.
2. Lewis I. The surgical treatment of carcinoma of the esophagus with special reference to a new operation for growths of the middle third. *Br J Surg* 1946;**34**:18-31.
3. McKeown K. Total three-stage oesophagectomy for cancer of the oesophagus. *Br J Surg* 1976;**63**:259.
4. Atkins BZ, Shah AS, Hutchenson KA, et al. Reducing hospital morbidity and mortality following esophagectomy. *Ann Thorac Surg* 2004;**78**:1170-6.
5. Braghetto I, Csendes A, Cardemil G, et al. Open transthoracic or transhiatal esophagectomy vs minimally invasive esophagectomy in terms of morbidity, mortality and survival. *Surg Endosc* 2006;**20**:1681-6.
6. Cuschieri A, Shimi S, Banting S. Endoscopic oesophagectomy through a right thoracoscopic approach. *J R Coll Surg Edinb* 1992;**37**:284-5.
7. Luketich J, Schauer P, Christie N. Minimally invasive esophagectomy. *Ann Thorac Surg* 2000;**70**:906-12.
8. Nguyen N, Schauer P, Luketich J. Combined laparoscopic and thoracoscopic approach to esophagectomy. *J Am Coll Surg* 1999;**188**:328-32.
9. Swanstrom L, Hansen P. Laparoscopic total esophagectomy. *Arch Surg* 1997;**132**:943-9.
10. Maloney JD, Weigel TL. Minimally invasive esophagectomy for malignant and premalignant diseases of the esophagus. *Surg Clin N Am* 2008;**88**:979-90.
11. Berrisford RG, Wajed SA, Sanders D, Rucklidge WM. Short-term outcomes following total minimally invasive oesophagectomy. *Br J Surg* 2008;**95**:602-10.
12. Wong J. Esophageal resection for cancer: the rationale of current practice. *Am J Surg* 1987;**153**:18-24.
13. Swanson SJ, Batirel HF, Bueno R, et al. Transthoracic esophagectomy with radical mediastinal and abdominal lymph node dissection and cervical esophagogastrostomy for esophageal carcinoma. *Ann Thorac Surg* 2001;**72**:1918-24: discussion 1924-1925.
14. Churchill ED, Sweet RH. Transthoracic resection of tumors of the stomach and esophagus. *Ann Surg* 1942;**115**:897.
15. Mathisen D, Grillo H, Hilgenberg A, et al. Transthoracic esophagectomy: A safe approach to carcinoma of the esophagus. *Ann Thorac Surg* 1988;**45**:137.
16. Hankins J, Attar S, McLaughlin J, et al. Carcinoma of the esophagus: A comparison of the results of transhiatal vs. transthoracic resection. *Ann Thorac Surg* 1989;**47**:700-5.
17. Pac M, Basoglu A, Keles M, et al. Transhiatal versus transthoracic esophagectomy for esophageal cancer. *J Thorac Cardiovasc Surg* 1993;**106**:205-9.
18. Stark S, Romberg M, Thomas J, et al. Transhiatal versus transthoracic esophagectomy for adenocarcinoma of the distal esophagus and cardia. *Am J Surg* 1996;**172**:478-82.
19. Rindani R, Martin C, Cox M. Transhiatal versus Ivor-Lewis oesophagectomy: is there a difference?. *Aust N Z J Surg* 1999;**69**:187-94.
20. Hulscher J, Tijssen J, Lanschot J. Transthoracic versus transhiatal resection for carcinoma of the esophagus: A meta-analysis. *Ann Thorac Surg* 2001;**72**:306-13.
21. Orringer MB, Marshall B, Chang AC, et al. Two thousand transhiatal esophagectomies: changing trends, lessons learned. *Ann Surg* 2007;**246**:363-74.
22. Wolff CS, Castillo SF, Larson DR, et al. Ivor Lewis approach is superior to transhiatal approach in retrieval of lymph nodes at esophagectomy. *Disease Esoph* 2008;**21**:328-33.
23. Ac Chang, Ji H, Birkmeyer NJ, Orringer MB, Birkmeyer JD. Outcomes after transhiatal and transthoracic esophagectomy for cancer. *Ann Thorac Surg* 2008;**85**:424-9.
24. Goldminc M, Maddern G, Le Prise E, Meunier B, Campion JP, Launois B. Oesophagectomy by a transhiatal approach or thoracotomy: A prospective randomized trial. *Br J Surg* 1993;**80**:367-76.
25. Chu K, Law S, Wong J, et al. A prospective randomized comparison of transhiatal and transthoracic resection for lower-third esophageal carcinoma. *Am J Surg* 1997;**174**:320-4.
26. Omloo JM, Lagarde SM, Hulscher JB, et al. Extended transthoracic resection compared with limited transhiatal resection for adenocarcinoma of the mid/distal esophagus. *Ann Surg* 2007;**246**:992-1001.
27. Hulscher J, Van Sandick J, Van Lanschot J. Extended transthoracic resection compared with limited transhiatal resection for adenocarcinoma of the esophagus. *N Engl J Med* 2002;**347**:1662-9.
28. Litle VR, Buenaventura PO, Luketich JD. Minimally invasive resection for esophageal cancer. *Surg Clin N Am* 2002;**82**:711-28.
29. Fabian T, Martin J, Katigbak M, McKelvey AA, Federico J. Thoracoscopic mobilization during minimally invasive esophagectomy: a head-to-head comparison of prone versus decubitus positions. *Surg Endosc* 2008;**11**:2485-9.
30. Bizekis G, Kent M, Luketich JD, Buenaventura PO, Landreneau R, Schuchert MJ, Alvelo-Rivera M. Initial experience with minimally invasive Ivor Lewis esophagectomy. *Ann Thorac Surg* 2006;**82**:402-7.
31. Benzoni E, Bresadola V, Terrosu G, Uzzau A, Cedolini C, Intini S, et al. Minimally invasive esophagectomy: a comparative study of transhiatal laparoscopic approach versus laparoscopic right transthoracic esophagectomy. *Surg Laparosc Endosc Percutan Tech* 2008;**2**:178-87.

32. Dapri G, Himpens J, Cadière GB. Minimally invasive esophagectomy for cancer: laparoscopic transhiatal procedure or thoracoscopy in prone position followed by laparoscopy?. *Surg Endosc* 2007;**4**:1060-9.
33. Galvani CA, Gorodner MV, Moser F, Jacobsen G, Chretien C, Espat NJ, et al. Robotically assisted laparoscopic transhiatal esophagectomy. *Surg Endosc* 2008;**1**:188-95.
34. Bonavina L, Incarbone R, Bona D, Peracchia A. Esophagectomy via laparoscopy and transmediastinal endodissection. *J Laparoendosc Adv Surg Tech* 2004;**14**:13-6.
35. Luketich JD, Alvelo-Rivera M, Buenaventura PO, et al. Minimally invasive esophagectomy: outcomes in 222 patients. *Ann Surg* 2003;**238**:486-94.
36. Bailey SH, Bull DA, Harpole DH, et al. Outcomes after esophagectomy: a ten-year prospective cohort. *Ann Thorac Surg* 2003;**75**:217-22.
37. Perry Y, Fernando HC, Buenaventura PO, Christie NA, Luketich JD. Minimally invasive esophagectomy in the elderly. *JSLS* 2002;**6**:299-304.
38. Nguyen NT, Follette DM, Wolfe BM, et al. Comparison of minimally invasive esophagectomy with transthoracic and transhiatal esophagectomy. *Arch Surg* 2000;**135**:920-5.
39. Law S, Fok M, Chu KM, Wong J. Thoracoscopic esophagectomy for esophageal cancer. *Surgery* 1997;**122**:8-14.
40. Bernabe KQ, Bolton JS, Richardson WS. Laparoscopic hand assisted vs open transhiatal esophagectomy: a case-control study. *Surg Endosc* 2005;**19**: 334-7.
41. Smithers BM, Gotley DC, Martin I, Thomas JM. Comparison of the outcomes between open and minimally invasive esophagectomy. *Ann Surg* 2007;**245**: 232-40.
42. Gemmill EH, McCulloch P. Systematic review of minimally invasive resection for gastro-oesophageal cancer. *Br J Surg* 2007;**94**:1461-7.
43. Altorki N, Girardi L, Skinner D. En bloc esophagectomy improves survival for stage III esophageal cancer. *J Thorac Cardiovasc Surg* 1997;**114**:948-56.
44. Hagen J, Peters J, DeMeester T. Superiority of extended en bloc esophagogastrectomy for carcinoma of the lower esophagus and cardia. *J Thorac Cardiovasc Surg* 1993;**106**:850-9.
45. Akiyama H, Tsurumaru M. Ono Y: Principles of surgical treatment for carcinoma of the esophagus. *Ann Surg* 1981;**194**:438-46.
46. Altorki N, Skinner D. Occult cervical nodal metastasis in esophageal cancer: preliminary results of three-field lymphadenectomy. *J Thorac Cardiovasc Surg* 1997;**113**:540-4.
47. Ando N, Ozawa S, Kitajima M. Improvement in the results of surgical treatment of advanced squamous esophageal carcinoma during 15 consecutive years. *Ann Surg* 2000;**232**:225-32.
48. Akiyama H, Tsurumaru M. Kajiyama Y: Radical lymph node dissection for cancer of the thoracic esophagus. *Ann Surg* 1994;**220**:364-72.
49. Nishimake T, Tanaka O, Suzuki T, et al. Patterns of lymphatic spread in thoracic esophageal cancer. *Cancer* 1994;**74**:4-11.
50. Altorki N, Kent M, Port J. Three-field lymph node dissection for squamous cell and adenocarcinoma of the esophagus. *Ann Surg* 2002;**236**:177-83.
51. Orringer M, Marshall B, Iannettoni M. Transhiatal esophagectomy: clinical experience and refinements. *Ann Surg* 1999;**230**:392-403.
52. Rizk N, Venkatraman E, Park B, et al. The prognostic importance of the number of involved lymph nodes in esophageal cancer: implications for revisions of the American Joint Committee on Cancer staging system. *J Thorac Cardovasc Surg* 2006;**132**:1374-81.
53. Greenstein A, Litle VR, Swanson SJ, et al. Effect of the number of lymph nodes sampled on postoperative survival of lymph node–negative esophageal cancer. *Cancer* 2008;**112**:1239-46.
54. Peyre CG, Hagen JA, DeMeester SR, et al. The number of lymph nodes removed predicts survival in esophageal cancer: an international study on the impact and extent of surgical resection. *Ann Surg* 2008;**248**:549-56.
55. Altorki NK, Zhou XK, Stiles B, et al. Total number of resected lymph nodes predicts survival in esophageal cancer. *Ann Surg* 2008;**248**:221-6.
56. Coleman J, Searless J, Jurkiewicz M, et al. Ten years experience with the free jejunal autograft. *Am J Surg* 1987;**154**:394-8.
57. McConnel R, Hester R, Jurkiewicz M, et al. Free jejunal grafts for reconstruction of pharynx and cervical esophagus. *Arch Otolaryngol* 1981;**107**:476-81.
58. Earlam R, Cunha-Melo J. Oesophageal squamous cell carcinoma: I. A critical review of surgery. *Br J Surg* 1980;**67**:381-90.
59. Giuli R, Gignoux M. Treatment of carcinoma of the esophagus. Retrospective study of 2400 patients. *Ann Surg* 1980;**192**:44-52.
60. Muller J, Erasmi H, Pichlmaier H, et al. Surgical therapy of oesophageal carcinoma. *Br J Surg* 1990;**77**:845-57.
61. Ellis H, Krasna M. Esophagogastrectomy for carcinoma of the esophagus and cardia: A comparison of findings and results after standard resection in three consecutive eight-year intervals with improved staging criteria. *J Thorac Cardiovasc Surg* 1997;**113**:836-46.
62. Luft H, Bunker J, Enthoven A. Should operations be regionalized? The empirical relation between surgical volume and mortality. *N Engl J Med* 1979;**25**:1364-9.
63. Chang AC, Birkmeyer JD. The volume-performance relationship in esophagectomy. *Thorac Surg Clinic* 2006;**16**:87-94.
64. Birkmeyer JD, Siewers AE, Finlayson EVA, et al. Hospital volume and surgical mortality in the United states. *N Engl J Med* 2002;**15**:1128-37.
65. Birkmeyer JD, Stukel TA, Siewers AE, et al. Surgeon volume and operative mortality in the United States. *N Engl J Med* 2003;**349**:2117-27.
66. Finlayson E, Fan Z, Birkmeyer JD. Outcomes in octogenarians undergoing high-risk cancer operations: a national study. *J Am Coll Surg* 2007;**205**:729-34.
67. Urschel J. Esophagogastrostomy anastomotic leaks complicating esophagectomy: A review. *Am J Surg* 1995;**169**:634-9.
68. Patil P, Patel S, Desai P. Cancer of the esophagus: esophagogastric anastomotic leak—a retrospective study of predisposing factors. *J Surg Oncol* 1992;**49**: 163-7.
69. Law S, Fok M, Wong J, et al. Comparison of hand-sewn and stapled esophagogastric anastomosis after esophageal resection for cancer. A prospective randomized controlled trial. *Ann Surg* 1997;**226**:169-73.
70. Behzadi A, Nichols FC, Cassivi SD, et al. Esophagogastrectomy: influence of stapled vs. hand-sewn anastomosis on outcome. *J Gastrointest Surg* 2005;**9**:1031-42.
71. Martin LW, Swisher SG, Hofstetter W, et al. Intrathoracic leaks following esophagectomy are no longer associated with increased mortality. *Ann Surg* 2005;**242**:392-9.
72. Sarela AI, Tolan DJ, Harris K, et al. Anastomotic leakage after esophagectomy for cancer: a mortality-free experience. *J Am Coll Surg* 2008;**206**:516-23.
73. Kauer WK, Stein HJ, Dittler HJ, Siewert JR. Stent implantation as a treatment option in patients with thoracic anastomotic leaks after esophagectomy. *Surg Endosc* 2008;**22**:50-3.
74. Tuebergen D, Rijcken E, Mennigen R, Hopkins AM, Senninger N, Bruewer MJ. Treatment of thoracic esophageal anastomotic leaks and esophageal perforations with endoluminal stents: efficacy and current limitations. *Gastrointest Surg* 2008;**7**:1168-76.
75. Freeman RK, Ascioti AJ, Wozniak TC. Postoperative esophageal leak management with the Polyflex esophageal stent. *J Thorac Cardiovasc Surg* 2007;**2**:333-8.
76. Schubert D, Scheidbach H, Kuhn R, Wex C, Weiss G, Eder F, et al. Endoscopic treatment of thoracic esophageal anastomotic leaks by using silicone-covered, self-expanding polyester stents. *Gastrointest Endosc* 2005;**7**:891-6.
77. Vigneswaran W, Trastek V, Pairolero P. Transhiatal esophagectomy for carcinoma of the esophagus. *Ann Thorac Surg* 1993;**56**:838-46.
78. Mk Ferguson, Durkin AE. Preoperative prediction of the risk of pulmonary complications after esophagectomy for cancer. *J Thorac Cardiovasc Surg* 2002;**1223**:661-9.
79. Avendano CE, Flume PA, Silvestri GA, et al. Pulmonary complications after esophagectomy. *Ann Thorac Surg* 2002;**73**:922-6.
80. Cope C, Kaiser L. Management of unremitting chylothorax by percutaneous embolization and blockage of retroperitoneal lymphatic vessels in 42 patients. *J Vasc Interv Radiol* 2002;**13**:1139-48.
81. Ferguson MK, Martin TR, Reeder LB, et al. Mortality after esophagectomy: risk factor analysis. *World J Surg* 1997;**21**:599-604.
82. Ritchie AJ, Whiteside M, Tolan M, et al. Cardiac dysrhythmia in total thoracic oesophagectomy. A prospective study. *Eur J Cardiothoracic Surg* 1993;**7**: 420-2.
83. Murthy SC, Law S, Whooley BP, et al. Atrial fibrillation after esophagectomy is a marker for postoperative morbidity and mortality. *J Thorac Cardiovasc Surg* 2003;**126**:1162-7.
84. Malhotra SK, Kaur RP, Gupta NM, et al. Incidence and types of arrhythmia after mediastinal manipulation during transhiatal esophagectomy. *Ann Thorac Surg* 2007;**82**:298-302.
85. Whooley BP, Law S, Murthy SC, et al. Analysis of reduced death and complication rates after esophageal resection. *Ann Surg* 2001;**233**:338-44.
86. Law S, Wong KH, Kwok KF, et al. Predictive factors for postoperative pulmonary complications and mortality after esophagectomy for cancer. *Ann Surg* 2004;**240**:791-800.
87. Sedrakyan A, Treasure T, Browne J, et al. Pharmacologic prophylaxis for postoperative atrial tachyarrhythmias in general thoracic surgery: evidence from randomized clinical trials. *J Thorac Cardiovasc Surg* 2005;**129**:997-1005.
88. Devereaux PJ, Yang H, Guyatt GH, et al. POISE Trial Investigators. Rationale, design, and organization of the PeriOperative Ischemic Evaluation (POISE) trial: a randomized controlled trial of metoprolol vs placebo in patients undergoing noncardiac surgery. *Am Heart J* 2006;**152**:223-30.
89. Honkoop P, Siersema P, van Blankenstein M, et al. Benign anastomotic strictures after transhiatal esophagectomy and cervical esophagogastrotomy: Risk factors and management. *J Thorac Cardiovasc Surg* 1996;**111**:1141-6.

90. Dewar L, Gelfand G, Finley R. Factors affecting cervical anastomotic leak and stricture formation following esophagogastrectomy and gastric tube interposition. *Am J Surg* 1992;**163**:484-9.
91. Pierie J, de Graaf P, Poen H, et al. Incidence and management of benign anastomotic stricture after cervical oesophagogastrostomy. *Br J Surg* 1993;**80**:471-4.
92. Orringer M, Lemmer J. Early dilatation in the treatment of esophageal disruption. *Ann Thorac Surg* 1986;**42**:536-9.
93. Blackmon SH, Correa AM, Wynn B, et al. Propensity-matched analysis of three techniques for intrathoracic esophagogastric anastomosis. *Ann Thorac Surg* 2007;**83**:1805-13.
94. Martin RE, Letsos P, Taves DH, Inculet RI, Johnston H, Preiksaitis HG. Oropharyngeal dysphagia in esophageal cancer before and after transhiatal esophagectomy. *Dysphagia* 2001;**16**:23-31.
95. Koh P, Turnbull G, Attia E, Le Brun P, Casson AG. Functional assessment of the cervical esophagus after gastric transposition and cervical esophagogastrostomy. *Eur J Cardiothorac Surg* 2004;**25**:480-5.
96. Barthel JS, Kelley ST, Klapman JB. Management of persistent gastroesophageal anastomotic strictures with removable self-expandable polyester silicon-covered (Polyflex) stents: an alternative to dilation. *Gastrointest Endosc* 2008;**67**:546-52.
97. Romagnoli R, Bechi P, Salizzoni M. Combined 24-hour intraluminal pH and bile monitoring of the denervated whole stomach as an esophageal substitute. *Hepatogastroenterology* 1999;**46**:86-91.
98. Turnball A, Ginsberg R. Options in the surgical treatment of esophageal carcinoma. *Chest Surg Clin North Am* 1994;**4**:315-29.
99. Dragstedt L, Camp E. Follow up of gastric vagotomy alone in the treatment of peptic ulcer. *Gastroenterology* 1948;**11**:460-5.
100. Gupta M, Chattopadhyay T, Sharma L. Emptying of the intrathoracic stomach with and without pyloroplasty. *Am J Gastroenterol* 1989;**84**:921-3.
101. Huang G, Zhang D, Zhang D. A comparative study of resection of carcinoma of the esophagus with and without pyloroplasty. In: DeMeester T, Skinner D, editors. *Esophageal Disorders*. Pathophysiology. New York: Raven Press; 1985, p. 383-8.
102. Fok M, Cheng S, Wong J. Pyloroplasty versus no drainage in gastric replacement of the esophagus. *Am J Surg* 1991;**162**:447-52.
103. Law S, Cheung M, Wong J. Pyloroplasty and pyloromyotomy in gastric replacement of the esophagus after esophagectomy: a randomized controlled trial. *J Am Coll Surg* 1997;**184**:630-6.
104. Kim J, Lee H, Kim MS, Lee JM, et al. Balloon dilation of the pylorus for delayed gastric emptying after esophagectomy. *Eur J Cardiothorac Surg* 2008;**33**:1105-11.
105. Bemelman W, Taat C, Slors F. Delayed postoperative emptying after esophageal resection is dependent on the size of the gastric substitute. *J Am Coll Surg* 1995;**180**:461-4.
106. Tam P, Cheung H, Wong J, et al. Local recurrences after subtotal esophagectomy for squamous cell carcinoma. *Ann Surg* 1987;**205**:189-94.
107. Siu K, Cheung H, Wong J. Shrinkage of the esophagus after resection for carcinoma. *Ann Surg* 1986;**203**:173-6.
108. Papachristou D. Histologically positive esophageal margin in the surgical treatment of gastric cancer. *Am J Surg* 1980;**139**:711.
109. Urba S, Orringer M, Turrisi A. Randomized trial of preoperative chemoradiation versus surgery alone in patients with locoregional esophageal carcinoma. *J Clin Oncol* 2001;**19**:305-13.
110. Bosset J, Gignoux M, Triboulet J. Chemoradiotherapy followed by surgery compared with surgery alone in squamous-cell cancer of the esophagus. *N Engl J Med* 1997;**337**:161-7.
111. Walsh T, Noonan N, Hennessy T. A comparison of multimodal therapy and surgery for esophageal adenocarcinoma. *N Engl J Med* 1996;**335**:462-7.

CHAPTER 39
Neoadjuvant and Adjuvant Therapy for Esophageal Cancer
G. Kwame Yankey and Mark J. Krasna

Staging Modalities
Multimodality Therapy Approaches to Surgical Management
  Neoadjuvant Radiotherapy
  Neoadjuvant Chemotherapy
Neoadjuvant Chemoradiotherapy
Postoperative Adjuvant Therapy
  Adjuvant Radiotherapy
  Adjuvant Chemotherapy
  Adjuvant Chemoradiotherapy
Nonsurgical Management
  Radiotherapy
  Chemoradiotherapy
Treatment of Esophageal Cancer by Stage
Conclusion

Esophageal cancer is the sixth most common malignant neoplasm in the world. Historically, squamous cell carcinoma of the esophagus has been prevalent in patients with heavy alcohol and smoking abuse. During the past 20 years, adenocarcinoma of the distal esophagus and the gastroesophageal junction has increased in incidence about 10- to 20-fold in North America and Europe, replacing squamous cell carcinoma as the most common esophageal malignant neoplasm.[1] Chronic gastroesophageal reflux disease, Barrett's dysplasia, obesity, and smoking have been shown to be risk factors associated with esophageal adenocarcinoma.

Esophageal cancer is usually diagnosed late in its course, when symptoms appear. Most patients in the United States present with stage IIB, III, or IV. The diagnosis is made with upper endoscopy and biopsy. Pretreatment staging is performed to determine tumor (T), node (N), and metastasis (M) status. T status can be predicted by endoscopic ultrasonography (EUS), computed tomography (CT), and bronchoscopy. M status can be predicted by CT and positron emission tomography (PET). N status can be predicted reliably by video-assisted thoracoscopy and laparoscopy.

Surgery, chemoradiotherapy, and a combination of these techniques are the treatments for locally advanced esophageal cancer. The 5-year survival with multimodality treatment of esophageal cancer is about 20%. However, despite a large number of clinical trials and retrospective reviews, no treatment modality has proved superior. Current trials have focused on adding chemotherapy with or without radiation to resection to down-stage the primary tumor, to eliminate micrometastases, and to improve overall survival.

STAGING MODALITIES

One of the challenges in the management of esophageal cancer is the lack of clear prognostic data based on clinical staging. Most results are presented as part of pathologic staging results. Noninvasive tests routinely used in staging of esophageal cancer include esophagogastroduodenoscopy, CT, and recent advances in PET.

CT scan of the thorax and abdomen should be performed to stage the tumor, lymph node metastases, and distant metastases.[2] Whereas CT is highly effective in the assessment of mediastinal esophageal carcinomas, it is less helpful in the staging of cervical or gastroesophageal junction carcinomas. Metastasis to celiac lymph nodes occurs most frequently with distal esophageal neoplasms (75%) and is present in nearly one third of patients with tumors of the proximal esophagus. Absence of fat planes is most often observed where the esophagus is in contact with the aorta, trachea, left main-stem bronchus, and left atrium. CT is very accurate in determining the presence of liver and adrenal gland metastasis.

EUS, one of the newer modalities for staging of esophageal cancer, uses the technologies of flexible endoscopy and ultrasonic imaging.[3] By virtue of its ability to depict the various histologic layers of the esophageal wall and periesophageal tissues, EUS has proved useful in staging of esophageal cancer. EUS seems to be more accurate than CT in the diagnosis of very early or advanced stage of disease. Lymph nodes at a distance of more than 2 cm from the esophageal lumen cannot be imaged because of the very limited penetration depth of ultrasound. Tumor invasion into the tracheobronchial system should be further evaluated by bronchoscopy with transbronchial fine-needle aspiration (FNA) for confirmation of the diagnosis.

PET has been used to detect and to stage esophageal cancer. Block and coworkers[4] compared CT and PET in staging of esophageal cancer. Among 58 patients, the uptake of fluorodeoxyglucose was increased at the site of the primary tumor in 56 patients. PET identified metastatic disease in 17 patients, whereas CT detected metastases in only five. Pathologic lymph node metastases were found in 21 patients. These nodes were detected by PET in 11 patients and by CT in six. For CT and PET together, the accuracy is nearly 92%. Luketich and associates[5] found that for distant metastases, the sensitivity, specificity, and accuracy of PET were 88%, 93%, and 91%, respectively. For local-regional nodal metastases, the sensitivity, specificity, and accuracy were 45%, 100%, and 48%, respectively, suggesting that small local-regional nodal metastases cannot be identified by current PET technology. Recently, there has been additional interest in the utility of PET after neoadjuvant therapy as a means of predicting response to therapy. The predictive values for predicting microscopic residual disease remain wanting at present.

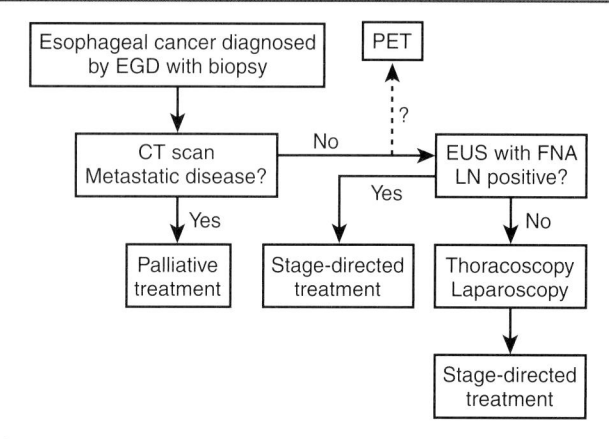

Figure 39-1
Proposed staging algorithm for esophageal cancer. CT, computed tomography; EGD, esophagogastroduodenoscopy; EUS, endoscopic ultrasonography; FNA, fine-needle aspiration; LN, lymph node; PET, positron emission tomography.

The use of EUS-guided FNA was reported in the diagnosis of esophageal cancer recurrence after distal esophageal resection and as a way of identifying and confirming mediastinal lymph node involvement, which is often crucial in planning the strategy of treatment, particularly before surgery. This advance has resulted in a change of our use of thoracoscopic and laparoscopic staging in esophageal cancer. EUS-FNA is currently able to achieve accurate lymph node staging in approximately 75% of patients (Fig. 39-1).

Many surgical studies show significant stratification of survival after resection of esophageal cancer based on accurate pathologic staging. Preoperative minimally invasive surgical staging in esophageal cancer may solve this problem just as the successful use of mediastinoscopy did in preoperative staging for lung cancer. Murray and associates[6] first reported their experience with minimally invasive surgical staging for esophageal cancer in 1977. With use of mediastinoscopy and mini-laparotomy, seven patients had positive lymph nodes by mediastinoscopy and 16 had celiac lymph nodes identified. Dagnini and colleagues[7] did routine laparoscopy in 369 patients with esophageal cancer and noted intra-abdominal metastases in 14% and celiac lymph node metastases in 9.7%.

With advances in thoracoscopic and laparoscopic techniques, thoracoscopy and laparoscopy have been used for staging of esophageal cancer. Successful combined thoracoscopy and laparoscopy for staging of disease in the chest and abdomen was evaluated in a follow-up series from three institutions of the Cancer and Leukemia Group B (CALGB) with an accuracy of more than 90%.[8] A more recent report of 65 patients showed a 94% accuracy with laparoscopy and 91% accuracy with thoracoscopy in esophageal cancer staging. This study also demonstrated that clinical stage evaluation based on noninvasive diagnostic methods including CT, MRI, and EUS may be used to guide surgeons to focus on the suspicious areas for the highest-yield biopsy targets in thoracoscopic and laparoscopic staging.[9] The main advantage of the thoracoscopic and laparoscopic staging procedure is that it provides greater accuracy in evaluation of regional and celiac lymph nodes. Such information is important in stratification of patients and selection of therapy, especially in the setting of new treatment protocols. Furthermore, the histologic status of mediastinal and abdominal lymph nodes is critical for the design of the field for irradiation. It allows dose delivery to be maximized to areas of known disease while minimizing dose to surrounding sensitive, normal tissue.[10]

MULTIMODALITY THERAPY APPROACHES TO SURGICAL MANAGEMENT

Neoadjuvant Radiotherapy

Preoperative radiation therapy is designed to reduce the tumor size and risk of tumor spread during surgical manipulation. Five published randomized trials compared neoadjuvant radiation followed by surgery versus surgery alone. None of the trials demonstrated survival benefit with preoperative radiation with the exception of the study by Nygaard and coworkers.[11] The study by Nygaard has been widely criticized for using different doses and fractionation schedules and cross-analysis of the results from four different treatment groups. A meta-analysis from the Esophageal Cancer Collaborative Group concluded that survival is not improved with neoadjuvant radiotherapy and should not be recommended for patients for whom surgical resection is indicated.

Neoadjuvant Chemotherapy

The purported benefit of preoperative chemotherapy is the elimination of micrometastases, down-staging of the tumor, reduction of tumor recurrences, and improved surgical resectability. In patients with localized, resectable tumors, chemotherapy-related toxicity can occasionally result in prolonged delay or even cancellation of planned surgical resection, risking further spread of disease. The resulting need for careful selection of patients for participation in clinical trials of preoperative chemotherapy can bias treatment results. Chemotherapy is usually given in a combination of two or more drugs; cisplatin and 5-fluorouracil are the most frequently used agents. Other agents active against metastatic esophageal cancer with radiosensitization include bleomycin, mitomycin C, carboplatin, and taxol.

Several randomized prospective trials comparing neoadjuvant chemotherapy plus surgery with surgical resection alone have been published with mixed results (Table 39-1). The two largest trials were conducted in the United States and United Kingdom by the multicenter North American Intergroup (INT 0113) and the U.K. Medical Research Council Group (MRC OE02), respectively. The U.S. Intergroup randomized 467 patients with resectable esophageal adenocarcinoma (54%) and squamous cell carcinoma (46%). The study compared three cycles of neoadjuvant cisplatin and 5-fluorouracil followed by surgery and additional chemotherapy (cisplatin and 5-fluorouracil) with surgery alone. The results reported by Kelsen and associates[12] showed that 2-year survival rates were 35% and 37% without a statistically significant difference in the overall survival between the two treatment groups. The MRC group randomized 802 patients with resectable esophageal adenocarcinoma (67%) and squamous cell carcinoma (33%) to two cycles of cisplatin and 5-fluorouracil plus surgery and surgery alone. An intent-to-treat analysis indicated that patients who received preoperative chemotherapy had a significant median (17.2 months versus 13.3 months) and 2-year (43% versus 34%) improvement in the survival rate.[13] Although the neoadjuvant chemotherapy arm had a survival advantage, the survival

Table 39-1
Randomized Trials of Neoadjuvant Chemotherapy Versus Surgery Alone in Resectable Esophageal Carcinoma

Study	Year	No.	CT	pCR (%)	Median Survival (months) S	Median Survival (months) CT + S	Survival S	Survival CT + S
Law	1997	147	CDDP, 5-FU	6.7	13	16.8	2 yr: 31%	2 yr: 44%
Kok	1997	160	CDDP, eto	8.6	11	18.5	NS	NS
Kelsen	1998	467	CDDP, 5-FU	2.5	16.1	14.9	2 yr: 37%	2 yr: 35%
Ancona	2001	96	CDDP, 5-FU	12.8	24	25	3 yr: 41%	3 yr: 44%
MRC	2002	802	CDDP, 5-FU	NS	13.3	17.2	2 yr: 34%	2 yr: 43%

CDDP, cisplatin; CT, chemotherapy; CT + S, neoadjuvant chemotherapy and surgery; eto, etoposide; 5-FU, 5-fluorouracil; NS, not stated; pCR, pathologic complete response; S, surgery alone.

Table 39-2
Randomized Trials of Neoadjuvant Chemoradiotherapy Versus Surgery Alone in Resectable Esophageal Cancer

Study	Year	No.	Preoperative CT	Preoperative RT (Gy)	pCR (%)	Median Survival (months) S	Median Survival (months) CRT + S	Survival at 3 Years (%) S	Survival at 3 Years (%) CRT + S
Nygaard	1992	88	cis, bleo	35	NS	6	7	9	17
Le Prise	1994	86	cis, FU	20	10	10	11	14	19
Apinop	1994	69	cis, FU	40	2	7	10	20	26
Walsh	1996	113	cis, FU	40	22	11	16	6	32
Bosset	1997	282	cis	37	20	18	19	34	36
Urba	2001	100	cis, FU, V	45	28	18	17	16	30
Burmeister	2005	200	cis, FU	35	15	19	22	—	—

bleo, bleomycin; cis, cisplatin; CRT + S, neoadjuvant chemoradiotherapy and surgery; CT, chemotherapy; FU, 5-fluorouracil; pCR, pathologic complete response; RT, radiotherapy; S, surgery alone; V, vinblastine.

data for 3 and 5 years are not yet available. It is unclear why the survival rate in the chemotherapy arm from this study is different from that of the U.S. Intergroup trial; further details from the U.K. MRC trial are worth reviewing. In the United States, preoperative chemotherapy is considered investigational and not the standard of care in management of esophageal cancer.

Neoadjuvant Chemoradiotherapy

Several trials have shown that neoadjuvant radiotherapy and chemotherapy alone do not improve overall long-term survival of patients with esophageal cancer, but the addition of radiation to a chemotherapeutic regimen before esophagectomy can down-stage the primary tumor, increase the resectability rate, eliminate or minimize micrometastases, and improve overall survival.

Chemotherapeutic agents such as cisplatin, 5-fluorouracil, bleomycin, mitomycin C, carboplatin, and taxol are radiosensitizers. When they are given concurrently with radiation, a synergistic effect is provided.

Several clinical trials have been conducted in which chemoradiotherapy was given before surgery to take advantage of the radiosensitizing benefits. Seven randomized prospective trials comparing neoadjuvant chemoradiotherapy plus surgery with surgical resection alone have been published (Table 39-2). With the exception of the study by Walsh, none of the trials demonstrated survival benefit from neoadjuvant chemoradiotherapy compared with surgery alone.

In 1996, Walsh and colleagues[14] from Ireland randomized 113 patients with adenocarcinoma to receive preoperative cisplatin and 5-fluorouracil with radiotherapy (58 patients) or surgery alone (55 patients). An intent-to-treat analysis indicated that patients who received preoperative chemoradiotherapy had a median survival of 16 months versus 11 months for the group treated with surgery alone and a 3-year survival rate of 32% versus 6%, respectively. The difference reached a statistical significance at 3 years ($P = .01$), and this trial remained one of the few to show survival advantage to preoperative chemoradiotherapy. This trial has been criticized for the extremely low 3-year survival rate of the surgery-alone control group, which is lower than that of the U.S. Intergroup

Table 39-3
Randomized Trials of Adjuvant Radiation Therapy Versus Surgery Alone in Resectable Esophageal Cancer

Study	Year	No.	RT (cGy)	Mortality (%)	Median Survival (months)	Survival at 3 Years (%)
Teniere	1991	102	4500-5500	1	18	26
		119	0	0	18	24
Fok	1993	30	4900	0	15	24
		30	0	0	21	28
Zieren	1995	33	5600	0	NA	22
		35	0	0	NA	20

RT, radiotherapy.

trial (23%). There were some concerns about the reliability of the results. The concerns were focused on the nonuniform systemic staging, large number of withdrawals, inclusion of patients who underwent inadequate surgical resections, and flawed statistical analysis.

Given the conflicting results of various randomized trials to address the role of preoperative chemoradiotherapy, the U.S. Intergroup developed a prospective randomized trial (CALGB C9781) in 1998. The patients were randomized to receive surgery alone or two cycles of cisplatin and 5-fluorouracil with concurrent radiotherapy followed by surgery. Five hundred patients were targeted to enroll with 3 years of follow-up; the primary endpoint was the overall survival. The trial was closed prematurely after 2 years because of lack of accrual, and a total of 56 patients were entered in the study. Results from the CALGB C9781 were presented at the American Society of Clinical Oncology symposium at San Francisco in January 2006. An intent-to-treat analysis showed a median survival of 4.5 years versus 1.8 years in favor of trimodality therapy (log rank P = .020). The 5-year survival was 39% versus 16% in favor of trimodality therapy, with analysis of progression-free survival under way.[15]

Various meta-analyses of published randomized trials have been performed in an attempt to clarify the survival advantage of neoadjuvant chemoradiotherapy. Greer and colleagues[16] analyzed six trials with a total of 738 patients, and only one of six showed a statistically significant survival benefit. The composite analysis showed a relative ratio of death of 0.86 (95% confidence interval [CI], 0.74-1.01) in favor of trimodality therapy. Fiorica and coworkers[17] analyzed six trials with a total of 768 patients, and the 3-year odds ratio for mortality (0.53) favored trimodality treatment. Urschél and Vasan[18] analyzed nine trials with 1116 patients, and the 3-year odds ratio for survival (0.66) favored trimodality.

The cumulative data from various trials and institutional experiences serve to suggest that neoadjuvant chemoradiotherapy followed by surgical resection provides more survival benefit than surgery alone. In many esophageal centers in the United States, trimodality therapy is the standard of care for locally advanced esophageal cancer (stage IIB-III).

Various trials have indicated that patients who have a pathologic complete response survive longer than do patients who have surgery alone and incomplete responders who received preoperative chemoradiotherapy (64% vs. 19% at 3 years, respectively, in the Urba trial[19]). However, increasing evidence from studies suggests that incomplete pathologic responders not only derive no benefit from neoadjuvant chemoradiotherapy but in fact have a worse prognosis than those who undergo surgical resection. Several studies are under way to determine the most applicable regimen that is needed to raise the pathologic complete response rate and the predictors for response to treatment to improve selection of patients for the chemoradiotherapy regimen.

POSTOPERATIVE ADJUVANT THERAPY

Adjuvant Radiotherapy

Radiotherapy after esophagectomy has been suggested to sterilize occult micrometastases and therefore increase cure rate and prolong survival. Three published prospective randomized trials compared adjuvant radiotherapy after surgery with surgery alone (Table 39-3). The data from these studies indicated that postoperative radiation after curative esophagectomy for cancer provided no overall survival benefit but may be harmful from the significant side effects from the radiation. A study published by Xiao and coworkers[20] in 2003 randomized 495 patients with esophageal cancer to surgery plus adjuvant radiotherapy or surgery alone. The study showed that the overall 5-year survival rate for the surgery plus radiotherapy versus surgery-alone group was 41.3% versus 31.7%, respectively, concluding that adjuvant radiotherapy provides a better survival rate than surgery alone does. The reliability of the results has been questioned because of the statistical analysis of the patients, the skewed distribution of patients, and the large number of and the rationale for withdrawals from the study.

Adjuvant Chemotherapy

There has been only one published prospective randomized trial comparing adjuvant chemotherapy with surgery alone in resectable esophageal cancer by Ando and colleagues[21] in 1997. The study was conducted by the Japanese Cooperative Oncology Group, and the group used cisplatinum and vindesine as the postoperative treatment after esophagectomy. Of the 205 patients randomized, 100 had surgery alone and 105 had adjuvant chemotherapy, with a median follow-up of 59 months. The 5-year survival was 45% for surgery alone versus

48% for the surgery and chemotherapy group. There was no significant difference in the median survival and 5-year survival. This study suggested that adjuvant chemotherapy after resectable esophageal cancer provided no survival benefit.

Adjuvant Chemoradiotherapy

A prospective randomized trial comparing adjuvant chemoradiotherapy with surgery alone in locoregionally advanced esophageal cancer was published by Rice and associates[22] in 2003. Eighty-three patients were randomized (31 received adjuvant therapy and 52 received surgery alone). The risk-unadjusted median survival and 4-year survival for those receiving adjuvant chemoradiotherapy versus esophagectomy alone were 28 months versus 14 months and 44% versus 17%, respectively. The data from the study indicate that adjuvant chemoradiotherapy provides an overall survival benefit for patients with locoregionally advanced esophageal cancer.

NONSURGICAL MANAGEMENT

Radiotherapy

Radiation has been used primarily to palliate symptoms of pain, bleeding, and dysphagia in patients with unresectable advanced esophageal cancer and comorbid medical conditions. The radiotherapy regimen for palliation varies from 30 Gy to 60 Gy for a period of 2 to 6 weeks, depending on the patient's performance. Given the poor survival benefit of radiotherapy alone for esophageal cancer (median survival of 6 months), it is used in combination with concurrent chemotherapy.

Chemoradiotherapy

Various randomized trials have been conducted to determine the survival benefit of concurrent chemoradiotherapy versus radiotherapy in nonsurgical management of advanced esophageal cancer. A prospective trial, the Intergroup study RTOG 85-01, published by al-Sarraf and colleagues,[23] randomized 123 patients with locally advanced esophageal cancer into chemoradiotherapy (61 patients) and radiotherapy-alone groups. The median survival and 5-year survival for patients who received chemoradiotherapy versus radiotherapy was 14 months versus 9 months and 26% versus 0%, respectively. The patients who received concurrent chemoradiotherapy had a significant improvement in median survival and 5-year survival, although there was a high local failure rate of about 45%. On the basis of these data and other published studies, the standard of care for nonsurgical management of advanced esophageal cancer is concurrent chemoradiotherapy.[23]

TREATMENT OF ESOPHAGEAL CANCER BY STAGE

The success rate for treatment of esophageal cancer with surgery alone is related to the disease stage. For most patients with localized esophageal cancer, surgical resection affords the best chance for local control and the best means of palliation of dysphagia. In all but the earliest stages of esophageal cancer (T1N0M0 or T2N0M0), however, both local and systemic recurrence of disease is common when surgical resection is performed as the sole treatment modality. For locally advanced lesions, surgery alone with complete resection of all grossly apparent disease is associated with 5-year survival rarely exceeding 20%.

If the depth of tumor invasion is limited to the submucosa without regional lymph node involvement or distant metastases (T1N0M0), the majority of patients undergoing complete resection will survive 5 years. Especially in this subgroup, data suggest that the incidence of unexpected lymph node metastasis is quite rare. This avoids the morbidity of giving chemoradiation as well as the increased perioperative risks after this treatment if resection is later undertaken. Survival after resection alone ranges from 60% to 90%, depending on the actual layer that is invaded by the tumor. As radical lymph node dissection is of lowest benefit here, a transhiatal esophagectomy[24] or (with a very short, distal lesion) a standard left transthoracic approach[25] can be used. Recent reports on laparoscopic mucosal stripping or laparoscopic thoracoscopic esophagectomy suggest that additional surgical alternatives are possible for these patients.[26,27] If surgery is not being contemplated, chemoradiation per the RTOG protocol should be given as definitive nonsurgical therapy.

Stage II and stage III esophageal cancer includes T1 tumors and T2 tumors with lymph node involvement and T3 tumors with or without lymph node spread. In the majority of these lesions, combination therapy with preoperative chemoradiation or postoperative adjuvant chemotherapy or radiotherapy has shown advantages in terms of local control and occasionally survival.

CONCLUSION

The cumulative literature appears to suggest that neoadjuvant chemoradiotherapy for esophageal carcinoma provides a survival advantage, particularly with down-staging to pathologic complete response status for patients with locally advanced esophageal cancer (nodal or full-thickness esophageal involvement), although the results of randomized, controlled trials are conflicting. There are trials under way investigating various combinations of preoperative chemotherapy and radiation to increase the chances of a pathologic complete response found at esophagectomy. Patients with pathologic complete response after neoadjuvant therapy have a consistent and significant survival benefit, and pathologic complete response has become the surrogate marker for survival after neoadjuvant chemoradiotherapy. The current standard of care is surgery for resectable disease, with a 5-year survival of 15% to 20%. A stage-specific approach is warranted.

Data from various randomized, controlled trials indicate a significant survival advantage for concurrent chemoradiotherapy for nonsurgical patients compared with radiotherapy alone. Concurrent chemoradiotherapy is currently the standard of care for nonsurgical patients with advanced esophageal carcinoma.

REFERENCES

1. Blot WJ, Devesa SS, Kneller RW, et al. Rising incidence of adenocarcinoma of the esophagus and gastric cardia. *JAMA* 1991;**265**:1287-9.
2. Inculet RI, Keller SM, Dwyer A, Roth JA. Evaluation of noninvasive tests for the preoperative staging of carcinoma of the esophagus: a prospective study. *Ann Thorac Surg* 1985;**40**(6):561-5.
3. Tio TL, Coene PP, den Hartog Jager FC, et al. Preoperative TNM classification of esophageal carcinoma by endosonography. *Hepato gastroenterology* 1990;**37**(4):376-81.

4. Block MI, Patterson GA, Sundaresan RS, et al. Improvement in staging of esophageal cancer with the addition of positron emission tomography. *Ann Thorac Surg* 1997;**64**(3):770-6.
5. Luketich JD, Schauer PR, Meltzer CC, Landreneau RJ, Urso GK, Townsend DW, et al. Role of positron emission tomography in staging esophageal cancer. *Ann Thorac Surg* 1977;**64**(3):765-9.
6. Murray GF, Wilcox BR, Starek PJ. The assessment of operability of esophageal carcinoma. *Ann Thorac Surg* 1977;**23**:393-9.
7. Dagnini G, Caldironi MW, Marin G, Buzzaccarini O, Tremolada C, Ruol A. Laparoscopy in abdominal staging of esophageal carcinoma. Report of 369 cases. *Gastrointest Endosc* 1986;**32**(6):400-2.
8. Krasna MJ, Reed C, Hollis D, Luketich JD, DeCamp M, Mayer R, Sugarbaker D. CALGB Thoracic Surgeons. CALGB 9380: a prospective trial of the feasibility of thoracoscopy/laparoscopy in staging esophageal cancer. *Ann Thorac Surg* 2001;**71**:1073-9.
9. Krasna MJ, Jiao X, Mao Y, Sonett J, Gamliel Z, Kwong K, et al. Thoracoscopy/laparoscopy in the staging of esophageal cancer: Maryland experience. *Surg Laparos. Endosc Percutan Tech* 2002;**12**(4):213-8.
10. Suntharalingam M, Haas ML, Sonett JR, Doyle LA, Hausner PF, Schuetz J, et al. Accurate lymph node assessment prior to trimodality therapy for esophageal carcinoma. *Cancer J* 2001;**7**(6):509-15.
11. Nygaard K, Hagen S, Hansen HS, Hatlevoll R, Hultborn R, Jakobsen A, et al. Pre-operative radiotherapy prolongs survival in operable esophageal carcinoma: a randomized, multicenter study of pre-operative radiotherapy and chemotherapy. The second Scandinavian trial in esophageal cancer. *World J Surg* 1992;**16**:1104-9.
12. Kelsen DP, Ginsberg R, Pajak TF, et al. Chemotherapy followed by surgery compared with surgery alone for localized esophageal cancer. *N Engl J Med* 1996;**335**:462-7.
13. Medical Research Council Oesophageal Cancer Working Group. Surgical resection with or without preoperative chemotherapy in oesophageal cancer: a randomized controlled trial [see comment]. *Lancet* 2002;**359**:1727-33.
14. Walsh TN, Noonan N, Hollywood D, et al. A comparison of multimodality therapy and surgery for esophageal adenocarcinoma. *N Engl J Med* 1996;**335**:462-7.
15. Tepper J, Krasna M, Niedzwiecki D, Hollis D, Reed C, Goldberg R, et al. Phase III trial of trimodality therapy with cisplatin, fluorouracil, radiotherapy, and surgery compared with surgery alone for esophageal cancer: CALGB 9781. *J Clin Oncol* 2008;**26**:1086-92.
16. Greer SE, Goodney PP, Sutton JE, Birkmeyer JD. Neoadjuvant chemoradiotherapy for esophageal carcinoma: a meta-analysis. *Surgery* 2005;**137**(2):172-7.
17. Fiorica F, Di Bona D, Schepis F, Licata A, Shahied L, Venturi A, et al. Preoperative chemoradiotherapy for oesophageal cancer: a systematic review and meta-analysis. *Gut* 2004;**53**:925-30.
18. Urschel JD, Vasan H. A meta-analysis of randomized controlled trials that compared neoadjuvant chemoradiation and surgery to surgery alone for resectable esophageal cancer. *Am J Surg* 2003;**185**(6):538-43.
19. Urba SG, Orringer MB, Turrisi A, Iannettoni M, Forastiere A, Strawderman M. Randomized trial of preoperative chemoradiation versus surgery alone in patients with locoregional esophageal carcinoma. *J Clin Oncol* 2001;**19**:305-13.
20. Xiao ZF, Yang ZY, Liang J, Miao YJ, Wang M, Yin WB, et al. Value of radiotherapy after radical surgery for esophageal cancer: a report of 495 patients. *Ann Thorac Surg* 2003;**75**:331-6.
21. Ando N, Iizuka T, Kakegawa T, Isono K, Watanabe H, Ide H, et al. A randomized trial of surgery with and without chemotherapy for localized squamous carcinoma of the thoracic esophagus: the Japan Clinical Oncology Group Study. *J Thor Cardiovasc Surg* 1997;**114**:205-9.
22. Rice TW, Adelstein DJ, Chidel MA, Rybicki LA, DeCamp MM, Murthy SC, Blackstone EH. Benefit of postoperative adjuvant chemoradiotherapy in locoregionally advanced esophageal carcinoma. *J Thorac Cardiovasc Surg* 2003;**126**:1590-6.
23. al-Sarraf M, Martz K, Herskovic A, Leichman L, Brindle JS, Vaitkevicius VK, et al. Progress report of combined chemoradiotherapy versus radiotherapy alone in patients with esophageal cancer: an intergroup study. *J Clin Oncology* 1997;**15**(1):277-84.
24. Rice TW, Mason DP, Murthy SC, Zuccaro Jr G, Adelstein DJ, Rybicki LA, Blackstone EH. T2N0M0 esophageal cancer. *J Thorac Cardiovasc Surg* 2007;**133**(2):317-24.
25. Krasna MJ. Left transthoracic esophagectomy. *Chest Surg Clin N Am* 1995;**5**:543-54.
26. DeMeester SR. New options for the therapy of Barrett's high-grade dysplasia and intramucosal adenocarcinoma: endoscopic mucosal resection and ablation versus vagal-sparing esophagectomy. *Ann Thorac Surg* 2008;**85**(2):S747-50.
27. Schuchert MJ, Luketich JD, Landreneau RJ, Kilic A, Gooding WE, Alvelo-Rivera M, et al. Minimally-invasive esophagomyotomy in 200 consecutive patients: factors influencing postoperative outcomes. *Ann Thorac Surg* 2008;**85**(5):1729-34.

M. Mediastinum

CHAPTER 40
Mediastinal Anatomy and Mediastinoscopy

Varun Puri and Bryan F. Meyers

Mediastinal Anatomy
Potential Spaces in the Mediastinum
Mediastinal Lymph Node Anatomy
Indications for Mediastinal Lymph Node Assessment
Preoperative Evaluation

Surgical Technique
High Paratracheal Dissection
Lower Paratracheal Dissection
Carinal Dissection
Node Biopsy Technique and Closure of the Incision

Management of Major Bleeding
Extended Mediastinoscopy
Complications
Endoscopic Techniques for Mediastinal Lymph Node Assessment

MEDIASTINAL ANATOMY

The anatomic boundaries of the mediastinum include the thoracic inlet superiorly, the diaphragm inferiorly, the sternum anteriorly, the spine posteriorly, and the pleural spaces bilaterally. It is convenient to divide the mediastinum into anatomic compartments that provide pathologic correlation. Many such schema are available, but only a few are in common use.

A classic description divides the mediastinum into four compartments: superior, anterior, middle, and posterior (Fig. 40-1). The superior mediastinum includes all structures from the thoracic inlet superiorly to a line drawn from the lower edge of the manubrium to the lower edge of the fourth thoracic vertebra. The inferior mediastinum, which lies inferior to this line, is subsequently divided into the anterior, middle, and posterior compartments. The boundary between the anterior and middle compartments is the anterior pericardium; between the middle and posterior compartments is the posterior aspect of the tracheal bifurcation, pulmonary vessels, and pericardium. Another system combines the anterior and superior compartments into an anterosuperior compartment, thus creating three compartments. With either of these systems, structures can be contained within two separate compartments. For example, in the four-compartment model, the upper portions of the trachea and esophagus are contained within the superior mediastinum; the lower portions are contained within the middle and posterior mediastinum.

Shields proposed a simpler three-compartment model consisting of an anterior compartment, middle (or visceral) compartment, and posterior compartment (paraventral sulcus) (Fig. 40-2).[1] All three compartments are bounded inferiorly by the diaphragm, laterally by the pleural space, and superiorly by the thoracic inlet. The anterior compartment is bounded anteriorly by the sternum and posteriorly by the great vessels and pericardium and contains the thymus, internal mammary vessels, areolar and adipose tissue, and potentially pathologic structures such as ectopic parathyroid tissue or a retrosternal goiter. The middle mediastinum is bounded posteriorly by the ventral surface of the thoracic spine; it occupies the entire thoracic inlet and contains the majority of mediastinal structures, namely, the great vessels, heart, pericardium, trachea, proximal main-stem bronchi, vagus nerves, phrenic nerves, esophagus, thoracic duct, descending aorta, and azygos venous system. The posterior compartment (paraventral sulcus) consists of potential spaces along the thoracic vertebrae that contain the sympathetic chain, proximal portions of the intercostal neurovascular bundles, thoracic spinal ganglia, and distal azygos vein. Whereas some anatomists may argue that the paraventral sulci are not truly a mediastinal space, they often harbor disease that is classically considered in the posterior

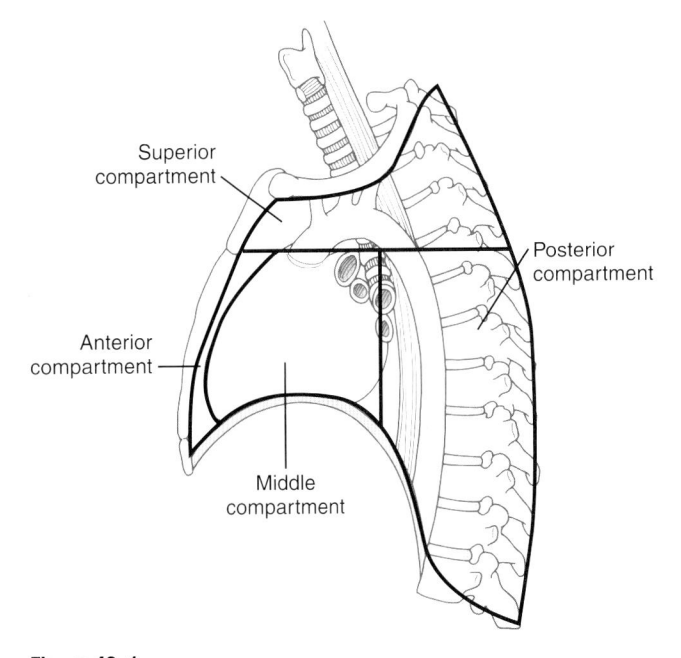

Figure 40–1
Four-compartment model of the mediastinum.

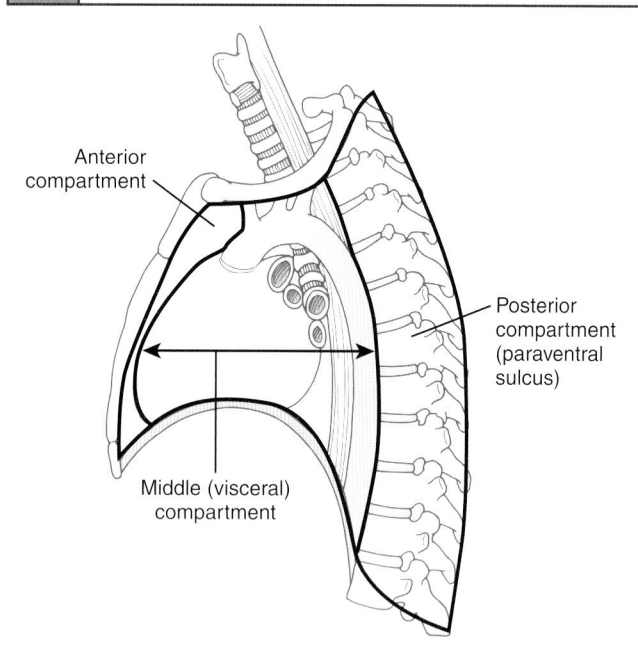

Figure 40–2
Three-compartment model of the mediastinum.

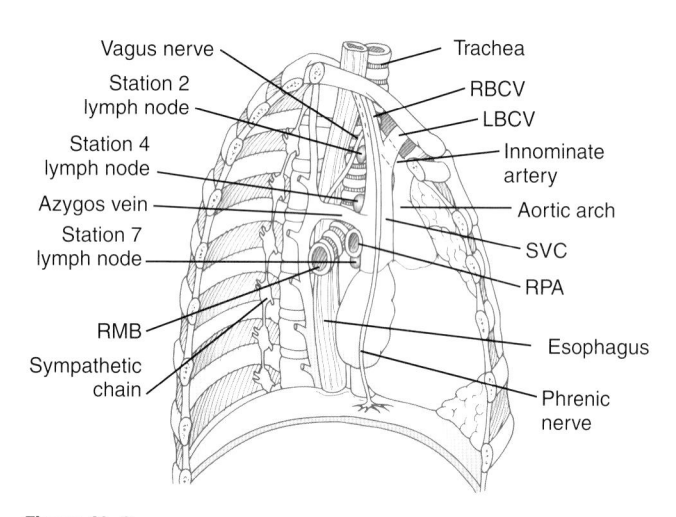

Figure 40–3
Right mediastinal view. LBCV, left brachiocephalic vein; RBCV, right brachiocephalic vein; RMB, right main bronchus; RPA, right pulmonary artery; SVC, superior vena cava.

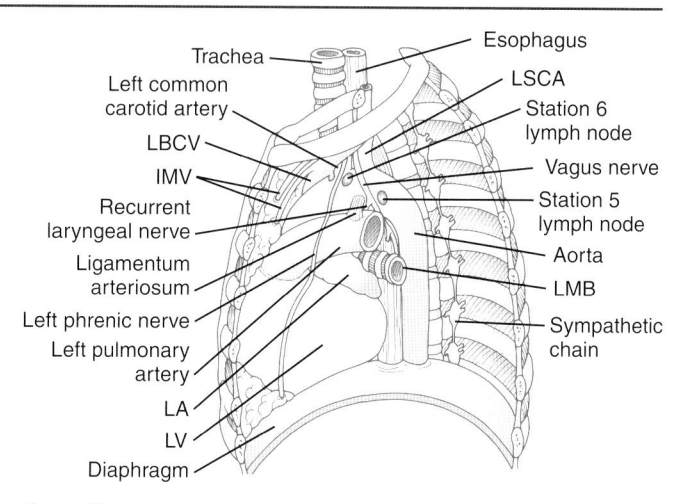

Figure 40–4
Left mediastinal view. IMV, internal mammary vessels; LA, left atrium; LBCV, left brachiocephalic vein; LMB, left main bronchus; LSCA, left subclavian artery; LV, left ventricle.

mediastinum (neurogenic tumors). Detailed sagittal views of mediastinal anatomy are depicted in Figures 40-3 and 40-4.

POTENTIAL SPACES IN THE MEDIASTINUM

For ease of communication in describing pathologic change, most commonly lymph node enlargement, several potential mediastinal spaces are described. The pretracheal space is a triangular space bounded anterolaterally by the superior vena cava and right brachiocephalic vein on the right, the aorta and pericardium on the left, and the trachea posteriorly. The pretracheal space is contiguous inferiorly with the subcarinal space, which is bounded superiorly by the carina, laterally by the main-stem bronchi, anteriorly by the pulmonary artery, and posteriorly by the esophagus (see Fig. 40-3). The pretracheal and subcarinal spaces are routinely explored in mediastinoscopy. The aortopulmonary window is the space bounded superiorly by the aortic arch, medially by the trachea and esophagus, inferiorly by the pulmonary artery, and laterally by the pleura. This space contains lymph nodes, the ligamentum arteriosum, and the left recurrent laryngeal nerve (see Fig. 40-4). Routine cervical mediastinoscopy does not access this space, but anterior mediastinotomy (Chamberlain procedure), extended cervical mediastinoscopy, and thoracoscopy or thoracotomy provide access to the aortopulmonary window.

MEDIASTINAL LYMPH NODE ANATOMY

Since the adoption of a common thoracic regional lymph node classification by the American Joint Committee and the Union Internationale Contre le Cancer in 1997, the system, often referred to as the Mountain and Dresler chart, has found widespread acceptance (Fig. 40-5).[2] This system classifies lymph nodes into 14 stations, of which stations 1 through 9 are contained within the mediastinal pleura and thus are mediastinal lymph nodes. Lymph node stations 2, 4, and 7, depicted in Figure 40-3, are the only nodal stations accessible by standard mediastinoscopy; stations 5 and 6, depicted in Figure 40-4, require an alternative approach like extended mediastinoscopy or anterior mediastinotomy.

INDICATIONS FOR MEDIASTINAL LYMPH NODE ASSESSMENT

The most common indication for assessment of mediastinal lymph nodes remains non–small cell lung cancer. Other indications include mediastinal lymphadenopathy of unknown etiology, mediastinal masses, primary tracheal tumors, and occasional esophageal tumors. The increasing use of modern imaging techniques including high-resolution computed tomography and positron emission tomography has led to a more selective strategy in invasive mediastinal lymph node assessment, especially for stage I non–small cell lung cancer. This stems from the fact that the sensitivity and negative predictive value of positron emission tomography approach

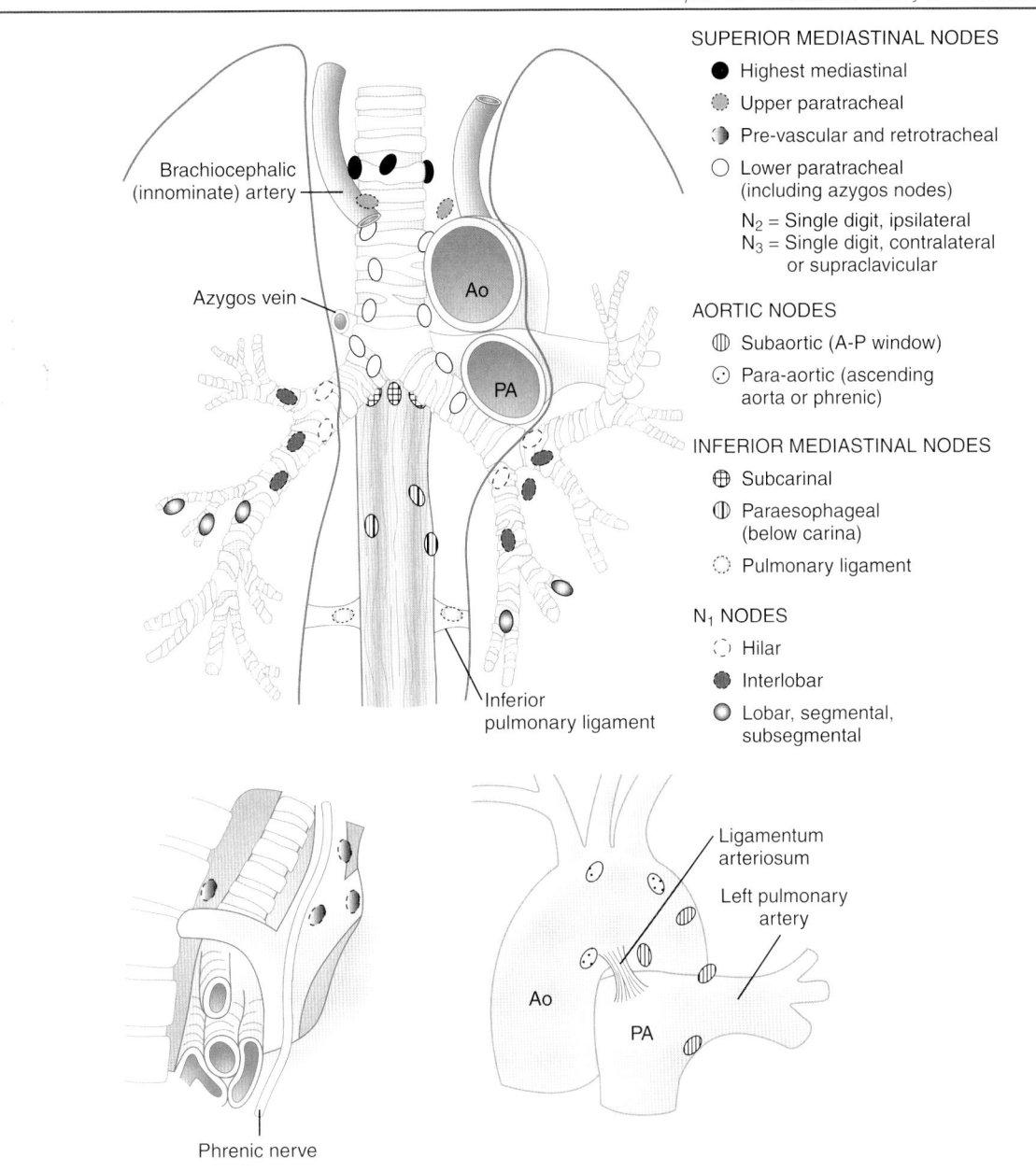

Figure 40–5
Regional lymph node stations for lung cancer staging. Ao, aorta; A-P, aortopulmonary; PA, pulmonary artery. *(From Mountain CF, Dresler CM. Regional lymph node classification for lung cancer staging. Chest 1997;111:1718-23.)*

SUPERIOR MEDIASTINAL NODES
- Highest mediastinal
- Upper paratracheal
- Pre-vascular and retrotracheal
- Lower paratracheal (including azygos nodes)

N_2 = Single digit, ipsilateral
N_3 = Single digit, contralateral or supraclavicular

AORTIC NODES
- Subaortic (A-P window)
- Para-aortic (ascending aorta or phrenic)

INFERIOR MEDIASTINAL NODES
- Subcarinal
- Paraesophageal (below carina)
- Pulmonary ligament

N_1 NODES
- Hilar
- Interlobar
- Lobar, segmental, subsegmental

those of cervical mediastinoscopy in a review of the literature (Table 40-1).[3,4]

The European Society of Cardiothoracic Surgery has provided recommendations for mediastinal lymph node assessment in preoperative staging of non–small cell lung cancer (Fig. 40-6).[4]

In addition, a cost-effectiveness analysis concluded that patients with clinical stage I lung cancer staged by computed tomography and positron emission tomography benefit little from mediastinoscopy.[5] Other views of the most efficient strategy for staging of the mediastinum exist, and results from ongoing trials of cervical mediastinoscopy will further refine its indications in the near future. An argument offered by some for routine cervical mediastinoscopy in non–small cell lung cancer is maintenance of familiarity with the technique and its minimal morbidity in experienced hands, but maintenance of familiarity with a procedure that is rarely needed is a questionable defense for its routine use.

Other, less-common indications for mediastinoscopy include drainage of bronchogenic cysts, abscess drainage, identification of ectopic parathyroid tissue, and tissue sampling for causes of superior vena cava syndrome.

PREOPERATIVE EVALUATION

Standard preoperative evaluation in a patient undergoing mediastinoscopy must include a history and physical examination. Special considerations include history of neck or chest surgery, such as permanent tracheostomy, or coexistent pathologic process such as a large goiter or aneurysms of the aortic

Table 40-1

Relative Performance of Various Modalities of Mediastinal Lymph Node Assessment

	Sensitivity (%)	Specificity (%)	NPV (%)	PPV (%)	Prevalence (%)
CT	57	82	83	56	28
PET	84	89	93	79	32
Blind TBNA	76	96	71	100	70
EUS-FNA	88	91	77	98	69
Mediastinoscopy	81	100	91	100	37

EUS-FNA, endoscopic esophageal ultrasound-guided fine-needle aspiration; NPV, negative predictive value; PPV, positive predictive value; prevalence: proportion of patients with metastatic mediastinal nodes in the study cohorts; TBNA, transbronchial needle aspiration.
From De Leyn, Lardinois D, Van Schil PE, et al. ESTS guidelines for preoperative lymph node staging for non–small cell lung cancer. Eur J Cardiothorac Surg 2007;32:1-8.

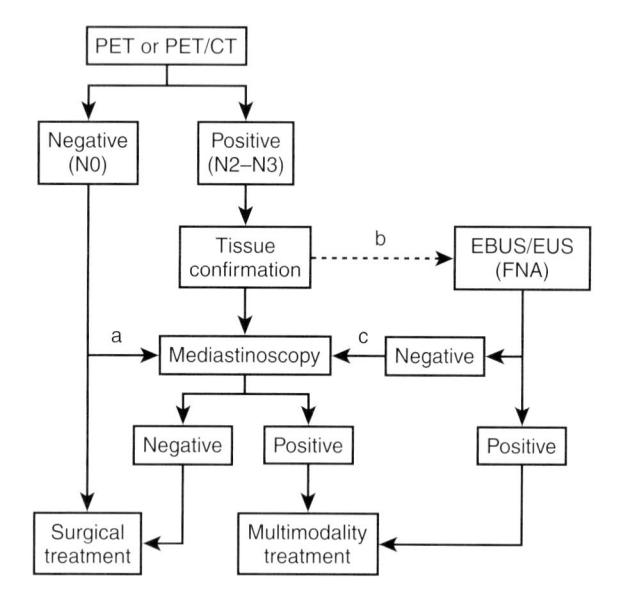

a: In central tumors, tumors with low FDG uptake, tumors with LNs ≥1.6 cm and/or PET N1 disease invasive staging remains indicated
b: Endoscopic techniques are minimally invasive and can be the first choice
c: Due to its higher NPV mediastinoscopy remains indicated

EUS: endoscopic esophageal ultrasound
EBUS: endobronchial ultrasound
NPV: negative predictive value
N0: LN <1 cm

Figure 40-6
The proposed algorithm to follow for primary mediastinal staging when positron emission tomography (PET) or positron emission tomography–computed tomography (PET/CT) is available. FDG, fluorodeoxyglucose; LN, lymph node. (From De Leyn P, Lardinois D, Van Schil PE, et al. ESTS guidelines for preoperative lymph node staging for non–small cell lung cancer. Eur J Cardiothorac Surg 2007;32:1-8.)

arch or innominate artery, which may prevent access to the pretracheal space. Prior neck or sternal incisions, including prior mediastinoscopy, may complicate the initial dissection but are not absolute contraindications to the procedure. Significant vascular calcification in the innominate artery may increase the risk of embolic events as this vessel is manipulated during the procedure. In addition, total atherosclerotic occlusion of the left common carotid artery may predispose patients to stroke if the innominate artery supplying the right common carotid artery is compressed by the mediastinoscope. The evaluation should also note cervical spine arthritis as significant neck extension is required for the procedure. Patients should undergo laboratory workup as for any general anesthetic and should have a type and crossmatch in place for the possibility of a blood transfusion.

SURGICAL TECHNIQUE

Standard cervical mediastinoscopy involves access of the middle mediastinal structures through a lighted hollow metal mediastinoscope introduced through a cervical incision. Recent innovations use fiberoptics and a television monitor to allow all members of the surgical team to see the anatomy simultaneously. This addition probably enhances safety and speeds the learning curve for trainees. Large-bore venous access is warranted, and many anesthetists routinely place a right radial arterial catheter to monitor blood pressure and to watch for innominate artery compression during the procedure. Alternatively, some centers use a pulse oximeter probe on the right hand. Once patients are intubated, they are placed in the supine position with the neck gently hyperextended, but not so much that the head is "floating," with an inflatable bag or rolled blanket placed behind the shoulders (Fig. 40-7).

The endotracheal tube is brought out to the patient's right and kept as lateral and low in profile as possible to allow the surgeon to insert the mediastinoscope directly over the patient's chin in the midline. Care must be taken to avoid turning the patient's chin to the side as this results in an off-center incision, which makes subsequent dissection more difficult and also produces a suboptimal cosmetic result.

The entire sternum and anterior cervical areas are prepared and draped to facilitate a sternotomy if massive bleeding is encountered. A 2.5-cm transverse incision is made one fingerbreadth above the sternal notch, and the platysma is divided in the line of the skin incision. The midline raphe between the strap muscles is opened vertically, and dissection is carried down to the trachea. On occasion, one needs to divide a low-lying thyroid isthmus or a thyroidea ima artery to reach the trachea. The pretracheal fascia is divided, and blunt finger dissection is undertaken to develop a plane anterior to the trachea in a caudal direction. A high-riding innominate artery can be

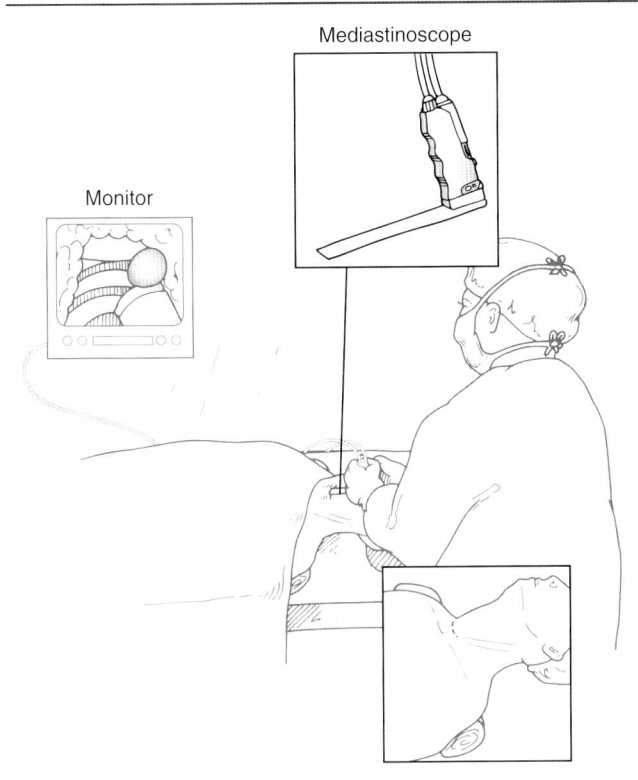

Figure 40–7
Patient and equipment positioning for videomediastinoscopy. The surgeon is shown looking across the operative field at the video monitor. *Top inset,* Diagram of a videomediastinoscope. *Bottom inset,* View of the patient's neck in extension, the incision site, and the support behind the patient's shoulders.

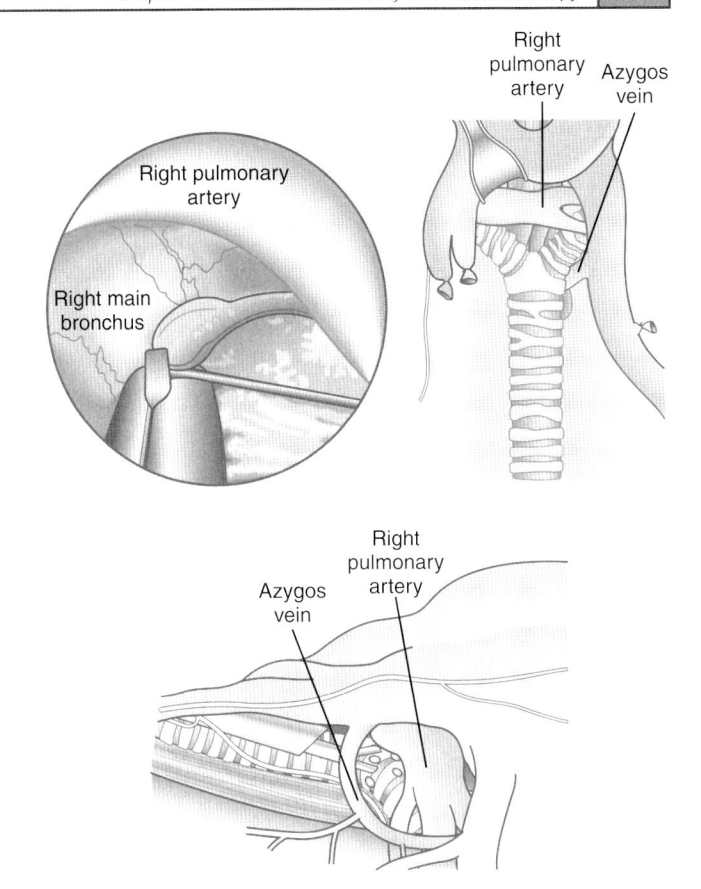

Figure 40–8
Enhanced visualization with cervical videomediastinoscopy. *(From De Leyn P, Lardinois D, Van Schil PE, et al. ESTS guidelines for preoperative lymph node staging for non–small cell lung cancer. Eur J Cardiothorac Surg 2007;32:1-8.)*

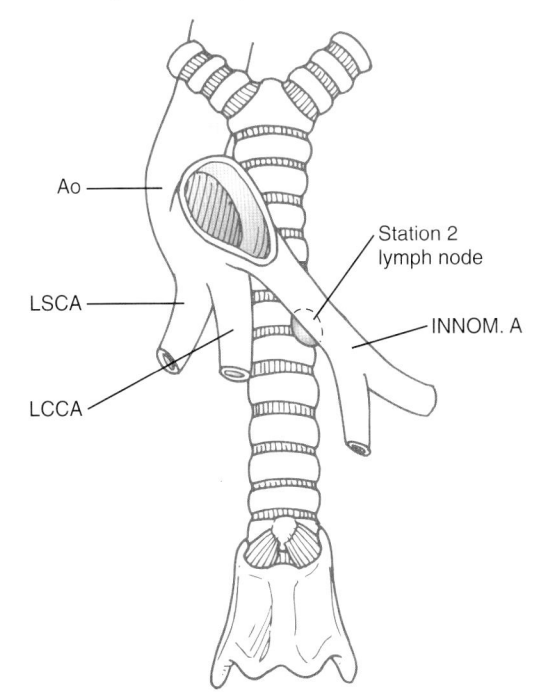

Figure 40–9
Anatomic structures at the high paratracheal level as seen from the surgeon's position standing at the patient's head. Ao, aorta; INNOM. A, innominate artery; LCCA, left common carotid artery; LSCA, left subclavian artery.

seen in aneurysmal disease, in the setting of an enlarged station 2 (right) lymph node, or as an anatomic variant. The preoperative computed tomographic scan can provide a clue to this situation and help avoid injury to the vessel during the initial dissection. The surgeon can obtain useful information during initial finger dissection of the pretracheal space, including the exact location of the ascending aorta and the angle and level at which the innominate artery crosses the field. In addition, firm pathologic lymph nodes alongside the distal trachea may be identified and partially dissected free of surrounding tissue.

The mediastinoscope is now inserted into the pretracheal plane that has been created (see Fig. 40-7). A standard mediastinoscope is a hollow lighted metal tube that permits only one individual to visualize the operative field. The introduction of videomediastinoscopy (Fig. 40-8; see also Fig. 40-7) has permitted all members of the team to visualize the operative field. This provides educational benefit, improves participation in the procedure (including anticipation of the surgeon's needs), and allows better supervision during training. In addition, magnification, improved optics, and superior lighting have improved anatomic visualization (see Fig. 40-8). With a first assistant stabilizing the scope, the videomediastinoscope can be used by the surgeon to introduce two instruments into the field for bimanual dissection and hemostasis.

HIGH PARATRACHEAL DISSECTION

The major anatomic landmark of the high paratracheal level is the innominate artery (Figs. 40-9 and 40-10), which is seen as a pulsatile structure crossing anterior to the trachea. Station

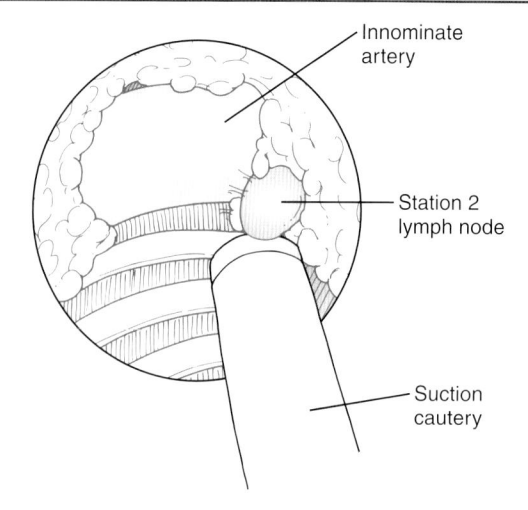

Figure 40–10
View through the mediastinoscope at the high paratracheal level. Note the tracheal rings posteriorly and the innominate artery anteriorly. Also note the suction cautery dissection through the pretracheal fascia to allow the underlying station 2 lymph node located to the right of the trachea to bulge into the operative field.

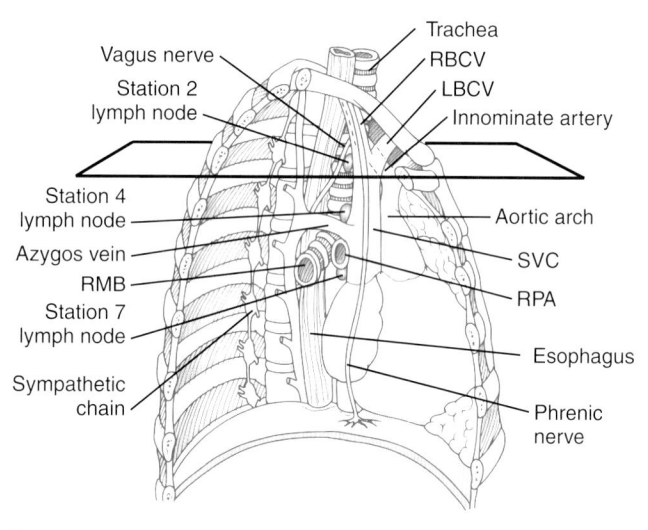

Figure 40–11
Right mediastinal view. The plane traverses the mediastinal structures at the high paratracheal station 2 lymph node level. LBCV, left brachiocephalic vein; RBCV, right brachiocephalic vein; RMB, right main bronchus; RPA, right pulmonary artery; SVC, superior vena cava.

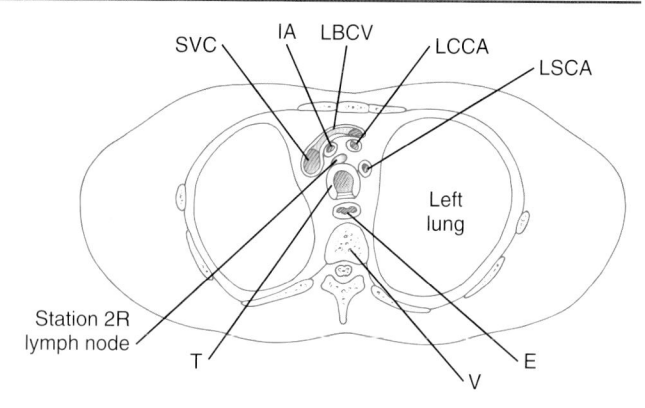

Figure 40–12
Transverse view of mediastinal structures at the high paratracheal level. E, esophagus; IA, innominate artery; LBCV, left brachiocephalic vein; LCCA, left common carotid artery; LSCA, left subclavian artery; SVC, superior vena cava; T, trachea; V, vertebra.

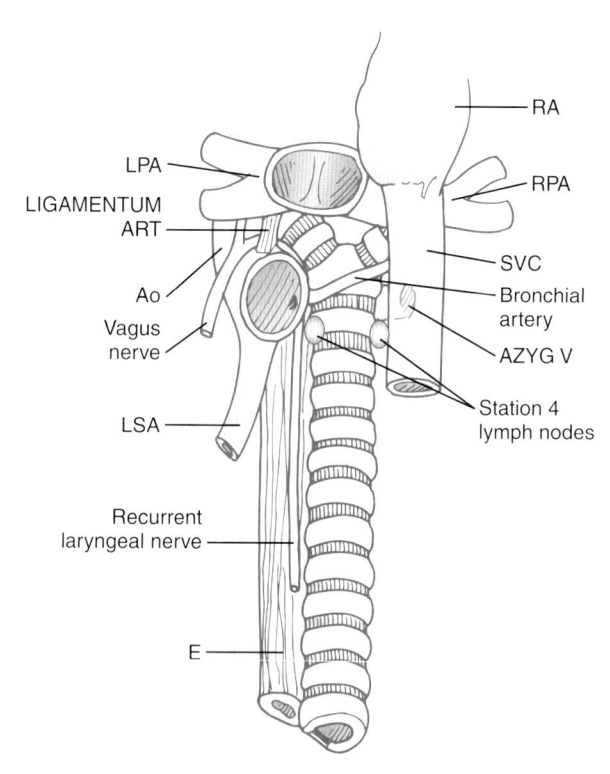

Figure 40–13
Anatomic structures at the lower paratracheal level as seen from the surgeon's position standing at the patient's head. Ao, aorta; AZYG V, azygos vein; E, esophagus; LIGAMENTUM ART, ligamentum arteriosum; LPA, left pulmonary artery; LSA, left subclavian artery; RA, right atrium; RPA, right pulmonary artery; SVC, superior vena cava.

2 lymph nodes lie to the left and right of the trachea at this level. Correlation of the endoscopic view at the station 2 lymph node level with sagittal anatomic structures as seen from the right chest is shown in Figure 40-11. Correlation of the endoscopic view with a transverse view of the mediastinal structures at this high paratracheal level is seen in Figure 40-12.

The operator's initial view of the paratracheal tissue often shows no obvious nodal tissue. Subsequent blunt dissection through the pretracheal tissue plane, assisted by careful use of the suction cautery tip, usually exposes the underlying lymph nodes. Dark pigmentation facilitates recognition of lymph nodes. It is recommended that lymph node dissection be carried out to the point that the node bulges into the operative field (see Fig. 40-10). This technique helps prevent inadvertent biopsy of other dark paratracheal structures, such as the vena cava or the right brachiocephalic vein, which do not bulge into the field. In other words, lymph nodes should be recognized as three-dimensional structures; major veins remain two-dimensional dark surfaces after the dissection.

LOWER PARATRACHEAL DISSECTION

Dissection inferior to the innominate artery reaches the lower paratracheal area and station 4 lymph nodes, which lie to the right and left of the trachea cephalad to the carina (Fig. 40-13). After blunt dissection of the paratracheal tissue permitting the

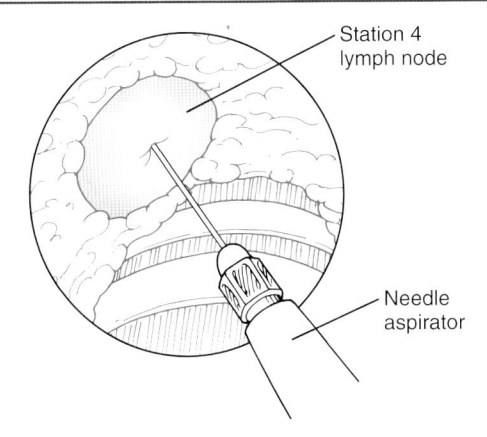

Chapter 40   Mediastinal Anatomy and Mediastinoscopy

Figure 40–14
View through the mediastinoscope at the lower paratracheal level. Note the use of an aspirating needle to rule out a vascular structure before biopsy of the suspected lymph node.

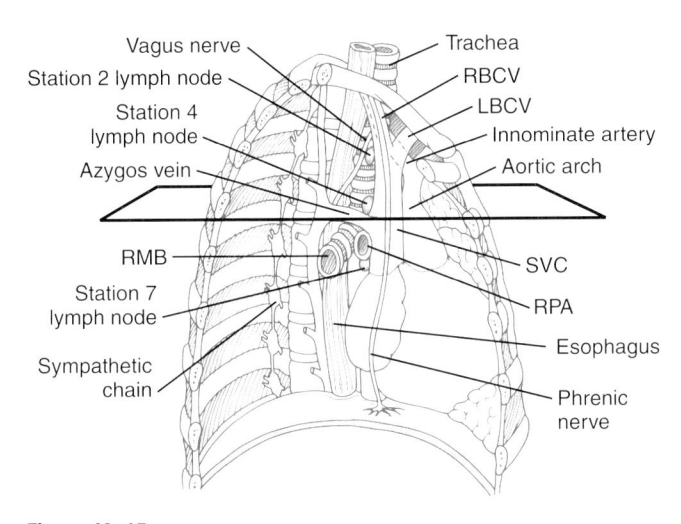

Figure 40–15
Right mediastinoscopic view with plane passing through the mediastinal structures located at the lower paratracheal level. LBCV, left brachiocephalic vein; RBCV, right brachiocephalic vein; RMB, right main bronchus; RPA, right pulmonary artery; SVC, superior vena cava.

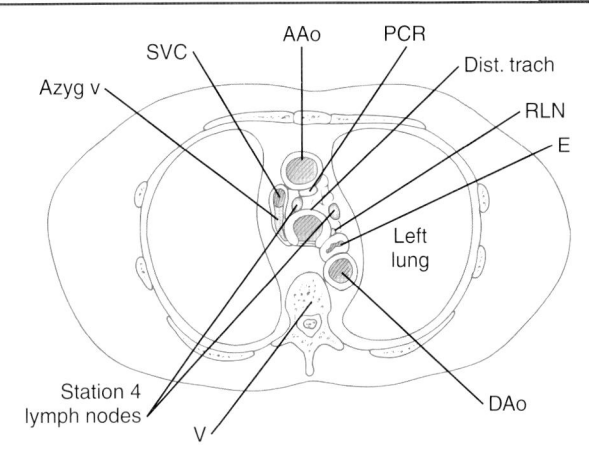

Figure 40–16
Transverse view of mediastinal structures at the lower paratracheal level. The pericardial recess (PCR) is a fluid-containing structure often mistaken for a lower mediastinal lymph node. The attenuated conformation of the structure along the outer wall of the ascending aorta (AAo) is a clue to its being a fluid-filled structure and not a node. Azyg v, azygos vein; DAo, descending aorta; Dist. trach, distal trachea; E, esophagus; RLN, recurrent laryngeal nerve; SVC, superior vena cava; V, vertebra.

nodes to bulge into the operative field, if there is any question about whether the tissue to undergo biopsy is a lymph node, it is wise to aspirate the tissue first with a small-bore needle to rule out a vascular structure (Fig. 40-14). This maneuver, which can be used at any level, may also alert the operator to the presence of a major blood vessel lying immediately beneath the node to be sampled. This is important as inflammatory or malignant adhesions between the lymph node and the underlying major vessel can lead to avulsion injury to the vessel during vigorous lymph node biopsy. The structures lying to the right of the trachea at this level include—in addition to the lymph nodes—the azygos vein, the superior vena cava, the mediastinal pleura, and the adjacent right upper lobe of the lung. The pleura can appear pigmented like a node, but the lung is characteristically seen to move behind the pleura with respiration. Structures lying to the left of the trachea at this level are the aortic arch, the left recurrent laryngeal nerve, a bronchial artery branch from the aorta, and the esophagus. The esophagus lies posterior and to the left of the trachea at this level and can be mistaken for a white tumor-filled lymph node. It can be recognized by the longitudinal muscle fibers of its outer muscular layer.

The use of electrocautery should be avoided in the left lower paratracheal region to prevent inadvertent injury to the esophagus and the rarely visualized left recurrent laryngeal nerve lying in the tracheoesophageal groove. If esophageal injury is identified, the esophagus should immediately be repaired through a right or left thoracotomy. Most surgeons prefer a right thoracotomy to repair the esophagus at this level. However, if there is preexisting lung disease in the left chest, a left thoracotomy may be used to address both. The site of esophageal injury usually lies directly medial to the aortic arch.

Correlation of the sagittal and transverse anatomy at the station 4 lymph node level is shown in Figure 40-15 and Figure 40-16, respectively.

CARINAL DISSECTION

The major anatomic landmarks of carinal dissection are widening of the trachea, the triangular tracheal cartilage at the carina, the proximal left main bronchus, and the right pulmonary artery crossing anteriorly (Fig. 40-17). Because of its more posterior takeoff from the trachea, the proximal right main bronchus may be difficult to identify. The mediastinoscopic view of structures at the carinal level is depicted in Figure 40-18.

Identification of the triangular cartilage of the distal trachea helps identify the level and prevents misidentification of the proximal left main bronchus as the trachea. Dissection at the carinal level must be performed with meticulous attention paid to the location of the right pulmonary artery. This pulsatile structure passes transversely across the field anterior to the airway. Extensive blunt dissection of the suspected nodal tissue followed by needle aspiration before biopsy is vital (see Fig. 40-18).

Correlation of the endoscopic view at the carinal station 7 lymph node level with anatomic structures as seen sagittally

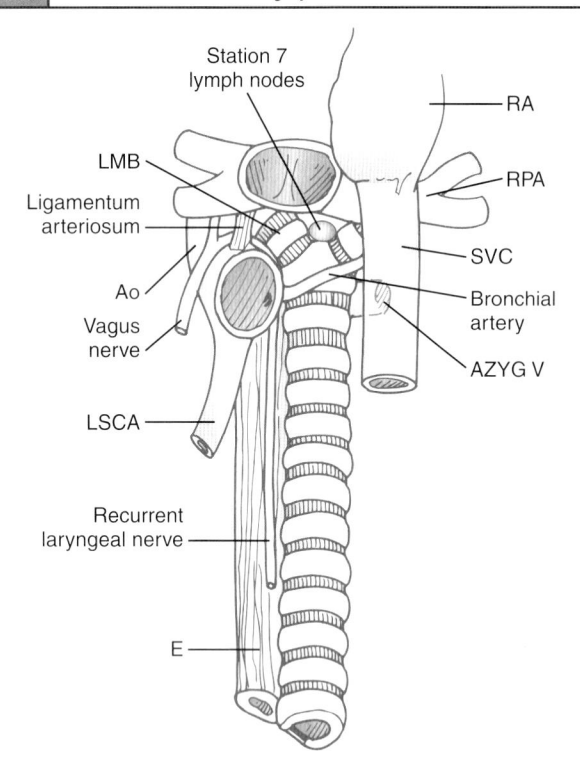

Figure 40–17
Anatomic structures at the carinal level as seen from the surgeon's perspective standing at the patient's head. Ao, aorta; AZYG V, azygos vein; E, esophagus; LMB, left main bronchus; LSCA, left subclavian artery; RA, right atrium; RPA, right pulmonary artery; SVC, superior vena cava.

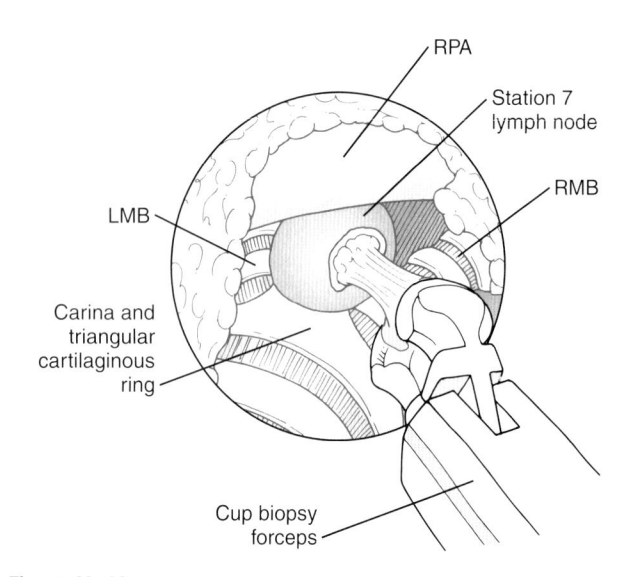

Figure 40–18
View through the mediastinoscope at the carinal level. Note the widened tracheal diameter and the triangular tracheal cartilage just proximal to the subcarinal tissue containing station 7 lymph nodes. After blunt dissection and needle aspiration, as described earlier, a nodal biopsy is illustrated with a cup biopsy forceps. LMB, left main bronchus; RMB, right main bronchus; RPA, right pulmonary artery.

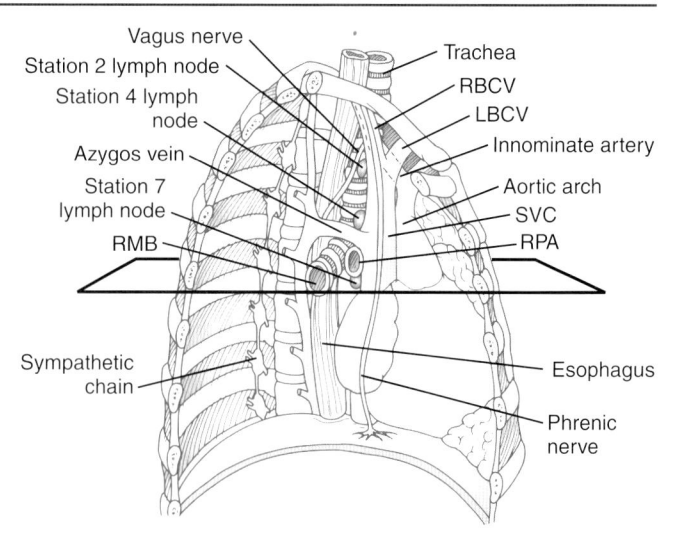

Figure 40–19
Right mediastinal view with a plane passing through the structures located at the subcarinal level. LBCV, left brachiocephalic vein; RBCV, right brachiocephalic vein; RMB, right main bronchus; RPA, right pulmonary artery; SVC, superior vena cava.

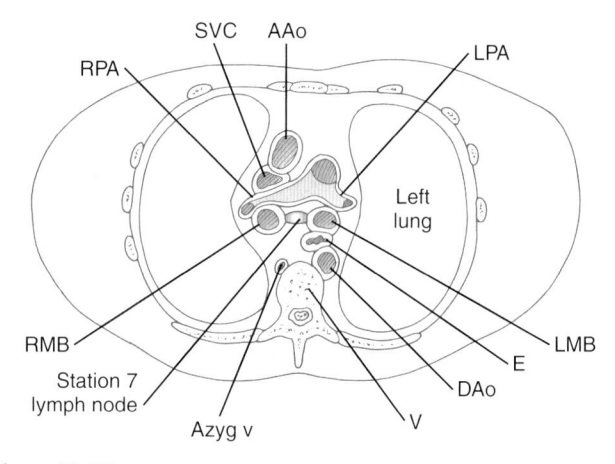

Figure 40–20
Transverse view of mediastinal structures at the subcarinal level. AAo, ascending aorta; Azyg v, azygos vein; DAo, descending aorta; E, esophagus; LMB, left main bronchus; LPA, left pulmonary artery; RMB, right main bronchus; RPA, right pulmonary artery; SVC, superior vena cava; V, vertebra.

from the right chest is shown in Figure 40-19. The transverse sectional anatomy at this level is shown in Figure 40-20.

NODE BIOPSY TECHNIQUE AND CLOSURE OF THE INCISION

As previously discussed, mediastinal node biopsy is initiated by dissection through the pretracheal fascia with a blunt suction cautery instrument (see Fig. 40-10). Next, the suspected lymph node is aspirated with a needle to confirm that it is not a vascular structure (see Fig. 40-14). Finally, a biopsy specimen is taken with a biopsy forceps (see Fig. 40-18). Often, the first biopsy removes only the outer capsule of the node and exposes the underlying parenchyma, which can then be further sampled. If no node is seen at the desired station, it is often helpful to withdraw the mediastinoscope slightly and even to rotate it to see tissue lying more anterior or anterolateral to the trachea. These areas may reveal nodal tissue with further dissection. After biopsy, hemostasis is achieved with electrocautery or with temporary packing with long length gauze. Close attention must be paid to hemostasis throughout the procedure to maintain a clear field of vision. For a mild persistent ooze, withdrawal of the mediastinoscope a short distance and waiting will often achieve hemostasis as a result of simple tissue apposition. Rarely, an endoscopic clip applier may be used to address a visible bleeding vessel. Once hemostasis has been achieved at all levels, the mediastinoscope is removed and the wound is closed in several layers. The strap muscles are reapproximated with interrupted sutures vertically in the midline, the platysma muscle transversely; the skin is closed with a subcuticular suture. We obtain postprocedure chest radiographs of all patients to ensure the absence of a pneumothorax or other visible abnormality. The patient can subsequently be discharged to home after standard postanesthesia care. Alternatively, after mediastinoscopy, the patient may be repositioned for tumor resection under the same anesthesia after frozen section evaluation of the lymph nodes by a pathologist.

MANAGEMENT OF MAJOR BLEEDING

A well-organized plan helps to deal with the possibility of major bleeding during mediastinoscopy. The first thing that is likely to happen is a complete loss of visualization. We recommend leaving the mediastinoscope in place and immediately packing the operative field with long gauze. This maneuver will temporarily contain most hemorrhage except that from systemic arteries. Attention is then turned to volume resuscitation and blood replacement if necessary. Waiting several minutes and then removing the packing often accomplishes hemostasis. If not, repeated packing preceded by a topical hemostatic agent such as oxidized cellulose can control venous and minor arterial bleeding without having to resort to median sternotomy or thoracotomy. Aortic, innominate artery, and bronchial artery injury adjacent to the aorta and major pulmonary artery injuries will not be contained with packing. Management should start with compression of the vessel with the mediastinoscope or removal of the mediastinoscope and compression of the vessel against the sternum with one's finger until either a median sternotomy (preferable in most situations) or a thoracotomy can be performed to allow direct vascular control.

EXTENDED MEDIASTINOSCOPY

We use the term *extended mediastinoscopy* to encompass techniques that go beyond the routine assessment of station 2, 4, and 7 lymph nodes in the mediastinum. A common misconception is that routine mediastinoscopy permits evaluation of the anterior mediastinum. However, a variation of mediastinoscopy known as extended cervical mediastinoscopy has been described that can access the anterior mediastinum as well as station 5 and 6 nodes in the aortopulmonary window (see Fig. 40-5). This procedure is started through the same cervical incision, but the surgeon subsequently creates a plane anterior to the innominate artery and posterior to the left brachiocephalic vein. Although it has been described, it is rarely done, however, because of the inherent difficulty of the procedure involving dissection of major vessels in a confined anatomic space and the easy accessibility to the aortopulmonary window by an anterior mediastinotomy or thoracoscopy. In addition, the belief among many thoracic surgeons is that tumors of the left upper lobe with involvement of nodes in stations 5 and 6 (if limited to intracapsular spread and in the absence of other mediastinal node involvement) have a better prognosis with surgical resection than do tumors in other lobes with mediastinal node involvement and therefore do not have to be staged before lung resection.

Transcervical extended mediastinal lymphadenectomy (TEMLA) is a recently described surgical procedure for staging of the mediastinal lymph nodes in patients with non–small cell lung cancer.[6] The operation is performed through a 5- to 8-cm collar incision in the neck and enables complete removal of all mediastinal nodal stations except for the pulmonary ligament nodes (station 9) and the most distal left paratracheal nodes (station 4L). In general, TEMLA is an open procedure performed partly with mediastinoscopy-assisted and videothoracoscopy-assisted techniques. Operative technique of TEMLA includes elevation of the sternal manubrium with a special retractor and bilateral visualization of the laryngeal recurrent and vagus nerves. The stated benefits include a higher sensitivity and specificity compared with standard mediastinoscopy or videomediastinoscopy.

Video-assisted mediastinoscopic lymphadenectomy (VAMLA) is a mediastinoscopic dissection technique proposed for a radical mediastinal assessment and as an adjunct to open lymphadenectomy at the time of pulmonary resection.[7] VAMLA dissection includes the en bloc resection of the subcarinal, right paratracheal, right tracheobronchial, and pretracheal compartments and dissection and lymphadenectomy of the left-sided tracheobronchial and paratracheal compartments. A specialized mediastinoscope with spreadable blades is used. All of these modifications to cervical mediastinoscopy have been recently described, but few have made their way into routine practice in the mainstream.

COMPLICATIONS

Mediastinoscopy is a safe procedure when it is performed by experienced surgeons with a knowledge of the surrounding mediastinal structures and a systematic deliberate method of tissue biopsy. Meticulous attention to hemostasis can help prevent subsequent bigger problems. A large series[8] of more than 2000 procedures described a morbidity rate of 0.6% and a mortality rate of 0.2%. Possible major complications include major vessel hemorrhage (aorta, innominate artery, pulmonary artery, bronchial artery, vena cava, azygos vein), esophageal perforation, and stroke secondary to innominate artery compression in the setting of severe atherosclerosis. Other complications include left recurrent laryngeal nerve injury, pneumothorax, wound infection, and, rarely, tumor seeding of the neck incision.

ENDOSCOPIC TECHNIQUES FOR MEDIASTINAL LYMPH NODE ASSESSMENT

The increasing evidence of the accuracy of endobronchial ultrasound–transbronchial needle aspiration (EBUS-TBNA) in diagnosis of mediastinal adenopathy with suspected lung cancer has led to its increasing application in the preoperative

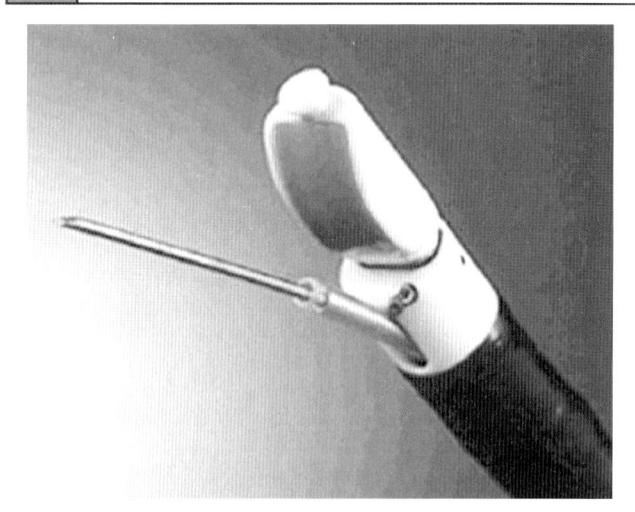

Figure 40–21
Image of the distal tip of a dedicated EBUS-TBNA bronchoscope. The needle exits obliquely so the puncture site can be within the EBUS view. *(From Ernst A, Feller-Kopman D, Herth FJ. Endobronchial ultrasound in the diagnosis and staging of lung cancer and other thoracic tumors. Semin Thorac Cardiovasc Surg 2007;19:201-5.)*

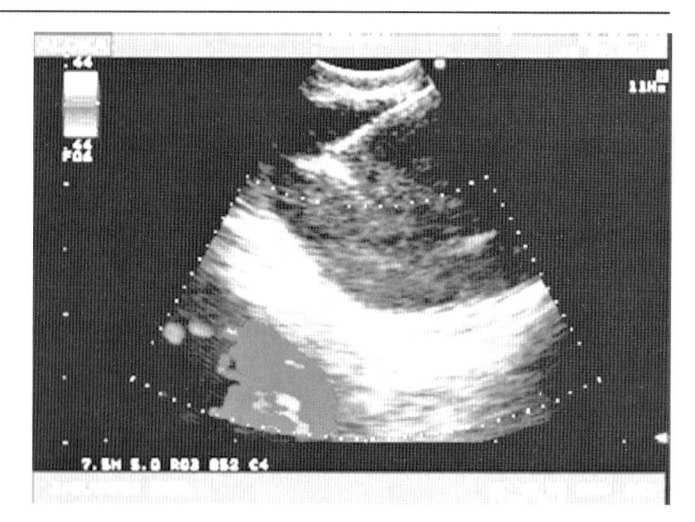

Figure 40–22
EBUS-guided puncture of a node in 10R position. The needle is clearly visible within the lesion. The system also allows color Doppler assessment of unclear structures. *(From Ernst A, Feller-Kopman D, Herth FJ. Endobronchial ultrasound in the diagnosis and staging of lung cancer and other thoracic tumors. Semin Thorac Cardiovasc Surg 2007;19:201-5.)*

setting. The recent development of a dedicated EBUS bronchoscope with a working channel that enables real-time imaging for TBNA has made the procedure technically easier. It uses an integrated curvilinear scanner at 7.5 MHz that produces a view through the bronchial wall into the mediastinal structures, similar to that produced by the instruments used by gastroenterologists (Fig. 40-21).[9] A dedicated needle system is attached to the scope and advanced through the working channel. The needle, when advanced, can now be seen in real time (Fig. 40-22).[9]

The EBUS-TBNA bronchoscope handles differently from a conventional bronchoscope as the distal end is thicker and stiffer. The forward view is oblique instead of 0 degrees. In addition, the white light image is darker. Once it is mastered, this endoscope allows lymph node biopsies under real-time ultrasound guidance. EBUS has access to all of the mediastinal lymph nodes except the subaortic and paraesophageal lymph nodes (stations 5, 6, 8, and 9). Hilar lymph nodes (stations 10, 11, and part of 12) are also approachable. Transesophageal endoscopic ultrasound–fine needle aspiration (EUS-FNA) has also been used in conjunction with EBUS-TBNA in mediastinal lymph node assessment.[10] EBUS has better access to anterior and superior mediastinal lymph nodes, whereas EUS has better access to posterior and inferior mediastinal lymph nodes. By combining EBUS-TBNA and EUS-FNA, most of the mediastinum can be evaluated.[11]

An additional role for these endoscopic techniques is in the setting of mediastinal reassessment after induction therapy when the initial diagnosis of N2 disease was made at mediastinoscopy. Although re-mediastinoscopy has been well described, it remains a technically difficult and potentially dangerous procedure. Mediastinal reassessment affects the decision to operate in this setting. Alternatively, if surgery is considered an option after induction therapy, we prefer to establish the initial diagnosis of histologic N2 disease by EBUS and use mediastinoscopy for restaging. It is strongly recommended that thoracic surgeons gain expertise in endoscopic assessment of mediastinal adenopathy.

REFERENCES

1. Shields TW. The mediastinum, its compartments and the mediastinal lymph nodes. In *General thoracic surgery*. 5th ed. Philadelphia: Lippincott Williams & Wilkins; 2000.
2. Mountain CF, Dresler CM. Regional lymph node classification for lung cancer staging. *Chest* 1997;**111**:1718-23.
3. Toloza EM, Harpole L, Detterbeck F, McCrory DC. Invasive staging of non–small cell lung cancer: a review of the current evidence. *Chest* 2003;**123**(1 Suppl):157S-66S.
4. De Leyn P, Lardinois D, Van Schil PE, et al. ESTS guidelines for preoperative lymph node staging for non–small cell lung cancer. *Eur J Cardiothorac Surg* 2007;**32**:1-8.
5. Meyers BF, Haddad F, Siegel BA, et al. Cost-effectiveness of routine mediastinoscopy in computed tomography– and positron emission tomography–screened patients with stage I lung cancer. *J Thorac Cardiovasc Surg* 2006;**131**:822-9.
6. Zielinski M. Transcervical extended mediastinal lymphadenectomy: results of staging in two hundred fifty-six patients with non–small cell lung cancer. *J Thorac Oncol* 2007;**2**:370-2.
7. Witte B, Hürtgen M. Video-assisted mediastinoscopic lymphadenectomy (VAMLA). *J Thorac Oncol* 2007;**2**:367-9.
8. Hammond ZT, Anderson RC, Meyers BF, et al. The current role of mediastinoscopy in the evaluation of thoracic disease. *J Thorac Cardiovasc Surg* 1999;**118**:894-9.
9. Ernst A, Feller-Kopman D, Herth FJ. Endobronchial ultrasound in the diagnosis and staging of lung cancer and other thoracic tumors. *Semin Thorac Cardiovasc Surg* 2007;**19**:201-5.
10. Rintoul RC, Skwarski KM, Murchison JT, Wallace WA, Walker WS, Penman ID. Endobronchial and endoscopic ultrasound-guided real-time fine-needle aspiration for mediastinal staging. *Eur Respir J* 2005;**25**:416-21.
11. Wallace MB, Pascual JM, Raimondo M, et al. Minimally invasive endoscopic staging of suspected lung cancer. *JAMA* 2008;**299**:540-6.

CHAPTER 41
Anterior Mediastinal Masses
Chuong D. Hoang, John C. Kucharczuk, and Joseph B. Shrager

Thymic Tumors
  Thymoma
    Pathology
    Classification
    Presentation
    Association with Myasthenia Gravis
    Association with Other Diseases
    The Anterior Mediastinal Mass That Might Be Thymoma
    Treatment
    Outcome
  Thymic Carcinoma
  Neuroendocrine Tumors of the Thymus

Other Abnormalities of the Thymus
  Hyperplasia
  Thymolipoma
  Thymic Cysts
Germ Cell Tumors
  Benign Mediastinal Teratoma
  Malignant Mediastinal Germ Cell Tumors
Lymphomas
Substernal Thyroid
Hyperfunctioning Mediastinal Parathyroid Adenoma
Surgical Approaches to Biopsy

Chamberlain Procedure (Anterior Mediastinotomy)
Transcervical Biopsy (Cervical Mediastinotomy)
Thoracoscopic Biopsy
Extended Mediastinoscopy
Therapeutic Surgical Procedures: Techniques of Thymectomy
Thymectomy by Median Sternotomy
Transcervical Thymectomy
"Maximal" Thymectomy: Trans-sternal and Transcervical
Thoracoscopic Thymectomy
Summary

Although the anatomy of the mediastinum is presented in detail elsewhere in this book, it is reviewed here from a thoracic surgical perspective, to highlight the radiographic and surgical anatomic subdivisions of the mediastinum that have been proposed. The simplest and most commonly used description is the three-compartment model proposed by Shields.[1] He divided the mediastinum into the anterior compartment, the middle (or visceral) compartment, and the posterior (or paravertebral) compartment. The anatomic limits of each compartment are shown in Figure 41-1, and the structures contained within each compartment are listed in Table 41-1. Locating a mass in the anterior mediastinum allows a differential diagnosis to be generated based on the knowledge of the normal structures in that compartment. From the perspective of thoracic surgery, this approach best allows the appropriate diagnostic and therapeutic procedures to be selected.

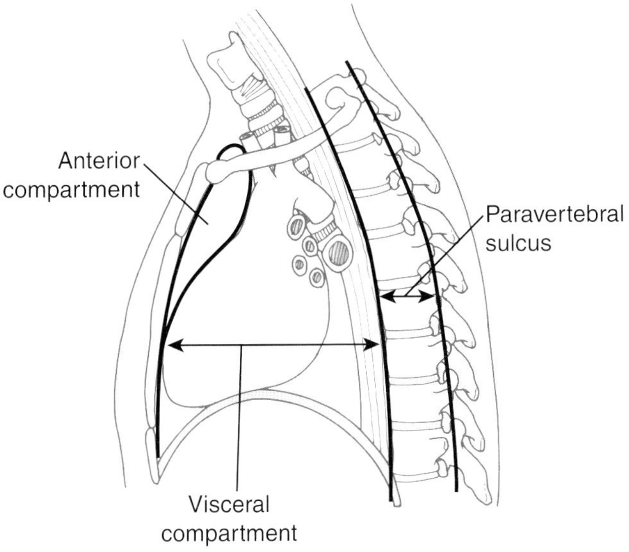

Table 41-2 is an extensive list of the pathologies that can appear as a mass in the anterior mediastinal compartment. By far, the four most common are thymoma, lymphoma, teratoma, and germ cell tumor.

THYMIC TUMORS

Lesions of the thymus account for approximately 50% of anterior mediastinal masses in adults and are thus of great importance. Although lymphomas and germ cell tumors of the anterior mediastinum often involve the thymus or actually arise from cells within the thymus (or both), these are most appropriately discussed as a group separate from thymic tumors and are usually classified separately. The thymic masses discussed in this section, then, are listed in Box 41-1.

Thymoma

Thymomas are the most common thymic tumor, and approximately 95% are located in the anterior mediastinum. They are of surgical interest both because excision is the primary therapy and because of their interesting association with myasthenia gravis (MG), a disease the clinical course of which can be favorably influenced by thymectomy.

Thymomas may be completely encapsulated or invasive. Large series have demonstrated the incidence of encapsulated lesions to be between 40% and 70% and that of microscopic or grossly invasive lesions to be between 30% and 60%. Although local invasion is usually limited to the capsule or to immediately adjacent structures, spread to more distant sites within the chest does occur, particularly to the pleura, diaphragm, and mediastinal lymph nodes. Aggressive thymomas have been reported to be associated with distant metastases in as many as 30% of patients at high-level referral centers,[2] but most broad studies report distant metastasis to be rare (<5%).

Figure 41-1
Three-compartment division of the mediastinum as proposed by Shields. *(From Shields TW. General thoracic surgery. 2nd ed. Philadelphia: Lea & Febiger; 1983, with permission.)*

Table 41-1

Components of Mediastinal Compartments* as Proposed by Shields

Anterior	Visceral (middle)	Paravertebral (posterior)
Thymus	Pericardium/heart	Sympathetic chain
Internal thoracic vessels	Great vessels	Proximal intercostals: nerve, artery, and vein
Internal thoracic lymph nodes	Trachea	Posterior paraesophageal lymph nodes
Prevascular lymph nodes	Proximal right and left main-stem	Intercostal lymph nodes
Fat and connective tissue	Esophagus	
	Phrenic nerve Thoracic duct Proximal azygos vein Pretracheal lymph nodes (levels 2, 4, and 7) Pleuropericardial lymph nodes Fat and connective tissue	

*The nodal basin draining the anterior chest wall and female breast lie in the anterior compartment, whereas the majority of those draining the lung and important in lung cancer staging lie in the visceral compartment.
From Shields TW. General thoracic surgery. 2nd ed. Philadelphia: Lea & Febiger; 1983, with permission.

Table 41-2

Mass Lesion in the Anterior Mediastinal Compartment: Differential Diagnosis

Neoplastic

Thyroid
    Substernal goiter
    Ectopic thyroid tissue
Thymus
    Thymic hyperplasia
    Thymoma
    Thymic carcinoma
    Thymic carcinoid
    Thymic small cell carcinoma
    Thymic cysts
    Thymolipoma
Teratoma
    Mature teratoma
    Immature teratoma
    Teratoma with malignant component
Lymphoma
Ectopic parathyroid with adenoma
Germ cell tumors
    Seminoma
    Nonseminomatous
        Yolk sac tumors
        Embryonal carcinoma
        Choriocarcinoma lymphangioma
Hemangioma
Lipoma
Liposarcoma
Fibroma
Fibrosarcoma
Cervicomediastinal hygroma

Infectious

Acute descending necrotizing mediastinitis
    Extension of deep cervical bacterial infection into the anterior compartment, with abscess formation and sepsis
Subacute mediastinitis
    Fungal, mycobacterial, actinomycotic, or histoplasmotic infection causing an inflammatory mass in the anterior mediastinum

Vascular

Aneurysm of the aortic arch with projection into the anterior mediastinum
Innominate vein aneurysm
Superior vena cava aneurysm
Dilation of the superior vena cava (with anomalous pulmonary venous return)
Persistent left superior vena cava

Pathology

Thymomas are derived from thymic epithelial cells, but most contain varying mixes of epithelial cells and lymphocytes.[3] Traditional histologic classifications have therefore grouped thymomas according to cytologic make-up: (1) predominantly lymphocytic, (2) predominantly epithelial, and (3) mixed.[4] There is also a recognized spindle cell variant of the epithelial subtype. Approximately 50% of the tumors are of the mixed variety, with the remainder split between the epithelial and lymphocytic subtypes. Unfortunately, these subtypes have little prognostic significance, other than the generally better prognosis of the spindle cell variant, and thus more recent investigators have proposed alternative histologic classification schemes (see later).

Of clinical significance is the fact that it may be more difficult to establish the diagnosis of thymoma from a small sample (e.g., by needle biopsy) of a lymphocyte-predominant thymoma versus the other subtypes because of its microscopic similarity to lymphoma. Immunohistochemical staining for cytokeratin often helps in making the diagnosis, as antibodies to this protein are present in 95% to 100% of thymomas.[5] Chromogranin staining allows differentiation between thymoma and thymic carcinoid (the former being negative and the latter positive for chromogranin).

Classification

No TNM classification has been found to be of value for staging thymomas.

The most widely used clinical classification scheme is that proposed by Masaoka and colleagues in 1981[6] (Table 41-3). This scheme takes into account the gross presence or absence of encapsulation and fixation or invasion into adjacent structures as identified at the time of surgery. It also recognizes the fact that a grossly well-encapsulated tumor may be found to have invasion through the capsule at microscopic examination. In the years since it was originally proposed,

Box 41-1
Thymic Masses

- Thymic hyperplasia
- Thymoma
- Thymic carcinoma
- Thymic neuroendocrine tumors
  - Carcinoid
  - Small cell carcinoma
- Thymic cysts (not rhizomatous)
- Thymolipoma
- Metastases to the thymus

Table 41-3
Classification Schemes for Thymoma

	Masaoka	WHO*
Stage I	Encapsulated, tumor may invade into, but not through capsule microscopically.	Type A (spindle cell, medullary)
Stage II		Type AB (mixed)
IIa	Macroscopic invasion into thymus or fat or adherent to but not through pleura or pericardium	Type B
IIb	Microscopic trans-capsular invasion	B1 (lymphocyte-rich, predominantly cortical)
Stage III	Macroscopic invasion of neighboring organs (pericardium, great vessels, lung)	B2 (cortical)
Stage IV		B3 (epithelial, well-differentiated thymic carcinoma)
IV A	Pleural or pericardial dissemination	Type C (thymic carcinoma)
IV B	Lymphogenous or hematogenous mets	

*In the World Health Organization (WHO) column, terms in parentheses represent nomenclature from previous histologic classifications that most closely approximate the current classification category.

the Masaoka system or later variations of it have been found to have prognostic significance by numerous authors.

In 1985, Marino and Muller-Hermelink[7] proposed a histologic classification that has come to be known as the Muller-Hermelink (MH) classification. This scheme divides thymomas into cortical, medullary, and mixed types. The cortical type contains medium to large epithelial cells of characteristic appearance, and usually abundant lymphocytes. The medullary type contains small to medium cells with different features and fewer lymphocytes. The former tend to be of higher clinical stage, whereas the latter tend to be of lower invasiveness. Many investigators have generated data in support of the prognostic significance of the MH classification,[8-11] showing that the medullary type has the best and the cortical type the least favorable prognosis. The World Health Organization (WHO) has adopted a classification system based on the MH criteria (see Table 41-3).[12] It has been suggested that such histologic systems be used in combination with a Masaoka-type staging system to provide more precise prognostic information.

Presentation

Most patients with thymomas present at an age older than 40 years. There is no major predominance in men or women. About 50% of patients are asymptomatic; the remaining patients present with either local symptoms (pain, dyspnea, cough, hoarseness) resulting from locally invasive tumors, or systemic symptoms of one of the associated systemic diseases.

Association with Myasthenia Gravis

Patients with thymomas may present with a number of associated diseases, largely autoimmune in etiology, but the most common associated illness is myasthenia gravis. Accumulated experience suggests that 5% to 15% of patients with MG are found to have thymomas, and that 30% to 50% of thymomas are associated with clinical MG. Notably, the disease may develop later, even after thymoma resection, if it is not present at the time of discovery of the thymic tumor. For this reason, it is essential that a complete thymectomy be performed as part of the resection of any anterior mediastinal tumor that may be a thymoma. As MG is an autoimmune disease caused by anti-acetylcholine receptor (anti-AChR) antibodies, its relationship to thymoma and treatment by thymectomy appears to be related to the role of the thymus in the creation of these antibodies.[13,14]

This association has a long and very interesting history that is beyond the scope of this chapter. Highlights, however, include the first description by Schumacher and Roth in 1912 of improvement in MG after thymectomy[15]; the more systematic evaluation of this concept by Blalock and coworkers in the late 1930s[16]; and the subsequent controversy over whether the morbidity and mortality of the procedure justified the chances of a remission from MG. Only in the late 1960s and 1970s did thymectomy for MG in the absence of thymoma gain wide acceptance, as improvements in perioperative care reduced the morbidity of the procedure and the benefits became clearer. Although convincing data suggest that patients with MG who are treated with thymectomy have a higher remission rate than historical controls treated by medication alone, there has never been a randomized study to definitively establish this concept. Just such a study is, however, now ongoing, sponsored by the National Institute of Neurological Disorders and Stroke.

Association with Other Diseases

Box 41-2 lists MG and the other systemic, autoimmune disorders most commonly associated with thymoma. Two percent to 15% of patients with thymoma suffer from some type of cytopenia. The most common type is pure red cell aplasia, thought to result from an abnormal IgG antibody that inhibits red cell synthesis. Most patients with this disease have the favorable, spindle-cell type of thymoma.[17] Approximately one third of patients with aplasia demonstrate improvement after thymectomy.[18] Hypogammaglobulinemia occurs in less than 5% of patients with thymoma, principally older patients. This disease generally does not respond to thymectomy, and the prognosis is poor. Of the other autoimmune disorders that occur in association with thymoma in lower frequencies, lupus appears to be the most common; again, resection does not appear to have an impact on the clinical course.

The Anterior Mediastinal Mass That Might Be Thymoma

Imaging

Radiologic studies play a central role in the evaluation of thymoma. Because many patients are asymptomatic at presentation, a widened mediastinum or loss of the normal anterior clear space on the lateral film of a routine chest radiograph may be the first sign of disease. In such a patient, a computed tomogram (CT) of the chest with intravenous contrast should be obtained as the next step. Patients who present with MG or another of the disorders that may be associated with thymoma should also have a chest CT.

Although no CT appearance is diagnostic of thymoma, a well-circumscribed, solid anterior mediastinal mass in an adult older than 40 years, without low-density areas that suggest the cystic and fatty components of a teratoma, is very likely to be a thymoma (Figs. 41-2 and 41-3). The presence of calcification is not particularly helpful, as both thymomas and teratomas may contain calcium. In some cases, lymphoma will be the obvious diagnosis on the basis of adenopathy outside the anterior mediastinum, but in the absence of this finding, differentiating a thymoma from a lymphoma may be difficult. It is often possible to suspect one over the other only on the basis of the thymoma patient's typically more advanced age. Magnetic resonance imaging (MRI) provides useful additional information only when the fluid or fatty nature of a component of the tumor is not clearly defined by CT, or when a vascular structure (e.g., an aneurysm) is suspected and has not been clearly ruled out by the contrast CT study.

The chest CT also provides information about a putative thymoma's local and regional spread. Loss of planes between the tumor and normal structures may suggest direct invasion, and visceral or parietal pleural deposits may be visible as well. The presence of such signs of local aggressiveness might steer the surgeon toward biopsy rather than resection, given the recent data suggesting improved results with neoadjuvant chemoradiotherapy before operation in aggressive thymoma and thymic carcinoma.[19-21] The role of positron emission tomography (PET) in thymic tumors is not well defined. It has

---

Box 41–2
Systemic Diseases Most Commonly Associated with Thymoma

- Myasthenia gravis
- Cytopenias (most commonly, red cell hypoplasia)
- Nonthymic malignancies
- Hypogammaglobulinemia
- Systemic lupus erythematosus
- Polymyositis
- Rheumatoid arthritis
- Thyroiditis
- Sjögren's syndrome
- Ulcerative colitis

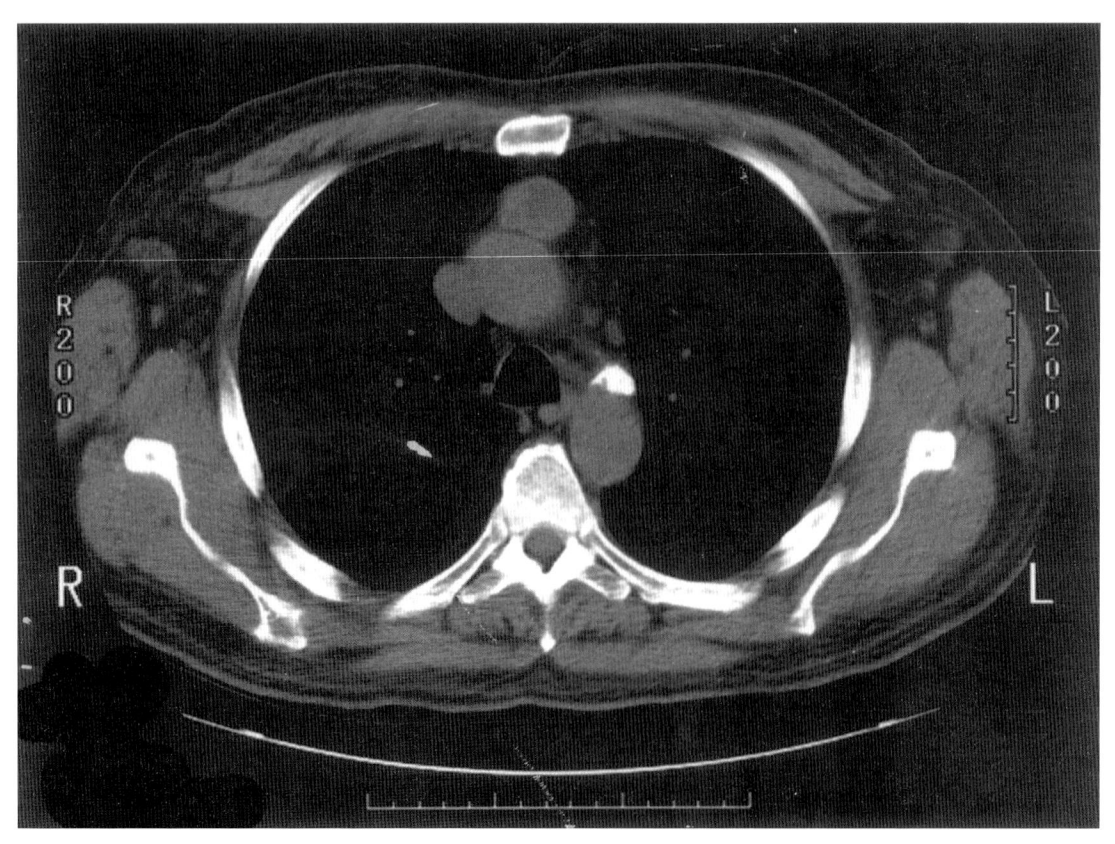

Figure 41–2
Characteristic CT appearance of a noninvasive thymoma: a well-circumscribed, solid anterior mediastinal mass.

recently been shown that PET may be useful for predicting the grade of malignancy according to histologic subtype.[22]

Serum Studies

All male patients with an anterior mediastinal mass should have serum testing for α-fetoprotein (AFP), β-human chorionic gonadotropin (β-hCG), and lactic dehydrogenase (LDH). Although these levels are normal in patients with mature teratoma, those with malignant germ cell tumors have significant elevations; thus the clinician should establish this diagnosis and rule out thymoma.

Evaluation for Myasthenia Gravis

All patients with suspected thymoma should be carefully questioned about muscle weakness or ocular signs of MG. The diagnosis of MG requires a characteristic history or physical findings, or both, as well as two positive diagnostic tests. Diagnostic testing for MG includes pharmacologic, serologic, and electrodiagnostic studies. Unfortunately, no single diagnostic test can rule out MG with certainty in patients with thymoma. If there is the slightest suggestion of MG on initial presentation, the patient should undergo additional testing preoperatively under the direction of an experienced neurologist.

Depending on the disease severity, patients with MG may require medical optimization before surgery by some combination of cholinesterase inhibitors, steroids, gamma globulin, and plasmapheresis. Additionally, drugs that may exacerbate the symptoms of MG must be avoided (e.g., aminoglycosides, certain inhalation anesthetics, and iodinated radiographic contrast). Establishing the preoperative forced vital capacity (FVC) for comparison postoperatively can be useful for determining the appropriateness of extubation in patients with MG after general anesthesia. We generally require a minimum FVC of 10 mL/kg before extubation.

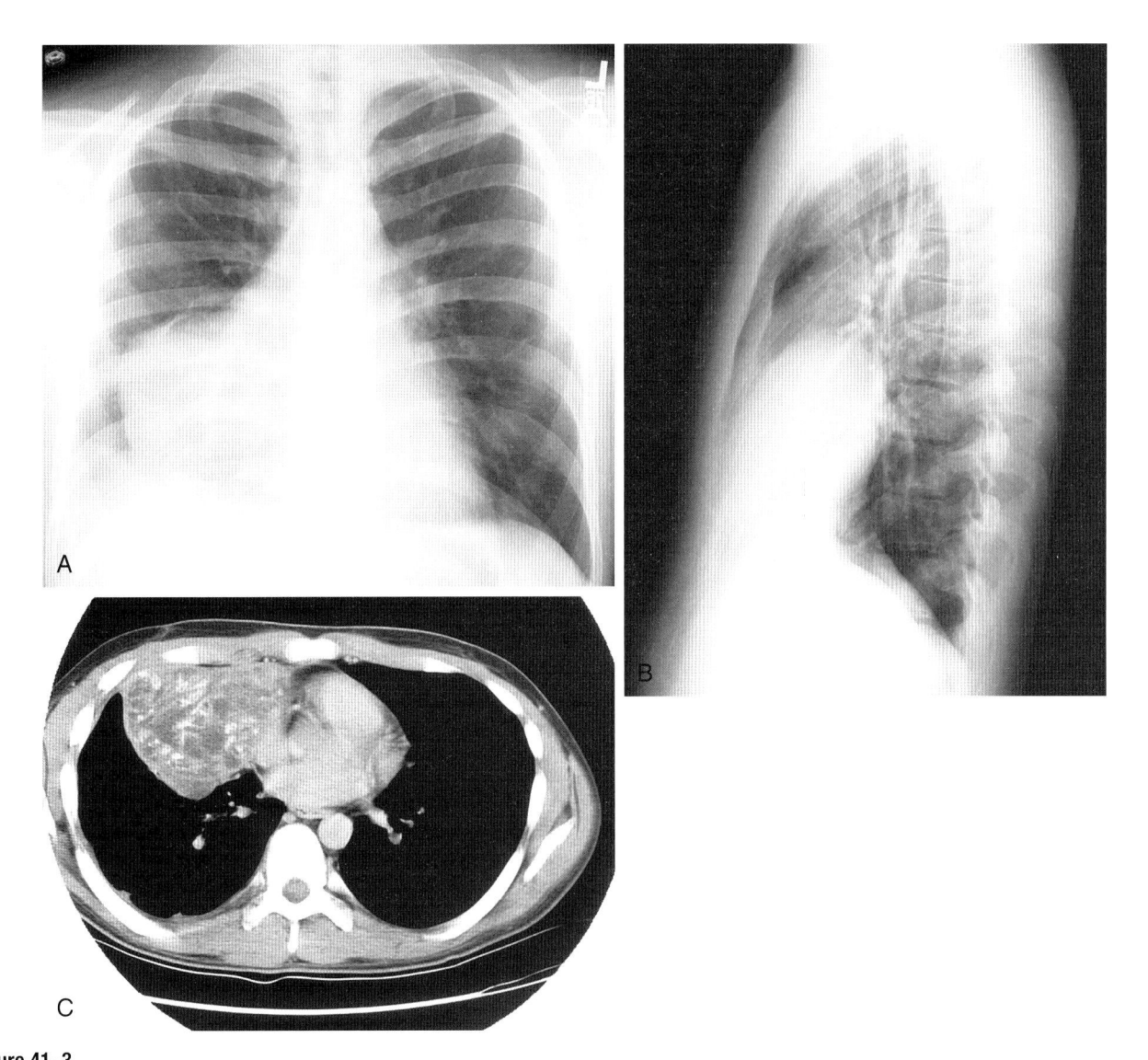

Figure 41-3
Posteroanterior (**A**) and lateral (**B**) chest radiographs from a 21-year-old man show a large mediastinal mass adjacent to the right cardiac border. This appearance is characteristic of a mediastinal teratoma. The CT scan (**C**) shows a complex cystic mass with solid components including fat and calcification consistent with a diagnosis of teratoma. In the absence of metastatic disease, the final differentiation between teratoma and teratocarcinoma can be made only by pathologic review. (**A** and **B** courtesy of Wallace T. Miller Jr, MD, Hospital of the University of Pennsylvania, Philadelphia.)

Biopsy

Typically, the clinician proceeds directly to resection of a discrete anterior mediastinal mass in any of the following situations: (1) the CT or MRI shows features consistent with teratoma; (2) the patient is older than 40 years, without clinical signs or symptoms of lymphoma and with normal AFP and β-hCG; or (3) the mass is associated with MG. In most other instances, biopsy is indicated, because despite the history, physical examination, imaging, and serum studies, one is still left with a mass that could represent thymoma, lymphoma, or teratoma.

There is controversy over whether the biopsy should be done by thin- or core-needle biopsy, anterior mediastinotomy (Chamberlain procedure), transcervical mediastinotomy, or video-assisted thoracoscopic surgery (VATS) (see Surgical Approaches to Biopsy, later). Needle biopsy has the disadvantage that optimal tissue may not be obtained, and the availability of pathologists adept at differentiating lymphoma from thymoma and among the various types of lymphoma by cytology and flow-cytometry is required. Although mediastinotomy almost always provides adequate tissue for diagnosis, there is a theoretical risk (unproven) that thymoma cells may be spread, rendering a previously contained tumor less clearly resectable (an even greater concern for VATS). We favor mediastinotomy when lymphoma is the leading clinical diagnosis, but we believe that needle biopsy is required for tumors that are more likely to be thymoma or germ cell tumor (e.g., aggressive thymoma in which neoadjuvant protocols might be considered).

Treatment

Surgery

Complete surgical resection along with complete thymectomy is the optimal management for thymoma that is not known preoperatively to be invasive. The technique is detailed later in this chapter.

Adjuvant Therapies

For aggressive thymomas, neoadjuvant chemotherapy before resection should be considered. The response rate to these regimens, which generally contain cisplatin, is high, and the rate of complete resection appears to be improved by such an approach. These patients should probably also receive postoperative radiotherapy.

Postoperative radiation therapy is certainly indicated in cases of incomplete resection and after complete resection of Masaoka stage III thymomas. As the rate of recurrence of completely resected stage I tumors is less than 5%, these patients are generally not considered for adjuvant radiation. Adjuvant radiotherapy for completely resected stage II thymoma is more controversial. We[23] and others[24] have presented data that strongly suggest that postoperative radiotherapy is not indicated in stage II disease.

Outcome

The outcome for patients with thymoma is stage specific. Patients with completely resected Masaoka stage I thymomas have an excellent prognosis, with an expected recurrence rate of less than 5%. Their 10- and 20-year survival rates are 99% and 90%, respectively.[25] As the stage increases, the recurrence rates increase and the survival rates decrease. Patients with stage II thymomas treated by complete resection with or without postoperative radiation therapy have recurrence rates as high as 20%.[24,26] The 5- and 10-year survival rates are 70% to 90% and 55% to 85%, respectively.[26,27] Long-term data from Japan show improvement in the 10- and 20-year survival rates to 94% and 90%, respectively.[25] The 5-year survival rates for patients with stage III tumors drops to about 50%.[28] It is uncertain whether patients with advanced stage III and IV disease who undergo tumor debulking have an improved prognosis compared with those who undergo biopsy alone. The M. D. Anderson Cancer Center, in Houston, reported their results in a patient cohort (N = 22) with advanced-stage thymoma in a recent phase II study evaluating tumor resectability after induction chemotherapy followed by surgical resection, radiation therapy, and consolidation chemotherapy.[29] With a median follow-up time of 50 months, 18 of 19 patients who completed the multidisciplinary approach were disease free. The progression-free survival rates were 77% at 5 years and 77% at 7 years.

Historically the presence of thymoma was believed to adversely affect the outcome after thymectomy for MG. Several modern studies, however, suggest that this is not the case. A review from the Toronto General Hospital revealed no significant difference in the complete response rate or postoperative Osserman grade of patients with MG undergoing thymectomy, with or without thymoma.[30] The complete remission rate of MG at 5 years after thymectomy was 36% with or without thymoma.

Thymic Carcinoma

Thymic carcinomas are rare invasive epithelial malignancies. A clinicopathologic study of 60 cases of thymic carcinoma revealed an overall 5-year survival of 33%.[31] Histologically, this group consists of a number of different cell types. They are unified, however, by their unequivocal malignant appearance on light microscopy. Although there is no formalized staging system, division of patients into those with low-grade histology and those with high-grade histology does have prognostic significance. Low-grade tumors include squamous, mucoepidermoid, and basaloid carcinomas. The high-grade tumors include sarcomatoid and clear cell carcinoma. The median survival time for patients with low-grade histology is 29 months, compared with 11 months for patients with high-grade histology.[32] Effective therapy of thymic carcinoma requires a multimodality approach, which typically includes induction therapy followed by resection, with postoperative radiation therapy if it was not included preoperatively. Unfortunately, most patients have recurrence, either locally or at distant sites, and die of their disease. Multiple neoadjuvant chemotherapy protocols have been proposed for patients presenting with clearly unresectable disease. To date, the numbers are too small and the results too variable to determine if this approach converts these patients into operative candidates or affects their overall outcome.[33]

Neuroendocrine Tumors of the Thymus

Neuroendocrine tumors of the thymus include thymic carcinoid and small cell carcinoma of the thymus. These tumors are related biochemically by the presence of APUD (amine precursor uptake and decarboxylation) cells and may actually represent a spectrum of the same abnormality.

Thymic carcinoid occurs more frequently in men than in women. One third of patients present with Cushing syndrome because of ectopic adrenocorticotropic hormone (ACTH) production. This portends a very poor prognosis. The treatment of thymic carcinoid is complete excision, and the overall cure rate is very low. The role of multimodality therapy is undefined.

Small cell carcinoma of the thymus is very uncommon. A 20-year review of extrapulmonary small cell carcinoma at the Mayo Clinic revealed only three cases out of a total of 54 patients.[34] This tumor, however, is very aggressive. It is treated with chemotherapy alone or in combination with radiation. Like small cell carcinoma of the lung, it is usually responsive to initial chemotherapy, but the response is often not durable.

Other Abnormalities of the Thymus

Hyperplasia

The infant thymus is a large triangular shaped gland that occupies a significant portion of the anterior mediastinum. In contrast, the adult thymus is an involuted organ consisting mostly of adipose tissue surrounded by a capsule. In true thymic hyperplasia, the gland is enlarged in both size and weight (for the patient's age). Histologically the gland appears normal. The presentation of thymic hyperplasia is along a spectrum ranging from the incidentally discovered mass to one causing respiratory compromise due to massive enlargement with tracheal compression. It can be seen in association with other disorders, such as MG, and can occur after severe illness—the so-called thymic rebound.

Thymolipoma

Thymolipomas are distinguished from simple mediastinal lipomas by their location in the thymic capsule. Histologically, these neoplasms contain mature adipose cells as well as normal thymic components. Interestingly, thymolipomas can be associated with thymic paraneoplastic syndromes such as red cell aplasia, aplastic anemia, and hypogammaglobulinemia (see previous discussion). The treatment of thymolipoma is excision.

Thymic Cysts

Mediastinal thymic cysts account for less than 0.2% of anterior mediastinal masses.[35] They are often asymptomatic and are usually discovered incidentally. Most are unilocular, and they must contain thymic tissue within the cyst wall to confirm the diagnosis. As a unique entity, they are inconsequential and completely benign. Removal is indicated to rule out other entities, such as thymoma with cystic components (i.e., cystic thymoma) and Hodgkin's disease. Excision yields a definitive diagnosis and completes treatment.

GERM CELL TUMORS

Germ cell tumors comprise a group of neoplasms that usually arise in gonadal tissue. The anterior mediastinum is the most common location for the occurrence of extragonadal germ cell tumors, which account for 15% to 20% of all anterior mediastinal masses. These tumors are divided into benign and malignant lesions.

Benign Mediastinal Teratoma

Benign mediastinal teratoma accounts for 60% of mediastinal germ cell tumors. It is usually asymptomatic in the adult. Children are more likely to present with symptoms caused by airway compression. On CT scan, the mass is well circumscribed and may contain calcification. It usually shows variable enhancement because of the presence of different tissue types including fat, muscle, bone, and cystic components (see Fig. 41-3). Curative treatment consists of complete excision via median sternotomy. Thoracosternotomy may be required for giant tumors.

Malignant Mediastinal Germ Cell Tumors

The malignant mediastinal germ cell tumors are divided into seminomatous and nonseminomatous tumors. Seminomas account for 40% of these tumors, and the nonseminomas account for 60%. The nonseminomas include embryonal cell carcinoma, choriocarcinoma, yolk sac tumors, and teratocarcinomas. These are generally diffuse, not discrete, anterior mediastinal masses.

The malignant germ cell tumors are much more common in males but they have been reported in females.[36] The preoperative evaluation of these patients includes a complete physical examination, and testicular examination in male patients. Radiographic studies should include a chest radiograph as well as a CT scan of the chest, abdomen, and pelvis. Serum AFP, β-hCG, and LDH levels should be obtained. Patients with pure seminoma have normal AFP. Those with any elevation in AFP or a marked elevation in β-hCG have mixed tumors containing both seminomatous and nonseminomatous elements. The differentiation between the seminomatous and nonseminomatous germ cell tumors has important prognostic and therapeutic implications. Like testicular seminomas, the pure mediastinal germ cell seminomas are extremely radiosensitive and are treated with radiation therapy. After radiation, about 80% of patients with pure seminoma are cured.[37] Residual masses greater than 3 cm should be resected.

Patients with nonseminomas have elevated AFP, β-hCG, and LDH levels. After confirmation by needle biopsy, they are usually treated with three-drug chemotherapy (bleomycin, etoposide, and cisplatin). Traditionally, surgical resection is reserved for a residual mass after treatment, with normalization of serum markers (this indirectly suggests a response from the tumor, translating to a greater chance of complete resectability). Recently, researchers at Indiana University reviewed their 25-year experience with treated mediastinal nonseminomatous germ cell tumors in 158 patients.[38] With a median follow-up of 34 months, they reported a 62% overall survival. Multivariate analysis revealed that, among other variables, pathologically identified complete tumor necrosis after chemotherapy was an independent predictor of survival. Operative risks for nonseminomatous germ cell tumors appear to be improved with the use of chemotherapy regimens that did not contain bleomycin. Data from Memorial Sloan-Kettering[39] and other institutions[40] suggest that all patients with a residual mass after chemotherapy should undergo resection even if their markers remain elevated. These studies revealed that post-chemotherapy serum marker levels correlated poorly with pathologic evidence of disease. Further there were no effective second-line chemotherapy regimens and long-term survival differences did not exist in patients with presurgical elevated markers versus patients with normal markers.

LYMPHOMAS

Both Hodgkin's disease and non-Hodgkin's lymphomas can appear as anterior mediastinal masses. The diagnosis is usually suspected on clinical history and CT scan. We recommend surgical biopsy over needle biopsy as the most efficient method of obtaining a precise diagnosis when lymphoma is suspected (see previous discussion). Surgical approaches to biopsy include cervical mediastinoscopy, anterior mediastinotomy, and, less commonly, thoracoscopy. It is imperative that the surgeon work in conjunction with the pathologist at the time of surgery to ensure that adequate tissue is obtained. The diagnosis of Hodgkin's disease is confirmed by the presence of Reed-Sternberg cells. The diagnosis and characterization of the non-Hodgkin's lymphoma rely on both light microscopy and cell surface markers. Flow cytometry requires fresh (unfixed) tissue, so the surgeon must ensure that not all of the biopsy tissue is placed in formalin.

Controversy persists over the sensitivity and specificity of the CT scan, gallium scan, and PET scan in determining the composition of residual masses after chemotherapy and radiotherapy for lymphomas. Some advocate multiple core-needle biopsies in this setting, but this is subject to sampling error. The only definitive method of determining the composition of a residual mass is surgical biopsy or resection, and either may rarely be indicated.

SUBSTERNAL THYROID

Substernal thyroid and ectopic thyroid tissue can appear as an anterior mediastinal mass. In most cases of substernal thyroid, an enlarged thyroid gland is palpable in the neck. Often, a chest radiograph shows deviation of the trachea. We have found that a CT scan without contrast is the single most useful test in differentiating substernal thyroid from other mediastinal masses. Because of its iodine content, substernal thyroid tissue shows enhancement on a noncontrast CT scan and usually confirms the diagnosis. The majority of substernal thyroids are goiters, but a benign process and a malignant one cannot be differentiated radiographically. The vast majority of substernal goiters are removed via a cervical approach. This is possible because the blood supply of the superior and inferior thyroid arteries originate in the neck. In some instances, a partial sternal split is required to provide adequate room for delivery of the gland from its substernal location. Infrequently, tracheal resection with primary anastomosis is required to correct tracheomalacia caused by compression, or by direct tracheal invasion in the case of malignant substernal thyroid neoplasms. This should be performed as a single-stage operation at the time of thyroid resection.

HYPERFUNCTIONING MEDIASTINAL PARATHYROID ADENOMA

Ectopic parathyroid glands can be located in the mediastinum. These patients present with primary hyperparathyroidism after an unsuccessful neck exploration. Before proceeding with mediastinal exploration, localizing studies are performed. Technetium-99m-sestamibi scintigraphy is the most useful study to localize hyperfunctioning ectopic parathyroid adenomas in the mediastinum. This study can also be performed as a subtraction study with iodine-123. Nonfunctional anatomic studies such as MRI may reveal a well-defined mass, but they are usually small (<3 cm).

The treatment for an ectopic mediastinal parathyroid adenoma is resection. This is performed via a transcervical approach, via a median sternotomy, or, in experienced hands, thoracoscopically. Resection involves removal of the thymus and surrounding fat to include the adenoma. Intraoperative use of rapid parathormone levels confirms the successful localization and removal of the adenoma. The presence of parathyroid tissue should also be confirmed by frozen section examination. If the transcervical approach is selected and there is no normalization of intraoperative parathyroid hormone, or if parathyroid tissue cannot be confirmed pathologically, the surgeon should convert to a median sternotomy.

SURGICAL APPROACHES TO BIOPSY

Chamberlain Procedure (Anterior Mediastinotomy)

This procedure is usually performed under general anesthesia, but it can be performed under local anesthesia if required. The patient is placed in the supine position with arms tucked. A 5-cm, horizontally oriented incision is made just lateral to the sternomanubrial joint over the second costal cartilage. The pectoralis muscle fibers are split from the sternochondral to the costochondral junction. The second cartilage is removed subperichondrially, and the pleura is gently swept laterally to avoid inadvertent pneumothorax. Care is taken to avoid injury to the internal thoracic artery and vein, but sometimes they must be divided to gain sufficient exposure. Biopsy is performed under direct vision with a scalpel or biopsy forceps. During closure, the perichondrium should be reapproximated to promote regrowth of a normal-shaped cartilage.

Transcervical Biopsy (Cervical Mediastinotomy)

Transcervical biopsy is performed through a transcervical collar type incision. The technique is identical to that described later for transcervical thymectomy, and it is facilitated by use of the Cooper retractor. Once exposure is obtained, tissue can be procured directly with biopsy forceps or scalpel. We have found this approach to be particularly useful to biopsy lesions directly beneath the sternum that would be difficult to reach by a Chamberlain procedure and thus might ultimately require a sternotomy.[41]

Thoracoscopic Biopsy

VATS can be used for biopsy of anterior mediastinal masses, but in most situations there are easier and more direct approaches. The anterior mediastinum can be reached from either the left or the right thorax, and the side should be selected on the basis of the predominant location of the mass. A 30-degree thoracoscope facilitates visualization of the anterior mediastinum. The thoracoscope is introduced through the fourth intercostal space in the posterior axillary line. Next, one or two working ports are created somewhat more anteriorly. Port placement is important while working in the anterior mediastinal compartment. Significant experience is required to avoid "clashing" of instruments by inappropriately placed port sites.

From the right thorax, the anterior compartment can be reached by incising the pleura anterior to the phrenic nerve as it runs along the superior vena cava. The connective tissue is gently swept away and the anterior mediastinal compartment entered. The lesion should be identified both visually and by tactile sensation before biopsy. Working on the left side can be more difficult because of the proximity of the major vessels of the visceral compartment (the aorta and its branches). Nevertheless, creating an incision anterior to the phrenic nerve allows access.

In our opinion, the VATS approach is more cumbersome and associated with greater risks than either the anterior mediastinotomy or the transcervical approaches. Dissection around the phrenic nerves can result in temporary or permanent dysfunction. Spillage of tumor during biopsy may cause inadvertent contamination of the pleural space. Finally, this approach requires single-lung ventilation, which adds an additional level of complexity to the anesthetic management, especially in patients with large masses and tracheal compression.

Extended Mediastinoscopy

In 1987, Ginsberg and colleagues reported the use of extended cervical mediastinoscopy in the staging of lung cancer.[42] This advanced technique allows placement of a mediastinoscope into the anterior compartment through a standard cervical mediastinoscopy incision. This involves the creation of a tunnel between the origin of the innominate artery and the left carotid. The tunnel is created by careful digital dissection, the mediastinoscope is then reinserted and advanced anteriorly toward the left into the tunnel, and the target lesion is clearly identified before biopsy. This technique requires considerable experience and carries the risk of significant bleeding because of the proximity of the aorta and pulmonary artery. Unless the surgeon has been specifically trained in this technique, most anterior mediastinal masses are more safely and easily approached via anterior or cervical mediastinotomy, as described previously.

THERAPEUTIC SURGICAL PROCEDURES: TECHNIQUES OF THYMECTOMY

The main surgical procedure carried out for tumors of the anterior mediastinum is thymectomy, as thymoma is the most common tumor in this area and demands complete extirpation of the gland. Only if there is a preoperative suspicion of a tumor other than thymoma (generally a teratoma) should the surgeon attempt to explore the anterior mediastinum and resect the tumor alone without the adjoining thymus. In this circumstance, a frozen section should always be obtained to confirm the preoperative diagnosis so as not to inadvertently perform less than a complete thymectomy for thymoma.

Thymectomy by Median Sternotomy

Median sternotomy is the most widely employed approach to thymectomy. Although a full sternotomy is typical, partial upper sternotomy with extension of the bony incision into the third or fourth intercostal space also has its advocates.[43] Adjacent structures to which the tumor is adherent must be resected en bloc. This often includes pleura, pericardium, and, in more aggressive tumors, the innominate vein (which may be resected without reconstruction), the superior vena cava (requiring reconstruction), and/or lung. Although historically the recommendation has been that both pleural spaces be widely opened, we hold that this should be done only on the side on which the tumor is adherent to the pleura, as opening an uninvolved hemithorax quite likely increases the risk of spread to that pleural space, with no obvious benefit. In all procedures, the upper and lower thymic poles are traced as far into the neck and down toward the diaphragm as necessary to ensure complete resection, and all fatty tissue between the phrenic nerves is included in the resection.

Transcervical Thymectomy

We have reported that noninvasive thymomas less than 4 cm in diameter may be completely resected along with the thymus by a transcervical approach.[41] However, when using this approach, the surgeon must have a low threshold for conversion to sternotomy if any suggestion of gross invasion is encountered. In fact, patients should be followed longer before this approach is widely applied for even small thymomas. Strong evidence exists, on the other hand, that in the absence of thymoma, transcervical thymectomy (TCT) provides results very similar to more aggressive thymectomy approaches in the treatment of MG.[44] Table 41-4 lists results of large modern studies of the various approaches to thymectomy for MG. Note that there is no dramatic difference in complete MG remission rates between the proposed approaches to thymectomy.

TCT and transcervical approaches to other masses in the anterior mediastinum are performed through a 5-cm curvilinear incision in the jugular notch. Details of the procedure have been described elsewhere.[45] In brief, after dissection of the two cervical poles, they are each tied with a silk suture and used for traction to aid in dissection of the remainder of the gland. After branches from the innominate vein to the gland are ligated and divided, a Cooper thymectomy retractor (Pilling Co., Fort Washington, PA) is used to maximally lift the sternum as an inflatable bag beneath the shoulders is deflated. Extracapsular removal of the entire gland then proceeds by primarily blunt dissection within the mediastinum by the operator, seated at the head of the table and using a headlight (Fig. 41-4). The resection includes the bulk of the extra-thymic mediastinal fat between the phrenic nerves and down to the diaphragm. The procedure does not remove the pleurae or the fat directly apposed to the pleurae, tissue posterior to the phrenic nerves, or other areas where ectopic thymic tissue has been described. No drains are left in place. Patients are generally discharged late on the day of surgery.

"Maximal" Thymectomy: Trans-sternal and Transcervical

Jaretzki and a few others have for many years advocated "maximal" thymectomy for MG, involving a cervical incision in addition to median sternotomy and requiring extensive neck and mediastinal dissection to investigate all areas where aberrant thymic tissue has been described.[46] Although Jaretzki has argued in favor of this approach, the evidence that this extensive operation provides better control of MG than even the least invasive transcervical approach is controversial (see Table 41-4) and has not convinced many to adopt this procedure.

Table 41-4
Large Studies of Myasthenia Gravis Response Rates after Thymectomy by Three Surgical Approaches*

	Authors (ref)	Crude complete remission rate (%)	Mean follow-up (yr)	Kaplan-Meier 5-yr remission rate (%)
Maximal transcervical and trans-sternal	Ashour et al (51)	35	1.7	NA
	Jaretzki et al (52)	46	3.4	50
	Busch et al (53)	19	7.7	NA
	Klein et al (54)	40	5.0	NA
Trans-sternal	Budde et al (55)	21	4.3	NA
	Durelli et al (56)	NA	5.0	30
	Masaoka et al (57)	40/45	5.0/20.0	NA
	Mulder et al (58)	36	3.6	NA
	Stern et al (59)	50	6.8	NA
	Huang et al (60)	58	8.5	NA
	Kattach et al (61)	17	4.5	NA
Extended transcervical†	Bril et al (62)	44	8.4	NA
	Calhoun et al (63)	35	5.0	NA
	de Perrot et al (64)	41	4.1	30
	Shrager et al (44)	37 (29)‡	4.4	43 (33)‡

*Includes only studies in the past 20 years in the English-language literature that represent a pure series of one type of procedure with at least 48 adult patients and that report complete remission rates and mean follow-up.
†Includes only studies representing pure series of extended TCT using the Cooper thymectomy retractor.
‡Values in parentheses represent the most restrictive definition of a complete response.
NA, not applicable.

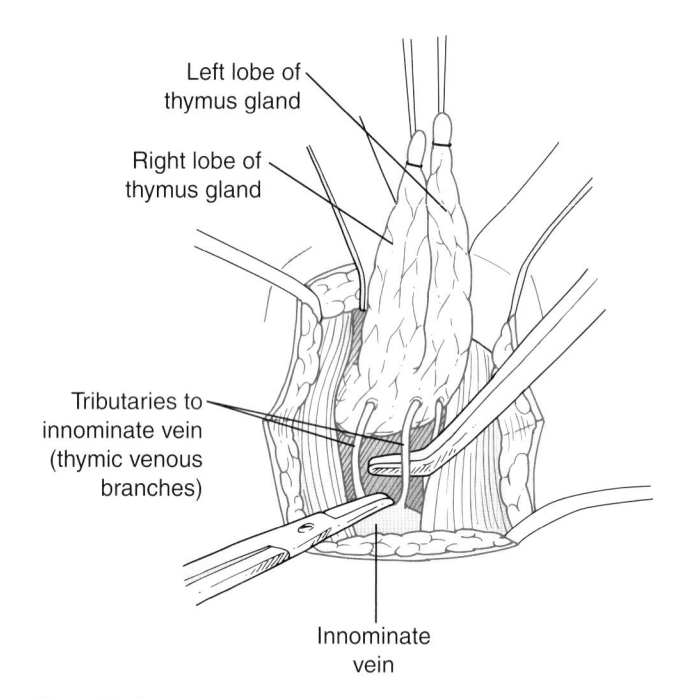

Figure 41-4
Technique of transcervical thymectomy. The surgeon's view from the head of the table shows the ligated upper thymic poles retracted anteriorly while the branches into the thymus from the innominate vein are controlled. *(From Kaiser LR. Atlas of general thoracic surgery. St Louis: Mosby-Year Book; 1997, with permission.)*

Thoracoscopic Thymectomy

A number of thoracoscopic approaches to thymectomy have been described that appear to allow complete thymectomy to be performed.[47,48] Approaches that combine the thoracoscopic and transcervical techniques with sternal lifting have also been reported.[49] However, there is no doubt that intercostal, thoracoscopic port incisions are more painful than a small incision in the jugular notch as performed for TCT. Thus, there would appear to be little reason to use thoracoscopy in lieu of or in addition to the transcervical approach unless it can be demonstrated that this allows more complete resection of thymic tissue and results in higher complete responses in MG. This is very unlikely when even "maximal" thymectomy does not result in markedly higher response rates than TCT. Shigemura and colleagues[50] performed a prospective trial on 20 patients to compare the efficacy of various thoracoscopic approaches with and without an open transcervical approach, and they concluded that a strictly VATS approach resulted in incomplete gland removal.

Summary

We have reviewed the various anterior mediastinal masses with particular regard to their presentation, diagnosis, and management. The association of thymic disease and myasthenia gravis has been emphasized. Surgical approaches to biopsy and resection of anterior mediastinal masses, including their potential advantages and disadvantages, have been described.

The appropriate management of anterior mediastinal masses requires flexibility and versatility on the part of the surgeon with regard to the method selected in each patient for biopsy or resection.

REFERENCES

1. Shields TW. The mediastinum, its compartments, and the mediastinal lymph nodes. In: Shields TW, LoCicero J, Ponn RB, editors. *General Thoracic Surgery*. Philadelphia: Lippincott Williams & Wilkins; 2000. p. 2343–6.
2. Batata MA, Martini N, Huvos AG, et al. Thymomas: clinicopathologic features, therapy, and prognosis. *Cancer* 1974;**34**:389-96.
3. McKenna WG. Malignancies of the thymus. In: Roth JA, Ruckdeschel JC, Weisenburger TH, editors. Thoracic Oncology. Philadelphia: WB Saunders; 1989. p. 1.
4. Lewis JE, Wick MR, Scheithauer BW, et al. Thymoma: a clinicopathologic review. *Cancer* 1987;**60**:2727-43.
5. Hirokawa K, Utsuyama M, Moriizumi E, et al. Immunohistochemical studies in human thymomas: localization of thymosin and various cell marker. *Virchows Arch B Cell Pathol Incl Mol Pathol* 1988;**55**:371-80.
6. Masaoka A, Monden Y, Nakahara K, et al. Follow-up study of thymomas with special reference to their clinical stages. *Cancer* 1981;**48**:2485-92.
7. Marino M, Muller-Hermelink HK. Thymoma and thymic carcinoma: relation of thymoma epithelial cells to the cortical and medullary differentiation of thymus. *Virchows Arch A Pathol Anat Histopathol* 1985;**407**:119-49.
8. Pescarmona E, Giardini R, Brisigotti M, et al. Thymoma in childhood: a clinicopathological study of five cases. *Histopathology* 1992;**21**:65-8.
9. Quintanilla-Martinez L, Wilkins EW Jr, Choi N, et al. Thymoma: histologic subclassification is an independent prognostic factor. *Cancer* 1994;**74**:606-17.
10. Rendina EA, Pescarmona EO, Venuta F, et al. Thymoma: a clinico-pathologic study based on newly developed morphologic criteria. *Tumori* 1988;**74**:79-84.
11. Ricci C, Rendina EA, Pescarmona EO, et al. Correlations between histological type, clinical behaviour, and prognosis in thymoma. *Thorax* 1989;**44**:455-60.
12. Okumura M, Ohta M, Tateyama H, et al. The World Health Organization histologic classification system reflects the oncologic behavior of thymoma: a clinical study of 273 patients. *Cancer* 2002;**94**:624-32.
13. Drachman DB. Myasthenia gravis. *N Engl J Med* 1994;**330**:1797-810.
14. Simpson JA. The thymus in the pathogenesis and treatment of myasthenia gravis. In: Satoyoshi E, editor. *Myasthenia Gravis Pathogenesis and Treatment*. Tokyo: University of Tokyo Press; 1981. p. 301–7.
15. Schumacher ED, Roth P. Thymectomie bei einem Fall von Morbus basedowi mit Myasthenia. *Mitteil Grenzgebieten Med Chir* 1912;**25**:746.
16. Blalock A, Harvey AM, Ford FR. The treatment of myasthenia gravis by removal of the thymus gland. *JAMA* 1941;**117**:1529-33.
17. Beard ME, Krantz SB, Johnson SA, et al. Pure red cell aplasia. *Q J Med* 1978;**47**:339-48.
18. Zeok JV, Todd EP, Dillon M, et al. The role of thymectomy in red cell aplasia. *Ann Thorac Surg* 1979;**28**:257-60.
19. Berruti A, Borasio P, Roncari A, et al. Neoadjuvant chemotherapy with Adriamycin, cisplatin, vincristine and cyclophosphamide (ADOC) in invasive thymomas: results in six patients. *Ann Oncol* 1993;**4**:429-31.
20. Macchiarini P, Chella A, Ducci F, et al. Neoadjuvant chemotherapy, surgery, and postoperative radiation therapy for invasive thymoma. *Cancer* 1991;**68**:706-13.
21. Venuta F, Rendina EA, Pescarmona EO, et al. Multimodality treatment of thymoma: a prospective study. *Ann Thorac Surg* 1997;**64**:1585-91:discussion 1591-2.
22. Endo M, Nakagawa K, Ohde Y, et al. Utility of (18)FDG-PET for differentiating the grade of malignancy in thymic epithelial tumors. *Lung Cancer* 2008;**61**:350-5.
23. Singhal S, Shrager JB, Rosenthal DI, et al. Comparison of stages I-II thymoma treated by complete resection with or without adjuvant radiation. *Ann Thorac Surg* 2003;**76**:1635-41:discussion 1641-2.
24. Mangi AA, Wright CD, Allan JS, et al. Adjuvant radiation therapy for stage II thymoma. *Ann Thorac Surg* 2002;**74**:1033-7.
25. Okumura M, Miyoshi S, Takeuchi Y, et al. Results of surgical treatment of thymomas with special reference to the involved organs. *J Thorac Cardiovasc Surg* 1999;**117**:605-13.
26. Nakahara K, Ohno K, Hashimoto J, et al. Thymoma: results with complete resection and adjuvant postoperative irradiation in 141 consecutive patients. *J Thorac Cardiovasc Surg* 1988;**95**:1041-7.
27. Blumberg D, Port JL, Weksler B, et al. Thymoma: a multivariate analysis of factors predicting survival. *Ann Thorac Surg* 1995;**60**:908-13:discussion 914.
28. Ciernik IF, Meier U, Lutolf UM. Prognostic factors and outcome of incompletely resected invasive thymoma following radiation therapy. *J Clin Oncol* 1994;**12**:1484-90.
29. Kim ES, Putnam JB, Komaki R, et al. Phase II study of a multidisciplinary approach with induction chemotherapy, followed by surgical resection, radiation therapy, and consolidation chemotherapy for unresectable malignant thymomas: final report. *Lung Cancer* 2004;**44**:369-79.
30. de Perrot M, Liu J, Bril V, et al. Prognostic significance of thymomas in patients with myasthenia gravis. *Ann Thorac Surg* 2002;**74**:1658-62.
31. Suster S, Rosai J. Thymic carcinoma: a clinicopathologic study of 60 cases. *Cancer* 1991;**67**:1025-32.
32. Ogawa K, Toita T, Uno T, et al. Treatment and prognosis of thymic carcinoma: a retrospective analysis of 40 cases. *Cancer* 2002;**94**:3115-9.
33. Lucchi M, Mussi A, Basolo F, et al. The multimodality treatment of thymic carcinoma. *Eur J Cardiothorac Surg* 2001;**19**:566-9.
34. Galanis E, Frytak S, Lloyd RV. Extrapulmonary small cell carcinoma. *Cancer* 1997;**79**:1729-36.
35. Wychulis AR, Payne WS, Clagett OT, et al. Surgical treatment of mediastinal tumors: a 40 year experience. *J Thorac Cardiovasc Surg* 1971;**62**:379-92.
36. Mayordomo JI, Paz-Ares L, Rivera F, et al. Ovarian and extragonadal malignant germ-cell tumors in females: a single-institution experience with 43 patients. *Ann Oncol* 1994;**5**:225-31.
37. Clamon GH. Management of primary mediastinal seminoma. *Chest* 1983;**83**:263-7.
38. Kesler KA, Rieger KM, Hammoud ZT, et al. A 25-year single institution experience with surgery for primary mediastinal nonseminomatous germ cell tumors. *Ann Thorac Surg* 2008;**85**:371-8.
39. Vuky J, Bains M, Bacik J, et al. Role of postchemotherapy adjunctive surgery in the management of patients with nonseminoma arising from the mediastinum. *J Clin Oncol* 2001;**19**:682-8.
40. Schneider BP, Kesler KA, Brooks JA, et al. Outcome of patients with residual germ cell or non-germ cell malignancy after resection of primary mediastinal nonseminomatous germ cell cancer. *J Clin Oncol* 2004;**22**:1195-200.
41. Deeb ME, Brinster CJ, Kucharzuk J, et al. Expanded indications for transcervical thymectomy in the management of anterior mediastinal masses. *Ann Thorac Surg* 2001;**72**:208-11.
42. Ginsberg RJ, Rice TW, Goldberg M, et al. Extended cervical mediastinoscopy: a single staging procedure for bronchogenic carcinoma of the left upper lobe. *J Thorac Cardiovasc Surg* 1987;**94**:673-8.
43. Nichols FC, Trastek VF. Thymectomy (sternotomy). In: Kaiser LR, Kron IL, Spray TL, editors. *Mastery of Cardiothoracic Surgery*. Philadelphia: Lippincott Williams & Wilkins; 2007. p. 100–106.
44. Shrager JB, Nathan D, Brinster CJ, et al. Outcomes after 151 extended transcervical thymectomies for myasthenia gravis. *Ann Thorac Surg* 2006;**82**:1863-9.
45. Kaiser LR. Transcervical thymectomy. In: Kaiser LR, editor. *Atlas of General Thoracic Surgery*. St Louis: Mosby-Year Book; 1997. p. 152–7.
46. Jaretzki A 3rd, Wolff M. "Maximal" thymectomy for myasthenia gravis: Surgical anatomy and operative technique. *J Thorac Cardiovasc Surg* 1988;**96**:711-6.
47. Mineo TC, Pompeo E, Lerut TE, et al. Thoracoscopic thymectomy in autoimmune myasthenia: results of left-sided approach. *Ann Thorac Surg* 2000;**69**:1537-41.
48. Yim AP, Kay RL, Ho JK. Video-assisted thoracoscopic thymectomy for myasthenia gravis. *Chest* 1995;**108**:1440-3.
49. Takeo S, Sakada T, Yano T. Video-assisted extended thymectomy in patients with thymoma by lifting the sternum. *Ann Thorac Surg* 2001;**71**:1721-3.
50. Shigemura N, Shiono H, Inoue M, et al. Inclusion of the transcervical approach in video-assisted thoracoscopic extended thymectomy (VATET) for myasthenia gravis: a prospective trial. *Surg Endosc* 2006;**20**:1614-8.
51. Ashour MH, Jain SK, Kattan KM, et al. "Maximal thymectomy for myasthenia gravis. *Eur J Cardiothorac Surg* 1995;**9**:461-4.
52. Jaretzki A 3rd, Penn AS, Younger DS, et al. Maximal" thymectomy for myasthenia gravis: results. *J Thorac Cardiovasc Surg* 1988;**95**:747-57.
53. Busch C, Machens A, Pichlmeier U, et al. Long-term outcome and quality of life after thymectomy for myasthenia gravis. *Ann Thorac Surg* 1996;**224**:225-32.
54. Klein M, Heidenreich F, Madjlessi F, et al. Early and late results after thymectomy in myasthenia gravis: a retrospective study [correction of analysis]. *Thorac Cardiovasc Surg* 1999;**47**:170-3.
55. Budde JM, Morris CD, Gal AA, et al. Predictors of outcome in thymectomy for myasthenia gravis. *Ann Thorac Surg* 2001;**72**:197-202.
56. Durelli L, Maggi G, Casadio C, et al. Actuarial analysis of the occurrence of remissions following thymectomy for myasthenia gravis in 400 patients. *J Neurol Neurosurg Psychiatry* 1991;**54**:406-11.
57. Masaoka A, Yamakawa Y, Niwa H, et al. Extended thymectomy for myasthenia gravis patients: a 20-year review. *Ann Thorac Surg* 1996;**62**:853-9.
58. Mulder DG, Graves M, Herrmann C. Thymectomy for myasthenia gravis: recent observations and comparisons with past experience. *Ann Thorac Surg* 1989;**48**:551-5.

59. Stern LE, Nussbaum MS, Quinlan JG, et al. Long-term evaluation of extended thymectomy with anterior mediastinal dissection for myasthenia gravis. *Surgery* 2001;**130**:774-8:discussion 778-80.
60. Huang CS, Hsu HS, Huang BS, et al. Factors influencing the outcome of transsternal thymectomy for myasthenia gravis. *Acta Neurol Scand* 2005;**112**: 108-14.
61. Kattach H, Anastasiadis K, Cleuziou J, et al. Transsternal thymectomy for myasthenia gravis: surgical outcome. *Ann Thorac Surg* 2006;**81**:305-8.
62. Bril V, Kojic J, Ilse WK, et al. Long-term clinical outcome after transcervical thymectomy for myasthenia gravis. *Ann Thorac Surg* 1998;**65**:1520-2.
63. Calhoun RF, Ritter JH, Guthrie TJ, et al. Results of transcervical thymectomy for myasthenia gravis in 100 consecutive patients. *Ann Surg* 1999;**230**: 555-9:discussion 559-61.
64. de Perrot M, Bril V, McRae K, et al. Impact of minimally invasive trans-cervical thymectomy on outcome in patients with myasthenia gravis. *Eur J Cardiothorac Surg* 2003;**24**:677-83.

CHAPTER 42
The Middle Mediastinum
Zane T. Hammoud and Michael J. Liptay

Contents of the Middle Mediastinum
Diagnostic Modalities
  Imaging
  Invasive Techniques
    Percutaneous Biopsy
    Endoscopic Ultrasound and Endobronchial Ultrasound

    Cervical Mediastinoscopy and Anterior Mediastinotomy
    Video-Assisted Thoracoscopic Surgery
    Other Techniques
Specific Diseases
  Lymph Node Diseases
  Tracheal Disorders

Pericardial Disorders
Mediastinal Infections

The mediastinum is bounded laterally by the two pleural spaces. Within this space are located the tracheobronchial tree, the heart and great vessels, a portion of the gastrointestinal tract, and a portion of the lymphatic system. Superiorly the mediastinum is bordered by the thoracic inlet, and inferiorly it is bordered by the thoracic surface of the diaphragm. The sternum serves as the anterior border of the mediastinum, and the spine is the posterior border. Also, the superior aspect of the mediastinum is in communication with the inferior aspect of the neck; thus, disorders involving the neck may also involve the mediastinum. Because of the various major structures located in it, the mediastinum is frequently the site of pathologic conditions involving those structures. Therefore, a thorough understanding of the mediastinum and its contents is required of any surgeon who treats any of the conditions that involve or are located in this space.

For practical purposes, the mediastinum is usually considered to be divided into four compartments. The superior compartment is located above an imaginary line drawn from the angle of Louis to the inferior aspect of the fourth thoracic vertebra. This compartment contains all of the structures that run through the thoracic inlet. The anterior compartment is defined as that space between the posterior aspect of the sternum and the anterior surfaces of the pericardium and great vessels. The posterior compartment extends from the posterior aspect of the pericardium to the anterior longitudinal ligament; in this compartment lie the descending thoracic aorta, the esophagus, and the sympathetic chain. The middle, or visceral, compartment is bounded anteriorly and posteriorly by the pericardium, and it contains the pericardium and its contents, major portions of the tracheobronchial tree, and lymphatics. Although the division of the mediastinum into these four compartments is anatomically and surgically convenient, structures predominantly located in one compartment may also be in another compartment. Other anatomic models (e.g., a three-compartment model and a three-zone model) exist. This chapter focuses on structures located in the middle compartment and discusses the pathologic disorders that affect structures therein.

CONTENTS OF THE MIDDLE MEDIASTINUM

Lymphatics. The middle mediastinum contains a rich network of lymphatic vessels and lymph nodes that primarily drain the lungs and esophagus. These include lymph nodes in the paratracheal and subcarinal positions. In addition, minor lymph node groups are located on the pericardium.

Trachea. The intrathoracic trachea as well as the proximal main-stem bronchi are located in the middle mediastinum.

Pericardium and contents. The entire pericardium, phrenic nerves, heart, and the ascending aorta and proximal arch are all located in the middle mediastinum.

DIAGNOSTIC MODALITIES
Imaging

The chest radiograph often provides the first glimpse of a possible abnormality in the mediastinum. For example, it may suggest mediastinal or hilar adenopathy. Narrowing or deviation of the tracheobronchial tree, enlargement of the pericardial silhouette, and calcification or enlargement of the great vessels are other abnormalities that may initially be seen radiographically (Fig. 42-1A). However, because of its limited resolution, the chest film often does not provide adequate information about specific mediastinal pathology. Further radiographic assessment by other modalities is necessary for a more accurate assessment.

Computed tomography (CT), often with intravenous or oral contrast, is indicated when mediastinal pathology is suspected on the basis of the chest film (see Fig 42-1B) or clinically. High-resolution spiral CT, with cross-sectional imaging of structures at intervals as narrow as 1 mm, is the radiologic modality of choice for imaging the middle mediastinum. All structures located in the middle mediastinum can be seen by CT. In addition, the relationship of these structures to other nearby structures can be delineated. Three-dimensional CT images can be reconstructed using computerized programs without the need for additional radiation. These reconstructions can be particularly useful for detailed assessment of structures, such as the trachea, located in the middle mediastinum.

Magnetic resonance imaging (MRI) may at times provide additional information in the assessment of middle mediastinal pathology. Advantages of MRI include its ability to differentiate between vascular, solid, and fluid elements in a given mass. However, MRI is most likely to be useful in the evaluation of posterior mediastinal masses (e.g., paravertebral tumors).

Positron emission tomography (PET) is a valuable tool for evaluating mediastinal pathology, especially mediastinal lymph node involvement in neoplasms (e.g., lung cancer). The degree of uptake of fluorodeoxyglucose (FDG) labeled

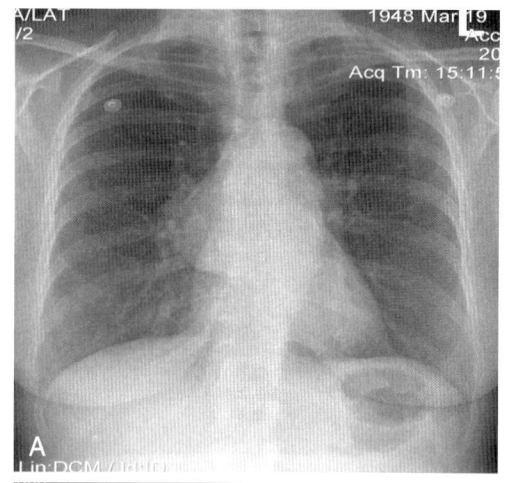

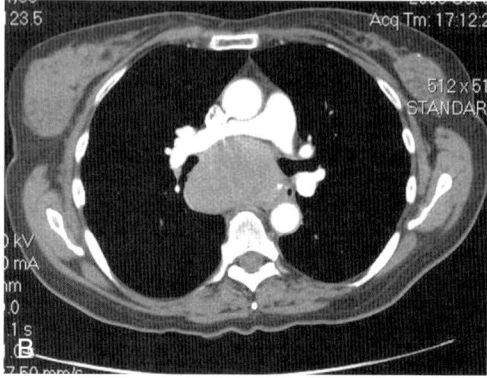

Figure 42–1
A, Posteroanterior chest radiograph of a 55-year-old woman with chest heaviness and mild dysphagia to solids. A large middle mediastinal mass is noted. **B,** CT scan demonstrates a subcarinal mass. Differential diagnosis includes adenopathy (lymphoma), and bronchogenic or esophageal duplication cyst. Resection revealed a plasmacytoma.

with radioactive fluoride (^{18}F) is a surrogate marker of the degree of metabolic activity in a cell. However, PET is limited, because it is difficult to distinguish between increased metabolic activity caused by tumor and that caused by inflammation. Furthermore, as PET does not provide an anatomic scan, the precise location of the increased metabolic activity may not be discernable. However, fusion of PET with CT (CT-PET) has allowed a more precise assessment of anatomy.[1]

Conventional ultrasonography is of limited value in the evaluation of middle mediastinal pathology, although it may help in determining whether a mass is cystic or solid. However, transesophageal endoscopic ultrasonography (EUS) has emerged as a valuable tool for the evaluation of certain mediastinal pathology, especially lymph nodes.[2] Other modalities, such as leukocyte scintigraphy, lymphoscintigraphy, and metaiodobenzylguanidine (MIBG) scanning, have limited and very specific indications in the evaluation of pathology in the middle mediastinum.

Invasive Techniques

Percutaneous Biopsy

Tissue from masses located in the middle mediastinum can often be obtained percutaneously. Most commonly, either ultrasound or CT is used to guide the operator. Both fine-needle biopsy and core needle biopsy can be performed. These techniques offer the advantage of obtaining adequate tissue for diagnosis using only local anesthesia and on an outpatient basis. Success rates, particularly with core needle biopsy, are excellent in experienced hands. The disadvantage of these techniques is the possibility of obtaining an inadequate amount of tissue for diagnosis or failure to make a diagnosis in masses that are relatively small.

Endoscopic Ultrasound and Endobronchial Ultrasound

EUS and endobronchial ultrasound (EBUS) are used with increasing frequency to obtain tissue from the mediastinum. EUS is more useful for the evaluation of masses near the esophagus, such as in the subcarinal space. With EUS, both fine-needle and core biopsy specimens may be obtained with minimal morbidity on an outpatient basis. EBUS-guided fine-needle aspiration can be used to obtain tissue from masses located near the major airways (e.g., lymph nodes).[3] This modality is increasingly used in the mediastinal staging of lung cancer, but it can also be used to obtain tissue from other middle mediastinal masses that encroach on the airways.

Cervical Mediastinoscopy and Anterior Mediastinotomy

Cervical mediastinoscopy is the gold standard for the evaluation of mediastinal pathology. In experienced hands, the procedure can be performed with low morbidity. It offers the advantage of obtaining a large amount of tissue from several locations, such as mediastinal lymph nodes. On occasion, an anterior mediastinotomy (Chamberlain procedure) may be necessary to obtain tissue—for example, when a mediastinal mass is located predominantly on one side of the mediastinum. The primary disadvantages of these two techniques are that they require a small incision and general anesthesia. However, with either technique, a histologic diagnosis can be obtained in a majority of cases.

Video-Assisted Thoracoscopic Surgery

The use of video-assisted thoracoscopic surgery (VATS) in the diagnosis and management of thoracic conditions has gained widespread acceptance. The VATS approach allows the surgeon to visualize the entire pleural space and ipsilateral mediastinum. Using VATS and dedicated instruments, tissue can be obtained from nearly all mediastinal compartments. In addition, some middle mediastinal masses (e.g., bronchogenic cysts) may be effectively managed by VATS techniques. The principal disadvantages of the VATS approach are that they require general anesthesia and single-lung ventilation. However, VATS has emerged as a powerful tool in the armamentarium of the thoracic surgeon.[4]

Other Techniques

Rarely, other attempts fail, or the preceding procedures cannot be used in a specific instance. Then, a thoracotomy or sternotomy may be necessary to obtain tissue to establish a histologic diagnosis of a middle mediastinal mass.

SPECIFIC DISEASES

Lymph Node Diseases

Enlargement of lymph nodes located in the middle mediastinum is seen in a wide variety of disorders. Metastasis from lung cancer is the most common cause of malignant mediastinal

Table 42-1

Histologic Diagnoses of Patients with Benign Mediastinal Adenopathy

Diagnosis	Patients (n)	Patients (%)
Noncaseating granuloma	130	63
Follicular reactive hyperplasia	20	10
Caseating granuloma	16	8
Anthracosis	11	5
Other	29	14
Total	206	100

From Hammoud ZT, Anderson RC, Meyers BF, et al. The current role of mediastinoscopy in the evaluation of thoracic disease. J Thorac Cardiovasc Surg 1999;118(5):894-9.

adenopathy. Lymph nodes located in the paratracheal area (levels 2 and 4), the tracheobronchial angle (level 10), and the subcarinal space (level 7) may be involved. When infiltrated by malignancy, these lymph nodes may appear enlarged on imaging studies such as CT or, even when not enlarged, may demonstrate uptake of FDG with PET. Other malignancies may also metastasize to these lymph nodes. Such malignancies include primarily intrathoracic cancers (e.g., cancers of the esophagus and trachea) and mesothelioma. In addition, malignancies located primarily outside the thoracic cavity, such as cancers of the pancreas and liver, may also metastasize to lymph nodes located in the middle mediastinum.

Lymphoma may also occur with mediastinal adenopathy. Rarely, these are primary mediastinal lymphomas. However, both Hodgkin's disease and non-Hodgkin's lymphoma, when generalized, may involve lymph nodes located primarily in the middle mediastinum. Typically, however, mediastinal lymphomas occur with anterior mediastinal masses. Lymphangiomas are other rare causes of middle mediastinal adenopathy.

Among the benign disorders that manifest with middle mediastinal adenopathy, inflammatory and infectious causes predominate (Table 42-1). Sarcoidosis is one of the most common causes of benign mediastinal adenopathy. Most commonly, this is seen on a CT scan as hilar adenopathy or as diffuse mediastinal adenopathy. A definitive diagnosis is made by obtaining tissue for histologic confirmation or by the finding of elevated levels of angiotensin-converting enzyme in the appropriate clinical setting. Histoplasmosis is a common cause of mediastinal adenopathy, particularly in regions around the Mississippi River. This fungal infection has a spectrum of disease manifestations in the thoracic cavity, including benign adenopathy (with characteristic calcification), broncholithiasis, granuloma formation, and mediastinal fibrosis. Other fungal infections that may be seen in certain regions include cryptococcosis and coccidioidomycosis. Mycobacterial infections, both tuberculous and nontuberculous, may present with hilar and mediastinal adenopathy as well. As in malignant disease, involvement of mediastinal lymph nodes can occur secondary to a primarily parenchymal process, such as bacterial or viral pneumonia.

Other rare causes of middle mediastinal adenopathy include fulminant congestive heart failure, which can lead to enlargement of lymph nodes in the mediastinum. Giant lymph node hyperplasia or Castleman's disease is commonly a solitary lesion but may have a multicentric appearance. Although this disease can be found anywhere, the majority (70%) of cases originate in the thorax.[5] The etiology of giant lymph node hyperplasia is unknown, and patients are typically asymptomatic.

Tracheal Disorders

The trachea is a tubular structure that connects the larynx with the bronchi. In the average adult, it measures 11 to 13 cm in length. The trachea begins at the cricoid, the only circumferential cartilaginous ring, and ends at the bifurcation into the right and left main-stem bronchi. The intrathoracic portion of the trachea as well as both main-stem bronchi course through the middle mediastinum and may be involved in a variety of disorders. Primary tumors of the trachea, such as squamous cell carcinoma and adenoid cystic carcinoma, may involve any portion of the airway but are usually seen in the intrathoracic portions. Other diseases, such as amyloidosis and Wegener's granulomatosis, may also involve the trachea. Tracheomalacia, which may be congenital or secondary to other disorders such as chronic obstructive pulmonary disease, can involve the intrathoracic trachea as well as the main-stem bronchi. Bronchogenic cysts are the most common congenital foregut cysts.[6] Approximately 80% of bronchogenic cysts are located in the middle mediastinum, most commonly in close proximity to the carina and main-stem bronchi. These cysts may be incidental findings on imaging studies, or the patients may present with various symptoms, resulting, for example, from compression secondary to the size of the cyst. Resection is recommended.

Pericardial Disorders

The pericardial sac serves multiple purposes, including mechanical protection of the heart and lubrication of cardiac movement. It also has an influence on the mechanical properties of cardiac function. The most common condition affecting the pericardium is an effusion. The presence of a pericardial effusion may lead to the compromise of cardiac function, particularly diastolic filling. The subsequent hemodynamic compromise (tamponade) can be fatal if not treated. The most common cause of pericardial effusion is malignancy, which accounts for more than 75% of cases, with cancer of lung and breast predominating.[7] Other causes of pericardial effusion include myocardial infarction, cardiac surgery, and trauma. Treatment, when indicated, involves drainage by either pericardiocentesis or the creation of a pericardial window.

Pericarditis can be caused by a wide variety of disorders, including connective tissue disorders, uremia, infection, malignancy, and cardiac surgery. Treatment generally consists of medical management of the underlying condition and often involves analgesia and anti-inflammatory medication. When pericarditis is severe or when there are multiple episodes of acute pericarditis, the condition can progress to a chronically diseased pericardium that constricts cardiac function by impairing diastolic filling. Such constrictive pericarditis often requires surgical resection of the pericardium to allow the heart to function properly.

Pericardial cysts are rare lesions thought to arise during embryonic development. They are most commonly found in the right cardiophrenic angle. They rarely cause symptoms and are most commonly detected on a routine chest film. Treatment consists of percutaneous drainage or surgical resection. Pericardial neoplasms are very rare—mesothelioma is the most common primary pericardial neoplasm. Metastatic neoplasms to the pericardium (e.g., from lung, breast, prostate, and lymphoma) are far more common than primary tumors.

Mediastinal Infections

Acute mediastinal infection is relatively rare. Most instances result from processes that involve the mediastinum secondarily, such as esophageal perforation, sternal infections after sternotomy, and tonsillar or odontogenic abscess. The most common cause of esophageal perforation is iatrogenic (e.g., after endoscopy). However, spontaneous perforation, as well as injury incurred during other intrathoracic procedures, may occur. Esophageal perforation leads to contamination of the middle mediastinum by oropharyngeal secretions, which may result in a spectrum of clinical presentations such as abscess formation or sepsis syndrome secondary to mediastinitis. Treatment depends on the location of the perforation, the timing of presentation, and the clinical condition of the patient. Most commonly, treatment involves wide drainage, débridement of necrotic tissue, and primary repair of the perforation.

Infections after sternotomy may contaminate the middle mediastinum with skin flora. Most commonly, such infections occur after cardiac surgical procedures. Risk factors include diabetes, re-do sternotomy, and harvesting of bilateral internal mammary arteries. Treatment includes prompt surgical débridement of devitalized tissue and bone, with possible muscle flap coverage.

Descending necrotizing mediastinitis occurs when oropharyngeal bacterial flora gain access to the middle mediastinum via the pretracheal, retrovisceral spaces or along the carotid sheaths following natural tissue planes. Such infections typically occur secondary to odontogenic abscess as a result of poor oral hygiene. Treatment generally consists of surgical drainage, most commonly through the neck, and systemic antibiotics. The underlying cause should be treated promptly.

Fibrosing mediastinitis is a rare, benign disorder characterized by the proliferation of fibrous tissue in the mediastinum. This is most commonly caused by an abnormal immunologic response to fungal infections, particularly histoplasmosis.[8] In its most severe form, the fibrotic process encases mediastinal structures such as the airway, superior vena cava, and pulmonary arterial branches, leading to compression of these structures with resultant symptoms. Treatment, when necessary, centers on relief of symptoms. Because of the dense fibrosis, surgical intervention is often quite challenging.

REFERENCES

1. Cerfolio RJ, Ojha B, Bryant A, Raghuveer V, Mountz J, Bartolucci A. The accuracy of integrated PET-CT compared with dedicated PET alone for the staging of patients with nonsmall cell lung cancer. *Ann Thorac Surg* 2004;**78**:1017-23.
2. Hunerbein M, Ghadimi BM, Haensch W, Schlag PM. Transesophageal biopsy of mediastinal and pulmonary tumors by means of endoscopic ultrasound guidance. *J Thorac Cardiovasc Surg* 1998;**116**:554-9.
3. Yasufuku K, Nakajima T, Chiyo M, Sekine Y, Shibuya K, Fujisawa T. Endobronchial ultrasonography: current status and future directions. *J Thorac Oncol* 2007;**2**(10):970-9.
4. Keleman JJ, Naunheim KS. Minimally invasive approaches to mediastinal neoplasms. *Semin Thorac Cardiovasc Surg* 2000;**12**:301-6.
5. Shahidi H, Myers JL, Kvale PA. Castleman's disease. *Mayo Clin Proc* 1995;**70**:969-77.
6. Ribet ME, Copin MC, Gosselin B. Bronchogenic cysts of the mediastinum. *J Thorac Cardiovasc Surg* 1995;**109**:1003-10.
7. Gasper WJ, Jamshidi R, Theodore PR. Palliation of thoracic malignancies. *Surg Oncol* 2007;**16**(4):259-65.
8. Wheat LJ, Conces D, Allen SD, Blue-Hnidy D, Loyd J. Pulmonary histoplasmosis syndromes: recognition, diagnosis, and management. *Semin Respir Crit Care Med* 2004;**25**(2):129-44.

CHAPTER 43
The Posterior Mediastinum
Larry R. Kaiser and Dhruv Singhal

Anatomy
Epidemiology
Diagnosis
Surgical Approaches to the Posterior Mediastinum
Lesions of the Mediastinum
Neurogenic Tumors
Esophageal Masses
Cysts of the Posterior Mediastinum
Bronchogenic Cysts
Gastroenteric Cysts
Neuroenteric Cysts
Other Masses of the Posterior Mediastinum
Infections of the Mediastinum
Summary

The posterior mediastinum is an anatomically diverse region with visceral organs, major vessels, large neural structures, and important lymphatic vessels. Lesions that originate in the mediastinum are rare compared with diverse lesions that can involve the mediastinum secondarily. Lesions contained within it are primarily tumors of neurogenic origin. Less common is a potpourri of lesions including vascular tumors, mesenchymal tumors, and lymphatic lesions.

ANATOMY

The posterior mediastinum, also called the paravertebral compartment, is a defined space between the posterior pericardium and the anterior spinal ligament including the paravertebral gutters. According to the traditional four-compartment model, the mediastinum is divided into anterior, middle, posterior, and superior compartments. The posterior mediastinum is bounded superiorly by the inferior border of the T4 vertebral body.[1,2]

In the traditional three-compartment model without a superior division, the entire length of the spine is included in the posterior mediastinum.[2] The diaphragm is the common inferior border for all three compartments. Within these boundaries, the posterior mediastinum contains the esophagus, descending aorta, sympathetic chain and vagus nerves, thoracic duct, azygos and hemiazygos veins, fat, and lymph nodes (Fig. 43-1).[1]

EPIDEMIOLOGY

Great differences exist between children and adults with respect to the location of mediastinal masses.[3] In adults, 65% of the lesions arise in the anterosuperior, 10% in the middle, and 25% in the posterior compartments; this distribution is reversed in children, in whom 25% of lesions arise in the anterosuperior, 10% in the middle, and 65% in the posterior compartments. In general, the incidence of posterior mediastinal lesions is higher in children, whereas anterior lesions predominate in adults.

DIAGNOSIS

Approximately 50% of posterior mediastinal lesions are asymptomatic and are detected on chest radiographs taken for unrelated reasons. As a rough guideline, the absence of symptoms suggests that a lesion is benign, whereas the presence of symptoms suggests malignancy.

The percentage of patients with symptoms from mediastinal masses precisely parallels or equals the percentage of malignant lesions. In adults, 50% to 60% of lesions are symptomatic, whereas the percentage of symptomatic lesions is higher in children (60% to 80%). Because the incidence of symptoms parallels the incidence of malignant lesions, a child with a mediastinal mass is considerably more likely to have a malignant neoplasm than is an adult with a mediastinal mass.

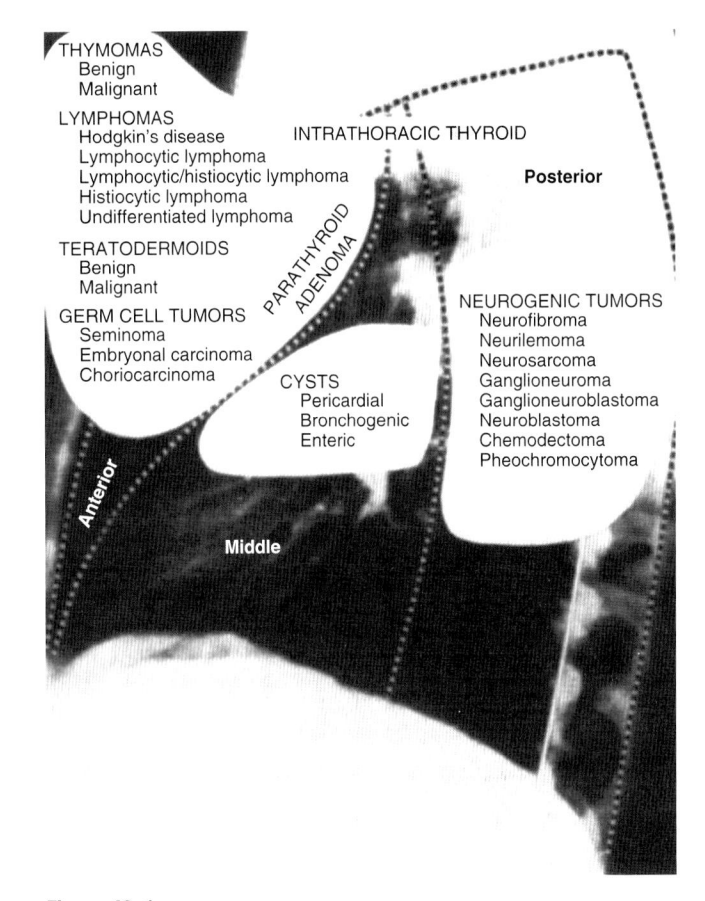

Figure 43–1
Lateral chest film divided into three anatomic subdivisions with the most common location of the tumors and cysts. (From Davis RD Jr, Sabiston DC Jr. Primary mediastinal cysts and neoplasms. In: Sabiston DC Jr, editor. *Essentials of surgery.* Philadelphia: WB Saunders; 1987.)

When a posterior mediastinal mass is discovered, a detailed history and physical examination are useful, particularly in patients with rarer symptoms (e.g., hoarseness and Horner's syndrome). The age of the patient can also narrow the diagnostic possibilities.

Computed tomography (CT) is the imaging modality of choice for the posterior mediastinum because of its ability to localize masses and to determine somewhat the extent of invasion. CT can often distinguish among the various masses and identify their origin, allowing correct diagnosis based on radiographic imaging.[4] Although magnetic resonance imaging (MRI) has been cited as useful in particular circumstances, such as with dumbbell tumors, cysts, and extramedullary hematopoiesis, CT remains the superior imaging modality for most posterior mediastinal masses.[5] Mediastinal sonography, although less expensive and comparable to CT in the diagnosis of many mediastinal masses, is not useful in the posterior mediastinum.[6]

The decision to sample a mediastinal mass is not straightforward. Biopsy before resection is not necessary in some cases and potentially harmful in others. The likelihood of a positive finding on biopsy depends on the presence of local symptoms and the location and extent of the lesion. Lesions in the posterior mediastinum require either fine-needle aspiration (CT guided) or a thoracoscopic approach.[7,8] If these procedures are not possible because of location in the paravertebral gutters, a limited posterolateral thoracotomy should be used to obtain adequate tissue for diagnosis.[9,10]

SURGICAL APPROACHES TO THE POSTERIOR MEDIASTINUM

Multiple standard approaches have been described to reach the posterior mediastinum. These include cervical, paravertebral, thoracotomy, transabdominal, and thoracoscopic (Fig. 43-2).

The cervical approach is accomplished through an incision along the anterior border of the sternocleidomastoid muscle. For lesions that are in the superior portion of the posterior mediastinum, incision of the buccopharyngeal fascia allows one to enter the peripharyngoesophageal space. When lower posterior mediastinal masses need to be reached, the paravertebral approach may be used by resecting posterior segments of one or more ribs and entering the retropleural plane that leads to the posterior mediastinum. Standard posterolateral thoracotomy, the most commonly employed approach, provides excellent access to the posterior mediastinum; the location of the lesion determines the intercostal space to be entered.

The posterior mediastinum can also be accessed transabdominally through the esophageal hiatus in various antireflux procedures, in hiatal hernia repairs, and during the transhiatal esophagectomy. A combined cervical approach with transabdominal mobilization allows the surgeon to remove the esophagus extrapleurally without traversing the pleural cavities or bony thorax.[11]

Currently, the decision to perform thoracoscopic surgery for posterior mediastinal lesions remains dependent on the surgeon's experience and comfort with video-assisted procedures; but for biopsy, this should be the procedure of choice.[8,12,13] Zierold and Halow[14] conducted a retrospective review that described use of thoracoscopic approaches for posterior mediastinal neurogenic masses. A total of 29 patients

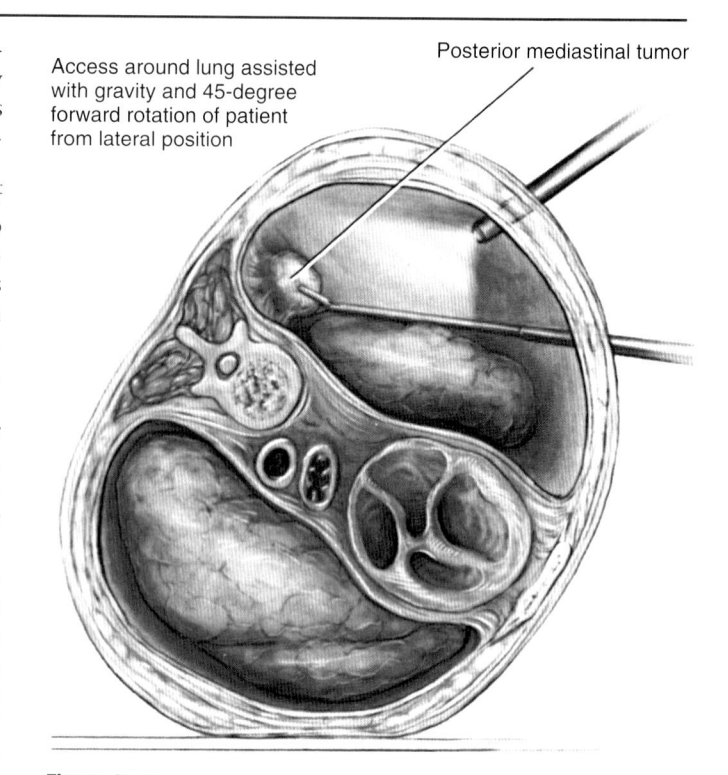

Figure 43-2
Thoracoscopic resection of a posterior mediastinal tumor. *(Reprinted with permission from Davis RD Jr, Sabiston DC Jr. Textbook of surgery. Philadelphia: WB Saunders; 1997. p. 1915.)*

(13 men, 16 women), aged 26 to 68 years, who underwent a thoracoscopic resection were identified. Preoperative imaging included chest radiography and CT in all patients and MRI in 15 of 29 patients (52%). All tumors were located in the posterior mediastinum without preoperative evidence of invasion or malignancy. Conversion to an open procedure was required in 12 of 29 (41%) patients (mini-thoracotomy in 11, posterolateral thoracotomy in 1). Tumor size necessitating conversion to an open procedure (mean = 4.79 cm) and tumor size amenable to thoracoscopy alone (mean = 3.84 cm) were not significantly different ($P < .09$). They concluded that thoracoscopic resection could be performed successfully, regardless of tumor type or size; however, malignant lesions, local invasion, and tumors larger than 5 cm may require an open procedure. Cardillo and associates[15] recently detailed their experience with 93 patients who underwent resection of a posterior mediastinal neurogenic tumor. The tumor was resected with a videothoracoscopic approach in 57 patients; 44 underwent video-assisted thoracoscopic surgery only, and 13 required conversion to an open approach. Mean operative time was significantly shorter in the video-assisted thoracoscopic surgery group, as was the median postoperative hospital stay and postoperative pain. At a mean follow-up of 73 months, no recurrences were noted.

The standard surgical approach involves a posterolateral thoracotomy incision and exposure of the posterior mediastinum. The tumor is always in a paravertebral location, and the exposure involves first incision of the overlying pleura and then dissection of the lesion away from the surrounding structures. Rarely is there any invasion of vertebral bodies, but it is important to recognize any involvement at the level of a neural foramen manifested by widening of the foramen and an inability to recognize a discrete nerve root. Involvement of the neural foramen should be suspected on the basis of preoperative imaging, specifically MRI, but at times this may become apparent only at the time of operation. Tumors arising from the sympathetic chain require segmental resection of the chain. Care should be taken to avoid unnecessary resection of segmental vessels that course along the vertebral bodies.

Once the pleura overlying the lesion has been incised, mobilization of the tumor proceeds expeditiously with a combination of sharp and blunt dissection. Complete resection can always be accomplished. Often, the procedure may start with videothoracoscopic visualization of the tumor; if mobilization is feasible, the tumor can be removed through a small incision. However, if mobilization proves difficult by the videothoracoscopic approach, there should be no hesitation in converting to an open procedure. This is especially important with lesions located at the apex of the chest.

> **Box 43-1**
> **Origin of Neurogenic Tumors in the Posterior Mediastinum**
>
> **Intercostal nerve tumors**
> Neurofibroma
> Neurilemoma
> Neurofibrosarcoma
> Neurosarcoma
>
> **Sympathetic ganglia tumors**
> Ganglioma
> Ganglioneuroblastoma
> Neuroblastoma
>
> **Paraganglia cell tumors**
> Paraganglioma (pheochromocytoma)

LESIONS OF THE MEDIASTINUM

Neurogenic Tumors

Neurogenic tumors of the thorax commonly occur in the posterior mediastinum and primarily affect young adults and children.[16] In recent decades, although these tumors continue to be the most common malignant neoplasm in children, they have become less common than tumors of the anterior mediastinum (thymomas or lymphomas) in adults. They now represent approximately 15% of all mediastinal masses in adults. Furthermore, in adults, the malignancy rate of neurogenic tumors is less than 10%. In children, fully 50% of these lesions are malignant.[16] Takeda and colleagues[17] reviewed their experience with 146 patients with intrathoracic neurogenic tumors treated during a 50-year period. In this series, there were 60 pediatric patients and 86 adults. There were 51 ganglioneuromas, 37 schwannomas, 30 neurofibromas, 18 neuroblastomas, 5 ganglioblastomas, and 5 others. Of these lesions, 136 were located in the posterior mediastinum, but only 13 patients (8.9%) had intraspinal extension of tumor; 84% of adults and 60% of children were asymptomatic at the time of presentation and 20.5% of the lesions were malignant, these occurring predominantly in the first 5 years of life.

Neurogenic tumors originate from embryonic neural crest cells around the spinal ganglia and from either sympathetic or parasympathetic components (Box 43-1). The differential diagnosis for neurogenic tumors arising from the intercostal nerves includes neurofibroma, neurilemoma, and neurogenic sarcoma. Sympathetic ganglia tumors include ganglioneuroma, ganglioneuroblastoma, and neuroblastoma. Pheochromocytomas can occur from paraganglia cells. Neurogenic tumors rarely arise from the phrenic and vagus nerves.

Neurogenic tumors can be benign or malignant. Benign lesions are classified as either neurilemoma (schwannoma) or neurofibroma. Neurilemomas are more common than neurofibromas. Of patients with nerve sheath tumors, 25% to 40% have multiple neurofibromatosis (von Recklinghausen's disease). Malignant tumors (neurogenic sarcomas or malignant schwannomas) are unusual. The incidence of malignancy is greater in tumors in patients with von Recklinghausen's disease (10% to 20%).

Patients with benign lesions are often asymptomatic as opposed to patients with malignant tumors, who frequently manifest symptoms of spinal cord compression or have cough, dyspnea, chest wall pain, and hoarseness. Horner's syndrome due to involvement of the superior cervical ganglion of the sympathetic chain is an unusual presentation. Most patients with neurogenic tumors are asymptomatic, so the initial diagnosis is usually made on the basis of findings noted on a chest radiograph done for some other reason. A rare patient may present with a pheochromocytoma or a chemically active neuroblastoma or ganglioneuroma. In all symptomatic patients, especially those with a history of significant hypertension or hypermetabolism, serum catecholamine levels and 24-hour urine levels of homovanillic acid and vanillylmandelic acid should be determined. If these levels are elevated, suggesting pheochromocytoma, preoperative α-adrenergic blockers and at times a beta-blocker need to be administered to avoid perioperative complications from episodic catecholamine release during tumor manipulation.

Neurogenic tumors that arise from intercostal nerves are typically neurilemomas or neurofibromas.[18] Neurilemomas (schwannomas) are the most common neurogenic tumors.[19,20] On histologic examination, they appear as well-encapsulated, firm, gray-tan masses.[21] They tend to occur in one of two morphologic patterns: either an organized architecture with a cellular palisading pattern of growth (Antoni's type A) or a loose reticular pattern (Antoni's type B).[22] Neurofibromas are poorly encapsulated, with a random arrangement of spindle-shaped cells.[23] Associated with neurofibromatosis type 1, these tumors tend to form in the paravertebral gutters (Fig. 43-3). Both neurilemomas and neurofibromas can occur as manifestations of von Recklinghausen's disease and can degenerate into neurosarcoma if they are left untreated.

Neuroblastoma, ganglioneuroblastoma, and ganglioneuroma are tumors of the sympathetic nervous system that arise from primitive sympathetic ganglia and are referred to collectively as neuroblastic tumors.[24] They arise wherever sympathetic tissue exists and may be seen in the neck, posterior mediastinum, adrenal gland, retroperitoneum, and pelvis. The three tumors differ in their degree of cellular and extracellular maturation; immature tumors tend to be aggressive and occur in younger patients (median age, just under 2 years), whereas mature tumors occur in older children (median age, approximately 7 years) and tend to behave in a benign fashion.[24]

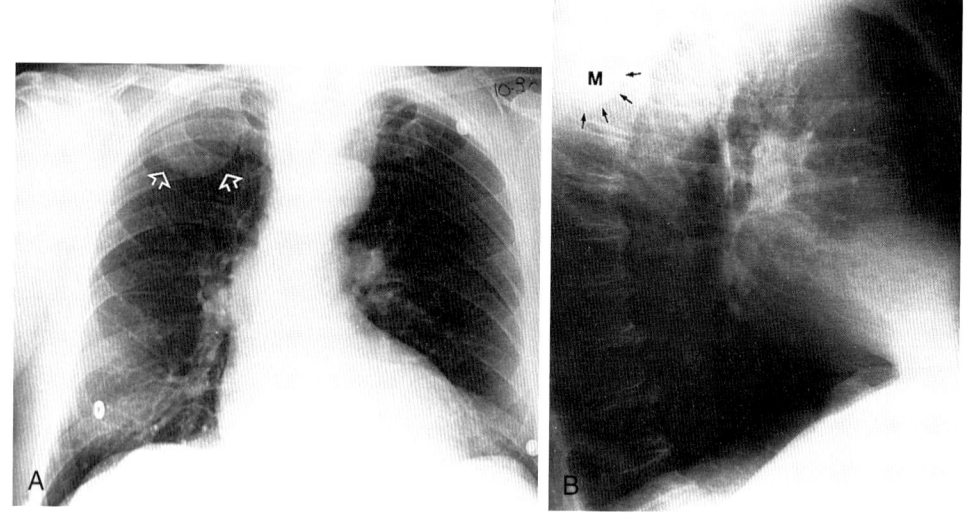

Figure 43–3
Posteroanterior and lateral chest radiographs: neurofibroma. **A,** A large mass projects in the right apex *(arrows)*. It has a smooth, sharp inferior margin. The superior margin makes broad contact with the chest wall, forming obtuse angles. These findings suggest that the mass did not arise in the lung parenchyma. **B,** The lateral chest view demonstrates a barely perceptible mass projecting far posterior behind the anterior margin of the vertebra (M, *arrows*). The location suggests a neurogenic mass. *(Reprinted with permission from Meholic A, Ketai L, Lofgren R. Hilum and mediastinum. In: Meholic A, Ketai L, Lofgren R, editors.* Fundamentals of chest radiology. *Philadelphia: WB Saunders; 1996. p. 217.)*

Ganglioneuromas usually manifest as a benign tumor composed of gangliocytes and mature stroma. They usually appear at an early age located in the paravertebral region and are the most common neurogenic tumors occurring in childhood. Ganglioneuroblastomas are composed of both mature gangliocytes and immature neuroblasts and have intermediate malignant potential.[25]

Neuroblastomas are also seen in children; more than 75% of the cases occur in children younger than 4 years. On histologic examination, these tumors are composed of small, round immature cells organized in a rosette pattern. They are highly invasive, and by the time diagnosis is made, they have often metastasized to the regional lymph nodes, bone, brain, liver, and lung. Interestingly, however, they may, in certain patients, have a relatively benign course, even when metastatic. Symptoms at time of diagnosis typically include cough, dysphagia, chest pain, and occasionally paraplegia. At times, they may manifest with paraneoplastic syndromes such as profuse watery diarrhea secondary to vasoactive intestinal protein syndrome, opsoclonus-polymyoclonus syndrome, and pheochromocytoma-like syndrome. Features such as DNA content, tumor proto-oncogenes, and catecholamine synthesis influence prognosis, and their presence or absence aids in categorizing patients with neuroblastoma as high, intermediate, or low risk. Treatment consists of resection and, usually, chemotherapy. Despite recent advances in treatment, including bone marrow transplantation, neuroblastoma in most patients remains a relatively lethal tumor, accounting for 10% of pediatric cancers but 15% of cancer deaths in children.[24]

A CT scan can help elucidate the tumor type and extent of tumor involvement (Figs. 43-4 and 43-5).[5,24] Neurogenic tumors from peripheral nerves appear as well-defined round or oval masses that are noncalcified in the paravertebral gutter. Neurilemomas have variable enhancement with either homogeneity or heterogeneity.[26] With enhanced CT, these tumors demonstrate variable attenuation, depending on their histology. Neurofibromas are usually homogeneous, low-attenuation lesions on unenhanced CT. Enhanced CT demonstrates homogeneous enhancement or early central blush. Malignant nerve sheath tumors show variable attenuation.[22]

Tumors arising from the sympathetic chain expand along the spinal axis, making them difficult to detect on a lateral view. Sympathetic chain tumors do not demonstrate calcification or bone changes. Characteristic radiographic findings of ganglioneuromas include oblong homogeneous low-attenuation lesions on both enhanced and unenhanced CT. Neuroblastomas appear as aggressive soft tissue lesions with calcification. Ganglioneuroblastomas appear with combined radiographic features of both ganglioneuromas and neuroblastomas. On CT, paragangliomas characteristically appear in the aortopulmonary window with high enhancement after administration of contrast medium.[22]

Tumors located in the posterior mediastinum that extend into the spinal canal through the intervertebral foramen are referred to as *dumbbell tumors.* Preoperative determination of intraspinal involvement of a neurogenic tumor is critical as surgical intervention mandates a combined surgical-neurosurgical procedure to avoid bleeding within the spinal canal that could lead to spinal cord compression.[27-30] This can be addressed by obtaining an MRI study looking for tumor within the spinal canal. These patients rarely may present with symptoms of spinal cord compression. About 10% of patients with neurogenic tumors have extension through a vertebral foramen. Although most of these lesions are benign, approximately 1% to 2% are malignant. MRI typically shows a smoothly rounded, homogeneous density abutting the vertebral column.

If a decision is made to obtain tissue, percutaneous fine-needle aspiration biopsy is an appropriate modality to confirm a diagnosis of a neurogenic tumor. A biopsy specimen that reveals a spindle cell neoplasm with characteristic radiographic findings is diagnostic of a neurogenic tumor. Biopsy specimens that demonstrate a combination of spindle cells and ganglion cells are diagnostic of ganglioneuromas. Immunohistochemical

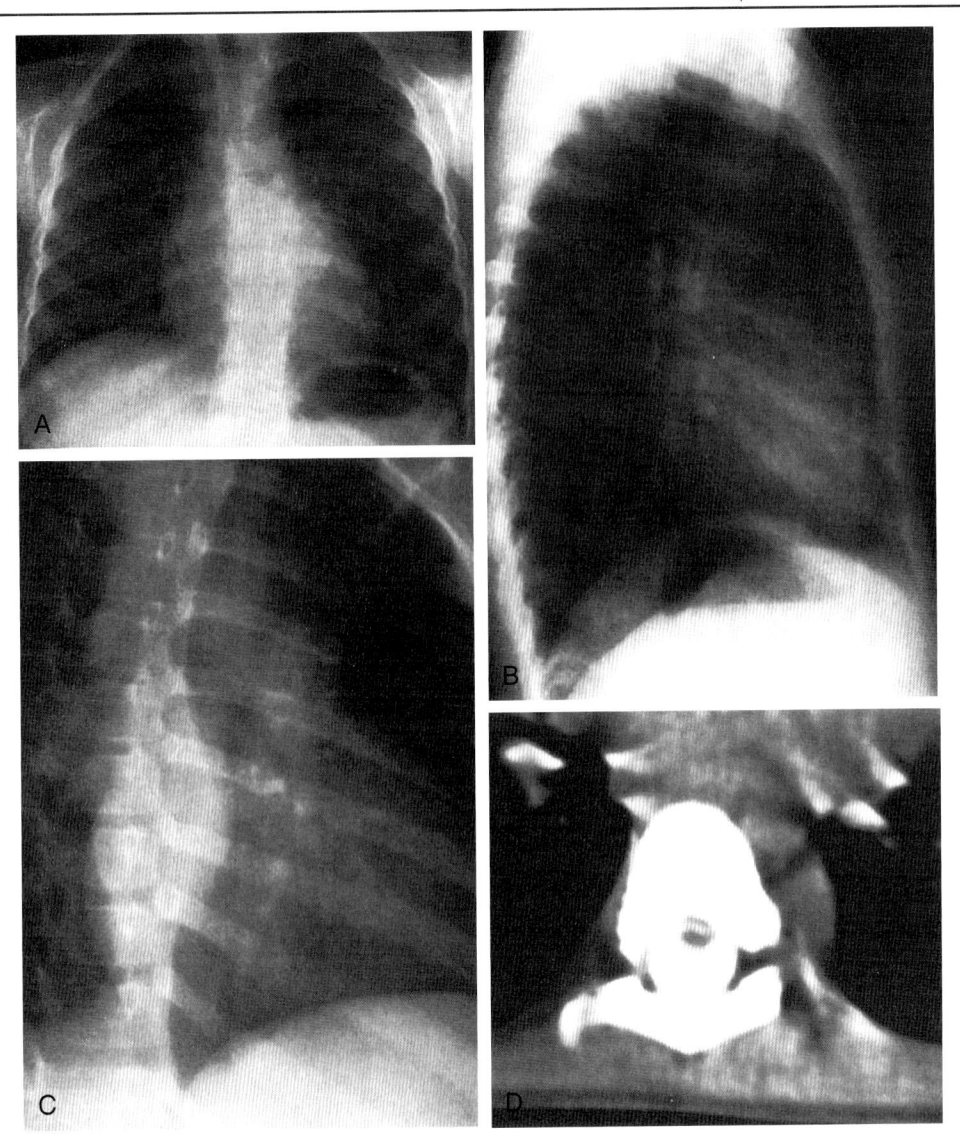

Figure 43–4
A to C, Chest films of a ganglioneuroblastoma. D, CT image of tumor extension into the spinal column.

analysis can cinch the diagnosis, particularly with molecular markers such as S-100 tumor antigen.[31,32]

Surgical intervention is the standard of care for neurogenic tumors; thus, biopsy should be performed only if the results will alter therapy. Traditionally, surgical resection of a posterior mediastinal neurogenic tumor was accomplished through a posterolateral thoracotomy, and this remains an excellent and safe approach. Recent improvements in video-assisted thoracoscopic surgery have allowed minimally invasive approaches to diagnosis and treatment of many tumors in the posterior mediastinum.[33] Advantages of thoracoscopic surgery compared with the classic thoracotomy operation include decreased operative time, decreased average length of postoperative hospitalization, and in many patients less postoperative pain.[34] Benign intrathoracic tumors are ideal lesions for resection by a video-assisted technique.

Thoracoscopic resection of posterior mediastinal neurogenic tumors can be performed successfully regardless of tumor type or size. However, malignant transformation, local invasion, and tumors larger than 5 cm are characteristics that increase the likelihood of requiring conversion to an open procedure.[14]

The standard surgical approach involves a posterolateral thoracotomy incision and exposure of the posterior mediastinum. The tumor is always found in a paravertebral location, and the resection is begun first by incision of the overlying pleura and then with a combination of sharp and blunt dissection, removing the lesion from the underlying vertebral bodies. Rarely is there any invasion of the bony vertebral body, but it is important to recognize any involvement of a neural foramen. If, in dissecting at the origin of the involved nerve root, it appears that the neural foramen is widened, this may indicate that the tumor is present within the spinal canal. If the foramen is widened, it is best to have a neurosurgeon perform a foraminotomy to ensure complete excision of the lesion and to ensure that tumor is either not left in the canal or divided, causing bleeding within the canal. The involved nerve root itself is routinely taken as part of the resection, although at times a portion of the root may be spared as long

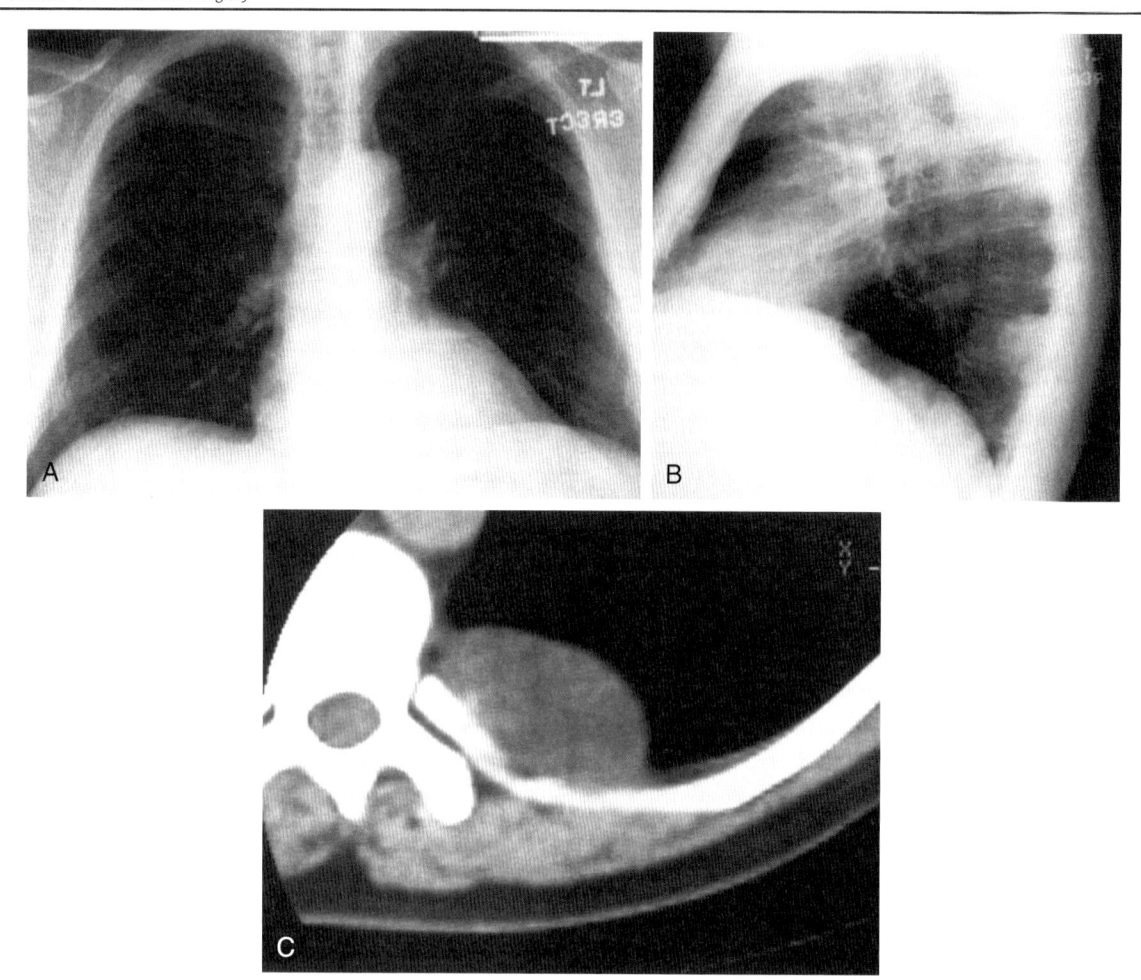

Figure 43–5
A and B, Chest films of a neurofibroma occurring in the posterior mediastinum. C, CT imaging better delineates the anatomic location of the mass and shows the absence of widening of the spinal foramen. This indicates that an intraspinal component to this tumor is unlikely.

as the tumor is completely resected. Some of these tumors arise from the sympathetic chain, and it is important to recognize this and to resect that portion of the sympathetic chain. Care should be taken to avoid resection of segmental vessels, if possible.

Once the pleura has been incised, it is usually easy to mobilize these lesions with a combination of sharp and blunt dissection. Complete resection can be accomplished in essentially all cases. The procedure often may start with videothoracoscopic visualization of the tumor and mobilization, and the tumor can be removed through a small incision in the skin. However, if mobilization proves difficult by the videothoracoscopic approach, there should be no hesitation about converting to an open procedure. This is especially important with lesions at the thoracic outlet.

When it is known that there is tumor involvement within the spinal canal, a well-described approach is a one-stage removal of the tumor performed through a posterolateral thoracotomy combined with transthoracic partial laminectomy.[35] This surgical approach avoids two incisions and limits traction on the spinal cord.[36] Alternatively, an initial posterior approach to the spine with laminectomy and removal of that portion of tumor within the canal can be immediately followed by thoracotomy with resection of the intrathoracic paravertebral tumor.

A more recently described procedure avoids a thoracotomy and invasion of the parietal pleura and uses a dorsal approach to perform a laminectomy with resection of a small portion of the neighboring rib head and neck.[37] In either case, once a dumbbell tumor has been recognized, a combined two-team approach with thoracic surgeons and neurosurgeons working together to perform a one-stage removal is the procedure of choice.[30,38]

The prognosis of primary neurogenic mediastinal tumors varies with their histopathology. Patients with benign neurogenic tumors have an excellent prognosis with complete surgical excision; patients with malignant neurogenic tumors still have poor long-term survival prospects.[16] Recurrence of a benign lesion is unusual.[39] Kang[40] reviewed the results of surgical treatment of 38 children with malignant mediastinal neurogenic tumors seen during an 18-year period. There were 23 (60.5%) neuroblastomas, 14 (36.8%) ganglioneuroblastomas, and 1 malignant neuroepithelioma. The mean age for the series was 3.4 ± 3.0 years, and 26 of the patients were symptomatic at presentation. Complete gross resection was possible in 30 patients, with 5-year survival of 95.2% for localized tumors and 52.5% for stage IV tumors.

With regard to neuroblastomas, spontaneous regression has been reported. Stage I (noninvasive) neuroblastomas are managed by resection alone, whereas stage II lesions (locally invasive on same side of midline) require postoperative

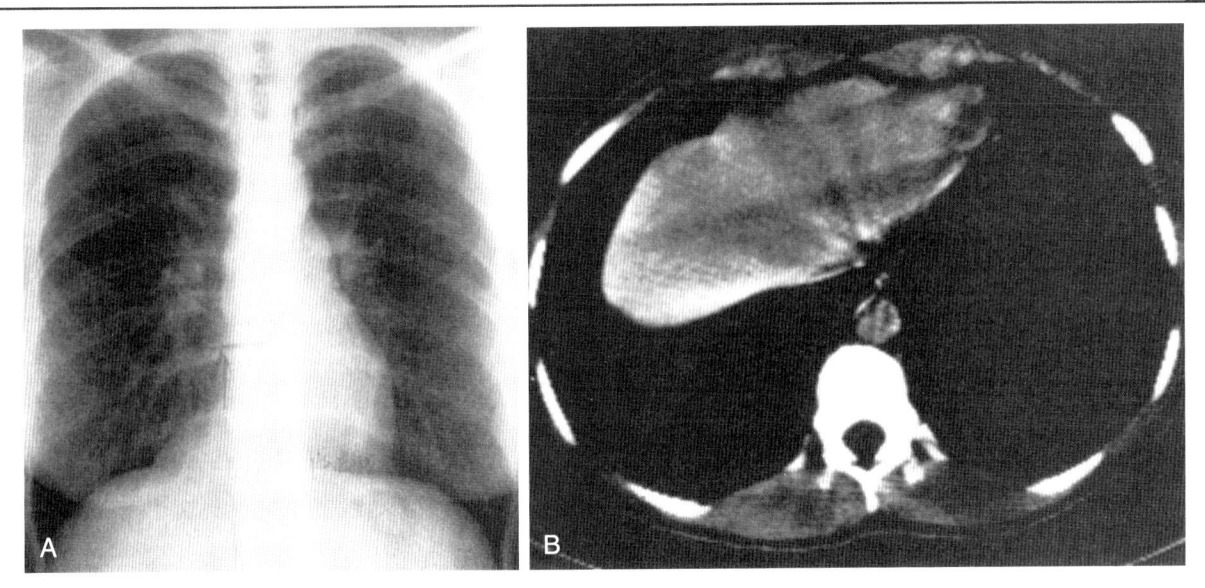

Figure 43–6
A, Chest film of a pericardial cyst in the right pericardiophrenic angle. B, CT image shows the characteristic nearer attenuation of the mass and the typical anatomic location.

irradiation. Stage III lesions (invasive across the midline) and stage IV lesions (systemic metastasis) require multimodality treatment including debulking, radiation therapy, chemotherapy, and a second-look operation. Children younger than 1 year tend to have an excellent prognosis; in older children, poorer prognosis is directly proportional to age.

Esophageal Masses

Esophagus-related posterior mediastinal masses include neoplasms, esophageal cysts,[41] diverticula, hiatal hernias, megaesophagus, and esophageal varices.[42]

Esophageal disease rarely appears on chest radiographs. Plain chest radiography is frequently normal in patients with esophageal carcinoma. Subtle abnormalities are sometimes present, including a retrocardiac mass, abnormal azygoesophageal recess interface, widened mediastinum, widened retrotracheal stripe, and esophageal air–fluid level. Hiatal hernia is the most common esophageal pathologic process detected on the chest radiograph. As with other posterior mediastinal disease, CT is reliable in predicting tumor size and assessing invasion of the mediastinum and tracheobronchial tree as well as spread of esophageal carcinoma to the liver, adrenals, and upper abdominal lymph nodes.

Endoscopic ultrasonography has become the most accurate imaging modality for locoregional cancer staging of the esophagus. Fine-needle aspiration capabilities have added a whole new level of accuracy in nodal staging, with reported numbers in the 90% range for luminal disease.[43] Transesophageal echocardiography is effective at detecting mediastinal masses, although it should be used in conjunction with CT or MRI for more thorough evaluation. Transesophageal echocardiography can demonstrate impingement of the left atrium or ventricle, which is a common occurrence with posterior masses. Echocardiographers need to be aware of a type of posterior mediastinal encroachment that is common with gastric or esophageal disease; this typically has two-dimensional echo features that may simulate a left atrial mass.[44]

Upper gastrointestinal barium examinations identify some type of hiatal hernia, usually a sliding type, in as many as 15% of symptomatic patients.[45] This is discussed in detail in the following chapters. The barium swallow also remains the most useful study to clarify the nature of a retrocardiac mass, such as a pseudotumoral venous collateral.[46] A complete discussion of esophageal cancer can be found in subsequent chapters.

Cysts of the Posterior Mediastinum

Mediastinal cysts form a group of uncommon benign lesions of congenital origin. Cystic lesions of the posterior mediastinum are relatively rare and include bronchogenic, hydatid,[47] enteric, intramural esophageal, and neuroenteric cysts. Thoracic CT is the most effective method for preoperative diagnosis of posterior mediastinal cysts (Fig. 43-6).[48]

The significant controversy regarding these cysts is whether to manage them with observation or surgical resection. They are benign lesions in which operation can be performed with a low morbidity and mortality rate, enabling the surgeon to rule out malignant transformation and to offer a definitive cure.[48] Reports of uneventful operative courses without recurrence for mediastinal cysts are readily available.[49,50]

Bronchogenic Cysts

Mediastinal cysts constitute 20% of all mediastinal masses, and bronchogenic cysts make up 60% of all mediastinal cysts.[9,48,51-53] They are part of the spectrum of bronchopulmonary foregut abnormalities that include extralobar and intralobar sequestration and congenital cystic adenomatoid malformations of the lung.

Cystic lesions can be located in the lung parenchyma or mediastinum. On histologic examination, bronchogenic cysts demonstrate a lining composed of ciliated columnar epithelium. The cyst wall may be composed of cartilage, mucus glands, and smooth muscle. They rarely communicate with the tracheobronchial tree.

Symptoms are present in the occasional patient, usually from compression of adjacent structures or recurrent infection. Paraesophageal bronchogenic cysts often are noted incidentally in the posterior mediastinum during routine chest radiography. If the diagnosis of a bronchogenic cyst is made preoperatively and patients are asymptomatic, observation is an appropriate course. If there is any question of malignant transformation based on radiographic appearance, positive results of cytology, or evidence of enlargement or recurrence, the lesion should be resected. The presence of symptoms—especially pain, cough, or hemoptysis—suggests the advisability of resection. Barium swallow study may identify the source of dysphagia due to external compression. The presence of an air–fluid level may indicate communication with the bronchopulmonary tree (rare) and the likelihood of recurrent infection and indicates that resection is in order. Once a bronchogenic cyst has become infected, the infection is difficult to eradicate and the lesion should be resected.[54]

Symptoms tend to develop with time, and resection at an asymptomatic stage may be best in healthy subjects. Video-assisted techniques provide an ideal approach for resection of these benign lesions. Depending on location, specifically if they are in the superior mediastinum, many of these may be resected through the mediastinoscope.[55] Martinod and coworkers[52] reported their 3- to 7-year experience with thoracoscopic resection in 10 patients with posterior mediastinal bronchogenic cysts. The average cyst size was 4.9 cm, and the largest diameter was 10 cm. There were no operative deaths and no postoperative complications. Long-term follow-up (range, 4.5 to 7.5 years) showed no late complications and no recurrence.

Gastroenteric Cysts

Gastroenteric or duplication cysts are periesophageal lesions that form from the posterior division of the primitive foregut. They may cause a middle or posterior mediastinal mass, particularly in the young. They occur within or adjacent to the wall of the esophagus. Communication with the upper gastrointestinal tract is uncommon.

On histologic examination, duplication cysts are lined by nonkeratinizing squamous, ciliated columnar, gastric, or small intestinal epithelium. In distinguishing bronchogenic from esophageal cysts, the lining epithelium is not helpful, but the presence of two muscle layers in esophageal cysts and bronchial glands or bronchial cartilage in bronchogenic cysts enables categorization in the majority of cases.[50]

Patients may present with a variety of symptoms, but these lesions are usually asymptomatic. Respiratory compromise with cough, dyspnea, recurrent pulmonary infections, and chest pain is not that uncommon. If gastric mucosa is present, perforation into the esophagus can cause hematemesis, or erosion into the adjacent lung parenchyma can develop into an abscess. These complications are exceedingly rare with these lesions.

Diagnosis is facilitated by the use of esophageal ultrasonography, chest CT, or contrast studies of the upper gastrointestinal tract.[41] Technetium Tc 99m scanning can be used to look for ectopic gastric mucosa. Resection is the therapy of choice, whether by thoracoscopic or open technique. Many of these lesions are amenable to a minimally invasive thoracoscopic approach that still allows complete resection. Posterolateral thoracotomy is the procedure of choice when greater exposure is required. The question always arises as to whether it is necessary to resect these benign lesions. Certainly, if the lesion is producing compressive symptoms or is infected, resection is indicated; it is the asymptomatic lesion discovered incidentally that poses the question of whether resection is indicated. It is often unclear if the lesion is truly cystic because the cyst contents become so inspissated as to appear solid. When the cystic nature of the lesion is unclear, a case can be made for resection, especially through a minimally invasive approach. Observation may be the approach chosen for those asymptomatic lesions that are clearly cystic.

Neuroenteric Cysts

Neuroenteric cysts make up 5% to 10% of foregut lesions. They occur in infants younger than 1 year and are uncommon in adults.[49] They have a connection to the meninges, usually by a stalk, and are associated with congenital defects of the thoracic spine. Neuroenteric cysts possess endodermal and ectodermal or neurogenic elements. They develop because of failure of separation of the notochord from the primitive gut. A CT scan showing a cystic mediastinal lesion associated with a vertebral abnormality such as congenital scoliosis, hemivertebrae, or spina bifida should prompt consideration of a diagnosis of neuroenteric cyst.

Other Masses of the Posterior Mediastinum

Primary or metastatic tumors of the thoracic spine may also appear as a posterior mediastinal paravertebral mass. Lymphomas, particularly Hodgkin's disease, may involve the posterior parietal group of lymph nodes and produce a fusiform paravertebral soft tissue mass. Infections such as tuberculosis can result in a paravertebral mass, as can a post-traumatic hematoma. A descending thoracic aortic aneurysm is an important lesion that can masquerade as a mediastinal neoplasm.

Extramedullary hematopoiesis, a compensatory response to insufficient bone marrow blood cell production, is a rare cause of a paravertebral mass.[56] The preferred sites of extramedullary hematopoietic involvement are the spleen, liver, and lymph nodes.[56] However, in hereditary spherocytosis, for example, the posterior paravertebral mediastinum is also commonly involved. Extramedullary hematopoietic tumors can occur without severe chronic hemolytic anemia. Therefore, this lesion must be considered in the differential diagnosis of a posterior mediastinal mass in patients even without clinical evidence of anemia.[57] Earlier reports demonstrated the utility of a conventional chest radiograph and CT scan of the thorax for diagnosis without biopsy or thoracotomy.[58] Later reports clarify the superiority of MRI in identifying intrathoracic extramedullary hematopoiesis, although it usually is used in conjunction with CT because of specific limitations.[56,59]

Castleman's disease (giant lymph node hyperplasia) is characterized by mass lesions that are vascular tumors often surrounded by lymphadenopathy (Fig. 43-7).[60,61] This arrangement makes CT useful diagnostically because CT may reveal lymphadenopathy surrounding an encapsulated mass that enhances brightly and is distinct from the aorta. The term is applied to three lesions that are histologically distinct: hyaline vascular, plasma cell, and generalized. The first two

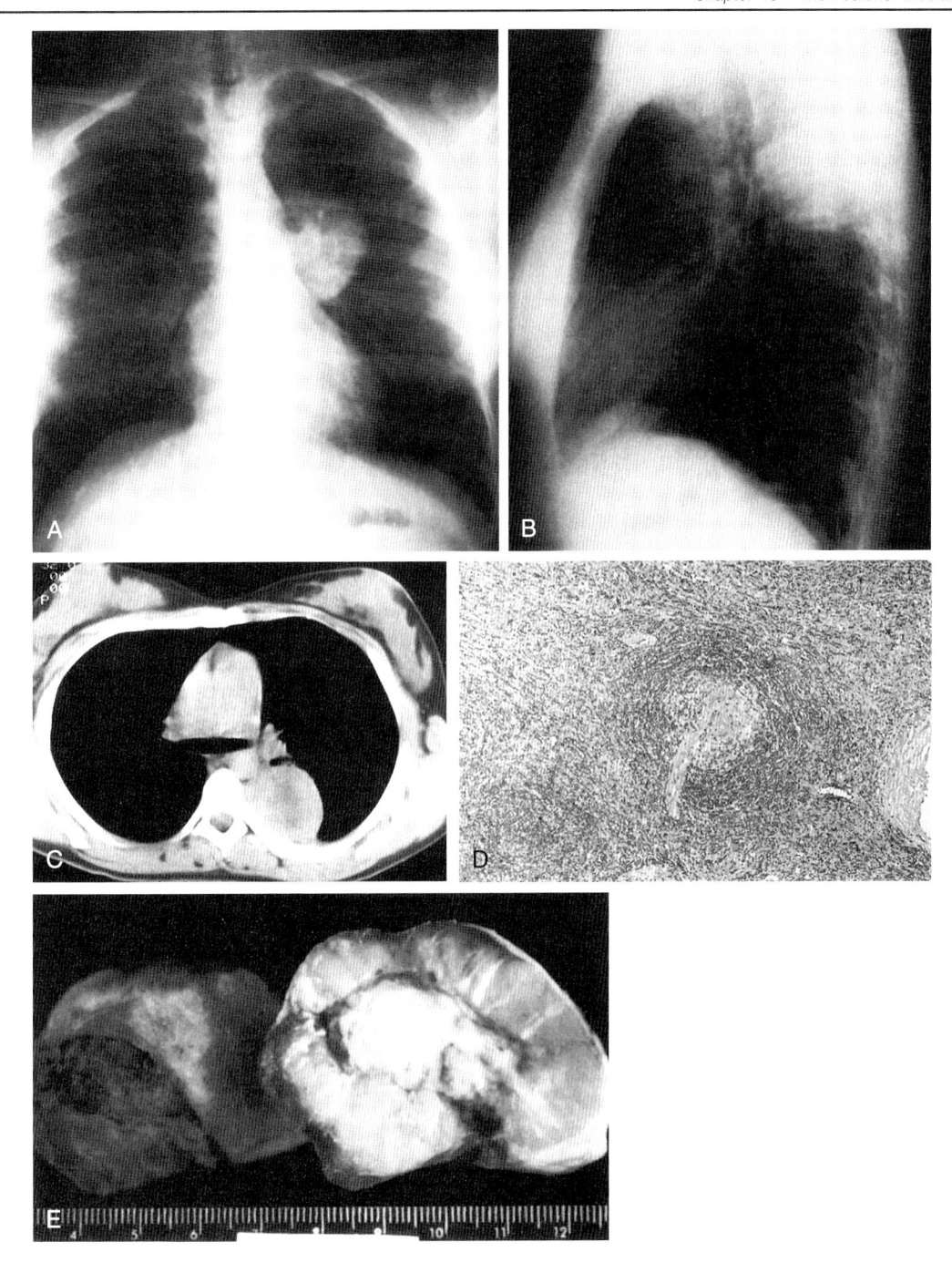

Figure 43-7
A and B, Chest films of a giant lymph node hyperplasia (Castleman's disease) that occurs in the posterior mediastinum. C, CT image of the tumor is similar to a neurogenic tumor. D, Photomicrograph of the tumor shows the small hyaline follicles and interfollicular capillary proliferation that are characteristic of the hyaline vascular form. E, Photograph of a gross specimen.

represent localized disease, whereas the third refers to multicentric (generalized) disease.

Hyaline vascular Castleman's disease accounts for 90% of cases. It is a localized lesion usually found incidentally in asymptomatic patients. Castleman's disease manifesting as a spinal epidural mass lesion with cord compression has been reported.[62] Surgical excision is the treatment of choice; radiotherapy has not been effective. The plasma cell variant, also localized, is much less common. Patients are much more likely to have symptoms and to present with fever, fatigue, weight loss, and hemolytic anemia. The sedimentation rate is often high and associated with hypergammaglobulinemia, which results from the production of interleukin-6 by the hyperplastic lymph nodes. Resection is the treatment of choice.

Generalized or multicentric Castleman's disease has the histologic features of both localized forms. The disease occurs in older patients, who typically present with severe systemic symptoms, generalized lymphadenopathy, and hepatosplenomegaly. The mortality from this disease is 50%, and the median survival is 27 months. Progression to lymphoma is common (Fig. 43-8). The diagnosis of lymphoma is made from biopsy, and treatment is directed at management of the lymphoma.

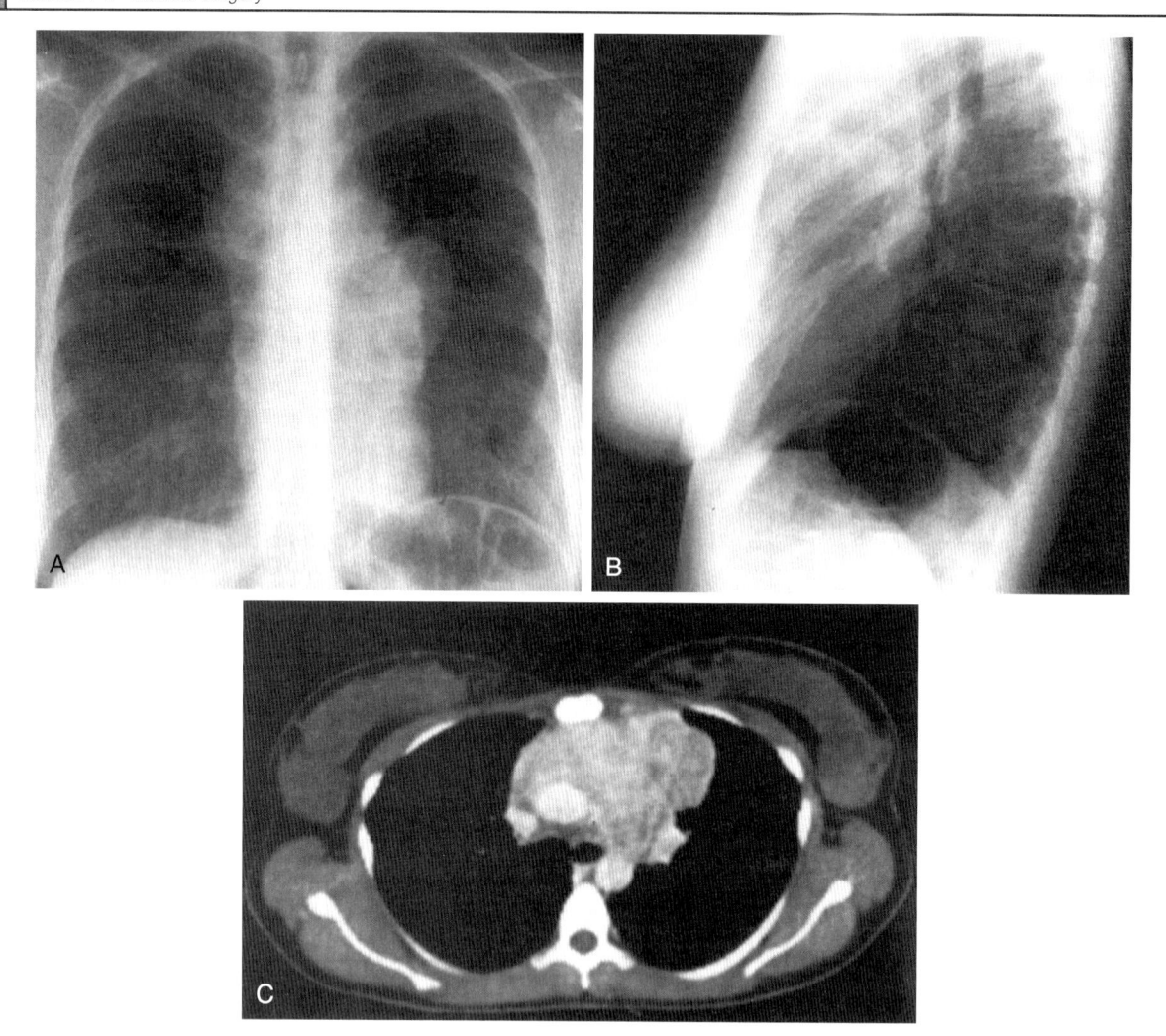

Figure 43–8
A and **B**, Chest films of a large B-cell non-Hodgkin's lymphoma that involves the anterosuperior mediastinum. **C**, CT image shows the involvement of the mediastinal structures by the lymphoma.

Other rare causes of a primary posterior mediastinal mass usually occuring in the paravertebral sulci include angiomyolipoma,[63,64] extralobar pulmonary sequestration,[65] neuroendocrine carcinoma,[66] mediastinal ependymomas,[67] cellular hemangiomas,[68] melanotic paraganglioma,[69] and mediastinal extension of a pancreatic pseudocyst.

INFECTIONS OF THE MEDIASTINUM

Descending necrotizing mediastinitis is a potentially fatal condition in its acute or chronic form that can involve the posterior mediastinum.[70] Acute mediastinitis most commonly occurs after postoperative infection or esophageal perforation. The organism most commonly isolated is *Staphylococcus*. In acute mediastinitis, the patient presents with the typical signs of infection, including fever, tachycardia, and leukocytosis. Subcutaneous emphysema resulting from esophageal perforation may be another clue to an infectious source.[70,71] In chronic mediastinitis, the etiology is a granulomatous infection. When the granulomas rupture, the contents lead to a fibrotic reaction.

The posterior mediastinum is more susceptible to infection than the other compartments of the thorax are. Anatomically, this is explained by the relative accessibility of the posterior mediastinum to the neck and abdomen. Inferiorly, the hiatus for the inferior vena cava and the hiatus for the aorta traversing the diaphragm are well sealed. However, the esophageal hiatus, which is most posterior, is not closed as well and provides a track between the posterior mediastinum and the abdominal cavity. Similarly, infections from the head and neck have easier access to the posterior mediastinum. The more anterior fascial planes that come down from the neck terminate before reaching the mediastinal compartments. There are two posterior spaces that directly communicate with the pharynx and neck and mediastinum. The first space is located between the visceral fascia and the alar fascia and is termed the *danger space* because of its direct communication with the posterior mediastinum. The second space is located between the prevertebral fascia and the vertebral bodies, allowing communication of vertebral infections.[70]

Not surprisingly, abscesses in the posterior mediastinum are more frequent than those in the anterior compartment. Although primary infection is possible, most infections are secondary and the source usually is readily apparent. Most common signs of posterior mediastinal abscess are pain, dysphagia, cough, and dyspnea. The pain occurs most often on

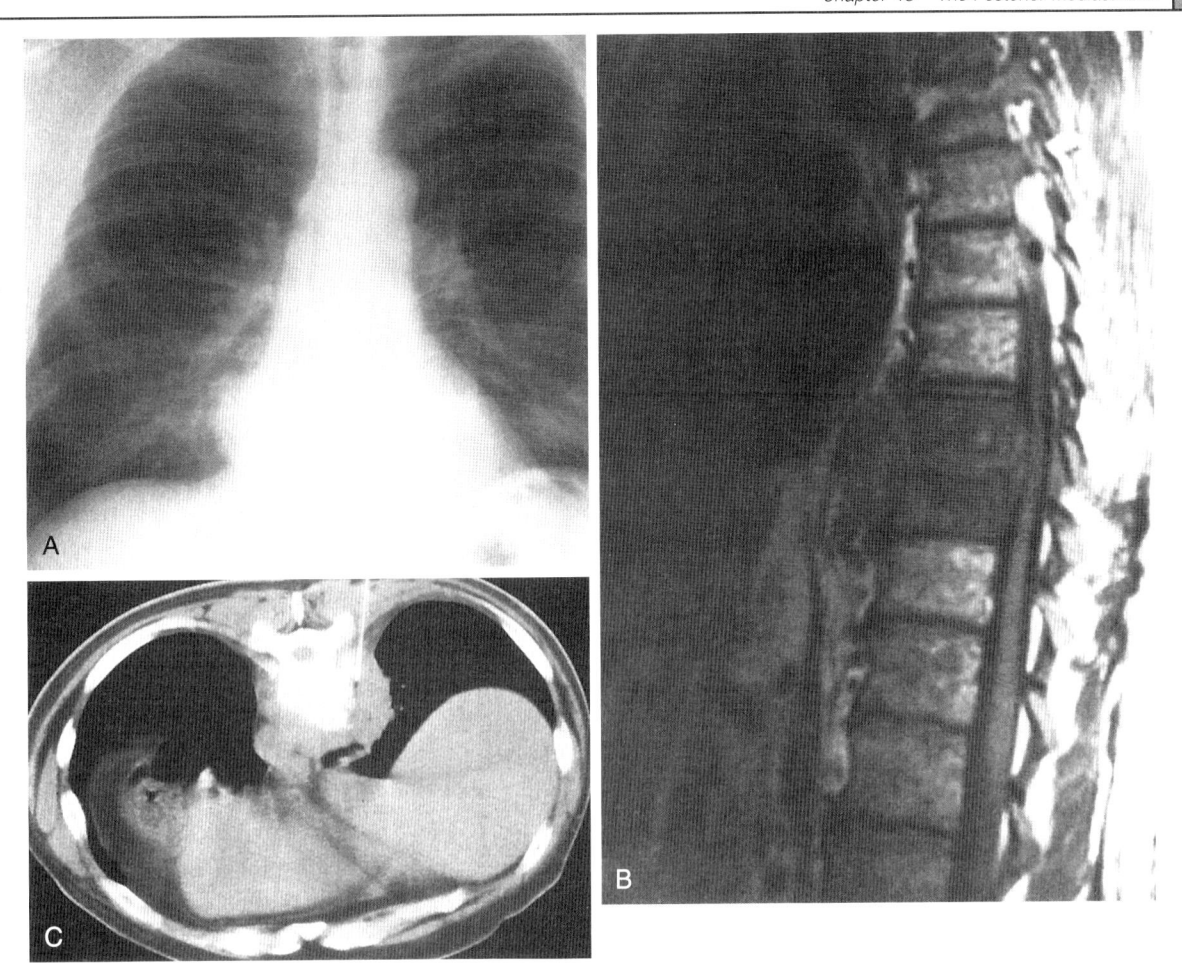

Figure 43–9
Paraspinous abscess in a 45-year-old man with AIDS and a systemic infection. **A,** Frontal chest radiograph demonstrates a mass behind the right side of the heart. **B,** Spinal MRI demonstrates reduced intensity in two vertebral bodies with posterior and anterior masses. **C,** CT-guided aspiration of the mass demonstrated a paraspinous *Staphylococcus aureus* infection. *(Reprinted with permission from Gamsu G. The mediastinum. In: Moss AA, Gamsu G, Genant HK, editors. Computed tomography of the body, 2nd ed, vol 1. Philadelphia: WB Saunders; 1992. p. 83.)*

swallowing and coughing, and it is felt posteriorly in the interscapular region or may radiate anteriorly. The symptoms are due to encroachment on the esophagus and trachea in the upper part of the chest. Esophageal perforation is the most common cause of a posterior mediastinal abscess. Another cause of posterior mediastinal abscess is extension of infection from the oropharynx, spine, lung pleura, or abdominal cavity.

CT scan may demonstrate an air–fluid level or mediastinal air (Fig. 43-9). Nonsurgical management includes intravenous antibiotics, but surgical intervention usually is required on an urgent basis. Surgical intervention includes wide opening of the mediastinal compartment by incision of the pleura followed by débridement, irrigation, drainage, and closure of the esophageal perforation with or without a muscle flap. In diffuse mediastinitis involving the posterior mediastinum, pericarditis or bilateral exudative pleuritis may be present.

Summary

Lesions of the posterior mediastinum most commonly are neurogenic in origin and usually are benign in adults. Despite this recognition, surgical intervention commonly is required. Minimally invasive surgical approaches may provide additional justification for removal of these lesions before they become symptomatic.

REFERENCES

1. Esposito C, Romeo C. Surgical anatomy of the mediastinum. *Semin Pediatr Surg* 1999;**8**:50-3.
2. Ronson RS, Duarte I, Miller JI. Embryology and surgical anatomy of the mediastinum with clinical implications. *Surg Clin North Am* 2000;**80**:157-69, x-xi.
3. Saenz NC, Schnitzer JJ, Eraklis AE, et al. Posterior mediastinal masses. *J Pediatr Surg* 1993;**28**:172-6.
4. Kawashima A, Fishman EK, Kuhlman JE, et al. CT of posterior mediastinal masses. *Radiographics* 1991;**11**:1045-67.
5. LeBlanc J, Guttentag AR, Shepard JA, et al. Imaging of mediastinal foregut cysts. *Can Assoc Radiol J* 1994;**45**:381-6.
6. Wernecke K, Diederich S. Sonographic features of mediastinal tumors. *AJR Am J Roentgenol* 1994;**163**:1357-64.
7. Bressler EL, Kirkham JA. Mediastinal masses: alternative approaches to CT-guided needle biopsy. *Radiology* 1994;**191**:391-6.
8. Kelemen JJ 3rd, Naunheim KS. Minimally invasive approaches to mediastinal neoplasms. *Semin Thorac Cardiovasc Surg* 2000;**12**:301-6.
9. Divisi D, Battaglia C, Crisci R, et al. Diagnostic and therapeutic approaches for masses in the posterior mediastinum. *Acta Biomed Ateneo Parmense* 1998;**69**:123-8.
10. Nordenstrom B. Paravertebral approach to the posterior mediastinum for mediastinography and needle biopsy. *Acta Radiol Diagn (Stockh)* 1972;**12**:298-304.

11. Chowbey PK, Vashistha A, Khullar R, et al. Laparoscopic excision of a lower posterior mediastinal paraspinal mass: technique and feasibility of the laparoscopic approach. *Surg Laparosc Endosc Percutan Tech* 2002;**12**:378-81:discussion 381-382.
12. Kumar A, Kumar S, Aggarwal S, et al. Thoracoscopy: the preferred approach for the resection of selected posterior mediastinal tumors. *J Laparoendosc Adv Surg Tech A* 2002;**12**:345-53.
13. Partrick DA, Rothenberg SS. Thoracoscopic resection of mediastinal masses in infants and children: An evaluation of technique and results. *J Pediatr Surg* 2001;**36**:1165-7.
14. Zierold D, Halow KD. Thoracoscopic resection as the preferred approach to posterior mediastinal neurogenic tumors. *Surg Laparosc Endosc Percutan Tech* 2000;**10**:222-5.
15. Cardillo G, Carleo F, Khalil MW, et al. Surgical treatment of benign neurogenic tumours of the mediastinum: a single institution report. *Eur J Cardiothorac Surg* 2008;**34**:1210-4.
16. Reeder LB. Neurogenic tumors of the mediastinum. *Semin Thorac Cardiovasc Surg* 2000;**12**:261-7.
17. Takeda S, Miyoshi S, Minami M, Matsuda H. Intrathoracic neurogenic tumor—50 years' experience in a Japanese institution. *Eur J Cardiothorac Surg* 2004;**26**:807-12.
18. Marchevsky AM. Mediastinal tumors of peripheral nervous system origin. *Semin Diagn Pathol* 1999;**16**:65-78.
19. Penkrot RJ, Bolden R. Thoracic neurilemmoma: case report and review of the world literature. *J Comput Tomogr* 1985;**9**:13-5.
20. Strollo DC, Rosado-de-Christenson ML, Jett JR. Primary mediastinal tumors: part II. Tumors of the middle and posterior mediastinum. *Chest* 1997;**112**:1344-57.
21. Al Refai M, Brunelli A. Fianchini A: Giant schwannoma of the posterior mediastinum. *Chest* 1999;**115**:907-8.
22. Lee JY, Lee KS, Han J, et al. Spectrum of neurogenic tumors in the thorax: CT and pathologic findings. *J Comput Assist Tomogr* 1999;**23**:399-406.
23. Mondal A. Cytopathology of neuroblastoma, ganglioneuroblastoma and ganglioneuroma. *J Indian Med Assoc* 1995;**93**:340-3.
24. Lonergan GJ, Schwab CM, Suarez ES, et al. Neuroblastoma, ganglioneuroblastoma, and ganglioneuroma: radiologic-pathologic correlation. *Radiographics* 2002;**22**:911-34.
25. Adam A, Hochholzer L. Ganglioneuroblastoma of the posterior mediastinum: a clinicopathologic review of 80 cases. *Cancer* 1981;**47**:373-81.
26. Moon WK, Im JG, Han MC. Malignant schwannomas of the thorax: CT findings. *J Comput Assist Tomogr* 1993;**17**:274-6.
27. Buchfelder M, Nomikos P, Paulus W, et al. Spinal-thoracic dumbbell meningioma: a case report. *Spine* 2001;**26**:1500-4.
28. Heltzer JM, Krasna MJ, Aldrich F, et al. Thoracoscopic excision of a posterior mediastinal "dumbbell" tumor using a combined approach. *Ann Thorac Surg* 1995;**60**:431-3.
29. Liu HP, Yim AP, Wan J, et al. Thoracoscopic removal of intrathoracic neurogenic tumors: a combined Chinese experience. *Ann Surg* 2000;**232**:187-90.
30. Yuksel M, Pamir N, Ozer F, et al. The principles of surgical management in dumbbell tumors. *Eur J Cardiothorac Surg* 1996;**10**:569-73.
31. Dillon KM, Hill CM, Cameron CH, et al. Mediastinal mixed dendritic cell sarcoma with hybrid features. *J Clin Pathol* 2002;**55**:791-4.
32. Moran CA, Suster S, Fishback N, et al. Mediastinal paragangliomas. A clinicopathologic and immunohistochemical study of 16 cases. *Cancer* 1993;**72**:2358-64.
33. Naunheim KS. Video thoracoscopy for masses of the posterior mediastinum. *Ann Thorac Surg* 1993;**56**:657-8.
34. Watanabe M, Takagi K, Aoki T, et al. [Thoracoscopic resection of mediastinal tumors.]. *Nippon Kyobu Geka Gakkai Zasshi* 1994;**42**:1016-20.
35. Suganuma H, Nakamura H, Sugiyama H, et al. [A case of dumbbell neurogenic tumors of the mediastinum.]. *Kyobu Geka* 1989;**42**:827-30.
36. Vasilakis D, Papaconstantinou C, Aletras H. Dumb-bell intrathoracic and intraspinal neurofibroma. Report of a case. *Scand J Thorac Cardiovasc Surg* 1986;**20**:171-3.
37. Osada H, Aoki H, Yokote K, et al. Dumbbell neurogenic tumor of the mediastinum: a report of three cases undergoing single-staged complete removal without thoracotomy. *Jpn J Surg* 1991;**21**:224-8.
38. Viard H, Sautreaux JL, Cougard P, et al. [Dumbbell neurogenic tumors of the posterior mediastinum. Apropos of five cases.]. *Ann Chir* 1991;**45**:699-703.
39. Schmezer A, Reinosch W, Laqua D, et al. [Thoracic neurinoma: a rare tumor of the posterior mediastinum.] *Chirurg* 1996;**67**:90-2.
40. Kang CH, Kim YT, Jeon S, et al. Surgical treatment of malignant mediastinal neurogenic tumors in children. *Eur J Cardiothorac Surg* 2007;**31**:725-30.
41. Hara M, Arakawa T, Ogino H, et al. A case of isolated esophageal cyst in the posterior mediastinum. *Radiat Med* 2001;**19**:161-4.
42. Basheda SG, O'Donovan P, Golish JA. Giant esophageal varices. An unusual cause of a posterior mediastinal mass. *Chest* 1993;**103**:1284-5.
43. Waxman I, Dye CE. Interventional endosonography. *Cancer J* 2002;**8**(Suppl. I):S113-123.
44. D'Cruz IA, Feghali N, Gross CM. Echocardiographic manifestations of mediastinal masses compressing or encroaching on the heart. *Echocardiography* 1994;**11**:523-33.
45. Hashemi M, Sillin LF, Peters JH. Current concepts in the management of paraesophageal hiatal hernia. *J Clin Gastroenterol* 1999;**29**:8-13.
46. Moult PJ, Waite DW, Dick R. Posterior mediastinal venous masses in patients with portal hypertension. *Gut* 1975;**16**:57-61.
47. Karnak I, Ciftci AO, Tanyel FC. Hydatid cyst: an unusual etiology for a cystic lesion of the posterior mediastinum. *J Pediatr Surg* 1998;**33**:759-60.
48. Zambudio AR, Lanzas JT, Calvo MJ, et al. Non-neoplastic mediastinal cysts. *Eur J Cardiothorac Surg* 2002;**22**:712-6.
49. Kumar R, Nayak SR. Unusual neuroenteric cysts: diagnosis and management. *Pediatr Neurosurg* 2002;**37**:321-30.
50. Salyer DC, Salyer WR, Eggleston JC. Benign developmental cysts of the mediastinum. *Arch Pathol Lab Med* 1977;**101**:136-9.
51. Itoh H, Shitamura T, Kataoka H, et al. Retroperitoneal bronchogenic cyst: report of a case and literature review. *Pathol Int* 1999;**49**:152-5.
52. Martinod E, Pons F, Azorin J, et al. Thoracoscopic excision of mediastinal bronchogenic cysts: results in 20 cases. *Ann Thorac Surg* 2000;**69**:1525-8.
53. Yang SW, Linton JA, Ryu SJ, et al. Retroperitoneal multilocular bronchogenic cyst adjacent to adrenal gland. *Yonsei Med J* 1999;**40**:523-6.
54. Roberts JR, Smythe WR, Weber RW, et al. Thoracoscopic management of descending necrotizing mediastinitis. *Chest* 1997;**112**:850-4.
55. Smythe WR, Bavaria JE, Kaiser LR. Mediastinoscopic subtotal removal of mediastinal cysts. *Chest* 1998;**114**:614-7.
56. Granjo E, Bauerle R, Sampaio R, et al. Extramedullary hematopoiesis in hereditary spherocytosis deficient in ankyrin: a case report. *Int J Hematol* 2002;**76**:153-6.
57. De Montpreville VT, Dulmet EM, Chapelier AR, et al. Extramedullary hematopoietic tumors of the posterior mediastinum related to asymptomatic refractory anemia. *Chest* 1993;**104**:1623-4.
58. Falappa P, Danza FM, Leone G, et al. Thoracic extramedullary hematopoiesis: evaluation by conventional radiology and computed tomography. *Diagn Imaging* 1982;**51**:19-24.
59. Tamburrini O, Della Sala M, Mancuso PP, et al. [The diagnostic imaging of intrathoracic extramedullary hematopoiesis.]. *Radiol Med (Torino)* 1992;**84**:582-6.
60. Hummel P, Benjamin V, Zagzag D. 28-year-old woman with neck and back pain. *Brain Pathol* 2002;**12**:395-7:2002.
61. Olscamp G, Weisbrod G, Sanders D, et al. Castleman disease: unusual manifestations of an unusual disorder. *Radiology* 1980;**135**:43-8.
62. Kachur E, Ang LC, Megyesi JF. Castleman's disease and spinal cord compression: case report. *Neurosurgery* 2002;**50**:399-402:discussion 402-403.
63. Fukuzawa J, Shimizu T, Sakai E, et al. [Case report of angiomyolipoma of the posterior upper mediastinum.]. *Nihon Kyobu Shikkan Gakkai Zasshi* 1992;**30**:464-7.
64. Kim YH, Kwon NY, Myung NH, et al. A case of mediastinal angiomyolipoma. *Korean J Intern Med* 2001;**16**:277-80.
65. Kamiyoshihara M, Kawashima O, Sakata S, et al. Extralobar pulmonary sequestration in the posterior mediastinum. *Scand Cardiovasc J* 2001;**35**:157-8.
66. Horie Y, Kato M. Neuroendocrine carcinoma of the posterior mediastinum: a possible primary lesion. *Arch Pathol Lab Med* 1999;**123**:933-6.
67. Wilson RW, Moran CA. Primary ependymoma of the mediastinum: a clinicopathologic study of three cases. *Ann Diagn Pathol* 1998;**2**:293-300.
68. Parker JR, Knott-Craig C, Min KW, et al. Cellular hemangioma of the posterior mediastinum: unusual presentation of a rare vascular neoplasm. *J Okla State Med Assoc* 1997;**90**:7-9.
69. Hofmann WJ, Wockel W, Thetter O, et al. Melanotic paraganglioma of the posterior mediastinum. *Virchows Arch* 1995;**425**:641-6.
70. Endo S, Murayama F, Hasegawa T, et al. Guideline of surgical management based on diffusion of descending necrotizing mediastinitis. *Jpn J Thorac Cardiovasc Surg* 1999;**47**:14-9.
71. Nomori H, Horio H, Kobayashi R. Descending necrotizing mediastinitis secondary to pharyngitis. A case report. *Scand Cardiovasc J* 1997;**31**:233-5.

CHAPTER 44
Surgical Treatment of Hyperhidrosis
Steven M. Keller

Clinical Presentation
Epidemiology
Autonomic Nervous System: Anatomy and Function
Treatment
  Nonoperative
  Surgical
    Operative Procedure for Hyperhidrosis
    Results of Endoscopic Thoracic Sympathicotomy
Complications and Sequelae of Surgery
  Immediate
  Chronic
    Compensatory Sweating
    Cardiopulmonary Complications
    Other
  Treatment of Complications
Summary

Hyperhidrosis is commonly defined as sweating in excess of physiologic requirements. Perhaps the earliest recognition of this disorder was by Charles Dickens, whose portrayal of Uriah Heep in *David Copperfield* describes accurately the clinical presentation of palmar hyperhidrosis.[1,2] "I saw Uriah Heep shutting up the office, and, feeling friendly towards everybody, went in and spoke to him, and at parting, gave him my hand. But oh, what a clammy hand this was! As ghostly to the touch as to the sight! I rubbed mine afterwards, to warm it, and to rub his off."

Patients are referred to the thoracic surgeon because of inordinate sweating of the palms, face, or axilla. Less commonly, patients complain of severe facial sweating. Multiple prior evaluations by internists and dermatologists are common.

The earliest sympathectomy undertaken specifically for treatment of hyperhidrosis was performed in Europe by Kotzareff in 1920.[3] The first sympathectomy for treatment of hyperhidrosis in the United States was accomplished in 1932 by Adson and colleagues.[4] The earliest thoracoscopic sympathectomy was performed in 1939 for treatment of hypertension.[5] The first thoracoscopic sympathectomy for treatment of hyperhidrosis was reported in 1978.[6] Paravertebral, supraclavicular, transaxillary, and transthoracic approaches have also been used to gain access to the sympathetic chain. Significant interest and large volumes of cases did not occur, however, until the availability of video-assisted thoracic surgery.

CLINICAL PRESENTATION

The typical patient gives a history of palmar and plantar sweating since early childhood. Parents may report that excessive wetness of the hands and feet was present during infancy. Patients commonly report having been teased by other children, who would not want to hold their hands, and having been berated by teachers for submitting assignments that were wet and smudged. Puddles are left on computer and piano keyboards. As patients enter adulthood, their wet hands adversely affect social interaction and influence career choice.

Sweating is intermittent and occurs at times of both apparent calm and obvious stress.[7] Sweating is usually worse during the summer months. Although the degree of hyperhidrosis varies, sweating is much greater than the dampness associated with stress. A dry hand may become soaking wet within minutes. Perspiration forms on the volar surface of the fingers and on the thenar and hypothenar eminences, and it fills the palmar skin folds (Fig. 44-1). Sweat may actually run down the arm and drip to the floor.

Nearly all patients with palmar hyperhidrosis also suffer from plantar hyperhidrosis, the degree and timing of which parallels that manifested in the hands. Patients walking barefoot leave tracks as if they were walking out of the shower. Footwear is ruined by the constant moistness. Open-toe sandals are impossible to wear because the wet feet slip. Despite the frequent moistness, fungal infections are rare. As many as 50% of patients with palmar and plantar hyperhidrosis also suffer from concomitant axillary hyperhidrosis that causes garment staining and odor (bromhidrosis).[1,6,8-13] Isolated

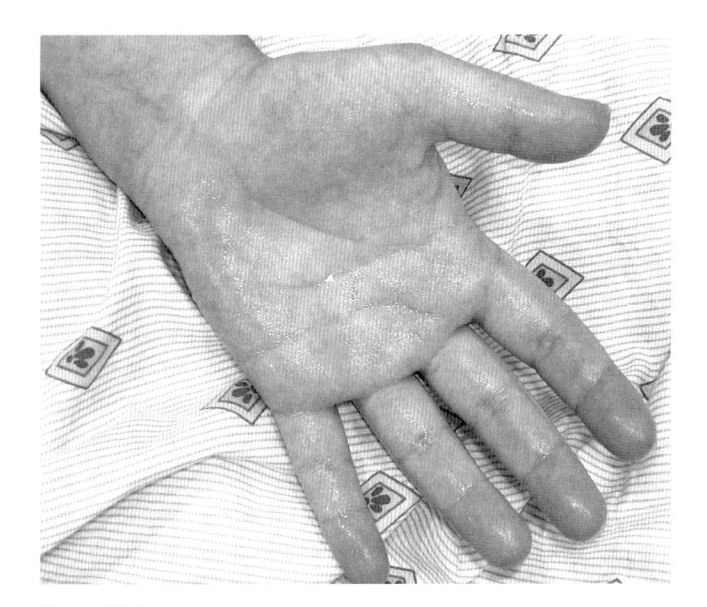

Figure 44-1
Typical appearance of palmar hyperhidrosis. Note wetness on the thenar and hypothenar eminences and on the palmar surface of distal phalanges.

axillary hyperhidrosis is a frequent complaint. Severe facial sweating is much less common.

In addition to altering their life style to avoid direct or indirect hand contact, sufferers from hyperhidrosis develop other coping mechanisms. A handkerchief or tissue is always in hand. They frequently wipe their hands on their clothing. In social situations, a cold drink is ever present to provide a reason for their cold wet hand or an excuse for the need to wipe their hand before a handshake.

The diagnosis of hyperhidrosis is based on patient history and physical examination. One expert multispecialty working group defined hyperhidrosis as focal sweating of greater than 6 months' duration that fulfills at least two of the following criteria: it is bilateral and symmetric, it impairs daily activities, it occurs at least weekly, the age of onset is less than 25 years, there is a family history, and focal sweating ceases during sleep.[14] There are currently no accepted objective definitions of palmar hyperhidrosis, but some have suggested that focal axillary sweat production of greater than 50 to 100 mg/5 min is diagnostic of axillary hyperhidrosis.[14]

EPIDEMIOLOGY

The prevalence of palmar and plantar hyperhidrosis was estimated as 0.6% to 1%[1] in a study of Israeli army recruits. Based on a survey of 13,000 college and high school students, investigators from Asia reported a prevalence of 4.6%.[12] A recent survey of 150,000 U.S. households yielded a hyperhidrosis prevalence of 2.8%.[11] Generalized hyperhidrosis may be associated with thyrotoxicosis, neurologic diseases, and rare inherited disorders. Patients with classic palmar, plantar, and axillary hyperhidrosis do not have concomitant illnesses.

A familial history of hyperhidrosis has been obtained in as many as 65% of patients who have undergone thoracoscopic sympathectomy.[1,10,12,15] Detailed kindred information provided by 49 affected individuals has led to the conclusion that the disease allele is actually present in 5% of the population, and that having one or two copies of the allele results in hyperhidrosis in 25% of carriers.[15] Investigators have localized hyperhidrosis associated genes to chromosomes 14[16] and 5.[17]

AUTONOMIC NERVOUS SYSTEM: ANATOMY AND FUNCTION

The autonomic nervous system is responsible for thermoregulation. Although both the sympathetic and parasympathetic components may contribute to sweating, the sympathetic nervous system primarily controls extremity sweating. Impulses originating in the hypothalamus reach preganglionic fibers located in the lateral horn of the ventral root of the spinal column.[18] These myelinated fibers exit the ventral root and travel a brief distance through the spinal nerve before exiting as the white rami communicantes to join the paravertebral ganglia of the sympathetic chain. The nerve may immediately establish a synapse with an unmyelinated postganglionic fiber, which returns to the spinal nerve as the gray ramus communicantes, or it may ascend a variable distance within the sympathetic chain before synapsing with a postganglionic fiber. The postganglionic nerve often travels a great distance before arriving at its target organ.

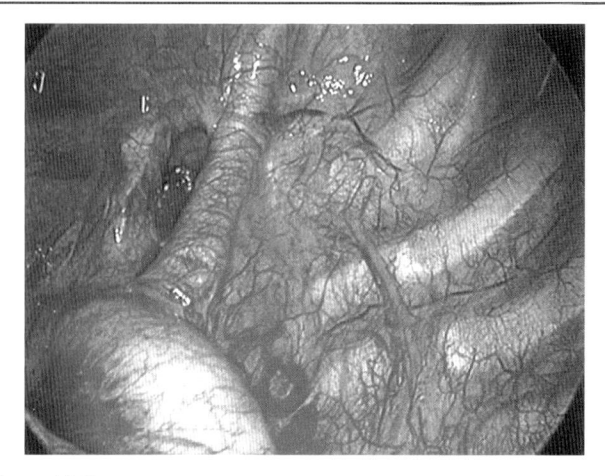

Figure 44–2
Left sympathetic chain.

The preganglionic sympathetic fibers responsible for sudomotor (sweating) activity in the hand are thought to arise from spinal segments T3 to T6. They converge on the T2 and T3 ganglia, where postganglionic fibers ascend to reach the hand via connections of the stellate ganglia to the brachial plexus.[19] The precise spinal levels responsible for palmar sweating have not been defined, but T2 has been thought to be the common pathway. Release of acetylcholine from the postganglionic neurons stimulates the eccrine sweat glands.

The sympathetic chain descends vertically in the thorax over the rib heads (Fig. 44-2), and rarely it is found between the medial border of the rib head and the longus colli muscle.[20,21] The sympathetic ganglia are located approximately 2 mm cranial to the midportion of the underlying vertebral body.[22] For example, the T2 ganglion is located between the heads of the second and third ribs. In addition to the orderly arrangement of the sympathetic nerves, Kuntz identified inconstant sympathetic branches from the second intercostal nerve to the first intercostal nerve (and hence brachial plexus) that bypassed the stellate ganglia.[23] The physiologic function of these nerves is unclear.

Whether hyperhidrosis represents focal dysfunction of the autonomic nervous system or is emblematic of a more global abnormality remains unknown. Resting palmar sweat production at room temperature is twice normal (Fig. 44-3).[24] The sudomotor skin response is enhanced as a result of shortened nerve recovery time.[25] Abnormal sensory processing is suggested by a decrease in spatial discrimination thresholds that did not improve under conditions of sensory deprivation.[26] These findings (i.e., the absence of plastic cortical somatocellular changes) suggest a lack of inhibition of the hypothalamus. Palmar sweat production in response to stress is greatly increased (see Fig. 44-3). When compared with the responses in unaffected controls, pulmonary function and resting cardiac function in the supine position are normal.[27-30] Circulating plasma catecholamine levels are within normal limits.[31] However, peak exercise heart rate and resting heart rate in the standing position are increased.[27,28] Other investigators have suggested that concomitant abnormalities of the parasympathetic system contribute to hyperhidrosis.[32,33]

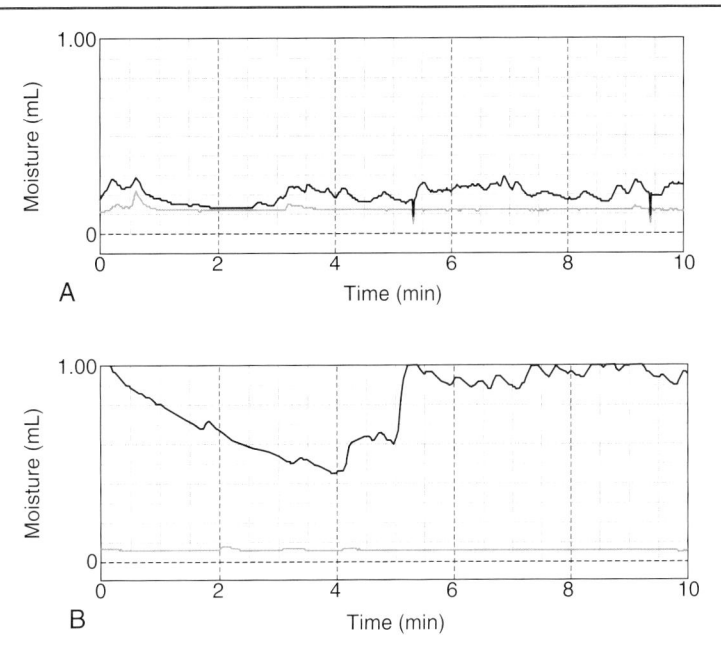

Figure 44–3
A, Normal sweat response. After attachment of the measuring device (Skin Moisture Meter SKD 2000, Skinos, Ltd, Japan), the patient reaches baseline. Sweating increases as autonomic stimulation begins. The subject does not return to baseline. **B,** Abnormal sweat response. Attachment of the measuring device causes anxiety and the baseline never reaches normal. The response to the stimulus is many times greater than in the normal subject. In both **A** and **B:** *Upper line,* thenar eminence; *lower line,* forehead.

TREATMENT

Nonoperative

Aluminum chloride hexahydrate 20% anhydrous ethyl alcohol solution (Drysol) has been used as initial therapy for palmar and plantar hyperhidrosis. The solution is applied daily to the affected area before sleep and is covered in plastic wrap to prevent damage to clothing or bedding. Application frequency is decreased once the desired anhidrosis is obtained. Side effects include rash and paradoxical hyperhidrosis. Efficacy has not been assessed in a controlled trial, and many patients report therapeutic failure.

Iontophoresis—placement of the hands or feet in a tap water solution through which an electric current flows—is another treatment that has been used for hyperhidrosis. The precise mechanism responsible for the elimination of sweat production is unknown. A battery-operated device is commercially available (Drionic). Control of palmar hyperhidrosis was reported in 82% of 112 patients who underwent eight daily 15-minute treatments.[34] The mean remission time was 35 days. Tingling, erythema, and vesicle formation were undesirable side effects.

The neurotoxin botulinum toxin A (Botox) stops sweat production by blocking the release of acetylcholine from the postganglionic nerve end. A randomized trial has demonstrated efficacy of this treatment for axillary hyperhidrosis.[35] Other investigators have reported success for palmar hyperhidrosis using 20 to 30 intradermal injections.[36-38] Median duration of sweat control varies between 6 and 9 months. Weakness of the intrinsic muscle of the hand, manifested by a decrease in the thumb–index finger pinch strength, has been reported in 25% to 60% of patients.

Oral anticholinergic medications such as glycopyrrolate and oxybutynin have been employed to block the stimulation of the sweat gland caused by the release of acetylcholine from the postganglionic sympathetic nerve fiber. One published report claimed a response of 79% in patients treated with glycopyrrolate.[39] Dry mouth, blurry vision, and constipation are common side effects.

Surgical

The goal of surgery is to interdict the sympathetic nerve innervation to the hand, axilla, or face. Disruption of the sympathetic chain can be accomplished by transection, by resection of ganglia, or by application of clips. The thoracic level at which interruption is necessary to achieve the desired anhidrosis while simultaneously minimizing systemic side effects is not precisely known and remains controversial. Interpretation of the voluminous literature is complicated by a plethora of inconsistent terms used to describe the operative procedures. For example, sympathectomy has been employed to describe both transection of the sympathetic chain and actual removal or ablation of the ganglion. The following recently proposed definitions seem reasonable[40]:

- Sympathectomy: removal or ablation of a sympathetic ganglion, accompanied by transection of the sympathetic chain above and below the ganglion
- Sympathicotomy: transection of the sympathetic chain at the indicated level
- Clipping: application of a clip at a specific level
- Blocking: placement of clips above and below the cited ganglion

Traditionally, palmar hyperhidrosis has been treated by transecting the sympathetic chain over the second and third ribs. If concomitant axillary hyperhidrosis was present, the sympathetic chain was also transected over the fourth rib. In the absence of palmar hyperhidrosis, axillary sweating was treated by transecting the sympathetic chain over the third and fourth ribs. Some authors believe that palmar hyperhidrosis can be effectively treated by limiting the transection to the level of the third rib.[41] Others have demonstrated equivalent results by transecting or clipping the sympathetic chain at T3-4.[10,42] Yet other surgeons have reported success with T4-5 sympathicotomy.[43]

Four phase III trials have been performed, three comparing different levels for palmar hyperhidrosis and one for isolated axillary hyperhidrosis. Sixty patients with palmar hyperhidrosis were randomized to either T2-3 or T3-4 sympathicotomy.[44] The single patient who did not experience complete resolution of symptoms was in the T3-4 group. However, the patients in the T3-4 group reported less severe compensatory sweating. In a second study, 232 patients were randomized to either T3 sympathicotomy or T2-to-T4 sympathicotomy.[41] All patients had resolution of symptoms, but patients in the T3 cohort had fewer instances of severe compensatory sweating and were more likely to be satisfied with the results of surgery. Finally, 25 patients underwent unilateral ablation of the T2 ganglion and contralateral ablation of the T2-3 ganglia.[45] The procedures were equally effective. Compensatory sweating was mild and did not differ between the two sides. Sixty-two patients with isolated axillary hyperhidrosis were randomly assigned to either T3-4 or T4 sympathectomy.[46] All patients reported resolution of symptoms. However, the T4 cohort had a lower incidence of compensatory sweating (57% versus 91%).

Regardless of the surgical technique, correct identification of the anatomic level is crucial. The second rib is generally the most proximal rib that can be seen in the thorax and can be reliably identified by a vertical, descending arterial branch that crosses the rib 1 cm lateral to the sympathetic chain.[47] This arterial branch originates from the subclavian artery and forms the second intercostal artery (Fig. 44-4A). The first intercostal space is covered by a fat pad, and the first rib is generally not visible from within the thorax. Additional landmarks are the azygos vein, which lies at the level of the fifth interspace, and the aortic arch, which reaches to the fourth interspace. The rib number can be determined with certainty by obtaining an intraoperative radiograph after a metallic marker has been introduced into the chest and placed over a rib.

Bilateral endoscopic thoracic sympathicotomy is the surgical procedure of choice for the surgical treatment of palmar hyperhidrosis. Hospitalization is not necessary, and the results are uniformly excellent. Virtually all patients will have dry, warm hands. Axillary and facial sweating may also be treated in a similar manner, although the prevailing sense is that isolated axillary hyperhidrosis is best treated with Botox injections. The details of the operation are determined by the level at which the sympathetic chain is clipped or transected.

Operative Procedure for Hyperhidrosis

After induction of general anesthesia, the arms are abducted 90 degrees. The head of the operating table is elevated or the table flexed into the semi-Fowler's position to help the lungs fall away from the apex. A double-lumen endotracheal tube is not necessary. A 1-cm incision is made over the third interspace in the anterior axillary line just lateral to the pectoralis major muscle (Fig. 44-5). Carbon dioxide (600 cc to 1200 cc) is insufflated, a 10-mm trocar is introduced, and the operating thoracoscopic (Karl Storz 26037 AA) is inserted. The

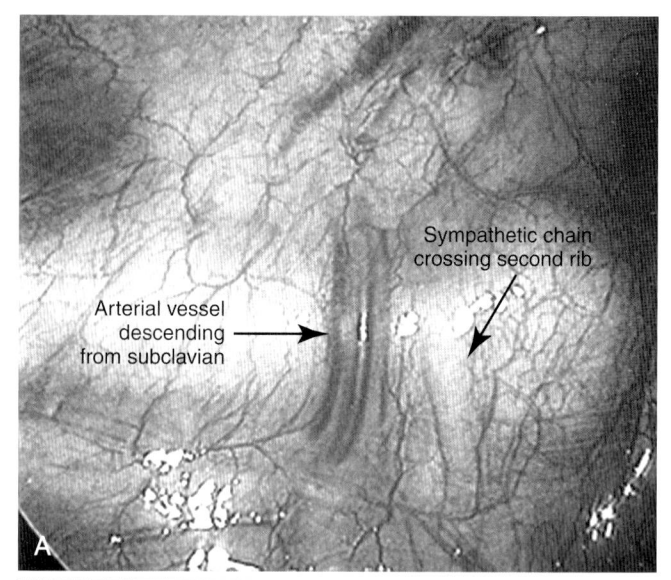

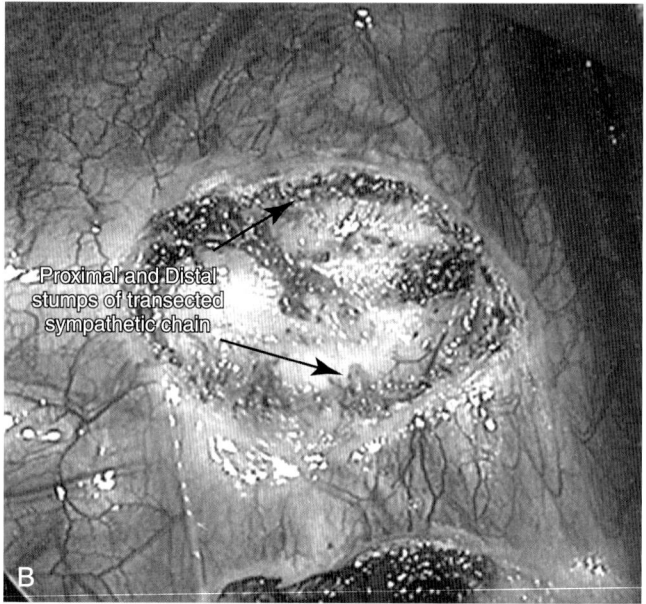

Figure 44–4
A, Descending vessels crossing the right second rib lateral to the sympathetic chain. **B,** After transection of the sympathetic chain, its proximal and distal stumps are visible.

sympathetic chain is visualized crossing the rib heads, and the ribs are correctly numbered. A cautery device is introduced via the operating thoracoscope and the sympathetic chain transected at the desired levels (see Fig. 44-4B). Hemostasis is ascertained, and the lung is inflated under direct vision as the trocar is withdrawn. The wound is closed and the identical procedure repeated in the contralateral thorax. A chest radiograph is obtained in the recovery room. Small apical pneumothoraces that do not require chest tubes are common. The patient is discharged when awake and comfortable.

Variations of the procedure are numerous and include: intermittent apnea instead of CO_2 gas, harmonic scalpel in place of electrocautery, and clips as an alternative to transection. If clips are utilized, two 5 mm ports are necessary, the first for the 5 mm thoracoscope and the second for the automatic clip applier. Investigators who have access to 2 millimeter diameter scopes

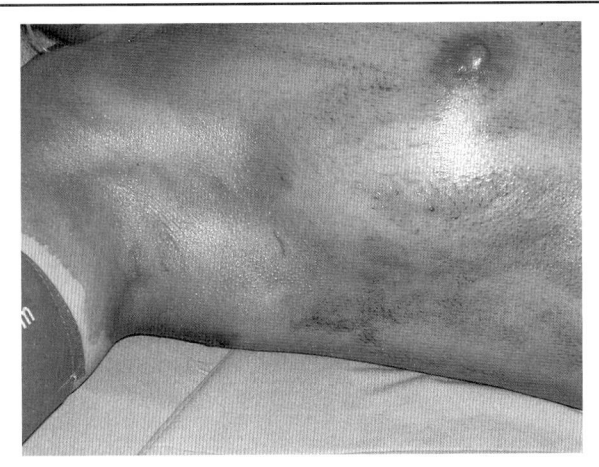

Figure 44–5
The patient is placed in the supine position with both arms perpendicular to the torso. A 1-cm incision is made lateral to the pectoralis major muscle at the level of the axillary hairline.

and cautery instruments have described smaller incisions.[48] Intraoperative palmar skin temperature and finger blood monitoring provide documentation of successful operation.[49,50]

Results of Endoscopic Thoracic Sympathicotomy

Virtually all patients report cure of palmar hyperhidrosis after endoscopic thoracic sympathicotomy.[6,9,10,42,48,51-56] Recurrence during the next few years is reported as 1% to 3%.[5,33,41] Quality-of-life questionnaires consistently demonstrate that more than 85% of patients are satisfied with the results of the surgery.[6,10,48,56-60] Treatment of axillary and craniofacial hyperhidrosis is somewhat less successful. Common reasons for dissatisfaction include compensatory sweating and recurrence.

Plantar sweating frequently abates after interruption of the T2-3 ganglia.[61] An increase in plantar skin temperature and a decrease in the sympathetic skin responses are measurable.[62] Similar results were reported after blocking the T4 ganglion by placing clips over the fourth and fifth ribs.[60] The anatomic basis for this unexpected but desirable response is unexplained.

Early treatment failures resulted from an inability to visualize the sympathetic chain because of extensive pulmonary–chest wall adhesions, an inability to access the sympathetic chain because of overlying vessels, and misidentification of the sympathetic chain.[63] The role of the Kuntz nerves is uncertain. Recurrent palmar hyperhidrosis may result from incomplete nerve interruption and nerve regeneration. Endoscopic reoperation is feasible, although the surgeon must be familiar with distorted intrathoracic anatomy and be prepared to perform a thoracotomy.[63]

COMPLICATIONS AND SEQUELAE OF SURGERY

Immediate

After surgery, patients commonly complain of incisional and retrosternal pain that is exacerbated by cough or deep breathing. Narcotic analgesics are generally necessary, but the most severe pain abates within 48 hours. Patients return to work or school 3 to 7 days after surgery. Anhidrosis occurs over the upper chest and face.

Postoperative bleeding is a rare complication of endoscopic thoracic sympathicotomy and can occur from injury to either intrathoracic or extrathoracic structures. The former include the intercostal vasculature and venous branches that occasionally cross the sympathetic chain. Rarely, injury to a major arterial or venous vessel is caused by misplacement of the trocar or cautery. Bleeding from a chest wall muscle or vessel may track into the pleural space and cause an unsuspected hemothorax. Repeat chest radiograph is necessary if there is unexplained hypotension. Infection is exceedingly uncommon.

Horner's syndrome (ptosis, miosis, and anhidrosis) occurs in less than 1% of patients and results from damage to the sympathetic nerves that pass through the stellate ganglia.[9,10,56,64] Nerve injury may occur as the result of misidentification of the nerve level or the proximal transmission of cautery heat. Ptosis is immediate and frequently permanent.

Chronic

Compensatory Sweating

After successful operation, as many as 75% of patients report sweating on regions of the torso that had been previously dry.[1,6,10,48,56,62,64,65] Although this is usually no more than an annoyance, as many as 3% of patients are plagued by sweating of the chest, thighs, and legs that is as severe as the original palmar sweating. This compensatory sweating is the most common and usually the most serious sequela of thoracic sympathicotomy. Although the cause remains obscure, compensatory sweating has been correlated with a body mass index of 25 or greater.[66] Other investigators have correlated compensatory sweating with the magnitude of finger temperature and blood flow increase after interruption of the sympathetic chain.[67] One investigator performed a temporary block of the sympathetic chain by injecting the planned sympathicotomy site (or sites) with Marcaine.[68] If compensatory sweating was severe, definitive surgery was not performed. However, this novel approach involves two separate thoracoscopic procedures.

Once established, the degree of compensatory sweating usually does not change.[69] Despite compensatory sweating, the majority of patients remain satisfied with the results of surgery. Gustatory sweating has been reported in as many as 73% of patients.[1,6,9,10,56,70]

Postoperative truncal and lower extremity sweating has been explained as the thermoregulatory response to the anhidrosis of the rostral chest and upper extremities. Attempts to ameliorate compensatory sweating by transecting only the rami and leaving the sympathetic chain intact resulted in an increased recurrence of palmar sweating and no change in the incidence of compensatory sweating.[71] Interruption of the sympathetic chain at fewer levels, thus sparing some of the sympathetic sweating fibers, has been proposed. However, limiting the sympathicotomy to the T2 ganglion appears to have no demonstrable effect on the occurrence of compensatory sweating[10,48,54,56,64] when compared with interruption of both T2 and T3.[6,9,52]

Although interruption of the T2 ganglion has been thought necessary to achieve dry palms, this concept may not be correct. Sympathetic fibers to the hand originate from T2 to T10,[72] but the relative contribution to sweating from each spinal level is not known. Twenty-eight patients who underwent interruption of only the T3 ganglion achieved dry hands, and none developed compensatory sweating.[13] Interruption of the T4 ganglion was performed in 165 patients who suffered from palmar and axillary hyperhidrosis. Compensatory sweating was rare and mild, with only one patient reporting persistent palmar sweating.[73]

If the success of a more caudal sympathicotomy is confirmed, the current understanding of upper extremity sympathetic innervation and activity will require reassessment. Although sympathetic fibers from the T2 and T3 spinal levels contribute fibers to the upper extremity, palmar sweating may be determined by sympathetic input originating distal to T4. Interruption at the T4 level would eliminate palmar sweating while leaving the remaining upper extremity sympathetic innervation intact without the need for thermoregulatory compensation.[51,53]

Cardiopulmonary Complications

Sympathetic fibers to the heart pass through the upper thoracic ganglia. After T2 sympathicotomy, the heart rate at rest and with peak exercise is reduced by 13% and 7%, respectively.[27] However, exercise capacity and the cardiorespiratory response to exercise remain unchanged.[28] After T2-3 sympathicotomy, resting heart rate has been reported to decrease 14% and at peak exercise 6%.[74] Peak oxygen uptake and exercise performance capacity were unchanged. Severe bradycardia has been reported. Shortening of the QTc interval has also been documented.[75]

The lungs also receive sympathetic innervation via the thoracic ganglia. Interruption of the upper thoracic ganglia results in subclinical alterations in some pulmonary function tests.[30,76]

Other

In addition to readily documented physical alterations and objectively measured cardiopulmonary effects, a number of patients have complained of vague, though sometimes severe, symptoms that have been difficult to assess and quantify. Although not generally documented in published reports, they have been the topics of bitter discussion in internet chat rooms and blogs. Among these symptoms are severe malaise, orthostatic changes, and a causalgia type of arm pain. The relationship to sympathicotomy or sympathectomy remains unexplained and deserves more in-depth investigation.

Treatment of Complications

The occurrence of severe compensatory sweating spurred the development of a potentially reversible procedure—interruption of the sympathetic chain by application of nerve-compressing clips[77]. Clips placed on the sympathetic chain cranial to consecutive ribs will isolate the intervening ganglia. Palmar hyperhidrosis is controlled as effectively with clipping as by sympathetic chain transection.[10,42] Removal of the clips at a second operation has resulted in return of palmar sweating and decrease of compensatory sweating in as many as 60% of patients.[10,77] Successful reconstruction of the severed sympathetic chain with a sural nerve graft has been reported.[78]

Summary

Before proceeding with surgery, patients should have some trial of nonoperative therapy. The length of time and financial resources dedicated to nonoperative treatments, as well as the number and variety of treatments attempted, depends on the patient and the severity of the hyperhidrosis. Although hyperhidrosis is the cause of significant personal and social discomfort, it is not a fatal illness. Therefore, it is incumbent on the surgeon to explain in detail both the risks of surgery and the potential sequelae of sympathicotomy. The patient must understand the various surgical options and that the procedure is most likely not reversible.

Compensatory sweating remains the most serious undesired consequence of thoracic sympathicotomy. A more detailed understanding of the autonomic nervous system is crucial to eliminate this potentially debilitating side effect. Clinical trials utilizing standardized operative procedures and outcomes measurements are required to document the results of novel surgical approaches.

REFERENCES

1. Adar R, Kurchin A, Zweig A, Mozes M. Palmar hyperhidrosis and its surgical treatment: a report of 100 cases. Ann Surg 1977;**186**:34-41.
2. Amir M, Arish A, Weinstein Y, Pfeffer M, Levy Y. Impairment in quality of life among patients seeking surgery for hyperhidrosis (excessive sweating): preliminary results. Isr J Psychiatry Relat Sci 2000;**37**:25-31.
3. Kotzareff A. Résection partielle du trone sympathique cervical droit pour hyperhidrose unilatérale. Rev Med Suisse Rom 1920;**40**:111-3.
4. Adson AW, Craig WM, Brown GE. Essential hyperhidrosis cured by sympathetic ganglionectomy and trunk resection. Arch Surg 1935;**31**:794-806.
5. Hughes J. Endothoracic sympathectomy. Proc R Soc Med 1942;**35**:585-6.
6. Kux M. Thoracic endoscopic sympathectomy in palmar and axillary hyperhidrosis. Arch Surg 1978;**113**:264-6.
7. Krogstad AL, Mork C, Pienchnik SK. Daily pattern of sweating and response to stress and exercise in patients with palmar hyperhidrosis. Br J Dermatol 2006;**154**:1118-22.
8. Herbst F, Plas EG, Fugger R, Fritsch A. Endoscopic thoracic sympathectomy for primary hyperhidrosis of the upper limbs. Ann Surg 1994;**220**:86-90.
9. Neumayer C, Bischof G, Fugger R, Imhof M, Jakesz R, Plas EG, et al. Efficacy and safety of thoracoscopic sympathicotomy for hyperhidrosis of the upper limb. Ann Chirurg Gyn 2001;**90**:195-9.
10. Reisfeld R, Nguyen R, Pnini A. Endoscopic thoracic sympathectomy for hyperhidrosis. Surg Laparosc Endosc Percutan Tech 2002;**12**:255-67.
11. Strutton DR, Kowalski JW, Glaser DE, Stang PE. US prevalence of hyperhidrosis and impact on individuals with axillary hyperhidrosis: results from a national survey. J Am Acad Dermatol 2004;**51**:241-8.
12. Tu YR, Li X, Lin M, et al. Epidemiological survey of primary palmar hyperhidrosis in adolescent in Fuzhou of People's Republic of China. Eur J Cardiothorac Surg 2007;**31**:737-9.
13. Riet M, Smet AA, Kuiken H, Kazemier G, Bonjer HJ. Prevention of compensatory hyperhidrosis after thoracoscopic sympathectomy for hyperhidrosis. Surg Endosc 2001;**15**:1159-62.
14. Hornberger J, Grimes K, Naumann M, et al. Recognition, diagnosis and treatment of primary focal hyperhidrosis. J Am Acad Dermatol 2004;**51**:274-86.
15. Ro KM, Cantor RM, Lange KL, Ahn SS. Palmar hyperhidrosis: evidence of genetic transmission. J Vasc Surg 2002;**35**:386-8.
16. Higashimoto I, Yoshiura K, Hirakawa N, et al. Primary palmar hyperhidrosis locus maps to 14q11.2-q13. Am J Med Genet 2006;**140A**:567-72.
17. Cantor-Chiul RM, Chandra F, Dorrani N, Swatling C, Glaser D, Ahn S. Evidence of a hyperhidrosis risk gene at 5q11.2. Abstract #1706, presented at the annual meeting of The American Society of Human Genetics, October 10, 2006, New Orleans, LA. Available at www.ashg.org/genetics/ashg/annmeet/2006.
18. Hamill RW. Peripheral autonomic nervous system. In: Robertson D, Low PA, Polinsky RJ, editors. Primer on the Autonomic Nervous System. San Diego: Academic Press; 1996, 12–25.
19. Schiller Y. The anatomy and physiology of the sympathetic innervations to the upper limbs. Clin Auton Res 13 (suppl 1):I/2-I/5 2003.
20. Kim do H, Hong YJ, Hwang JJ, Kim KD. Lee DY. Topographical considerations under video-scope guidance in the T3,4 levels sympathetic surgery. Eur J Cardiothorac Surg 2008;**33**:786-9.
21. Wang Y-C, Sun M-H, Lin C-W, Chen Y-J. Anatomical location of T2-3 sympathetic trunk and Kuntz nerve determined by transthoracic endoscopy. J Neurosurg 2002;**96**(Suppl. 1):68-72.
22. Yarzebski JL, Wilkinson HA. T2 and T3 sympathetic ganglia in the adult human: a cadaver and clinical-radiographic study and its clinical application. Neurosurgery 1987;**21**:339-42.
23. Kuntz A. Distribution of the sympathetic rami to the brachial plexus. Arch Surg 1927;**15**:871-7.

24. Bonde P, Nwaejike N, Fullerton C, Allen J, Mcguigan J. An objective assessment of the sudomotor response after thoracoscopic sympathectomy. *J Thorac Cardiovasc Surg* 2008;**135**:635-41.
25. Manca D, Valls-Solé J, Callejas MA. Excitability recovery curve of the sympathetic skin response in healthy volunteers and patients with palmar hyperhidrosis. *Clin Neurophysiol* 2000;**111**:1767-70.
26. Leon-Sarmiento FE, Hernandez HG, Schroeder N. Abnormal tactile discrimination and somatosensory plasticity in familial primary hyperhidrosis. *Neurosci Lett* 2008;**441**:332-4.
27. Noppen M, Herregodts P, Dendale P, D'Haens J, Vincken W. Cardiopulmonary exercise testing following bilateral thoracoscopic sympathicolysis in patients with essential hyperhidrosis. *Thorax* 1995;**50**:1097-100.
28. Noppen M, Dendale P, Hagers Y, Herregodts P, Vincken W, D'Haens J. Changes in cardiocirculatory autonomic function after thoracoscopic upper dorsal sympathicolysis for essential hyperhidrosis. *J Auton Nerv Syst* 1996;**60**:115-20.
29. Noppen MP, Vincken WG. Partial pulmonary sympathetic denervation by thoracoscopic D2-D3 sympathicolysis for essential hyperhidrosis: effect on the pulmonary diffusion capacity. *Resp Med* 1997;**91**:537-45.
30. Tseng M-Y, Tseng J-H. Thoracoscopic sympathectomy for palmar hyperhidrosis: effects on pulmonary function. *J Clin Neurosci* 2001;**8**:539-41.
31. Noppen M, Sevens C, Gerlo E, Vincken W. Plasma catecholamine concentrations in essential hyperhidrosis and effects of thoracoscopic D2-D3 sympathicolysis. *Eur J Clin Invest* 1997;**27**:202-5.
32. Birner P, Heinzl H, Schindl M, Pumprla J, Schnider P. Cardiac autonomic function in patients suffering from primary focal hyperhidrosis. *Eur Neurol* 2000;**44**:112-6.
33. Kaya D, Karaca S, Barutcu I, Esen AM, Kulac M, Esen O. Heart rate variability in patients with essential hyperhidrosis: dynamic influence of sympathetic and parasympathetic maneuvers. *Ann Noninvasive Electrocardiol* 2005;**10**:1-6.
34. Karakoç Y, Aydermir EH, Kalkan T, Ünal G. Safe control of palmoplantar hyperhidrosis with direct electric current. *Int J Derm* 2002;**41**:602-5.
35. Heckmann M, Ceballos-Baumann AO, Plewig G. for the Hyperhidrosis Study Group. Botulinum Toxin A for axillary hyperhidrosis (excessive sweating). *N Engl J Med* 2001;**344**:488-93.
36. Lowe NJ, Yamauchi PS, Lask GP, et al. Efficacy and safety of botulinum toxin type A in the treatment of palmar hyperhidrosis: a double blind randomized placebo controlled study. *Dermatol Surg* 2002;**28**:822-7.
37. Schnider P, Binder M, Auff E, et al. Double-blind trial of botulinum A toxin for the treatment of focal hyperhidrosis of the palm. *Br J Dermatol* 1997;**136**:548-52.
38. Yamashita N, Shimizu H, Kawada M, et al. Local injection of botulinum toxin A for palmar hyperhidrosis: Usefulness and efficacy in relation to severity. *J Dermatol* 2008;**35**:325-9.
39. Bajaj V, Langtry JA. Use of oral glycopyrronium bromide in hyperhidrosis. *Br J Dermatol* 2007;**157**:118-21.
40. Wexler B, Luketich JD, Shende MR. Endoscopic thoracic sympathectomy: at what level should you perform surgery? *Thorac Surg Clin* 2008;**18**:183-91.
41. Li X, Tu YR, Lin M, Lai FC, Chen JF, Dai ZJ. Endoscopic thoracic sympathectomy for palmar hyperhidrosis: a randomized control trial comparing T3 and T2-4 ablation. *Ann Thorac Surg* 2008;**85**:1747-52.
42. Reisfeld R. Sympathectomy for hyperhidrosis: Should we place the clamps at T2-T3 or T3-T4? *Clin Auton Res* 2006;**16**:384-9.
43. Mahdy T, Youssef T, Elmonem HA, Omar W, Elateef AA. T4 sympathectomy for palmar hyperhidrosis: Looking for the right operation. *Surgery* 2008;**143**:784-9.
44. Yazbek G, Wolosker N, de Campos JRM, Kauffman P, Ishy A, Puech-Leao P. Palmar hyperhidrosis: which is the best level of denervation using video-assisted thoracoscopic sympathectomy: T2 or T3 ganglion? *J Vasc Surg* 2005;**42**:281-5.
45. Katara AN, Domino JP, Cheah WK, So SB, Ning C, Lomanto D. Comparing T2 and T2-T3 ablation in thoracoscopic sympathectomy for palmar hyperhidrosis: a randomized control trial. *Surg Endosc* 2007;**21**:1768-71.
46. Munia MAS, Wolosker N, Kauffman P, de Campos JR, Puech-Leao P. A randomized trial of T3-T4 versus T4 sympathectomy for isolated axillary hyperhidrosis. *J Vasc Surg* 2007;**45**:130-3.
47. Chiou TSM, Liao K-K. Orientation landmarks of endoscopic transaxillary T-2 sympathectomy for palmar hyperhidrosis. *J Neurosurg* 1996;**85**:310-5.
48. Lee DY, Yoon YH, Shion HK, Kim HK, Hong YJ. Needle thoracic sympathectomy for essential hyperhidrosis: intermediate-term follow-up. *Ann Thorac Surg* 2000;**69**:251-3.
49. Klodell CT, Lobato EB, Willert JL, Gravenstein N. Oximetry-derived perfusion index for intraoperative identification of successful thoracic sympathectomy. *Ann Thorac Surg* 2005;**80**:467-70.
50. Sáiz-Sapena N, Vanaclocha V, Panta F, Kadri C, Torres W. Operative monitoring of hand and axillary temperature during endoscopic superior thoracic sympathectomy for the treatment of palmar hyperhidrosis. *Eur J Surg* 2000;**166**:65-9.
51. Chou SH, Kao EL, Lin CC, Chang YT, Huang MF. The importance of classification in sympathetic surgery and a proposed mechanism for compensatory hyperhidrosis: experience with 646 cases. *Surg Endosc* 2006;**20**:1749-53.
52. Gossot D, Kabiri H, Caliandro R, Debrosse D, Girard P, Grunenwald D. Early complications of thoracic endoscopic sympathectomy: a prospective study of 940 procedures. *Ann Thor Surg* 2001;**71**:1116-9.
53. Lin C-C, Telaranta T. Lin-Telaranta classification: the importance of different procedures for different indications in sympathetic surgery. *Ann Chirurg Gyn* 2001;**90**:161-6.
54. Lin T-S, Fang H-Y. Transthoracic endoscopic sympathectomy in the treatment of palmar hyperhidrosis-with emphasis on perioperative management (1,360 case analyses). *Surg Neurol* 1999;**52**:453-7.
55. Moya J, Ramos R, Villalonga R, et al. Thoracic sympathicolysis for primary hyperhidrosis: a review of 918 procedures. *Surg Endosc* 2006;**20**:598-602.
56. Rex LO, Drott C, Claes G, Gothberg G, Dalman P. The Borås experience of endoscopic thoracic sympathicotomy for palmar, axillary, facial hyperhidrosis and facial blushing. *Eur J Surg* 1998;**164**(Suppl 580):23-6.
57. Boley TM, Belangee KN, Markwell S, Hazelrigg SR. The effect of thoracoscopic sympathectomy on quality of life and symptom management of hyperhidrosis. *J Am Coll Surg* 2007;**204**:435-8.
58. de Campos JRM, Kauffman P, de Campos Werebe E, et al. Quality of life, before and after thoracic sympathectomy: report on 378 operated patients. *Ann Thorac Surg* 2003;**76**:886-91.
59. Kumagai K, Kawase H, Kawanishi M. Health-related quality of life after thoracoscopic sympathectomy for palmar hyperhidrosis. *Ann Thorac Surg* 2005;**80**:461-6.
60. Neumayer C, Panhofer P, Zacherl J, Bischof G. Effect of endoscopic thoracic sympathetic block on plantar hyperhidrosis. *Arch Surg* 2005;**140**:676-80.
61. Wolosker N, Yazbek G, de Campos JRM, Kauffman P, Ishy A, Puech-Leao P. Evaluation of plantar hyperhidrosis in patients undergoing video-assisted thoracoscopic sympathectomy. *Clin Auton Res* 2007;**17**:172-6.
62. Chen H-J, Liang C-L, Lu K. Associated changes in plantar temperature and sweating after transthoracic endoscopic T2-3 sympathectomy for palmar hyperhidrosis. *J Neurosurg* 2001;**95**(Suppl. 1):58-63.
63. Lin T-S. Video-assisted thoracoscopic "resympathicotomy" for palmar hyperhidrosis: analysis of 42 cases. *Ann Thorac Surg* 2001;**72**:895-8.
64. Lin T-S, Kuo S-J, Chou M-C. Uniportal endoscopic thoracic sympathectomy for treatment of palmar and axillary hyperhidrosis: analysis of 2000 cases. *Neurosurgery* 2002;**51**(Suppl. 2):84-7.
65. Lin T-S. Transthoracic endoscopic sympathectomy for palmar and axillary hyperhidrosis in children and adolescents. *Pediatr Surg Int* 1999;**15**:475-8.
66. de Campos JRB, Wolosker N, Takeda FR, et al. The body mass index and level of resection: predictive factors for compensatory sweating after sympathectomy. *Clin Auton Res* 2005;**15**:116-20.
67. Fujita T, Mano M, Nishi H, Shimizu N. Intraoperative prediction of compensatory sweating for thoracic sympathectomy. *Jpn J Thorac Cardiovasc Surg* 2005;**53**:481-5.
68. Miller DL, Force SD. Temporary thoracoscopic sympathetic block for hyperhidrosis. *Ann Thorac Surg* 2008;**85**:1211-6.
69. Steiner Z, Kleiner O, Hershkovitz Y, Mogilner J, Cohen Z. Compensatory sweating after thoracoscopic sympathectomy: an acceptable trade-off. *J Pediatr Surg* 2007;**42**:1238-42.
70. Licht PB, Pilegaard HK. Gustatory side effects after thoracoscopic sympathectomy. *Ann Thorac Surg* 2006;**81**:1043-7.
71. Gossot D, Toledo L, Fritsch S, Célérier M. Thoracoscopic sympathectomy for upper limb hyperhidrosis: looking for the right operation. *Ann Thorac Surg* 1997;**64**:975-8.
72. Ray BS, Hinsey JC, Geohegan WA. Observations on the distribution of the sympathetic nerves to the pupil and upper extremity as determined by stimulation of the anterior roots in man. *Ann Surg* 1943;**118**:647-55.
73. Lin C-C, Wu H-H. Endoscopic T4 sympathetic block by clamping (ESB4) in treatment of hyperhidrosis palmaris et axillaries-experiences of 165 cases. *Ann Chirurg Gyn* 2001;**90**:167-9.
74. Inbar O, Leviel D, Shwartz I, Paran H, Whipp BJ. Thoracic sympathectomy and cardiopulmonary response to exercise. *Eur J Appl Physiol* 2008;**104**:79-86.
75. Papa MZ, Schneiderman J, Tucker E, Bass A, Drori Y, Adar R. Cardiovascular changes after bilateral upper dorsal sympathectomy. *Ann Surg* 1986;**204**:715-8.
76. Vigil L, Calaf N, Codina E, Fibla JJ, Gomez G, Casan P. Video-assisted sympathectomy for essential hyperhidrosis: effects on cardiopulmonary function. *Chest* 2005;**128**:2702-5.
77. Lin C-C, Mo L-R, Lee L-S, Ng S-M, Hwang M-H. Thoracoscopic T2-sympathetic block by clipping: a better and reversible operation for treatment of hyperhidrosis palmaris—experience with 326 cases. *Eur J Surg* 1998;**164**(Suppl 580):13-6.
78. Telaranta T. Secondary sympathetic chain reconstruction after endoscopic thoracic sympathicotomy. *Eur J Surg Suppl* 1998(580):17-8.

N. The Future

CHAPTER 45

The Use of Genetic Science in Thoracic Disease

Jonathan D'Cunha and Michael A. Maddaus

Mechanisms of Carcinogenesis and Metastasis
Molecular Markers: Current Concepts
Microarray Analysis of Primary Tumors
Molecular Detection of Occult Micrometastases
Detection of Molecular Markers in Blood
Proteomics: The Analysis of Tumor Protein Expression Profiles
Tumor Marker Panels
Personalized Oncology
Summary

A revolution in biotechnology is upon us: the days of predicting a patient's risk of cancer recurrence and of mortality according to observations (e.g., degree of atypia, number of observed mitoses) are veering toward the realm of history. Although molecular diagnostic and analytic technologies are in their infancy, their application to the analysis of tumor genetics and detection of occult cancer cells is being assessed in many current studies. Furthermore, advances in molecular approaches to thoracic disease over the past several years have made targeted therapy for an individual patient a reality. This chapter begins with a brief review of pathogenic and metastatic mechanisms, and then it highlights seven prominent areas of molecular diagnosis in lung cancer and other thoracic cancers: (1) molecular markers, (2) microarray analysis of primary tumor, (3) molecular detection of occult micrometastases, (4) detection of molecular markers in blood, (5) proteomics (the analysis of tumor-protein expression profiles), (6) tumor marker panels, and (7) personalized oncology.

MECHANISMS OF CARCINOGENESIS AND METASTASIS

The process of tumorigenesis and progression to metastasis is incompletely understood. Nonetheless, certain insights have guided investigators in developing our current understanding of the overall process as a normal cell develops into a malignant cell, providing the basis of and rationale for the molecular diagnosis of thoracic cancers.

Progression of normal bronchial or esophageal epithelium to overt carcinoma is the result of a series of acquired genetic alterations that are under the influence of multiple environmental, biologic, and molecular processes. Non–small cell lung cancer (NSCLC) illustrates many features of this complex relationship. NSCLC pathogenesis is clearly influenced by carcinogens such as those in tobacco smoke. The critical control points in this sequence of malignant degeneration include various proto-oncogenes and tumor suppressor genes. Several studies have demonstrated that genetic abnormalities occur early in the process and remain persistent even after cessation of smoking or even with more limited exposure to carcinogen.[1,2] In fact, the development of tumors may occur with either the activation or the deletion of those critical regulatory genes. A number of genetic abnormalities have been identified frequently in early-stage lung cancers, such as mutations in the p53 tumor suppressor gene, mutations in the K-ras proto-oncogene, hypermethylation of the p16 tumor suppressor gene promoter, and loss of heterozygosity in chromosomal regions of importance.[1] Those genetic events set the stage for the development of metastatic deposits of tumor.

Tumor metastasis is an equally complex series of molecular events. The fundamental steps required for metastasis include ongoing local tumor proliferation, angiogenesis,[3,4] invasion, dissemination, and implantation.[5,6] According to the prevailing model of tumor dissemination, this capability is acquired relatively late in a stepwise process of tumor progression. Initially, certain cells of the nascent tumor with advantageous growth characteristics are further selected to become the progenitors of successor cells that may predominate the tumor mass. These advantageous phenotypes must include self-sufficiency in growth signals, resistance to antigrowth signals, limitless replication capability, sustained angiogenesis, and evasion of apoptosis.[7] Subsequently, individual cells in these large populations acquire additional unique mutations conferring the rare capability to undergo the metastatic cascade. Only a subset of cells in the primary tumor will attain this phenotype after successive genetic aberrations.[8,9] Thus, any primary tumor mass comprises heterogeneous cell populations diverse in genotype and biologic behavior. At the molecular level, a number of genes have been implicated in each of the distinct steps of metastasis, but the precise mechanisms remain incompletely understood. An increasing body of evidence supports the idea that a tumor has the capacity to grow from a small number of cells that have the ability to self-renew and differentiate. These cells are termed cancer stem cells. Even this general understanding of carcinogenesis and metastasis can lead to rational approaches that help us develop and interpret the genetic analysis of thoracic malignancies.

MOLECULAR MARKERS: CURRENT CONCEPTS

A molecular marker is a biological molecule found in blood, other body fluids, or tissues that is a sign of cancer. A molecular marker may be used to identify, stage, or guide treatment decisions for a particular tumor. In studying thoracic malignancies, we might hope that a particular tumor would have a single, discrete molecular marker, but it is not surprising that, as complex as tumor genetics is, a tumor most likely has a molecular fingerprint of several markers. Thus, no single molecular marker can be predictive. Thinking in terms of a *panel* of molecular markers is more appropriate in attempting to classify and treat thoracic malignancies (see Tumor Marker Panels, later).

The ability of malignant cells to proliferate and metastasize can be ascribed to specific genetic alterations of a particular tumor cell type. There are specific relationships for a particular solid organ tumor, but in general, thoracic malignancies follow the same general trends followed by other tumor types. Many investigations have been launched in quest of numerous genetic markers in thoracic malignancies, with NSCLC being a representative malignancy model. The molecular complexities of tumors are not to be underestimated; genetic alterations at the DNA, RNA, and protein levels all account for the biology of the tumor cell. Thus, it is important to gain insight into all of these levels to better understand a particular molecular marker.

DNA-based markers include single nucleotide polymorphisms (SNPs), chromosomal translocations, changes in DNA copy number, DNA microsatellite instability, and differential promoter methylation. In addition to these DNA aberrations, mutations in oncogenes, tumor suppressor genes, and mismatch repair genes can occur. Identification of these altered genes may yield a molecular marker that can be investigated and potentially used clinically. For example, several oncogenes with mutations are known to be predictive of prognosis in patients with NSCLC (K-*ras*, *p53*, cyclin-dependent kinase inhibitor A, retinoblastoma gene).[10-16] *MYC* (2.5-10%), cyclin D1 (5%), and epidermal growth factor receptor (EGFR) (6%) are amplified and overexpressed in patients with NSCLC. C-*erbB2* or *BCL2* overexpression is involved in 25% of cases.[17] Other important considerations at the DNA level include the epigenetic regulation of transcription and translation, which may lead to carcinogenesis. Recently, gene silencing by CpG methylation has received a fair amount of attention: identifying hypermethylated DNA may help characterize malignancy in the sputum or in bronchoalveolar lavage fluid. SNPs are another area of intense investigation for human lung cancer. A recent study of the 250K SNP array from Affymetrix (Santa Clara, CA) focused on evaluating copy number changes in 371 adenocarcinomas of the lung. Of the 57 recurrent alterations found, many had not been previously discovered.[18] It is through investigations such as this that novel candidate markers are being identified.

RNA-based markers include genes that are overexpressed or underexpressed as transcripts of regulatory RNAs (micro RNAs).[19] Differentially expressed genes in a particular tumor are detectable for thoracic malignancies such as NSCLC or esophageal cancer in the lymph nodes and serum of patients. No one single marker has proved ideal as a predictor of cancer. Recent efforts have focused on a panel of markers for most thoracic malignancies. Patterns of markers can more accurately predict cancer than a single molecule can, but choosing which genes to include in an analysis requires a multidisciplinary integration of biostatistics and bioinformatics. We await the results of large prospective studies evaluating various markers. MicroRNAs (miRNAs) are an abundant class of small non-protein-coding RNAs that function as negative gene regulators in the cell. Investigations have suggested that a single miRNA could bind to a number of mRNA targets; these targets could be implicated in cellular transformation and oncogenesis. This area of investigation is new, but it has already been shown that miRNA expression profiles can be used to classify human cancers.[20] In lung cancer, miRNA expression profiles and specific miRNAs have been shown to correlate with prognosis and survival.[19,21] The emerging findings on miRNAs are very exciting; further development is needed, along with integration with other molecular marker technology.

Protein-based markers include tumor proteins expressed on the cell surface or shed into serum. Proteomics (described later) is the genome-wide study of these peptides. Such markers or panels of markers hold great predictive promise, both alone and in combination with other markers. Again, no single protein or peptide will be the sole tag for a particular malignancy, but a panel of markers for detection and for monitoring response to therapy is a potential reality.

MICROARRAY ANALYSIS OF PRIMARY TUMORS

The exact molecular basis for tumorigenesis and metastasis in patients with thoracic cancers is unknown. Much of the control for this complex process takes place at the level of transcription, so significant insight into cellular function (of either tumor cells or normal cells) may be gained by globally assessing gene expression. Until recently, investigators were limited to the analysis of a finite number of genes in any particular experiment. The sequencing of the human genome, however, has heralded a new era in the investigation of cancer biology. Advanced tools have rapidly evolved to analyze complex genomes in a comprehensive way. A principal technology in this new era is the DNA microarray, which enables simultaneous analysis of the entire population of cellular genetic transcripts (gene expression profiling) in a given physiologic or pathologic state. Although the DNA microarray has not reached its full potential, it has shown promise in deciphering the biological complexities of cancer. The following section discusses the biological and clinical impact of microarray profiling studies in patients with lung and esophageal cancer.

Briefly, a DNA microarray comprises multiple, gene-specific polynucleotides (probes) arranged along exact coordinates of a two-dimensional grid (array), individually immobilized to a single substrate.[22] Total RNA pools from experimental or reference specimens are reverse-transcribed to fluorescence-labeled complementary DNA (cDNA) before incubation with the microarray (Fig. 45-1A). This process allows simultaneous quantitation of the relative (experimental versus reference) amount of messenger RNA (mRNA) transcripts. The number (which may be hundreds of thousands) of immobilized microarray probes determines the amount of gene expression information returned from each microarray experiment. This method depends on the highly sensitive and specific hybridization between complementary strands of nucleic acids.

Microarray platforms are of two general types: cDNA and oligonucleotide. Typically, the cDNA microarray contains hundreds to tens of thousands of long, polymerase chain reaction–derived representations of specific genes (about 600 to 2400 base pairs). In contrast, the oligonucleotide microarray

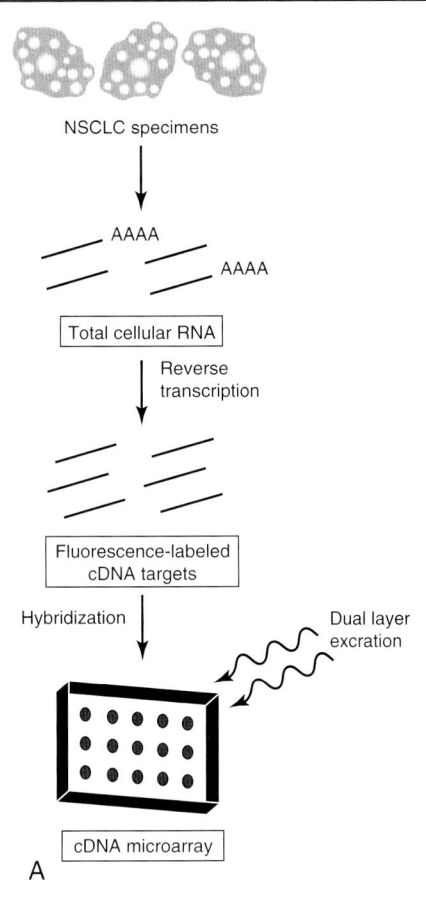

Figure 45–1
Principles of complementary DNA (cDNA) microarray processing. **A,** The main components of a microarray experiment. NSCLC, non–small cell lung cancer.

(Continued)

contains tens of thousands to hundreds of thousands of 25-mer oligonucleotides complementary to unique gene sequences, directly deposited by light-directed chemical synthesis.[23] Currently, no consensus exists as to the ideal type of microarray platform. Each has distinct advantages and drawbacks that are beyond the scope of this discussion. In general, the data sets derived from each platform are identical; each allows for large-scale analysis of gene expression in biologic specimens from a single experiment. Functionally, most investigators have gravitated toward the Affymetrix-type chip.

The vast amounts of data generated by microarray analyses have necessitated evolution in bioinformatics—a field concerned with the acquisition, storage, display, and analysis of genome-wide expression data. So many options are now available for analysis or data mining that choosing among them is challenging. The predominant analytic method in current use is a family of algorithms referred to as cluster analysis. For example, one specific type of algorithm is hierarchical clustering. The term *cluster analysis* generally applies to methods for organizing multivariate data into groups with similar patterns, so that they may impart additional information about certain genes and the study specimens (see Fig. 45-1B).[24] Overall, data analysis can be divided into four common themes: detection of differential gene expression, pattern discovery, prediction of specimen characteristics, and inference of molecular pathways and networks. The existing microarray literature on lung and esophageal cancers has addressed the first three of those four themes of analysis and has reported analyses and hypotheses regarding the molecular pathways and networks of importance.

Initial NSCLC microarray profiling studies were conducted either on cell culture systems[25,26] or on matched tumor versus nontumor specimens,[27,28] to identify genes with significantly altered expression levels. Many of the genes differentially expressed in tumor specimens were involved in cell cycle regulation, cell metabolism and signaling, or apoptosis; the findings of those initial NSCLC microarray profiling studies were consistent with the findings of studies in the broader cancer literature. However, some genes were identified that were not commonly associated with NSCLC: they suggest previously unrecognized mechanisms in tumorigenesis, or perhaps they represent novel therapeutic targets (or both).

The most interesting recent investigations have focused on patients with early-stage NSCLC. This focus has been clearly advantageous because including patients with more advanced disease adds many clinical variables that complicate their prognosis. Several groups have been able to identify gene expression profiles between 22 and 50 genes that can separate otherwise identical tumors in terms of disease-free survival and overall survival rates after potentially curative resection.[29-32] Bhattacharjee and colleagues studied 186 NSCLC tumors using a clustering technique specialized for gene pattern discovery; they identified four distinct, novel subgroups of adenocarcinomas according to gene expression profiles[30] and concluded that lung cancer diagnosis could be improved by integrating expression profile data.

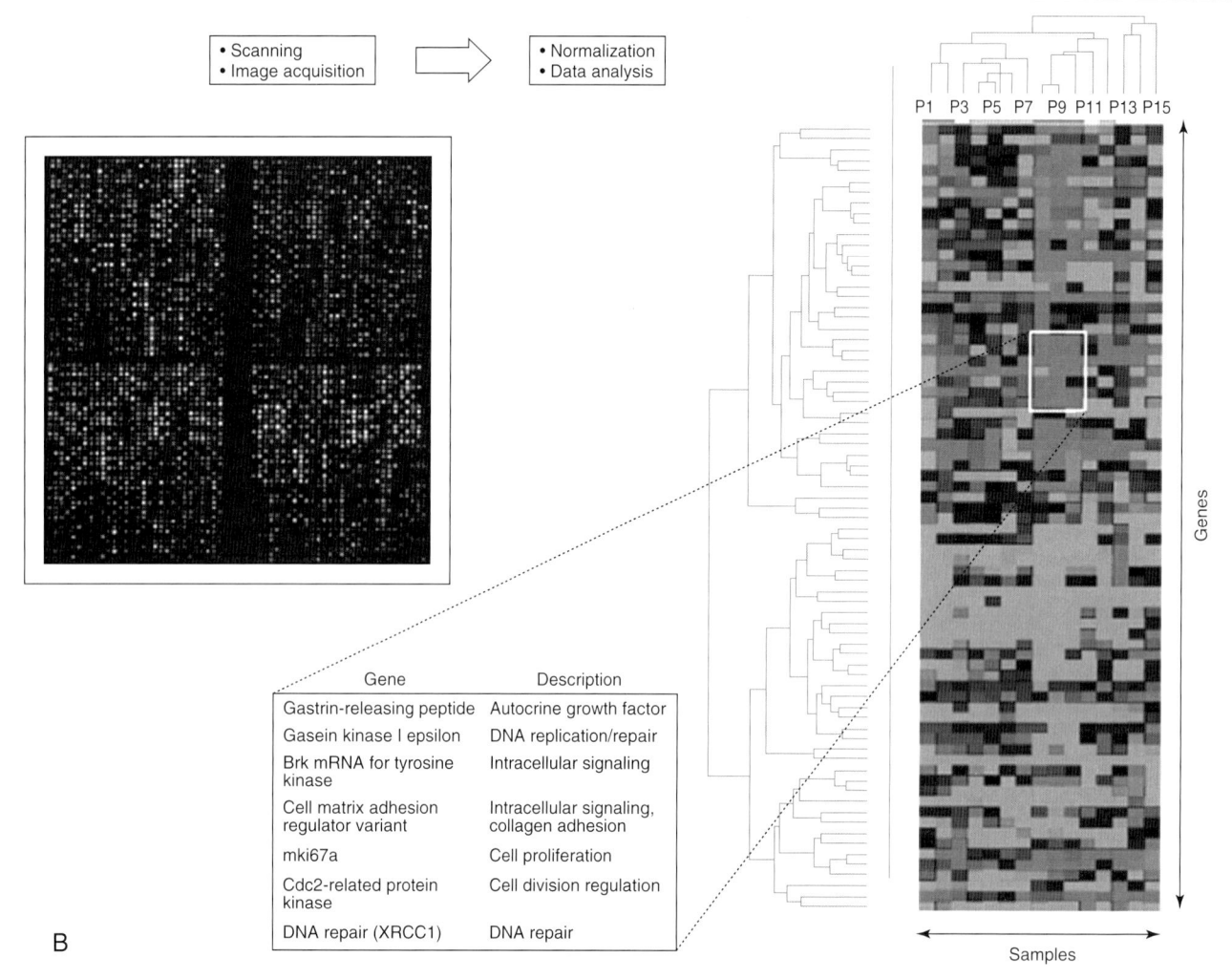

Figure 45–1, cont'd
B, The main steps in microarray data acquisition and analysis. Dual-channel fluorescence for each gene spotted onto the microarray is detected by a confocal scanning microscope. Computer software merges and converts these data into a graphic image. Gene expression data are analyzed with sophisticated algorithms. Shown is an example of a two-dimensional hierarchical cluster analysis. Gene expression ratios are color coded (*red*, overexpression; *green*, underexpression; *black*, no change) to reflect relative mRNA transcript abundance. (See color version in the online edition through Expert Consult.)

Beer and colleagues constructed a risk index based on a set of 50 genes identified by hierarchical clustering and univariate Cox analysis that could predict survival in early-stage lung adenocarcinoma patients.[29] Members of the gene set included genes not previously associated with survival, suggesting novel therapeutic targets. They stated that a gene set predictive of survival in early-stage adenocarcinoma might identify a high-risk subgroup who could benefit from adjuvant therapy.

Kikuchi and coworkers microdissected individual cancer cells from 37 NSCLC tumors before performing microarray analysis to identify novel tumorigenesis genes as well as genes related to chemosensitivity.[33] Their subset cluster analysis of 18 specimens identified 40 genes whose expression levels could discriminate gross, pathologically confirmed lymph node metastasis.[33] They speculated that such gene profile–based characteristics of NSCLC tumors could eventually guide personalized therapies for patients.

Regardless of the study, larger-scale prospective studies are required. Some overlap occurred between profiles in the studies described here, but there were also some distinct differences that may be attributed to varying microarray technique, samples, and statistical methods. To resolve some of these issues, the National Cancer Institute issued a Director's Challenge recently, which led to the first dataset whose main aim was to establish uniformity across different subject populations and different laboratories. Through a highly coordinated effort, the authors recently reported their results of their large, training-testing, multisite, blinded validation study. They were able to characterize the performance of several prognostic models by reviewing the gene expression profiles for 442 lung adenocarcinomas.[34] Their models performed best when microarray data were combined with basic clinical variables of tumor stage, patient age, and patient sex. This was able to predict overall survival in the study population. Furthermore, their results support the combined use of clinical and molecular information in the prognostic modeling of early-stage NSCLC.

Microarray studies of esophageal tumors have been generally small in terms of the number of tumors analyzed, but some early insights have been noteworthy. Selaru and colleagues used hierarchical cluster analysis in an attempt to classify esophageal tumor specimens by gene expression profiles. As predicted, they found that specimens from patients with Barrett's esophagus and from patients with esophageal cancer clustered separately.[35] In addition, they were able to accurately subgroup squamous cell carcinomas and adenocarcinomas by comparing cluster analysis findings with histopathologic subtypes.

Other investigators have used microarray analysis to gain insight into the progression of esophageal tumors from dysplasia to metastasis. Using a cancer gene–specific microarray of 588 genes, Zhou and coworkers identified sets of differentially expressed genes in normal esophageal mucosa, basal cell hyperplasia, high-grade dysplasia, carcinoma in situ, and overt cancer.[36] Their analysis showed that two genes ($P_{160}ROCK$ and JNK_2) in particular may play an important role in carcinogenesis. Their results are potentially powerful, because they evaluated gene expression across different stages of carcinogenesis. In their analysis, the $P_{160}ROCK$ gene (a member of the family of Rho-associated serine/threonine kinase isoenzymes that regulate cell motility and morphologic changes) was dramatically upregulated in the tissues with high-grade dysplasia. Thus, its activation may be one of the early events in carcinogenesis of esophageal tumors.

Further, Wang and colleagues used transcriptional profiling with microarrays of esophageal tissues at various stages of carcinogenesis from patients with Barrett's esophagus and esophageal adenocarcinoma.[37] They identified 36 genes that were differentially modulated according to microarray data in Barrett's neoplastic progression; 12 genes were significantly differentially expressed in cancer-associated Barrett's, a gene set that they hypothesized represents a biomarker profile for adenocarcinoma at early stages.

Additionally, Kihara and coworkers analyzed the expression profiles of 20 surgically resected esophageal tumors in patients treated with adjuvant therapy.[38] They identified a profile of 52 genes that were correlated with patient's prognosis, and they found that the gene set accurately predicted the chemosensitivity and chemoresistance of the tumors to various agents. From this gene set, they obtained a "drug response score" that correlated significantly with prognosis.

More recently, others have performed similar analyses in patients with squamous cell carcinoma of the esophagus, with the goal of identifying novel markers for prognosis and treatment.[39] The investigation of esophageal cancer has substantially progressed in the past few years, but it remains hampered by the lack of studies with large numbers of specimens and the lack of a unified commitment to standardization (as compared with the large studies of NSCLC). Prospective verification of genes and predictive models is also needed in studies of esophageal cancer.

Mesothelioma is another malignancy that has been the target of gene expression analysis, although relatively few studies have evaluated it to date, in part because of its rare incidence and because of the difficulty in acquiring suitable tissue for analysis. Most reported studies have been performed on malignant pleural mesothelioma (MPM) cell lines and have provided only descriptive data. Our group at the University of Minnesota has attempted to make some sense of this by incorporating primary tumor specimens into the array analysis with hierarchical clustering.[40] In our analysis, we identified several genes associated with MPM and also noted matriptase overexpression (826-fold)—clues to the mechanisms of oncogenic transformation. Not surprisingly, other investigators have performed similar studies with alternative findings, which highlights the inherent variability of the approach used. Still other groups have expanded the analysis of primary tumor specimens. Gordon comprehensively reviewed the mesothelioma studies,[41] and Gordon and coworkers highlighted the recent attempts at translating microarray data into clinically relevant prognostic information.[42,43] They used a gene expression ratio–based prognostic analysis of MPM tissues in an attempt to predict and validate the clinical outcome in 39 independent MPM tumor specimens. They theorized that using such gene ratios to translate gene expression data into easily reproducible, statistically validated clinical tests will help facilitate clinical decision making in the future.

MOLECULAR DETECTION OF OCCULT MICROMETASTASES

The detection of regional thoracic lymph node metastases by routine histopathologic analysis portends a significantly diminished patient survival rate, usually secondary to the later development of systemic metastases in NSCLC. However, even with N0 status, the 5-year survival rate of patients with T1 and T2 tumors combined is about 60% to 70%, indicating that the undetected presence of occult micrometastases (OM) in either lymph nodes or other systemic sites might be clinically significant. The ability to accurately detect OM would allow better prediction of the risk of tumor recurrence and of death, as well as the use of targeted adjuvant therapy in high-risk patients. The term *occult micrometastases* has been criticized by some as ambiguous, but it is now commonly used, even though it has been suggested that a better term would be *occult tumor cells*.[44] In this chapter, we will use OM.

Two techniques are primarily used to detect OM: immunohistochemistry (IHC) (Fig. 45-2) and polymerase chain reaction (PCR) (Fig. 45-3). With respect to IHC, several groups have investigated the utility of antibodies (Abs) to various tumor markers in detecting OM in the lymph nodes of patients with surgically resected stage I NSCLC. Such Abs include, for example, anti-cytokeratin monoclonal Abs (mAbs) (MNF116, CAM5.2, and AE1/AE3), Ber-Ep4 (an epithelial cell–specific mAb), and anti-p53 mAb. Detection rates have varied widely, with a change in nodal status occurring in 4% to 58% of lymph nodes. Of the six largest studies, four showed a direct correlation between positive IHC results and an increased risk of cancer relapse (Table 45-1). Two clinical trials, the Cancer and Leukemia Group B (CALGB) 9761 and the American College of Surgeons Oncology Group, are in the process of defining, in a prospective, multi-institutional manner, the relationship between lymph node OM detected by IHC and systemic tumor recurrence. Preliminary analysis of CALGB 9761 IHC results demonstrated an upstaging of 11% of the 178 patients.[45] Final analysis of the results of the CALGB 9761 trial is currently being performed.

The detection of individual tumor cells in patients' bone marrow is another area of active interest. Passlick's group has demonstrated that IHC is a valid and reliable approach for detecting occult disseminated tumor cells in bone marrow.[46] Using cytokeratin IHC, several groups have demonstrated a 22% to 59% incidence of bone marrow micrometastases in NSCLC.[46-49] An increasing number of published articles have elucidated the potential prognostic importance of this finding.[46,47,49,50]

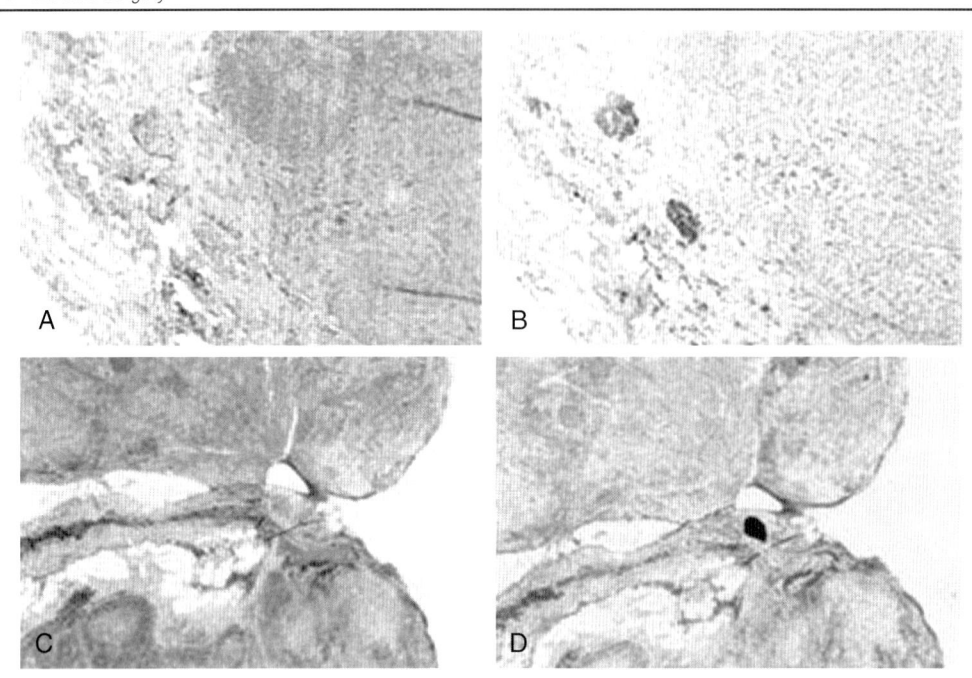

Figure 45–2
Two lymph nodes with tumor detected by immunohistochemistry (IHC) but not by routine hematoxylin and eosin stain (H&E). *Top:* The first lymph node, stained by H&E **(A)** and for cytokeratin by IHC **(B)**. *Bottom:* The second lymph node, stained by H&E **(C)** and for cytokeratin by IHC **(D)**. *(Adapted with permission from Vollmer RT, Herndon JE 2nd, D'Cunha J, et al.* Clin Cancer Res *2003;**9**:5630-5635.)*

Using IHC to detect OM has two main drawbacks: (1) the need for visual detection of OM deposits by a human operator and (2) the inability to test the entire nodal specimen, unless it is available for processing onto slides that can then be stained and reviewed. The use of PCR-based assays to detect tumor cell molecules, most typically tumor-related mRNA, overcomes those two drawbacks. To date, most NSCLC studies have focused on identifying the markers that would serve as suitable surrogates for the presence of viable tumor cells, and on defining the application of the technique.

In the past 10 years, a number of studies of several different malignancies have used reverse transcriptase-PCR (RT-PCR) to detect micrometastatic disease, including thoracic tumors such as NSCLC. RT-PCR detects micrometastatic disease by identifying an appropriate tumor marker. A number of molecular markers have been investigated in patients with NSCLC. Apo-mucin type 1 (MUC1) mRNA, a mucopolysaccharide gene associated with epithelial tissues, was the first marker used in NSCLC lymph nodes to identify micrometastatic disease in patients with surgically resected NSCLC.[51] Subsequent studies have revealed the ubiquitousness of MUC1 mRNA in many tissues, diminishing its value as a tumor marker[52-54] (and Maddaus and D'Cunha, unpublished data). Other markers need to be identified in patients with NSCLC.

Carcinoembryonic antigen (CEA) has emerged as a potentially suitable NSCLC tumor marker from a number of RT-PCR–based studies.[55-58] Collectively, those studies demonstrated that CEA has relatively high specificity (mRNA transcripts were detectable in almost all epithelial cells, including cancer cells, but not in nonepithelial cells) and a relatively high sensitivity (it detected one malignant cell in up to 10^6 normal cells). Our group, within the CALGB 9761 trial, used RT-PCR to examine the potential of CEA as a marker of OM in lymph nodes of patients with early-stage NSCLC; our results definitively expanded on previous findings.[59] Standard and quantitative real-time RT-PCR for CEA detected OM in patients with stage I NSCLC at similar rates, with both methods upstaging patients in about 50% of cases.

A potential shortcoming of OM detection by both IHC and RT-PCR is the binary (yes-or-no) result regarding the presence or absence of OM. Although predictive of an increased risk of tumor recurrence, simple yes-or-no results fail to further stratify risk. Studies of N2 disease detected by hematoxylin and eosin (H&E) staining revealed significant survival differences between patients with lymph nodes replaced by tumors and patients with microscopic disease found incidentally after surgical resection.[60] Similarly, rates of tumor recurrence and of survival in patients with lymph nodes negative by H&E although they harbor OM may also be related to the number of micrometastatic tumor cells present.

A possible solution may be the use of quantitative real-time RT-PCR (QRT-PCR), a technology now broadly available.[61] QRT-PCR, unlike other approaches to quantifying PCR products, requires no post-PCR product manipulation (such as gel electrophoresis). Moreover, QRT-PCR enables rapid processing of many samples (96 reactions in 3 to 4 hours). QRT-PCR uses a target molecule–specific oligonucleotide probe (in this case to CEA mRNA) with a covalently attached fluorescent reporter and quencher dye. When the probe is intact, the quenching dye absorbs the fluorescent energy of the reporter dye. If the target molecule of interest is present, the specific oligonucleotide probe anneals to it. During the PCR extension phase, the fluorescent probe is cleaved by the exonuclease activity of Taq DNA polymerase, thus increasing the reporter dye's emission. Curves plotting the relative fluorescence change against the PCR cycle number are constructed, and the point of increase in fluorescence above

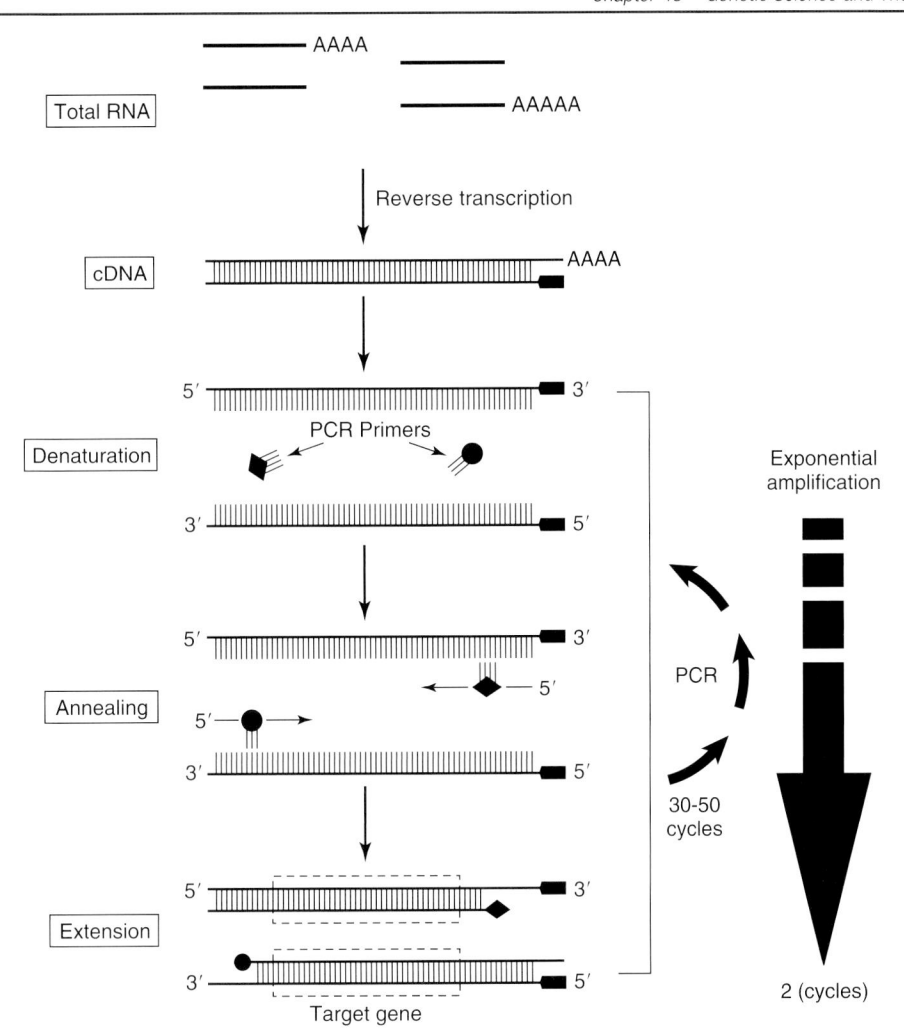

Figure 45-3
Principles involved in reverse transcriptase–polymerase chain reaction (RT-PCR). RNA from an experimental source is converted to complementary DNA (cDNA). PCR amplification (with gene-specific primers) proceeds in three steps, resulting in the amplification of the gene of interest.

background is calculated; from this calculation, the threshold cycle (C_T) is determined. Because C_T values decrease linearly with increasing target molecule quantity in the input sample, they provide a quantitative measurement.

The potential application of QRT-PCR was demonstrated in the same group of 53 patients in our CALGB 9761 study cited previously: of 232 lymph nodes, 59 (25.4%) were positive by QRT-PCR for CEA mRNA. Estimates of the quantity of micrometastatic cells in those 59 nodes ranged from 1.1×10^3 to 3.2×10^5 cells per lymph node station (median, 7190 tumor cells per lymph node station). The increased sensitivity of this molecular approach (versus the standard H&E analysis) accounted for the additional seven patients whose tumors were upstaged. Others have subsequently confirmed our findings and suggested a prognostic relationship.[62,63] The prognostic importance of OM in NSCLC awaits the conclusion of the CALGB 9761 (manuscript in preparation).

Numerous other markers have been investigated in NSCLC by QRT-PCR, including cytokeratin 7, cytokeratin 19, KS1/4, LUNX, and PDEF. This list of markers is not meant to be all-inclusive but rather to highlight the fact that many markers exist. The single-institution studies of such markers have looked at limited numbers of patients, yet the vast majority of those reports suggested some prognostic significance.[64,65] KS1/4 is an intriguing marker because it has a very high specificity for lung cancer.[66] KS1/4 is a gene that encodes a glycoprotein expressed in epithelial cells recognized by the monoclonal antibody Ber-EP4. Monoclonal antibodies to Ber-EP4 (such as edrecolomab) have been used in IHC studies of NSCLC lymph nodes to identify micrometastatic disease. Furthermore, antibodies to Ber-EP4 have shown predictive promise in clinical trials for patients with colorectal cancer. Using edrecolomab, 189 patients with resected stage III colorectal cancer had a 32% increase in overall survival rate, as compared with the no-treatment arm ($P < .01$), and a decreased tumor recurrence rate ($P < .04$).[67] Those results raise both staging and therapeutic issues.

An analogous approach has been used to evaluate the lymph nodes of patients with esophageal cancer. In esophageal cancer, lymph node involvement is the strongest predictor of recurrence and poor outcome. As with studies evaluating the prognostic importance of IHC-detected NSCLC micrometastases, the prognostic importance of IHC-detected lymph node involvement in patients with esophageal cancer has varied.[68-72] This variation underscores one of the potential

Table 45-1
Prognostic Studies to Detect Micrometastatic Disease in Patients with NSCLC

Authors (ref)	Antibody	Patients (N)	Number of positive patients (%)	Survival impact?
Chen et al. (107)	Polyclonal antikeratin	65	38 (58)	Yes
Passlick et al. (108)	Ber-Ep4	70	11 (16)	Yes
Dobashi et al. (109)	p53	31	14 (45)	Yes
Nicholson et al. (110)	MNF116	49	3 (6)	No
Maruyama et al. (111)	CAM5.2	44	31 (70)	Yes
Goldstein et al. (112)	AE1/AE3	80	3 (4)	No
Ohta et al. (113)	VEGF	181	44 (24)	Yes
Gu et al. (114)	AE1/AE3 and p53	49	22 (45)	Yes
Osaki et al. (115)	AE1/AE3	115	32 (28)	Yes
Marchevsky et al. (116)	AE1/AE3	33	5 (15)	No
Rena et al. (117)	AE1/AE3	87	14 (16)	No

NSCLC, non–small cell lung cancer.

pitfalls of IHC—namely, sampling error from evaluating only a limited number of sections of the lymph node.

Luketich's group (Godfrey and colleagues) used QRT-PCR to detect micrometastases in 387 lymph nodes from 30 histologically node-negative patients.[73] In their report focusing on primary adenocarcinomas, CEA expression was used to identify 11 additional patients who had micrometastases. Of those 11 patients, 9 suffered disease recurrence. The Kaplan-Meier analysis demonstrated that QRT-PCR–positive lymph nodes correlated with a significantly lower disease-free survival rate ($P < .0001$) and a significantly lower overall survival ($P < .0006$). Other similar studies have followed, including one that evaluated over 39 different markers in esophageal adenocarcinoma from Luketich's group.[74] Finally, Inoue and colleagues used CEA RT-PCR in 57 patients with esophageal carcinoma (primarily squamous cell, histologically) to show that CEA-positive cells could be detected in 70% of patients.[75] Their study lacked prognostic significance, however, as did a similar study with 48 patients who had squamous cell histology.[76]

DETECTION OF MOLECULAR MARKERS IN BLOOD

The use of genetic science to help patients with thoracic cancer has raised hopes of finding an appropriate, clinically useful screening test. Screening peripheral blood is appealing; it is easily accessible, and the minimal overall change in blood volume may enable quantitative measurement. Moreover, many cancer patients end up with metastatic disease. Thus, early detection and correlation with response to initial therapy is particularly attractive. Reproducibly and accurately detecting circulating tumor cells (CTCs) is challenging, but this clearly could be beneficial in diagnosis, in risk stratification, in prediction of recurrence, in new therapies, and in gauging of the response to therapy. Of the several challenges in the detection of CTCs, the first is to identify an appropriate marker. Second, the method should be able to detect one CTC in 10^6 circulating cells. Not surprisingly, most approaches have involved an enrichment step from peripheral blood, followed by RT-PCR. One of the biggest limitations in this area is the signal-to-noise ratio—that is, the problem of differentiating meaningful information from background gene expression.

It has been known for years that CTCs are detectable in patients with very-early-stage NSCLC, although detection is more frequent in patients with advanced disease.[77] A number of investigators have used RT-PCR to detect circulating tumor cells in patients with NSCLC; such assays originally focused on a limited number of tumor-derived mRNA molecules, such as EGFR[78] and CEA,[57] but the focus has expanded with increased research in this area. Kurusu and associates used RT-PCR to detect CEA mRNA in blood samples from patients with NSCLC, preoperatively and then 2 to 3 weeks after surgical resection.[57] Preliminary in vitro studies demonstrated that the sensitivity of their assay for tumor cell detection was 10 NSCLC cancer cells in 10^6 peripheral blood leukocytes. Of 103 preoperative blood samples, 62 (60%) were positive by CEA mRNA analysis; of those 62 samples, 27 (44%) remained positive postoperatively, whereas 35 (56%) became negative. No difference in the rate of detection was seen between adenocarcinomas and squamous cell carcinomas. Of 41 patients with a negative preoperative blood test, only 2 had a positive postoperative blood test. Important features of the Kurusu study included the following: (1) the clear correlation between a positive preoperative blood test and postoperative pathologic stage, (2) the high rate of positive preoperative blood tests among patients with "early" stage IA and IB NSCLC who went on to develop disease postoperatively, and (3) the correlation between persistent postoperative blood positivity and postoperative stage, suggesting persistent but undetected systemic disease.

Like NSCLC, esophageal cancer has several reports examining the potential clinical utility of CTCs. In 2006, Setoyama and colleagues retrospectively investigated the clinical significance of peripheral blood CTCs in the postoperative period after curative esophagectomy by using CEA QRT-PCR.[79] Of the 106 patients in their study, 34 had recurrent disease. Of those, 26 patients (77%) were CEA QRT-PCR positive. Eight patients who developed recurrent disease were CEA QRT-PCR negative. Patients positive for CEA mRNA experienced significantly shorter disease-free intervals (29.7% versus 88.4%, $P < .001$). In multivariate analysis, CEA mRNA positivity was an independent factor for disease-free interval. Liu and colleagues also sought to examine the clinical utility of CTCs in perioperative blood samples.[80] Using a similar quantitation system to that developed by us for NSCLC, CEA QRT-PCR was used to detect as few as three tumor cells per milliliter of peripheral blood. Further, their analysis of 53 patients with esophageal cancer showed a significant increase of CTCs in the blood after esophagectomy. The authors' data suggested that CTC in the peripheral blood was related to the development of subsequent metastases.

Recently, Xi and colleagues tackled this marker problem head-on.[81] No single marker provides adequate sensitivity by itself. Thus, these investigators sought to determine the optimal marker combinations for detection of CTCs. They used QRT-PCR to test the expression of selected potential markers in tissue samples from a number of solid-organ malignancies (breast, colon, esophageal, head and neck, lung, and melanoma). Of the 52 potential markers that were screened, three to eight useful markers were identified for each tumor type. In their report, they identified combinations that had a minimum of 1000-fold higher expression in tumors when compared with normal blood. For esophageal cancer, CEA, CK7, CK19, TACSTD1, CK20, and TM4SF3 were tested, with CK7 and TM4SF3 being the best combination. For NSCLC, CEA, CK7, CK19, EGFR, LUNX, SCCA, SFTPB, and TACSDT1 were tested, with CK7, EGFR, SCCA, and SFTPB being the best combination. Although the study has clear strengths, there was no prognostic validation of markers performed. Future studies should address this prospectively in the cooperative group setting.

Detection of tumor markers in blood is not limited to nucleic acids. For a number of years, there has been interest in identifying abnormal proteins, peptides, and autoantibodies. Despite a large initiative to identify a suitable protein marker, no study has yet yielded promising results using existing markers.[82-85] Efforts to detect serum autoantibodies have been more promising. Abnormally expressed and structurally altered proteins may elicit the production of autoantibodies in patients with lung cancer. Anti-p53 antibodies have been found in the sera of patients with lung cancer containing p53 mutations.[86] Mitsudomi and colleagues identified anti-p53 antibodies in more than 20% of 188 patients with NSCLC.[87] In addition, several other autoantibodies have recently been identified as potential markers for lung cancer detection, including antiglycosylated annexins I and anti-p40 antibodies.[88a] Brichory and coworkers[88] found that antibodies to glycosylated annexins I and II were present in 60% of patients with lung adenocarcinomas and in 33% of patients with squamous cell carcinomas. Such studies have served as the basis for the future development of biochips that may provide molecular profiles of the antibody response to tumor antigens in patients with thoracic cancer.[89]

PROTEOMICS: THE ANALYSIS OF TUMOR PROTEIN EXPRESSION PROFILES

The sequencing of the human genome paved the way for understanding the functionality of complex biological systems, and genomics will no doubt lead to major advances in medicine and cancer biology in the near future. Proteomics promises to be a powerful tool to study translational lung cancer research. As this area has evolved, it is seen as being complementary to the other genetic approaches described in this chapter.

Proteomics encompasses many platform technologies for protein separation and identification. Its major challenge is the vastly increased complexity of the human proteome, as compared with the genome. Proteomic analysis of cancer specimens entails a number of variations. Analysis of tissue biopsies is far more complicated and challenging, given the heterogeneous nature of the samples. Most proteomic approaches have employed homogenization of the sample of interest, with subsequent separation of proteins by two-dimensional polyacrylamide gel electrophoresis (2D PAGE).[90] Particular proteins of interest are identified as "spots" on these gels and then eluted from the gel by various techniques. The protein's identity is then determined using mass spectrometry and proteomic databases.[91]

In contrast to other molecular approaches, studies in lung cancer proteomics have led the way among investigations of solid-organ tumors.[57] With lung cancer as the backdrop for translational investigations using proteomic approaches, Hanash and colleagues[92] analyzed more than 1000 lung cancer–related samples, using 2D PAGE in combination with mass spectroscopy. They compiled a lung cancer proteomic database integrating protein and gene expression data. Their ultimate goals are to identify novel biomarkers for the early detection of lung cancer, to develop novel classification of tumors, and to reveal targets for future therapeutic intervention.[92-94] Analysis of the gene expression and protein expression patterns in parallel allowed them to directly compare gene and protein expression in the same tumor set. They analyzed 165 protein spots representing protein products of 98 genes in 76 lung adenocarcinomas using 2D PAGE. On essentially the same set of samples, they performed microarray analysis. Interestingly, of the 98 genes, only 21 showed a significant correlation between protein and mRNA levels. As an extension of their studies, they identified specific cytokeratin isoforms that were predictive of survival in patients with lung cancer.[94]

Not surprisingly, many others have updated studies in this area. Seike and colleagues performed proteomic studies on lung cancer cell lines to elucidate signatures for the histologic phenotype (NSCLC and small cell lung cancer).[95] In their study, 32 different proteins were identified from lung cancer cell lines and signatures for the histologic subtypes identified. This approach was then used to correctly classify isolated cancer cells into three histologic groups (squamous, adenocarcinoma, other subtypes) based on their protein signatures. Furthermore, fatty acid–binding protein 5 (FABP5) was considered the most informative spot for discriminating between adenocarcinomas and squamous cell carcinomas.

The next step is to identify the proteomic signature that has prognostic significance in NSCLC. Yanagisawa and colleagues attempted to address this by deriving a 25-signal proteomic signature in stage I NSCLC patients.[96] Their analysis was somewhat complex. From the 174 NSCLC patients who underwent surgical resection, the authors used 116 NSCLC specimens as a training set and then performed an independent, blinded validation set of 58 NSCLC specimens. Normal lung specimens were included also. Among the stage I NSCLC patients studied in the validation set, the signature was predictive of overall survival and relapse-free survival in patients who had a high-risk signature ($P < .001$).

In the lung cancer arena, the newest frontiers involve studying the alteration in the proteome at the genetic or epigenetic level. For example, gene products of the FANC family are regulated by DNA hyper-methylation and are frequently altered in patients with lung cancer, leading to variable sensitivity to platinum-based therapies. This is being studied in a phase 3 trial of NSCLC to identify whether alterations in methylation of FANC family proteins might be helpful in guiding adjuvant therapy for NSCLC.

TUMOR MARKER PANELS

Thoracic malignancies, like many tumors, cannot be characterized in full by a single molecular marker. Each tumor may have its own molecular fingerprint. As we move toward refining staging and treatment according to molecular markers, a panel of molecular markers for specific tumors (and possibly tumor subtype) is likely to be analyzed routinely, allowing refinement of the sensitivity and specificity of risk prediction.

Kwiatkowski and coworkers evaluated 244 patients with stage I NSCLC in an effort to identify variables predicting risk of tumor recurrence.[97] Variables included the following: adenocarcinoma solid tumor with mucin subtype, tumor diameter 4 cm or greater, lymphatic invasion, p53 expression, K-*ras* mutation, and the absence of H-*ras* p21 expression. Their data inspired them to propose a molecular tumor subclassification. Patient survival rates at 5 years correlated inversely with the number of prognostic variables as follows: one or two factors, 87%; three factors, 58%; and four or more factors, 21%.

D'Amico and colleagues proposed a molecular model system consisting of five biologic markers involved in various parts of the metastatic process: growth regulation, cell cycle regulation, apoptosis, angiogenesis, and metastatic adhesion factor.[98] In a multivariable analysis of 408 patients with stage I NSCLC, they found that five biological factors were predictive: erbB-2, RB, p53, factor VIII staining for angiogenesis, and CD-44. Using their system, patients were substratified by survival at 5 years as follows: zero to one marker, 77% survival; two markers, 62% survival; and three to five markers, 49% survival.

Gordon and coworkers[99] expanded on this concept by demonstrating the diagnostic superiority of a small panel of tumor-associated genes whose expression levels can be used to calculate a set of gene expression ratios for any particular sample. They identified significant genes by microarray analysis of 150 NSCLC tumors compared with 31 malignant mesothelioma samples. Using six genes to calculate three sets of gene expression ratios (calretinin/claudin-7, VAC-β/TACSTD1, and MRC OX-2/TITF-1), they were able to correctly classify 99% of tumors by type. After refining their methodology, they identified a panel of eight genes and calculated a set of four gene expression ratios that accurately predicted treatment-related clinical outcome ($P = .0035$) for 29 patients with malignant mesothelioma.[42]

Not surprisingly, studies in the area of serum biomarkers have been extended to the field of proteomics. One of the more exciting potentials of molecular approaches to thoracic oncology is in the application of these technologies to early diagnosis. Patz and coworkers recently published their study, which identified four serum proteins (CEA, retinol binding protein, alpha-1-antitrypsin, and squamous cell carcinoma antigen) that identified patients who had lung cancer.[100] This approach may eventually be clinically useful as an adjunct for approaching those difficult cases involving patients with pulmonary nodules that are indeterminate, or for potentially predicting those individuals at high risk for lung cancer.

More recently, the concept of testing lymph nodes and peripheral blood with a panel of molecular markers has been increasingly applied. This has been performed for a number of solid organ tumors, and a model for this was nicely presented in esophageal cancer by Luketich's group (Xi and colleagues), who identified a panel of molecular markers useful in patients with esophageal adenocarcinoma; the panel initially included 39 genes from their literature and database searches.[81] They did molecular testing by calculating the median relative expression to refine these 39 genes down to six genes of variable expression (*TACSTD1*, *CK7*, *CK19*, *CK20*, *CEA*, and *Villin 1*). They found a more robust classification with sets of markers than with the individual markers alone. In particular, *TACSTD1* with *CK19* was the best marker combination, with an accuracy of 98% (*TACSTD1*) and 97% (*CK19*). Of 34 patients with esophageal adenocarcinoma, five had positive lymph nodes by multimarker QRT-PCR analysis; this finding correlated with a worse disease-free survival rate ($P = .0023$).

PERSONALIZED ONCOLOGY

It might be expected that as molecular approaches to thoracic malignancies evolve and become more sophisticated, we would see the potential applied to the field of targeted therapeutics. The expression of specific markers may highlight a particular signaling pathway of interest that can characterize how a patient might respond to a particular treatment regimen. Furthermore, the integration of the concepts expressed earlier in this chapter lead to this new frontier in molecular oncology. Many investigators have recognized this, and numerous studies are evaluating the immense promise in this area.

Brooks and colleagues prospectively evaluated this in a study of stage III NSCLC patients (confirmed pathologically) treated with vinorelbine and external beam radiation between 1996 and 2001. In their analysis, they included markers for apoptosis (p53, bcl-2), drug sensitivity (multidrug resistance, glutathione S-transferase), growth factors (EGFR, erbB-2), and mismatch repair genes (*hMLH1*, *hMLH2*). They evaluated histologically positive mediastinal lymph nodes via immunohistochemistry. Multivariable analysis of marker-associated overexpression of p53 and low expression of hMSH2 was associated with poor treatment response and death from cancer.[101]

Many new targeted agents such as gefitinib (Iressa) or erlotinib (Tarceva) are clinically effective when the targeted marker is mutated or overexpressed.[102-105] It would not be surprising if, as we understand more about molecular markers and their expression, we find that this field complements tumor classification. To this end, somatic mutations in the tyrosine-kinase domain of EGFR have recently been shown to be predictive of the increased efficacy of gefitinib in NSCLC patients. Mutations in both *erbB1* (EGFR) and *erbB2* (Her2/neu) have been identified, and their effects on prognosis and response to targeted therapies are an active area of investigation. Indeed, the study of mutations in the EGFR pathway has promise in lung cancer prognosis and potential response to therapy. At our institution, we are beginning to incorporate these considerations into empirical salvage therapy for patients (women, nonsmokers, with adenocarcinomas), but soon these considerations will be paramount in therapy initiation.

Such an approach has recently been reported by Potti and colleagues and may be a key piece in establishing a personalized approach to adjuvant lung cancer therapy.[106] In their investigations, they made use of clinical variables and multiple gene expression profiles from two large multicenter cooperative group studies of early-stage lung cancer (CALGB 9761 and ACOSOG Z003), to validate the predictive model of recurrence and death that they originally derived from a single-institution tumor bank. From these investigations in 89 patients, they were able to reclassify stage IA patients, and they identified a subset of higher-risk patients who would be appropriate for additional adjuvant chemotherapy. Their model appears to predict overall survival in stage 1 NSCLC patients more accurately than the standard H&E based staging system. Overall, this model had predictive accuracies of 72% (ACOSOG Z0030) and 79% (CALGB 9761). Their model, which they call the "lung metagene model," has the potential to increase the precision of predicting a patient's risk of disease recurrence, and to guide decisions based on adjuvant therapy in early-stage NSCLC. The challenge of this approach will be to validate it through prospective, randomized trials run in the cooperative oncology groups.

Summary

Translational research in thoracic cancers will use the entire armamentarium of molecular biology, including genomics and proteomics. Currently, the TNM stage is the most important predictor of patient survival. In the new era of molecular analysis of solid-organ tumors, it is highly likely that molecular subclassification strategies will add depth and refinement to our predictive ability. Many studies have already suggested important molecular markers, but those markers must be tested in large prospective studies with homogeneous groups of patients, so that clinicians can use the overall predictive ability of individual markers. These studies will also serve as the framework for what is even more important: the rational design of molecularly targeted therapies. The future of genetic science for patients with thoracic cancer lies in our ability to use both the current and the novel assays of the future, and their markers, to identify patients at risk for early recurrence. In addition, markers must be used as molecular handles, so that novel compounds can target their functional pathways. A targeted approach is likely to have a dramatic, positive impact on prognosis and survival.

Acknowledgements

We are grateful to Mary Knatterud for her expert editorial remarks on this chapter, and to Lisa D'Cunha for her medical illustrations. Chuong Hoang was a previous contributor to this work.

REFERENCES

1. Mao L, Lee JS, Kurie JM, et al. Clonal genetic alterations in the lungs of current and former smokers. *J Natl Cancer Inst* 1997;**89**:857-62.
2. Wistuba II, Montellano FD, Milchgrub S, et al. Deletions of chromosome 3p are frequent and early events in the pathogenesis of uterine cervical carcinoma. *Cancer Res* 1997;**57**:3154-8.
3. Folkman J. Tumor angiogenesis: therapeutic implications. *N Engl J Med* 1971;**285**:1182-6.
4. Folkman J. Angiogenesis in cancer, vascular, rheumatoid and other disease. *Nat Med* 1995;**1**:27-31.
5. Stetler-Stevenson WG, Kleiner DE Jr. Molecular biology of cancer: invasion and metastasis. In: DeVita VT Jr, Hellman S, Rosenberg SA, editors. Cancer: principles and practice of oncology. Philadelphia: Lippincott, Williams and Wilkins; 2001, p 123.
6. Yokota J. Tumor progression and metastasis. *Carcinogenesis* 2000;**21**:497-503.
7. Hanahan D, Weinberg RA. The hallmarks of cancer. *Cell* 2000;**100**:57-70.
8. Fidler IJ, Poste G. The cellular heterogeneity of malignant neoplasms: implications for adjuvant chemotherapy. *Semin Oncol* 1985;**12**:207-21.
9. Poste G, Fidler IJ. The pathogenesis of cancer metastasis. *Nature* 1980;**283**:139-46.
10. Eberhard DA, Johnson BE, Amler LC, et al. Mutations in the epidermal growth factor receptor and in KRAS are predictive and prognostic indicators in patients with non-small-cell lung cancer treated with chemotherapy alone and in combination with erlotinib. *J Clin Oncol* 2005;**23**:5900-9.
11. Esposito V, Baldi A, De Luca A, et al. Cell cycle related proteins as prognostic parameters in radically resected non-small cell lung cancer. *J Clin Pathol* 2005;**58**:734-9.
12. Gessner C, Liebers U, Kuhn H, et al. BAX and p16INK4A are independent positive prognostic markers for advanced tumour stage of nonsmall cell lung cancer. *Eur Respir J* 2002;**19**:134-40.
13. Mascaux C, Iannino N, Martin B, et al. The role of RAS oncogene in survival of patients with lung cancer: a systematic review of the literature with meta-analysis. *Br J Cancer* 2005;**92**:131-9.
14. Nigro JM, Baker SJ, Preisinger AC, et al. Mutations in the p53 gene occur in diverse human tumour types. *Nature* 1989;**342**:705-8.
15. Passlick B, Izbicki JR, Haussinger K, Thetter O, Pantel K. Immunohistochemical detection of P53 protein is not associated with a poor prognosis in non-small-cell lung cancer. *J Thorac Cardiovasc Surg* 1995;**109**:1205-11.
16. Wang J, Lee JJ, Wang L, et al. Value of p16INK4a and RASSF1A promoter hypermethylation in prognosis of patients with resectable non-small cell lung cancer. *Clin Cancer Res* 2004;**10**(18 Pt 1):6119-25.
17. Salgia R, Skarin AT. Molecular abnormalities in lung cancer. *J Clin Oncol* 1998;**16**:1207-17.
18. Weir BA, Woo MS, Getz G, et al. Characterizing the cancer genome in lung adenocarcinoma. *Nature* 2007;**450**:893-8.
19. Yanaihara N, Caplen N, Bowman E, et al. Unique microRNA molecular profiles in lung cancer diagnosis and prognosis. *Cancer Cell* 2006;**9**:189-98.
20. Lu J, Getz G, Miska EA, et al. MicroRNA expression profiles classify human cancers. *Nature* 2005;**435**:834-8.
21. Hu Z, Chen J, Tian T, et al. Genetic variants of miRNA sequences and non-small cell lung cancer survival. *J Clin Invest* 2008;**118**:2600-8.
22. Southern E, Mir K, Shchepinov M. Molecular interactions on microarrays. *Nat Genet* 1999;**21**(Suppl. 1):5-9.
23. Lipshutz RJ, Fodor SP, Gingeras TR, Lockhart DJ. High density synthetic oligonucleotide arrays. *Nat Genet* 1999;**21**(Suppl. 1):20-4.
24. Quackenbush J. Computational analysis of microarray data. *Nat Rev Genet* 2001;**2**:418-27.
25. Chen JJ, Peck K, Hong TM, et al. Global analysis of gene expression in invasion by a lung cancer model. *Cancer Res* 2001;**61**:5223-30.
26. Gemma A, Takenaka K, Hosoya Y, et al. Altered expression of several genes in highly metastatic subpopulations of a human pulmonary adenocarcinoma cell line. *Eur J Cancer* 2001;**37**:1554-61.
27. Goodwin LO, Mason JM, Hajdu SI. Gene expression patterns of paired bronchioloalveolar carcinoma and benign lung tissue. *Ann Clin Lab Sci* 2001;**31**:369-75.
28. Wang KK, Liu N, Radulovich N, et al. Novel candidate tumor marker genes for lung adenocarcinoma. *Oncogene* 2002;**21**:7598-604.
29. Beer DG, Kardia SL, Huang CC, et al. Gene-expression profiles predict survival of patients with lung adenocarcinoma. *Nat Med* 2002;**8**:816-24.
30. Bhattacharjee A, Richards WG, Staunton J, et al. Classification of human lung carcinomas by mRNA expression profiling reveals distinct adenocarcinoma subclasses. *Proc Natl Acad Sci U S A* 2001;**98**:13790-5.
31. Garber ME, Troyanskaya OG, Schluens K, et al. Diversity of gene expression in adenocarcinoma of the lung. *Proc Natl Acad Sci U S A* 2001;**98**:13784-9.

32. Wigle DA, Jurisica I, Radulovich N, et al. Molecular profiling of non-small cell lung cancer and correlation with disease-free survival. *Cancer Res* 2002;**62**:3005-8.
33. Kikuchi T, Daigo Y, Katagiri T, et al. Expression profiles of non-small cell lung cancers on cDNA microarrays: identification of genes for prediction of lymph-node metastasis and sensitivity to anti-cancer drugs. *Oncogene* 2003;**22**: 2192-205.
34. Shedden K, Taylor JM, Enkemann SA, et al. Gene expression-based survival prediction in lung adenocarcinoma: a multi-site, blinded validation study. *Nat Med* 2008;**14**:822-7.
35. Selaru FM, Zou Y, Xu Y, et al. Global gene expression profiling in Barrett's esophagus and esophageal cancer: a comparative analysis using cDNA microarrays. *Oncogene* 2002;**21**:475-8.
36. Zhou J, Zhao LQ, Xiong MM, et al. Gene expression profiles at different stages of human esophageal squamous cell carcinoma. *World J Gastroenterol* 2003; **9**:9-15.
37. Wang S, Zhan M, Yin J, et al. Transcriptional profiling suggests that Barrett's metaplasia is an early intermediate stage in esophageal adenocarcinogenesis. *Oncogene* 2006;**25**:3346-56.
38. Kihara C, Tsunoda T, Tanaka T, et al. Prediction of sensitivity of esophageal tumors to adjuvant chemotherapy by cDNA microarray analysis of gene-expression profiles. *Cancer Res* 2001;**61**:6474-9.
39. Yamabuki T, Daigo Y, Kato T, et al. Genome-wide gene expression profile analysis of esophageal squamous cell carcinomas. *Int J Oncol* 2006;**28**:1375-84.
40. Hoang CD, D'Cunha J, Kratzke MG, et al. Gene expression profiling identifies matriptase overexpression in malignant mesothelioma. *Chest* 2004;**125**: 1843-52.
41. Gordon GJ. Transcriptional profiling of mesothelioma using microarrays. *Lung Cancer* 2005;**49**(Suppl. 1):S99-103.
42. Gordon GJ, Jensen RV, Hsiao LL, et al. Using gene expression ratios to predict outcome among patients with mesothelioma. *J Natl Cancer Inst* 2003;**95**: 598-605.
43. Gordon GJ, Rockwell GN, Godfrey PA, et al. Validation of genomics-based prognostic tests in malignant pleural mesothelioma. *Clin Cancer Res* 2005;**11**:4406-14.
44. Coello MC, Luketich JD, Litle VR, Godfrey TE. Prognostic significance of micrometastasis in non-small-cell lung cancer. *Clin Lung Cancer* 2004; **5**:214-25.
45. Vollmer RT, Herndon JE 2nd, D'Cunha J, et al. Immunohistochemical detection of occult lymph node metastases in non-small cell lung cancer: anatomical pathology results from Cancer and Leukemia Group B Trial 9761. *Clin Cancer Res* 2003;**9**:5630-5.
46. Passlick B, Kubuschok B, Izbicki JR, Thetter O, Pantel K. Isolated tumor cells in bone marrow predict reduced survival in node-negative non-small cell lung cancer. *Ann Thorac Surg* 1999;**68**:2053-8.
47. Chen YH, Gao W, Zhou T, et al. Detection of bone marrow micrometastasis. *Hybridoma* 1999;**18**:465-6.
48. Cote RJ, Beattie EJ, Chaiwun B, et al. Detection of occult bone marrow micrometastases in patients with operable lung carcinoma. *Ann Surg* 1995;**222**:423-5:415-423; discussion.
49. Ohgami A, Mitsudomi T, Sugio K, et al. Micrometastatic tumor cells in the bone marrow of patients with non-small cell lung cancer. *Ann Thorac Surg* 1997;**64**:363-7.
50. Pantel K, Izbicki J, Passlick B, et al. Frequency and prognostic significance of isolated tumour cells in bone marrow of patients with non-small-cell lung cancer without overt metastases. *Lancet* 1996;**347**:649-53.
51. Salerno CT, Frizelle S, Niehans GA, et al. Detection of occult micrometastases in non-small cell lung carcinoma by reverse transcriptase-polymerase chain reaction. *Chest* 1998;**113**:1526-32.
52. Bostick PJ, Chatterjee S, Chi DD, et al. Limitations of specific reverse-transcriptase polymerase chain reaction markers in the detection of metastases in the lymph nodes and blood of breast cancer patients. *J Clin Oncol* 1998;**16**:2632-40.
53. Brugger W, Buhring HJ, Grunebach F, et al. Expression of MUC-1 epitopes on normal bone marrow: implications for the detection of micrometastatic tumor cells. *J Clin Oncol* 1999;**17**:1535-44.
54. Dent GA, Civalier CJ, Brecher ME, Bentley SA. MUC1 expression in hematopoietic tissues. *Am J Clin Pathol* 1999;**111**:741-7.
55. Castaldo G, Tomaiuolo R, Sanduzzi A, et al. Lung cancer metastatic cells detected in blood by reverse transcriptase-polymerase chain reaction and dot-blot analysis. *J Clin Oncol* 1997;**15**:3388-93.
56. Fujita J, Ueda Y, Bandoh S, Namihira H, Ishii T, Takahara J. A case of leptomeningeal metastasis from lung adenocarcinoma diagnosed by reverse transcriptase-polymerase chain reaction for carcinoembryonic antigen. *Lung Cancer* 1998;**22**:153-6.
57. Kurusu Y, Yamashita J, Ogawa M. Detection of circulating tumor cells by reverse transcriptase-polymerase chain reaction in patients with resectable non-small-cell lung cancer. *Surgery* 1999;**126**:820-6.
58. Yamashita JI, Kurusu Y, Fujino N, Saisyoji T, Ogawa M. Detection of circulating tumor cells in patients with non-small cell lung cancer undergoing lobectomy by video-assisted thoracic surgery: a potential hazard for intraoperative hematogenous tumor cell dissemination. *J Thorac Cardiovasc Surg* 2000;**119**:899-905.
59. D'Cunha J, Corfits AL, Herndon JE 2nd, et al. Molecular staging of lung cancer: real-time polymerase chain reaction estimation of lymph node micrometastatic tumor cell burden in stage I non-small cell lung cancer—preliminary results of Cancer and Leukemia Group B Trial 9761. *J Thorac Cardiovasc Surg* 2002;**123**:484-91:discussion 491.
60. Luke WP, Pearson FG, Todd TR, Patterson GA, Cooper JD. Prospective evaluation of mediastinoscopy for assessment of carcinoma of the lung. *J Thorac Cardiovasc Surg* 1986;**91**:53-6.
61. Gibson UE, Heid CA, Williams PM. A novel method for real time quantitative RT-PCR. *Genome Res* 1996;**6**:995-1001.
62. Maeda J, Inoue M, Okumura M, et al. Detection of occult tumor cells in lymph nodes from non-small cell lung cancer patients using reverse transcription-polymerase chain reaction for carcinoembryonic antigen mRNA with the evaluation of its sensitivity. *Lung Cancer* 2006;**52**:235-40.
63. Nosotti M, Falleni M, Palleschi A, et al. Quantitative real-time polymerase chain reaction detection of lymph node lung cancer micrometastasis using carcinoembryonic antigen marker. *Chest* 2005;**128**:1539-44.
64. Le Pimpec-Barthes F, Danel C, Lacave R, et al. Association of CK19 mRNA detection of occult cancer cells in mediastinal lymph nodes in non-small cell lung carcinoma and high risk of early recurrence. *Eur J Cancer* 2005; **41**:306-12.
65. Wang XT, Sienel W, Eggeling S, et al. Detection of disseminated tumor cells in mediastinoscopic lymph node biopsies and lymphadenectomy specimens of patients with NSCLC by quantitative RT-PCR. *Eur J Cardiothorac Surg* 2005;**28**:26-32.
66. Wallace MB, Block MI, Gillanders W, et al. Accurate molecular detection of non-small cell lung cancer metastases in mediastinal lymph nodes sampled by endoscopic ultrasound-guided needle aspiration. *Chest* 2005;**127**: 430-7.
67. Schwartzberg LS. Clinical experience with edrecolomab: a monoclonal antibody therapy for colorectal carcinoma. *Crit Rev Oncol Hematol* 2001;**40**:17-24.
68. Izbicki JR, Hosch SB, Pichlmeier U, et al. Prognostic value of immunohistochemically identifiable tumor cells in lymph nodes of patients with completely resected esophageal cancer. *N Engl J Med* 1997;**337**: 1188-94.
69. Komukai S, Nishimaki T, Watanabe H, Ajioka Y, Hatakeyama ST. Significance of immunohistochemically demonstrated micrometastases to lymph nodes in esophageal cancer with histologically negative nodes. *Surgery* 2000;**127**: 40-6.
70. Nakamura T, Ide H, Eguchi R, Hayashi K, Ota M, Takasaki K. Clinical implications of lymph node micrometastasis in patients with histologically node-negative (pN0) esophageal carcinoma. *J Surg Oncol* 2002;**79**:224-9.
71. Sato F, Shimada Y, Li Z, Watanabe G, Maeda M, Imamura M. Lymph node micrometastasis and prognosis in patients with oesophageal squamous cell carcinoma. *Br J Surg* 2001;**88**:426-32.
72. Tabira Y, Yasunaga M, Sakaguchi T, Yamaguchi T, Okuma T, Kawasuji M. Outcome of histologically node-negative esophageal squamous cell carcinoma. *World J Surg* 2002;**26**:1446-51.
73. Godfrey TE, Raja S, Finkelstein SD, Gooding WE, Kelly LA, Luketich JD. Prognostic value of quantitative reverse transcription-polymerase chain reaction in lymph node-negative esophageal cancer patients. *Clin Cancer Res* 2001;**7**:4041-8.
74. Xi L, Luketich JD, Raja S, et al. Molecular staging of lymph nodes from patients with esophageal adenocarcinoma. *Clin Cancer Res* 2005;**11**:1099-109.
75. Inoue H, Kajiyama Y, Tsurumaru M. Clinical significance of bone marrow micrometastases in esophageal cancer. *Dis Esophagus* 2004;**17**:328-32.
76. Natsugoe S, Nakashima S, Nakajo A, et al. Bone marrow micrometastasis detected by RT-PCR in esophageal squamous cell carcinoma. *Oncol Rep* 2003;**10**:1879-83.
77. Mao L. Recent advances in the molecular diagnosis of lung cancer. *Oncogene* 2002;**21**:6960-9.
78. De Luca A, Pignata S, Casamassimi A, et al. Detection of circulating tumor cells in carcinoma patients by a novel epidermal growth factor receptor reverse transcription-PCR assay. *Clin Cancer Res* 2000;**6**:1439-44.
79. Setoyama T, Natsugoe S, Okumura H. Carcinoembryonic antigen messenger RNA expression in blood predicts recurrence in esophageal cancer. *Clin Cancer Res* 2006;**12**:5972-7.

80. Liu Z, Jiang M, Zhao J, Ju H. Circulating tumor cells in perioperative esophageal cancer patients: quantitative assay system and potential clinical utility. *Clin Cancer Res* 2007;**13**:2992-7.
81. Xi L, Nicastri DG, El-Hefnawy T, Hughes SJ, Luketich JD, Godfrey TE. Optimal markers for real-time quantitative reverse transcription PCR detection of circulating tumor cells from melanoma, breast, colon, esophageal, head and neck, and lung cancers. *Clin Chem* 2007;**53**:1206-15.
82. Foa P, Fornier M, Miceli R, et al. Preoperative CEA, NSE, SCC, TPA and CYFRA 21.1 serum levels as prognostic indicators in resected non-small cell lung cancer. *Int J Biol Markers* 1999;**14**:92-8.
83. Karnak D, Ulubay G, Kayacan O, Beder S, Ibis E, Oflaz G. Evaluation of Cyfra 21-1: a potential tumor marker for non-small cell lung carcinomas. *Lung* 2001;**179**:57-65.
84. Salgia R, Harpole D, Herndon JE 2nd, Pisick E, Elias A, Skarin AT. Role of serum tumor markers CA 125 and CEA in non-small cell lung cancer. *Anticancer Res* 2001;**21**(2B):1241-6.
85. Tas F, Aydiner A, Topuz E, Yasasever V, Karadeniz A, Saip P. Utility of the serum tumor markers: CYFRA 21.1, carcinoembryonic antigen (CEA), and squamous cell carcinoma antigen (SCC) in squamous cell lung cancer. *J Exp Clin Cancer Res* 2000;**19**:477-81.
86. Iizasa T, Fujisawa T, Saitoh Y, Hiroshima K, Ohwada H. Serum anti-p53 autoantibodies in primary resected non-small-cell lung carcinoma. *Cancer Immunol Immunother* 1998;**46**:345-9.
87. Mitsudomi T, Suzuki S, Yatabe Y, et al. Clinical implications of p53 autoantibodies in the sera of patients with non-small-cell lung cancer. *J Natl Cancer Inst* 1998;**90**:1563-8.
88. Brichory FM, Misek DE, Yim AM, Krause MC, Giordano TJ, Beer DG, Hanash SM. An Immune response manifested by the common occurrence of annexins I and II autoantibodies and high circulating levels of IL-6 in lung cancer. *Proc Natl Acad Sci USA.* 2001 Aug14;**98(17)**:9824-9.
88a. Yamaguchi K, Patturajan M, Trink B, et al. Circulating antibodies to p40 (AIS) in the sera of respiratory tract cancer patients. *Int J Cancer* 2000;**89**:524-8.
89. Celis JE, Gromov P. Proteomics in translational cancer research: toward an integrated approach. *Cancer Cell* 2003;**3**:9-15.
90. O'Farrell PH. High resolution two-dimensional electrophoresis of proteins. *J Biol Chem* 1975;**250**:4007-21.
91. MacCoss MJ, Wu CC, Yates JR 3rd. Probability-based validation of protein identifications using a modified SEQUEST algorithm. *Anal Chem* 2002;**74**:5593-9.
92. Hanash S, Brichory F, Beer D. A proteomic approach to the identification of lung cancer markers. *Dis Markers* 2001;**17**:295-300.
93. Chen G, Gharib TG, Huang CC, et al. Proteomic analysis of lung adenocarcinoma: identification of a highly expressed set of proteins in tumors. *Clin Cancer Res* 2002;**8**:2298-305.
94. Gharib TG, Chen G, Wang H, et al. Proteomic analysis of cytokeratin isoforms uncovers association with survival in lung adenocarcinoma. *Neoplasia* 2002;**4**:440-8.
95. Seike M, Kondo T, Fujii K, et al. Proteomic signatures for histological types of lung cancer. *Proteomics* 2005;**5**:2939-48.
96. Yanagisawa K, Tomida S, Shimada Y, Yatabe Y, Mitsudomi T, Takahashi TA. 25-signal proteomic signature and outcome for patients with resected non-small-cell lung cancer. *J Natl Cancer Inst* 2007;**99**:858-67.
97. Kwiatkowski DJ, Harpole Jr DH, Godleski J, et al. Molecular pathologic substaging in 244 stage I non-small-cell lung cancer patients: clinical implications. *J Clin Oncol* 1998;**16**:2468-77.
98. D'Amico TA, Massey M, Herndon JE 2nd, Moore MB, Harpole DH Jr. A biologic risk model for stage I lung cancer: immunohistochemical analysis of 408 patients with the use of ten molecular markers. *J Thorac Cardiovasc Surg* 1999;**117**:736-43.
99. Gordon GJ, Jensen RV, Hsiao LL, et al. Translation of microarray data into clinically relevant cancer diagnostic tests using gene expression ratios in lung cancer and mesothelioma. *Cancer Res* 2002;**62**:4963-7.
100. Patz EF Jr, Campa MJ, Gottlin EB, Kusmartseva I, Guan XR, Herndon JE 2nd. Panel of serum biomarkers for the diagnosis of lung cancer. *J Clin Oncol* 2007;**25**:5578-83.
101. Brooks KR, To K, Joshi MB, et al. Measurement of chemoresistance markers in patients with stage III non-small cell lung cancer: a novel approach for patient selection. *Ann Thorac Surg* 2003;**76**:187-93:discussion 193.
102. Birnbaum A, Ready N. Gefitinib therapy for non-small cell lung cancer. *Curr Treat Options Oncol* 2005;**6**:75-81.
103. Kris MG, Natale RB, Herbst RS, et al. Efficacy of gefitinib, an inhibitor of the epidermal growth factor receptor tyrosine kinase, in symptomatic patients with non-small cell lung cancer: a randomized trial. *JAMA* 2003;**290**:2149-58.
104. Lynch TJ, Bell DW, Sordella R, et al. Activating mutations in the epidermal growth factor receptor underlying responsiveness of non-small-cell lung cancer to gefitinib. *N Engl J Med* 2004;**350**:2129-39.
105. Sakurada A, Shepherd FA, Tsao MS. Epidermal growth factor receptor tyrosine kinase inhibitors in lung cancer: impact of primary or secondary mutations. *Clin Lung Cancer* 2006;**7**(4 Suppl.):S138-44.
106. Potti A, Mukherjee S, Petersen R, et al. A genomic strategy to refine prognosis in early-stage non-small cell lung cancer. *N Engl J Med* 2006;**355**:570-80.
107. Chen ZL, Perez S, Holmes EC, et al. Frequency and distribution of occult micrometastases in lymph nodes of patients with non-small-cell lung carcinoma. *J Natl Cancer Inst* 1993;**85**:493-8.
108. Passlick B, Izbicki JR, Kubuschok B, Thetter O, Pantel K. Detection of disseminated lung cancer cells in lymph nodes: impact on staging and prognosis. *Ann Thorac Surg* 1996;**61**:177-82:discussion 183.
109. Dobashi K, Sugio K, Osaki T, Oka T, Yasumoto K. Micrometastatic P53-positive cells in the lymph nodes of non-small-cell lung cancer: prognostic significance. *J Thorac Cardiovasc Surg* 1997;**114**:339-46.
110. Nicholson AG, Graham AN, Pezzella F, Agneta G, Goldstraw P, Pastorino U. Does the use of immunohistochemistry to identify micrometastases provide useful information in the staging of node-negative non-small cell lung carcinomas? *Lung Cancer* 1997;**18**:231-40.
111. Maruyama R, Sugio K, Mitsudomi T, Saitoh G, Ishida T, Sugimachi K. Relationship between early recurrence and micrometastases in the lymph nodes of patients with stage I non-small-cell lung cancer. *J Thorac Cardiovasc Surg* 1997;**114**:535-43.
112. Goldstein NS, Mani A, Chmielewski G, Welsh R, Pursel S. Immunohistochemically detected micrometastases in peribronchial and mediastinal lymph nodes from patients with T1, N0, M0 pulmonary adenocarcinomas. *Am J Surg Pathol* 2000;**24**:274-9.
113. Ohta Y, Oda M, Wu J, et al. Can tumor size be a guide for limited surgical intervention in patients with peripheral non-small cell lung cancer? assessment from the point of view of nodal micrometastasis. *J Thorac Cardiovasc Surg* 2001;**122**:900-6.
114. Gu CD, Osaki T, Oyama T, et al. Detection of micrometastatic tumor cells in pN0 lymph nodes of patients with completely resected nonsmall cell lung cancer: impact on recurrence and survival. *Ann Surg* 2002;**235**:133-9.
115. Osaki T, Oyama T, Gu CD, et al. Prognostic impact of micrometastatic tumor cells in the lymph nodes and bone marrow of patients with completely resected stage I non-small-cell lung cancer. *J Clin Oncol* 2002;**20**:2930-6.
116. Marchevsky AM, Qiao JH, Krajisnik S, Mirocha JM, McKenna RJ. The prognostic significance of intranodal isolated tumor cells and micrometastases in patients with non-small cell carcinoma of the lung. *J Thorac Cardiovasc Surg* 2003;**126**:551-7.
117. Rena O, Carsana L, Cristina S, et al. Lymph node isolated tumor cells and micrometastases in pathological stage I non-small cell lung cancer: prognostic significance. *Eur J Cardiothorac Surg* 2007;**32**:863-7.

CHAPTER 46
Innovative Therapy and Technology

Joseph J. Wizorek, Arjun Pennathur, Neil A. Christie, Hiran C. Fernando, and James D. Luketich

Radiofrequency Ablation
  Patient Selection
  Operative Technique
  Treatment Response
  Clinical Results
Stereotactic Radiosurgery
  Techniques
  Patient Selection
  Results
  Summary
Microwave Ablation
Chemoperfusion of the Pleural Cavity
Implications for Thoracic Surgical Oncologists
  Summary

Lung cancer remains the number one cause of cancer-related deaths in men and women, and the incidence continues to rise with approximately 175,000 new cases diagnosed annually in the United States.[1] In this chapter, we review several innovative therapies for the treatment of bronchogenic and metastatic lung tumors. Application of these new therapies continues to evolve, and in most cases, surgical resection remains the mainstay of therapy. However, most patients with non–small cell lung carcinoma (NSCLC) present with advanced disease, and many with early-stage disease are unable to tolerate pulmonary resection because of compromised cardiopulmonary function.[2] The new alternatives to traditional surgical treatment allow additional options when surgery is not clearly of benefit or when the patient is not a candidate for traditional resection. Like other recent advances, such as videothoracoscopy, these new less-invasive approaches may allow surgeons to treat patients with thoracic malignant neoplasms even in the setting of marginal pulmonary reserve.[3]

The two principal nonoperative modalities are radiofrequency ablation and stereotactic radiosurgery. Another ablative modality, microwave ablation, is also being evaluated, although current clinical experience is limited with this novel approach. The main goal of these less-invasive therapies is to locally destroy the pulmonary or thoracic neoplasm while preserving the surrounding normal tissues. Also discussed in this chapter is the role of intrathoracic chemoperfusion for malignant neoplasms with a propensity for local pleural recurrence.

It is important that thoracic surgical oncologists stay abreast of these new therapies, design clinical trials, and critically evaluate and report the results. The introduction of new technology should not change the paradigm of who treats thoracic malignant neoplasms. Failure of surgeons to adapt to this new technology will lead to fragmentation in the care of the patient with a thoracic malignant neoplasm. In addition, most localized thoracic malignant neoplasms should still be treated surgically, and failure to involve an experienced thoracic surgical oncologist in the design of clinical trials will lead to compromised patient care.

RADIOFREQUENCY ABLATION

Radiofrequency ablation (RFA) uses high-frequency alternating current to heat and coagulate tissue. RFA systems have three components: (1) a generator, (2) an active electrode that is placed within the tumor, and (3) a dispersive electrode (Bovie pad) placed on the thighs of the patient (Fig. 46-1). As the radiofrequency energy moves from the active electrode to

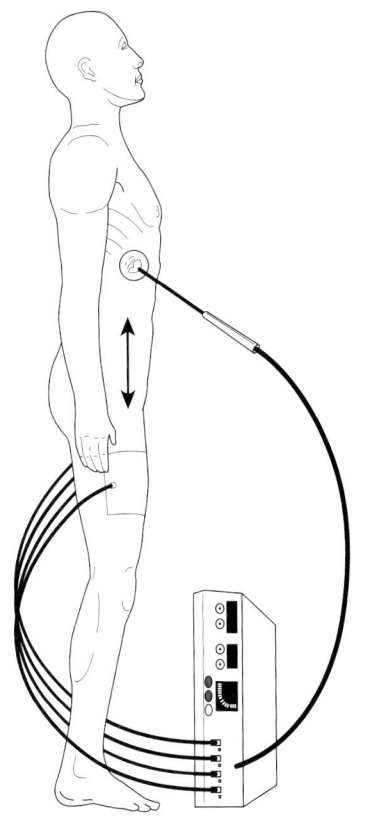

Figure 46–1
The radiofrequency ablation system.

the dispersive electrode and back, ions within the tissue oscillate with the changing direction of the current, resulting in frictional heating of the tissue. As the temperature within the tissue rises to more than 60°C, cell death occurs because of protein denaturation and coagulation necrosis. Moreover, the dispersion of energy beyond the vicinity of the active electrode is minimal, allowing focused delivery of energy to the target lesion with minimal injury to the surrounding normal tissue. The goal of RFA in the treatment of lung tumors is complete coagulation necrosis of the lesion with a small rim of extension into adjacent normal pulmonary parenchyma.

Most experience with RFA has been in the treatment of liver tumors, both as an adjunct to resection and as primary therapy. Because of lower complication rates, RFA has supplanted other less-invasive modalities (e.g., cryotherapy).[4,5] In a large international multicenter study of 2320 patients who underwent percutaneous RFA for malignant liver neoplasms, mortality was 0.3%, and the overall complication rate was 7.1%.[6]

Several centers around the world have published reports demonstrating the safety and feasibility of RFA for lung tumors.[7,8] Animal models, to investigate the feasibility of RFA for the treatment of lung tumors, have been used to develop treatment algorithms for humans. In a study by Goldberg and colleagues[9] with a rabbit model of lung sarcoma, seven lesions were treated with RFA for 6 minutes at 90°C, and the remaining four tumors were left untreated as controls. The authors noted computed tomography (CT) evidence of coagulation necrosis surrounding the tumor, manifested radiographically by increased opacity enveloping the lesion. This was followed temporally by the development of central tissue attenuation consistent with cavitation. Histologic analysis revealed that at least 95% of the tumor nodules were necrotic, although some rabbits (43%) had residual tumor nests at the periphery of the tumor. Pneumothorax was the only procedure-related complication, occurring in 29% of treated rabbits and 25% of controls. In another study, Miao and colleagues[10] implanted VX2 sarcomas into the lungs of 18 rabbits (12 treated and 6 controls). The lesions were then treated with RFA for 60 seconds with a cooled-tip electrode. Absolute tumor eradication was achieved in 33% of the rabbits. A partial response was observed in 41.6% of rabbits that survived longer than 3 months. On histopathologic evaluation, the ablated lesions retained their fundamental tissue architecture with evidence of coagulation necrosis. Surrounding edema and inflammation were noted in the normal adjacent pulmonary parenchyma. One to 3 months after treatment, the ablated tumor became an atrophied nodule of coagulation necrosis within a fibrotic capsule.

The timing and progression of these postablation changes become important issues in evaluating postprocedure treatment response in patients with pulmonary tumors. Some investigators have performed RFA followed by resection to evaluate the efficacy of the ablation procedure. In one multicenter study of 15 patients, ablation was possible in 13 cases.[11] In these 13 patients, median tumor kill was 70%, with seven patients achieving 100% ablation. Five of the final six cases exhibited 100% ablation, suggesting mastery of the learning curve for the technique. Nguyen and colleagues[12] published the results of an ablate-and-resect study in which vital immunohistochemical stains were used to assess tumor cell viability. In seven tumors studied with this technique, more than 80% nonviability was documented. Three patients (38%) demonstrated 100% nonviability. All three tumors were less than 2 cm in diameter. A single ablation with either a 3- or 3.5-cm active electrode was performed, such that the larger tumors may have been inadequately ablated. More recently, Schneider and colleagues[13] reported their series of ablate-and-resect pulmonary metastasectomies. Eighteen patients underwent RFA and subsequent thoracotomy and resection for 18 diverse solid tumor metastases. Lesion size ranged from 0.7 to 2.5 cm. The resected specimens were evaluated for tumor viability with immunohistochemistry. Complete ablation was achieved in 39%. More than 90% ablation was achieved in 50% of the resected lesions, and the authors considered this to be a successful ablation, asserting that subsequent growth of the residual lesion (had it not been resected) was unlikely. An incomplete ablation was documented in the remaining 11%. These studies demonstrate that although RFA can produce effective ablation, 100% tumor cell death is not universally achieved, and resection remains the treatment of choice for those able to tolerate surgical intervention.

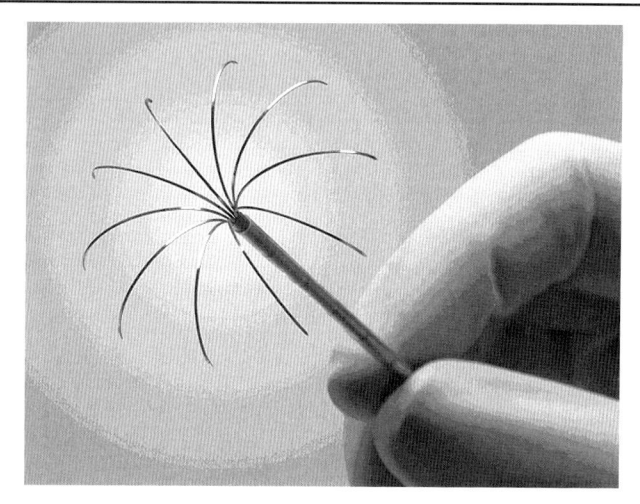

Figure 46–2
The Boston Scientific LeVeen needle electrode.

Currently, three U.S. Food and Drug Administration–approved devices are available for the performance of RFA: Boston Scientific (Boston, MA), RITA (Mountain View, CA), and Valley Laboratory (Boulder City, CO). The Boston Scientific device is an impedance-based system in which the endpoint of treatment is determined by a significant rise in tissue impedance, indicating an inability of the target lesion to maintain further conduction and, therefore, ablation. The RITA and Valley Laboratory systems are temperature-based devices that elevate the tumor temperature to predetermined lethal levels for a designated time. The Boston Scientific and RITA active probes both consist of an expandable needle system (Fig. 46-2 and 46-3); the Valley Laboratory system consists of either a single needle or three parallel needles (Fig. 46-4) that are placed within the tumor. The Valley Laboratory (VL) electrode consists of a proximal insulated portion and a distal uninsulated active tip. The electrode is irrigated with a continuous infusion of cold saline and for this reason is sometimes referred to as a *cool-tip electrode*. The dissolved saline ions enhance conduction and therefore, theoretically, decrease the required time to achieve effective ablation.

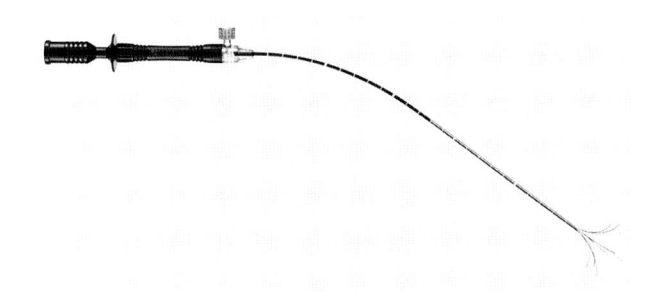

Figure 46–3
The RITA electrode.

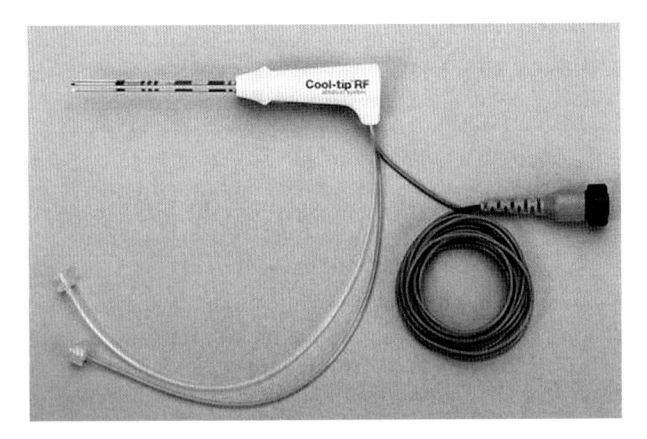

Figure 46–4
The Valley Laboratory (VL) probe.

Two animal studies comparing the relative efficacy of the various probes report disparate results. Pereira and colleagues[14] reported significantly better ablation lengths and volumes with the VL cool-tip probes compared with the expandable probes in a pig model of RFA. Conversely, Denys and coworkers[15] achieved larger volumes and more spherical ablation zones with the expandable probes compared with the VL cool-tip probe. A recent Japanese report of RFA for treatment of 342 pulmonary tumors in 128 patients cites tumor size greater than 2 cm and use of the single-needle VL probe to be associated with local progression on multivariate analysis. The single-needle VL probe was used for 195 of the ablation procedures, the Boston Scientific probe for 142; five of the procedures were performed with the VL cluster probes.[16]

Patient Selection

For NSCLC, RFA should be reserved for patients diagnosed as stage I who are believed to be at increased risk for pulmonary resection or for those who refuse surgery. On occasion, RFA may be a reasonable therapy for a medically inoperable patient with more advanced cancer (e.g., satellite nodules) localized to the lung.[17] The efficacy of RFA is low for nodules of more than 5 cm in diameter. RFA is also not recommended for lesions abutting the mediastinum.[18] Other patients who may be considered for treatment with RFA include those with advanced-stage disease who have responded to definitive radiation therapy and chemotherapy but have a persistent solitary peripheral focus of cancer and those who present with a recurrent isolated cancer after previous lung resection. RFA is also a suitable option for some patients with limited peripheral pulmonary metastases. Like resection, this treatment should be reserved for those patients with a limited number of metastases, disease localized to the chest, or controlled or controllable primary sites and only for those patients who are believed to be at increased operative risk for resection of their pulmonary metastases. In some situations, complete resection of all pulmonary metastases is not possible, and RFA can be used as an adjunct intraoperatively. We have certainly found RFA to be of use in the situation in which a wedge resection of a peripheral nodule was performed and resection of other nodules would have required a lobectomy or pneumonectomy. To preserve pulmonary parenchyma, some of these tumors were treated with intraoperative RFA through open thoracotomy. Table 46-1 outlines suggested selection criteria for the use of RFA.

Table 46–1
Selection Criteria for Radiofrequency Ablation

Inclusion Criteria	Exclusion Criteria
NSCLC stage I or II*; poor surgical candidate	Tumor abutting hilum or large pulmonary vessel
NSCLC stage IIIB (satellite nodule in same lobe) or stage IV (nodule in another lobe or lung); poor surgical candidate	Malignant effusion
Stage IIIA or IV with solitary pulmonary nodule remaining after standard therapies	Pulmonary hypertension
Pulmonary metastases; primary disease controlled or controllable; poor surgical candidate	More than three tumors in one lung
Target lesion ≤5 cm	Target lesion >5 cm

*Patients with stage II should receive additional therapy because N1 disease will not be treated with radiofrequency ablation.
NSCLC, non–small cell lung carcinoma.

Operative Technique

In our initial experience, RFA was performed through an open thoracotomy. This approach provides the most controlled method for RFA application but negates the most attractive attribute of the technology, that is, its nonoperative applicability. Surgical resection remains the standard of care for early-stage NSCLC. RFA should be used as an adjunct to surgery or as a suboptimal substitute in patients unable or unwilling to undergo resection. Situations may arise, such as that described previously, in which a patient presents with two or more tumors, some amenable to resection and others to RFA. Although video-assisted thoracoscopic surgery (VATS) has been postulated to be an attractive approach for the application of RFA, optimal needle deployment within the tumor in the setting of a collapsed lung is often difficult.

The most common method of pulmonary RFA entails percutaneous CT-guided administration. Either general or local anesthesia can be used in performing CT-guided RFA. Our preference has been to use general anesthesia.[19] This allows needle deployment, ablation, and biopsies (if required) to be

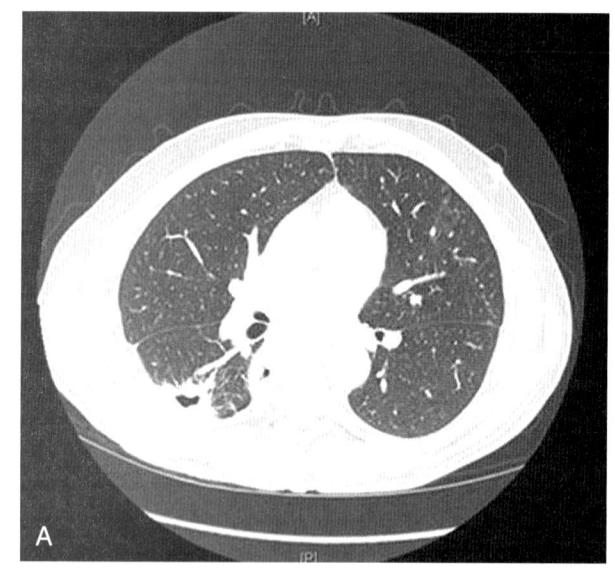

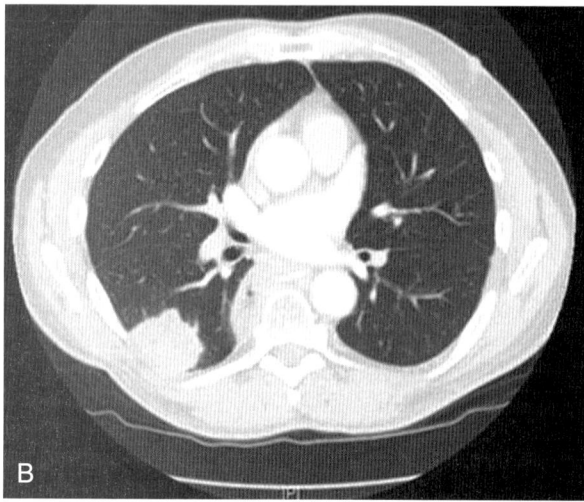

Figure 46–5
Radiographic evidence of tumor ablation. **A,** Before ablation. **B,** Three months after ablation; note central cavitation and overall decrease in size.

performed in a more controlled manner. In addition, some patients with cardiopulmonary compromise may have difficulty maintaining optimal body position if awake or sedated. Positioning of the patient is extremely important during CT-guided RFA. We prefer to position the patient in such a way that the target lesion is accessed with minimal penetration of normal lung parenchyma. This decreases the risks of hemorrhage and prolonged air leak. Positioning is also important to ensure adequate clearance of the RFA probe within the scanner. The maximum number of lesions that can be ablated in a single setting is debatable. As a general rule, however, ablation of more than three lesions in one setting is not recommended.

Treatment Response

RFA incites an inflammatory response that may persist for up to 3 months, making it difficult to determine radiographically whether the mass represents scar or viable cancer. The mass may initially appear larger on radiographic imaging and then subsequently decrease in size. Ablated lesions may demonstrate central cavitation (Fig. 46-5) or develop bubble lucencies, both of which are radiographic indicators of effective ablation. Other centers have used CT densitometry protocols to evaluate for persistent or recurrent disease.[20] Densitometry involves the injection of contrast material and subsequent CT images of the ablated nodule at 0, 45, 180, and 300 seconds after the injection of contrast material. Lesions larger than 9 mm that enhance to 15 Hounsfield units or more after 1 minute are suggestive of cancer. These densitometry techniques are time-consuming and typically valuable only for those patients with single tumor nodules. We have modified the Response Evaluation Criteria in Solid Tumors to evaluate treatment responses objectively (Table 46-2).[18] CT scans are obtained at 3-month intervals to assess lesion size and characteristics. Whenever possible, positron emission tomography (PET) scans are also obtained to aid in the determination of tumor response. The American College of Surgeons Oncology Group is accruing patients in a multicenter study evaluating RFA in high-risk patients with stage IA NSCLC. This study (Z4033) will address such issues as response assessment by standardizing the follow-up protocol used by the various study sites. Follow-up assessment will include CT (size criteria and densitometry) and serial PET scans.

Clinical Results

In our initial experience with RFA at the University of Pittsburgh, we treated 33 tumors in 18 patients.[18] Tumors included metastatic carcinoma ($n = 8$), sarcoma ($n = 5$), and NSCLC ($n = 5$). The mean age was 60 years (range, 27 to 95 years). Our principal finding was the lack of effectiveness in treating tumors larger than 5 cm. Using the Response Evaluation Criteria in Solid Tumors, we found that a radiographically determined response rate of 66% was seen for tumors of 5 cm or less compared with only 33% in patients with tumors larger than 5 cm. A multicenter study summarizing the results of 493 patients undergoing RFA of pulmonary nodules concluded that RFA is safe, with negligible morbidity and mortality (0.4%), and is associated with a gain in quality of life.[21] We have also reported the results of RFA in a series of 18 patients with NSCLC.[22] A total of 21 tumors were treated. Most patients ($n = 9$) had stage I NSCLC. There were four patients with stage IV cancer, including three patients with recurrences after previous lobectomy and one patient with a synchronous liver metastasis that was also treated with RFA. The median tumor diameter was 2.8 cm (range, 1.2 to 4.5 cm). Morbidity was minor in most cases but occurred in 55.6% of patients. The most common complication was pneumothorax (38.9%), which resolved with pigtail catheter drainage within 24 hours in most cases. At a median follow-up of 14 months, 83.3% of the patients were alive. Local progression occurred in 38.1% of the ablated nodules. For stage I cancer, the mean progression-free interval was 17.6 months; the median progression-free interval was not reached. Although this is a small study, these results compare favorably with standard methods of external beam radiation, in which local progression is seen in more than 50% of cases.[23]

More recently, we updated our experience with RFA for the treatment of stage I NSCLC.[24] Nineteen patients underwent RFA during a 3-year period. Median age was 78 years (range, 68 to 88 years). Initial complete response was observed in two patients (10.5%), partial response in 10 (53%), and stable disease in five (26%). Early progression occurred

Table 46-2
Modified Response Evaluation Criteria in Solid Tumors

Response	CT Mass Size	CT Mass Quality	PET
Complete (two of the following)	Lesion disappearance (scar) less than 25% of original size	Cyst or cavity formation Low density of entire lesion	SUV < 2.5
Partial (one of the following)	Decrease of more than 30% in the LD of target lesion	Central necrosis or central cavitation with liquid density	Decreased SUV or area of FDG uptake
Stable lesion (one of the following)	Decrease of less than 30% in the LD of target lesion	Mass solid appearance, no central necrosis or cavitation	Unchanged SUV or area of FDG uptake
Progression (two of the following)	Increase of more than 20% in the LD of target lesion	Solid mass, invasion of adjacent structures	Higher SUV or larger area of FDG uptake

FDG, fluorodeoxyglucose; LD, largest diameter; SUV, standard uptake value of [^{18}F]-FDG on PET scan.

in two patients (10.5%). During follow-up, local progression occurred in eight nodules (42%), and the median time to progression was 27 months. There was no procedure-related mortality, although six deaths occurred during follow-up. The median follow-up in the remaining patients was 23 months. The probability of survival at 1 year was estimated to be 95% (95% confidence interval [CI], 0.68-0.91), and the median survival was not reached.

Lanuti and colleagues[25] have recently published their mid-term results of a series of 31 nonsurgical patients with NSCLC who underwent a total of 38 percutaneous RFA treatments. There were no 30-day mortalities. Five patients developed pneumothorax; three required chest tubes. Six patients developed pneumonia within 4 weeks of treatment; all resolved with oral antibiotics. There were eight cases of postprocedure pleural effusion. These are typical morbidities. The authors note, however, one patient who developed transient laryngeal nerve injury after ablation of a left upper lobe lesion abutting the mediastinum. We reiterate that RFA should not be applied to central lesions. Tumor size ranged from 0.8 to 4.4 cm. Local recurrence was assessed by CT and PET and found in 31.5% of all treated tumors but in 50% of tumors larger than 3.0 cm, 44.4% of tumors 2.0 to 3.0 cm, and 21.7% of tumors smaller than 2.0 cm. Survival at median follow-up of 17 months was 74%, and overall survival was 30 months.

The RAPTURE study[26] was a prospective, intention-to-treat, single-arm, multicenter, international clinical trial designed to validate the feasibility and safety of RFA for pulmonary tumors as well as to assess efficacy; 106 patients with 183 tumors were treated with 137 RFA treatments. All patients were deemed to be nonsurgical candidates. The authors reported a 99% technical success rate. There were no mortalities. Pneumothorax requiring chest tube evacuation developed in 27 patients. Pleural effusions occurred in 15 patients, four requiring drainage. Tumor sizes ranged from 0.5 to 3.4 cm. Pulmonary function was assessed before the procedure and then at 1, 3, 6, and 12 months after the procedure and was not significantly changed. Of the 85 patients who could be assessed for tumor response, 88% exhibited complete response to treatment at 1 year. Local progression was noted in 12%. Overall survival was 70%, and cancer-specific survival was 92% at 1 year.

These results demonstrate feasibility and safety of RFA for pulmonary tumors not amenable to surgical resection. Further critical evaluation of ongoing clinical trials will aid in defining the impact of RFA on long-term tumor control and its potential applicability for larger tumors and more advanced disease.

STEREOTACTIC RADIOSURGERY

External beam radiation therapy is commonly used to treat NSCLC when surgical resection is not possible. Unfortunately, cure is rare, local progression is common, and morbidity can be significant. Qiao and associates[27] summarized results from 18 studies reporting external beam radiation for stage I NSCLC. The mean 3-year and 5-year survivals were 34% and 21%, respectively. In one study of 71 node-negative patients who received at least 60 Gy of external beam radiation to their primary tumors, 3-year and 5-year survivals were only 19% and 12%.[28]

In another study of radiation therapy in 60 patients with stage I or stage II NSCLC, local progression was documented in 53% of patients with a median progression-free survival of 18.5 months and an overall median survival of only 20 months.[23] Higher radiation doses seem to enhance local tumor control.[29] Bradley and colleagues[30] showed that patients receiving more than 70 Gy had better local control and cancer-specific survival than did those treated with lower doses. Increased doses of radiation, however, result in increased toxicity and damage to the surrounding pulmonary parenchyma. Radiation fibrosis seems to depend on the volume of lung irradiated above a threshold of 20 to 30 Gy.[31] Pulmonary toxicity is the major morbidity associated with external beam radiation treatment of NSCLC. Radiation pneumonitis is a potentially life-threatening sequela and occurred in 8.3% of patients treated with definitive radiotherapy.[23]

Techniques

Stereotactic radiosurgery (SRS) is a relatively new approach that enables the selective delivery of an intense dose of high-energy radiation to a precise target volume. The improved accuracy is achieved through computer-controlled spatial localization of the tumor and delivery of multiple cross-fired beams of radiation that converge on the tumor, minimizing injury to surrounding normal tissue. In many centers, this technology has become standard treatment for intracranial tumors (gamma knife). Unlike in the brain, however, respiratory motion imposes technical difficulties for the precise delivery of radiation to lung tumors. These respiratory displacements are greatest near the diaphragm and are less significant near the lung apices and adjacent to the carina. Several techniques are available to minimize the effects of respiratory motion on the precise delivery of the concentrated radiation. One approach is to use breath-holding techniques, often in combination with an abdominal compression device, to limit the ability of the diaphragm to move caudally.[32]

At the University of Pittsburgh, we have used the CyberKnife Stereotactic Radiosurgery System (Accuray, Sunnyvale, CA), a frameless SRS.[33] The CyberKnife system consists of a linear accelerator radiation source that is mounted on a robotic arm (Fig. 46-6). Before initiation of treatment, two to four small gold fiducials are implanted in the pulmonary parenchyma around the periphery of the tumor. This is accomplished either percutaneously by CT guidance or transbronchially under fluoroscopic guidance. At the time of therapy, cameras on the CyberKnife system use these markers to localize the tumor in space. The CyberKnife Synchrony option records respiratory motion and combines these data with the fiducial images to optimize precise radiation delivery for any point of the respiratory cycle. A major advantage with this system over those involving breath-holding and immobilization techniques is that the treatment times are shorter and therefore better tolerated by patients, who often have some degree of cardiopulmonary compromise (Fig. 46-7).

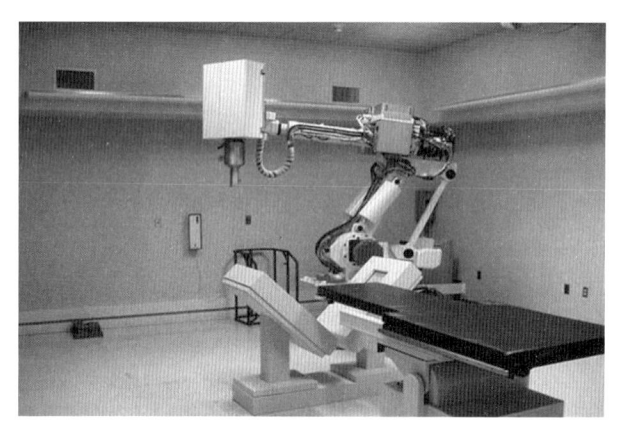

Figure 46–6
CyberKnife stereotactic robotic radiosurgery system.

Patient Selection

Patient selection is virtually identical to that for RFA. One advantage of SRS, however, is that central tumors can be safely treated. In addition, we have found that osteosarcomas can be extremely difficult to penetrate with the RFA needle. Because SRS requires fiducials to be positioned close to a tumor, rather than within it, SRS may be a better option for the treatment of metastatic osteosarcomas.

Results

Whyte and coworkers[34] published the first results of SRS with the CyberKnife system for the treatment of lung tumors. This study included 23 patients from two institutions. Respiratory

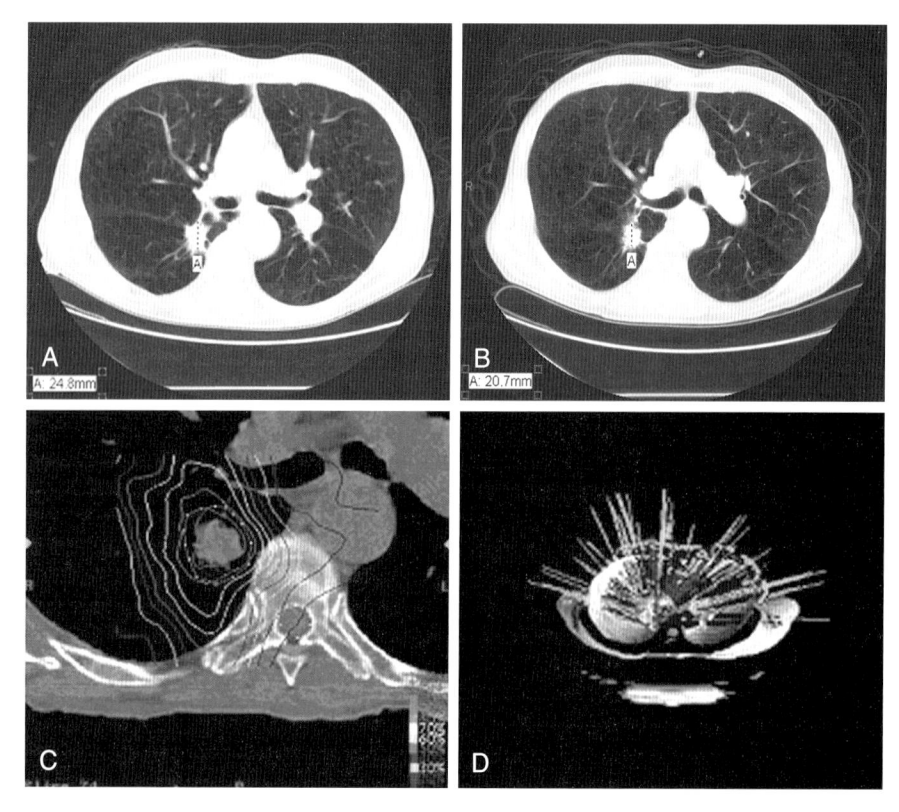

Figure 46–7
CT scans of right lung squamous carcinoma treated with CyberKnife (20 Gy single fraction). **A,** Before CyberKnife treatment. **B,** Three months after treatment; tumor size is decreased. **C,** Radiation plan with isodose mapping. **D,** Radiation paths.

gating was used in 14 patients and breath-holding in 9 patients. A single fraction of 15 Gy was used. Three patients developed pneumothorax after fiducial placement. There was no radiation esophagitis or clinically apparent radiation pneumonitis. At a mean follow-up of 7 months, two patients (8.6%) had a complete response, 15 (65.2%) had a partial response, four (17.4%) had stable disease, and two (8.7%) had evidence of progression.

In our initial experience at the University of Pittsburgh, 32 patients (27 with NSCLC and 5 with pulmonary metastases) were treated with SRS by the CyberKnife system.[33] Patients were treated with 20 Gy in a single fraction. The radiobiology of SRS (by virtue of a high single focused dose) is different from that of external beam radiation. The biologically effective dose is much higher.[35] Biological equivalent dose (BED10) is based on the linear-quadratic equation and allows dose comparison among different institutions. BED10 = nd (1 + d/[α/β]), where n is number of fractions, d is dose per fraction, and the α/β ratio value is unique to each tissue type (α/β = 3 for normal lung parenchyma, α/β = 10 for tumors).[36]

It has been shown that higher biologically effective doses improve local progression-free survival.[37,38] In our initial protocol, the 20-Gy dose was equivalent to a BED10 of 60 to 70 Gy with standard techniques.[33] After SRS in the 32 patients, an initial complete response was seen in seven (22%), partial response in 10 (31%), stable disease in nine (28%), and progression in five (16%). The probability of 1-year overall survival for the entire group and for patients assigned to stage I was 78% (95% CI, 65-0.94) and 91% (95% CI, 75-1), respectively. Both of these studies demonstrate the safety and feasibility of SRS; however, results are still inferior to pulmonary resection.

One issue that is being investigated is whether increasing the SRS dose improves outcomes. Timmerman and colleagues[32] have previously reported the results of a dose escalation study in 37 patients with stage I NSCLC. A breath-holding technique with abdominal compression was used. In this series, the dose was escalated from 20 to 60 Gy in three fractions. Complete response was seen in 27% of patients and a partial response in 60%. At a median follow-up of 15 months, six patients (16.2%) had experienced local failure. All six received lower than 18 Gy, supporting the concept of dose escalation. The same group published a follow-up study.[39] In patients with stage I NSCLC, tumors were stratified into T1[19] and T2.[29] Dose-limiting toxicity included bronchitis, pericardial effusion, hypoxia, and pneumonitis. Local failure occurred in four (21%) of the T1 tumors and six (21%) of the T2 tumors. In the T1 tumors, eight patients (42%) had regional or distant recurrence (or both). In the T2 tumors, six patients (21%) had regional or distant recurrence.

Several additional case series have also been published.[40-43] A recently published review by Nguyen and colleagues[36] compared effectiveness and morbidity of the published VATS lobectomy data (19 studies, 3988 patients) with the published SRS data (24 studies, 1485 patients) for early-stage NSCLC. The SRS data were further subgrouped into those studies that reported a BED10 of at least 100 Gy (14 studies, 969 patients) and those with a reported BED10 of less than 100 Gy (10 studies, 516 patients). Local control and survival were comparable for those studies that used a BED10 of 100 Gy or more. Mortality was 1% for the VATS group, 0.6% for the SRS group with more than 100 Gy, and 0% for the SRS group with less than 100 Gy. All of the SRS mortalities (six patients) were noted to be from a single study that used a BED10 of 180 Gy to centrally located tumors. Morbidity was 16% for the VATS group (prolonged air leak, arrhythmia, pneumonia, stroke, pulmonary embolism) versus 5% for the entire SRS group (grade 3-4 pneumonitis, rib fractures, pleural effusion). VATS 2- to 5-year survival ranged from 60% to 96%. Actuarial survival ranged from 42% to 91% for the SRS group with more than 100 Gy and from 24% to 90% for the SRS group with less than 100 Gy. Local control, although not reported in all studies, ranged from 88% to 100% for the VATS group, 74% to 100% for the SRS group with more than 100 Gy, and 57% to 91% for the SRS group with less than 100 Gy. The authors note that SRS is feasible, safe, and associated with minimal morbidity, and delivery of more than 100 Gy appears comparable to VATS lobectomy with respect to local control.[36] We have modified our initial protocol of delivering a single 20-Gy fraction to now include a second fraction to achieve a BED10 of more than 100 Gy.

Onishi and colleagues[44] reported the Japanese multi-institutional SBRT data. Ninety-nine patients who were surgical candidates but refused surgery underwent SRS. The 5-year overall survival was 88.4% for those patients treated with more than 100 Gy SRS and 69.4% for those treated with less than 100 Gy. Multi-institutional phase II studies of SRS in the treatment of potentially resectable stage I NSCLC are under way in Japan (JCOG0403) and the United States (RTOG0236). An international multicenter randomized study to address the role of SRS in the treatment of operable stage I NSCLC is the logical next step (RTOG 0618).

Summary

Neither of these novel treatment modalities (RFA or SRS) is as effective as resection. RFA ablates lesions from the inside out, with treatment failures typically seen at the periphery of the lesion. SRS, on the other hand, can be configured to deliver a lethal dose to the entire target volume, usually encompassing a small amount of normal lung parenchyma surrounding the lesion. At the University of Pittsburgh, we now routinely place fiducial markers during RFA for lesions larger than 3 cm or for asymmetric lesions in which a uniform ablation is not likely to be achieved. During follow-up, if persistent tumor is suspected, it can be re-treated with either another RFA application or SRS. We use CyberKnife more often than RFA for such scenarios.

MICROWAVE ABLATION

Microwave ablation (MWA) is a relatively recent, promising, novel tumor ablation modality. Microwaves comprise the zone of electromagnetic radiation between 900 and 2450 MHz. The sinus waves possess electrical properties, with the charge changing from positive to negative as the wave travels from peak to trough. As microwave radiation interacts with water, the individual polar molecules oscillate, flipping back and forth with the changing charge of the microwave. Because of the high-frequency electromagnetic radiation, the water molecules change direction 2 to 5 billion times per second. The resulting friction produces heat. This dielectric heating can be of sufficient magnitude to coagulate protein and to cause cell death.[45,46]

Like RFA, MWA is amenable to percutaneous and open approaches. In general, a microwave antenna is inserted into a target lesion by CT guidance in much the same way as the RFA probe is. The antenna is insulated throughout most of its length, with a variable length of exposed tip. The antenna is connected to a microwave generator that emits an electromagnetic wave. This leads to excitation of water molecules, subsequent friction and heat generation, and ultimately coagulation necrosis. Unlike in RFA, a dispersive electrode is not necessary. Moreover, multiple antennae can be activated simultaneously (multiple active antennae per lesion or treatment of multiple lesions simultaneously). MWA does not cause tissue boiling or charring, which can occur with RFA. Charring limits current conduction and compromises uniform ablation. Boiling limits the maximal attainable temperature. MWA may allow temperatures within the targeted lesions to be driven higher, resulting in a larger ablation zone in a shorter time.[46]

As with RFA, most clinical experience with MWA has been in the treatment of liver tumors.[46-48] MWA has been compared with RFA (using the RITA system) in a hepatic porcine model.[48a] Nineteen pigs were sacrificed at 0, 2, and 28 days after ablation. To quantitate the heat-sink effect of blood vessels on ablation, the investigators created a deflection score. This was defined by measuring the diameter of the zone of ablation at a blood vessel (>3 mm) and the diameter of the ablation zone adjacent to the same blood vessel. The percentage difference between those diameters is the deflection score. The deflection score was significantly less ($P < .02$) after MWA (3.6%) compared with RFA (17%). The ablation zone was significantly greater ($P < .01$) in the long axis after MWA (3.6 cm) than with RFA (2.2 cm). There were no differences, however, in short axis measurement or tumor volume. The differences in length of ablation may have been related to the protocol design. For MWA, a 3.6-cm electrode was used; whereas for RFA, deployment of the RITA probe was only 3.0 cm. Shibata and associates[47] performed a randomized comparison of MWA ($n = 36$) and RFA ($n = 36$) for small hepatocellular carcinomas. There were no significant differences noted in the rates of initial therapeutic effect, complications, or residual disease.

Clinical experience with MWA for the treatment of lung tumors is limited. Feng and coworkers[49] reported the application of MWA to 28 lung tumors in 20 patients. A response of 50% or more was noted in 13 of the nodules (46.4%) and a complete response in three (10.7%). No significant complications were noted. An ablate-and-resect study was performed by Simon and coauthors.[46] Patients underwent MWA before planned resection. The mean tumor diameter was 3 cm (range, 2 to 5.5 cm), with an average tumor volume of 7.1 cm³. The maximum ablation achieved was 4 cm (3 to 5 cm), with a tumor volume of 23.4 cm³.

Wolf and coworkers[50] recently published their retrospective experience in using MWA to treat 82 lung tumors (primary NSCLC and metastases) in 50 patients by CT guidance. Tumor size was 3.5 ± 1.6 cm. A single antenna was used for lesions of 2 cm or smaller; multiple antennae were used to treat lesions larger than 2 cm. Follow-up evaluation consisted of CT and PET imaging. There were no procedure-related mortalities. Morbidities included acute respiratory distress syndrome (two patients, 1% of ablations), cutaneous burns (three patients, 2%), pneumothorax (66 patients, 44%; 27 patients required tube evacuation), minor hemoptysis (six patients, 4%), and pneumonia (three patients, 2%). At mean follow-up of 10 months, 48% had residual or recurrent disease. Local control at 1 year was 67%; time to first recurrence was 16.2 months. Actuarial survival was 65%, 55%, and 45% at 1, 2, and 3 years, respectively. Cancer-specific survival was 83%, 73%, and 61% at 1, 2, and 3 years, respectively. Tumor size of more than 3 cm was not associated with decreased local control or survival. Radiographic evidence of postablation lesion cavitation was associated with reduced cancer-specific mortality.

MWA promises higher intratumoral temperatures, larger ablation zones, faster treatment times, and more uniform convection profiles than RFA. Additional experience with this modality along with refinements in equipment and techniques is necessary before the role of MWA can be established in the treatment of early-stage lung cancer.

CHEMOPERFUSION OF THE PLEURAL CAVITY

The results of surgical therapy alone or combined with traditional chemotherapy or radiation therapy have been disappointing for patients with malignant pleural extension from malignant mesothelioma, thymic malignant neoplasms, and NSCLC. The standard of care for most of these malignant neoplasms continues to evolve. One strategy is to surgically remove all gross disease (cytoreduction) and then bathe the hemithorax with cytotoxic agents (chemoperfusion). The advantage of this approach is the direct exposure of any residual microscopic disease to a higher drug concentration than that achievable by conventional (systemic) chemotherapy while also minimizing the toxic systemic side effects. Adding hyperthermia to this strategy has been shown in some studies to increase the local tissue and cellular concentrations of the chemotherapeutic agent compared with normothermic perfusion.[51] The drug most commonly reported for use in intrapleural hyperthermic chemoperfusion is cisplatinum. Additional proposed mechanisms of synergy between cisplatinum perfusion and hyperthermia include a significant enhancement of the DNA cross-linking effect of the drug and heat-induced inhibition of DNA repair.[52]

Most of the experience with intraoperative hyperthermic chemoperfusion has been in the treatment of intraperitoneal malignant neoplasms.[51-53] A few centers have published results of nonrandomized trials of cytoreductive surgery followed by intraoperative hyperthermic intrathoracic perfusion chemotherapy. In most centers, this application is limited to clinical trials, with the majority of the experience being reported for patients with malignant mesothelioma and, to a lesser degree, thymic malignant neoplasms. Limited data exist for the application of chemoperfusion for the treatment of stage IIIB NSCLC. Although a cautionary note must be added about efficacy, these reports have demonstrated feasibility and some optimism that local control and, in some cases, survival may be better compared with historical controls.

The optimal temperature of the perfusate is unknown, but temperatures higher than 43°C may be associated with an increased risk of pulmonary edema if the ipsilateral lung remains in situ, for example, after pleurectomy alone. In the case of extrapleural pneumonectomy, perfusion at the same operative setting as the resection may lead to an increased risk of postpneumonectomy pulmonary edema due to the aggressive hydration that is routinely administered to minimize the renal toxicity of cisplatinum. In our protocol, if extrapleural pneumonectomy is performed, we delay hyperthermic chemoperfusion with cisplatinum for 4 days. If the contralateral lung is functioning well at that point and there is minimal oxygen requirement, we return to the operating room and hydrate the patient aggressively to induce a diuresis. We then perform the hyperthermic chemoperfusion at 43°C for 2 hours with videothoracoscopic access.

In one report, Yellin and colleagues[53] described the results of hyperthermic pleural perfusion with cisplatinum in a heterogeneous group of patients with malignant pleural involvement. This group of 26 patients included seven with malignant mesothelioma, seven with stage IVA thymoma, four with thymic carcinoma, one with chest wall sarcoma, three with NSCLC, two with metastatic sarcoma, and two with metastatic carcinoma (one ovarian, one squamous of unknown origin). Surgical resection of all gross disease was attempted with resection and pleurectomy in 10, extrapleural pneumonectomy in eight, and incomplete resections in the other patients. Hyperthermic chemoperfusion was performed with cisplatinum at various concentrations at an infusion temperature of 42°C for 1 hour. Intrapleural temperatures ranged from 40.1°C to 41.5°C with a maximal systemic temperature of 38°C. Creatinine clearance remained unchanged in all patients, and no significant hematologic toxicities were reported. The most notable postoperative complication was empyema, which occurred in four of 26 patients (15%). There was one postoperative death from a gastric herniation, apparently unrelated to the chemoperfusion. Complete ipsilateral pleuropulmonary control of disease was reported in 17 of 24 (71%) assessable patients. Overall 3-year survival was 44% in this group of patients, which, as noted, was better than the expected survival based on historical controls.

In a report by de Bree and colleagues[54] from the Netherlands Cancer Institute, cytoreductive surgery was performed for 11 patients with malignant mesothelioma and three patients with pleural thymoma metastases. This was followed by hyperthermic chemoperfusion of the pleural cavity with a combination of doxorubicin (Adriamycin) and cisplatin. In the thymoma group, four perfusions were performed for three patients. Complications included one grade 2 nephrotoxicity and one wound dehiscence. At an early follow-up of 18 months, all three patients were alive and free of disease. In a follow-up comment, however, two of the patients suffered disease recurrence.[55] In the mesothelioma group, at a mean follow-up of 7 months, there were three recurrences, with two of the patients dying of contralateral and peritoneal disease.

The same group recently reported a comparison of 22 patients with stage I mesothelioma treated with cytoreductive surgery and hyperthermic chemoperfusion with another 15 mesothelioma patients treated with extrapleural pneumonectomy and postoperative hemithoracic radiation to 54 Gy (no chemoperfusion). The chemoperfusion group suffered the only postoperative mortalities (two, 9%), more complications (70% versus 53%), and shorter survival (11 months versus 29 months; P = NS). Local control was 67% versus 20% for the extrapleural pneumonectomy–radiation therapy group and the hyperthermic chemoperfusion group, respectively. Median time to local recurrence was not reached in the extrapleural pneumonectomy–radiation therapy group and was 9 months in the chemoperfusion group (P = .003). Although it is feasible, and with results not unlike those of historical controls, hyperthermic chemoperfusion was associated with significantly greater morbidity and shorter term of local control than in a contemporary cohort that underwent a simpler therapeutic regimen.[56]

Richards and associates,[57] however, recently reported their experience of 44 patients with malignant pleural mesothelioma who underwent resection followed by intraoperative intracavitary chemoperfusion with escalating doses of cisplatinum. They report an 11% mortality, dose-limiting renal toxicity with a dose of 250 mg/m^2 (9%), atrial fibrillation (32%), acute respiratory distress syndrome (11%), pneumonia (9%), and deep venous thrombosis (9%). A significant difference in survival was seen between those patients receiving low-dose hyperthermic chemoperfusion (50 to 150 mg/m^2; median survival, 6 months) and those receiving higher but not toxic doses (175 to 250 mg/m^2; median survival, 18 months).

The role of intracavitary chemotherapy with or without hyperthermia for thoracic malignant neoplasms with pleural involvement remains unclear. Further clinical trials will be required to determine the ideal candidates, the optimal chemotherapeutic agents, and the timing and temperature of the perfusate. Logical requirements for inclusion of patients in these treatment protocols include disease confined to one pleural cavity with no extrathoracic metastases and that gross removal of all local disease is achievable.

IMPLICATIONS FOR THORACIC SURGICAL ONCOLOGISTS

With the advent of percutaneous ablation techniques for the treatment of early-stage lung cancer, controversy has emerged about the optimal approach in treating these patients. These issues are driven by the emergence of novel technology that spans the practice venues of several disciplines; by interventional radiologists and pulmonologists eager to implement these techniques; by thoracic surgical oncologists reluctant to relinquish management of the cancer patient; by the patient's natural tendency to seek out less-invasive interventions; and by the detection of smaller, earlier, and more easily treatable lesions. A primary issue relates to who should be performing these procedures: experienced interventional radiologists with surgical "backup," surgeons with extensive experience in minimally invasive and percutaneous CT-guided techniques, or a combined approach whereby the radiologist performs the biopsy and the surgeon performs the ablation. A variety of scenarios have occurred at different centers based on institutional and departmental biases and the available expertise and interest of the surgical and radiology staff. A similar procedural evolution occurred with the implementation of VATS techniques. The Society of Thoracic Surgeons/American Association for Thoracic Surgery position statement on VATS has recommended that such procedures be performed by surgeons familiar with open thoracic surgical approaches and the management of their complications. The surgeon must have the judgment, training, and capability to proceed to an open thoracic procedure if necessary and should personally guide the preoperative and postoperative care of the patient.[58] Although some interventional radiologists may have the experience and ability to perform difficult percutaneous interventions, there is great variability in their clinical training, and many may have never studied or treated patients with lung cancer. Conversely, many thoracic surgeons have dedicated their entire training and career to treating lung cancer and perform minimally invasive and percutaneous procedures on a daily basis. Thoracic surgeons are specifically trained in the areas of pulmonary physiology and oncology, are personally capable of managing procedure-related complications, are involved in the primary and follow-up care of patients with cancer, and have developed a historical association with consultants in the management of this disease.

There is no doubt, however, that complacency of thoracic surgical leadership can lead to a critical deficiency in embracing and incorporating these new techniques in a timely manner, resulting in a loss of control of these modalities and potentially the patients themselves.

Credentialing is also an important and controversial issue. Hospital administration and departmental guidelines have to be established to identify those physicians approved to conduct these procedures. Surgeons need to complete a dedicated didactic session covering the basic knowledge base and techniques, in conjunction with a period of proctorship until proficiency is demonstrated after performing a prescribed number of supervised interventions. Currently, there are no nationally accepted standards for the credentialing of surgeons to perform RFA within the chest. Gaining access to a CT scanner can also be a complicated process. Operating rooms with built-in CT scanners offer the ideal environment for performing these procedures. The necessary surgical equipment and staff are on hand, making the procedure safer and more efficient. If the procedures must be performed in the radiology suite, negotiations must be performed for scheduling. The room must be capable of supporting an anesthesia circuit, with built-in oxygen and suction. All supplies related to the procedure must be stored on site or in a portable cart. Quality assurance programs must be implemented to ensure optimal patient outcomes, with a database monitoring treatment morbidity and mortality profiles. Thoracic surgeons are best suited to make the decision as to which surgical or ablative modality is to be used in any given clinical setting. Whether to use an open, thoracoscopic, or percutaneous technique to manage a patient with a small pulmonary nodule requires careful judgment and expertise with each technique to ensure an optimal oncologic outcome. Certainly, percutaneous therapeutic modalities will ultimately have a role in high-risk patients with compromised lung function.

Decision-making can be even more complex in managing patients with difficult lesions, such as ground-glass opacities. These lesions tend to be small and slow growing and have a more indolent natural history. Many of these lesions may represent carcinoma in situ or minimally invasive cancers for which anatomic resection with or without lymph node dissection may not be necessary.[59] The use of percutaneous ablative techniques in this setting may represent an ideal application of the technology.

As these innovative techniques are developed and refined, careful attention must be paid to several important pitfalls, including over-application in the setting of indeterminate solitary pulmonary nodules, inappropriate or inadequate management of small to medium-sized lung cancer, inappropriate interventions directed toward metastatic disease, and risk of inadequate staging before intervention. To avoid these pitfalls, thoracic surgeons should maintain a leadership position in the deployment of these techniques for the treatment of patients with thoracic malignant neoplasms.

Summary

RFA and SRS have been demonstrated to be safe with reasonable efficacy in the treatment of small lung tumors. It is unclear which option is the more effective in the treatment of NSCLC, with both RFA and SRS demonstrating similar early response and progression rates. RFA can be performed in one treatment session, whereas it now seems that SRS is more effective if larger doses of radiation over two to three fractions are performed. RFA is not recommended for centrally based tumors. There are also some tumors (e.g., small apical tumors, posteriorly positioned tumors close to the diaphragm, and tumors close to the scapula) that may be difficult to impale percutaneously. Such patients are more optimally treated with SRS. In certain circumstances, a combined approach may be beneficial (RFA and SRS).

Experience with MWA is currently too limited to assess its value in the armamentarium against lung cancer, but its potential is promising. Treatment times and heat-sink effect may be less with respect to RFA. This may prove to be protective, minimizing the necrosis of large blood vessel and reducing the risk of fatal hemoptysis. Future studies need to address long-term outcomes by use of standardized assessments of treatment response between centers. Comparisons between different RFA and SRS systems must be undertaken to delineate the optimal use of these strategies in the treatment of early-stage lung cancer. Until long-term data with these ablative techniques become available, surgical resection should be performed when it is clinically possible.

Although surgical resection remains the gold standard for local control of pulmonary malignant neoplasms, newer technologies such as radiofrequency ablation and stereotactic radiosurgery hold the potential for less-invasive treatment in the future. We anticipate that these newer less-invasive techniques will complement existing minimally invasive surgical treatments and may further ease the burden of treatment and also ultimately improve survival in selected high-risk patients with pulmonary tumors. Critical appraisal of these techniques during the next decade will establish their role, and the thoracic surgical oncologist must remain abreast of the evolving technology and play an active leadership role in its evaluation.

REFERENCES

1. Jemal A, Siegel R, Ward E, et al. Cancer statistics, 2006. *CA Cancer J Clin* 2006;**56**:106-30.
2. Bach PB, Cramer LD, Warren JL, et al. Racial differences in the treatment of early stage non–small cell lung cancer. *N Engl J Med* 1999;**341**:1198-205.
3. McKenna RJ, Houck W, Fuller CB. Video-assisted thoracic surgery lobectomy: experience with 100 cases. *Ann Thorac Surg* 2006;**81**:421-6.
4. Sutherland LM, Williams JA, Padbury RT, et al. Radiofrequency ablation of liver tumors: a systematic review. *Arch Surg* 2006;**141**(2):181-90.
5. Jungraithmayr W, Burger D, Olschewski M, et al. Cryoablation of malignant liver tumors: results of a single center study. *Hepatobiliary Pancreat Dis Int* 2005;**4**(4):554-60.
6. Livraghi T, Solbiati L, Meloni MF, et al. Treatment of focal liver tumors with percutaneous radio-frequency ablation: complications encountered in a multicenter study. *Radiology* 2003;**226**:441-51.
7. Dupuy DE, Zagoria RJ, Akerley W, et al. Percutaneous radiofrequency ablation of malignancies in the lung. *AJR Am J Roentgenol* 2000;**174**(1):57-9.
8. Schaefer O, Lohrman C, Langer M. CT guided radiofrequency ablation of a bronchogenic carcinoma. *Br J Radiol* 2003;**76**:268-70.
9. Goldberg SN, Gazelle GS, Compton CC, et al. Radiofrequency tissue ablation of VX2 tumor nodules in the rabbit lung. *Acad Radiol* 1996;**3**:929-35.

10. Miao Y, Ni Y, Bosmans H, et al. Radiofrequency ablation for eradication of pulmonary tumor in rabbits. *J Surg Res* 2001;**99**:265-71.
11. Yang S, Whyte R, Askin F, et al. Radiofrequency ablation of primary and metastatic lung tumors: analysis of an ablate and resect study. Presented at the American Association for Thoracic Surgery 82nd Annual Meeting, Washington, DC, May 5-8, 2002.
12. Nguyen CL, Scott WJ, Young NA, et al. Radiofrequency ablation of primary lung cancer: results from an ablate and resect pilot study. *Chest* 2005;**128**:3507-11.
13. Schneider T, Warth A, Herpel E, et al. Intraoperative radiofrequency ablation of lung metastases and histologic evaluation. *Ann Thorac Surg* 2009;**87**:379-84.
14. Pereira PL, Trubenbach J, Schenk M, et al. Radiofrequency ablation: in vivo comparison of four commercially available devices in pig livers. *Radiology* 2004;**232**:482-90.
15. Denys AL, De Baere T, Kuoch V, et al. Radiofrequency tissue ablation of the liver: in vivo and ex vivo experiments with four different systems. *Eur Radiol* 2003;**13**:2346-52.
16. Hiraki T, Sakurai J, Tsuda T, et al. Risk factors for local progression after percutaneous radiofrequency ablation of lung tumors: evaluation based on a preliminary review of 342 tumors. *Cancer* 2006;**107**:2973-80.
17. Battafarano RJ, Meyers BF, Guthrie TJ, et al. Surgical resection of multifocal non–small cell lung cancer is associated with prolonged survival. *Ann Thorac Surg* 2002;**74**:988-93.
18. Herrera LJ, Fernando HC, Perry Y, et al. Radiofrequency ablation of pulmonary malignant tumors in non-surgical candidates. *J Thorac Cardiovasc Surg* 2003;**125**:29-937.
19. Hoffman RT, Jacobs TF, Lubienski A, et al. Percutaneous radiofrequency ablation of pulmonary tumors—is there a difference between treatment under general anaesthesia and under conscious sedation? *Eur J Radiology* 2006;**59**:168-74.
20. Suh RD, Wallace AB, Sheehan RE, et al. Unresectable pulmonary malignancies: CT guided percutaneous radiofrequency ablation. Preliminary results. *Radiology* 2003;**229**:821-9.
21. Steinke K, Sewell PE, Dupuy D, et al. Pulmonary radiofrequency ablation: an international study survey. *Anticancer Res* 2004;**24**:339-43.
22. Fernando HC, De Hoyos A, Landreneau RJ, et al. Radiofrequency ablation for the treatment of nonsmall cell lung cancer in marginal surgical candidates. *J Thorac Cardiovasc Surg* 2005;**129**:639-44.
23. Zierhut D, Bettscheider C, Schubert K, et al. Radiation therapy of stage I and II non–small cell lung cancer. *Lung Cancer* 2001;**34**:S39-43.
24. Pennathur A, Luketich JD, Abbas G, et al. Radiofrequency ablation for treatment of stage I non–small cell lung cancer in high-risk patients. *J Thorac Cardiovasc Surg* 2007;**134**:857-64.
25. Lanuti M, Sharma A, Digumarthy S, et al. Radiofrequency ablation for treatment of medically inoperable stage I non–small cell lung cancer. *J Thorac Cardiovasc Surg* 2009;**137**:160-6.
26. Lencioni R, Crocetti L, Cioni R, et al. Response to radiofrequency ablation of pulmonary tumors: a prospective, intention-to-treat, multicentre clinical trial (the RAPTURE study). *Lancet Oncology* 2008;**9**:621-8.
27. Qiao X, Tullgren O, Lax I, et al. The role of radiotherapy in treatment of stage I non–small cell lung cancer. *Lung Cancer* 2003;**41**:1-1.
28. Kupelian PA, Komaki R, Allen P. Prognostic factors in the treatment of node-negative non–small cell lung carcinoma with radiation alone. *Int J Radiat Oncol Biol Phys* 1996;**36**:607-13.
29. Bauermann M, Appold S, Peterson S, et al. Dose and fractionation concepts in the primary radiotherapy of non–small cell lung cancer. *Lung Cancer* 2001;**33**(Suppl):S35-45.
30. Bradley JD, Ieumwananonthachai N, Purdy JA, et al. Gross tumor volume, critical prognostic factor in patients with three-dimensional conformal radiation therapy for non–small cell lung cancer. *Int J Radiat Oncol Biol Phys* 2002;**52**(1):49-57.
31. Abratt RP, Morgan GW. Lung toxicity following chest irradiation in patients with lung cancer. *Lung Cancer* 2002;**35**(2):103-9.
32. Timmerman R, Papiez L, McGarry R, et al. Extracranial stereotactic radioablation: results of a phase I study in medically inoperable stage I non–small cell lung cancer. *Chest* 2003;**124**:1946-55.
33. Pennathur A, Luketich JD, Burton S, et al. Stereotactic radiosurgery for the treatment of lung neoplasm: initial experience. *Ann Thorac Surg* 2007;**83**:1820-5.
34. Whyte RI, Crownover R, Murphy MJ, et al. Stereotactic radiosurgery for lung tumors: preliminary report of a phase I trial. *Ann Thorac Surg* 2003;**75**:1097-101.
35. Timmerman RD, Papiez L, et al. The Song/Kavanagh/Benedict: Article reviewed. *Oncology* 2004;**18**:1430-5.
36. Nguyen NP, Garland L, Welsh J, et al. Can stereotactic fractionated radiation therapy become the standard of care for early stage non–small cell lung carcinoma? *Cancer Treat Rev* 2008;**34**:719-27.
37. Timmerman R, Galvin J, Michalski J, et al. Accreditation and quality assurance for radiation therapy oncology group: multicenter clinical trials using stereotactic body radiation therapy in lung cancer. *Acta Oncologica* 2006;**45**:779-86.
38. Martel M, Ten Haken R, Hazuka M, et al. Estimation of tumor control probability from 3-D dose distributions of non–small cell lung cancer patients. *Lung Cancer* 1999;**24**:31-7.
39. McGarry RC, Papiez L, Williams M, et al. Stereotactic body radiation therapy of early-stage nonsmall cell lung carcinoma: phase I study. *Int J Radiat Oncol Biol Phys* 2005;**63**:1010-5.
40. Timmerman RD, Park C, Kavanagh BD. The North American experience with stereotactic body radiation therapy in non–small cell lung cancer. *J Thorac Oncology* 2007;**2**(Suppl. 3):S101-12.
41. Brown WT, Wu X, Amendola B, et al. Treatment of early non–small cell lung cancer, stage IA, by image-guided robotic stereotactic radioablation—CyberKnife. *Cancer J* 2007;**13**:87-94.
42. Baumann P, Nyman J, Lax I, et al. Factors important for efficacy of stereotactic body radiotherapy of medically inoperable stage I lung cancer. A retrospective analysis of patients treated in the Nordic countries. *Acta Oncologica* 2006;**45**:787-95.
43. Brown WT, Wu X, Fowler JF, et al. Lung metastases treated by CyberKnife image-guided robotic stereotactic radiosurgery at 41 months. *South Med J* 2008;**101**:376-82.
44. Onishi H, Shirato H, Hiraoka M, et al. Hypofractionated stereotactic radiotherapy for stage I non–small cell lung cancer: updated results of 257 patients in a Japanese multi-institutional study. *J Thorac Oncol* 2007;**2**:S94-100.
45. Furukawa K, Toyoaki M, Kato Y, et al. Microwave coagulation therapy in canine peripheral lung tissue. *J Surg Res* 2005;**123**:245-50.
46. Simon CS, Dupuy DE, Mayo-Smith WW. Microwave ablation: principles and applications. *Radiographics* 2005;**25**:S69-83.
47. Shibata T, Limuro Y, Yammoto Y, et al. Small hepatocellular carcinoma: comparison of radiofrequency ablation and percutaneous microwave coagulation therapy. *Radiology* 2002;**223**:331-7.
48. Lu MD, Chen JW, Xie XY, et al. Hepatocellular carcinoma: US-guided percutaneous microwave coagulation therapy. *Radiology* 2001;**221**:167-72.
48a. Wright AS, Sampson LA, Warner TF, et al. Radiofrequency versus microwave ablation in a hepatic porcine model. *Radiology* 2005;**236**:132-39.
49. Feng W, Liu W, Liu C, et al. Percutaneous microwave coagulation therapy for lung cancer. *Zhonghua Zhong Liu Za Zhi* 2002;**24**:388-90.
50. Wolf FJ, Grand DJ, Machan JT, et al. Microwave ablation of lung malignancies: effectiveness, CT findings, and safety in 50 patients. *Radiology* 2008;**247**:871-9.
51. Witkamp AJ, de Bree E, Zoetmulder FA. Rationale and techniques of intraoperative hyperthermic intraperitoneal chemotherapy. *Cancer Treat Rev* 2001;**27**:365-75.
52. Kodama K, Doi O, Tatsuta M, et al. Development of postoperative intrathoracic chemo-thermotherapy for lung cancer with objective of improving local cure. *Cancer* 1989;**64**:1422-8.
53. Yellin A, Simansky DA, Paley M, et al. Hyperthermic pleural perfusion with cisplatin: Early clinical experience. *Cancer* 2001;**92**:2197-203.
54. de Bree E, van Ruth S, Baas P, et al. Cytoreductive surgery and intraoperative hyperthermic chemotherapy in patients with malignant pleural mesothelioma or pleural metastases of thymoma. *Chest* 2002;**121**:480-7.
55. de Bree E, van Ruth S, Rutgers EJ, et al. Reoperation combined with intraoperative hyperthermic intrathoracic perfusion chemotherapy for pleural recurrence of thymoma. Letter to the editor. *J Surg Oncol* 2002;**80**:224-5.
56. van Sandick J, Kappers I, Baas P, et al. Surgical treatment in the management of malignant pleural mesothelioma: a single institution's experience. *Ann Surg Onc* 2008;**15**(6):1757-64.
57. Richards WG, Zellos L, Bueno R, et al. Phase I to II study of pleurectomy/decortication and intraoperative intracavitary hyperthermic cisplatin lavage for mesothelioma. *J Clin Oncol* 2006;**24**:1561-7.
58. McNeally MF, Lewis RJ, Anderson RJ, et al. Statement of the STS/ AATS joint committee on thoracoscopy and video-assisted thoracic surgery. *J Thorac Cardiovasc Surg* 1992;**104**(1):1.
59. Noguchi M, Morikawa A, Kawasaki M, et al. Small adenocarcinoma of the lung: histologic characteristics and prognosis. *Cancer* 1995;**75**(12):2844-52.

Section 2

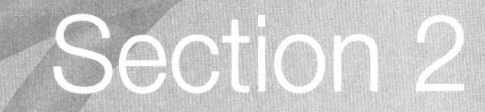

Adult Cardiac Surgery

Basic Science

Diagnostic Procedures

Medical- and Catheter-Based Treatment of Cardiovascular Disease

Perioperative and Intraoperative Care of the Cardiac Surgical Patient

Surgical Management of Aortic Disease

Surgical Management of Valvular Heart Disease

Management of Cardiac Arrhythmias

Surgical Treatment of Coronary Artery Disease and Its Complications

Surgical Management of Heart Failure

A. Basic Science

CHAPTER 47

Surgical Anatomy of the Heart

Andrew C. Cook, Benson R. Wilcox, and Robert H. Anderson

Location of the Heart
Morphologically Right Atrium
Morphologically Left Atrium
Morphologically Right Ventricle
Morphologically Left Ventricle
Aorta
Pulmonary Trunk and Branch Pulmonary Arteries
Coronary Arteries and Veins

In this chapter, we provide a brief overview of cardiac structure as it is relevant for the cardiac surgeon. We describe the heart as it is located in the body in its anatomic, or attitudinally correct, position.[1] Whenever possible, however, we illustrate the cardiac components as they would be viewed by the surgeon during an operative procedure, whether the pictures were taken in the operating room or are of anatomic specimens.[2] However, in some instances, information is best presented with the heart photographed in a nonsurgical orientation. When this occurs, it is clearly stated.

LOCATION OF THE HEART

Regardless of the surgical approach, the surgeon who enters the mediastinum is confronted by the heart enclosed in its pericardial sac. The sac is freestanding around the atrial chambers and the ventricles, but it becomes adherent to the adventitial coverings of the great arteries and veins at their entrances to and exits from the heart, where these attachments close the pericardial cavity. The pericardial cavity is contained between the two layers of the serous pericardium, a thin-walled sac folded on itself within the fibrous cavity. The inner layer, or epicardium, is firmly attached to the myocardium, whereas the outer layer is adherent to the fibrous pericardium. The pericardial cavity, therefore, is the space between the inner lining of the fibrous pericardium and the surface of the heart (Fig. 47-1). By virtue of the shape of the cardiac chambers and the great arteries, there are two recesses within this cavity that are lined by serous pericardium. The first is the transverse sinus, a horseshoe-shaped space behind the great arteries and in front of the atria (Fig. 47-2). Laterally on each side, the ends of the transverse sinus are in free communication with the rest of the pericardial cavity. The second pericardial recess is the oblique sinus, a blind-ending cavity behind the left atrium (Fig. 47-3).

Most of the cardiac surface facing the surgeon is occupied by the so-called right heart, which in reality is anterior. Thus, the surgeon is confronted by the extensive appendage of the right atrium, receiving the superior caval vein at its superior border. To the left are the aorta and the pulmonary trunk, exiting from the base of the heart and extending in a superior direction, with the aortic root in an inferior and rightward position. When the aortic root is not in this "normal" relationship, the ventriculoarterial connections are almost always abnormal. The morphologically right appendage has a characteristic shape, being triangular and possessing a broad junction with its venous component (Fig. 47-4). The morphologically left appendage may not be seen immediately. If searched for, it is found as a tubular, meandering structure at the left border of the pulmonary trunk (Fig. 47-5), having a narrow junction with the rest of the atrium.

The ventricular mass then extends to the cardiac apex, which normally reaches into the left hemithorax. The overall cardiac silhouette is usually positioned with one third of its bulk to the right and two thirds to the left of the midline (Fig. 47-6). An anomalous position of either the ventricular mass or the apex is highly suggestive of the presence of congenital cardiac malformations, although not always. In shape, the ventricular mass is a three-sided pyramid, having (1) diaphragmatic, (2) anterior or sternocostal, and (3) left or pulmonary surfaces. The margin between the first two surfaces is sharp, so it is called the acute margin. The transition between the sternocostal and pulmonary surfaces is more gradual and rounded.

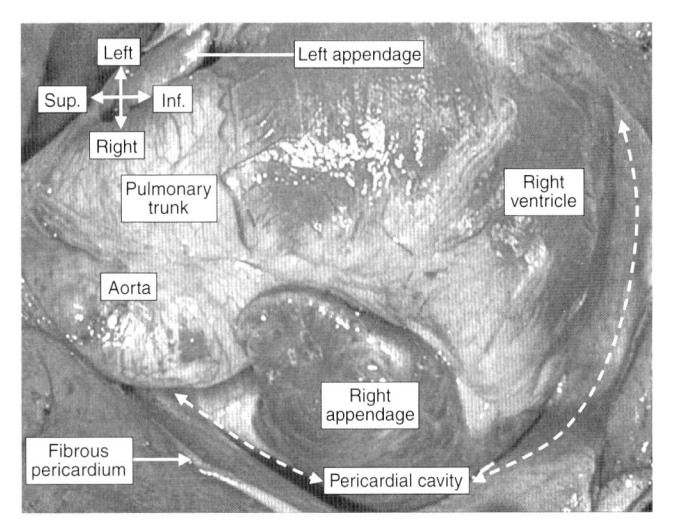

Figure 47-1
The heart is shown as seen by the surgeon through a median sternotomy. The pericardial cavity has been opened and is between the fibrous pericardium and the epicardium. The compass shows the orientation. (See color version in the online edition through Expert Consult.) *(Copyright for the original illustration from which this figure was prepared belongs to Benson R. Wilcox, Andrew C. Cook, and Robert H. Anderson.)*

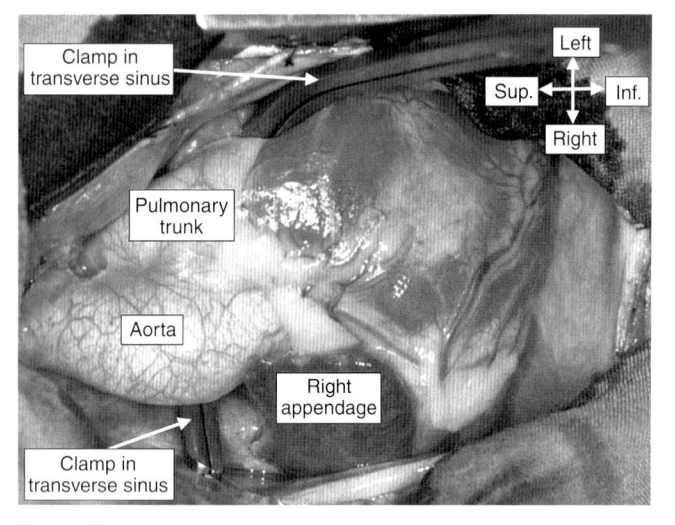

Figure 47–2
With the pericardium opened in the operating room, the surgical clamp has been passed through the transverse sinus of the pericardium, which is between the back of the arterial trunks and the front of the atrial chambers. (See color version in the online edition through Expert Consult.) *(Copyright for the original illustration from which this figure was prepared belongs to Benson R. Wilcox, Andrew C. Cook, and Robert H. Anderson.)*

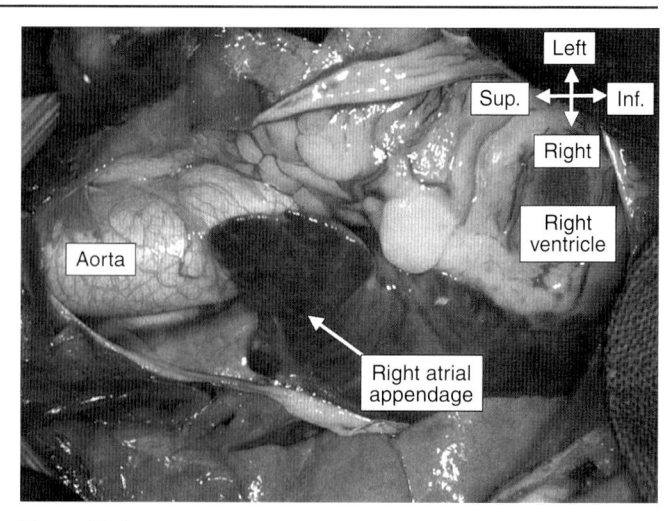

Figure 47–4
This picture of the heart, as seen in the operating room through a median sternotomy, shows the typical triangular appearance of the morphologically right atrial appendage. (See color version in the online edition through Expert Consult.) *(Copyright for the original illustration from which this figure was prepared belongs to Benson R. Wilcox, Andrew C. Cook, and Robert H. Anderson.)*

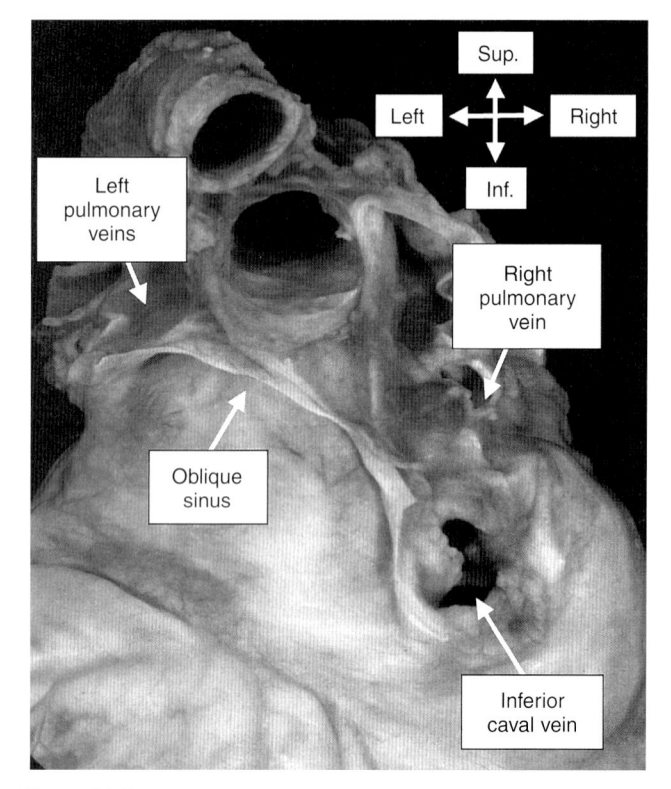

Figure 47–3
This anatomic specimen has been removed from the body and is viewed from behind, with the apex pointing down. The oblique sinus of the pericardium is seen between the pericardial reflections around the pulmonary veins and the inferior caval vein. (See color version in the online edition through Expert Consult.) *(Copyright for the original illustration from which this figure was prepared belongs to Benson R. Wilcox, Andrew C. Cook, and Robert H. Anderson.)*

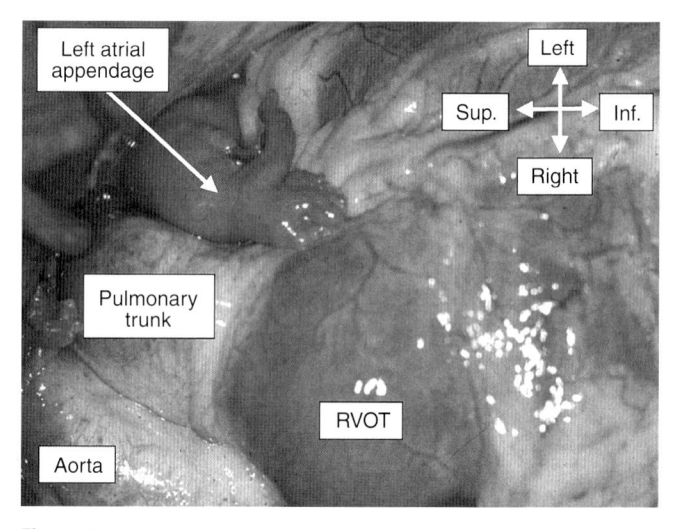

Figure 47–5
In this picture, with the pericardium opened through a median sternotomy, the heart has been rotated slightly to show the typical tubular configuration of the morphologically left atrial appendage. RVOT, right ventricular outflow tract. (See color version in the online edition through Expert Consult.) *(Copyright for the original illustration from which this figure was prepared belongs to Benson R. Wilcox, Andrew C. Cook, and Robert H. Anderson.)*

For the surgeon, it is the pulmonary surface that is considered to be the obtuse margin, as it is irrigated by the obtuse marginal arteries (Fig. 47-7). The greater part of the anterior surface of the ventricular mass is occupied by the morphologically right ventricle. Its left border is marked by the anterior interventricular, or descending, branch of the left coronary artery, and its right border is marked by the right coronary artery, which runs obliquely in the atrioventricular groove.

Appreciating the surface anatomy of the heart is helpful in determining the most appropriate site for an incision to gain

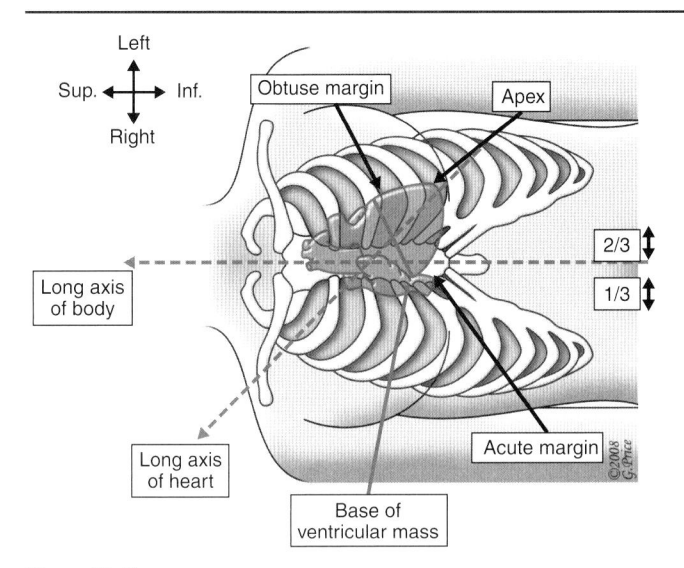

Figure 47–6
The cardiac structure placed in the context of the chest as would be seen by a surgeon standing on the right side of the operating table. Note that in the usual situation, two thirds of the cardiac silhouette are positioned to the left of the midline. *(Copyright for the original diagram from which this figure was prepared belongs to Benson R. Wilcox, Andrew C. Cook, and Robert H. Anderson.)*

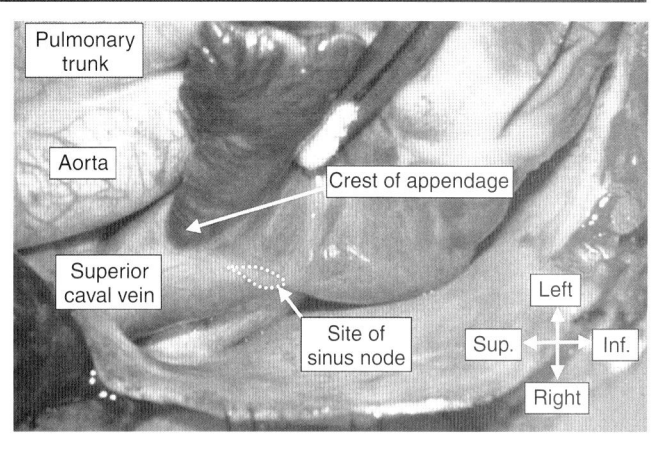

Figure 47–8
In this picture, taken in the operating room, the surgeon has reflected the atrial appendage to show the location of the terminal groove and the crest of the appendage. Note the site of the sinus node *(dotted lines)*. (See color version in the online edition through Expert Consult.) *(Copyright for the original illustration from which this figure was prepared belongs to Benson R. Wilcox, Andrew C. Cook, and Robert H. Anderson.)*

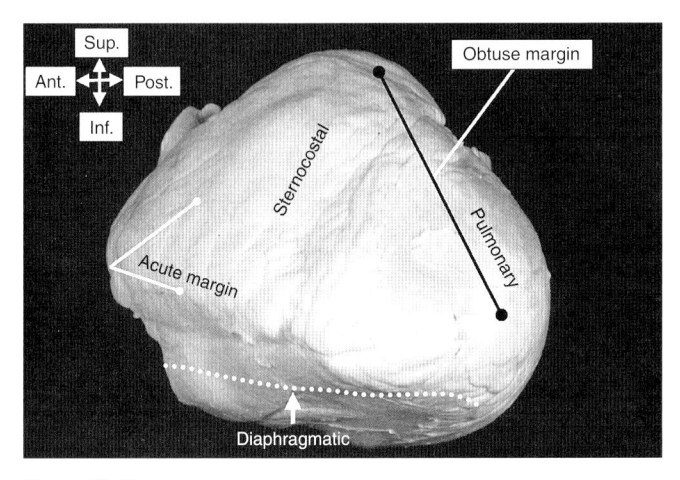

Figure 47–7
This heart has been removed from the thorax and is viewed from the apex, looking toward the base of the ventricular mass. It shows the surfaces of the ventricular mass and the locations of the acute and obtuse margins. (See color version in the online edition through Expert Consult.) *(Copyright for the original illustration from which this figure was prepared belongs to Benson R. Wilcox, Andrew C. Cook, and Robert H. Anderson.)*

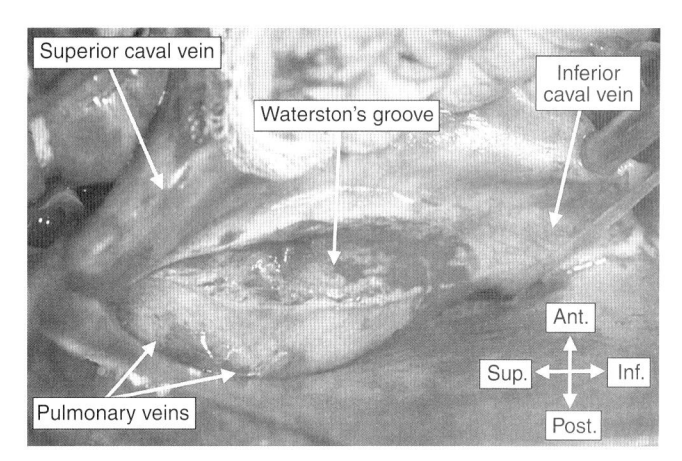

Figure 47–9
In this picture, showing the view through a median sternotomy, the surgeon has incised through the epicardium covering Waterston's groove, showing the base of the deep fold between the systemic venous tributaries and the right pulmonary veins. (See color version in the online edition through Expert Consult.) *(Copyright for the original illustration from which this figure was prepared belongs to Benson R. Wilcox, Andrew C. Cook, and Robert H. Anderson.)*

access to a given cardiac chamber.[2] For example, the relatively bloodless outlet portion of the right ventricle just beneath the origin of the pulmonary trunk affords ready access to the ventricular cavity. The important landmark for the right atrium is the terminal groove, or sulcus terminalis, which marks the border between the appendage and the venous component (Fig. 47-8). The sinus node is typically located in this groove, usually laterally in the superior cavoatrial junction inferior to the crest of the appendage. Posterior and parallel to the terminal groove is a second, deeper groove between the right atrium and the right pulmonary veins. Dissections into this deep interatrial groove, also known as Waterston's or Sondergaard's groove, permit incisions to be made into the left atrium (Fig. 47-9).

MORPHOLOGICALLY RIGHT ATRIUM

The right atrium has three components: the appendage, the venous sinus receiving the systemic venous return, and the vestibule. It is separated from the left atrium by the septum. As mentioned, the junction between the appendage and the venous sinus is marked externally by the prominent terminal groove. Internally, the groove corresponds with the position of the terminal crest (crista terminalis), which gives origin to

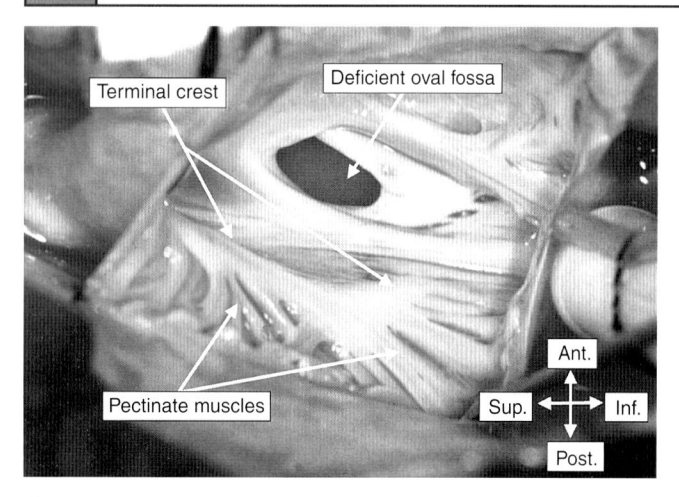

Figure 47-10
Opening the right atrial appendage in this patient with a defect in the oval fossa reveals the markedly different configuration of the endocardial surfaces of the pectinated appendage as opposed to the smooth-walled systemic venous sinus. The pectinate muscles originate from the terminal crest, marked externally by the terminal groove (see Fig. 47-7). (See color version in the online edition through Expert Consult.) *(Copyright for the original illustration from which this figure was prepared belongs to Benson R. Wilcox, Andrew C. Cook, and Robert H. Anderson.)*

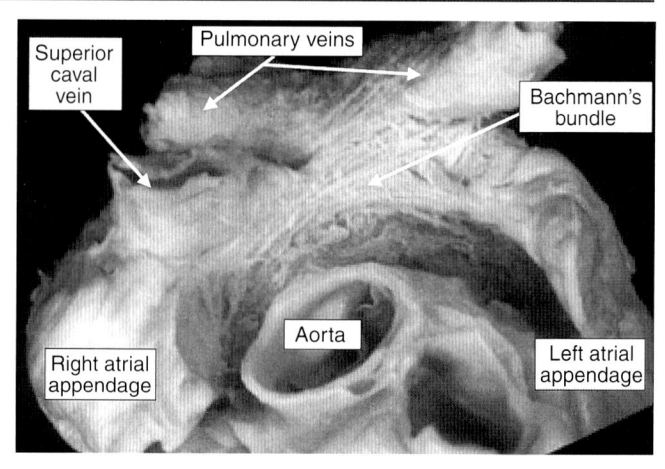

Figure 47-12
The heart has been photographed from in front, after the epicardium has been removed from the surface of the anterosuperior interatrial groove. Note the broad sweep of parallel fibers that extend from the crest of the atrial appendage in front of the superior caval vein toward the left atrial appendage. This is Bachmann's bundle. (See color version in the online edition through Expert Consult.) *(Copyright for the original illustration from which this figure was prepared belongs to Benson R. Wilcox, Andrew C. Cook, and Robert H. Anderson.)*

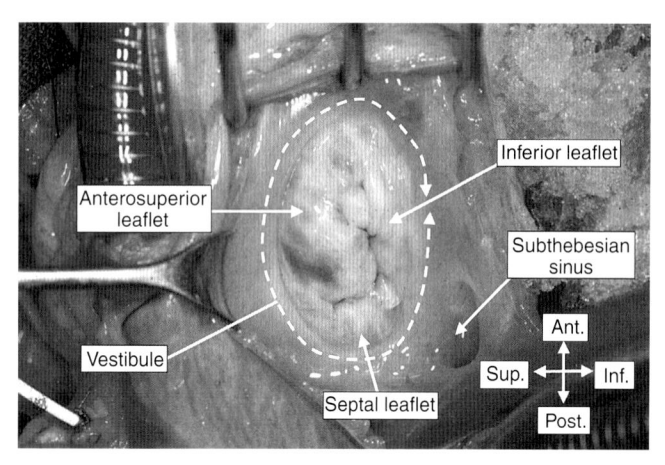

Figure 47-11
The right atrium has been opened to show the smooth vestibule of the tricuspid valve. The three leaflets of the valve are positioned septally, anterosuperiorly, and inferiorly. Note the extensive subthebesian sinus, often described as subeustachian when the heart is viewed in attitudinally incorrect fashion. (See color version in the online edition through Expert Consult.) *(Copyright for the original illustration from which this figure was prepared belongs to Benson R. Wilcox, Andrew C. Cook, and Robert H. Anderson.)*

the pectinate muscles of the appendage (Fig. 47-10). Significantly, the pectinate muscles within the appendage encircle the full extent of the third component, the vestibule, which is the smooth muscle encircling the orifice of the tricuspid valve (Fig. 47-11). This extensive array of pectinate muscles serves to identify an atrium as being morphologically right even when abnormally located, or when duplicated as seen in isomerism.[3] Superiorly and anteriorly, the appendage terminates in a prominent crest that forms the summit of the terminal groove, and that continues in the transverse sinus behind the aorta across the interatrial groove as Bachmann's bundle (Fig. 47-12). The sinus node lies in the terminal groove in an immediately subepicardial position. It is a spindle-shaped structure that usually lies to the right of the crest—that is, lateral to the superior cavoatrial junction. In about one tenth of cases, the node extends across the crest into the interatrial groove, draping itself across the cavoatrial junction in horseshoe fashion.[4] For the surgeon, the artery to the sinus node is also of significance. It is a branch of the right coronary artery in about 55% of individuals and a branch of the circumflex artery in the remainder.[5] Regardless of its origin, it usually courses through the anterior interatrial groove toward the superior cavoatrial junction, frequently running within the atrial myocardium. Having reached the cavoatrial junction, the artery may cross the crest of the appendage, course retrocavally, or even divide to form an arterial circle around the junction.

On first sight, when inspecting the internal morphology of the right atrium, there appears to be an extensive septal surface between the orifices of the caval veins and the orifice of the tricuspid valve. The apparent extent of this septum is spurious.[6,7] The true septum between the right and left atrial chambers is formed by the floor of the oval fossa (derived from the fetal flap valve), and its adjacent anteroinferior muscular rim.[6] The extensive superior rim, or the so-called septum secundum, is formed by a deep interatrial fold extending between the systemic and the pulmonary veins (Fig. 47-13). The larger part of the anterior atrial wall is folded around the aortic root. That the margins of the true atrial septum are limited is of major surgical importance, as it is easy to pass outside the heart when attempting to gain access to the left atrium through a right atrial approach.

In addition to the position of the sinus node, and the extent of the atrial septum, the other major area of surgical significance in the right atrium is the site of the atrioventricular node. This is contained within the triangle of Koch (Fig. 47-14).

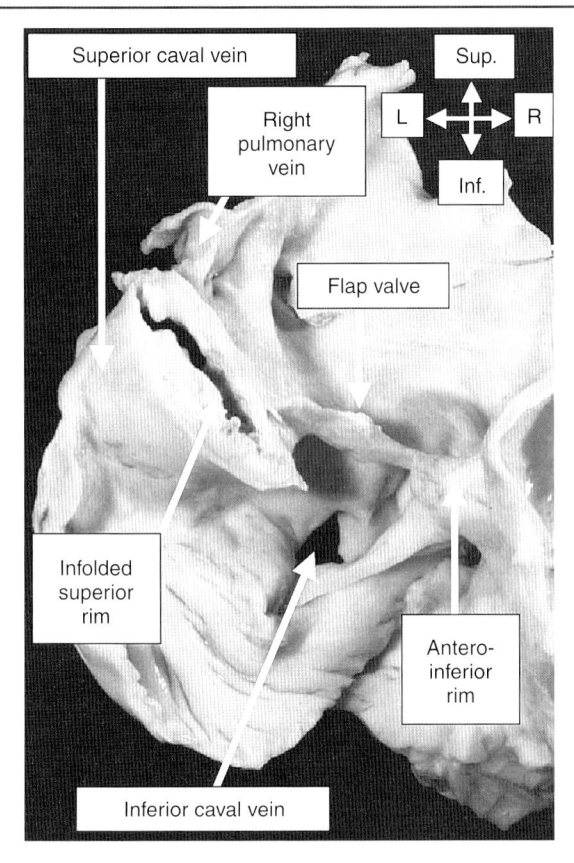

Figure 47–13
This heart has been sectioned in four-chamber fashion through the oval fossa. The section shows that the so-called septum secundum is no more than the infolded atrial walls between the tributaries of the systemic venous sinus and the right pulmonary veins. The true septal structures are the floor of the oval fossa (flap valve) and its hinge point from the anteroinferior rim. *(Copyright for the original illustration from which this figure was prepared belongs to Benson R. Wilcox, Andrew C. Cook, and Robert H. Anderson.)*

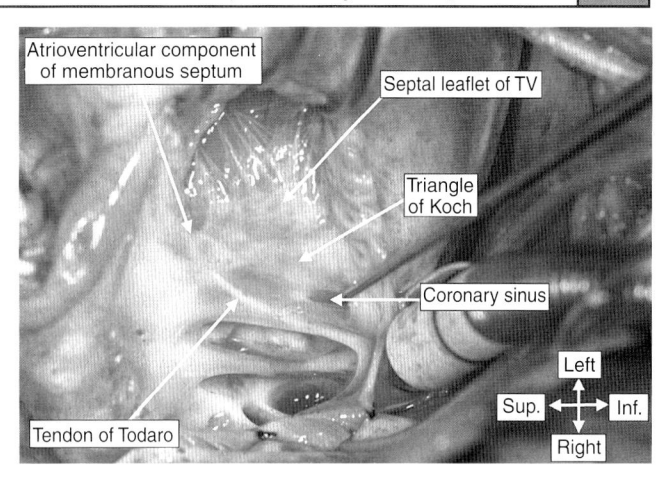

Figure 47–14
The right atrium has been opened via a median sternotomy to show the landmarks of the triangle of Koch. In this patient, the continuation of the eustachian valve through the tendon of Todaro is clearly seen, with the tendon inserting into the atrioventricular component of the central fibrous body. (See color version in the online edition through Expert Consult.) *(Copyright for the original illustration from which this figure was prepared belongs to Benson R. Wilcox, Andrew C. Cook, and Robert H. Anderson.)*

This important landmark is demarcated by the tendon of Todaro, the attachment of the septal leaflet of the tricuspid valve, and the orifice of the coronary sinus.[8] The tendon of Todaro is a fibrous structure formed by the union of the eustachian and thebesian valves. The fibrous extension of these two valvar remnants buries itself in the tissue separating the oval fossa from the mouth of the coronary sinus, and it runs medially as the tendon of Todaro, which inserts into the central fibrous body. The entire atrial component of the axis of atrioventricular conduction tissues is contained within the confines of the triangle of Koch. If, in hearts with normal segmental connections, this area is scrupulously avoided during surgical procedures, the atrioventricular conduction tissues will not be damaged. The node itself, located in the smooth atrial musculature of the triangle, is some distance above the hinge point of the septal leaflet of the tricuspid valve. The atrioventricular bundle, however, penetrates more or less directly at the apex of the triangle of Koch.

Much has been written in recent years about the role of "specialized" pathways of tissue in conduction of the sinus impulse to the atrioventricular node.[9,10] It can now be stated with certainty that there are no insulated or isolated tracts of specialized conduction tissue extending between the nodes that can be avoided surgically, as is possible with the penetrating and branching atrioventricular bundles.[11] The major muscle bundles of the atrial chambers serve as preferential pathways of conduction, but the course of these preferential pathways is dictated by the overall geometry of the chambers. Ideally, prominent muscle bundles, such as the terminal crest or the superior rim of the oval fossa, should be preserved during atrial surgery. But even if they cannot be preserved, the surgeon can be sure that internodal conduction will continue as long as some strand of atrial myocardium connects the nodes, provided that the arterial supply to the nodes, or the nodes themselves, are not traumatized. The key to avoidance of postoperative atrial arrhythmias, therefore, is the fastidious preservation of the sinus and atrioventricular nodes and their arteries.[2]

The central fibrous body touches on three of the four cardiac chambers, but it is in the right atrium that it becomes first, and perhaps most clearly, evident to the surgeon (see Fig. 47-14). Rather than being a specific body, it is better conceptualized as an area in the heart where the membranous septum and the leaflets of the atrioventricular and aortic valves join in fibrous continuity. When viewed from the left heart (Fig. 47-15), it is possible to assess its proximity to the aortic and mitral valves and to the left bundle branch of the conduction axis. Because of this intimate relationship to so many important structures in the heart, the central fibrous body acts as an anatomic focal point for the cardiac surgeon.[2]

The vestibule of the atrium, surrounding the orifice of the tricuspid valve, is continuous with both the venous component and the appendage of the right atrium. Its anterosuperior part overlies the anteroseptal commissure of the tricuspid valve and continues along the supraventricular crest of the right ventricle. The posteroinferior component extends beneath the orifice of the coronary sinus, where there is usually an extensive trabeculated diverticulum found behind the sinus, the so-called post-eustachian sinus of Keith.

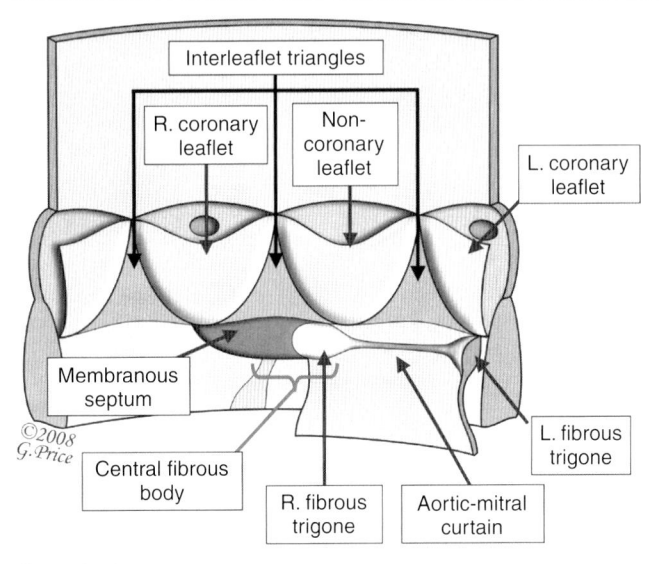

Figure 47–15
The left ventricular aspect of the aortic root, illustrating the various components of the fibrous skeleton. The area of fibrous continuity between the leaflets of the aortic and mitral valves is thickened at both ends to form the so-called fibrous trigones. As can be seen, the right trigone is then continuous with the membranous septum, these structures forming the central fibrous body. Note that the membranous septum itself continues upward to the sinutubular junction as one of the fibrous interleaflet triangles of the aortic root. Note also the location of the left bundle branch. (See Fig. 47-26.) *(Copyright for the original diagram from which this figure was prepared belongs to Benson R. Wilcox, Andrew C. Cook, and Robert H. Anderson.)*

Figure 47–16
The morphologically left atrium is photographed from its left side to show the component parts. Note the extensive body, which also receives the septal aspect of the chamber. (See color version in the online edition through Expert Consult.) *(Copyright for the original illustration from which this figure was prepared belongs to Benson R. Wilcox, Andrew C. Cook, and Robert H. Anderson.)*

MORPHOLOGICALLY LEFT ATRIUM

Because of its position, only the appendage of the left atrium may be immediately evident to a surgeon on exposing the heart. Like the right atrium, the left atrium has a venous component, an appendage, and a vestibule, and is separated from its partner by the septum. In addition, the left atrium possesses a well-formed body, forming the dome of the atrium when the veins are connected anomalously, as in totally anomalous pulmonary venous connection. Unlike that of the right atrium, however, the venous component of the left atrium is considerably larger than the appendage, and the narrow junction between these two parts is not marked by either a terminal groove or a crest (Fig. 47-16). The pectinate muscles are confined within the appendage, and again, unlike on the right side, they do not extend around the vestibule.[3] This difference in the extent of the pectinate muscles always permits the morphologically right appendage to be distinguished from the morphologically left structure. Because of its posterior position and its firm anchorage by the four pulmonary veins, direct access to the left atrium can be difficult, so surgeons must use their knowledge of anatomy to gain the best exposure of the cavity. Probably the most popular route is an incision made just posterior to the interatrial groove. As described, this extensive infolding between the right pulmonary veins and the systemic veins produces the superior rim of the oval fossa. A posteriorly directed incision along this groove takes the surgeon directly into the left atrium. Because the infolding of the interatrial groove also forms the superior border of the oval fossa, much the same access can be gained by approaching through the right atrium and incising just

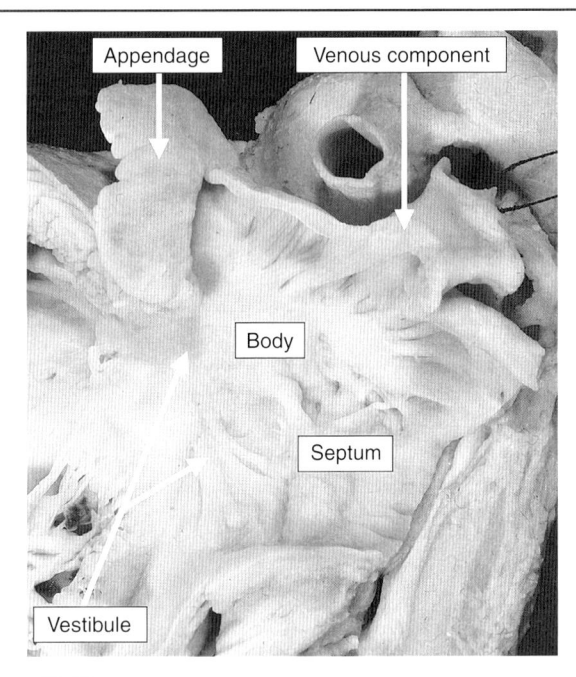

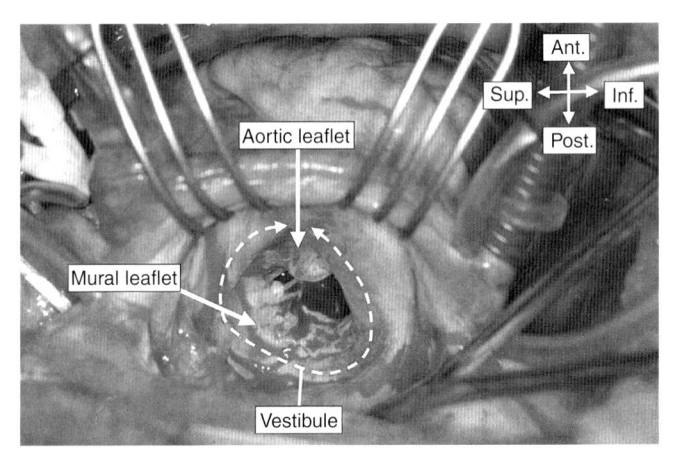

Figure 47–17
The left atrium is photographed in the operating room through an incision made in the dome. Note the vestibule of the mitral valve, which has aortic and mural leaflets. (See color version in the online edition through Expert Consult.) *(Copyright for the original illustration from which this figure was prepared belongs to Benson R. Wilcox, Andrew C. Cook, and Robert H. Anderson.)*

superiorly within the fossa. A further approach to the left atrium is the so-called superior approach, incising directly through the roof.

Once access is gained to the left atrium, the small size of the opening of the appendage is apparent, lying to the left of the mitral orifice as viewed by the surgeon. The greater part of the pulmonary venous atrium is usually located inferiorly, away from the operative field, and the vestibule of the mitral orifice dominates the picture (Fig. 47-17). The septal aspect is

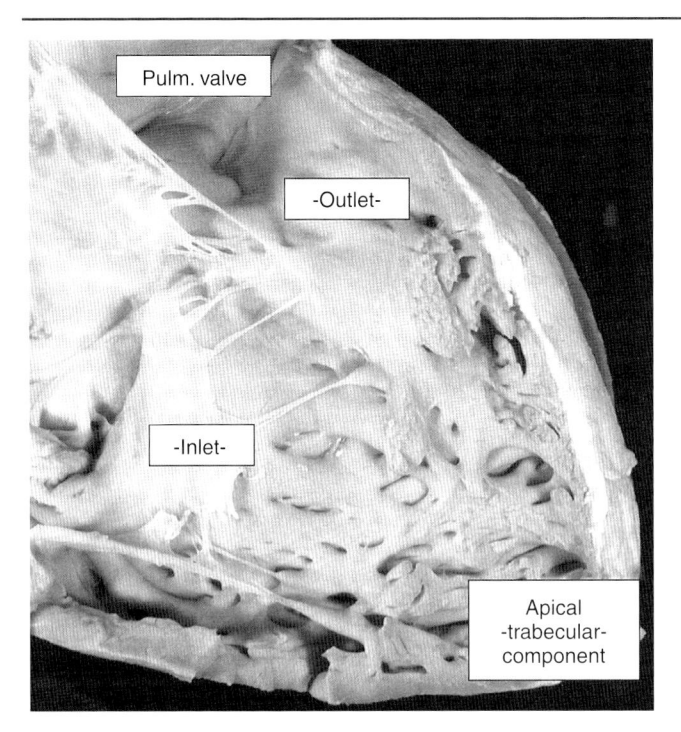

Figure 47-18
The morphologically right ventricle is opened in clam-like fashion and the septal surface is photographed to show its three component parts. *(Copyright for the original illustration from which this figure was prepared belongs to Benson R. Wilcox, Andrew C. Cook, and Robert H. Anderson.)*

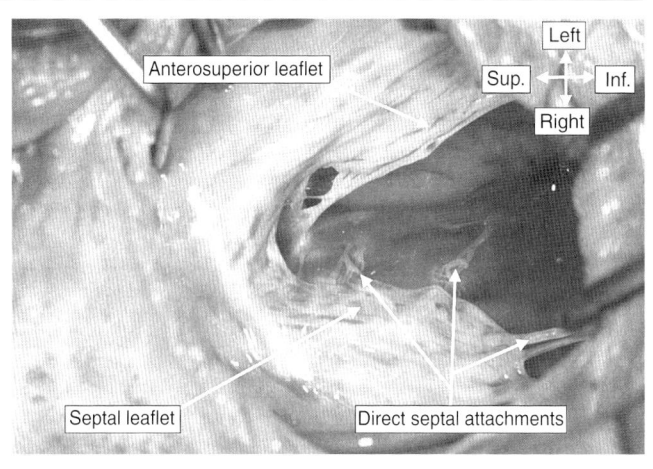

Figure 47-19
The tricuspid valve is seen through the right atrium in the operating room. Note the tendinous cords that attach the septal leaflet directly to the septum. This is the most characteristic morphologic feature of the tricuspid valve. (See color version in the online edition through Expert Consult.) *(Copyright for the original illustration from which this figure was prepared belongs to Benson R. Wilcox, Andrew C. Cook, and Robert H. Anderson.)*

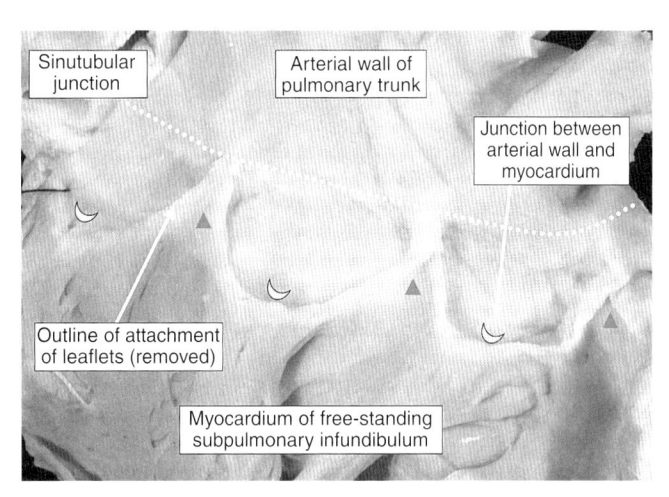

Figure 47-20
The pulmonary outflow tract has been opened and the leaflets of the pulmonary valve have been removed, showing their initial semilunar attachment. The most distal attachment is to the sinutubular junction *(dotted line)*, and, proximally, the hinge point incorporates right ventricular musculature into the base of each pulmonary valvar sinus *(gray crescents)*. Fibrous triangles making up the wall of the pulmonary trunk *(red triangles)* are incorporated into the ventricular outflow tract. (See color version in the online edition through Expert Consult.) *(Copyright for the original illustration from which this figure was prepared belongs to Benson R. Wilcox, Andrew C. Cook, and Robert H. Anderson.)*

anterior, exhibiting the typically roughened flap-valve aspect of its left side (see Fig. 47-16). The large sweep of tissue between the flap-valve of the septum and the opening of the appendage is the internal aspect of the deep anterior interatrial groove.

MORPHOLOGICALLY RIGHT VENTRICLE

Understanding of ventricular morphology is greatly aided by considering the ventricles in terms of three components (Fig. 47-18), rather than in terms of the traditional sinus and conus parts. The three portions are the inlet, trabecular, and outlet parts.[12] The inlet portion of the right ventricle contains, and is limited by, the tricuspid valve and its tension apparatus. The leaflets of the valve are positioned septally, inferiorly (or murally), and anterosuperiorly. The most constant distinguishing feature of the valve is the direct attachments to the septum of the cords of its septal leaflet (Fig. 47-19). The trabecular component of the right ventricle extends out to the apex, where its wall is particularly thin and is especially vulnerable to perforation by cardiac catheters and pacemaker electrodes. The outlet component of the right ventricle is a complete muscular structure, the infundibulum, which supports the pulmonary valve. The three leaflets of the pulmonary valve do not have a ring or an annulus. Instead, they are attached to the infundibular musculature in semilunar fashion (Fig. 47-20), the semilunar hinge-points crossing the anatomic ventriculoarterial junction, which does form a complete ring, as does the sinutubular junction.[13] The basal attachments of the leaflets are attached in the ventricle, upstream relative to the anatomic ventriculoarterial junction, whereas the peripheral attachments are to the arterial sinutubular junction. The overall valvar structure, therefore, takes the form of a three-pointed coronet (Fig. 47-21).

A distinguishing feature of the right ventricle is the prominent muscular shelf separating the tricuspid and pulmonary valves: the supraventricular crest. Although at first sight it looks like a large muscle bundle, much of the crest is no more than the infolded inner heart curve. Incisions, or deep sutures through this part, run into the transverse sinus and right atrioventricular groove and can jeopardize the right coronary artery.[14] The distal part of the crest is continuous with the freestanding subpulmonary infundibulum, the presence of this muscular sleeve permitting the valve to be removed and used as an autograft in the Ross procedure (Fig. 47-22). The body of the supraventricular crest inserts between the limbs of a prominent and important right ventricular septal trabeculation. This structure, called the septomarginal trabeculation, has superior and inferior limbs that clasp the crest. The superior limb runs up to the attachment of the leaflets of the pulmonary valve, whereas the inferior limb extends backward inferior to the interventricular component of the membranous septum. The characteristic medial papillary muscle (see Fig. 47-22) usually arises from this inferior limb, and a line extending from the muscle to the apex of the triangle of Koch marks the location of the atrioventricular conduction axis. The body of the septomarginal trabeculation runs to the apex of the ventricle, where it breaks up into a sheath of smaller trabeculations. Some of these mingle into the trabecular portion, and some support the tension apparatus of the tricuspid valve. Two trabeculations may be particularly prominent. One becomes the anterior papillary muscle of the tricuspid valve, and the other extends from the septomarginal trabeculation to the papillary muscle, forming the moderator band. Other significant right ventricular trabeculations are usually found in the transitional zone to the infundibulum. Variable in number, these are the septoparietal trabeculations (Fig. 47-23).

It is the coarseness of the apical trabeculations that is the most constant feature of the morphologically right ventricle when the chamber is malformed. In the normal heart, a number of morphologic differences exist between the two ventricles, including the arrangement of the leaflets of the atrioventricular valves and their tension apparatus, their shape, the thickness of their walls, and the configuration of the outflow tracts. These features, however, can be altered or lacking in the congenitally abnormal heart. When making the final arbitration, therefore, it is important to follow the "morphological method" introduced by Van Praagh and his colleagues,[15] which states that one variable feature should not be defined on the basis of another feature that is itself variable. When distinguishing ventricular morphology, therefore, it is necessary to rely on the contrast between the coarse trabeculations of the right ventricle and those that are much finer in the apical part of the left ventricle.

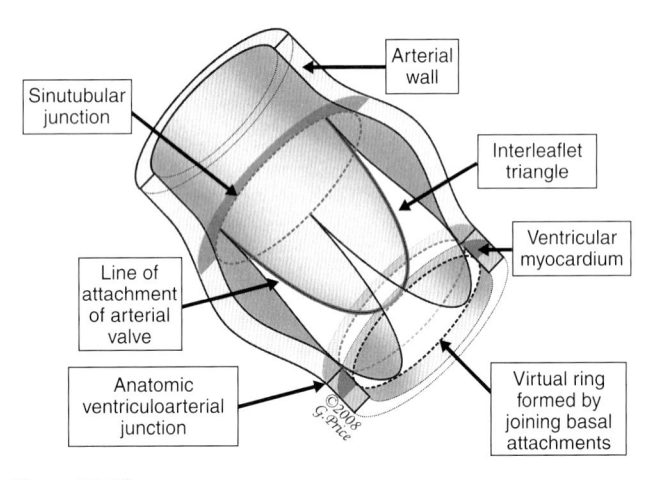

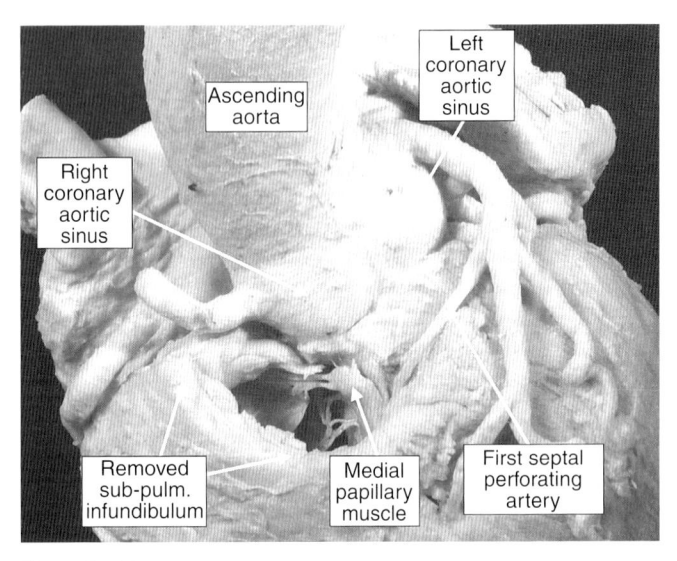

Figure 47–22
The freestanding sleeve of subpulmonary infundibular musculature has been removed in this anatomic specimen, as the surgeon would remove the pulmonary valve during the Ross procedure. The dissection has not impinged on the cavity of the left ventricle. Note the location of the medial papillary muscle and the first septal perforating artery. *(Copyright for the original illustration from which this figure was prepared belongs to Benson R. Wilcox, Andrew C. Cook, and Robert H. Anderson.)*

Figure 47–21
The idealized three-dimensional arrangement of the arterial valves. There is no ringlike "annulus" supporting the valvar leaflets. Instead, the leaflets are attached within the arterial root in crownlike fashion. *(Copyright for the original diagram from which this figure was prepared belongs to Robert H. Anderson, Benson R, Wilcox, and Andrew C. Cook.)*

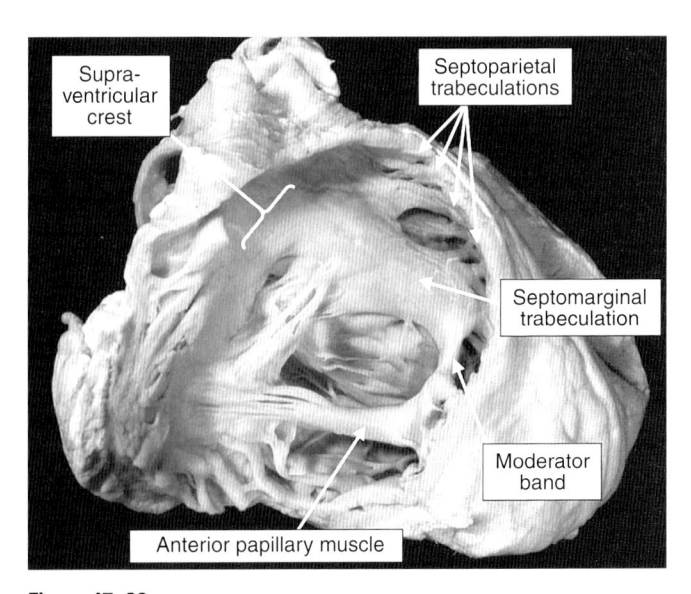

Figure 47–23
This heart, seen in anatomic orientation, has been prepared by windowing the anterior wall of the right ventricle. The dissection reveals the continuation of the septomarginal trabeculation through the moderator band to the anterior papillary muscle, and shows well the multiple septoparietal trabeculations. *(Copyright for the original illustration from which this figure was prepared belongs to Benson R. Wilcox, Andrew C. Cook, and Robert H. Anderson.)*

MORPHOLOGICALLY LEFT VENTRICLE

The left ventricle is also conveniently considered in terms of inlet, trabecular, and outlet components (Fig. 47-24), although in contrast to the right ventricle, the inlet and outlet components overlap considerably in the morphologically left ventricle. The inlet component surrounds, and is limited by, the mitral valve and its tension apparatus. The two leaflets of the mitral valve, supported by two prominent papillary muscle groups and their commissural cords, and closing along a solitary zone of apposition, have widely different appearances (Fig. 47-25). The aortic leaflet is short, squat, and relatively square. This leaflet, which is in fibrous continuity with two of the leaflets of the aortic valve, is best termed the aortic leaflet, because it is not strictly in either an anterior or a superior position. The other leaflet is much shallower, and its junctional attachment is more extensive, being connected to the parietal part of the left atrioventricular junction. It is accurately termed the mural leaflet. Because the aortic leaflet of the mitral valve also forms part of the outlet of the left ventricle (Fig. 47-26), the distinction between inlet and outlet is somewhat blurred. The papillary muscles of the valve, located in anteroinferior and posterosuperior positions, are close to each other at their origin. The muscles are usually described as being posteromedial and anterolateral, but this is wrong, reflecting the penchant of previous anatomists, and others, to describe the heart as though positioned on its apex.[1] Unlike those of the tricuspid valve, the leaflets of the mitral valve have no direct septal attachments, the deep posterior diverticulum of the subaortic outflow tract displacing the aortic leaflet of the mitral valve away from the septum (see Fig. 47-26). The trabecular component of the left ventricle extends to the ventricular apex and has characteristically fine trabeculations (see Fig. 47-24).

As in the right ventricle, the apical myocardium is surprisingly thin. This feature is important to the cardiac surgeon who has reason to place catheters and electrodes in the right ventricle or drainage tubes in the left side.[2] Immediate perforation, or delayed rupture, may occur. The outlet component of the left ventricle supports the aortic valve. Unlike its right ventricular counterpart, it is not a complete muscular structure. The septal wall is largely composed of muscle, but the membranous septum forms part of the subaortic outflow tract. The posterior

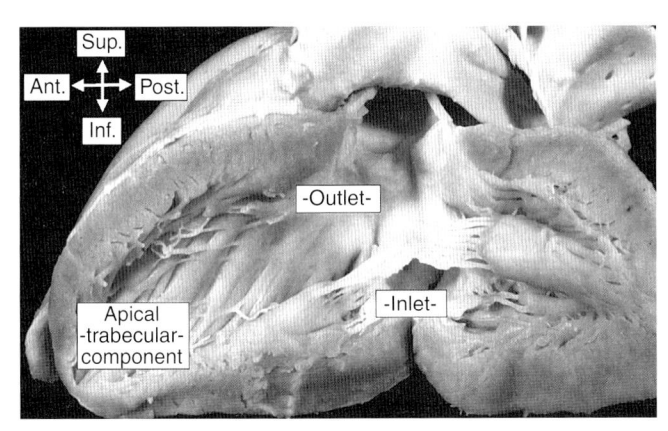

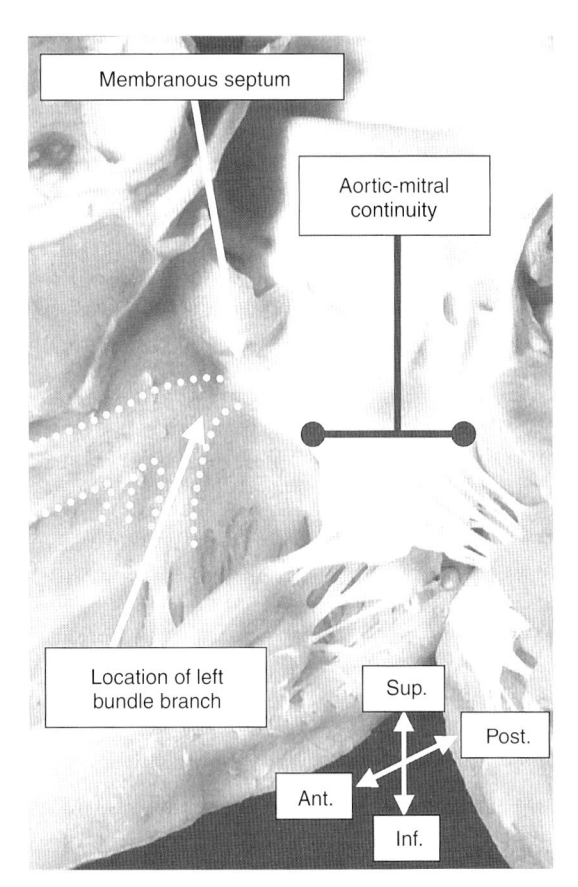

Figure 47-24
The morphologically left ventricle is opened in clam-like fashion to show its three component parts. *(Copyright for the original illustration from which this figure was prepared belongs to Benson R. Wilcox, Andrew C. Cook, and Robert H. Anderson.)*

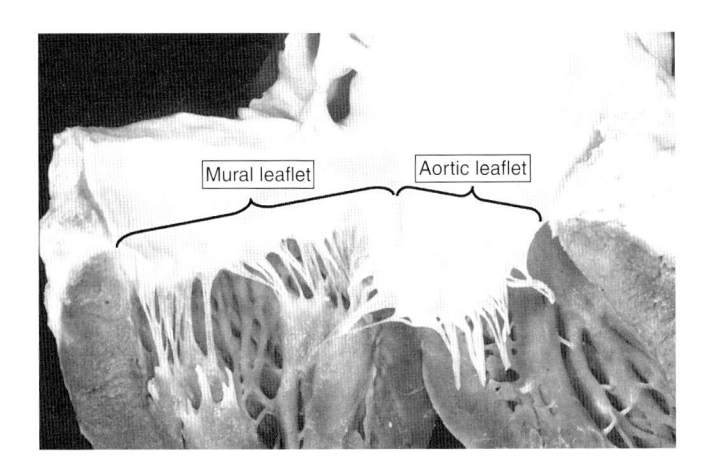

Figure 47-25
The heart has been opened through the left atrioventricular junction, and it has been spread to show the difference in structure between the aortic and mural leaflets of the mitral valve. *(Copyright for the original illustration from which this figure was prepared belongs to Benson R. Wilcox, Andrew C. Cook, and Robert H. Anderson.)*

Figure 47-26
The specimen is opened through the left ventricular outflow tract, showing the relationship of the left bundle branch to the membranous septum and the aortic root. Note the region of aortic to mitral valvar fibrous continuity. (See color version in the online edition through Expert Consult.) *(Copyright for the original illustration from which this figure was prepared belongs to Benson R. Wilcox, Andrew C. Cook, and Robert H. Anderson.)*

portion of the outflow tract is composed of the fibrous curtain joining the apparatus of the aortic valve to the aortic leaflet of the mitral valve (see Fig. 47-26). As with the pulmonary valve, the leaflets of the aortic valve are hinged in semilunar fashion, with the peripheral attachments supported at the sinutubular junction, whereas the most basal parts take origin from ventricular structures. The overall arrangement is crownlike (see Fig. 47-21), rather than forming an annulus.[13,16]

The muscular septal surface of the outflow tract is characteristically smooth, and down this surface cascades the fanlike left bundle branch. The landmark of the descent of the left bundle branch is the membranous septum immediately beneath the zone of apposition between the right coronary and noncoronary leaflets of the aortic valve (see Fig. 47-15). The bundle descends, initially, as a relatively narrow solitary fascicle, but soon it divides into three interconnected fascicles that radiate into anterior, septal, and posterior divisions. The interconnecting radiations do not fan out to any degree until the bundle itself has descended to between one third and one half the length of the septum.

AORTA

The ascending aorta begins at the distal extremity of the three aortic sinuses, the sinutubular junction, which lies at the line of opening of the free edge of the leaflets of the aortic valve. It runs its short course passing superiorly, obliquely to the right, and slightly forward toward the sternum. It is contained within the fibrous pericardial sac, so its surface is covered with serous pericardium. Its anterior surface abuts directly on the pulmonary trunk, which is also covered with serous pericardium. The two vessels together make up the vascular pedicle of the heart. The ascending aorta is related anteromedially to the right atrial appendage, and posterolaterally to the right ventricular outflow tract and the pulmonary trunk. Extrapericardially, the thymus gland lies between it and the sternum. The medial wall of the right atrium, the superior caval vein, and the right pleura relate to its right side. On the left, its principal relationship is with the pulmonary trunk. Posterior to the ascending aorta is the transverse sinus of the pericardium, which separates it from the "roof" of the left atrium and the right pulmonary artery.

The arch of the aorta begins at the superior attachment of the pericardial reflection just proximal to the origin of the brachiocephalic artery (Fig. 47-27). It continues superiorly briefly before coursing posteriorly and to the left, crossing the lateral aspect of the distal trachea and finally terminating on the lateral aspect of the vertebral column. Here it is tethered by the parietal pleura and the arterial ligament. During its course, it gives off the brachiocephalic, the left common carotid, and the left subclavian arteries. Bronchial arteries may arise from the arch and can be particularly troublesome if not carefully identified in the presence of aortic coarctation. The left phrenic and vagus nerves run over the anterolateral aspect of the arch just beneath the mediastinal pleura. The left recurrent laryngeal nerve takes origin from the vagus and curls superiorly around the arterial ligament before passing on to the posteromedial side of the arch. Here, the arch relates to the tracheal bifurcation and esophagus on its medial border, but also to the left main bronchus and the left pulmonary artery inferiorly.

The descending, or thoracic, aorta continues from the arch, running an initial course lateral to the vertebral bodies

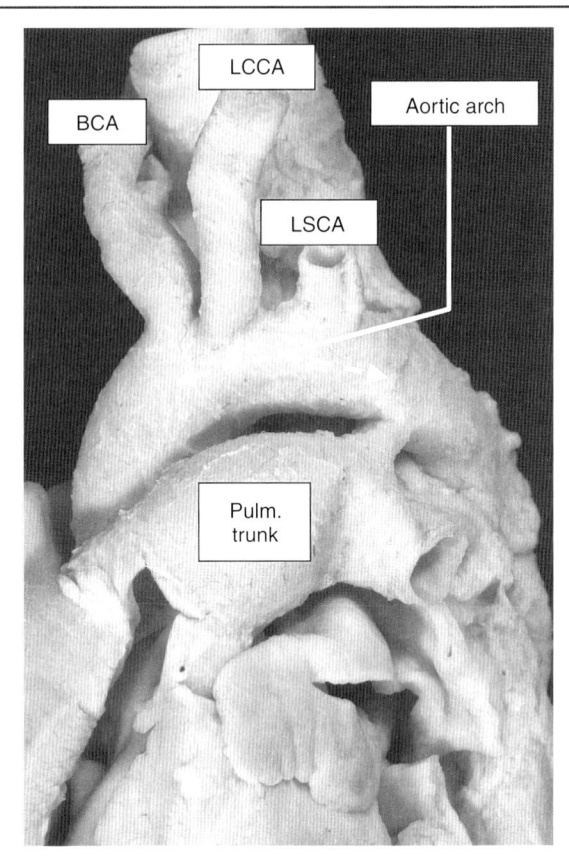

Figure 47–27
The heart has been photographed from the left side in anatomic position to show the normal structure of the great arteries and the arterial duct. BCA, brachiocephalic artery; LCCA, left common carotid artery; LSCA, left subclavian artery. *(Copyright for the original illustration from which this figure was prepared belongs to Benson R. Wilcox, Andrew C. Cook, and Robert H. Anderson.)*

and reaching an anterior position at its termination. It gives off many branches to the organs of the thorax throughout its course, as well as the prominent lower nine pairs of intercostal arteries. These latter vessels are of critical concern for the cardiac surgeon. In coarctation of the aorta, they serve as primary collateral vessels to bypass the obstructed aorta, accounting for the rib notching seen in older children with this lesion. These vessels, and their branches to the chest wall, can be a source of troublesome bleeding if not properly secured when operating on such patients. Also, the surgeon must remember that the dorsal branches of the intercostal vessels contribute a spinal branch that is important in supplying blood to the spinal cord. Because it is difficult to predict exactly from where these vital branches will arise, the surgeon must make every attempt to protect their origin from permanent occlusion. The important bronchial arteries (Fig. 47-28) also arise from the descending segment of the thoracic aorta. These vessels can become dilated in the presence of pulmonary atresia, when they serve as a source of pulmonary vascular supply.

PULMONARY TRUNK AND BRANCH PULMONARY ARTERIES

The pulmonary trunk is a short vessel, usually less than 5 cm in length in the adult (Fig. 47-29). It is completely contained within the pericardium and, like its running mate, the

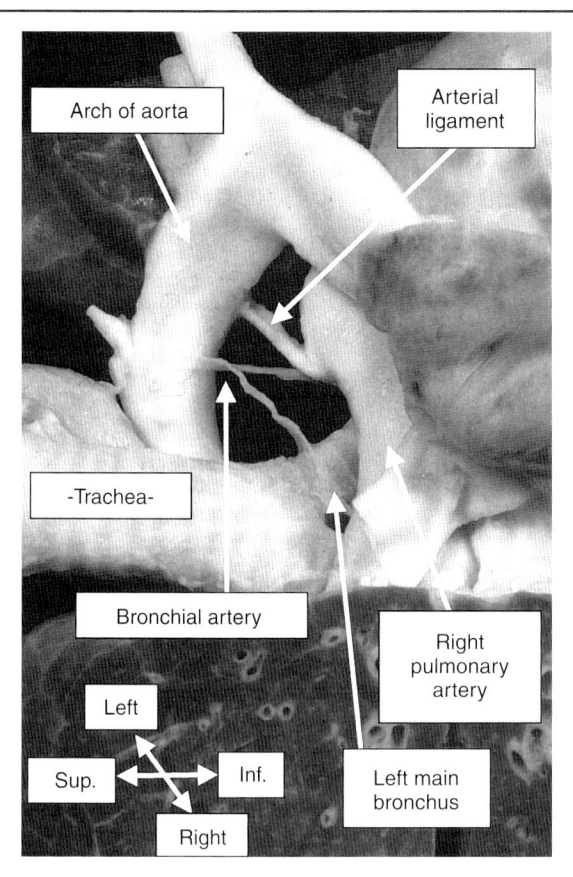

Figure 47–28
This heart is positioned as it might be seen by the surgeon working through a median sternotomy. The aortic arch is deflected forward and has been dissected to show the origin of the bronchial arteries. Note that the arterial duct in this specimen has become ligamentous. *(Copyright for the original illustration from which this figure was prepared belongs to Benson R. Wilcox, Andrew C. Cook, and Robert H. Anderson.)*

Figure 47–29
This view of the heart through a median sternotomy shows the extent of the pulmonary trunk, the surgeon having encircled the trunk with a tape. Note the circular ventriculoarterial junction. (See color version in the online edition through Expert Consult.) *(Copyright for the original illustration from which this figure was prepared belongs to Benson R. Wilcox, Andrew C. Cook, and Robert H. Anderson.)*

CORONARY ARTERIES AND VEINS

The coronary circulation is made up of the coronary arteries and veins together with the lymphatics of the heart. Because the lymphatics are of very limited significance to operative anatomy, they are not discussed further. The coronary arteries are the first branches of the ascending portion of the aorta, arising from the aortic root immediately above its attachment to the heart. Normally, there are three sinuses at the aortic root, but only two coronary arteries. The sinuses can be named, therefore, according to whether they give rise to an artery, the normal arrangement being a right coronary, left coronary, and noncoronary sinus (Fig. 47-30). In this respect, the terms *right* and *left* refer to the coronary sinuses giving rise to the right and left coronary arteries, rather than to the position of the sinuses relative to the right-left coordinates of the body. This is important because in the normal heart, the aortic root is obliquely situated, whereas in malformed hearts, the root is frequently abnormally situated. Whatever the position of the aortic root, however, the two coronary arteries, when two are present, almost always take origin from those aortic sinuses that face the sinuses of the pulmonary trunk. Because of this, it is more convenient, and more accurate, to term these sinuses the left-hand- and right-hand-facing sinuses, taking as the point of reference the observer standing within the nonfacing sinus and looking toward the pulmonary trunk (Fig. 47-31). This convention, introduced by the group from Leiden,[17] holds true irrespective of the relationships of the arterial trunks.

The coronary arteries usually arise from the aortic sinuses beneath the sinutubular junction. Deviations of origins relative to the junction are not uncommon and are considered abnormal only when they deviate by a distance greater than 1 cm. According to Bader,[18] this occurs in 3.5% of hearts. The arterial opening can be deviated either toward the ventricle, so that the artery arises deep within the aortic sinus, or toward the aortic arch, so that the origin is outside the sinus. Such displacement may lead to the artery's taking an oblique course through the aortic wall, thus called an intramural course,

ascending aorta, is covered with a layer of serous pericardium except where the two vessels abut each other in the vascular pedicle. It takes origin from the most anterior aspect of the heart, lying just behind the lateral edge of the sternum and the second left intercostal space, superior and to the left of the aortic root. Initially, the pulmonary trunk overlies the aorta and the left coronary artery, but it soon moves to a side-by-side relationship with the ascending aorta. The left coronary artery turns abruptly anteriorly to lie between the left atrial appendage and the pulmonary trunk. The arterial ligament extends from the aortic arch to the very end of the pulmonary trunk as the latter divides into left and right pulmonary arteries. The left pulmonary artery courses superior to the left main-stem bronchus and laterally in front of the descending aorta before it sends branches to the hilum of the lung. The right pulmonary artery is somewhat longer than the left, having to traverse the mediastinum beneath the aortic arch, and then behind the superior caval vein, to reach the hilum of the lung. It lies in a posteroinferior position relative to the azygos vein, and is anterior to the left main bronchus. The right pulmonary artery often branches before reaching the lateral wall of the superior caval vein posterior to the transverse sinus of the pericardium. In this situation, a large upper lobar branch may be mistaken for the right pulmonary artery itself.

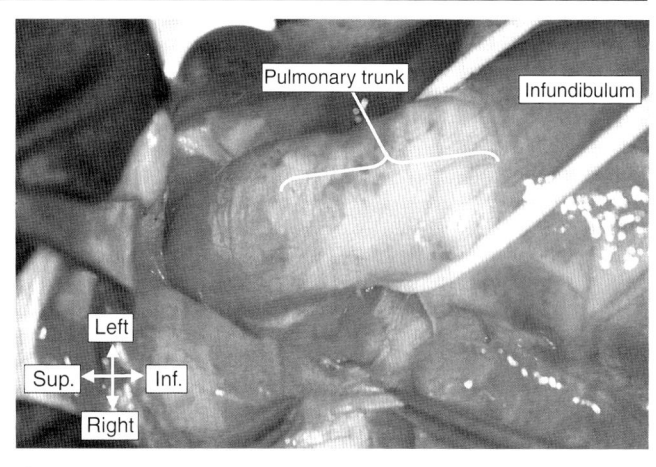

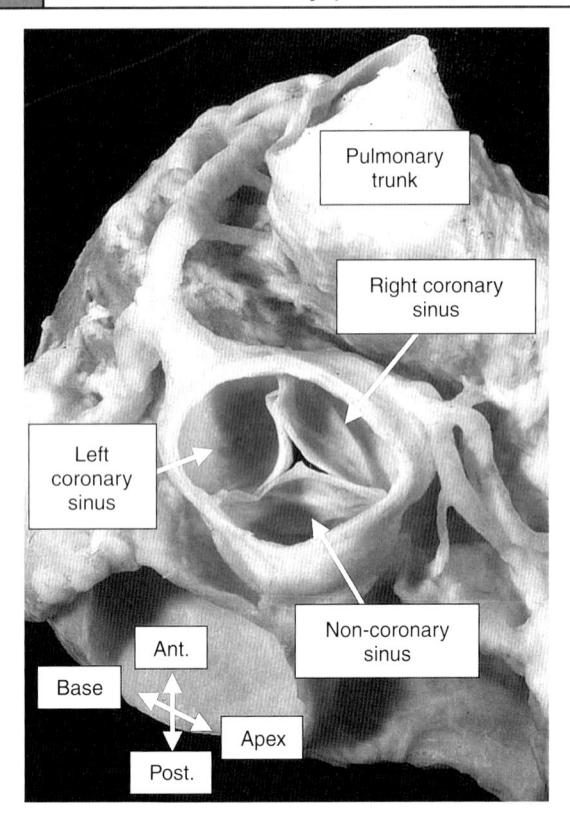

Figure 47-30
The aorta has been removed at the level of the sinutubular junction, and the heart is photographed from above and from the right. The dissection shows the origin of the coronary arteries from the two aortic sinuses adjacent to the pulmonary trunk. Note again the circular anatomic ventriculoarterial junction between the pulmonary trunk and the right ventricular infundibular musculature (compare with Fig. 47-29). *(Copyright for the original illustration from which this figure was prepared belongs to Benson R. Wilcox, Andrew C. Cook, and Robert H. Anderson.)*

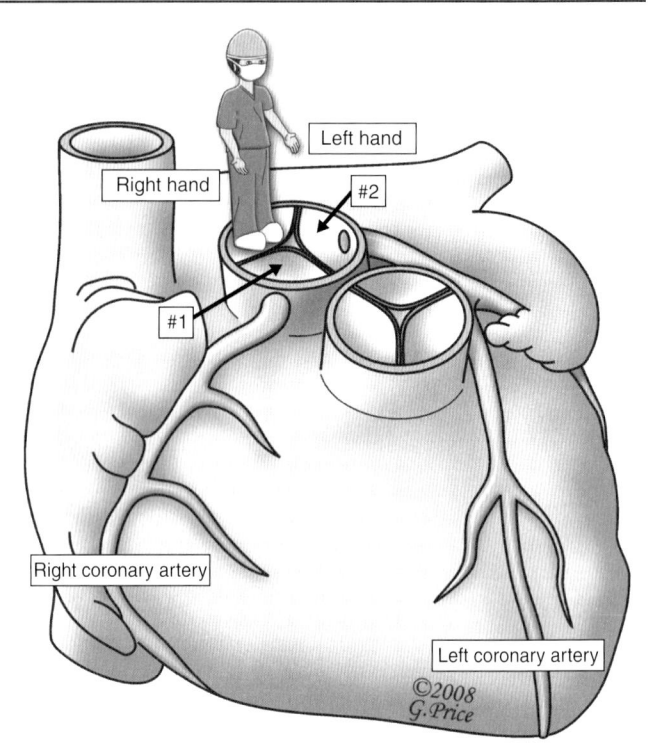

Figure 47-31
From the stance of the surgeon, the two aortic sinuses supporting the coronary arteries are to the right- and left-hand sides. Conventionally, the right-hand sinus is considered sinus #1. In the normal heart, this sinus gives rise to the right coronary artery. The convention of naming the sinuses holds, regardless of the interrelationships of the arterial trunks. *(Copyright for the original diagram from which this figure was prepared belongs to Benson R. Wilcox, Andrew C. Cook, and Robert H. Anderson.)*

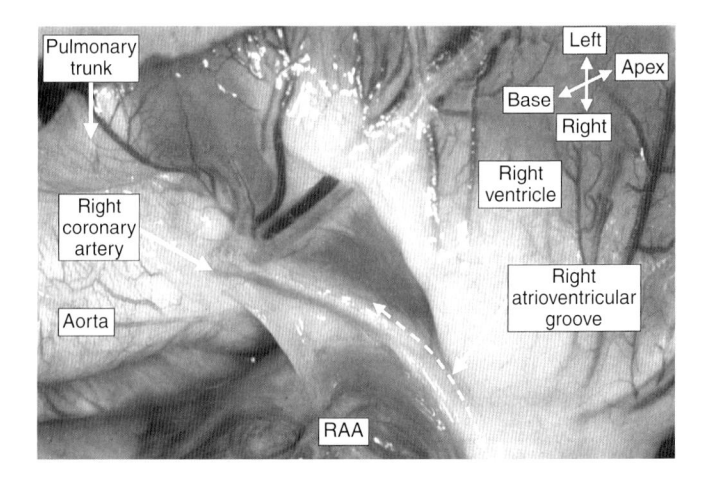

Figure 47-32
This picture, taken in the operating room through a median sternotomy, shows the aortic origin of the right coronary artery. RAA, right atrial appendage. (See color version in the online edition through Expert Consult.) *(Copyright for the original illustration from which this figure was prepared belongs to Benson R. Wilcox, Andrew C. Cook, and Robert H. Anderson.)*

which introduces the potential for luminal narrowing and disturbances in myocardial perfusion, particularly when the deviated origin is intimately related to a valvar commissure.[19]

The left coronary artery almost always takes origin from a single orifice in the left-hand-facing sinus. In contrast, in about half of all hearts, there are two orifices in the right-hand-facing sinus. In such instances, the orifices are unequal in size, the larger giving rise to the main trunk of the right coronary artery, whereas the considerably smaller second orifice usually gives rise to an infundibular artery, or rarely to the artery supplying the sinus node. The coronary arteries can also arise, though rarely, from a solitary orifice, usually within the right-hand-facing sinus.

The epicardial course of the major coronary arteries follows the atrioventricular and interventricular grooves. The right coronary artery emerges from the right-hand-facing aortic sinus and immediately enters the right atrioventricular groove (Fig. 47-32). In approximately 90% of cases, this artery gives rise to the so-called posterior descending artery at the crux, the artery in reality being positioned inferiorly rather than posteriorly. In a good proportion of these cases, the artery then continues beyond the crux, and it supplies downgoing branches to the diaphragmatic surface of the left ventricle. This is called right coronary arterial dominance (Fig. 47-33). As the artery encircles the tricuspid orifice, it is most closely related to the origin of the valvar attachments near the takeoff of its acute marginal branch. Other important branches also take origin from this encircling segment of the artery. Immediately after its origin, the artery gives rise

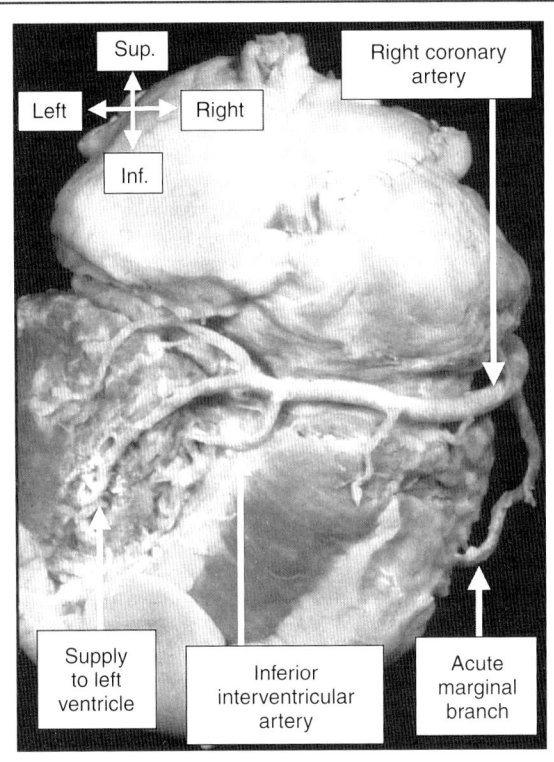

Figure 47–33
The heart has been removed from the thorax and is positioned on its apex. The dissection shows a right dominant coronary artery. (Copyright for the original illustration from which this figure was prepared belongs to Benson R. Wilcox, Andrew C. Cook, and Robert H. Anderson.)

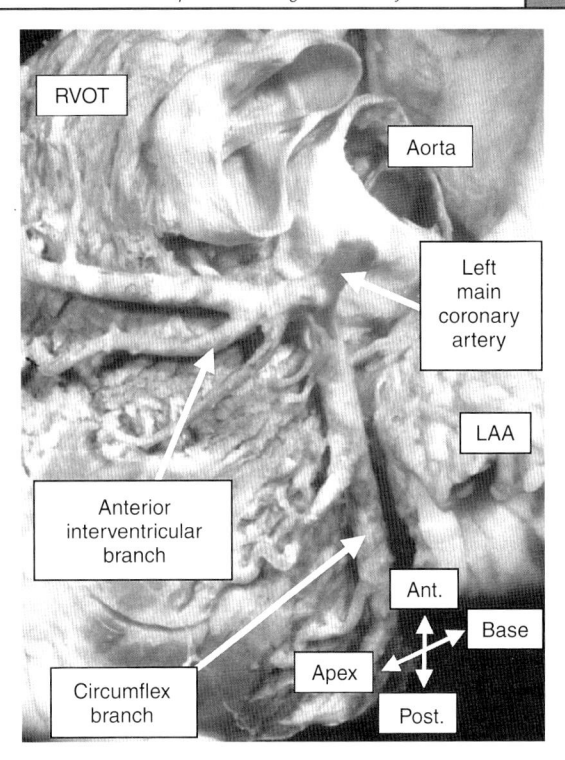

Figure 47–34
This dissection, with the heart positioned in anatomic position and photographed from the left side, shows the branches of the main stem of the left coronary artery. LAA, left atrial appendage; RVOT, right ventricular outflow tract. (See color version in the online edition through Expert Consult.) (Copyright for the original illustration from which this figure was prepared belongs to Benson R. Wilcox, Andrew C. Cook, and Robert H. Anderson.)

to downgoing infundibular branches, one of which may also arise by a separate orifice. In just over half the cases, the right coronary artery also gives rise to the artery to the sinus node. Very rarely, but of major significance when present, the nodal artery can arise laterally from the right coronary artery, coursing over the lateral margin of the appendage to reach the terminal groove.[2]

The main stem of the left coronary artery emerges from the left-hand-facing sinus between the pulmonary trunk and the left atrial appendage. It is a very short structure, rarely extending beyond 1 cm before branching into its anterior interventricular and circumflex branches (Fig. 47-34). In some hearts, the main stem trifurcates, with an intermediate branch present between the two main branches. The intermediate branch supplies the obtuse margin of the left ventricle. The anterior interventricular artery runs within the anterior interventricular groove, giving off diagonal branches to the obtuse margin, and the important perforating branches that pass inferiorly into the septum. The first major septal perforating branch is particularly important (see Fig. 47-22), as it is at major risk when the pulmonary valve is removed for use as a homograft.[20] The interventricular artery then continues toward the apex, and it frequently curves under the apex onto the diaphragmatic surface of the ventricles. The circumflex branch of the left coronary artery passes backward to run in relationship with the mitral orifice. It is most closely related to the orifice when it gives rise to the inferior interventricular artery at the crux, a so-called dominant left coronary artery (Fig. 47-35). A dominant left coronary artery, however, is found in only

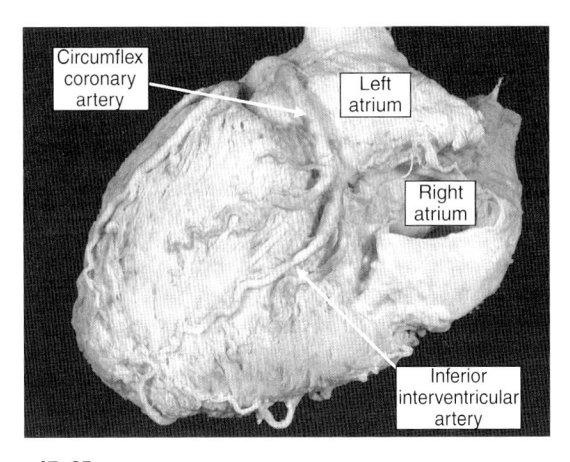

Figure 47–35
In this heart, which is positioned in anatomic orientation but photographed from its diaphragmatic aspect, it is the circumflex coronary artery that is dominant (compare with Fig. 47-33). (Copyright for the original illustration from which this figure was prepared belongs to Benson R. Wilcox, Andrew C. Cook, and Robert H. Anderson.)

about 10% of cases. When the left coronary is not dominant, the circumflex artery usually terminates by supplying downgoing branches to the pulmonary surface of the left ventricle. In roughly 45% of normal individuals, the circumflex artery also gives rise to the artery that supplies the sinus node.

Throughout much of their epicardial course, the arteries and their accompanying veins are encased in epicardial

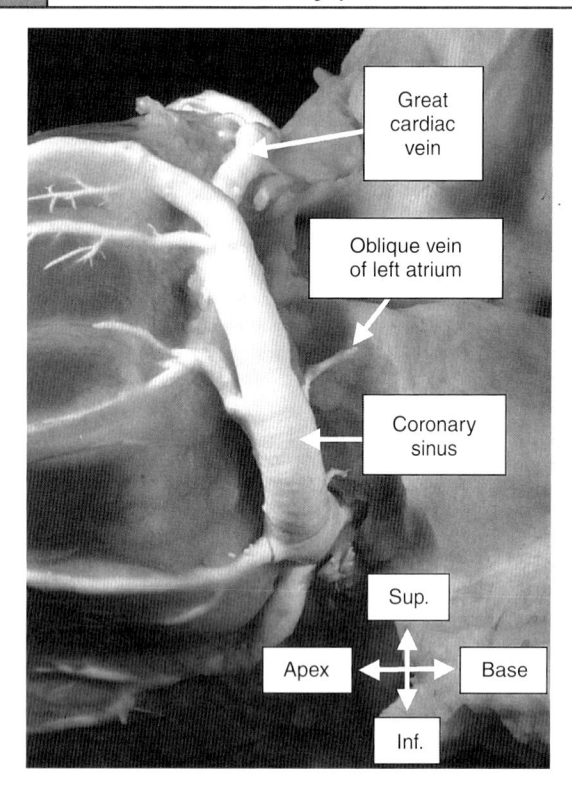

Figure 47–36
This specimen has been prepared by filling the coronary sinus with Silastic. The heart is positioned to show its diaphragmatic aspect. The coronary sinus is formed at the union of the great cardiac vein with the oblique vein of the left atrium. (See color version in the online edition through Expert Consult.) *(Copyright for the original illustration from which this figure was prepared belongs to Benson R. Wilcox, Andrew C. Cook, and Robert H. Anderson.)*

adipose tissue. In some hearts, the myocardium itself may form a "bridge" over segments of the artery. The role of these bridges in the development of coronary arterial disease is not clear. They can certainly be an impediment to surgeons in their effort to isolate the artery.

The coronary veins drain blood from the myocardium to the right atrium. The smaller veins—namely, the anterior and the so-called small cardiac veins—drain directly to the cavity of the atrium. They are not of surgical significance. The larger veins accompany the major arteries and are the tributaries of the coronary sinus. The great cardiac vein runs alongside the anterior interventricular (left anterior descending) artery. It encircles the mitral orifice to enter the posterior and leftward margin of the atrioventricular groove, becoming the coronary sinus as it receives the oblique vein of the left atrium (Fig. 47-36). The coronary sinus then runs within the groove, lying between the left atrial wall and the ventricular myocardium, before draining into the right atrium. At the crux, the sinus receives the middle cardiac vein, which has ascended with the inferior interventricular (posterior descending) artery, and the small cardiac vein, which has encircled the tricuspid orifice in company with the right coronary artery. Occasionally, these latter two veins drain directly to the right atrium. The orifice of the coronary sinus is guarded by the thebesian valve, which, on very rare occasions, may be imperforate. Valves are also found in the cardiac veins. That found in the great cardiac vein where it turns around the pulmonary surface is most constant and is called the valve of Vieussens.

Acknowledgments

The research on which this chapter is based was supported by grants from the British Heart Foundation. Research at the Institute of Child Health and Great Ormond Street Hospital for Children NHS Trust benefits from R&D funding received from the NHS Executive.

REFERENCES

1. Cook AC, Anderson RH. Attitudinally correct nomenclature [editorial]. *Heart* 2002;**87**:503-6.
2. Wilcox BR, Anderson RH. *Surgical Anatomy of the Heart.* ed 2 London: Gower Medical; 1992.
3. Uemura H, Ho SY, Devine WA, et al. Atrial appendages and venoatrial connections in hearts from patients with visceral heterotaxy. *Ann Thorac Surg* 1995;**60**:561-9.
4. Anderson KR, Ho SY, Anderson RH. The location and vascular supply of the sinus node in the human heart. *Br Heart J* 1979;**41**:28-32.
5. James TN. *Anatomy of the Coronary Arteries.* New York: Hoeber; 1961, 103-106.
6. Anderson RH, Webb S, Brown NA. Clinical anatomy of the atrial septum with reference to its developmental components. *Clin Anat* 1999;**12**:362-74.
7. Sweeney LJ, Rosenquist GC. The normal anatomy of the atrial septum in the human heart. *Am Heart J* 1979;**98**:194-9.
8. Anderson RH, Ho SY. Architecture of the sinus node, the atrioventricular conduction axis, and the internodal myocardium. *J Cardiovasc Electrophysiol* 1998;**9**:1233-48.
9. Isaacson R, Titus JL, Merideth J, et al. Apparent interruption of atrial conduction pathways after surgical repair of transposition of the great arteries. *Am J Cardiol* 1972;**30**:533-5.
10. James TN. The connecting pathways between the sinus node and the A-V node and between the right and the left atrium in the human heart. *Am Heart J* 1963;**66**:498-508.
11. Janse MJ, Anderson RH. Internodal atrial specialised pathways—fact or fiction? *Eur J Cardiol* 1974;**2**:117-37.
12. Anderson RH, Becker AE. *Cardiac Anatomy: an Integrated Text and Colour Atlas.* ed 1 London: Gower Medical; 1980, 3.2-3.3.
13. Anderson RH. Clinical anatomy of the aortic root. *Heart* 2000;**84**:670-3.
14. McFadden PM, Culpepper WS, Ochsner JL. Iatrogenic right ventricular failure in tetralogy of Fallot repairs: reappraisal of a distressing problem. *Ann Thorac Surg* 1982;**33**:400-2.
15. Van Praagh R, David I, Wright GB, Van Praagh S. Large RV plus small LV is not single RV. *Circulation* 1980;**61**:1057-8.
16. Anderson RH, Devine WA, Ho SY, et al. The myth of the aortic annulus: the anatomy of the subaortic outflow tract. *Ann Thorac Surg* 1991;**52**:640-6.
17. Gittenberger-de Groot AC, Sauer U, Oppenheimer-Dekker A, Quaegebeur J. Coronary arterial anatomy in transposition of the great arteries: a morphologic study. *Pediatr Cardiol* 1983;**4**(Suppl I):15-24.
18. Bader G. Beitrag zur Systematik und Haufigkeit der Anomalien der Coronararterien des Menschen. *Virch Arch Pathol Anat* 1963;**337**:88-96.
19. Gittenberger-de Groot AC, Sauer U, Quaegebeur J. Aortic intramural coronary artery in three hearts with transposition of the great arteries. *J Thorac Cardiovasc Surg* 1986;**91**:566-71.
20. Hosseinpour AR, Anderson RH, Ho SY. The anatomy of the septal perforating arteries in normal and congenitally malformed hearts. *J Thorac Cardiovasc Surg* 2001;**121**:1046-52.

CHAPTER 48
Vascular Physiology
Basel Ramlawi and Frank W. Sellke

Vascular Resistance
Regulation of Microvascular Tone
  Intrinsic and Extrinsic Vasomotor Control
  Role of the Endothelium
  Role of Metabolism and Autoregulation
  Flow-Induced Dilation
Neurohumoral Influence on Microcirculation
Intrinsic Myogenic Tone
Impact of Extravascular and Humoral Forces on the Microcirculation
Role of Venules in Vascular Resistance
Endothelial Factors in Vascular Growth and Response to Injury
Impact of Disease States on Coronary Circulation
Pulmonary Vascular Physiology
Summary

Myocardial and pulmonary perfusion are regulated by a complex array of influences intrinsic and extrinsic to the vasculature and may be influenced by obstructive atherosclerotic lesions or, in the case of pulmonary hypertension, fibromuscular changes in the blood vessels. A basic understanding of vascular tone and the influences in various disease states that may change vasomotor regulation is necessary to optimize patient care. Surgical decisions are generally made on the basis of the anatomy of large arteries. Whereas the presence of obstructive lesions and vasomotor state of these vessels can affect myocardial, pulmonary, or other organ perfusion, it is the microcirculation that has a more significant role in the regulation of blood flow under normal circumstances. Much has been learned over the past 20 or 30 years that has increased our understanding of the regulation of blood vessels and organ perfusion in health and in disease states.

Many cell types make up the walls of blood vessels. Endothelial cells make up the inner layer. This intimal endothelial layer is surrounded by a variable number of layers of smooth muscle cells comprising the medial layer. The adventitial layer surrounds the vascular smooth muscle layers. This last layer is responsible for providing structural integrity to the blood vessel, particularly larger arteries. Initially, the endothelium was thought to serve mainly as a barrier to the diffusion of macromolecules, but recently much has been learned about the pivotal role it plays in vascular function, regulation of vascular tone, and control of local blood flow.[1] Smooth muscle cells also control vascular tone via humoral vasoactive factors, neural mediators, or local paracrine factors (Fig. 48-1).

The classification of microvessels based on structural characteristics is rather arbitrary, and there is a lack of uniformity in the definitions of microvascular segments such as small arteries, arterioles, venules, and so on. The transition between these segments is gradual and there is no clear demarcation between them. In general, microvessels are defined as vessels less than 300 μm in internal diameter. Capillaries are the smallest blood vessels, defined as vessels whose walls are composed of only endothelial tubes. The microvessels through which blood flows toward capillaries are arterial microvessels, and those that drain from capillaries are venous microvessels.[2] Arterial microvessels usually have three coats—a thin tunica intima; a relatively thick tunica media, composed of one to several layers of smooth muscle cells disposed circumferentially; and a tunica adventitia, made up of fibrous elements and fibroblasts.

Venous microvessels collect the blood from capillaries and have thinner vascular walls than arterial microvessels. Venules, 50 μm in diameter, do not possess smooth muscle cell layers. Smaller venules have only endothelial cells and pericytes; because these venules are the most permeable, they play an important role in substance exchange.

The various vascular beds in the body possess many similarities and subtle differences. The regulation of myocardial perfusion depends on many intrinsic and extrinsic factors that may be affected by atherosclerotic lesions. In the coronary circulation, it has been shown that vasomotor regulation of vessels, in addition to the actual anatomy, plays an important role in coronary perfusion and operative decision making. Blood flow is also largely dependent on the resistance generated by the microcirculation. Although early vasomotor regulation studies consisted of indirect assessments using measurements of flow and calculations of resistance, more recent investigations into the properties of the intact coronary circulation have yielded much information, as have modern methods of analysis for interpretation of physiologic data.[3-6]

The microcirculation possesses unique features that allow it to respond to the dynamic changes in nutrient requirements and to interact with surrounding tissue. This chapter focuses on issues relating to the regulation of vascular tone, with an emphasis on coronary and pulmonary microcirculations.

VASCULAR RESISTANCE

An understanding of vascular resistance is important, as it is these resistance vessels that cause pressure losses and are responsible for regulation of perfusion. Initially, it was thought that the precapillary arterioles were responsible for vascular resistance, with little resistance involvement by the vessels larger than 25 to 50 μm in diameter. Subsequent work revealed that over half of total vascular resistance is caused by vessels larger than 100 μm, and this can be observed in vessels larger than 300 μm.[7,8] Also, contrary to previous belief, the venous circulation, under similar conditions of vasodilation, may account for up to 30% of vascular resistance. Figure 48-2 shows that under the vasodilatory effects of dipyridamole, larger arteries and veins assume a greater role in resistance.[8,9] Similarly, ischemia results in a significant redistribution of vascular resistance.[9] This reveals that the distribution of vascular resistance is dynamic and is dependent on vascular tone, among other factors.

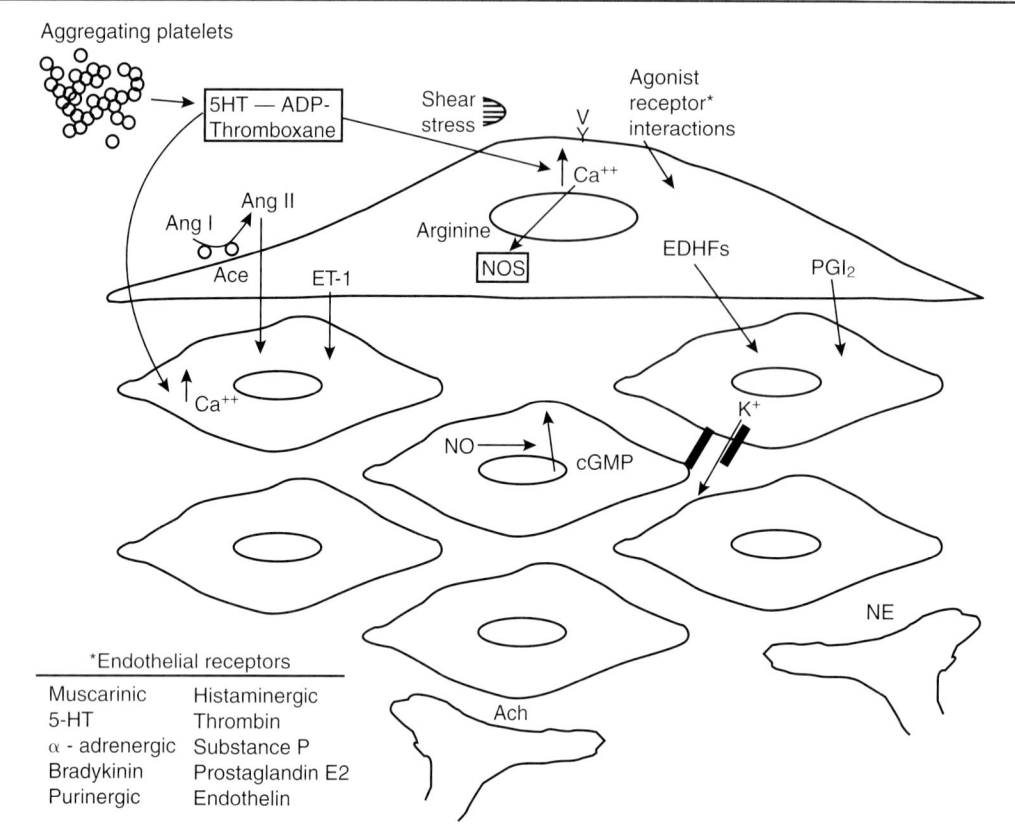

Figure 48-1
Regulation of vascular tone by factors released from the endothelium, activated platelets and leukocytes, neuronally released factors, and circulating substances. Ace, angiotensin converting enzyme; Ach, acetylcholine; ADP, adenosine diphosphate; Ang, angiotensin; cGMP, cyclic guanosine monophosphate; EDHF, endothelium-derived hyperpolarizing factor; ET, endothelin; 5HT, 5-hydroxytryptamine (serotonin); NE, norepinephrine; NO, nitric oxide; NOS, nitric oxide synthase; PGI_2, prostaglandin I_2.

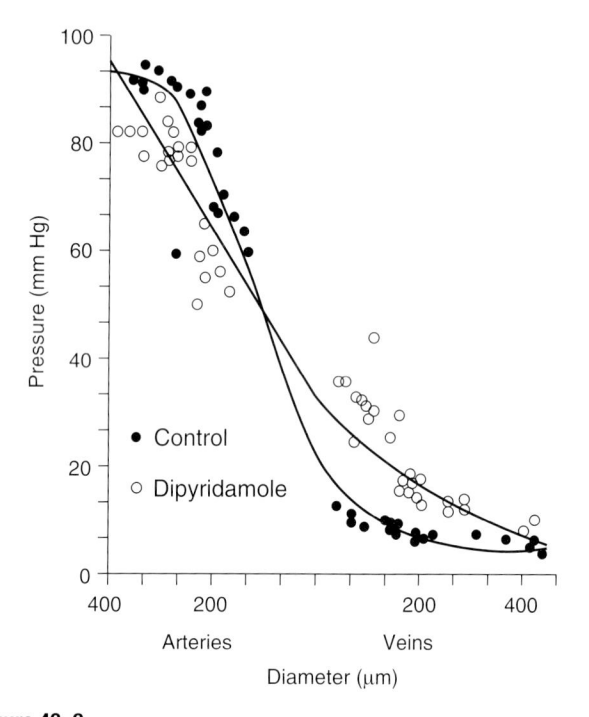

Figure 48-2
Intravascular pressures in the coronary microcirculation under basal conditions and during vasodilation with dipyridamole. The distribution of vascular resistance is not static. Instead, the size of the vessels regulating vascular tone depends on the tone of the vasculature. *(Adapted from Chilian WM, Layne SM, Klausner EC, et al. Am J Physiol 1989;***256***:H383-90.)*

The redistribution of microvascular resistance may change the myogenic tone in each microvascular segment because the luminal pressure in a certain vascular segment is determined by the systemic pressure and the relative distribution of vascular resistance. That is, when resistance is shifted upstream by dilation of small arterioles, for instance, the luminal pressure in the upstream microvessels decreases, resulting in myogenic dilation. The changes in the venular pressure caused by the resistance redistribution may also critically affect the substance exchange capacity and edema formation.

In the coronary circulation, pressure losses are also caused by vessels as they course from the epicardium through the myocardium.[10] This is accentuated further in the setting of cardiac hypertrophy. Such a phenomenon is particularly relevant clinically, as it plays a role in explaining the pathophysiology of subendocardial infarcts, as shown in Figure 48-3. The hypertrophied pathologic state causes a decrease in the perfusion pressure of the subendocardium, predisposing it to ischemia and infarction.[11]

REGULATION OF VASCULAR TONE

Intrinsic and Extrinsic Vasomotor Control

Vessels possess intrinsic control mechanisms for maintaining the homeostasis of the local microenvironment in the face of stress. Vasomotor tone regulation is a complex process that is influenced by the intrinsic properties of the vessel wall, by local innervation, and by substances from surrounding parenchymal

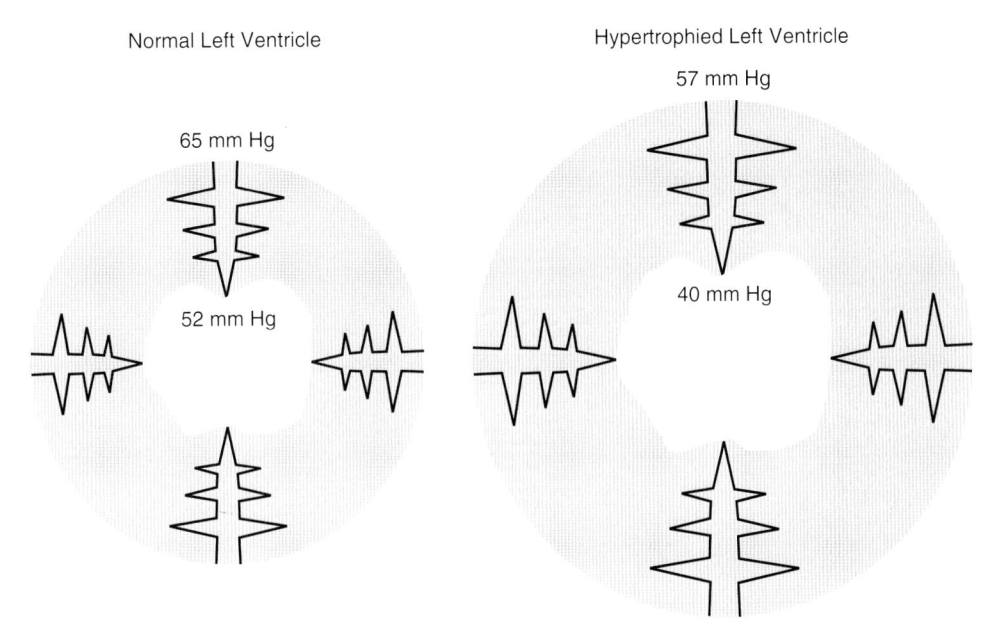

Figure 48–3
Transmural losses of coronary perfusion pressure in normal and hypertrophied hearts. Pressures were measured using micropuncture–servo null techniques in hearts perfused via the left main coronary artery at 100 mm Hg. *(Adapted from Fujii M, Nuno DW, Lamping KG, et al.* Circ Res *1992;71:120-6.)*

tissue. Properties intrinsic to the vessel wall and interactions with adjacent tissues work together to promote metabolic regulation and autoregulation. Endothelial regulation of vasomotor tone is also critically involved in organ perfusion. Vascular responses to endogenous substances are summarized in Figure 48-4. All of these factors play an especially significant role in the setting of microvascular tone.[2]

On the basis of in vitro observations, Jones and colleagues found that larger arterioles are more sensitive to shear stress than myogenic factors, whereas small microvessels are more sensitive to metabolic factors.[12] Based on this they proposed three distinct microdomains that are governed by distinct forms of regulation. They have divided the arterial microvessels into (1) small arterioles (<50 μm), which are most sensitive to metabolic mediators; (2) intermediate arterioles (50 to 80 μm), where myogenic mechanisms predominate; and (3) large arterioles (80 to 150 μm), where flow-induced dilation most potently occurs. This model provides insight for understanding the regulation of microvessels, although there is undoubtedly overlap among these three components.

Jones and colleagues hypothesized that the longitudinal disposition of these three microdomains may enable the integrated adjustment of flow conductance in the face of various influences, such as increased metabolism, a reduction in perfusion pressure, and so on, by affecting other microdomains together.[12] For example, the dilation of small arterioles by augmented metabolism produces a decrease in luminal pressure in upstream microvessels, leading to the dilation of intermediate arterioles by decreasing the myogenic tone. These microvascular dilations could produce an increase in shear stress and could result in enhanced flow-induced dilation in large arterioles. As a result, all sizes of arterial microvessels dilate in response to the metabolic stimulation. The marked longitudinal heterogeneity of microvascular responses may be at least partly explained by this microdomain hypothesis.

Role of the Endothelium

The endothelium plays a pivotal role in vasomotor tone regulation. Many substances can affect tone via endothelium-mediated mechanisms. Endothelial cells also release several substances that affect coronary resistance, such as nitric oxide (NO•), prostaglandins, a hyperpolarizing factor, endothelin, and reactive oxygen species (ROS). These are summarized in Figure 48-5. As the major regulatory molecule, NO is produced by a constitutively expressed enzyme known as endothelial nitric oxide synthase (eNOS or NOS-3). NO is formed as a result of a series of electron transfers from NADPH to the flavins FAD and FMN on the reductase domain, and electron transfer to a prosthetic heme group in the oxygenase domain. When heme reduction occurs, arginine is catalyzed to citrulline and nitric oxide. The NO• formed diffuses to underlying vascular smooth muscle, where its actions include stimulation of soluble guanylate cyclase, increasing the level of cyclic guanosine monophosphate (cGMP) and prompting vasodilation via activation of cGMP-dependent protein kinase.[13] Although binding of calcium/calmodulin is a prerequisite for activity of eNOS, other events, such as phosphorylation,[14] membrane binding,[15] binding of eNOS with heat-shock protein 90, and association with the integral membrane protein caveolin,[16] can also modulate NOS activity. Also, NO• may undergo reactions with thiol-containing compounds to form biologically active nitroso molecules.[17]

Although eNOS is expressed constitutively, it undergoes important gene expression regulation by factors such as shear stress, endothelial cell growth, hypoxia, exposure to oxidized

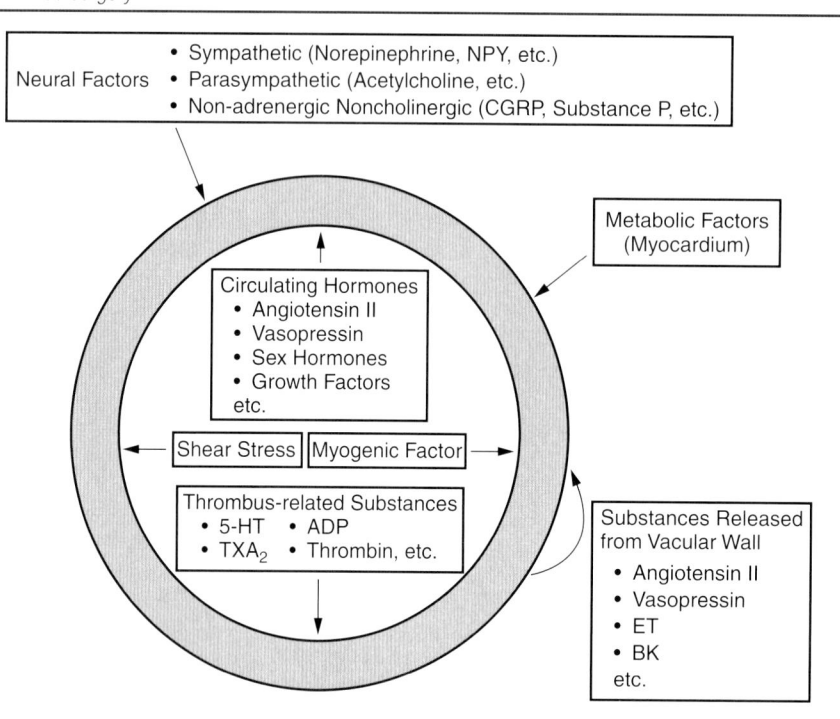

Figure 48–4
Factors that influence microvascular tone. ADP, adenosine diphosphate; BK, Ca^{2+}-activated K^+; CGRP, calcitonin gene-related peptide; ET, endothelin; 5HT, 5-hydroxytryptamine (serotonin); NPY, neuropeptide Y; TXA_2, thromboxane A_2. *(Adapted from Komaru T, Kanatsuka H, Shirato K. Pharmacol Ther 2000;**86**:217-61.)*

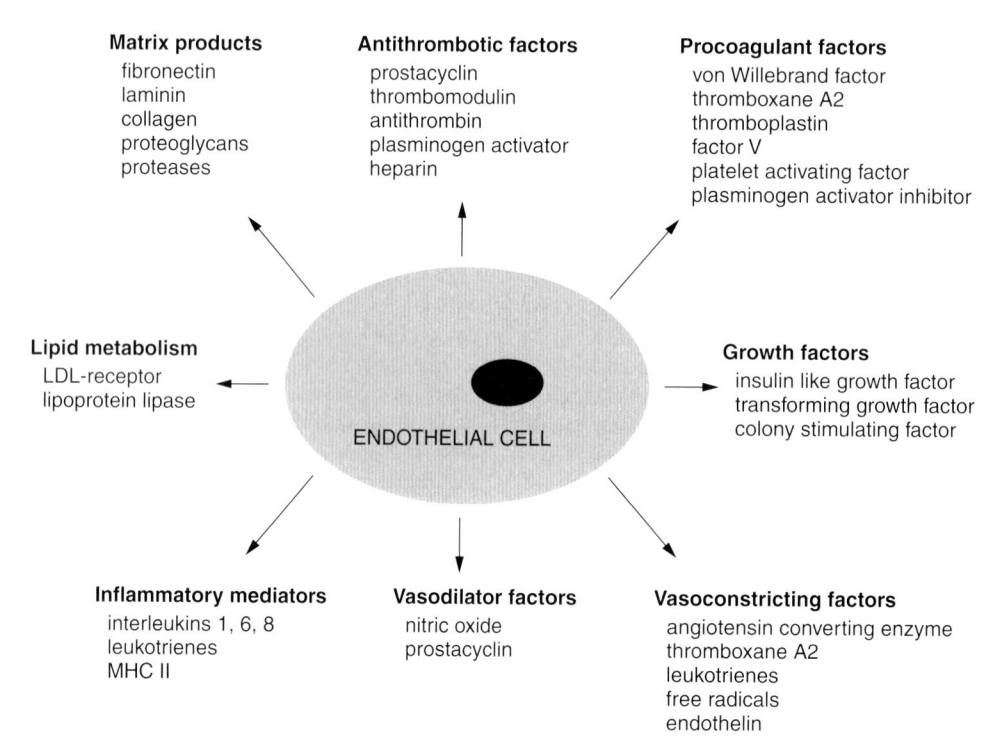

Figure 48–5
Endothelial cells have both metabolic and synthetic functions. Through the secretion of a large variety of mediators they are able to influence cellular function throughout the body. LDL, low-density lipoprotein; MHC, major histocompatibility complex. *(Adapted from Galley HF, Webster NR. Physiology of the endothelium. Br J Anaesth 2004;**93**:105-13.)*

low-density lipoprotein, and exposure to cytokines.[18-20] In the coronary circulation, the release of NO• confers a state of basal vasodilation. Hence, administration of NO synthase antagonists produces an increase in resting coronary resistance. On the other hand, when substances such as acetylcholine and bradykinin are administered, coronary microvessels of all sizes dilate. Endothelial NO production is affected by a variety of mechanisms in many disease states. The signal transduction pathways through which NO acts are summarized in Figure 48-6. It is likely that the most important pathway involves activation of soluble guanylate cyclase, which catalyzes the formation of cGMP from guanidine triphosphate. The cGMP serves as an allosteric regulator of the enzyme cGMP-dependent protein kinase (PKG). PKG phosphorylates contractile proteins and ion channels, decreasing intracellular calcium and the sensitivity of contractile proteins to intracellular calcium. The binding of NO to cytochrome oxidase in the mitochondria leads to regulation of oxygen consumption and in turn may affect oxygen demand. Similarly, the receptors of atrial natriuretic peptide (ANP) and brain natriuretic peptide (BNP) are also particulate forms of guanylate cyclases, and these substances produce vasodilation via similar pathways. NO is also released in response to sodium nitroprusside and organic nitrates.

Although NO is the major regulator of vascular tone, there are other factors that modulate endothelium-dependent vascular tone in coronary, pulmonary, and peripheral circulations. Endothelium-derived hyperpolarizing factor (EDHF) is an example. The endothelium-dependent hyperpolarization of vascular smooth muscle is mediated by the opening of a calcium-dependent potassium channel or by activating Na/K-ATPase. The role of the various EDHFs probably varies depending on the vessel size, the species, and the vascular bed under consideration. When the vascular smooth muscle is hyperpolarized, voltage-sensitive calcium channels are closed, leading to a reduction in intracellular calcium. Several different EDHFs exist, such as epoxyeicosatrienoic acid (EET), a cytochrome p450 metabolite of arachidonic acid. Other possible EDHFs include potassium and hydrogen peroxide. Prostaglandin synthesis by the endothelium also contributes to modulation of tone in the microcirculation. The predominant prostaglandin produced by endothelial cells is prostacyclin (PGI_2). There is substantial interaction between nitric oxide, EDHF, and prostacyclin. A major stimulus for release of prostacyclin, NO, and EDHF is shear stress, or the tangential force of fluid as it flows over the endothelium, resulting in flow-dependent vasodilation. Interestingly, the importance of nitric oxide seems to decline and the role of the EDHF increases as

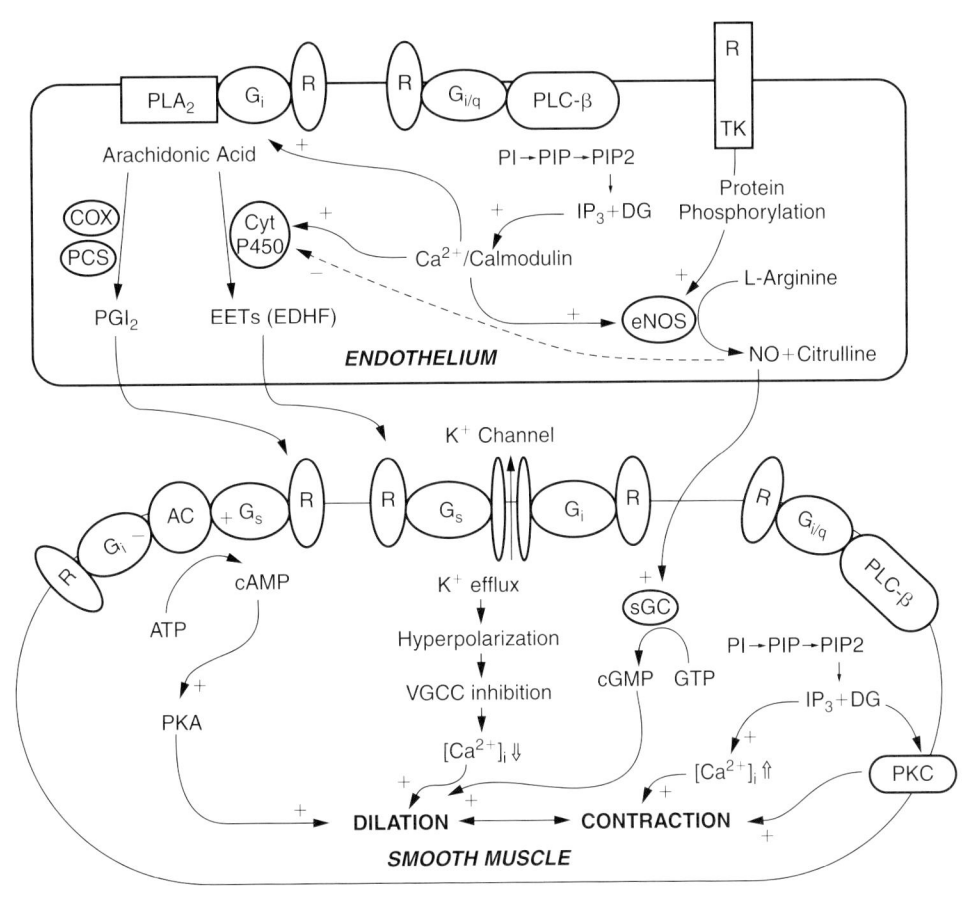

Figure 48–6
Signal transduction pathways for the vascular responses to agonists. Nitric oxide (NO), prostaglandin I_2 (PGI_2), and endothelium-derived hyperpolarizing factor (EDHF) are important for the cross-talk between the endothelium and the vascular smooth muscle. AC, adenylyl cyclase; COX, cyclooxygenase; Cyt P450, cytochrome P450; DG, diacylglycerol; eNOS, endothelial nitric oxide synthase; Gi, Gi-protein; Gq, Gq protein; PCS, prostacyclin synthase; PI, phosphatidylinositol; PIP, phosphatidylinositol 4-phosphate; PIP2, phosphatidylinositol 4,5-bisphosphate; PKA, protein kinase A; PLA_2, phospholipase A_2; PLC, phospholipase C; R, receptors; TK, tyrosine kinase; VGCC, voltage-gated Ca^{2+} channel. (Adapted from Komaru T, Kanatsuka H, Shirato K. Pharmacol Ther 2000;86:217-61.)

blood vessels decrease in size. Consequently, the production of EDHF may increase when nitric oxide is low. The interaction of endothelial cells with vascular smooth muscle cells and the intermediates involved is outlined in Figure 48-7.

Role of Metabolism and Autoregulation

The ability of a vascular bed to adjust its tone to maintain a constant flow during changes in perfusion pressure is termed autoregulation.[21] This process is most effective in the coronary circulation when pressure is between 40 and 160 mm Hg. The subendocardium and the subepicardium differ in the range of pressures over which autoregulation can be observed: in the subendocardium, flow begins to decrease at pressures of less than 70 to 75 mm Hg, whereas this happens at significantly lower pressures in the superficial layers of the myocardium.[22] Clinically, systemic arterial hypertension affects the range over which autoregulation occurs in the subendocardium, such that flow begins to decline at even higher pressures. Such a change in subendocardial perfusion pressure in the setting of hypertrophic myocardium increases the likelihood of subendocardial ischemia. Also, patients with systemic hypertension may have an increased lower limit of autoregulation and thus may suffer brain ischemia during surgery, or at other times even at pressures sufficient to sustain adequate perfusion in patients with normal blood pressure.

With regard to both autoregulation and metabolic vascular regulation, the predominant changes in vasomotor tone occur in vessels less than 100 μm in diameter. The rate of oxygen consumption in the myocardium is closely related to myocardial perfusion via coronary microvascular tone. As the myocardial oxygen requirements increase, coronary flow rises in response. Mostly, this is because the ability of the myocardium to extract additional oxygen to meet increased demand is limited, because myocardial oxygen extraction is near maximum even under resting conditions.

Flow-Induced Dilation

Flow-induced dilation is a ubiquitous phenomenon of blood vessels in various organs and animals, including humans.[2,23,24] Flow-induced dilation plays important physiologic roles in the following ways: (1) it protects the vessel wall against friction induced injury, (2) it prevents the vascular steal phenomenon by dilating upstream vessels when there is focal hyperemia, (3) it reduces the heterogeneity of flow distribution, and (4) it buffers the pressure distribution if there are rapid pressure changes.

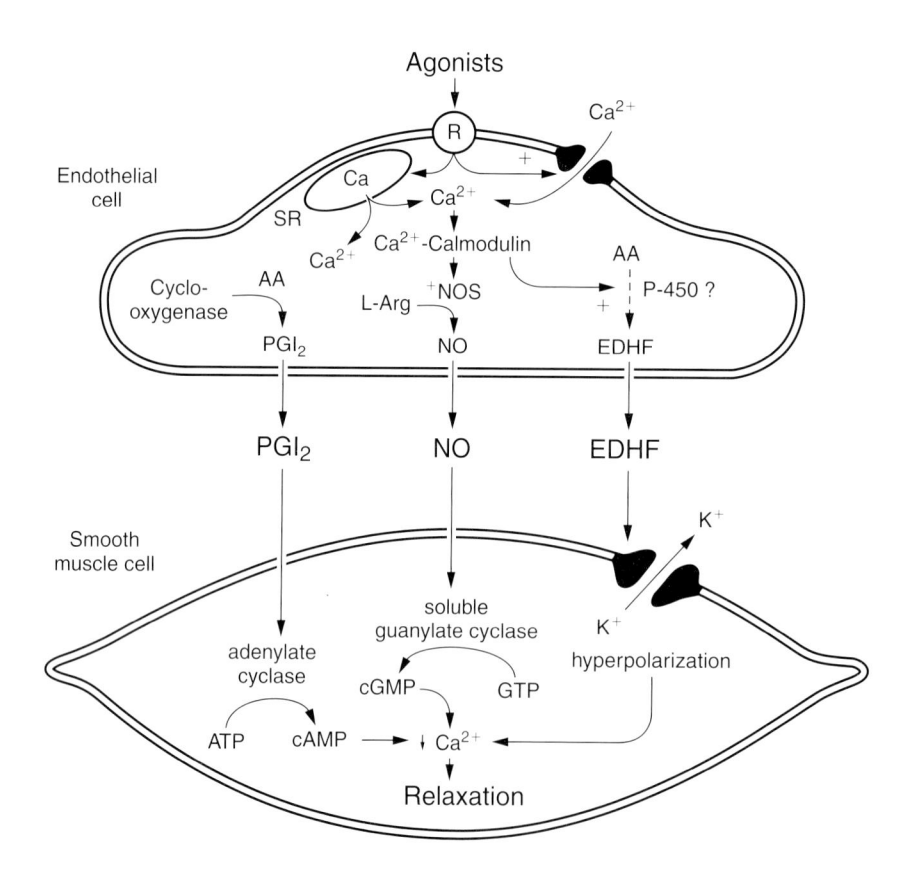

Figure 48–7
Role of the increase in cytosolic calcium concentration in the release of endothelium-derived relaxing factors (EDRF). Endothelial receptor activation induces an influx of calcium into the cytoplasm of the endothelial cell; after interaction with calmodulin, NO-synthase and cyclooxygenase are activated, leading to the release of endothelium-derived hyperpolarizing factor (EDHF). NO causes relaxation by activating the formation of cyclic GMP (cGMP) from GTP. EDHF causes hyperpolarization and relaxation by opening K$^+$ channels. Prostacyclin (PGI$_2$) causes relaxation by activating adenylate cyclase (AC), which leads to the formation of cyclic AMP (cAMP). Any increase in cytosolic calcium (including that induced by the calcium ionophore A23187) causes the release of relaxing factors. When agonists activate the endothelial cells, an increase in inositol phosphate may contribute to the increase in cytoplasmic Ca^{2+} by releasing it from the sarcoplasmic reticulum (SR). *(Adapted from Vanhoutte PM, Boulanger CM, Vidal M, Mombouli JV. Endothelium-derived mediators and the renin-angiotensin system. In: Robertson JIS, Nicholls MG, editors. The renin-angiotensin system. London: Gower Medical; 1993, with permission).*

Flow is sensed by endothelial cells through as yet unidentified mechanoreceptors. In contrast to the myogenic response, the endothelium is required for flow-induced dilation. Regulation of flow-mediated vasodilation is controversial, and both NO and prostaglandins have been shown to be involved, at least in porcine coronary arterioles.[25,26] The exact mechanism of regulation may depend on age, vessel size, and the vascular bed under consideration. A possible flow-induced arteriolar dilation mechanism is summarized in Figure 48-8.

Autoregulation is mediated by the actions of several factors such as NO, EDHF, and adenosine. Removal of a particular factor does not prevent autoregulation, as the other factors seem to take over its function. Adenosine and hydrogen peroxide also cause hyperpolarization of vascular smooth muscle. From the work of Duncker and colleagues, and others, we now know that several factors work together to influence metabolic regulation and autoregulation, leading to adequate regulation of coronary vascular tone despite interruption of any particular pathway.[21]

Neurohumoral Influence on Microcirculation

The coronary arterial system is densely innervated with the sympathetic and parasympathetic nervous systems.[27] Neurotransmitters released from nervous tissues and a wide variety of humoral substances significantly affect the microvascular tone. Neurohumoral factors have an effect on coronary microvascular tone, and together with myogenic, flow-induced, and local metabolic controls, they participate in determining the coronary vascular resistance necessary for oxygen and nutrition supply to the myocardium (see Fig. 48-4).

The role of the autonomic sympathetic and parasympathetic nervous systems is important in regulation of coronary perfusion. In vivo, the vascular response to sympathetic stimulation is mediated by both α-adrenergic and β-adrenergic receptors. In the coronary circulation, the predominant receptor subtype seems to be the β-adrenergic receptor.[28] For example, direct sympathetic nerve stimulation stimulates coronary vasodilation and an increase in coronary flow. If β-adrenergic antagonists are administered, a transient vasoconstriction can be observed.[28] When coronary microvessels are studied in vitro, α-adrenergic stimulation has minimal contractile effects. When selective $α_2$-adrenergic stimulation is applied using pharmacologic stimuli, there is rather potent vasodilation of all sizes of coronary microvessels, predominantly the result of the release of endothelium-derived nitric oxide (NO•). β-Adrenergic stimulation produces a potent relaxation of all coronary arteries, but especially of small-resistance vessels.[28] Also, $β_2$-adrenergic receptor subtype predominates in vessels less than 10 μm in diameter in in vitro studies, whereas a mixed $β_1$- and $β_2$-adrenergic receptor population controls vascular resistance in in vivo studies.[28] On the other hand, larger coronary vessels are regulated by a mixed $β_1$- and $β_2$-adrenoceptor subtype population. Activation of cholinergic receptors by either vagal stimulation or the infusion of acetylcholine produces uniform vasodilation of coronary vessels.[29] This vasodilation is predominantly mediated by endothelium-derived NO•, although release of EDHF[30] and release of prostaglandin substances may contribute.[31] The coronary flow increase by vagal stimulation could be blunted by a metabolically mediated flow decrease caused by a decrease in the heart rate and myocardial contractility.[32]

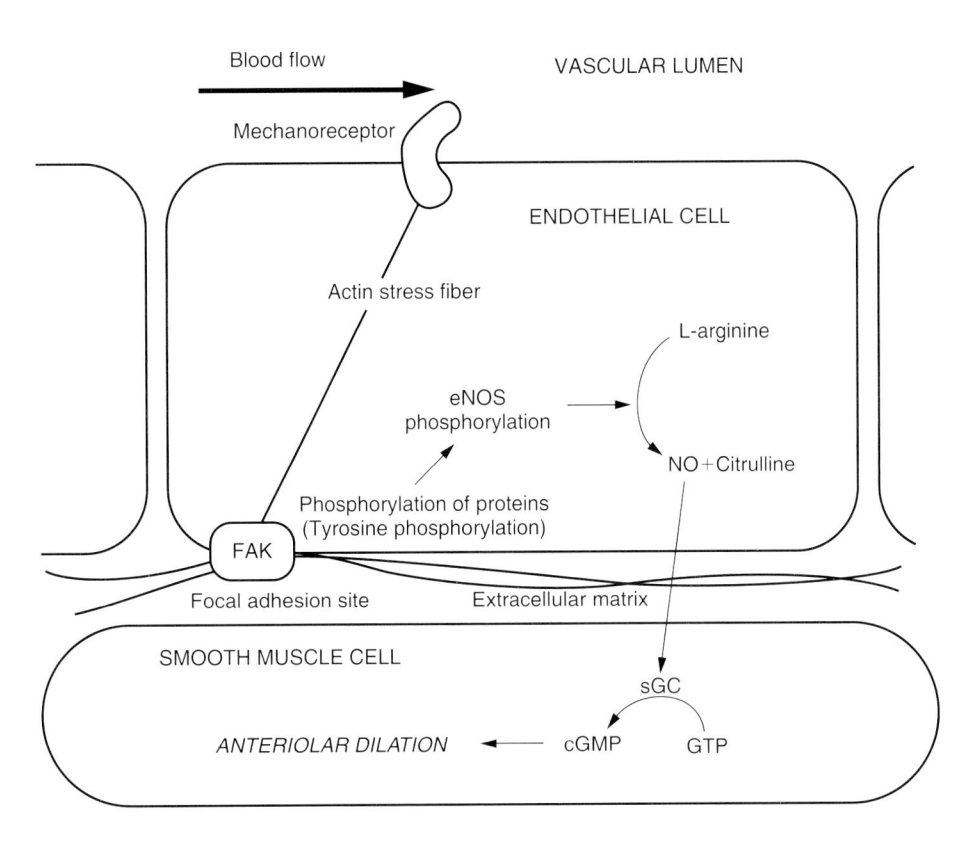

Figure 48–8
Possible signal transduction pathway for the flow-induced arteriolar dilation, which is mediated by mechanotransduction via actin stress fibers, and the subsequent activation of the focal adhesion kinase and endothelial nitric oxide synthase (eNOS) phosphorylation. FAK, focal adhesion kinase; sGC, soluble guanylyl cyclase. *(Adapted from Komaru T, Kanatsuka H, Shirato K.* Pharmacol Ther *2000;***86***:217-61.)*

Other neurotransmitters that act on the coronary circulation include neuropeptide Y (NPY), which is mainly released with norepinephrine as a co-transmitter from sympathetic postganglionic nerve terminals upon intense sympathetic activation.[2,33] Intracoronary application of NPY markedly decreases coronary flow, producing myocardial ischemia without large coronary artery constriction.[34,35] These results point to its potent and specific constrictor effects on coronary microvessels. Also, substance P, a potent vasodilator whose effect is dependent on the endothelium, is contained in perivascular nerve fibers and sensory ganglia.[36]

Intrinsic Myogenic Tone

Myogenic contraction is observed when applying luminal pressure to microvessels, which causes development of intrinsic vascular tone, as shown by elevated wall tension or a decrease in vessel diameter. The microcirculation possesses this intrinsic myogenic tone response, which also contributes to maintaining basal vascular tone and autoregulation.[37] Myogenic microvascular control is endothelium independent, and it is likely to play a critical role in determining the basal tone and in maintaining the intraluminal pressure of the downstream exchange vessels within a physiologic level.[38,39] In the myocardium, myogenic responses to increases in pressure are greater in subepicardial microvessels than in vessels from the subendocardium. Also, myogenic tone may be reduced during inflammatory states when increased expression of iNOS causes altered myocardial perfusion. Increases in myogenic tone, which occur during stretch of vascular smooth muscle, are associated with an increase in inositol 1,4,5-trisphosphate, presumably because of activation of phospholipase C.[37,40,41] Also, the myogenic tone mediator 20-HETE produces constriction of vascular smooth muscle by promoting Ca^{2+}-activated K^+ (BK) channel inhibition. This induces depolarization and increases levels of $[Ca^{2+}]_i$. This effect is most likely caused by activation of L-type Ca^{2+} channels or the activation of protein kinase C (PKC) and inhibition of the Na/K-ATPase.[42] Other mediators probably involved in the myogenic tone response include mitogen-activated protein (MAP) kinases and Rho protein. The downstream mediator Rho kinase may modulate myogenic tone by regulation of the actin cytoskeleton. One potential therapeutic agent for treatment of hypertension and coronary spasm is the use of Rho kinase inhibitors. A summary of possible mechanisms of myogenic tone is shown in Figure 48-9.

Impact of Extravascular and Humoral Forces on the Microcirculation

In the setting of pathologic processes such as ischemia leading to decreased tissue compliance or increased tissue edema, extravascular forces play an especially important role. For example, collateral perfusion is particularly sensitive to changes in heart rate (more frequent extravascular compression) and ventricular diameter (stretch).[6,43] The coronary circulation is particularly unique in that it is exposed to a large number of extravascular forces produced by contraction of adjacent myocardium and intraventricular pressures. Of relevance to the concept of extravascular forces is the idea that these might collapse coronary vessels under certain circumstances. Of note, flow through the epicardial coronary arteries halted when aortic pressure fell to levels ranging from 25 to 50 mm Hg, raising the possibility that extravascular forces might be sufficiently high to collapse vessels when intraluminal pressures declined to values below this critical value.[44] Flow in the coronary microcirculation continued even when the arterial driving pressure was minimally higher than coronary venous pressure. Based on modeling and various experimental interventions, it was determined that the decrease of antegrade blood flow in larger upstream vessels associated with continued forward flow in microvessels was probably the result of capacitance in the coronary circulation.[45] Kanatsuka and colleagues used a floating microscope to visualize epicardial capillaries and were able to show that red cells continued to flow, even after perfusion had stopped in the more proximal vessels.[46] Using this approach, they showed that the pressure at which flow stops in the epicardial coronary microvessels was only a few millimeters of mercury higher than right atrial pressure.[46] Also, when ventricular diastolic pressure is high, vessels deeper in the subendocardium might be made to collapse by pressure transmitted from the ventricular chamber. In contrast, coronary epicardial vessels do not close at any pressure. It therefore seems likely that the concept of "critical closing pressure" is not applicable to all vessels in the coronary circulation.

The response of the coronary microcirculation to humoral agents differs with vessel size and location. Endothelin-1 produces vasoconstriction when administered to the adventitial surfaces of coronary microvessels. The degree of constriction produced by endothelin-1 is inversely related to the size of the vessels. In contrast, when endothelin-1 is administered intraarterially, vasodilation occurs, presumably via release of nitric oxide.[29,31] Also, serotonin constricts vessels less than 100 μm in diameter, whereas it causes vasodilation of smaller arteries.[47] Vasopressin, on the other hand, produces greater constriction of microvessels less than 100 μm in diameter than it produces in larger microvessels.[47,48] In the larger epicardial coronary arteries, vasopressin predominantly causes vasodilation.

Role of Venules in Vascular Resistance

Control of vasomotor regulation differs between the venous and arterial microcirculations, and certain reactions to pathologic stimuli occur preferentially on one side of the capillary bed. Therefore, consideration of the venous circulation apart from the arterial circulation is needed. Venules have considerable importance under conditions of vascular dilation, such as during exercise, metabolic stress, or reperfusion after myocardial ischemia.[9] The venous circulation may influence myocardial stiffness and relaxation properties of the heart. Veins also respond differently to agonists and neuronal stimulation compared with arteries in the same vascular bed.[31,49] Also, venules are the initiating site of neutrophil adherence and transmigration, whereas arterioles seldom manifest these initial changes in the inflammatory response.[50] Ischemia-reperfusion has been determined to cause endothelial dysfunction in veins, but, under similar conditions, arterioles appear to be more susceptible to a reduction in endothelium-dependent relaxation than are coronary venules, despite the fact that leukocytes preferentially adhere to venular rather than to arterial endothelial cells.[51] In addition, complement fragment C5a causes neutrophil adherence in venules but not in arterioles, suggesting that different mechanisms mediate neutrophil-endothelial adherence in the two vessel types.[52]

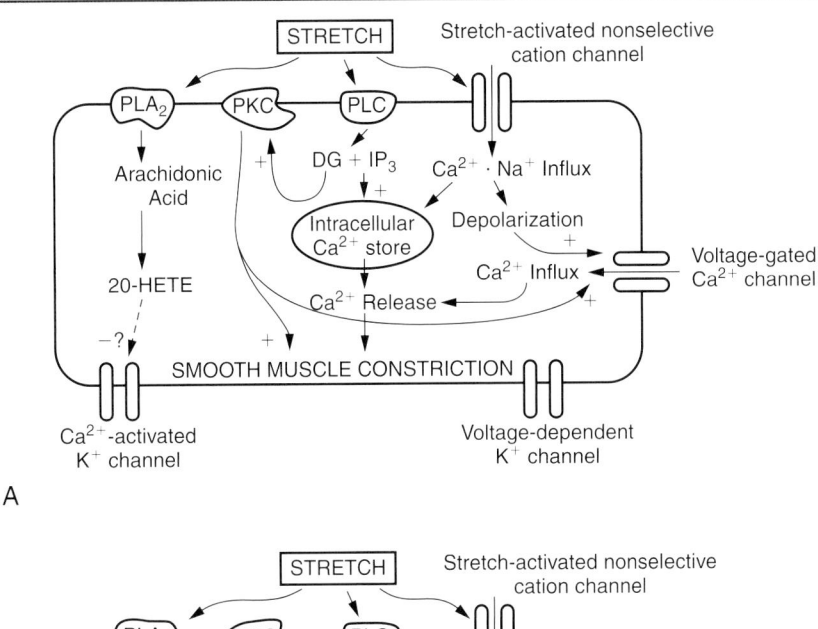

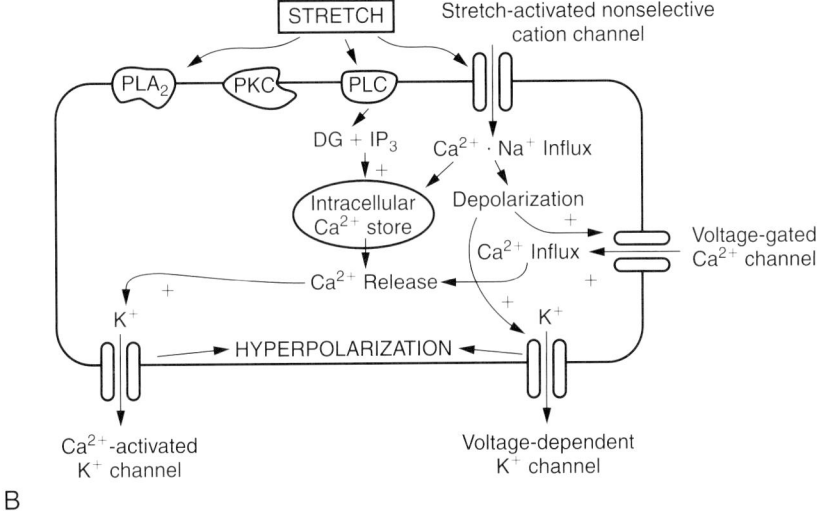

Figure 48–9
Schematic illustrations for the possible mechanisms of the myogenic constriction (**A**) and its compensatory mechanisms (**B**). DG, diacylglycerol; 20-HETE, 20-hydroxyeicosatetraenoic acid; IP$_3$, inositol 1,4,5-trisphosphate; PKC, protein kinase C; PLA$_2$, phospholipase A$_2$; PLC, phospholipase C. (Adapted from Komaru T, Kanatsuka H, Shirato K. Pharmacol Ther 2000;86:217-61.)

ENDOTHELIAL FACTORS IN VASCULAR GROWTH AND RESPONSE TO INJURY

It is important to identify the role of nitric oxide and nitric oxide–related factors in vascular development (Fig. 48-10). Nitric oxide inhibits vascular smooth muscle proliferation via apoptosis. Animal models have shown that treatment with L-nitroarginine methyl ester (L-NAME), an inhibitor of NO formation, markedly increases neointimal development after vascular injury.[53] Also, local transfection with the eNOS cDNA reduces the intimal proliferation that follows balloon injury.[54] The vascular response to injury is enhanced in mice deficient in eNOS.[55,56] Thus, NO and cGMP-elevating agents inhibit the growth of fibroblasts and vascular smooth muscle. This effect of NO on vascular smooth muscle growth is mediated by cGMP and can be mimicked by cGMP analogs such as atrial natriuretic factor.[56,57]

NO plays an important role in supporting the process of angiogenesis, as endothelial cells do not seem to be sensitive to the growth-inhibitory effects of nitric oxide. In fact, vascular endothelial growth factor (VEGF)-1 actions during angiogenesis are mediated by NO. Endothelial cells in the proliferative phase have a sixfold increase in eNOS expression compared with confluent ones, and eNOS knockout mice have little VEGF activity.[19] During the vascular injury response, this feed-forward condition promotes vascular growth, because while endothelial cells are proliferating to form new blood vessels, the high levels of NO promote tube formation. Similarly, in response to the denudation injury, proliferating endothelial cells increase NO production during the growth period to compensate for the lack of endothelial cells in the denuded area while also decreasing platelet adhesion and vascular smooth muscle proliferation in that same area. Moreover, endothelial progenitor cells (EPCs) from the bone marrow play a role in repair of denuded vessels as well as angiogenesis. Although not completely elucidated, circulating EPCs seem to vary in quantity from one patient to the next, depending on the presence of common risk factors such as diabetes (decreased amount) or lipid-lowering drugs such as HMG-Co A reductase inhibitors (increased amount).

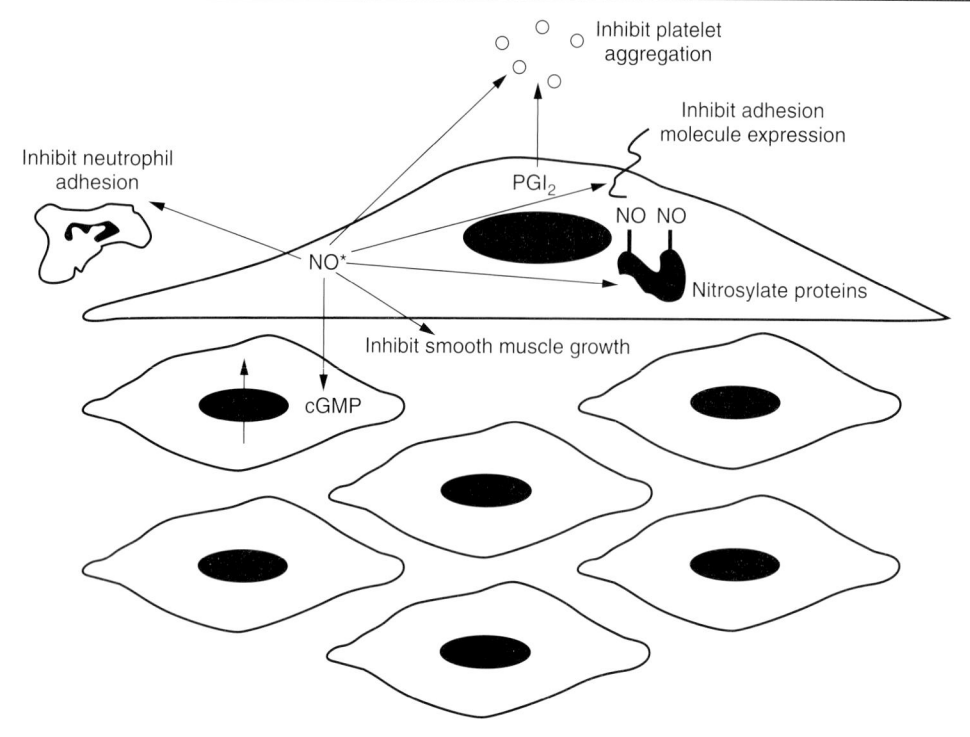

Figure 48–10
Schematic representation of endothelium and vascular smooth muscle, demonstrating the multifaceted roles of nitric oxide released from the endothelium in the modulation of vascular function, structure, and the response to injury. cGMP, cyclic guanidine monophosphate; PGI_2, prostacyclin.

IMPACT OF DISEASE STATES ON CORONARY CIRCULATION

Coronary microvascular homeostasis may be adversely affected in disease states through variation in the vessels' diameter, quantity, or responsiveness to humoral factors. Vasomotor tone reliant on endothelial function is particularly vulnerable to pathologies such as atherosclerosis, hyperlipidemia, diabetes, and the aging process. This mechanism is highlighted in Figure 48-11. The mechanisms underlying these abnormal endothelium-dependent responses are most likely multifactorial. Factors responsible include abnormalities of G-protein signaling, resulting in reduced activation of eNOS in response to endothelial cell receptor activation; an alteration of levels of the critical cofactor for eNOS tetrahydrobiopterin; and an overproduction of asymmetric dimethylarginine (ADMA), which acts as an antagonist for the eNOS substrate L-arginine. It has been shown that oxidative stress (via increased production of vascular superoxide $O_2^{-\bullet}$) is particularly increased in the presence of common risk factors. Such an increase in oxidative stress will cause a reduction in endothelium-dependent vasodilation.

It is accepted that diseases that affect endothelium-dependent vascular dilation have an impact on the coronary microcirculation as well as on larger vessels. Experiments have demonstrated that in coronary microvessels from monkeys fed a high-cholesterol diet for 18 months, relaxation in response to acetylcholine and bradykinin was dramatically impaired, and sometimes paradoxical constrictions were even produced.[58] Similar findings of diet-induced atherosclerosis have been made in other animal models. Subsequent studies performed using in vivo techniques showed that vasoconstriction caused by serotonin and ergonovine (both known to be modulated by the endothelium) was markedly enhanced in the coronary microcirculation of hypercholesterolemic monkeys.[59] These findings are impressive because the coronary microcirculation is spared from the development of overt atherosclerosis. Therefore, in the setting of a risk factor for atherosclerosis, endothelial dysfunction occurs, leading to an abnormal vascular response. It was then demonstrated in humans with hypercholesterolemia that diminished flow responses to acetylcholine were restored with reduction of cholesterol levels.[60] Similar observations have been made either in humans or in experimental models of hypertension,[61] ischemia-reperfusion,[52,62] and diabetes.[63] It has been suggested that this endothelial dysfunction plays a role in the development of clinical symptoms despite normal coronary anatomy.

Impaired endothelium-dependent vasodilation also has been linked to increased cardiovascular events. The loss of NO in cardiovascular disease not only leads to a decrease in vasodilation but also predisposes to atherosclerotic lesion formation and vascular smooth muscle proliferation. NO also has antioxidant properties and prevents adhesion molecule expression by endothelial cells. An example of relevance to the clinical setting is the endothelial changes in the coronary microcirculation after cardioplegic arrest and cardiopulmonary bypass during cardiac surgery.[64] In this setting, endothelial dysfunction persists for some time after cardiopulmonary bypass, and normalizes thereafter. This has important clinical implications, as it is common for patients undergoing coronary artery bypass grafting, with seemingly complete coronary revascularization, to exhibit signs of myocardial ischemia during the hours after surgery—most likely caused by endothelial dysfunction.

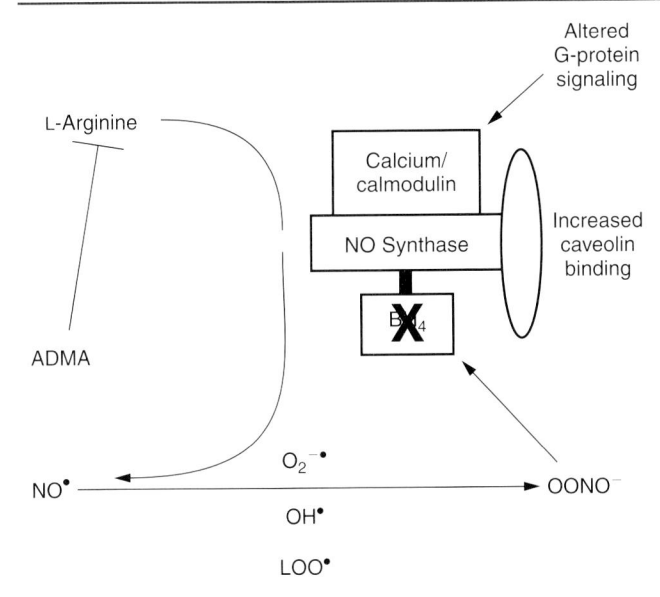

Figure 48–11
Reduced production and bioreactivity of endothelium-derived nitric oxide (NO) in the setting of atherosclerosis, diabetes, and many other pathologic conditions. Asymmetrical dimethylarginine (ADMA) acts as an antagonist of l-arginine. Superoxide and other oxygen free radicals may interfere with NO availability in conditions of increased oxidant stress. The peroxynitrite radical (OONO•) may inhibit tetrahydrobiopterin (BH_4), a cofactor for nitric oxide synthase (NOS). LOO•, peroxyl radical.

Collateral vessels in the coronary circulation are particularly important in coronary disease. They allow for normal resting perfusion to a region of the myocardium that is served by an occluded vessel, albeit at a lower perfusion pressure. However, the coronary arterioles nourished by collaterals develop markedly abnormal vascular reactivity—for example, impaired endothelium-dependent vascular relaxations and enhanced constrictions to vasopressin.[48] Possible mechanisms of this impaired microvascular endothelium-dependent relaxation in the collateral-dependent region may involve changes in shear stress, pulsatile flow in the collateral-dependent microvasculature, or intracellular calcium levels. Such changes may cause disturbance in microvascular tone during a disease state.[18]

It has been also found that treatment of collateral-dependent vessels with angiogenic growth factors may enhance endothelium-dependent relaxation, in addition to improving other aspects of cardiac performance. In patients suffering from disease not amenable to current intervention techniques (e.g., surgical coronary grafting or percutaneous techniques), direct treatment with angiogenic factors can theoretically be the basis for a clinical improvement. Several animal studies have demonstrated that therapeutic angiogenic interventions, in the setting of chronic ischemia, are associated with an improvement in myocardial perfusion and endothelium-dependent vasodilation in the area supplied by collaterals.[65-67] These studies used growth factors such as VEGF, fibroblast growth factor (FGF)-1, or FGF-2 placed in the perivascular area. Possible mechanisms through which these factors act include FGF-2- and VEGF-induced release of NO, which improves collateral perfusion and decreases tissue ischemia.[68] In addition, it has been shown that during periods of chronic ischemia there occurs an upregulation of FGF-2 and VEGF receptors. This finding is consistent with results showing that after administration of growth factors, endothelium-dependent relaxation occurs in the collateral-dependent region but not in myocardium perfused via the original vessels.[69] Also, these growth factors may stimulate the release of bone-marrow-derived endothelial progenitor cells that promote collateral growth and endothelial function at the treated sites. Unfortunately, clinical trials to date have not demonstrated much benefit with growth factor therapy in patients.

Clinically, patients suffering from ventricular hypertrophy often complain of angina-like symptoms. Animal and human studies have demonstrated that cardiac hypertrophy causes a reduction in the maximal capacity of the coronary circulation to dilate in response to either reactive hyperemia or pharmacologic stimuli.[5,61,70] One possible cause for this abnormal response may be a mismatch between the elevated myocardial mass and the relatively reduced coronary microcirculation. Peak flow normalized to myocardial mass may be reduced because of this relative paucity of coronary arterioles, because as the myocardium hypertrophies, the coronary resistance circulation may not increase enough to keep pace with the larger muscle mass. Another possible mechanism of impaired vasodilator responses may be explained by endothelial dysfunction, because many of the diseases associated with myocardial hypertrophy are also associated with a loss of endothelial NO production.

In normal hearts, there is a linear relationship between the diameter of an epicardial coronary artery and the mass of myocardium perfused. Interestingly, epicardial coronary arteries do not enlarge to the same extent as the myocardium hypertrophies, so that for any diameter coronary artery, the amount of myocardium perfused is increased twofold. This phenomenon is particularly relevant in the presence of a coronary stenosis, where a small lesion that is otherwise considered minimal becomes flow limiting in a hypertrophic state.

PULMONARY VASCULAR PHYSIOLOGY

The pulmonary vascular response has unique characteristics that distinguish it from other vascular beds. The normal pulmonary circulation is a low-pressure, low-resistance circuit with little or no resting tone. In contrast to the systemic circulation, where neural and humoral mechanisms predominate, the pulmonary circulation is under the control of both active factors that affect vascular smooth muscle tone (e.g., autonomic nerves, humoral factors, gasses), and passive factors (e.g., cardiac output, left atrial pressure, airway pressure).[71]

In a normal state, unlike systemic arteries, pulmonary arteries have a much thinner smooth muscle layer, which is consistent with a low-pressure system. Small pulmonary arteries are the main effectors of pulmonary vascular resistance, such as hypoxic pulmonary vasoconstriction. Also, the pulmonary capillary bed and the systemic capillary bed respond differently. Pulmonary veins are similar in structure to pulmonary arteries but have less smooth muscle and may be regulated differently. Constriction of pulmonary arteries results in elevated pulmonary artery pressure, which increases the pressure on the right side of the heart, whereas constriction of pulmonary veins increases pulmonary capillary pressure, and this could result in pulmonary edema. With disease, the structure of pulmonary vessels may change significantly. With a chronic increase in pulmonary vascular pressure, there is a structural

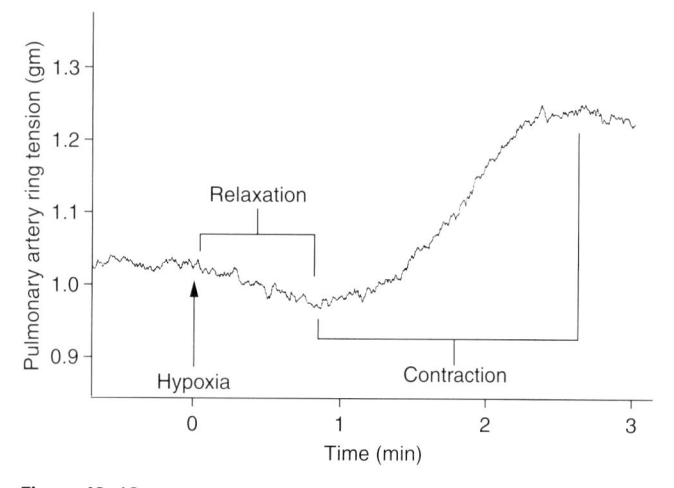

Figure 48-12
Actual tracing of isolated pulmonary artery response to hypoxia. Isolated rat pulmonary artery, supported between steel wires in a 37° C organ bath containing modified Henseleit solution and connected to a force transducer, was contracted with phenylephrine (10^{-7} M) and gassed with 95% oxygen, 5% carbon dioxide (hypoxia). The resulting tension tracing exhibits relaxation preceding a transient vascular contraction. *(Adapted from Tsai BM, Wang M, Turrentine MW, Mahomed Y, Brown JW, Meldrum DR.* Ann Thorac Surg *2004;78:360-8.)*

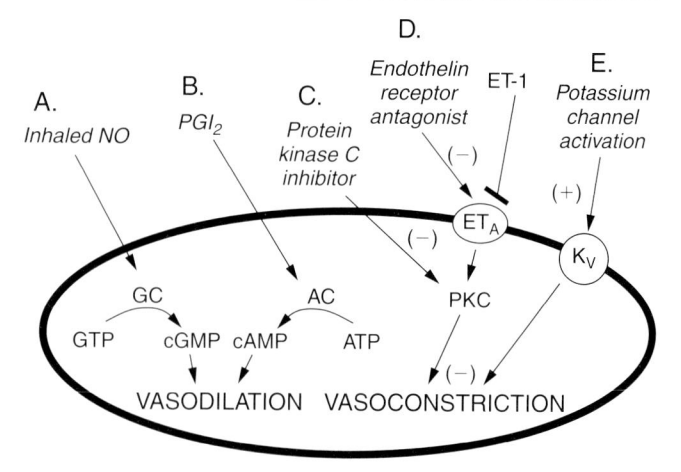

Figure 48-13
Therapeutic strategies for blocking hypoxic pulmonary vasoconstriction. (A) Inhaled nitric oxide (NO) and (B) prostacyclin (PGI_2) activate guanylate cyclase (GC) and adenylate cyclase (AC), respectively, to cause vasodilation. (C) Protein kinase C (PKC) inhibitors prevent protein kinase C–mediated vasoconstriction. (D) Endothelin receptor (ET_A, ET_B) antagonists prevent endothelin-1 (ET-1) from binding to ET_A, thus inhibiting vasoconstriction. (E) Potassium channel activation prevents calcium-dependent vasoconstriction. ATP, adenosine triphosphate; cAMP, adenosine 3′,5′-cyclic monophosphate; cGMP, guanidine 3′,5′-cyclic monophosphate; GTP, guanosine triphosphate; Kv, voltage gated potassium channel. *(Adapted from Tsai BM, Wang M, Turrentine MW, Mahomed Y, Brown JW, Meldrum DR.* Ann Thorac Surg *2004;78:360-8.)*

remodeling, with fibrosis, particularly in the intimal layer, and increased size of the smooth muscle layer, which results in a marked alteration in control mechanisms.[71]

A unique characteristic of the pulmonary circulation is its response to hypoxia. Pulmonary arteries contract when oxygen tension is acutely decreased (Fig. 48-12), unlike systemic vessels, which dilate in response to hypoxia. This phenomenon, called hypoxia-induced pulmonary vasoconstriction (HPV) is an important mechanism that aids in matching ventilation with perfusion by directing blood flow from poorly ventilated regions of the lung to areas with normal or relatively high ventilation.[72] Although acute HPV benefits gas exchange and maximizes oxygenation of venous blood in the pulmonary artery, sustained HPV or chronic exposure to hypoxia is a major cause of the elevated pulmonary vascular resistance and pulmonary arterial pressure in patients with pulmonary arterial hypertension associated with hypoxic cardiopulmonary diseases.[73] Chronic vasoconstriction leads to vascular remodeling, pulmonary hypertension, and possibly cor pulmonale. Patients with chronic obstructive pulmonary disease, for example, are usually hypoxemic and may fall into this category. Similarly, pulmonary vasoconstriction presents a challenge in pediatric patients with congenital heart disease, as they are particularly susceptible to developing pulmonary hypertensive crises after cardiac interventions.[74] Also, pulmonary vascular resistance is often increased after lung transplantation.[75] Hypoxia is a potent vasoconstrictive stimulus in these patients.[76]

Although the exact mechanism of HPV remains unclear, many believe that it is probably related to the activation or inhibition of calcium channels in the pulmonary vascular smooth muscle that leads to contraction.[77,78] This hypothesis is supported by increasing evidence that an increase in cytosolic calcium appears to be an important factor in HPV development.[79] Also, hypoxia has been shown to block the outward flow of potassium, which results in membrane depolarization.[80] Agents that open potassium channels have been shown to decrease HPV.[77] Alternatively, HPV may also be related to the inhibition or secretion of an unknown endogenous mediator that results in vasoconstriction.[73] Pulmonary venous hypertension causes pulmonary endothelial dysfunction characterized by reduced bioavailability of nitric oxide and increased formation of vasoconstrictors such as endothelin 1 and thromboxane A_2.[81,82] Pulmonary venous hypertension may therefore increase pulmonary vasoconstriction and remodeling and cause an increase in pulmonary vascular resistance.[83,84] Lung vascular responses may further increase pulmonary arterial pressure in congestive heart failure and augment the risk for right ventricular failure.

Aside from oxygen, agents used as potential therapies for HPV include inhaled NO, prostaglandins, endothelin receptor antagonists, protein kinase C inhibitors, and potassium channel activators (Fig. 48-13). Inhaled vasodilators are now thought to circumvent potentially deleterious systemic side effects by acting predominantly on the pulmonary circulation (e.g., epoprostenol or the phosphodiesterase-3 inhibitor milrinone).[85,86]

Summary

This chapter provided an overview of some of the newer concepts regarding physiologic and pathophysiologic control of vascular tone. Properties of peripheral vessels cannot be extrapolated to the coronary or pulmonary circulation. Similarly, properties of one size or class of coronary microvessel cannot be generalized. Certainly the technology used in more recent studies is dramatically changed from that of older ones. Although we attempted to focus on studies that directly examined the microvasculature using the newer technology (in vitro preparations or in situ observations), it was also important to present classical studies of the intact circulation performed in intact animals or isolated hearts. Newer research questions have necessitated the use of more basic techniques, including cell culture and molecular biological approaches. A recent development has been the ability to make many in vivo hemodynamic measurements in human subjects in the catheterization laboratory, thus obviating the need the expenses of flow studies in large animals. As the field of vascular biology grows, we will continue to validate our observations in the intact circulation of our patients and to translate this basic science to the clinical setting.

REFERENCES

1. Furchgott RF, Zawadzki JV. The obligatory role of endothelial cells in the relaxation of arterial smooth muscle by acetylcholine. *Nature* 1980;**288**:373-6.
2. Komaru T, Kanatsuka H, Shirato K. Coronary microcirculation: physiology and pharmacology. *Pharmacol Ther* 2000;**86**:217-61.
3. Feigl EO. Coronary physiology. *Physiol Rev* 1983;**63**:1-205.
4. Hoffman JI. Transmural myocardial perfusion. *Prog Cardiovasc Dis* 1987;**29**:429-64.
5. Marcus ML. *The Coronary Circulation in Health and Disease*. New York: McGraw-Hill; 1983.
6. Schaper W. *The Pathophysiology of Myocardial Perfusion*. New York: Elsevier/North-Holland Biomedical Press; 1979.
7. Nellis SH, Liedtke AJ, Whitesell L. Small coronary vessel pressure and diameter in an intact beating rabbit heart using fixed-position and free-motion techniques. *Circ Res* 1981;**49**:342-53.
8. Chilian WM, Eastham CL, Marcus ML. Microvascular distribution of coronary vascular resistance in beating left ventricle. *Am J Physiol* 1986;**251**:H779-88.
9. Chilian WM, Layne SM, Klausner EC, Eastham CL, Marcus ML. Redistribution of coronary microvascular resistance produced by dipyridamole. *Am J Physiol* 1989;**256**:H383-90.
10. Chilian WM. Microvascular pressures and resistances in the left ventricular subepicardium and subendocardium. *Circ Res* 1991;**69**:561-70.
11. Fujii M, Nuno DW, Lamping KG, Dellsperger KC, Eastham CL, Harrison DG. Effect of hypertension and hypertrophy on coronary microvascular pressure. *Circ Res* 1992;**71**:120-6.
12. Jones CJ, Kuo L, Davis MJ, Chilian WM. Regulation of coronary blood flow: coordination of heterogeneous control mechanisms in vascular microdomains. *Cardiovasc Res* 1995;**29**:585-96.
13. Murad F. Cyclic guanosine monophosphate as a mediator of vasodilation. *J Clin Invest* 1986;**78**:1-5.
14. Corson MA, James NL, Latta SE, Nerem RM, Berk BC, Harrison DG. Phosphorylation of endothelial nitric oxide synthase in response to fluid shear stress. *Circ Res* 1996;**79**:984-91.
15. Venema RC, Sayegh HS, Arnal JF, Harrison DG. Role of the enzyme calmodulin-binding domain in membrane association and phospholipid inhibition of endothelial nitric oxide synthase. *J Biol Chem* 1995;**270**:14705-11.
16. Michel JB, Feron O, Sacks D, Michel T. Reciprocal regulation of endothelial nitric-oxide synthase by Ca2+-calmodulin and caveolin. *J Biol Chem* 1997;**272**:15583-6.
17. Myers PR, Minor RL Jr, Guerra R Jr, Bates JN, Harrison DG. Vasorelaxant properties of the endothelium-derived relaxing factor more closely resemble S-nitrosocysteine than nitric oxide. *Nature* 1990;**345**:161-3.
18. Uematsu M, Ohara Y, Navas JP, Nishida K, Murphy TJ, Alexander RW, et al. Regulation of endothelial cell nitric oxide synthase mRNA expression by shear stress. *Am J Physiol* 1995;**269**:C1371-8.
19. Arnal JF, Yamin J, Dockery S, Harrison DG. Regulation of endothelial nitric oxide synthase mRNA, protein, and activity during cell growth. *Am J Physiol* 1994;**267**:C1381-8.
20. McQuillan LP, Leung GK, Marsden PA, Kostyk SK, Kourembanas S. Hypoxia inhibits expression of eNOS via transcriptional and posttranscriptional mechanisms. *Am J Physiol* 1994;**267**:H1921-7.
21. Duncker DJ, van Zon NS, Ishibashi Y, Bache RJ. Role of K+ ATP channels and adenosine in the regulation of coronary blood flow during exercise with normal and restricted coronary blood flow. *J Clin Invest* 1996;**97**:996-1009.
22. Boatwright RB, Downey HF, Bashour FA, Crystal GJ. Transmural variation in autoregulation of coronary blood flow in hyperperfused canine myocardium. *Circ Res* 1980;**47**:599-609.
23. Pohl U, Holtz J, Busse R, Bassenge E. Crucial role of endothelium in the vasodilator response to increased flow in vivo. *Hypertension* 1986;**8**:37-44.
24. Drexler H, Zeiher AM, Wollschlager H, Meinertz T, Just H, Bonzel T. Flow-dependent coronary artery dilatation in humans. *Circulation* 1989;**80**:466-74.
25. Jimenez AH, Tanner MA, Caldwell WM, Myers PR. Effects of oxygen tension on flow-induced vasodilation in porcine coronary resistance arterioles. *Microvasc Res* 1996;**51**:365-77.
26. Kuo L, Chilian WM, Davis MJ. Interaction of pressure- and flow-induced responses in porcine coronary resistance vessels. *Am J Physiol* 1991;**261**:H1706-15.
27. Young MA, Knight DR, Vatner SF. Autonomic control of large coronary arteries and resistance vessels. *Prog Cardiovasc Dis* 1987;**30**:211-34.
28. Wang SY, Friedman M, Johnson RG, Weintraub RM, Sellke FW. Adrenergic regulation of coronary microcirculation after extracorporeal circulation and crystalloid cardioplegia. *Am J Physiol* 1994;**267**:H2462-70.
29. Lamping KG, Chilian WM, Eastham CL, Marcus ML. Coronary microvascular response to exogenously administered and endogenously released acetylcholine. *Microvasc Res* 1992;**43**:294-307.
30. Hammarstrom AK, Parkington HC, Coleman HA. Release of endothelium-derived hyperpolarizing factor (EDHF) by M3 receptor stimulation in guinea-pig coronary artery. *Br J Pharmacol* 1995;**115**:717-22.
31. Sellke FW, Dai HB. Responses of porcine epicardial venules to neurohumoral substances. *Cardiovasc Res* 1993;**27**:1326-32.
32. Van Winkle DM, Feigl EO. Acetylcholine causes coronary vasodilation in dogs and baboons. *Circ Res* 1989;**65**:1580-93.
33. Gu J, Polak JM, Adrian TE, Allen JM, Tatemoto K, Bloom SR. Neuropeptide tyrosine (NPY): a major cardiac neuropeptide. *Lancet* 1983;**1**:1008-10.
34. Clarke JG, Davies GJ, Kerwin R, Hackett D, Larkin S, Dawbarn D, et al. Coronary artery infusion of neuropeptide Y in patients with angina pectoris. *Lancet* 1987;**1**:1057-9.
35. Maturi MF, Greene R, Speir E, Burrus C, Dorsey LM, Markle DR, et al. Neuropeptide-Y. A peptide found in human coronary arteries constricts primarily small coronary arteries to produce myocardial ischemia in dogs. *J Clin Invest* 1989;**83**:1217-24.
36. Mione MC, Ralevic V, Burnstock G. Peptides and vasomotor mechanisms. *Pharmacol Ther* 1990;**46**:429-68.
37. Kuo L, Davis MJ, Chilian WM. Myogenic activity in isolated subepicardial and subendocardial coronary arterioles. *Am J Physiol* 1988;**255**:H1558-62.
38. Davis MJ. Microvascular control of capillary pressure during increases in local arterial and venous pressure. *Am J Physiol* 1988;**254**:H772-84.
39. Kuo L, Chilian WM, Davis MJ. Coronary arteriolar myogenic response is independent of endothelium. *Circ Res* 1990;**66**:860-6.
40. Narayanan J, Imig M, Roman RJ, Harder DR. Pressurization of isolated renal arteries increases inositol trisphosphate and diacylglycerol. *Am J Physiol* 1994;**266**:H1840-5.
41. Osol G, Laher I, Cipolla M. Protein kinase C modulates basal myogenic tone in resistance arteries from the cerebral circulation. *Circ Res* 1991;**68**:359-67.
42. Miller FJ Jr, Dellsperger KC, Gutterman DD. Myogenic constriction of human coronary arterioles. *Am J Physiol* 1997;**273**:H257-64.
43. Conway RS, Kirk ES, Eng C. Ventricular preload alters intravascular and extravascular resistances of coronary collaterals. *Am J Physiol* 1988;**254**:H532-41.
44. Bellamy RF. Diastolic coronary artery pressure-flow relations in the dog. *Circ Res* 1978;**43**:92-101.
45. Eng C, Jentzer JH, Kirk ES. The effects of the coronary capacitance on the interpretation of diastolic pressure-flow relationships. *Circ Res* 1982;**50**:334-41.
46. Kanatsuka H, Ashikawa K, Komaru T, Suzuki T, Takishima T. Diameter change and pressure—red blood cell velocity relations in coronary microvessels during long diastoles in the canine left ventricle. *Circ Res* 1990;**66**:503-10.
47. Lamping KG, Kanatsuka H, Eastham CL, Chilian WM, Marcus ML. Nonuniform vasomotor responses of the coronary microcirculation to serotonin and vasopressin. *Circ Res* 1989;**65**:343-51.
48. Sellke FW, Quillen JE, Brooks LA, Harrison DG. Endothelial modulation of the coronary vasculature in vessels perfused via mature collaterals. *Circulation* 1990;**81**:1938-47.
49. Klassen GA, Armour JA. Epicardial coronary venous pressures: autonomic responses. *Can J Physiol Pharmacol* 1982;**60**:698-706.
50. Yuan Y, Mier RA, Chilian WM, Zawieja DC, Granger HJ. Interaction of neutrophils and endothelium in isolated coronary venules and arterioles. *Am J Physiol* 1995;**268**:H490-8.
51. Lefer DJ, Nakanishi K, Vinten-Johansen J, Ma XL, Lefer AM. Cardiac venous endothelial dysfunction after myocardial ischemia and reperfusion in dogs. *Am J Physiol* 1992;**263**:H850-6.
52. Piana RN, Wang SY, Friedman M, Sellke FW. Angiotensin-converting enzyme inhibition preserves endothelium-dependent coronary microvascular responses during short-term ischemia-reperfusion. *Circulation* 1996;**93**:544-51.

53. Cayatte AJ, Palacino JJ, Horten K, Cohen RA. Chronic inhibition of nitric oxide production accelerates neointima formation and impairs endothelial function in hypercholesterolemic rabbits. *Arterioscler Thromb* 1994;**14**:753-9.
54. von der Leyen HE, Gibbons GH, Morishita R, Lewis NP, Zhang L, Nakajima M, et al. Gene therapy inhibiting neointimal vascular lesion: in vivo transfer of endothelial cell nitric oxide synthase gene. *Proc Natl Acad Sci U S A* 1995;**92**:1137-41.
55. Moroi M, Zhang L, Yasuda T, Virmani R, Gold HK, Fishman MC, Huang PL. Interaction of genetic deficiency of endothelial nitric oxide, gender, and pregnancy in vascular response to injury in mice. *J Clin Invest* 1998;**101**:1225-32.
56. Yu SM, Hung LM, Lin CC. cGMP-elevating agents suppress proliferation of vascular smooth muscle cells by inhibiting the activation of epidermal growth factor signaling pathway. *Circulation* 1997;**95**:1269-77.
57. Itoh H, Pratt RE, Ohno M, Dzau VJ. Atrial natriuretic polypeptide as a novel antigrowth factor of endothelial cells. *Hypertension* 1992;**19**:758-61.
58. Sellke FW, Armstrong ML, Harrison DG. Endothelium-dependent vascular relaxation is abnormal in the coronary microcirculation of atherosclerotic primates. *Circulation* 1990;**81**:1586-93.
59. Chilian WM, Dellsperger KC, Layne SM, Eastham CL, Armstrong MA, Marcus ML, Heistad DD. Effects of atherosclerosis on the coronary microcirculation. *Am J Physiol* 1990;**258**:H529-39.
60. Drexler H, Zeiher AM, Meinzer K, Just H. Correction of endothelial dysfunction in coronary microcirculation of hypercholesterolaemic patients by L-arginine. *Lancet* 1991;**338**:1546-50.
61. Treasure CB, Klein JL, Vita JA, Manoukian SV, Renwick GH, Selwyn AP, et al. Hypertension and left ventricular hypertrophy are associated with impaired endothelium-mediated relaxation in human coronary resistance vessels. *Circulation* 1993;**87**:86-93.
62. Quillen JE, Sellke FW, Brooks LA, Harrison DG. Ischemia-reperfusion impairs endothelium-dependent relaxation of coronary microvessels but does not affect large arteries. *Circulation* 1990;**82**:586-94.
63. Matsunaga T, Okumura K, Ishizaka H, Tsunoda R, Tayama S, Tabuchi T, Yasue H. Impairment of coronary blood flow regulation by endothelium-derived nitric oxide in dogs with alloxan-induced diabetes. *J Cardiovasc Pharmacol* 1996;**28**:60-7.
64. Sellke FW, Shafique T, Schoen FJ, Weintraub RM. Impaired endothelium-dependent coronary microvascular relaxation after cold potassium cardioplegia and reperfusion. *J Thorac Cardiovasc Surg* 1993;**105**:52-8.
65. Bauters C, Asahara T, Zheng LP, Takeshita S, Bunting S, Ferrara N, et al. Recovery of disturbed endothelium-dependent flow in the collateral-perfused rabbit ischemic hindlimb after administration of vascular endothelial growth factor. *Circulation* 1995;**91**:2802-9.
66. Harada K, Friedman M, Lopez JJ, Wang SY, Li J, Prasad PV, et al. Vascular endothelial growth factor administration in chronic myocardial ischemia. *Am J Physiol* 1996;**270**:H1791-802.
67. Sellke FW, Wang SY, Friedman M, Harada K, Edelman ER, Grossman W, Simons M. Basic FGF enhances endothelium-dependent relaxation of the collateral-perfused coronary microcirculation. *Am J Physiol* 1994;**267**:H1303-11.
68. Sellke FW, Wang SY, Stamler A, Lopez JJ, Li J, Simons M. Enhanced microvascular relaxations to VEGF and bFGF in chronically ischemic porcine myocardium. *Am J Physiol* 1996;**271**:H713-20.
69. Rapps JA, Jones AW, Sturek M, Magliola L, Parker JL. Mechanisms of altered contractile responses to vasopressin and endothelin in canine coronary collateral arteries. *Circulation* 1997;**95**:231-9.
70. Marcus ML, Harrison DG, Chilian WM, Koyanagi S, Inou T, Tomanek RJ, et al. Alterations in the coronary circulation in hypertrophied ventricles. *Circulation* 1987;**75**:I19-25.
71. Barnes PJ, Liu SF. Regulation of pulmonary vascular tone. *Pharmacol Rev* 1995;**47**:87-131.
72. Mauban JR, Remillard CV, Yuan JX. Hypoxic pulmonary vasoconstriction: role of ion channels. *J Appl Physiol* 2005;**98**:415-20.
73. Tsai BM, Wang M, Turrentine MW, Mahomed Y, Brown JW, Meldrum DR. Hypoxic pulmonary vasoconstriction in cardiothoracic surgery: basic mechanisms to potential therapies. *Ann Thorac Surg* 2004;**78**:360-8.
74. Hopkins RA, Bull C, Haworth SG, de Leval MR, Stark J. Pulmonary hypertensive crises following surgery for congenital heart defects in young children. *Eur J Cardiothorac Surg* 1991;**5**:628-34.
75. Robin ED, Theodore J, Burke CM, Oesterle SN, Fowler MB, Jamieson SW, et al. Hypoxic pulmonary vasoconstriction persists in the human transplanted lung. *Clin Sci (Lond)* 1987;**72**:283-7.
76. Waldman JD, Lamberti JJ, Mathewson JW, Kirkpatrick SE, Turner SW, George L, Pappelbaum SJ. Congenital heart disease and pulmonary artery hypertension. I. Pulmonary vasoreactivity to 15% oxygen before and after surgery. *J Am Coll Cardiol* 1983;**2**:1158-64.
77. Barman SA. Potassium channels modulate hypoxic pulmonary vasoconstriction. *Am J Physiol* 1998;**275**:L64-70.
78. Jabr RI, Toland H, Gelband CH, Wang XX, Hume JR. Prominent role of intracellular Ca2+ release in hypoxic vasoconstriction of canine pulmonary artery. *Br J Pharmacol* 1997;**122**:21-30.
79. Woodmansey PA, Zhang F, Channer KS, Morice AH. Effect of the calcium antagonist amlodipine on the two phases of hypoxic pulmonary vasoconstriction in rat large and small isolated pulmonary arteries. *J Cardiovasc Pharmacol* 1995;**25**:324-9.
80. Gelband CH, Gelband H. Ca2+ release from intracellular stores is an initial step in hypoxic pulmonary vasoconstriction of rat pulmonary artery resistance vessels. *Circulation* 1997;**96**:3647-54.
81. Christman BW, McPherson CD, Newman JH, King GA, Bernard GR, Groves BM, Loyd JE. An imbalance between the excretion of thromboxane and prostacyclin metabolites in pulmonary hypertension. *N Engl J Med* 1992;**327**:70-5.
82. Cody RJ, Haas GJ, Binkley PF, Capers Q, Kelley R. Plasma endothelin correlates with the extent of pulmonary hypertension in patients with chronic congestive heart failure. *Circulation* 1992;**85**:504-9.
83. Moraes DL, Colucci WS, Givertz MM. Secondary pulmonary hypertension in chronic heart failure: the role of the endothelium in pathophysiology and management. *Circulation* 2000;**102**:1718-23.
84. Delgado JF, Conde E, Sanchez V, Lopez-Rios F, Gomez-Sanchez MA, Escribano P, et al. Pulmonary vascular remodeling in pulmonary hypertension due to chronic heart failure. *Eur J Heart Fail* 2005;**7**:1011-6.
85. Lamarche Y, Perrault LP, Maltais S, Tetreault K, Lambert J, Denault AY. Preliminary experience with inhaled milrinone in cardiac surgery. *Eur J Cardiothorac Surg* 2007;**31**:1081-7.
86. Hentschel T, Yin N, Riad A, Habbazettl H, Weimann J, Koster A, et al. Inhalation of the phosphodiesterase-3 inhibitor milrinone attenuates pulmonary hypertension in a rat model of congestive heart failure. *Anesthesiology* 2007;**106**:124-31.

CHAPTER 49
Physiology of the Myocardium
R. John Solaro and Margaret V. Westfall

The Integrative Biology of the Myocardium
Cardiac Dynamics in Exercise
Molecular Cellular Biology
Sarcomere Mechanics

Excitation–Contraction Coupling
Modulation of Excitation–Contraction
 Coupling by Phosphorylation
Cross-Bridges and Stroke Volume

Cellular Biology of Contractility
Cellular Biology of Afterload
Cellular Biology of Cell Length
Cardiac Function Curves

THE INTEGRATIVE BIOLOGY OF THE MYOCARDIUM

The essential function of the muscles that make up the myocardium is to transfer to the arteries the volume of blood added to the ventricular chambers during diastole.[1] This transfer must occur within the narrow limits of end-diastolic pressures and must produce a flow of materials to the organs that matches the needs of the cells. By *needs*, we mean matching the flow of oxygen, which is consumed by the cells at a rate greater than all other materials, to the demand for oxygen. By supplying the tissues' oxygen needs, the demand for all other substances in blood is met. An inevitable consequence of the work done during exercise is an increase in oxygen consumption, and with linear incremental increases in oxygen consumption there are linear incremental increases in cardiac output (CO) to match the increases in venous return (VR). The tight coupling of oxygen demand to CO and VR indicates a regulatory system that is able to sense the tissue oxygen needs, and to engage control mechanisms that adjust the CO. In this chapter, we are concerned with the role of the myocardium in the task of the cardiovascular system to couple oxygen demand to oxygen supply.

In accomplishing this task, the activity of the myocardium must vary over a wide range of short-term regulation (seconds, minutes, and hours) and of long-term regulation (days, weeks, and years). In the short term, during the course of a normal day as tissue oxygen demands and hence cardiac output changes from sleep to strong exercise, variations in activity of the myocardium occur by both intrinsic and extrinsic control mechanisms. The major intrinsic regulator is the Frank-Starling mechanism, in which the pressure developed by the ventricle increases as the end-diastolic volume increases. Extrinsic regulators of the myocardium include the autonomic nerves of the sympathetic and parasympathetic systems, and humoral factors including catecholamines, thyroid hormone, and insulin. In long-term regulation, the activity of the myocardium is more permanently changed in response to chronic changes in oxygen demand associated with frequent bouts of chronic exercise and altered states of the pump and vascular system associated with aging and various long-standing pathologies. In this long-term regulation, the size of the cells making up the ventricular myocardium changes (i.e., hypertrophy or atrophy, without a change in cell number). The cells are remodeled by alterations in subcellular mechanisms regulating contraction and relaxation. This long-term regulation occurs physiologically with normal development of the heart from the immature to the mature myocardium, with normal physiologic aging, and with acquired or inherited pathologies that directly or indirectly affect the function of the myocardium.[2,3] In this chapter, we focus on current concepts and theories of the cellular, subcellular, and molecular mechanisms for short-term regulation of the myocardium. These mechanisms are constrained to account for the dynamic and steady-state functional properties of the heart. Changes in flow and ventricular volumes during an episode of exercise reveal these functional properties.

CARDIAC DYNAMICS IN EXERCISE

Figure 49-1 displays changes in heart rate (HR), CO, stroke volume (SV), and ventricular volumes of a young healthy adult during a bout of exercise on a stationary bike. The measurements were made before and after administration of propranolol, a β-adrenergic blocking agent. Note that in the control condition, CO increased with workload, but end-diastolic volume (EDV) remained rather constant even though CO nearly tripled. SV increased and end-systolic volume (ESV) decreased. These data show that the increased VR that occurs in exercise is handled by the heart largely by increases in HR and decreases in ESV. Elevations in EDV as a mechanism to increase CO are not favorable because of the increased energy cost according to the law of LaPlace.[1] A decrease in ESV provides an important mechanism for matching CO to increased VR without increases in EDV. As we will show, this reduction in ESV at constant EDV can be one measure of the contractile ability of the cells of the heart—that is, the contractility or inotropic state of the heart. After blockade of adrenergic β-receptors with propranolol, there is a blunting of the ability of the sympathetic nervous system to influence the heart. However, CO still increased about threefold. This is testimony to the ability of the cardiovascular system to match the CO to the increased tissue oxygen needs without sympathetic nervous system control mechanisms. However, the increase in CO in the presence of propranolol did not occur without cost. One cost was that the increase in HR was

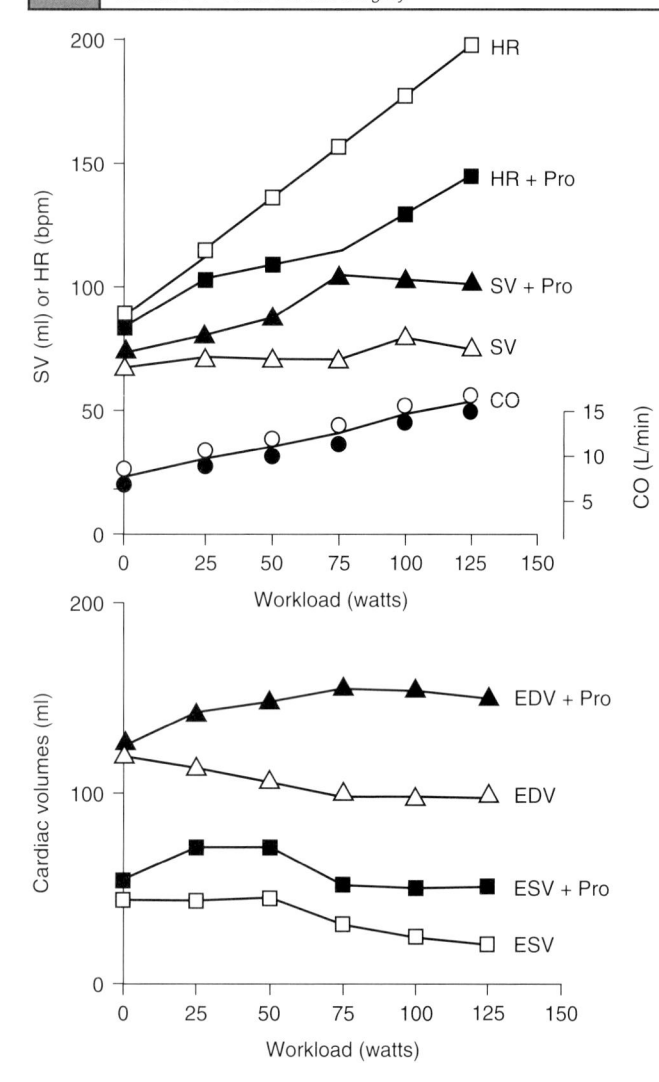

Figure 49–1
Dependence of heart rate (HR), cardiac output (CO), and left ventricular volumes on workload in a bout of exercise. The experiments were carried on a healthy young man before and after the administration of propranolol, a β-adrenergic blocking agent. See text for description. EDV, end-diastolic volume; ESV, end-systolic volume; Pro, propranolol; SV, stroke volume. *(Data courtesy of Dr. Edward Lakatta.)*

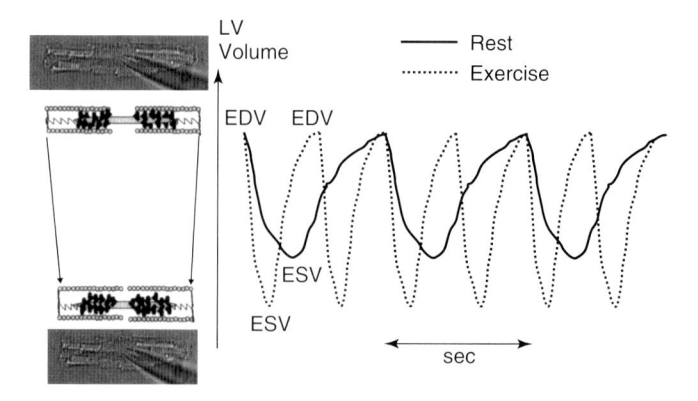

Figure 49–2
Time dependence of left ventricular (LV) volume before and during exercise. Note the reduction in cycle time associated with the increased heart rate. The left panel depicts how the change in volume reflects a change in sarcomere length and cell length of ventricular myocytes making up the ventricular chamber. EDV, end-diastolic volume; ESV, end-systolic volume.

reduced. With a decrease in HR and a constant CO, the SV had to be elevated (CO = SV × HR). The increase in SV occurred largely because of an increase in EDV. Increases in EDV present a threat to the economy of contraction, and they may also stimulate hypertrophic signaling pathways as a result of cell stretch.[2,3] These effects of propranolol indicate an important role of the β-receptors and the sympathetic nervous system in regulation of the ability of the heart to maintain CO with little or no change in EDV. Figure 49-2 depicts the dynamics of cardiac function with data relating time dependence of left ventricular volume before and after an episode of exercise. These data demonstrate not only the decrease in ESV with little change in EDV but also enhanced dynamics and abbreviation of the contraction–relaxation cycle. The abbreviation of cardiac cycle time is critical for the maintenance of cardiac filling during the fast HR that occurs with exercise. Figure 49-2 also illustrates that the volume changes are associated with shortening of the cells making up the left ventricular chamber, and that the changes in cell length reflect changes in sarcomere length. We discuss next the molecular and cellular mechanisms responsible for maintenance of CO with elevations of VR with minimal change in EDV.

MOLECULAR CELLULAR BIOLOGY

Figure 49-3 depicts cellular structures involved in excitation, contraction, and relaxation. Tight junctions of low electrical resistance connect heart cells.[4,5] When one cell is activated (depolarized), all cells become activated. Therefore, unlike skeletal muscle, the heart does not recruit motor units to regulate contraction. Instead, regulation is at the level of the cells themselves. There are mechanisms that permit regulation of the activity of each cell to meet varying demands on the circulation. We will therefore concentrate now on understanding overt left ventricular cardiac function in terms of the properties of the cardiac myocytes. The objectives are to understand the following:

- The molecular and cellular mechanisms responsible for the changes in wall tension and ventricular volume that occur in the transition from diastole to systole
- The regulatory devices used by the heart to ensure ejection of an SV equal to the LV at optimal EDV during basal physiologic states and during exercise
- The mechanisms that ensure that dynamics of the heart beat are tuned to match the prevailing frequency, the HR

SARCOMERE MECHANICS

Sarcomeres are the fundamental structural units responsible for the ability of myocardial cells to shorten and generate forces (Fig. 49-4, and see Fig. 49-3). Side arms of the myosin molecules (cross-bridges) that make up the thick filament are molecular motors that also hydrolyze ATP. Light chains on the myosin head, which are different in ventricles and atria, appear to regulate the rate of the ATP hydrolysis. A thick filament–associated protein (called myosin-binding protein C, or C-protein) may be important in regulating the radial movement of the cross-bridge. C-protein also binds to titin,

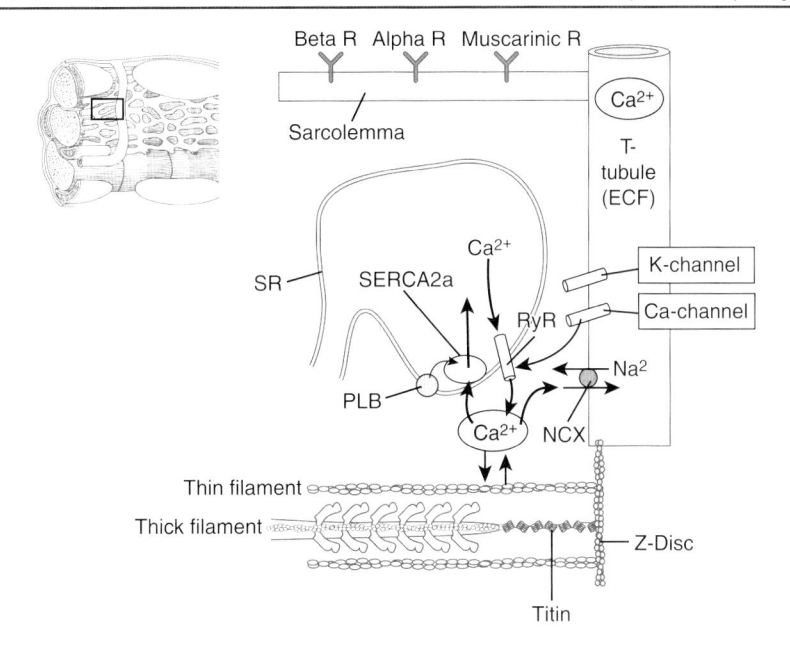

Figure 49–3
Microscopic view of a portion of a myocardial cell illustrating structures critical to excitation–contraction coupling. The T-tubule–containing channels and transporters are shown as an invagination of the surface membrane (or sarcolemma), which contains surface α- and β-receptors for norepinephrine, epinephrine, and muscarinic receptors for acetylcholine. Also shown is the sarcoplasmic reticulum (SR), an internally enclosed network of tubules in which high concentrations of Ca^{2+} are stored in diastole. With electrical excitation of the cell, Ca^{2+} channels open and the small release of Ca^{2+} into the cytoplasm induces Ca^{2+} release from the SR through ryanodine receptors (RyR2; SR Ca^{2+} release channels). Ca^{2+} moves to the myofilaments (shown as a half-sarcomere; see Fig. 49-4) and activates contraction. Ca^{2+} is removed from the cytoplasm by an SR Ca^{2+}-activated Mg-ATPase (SERCA2a) and exchanged for Na^+ by the action of the Na^+/Ca^{2+} exchange protein (NCX) in the sarcolemma. Phospholamban (PLB) inhibits transport of Ca^{2+} by SERCA2a, and the inhibition is released when PLB becomes phosphorylated. See the text for details. ECF, extracellular fluid.

a long structural protein that extends from the center of the sarcomere to the Z-disc. This interaction is of significance in cross-bridge function and in the generation of passive tension. The reaction of the myosin cross-bridges with the actins of the thin filaments generates active cellular force, shortening, and power.[6,7] The basic reaction cycle includes an attachment step; a movement of the lever arm of the myosin head, which impels the thin filament in each half-sarcomere to slide toward the center; and a detachment step, which completes the cycle.[6] Figure 49-4 displays the cross-bridge in diastole (left) and at the end of the power stroke (right). The energy for these movements comes from the hydrolysis of one molecule of Mg-ATP during each cycle. In diastole, the cross-bridges contain bound Mg-ADP and inorganic phosphate (P_i), which has been generated from the splitting of Mg-ATP on the surface of the myosin head, poising it for reaction with actin. As actin sites become available, the cross-bridge attaches and enters into a catalytic cycle in which the release of P_i and Mg-ADP, together with isomerization of the cross-bridge, induces a progressive change in mechanical state of the cross-bridge, leading to thin-filament sliding. The terminal state is a strongly bound so-called rigor cross-bridge that is free of P_i and nucleotide. Detachment requires binding of Mg-ATP, which is quickly split, without release of products, so that the cycle may begin again if actins remain accessible. Each actin–cross-bridge reaction cycle is therefore powered by the hydrolysis of Mg-ATP.

Ca^{2+} binding triggers conformational changes and movements of the thin-filament proteins troponin (Tn, a heterotrimeric protein complex) and tropomyosin (Tm) that switch on the actin–cross-bridge reaction.[3,8] Figures 49-4 and 49-5 illustrate the steps in this process. In diastole, Tn and Tm are situated on the thin filament in positions that hinder the actin–cross-bridge reaction. Tn and Tm are held in this position largely through the tethering action of troponin I (TnI). TnI is an inhibitory protein of the Tn complex, which binds tightly to actin through a highly basic peptide, to the C-terminal end of TnT, the Tm binding unit of Tn, and the C-terminal lobe of troponin C (TnC), the Ca^{2+} receptor protein. This inhibitory property of TnI is amplified by virtue of these multiple protein–protein interactions to immobilize the long α-helical Tm in a blocking position that encompasses many actins along the thin filament. When released into the myofilament space by mechanisms summarized later, Ca^{2+} binds to a single regulatory site on the N-terminal lobe of TnC, the Ca^{2+} receptor protein in the heterotrimeric Tn complex. Ca^{2+} binding to the C-lobe exposes a "sticky patch" of hydrophobic amino acids that promotes binding of TnC to the inhibitory peptide and C-terminal regions of TnI. This reaction releases the inhibitory peptide from actin and leads to a pivoting of the Tn complex on the thin filament, with TnT acting as a lever to move Tm from its blocking position on the thin filament. An important aspect of the transition from diastole to systole is that the reaction of cross-bridges with the thin filament can itself promote more actin–cross-bridge reactions by cooperative feedback mechanisms. It is apparent that cross-bridge binding may enhance the affinity of TnC for Ca^{2+} as well as

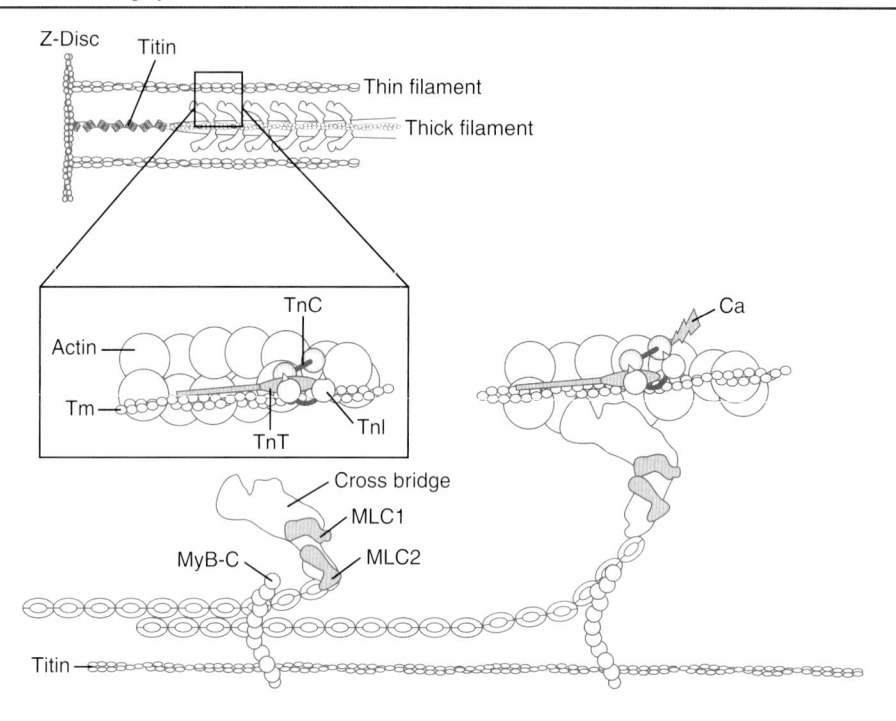

Figure 49–4
Illustration of a cardiac myocyte half-sarcomere showing a regulatory unit in diastole and systole. Microscopic view shows that the regulatory unit consists of seven actins, one tropomyosin (Tm), and one heterotrimeric troponin complex, which consists of a Ca^{2+}-binding protein (TnC), an inhibitory protein (TnI), and a Tm-binding protein (TnT). Although not shown here, the thin filament in a half-sarcomere contains approximately 30 regulatory units. The action of cross-bridges, discussed further in the text, in each half-sarcomere impels the thin filaments toward the center of the sarcomere by a reaction with actin powered by ATP hydrolysis. Cross-bridges are impeded from reacting with the thin filament by tropomyosin and troponin. Ca^{2+} binding to a regulatory lobe of troponin C releases the thin filament from this inhibition. See the text for a further description. Myosin-binding protein C (MyB-C) and myosin light chains (MLC1 and MLC2) modulate cross-bridge activity. Titin is a major structural protein responsible for passive tension.

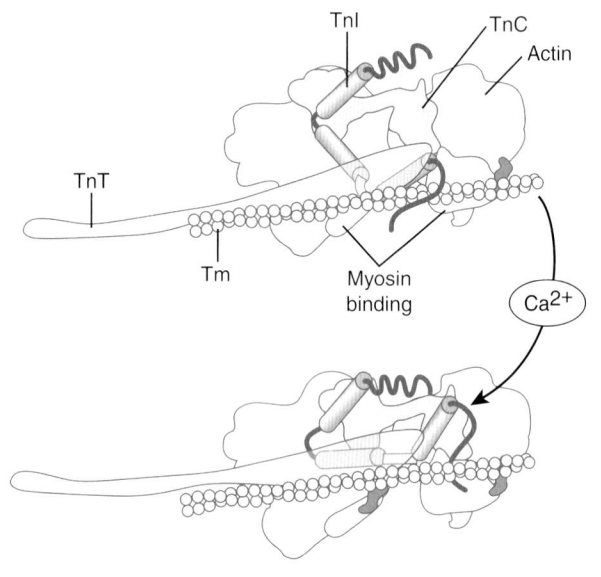

Figure 49-5
Molecular mechanism of thin filament activation by Ca^{2+}. In diastole, tropomyosin (Tm) and troponin (Tn) act to impede the thin filament–cross-bridge reaction by steric and allosteric effects on the actin sites that react with myosin. TnI, the inhibitory protein, binds tightly to actin through an inhibitory peptide (Ip). With Ca^{2+} binding to troponin C (TnC), a strong attraction between the Ip and C-terminal regions of Tn is promoted, resulting in movement of the Ip of TnI away from the actin-binding site, a release of TnT, and a movement of Tm, exposing regions of actin that react with myosin cross-bridges also. See text for further discussion.

moving Tm farther away from the region of actin that reacts with the cross-bridges.

At this stage, it is important to understand that the number of cross-bridges reacting with the thin filaments determines the force generated by the sarcomere. An important determinant of the number of cross-bridges reacting with the thin filaments is the amount of Ca^{2+} released to the myofilaments and, thus, the relative occupation of sarcomeric TnC proteins with Ca^{2+} (in the basal state, this is about 20% to 25% of the total TnC).[8] Other important determinants of the number of cross-bridges reacting with the thin filaments are the sarcomere length[9] and the load (velocity of shortening).[6] We will discuss the mechanisms by which each of these variables affects the number of cycling cross-bridges.

Molecular springs interlaced with the thin and thick filaments form elastic elements in the sarcomere that determine passive elastic properties of the cell and have a possible role in active contraction of the cells.[10] A major elastic element is the giant protein titin (Fig. 49-3), which is a long and flexible protein extending from the Z-disc to the midline of the sarcomere. As illustrated in Figure 49-3, titin has a region near the Z-disc that is coiled much like a spring. There is accumulating and solid evidence that when the sarcomere is stretched, titin elongates, giving rise to passive tension. Moreover, there is evidence that when the sarcomere shortens, the titin spring imposes a restoring force that is likely to be important in early diastole. Regions of titin in the thin filament–thick filament overlap zone also interact with myosin-binding protein C, a thick filament–associated protein that binds to the head/neck

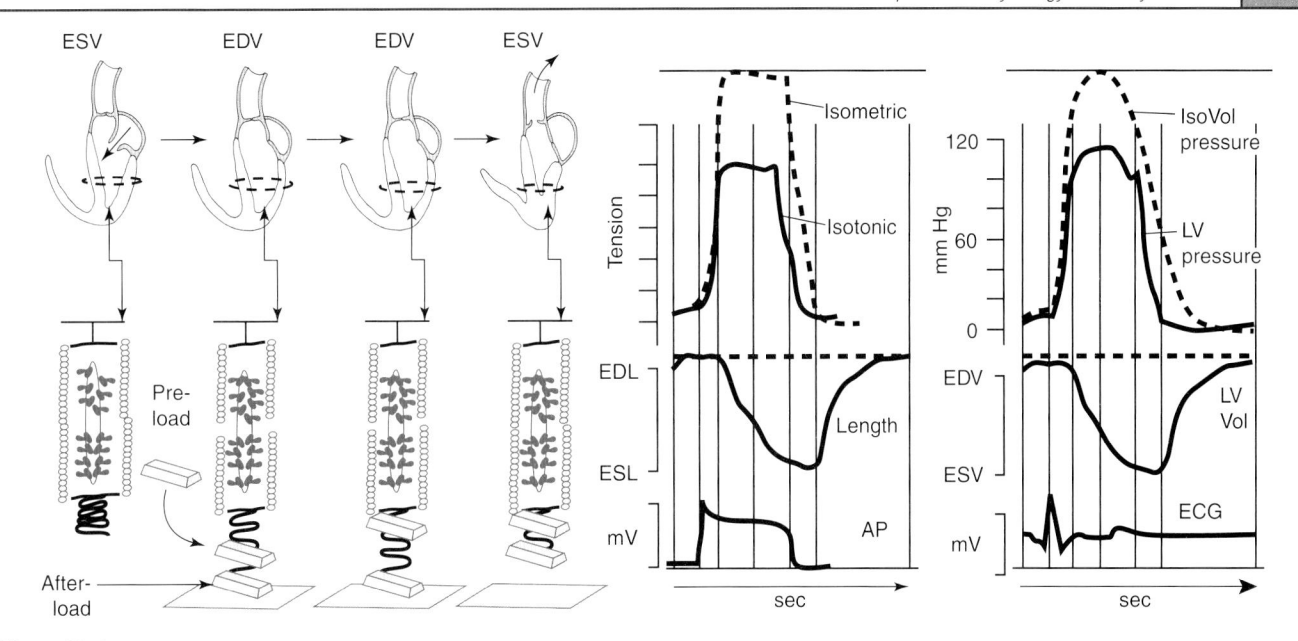

Figure 49–6
Relationships between ventricular states in the cardiac cycle and the mechanics of isolated muscle preparations. The cycle begins on the left at an end-systolic volume (ESV) and end-systolic (ES) sarcomere length. In the linear muscle setup, the analog of end-diastolic volume (EDV) is a weight, the preload, added prior to activation. The addition of the preload establishes sarcomere length. The load the sarcomere discovers it must lift is not seen until after activation, and it is the afterload that is supported on the platform. With activation as triggered by the action potential (AP) and measured as the electrocardiogram (ECG), force-generating cross-bridges react with actin, developing tension isometrically until the tension developed matches the afterload. At that point, the sarcomere shortens with a velocity appropriate to the number of reacting cross-bridges to the load. This sarcomeric activity is reflected in the ventricle as an increase in wall tension, isovolumic (IsoVol) pressure development followed by opening of the aortic valve, and ejection of blood against the rising pressure in the aorta. *Dashed lines* represent measurements in which muscle length was held constant, or in which the aorta was clamped to produce an isovolumic beat. The peak amplitude of pressure or tension provides a measure of contractility. EDL, end-diastolic length; ESL, end-systolic length; LV, left ventricular.

region of myosin. Thus, the conformational changes in titin may also affect cross-bridge disposition. Although not depicted in Figure 48-3, the Z-disc of the sarcomere not only anchors the thin filaments but also links sarcomeres in series by interactions between titin and the thin filaments. There are also lateral connections linking the sarcomere to the surface membrane. In addition to its role in force transmission, the Z-disc is emerging as a locus of communication in the cells. The Z-disc appears as a crossroad for interactions among many diverse proteins including channels, kinases, and phosphatases, and cytoskeletal elements that connect to the nucleus as well as to a network of cytoskeletal proteins and membrane proteins at focal adhesion complexes.[10]

We will use Figure 49-6, which relates the circumferential shortening associated with the heartbeat to sarcomeric activity, to discuss the cellular and sarcomeric correlates of preload, afterload, and contractility. Thus, in Figure 49-6, we relate the contraction–relaxation cycle of the heart beat to events in a single sarcomere; mechanical changes that occur in the active and passive elements of the sarcomere are related to the beat of the heart. The sarcomere is depicted as a contractile element in series with a passive spring that is a lumped elastic element (collagen, titin, and cytoskeletal proteins). A load attached to the end of the sarcomere establishes the sarcomere length before activation and is termed the preload. The preload stretches the sarcomere to its diastolic length; the correlate of the preload in the ventricle is the EDV. In the ventricle, an end-diastolic pressure (EDP) develops as the passive springs are stretched.

Figure 49-6 also illustrates the sarcomere with an attached afterload. This is a load that the sarcomere does not "see" until after activation. The correlate of afterload in the ventricle is the aortic pressure. With cellular excitation, Ca^{2+} is released into the myofilament space, the cross-bridges in the sarcomere react with actin sites on thin filaments, and the cell develops tension, shortens, and stretches the elastic element. As tension increases, the afterload is lifted, and the muscle cell shortens. The sarcomere will shorten as long as it can develop tension equal to the afterload. As excitation wanes, the cell returns to the diastolic state, ready for another cycle. Figure 49-6 also shows records of the isotonic twitch (the load is constant) and the ventricular pressure. The correlate of cellular tension is the pressure (by the law of LaPlace, where wall tension = pressure × radius of curvature ÷ [2 × wall thickness]), and the correlate of cellular length is the ventricular volume. In fact, the aortic pressure is increasing during ejection, and, thus, strictly speaking, afterload is not constant. This is referred to as an auxotonic twitch.

The concept of contractility is illuminated by repeating this sequence of events but with the sarcomere held isometric (dashed lines in Figure 49-6). In this case, the sarcomere cannot lift the load and develops the maximum isometric tension possible at the particular length, established by the preload and the extent of availability of thin filament sites for reaction with cross-bridges. The peak amplitude of isometric tension is a measure of contractility, one definition of which is maximum tension when the sarcomeres are neither lengthening nor shortening. The peak tension in the isometric twitch reflects

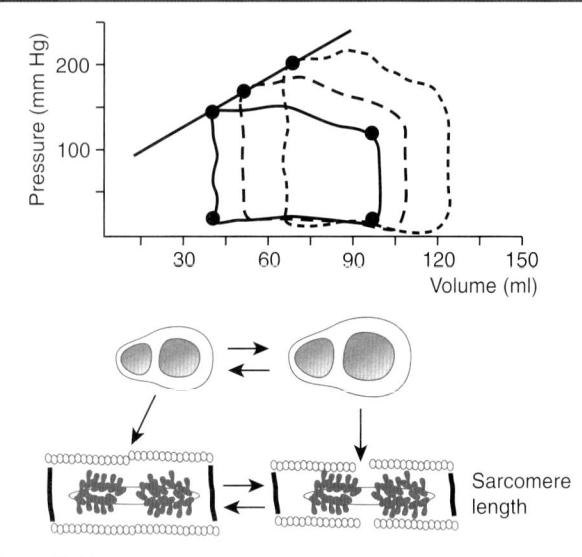

Figure 49-7
Pressure–volume (P-V) relationships of the left ventricle at varying end-diastolic volumes generated by infusion of blood or saline into the circulation. The P-V loops represent data obtained in human subjects in a resting condition. End-systolic pressure (ESP) points are shown as *filled circles*. These points represent a state in which the ventricle is neither lengthening nor shortening, and is developing the peak pressure (tension) at that particular ventricular volume (sarcomere length). Thus, points on the volume-ESP relationship reflect the length tension properties of the muscle cells. The relationship between these points and a circumferential array of ventricular cells and the length of the sarcomere is schematically shown to illustrate that the P-V loop is rooted in a complex relationship between sarcomere length and ventricular geometry. See the text and Covell and Ross (reference 1) for further discussion.

in part the amount of Ca^{2+} delivered to the myofilaments, and in part the sarcomere length. As we will see, the amount of Ca^{2+} is a regulated variable in heart muscle cells; thus, peak tension or contractility in the isometric twitch could increase or decrease. In animal experiments, this measure of contractility can be determined in beating hearts as well.[1] The approach is to transiently cross-clamp the aorta, which in effect makes resistance and therefore afterload infinite. Dashed lines in the right panel of Figure 49-6 show an isovolumic beat of the ventricle. The peak pressure in this isovolumic beat is a measure of the contractility in the same way that peak tension is a measure of contractility in the sarcomere.

How can contractility be measured in humans without doing the drastic invasive procedure of clamping the aorta? And how does this present definition of contractility relate to the previous indication that contractility is related to end-systolic length and thus end-systolic pressure (ESP) of the sarcomeres? The answers to both these questions are couched in terms of the pressure-volume loop (P-V loop) of the left ventricular beat. Figure 49-7 shows the dependence of ventricular pressure on ventricular volume during cardiac cycles occurring at three different afterloads. The figure also illustrates that the cross-sectional area of the ventricles at the ESV and the EDV is associated with changes in sarcomere length of the cells. In a beat, the volume added during diastole (loading volume) stretches the sarcomeres from the ESV to establish the end-diastolic cell length and EDV. With electrical activation, Ca^{2+} is released into the myofilament space. The sarcomeres develop tension isometrically (isovolumic pressure development) until the cell tension produces a pressure greater than the aortic pressure (the afterload); the valve opens and blood is ejected from the ventricle. The ejection continues with shortening of the sarcomeres to a point at which the pressure developed in the ventricle no longer exceeds the afterload. At this ESP point, the valve closes with the waning of electrical activation and restoration of diastolic Ca^{2+}, and pressure falls isovolumically. The ESP is thus a point in which the sarcomeres are no longer shortening or lengthening. ESP is, in effect, a point essentially reflecting isometric tension—that is, a measure of contractility. The ESP points can be varied by varying afterload, as displayed in Figure 49-7 with the dashed P-V loops. Afterload was increased in this example by rapidly increasing the loading volume through an increase in VR. As discussed later, these ESP points reflect isovolumic pressure or isometric cellular tension and are points on the sarcomere length–tension relationship. A line connecting these points represents a constant state of contractility. The pressure or tension is different at each of the points because the muscle and sarcomere length has changed, not because the contractility has changed. Each beat depicted in Figure 49-7 thus occurred with essentially the same amount of Ca^{2+} released to the myofilaments. The increase in ESP with increases in ventricular volume is the essence of Starling's law of the heart, also known as the Frank-Starling relationship.[1,9]

The ESP also reflects the extent of shortening, as previously discussed. Imagine, as we will consider later, that the contractility increases. The ESP–volume relationship will shift up and to the left, and thus at a given afterload the sarcomere will be able to shorten farther than at the previous level. Circumferential shortening will occur to a greater extent, and the SV will be increased for a given afterload. We take this concept up again after describing the cellular mechanisms by which contractility can be altered.

EXCITATION–CONTRACTION COUPLING

With the realization that Ca^{2+} ions trigger and regulate the number of actin–cross-bridge reactions, it is easy to understand that switching the heart beat on and off must involve cellular mechanisms that provide and remove Ca^{2+} ions to and from troponin C. Figure 49-8 shows evidence that during a beat of the cells, there is transient increase in intracellular Ca^{2+}. Adult mammalian myocardial cells have evolved elaborate membranous structures and membrane proteins to keep Ca^{2+} away from the myofilaments during diastole, and to provide Ca^{2+} to the myofilaments during systole.[4,11,12] The myofilaments are surrounded by a reticulum of tubular membranes, called the sarcoplasmic reticulum (SR). These tubules form an internally enclosed compartment that is not contiguous with the extracellular fluid and that contains a number of proteins that regulate the storage, release, and reuptake of Ca^{2+}. As illustrated in Figure 49-3, the surface membrane or sarcolemma of ventricular myocytes plunges into the cellular interior and forms the T-tubules. These invaginations occur along the length of the cell in register with each of the sarcomeres. The T-tubules serve to bring the extracellular fluid, as well membrane ion channels, transporters, and exchangers, into the depths of the cell interior. The T-tubules are in proximity to the terminal swellings of the SR that are the main storage depots for Ca^{2+} during diastole.

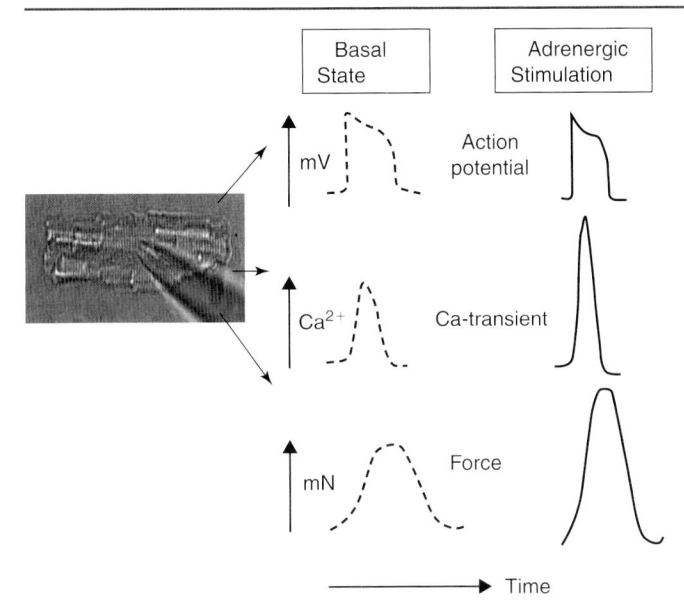

Figure 49–8
Schematic of action potential, intracellular transient change in Ca^{2+}, and isometric tension of a single cardiac myocyte in a basal state and during stimulation with an adrenergic agonist. The effects of adrenergic stimulation are an abbreviation of the action potential and an increase in the amplitude and dynamics of both the Ca^{2+} transient and the twitch tension.

Integrated activity of proteins and protein complexes in the sarcolemma (SL), the T-tubules, the SR, and the myofilaments makes up the essential elements of a process known as excitation–contraction coupling, whereby electrical impulses arriving at the cell are coupled to a release of Ca^{2+} and to the promotion of the actin–cross-bridge reaction.[4,11,12] Measurements of cellular processes of membrane potential, intracellular Ca^{2+}, and tension are displayed in Figure 49-8. The triggering event is action potential depolarization of the SL and the ensuing depolarization of the sarcolemmal T-tubule. This excitatory process initiates activation of voltage-dependent, L-type Ca^{2+} channels (also known as dihydropyridine receptors), which are primarily clustered within the T-tubules at the sarcolemmal–SR junction. The transverse tubules of the SR contain Ca^{2+} release channels. These channels are also known as ryanodine receptors (RyR2, cardiac isoform) because of their ability to bind this alkaloid. Depolarization-induced influx of Ca^{2+} current (I_{Ca}) through the L-type channels contributes approximately 20% to 25% of the free Ca^{2+} in a cardiac twitch. Equally important, I_{Ca} is proposed to act locally to trigger the release of SR Ca^{2+} via the SR Ca^{2+} release channels. The release of Ca^{2+} through the RyRs contributes the remaining 75% to 80% of Ca^{2+} necessary for cardiac contraction. The process of coupling between the influx of Ca^{2+} via I_{Ca} and Ca^{2+} release from the RyR2 is known as Ca^{2+}-induced Ca^{2+} release (CICR). The gating of the RyR2 by I_{Ca} is the essence of CICR. Experiments employing fluorescent indicators that sense Ca^{2+} have revealed the activity of local clusters of RyR receptors. These experiments demonstrate elementary events known as Ca^{2+} sparks that reflect the activity of small groups of RyRs. Enhanced I_{Ca} increases localized Ca^{2+} accumulation, which increases Ca^{2+} spark frequency and produces a graded stimulation of RyR Ca^{2+} release from the SR. Release into the cytosol increases the local concentration of Ca^{2+} surrounding the myofilaments and promotes Ca^{2+} binding to TnC on the thin filaments. The reaction of Ca^{2+} with TnC triggers the protein–protein interactions that release regulatory units of the thin filament from an inhibited state (see Figs 49-4 and 49-5). During a beat of the heart in a basal physiologic state, the amount of Ca^{2+} delivered to the myofilaments is sufficient to activate only about 20% to 25% of the regulatory units. The 75% of actin–cross-bridge reactions that remain available for increases in contractility form a molecular basis for what is commonly referred to as cardiac reserve.

As illustrated in Figure 49-8, the elevation in Ca^{2+} levels observed during systole is transient, with SL and SR proteins working to sequester Ca^{2+} and return it to baseline levels in the return to diastole.[4,11,12] In the steady-state contraction–relaxation cycle, an equal efflux must match the influx of Ca^{2+}. In human hearts, this sequestration process involves two major cellular pumps. The majority of Ca^{2+} (70%) is resequestered into the SR via Ca^{2+} pumps (sarcoendoplasmic reticulum Ca^{2+} pump; SERCA2a isoform) present on the longitudinal tubules of the SR. SERCA2a is a Ca^{2+}-activated Mg-ATPase that couples Mg-ATP hydrolysis to the active transport of Ca^{2+} from the cytoplasmic space into the SR. A high-capacity, low-affinity Ca^{2+} binding protein, known as calsequestrin, serves as a sink for Ca^{2+} in the interior of the SR. Most of the remaining Ca^{2+} is removed from the cell via the SL Na^+/Ca^{2+} exchanger (NCX) operating in the inward mode (inward $I_{Na/Ca}$). Relatively small and slow processes for Ca^{2+} efflux from the cytosol include transport via a sarcolemmal Ca^{2+} pump and transport into the mitochondrial space.[9] The proportion of Ca^{2+} flux through the NCX and these slow processes is species dependent, with a lower proportion of Ca^{2+} handled by these mechanisms in rodents than in humans. This species difference requires consideration when applying results obtained in rodent studies to human cardiac function.[4]

MODULATION OF EXCITATION–CONTRACTION COUPLING BY PHOSPHORYLATION

The autonomic nervous system is the major regulator of the amount of Ca^{2+} delivered to the myofilaments.[4,11,12] The myocardium has evolved an elaborate signaling cascade to link adrenergic and cholinergic neural activity as well as blood levels of neurohumors such as epinephrine and acetylcholine to modulation of cellular Ca^{2+} fluxes. As illustrated in Figure 49-9, binding of neurotransmitters, neurohumors, or pharmacologic agonists to adrenergic or cholinergic receptors triggers the cascade. GTP-binding proteins, known collectively as G-proteins, transduce receptor binding to an alteration of the enzyme activity of adenylyl cyclase, which is responsible for the generation of cyclic AMP (cAMP) from ATP. Stimulatory G-proteins (G_s) linked to adrenergic β-receptors promote the formation of cAMP, whereas inhibitory G-proteins (G_i) inhibit adenylyl cyclase and may also activate phosphatases. cAMP activates protein kinase A (PKA), which phosphorylates key proteins that regulate the entry and exit of Ca^{2+} from the myofilament space. In the case of SR, the PKA substrate is phospholamban (PLB), a small proteolipid that, when dephosphorylated, inhibits the activity of SERCA2a (Fig. 49-9 and see Fig. 49-3). PLB is also

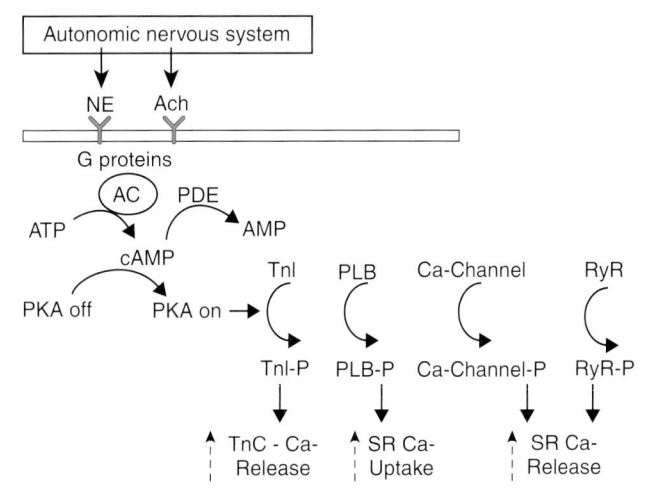

Figure 49–9
Schematic representation of autonomic signal transduction and signaling in cardiac muscle cells. With binding of neurotransmitters acetylcholine (Ach) and norepinephrine (NE) to the receptors indicated, there is an activation of adenylyl cyclase (AC), elaboration of cAMP, and activation of protein kinase A (PKA). Levels of cAMP are also regulated by the activity of phosphodiesterases (PDE) that convert cAMP to AMP. PKA phosphorylates troponin I (TnI), phospholamban (PLB), Ca^{2+} channel subunits, and ryanodine receptors (RyR), as well as K channels (not shown). These phosphorylations elicit effects on Ca^{2+} uptake and release into the cytoplasmic space, resulting in increased contractility and dynamics of contraction and relaxation. Separate enzymes called phosphatases catalyze dephosphorylation. See text for further discussion.

a substrate for Ca^{2+}-activated calmodulin-dependent kinase (CAMK).[4,11] This Ca^{2+}-dependent phosphorylation appears important in a "staircase" effect, in which force generated by the myocardium increases with HR. With the increased frequency, there is a higher Ca^{2+} influx because of increased amplitude and delayed inactivation of I_{Ca}. Phosphorylation of PLB by either PKA or CAMK depresses the PLB-SERCA2a interaction and releases Ca^{2+} pumping activity from inhibition; Ca^{2+} affinity of the pump increases, without changes in the maximal Ca^{2+} transport velocity. This increase in Ca^{2+} uptake increases Ca^{2+} loaded into the SR and induces an accelerated relaxation of the myocytes. This increase in rate of Ca^{2+} removal from the cytoplasm and myofilaments accounts in large part for the enhanced relaxation and abbreviated contraction–relaxation cycle during adrenergic stimulation. The enhanced relaxation also depends on PKA-dependent phosphorylation of TnI.[3,8,13] The phosphorylation of TnI at PKA sites enhances Ca^{2+} release from TnC and speeds up cross-bridge cycling rate.[8] These consequences of PLB and TnI phosphorylation are critical to the ability of the heart to tune its activity cycle to the fast heart rates during adrenergic stimulation and to accommodate the increasing VR without a significant change in EDV (see Figs. 49-1 and 49-2). A subunit in the oligomeric assembly of proteins that makes up the L-type Ca^{2+} channel of the heart is also a substrate for PKA.[4] Phosphorylation enhances the probability that the channel will open upon depolarization, but it does not affect the unitary conductance. This increase in the trigger for Ca^{2+} release, together with the increased Ca^{2+} loading associated with PLB phosphorylation, essentially accounts for the increase in the systolic Ca^{2+} transient (see Fig. 49-8). Regulation of the release of Ca^{2+} through SR RyRs by PKA and by CAMK also provides a mechanism to control delivery of Ca^{2+} to the myofilaments and thus to control contractility by an increase in the open probability of the Ca^{2+} release channel. The amount of Ca^{2+} loaded within the SR lumen is a critical factor influencing RyR Ca^{2+} release. Increases in SR Ca^{2+} content generally stimulate the frequency and amplitude of Ca^{2+} sparks, and decreases in content reverse these trends. The duration of the cardiac action potential is also abbreviated with adrenergic stimulation (see Fig. 49-8). This appears because of PKA-dependent phosphorylation of one form of the K channel important in determination of the duration of the action potential.[14] Separate enzymes called phosphatases, which are controlled by a poorly understood regulatory pathway, catalyze dephosphorylation and restoration of the basal state.

CROSS-BRIDGES AND STROKE VOLUME

In connecting the molecular and cellular properties of the heart to cardiac output, we use the premise that the stroke volume ultimately depends on the actin–myosin interaction. Up to now, we have discussed the determinants of SV in terms of contractility, afterload, and preload. We now discuss the relationships between contractility, afterload, and preload as determinants of the number and rate of cycling of force-generating cross-bridges reacting with the thin filaments. The following equation serves to illustrate the progression of this analysis from active cross-bridges, which determine the systolic change in cell length and tension, to SV and to CO:

$$CO = HR \times SV \leftarrow (\text{change in LV volume and pressure})$$
$$\uparrow$$
$$(\text{change in cell tension and length})$$

The cellular properties of length and tension are related in a highly complex manner to LV pressure and volume.[1] However, an understanding of how systolic cross-bridges determine cell tension and shortening sets the stage for understanding the geometric considerations that relate these properties to the ventricular chamber.[1,15]

CELLULAR BIOLOGY OF CONTRACTILITY

Changes in the amount of Ca^{2+} delivered to the myofilaments, which recruit spare actin–cross-bridge reactions, may occur by the following:

- Changes in the intracellular Ca^{2+} and activity of the autonomic nervous system that releases neurohumors, which alter the state of phosphorylation of the regulatory proteins in the cells as described earlier.
- Changes in the chemical environment of the cells. One example is the accumulation of metabolic wastes that occurs during a reduction in coronary flow and that results in acidosis.
- Changes in HR. With increases in HR, the SR fills to a greater extent with Ca^{2+}, through phosphorylations involving Ca^{2+} calmodulin–dependent kinases.

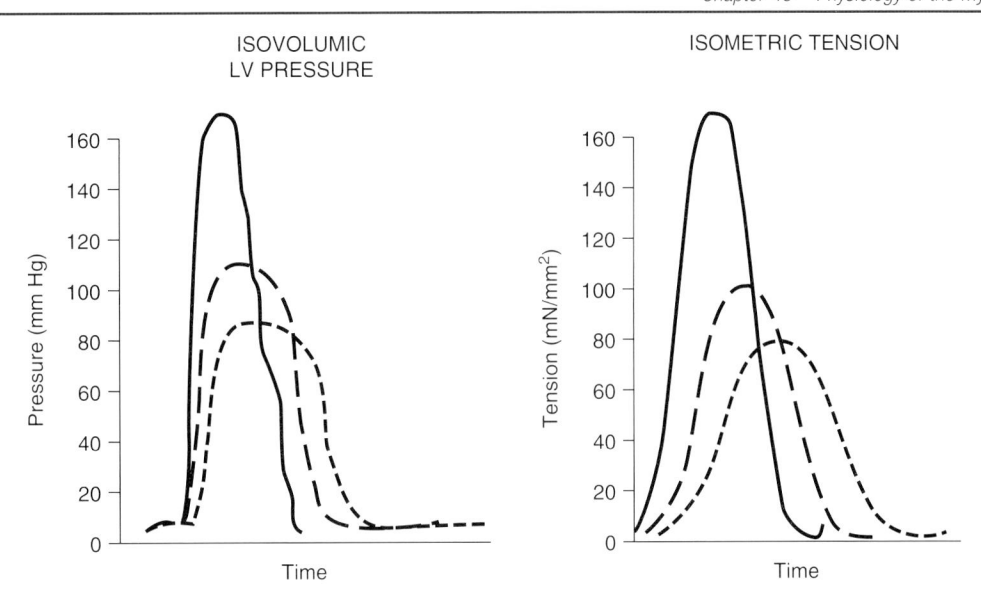

Figure 49–10
Comparison of isovolumic beats and isometric twitches at three levels of contractility. Peak amplitude of tension or pressure under these conditions provides a measure of contractility or inotropic state of the heart. Maximum rates of pressure development (+dp/dt$_{max}$) also provide a measure of contractility. Even though pressures are not developed isovolumically during normal beats, +dp/dt$_{max}$ remains a useful index of contractility. LV, left ventricular.

- Administration of pharmacologic agents. Drugs that affect contractility are known as inotropic agents. Some agents such as dobutamine mimic adrenergic neurotransmitters, and some agents such as digitalis indirectly increase Ca^{2+} loading into the SR by inhibiting Na^+/K^+-ATPase, reducing the Na gradient, and thus inhibiting Ca^{2+} extrusion through the Na^+/Ca^{2+} exchanger. There are inotropic agents that inhibit breakdown of cAMP by an inhibition of phosphodiesterase activity, whereas other agents, known as Ca^{2+} sensitizers, activate the sarcomere directly.[16]

Figure 49-10 shows a recording of ventricular pressure and of tension developed by ventricular papillary muscles. In precise determinations of contractility, it is important that afterload and preload remain constant. Both of these constraints are met if the pressure is developed at constant LV volume or the tension is developed at constant muscle length. In this case, peak pressure or tension would be expected to vary with the amount of Ca^{2+} delivered to the myofilaments, as would occur with variations in sympathetic nervous system stimulation, for example. Note that the rate of increase in the pressure also varies with contractility. The time derivative of the pressure trace gives the maximum rate of pressure rise (+dp/dt) and fall (–dp/dt), both of which are useful indices of contractility in the clinic, even though afterload and preload are not strictly controlled. Ejection fraction (SV/EDV) is also an index of contractility, as is the ratio of end-systolic to end-diastolic dimensions obtained from echocardiographic assessment of cardiac function.

CELLULAR BIOLOGY OF AFTERLOAD

Cardiac muscle cells lift light loads faster than heavier loads, according to a general characteristic property of striated muscle known as the force–velocity relationship.[6] The velocity of shortening approaches a maximum value (V_{max}) as the load approaches zero, velocity is zero at the maximum load, and the cells develop maximum isometric tension under the particular conditions. As load increases between these extremes, the rate of thin-filament sliding decreases, permitting a longer time for the cross-bridges to react. By this mechanism, the number of cycling cross-bridges is matched to the load that the muscle discovers it must lift. As discussed in the context of Figure 49-6, at the isometric extreme (zero velocity), the level of Ca^{2+} activation determines maximum tension. It is also apparent that Ca^{2+} also increases V_{max} by increasing the rate that the cross-bridges enter the force-generating state. Thus, the force–velocity relationship shifts with increases or decreases in contractility.

CELLULAR BIOLOGY OF CELL LENGTH

We now explicitly relate the sarcomere length tension properties of the cardiac muscle cells to the pressure–volume relationship. Figure 49-11 displays the entire relationship between sarcomere length and the active and passive (resting) tension. Active tension rises and falls from an optimal value, whereas passive tension rises exponentially. The rise in passive tension, which would elevate diastolic LV pressure, is so steep in heart cells as to disallow filling of the ventricle to sarcomere lengths greater than 2.2 μm. In other words, during diastole, atrial pressures cannot rise high enough to fill the ventricles to a volume that produces sarcomere lengths exceeding 2.2 μm. Thus, in the physiologic state, considerations of the length–tension relationships, and therefore the volume–pressure relationships of the heart, are restricted to the operating range illustrated in Figure 49-11. To measure the length–tension relationship, the muscle cells are stretched at rest to various sarcomere lengths and held isometric. The cells develop a passive tension as they are stretched. At each length, the cells are stimulated to give a measure of the total isometric tension at that particular sarcomere length. Two

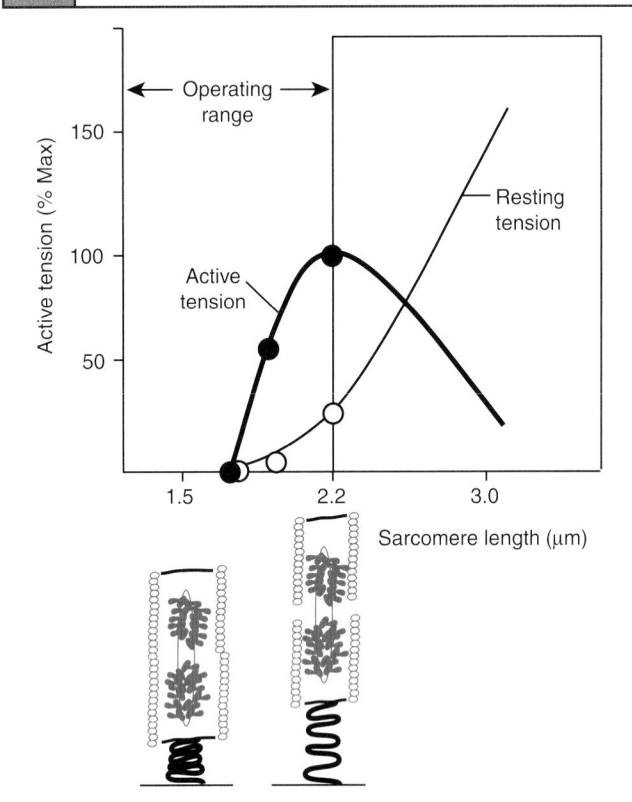

Figure 49–11
Dependence of tension on sarcomere length. Three measurements are shown in which a linear muscle preparation (papillary muscle or trabecula) was stretched from its equilibrium length, and determinations of resting (passive) and total active force were made. Active tension is the difference between total tension and passive tension. Beyond a sarcomere length of 2.2 μm, resting tension rises to high levels that are nonphysiologic, as discussed in the text. Thus, the cells never operate beyond the working range into the *panel*. Two sarcomeres, depicted at the extremes of the length–tension relationship, illustrate the stretching of passive springs in titin and the change in overlap of the thin and thick filaments.

such lengths are illustrated in Figure 49-11. At the shorter length, there is no passive tension and maximum developed tension is essentially zero because of the double overlap of thin filaments. At the optimal sarcomere length, active tension (the difference between total and passive tension) is at an optimum. Some resting tension exists at this sarcomere length as passive elements (notably titin) in the sarcomere and extracellular matrix are stretched. At the optimal sarcomere length of 2.2 μm, there is maximal overlap between the thick filament cross-bridges and the thin filaments.

In Figure 49-12, we show how the working range of the length–tension relationship relates to the pressure–volume relationship of the left ventricle. The basic premise is that cell and sarcomere lengths track the change in ventricular volumes, and ventricular pressure tracks changes in cell tension. Thus, one can imagine the generation of the volume–pressure relationship by an approach similar to that for generation of the length–tension relationship. In this case, although EDV is incrementally increased, EDP is measured at each volume, as is peak systolic isovolumic pressure. Figure 49-12 indicates an association of each ventricular volume with a particular sarcomere length. Important points are the following:

- Measurements of the relationship between, on the one hand, cell length and tension and, on the other, ventricular volume and isovolumic peak systolic pressure, are made at constant contractility. The basal inotropic state represents about 20% to 25% of the maximal inotropic state.
- A line connecting the peak systolic pressure points determined at constant volumes is a measure of contractility. These systolic pressure points are essentially the same ESP points inscribed by variations in afterload (see Fig. 49-7). As we mentioned, the ESP represents a point at which the cells are neither lengthening nor shortening.
- The position of the ESP–volume relationship is a critical determinant of ESV and thus of the ability of the ventricle to eject blood.
- Figure 49-12 indicates that this position changes with an increase in contractility, which we now picture as an increase in Ca^{2+} activation of the cells that results in an increase in peak systolic pressure at a particular ventricular volume. This relationship between ventricular volume and pressure was recognized by Otto Frank and Ernest Starling over 100 years ago and is commonly referred to as the Frank-Starling relationship or Starling's law of the heart.

Despite this long-standing knowledge of Starling's law, the molecular mechanism responsible for the shape of the ESP–volume relationship remains unclear.[9] The relationship is steeper than one would expect from simple geometric considerations of filament overlap. There is excellent evidence that this relatively steep relationship is the result of a length dependence of Ca^{2+} activation.[9] Measurement of myofilament response to Ca^{2+} demonstrated a decrease in Ca^{2+} sensitivity as the sarcomere become shorter. Thus, at a constant level of systolic Ca^{2+}, we would expect the sarcomeres to be more sensitive to Ca^{2+} as their length increases. This results in a steeper length–tension relationship that would occur with no change in Ca^{2+} sensitivity. Length-dependent changes in interfilament spacing, radial movements of cross-bridges away from the thick filament proper, and cross-bridge–dependent activation of the myofilaments have all been invoked as mechanisms for length-dependent activation.[9]

CARDIAC FUNCTION CURVES

So far, we have depicted regulation of CO as relationships between workload, HR, and ventricular volumes (see Fig. 49-1), as relationships between time and ventricular volume changes (see Fig. 49-2), and as a relationship between ventricular volume and ventricular pressure (see Fig. 49-7). We now consider another view of regulation of cardiac output as so-called Starling curves or the Starling relationship, or simply cardiac function curves. These curves relate some measure of ventricular filling such as EDV or EDP to some measure of ejection, SV, or CO. Figure 49-13A depicts the transition from determinations of SV from pressure–volume loops at constant contractility and afterload to a relationship between EDV and SV. Three beats are shown at different preloads. The function curve thus provides a relationship between EDV and SV at constant afterload and contractility. Figure 49-13B indicates the shift in the cardiac function

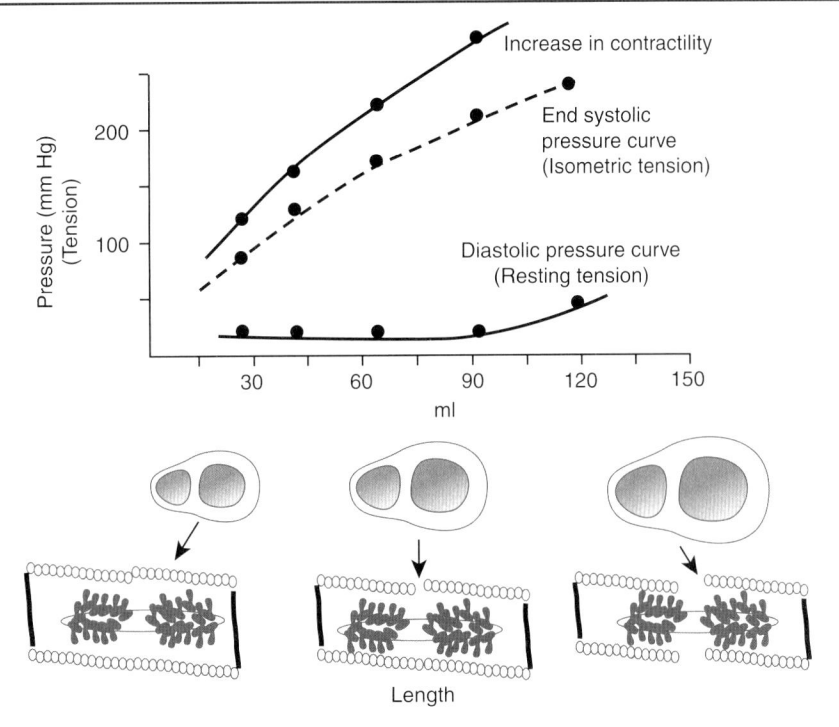

Figure 49–12
Generation of systolic and diastolic pressure curves from steady-state measurements of isovolumic pressure development over a range of end-diastolic volumes. Points on the curves were generated by plotting the peak diastolic and systolic pressures at each ventricular volume in hearts with cross-clamped aortas (as in Fig. 49-6). The correlation of ventricular volume with sarcomere length and of ventricular pressure with tension emphasizes that the dependence of pressure on volume is rooted in the length–tension relationship of cardiac sarcomeres.

curve as a result of an elevated afterload. In this case, the pressure–volume loops show the same SV, which is achieved at an elevated EDV. Figure 49-13C indicates the shift in the cardiac function curve as a result of increased contractility. The pressure–volume loops show the same SV, which is achieved at a lower EDV and ESV. One imagines the same shift for all the preloads indicated in Figure 49-13A. With knowledge of the HR, it is possible to convert the EDV-SV relationship to a relationship between EDV and CO. Effects of increases and decreases in afterload and contractility on the relationship between EDV and CO and SV are illustrated in Figure 49-14.

The exact cardiac function that is operative in the heart at any particular time reflects the integrated effects of many factors. These include the determinants of afterload (blood pressure) and of contractility, changes in HR, levels of autonomic nervous system activity and circulating neurohumors, the intracellular and cellular chemical environment (anoxia, hypoxia, acidosis, hypercapnia, metabolites), and the presence of pharmacologic agents that affect afterload or contractility. The EDV is determined by the flow of blood back to the heart, which in turn is determined by the total blood volume, the venous tone, resistance to flow, the pumping actions of muscle, and the intrathoracic pressure. The integrated effects of these determinants of cardiac function in the physiologic state are revealed in the exercise episode depicted in Figure 49-1. Pathophysiologic states may be understood in terms of a breakdown of these physiologic control mechanisms.[16,17] For example, in heart failure, the SR Ca^{2+} load may be diminished by reduced expression of SERCA2a. There may also be alterations in myofilament response to Ca^{2+}. The ultimate effect of these changes is a reduction in contractility, much like that simulated by β-adrenergic blockade in the data shown in Figure 49-1. With elevations in EDV, heart cells are stimulated to grow but the growth becomes maladaptive and failure ensues as remodeling occurs. Detailed discussion of these events is beyond the scope of this chapter, but it is clear that an understanding of cardiac pathophysiology begins with an understanding of the physiology of the myocardium.[16,17]

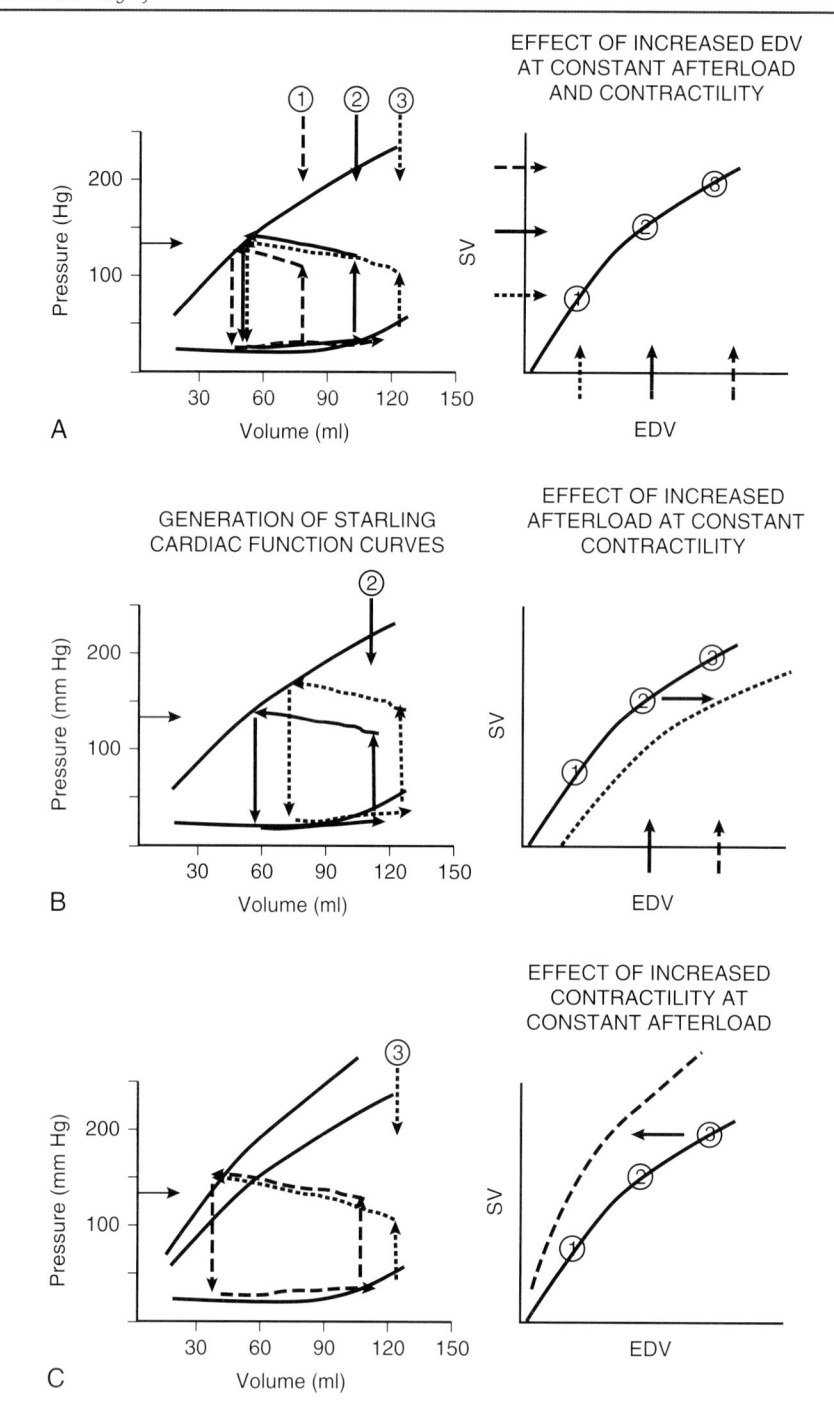

Figure 49–13
Generation of Starling cardiac function curves from pressure–volume relationships. **A,** Three beats (1, 2, 3) are shown with increases in preload at constant contractility and afterload. A plot of stroke volume (SV) at each of the end-diastolic volumes (EDV) associated with each beat generates a common form of the cardiac function curve or Starling relationship. **B,** Change in steady-state pressure–volume loop after an increase in afterload. Only beat 2 from **A** is shown for illustrative purposes, but a similar shift in the cardiac function would occur at all EDVs. **C,** Change in steady-state pressure–volume loop after an increase in contractility. Only beat 3 from **A** is shown for illustrative purposes, but a similar shift in the cardiac function would occur at all EDVs.

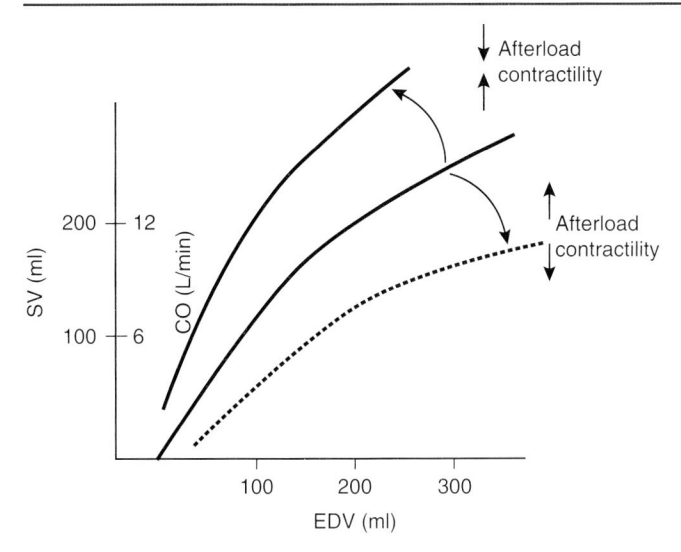

Figure 49–14
Effect of alterations in afterload and contractility on the cardiac function curve. Each curve represents a state of constant contractility and afterload. Shifts in the cardiac function curve from a physiologic basal state *(central solid line)* occur with changes in afterload and contractility. CO, cardiac output; EDV, end-diastolic volume; SV, stroke volume.

REFERENCES

1. Covell JW, Ross J Jr. Systolic and diastolic function (mechanics) of the intact heart. In: Page E, Fozzard H, Solaro RJ, editors. *Handbook of physiology.* New York: Oxford University Press; 2002, Section 2: The cardiovascular system, vol. 1, The heart. p. 741-85.
2. Frey N, Olson E. Cardiac hypertrophy: the good, the bad, and the ugly. *Annu Rev Physiol* 2003;**65**:45-79.
3. Solaro RJ, Wolska BM, Arteaga G, et al. Modulation of thin filament activity in long and short term regulation of cardiac function. In: Solaro RJ, Moss RL, editors. *Molecular control mechanisms in striated muscle contraction.* Boston: Kluwer Academic; 2002. p. 291-327.
4. Bers DM. *Excitation-contraction coupling and cardiac contractile force.* 2nd ed. Boston: Kluwer Academic; 2001.
5. Spray DC, Suadicani SO, Srinivas M, et al. Gap junctions in the cardiovascular system. In: Page E, Fozzard H, Solaro RJ, editors. *Handbook of physiology.* New York: Oxford University Press; 2002, Section 2: The cardiovascular system, vol. 1, The heart. p. 169-212.
6. Homsher E. Determinants of unloaded shortening velocity in striated muscle. In: Solaro RJ, Moss RL, editors. *Molecular control mechanisms in striated muscle contraction.* Boston: Kluwer Academic; 2002. p. 417-42.
7. Walker JW. Kinetics of the actin-myosin interaction. In: Page E, Fozzard H, Solaro RJ, editors. *Handbook of physiology.* New York: Oxford University Press; 2002, Section 2: The cardiovascular system, vol. 1, The heart. p. 240-63.
8. Solaro RJ. Modulation of cardiac myofilament activity by protein phosphorylation. In: Page E, Fozzard H, Solaro RJ, editors. *Handbook of physiology.* New York: Oxford University Press; 2002, Section 2: The cardiovascular system, vol. 1: The heart. p. 264-300.
9. Fuchs F. The Frank-Starling relationship: cellular and molecular mechanisms. In: Solaro RJ, Moss RL, editors. *Molecular control mechanisms in striated muscle contraction.* Boston: Kluwer Academic; 2002. p. 379-416.
10. Clark KA, Mittal B, Sanger JM, Sanger JW. Striated muscle cyto-architecture: an intricate web of form and function. *Annu Rev Cell Dev Biol* 2002;**18**:637-706.
11. Tada M, Toyofuku T. Cardiac sarcoplasmic reticulum Ca^{2+}-ATPase. In: Page E, Fozzard H, Solaro RJ, editors. *Handbook of physiology.* New York: Oxford University Press; 2002, Section 2: The cardiovascular system, vol. 1, The heart. p. 301-34.
12. Trafford AW, Eisner DA. Excitation-contraction coupling in cardiac muscle. In: Solaro RJ, Moss RL, editors. *Molecular control mechanisms in striated muscle contraction.* Boston: Kluwer Academic; 2002. p. 48-89.
13. Westfall MV, Metzger JM. Troponin I isoforms and chimeras: tuning the molecular switch of cardiac contraction. *News Physiol Sci* 2001;**16**:278-81.
14. Thomas D, Zhang W, Karle C, et al. Deletion of protein kinase A phosphorylation sites in the HERG potassium channel inhibits activation shift by protein kinase A. *J Biol Chem* 1999;**274**:27457-62.
15. Solaro RJ. Integration of myofilament response to Ca^{2+} with cardiac pump regulation and pump dynamics. *Adv Physiol Ed* 1999;**22**:S155-63.
16. Rice CL, Solaro RJ, et al. Support of the failing heart. In: Wilmore DW, Cheung LY, Harken AH, editors. *ACS surgery principles and practice.* New York: WebMD; 2002. p. 1391-400.
17. Katz AM. A modern view of heart failure: practical applications of cardiovascular physiology. In: Page E, Fozzard H, Solaro RJ, editors. *Handbook of physiology.* New York: Oxford University Press; 2002, Section 2: The cardiovascular system, vol. 1: The heart. p. 786-804.

CHAPTER 50
Ventricular Mechanics
Mark Ratcliffe, Arthur Wallace, and Julius Guccione

Structure of Ventricular Tissue
  Myocyte Orientation
  Laminar Organization of Myocardium
  Extracellular Matrix
The Cardiac Cycle
  Electromechanical Activation
  Cardiac Cycle per se
  The Pressure–Volume Loop
Determinants of Left Ventricular Filling
  Pressure–Volume Analysis
  End-Diastolic Pressure–Volume Relationship
  Myocardial Stiffness
  Myocyte Relaxation
  Left Ventricular Torsion and Recoil
  Ventricular Suction
  Echocardiographic Measures of Diastolic Function

  Atrial Contraction
  Diastolic Dysfunction from Myocardial Ischemia
  Diastolic Dysfunction from Hypertrophy
Systolic Function and End-Systolic Elastance
  Cardiac Output and Cardiac Index
  The Swan-Ganz Catheter
  Ejection Fraction
  The End-Systolic Pressure–Volume Relationship
  Systolic Dysfunction from Myocardial Ischemia
Pump Function
  The Frank-Starling Relationship
  The Force Frequency Relationship

Non-Starling Regulation of Blood Pressure and Cardiac Output
Myocardial Energy Expenditure and Efficiency
  Determinants of Myocardial Energy Consumption
Afterload and Ventriculoarterial Coupling
Regional Strain
  Tissue Doppler
  Magnetic Resonance Imaging
Regional Stress and the Finite-element Method
Ventricular Interaction and Pericardium
  Ventricular Interaction
  Pericardium

In Chapter 49, the myocardium at the cellular and subcellular level was considered. In this chapter, we will look at the mechanics of the heart at the tissue and organ level. We will focus primarily on the left ventricle, but short discussions of left atrial function as it relates to left ventricular (LV) filling and ventricular interaction will be included. First, we will review several important myocardial structural elements, an understanding of which is necessary to appreciate function during active contraction (systole), relaxation, and filling (diastole). Next, we will review the cardiac mechanical and flow events that comprise the cardiac cycle. We will then cover diastolic and systolic function, with an emphasis on pressure–volume analysis. A discussion of pump function, myocardial energy expenditure, and myocardial efficiency will follow. The finite-element method will be briefly discussed as a means to calculate regional contractility and stress. Furthermore, in each section, we will consider the effect that common clinical conditions such as ventricular hypertrophy and myocardial ischemia have on ventricular function. Where appropriate, we will briefly describe state-of-the-art methods used to measure regional and global LV function.

STRUCTURE OF VENTRICULAR TISSUE

The tissue level structure of the myocardium is intimately related to systolic and diastolic function. For example, myocyte orientation determines the LV torsion that occurs during active contraction and the subsequent untwisting that occurs during relaxation and filling. The extracellular matrix (ECM) is an important determinant of LV diastolic compliance.

Myocyte Orientation

The orientation of myofibers is complex, with variation across both the LV wall and in different LV regions. The orientation of myofibers was first quantified by Streeter and colleagues,[1-4] who measured myocyte orientation in tangential sections obtained across the LV wall of the dog heart and found a smooth transition in the helix angle (in the tangential plane relative to the horizontal) from the epicardium (–60 degrees) to the endocardium (+60 degrees). Myofiber orientation data collected by Streeter are displayed in Figure 50-1.[1] Other studies using this histologic sampling confirmed his results in different species.[2-6]

Recent advances in magnetic resonance imaging (MRI) now allow rapid and nondestructive assessment of muscle fibers throughout the entire heart. Magnetic resonance diffusion tensor imaging exploits the anisotropic diffusion of water through ordered tissues. This method has been correlated with histologically measured fiber angles[2-4] and has been used to thoroughly map the fiber orientation in the entire left ventricle of a normal rabbit, goat, sheep, and human.[2,3]

Laminar Organization of Myocardium

The laminar nature of the myocardium has been appreciated since the 1800s.[2] Adjacent myocytes are organized into sheets, or lamina, that are three to four cells thick.[3,4] Furthermore, there are extensive cleavage planes between sheets[3,4] that are most apparent in the midwall of the left ventricle where the planes are radially oriented. The laminar organization of the left ventricle has been recently championed by Torrent-Guasp's group,[3] who suggested that the left ventricle consisted of a single folded myocardial band. Alternatively, Lagrice and colleagues proposed a finite-element–based mathematical model that represents sheet geometry.[4] A diagram of the laminar architecture of the myocardium is shown in Figure 50-2.[4]

Extracellular Matrix

The ECM is an important determinant of LV diastolic compliance. Scanning electron microscopy of the ECM demonstrates an extensive network of collagen fibers that are organized

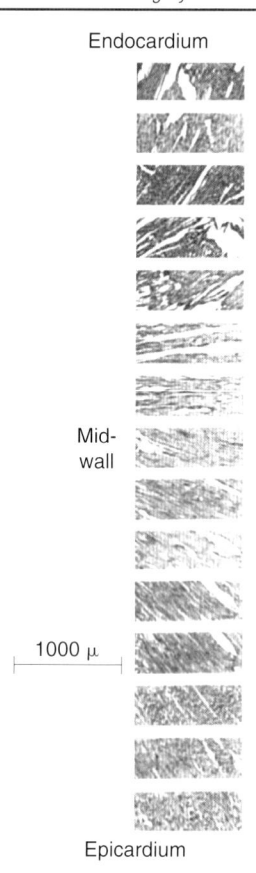

Figure 50–1
Photomicrographs of myocardial fiber orientation. *(From Streeter DD Jr, Hanna WT. Circ Res 1973;33[6]:656–64.)*

into three primary components.[5] Briefly, the endomysium surrounds individual cells and groups of cells, and the epimysium surrounds entire muscle groups.[6] Perimysial fibers that connect groups of cells can be seen in Figure 50-2A. Perimysial fibers associated with papillary muscle myocardium have a coiled shape that may play an important role in papillary muscle strength and stiffness.[7]

THE CARDIAC CYCLE

Electromechanical Activation

The rhythmic electrical activation of the heart normally begins at the sinoatrial node. Electrical activation spreads rapidly over the atria, initiating atrial contraction. There is a delay while electrical activation moves slowly through the atrioventricular node. The electrical activation then propagates rapidly along the bundle of His, and then the right and left bundle branches and the sub-branches (Purkinje fibers) before initiating a coordinated ventricular contraction. The excitation of the ventricles results in the QRS complex of the electrocardiogram.

Cardiac Cycle per se

Plots of the electrocardiogram (ECG) and of the left atrial, LV, and aortic pressures during the cardiac cycle are schematically illustrated in Figure 50-3. Depolarization and contraction of the left ventricle raises intracavitary LV pressure. First, this causes the mitral valve to close. When LV pressure exceeds the pressure in the aorta, the aortic valve opens and pressurized blood is ejected into the aorta.

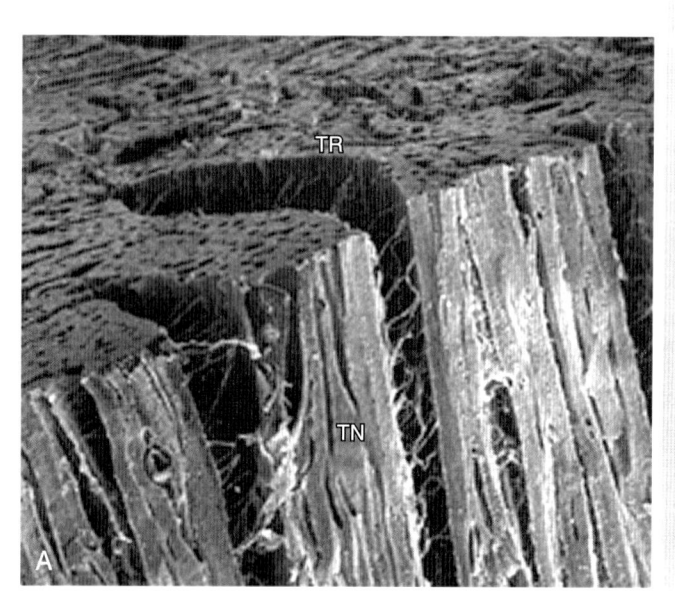

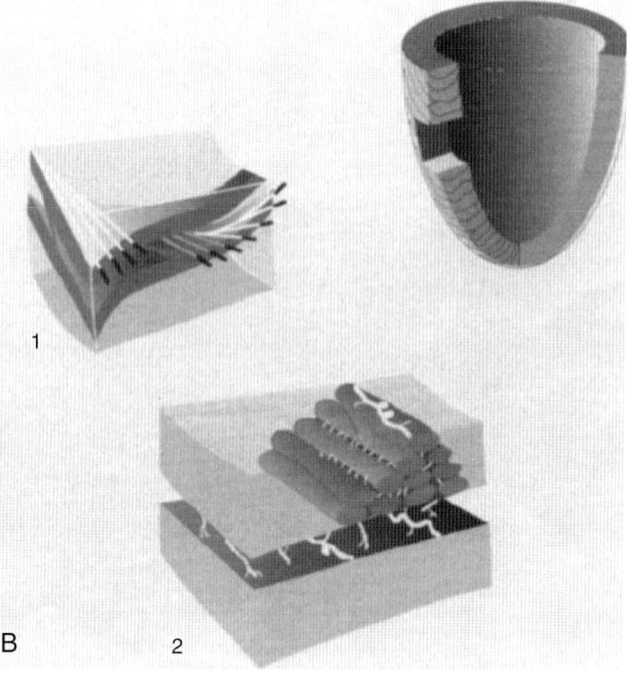

Figure 50–2
A, Scanning electron microscope image of a left ventricular, midanterior midwall. Tangential (TN) and transverse (TR) surfaces are shown. B, Schematic of cardiac microstructure. Transmural segment (1) contains layers of tightly coupled myocytes. These layers run in an approximately radial direction, and there are circumferential and tangential muscle branches between adjacent layers. Orientations of muscle fiber axes are indicated. 2, cellular arrangement. Fine lines, components of extracellular collagen matrix. *(From Legrice IJ, Hunter PJ, Smaill BH. Am J Physiol 1997;272[5 Pt 2]: H2466–76.)*

Chapter 50 Ventricular Mechanics | 741

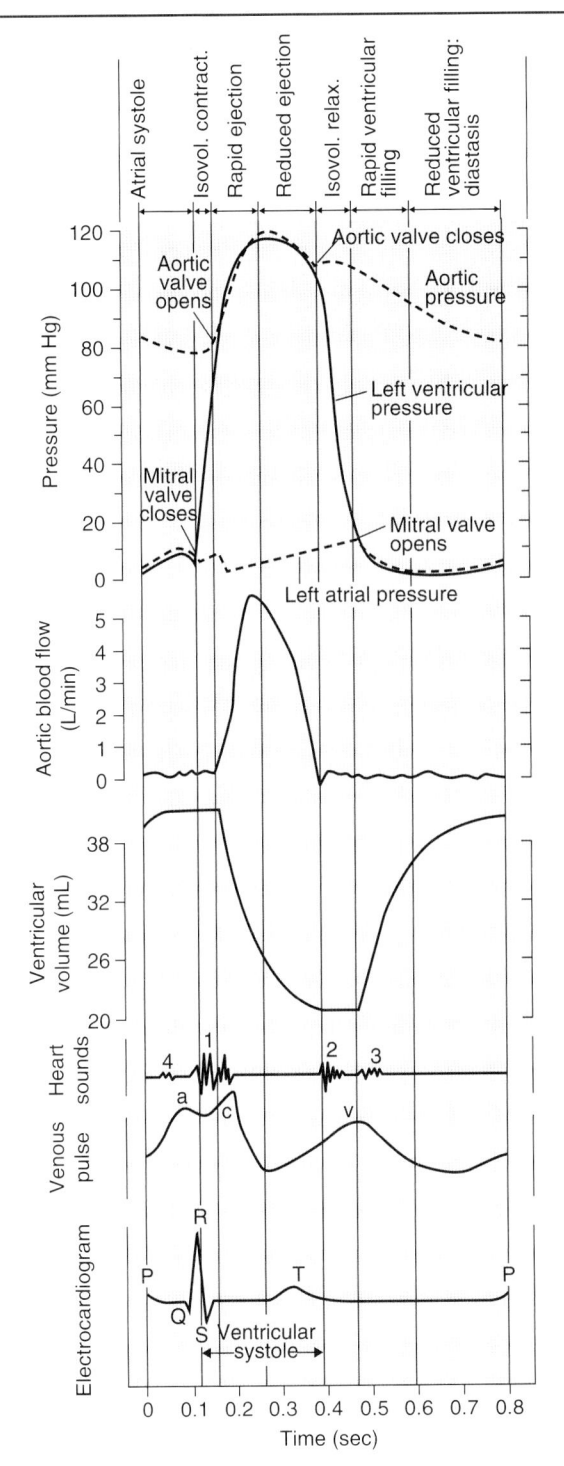

Figure 50-3
The cardiac cycle. *(Adapted from Hurst JW, Logue RB: The heart. 2nd ed. New York: McGraw-Hill; 1970, p. 76, and from Notomi Y, Martin-Miklovic MG, Oryszak SJ, et al. Circulation 2006;**113**[21]: 2524-33.)*

At the end of ejection, LV pressure falls below aortic pressure and the aortic valve closes. Relaxation of the myocytes is locally initiated and not directly coordinated by the conduction system. As the myocytes relax, the pressure drops in the ventricle. When LV pressure falls below the pressure in the atria, the mitral valve opens and filling begins.

The Pressure–Volume Loop

Pressure and volume of the left ventricle are plotted as shown in Figure 50-4A. Active contraction (systole) begins at the bottom right corner of the loop. Contraction is isovolumic until the aortic valve opens at the top right corner and the ventricle ejects. The end of systole occurs at the upper left hand corner of the loop.

Diastole is initially isovolumic until the mitral valve opens at the bottom left corner and ventricular filling begins. Ventricular filling begins at the bottom left hand corner of the loop, where it is broken into a period of early, rapid filling; slow filling (diastasis); and filling associated with atrial systole. The end of filling is the end of diastole (bottom right corner of the loop).

DETERMINANTS OF LEFT VENTRICULAR FILLING

Pressure–Volume Analysis

Pressure–volume analysis of the cardiac cycle is a cornerstone of LV mechanics. Pressure–volume analysis was initially described in 1895 by Otto Frank,[8] but the analysis was limited by the lack of suitable methods to measure LV pressure and volume. In the 1960s, interest in pressure–volume analysis was renewed with the development of methods such as cineangiography[9] and echocardiography[10] that could measure ventricular volume in vivo.[11]

Cardiac imaging methods have advanced substantially. The imaging method most widely used for studying the heart is still echocardiography, which can also be used to measure flow velocities (or at least the component of velocity along the line of the ultrasound beam), through the Doppler effect.[12]

MRI provides high-quality, spatially registered images that can be used to calculate volumes. MRI is the gold standard for cardiac global function volume measurements.[13] Although recent advances have been made in imaging quality and speed with computed tomography (CT), MRI provides better temporal resolution, and it does not risk radiation exposure and potentially harmful contrast agents.[13] Because CT, MRI, and three-dimensional (3D) echocardiography build collated data sets from multiple cardiac cycles, they can be used only when the rhythm is regular and the hemodynamic properties are in steady state.

The conductance catheter is best for real-time volume measurement during changes in LV preload or afterload.[14] However, its inability to measure absolute ventricular volume because of parallel conductance is a limitation of the method.[14]

Pressure–volume loops remain similar unless loading or the strength of contraction (contractility) is changed. If preload or afterload is changed—for example, by clamping the vena cava or aorta while contractility remains the same—a family of curves is generated. The end-diastolic and end-systolic points subtend two lines. The end-diastolic line, referred to as the end-diastolic pressure–volume relationship (EDPVR) or ventricular compliance curve, is typically curvilinear. A typical EDPVR relationship is displayed in Figure 50-5A. The end-systolic line, referred to as the end-systolic pressure–volume relationship (ESPVR) or end-systolic elastance, is nearly straight. The ESPVR relationship will be discussed further.

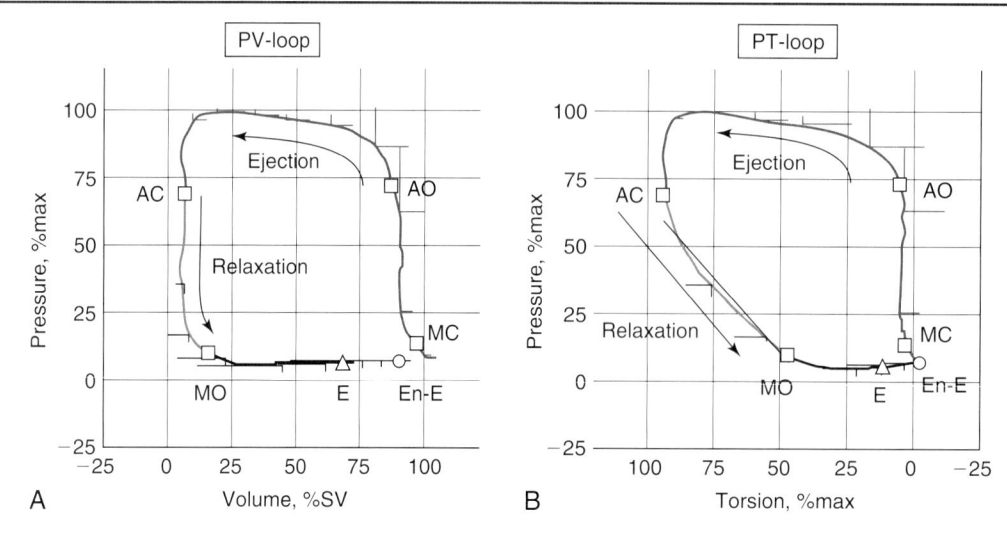

Figure 50–4
A, The pressure–volume (PV) (work) loop of the left ventricle. **B,** Loops during variable load (vena caval occlusion) and associated systolic and diastolic chamber stiffness curves. MC/MO, mitral valve closing/opening; AC/AO, aortic valve closing/opening; E, peak; En-E, end of filling. *(From Notomi Y, Martin-Miklovic MG, Oryszak SJ, et al. Circulation 2006;**113**[21]:2524–33.)*

End-Diastolic Pressure–Volume Relationship

The EDPVR (or left ventricular compliance) is typically described by an exponential relationship,[11]

$$P_{ED} = A + Be^{\alpha V_{ED}}, \quad (1)$$

where P is left ventricular pressure, V is left ventricular volume, ED is end-diastole, A is an offset in left ventricular pressure, and B and α are diastolic stiffness constants. A shift of the EDPVR curve up and to the left represents an increase in diastolic chamber stiffness (i.e., a decrease in compliance). A shift of the curve down or to the right means that diastolic chamber stiffness is decreased (i.e., an increase in compliance).

Statistical comparison of EDPVR between subjects before and after interventions is an issue. A t-test is not appropriate because it fails to take colinearity into account.[15,16] As seen in Equation 2, a logarithmic transformation allows the use of multiple linear regression, but the offset term (A) must be removed[15,16]:

$$\ln[P_{ED}] = \ln[B] + \alpha(V_{ED}), \quad (2)$$

where P is left ventricular pressure, V is left ventricular volume, ED is end-diastole, A is an offset in left ventricular pressure, and B and α are diastolic stiffness constants.

Box 50-1 has a short list of mechanical factors that combine to determine the EDPVR.

Myocardial Stiffness

Myocyte and ECM stiffness (discussed earlier) are determinants of global LV diastolic function. The passive stiffness of the myocyte is dependent on the giant intracellular protein titin. As discussed in Chapter 49 (see Fig. 49-3), the Z-line (or Z-disc) is the center point of the I band and the attachment point of actin (thin filament). The M-line is the center point of the A band (myosin; thick filaments). Titin molecules extend from the Z-line to the M-line.[17] Successive titin molecules are in head-to-head and tail-to-tail arrangements, creating a continuous protein structure that extends the entire length of the myocyte. The majority of titin's I band region is extensible and functions as a molecular spring that develops a restoring force when the cell is stretched[17] or compressed.[18] A diagram showing the structure of titin is seen in Figure 50-6.[18]

Myocyte Relaxation

LV relaxation, a component of early diastolic filling, is an energy-dependent process involving the removal of Ca^{2+} from troponin-C, followed by the dissociation of actin and myosin cross-bridges, thus allowing the myofibrils to relax and to return to their original end-diastolic length.[19] A typical LV relaxation curve is seen in Figure 50-5B.[20]

LV relaxation is classically evaluated by the exponential time constant of isovolumic relaxation (T), requiring cardiac catheterization to measure LV pressure.

$$P[t] = P_0 e^{-\frac{t}{T}}, \quad (3)$$

where P is left ventricular pressure, P_0 is the pressure at the time of dP/dt_{min}, t is time after dP/dt_{min}, and T is the time constant of isovolumic pressure fall.[21] Figure 50-5B demonstrates how relaxation pressure (see Equation 3) can be subtracted from actual diastolic pressure data to obtain a corrected pressure.[20]

Left Ventricular Torsion and Recoil

The myofiber architecture described previously (see Structure of Ventricular Tissue) causes the left ventricle to undergo torsion during systole. The magnitude of torsion is a function of myocyte contractility.[22] As myocyte contraction and torsion occur, extracellular collagen matrix[23] and intracellular titin are compressed.[17] Untwisting occurs in early diastole, with 40% of the left ventricle untwisting during isovolumic relaxation (see Fig. 50-4B).[24]

LV untwisting continues during ventricular filling. Mitral valve opening is immediately followed by the development of a pressure gradient between the LV apex and base,[25]

Box 50-1
Factors That Affect the End-Diastolic Pressure–Volume Relationship

- Myocardial (myocyte and extracellular matrix) passive stiffness
- Myocyte relaxation
- Ventricular suction
- Ventricular interaction
- Pericardium

a negative LV pressure (to the right of the gray bar), is shown in Figure 50-7.[30]

It is now thought that ventricular suction is caused by LV untwisting and the elastic recoil of the compressed myocytes in early diastole. The concept is that end-systolic volume is smaller than the diastolic equilibrium volume.[31] As a consequence, depending on the time course of myocyte relaxation, the left ventricle generates the negative intracavitary pressure described earlier. In short, ventricular suction helps to draw blood into the chamber across the mitral valve.

Echocardiographic Measures of Diastolic Function

Most clinical measurements of diastolic function focus on echocardiographic Doppler transmitral blood-flow patterns. Normally, early flow (E wave) is higher than that associated with atrial contraction (A wave). Mitral flow patterns are displayed in Figure 50-8.[32] Diastolic dysfunction is typically associated with a reversal of the E-to-A ratio.[33] However, the E-to-A ratio in dilated cardiomyopathy may range between complete A-wave dominance, which suggests decreased ventricular compliance, and a "pseudonormalized" pattern (E-wave dominance).[34] Mitral flow patterns are difficult to interpret, however, because of confounding factors, including atrial pressure, ventricular relaxation time, and mitral regurgitation.[35] In addition, aging is associated with a decrease in the E-to-A ratio, possibly related to increasing myocardial fibrosis with age.[36] Abnormal mitral flow patterns are also seen in Figure 50-8.[32]

Atrial Contraction

The atrial contraction near the end of ventricular diastole augments the final filling of the ventricle before the next ventricular contraction.[37]

Diastolic Dysfunction from Myocardial Ischemia

Acute coronary occlusion causes the EDPVR to shift up and to the left.[38] It was initially thought that the change in EDPVR was caused by an increase in myocardial passive stiffness. However, it is now thought that the change in EDPVR is secondary to increased right ventricular pressure mediated by an intact pericardium (see Ventricular Interaction and Pericardium, later).[39] Anterior myocardial ischemia is also associated with a decrease in the pressure gradient between the LV apex and base that normally occurs during the rapid filling phase of diastole. The mechanism is thought to be loss of LV torsion resulting from reduced myocardial contractility, and the subsequent inability to store energy that would be released during elastic recoil.[25]

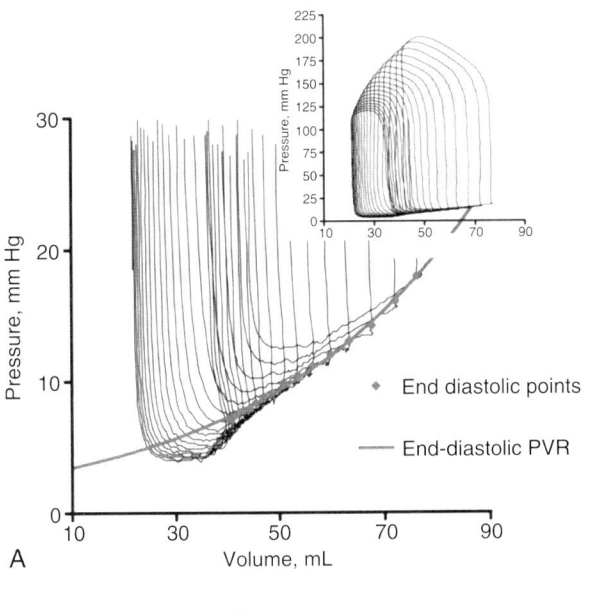

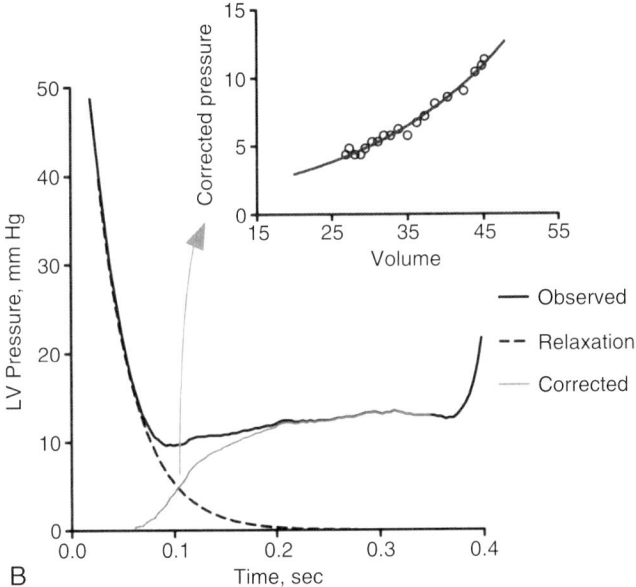

Figure 50-5
Characterization of end-diastolic pressure–volume relationship (EDPVR) by multiple-beat (**A**) and relaxation-corrected single-beat (**B**) methods. Note that the graph in A is expanded from the complete pressure volume loop data (insert). LV, left ventricular. *(From Jaber WA, Lam CS, Meyer DM, Redfield MM. Am J Physiol Heart Circ Physiol 2007;**293**[5]: H2738-46.)*

which determines early LV filling.[26] The rate of untwisting is a predictor of the pressure gradient between the LV apex and base, as well as of the time constant of diastolic relaxation.[27] Finally, the rate of recoil is a preload-independent assessment of LV relaxation.[28]

Ventricular Suction

The presence of negative intracavitary LV pressure in early diastole was shown in a series of elegant experiments by Meisner and colleagues[29] and Yellin and coworkers,[30] in which a Starr Edwards mitral prosthesis was modified to close during diastolic filling. Data from one of Yellin's experiments, in which mitral valve occlusion caused

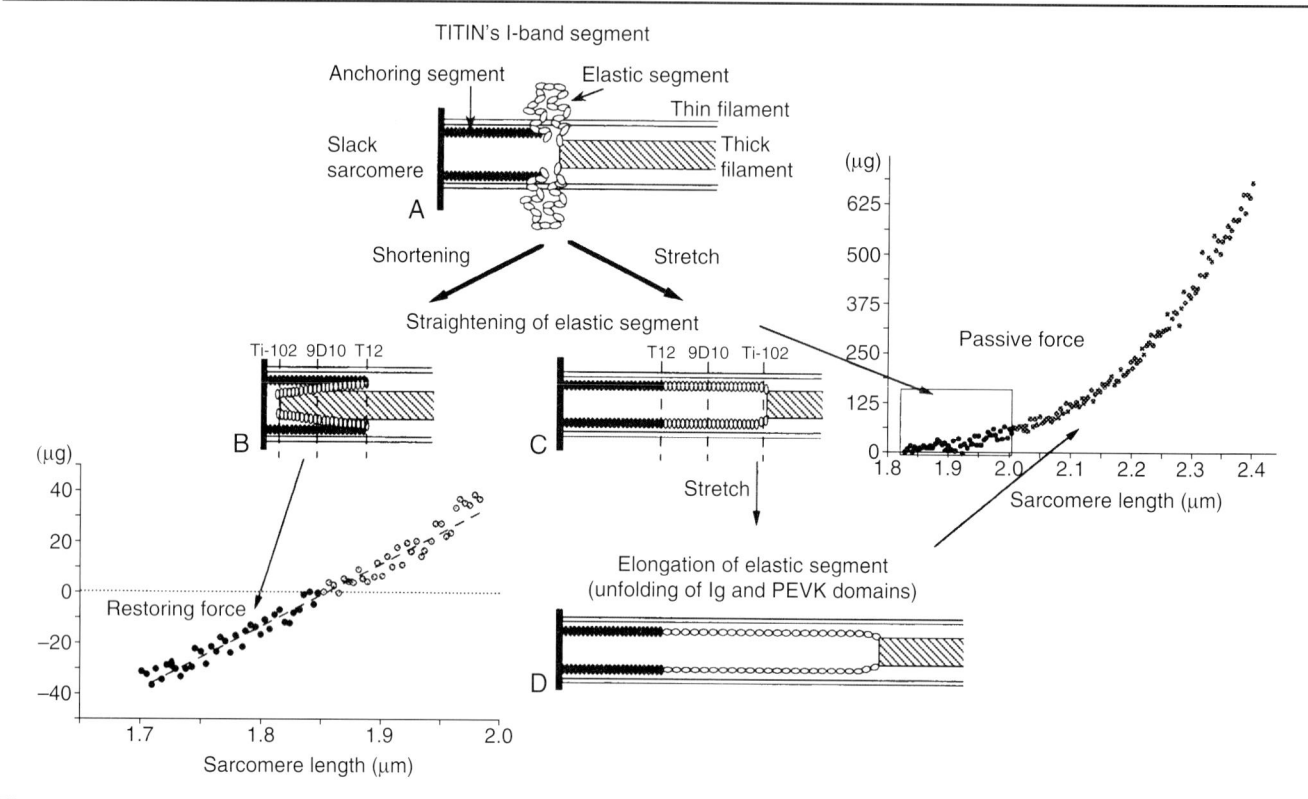

Figure 50–6
Working hypothesis of how titin generates both passive and restoring forces. *(From Helmes M, Trombitas K, Granzier H. Circ Res 1996;**79**[3]:619-26.)*

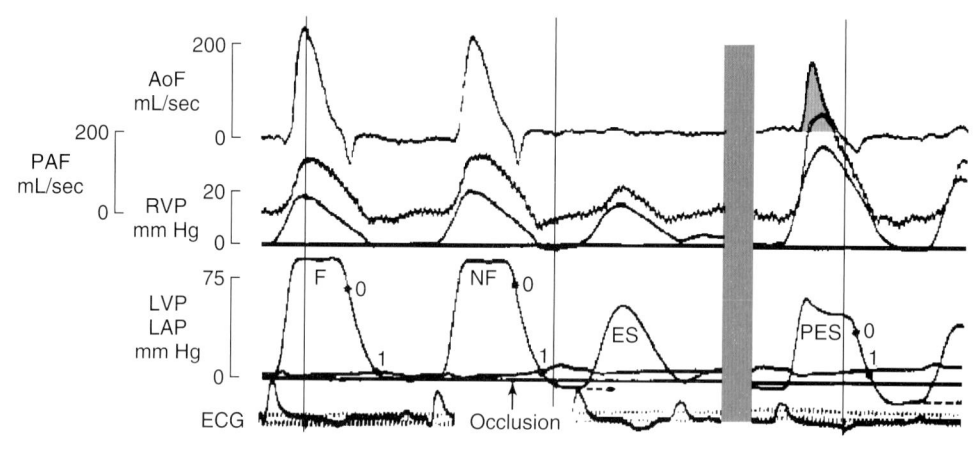

Figure 50–7
Oscillographic record of hemodynamic response to mitral valve occlusion. AoF, aortic flow; RVP, right ventricular pressure; LVP, left ventricular pressure; LAP, left atrial pressure. Note that LVP during diastole is negative after occlusion of the mitral valve (gray bar). *(From Yellin EL, Hori M, Yoran C, Sonnenblick EH, Gabbay S, Frater RW. Am J Physiol 1986;**250**[4 Pt 2]:H620-9.)*

Patients with dilated cardiomyopathy show abnormally low diastolic suction.[40] The mechanism may be similar.

Diastolic Dysfunction from Hypertrophy

Concentric hypertrophy is hypertrophy of the left ventricle in which the ratio of wall thickness to ventricular radius is increased.[41] It is commonly caused by hypertension and aortic stenosis. The cause of diastolic dysfunction in concentric hypertrophy is thought to be an increase in myocardial stiffness rather than a change in myocardial relaxation or recoil.[42] In patients with aortic stenosis, diastolic dysfunction is found in approximately 50% of the patients with normal systolic ejection performance and in 100% of the patients with depressed function.[43]

SYSTOLIC FUNCTION AND END-SYSTOLIC ELASTANCE

Cardiac Output and Cardiac Index

The simplest and most common measures of systolic function are cardiac output (CO) and ejection fraction. Briefly, the difference between the volume at end-diastole (ED) and end-systole (ES) is the stroke volume (SV),

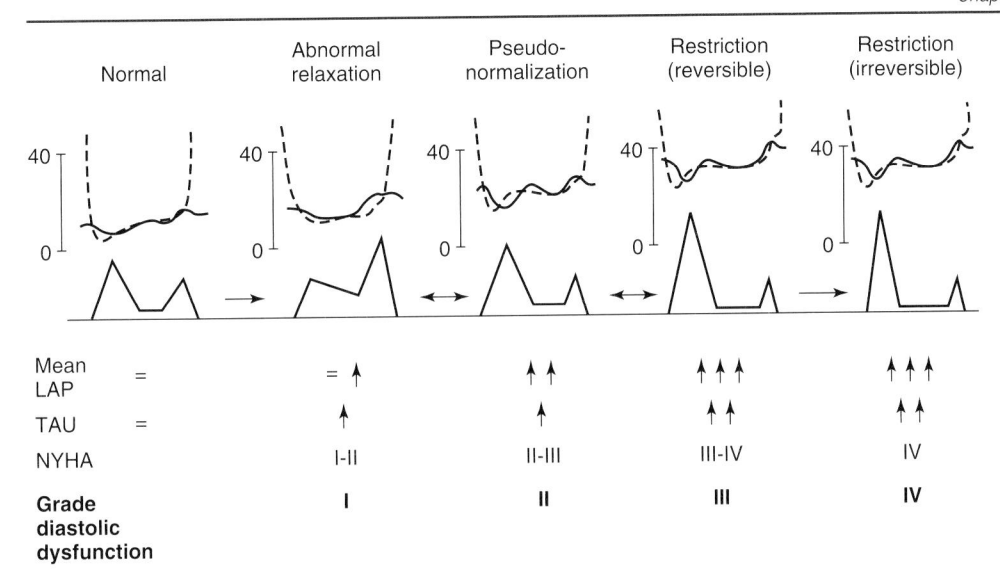

Figure 50–8
Diagram of a proposed grading system for diastolic dysfunction based on the progression of disease patterns in patients with cardiac disease. LAP, left atrial pressure; Tau, time constant of left ventricular relaxation (see Equation 3); NYHA, New York Heart Association class. *(From Nishimura RA, Tajik AJ. J Am Coll Cardiol 1997;30[1]:8-18.)*

$$SV = V_{ED} - V_{ES}, \quad (4)$$

and the cardiac output is the stroke volume multiplied by the heart rate (HR):

$$CO = HR \times SV \quad (5)$$

To account for the differences to be expected in the values of the CO for different-sized subjects, we can use the cardiac index (CI), which scales the cardiac output for body surface area (BSA):

$$CI = CO / BSA \quad (6)$$

The Swan-Ganz Catheter

The indicator dilution technique is widely used to estimate CO and thermodilution, and the Swan-Ganz catheter is the most common method of indicator dilution.[44] Briefly, a room-temperature bolus of saline is injected into the right atrium through the proximal port of the Swan-Ganz catheter. A thermistor in the tip of the catheter measures the change in temperature as the bolus of saline is carried through the pulmonary artery.[44] Thermodilution cardiac output compares favorably with measurement of cardiac output using the Fick principle.[45]

The Swan-Ganz catheter is used in many cardiac surgery units. However, there has been recent controversy over the risk benefit of the device.[46] Complications, including right ventricular perforation and pulmonary artery rupture, occur in 0.1% of patients.[47] A recent meta-analysis found the odds ratio to be 1.0.[48]

Ejection Fraction

The ratio of the SV to the ED volume is the ejection fraction (EF):

$$EF = SV / V_{ED} \quad (7)$$

Both cardiac output and ejection fraction are sensitive to afterload. Specifically, the greater the afterload (resistance to flow), the lower the CO and EF will be. Also, procedures and operations that alter ventricular size and material properties can cause an increase in ejection fraction that does not represent a true increase in ventricular pump function. This point has been made by Dickstein and colleagues[49] in regard to Batista's operation and by Wall and colleagues[50] in regard to cell transplantation. It is therefore incorrect to conclude that when a surgical procedure increases ejection fraction, pump function has improved.

The End-Systolic Pressure–Volume Relationship

Suga, Sagawa, and coworkers, and others, developed the ESPVR concept and suggested that it could be used as an index of global ventricular contractility.[51-56] In principle, the measurement of ESPVR is straightforward. It requires only the acquisition of ventricular pressure–volume (PV) loops at two or more preload or afterload conditions. The end-systolic points on these PV loops are identified, and a line is drawn through them; the slope of this line is the end-systolic (peak) elastance, or E_{ES}.[51-56] The ESPVR is of great value because it is inherently load independent. However, it must be recognized that the ESPVR is not pump function per se, as it does not take diastolic function into consideration. As with EF, this point has been made by Dickstein and colleagues with regard to Batista's operation.[49]

E_{ES} is typically described by the following equation:

$$P_{ES} = E_{ES}(V_{ES} - V_0), \quad (8)$$

where ES is end-systole, and E_{ES} and V_0 are the slope and volume intercept of the ESPVR curve, respectively.[54] Note that a shift of the ESPVR curve up and to the left represents an improvement in systolic chamber stiffness. As an example, the effect of epinephrine on the ESPVR is seen in Figure 50-9 (dashed line). A shift of the curve down or to the right means that systolic function is worse. Note that both the slope and the intercept can change.[11]

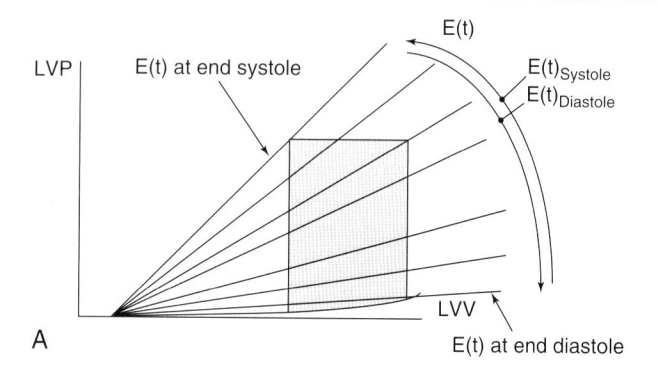

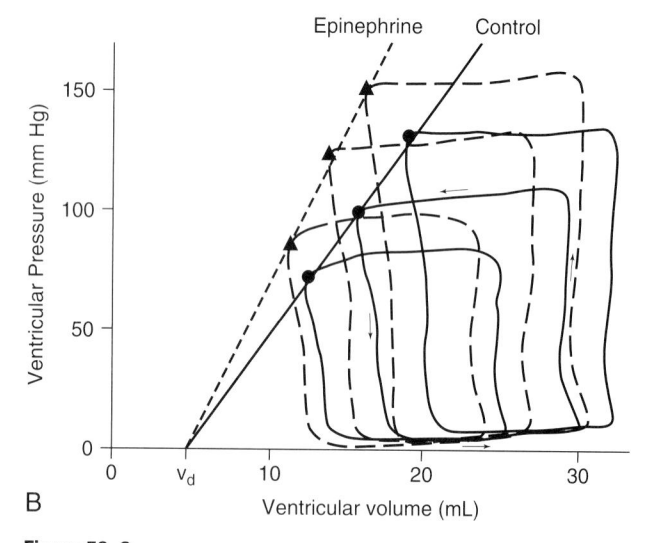

Figure 50-9
A, The time varying elastance E(t) concept and graph of the end-systolic pressure–volume relationship (ESPVR), with and without catecholamine effect. **B,** A graph of left ventricular pressure–volume loops of a denervated heart. *(From Suga H, Sagawa K, Shoukas AA. Circ Res 1973;32[3]:314-22.)*

Systolic Dysfunction from Myocardial Ischemia

Myocardial ischemia and infarction result in loss of contractile function of the involved myocytes. As a consequence, the ESPVR curve moves to the right.[57]

PUMP FUNCTION

The Frank-Starling Relationship

Cardiac output is regulated by intrinsic cardiac and extrinsic regulatory mechanisms. The Frank-Starling relationship is the principal intrinsic cardiac regulatory mechanism. In 1914, Patterson and Starling described the relationships between stroke volume and end-diastolic volume, and between stroke volume and end-diastolic pressure.[58,59] Starling's work was remarkable in that he did not possess cardiac imaging and relied on the displacement of water in a cylindrical container surrounding the heart as a measure of LV volume. The relationship between stroke volume and end-diastolic pressure is typically referred to as the Frank-Starling relationship or Starling's law.

The molecular determinants of the Frank-Starling relationship are discussed in Chapter 49. Briefly, the magnitude of the force generated by the myocytes is dependent on their initial length at the time of initiation of the contraction, as described by the Frank-Starling law. The general shape of the Frank-Starling relationship is shown in Figure 50-10.[60] No specific mathematical relationship exists, although a quadratic polynomial function has been used to approximate the relationship.[61] A shift of the Frank-Starling curve up and to the left reflects an improvement in pump function. A shift of the curve down and to the right implies that pump function is worse.

More recently, the relationship between stroke work and end-diastolic volume has been recommended by Glower and colleagues because of its linear nature[60] (see Fig. 50-10):

$$SW = M_W(V_{ED} - V_W), \quad (9)$$

where M_W and V_W are the slope and intercept, respectively, of the preload recruitable stroke work relationship.[60] Stroke work (SW) is defined as follows:

$$SW = \int_{ED}^{ES} P(V)dV - \int_{ES}^{ED} P(V)dV \approx P_{Max}SV, \quad (10)$$

where ED is end-diastole, ES is end-systole, P is left ventricular pressure, V is left ventricular volume, and SV is stroke volume. Note that two types of work must be considered. The integral from end-diastole to end-systole gives the work performed by the heart during ventricular ejection. Once the mitral valve opens, the vasculature performs work on the ventricle during ventricular filling. The integral of the pressure–volume plot under the end-diastolic pressure–volume relationship gives the work performed by the vasculature on the ventricle.

The Force Frequency Relationship

The effect of contraction frequency on myocardial force generation is known as the force frequency relationship, or as then staircase or treppe phenomenon.[62,63] Specifically, in isolated cat papillary muscle, developed force increases substantially when contraction is increased from 20 to 200 beats per minute.[64] The effect is thought to be secondary to an increase in intracellular Ca^{2+} concentration.

The force frequency relationship is operative in normal human hearts.[65] However, the effect of heart rate on E_{ES}[66] in patients with hypertrophic cardiomyopathy and on tension development in muscle strips from patients with dilated cardiomyopathy[65] is absent.

NON-STARLING REGULATION OF BLOOD PRESSURE AND CARDIAC OUTPUT

Extrinsic regulatory mechanisms of the cardiac output are mediated by the autonomic nervous system and include effects on heart rate and ventricular contractility. Efferent sympathetic fibers that originate in the upper thoracic and lower cervical segments of the spinal cord synapse with postganglionic fibers in the stellate and middle cervical ganglia. Postganglionic sympathetic fibers join parasympathetic fibers to form the cardiac plexus before they course to the heart. Preganglionic parasympathetic fibers course in the vagus nerves to synapse with postganglionic fibers from cells in the epicardium of the heart.[67] Sympathetic activity increases heart rate, and parasympathetic activity decreases heart rate. Parasympathetic activity usually predominates.

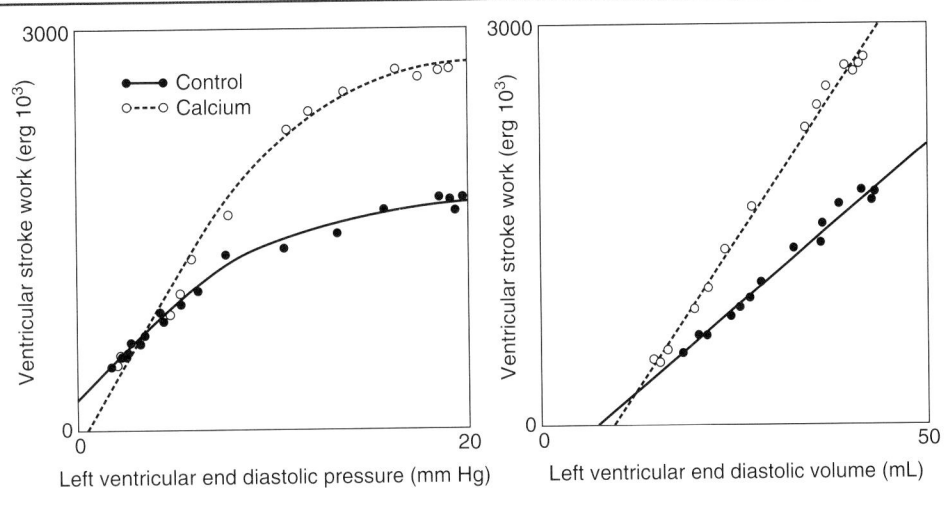

Figure 50–10
Effects of calcium infusion on stroke work versus end-diastolic pressure *(left)* and stroke work versus end-diastolic volume *(right)*. *(From Glower DD, Spratt JA, Snow ND, Kabas JS, Davis JW, Olsen CO, et al. Circulation 1985;**71**:944-1009.)*

Pressure and volume receptors provide input to two important heart rate regulatory mechanisms, the baroreceptor[68] and Bainbridge reflexes.[69] An increase in systemic blood pressure stimulates baroreceptors in the carotid sinus and aortic arch, which increases parasympathetic tone, causing the heart rate to decrease.[68] This is called the baroreceptor reflex. In contrast, an increase in circulating blood volume stimulates stretch receptors in the atria, increasing sympathetic tone and causing heart rate to increase (the Bainbridge reflex).[69] The resultant change in heart rate is the sum of the competing reflexes.

In addition, the autonomic nervous system alters atrial and ventricular contractility. Stimulation of cardiac sympathetic fibers have been shown to effectively double LV pressure and the rate of pressure change in the isolated dog heart.[70] In contrast to the effect on heart rate, the effect of sympathetic output on contractility is stronger than that of parasympathetic activity.

A variety of circulating hormones affect cardiac contractility. The best example is epinephrine, which is released from the adrenal medulla into the circulation as part of the body's fight-or-flight reaction to danger or other stress (see Fig. 50-9B). Other circulating hormones that increase contractility include thyroid hormone,[71] insulin,[72] and glucagon.[73]

MYOCARDIAL ENERGY EXPENDITURE AND EFFICIENCY

Determinants of Myocardial Energy Consumption

Because cardiac energy metabolism is aerobic, myocardial oxygen consumption (MVO_2) should be proportional to myocardial energy expenditure. A number of investigators have proposed models that explain the energy expenditure of the ventricle.[74-76] Braunwald, in pioneering work that began in the 1950s, found that wall tension[74] and contractility[75] were determinants of MVO_2. The tension time index concept of Braunwald has been expanded by Weber and others to become the integral of systolic stress.[77] It should be noted that the work of Braunwald in this area is the cornerstone of our treatment of myocardial ischemia with afterload reduction and reduction of heart rate with β-blockers.

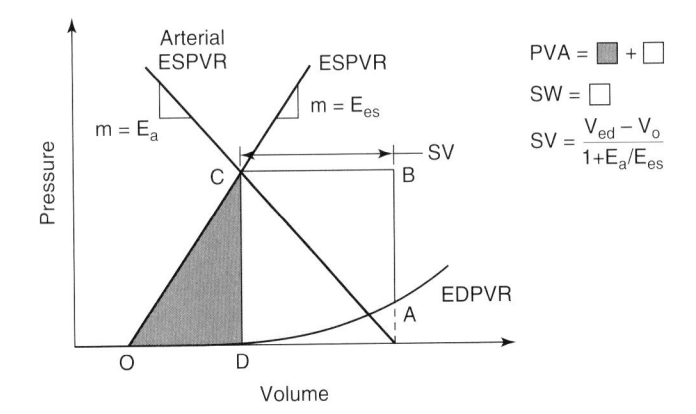

Figure 50–11
Model of myocardial energy expenditure based on pressure–volume analysis. *Gray triangle*, potential energy; ESPVR, end-systolic pressure–volume relationship; PVA, pressure–volume area; SV, stroke volume; SW, stroke work. A is the end of diastole; B, the start of ejection; C, the end of systole; and D, the end of isovolumic relaxation. Please see the section on Afterload and ventriculoarterial coupling for an explanation of the Arterial ESPVR, E_A. *(From Suga H. Am J Physiol 1979;**236**[3]: H498-505.)*

Suga and colleagues proposed a model of myocardial energy expenditure based on pressure–volume analysis.[78] They used an isolated heart preparation in which the left ventricle ejected against a variable afterload, to study the relationship between stroke work, potential energy, and myocardial oxygen consumption.[78] Interestingly, they found a very close relationship between ventricular energetics described by the pressure–volume analysis and the oxygen consumption. Specifically, they found that total oxygen consumption per beat was proportional to the sum of the potential energy (Fig. 50-11, triangle ODC) and stroke work (Fig. 50-11, pressure–volume loop ABCD).

$$PVA = [SW + PE]\alpha MVO_2, \qquad (11)$$

where PVA is the pressure–volume area, SW is the stroke work, PE is the potential energy, and MVO_2 is the myocardial oxygen consumption.[78]

The efficiency of ventricular function can be calculated by the ratio of external work divided by total energy consumed per beat. Total work is equal to the total energy consumed per beat. The total energy consumed per beat is equal to the sum of the external work and the potential energy per beat. The efficiency is therefore the work of the pump divided by the total oxygen consumed per beat, or

$$\text{efficiency} = SW/MV_{O_2} \quad (12)$$

All changes in SW/MV_{O_2} (efficiency) can be accounted for by the relative changes in E_{ES} and E_A in the LV pressure–volume diagram.[79]

AFTERLOAD AND VENTRICULOARTERIAL COUPLING

Optimal vascular function is essential to optimal ventricular performance. Impedance is the opposition of a system to a driving function. Maximal energy transfer of a system is achieved when the output impedance of the source equals the input impedance of the load.

The impedance of the heart can be described by the pressure–volume relationship. The end-systolic pressure–volume relationship describes the output impedance of the heart. Sunagawa and colleagues developed a formula that gives the SV for a given preload as a function of systolic ventricular properties (ESPVR$_i$, E_{ES}, V_{0},) and the arterial elastance (E_A).[80] The model included the vascular system as a modified Windkessel element, and E_A is a lumped parameter characterization of the impedance of the Windkessel element.[81] The equation is as follows:

$$SV = \frac{V_{ED} - V_0}{1 + \frac{E_A}{E_{ES}}}, \quad (13)$$

where SV is stroke volume, V is LV volume, ED is end-diastole, V_0 and E_{ES} are the intercept and slope of the ESPVR relationship, and E_A is the arterial elastance. Please see Figure 50-11 for a graphic representation of E_A.

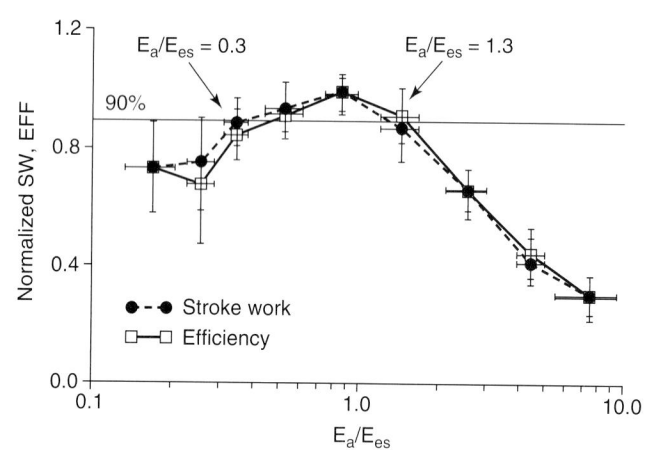

Figure 50–12
Average normalized stroke work (SW) and SW per myocardial oxygen consumption (MVo$_2$) as a function of the curve from graphing arterial elastance (E_a) against the slope of the end-systolic pressure–volume relationship (E_{es}). EFF, efficiency. (From De Tombe PP, Jones S, Burkhoff D, Hunter WC, Kass DA. Am J Physiol 1993;**264**[6 Pt 2]:H1817-24.)

Burkoff and Sagawa extended the SV/E_A relationship (Equation 13)[80] to include SW, MV$_{O_2}$, and ventricular efficiency.[81] That model predicted that SW would be maximal when E_A = E_{ES} (E_A/E_{ES} = 1).[81] The afterload that results in the greatest efficiency is always less than that which provides the maximum SW.[81] Because of concern that the optimal E_A/E_{ES} for stroke volume and efficiency occurred at different points, De Tombe and colleagues measured stroke work in isolated hearts and found that maximal stroke work occurred at E_A/E_{ES} = 0.80, but that efficiency was maximal at E_A/E_{ES} = 0.70 (Fig. 50-12). However, there was a significant range of E_A/E_{ES} values where both stoke work and efficiency were greater than 90% of their maximum values.[82] Thus, impedance matching between the LV and the arterial system does seem to be important.

E_A/E_{ES} has subsequently been measured in patients with dilated cardiomyopathy. E_A/E_{ES} was 3.24 but was decreased to 1.86 when the patients were given dobutamine, and to 1.78 with afterload reduction.[83] This study shows that impedance matching in the hypertrophied and failing heart is far from optimal, and it lays the groundwork for afterload reduction therapy.

REGIONAL STRAIN

Regional measures of cardiac function can also be obtained from imaging. Projection imaging gives information only about the motion of the portion of the wall at the edge of the heart in the particular projection used to make the image. Tomographic imaging provides wall motion information all around the heart, although it is less reliable where the plane of the image intersects the wall obliquely (e.g., near the apex or base of the heart in short-axis imaging). Although imaging of the ventricular cavity provides information only about the motion of the endocardial surface of the wall, tomographic imaging provides images of both endocardial and epicardial surfaces, permitting measurement of wall thickening. A limitation of both approaches involves the uncertainty of how to account for the contribution of the motion of the heart as a whole to the local wall motion. The motion in the imaging plane may be approximately compensated for by subtracting the motion of the centroid of the ventricle. However, the through-plane motion of the curved heart wall can still lead to apparent changes in wall motion or thickening that are just reflections of the changing location of the intersection of the heart with the spatially fixed imaging plane.

The lack of recognizable features that can be tracked within the heart wall means that conventional imaging is limited to assessing the radial component of the heart wall motion, only at the surfaces of the wall. Using invasive techniques, we can imbed material markers in the wall, such as small metal beads or ultrasound crystals, whose position can be tracked as the heart moves.[23,84,85] However, in addition to the invasive nature of these procedures, which pose some risk and can alter the local motion of the wall, only a limited number of such markers can be tracked in the heart of a given subject, limiting the sampling density of tracked points in the wall.

Tissue Doppler

Echocardiography can provide some information on intramural motion through the use of the Doppler effect to track the velocity (or the component of velocity along the line of the ultrasound beam) of the tissue of the wall. The gradient of the velocity gives the rate of tissue deformation, or a one-dimensional component of the strain rate, along the ultrasound beam. It would be necessary to integrate this over time to estimate the total deformation over the cardiac cycle. In addition to the limited spatial component information available from the Doppler effect, there is still the uncertainty of how to account for the through-plane motion.

Magnetic Resonance Imaging

MRI has several advantages as a method for noninvasive assessment of within-wall cardiac motion, including the potential to recover the full 3D motion pattern in the heart wall. Two approaches have been used to study intramural motion with MRI—magnetization tagging and phase shifts. Magnetization tagging uses the ability of modified MRI techniques to noninvasively create localized perturbations of the tissue magnetization (e.g., with spatial modulation of magnetization [SPAMM])[86-88] to noninvasively produce MR-visible landmarks in the heart wall. These persist for times on the order of tissue T1 relaxation times, so they can be tracked over the cardiac cycle; we can then produce a new set of such tags at a consistent phase of each cardiac cycle. The tags provide a direct marker for the displacement of the underlying tissue in the image plane, as they move exactly the same way. For tags created as sheets of altered magnetization initially perpendicular to the image plane, the intersection of these sheets with the image plane appear as dark lines in the images of the heart wall; motion of these lines shows the local one-dimensional component of the motion perpendicular to the originally tagged plane, even in the presence of through-plane motion. Phase-shift approaches to studying the intramural motion use the phase shift of the received signal that can be produced by motion along modified magnetic field gradients used in MRI. The phase shift is typically dependent on the motion between two times, effectively giving a measure of the velocity if those times are close together, or a measure of the interval displacement if they are farther apart. In using the velocity mode, the results must be integrated to find the net displacement, whereas in the interval displacement mode, the results for different intervals must still be combined to find the full motion over the cardiac cycle. In either case, additional reference images must also be obtained to correct for other possible (nonmotion) sources of phase shifts.

From a suitable set of data on the regional motion in the heart wall, derived from either multiplanar tagged MRI or phase-shift MRI sensitized to motion in multiple directions, full 3D motion of the heart wall can be reconstructed. This generally requires some sort of interpolation to fill in the gaps in the image-derived data because of the finite density of spatial sampling of the motion in the images. Finite-element methods are one way to carry out this 3D motion reconstruction.

Given 2D or 3D data on the motion of (and in) the heart wall, there are several ways to quantitatively characterize the motion. The material-point correspondence data provided by tagged MRI permit us to map the serial displacements of each point in the wall; this can be considered as a set of vectors over time, linking corresponding locations of each material point (a Lagrangian representation of the motion). The velocity data provided by phase-shift MRI could be used to follow the serial evolution of velocity vectors at each spatial location in the images (a Eulerian representation of the motion). The velocities must be integrated over time to recover the displacements, a process that is subject to cumulative error because of the integration of noise or other errors in the measurements.[89-91]

Although the displacement and velocity are useful to describe the motion of material points, we are also interested in characterizing the motion of the material neighborhood around each such point. In addition to the "rigid body" components of the motion, its deformation (or strain) can be characterized. Strain is defined as the fractional change in length, caused by the motion, of a material line segment initially oriented along a given direction in the tissue:

$$\varepsilon = \frac{l - l_0}{l_0}, \qquad (14)$$

where ε is the strain, l is the deformed length, and l_0 is the initial length.

However, strain is a more complex quantity than the displacement and cannot be adequately described by a vector but rather must be described with a tensor of rank two. For example, at a given location in the wall, the tissue may be lengthening in the radial direction while at the same time it is shortening in the circumferential and longitudinal directions. The local radial, circumferential, and longitudinal strains provide a useful and intuitive way to characterize the deformation. Another potential choice of strains would be along and perpendicular to the local muscle fiber orientation in the wall. In general, for a given set of initial orientations of material line segments in the tissue, the angle between the segments will also change because of the motion (i.e., shear); the shears between the pairs of initial directions are also needed to fully characterize the deformation. For example, the shear between the longitudinal and circumferential directions is a measure of the local torsion of the heart wall around the long axis of the ventricle. However, there will always be a set of three mutually orthogonal initial directions in the tissue at each location that will remain as such after motion—the eigenvectors, or principal directions of the deformation. One of these directions will lie along the direction of the greatest lengthening and another will lie along the direction of greatest shortening; the strains along these directions of the eigenvectors are called the principal strains. The principal strains and their directions provide a description of the deformation that is independent of the choice of reference frame.

REGIONAL STRESS AND THE FINITE-ELEMENT METHOD

The distributions of stress in the ventricles of the heart are determined by (1) the 3D geometry and tissue structure of the ventricular walls, (2) the boundary conditions imposed by the ventricular cavity and pericardial pressures and structures, such as the fibrous valve ring skeleton at the base of the ventricles, and (3) the 3D mechanical properties of the myofibers and their collagen interconnections in the relaxed and actively contracting states. Formulating a mathematical model for predicting the distributions of wall stress in such a complex and constantly changing mechanical system is clearly very difficult, but there are important reasons to attempt this. An accurate model of the mechanics of the ventricular myocardium would provide a sound basis for interpreting the complex regional changes in cardiac function that occur in pathologic conditions such as ischemic heart disease,[92,93] in terms of changes in the local properties of the tissue. Knowledge of the stress distributions in the intact myocardium would also provide valuable insight into normal ventricular function, because regional coronary blood flow,[94] myocardial oxygen consumption,[74] hypertrophy, and remodeling[95,96] are all influenced by ventricular wall stress.[97]

To keep the problem mathematically tractable, many workers have developed models of left ventricular mechanics using simple geometric approximations, such as thin-walled spheres,[98] thin-walled ellipsoids,[99-103] thick-walled ellipsoids,[99-102,104,105] thick-walled spheres,[106-111] thick-walled cylinders,[94,112-119] solids of revolution,[120] and noncircular cylinders.[121] However, the analyses made by these models also make other simplifying assumptions about the material behavior of the heart muscle and the governing equations of motion.

The most common thin walled model is the law of LaPlace:

$$P = T_1/r_1 + T_2/r_2, \quad (15)$$

where P is intracavitary pressure, r_1 and r_2 are the greatest and least (principal) radii of curvature of the membrane, and T_1 and T_2 are the tensions in the membrane along the corresponding directions.[122] Notably, the LaPlace stress law assumes a thin-walled sphere (i.e., the ratio of wall thickness to radius is small). Hence, tension is calculated, not stress. Even with this assumption, predicted stress is thought to be accurate.[123]

More sophisticated formulas try to take the finite thickness of the wall explicitly into account. One of the most common is the following equation developed by Janz:

$$\bar{\sigma}_{\theta\alpha} = P \frac{\Delta A_C}{\Delta A_W}, \quad (16)$$

where $\bar{\sigma}_{\theta\alpha}$ is average circumferential stress, A_C is the area of the cavity, and A_W is the area of the wall (Fig. 50-13).[120]

Such approximations generally neglect the anisotropy of the material properties of the heart wall. In addition, they generally neglect the presence of significant residual stresses in the wall, even in the absence of pressure differences (the unloaded state), as manifested experimentally by the springing open of an incision into the heart wall even in the absence of contraction or pressurized blood in the chamber.[120,124]

Stress in the ventricular wall cannot be measured.[125] As a consequence, the stresses predicted by models of ventricular mechanics cannot be directly verified. Nevertheless, experimental measurements of myocardial strains have been used for model validation. Arts and coworkers[114] compared the deformations predicted by their cylindrical model of the ejecting left ventricle with systolic strains. These were measured on the epicardium of open-chest canines using a triangular arrangement of inductance gauges. Guccione and associates[126] used experimental measurements of myocardial strains to validate a thick-walled cylindrical model of the passive left ventricle that employed finite deformation theory and a 3D constitutive equation referring to a system of fiber coordinates. By optimizing material parameters, the model was able to reproduce the circumferential, longitudinal, and torsional

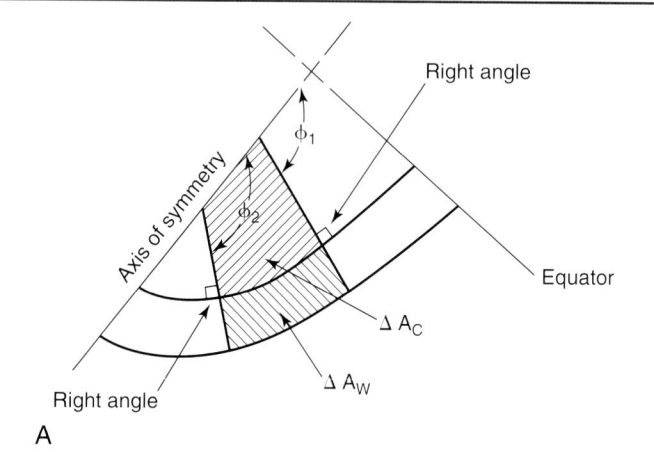

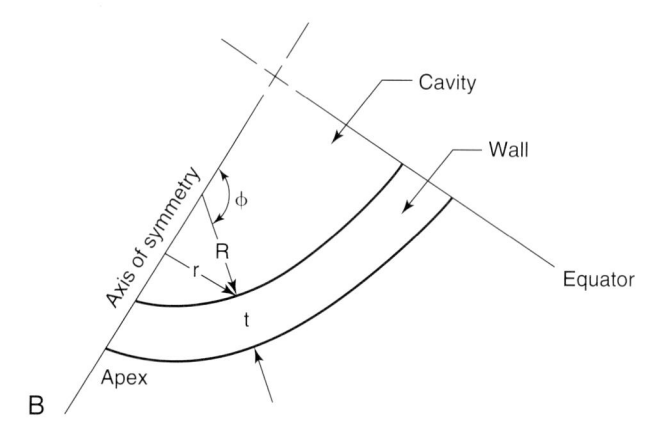

Figure 50-13
Estimation of local myocardial stress using geometric approximations. R, the meridional radius of curvature at the cavity surface; r, circumferential radius of curvature at the cavity surface; t, wall thickness. (From Janz RF. Am J Physiol 1982;**242**[5]:H875-81.)

epicardial strains that had been measured in the isolated arrested dog heart. However, cylindrical models are probably confined, at best, to describing the mechanics of a narrow equatorial cross-section of the left ventricular wall. Such simple models are not suitable for analyzing the nonhomogeneous effects of 3D variations in the geometry, fiber orientations, and mechanical properties of the heart.

As early as 1906, researchers first began suggesting the solution of continuum mechanics problems by modeling the body with a lattice of elastic bars and employing frame analysis methods (see Cook[127]). In 1941, Courant recognized piecewise polynomial interpolation over triangular subregions as a Rayleigh-Ritz solution of a variational problem. Because there were no computers at the time, neither approach was practical, and Courant's work was largely forgotten until a new generation of engineers independently developed it. By 1953, structural engineers were solving matrix stiffness equations with digital computers. The widespread use of finite-element methods in engineering began with the classic papers by Turner and colleagues[128] and Argyris and Kelsey.[129] The term *finite element* was coined in 1960, and the method began to be recognized as mathematically rigorous by 1963.

Many finite-element models of ventricular mechanics have been proposed, although most do not include the nonlinear kinematic terms associated with large deformations, because an iterative solution of the nonlinear governing equations at each

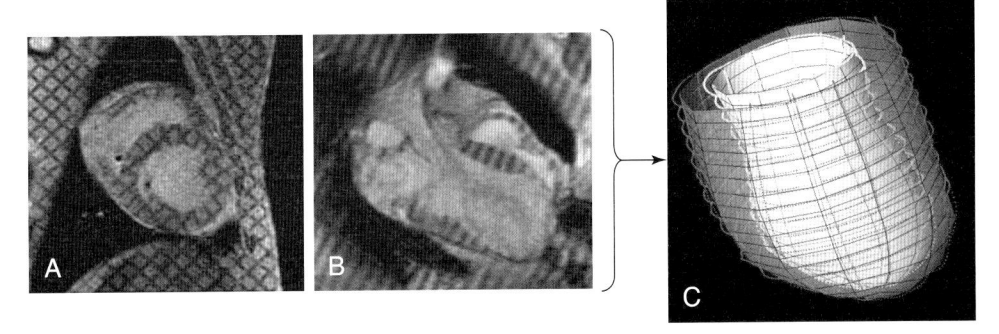

Figure 50–14
Finite-element model from in vivo magnetic resonance image. Endocardial and epicardial contours from both short (A) and long-axis views (B) are used to create the 3D finite element model geometry (C). Tag-deformation (A and B) is used to validate myocardial strain predictions from the finite element model. *(From Janz RF. Am J Physiol 1982;**242**[5]:H875-81.)*

load step is required. The importance of adopting nonlinear finite deformation theory for the analysis was demonstrated by Janz and colleagues.[130] A few finite-element modeling studies of the left ventricle have validated stress calculations by showing good agreement with myocardial strain measured with implanted markers.[124,131-133] However, this is invasive and is limited to few simultaneous LV locations (usually only two). With advancements in MRI, myocardial strain can be quantified noninvasively throughout the left ventricle with tagged MRI.[134,135] In a pioneering study, Moulton and coworkers[136] used tagged MRI to determine isotropic, diastolic material properties in a 2D finite-element analysis of beating canine hearts. Using a more realistic material law, Okamoto and associates[137] determined anisotropic myocardial material properties in a 3D finite-element model using tagged MRI. However, the experimental preparation and loading conditions were not physiologic and therefore did not create significant transverse shear strain. Since then, Guccione and colleagues[138] have successfully modeled end-isovolumic systole in an ovine model of myocardial infarction and determined material parameters that reproduced circumferential stretching (as measured with 2D tagged MRI) in the infarcted border zone. This finite-element study successfully revealed that the mechanism of circumferential stretching in the infarct border zone during isovolumic systole is related to impaired contractile function in that region.

Our state-of-the-art finite-element model is built on the laws of large deformation continuum mechanics and has been described previously.[138,139] In short, the passive myocardium is modeled by a strain energy function, W, that is anisotropic relative to the local fiber direction:

$$W = 0.5C(e^Q - 1), \quad (17)$$

where

$$Q = [b_f E_{11}^2 + b_t(E_{22}^2 + E_{33}^2 + E_{23}^2 + E_{32}^2) + b_{fs}(E_{12}^2 + E_{21}^2 + E_{13}^2 + E_{31}^2)], \quad (18)$$

where E_{11} is fiber strain, E_{22} is cross-fiber in-plane strain, E_{33} is radial strain, E_{23} is shear in the transverse plane, and E_{12} and E_{13} are shear strain in the fiber–cross-fiber and fiber–radial coordinate planes, respectively, and where $C = 0.88$ kPa, $b_f = 18.48$, $b_t = 3.58$, and $b_{fs} = 1.627$.[140]

Active contraction is simulated by adding stress in the muscle fiber direction defined by a time-varying elastance model.[138] For end-systole, this reduces to the following equation:

$$T_0 = T_{max} \frac{Ca_0^2}{Ca_0^2 + ECa_{50}^2} C_t, \quad (19)$$

where T_{max} is the maximum isometric tension achieved at the longest sarcomere length and maximum peak intracellular calcium concentration $(Ca_0)_{max}$:

$$C_t = \frac{1}{2}[1 - \cos(\omega)], \omega = \Pi \frac{0.25 + t_r}{t_r}, \ t_r = ml + b, \quad (20)$$

where m and b are constants. Length-dependent calcium sensitivity is given by

$$ECa_{50}^2 = \frac{(Ca_0)_{max}^2}{\exp[B(l-l_0)]-1}, \text{ and } l = l_R\sqrt{2E_{11}^2 + 1} \quad (21)$$

where B is a constant, l_0 is the sarcomere length at which no active tension develops, and l_R is the stress-free sarcomere length. Active material parameters were set to the following values as previously described[138]: $T_{max} = 135.7$ kPa, $Ca_0 = 4.35$ µmol/L, $(Ca_0)_{max} = 4.35$ µmol/L, $m = 1.0489$ sec/µm, $b = -1.429$ sec, $B = 4.75$ µm^{-1}, and $l_0 = 1.58$ µm; l_R is assumed to vary linearly from 1.78 µm at the endocardium to 1.91 µm at the epicardium, in accordance with experimental observations of Rodriguez and coworkers.[141]

Finite-element modeling can be used to calculate myocardial stress and contractility. For example, we used tagged MRI to validate finite-element models of LV aneurysm.[142] Five sheep underwent anteroapical myocardial infarction (25% of LV mass) and 22 weeks later underwent tagged MRI. Figure 50-14 shows a representative finite-element model of the left ventricle that was formed using in vivo geometry from MRI, LV pressure measurements, and myofiber helix angles measured with diffusion tensor MRI. Systolic material parameters were determined that enabled finite-element models to reproduce midwall, systolic myocardial strains from tagged MRI (630 ± 187 strain comparisons per animal).[142] Figure 50-15 shows the calculated systolic stress. In the infarct border zone, end-systolic midwall stress was elevated in both fiber (24.2 ± 2.7 to 29.9 ± 2.4 kPa; $P < .01$) and cross-fiber (5.5 ± -0.7 to 11.7 ± 1.3 kPa; $P = .02$) directions relative to noninfarct regions. Stress calculations from these validated models

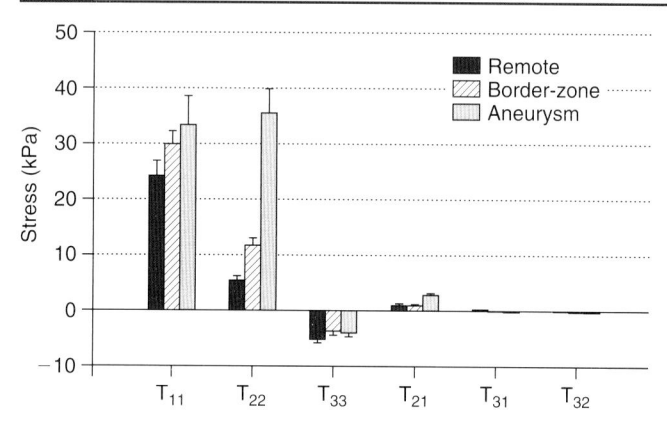

Figure 50-15
End-systolic midwall fiber (T11), cross fiber (T22), radial (T33), and shear stresses (T21, T31, and T32) at normalized afterload. Aneurysm is the infarct proper, borderzone is the infarct borderzone, and remote is the area remote from the infarct. (From Walker JC, Ratcliffe MB, Zhang P, Wallace AW, Hsu EW, Saloner DA, et al.[142])

show a 24% increase in fiber stress and a 115% increase in cross-fiber stress in the borderzone relative to remote regions, which may contribute to LV remodeling.[142]

VENTRICULAR INTERACTION AND PERICARDIUM

Ventricular Interaction

The right ventricle can affect or interact with the performance of the left ventricle, and vice versa.[143,144] Interaction occurs in two ways. First, the ventricles are connected in series, and a change in output of one affects the other (series interaction). In addition, direct ventricular interaction occurs because the right and left ventricles are mechanically connected through the interventricular septum. Determining the relative effects of series and direct interaction can be difficult. Slinker and Glantz used a statistical approach,[145] Baker and coworkers used right heart bypass,[146] and Slater and colleagues[147] used an isolated heart preparation to determine the relative contribution of series and direct ventricular interaction.

Ventricular interaction analysis is divided into diastolic interaction[145] and systolic interaction.[147-149] With an intact pericardium, Slinker and Glantz determined that direct ventricular interaction is half as important as a series interaction at end-diastole.[145] Concentric hypertrophy, presumably because the septum is thicker, further reduces the effect of direct diastolic interaction.[150]

Ventricular interaction during systole has been measured by causing abrupt changes in right or left ventricular load and measuring the performance of the other ventricle. The ratio of pressure change or gain is usually reported. Typical right-to-left gain is 10%.[149] Typical left-to-right gain is 4%.[149] Systolic interaction is increased substantially in dilated cardiomyopathy with a right-to-left gain of 22% in isolated perfused heart excised at heart transplantation.[147]

Pericardium

The heart is invested by the pericardium. This is a double-layered fibrous sac that is flexible but not stretchy. The inner (visceral) layer is effectively part of the epicardial aspect of the heart, whereas the outer (parietal) layer fits closely around the heart with a potential space between. Normally, the layers are separated only by a thin film of fluid, which acts as a lubricant so that the two surfaces can slide freely. The pericardium is, in turn, surrounded by the intrathoracic cavity, which is normally at subatmospheric pressure, which may help with venous return to the right side of the heart. In terms of the effect of myocardial ischemia on diastolic dysfunction,[39] the pericardium plays an important role in mediating the mechanical effect between ventricles and between atria and ventricles.[151]

Acknowledgement

We acknowledge the use of content written by the previous author, Leon Axel.

REFERENCES

1. Streeter DD Jr, Hanna WT. Engineering mechanics for successive states in canine left ventricular myocardium. II. Fiber angle and sarcomere length. *Circ Res* 1973;**33**(6):656-64.
2. Pettigrew J. On the arrangement of the muscular fibres in the ventricles of the vertebrate heart, with physiological remarks. *Phil Trans* 1864;**154**:445-500.
3. Kocica MJ, Corno AF, Carreras-Costa F, Ballester-Rodes M, Moghbel MC, Cueva CN, et al. The helical ventricular myocardial band: global, three-dimensional, functional architecture of the ventricular myocardium. *Eur J Cardiothorac Surg* 2006;**29**(Suppl. 1):S21-40.
4. Legrice IJ, Hunter PJ, Smaill BH. Laminar structure of the heart: a mathematical model. *Am J Physiol* 1997;**272**(5 Pt 2):H2466-76.
5. Borg TK, Caulfield JB. The collagen matrix of the heart. *Fed Proc* 1981;**40**(7):2037-41.
6. Robinson TF, Cohen-Gould L, Factor SM, Eghbali M, Blumenfeld OO. Structure and function of connective tissue in cardiac muscle: collagen types I and III in endomysial struts and pericellular fibers. *Scanning Microsc* 1988;**2**(2):1005-15.
7. Robinson TF, Geraci MA, Sonnenblick EH, Factor SM. Coiled perimysial fibers of papillary muscle in rat heart: morphology, distribution, and changes in configuration. *Circ Res* 1988;**63**(3):577-92.
8. Frank O. Zur dynamik des herzmuskels. *Z Biol* 1895;**32**:370-447.
9. Dodge HT, Sandler H, Ballew DW, Lord Jr JD. The use of biplane angiocardigraphy for the measurement of left ventricular volume in man. *Am Heart J* 1960;**60**:762-76.
10. Fortuin NJ, Pawsey CG. The evaluation of left ventricular function by echocardiography. *Am J Med* 1977;**63**:1-9.
11. Burkhoff D, Mirsky I, Suga H. Assessment of systolic and diastolic ventricular properties via pressure-volume analysis: a guide for clinical, translational, and basic researchers. *Am J Physiol Heart Circ Physiol* 2005;**289**(2):H501-12.
12. Feigenbaum H, Armstrong WF, Ryan T. *Echocardiography*. Philadelphia: Lippincott Williams & Wilkins; 2004.
13. Dilsizian V, Pohost GM, editors. Cardiac CT, PET and MR. Malden MA: Wiley-Blackwell; 2006.
14. Baan J, Van der Velde E, De Bruin H, Smeenk G, Koops J, Van Dijk A, et al. Continuous measurement of left ventricular volume in animals and humans by conductance catheter. *Circulation* 1984;**70**:812-23.
15. Slinker BK, Glantz SA. Multiple regression for physiological data analysis: the problem of multicollinearity. *Am J Physiol* 1985;**249**(1 Pt 2):R1-12.
16. Slinker BK, Glantz SA. Multiple linear regression is a useful alternative to traditional analyses of variance. *Am J Physiol* 1988;**255**(3 Pt 2):R353-67.
17. Granzier H, Wu Y, Siegfried L, LeWinter M. Titin: physiological function and role in cardiomyopathy and failure. *Heart Fail Rev* 2005;**10**(3):211-23.
18. Helmes M, Trombitas K, Granzier H. Titin develops restoring force in rat cardiac myocytes. *Circ Res* 1996;**79**(3):619-26.
19. Hinken AC, Solaro RJ. A dominant role of cardiac molecular motors in the intrinsic regulation of ventricular ejection and relaxation. *Physiology (Bethesda)* 2007;**22**:73-80.
20. Jaber WA, Lam CS, Meyer DM, Redfield MM. Revisiting methods for assessing and comparing left ventricular diastolic stiffness: impact of relaxation, external forces, hypertrophy, and comparators. *Am J Physiol Heart Circ Physiol* 2007;**293**(5):H2738-46.

21. Weiss JL, Frederiksen JW, Weisfeldt ML. Hemodynamic determinants of the time-course of fall in canine left ventricular pressure. *J Clin Invest* 1976;**58**(3):751-60.
22. Buchalter MB, Rademakers FE, Weiss JL, Rogers WJ, Weisfeldt ML, Shapiro EP. Rotational deformation of the canine left ventricle measured by magnetic resonance tagging: effects of catecholamines, ischaemia, and pacing. *Cardiovasc Res* 1994;**28**(5):629-35.
23. Waldman LK, Nosan D, Villarreal F, Covell JW. Relation between transmural deformation and local myofiber direction in canine left ventricle. *Circ Res* 1988;**63**(3):550-62.
24. Notomi Y, Martin-Miklovic MG, Oryszak SJ, Shiota T, Deserranno D, Popovic ZB, et al. Enhanced ventricular untwisting during exercise: a mechanistic manifestation of elastic recoil described by Doppler tissue imaging. *Circulation* 2006;**113**(21):2524-33.
25. Courtois M, Kovacs SJ, Ludbrook PA. Physiological early diastolic intraventricular pressure gradient is lost during acute myocardial ischemia. *Circulation* 1990;**81**(5):1688-96.
26. Little WC. Diastolic dysfunction beyond distensibility: adverse effects of ventricular dilatation. *Circulation* 2005;**112**(19):2888-90.
27. Notomi Y, Popovic ZB, Yamada H, Wallick DW, Martin MG, Oryszak SJ, et al. Ventricular untwisting: a temporal link between left ventricular relaxation and suction. *Am J Physiol Heart Circ Physiol* 2008;**294**(1):H505-13.
28. Dong SJ, Hees PS, Siu CO, Weiss JL, Shapiro EP. MRI assessment of LV relaxation by untwisting rate: a new isovolumic phase measure of tau. *Am J Physiol Heart Circ Physiol* 2001;**281**(5):H2002-9.
29. Meisner JS, Nikolic S, Tamura T, Tamura K, Frater RW, Yellin EL. Development and use of a remote-controlled mitral valve. *Ann Biomed Eng* 1986;**14**(4):339-49.
30. Yellin EL, Hori M, Yoran C, Sonnenblick EH, Gabbay S, Frater RW. Left ventricular relaxation in the filling and nonfilling intact canine heart. *Am J Physiol* 1986;**250**(4 Pt 2):H620-9.
31. Gilbert JC, Glantz SA. Determinants of left ventricular filling and of the diastolic pressure-volume relation. *Circ Res* 1989;**64**(5):827-52.
32. Nishimura RA, Tajik AJ. Evaluation of diastolic filling of left ventricle in health and disease: Doppler echocardiography is the clinician's Rosetta Stone. *J Am Coll Cardiol* 1997;**30**(1):8-18.
33. Wiegers S, Plappert T, St John Sutton M. Role of echocardiography in the diagnosis and treatment of cardiomyopathies. In: *Heart failure: scientific principles and clinical practice*. Poole-Wilson P, editor. New York: Churchill Livingstone; 1997. p. 461-87.
34. Pinamonti B, Di Lenarda A, Sinagra G, Camerini F. Restrictive left ventricular filling pattern in dilated cardiomyopathy assessed by Doppler echocardiography: clinical, echocardiographic and hemodynamic correlations and prognostic implications. Heart Muscle Disease Study Group. *J Am Coll Cardiol* 1993;**22**(3):808-15.
35. Vanoverschelde JL, Raphael DA, Robert AR, Cosyns JR. Left ventricular filling in dilated cardiomyopathy: relation to functional class and hemodynamics. *J Am Coll Cardiol* 1990;**15**(6):1288-95.
36. Bryg RJ, Williams GA, Labovitz AJ. Effect of aging on left ventricular diastolic filling in normal subjects. *Am J Cardiol* 1987;**59**(9):971-4.
37. Toma Y, Matsuda Y, Moritani K, Ogawa H, Matsuzaki M, Kusukawa R. Left atrial filling in normal human subjects: relation between left atrial contraction and left atrial early filling. *Cardiovasc Res* 1987;**21**(4):255-9.
38. Bertrand ME, Lablanche JM, Fourrier JL, Traisnel G, Mirsky I. Left ventricular systolic and diastolic function during acute coronary artery balloon occlusion in humans. *J Am Coll Cardiol* 1988;**12**(2):341-7.
39. Kass DA, Midei M, Brinker J, Maughan WL. Influence of coronary occlusion during PTCA on end-systolic and end-diastolic pressure-volume relations in humans. *Circulation* 1990;**81**(2):447-60.
40. Yotti R, Bermejo J, Antoranz JC, Desco MM, Cortina C, Rojo-Alvarez JL, et al. A noninvasive method for assessing impaired diastolic suction in patients with dilated cardiomyopathy. *Circulation* 2005;**112**(19):2921-9.
41. Grossman W, Jones D, McLaurin LP. Wall stress and patterns of hypertrophy in the human left ventricle. *J Clin Invest* 1975;**56**(1):56-64.
42. Kass DA, Wolff MR, Ting CT, Liu CP, Chang MS, Lawrence W, et al. Diastolic compliance of hypertrophied ventricle is not acutely altered by pharmacologic agents influencing active processes. *Ann Intern Med* 1993;**119**(6):466-73.
43. Hess OM, Villari B, Krayenbuehl HP. Diastolic dysfunction in aortic stenosis. *Circulation* 1993;**87**(Suppl. 5):IV73-6.
44. Ganz W, Swan HJ. Measurement of blood flow by thermodilution. *Am J Cardiol* 1972;**29**(2):241-6.
45. Lehmann KG, Platt MS. Improved accuracy and precision of thermodilution cardiac output measurement using a dual thermistor catheter system. *J Am Coll Cardiol* 1999;**33**(3):883-91.
46. Sandham JD, Hull RD, Brant RF, Knox L, Pineo GF, Doig CJ, et al. A randomized, controlled trial of the use of pulmonary-artery catheters in high-risk surgical patients. *N Engl J Med* 2003;**348**(1):5-14.
47. Bossert T, Gummert JF, Bittner HB, Barten M, Walther T, Falk V, et al. Swan-Ganz catheter-induced severe complications in cardiac surgery: right ventricular perforation, knotting, and rupture of a pulmonary artery. *J Card Surg* 2006;**21**(3):292-5.
48. Shah MR, Hasselblad V, Stevenson LW, Binanay C, O'Connor CM, Sopko G, et al. Impact of the pulmonary artery catheter in critically ill patients: meta-analysis of randomized clinical trials. *JAMA* 2005;**294**(13):1664-70.
49. Dickstein M, Spotnitz H, Rose E, Burkhoff D. Heart reduction surgery: an analysis of the impact on cardiac function. *J Thorac Cardiovasc Surg* 1997;**113**:1032-40.
50. Wall ST, Walker JC, Healy KE, Ratcliffe MB, Guccione JM. Theoretical impact of the injection of material into the myocardium: a finite element model simulation. *Circulation* 2006;**114**(24):2627-35.
51. Grossman W, Braunwald E, Mann T, McLaurin LP, Green LH. Contractile state of the left ventricle in man as evaluated from end-systolic pressure-volume relations. *Circulation* 1977;**56**(5):845-52.
52. Monroe RG, French GN. Left ventricular pressure-volume relationships and myocardial oxygen consumption in the isolated heart. *Circ Res* 1961;**9**:362-74.
53. Sagawa K. The ventricular pressure-volume diagram revisited. *Circ Res* 1978;**43**(5):677-87.
54. Suga H, Sagawa K. Instantaneous pressure-volume relationships and their ratio in the excised, supported canine left ventricle. *Circ Res* 1974;**35**(1):117-26.
55. Suga H, Sagawa K, Kostiuk DP. Controls of ventricular contractility assessed by pressure-volume ratio, Emax. *Cardiovasc Res* 1976;**10**(5):582-92.
56. Suga H, Sagawa K, Shoukas AA. Load independence of the instantaneous pressure-volume ratio of the canine left ventricle and effects of epinephrine and heart rate on the ratio. *Circ Res* 1973;**32**(3):314-22.
57. Kass DA. Clinical ventricular pathophysiology: a pressure volume view. In: Warltier DC, editor. *Ventricular function (A Society of Cardiovascular Anesthesiologists monograph)*. Baltimore: Williams and Wilkins; 1996.
58. Patterson S, Piper H, Starling E. The regulation of the heart beat. *J Physiol (London)* 1914;**48**:465-513.
59. Patterson S, Starling E. On the mechanical factors which determine the output from the ventricles. *J Physiol (London)* 1914;**48**:357-79.
60. Glower DD, Spratt JA, Snow ND, Kabas JS, Davis JW, Olsen CO, et al. Linearity of the Frank-Starling relationship in the intact heart: the concept of preload recruitable stroke work. *Circulation* 1985;**71**:944-1009.
61. Ratcliffe MB, Hong J, Salahieh A, Ruch S, Wallace AW. The effect of ventricular volume reduction surgery in the dilated, poorly contractile left ventricle: a simple finite element analysis. *J Thorac Cardiovasc Surg* 1998;**116**(4):566-77.
62. Dale AS. The staircase phenomenon in ventricular muscle. *J Physiol* 1932;**75**(1):1-6.
63. Palomeque J, Vila Petroff MG, Mattiazzi A. Pacing staircase phenomenon in the heart: from Bodwitch to the XXI century. *Heart Lung Circ* 2004;**13**(4):410-20.
64. Koch-Weser J, Blinks JR. The influence of the interval between beats on myocardial contractility. *Pharmacol Rev* 1963;**15**:601-52.
65. Mulieri LA, Leavitt BJ, Hasenfuss G, Allen PD, Alpert NR. Contraction frequency dependence of twitch and diastolic tension in human dilated cardiomyopathy (tension-frequency relation in cardiomyopathy). *Basic Res Cardiol* 1992;**87**(Suppl. 1):199-212.
66. Liu CP, Ting CT, Lawrence W, Maughan WL, Chang MS, Kass DA. Diminished contractile response to increased heart rate in intact human left ventricular hypertrophy: systolic versus diastolic determinants. *Circulation* 1993;**88**(4 Pt 1):1893-906.
67. Grimm DR. Neurally mediated syncope: a review of cardiac and arterial receptors. *J Clin Neurophysiol* 1997;**14**(2):170-82.
68. Daly I, Verney E. The localization of receptors involved in the reflex regulation of the heart rate. *J Physiol* 1927;**62**:330-40.
69. Bainbridge F. The influence of venous filling upon the rate of the heart. *J Physiol* 1915;**50**:65-84.
70. Levy MN, Ng ML, Zieske H. Cardiac and respiratory effects of aortic arch baroreceptor stimulation. *Circ Res* 1966;**19**(5):930-9.
71. Muller A, Zuidwijk MJ, Simonides WS, van Hardeveld C. Modulation of SERCA2 expression by thyroid hormone and norepinephrine in cardiocytes: role of contractility. *Am J Physiol* 1997;**272**(4 Pt 2):H1876-85.
72. Muller JE, Mochizuki S, Koster JK Jr, Collins JJ Jr, Cohn LH, Neely JR. Insulin therapy for depressed myocardial contractility after prolonged ischemia. *Am J Cardiol* 1978;**41**(7):1215-21.
73. Puri PS, Bing RJ. Effects of glucagon on myocardial contractility and hemodynamics in acute experimental myocardial infarction: basis for its possible use in cardiogenic shock. *Am Heart J* 1969;**78**(5):660-8.
74. Sarnoff SJ, Braunwald E, Welch GH Jr, Case RB, Stainsby WN, Macruz R. Hemodynamic determinants of oxygen consumption of the heart with special reference to the tension-time index. *Am J Physiol* 1958;**192**(1):148-56.

75. Klocke FJ, Kaiser GA, Ross J Jr, Braunwald E. Mechanism of increase of myocardial oxygen uptake produced by catecholamines. *Am J Physiol* 1965;**209**(5):913-8.
76. Braunwald E. Thirteenth Bowditch lecture: the determinants of myocardial oxygen consumption. *Physiologist* 1969;**12**(2):65-93.
77. Weber KT, Janicki JS. Myocardial oxygen consumption: the role of wall force and shortening. *Am J Physiol* 1977;**233**(4):H421-30.
78. Suga H. Total mechanical energy of a ventricle model and cardiac oxygen consumption. *Am J Physiol* 1979;**236**(3):H498-505.
79. Nozawa T, Yasumura Y, Futaki S, Tanaka N, Uenishi M, Suga H. Efficiency of energy transfer from pressure-volume area to external mechanical work increases with contractile state and decreases with afterload in the left ventricle of the anesthetized closed-chest dog. *Circulation* 1988;**77**(5):1116-24.
80. Sunagawa K, Maughan WL, Burkhoff D, Sagawa K. Left ventricular interaction with arterial load studied in isolated canine ventricle. *Am J Physiol* 1983;**245**(5 Pt 1):H773-80.
81. Burkhoff D, Sagawa K. Ventricular efficiency predicted by an analytical model. *Am J Physiol* 1986;**250**(6 Pt 2):R1021-7.
82. De Tombe PP, Jones S, Burkhoff D, Hunter WC, Kass DA. Ventricular stroke work and efficiency both remain nearly optimal despite altered vascular loading. *Am J Physiol* 1993;**264**(6 Pt 2):H1817-24.
83. Ishihara H, Yokota M, Sobue T, Saito H. Relation between ventriculoarterial coupling and myocardial energetics in patients with idiopathic dilated cardiomyopathy. *J Am Coll Cardiol* 1994;**23**(2):406-16.
84. Hashima AR, Young AA, McCulloch AD, Waldman LK. Nonhomogeneous analysis of epicardial strain distributions during acute myocardial ischemia in the dog. *J Biomech* 1993;**26**(1):19-35.
85. Villarreal FJ, Lew WY, Waldman LK, Covell JW. Transmural myocardial deformation in the ischemic canine left ventricle. *Circ Res* 1991;**68**(2):368-81.
86. Park J, Metaxas D, Axel L. Analysis of left ventricular wall motion based on volumetric deformable models and MRI-SPAMM *Med Image Anal* 1996;**1**(1):53-71.
87. Park J, Metaxas DN, Axel L. Complete left ventricular wall motion estimation from cascaded MRI-SPAMM data. *Stud Health Technol Inform* 1998;(52 Pt 2):1063-5.
88. Park J, Metaxas DN, Axel L, Yuan Q, Blom AS. Cascaded MRI-SPAMM for LV motion analysis during a whole cardiac cycle. *Int J Med Inform* 1999;**55**(2):117-26.
89. Greve JM, Les AS, Tang BT, Draney Blomme MT, Wilson NM, Dalman RL, et al. Allometric scaling of wall shear stress from mice to humans: quantification using cine phase-contrast MRI and computational fluid dynamics. *Am J Physiol Heart Circ Physiol* 2006;**291**(4):H1700-8.
90. Isoda H, Hirano M, Takeda H, Kosugi T, Alley MT, Markl M, et al. Visualization of hemodynamics in a silicon aneurysm model using time-resolved, 3D, phase-contrast MRI. *AJNR Am J Neuroradiol* 2006;**27**(5):1119-22.
91. Yamashita S, Isoda H, Hirano M, Inagawa S, Takehara Y, et al. Visualization of hemodynamics in intracranial arteries using time-resolved three-dimensional phase-contrast MRI. *J Magn Reson Imaging* 2007;**25**(3):473-8.
92. Lew WY. Influence of ischemic zone size on nonischemic area function in the canine left ventricle. *Am J Physiol* 1987;**252**(5 Pt 2):H990-7.
93. Theroux P, Ross J Jr, Franklin D, Covell JW, Bloor CM, Sasayama S. Regional myocardial function and dimensions early and late after myocardial infarction in the unanesthetized dog. *Circ Res* 1977;**40**(2):158-65.
94. Jan KM. Distribution of myocardial stress and its influence on coronary blood flow. *J Biomech* 1985;**18**(11):815-20.
95. Alpert NR, editor. *Cardiac hypertrophy*. New York: Academic Press; 1971.
96. Fung Y. *Biomechanics: circulation*. New York: Springer-Verlag; 1997.
97. Yin FC. Ventricular wall stress. *Circ Res* 1981;**49**(4):829-42.
98. Woods RH. A few applications of a physical theorem to membranes in the human body in a state of tension. *J Anat Physiol* 1892;**26**(Pt 3):362-70.
99. Ghista DN, Sandler H. An analytic elastic-viscoelastic model for the shape and the forces in the left ventricle. *J Biomech* 1969;**2**(1):35-47.
100. Mirsky I. Left ventricular stresses in the intact human heart. *Biophys J* 1969;**9**(2):189-208.
101. Mirsky I. Effects of anisotropy and nonhomogeneity on left ventricular stresses in the intact heart. *Bull Math Biophys* 1970;**32**(2):197-213.
102. Wong AY, Rautaharju PM. Stress distribution within the left ventricular wall approximated as a thick ellipsoidal shell. *Am Heart J* 1968;**75**(5):649-62.
103. Walker ML, Hawthorne EW, Sandler H. Methods for assessing performance for the intact hypertrophied heart. In: Alpert NR, editor. *Cardiac hypertrophy*. New York: Academic Press; 1971. p. 387-405.
104. Beyer R, Sideman S. The dynamic twisting of the left ventricle: a computer study. *Ann Biomed Eng* 1986;**14**:547-62.
105. van den Broek JH, van den Broek MH. Application of an ellipsoidal heart model in studying left ventricular contractions. *J Biomech* 1980;**13**(6):493-503.
106. Abe H, Nakamura T. Finite deformation model for the mechanical behavior of left ventricular wall muscles. *Math Modeling* 1982;**3**:143-52.
107. Demiray H. Stresses in ventricular wall. *ASME J Appl Mech* 1976;**43**:194-7.
108. Mirsky I. Ventricular and arterial wall stresses based on large deformation analyses. *Biophys J* 1973;**13**(11):1141-59.
109. Moriarty TF. The law of Laplace: its limitations as a relation for diastolic pressure, volume, or wall stress of the left ventricle. *Circ Res* 1980;**46**:321-31.
110. Shivakumar PN, Man C-S, Rabkin SW. Modeling of the heart and pericardium at end-diastole. *J Biomech* 1989;**22**:201-9.
111. Vito RP. The role of the pericardium in cardiac mechanics. *J Biomech* 1979;**12**(8):587-92.
112. Arts T, Reneman RS. Dynamics of left ventricular wall and mitral valve mechanics: a model study. *J Biomech* 1989;**22**(3):261-71.
113. Arts T, Reneman RS, Veenstra PC. A model of the mechanics of the left ventricle. *Ann Biomed Eng* 1979;**7**(3-4):299-318.
114. Arts T, Veenstra PC, Reneman RS. Epicardial deformation and left ventricular wall mechanisms during ejection in the dog. *Am J Physiol* 1982;**243**(3):H379-90.
115. Chadwick RS. Mechanics of the left ventricle. *Biophys J* 1982;**39**(3):279-88.
116. Feit TS. Diastolic pressure-volume relations and distribution of pressure and fiber extension across the wall of a model left ventricle. *Biophys J* 1970;**26**:71-83.
117. Ohayon J, Chadwick RS. Theoretical analysis of the effects of a radial activation wave and twisting motion on the mechanics of the left ventricle. *Biorheology* 1988;**25**(3):435-47.
118. Tozeren A. Static analysis of the left ventricle. *J Biomech Eng* 1983;**105**(1):39-46.
119. van den Broek JH, van der Gon JJ. A model study of isovolumic and non-isovolumic left ventricular contractions. *J Biomech* 1980;**13**(2):77-87.
120. Janz RF. Estimation of local myocardial stress. *Am J Physiol* 1982;**242**(5):H875-81.
121. Janz RF, Ozpetek S, Ginzton LE, Laks MM. Regional stress in a noncircular cylinder. *Biophys J* 1989;**55**(1):173-82.
122. Fung YC. *Biomechanics: motion, flow, stress, and growth*. New York: Springer Verlag; 1990.
123. Florenzano F, Glantz SA. Left ventricular mechanical adaptation to chronic aortic regurgitation in intact dogs. *Am J Physiol* 1987;**252**(5 Pt 2):H969-84.
124. Omens JH, MacKenna DA, McCulloch AD. Measurement of strain and analysis of stress in resting rat left ventricular myocardium. *J Biomech* 1993;**26**(6):665-76.
125. Huisman RM, Elzinga G, Westerhof N, Sipkema P. Measurement of left ventricular wall stress. *Cardiovasc Res* 1980;**14**(3):142-53.
126. Guccione JM, McCulloch AD, Waldman LK. Passive material properties of intact ventricular myocardium determined from a cylindrical model. *J Biomech Eng* 1991;**113**(1):42-55.
127. Cook RD. *Concepts and applications of finite elements analysis*. New York: John Wiley & Sons; 1981.
128. Turner MJ, Clough RW, Matin HC, Topp LJ. Stiffness and deflection analysis of complex structures. *J Aero Sci* 1956;**9**:805-23.
129. Argyris JH, Kelsey S, editors. *Energy theorems and structural analysis*. London: Butterworths; 1960.
130. Janz RF, Kubert BR, Moriarty TF, Grimm AF. Deformation of the diastolic left ventricle: II. Nonlinear geometric effects. *J Biomech* 1974;**7**(6):509-16.
131. Bovendeerd PH, Arts T, Delhaas T, Huyghe JM, van Campen DH, Reneman RS. Regional wall mechanics in the ischemic left ventricle: numerical modeling and dog experiments. *Am J Physiol* 1996;**270**(1 Pt 2):H398-410.
132. Usyk TP, Mazhari R, McCulloch AD. Effect of laminar orthotopic myofiber architecture on regional stress and strain in the canine left ventricle. *J Elasticity* 2000;**61**:143-64.
133. Vetter FJ, McCulloch AD. Three-dimensional stress and strain in passive rabbit left ventricle: a model study. *Ann Biomed Eng* 2000;**28**(7):781-92.
134. Denney TS Jr, Gerber BL, Yan L. Unsupervised reconstruction of a three-dimensional left ventricular strain from parallel tagged cardiac images. *Magn Reson Med* 2003;**49**(4):743-54.
135. Ozturk C, McVeigh ER. Four-dimensional B-spline based motion analysis of tagged MR images: introduction and in vivo validation. *Phys Med Biol* 2000;**45**(6):1683-702.
136. Moulton MJ, Creswell LL, Downing SW, Actis RL, Szabo BA, Pasque MK. Myocardial material property determination in the in vivo heart using magnetic resonance imaging. *Int J Card Imaging* 1996;**12**(3):153-67.
137. Okamoto RJ, Moulton MJ, Peterson SJ, Li D, Pasque MK, Guccione JM. Epicardial suction: a new approach to mechanical testing of the passive ventricular wall. *J Biomech Eng* 2000;**122**(5):479-87.
138. Guccione JM, Moonly SM, Moustakidis P, Costa KD, Moulton MJ, Ratcliffe MB, et al. Mechanism underlying mechanical dysfunction in the border zone of left ventricular aneurysm: a finite element model study. *Ann Thorac Surg* 2001;**71**(2):654-62.
139. Costa KD, Hunter PJ, Wayne JS, Waldman LK, Guccione JM, McCulloch AD. A three-dimensional finite element method for large elastic deformations of ventricular myocardium: II. Prolate spheroidal coordinates. *J Biomech Eng* 1996;**118**(4):464-72.

140. Guccione JM, Costa KD, McCulloch AD. Finite element stress analysis of left ventricular mechanics in the beating dog heart. *J Biomech* 1995;**28**(10):1167-77.
141. Rodriguez EK, Omens JH, Waldman LK, McCulloch AD. Effect of residual stress on transmural sarcomere length distributions in rat left ventricle. *Am J Physiol* 1993;**264**(4 Pt 2):H1048-56.
142. Walker JC, Ratcliffe MB, Zhang P, Wallace AW, Hsu EW, Saloner DA, et al. Magnetic resonance imaging-based finite element stress analysis after linear repair of left ventricular aneurysm. *J Thorac Cardiovasc Surg* 2008:**135**: 1094–102.
143. Elzinga G, van Grondelle R, Westerhof N, van den Bos GC. Ventricular interference. *Am J Physiol* 1974;**226**(4):941-7.
144. Santamore WP, Lynch PR, Meier G, Heckman J, Bove AA. Myocardial interaction between the ventricles. *J Appl Physiol* 1976;**41**(3):362-8.
145. Slinker B, Glantz S. End-systolic and end-diastolic ventricular interaction. *Am J Physiol* 1986;**251**:H1062-75.
146. Baker AE, Dani R, Smith ER, Tyberg JV, Belenkie I. Quantitative assessment of independent contributions of pericardium and septum to direct ventricular interaction. *Am J Physiol* 1998;**275**(2 Pt 2):H476-83.
147. Slater JP, Lipsitz EC, Chen JM, Levin HR, Oz MC, Goldstein DJ, et al. Systolic ventricular interaction in normal and diseased explanted human hearts. *J Thorac Cardiovasc Surg* 1997;**113**(6):1091-9.
148. Santamore WP, Burkhoff D. Hemodynamic consequences of ventricular interaction as assessed by model analysis. *Am J Physiol* 1991;**260**(1 Pt 2): H146-57.
149. Yamaguchi S, Harasawa H, Li KS, Zhu D, Santamore WP. Comparative significance in systolic ventricular interaction. *Cardiovasc Res* 1991;**25**(9):774-83.
150. Slinker BK, Chagas AC, Glantz SA. Chronic pressure overload hypertrophy decreases direct ventricular interaction. *Am J Physiol* 1987;**253**(2 Pt 2):H347-57.
151. Maruyama Y, Ashikawa K, Isoyama S, Kanatsuka H, Ino-Oka E, Takishima T. Mechanical interactions between four heart chambers with and without the pericardium in canine hearts. *Circ Res* 1982;**50**(1):86-100.

CHAPTER 51
Blood Coagulation, Transfusion, and Conservation
Jerrold H. Levy, Marie Steiner, and Kenichi A. Tanaka

Normal Hemostatic Mechanisms
Inhibiting Hemostasis: Anticoagulation
 Heparin
  Protamine Administration for Heparin Reversal
 Low-Molecular-Weight Heparin
 Fondaparinux
 Warfarin
 New Oral Anticoagulants
 Heparin-Induced Thrombocytopenia and New Anticoagulants
Acquired Platelet Dysfunction
Hemostatic Testing
 Risk Factors for Bleeding
  Patient-Related Causes of Bleeding

Physician-Related Causes of Bleeding
Procedure-Related Causes of Bleeding
Drug-Related Causes of Bleeding
Transfusion Therapy and Transfusion Guidelines
 Red Blood Cells
 Fresh-Frozen Plasma
 Cryoprecipitate
 Massive Transfusion
Adverse Effects of Transfusions
 Transfusion-Related Acute Lung Injury
 Mechanical Blood Conservation Strategies
 Preoperative Autologous Donation
 Acute Normovolemic Hemodilution

Platelet Plasmapheresis
Red Blood Cell Scavenging Techniques
Prohemostatic Agents Used in Surgery
 Antifibrinolytic Agents
  Lysine Analogs: Epsilon Aminocaproic Acid and Tranexamic Acid
 Aprotinin
 Protamine
 Desmopressin
 Fibrinogen
 Recombinant Factor VIIa
 Reversal of Vitamin K Antagonist–Associated Coagulopathy
 Topical Hemostatic Agents
Summary

After cardiac surgery, patients may exhibit hemostatic abnormalities, both quantitative and qualitative. However, preexisting and acquired problems also contribute to bleeding. The increasing use of antiplatelet agents (e.g., clopidogrel [Plavix]) and anticoagulation agents contributes to a compromised preoperative hemostatic state that is exacerbated by the tissue injury associated with surgery.[1] This complex hemostatic alteration is further complicated by heparin and cardiopulmonary bypass (CPB), which result in additional acquired defects in hemostatic mechanisms.[2] Furthermore, with massive bleeding, dilutional hemostatic changes and hypothermia can also occur, and these also contribute to coagulopathy.

Managing bleeding after cardiac surgery requires many preventive and therapeutic considerations.[3,4] In high-risk patients, intraoperative measures to prevent bleeding can be used to prevent the adverse effects of CPB and mediastinal suctioning that can produce hemostatic abnormalities.[1] Furthermore, tissue injury and increases in stress response can activate fibrinolysis, which produces hemostatic disorders. Pharmacologic therapies to reduce bleeding and the need for allogeneic transfusions have been extensively studied in cardiac surgery and will be reviewed here. These therapies are based on reversing the defects associated with coagulopathy.

Preoperative interventions to reduce blood transfusion begin with identification of high-risk patients who should receive preoperative and perioperative blood conservation measures and for whom antithrombotic drugs should be limited (Box 51-1). Perioperative blood conservation interventions include use of antifibrinolytic drugs, selective use of off-pump coronary artery bypass graft surgery, routine use of a cell-saving device, and implementation of appropriate transfusion modalities. An important intervention is a multimodality

Box 51-1
Predictors of Postoperative Bleeding in Cardiothoracic Surgery

- Advanced age
- Small body size or preoperative anemia (low red blood cell volume)
- Antiplatelet or antithrombotic drugs
- Prolonged operation (e.g., cardiopulmonary bypass time—high correlation with operation)
- Emergency operation
- Other comorbidities (congestive heart failure, chronic obstructive pulmonary disease, hypertension, peripheral vascular disease, renal failure)

From Ferraris VA, Ferraris SP, Saha SP, et al. Ann Thorac Surg 2007;**83**:S27-86.

blood conservation program that is institution based, that is accepted by all health-care providers, and that involves well-thought-out algorithms to guide transfusion decisions. In this chapter, we focus on coagulation changes that occur in cardiac surgery, therapies to prevent and treat bleeding when it occurs, and blood conservation strategies. Recent concepts in understanding pharmacologic agents are reviewed.

NORMAL HEMOSTATIC MECHANISMS

The vascular endothelium, which plays a major role in preventing clotting (Fig. 51-1), is a nonthrombogenic surface that secretes various substances to prevent coagulation from occurring. Prostacyclin (PGI_2), tissue plasminogen activator

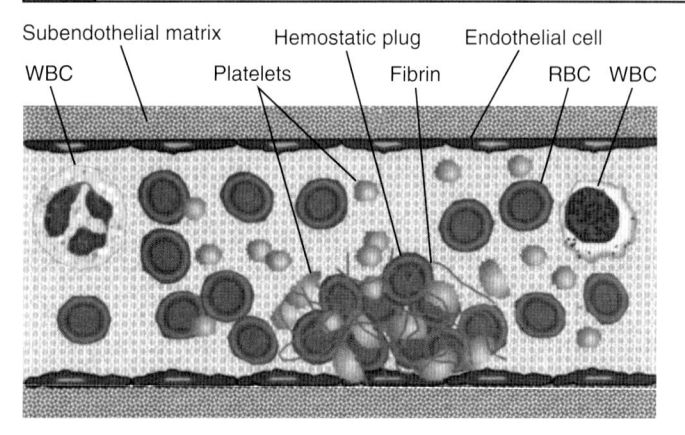

Figure 51–1
Clot formation and hemostatic balance. Hemostasis refers to the prevention of blood loss. Techniques include vasoconstriction, and coagulation by cellular and other factors. Undue bleeding is controlled and the fluidity of the blood is maintained by counterbalances in the coagulation and fibrinolytic systems. Blood vessel injury or disruption, platelet defects, abnormalities of the normally circulating anticoagulants, and fibrinolytic mechanisms may upset the balance between fibrinolysis and coagulation. Blood normally circulates through endothelium-lined vessels without coagulation or platelet activation occurring, and without appreciable hemorrhage. Injury to the endothelial cells triggers the hemostatic process, which begins with tissue factor liberation, the exposing of subendothelial proteins such as collagen, and the attachment (adhesion) of platelets to the damaged endothelium, sometimes via a von Willebrand's factor bridge. The platelets then change form (activate) and release factors that stimulate the clotting process. They also bind together (aggregate). At the same time, plasma proteins may react with elements in the subendothelium, activating the contact phase of coagulation. Exposed fibroblasts and macrophages present tissue factor, a membrane protein, to the blood at the injured site, thereby triggering the extrinsic phase of blood coagulation. Under normal conditions, hemostasis protects the individual from massive bleeding secondary to trauma. In abnormal states, life-threatening bleeding can occur or thrombosis can occlude the vascular tree. Factors that influence hemostasis include (1) vascular extracellular matrix and alterations in endothelial reactivity, (2) platelets, (3) coagulation proteins, (4) inhibitors of coagulation, and (5) fibrinolysis. RBC, red blood cell; WBC, white blood cell.

(tPA), heparan sulfate, antithrombin III, protein C, and endothelium-derived relaxing factor (EDRF) are expressed or secreted to inhibit platelet activation and fibrin formation, and to provide vascular patency.[5] However, if a blood vessel is cut or otherwise damaged, tissue factor and other molecular promoters are released or exposed to provide a thrombotic surface. Exposure of subendothelial vascular basement membrane activates platelets, and expression of tissue factor also activates the thrombin generation and cellular amplification.[6] Another important mechanism for the initiation of the coagulation cascade is platelet activation. Receptors on platelets bind to the damaged blood vessel by forming a bridge with von Willebrand's factor (vWF) to initiate platelet adhesion.[7] Once platelets adhere, they undergo surface receptor changes that cause platelets to aggregate. Once platelets aggregate, they expose factors on their surfaces that provide a template for additional initiation of the coagulation cascade and formation of the early hemostatic plug. Platelets play vital roles in maintaining vascular hemostasis. Any abnormality in platelet number or function poses significant risk for postoperative coagulopathy.

INHIBITING HEMOSTASIS: ANTICOAGULATION

Heparin

Heparin is the primary agent used to prevent clotting during cardiovascular surgery. It is isolated from porcine intestine (previously from beef lung), where it is bound to histamine and stored in mast cell granules. When heparin is isolated, the purification results in a heterogeneous mixture of molecules. Heparin is an acidic molecule with side groups, either sulfates or N-acetyl groups, attached to individual sugar groups; these molecular aspects are important for producing its anticoagulant activity.[8,9] Heparin acts as an anticoagulant by binding to antithrombin III (AT), enhancing the rate of thrombin-AT complex formation by 1000 to 10,000 times. Other factors in the clotting cascade, including factor Xa, are also inhibited by AT.[9] Anticoagulation thus depends on the presence of adequate amounts of circulating AT.

Heparin anticoagulation can be reversed immediately by removing heparin from AT with the highly basic molecule protamine. Heparin also binds to a number of other blood and endothelial proteins.[8] Each of these can potentially influence the ability of heparin to act as an anticoagulant, and each may, along with AT levels, affect heparin dose responses in patients. Heparin can also produce platelet dysfunction after acute or constant administration, especially with high-dose administration during cardiac surgery. Severe adverse reactions to heparin include immune reactions (e.g., hypersensitivity) and the perhaps better-recognized heparin-induced thrombocytopenia (see later).

In January 2008, the Food and Drug Administration received reports of clusters of acute hypersensitivity reactions in patients undergoing dialysis. The Centers for Disease Control and Prevention identified heparin as a common feature of the cases, leading to a recall of particular lots. However, after the initial recall, reports of allergic-type reactions in patients in other clinical settings continued. The contaminant was recently identified as an unusual oversulfated form of chondroitin sulfate (OSCS), representing up to nearly 30% by weight in suspect lots of heparin.[10] Highly charged molecules like this can activate enzymatic cascades in plasma. Contaminated lots of unfractionated heparin were found to activate the kinin-kallikrein pathway to produce vasodilation via contact activation.[10]

Protamine Administration for Heparin Reversal

Protamine, the primary heparin-neutralizing agent, is a basic polypeptide isolated from salmon sperm. Composed mostly of arginine, protamine can immediately reverse the anticoagulation effect of unfractionated heparin by a nonspecific acid–base (polyanionic-polycationic) interaction. Different methods can be used to calculate the reversal dose of protamine, but a useful approximation is to use 1.0 to 1.3 mg protamine for each 100 units of unfractionated heparin initially administered.[8] Protamine has the potential to function as an anticoagulant, when excessive doses have been administered (Fig. 51-2).[11] Additional considerations about protamine and its potential adverse effects will be considered later.

Low-Molecular-Weight Heparin

Low-molecular-weight heparin (LMWH) is a derivative of unfractionated heparin, whose fragments have a mean molecular weight of approximately 5000 daltons. LMWH fragments

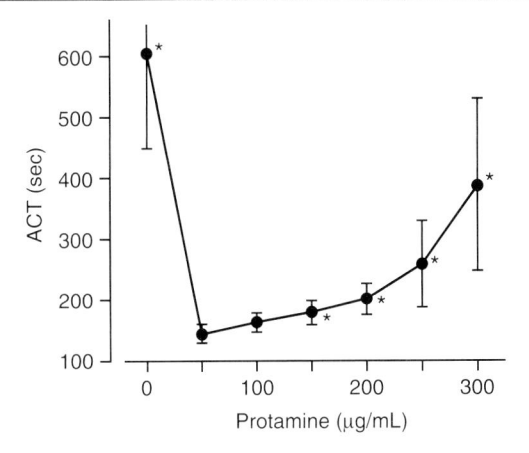

Figure 51–2
Excess protamine (i.e., at a dosage higher than that required to reverse systemic anticoagulation) contributes to elevations in activated clotting time (ACT). Protamine overdosage should be strictly avoided. *(From Mochizuki T, Olson PJ, Szlam F, Ramsay JG, Levy JH:* Anesth Analg *1998;***87***:781-5.)*

of less than 18 saccharides retain the critical pentasaccharide sequence needed for formation of the Xa:antithrombin complex.[12] It has been suggested that LMWHs provide a therapeutic benefit because factor Xa generation occurs several steps earlier in the coagulation cascade than thrombin generation; inhibition of Xa has a marked effect on the later steps in coagulation. Although the use of LMWH is rapidly increasing in cardiovascular medicine because of its long half-life and ease of dosing, it may pose a problem for cardiac surgical patients because commonly used hemostatic tests are not affected by it. Furthermore, because LMWHs are not readily reversible with protamine, they are not suitable anticoagulants for CPB.

Fondaparinux

Fondaparinux (Arixtra), a synthetic pentasaccharide with a duration of action longer than that of LMWH, selectively binds antithrombin and causes rapid and predictable inhibition of factor Xa.[13] Fondaparinux is more effective than enoxaparin in preventing venous thrombosis in patients undergoing orthopedic surgery, and it is similar in effectiveness to enoxaparin or unfractionated heparin in patients with pulmonary embolism.[14] Pilot trials involving patients with acute coronary syndromes and patients undergoing percutaneous coronary intervention suggest that fondaparinux may be as effective as enoxaparin, or safer than unfractionated heparin.[15] The Fifth Organization to Assess Strategies in Acute Ischemic Syndromes (OASIS-5; NCT00139815) trial compared the efficacy and safety of fondaparinux and enoxaparin (Lovenox, Sanofi-Aventis) in high-risk patients with unstable angina or myocardial infarction without ST-segment elevation.[15] The result of this study indicated that fondaparinux reduces the risk of ischemic events as effectively as enoxaparin does, but with lesser risk of major bleeding.

Warfarin

Warfarin, a member of the family of drugs known as vitamin K antagonists, is the most widely available oral anticoagulant. It has major limitations, including slow onset and offset and a narrow therapeutic window, and its metabolism is affected by diet, concomitant drugs, and genetic polymorphisms, and thus it requires careful monitoring.[16] Warfarin is a vitamin K analog that interferes with the transformation of coagulation factors to an active form. Vitamin K is required in the post-translational carboxylation required for the synthesis of active coagulation factors II, VII, IX, and X. Without vitamin K, these coagulation factors are incapable of chelating calcium, which is required for their binding to phospholipid membranes during the normal clotting process. The resultant deficient clotting factor activities decrease prothrombin activation. Warfarin also inhibits the carboxylation of protein C and protein S, thus impairing the function of the natural inhibitory anticoagulant proteins. Warfarin is often a mainstay in preventing thromboembolic complication in patients with prosthetic heart valves, atrial fibrillation, atrial mural thrombi, deep vein thrombosis, or prior pulmonary embolic problems. Warfarin is rapidly absorbed from the gastrointestinal tract, with peak plasma concentrations reached 1 to 4 hours after ingestion; the anticoagulant effect of the coumarin becomes visible only after a significant decrease in the concentration of normal vitamin K–dependent clotting factors.[8] Because these clotting factors have half-lives of various durations, warfarin therapy is typically initiated in combination with a heparin anticoagulant until the level of the factor with the longest half-life, factor II, has been reduced.

New Oral Anticoagulants

Ximelagatran, the first oral anticoagulant, was withdrawn from the market in Europe because of organ toxicity. Newer oral anticoagulants in advanced stages of clinical development are directed against the active site of factor Xa or thrombin, the enzymes responsible for thrombin generation and fibrin formation, respectively.[16] Rivaroxaban and apixaban target factor Xa, whereas dabigatran etexilate inhibits thrombin. Rivaroxaban is a small molecule directed against the active site of factor Xa. After oral administration, it is absorbed in the stomach and small intestine with a bioavailability of 60% to 80%. Peak plasma levels are achieved in 3 hours, and the drug circulates with a half-life of 9 hours.[16]

Heparin-Induced Thrombocytopenia and New Anticoagulants

Heparin-induced thrombocytopenia (HIT) is an adverse, potentially life-threatening, effect of heparin, produced by antibodies (IgG) to the composite of heparin–platelet factor 4 (PF4) that leads to the formation of immune complexes.[17] These immune complexes bind to platelets via platelet Fc-receptors (CD 32), producing intravascular platelet activation, thrombocytopenia, and platelet activation with potential thromboembolic complications that can result in limb loss or death.[17] HIT can occur after 5 to 10 days of heparin therapy, but it may occur earlier in cases of occult heparin exposure from prior hospitalizations or in the cardiac catheterization laboratory. HIT develops in 1% to 3% of heparin-treated patients.[18]

The antibodies that mediate HIT (i.e., heparin–PF4 antibodies) occur more often than the overt disease itself and, even without thrombocytopenia, are themselves associated with increased thrombotic morbidity and mortality.[18] HIT should be suspected whenever the platelet count drops more than 50%

from baseline after starting heparin (or sooner if there was prior heparin exposure), or when new thrombosis occurs during, or soon after, heparin treatment, with other causes excluded. When HIT is strongly suspected, with or without complicating thrombosis, heparins should be discontinued, and a fast-acting, nonheparin alternative anticoagulant, such as a direct thrombin inhibitor (argatroban or r-hirudin) or danaparoid, should be initiated immediately.[18,19]

As noted previously, even without inducing thrombocytopenia, heparin-PF4 antibodies may increase morbidity or mortality in various patient populations. In patients with, versus without, heparin-PF4 antibodies, regardless of the platelet count, there are significant increases in the hospitalization and in-hospital mortality after cardiac surgery[20] and other surgeries. Despite their association with long-term adverse effects, circulating heparin-PF4 antibodies are transient, although they are very likely recurrent with repeated heparin exposure. The agents currently recommended or approved for typical use in patients with HIT are the direct thrombin inhibitors, specifically argatroban, or danaparoid.[19] For cardiac surgery, bivalirudin has emerged as the agent most studied in this setting, for on- or off-pump surgery.[21,22] For patients who have HIT and are under intensive care, fondaparinux is a potential alternative for prophylaxis, and eventually the patient should be switched to warfarin when long-term anticoagulation is desired.[17]

ACQUIRED PLATELET DYSFUNCTION

Antiplatelet agents are the primary therapy for patients with atherosclerotic vascular disease and coronary artery disease; this therapy is consistent with the role of platelets in atherosclerosis.[23] Treatment with aspirin reduces the incidence of occlusive arterial vascular events. Aspirin irreversibly acetylates cyclooxygenase and thereby prevents formation of thromboxane A_2, a prostaglandin that mediates the activation of more platelets. Clopidogrel is a thienopyridine that inhibits the P2Y12 receptor, and it is widely used in patients with atherosclerotic vascular disease and in patients who do not tolerate aspirin.[23] The combination of aspirin plus clopidogrel is recommended after coronary stenting and for up to 9 months in patients with acute coronary syndrome.[23] These drugs and other anticoagulant therapies are associated with excessive intraoperative and postoperative bleeding, as well as resultant transfusions, in most but not all situations.[24-26] Patients with thrombocytopenia or with qualitative platelet defects (e.g., renal failure, von Willebrand's disease) may be at greater risk for bleeding. Discontinuation of antiplatelet and antithrombotic drugs before cardiac surgery in these high-risk patients should be considered.

Clopidogrel and aspirin therapy result in a higher rate of postoperative bleeding, the use of more transfused blood products, and a higher rate of reexploration for mediastinal hemorrhage during emergency coronary artery bypass grafting surgery (CABG).[27-29] Joint guidelines from the American College of Cardiology and the American Heart Association (ACC/AHA) and the current guidelines from the Society of Thoracic Surgeons (STS) recommend stopping adenosine diphosphate (ADP) inhibitors 5 to 7 days before cardiac operations, if possible, recognizing that operations sooner than 5 days in patients on ADP inhibitors risk increased perioperative bleeding and transfusions and possibly worse long-term outcomes.[30] However, in patients with drug-eluting stents, the abrupt discontinuation of platelet inhibitors may also increase the risk for thrombotic events, and there is little evidence to guide therapy in this situation; discussion with all members of the cardiovascular team—cardiologists, cardiac surgeons, anesthesiologists, and the operating team—is warranted. New shorter-acting antiplatelet agents under investigation (e.g., cangrelor) may offer an important therapy, but for now, changing to a glycoprotein (GP) IIb/IIIa inhibitor or to a direct thrombin inhibitor may be an alternative.[24]

Additional therapeutic agents may produce platelet dysfunction. Platelet glycoprotein (GP) IIb/IIIa complexes are important in platelet-mediated thrombus formation and have been used as therapeutic strategies to treat acute coronary thromboses, probably less commonly because of the increased use of clopidogrel.[31] Three different GP IIb/IIIa antagonists are available, and they differ in antagonist affinity, reversibility, and receptor specificity. GP IIb/IIIa (IIbβ3) is a receptor on platelets that binds to key hemostatic proteins, including fibrinogen and vWF, to allow cross-linking of platelets and platelet aggregation. By blocking this final common pathway using GP IIb/IIIa antagonists, these drugs function as inhibitors of platelet participation in acute thrombosis.

Various antagonists of GP IIb/IIIa are available. The first of these agents, the monoclonal antibody abciximab (ReoPro), has been approved for use in percutaneous coronary intervention. Tirofiban (Aggrastat), a nonpeptide, is approved for treatment of acute coronary syndromes (unstable angina or non-Q-wave myocardial infarction) and eptifibatide (Integrilin), a peptide, for use in both percutaneous coronary intervention and acute coronary syndromes. The shorter-acting agents, tirofiban and eptifibatide, are used during coronary intervention. The longer-acting agent, abciximab, is used with decreasing frequency because of its long half-life and potential for thrombocytopenia and bleeding.

HEMOSTATIC TESTING

Hemostatic testing is often used preoperatively to identify patients at risk for bleeding and to better define the specific defect producing bleeding. Although platelet dysfunction is a major cause of bleeding after cardiac surgery, appropriate laboratory evaluation of platelet dysfunction is not widely available. Hemostatic testing would help identify the best pharmacologic and transfusion-based therapy, but most platelet function tests available for point-of-care testing or in the laboratory have not been suitably validated for cardiac surgical patients, and non-point-of-care testing is not readily available. Furthermore, dilutional thrombocytopenia may affect the test results. Better tests of platelet dysfunction are needed to more accurately diagnose the underlying disorder in this patient population.[32]

Despite the lack of studies supporting platelet function tests in the perioperative management of cardiac surgical patients, many studies have shown that using algorithms based on point-of-care coagulation tests can decrease bleeding and transfusion requirements after cardiac surgery. An important caution is that hemostatic tests may be abnormal in patients who are not bleeding. Transfusion algorithms can be used to guide intraoperative transfusion and may prevent or decrease the empiric administration of hemostatic factors.[33] Cardiac surgery services should use transfusion guidelines based on laboratory-guided algorithms, and the possible benefits of point-of-care testing should be tested against this standard.

Risk Factors for Bleeding

Although most studies do not distinguish between red blood cell transfusion and hemostatic factor transfusion, Ferraris and colleagues[24] summarized the variables associated with increased transfusion requirements caused by patient-related, procedure-related, and process-related factors in their inclusive review. They identified a high-risk profile associated with increased postoperative blood transfusion, and six variables stand out as important indicators of bleeding risk: (1) advanced age, (2) low preoperative red blood cell volume (related to preoperative anemia or small body size), (3) preoperative antiplatelet or antithrombotic drugs, (4) reoperative or complex procedures, (5) emergency operations, and (6) noncardiac patient comorbidities. Risk factors are summarized at the *Annals of Thoracic Surgery* website, available at http://ats.ctsnetjournals.org/cgi/content/full/83/5_Supplement/S27.

Patient-Related Causes of Bleeding

Patients at greater risk for bleeding include those with acquired or congenital coagulopathies, those scheduled for complex procedures (e.g., combined valve and coronary revascularization, aortic dissection with deep hypothermic circulatory arrest), those having repeat cardiac procedures, those with sepsis with thrombocytopenia, and those who are Jehovah's Witnesses. There is evidence that certain patients have an accentuated response to antiplatelet drugs.[34] Patients with thrombocytopenia from whatever cause (defined as a platelet count below 50,000) are at high risk for excessive bleeding after CABG, but this depends on the variety of platelet dysfunction and is difficult to measure. Patients with preoperative anemia have a lower starting red blood cell mass going into surgery, and anemia can contribute in complex ways to bleeding. Patients with other congenital or acquired qualitative platelet defects, such as von Willebrand's disease, Bernard-Soulier syndrome, and Glanzmann's thrombasthenia, are at increased risk for bleeding.[24] Acquired qualitative defects occur with hepatic and renal failure and are commonly drug induced.

Physician-Related Causes of Bleeding

Another factor in surgical bleeding, and thus blood transfusion, is the surgeon. Surgical practices differ widely and influence morbidity and mortality.[35] Differences in CPB practices, such as time on bypass, can affect platelet function and perioperative bleeding. Surgeons define therapy differently, and even their different degrees of exploration for excessive postoperative hemorrhage contribute to variability in transfusion practices.[36] Furthermore, transfusion practices vary among centers.[24,37,38]

Procedure-Related Causes of Bleeding

Certain procedure-related factors increase risk for bleeding and perioperative morbidity and mortality. Repeat procedures have higher transfusion rates, and the type and urgency of the surgery are independent predictors for transfusion.[39-42] CPB also influences platelet function and coagulation.[42] Although off-pump cardiac surgery is associated with an overall reduction in transfusion, these patients, because of the extensive surgery, blood loss, and hemodilution, can also need transfusion.[43,44] Complex, long procedures (e.g., bilateral internal mammary artery grafts, aortic valve replacement with a pulmonary autograft [Ross procedure], surgery related to ventricular-assist devices or artificial hearts) are associated with greater risk for bleeding.[24]

Drug-Related Causes of Bleeding

Therapy for the prevention or treatment of cardiovascular disease involves maximizing platelet function, inhibiting clot formation, and causing clots to lyse. When patients who need surgery are on these agents, there is a greater risk for bleeding.[24] However, this may not be the case for patients who are on warfarin and undergoing CPB, because of better thrombin inhibition.[45] Ferraris and coworkers note that preoperative antiplatelet and anticoagulant treatment as prophylaxis for coronary occlusive disease is associated with excessive intraoperative and postoperative bleeding (with resultant transfusion) in most but not all situations, so this aspect of preoperative medication regimens must be managed for maximal cardioprotective benefit while minimizing risk for hemorrhagic complications.[24] As mentioned, clopidogrel and aspirin therapy result in higher postoperative bleeding, use of more transfused blood products, and a higher rate of reexploration for mediastinal hemorrhage during emergency CABG[27-29] (see Acquired Platelet Dysfunction, earlier, for ACC/AHA and STS guidelines).

TRANSFUSION THERAPY AND TRANSFUSION GUIDELINES

The appropriate use of either red blood cell transfusions or platelet components for cardiac surgical patients continues to be defined. Physicians make transfusion decisions on the basis of limited objective data, using clinical judgment and what they learned in their training. Guidelines and transfusion algorithms for the management of bleeding in cardiac surgical patients have been reported.[40,46] Bleeding and reexploration in cardiac surgery are consistently associated with adverse outcomes.[47-49] As a result, patients with bleeding are often transfused. However, the lack of consistent evidence-based medicine supporting the decision to transfuse is illustrated by the wide ranges in the rates of blood product use in patients undergoing CABG: from 3% to 83% for red cell products, and from 0% to 40% for platelets.[37,38]

Unfortunately, most physicians have difficulty following the guidelines and often resort to empiric therapy, often because laboratory tests take too much time, are difficult to obtain, or cannot identify platelet defects, or because of concern about later getting blood products from the blood bank in a timely fashion. Transfusion algorithms have been developed using institution-derived transfusion practices with point-of-care testing to guide therapeutic approaches to bleeding and transfusion. In randomized studies, the use of point-of-care testing and transfusion algorithms decreases the rate of transfusions and improves hemostasis.[50-53] Although different point-of-care tests were used in the studies, it is unclear whether the algorithms developed for guiding transfusion

> **Box 51–2**
> **Guidelines for Transfusion of Red Blood Cells, Platelets, Fresh-Frozen Plasma, and Cryoprecipitate**
>
> - The risks of bleeding in surgical patients are determined by the extent and surgery, the capacity to control bleeding, the expected rate of bleeding, and the outcomes of uncontrolled bleeding.
> - Red blood cell (RBC) transfusions should not be dictated by a single hemoglobin trigger but instead should be based on the patient's risks of developing complications of inadequate oxygenation. RBC transfusion is rarely indicated when the hemoglobin concentration is greater than 10 g/dL and is almost always indicated when it is less than 6 g/dL. The indications for autologous transfusion may be more liberal than for allogeneic transfusion.
> - Prophylactic platelet transfusion is ineffective when thrombocytopenia is the result of increased platelet destruction. Surgical patients with microvascular bleeding usually need platelet transfusion if the platelet count is less than 50×10^9/L, and rarely if it is greater than 100×10^9/L.
> - Fresh-frozen plasma is indicated for urgent reversal of warfarin therapy, correction of known coagulation factor deficiencies for which specific concentrates are unavailable, and correction of microvascular bleeding when prothrombin and partial thromboplastin times are greater than 1.5 times normal. It is contraindicated for increase of plasma volume or albumin concentration.
> - Cryoprecipitate should be considered for patients with von Willebrand's disease unresponsive to desmopressin, bleeding patients with von Willebrand's disease, and bleeding patients with fibrinogen levels below 80 to 100 mg/dL. (We believe, however, the fibrinogen level should be higher. See text, Fibrinogen.)

*Modified from Practice Guidelines for Blood Component Therapy. Anesthesiology 1994;**84**:732-47.*

and the multidisciplinary approach are more important than the point-of-care testing used because empiric transfusions are eliminated. Ferraris and colleagues note that a multimodality approach is more important than the individual components of the process.[24,25]

The American Society of Anesthesiologists (ASA) established the Task Force on Blood Component Therapy to develop evidence-based indications for transfusing red blood cells, platelets, fresh-frozen plasma, and cryoprecipitate in perioperative settings.[54] Guidelines were developed according to an exact methodology. The recommendations of the task force (see www.asahq.org/publicationsAndServices/transfusion.pdf) are listed in Box 51-2. These guidelines are recommendations, but there are concerns about specific blood components for cardiac surgical patients, as discussed in the following paragraphs.

Red Blood Cells

Unfortunately, there is no red cell transfusion standard based on a single minimum acceptable hemoglobin for all patients. Chronic anemia is better tolerated than acute anemia, but with acute anemia, compensatory mechanisms that increase cardiac output and improve oxygen transport depend on the patient's cardiovascular reserve, which may be diminished in cardiac surgical patients with heart failure or flow-restricting lesions. Factors to be considered before transfusing red blood cells (RBCs) include intravascular volume status, ongoing rate and amount of active bleeding, and the need for augmented oxygen transport (e.g., after cardiac surgery requiring multiple inotropes and an intra-aortic balloon pump, patients who are anemic may need RBCs). Thus, the need for transfusion must balance the risks against the need for oxygen-carrying capacity in recovery from trauma, surgery, or illness, as noted in the ASA guidelines for perioperative blood transfusion and adjuvant therapies.[55] The task force noted in its recommendations that a transfusion of "red blood cells should usually be administered when the hemoglobin concentration is low (e.g., less than 6 g/dL in a young, healthy patient), especially when the anemia is acute. Red blood cells are usually unnecessary when the hemoglobin concentration is more than 10 g/dL. These conclusions may be altered in the presence of anticipated blood loss" or active critical or target organ (i.e., myocardium, central nervous system, or renal) ischemia. "Determining whether intermediate hemoglobin concentrations (i.e., 6-10 g/dL) justify or require RBC transfusion should be based on any ongoing indication of organ ischemia, potential or actual ongoing bleeding (rate and magnitude), the patient's intravascular volume status, and the patient's risk factors for complications of inadequate oxygenation. These risk factors include a low cardiopulmonary reserve and high oxygen consumption."[55] Hemoglobin triggers for transfusion are not to be taken as absolute indications, and cardiac patients should be transfused if signs or symptoms of inadequate myocardial oxygenation are present. One important aspect of adverse events associated with RBC transfusions may relate to the age of the RBCs transfused, although large prospective randomized clinical trials remain to be conducted.[56-58]

Fresh-Frozen Plasma

After RBCs and platelets are removed from a unit of blood, plasma remains. That 170 to 250 mL, containing blood coagulation factors, fibrinogen, and other plasma proteins, is then frozen and can be stored for up to 1 year. Before being administered, the fresh-frozen plasma (FFP) must be thawed in a waterbath at 37° C, which takes about 30 minutes. After thawing, a unit of FFP is stored at 1° to 6° C and is transfused within 24 hours. FFP should be administered through a component administration set with a 170-micron filter. If not used within 24 hours, it can be relabeled as thawed plasma and stored at 1° to 6° C for an additional 4 days. Thawed plasma maintains normal levels of all factors except factor V, which falls to 80% of normal, and factor VIII (FVIII), which falls to 60% of normal.[59] Because these levels are above the in vivo threshold for normal hemostatic function, and FVIII is an acute-phase reactant, thawed plasma *can* be used as a substitute for FFP.[59]

FFP is traditionally used for treating bleeding resulting from coagulopathies that involve a prolongation of either activated partial thromboplastin time (aPTT) or prothrombin time and International Normalized Ratio (PT/INR) greater than 1.5 times normal, or a coagulation factor assay of less than 25%.[55] FFP is often used to reverse the effect of warfarin before surgery or during active bleeding episodes (see Reversal of Vitamin K Antagonist–Associated Coagulopathy, later). When FFP is indicated, it should be administered in a dosage calculated to achieve a minimum of 30% of plasma factor concentration. A dosage of 10 to 15 mL/kg of FFP generally results in a rise of most coagulation proteins by 25% to 30%

(or increases in 0.25 to 0.3 U/mL), although a dosage of 5 to 8 mL/kg may be adequate if needed to urgently reverse warfarin anticoagulation, but this varies with the initial levels of the vitamin K–dependent coagulation factors.[55] FFP is also part of a transfusion algorithm for post-traumatic bleeding.

FFP is overused in cardiac surgery, often because of empiric decisions. A major cause of bleeding after cardiac surgery is platelet dysfunction. Furthermore, the PT and partial thromboplastin time (PTT), which are widely used to evaluate bleeding, have never been demonstrated to reflect bleeding in cardiac surgical patients. Finally, the PT and PTT can be abnormal even in patients who are not bleeding.

Cryoprecipitate

Cryoprecipitate consists of the insoluble proteins that precipitate when FFP is thawed at 1° to 6° C. The residual volume (approximately 15 mL) after the FFP is used is refrozen and stored. Cryoprecipitate contains therapeutic amounts of factor VIII:C, factor XIII, vWF, and fibrinogen. Each bag of cryoprecipitate contains 80 to 100 units of factor VIII:C, 150 to 200 mg of fibrinogen, and significant amounts of factor XIII and vWF, including high-molecular-weight multimers. Cryoprecipitate is used to increase fibrinogen levels depleted after massive hemorrhage or coagulopathy, and for the treatment of congenital or acquired factor XIII deficiency.

In Europe, specific fibrinogen concentrates are available for fibrinogen replacement therapy. However, one unit of cryoprecipitate per 10 kg of body weight increases plasma fibrinogen by roughly 50 to 70 mg/dL without contributing to consumption or massive bleeding.[60,61] The minimum hemostatic level of fibrinogen is traditionally suggested to be around 100 mg/dL, but normal fibrinogen levels are 200 mg/dL and higher, and these higher levels of fibrinogen may be important for clot formation (see Fibrinogen, later). Because cryoprecipitate does not contain factor V, it should not be the sole replacement therapy for patients with disseminated intravascular coagulopathy, which is almost always associated with various factor deficiencies and thrombocytopenia, as noted in the guidelines from the American Association of Blood Banking (AABB) (Available at www.AABB.org). Because fibrinogen is an important determinant of hemostatic function and clot strength, fibrinogen levels should be routinely evaluated in bleeding patients, especially after multiple transfusions. Hypofibrinogenemia itself can cause a prolonged PT and PTT, and FFP transfusion alone may not provide sufficient repletion. Cryoprecipitate is probably underutilized in cardiac surgical patients who are bleeding and refractory to standard FFP and platelets.

Massive Transfusion

Massive transfusion is defined as the acute replacement of more than one blood volume, or the use of more than 10 units of packed RBCs within several hours. In the acute clinical setting, the transfusion of four or more red cell units within 1 hour when ongoing need is foreseeable, or replacing 50% of the total blood volume within 3 hours, may be more appropriate.[61,62] The most common clinical situation leading to massive transfusion is extensive trauma; however, massive transfusion may also occur in nontrauma settings during surgical procedures causing large blood loss, especially after cardiothoracic surgery.[61,62] Extensive information has been learned from the Iraq war in this area.[63-65] Blood transfusion is a main therapy option for treating acute hemorrhage. However, for trauma patients, ideal repletion is with fresh whole blood, which is not widely available. The etiology of coagulopathy during massive transfusion is complex and involves dilutional factors, hypothermia, tissue hypoperfusion/ischemia, acidosis, and potential disseminated intravascular coagulation; this syndrome may occur in cardiac surgical patients, too. Treatment of the coagulopathy should include volume replacement, normothermia, resolution of acid–base abnormalities and blood component therapy, and correction of hypocalcemia. Because of fibrinolysis, an antifibrinolytic should be considered for the cardiac surgical patient. The role of off-label use of recombinant activated factor VII (see Recombinant Factor VIIa, later) to manage bleeding that cannot be controlled by conventional measures is still evolving.

ADVERSE EFFECTS OF TRANSFUSIONS

The risks of allogeneic transfusion extend beyond viral transmission and include allergy, alloimmunization, bacterial sepsis, graft-versus-host disease, transfusion-related acute lung injury (TRALI), renal failure, volume overload, and immunosuppression.[66-68] Beside possible bacterial contamination, platelet concentrates for transfusions contain a high concentration of donor white blood cells, which can produce multiple adverse effects. Cytokines, such as interleukins 6 (IL-6) and 8 (IL-8), tissue necrosis factor alpha (TNFα), and other inflammatory mediators especially concentrated in platelet products could contribute to adverse outcomes.

Platelet concentrates without leukodepletion have been found to be a proinflammatory mixture.[69] Although similar work has not been performed with platelet transfusion, the levels of cytokines, TNFα, IL-6, and IL-8 are increased 100- to 1000-fold over baseline in platelet products.[69] As complement and cytokines depress platelet function and increase the release of tPA, the large influx of proinflammatory mediators from platelet transfusion might mitigate some of the procoagulant function of platelets, increase bleeding, or make platelet transfusions ineffective.[70]

Even though active white cells are responsible for forming the high levels of complement and cytokine factors, leukoreduction may be only partially effective in reducing the immunosuppressive effects of platelets.[71] In red cell transfusion, leukoreduction may affect T-cell activation and expression of key immune molecules on the surface of white cells.[72] Other mechanisms of immunosuppression not affected by leukoreduction may come into play. The presence of free, nonprotein-bound iron leads to the activation of white cells (whether allogeneic or autologous).[73] Furthermore, leukoreduced platelet units that are stored at room temperature today may increase the number of septic platelet transfusion units. The effect of bacterial cell wall material on the systemic proinflammatory processes seen during CPB is not clear.

Platelet transfusions have long been known to possess a storage lesion leading to decreased effectiveness compared with native circulating platelets.[74] Large percentages of platelets may already be hemostatically "dead" and functioning only as cellular shells. This lack of normal cellular activity and regulation may play some role in increasing adverse events. For example, infusion of a platelet product into a patient with an embolic nidus could potentiate thrombus or cerebral infarction. Similarly, a prothrombotic potential in a reperfused coronary or cerebral artery could promote thrombus generation if platelet transfusion were additive to thrombotic tendencies. This is best reflected by a study demonstrating that platelet transfusions were associated with infection, vasopressor use, respiratory medication use, stroke, and death.[69]

Transfusion-Related Acute Lung Injury

TRALI is one of the most life-threatening adverse effects of transfusion. Although the true incidence of TRALI is unknown, it is the leading cause of transfusion-related death according to the United States Food and Drug Administration (FDA).[75] Clinical presentation of TRALI, in its severe form, is indistinguishable from adult respiratory distress syndrome (ARDS) and is characterized by acute onset (within minutes, to 1 to 2 hours after transfusion), bilateral pulmonary infiltrates, and hypoxia without evidence of heart failure.[66,76,77] TRALI may resolve faster and has a lower mortality rate than ARDS. TRALI usually develops within 6 hours (most often less than 2 hours) of a transfusion, usually resolves within 24 to 48 hours, and has a mortality rate of around 5% to 10%, whereas ARDS does not usually develop until at least 24 hours after exposure to a risk factor, has a duration often longer than 72 hours, and has a mortality approaching 30% to 60%.[66] Because of increasing awareness and identification of TRALI, and also because of decreases in the incidence of infectious and hemolytic complications of transfusions, TRALI is now a primary cause of transfusion-associated mortality reported to the FDA and has become a frequent cause of transfusion-related morbidity.[78] It can occur after the transfusion of RBCs, but it is most often seen after transfusion of the plasma-containing blood components such as FFP and platelets. TRALI can be confused with other transfusion- and non-transfusion-related events such as anaphylaxis, hemolysis, circulatory overload, and cardiac failure, as patients present with acute shock, florid pulmonary edema, and pulmonary hypertension.[79,80] Risk estimates suggest it occurs once in 8000 to 70,000 transfused units.[66]

Depending on the causative factor in the transfused component and the inflammatory state of the pulmonary circulation after cardiac surgery, two different (but at times complementary and overlapping) pathogenic mechanisms are thought to cause TRALI: the classic antibody-mediated for most, and the two-hit inflammatory insult for some.[66,79,81] Most cases of TRALI are caused by passive transfer of donor-related antileukocytic antibodies directed at human leukocyte antigen (HLA) or granulocyte-specific antigens on the patient's leukocytes.[66] This promotes priming and activation of a patient's granulocytes, leading to their pulmonary sequestration and release of proteases, oxidants, and leukotrienes, which cause alveolar epithelial and microvascular endothelial damage, resulting in increased permeability and an eventual development of noncardiogenic pulmonary edema. The two-hit model of TRALI is similar to that which has been proposed to cause ARDS. With TRALI, however, the specific causative agent in the blood component is unknown, although there is growing evidence associating bioactive factors or white cell priming lipids, CD40 ligand released by platelets, or several reactive lipid-like substances accumulating in red blood cells or platelets during storage. These compounds, called biological response modifiers, can be the first pulmonary insult but are more likely the second. The first insult or hit is generally a systemic inflammatory condition secondary to major surgery, sepsis, trauma or pulmonary aspiration that causes activation of the pulmonary endothelium and polymorphonuclear lymphocytes (PMN) priming, leading to their sequestration in the pulmonary vasculature. The second hit occurs when the primed PMNs are activated by the biological response modifiers in the transfused component.

Therapy for TRALI is supportive. Suspected cases of TRALI should be reported to the hospital transfusion service so as to begin an investigation, including testing of associated donors for antileukocytic and antiplatelet antibodies and typing recipients for HLA antigens (i.e., via leukocytes in a pretransfusion blood specimen or buccal swab technique). If donor antileukocytic antibodies that react specifically to the patient's leukocytes are found, avoiding future transfusion of plasma-containing components from this donor is recommended. The patient, however, is not at an increased risk for future TRALI reactions with future transfusion.

Mechanical Blood Conservation Strategies

Preoperative Autologous Donation

Preoperative autologous donation has been reported for cardiac and noncardiac surgical patients. It is not feasible, however, when surgery is urgent, and its cost-effectiveness has been questioned. Hospitals and blood banks need specific procedures to draw and save blood for a patient's subsequent surgery. For patients with a critical cardiac disease, the potential for volume shifts and hemodynamic instability are concerns. The AABB guidelines for preoperative autologous donation suggest that no more than 450 mL or 12% of estimated blood volume should be withdrawn at one time, and the patient's hemoglobin concentration should be 11 g/dL or greater at the time of donation. Donations should not be performed more often than every third day. Autologous donation is performed with preoperative erythropoietin to boost the red blood cell mass, but this technique needs additional weeks to be effective.

Acute Normovolemic Hemodilution

Autologous blood (15% to 20% of blood volume) may be collected in the operating room before surgery, with accompanying intravascular volume expansion to maintain normovolemia. This technique is often performed in patients with normal to higher red cell masses and calculated intravascular volumes. Reports have shown a 20% to 58% decrease in allogeneic transfusion when autologous blood is re-transfused after CPB.[58]

Platelet Plasmapheresis

Platelet-rich plasma (PRP) plasmapheresis has been used after CPB. RBCs are usually returned via a large-bore central venous access catheter. Autologous PRP is re-transfused after heparin neutralization. The efficacy of this technique is not well established, and it is not commonly practiced.[16,45,52]

Red Blood Cell Scavenging Techniques

RBC salvage is commonly used during cardiac surgery. Shed blood is removed from the surgical field and mixed with an anticoagulant (heparin or citrate). RBCs are separated from

> **Box 51-3**
> **Pharmacologic Prohemostatic Agents**
>
> - Aprotinin
> - Lysine analogs
> - Protamine
> - Desmopressin (DDAVP)
> - Recombinant factor VIIa (rFVIIa, NovoSeven)
> - Purified protein concentrates
> - Fibrinogen/factor XIII
> - Fibrin glue/topical thrombin

From www.BleedingWeb.com with permission.

plasma and other formed elements by centrifugation and washed with saline. Salvaged, processed blood is a pure RBC product with a hematocrit between 50% and 60%. Clinicians sometimes send the blood remaining in the extracorporeal circuit to the cell salvage system after the patient is separated from cardiopulmonary bypass; however, this type of processing removes platelets and coagulation factors.

PROHEMOSTATIC AGENTS IN SURGERY

Although transfusion of banked blood products is the standard therapeutic approach to surgical bleeding,[67,69,82] few studies have demonstrated the effectiveness of this procedure.[83] Multiple systemic and topical prohemostatic agents are also used during cardiac surgery (Box 51-3). One of the unique aspects in this patient population is the ability to preemptively treat for potential bleeding problems, specifically with antifibrinolytic agents. Prohemostatic agents are reviewed next.

Antifibrinolytic Agents

Tissue injury during surgery and CPB produces direct and indirect activation of complex hemostatic pathways that produce fibrinolysis.[84,85] Extensive research has been published on the use of aprotinin and lysine-analog antifibrinolytics to modify the adverse effects of CPB in adults and pediatric patients.[86-88] The efficacy of these agents in decreasing bleeding (and resultant transfusion) is well established, as noted by the 2007 guidelines published by the STS and the Society of Cardiovascular Anesthesiologists.[24] Although the safety and efficacy of aprotinin have been extensively studied in randomized placebo controlled studies,[88] recent reports from observational databases have posed questions.[89,90]

Lysine Analogs: Epsilon Aminocaproic Acid and Tranexamic Acid

The synthetic lysine analogs epsilon aminocaproic acid (EACA or Amicar) and tranexamic acid (TA) inhibit fibrinolysis by attaching to the lysine binding site of the plasmin (ogen) molecule, displacing plasminogen from fibrin.[5] Levi and colleagues[91] reported a meta-analysis of all randomized controlled trials of the three most often used pharmacologic strategies to decrease perioperative blood loss (aprotinin, lysine analogs [EACA and TA], and desmopressin). Studies were included if they reported at least one clinically relevant outcome (mortality, rethoracotomy, proportion of patients receiving a transfusion, or perioperative myocardial infarction) as well as perioperative blood loss. In addition, a separate meta-analysis was done for studies on complicated cardiac surgery. Seventy-two trials (8409 patients) met the inclusion criteria. Treatment with aprotinin decreased mortality almost twofold (odds ratio [OR], 0.55; 95% confidence interval [CI], 0.34-0.90) compared with placebo. Treatment with aprotinin and with lysine analogs decreased the frequency of surgical reexploration (OR, 0.37; 95% CI, 0.25-0.55, and OR, 0.44; 95% CI, 0.22-0.90, respectively). These two treatments also significantly decreased the proportion of patients receiving any allogeneic blood transfusion. The use of desmopressin resulted in a small decrease in perioperative blood loss but was not associated with a favorable effect on other clinical outcomes. Aprotinin and lysine analogs did not increase the risk of perioperative myocardial infarction; however, desmopressin was associated with a 2.4-fold increase in the risk of this complication.[91]

From the Cochrane Database, Henry and associates reported an evaluation of randomized controlled trials of antifibrinolytic drugs in adults scheduled for nonurgent surgery. Two reviewers independently assessed trial quality and extracted data.[92] They found 61 trials of aprotinin (7027 participants). Aprotinin reduced the rate of RBC transfusion by a relative 30% (relative risk [RR], 0.70; 95% CI, 0.64-0.76). The average absolute risk reduction (ARR) was 20.4% (95% CI, 15.6-25.3). On average, aprotinin use saved 1.1 units of RBCs (95% CI, 0.69-1.47) in those needing transfusion. Aprotinin also significantly reduced the need for reoperation because of bleeding (RR, 0.40; 95% CI, 0.25-0.66). However, they did not report added decreases in transfusion factors (i.e., platelets). They also found 18 trials of TA (1342 participants). TA reduced the rate of RBC transfusion by a relative 34% (RR, 0.66; 95% CI, 0.54-0.81). This represented an ARR of 17.2% (95% CI, 8.7%-25.7%). TA use resulted in a savings of 1.03 units of RBCs (95% CI, 0.67-1.39) in those needing transfusion. They found four trials of EACA use (208 participants). EACA use resulted in a statistically nonsignificant decrease in RBC transfusion (RR, 0.48; 95% CI, 0.19-1.19). Eight trials made head-to-head comparisons between TA and aprotinin. There was no significant difference between the two drugs in the rate of RBC transfusion: RR was 1.21 (95% CI, 0.83-1.76) for TA compared with aprotinin. They also reported that aprotinin did not seem to be associated with an excess risk of adverse effects, including thromboembolic events (RR, 0.64; 95% CI; 0.31-1.31) and renal failure (RR, 1.19; 95% CI, 0.79-1.79). However, they did note the lack of safety data available for TA and EACA. The authors infer that aprotinin reduces the need for red cell transfusion, and the need for reoperation because of bleeding, without serious adverse effects. Although they noted similar trends were seen with TA and EACA, they reported that "the data were rather sparse." The evidence reviewed supported the use of aprotinin in cardiac surgery. They also suggested that further small trials of this drug are not warranted.

Pediatric Patients

Eaton reviewed 11 comparative studies (more than 1000 patients) of lysine analogs in pediatric heart surgery, 340 patients receiving EACA and 404 receiving TA.[86] Most were prospective, randomized, controlled trials. Interestingly, well over half of the studied patients were from a single center. Two studies[93,94] including All India Institute studies[94] included 750 cyanotic patients exclusively. Two studies involved EACA,[94,95] three involved TA,[93,96,97] and one compared both drugs.[98] All six studies showed efficacy of antifibrinolytic treatment in decreasing bleeding and transfusion. The 24-hour blood loss was decreased by 11% to 44%, and treated patients received 20% to 50% less blood than controls. In addition, sternal closure times were reduced by 6 to 25 minutes, and reexploration rates were improved by 50% to 100%. The benefit of antifibrinolytic treatment is less clear in reoperations. Thus, both EACA and TA appear effective in reducing bleeding and transfusion in cyanotic patients, but the efficacy in other high-risk and mixed populations is not as well proved. See Eaton's review for details.[86]

Aprotinin

Aprotinin is a protease inhibitor that attenuates many aspects of the inflammatory responses to CPB.[5,99] Over 70 randomized controlled trials, with 20 to 796 patients each (median, 75), confirmed the efficacy of aprotinin for limiting the need for transfusions in patients undergoing cardiac surgery.[100] Aprotinin had been the only the FDA-approved pharmacologic treatment for reducing the need for blood transfusion in patients undergoing CABG surgery. Aprotinin's efficacy has been reported for about 7000 patients, including several meta-analyses of randomized, double-blind clinical studies.[101] Levi and coworkers performed a meta-analysis of 3212 patients from 26 studies and noted that treatment with aprotinin decreased mortality almost twofold (OR, 0.55; 95% CI, 0.34-0.90) when compared with placebo, which was confirmed in a separate analysis of complex cardiac surgery patients.[102] These studies also reported that aprotinin reduced reexploration for bleeding.[102]

Another review of randomized controlled trials evaluated mortality, myocardial infarction (MI), renal failure, stroke, and atrial fibrillation in CABG trials of 3887 patients studying aprotinin.[103] Aprotinin reduced transfusions (RR, 0.61; 95% CI, 0.58-0.66) compared with placebo and was not associated with increased mortality (RR, 0.96; 95% CI, 0.65-1.40), MI (RR, 0.85; 95% CI, 0.63-1.14), or renal failure (RR, 1.01; 95% CI, 0.55-1.83).[103]

Any drug or blood product that decreases bleeding and transfusion requirements has the potential to affect grafted vessel patency, but three studies did not show significant differences in patency at postoperative examination.[104-106] In the largest study of patients undergoing cardiac catheterization after surgery, the effects of aprotinin on graft patency, prevalence of MI, and blood loss was studied in patients undergoing primary coronary surgery with CPB (IMAGE study).[107] Patients from 13 international sites were randomized to receive aprotinin (n = 436) or placebo (n = 434). Graft angiography was performed a mean of 10.8 days after the operation. Electrocardiograms, cardiac enzymes, and blood loss and replacement were evaluated. In 796 assessable patients, aprotinin reduced thoracic drainage volume by 43% (P < .0001) and need for RBC administration by 49% (P < .0001). Among 703 patients with assessable saphenous vein grafts, occlusions occurred in 15.4% of aprotinin-treated patients and 10.9% of patients receiving placebo (P = .03). After adjusting risk factors associated with vein graft occlusion, the aprotinin versus placebo risk ratio decreased from 1.7 to 1.05 (95% CI, 0.6 to 1.8). These factors included female sex, lack of prior aspirin therapy, small and poor distal vessel quality, and possible use of aprotinin-treated blood as excised vein perfusate. At U.S. sites, patients had characteristics more favorable for graft patency, and occlusions occurred in 9.4% of the aprotinin group and 9.5% of the placebo group (P = .72). At Danish and Israeli sites, where patients had more adverse characteristics, occlusions occurred in 23.0% of aprotinin- and 12.4% of placebo-treated patients (P = .01). Aprotinin did not affect the occurrence of MI (aprotinin, 2.9%; placebo, 3.8%) or mortality (aprotinin, 1.4%; placebo, 1.6%).

Sedrakyan and colleagues evaluated clinical outcomes (mortality, MI, renal failure, stroke, atrial fibrillation) in patients undergoing CABG who received aprotinin, by performing a quantitative review of randomized controlled trials.[103] They evaluated MEDLINE, EMBASE, and PHARMLINE (1988 to 2001), and reference lists of relevant articles were searched for CABG studies. Criteria for data inclusion were as follows: (1) random allocation of study treatments, (2) placebo control, (3) enrollment of only those patients undergoing CABG, (4) no combination with another experimental medication or device, and (5) prophylactic and continuous intraoperative use. Data from 35 CABG trials (N = 3879) confirmed that aprotinin reduces transfusions (RR, 0.61; 95% CI, 0.58-0.66) relative to placebo, with a 39% risk reduction. Aprotinin therapy was not associated with increased or decreased mortality (RR, 0.96; 95% CI, 0.65-1.40), MI (RR, 0.85; 95% CI, 0.63-1.14), or renal failure (RR, 1.01; 95% CI, 0.55-1.83) risk, but it was associated with a reduced risk of stroke (RR, 0.53; 95% CI, 0.31-0.90) and a trend toward reduced atrial fibrillation (RR, 0.90; 95% CI, 0.78-1.03). The authors inferred that concerns that aprotinin therapy is associated with increased mortality, MI, or renal failure risk is not supported by data from published, randomized, placebo-controlled clinical trials. Evidence for a reduced risk of stroke and a tendency toward reduction of atrial fibrillation event was observed in patients who received aprotinin.

Studies in Pediatric Cardiac Surgery

The 14 randomized controlled trials (RCTs)[93,94,108-119] of aprotinin use in pediatric cardiac surgery include heterogeneous populations, small numbers of subjects resulting in low statistical power, variable CPB or surgical techniques, differences in surgical outcomes, and variability of dosing.[86] Aprotinin-treated patients have lower blood loss and transfusion compared with controls, but the differences are not consistently statistically significant. Five of the 14 RCTs have shown a decrease in bleeding,[93,94,113,115,118] and six showed a decrease in at least one measure of transfusion with aprotinin treatment.[93,94,112,114,116,118] In contrast, Boldt and associates have published three RCTs showing no benefit of aprotinin treatment.[108-110] The published RCTs of aprotinin in the pediatric population, however, have all involved infants and older children with a wide variety of diagnoses, both cyanotic and noncyanotic. Neonates, reoperations, and complex and simple operations are represented in variable proportion. This is important because of the variability in risks for bleeding and transfusion in such a mixed population.

Miller and coworkers[116] report an interesting study of 45 high-risk infants and children undergoing repeat sternotomy for various indications, 40% having Glenn shunts or Fontan surgery. Patients were randomized to receive high-dose or low-dose aprotinin, or no treatment. Although there was no difference in bleeding, fewer patients receiving high-dose aprotinin required transfusion of FFP and platelets in the operating room, chest closure time was shorter, and overall bleeding-related costs were significantly reduced. Miller and colleagues[116] and Carrel and coworkers,[120] in their previously discussed studies, found aprotinin effective only in the high-dose groups. See Eaton's review for details.[86]

Adverse Effects

Anaphylaxis

Aprotinin is a polypeptide, and anaphylactic reactions to it have been described. The risk of anaphylaxis is reported as 2.7% in reexposed patients from several studies.[121-124] Beierlein and colleagues reviewed literature from 1963 to 2003 and noted 124 cases of aprotinin-induced anaphylaxis, with 11 deaths, reported in 61 publications.[121] The reexposure interval was less than 3 months in 72% (38 of 53 patients). Dietrich and associates reported adverse reactions after reexposure in cardiac surgery between 1988 and 1995.[122] There were 248 reexposures to aprotinin in 240 patients: 101 adult and 147 pediatric cases, with a reexposure time of 344 days (interquartile range, 1039). They noted seven reactions to aprotinin (2.8% incidence). Reexposure in less than 6 months had a higher incidence of adverse reactions (5 of 111 [4.5%] versus 2 of 137 [1.5%], $P < .05$), and two patients reacted to a test dose of 10,000 kallikrein inhibitor units (KIU).

An aprotinin test dose may also cause anaphylaxis.[123] After 248 aprotinin reexposures, there were seven reactions; four patients had received test doses, and two showed no response to the test dose but developed anaphylaxis during the initial loading dose.[122] Additional reports note that three of 121 patients developed anaphylaxis after aprotinin reexposure; two of these three did not react to the test dose but developed anaphylaxis within 5 minutes after the first loading dose.[123] The three patients had also been pretreated for anaphylaxis with antihistamines and corticosteroids, therapy that may have varied the onset of the reactions.[123] The risk for anaphylaxis is increased in patients with prior aprotinin exposure, and a history of exposure should be determined before aprotinin administration. The risk for a fatal reaction appears to be greater on reexposure within 12 months, as suggested by new FDA guidelines. Test doses and first loading doses that involve reexposure should be performed only when cannulation can be rapidly performed. Aprotinin is removed from marketing in most countries.

Renal Effects

Aprotinin is rapidly eliminated by renal excretion, with a half-life of about 5 hours. It may also have a transient effect on the proximal tubule cells or alter intrarenal blood flow through inhibition of renin and kallikrein activity. However, clinical studies reported by Lemmer and coworkers showed no adverse effects of aprotinin on postoperative renal function.[125] Added studies based on observational data have shown increases in creatinine, but in one study the risk of renal dysfunction with aprotinin was the same as that with FFP (OR, 2.4 versus 2.4).[90]

More Recent Studies of Aprotinin

Observational studies of aprotinin published in 2006 and 2007 suggested that "the association between aprotinin and serious end-organ damage indicates that continued use is not prudent."[90,126] In response to these reports and another observational study,[127] the FDA conducted two advisory meetings to review the risk–benefit profile of an aprotinin injection (Trasylol) to reduce bleeding in CABG surgery (see the FDA website, www.FDA.gov, and the Trasylol website, www.trasylol.com/press_release.htm). As reported on the FDA website, "On October 19, 2007, FDA was notified of a Data Safety Monitoring Board's (DSMB) recommendation to stop patient enrollment in an independent Canadian study, the aprotinin treatment group arm of the Blood Conservation Using Antifibrinolytics (BART), a randomized trial in a cardiac surgery population study." The report added that preliminary findings suggest that, compared with the antifibrinolytic drugs EACA and TA, "Aprotinin increases the risk of death" (www.fda.gov/cder/drug/early_comm/aprotinin.htm). The report continued, "The BART study was designed to test the hypothesis that aprotinin was superior to epsilon-aminocaproic acid and tranexamic acid in decreasing the occurrence of massive bleeding associated with cardiac surgery. The study had planned to enroll nearly 3000 adult Canadian patients who were to undergo various types of cardiac surgery that placed them at high risk for bleeding. Information from the interim analyses performed by the DSMB is limited, but FDA has been informed that: the 30-day mortality in the aprotinin group nearly had reached conventional statistical significance at the interim analysis, when compared with either epsilon-aminocaproic acid or tranexamic acid; a trend toward increased mortality in the aprotinin group had been observed throughout the study; the use of aprotinin was associated with less serious bleeding than either of the comparator drugs; however, more deaths due to hemorrhage had been observed among patients receiving aprotinin; the DSMB concluded that continued enrollment of patients into the aprotinin group was unlikely to significantly change the study findings."

The FDA further noted, "Additional data collection and analyses must be performed to more thoroughly assess the findings from the BART study. However, these preliminary data support the findings from observational studies that also suggested increased risks for mortality when aprotinin was compared with other antifibrinolytic drugs. These observational studies were discussed at a September 12, 2007, joint meeting of the Cardiovascular and Renal Drugs and Drug Safety and Risk Management Advisory Committees. In light of the preliminary BART study findings, FDA anticipates reevaluation of the overall risks and benefits of Trasylol. This reevaluation may result in the need to revise the labeling or other regulatory actions. Until this process has been completed, health-care providers who are considering use of Trasylol should be aware of the risks and benefits described in the labeling for Trasylol and the accumulating data suggesting Trasylol administration increases the risk for death compared to other antifibrinolytic drugs."

On November 5, 2007, the FDA announced, "At the agency's request, Bayer Pharmaceuticals Corporation had agreed to a marketing suspension of aprotinin (Trasylol) a drug used to control bleeding during heart surgery, pending detailed review of preliminary results from a Canadian study that suggested an increased risk for death" (www.fda.gov/bbs/topics/NEWS/2007/NEW01738.html). They noted, "FDA requested the suspension in the interest of patient safety based on the serious nature of the outcomes suggested in the preliminary data. FDA has not yet received full study data but expects to act quickly with Bayer, the study's researchers at the Ottawa Health Research Institute, and other regulatory agencies to undertake a thorough analysis of data to better understand the risks and benefits of Trasylol. There are not many treatment options for patients at risk for excessive bleeding during cardiac surgery. Thus, FDA is working with Bayer to phase Trasylol out of the marketplace in a way that does not cause shortages of other drugs used for this purpose. Until FDA can review the data from the terminated study it is not possible to determine and identify a population of patients undergoing cardiac surgery for which the benefits of Trasylol outweigh the risks. Understanding that individual doctors may identify specific cases where benefit outweighs risk, FDA is committed to exploring ways for those doctors to have continued, limited access to Trasylol."

In 2008, more observational studies were published.[127,128] Data on 10,275 consecutive patients undergoing surgical coronary revascularization at Duke University Medical Center between 1996 and 2005 were fit to a logistic-regression model predicting each patient's likelihood of receiving aprotinin based on preoperative characteristics, and to models predicting long-term survival (up to 10 years) and decline in renal function, as measured by increases in serum creatinine levels.[128] They report that 1343 patients (13.2%) received aprotinin, 6776 patients (66.8%) received aminocaproic acid, and 2029 patients (20.0%) received no antifibrinolytic therapy. All patients underwent CABG, and 1181 patients (11.5%) underwent combined coronary-artery bypass grafting and valve surgery. In the risk-adjusted model, survival was worse among patients treated with aprotinin, with a main-effects hazard ratio for death of 1.32 (95% CI, 1.12-1.55) for the comparison with patients receiving no antifibrinolytic therapy (P = .003) and 1.27 (95% CI, 1.10-1.46) for the comparison with patients receiving aminocaproic acid (P = .004). Compared with the use of aminocaproic acid or no antifibrinolytic agent, aprotinin use was also associated with a larger risk-adjusted increase in the serum creatinine level (P < .001) but not with a greater risk-adjusted incidence of dialysis (P = .56). Interestingly, aprotinin is commonly used in high-risk patients who are already at a greater risk for adverse events. Furthermore, statisticians note that odds ratios of less than 2.0 can be statistically significant but may not be clinically relevant.

Another study used electronic administrative records of the Premier Perspective Comparative Database to evaluate hospitalized patients with operating-room charges for the use of aprotinin (33,517 patients) or aminocaproic acid (44,682 patients) on the day CABG was performed.[127] In all, 1512 of the 33,517 aprotinin recipients (4.5%) and 1101 of the 44,682 aminocaproic acid recipients (2.5%) died. After adjustment for 41 characteristics of patients and hospitals, the estimated risk of death was 64% higher in the aprotinin group than in the aminocaproic acid group (RR, 1.64; 95% CI, 1.50-1.78). In the first 7 days after surgery, the adjusted relative risk of in-hospital death in the aprotinin group was 1.78 (95% CI, 1.56-2.02). The relative risk in a propensity-score-matched analysis was 1.32 (95% CI, 1.08-1.63). In the instrumental-variable analysis, the use of aprotinin was found to be associated with an excess risk of death of 1.59 per 100 patients (95% CI, 0.14-3.04). This is also an observational database, where the decision to use a drug based on cardiac surgeon or other members of the team is usually based on risks for bleeding and other associated risks as well.

The BART study,[129] as previously mentioned, was designed to determine whether aprotinin was superior to either TA or EACA in decreasing massive postoperative bleeding and other clinically important consequences. The Canadian study was a multicenter, blinded trial that randomly assigned 2331 high-risk cardiac surgical patients to receive aprotinin (781 patients), TA (770), or EACA (780). The primary outcome was massive postoperative bleeding. Secondary outcomes included death from any cause at 30 days. The trial was terminated early because of a trend toward a higher rate of death in patients receiving aprotinin. A total of 74 patients (9.5%) in the aprotinin group had massive bleeding, as compared with 93 (12.1%) in the TA group and 94 (12.1%) in the EACA group (RR in the aprotinin group for both comparisons, 0.79; 95% CI, 0.59-1.05). At 30 days, the rate of death from any cause was 6.0% in the aprotinin group, as compared with 3.9% in the TA group (RR, 1.55; 95% CI, 0.99-2.42) and 4.0% in the EACA group (RR, 1.52; 95% CI, 0.98-2.36). The relative risk of death in the aprotinin group, as compared with that in both groups receiving lysine analogs, was 1.53 (95% CI, 1.06-2.22).[129] Of interest was the lack of renal dysfunction in the aprotinin-treated patients.

Protamine

Protamine, a polypeptide composed of about 70% arginine residues, has a high pKa and thus can reverse the acidic molecule heparin by a simple acid–base interaction.[130] (Protamine does not reverse low-molecular-weight heparin.) After administration, protamine rapidly reverses heparin, as noted by the return of activated clotting times and by the marked elevations in plasma concentrations of prothrombin fragment 1.2, thrombin–antithrombin complex, and fibrin monomer.

Potential adverse reactions of protamine include anaphylaxis, acute pulmonary vasoconstriction and right ventricular failure, and hypotension.[130] Reported reactions range from minimal cardiovascular effects to life-threatening cardiovascular collapse. Life-threatening reactions to protamine probably represent true anaphylactic or allergic manifestations, mediated by immunospecific antibodies. Patients with diabetes are at increased risk for adverse reactions because of the presence of neutral protamine Hagedorn (NPH), which contains insulin and protamine and causes increased protamine sensitization.[130]

Stewart and colleagues reported a 27% incidence of reactions after cardiac catheterization in insulin-dependent diabetics who were also receiving NPH insulin preparations.[131] Other reports, however, do not corroborate those extreme results. In a study of 1551 cardiac surgery patients, we reported that the incidence of reactions to protamine was one in 50 among patients with NPH-insulin–dependent diabetes, compared with one in 1501 among the non-NPH-insulin–dependent patients with diabetes.[132] A subsequent, prospective study found that reactions occurred in less than 1% of patients (1/160) with NPH-insulin–dependent diabetes.[133] Individuals reported at risk for protamine reactions include those with vasectomy, those with multiple drug allergies, and those with prior protamine exposure.[130] Levy and associates reported that the incidence of life-threatening reactions in cardiac surgical patients ranges from 0.6% to 2% in patients at risk.[132,133] Life-threatening reactions to protamine represent true allergic reactions. Currently, there are no clinically available alternatives to protamine.

Desmopressin

Desmopressin (DDAVP), the V_2 analog of arginine vasopressin, stimulates the release of ultra-large multimers of von Willebrand's factor from endothelial cells. Desmopressin increases vWF and associated factor VIII levels. It induces release of normal vWF from cellular compartments.[100,134-136] Von Willebrand's disease (VWD) is the most common inherited bleeding disorder, and it is caused by quantitative (types 1 and 3) or qualitative (type 2) defects of vWF.[137] Desmopressin is the treatment for type 1 VWD. In type 3 and in severe forms of types 1 and 2 VWD, desmopressin response may be insufficient or ineffective, and plasma-derived, virally inactivated vWF concentrates should be used for bleeding, surgery, and secondary long-term prophylaxis.[137] Desmopressin should be administered in normal saline by slow intravenous infusion at a dosage of 0.3 μg/kg to avoid hypotension.[138,139] An initial study reported that desmopressin reduced blood loss and transfusion needs by around 30% during complex cardiac surgery.[140-142] Later attempts to reproduce these findings were variable, and most did not confirm the marked benefit originally reported.[139,143] Mannucci noted that 18 trials of desmopressin in 1295 patients undergoing cardiac surgery showed a small effect on perioperative blood loss (median decrease, 115 mL).[136] Although desmopressin helps to reduce perioperative bleeding, its effect is too small to influence other, more clinically relevant outcomes such as the need for transfusion and reoperation. Levi and coworkers noted that the number of myocardial infarctions in patients receiving received desmopressin was twice that among patients who received placebo, with no improvement in clinical outcomes.[102] However, another review, evaluating 16 trials of desmopressin in cardiac surgery and in other high-risk operations, showed that the rate of thrombosis did not differ significantly between patients who received desmopressin and patients who received placebo (3.4% versus 2.7%).[144]

Fibrinogen

Fibrinogen is an important and often neglected coagulation factor that plays a major role in producing effective clot in surgical patients. Furthermore, levels represent an important predictor of perioperative bleeding.[83,145] Blome and colleagues reported that the fibrinogen level after CPB was inversely correlated with postoperative chest tube drainage volume, but bleeding was not correlated with platelet count, prothrombin time, or activated partial thromboplastin time.[146] Similarly, after childbirth, decreased fibrinogen levels are reported to adversely affect the severity of postpartum bleeding. During the third trimester of pregnancy, fibrinogen levels are elevated to greater than 400 mg/dL. For each 100 mg/dL decrease in fibrinogen level in parturient women, odds for bleeding were 2.63-fold higher.[147] These clinical data highlight the critical role of fibrinogen in the prevention of excessive bleeding. Adequate plasma levels (about 200 mg/dL) need to be

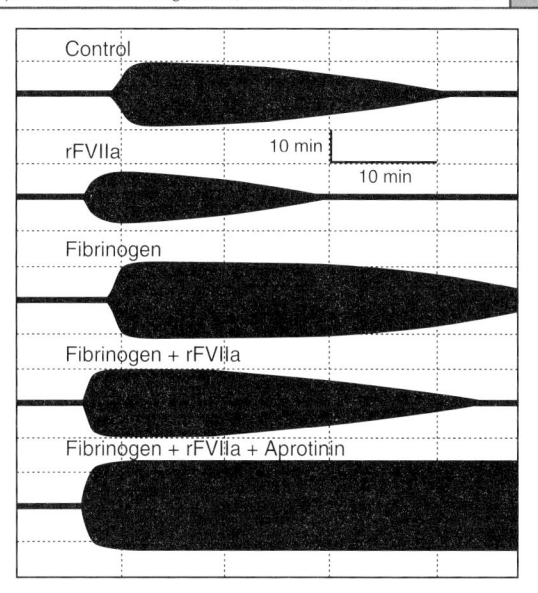

Figure 51-3
Thromboelastography recordings obtained with the ROTEM device after the addition of recombinant factor VIIa (rFVIIa) or fibrinogen in the presence of tissue-type plasminogen activator in plasma. Tissue-type plasminogen activator was added to stimulate fibrinolysis. Final concentration of rFVIIa, 1.5 μg/mL; final concentration of fibrinogen, 100 mg/dL. The maximal clot firmness (the width of the clot tracing) was improved only after the addition of fibrinogen. The onset of clotting was shorter after the addition of rFVIIa, but the extent of lysis (i.e., decreased clot firmness) was increased in contrast to the samples with fibrinogen. Fibrinolysis was observed after the addition of rFVIIa and fibrinogen, and the clot structure was improved after the addition of an antifibrinolytic aprotinin.[148]

achieved before administering other procoagulant interventions (e.g., FVIIa). Fibrinogen can be efficiently repleted by human plasma–derived fibrinogen concentrate (Fig. 51-3); otherwise, fibrinogen-rich cryoprecipitate can be given (one unit per 10 kg increases fibrinogen by 50 to 70 mg/dL). In Europe, fibrinogen concentrates are available and cryoprecipitate is not used.[148]

Recombinant Factor VIIa

Recombinant FVIIa (rFVIIa) is an important example of applying recombinant technology—the synthesizing of large quantities of molecules that are critical for specific biological functions. Although multiple mechanisms for its efficacy have been described, rFVIIa is thought to act locally at the site of tissue and vascular-wall injury by binding to exposed tissue factor, forming small amounts of thrombin that are sufficient to activate platelets.[149] The activated platelet surface can then form a template on which rFVIIa directly or indirectly mediates further activation of coagulation, eventually forming much more thrombin and leading to the conversion of fibrinogen to fibrin.[146,147,150,151] In perioperative patients, rFVIIa is a novel, off-label approach to treating refractory bleeding because it is approved for treating bleeding in patients with hemophilia who had antibodies inactivating factor VIII or IX.[148] Increasing numbers of reports described its use in patients after major hemorrhage from surgery, trauma, or other causes. Recent studies have evaluated rFVIIa for treating spontaneous intracranial hemorrhage.

> **Box 51-4**
> **Rescue Therapy with Off-Label rFVIIa in the Perioperative Setting**
>
> - Severe (1 L/hr) or life-threatening (e.g., central nervous system) bleeding without surgical source of bleeding
> - Marginal response to routine hemostatic therapy (e.g., platelets, fresh-frozen plasma, cryoprecipitate, desmopressin)
> - Judicious use with cerebrovascular disease, disseminated intravascular coagulopathy, or ongoing activation (as with cardiopulmonary bypass)
> - Consider lower dose (30 µg/kg)
> - Patients who have multiple antibodies, or platelets or factors are not available
> - Patients who are hemodynamically unable to tolerate repletion volume

Modified from Levy JH. Transfusion 2008;**48**:31S-8; Goodnough LT, Lublin DM, Zhang L, Despotis G, Eby C. Transfusion 2004;**44**:1325-31; and Despotis G, Avidan M, Lublin DM. Ann Thorac Surg 2005;**80**:3-5.

> **Box 51-5**
> **Topical Hemostatic Agents**
>
> - Gelatin sponge: Gelfoam, purified pork skin gelatin (Jello)
> - Oxidized regenerated cellulose: Surgicel or Oxycel, from (plant-based) alpha-cellulose, in knit or microfibrillar form
> - Microfibrillar collagen: Avitene (collagen derived from bovine skin)
> - Topical thrombin: bovine derived, human, and human recombinant (Recothrom)
> - Fibrin sealants: Tisseel/CoSeal (human fibrinogen, bovine thrombin, aprotinin)

From BleedingWeb.com, with permission.

Controlled clinical trials report that the incidence of thrombotic complications among patients who received rFVIIa was relatively low and similar to that among patients who received placebo.[152] However, most case reports that involve administering rFVIIa as rescue therapy (Box 51-4) include patients who have impaired coagulation, have received multiple transfusions, and are at a high risk for adverse events. The complex role that transfusion therapy has in producing adverse outcomes is increasingly being noted in the literature. A report using the FDA MedWatch database noted thromboembolic events in patients with diseases other than hemophilia in whom rFVIIa was used on an off-label basis, and it included 54% of the events as arterial thrombosis (e.g., stroke or acute myocardial infarction).[153] Venous thromboembolism (mostly, venous thrombosis or pulmonary embolism) occurred in 56% of patients. In 72% of the 50 reported deaths, thromboembolism was considered the probable cause. It is not clear to what extent the clinical conditions requiring the use of rFVIIa may have contributed to the risk of thrombosis.[100] However, Mannucci and Levi noted that rFVIIa has expanded the treatment options for acute hemorrhage in patients with conditions other than hemophilia.[100]

Other major issues about rFVIIa include costs and dosing. Randomized clinical trials are underway to study this agent in various surgical populations. This drug has also seen widespread use in battlefield conditions in Iraq.

Reversal of Vitamin K Antagonist–Associated Coagulopathy

After stopping therapy with vitamin K antagonists, the anticoagulant effect requires days to return to baseline, but it can be more rapidly reversed by agents including vitamin K, FFP, and other, novel pharmacologic therapies. When warfarin therapy needs to be reversed, patients are given vitamin K at doses of 10 to 20 mg orally or intramuscularly, and the prothrombin time is usually reversed in 24 hours if the patient does not have underlying liver disease. Alternatively, in patients requiring urgent surgery, the anticoagulation effects can be reversed by giving FFP, starting with 2 units and then more as required.[8]

Older, critically ill patients with complex diagnoses often receive warfarin and derivative agents for thromboembolic prophylaxis of atrial fibrillation or valvular heart disease. Prohemostatic agents are often needed to urgently reverse the anticoagulant effect of these drugs in the perioperative setting. Treatments available for reversal include vitamin K, FFP, prothrombin complex concentrates (PCCs), and rFVIIa. Warfarin reversal is emerging as a major indication for FFP in tertiary hospitals.[154] PCCs were originally developed for repleting factor IX in hemophilia B, and thus they contain a standardized amount of factor IX along with various amounts of other vitamin K–dependent factors (prothrombin, FVII, factor X, proteins C and S). PCCs are recommended in guidelines as primary treatment for reversal in patients with life-threatening bleeding and an elevated INR, and rFVIIa may be considered as an alternative.[155] Evidence suggests that PCCs offer quicker INR correction than FFP, and better bleeding control; they also have a lower infusion volume and are more readily available without crossmatching.[156-158] Although there are historical concerns regarding potential thrombotic risk with PCCs, present-day PCCs are much improved.[158] Clinical data suggest that the benefits of rFVIIa over FFP may be similar to those of PCCs; however, preclinical comparisons suggest that PCCs are more effective in correcting coagulopathy.[48,158] Although many patients requiring rapid reversal of warfarin are currently treated with FFP, PCC should be considered as an alternative therapy in this setting.

Topical Hemostatic Agents

Topical agents used as adjunctive measures to promote surgical hemostasis include microfibrillar collagen, bovine collagen–based composite mixed with autologous plasma, and fibrin sealants (Box 51-5). Gelatin sponge, or Gelfoam, is purified pork skin gelatin that is intended to augment contact activation and hemostasis. Gelatin substances absorb many times their weight in blood. Gelfoam can be applied dry, directly to the bleeding surface, and pressure applied, or wet in saline. Oxidized regenerated cellulose, also known as Surgicel or Oxycel, is derived from alpha-cellulose and is plant based. Surgicel is in "knit form" and Oxycel comes in a microfibrillar form. These cellulose derivatives are acidic and are thought to cause some small-vessel contraction as well as contact activation, and thus need an intact hemostatic system to work. These agents are applied dry and absorb within

4 to 8 weeks. Microfibrillar collagen (Avitene) is derived from bovine skin. It is commonly used in a light flour form but is also available in a nonwoven web form. This collagen preparation binds avidly to blood surfaces, so a relatively dry field is not necessary to apply it. It causes less swelling than Gelfoam. Like the other agents, it enhances contact activation. Collagen sponges derived from bovine Achilles tendon or bovine skin are similar to Avitene and work the exact way.

The other types of hemostatic agents based on topical thrombin are used alone or in combination. In 1999, FloSeal, an agent that consists of bovine thrombin plus cross-linked gelatin granules mixed together, became available. Fibrin sealants, including Tisseel and CoSeal, are combinations of purified human fibrinogen, bovine or human thrombin, and an antifibrinolytic agent to prevent clot lysis.[159] These agents need a relatively dry field to work. Also, in some institutions, autologous fibrin sealants are created by taking fibrinogen and thrombin from the patient's plasma, or platelet gels are created from the patient's platelets.

A major problem of bovine thrombin is that a patient may produce antibodies that cross-react with thrombin and factor V to produce complications ranging from anaphylaxis to bleeding.[160-166] As a result, human thrombin, both purified and recombinant, has been developed. Human thrombin is available as Evithrom, and recombinant thrombin as Recothrom.[167] Although human thrombin is extensively purified, the label still warns that there is a risk of transmitting infectious agents such as viruses and, theoretically, the Creutzfeldt-Jakob disease agent.

Gelfoam, Surgicel, Avitene, and the collagen sponges can be stored at room temperature and are ready to use. FloSeal requires a 2- to 5-minute preparation time. Fibrin sealants, however, are kept in cold storage and thawed prior to use; preparation time can be 20 or 30 minutes.

SUMMARY

Cardiac surgical patients are at significant risk for bleeding, and some may need a transfusion. Risk factors include advanced age, low preoperative red blood cell volume (preoperative anemia or small body size), use of preoperative antiplatelet or antithrombotic drugs, reoperative or complex procedures, emergency operations, and noncardiac comorbidities. Perioperative interventions can reduce bleeding and the need for transfusion. Evidence-based blood conservation techniques include the following:

- Drugs that increase preoperative blood volume (e.g., erythropoietin) or decrease postoperative bleeding (e.g., antifibrinolytics)
- Devices that conserve blood (e.g., intraoperative blood salvage and blood-sparing techniques), and off-pump CABG surgery
- Interventions that protect the patient's own blood from the stress of operation (e.g., autologous pre-donation and normovolemic hemodilution)
- Institution-specific blood transfusion algorithms supplemented with point-of-care testing

Most important is for institutions to have a multimodality blood conservation program that combines all of these techniques, that is accepted by all health-care providers, and that involves transfusion algorithms to guide decisions.

REFERENCES

1. Despotis GJ, Avidan MS, Hogue Jr CW. Mechanisms and attenuation of hemostatic activation during extracorporeal circulation. *Ann Thorac Surg* 2001;**72**:S1821-31.
2. Levy JH, Tanaka KA, Steiner ME. Evaluation and management of bleeding during cardiac surgery. *Curr Hematol Rep* 2005;**4**:368-72.
3. Levy JH, Despotis GJ. Transfusion and hemostasis in cardiac surgery. *Transfusion* 2008;**48**:1S.
4. Levy JH. Pharmacologic methods to reduce perioperative bleeding. *Transfusion* 2008;**48**:31S-8S.
5. Levy JH. Pharmacologic preservation of the hemostatic system during cardiac surgery. *Ann Thorac Surg* 2001;**72**:S1814-20.
6. Hoffman M, Monroe 3rd DM. A cell-based model of hemostasis. *Thromb Haemost* 2001;**85**:958-65.
7. Despotis GJ, Avidan MS, Hogue Jr CW. Mechanisms and attenuation of hemostatic activation during extracorporeal circulation. *Ann Thorac Surg* 2001;**72**:S1821-31.
8. Despotis GJ, Gravlee G, Filos K, Levy J. Anticoagulation monitoring during cardiac surgery: a review of current and emerging techniques. *Anesthesiology* 1999;**91**:1122-51.
9. Levy JH. Novel intravenous antithrombins. *Am Heart J* 2001;**141**:1043-7.
10. Kishimoto TK, Viswanathan K, Ganguly T, Elankumaran S, Smith S, Pelzer K, et al. Contaminated heparin associated with adverse clinical events and activation of the contact system. *N Engl J Med* 2008;**358**(23):2457-67.
11. Mochizuki T, Olson PJ, Szlam F, Ramsay JG, Levy JH. Protamine reversal of heparin affects platelet aggregation and activated clotting time after cardiopulmonary bypass. *Anesth Analg* 1998;**87**:781-5.
12. Weitz JI. Low-molecular-weight heparins. *N Engl J Med* 1997;**337**:688-98.
13. Weitz JI, Hirsh J. New anticoagulant drugs. *Chest* 2001;**119**:95S-107S.
14. Buller HR, Davidson BL, Decousus H, Gallus A, Gent M, Piovella F, et al. Subcutaneous fondaparinux versus intravenous unfractionated heparin in the initial treatment of pulmonary embolism. *N Engl J Med* 2003;**349**:1695-702.
15. Mehta SR, Granger CB, Eikelboom JW, Bassand JP, Wallentin L, Faxon DP, et al. Efficacy and safety of fondaparinux versus enoxaparin in patients with acute coronary syndromes undergoing percutaneous coronary intervention: results from the OASIS-5 trial. *J Am Coll Cardiol* 2007;**50**:1742-51.
16. Eikelboom JW, Weitz JI. A replacement for warfarin: the search continues. *Circulation* 2007;**116**:131-3.
17. Warkentin TE. Heparin-induced thrombocytopenia: pathogenesis and management. *Br J Haematol* 2003;**121**:535-55.
18. Levy JH, Tanaka KA, Hursting MJ. Reducing thrombotic complications in the perioperative setting: an update on heparin-induced thrombocytopenia. *Anesth Analg* 2007;**105**:570-82.
19. Warkentin TE, Greinacher A. Heparin-induced thrombocytopenia: recognition, treatment, and prevention: the Seventh ACCP Conference on Antithrombotic and Thrombolytic Therapy. *Chest* 2004;**126**:311S-37S.
20. Bennett-Guerrero E, Slaughter TF, White WD, Welsby IJ, Greenberg CS, El-Moalem H, Ortel TL. Preoperative anti-PF4/heparin antibody level predicts adverse outcome after cardiac surgery. *J Thorac Cardiovasc Surg* 2005;**130**:1567-72.
21. Dyke CM, Koster A, Veale JJ, Maier GW, McNiff T, Levy JH. Preemptive use of bivalirudin for urgent on-pump coronary artery bypass grafting in patients with potential heparin-induced thrombocytopenia. *Ann Thorac Surg* 2005;**80**:299-303.
22. Merry AF, Raudkivi PJ, Middleton NG, McDougall JM, Nand P, Mills BP, et al. Bivalirudin versus heparin and protamine in off-pump coronary artery bypass surgery. *Ann Thorac Surg* 2004;**77**:925-31:discussion 931.
23. Schneider DJ, Sobel BE. Conundrums in the combined use of anticoagulants and antiplatelet drugs. *Circulation* 2007;**116**:305-15.
24. Ferraris VA, Ferraris SP, Saha SP, Hessel 2nd EA, Haan CK, Royston BD, et al. Perioperative blood transfusion and blood conservation in cardiac surgery: the Society of Thoracic Surgeons and The Society of Cardiovascular Anesthesiologists clinical practice guideline. *Ann Thorac Surg* 2007;**83**:S27-86.
25. Ferraris VA, Gildengorin V. Predictors of excessive blood use after coronary artery bypass grafting: a multivariate analysis. *J Thorac Cardiovasc Surg* 1989;**98**:492-7.
26. Pothula S, Sanchala VT, Nagappala B, Inchiosa Jr MA. The effect of preoperative antiplatelet/anticoagulant prophylaxis on postoperative blood loss in cardiac surgery. *Anesth Analg* 2004;**98**:4-10.
27. Yende S, Wunderink RG. Effect of clopidogrel on bleeding after coronary artery bypass surgery. *Crit Care Med* 2001;**29**:2271-5.
28. Hongo RH, Ley J, Dick SE, Yee RR. The effect of clopidogrel in combination with aspirin when given before coronary artery bypass grafting. *J Am Coll Cardiol* 2002;**40**:231-7.

29. Ray JG, Deniz S, Olivieri A, Pollex E, Vermeulen MJ, Alexander KS, et al. Increased blood product use among coronary artery bypass patients prescribed preoperative aspirin and clopidogrel. *BMC Cardiovasc Disord* 2003;**3**:3.
30. Braunwald E, Antman EM, Beasley JW, Califf RM, Cheitlin MD, Hochman JS, et al. ACC/AHA 2002 guideline update for the management of patients with unstable angina and non-ST-segment elevation myocardial infarction—summary article: a report of the American College of Cardiology/American Heart Association task force on practice guidelines (Committee on the Management of Patients With Unstable Angina). *J Am Coll Cardiol* 2002;**40**:1366-74.
31. Levy JH, Smith PK. Platelet inhibitors and cardiac surgery. *Ann Thorac Surg* 2000;**70**:S1-2.
32. Despotis GJ, Skubas NJ, Goodnough LT. Optimal management of bleeding and transfusion in patients undergoing cardiac surgery. *Semin Thorac Cardiovasc Surg* 1999;**11**:84-104.
33. Avidan MS, Alcock EL, Da Fonseca J, Ponte J, Desai JB, Despotis GJ, Hunt BJ. Comparison of structured use of routine laboratory tests or near-patient assessment with clinical judgement in the management of bleeding after cardiac surgery. *Br J Anaesth* 2004;**92**:178-86.
34. Ferraris VA, Ferraris SP, Joseph O, Wehner P, Mentzer Jr RM. Aspirin and postoperative bleeding after coronary artery bypass grafting. *Ann Surg* 2002;**235**:820-7.
35. Ott E, Mazer CD, Tudor IC, Shore-Lesserson L, Snyder-Ramos SA, Finegan BA, et al. Coronary artery bypass graft surgery—care globalization: the impact of national care on fatal and nonfatal outcome. *J Thorac Cardiovasc Surg* 2007;**133**:1242-51.
36. Munoz JJ, Birkmeyer NJ, Dacey LJ, Birkmeyer JD, Charlesworth DC, Johnson ER, et al. Trends in rates of reexploration for hemorrhage after coronary artery bypass surgery. Northern New England Cardiovascular Disease Study Group. *Ann Thorac Surg* 1999;**68**:1321-5.
37. Stover EP, Siegel LC, Parks R, Levin J, Body SC, Maddi R, et al. Variability in transfusion practice for coronary artery bypass surgery persists despite national consensus guidelines: a 24-institution study. Institutions of the Multicenter Study of Perioperative Ischemia Research Group. *Anesthesiology* 1998;**88**:327-33.
38. Johnson RG, Thurer RL, Kruskall MS, Sirois C, Gervino EV, Critchlow J, Weintraub RM. Comparison of two transfusion strategies after elective operations for myocardial revascularization. *J Thorac Cardiovasc Surg* 1992;**104**:307-14.
39. Moskowitz DM, Klein JJ, Shander A, Cousineau KM, Goldweit RS, Bodian C, et al. Predictors of transfusion requirements for cardiac surgical procedures at a blood conservation center. *Ann Thorac Surg* 2004;**77**:626-34.
40. Karkouti K, Cohen MM, McCluskey SA, Sher GD. A multivariable model for predicting the need for blood transfusion in patients undergoing first-time elective coronary bypass graft surgery. *Transfusion* 2001;**41**:1193-203.
41. Karkouti K, Wijeysundera DN, Yau TM, Beattie WS, Abdelnaem E, McCluskey SA, et al. The independent association of massive blood loss with mortality in cardiac surgery. *Transfusion* 2004;**44**:1453-62.
42. Despotis GJ, Filos KS, Zoys TN, Hogue Jr CW, Spitznagel E, Lappas DG. Factors associated with excessive postoperative blood loss and hemostatic transfusion requirements: a multivariate analysis in cardiac surgical patients. *Anesth Analg* 1996;**82**:13-21.
43. Wijeysundera DN, Beattie WS, Djaiani G, Rao V, Borger MA, Karkouti K, Cusimano RJ. Off-pump coronary artery surgery for reducing mortality and morbidity: meta-analysis of randomized and observational studies. *J Am Coll Cardiol* 2005;**46**:872-82.
44. Cheng DC, Bainbridge D, Martin JE, Novick RJ. Does off-pump coronary artery bypass reduce mortality, morbidity, and resource utilization when compared with conventional coronary artery bypass? A meta-analysis of randomized trials. *Anesthesiology* 2005;**102**:188-203.
45. Dietrich W, Dilthey G, Spannagl M, Richter JA. Warfarin pretreatment does not lead to increased bleeding tendency during cardiac surgery. *J Cardiothorac Vasc Anesth* 1995;**9**:250-4.
46. Goodnough LT, Despotis GJ, Hogue Jr CW, Ferguson Jr TB. On the need for improved transfusion indicators in cardiac surgery. *Ann Thorac Surg* 1995;**60**:473-80.
47. Unsworth-White MJ, Herriot A, Valencia O, Poloniecki J, Smith EE, Murday AJ, et al. Resternotomy for bleeding after cardiac operation: a marker for increased morbidity and mortality. *Ann Thorac Surg* 1995;**59**:664-7.
48. Moulton MJ, Creswell LL, Mackey ME, Cox JL, Rosenbloom M. Reexploration for bleeding is a risk factor for adverse outcomes after cardiac operations. *J Thorac Cardiovasc Surg* 1996;**111**:1037-46.
49. Dacey LJ, Munoz JJ, Baribeau YR, Johnson ER, Lahey SJ, Leavitt BJ, et al. Reexploration for hemorrhage following coronary artery bypass grafting: incidence and risk factors. Northern New England Cardiovascular Disease Study Group. *Arch Surg* 1998;**133**:442-7.
50. Nuttall GA, Oliver WC, Santrach PJ, Bryant S, Dearani JA, Schaff HV, Ereth MH. Efficacy of a simple intraoperative transfusion algorithm for nonerythrocyte component utilization after cardiopulmonary bypass. *Anesthesiology* 2001;**94**:773-81:discussion 5A-6A.
51. Avidan MS, Alcock EL, Da Fonseca J, Ponte J, Desai JB, Despotis GJ, Hunt BJ. Comparison of structured use of routine laboratory tests or near-patient assessment with clinical judgement in the management of bleeding after cardiac surgery. *Br J Anaesth* 2004;**92**:178-86.
52. Despotis GJ, Grishaber JE, Goodnough LT. The effect of an intraoperative treatment algorithm on physicians' transfusion practice in cardiac surgery. *Transfusion* 1994;**34**:290-6.
53. Shore-Lesserson L, Manspeizer HE, DePerio M, Francis S, Vela-Cantos F, Ergin MA. Thromboelastography-guided transfusion algorithm reduces transfusions in complex cardiac surgery. *Anesth Analg* 1999;**88**:312-9.
54. Practice Guidelines for Blood Component Therapy. A Report by the American Society of Anesthesiologists Task Force on Blood Component Therapy. *Anesthesiology* 1994;**84**:732-47.
55. Practice guidelines for perioperative blood transfusion and adjuvant therapies. an updated report by the American Society of Anesthesiologists Task Force on Perioperative Blood Transfusion and Adjuvant Therapies. *Anesthesiology* 2006;**105**:198-208.
56. Koch CG, Li L, Sessler DI, Figueroa P, Hoeltge GA, Mihaljevic T, Blackstone EH. Duration of red-cell storage and complications after cardiac surgery. *N Engl J Med* 2008;**358**:1229-39.
57. Koch CG, Li L, Van Wagoner DR, Duncan AI, Gillinov AM, Blackstone EH. Red cell transfusion is associated with an increased risk for postoperative atrial fibrillation. *Ann Thorac Surg* 2006;**82**:1747-56.
58. Koch CG, Khandwala F, Li L, Estafanos FG, Loop FD, Blackstone EH. Persistent effect of red cell transfusion on health-related quality of life after cardiac surgery. *Ann Thorac Surg* 2006;**82**:13-20.
59. Downes KA, Wilson E, Yomtovian R, Sarode R. Serial measurement of clotting factors in thawed plasma stored for 5 days. *Transfusion* 2001;**41**:570.
60. Leslie SD, Toy PT. Laboratory hemostatic abnormalities in massively transfused patients given red blood cells and crystalloid. *Am J Clin Pathol* 1991;**96**:770-3.
61. Hardy JF, de Moerloose P, Samama CM. Massive transfusion and coagulopathy: pathophysiology and implications for clinical management. *Can J Anaesth* 2006;**53**:S40-58.
62. Karkouti K, O'Farrell R, Yau TM, Beattie WS. Prediction of massive blood transfusion in cardiac surgery. *Can J Anaesth* 2006;**53**:781-94.
63. Schreiber MA, Perkins J, Kiraly L, Underwood S, Wade C, Holcomb JB. Early predictors of massive transfusion in combat casualties. *J Am Coll Surg* 2007;**205**:541-5.
64. McLaughlin DF, Niles SE, Salinas J, Perkins JG, Cox ED, Wade CE, Holcomb JB. A predictive model for massive transfusion in combat casualty patients. *J Trauma* 2008;**64**:S57-63:discussion S63.
65. Perkins JG, Schreiber MA, Wade CE, Holcomb JB. Early versus late recombinant factor VIIa in combat trauma patients requiring massive transfusion. *J Trauma* 2007;**62**:1099-101:1095-9; discussion.
66. Sheppard CA, Logdberg LE, Zimring JC, Hillyer CD. Transfusion-related acute lung injury. *Hematol Oncol Clin North Am* 2007;**21**:163-76.
67. Spiess BD. Risks of transfusion: outcome focus. *Transfusion* 2004;**44**:4S-14S.
68. Despotis GJ, Zhang L, Lublin DM. Transfusion risks and transfusion-related pro-inflammatory responses. *Hematol Oncol Clin North Am* 2007;**21**:147-61.
69. Spiess BD, Royston D, Levy JH, Fitch J, Dietrich W, Body S, et al. Platelet transfusions during coronary artery bypass graft surgery are associated with serious adverse outcomes. *Transfusion* 2004;**44**:1143-8.
70. Cicala C, Cirino G. Linkage between inflammation and coagulation: an update on the molecular basis of the crosstalk. *Life Sci* 1998;**62**:1817-24.
71. Ferrer F, Rivera J, Corral J, Gonzalez-Conejero R, Lozano ML, Vicente V. Evaluation of pooled platelet concentrates using prestorage versus poststorage WBC reduction: impact of filtration timing. *Transfusion* 2000;**40**:781-8.
72. van de Watering L, Brand A. Independent association of massive blood loss with mortality in cardiac surgery. *Transfusion* 2005;**45**:1235-6:1235; author reply.
73. Moison RM, Bloemhof FE, Geerdink JA, de Beaufort AJ, Berger HM. The capacity of different infusion fluids to lower the prooxidant activity of plasma iron: an important factor in resuscitation? *Transfusion* 2000;**40**:1346-51.
74. Blumberg N, Heal JM, Hicks Jr GL, Risher WH. Association of ABO-mismatched platelet transfusions with morbidity and mortality in cardiac surgery. *Transfusion* 2001;**41**:790-3.
75. Goldman M, Webert KE, Arnold DM, Freedman J, Hannon J, Blajchman MA. TRALI Consensus Panel. Proceedings of a consensus conference: towards an understanding of TRALI. *Transfusion Med Rev* 2005;**19**:2-31.

76. Moore SB. Transfusion-related acute lung injury (TRALI): clinical presentation, treatment, and prognosis. *Crit Care Med* 2006;**34**:S114-7.
77. Kleinman S. A perspective on transfusion-related acute lung injury two years after the Canadian Consensus Conference. *Transfusion* 2006;**46**:1465-8.
78. Mair DC, Hirschler N, Eastlund T. Blood donor and component management strategies to prevent transfusion-related acute lung injury (TRALI). *Crit Care Med* 2006;**34**:S137-43.
79. Silliman CC, Ambruso DR, Boshkov LK. Transfusion-related acute lung injury. *Blood* 2005;**105**:2266-73.
80. Levy JH, Adkinson Jr NF. Anaphylaxis during cardiac surgery: implications for clinicians. *Anesth Analg* 2008;**106**:392-403.
81. Silliman CC, Kelher M. The role of endothelial activation in the pathogenesis of transfusion-related acute lung injury. *Transfusion* 2005;**45**:109S-16S.
82. Spiess BD. Transfusion of blood products affects outcome in cardiac surgery. *Semin Cardiothorac Vasc Anesth* 2004;**8**:267-81.
83. Levy JH. Massive transfusion coagulopathy. *Semin Hematol* 2006;**43**:S59-63.
84. Levy JH, Tanaka KA. Inflammatory response to cardiopulmonary bypass. *Ann Thorac Surg* 2003;**75**:S715-20.
85. Paparella D, Brister SJ, Buchanan MR. Coagulation disorders of cardiopulmonary bypass: a review. *Intensive Care Med* 2004;**30**:1873-81.
86. Eaton MP. Antifibrinolytic therapy in surgery for congenital heart disease. *Anesth Analg* 2008;**106**:1087-100.
87. Munoz JJ, Birkmeyer NJ, Birkmeyer JD, O'Connor GT, Dacey LJ. Is epsilon-aminocaproic acid as effective as aprotinin in reducing bleeding with cardiac surgery? A meta-analysis. *Circulation* 1999;**99**:81-9.
88. Sedrakyan A, Treasure T, Elefteriades JA. Effect of aprotinin on clinical outcomes in coronary artery bypass graft surgery: a systematic review and meta-analysis of randomized clinical trials. *J Thorac Cardiovasc Surg* 2004;**128**:442-8.
89. Karkouti K, Beattie WS, Dattilo KM, McCluskey SA, Ghannam M, Hamdy A, et al. A propensity score case-control comparison of aprotinin and tranexamic acid in high-transfusion-risk cardiac surgery. *Transfusion* 2006;**46**:327-38.
90. Mangano DT, Tudor IC, Dietzel C. The risk associated with aprotinin in cardiac surgery. *N Engl J Med* 2006;**354**:353-65.
91. Levi M, Cromheecke ME, de Jonge E, Prins MH, de Mol BJ, Briet E, Buller HR. Pharmacological strategies to decrease excessive blood loss in cardiac surgery: a meta-analysis of clinically relevant endpoints. *Lancet* 1999;**354**:1940-7.
92. Henry DA, Moxey AJ, Carless PA, O'Connell D, McClelland B, Henderson KM, et al. Anti-fibrinolytic use for minimising perioperative allogeneic blood transfusion. *Cochrane Database Syst Rev* 2001(4):CD001886.
93. Bulutcu FS, Ozbek U, Polat B, Yalcin Y, Karaci AR, Bayindir O. Which may be effective to reduce blood loss after cardiac operations in cyanotic children: tranexamic acid, aprotinin or a combination? *Paediatr Anaesth* 2005;**15**:41-6.
94. Chauhan S, Kumar BA, Rao BH, Rao MS, Dubey B, Saxena N, Venugopal P. Efficacy of aprotinin, epsilon aminocaproic acid, or combination in cyanotic heart disease. *Ann Thorac Surg* 2000;**70**:1308-12.
95. Rao BH, Saxena N, Chauhan S, Bisoi AK, Venugopal P. Epsilon aminocaproic acid in paediatric cardiac surgery to reduce postoperative blood loss. *Indian J Med Res* 2000;**111**:57-61.
96. Chauhan S, Bisoi A, Kumar N, Mittal D, Kale S, Kiran U, Venugopal P. Dose comparison of tranexamic acid in pediatric cardiac surgery. *Asian Cardiovasc Thorac Ann* 2004;**12**:121-4.
97. Chauhan S, Bisoi A, Modi R, Gharde P, Rajesh MR. Tranexamic acid in paediatric cardiac surgery. *Indian J Med Res* 2003;**118**:86-9.
98. Chauhan S, Das SN, Bisoi A, Kale S, Kiran U. Comparison of epsilon aminocaproic acid and tranexamic acid in pediatric cardiac surgery. *J Cardiothorac Vasc Anesth* 2004;**18**:141-3.
99. Levy JH. Hemostatic agents. *Transfusion* 2004;**44**:58S-62.
100. Mannucci PM, Levi M. Prevention and treatment of major blood loss. *N Engl J Med* 2007;**356**:2301-11.
101. Royston D, Chhatwani A. Safety aspects of aprotinin therapy in cardiac surgery patients. *Expert Opin Drug Saf* 2006;**5**:539-52.
102. Levi M, Cromheecke ME, de Jonge E, Prins MH, de Mol BJ, Briet E, Buller HR. Pharmacological strategies to decrease excessive blood loss in cardiac surgery: a meta-analysis of clinically relevant endpoints. *Lancet* 1999;**354**:1940-7.
103. Sedrakyan A, Treasure T, Elefteriades JA. Effect of aprotinin on clinical outcomes in coronary artery bypass graft surgery: a systematic review and meta-analysis of randomized clinical trials. *J Thorac Cardiovasc Surg* 2004;**128**:442-8.
104. Bidstrup BP, Underwood SR, Sapsford RN, Streets EM. Effect of aprotinin (Trasylol) on aorta-coronary bypass graft patency. *J Thorac Cardiovasc Surg* 1993;**105**:147-52:discussion 153.
105. Havel M, Grabenwoger F, Schneider J, Laufer G, Wollenek G, Owen A, et al. Aprotinin does not decrease early graft patency after coronary artery bypass grafting despite reducing postoperative bleeding and use of donated blood. *J Thorac Cardiovasc Surg* 1994;**107**:807-10.
106. Lemmer Jr JH, Stanford W, Bonney SL, Breen JF, Chomka EV, Eldredge WJ, et al. Aprotinin for coronary bypass operations: efficacy, safety, and influence on early saphenous vein graft patency—a multicenter, randomized, double-blind, placebo-controlled study. *J Thorac Cardiovasc Surg* 1994;**107**:551-3:543-51; discussion.
107. Alderman EL, Levy JH, Rich JB, Nili M, Vidne B, Schaff H, et al. Analyses of coronary graft patency after aprotinin use: results from the International Multicenter Aprotinin Graft Patency Experience (IMAGE) trial.[see comment]. *J Thorac Cardiovasc Surg* 1998;**116**:716-30.
108. Boldt J, Knothe C, Zickmann B, Wege N, Dapper F, Hempelmann G. Aprotinin in pediatric cardiac operations: platelet function, blood loss, and use of homologous blood. *Ann Thorac Surg* 1993;**55**:1460-6.
109. Boldt J, Knothe C, Zickmann B, Wege N, Dapper F, Hempelmann G. Comparison of two aprotinin dosage regiments in pediatric patients having cardiac operations. *J Thorac Cardiovasc Surg* 1993;**105**:705-11.
110. Boldt J, Zickmann B, Schindler E, Welters A, Dapper F, Hempelmann G. Influence of aprotinin on the thrombomodulin/protein C system in pediatric cardiac operations. *J Thorac Cardiovasc Surg* 1994;**107**:1215-21.
111. Davies MJ, Allen A, Kort H, Weerasena NA, Rocco D, Paul CL, et al. Prospective, randomized, double-blind study of high-dose aprotinin in pediatric cardiac operations. *Ann Thorac Surg* 1997;**63**:497-503.
112. D'Errico CC, Shayevitz JR, Martindale SJ, Mosca RS, Bove EL. The efficacy and cost of aprotinin in children undergoing reoperative open heart surgery. *Anesth Analg* 1996;**83**:1193-9.
113. Dietrich W, Mossinger H, Spannagl M, Jochum M, Wendt P, Barankay A, et al. Hemostatic activation during cardiopulmonary bypass with different aprotinin dosages in pediatric patients having cardiac operations. *J Thorac Cardiovasc Surg* 1993;**105**:712-20.
114. Herynkopf F, Lucchese F, Pereira E, Kalil R, Prates P, Nesralla IA. Aprotinin in children undergoing correction of congenital heart defects: a double-blind pilot study. *J Thorac Cardiovasc Surg* 1994;**108**:517-21.
115. Huang H, Ding W, Su Z, Zhang W. Mechanism of the preserving effect of aprotinin on platelet function and its use in cardiac surgery. *J Thorac Cardiovasc Surg* 1993;**106**:11-8.
116. Miller BE, Tosone SR, Tam VK, Kanter KR, Guzzetta NA, Bailey JM, Levy JH. Hematologic and economic impact of aprotinin in reoperative pediatric cardiac operations. *Ann Thorac Surg* 1998;**66**:535-40:discussion 541.
117. Seghaye CM, Duchateau J, Grabitz GR, Jablonka K, Wenzl T, Marcus C, et al. Influence of low-dose aprotinin on the inflammatory reaction due to cardiopulmonary bypass in children. *Ann Thorac Surg* 1996;**61**:1205-11.
118. Mossinger H, Dietrich W, Braun SL, Jochum M, Meisner H, Richter JA. High-dose aprotinin reduces activation of hemostasis, allogeneic blood requirement, and duration of postoperative ventilation in pediatric cardiac surgery. *Ann Thorac Surg* 2003;**75**:430-7.
119. Wippermann CF, Schmid FX, Eberle B, Huth RG, Kampmann C, Schranz D, Oelert H. Reduced inotropic support after aprotinin therapy during pediatric cardiac operations. *Ann Thorac Surg* 1999;**67**:173-6.
120. Carrel TP, Schwanda M, Vogt PR, Turina MI. Aprotinin in pediatric cardiac operations: a benefit in complex malformations and with high-dose regimen only. *Ann Thorac Surg* 1998;**66**:153-8.
121. Beierlein W, Scheule AM, Dietrich W, Ziemer G. Forty years of clinical aprotinin use: a review of 124 hypersensitivity reactions. *Ann Thorac Surg* 2005;**79**:741-8.
122. Dietrich W, Spath P, Ebell A, Richter JA. Prevalence of anaphylactic reactions to aprotinin: analysis of two hundred forty-eight reexposures to aprotinin in heart operations. *J Thorac Cardiovasc Surg* 1997;**113**:194-201.
123. Dietrich W, Spath P, Zuhlsdorf M, Dalichau H, Kirchhoff PG, Kuppe H, et al. Anaphylactic reactions to aprotinin reexposure in cardiac surgery: relation to antiaprotinin immunoglobulin G and E antibodies. *Anesthesiology* 2001;**95**:64-71.
124. Jaquiss RD, Huddleston CB, Spray TL. Use of aprotinin in pediatric lung transplantation. *J Heart Lung Transplant* 1995;**14**:302-7.
125. Lemmer Jr JH, Stanford W, Bonney SL, Chomka EV, Karp RB, Laub GW, et al. Aprotinin for coronary artery bypass grafting: effect on postoperative renal function. *Ann Thorac Surg* 1995;**59**:132-6.
126. Mangano DT, Miao Y, Vuylsteke A, Tudor IC, Juneja R, Filipescu D, et al. Mortality associated with aprotinin during 5 years following coronary artery bypass graft surgery. *JAMA* 2007;**297**:471-9.
127. Schneeweiss S, Seeger JD, Landon J, Walker AM. Aprotinin during coronary-artery bypass grafting and risk of death. *N Engl J Med* 2008;**358**:771-83.
128. Shaw AD, Stafford-Smith M, White WD, Phillips-Bute B, Swaminathan M, Milano C, et al. The effect of aprotinin on outcome after coronary-artery bypass grafting. *N Engl J Med* 2008;**358**:784-93.

129. Fergusson DA, Hebert PC, Mazer CD, Fremes S, MacAdams C, Murkin JM, et al. A comparison of aprotinin and lysine analogues in high-risk cardiac surgery. *N Engl J Med* 2008;**358**:2319-31.
130. Levy JH, Adkinson Jr NF. Anaphylaxis during cardiac surgery: implications for clinicians. *Anesth Analg* 2008;**106**(2):392-403.
131. Stewart WJ, McSweeney SM, Kellett MA, Faxon DP, Ryan TJ. Increased risk of severe protamine reactions in NPH insulin-dependent diabetics undergoing cardiac catheterization. *Circulation* 1984;**70**:788-92.
132. Levy JH, Zaidan JR, Faraj B. Prospective evaluation of risk of protamine reactions in patients with NPH insulin-dependent diabetes. *Anesth Analg* 1986;**65**:739-42.
133. Levy JH, Schwieger IM, Zaidan JR, Faraj BA, Weintraub WS. Evaluation of patients at risk for protamine reactions. *J Thorac Cardiovasc Surg* 1989;**98**:200-4.
134. Mannucci PM. Treatment of von Willebrand's disease. *N Engl J Med* 2004;**351**:683-94.
135. Mannucci PM. *Hemostatic drugs. N Engl J Med* 1998;**339**:245-53.
136. Mannucci PM. Desmopressin (DDAVP) in the treatment of bleeding disorders: the first 20 years. *Blood* 1997;**90**:2515-21.
137. Federici AB, Mannucci PM. Management of inherited von Willebrand disease in 2007. *Ann Med* 2007;**39**:346-58.
138. Frankville DD, Harper GB, Lake CL, Johns RA. Hemodynamic consequences of desmopressin administration after cardiopulmonary bypass. *Anesthesiology* 1991;**74**:988-96.
139. Rocha E, Llorens R, Paramo JA, Arcas R, Cuesta B, Trenor AM. Does desmopressin acetate reduce blood loss after surgery in patients on cardiopulmonary bypass? *Circulation* 1988;**77**:1319-23.
140. Salzman EW, Weinstein MJ, Reilly D, Ware JA. Adventures in hemostasis: desmopressin in cardiac surgery. *Arch Surg* 1993;**128**:212-7.
141. Salzman EW, Weinstein MJ, Weintraub RM, Ware JA, Thurer RL, Robertson L, et al. Treatment with desmopressin acetate to reduce blood loss after cardiac surgery: a double-blind randomized trial. *N Engl J Med* 1986;**314**:1402-6.
142. Weinstein M, Ware JA, Troll J, Salzman E. Changes in von Willebrand factor during cardiac surgery: effect of desmopressin acetate. *Blood* 1988;**71**:1648-55.
143. de Prost D, Barbier-Boehm G, Hazebroucq J, Ibrahim H, Bielsky MC, Hvass U, et al. Desmopressin has no beneficial effect on excessive postoperative bleeding or blood product requirements associated with cardiopulmonary bypass. *Thromb Haemost* 1992;**68**:106-10.
144. Mannucci PM, Carlsson S, Harris AS. Desmopressin, surgery and thrombosis. *Thromb Haemost* 1994;**71**:154-5.
145. Nielsen VG, Levy JH. Fibrinogen and bleeding: old molecule, new ideas. *Anesth Analg* 2007;**105**:902-3.
146. Blome M, Isgro F, Kiessling AH, Skuras J, Haubelt H, Hellstern P, Saggau W. Relationship between factor XIII activity, fibrinogen, haemostasis screening tests and postoperative bleeding in cardiopulmonary bypass surgery. *Thromb Haemost* 2005;**93**:1101-7.
147. Charbit B, Mandelbrot L, Samain E, Baron G, Haddaoui B, Keita H, et al. The decrease of fibrinogen is an early predictor of the severity of postpartum hemorrhage. *J Thromb Haemost* 2007;**5**:266-73.
148. Tanaka KA, taketomi T, Szlam F, Calatzis A, Levy JH. Improved clot formation by combined administration of activated factor VII (Novo Seven) and fibrinogen (Haemo complettan P). *Anesth Analg* 2008;**106**:732-8.
149. Roberts HR, Monroe DM, White GC. The use of recombinant factor VIIa in the treatment of bleeding disorders. *Blood* 2004;**104**:3858-64.
150. ten Cate H, Bauer KA, Levi M, Edgington TS, Sublett RD, Barzegar S, et al. The activation of factor X and prothrombin by recombinant factor VIIa in vivo is mediated by tissue factor. *J Clin Invest* 1993;**92**:1207-12.
151. Butenas S, Brummel KE, Branda RF, Paradis SG, Mann KG. Mechanism of factor VIIa-dependent coagulation in hemophilia blood. *Blood* 2002;**99**:923-30.
152. Levy JH, Fingerhut A, Brott T, Langbakke IH, Erhardtsen E, Porte RJ. Recombinant factor VIIa in patients with coagulopathy secondary to anticoagulant therapy, cirrhosis, or severe traumatic injury: review of safety profile. *Transfusion* 2006;**46**:919-33.
153. O'Connell KA, Wood JJ, Wise RP, Lozier JN, Braun MM. Thromboembolic adverse events after use of recombinant human coagulation factor VIIa. *JAMA* 2006;**295**:293-8.
154. Ozgonenel B, O'Malley B, Krishen P, Eisenbrey AB. Warfarin reversal emerging as the major indication for fresh frozen plasma use at a tertiary care hospital. *Am J Hematol* 2007;**82**:1091-4.
155. Dager WE, King JH, Regalia RC, Williamson D, Gosselin RC, White RH, et al. Reversal of elevated international normalized ratios and bleeding with low-dose recombinant activated factor VII in patients receiving warfarin. *Pharmacotherapy* 2006;**26**:1091-8.
156. Lankiewicz MW, Hays J, Friedman KD, Tinkoff G, Blatt PM. Urgent reversal of warfarin with prothrombin complex concentrate. *J Thromb Haemost* 2006;**4**:967-70.
157. Kessler CM. Urgent reversal of warfarin with prothrombin complex concentrate: where are the evidence-based data? *J Thromb Haemost* 2006;**4**:963-6.
158. Dickneite G. Prothrombin complex concentrate versus recombinant factor VIIa for reversal of coumarin anticoagulation. *Thromb Res* 2007;**119**:643-51.
159. Schenk 3rd WG, Burks SG, Gagne PJ, Kagan SA, Lawson JH, Spotnitz WD. Fibrin sealant improves hemostasis in peripheral vascular surgery: a randomized prospective trial. *Ann Surg* 2003;**237**:871-6:discussion 876.
160. Ortel TL, Mercer MC, Thames EH, Moore KD, Lawson JH. Immunologic impact and clinical outcomes after surgical exposure to bovine thrombin. *Ann Surg* 2001;**233**:88-96.
161. Lawson JH, Lynn KA, Vanmatre RM, Domzalski T, Klemp KF, Ortel TL, et al. Antihuman factor V antibodies after use of relatively pure bovine thrombin. *Ann Thorac Surg* 2005;**79**:1037-8.
162. Lawson JH. The clinical use and immunologic impact of thrombin in surgery. *Semin Thromb Hemost* 2006;**1**(32 Suppl):98-110.
163. Pope M, Johnston KW. Anaphylaxis after thrombin injection of a femoral pseudoaneurysm: recommendations for prevention. *J Vasc Surg* 2000;**32**:190-1.
164. Rothenberg DM, Moy JN. Anaphylactic reaction to topical bovine thrombin. *Anesthesiology* 1993;**78**:779-82.
165. Tadokoro K, Ohtoshi T, Takafuji S, Nakajima K, Suzuki S, Yamamoto K, et al. Topical thrombin-induced IgE-mediated anaphylaxis: RAST analysis and skin test studies. *J Allergy Clin Immunol* 1991;**88**:620-9.
166. Wai Y, Tsui V, Peng Z, Richardson R, Oreopoulos D, Tarlo SM. Anaphylaxis from topical bovine thrombin (Thrombostat) during haemodialysis and evaluation of sensitization among a dialysis population. *Clin Exp Allergy* 2003;**33**:1730-4.
167. Chapman WC, Lockstadt H, Singla N, Kafie FE, Lawson JH. Phase 2, randomized, double-blind, placebo-controlled, multicenter clinical evaluation of recombinant human thrombin in multiple surgical indications. *J Thromb Haemost* 2006;**4**:2083-5.
168. Goodnough LT, Lublin DM, Zhang L, Despotis G, Eby C. Transfusion medicine service policies for recombinant factor VIIa administration. *Transfusion* 2004;**44**:1325-31.
169. Despotis G, Avidan M, Lublin DM. Off-label use of recombinant factor VIIA concentrates after cardiac surgery. *Ann Thorac Surg* 2005;**80**:3-5.

B. Diagnostic Procedures

CHAPTER 52

Coronary Angiography: Valve and Hemodynamic Assessment

Yuri B. Pride and Lawrence A. Garcia

Diagnostic Catheterization Techniques
  Indications
  Contraindications
  Complications
Angiography
  Left Coronary Angiography
  Right Coronary Angiography
  Coronary Anomalies
  Angiographic Projections
    Left Main Coronary Artery
    Left Anterior Descending and Diagonal Arteries
    Left Circumflex Artery

    Right Coronary Artery
    Graft Angiography
Hemodynamics
  Principles
  Right Heart Catheterization
  Pressure Waveforms
    Right Atrium
    Right Ventricle
    Pulmonary Artery
    Pulmonary Capillary Wedge Pressure (Left Atrium)
    Systemic Arterial Pressure
  Cardiac Output

Shunts
  Left-to-Right Shunts
  Right-to-Left Shunts
  Bidirectional Shunts
Assessment of Vascular Resistance
Valve Assessment
  Aortic Stenosis
  Aortic Regurgitation
  Mitral Stenosis
  Mitral Regurgitation
  Pericardial Disease

After the first intravascular catheter was placed by Forsmann in the 1920s,[1] techniques to achieve vascular access developed rapidly. Sones and coworkers performed the first selective diagnostic coronary catheterization in 1956.[2,3] In 1977, Grüntzig performed the first coronary angioplasty.[4,5] Angioplasty and the placement of intravascular stents has now become the predominant form of catheter-based intervention in all major vascular beds.

Coronary artery disease (CAD) is the leading cause of death in the United States,[6] and this has remained relatively unchanged over the past several decades despite improvements in primary and secondary prevention and the management of acute coronary syndromes, including rapid reperfusion for ST-segment myocardial infarction.[7] In addition to having high mortality, CAD is a significant cause of morbidity in the United States, with increasing rates of congestive heart failure (CHF) noted over the past decade.[8]

Access for right or left heart catheterizations can be performed via the brachial, radial, or femoral artery.[9-13] Other potential but less commonly used sites include direct cutdown (brachial or femoral) and, in rare instances, direct left ventricular (LV) puncture.[14]

DIAGNOSTIC CATHETERIZATION TECHNIQUES

Indications

The most common reason to perform coronary angiography is to assess for the presence of clinically suspected CAD.[15-19] Diagnostic angiography is also performed when a percutaneous intervention or surgical revascularization might be planned, or when valve replacement or repair or percutaneous procedures are planned. The risk-to-benefit ratio should be determined prior to angiography to identify patients who will benefit most from imaging.

Contraindications

The principal contraindications to coronary angiography include bleeding diathesis, renal failure (true or impending), fever, ongoing infection, and severe anemia (Box 52-1). Also, uncontrolled or uncorrected hypokalemia, hyperkalemia, digoxin toxicity, severe allergy to contrast dyes, and overanticoagulation with an international normalized ratio (INR) of greater than 1.8 (although for radial access, this may not be a contraindication) are considered relative contraindications to catheterization.

Box 52-1
Relative Contraindications to Cardiac Catheterization and Angiography

- Bleeding diathesis, or inability to take aspirin or an adenosine diphosphate (ADP) inhibitor
- Concurrent febrile illness
- Severe renal insufficiency or anuria without dialysis planned
- Severe allergy to contrast agents
- Severe hypokalemia or digitalis toxicity
- Severe hypertension or ongoing unstable coronary syndrome

Table 52-1

Possible Complications of Peripheral Catheterization

Complication	Rate (%)
Vascular access dissection or perforation	0.1-0.2
Bleeding/hematoma	1.5-2.0
Allergic reaction	0.5-2.0
Vasovagal events	1.0-2.0
Death	0.1-0.2

Complications

Complications of coronary angiography primarily involve vascular access site complications. Catheter manipulation in atherosclerotic vessels may lead to emboli (thrombus, atherosclerotic debris, calcium, or air) or clot formation, potentially leading to stroke, myocardial infarction (MI), worsening renal function, or CHF (Table 52-1). Pseudoaneurysm or other vascular access complications may be as high as 3%[20] in patients with severe peripheral arterial occlusive disease.

ANGIOGRAPHY

Coronary angiography is performed by selective injection. In rare instances, nonselective coronary imaging is still performed, but this is usually to find the ostia of coronary arteries or bypass grafts.

The most common access for coronary angiography is the femoral artery, although brachial, radial, and axillary approaches are also used. The most common method of cannulation of the vessel is the Seldinger technique.[21] In this method, the vessel is punctured and a guide wire, usually J-tipped, is advanced into the vessel.[22,23] This wire then serves as a rail over which the dilator and sheath enter the vessel.

Once access is obtained, the sheath acts as an entry point for passage and exchange of catheters and devices over the J wire. Various preshaped coronary catheters and bypass graft catheters are available for coronary and bypass graft or conduit angiography. Once a catheter is advanced into the aorta, it is positioned either in the ascending aorta or in the descending aorta for clearing and flushing. The guide wire is withdrawn and the catheter is connected to a manifold system that allows, in a closed system, the ability to transduce the pressure at the tip of the catheter and allow contrast injections without reconnecting a second apparatus or device. Once the catheter is cleared, it is advanced with pressure monitoring into the ostia of the coronary artery. If the pressure waveform dampens, this suggests either an ostial coronary artery lesion or an unfavorable angle of the catheter. Care should always be taken with engagement and injection into any arterial conduit, so as to avoid dissection or lifting of lesion flaps in proximal atheromas. Contrast may be carefully injected to identify a proximal lesion or problem with the dampened waveform. At times, the original catheter may be downsized (5-French for a 6-Fr diagnostic catheter); small-volume contrast injection under cine or nonselective angiography may define the anatomy.

Left Coronary Angiography

In cannulating the left main coronary ostium, a complete and safe study should be ensured by taking care to confirm that the pressure tracing is not dampened or ventricularized. Normally, a preshaped catheter such as a Judkins left 4 catheter (JL4) is used as a default catheter for left coronary angiography. It is successful in engaging the left main ostium approximately 80% of the time. If the aortic root is dilated or narrow, this can usually be accommodated with longer or shorter catheters (JL6 or JL3.5). In addition, if the anatomy is altered, with a left main origin that is posterior, an Amplatz catheter may be used to cannulate the ostium of the left main. The coronary anatomy is defined with contrast injections of 8 to 10 mL during cine runs. The angles taken during angiography allow three-dimensional reconstruction of the anatomy using orthogonal views to see the arteries in multiple planes. The left system begins with the left main, which then terminally bifurcates into the left anterior descending (LAD) and left circumflex (LCX) coronary arteries. In approximately one third of patients, the left main terminally trifurcates into the LAD, the LCX, and an intermediate branch (ramus intermedius) supplying much of the left ventricular free wall.[24] The LAD gives off septal arteries as it courses down the interventricular groove, as well as various diagonal arteries supplying the anterolateral free wall of the left ventricle. The LCX gives off marginal arteries as it courses in the atrioventricular (AV) groove. The marginal arteries supply the lateral free wall of the left ventricle (Fig. 52-1).

Right Coronary Angiography

The right coronary artery (RCA) is usually engaged with a Judkins right 4-cm catheter (JR4). The RCA courses in the interventricular groove and gives off acute marginal and right ventricular branches that supply the right ventricular (RV) free wall. The RCA terminally bifurcates at the crux to form the right posterior descending and right posterolateral coronary arteries, which supply the inferior and inferolateral segments of the left ventricle, respectively. The right posterior descending artery courses in the posterior interventricular septum, supplying the septum as well (see Fig. 52-1).

The dominance of the coronary circulation depends on which artery supplies the posterior circulation—namely, the posterior descending artery or the posterolateral artery.[25] About two thirds of the population is right-dominant (the RCA provides both of these branches), 25% is codominant (the RCA supplies the posterior descending artery and the LCX gives off the posterolateral artery), and 15% is left-dominant (the LCX provides both of these branches).[25]

Coronary Anomalies

Several coronary anomalies exist. Most are anatomic variants, such as dual ostia for the LAD and LCX. Others may be congenital, such as those involving the origin of the LCX from the RCA (Fig. 52-2).[26-32] Most congenital anomalies, such as these, have little impact on coronary circulation. However, in the case of the LAD originating from the RCA or right coronary cusp and coursing posteriorly, there is an associated increased mortality, usually secondary to arrhythmias and ischemia.[29,31]

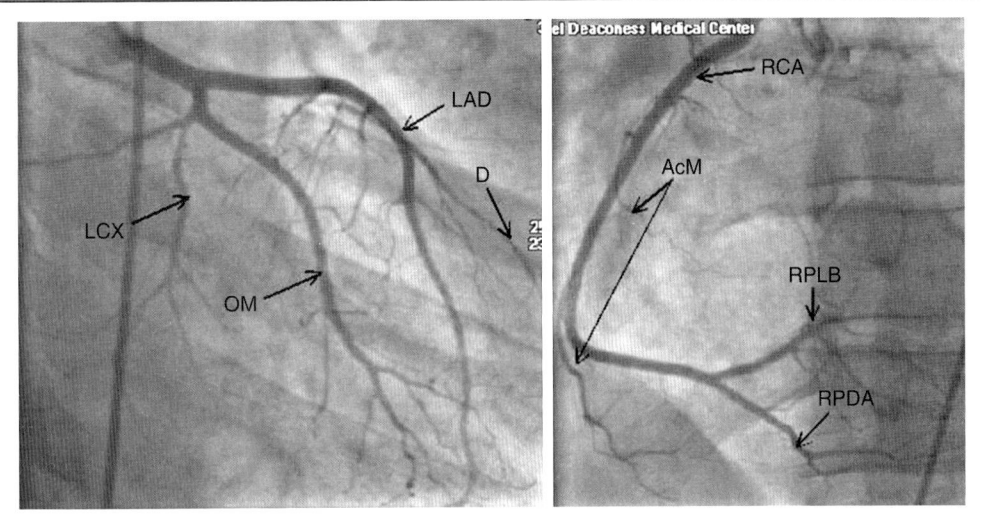

Figure 52-1
Coronary angiographs of the left *(left)* and right *(right)* coronary arteries. AcM, acute marginal artery; D, diagonal artery; LAD, left anterior descending artery; LCX, left circumflex artery; OM, obtuse marginal artery; RCA, right coronary artery; RPDA, right posterior descending artery; RPLB, right posterolateral branch artery.

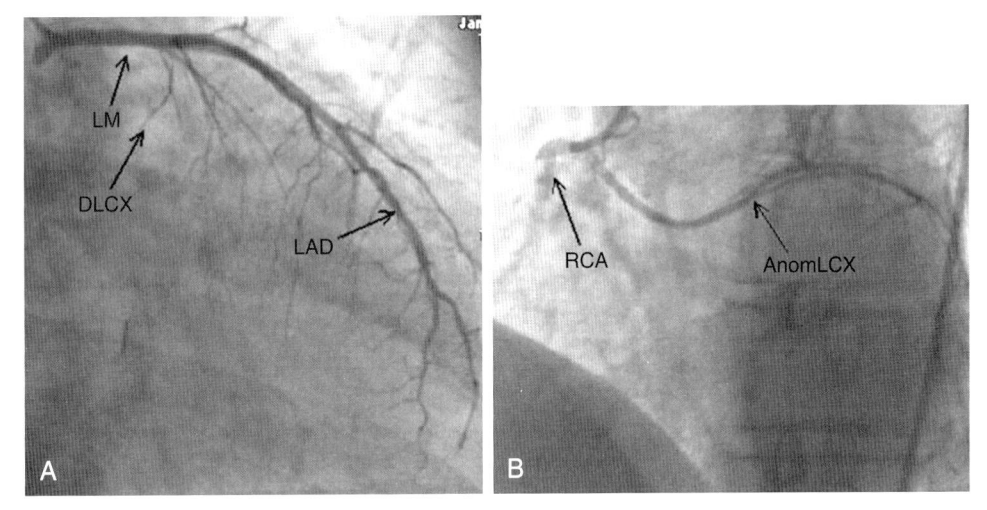

Figure 52-2
A, Long left main coronary artery (LM) with a diminutive left circumflex artery (DLCX). **B,** Anomalous left circumflex artery (AnomLCX) arising from the right coronary artery (RCA) seen in a right anterior oblique view. LAD, left anterior descending artery.

Angiographic Projections

When performing angiography in the coronary circulation, as when performing any other angiography, it is necessary to obtain multiple views in various orthogonal planes of a vessel to fully and clearly define all its segments. Without orthogonal angulation, an inexperienced eye might not see a significant coronary lesion. Generally, all views are reported by convention with left or right angulation first, followed by the cranial or caudal angulation. For example, a 30/25 left anterior oblique (LAO)/cranial is 30 degrees LAO with 25 degrees of cranial angulation.

All major coronary arteries lie in one of two planes: the interventricular septum or the AV groove (Fig. 52-3). The image projections are designed to display the intended anatomy in profile. For example, the right posterior descending artery coursing along the interventricular septum and the inferior wall is best seen with the interventricular septum in its longest profile, the flat right anterior oblique (RAO) projection. On the other hand, the LCX, which courses along the AV groove, is best visualized in the anteroposterior (AP) or RAO caudal projection, looking at the AV groove in profile.

Left Main Coronary Artery

The left main coronary artery is best seen in a shallow LAO with slight caudal projection for its middle and distal segments, and with some cranial angulation for its proximal or ostial segment. Another helpful view is the steep LAO/caudal (also called the spider view) of the terminal left main bifurcation. This last view is not helpful with a horizontally positioned heart, and for these patients it may be best viewed with a steep RAO/caudal view.

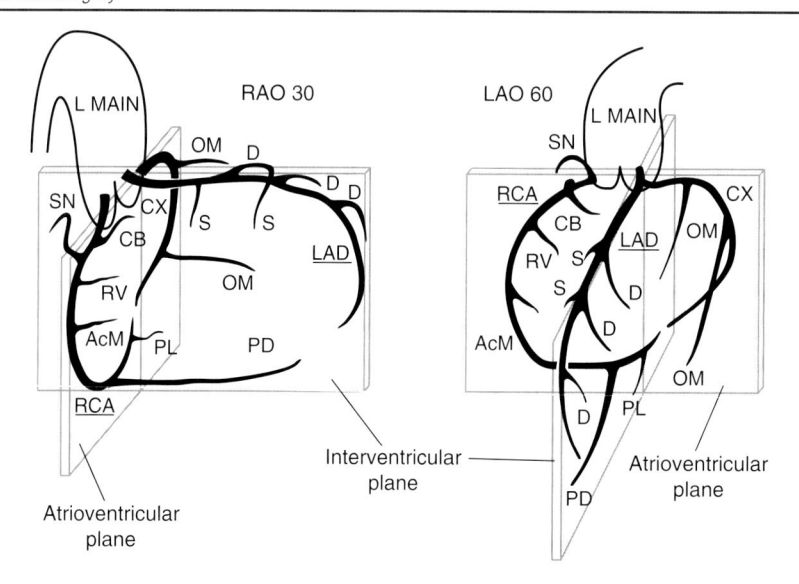

Figure 52-3
Representation of coronary anatomy in relationship to the interventricular and atrioventricular valve planes as seen in two views: right anterior oblique (RAO) and left anterior oblique (LAO). Coronary branches are as follows: AcM, acute marginal; CB, conus branch; CX, circumflex; D, diagonal; L Main, left main; LAD, left anterior descending; OM, obtuse marginal; PD, posterior descending; PL, posterolateral left ventricular; RCA, right coronary; RV, right ventricular; S, septal; SN, sinus node. *(Used with permission from Coronary angiography. In: Baim DS, Grossman W, editors.* Grossman's cardiac catheterization, angiography, and intervention. *6th edition. Philadelphia: Lippincott Williams and Wilkins; 2000.)*

Left Anterior Descending and Diagonal Arteries

The course of the LAD is anterior and inferior to the left main. It then enters the interventricular groove and courses to the apex of the heart. No one view is best for the entire course of the LAD. The proximal LAD is best seen in the steep LAO projections with cranial angulation. The middle and distal segments are generally best visualized with LAO and RAO with some caudal angulation. In some cases, when the proximal LAD is not well seen (horizontal heart), an RAO/cranial of 30 degrees each is sufficient to open the proximal LAD and bifurcation with the LCX.

The diagonal arteries, the major branches of the LAD, course off the LAD toward the lateral free wall of the left ventricle. The best view for most of the diagonal arteries, their origin, and their distal segments is usually a steep LAO with steep cranial angulation (50/45-50). In some cases, the first diagonal artery is the only diagonal artery given by the LAD. This vessel then supplies the entire diagonal system (we sometimes refer to this as a twin LAD, given the importance of this vessel to epicardial blood flow).

Left Circumflex Artery

The LCX is best seen in caudal projections. The proximal portion of the LCX is best seen in the RAO/caudal angulation. This angle also serves to show the marginal arteries, as well. The alternative for the mid segment of the LCX and marginal arteries is the steep LAO/caudal (spider view). In obese patients, this view can be challenging, as the x-ray has to penetrate extra tissue, so the image may be distorted, dark, or hazy.

Right Coronary Artery

The RCA enters the anterior AV groove and courses distally. The proximal segment of the RCA is best seen in the flat LAO angulation. If the ostium of the RCA is of interest, then a steep (50-degree) LAO projection is best. The mid segment of the RCA is best seen in the LAO and flat RAO projections. The crux, or distal RCA, and the proximal portions of the right posterior descending and right posterolateral arteries are best seen with an AP or slight LAO with 20 to 30 degrees of cranial angulation. The middle and distal segments of the right posterior descending artery are best visualized with a flat RAO projection.

Graft Angiography

Commonly, saphenous vein grafts to the right and left coronary circulations arise from the anterior surface of the aorta several centimeters from the sinus of Valsalva. RCA grafts generally arise from the right anterior aorta and the left system grafts commonly arise from the left anterior side of the aorta, with the LAD grafts usually being lower than the LCX grafts. In many cases, the surgeon may place a ring at the origin of a graft that can greatly reduce the chance of missing a graft because one cannot cannulate or find it. The best views for the LAD/diagonal grafts are flat LAO and RAO projections to visualize the graft in its greatest profile. The distal (native) vessel is then imaged with some cranial or caudal projection to define all its segments after the distal anastomosis according to the vessel of interest (i.e., cranial for the LAD, and caudal for the LCX). These images are usually easier to obtain and evaluate because there is less overlap of other coronary anatomy to deal with. However, the ability to view well the origin or distal anastomosis may be challenging for some grafts. The RCA grafts are usually best seen with flat LAO and RAO projections. Again, after the graft has been imaged, the native vessel is imaged with some cranial or caudal angulation to fully define the anatomy after the distal anastomosis (Fig. 52-4).

Since the mid 1990s, the internal mammary artery (IMA) has increasingly been the conduit of choice for the LAD and in some cases for the RCA because of the high patency of

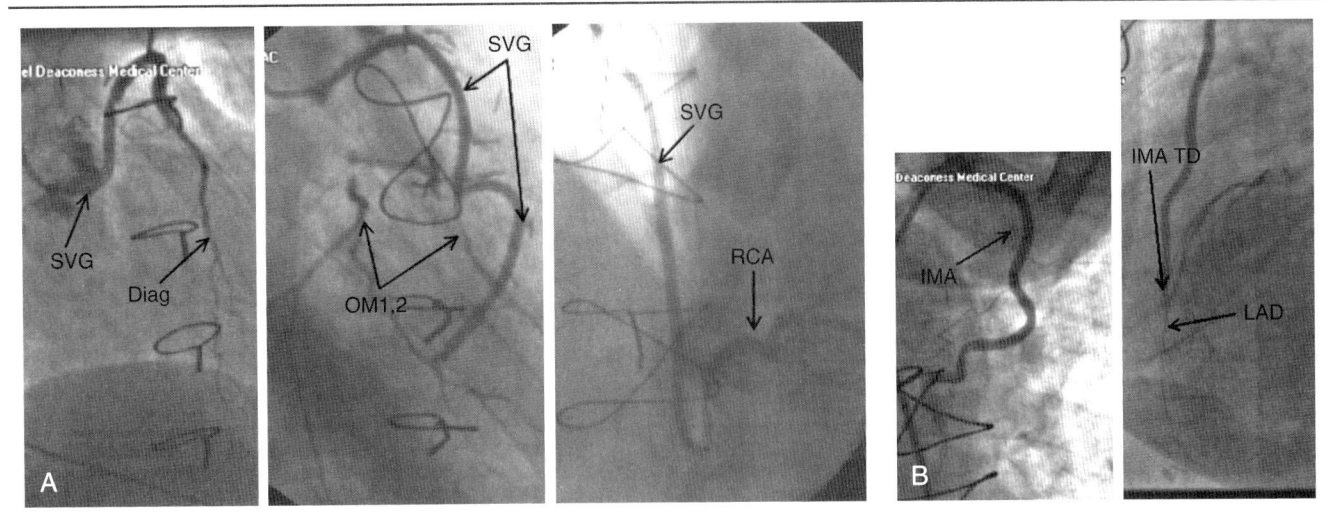

Figure 52-4
A, Graft angiography. Diag, diagonal artery; OM1,2, obtuse marginal arteries 1 and 2; RCA, right coronary artery; SVG, saphenous vein graft.
B, Internal mammary artery (IMA) angiography. IMA TD, IMA touchdown; LAD, left anterior descending artery.

these conduits.[33] Generally, the IMA is cannulated after the subclavian artery is engaged with the preformed catheter and J wire. The catheter is advanced and cleared. Then, the catheter is withdrawn and a gentle counterclockwise torque is applied until the catheter engages the origin of the left IMA (LIMA). Once the vessel is engaged, the catheter is given a gentle clockwise torque to remove any excess tension on the catheter.[34] The views for angiography for the LIMA are generally AP or slight RAO/cranial (0-20/40) for the proximal and mid segments of the graft, and steep flat LAO to lateral projection for the anastomosis of the LIMA with the LAD. The right IMA conduit is similarly engaged from the right subclavian artery. The views for the mid segment, origin, and anastomosis are, generally, flat LAO with some cranial and steep AP cranial, respectively (see Fig. 52-4).

HEMODYNAMICS

Principles

The hemodynamic assessment performed during coronary angiography is as integral a part of the procedure as is the imaging of the coronary vasculature. At any given moment, the hemodynamics reflect a culmination and interaction between various ongoing dynamic processes determining cardiac output, coronary artery disease, left ventricular function, systemic metabolic needs, and systemic and pulmonary pressures.[35,36] Hemodynamic measurements (vessel or ventricular pressures), measurement of cardiac output, and the evaluation of shunts are an integral part of diagnostic coronary evaluation. All pressures should be measured with a transducer that will allow direct real-time measurements. An important element for this process is the establishment of a zero reference. The reference is usually accepted as the mid chest level in the anterior-posterior direction.

Right Heart Catheterization

The measurement of right heart (RH) pressures and oxygen saturations is a very good and easy method of obtaining the current cardiovascular status. Cardiac output (CO) is the flow of blood from the heart to the body and is reported in liters per minute. To standardize this number for a patient's size, these units are divided by the patients body surface area (BSA), which leads to the cardiac index (CI) in liters per minute per meter squared.

During the RH catheterization (RHC), oxygen saturations should be obtained from the superior vena cava (SVC), right atrium, right ventricle, pulmonary artery (PA), and pulmonary capillary wedge pressure (PCWP) positions. When obtained with an arterial saturation, the CO or CI can be calculated, and it allows possible shunt evaluation (see Shunts, later).

Pressure tracings are obtained at each level of the advancement of the RH catheter. Normal values for the RH and systemic arterial (left ventricular) pressures are shown in Table 52-2 and Figure 52-5. Since the introduction of the balloon-tipped RH catheter,[37] RHC has become very common in the catheterization laboratory.

Pressure Waveforms

Right Atrium

The *a* wave occurs during atrial systole, which occurs after the P wave on the surface electrocardiogram (ECG). During atrial diastole, there is a decline in the pressure waveform, which corresponds to the *x* descent. In the ventricle below, as systole begins, the *x* descent may be interrupted by a movement of the tricuspid valve. This is termed the *c* wave, with the remainder of the *x* descent called *x'*. As ventricular systole progresses and forward flow occurs, the tricuspid valve is closed, and filling of the right atrium results in the *v* wave. Ultimately, ventricular relaxation occurs, the tricuspid valve opens, and atrial pressure falls as blood flows from the right atrium to the right ventricle. This corresponds to the *y* descent.

Right Ventricle

RV pressure rises with ventricular systole. As diastole commences, the pulmonic valve closes and a rapid decline in pressure is noted. After the tricuspid valve opens, there is rapid filling of the ventricle and a slow increase in its pressure. With

Table 52–2
Normal Cardiac Pressures and Values

Chamber	a Wave	v Wave	Mean	Systolic	End Diastolic	Mean
Right atrium	2-8*	2-8	0-6	—	—	—
Right ventricle	—	—	—	15-30	0-8	—
Pulmonary artery	—	—	—	15-30	4-12	8-16
Pulmonary capillary wedge pressure	3-15	3-10	1-10	—	—	—
Left ventricle	—	—	—	100-140	3-12	—
Aorta	—	—	—	100-140	60-90	70-110

*All measurements in millimeters of mercury.

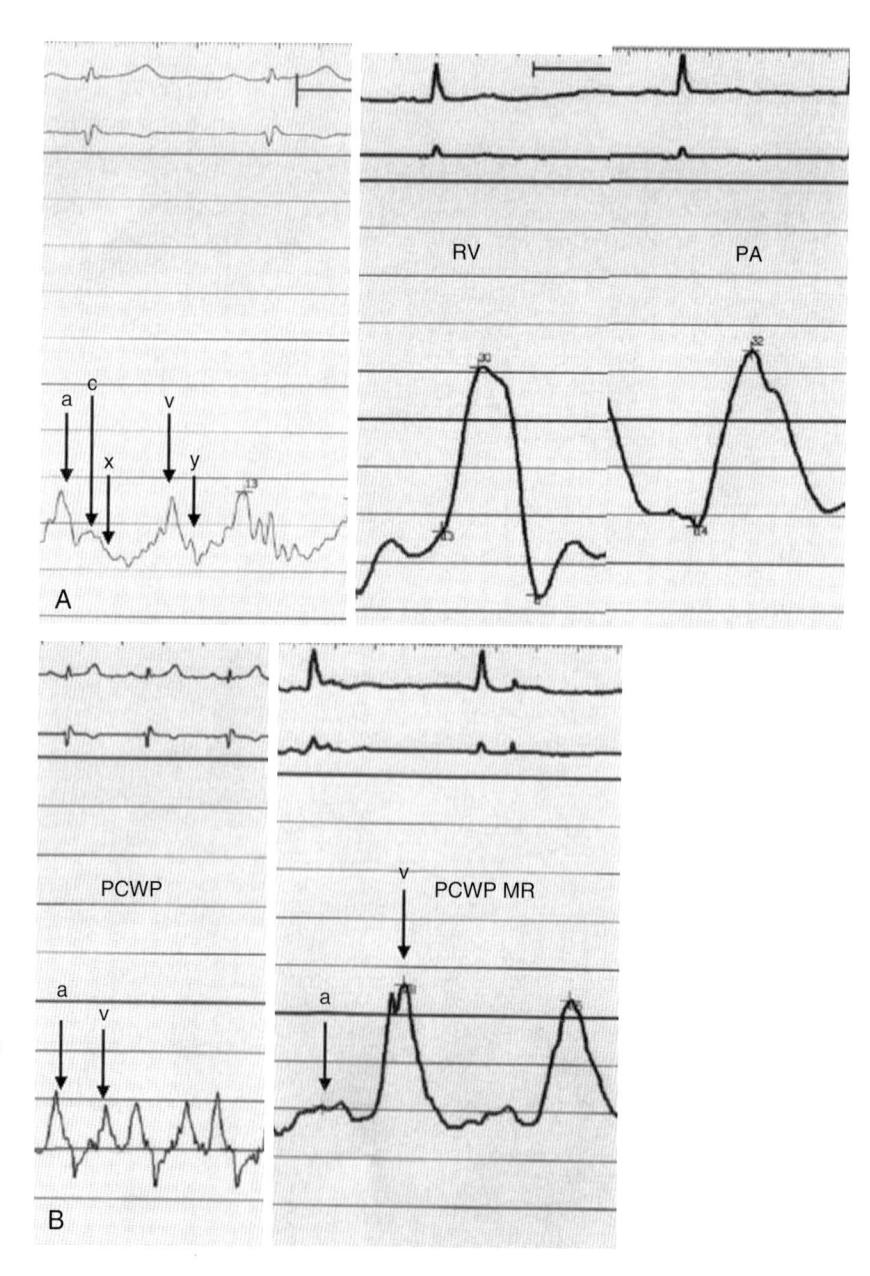

Figure 52–5
A, Right heart pressure tracings of right atrium (RA), right ventricle (RV), and pulmonary artery (PA). Waves: *a,* from atrial systole; *c,* from closed tricuspid valve and ventricular systole slightly pushing the valve into the atrium; *v,* from ventricular systole; *x,* descent with atrial diastole; *y,* descent from atrial emptying after ventricular systole. **B,** Right heart pressure tracings. PCWP, pulmonary (artery) capillary wedge pressure; PCWP MR, PCWP tracing with substantial mitral regurgitation; a, *a* wave; v, *v* wave.

atrial systole, the final pressure recorded is the end-diastolic pressure.

Pulmonary Artery

In the pulmonary artery, after ventricular systole opens the pulmonic valve, there is a rise in the systolic pressure. As diastole commences, the pressure declines. With closure of the pulmonic valve, the diastolic pressure plateaus to a higher degree than in the ventricle. The diastolic pressure of the PA correlates closely with the left atrial (LA) pressure and PCWP.

Pulmonary Capillary Wedge Pressure (Left Atrium)

With the use of balloon tipped catheters, a wedge position, in which the catheter is wedged into a distal vessel, can transduce pressure from the downstream circulation—namely, the left atrium.[38] This maneuver is performed with relative ease and allows an indirect measure of LA pressures without need for trans-septal puncture. Many studies have validated PCWP as a surrogate for LA pressure in the evaluation of mitral stenosis.[38-40]

Systemic Arterial Pressure

The arterial pressure waveform begins with LV systole. Once the aortic valve opens, systolic pressure rises precipitously. As ventricular diastole begins and pressures fall, the aortic valve closes and the aortic pressure declines. An interruption in the pressure tracing corresponds to the aortic valve closure. This phenomenon is denoted by the dicrotic notch on the arterial waveform. Depending on the patency of the aortic valve and the compliance of the aorta, the usual pulse pressure is 45 to 50 mm Hg. In noncompliant aortic systems (e.g., in older patients with calcified vessels) or in aortic regurgitation, there is a wide pulse pressure (see Fig. 52-5).

Cardiac Output

Cardiac output, the amount of blood sent to deliver enough oxygen, glucose, and nutrients to the body, is expressed in liters per minute. This measurement can be obtained through several methods, such as the Fick, thermodilution, or dye method.[41-44] The Fick method is the most commonly used in our cardiac catheterization laboratory.[42] It assumes that the rate at which oxygen is consumed is a function of the rate of blood flow and the rate of oxygen loading by the red blood cells. By measuring the difference in the oxygen content in the arterial and mixed venous circulation (A-V O_2 difference) and the oxygen consumption, CO can be calculated:

$$CI (L/min) = O_2 \text{ consumption} (mL/min/m^2) \div A - V O_2 \text{ difference}$$

The normal oxygen consumption index ranges from 110 to 150 mL/min/m². In our laboratory, we assume an oxygen consumption index of 125 mL/min/m² (110 mL/min/m² for older women). This must then be multiplied by the subject's BSA in meters squared, to arrive at the oxygen consumption, thus allowing determination of the cardiac output. If we do not multiply by the BSA, we have the cardiac index.

Table 52-3
Normal Values

Reference Point	Value
Oxygen consumption index (mL/min/m²)	110-150
A-V O_2 difference (mL/L)	30-50
Cardiac output (CO)	2.5-4.2
Cardiac index (CI)	2.0-3.0
Resistances	
Pulmonary vascular resistance (PVR)	20-130
Systemic vascular resistance (SVR)	700-1600

The more reliable way to determine the O_2 consumption is by direct measurement. This can be done by using the Douglas bag, in which the oxygen content of expired air is compared with the oxygen content in the ambient air, and thus oxygen consumption is calculated. It can also be done by using a metabolic rate meter[43]; here, the patient breathes into a container that has O_2 and CO_2 sensors that measure the expired content of O_2 and CO_2, and the oxygen consumption is calculated. To calculate the A-V O_2 difference, we need the arterial oxygen saturation, the most mixed venous oxygen saturation (PA saturation, assuming no shunts), and the hemoglobin (Hgb) concentration:

$$A - V O_2 \text{ difference} = P_A (\% sat) - P_a (\% sat)(Hgb \text{ in } g/dL) (1.36 mL O_2/g Hgb),$$

where P_A is the oxygen saturation in the peripheral arterial circulation (assumed to be the same as in the LV or pulmonary vein), P_a is the oxygen saturation in the PA, Hgb is the hemoglobin concentration in the blood, and 1.36 is the correction factor for the ability of fully saturated hemoglobin to carry oxygen.

The cardiac index can then be calculated:

$$CI = O_2 \text{ consumption (assumed or directly measured)} \div A - V O_2 \text{ difference}$$

Once calculated, the CI can be multiplied by the BSA to determine the CO (Table 52-3).

SHUNTS

When the flow of blood in the heart enters another chamber without traversing a valve, a shunt is present. Evaluation, detection, and localization of intracardiac shunts are an integral part of the diagnostic coronary and RH catheterizations.

Left-to-Right Shunts

The typical left-to-right shunt seen in the catheterization laboratory is an atrial septal defect (ASD). Other causes of left-to-right shunting are patent foramen ovale (PFO), ventricular septal defect (VSD) (Fig. 52-6), and patent ductus arteriosus

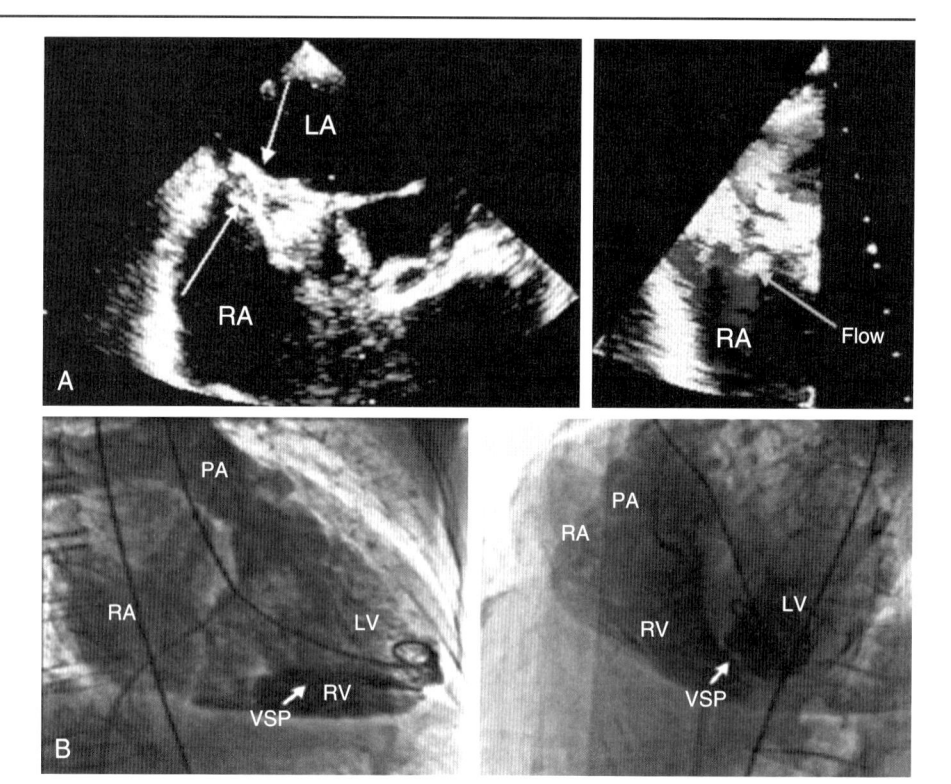

Figure 52–6
A, Atrial septal defect noted from transesophageal echocardiography in both two-dimensional and color flow Doppler images. **B,** Ventricular septal defect noted in ventriculography from right and left anterior oblique projections. LA, left atrium; LV, left ventricle; PA, pulmonary artery; RA, right atrium; RV, right ventricle; VSP, ventricular septal perforation.

(PDA). In each of these there is a step-up in oxygen saturation at a different level of the RHC. For the ASD, this occurs in the right atrium; for the VSD it is in the right ventricle, and for the PDA it is in the PA. The key to understanding and quantifying the shunt is determining where the most mixed venous sample can be obtained. In the case of an ASD, it is a combination of the superior vena cava (SVC) and the inferior vena cava (IVC); for a VSD it is the right atrium, and for a PDA it is the right ventricle.

In a shunt evaluation, oximetry is the method by which the right heart chambers or vessels are evaluated. Early work by Dexter and colleagues[45] defined what we use today for maximal changes in each RH chamber for oxygen saturations. In general, a maximal change of 8% from the SVC to the PA is considered sufficiently significant to evaluate further for the presence of an intracardiac shunt.

If a shunt is suspected, oximetry is performed. Once the data are collected, it is important to quantify the amount of the shunt. The pulmonary and systemic blood flows and the magnitude of the left-to-right shunt should be calculated. Pulmonary blood flow (Q_p) is calculated by the following formula:

$$Q_P = O_2 \text{ consumption (mL/min)} \div [(P_V O_2) - (P_A O_2)]$$

Systemic blood flow (Q_s) is calculated by the following formula:

$$Q_S = O_2 \text{ consumption (mL/min)} \div [(S_A O_2) - (M_V O_2)],$$

where $M_V O_2$ denotes the mixed venous oxygen concentration.

The Q_P/Q_S is the ratio of the relative blood flows in the pulmonary and systemic circulations, which can then be reduced to

$$Q_P/Q_S = (S_A O_2) - (M_V O_2) \div [(P_V O_2) - (P_A O_2)]$$

The $M_V O_2$ is a value of the average oxygen concentration from the right atrium for VSD, from the right ventricle for PDA, and for an ASD it is a derived number from the Flamm equation,[41] where $M_V O_2 = [3 \text{ (SVC)} + 1 \text{ (IVC)}] \div 4$.

A Q_P/Q_S greater than 2.0 is considered high and signals possible surgical correction or percutaneous closure. Values between 1.5 and 2.0 are intermediate, and surgical or percutaneous closure may be pursued if there is low surgical risk, or if symptoms for percutaneous closure (Fig. 52-7) are present (cryptogenic stroke for ASD or PFO). A ratio of less than 1.0 suggests a right-to-left shunt.

Right-to-Left Shunts

Any significant right-to-left shunt is generally detected early without catheterization, as the patient usually has cyanosis or arterial hypoxemia. The oximetric evidence is a Q_P/Q_S of less than 1.0. Usually, a ratio of less than 0.7 is considered critical, and less than 0.3 is not compatible with life.

Regardless of the cause, the basis for evaluation of the site of the right-to-left shunt may be analyzed if the PV, LA, LV, and aortic saturations can be obtained. When the shunt is extra-anatomic from the pulmonary circulation, the site of stepdown is the site of the shunt. For example, if the stepdown occurs in the LV, there is a VSD. Unfortunately, this would require entering the left atrium, which may be difficult in some patients.

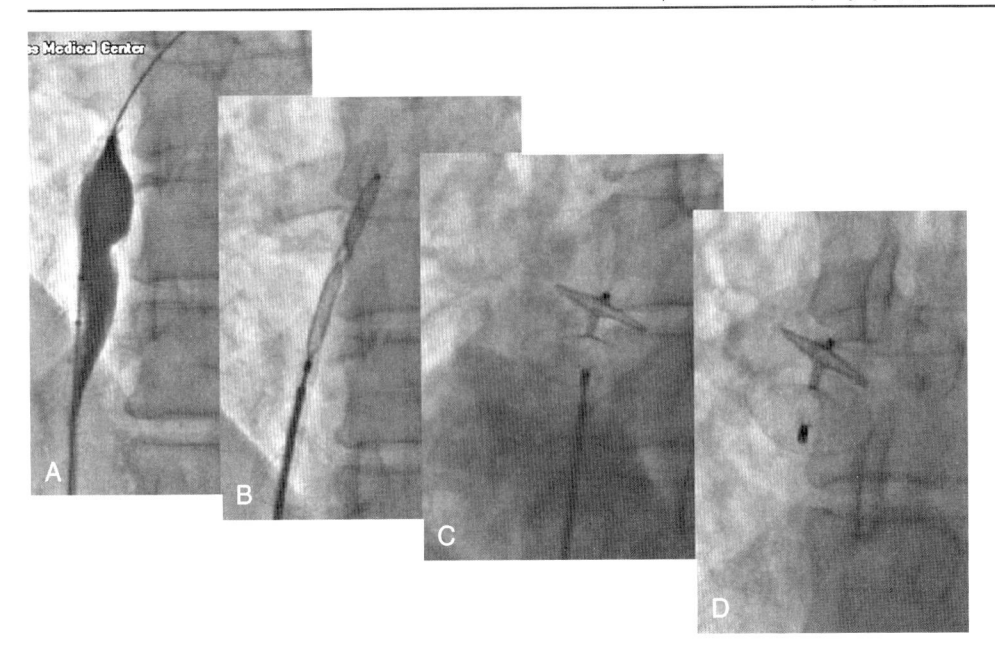

Figure 52–7
Closure device for patent foramen ovale or atrial septal defect (Amplatzer, Amplazter Ind., Chicago). **A,** Sizing balloon in the canal of the atrial defect. **B,** Constrained device in the Mullins sheath (Cook Inc., Bloomington, IN). **C,** Deployed device without release. **D,** Final release of device.

Bidirectional Shunts

If there is evidence of both left-to-right and right-to-left shunting, a formula comparing the effective blood flow (Q_{eff}) is used. This flow rate is the hypothetical flow in the absence of any shunting:

$$Q_{eff} = O_2 \text{ consumption (mL/min)} \div [(P_VO_2) - (M_VO_2)]$$

Then the left-to-right and right-to-left shunts are $Q_P - Q_{eff}$ and $Q_{eff} - Q_S$, respectively.

ASSESSMENT OF VASCULAR RESISTANCE

Vascular resistance is calculated by dividing the pressure gradient across the vascular bed in question by the blood flow through it. In essence, there are two major vascular beds, systemic and pulmonary. For systemic vascular resistance (SVR),

$$SVR = (\text{mean arterial pressure} - \text{right atrial pressure}) \div CO.$$

For pulmonary vascular resistance (PVR):

$$PVR = (\text{PA pressure} - \text{PCWP} [\text{LA pressure}]) \div CO.$$

Normal values for the SVR and PVR are listed in Table 52-3. A high SVR is seen in patients with systemic hypertension, hypovolemia, significant blood loss, and CHF. A low SVR is seen with high fevers, sepsis, thyrotoxicosis, or arteriovenous fistulae.

VALVE ASSESSMENT

The assessment of valvular abnormalities is an integral part of any catheterization. During a routine right and left heart catheterization, diagnostic information may be derived for all four valves in the heart. The principal valvular anomalies that require interrogation and potential surgical repair are aortic stenosis (AS), aortic regurgitation (AR), mitral stenosis (MS), mitral regurgitation (MR), and, in some cases, severe tricuspid regurgitation (TR).

Aortic Stenosis

Generally, hemodynamically significant AS is secondary to primary valve pathology (congenital bicuspid aortic valve) or to valve degeneration (calcific AS).[46-49] Patients referred for catheterization for evaluation of AS generally have one of the following indications for the procedure: syncope, angina, or LV dysfunction. However, catheterization is recommended for hemodynamic measurements for the assessment of severity of AS if the results of noninvasive tests are equivocal or if there is discordance between the clinical assessment and the results of noninvasive tests.[50]

To determine the significance of AS, simultaneous measurements of pressure across the aortic valve must be performed. To best achieve this, a catheter is passed into the LV cavity, and the systolic pressure in the LV cavity is compared with a simultaneous pressure measurement in the ascending aorta. However, it is difficult to place a long sheath at the level of the sinus of Valsalva to measure direct pressure differences from the LV to the ascending aorta. Therefore, a catheter is placed in the abdominal aorta and zeroed with a catheter placed in the ascending aorta to determine any pressure difference or augmentation for simultaneous pressure recordings from the LV and the aorta.

Entering the LV in a retrograde fashion can be quite challenging in some patients with AS. The deformities of the valve apparatus and calcific buildup make entering the orifice of the aortic valve very difficult. It is common to attempt to cross the aortic valve with the pigtail catheter in a retrograde fashion without the use of a wire. If this method fails, an attempt can be made to probe the aortic valve with a straight wire extended from the tip of the pigtail catheter while changing the orientation of the catheter to adjust the area probed by the wire, and with gentle retraction of the catheter to adjust the anterior-posterior orientation of the wire. If the pigtail catheter does not provide an adequate orientation despite these maneuvers, then a JR4 or Amplatz left 1 catheter, among others (e.g., a Feldman catheter), may improve the orientation of the wire and eventually allow passage into the LV.

Once the LV is entered, simultaneous pressures should be measured. These pressures must be obtained along with a simultaneous CO. In our laboratory, it is routine to obtain a simultaneous PCWP tracing to evaluate the mitral valve also at this time. Once the CO is obtained, the aortic valve may be calculated using the Gorlin equation,[51] as follows:

$$\text{Aortic valve area (cm}^2) = [CO/(DFP \text{ or } SEP)(HR)] \ C(\sqrt{P}),$$

where DFP or SEP is diastolic filling period or systolic ejection period, HR is heart rate in beats/min, C is an empirical constant (44.3 for aortic and tricuspid valves, and 37.7 for the mitral valve), and P is the pressure gradient in millimeters of mercury.

In the Gorlin equation, heart rate and systolic ejection periods are generally similar among most patients. Therefore, an alternative equation, the Hakki formula, has been suggested.[47] Here, the aortic valve area can be estimated by dividing the CO by the square root of the peak-to-peak gradient (P):

$$\text{Valve area} = CO \ \sqrt{P}$$

AS is considered severe when the valve area is less than 1.0 cm², and it is critical when the valve area is less than 0.7 cm².[50] Indications for aortic valve replacement include symptomatic severe AS; severe AS in the setting of coronary artery bypass graft, aortic root, or other valvular surgery; and severe AS in the setting of a depressed left ventricular ejection (<50%).[50] Aortic valve replacement is considered reasonable for patients with moderate AS undergoing other cardiac or aortic surgery.[50] If aortic valve replacement is contraindicated because of other medical comorbidities, an aortic valvuloplasty may be considered (see elsewhere in this text). However, the long-term outcomes from aortic valve dilation are poor, with recurrence being the rule and not the exception.

Aortic Regurgitation

Aortic regurgitation is the result of an incompetent aortic valve. This dynamic process allows blood to enter the LV cavity in diastole in a retrograde fashion across the aortic valve. The consequence of the regurgitant fraction is an increased demand on the LV to maintain an adequate CO in addition to the regurgitant volume. The magnitude of the regurgitant volume depends on the size of the orifice in the aortic valve and the pressure difference between the aorta and LV in diastole. The principal causes of AR are primary diseases of the valve (rheumatic or endocarditis) and of the aortic root (aneurysm, syphilis, ankylosing spondylitis).[52-58]

The clinical signs of chronic AR begin with a widened pulse pressure on noninvasive measurements. The patient with chronic AR may also have several clinical signs on physical examination: Quincke's pulses (nailbed capillary pulsations), Duroziez's sign (systolic murmur over the femoral artery when compressed proximally, and diastolic murmur when compressed distally), Corrigan's pulse (water-hammer pulsation with early rise then collapse), the Austin-Flint murmur (early closure of the mitral valve from AR, simulating MS), or de Musset's sign (head bobbing with each cardiac cycle).

Preoperative evaluation of patients with chronic AR includes coronary angiography and evaluation of LV function. If the patient is mildly symptomatic or symptomatic on exercise testing, or if there is any deterioration of LV function, then there is consensus that an aortic valve replacement is warranted.[50,52,54,59] Replacement of the valve before any deterioration of LV function is the goal in AR.[52]

Mitral Stenosis

Mitral stenosis is almost invariably caused by rheumatic heart disease. The fusion of the mitral apparatus is either from the commissure at the cusps, subvalvular at the cusps, or a combination of these.[59-62] In adults, the normal valve area is between 4 and 6 cm². When the valve area is less than 2 cm², the mitral stenosis is considered mild; less than 1 cm² is considered critical mitral stenosis. Because the hemodynamic result of chronic mitral stenosis is elevated pulmonary pressure, the typical feature of severe and critical mitral stenosis is dyspnea with exertion.

Determining the gradient across the mitral valve can be accomplished in two ways. First, the LA pressure can be measured directly, through a transeptal approach into the left atrium from the right atrium. This is the most accurate method of determining the LA pressure compared with the left ventricular pressure. The most significant problem with this approach is the inherent risk associated with performing a transeptal puncture (aortic puncture, PA puncture). A lower-risk approach that has been validated is to obtain a confirmed PCWP through a right heart catheterization at the time of simultaneous LV tracings. With this method, the mitral valve can be reliably evaluated, and the hemodynamic significance of its stenosis for valvuloplasty or surgical repair or replacement can be discerned.

The procedure for hemodynamic assessment of mitral stenosis in the catheterization laboratory is generally to obtain access in both the femoral artery and vein. A RHC is performed and a confirmed PCWP obtained. Confirming the PCWP by measuring oxygen saturation confirms the pulmonary vein samples for the valve area CO calculation. A pigtail catheter is placed into the LV cavity and a simultaneous tracing of LV pressure and PCWP are obtained. A gradient less than 5 mm Hg at the time of the catheterization may allow the Gorlin equation to have a significant error in the true valve area. The patient should then be placed under hemodynamic stress, either via exercise, medication, or atrial pacing, to increase the atrial gradient. Once the maximal gradient is confirmed, and the diastolic filling periods and CO are obtained, the valve area can be calculated with the Gorlin equation. Likewise, as with AS, the Hakki formula, if calculated under adequate conditions of heart rate and CO, may approximate the mitral valve area by taking the CO and dividing by the square root of the gradient.

Mitral Regurgitation

Mitral regurgitation may be the consequence of disruptions of the mitral leaflets, annulus, or subvalvular apparatus, including the chordae and papillary musculature.[63-66] Generally, mitral leaflet abnormalities result from rheumatic heart disease, chronic mitral valve prolapse, or bacterial endocarditis. Other causes include systemic diseases, such as systemic lupus erythematosus. When the mitral annulus becomes dilated as a consequence of LV dilation, the annulus may not allow coaptation of the mitral cusps, with MR as the result. Furthermore, if the annulus becomes calcified, the ability to constrict with ventricular contraction is impaired, and MR may result. Last, chordal and subchordal structures (papillary muscles) may be congenitally short or long or fibrotic, they may rupture as a result of ischemic or infectious myonecrosis, or they may be dysfunctional as a result of ischemia. Any of these clinical scenarios may not allow optimal tethering of the valvular apparatus in systole, thus resulting in MR.

Ischemic MR is one special case of significant mitral regurgitation.[67-69] The posterior papillary musculature has a single blood supply (usually the LCX). Thus, with an acute coronary syndrome involving the marginal circulation of the LCX, potentially significant and acute MR may ensue, with resultant CHF.

In the cardiac catheterization laboratory, significant MR is assessed with left ventriculography. In the RAO projection, the left ventricle and left atrium are seen in profile. Therefore, any MR can be assessed and quantified. In the tracing, mild MR (1+) is that which appears but promptly clears before the next cardiac cycle. Mild to moderate MR (2+) is that which appears and clears after the next cycle or does not opacify as darkly as the left ventricle. Moderate to severe MR (3+) is that which appears and does not clear with subsequent cardiac cycles and is opacified as deeply as the left ventricle. Finally, severe MR (4+) is that which appears and does not clear with subsequent cardiac cycles and is opacified more deeply than the left ventricle.

The clinical indication for repair or replacement is based on the hemodynamic assessment, left ventricular size, and other comorbidities (e.g., atrial fibrillation).[50]

Pericardial Disease

The pericardium forms a cavity that is held firmly in place via attachments to the sternum and the vertebral bodies, and with the diaphragm it holds the heart in its place in the chest despite different body positions.[70] The pericardium has two layers: an inner (visceral) layer intimately associated with the surface of the heart, and an outer (parietal) layer that is the continuation of the visceral pericardium as it reflects on itself. The parietal pericardium is fibrous, and the visceral pericardium is smooth, made up of a single layer of mesothelial cells. In the pericardial space is usually about 50 mL of clear, ultrafiltrate fluid that acts as a lubricant to reduce any friction between the heart and the surrounding pericardium. Various pathophysiologic processes affect the pericardium.[71-76]

Normal pericardial pressures are zero or negative, and thus they have only a small effect on cardiac distending pressures. Two pericardial abnormalities are encountered in the catheterization laboratory: acute pericarditis and constrictive pericarditis.

Acute pericarditis is caused by inflammation of the pericardium that results in chest pain, possible pericardial friction rub, and ECG abnormalities.[77] Etiologies of acute pericarditis include infectious, idiopathic, and uremic, or it may be secondary to neoplasm or trauma. The principal indication for evaluating a patient with pericarditis in the catheterization laboratory is the presence of an effusion requiring pericardial drainage or sampling (Fig. 52-8).

Various ECG signs of acute pericarditis and a pericardial effusion are nonspecific ST-segment abnormalities, usually diffuse elevation up to 1 to 2 mm, and PR-segment depression. Also, because the heart may swing with each cardiac cycle in the fluid space of the effusion, electrical alternans may be seen if there is a large effusion. Once the pericardial effusion is suspected, it can be readily detected with echocardiography. Clinical signs of a significant pericardial effusion may be noted on the physical examination. One of the consequences of a large or acute pericardial effusion is cardiac tamponade. In tamponade, an increase in intrapericardial pressure causes an elevation of intracardiac pressures (equalization of pressures), abnormalities of the jugular venous pressures, progressive limitation of ventricular diastolic filling, and, ultimately, a reduction of stroke volume and CO. Given this constellation of hemodynamic effects, the clinical findings of a patient in impending or fulminant tamponade are tachycardia, a large pulsus paradoxus, and abnormalities of the jugular venous pulsations. If clinical signs or echocardiographic findings lead to a suspicion of tamponade, a pericardial drain should be placed.

In the catheterization laboratory, the pericardial space is usually approached from just left of the subxyphoid, with the needle directed toward the patient's left shoulder. It is our practice to begin with a RHC to evaluate PCWP and then return the catheter to the right atrium and access an arterial system (usually the femoral artery). Right atrial (central venous) pressures should demonstrate blunted x and prominent y descents. We then enter the pericardial space, with an alligator clip attached to the needle, to allow us to see if we come in contact with the epicardium (an injury current, or ST-segment elevation, will be seen). Once entered, the needle is transduced with and compared with a catheter in the right atrium. If tamponade is present, the pressures should be similar and track each other. At this time, samples should be taken for laboratory evaluation of the pericardial fluid (e.g., electrolytes, pH, cultures). A J-tipped wire is then advanced into the space. Over this wire, a dilator is advanced and, ultimately, a drain placed. Aspiration of the effusion follows, with intermittent hemodynamic assessments. As the effusion is drained, the pericardial pressure should return to zero or negative, with a resultant decline in right atrial pressure. The drain should be left in place until the drainage falls below 30 mL over 24 hours.

Constrictive pericarditis is usually a uniform scarring of the pericardium that causes restriction of diastolic filling of the heart.[78] It most commonly follows acute pericarditis. After the initial event, there is fibrin deposition and scarring of the pericardium, ultimately leading to the uniform restriction of diastolic filling. The differentiation of constrictive pericarditis from restrictive myocardial disease remains difficult, and the diagnosis can remain equivocal even after extensive noninvasive and invasive evaluations.[79-82]

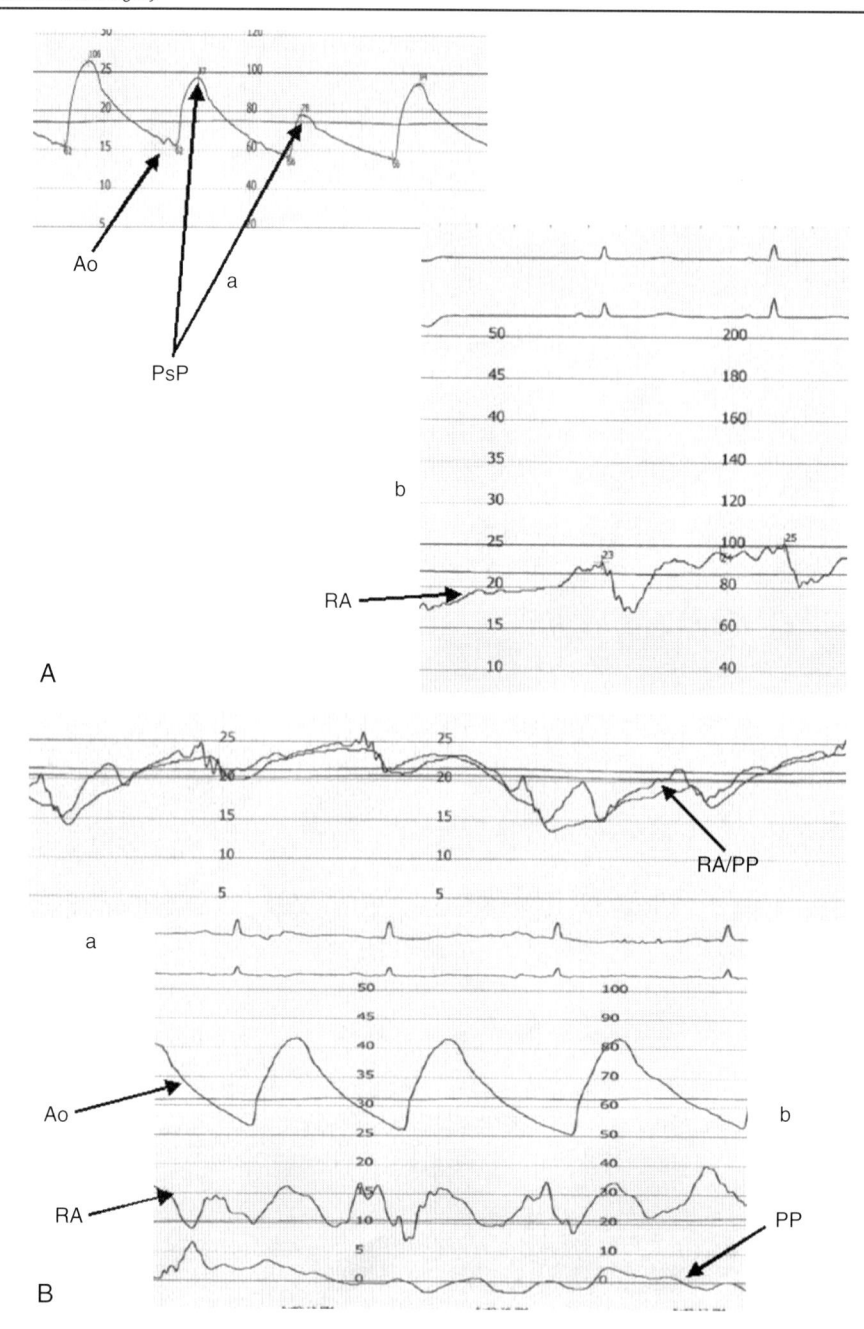

Figure 52-8
Hemodynamics of tamponade. **A,** Aortic pressure (a). Pulsus paradoxus (PsP) of greater than 20 mm Hg is seen *(arrows)*. Right atrial (RA) pressure pre-pericardiocentesis (b). **B,** Pericardial and right atrial pressure pre-pericardiocentesis and drainage (a). Note the "tracking" of the RA pressure with the pericardial pressure (RA/PP). Hemodynamics of aorta (Ao), right atrium (RA), and pericardial space (PP) after evacuation of 400 mL fluid (b). Note the loss of significant pulsus, and the separation of the pericardial and RA pressure tracings.

There is an elevation and equalization of the diastolic pressure in all four cardiac chambers. The central venous pressure shows a prominent x and y descent, frequently appearing as a W waveform. Moreover, the right and left ventricular tracings reveal diastolic equalization with the classic dip and plateau of ventricular filling. There is rapid ventricular filling in early diastole, hence the dip, and slow or negligible filling in late diastole, hence the plateau. It is important to remember that if ventricular filling is low, such as in hypovolemia, the classic patterns may not be seen. We recommend a volume load to raise the right atrial pressure to fully evaluate the prospect of constrictive pericarditis. Another hemodynamic effect of a uniform constriction to cardiac filling is the lack of transmitted intrathoracic pressures to the pericardium and heart chambers. Thus, in constrictive pericarditis, with inspiration, systemic venous and right atrial pressures do not fall and may actually increase. This is Kussmaul's sign (Fig. 52-9).[83]

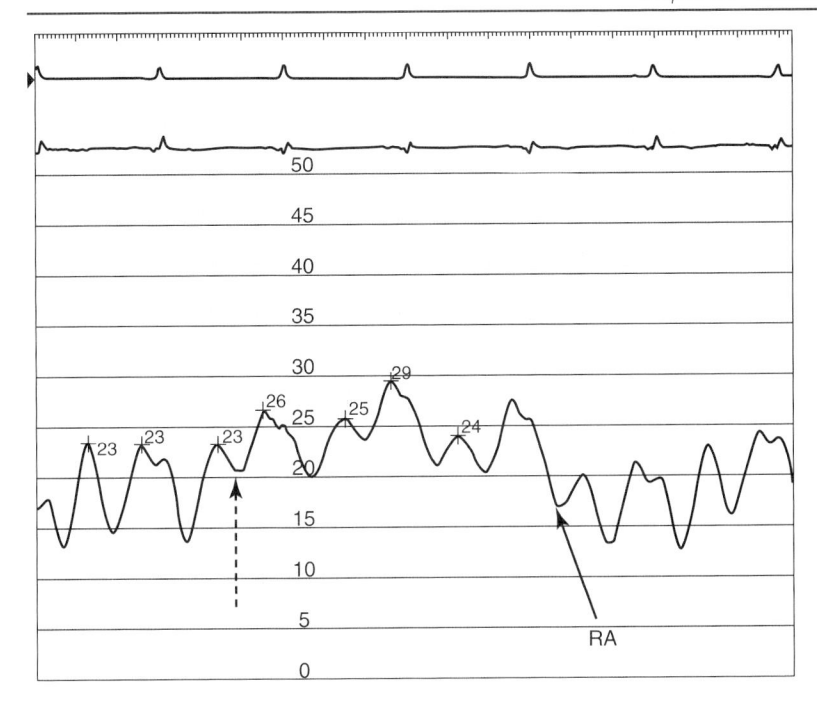

Figure 52–9
Right atrial pressure tracing from patient with constrictive pericarditis. Kussmaul's sign is evident during inspiration *(dashed arrow)*. RA, right atrium.

REFERENCES

1. Forssman W. Die Sondierung des rechten Herzens. *Klin Wochenschr* 1929;**8**:2085.
2. Sones FM, Shirley EK. Cine coronary arteriography. *Mod Concepts Cardiovasc Dis* 1962;**31**:735-8.
3. Sones FM, Shirley EK, Proudfit WL, Wescott RN. Cine coronary arteriography. *Circulation* 1959;**20**:773.
4. Grüntzig AR. Perkutane Dilatation von Coronarstenosen-Beschreibung eines neuen Kathetersystems. *Klin Wochenschr* 1976;**54**:543.
5. Grüntzig AR, Turina MI, Schneider JA. Experimental percutaneous dilatation of coronary artery stenosis. *Circulation* 1976;**54**:81.
6. Rosamond W, Flegal K, Friday G, et al. Heart disease and stroke statistics—2007 update: a report from the American Heart Association Statistics Committee and Stroke Statistics Subcommittee. *Circulation* 2007;**115**:e69-171.
7. Antman EM, Hand M, Armstrong PW, et al. 2007 Focused update of the ACC/AHA 2004 Guidelines for the Management of Patients with ST-Elevation Myocardial Infarction: a report of the American College of Cardiology/American Heart Association Task Force on Practice Guidelines: developed in collaboration with the Canadian Cardiovascular Society endorsed by the American Academy of Family Physicians: 2007 Writing Group to Review New Evidence and Update the ACC/AHA 2004 Guidelines for the Management of Patients with ST-Elevation Myocardial Infarction, Writing on Behalf of the 2004 Writing Committee. *Circulation* 2008;**117**:296-329.
8. McCullough PA, Philbin EF, Spertus JA, Kaatz S, Sandberg KR, Weaver WD. Confirmation of a heart failure epidemic: findings from the Resource Utilization among Congestive Heart Failure (REACH) study. *J Am Coll Cardiol* 2002;**39**:60-9.
9. Brock R, Milstein BB, Ross DN. Percutaneous left ventricular puncture in the assessment of aortic stenosis. *Thorax* 1956;**11**:163-71.
10. Campeau L. Percutaneous radial artery approach for coronary angiography. *Cathet Cardiovasc Diagn* 1989;**16**:3-7.
11. Fergusson DJ, Kamada RO. Percutaneous entry of the brachial artery for left heart catheterization using a sheath: further experience. *Cathet Cardiovasc Diagn* 1986;**12**:209-11.
12. Hillis LD. Percutaneous left heart catheterization and coronary arteriography using a femoral artery sheath. *Cathet Cardiovasc Diagn* 1979;**5**:393-9.
13. Nguyen T, Saito S, Grines C. Vascular access. *J Interv Cardiol* 2002;**15**:163-6.
14. Semple T, McGuiness JB, Gardner H. Left heart catheterization by direct ventricular puncture. *Br Heart J* 1968;**30**:402-6.
15. Effects of tissue plasminogen activator and a comparison of early invasive and conservative strategies in unstable angina and non-Q-wave myocardial infarction. Results of the TIMI IIIB Trial. Thrombolysis in Myocardial Ischemia. *Circulation* 1994;**89**:1545-56.
16. Braunwald E, Gorlin R, McIntosh HD, Ross RS, Rudolph AM, Swan HJ. Cooperative study on cardiac catheterization: summary. *Circulation* 1968;**37**:III93-101.
17. Davies RF, Goldberg AD, Forman S, et al. Asymptomatic Cardiac Ischemia Pilot (ACIP) study two-year follow-up: outcomes of patients randomized to initial strategies of medical therapy versus revascularization. *Circulation* 1997;**95**:2037-43.
18. Kadir S. Regional anatomy of the thoracic aorta. In: Kadir S, editor. *Atlas of normal and variant angiographic anatomy.* Philadelphia: WB Saunders; 1991.
19. van Miltenburg-van Zijl AJ, Simoons ML, Veerhoek RJ, Bossuyt PM. Incidence and follow-up of Braunwald subgroups in unstable angina pectoris. *J Am Coll Cardiol* 1995;**25**:1286-92.
20. Arora N, Matheny ME, Sepke C, Resnic FS. A propensity analysis of the risk of vascular complications after cardiac catheterization procedures with the use of vascular closure devices. *Am Heart J* 2007;**153**:606-11.
21. Seldinger SI. Catheter replacement of the needle in percutaneous arteriography: a new technique. *Acta Radiol* 1953;**39**:368-76.
22. Barry WH, Levin DC, Green LH, Bettman MA, Mudge Jr GH, Phillips D. Left heart catheterization and angiography via the percutaneous femoral approach using an arterial sheath. *Cathet Cardiovasc Diagn* 1979;**5**:401-9.
23. Judkins M, Kidd HJ, Frische LH, Dotter CT. Lumen-following safety J-guide for catheterization of tortuous vessels. *Radiology* 1967;**88**:1127-30.
24. Halon DA, Sapoznikov D, Lewis BS, Gotsman MS. Localization of lesions in the coronary circulation. *Am J Cardiol* 1983;**52**:921-6.
25. Kaimkhani ZA, Ali MM, Faruqi AM. Pattern of coronary arterial distribution and its relation to coronary artery diameter. *J Ayub Med Coll Abbottabad* 2005;**17**:40-3.
26. Angelini P. Normal and anomalous coronary arteries: definitions and classification. *Am Heart J* 1989;**117**:418-34.
27. Rapp AH, Hillis LD. Clinical consequences of anomalous coronary arteries. *Coron Artery Dis* 2001;**12**:617-20.
28. Roberts WC, Kragel AH. Anomalous origin of either the right or left main coronary artery from the aorta without coursing of the anomalistically arising artery between aorta and pulmonary trunk. *Am J Cardiol* 1988;**62**:1263-7.
29. Roberts WC, Siegel RJ, Zipes DP. Origin of the right coronary artery from the left sinus of Valsalva and its functional consequences: analysis of 10 necropsy patients. *Am J Cardiol* 1982;**49**:863-8.
30. Safi AM, Rachko M, Tang A, Ketosugbo A, Kwan T, Afflu E. Anomalous origin of the left main coronary artery from the right sinus of Valsalva: disabling angina and syncope with noninterarterial courses—case report of two patients. *Heart Dis* 2001;**3**:24-7.
31. Serota H, Barth 3rd CW, Seuc CA, Vandormael M, Aguirre F, Kern MJ. Rapid identification of the course of anomalous coronary arteries in adults: the "dot and eye" method. *Am J Cardiol* 1990;**65**:891-8.
32. Yamanaka O, Hobbs RE. Coronary artery anomalies in 126,595 patients undergoing coronary arteriography. *Cathet Cardiovasc Diagn* 1990;**21**:28-40.
33. Goldman S, Zadina K, Moritz T, et al. Long-term patency of saphenous vein and left internal mammary artery grafts after coronary artery bypass surgery: results from a Department of Veterans Affairs Cooperative Study. *J Am Coll Cardiol* 2004;**44**:2149-56.

34. Kuntz RE, Baim DS. Internal mammary angiography: a review of technical issues and newer methods. *Cathet Cardiovasc Diagn* 1990;**20**:10-6.
35. Dexter L, Whittenberger JL, Haynes FW, Goodale WT, Gorlin R, Sawyer CG. Effect of exercise on circulatory dynamics of normal individuals. *J Appl Physiol* 1951;**3**:439-53.
36. Guyton RE, Jones EC, Coleman TG. *Cardiac output and its regulation: circulatory physiology*. Philadelphia: WB Saunders; 1973.
37. Swan HJ, Ganz W, Forrester J, Marcus H, Diamond G, Chonette D. Catheterization of the heart in man with use of a flow-directed balloon-tipped catheter. *N Engl J Med* 1970;**283**:447-51.
38. Lange RA, Moore Jr DM, Cigarroa RG, Hillis LD. Use of pulmonary capillary wedge pressure to assess severity of mitral stenosis: is true left atrial pressure needed in this condition? *J Am Coll Cardiol* 1989;**13**:825-31.
39. Alpert JS. The lessons of history as reflected in the pulmonary capillary wedge pressure. *J Am Coll Cardiol* 1989;**13**:830-1.
40. Nishimura RA, Rihal CS, Tajik AJ, Holmes Jr DR. Accurate measurement of the transmitral gradient in patients with mitral stenosis: a simultaneous catheterization and Doppler echocardiographic study. *J Am Coll Cardiol* 1994;**24**:152-8.
41. Fegler G. Measurement of cardiac output in anaesthetized animals by a thermodilution method. *Q J Exp Physiol Cogn Med Sci* 1954;**39**:153-64.
42. Fick A. Uber die Messung des Blutquantums in den Herzventrikeln. *Sitz der Physik-Med ges Wurtzberg* 1870.
43. Lange RA, Dehmer GJ, Wells PJ, et al. Limitations of the metabolic rate meter for measuring oxygen consumption and cardiac output. *Am J Cardiol* 1989;**64**:783-6.
44. Stewart GN. Researches on the circulation time and on the influences which affect it. *J Physiol* 1897;**22**:159-83.
45. Dexter L, Haynes FW, Burwell CS, Eppinger EC, Sagerson RP, Evans JM. Studies of congenital heart disease. II: The pressure and oxygen content of blood in the right auricle, right ventricle, and pulmonary artery in control patients, with observations on the oxygen saturation and source of pulmonary "capillary" blood. *J Clin Invest* 1947;**26**:554-60.
46. Braunwald E, Goldblatt A, Aygen MM, Rockoff SD, Morrow AG. Congenital aortic stenosis: I. Clinical and hemodynamic findings in 100 patients, and II. Surgical treatment and the results of operation. *Circulation* 1963;**27**:426-62.
47. Moller JH, Nakib A, Eliot RS, Edwards JE. Symptomatic congenital aortic stenosis in the first year of life. *J Pediatr* 1966;**69**:728-34.
48. Roberts WC. Valvular, subvalvular and supravalvular aortic stenosis: morphologic features. *Cardiovasc Clin* 1973;**5**:97-126.
49. Selzer A. Changing aspects of the natural history of valvular aortic stenosis. *N Engl J Med* 1987;**317**:91-8.
50. Bonow RO, Carabello BA, Kanu C, et al. ACC/AHA 2006 guidelines for the management of patients with valvular heart disease: a report of the American College of Cardiology/American Heart Association Task Force on Practice Guidelines (writing committee to revise the 1998 Guidelines for the Management of Patients with Valvular Heart Disease): developed in collaboration with the Society of Cardiovascular Anesthesiologists: endorsed by the Society for Cardiovascular Angiography and Interventions and the Society of Thoracic Surgeons. *Circulation* 2006;**114**:e84-231.
51. Gorlin R, Gorlin SG. Hydraulic formula for calculation of the area of the stenotic mitral valve, other cardiac valves, and central circulatory shunts. I. *Am Heart J* 1951;**41**:1-29.
52. Borer JS, Herrold EM, Hochreiter CA, et al. Aortic regurgitation: selection of asymptomatic patients for valve surgery. *Adv Cardiol* 2002;**39**:74-85.
53. Girardi LN. Surgical approaches when aortic regurgitation is associated with aortic root disease. *Adv Cardiol* 2002;**39**:86-92.
54. Hoit BD. Medical treatment of valvular heart disease. *Curr Opin Cardiol* 1991;**6**:207-11.
55. Lautermann D, Braun J. Ankylosing spondylitis: cardiac manifestations. *Clin Exp Rheumatol* 2002;**20**:S11-5.
56. Levine AJ, Dimitri WR, Bonser RS. Aortic regurgitation in rheumatoid arthritis necessitating aortic valve replacement. *Eur J Cardiothorac Surg* 1999;**15**:213-4.
57. Ward C. Clinical significance of the bicuspid aortic valve. *Heart* 2000;**83**:81-5.
58. Yener N, Oktar GL, Erer D, Yardimci MM, Yener A. Bicuspid aortic valve. *Ann Thorac Cardiovasc Surg* 2002;**8**:264-7.
59. Boon NA, Bloomfield P. The medical management of valvar heart disease. *Heart* 2002;**87**:395-400.
60. Bruce CJ, Nishimura RA. Clinical assessment and management of mitral stenosis. *Cardiol Clin* 1998;**16**:375-403.
61. Hasegawa R, Kitahara H, Watanabe K, Kuroda H, Amano J. Mitral stenosis and regurgitation with systemic lupus erythematosus and antiphospholipid antibody syndrome. *Jpn J Thorac Cardiovasc Surg* 2001;**49**:711-3.
62. Waller BF. *Rheumatic and nonrheumatic conditions producing valvular heart diseases*. Philadelphia: FA Davis; 1986.
63. Enriquez-Sarano M, Orszulak TA, Schaff HV, Abel MD, Tajik AJ, Frye RL. Mitral regurgitation: a new clinical perspective. *Mayo Clin Proc* 1997;**72**:1034-43.
64. Fenster MS, Feldman MD. Mitral regurgitation: an overview. *Curr Probl Cardiol* 1995;**20**:193-280.
65. Irvine T, Li XK, Sahn DJ, Kenny A. Assessment of mitral regurgitation. *Heart* 2002:88:(Suppl. 4):iv11-9.
66. Otto CM. Timing of surgery in mitral regurgitation. *Heart* 2003;**89**:100-5.
67. Birnbaum Y, Chamoun AJ, Conti VR, Uretsky BF. Mitral regurgitation following acute myocardial infarction. *Coron Artery Dis* 2002;**13**:337-44.
68. Cohn LH. Mitral valve repair for ischemic mitral regurgitation. *Adv Cardiol* 2002;**39**:153-6.
69. Iung B. Management of ischaemic mitral regurgitation. *Heart* 2003;**89**:459-64.
70. Wilcox BR, Anderson RH. *Surgical anatomy of the heart*. New York: Raven Press; 1985.
71. Aikat S, Ghaffari S. A review of pericardial diseases: clinical, ECG and hemodynamic features and management. *Cleve Clin J Med* 2000;**67**:903-14.
72. Fowler NO. Pericardial disease. *Heart Dis Stroke* 1992;**1**:85-94.
73. Maisch B. Pericardial diseases, with a focus on etiology, pathogenesis, pathophysiology, new diagnostic imaging methods, and treatment. *Curr Opin Cardiol* 1994;**9**:379-88.
74. Roberts WC, Spray TL. Pericardial heart disease. *Curr Probl Cardiol* 1977;**2**:1-71.
75. Vasquez A, Butman SM. Pathophysiologic mechanisms in pericardial disease. *Curr Cardiol Rep* 2002;**4**:26-32.
76. Zhang S, Kerins DM, Byrd 3rd BF. Doppler echocardiography in cardiac tamponade and constrictive pericarditis. *Echocardiography* 1994;**11**:507-21.
77. Lange RA, Hillis LD. Clinical practice: acute pericarditis. *N Engl J Med* 2004;**351**:2195-202.
78. Goldstein JA. Cardiac tamponade, constrictive pericarditis, and restrictive cardiomyopathy. *Curr Probl Cardiol* 2004;**29**:503-67.
79. Hatle LK, Appleton CP, Popp RL. Differentiation of constrictive pericarditis and restrictive cardiomyopathy by Doppler echocardiography. *Circulation* 1989;**79**:357-70.
80. Ling LH, Oh JK, Schaff HV, et al. Constrictive pericarditis in the modern era: evolving clinical spectrum and impact on outcome after pericardiectomy. *Circulation* 1999;**100**:1380-6.
81. Oh JK, Hatle LK, Seward JB, et al. Diagnostic role of Doppler echocardiography in constrictive pericarditis. *J Am Coll Cardiol* 1994;**23**:154-62.
82. Vaitkus PT, Kussmaul WG. Constrictive pericarditis versus restrictive cardiomyopathy: a reappraisal and update of diagnostic criteria. *Am Heart J* 1991;**122**:1431-41.
83. Meyer TE, Sareli P, Marcus RH, Pocock W, Berk MR, McGregor M. Mechanism underlying Kussmaul's sign in chronic constrictive pericarditis. *Am J Cardiol* 1989;**64**:1069-72.

CHAPTER 53
Applications of Cardiovascular Magnetic Resonance and Computed Tomography in Cardiovascular Diagnosis

Thomas H. Hauser, Susan B. Yeon, and Warren J. Manning

Imaging Principles and Approaches
Challenges of Cardiac Imaging
Imaging Comparisons
Imaging Precautions
Clinical Applications
   Diseases of the Thoracic Aorta
      Aortic Aneurysm
      Aortic Dissection
      Aortic Intramural Hematoma
      Sinus of Valsalva Aneurysm

      Atherosclerotic Plaque and Aortic
         Penetrating Ulcer
      Takayasu's Arteritis
      Congenital Aortic Anomalies
      Thoracic Trauma
   Cardiac Imaging
      Ventricular Structure and Function
      Identification of Myocardial Scar and
         Ischemia
      Congenital Heart Disease

      Cardiac and Paracardiac Masses
      Pericardial Disease
      Valvular Heart Disease
      Cardiomyopathies
      Coronary Artery Imaging
The Future Role of Cardiovascular
   Magnetic Resonance and Computed
   Tomography

Cardiovascular magnetic resonance (CMR) and cardiovascular computed tomography (CCT) are increasingly used in the diagnosis and management of cardiovascular disease.[1-3] Both of these imaging modalities have overcome similar challenges posed by cardiac and respiratory motion and the demand for high temporal and spatial resolution to enable noninvasive imaging that aids in the diagnosis and management of a variety of cardiovascular disorders. In addition, CMR and CCT have unique capabilities that permit great flexibility, precision, and reproducibility in the acquisition and display of anatomic and functional data that are useful for surgical diagnosis, planning, and follow-up.

IMAGING PRINCIPLES AND APPROACHES

CMR imaging is performed with the use of static and dynamic magnetic fields and does not employ any ionizing radiation. Images are generated from induced radiofrequency signals arising from water and fat protons in the body. Differences in proton density, magnetic relaxation times (T1, longitudinal relaxation time; T2, transverse relaxation time), blood flow, and other parameters produce intrinsic signal contrast among tissues. CMR approaches can be broadly classified into spin echo (black blood) and gradient echo (bright blood) sequences, often modified with prepulses. Spin echo imaging is particularly useful for defining anatomic structure and tissue characterization (e.g., fat replacement or iron deposition).

Gradient echo techniques can produce single-shot (displaying a single phase during the cardiac cycle) or cine (displaying multiple phases at one level during the cardiac cycle) images. Cine images demonstrate motion of structures (such as cardiac chambers and valves) during the cardiac cycle, permitting qualitative and quantitative assessment of motion. Both spin echo and gradient echo CMR techniques are flow sensitive. Because of the inherent contrast between the blood pool and surrounding tissue, administration of an exogenous CMR contrast agent is generally not required for general evaluation of cardiac anatomy. However, administration of an extracellular magnetic resonance–specific intravenous contrast agent, such as gadolinium–diethylenetriaminepentaacetic acid (Gd-DTPA), enables certain applications such as contrast-enhanced magnetic resonance angiography (CE-MRA) and assessment of myocardial perfusion and viability. Gadolinium induces T1 shortening, which is detected as increased signal in contrast-enhanced T1-weighted images (the signal enhancement is not linearly related to contrast agent concentration). Flow velocity encoding (also known as phase contrast) is an additional CMR modality that enables quantitation of blood flow. This method enables determination of regurgitant fraction and shunt flows.

CCT uses ionizing radiation to generate images based on the attenuation of the tissues of the body. Today, CCT is typically performed with third-generation multislice scanners. These CCT units are arranged with a radiation tube opposed to a series of detectors attached to a gantry that rapidly rotate as the patient is advanced through the scanner. The detector arrays typically obtain 4, 8, 16, 32, 40, 64, 256, or 320 axial slices during a single rotation of the gantry. A higher number of slices permits greater coverage with each rotation of the gantry, allowing shorter imaging times, less contrast material, and potentially less radiation exposure. Cardiac imaging is usually performed with 64-, 256-, or 320-slice machines. Images can be acquired in one of two modes: helical (or spiral) or step-and-shoot. In the helical mode, data are acquired in a helical path as the patient is advanced through the scanner. The speed at which the patient is advanced through the scanner is called the pitch. A high pitch (faster speed) is associated with a lower radiation exposure; low pitch (slower speed) is associated with a higher radiation exposure. Cardiac imaging is generally performed with a relatively low pitch. The radiation exposure can be reduced somewhat by electrocardiogram (ECG) dose modulation, varying the intensity of radiation exposure during the cardiac cycle. With the step-and-shoot mode, imaging is performed without advancing the patient through the gantry. After each acquisition, the patient is then advanced a fixed distance, and images are obtained contiguous to the prior image data set. This is repeated until the entire area to be imaged is covered. Imaging can be completed in one or two steps with 256- and 320-slice machines.

CHALLENGES OF CARDIAC IMAGING

CMR and CCT have faced similar challenges posed by cardiac and respiratory motion and requirements for high temporal, spatial, and contrast resolution.

The acquisition of most cardiac images requires gating or triggering during a specific portion of the cardiac cycle. Thus, imaging is usually performed during regular sinus rhythm. The duration of image acquisition with CCT is generally less than 10 to 15 seconds, allowing breath-holding to be used for suppression of respiratory motion. Although breath-holding can also be used for most CMR acquisitions, free-breathing navigator gating is sometimes used for longer image acquisitions. Navigator gating is a CMR technique that identifies the interface between the lung and diaphragm, most commonly at the dome of the right hemidiaphragm. Data about the position of the lung-diaphragm interface from the navigator can then be used for respiratory gating.

High temporal resolution is needed to take advantage of these gating techniques. CMR can typically be performed with very high temporal resolution, with CMR data acquired in less than 40 msec. The temporal resolution of CCT is limited by gantry rotation speed. Typical gantry rotation speeds are 330 to 400 msec per rotation. The use of half-cycle reconstruction allows an image to be acquired in one half-rotation, with an effective temporal resolution of approximately 165 to 200 msec. Intravenous or oral beta-blockers are typically administered for coronary artery CCT to prolong the period of diastasis during which the coronary artery can best be imaged. The temporal resolution of CCT can be improved to approximately 83 msec with dual source technology, in which two sets of radiation tubes and detectors are mounted on the gantry. Each set acquires data over one quarter-rotation, and the data are combined to form a single image. Multicycle reconstruction can also be used to improve the temporal resolution of CCT to approximately 40 msec by acquiring data for a single image over multiple cardiac cycles, but this is infrequently used because of the requirement for a very low pitch and a resultant very high radiation exposure.

The development of high spatial resolution has also been important for CMR and CCT, particularly for coronary artery imaging. Spatial resolution of CMR has been improved with specific imaging sequences that increase acquisition time and with imaging at higher field strengths (e.g., 3 T) and is typically 1 to 2 mm in-plane spatial resolution, whereas the spatial resolution of CCT has improved with the development of smaller detectors. Routine CCT generally has a higher spatial resolution compared with CMR, with isotropic spatial resolution of 0.5 mm. Although this spatial resolution is technically achievable by CMR, scan length would be further prolonged and image quality would suffer from reduced signal-to-noise ratio.

Image contrast for CMR is generally created with specific imaging sequences and prepulses. The use of a contrast agent is generally not required except for specific applications as noted before. CCT does not have the inherent contrast resolution of CMR; thus, iodinated contrast material is typically required for imaging. The timing of administration of the contrast agent relative to image acquisition is critical in producing high-quality images. Imaging is typically performed during passage of contrast material in the ascending aorta and coronary arteries. The correct timing is determined by a small timing bolus given just before imaging or by automated detection of contrast material in the ascending or descending aorta. A similar process is used for CE-MRA.

IMAGING COMPARISONS

The advantages and limitations of CMR and CCT complement those of other imaging techniques, such as echocardiography, x-ray angiography, and radionuclide imaging. Compared with echocardiography and radionuclide imaging, CMR and CCT offer superior anatomic scope and spatial resolution. CMR is the reference standard for evaluation of left ventricular cavity size, systolic function, and mass, providing highly reproducible measures and enhancing noninvasive follow-up of disease processes.[4] CCT measures of left ventricular cavity size and systolic function compare favorably with CMR.[5] In contrast to echocardiography and nuclear imaging, CMR permits unrestricted image acquisition orientation, which can be readily adjusted to particular patient and study requirements. CCT acquisitions are always in the axial plane. Isotropic resolution facilitates post-processing reconstruction in any desired orientation. There is also much advanced post-processing software for CCT. In contrast, echocardiography offers the advantages of portability, lower cost, lack of ionizing radiation, widespread availability, greater ease of patient monitoring, and greater sensitivity for structures with chaotic motion, such as vegetations. Whereas CMR and CCT myocardial perfusion techniques have been shown to provide useful qualitative and quantitative data, they have not yet been clinically validated to provide the diagnostic and prognostic information proven for radionuclide techniques. Further comparisons between CMR, CCT, and other techniques will be made in the following sections dealing with specific types of examinations.

IMAGING PRECAUTIONS

Precautions generally applicable to magnetic resonance imaging are applicable to CMR. Before imaging, all patients must undergo detailed screening for any potential contraindications to magnetic resonance scanning. In addition to general concerns of metallic implants and severe claustrophobia, patients should be screened for the presence of any incompatible material. Excluded devices include some that are relatively common among those with cardiovascular disease, such as pacemakers, retained permanent pacemaker leads, and implantable cardioverters-defibrillators. Bioprosthetic and mechanical heart valves, sternotomy wires, thoracic vascular clips, and intracoronary stents are generally considered CMR safe at field strengths up to 3 T (see www.mrisafety.com), although they may produce local artifacts that reduce image quality.[6]

Because of bulk cardiac motion during systole and diastole, most CMR protocols require ECG triggering with images composed from data collected during multiple successive cardiac cycles. Despite this, good functional image quality can frequently be obtained among patients with atrial fibrillation,[7] although image quality may be impaired among subjects with frequent and irregular premature beats. Among patients with irregular rhythms, non–ECG-gated real-time imaging CMR (which permits real-time image acquisition analogous to two-dimensional echocardiography but at lower spatial and temporal resolutions than those attained with a gated CMR technique) can provide useful information.[8] CCT data are generally of poor quality in the setting of atrial fibrillation and frequent ectopy,[9,10] although acquisitions with 256- or 320-slice machines over a single heart beat may provide better image quality.

All subjects require appropriate monitoring during the imaging study. Basic monitoring modalities include ECG monitoring for rate and rhythm (CMR magnetic fields distort ST segment appearance, rendering it uninterpretable), intercom voice contact, and visualization (by direct view or camera). For patients requiring greater intensity of monitoring, automated cuff blood pressure monitoring and pulse oximetry can be added.

As noted earlier, CMR generally does not require the use of an exogenous contrast agent. When needed, however, gadolinium-containing CMR contrast agents have a much more favorable safety profile in regard to both nephrotoxicity and anaphylaxis compared with iodinated agents used in x-ray angiography and computed tomography.[11] Administration of gadolinium contrast to patients with severe renal dysfunction may result in nephrogenic systemic fibrosis, a very rare but severe disorder that may result in death.[12,13] Patients are typically screened with a questionnaire to identify those who may potentially have renal disease and who require a determination of the estimated glomerular filtration rate. Patients with mild renal impairment (estimated glomerular filtration rate of 30 to 60 mL/kg/1.73 m^2) can be imaged with a reduced dose of contrast agent. Alternative imaging modalities are usually used in those patients with moderate to severe renal dysfunction (estimated glomerular filtration rate of less than 30 mL/kg/1.73 m^2), especially in the setting of dialysis therapy.

Because of the general requirement for iodinated contrast agents, CCT must be performed with caution in patients with diabetes or mild renal insufficiency. Alternative noninvasive imaging methods are preferable in the setting of moderate to severe renal insufficiency unless dialysis has already been instituted. The use of saline, bicarbonate solution, and N-acetylcysteine may reduce the incidence of acute renal failure due to iodinated contrast material[14-16] but may not be effective in patients with severe renal dysfunction.[17,18]

Radiation exposure is a significant consideration in the use of CCT. Typical helical acquisitions with a 64-slice machine are associated with an effective dose of 15 to 21 mSv, which is associated with a nontrivial risk of cancer that is higher in women and in younger patients.[19] Dose modulation (reducing the radiation dose during ventricular systole) reduces the effective dose to 5 to 10 mSv.[19] Imaging with lower energy radiation reduces the dose an additional 15% to 20%.[20] Prospective gating with use of a step-and-shoot mode of imaging is associated with a relatively low radiation exposure of 4 to 6 mSv, but it does not perform imaging over the entire cardiac cycle.[21] Increasing awareness of the radiation exposure associated with CCT has led to the adoption of one or more of these techniques at most centers. For middle-aged and younger patients with chronic disorders, potential radiation exposure for the expected multiple tests over their lifetimes should be considered.

CLINICAL APPLICATIONS

Diseases of the Thoracic Aorta

CMR and CCT are widely used clinically for the assessment of thoracic aortic aneurysm and dissection. With CMR, the structure of the aorta is delineated by a combination of the following protocol components in the transverse, coronal, sagittal, and oblique planes: (1) ECG-gated spin echo imaging, which reveals the aortic wall with rapidly flowing blood appearing black and thrombus and slowly moving blood appearing gray; (2) ECG-gated steady-state free precession (SSFP) imaging, which produces bright blood images in single-shot as well as in cine acquisitions; and (3) three-dimensional (3D) CE-MRA with a gradient echo acquisition. Temporally resolved CE-MRA is particularly useful to minimize motion artifacts that would otherwise cause nondiagnostic or false-positive results. With CCT, imaging of the aorta involves a larger image acquisition volume to include the entire thoracic aorta and can be performed with or without ECG gating. Gating is preferred for the evaluation of dissection to avoid motion artifacts that can mimic a dissection flap.[21]

Aortic Aneurysm

CMR and CCT are also superior methods for identification of true and false thoracic aortic aneurysms. In true aneurysms, the aneurysmal aortic wall is composed of intima, media, and adventitia. False aneurysms represent a contained rupture of the intima and media, with only the adventitia and periadventitial connective tissue limiting the hemorrhage (Fig. 53-1). False aneurysms generally have a narrow "neck" or communication with the main aortic lumen. True aneurysms are more commonly fusiform (bulge aligned along the long axis of the aorta; Fig. 53-2) than saccular (sacklike bulge extending from a side of the aortic wall). CE-MRA reveals the presence and extent of these lesions as well as any associated thrombus. CCT is recommended as the imaging modality of choice for most patients in the assessment of acute disease; 3D CE-MRA is recommended for most patients with chronic disease.[22] As with aortic dissection, advantages of CMR and CCT assessment compared with x-ray angiography include the capability to evaluate for associated complications, such as hemopericardium and left ventricular dysfunction. CMR can also assess for the presence of associated aortic regurgitation. After composite graft replacement of the ascending aorta, CMR is useful for detection of postoperative complications, such as leakage or hematoma formation.[23,24]

Aortic Dissection

CMR and CCT, along with transesophageal echocardiography (TEE), are the primary methods used to diagnose and to monitor patients with acute or chronic aortic dissection. Because each of these imaging modalities has high diagnostic accuracy for dissection, the selection among these methods is generally governed by the condition of the patient, institutional access, and local expertise. Both CMR and CCT offer a good combination of sensitivity and specificity (sensitivity above 95% and specificity above 90%) for dissection[25] and provide information about involvement of major branch vessels and all segments of the aorta, unlike TEE, which is limited to the thoracic aorta and by the adequacy of acoustic windows (particularly for the segment of ascending aorta anterior to the trachea). All three methods provide useful information about pericardial involvement. CMR can also assess aortic valve integrity, as can TEE. The main disadvantages of CMR in the acute setting are potential obstacles to continuous monitoring and care of an unstable patient during transport and performance of the study and the requirement that the patient remain motionless during the examination. CCT is frequently available in the emergency department and is therefore the most common initial imaging modality chosen to diagnose acute aortic dissection.[26] However, CMR is considered the imaging procedure of choice[27] for serial follow-up of the medically or surgically treated patient with dissection according to the recommendations of the task force on aortic dissection of the European Society of Cardiology (which have been endorsed by the American College of Cardiology) because of the lack of radiation exposure.[28] Follow-up is recommended after hospital discharge at 1 month, 3 months, 6 months, 12 months, and yearly thereafter.[28] Accurate interpretation of postoperative images requires knowledge of the surgical procedure performed and the expected range of routine postoperative sequelae, including thickening around the graft and presence of thrombus outside the graft and within the native aortic wrap.[29]

CCT aortic assessment is typically completed in less than 1 minute and often in less than 30 seconds; CMR aortic assessment can often be completed within 20 minutes. Both can display the location and extent of dissection identified as an intimal flap separating true and false aortic lumens along with sites of intraluminal communication and can readily assess involvement of the aortic root, arch vessels, and renal arteries (see Fig. 53-2). CMR spin echo images may identify relatively bright regions within the true or false lumen attributable to stagnant blood flow or thrombus. Gradient echo images demonstrate flap motion and blood flow in the true and false lumens. 3D CE-MRA is highly sensitive for dissection[30] and can be implemented with subsecond temporal resolution to obviate the need for a breath hold (Fig. 53-3).[31] Alternatively, SSFP imaging without administration of an exogenous contrast

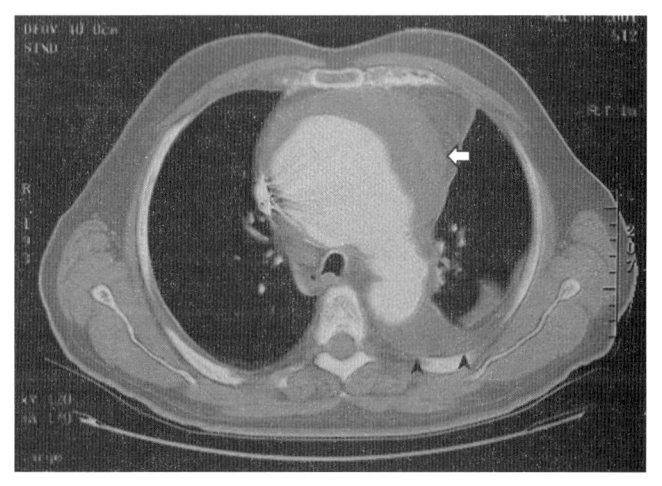

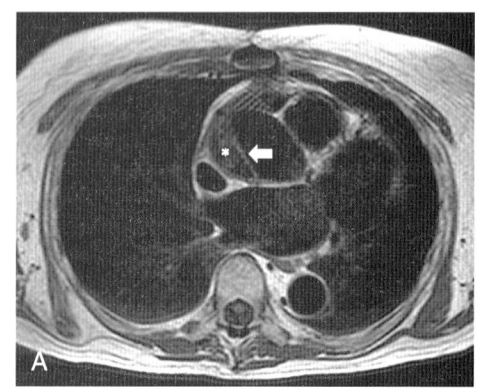

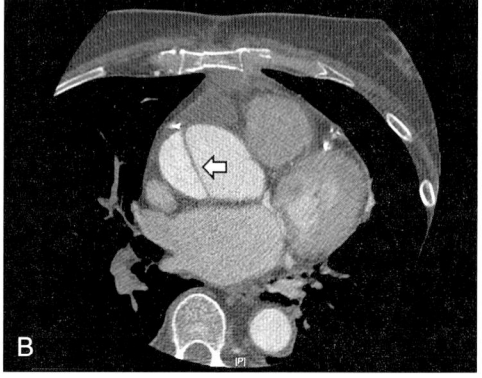

Figure 53–1
Ruptured aorta. Non–ECG-gated contrast-enhanced CCT axial image of the aorta at the level of the aortic arch. There is a contained rupture of the ascending aorta with blood and thrombus filling the mediastinum *(white arrow)* and a hemorrhagic left pleural effusion *(black arrowheads)*.

Figure 53–2
Aortic dissection. Axial images of aortic dissection from the same patient. **A,** T1-weighted spin echo CMR shows a dissection flap *(arrow)* in the ascending aorta. Note the increased signal in the false lumen *(asterisk)* due to slow blood flow. **B,** ECG-gated contrast-enhanced CCT axial image at the same location as the CMR image. The dissection flap *(arrow)* is again identified in the ascending aorta.

agent can be accomplished within 4 minutes and may suffice (Fig. 53-4).[32] Left ventricular function and involvement of the proximal coronary arteries can be assessed by CCT with a gated acquisition or CMR with additional cine and coronary imaging. CMR can also assess the presence of aortic regurgitation (by cine imaging of the left ventricular outflow tract) and the size of the regurgitant fraction (by a phase velocity encoding acquisition at the base of the aortic root).

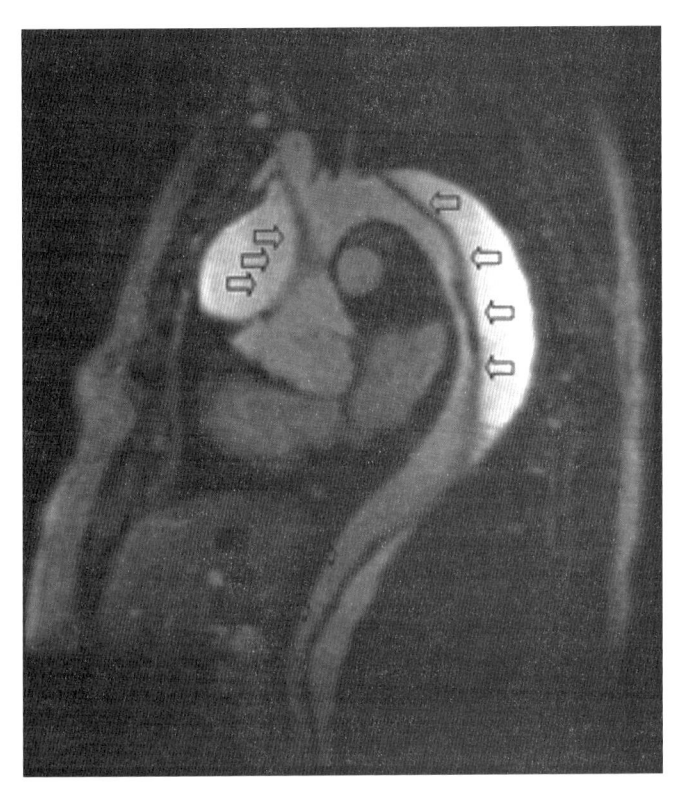

Figure 53–3
Aortic dissection. The three-dimensional contrast-enhanced CMR oblique image of the thoracic aorta demonstrates a DeBakey classification type 1 dissection (arrows) involving the ascending and descending thoracic aorta.

Aortic Intramural Hematoma

Intramural hematoma can be identified by a localized thickening, frequently crescentic or circular, within the wall of the aorta, interposed between intima and media, with characteristics of an acute or subacute collection of blood.[33] Whereas both CMR and CCT can identify intramural hematoma,[34] CMR has been found to be superior to CCT in distinguishing acute intramural hematoma from atherosclerotic plaque and chronic intraluminal thrombus.[35] Acute hemorrhage appears isointense or more intense compared with the aortic wall on T1-weighted images and displays high signal intensity on T2-weighted images.[33,36] In contrast, subacute hemorrhage displays high signal intensity on T1 images and less signal intensity on T2 images. The layer of displaced calcified intima overlying the hematoma generally produces a relatively smooth surface concave to the lumen (crescent shape), which may help distinguish this entity from protuberant, frequently irregularly shaped atherosclerotic plaque.

Sinus of Valsalva Aneurysm

A sinus of Valsalva aneurysm is often first suspected on transthoracic echocardiography and can be readily visualized by CCT, CMR, and TEE as an enlargement or outpouching (frequently creating a "windsock" appearance) of a sinus of the aortic root. CMR and echocardiography offer the advantage of providing information about blood flow (e.g., rupture of the aneurysmal sinus into an adjacent chamber) in addition to anatomy (Fig. 53-5). Shunt flow through the rupture is generally present both in diastole and in systole. The magnitude of the shunt may be calculated by flow velocity encoding data.

Atherosclerotic Plaque and Aortic-Penetrating Ulcer

CMR, CCT, and TEE can provide qualitative and quantitative information about the presence, thickness, and distribution of atherosclerotic plaque in the aorta.[37-39] Complex plaque is generally defined as protuberant plaque at least 4 mm in thickness or plaque with mobile elements because plaque with these

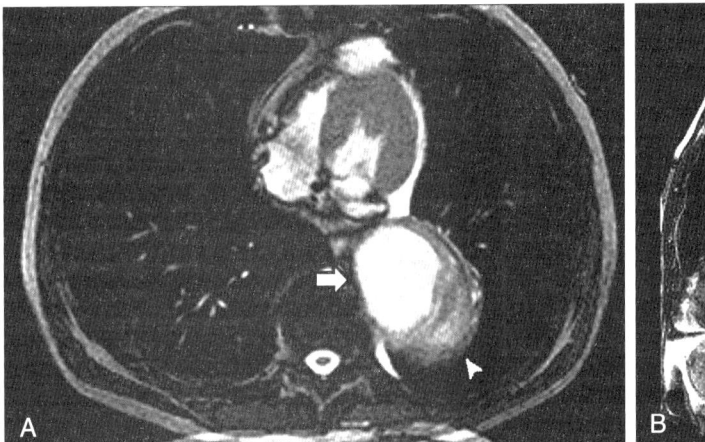

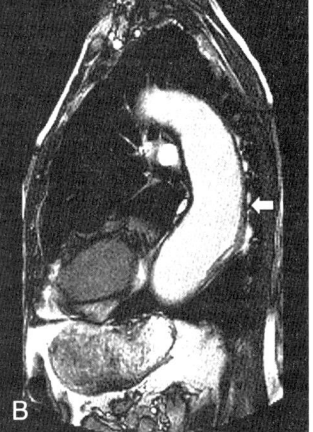

Figure 53–4
Aortic aneurysm. Non–contrast-enhanced CMR in the transverse (A) and oblique sagittal (B) imaging planes of a patient with a descending thoracic aortic aneurysm (arrow) partially filled with thrombus (arrowhead). Each image was acquired in less than 1 second with the SSFP sequence without the administration of an exogenous contrast agent. (Courtesy of Tim Leiner, MD, PhD.)

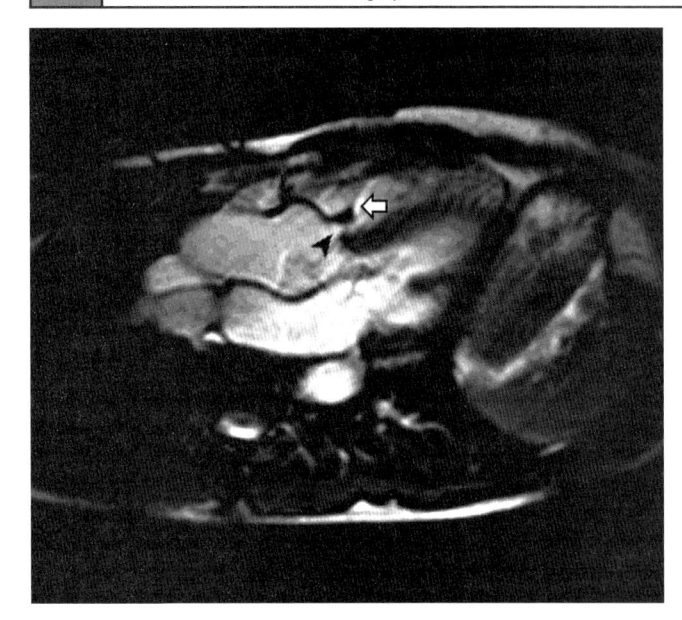

Figure 53-5
Sinus of Valsalva aneurysm. SSFP cine CMR image of a ruptured sinus of Valsalva aneurysm *(arrowhead)* with signal void *(arrow)* in the right ventricle from associated turbulent flow.

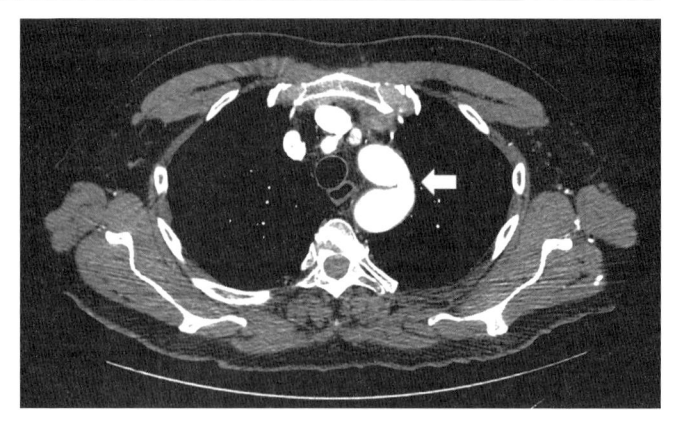

Figure 53-6
Aortic coarctation. Non–ECG-gated contrast-enhanced axial CCT image at the level of the aortic arch shows severe narrowing of the aorta *(arrow)*.

characteristics is associated with embolic risk.[40] Plaque thickness can readily be ascertained by CMR or CCT, although overlying mobile elements are best assessed by TEE because of their chaotic motion and relatively small size.[41] Ascending aortic plaque is a predictor of adverse cerebral outcomes after coronary artery bypass grafting. Preoperative (CMR or CCT) or intraoperative (TEE) identification of such plaque may prompt alteration in surgical strategy or technique.[40,42]

Aortic ulceration occurs in regions of atherosclerotic plaque. Penetrating ulcers are described as those breaching the internal elastic lamina with associated hematoma formation in the media.[43,44] CMR and CCT images visualize the position and shape of such ulcers and accompanying adjacent intramural hematoma.[35,39,41] Penetrating ulcers are also frequently associated with aortic aneurysm formation.[44,45] Associated chest or back pain is a significant risk factor for progression to pseudoaneurysm or free rupture.[44]

Takayasu's Arteritis

Takayasu's arteritis is a chronic idiopathic vasculitis that primarily affects the aorta and its branches. It is most prevalent among Asian women younger than 40 years.[46,47] The aortic arch (or distal aorta) and its branches as well as the pulmonary arteries have characteristically tapered narrowings or occlusions with areas of dilatation. The availability of noninvasive imaging is important among these patients, who require long-term follow-up to guide medical and surgical therapy. These lesions have been traditionally detected by conventional x-ray angiography, but CMR and CCT can accurately display these lesions and also provide information about a vessel wall abnormality.[48,49] CMR is generally preferred because of the need for repeated imaging in these younger subjects. Evidence of vessel wall edema is common but does not correlate well with subsequent lesion development.[50] Therefore, the current role of imaging in this disease is to identify the characteristic angiographic lesions.[49]

Congenital Aortic Anomalies

Both CMR and CCT can readily identify and characterize aortic coarctation, patent ductus arteriosus, and other congenital abnormalities involving the great vessels. The choice is based on local expertise or availability and issues related to the patient's age and renal function.

Aortic coarctation is characterized by a ridge of medial thickening and intimal hyperplasia along the posterolateral aortic wall. Coarctation most commonly presents just distal to the left subclavian, occurring more rarely just proximal to the left subclavian. Anatomic assessment with CMR or CCT reveals the location of the coarctation and associated collaterals, usually assessed in an oblique sagittal view aligned with the descending and ascending thoracic aorta (Fig. 53-6).[51] Typical CMR protocols use spin echo, gradient echo, or CE-MRA techniques.[52,53] Additional cardiac lesions that frequently accompany coarctation can also be identified, including bicuspid aortic valve (imaged in cross section) and ventricular septal defect (imaged in a horizontal long-axis or four-chamber view). Imaging is also useful for follow-up after surgical repair or balloon angioplasty,[52,54] and routine CMR follow-up has been recommended.[55] Potential complications that may be visualized include renarrowing and aneurysm or pseudoaneurysm at the repair site.

Whereas patent ductus arteriosus can usually be identified by transthoracic echocardiography, CMR or CCT may be useful when echocardiographic images are nondiagnostic due to poor acoustic windows.[56,57] For both patent ductus arteriosus and atrial or ventricular septal defects, CMR can provide an assessment of the pulmonic-to-systemic flow ratio (Qp/Qs) by applying the flow velocity encoding technique.[58]

CMR imaging is usually preferred to CCT for evaluation of congenital aortic anomalies because of concerns about radiation exposure in these generally younger patients and the potential need for serial studies in this population.

Thoracic Trauma

Chest radiography and CCT are generally the initial imaging modalities for assessment of acute thoracic trauma. In addition to providing information about the thoracic aorta, CCT also provides a comprehensive assessment of the thoracic anatomy, including the chest wall, mediastinum, diaphragm, and vertebrae. CMR may be useful for assessment

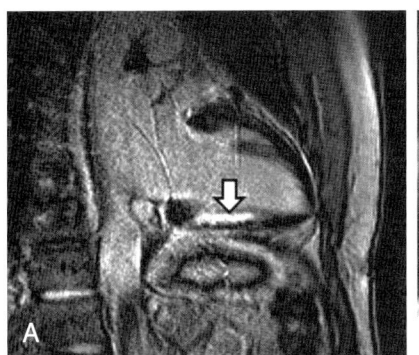

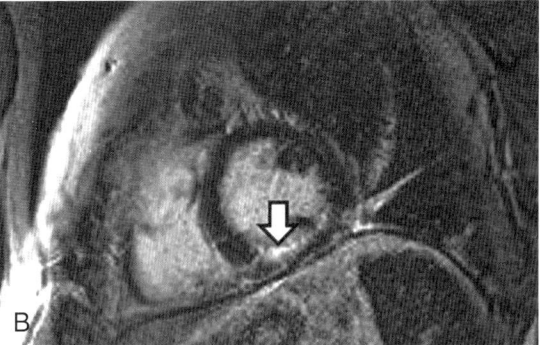

Figure 53-7
Late gadolinium enhancement CMR two-chamber (**A**) and mid-ventricular short-axis (**B**) views in a patient with an inferior myocardial infarction. The region of late contrast enhancement *(arrows)* corresponds to scar.

of diaphragmatic, mediastinal, and aortic injury if computed tomographic scanning results are equivocal and for characterizing post-traumatic masses such as hematomas.[59]

Cardiac Imaging

Ventricular Structure and Function

CMR is the reference standard for the quantitative assessment of left and right ventricular chamber sizes, systolic function, and mass, with greater reproducibility than is available with other techniques.[4] Gender-specific normal reference values for CMR left ventricular mass, volumes, and ejection fraction have been defined and may be sequence dependent.[60,61] A set of breath-hold two-chamber, four-chamber, and short-axis cine images (acquired with a pulse sequence like SSFP) spanning the ventricles can be acquired within 10 minutes *without* use of an exogenous contrast agent. SSFP techniques provide superior endocardial border definition, thereby enabling use of semiautomated techniques for image analysis. Regional systolic function can be assessed by examining segmental wall motion and thickening. A 17-segment model common to echocardiography and nuclear cardiology is recommended.[62,63] In addition, CMR tagging methods may be useful in characterizing focal abnormalities and myocardial twist.[64]

The evaluation of left ventricular cavity size and systolic function with CCT requires acquisition of images throughout the cardiac cycle. This typically requires a helical acquisition, with or without dose modulation, and iodinated contrast material. Images are then reconstructed at 5% or 10% intervals over the entire cardiac cycle, with perhaps superior results with 5% intervals.[65] The entire 3D volume is reconstructed and can be displayed as a cine, but most centers choose to evaluate two-dimensional slices in the two-chamber, four-chamber, and short-axis orientations. Semiautomated algorithms for the quantitative evaluation of left ventricular cavity size and systolic function compare favorably with CMR.[5] Assessment of the right ventricle is more difficult because the passage of contrast material through the heart is timed to maximize opacification of the left side of the heart, such that the right ventricle cannot be adequately assessed in at least 25% of subjects.[66]

Left and right ventricular function has been most commonly assessed clinically by transthoracic echocardiography because of its wide availability and relative ease of use. Echocardiographic assessment is frequently limited by variability of views and suboptimal image quality and generally remains only qualitative. CMR and CCT offer advantages compared with echocardiography in providing uniformly superior image quality and in the quantification of both systolic function and cavity size.

Identification of Myocardial Scar and Ischemia

Among patients with resting regional left ventricular systolic dysfunction, identification of the presence and distribution of scar and viable myocardium within dysfunctional regions has important prognostic and therapeutic implications. A late gadolinium enhancement CMR technique has proved highly sensitive for determining the presence and spatial extent of acute and chronic myocardial infarction identified as regions of hyperenhancement (Fig. 53-7).[67-69] For heart failure patients with ischemic heart disease, CMR identification of scar closely agrees with positron emission tomography data.[70] Among patients with stable coronary artery disease undergoing mechanical revascularization by coronary artery bypass graft surgery or percutaneous intervention, the transmural and segmental extent of left ventricular scar detected by CMR is a strong negative predictor for regional and global recovery of systolic function after revascularization.[71] Analogous to transthoracic echocardiographic methods, low-dose dobutamine CMR also provides viability assessment.[72]

Pharmacologic CMR stress testing is useful for assessment of ischemia by induction of either wall motion abnormalities (dobutamine) or perfusion defects (vasodilator). Dobutamine CMR is superior to dobutamine echocardiography for the detection of ischemia-induced wall motion abnormalities,[73] but CMR perfusion techniques for assessment of myocardial ischemia with contrast enhancement are currently used only at specialized centers.[74,75]

CCT applications for the detection of scar and evaluation of myocardial perfusion are in development[76] but currently limited because of relatively high radiation exposures.

Congenital Heart Disease

CMR plays an important role in the diagnosis and management of simple and complex congenital heart disease.[77] The lack of ionizing radiation exposure is of particular

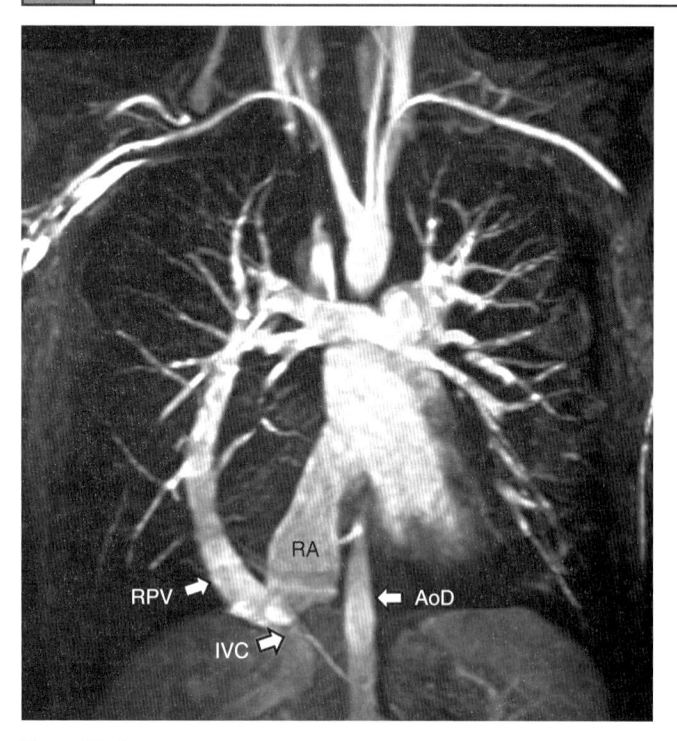

Figure 53–8
Scimitar syndrome. The scimitar syndrome is a rare form of partial anomalous pulmonary venous connection in which the entire right lung drains into the inferior vena cava. This contrast-enhanced CMR coronal maximal intensity projection in the anterior-posterior orientation shows the typical findings of the scimitar syndrome. The single right pulmonary vein (RPV) enters the inferior vena cava (IVC). The right atrium (RA) and descending aorta (AoD) are also shown. *(Courtesy of Andrew Powell, MD.)*

importance for these patients, who often undergo numerous monitoring tests during their lifetime. Its capabilities are complementary to those of echocardiography and cardiac catheterization in patients with congenital heart disease. CMR is particularly useful among children and adults with suboptimal acoustic windows[78] and those with complex lesions. CMR can effectively identify the location, orientation, and relationships between the venae cavae, cardiac chambers, valves, great vessels, and pulmonary veins. Anatomic structure can be displayed in tomographic views and in 3D reconstructions, which are particularly helpful in delineating complex spatial relationships (Fig. 53-8). In addition, phase contrast scans can be used for measurement of flow and thus quantify the magnitude of shunts associated with atrial and ventricular septal defects (Fig. 53-9).[79] Aortic forward and regurgitant flow can be quantified by phase contrast imaging in an axial (or oblique) plane transverse to the long axis of the ascending aorta. Similarly, phase contrast imaging in a cross-sectional slice of the proximal main pulmonary artery (oblique, generally near-coronal view) enables quantification of pulmonary artery forward and regurgitant flows. Thus, the ratio of pulmonary and aortic (forward) flows (Qp/Qs) can be calculated to identify and to quantify a significant (Qp/Qs > 1.5) intracardiac shunt.[79] CMR is particularly helpful for quantitation of right ventricular size and function important for clinical assessment of many types of congenital heart disease.[80]

CCT has similar utility in the assessment of the anatomy of the heart and great vessels in congenital heart disease. CMR is generally preferred in the assessment of congenital heart disease in children and young adults because of the greater risk of radiation exposure in this population. However, CCT can be helpful in the evaluation or follow-up of congenital heart disease in the adult population and in patients with a contraindication to CMR imaging.[81] Application of CCT in this setting requires careful attention to the reduction of radiation exposure and the timing of administration of contrast material to delineate the anatomy of interest.

Cardiac and Paracardiac Masses

CMR and CCT can readily delineate cardiac and paracardiac masses, such as tumors, myxomas, and thrombi. A particular benefit of both methods is for masses that extend outside the heart. Intracardiac masses are usually initially detected by transthoracic echocardiography and frequently are effectively characterized by echocardiography alone. When echocardiographic images are suboptimal or do not adequately define the extent of the mass, further imaging with CMR or CCT is useful to further define the characteristics and spatial extent of the mass within and beyond the cardiac borders. There are few data about the utility of CCT or CMR in the assessment of cardiac tumors because they are relatively rare. CMR may be more sensitive than echocardiography for detection of intracardiac and paracardiac involvement with lymphoma.[82] The 3D characterization of the mass is often helpful for surgical planning. Characterization of masses based on T1-weighted, T2-weighted, cine CMR, and post-contrast imaging is useful (Fig. 53-10).[83]

CMR offers additional advantages of being able to demonstrate specific tissue characteristics. Fat suppression techniques can aid in the diagnosis of lipomatous hypertrophy of the interatrial septum, resulting in thickening of the septum with relative sparing in the region of the fossa ovalis. The diagnosis is generally made by echocardiography alone, but marked focal septal thickening may suggest an atrial mass (thrombus or tumor). Fatty deposits may extend beyond the septum to surrounding pericardial deposits and occasionally cause deformation of the adjacent superior vena cava (Fig. 53-11). On T1-weighted images, the fatty tissue produces a characteristically high signal intensity (bright) that is selectively suppressed with a fat suppression sequence.

Thrombus is generally suspected by the appearance of a mass in a region of blood stasis (such as an aneurysmal or akinetic left ventricular apex) on either CMR or CCT.[84] The appearance of thrombus on CMR varies with the time. Early thrombus is seen as a region of high signal intensity on T1- and T2-weighted images. After 1 to 2 weeks, higher signal intensity may be noted on T1-weighted images and decreased signal intensity on T2-weighted images. Chronic thrombi have low signal intensity, with even greater signal loss in regions of calcification. Late gadolinium enhancement CMR may also define thrombi as a signal void lining the left ventricular cavity adjacent to hyperenhanced myocardial infarction and surrounding blood pool.[85]

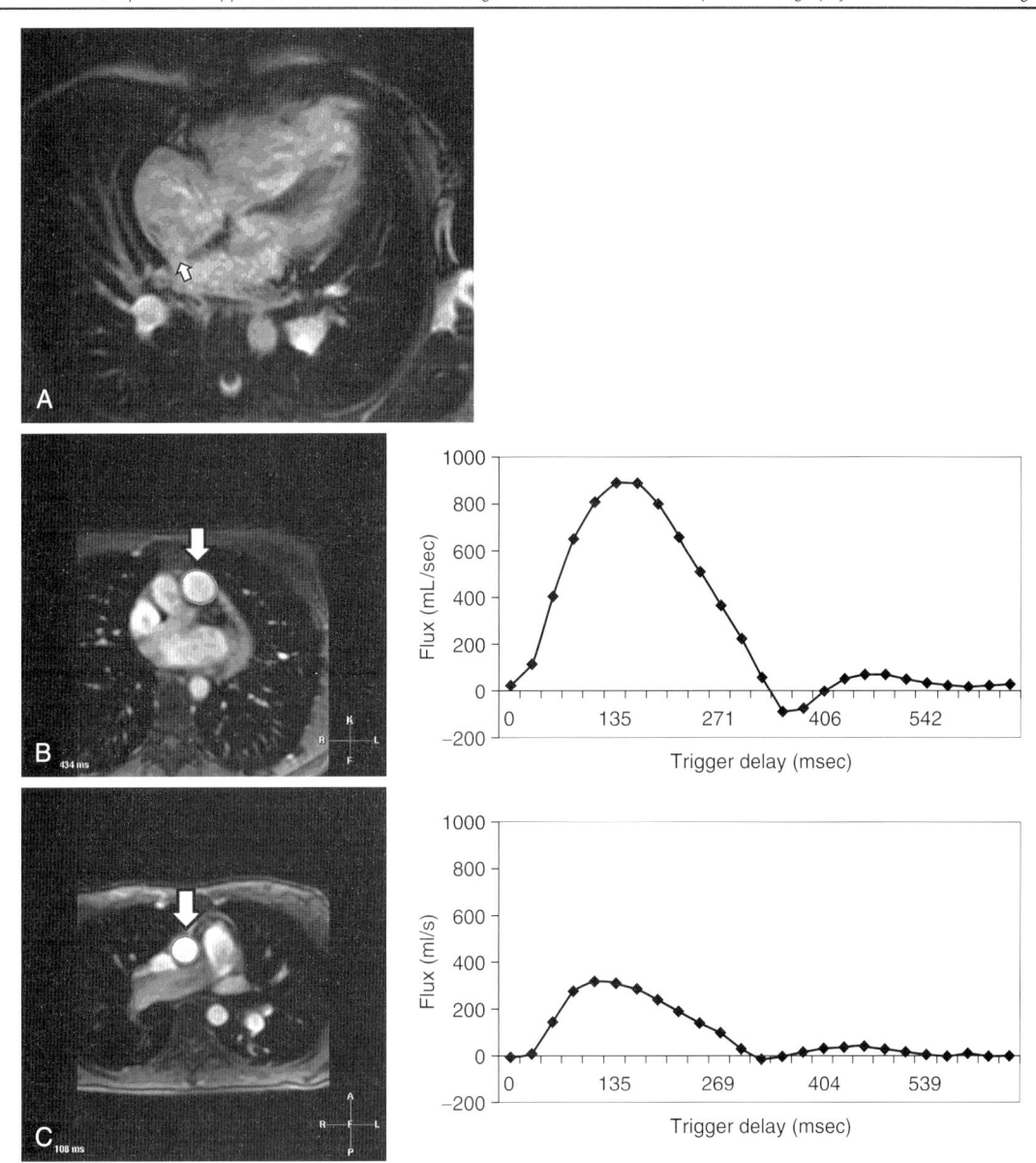

Figure 53–9
Sinus venosus atrial septal defect. **A,** Four-chamber SSFP cine CMR image of a sinus venosus atrial septal defect *(arrow)*. Phase velocity CMR at the level of the pulmonary artery (**B,** *arrow*) and aortic root (**C,** *arrow*) and corresponding flux contours indicate a pulmonary-to-systemic shunt ratio (Qp/Qs) of 3.0.

Pericardial Disease

CMR and CCT imaging capabilities, including a wide field of view, enable it to readily identify pericardial masses and cysts, pericardial effusion, and pericardial thickening. With CMR, a pericardial effusion has low signal intensity (relatively dark) on T1-weighted images and high signal intensity (bright) on T2-weighted and gradient echo scans. Late gadolinium enhancement CMR demonstrates marked enhancement of the pericardium in patients with acute pericarditis (Fig. 53-12).[86,87] With CCT, pericardial effusion has an intermediate attenuation that stands apart from the low-attenuation visceral and parietal pericardial fat (Fig. 53-13). Iodinated contrast material is not typically required to assess the pericardium with CCT. Both CCT and CMR are particularly useful for the identification of loculated effusions and accompanying pericardial masses or pericardial thickening.

CMR and CCT can also be useful in the diagnosis of constrictive pericarditis (Fig. 53-14).[88,89] Whereas the diagnosis requires clinical assessment for constrictive physiology, both imaging modalities can effectively identify focal regions of pericardial thickening characteristic of this disorder. CCT is preferred for identification of pericardial calcifications (which lack signal by CMR; Fig. 53-15).[88] On spin echo CMR images, normal pericardial thickness is 3 mm or less. Among patients with pericardial constriction, the CMR pericardial thickness is generally more than 6 mm,[89] with 4 to 6 mm being intermediate. Pericardial thickening associated

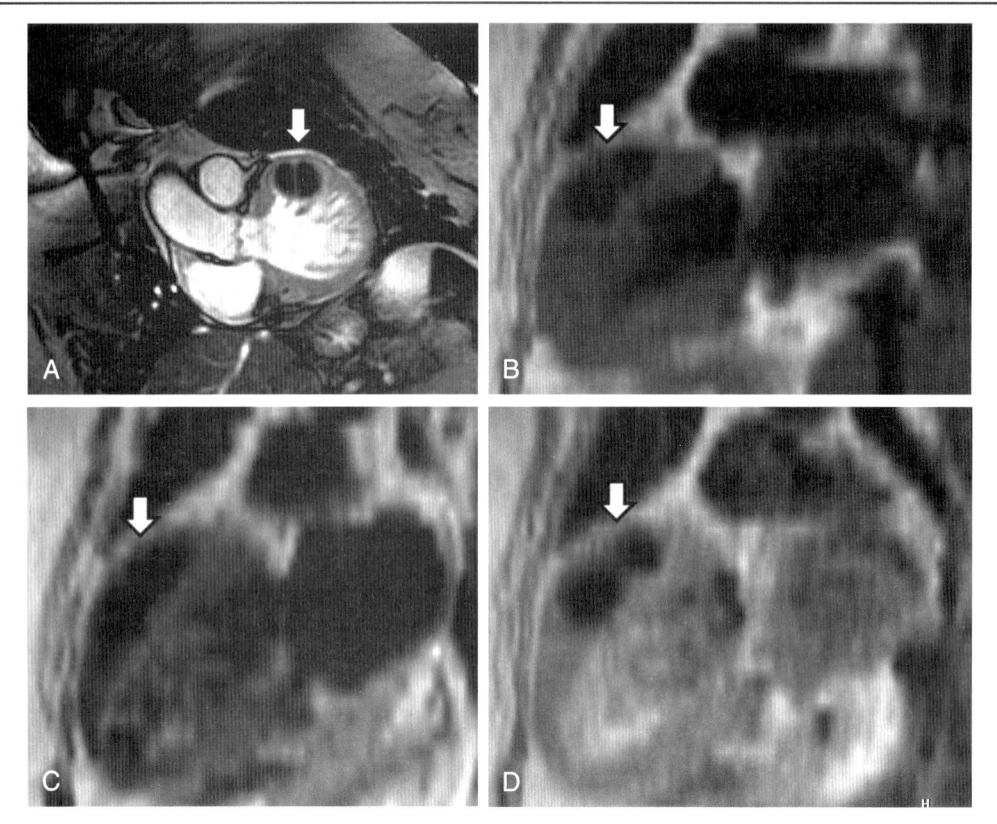

Figure 53–10
Myocardial fibroma. **A,** SSFP cine CMR image of the left ventricular outflow tract shows a well-circumscribed intramyocardial mass with low signal *(arrow)*. The mass had low signal on T1 weighting **(B)**, T2 weighting **(C)**, and T1 weighting after administration of contrast material **(D)** on spin echo imaging in the two-chamber view *(arrows)*, indicating calcification of the mass. These findings are consistent with a fibroma.

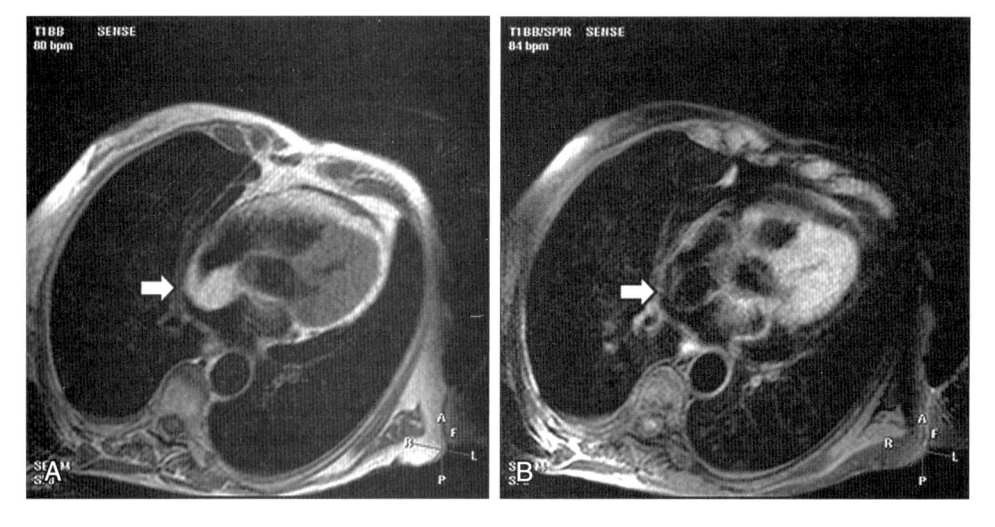

Figure 53–11
Lipomatous septal hypertrophy. Axial T1-weighted CMR spin echo image demonstrates high signal and focal thickening of the atrial septum **(A)** with signal loss after fat suppression **(B)** consistent with lipomatous hypertrophy.

with constriction is frequently focal, so identifying the location of thickening may be important to the surgical approach.[90,91] Spin echo images instead of gradient echo images should be used to assess pericardial thickness because the latter may overestimate pericardial thickness and fail to distinguish between patients with and without constriction.[92] ECG-gated acquisitions are useful for demonstration of abnormal early diastolic septal motion characteristic of constriction. CMR tagging methods are useful in identifying regions of parietal to visceral pericardial adherence.[93] In these areas,

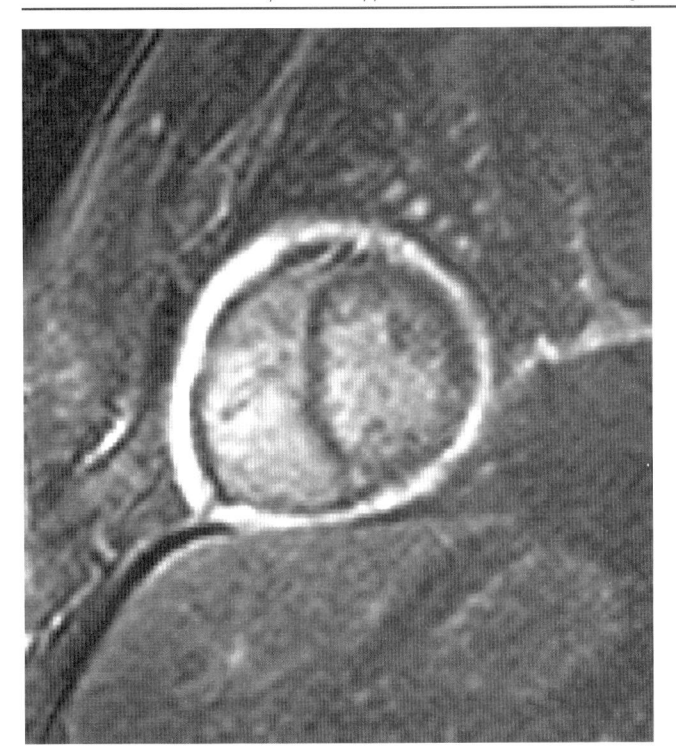

Figure 53–12
Pericarditis. Late gadolinium enhancement CMR image in the short-axis view at the level of the mid ventricle shows circumferential enhancement of the pericardium.

Figure 53–13
Pericardial effusion. Non-gated CCT image with a moderate pericardial effusion predominantly in the dependent portion of the pericardium *(asterisk)*, but also visible as a thin line at the anterior aspect of the heart *(arrowhead)*.

lack of free sliding between the pericardial layers during the cardiac cycle is visualized as persistent continuity in tag lines crossing the pericardial interface (lines deform but do not break).

Valvular Heart Disease

Although echocardiography is used most commonly in clinical practice for assessment of valvular morphology and stenosis, CMR offers specific advantages for the quantitative assessment of valvular regurgitation. Valvular regurgitation can be detected as a flow disturbance (signal void) on cine images, although the magnitude of the signal void is reduced with gradient echo and SSFP images with shorter echo times. Importantly, flow velocity encoding is a powerful technique for quantifying the regurgitant volume (Fig. 53-16). Flow velocity encoding (phase contrast) scans of the aortic root in axial or oblique (near-axial) cross-sectional views enable quantitation of aortic forward and regurgitant flows. The difference between left ventricular stroke volume (derived from summation of discs method applied to a contiguous stack of short-axis images spanning the left ventricle) and forward aortic flow is a quantitative measure of mitral regurgitation. The regurgitant fraction can be calculated as the ratio of the regurgitant volume to total stroke volume. By use of these techniques, CMR and echocardiography have good agreement in the assessment of mitral and aortic regurgitation. Analogous methods can be performed for pulmonary and tricuspid regurgitation.

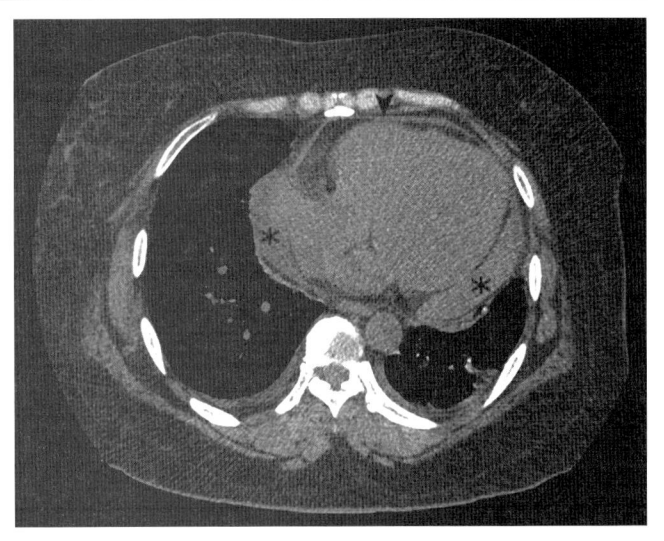

Cross-sectional and longitudinal views of the valves can be used to characterize valve deformities and stenoses (Fig. 53-17). CCT and CMR measures of aortic stenosis agree closely with both transthoracic and transesophageal echocardiography measurements.[94] Flow velocity encoding techniques may be useful in estimated valve gradients, although this application has not yet been fully validated.[95]

Cardiomyopathies

CMR and CCT are both useful in characterizing biventricular structure and function among patients with cardiomyopathy. The high reproducibility of these measures of ventricular size and function makes them a valuable tool for quantitative serial assessment among patients with dilated cardiomyopathy.

Among patients with hypertrophic cardiomyopathy, CMR and CCT can accurately delineate the distribution of hypertrophy among ventricular segments free of limitations (such as foreshortening of the apex and off-axis views) encountered by echocardiography. Thus, these imaging modalities are particularly helpful in identification of asymmetrical or apical hypertrophy (Fig. 53-18) and apical aneurysms.[96] Among patients with hypertrophic cardiomyopathy, late gadolinium enhancement CMR frequently identifies regions of myocardial fibrosis, which generally occurs at the junction of the interventricular septum with the right ventricular free wall.[97]

CMR provides unique information for certain specific types of cardiomyopathy. Late gadolinium enhancement images may detect focal myocardial abnormalities associated with sarcoidosis.[98] Hemochromatosis with myocardial iron deposition and left ventricular dysfunction is associated with

Figure 53-14
Effusive-constrictive pericarditis. Axial dual inversion T1-weighted (A) and cine SSFP (B) CMR images of a patient with effusive-constrictive pericarditis. Pericardial fluid appears relatively bright; pericardium and organized material appear dark. The end-systolic tagged four-chamber image (C) demonstrates tethering of pericardial elements to the right ventricular *(arrow)* and left ventricular *(arrowhead)* walls.

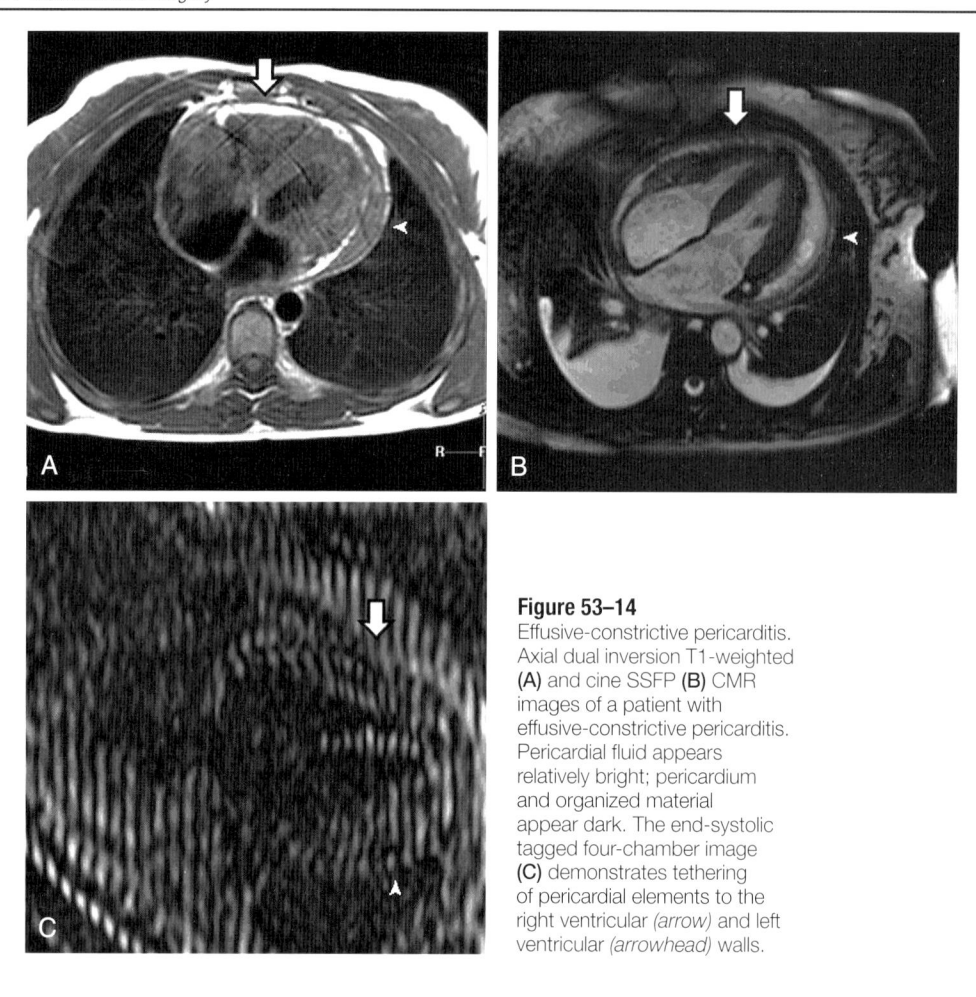

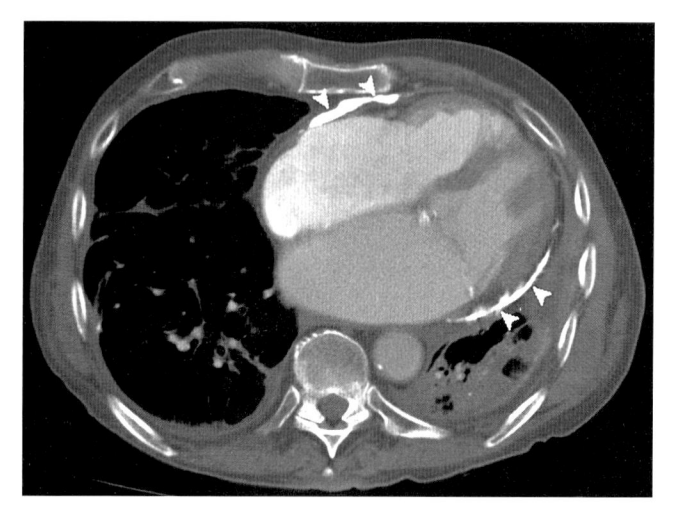

Figure 53-15
Non–ECG-gated contrast-enhanced axial CCT image of a patient with pericardial constriction and pericardial calcification *(arrowheads)*.

a depressed $T2^*$.[99] CMR serves as a cornerstone for diagnosis of arrhythmogenic right ventricular dysplasia to determine right ventricular cavity size, to evaluate global and regional right ventricular free wall function, and to detect any fibrofatty infiltration of myocardium, although the specificity and sensitivity of these findings have not been fully defined (Fig. 53-19).[100]

CMR and CCT may also be useful for discriminating between ischemic and nonischemic causes of cardiomyopathy. CMR can identify scar suggestive of prior infarction as well as assess coronary artery disease,[101] with a high predictive value for excluding left main or three-vessel coronary disease.[102] CCT also has good accuracy for excluding left main or three-vessel disease.[103]

Coronary Artery Imaging

Noninvasive coronary artery imaging is technically demanding, with maximal demands on spatial, temporal, and contrast resolution. At experienced centers, coronary MRA can effectively identify significant stenoses in the proximal to mid native coronary arteries.[102] Current imaging protocols incorporate methodology to suppress the effects of cardiac motion and respiratory motion.[104] Cardiac motion is addressed through robust ECG signal detection to trigger gating and customized adjustment of the acquisition window. Respiratory motion artifacts are suppressed by CMR navigators or prolonged breath holds.[105] A 3D acquisition is employed to enhance the signal-to-noise ratio, although the signal-to-noise ratio is somewhat diminished by the prepulses required to optimize the contrast-to-noise ratio. To enhance contrast between blood in the coronaries and the

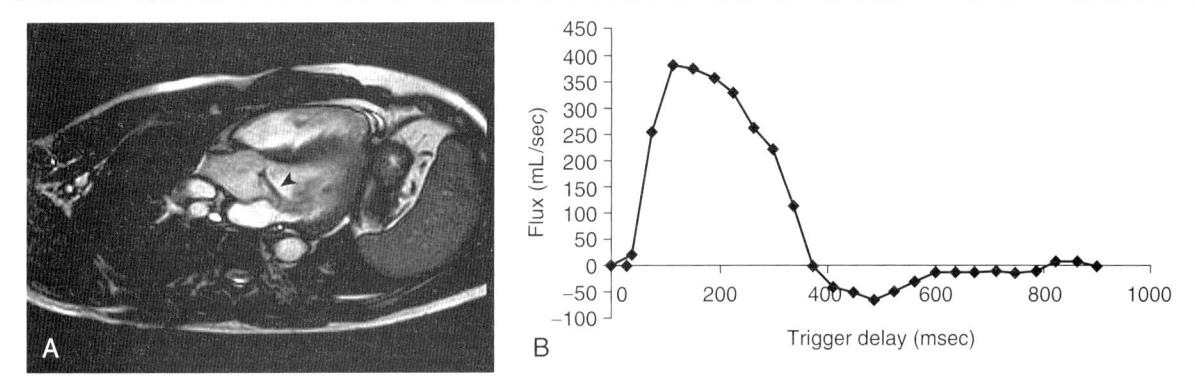

Figure 53–16
Aortic regurgitation. **A,** SSFP cine CMR image of the left ventricular outflow tract shows an eccentric jet of turbulent flow indicating aortic regurgitation *(arrowhead)*. **B,** Flow contour from a phase contrast acquisition in the aortic root just above the aortic valve indicates significant negative diastolic flow.

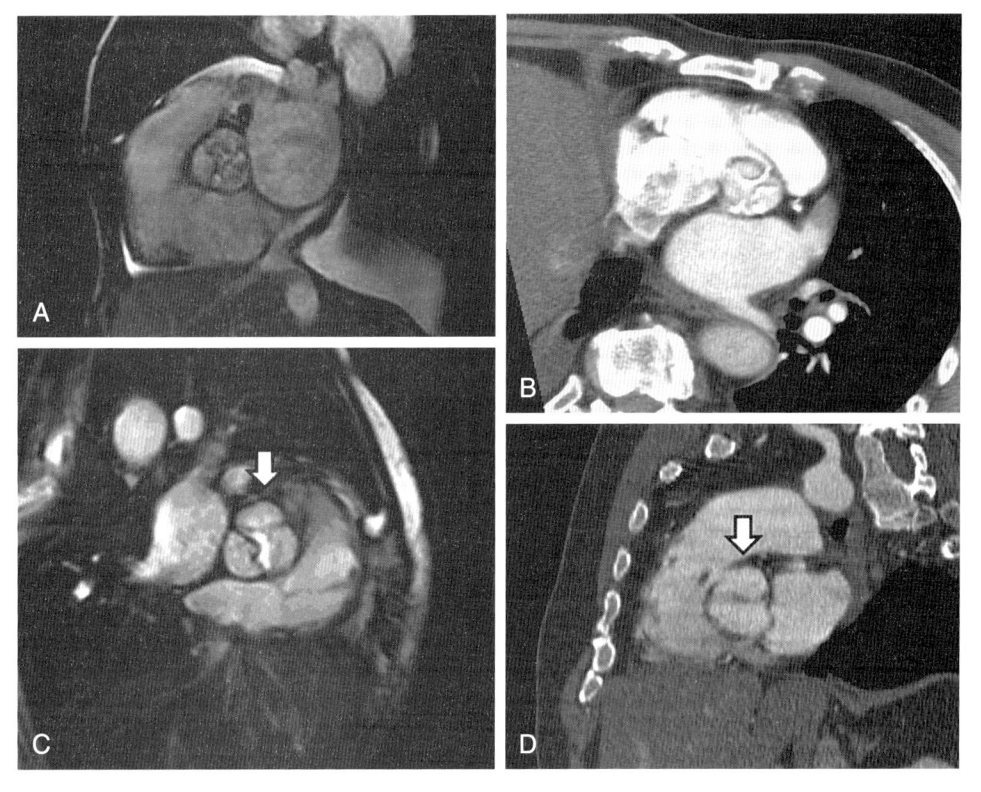

Figure 53–17
Aortic valve disease. SSFP cine CMR (**A**) and CCT (**B**) images of a trileaflet, calcified, and stenotic aortic valve in short axis.

surrounding myocardium and epicardial fat, a T2-weighted preparation prepulse and a frequency-selective fat-saturation prepulse are applied. In a multicenter study of patients referred for elective x-ray coronary angiography, coronary MRA had a 72% accuracy in diagnosis of coronary artery disease (defined as ≥50% diameter stenosis on x-ray angiography; Fig. 53-20).[102] The accuracy of coronary artery CMR for diagnosis of left main coronary artery disease or three-vessel disease was 87%. Of note, the negative predictive value of MRA for left main or three-vessel disease was 97% to 100%. Whole heart techniques, which acquire a 3D imaging volume of the entire heart in a manner analogous to CCT, are increasingly popular with promising results.[106,107] A preliminary multicenter trial report evaluating this technique suggests promising results.[108] High-field (3-T) coronary artery CMR with a gadolinium-based contrast agent also appears promising.[109]

CCT has shown tremendous promise in the evaluation of native vessel coronary artery disease. Multiple single-center studies have demonstrated sensitivities and specificities in the range of 90%, with superior results for 64-slice technology, the current standard. Although an initial multicenter trial with 16-slice technology had good sensitivity of 94% with a specificity of 52%,[110] two large 64-slice

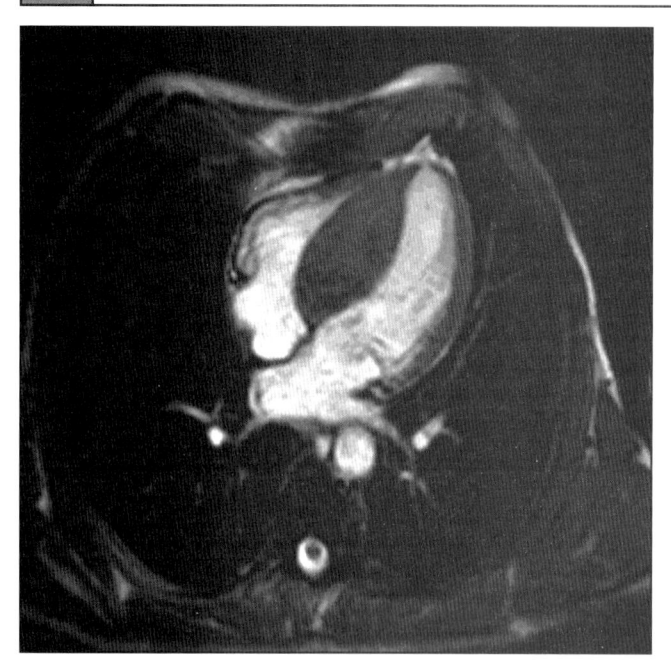

Figure 53–18
Hypertrophic cardiomyopathy. SSFP cine CMR four-chamber image in a patient with hypertrophic cardiomyopathy with asymmetrical septal hypertrophy.

multicenter trials have recently shown sensitivities in the range of 85% to 94% with specificities of 83% to 90% (Fig. 53-21).[111,112] These trials have generally been performed in high-risk patients with abnormal stress test results. Further trials are needed to clarify the future clinical role of CCT for the detection of coronary artery disease. Epicardial calcium is associated with the development of coronary atherosclerosis and is a marker of increased risk for adverse events associated with coronary artery disease.[113] The presence of epicardial calcium is a well-recognized limitation for coronary artery CCT, with an exaggerated appearance on imaging (frequently referred to as blooming) that interferes with the accurate determination of coronary artery stenosis.

Several studies have directly compared CCT with coronary artery CMR for the detection of coronary artery disease. Overall, these studies have suggested near-equivalence of the current methods when *interpretable* segments are considered and superiority for 64-slice multidetector computed tomography for patients with lower calcium scores with intention-to-diagnose analyses.[114-117]

The accuracy of CCT and CMR for graft vessel disease is generally superior to that for the detection of native vessel disease because the grafts are larger and move less, reducing the technical demands of imaging. However, local image artifacts due to associated implanted metallic objects (such as hemostatic clips, stainless steel graft markers, and sternal wires) may interfere with adequate graft visualization, causing signal dropout with CMR and beam hardening artifacts with CCT (Fig. 53-22).[104] In spite of these limitations, various investigators have demonstrated a sensitivity of 88% to 98% and a specificity of 72% to 100% for CMR detection of coronary artery bypass graft patency.[118-123] Langerak and colleagues suggest that a high-resolution navigator-gated 3D CMR approach can yield not only high sensitivity and specificity for graft occlusion (83% and 98% to 100%, respectively) but also fairly high sensitivity and specificity for graft stenosis of 70% or more (73% and 80% to 87%, respectively).[124] These investigators have found an even higher sensitivity and specificity for graft stenosis of 70% or more (87% to 100% and 84% to 100%, respectively) with use of a flow velocity encoding protocol.[125] CCT has proved to be similarly accurate in the evaluation of graft vessel disease, with sensitivities and specificities exceeding 95%.[126]

The most common clinical use of coronary artery CMR is for the identification and characterization of anomalous coronary arteries. Studies comparing coronary artery CMR with conventional x-ray coronary angiography reveal equivalent to superior accuracy in the identification of anomalous coronary arteries.[127-130] Because coronary artery CMR demonstrates the origin and course of each coronary artery in 3D relation to the great vessels, it can resolve spatial ambiguity sometimes encountered in interpreting conventional projection x-ray coronary angiographic images.[127,129,130] Coronary artery CMR is particularly helpful in identifying whether the anomalous artery courses between the aorta and the pulmonary artery (Fig. 53-23), a malignant configuration associated with sudden death and myocardial infarction among young adults.[131] In addition, among patients undergoing cardiac surgery for repair or palliation of other congenital defects, it may be important to identify and to define any coincident anomalous coronary arteries to avoid inadvertent iatrogenic injury.[128] Whereas CCT is also good at detecting the presence and course of anomalous coronary arteries, CMR is generally preferred because of the lack of radiation in this generally younger population.

Data on the determination of prognosis in patients with coronary atherosclerosis or obstructive disease are beginning to emerge. Coronary artery calcification, most commonly quantified with the Agatston score, is predictive of future coronary adverse events and is superior to traditional risk factors alone.[113] Implementation of coronary calcium imaging has been hindered by a lack of a therapy tied to this finding to reduce event rates. CCT also has prognostic information. Patients with obstructive disease, compared with those with nonobstructive or no disease, have a worse prognosis that further worsens with the number of vessels involved.[132]

THE FUTURE ROLE OF CARDIOVASCULAR MAGNETIC RESONANCE AND COMPUTED TOMOGRAPHY

CMR and CCT technologies continue to evolve, with promising results. Advances in CCT have been focused on increasing the number of detectors, faster gantry speeds, and algorithms to decrease radiation exposure. Advances in CMR have been focused on higher field strengths, faster imaging with use of parallel acquisitions, and novel contrast agents. Both technologies are likely to continue to advance rapidly, with their clinical roles defined by multicenter trials.

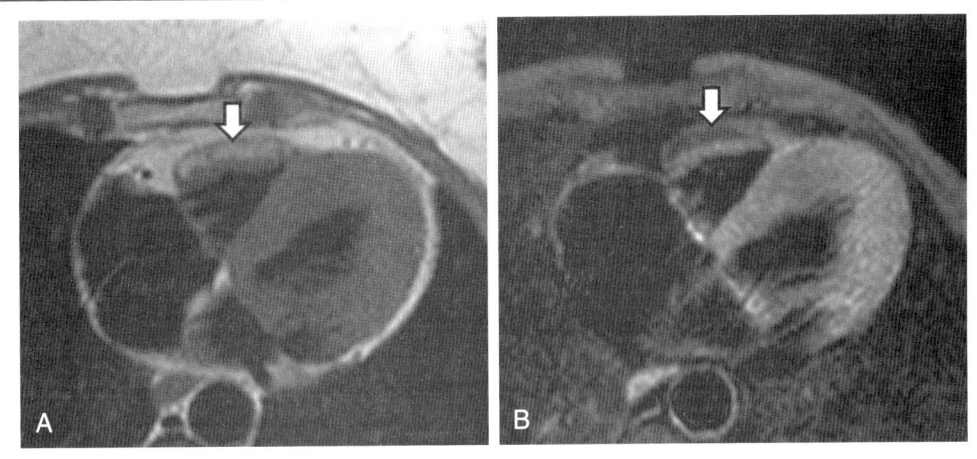

Figure 53–19
Arrhythmogenic right ventricular cardiomyopathy. Spin echo CMR without **(A)** and with **(B)** a fat suppression prepulse. There is bright signal in the free wall of the right ventricle that suppresses with fat suppression *(arrows)*.

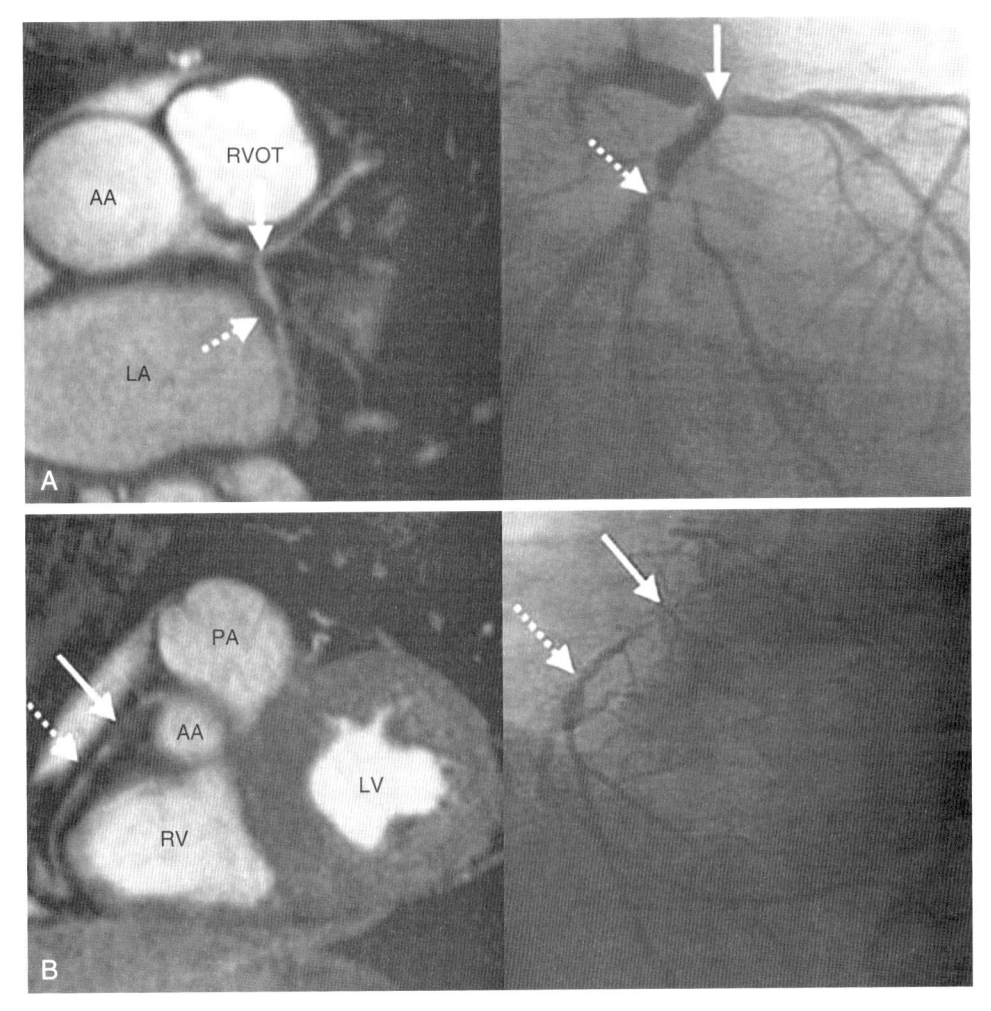

Figure 53–20
Coronary artery disease. **A,** Coronary CMR image with a three-dimensional gradient echo sequence *(left)* and a corresponding x-ray coronary angiogram *(right)* indicate a severe lesion at the bifurcation of the left main coronary artery *(solid arrows)* and a more distal focal stenosis of the proximal left circumflex coronary artery *(broken arrows)*. **B,** Coronary CMR image *(left)* and a corresponding x-ray angiogram *(right)* indicate two stenoses of the proximal *(solid arrows)* and middle *(broken arrows)* right coronary artery. AA, ascending aorta; LA, left atrium; RVOT, right ventricular outflow tract; PA, pulmonary artery; RV, right ventricle; LV, left ventricle. *(From Kim WY, Danias PG, Stuber M, et al. Three-dimensional coronary magnetic resonance angiography for the detection of coronary stenoses. N Engl J Med 2001;**345**:1863-1869, with permission.)*

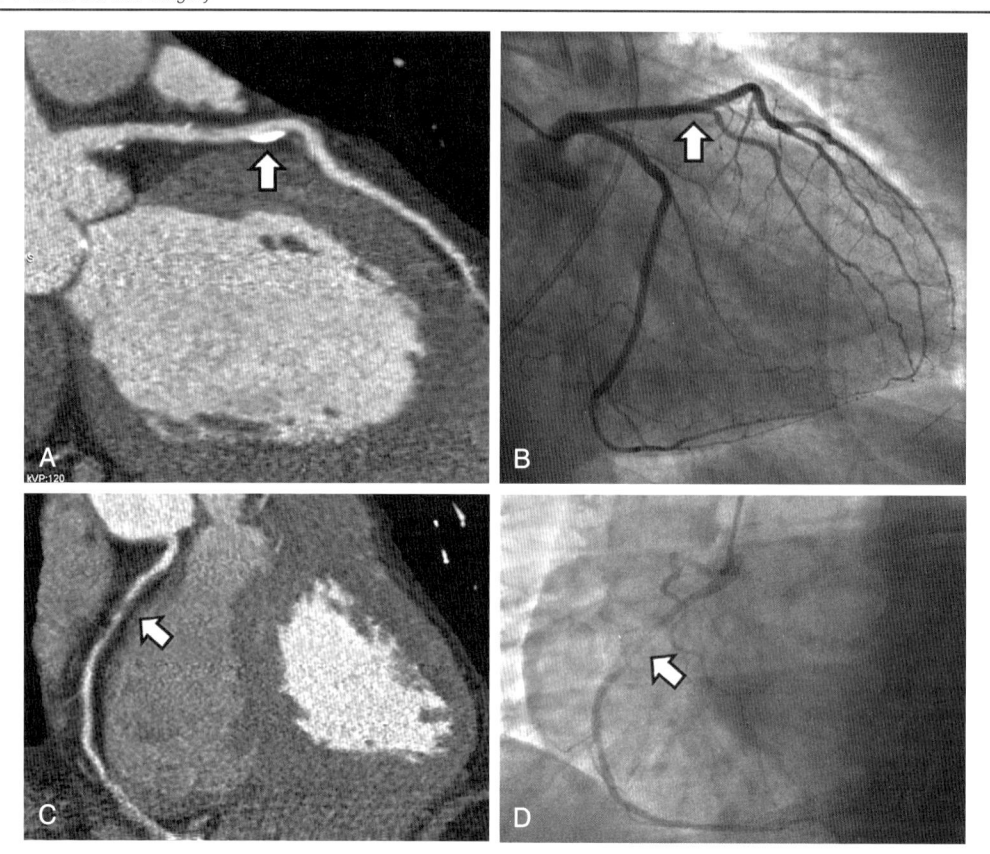

Figure 53-21
Coronary artery disease. **A,** Curved multiplanar reformation CCT image of the left anterior descending coronary artery shows a calcified plaque *(arrow)* without stenosis. **B,** Invasive x-ray angiography confirmed the absence of stenosis, with the plaque present as a subtle indentation of the lumen *(arrow)*. **C,** Curved multiplanar reformation CCT image of the right coronary artery showing a noncalcified plaque with severe stenosis *(arrow)*. **D,** Invasive x-ray angiography confirmed the presence of severe stenosis *(arrow)*.

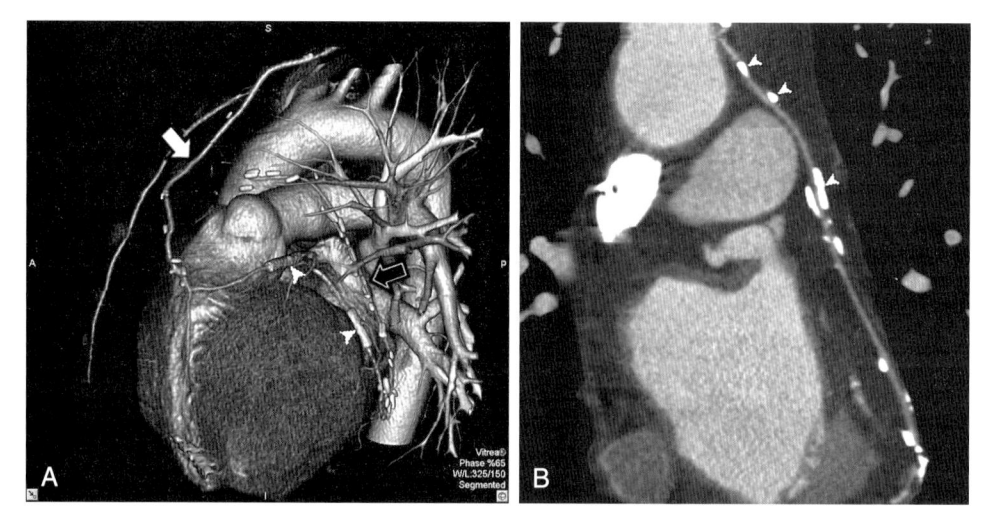

Figure 53-22
Bypass grafts. **A,** A three-dimensional volume-rendered CCT image of a left internal mammary graft to the left anterior descending coronary artery *(white arrow)* and a reverse saphenous vein graft to an obtuse marginal graft *(black arrow)*. Note the stents in the native coronary vessels *(arrowheads)*. **B,** Curved multiplanar CCT image of the left internal mammary graft to the left anterior descending coronary artery in the same patient, demonstrating multiple surgical clips *(arrowheads)*.

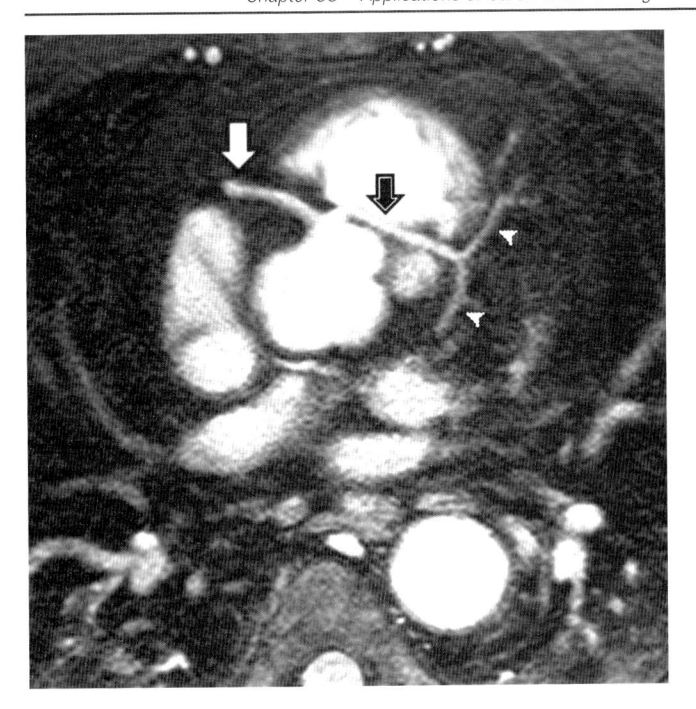

Figure 53–23
Anomalous coronary artery. The three-dimensional coronary CMR image reformatted in the axial plane indicates an anomalous origin of the left main coronary artery *(black arrow)* from the right sinus of Valsalva. The left coronary artery courses between the aorta and the main pulmonary artery (malignant form) before bifurcating into the left anterior descending and left circumflex arteries *(arrowheads)*. The right coronary artery *(white arrow)* originates normally from the right sinus of Valsalva.

REFERENCES

1. Budoff MJ, Shinbane JS. *Cardiac CT imaging: diagnosis of cardiovascular disease.* London: Springer Verlag; 2006.
2. Higgins CB, De Roos A, editors. *Cardiovascular MRI and MRA.* Lippincott Williams & Wilkins; 2002.
3. Manning WJ, Pennell DJ. *Cardiovascular magnetic resonance.* London: Churchill Livingstone; 2009.
4. Bellenger NG, Burgess MI, Ray SG, et al. Comparison of left ventricular ejection fraction and volumes in heart failure by echocardiography, radionuclide ventriculography and cardiovascular magnetic resonance; are they interchangeable? *Eur Heart J* 2000;**21**:1387-96.
5. Sugeng L, Mor-Avi V, Weinert L, et al. Quantitative assessment of left ventricular size and function: side-by-side comparison of real-time three-dimensional echocardiography and computed tomography with magnetic resonance reference. *Circulation* 2006;**114**:654-61.
6. Hartnell GG, Spence L, Hughes LA, Cohen MC, Saouaf R, Buff B. Safety of MR imaging in patients who have retained metallic materials after cardiac surgery. *AJR Am J Roentgenol* 1997;**168**:1157-9.
7. Hundley WG, Meshack BM, Willett DL, et al. Comparison of quantitation of left ventricular volume, ejection fraction, and cardiac output in patients with atrial fibrillation by cine magnetic resonance imaging versus invasive measurements. *Am J Cardiol* 1996;**78**:1119-23.
8. Schalla S, Nagel E, Lehmkuhl H, et al. Comparison of magnetic resonance real-time imaging of left ventricular function with conventional magnetic resonance imaging and echocardiography. *Am J Cardiol* 2001;**87**:95-9.
9. Wolak A, Gutstein A, Cheng VY, et al. Dual-source coronary computed tomography angiography in patients with atrial fibrillation: initial experience. *J Cardiovasc Comput Tomogr* 2008;**2**:172-80.
10. Tsiflikas I, Drosch T, Brodoefel H, et al. Diagnostic accuracy and image quality of cardiac dual-source computed tomography in patients with arrhythmia. *Int J Cardiol* 2009 Feb 24:[Epub ahead of print].
11. Prince MR, Arnoldus C, Frisoli JK. Nephrotoxicity of high-dose gadolinium compared with iodinated contrast. *J Magn Reson Imaging* 1996;**6**:162-6.
12. Perez-Rodriguez J, Lai S, Ehst BD, Fine DM, Bluemke DA. Nephrogenic systemic fibrosis: incidence, associations, and effect of risk factor assessment—report of 33 cases. *Radiology* 2009;**250**:371-7.
13. Kallen AJ, Jhung MA, Cheng S, et al. Gadolinium-containing magnetic resonance imaging contrast and nephrogenic systemic fibrosis: a case-control study. *Am J Kidney Dis* 2008;**51**:966-75.
14. Merten GJ, Burgess WP, Gray LV, et al. Prevention of contrast-induced nephropathy with sodium bicarbonate: a randomized controlled trial. *JAMA* 2004;**291**:2328-34.
15. Pannu N, Wiebe N, Tonelli M. Prophylaxis strategies for contrast-induced nephropathy. *JAMA* 2006;**295**:2765-79.
16. Liu R, Nair D, Ix J, Moore DH, Bent S. *N*-Acetylcysteine for the prevention of contrast-induced nephropathy. A systematic review and meta-analysis. *J Gen Intern Med* 2005;**20**:193-200.
17. Brar SS, Shen AY, Jorgensen MB, et al. Sodium bicarbonate vs sodium chloride for the prevention of contrast medium–induced nephropathy in patients undergoing coronary angiography: a randomized trial. *JAMA* 2008;**300**:1038-46.
18. Maioli M, Toso A, Leoncini M, et al. Sodium bicarbonate versus saline for the prevention of contrast-induced nephropathy in patients with renal dysfunction undergoing coronary angiography or intervention. *J Am Coll Cardiol* 2008;**52**:599-604.
19. Einstein AJ, Henzlova MJ, Rajagopalan S. Estimating risk of cancer associated with radiation exposure from 64-slice computed tomography coronary angiography. *JAMA* 2007;**298**:317-23.
20. Hausleiter J, Meyer T, Hadamitzky M, et al. Radiation dose estimates from cardiac multislice computed tomography in daily practice: impact of different scanning protocols on effective dose estimates. *Circulation* 2006;**113**:1305-10.
21. Maruyama T, Takada M, Hasuike T, Yoshikawa A, Namimatsu E, Yoshizumi T. Radiation dose reduction and coronary assessability of prospective electrocardiogram-gated computed tomography coronary angiography: comparison with retrospective electrocardiogram-gated helical scan. *J Am Coll Cardiol* 2008;**52**:1450-5.
22. Hartnell GG. Imaging of aortic aneurysms and dissection: CT and MRI. *J Thorac Imaging* 2001;**16**:35-46.
23. Fattori R, Descovich B, Bertaccini P, et al. Composite graft replacement of the ascending aorta: leakage detection with gadolinium-enhanced MR imaging. *Radiology* 1999;**212**:573-7.
24. Lange C, Odegard A, Lundbom J, Hatlinghus S, Myhre HO. Type III endoleak from a thoracic aortic stent-graft. *J Endovasc Ther* 2002;**9**:535-8.
25. Sommer T, Fehske W, Holzknecht N, et al. Aortic dissection: a comparative study of diagnosis with spiral CT, multiplanar transesophageal echocardiography, and MR imaging. *Radiology* 1996;**199**:347-52.
26. Hagan PG, Nienaber CA, Isselbacher EM, et al. The International Registry of Acute Aortic Dissection (IRAD): new insights into an old disease. *JAMA* 2000;**283**:897-903.
27. Schmidta M, Theissen P, Klempt G, et al. Long-term follow-up of 82 patients with chronic disease of the thoracic aorta using spin-echo and cine gradient magnetic resonance imaging. *Magn Reson Imaging* 2000;**18**:795-806.
28. Erbel R, Alfonso F, Boileau C, et al. Diagnosis and management of aortic dissection. *Eur Heart J* 2001;**22**:1642-81.
29. Rofsky NM, Weinreb JC, Grossi EA, et al. Aortic aneurysm and dissection: normal MR imaging and CT findings after surgical repair with the continuous-suture graft-inclusion technique. *Radiology* 1993;**186**:195-201.
30. Krinsky GA, Rofsky NM, DeCorato DR, et al. Thoracic aorta: comparison of gadolinium-enhanced three-dimensional MR angiography with conventional MR imaging. *Radiology* 1997;**202**:183-93.
31. Finn JP, Baskaran V, Carr JC, et al. Thorax: low-dose contrast-enhanced three-dimensional MR angiography with subsecond temporal resolution—initial results. *Radiology* 2002;**224**:896-904.
32. Pereles FS, McCarthy RM, Baskaran V, et al. Thoracic aortic dissection and aneurysm: evaluation with nonenhanced true FISP MR angiography in less than 4 minutes. *Radiology* 2002;**223**:270-4.
33. Murray JG, Manisali M, Flamm SD, et al. Intramural hematoma of the thoracic aorta: MR image findings and their prognostic implications. *Radiology* 1997;**204**:349-55.
34. Salvolini L, Renda P, Fiore D, Scaglione M, Piccoli G, Giovagnoni A. Acute aortic syndromes: role of multi-detector row CT. *Eur J Radiol* 2008;**65**:350-8.
35. Yucel EK, Steinberg FL, Egglin TK, Geller SC, Waltman AC, Athanasoulis CA. Penetrating aortic ulcers: diagnosis with MR imaging. *Radiology* 1990;**177**:779-81.
36. Nienaber CA, von Kodolitsch Y, Petersen B, et al. Intramural hemorrhage of the thoracic aorta. Diagnostic and therapeutic implications. *Circulation* 1995;**92**:1465-72.
37. Fayad ZA, Nahar T, Fallon JT, et al. In vivo magnetic resonance evaluation of atherosclerotic plaques in the human thoracic aorta: a comparison with transesophageal echocardiography. *Circulation* 2000;**101**:2503-9.

38. Chan SK, Jaffer FA, Botnar RM, et al. Scan reproducibility of magnetic resonance imaging assessment of aortic atherosclerosis burden. *J Cardiovasc Magn Reson* 2001;**3**:331-8.
39. Ibanez B, Cimmino G, Benezet-Mazuecos J, et al. Quantification of serial changes in plaque burden using multi-detector computed tomography in experimental atherosclerosis. *Atherosclerosis* 2009;**202**:185-91.
40. Tunick PA, Kronzon I. Atheromas of the thoracic aorta: clinical and therapeutic update. *J Am Coll Cardiol* 2000;**35**:545-54.
41. Kutz SM, Lee VS, Tunick PA, Krinsky GA, Kronzon I. Atheromas of the thoracic aorta: A comparison of transesophageal echocardiography and breath-hold gadolinium-enhanced 3-dimensional magnetic resonance angiography. *J Am Soc Echocardiogr* 1999;**12**:853-8.
42. Gillinov AM, Lytle BW, Hoang V, et al. The atherosclerotic aorta at aortic valve replacement: surgical strategies and results. *J Thorac Cardiovasc Surg* 2000;**120**:957-63.
43. Hayashi H, Matsuoka Y, Sakamoto I, et al. Penetrating atherosclerotic ulcer of the aorta: imaging features and disease concept. *Radiographics* 2000;**20**:995-1005.
44. Troxler M, Mavor AI, Homer-Vanniasinkam S. Penetrating atherosclerotic ulcers of the aorta. *Br J Surg* 2001;**88**:1169-77.
45. Tittle SL, Lynch RJ, Cole PE, et al. Midterm follow-up of penetrating ulcer and intramural hematoma of the aorta. *J Thorac Cardiovasc Surg* 2002;**123**:1051-9.
46. Arend WP, Michel BA, Bloch DA, et al. The American College of Rheumatology 1990 criteria for the classification of Takayasu arteritis. *Arthritis Rheum* 1990;**33**:1129-34.
47. Kerr GS, Hallahan CW, Giordano J, et al. Takayasu arteritis. *Ann Intern Med* 1994;**120**:919-29.
48. Yamada I, Numano F, Suzuki S. Takayasu arteritis: evaluation with MR imaging. *Radiology* 1993;**188**:89-94.
49. Yamada I, Nakagawa T, Himeno Y, Kobayashi Y, Numano F, Shibuya H. Takayasu arteritis: diagnosis with breath-hold contrast-enhanced three-dimensional MR angiography. *J Magn Reson Imaging* 2000;**11**:481-7.
50. Tso E, Flamm SD, White RD, Schvartzman PR, Mascha E, Hoffman GS. Takayasu arteritis: utility and limitations of magnetic resonance imaging in diagnosis and treatment. *Arthritis Rheum* 2002;**46**:1634-42.
51. Haramati LB, Glickstein JS, Issenberg HJ, Haramati N, Crooke GA. MR imaging and CT of vascular anomalies and connections in patients with congenital heart disease: significance in surgical planning. *Radiographics* 2002;**22**:337-47, discussion 348-9.
52. Riquelme C, Laissy JP, Menegazzo D, et al. MR imaging of coarctation of the aorta and its postoperative complications in adults: assessment with spin-echo and cine-MR imaging. *Magn Reson Imaging* 1999;**17**:37-46.
53. Godart F, Labrot G, Devos P, McFadden E, Rey C, Beregi JP. Coarctation of the aorta: comparison of aortic dimensions between conventional MR imaging, 3D MR angiography, and conventional angiography. *Eur Radiol* 2002;**12**:2034-9.
54. Hager A, Kaemmerer H, Hess J. Comparison of helical CT scanning and MRI in the follow-up of adults with coarctation of the aorta. *Chest* 2005;**127**:2296.
55. Therrien J, Thorne SA, Wright A, Kilner PJ, Somerville J. Repaired coarctation: a "cost-effective" approach to identify complications in adults. *J Am Coll Cardiol* 2000;**35**:997-1002.
56. Chien CT, Lin CS, Hsu YH, Lin MC, Chen KS, Wu DJ. Potential diagnosis of hemodynamic abnormalities in patent ductus arteriosus by cine magnetic resonance imaging. *Am Heart J* 1991;**122**:1065-73.
57. Lee EY, Siegel MJ, Hildebolt CF, Gutierrez FR, Bhalla S, Fallah JH. MDCT evaluation of thoracic aortic anomalies in pediatric patients and young adults: comparison of axial, multiplanar, 3D images. *AJR Am J Roentgenol* 2004;**182**:777-84.
58. Petersen SE, Voigtlander T, Kreitner KF, et al. Quantification of shunt volumes in congenital heart diseases using a breath-hold MR phase contrast technique—comparison with oximetry. *Int J Cardiovasc Imaging* 2002;**18**:53-60.
59. Mirvis SE, Shanmuganathan K. MR imaging of thoracic trauma. *Magn Reson Imaging Clin N Am* 2000;**8**:91-104.
60. Salton CJ, Chuang ML, O'Donnell CJ, et al. Gender differences and normal left ventricular anatomy in an adult population free of hypertension. A cardiovascular magnetic resonance study of the Framingham Heart Study Offspring cohort. *J Am Coll Cardiol* 2002;**39**:1055-60.
61. Alfakih K, Thiele H, Plein S, Bainbridge GJ, Ridgway JP, Sivananthan MU. Comparison of right ventricular volume measurement between segmented k-space gradient-echo and steady-state free precession magnetic resonance imaging. *J Magn Reson Imaging* 2002;**16**:253-8.
62. Nagel E, Lorenz C, Baer F, et al. Stress cardiovascular magnetic resonance: consensus panel report. *J Cardiovasc Magn Reson* 2001;**3**:267-81.
63. Nagel E, Lehmkuhl HB, Bocksch W, et al. Noninvasive diagnosis of ischemia-induced wall motion abnormalities with the use of high-dose dobutamine stress MRI: comparison with dobutamine stress echocardiography. *Circulation* 1999;**99**:763-70.
64. Reichek N. MRI myocardial tagging. *J Magn Reson Imaging* 1999;**10**:609-16.
65. Mahnken AH, Hohl C, Suess C, et al. Influence of heart rate and temporal resolution on left-ventricular volumes in cardiac multislice spiral computed tomography: a phantom study. *Invest Radiol* 2006;**41**:429-35.
66. Raman SV, Shah M, McCarthy B, Garcia A, Ferketich AK. Multi-detector row cardiac computed tomography accurately quantifies right and left ventricular size and function compared with cardiac magnetic resonance. *Am Heart J* 2006;**151**:736-44.
67. Kim RJ, Fieno DS, Parrish TB, et al. Relationship of MRI delayed contrast enhancement to irreversible injury, infarct age, and contractile function. *Circulation* 1999;**100**:1992-2002.
68. Simonetti OP, Kim RJ, Fieno DS, et al. An improved MR imaging technique for the visualization of myocardial infarction. *Radiology* 2001;**218**:215-23.
69. Wagner A, Mahrholdt H, Holly TA, et al. Contrast-enhanced MRI and routine single photon emission computed tomography (SPECT) perfusion imaging for detection of subendocardial myocardial infarcts: an imaging study. *Lancet* 2003;**361**:374-9.
70. Klein C, Nekolla SG, Bengel FM, et al. Assessment of myocardial viability with contrast-enhanced magnetic resonance imaging: comparison with positron emission tomography. *Circulation* 2002;**105**:162-7.
71. Kim RJ, Wu E, Rafael A, et al. The use of contrast-enhanced magnetic resonance imaging to identify reversible myocardial dysfunction. *N Engl J Med* 2000;**343**:1445-53.
72. Wellnhofer E, Olariu A, Klein C, et al. Magnetic resonance low-dose dobutamine test is superior to SCAR quantification for the prediction of functional recovery. *Circulation* 2004;**109**:2172-4.
73. Mandapaka S, Hundley WG. Dobutamine cardiovascular magnetic resonance: a review. *J Magn Reson Imaging* 2006;**24**:499-512.
74. Al-Saadi N, Nagel E, Gross M, et al. Noninvasive detection of myocardial ischemia from perfusion reserve based on cardiovascular magnetic resonance. *Circulation* 2000;**101**:1379-83.
75. Ibrahim T, Nekolla SG, Schreiber K, et al. Assessment of coronary flow reserve: comparison between contrast-enhanced magnetic resonance imaging and positron emission tomography. *J Am Coll Cardiol* 2002;**39**:864-70.
76. Blankstein R, Okada DR, Rocha-Filho JA, Rybicki FJ, Brady TJ, Cury RC. Cardiac myocardial perfusion imaging using dual source computed tomography. *Int J Cardiovasc Imaging* 2009 Feb 20:[Epub ahead of print].
77. Nienaber CA, Rehders TC, Fratz S. Detection and assessment of congenital heart disease with magnetic resonance techniques. *J Cardiovasc Magn Reson* 1999;**1**:169-84.
78. The clinical role of magnetic resonance in cardiovascular disease. Task Force of the European Society of Cardiology, in collaboration with the Association of European Paediatric Cardiologists. *Eur Heart J* 1998;**19**:19-39.
79. Beerbaum P, Korperich H, Barth P, Esdorn H, Gieseke J, Meyer H. Noninvasive quantification of left-to-right shunt in pediatric patients: phase-contrast cine magnetic resonance imaging compared with invasive oximetry. *Circulation* 2001;**103**:2476-82.
80. Helbing WA, Bosch HG, Maliepaard C, et al. Comparison of echocardiographic methods with magnetic resonance imaging for assessment of right ventricular function in children. *Am J Cardiol* 1995;**76**:589-94.
81. Cook SC, Raman SV. Multidetector computed tomography in the adolescent and young adult with congenital heart disease. *J Cardiovasc Comput Tomogr* 2008;**2**:36-49.
82. Tesoro-Tess JD, Biasi S, Balzarini L, et al. Heart involvement in lymphomas. The value of magnetic resonance imaging and two-dimensional echocardiography at disease presentation. *Cancer* 1993;**72**:2484-90.
83. Patel RAG, Schietinger BJ, Kramer CM. Cardiac masses. In: Manning WJ, editor. *Atlas of cardiovascular magnetic resonance*. Philadelphia: Springer; 2009. p. 97-104.
84. Stanford W, Rooholamini SA, Galvin JR. Ultrafast computed tomography for detection of intracardiac thrombi and tumors. In: Elliott LP, editor. *Cardiac imaging in infants, children, and adults*. Philadelphia: JB Lippincott; 2001. p. 494-500.
85. Mollet NR, Dymarkowski S, Volders W, et al. Visualization of ventricular thrombi with contrast-enhanced magnetic resonance imaging in patients with ischemic heart disease. *Circulation* 2002;**106**:2873-6.
86. Taylor AM, Dymarkowski S, Verbeken EK, Bogaert J. Detection of pericardial inflammation with late-enhancement cardiac magnetic resonance imaging: initial results. *Eur Radiol* 2006;**16**:569-74.
87. Yeon SB, Oyama N. The pericardium: anatomy and spectrum of disease. In: Manning WJ, Pennell DJ, editors. *Cardiovascular magnetic resonance*. Philadelphia: Churchill Livingstone; 2009.
88. Robles P, Rubio A, Olmedilla P. Value of multidetector cardiac CT in calcified constrictive pericarditis for pericardial resection. *Heart* 2006;**92**:1112.
89. Masui T, Finck S, Higgins CB. Constrictive pericarditis and restrictive cardiomyopathy: evaluation with MR imaging. *Radiology* 1992;**182**:369-73.

90. Breen JF. Imaging of the pericardium. *J Thorac Imaging* 2001;**16**:47-54.
91. Reinmuller R, Gurgan M, Erdmann E, Kemkes BM, Kreutzer E, Weinhold C. CT and MR evaluation of pericardial constriction: a new diagnostic and therapeutic concept. *J Thorac Imaging* 1993;**8**:108-21.
92. Hartnell GG, Hughes LA, Ko JP, Cohen MC. Magnetic resonance imaging of pericardial constriction: comparison of cine MR angiography and spin-echo techniques. *Clin Radiol* 1996;**51**:268-72.
93. Kojima S, Yamada N, Goto Y. Diagnosis of constrictive pericarditis by tagged cine magnetic resonance imaging. *N Engl J Med* 1999;**341**:373-4.
94. Pouleur AC, le Polain de Waroux JB, Pasquet A, Vanoverschelde JL, Gerber BL. Aortic valve area assessment: multidetector CT compared with cine MR imaging and transthoracic and transesophageal echocardiography. *Radiology* 2007;**244**:745-54.
95. Kilner PJ, Manzara CC, Mohiaddin RH, et al. Magnetic resonance jet velocity mapping in mitral and aortic valve stenosis. *Circulation* 1993;**87**:1239-48.
96. Maron MS, Finley JJ, Bos JM, et al. Prevalence, clinical significance, and natural history of left ventricular apical aneurysms in hypertrophic cardiomyopathy. *Circulation* 2008;**118**:1541-9.
97. Choudhury L, Mahrholdt H, Wagner A, et al. Myocardial scarring in asymptomatic or mildly symptomatic patients with hypertrophic cardiomyopathy. *J Am Coll Cardiol* 2002;**40**:2156-64.
98. Shimada T, Shimada K, Sakane T, et al. Diagnosis of cardiac sarcoidosis and evaluation of the effects of steroid therapy by gadolinium-DTPA–enhanced magnetic resonance imaging. *Am J Med* 2001;**110**:520-7.
99. Anderson LJ, Holden S, Davis B, et al. Cardiovascular T2-star (T2*) magnetic resonance for the early diagnosis of myocardial iron overload. *Eur Heart J* 2001;**22**:2171-9.
100. Corrado D, Fontaine G, Marcus FI, et al. Arrhythmogenic right ventricular dysplasia/cardiomyopathy: need for an international registry. Study Group on Arrhythmogenic Right Ventricular Dysplasia/Cardiomyopathy of the Working Groups on Myocardial and Pericardial Disease and Arrhythmias of the European Society of Cardiology and of the Scientific Council on Cardiomyopathies of the World Heart Federation. *Circulation* 2000;**101**:E101-6.
101. McCrohon JA, Moon JC, Prasad SK, et al. Differentiation of heart failure related to dilated cardiomyopathy and coronary artery disease using gadolinium-enhanced cardiovascular magnetic resonance. *Circulation* 2003;**108**:54-9.
102. Kim WY, Danias PG, Stuber M, et al. Coronary magnetic resonance angiography for the detection of coronary stenoses. *N Engl J Med* 2001;**345**:1863-9.
103. Andreini D, Pontone G, Pepi M, et al. Diagnostic accuracy of multidetector computed tomography coronary angiography in patients with dilated cardiomyopathy. *J Am Coll Cardiol* 2007;**49**:2044-50.
104. Manning WJ, Stuber M, Danias PG, Botnar RM, Yeon SB, Aepfelbacher FC. Coronary magnetic resonance imaging: current status. *Curr Probl Cardiol* 2002;**27**:275-333.
105. Gay SB, Sistrom CL, Holder CA, Suratt PM. Breath-holding capability of adults. Implications for spiral computed tomography, fast-acquisition magnetic resonance imaging, and angiography. *Invest Radiol* 1994;**29**:848-51.
106. Sakuma H, Ichikawa Y, Chino S, Hirano T, Makino K, Takeda K. Detection of coronary artery stenosis with whole-heart coronary magnetic resonance angiography. *J Am Coll Cardiol* 2006;**48**:1946-50.
107. Sato Y, Komatsu S, Matsumoto N, et al. Whole heart coronary magnetic resonance angiography for the detection of coronary artery stenosis and atherosclerotic coronary artery plaque in a patient with unstable angina. *Int J Cardiol* 2007;**115**:262-4.
108. Kato S, Sakuma H, Ishida N, et al. Assessment of coronary artery disease using magnetic resonance coronary angiography: a multicenter trial. *Circulation* 2008;**118**:S778.
109. Yang Q, Li K, Bi X, et al. 3T contrast-enhanced whole heart coronary MRA using 32-channel cardiac coils for detection of coronary artery disease. *J Cardiovasc Magn Reson* 2009;**11**:5.
110. Garcia MJ, Lessick J, Hoffmann MH. Accuracy of 16-row multidetector computed tomography for the assessment of coronary artery stenosis. *JAMA* 2006;**296**:403-11.
111. Miller JM, Rochitte CE, Dewey M, et al. Diagnostic performance of coronary angiography by 64-row CT. *N Engl J Med* 2008;**359**:2324-36.
112. Budoff MJ, Dowe D, Jollis JG, et al. Diagnostic performance of 64-multidetector row coronary computed tomographic angiography for evaluation of coronary artery stenosis in individuals without known coronary artery disease: results from the prospective multicenter ACCURACY (Assessment by Coronary Computed Tomographic Angiography of Individuals Undergoing Invasive Coronary Angiography) trial. *J Am Coll Cardiol* 2008;**52**:1724-32.
113. Detrano R, Guerci AD, Carr JJ, et al. Coronary calcium as a predictor of coronary events in four racial or ethnic groups. *N Engl J Med* 2008;**358**:1336-45.
114. Kefer J, Coche E, Legros G, et al. Head-to-head comparison of three-dimensional navigator-gated magnetic resonance imaging and 16-slice computed tomography to detect coronary artery stenosis in patients. *J Am Coll Cardiol* 2005;**46**:92-100.
115. Maintz D, Ozgun M, Hoffmeier A, et al. Whole-heart coronary magnetic resonance angiography: value for the detection of coronary artery stenoses in comparison to multislice computed tomography angiography. *Acta Radiol* 2007;**48**:967-73.
116. Dewey M, Teige F, Schnapauff D, et al. Noninvasive detection of coronary artery stenoses with multislice computed tomography or magnetic resonance imaging. *Ann Intern Med* 2006;**145**:407-15.
117. Liu X, Zhao X, Huang J, et al. Comparison of 3D free-breathing coronary MR angiography and 64-MDCT angiography for detection of coronary stenosis in patients with high calcium scores. *AJR Am J Roentgenol* 2007;**189**:1326-32.
118. Rubinstein RI, Askenase AD, Thickman D, Feldman MS, Agarwal JB, Helfant RH. Magnetic resonance imaging to evaluate patency of aortocoronary bypass grafts. *Circulation* 1987;**76**:786-91.
119. Jenkins JP, Love HG, Foster CJ, Isherwood I, Rowlands DJ. Detection of coronary artery bypass graft patency as assessed by magnetic resonance imaging. *Br J Radiol* 1988;**61**:2-4.
120. Galjee MA, van Rossum AC, Doesburg T, van Eenige MJ, Visser CA. Value of magnetic resonance imaging in assessing patency and function of coronary artery bypass grafts. An angiographically controlled study. *Circulation* 1996;**93**:660-6.
121. White RD, Pflugfelder PW, Lipton MJ, Higgins CB. Coronary artery bypass grafts: evaluation of patency with cine MR imaging. *AJR Am J Roentgenol* 1988;**150**:1271-4.
122. Aurigemma GP, Reichek N, Axel L, Schiebler M, Harris C, Kressel HY. Noninvasive determination of coronary artery bypass graft patency by cine magnetic resonance imaging. *Circulation* 1989;**80**:1595-602.
123. Engelmann MG, Knez A, von Smekal A, et al. Non-invasive coronary bypass graft imaging after multivessel revascularisation. *Int J Cardiol* 2000;**76**:65-74.
124. Langerak SE, Vliegen HW, de Roos A, et al. Detection of vein graft disease using high-resolution magnetic resonance angiography. *Circulation* 2002;**105**:328-33.
125. Langerak SE, Vliegen HW, Jukema JW, et al. Value of magnetic resonance imaging for the noninvasive detection of stenosis in coronary artery bypass grafts and recipient coronary arteries. *Circulation* 2003;**107**:1502-8.
126. Malagutti P, Nieman K, Meijboom WB, et al. Use of 64-slice CT in symptomatic patients after coronary bypass surgery: evaluation of grafts and coronary arteries. *Eur Heart J* 2007;**28**:1879-85.
127. Post JC, van Rossum AC, Bronzwaer JG, et al. Magnetic resonance angiography of anomalous coronary arteries. A new gold standard for delineating the proximal course? *Circulation* 1995;**92**:3163-71.
128. Taylor AM, Thorne SA, Rubens MB, et al. Coronary artery imaging in grown up congenital heart disease: complementary role of magnetic resonance and x-ray coronary angiography. *Circulation* 2000;**101**:1670-9.
129. Vliegen HW, Doornbos J, de Roos A, Jukema JW, Bekedam MA, van der Wall EE. Value of fast gradient echo magnetic resonance angiography as an adjunct to coronary arteriography in detecting and confirming the course of clinically significant coronary artery anomalies. *Am J Cardiol* 1997;**79**:773-6.
130. Bunce NH, Lorenz CH, Keegan J, et al. Coronary artery anomalies: assessment with free-breathing three-dimensional coronary MR angiography. *Radiology* 2003;**227**:201-8.
131. Basso C, Maron BJ, Corrado D, Thiene G. Clinical profile of congenital coronary artery anomalies with origin from the wrong aortic sinus leading to sudden death in young competitive athletes. *J Am Coll Cardiol* 2000;**35**:1493-501.
132. Ostrom MP, Gopal A, Ahmadi N, et al. Mortality incidence and the severity of coronary atherosclerosis assessed by computed tomography angiography. *J Am Coll Cardiol* 2008;**52**:1335-43.

CHAPTER 54

Nuclear Cardiology and Positron Emission Tomography in the Assessment of Patients with Cardiovascular Disease

Brian G. Abbott and Barry L. Zaret

General Principles
Radioactive Tracers
Equipment and Procedures
Stable Coronary Artery Disease
Stress Testing in Detection of CAD
Exercise Stress Testing
Exercise Stress Myocardial Perfusion Imaging
Pharmacologic Stress Myocardial Perfusion Imaging
Prognosis and Risk Stratification
Stable Angina

Medical Therapy versus Revascularization
Preoperative Evaluation for Noncardiac Surgery
Acute Coronary Syndrome
Territory at Risk and Infarct Size
Rest MPI for Acute Coronary Syndrome
Risk Stratification after Myocardial Infarction
Assessment of Myocardial Viability
Left Ventricular Ejection Fraction and Prognosis
Positron Emission Tomography and SPECT for Determining Viability

Positron Emission Tomography
Quantitative Methods
Single-Photon Emission Computed Tomography
Thallium
Technetium-Labeled Agents
Prognostic Implications of Viability Assessment
Evaluation of Patients after Revascularization
Future Directions

Nuclear cardiology involves the imaging of the distribution of cardiac radiopharmaceutical agents to characterize physiologic and pathophysiologic processes in the heart. The ability to image myocardial perfusion function and metabolism noninvasively with nuclear techniques has led to the development of a field that has been validated extensively and provides powerful diagnostic and prognostic information in the management of patients with known or suspected coronary artery disease (CAD). Moreover, nuclear cardiology procedures have been employed widely in the evaluation of patients before cardiac and noncardiac surgery. This chapter provides an overview of the concepts and techniques used in nuclear cardiology, and it summarizes its role in the assessment of patients with stable coronary disease or acute coronary syndromes, and in the determination of myocardial viability in patients considered for revascularization. As a complete discussion of the technical and procedural aspects of nuclear cardiology is beyond the scope of this chapter, the central focus will be on the use of nuclear cardiology in patients with known or suspected CAD, with an emphasis on patients undergoing cardiac surgery. For a more detailed discussion, the reader is referred to other, more comprehensive reviews.[1,2]

General Principles

Nuclear cardiology has been dominated by radionuclide myocardial perfusion imaging (MPI) as a means to evaluate patients with known or suspected coronary disease. MPI is performed to evaluate diagnostically patients with symptoms suggestive of myocardial ischemia, and to risk-stratify patients with known CAD. Radionuclide MPI plays a central role in the evaluation of the cardiac patient and is in widespread clinical use, with more than 7 million MPI procedures performed in the United States annually.[3]

Myocardial perfusion is governed during resting conditions by the coronary resistance vessels. During periods of increased work, such as during exercise, flow is increased to balance the metabolic demands of the myocardium. This is achieved by vasodilation of the resistance vessels, which reduces vascular resistance in the coronary arterial bed. In stenotic, atherosclerotic coronary arteries, resting flow is maintained by decreasing the downstream vascular resistance. Although this compensation maintains flow under resting conditions, a critical stenosis (>50% to 70% narrowing of the lumen) impairs coronary flow reserve, or the ability of the artery to increase flow appropriately during periods of increased demand.

Radioactive Tracers

Myocardial perfusion is imaged with the use of radiopharmaceutical agents that accumulate rapidly in the myocardium in proportion to myocardial blood flow. The most commonly used radiotracers currently are the technetium-99m (^{99m}Tc)-labeled compounds sestamibi and tetrofosmin, and, to a lesser extent, thallium-201 (^{201}Tl). When injected intravenously, these tracers are extracted from the blood pool and accumulate in cells, including myocytes, that have an intact cell membrane and are metabolically active. ^{99m}Tc-sestamibi and tetrofosmin are lipophilic cationic complexes that are taken up by myocytes across mitochondrial membranes, but at equilibrium they are retained in the mitochondria because of their large negative transmembrane potential. ^{201}Tl is transported in the same manner potassium is, across the myocyte sarcolemmal membrane via the Na/K-ATPase transport system. Because the retention of radiotracer is proportional to myocardial flow, the amount of tracer uptake is a surrogate visualized representation of regional myocardial perfusion. The tracers used are radioactive isotopes that undergo radioactive decay over a short period of time.

Equipment and Procedures

As the accumulated radiotracer decays, photons are emitted, and as they exit the body, they can be detected using a specialized gamma camera. MPI relies on single-photon emission computed tomography (SPECT) techniques to acquire and ultimately display the perfusion distribution obtained from the radiotracer uptake. After the radiopharmaceutical is injected, the patient lies supine on the SPECT camera table and is positioned in the gantry of the camera. The photons emitted from the heart are then detected via large crystals or solid-state detectors in the SPECT camera as it revolves around the patient.

As the camera detector moves around the patient, emitted photons interact with the camera's crystal and produce scintillations of light that represent the spatial distribution of radioactivity in the patient. The emitted "counts" localized to each region of the myocardium are then stored digitally. This three-dimensional representation of the myocardial perfusion is then processed and reconstructed using computer algorithms to display the acquired information in a series of slices, oriented in the short axis and in the horizontal and vertical long axes of the left ventricle. The slices are then displayed on a computer screen for visual inspection of regional myocardial perfusion as well as computer quantification of tracer uptake. The stress images, acquired after injection of radiotracer during exercise or pharmacologic stress (described later in detail) are displayed adjacent to images acquired at rest, permitting direct comparison of perfusion in the two imaging states. The maximal uptake of radiotracer in the heart is used to represent normal perfusion, and the rest of the counts are considered as relative uptakes to this maximum. As shown in Figure 54-1, a regional perfusion defect on the stress images that is not present on the resting study is considered to be "reversible" and consistent with stress-induced ischemia in that vascular territory. A defect that persists on stress and rest is deemed "fixed" and representative of scar or prior myocardial infarction. Quantitative programs are commonly used to assess the extent and severity of each defect, and this information is then incorporated into the final interpretation of regional myocardial perfusion. The perfusion images are also obtained in concert with electrocardiographic (ECG) gating, which stores the counts with respect to the timing of the cardiac cycle. By gating the acquisition to the R-R interval of the ECG, images from each frame can be summed and displayed as a cine movie of the left ventricle contracting from diastole to systole. Performing gated SPECT facilitates measurement of left ventricular (LV) ejection fraction (LVEF) and LV volumes by automated computer algorithms, as well as by visual inspection of the movie for regional wall motion and thickening (Fig. 54-2).[4]

A typical SPECT MPI protocol involves the performance of exercise, typically on a treadmill or bicycle, or alternatively a pharmacologic stressor, such as adenosine, dipyridamole, regadenoson, or dobutamine, for patients unable to perform physical exercise. The radiotracer is injected at peak stress and the stressor is then continued for an additional 1 to 2 minutes to maximize myocardial extraction of the circulating tracer. Imaging is performed 30 to 60 minutes later for sestamibi or tetrofosmin, as these agents have only minimal redistribution or washout from the myocardium. The initial imaging can be either at rest or at stress, and both studies can be performed on the same day depending on the patient's weight. Although ^{201}Tl is used less commonly for stress MPI, it is commonly used for rest imaging in a dual-isotope protocol. In this protocol, ^{201}Tl is injected for resting imaging, followed immediately by stress perfusion imaging with a ^{99m}Tc agent, thus obviating the need to wait 2 to 3 hours for the first dose to decay.[5] Thus, imaging time is reduced and patient throughput is increased. Recent advances in camera technology and processing have facilitated faster image acquisition and the use of lower dosages of radiopharmaceuticals.

STABLE CORONARY ARTERY DISEASE

Stress Testing in the Detection of CAD

Nuclear cardiology is a central part of the evaluation of patients with suspected or proven coronary artery disease. The ability of SPECT myocardial perfusion imaging to detect CAD in patients with symptoms suggestive of ischemic heart disease has been validated extensively.

Exercise Stress Testing

Exercise stress testing without adjunct noninvasive imaging is frequently used as the initial screening test in patients without known coronary artery disease who present with chest pain syndromes or symptoms suggestive of ischemia. The premise of exercise stress testing is that the increased myocardial oxygen demand during exercise will produce clinical signs of ischemia (angina, ECG changes) in the setting of a flow-limiting stenosis that impairs myocardial blood supply. The diagnostic performance of this test varies greatly depending on the pretest likelihood of the population being studied. In patients with an intermediate pretest probability of CAD on the basis of symptoms and risk factors, exercise treadmill testing is useful as an initial screening test. However, the overall sensitivity of treadmill exercise testing is approximately 70%. A meta-analysis of more than 24,000 patients undergoing exercise stress testing and coronary angiography observed a mean sensitivity of 68% and a mean specificity of 77%. Accuracy was greatest in patients with multivessel coronary disease and those with left main or three-vessel coronary artery disease.[6]

Exercise Stress Myocardial Perfusion Imaging

Because exercise treadmill testing relies on changes in the 12-lead ECG as a surrogate of ischemia, the accuracy of the test is highly dependent on the baseline electrocardiogram. Abnormalities such as previous myocardial infarction (Q waves or left bundle branch block) or ST-T wave changes

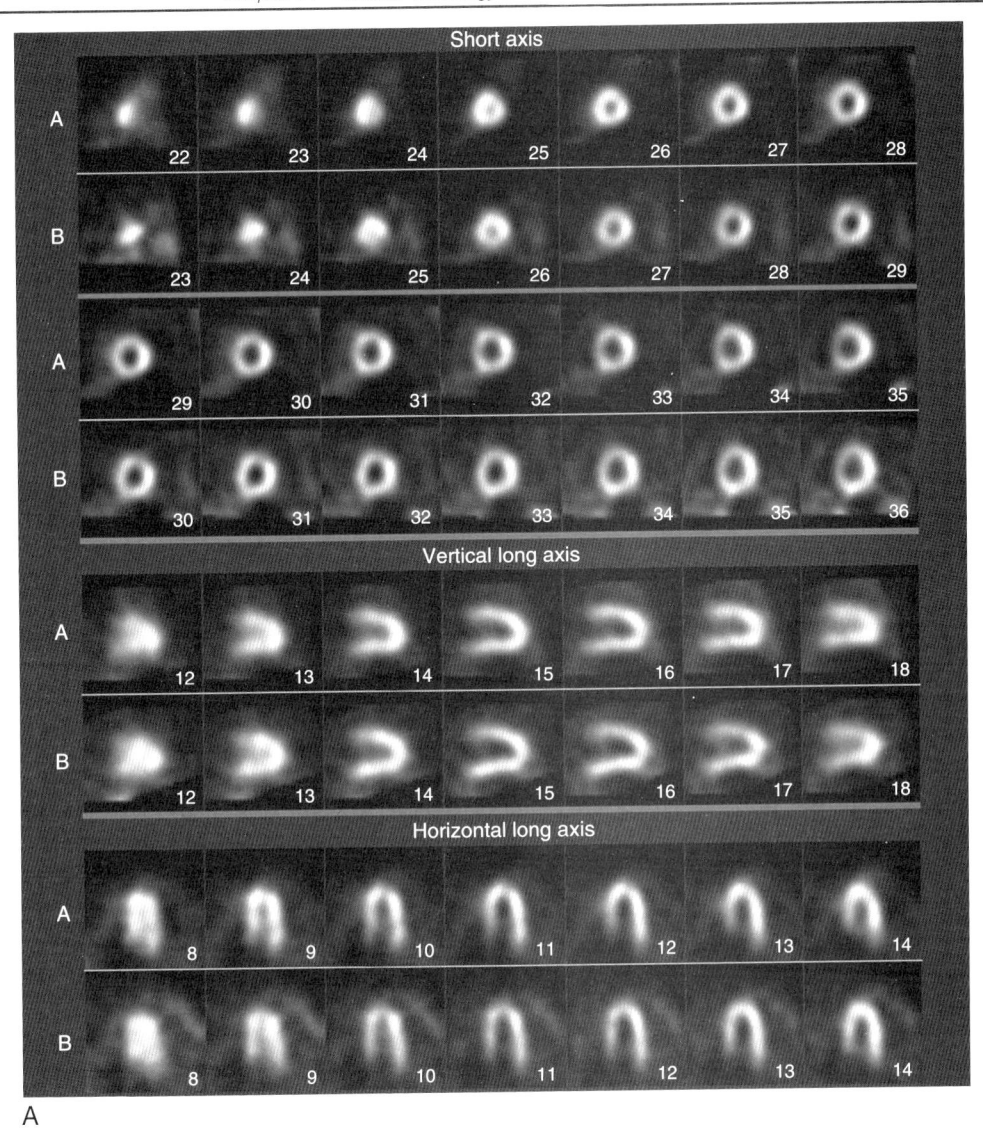

Figure 54-1
Visual display of SPECT myocardial perfusion images. The stress study (rows labeled A) is shown immediately above the rest study (rows labeled B) for comparison. There are three representations of the same imaging procedure, each oriented differently: short-axis slices from apex to mid-ventricle and mid-ventricle to base *(top)*, vertical long-axis slices from septum to lateral wall *(middle)*, and horizontal long-axis slices from inferior to anterior wall *(bottom)*. **A,** Normal study in grayscale, with uniform uptake of radiotracer on stress and rest.

resulting from left ventricular hypertrophy or therapy with digoxin, hamper the ability to interpret ischemic changes accurately during exercise. In patients with an abnormal ECG, myocardial perfusion imaging adds significant diagnostic accuracy to the treadmill test for detecting CAD. Large studies have consistently shown that SPECT myocardial perfusion imaging with technetium-labeled agents, such as sestamibi, yields a greater than 90% sensitivity for the detection of coronary artery disease.[7-9] False-negative scans tend to occur in the setting of single-vessel disease (particularly in the left circumflex artery distribution), a mild degree of stenosis (<70% occluded), or when the patient is unable to achieve the target heart rate or is taking antianginal therapy. These studies have also observed that the specificity of stress SPECT imaging is in the range of 68%. The less optimal specificity can be attributed to both referral bias (performing angiography in only those patients with abnormal scans), as well as false-positive scans with defects resulting from artifacts produced by soft tissue attenuation (diaphragm, breast) or patient motion.

Contemporary imaging techniques that employ ECG gating have facilitated the simultaneous assessment of myocardial perfusion and function. Examination of regional wall motion and thickening enhances the evaluation of a suspect area of hypoperfusion by providing the ability to distinguish true myocardial scarring from attenuation. Specificity can also be enhanced with the use of attenuation correction. These algorithms incorporate additional data obtained from an external radioactive source or computed tomography to create a soft tissue attenuation image of the chest, and then adjust the regional counts on the emission scan to correct for the loss of counts resulting from attenuation from overlying breast, diaphragm, and chest wall structures.[10]

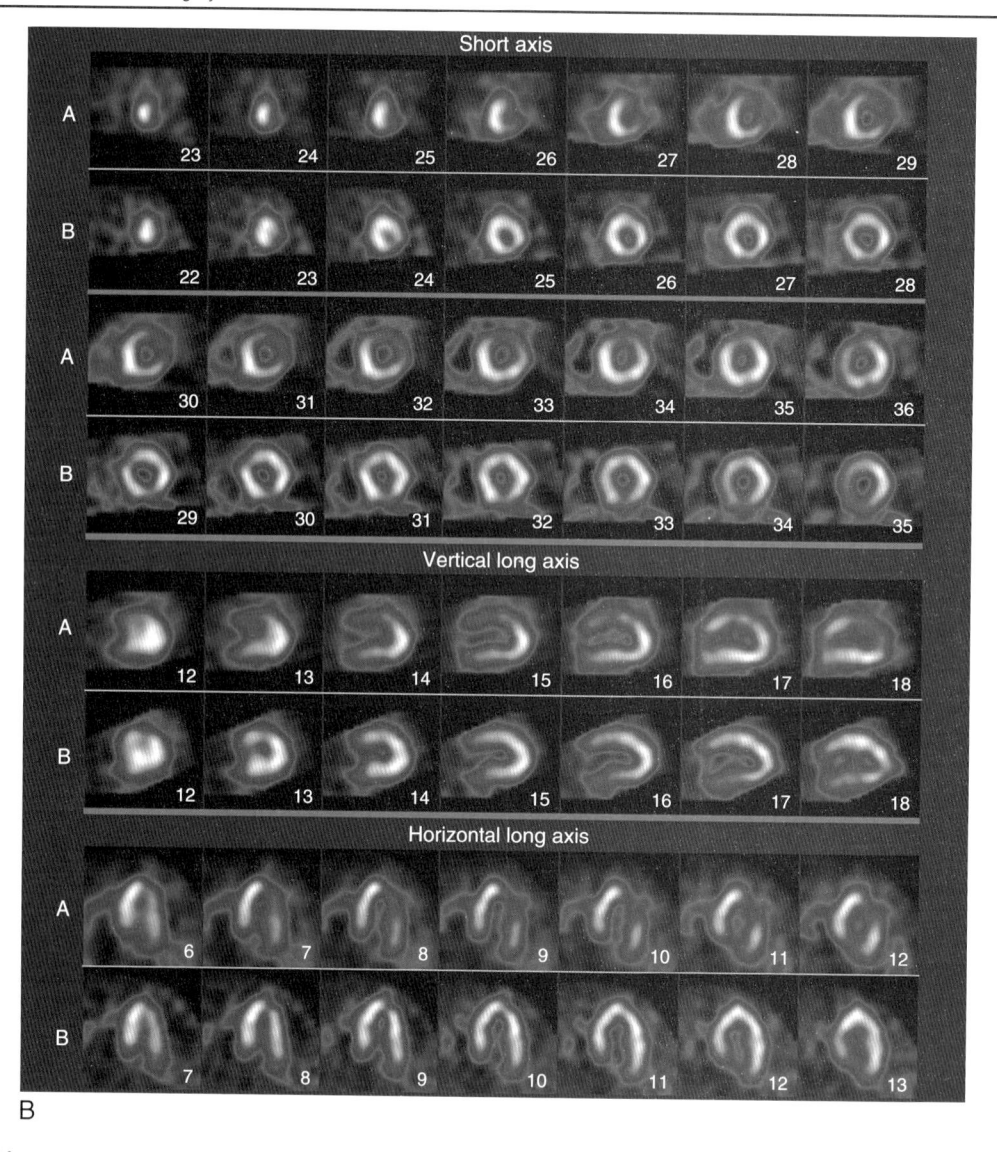

Figure 54–1, cont'd
B, Color-enhanced study in which the stress images demonstrate a perfusion defect in the anterolateral wall, as evidenced by less radiotracer accumulation relative to other regions of the left ventricle. As the corresponding rest images show normal perfusion throughout the myocardium, the perfusion defect is considered "reversible," consistent with ischemia.

Pharmacologic Stress Myocardial Perfusion Imaging

As many patients are unable to perform physical exercise to a workload adequate for a diagnostic exercise stress test, myocardial perfusion imaging performed after pharmacologic stress is used frequently as an alternative. This is typically performed after the intravenous infusion of a vasodilator, such as dipyridamole, adenosine, or regadenoson, or after administration of the inotrope dobutamine. Dipyridamole stimulates the release of endogenous adenosine in the distal coronary vasculature, which then binds adenosine receptors in the vasculature, producing the desired effect of coronary artery vasodilation, as well as undesirable effects such as flushing, bronchospasm, headache, and even transient heart block. This vasodilation of the resistance vessels increases myocardial blood flow, mimicking the effects of physical exercise.

Dipyridamole is typically administered intravenously as a bolus injection over a period of 4 minutes, with peak effect occurring at 8 minutes, at which time the radiotracer is injected.[11] A 4- to 6-minute continuous infusion of intravenous adenosine is now used more commonly.[12,13] Both agents are equally effective in increasing myocardial blood flow threefold to fivefold over rest, which is similar to that produced by exercise. Although adenosine tends to achieve maximal flow in more patients than dipyridamole, side effects are more common with adenosine. Regadenoson is a new adenosine A_{2A} receptor agonist that selectively increases coronary blood flow without producing side effects, such as hypotension, atrioventricular block, chest pain, and flushing, which are common with adenosine and dipyridamole.[14-16] Regadenoson can be used as an alternative stressor in patients with lung disease, because its receptor

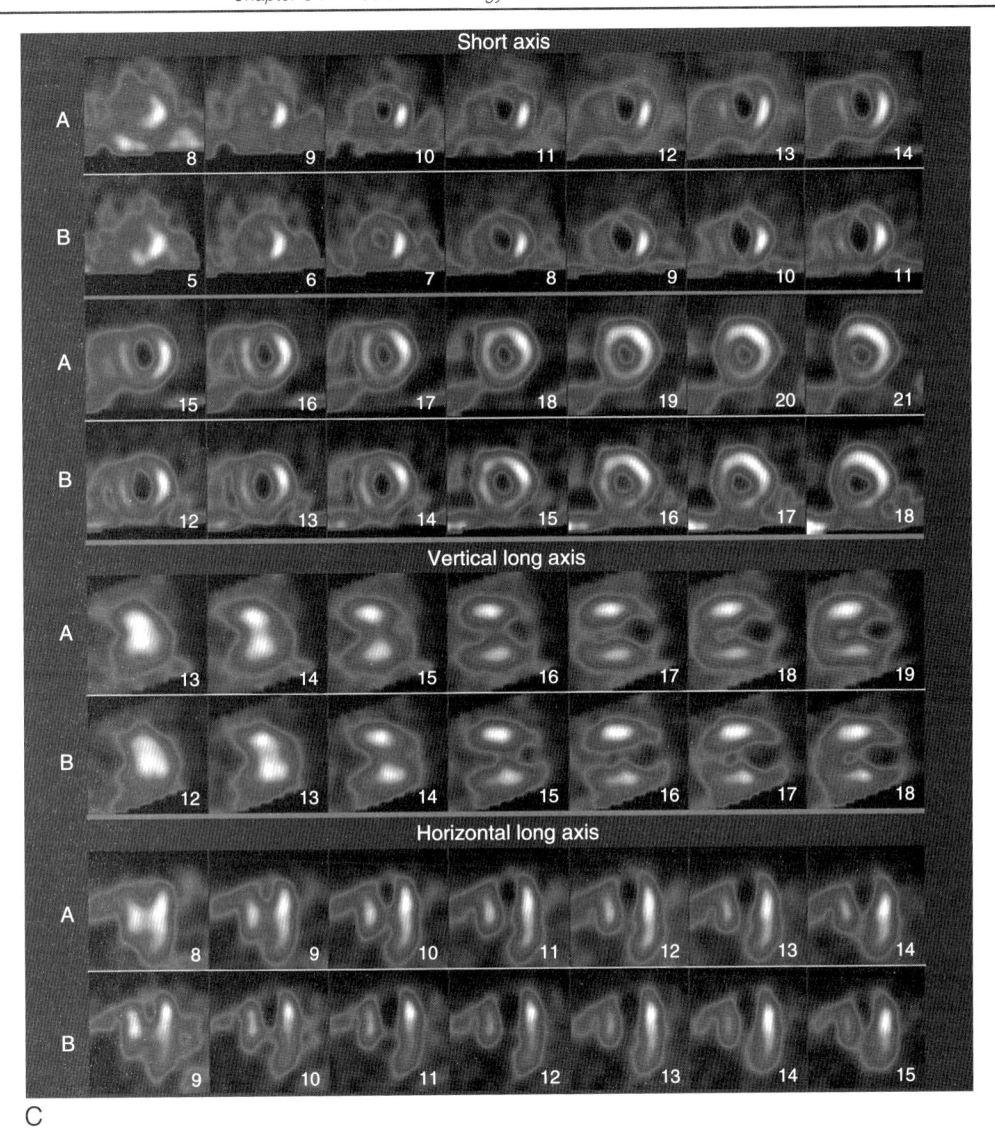

Figure 54-1, cont'd
C, These SPECT images demonstrate large perfusion defects in the anteroseptal, inferoseptal, and apical regions, which are present on both the stress and rest images. Because these defects do not show any change from stress to rest, they are termed "fixed" defects, consistent with scar (i.e., prior myocardial infarction).

selectivity may avoid the bronchospasm that can occur with other vasodilators.[17,18]

An intravenous infusion of dobutamine is also effective for pharmacologic stress. It is typically used as an alternative to vasodilator stress in patients with bronchospasm and pulmonary disease. The dobutamine infusion produces increased myocardial oxygen demand by increasing heart rate, blood pressure, and myocardial contractility.[19]

All of the currently used pharmacologic stress agents have similar abilities to produce flow heterogeneity and corresponding perfusion defects in the presence of a significant (>50% to 70%) stenosis of a coronary artery. A meta-analysis of dipyridamole SPECT imaging demonstrated a sensitivity of 89% and specificity of 65% for the detection of coronary artery disease. Dipyridamole and adenosine tests had essentially similar sensitivities and specificities. The sensitivity of dobutamine SPECT imaging in detecting CAD is approximately 80%, which is slightly lower than that of the vasodilator agents.[20]

Prognosis and Risk Stratification

Stable Angina

The goals of stress testing extend beyond the detection of coronary artery disease alone. For stress testing information to be useful, results must reliably identify patients of sufficiently low risk that further evaluation or intervention can be safely avoided, while also providing additional information to the clinical risk assessment when results are abnormal. The ability of both exercise and pharmacologic MPI to add incremental prognostic information to the clinical risk assessment in patients with known CAD has been evaluated in thousands of patients.[21] Several large studies of patients with known or suspected CAD, including both men and women, have

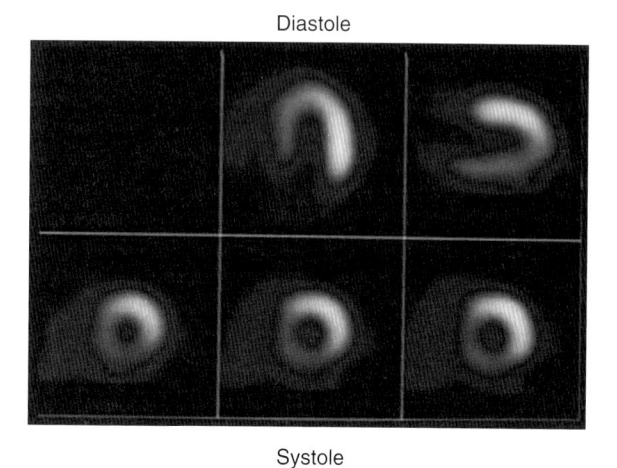

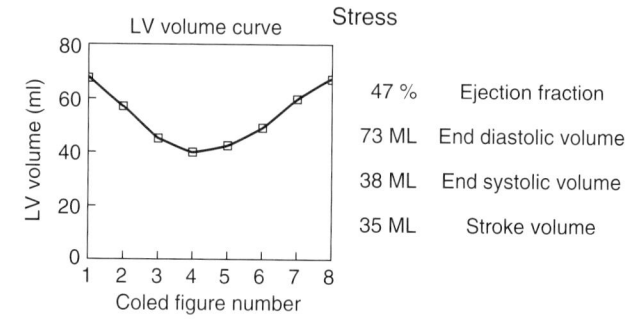

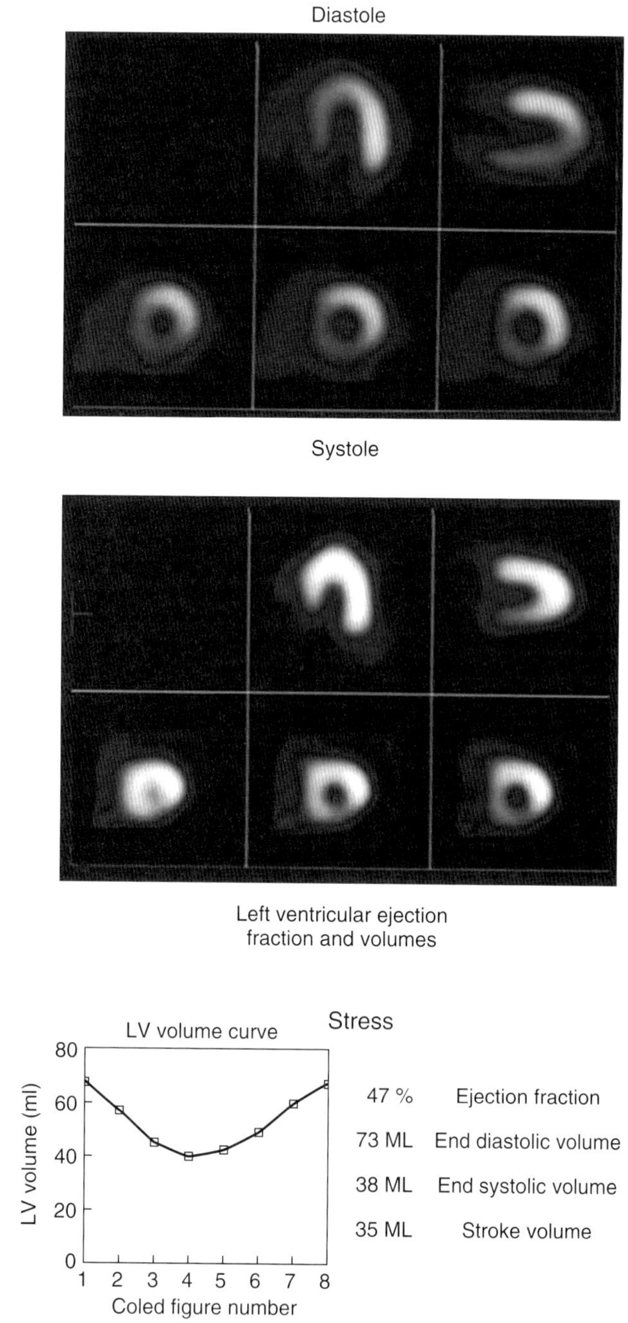

Figure 54-2
Gated SPECT still-frame images of diastole and systole. During SPECT image acquisition, the acquired images can be stored in relationship to the cardiac cycle using the R-R interval of the electrocardiogram. The resulting images that are "gated" to the cardiac cycle can then be viewed as a cine-loop from diastole to systole. Moreover, these data can be used to calculate left ventricular (LV) volumes during diastole and systole, as well as the corresponding left ventricular ejection fraction (diastole-systole).

Box 54–1
Stress Testing Variables Associated with Worse Prognosis

Perfusion Parameters
- Multivessel disease pattern
- Large reversible (ischemic) defect
- Large scar, >14% of left ventricle
- Transient left ventricular dilation with stress
- Right ventricular uptake
- Resting left ventricular dysfunction
- Pulmonary uptake of thallium-201

Nonperfusion Parameters
- Poor exercise capacity
- Angina at low workload
- Dynamic ST-segment depression ≥ 3 mm with exercise
- Exercise-induced ventricular arrhythmias
- Vasodilator stress-induced ST-segment depression ≥ 1 mm
- Hypotensive blood pressure response

demonstrated the incremental prognostic value of a normal MPI.[22-26]

Perhaps of greatest clinical usefulness is that these studies have consistently shown that patients with a normal MPI have a subsequent annual rate of cardiac death and nonfatal myocardial infarction (MI) of less than 1%, even patients with known CAD.[27,28] When the results are abnormal, the SPECT scan provides incremental prognostic information beyond that obtained by clinical, ECG, and stress testing combined. Moreover, the value of SPECT MPI in determining prognosis is such that the information obtained from subsequent coronary angiography does not provide any incremental prognostic information beyond that obtained by the SPECT results.[29,30] The increase in the risk of hard events increases in proportion to the severity and extent of the perfusion defect when assessed by semiquantitative methods or automated quantitative approaches. The degree of ischemia on SPECT is associated with an increase in the short-term incidence of nonfatal MI, whereas scar size is more predictive of cardiac death.[28] Important stress MPI variables that are predictive of future cardiac events include defects in more than one vascular territory (multivessel disease), transient left ventricular cavity dilation during stress,[31] and increased pulmonary uptake of radiotracer[32,33] (suggesting increased LV filling pressures), as well as other parameters outlined in Box 54-1. The prognostic ability of stress MPI is also enhanced by inclusion of ECG-gated SPECT, which permits assessment of LV global systolic performance, the most potent predictor of event-free survival, as well as analysis of regional wall motion and LV volumes.[34-36]

Medical Therapy versus Revascularization

One of the most important contributions of stress MPI in the clinical evaluation of patients with known or suspected CAD is the ability to provide prognostic information that can be used to guide further testing and therapies. Because the extent and severity of ischemia on a stress MPI study is directly proportional to the risk of future cardiac events, this information can be incorporated into the decision-making process concerning medical or revascularization therapies for a given patient. Patients with mild ischemic defects that are not high risk can generally be safely treated medically, whereas higher-risk findings (transient ischemic dilation, multivessel disease pattern, large territory at risk) should be strongly considered for more invasive evaluation and a lower threshold for revascularization. A 3-year follow-up study of patients with mild to moderate defects on stress SPECT myocardial perfusion imaging treated with medical therapy noted a 2% incidence of cardiac death or nonfatal infarction and less than a 5% rate of revascularization, suggesting that SPECT imaging is highly useful in identifying patients with CAD who have a sufficiently low risk for events that revascularization is not necessary.[37]

In contrast, the benefit of revascularization over medical therapy has been characterized in patients with high-risk stress SPECT MPI findings. Hachamovitch and colleagues[28] followed 5183 patients after stress MPI for a mean of 2 years, and found that the rates of MI and cardiac death did not differ substantially between patients treated with medical therapy or revascularization after a normal or mildly abnormal scan. However, patients with severely abnormal scans had a significantly higher annualized cardiac death rate when treated medically (4.6% deaths per year) compared with those referred for revascularization (1.3% per year) (Fig. 54-3). Patients with a greater ischemic burden on imaging were also found to benefit more from revascularization than medical therapy, with serial imaging studies showing a greater reduction in reversible defect size in those treated with revascularization. A subsequent observational study of 10,627 consecutive patients with no prior infarct or revascularization demonstrated a survival advantage in patients with no or mild ischemia treated with medical therapy, with revascularization having prognostic benefit beyond medical therapy in patients with moderate to severe ischemia.[38] More recently, the Clinical Outcomes Utilizing Revascularization and Aggressive Drug Evaluation (COURAGE) trial[39] showed no difference in the incidence of death or myocardial infarction in 2287 patients with stable angina randomized to optimal medical therapy or percutaneous revascularization. A substudy of this trial showed that the addition of percutaneous revascularization to optimal medical therapy resulted in more effective reduction of ischemia than medical therapy alone, with less angina.[40] Moreover, regardless of treatment assignment, the degree of residual ischemia on follow-up perfusion imaging was proportional to the risk of subsequent cardiac events. Thus, it appears that revascularization can be employed selectively in patients with CAD based on the extent and severity of the ischemic burden. Patients with low-risk findings can be treated medically, whereas more extensive ischemia is best treated with more aggressive interventions.

These principles have been shown to have a favorable impact in terms of both patient outcomes and cost when applied clinically. Several large studies have focused on the clinical use of stress MPI to guide patient management and have shown that referral for coronary angiography is accordingly low (about 3.5%) after a normal stress MPI, but referrals increase to 60% when the stress MPI is moderately to severely abnormal.[28,41,42] This demonstrates that clinicians can incorporate MPI into their practice appropriately, particularly when deferring further invasive evaluation when the MPI is normal. The use of stress MPI to guide patient management has also been demonstrated to be cost effective.

An "ischemia-guided" approach to managing patients with CAD has been shown to optimize the use of angiography and subsequent revascularization procedures.[43] The Economics of Noninvasive Diagnosis (END) study[44,45] compared differences in cost for 11,372 consecutive patients referred for either stress MPI or cardiac catheterization as the initial approach. Not only were the rates of subsequent myocardial infarction the same in the two groups, costs were significantly higher for the direct cardiac catheterization group as compared with the MPI ischemia-guided approach. Moreover, patients sent directly to cardiac catheterization were more likely to be treated with coronary revascularization in all subsets of risk when compared with those undergoing stress MPI initially. The ischemia-guided approach to stable angina was found to be less costly, with less interventions and similar cardiac event rates. These cost differences can be directly attributed to a decrease in apparently unnecessary procedures in patients with negative MPI results.

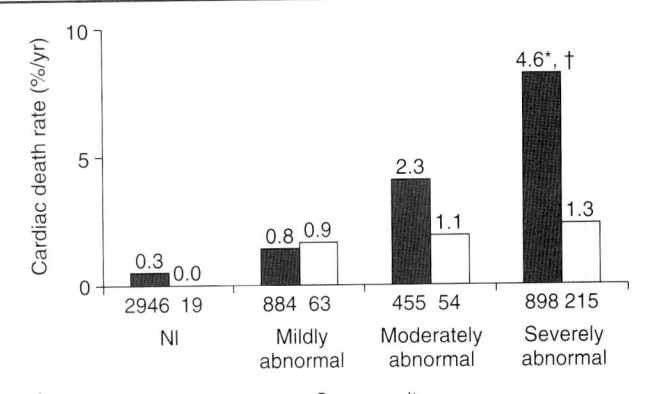

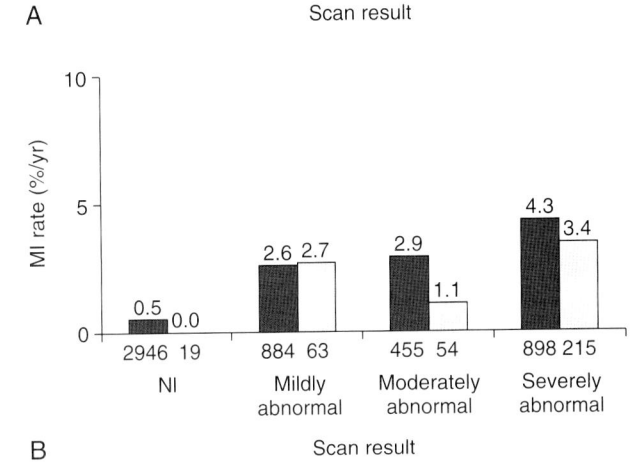

Figure 54–3
SPECT myocardial perfusion imaging and prognosis. This large retrospective analysis of patients undergoing stress SPECT myocardial perfusion imaging demonstrates the incremental prognostic information obtained with the imaging results. The annualized incidence of cardiac death (**A**) and myocardial infarction (MI) (**B**) is displayed for patients treated medically (solid columns) and those undergoing revascularization (gray columns) with respect to the myocardial perfusion image result. Annualized cardiac events were low (<1%) in both groups with normal SPECT studies. However, event rates increased with respect to the degree of SPECT abnormality. Survival was significantly improved in those with severely abnormal scans who underwent revascularization. *$P < .01$ compared with patients undergoing revascularization early after nuclear testing; †$P < .001$ compared with patients treated with medical therapy after nuclear testing; Abnl, abnormal; Nl, normal. (Reprinted with permission from Hachamovitch R, Berman DS, Shaw LJ, et al. Circulation **97**:535-43, 1998.)

Preoperative Evaluation for Noncardiac Surgery

Perioperative cardiac events are an important cause of morbidity and mortality during and after noncardiac surgery, and they occur in more than 2% of patients undergoing these procedures. Much of this risk can be assessed preoperatively via clinical evaluation (a history of coronary artery or cerebrovascular disease, congestive heart failure, renal insufficiency, insulin-requiring diabetes, or high-risk surgical procedure) to identify patients at high risk for cardiac complications who might benefit from risk-reduction strategies (specific perioperative medical therapy or revascularization) and patients having sufficiently low risk that further evaluation before surgery is not necessary.[46] However, patients with an intermediate risk for cardiac complications may benefit from further noninvasive testing to identify ischemia and provide further risk stratification prior to surgery.[47] Provocative testing for ischemia is typically performed in such patients. However, exercise testing is not always feasible for patients with pulmonary disease or low exercise capacity, and in particular for those undergoing orthopedic or vascular surgery. Pharmacologic stress MPI has been shown to add significant information to preoperative risk stratification.[48] It is recommended for those patients with intermediate clinical risk predictors (prior MI, diabetes, renal insufficiency), for those who have poor functional capacity, and for those undergoing a high-risk surgical procedure (emergent surgery, aortic or peripheral vascular surgery, prolonged procedures with anticipated large blood loss or volume shifts). When results of stress MPI are normal, the incidence of perioperative cardiac events has been shown to be approximately 1% for all procedures, including major vascular surgery.[49] Although the severity and extent of ischemia remains an important predictor of adverse cardiac events during and after surgery, recent studies have shown that revascularization before noncardiac surgery does not appear to affect later outcome in terms of death and nonfatal myocardial infarction.[50]

ACUTE CORONARY SYNDROME

Territory at Risk and Infarct Size

Resting MPI has been used to determine the territory at risk during an acute coronary syndrome, and it can be used to assess the extent of myocardial salvage achieved with reperfusion strategies.[51] Radiopharmaceuticals labeled with ^{99m}Tc can be injected at rest in the setting of an acute ST-segment elevation myocardial infarction on presentation. After initial treatment and stabilization with either pharmacologic or mechanical reperfusion, perfusion images can be acquired that represent the initial myocardial area at risk *during* the coronary occlusion. These images are then compared with those acquired at rest after a subsequent injection *after* reperfusion. The difference in the size of the defect between these two scans is the salvage index, representing the degree of myocardium that was rescued by reperfusion (i.e., the initial territory at risk minus the ultimate scar).[52,53] Although this methodology is not used widely in clinical practice, it is a useful tool in the evaluation of therapies used in the treatment of acute MI. The salvage index has been validated as a surrogate marker of patient outcome, and it provides a quantitative means of comparing the efficacy of therapeutic strategies.[54] The use of the infarct size, territory at risk, and the salvage index has played a central role in trials focusing on the efficacy of angioplasty[52,55] and thrombolysis.[56] This methodology can also assist in determining important clinical factors associated with reperfusion outcome, such as time to reperfusion.[55]

Myocardial infarct size can be measured quantitatively after MI and has been shown to be highly predictive of poor outcome.[53,54,57,58] The ischemic burden on cardiac stress SPECT imaging is associated with future nonfatal myocardial infarction, whereas fixed perfusion defects and a depressed ejection fraction are predictive of future cardiac death.[59] Quantification of the infarct size as a percentage of the left ventricle is an effective way to risk-stratify a patient's risk for cardiac death in the near term. Studies using ^{99m}Tc SPECT after acute MI have observed that mortality within the subsequent 24 months was approximately 8% if the infarct encompassed more than 12% to 14% of the left ventricle.[58,60]

Rest MPI for Acute Coronary Syndrome

The triage of patients who present to the emergency department with acute chest pain is a substantial diagnostic challenge. Radionuclide myocardial perfusion imaging has been shown to have favorable diagnostic and prognostic value in this setting, with an excellent sensitivity for detecting acute MI that is not recognized by other testing modalities (e.g., serum markers, ECG).[61-65] A major advantage of a triage protocol that employs rest SPECT MPI is that ischemia or infarction can be detected earlier than with serum markers. A patient with chest pain and an ECG that is normal or nondiagnostic for ischemia or infarction can be injected in the emergency department, and then imaged in 30 to 60 minutes. Several observational and randomized studies have repeatedly shown that a normal resting perfusion imaging study has a negative predictive value of greater than 99% to exclude MI, and that defects at rest are associated with a higher incidence of death and MI at 30 days.[64-67] Thus, a normal resting MPI in a patient with chest pain essentially excludes acute MI and is predictive of a sufficiently low risk of near-term adverse cardiac events that the patient can be discharged home. Furthermore, an abnormal study is associated with a worse near-term outcome, and hospitalization is warranted (Fig. 54-4). Once MI or unstable angina has been excluded, provocative testing can be performed, with or without MPI, to identify stress-induced ischemia. Protocols that use immediate rest MPI to exclude an acute coronary syndrome, and subsequent stress testing to evaluate for significant CAD have demonstrated both reductions in unnecessary hospitalizations and cost savings compared with routine care.[68]

Risk Stratification after Myocardial Infarction

Stress MPI has been shown to have excellent diagnostic value in patients after an acute myocardial infarction (AMI). Dipyridamole vasodilator stress MPI early after AMI is highly predictive of future cardiac events. In fact, recent studies have found that the most important predictors of future cardiac death and recurrent MI are the extent and severity of degree of the reversible (ischemic) myocardial perfusion defect. Bateman and colleagues[69] reported the results of a multicenter trial that randomized 451 patients after a first acute infarction to either early (hospital day 2 to 4) dipyridamole stress MPI or routine predischarge (hospital day 6 to 12) submaximal exercise MPI.

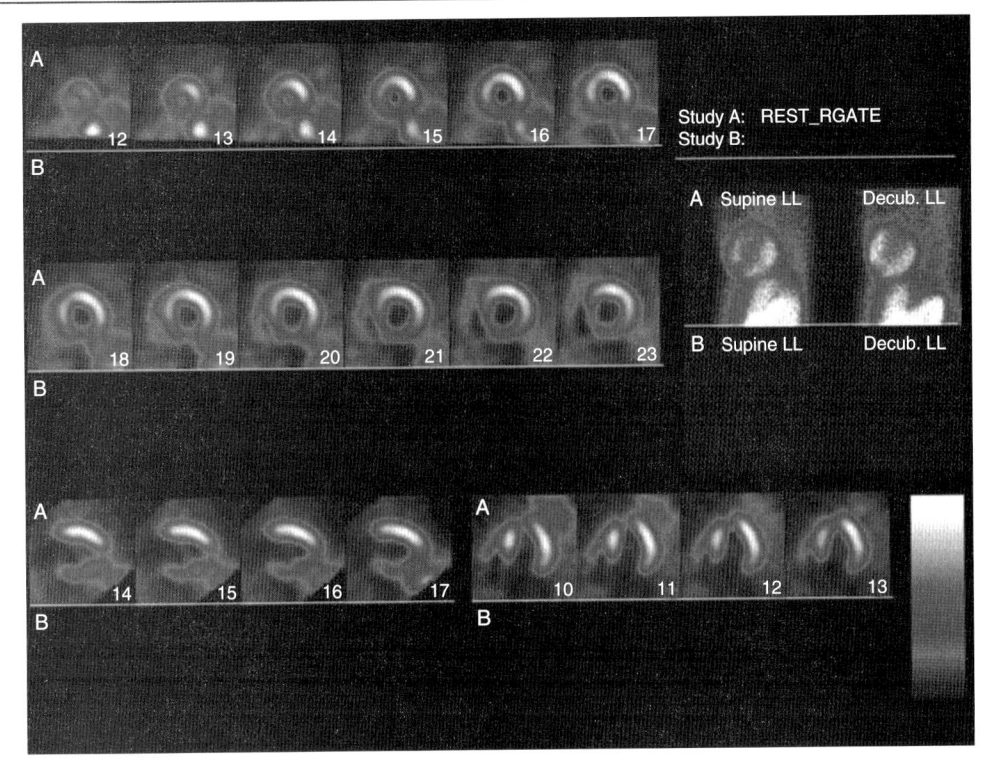

Figure 54–4
Rest SPECT myocardial perfusion imaging during ongoing chest pain in a patient with a normal electrocardiogram. Injection of radiotracer during ongoing chest pain and subsequent imaging 45 minutes later demonstrates a moderate-sized area of decreased perfusion in the inferior wall. The patient was brought directly to cardiac catheterization, and coronary angiography demonstrated a 95% stenosis of the right coronary artery that was treated with angioplasty and intracoronary stenting.

The extent and severity of the stress defect and the degree of defect reversibility were found to be the most important predictors of cardiac death and recurrent myocardial infarction. The early use of pharmacologic stress perfusion imaging after acute infarction was more predictive of early and late cardiac events, and provided greater incremental diagnostic and prognostic value than predischarge submaximal exercise perfusion imaging. One major advantage of this approach is that management decisions can made much earlier in the hospital course after an uncomplicated AMI. More recently, the INSPIRE trial showed that MPI performed early after AMI in appropriate patients can safely and reliably identify patients with findings of low risk or lack of inducible ischemia who would be unlikely to benefit from an invasive approach, as well as those with extensive ischemia in whom intensive anti-ischemic medical or interventional therapies are appropriate. Thus, noninvasive imaging as an initial strategy for categorizing risk and triaging for subsequent care of stable survivors of MI who have not undergone acute coronary angiography seems reasonable.[70]

ASSESSMENT OF MYOCARDIAL VIABILITY

Left Ventricular Ejection Fraction and Prognosis

Numerous studies have demonstrated that left ventricular systolic performance is a powerful and independent predictor of mortality in patients both with and without CAD. When the left ventricular ejection fraction becomes depressed after MI or with chronic ischemic heart disease, the risk of sudden cardiac death increases substantially.[34,71-73]

Data from the Thrombolysis in Myocardial Infarction (TIMI) trials indicated that the prognostic significance of LVEF assessment was also maintained after thrombolysis, although the overall mortality was lower than in the prethrombolytic era.[74] The powerful prognostic significance of resting LVEF assessed by radionuclide angiography is also important in patients treated with thrombolysis or primary angioplasty.[71,75] Not only is resting LVEF the strongest predictor of 6-month mortality but it is also predictive of ventricular arrhythmias and sudden death in a similar group of patients. The prognostic significance of LVEF in patients with chronic coronary artery disease is also well established and is independent of the extent of anatomic disease.[76]

All of the available techniques used to assess left ventricular function, including nuclear techniques such as radionuclide angiography and gated SPECT, as well as two- and three-dimensional echocardiography, contrast ventriculography, and magnetic resonance imaging, provide similar prognostic information in patients with MI and chronic CAD. Radionuclide angiography is a highly accurate, widely validated, and reproducible technique, making it a useful tool when serial measurements of LVEF are required. Nonetheless, two-dimensional resting echocardiography, gated SPECT MPI, and magnetic resonance imaging are replacing radionuclide angiography for the assessment of LVEF. Ejection fractions assessed by gated SPECT stress MPI provide incremental prognostic information beyond the perfusion imaging results. In a study of 1680 patients undergoing stress MPI, patients with a gated SPECT LVEF of greater than 45% had low mortality rates (<1% per year), even when associated with severe perfusion defects. However, patients with an LVEF of less than 45% on gated SPECT had a mortality rate of 9.2% per year, even if only mild or moderate perfusion abnormalities were present.[77] This underscores the importance of LVEF in determining prognosis, and the need to pursue aggressive medical and surgical strategies in patients with depressed LVEF. Gated SPECT indices of end-diastolic and end-systolic volumes consistent with LV dilation have also been shown to add prognostic value in predicting cardiac death and nonfatal MI independent of the perfusion abnormalities on the scan.[34]

Positron Emission Tomography and SPECT for Determining Myocardial Viability

Because LVEF is a major determinant of survival in patients with ischemic heart disease, therapeutic strategies that might improve systolic performance, and thereby improve survival, have been widely studied. Patients with chronic CAD and patients after AMI are two important groups at risk for the development of left ventricular dysfunction. However, the left ventricular systolic dysfunction is not always the result of scarring and fibrosis of the myocardium: it may be the result of the repetitive or chronic myocardial ischemia. Thus, LV dysfunction at rest may not necessarily be irreversible. The evaluation of patients with ischemic cardiomyopathies caused by chronic CAD or MI becomes important in selecting patients who might have reversible dysfunction and who might benefit from coronary revascularization.

Ischemic myocardial dysfunction is produced by four pathophysiologic processes. After MI, the myocardium in the vascular territory served by an acutely occluded culprit artery may undergo necrosis and scarring, leading to extensive fibrosis and subsequent regional dysfunction. With an acute coronary syndrome, if myocardial blood flow is restored either spontaneously or with a therapeutic reperfusion strategy such as angioplasty or thrombolysis, regional contractile dysfunction may occur even without myocardial necrosis, a state which has been termed *stunning*. This postischemic dysfunction after a transient period of ischemia followed by reperfusion is characterized by normal flow but reduced function in the absence of myocardial scarring. Regional dysfunction may also be observed in chronic CAD, with reductions in blood flow presumably occurring more slowly. The contractile impairment is thought to result from a compensatory downregulation of function during prolonged periods of myocardial hypoperfusion, a concept termed *hibernation*. Left ventricular dysfunction may also deteriorate as a result of *remodeling*, characterized by histologic and biochemical changes in the myocardium as a result of an ischemic insult.

Myocardial viability was initially defined as the ability to recover global or regional left ventricular function after revascularization. In this paradigm, treatment of repetitive or chronic ischemia, defined pathologically as stunning and hibernation, respectively, was deemed responsible for the improvement in contractility. Thus, the ability to identify dysfunctional but viable myocardium resulting from these pathologic states became important when considering a patient for potential revascularization.

Although recovery of function may be an important goal of revascularization, the central goal of assessing myocardial viability is to predict outcome with therapy—that is, to differentiate patients with potentially reversible left ventricular dysfunction whose prognosis may be improved with revascularization from those with large areas of infarct or scar who may not benefit (or may even do worse) with surgery. Thus, viability assessment provides better insight into the risk-to-benefit ratio in patients with ischemic LV dysfunction by effectively differentiating between those with a significant amount of viable myocardium who are at increased risk if treated medically, and those who would be at high risk with either treatment.

At present, a number of diagnostic approaches exist for assessing myocardial viability in patients with ischemic cardiomyopathy. The major nuclear cardiology modalities to determine viability include techniques that assess cell membrane integrity, regional perfusion, or myocardial metabolism.

Viability assessments are typically performed in a particular subset of patients—namely, those with known CAD and left ventricular systolic dysfunction who are potential candidates for surgical revascularization. Most viability assessment is performed in patients with chronic ischemic cardiomyopathies, or after acute MI, because as many as 50% of patients with prior myocardial infarction will have residual viable myocardium.[78] The methods used for viability assessment are similar to those used for prognostic assessment in patients with CAD. Thus, protocols used for stress MPI can be easily modified to obtain information regarding viability. However, if the assessment of viability is the principal clinical question, a protocol designed to specifically assess viability should be used. When the question of myocardial viability is primary, however, it is best to follow a specific viability imaging protocol. The nuclear cardiology techniques that have been validated extensively in the assessment of myocardial viability include the use of positron emission tomography (PET) imaging of myocardial metabolism, and resting SPECT perfusion imaging of ^{201}Tl and the ^{99m}Tc-labeled tracers sestamibi and tetrofosmin.

Positron Emission Tomography

Positron emission tomography has been extensively evaluated as a noninvasive imaging modality for viability assessment. PET viability studies involve the determination and comparison of both myocardial blood flow and the metabolic status of the myocardium.[79] Perfusion is usually assessed with ^{13}N-labeled NH_3, and glucose utilization is typically assessed with ^{18}F-fluorodeoxyglucose (FDG), which when taken up by the myocardium reflects glucose transport across the myocyte membrane. FDG accumulates in myocytes in proportion to glucose uptake, but it undergoes phosphorylation by hexokinase to FDG-6-phosphate in the first step of glycolysis. FDG-6-phosphate is a form of deoxyglucose that becomes trapped in the myocyte and is not metabolized further. Thus, FDG uptake reflects exogenous glucose utilization. Normal myocardium preferentially utilizes fatty acids for energy, but it switches to increased glucose utilization during periods of ischemia. In myocardial regions with ischemic dysfunction, myocardial glucose uptake may be increased, and thus FDG uptake is enhanced, reflecting viability. On the other hand, FDG does not accumulate in areas of fibrosis or scar. FDG uptake is then compared with resting perfusion imaging. Perfusion and metabolism are considered matched if areas of preserved flow show normal metabolic activity, and areas of reduced flow have diminished FDG uptake (scar). However, perfusion and metabolism may be discordant, or mismatched. In this scenario, FDG uptake is present in areas of hypoperfusion, indicating that despite

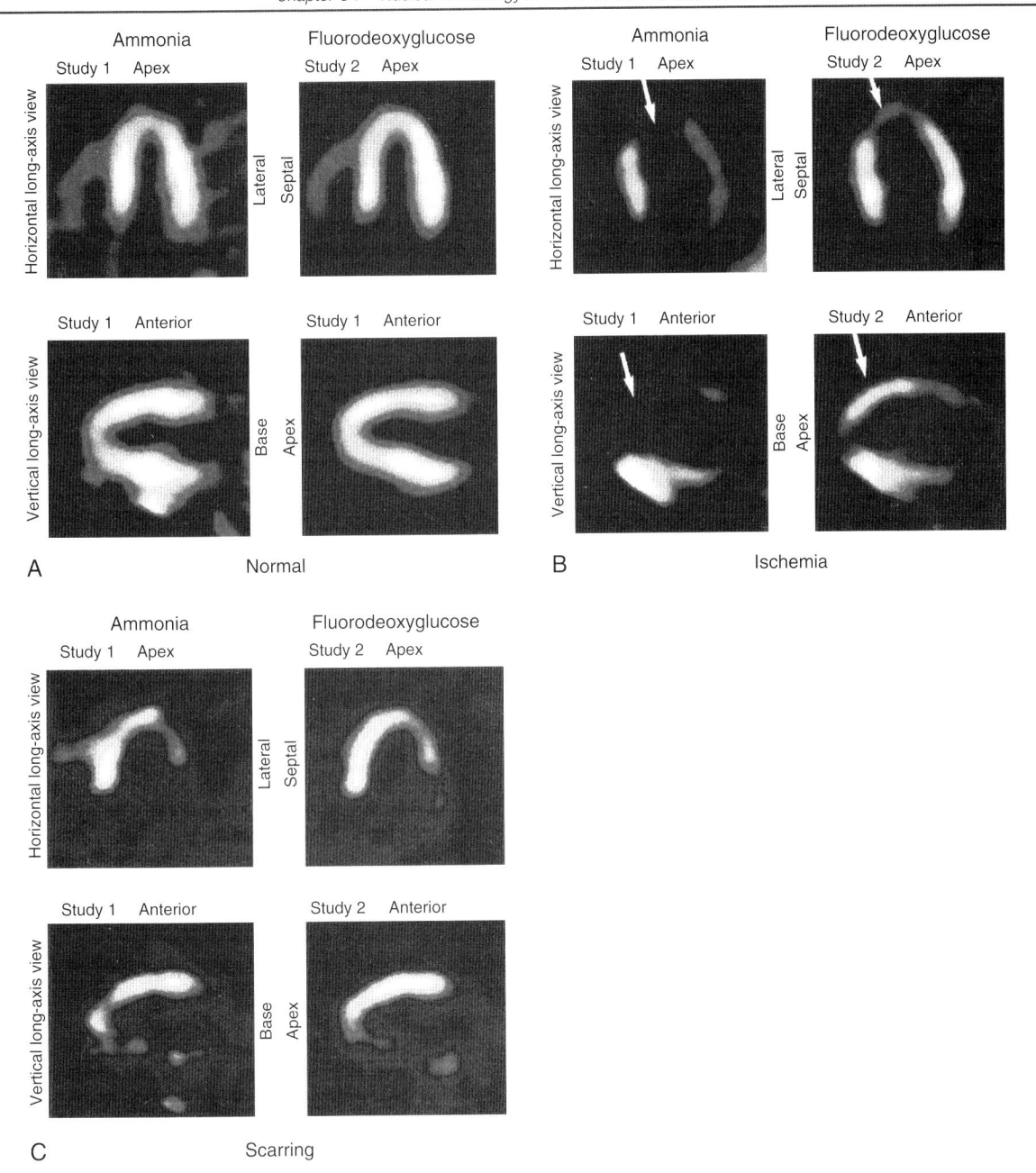

Figure 54–5

A positron emission tomography (PET) viability study. For each panel of four views, perfusion imaging with ^{13}N-labeled ammonia uptake is on the left, and metabolic imaging with [^{18}F]fluorodeoxyglucose (FDG) uptake is on the right. The upper row of each panel is the horizontal long-axis slice with the apex at the top, and the lower row is a vertical long-axis slice with the apex pointing to the left. The yellow and white areas are sites of maximal activity, and the blue areas are sites of minimal activity. The red areas indicate intermediate activity. **A,** Normal images. **B,** An example of ischemia and viable tissue. **C,** An example of myocardial scarring. Note the homogeneous uptake of both ammonia and FDG in the normal study. In the presence of ischemia (**B**), there is a mismatch *(arrows)*, with decreased perfusion and augmented metabolic activity in the apex and the anterior wall. With scarring (**C**), there is equally decreased uptake of FDG and ammonia in the inferior and lateral walls. A, anterior wall; I, inferior wall; L, lateral wall; S, septum. (see color version in the online edition through Expert consult.)

decreased blood flow, the myocardium is still metabolically active, hence viable. This mismatched defect is most predictive of functional recovery after revascularization (Fig. 54-5).

Quantitative Methods

The clinical assessment of myocardial viability using FDG is based predominantly on comparison of its qualitative or semiquantitative uptake relative to a myocardial perfusion tracer. Quantification of myocardial glucose utilization is possible but requires kinetic modeling of transmembrane transport and phosphorylation to adjust for the behavior of injected FDG in relation to endogenous glucose.[80] Another quantitative approach is the assessment of myocardial glucose utilization, using dynamic PET acquisitions and sequential arterial blood sampling to measure fractional ^{18}F-FDG uptake in relation to the delivered dose.

Perhaps of greater importance is the ability of cardiac PET to determine absolute myocardial blood flow using tracer kinetic models. Quantitative myocardial blood flow can be measured with dynamic imaging of ^{13}N-ammonia, rubidium-82 (^{82}Rb), or $H_2^{15}O$. These agents can be used to determine regional myocardial blood flow. Flow can be measured at rest and after pharmacologic vasodilation to determine the myocardial blood flow reserve (the ratio of maximal flow to resting flow). Reduction in coronary flow reserve has proved useful in the assessment of stenosis severity (flow limitation) in CAD,[81-84] in patients with no known CAD but with risk factors,[85] and to evaluate changes in flow after medical treatment of such CAD risk factors as hyperlipidemia,[86,87] diabetes,[88] and smoking.[89]

Flow reserve is also useful in differentiating viable from nonviable myocardium, as a certain degree of myocardial blood flow is necessary to maintain myocyte viability. In the setting of a functionally significant coronary artery stenosis, the vasculature distal to the lesion may retain the ability to vasodilate and thus increase regional myocardial blood flow. Regions of myocardium that can achieve this must therefore be viable. Flow reserve has been studied as a surrogate for myocardial viability in patients with previous infarction and chronic coronary artery disease.[90]

Single-Photon Emission Computed Tomography

Thallium

Thallium-201 (^{201}Tl) has been used as a tracer to assess both regional blood flow and myocardial viability.[78] Like potassium, it is actively transported across the myocyte sarcolemmal membrane via the Na/K-ATPase, and it is extracted from the blood in proportion to myocardial blood flow. Cellular extraction is diminished only when there is irreversible injury to the myocyte, making ^{201}Tl an attractive agent for imaging pathophysiologic conditions such as chronic hypoperfusion and postischemic dysfunction. Because retention of thallium in the myocardium corresponds to cell membrane integrity, regional uptake of thallium corresponds to viable myocardium. Thus, decreased myocardial uptake early after injection of ^{201}Tl can be the result of reduced regional blood flow or infarction. After injection, ^{201}Tl redistributes in the myocardium by continuous exchange between the myocardium and the extracardiac compartments (interstitium, blood pool), driven by the concentration gradient of the tracer and by intact myocyte viability. Imaging after redistribution shows less regional heterogeneity of initial ^{201}Tl distribution, thereby reducing the relative difference between the ischemic and normal regions. An increase in regional ^{201}Tl activity on the redistribution images is indicative of myocardium that has reduced flow, but more importantly of myocardium that has intact cellular integrity and thus viability. Thus, ^{201}Tl redistribution has been used to distinguish viable from scarred myocardium. ^{201}Tl can be imaged at rest and again 4 hours later to assess redistribution, or by using another injection if part of a stress MPI protocol. Viability can also be assessed quantitatively with ^{201}Tl. The presence of ^{201}Tl uptake greater than 50% to 60% of maximum is predictive of functional recovery in the majority of segments. Moreover, the final thallium uptake with redistribution appears to be more important than the degree of change from rest to redistribution in predicting recovery.[91,92]

Technetium-Labeled Tracers

Technetium agents, currently used more than thallium for stress MPI, also provide insight into the viability of the myocardium. The ability to determine viability from an initial stress-rest MPI study with technetium often obviates the need for further testing with PET or thallium protocols. Uptake and retention of the technetium perfusion tracers sestamibi and tetrofosmin require that the myocyte cell and mitochondrial membranes be intact. Thus, tracer accumulation indicates cellular integrity and reflects cellular viability.[93] Computer-assisted quantitative analysis of regional myocardial uptake of sestamibi has been shown to improve accuracy in predicting functional recovery after revascularization, and as with ^{201}Tl, tracer uptake greater than 50% of peak is suggestive of myocardial viability.[94] The administration of nitrates to enhance resting blood and hence tracer uptake has also been studied with ^{99m}Tc-labeled agents, because it has been questioned whether sestamibi, when compared with PET imaging, leads to an underestimate of viability.[95,96] Assessment of metabolism for viability with FDG can also be performed using SPECT systems with special equipment (high-energy collimators or coincidence detection).[97]

Prognostic Implications of Viability Assessment

Despite recent advances in medical and antiarrhythmic device therapy for heart failure, patients with ischemic cardiomyopathy and congestive heart failure continue to have a poor prognosis.[98] Many of these patients would benefit from orthotopic heart transplant, but donor organ supply is limited. In 2007, with more than 3000 transplant candidates, just over 2200 transplants were performed, and 15% of candidates died waiting for a donor organ.[99] With such limited access to transplantation, and to improve survival in these patients, surgical revascularization is often considered. The selection of appropriate patients for surgical revascularization is largely based on early surgical survival studies that provided insight into which patients obtain the most benefit from surgical revascularization. The Veterans Administration Cooperative Trial[100] and the Coronary Artery Surgery Study[101] both demonstrated that patients with significant left main or multivessel CAD and depressed ejection fraction (35% to 50%) had better survival with revascularization than medical therapy. Not unexpectedly, these patients often have a high perioperative mortality with coronary artery bypass grafting (CABG).[102-104] Assessment of viability may be useful in these patients to balance the potential benefits of revascularization with the risk of the procedure.[105-107]

The potential to improve ventricular function (and moreover survival) with revascularization necessitates an evaluation for hibernating myocardium in most patients with left ventricular dysfunction, especially those without angina. However, viability testing may not be necessary if the patient has angina pectoris or if initial testing revealed stress-induced ischemia. The clinical endpoints commonly used in viability assessment include recovery of regional or global ventricular function, and improvement in symptoms or survival. Most studies focusing on the assessment of myocardial viability have used improvement in ventricular function with revascularization as the clinical endpoint. Although useful in comparing the accuracy of the various techniques to determine viability, functional improvement has been used largely as a surrogate for outcome because of the relationship between left ventricular function and outcome. Many studies have focused on the ability of viability assessment to predict functional recovery with revascularization, but relatively few have used survival and outcomes as an endpoint. The prognostic implications of PET perfusion–metabolism mismatch and the presence of viability on imaging with thallium or sestamibi have been demonstrated in several studies that have shown similar findings.[79,107,108] Patients with perfusion–metabolism mismatch have a very high mortality when managed medically, and a much lower mortality if revascularized. On the other hand, those with matched defects, indicating scar, had no such difference in outcomes between medical and surgical management. Although the methods included a combination of techniques and outcomes (death, nonfatal MI, unstable angina, need for transplant or revascularization), this distinction is not subtle. Patients with demonstrated viability had an annual event rate of 27% if treated medically, compared with 6% in similar patients who underwent coronary revascularization.[109] However, patients with matched defects suggesting no viability had similar event rates with medical or surgical treatment. This dichotomy in outcomes underscores the prognostic implication of determining viability.

A meta-analysis of pooled data from 24 studies of viability using all currently used techniques and encompassing over 3000 patients further illustrates this point.[107] In patients with ischemic cardiomyopathy (mean LVEF, 32% ± 8%), those with demonstrated viability had an annual mortality of 3.2% if treated with revascularization and 16% if treated medically. Those without viability had essentially similar outcomes (7.7% versus 6.2% mortality, respectively). This recent analysis provides further evidence that the preoperative determination of viability provides information regarding not only functional recovery but improvement in survival as well. Results from the recently completed Positron Emission Tomography and Recovery following Revascularization-2 (PARR-2) trial showed a trend toward improved 1-year outcome when PET-FDG–guided therapy was used compared with standard care.[110] It is unclear whether the improvement in outcome with revascularization is entirely the result of improvement in LVEF after surgery. Samady and coworkers[111] examined survival after CABG in 104 patients, with an assessment of function before and after surgical revascularization. Outcomes were similar in patients irrespective of whether the LVEF improved after CABG, suggesting that revascularization of ischemic myocardium, even without improvement in ventricular function, may prevent future infarction and death. Of note, no formal viability assessment was performed in the majority of these patients.

On the basis of studies such as these, some have advocated revascularization for all patients with ischemic cardiomyopathy, asserting that hibernating myocardium should be suspected in all patients with CAD and LV dysfunction. However, others maintain that preoperative viability assessment provides an opportunity to balance the potential benefit from surgical revascularization against the risks of the procedure. The Surgical Treatments for Ischemic Heart Disease (STICH) trial,[112] a study of 2136 patients randomized to optimal medical therapy, surgical revascularization, or ventricular restoration (or combinations of these) has recently completed enrollment, and the results may elucidate the best treatment approach for patients with ischemic cardiomyopathy and heart failure.

EVALUATION OF PATIENTS AFTER REVASCULARIZATION

Despite technical advances, the effectiveness of both percutaneous and surgical revascularization procedures is limited by restenosis and vein graft closure, respectively.

Progression of the underlying atherosclerosis or development of new stenoses can cause recurrent ischemia, manifesting as recurrence of symptoms, congestive heart failure resulting from LV dysfunction, MI, or cardiac death. Symptom status is not a reliable predictor of stenosis after coronary angioplasty, as evidenced by the subjects (up to 25%) who have silent ischemia on treadmill testing.[36] However, routine exercise treadmill testing is not currently advocated after coronary angioplasty, as it does not reliably detect restenosis.[34] SPECT imaging has been demonstrated to accurately detect restenosis, particularly in the 3- to 9-month window of greatest risk for restenosis, with positive and negative predictive values of approximately 90%.[80] A recent study demonstrated that ^{201}Tl stress defect size was predictive of cardiac death and MI, even up to 3 years after percutaneous transluminal coronary angioplasty (PTCA).[49] Further study is necessary to evaluate if routine stress MPI after angioplasty indeed alters prognosis, particularly in asymptomatic patients, and in high-risk subsets of patients (e.g., those with decreased LV function, multivessel or proximal left anterior descending artery disease, diabetes, renal failure) after angioplasty. The prognostic value of SPECT MPI after CABG has been studied in more than 2000 patients, and the results have consistently demonstrated that the finding of reversible defects on stress SPECT MPI is a strong predictor of worse cardiac outcome in symptomatic subjects early (in 1 to 5 years) after CABG, and in all subjects more than 5 years after surgical revascularization.

FUTURE DIRECTIONS

Although the cornerstone of nuclear cardiology has been myocardial perfusion imaging with SPECT and PET techniques, the field is rapidly expanding in many arenas. Recent technologic advances in hardware and processing have led to the ability to acquire scans in a fraction of the time needed with conventional cameras. These advances will improve image quality and reduce both imaging time and radiation exposure. The emerging field of cardiac computed tomography (CT) and CT angiography has also led to the development of hybrid cameras, such as PET/CT and SPECT/CT, which will ultimately permit synthesis of the anatomic data from CT with the perfusion data from perfusion imaging, which will facilitate the simultaneous assessment of the ischemic burden produced by a given coronary artery stenosis. Novel radiotracers currently under investigation include the fatty acid analog iodine-123-BMIPP, which appears to hold promise as a marker of recent myocardial ischemia with "ischemic memory" that may last up to 30 hours after an episode of cardiac chest pain.[113] Another new tracer being studied, iodine-123-metaiodobenzylguanidine (MIBG), is a marker of cardiac adrenergic activity, and thus can be helpful in determining both response to medical therapy and prognosis in patients with LV dysfunction and heart failure,[114] as well as in predicting which patients might benefit from an implantable cardiac defibrillator. Both myocardial perfusion imaging and gated blood-pool imaging with phase analysis can be used to assess ventricular desynchrony that might be amenable to cardiac resynchronization therapies.[115]

Other areas currently under investigation include the concept of molecular imaging[116] of a variety of targets including angiotensin receptors,[117] matrix metalloproteinases,[118,119] integrins,[120,121] and other processes involved in angiogenesis.[122] Advances in PET imaging[123,124] with new fluoride-18-labeled agents[125] and the further validation of Rb-82 perfusion,[126] as well as improvements in SPECT technology, may well enhance the ability to image novel processes, as well as to reduce both imaging time and radiation exposure.[127] Such new approaches will undoubtedly contribute to the clinical usefulness of nuclear cardiology imaging techniques in the evaluation and management of patients with known or suspected heart disease.

REFERENCES

1. Beller GA, Zaret BL. Contributions of nuclear cardiology to diagnosis and prognosis of patients with coronary artery disease. *Circulation* 2000;**101**: 1465-78.
2. Russell RR 3rd, Zaret BL. Nuclear cardiology: present and future. *Current Problems in Cardiology* 2006;**31**:557-629.
3. Arlington Medical Resources I. The myocardial perfusion study market guide. 2007.
4. Hansen CL, Goldstein RA, Akinboboye OO, et al. Myocardial perfusion and function: single photon emission computed tomography. *Journal of Nuclear Cardiology* 2007;**14**:e39-60.
5. Hachamovitch R. Clinical application of rest thallium-201/stress technetium-99m sestamibi dual isotope myocardial perfusion single-photon emission computed tomography. *Cardiology in Review* 1999;**7**:83-91.
6. Gianrossi R, Detrano R, Mulvihill D, et al. Exercise-induced ST depression in the diagnosis of coronary artery disease: a meta-analysis. *Circulation* 1989;**80**: 87-98.
7. Fleischmann KE, Hunink MG, Kuntz KM, et al. Exercise echocardiography or exercise SPECT imaging? a meta-analysis of diagnostic test performance [see comment]. *JAMA* 1998;**280**:913-20.
8. Berman DS, Shaw LJ, Hachamovitch R, et al. Comparative use of radionuclide stress testing, coronary artery calcium scanning, and noninvasive coronary angiography for diagnostic and prognostic cardiac assessment. *Seminars in Nuclear Medicine* 2007;**37**:2-16.
9. Johansen A, Hoilund-Carlsen PF, Christensen HW, et al. Diagnostic accuracy of myocardial perfusion imaging in a study population without post-test referral bias [see comment]. *Journal of Nuclear Cardiology* 2005;**12**:530-7.
10. Bateman TM, Cullom SJ. Attenuation correction single-photon emission computed tomography myocardial perfusion imaging. *Seminars in Nuclear Medicine* 2005;**35**:37-51.
11. Klocke FJ, Baird MG, Lorell BH, et al. ACC/AHA/ASNC guidelines for the clinical use of cardiac radionuclide imaging—executive summary: a report of the American College of Cardiology/American Heart Association Task Force on Practice Guidelines (ACC/AHA/ASNC Committee to Revise the 1995 Guidelines for the Clinical Use of Cardiac Radionuclide Imaging). *Journal of the American College of Cardiology* 2003;**42**:1318-33.
12. Bokhari S, Ficaro EP, McCallister BD Jr. Adenosine stress protocols for myocardial perfusion imaging. *Journal of Nuclear Cardiology* 2007;**14**:415-6.
13. O'Keefe JH Jr, Bateman TM, Handlin LR, et al. Four- versus 6-minute infusion protocol for adenosine thallium-201 single photon emission computed tomography imaging. *American Heart Journal* 1995;**129**:482-7.
14. Iskandrian AE, Bateman TM, Belardinelli L, et al. Adenosine versus regadenoson comparative evaluation in myocardial perfusion imaging: results of the ADVANCE phase 3 multicenter international trial. *Journal of Nuclear Cardiology* 2007;**14**:645-58.
15. Hendel RC, Bateman TM, Cerqueira MD, et al. Initial clinical experience with regadenoson, a novel selective A2A agonist for pharmacologic stress single-photon emission computed tomography myocardial perfusion imaging [see comment]. *Journal of the American College of Cardiology* 2005;**46**:2069-75.
16. Cerqueira MD, Nguyen P, Staehr P, et al. Effects of age, gender, obesity, and diabetes on the efficacy and safety of the selective A2A agonist regadenoson versus adenosine in myocardial perfusion imaging: integrated ADVANCE-MPI trial results. *J Am Coll Cardiol Cardiovasc Imaging* 2008;**1**:307-16.
17. Thomas GS, Tammelin BR, Schiffman GL, et al. Safety of regadenoson, a selective adenosine A2A agonist, in patients with chronic obstructive pulmonary disease: a randomized, double-blind, placebo-controlled trial (RegCOPD trial). *Journal of Nuclear Cardiology* 2008;**15**:319-28.
18. Leaker BR, O'Connor B, Hansel TT, et al. Safety of regadenoson, an adenosine A2A receptor agonist for myocardial perfusion imaging, in mild asthma and moderate asthma patients: a randomized, double-blind, placebo-controlled trial. *Journal of Nuclear Cardiology* 2008;**15**:329-36.
19. Navare SM, Katten D, Johnson LL, et al. Risk stratification with electrocardiographic-gated dobutamine stress technetium-99m sestamibi single-photon emission tomographic imaging: value of heart rate response and assessment of left ventricular function [see comment]. *Journal of the American College of Cardiology* 2006;**47**:781-8.
20. Kim C, Kwok YS, Heagerty P, et al. Pharmacologic stress testing for coronary disease diagnosis: a meta-analysis. *American Heart Journal* 2001;**142**:934-44.
21. Iskander S, Iskandrian AE. Risk assessment using single-photon emission computed tomographic technetium-99m sestamibi imaging. *Journal of the American College of Cardiology* 1998;**32**:57-62.
22. Metz LD, Beattie M, Hom R, et al. The prognostic value of normal exercise myocardial perfusion imaging and exercise echocardiography: a meta-analysis [see comment]. *Journal of the American College of Cardiology* 2007;**49**:227-37.
23. Hachamovitch R, Hayes S, Friedman JD, et al. Determinants of risk and its temporal variation in patients with normal stress myocardial perfusion scans: what is the warranty period of a normal scan? *Journal of the American College of Cardiology* 2003;**41**:1329-40.
24. Bateman TM. Clinical relevance of a normal myocardial perfusion scintigraphic study. American Society of Nuclear Cardiology. *Journal of Nuclear Cardiology* 1997;**4**:172-3.
25. Amanullah AM, Berman DS, Hachamovitch R, et al. Identification of severe or extensive coronary artery disease in women by adenosine technetium-99m sestamibi SPECT. *American Journal of Cardiology* 1997;**80**:132-7.
26. Hachamovitch R. Prognostic characterization of patients with mild coronary artery disease with myocardial perfusion single photon emission computed tomography: validation of an outcomes-based strategy [comment]. *Journal of Nuclear Cardiology* 1998;**5**:90-5.
27. Hachamovitch R, Berman DS, Kiat H, et al. Incremental prognostic value of adenosine stress myocardial perfusion single-photon emission computed tomography and impact on subsequent management in patients with or suspected of having myocardial ischemia. *American Journal of Cardiology* 1997;**80**:426-33.
28. Hachamovitch R, Berman DS, Shaw LJ, et al. Incremental prognostic value of myocardial perfusion single photon emission computed tomography for the prediction of cardiac death: differential stratification for risk of cardiac death and myocardial infarction [erratum appears in Circulation 1998;98(2):190]. *Circulation* 1998;**97**:535-43.
29. Kwok JMF, Christian TF, Miller TD, et al. Incremental prognostic value of exercise single-photon emission computed tomographic (SPECT) thallium 201 imaging in patients with ST-T abnormalities on their resting electrocardiograms. *American Heart Journal* 2005;**149**:145-51.
30. Iskandrian AS, Chae SC, Heo J, et al. Independent and incremental prognostic value of exercise single-photon emission computed tomographic (SPECT) thallium imaging in coronary artery disease. *Journal of the American College of Cardiology* 1993;**22**:665-70.
31. Abidov A, Germano G, Berman DS. Transient ischemic dilation ratio: a universal high-risk diagnostic marker in myocardial perfusion imaging [comment]. *Journal of Nuclear Cardiology* 2007;**14**:497-500.
32. Hansen CL, Sangrigoli R, Nkadi E, et al. Comparison of pulmonary uptake with transient cavity dilation after exercise thallium-201 perfusion imaging. *Journal of the American College of Cardiology* 1999;**33**:1323-7.
33. Jain D, Thompson B, Wackers FJ, et al. Relevance of increased lung thallium uptake on stress imaging in patients with unstable angina and non-Q wave myocardial infarction: results of the Thrombolysis in Myocardial Infarction (TIMI)-IIIB study. *Journal of the American College of Cardiology* 1997;**30**:421-9.
34. Sharir T, Kang X, Germano G, et al. Prognostic value of poststress left ventricular volume and ejection fraction by gated myocardial perfusion SPECT in women and men: gender-related differences in normal limits and outcomes. *Journal of Nuclear Cardiology* 2006;**13**:495-506.
35. Iskandrian AE, Heo J, Mehta D, et al. Gated SPECT perfusion imaging for the simultaneous assessment of myocardial perfusion and ventricular function in the BARI 2D trial: an initial report from the Nuclear Core Laboratory. *Journal of Nuclear Cardiology* 2006;**13**:83-90.

36. Abidov A, Germano G, Hachamovitch R, et al. Gated SPECT in assessment of regional and global left ventricular function: major tool of modern nuclear imaging. *Journal of Nuclear Cardiology* 2006;**13**:261-79.
37. O'Keefe JH Jr, Bateman TM, Ligon RW, et al. Outcome of medical versus invasive treatment strategies for non-high-risk ischemic heart disease [see comment]. *Journal of Nuclear Cardiology* 1998;**5**:28-33.
38. Hachamovitch R, Hayes SW, Friedman JD, et al. Comparison of the short-term survival benefit associated with revascularization compared with medical therapy in patients with no prior coronary artery disease undergoing stress myocardial perfusion single photon emission computed tomography. *Circulation* 2003;**107**:2900-7.
39. Boden WE, O'Rourke RA, Teo KK, et al. Optimal medical therapy with or without PCI for stable coronary disease [see comment]. *New England Journal of Medicine* 2007;**356**:1503-16.
40. Shaw LJ, Berman DS, Maron DJ, et al. Optimal medical therapy with or without percutaneous coronary intervention to reduce ischemic burden: results from the Clinical Outcomes Utilizing Revascularization and Aggressive Drug Evaluation (COURAGE) trial nuclear substudy. *Circulation* 2008;**117**:1283-91.
41. Bateman TM, O'Keefe JH Jr, Dong VM, et al. Coronary angiographic rates after stress single-photon emission computed tomographic scintigraphy. *Journal of Nuclear Cardiology* 1995;**2**:217-23.
42. Hachamovitch R, Berman DS, Kiat H, et al. Exercise myocardial perfusion SPECT in patients without known coronary artery disease: incremental prognostic value and use in risk stratification. *Circulation* 1996;**93**:905-14.
43. Hachamovitch R, Berman DS. The use of nuclear cardiology in clinical decision making. *Seminars in Nuclear Medicine* 2005;**35**:62-72.
44. Shaw LJ, Hachamovitch R, Berman DS, et al. The economic consequences of available diagnostic and prognostic strategies for the evaluation of stable angina patients: an observational assessment of the value of precatheterization ischemia. Economics of Noninvasive Diagnosis (END) Multicenter Study Group. *Journal of the American College of Cardiology* 1999;**33**:661-9.
45. Shaw LJ, Hachamovitch R, Heller GV, et al. Noninvasive strategies for the estimation of cardiac risk in stable chest pain patients. The Economics of Noninvasive Diagnosis (END) Study Group. *American Journal of Cardiology* 2000;**86**:1-7.
46. American College of Cardiology/American Heart Association Task Force on Practice G, American Society of E, American Society of Nuclear C, et al. ACC/AHA 2007 guidelines on perioperative cardiovascular evaluation and care for noncardiac surgery: executive summary: a report of the American College of Cardiology/American Heart Association Task Force on Practice Guidelines (Writing Committee to Revise the 2002 Guidelines on Perioperative Cardiovascular Evaluation for Noncardiac Surgery). *Anesthesia & Analgesia* 2008;**106**:685-712.
47. Hashimoto J, Nakahara T, Bai J, et al. Preoperative risk stratification with myocardial perfusion imaging in intermediate and low-risk non-cardiac surgery. *Circulation Journal* 2007;**71**:1395-400.
48. Brown KA. Advances in nuclear cardiology: preoperative risk stratification. *Journal of Nuclear Cardiology* 2004;**11**:335-48.
49. Hoeks SE, Schouten O, van der Vlugt MJ, et al. Preoperative cardiac testing before major vascular surgery. *Journal of Nuclear Cardiology* 2007;**14**:885-91.
50. McFalls EO, Ward HB, Moritz TE, et al. Coronary-artery revascularization before elective major vascular surgery [see comment]. *New England Journal of Medicine* 2004;**351**:2795-804.
51. Haronian HL, Remetz MS, Sinusas AJ, et al. Myocardial risk area defined by technetium-99m sestamibi imaging during percutaneous transluminal coronary angioplasty: comparison with coronary angiography. *Journal of the American College of Cardiology* 1993;**22**:1033-43.
52. Stone GW, Dixon SR, Grines CL, et al. Predictors of infarct size after primary coronary angioplasty in acute myocardial infarction from pooled analysis from four contemporary trials. *American Journal of Cardiology* 2007;**100**:1370-5.
53. Gibbons RJ, Valeti US, Araoz PA, et al. The quantification of infarct size. *Journal of the American College of Cardiology* 2004;**44**:1533-42.
54. Gibbons RJ, Miller TD, Christian TF. Infarct size measured by single photon emission computed tomographic imaging with (99m)Tc-sestamibi: a measure of the efficacy of therapy in acute myocardial infarction. *Circulation* 2000;**101**:101-8.
55. Brodie BR, Webb J, Cox DA, et al. Impact of time to treatment on myocardial reperfusion and infarct size with primary percutaneous coronary intervention for acute myocardial infarction (from the EMERALD trial). *American Journal of Cardiology* 2007;**99**:1680-6.
56. Bruce CJ, Christian TF, Schaer GL, et al. Determinants of infarct size after thrombolytic treatment in acute myocardial infarction. *American Journal of Cardiology* 1999;**83**:1600-5.
57. Fieno DS, Thomson LEJ, Slomka P, et al. Quantitation of infarct size in patients with chronic coronary artery disease using rest-redistribution Tl-201 myocardial perfusion SPECT: correlation with contrast-enhanced cardiac magnetic resonance [see comment]. *Journal of Nuclear Cardiology* 2007;**14**:59-67.
58. Miller TD, Hodge DO, Sutton JM, et al. Usefulness of technetium-99m sestamibi infarct size in predicting posthospital mortality following acute myocardial infarction. *American Journal of Cardiology* 1998;**81**:1491-3.
59. Sharir T, Germano G, Kang X, et al. Prediction of myocardial infarction versus cardiac death by gated myocardial perfusion SPECT: risk stratification by the amount of stress-induced ischemia and the poststress ejection fraction. *Journal of Nuclear Medicine* 2001;**42**:831-7.
60. Miller TD, Piegas LS, Gibbons RJ, et al. Role of infarct size in explaining the higher mortality in older patients with acute myocardial infarction. *American Journal of Cardiology* 2002;**90**:1370-4.
61. Kaul S, Senior R, Firschke C, et al. Incremental value of cardiac imaging in patients presenting to the emergency department with chest pain and without ST-segment elevation: a multicenter study. *American Heart Journal* 2004;**148**:129-36.
62. Kontos MC. Myocardial perfusion imaging in the acute care setting. *Journal of Nuclear Cardiology* 2007;**14**:S125-32.
63. Kontos MC, Tatum JL. Imaging in the evaluation of the patient with suspected acute coronary syndrome. *Cardiology Clinics* 23:517-30
64. Heller GV, Stowers SA, Hendel RC, et al. Clinical value of acute rest technetium-99m tetrofosmin tomographic myocardial perfusion imaging in patients with acute chest pain and nondiagnostic electrocardiograms [see comment]. *Journal of the American College of Cardiology* 1998;**31**:1011-7.
65. Udelson JE, Beshansky JR, Ballin DS, et al. Myocardial perfusion imaging for evaluation and triage of patients with suspected acute cardiac ischemia: a randomized controlled trial [see comment] [erratum appears in JAMA 2003;289(2):178]. *JAMA* 2002;**288**:2693-700.
66. Abbott BG, Wackers FJ. Use of radionuclide imaging in acute coronary syndromes. *Current Cardiology Reports* 2003;**5**:25-31.
67. Kontos MC, Jesse RL, Anderson FP, et al. Comparison of myocardial perfusion imaging and cardiac troponin I in patients admitted to the emergency department with chest pain. *Circulation* 1999;**99**:2073-8.
68. Radensky PW, Hilton TC, Fulmer H, et al. Potential cost effectiveness of initial myocardial perfusion imaging for assessment of emergency department patients with chest pain. *American Journal of Cardiology* 1997;**79**:595-9.
69. Bateman TM, Berman DS, Heller GV, et al. American Society of Nuclear Cardiology position statement on electrocardiographic gating of myocardial perfusion SPECT scintigrams. *Journal of Nuclear Cardiology* 1999;**6**:470-1.
70. Mahmarian JJ, Shaw LJ, Filipchuk NG, et al. A multinational study to establish the value of early adenosine technetium-99m sestamibi myocardial perfusion imaging in identifying a low-risk group for early hospital discharge after acute myocardial infarction. *Journal of the American College of Cardiology* 2006;**48**:2448-57.
71. Burns RJ, Gibbons RJ, Yi Q, et al. The relationships of left ventricular ejection fraction, end-systolic volume index and infarct size to six-month mortality after hospital discharge following myocardial infarction treated by thrombolysis. *Journal of the American College of Cardiology* 2002;**39**:30-6.
72. Ndrepepa G, Mehilli J, Martinoff S, et al. Evolution of left ventricular ejection fraction and its relationship to infarct size after acute myocardial infarction [see comment] [erratum appears in J Am Coll Cardiol 2007;50(17):1733]. *Journal of the American College of Cardiology* 2007;**50**:149-56.
73. Alegria JR, Miller TD, Gibbons RJ, et al. Infarct size, ejection fraction, and mortality in diabetic patients with acute myocardial infarction treated with thrombolytic therapy. *American Heart Journal* 2007;**154**:743-50.
74. Zaret BL, Wackers FJ, Terrin ML, et al. Value of radionuclide rest and exercise left ventricular ejection fraction in assessing survival of patients after thrombolytic therapy for acute myocardial infarction: results of Thrombolysis in Myocardial Infarction (TIMI) phase II study. The TIMI Study Group. *Journal of the American College of Cardiology* 1995;**26**:73-9.
75. Gosselink AT, Liem AL, Reiffers S, et al. Prognostic value of predischarge radionuclide ventriculography at rest and exercise after acute myocardial infarction treated with thrombolytic therapy or primary coronary angioplasty. The Zwolle Myocardial Infarction Study Group. *Clinical Cardiology* 1998;**21**:254-60.
76. Mock MB, Ringqvist I, Fisher LD, et al. Survival of medically treated patients in the coronary artery surgery study (CASS) registry. *Circulation* 1982;**66**:562-8.
77. Sharir T, Germano G, Kavanagh PB, et al. Incremental prognostic value of post-stress left ventricular ejection fraction and volume by gated myocardial perfusion single photon emission computed tomography. *Circulation* 1999;**100**:1035-42.
78. Bonow RO, Dilsizian V. Thallium 201 for assessment of myocardial viability [see comment]. *Seminars in Nuclear Medicine* 1991;**21**:230-41.
79. Schinkel AFL, Poldermans D, Elhendy A, et al. Assessment of myocardial viability in patients with heart failure. *Journal of Nuclear Medicine* 2007;**48**:1135-46.
80. Knuuti MJ, Nuutila P, Ruotsalainen U, et al. The value of quantitative analysis of glucose utilization in detection of myocardial viability by PET. *Journal of Nuclear Medicine* 1993;**34**:2068-75.

81. Roelants V, Bol A, Bernard X, et al. Direct comparison between 2-dimensional and 3-dimensional PET acquisition modes for myocardial blood flow absolute quantification with O-15 water and N-13 ammonia. *Journal of Nuclear Cardiology* 2006;13:220-4.
82. Chareonthaitawee P, Christenson SD, Anderson JL, et al. Reproducibility of measurements of regional myocardial blood flow in a model of coronary artery disease: comparison of H2150 and 13NH3 PET techniques. *Journal of Nuclear Medicine* 2006;47:1193-201.
83. Kitsiou AN, Bacharach SL, Bartlett ML, et al. 13N-ammonia myocardial blood flow and uptake: relation to functional outcome of asynergic regions after revascularization. *Journal of the American College of Cardiology* 1999;33:678-86.
84. Di Carli MF, Hachamovitch R, Berman DS. The art and science of predicting postrevascularization improvement in left ventricular (LV) function in patients with severely depressed LV function [comment]. *Journal of the American College of Cardiology* 2002;40:1744-7.
85. Dorbala S, Hassan A, Heinonen T, et al. Coronary vasodilator reserve and Framingham risk scores in subjects at risk for coronary artery disease. *Journal of Nuclear Cardiology* 2006;13:761-7.
86. Gould KL, Martucci JP, Goldberg DI, et al. Short-term cholesterol lowering decreases size and severity of perfusion abnormalities by positron emission tomography after dipyridamole in patients with coronary artery disease. A potential noninvasive marker of healing coronary endothelium [see comment]. *Circulation* 1994;89:1530-8.
87. Czernin J, Barnard RJ, Sun KT, et al. Effect of short-term cardiovascular conditioning and low-fat diet on myocardial blood flow and flow reserve. *Circulation* 1995;92:197-204.
88. Yokoyama I, Momomura S, Ohtake T, et al. Reduced myocardial flow reserve in non-insulin-dependent diabetes mellitus [see comment]. *Journal of the American College of Cardiology* 1997;30:1472-7.
89. Czernin J, Sun K, Brunken R, et al. Effect of acute and long-term smoking on myocardial blood flow and flow reserve. *Circulation* 1995;91:2891-7.
90. Marzullo P, Parodi O, Sambuceti G, et al. Residual coronary reserve identifies segmental viability in patients with wall motion abnormalities. *Journal of the American College of Cardiology* 1995;26:342-50.
91. Bax JJ, Wijns W, Cornel JH, et al. Accuracy of currently available techniques for prediction of functional recovery after revascularization in patients with left ventricular dysfunction due to chronic coronary artery disease: comparison of pooled data. *Journal of the American College of Cardiology* 1997;30:1451-60.
92. Udelson JE, Bonow RO, Dilsizian V. The historical and conceptual evolution of radionuclide assessment of myocardial viability. *Journal of Nuclear Cardiology* 2004;11:318-34.
93. Sciagra R, Pellegri M, Pupi A, et al. Prognostic implications of Tc-99m sestamibi viability imaging and subsequent therapeutic strategy in patients with chronic coronary artery disease and left ventricular dysfunction. *Journal of the American College of Cardiology* 2000;36:739-45.
94. Maes AF, Borgers M, Flameng W, et al. Assessment of myocardial viability in chronic coronary artery disease using technetium-99m sestamibi SPECT: correlation with histologic and positron emission tomographic studies and functional follow-up. *Journal of the American College of Cardiology* 1997;29:62-8.
95. Slart RHJA, Agool A, van Veldhuisen DJ, et al. Nitrate administration increases blood flow in dysfunctional but viable myocardium, leading to improved assessment of myocardial viability: a PET study. *Journal of Nuclear Medicine* 2006;47:1307-11.
96. He Z-X, Yang M-F, Liu X-J, et al. Association of myocardial viability on nitrate-augmented technetium-99m hexakis-2-methoxylisobutyl isonitrile tomography and intermediate-term outcome in patients with prior myocardial infarction and left ventricular dysfunction. *American Journal of Cardiology* 2003;92:696-9.
97. Slart RHJA, Bax JJ, de Boer J, et al. Comparison of 99mTc-sestamibi/18FDG DISA SPECT with PET for the detection of viability in patients with coronary artery disease and left ventricular dysfunction. *European Journal of Nuclear Medicine & Molecular Imaging* 2005;32:972-9.
98. Mosterd A, Hoes AW. Clinical epidemiology of heart failure. *Heart* 2007;93:1137-46.
99. Scientific Registry of Transplant Recipients. Available at www.ustransplant.org/national_stats.aspx, accessed 2/5/09.
100. Eleven-year survival in the Veterans Administration randomized trial of coronary bypass surgery for stable angina. The Veterans Administration Coronary Artery Bypass Surgery Cooperative Study Group. *New England Journal of Medicine* 1984;311:1333-9.
101. Killip T, Passamani E, Davis K. Coronary artery surgery study (CASS): a randomized trial of coronary bypass surgery—eight years' follow-up and survival in patients with reduced ejection fraction. *Circulation* 1985;72:V102-9.
102. Kron IL, Flanagan TL, Blackbourne LH, et al. Coronary revascularization rather than cardiac transplantation for chronic ischemic cardiomyopathy. *Annals of Surgery* 1989;210:348-52:discussion 352-4.
103. Caines AEB, Massad MG, Kpodonu J, et al. Outcomes of coronary artery bypass grafting versus percutaneous coronary intervention and medical therapy for multivessel disease with and without left ventricular dysfunction. *Cardiology* 2004;101:21-8.
104. Ghose T, Thompson RC. Revascularization for patients with severe coronary artery disease and left ventricular dysfunction. *Current Cardiology Reports* 2006;8:255-60.
105. Liao L, Cabell CH, Jollis JG, et al. Usefulness of myocardial viability or ischemia in predicting long-term survival for patients with severe left ventricular dysfunction undergoing revascularization. *American Journal of Cardiology* 2004;93:1275-9.
106. Sciagra R, Leoncini M, Cannizzaro G, et al. Predicting revascularization outcome in patients with coronary artery disease and left ventricular dysfunction (data from the SEMINATOR study). *American Journal of Cardiology* 2002;89:1369-73.
107. Allman KC, Shaw LJ, Hachamovitch R, et al. Myocardial viability testing and impact of revascularization on prognosis in patients with coronary artery disease and left ventricular dysfunction: a meta-analysis [see comment]. *Journal of the American College of Cardiology* 2002;39:1151-8.
108. Camici PG, Prasad SK, Rimoldi OE. Stunning, hibernation, and assessment of myocardial viability. *Circulation* 2008;117:103-14.
109. Iskander S, Iskandrian AE. Prognostic utility of myocardial viability assessment. *American Journal of Cardiology* 83:696-702
110. Beanlands RSB, Nichol G, Huszti E, et al. F-18-fluorodeoxyglucose positron emission tomography imaging-assisted management of patients with severe left ventricular dysfunction and suspected coronary disease: a randomized, controlled trial (PARR-2) [see comment]. *Journal of the American College of Cardiology* 2007;50:2002-12.
111. Samady H, Elefteriades JA, Abbott BG, et al. Failure to improve left ventricular function after coronary revascularization for ischemic cardiomyopathy is not associated with worse outcome. *Circulation* 1999;100:1298-304.
112. The STICH Trial.
113. Inaba Y, Bergmann SR. Diagnostic accuracy of beta-methyl-p-[123I]-iodophenyl-pentadecanoic acid (BMIPP) imaging: a meta-analysis. *Journal of Nuclear Cardiology* 2008;15:345-52.
114. Sugiura T, Takase H, Toriyama T, et al. Usefulness of Tc-99m methoxyisobutylisonitrile scintigraphy for evaluating congestive heart failure. *Journal of Nuclear Cardiology* 2006;13:64-8.
115. Zaret BL. Cardiac imaging and cardiac resynchronization therapy: time to get in phase. *J Am Coll Cardiol Cardiovasc Imaging* 2008;1:614-6.
116. Sinusas AJ. Cardiovascular molecular imaging. *Journal of Nuclear Medicine* 2007;48:26N-7.
117. Aras O, Messina SA, Shirani J, et al. The role and regulation of cardiac angiotensin-converting enzyme for noninvasive molecular imaging in heart failure. *Current Cardiology Reports* 2007;9:150-8.
118. Chung G, Sinusas AJ. Imaging of matrix metalloproteinase activation and left ventricular remodeling. *Current Cardiology Reports* 2007;9:136-42.
119. Su H, Spinale FG, Dobrucki LW, et al. Noninvasive targeted imaging of matrix metalloproteinase activation in a murine model of postinfarction remodeling. *Circulation* 2005;112:3157-67.
120. Zhang J, Krassilnikova S, Gharaei AA, et al. Alphavbeta3-targeted detection of arteriopathy in transplanted human coronary arteries: an autoradiographic study. *FASEB Journal* 2005;19:1857-9.
121. Sadeghi MM, Krassilnikova S, Zhang J, et al. Detection of injury-induced vascular remodeling by targeting activated alphavbeta3 integrin in vivo. *Circulation* 2004;110:84-90.
122. Sinusas AJ. Targeted imaging offers advantages over physiological imaging for evaluation of angiogenic therapy. *J Am Coll Cardiol Cardiovasc Imaging* 2008;1:511-4.
123. Di Carli MF, Hachamovitch R. Hybrid PET/CT is greater than the sum of its parts. *Journal of Nuclear Cardiology* 2008;15:118-22.
124. Di Carli MF, Dorbala S, Curillova Z, et al. Relationship between CT coronary angiography and stress perfusion imaging in patients with suspected ischemic heart disease assessed by integrated PET-CT imaging. *Journal of Nuclear Cardiology* 2007;14:799-809.
125. Yalamanchili P, Wexler E, Hayes M, et al. Mechanism of uptake and retention of F-18 BMS-747158-02 in cardiomyocytes: a novel PET myocardial imaging agent [see comment]. *Journal of Nuclear Cardiology* 2007;14:782-8.
126. Sampson UK, Dorbala S, Limaye A, et al. Diagnostic accuracy of rubidium-82 myocardial perfusion imaging with hybrid positron emission tomography/computed tomography in the detection of coronary artery disease. *Journal of the American College of Cardiology* 2007;49:1052-8.
127. Borges-Neto S, Pagnanelli RA, Shaw LK, et al. Clinical results of a novel wide beam reconstruction method for shortening scan time of Tc-99m cardiac SPECT perfusion studies. *Journal of Nuclear Cardiology* 2007;14:555-65.

CHAPTER 55
Diagnostic Echocardiography (Ultrasound Imaging in Cardiovascular Diagnosis)
Rosario V. Freeman and Catherine M. Otto

Basic Principles
Ultrasound Imaging Modalities
Doppler Echocardiography
Ventricular Function
  Systolic Function
  Diastolic Function
Ischemic Heart Disease
  Stress Testing for Coronary Disease
  Complications of Acute Myocardial Infarction

Cardiac Masses
Cardiomyopathies
  Congestive Heart Failure
  Hypertrophic and Restrictive Cardiomyopathy
  Cardiac Transplantation
Pericardial and Constrictive Heart Disease
Valvular Heart Disease
  Aortic Stenosis
  Aortic Regurgitation

Mitral Stenosis
Mitral Regurgitation
Tricuspid Valve Disease
Prosthetic Valves
Endocarditis
Aortic Disease
Congenital Heart Disease

Echocardiography has broad utility in the diagnosis and management of cardiovascular disease. Advances in image quality and Doppler quantitation allow real-time, precise anatomic definition and physiologic interrogation of cardiac and vascular structures with minimal risk and discomfort for the patient. Common clinical applications of echocardiography include assessment of myocardial and valvular function, identification of structural abnormalities, and optimization of timing for surgical intervention.[1-4] Echocardiography use has expanded beyond the diagnostic laboratory to include the intensive care unit, emergency department, operating room, and electrophysiology and cardiac catheterization laboratories. This chapter reviews the basic principles of ultrasound imaging and Doppler quantitation. A discussion of the application of echocardiography for a range of cardiovascular diseases is then presented.[5]

BASIC PRINCIPLES

Echocardiographic images are generated from analyses of reflected ultrasound waves. Ultrasound waves are high in frequency, above 20 kHz, beyond the audible sound wave range. A transducer produces ultrasound waves that reflect off tissue boundaries and are received back by the transducer. Reflected waves take longer to return from structures farther from the transducer than from nearby structures. Complex analysis of the intensity and timing of the reflected ultrasound waves provides image generation. Factors that affect image generation include ultrasound beam refraction through different physical media, absorption of ultrasound energy by intervening tissue (attenuation), and disarrayed beam reflection, termed scatter.[1,2] Image artifacts may be generated if reflected ultrasound waves "re-reflect" on internal structures, delaying the time for some of the reflected ultrasound waves to return to the transducer. Proper interpretation of echocardiographic images should account for potential ultrasound artifacts. Propagation of ultrasound waves is optimal through liquid medium, such as blood. Air and bone cause significant acoustic impedance, with resulting poor ultrasound penetration. Therefore, intrathoracic air, intervening ribs, and surface bandages between the transducer and the heart result in suboptimal image generation. Transducers of different size, type, and frequency are available to optimize image quality.

ULTRASOUND IMAGING MODALITIES

Echocardiographic examinations include use of several ultrasound modalities. The basic imaging format is real-time two-dimensional imaging that sweeps an ultrasound beam across an imaging tomographic plane to provide images at a frame rate of about 30 frames per second. For transthoracic echocardiography (TTE), the transducer is placed on the body surface, and images are taken after standard image planes are optimized (Fig. 55-1).[6] Technological advances now allow decreased size of ultrasound systems with increased portability. Although most diagnostic echocardiography still requires full ultrasound systems, smaller, hand-held devices are increasingly available for preliminary diagnostic testing in intensive care units, emergency departments, and similar clinical settings.

M-mode (motion) is produced by display of signals from a single ultrasound beam against the time dimension (Fig. 55-2). Temporal resolution is improved because time for the imaging sweep is not necessary for M-mode image generation. M-mode is useful for finite measurement of cardiac dimensions and timing of events, such as valve opening and closing.

Transesophageal echocardiography (TEE) is a semi-invasive procedure in which the transducer is mounted on a flexible endoscope and positioned in the esophagus and stomach. Manipulation of the TEE probe is constrained by esophageal anatomy, and oblique TEE image planes may hinder acquisition

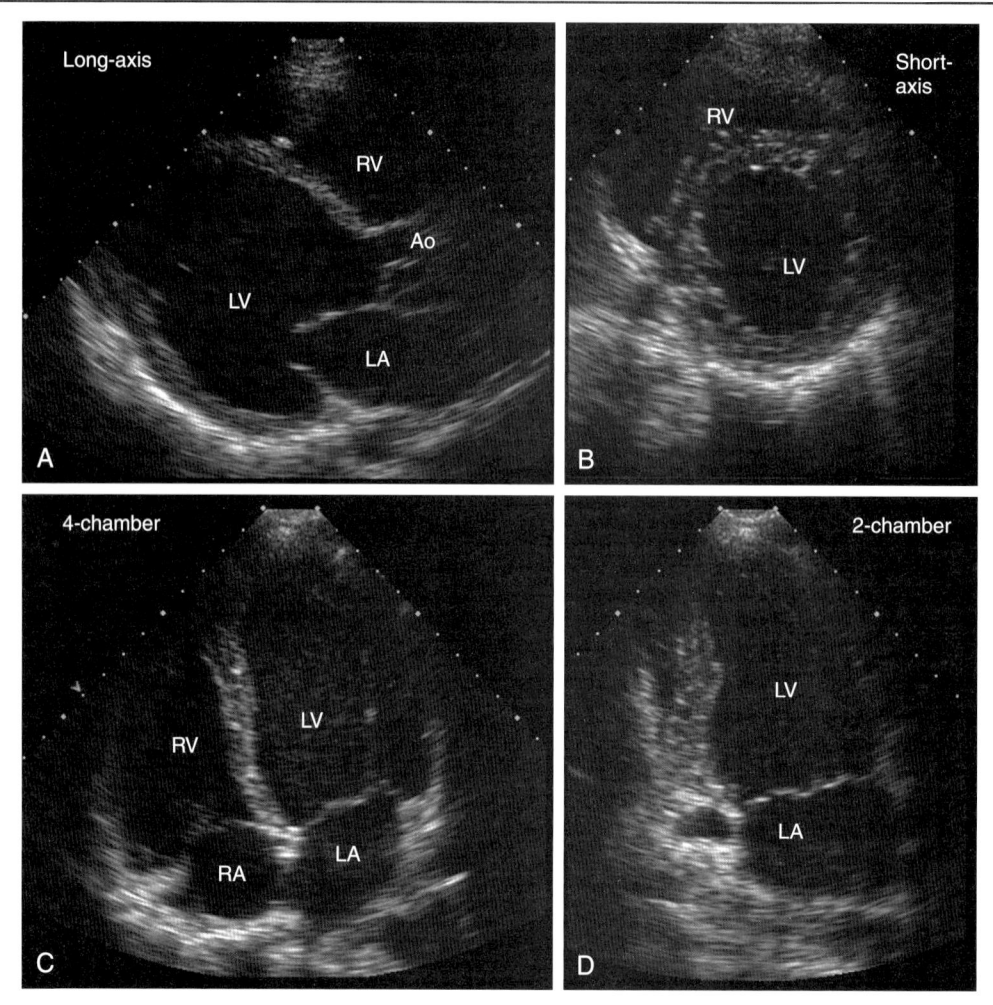

Figure 55-1
A, Parasternal long-axis view in a patient with dilated cardiomyopathy shows the anteroseptum and posterior wall of the left ventricle. Mitral and aortic valves are also well seen in this view. **B,** Parasternal short-axis view in a different patient shows a cross section through the midportion of the right and left ventricles. **C,** Apical four-chamber view shows the lateral and inferoseptal walls of the left ventricle and the free wall of the right ventricle. **D,** Apical two-chamber view shows anterior and inferior walls of the left ventricle.

of correct cardiac dimensions. However, image resolution for TEE is significantly improved over TTE because of the lack of intervening air or bone. Placement of the TEE transducer in the esophagus permits better visualization of posterior cardiac structures, such as the mitral valve, left atrium, left atrial appendage, interatrial septum, and thoracic aorta. TEE is more accurate than TTE imaging for identification of valvular vegetations, complications of endocarditis, and aortic disease and for evaluation of mitral valve abnormalities. TEE is used to identify left atrial thrombus as a potential cardiac source of distal embolic disease and to exclude thrombus before direct current cardioversion for atrial fibrillation.[7] In the intensive care unit, TEE has been used in determining the cause of unexplained hypotension[8] and is helpful in evaluating patients at increased risk for ischemia, hypovolemia, and pericardial tamponade after cardiac surgery.[9] However, TEE usually requires conscious sedation to reduce the patient's discomfort, with additional monitoring and nursing support.

Contrast echocardiography is performed in conjunction with standard two-dimensional imaging to opacify intracardiac chambers. Contrast agents include intravenous agitated saline, used to opacify the right-sided heart chambers for detection of intracardiac shunts (Fig. 55-3), and commercially made microbubble agents that traverse the pulmonary bed to provide left-sided heart opacification. When image quality is suboptimal, opacification of the left-sided cardiac chambers enhances endocardial border definition to aid in wall motion analysis (Fig. 55-4).[10] Although transpulmonary contrast agents have the potential to provide information on myocardial perfusion, this methodology is still in development.[11,12]

Epicardial intraoperative echocardiography is performed by placing the transducer directly on the heart during cardiac surgery. This modality is used when anterior structures are suboptimally seen through a transesophageal approach. Intravascular ultrasound imaging is performed through a percutaneously placed intravascular catheter. The most common use of this technique is intracoronary transducer placement to assist in plaque characterization and assessment of stenosis severity. Intracardiac transducers are also placed percutaneously and are used in the catheterization and electrophysiology laboratories for peri-procedural aid in catheter placement. Three-dimensional (3D) echocardiography improves spatial resolution, but increased time requirements

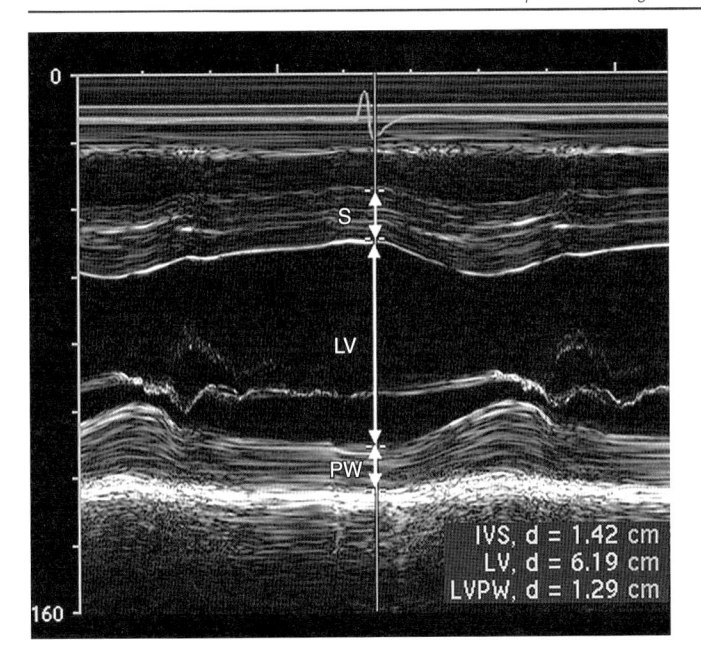

Figure 55–2
M-mode tracing from a patient with aortic regurgitation and a dilated left ventricle. Left ventricular wall thickness and chamber size are shown throughout the cardiac cycle. Diastolic measurements of the septum (S), left ventricular chamber size (LV), and posterior wall (PW) are shown. In the mid left ventricular cavity, the mitral valve can be seen opening during diastole and closing during systole.

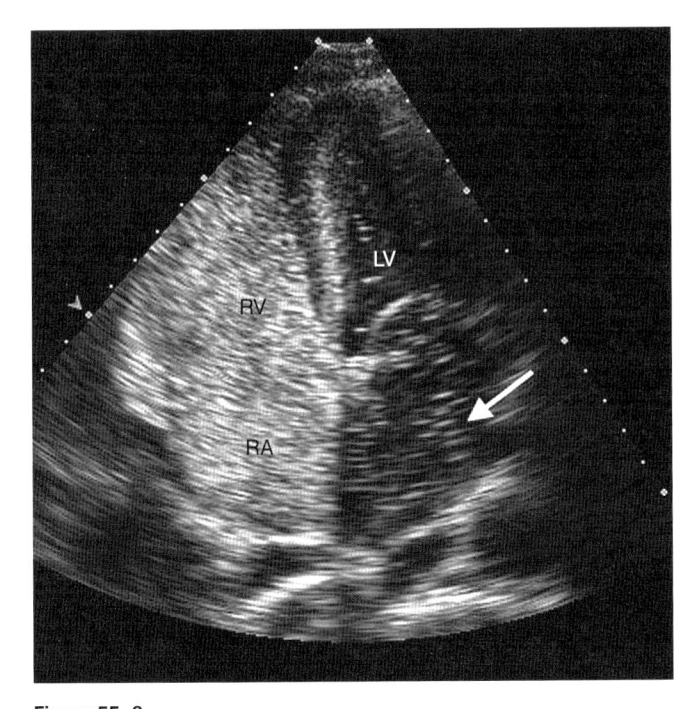

Figure 55–3
Opacification of the right atrium and right ventricle with intravenous agitated saline. An interatrial shunt is demonstrated by right-to-left shunting across the intra-atrial septum with bubbles (arrow) identified in the left atrium and left ventricle within three cardiac cycles.

for 3D image acquisition and processing decrease utility of 3D imaging for routine imaging.[13] The greatest utility for 3D echocardiography is in imaging of the interatrial septum and mitral valve for guidance on anatomy and amenability for reparative intervention.

DOPPLER ECHOCARDIOGRAPHY

Doppler echocardiography uses the principle that reflected sound from a moving object returns with a different frequency than transmitted frequencies. This frequency "shift" allows evaluation of flow direction and velocity (higher velocities create larger Doppler shifts).[1,2] With pulsed wave Doppler, the transducer alternates between sending and receiving signals, sampling blood velocities at a specified depth along the ultrasound beam. There is a limited measurable maximum velocity with pulsed wave Doppler, the Nyquist limit, beyond which the signal aliases and peak velocity cannot be accurately measured. With continuous wave Doppler, the transducer continuously transmits and receives signals along the entire length of the ultrasound beam. Although the specific depth origin of the continuous wave Doppler velocity cannot be localized, signal aliasing does not occur, and higher blood velocities, such as in stenotic valves, can be measured.

Pulsed wave and continuous wave Doppler velocity data are displayed as a graph of velocity versus time, with signal strength displayed by a decibel gray scale. By convention, frequency shifts toward the transducer are shown above the baseline. The velocity-time integral is the integral of blood flow velocity over time, measured in distance. The shape, timing, and density of spectral Doppler images provide valuable qualitative evaluation of blood flow, and increased jet density suggests increased flow volume. Rapid equalization of pressure gradients between two cardiac chambers leads to steeper jet slopes (Fig. 55-5). Color flow Doppler is a form of pulsed wave Doppler whereby velocities are sampled along multiple scan lines in a sector, color coded, and then superimposed on a two-dimensional image. By convention, flow away from the transducer is blue, and flow toward the transducer is red.

Combined with qualitative measures, Doppler echocardiography allows quantitation of valve stenosis and regurgitation severity, cardiac stroke volume, ventricular systolic and diastolic function, and intracardiac pressure. Three basic Doppler principles are used in clinical practice: (1) flow quantitation (stroke volume calculation), (2) continuity of flow (continuity equation), and (3) pressure-velocity (Bernoulli's equation).

Stroke volume (SV) traversing a cardiac orifice is the product of the cross-sectional area (CSA) at that point and the velocity-time integral (VTI_{FLOW}).

$$SV = CSA \times VTI_{FLOW}$$

Cross-sectional area, assuming a circular orifice, is calculated by measuring the diameter at the point of interest (area = πr^2). The velocity-time integral is obtained from spectral Doppler interrogation. The principle of continuity of flow describes the concept that the stroke volume passing just proximal to an orifice (SV_{pre}) is the same as the stroke volume passing through the orifice ($SV_{orifice}$). The most common application of the continuity equation is in aortic valve area measurement for stenosis, in which the stroke volume (SV_{pre}) is measured at the left ventricular outflow tract.

When a blood flow stream narrows (i.e., in traversing a valvular orifice), flow velocity (V) increases in proportion to the degree of narrowing. Increases in velocity are correlated with increased pressure gradients across an orifice. This relationship is described by the Bernoulli equation (pressure-velocity

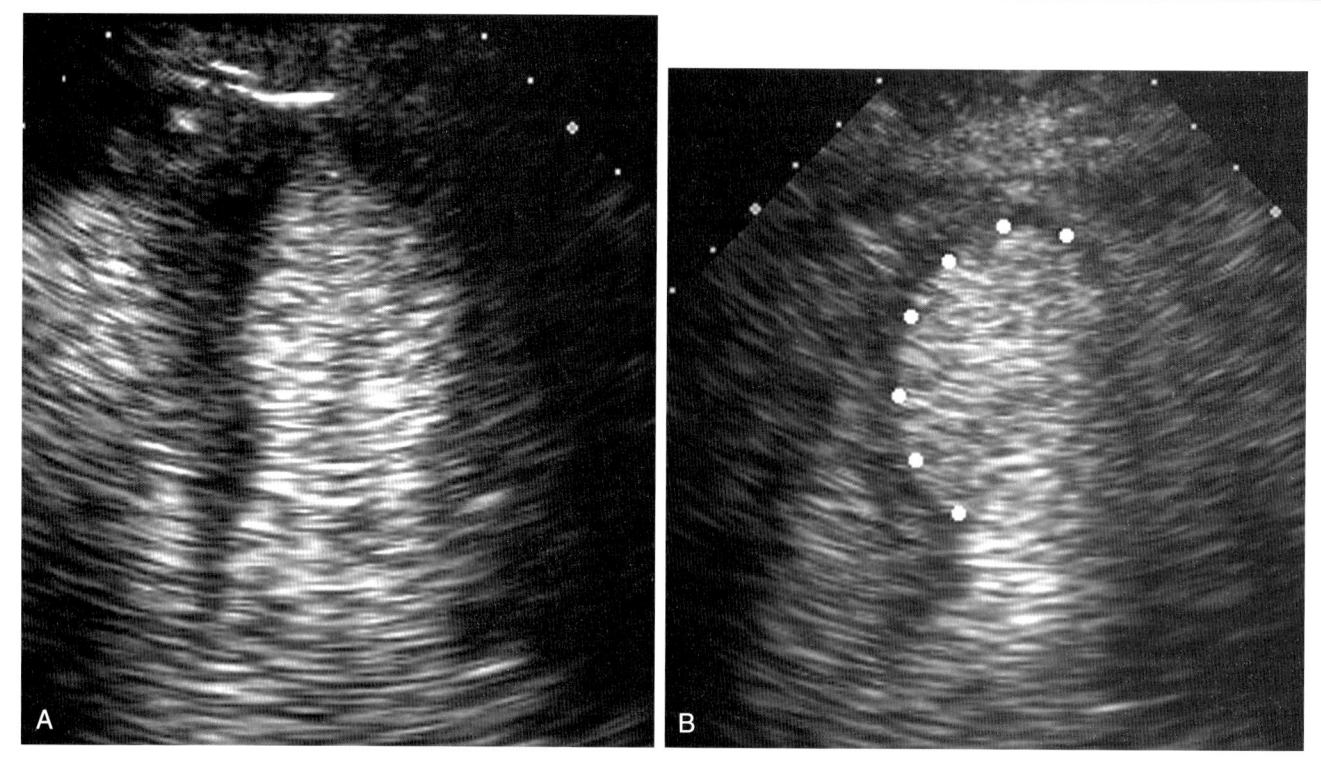

Figure 55-4
Abnormal stress echocardiogram with images of the apical four-chamber view taken at rest **(A)** and after administration of dobutamine **(B)**. Intravenous administration of a transpulmonary microbubble contrast agent is used to opacify the left ventricular chamber. After administration of dobutamine, a wall motion abnormality is evidenced by hypokinesis with thinning and contour change in the apex and distal septum of the left ventricle (*dots,* **B**).

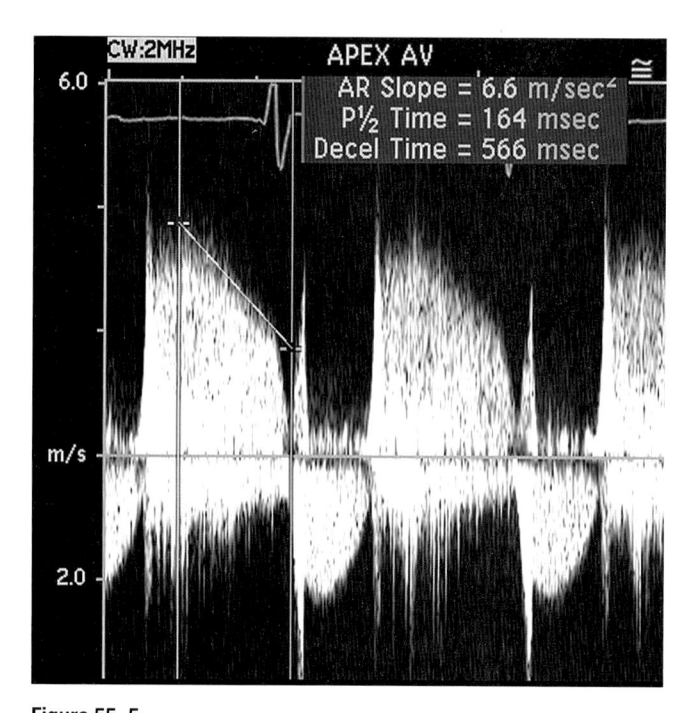

Figure 55-5
Spectral Doppler tracing of a patient with severe aortic regurgitation. In this patient, the density of regurgitant flow (toward the transducer, shown above the baseline) is nearly equal to anterograde flow (from the transducer, shown below the baseline). There is a relatively steep aortic regurgitant Doppler slope, 6.6 m/sec^2, which suggests rapid equalization of pressures between the aorta and left ventricle.

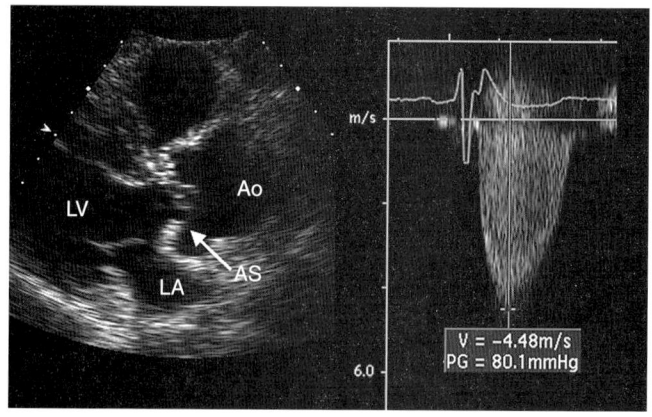

Figure 55-6
Severe aortic stenosis (AS), evidenced by thickened, calcified aortic valve leaflets seen on the parasternal long-axis view. On continuous Doppler imaging across the aortic valve, the peak velocity (V) is 4.5 m/sec, corresponding to a peak gradient (PG) of 80 mm Hg by the simplified Bernoulli equation.

relationship). Ignoring the effects of viscous loss and local red blood cell acceleration, the relationship is simplified to

$$\Delta P = 4V^2$$

Estimation of transvalvular pressure gradients is a common application of the simplified Bernoulli equation (Fig. 55-6).

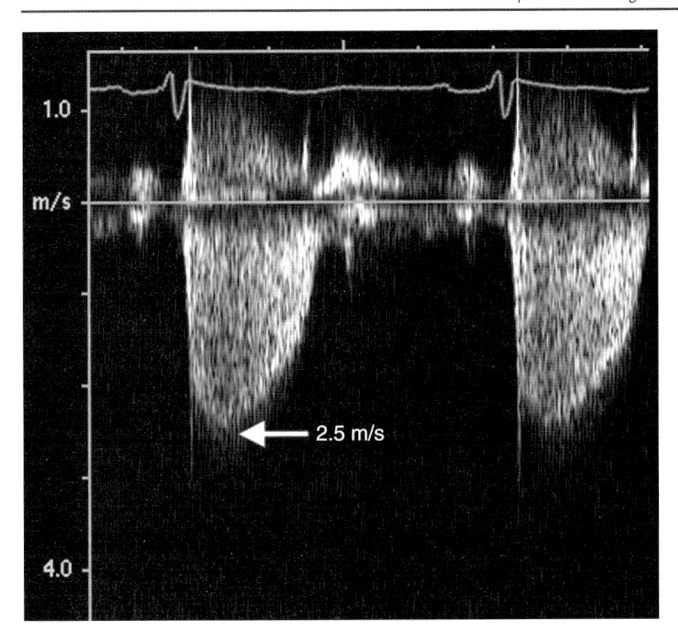

Figure 55–7
The peak pressure gradient is calculated with the peak velocity from the continuous Doppler tracings of the tricuspid regurgitant jet by use of the simplified Bernoulli equation. Peak velocity is 2.5 m/sec, which corresponds to a peak pressure gradient (right ventricular systolic pressure) of 25 mm Hg. The pulmonary arterial systolic pressure is obtained by adding the estimated right atrial pressure (see Fig. 55-1) to the peak gradient.

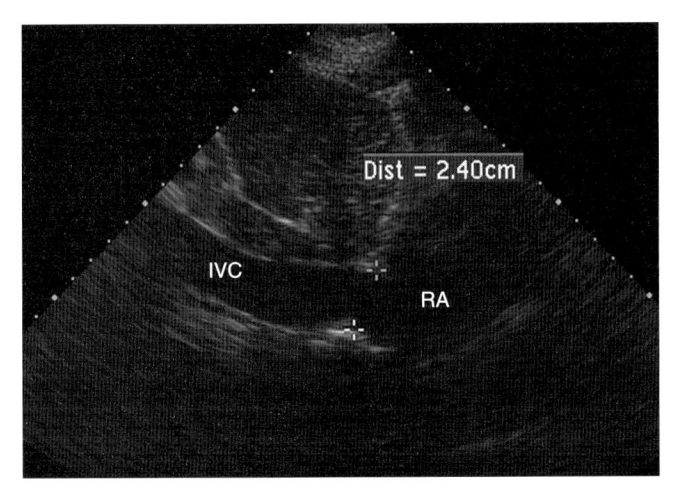

Table 55–1
Right Atrial Pressure Estimation

Inferior Vena Cava Diameter	Change in Diameter with Inspiration	Right Atrial Pressure Estimation
Less than 1.5 cm	Collapse	0-5 mm Hg
Between 1.5 and 2.5 cm	Decrease in diameter > 50%	5-10 mm Hg
Between 1.5 and 2.5 cm	Decrease in diameter < 50%	10-15 mm Hg
More than 2.5 cm	Decrease in diameter < 50%	15-20 mm Hg
More than 2.5 cm	No change	>20 mm Hg

Figure 55–8
Inferior vena cava (IVC) diameter at rest in a patient with mildly increased right atrial pressures.

Another common application is estimation of pulmonary arterial pressures. The pressure gradient between the right ventricle and right atrium is calculated with the systolic velocity from the tricuspid regurgitant jet (Fig. 55-7). In the absence of pulmonary stenosis, pulmonary arterial systolic pressure is equal to the sum of right ventricular systolic pressure and right atrial pressure. Right atrial pressure is obtained by examining inferior vena cava diameter at rest and with inspiration, measured at 2 cm from the junction to the right atrium (Fig. 55-8 and Table 55-1). Measurement of pulmonary arterial systolic pressure is widely applicable as 90% of individuals have some degree of tricuspid regurgitation. Another application of the pressure-velocity relationship is calculation of the change in intraventricular pressure over time (a measure of systolic function).

Echocardiography is the method of choice for the noninvasive evaluation of valvular regurgitation.[14,15] Color Doppler mapping is helpful for visualization of the jet origin and direction. Measurement of the narrowest jet width on color Doppler imaging (vena contracta) at or just distal to the regurgitant orifice is a simple measure that correlates with regurgitation severity and is less affected by eccentric regurgitant jets (Fig. 55-9). Accuracy in measuring the vena contracta is crucial as small errors lead to inaccurate assessment of regurgitation severity. Another qualitative marker of regurgitation severity is flow reversal of the Doppler signal in adjacent upstream vascular structures, seen when regurgitation severity is moderate or greater. Quantitative measures of regurgitant severity are recommended for clinical decision making and are discussed in the later section on valve disease. Recommended quantitative approaches include the proximal isovelocity surface area approach[16] and comparison of volume flow rate across the regurgitant valve with that of a normal valve.[15]

VENTRICULAR FUNCTION

Systolic Function

Two-dimensional echocardiographic imaging allows assessment of global and regional left ventricular systolic function. Diameter measurements of left ventricular chamber dimension at end-systole and at end-diastole by either two-dimensional or M-mode imaging are accurate and reproducible. Fractional shortening, the diastolic to systolic change in internal chamber dimension divided by the end-diastolic dimension, is a measure of systolic function, with a normal range of 25% to 45%. However, global systolic function is more precisely described by ejection fraction (EF), which uses end-diastolic volume (EDV) and end-systolic volume (ESV).[6] Volumes are calculated from endocardial border tracings in two orthogonal views by geometric formulas (Fig. 55-10). The most commonly applied algorithm is the biplane apical summation of discs method. Accuracy in ejection fraction measurement depends on adequate endocardial definition. Because the left

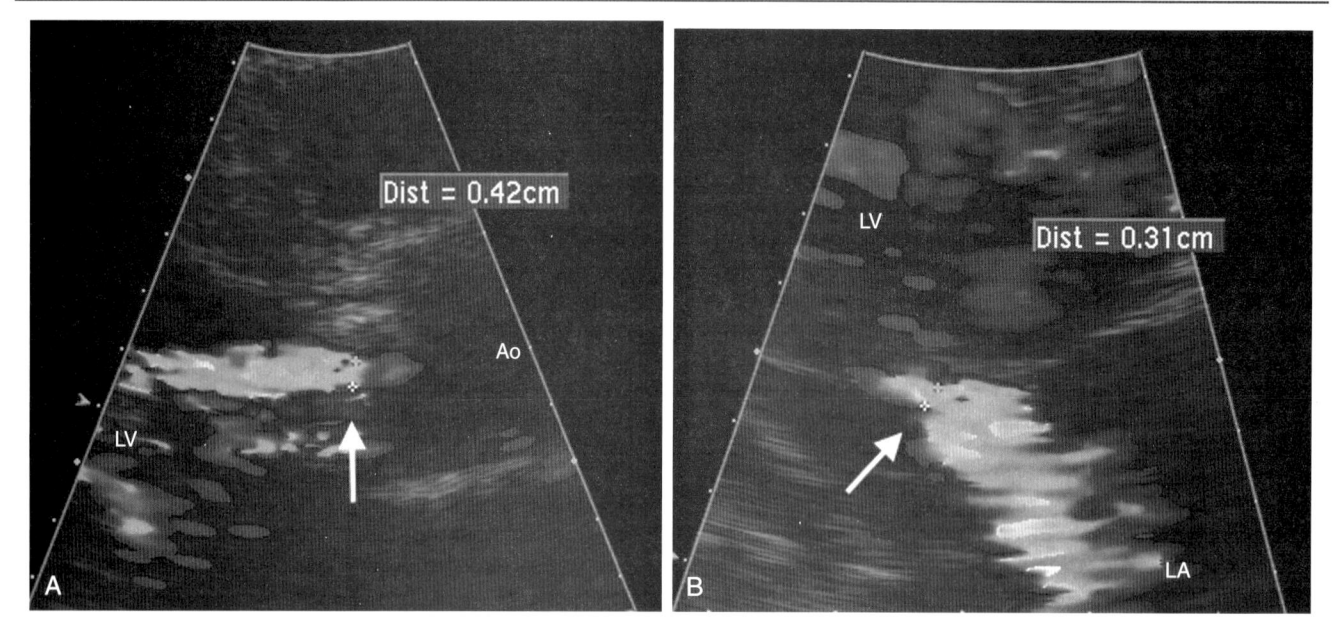

Figure 55–9
Vena contracta (arrow), the narrowest portion of the jet just distal to the regurgitant orifice for aortic valve **(A)** and mitral valve **(B)** regurgitation.

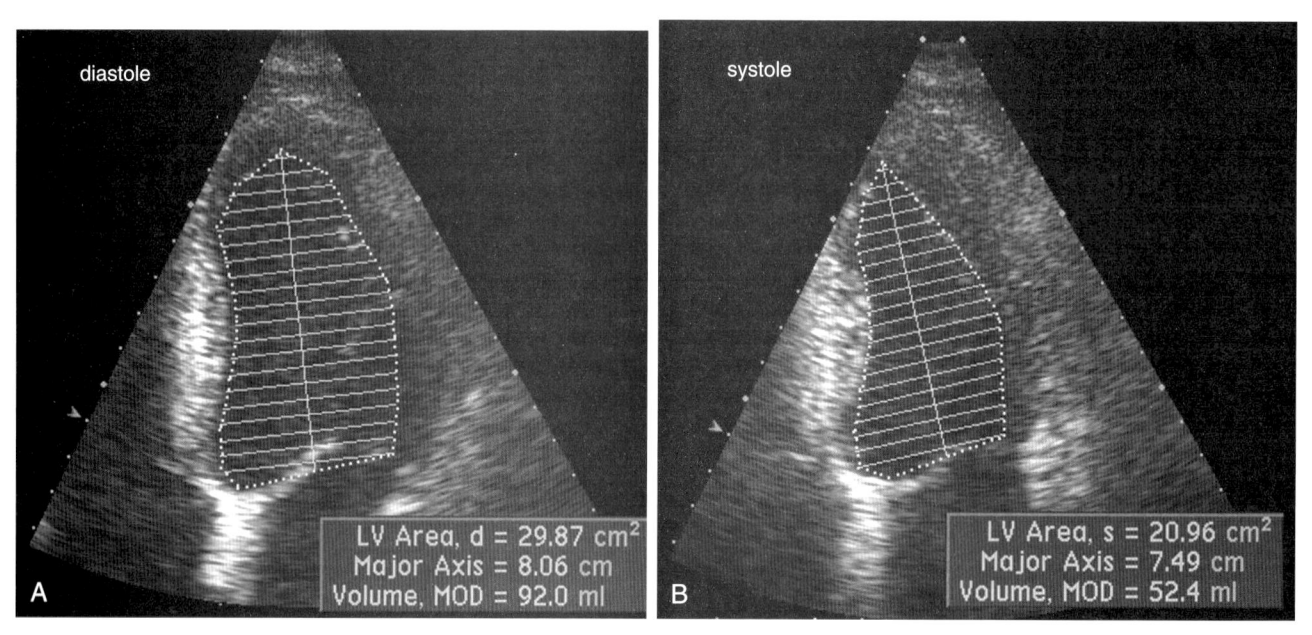

Figure 55–10
Endocardial border tracings of the left ventricle in the apical four-chamber view during diastole **(A)** and systole **(B)** are used to calculate left ventricular volumes. With use of the same left ventricular volume calculation for the apical two-chamber view, ejection fraction is calculated by the apical biplane method of discs algorithm.

ventricle is assumed to be bullet shaped and symmetrical, standard, nonoblique imaging planes are needed for optimal measurement.

$$EF = 100\% \times (EDV - ESV)/EDV$$

Echocardiographic ejection fraction measurement is comparable to other diagnostic modalities, such as nuclear imaging and angiography, and offers advantages of a rapid, reproducible, and noninvasive test. Calculation of ejection fraction is more challenging with segmental wall motion abnormalities and with arrhythmia, in which variability in cardiac cycle length affects beat-to-beat left ventricular volumes. Patients with conduction delay or who have previously undergone cardiac surgery may have dyssynchronous activation of the interventricular septum. When image quality precludes endocardial border tracing, qualitative assessment by an experienced reader is a reasonable alternative. Visual estimates of ejection fraction are usually reported in increment ranges of 5% or 10% (e.g., 50% to 55% or 20% to 30%).

A Doppler-derived measure of left ventricular systolic function uses the early systolic rate of velocity increase in the

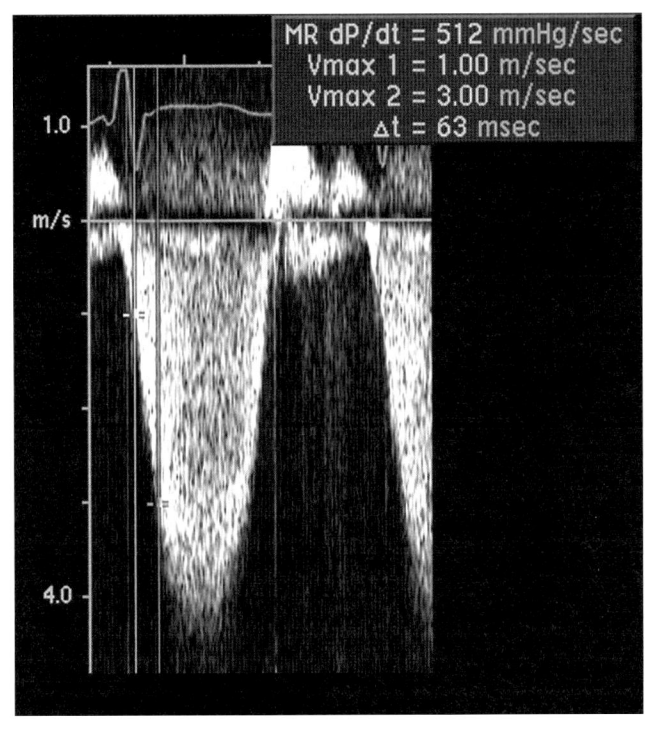

Figure 55-11
Continuous wave Doppler tracings of the mitral regurgitant jet showing a decreased rate of rise to the peak left ventricular cavity pressure during early systole in a patient with severely reduced left ventricular systolic dysfunction and ejection fraction of 25% (dP/dt). With normal systolic function, the change in rate of rise in pressure over time should be more than 1000 mm Hg/sec.

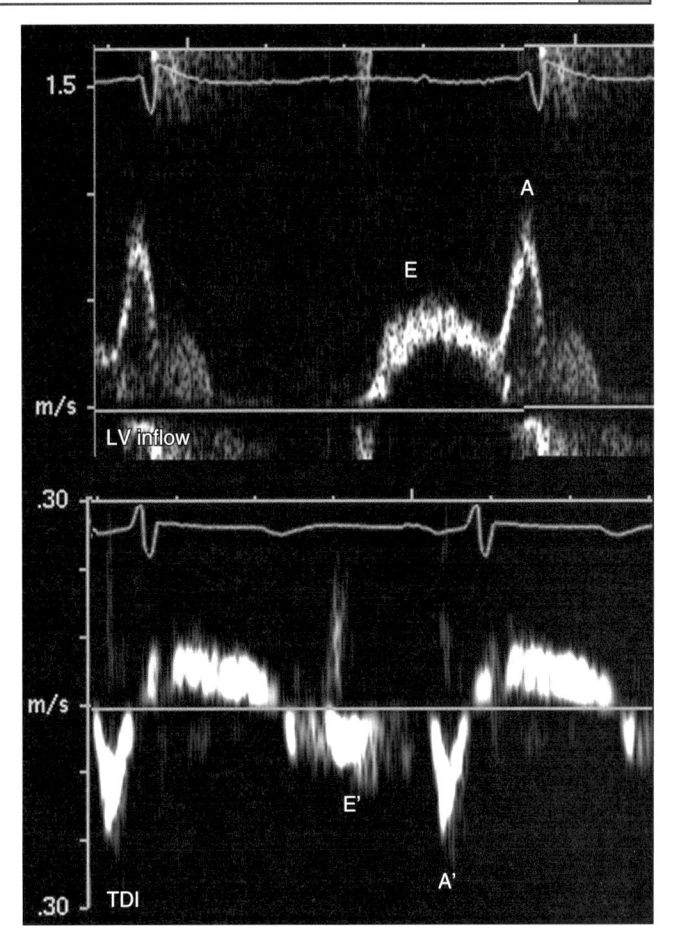

Figure 55-12
Doppler indices for mild diastolic dysfunction. With impaired ventricular relaxation, peak early mitral inflow velocity is decreased. There is increased reliance on atrial contribution to ventricular filling with reversal of the E:A ratio on the left ventricular (LV) inflow tracing. A ratio of LV inflow E wave to tissue Doppler velocity (TDI) E' wave (E:E' ratio) below 8 implies normal left atrial pressure. In this case, E:E' = 0.6/0.01 = 6.

mitral regurgitant jet, a relatively load independent measure of contractility (Fig. 55-11). The transmitral pressure gradient is measured at two points on the velocity curve. The slope of the mitral regurgitant jet between these two points represents the rate of change in left ventricular pressure over time (dP/dt). A normal dP/dt is more than 1000 mm Hg/sec; a lower dP/dt slope is concordant with a delay in left ventricular systolic pressure generation and depressed left ventricular function.

Right ventricular function is usually reported qualitatively, on a scale of normal to mildly, moderately, or severely depressed. Quantitative measures of right ventricular function are difficult because, as opposed to the left ventricle, geometric assumptions of symmetry are not valid. The right ventricular free wall "wraps" around the left ventricle, forming a crescent-shaped chamber. Multiple views of the right ventricle are often needed to provide a reasonable assessment of global systolic function.

Diastolic Function

Diastole comprises four phases: (1) isovolumic relaxation; (2) atrioventricular valve opening with passive early rapid ventricular filling; (3) diastasis, or deceleration of passive left ventricular filling due to equalization of atrial and ventricular pressures; and (4) late active ventricular filling due to atrial contraction. Several echocardiographic parameters are used to evaluate diastolic function.[17,18] Increased left atrial chamber size is a surrogate measure of increased left atrial (and left ventricular end-diastolic) pressures. Pulsed wave Doppler diastolic indices include evaluation of left ventricular inflow velocities with early E wave filling and the atrial contribution to filling (A wave). The time for the E wave deceleration and isovolumic relaxation time are measures of ventricular relaxation.

In normal, young individuals, early filling is the dominant component to ventricular filling, with atrial contraction contributing less than 20% to total filling volume. The E wave is dominant, with an E:A ratio above 1.0. With aging, ventricular stiffness increases with delay of myocardial relaxation and increased relative contribution of atrial contraction (impaired relaxation; Fig. 55-12). This is manifested as reversal of the E and A velocities and an E:A ratio of less than 1. In advanced diastolic dysfunction, decreased ventricular compliance leads to rapid equalization of the transmitral diastolic pressure gradient. With increased left ventricular end-diastolic pressure, the atrial contribution to ventricular filling is relatively small. This is manifested as a reversal of the transmitral filling pattern with an E:A ratio above 2, a steep deceleration slope, and a shortened isovolumic relaxation time (Fig. 55-13). Although patients in transition from an impaired relaxation pattern to a restrictive pattern have decreased ventricular compliance, the E:A ratio may appear normal, making interpretation of diastolic

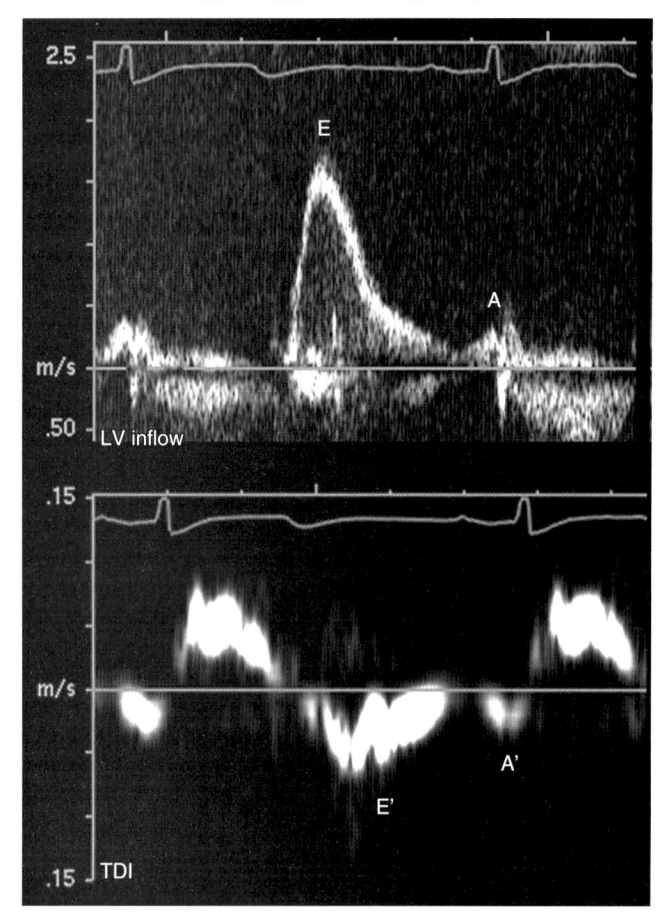

Figure 55-13
With advanced diastolic dysfunction (restrictive filling), there is decreased ventricular compliance. Higher left atrial pressures drive transmitral filling with a higher, early peaked E wave and E:A ratio above 2. The E:E' ratio is above 12 with prolongation and higher peak velocities of the pulmonary venous A wave. A ratio of left ventricular (LV) inflow E wave to tissue Doppler velocity (TDI) E' wave (E:E' ratio) above 15 implies elevated left atrial pressure. In this case, E:E' = 1.7/0.07 = 24.

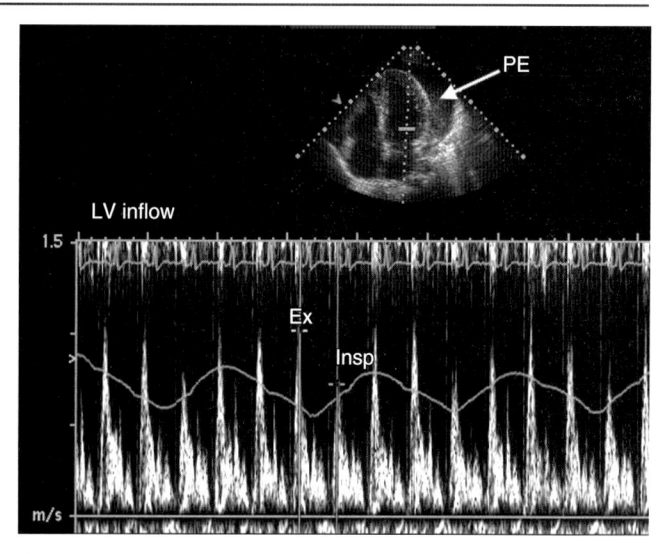

Figure 55-14
Pericardial effusion (PE) in a patient with dyspnea. The transmitral pulsed Doppler tracing demonstrates respiratory variation in flow. Ex, expiration; Insp, inspiration.

indices difficult. Loading conditions (heart rate, volume overload, mitral regurgitation) affect left atrial pressure and transmitral gradients. Mitral inflow evaluation repeated during a Valsalva maneuver (transient preload decrease) may unmask diastolic dysfunction, aiding in diagnosis.

Tissue Doppler interrogation at the septum and lateral wall just below the mitral anulus allows evaluation of myocardial diastolic motion. Myocardial early (E') and atrial (A') waves correspond to mitral E and A waves but are less sensitive to atrial loading conditions than mitral inflow (see Figs. 55-12 and 55-13). The ratio of transmitral E to myocardial E' is a surrogate measure of left ventricular filling pressure. An E:E' ratio below 8 suggests normal left atrial pressure, and a ratio above 15 suggests increased left atrial pressure. A ratio between 8 and 15 is indeterminate, and other indices should be used for diastolic assessment.

Abnormalities in diastolic indices can also be seen with extracardiac constraint of ventricular filling, such as in constrictive pericarditis or tamponade. Normal right ventricular filling demonstrates mild respiratory variation in transtricuspid velocities. On inspiration, there is an increase in systemic venous return and a transient increase in velocities, with normal magnitude increase less than 20%. Because left atrial filling is not respiratory dependent, transmitral velocities do not normally vary with respiration. With pericardial tamponade and chronic pulmonary disease, exaggerated inspiratory-expiratory respiratory variation in the transtricuspid and transmitral velocities can be seen (Fig. 55-14).

ISCHEMIC HEART DISEASE

Direct visualization of coronary anatomy beyond the coronary ostia is rarely possible with echocardiography. However, echocardiography allows real-time visualization of the effects of coronary perfusion on endocardial motion and wall thickening. With impaired coronary blood flow, segmental wall motion abnormalities are seen in the affected myocardial region. Myocardial responses to ischemia include *hypokinesis*, myocardial thickening with relatively less inward motion than the rest of the myocardium; *akinesis*, absence of thickening or inward motion; and *dyskinesis*, thinned and infarcted myocardium with paradoxical outward systolic motion.

Myocardial response to ischemia is proportionate to the severity of ischemia, with hypokinesis progressing to akinesis in more severe cases. Although acutely infarcted myocardium appears hypokinetic, wall thickness may be normal as postinfarction remodeling has not yet occurred. In patients with an acute ST elevation infarction, myocardial segments subject to prolonged ischemia are likely to remain hypocontractile long term, whereas segments subject to only a short duration of coronary flow limitation may eventually return to a normal contractile state. Postinfarction myocardial dysfunction that subsequently returns to normal is termed stunned myocardium. Irreversibly infarcted regions usually appear thinned and akinetic with persistent akinetic or dyskinetic wall motion on long-term evaluation.

Echocardiography is useful in detection of coronary disease in patients with chest pain symptoms. In patients with active chest discomfort, the absence of regional wall motion abnormalities on a resting study is an effective means of ruling out acute ischemia (negative predictive accuracy ~95%).[5] In the operating room, intraoperative TEE allows continuous monitoring of cardiac function and has been used during coronary revascularization, during valvular surgery, and in noncardiac surgery to monitor patients at high risk of cardiac events. TEE has also proved useful for the evaluation of cardiac function in the hemodynamically unstable patient when ischemia is suspected but transthoracic windows are suboptimal.

Takotsubo cardiomyopathy, or transient apical ballooning syndrome, is a newly recognized acute, ischemic cardiac syndrome. Clinical presentation is acute chest pain or dyspnea that follows a significant emotional or physiologic stress. The clinical manifestation is transient akinesis of the apical and mid left ventricular segments with regional wall motion abnormalities that extend beyond a single epicardial coronary arterial distribution. This condition is rare, with a strong predominance of women (>90%). Angiography demonstrates absence of obstructive coronary disease or acute plaque rupture. Outcome is generally good, and ventricular functional recovery is likely with supportive care.[19,20]

Stress Testing for Coronary Disease

Stress echocardiography is useful for initial diagnosis of coronary disease, monitoring of disease progression in patients with known coronary lesions, and evaluation of the functional significance of residual lesions after revascularization. Stress echocardiography provides direct, real-time visualization of myocardial function, allowing diagnosis of induced myocardial ischemia in a controlled setting.[21,22] Accuracy for stress echocardiography to determine the extent and location of myocardial ischemia is excellent, and it is particularly useful when baseline electrocardiographic abnormalities render standard exercise electrocardiography testing nondiagnostic. The addition of echocardiographic images at rest and at peak stress increases both sensitivity and specificity over standard exercise electrocardiography. Various exercise (treadmill or bicycle ergometer) and nonexercise (pharmacologic—dobutamine) cardiac stressors are used. Images are acquired at rest and at peak stress. For treadmill protocols, images are acquired immediately after stress because of imaging difficulties while the patient is upright on the treadmill. Resting and stress imaging data are then integrated with electrocardiographic data, exercise tolerance, and the patient's symptoms for final interpretation. With use of standard views of the left ventricle, side-by-side comparison of the rest and stress digital images identifies new wall motion abnormalities (see Fig. 55-4). Ischemia diagnosis is dependent on accurate evaluation of segmental wall motion and visualization of interval change from the rest images. As a consequence, diagnosis of ischemia is often more difficult in patients with preexisting coronary artery disease and resting abnormalities. When endocardial definition is suboptimal, intravenous contrast agents can be used to opacify the left ventricular cavity and to aid in endocardial border definition. Results of stress echocardiography testing offer long-term prognostic information.[23-25]

In the absence of a significant coronary narrowing, the myocardial response to stress is augmentation of systolic function with *hyperdynamic* motion. Flow-limiting coronary lesions are associated with systolic dysfunction in the myocardial region distal to the lesion. In noninfarcted myocardium, systolic function is preserved if coronary blood flow is adequate to meet oxygen demand at rest. The ischemic effect on ventricular wall motion and thickening is proportional to the severity of impaired coronary blood flow. For intermediate-range lesions (50% to 60% stenosed) or single-vessel disease in which only a few myocardial segments are affected, ischemic abnormalities may be subtle or transient. With cessation of the stressor and restoration of adequate coronary flow, wall motion returns to normal. A submaximal test result or prolonged delay in obtaining stress images after exercise lowers test sensitivity, because provocation of ischemia is dependent on reaching an adequate workload, and detection of ischemia requires that the abnormality persist long enough for image recording.

Exercise stress echocardiography is usually performed following a standard symptom-limited protocol to achieve as high a workload as possible. Pharmacologic stressors such as dobutamine are alternatives to exercise when testing cannot be performed because of physical limitation or when exercise response may be limited, such as in post–cardiac transplantation patients, with denervated hearts, to monitor for transplant vasculopathy. Dobutamine is typically initiated at 10 μg/kg/min and is incrementally increased at 3-minute intervals to a maximum of 40 μg/kg/min. If target heart rate (85% of the patient's maximum predicted heart rate) is not achieved, atropine can be additionally administered.

Complications of Acute Myocardial Infarction

Echocardiography is the diagnostic tool of choice to evaluate for complications of myocardial infarction. Two-dimensional imaging allows assessment of myocardial dysfunction and regional wall motion abnormalities. For patients with congestive heart failure, assessment of residual left ventricular systolic function and estimation of pulmonary pressures can be performed. Mitral regurgitation is a common complication of ischemic disease. In patients with regional wall motion abnormalities and left ventricular chamber enlargement, significant mitral regurgitation can result from distortion of the mitral subvalvular apparatus. Mitral regurgitation can also occur as a direct result of papillary muscle ischemia, rupture of a necrotic papillary muscle head, and infarct scarring with tethering of the subvalvular apparatus.

Myocardial necrosis with ventricular rupture can be identified both in the free wall and in the interventricular septum by a combination of two-dimensional and Doppler techniques. A ventricular septal defect is identified by characteristic color flow and continuous wave Doppler flow across the defect. A ventricular free wall rupture that is contained is termed a pseudoaneurysm (Fig. 55-15). Pseudoaneurysms often have an abrupt transition from normal myocardial tissue to the aneurysmal dilation and thrombus within the pseudoaneurysm. Myocardial infarction with ventricular wall thinning can also lead to focal dilation and true aneurysm formation. Like pseudoaneurysms, thrombi can form within ventricular aneurysms and pose a risk of distal embolization.

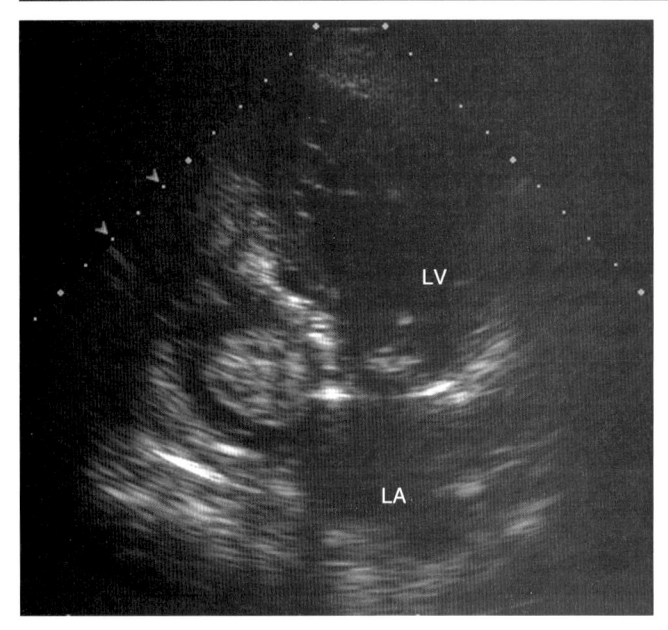

Figure 55-15
Pseudoaneurysm in a patient with a prior ST elevation inferior myocardial infarction. The inferior wall of the left ventricle appears thinned and bright. There is a rupture of the base of the heart with a large pseudoaneurysm adjacent to the left ventricle. Within the pseudoaneurysm is a large spherical thrombus.

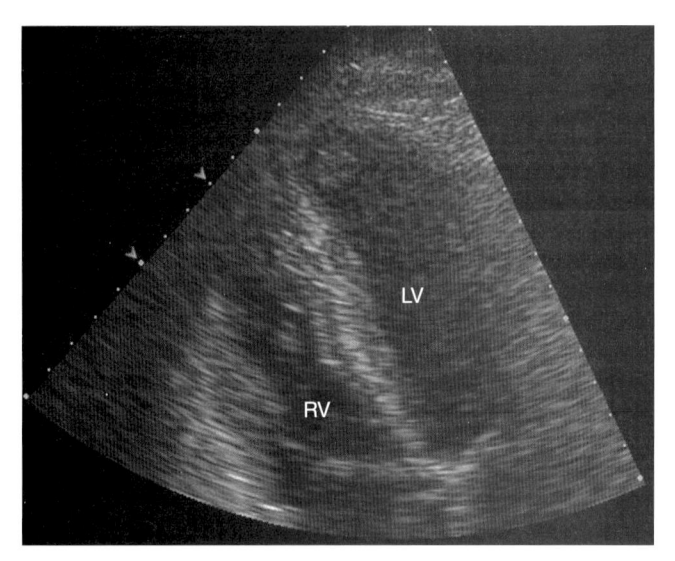

Figure 55-16
Small apical thrombus in the left ventricle of a patient with a recent anteroapical myocardial infarction.

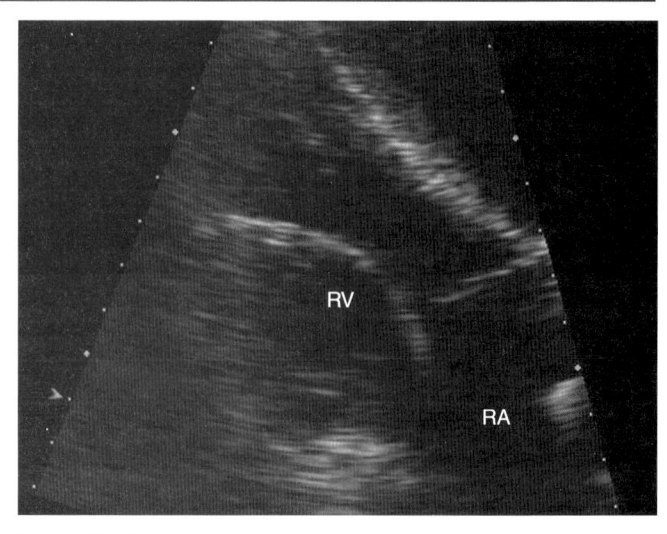

Figure 55-17
Right ventricular pacer lead seen crossing the tricuspid valve into the right ventricle.

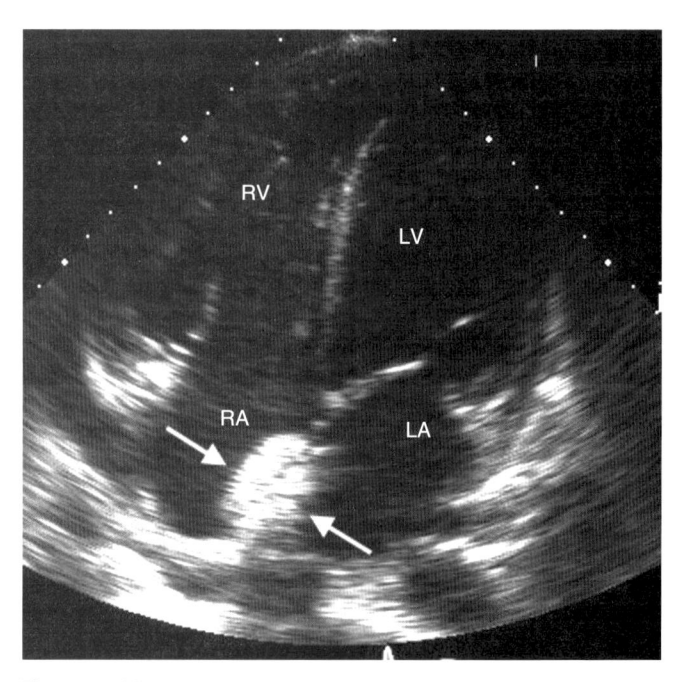

Figure 55-18
Atrial septal defect closure device that was placed percutaneously. The prosthetic material appears bright and echogenic and spans the interatrial septum (arrows).

Mural thrombi occur primarily in anterior and apical infarctions and are less frequent with early revascularization (Fig. 55-16). Right ventricular infarction is most often associated with inferior myocardial infarctions and is diagnosed on echocardiography by evaluation of right ventricular size and systolic function. A cause of hypoxemia after inferior myocardial infarction is increased right-sided pressures with resulting right-to-left shunting across a patent foramen ovale. This can be diagnosed by TEE evaluation of the intra-atrial septum with a contrast study using agitated saline. A similar phenomenon has been described in postoperative hypoxemic patients with increased right atrial pressure.[26]

CARDIAC MASSES

Image resolution of echocardiography is excellent, with cardiac masses as small as 1 to 2 mm in diameter visualized. If there is concern for a cardiac mass, it is important to correlate any findings with the clinical history to correctly identify expected material such as pacing wires, central venous catheters, prosthetic valves, and intracardiac devices (Figs. 55-17 to 55-19). In addition, possible cardiac masses seen on echocardiography should be scrutinized carefully to exclude ultrasound artifact and normal structural variants. Commonly encountered cardiac masses include normal structures, tumors,

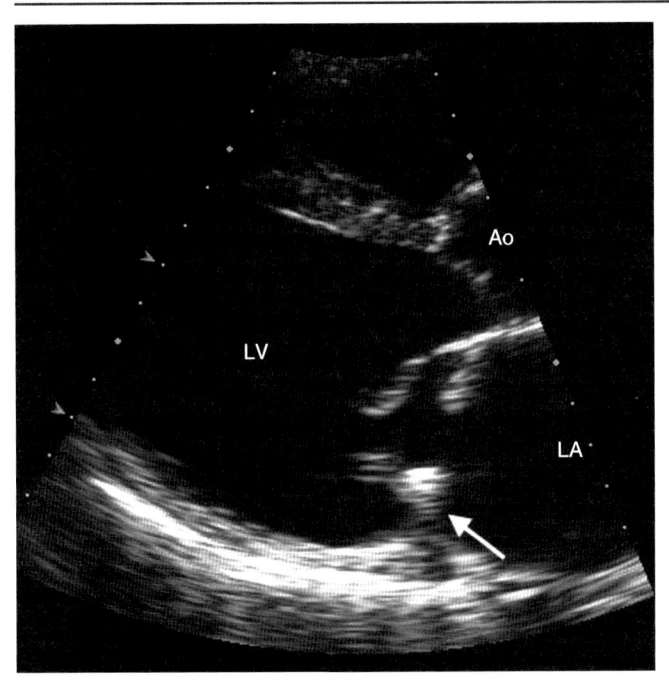

Figure 55-19
Ischemic heart disease with thinning and scarring of the posterior wall. There is a cross section of a prosthetic mitral anuloplasty ring seen adjacent to the mitral valve leaflets (arrow).

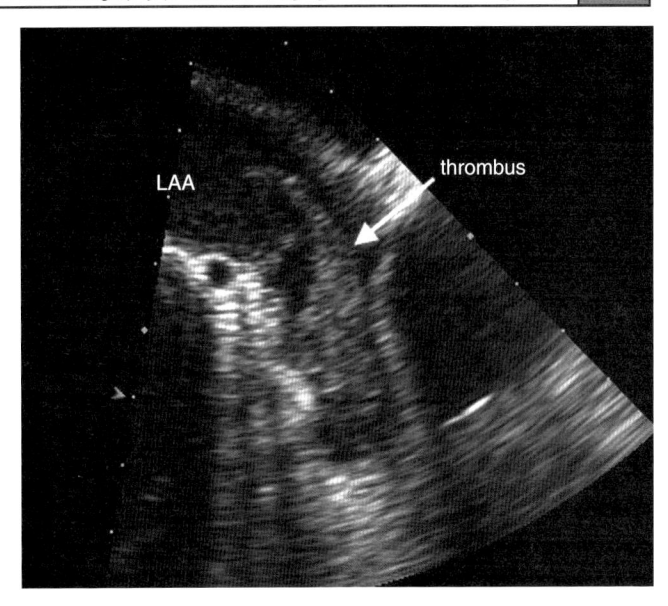

Figure 55-20
Imaged by TEE, an atrial thrombus is seen in the left atrial appendage (arrow) in a patient with atrial fibrillation undergoing evaluation for elective cardioversion. Low-velocity blood flow is evidenced by the spontaneous echo contrast seen at the ostia of the left atrial appendage (LAA).

thrombi, and vegetations. These categories are not mutually exclusive (i.e., a lesion may consist of coexistent vegetations and thrombi).

Thrombi tend to occur in intracardiac regions of blood stasis and decreased flow. In the left ventricle, these regions are usually at the sites of prior infarcts that are aneurysmal and hypokinetic, most commonly at the left ventricular apex. The sensitivity and specificity of TTE echocardiography for left ventricular apical thrombi are approximately 95% and 88%, respectively. For transesophageal imaging, transducer placement is obligatorily constrained by esophageal anatomy, and the true apex is often not in view, decreasing diagnostic accuracy for apical thrombi. In the left atrium, thrombi occur most often in the atrial appendage in patients in atrial fibrillation or flutter but can also occur in patients in sinus rhythm and with lower atrial blood velocities, such as with mitral stenosis. Findings suggestive of low-velocity blood flow, such as spontaneous echo contrast, are associated with thrombus formation. Because the anatomic position of the left atrial appendage is posterior, thrombi are more optimally seen with TEE imaging, in which the transducer images from behind the heart (Fig. 55-20). The sensitivity and specificity of TEE to detect left atrial thrombus are very high, nearing 100%, but care is needed to visualize the appendage in at least two image planes for a definitive diagnosis. The pulmonary artery is difficult to image beyond the bifurcation. Therefore, echocardiography is a poor diagnostic tool for pulmonary embolism.[27] Rarely, large pulmonary emboli can be imaged in the main pulmonary artery. Often, the only evidence of a large pulmonary embolism is right ventricular dysfunction.

In patients with a systemic embolic event, echocardiography identifies a potential cardiac source of the embolus in up to 30% of cases. Echocardiographic findings associated with increased risk of embolism include left-sided thrombi, valvular masses (endocarditis), and aortic atherosclerotic disease.

Although image quality to evaluate for these abnormalities is improved with transesophageal imaging, TEE is more invasive, and the risks of the procedure have to be weighed against the benefits of a more definitive diagnosis.[28] In addition, systemic embolism may occur if there is paradoxical embolism through an interatrial shunt, such as an atrial septal defect or patent foramen ovale (Fig. 55-21). A patent foramen ovale is not diagnostic for systemic embolism, as this is a common finding, present in approximately 20% of the general population. However, outcome studies in patients with cerebrovascular events do suggest an association between stroke and a patent foramen ovale. Clinical trials are currently under way to determine the benefit of patent foramen ovale closure. A patent foramen ovale may be seen by color Doppler imaging, but more definitive echocardiographic diagnosis is made with infusion of agitated saline (see Fig. 55-3). The interatrial shunt should be seen within three cardiac cycles after opacification of the right atrium. A Valsalva maneuver during injection of the contrast agent may be needed to transiently increase right atrial pressure. Saline contrast that appears later than five cardiac cycles may signify an intrapulmonary shunt.

Valvular vegetations are identified on echocardiography as independently mobile masses attached to the upstream side of cardiac valves (e.g., the ventricular side of the aortic valve or the left atrial side of the mitral valve). Vegetations are most often due to infective endocarditis. However, the differential also includes nonbacterial thrombotic endocarditis and benign masses such as papillary fibroelastomas. Other intracardiac attachment sites for vegetations are indwelling catheters or pacer leads and congenital abnormalities such as ventricular septal defects.

Most tumors in the heart are noncardiac in origin. The most common metastatic tumors to the heart are lung, breast, lymphoma, leukemia, stomach, and melanoma. Metastatic involvement includes direct invasion of the pericardium, distant

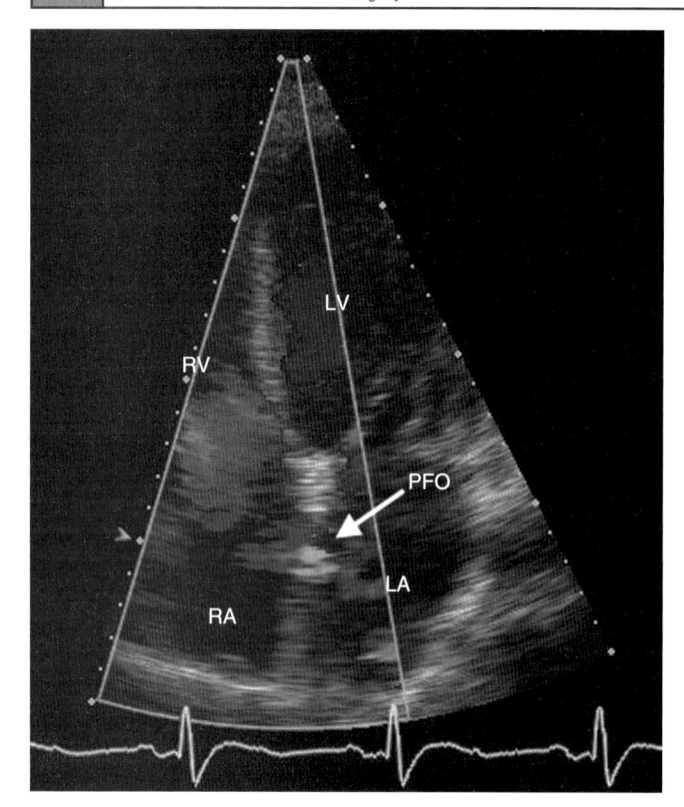

Figure 55-21
Color Doppler imaging shows left-to-right flow across the interatrial septum, consistent with a patent foramen ovale (PFO). (See color version in the online edition through ExpertConsult.)

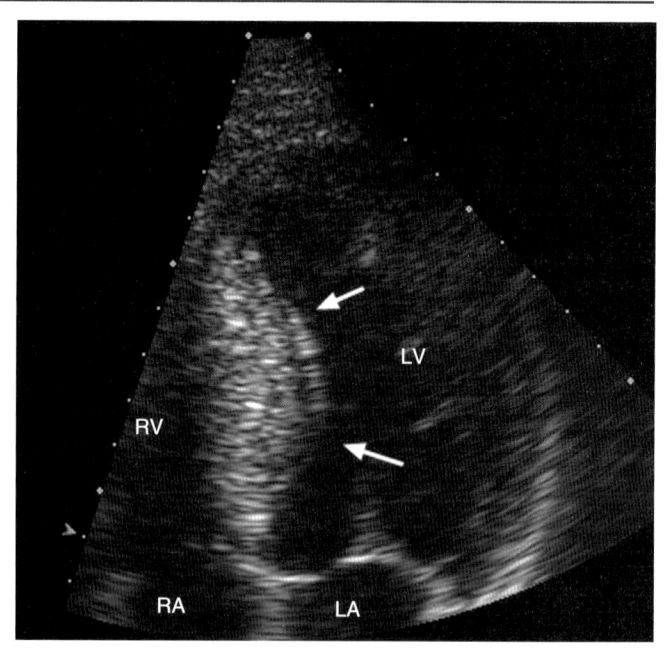

Figure 55-22
Prominent hypertrophy of the interventricular septum *(arrows)* in a patient with hypertrophic cardiomyopathy seen on the apical four-chamber view.

metastasis with pericardial or intramyocardial masses, and, in rare cases, endocardial masses. In the case of renal cell carcinoma, direct extension through the inferior vena cava into the right atrium may be seen. Primary cardiac tumors in the heart are rare, and the majority of these are benign. Atrial myxoma, the most common primary tumor, is often found incidentally during transthoracic imaging.

CARDIOMYOPATHIES

Congestive Heart Failure

Echocardiography is valuable for the assessment of left and right ventricular systolic and diastolic function, measurement of chamber size and wall thickness, visualization of valve anatomy and function, and clinical evaluation of hemodynamic status in patients with heart failure. In addition, echocardiography may identify a reversible cause of heart failure, such as valve stenosis or regurgitation. Congestive heart failure due to ischemic heart disease may be recognized on the basis of regional myocardial dysfunction. However, end-stage ischemic disease may result in global biventricular dysfunction, indistinguishable from a primary cardiomyopathy.

Nonischemic dilated cardiomyopathy is characterized by cardiac chamber enlargement and systolic dysfunction (see Fig. 55-1A). Systolic dysfunction is typically global in nature, but some heterogeneity in regional function may be observed. Ventricular dilation may tether the mitral subvalvular apparatus, resulting in significant mitral regurgitation. Systolic dysfunction and chronic volume overload can also lead to secondary pulmonary hypertension. Although systolic dysfunction is typically the dominant finding, diastolic dysfunction, with increased myocardial wall stress and intracardiac pressures, is also present. Diagnostic indices for dilated cardiomyopathy include systolic and diastolic function, valvular function, and pulmonary pressure estimates. Additional measurements of left ventricular mass, Doppler-derived dP/dt, and ejection fraction provide prognostic information.[29]

Hypertrophic and Restrictive Cardiomyopathy

Hypertrophic cardiomyopathy is characterized by abnormal myocardial thickening. The most common form of hypertrophic cardiomyopathy is asymmetrical thickening of the basal interventricular septum (Fig. 55-22). In advanced cases, septal thickening can cause obstruction of left ventricular outflow.[30] Severity of left ventricular outflow obstruction may be altered by different loading conditions, with decreased intracardiac volume transiently increasing the severity of obstruction (as seen with the Valsalva maneuver). Additional findings may include systolic motion of the anterior mitral valve leaflet and chordae into the left ventricular outflow tract. Faulty systolic coaptation of the mitral valve results in posteriorly directed regurgitation. In patients with significant outflow obstruction, pressure gradients in the left ventricular outflow tract can be measured. Other variants of hypertrophy include diffuse, concentric, and apical.

Echocardiography is diagnostic for hypertrophic cardiomyopathy. In patients with hypertrophic cardiomyopathy, echocardiography is used to monitor outflow tract gradients and to evaluate mitral regurgitation. This information assists in timing of surgical or percutaneous myomectomy intervention and is used in the cardiac catheterization laboratory to guide percutaneous septal ablation procedures. Intraoperative TEE imaging is used to guide surgical myomectomy and can aid in monitoring for procedural complications, such as ventricular septal defect.³¹ Because hypertrophic cardiomyopathy is associated with angina, arrhythmia, and sudden cardiac death, echocardiographic screening of family members of affected individuals is recommended.

Restrictive cardiomyopathy is uncommon and is typically caused by one of several infiltrative disease processes, such as sarcoidosis and amyloidosis. Diastolic function is impaired, with evidence of decreased left ventricular compliance and a restrictive mitral inflow filling pattern.³⁰ Systolic function is usually preserved in the earlier stages of the disease. Echocardiographic findings may include increased myocardial wall thickness, biatrial enlargement, and elevation in pulmonary arterial systolic pressures. However, these findings are not uniformly present, making restrictive cardiomyopathy difficult to diagnose definitively.

Cardiac Transplantation

Echocardiography is beneficial to reassess left ventricular function and to optimize intravascular volume status. In end-stage cardiac disease, echocardiography is used in decision making and clinical management for left ventricular assist devices or biventricular assist devices. For these devices, significant aortic regurgitation, severe mitral stenosis, or interatrial shunts may adversely affect optimal device performance. Evaluation can be made for functional issues, including peri-device hematoma, thrombus, and right ventricular function, but acoustic shadowing from the device makes a complete assessment difficult. Doppler interrogation of device cannulas allows assessment for partial occlusion or leakage. Echocardiographic imaging allows optimal placement of newer, percutaneously placed flow cannulas.

After cardiac transplantation, echocardiography is useful to monitor for biventricular function, pericardial effusion, and pulmonary hypertension and to assist in bioptome placement during cardiac biopsies. Cardiac organ rejection is evidenced by myocardial thickening and diastolic dysfunction in the initial stages, progressing eventually to systolic dysfunction.³² Normal echo findings after cardiac transplantation include biatrial enlargement from suturing of the residual native atria to the transplanted heart. The suture line may be discerned as a linear echodensity along the mid-atrial wall. Doppler tracings along the aortic and pulmonic connections allow assessment of anastomotic stenoses. For long-term follow-up after transplantation, dobutamine echocardiography has shown increased sensitivity over other stress testing modalities to screen for transplant vasculopathy.³³

PERICARDIAL AND CONSTRICTIVE HEART DISEASE

The pericardium is a thin, dense structure that forms an enclosed space around the heart. The pericardium is difficult to image because it is thin and often directly in contact with other mediastinal structures, but it may be seen if fluid that is echolucent is located adjacently. A small amount of pericardial fluid is a normal finding. Other pericardial findings by echocardiography include fibrinous stranding, tumors, and hematoma.

Large amounts of pericardial fluid are abnormal and can cause external cardiac compression, or tamponade. The size of a pericardial fluid collection alone does not dictate hemodynamic significance. When pericardial fluid accumulates slowly, more than a liter can be contained in the pericardial space at

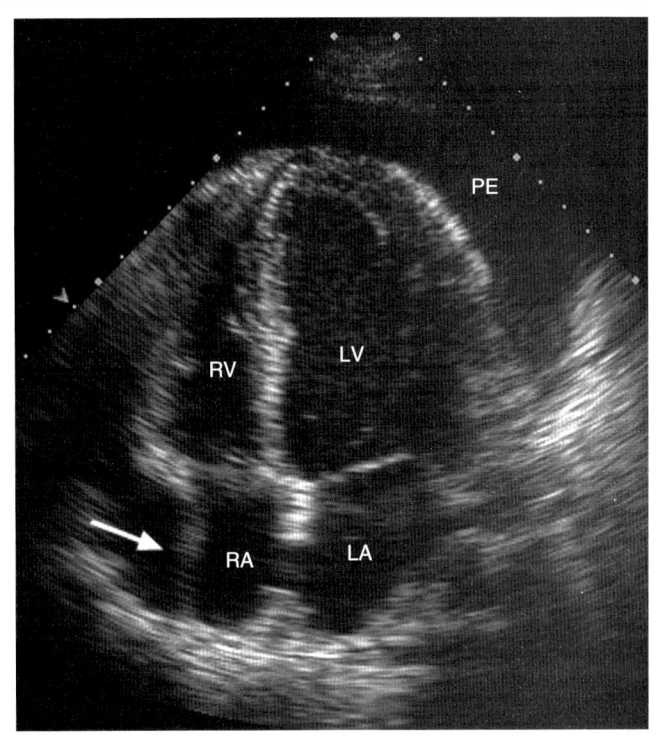

Figure 55–23
Circumferential pericardial effusion (PE). There is right atrial systolic collapse seen on the apical four-chamber view (arrow).

a low pressure with few overt clinical signs. However, if fluid accumulates rapidly, intrapericardial pressures may exceed intracardiac pressure with only a small fluid volume, leading to hemodynamic compromise or tamponade physiology. Echocardiographic findings in tamponade include systolic collapse of the right atrial free wall and diastolic collapse of the right ventricular free wall (atria, lower pressure chambers, are usually affected before ventricles) due to increased intrapericardial pressure³⁴ (Fig. 55-23). However, if there is right ventricular hypertrophy or pulmonary hypertension, higher intracardiac pressures may negate chamber collapse. Other echocardiographic findings include inferior vena cava dilation and exaggerated respiratory variation in flows (>25%) across the atrioventricular valves. However, in the patient with clinical signs of tamponade and a large pericardial effusion, absence of echocardiographic markers for tamponade does not exclude the diagnosis. Echocardiographic quantification and localization of pericardial fluid guide clinical decision making regarding approach and feasibility of surgical versus percutaneous pericardial drainage procedures.

Focal tamponade due to a loculated fluid collection may occur. After cardiothoracic surgery, focal hematomas posterior and adjacent to the right atrium may impede right atrial inflow. In these patients, suboptimal acoustic windows caused by limitations in positioning of the patient or surface bandages often limit image quality. Therefore, heightened suspicion, particularly in postoperative patients with hemodynamic instability, is recommended. If image quality is suboptimal, transesophageal imaging may be needed.

Pericarditis, an inflammatory condition involving the pericardium, classically presents with chest pain, diffuse ST elevation on electrocardiography, and auscultated rub. Concurrent pericardial effusion may or may not be present. Pericardial thickening can occur, but it may be difficult to image directly by echocardiography. With recurrent pericarditis, the pericardium can become thickened and adherent to the myocardium, causing impaired cardiac filling or "constriction." Other causes of constriction include radiation therapy, prior trauma, and prior cardiac surgery. Exaggerated septal motion during the cardiac cycle signifies equalization of diastolic pressures in the cardiac chambers. Biventricular size and systolic function are usually preserved. Supporting echocardiographic findings include increased central venous pressure (inferior vena cava dilation), prominent y descent on hepatic vein Doppler tracings, and restrictive filling pattern on transmitral Doppler interrogation with rapid early diastolic filling.

Differentiation between pericardial constriction and restrictive cardiomyopathy can be challenging.[35] Both conditions have increased central venous pressures, usually with preserved systolic function. For restrictive cardiomyopathy, biatrial enlargement and pulmonary hypertension tend to be more prominent findings. For pericardial constriction, marked respiratory variation in ventricular filling is more common, but it is not definitive. Often, supplementary diagnostic tests are needed to differentiate the diagnoses. These include chest tomography and magnetic resonance imaging, which allow measurement of pericardial wall thickness; simultaneous left- and right-sided pressure tracings with volume loading in the cardiac catheterization laboratory to aid in the diagnosis; and myocardial biopsy for detection of infiltrative myocardial disease.

VALVULAR HEART DISEASE

Echocardiography is invaluable for assessment of valvular anatomy and function.[36] Echocardiographic imaging has supplanted the need for invasive valvular diagnostics in the catheterization laboratory in most patients. Serial echocardiographic studies are used to monitor for onset of adverse hemodynamic effects of valve dysfunction on cardiac function and pulmonary pressures.

Aortic Stenosis

Echocardiography allows identification of the cause of aortic stenosis and assessment of valve hemodynamics. Patients with aortic stenosis of a trileaflet valve tend to present later (sixth or seventh decade of life) than do patients with aortic stenosis of a bicuspid valve (fourth or fifth decade of life). In patients with severe stenosis, leaflet calcification may hinder definitive identification of the number of leaflets. Another less common cause of aortic stenosis is rheumatic valve disease, with echocardiographic findings of commissural fusion and concurrent mitral valve involvement.

Aortic stenosis severity is evaluated by peak instantaneous transaortic velocities acquired from continuous Doppler ultrasound tracings. Several acoustic windows should be used to ensure that the maximal velocity is recorded (see Fig. 55-6). A velocity of more than 4 m/sec indicates severe stenosis, and a velocity of 2.5 to 3 m/sec indicates mild stenosis. Velocities of less than 2.5 m/sec are not hemodynamically significant. Peak transaortic pressure gradients are calculated by the simplified Bernoulli equation. Because transvalvular pressure gradients vary with volume flow rate, higher pressure gradients and flow velocities will be recorded in the setting of increased stroke volume (i.e., aortic regurgitation), and lower pressure gradients and velocities will be recorded when flow rates are decreased (i.e., left ventricular systolic dysfunction). Aortic valve area (AVA) is calculated by the continuity equation, whereby the cross-sectional area (CSA) of the left ventricular outflow tract (LVOT) is calculated from the diameter in the parasternal long-axis view, the velocity-time integrals in the left ventricular outflow tract are obtained with pulsed Doppler from an apical view, and the aortic signal is the highest velocity signal recorded with continuous Doppler.

$$AVA = (CSA_{LVOT} \times VTI_{LVOT})/VTI_{AV}$$

For routine clinical use, this equation can be simplified further by substituting peak velocities (V) in place of the velocity-time integral measurements:

$$AVA = (CSA_{LVOT} \times V_{LVOT})/V_{AV}$$

A valve area of less than 1.0 cm² indicates severe stenosis, and a valve area of 1.0 to 1.5 cm² is consistent with moderate stenosis. Diagnostic limitations for echocardiography in evaluating aortic stenosis include measurement variability, optimal alignment of the ultrasound beam to maximize transaortic velocities, and accurate measurement of the left ventricular outflow tract diameter for cross-sectional area calculation.

Increased afterload in aortic stenosis leads to an increase in myocardial wall stress with left ventricular hypertrophy and impaired diastolic filling. Systolic dysfunction is not common but can occur in the late stages of the disease. In patients under consideration for surgical intervention for aortic stenosis, preoperative transthoracic imaging should be completed to fully assess disease severity. Transesophageal imaging is usually less optimal for diagnostic evaluation as it is limited by the inability to optimally align the ultrasound beam for Doppler interrogation of the aortic valve. Direct planimetry of the valve orifice is relatively limited by the nonplanar anatomy of the aortic valve, acoustic shadowing, and beam width artifact from valve calcification.

Aortic Regurgitation

Echocardiography allows determination of the cause of aortic regurgitation.[15] Common causes include bicuspid aortic valve, endocarditis, and aortic root dilation. The aortic valve and proximal ascending aorta are generally well visualized by TTE (Fig. 55-24), which can aid in surgical planning by determining whether regurgitation is due to aortic root disease or primary valve dysfunction. Doppler echocardiography has high sensitivity and specificity for detecting regurgitation. Regurgitation is qualitatively evaluated as mild, moderate, or severe on the basis of the size of the color flow jet relative to the left ventricular outflow tract. With greater than moderate regurgitation, Doppler interrogation of flow in the descending thoracic and proximal abdominal aorta may show holodiastolic flow reversal (Fig. 55-25). The density of the continuous wave Doppler signal relative to anterograde flow is another measure of regurgitant severity. With acute or severe regurgitation, early diastolic equalization of aortic and left ventricular pressures may lead to a steep diastolic deceleration slope of the Doppler envelope and, in severe cases, a late diastolic velocity

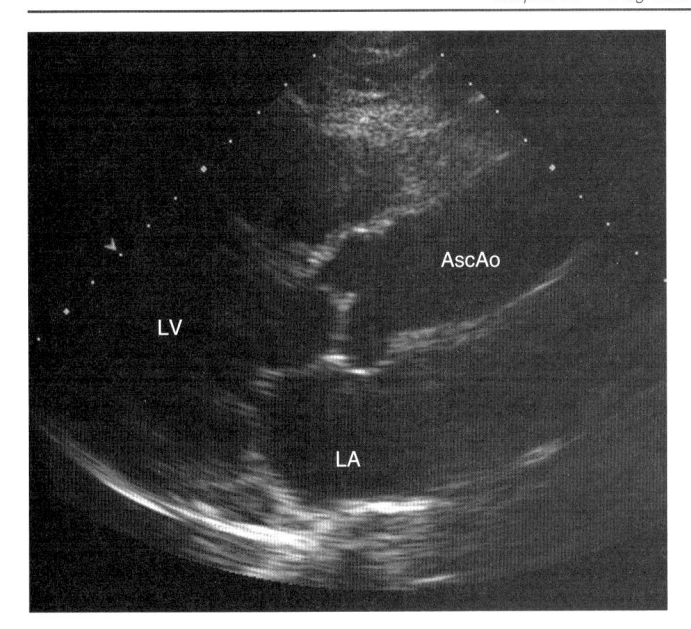

Figure 55-24
Normal-caliber proximal ascending aorta as seen from the parasternal long-axis view.

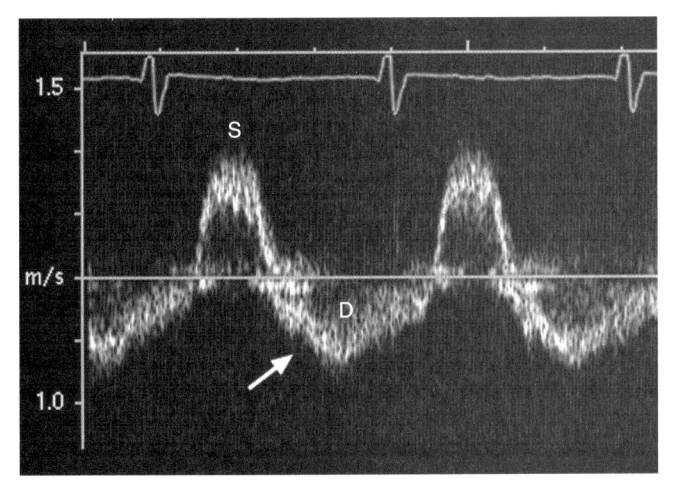

Figure 55-25
Continuous Doppler ultrasound imaging of the abdominal aorta demonstrates anterograde aortic flow during systole (S) and holodiastolic flow reversal during diastole (D), consistent with severe aortic regurgitation *(arrow)*.

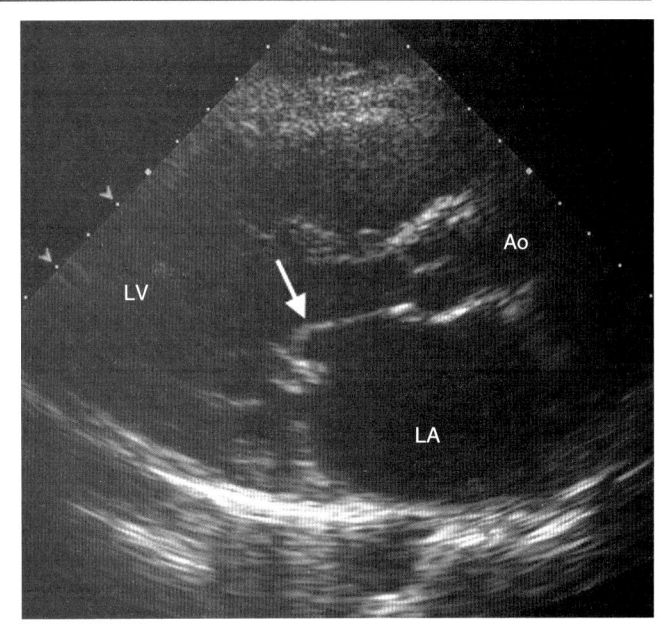

Figure 55-26
Rheumatic mitral valve stenosis. Imaging from the parasternal long-axis view demonstrates calcification of the mitral valve. There is restricted opening of the valve with diastolic doming of the anterior leaflet *(arrow)*.

that approaches zero (see Fig. 55-5). Eccentric regurgitant jets directed posteriorly may restrict diastolic opening of the anterior mitral valve leaflet. Quantitative evaluation of regurgitant severity is possible by measuring the jet vena contracta or calculating the regurgitant orifice area (see Fig. 55-9).

With significant, chronic aortic regurgitation, ventricular chamber enlargement or dysfunction due to the increased hemodynamic load may occur. These patients usually develop cardiopulmonary symptoms such as dyspnea, decreased exercise tolerance, and congestive heart failure that require valve replacement. In asymptomatic patients, serial echocardiography is recommended to monitor regurgitation severity and ventricular size and function. Surgery is recommended once an adverse hemodynamic effect on ventricular size or function has occurred, evidenced by a fall in ejection fraction below 50%, a left ventricular end-systolic diameter that exceeds 55 mm, or an end-diastolic diameter that exceeds 70 mm.

Mitral Stenosis

Mitral stenosis is almost always due to rheumatic valve disease. The echocardiographic appearance of a rheumatic mitral valve includes commissural fusion, leaflet thickening, calcification, and restricted leaflet motion (Fig. 55-26). The mitral valve appears "domed" in diastole because of the inability to open fully. In severe cases, the subvalvular apparatus is also affected with chordal thickening and fusion. Other rare causes of mitral stenosis are severe mitral anular calcification and left ventricular inflow obstruction from a vegetation or myxoma. Patients with moderate mitral stenosis (mean gradients, 5 to 10 mm Hg) may be asymptomatic at rest but develop dyspnea with increased cardiac demand, such as exercise or pregnancy. Progressive obstruction of mitral inflow leads to increased left atrial pressure and dilation, increasing the propensity for development of atrial fibrillation.

Peak and mean mitral pressure gradients are estimated from transmitral velocities by applying the Bernoulli equation. Mitral valve area (MVA) can be calculated from the empirically derived equation MVA = 220/PHT, where PHT (pressure half-time) is the time duration for the peak early mitral inflow pressure gradient to drop by half. Because of the quadratic pressure-velocity relationship described in the Bernoulli equation, in which the pressure change equals $4 V_{max}^2$, PHT is also the time duration for early mitral inflow velocity to decrease by $V_{max}/2^{1/2}$. Planimetry of the mitral valve orifice in a parasternal short-axis view is another accurate and reproducible measurement for mitral valve area (Fig. 55-27). Patients with significant mitral stenosis often have pulmonary hypertension, which can be estimated echocardiographically from the peak velocity of the tricuspid

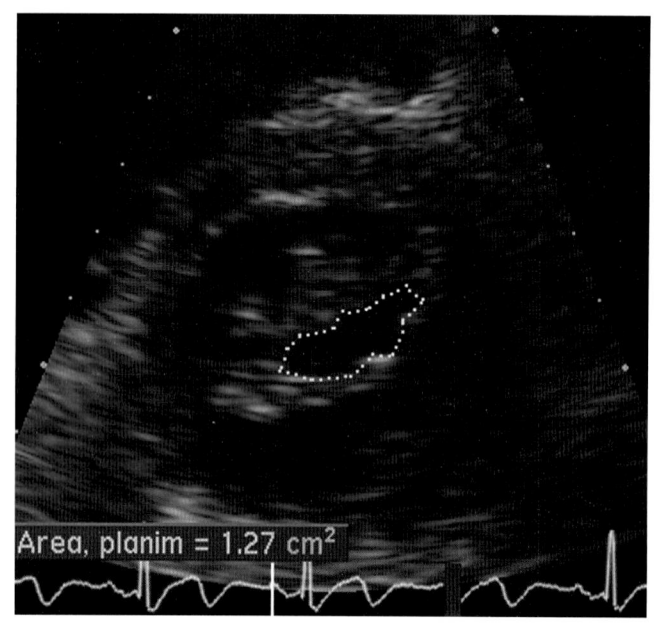

Figure 55-27
Rheumatic mitral valve stenosis. Imaging from the parasternal short-axis view allows direct planimetry of the valve opening (area = 1.3 cm²).

Figure 55-28
Myxomatous disease of the mitral valve with redundant mitral valve leaflets and systolic prolapse of the midportion into the left atrium beyond the level of the mitral valve anulus. In this patient, prolapse of the posterior mitral leaflet is more prominent than the anterior leaflet (arrow).

regurgitant jet as described previously. Evaluation of coexisting mitral regurgitant severity also is important. When clinical symptoms seem discrepant with the hemodynamic severity of mitral stenosis, exercise testing with Doppler measurement of the rise in pulmonary pressures may be a helpful adjunct.

Echocardiography is used for selection of candidates for percutaneous or surgical valvotomy. Valve characteristics that favor a successful valvotomy include pliable mitral valve leaflets, minimal commissural fusion, and minimal valvular or subvalvular calcification. Percutaneous valvuloplasty is not performed if anatomy is unfavorable or if pre-procedure TEE demonstrates a left atrial appendage thrombus or there is moderate or severe mitral regurgitation. Conditions that require mitral valve replacement or surgical repair for mitral stenosis include significant mitral regurgitation, other valvular disease, and concurrent coronary disease.

Mitral Regurgitation

The first step in echocardiographic evaluation of mitral regurgitation is determination of the cause and mechanism of regurgitation. Common causes of primary mitral valve dysfunction with regurgitation are mitral valve prolapse, endocarditis, and rheumatic disease. Secondary or functional regurgitation of an otherwise anatomically normal mitral valve can occur with leaflet tethering or dilation of the mitral valve anulus and is usually a consequence of ischemic myocardial dysfunction or dilated cardiomyopathy. Echocardiography is integral to visualization of leaflet anatomy, assessment of ventricular geometry, and estimation of pulmonary pressures. Transthoracic imaging may be supplemented by TEE if images are suboptimal. In mitral valve prolapse, echocardiography reveals thickened and redundant leaflets (Fig. 55-28). Leaflet prolapse of more than 2 mm above the base of the mitral valve leaflets into the left atrium is diagnostic.

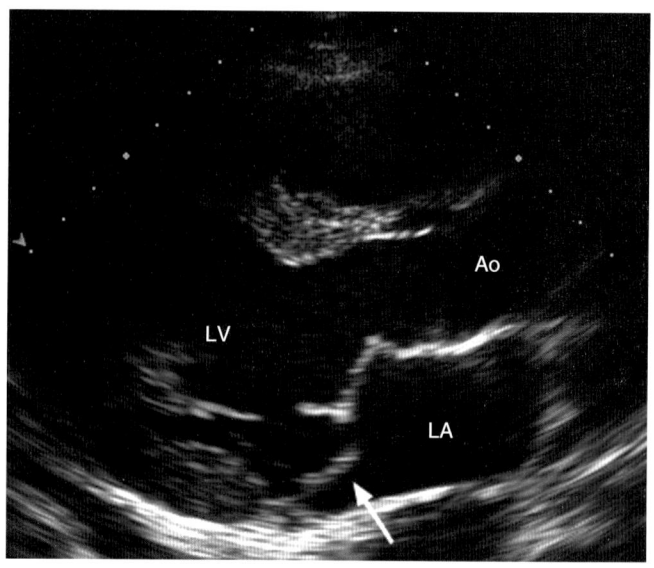

Color Doppler mapping allows visualization and assessment of the regurgitant jet flow disturbance, jet size, direction, and jet eccentricity. Color Doppler imaging has a high sensitivity and specificity for detection of mitral regurgitation, a small degree of which is present in up to 80% of normal individuals. By color Doppler mapping, regurgitant flow disturbances in the left atrium range from a small localized area adjacent to the valve (mild regurgitation) to a large flow disturbance that fills the entire left atrium (severe regurgitation). Measurement of the vena contracta at the regurgitant orifice correlates with severity, even with eccentric jets (see Fig. 55-9). The shape and direction of the regurgitant jet aid in establishing the mechanism of valve dysfunction. For example, posterior mitral valve leaflet prolapse is usually associated with an anteriorly directed regurgitant jet. Eccentric jets that adhere to the atrial wall typically appear smaller than centrally directed jets. Evaluation of the jet from at least two orthogonal views with careful adjustment of instrument settings is essential.

Greater regurgitation severity leads to increased left atrial pressures and velocity of regurgitant flow. Doppler evaluation of the peak early inflow velocity (E wave) and the shape and intensity of the continuous wave Doppler envelope provide added data on regurgitation severity; worsened regurgitation shows higher, denser jets. Another qualitative measure of mitral regurgitant severity is systolic flow reversal of the Doppler signal in the pulmonary veins in patients in normal sinus rhythm (Fig. 55-29).

Quantitative evaluation of regurgitation severity is possible by measurement of the regurgitant volume by use of the proximal isovolumic surface area and calculation of the regurgitant orifice area. The proximal isovelocity surface area (PISA) calculation assumes that flow accelerates in a laminar fashion toward a regurgitant orifice, forming concentric "hemispheres" of isovelocity (Fig. 55-30).[16] The effective regurgitant orifice area can be calculated once hemisphere surface area, blood velocity at that hemisphere (aliasing velocity), and orifice

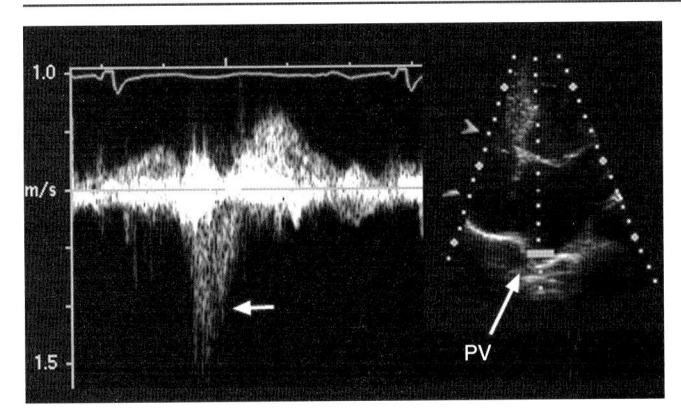

Figure 55–29
Pulmonary vein tracing in a patient with mitral valve prolapse and significant mitral regurgitation. The Doppler cursor is positioned in the right upper pulmonary vein (PV, *right*). The spectral Doppler tracing shows mid-late systolic flow reversal that is directed away from the transducer *(arrow, left)*.

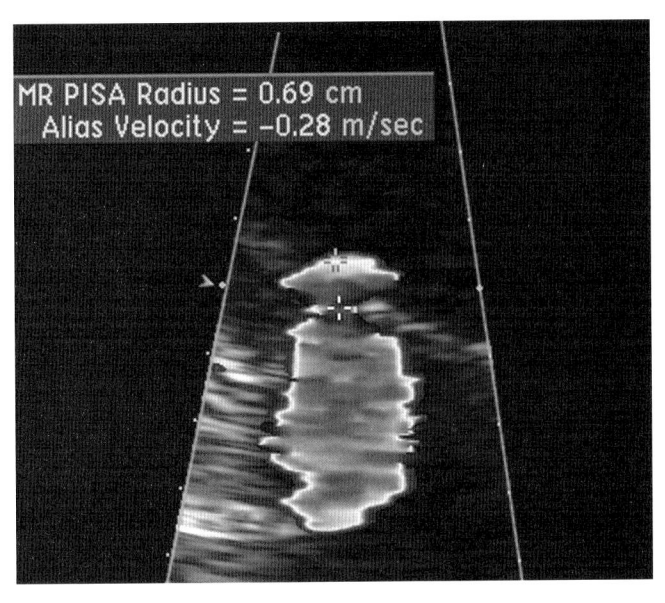

Figure 55–30
Regurgitation severity quantification by proximal isovelocity surface area (PISA) method. As blood flow approaches a regurgitant orifice, velocity increases, forming concentric isovelocity hemispheres. The aliasing blood velocity, measured at the hemisphere margin, and the radius provide data on the regurgitant instantaneous flow rate and the effective regurgitant orifice area. The PISA calculations are less accurate with eccentric regurgitant jets.

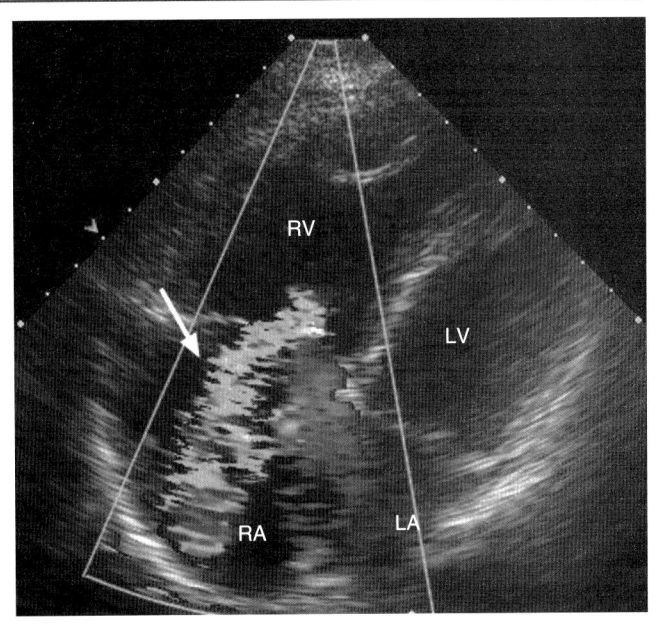

Figure 55–31
Patient with primary pulmonary hypertension imaged from the apical four-chamber view. There is severe right ventricular enlargement with tricuspid anular dilatation and poor tricuspid valve leaflet coaptation. Color Doppler imaging demonstrates moderate tricuspid regurgitation *(arrow)*. (See color version in the online edition through Expert Consult.)

regurgitant velocity are measured. Calculation of the effective regurgitant orifice area by PISA is more accurate when the regurgitant orifice is circular and the jet is not eccentric. Another method of assessing regurgitation severity is to compare anterograde volume across the regurgitant valve (includes anterograde and regurgitant flow) with flow across a competent valve (the difference equals the regurgitant volume), allowing calculation of regurgitant fraction and effective orifice area. Quantitative gradation of regurgitation by the American Society of Echocardiography is now incorporated in the American Heart Association/American College of Cardiology guidelines on valvular heart disease.[14,15] Reporting of quantitative measures is preferred as color Doppler measures of regurgitant jet size and flow disturbance alone are often subject to transducer frequency and instrument settings.

As with aortic regurgitation, progressive regurgitant volume and increased hemodynamic cardiac load can lead to ventricular chamber enlargement or dysfunction. Serial and echocardiographic measures of ventricular size and systolic function serve as the primary determinants of the timing of intervention for chronic mitral regurgitation. In asymptomatic patients, surgery is recommended with left ventricular end-systolic diameter of more than 40 mm, ejection fraction below 60%, onset of atrial fibrillation, or pulmonary hypertension.

With increased expertise in mitral valve repair and improved outcomes, some experienced surgical centers advocate earlier mitral valve repair, even in those with normal ventricular size and function, when the likelihood of a successful repair exceeds 90%. Early intervention mandates a careful echocardiographic evaluation to ensure that regurgitation is severe by established guidelines (effective regurgitant orifice area ≥ 0.4 cm^2, regurgitant volume ≥ 60 mL, regurgitant fraction $\geq 50\%$). Close collaboration between the echocardiographer and cardiac surgeon is needed to evaluate the likelihood of mitral valve repair. During surgery, intraoperative TEE is used to evaluate adequacy of repair and to identify residual mitral regurgitation after repair.

Tricuspid Valve Disease

Most right-sided valvular disease in adults is secondary to left-sided heart dysfunction. Trace to mild regurgitation of both the tricuspid and pulmonic valves is a normal finding seen in more than 80% of normal adults. Significant functional tricuspid regurgitation may be due to pulmonary hypertension (>55 mm Hg), often with concurrent right ventricular and anular dilation (Fig. 55-31).[37] Other causes of tricuspid

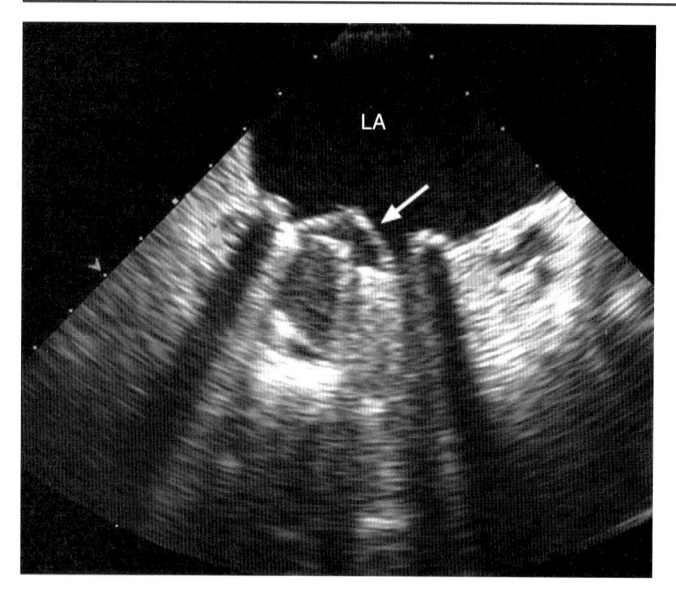

Figure 55-32
St. Jude mechanical prosthesis (arrow) in the mitral position demonstrating acoustic shadowing of the left ventricle when TEE is used. In patients with mitral prostheses, TEE is often required to definitively evaluate for valve dysfunction, endocarditis, and regurgitation into the left atrium.

regurgitation include endocarditis, carcinoid disease, mediastinal irradiation, and injury after pacer lead placement. Echocardiographic features of carcinoid include tricuspid leaflet calcification, thickening, and retraction. A congenital cause of tricuspid regurgitation is Ebstein's anomaly, with apical displacement of the tricuspid septal leaflet and poor leaflet coaptation. Severe tricuspid regurgitation results in a wide vena contracta (>7 mm) and systolic flow reversal in the hepatic veins (imaged from the subcostal view). With progressive, right-sided volume overload, the right ventricle may become dilated, hypertrophied, and hypokinetic.

Prosthetic Valves

Prosthetic valves fall into two main classes, bioprosthetic and mechanical valves. Because of the sewing ring and struts in prosthetic valves, the functional valve area of prosthetic valves is smaller than that of native valves, resulting in relatively higher anterograde velocities. Knowledge of the individual flow dynamics of the different valve types is important to discriminate normal from abnormal transvalvular flow and function. Flow profiles differ between the different mechanical valve types and also vary by valve size. Optimal echocardiographic evaluation is often hindered by valve positioning, reverberations from artificial materials that hinder visualization of the valve occluders, and acoustic shadowing from artificial materials incorporated into the valves in the far field (Fig. 55-32). This is particularly problematic in evaluating mitral prostheses for regurgitation because of the valve's relatively posterior position and shadowing of the left atrium. TEE (which images from posterior to the heart and provides improved image quality) is often needed for a more definitive assessment of a prosthetic valve.[38]

For any prosthetic valve, it is not uncommon to see a small amount of regurgitant valvular flow. Tiny paravalvular regurgitant jets may be seen in the immediate postoperative period and usually resolve over time. Expected transvalvular velocities, areas, and gradients are dependent on valve size, patient size, valve type, and valve position. Flow hemodynamics and color Doppler pattern are dependent on the type of valve placed. With a single tilting disc valve, there is an asymmetrical flow profile with major and minor anterograde flow identified and an eccentric, small regurgitant jet. Bileaflet mechanical valves have complex fluid dynamics with anterograde flow seen through two minor orifices corresponding to each leaflet and one central major orifice. During valve closure, two small, central intersecting regurgitant jets are normally seen. Because of the absence of prosthetic material, the appearance of homograft and stentless tissue aortic valves may be echocardiographically indistinguishable from native valves. Anterograde flow velocities of stentless valves are more similar to those of native valves, and only trivial regurgitation is expected.

Estimation of transvalvular gradients is relatively reliable for bioprosthetic valves. However, with mechanical valves, flow is heterogeneous across the entire orifice face, and high local velocities at the smaller leaflet orifices may lead to overestimation of the transvalvular gradient.

Because prosthetic valve hemodynamics vary by the patient's habitus and the type of valve, a baseline echocardiogram relatively soon (2 to 3 months) after surgery is recommended. After this, serial echocardiographic examinations are typically not necessary to identify subsequent interval changes in function unless the patient develops new cardiopulmonary symptoms or valve dysfunction is suspected.

Complications of mechanical valves, including endocarditis and pannus or thrombus that impairs disc motion, can be accurately diagnosed by echocardiography. Because of improved image quality and more optimal transducer placement, TEE is nearly always needed in the evaluation of prosthetic valve dysfunction, often in combination with data from transthoracic imaging.

Endocarditis

Used in combination with clinical and bacteriologic data, echocardiography provides invaluable information in the evaluation for endocarditis.[39] The risk of endocarditis is highest in patients with valve prostheses, native valve disease, congenital heart disease, or a clinical risk factor (e.g., intravenous drug use). Major echocardiographic diagnostic criteria include echodense masses adherent to valve leaflets or endocardial surfaces, paravalvular abscesses, and prosthetic valve dehiscence. Vegetations typically appear as irregular masses of varying sizes attached to the affected valve (Fig. 55-33).

When endocarditis is suspected on the basis of predisposing factors, fever, sepsis, or embolic events, TTE is the initial procedure of choice because of lower cost and risk to the patient. TTE allows better manipulation of the transducer to evaluate possible fistulas and abnormal communications. Although the specificity of TTE is adequate, ranging from 91% to 98%, the sensitivity of TTE is relatively poor (ranging from 36% to 90%), with more studies at the lower end of the spectrum. Therefore, in patients with a normal transthoracic study but in whom clinical suspicion for endocarditis is significant, TEE should also be performed.[40] Diagnostic accuracy of TEE is higher, and TEE more readily images complications

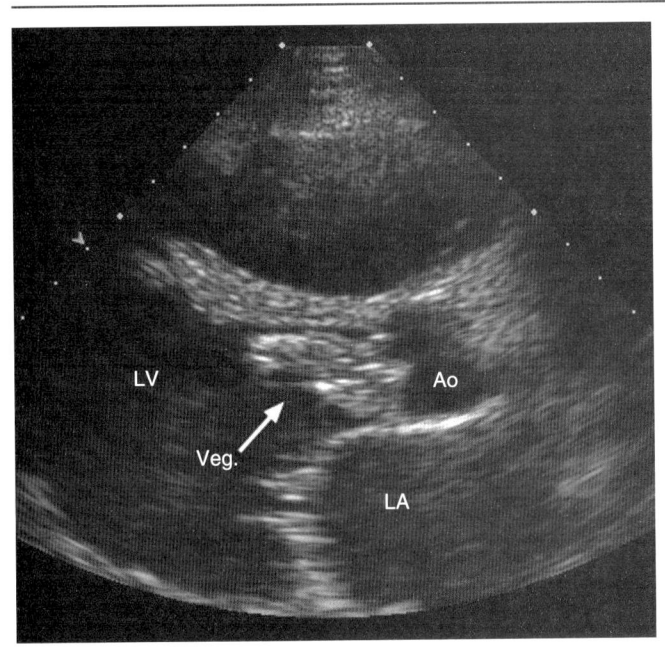

Figure 55-33
Native aortic valve endocarditis in a patient who presented with severe aortic regurgitation and cardiogenic shock. There is a large, mobile vegetation adherent to the aortic valve that prolapses into the left ventricular outflow tract *(arrow)*.

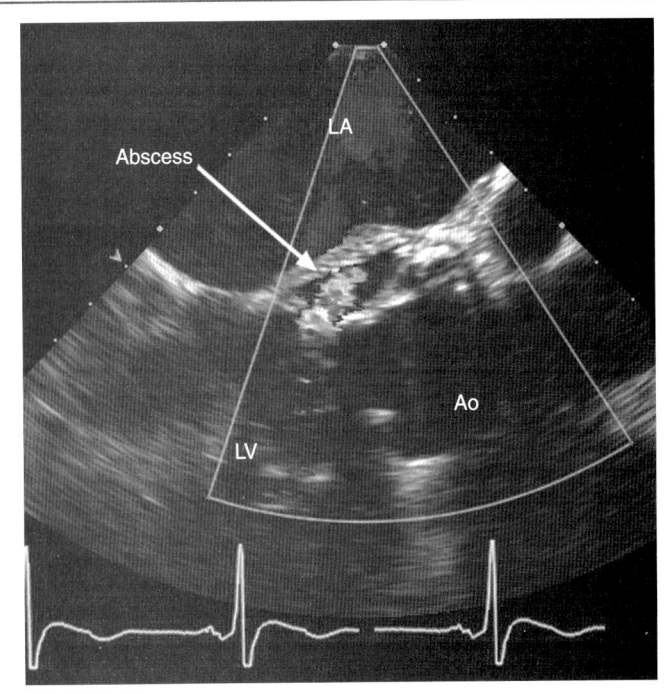

Figure 55-34
Pseudoaneurysm of the mitral-aortic intervalvular fibrosa *(arrow)* in a patient with a mechanical aortic valve, as imaged by TEE. Systolic flow is seen by color Doppler imaging from the pseudoaneurysm into the left ventricular outflow tract. (See color version in the online edition through ExpertConsult.)

of endocarditis. However, TEE does carry the inherent risks of conscious sedation and of the procedure itself. Regardless, if the initial echocardiographic evaluation for endocarditis is normal but clinical suspicion remains high, repeated echocardiography should be considered because a subsequent study may be abnormal with disease progression.

Limitations of echocardiography for endocarditis include the inability to distinguish between acute and chronic lesions and between vegetations and thrombus; the inability to differentiate reverberations from calcifications or prosthetic materials; and the inability to identify nonbacterial thrombotic lesions, as can be seen in systemic lupus erythematosus. False-positive findings include normal leaflet thickening, Lambl's excrescences on the aortic valve, mitral leaflet redundancy resulting from myxomatous disease, partial flail leaflets, leaflet calcification, and degenerative changes.

Common complications of endocarditis include involvement of other valves, leaflet perforation, paravalvular abscess, fistula development, and coronary embolization. Valve dysfunction associated with endocarditis usually leads to regurgitation; stenosis is rare. As with native valves, endocarditis of a bioprosthetic valve is often evidenced by a vegetation. With mechanical valves, vegetations are less common. Instead, infection often causes valve instability, with dehiscence, paravalvular leak, or paravalvular abscess. Paravalvular abscesses usually appear as an echolucency adjacent to the valve anulus. A paravalvular abscess in the aortic position may extend to the anterior mitral valve leaflet with involvement of the mitral-aortic intervalvular fibrosa (Fig. 55-34). Because of its communication with the left ventricular cavity, flow into and out of the pseudoaneurysm can be demonstrated by color Doppler imaging. Infection that involves the aortic sinuses can lead to sinus of Valsalva aneurysm and rupture; Doppler interrogation demonstrates flow into the cardiac chamber adjacent to the affected sinus. TEE is usually needed in the evaluation of prosthetic valve endocarditis because of improved image quality.

AORTIC DISEASE

TTE is reasonably reliable in imaging of aortic anatomy throughout most of the thoracic and proximal abdominal aorta (see Fig. 55-24).[41] Standard aortic diameter measurements can be taken from the aortic valve anulus, sinuses, sinotubular junction, ascending aorta, arch, and descending thoracic aorta. Nonoblique imaging is essential for accurate measurement of internal aortic dimensions at end-diastole. Image resolution with TTE is often limited by the aorta's posterior position and overlying air-filled structures, such as the trachea and lungs. In addition, distance from the chest wall to the aorta hinders optimal image resolution. Therefore, TEE, with the shorter distance between the transducer and the aorta, the use of a higher frequency transducer, and the better ultrasound penetration, is often needed to complete a full echocardiographic evaluation of the aorta. Computed tomography and magnetic resonance imaging allow better spatial imaging of the aorta, particularly with 3D rendering. However, echocardiography allows imaging in the absence of radiation or contrast exposure, without imaging constraints in those with implanted metallic devices (such as pacemakers). Echocardiography also has the advantage of being a portable modality and allowing identification of concurrent pericardial fluid and aortic regurgitation. Importantly, with echocardiography, data are readily available as limited imaging of the aorta is routinely performed on most transthoracic echocardiographic studies.

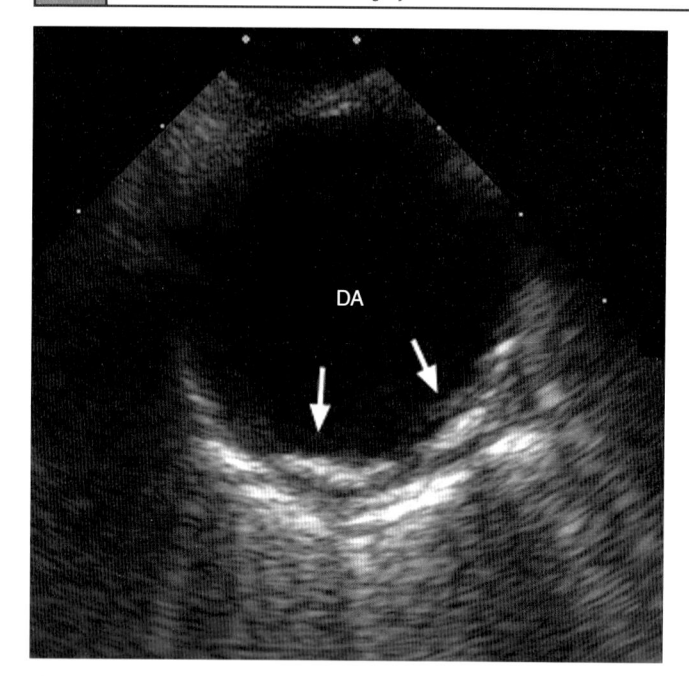

Figure 55–35
Mild atherosclerosis of the descending thoracic aorta (DA) imaged by TEE. Calcification within the atherosclerotic plaque causes acoustic shadowing distally in the far field.

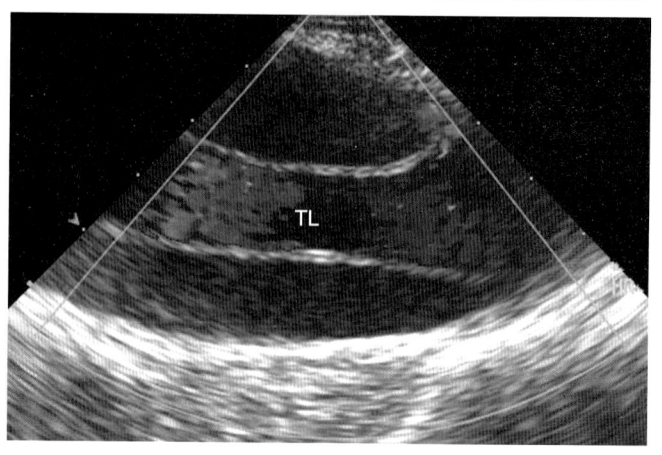

Figure 55–36
A dissection flap is seen within an enlarged aorta, imaged by TEE. The true lumen (TL) is visualized by color Doppler imaging. (See color version in the online edition through Expert Consult.)

Asymptomatic dilation of the ascending aorta is associated with atherosclerosis, systemic hypertension, bicuspid aortic valves, and Marfan disease. Marfan disease is associated with dilation of the aortic sinuses with effacement of the sinotubular junction. Patients with aneurysmal dilation of the sinuses or ascending aorta are at increased risk for dissection and aortic rupture. Therefore, serial echocardiographic examinations monitor for progressive enlargement to time referral for prophylactic surgical repair.

Atherosclerotic disease is more easily evaluated with TEE, which can readily image the severity and extent of disease along the length of the thoracic and proximal abdominal aorta (Fig. 55-35). Common findings include atherosclerotic plaques, ulceration, associated dilation, and adherent mobile thrombi, which are all considered potential sources of distal embolic disease. Intraoperative use of TEE or epiaortic scanning with a sterile transducer to localize atherosclerotic plaques directs optimal placement of the aortic cannula for the arterial bypass circuit and for aortic cross-clamping.

In aortic dissection, the flap appears as a thin, mobile echodensity within the aortic lumen (Fig. 55-36). The false lumen may contain thrombus, may be localized, or may propagate distally. Color flow Doppler imaging may be used to identify entrance and exit points to the false lumen. Associated findings with dissection can include intramural hematoma, extension of the dissection into the branch vessels or a coronary artery with resulting regional wall motion abnormalities, pericardial or pleural effusion, aortic root dilatation, and flail aortic leaflet with aortic regurgitation. Predisposing factors for aortic dissection include congenital aortic valve disease, aneurysm, and atherosclerotic disease. The sensitivity of TTE for detection of aortic dissection ranges between 29% and 80% and is limited by beam width artifacts and reverberations, which increase false-positive results. The specificity of TTE is also low because of difficulty in imaging the posteriorly located aorta. In the hands of an experienced operator, TEE provides improved image quality and more complete evaluation of the length of the thoracic aorta, with sensitivity and specificity approaching 100%. TEE is also used intraoperatively to evaluate effectiveness of surgical repair and residual defects. After surgical intervention, serial echocardiography is used to monitor for recurrent disease, to evaluate the proximal and distal graft anastomotic sites, and to assess prosthetic valvular function. TEE, computed tomography, and cardiac magnetic resonance imaging have equivalent diagnostic accuracy for aortic dissection. The choice of imaging modality in each patient depends on prompt availability and the differential diagnosis in each patient.

CONGENITAL HEART DISEASE

Echocardiography is a key diagnostic modality in patients with congenital heart disease.[42] Indications for echocardiography include diagnosis, monitoring for hemodynamic progression of lesions on cardiac function, and anatomic definition and guidance for palliative or reparative interventions. Echocardiography accurately detects intracardiac shunts by Doppler interrogation and by contrast studies in which agitated saline is injected intravenously. By comparison of the volume flow rates across the pulmonic and aortic valves, quantitation of the pulmonic-to-systemic shunt ratio can also be provided.

For atrial septal defects, echocardiography permits distinction between secundum, primum, and sinus venosus defects with demonstration of left-to-right flow across the atrial septum on color Doppler flow imaging. Other findings associated with an atrial septal defect can include right-sided heart enlargement, hypertrophy, and pulmonary hypertension. Three-dimensional echocardiography allows improved spatial resolution of the interatrial septum and aids in decision making regarding size and placement of the defect for percutaneous versus surgical closure. Ventricular septal defects can be identified by Doppler flow across the interventricular septum. In adults, most encountered defects are small, with high-velocity left-to-right systolic flow and a relatively small shunt volume. Larger, chronic shunts may result in pulmonary hypertension, right ventricular enlargement, and hypertrophy.

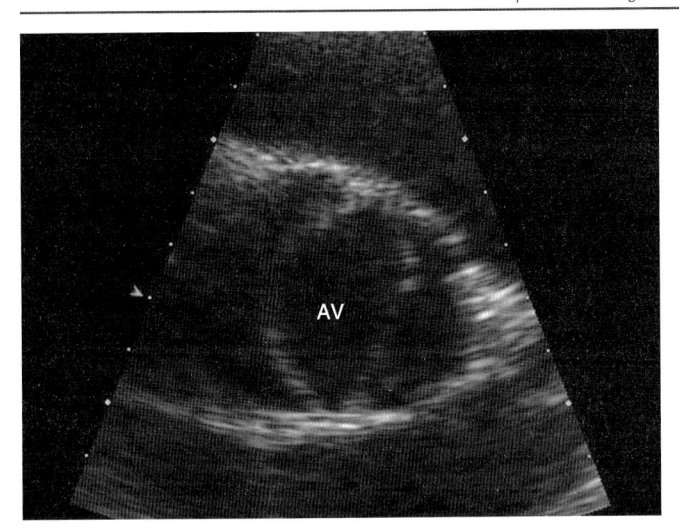

Figure 55–37
Parasternal short-axis view of a bicuspid aortic valve (AV), showing a linear anterior-posterior valve opening during systole.

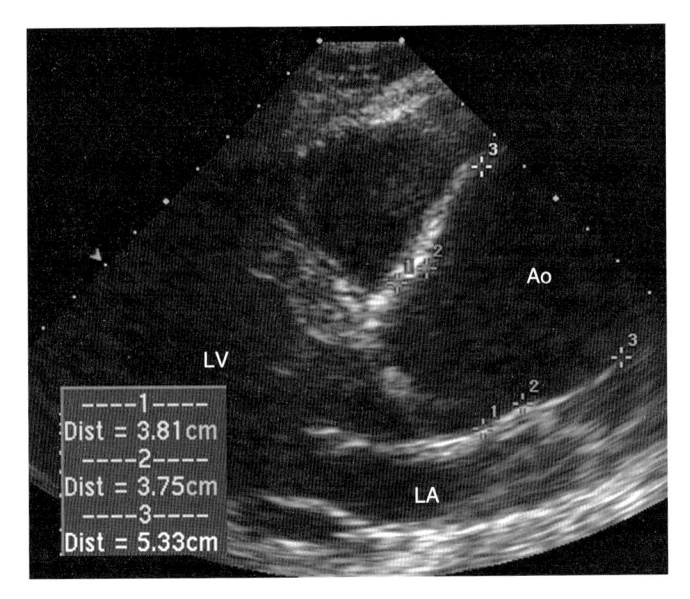

Figure 55–38
Dilation of the aortic root and ascending aorta in a patient with a bicuspid aortic valve. Measurements are taken at the coronary sinuses (1), sinotubular junction (2), and proximal ascending aorta (3).

Bicuspid aortic valves are the most commonly occurring congenital abnormality (Fig. 55-37). Aortic root dilation is common in these patients, and serial echocardiography is indicated to monitor for progressive valve dysfunction and aortic dilation (Fig. 55-38). In patients with aortic coarctation, transthoracic imaging can demonstrate the aortic narrowing. Doppler examination of the thoracic aorta shows increased anterograde flow velocity in the region of the coarctation, with anterograde aortic flow that persists into diastole. Another congenital abnormality of the aorta seen by Doppler echocardiography is patent ductus arteriosus. With a patent ductus arteriosus, color Doppler imaging may show the communication between the pulmonary artery and aorta; if shunt flow into the pulmonary artery is large enough, it may demonstrate aortic diastolic flow reversal.

The most common complex congenital heart disease seen in the adult population is tetralogy of Fallot. Most patients with tetralogy of Fallot have undergone surgical repair with ventricular septal defect closure and enlargement–patch repair of the right ventricular outflow tract. Serial echocardiography is performed to monitor for pulmonic regurgitation related to the transanular pulmonic patch. These patients often require repeated surgical intervention once serial echocardiographic evaluation documents adverse effect on right ventricular size and systolic function. In patients with previous surgical repair of complex congenital heart disease, echocardiography is a key tool in monitoring for long-term complications of prior palliative or corrective surgeries, such as interatrial baffle leak or stenosis in patients with transposition of the great arteries. With knowledge of the previous surgical procedures and a careful and meticulous examination, anatomy and physiology are usually well demonstrated with echocardiography. However, in complex cases, other imaging procedures, including magnetic resonance imaging and cardiac catheterization, may be needed for complete evaluation of the patient. Prior operative reports often greatly assist the echocardiographer in interpreting the nature of congenital repair and in identifying complications.

REFERENCES

1. Feigenbaum H. *Echocardiography*. 6th ed Philadelphia: Lippincott Williams & Wilkins; 2004.
2. Otto CM. *Textbook of Clinical Echocardiography*. 4th ed Philadelphia: WB Saunders; 2009.
3. Otto CM. *The Practice of Clinical Echocardiography*. 3rd ed Philadelphia: WB Saunders; 2007.
4. Douglas PS, Khandheria B, Stainback RF, et al. ACCF/ASE/ACEP/ASNC/SCAI/SCCT/SCMR 2007 appropriateness criteria for transthoracic and transesophageal echocardiography: a report of the American College of Cardiology Foundation Quality Strategic Directions Committee Appropriateness Criteria Working Group, American Society of Echocardiography, American College of Emergency Physicians, American Society of Nuclear Cardiology, Society for Cardiovascular Angiography and Interventions, Society of Cardiovascular Computed Tomography, and the Society for Cardiovascular Magnetic Resonance endorsed by the American College of Chest Physicians and the Society of Critical Care Medicine. *J Am Coll Cardiol* 2007;**50**(2):187-204.
5. Cheitlin MD, Armstrong WF, Aurigemma GP, et al. ACC/AHA/ASE Guideline Update for the Clinical Application of Echocardiography: summary article. A report of the American College of Cardiology/American Heart Association Task Force on Practice Guidelines (ACC/AHA/ASE) Committee to Update the 1997 Guidelines for the Clinical Application. *J Am Soc Echocardiogr* 2003;**16**:1091-110.
6. Lang R, Bierig M, Devereux R, et al. Recommendations for chamber quantification: a report from the American Society of Echocardiography's Guidelines and Standard Committee and the Chamber Quantification Writing Group. *J Am Soc Echocardiogr* 2005;**18**:1440-63.
7. Klein AL, Grimm RA, Murray RD, Apperson-Hansen C, Asinger RW, Black IW, et al. Assessment of Cardioversion Using Transesophageal Echocardiography Investigators. use of transesophageal echocardiography to guide cardioversion in patients with atrial fibrillation. *N Engl J Med* 2001;**344**:1411-20.
8. Khoury AF, Afridi I, Quinones MA, Zoghbi WA. Transesophageal echocardiography in critically ill patients: feasibility, safety, and impact on management. *Am Heart J* 1994;**124**:1363-71.
9. Russo AM, O'Connor WH, Waxman HL. Atypical presentations and echocardiographic findings in patients with cardiac tamponade occurring early and late after cardiac surgery. *Chest* 1993;**104**:71-8.
10. Dolan MS, Riad K, El-Shafei A, Puri S, Tamirisa K, Bierig M, et al. Effect of intravenous contrast for left ventricular opacification and border definition on sensitivity and specificity of dobutamine stress echocardiography compared with coronary angiography in technically difficult patients. *Am Heart J* 2001;**142**:908-15.
11. Main ML, Magalski A, Morris BA, et al. Combined assessment of microvascular integrity and contractile reserve improves differentiation of stunning and necrosis after acute anterior wall myocardial infarction. *J Am Coll Cardiol* 2002;**40**:1079-84.

12. Jeetley P, Hickman M, Kamp O, Lang RM, Thomas JD, Vannan MA, et al. Myocardial contrast echocardiography for the detection of coronary artery stenosis: a prospective multicenter study in comparison with single-photon emission computed tomography. *J Am Coll Cardiol* 2006;**47**(1):141-5.
13. Hung J, Lang R, Flachskampf F, et al. 3D echocardiography: a review of the current status and future directions. *J Am Soc Echocardiogr* 2007;**20**:213-33.
14. Quinones MA, Otto CM, Stoddard M, Waggoner A, Zoghbi WA. Recommendations for quantification of Doppler echocardiography: a report from the Doppler Quantification Task Force of the Nomenclature and Standards Committee of the American Society of Echocardiography. *J Am Soc Echocardiogr* 2002;**15**:167-84.
15. Zoghbi WA, Enriquez-Sarano M, Foster E, et al. Recommendations for evaluation of the severity of native valvular regurgitation with two-dimensional and Doppler echocardiography: a report from the Doppler Quantification Task Force of the Nomenclature and Standards Committee of the American Society of Echocardiography. *J Am Soc Echocardiogr* 2003;**16**:777-802.
16. Pu M, Prior DL, Fan X, Asher CR, Vasquez C, Griffin BP, Thomas JD. Calculation of mitral regurgitant orifice area with use of a simplified proximal convergence method: initial clinical application. *J Am Soc Echocardiogr* 2001;**14**:180-5.
17. Gilman G, Nelson TA, Hansen WH, Khandheria BK, Ommen SR. Diastolic function: a sonographer's approach to the essential echocardiographic measurements of left ventricular diastolic function. *J Am Soc Echocardiogr* 2007;**20**(2):199-209.
18. Lester SJ, Tajik AJ, Nishimura RA, Oh JK, Khandheria BK, Seward JB. Unlocking the mysteries of diastolic function: deciphering the Rosetta Stone 10 years later. *J Am Coll Cardiol* 2008;**51**(7):679-89.
19. Dec GW. Recognition of the apical ballooning syndrome in the United States. *Circulation* 2005;**111**(4):388-90.
20. Sharkey SW, Lesser JR, Zenovich AG, et al. Acute and reversible cardiomyopathy provoked by stress in women from the United States. *Circulation* 2005;**111**(4):472-9.
21. Pellikka PA. Stress echocardiography for the diagnosis of coronary artery disease: progress towards quantification. *Curr Opin Cardiol* 2005;**20**(5):395-8.
22. Armstrong WF, Zoghbi WA. Stress echocardiography: current methodology and clinical applications. *J Am Coll Cardiol* 2005;**45**(11):1739-47.
23. Sicari R, Pasanisi E, Venneri L, Landi P, Cortigiani L, Picano E. Echo Persantine International Cooperative (EPIC) Study Group; Echo Dobutamine International Cooperative (EDIC) Study Group. Stress echo results predict mortality: a large-scale multicenter prospective international study. *J Am Coll Cardiol* 2003;**41**(4):589-95.
24. Yao SS, Qureshi E, Sherrid MV, Chaudhry FA. Practical applications in stress echocardiography: risk stratification and prognosis in patients with known or suspected ischemic heart disease. *J Am Coll Cardiol* 2003;**42**(6):1084-90.
25. Arruda-Olson AM, Juracan EM, Mahoney DW, McCully RB, Roger VL, Pellikka PA. Prognostic value of exercise echocardiography in 5,798 patients: is there a gender difference? *J Am Coll Cardiol* 2002;**39**(4):625-31.
26. Silver MT, Lieberman EH, Thibault GE. Refractory hypoxemia in inferior myocardial infarction from right-to-left shunting through a patent foramen ovale: a case report and review of the literature. *Clin Cardiol* 1994;**17**:627-30.
27. Miniati M, Monti S, Pratali L, Di Ricco G, Marini C, Formichi B, et al. Value of transthoracic echocardiography in the diagnosis of pulmonary embolism: results of a prospective study in unselected patients. *Am J Med* 2001;**110**:528-35.
28. Manning WJ. Role of transesophageal echocardiography in the management of thromboembolic stroke. *Am J Cardiol* 1997;**80**(4C):19D-28D.
29. Kolias TJ, Aaronson KD, Armstrong WF. Doppler-derived dP/dt and –dP/dt predict survival in congestive heart failure. *J Am Coll Cardiol* 2002;**36**:1594-9.
30. Tam JW, Shaikh N, Sutherland E. Echocardiographic assessment of patients with hypertrophic and restrictive cardiomyopathy: imaging and echocardiography. *Curr Opin Cardiol* 2002;**17**:470-7.
31. Ommen SR, Park SH, Click RL, Freeman WK, Schaff HV, Tajik AJ. Impact of intraoperative transesophageal echocardiography in the surgical management of hypertrophic cardiomyopathy. *Am J Cardiol* 2002;**90**:1022-4.
32. Burgess MI, Bhattacharyya A, Ray SG. Echocardiography after cardiac transplantation. *J Am Soc Echocardiogr* 2002;**15**:917-25.
33. Spes CH, Klauss V, Mudra H, Schnaack SD, Tammen AR, Rieber J, et al. Diagnostic and prognostic value of serial dobutamine stress echocardiography for noninvasive assessment of cardiac allograft vasculopathy: a comparison with coronary angiography and intravascular ultrasound. *Circulation* 1999;**100**:509-15.
34. Wann S, Passen E. Echocardiography in pericardial disease. *J Am Soc Echocardiogr* 2008;**21**(1):7-13.
35. Asher CR, Klein AL. Diastolic heart failure: restrictive cardiomyopathy, constrictive pericarditis, and cardiac tamponade: clinical and echocardiographic evaluation. *Cardiol Rev* 2002;**10**:218-29.
36. Bonow RO, Carabello BA, Kanu C, de Leon Jr AC, Faxon DP, Freed MD, et al. ACC/AHA 2006 guidelines for the management of patients with valvular heart disease: a report of the American College of Cardiology/American Heart Association Task Force on Practice Guidelines: developed in collaboration with the Society of Cardiovascular Anesthesiologists: endorsed by the Society for Cardiovascular Angiography and Interventions and the Society of Thoracic Surgeons. *Circulation* 2006(5):114:e84–231.
37. Bossone E, Duong-Wagner TH, Paciocco G, Oral H, Ricciardi M, Bach DS, et al. Echocardiographic features of primary pulmonary hypertension. *J Am Soc Echocardiogr* 1999;**12**:655-62.
38. Bach DS. Transesophageal echocardiographic (TEE) evaluation of prosthetic valves. *Cardiol Clin* 2000;**18**:751-71.
39. Sachdev M, Peterson GE, Jollis JG. Imaging techniques for diagnosis of infective endocarditis. *Infect Dis Clin North Am* 2002;**16**:319-37.
40. Ryan EW, Bolger AF. Transesophageal echocardiography (TEE) in the evaluation of infective endocarditis. *Cardiol Clin* 2000;**18**:773-87.
41. Goldstein SA, Mintz GS, Lindsay Jr J. Aorta: comprehensive evaluation by echocardiography and transesophageal echocardiography. *J Am Soc Echocardiogr* 1993;**6**:634-59.
42. Linker DT. *Practical Echocardiography of Congenital Heart Disease: From Fetus to Adult.* Seattle: Churchill Livingstone; 2000.

C. Medical- and Catheter-Based Treatment of Cardiovascular Disease

CHAPTER 56

Interventional Cardiology

Riya S. Chacko, Joseph P. Carrozza Jr., Duane S. Pinto

Historical Perspective
Percutaneous Coronary Intervention
  Procedures
    PCI for Unstable Angina and Non-ST-Segment Myocardial Infarction
    PCI for ST-Elevation Myocardial Infarction
    PCI for Chronic Stable Angina
      Multivessel PCI
      Left Main-Stem Disease
    Elective PCI and Noncardiac Surgery
Complications of Percutaneous Coronary Intervention
  Death
  Emergency Bypass Surgery

Myocardial Infarction
Vascular Complications and Hemorrhagic Complications
Contrast Nephropathy
Anaphylactoid Reactions
Restenosis
Advanced Technology in Percutaneous Coronary Intervention
  Drug-Eluting Stents
  Atherectomy Devices
  Thrombectomy and Distal Protection
  Intravascular Ultrasound
  Catheter-Based Therapy after Bypass
  Hybrid Coronary Revascularization

Pharmacology
  Surgical Considerations for Anticoagulation
Noncoronary Interventional Cardiac Procedures
  Balloon Mitral Valvuloplasty
  Balloon Aortic Valvuloplasty
  Percutaneous Endovascular Valve Replacement
  Ethanol Septal Ablation for Hypertrophic Obstructive Cardiomyopathy
  Closure of Patent Foramen Ovale and Atrial Septal Defect
  Percutaneous Circulatory-Assist Devices

Interventional cardiology is a subspecialty of medicine that treats a variety of cardiovascular disorders using catheter-based therapeutics. Despite its humble beginnings in 1977, interventional cardiology now includes an array of procedures and techniques for the treatment of ischemic, valvular, and congenital heart disorders. The growth and maturation of the discipline have closely paralleled the rapid influx of new technologies and pharmacotherapeutics. This chapter will review the historical development in interventional cardiology, indications and techniques, and the evolution of the devices and medications used during these procedures.

HISTORICAL PERSPECTIVE

After the refinement of diagnostic coronary angiographic catheters by Sones, Judkins, and Abrahms in the 1950s, the radiologist Charles Dotter performed the first endovascular dilation of a stenotic artery for therapeutic purposes in 1964.[1] Peripheral arterial lesions were treated with progressive co-axial catheter dilation to improve blood flow. Complications including hematoma formation and distal embolization were common, and this technique, referred to as "dottering," did not gain favor in the United States. However, European investigators continued to study and modify the technique. One such physician, Andreas Gruentzig, modified the Dotter multiple catheter system and developed a double-lumen catheter with a distensible balloon on the end that provided circumferential rather than coaxial pressure on the atherosclerotic plaque. However, inflation of the angioplasty balloon within the atherosclerotic plaque led to fissuring and cracking of the intima with stretching of the media and adventitia (Fig. 56-1).

Gruentzig performed the first *peripheral* balloon angioplasty in 1974 and then the first human coronary angioplasty in the operating room during elective coronary artery bypass surgery. When Gruentzig performed the first *percutaneous* transluminal coronary angioplasty (PTCA) in September 1977, the discipline of interventional cardiology was born.[2]

Initially, balloon angioplasty was offered as an alternative to bypass surgery in symptomatic patients with focal, proximal stenoses. Dilation of these arteries was usually associated with significant improvement in angina and in objective measures of ischemia.[3] However, the application of PTCA was limited to a small fraction of coronary lesions, as first-generation fixed-wire balloons lacked the ability to be steered and the profile needed to traverse distal and tortuous vessels. Easier to use over-the-wire and rapid-exchange systems began to replace the initial fixed balloon-on-wire system developed by Gruentzig. The development of conformable, low-profile balloons facilitated dilation of distal lesions in tortuous and calcified vessels.

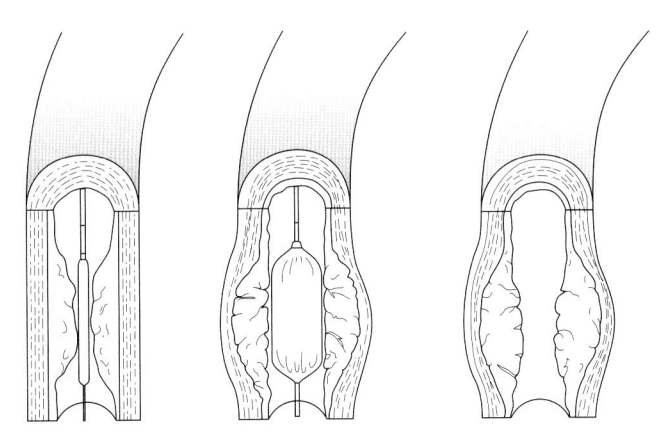

Figure 56-1
Mechanism of lumen enlargement with angioplasty. *(From Willerson JT, editor. Treatment of heart diseases. New York: Hower medical, 1992.)*

The major limitations of balloon angioplasty—abrupt vessel closure and restenosis—were addressed by the development of new devices in the late 1980s and early 1990s. With the introduction of atherectomy devices, laser balloon catheters, and endovascular stents, the more generic term *percutaneous coronary intervention* (PCI) replaced PTCA and referred to any catheter-based procedure intended to enlarge the lumen of a stenotic vessel. Athero-ablative techniques such as directional and rotational atherectomy and excimer laser angioplasty were marketed initially as replacements for balloon angioplasty. Although these techniques improved technical success in certain high-risk subsets such as fibrocalcific and bifurcation stenoses, they were technically difficult to perform, did not have a major impact on restenosis, and have largely been abandoned as stand-alone therapies.

The widespread use of endovascular prostheses, or stents, unequivocally improved the acute safety and long-term efficacy of catheter-based treatment. As a result, over 1 million PCIs are now performed each year in the United States to alleviate symptoms and reduce adverse cardiac events.[4] Stents were originally approved to seal dissection flaps and reverse acute vessel closure after PTCA by inhibiting elastic recoil in the arterial wall. The Gianturco-Roubin coil stent was the first such device approved in the United States, and it was approved on the basis of its ability to stabilize dissections and thus reduce the incidence of abrupt vessel closure and early complications.[5] In 1994, the balloon-expandable Palmaz-Schatz slotted tube stent was approved for elective use after two randomized trials showed significant reductions in angiographic restenosis.[6,7]

Thus, by the end of the millennium, stents became the default technology for catheter-based therapy, with 70% to 80% of all patients undergoing PCI receiving a stent. Despite the salutary effects of stents, restenosis still occurred in 10% to 30% of patients, who usually presented with recurrent ischemia, leading to repeat revascularization procedures. The use of adjunctive intravascular brachytherapy after balloon dilation of in-stent restenosis greatly reduced the need for subsequent revascularization procedures in patients who suffered restenosis despite stents, but it was associated with no significant impact on long-term outcome. As a result, this technology has been largely abandoned for use in coronary arteries.

In 2004, the U.S. Food and Drug Administration (FDA) approved the use of drug-eluting stents (DESs) that elute either sirolimus or paclitaxel into the vessel directly from a polymeric coating on the stent. The introduction of this technology dramatically reduced restenosis rates. Some of the initial enthusiasm for the DES was tempered by reports suggesting a higher incidence of very late stent thrombosis with DESs compared with bare metal stents (BMSs). This led to a more individualized approach to DES usage, with a BMS used in patients who had a high risk of hemorrhage or poor compliance with dual antiplatelet therapy. Presently, a DES is used in approximately 60% to 70% of all PCIs in the United States. Second-generation DESs featuring newer drugs, polymers, and stent delivery systems are now approved for use.

PERCUTANEOUS CORONARY INTERVENTION PROCEDURES

Coronary intervention, like diagnostic angiography, begins with placement of a vascular access sheath in the femoral, brachial, or radial artery. Although choice of the access site is at the discretion of the operator, over 95% of interventional procedures are performed via the femoral approach.[8] Radial or brachial arterial access may be preferable in certain circumstances such as iliofemoral occlusion, the presence of abdominal aortic aneurysm, recent femoral–popliteal bypass grafting, unfavorable body habitus, coagulopathy, or patient preference. Procedural success rates are comparable across all access sites, but radiation exposure and procedure times are slightly longer with brachial or radial procedures. Bleeding and vascular complications may be lower with brachial and radial access.[9]

Arterial access is obtained via percutaneous puncture of the anterior wall of the artery with a hollow needle.[10] A guide wire is advanced through the lumen of the needle to the aorta, and the needle is removed. A vascular sheath is then inserted over this wire. Large-lumen guiding catheters are then advanced through the arterial sheath and over the guide wire to the ascending aorta. The guide wire is removed, and selective cannulation of the coronary arteries or bypass conduits is undertaken. If a stenosis is repaired, a 0.014-inch wire is used to traverse the stenosis, and the equipment used to treat the stenosis is advanced coaxially over this wire into the vessel (Fig. 56-2).

PCI for Unstable Angina and Non-ST-Segment Myocardial Infarction

Current guidelines support the use of an early invasive management strategy for patients with unstable angina (UA) or non-ST-segment myocardial infarction (NSTEMI) who are at moderate or high risk for reinfarction or death, such as those with positive cardiac biomarkers, ST-segment changes on 12-lead electrocardiogram, or clinical parameters such as congestive heart failure, refractory angina, or arrhythmia.[11] A recent meta-analysis supported the use of an invasive

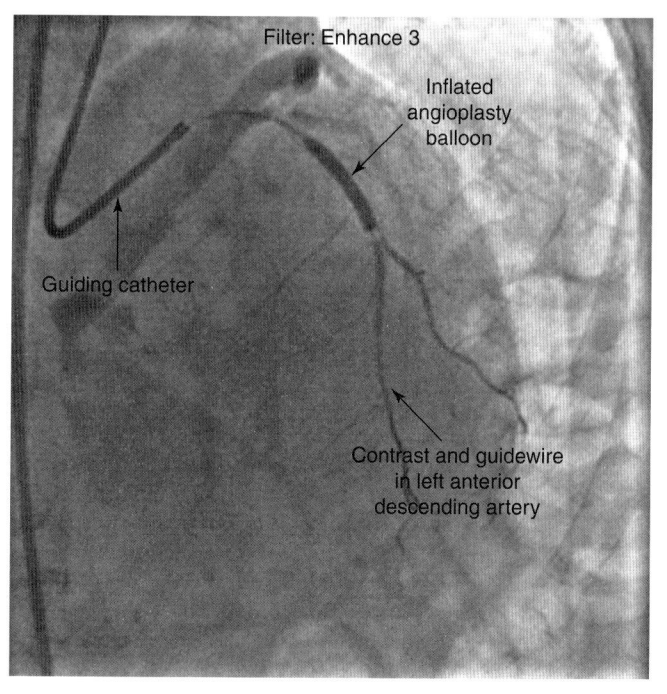

Figure 56–2
Angiogram during percutaneous coronary intervention of the left anterior descending artery.

strategy in high- and low-risk men, and in women only if serum biomarkers were elevated.[12] This strategy involves early administration of antithrombotic and antiplatelet medications as well as early angiography for further risk stratification. When the coronary anatomy is suitable, revascularization with coronary artery bypass grafting (CABG) or PCI is performed unless there is a strong contraindication. Typically, among moderate- and high-risk patients undergoing angiography for UA or NSTEMI, approximately 30% are managed without revascularization, 55% to 60% with PCI, and 10% to 15% with CABG.[13] Those at low clinical risk can be treated with a selective invasive strategy, and revascularization can be used for those with high-risk noninvasive test results or recurrent symptoms. One large randomized trial found that monotherapy with the direct thrombin inhibitor bivalirudin was not inferior to the combination of heparin and a platelet glycoprotein (GP) IIb/IIIa receptor blocker for patients with acute coronary syndromes undergoing PCI.[13]

PCI for ST-Elevation Myocardial Infarction

The benefits of mechanical or pharmacologic reperfusion therapy in the setting of acute ST-segment elevation myocardial infarction (STEMI) are well established. PCI has been shown to effectively reestablish normal epicardial coronary perfusion in greater than 90% of patients. Long-term patency rates exceed 85%, and both the risk of reinfarction and death are significantly reduced with PCI compared with fibrinolytic therapy.[1,14-16] Even if transport to a facility equipped for immediate PCI is required, catheter-based revascularization has been shown to have superior outcomes when compared with fibrinolytic therapy, assuming the artery can be opened expeditiously at an experienced center.[17] Patients who develop cardiogenic shock in the setting of acute myocardial infarction (MI) also seem to benefit from immediate revascularization with PCI or CABG. Improved survival at 6 months has been shown in a randomized trial comparing immediate revascularization, using either PCI or CABG, with initial medical stabilization using fibrinolytic therapy or delayed revascularization (or both). However, in the subset of patients older than 75 years who had acutely infarcted, reduced survival was noted when immediate revascularization was used, compared with medical stabilization followed by delayed revascularization.[18] Fibrinolytic therapy fails to restore normal blood flow in greater than 50% of patients, and PCI may also be indicated as salvage therapy in such cases. In those with persistent symptoms or persistent electrocardiographic evidence of ongoing infarction, "rescue" PCI has been shown to result in improved arterial patency with reductions in infarct size, early heart failure, and mortality.[19,20]

In comparison with PTCA alone, PCI with stent placement significantly reduces the incidence of death and ischemic target vessel revascularization, and the benefit is maintained for up to 5 years in patients with acute MI.[21-23] Current guidelines support a 90-minute door-to-balloon time.[24] Delays to reperfusion with PCI further decrease the mortality benefit of PCI over fibrinolysis, especially in higher-risk patients who present earlier in the MI period.[25] The term *facilitated* PCI refers to the use of fibrinolytics with or without GPIIb/IIIa inhibitors prior to PCI. Facilitated PCI has been associated with improved angiographic results prior to PCI, but not after PCI, and also with a significantly increased risk of bleeding, without a proven mortality benefit.[26] Therefore, there is not yet a proven beneficial role of facilitated PCI in STEMI.[27]

PCI for Chronic Stable Angina

Although medical therapy is preferred in patients with minimal symptoms and only a small area of ischemic myocardium, patients with large amounts of ischemic but viable myocardium in jeopardy have better anginal control if coronary revascularization is performed. Patients who are asymptomatic or whose symptoms can be controlled with medications, but who have high-risk noninvasive test findings have been shown to have lower rates of death or MI when treated with revascularization than when given medical therapy.[28,29]

The Clinical Outcomes Utilizing Revascularization and Aggressive Drug Evaluation (COURAGE) trial found that in the initial management of stable coronary artery disease, PCI and medical management did not significantly differ in their reduction of death, MI, or adverse cardiovascular events.[30] By 5 years, there was no significant difference in angina symptoms, although PCI was associated with earlier palliation of angina. The American College of Cardiology/American Heart Association (ACC/AHA) guidelines for percutaneous coronary intervention, however, suggest that asymptomatic or minimally symptomatic patients with coronary lesions that are 50% stenosed or greater in one or two arteries undergo PCI if there is a high likelihood of success and a low risk of morbidity and mortality, and if the arteries supply a moderate or large area of viable myocardium.[28,31] Thus, the decision to undergo elective PCI is based on the degree of myocardium at risk and failure of initial medical therapy.

Multivessel PCI

The comparative usefulness of multivessel PCI or CABG has been the subject of significant debate. Whether to perform PCI or CABG is often based on the severity and extent of disease, as well as on patient risk factors. Perceived benefits of CABG compared with PCI are described in Box 56-1. Various lesion subsets have been evaluated in registries that suggest a benefit for CABG compared with PTCA in patients with three-vessel disease

---

Box 56–1
Benefits of Coronary Artery Bypass Graft Surgery and Benefits of Percutaneous Coronary Intervention

Coronary Artery Bypass Graft
- Fewer subsequent procedures and hospitalizations
- More complete symptom relief at 1 and 3 years
- More complete initial revascularization
- Improved survival in diabetic patients

Percutaneous Coronary Intervention
- No excess mortality up to 5 years (except diabetics)
- Most patients asymptomatic at 1- and 3-year follow-ups
- Quicker recovery from initial procedure
- With stents, 80% to 90% of patients do not require coronary artery bypass graft surgery
- Lower cost, especially with stents

or severe stenosis of the proximal left anterior descending (LAD) artery (Fig. 56-3).[32] Randomized comparisons have been performed of CABG and PTCA (Table 56-1). The largest was the Bypass Angioplasty Revascularization Investigation (BARI) trial, which demonstrated that 5-year survival and survival free of Q-wave myocardial infarction did not differ significantly between the PTCA and CABG groups (86.3% versus 89.3%, and 78.4% versus 80.4%, respectively; $P = .19$). On the other hand, patients randomized to CABG were much less likely to require repeat revascularization. At 5-year follow-up, 54% of those assigned to PTCA had undergone additional revascularization procedures, compared with only 8% of the patients assigned to CABG. Nonetheless, 69% of patients initially assigned to PTCA avoided CABG over a 5-year period.[33] All of the other trials comparing PTCA and CABG have shown similar results with a fourfold to 10-fold-higher likelihood of repeat revascularization after initial PTCA, but no significant differences in mortality or MI.

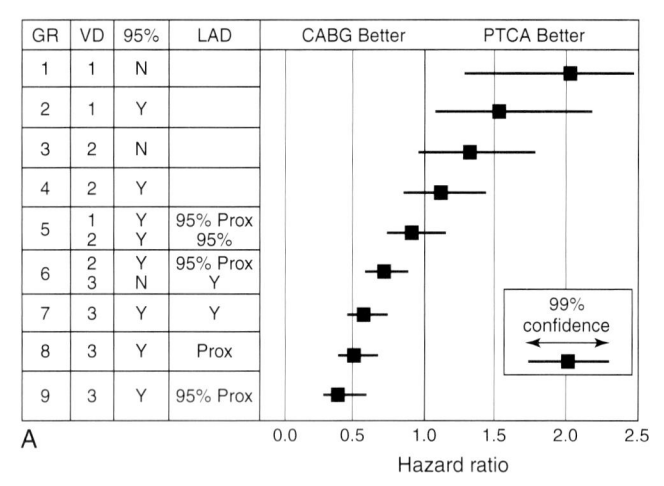

A meta-analysis of the randomized PTCA and CABG trials including 3371 patients (BARI was excluded as it was unpublished at the time)[34] reported that there were no significant differences in mortality or MI. Rates of repeat revascularization were significantly higher with PTCA, particularly during the first year of follow-up. Rates of angina were also higher at years 1 and 3 with PTCA, but the relative advantage of CABG diminished over time.[35,36]

Although the randomized trials have not demonstrated differences in mortality between PTCA and CABG, CABG may provide an important advantage for diabetic patients.[37] This finding is based primarily on the diabetic subgroup from the BARI trial ($n = 353$). At 5-year follow-up, all-cause mortality was 19.4% in the 180 patients assigned to CABG, and 34.5% among the 173 patients assigned to PCI ($P = .003$). Somewhat different results have been observed in registry studies, which provide important additional insight to the randomized controlled trials as only a very small percentage of all eligible patients were enrolled in the trials.[38] For example, in a registry of patients who were screened but not randomized in the BARI trial, long-term follow-up demonstrated no significant difference in mortality between diabetic patients undergoing CABG and those assigned to PCI.[39,39a] In contrast to the randomized trial, patients in the BARI registry had their initial revascularization strategy chosen by their physicians.

In the BARI registry, nearly twice as many patients were selected for PTCA ($n = 1189$) as CABG ($n = 625$), and as in the randomized trial, mortality at 7 years was similar for PTCA (13.9%) and CABG (14.2%) ($P = .66$). Seven-year mortality was higher for patients undergoing PTCA in the randomized trial than in the registry (19.1% versus 13.9%, $P < .01$) but not for those undergoing CABG (15.6% versus 14.2%, $P = .57$). The BARI registry data thus suggest that physicians were able to select patients for PTCA without compromising long-term survival either in the overall population or in treated diabetics.

Several studies have examined outcomes of multivessel BMS placement compared with CABG (see Table 56-1). Meta-analysis of the four major randomized trials comparing BMS and CABG reveals a 5-year safety profile for PCI that is similar to that for CABG. Lower repeat revascularization rates were found among the CABG patients (29.0% versus 7.9%, respectively; hazard ratio, 0.23; 95% confidence interval, 0.18-0.29; $P < .001$) (Fig. 56-4, Panel A) with no difference in rates of death, stroke, or MI (see Fig. 56-4, Panel B). No subgroup, including diabetic patients and those presenting with 3-vessel disease, was found to have a selective benefit with CABG.[40]

It was postulated that reductions in repeat revascularization rates associated with the DES would lower adverse events after multivessel PCI sufficiently to favor this strategy over CABG. Nevertheless, the optimal treatment for patients

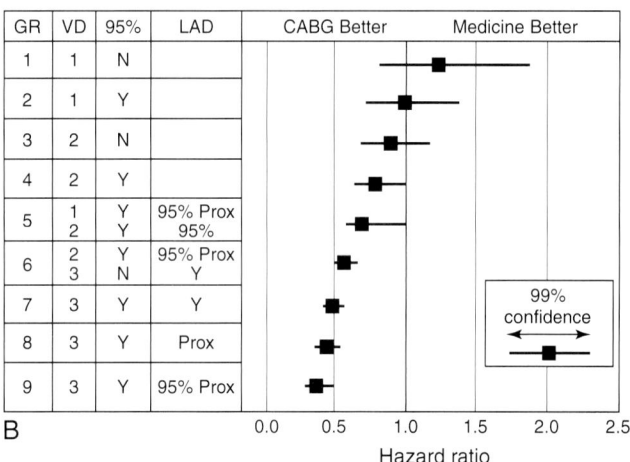

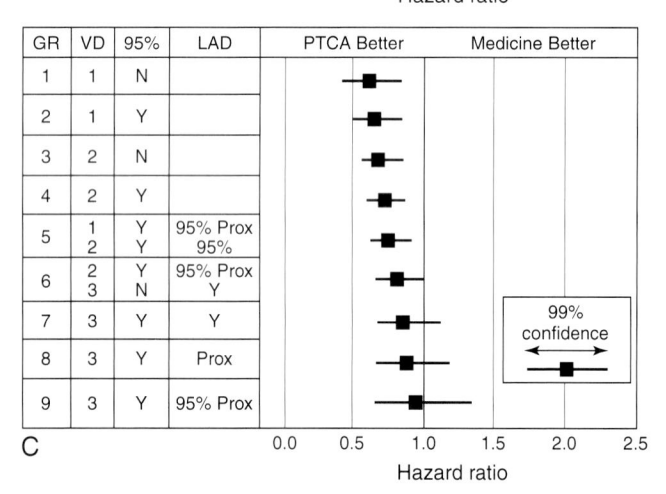

Figure 56–3
Adjusted hazard (mortality) ratios comparing coronary artery bypass grafting (CABG), percutaneous transluminal coronary angioplasty (PTCA), and medical therapy for nine coronary anatomy severity groups (GR). **A,** CABG versus PTCA. **B,** CABG versus medical therapy. **C,** PTCA versus medical therapy. *(From Jones RH, Kesler K, Phillips HR, et al.* J Thorac Cardiovasc Surg *1996;**111**:1013, with permission.)*

Table 56–1

Randomized Clinical Trials Comparing Coronary Artery Bypass Grafting (CABG) and Percutaneous Coronary Intervention (PCI)*

Trial	Patients (N)	Clinical Eligibility Criteria	Angiographic Eligibility Criteria	Endpoints	Comment
PTCA versus CABG Trials					
RITA	1011	Revascularization indicated and equivalent by PTCA or CABG	One, two, or three vessels > 50% stenotic; equivalent revascularization possible	Death, nonfatal MI, repeat revascularization, exercise test performance, angina control, LV function	45% had single-vessel disease
GABI	359	Revascularization indicated and equivalent by PTCA or CABG with age < 76 yr	Two or three vessels with ≥70% stenosis	Death, nonfatal MI, exercise test performance, angina control	IMA used in only 37% of CABG patients; >80% of patients had two-vessel disease
EAST	392	Revascularization indicated and equivalent by PTCA or CABG	Two or three vessels with ≥50% stenosis	Death, nonfatal MI, angiographic assessment, repeat revascularization, thallium-201 perfusion, quality of life, resource utilization	Repeat revascularization in 5.4% of PTCA group compared with 13% of patients having CABG
CABRI	1054	Revascularization indicated and equivalent by PTCA or CABG; evidence of ischemia necessary	Two or three vessels with ≥50% stenosis	Death, nonfatal MI, angiographic assessment, exercise test performance, angina control, heart failure	Complete revascularization with PTCA was not required
ERACI	127	Revascularization indicated and equivalent by PTCA or CABG	Two or three vessels with ≥70% stenosis	Death, nonfatal MI, repeat revascularization, angina control	Similar in-hospital and 1-yr survival and freedom from MI; less angina and fewer repeat procedures with CABG
BARI	1829	Revascularization indicated and equivalent by PTCA or CABG; stable or unstable angina pectoris or proven silent ischemia, with age 17 to 79 yr	Two or three vessels with ≥50% stenosis supplying two or three of the major myocardial territories	Death, nonfatal MI, repeat revascularization, exercise test performance, angina control, heart failure, LV function, resource utilization, quality of life	Overall survival similar with PTCA and CABG, but the late survival of treated diabetic patients better with CABG when IMA grafts were used
Multivessel Stenting versus CABG Trials					
ARTS	1205	Revascularization indicated and equivalent by PTCA or CABG; stable or unstable angina pectoris or proven silent ischemia	Two or three vessels with ≥50% stenosis supplying two or three of the major myocardial territories	Death, stroke, nonfatal MI, repeat revascularization, all-cause mortality, angina control, resource utilization	No significant difference between PCI and CABG in terms of death, stroke, or MI; PCI was associated with a greater need for repeat revascularization
ERACI-II	450	Revascularization indicated and equivalent by PTCA or CABG; stable or unstable angina pectoris or proven silent ischemia	Two or three vessels with ≥70% stenosis in one vessel and >50% stenosis supplying two or three of the major myocardial territories	Composite of all-cause mortality, nonfatal Q-wave MI, stroke or repeat revascularization within 30 days	Better survival and freedom from MI with PCI and with CABG; repeat revascularization higher in PCI group
SOS	988	Revascularization indicated and equivalent by PTCA or CABG; stable or unstable angina pectoris or proven silent ischemia	Two or three vessels with significant stenosis in one vessel and >50% stenosis supplying two or three of the major myocardial territories	Composite of death or nonfatal MI or all-cause mortality; repeat revascularization, angina control, LV function, resource utilization	Significantly higher number of repeat revascularizations with PCI; no difference in composite measure of death and Q-wave MI; fewer deaths in the CABG group

(Continued)

Table 56-1
Randomized Clinical Trials Comparing Coronary Artery Bypass Grafting (CABG) and Percutaneous Coronary Intervention (PCI)*—cont'd

Trial	Patients (N)	Clinical Eligibility Criteria	Angiographic Eligibility Criteria	Endpoints	Comment
AWESOME	454	Revascularization indicated and equivalent by PTCA or CABG and risk factors for adverse outcome with CABG	Two or three vessels with significant stenosis	Death	Comparable survival between PCI and CABG in patients with medically refractory myocardial ischemia, with higher repeat revascularization in PCI group
MASS-II	611	Revascularization indicated and equivalent by PTCA or CABG; stable angina pectoris or proven silent ischemia	Two or three vessels with ≥70% stenosis	Cardiac death, nonfatal acute MI, and unstable angina	Included medical therapy arm; no difference in cardiac death or MI among patients in the CABG, medical, or PCI therapy groups; significantly greater need for repeat revascularization in patients who underwent PCI

IMA, internal mammary artery; LV, left ventricular; MI, myocardial infarction; PTCA, percutaneous transluminal coronary angioplasty.
Adapted from Smith Jr SC, Feldman TE, Hirshfeld Jr JW, et al. ACC/AHA/SCAI 2005 Guideline Update for Percutaneous Coronary Intervention: a report of the American College of Cardiology/American Heart Association Task Force on Practice Guidelines (ACC/AHA/SCAI Writing Committee to Update the 2001 Guidelines for Percutaneous Coronary Intervention). J Am Coll Cardiol 2006;47:e1-121.
*see references 5-7, 21, 23, 26, 27, 29, 30, 33, 36-39, 42-45, 63, 71, 75, 76, 77, 84-86, 89, 90, 98-101, 103-108, 121, 134, 166, 172.

with multivessel disease remains uncertain. Registry data suggest equivalent outcomes with the DES and CABG among nondiabetic patients but a continued advantage for CABG among diabetic patients.[41] The Synergy between Percutaneous Coronary Intervention with TAXUS and Cardiac Surgery (SYNTAX) trial reported low repeat revascularization rates at 1 year among patients receiving the paclitaxel-eluting stent, compared with CABG.[42] There was no statistically significant difference in risk of death (4.3% versus 3.5%, respectively; $P = .37$) or heart attack (4.8% versus 3.2%, respectively; $P = .11$). The risk of stroke was significantly greater for bypass surgery (0.6% for PCI versus 2.2% for bypass; $P = .003$). The combined endpoint of myocardial infarction, stroke, death, or revascularizaton was higher with PCI (17.8% versus 12.1%; $P = .0015$), mainly driven by differences in rates of repeat revascularization (13.7% versus 5.9%; $P < .05$).[42] For patients with two- and three-vessel coronary artery disease, a large, observational registry from New York State found a lower incidence of death and MI for those undergoing CABG than for those receiving a DES.[43] However, as with all observational studies, unmeasured confounders may have had an impact on the results. The FREEDOM (Future Revascularization Evaluation in Patients with Diabetes Mellitus: Optimal Management of Multivessel Disease) trial is an ongoing study evaluating DESs or CABG for diabetic patients with multivessel disease.[44]

Left Main-Stem Disease

Stent placement in the left main coronary artery (LMCA) can be performed with high rates of procedural success. As is the case with multivessel PCI, PCI of the LMCA is associated with higher rates of repeat revascularization. The DES has rapidly and largely replaced bare metal stents for PCI of the unprotected left main. However, PCI is still chosen less frequently than CABG for unprotected left main revascularization. Registries describing outcomes after DES implantation or CABG for LMCA stenosis have demonstrated higher rates of repeat revascularization with PCI and lower mortality rates with CABG.[43,45] It is unknown whether differences in patient risk and angiographic parameters affect these results. In most cases, CABG should be performed for those with LMCA disease who are candidates for surgery.[46]

Elective PCI and Noncardiac Surgery

The incidence of perioperative cardiac events ranges from 2% to 6%, depending on the type of surgery performed and the patient's clinical risk factors. Most studies have focused on patients requiring vascular surgery. It is currently recommended that patients with three or more clinical risk factors and poor functional capacity (class IIa) may undergo further testing before vascular surgery. Those with one or two clinical risk factors and poor functional capacity undergoing intermediate-risk surgery or who have good functional capacity prior to vascular surgery (class IIb) may also undergo testing.[47] The current ACC guidelines recommend PCI only for those who would receive a benefit of revascularization independent of surgery. Further cardiac testing is recommended prior to surgery only if it will change management.[48] Moreover, surgery soon after PCI may be associated with adverse outcomes. Because uninterrupted antiplatelet therapy is necessary after stent implantation, bleeding complications may result in the perioperative period, or there may be catastrophic consequences caused by stent thrombosis resulting from discontinuation

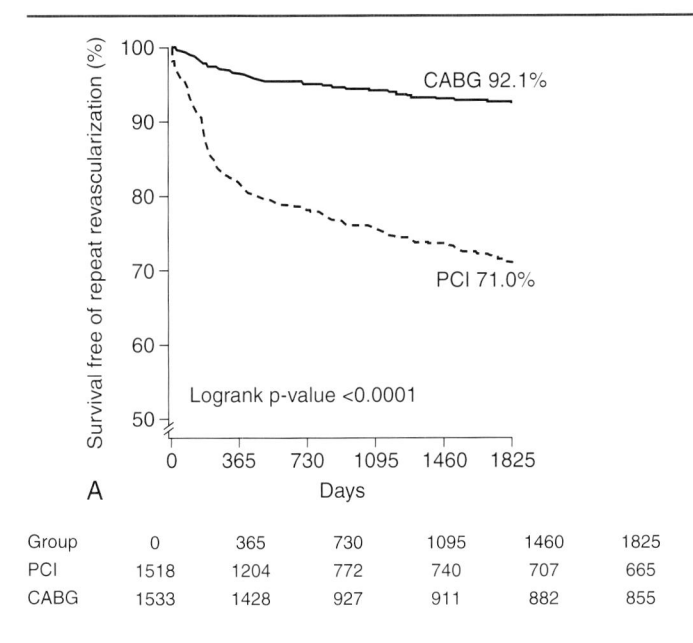

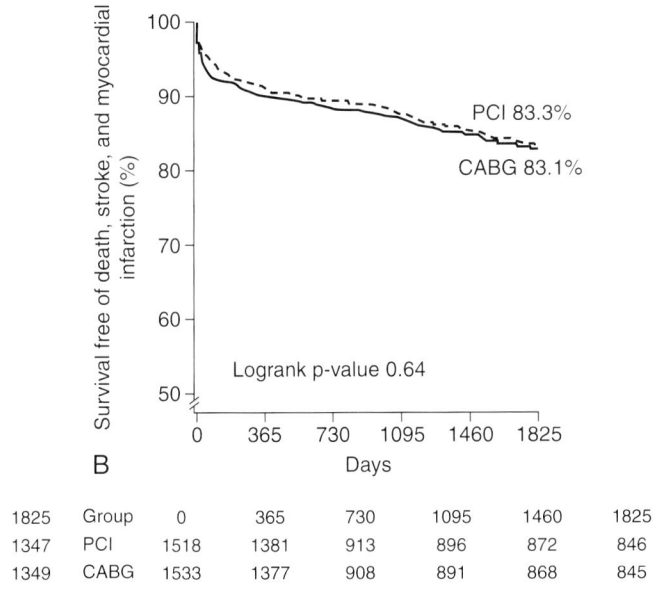

Figure 56–4
Kaplan-Meier event-free survival analysis of repeat revascularization (**A**), and death, stroke, or myocardial infarction (**B**). CABG, coronary artery bypass graft surgery; PCI, percutaneous coronary intervention.

of antiplatelet medications or from a hypercoagulable state induced by surgery.

In a small cohort of 192 patients, the highest risk of cardiovascular events in the postoperative period occurred in those who discontinued clopidogrel prematurely after PCI (30.7% versus 0%, $P = .026$).[49] Moreover, early surgery (at less than 6 weeks) after BMS placement has been associated with a higher incidence of adverse events such as death and MI[50] and should be avoided when possible. Current guidelines suggest that after BMS placement, dual antiplatelet therapy (aspirin plus clopidogrel) should be administered for at least 1 month (or a minimum of 2 weeks if significant bleeding occurs), and for 3 months after sirolimus, and for 6 months after paclitaxel-coated stents, with a suggested duration of at least 1 year for all three (class Ib).[28,31,51]

COMPLICATIONS OF PERCUTANEOUS CORONARY INTERVENTION

Death

Mortality can occur during PCI from a variety of complications, including anaphylactoid reactions, acute MI, pericardial tamponade, stroke, or vascular trauma. Since stents have been used, mortality rates associated with elective coronary intervention have fallen to less than 0.3%.[52,53] Patients at higher risk include older adults, those undergoing emergency PCI or PCI on saphenous vein grafts, and those with decompensated heart failure or reduced cardiac ejection fraction, end-stage renal disease, cardiogenic shock, or acute MI.[14,54]

Emergency Bypass Surgery

Although technical improvement made PTCA success rates reach approximately 60%,[15] successful PTCA was limited by an inability to expand balloons in fibrocalcific lesions. In addition, the barotrauma associated with dilation of stenotic lesions may lead to medial dissection and many of the complications of angioplasty. Abrupt vessel closure occurs in approximately 5% of cases and is caused by a combination of factors including arterial dissection, vascular recoil, vasospasm, and thrombosis. Flow-limiting dissections and thrombosis were treated with prolonged balloon inflations and aggressive anticoagulation, but despite these treatments, emergency bypass surgery was required in almost 50% of cases of abrupt vessel closure. In the pre-stent era, emergency surgery was required in approximately 3% to 5% of procedures,[15] with significantly greater morbidity and mortality than seen with elective bypass surgery.[55-57] Cardiac tamponade may develop on occasion because of vessel perforation with the coronary guide wire or with balloon dilation.

The widespread use of stents has led to an evolution of the role of the cardiac surgeon in managing acute complications of PCI. During the initial development of PTCA, immediate surgical backup was necessary, because not infrequently, acute vessel closure necessitated urgent surgical revascularization. The incidence of emergency cardiac surgery for failed PTCA was approximately 5% to 7% in the 1990s.[58,59] The need for emergency surgery has fallen dramatically in recent years, however, paralleling improvements in stent technology and pharmacologic therapy, and it now occurs in less than 1% of cases.[18,60] Registry data support the safety of elective PCI in community hospitals without the presence of cardiac surgery backup for low-risk patients.[61,62] Although the incidence of emergency surgery is low, the ACC/AHA guidelines for PCI do not support the performance of elective PCI without surgical backup.[28] A large, prospective trial, MASS-COMM, is currently randomizing patients in Massachusetts to PCI in a hospital without on-site surgical backup versus PCI at an institute with on-site surgical backup.

The improvements in immediate PCI outcomes and the recognition of improved survival with PCI performed in the setting of acute MI have led to the development of programs performing primary PCI without surgical backup. The C-PORT study confirmed the safety of primary PCI without surgical backup.[63]

It is well known that operator experience and hospital volume play an important role in these cases, as PCI for acute MI is often more technically demanding than routine PCI.

Various studies have correlated both limited operator experience (<75cases/yr) and low hospital volume (<200 cases/yr) with less favorable outcomes for primary PCI.[64-66]

PCI for acute MI at institutions without surgical backup is currently performed, and published guidelines consist of requirements for operator and hospital volume, ready availability of necessary interventional and hemodynamic monitoring equipment, rigorous quality assurance, and a formalized protocol for immediate (<1 hour) transfer for emergency CABG.[28] Certain lesion subsets that would ordinarily be attempted by operators with onsite surgical backup are proscribed when surgical backup is not available. Because of the risk of catheter injury to the left main artery, culprit stenoses (i.e., occluded 60% or more) that are downstream from a lesion in the left main coronary artery should be avoided. When there is normal flow in the infarct artery, and either the patient has three-vessel disease or the culprit lesion is long or angulated, PCI should be avoided as well. High-grade left main coronary disease or hemodynamic instability should prompt rapid transfer to an institution equipped to perform bypass surgery, preferably after placement of an intra-aortic balloon counterpulsation device.[28]

Emergency bypass surgery is performed mainly for persistent abrupt vessel closure, extensive vessel dissection, unstable left main coronary artery stenosis or injury, uncontrolled vessel perforation, and cardiac tamponade. The Society of Thoracic Surgeons reported an operative mortality that exceeds 5% for patients requiring emergency bypass surgery within 6 hours of PTCA.[60,67] Although the frequency of emergency surgery continues to fall, and surgical technique and postprocedure management continue to improve, patient outcomes continue to be significantly worse than for elective surgery. The poor outcomes in this population are not unexpected, because as PCI has improved, the patients who cannot be salvaged and require emergency surgery comprise a population with more unfavorable risk factors and comorbidities. Considerations such as conduit selection, myocardial protection, and the need for coronary artery repair make the surgical procedure technically demanding.

Myocardial Infarction

Although Q-wave MI occurs in less than 1% of patients, the incidence of postprocedure myonecrosis (as measured by elevation of cardiac markers such as creatinine phosphokinase [CPK]-MB and troponins) may be found in almost one third of patients and is more common after atherectomy procedures, and after PCI performed in thrombus-containing lesions, in the setting of acute coronary syndromes, or for treatment of saphenous vein graft disease.[68-70] Periprocedural myocardial infarction may result from acute vessel closure, perforation, or, most commonly, embolization of thrombus or atheroma.

Other complications of coronary intervention include arrhythmias, stroke caused by spontaneous intracerebral hemorrhage with anticoagulation, and stroke caused by embolic debris or equipment from catheters, arteries, cardiac chambers, or valves.

Vascular Complications and Hemorrhagic Complications

The use of antithrombotic, fibrinolytic, and antiplatelet agents, as well as aggressive anticoagulation and prolonged sheath placement is associated with an increase in vascular complications.[71] Impaired coagulation and the need for larger-lumen catheters for coronary intervention (typically 6 to 8 French) lead to more frequent access-site complications compared with simple diagnostic angiography. Complications include hematoma (1% to 5%), retroperitoneal hemorrhage, and pseudoaneurysm (1%) formation.[72] Patients with significant peripheral vascular disease are at higher risk for such complications. Infrequent (<1%) complications include arteriovenous fistula formation, infection, cholesterol embolization, and vascular occlusion. Femoral access-site complications requiring surgical repair or transfusion occur in 2% to 5% of cases. Traditionally, surgery was performed to close pseudoaneurysms greater than 2 cm in diameter because of significant risk of spontaneous rupture. Ultrasound-guided injection of thrombin into the pseudoaneurysm has obviated the need for open surgical repair. Surgical exploration is undertaken for repair of fistulae and arterial lacerations, and in cases of arterial occlusion and uncontrolled bleeding leading to hemodynamic compromise.

Contrast Nephropathy

Nephropathy induced by contrast media used for angiography is an important clinical concern. The occurrence of contrast agent–induced nephropathy is associated with poorer clinical outcomes.[73,74] Although most of these cases are self-limited, a fraction of patients require short-term dialysis and some require permanent dialysis. The risk of occurrence is less than 1% overall. Patients with baseline renal insufficiency or diabetes, or those who receive large volumes of contrast material are at highest risk. The risk in this population is more than 35%.[73,74] Additional risk factors include dehydration, advanced age, large contrast volume, multiple myeloma, exposure to nephrotoxic drugs, congestive heart failure, and liver disease.

The risk of contrast agent–induced nephropathy can be reduced by hydration, with either normal saline or sodium bicarbonate, before and after the procedure. Forced diuresis, calcium antagonists, dopamine, and atrial natriuretic peptide have not been shown to be beneficial.[75,76] The use of an iso-osmolar contrast agent, iodixanol, was compared with a low-osmolar contrast agent, iohexol, in high-risk patients, and was shown to reduce the incidence of contrast-induced nephropathy.[77] There is evidence that acetylcysteine, selective dopamine-1 receptor agonists, and theophylline may be beneficial in some cases, but the role for these agents requires further study.[75,78,79]

Anaphylactoid Reactions

The term *anaphylaxis* is reserved for allergic, IgE-mediated immediate hypersensitivity reactions. *Anaphylactoid* reactions are clinically similar to anaphylaxis but are not IgE-mediated. Both anaphylaxis and anaphylactoid reactions can produce immediate, potentially life-threatening systemic reactions because of the massive release of mediators such as histamine from mast cells and basophils.

The incidence of death from contrast media complications in the catheterization laboratory is estimated at 1 death per 55,000. Mild cases may be associated with a variety of symptoms such as itching, urticaria, flushing, cough, sneezing, wheezing, abdominal cramps, diarrhea, headache, back and chest pain, nausea, vomiting, fever, and chills. More severe reactions lead to dyspnea, a sense of impending doom, and hypotension, potentially resulting in cardiovascular collapse and death. Depending on the severity of the clinical findings, patients may require treatment with catecholamines, antihistamines, corticosteroids, or intravenous fluids. In patients with prior reactions, pretreatment with corticosteroids and diphenhydramine, and the use of nonionic contrast media have significantly reduced the potential of recurrent reaction.[80]

Restenosis

Despite successful initial luminal enlargement, the Achilles' heel of balloon angioplasty has always been restenosis. After the acute arterial injury that is a prerequisite for luminal enlargement, a complex interaction between the vessel and blood elements occurs. Although these processes are often viewed as pathologic, they actually recapitulate all of the elements of wound healing. Immediately after balloon dilation, 20% to 30% of the initial gain may be lost because of vascular recoil. Platelets, neutrophils, and macrophages adhere to the site of injury, resulting in an inflammatory response and secretion of a variety of mitogens. Many of these growth factors, such as platelet-derived growth factor, stimulate a change in smooth muscle cells from a contractile to a proliferative phenotype. Matrix metalloproteinases promote smooth muscle cell migration from the media to the intima. The combination of smooth muscle cell proliferation, neointimal hyperplasia, and elastic recoil (i.e., negative remodeling) is a ubiquitous process that in most vessels results in mild to moderate renarrowing; however, in 20% to 50% of patients without stents, it may result in a clinically significant restenosis that may continue for 6 to 12 months.

Although angiographic restenosis may be silent clinically, many patients present with recurrent angina or provocable ischemia during functional testing. It is now recognized that restenosis may not be clinically benign: about 10% of patients with restenosis present with acute MI.[81] Risk factors for restenosis after PTCA have been well documented (Table 56-2). In large populations, late lumen loss follows a near-Gaussian distribution, with approximately 50% of the initial gain in lumen diameter lost by 6 to 8 months.[82] The slope of the gain–loss relationship is approximately 0.5, and it is similar across all devices used for PCI. The reduction in restenosis rates observed after BMS placement is entirely explained by the ability of these stents to safely maximize acute gain, thereby allowing greater tolerance for late loss. The DES also decreased neointimal and smooth muscle cell growth, reducing late loss as well, in addition to the greater acute gain seen with the BMS.

Nevertheless, restenosis remained a problem in interventional cardiology, with rates ranging from 12% to greater than 50% in certain subgroups with the BMS (see Table 56-2).[17,83] The advent of the DES introduced local drug delivery from a polymer-coating on the stent consisting of anti-inflammatory and antiproliferative medications with a slow controlled release that effectively reduced the incidence of restenosis from 30% to less than 10%.[84-86] Restenosis after DES placement is generally treated with repeat PCI, with or without another DES, or with CABG.

ADVANCED TECHNOLOGY IN PERCUTANEOUS CORONARY INTERVENTION

Drug-Eluting Stents

Drug-eluting stents were approved for use in 2004 for the treatment of symptomatic ischemic disease in discrete de novo lesions of less than 30 mm long in native coronary arteries with a reference luminal diameter between 2.5 and 3.5 mm for the Cypher (sirolimus-coated stent), and less than 28 mm long in native arteries between 2.5 and 3.75 mm in diameter for the Taxus (paclitaxel-coated stent). As mentioned, with local delivery of polymer coatings eluting either paclitaxel, sirolimus, zotarolimus, or everolimus, smooth muscle cell proliferation and neointimal hyperplasia are inhibited, and the incidence of restenosis is drastically reduced. These drugs inhibit neointimal and smooth muscle cell proliferation by either cytostatic or cytocidal inhibition of the cell cycle. Drugs from the "limus" family also have anti-inflammatory and antimigratory properties. Currently, 60% to 70% of coronary stents are DESs. Many studies have shown a sustained, long-term benefit of DES over BMS in reducing target-lesion revascularization.[87-90]

Off-label DES implantation is estimated by the FDA to account for 60% of its current use. Off-label uses include stenting in bifurcation stenoses, ostial or totally occluded lesions, bypass grafts, lesions longer than 30 mm, vessels smaller in diameter than 2.5 mm or larger than 3.5 to 3.75 mm, left main stenosis, or restenosis. The FDA currently concludes that off-label use of a DES may be associated with increased risks compared with a BMS, but recent studies suggest that these higher-risk lesions may actually benefit to a greater degree than on-label uses.[91,92]

A major concern with the use of a DES is the development of stent thrombosis. Stent thrombosis is classified as early (0 to 30 days), late (31 to 365 days), or very late (greater than 365 days), with a level of certainty defined as either probable, possible, or definite. Definite stent thrombosis requires angiographic or autopsy-based evidence of thrombus or occlusion. Probable stent thrombosis is defined as unexplained death within 30 days of PCI, or acute MI in the territory of the stented lesion. Finally, possible stent thrombosis includes all unexplained deaths occurring after 30 days of the index procedure.[93]

Table 56–2
Risk Factors for Restenosis

Patient Factors	Lesion Factors	Technical Factors
Diabetes	Small vessels	High residual post-treatment stenosis
End-stage renal disease	Left anterior descending location	
Unstable coronary syndrome	Long lesions	
	Prior restenosis Ostial location Bifurcation	

Initial pivotal studies showed the incidence of stent thrombosis to be low (0.6% for DES and 0.8% for BMS),[84,85] with no significant difference in stent thrombosis between BMS and DES. Studies have shown similar rates of stent thrombosis in the first year when comparing BMS and DES but then a not statistically significant trend toward increased rates of stent thrombosis with the DES.[94-96] Because of concern that the premature disruption of dual antiplatelet therapy may increase the risk for late in-stent thrombosis, current guidelines recommend uninterrupted dual antiplatelet therapy for at least 3 months for the sirolimus-eluting stent and 6 months for the paclitaxel-eluting stent, and preferably 1 year of uninterrupted therapy. It is recommended that clopidogrel be continued for at least 1 month in those receiving a BMS (minimum of 2 weeks if there is an increased risk of bleeding) and ideally up to 6 months.[51]

Atherectomy Devices

Atherectomy devices were designed to achieve luminal enlargement by plaque removal rather than dissection and vascular stretching. Directional coronary atherectomy involved a cup-shaped cutter housed in a rigid cylinder in which a window was etched. A balloon was attached to the opposite wall of the cylinder. During balloon inflation, the atheroma was directed into the housing, shaved by the rotating cutter, and compressed into the nose cone for removal. This device was used successfully for treatment of bifurcation, ostial, eccentric, and ulcerated lesions. However, because of technical difficulty and a high incidence of periprocedural MI, directional coronary atherectomy is no longer available.

Rotational atherectomy (RA, or PTCRA) incorporates a nickel-plated, brass burr coated with diamond chips on its leading edge (Fig. 56-5). The burr is rotated at 140,000 to 200,000 revolutions per minute, and using the principle of differential cutting, pulverizing plaque into 5- to 12-micron particles. These particles are cleared by the reticuloendothelial system. Rotational atherectomy is currently used as an "enabling device" prior to PTCA or stenting, to improve vascular compliance in undilatable devices or to debulk heavily calcified plaque.

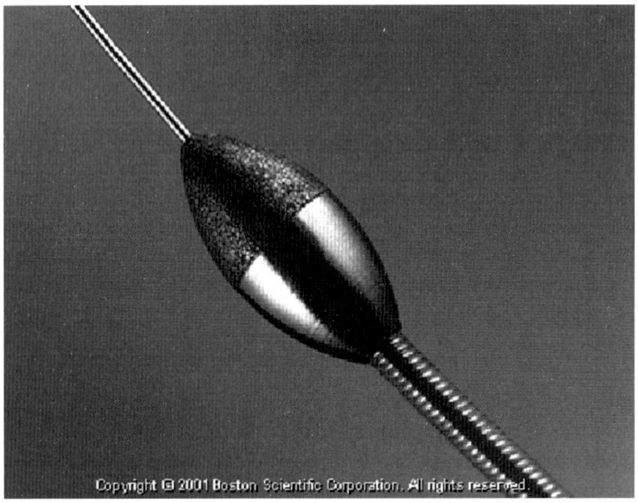

Figure 56–5
Rotational atherectomy catheter. *(Courtesy of Boston Scientific, Inc., Natick, MA.)*

Thrombectomy and Distal Protection

Treatment of thrombus-containing lesions has always been a challenge for the interventional cardiologist. Intraluminal thrombus is associated with a higher risk of periprocedural complications.[97] Current thrombectomy devices use a variety of techniques including transluminal extraction using a rotating helical auger at the tip of the catheter in conjunction with a luminal suction to remove clots, or using an aspiration device, the Angiojet (Possis Medical, Minneapolis, MN), or simple suction thrombectomy using a variety of hollow-lumen catheters.

The Vein Graft AngioJet Study (VEGAS)-II trial compared intracoronary fibrinolysis with thrombectomy and demonstrated a reduction in 30-day major adverse cardiac events with thrombectomy compared with prolonged infusion of urokinase.[98] Despite effective thrombectomy, distal embolization remains common during treatment of saphenous vein graft disease and in the setting of acute coronary syndromes. This observation is best explained by the finding that atheroembolism frequently occurs during manipulation of friable atheroma. This has led to the development of other interventional devices aimed at reducing distal embolization of plaque and thrombus during intervention on high-risk lesions. The PercuSurge GuardWire is a "balloon occlusion protection" device that uses a coronary guide wire with a hollow hypotube that allows inflation of an occlusion balloon at the end of the wire. Inflation creates a static column of blood in the vessel, trapping any debris liberated during balloon inflation or stent deployment. A sump catheter is then advanced over the wire and used to aspirate the static column of blood and debris. The Saphenous Vein Graft Angioplasty Free of Emboli Randomized trial (SAFER) demonstrated a 50% reduction in periprocedural MI for patients randomized to the GuardWire compared with conventional systems during intervention on saphenous vein bypass grafts. These devices are approved only for use during saphenous vein graft intervention and have not been proved beneficial in native coronary arteries.[99-101]

Second-generation devices employ balloon occlusion devices combined with a flush and extraction mechanism and filters mounted at the end of the wire to trap embolized material. The latter have the theoretical advantage over the distal protection balloons that antegrade blood flow can be preserved, limiting ischemic time resulting from occlusion.[102] Randomized comparisons of these devices demonstrated equivalent outcomes.[103,104]

The use of thrombectomy in acute MI remains controversial. The Thrombus Aspiration during Primary Percutaneous Coronary Intervention (TAPAS) study[105] showed improved myocardial perfusion, ST-segment resolution, and 1-year survival with manual thrombectomy.[106] In contrast, the Vacuum Aspiration Thrombus Removal (VAMPIRE) trial failed to show a mortality benefit with thrombus aspiration, but appropriate antiplatelet and antithrombotic therapy was not used in this study.[107]

As with manual thrombectomy, there is controversy regarding the value of mechanical thrombectomy. In the AiMI (AngioJet Rheolytic Thrombectomy in Patients Undergoing Primary Angioplasty for Acute Myocardial Infarction) trial, a total of 480 patients were randomized to rheolytic thrombectomy with AngioJet or conventional primary angioplasty. The primary endpoint was infarct size estimated by technetium-99m sestamibi. This trial showed a paradoxically larger infarct size and higher mortality in patients treated with thrombectomy than in those treated with conventional primary angioplasty.[108] Given the lack of a gold standard or an appropriately powered trial to evaluate reperfusion, there is conflicting evidence as to the effectiveness of thrombectomy in acute MI.

Intravascular Ultrasound

Intravascular ultrasound (IVUS) is an invasive tomographic imaging modality that provides visualization not only of the vessel lumen but also of the vessel itself, and therefore it can provide information regarding vessel cross-sectional area, plaque characteristics, and stent expansion, and it is helpful when angiography is inconclusive or inadequate. Newer IVUS devices allow in vivo histopathologic characterization. Techniques to identify vulnerable plaques using IVUS are currently in development.

Catheter-Based Therapy after Bypass

In the first year after bypass surgery, approximately 8% of patients require repeat revascularization because of a recurrence of ischemia.[109] Over time, the number of patients who develop recurrences of symptoms increases substantially. The recurrences result from saphenous vein graft (SVG) attrition in most instances, although progression of native vessel disease also contributes to recurrent ischemia. Approximately 7% of grafts fail in the first week, and another 15% to 20% in the first year. Thereafter, 1% to 2% per year fail during the first 5 to 6 years, and this increases to 3% to 5% per year in years 6 to 10 postoperatively.[110] At 10 years postoperatively, approximately half of all SVG conduits are occluded, and only half of the remaining patent grafts are free of significant disease.[28] Arterial conduit grafts, especially the left internal mammary, are relatively resistant to atherosclerosis. Because of the increase in morbidity associated with repeat CABG,[111] PCI, if technically possible, is the preferred strategy. Graft failure in the first month of surgery is usually the result of thrombosis resulting from nonlaminar flow,[112] whereas perianastomotic stenosis is usually the culprit 1 to 12 months after surgery and histologically resembles restenosis after PCI. The latter responds well to balloon dilation.

Ischemia occurring more than 1 year after surgery may result from progression of atherosclerotic disease in the native coronary vessels or accelerated atherosclerosis in bypass grafts.[113] As the disease in these grafts progresses, the plaques become diffuse and are often degenerated, bulky, and thrombotic. Vein graft atherosclerotic lesions often lack thick fibrous caps. PCI on these vessels is associated with substantial risk of distal embolization and periprocedural MI.[114] This risk may be reduced by the use of thrombectomy devices and embolic protection devices.[98,99] Even if PCI of an SVG is performed successfully without adverse events, recurrent ischemic events are common due to restenosis, and to rapidly progressive disease in the SVG and native vessels.[113] Such patients, particularly those without a patent arterial conduit to the LAD artery, should receive serious consideration for repeat surgical revascularization. A DES in vein grafts has been shown to reduce restenosis compared with a BMS, although the recently published[113a] RRISC (Reduction of Restenosis in Saphenous Vein Grafts with Cypher Sirolimus-Eluting Stent) trial reported an excess of late mortality with DES. Consensus guidelines have been published for PCI after CABG (Box 56-2).[51]

Hybrid Coronary Revascularization

Although bypass surgery has longer patency rates using left internal mammary artery (LIMA) grafts and decreased target lesion revascularization, the inherent limitations of vein graft conduits and improved outcomes with DES may require a multidisciplinary approach to revascularization. Therefore, these "hybrid revascularizations" use both stenting internal mammary grafting through a mini-thoracotomy or minimally invasive direct coronary artery bypass grafting (MIDCAB). In one study, the incidence of adverse cardiovascular events was decreased in the hybrid arm using DES compared with off-pump bypass surgery, both in the early postoperative period and at 1 year.[115] This approach requires further investigation.

Box 56-2

Recommendations for Percutaneous Coronary Intervention (PCI) in Patients with Prior Coronary Artery Bypass Graft (CABG) Surgery

Class I: Conditions for which there is evidence for and/or general agreement that the procedure or treatment is useful and effective

- Patients with early ischemia (usually within 30 days) after bypass surgery.
- It is recommended that distal embolic protection devices be used when technically feasible in patients undergoing PCI to saphenous vein grafts.

Class IIa: Conditions where there is conflicting evidence, but weight of evidence/opinion is in favor of usefulness/efficacy

- Patients with ischemia occurring 1 to 3 years postoperatively and preserved left ventricular function with discrete lesions in graft conduits.
- Disabling angina secondary to new disease in a native coronary circulation. (If angina is not typical, the objective evidence of ischemia should be obtained.)
- Patients with diseased vein grafts >3 years after bypass surgery.
- PCI is reasonable and technically feasible in patients with a patent left internal mammary artery graft who have clinically significant obstructions in other vessels.

Class III: Conditions for which there is evidence and/or general agreement that the procedure/treatment is not useful/effective, and in some cases may be harmful.

- PCI to chronic total vein graft occlusions.
- Patients with multivessel disease, failure of or multiple saphenous vein grafts, and impaired left ventricular function unless repeat CABG poses excessive risk due to severe comorbid conditions.

From Smith Jr SC, Feldman TE, Hirshfeld Jr JW, et al. ACC/AHA/SCAI 2005 Guideline Update for Percutaneous Coronary Intervention: a report of the American College of Cardiology/American Heart Association Task Force on Practice Guidelines (ACC/AHA/SCAI Writing Committee to Update the 2001 Guidelines for Percutaneous Coronary Intervention). J Am Coll Cardiol 2006;47:e1-121.

PHARMACOLOGY

Surgical Considerations for Anticoagulation

With current data, it is generally recommended that elective CABG be delayed for 5 to 7 days after the administration of clopidogrel to decrease the risk of blood loss.[116,117] The incidence of increased bleeding is associated with the use of either thienopyridines or GP IIb/IIIa inhibitors when urgent CABG is performed. However, no increase in operative bleeding was seen when GP IIb/IIIa inhibitors were discontinued at least 2 hours before surgery.[118-120] Other studies have shown that the bleeding risk associated with abciximab may be alleviated by platelet transfusions perioperatively. Platelet transfusion may reverse the effect of the GP IIb/IIIa receptor antagonist, abciximab, and reduce the incidence of bleeding.[121] Operation within 12 hours of fibrinolytic therapy for acute MI is associated with increased bleeding and transfusion, and a greater incidence of reoperation for perioperative bleeding.[122]

NONCORONARY INTERVENTIONAL CARDIAC PROCEDURES

Improvements in catheters, guide wires, balloons, stents, and other technologies have facilitated the use of catheter-based therapies and have allowed interventional cardiologists to treat noncoronary cardiac problems such as valvular, congenital, and other structural heart diseases that previously were the purview of surgical therapy only. In addition, the development of percutaneous assist devices allows the interventional cardiologist to treat the highest-risk patients with an added degree of safety.

Balloon Mitral Valvuloplasty

Inoue and coworkers in 1984 and Lock and colleagues in 1985 introduced percutaneous mitral balloon valvotomy (PMBV) for the treatment of selected patients with mitral stenosis.[123,124] A single deflated balloon or a double balloon is advanced from the venous access to the right atrium. Using a trans-septal approach, the balloon is advanced across the interatrial septum to the left atrium and then across the stenotic mitral valve. The balloon is inflated and rapidly deflated, fracturing calcifications of the leaflet tissue and separating fused commissures. Typically, the valve area increases from a critically stenotic value of less than 1.0 cm^2 to approximately 2.0 cm^2, a change associated in 80% to 95% of patients with a rapid reduction in left atrial pressure that is sufficient to produce substantial hemodynamic improvements, including a decrease in left atrial pressure and a 50% to 60% decrease in the transmitral pressure gradient, a reduction in pulmonary artery pressure, and an increase in cardiac output.

Patients are selected for PMBV on the basis of echocardiographic and clinical criteria. PMBV is a reasonable option for patients who are candidates for surgical commissurotomy. The salutary long-term results, lower costs, and the avoidance of thoracotomy make this procedure the treatment of choice in young patients with pliable, noncalcified mitral valves and no left atrial thrombus.[125] In addition, percutaneous valvotomy can be considered a palliative procedure in patients who have severe valve deformities and are poor surgical candidates. Mitral valve repair or replacement is usually preferred in symptomatic patients with severe subvalvular or calcific disease, or when left atrial thrombus or significant valvular regurgitation precludes safe balloon valvotomy. Closed commissurotomy is still performed in some developing nations where cost and lack of balloon catheters are continuing problems

The ACC/AHA task force published recommendations for PMBV in 2006[126] and recommended consideration of PMBV for patients who have exercise intolerance, severe pulmonary hypertension, no left atrial thrombus, a calculated effective mitral valve area of 1.5 cm^2 or less with trace or mild mitral regurgitation, and appropriate mitral anatomy as determined by echocardiography.

Echocardiography is an essential screening procedure in patients being considered for PMBV.[125] The extent of valvular and subvalvular deformity can be evaluated, and the likelihood of a successful result can be assessed. This can be accomplished by applying the Wilkins score, which scores from 0 to 4 for each of four factors: (1) the degree of leaflet rigidity, (2) the severity of leaflet thickening, (3) the amount of leaflet calcification, and (4) the extent of subvalvular thickening and calcification. The maximum score is 16; higher scores indicate more severe anatomic disease and a lower likelihood of a successful PMBV.[127]

The National Heart, Lung, and Blood Institute's Balloon Valvuloplasty Registry evaluated 736 patients older than 18 and treated with PMBV who were followed for 4 years. The actuarial survival rates at 1, 2, 3, and 4 years were 93%, 90%, 87%, and 84%, respectively. The event-free survival rates (freedom from death, mitral valve surgery, or repeat balloon valvotomy) at 1, 2, 3, and 4 years were 80%, 71%, 66%, and 60%, respectively.[128] The clinical and hemodynamic results of PMBV have been compared with the different forms of surgical correction: closed surgical valvotomy, and open and closed surgical commissurotomy. The outcome after PMBV was as good as or better than after surgery for patients who are candidates for valvotomy.[129,130] Long-term outcomes are actually improved in PMBV as compared with closed commissurotomy.[16,131]

Complications of PMBV include severe mitral regurgitation in 2% to 10% of patients, mitral valve restenosis, or formation of an atrial septal defect. After PMBV, up to 21% of patients develop recurrent heart failure due to mitral restenosis. Although most of these patients undergo mitral valve replacement, repeat balloon valvuloplasty is an alternative approach, especially in patients who are not good surgical candidates.[132] In addition, mitral valve restenosis after previous commissurotomy can be treated with PMBV. The immediate hemodynamic results and the long-term hemodynamics appear to be identical to those seen with balloon valvotomy in unoperated mitral stenosis.[133] Percutaneous mitral valve replacement has not yet been attempted in humans. However, percutaneous mitral valve repair has been attempted and is usually reserved for those with moderate-severe or severe mitral regurgitation. The Endovascular Valve Edge-to-Edge Repair Study (EVEREST) evaluated the trans-septal approach for applying a clip device (Evalve, Inc., Menlo Park, CA) to the mitral valve (Fig. 56-6). The trial reported an 85% freedom from adverse events rate at 30 days, and a freedom from valve surgery rate of 82% at 6 months.[134]

Balloon Aortic Valvuloplasty

Percutaneous balloon dilation can also be performed for aortic stenosis. Typically, one or more balloons are advanced across a stenotic valve in a retrograde manner and inflated to

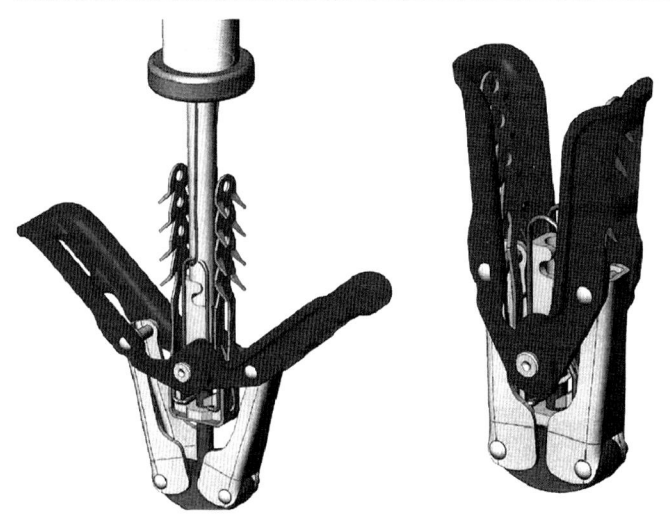

Figure 56–6
The MitraClip edge-to-edge mitral valve repair device (Evalve, Inc., Menlo Park, CA) consists of an outer guide catheter that is delivered to the left atrium trans-septally, 24 Fr proximally, and 22 Fr at the level of the interatrial septum. A clip delivery system is delivered through the guide catheter into the left atrium and over the mitral regurgitant jet. A U-shaped gripper attached to each arm secures the leaflets. General anesthesia and transesophageal echocardiography are required for this procedure. (From Feldman T, Wasserman HS, Herrmann HC, et al. Percutaneous mitral valve repair using the edge-to-edge technique: six month results of the *Everest* Phase I Clinical Trial. J Am Coll Cardiol 2005; **46**: 2134-40.)

Figure 56–7
Edwards Sapien stent-fixed transcatheter xenograft. Valve size and stent diameter is 23 mm. **A,** Outflow view. **B,** Lateral view. A 22- or 24-Fr catheter is used to access the femoral artery, and a balloon-expandable tubular slotted stainless steel stent with an equine pericardial trileaflet valve is deployed in the native aortic anulus in a retrograde manner through the aorta. (From Walther T, Falk V, Dewey T, et al. Valve-in-a-valve concept for transcatheter minimally invasive repeat xenograph implantation. J Am Coll Cardiol 2007; **50**: 56-60.)

dilate the valve.[135] This procedure has an important role in treating adolescents and young adults with congenital aortic stenosis. In patients with bicuspid or calcific valvular aortic stenosis, the mechanism of dilation is through fracture of calcific deposits in the valve leaflets as well as stretching of the annulus with separation of the calcified or fused commissures.[136] Although there is often immediate and significant reduction in the transvalvular pressure gradient, the post-valvotomy valve area rarely exceeds 1.0 cm^2. Despite this modest change in valve area, symptomatic improvement is usually seen.[137]

The role for this procedure is limited both by a high rate of serious complications (>10%) and by poor clinical durability.[137] Restenosis and clinical deterioration occur within 6 to 12 months in most patients, and, in contrast to the results after surgical aortic valve replacement, there is no impact on long-term survival. Thus, aortic valvuloplasty should not be considered a substitute for aortic valve replacement.[138-140] Aortic valvuloplasty can be performed in some cases as a bridge to surgery in hemodynamically unstable patients who are at high risk for aortic valve replacement, or in asymptomatic patients who require urgent noncardiac surgery. Aortic valvuloplasty may also be performed for palliation of congestive heart failure in patients with serious comorbidities and limited life expectancy.[140]

Percutaneous Endovascular Valve Replacement

High-risk patients who are not surgical candidates for valvular repair or replacement may be offered endovascular valve replacement as a nonsurgical alternative. Cribier and colleagues first described this method in humans via an antegrade trans-septal, transvenous approach in 1986,[141] and Webb and associates later described a similar approach using the femoral artery for retrograde percutaneous aortic valve replacement.[142]

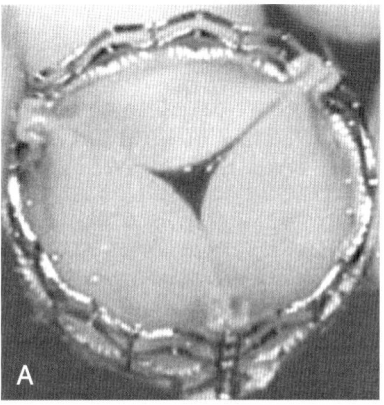

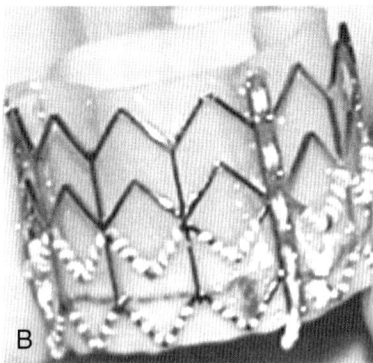

For this procedure, a large 22- or 24-Fr catheter is used to access the femoral artery, and a balloon-expandable, tubular, slotted stainless steel stent with an equine pericardial trileaflet valve, the Edwards Sapien valve, is deployed in the native aortic annulus in a retrograde manner through the aorta (Fig. 56-7). Webb and colleagues described outcomes after implantation in 50 patients. Valve implantation was successful in 86% of patients. Intraprocedural mortality was 2%. Mortality at 30 days was 12% when the logistic European System for Cardiac Operative Risk Evaluation risk score was 28%.[142]

Right ventricular burst pacing may be induced to create cardiac standstill during deployment to minimize cardiac motion. Reports show successful stent deployment in 86% of patients, with 30% of patients achieving a reduction in their New York Heart Association functional class.[142] The REVIVE trial, currently ongoing, is studying the use of percutaneous valve replacements in the aortic position in 27 patients. Initial results show a significant increase in LV function, valve area, and gradient.[143]

Potential complications of this approach are malposition of the stent, which may lead to valve embolization or cause coronary occlusion; significant vascular damage; access-site infections; and stroke. Intraprocedural mortality is close to 2%, with a 30-day mortality of 12%.[142] In the REVIVE trial, there was a 26% adverse event rate within the first 30 days, including tamponade, stroke, arrhythmia, urosepsis, and an unexplained death.[143] To minimize the vascular damage inevitable with the passage of large catheters through the iliac artery and aorta, a direct transapical approach has been developed and is under investigation. In this approach, a small chest wall incision is made, and the left ventricle is entered at the apex. The delivery sheath is advanced across the valve, and after valve deployment, the catheter is removed and the ventricular incision closed.

A transarterial retrograde approach has been used with the CoreValve ReValving System (Irvine, CA). This technology is currently under evaluation using an 18-Fr system with a self-expandable porcine pericardium bioprosthesis in a nitinol frame.[144]

Ethanol Septal Ablation for Hypertrophic Obstructive Cardiomyopathy

Nonsurgical septal reduction therapy, also called alcohol septal ablation, is a procedure whereby percutaneous obliteration of the first or second septal perforating coronary arteries is performed using absolute alcohol, which causes an iatrogenic septal infarct to reduce left ventricular outflow tract obstruction and thereby improve symptoms. The procedure itself entails placing a 0.014-inch guide wire into the major arterial supply of the septum, usually the first septal branch. Alcohol is injected through the lumen of an inflated angioplasty balloon into the septal branch, causing the infarction. Transient heart block is common, necessitating placement of a prophylactic pacing wire.[145]

Symptomatic patients with moderate to severe heart failure symptoms, an interventricular septal thickness of 18 mm or greater, a left ventricular outflow tract gradient at rest of at least 30 mm Hg, or an intraventricular gradient during provocation are potential candidates for this procedure.[146]

Septal reduction therapy has been shown to produce impressive reductions in outflow tract gradient and in symptoms. Significant reductions in pulmonary pressures, outflow tract gradient, and left ventricular hypertrophy and mass have been demonstrated.[147,148] Immediate hemodynamic results are comparable to those found with surgical myotomy or myectomy.[149-151] The most common complication of the procedure is the development of complete heart block, requiring a permanent pacemaker in approximately 7% to 14% of patients[152-154] up to 5 days after the procedure, right bundle branch block in 46%, and primary AV conduction delay in 56%.[145] The risk of complete heart block is increased with septal ablation in those with a baseline left bundle branch block, as ablation usually targets the basal septum, which lies closer to the right bundle. The reverse is true for septal myectomy.[145]

Other complications include the development of coronary dissection, ventricular arrhythmia, or unwanted MI. Reported results at 1 year follow-up continue to show benefit, especially in those older than 65,[155,156] and long-term efficacy data are currently being collected. The procedural complication rate for septal ablation is higher than for surgical myectomy, although the survival rates are similar.[153,154]

Closure of Patent Foramen Ovale and Atrial Septal Defect

Patent foramen ovale (PFO), present in roughly 25% of adults, is a persistent flaplike opening between the remnants of the atrial septum primum and the secundum. It can be demonstrated in almost 50% of patients younger than 55 years with cryptogenic stroke.[157,158] The presumed cause of stroke in these cases is paradoxical embolism, whereby venous thrombus is allowed to access the systemic circulation through the PFO during physiologic conditions when right atrial pressure exceeds left atrial pressure. Medical therapy with either warfarin or antiplatelet agents is the current standard of care for cryptogenic stroke in the patients with PFO, but despite its use, the risk of recurrent stroke remains high. Patients with PFO and paradoxical embolism have an approximately 3.5% yearly risk of recurrent cerebrovascular events.[159] Surgical closure has been effective in preventing recurrent stroke, but adequate randomized studies comparing anticoagulation, surgical closure, and percutaneous closure have not been performed.[160]

Because of the bleeding risks associated with chronic anticoagulant use, the costs of drugs and monitoring, and the desire of physicians and patients to avoid prolonged recovery and open-heart surgery, percutaneous closure can be offered as a less invasive option for stroke prevention in these patients. It has been employed in thousands of patients using a variety of occlusion devices. Procedural outcomes are excellent, and the stroke recurrence rate is less than 1% at follow-up exceeding 1 year.[161-163] The Amplatzer PFO occluder (AGA Medical Corp., Golden Valley, MN) (Fig. 56-8), and the CardioSEAL (NMT Medical, Boston, MA) were initially approved under a Humanitarian Device Exemption by the FDA for PFO closure. However, these devices are now available either as part of randomized trials for patients with first stroke and PFO, or in open-label registries restricted to patients with recurrent stroke despite medical therapy. No device is approved for PFO and atrial septal defect (ASD) closure after cryptogenic stroke, mainly because of a lack of sufficient data. At our institution, the procedure time is approximately 15 to 20 minutes using only fluoroscopic guidance and transthoracic confirmation of appropriate

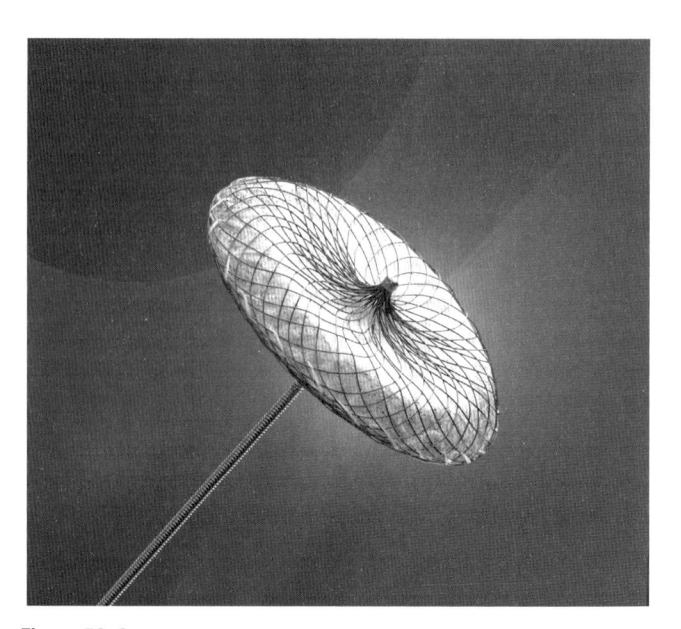

Figure 56–8
Amplatzer septal occlusion devices used for percutaneous closure. *(Courtesy of AGA Medical Corporation, Plymouth, MN.)*

positioning. Patients are required to take aspirin and clopidogrel as well as endocarditis prophylaxis for dental procedures for 6 to 12 months. Long-term anticoagulation is not required thereafter. One study found freedom from adverse events such as stroke, transient ischemic attack (TIA), or peripheral embolism to be as high as 97% at 2 years and 96% at 5 and 10 years.[164] Windecker and coworkers compared medical therapy with percutaneous PFO closure and found no significant difference in death, stroke, or TIA, but they did find a significant benefit with percutaneous closure in those who suffered more than one cerebrovascular event.[165] There is also a high prevalence of PFO in patients with classic migraine headaches, and one small randomized trial reported a reduction in migraine frequency after PFO closure.[166] Larger randomized trials are ongoing.

Although PFO represents a potential communication between the left and right atria, ASDs are congenital abnormalities characterized by a structural deficiency that leads to continuous, free communication between the atria. The defect is often asymptomatic until adulthood, but complications of an undetected lesion include irreversible pulmonary hypertension, right ventricular failure, atrial arrhythmias, paradoxical embolization, and cerebral abscess. These defects are generally repaired when the pulmonary-to-systemic flow ratio is 1.5 or greater, or in those where the defect leads to symptoms, embolism, or right ventricular dysfunction. Scuba divers with neurologic compression sickness and ASD also may be considered for closure. Those with ostium primum defects, sinus venosus defects, or defects with less than 4 mm of surrounding tissue or a stretched diameter of greater than 38 mm are better served by surgical rather than percutaneous closure. Percutaneous closure is usually performed using septal occlusion devices similar to those used for PFO closure. Adjunctive transesophageal echocardiographic or intracardiac echocardiography is often used to assist in sizing and placement. One multicenter nonrandomized study compared 154 patients who underwent surgical closure and 442 who had closure with an Amplatzer septal occluder device. Both methods had equal success rates, but percutaneous closure was associated with fewer complications (7.2% versus 24.0%; $P<.0001$) and shorter duration of hospitalization (1 versus 3 days).[167]

Endovascular ventricular septal defect (VSD) closure is under development. Initial studies have shown a postprocedural complete closure rate of 47%, which rose to 69.6% at 6 months and then 92.3% at 12 months using an Amplatzer VSD closure device in muscular VSDs.[168] Amplatzer VSD closure devices are also being studied for membranous VSDs, with complete closure demonstrated in phase I trials in 20 of 32 patients at 24 hours and 27 of 28 patients at 6-month follow-up.[169] Significant periprocedural complications (roughly 11.5%) have included device embolization and vascular and arrhythmogenic complications.[170] These investigational devices hold a promising future in the endovascular repair of congenital or post-MI ventricular defects.

Percutaneous Circulatory Assist Devices

The intra-aortic balloon pump (IABP) uses the principle of counterpulsation to increase diastolic blood flow to coronary arteries and to mechanically reduce the afterload on the heart during systole. This method was first described in 1952 in animals by Adrian and Arthur Kantrowitz.[171] The device consists of a double-lumen catheter from (7 to 9.5 Fr) with a 25- to 50-mL balloon at its distal end. The inner lumen monitors arterial blood pressure and the outer lumen allows the transfer of helium gas into the balloon. It is used in patients with cardiogenic shock or with mechanical complications of MI such as acute mitral regurgitation or VSD, or as a bridge for high-risk patients before bypass surgery.[172] The IABP is contraindicated in those with aortic regurgitation and significant peripheral vascular disease.

Left ventricular assist devices maintain partial or total circulatory support in cases of severe left ventricular failure, or temporarily during high-risk PCI. The Impella 2.5 device (Abiomed, Danvers, MA) is a catheter-mounted microaxial blood pump. It features a motorized pump that is inserted into the left ventricle through the aortic valve by means of the femoral artery. The pump produces a mean flow of 2.5 L/min and mechanically "unloads" the left ventricle (Fig. 56-9) by aspirating blood from the left ventricle and then expelling it into the aorta by means of a rotor-driven pump. Current FDA approval allows the Impella device to be used for 6 hours, but studies have shown it to be safe for up to 7 days in humans. Ongoing randomized trials are comparing Impella and IABP support for high-risk PCI or primary PCI performed in patients with cardiogenic shock. The TandemHeart (Cardiac Assist, Pittsburgh, PA) is a left atrial–to–femoral artery bypass system comprising a trans-septal cannula, arterial cannulae, and a centrifugal blood pump (Fig. 56-10). The pump can deliver flow rates up to 5.0 L/min at a maximum speed of 7500 rpm. TandemHeart has been shown to significantly reduce preload and to augment cardiac output. In a randomized comparison between the TandemHeart and IABP in patients with cardiogenic shock, the improved cardiac index afforded by the left ventricular assist device resulted in a more rapid decrease in serum lactate and improved renal function.[173]

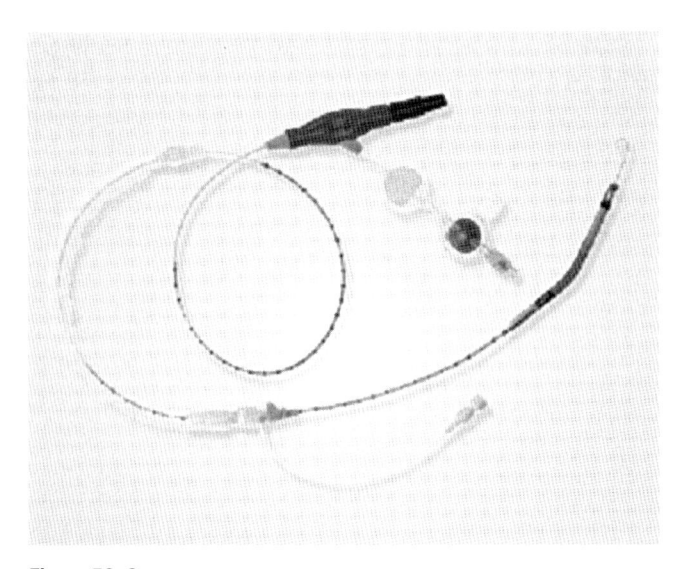

Figure 56-9
The Impella 2.5 device used for percutaneous cardiac support. A flow of up to 2.5 L/min can be provided by this device. *(Courtesy of Abiomed Corporation, Danvers, MA.)*

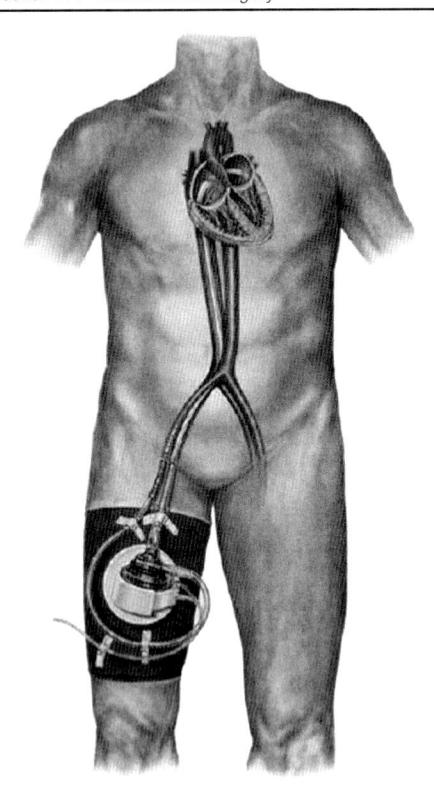

Figure 56–10
The TandemHeart percutaneous cardiac assist device (Cardiac Assist, Pittsburgh, PA). The catheter is advanced through the femoral vein and across the interatrial septum into the left atrium. Blood is removed and a pump returns oxygenated blood to the patient's systemic circulation through an arterial cannula. A flow of up to 5 L/min can be provided.

REFERENCES

1. Dotter CT, Judkins MP. Transluminal treatment of arteriosclerotic obstruction: description of a new technique and preliminary report of its application. *Circulation* 1964;**30**:654.
2. Gruentzig AR, Senning A, Siegenthaler WE. Nonoperative dilatation of coronary-artery stenosis: percutaneous transluminal coronary angioplasty. *N Engl J Med* 1979;**301**:61-8.
3. Bourassa MG, Wilson JW, Detre KM, Kelsey SF, Robertson T, Passamani ER. Long-term follow-up of coronary angioplasty: the 1977-1981 National Heart, Lung, and Blood Institute registry. *Eur Heart J* 1989;**10**(Suppl G):36-41.
4. King III SB, Smith Jr SC, Hirshfeld Jr JW, Jacobs AK, Morrison DA, Williams DO, et al. 2007 focused update of the ACC/AHA/SCAI 2005 Guideline Update for Percutaneous Coronary Intervention: a report of the American College of Cardiology/American Heart Association Task Force on Practice Guidelines: 2007 Writing Group to Review New Evidence and Update the ACC/AHA/SCAI 2005 Guideline Update for Percutaneous Coronary Intervention, Writing on Behalf of the 2005 Writing Committee. *Circulation* 2008;**117**:261-95.
5. George BS, Voorhees 3rd WD, Roubin GS, Fearnot NE, Pinkerton CA, Raizner AE, et al. Multicenter investigation of coronary stenting to treat acute or threatened closure after percutaneous transluminal coronary angioplasty: clinical and angiographic outcomes. *J Am Coll Cardiol* 1993;**22**:135-43.
6. Serruys PW, de Jaegere P, Kiemeneij F, Macaya C, Rutsch W, Heyndrickx G, et al. A comparison of balloon-expandable-stent implantation with balloon angioplasty in patients with coronary artery disease. Benestent Study Group. *N Engl J Med* 1994;**331**:489-95.
7. Fischman DL, Leon MB, Baim DS, Schatz RA, Savage MP, Penn I, et al. A randomized comparison of coronary-stent placement and balloon angioplasty in the treatment of coronary artery disease. Stent Restenosis Study Investigators. *N Engl J Med* 1994;**331**:496-501.
8. Noto Jr TJ, Johnson LW, Krone R, Weaver WF, Clark DA, Kramer Jr JR, Vetrovec GW. Cardiac catheterization 1990: a report of the Registry of the Society for Cardiac Angiography and Interventions (SCA&I). *Cathet Cardiovasc Diagn* 1991;**24**:75-83.
9. Kiemeneij F, Laarman GJ, Odekerken D, Slagboom T, van der Wieken R. A randomized comparison of percutaneous transluminal coronary angioplasty by the radial, brachial and femoral approaches: the access study. *J Am Coll Cardiol* 1997;**29**:1269-75.
10. Judkins MP. Selective coronary arteriography: a percutaneous transfemoral technique. *Radiology* 1967;**89**:815-24.
11. ACC/AHA 2007 Guidelines for the Management of Patients with Unstable Angina/Non-ST-Elevation Myocardial Infarction: a report of the American College of Cardiology/American Heart Association Task Force on Practice Guidelines (Writing Committee to Revise the 2002 Guidelines for the Management of Patients With Unstable Angina/Non-ST-Elevation Myocardial Infarction): Developed in Collaboration with the American College of Emergency Physicians, the Society for Cardiovascular Angiography and Interventions, and the Society of Thoracic Surgeons: Endorsed by the American Association of Cardiovascular and Pulmonary Rehabilitation and the Society for Academic Emergency Medicine. *Circulation* 2007;**116**:e148-304.
12. O'Donoghue M, Boden WE, Braunwald E, Cannon CP, Clayton TC, de Winter RJ, et al. Early invasive vs conservative treatment strategies in women and men with unstable angina and non-ST-segment elevation myocardial infarction: a meta-analysis. *JAMA* 2008;**300**:71-80.
13. Stone GW, McLaurin BT, Cox DA, Bertrand ME, Lincoff AM, Moses JW, et al. Bivalirudin for patients with acute coronary syndromes. *N Engl J Med* 2006;**355**:2203-16.
14. Schuhlen H, Kastrati A, Dirschinger J, Hausleiter J, Elezi S, Wehinger A, et al. Intracoronary stenting and risk for major adverse cardiac events during the first month. *Circulation* 1998;**98**:104-11.
15. Dorros G, Cowley MJ, Simpson J, Bentivoglio LG, Block PC, Bourassa M, et al. Percutaneous transluminal coronary angioplasty: report of complications from the National Heart, Lung, and Blood Institute PTCA. *Registry. Circulation* 1983;**67**:723-30.
16. Reyes VP, Raju BS, Wynne J, Stephenson LW, Raju R, Fromm BS, et al. Percutaneous balloon valvuloplasty compared with open surgical commissurotomy for mitral stenosis. *N Engl J Med* 1994;**331**:961-7.
17. Cutlip DE, Chauhan MS, Baim DS, Ho KK, Popma JJ, Carrozza JP, et al. Clinical restenosis after coronary stenting: perspectives from multicenter clinical trials. *J Am Coll Cardiol* 2002;**40**:2082-9.
18. Hasdai D, Berger PB, Bell MR, Rihal CS, Garratt KN, Holmes Jr DR. The changing face of coronary interventional practice: the Mayo Clinic experience. *Arch Intern Med* 1997;**157**:677-82.
19. Wijeysundera HC, Vijayaraghavan R, Nallamothu BK, Foody JM, Krumholz HM, Phillips CO, et al. Rescue angioplasty or repeat fibrinolysis after failed fibrinolytic therapy for ST-segment myocardial infarction: a meta-analysis of randomized trials. *J Am Coll Cardiol* 2007;**49**:422-30.
20. Gershlick AH, Stephens-Lloyd A, Hughes S, Abrams KR, Stevens SE, Uren NG, et al. Rescue angioplasty after failed thrombolytic therapy for acute myocardial infarction. *N Engl J Med* 2005;**353**:2758-68.
21. Grines CL, Cox DA, Stone GW, Garcia E, Mattos LA, Giambartolomei A, Brodie BR, et al. Coronary angioplasty with or without stent implantation for acute myocardial infarction. Stent Primary Angioplasty in Myocardial Infarction Study Group. *N Engl J Med* 1999;**341**:1949-56.
22. Mehta RH, Harjai KJ, Cox DA, Stone GW, Brodie BR, Boura J, et al. Comparison of coronary stenting versus conventional balloon angioplasty on five-year mortality in patients with acute myocardial infarction undergoing primary percutaneous coronary intervention. *Am J Cardiol* 2005;**96**:901-6.
23. Stone GW, Grines CL, Cox DA, Garcia E, Tcheng JE, Griffin JJ, et al. Controlled Abciximab and Device Investigation to Lower Late Angioplasty Complications (CADILLAC) Investigators. Comparison of angioplasty with stenting, with or without abciximab, in acute myocardial infarction. *N Engl J Med* 2002;**346**:957-66.
24. Antman EM, Anbe DT, Armstrong PW, Bates ER, Green LA, Hand M, et al. ACC/AHA guidelines for the management of patients with ST-elevation myocardial infarction: a report of the American College of Cardiology/American Heart Association Task Force on Practice Guidelines (Committee to Revise the 1999 Guidelines for the Management of Patients with Acute Myocardial Infarction). *J Am Coll Cardiol* 2004;**44**:671-719.
25. Pinto DS, Kirtane AJ, Nallamothu BK, Murphy SA, Cohen DJ, Laham RJ, et al. Hospital delays in reperfusion for ST-elevation myocardial infarction: implications when selecting a reperfusion strategy. *Circulation* 2006;**114**:2019-25.
26. Facilitated percutaneous coronary intervention for acute ST-segment elevation myocardial infarction. Results from the prematurely terminated Addressing the Value of Facilitated Angioplasty after Combination Therapy or Eptifibatide Monotherapy in Acute Myocardial Infarction (ADVANCE MI) trial. *Am Heart J* 2005;**150**:116-22.
27. Ellis SG, Tendera M, de Belder MA, van Boven AJ, Widimsky P, Janssens L, et al. the FINESSE Investigators. Facilitated PCI in patients with ST-elevation myocardial infarction. *N Engl J Med* 2008;**358**:2205-17.

28. Smith Jr SC, Feldman TE, Hirshfeld Jr JW, Jacobs AK, Kern MJ, King SB III, et al. ACC/AHA/SCAI 2005 Guideline Update for Percutaneous Coronary Intervention: a report of the American College of Cardiology/American Heart Association Task Force on Practice Guidelines (ACC/AHA/SCAI Writing Committee to Update the 2001 Guidelines for Percutaneous Coronary Intervention). *J Am Coll Cardiol* 2006;**47**:e1-121.
29. Davies RF, Goldberg AD, Forman S, Pepine CJ, Knatterud GL, Geller N, et al. Asymptomatic Cardiac Ischemia Pilot (ACIP) study two-year follow-up: outcomes of patients randomized to initial strategies of medical therapy versus revascularization. *Circulation* 1997;**95**:2037-43.
30. Boden WE, O'Rourke RA, Teo KK, Hartigan PM, Maron DJ, Kostuk WJ, et al. the COURAGE Trial Research Group. Optimal medical therapy with or without PCI for stable coronary disease. *N Engl J Med* 2007;**356**:1503-16.
31. Smith Jr SC, Dove JT, Jacobs AK, Kennedy JW, Kereiakes D, Kern MJ, et al. ACC/AHA guidelines of percutaneous coronary interventions (revision of the 1993 PTCA guidelines)—executive summary: a report of the American College of Cardiology/American Heart Association Task Force on Practice Guidelines (committee to revise the 1993 guidelines for percutaneous transluminal coronary angioplasty). *J Am Coll Cardiol* 2001;**37**:2215-39.
32. Jones RH, Kesler K, Phillips 3rd HR, Mark DB, Smith PK, Nelson CL, et al. Long-term survival benefits of coronary artery bypass grafting and percutaneous transluminal angioplasty in patients with coronary artery disease. *J Thorac Cardiovasc Surg* 1996;**111**:1013-25.
33. Five-year clinical and functional outcome comparing bypass surgery and angioplasty in patients with multivessel coronary disease. a multicenter randomized trial. Writing Group for the Bypass Angioplasty Revascularization Investigation (BARI) Investigators. *JAMA* 1997;**277**:715-21.
34. Pocock SJ, Henderson RA, Rickards AF, Hampton JR, King 3rd SB, Hamm CW, et al. Meta-analysis of randomised trials comparing coronary angioplasty with bypass surgery. *Lancet* 1995;**346**:1184-9.
35. Takagi H, Kawai N, Umemoto T. Meta-analysis of four randomized controlled trials on long-term outcomes of coronary artery bypass grafting versus percutaneous coronary intervention with stenting for multivessel coronary disease. *Am J Cardiol* 2008;**101**:1259-62.
36. Hueb W, Lopes NH, Gersh BJ, Soares P, Machado LAC, Jatene FB, et al. Five-Year Follow-Up of the Medicine, Angioplasty, or Surgery Study (MASS II): a randomized controlled clinical trial of 3 therapeutic strategies for multivessel coronary artery disease. *Circulation* 2007;**115**:1082-9.
37. Influence of diabetes on 5-year mortality and morbidity in a randomized trial comparing CABG and PTCA in patients with multivessel disease: the Bypass Angioplasty Revascularization Investigation (BARI). *Circulation* 1997;**96**:1761-9.
38. Kurbaan AS, Bowker TJ, Ilsley CD, Sigwart U, Rickards AF. Difference in the mortality of the CABRI diabetic and nondiabetic populations and its relation to coronary artery disease and the revascularization mode. *Am J Cardiol* 2001;**87**:947-50:A3.
39. Feit F, Brooks MM, Sopko G, Keller NM, Rosen A, Krone R, et al. Long-term clinical outcome in the Bypass Angioplasty Revascularization Investigation Registry: comparison with the randomized trial. BARI Investigators. *Circulation* 2000;**101**:2795-2802.
39a. Detre KM, Guo P, Holubkov R, et al. Coronary revascularization in diabetic patients : a comparison of the randomized and observational components of the bypass angioplasty revascularization investigation (BARI). *Circulation*. 1999;**99**:633-40.
40. Daemen J, Boersma E, Flather M, Booth J, Stables R, Rodriguez A, et al. Long-term safety and efficacy of percutaneous coronary intervention with stenting and coronary artery bypass surgery for multivessel coronary artery disease. a meta-analysis with 5-year patient-level data from the ARTS, ERACI-II, MASS-II, and SoS Trials. *Circulation* 2008;**118**(11):1146-54.
41. Javaid A, Steinberg DH, Buch AN, Corso PJ, Boyce SW, Pinto Slottow TL, et al. Outcomes of coronary artery bypass grafting versus percutaneous coronary intervention with drug-eluting stents for patients with multivessel coronary artery disease. *Circulation* 2007;**116**:200-6.
42. Serruys PW, Morice M-C, Kappetein AP, et al. Percutaneous coronary intervention versus coronary-artery bypass grafting for severe coronary artery disease. *N Engl J Med*. 2009;**360**:961-72.
43. Hannan EL, Wu C, Walford G, Culliford AT, Gold JP, Smith CR, et al. Drug-eluting stents vs. coronary-artery bypass grafting in multivessel coronary disease. *N Engl J Med* 2008;**358**:331-41.
44. Farkouh ME, Dangas G, Leon MB, Smith C, Nesto R, Buse JB, et al. Design of the Future Revascularization Evaluation in Patients with Diabetes Mellitus: Optimal Management of Multivessel Disease (FREEDOM) trial. *Am Heart J* 2008;**155**:215-23.
45. Seung KB, Park D-W, Kim Y-H, Lee S-W, Lee CW, Hong M-K, et al. Stents versus coronary-artery bypass grafting for left main coronary artery disease. *N Engl J Med* 2008;**358**:1781-92.
46. Carrozza Jr JP, Sellke FW. A 69-year-old woman with left main coronary artery disease. *JAMA* 2004;**292**:2506-14.
47. Poldermans D, Hoeks SE, Feringa HH. Pre-operative risk assessment and risk reduction before surgery. *J Am Coll Cardiol* 2008;**51**:1913-24.
48. Fleisher LA, Beckman JA, Brown KA, Calkins H, Chaikof EL, Fleischmann KE, et al. ACC/AHA 2007 Guidelines on Perioperative Cardiovascular Evaluation and Care for Noncardiac Surgery: a report of the American College of Cardiology/American Heart Association Task Force on Practice Guidelines (Writing Committee to Revise the 2002 Guidelines on Perioperative Cardiovascular Evaluation for Noncardiac Surgery). *Circulation* 2007;**116**:e418-500.
49. Schouten O, van Domburg RT, Bax JJ, de Jaegere PJ, Dunkelgrun M, Feringa HH, et al. Noncardiac surgery after coronary stenting: early surgery and interruption of antiplatelet therapy are associated with an increase in major adverse cardiac events. *J Am Coll Cardiol* 2007;**49**:122-4.
50. Kaluza GL, Joseph J, Lee JR, Raizner ME, Raizner AE. Catastrophic outcomes of noncardiac surgery soon after coronary stenting. *J Am Coll Cardiol* 2000;**35**:1288-94.
51. King Smith III SB, Smith Jr SC, Hirshfeld Jr JW, Jacobs AK, Morrison DA, Williams DO. 2007 Focused Update of the ACC/AHA/SCAI 2005 Guideline Update for Percutaneous Coronary Intervention. *J Am Coll of Cardiol* 2008;**51**:172-209.
52. Bredlau CE, Roubin GS, Leimgruber PP, Douglas Jr JS, King 3rd SB, Gruentzig AR. In-hospital morbidity and mortality in patients undergoing elective coronary angioplasty. *Circulation* 1985;**72**:1044-52.
53. Wyman RM, Safian RD, Portway V, Skillman JJ, McKay RG, Baim DS. Current complications of diagnostic and therapeutic cardiac catheterization. *J Am Coll Cardiol* 1988;**12**:1400-6.
54. Keeley EC, Velez CA, O'Neill WW, Safian RD. Long-term clinical outcome and predictors of major adverse cardiac events after percutaneous interventions on saphenous vein grafts. *J Am Coll Cardiol* 2001;**38**:659-65.
55. Andreasen JJ, Mortensen PE, Andersen LI, Arendrup HC, Ilkjaer LB, Kjoller M, Thayssen P. Emergency coronary artery bypass surgery after failed percutaneous transluminal coronary angioplasty. *Scand Cardiovasc J* 2000;**34**:242-6.
56. Reber D, Sendtner E, Tollenaere P, Birnbaum D. Emergency aortocoronary bypass grafting after failed percutaneous transluminal angioplasty versus elective bypass grafting. *J Cardiovasc Surg (Torino)* 1996;**37**:71-3.
57. Black AJ, Namay DL, Niederman AL, Lembo NJ, Roubin GS, Douglas Jr JS, King 3rd SB. Tear or dissection after coronary angioplasty: morphologic correlates of an ischemic complication. *Circulation* 1989;**79**:1035-42.
58. Greene MA, Gray Jr LA, Slater AD, Ganzel BL, Mavroudis C. Emergency aortocoronary bypass after failed angioplasty. *Ann Thorac Surg* 1991;**51**:194-9.
59. Taylor PC, Boylan MJ, Lytle BW, McCarthy P, Stewart RW, Loop FD, Cosgrove DM. Emergent coronary bypass for failed PTCA: a 10-year experience with 253 patients. *J Invasive Cardiol* 1994;**6**:97-8.
60. Seshadri N, Whitlow PL, Acharya N, Houghtaling P, Blackstone EH, Ellis SG. Emergency coronary artery bypass surgery in the contemporary percutaneous coronary intervention era. *Circulation* 2002;**106**:2346-50.
61. Frutkin AD, Mehta SK, Patel T, Menon P, Safley DM, House J, et al. Outcomes of 1,090 consecutive, elective, nonselected percutaneous coronary interventions at a community hospital without onsite cardiac surgery. *Am J Cardiol* 2008;**101**:53-7.
62. Paraschos A, Callwood D, Wightman MB, Tcheng JE, Phillips HR, Stiles GL, et al. Outcomes following elective percutaneous coronary intervention without on-site surgical backup in a community hospital. *Am J Cardiol* 2005;**95**:1091-3.
63. Aversano T, Aversano LT, Passamani E, Knatterud GL, Terrin ML, Williams DO, Forman SA. for the Atlantic Cardiovascular Patient Outcomes Research Team. Thrombolytic Therapy vs. Primary Percutaneous Coronary Intervention for Myocardial Infarction in Patients Presenting to Hospitals without On-site Cardiac Surgery: a randomized controlled trial. *JAMA* 2002;**287**:1943-51.
64. Canto JG, Every NR, Magid DJ, Rogers WJ, Malmgren JA, Frederick PD, et al. The volume of primary angioplasty procedures and survival after acute myocardial infarction. National Registry of Myocardial Infarction 2 Investigators. *N Engl J Med* 2000;**342**:1573-80.
65. Magid DJ, Calonge BN, Rumsfeld JS, Canto JG, Frederick PD, Every NR, Barron HV. Relation between hospital primary angioplasty volume and mortality for patients with acute MI treated with primary angioplasty vs thrombolytic therapy. *JAMA* 2000;**284**:3131-8.
66. McGrath PD, Wennberg DE, Dickens Jr JD, Siewers AE, Lucas FL, Malenka DJ, et al. Relation between operator and hospital volume and outcomes following percutaneous coronary interventions in the era of the coronary stent. *JAMA* 2000;**284**:3139-44.
67. Reinecke H, Fetsch T, Roeder N, Schmid C, Winter A, Ribbing M, et al. Emergency coronary artery bypass grafting after failed coronary angioplasty: what has changed in a decade? *Ann Thorac Surg* 2000;**70**:1997-2003.

68. Hong MK, Mehran R, Dangas G, Mintz GS, Lansky AJ, Pichard AD, et al. Creatine kinase-MB enzyme elevation following successful saphenous vein graft intervention is associated with late mortality. *Circulation* 1999;**100**:2400-5.
69. Kini A, Marmur JD, Kini S, Dangas G, Cocke TP, Wallenstein S, et al. Creatine kinase-MB elevation after coronary intervention correlates with diffuse atherosclerosis, and low-to-medium level elevation has a benign clinical course: implications for early discharge after coronary intervention. *J Am Coll Cardiol* 1999;**34**:663-71.
70. Kugelmass AD, Cohen DJ, Moscucci M, Piana RN, Senerchia C, Kuntz RE, Baim DS. Elevation of the creatine kinase myocardial isoform following otherwise successful directional coronary atherectomy and stenting. *Am J Cardiol* 1994;**74**:748-54.
71. Platelet glycoprotein IIb/IIIa receptor blockade and low-dose heparin during percutaneous coronary revascularization. The EPILOG Investigators. *N Engl J Med* 1997;**336**:1689-96.
72. Nasser TK, Mohler 3rd ER, Wilensky RL, Hathaway DR. Peripheral vascular complications following coronary interventional procedures. *Clin Cardiol* 1995;**18**:609-14.
73. McCullough PA, Wolyn R, Rocher LL, Levin RN, O'Neill WW. Acute renal failure after coronary intervention: incidence, risk factors, and relationship to mortality. *Am J Med* 1997;**103**:368-75.
74. Gruberg L, Mintz GS, Mehran R, Gangas G, Lansky AJ, Kent KM, et al. The prognostic implications of further renal function deterioration within 48 h of interventional coronary procedures in patients with pre-existent chronic renal insufficiency. *J Am Coll Cardiol* 2000;**36**:1542-8.
75. Tepel M, van der Giet M, Schwarzfeld C, Laufer U, Liermann D, Zidek W. Prevention of radiographic-contrast-agent-induced reductions in renal function by acetylcysteine. *N Engl J Med* 2000;**343**:180-4.
76. Solomon R, Werner C, Mann D, D'Elia J, Silva P. Effects of saline, mannitol, and furosemide on acute decreases in renal function induced by radiocontrast agents. *N Engl J Med* 1994;**331**:1416-20.
77. Aspelin P, Aubry P, Fransson S-G, Strasser R, Willenbrock R, Berg KJ. The NEPHRIC Study Investigators. Nephrotoxic effects in high-risk patients undergoing angiography. *N Engl J Med* 2003;**348**:491-9.
78. Madyoon H, Croushore L, Weaver D, Mathur V. Use of fenoldopam to prevent radiocontrast nephropathy in high-risk patients. *Catheter Cardiovasc Interv* 2001;**53**:341-5.
79. Huber W, Schipek C, Ilgmann K, Page M, Hennig M, Wacker A, et al. Effectiveness of theophylline prophylaxis of renal impairment after coronary angiography in patients with chronic renal insufficiency. *Am J Cardiol* 2003;**91**:1157-62.
80. Goss JE, Chambers CE, Heupler Jr FA. Systemic anaphylactoid reactions to iodinated contrast media during cardiac catheterization procedures: guidelines for prevention, diagnosis, and treatment. Laboratory Performance Standards Committee of the Society for Cardiac Angiography and Interventions. *Cathet Cardiovasc Diagn* 1995;**34**:99-104:discussion 105.
81. Lee MS, Pessegueiro A, Zimmer R, Jurewitz D, Tobis J. Clinical presentation of patients with in-stent restenosis in the drug-eluting stent era. *J Invasive Cardiol* 2008;**20**:401-3.
82. Kuntz RE, Gibson CM, Nobuyoshi M, Baim DS. Generalized model of restenosis after conventional balloon angioplasty, stenting and directional atherectomy. *J Am Coll Cardiol* 1993;**21**:15-25.
83. Kastrati A, Schomig A, Elezi S, Schuhlen H, Dirschinger J, Hadamitzky M, et al. Predictive factors of restenosis after coronary stent placement. *J Am Coll Cardiol* 1997;**30**:1428-36.
84. Moses JW, Leon MB, Popma JJ, Fitzgerald PJ, Holmes DR, O'Shaughnessy C, SIRIUS Investigators et al. Sirolimus-eluting stents versus standard stents in patients with stenosis in a native coronary artery. *N Engl J Med* 2003;**349**:1315-23.
85. Stone GW, Ellis SG, Cox DA, Hermiller J, O'Shaughnessy C, Mann JT. the TAXUS-IV Investigators et al. A polymer-based, paclitaxel-eluting stent in patients with coronary artery disease. *N Engl J Med* 2004;**350**:221-31.
86. Morice M-C, Serruys PW, Sousa JE, Fajadet J, Ban Hayashi E, Perin M. the RAVEL Study Group et al. A randomized comparison of a sirolimus-eluting stent with a standard stent for coronary revascularization. *N Engl J Med* 2002;**346**:1773-80.
87. Cutlip DE, Chhabra AG, Baim DS, Chauhan MS, Marulkar S, Massaro J, et al. Beyond restenosis: five-year clinical outcomes from second-generation coronary stent trials. *Circulation* 2004;**110**:1226-30.
88. Marzocchi A, Saia F, Piovaccari G, Manari A, Aurier E, Benassi A, et al. Long-term safety and efficacy of drug-eluting stents: two-year results of the REAL (Registro Angioplastiche dell'Emilia Romagna) multicenter registry. *Circulation* 2007;**115**:3181-8.
89. Morice MC, Serruys PW, Barragan P, Bode C, Van Es GA, Stoll HP, et al. Long-term clinical outcomes with sirolimus-eluting coronary stents: five-year results of the RAVEL trial. *J Am Coll Cardiol* 2007;**50**:1299-304.
90. Schampaert E, Moses JW, Schofer J, Schluter M, Gershlick AH, Cohen EA, et al. Sirolimus-eluting stents at two years: a pooled analysis of SIRIUS, E-SIRIUS, and C-SIRIUS with emphasis on late revascularizations and stent thromboses. *Am J Cardiol* 2006;**98**:36-41.
91. Jensen LO, Maeng M, Kaltoft A, Thayssen P, Hansen HH, Bottcher M, et al. Stent thrombosis, myocardial infarction, and death after drug-eluting and bare-metal stent coronary interventions. *J Am Coll Cardiol* 2007;**50**:463-70.
92. Marroquin OC, Selzer F, Mulukutla SR, Williams DO, Vlachos HA, Wilensky RL, et al. A comparison of bare-metal and drug-eluting stents for off-label indications. *N Engl J Med* 2008;**358**:342-52.
93. Cutlip DE, Windecker S, Mehran R, Boam A, Cohen DJ, van Es G-A, et al. on behalf of the Academic Research C. Clinical end points in coronary stent trials: a case for standardized definitions. *Circulation* 2007;**115**:2344-51.
94. Stone GW, Ellis SG, Colombo A, Dawkins KD, Grube E, Cutlip DE, et al. Offsetting impact of thrombosis and restenosis on the occurrence of death and myocardial infarction after paclitaxel-eluting and bare metal stent implantation. *Circulation* 2007;**115**:2842-7.
95. Mauri L, Hsieh W-H, Massaro JM, Ho KKL, D'Agostino R, Cutlip DE. Stent thrombosis in randomized clinical trials of drug-eluting stents. *N Engl J Med* 2007;**356**:1020-9.
96. Pfisterer M, Brunner-La Rocca HP, Buser PT, Rickenbacher P, Hunziker P, Mueller C, et al. Late clinical events after clopidogrel discontinuation may limit the benefit of drug-eluting stents: an observational study of drug-eluting versus bare-metal stents. *J Am Coll Cardiol* 2006;**48**:2584-91.
97. Mega JL, Morrow DA, Sabatine MS, Zhao XQ, Snapinn SM, DiBattiste PM, et al. Correlation between the TIMI risk score and high-risk angiographic findings in non-ST-elevation acute coronary syndromes: observations from the Platelet Receptor Inhibition in Ischemic Syndrome Management in Patients Limited by Unstable Signs and Symptoms (PRISM-PLUS) trial. *Am Heart J* 2005;**149**:846-50.
98. Kuntz RE, Baim DS, Cohen DJ, Popma JJ, Carrozza JP, Sharma S, et al. A trial comparing rheolytic thrombectomy with intracoronary urokinase for coronary and vein graft thrombus (the Vein Graft AngioJet Study [VeGAS 2]). *Am J Cardiol* 2002;**89**:326-30.
99. Baim DS, Wahr D, George B, Leon MB, Greenberg J, Cutlip DE, et al. Randomized trial of a distal embolic protection device during percutaneous intervention of saphenous vein aorto-coronary bypass grafts. *Circulation* 2002;**105**:1285-90.
100. Stone GW, Webb J, Cox DA, Brodie BR, Qureshi M, Kalynych A, et al. for the Enhanced Myocardial E, Recovery by Aspiration of Liberated Debris I. Distal microcirculatory protection during percutaneous coronary intervention in acute ST-segment elevation myocardial infarction: a randomized controlled trial. *JAMA* 2005;**293**:1063-72.
101. Cura FA, Escudero AG, Berrocal D, Mendiz O, Trivi MS, Fernandez J, et al. Protection of distal embolization in high-risk patients with acute ST-segment elevation myocardial infarction (PREMIAR). *Am J Cardiol* 2007;**99**:357-63.
102. Stone GW, Rogers C, Ramee S, White C, Kuntz RE, Popma JJ, et al. Distal filter protection during saphenous vein graft stenting: technical and clinical correlates of efficacy. *J Am Coll Cardiol* 2002;**40**:1882-8.
103. Stone GW, Rogers C, Hermiller J. A prospective randomized multicenter trial comparing distal protection during saphenous vein graft intervention with a filter-based device compared to balloon occlusion and aspiration: the FIRE trial. *J Am Coll Cardiol* 2003;**41**:43A.
104. Carrozza JJP, Mumma M, Breall JA, Fernandez A, Heyman E, Metzger C. Randomized evaluation of the TriActiv balloon-protection flush and extraction system for the treatment of saphenous vein graft disease. *J Am Coll Cardiol* 2005;**46**:1677-83.
105. Svilaas T, Vlaar PJ, van der Horst IC, Diercks GFH, de Smet BJGL, van den Heuvel AFM, et al. Thrombus aspiration during primary percutaneous coronary intervention. *N Engl J Med* 2008;**358**:557-67.
106. Vlaar PJ, Svilaas T, van der Horst IC, Diercks GF, Fokkema ML, de Smet BJ, et al. Cardiac death and reinfarction after 1 year in the Thrombus Aspiration during Percutaneous coronary intervention in Acute myocardial infarction Study (TAPAS): a 1-year follow-up study. *Lancet* 2008;**371**:1915-20.
107. Ikari Y, Sakurada M, Kosuma K. Upfront thrombus aspiration in primary coronary intervention for patients with ST-segment elevation acute myocardial infarction: report of the VAMPIRE (VAcuuM aspPiration thrombus REmoval) trial. *J Am Coll Cardiol Intv* 2008;**1**:424-31.
108. Ali A, Cox D, Dib N, Brodie B, Berman D, Gupta N, et al. Rheolytic thrombectomy with percutaneous coronary intervention for infarct size reduction in acute myocardial infarction: 30-day results from a multicenter randomized study. *J Am Coll Cardiol* 2006;**48**:244-52.
109. Cameron AA, Davis KB, Rogers WJ. Recurrence of angina after coronary artery bypass surgery: predictors and prognosis (CASS Registry). Coronary Artery Surgery Study. *J Am Coll Cardiol* 1995;**26**:895-9.

110. Johnson WD, Kayser KL, Pedraza PM. Angina pectoris and coronary bypass surgery: patterns of prevalence and recurrence in 3105 consecutive patients followed up to 11 years. *Am Heart J* 1984;**108**:1190-7.
111. Verheul HA, Moulijn AC, Hondema S, Schouwink M, Dunning AJ. Late results of 200 repeat coronary artery bypass operations. *Am J Cardiol* 1991;**67**:24-30.
112. Fitzgibbon GM, Kafka HP, Leach AJ, Keon WJ, Hooper GD, Burton JR. Coronary bypass graft fate and patient outcome: angiographic follow-up of 5,065 grafts related to survival and reoperation in 1,388 patients during 25 years. *J Am Coll Cardiol* 1996;**28**:616-26.
113. Piana RN, Moscucci M, Cohen DJ, Kugelmass AD, Senerchia C, Kuntz RE, et al. Palmaz-Schatz stenting for treatment of focal vein graft stenosis: immediate results and long-term outcome. *J Am Coll Cardiol* 1994;**23**:1296-304.
113a. Vermeersch P, Agostoni P, Verheye S, et al. Increased late mortality after sirolimus-eluting stents versus bare-metal stents in diseased saphenous vein grafts: results from the Randomized DELAYED RRISC Trial. *J Am Coll Cardiol* 2007;**50**:261-67.
114. Liu MW, Douglas Jr JS, Lembo NJ, King 3rd SB. Angiographic predictors of a rise in serum creatine kinase (distal embolization) after balloon angioplasty of saphenous vein coronary artery bypass grafts. *Am J Cardiol* 1993;**72**:514-7.
115. Kon ZN, Brown EN, Tran R, Joshi A, Reicher B, Grant MC, et al. Simultaneous hybrid coronary revascularization reduces postoperative morbidity compared with results from conventional off-pump coronary artery bypass. *J Thorac Cardiovasc Surg* 2008;**135**:367-75.
116. Kapetanakis EI, Medlam DA, Boyce SW, Haile E, Hill PC, Dullum MKC, et al. Clopidogrel administration prior to coronary artery bypass grafting surgery: the cardiologist's panacea or the surgeon's headache? *Eur Heart J* 2005;**26**:576-83.
117. Reichert MG, Robinson AH, Travis JA, Hammon JW, Kon ND, Kincaid EH. Effects of a waiting period after clopidogrel treatment before performing coronary artery bypass grafting. *Pharmacotherapy* 2008;**28**:151-5.
118. Lincoff AM, LeNarz LA, Despotis GJ, Smith PK, Booth JE, Raymond RE, et al. Abciximab and bleeding during coronary surgery: results from the EPILOG and EPISTENT trials. Improve Long-term Outcome with abciximab GP IIb/IIIa blockade. Evaluation of Platelet IIb/IIIa Inhibition in STENTing. *Ann Thorac Surg* 2000;**70**:516-26.
119. Lemmer Jr JH, Metzdorff MT, Krause Jr AH, Martin MA, Okies JE, Hill JG. Emergency coronary artery bypass graft surgery in abciximab-treated patients. *Ann Thorac Surg* 2000;**69**:90-5.
120. Dyke CM, Bhatia D, Lorenz TJ, Marso SP, Tardiff BE, Hogeboom C, Harrington RA. Immediate coronary artery bypass surgery after platelet inhibition with eptifibatide: results from PURSUIT. *Ann Thorac Surg* 2000;**70**:866-71.
121. The Clopidogrel in Unstable Angina to Prevent Recurrent Events Trial Investigators. Effects of clopidogrel in addition to aspirin in patients with acute coronary syndromes without ST-segment elevation. *N Engl J Med* 2001;**345**:494-502.
122. Barner HB, Lea 4th JW, Naunheim KS, Stoney Jr WS. Emergency coronary bypass not associated with preoperative cardiogenic shock in failed angioplasty, after thrombolysis, and for acute myocardial infarction. *Circulation* 1989;**79**:I152-9.
123. Lock JE, Khalilullah M, Shrivastava S, Bahl V, Keane JF. Percutaneous catheter commissurotomy in rheumatic mitral stenosis. *N Engl J Med* 1985;**313**:1515-8.
124. Inoue K, Owaki T, Nakamura T, Kitamura F, Miyamoto N. Clinical application of transvenous mitral commissurotomy by a new balloon catheter. *J Thorac Cardiovasc Surg* 1984;**87**:394-402.
125. Cohen DJ, Kuntz RE, Gordon SP, Piana RN, Safian RD, McKay RG, et al. Predictors of long-term outcome after percutaneous balloon mitral valvuloplasty. *N Engl J Med* 1992;**327**:1329-35.
126. Bonow RO, Carabello BA, Chatterjee K, de Leon Jr AC, Faxon DP, Freed MD, et al. ACC/AHA 2006 Guidelines for the Management of Patients with Valvular Heart Disease: a Report of the American College of Cardiology/American Heart Association Task Force on Practice Guidelines (Writing Committee to Revise the 1998 Guidelines for the Management of Patients With Valvular Heart Disease): developed in collaboration with the Society of Cardiovascular Anesthesiologists: endorsed by the Society for Cardiovascular Angiography and Interventions and the Society of Thoracic Surgeons. *Circulation* 2006;**114**:e84-231.
127. Abascal VM, Wilkins GT, O'Shea JP, Choong CY, Palacios IF, Thomas JD, et al. Prediction of successful outcome in 130 patients undergoing percutaneous balloon mitral valvotomy. *Circulation* 1990;**82**:448-56.
128. Dean LS, Mickel M, Bonan R, Holmes Jr DR, O'Neill WW, Palacios IF, et al. Four-year follow-up of patients undergoing percutaneous balloon mitral commissurotomy: a report from the National Heart, Lung, and Blood Institute Balloon Valvuloplasty Registry. *J Am Coll Cardiol* 1996;**28**:1452-7.
129. Ben Farhat M, Ayari M, Maatouk F, Betbout F, Gamra H, Jarra M, et al. Percutaneous balloon versus surgical closed and open mitral commissurotomy: seven-year follow-up results of a randomized trial. *Circulation* 1998;**97**:245-50.
130. Turi ZG, Reyes VP, Raju BS, Raju AR, Kumar DN, Rajagopal P, et al. Percutaneous balloon versus surgical closed commissurotomy for mitral stenosis: a prospective, randomized trial. *Circulation* 1991;**83**:1179-85.
131. Farhat MB, Ayari M, Maatouk F, Betbout F, Gamra H, Jarrar M, et al. Percutaneous balloon versus surgical closed and open mitral commissurotomy: seven-year follow-up results of a randomized trial. *Circulation* 1998;**97**:245-50.
132. Pathan AZ, Mahdi NA, Leon MN, Lopez-Cuellar J, Simosa H, Block PC, et al. Is redo percutaneous mitral balloon valvuloplasty (PMV) indicated in patients with post-PMV mitral restenosis? *J Am Coll Cardiol* 1999;**34**:49-54.
133. Iung B, Garbarz E, Michaud P, Mahdhaoui A, Helou S, Farah B, et al. Percutaneous mitral commissurotomy for restenosis after surgical commissurotomy: late efficacy and implications for patient selection. *J Am Coll Cardiol* 2000;**35**:1295-302.
134. Feldman T, Wasserman HS, Herrmann HC, Gray W, Block PC, Whitlow P, et al. Percutaneous mitral valve repair using the edge-to-edge technique: six-month results of the EVEREST phase I clinical trial. *J Am Coll Cardiol* 2005;**46**:2134-40.
135. Safian RD, Berman AD, Diver DJ, McKay LL, Come PC, Riley MF, et al. Balloon aortic valvuloplasty in 170 consecutive patients. *N Engl J Med* 1988;**319**:125-30.
136. Safian RD, Mandell VS, Thurer RE, Hutchins GM, Schnitt SJ, Grossman W, McKay RG. Postmortem and intraoperative balloon valvuloplasty of calcific aortic stenosis in elderly patients: mechanisms of successful dilation. *J Am Coll Cardiol* 1987;**9**:655-60.
137. Brady ST, Davis CA, Kussmaul WG, Laskey WK, Hirshfeld Jr JW, Herrmann HC. Percutaneous aortic balloon valvuloplasty in octogenarians: morbidity and mortality. *Ann Intern Med* 1989;**110**:761-6.
138. Rahimtoola SH. Catheter balloon valvuloplasty for severe calcific aortic stenosis: a limited role. *J Am Coll Cardiol* 1994;**23**:1076-8.
139. Lieberman EB, Bashore TM, Hermiller JB, Wilson JS, Pieper KS, Keeler GP, et al. Balloon aortic valvuloplasty in adults: failure of procedure to improve long-term survival. *J Am Coll Cardiol* 1995;**26**:1522-8.
140. Bonow RO, Carabello B, de Leon Jr AC, Edmunds Jr LH, Fedderly BJ, Freed MD, et al. Guidelines for the management of patients with valvular heart disease: executive summary: a report of the American College of Cardiology/American Heart Association Task Force on Practice Guidelines (Committee on Management of Patients with Valvular Heart Disease). *Circulation* 1998;**98**:1949-84.
141. Cribier A, Savin T, Saoudi N, Rocha P, Berland J, Letac B. Percutaneous transluminal valvuloplasty of acquired aortic stenosis in elderly patients: an alternative to valve replacement? *Lancet* 1986;**1**:63-7.
142. Webb JG, Pasupati S, Humphries K, Thompson C, Altwegg L, Moss R, et al. Percutaneous transarterial aortic valve replacement in selected high-risk patients with aortic stenosis. *Circulation* 2007;**116**:755-63.
143. Cribier A, Eltchaninoff H, Tron C, Bauer F, Agatiello C, Nercolini D, et al. Treatment of calcific aortic stenosis with the percutaneous heart valve: mid-term follow-up from the initial feasibility studies: the French experience. *J Am Coll Cardiol* 2006;**47**:1214-23.
144. Grube E, Ulrich G, Schuler G, Linke A, Bonan R, Serruys PW. Experience with CoreValve aortic valve replacement in patients with surgical aortic valve replacement. *J Am Coll Cardiol* 2008;**51**:B21-2.
145. Knight CJ. Alcohol septal ablation for obstructive hypertrophic cardiomyopathy. *Heart* 2006;**92**:1339-44.
146. Gietzen FH, Leuner CJ, Obergassel L, Strunk-Mueller C, Kuhn H. Role of transcoronary ablation of septal hypertrophy in patients with hypertrophic cardiomyopathy, New York Heart Association functional class III or IV, and outflow obstruction only under provocable conditions. *Circulation* 2002;**106**:454-9.
147. Nagueh SF, Lakkis NM, Middleton KJ, Killip D, Zoghbi WA, Quinones MA, Spencer 3rd WH. Changes in left ventricular diastolic function 6 months after nonsurgical septal reduction therapy for hypertrophic obstructive cardiomyopathy. *Circulation* 1999;**99**:344-7.
148. Park TH, Lakkis NM, Middleton KJ, Franklin J, Zoghbi WA, Quinones MA, et al. Acute effect of nonsurgical septal reduction therapy on regional left ventricular asynchrony in patients with hypertrophic obstructive cardiomyopathy. *Circulation* 2002;**106**:412-5.
149. Nagueh SF, Ommen SR, Lakkis NM, Killip D, Zoghbi WA, Schaff HV, et al. Comparison of ethanol septal reduction therapy with surgical myectomy for the treatment of hypertrophic obstructive cardiomyopathy. *J Am Coll Cardiol* 2001;**38**:1701-6.
150. Sitges M, Shiota T, Lever HM, Qin JX, Bauer F, Drinko JK, et al. Comparison of left ventricular diastolic function in obstructive hypertrophic cardiomyopathy in patients undergoing percutaneous septal alcohol ablation versus surgical myotomy/myectomy. *Am J Cardiol* 2003;**91**:817-21.
151. Firoozi S, Elliott PM, Sharma S, Murday A, Brecker SJ, Hamid MS, et al. Septal myotomy-myectomy and transcoronary septal alcohol ablation in hypertrophic obstructive cardiomyopathy: a comparison of clinical, haemodynamic and exercise outcomes. *Eur Heart J* 2002;**23**:1617-24.

152. Chang SM, Nagueh SF, Spencer 3rd WH, Lakkis NM. Complete heart block: determinants and clinical impact in patients with hypertrophic obstructive cardiomyopathy undergoing nonsurgical septal reduction therapy. *J Am Coll Cardiol* 2003;**42**:296-300.
153. Faber L, Welge D, Fassbender D, Schmidt HK, Horstkotte D, Seggewiss H. One-year follow-up of percutaneous septal ablation for symptomatic hypertrophic obstructive cardiomyopathy in 312 patients: predictors of hemodynamic and clinical response. *Clin Res Cardiol* 2007;**96**:864-73.
154. Seggewiss H, Rigopoulos A, Welge D, Ziemssen P, Faber L. Long-term follow-up after percutaneous septal ablation in hypertrophic obstructive cardiomyopathy. *Clin Res Cardiol* 2007;**96**:856-63.
155. Gietzen FH, Leuner CJ, Raute-Kreinsen U, Dellmann A, Hegselmann J, Strunk-Mueller C, Kuhn HJ. Acute and long-term results after transcoronary ablation of septal hypertrophy (TASH): catheter interventional treatment for hypertrophic obstructive cardiomyopathy. *Eur Heart J* 1999;**20**:1342-54.
156. Oomman A, Ramachandran P, Subramanyan K, Kalarickal MS, Osman MN. Percutaneous transluminal septal myocardial ablation in drug-resistant hypertrophic obstructive cardiomyopathy: 18-month follow-up results. *J Invasive Cardiol* 2001;**13**:526-30.
157. Di Tullio M, Sacco RL, Gopal A, Mohr JP, Homma S. Patent foramen ovale as a risk factor for cryptogenic stroke. *Ann Intern Med* 1992;**117**:461-5.
158. Lechat P, Mas JL, Lascault G, Loron P, Theard M, Klimczac M, et al. Prevalence of patent foramen ovale in patients with stroke. *N Engl J Med* 1988;**318**:1148-52.
159. Bridges ND, Hellenbrand W, Latson L, Filiano J, Newburger JW, Lock JE. Transcatheter closure of patent foramen ovale after presumed paradoxical embolism. *Circulation* 1992;**86**:1902-8.
160. Harvey JR, Teague SM, Anderson JL, Voyles WF, Thadani U. Clinically silent atrial septal defects with evidence for cerebral embolization. *Ann Intern Med* 1986;**105**:695-7.
161. Braun MU, Fassbender D, Schoen SP, Haass M, Schraeder R, Scholtz W, Strasser RH. Transcatheter closure of patent foramen ovale in patients with cerebral ischemia. *J Am Coll Cardiol* 2002;**39**:2019-25.
162. Martin F, Sanchez PL, Doherty E, Colon-Hernandez PJ, Delgado G, Inglessis I, et al. Percutaneous transcatheter closure of patent foramen ovale in patients with paradoxical embolism. *Circulation* 2002;**106**:1121-6.
163. Onorato E, Melzi G, Casilli F, Pedon L, Rigatelli G, Carrozza A, et al. Patent foramen ovale with paradoxical embolism: mid-term results of transcatheter closure in 256 patients. *J Interv Cardiol* 2003;**16**:43-50.
164. Wahl A, Kunz M, Moschovitis A, Nageh T, Schwerzmann M, Seiler C, et al. Long-term results after fluoroscopy-guided closure of patent foramen ovale for secondary prevention of paradoxical embolism. *Heart* 2008;**94**:336-41.
165. Windecker S, Wahl A, Nedeltchev K, Arnold M, Schwerzmann M, Seiler C, et al. Comparison of medical treatment with percutaneous closure of patent foramen ovale in patients with cryptogenic stroke. *J Am Coll Cardiol* 2004;**44**:750-8.
166. Dowson A, Mullen MJ, Peatfield R, Muir K, Khan AA, Wells C, et al. Migraine Intervention with STARFlex Technology (MIST) Trial: a prospective, multicenter, double-blind, sham-controlled trial to evaluate the effectiveness of patent foramen ovale closure with STARFlex septal repair implant to resolve refractory migraine headache. *Circulation* 2008;**117**:1397-404.
167. Du ZD, Hijazi ZM, Kleinman CS, Silverman NH, Larntz K. Comparison between transcatheter and surgical closure of secundum atrial septal defect in children and adults: results of a multicenter nonrandomized trial. *J Am Coll Cardiol* 2002;**39**:1836-44.
168. Holzer R, Balzer D, Cao Q-L, Lock K, Hijazi ZM. Device closure of muscular ventricular septal defects using the Amplatzer muscular ventricular septal defect occluder: immediate and mid-term results of a U.S. registry. *J Am Coll Cardiol* 2004;**43**:1257-63.
169. Fu Y-C, Bass J, Amin Z, Radtke W, Cheatham JP, Hellenbrand WE, et al. Transcatheter closure of perimembranous ventricular septal defects using the new Amplatzer membranous VSD occluder: results of the U.S. phase I trial. *J Am Coll Cardiol* 2006;**47**:319-25.
170. Butera G, Carminati M, Chessa M, Piazza L, Micheletti A, Negura DG, et al. Transcatheter closure of perimembranous ventricular septal defects: early and long-term results. *J Am Coll Cardiol* 2007;**50**:1189-95.
171. Kantrowitz A, Tjonneland S, Freed PS, et al. Initial clinical experience with intraaortic balloon pumping in cardiogenic shock. *JAMA* 1968;**203**:113-18.
172. Trost JC, Hillis LD. Intra-aortic balloon counterpulsation. *Am J Cardiol* 2006;**97**:1391-8.
173. Burkhoff D, Cohen H, Brunckhorst C, O'Neill WW. A randomized multicenter clinical study to evaluate the safety and efficacy of the TandemHeart percutaneous ventricular assist device versus conventional therapy with intraaortic balloon pumping for treatment of cardiogenic shock. *Am Heart J* 2006;**152**(469):e1-8.

CHAPTER 57

Medical Management of Acute Coronary Syndromes

Robert M. Califf

Pathophysiology of Acute Coronary
  Syndromes
  Inflammatory Response to Injury
    Plaque Rupture
    Role of Platelets in ACS
Diagnosis and Epidemiology of Acute
  Coronary Syndrome Subtypes
Initial Risk Stratification
Medical Versus Catheterization-Based
  Strategies

Guideline-Recommended Medical
  Management of non–ST-Segment
  Elevation Acute Coronary Syndromes
  Anti-ischemic Agents
  Antithrombotic Therapy
  Intravenous Antithrombin Therapy
  Intravenous Platelet Glycoprotein IIb/IIIa
    Inhibitors
  Beta-Blockers
  Angiotensin-Converting Enzyme Inhibitors

Statins
Guideline-Recommended Medical
  Management of ST-Segment Elevation
  Myocardial Infarction
  General Management
  Fibrinolytic Agents
Predischarge Risk Stratification
Acute Coronary Syndromes in Patients
  with Previous Bypass Surgery
Conclusion

The term *acute coronary syndromes* (ACS) refers to the spectrum of conditions compatible with acute myocardial ischemia, from unstable angina to acute myocardial infarction (MI). These disorders are a major cause of morbidity and mortality around the world. In the United States alone, more than 650,000 people will have a new ACS event every year, and another 450,000 will have a repeated occurence.[1] Just under half of these people will die of their ACS event. ACS also entails major financial costs; in 1998 alone, Medicare paid $10.6 billion in hospital costs for ACS.[1]

The adverse clinical and financial consequences of ACS may be exacerbated by a lack of adherence to practice guideline recommendations. Since 1980, the American College of Cardiology (ACC) and the American Heart Association (AHA) jointly have published guidelines for the treatment of various cardiovascular diseases. In 2002, the ACC/AHA issued revised guidelines for the management of patients with unstable angina or non–ST-segment elevation acute MI (NSTEMI),[2] the two conditions that together make up non–ST-segment elevation ACS (NSTE ACS). For ST-segment acute MI (STEMI, the remaining disorder of ACS), the guidelines were last updated in 2008.[3] Whenever possible, the recommendations given in this chapter reflect these practice guidelines, which represent a consensus of relevant professional societies and are meant to assist physicians in making the most appropriate, evidence-based decisions about the management of their patients in specific circumstances.

PATHOPHYSIOLOGY OF ACUTE CORONARY SYNDROMES

The various manifestations of ACS share a pathophysiologic origin. They usually begin with the disruption, through fissuring or rupture, of an atherosclerotic plaque within the wall of a coronary artery. This stimulates expression of tissue factor, which in turn stimulates platelet activation, the coagulation cascade, and thrombus formation within the arterial wall, partially or completely occluding the coronary artery. The resulting reduced or absent blood flow to the myocardium may or may not produce symptoms of ischemia. Increasingly, the importance of platelet-fibrin emboli and diffuse vascular inflammation with "downstream" smaller vessel obstruction has been recognized.

Inflammatory Response to Injury

Many investigators have advanced the theory that atherosclerosis is an inflammatory response to injury within the vessel wall. The atherosclerotic lesions that form within coronary vessels are products of this chronic inflammatory process.

Various risk factors cause inflammatory changes in the circulation and vessel wall, including excess low-density lipoprotein (LDL) cholesterol and oxidized LDL cholesterol, other sources of oxidative stress, cigarette smoking, hypertension, and diabetes mellitus. Recently, immune responses and viral infections have also been implicated, although these findings remain controversial.[1,2,4,5] In a sense, it can be argued that atherosclerosis is the common response to combinations of these insults. Most recently, the concept that vascular progenitor cells from the marrow play a role in vessel repair has garnered intense interest. As this stem cell function becomes less effective with aging, the inability to repair vascular damage after inflammation may prove a critical factor in the relationship between aging and atherosclerosis.

For patients who undergo percutaneous coronary intervention (PCI), the procedure itself can traumatize the vessel wall, but the response to this mechanical injury is more fibrotic. Therefore, ACS rarely occurs after PCI by plaque fissuring at the site of the PCI, except in the immediate peri-procedural period. In contrast, the lumen of saphenous vein grafts is prone to lipid-rich atheroma and superimposed diffuse thrombosis so that over time, vein grafts become sources of unstable atheromatous mass.

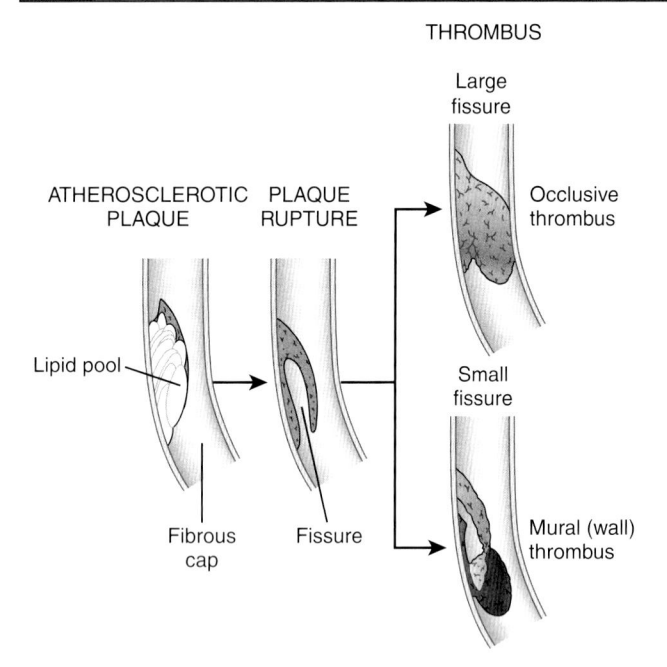

Figure 57-1
Pathophysiology of acute coronary syndromes. Rupture of an atherosclerotic plaque can lead to development of a mural (wall) thrombus or a partially or totally occlusive thrombus, resulting in ischemia.

Plaque Rupture

The most dangerous kind of plaque is a nonobstructive, lipid-rich plaque with a thin fibrous cap, often called vulnerable plaque, which is most prone to rupture. There may be gender differences in plaque behavior; women appear to be more prone than men to development of fissuring as opposed to rupture, with its correspondingly higher risk of nonocclusive thrombus (Fig. 57-1).

The degree of damage depends on the distribution of myocardium supplied by the affected artery; the degree of obstruction by the clot; the amount of small vessel obstructed by inflammation, thrombotic emboli, and vasoconstriction; and the extent of collateral flow. Even if the thrombus resulting from the original rupture does not obstruct the artery, smaller clots generated by the process (microemboli) can travel downstream to smaller arteries, occluding the microvasculature and causing myocardial necrosis.[6,7]

Most clinical signs of ACS reflect development of a clot large enough to cause ischemia, which can lead to myocardial necrosis with its ensuing risk of sudden death. Plaque rupture may cause no symptoms at all or may be characterized by exertion-related symptoms of ischemia (stable angina), unpredictable symptoms of ischemia without evidence of myocardial necrosis (unstable angina), signs of infarction without ST-segment elevation on the electrocardiogram (NSTEMI), signs of infarction with electrocardiographic changes such as ST-segment elevation (STEMI), or sudden death.

Angiographic and autopsy studies have shown that unstable angina and NSTEMI often reflect intermittent occlusion of coronary arteries with spontaneous recovery of blood flow to affected tissue (reperfusion).[8] Thrombotic occlusion is more persistent in STEMI because plaque damage is usually more severe or because collateral flow is absent.

Role of Platelets in ACS

Plaque rupture leads to vessel wall damage, which in turn stimulates the initiation of two pathways toward coagulation (Fig. 57-2). The intrinsic pathway of the coagulation cascade ultimately results in the production of thrombin. Thrombin is an enzyme that splits fibrinogen into fibrin monomers, which, when cross-linked, stabilize a platelet-rich thrombus by forming a net. Thrombin also amplifies the coagulation process by stimulating further thrombin generation. In addition, fibrin-bound thrombin activates (1) factor XIII, a plasma enzyme that stabilizes the linked fibrin threads, and (2) carboxypeptidase B, another enzyme that reduces the body's intrinsic fibrinolytic process.

The second pathway leading from plaque rupture to thrombosis begins when injury to the endothelium of the vessel (caused by plaque rupture or PCI) exposes collagen and von Willebrand's factor to the bloodstream. Platelets in the bloodstream quickly bind to von Willebrand's factor, forming a protective layer over the injured vessel wall. The bound platelets are then activated by collagen and undergo a conformational change, spewing vasoactive substances into the circulation. During this change, glycoprotein (GP) IIb/IIIa receptors are expressed on the platelet surface. Simultaneously, platelets release adenosine diphosphate and thromboxane, potent platelet stimulants, into the circulation. This release recruits and activates additional platelets. Fibrinogen in the bloodstream cross-links platelets through their GP IIb/IIIa receptors. Platelets start to aggregate, and a thrombus forms. Aspirin, ticlopidine, and clopidogrel inhibit some but not all portions of this pathway. GP IIb/IIIa inhibitors block the final step in thrombus formation by occupying GP IIb/IIIa receptors on platelets, thus preventing cross-linking of fibrinogen and aggregation of platelets.

These complementary pathways result in clot formation. In simple terms, platelet activation leads to expression of the GP IIb/IIIa receptor. Fibrin cross-links multiple platelets by binding simultaneously to two molecules of GP IIb/IIIa. The coagulation cascade leads to the production of fibrin, which binds the platelet thrombus into a resistant net.

DIAGNOSIS AND EPIDEMIOLOGY OF ACUTE CORONARY SYNDROME SUBTYPES

Patients with possible ACS are categorized by the presence or absence of persistent ST-segment elevation on electrocardiography and by the level of various biomarkers in their circulation (Fig. 57-3). This nomenclature is critical, because patients with persistent ST-segment elevation require lifesaving rapid reperfusion therapy, whereas no benefit of acute reperfusion therapy has been found in patients without ST-segment elevation. Patients with ACS but no persistent ST-segment elevation (and those with other electrocardiographic abnormalities) are retrospectively categorized as having unstable angina or NSTEMI, with or without Q waves, once the results of biomarker tests are available. This terminology is more descriptive than previous classifications in that it reflects the need for clinicians to make immediate therapeutic decisions once the medical history and electrocardiogram have been obtained. The epidemiology of ACS is changing, with more NSTE ACS and fewer STEMI cases being observed. These changes in the ACS population seem to reflect the aging of society

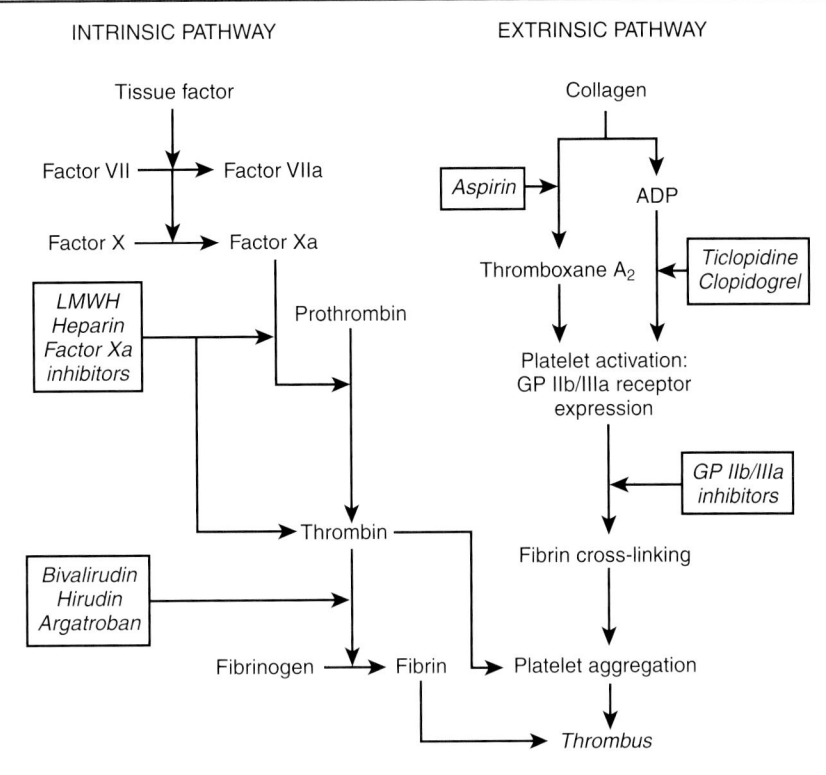

Figure 57–2
Role of platelets in thrombosis. Plaque rupture exposes tissue factor and collagen to the circulation, which stimulates intrinsic and extrinsic pathways to clotting. Medications that block various steps in these pathways are indicated in boxes. ADP, adenosine diphosphate; GP, glycoprotein; LMWH, low-molecular-weight heparin.

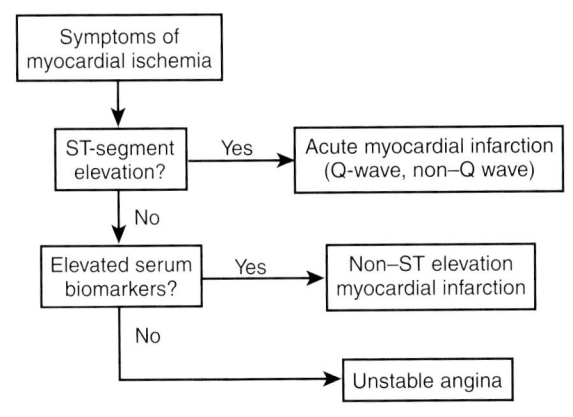

Figure 57–3
Categorization of patients with possible acute coronary syndromes. *(Modified from American Heart Association. Heart disease and stroke statistics—2003 update. Dallas: American Heart Association; 2003.)*

Table 57–1

Canadian Cardiovascular Society Classification of Anginal Symptoms[9]

Class	Description
I	No angina with ordinary activity; pain with strenuous exertion
II	Slight limitation of ordinary activity
III	Marked limitations of ordinary activity
IV	Pain with any physical activity; symptoms may occur at rest

(older patients have a higher proportion of NSTE ACS than STEMI) coupled with widespread use of effective secondary prevention measures that preclude the complete vessel occlusion required to produce STEMI. The adoption of troponin measurement as a standard of care has further expanded the population of NSTEMI patients who previously would have been classified as having unstable angina.

Unstable coronary syndromes may be classified according to the Canadian Cardiovascular Society classification, which grades symptoms from class I to class IV (Table 57-1).[9] This classification of angina is useful both prognostically and therapeutically. Patients with advanced Canadian Cardiovascular Society anginal symptoms have a higher risk of death from MI than do patients with more stable symptoms. There also is some suggestion that more potent therapies may be best suited to patients with the most advanced disease.

INITIAL RISK STRATIFICATION

Information from history, physical examination, electrocardiography, and biomarker tests is used to assign patients to one of four categories: noncardiac disorders, chronic stable angina, possible ACS, and definite ACS. This chapter is focused on the last two groups (Fig. 57-4).

Figure 57-5 shows an algorithm by which patients with symptoms of cardiac ischemia are treated at Duke University

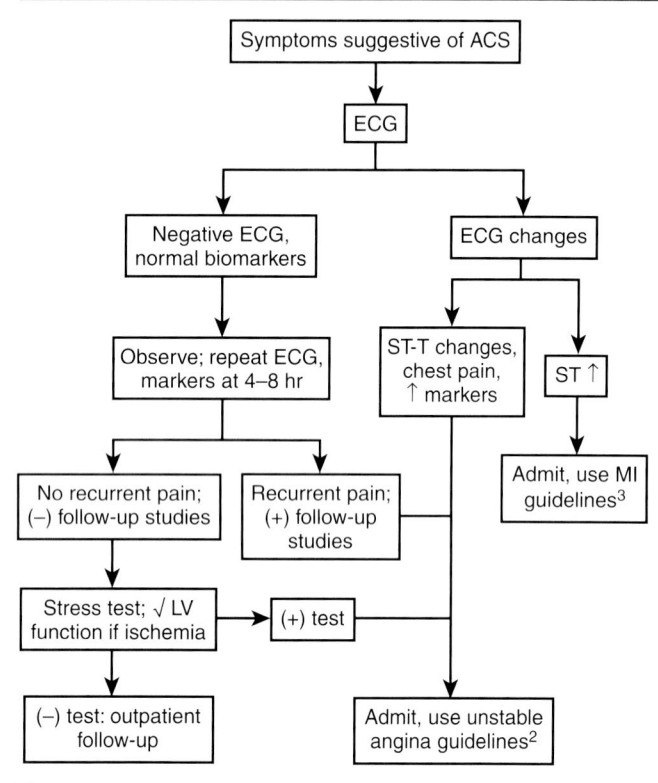

Figure 57–4
Evaluation and immediate management of patients with suspected acute coronary syndromes (ACS). ECG, electrocardiography; LV, left ventricular; MI, myocardial infarction.

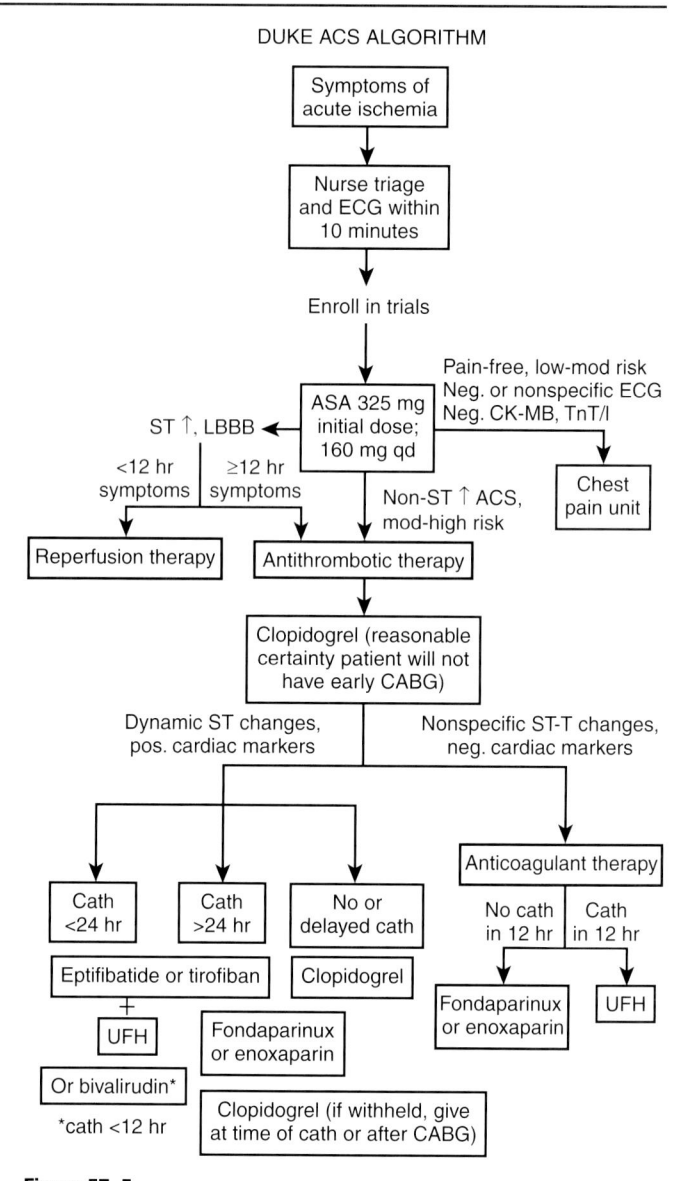

Figure 57–5
Algorithm for treatment of patients with symptoms of cardiac ischemia at Duke University Medical Center. ACS, acute coronary syndromes; ASA, aspirin; CABG, coronary artery bypass graft; CK-MB, creatine kinase MB isoenzyme; ECG, electrocardiography; LBBB, left bundle branch block; TnT/I, troponins T and I; UFH, unfractionated heparin.

Medical Center.[1] Patients with possible ACS are candidates for additional observation in a specialized facility (such as a chest pain unit).[10] Patients with definite ACS, as noted, are managed primarily according to the electrocardiographic pattern; those with ST-segment elevation are possible candidates for immediate reperfusion therapy and are managed according to American College of Cardiology and American Heart Association (ACC/AHA) practice guidelines for acute STEMI[3]; those without ST-segment elevation either undergo further observation or are admitted.[2] Patients with low-risk ACS and no transient ST-segment depression (≥0.05 mV) or T-wave inversions (≥0.2 mV), no positive cardiac markers or hemodynamic abnormalities, and no positive stress test result may be discharged and seen as outpatients.[1] This algorithm pertains to Duke University Medical Center only and should not be construed as presenting the definitive standard of care or containing diagnostic or therapeutic recommendations.

The prognosis of patients with NSTE ACS with positive markers or electrocardiographic abnormalities, contrary to the conventional wisdom, actually is worse than that of patients with acute STEMI; those with ST-segment depression, for example, have a mortality rate at 6 months of 8.9% compared with 6.8% for those with ST-segment elevation.[11] The risks of death and of death or MI at 30 days can be calculated for the general ACS population without STEMI according to a predictive model developed from the large Platelet Glycoprotein IIb/IIIa in Unstable Angina: Receptor Suppression Using Integrilin Therapy (PURSUIT) trial database (Fig. 57-6).[12] Perhaps not surprisingly, age, electrocardiographic pattern, and heart failure account for most of the risk. What is particularly useful about this model, however, is that use of these variables to determine early clinical risk also may allow us to predict which patients may derive the most benefit from more aggressive treatment.

For acute MI, the risk of death at 30 days was 7.0% in the Global Utilization of Streptokinase and TPA for Occluded Coronary Arteries (GUSTO-I) trial, the largest trial of fibrinolysis in MI to date.[13] (The rate had increased to 9.6% by 1 year.[14]) Among patients who died, the expected risk factors predominated; the most powerful of these were age, heart rate, hemodynamics, prior MI, and location of current MI. Figure 57-7 shows a nomogram for predicting 1-year mortality after MI among 30-day survivors, with use of the three most predictive baseline clinical, electrocardiographic, and in-hospital variables.[14] The only unexpected finding regarding risk factors predictive of mortality at 1 year versus 30 days was the poor long-term prognosis of black patients.[14] After adjustment for other prognostic factors, including revascularization,

		Score	
		Death	Death or MI
Age, yr	50	0	8 (11)
	60	2 (3)	9 (12)
	70	4 (6)	11 (13)
	80	6 (9)	12 (14)
Sex	Female	0	0
	Male	1	1
Worse CCS	0, I, II	0	0
past 6 weeks	III, IV	2	2
Heart rate, bpm	80	0	0
	100	1 (2)	0
	120	2 (5)	0
Systolic blood	120	0	0
pressure, mm Hg	100	1	0
	80	2	0
Heart failure	No	0	0
	Yes	3	2
ST depression	No	0	0
at baseline	Yes	3	1

Figure 57–6
Prediction of death or myocardial infarction (MI) at 30 days among patients with NSTE ACS in the PURSUIT trial. Separate points are assigned for the risk factors of age and heart rate, depending on whether the patient has unstable angina or MI (points for MI in parentheses). CCS, Canadian Cardiovascular Society. *(Reprinted with permission from Boersma E, Pieper KS, Steyerberg EW, et al. Predictors of outcomes in patients with acute coronary syndromes without persistent ST-segment elevation: results from an international trial of 9461 patients[12].)*

1. Find points for each marker	2. Sum points for all risk markers	3. Find risk for given point total	
Age, yr Points	Age _____	**Total points**	**Predicted survival (%)**
30 10		126	40
40 15	Prior MI _____	119	50
50 20		113	60
60 32	In-hospital	105	70
70 46	CHF/PE _____	94	80
80 59		77	90
90 73	Total _____	75	91
100 86		72	92
		69	93
Prior MI		65	94
No 0		61	95
Yes 18		56	96
		50	97
In-hospital CHF/PE		40	98
No 0		25	99
Yes 25			

Figure 57–7
Nomogram to predict 1-year survival in patients receiving fibrinolytic agents for myocardial infarction and surviving to days, with use of baseline clinical and electrocardiographic factors and in-hospital factors. CHF/PE, congestive heart failure or pulmonary edema; MI, myocardial infarction. *(Reprinted with permission from Califf RM, Pieper KS, Lee KL, et al. Prediction of 1-year survival after thrombolysis for acute myocardial infarction in the GUSTO-I trial[14].)*

black patients still had more than twice the risk of white patients for late mortality in GUSTO-I. Differential access to or use of secondary prevention measures may explain some of this disparity.

Cardiac biomarkers, especially the troponins, play an important role in risk stratification of patients with ACS, particularly those without ST-segment elevation. In the Global Use of Strategies To Open Occluded Coronary Arteries (GUSTO-IIa), for example, a positive troponin T result at baseline was highly predictive of 1-year mortality.[15] At 1 year, mortality among patients who were troponin positive at arrival was 14% compared with 5% among patients who were initially troponin negative. The Thrombolysis In Myocardial Infarction (TIMI) group has shown a strong association between baseline troponin I level and 42-day mortality in NSTE ACS.[16] Moreover, a positive baseline troponin T level can predict 1-year mortality in ACS, even after adjustment for other baseline clinical and electrocardiographic characteristics.[17]

Troponin levels also add predictive information even in the presence of STEMI.[15] Among patients with MI in the GUSTO-IIa trial, those with a positive baseline troponin T level had higher rates of death at 30 days (13% versus 4.7%), in-hospital repeated MI (91% versus 81%), and bypass surgery (16% versus 14%) compared with troponin-negative patients with STEMI.

Positive biomarkers predict not only which patients are at higher risk for adverse outcomes but also those who might benefit most from aggressive treatment. Lindahl and colleagues reported a greater benefit of dalteparin among baseline troponin T–positive patients (versus troponin T–negative) in the Fragmin In Unstable Coronary Artery Disease (FRISC) trial.[18] Other trials have shown preferential effects of GP IIb/IIIa inhibitors among patients with NSTE ACS who are troponin positive at baseline.[17-20] Finally, the benefits of an invasive versus a conservative mode of therapy may be greater for patients who are troponin positive on arrival.[21] Troponins appear to be a powerful tool for risk stratification and selection of aggressive medical and interventional therapies.

A biomarker of more recent interest is C-reactive protein. Although it is generally recognized as a marker of systemic inflammation and has recently been noted as a new risk marker for chronic coronary artery disease, the role of C-reactive protein in ACS has been less prominently discussed. In the recent GUSTO-IV ACS trial, elevated C-reactive protein level was a potent predictor of recurrent vascular events.[21]

Even more recently, several groups have shown the prognostic value of measurement of atrial natriuretic peptide and brain natriuretic peptide levels in patients with NSTE ACS.[22,23] This marker reflects atrial stretch, most often due to heart failure, in this population. Patients with elevated atrial natriuretic peptide and brain natriuretic peptide levels had a significantly increased risk of death during follow-up.

An approach that has gained in favor as data have accumulated is the "multimarker" strategy, initially introduced and recently confirmed in a randomized trial by Newby and colleagues.[24] This approach, which refers to the simultaneous use of troponin, creatine kinase (CK)–MB, and myoglobin, might be further enhanced by including C-reactive protein and brain natriuretic peptide in the mix of markers. In the future, arrays of protein biomarkers will likely be used to stratify prognosis, to determine preferred treatment alternatives, and to examine the biological impact of treatment for both research and clinical care.

MEDICAL VERSUS CATHETERIZATION-BASED STRATEGIES

Once a patient's risk has been estimated, the choices for management are split into two broad categories: medical management and catheter-based or surgical strategies. Table 57-2 details the definitive recommendations for early invasive

Table 57–2
Guideline Class IA Recommendations for Early Invasive Strategy (versus Medical Therapy Only) for Patients with NSTE ACS[2] and STEMI[3]

Characteristics	Treatment
NSTE ACS	
Angina that recurs; occurs at rest; occurs with heart failure symptoms, S_3 gallop, pulmonary edema, worsening rales, or new or worsening mitral regurgitation; or occurs with low-level activity despite intensive anti-ischemic therapy Elevated troponin (T or I) level New ST-segment depression High-risk findings on noninvasive stress test Left ventricular systolic function (ejection fraction <40% on noninvasive study) Hemodynamic instability Sustained ventricular tachycardia PCI within 6 months Prior bypass surgery	Early angiography, possible intervention
Left main disease,* candidate for bypass	Bypass
Three-vessel disease with ejection fraction <50%	Bypass
Multivessel disease including proximal left anterior descending coronary artery, ejection fraction <50%, or untreated diabetes	Bypass
Multivessel disease with ejection fraction >50%, no diabetes†	PCI
STEMI	
If able to be performed <12 hours after symptom onset or >12 hours if symptoms persist, if able to be performed <90 minutes at experienced centers‡	PCI
Persistent or recurrent symptomatic ischemia, spontaneous or induced, with or without electrocardiographic changes	PCI
Cardiogenic shock, severe pulmonary congestion, continuing hypotension, if able to be performed <18 hours after onset	PCI
Failed angioplasty with persistent pain or hemodynamic instability; suitable anatomy	Bypass
Persistent, recurrent, or refractory ischemia; suitable anatomy; not a candidate for PCI	Bypass
Surgical repair of ventricular septal defect of mitral valve insufficiency	Bypass

*50% diameter stenosis.
†Class/level of evidence I/A if severe angina persists despite medical therapy.
‡Operators performing more than 75 percutaneous coronary intervention (PCI) procedures per year; centers performing more than 200 procedures per year that have cardiac-surgery capability.
Modified from the ACC/AHA guidelines.[2,3]

approaches and procedures from the NSTE ACS and STEMI guidelines.[2,3] The bottom line for both STEMI and NSTE ACS is that for most patients with medium or high risk, catheterization is the critical component of treatment, which also should include medical therapy. Thus, medical therapy is seen not as an alternative to invasive evaluation and management but rather as an adjunctive but crucial component of the invasive strategy.

In general, for patients with NSTE ACS, medical management should be reserved only for those who are low risk, as evidenced by lack of electrocardiographic changes, hemodynamic abnormalities, or cardiac markers, and for patients in whom procedures are contraindicated. The FRISC II[25-26] and Treat Angina with Aggrastat and Determine the Cost of Therapy with Invasive or Conservative Strategies (TACTICS)–TIMI 18 trials[27] both have shown the superiority of an early invasive strategy versus a more conservative one. In FRISC II, however, randomization occurred after approximately 5 days of treatment with dalteparin. Thus, although the catheterization-based strategy appeared to benefit patients and dalteparin was beneficial during the waiting period, this approach is unlikely to be adopted because of the cost of prolonged observation. In the TACTICS–TIMI 18 trial, patients in the invasive arm underwent angiography much more rapidly than in FRISC II (median, 24 hours) with revascularization to follow. As with FRISC II, the invasive strategy was associated with significantly improved clinical outcomes. Also, in agreement with the troponin substudy of FRISC II,[25] the troponin-positive patients in TACTICS–TIMI 18 derived particular benefit from more aggressive management, showing an absolute 10% reduction in the primary endpoint (compared with an absolute 3.5% reduction for the trial population as a whole). Most recently, the third British Randomised Intervention Trial of Unstable Angina (RITA 3) also showed a benefit of early, aggressive intervention in this population.[28]

Recent trials in chronic stable coronary artery disease have shown only a modest symptomatic benefit for revascularization compared with modern medical therapy,[29,30] raising the question of whether the early interventional approach should be reassessed. Several major trials are ongoing, but until they provide results, the aggressive approach is still preferred in high-risk patients.

Primary PCI has become the standard of care for eligible STEMI patients treated at experienced centers. Bypass surgery becomes an option for those who are not candidates for PCI or for whom PCI has failed and for those who have persistent symptoms, unstable hemodynamics, or structural defects requiring concomitant cardiac surgery. Fibrinolysis remains the appropriate choice for patients who arrive at facilities with lower procedural volumes or that lack expertise for the invasive approach. Among patients with STEMI, medical management (without fibrinolysis or direct PCI) should be considered only for those with an absolute contraindication to both reperfusion approaches or for those with comorbid disease leading to an expressed desire to avoid life-prolonging interventions.

Given the rapid evolution of these guidelines toward the invasive approach to management, several organizational issues have become important. There is a considerable body of evidence showing that volume and expertise are critical in delivering acute invasive care to patients with ACS of both types. These findings point to the possibility of developing "ACS centers," similar to current trauma centers, so that well-prepared facilities can provide the best coordinated care.[31] An additional facet of this issue is the question of on-site surgery. The recently completed Cardiovascular Patient Outcomes Research Team (C-PORT) trial[32] found that direct PCI in sites without on-site surgery was superior to fibrinolysis with alteplase, although the trial was small and debate has arisen about whether these results are generalizable. Nevertheless, an increasing number of small hospitals are offering direct PCI for STEMI without on-site surgical backup. Arrangements should be in place at such institutions for rapid transfer of patients who need surgery, although the number of such cases continues to increase.

The role of surgery in this invasive approach remains subjective and poorly defined. In general, current guidelines recommend surgery for patients with three-vessel disease, left main disease, or concurrent structural defects (mitral regurgitation, septal defect). Despite the finding in the Bypass Angioplasty Revascularization Investigation (BARI) of the superiority of surgery over PCI in patients with diabetes mellitus,[33] referral patterns continue to favor PCI in diabetic patients unless the anatomy is considered technically prohibitive. Continuously emerging innovations such as drug-eluting stents, robotic surgery, and combined procedures make exact determination of the indication for PCI versus bypass surgery fluid at present.

GUIDELINE-RECOMMENDED MEDICAL MANAGEMENT OF NON–ST-SEGMENT ELEVATION ACUTE CORONARY SYNDROMES

In an ideal world, every clinical decision would be backed by firm evidence from large, adequately powered, randomized clinical trials. Such data exist for few clinical decisions, however. Table 57-3 lists the class I, level A recommendations ("almost always do it") and class III, level A recommendations ("never do it") from the ACC/AHA guidelines for NSTE ACS.[2,34] For most therapeutic decisions, physicians treating patients with ACS will not be able to rely on solid evidence.

Table 57–3
Guideline Recommendations for Medical Therapy in NSTE ACS[2,34]

Class IA (Recommended) Therapies
Immediate, continued antiplatelet therapy with aspirin; add or substitute clopidogrel if aspirin not tolerated or as appropriate
Platelet glycoprotein IIb/IIIa inhibition (plus aspirin or clopidogrel and heparin) if continued ischemia or other high-risk features
Subcutaneous low-molecular-weight or intravenous unfractionated heparin (plus aspirin or clopidogrel)
Platelet glycoprotein IIb/IIIa antagonist (plus aspirin or clopidogrel and heparin) if angiography and percutaneous intervention planned
Lipid-lowering drugs (statin) and diet if low-density lipoprotein level >130 mg/dL
Hypertension control to <130/85 mm Hg
Angiotensin-converting enzyme inhibitor for patients with heart failure, ejection fraction <40%, hypertension, or diabetes

Class IIIA (Not Recommended) Therapies
Immediate-release dihydropyridine calcium antagonist without beta-blockade
Thrombolytic therapy without ST-segment elevation, left bundle branch block, or true posterior infarction
Abciximab, if percutaneous intervention is not planned

Nevertheless, increasing support for the construct of "minimum necessary care" is accumulating from ongoing studies, and centers with excellent adherence to current guidelines have better patient outcomes.[34,35] It is also becoming clear that rates of adherence depend on institutional and group systems rather than on the attributes of individual providers.

Anti-ischemic Agents

Several therapies are thought by consensus groups to be valuable for initial management of ACS. One of these is bed rest with continuous electrocardiography for both arrhythmias and ongoing ischemia.[2] Also included is nitroglycerin, given sublingually, by spray, or intravenously. Patients should receive supplemental oxygen if they have evidence of respiratory distress or impaired oxygenation on pulse oximetry, and intravenous morphine can be valuable for relieving chest pain if nitroglycerin is ineffective.[2] Morphine also helps reduce anxiety and, correspondingly, the catecholamine surge that accompanies acute chest pain. The third advantage of intravenous morphine is that it dilates blood vessels, which could benefit patients with pulmonary congestion that might be aided through preload reduction.

Antithrombotic Therapy

Given that the pathophysiology of ACS involves thrombosis in response to vascular injury, it makes sense that the cornerstone of its medical management involves antithrombotic therapy. The key antithrombotic treatment for ACS—and for atherosclerotic coronary disease generally—is oral aspirin therapy.[36] In four randomized trials of aspirin versus placebo in patients with unstable angina,[37-40] there was an approximately 51% reduction in the risk of death at 30 days or more and a 47% reduction in the risk of death or MI with aspirin versus placebo. Further, the effect of aspirin therapy appears to be greatest among the highest risk patients (those with MI), with an estimated aggregate benefit of approximately 24 fewer deaths for every 1000 patients treated with 5 weeks of aspirin therapy.[41] For patients with unstable angina, there are about 50 fewer ischemic events at 6 months (vascular death, nonfatal MI, or nonfatal stroke) for every 1000 patients treated with aspirin versus placebo.[41] Aspirin also may have more than just an antiplatelet effect. In one study, patients with the highest plasma levels of C-reactive protein showed the greatest reduction in MI with aspirin treatment.[42] Another report noted that patients with chronic stable angina have increased levels of proinflammatory cytokines, which were reduced with aspirin treatment.[43]

Although the use of aspirin in ACS increases the risk of bleeding, there is a consensus that the benefits far outweigh the risks. Specifically, in patients undergoing bypass surgery, those treated with aspirin throughout the procedure show a dramatic reduction in postoperative ischemic events compared with those who did not receive aspirin throughout the procedure.[44]

For patients with either aspirin intolerance or true aspirin allergy, other oral antiplatelet agents may be valuable. In particular, a thienopyridine agent should be used for this subgroup of patients. The recent Clopidogrel in Unstable Angina to Prevent Recurrent Ischemic Events (CURE) trial provides the basis for use of dual antiplatelet strategy among patients with ACS.[45] In this study, 12,562 patients with NSTEMI were randomly assigned to receive aspirin plus placebo therapy or aspirin plus clopidogrel therapy. The primary endpoint of the trial was the composite of cardiovascular death, MI, or stroke. The incidence of the primary endpoint at a mean follow-up of 9 months was reduced from 11.5% in the aspirin-placebo group to 9.3% in the aspirin-clopidogrel group (relative risk reduction, 0.80; $P < .001$). The effect was focused on the incidence of MI, reducing this component from 6.7% to 5.2%. The risks of both major bleeding and transfusion were increased with combination therapy. The large CAPRIE trial supports the use of clopidogrel alone in high-risk patients.[46] This trial, which randomly assigned 19,185 patients with vascular disease (ischemic stroke, MI, peripheral arteriolar disease) to receive either aspirin or clopidogrel therapy, had a composite primary endpoint of vascular death, ischemic stroke, or nonfatal MI. With a mean follow-up of 1.9 years, the event rate was 5.32% with clopidogrel versus 5.83% for aspirin (relative risk reduction, 8.7%; 95% confidence interval, 0.3-16.5). The more recent CHARISMA trial[47] reinforces the view that dual antiplatelet therapy with aspirin and clopidogrel is beneficial in the acute and early chronic phase of ACS but may not be needed after the first year of treatment.

Bleeding in patients who undergo surgery after treatment with clopidogrel has been a contentious issue. Like aspirin, clopidogrel permanently impairs platelet function, but when it is used in conjunction with aspirin, the effect on surgical bleeding appears to be more profound than with aspirin alone. This has caused many to withhold clopidogrel in patients with ACS until the anatomy has been defined, so that such patients would not undergo surgery after clopidogrel treatment unless PCI failed. Others, meanwhile, argue that the clear benefits of clopidogrel when it is added to aspirin outweigh the bleeding risks incurred during surgery. Empiric analysis indicates that patients undergoing surgery more than 5 days after clopidogrel is discontinued no longer have an increased risk of bleeding. Several short-acting intravenous thienopyridine molecules are currently under development.[48,49] Their use is expected to improve the capability to manage operations much in the way that heparin is used for anticoagulation, with brief interludes to perform surgery.

Intravenous Antithrombin Therapy

Together with aspirin, intravenous or subcutaneous heparin has been a cornerstone of antithrombotic treatment of NSTE ACS, although the evidence is far from definitive.[50] Six randomized trials enrolling a combined total of only about 1300 patients have been done to date. They show a consistent trend toward a reduced incidence of death or MI during treatment with unfractionated heparin plus aspirin compared with aspirin alone ($P = .06$). The lack of statistical significance probably reflects the modest size of each individual trial and of the overall pooled population. This is partly why the ACC/AHA guideline recommendation for the use of heparin in NSTE ACS carries a grade of B for the supporting evidence.[2]

Heparin has several drawbacks as an antithrombotic agent. First, it binds to many plasma proteins present during atherosclerotic plaque rupture, making the drug less effective. Because the large size of the heparin molecule prevents deep penetration of thrombus, some thrombin in the ruptured plaque cannot be neutralized by heparin therapy. Heparin also requires an intermediary molecule, antithrombin III, making its pharmacodynamic effect less predictable. Adverse effects on platelets, including stimulation of platelet aggregation and development of the rare but sometimes fatal heparin-induced thrombocytopenia syndrome, also make heparin suboptimal in acute situations. Finally, the apparent "rebound effect" after discontinuation of heparin infusion, evidenced by a cluster of clinical effects occurring within hours afterward, can have serious implications for patients with unstable coronary syndromes.[51]

The low-molecular-weight heparins were developed to overcome some of the disadvantages of unfractionated heparin. They typically are given subcutaneously, appear to have a more stable dose response, are less resistant to uptake by circulating plasma proteins, and may be less likely to cause heparin-induced thrombocytopenia. Six moderate to large trials have randomly assigned patients with ACS to receive one of three different low-molecular-weight heparins or unfractionated heparin.[52-60] Together, the three trials of enoxaparin showed a clear advantage of this low-molecular-weight heparin over unfractionated heparin in reducing the composite endpoints of (1) death, MI, or recurrent ischemia and (2) death or MI (Table 57-4).[52-54] The most recent trials, the Aggrastat to Zocor (A to Z) and SYNERGY[61] studies, showed that in combination with a platelet GP IIb/IIIa inhibitor, enoxaparin again exhibited a trend toward superiority over unfractionated heparin.[54] This benefit, however, was achieved at the cost of a modest increase in the risk of bleeding.[52,53-59] A systematic overview[62] demonstrates these findings clearly (Fig. 57-8).

In the Fragmin in Unstable Coronary Artery Disease (FRIC) study of dalteparin[60] and the Fraxiparine in Ischaemic Syndrome (FRAXIS) trial of nadroparin,[63] no benefit over unfractionated heparin was observed. Because the various low-molecular-weight heparins have not been compared

Table 57-4
Clinical Efficacy of Enoxaparin in Randomized Trials of ACS

Study	N	Outcome Measure	Time of Measure (days)	Event Rate (%) Enoxaparin	Event Rate (%) Control
NSTE ACS					
ESSENCE[51]	3171	Death, infarction, recurrent ischemia	14	16.6	19.8
TIMI 11B[52]	3910	Death, infarction, urgent revascularization	43	17.3	19.7
A to Z[53]	3987	Death, reinfarction, refractory ischemia	7	8.4	9.4
STEMI					
ASENOX[55]	154	Death	30	7.1	8.2
Baird[56]	300	Death, reinfarction, readmission	90	26.0	36
ASSENT-3[57]	6116	Death, in-hospital reinfarction, in-hospital refractory ischemia	30	11.4	15.4
ASSENT-3 Plus[58]	1639	Death, in-hospital reinfarction, in-hospital refractory ischemia	30	14.2	17.4

directly, this heterogeneity in results may reflect the trials or the specific agents, but it seems prudent to recommend the use of enoxaparin for patients with ACS when a low-molecular-weight agent is chosen instead of unfractionated heparin.

Because low-molecular-weight heparins have a prolonged half-life and are given subcutaneously, surgical bleeding is a concern. This issue is particularly prominent in patients with renal dysfunction, because low-molecular-weight heparins are eliminated by the kidneys. Although a significant part of the activity of low-molecular-weight heparins is antagonized by protamine, studies raise the question of whether protamine has a detrimental effect on outcome.[64]

Three intravenous direct thrombin inhibitors—argatroban, lepirudin, and bivalirudin—have been approved for use in the United States. Argatroban and lepirudin are indicated for anticoagulant treatment of patients with heparin-induced thrombocytopenia, whereas bivalirudin is indicated for anticoagulant use in patients with ACS undergoing PCI. None is specifically approved as a primary anticoagulant for treatment of ACS, but lepirudin has been studied extensively in this group of patients,[65] and the pivotal trials that led to bivalirudin approval[66,67] enrolled patients with unstable angina and recent MI. A systematic registry[68] is assessing improvements in clinical outcomes with the direct thrombin inhibitors among patients with ACS and those requiring PCI, but more work is needed before any of these can be considered a cornerstone of therapy for patients with NSTE ACS.

A recent trial[69] compared treatment based on unfractionated or low-molecular-weight heparin with treatment based on bivalirudin in very high-risk ACS patients chosen for an early interventional approach. As in many other trials, bivalirudin resulted in fewer significant bleeding episodes. The combination of heparin and GP IIb/IIIa inhibitors resulted in nonsignificantly fewer acute ischemic events, so that the overall composite endpoint favored bivalirudin. Interestingly, 6-month mortality favored bivalirudin, whereas 1-year follow-up found no difference in total mortality.[70] Unfortunately, the combination of bivalirudin and a GP IIb/IIIa inhibitor seemed to result in more bleeding, with no further reduction in ischemic events. A trial with two arms (bivalirudin versus heparin plus GP IIb/IIIa inhibitor) found similar results in the STEMI populations.[71]

Fondaparinux is a synthetic direct factor Xa inhibitor that has been evaluated in both STEMI and NSTE ACS.[72] In both cases, fondaparinux exhibited a favorable profile of prevention of ischemic events and a lower rate of bleeding than did the comparator regimen. Uptake of this therapy has been limited by the finding that catheter-related thrombosis was higher in patients receiving fondaparinux treatment and by concerns that the trials were heavily weighted with patient enrollment in countries with developing economies (and therefore with correspondingly different patterns of practice).[73] Nevertheless, there is no debate about the fact that fondaparinux is a reasonable alternative antithrombotic strategy. Multiple ongoing trials are evaluating new direct thrombin inhibitors and factor Xa inhibitors that can be taken orally as well as intravenously.[74]

Intravenous Platelet Glycoprotein IIb/IIIa Inhibitors

Widespread awareness of the pivotal role that the platelet plays in the pathobiology of ACS led to development of GP IIb/IIIa inhibitors. These drugs have since become an important adjunctive therapy for patients with ACS. There are two basic categories of intravenous GP IIb/IIIa inhibitors: the monoclonal antibody and the small-molecule inhibitors. Three intravenous agents are approved for use in the

INTENTION-TO-TREAT POPULATION: EFFICACY ENDPOINTS AT 30 DAYS

A Death at 30 days

Trial	Events, No./Total (%) Enoxaparin	UFH	OR (95% CI)
ESSENCE	39/1607 (2.4)	49/1564 (3.1)	0.77 (0.51–1.18)
TIMI 11B	66/1953 (3.4)	71/1957 (3.6)	0.93 (0.66–1.31)
ACUTE II	8/315 (2.5)	4/210 (1.9)	2.29 (0.56–9.43)
INTERACT	9/380 (2.4)	15/366 (4.1)	0.58 (0.26–1.32)
A to Z	47/1853 (2.5)	33/1765 (1.9)	1.36 (0.87–2.13)
SYNERGY	160/4992 (3.2)	153/4983 (3.1)	1.04 (0.84–1.30)
Overall	329/11100 (3.0)	325/10845 (3.0)	1.00 (0.85–1.17)

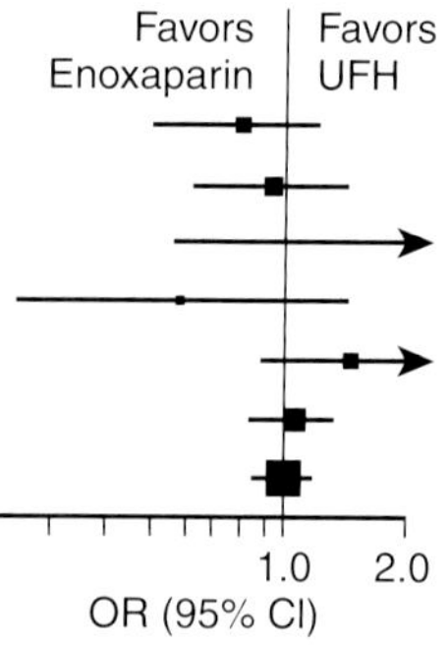

B Death or myocardial infarction at 30 days

Trial	Events, No./Total (%) Enoxaparin	UFH	OR (95% CI)
ESSENCE	94/1607 (5.8)	118/1564 (7.5)	0.76 (0.58–1.01)
TIMI 11B	145/1953 (7.4)	163/1957 (8.3)	0.88 (0.70–1.11)
ACUTE II	25/315 (7.9)	17/210 (8.1)	0.97 (0.51–1.83)
INTERACT	19/380 (5.0)	33/366 (9.0)	0.54 (0.30–0.96)
A to Z	137/1852 (7.4)	139/1768 (7.9)	0.94 (0.73–1.20)
SYNERGY	696/4992 (14.0)	722/4962 (14.5)	0.96 (0.86–1.07)
Overall	1116/11099 (10.1)	1192/10847 (11.0)	0.91 (0.83–0.99)

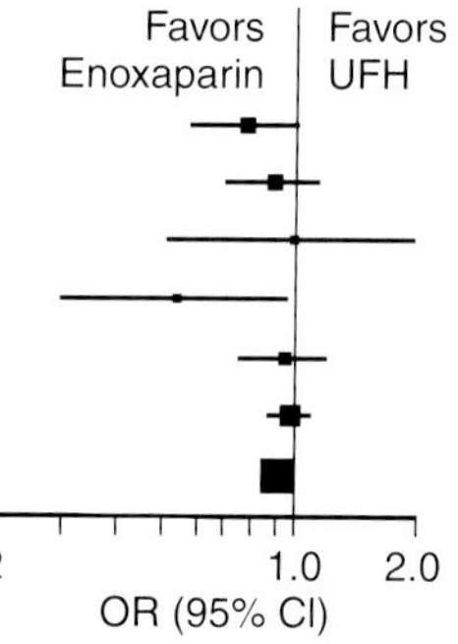

A

SAFETY ANALYSIS: TRANSFUSION UP TO 7 DAYS AFTER RANDOMIZATION

A Overall safety population

Trial	Events, No./Total (%) Enoxaparin	UFH	OR (95% CI)
ESSENCE	52/1578 (3.3)	58/1529 (3.8)	0.87 (0.59–1.26)
TIMI 11B	13/1938 (0.7)	13/455 (0.6)	1.17 (0.53–2.58)
INTERACT	10/380 (2.6)	12/366 (3.3)	0.80 (0.35–1.85)
SYNERGY	506/4148 (12.2)	566/4775 (11.8)	1.03 (0.91–1.17)
Overall	581/8044 (7.2)	647/8606 (7.5)	1.01 (0.89–1.14)

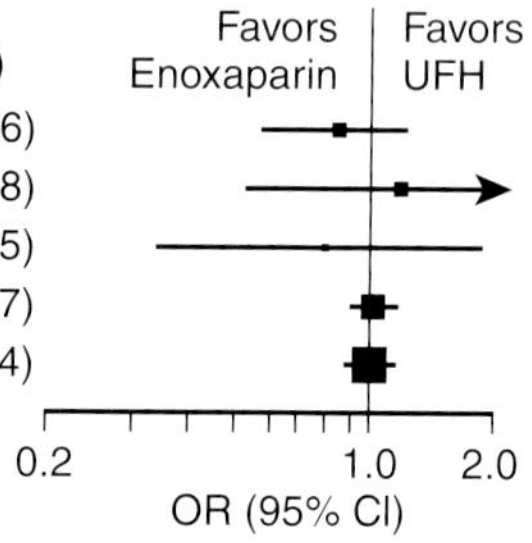

B No prerandomization therapy safety population

Trial	Events, No./Total (%) Enoxaparin	UFH	OR (95% CI)
ESSENCE	52/1578 (3.3)	58/1529 (3.8)	0.87 (0.59–1.26)
TIMI 11B	13/1248 (1.0)	7/1233 (0.6)	1.79 (0.73–4.37)
INTERACT	6/304 (2.0)	9/295 (3.1)	0.66 (0.24–1.80)
SYNERGY	137/1056 (13.0)	157/1158 (13.6)	0.95 (0.74–1.22)
Overall	208/4186 (5.0)	231/4215 (5.5)	0.94 (0.77–1.16)

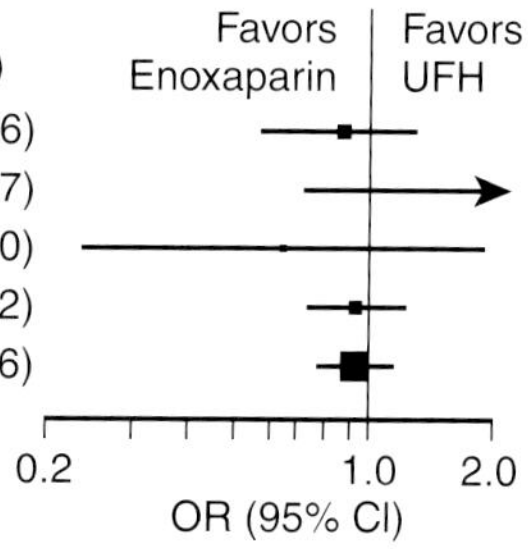

B

Figure 57–8
A, Efficacy of enoxaparin versus unfractionated heparin (UFH) in intention-to-treat population at 30 days. **B,** Safety of enoxaparin versus unfractionated heparin: transfusion up to 7 days after randomization. *(Reprinted with permission from Petersen JL, Mahaffey KW, Hasselblad V, et al. Efficacy and bleeding complications among patients randomized to enoxaparin or unfractionated heparin for antithrombin therapy in non–ST-segment elevation acute coronary syndromes: a systematic overview.[62])*

United States: the monoclonal antibody fragment abciximab; eptifibatide, a peptide inhibitor; and tirofiban, a peptidomimetic. These agents have many similarities but also many differences, including their molecular sizes, ease and speed of reversibility, selectivity, and antigenic properties.[75]

The use of GP IIb/IIIa inhibitors in PCI or NSTE ACS has seen some of the most intense research in acute cardiac care in the last decade. At least 14 major clinical trials have compared these agents with placebo in these settings, and almost 50,000 patients have been randomized. This very large data set allows us to draw inferences about the benefits and risks of this drug class.

There have been six moderate to large placebo-controlled trials of GP IIb/IIIa inhibitors in patients with ACS.[76] In the aggregate, the 30-day incidence of death or MI was reduced by a modest but statistically significant relative 9% with the use of these agents. In each of the five trials that studied either a peptide or peptidomimetic GP IIb/IIIa inhibitor, the estimated effect always favored the platelet inhibitor; whereas in the single large trial of abciximab, the opposite was true. These trials differed in study design, however, making direct comparisons inappropriate and potentially misleading. For example, three trials measured a primary endpoint of death or MI at 30 days (PARAGON-A, PURSUIT, and GUSTO-IV); the other three also included refractory ischemia (PRISM and PRISM-PLUS) or severe recurrent ischemia (PARAGON-B). PARAGON-B had a 30-day primary endpoint, but the two tirofiban trials had a much earlier primary endpoint (48 hours in PRISM and 7 days in PRISM-PLUS). Nonetheless, it appears prudent to recommend only the small-molecule compounds for initial "upstream" GP IIb/IIIa inhibition in appropriate patients, specifically, those considered high risk at initial evaluation. This includes patients (1) older than 65 years, (2) with prolonged or ongoing chest pain, (3) with chest pain at rest with ischemic electrocardiographic changes, (4) with hemodynamic instability (including evidence of heart failure), and (5) with elevated cardiac biomarkers (CK-MB or troponin).[2]

As with other antiplatelet agents, bleeding is increased with GP IIb/IIIa inhibitors, especially in the mucosal areas, including the gastrointestinal tract. There is no antidote to these agents, but their active half-life is relatively short, as the platelet is not irreversibly altered. Interesting data have emerged to indicate that patients undergoing bypass surgery may benefit from GP IIb/IIIa inhibition during the procedure.[77] Previous research shows that platelets are activated during cardiopulmonary bypass and a significant proportion of platelets stick to the bypass conduits and membranes; GP IIb/IIIa inhibitors reduce this effect. Furthermore, in patients who undergo urgent procedures after receiving GP IIb/IIIa inhibitors, clinical outcomes appear to be improved relative to those undergoing surgery without GP IIb/IIIa inhibition.[78] These findings must be examined in randomized clinical trials before routine treatment prior to surgery can be justified, but surgeons at least can be comfortable with proceeding when treatment already has occurred.

The use of GP IIb/IIIa inhibitors has declined in recent years, particularly as dual treatment with aspirin and a thienopyridine has been found to be effective. The large EARLY ACS trial[79] found that in the modern era of routine use of aspirin, thienopyridines, and effective anticoagulation, the use of GP IIb/IIIa inhibitors prior to entry into the catheterization laboratory did not add benefit, compared with assessing the anatomy with angiography and adding GP IIb/IIIa inhibitors after the decision was made to pursue high-risk PCI.

Beta-Blockers

All patients with ACS should be given a beta-blocker if such therapy is not contraindicated.[2] For patients in the acute phase of ischemia, an intravenous agent should be considered. Most of the data supporting beta-blockade in ACS reflects literature reporting on experiences with STEMI; most of it predates the reperfusion era. The largest experience with beta-blockers was the first International Study of Infarct Survival (ISIS) trial, which showed that mortality was reduced by approximately 15% with atenolol versus placebo treatment among 16,027 patients with suspected acute MI, many of whom did not have STEMI.[80] In a substudy of the TIMI IIIB trial, however, rates of reinfarction and recurrent ischemia were lower with immediate use of metoprolol versus delayed use; the study did not have adequate statistical power to assess mortality.[81] Nonetheless, the bulk of the evidence supports use of beta-blockade in all patients with ACS, unless there is an absolute contraindication, such as acute decompensated heart failure with various levels of bradycardia and heart block. Although other conditions, such as chronic lung disease, have been considered relative contraindications to beta-blockers, a recent evaluation of the Medicare database provides supportive evidence for a major benefit of beta-blockers even in patients with relative contraindications.[82]

Angiotensin-Converting Enzyme Inhibitors

There are no data to support the use of angiotensin-converting enzyme (ACE) inhibitors as acute therapy for NSTE ACS, but substantial evidence supports their relatively early use in MI and their long-term value in this population. A series of systematic overviews in which all known patient data have been combined into a single database provides definitive evidence of major benefit in patients with evidence of heart failure or left ventricular dysfunction.[83] Highly significant evidence for benefit in all MI patients was found in this overview, although the magnitude of the benefit was relatively small (5 lives saved per 1000 patients treated).

The Heart Outcomes Prevention Evaluation (HOPE) study, which compared ramipril and placebo in patients with vascular disease or high-risk characteristics such as diabetes, showed significantly improved clinical outcomes with ramipril.[84] The current guidelines therefore call for the use of ACE inhibitors in patients with ACS and heart failure, left ventricular dysfunction (ejection fraction <40%), hypertension, or diabetes. Additional large trials are evaluating ACE inhibitors in patients without left ventricular dysfunction to determine whether the HOPE findings can be validated with other ACE inhibitors or angiotensin receptor blockers.

For patients unable to tolerate ACE inhibitors because of cough (a common side effect of ACE inhibitors), angiotensin-receptor blockers appear to produce similar benefits without the side effects. To date, angiotensin receptor blockers cannot be recommended as substitutes for ACE inhibitors in most situations because they have not been proved superior in head-to-head trials; rather, they should be reserved for patients who cannot tolerate ACE inhibitors. However, a large amount of data now supports the concept that either choice is reasonable in the post-MI setting (VALIANT[85]) and in the chronic setting of left ventricular dysfunction (CHARM[86]); further, we now have firm data that angiotensin receptor blockers reduce cardiovascular events in patients who cannot tolerate ACE inhibitors (CHARM,[86,87]).

Statins

Cholesterol-lowering therapy reduces vascular events and mortality in patients with coronary artery disease and hypercholesterolemia[87] and in patients with mild cholesterol elevation (209 to 218 mg/dL) after MI and unstable angina.[89,90] In the Myocardial Ischemia Reduction with Aggressive Cholesterol Lowering (MIRACL) study, 3086 patients were randomly assigned to treatment with either atorvastatin (80 mg daily) or placebo 24 to 96 hours after ACS.[91] At 16 weeks, only 14.8% of treated patients had reached the primary endpoint of death, nonfatal MI, resuscitated cardiac arrest, or recurrent severe myocardial ischemia compared with 17.4% of the placebo-treated patients (P = .048). The risks of death, nonfatal MI, cardiac arrest, and worsening heart failure did not differ between the two groups, but treated patients had fewer strokes and less severe recurrent ischemia. The Lipid–Coronary Artery Disease (L-CAD) study randomly assigned patients with ACS (N = 126) to early treatment with pravastatin (alone or combined with cholestyramine or niacin) or usual care. At 24 months, the early-aggressive treatment group had significantly fewer clinical events than the usual care group (23% versus 52%; P = .005).[92] In a Swedish registry of approximately 20,000 patients, the adjusted relative risk of mortality was 25% lower in cardiac patients who started statin therapy before discharge.[93] However, several registries have failed to replicate these findings.[94] The evidence for safety nevertheless is substantial with early treatment, and continued long-term therapy is clearly much more likely when it is started in the hospital. The National Cholesterol Education Program 2 and the ACC/AHA guidelines for NSTE ACS therefore recommend a target LDL cholesterol level of less than 100 mg/dL, a low–saturated fat diet for people with an LDL cholesterol level of more than 100 mg/dL, and the addition of lipid-lowering therapy for those with an LDL cholesterol level of more than 130 mg/dL.[2,6,95]

Most recently, the PROVE-IT trial[96] randomly assigned ACS patients to either atorvastatin (80 mg/day) or pravastatin (40 mg/day) after initial symptomatic and hemodynamic stabilization. This produced a gradient in median LDL cholesterol levels from 95 mg/dL in patients treated with pravastatin to 62 mg/dL in patients treated with atorvastatin. A 16% reduction in major cardiac events was observed. This has pushed the target for LDL cholesterol level to less than 70 mg/dL in the view of many experts. In addition, achievement of a C-reactive protein level below 2.0 mg/dL was associated with a superior outcome in this trial.

GUIDELINE-RECOMMENDED MEDICAL MANAGEMENT OF ST-SEGMENT ELEVATION MYOCARDIAL INFARCTION

General Management

For the most part, medical management in acute STEMI closely follows medical treatment in NSTE ACS, except when fibrinolytic agents are used; the primary difference is the withholding of GP IIb/IIIa inhibitors if fibrinolytic agents are going to be given. Studies examining the use of such combination treatment in patients with MI have had disappointing results, although some role may be found in young patients at low risk for intracranial hemorrhage.[97,98]

Fibrinolytic Agents

The evidence that direct PCI is superior to fibrinolytic therapy for acute reperfusion in STEMI when both are available in competent hands is not definitive. Debate remains concerning three possible situations: when prehospital administration of fibrinolytic drugs is feasible[99]; when the patient must be transported a long distance or for a long time to receive access to direct PCI[100]; and when more than 6 hours have elapsed since symptom onset. Efforts to regionalize access to appropriate acute cardiac care should diminish the proportion of uncertain cases.[101] The Occluded Artery Trial[29] clarified that beyond the first 24 hours, opening of a recently totally occluded artery is not an emergency imperative.

When fibrinolytic therapy is needed, the four most commonly used agents are streptokinase, alteplase, reteplase, and tenecteplase. Table 57-5 presents a brief comparison of these agents.[102-108] The incidence of TIMI grade 3 (normal) blood flow at 90 minutes after treatment initiation ranges from 33% (with streptokinase) to 63% (with tenecteplase) when it is given with intravenous heparin. This knowledge is critical because early achievement of normal coronary blood flow has been linked with improved 30-day survival.[103] Tenecteplase has the added advantage of single-bolus dosing.

Table 57–5
Fibrinolytic Agents for STEMI

Agent	90-Minute TIMI Grade 3 Flow (%)	30-Day Mortality	In-Hospital Events	
			Any Stroke	Reinfarction
Streptokinase	33	7.4	1.4	4.0
Alteplase	54	6.3	1.6	4.0
Reteplase	59	7.5	1.6	4.2
Tenecteplase	55-63	6.2	1.8	4.1

*With intravenous heparin.
†Depending on weight.

The most significant complications of fibrinolytic therapy relate to bleeding risk. The rate of in-hospital intracranial hemorrhage has ranged from 0.57% with streptokinase to 0.93% with tenecteplase (both given with intravenous heparin).[104-106] Rates of serious or major bleeding rates follow this basic pattern, but the use of transfusions in these patients has decreased during the years. For example, the rate of transfusion among alteplase-treated patients in GUSTO-I (enrollment completed in 1993) was 10%[102]; by 1997, when GUSTO-III completed enrollment, it had decreased to 6.3%[106]; and by 1998, when ASSENT-2 completed enrollment, it was only 5.5%.[105] Thus, although the incidence of serious bleeding has not decreased, physicians appear to have become more judicious in their use of transfusions, perhaps because of increasing knowledge of the risks involved.[109]

PREDISCHARGE RISK STRATIFICATION

Patients with ACS should undergo continuous risk stratification—from the initial assessment, to the initial response to treatment, to the hospital course after leaving the intensive or cardiac care unit. Once the patient's condition has stabilized, if a conservative approach to intervention has been chosen, noninvasive stress testing by radionuclide imaging, echocardiography, or exercise or pharmacologic stress testing is recommended.[110-112] Such testing can detect ischemia in patients with a low likelihood of coronary disease and, more important, provide an integrated estimate of risk, including left ventricular function. With the results of noninvasive testing, other appropriate diagnostic and therapeutic measures can begin.

The choice of test should reflect patient characteristics, test availability, and expertise in interpretation. Because it is simple, inexpensive, and easy to perform and to interpret, the standard low-level exercise electrocardiographic stress test remains the test of choice for patients who are able to exercise and have no confounding factors on the resting electrocardiogram. Otherwise healthy patients with confounding electrocardiographic factors should undergo exercise testing with imaging. Patients who cannot exercise should undergo a pharmacologic stress test with imaging. Low-risk patients without symptoms for 12 to 24 hours can undergo a low-level exercise test (Bruce stage II). Patients without ischemic signs for 7 to 10 days can undergo a symptom-limited test.

In general, induction of ischemia at a low workload (≤ 6.5 metabolic equivalents [METs]) or a high-risk treadmill score (≥ 11)[113] implies severe impairment in coronary blood flow. Such results are associated with increased risks for adverse outcomes or severe angina after discharge. Barring contraindications, such patients generally merit referral for early angiography and possible revascularization. Conversely, achievement of a higher workload (>6.5 METs) without evidence of ischemia (low-risk treadmill score ≥ 5) correlates with lesser coronary artery obstruction and a better prognosis. Such patients often can be safely managed with a conservative approach. Ischemia developing above 6.5 METs may be associated with severe coronary artery obstruction, but unless patients have other high-risk markers (>0.2 mV ST-segment depression or elevation, decreased blood pressure, ST-segment shifts in multiple leads, or prolonged recovery of ST shifts), they also can be managed conservatively.

Recently, computed tomographic angiography has become available as a test to estimate the extent of angiographic disease. The most plausible use of this technology is in patients with acute symptoms but without definitive electrocardiographic abnormalities or elevated cardiac markers, although much more evidence is needed. In patients with definitive ACS, computed tomographic angiography might have utility in detecting severe three-vessel disease and left main disease, although no credible studies have yet been done in this indication.

ACUTE CORONARY SYNDROMES IN PATIENTS WITH PREVIOUS BYPASS SURGERY

Although bypass surgery improves survival and quality of life, many patients return with acute ACS events, particularly after 5 years of follow-up. In general, patients with prior bypass surgery have a worse prognosis when an ACS event occurs than do patients without prior surgery. Part of this increased risk is due to the advanced age of this population relative to patients without previous bypass grafting. Unfortunately, no clinical trials have specifically addressed the issue of management in post-bypass patients with ACS. Most large trials have included these patients, however, offering some opportunity to look at potential differences in retrospect.

In NSTE ACS, no difference in benefit has been observed for any of the standard therapies as a function of previous bypass surgery.[114-116] In STEMI, outcomes after fibrinolysis trend in the same direction for post-bypass patients as with others. When primary PCI is used as the method of reperfusion, identification of the infarct artery is difficult, and results of the procedure may be less successful.[117,118] When the bypass graft itself is the "culprit," the benefit of GP IIb/IIIa inhibitors is not clear.[118]

CONCLUSION

The field of ACS is now dominated by large, definitive clinical trials that have established a standard of care that is leading to better clinical outcomes. The criteria for surgical treatment of ACS continue to evolve, but the preferred status of the invasive approach and the emerging technological improvements in both PCI and surgery will likely lead to more revascularization procedures. Invasive therapy still must be coupled with the best medical therapy, as described.

REFERENCES

1. American Heart Association. *Heart Disease and Stroke Statistics—2003 Update*. Dallas: American Heart Association; 2003.
2. Braunwald E, Antman EM, Beasley JM, et al: ACC/AHA 2002 guideline update for the management of patients with unstable angina and non–ST-segment elevation myocardial infarction. Available at: http://www.acc.org/clinical/guidelines/unstable/incorporated/index.htm. Accessed 31 March 2003.
3. Pollack Jr CV, Antman EM, Hollander JE. American College of Cardiology; American Heart Association. 2007 focused update to the ACC/AHA guidelines for the management of patients with ST-segment elevation myocardial infarction: implications for emergency department practice. *Ann Emerg Med* 2008;**2008**(52):344-55el.
4. Libby P, Ridker PM. Novel inflammatory markers of coronary risk: theory versus practice. *Circulation* 1999;**100**:1148-50.
5. Danesh J. Coronary heart disease, Helicobacter pylori, dental disease, Chlamydia pneumoniae, and cytomegalovirus: meta-analyses of prospective studies. *Am Heart J* 1999;**138**:S434-7.

6. Roe MT, Ohman EM, Maas AC, et al. Shifting the open-artery hypothesis downstream: the quest for optimal reperfusion. *J Am Coll Cardiol* 2001;**37**:9-18.
7. Topol EJ, Yadav JS. Recognition of the importance of embolization in atherosclerotic vascular disease. *Circulation* 2000;**101**:570-80.
8. Fuster V, Badimon L, Badimon JJ, et al. The pathogenesis of coronary artery disease and the acute coronary syndromes. *N Engl J Med* 1992;**326**:242-50.
9. Campeau L. Grading of angina pectoris. *Circulation* 1976;**54**:522-3.
10. Newby LK, Storrow AB, Gibler WB, et al. Bedside multimarker testing for risk stratification in chest pain units: the CHest pain Evaluation by Creatine Kinase-MB, Myoglobin, And Troponin I (CHECKMATE) study. *Circulation* 2001;**103**:1832-7.
11. Savonitto S, Ardissino D, Granger CB, et al. Prognostic value of the admission electrocardiogram in acute coronary syndromes. *JAMA* 1999;**281**:707-13.
12. Boersma E, Pieper KS, Steyerberg EW, et al. Predictors of outcomes in patients with acute coronary syndromes without persistent ST-segment elevation: results from an international trial of 9461 patients. *Circulation* 2000;**101**:2557-67.
13. Lee KL, Woodlief LW, Topol EJ, et al. Predictors of 30-day mortality in the era of reperfusion for acute myocardial infarction: results from an international trial of 41,021 patients. *Circulation* 1995;**91**:1659-68.
14. Califf RM, Pieper KS, Lee KL, et al. Prediction of 1-year survival after thrombolysis for acute myocardial infarction in the GUSTO-I trial. *Circulation* 2000;**101**:2231-8.
15. Ohman EM, Armstrong PW, Christenson RH, et al. Cardiac troponin T levels for risk stratification in acute myocardial ischemia. *N Engl J Med* 1996;**335**:1333-41.
16. Antman EM, Tanasijevic MJ, Thompson B, et al. Cardiac-specific troponin I levels to predict the risk of mortality in patients with acute coronary syndromes. *N Engl J Med* 1996;**335**:1342-9.
17. Newby LK, Christenson RH, Ohman EM, et al. Value of serial troponin T measures for early and late risk stratification in patients with acute coronary syndromes. *Circulation* 1998;**98**:1853-9.
18. Lindahl B, Venge P, Wallentin Z. Troponin T identifies patients with unstable coronary artery disease who benefit from long-term antithrombotic protection. Fragmin in unstable coronary artery disease (FRISC) study group. *J Am coll Cardiol* 1997;**29**:43-8.
19. Heeschen C, Hamm CW, Goldmann B, et al. Troponin concentrations for stratification of patients with acute coronary syndromes in relation to therapeutic efficacy of tirofiban. *Lancet* 1999;**354**:1757-62.
20. Newby LK, Ohman EM, Christenson RH, et al. Benefit of glycoprotein IIb/IIIa inhibition in patients with acute coronary syndromes and troponin T–positive status: the PARAGON-B troponin T substudy. *Circulation* 2001;**103**:2891-6.
21. James SK, Armstrong P, Barnathan E, et al. Troponin and C-reactive protein have different relations to subsequent mortality and myocardial infarction after acute coronary syndrome. A GUSTO-IV substudy. *J Am Coll Cardiol* 2003;**41**:916-24.
22. Omland T, de Lemos JA, Morrow DA, et al. Prognostic value of N-terminal pro-atrial and pro-brain natriuretic peptide in patients with acute coronary syndromes. *Am J Cardiol* 2002;**89**:463-5.
23. Morrow DA, de Lemos JA, Blazing MA, et al. Prognostic value of serial B-type natriuretic peptide testing during follow-up of patients with unstable coronary artery disease. *JAMA* 2005;**294**:2866-71.
24. Newby LK, Storrow AB, Gibler WB, et al. Bedside multimarker testing for risk stratification in chest pain units: The chest pain evaluation by creatine kinase-MB, myoglobin, and troponin I (CHECKMATE) study. *Circulation* 2001;**103**:1832-7.
25. Kontny F. Improving outcomes in acute coronary syndromes: the FRISC II trial. *Clin Cardiol* 2002;**24**:I3-7.
26. FRISC II Investigators. Invasive compared with non-invasive treatment in unstable coronary-artery disease: FRISC II prospective randomised multicentre study. *Lancet* 1999;**354**:708-15.
27. Cannon CP, Weintraub WS, Demopoulos LA, et al. Comparison of early invasive and conservative strategies in patients with unstable coronary syndromes treated with the glycoprotein IIb/IIIa inhibitor tirofiban. *N Engl J Med* 2001;**344**:1879-87.
28. Fox KA, Poole-Wilson PA, Henderson RA, et al. Interventional versus conservative treatment for patients with unstable angina or non–ST-elevation myocardial infarction: the British Heart Foundation RITA 3 randomised trial. *Lancet* 2002;**360**:743-51.
29. Hochman JS, Lamas GA, Buller CE, et al. Coronary intervention for persistent occlusion after myocardial infarction. *N Engl J Med* 2006;**355**:2395-407.
30. Shaw LJ, Berman DS, Maron DJ, et al. Optimal medical therapy with or without percutaneous coronary intervention to reduce ischemic burden: results from the Clinical Outcomes Utilizing Revascularization and Aggressive Drug Evaluation (COURAGE) trial nuclear substudy. *Circulation* 2008;**117**:1283-91.
31. Califf RM, Faxon DP. Need for centers to care for patients with acute coronary syndromes. *Circulation* 2003;**107**:1467-70.
32. Aversano T, Aversano LT, Passamani E, et al. Thrombolytic therapy vs primary percutaneous coronary intervention for myocardial infarction in patients presenting to hospitals without on-site cardiac surgery: a randomized controlled trial. *JAMA* 2002;**287**:1943-51.
33. The BARI. Investigators: Comparison of coronary bypass surgery with angioplasty in patients with multivessel disease. *N Engl J Med* 1996;**335**:217-25.
34. Califf RM, Peterson ED, Gibbons RJ, et al. Integrating quality into the cycle of therapeutic development. *J Am Coll Cardiol* 2002;**40**:1895-901.
35. Peterson ED, Pollack CV, Roe MT, et al. Early use of glycoprotein IIb/IIIa inhibitors and outcomes in non–ST-elevation acute myocardial infarction: observations from NRMI-4. *J Am Coll Cardiol* 2002;**39**:303A.
36. Antiplatelet Trialists' Collaboration. Collaborative overview of randomised trials of antiplatelet therapy, I: prevention of death, myocardial infarction, and stroke by prolonged antiplatelet therapy in various categories of patients. *BMJ* 1994;**308**:81-106.
37. Cairns JA, Gent M, Singer J, et al. Aspirin, sulfinpyrazone, or both in unstable angina. Results of a Canadian multicenter trial. *N Engl J Med* 1985;**313**:1369-75.
38. Lewis Jr HD, Davis JW, Archibald DG, et al. Protective effects of aspirin against acute myocardial infarction and death in men with unstable angina. Results of a Veterans Administration Cooperative Study. *N Engl J Med* 1983;**309**:396-403.
39. Theroux P, Ouimet H, McCans J, et al. Aspirin, heparin, or both to treat acute unstable angina. *N Engl J Med* 1988;**319**:1105-11.
40. Wallentin. LC, for the Research Group on Instability in Coronary Artery Disease in Southeast Sweden: aspirin (75 mg/day) after an episode of unstable coronary artery disease: long-term effects on the risk for myocardial infarction, occurrence of severe angina and the need for revascularization. *J Am Coll Cardiol* 1991;**18**:1587-93.
41. Awtry EH, Loscalzo J. Aspirin. *Circulation* 2000;**101**:1206-18.
42. Ridker PM, Cushman M, Stampfer MJ, et al. Inflammation, aspirin, and the risk of cardiovascular disease in apparently healthy men [erratum published N Engl J Med 337:356, 1997]. *N Engl J Med* 1997;**336**:973-9.
43. Ikonomidis I, Andreotti F, Economou E, et al. Increased proinflammatory cytokines in patients with chronic stable angina and their reduction by aspirin. *Circulation* 1999;**100**:793-8.
44. Mangano DT. Aspirin and mortality from coronary bypass surgery. *N Engl J Med* 2002;**347**:1309-17.
45. The CURE. Trial Investigators: Effects of clopidogrel in addition to aspirin in patients with acute coronary syndromes without ST-segment elevation. *N Engl J Med* 2001;**345**:494-502.
46. The CAPRIE. Steering Committee: A randomised, blinded, trial of clopidogrel versus aspirin in patients at risk of ischaemic events (CAPRIE). *Lancet* 1996;**348**:1329-39.
47. Wang TH, Bhatt DL, Fox KA, et al. An analysis of mortality rates with dual-antiplatelet therapy in the primary prevention population of the CHARISMA trial. *Eur Heart J* 2007;**28**:2200-7.
48. Storey RF, Judge HM, Wilcox RG, et al. Inhibition of ADP-induced P-selectin expression and platelet-leukocyte conjugate formation by clopidogrel and the $P2Y_{12}$ receptor antagonist AR-C69931MX but not aspirin. *Thromb Haemost* 2002;**88**:488-94.
49. Greenbaum AB, Ohman EM, Gibson CM, et al. Preliminary experience with intravenous $P2Y_{12}$ platelet receptor inhibition as an adjunct to reduced-dose alteplase during acute myocardial infarction: results of the Safety, Tolerability and Effect on Patency in Acute Myocardial Infarction (STEP-AMI) angiographic trial. *Am Heart J* 2007;**154**:702-9.
50. Oler A, Whooley MA, Oler J, et al. Adding heparin to aspirin reduces the incidence of myocardial infarction and death in patients with unstable angina. A meta-analysis. *JAMA* 1996;**276**:811-5.
51. Bahit MC, Topol EJ, Califf RM, et al. Reactivation of ischemic events in acute coronary syndromes: results from GUSTO-IIb. *J Am Coll Cardiol* 2001;**37**:1001-7.
52. The ESSENCE. Study Group: A comparison of low-molecular-weight heparin with unfractionated heparin for unstable coronary artery disease. *N Engl J Med* 1997;**337**:447-52.
53. Antman EM, McCabe CH, Gurfinkel EP, et al. Enoxaparin prevents death and cardiac ischemic events in unstable angina/non–Q-wave myocardial infarction: results of the Thrombolysis In Myocardial Infarction (TIMI) 11B trial. *Circulation* 1999;**100**:1593-601.
54. Blazing MA, de Lemos JA, White HD, et al. Safety and efficacy of enoxaparin vs unfractionated heparin in patients with non–ST-segment elevation acute coronary syndromes who receive tirofiban and aspirin: a randomized controlled trial. *JAMA* 2004;**292**:55-64.
55. Wong GC, Giugliano RP, Antman EM. Use of low-molecular-weight heparins in the management of acute coronary artery syndromes and percutaneous coronary intervention. *JAMA* 2003;**289**:331-42.

56. Tatu-Chitoiu G, Teodorescu C, Dan M, et al. Efficacy and safety of a new streptokinase regimen with enoxaparin in acute myocardial infarction. *J Thromb Thrombolysis* 2003;**15**:171-9.
57. Baird SH, Menown IB, McBride SJ, et al. Randomised comparison of enoxaparin with unfractionated heparin following fibrinolytic therapy for acute myocardial infarction. *Eur Heart J* 2002;**23**:627-32.
58. The ASSENT-3 Investigators: Efficacy and safety of tenecteplase in combination with enoxaparin, abciximab, or unfractionated heparin: the ASSENT-3 randomised trial in acute myocardial infarction. *Lancet* 2001;**358**:605-13.
59. Wallentin L, Goldstein P, Armstrong PW, et al. Efficacy and safety of tenecteplase in combination with the low-molecular-weight heparin enoxaparin or unfractionated heparin in the prehospital setting: the Assessment of the Safety and Efficacy of a New Thrombolytic Regimen (ASSENT)–3 PLUS randomized trial in acute myocardial infarction. *Circulation* 2003;**108**:135-42.
60. Klein W, Buchwald A, Hillis SE, et al. Comparison of low-molecular-weight heparin with unfractionated heparin acutely and with placebo for 6 weeks in the management of unstable coronary artery disease [erratum published Circulation 97:413, 1998]. *Circulation* 1997;**96**:61-8.
61. Mahaffey KW, Cohen M, Garg J, et al. High-risk patients with acute coronary syndromes treated with low-molecular-weight or unfractionated heparin: outcomes at 6 months and 1 year in the SYNERGY trial. *JAMA* 2005;**294**: 2594-600.
62. Petersen JL, Mahaffey KW, Hasselblad V, et al. Efficacy and bleeding complications among patients randomized to enoxaparin or unfractionated heparin for antithrombin therapy in non–ST-segment elevation acute coronary syndromes: a systematic overview. *JAMA* 2004;**292**:89-96.
63. The FRAXIS. Study Group: Comparison of two treatment durations (6 days and 14 days) of a low molecular weight heparin with a 6-day treatment of unfractionated heparin in the initial management of unstable angina or non–Q wave myocardial infarction. *Eur Heart J* 1999;**20**:1553-62.
64. Stafford-Smith M, Lefrak EA, Qazi AG, et al. Efficacy and safety of heparinase I versus protamine in patients undergoing coronary artery bypass grafting with and without cardiopulmonary bypass. *Anesthesiology* 2005;**103**:229-40.
65. The OASIS-2 Investigators. Effects of recombinant hirudin (lepirudin) compared with heparin on death, myocardial infarction, refractory angina, and revascularisation procedures in patients with acute myocardial ischaemia without ST elevation: a randomised trial. *Lancet* 1999;**353**:429-38.
66. Bittl JA, Strony J, Brinker JA, et al. Treatment with bivalirudin (Hirulog) as compared with heparin during coronary angioplasty for unstable or postinfarction angina. *N Engl J Med* 1995;**333**:764-9.
67. Bittl JA, Chaitman BR, Feit F, et al. Bivalirudin versus heparin during coronary angioplasty for unstable or postinfarction angina: final report reanalysis of the Bivalirudin Angioplasty Study. *Am Heart J* 2001;**142**:952-9.
68. Granger CB. Strategies at patient care in acute coronary syndromes: rationale for the Global Registry of Acute Coronary Events (GRACE) Registry. *Am J Cardiol* 2000;**86**:4M-9M.
69. Stone GW, McLaurin BT, Cox DA, et al. Bivalirudin for patients with acute coronary syndromes. *N Engl J Med* 2006;**355**:2203-16.
70. White HD, Ohman EM, Lincoff AM, et al. Safety and efficacy of bivalirudin with and without glycoprotein IIb/IIIa inhibitors in patients with acute coronary syndromes undergoing percutaneous coronary intervention 1-year results from the ACUITY (Acute Catheterization and Urgent Intervention Triage strategY) trial. *J Am Coll Cardiol* 2008;**52**:807-14.
71. Stone GW, Witzenbichler B, Guagliumi G, et al. Bivalirudin during primary PCI in acute myocardial infarction. *N Engl J Med* 2008;**358**:2218-30.
72. Yusuf S, Mehta SR, Chrolavicius S, et al. Effects of fondaparinux on mortality and reinfarction in patients with acute ST-segment elevation myocardial infarction: the OASIS-6 randomized trial. *JAMA* 2006;**295**:1519-30.
73. Califf RM. Fondaparinux in ST-segment elevation myocardial infarction: the drug, the strategy, the environment, or all of the above? *JAMA* 2006;**295**: 1579-80.
74. Giugliano RP, Braunwald E. The year in non–ST-segment elevation acute coronary syndrome. *J Am Coll Cardiol* 2008;**52**:1095-103.
75. Lincoff AM, Califf RM, Topol EJ. Platelet glycoprotein IIb/IIIa receptor blockade in coronary artery disease. *J Am Coll Cardiol* 2000;**35**:1103-15.
76. Boersma E, Harrington RA, Moliterno DJ, et al. Platelet glycoprotein IIb/IIIa inhibitors in acute coronary syndromes: a meta-analysis of all major randomised clinical trials (erratum published Lancet 359:2120, 2002). *Lancet* 2002;**359**:189-98.
77. The PRISM-PLUS. Study Investigators: Inhibition of the platelet glycoprotein IIb/IIIa receptor with tirofiban in unstable angina and non–Q-wave myocardial infarction. *N Engl J Med* 1998;**338**:1488-97.
78. Dyke CM, Bhatia D, Lorenz TJ, et al. Immediate coronary artery bypass surgery after platelet inhibition with eptifibatide: results from PURSUIT. *Ann Thorac Surg* 2000;**70**:866-71.
79. Giugliano RP, White JA, Bode C, et al. Early versus delayed, provisional eptifibatide in acute coronary syndrome. *N Engl J Med* 2009;**360**:2176-90.
80. First International Study of Infarct Survival Collaborative Group. Randomised trial of intravenous atenolol among 16 027 cases of suspected acute myocardial infarction: ISIS-1. *Lancet* 1986;**2**:57-66.
81. The TIMI. IIIB Investigators: Effects of tissue plasminogen activator and a comparison of early invasive and conservative strategies in unstable angina and non–Q-wave infarction: results of the TIMI IIIB trial. *Circulation* 1994;**89**:1545-56.
82. Chen J, Radford MJ, Wang Y, et al. Effectiveness of beta-blocker therapy after acute myocardial infarction in elderly patients with chronic obstructive pulmonary disease or asthma. *J Am Coll Cardiol* 2001;**37**:1950-6.
83. Latini R, Maggioni AP, Flather M, et al. ACE inhibitor use in patients with myocardial infarction. Summary of evidence from clinical trials. *Circulation* 1995;**92**:3132-7.
84. The HOPE. Study Investigators: Effects of ramipril on cardiovascular and microvascular outcomes in people with diabetes mellitus: results of the HOPE study and MICRO-HOPE substudy. *Lancet* 2000;**355**:253-9.
85. Pfeffer MA, McMurray JJ, Velazquez EJ, et al. Valsartan, captopril, or both in myocardial infarction complicated by heart failure, left ventricular dysfunction, or both. *N Engl J Med* 2003;**349**:1893-906.
86. Young JB, Dunlap ME, Pfeffer MA, et al. Mortality and morbidity reduction with Candesartan in patients with chronic heart failure and left ventricular systolic dysfunction: results of the CHARM low-left ventricular ejection fraction trials. *Circulation* 2004;**110**:2618-26.
87. Granger CB, McMurray JJ, Yusuf S, et al. Effects of candesartan in patients with chronic heart failure and reduced left-ventricular systolic function intolerant to angiotensin-converting-enzyme inhibitors: the CHARM-Alternative trial. *Lancet* 2003;**362**:772-6.
88. The 4S Study Group: Randomised trial of cholesterol lowering in 4444 patients with coronary heart disease: the Scandinavian Simvastatin Survival Study (4S). *Lancet* 1994;**344**:1383-9.
89. The LIPID. Study Group: Prevention of cardiovascular events and death with pravastatin in patients with coronary heart disease and a broad range of initial cholesterol levels. *N Engl J Med* 1996;**339**:1349-57.
90. Sacks FM, Pfeffer MA, Moye LA, et al. The effect of pravastatin on coronary events after myocardial infarction in patients with average cholesterol levels. *N Engl J Med* 1996;**335**:1001-9.
91. Schwartz GG, Olsson AG, Ezekowitz MD, et al. Effects of atorvastatin on early recurrent ischemic events in acute coronary syndromes. The MIRACL Study: a randomized trial. *JAMA* 2001;**285**:1711-8.
92. Arntz HR, Agrawal R, Wunderlich W, et al. Beneficial effects of pravastatin (+/– cholestyramine/niacin) initiated immediately after a coronary event (the randomized Lipid-Coronary Artery Disease [L-CAD] Study). *Am J Cardiol* 2000;**86**:1293-8.
93. Stenestrand U, Wallentin L. Early statin treatment following acute myocardial infarction and 1-year survival. *JAMA* 2001;**285**:430-6.
94. Newby LK, Kristinsson A, Bhapkar MV, et al. Early statin initiation and outcomes in patients with acute coronary syndromes. *JAMA* 2002;**287**:3087-95.
95. National Cholesterol Education Program. *Second report of the Expert Panel on Detection, Evaluation, and Treatment of High Blood Cholesterol in Adults (Adult Treatment Panel II)*. Washington, DC: US Dept of Health and Human Services; 1993, NIH publication No. 93-3096.
96. Murphy SA, Cannon CP, Wiviott SD, et al. Effect of intensive lipid-lowering therapy on mortality after acute coronary syndrome (a patient-level analysis of the Aggrastat to Zocor and Pravastatin or Atorvastatin Evaluation and Infection Therapy–Thrombolysis in Myocardial Infarction 22 trials). *Am J Cardiol* 2007;**100**:1047-51.
97. The SPEED. Study Group: Trial of abciximab with and without low-dose reteplase for acute myocardial infarction. *Circulation* 2000;**101**:2788-94.
98. Topol EJ. Reperfusion therapy for acute myocardial infarction with fibrinolytic therapy or combination reduced fibrinolytic therapy and platelet glycoprotein IIb/IIIa inhibition: the GUSTO V randomised trial. *Lancet* 2001;**357**:1905-14.
99. Welsh RC, Travers A, Senaratne M, et al. Feasibility and applicability of paramedic-based prehospital fibrinolysis in a large North American center. *Am Heart J* 2006;**152**:1007-14.
100. Widimsky P, Budesinsky T, Vorac D, et al. Long distance transport for primary angioplasty vs immediate thrombolysis in acute myocardial infarction. Final results of the randomized national multicentre trial—PRAGUE-2. *Eur Heart J* 2003;**24**:94-104.
101. Jollis JG, Roettig ML, Aluko AO, et al. Implementation of a statewide system for coronary reperfusion for ST-segment elevation myocardial infarction. *JAMA* 2007;**298**:2371-80.
102. The GUSTO Investigators. An international randomized trial comparing four thrombolytic strategies for acute myocardial infarction. *N Engl J Med* 1993;**329**:673-82.
103. Simes RJ, Holmes Jr DR, Ross AM, et al. The link between the angiographic substudy and mortality outcomes in a large randomized trial of myocardial

103. reperfusion: the importance of early and complete infarct artery reperfusion. *Circulation* 1995;**91**:1923-8.
104. Gore JM, Granger CB, Sloan MA, et al. Stroke after thrombolytic therapy: mortality and functional outcomes in the GUSTO-I trial. *Circulation* 1995;**92**:2811-8.
105. The ASSENT-2 Investigators: Single-bolus tenecteplase compared with front-loaded alteplase in acute myocardial infarction: the ASSENT-2 double-blind randomised trial. *Lancet* 1999;**354**:716-22.
106. The GUSTO- III . Investigators: A comparison of reteplase with alteplase for acute myocardial infarction [erratum published N Engl J Med 338:546-547, 1998]. *N Engl J Med* 1997;**337**:1118-23.
107. Cannon CP, Gibson CM, McCabe CH, et al. TNK–tissue plasminogen activator compared with front loaded alteplase in acute myocardial infarction: results of the TIMI 10B trial. *Circulation* 1998;**98**:2805-14.
108. The RAPID II . Investigators: Randomized comparison of coronary thrombolysis achieved with double-bolus reteplase (recombinant plasminogen activator) and front-loaded, accelerated alteplase (recombinant tissue plasminogen activator) in patients with acute myocardial infarction. *Circulation* 1996;**94**:891-8.
109. Goodnough LT, Brecher ME, Kanter MH, et al. Transfusion medicine. Blood transfusion. *N Engl J Med* 1999;**340**:438-47.
110. Gibbons RJ, Balady GJ, Beasley JW, et al. ACC/AHA guidelines for exercise testing. *J Am Coll Cardiol* 1997;**30**:260-311.
111. Cheitlin MD, Alpert JS, Armstrong WF, et al. ACC/AHA guidelines for the clinical application of echocardiography. Developed in collaboration with the American Society of Echocardiography. *Circulation* 1997;**95**:1686-744.
112. Ritchie JL, Bateman TM, Bonow RO, et al. Guidelines for the clinical use of cardiac radionuclide imaging. Developed in collaboration with the American Society of Nuclear Cardiology. *J Am Coll Cardiol* 1995;**25**:521-47.
113. Mark DB, Shaw L, Harrell Jr FE, et al. Prognostic value of a treadmill exercise score in outpatients with suspected coronary artery disease. *N Engl J Med* 1991;**325**:849-53.
114. Labinaz M, Kilaru R, Pieper K, et al. Outcomes of patients with acute coronary syndromes and prior coronary artery bypass grafting: results from the platelet glycoprotein IIb/IIIa in unstable angina: receptor suppression using integrilin therapy (PURSUIT) trial. *Circulation* 2002;**105**:322-7.
115. Labinaz M, Sketch Jr MH, Ellis SG, et al. Outcome of acute ST-segment elevation myocardial infarction in patients with prior coronary artery bypass surgery receiving thrombolytic therapy. *Am Heart J* 2001;**141**:469-77.
116. Brilakis ES, de Lemos JA, Cannon CP, et al. Outcomes of patients with acute coronary syndrome and previous coronary artery bypass grafting (from the Pravastatin or Atorvastatin Evaluation and Infection Therapy [PROVE IT-TIMI 22] and the Aggrastat to Zocor [A to Z] trials). *Am J Cardiol* 2008;**102**:552-8:2008.
117. Grines CL, Westerhausen DR, Grines LL, et al. A randomized trial of transfer for primary angioplasty versus on-site thrombolysis in patients with high-risk myocardial infarction. *J Am Coll Cardiol* 2002;**39**:1713-9.
118. Mehta RH, Honeycutt E, Shaw LK, Glower D, Harrington RA, Sketch Jr MH. Clinical correlates of long-term mortality after percutaneous interventions of saphenous vein grafts. *Am Heart J* 2006;**152**:801-6.

CHAPTER 58
The Pharmacologic Management of Heart Failure
Eric H. Awtry and Wilson S. Colucci

Pathophysiology of Heart Failure
  Acute Heart Failure
  Chronic Heart Failure
Pharmacologic Agents Used in the Treatment of Heart Failure
  Specific Agents
    Diuretics
    Vasodilators

Neurohormonal Inhibiting Agents
Inotropic Agents
Other Agents
  Natriuretic Peptides
Approach to the Management of Heart Failure
  Initial Approach and Clinical Assessment

Pharmacologic Treatment of Chronic Compensated Systolic Heart Failure
Treatment of Decompensated Systolic Heart Failure
Treatment of Diastolic Heart Failure
Flash Pulmonary Edema
Perioperative Heart Failure

Heart failure has become an increasingly important cause of morbidity and mortality in the United States and in other industrialized nations. Despite improvement in heart failure treatment, its prevalence continues to rise, in large part as a result of the aging of the population and the improved survival of heart failure patients. In 2006, the most recent year for which statistics are available, the estimated prevalence of heart failure in the U.S. population was 5.7 million. In the same year, heart failure was listed as the primary diagnosis in almost 1.1 million hospital discharges, an increase of 26% since 1996. The economic impact is staggering, with a yearly cost of caring for these patients estimated at more than $37 billion, more than half of which is accounted for by direct hospital costs. Despite improvements in therapies, one in five patients will die within 1 year of the initial diagnosis with heart failure, and in the United States alone, heart failure is listed as the principal cause for almost 59,000 deaths annually and as a contributing cause in more than 292,000 deaths.

From a surgical standpoint, heart failure has a significant impact on perioperative morbidity and mortality. Preoperative heart failure is a strong predictor of adverse outcome in patients undergoing noncardiac surgery, and a history of heart failure or depressed left ventricular systolic function is an independent predictor of mortality after coronary artery bypass surgery. A thorough understanding of the pathophysiology and treatment of heart failure is therefore essential for those physicians who manage patients in the perioperative period. Effective preoperative management of heart failure may prevent perioperative decompensation, and rapid recognition and treatment of postoperative heart failure are essential to prevent progressive pulmonary congestion and organ hypoperfusion. For the well-compensated patient, an understanding of the medical management of chronic heart failure ensures continuation of appropriate therapy both perioperatively and at the time of hospital discharge.

This chapter focuses primarily on the various pharmacologic modalities available for the treatment of heart failure, including their mechanisms of action, benefits as shown in clinical trials, and suggested utility in the management of patients with acute and chronic heart failure. The use of many of these pharmacotherapies is based on our current understanding of the pathophysiologic mechanisms underlying heart failure. Therefore, a brief mechanistic overview is provided in an effort to place these therapies in a pathophysiologic context.

PATHOPHYSIOLOGY OF HEART FAILURE

Our understanding of the pathophysiology of heart failure has evolved dramatically during the past 2 decades. The traditional hemodynamic model, although still applicable in the setting of acutely decompensated heart failure, is less relevant in the setting of chronic heart failure, for which the concepts of progressive ventricular remodeling and neurohormonal activation have come to the forefront. These processes are briefly discussed here as they relate to the pharmacologic treatment of heart failure.

The term *heart failure* does not refer to a single entity; rather, it denotes a syndrome that is characterized by signs or symptoms of intravascular volume overload or manifestations of inadequate tissue perfusion. It is the end result of a variety of cardiac injuries and the ensuing pathologic remodeling that impair the heart's ability to fill with or to eject blood; it may originate from a wide range of disorders of the myocardium, pericardium, endocardium, or intracardiac valves (Table 58-1). Heart failure can be categorized pathophysiologically in several ways.

- *Left-sided heart failure* is characterized by signs and symptoms of pulmonary congestion (dyspnea, orthopnea, pulmonary rales, pleural effusions). *Right-sided heart failure* is characterized by peripheral congestion (elevated jugular venous pressure, peripheral edema, hepatic congestion).
- *Systolic heart failure* refers to that occurring in the setting of left ventricular systolic dysfunction (i.e., reduced ejection fraction). *Diastolic heart failure* refers to that resulting from impaired left ventricular diastolic filling despite normal left ventricular systolic function. These two abnormalities often coexist, although one usually predominates.

Table 58-1
Common Causes of Heart Failure

Myocardial
Ischemia or infarction
Viral myocarditis
Idiopathic cardiomyopathy
Hypertrophic cardiomyopathy
Hypertension
Toxins (alcohol, cocaine, chemotherapeutic agents)
Infiltrative diseases (amyloidosis, hemochromatosis)
Infectious (Lyme disease, Chagas' disease)
Peripartum cardiomyopathy
Thyroid dysfunction
Metabolic abnormalities (thiamine or selenium deficiency)
Valvular
Aortic stenosis
Aortic regurgitation
Mitral stenosis
Mitral regurgitation
Arrhythmic
Tachycardia-mediated cardiomyopathy
Pericardial
Constrictive pericarditis

Table 58-2
Clinical Classifications of Heart Failure

New York Heart Association Classification	
Class I	Symptoms only with greater than usual activity
Class II	Asymptomatic at rest but with symptoms during normal activities
Class III	Asymptomatic at rest but with symptoms during minimal exertion
Class IV	Symptoms at rest
American College of Cardiology/American Heart Association Classification	
Stage A	Patients with structurally normal hearts, asymptomatic, but at risk for the development of heart failure due to the presence of risk factors (e.g., hypertension, coronary artery disease, diabetes)
Stage B	Patients with structurally abnormal hearts (e.g., left ventricular systolic dysfunction, left ventricular hypertrophy, valvular dysfunction, prior myocardial infarction) but without symptoms of heart failure
Stage C	Patients with structurally abnormal hearts and current or prior symptoms of heart failure
Stage D	Patients with end-stage heart failure symptoms not responsive to standard therapy

- *Acute heart failure* denotes the sudden development of heart failure in the absence of preexisting cardiac dysfunction or the sudden decompensation in a patient with previously stable cardiac disease. This results from an abrupt alteration in cardiac structure or function (e.g., after an acute myocardial infarction or after valvular rupture) and is generally associated with clinical instability. *Chronic heart failure* results from a more indolent process of myocardial dysfunction and may be associated with less clinical severity because of the development of compensatory mechanisms (see later).
- *Low-output heart failure* is that resulting from a reduction in cardiac output (due to either systolic or diastolic dysfunction) and is usually characterized by venous congestion and increased arterial resistance (i.e., vasoconstriction). *High-output heart failure* occurs in the setting of increased cardiac output (e.g., thyrotoxicosis, anemia, beriberi, Paget's disease, arteriovenous fistulas) and is characterized by venous congestion and normal or reduced arterial resistance.
- *Backward heart failure* refers to the hypothesis that the manifestations of heart failure are primarily the result of an accumulation of fluid (and pressure) behind the failing ventricle. *Forward heart failure* proposes that heart failure results from a primary reduction in cardiac output with resultant organ hypoperfusion, sodium and water retention, and subsequent venous congestion. This is not as useful a distinction, as both mechanisms probably operate in the majority of patients with heart failure.

Heart failure may be classified symptomatically on the basis of its clinical severity (Table 58-2). Despite the varied causes and classifications of heart failure, the manifestations all reflect intravascular volume overload, inadequate tissue perfusion, or their combination. A thorough explanation of all these forms of heart failure is beyond the scope of this chapter. The following discussion, therefore, focuses primarily on left ventricular systolic failure in both the acute and chronic setting.

Acute Heart Failure

The response of the cardiovascular system to the onset of myocardial dysfunction and the pathophysiologic mechanisms underlying the subsequent progression to heart failure depends in large part on the acuity of the dysfunction. An acute cardiac insult results in a series of hemodynamic alterations that account for the clinical manifestations of left ventricular failure. This occurs irrespective of whether the initial insult depresses myocardial contractility (systolic dysfunction) or impairs ventricular filling (diastolic dysfunction). The cascade begins with a rise in left ventricular end-diastolic pressure. This elevated pressure is transmitted to the left atrium and subsequently to the pulmonary venous and capillary system. The increased intravascular pressure results in transudation of fluid into the pulmonary interstitium, where it interferes with gas exchange, resulting in hypoxemia and

Table 58-3
Compensatory Mechanisms in Heart Failure

Compensatory Response	Stimuli	Beneficial Effects	Adverse Effects	Potential Pharmacologic Interventions
Renin-angiotensin system activation	↓CO/BP ↓Renal blood flow ↑β-Adrenergic activity	Maintain vital organ perfusion through vasoconstriction and sodium retention	↑Afterload → worsened LV function Adverse LV remodeling (apoptosis, myocyte hypertrophy)	ACE inhibitors ARBs
Adrenergic activation	↓CO/BP	↑CO through ↑ in heart rate and contractility ↑BP	↑Ischemia ↑Afterload → worsened LV function ↑LVEDP → pulmonary congestion Adverse LV remodeling (apoptosis, myocyte hypertrophy)	β-Adrenergic blocking agents
Renal salt and water retention	↑Antidiuretic hormone ↑Norepinephrine ↑Angiotensin II ↑Aldosterone ↓Renal blood flow	↑Preload → ↑stroke volume and CO	Pulmonary and systemic congestion Adverse LV remodeling	Diuretics Aldosterone inhibitors ACE inhibitors, ARBs β-Adrenergic blocking agents
↑Natriuretic peptide secretion	Volume expansion (atrial stretch)	Diuresis Natriuresis Partial inhibition of renin-angiotensin system and norepinephrine	None known	Natriuretic peptides

ACE, angiotensin-converting enzyme; ARB, angiotensin receptor blocker; BP, blood pressure; CO, cardiac output; LV, left ventricular; LVEDP, left ventricular end-diastolic pressure.

dyspnea. In addition, there is often an associated reduction in cardiac output resulting in inadequate delivery of blood to the arterial system with resultant organ hypoperfusion.

The heart's response to these hemodynamic alterations is the activation of several compensatory mechanisms (Table 58-3). A rapid, generalized activation of the adrenergic system occurs and is associated with a withdrawal of parasympathetic tone. Direct sympathetic stimulation of the heart and β-adrenergically induced release of epinephrine and norepinephrine from the adrenal glands result in tachycardia and an increase in myocardial contractility, both of which serve to augment cardiac output. Catecholamine-induced peripheral arterial vasoconstriction redirects the available cardiac output away from relatively nonessential organs (i.e., skin, skeletal muscle, gut, kidney) and helps maintain sufficient blood pressure to ensure adequate perfusion of more vital organs (i.e., heart and brain). Furthermore, β-adrenergic stimulation of the juxtaglomerular apparatus in the kidneys results in the release of renin and activation of the renin-angiotensin system. The angiotensin II thus produced is a potent vasoconstrictor and acts in concert with the direct α-adrenergic stimulation of the vasculature to maintain blood pressure. The reduced renal blood flow from depressed cardiac output and redistribution of blood volume results in activation of renal baroreceptors. This further stimulates renin release and augments sympathetic activation, thereby contributing to vasoconstriction.

In addition to producing these hemodynamic alterations, acute heart failure is characterized by marked sodium and water retention. This occurs through a variety of mechanisms. Angiotensin II directly promotes the reabsorption of sodium in the proximal nephron and indirectly promotes the reabsorption of sodium from the distal nephron, this latter effect being mediated through angiotensin II–induced release of aldosterone from the adrenal cortex. Furthermore, angiotensin II and norepinephrine stimulate hypothalamic release of arginine vasopressin, resulting in further vasoconstriction and free water reabsorption. These changes produce an expansion of intravascular volume and augmentation of venous return, thereby increasing ventricular end-diastolic volume (*preload*). The increased preload results in an increase in stroke volume by the Frank-Starling mechanism (Fig. 58-1) and thereby helps support the cardiac output.

Chronic Heart Failure

In combination, the aforementioned mechanisms serve a compensatory role in acute heart failure, helping to maintain cardiac output and blood pressure to allow adequate perfusion of vital organs. These compensatory mechanisms may initially be adequate to allow clinical stability, and the patient may subsequently go through a stage of asymptomatic ventricular dysfunction, maintained in part by chronic stimulation of the adrenergic and renin-angiotensin systems. As heart failure progresses, the hemodynamic overload induces changes in the shape and size of the ventricle, a process known as *ventricular remodeling*. The specific changes that occur depend in part on the hemodynamic stressors facing the ventricle. In predominantly pressure-overloaded conditions (e.g., hypertension, aortic stenosis), there is a rise in systolic wall stress that results in left ventricular hypertrophy. If this hypertrophy is insufficient to normalize the wall stress, dilation occurs. Under conditions of volume overload (e.g., aortic or mitral insufficiency), there is

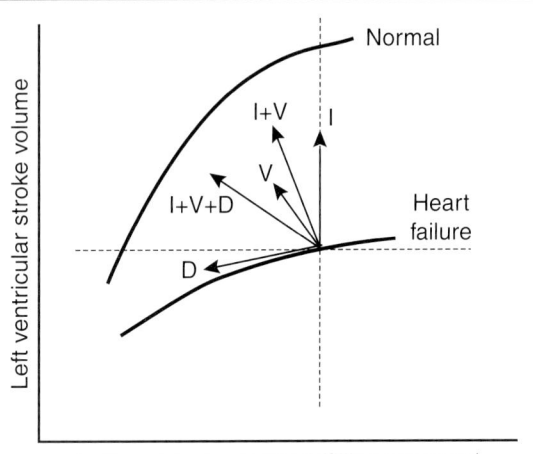

Figure 58-1
Frank-Starling curve with normal systolic function and with heart failure and the hemodynamic effect of pharmacologic therapy. In the normal setting, an increase in preload results in an increase in stroke volume. In heart failure, this relationship is blunted, and at any given stroke volume, the preload must be higher *(horizontal dotted line)*. Similarly, for any given preload, the stroke volume is lower *(vertical dotted line)*. Diuretic therapy (D) reduces preload without a significant effect on stroke volume, whereas inotropic therapy (I) augments stroke volume without an appreciable effect on preload. Vasodilator therapy (V) has moderate beneficial effects on both preload and stroke volume; however, the greatest effects are seen with combination therapy (I + V, I + V + D).

Table 58–4
Factors Involved in Ventricular Remodeling

Stimulants of Ventricular Remodeling	Molecular and Cellular Events That Mediate Ventricular Remodeling
Altered hemodynamic load (increased preload, afterload, wall stress)	Myocyte hypertrophy
β-Adrenergic stimulation	Myocyte loss (necrosis and apoptosis)
Activation of the renin-angiotensin system	Myocyte "slippage"
Inflammatory cytokines (e.g., tumor necrosis factor α, interleukins 1 and 6)	Transition to fetal myocyte phenotype
Vasoactive peptides (e.g., endothelin)	Neurohormonal activation
Oxidative stress	Fibroblast proliferation
	Alterations in the interstitial matrix
	Alterations in excitation-coupling

a rise in diastolic wall stress that induces ventricular dilation. This dilation in turn results in increased systolic wall stress (by the Laplace relationship) and subsequent hypertrophy. These hypertrophic changes help maintain systolic wall stress within a normal range and help preserve ventricular contractile function. However, with continued hemodynamic overload, there is progressive ventricular dilation, eventuating in the development of a dilated, spherical heart. This altered ventricular morphology produces less efficient ventricular contraction, may induce mitral regurgitation due to annular dilation and malcoaptation of the valve leaflets, and is associated with an adverse prognosis.

The stimuli that induce ventricular remodeling are varied and the mechanisms underlying the remodeling process are complex (Table 58-4). It appears that increased wall stress (resulting from ventricular dilation and increased afterload) and neurohormones (i.e., β-adrenergic and renin-angiotensin systems), vasoactive peptides (e.g., endothelin), and cytokines (e.g., tumor necrosis factor α) mediate remodeling. These factors may have direct effects on the cardiac myocytes or may act indirectly through stimulation of second-messenger systems and thereby induce a variety of changes in myocyte structure and function. On a cellular level, myocyte hypertrophy results from the replication of sarcomeres either in parallel (producing ventricular hypertrophy) or in series (producing ventricular dilation). Alterations in the expression of various contractile proteins occurs with reexpression of fetal genes and reduced expression of adult contractile genes, resulting in abnormalities of calcium handling and excitation-contraction coupling. Chronic stimulation of the sympathetic system is accompanied by a reduction in the density of β-adrenergic receptors in the myocardium and an uncoupling of the receptors from their intracellular mediators. This results in a blunted response of the failing myocardium to either endogenous (e.g., exercise) or exogenous (e.g., dopamine or dobutamine) adrenergic stimulation.

In addition to these alterations of the contractile apparatus within the myocytes, there is a progressive reduction in the number of myocytes, in part the result of apoptosis induced by the various stimuli of remodeling. Furthermore, changes occur in the extracellular matrix related to fibroblast proliferation, interstitial fibrosis, and increased expression of degradative enzymes such as matrix metalloproteinases. The last factor results in the loss of mechanical coupling of myocytes and may contribute to the remodeling process by facilitating "myocyte slippage" and, thereby, ventricular dilation.

As the remodeling process develops, the neurohormonal effects of the β-adrenergic and renin-angiotensin systems on the peripheral vasculature and renal salt and water handling continue. The intense vasoconstriction, while maintaining flow to vital organs, contributes to hypoperfusion of the kidneys and progressive renal dysfunction. The augmented preload and cardiac output resulting from sodium and water retention help maintain circulating blood volume and tissue perfusion. However, the associated increase in end-diastolic pressure and increased ventricular wall stress contribute to progressive ventricular remodeling and result in pulmonary and systemic venous hypertension and precipitation of congestive symptoms. Thus, these initially compensatory changes become deleterious in the chronic setting. The inhibition of these processes offers not only a mechanism for the treatment of heart failure but also the potential to reverse the adverse remodeling seen in the chronic state (see Table 58-3).

PHARMACOLOGIC AGENTS USED IN THE TREATMENT OF HEART FAILURE

The majority of pharmacologic agents used for the treatment of heart failure effect benefit either directly by interfering with the hemodynamic alterations described before or through inhibition of the neurohormonal activation underlying these alterations (see Fig. 58-1). These medications fall into several

Table 58-5
Diuretics Commonly Used in the Treatment of Heart Failure

Class and Examples	Daily Dose Range	Duration of Action	Adverse Effects (by class)
Loop diuretics			
Furosemide (Lasix)	20-480 mg PO 20-300 mg IV	4-6 hours	Hypokalemia, hyperuricemia, metabolic alkalosis, ototoxicity at high doses
Torsemide (Demadex)	5-40 mg PO	12 hours	
Bumetanide (Bumex)	0.5-5 mg PO	4-6 hours	
Ethacrynic acid (Edecrin)	25-100 mg PO	12 hours	
Thiazide diuretics			
Chlorothiazide (Diuril)	125-500 mg PO	6-12 hours	Hypokalemia, hyponatremia, hyperuricemia, hyperglycemia, hyperlipidemia
Hydrochlorothiazide (HydroDiuril)	12.5-50 mg PO	12-18 hours	
Chlorthalidone (Hygroton)	25-100 mg PO	24 hours	
Thiazide-like diuretics			
Metolazone (Zaroxolyn)	0.5-10 mg PO	24 hours	Hypokalemia, hypomagnesemia
Aldosterone inhibitors			
Spironolactone (Aldactone)	25 mg PO	8-12 hours	Hyperkalemia, nausea, gynecomastia (spironolactone)
Eplerenone	25-50 mg PO	4-6 hours	
Potassium-sparing diuretics			
Amiloride (Midamor)	5-10 mg PO	24 hours	Hyperkalemia when combined with angiotensin-converting enzyme inhibitor or angiotensin receptor blocker
Triamterene (Dyrenium)	50-100 mg PO	12 hours	

categories: diuretics, vasodilators, inotropic agents, and neurohormonal inhibitors. Diuretics act to reduce preload (leftward shift on the Frank-Starling curve), resulting in decreased filling pressures and improved congestive symptoms. Although this fall in preload may be associated with a reduction in stroke volume, this effect is minimal in patients with elevated filling pressures. Pure venodilators similarly reduce filling pressures and congestive symptoms and have minimal effect on stroke volume. Arterial vasodilators and inotropic agents predominantly augment cardiac output and thereby improve organ perfusion; arterial vasodilators act indirectly through a reduction in vascular resistance, whereas inotropic agents directly increase contractility and stroke volume. Although the increased cardiac output seen with these agents may result in a fall in filling pressures, the effect may be relatively modest. As a result of the differential effects of these agents, many patients with heart failure attain the greatest benefit from combination therapy. Neurohormonal inhibitors may have mixed hemodynamic effects. The blockade of adrenergic tone (beta-blockers) and inhibition of the renin-angiotensin system (angiotensin-converting enzyme [ACE] inhibitors, angiotensin receptor blockers [ARBs]) results in vasodilation and augmented cardiac output. These agents may also decrease preload and reduce filling pressures through a reduction in neurohormonally mediated renal sodium and water retention.

Specific Agents

Diuretics

Diuretics have long played an important role in the symptomatic treatment of heart failure (Table 58-5). The induced diuresis and natriuresis reduce extracellular volume and ventricular filling pressures, thereby ameliorating congestive symptoms. This effect occurs without a significant decrease in cardiac output or systemic blood pressure unless excessive diuresis and intravascular volume depletion occur. Whereas diuretics are beneficial in controlling symptoms and improving exercise capacity in patients with heart failure, with the exception of spironolactone, eplerenone diuretic use has not resulted in a decrease in mortality.

Loop diuretics act in the thick ascending limb of the loop of Henle, where they inhibit the Na^+-K^+-$2Cl^-$ transporter, resulting in increased delivery of sodium and water to the distal nephron. They also decrease the tonicity of the medullary interstitium and thereby limit the osmotic reabsorption of free water from the collecting tubules. Currently available loop diuretics include furosemide, bumetanide, torsemide, and ethacrynic acid. There is an increased risk of ototoxicity with ethacrynic acid; therefore, this agent should be reserved for patients who are allergic to or intolerant of other agents.

Furosemide is the loop diuretic most commonly used for the treatment of heart failure. For patients with mild to moderate congestive symptoms, it can be given orally at initial doses of 20 to 40 mg daily. Its bioavailability ranges from 40% to 70%, and gradual dose titration is frequently required. Furosemide has a relatively short half-life. Once renal tubular levels of the drug decline, avid sodium reabsorption occurs throughout the nephron, potentially limiting or preventing effective natriuresis. A twice-daily dosing regimen may therefore be required to produce adequate salt and water loss. In patients with more severe volume retention or decompensated heart failure, intravenous administration of furosemide (20 to 100 mg) may produce a more rapid and effective diuresis. The maximum intravenous dose is 300 mg; however, the risk of ototoxicity increases at such high doses. For patients who require frequent high doses of intravenous furosemide, a continuous infusion may produce a more effective diuresis and require a lower total daily dose. The infusion is usually started at 5 to 10 mg/hr and titrated as needed to obtain the desired effect. Bumetanide and torsemide have greater bioavailability than does furosemide (~80%) but have not demonstrated better efficacy and are significantly more expensive.

Thiazide diuretics act in the distal convoluted tubule, where they inhibit the Na^+-Cl^- cotransporter. Their efficacy is dependent on the delivery of sodium to the distal nephron; therefore, their diuretic effect is limited by sodium reabsorption from more proximal regions, as occurs during intravascular volume depletion or in low-flow states. In addition, they are ineffective when glomerular filtration rates fall below 30 mL/min. Thiazides may be useful as the sole diuretic in treatment of mild congestive symptoms; however, their predominant role in the management of more advanced heart failure is as an adjunct to other diuretic therapy in patients who exhibit diuretic resistance. Although several thiazides are available, the most frequently used are hydrochlorothiazide (12.5 to 50 mg daily) and metolazone (2.5 to 10 mg daily). These agents exhibit synergism with loop diuretics and should be given approximately 30 minutes before administration of furosemide, bumetanide, or torsemide.

Spironolactone is a competitive inhibitor of aldosterone in the distal convoluted tubule, whereas eplerenone is a selective aldosterone blocker. These agents stimulate a mild natriuresis and potassium reabsorption and may be most effective in patients with advanced heart failure, in whom marked activation of the renin-angiotensin-aldosterone system results in aldosterone levels as high as 20 times normal. In the Randomized Aldactone Evaluation Study (RALES), patients with moderate to severe congestive heart failure (NYHA class III-IV) were treated with spironolactone (25 to 50 mg daily) and had improved symptoms, reduced rates of hospitalization for heart failure, and 30% reduction in mortality. In the Eplerenone Post-Acute Myocardial Infarction Heart Failure Efficacy and Survival Study (EPHESUS), patients with acute myocardial infarction, left ventricular ejection fraction of 40% or less, and evidence of heart failure were treated with eplerenone (25 to 50 mg daily) and had a 15% reduction in mortality and significantly fewer episodes of heart failure. The mechanism of benefit of these agents is unlikely to be related to a diuretic effect as they are relatively weak diuretics. Rather, it probably reflects inhibition of aldosterone-induced myocardial fibrosis and ventricular remodeling. The major side effect of spironolactone is gynecomastia, which is not seen with eplerenone because of its selective mineralocorticoid blockade. The dose of these agents should not exceed 50 mg daily because of the risk of hyperkalemia, especially in patients with a serum creatinine concentration of 2.5 mg/dL or higher or when they are used in conjunction with an angiotensin-converting enzyme inhibitor or angiotensin receptor blocker for the treatment of heart failure.

Amiloride and triamterene inhibit the reabsorption of sodium in the distal convoluted tubule and proximal collecting duct, resulting in a mild natriuresis and reduction of the ionic gradient required for potassium secretion into the urine. These agents produce a mild diuresis without the potassium wasting seen with loop diuretics and thiazides and may be effective for the control of mild congestive symptoms. However, when they are given alone, they are not effective in maintaining a negative fluid balance in patients with advanced heart failure. In such patients, these agents may have benefit as part of a combination diuretic regimen, especially given their potassium-sparing properties.

Patients treated with diuretics require close monitoring of their renal function and serum electrolytes. Loop diuretics and thiazides can lead to profound hypokalemia and hypomagnesemia, especially when they are used in combination; spironolactone may result in hyperkalemia. In contrast to loop diuretics, thiazides do not alter the tonicity of the renal medullary interstitium and may produce significant hyponatremia due to the reabsorption of free water from the distal convoluted tubule in the face of a preserved interstitial gradient. In addition to these metabolic effects, thiazides may adversely affect serum lipid levels, and spironolactone may induce gynecomastia.

Vasodilators

Nitrovasodilators

Nitric oxide is formed by normal endothelial and smooth muscle cells throughout the vasculature and functions in both a paracrine and an autocrine fashion. Its primary mechanism of action involves an induced increase in intracellular cyclic guanosine monophosphate, which results in vascular smooth muscle relaxation. Nitrovasodilators such as sodium nitroprusside and organic nitrates (i.e., nitroglycerin) are metabolized to nitric oxide within the vasculature. They are potent vasodilators and, as such, are useful in the management of heart failure.

Nitroprusside is the sodium salt of nitric oxide and ferricyanide. It is a balanced vasodilator and produces both vasodilation and venodilation in both the systemic and pulmonary systems. These effects result in favorable hemodynamic changes, including a decrease in right atrial and pulmonary capillary wedge pressures (i.e., decreased preload), a reduction in pulmonary and systemic vascular resistance (i.e., decreased afterload), and an increase in stroke volume and cardiac output/index (Fig. 58-2). In contrast to other arterial vasodilators, nitroprusside does not cause a significant increase in heart rate, and its use is usually associated with a decrease in myocardial oxygen demand. Nitroprusside is useful for the management of heart failure associated with elevated filling pressures, low cardiac output, and high vascular resistance, as occurs in patients with decompensated systolic failure. It is also ideally suited for the management of heart failure associated with profound hypertension, acute mitral regurgitation, acute aortic insufficiency, or acute ventricular septal defect.

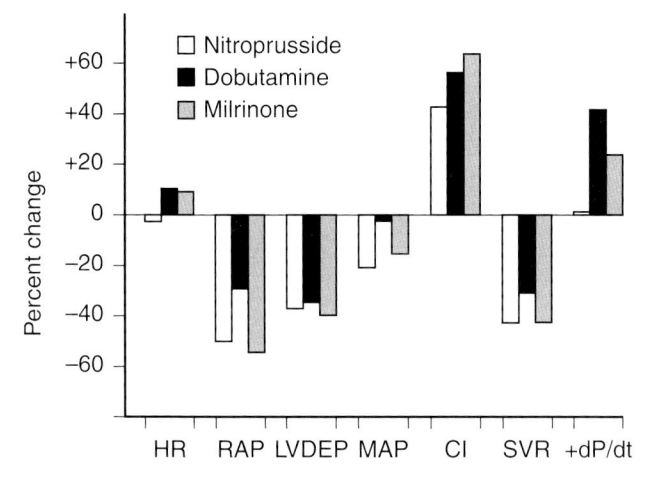

Figure 58–2
Comparative hemodynamic effects of maximally tolerated doses of nitroprusside, dobutamine, and milrinone in patients with severe heart failure. CI, cardiac index; dP/dt, change in pressure per change in time; HR, heart rate; LVEDP, left ventricular end-diastolic pressure; MAP, mean arterial pressure; RAP, right atrial pressure; SVR, systemic vascular resistance. *(Modified from Colucci WS, Wright RF, Jaski BE, et al. Milrinone and dobutamine in severe heart failure: differing hemodynamic effects and individual patient responsiveness. Circulation 1986;73:III175.)*

Nitroprusside is administered as a continuous infusion. Its onset of action is rapid (within 30 seconds), and it reaches peak effect within 2 minutes. Similarly, its effects completely resolve within 3 minutes of discontinuation of its infusion. Because of these rapid changes in hemodynamics, it is best administered under the guidance of pulmonary (i.e., Swan-Ganz catheter) and systemic arterial monitoring. The usual starting dose is 0.1 to 0.25 µg/kg/min. The dose may be titrated up by 0.25 µg/kg/min every 5 to 10 minutes until the desired effect is achieved or the maximum dose is reached (10 µg/kg/min). The use of nitroprusside may be limited by the development of hypotension, especially in patients with normal left ventricular systolic function or low filling pressures. Rapid cessation of nitroprusside may result in rebound hypertension, probably reflecting neurohormonal activation. Nitroprusside is metabolized in the vasculature to nitric oxide and cyanide; cyanide is further metabolized in the liver to thiocyanate, which is excreted by the kidneys. Accumulation of these toxic metabolites is more likely to occur when nitroprusside is infused at higher doses or for prolonged periods, especially in the setting of hepatic and renal dysfunction. Cyanide toxicity may be manifested as abdominal pain, confusion, or seizure and is usually preceded by lactic acidosis. Thiocyanate toxicity usually manifests as nausea, confusion, fatigue, psychosis, and, rarely, coma. If toxicity is suspected, the infusion should be discontinued and serum levels of the metabolites should be measured. Cyanide toxicity can be treated with sodium nitrite (300 mg) or sodium thiosulfate (12.5 g), but thiocyanate toxicity may require hemodialysis.

Nitroglycerin, like nitroprusside, is a potent vasodilator; however, it has dose-dependent effects in the arterial and venous systems. At low doses, it is a relatively selective venodilator, resulting in increased venous capacitance and decreased left and right ventricular filling pressures. At higher doses, it is also an arterial dilator and results in a fall in pulmonary and systemic vascular resistance, although less predictably and to a lesser extent than nitroprusside. Intravenous nitroglycerin is an effective agent in the management of acute decompensated heart failure characterized by increased filling pressures and elevated vascular resistance. In addition, nitroglycerin has a significant vasodilative effect on epicardial coronary arteries and may indirectly improve left ventricular function by improving blood flow to ischemic myocardium. It is thus an agent of choice in managing heart failure associated with acute myocardial ischemia or infarction.

Intravenous nitroglycerin is usually initiated at 20 µg/min and titrated up by 10 to 20 µg/min every 5 to 10 minutes until the desired hemodynamic effect is achieved or the maximum dose is reached (400 µg/min). Its effects are immediate and resolve rapidly after discontinuation of the infusion. Nitroglycerin may result in hypotension, especially at high doses and in patients with low filling pressures. Its use is commonly associated with a headache, occasionally requiring downtitration or discontinuance of the infusion. Nitrate tolerance frequently develops but can usually be overcome by increasing the infusion rate.

Hydralazine

Hydralazine is a direct vasodilator that causes relaxation of arteriolar smooth muscle by an unknown mechanism. It does not cause venodilation or dilation of epicardial coronary arteries; thus, its hemodynamic effects are primarily limited to a reduction in vascular resistance. Hydralazine is an effective antihypertensive agent, especially when it is used in combination with other agents. When it is administered to patients with congestive heart failure, it is most effective in combination with venodilating agents (e.g., organic nitrates). The combination of hydralazine and oral nitrates, when it is added to a regimen of digoxin and diuretics, has been shown in randomized trials to reduce mortality, to improve left ventricular systolic function, and to reduce symptoms in patients with heart failure. However, the benefit of this regimen on mortality and left ventricular function is less than that of ACE inhibitors. In general, hydralazine is not a first-line agent for the treatment of heart failure. Nonetheless, it should be considered in patients who are intolerant of ACE inhibitors because of allergy or renal insufficiency, and it is the agent of choice for afterload reduction in pregnant patients. In addition, it may offer further relief in patients with heart failure who remain symptomatic despite treatment with ACE inhibitors.

Hydralazine therapy is initiated at a dose of 10 mg four times daily and titrated upward as blood pressure tolerates to a maximum dose of 100 mg four times daily. Organic nitrates are given concurrently (i.e., isosorbide dinitrate, 30 to 160 mg daily). Hydralazine-induced vasodilation is associated with a baroreceptor-mediated increase in sympathetic activity, resulting in a reflex tachycardia, increased ventricular contractility, increased renin activity, and fluid retention. In patients with underlying coronary artery disease, the arteriolar dilation may result in a coronary steal phenomenon and, combined with the tachycardia, may precipitate myocardial ischemia. Coadministration with β-adrenergic blocking agents may prevent this complication; nonetheless, hydralazine should be used with caution in patients with an ischemia cardiomyopathy. Other side effects occur more frequently and include headaches, flushing, palpitations, nausea, and dizziness. A lupus-like syndrome occurs in 5% to 10% of patients and may require discontinuation of the drug.

Calcium Channel Blocking Agents

In general, the use of calcium channel blocking agents for the treatment of heart failure has been disappointing, despite the fact that they are relatively potent vasodilators. Verapamil and diltiazem have negative inotropic effects and may worsen symptoms in patients with systolic heart failure. However, these agents may improve diastolic function because of their rate-slowing effects and induced alterations in calcium homeostasis and thus may be beneficial in the treatment of diastolic heart failure. The first-generation dihydropyridine nifedipine has been associated with an increase in adverse effects, including a trend toward increased mortality in patients with systolic heart failure. This may relate to neurohormonal activation resulting from fluctuations in its hemodynamic effects, especially with short-acting formulations. Newer second-generation dihydropyridines, such as amlodipine and felodipine, appear to be safe in patients with heart failure but have not demonstrated significant benefit with regard to morbidity or mortality. Therefore, although these agents could be considered for the treatment of hypertension or angina in patients with left ventricular systolic dysfunction, calcium channel blocking agents in general should not be used for primary treatment of heart failure.

Neurohormonal Inhibiting Agents

Angiotensin-Converting Enzyme Inhibitors

ACE inhibitors have a variety of beneficial effects on the pathophysiologic mechanism of heart failure. Hemodynamically, ACE inhibitors are potent vasodilators and reduce both preload and afterload. The subsequent fall in intracardiac pressures and reduction in wall stress result in a decrease in myocardial oxygen demand, potentially reducing ischemia, and a decrease in the activity of the sympathetic nervous system, thereby reducing electrical instability. In addition, the ACE inhibitor–induced reduction in angiotensin as well as the subsequent reduction in adrenal aldosterone release may have direct effects on the extent of fibrosis and collagen deposition that characterize myocardial remodeling in heart failure. The effects of ACE inhibitors are primarily mediated by inhibition of the enzyme responsible for the conversion of angiotensin I to angiotensin II, thereby decreasing production of angiotensin II. However, some of the benefit of ACE inhibitors may result from their effects on the kinin system; ACE inhibitors decrease the degradation of kinins (e.g., bradykinin) and thereby enhance their vasodilative effects and potentiate kinin-mediated synthesis of vasodilative prostaglandins.

ACE inhibitors have been extensively studied in a wide variety of patients with heart failure and have almost universally demonstrated benefit in hemodynamics, symptoms, exercise capacity, hospitalization, and mortality. In the Cooperative North Scandinavian Enalapril Survival Study (CONSENSUS), patients with severe (NYHA class IV) heart failure who were already treated with digoxin and diuretics had a 40% reduction in mortality at 6 months when treated with enalapril. Patients with less-severe heart failure (NYHA class II-III and an ejection fraction ≤35%) were studied in the treatment arm of the SOLVD (Studies Of Left Ventricular Dysfunction) trial. In this trial, patients who were treated with enalapril had a 16% reduction in mortality and a 26% reduction in the risk of death or hospitalization for worsening heart failure. In the Acute Infarction Ramipril Efficacy study, patients with symptomatic heart failure, a recent myocardial infarction, and ejection fractions below 40% demonstrated a 27% decrease in mortality after 30 days of treatment with ramipril. Furthermore, several studies have demonstrated that asymptomatic patients with depressed ejection fractions (<35% to 40%) have reduced morbidity and mortality when treated with ACE inhibitors, although the magnitude of this benefit is less than that seen in patients with overt heart failure. Thus, the results of clinical trials with ACE inhibitors reveal a consistent benefit in patients with symptomatic heart failure or asymptomatic left ventricular dysfunction (Fig. 58-3).

A variety of ACE inhibitors are currently available (Table 58-6). These agents differ in regard to their plasma half-life, dosing regimen, and ability to inhibit ACE at the tissue level. However, available data suggest that the beneficial effects of these agents are a class effect and not dependent on individual pharmacologic characteristics. Nonetheless, in selecting an ACE inhibitor for the treatment of heart failure, preference should be given to those agents that have demonstrated efficacy in large-scale trials (enalapril, captopril, lisinopril, and ramipril). ACE inhibitors should be initiated at low doses,

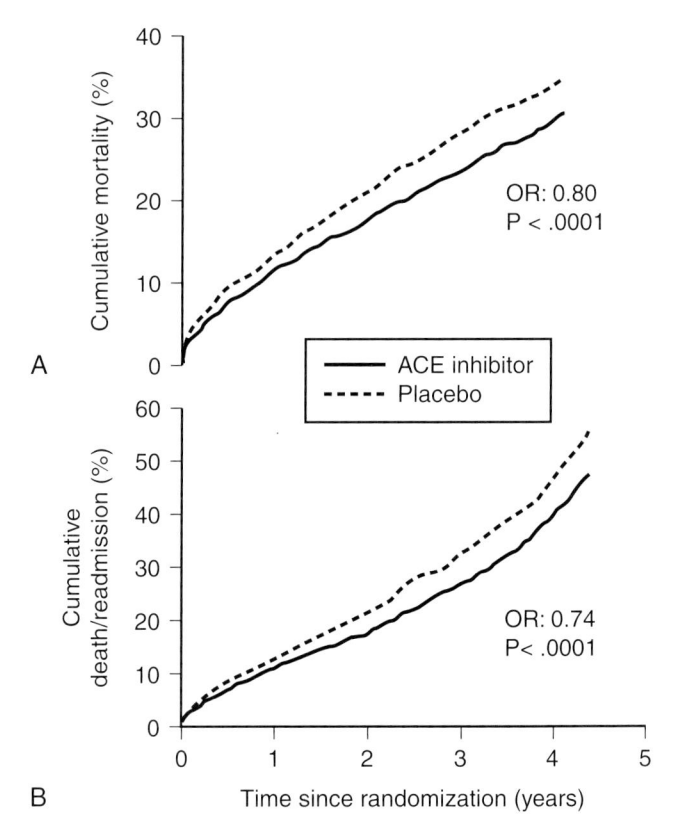

Figure 58-3
The effect of angiotensin-converting enzyme (ACE) inhibitors on the total mortality (**A**) and total mortality plus readmission for heart failure (**B**) in patients with heart failure or left ventricular systolic dysfunction. OR, odds ratio. *(Modified from Flather MD, Yusuf S, Kober L, et al. Long-term ACE-inhibitor therapy in patients with heart failure or left ventricular dysfunction: a systematic overview of data from individual patients.* Lancet *2000;355:1575-81.)*

especially in patients with hypotension before treatment. If initial doses are tolerated hemodynamically, the dose should be gradually titrated upward over several days to several weeks. In general, these agents should be titrated upward to goal doses as determined by clinical trials or to the highest dose that can be tolerated. Although lower doses may offer mortality benefit similar to that of higher doses, higher doses are associated with augmented symptom control. In patients with decompensated heart failure who cannot receive oral agents, intravenous enalaprilat can be used. Enalaprilat is the active form of the oral ACE inhibitor enalapril. When it is given intravenously, it is a balanced vasodilator resulting in a reduction in left and right ventricular filling pressures and vascular resistance.

Use of ACE inhibitors may be limited by the development of side effects. Hypotension is the most common adverse effect, occurs most frequently during the initiation of therapy, and is more common in patients who are volume depleted. It

Table 58–6
Oral Agents Commonly Used in the Treatment of Heart Failure

Class and Examples	Starting Dose	Target or Maximum Dose	Adverse Effects (by class)
Nitrovasodilators			
Isosorbide mononitrate (Imdur)	30 mg qd	120 mg qd	Headache; nitrate tolerance with continuous use
Isosorbide dinitrate	10 mg tid	30 mg tid	
Direct-acting vasodilators			
Hydralazine (Apresoline)	10 mg qid	100 mg qid	Reflex tachycardia, lupus-like syndrome
Angiotensin-converting enzyme inhibitors			
Captopril (Capoten)	6.25 mg tid	50 mg tid	Hypotension, cough, rash, angioedema, hyperkalemia
Enalapril (Vasotec)	2.5 mg bid	10-20 mg bid	Renal dysfunction (especially in patients with bilateral renal artery stenosis)
Lisinopril (Zestril, Prinivil)	2.5 mg qd	40 mg qd	
Ramipril (Altace)	2.5 mg qd	10 mg qd	
Quinapril (Accupril)	10 mg bid	40 mg qd	
Fosinopril (Monopril)	10 mg qd	40 mg qd	
Trandolapril (Mavik)	0.5 mg qd	8 mg qd	
Angiotensin receptor blockers			
Losartan (Cozaar)	50 mg qd	100 mg qd	Hyperkalemia
Candesartan (Atacand)	4 mg qd	32 mg qd	Renal dysfunction (especially in patients with bilateral renal artery stenosis)
Valsartan (Diovan)	80 mg qd	320 mg qd	
β-Adrenergic blocking agents			
Carvedilol (Coreg)	3.125 mg bid	25 mg bid	Bradycardia, hypotension, bronchospasm
Metoprolol (Toprol XL)	25 mg qd	200 mg qd	May worsen heart failure during initiation and titration
Bisoprolol (Zebeta)	1.25 mg qd	10 mg qd	
Inotropic agents			
Digoxin (Lanoxin)	0.125 mg qd	Serum digoxin level: 0.5-0.8 ng/mL	Nausea, bradycardia, heart block, ventricular tachyarrhythmias
Calcium channel blockers*			
Amlodipine (Norvasc)	2.5 mg qd	10 mg qd	Amlodipine: pedal edema
Verapamil (Calan, Verelan)	120 mg qd	480 mg qd	Verapamil and diltiazem: bradycardia, worsened systolic heart failure
Diltiazem (Cardizem, Dilacor)	120 mg qd	540 mg qd	

*Calcium channel blockers should not be routinely used for the treatment of systolic heart failure. Although amlodipine is safe in this setting, verapamil and diltiazem may worsen systolic heart failure, and their use is limited to the treatment of diastolic heart failure.

can usually be managed by reducing diuretic dosing and titrating the ACE inhibitor slowly. Moderate hypotension (systolic blood pressure > 85 mm Hg) can frequently be tolerated as long as organ hypoperfusion is not present. ACE inhibitors produce vasodilation of renal efferent arterioles and thereby reduce glomerular filtration rate. Worsening renal function can be seen in 5% to 30% of patients treated with these agents; the risks are significantly higher in patients with more severe heart failure and in those with bilateral renal artery stenosis. Hypokalemia may also occur, even in the absence of declining renal function. At least 5% to 10% of patients treated with ACE inhibitors develop a dry, nonproductive cough. This probably results from the inhibition of bradykinin metabolism and resolves with cessation of the drug. Less than 1% of patients develop angioedema when they are treated with ACE inhibitors. This can be life-threatening and precludes further use of the drug. Both the efficacy and side effect profile of ACE inhibitors are affected by volume status, and careful monitoring of volume and appropriate diuretic dosing are important. Volume overload will blunt the therapeutic effects of ACE inhibitors, and whereas dietary sodium restriction may enhance the response to ACE inhibitors, volume depletion will exaggerate their hypotensive effects.

Angiotensin Receptor Blocking Agents

ARBs differ from ACE inhibitors in that they inhibit the binding of angiotensin to its receptor rather than block its production. Theoretically, ARBs should be more effective at inhibiting the renin-angiotensin-aldosterone system as they block angiotensin produced by both ACE and non-ACE pathways; however, clinical trials of ARB therapy in heart failure have not demonstrated consistent superiority over ACE inhibitors. A meta-analysis of 17 trials comprising more than 12,000 patients demonstrated that ARBs were not superior to ACE inhibitors in reducing morbidity or mortality of patients with heart failure, although they appear to be beneficial in patients who are not already taking ACE inhibitors. The results of the Candesartan in Heart Failure Assessment of Reduction in Mortality and Morbidity (CHARM) trials have shed more light on this subject. These studies revealed that in patients with class II-IV heart failure and left ventricular ejection fraction of 40% or lower, treatment with the ARB candesartan results in clinically important reductions in mortality and hospitalization for heart failure. Importantly, the benefit was seen in patients who were intolerant of ACE inhibitors. Furthermore, in patients who were already receiving an optimal dose of an ACE inhibitor, the addition of candesartan produced additive clinical benefit.

ARBs have a risk of hypotension, renal dysfunction, and hyperkalemia similar to that of ACE inhibitors, and combination ARB and ACE inhibitor therapy is associated with an increased incidence of these adverse effects. The risk of angioedema appears to be decreased with ARBs compared with ACE inhibitors. In addition, because ARBs do not affect the kinin system, the incidence of cough is significantly less than that with ACE inhibitors. In general, ARBs are not yet considered first-line therapy for heart failure, although guidelines in this regard are evolving. ARBs are, however, a reasonable alternative in patients who are intolerant of ACE inhibitors because of the development of a persistent cough or angioedema and should be considered additive therapy in patients with persistent heart failure symptoms despite ACE inhibitor use.

β-Adrenergic Blocking Agents

The recent understanding of heart failure not only as a hemodynamic syndrome related to left ventricular systolic dysfunction but as a state of adverse neurohormone-mediated remodeling has prompted extensive investigation into the utility of beta-blocking agents in the treatment of heart failure. Basic studies have shown that these agents can inhibit the adverse effects of norepinephrine on the myocardium and result in upregulation of cardiac β-adrenergic receptors. The long-term administration of these agents is associated with a reversal of left ventricular remodeling, resulting in a decrease in left ventricular volume and an increase in ejection fraction with concomitant improvement in hemodynamics.

Large clinical trials encompassing more than 10,000 patients have demonstrated that these effects translate into significant clinical benefit. Although the enrollment criteria and the specific beta-blocking agent used varied among the trials, they all included patients with systolic heart failure (left ventricular ejection fraction of <35% to 45%) who were already being treated with a regimen of an ACE inhibitor and a diuretic, with or without digoxin. In sum, these trials demonstrated an approximately 35% reduction in mortality and 40% reduction in hospitalization due to heart failure in patients treated with beta-blocking agents. In addition, treatment with beta-blockers reduces symptoms of heart failure and improves exercise capacity, although these effects may not be evident for several weeks or months after initiation of treatment (Fig. 58-4).

Three beta-blocking agents are currently approved by the Food and Drug Administration for the treatment of systolic heart failure: metoprolol, carvedilol, and bisoprolol. Metoprolol and bisoprolol are β_1 receptor specific; carvedilol inhibits the β_1, β_2, and α_1 receptors and has both vasodilative and

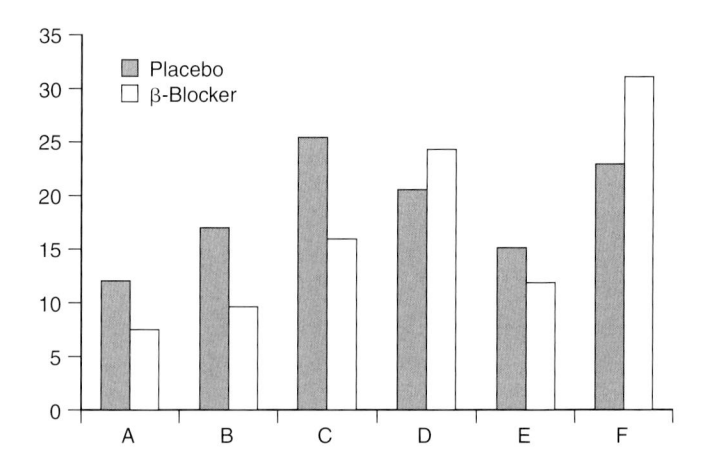

Figure 58–4
The effect of beta-blocker therapy on clinical endpoints in patients with heart failure. Data from trials using metoprolol, carvedilol, bucindolol, and nebivolol. HF, heart failure. Endpoints D and E refer to patients who improved or deteriorated by at least one class. Left ventricular ejection fraction (LVEF) was measured after at least 5 months of therapy and reflects an unweighted mean increase of 29% with beta-blocker therapy. *(Modified from Lechat P, Packer M, Chalon S, et al. Clinical effects of beta-adrenergic blockade in chronic heart failure: a meta-analysis of double-blind, placebo-controlled, randomized trials. Circulation 1998;98:1184-91.)*

antioxidant properties. The absolute magnitude of benefit is similar with these agents, and current trial data are inadequate to support use of one agent over another. Beta-blocker therapy for heart failure should be initiated at lower doses than is routinely used for the treatment of hypertension or angina and gradually titrated upward to doses that have demonstrated benefit in clinical trials (see Table 58-6).

Use of beta-blocking agents can be associated with significant adverse effects in patients with heart failure. The renal hemodynamic effect of these agents may result in volume retention, which in combination with their negative inotropic effect may cause an initial worsening of heart failure symptoms. This adverse effect is more common in patients who are volume overloaded before beta-blocker therapy and usually responds to an increase in diuretic dose. Hypotension is frequently seen after the initiation of beta-blockers and may limit use of these agents. This effect is more pronounced with carvedilol because of its peripheral vasodilating effects and can usually be managed with a reduction in dose or changing to a β_1 receptor–specific agent. Other frequent side effects include fatigue and bradycardia, both of which can usually be managed with reduction of the dose of beta-blocker or discontinuation of other atrioventricular nodal blocking agents (e.g., digoxin). Given the strength of the data supporting their use, beta-blockers should be administered to all patients with systolic heart failure who do not have a contraindication to their use. Nonetheless, beta-blockers should be avoided in patients with decompensated heart failure, symptomatic hypotension, or significant resting bradycardia or heart block in the absence of a permanent pacemaker.

Inotropic Agents

Digoxin

Digoxin is a cardiac glycoside and, as such, is a selective inhibitor of the membrane-bound Na^+/K^+-ATPase. The binding of digoxin to this enzyme results in increased intracellular calcium with a resultant augmentation of myocardial contractility. In general, the overall effect on global left ventricular systolic function is relatively small, with an average absolute increase in ejection fraction of 1% to 2%. Digoxin also affects the cardiac conduction system through increases in vagal tone and decreases in sympathetic tone. This results in decreased automaticity of the atria and atrioventricular nodal tissues and prolongation of the refractory period and reduction in conduction velocity of the atrioventricular node. The net result is a slowing of the atrial rate and blockade of the atrioventricular node.

Several clinical trials have evaluated the role of digoxin in the treatment of patients with heart failure. The Prospective Randomized Study Of Ventricular Failure and Efficacy of Digoxin (PROVED) and the Randomized Assessment of Digoxin on Inhibitors of Angiotensin-Converting Enzyme (RADIANCE) trials studied the effects of withdrawal of digoxin from clinically stable patients with class II or class III heart failure and systolic dysfunction. They found that withdrawal of digoxin was associated with a significant worsening of heart failure symptoms and deterioration of functional capacity. The Digitalis Investigation Group (DIG) trial evaluated the effect of starting digoxin in patients with systolic heart failure who were already receiving therapy with diuretics and ACE inhibitors. In this trial, digoxin use was associated with a decrease in the risk of hospitalization for heart failure but no change in overall mortality. Thus, digoxin can no longer be considered a first-line therapy for patients with heart failure; however, it appears useful in patients who remain symptomatic despite therapy with other agents. In this setting, the serum digoxin level should be maintained at 0.5 to 0.8 ng/mL, as higher doses may be associated with adverse outcomes.

Digoxin may also be useful in the control of supraventricular arrhythmias in patients with depressed left ventricular systolic function. When it is used in this setting, digoxin may be given as an initial load (0.25 mg orally or intravenously every 8 hours for 24 hours) followed by a single daily dose of 0.125 mg or 0.25 mg. When it is used for the treatment of heart failure, there is little value in a loading dose, and once-daily dosing is appropriate. Digoxin is excreted unchanged by the kidney, and its dose must be adjusted in the setting of renal failure. It has a relatively narrow therapeutic window, and intermittent monitoring of its serum level is required. Higher serum digoxin levels (>2.0 ng/mL) are associated with an increased risk of toxic side effects (Table 58-7), especially in the presence of hypokalemia or hypomagnesemia. Mild digoxin toxicity (ectopic beats, first-degree atrioventricular block, gastrointestinal symptoms) may only require withholding of the drug. More severe toxicity (profound bradycardia, high-degree atrioventricular block, ventricular tachyarrhythmias) requires administration of digoxin-specific antibodies. Hemodialysis is ineffective for the treatment of digoxin toxicity.

Dopamine

Dopamine is the immediate metabolic precursor of epinephrine and norepinephrine. It is an endogenous catecholamine that functions as an essential neurotransmitter and is involved in the central regulation of movement and in the regulation of the cardiovascular system. Exogenously administered dopamine does not cross the blood-brain barrier, and thus its effects are predominantly cardiovascular. The cardiovascular response to dopamine infusion is mediated by dopaminergic, β-adrenergic, and α-adrenergic receptors. At low doses (1 to 2 µg/kg/min), dopamine binds to dopaminergic receptors in

Table 58–7

Signs and Symptoms of Digoxin Toxicity

Nausea, vomiting, abdominal pain
Anorexia
Fatigue, malaise
Confusion, delirium
Visual changes (yellow vision, halo around visual field)
First-, second-, or third-degree heart block
Excessively low ventricular rate in atrial fibrillation
Paroxysmal atrial tachycardia (classically with associated heart block)
Premature ventricular depolarizations
Ventricular tachycardia

the renal, mesenteric, and peripheral vasculature, stimulating a rise in intracellular cyclic adenosine monophosphate (cAMP) and inducing vasodilation in these beds. Although it produces a mild fall in systemic vascular resistance, its main effect is to increase glomerular filtration rate, renal blood flow, and renal sodium excretion, thereby augmenting urine output. At intermediate doses (2 to 5 μg/kg/min), dopamine induces the release of norepinephrine from sympathetic nerve terminals in the heart and directly stimulates cardiac $β_1$-adrenergic receptors. This results in positive inotropic and chronotropic effects, augmenting cardiac output and causing tachycardia. Although intermediate-dose dopamine may be associated with increased systolic blood pressure, the systemic vascular resistance is usually unchanged because of renal and splanchnic vasodilation. At high doses of dopamine (5 to 15 μg/kg/min), α-adrenergic stimulation occurs, resulting in generalized vasoconstriction. A further rise in systolic blood pressure results; however, this occurs in association with an increase in systemic vascular resistance, which may suppress left ventricular systolic function because of the increase in afterload. In addition, at high doses, the α-adrenergic effects overcome the vasodilative effects in the renal and splanchnic vessels, and renal blood flow and urine output may decline.

The varied hemodynamic effects of dopamine make it a potentially useful agent for the treatment of heart failure in a variety of clinical settings. In the patient with congestion and oliguria but with adequate blood pressure, low-dose dopamine increases renal blood flow, thereby improving renal function, and augments urine output, thereby decreasing ventricular filling pressures. In the patient with cardiogenic shock, higher-dose dopamine is useful to maintain an adequate blood pressure. When the higher doses are used, patients must be monitored closely for signs of worsening heart failure; placement of a pulmonary arterial catheter is helpful in this regard. Although the increased systemic vascular resistance may be partially offset by the increase in cardiac contractility, in many patients, the ventricular filling pressures rise as a result of increased afterload. In addition, the venoconstricting effects augment venous return, thereby increasing ventricular preload. For these reasons, dopamine is not routinely used alone for inotropic support of the failing heart. Rather, for the treatment of patients with congestive heart failure, dopamine is often combined with another inotrope (e.g., dobutamine) or vasodilator (e.g., nitroprusside).

Although dopamine may have beneficial effects in some patients with congestive heart failure, there are few data to suggest an improvement in long-term outcomes. The use of dopamine is often limited by the development of tachycardia, which may precipitate ischemia in patients with coronary artery disease. Both supraventricular and ventricular arrhythmias may occur. In addition, dopamine may cause nausea, vomiting, and headaches and may precipitate myocardial ischemia. Marked vasoconstriction may result in digital gangrene, especially in patients with peripheral vascular disease, and ischemic skin necrosis may occur at sites of cutaneous infiltration.

Dobutamine

Dobutamine is a synthetic catecholamine that acts by direct stimulation of α- and β-adrenergic receptors and is available as a racemic mixture of its (+) and (−) stereoisomers. The (−) isomer is a potent $α_1$ receptor agonist and a relatively weak $β_1$ receptor agonist. The (+) isomer is a potent $β_1$ and $β_2$ receptor agonist and an $α_1$ receptor antagonist. The net effect is relatively selective $β_1$ receptor stimulation, resulting in augmentation of contractility and increased cardiac output. In contrast to the hemodynamic effects of dopamine, the inotropic effect of dobutamine is associated with relatively little increase in heart rate and with a modest reduction in left ventricular filling pressure and peripheral resistance. The latter effect results from $β_2$ receptor–mediated vasodilation. Dobutamine does not bind to dopamine receptors; thus, it does not result in renal or splanchnic vasodilation. Nonetheless, renal blood flow may increase as a reflection of increased cardiac output.

The hemodynamic effects of dobutamine make it an ideal agent for the treatment of decompensated heart failure, either alone or in combination with other inotropic or vasodilating agents. Dobutamine is usually started at a dose of 2.5 μg/kg/min and up-titrated in increments of 2.5 μg/kg/min as needed until an adequate therapeutic effect is obtained, adverse effects occur, or the maximum therapeutic dose is reached (15 to 20 μg/kg/min). Patients with more advanced heart failure may have a greater degree of β-receptor downregulation and require higher initial doses of dobutamine. Patients receiving chronic beta-blocker therapy may initially have relatively little inotropic response to dobutamine but a moderate vasopressor response resulting from the unmasking of $α_1$-adrenergic vasoconstriction in the presence of β-receptor blockade.

If an adequate therapeutic response is not achieved despite maximal doses of dobutamine, a second agent should be added. For patients with increased ventricular filling pressures and adequate systolic blood pressure, the addition of a diuretic and a vasodilator (such as nitroprusside) should be considered. Alternatively, a phosphodiesterase inhibitor such as milrinone (see later) may be of value in this setting by further augmenting cardiac output and vasodilation. Patients with congestive heart failure associated with hypotension may require the addition of a vasopressor (i.e., high-dose dopamine) to augment blood pressure and to allow effective diuresis.

Dobutamine has proved an effective agent in the management of hospitalized patients with congestive heart failure. In addition, intermittent administration of dobutamine to outpatients with severe heart failure has resulted in an improvement in patients' symptoms and may reduce hospital admissions. However, there has not been a demonstrable improvement in mortality in either setting. Continuous infusions of dobutamine are usually well tolerated for up to several days, although tolerance may develop and limit the efficacy of longer term infusion. Dobutamine administration is occasionally limited by the development of excess tachycardia; however, it is not uncommon to see a slight fall in the heart rate after dobutamine infusion due to withdrawal of sympathetic tone as the patient's hemodynamic status improves. Patients with a prior history of hypertension may have a marked hypertensive response to dobutamine; those with volume depletion may become hypotensive as a result of mild vasodilation. Like dopamine, dobutamine may precipitate atrial and ventricular arrhythmias and may aggravate myocardial ischemia.

Phosphodiesterase Inhibitors

Phosphodiesterase (PDE) is a membrane-bound enzyme that breaks down cAMP. It exists in several forms; PDE type 3 is the predominant isoform in cardiovascular issue. Milrinone and amrinone inhibit this enzyme and thereby result in increased cytosolic cAMP. This in turn results in increased myocardial contractility and augmentation of cardiac output. In the vasculature, these agents are potent vasodilators and venodilators, resulting in reductions in systemic and pulmonary vascular resistance (afterload) and in right- and left-sided filling pressures (preload).

The mixed hemodynamic effects of PDE inhibitors distinguish them from other inotropes or vasodilators. Compared with dobutamine, milrinone produces a greater reduction in systemic vascular resistance for a given increase in cardiac output. Similarly, compared with nitroprusside, milrinone produces a greater increase in cardiac output for a given reduction in systemic vascular resistance (Fig. 58-5). Thus, PDE inhibitors may be useful for the management of patients with decompensated heart failure that is characterized by reduced cardiac output, elevated systemic vascular resistance, and elevated filling pressures. PDE inhibitors also have antiplatelet effects and cause dilation of epicardial coronary arteries and bypass grafts. These properties, combined with the previously noted reductions in pulmonary arterial pressure and pulmonary vascular resistance, have given these agents an important role in the hemodynamic support of patients after cardiac surgery.

Amrinone (now renamed inamrinone) is less selective for the PDE3 isoenzyme, has a longer elimination half-life (2 to 3 hours versus 30 to 60 minutes), and is approximately 10-fold less potent than milrinone. In addition, it has been associated with significant thrombocytopenia in 10% of patients in whom it is administered. For these reasons, amrinone has fallen out of favor and milrinone has become the PDE inhibitor of choice for the management of decompensated heart failure. Milrinone is given as an initial loading dose (50 μg/kg over 10 minutes) followed by a continuous infusion (0.25 to 1.0 μg/kg/min). It is excreted predominantly by the kidney; in patients with renal failure, a 50% reduction in the infusion rate is required. Titration may be limited by the development of tachycardia and arrhythmias, both of which are mediated by the increase in cAMP. Because of the potent vasodilative properties of PDE inhibitors, they should be used with care in patients who have normal or low vascular resistance or filling pressures. These patients may be intolerant of the vasodilation, and marked hypotension may result.

Clinical trials have demonstrated the efficacy of intravenous milrinone in improving hemodynamics and reducing symptoms in hospitalized patients with decompensated heart failure. However, a mortality benefit has not been demonstrated, and when milrinone is administered routinely to patients with less-severe congestive heart failure (i.e., no evidence of end-organ hypoperfusion), it does not appear to offer benefit over usual treatment with ACE inhibitors and diuretics.

Other Agents

Natriuretic Peptides

Natriuretic peptides are naturally occurring peptides that are produced in low levels in the normal heart. Atrial natriuretic peptide (ANP) is produced in the atria, whereas brain natriuretic peptide (BNP; originally isolated from porcine brain tissue) is produced in the ventricles. In patients with heart failure, both ANP and BNP are secreted at high levels in response to increased intracardiac pressure and volume. These peptides act through a receptor-mediated guanosine monophosphate pathway in vascular smooth muscle cells and are degraded by neutral endopeptidase. They have potent balanced vasodilating actions resulting in decreased ventricular preload and afterload. In the kidney, these peptides cause vasodilation of the afferent arteriole, thereby increasing glomerular filtration rate, and inhibit sodium reabsorption in the renal collecting ducts and aldosterone secretion by the adrenal glands, thereby resulting in natriuresis and diuresis.

Nesiritide is a recombinant peptide that is identical to endogenous BNP and has both vasodilative and natriuretic properties. In addition, it antagonizes the renin-angiotensin-aldosterone system. When it is administered to patients with heart failure, nesiritide reduces right atrial and pulmonary capillary wedge pressures, decreases systemic vascular resistance, increases cardiac output, and produces a diuresis and natriuresis. Clinical studies have demonstrated persistent hemodynamic effects of prolonged (24- to 48-hour) infusions and improvements in clinical status that may be greater than those seen with intravenous nitroglycerin. Nesiritide is usually given as an initial bolus of 2 μg/kg followed by an infusion of 0.01 μg/kg/min. Its hemodynamic effects are apparent within 15 minutes and persist for up to 4 hours after discontinuation of the infusion. Nesiritide does not aggravate arrhythmias and has no toxic metabolites; however, significant and prolonged hypotension can occur with this agent and is the most common limiting factor. Furthermore, several recent meta-analyses have suggested an increased risk of death and worsened renal function after administration of nesiritide to patients with acutely decompensated heart failure. Thus, the use of nesiritide should be limited to the treatment of decompensated congestive heart failure characterized by volume overload and increased filling pressures in patients who are intolerant of inotropic agents and resistant to usual diuretics.

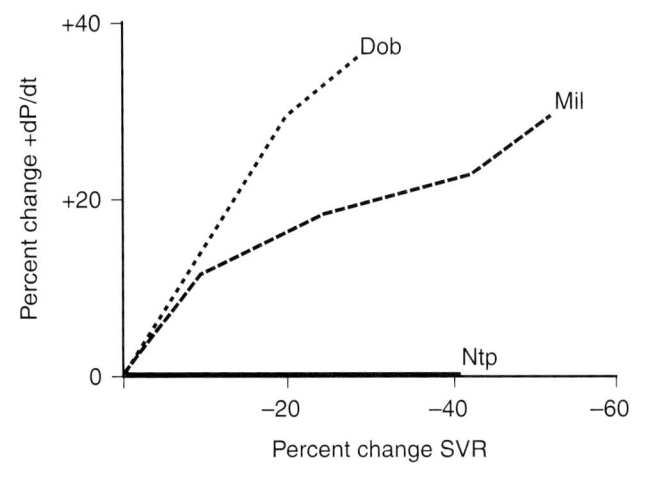

Figure 58–5
The relative effects of varying doses of nitroprusside (Ntp), dobutamine (Dob), and milrinone (Mil) on the peak positive dP/dt and systemic vascular resistance (SVR). *(Modified from Colucci WS, Wright RF, Jaski BE, et al. Milrinone and dobutamine in severe heart failure: differing hemodynamic effects and individual patient responsiveness. Circulation 1986;73:III175.)*

APPROACH TO THE MANAGEMENT OF HEART FAILURE

Initial Approach and Clinical Assessment

The treatment of heart failure is dependent on its recognition. Because heart failure may manifest in a variety of ways, the clinician must maintain a high index of suspicion, especially in the patient with a prior history of heart failure or with risk factors for the development of heart failure. Acute heart failure usually manifests dramatically with signs and symptoms of pulmonary and systemic congestion, at times associated with evidence of hypoperfusion (Table 58-8). In this setting, the clinical examination is usually striking and the diagnosis is rarely overlooked. Conversely, chronic heart failure may have a more indolent course, and the associated dyspnea, fatigue, and edema may be mistaken for other noncardiac conditions. In addition, the physical examination of patients with chronic heart failure may be somewhat misleading in that they often have clear lung fields despite having significantly elevated filling pressures.

The initial evaluation of the patient with heart failure should include an assessment of the disease severity. The most common classification in this regard is that devised by the New York Heart Association (see Table 58-2), which categorizes patients with symptomatic heart failure on the basis of their functional level. A broader classification scheme has recently been proposed by the American College of Cardiology/American Heart Association and includes patients with structurally normal hearts but at risk for development of heart failure (stage A), those with asymptomatic structural heart disease (stage B), those with overt heart failure (stage C), and those with severe heart failure that requires specialized care such as mechanical assistance or transplantation (stage D). Although the functional class may vary over time, these classifications remain useful because they provide an objective measure by which to follow disease progression and response to therapy. The choice of specific therapies is, in part, additionally dependent on disease severity. Patients with severe decompensated heart failure require the rapid administration of intravenous pharmacologic therapy to reduce pulmonary congestion, to augment perfusion of vital organs, and to attain hemodynamic stability. Conversely, patients with chronic compensated heart failure can frequently be treated with oral medications with the goal of controlling symptoms, improving functional capacity, and reducing long-term mortality.

In addition to the initiation of pharmacologic therapy, the initial approach to the care of the patient with heart failure should always include a thorough evaluation of the etiology of heart failure and a careful search for aggravating or precipitating factors (Table 58-9). Although the history and physical examination may provide clues to the underlying cardiac abnormality, a formal assessment of cardiac function by echocardiography should be performed in all patients presenting with new or significantly worsened heart failure. This test permits identification and characterization of pericardial, myocardial, and valvular disease and allows the quantification of left ventricular systolic and diastolic function. Initial laboratory evaluation should also include a chest radiograph (to assess cardiac size, pulmonary congestion, and structural intrathoracic abnormalities), electrocardiogram (to evaluate for evidence of ischemic heart disease or ventricular hypertrophy), complete blood count, electrolyte values, thyroid function tests, and assessment of renal function.

All patients with heart failure should be counseled about lifestyle modifications that may help alleviate their symptoms. This includes moderate sodium restriction (≤2 g sodium daily); compliance with treatment regimens; and avoidance of alcohol, cigarettes, and nonsteroidal anti-inflammatory agents. Most heart failure patients do not require fluid restriction, but close monitoring of weight is essential for the early recognition of volume retention.

Pharmacologic Treatment of Chronic Compensated Systolic Heart Failure

Patients with chronic compensated heart failure represent a spectrum of patients ranging from those with asymptomatic left ventricular dysfunction to those with previously

Table 58-8
Signs and Symptoms of Heart Failure

Evidence of Congestion	Evidence of Hypoperfusion
Symptoms	**Symptoms**
Orthopnea	Fatigue, weakness
Dyspnea on exertion	Confusion
Paroxysmal nocturnal dyspnea	Symptomatic hypotension
Anorexia, nausea	
Signs	**Signs**
Pulmonary rales	Cool extremities
Elevated jugular venous pressure	Mottled extremities
Hepatojugular reflux	Narrowed pulse pressure
Edema	Worsening renal insufficiency
Ascites	Progressive hyponatremia
Loud S_3	Cheyne-Stokes respirations

Table 58-9
Potential Aggravating Factors Contributing to Decompensation in Chronic Heart Failure

Myocardial ischemia or infarction
Systemic hypertension
Tachyarrhythmias (ventricular or supraventricular)
Superimposed valvular heart disease
Exacerbation of underlying lung disease
Pulmonary embolism
Infection
Thyroid disease
Anemia
Medication noncompliance
Dietary indiscretions (excessive salt and water intake)
Excessive alcohol use

decompensated heart failure who have responded to medical therapy. The goals of treatment in this population include maintenance of a symptom-free state, improvement in functional capacity, prevention of decompensation, and reduction of mortality. Several individual classes of medications have proven efficacy in this regard (Table 58-10), although in general, most patients with systolic heart failure require multidrug therapy.

All patients with left ventricular systolic dysfunction should receive treatment with an ACE inhibitor as these agents improve mortality of patients with all classes of heart failure and delay the onset of symptoms in patients with asymptomatic left ventricular dysfunction. Therapy should be initiated at low doses and slowly titrated upward if it is tolerated (i.e., systolic blood pressure >90 mm Hg, no symptoms of hypotension) to doses that have been proved efficacious in randomized trials (see Table 58-6). Renal function should be monitored closely, especially in patients with concomitant vascular disease. Other vasodilators should be considered in patients with symptomatic heart failure who are unable to tolerate ACE inhibitors because of side effects. Whereas ARBs should not be used as first-line therapy for heart failure, they are the preferred agents for patients who develop cough with ACE inhibitors. Patients who develop progressive renal insufficiency or hyperkalemia with ACE inhibitors are equally likely to develop these complications with ARBs; these agents should not be used in this setting. The combination of hydralazine and nitrates is a less effective regimen than ACE inhibitors but is a reasonable alternative in patients who are intolerant of these agents or ARBs.

All patients with class II-IV heart failure should also receive a beta-blocker as these agents provide a marked mortality benefit. Care must be taken to ensure that patients are hemodynamically stable and euvolemic before beta-blocker therapy is started because initiation of beta-blockade may be associated with orthostatic hypotension and worsening of heart failure symptoms. These agents should always be started at low doses (see Table 58-6), titrated very slowly (increasing dose every 2 weeks), and avoided in patients who recently required intravenous diuretics or inotropic agents. They should also be avoided in patients with a heart rate below 60 beats per minute, systolic blood pressure of less than 100 mm Hg, or evidence of atrioventricular block, and they should be used with care in patients with bronchospastic lung disease. Most patients with heart failure who receive beta-blocker therapy should be concomitantly treated with diuretics, especially those patients with current or recent volume retention. If heart failure symptoms worsen after beta-blockers are started, diuretic therapy should be initiated or increased and usually allows continued beta-blocker use. In general, beta-blocker therapy should not be initiated during the hospitalization of patients with decompensated heart failure; rather, it should be started on an outpatient basis once a stable medical regimen has been established. It is generally preferable to initiate ACE inhibitor therapy before beta-blocker therapy as ACE inhibitors result in rapid relief of symptoms and may facilitate the initiation of beta-blockade.

Patients with symptoms or signs of congestion may respond to afterload-reducing therapy alone; however, most require the addition of a diuretic. Loop diuretics such as furosemide are preferred as they are more effective than thiazide diuretics, especially in patients with renal insufficiency (serum creatinine concentration >2.5 mg/dL). If volume overload persists despite upward titration of the loop diuretic, addition of a thiazide (e.g., metolazone, 2.5 mg orally given 30 minutes before the loop diuretic) should be considered and provides effective combination therapy. This combination can lead to profound potassium and magnesium wasting and requires close monitoring of serum electrolytes. Spironolactone (25 to 50 mg daily) should be added to the regimen of patients with class IV heart failure as it provides a mortality benefit in this setting.

Digoxin should be considered in any patient who continues to have symptomatic heart failure despite treatment with an ACE inhibitor and beta-blocker. Although this agent has not demonstrated a mortality benefit in any class of heart failure, when it is used as part of a multidrug regimen, it is useful for controlling symptoms and reducing hospital admissions. It may be particularly beneficial in patients with atrial fibrillation, in whom improved heart rate control may lead to symptomatic improvement.

Table 58-10
Beneficial Effects of Oral Pharmacotherapy for Chronic Heart Failure

Medication	Improves Mortality	Improves Symptoms	Reduces Recurrent Heart Failure	Heart Failure Class for Which Treatment Is Indicated
Angiotensin-converting enzyme inhibitors	Yes	Yes	Yes	Class I-IV*
Beta-blockers	Yes	Yes	Yes	Class II-IV
Hydralazine	Yes	Yes	No	Class II-IV†
Spironolactone	Yes	Yes	No	Class III-IV
Diuretics	No	Yes	No	Class II-IV
Digoxin	No	Yes	Yes	Class II-IV

*Also indicated in patients with asymptomatic left ventricular systolic dysfunction.
†Not a first-line drug but should be considered in patients who are intolerant of angiotensin-converting enzyme inhibitors.

Treatment of Decompensated Systolic Heart Failure

Patients with chronic systolic heart failure may have periods of relative stability interrupted by periods of decompensation. These periods of decompensation may be precipitated by medication noncompliance, dietary indiscretion (i.e., excessive sodium or water intake), or progression of the underlying myopathic process. The patient often reports a gradual worsening of symptoms or progressive weight gain during the course of several days, although the clinical presentation may appear relatively acute.

Patients with decompensated heart failure may present with hemodynamic instability and usually have evidence of systemic and pulmonary congestion with or without evidence of decreased organ perfusion. Although pulmonary arterial catheterization is sometimes necessary to precisely define the hemodynamic derangement, many patients with decompensated heart failure can be adequately evaluated on the basis of their clinical history and physical examination findings, specifically whether they have evidence of pulmonary or systemic congestion or organ hypoperfusion. Congestion may be evidenced by an elevation in the jugular venous pressure, the presence of pulmonary rales, or peripheral edema. These patients are usually dyspneic with minimal exertion or even at rest and often report increased orthopnea and paroxysmal nocturnal dyspnea. Hypoperfusion may be manifested as cold extremities, mottled skin, cyanosis, mental obtundation, or declining renal function. Measurement of the pulse pressure (the difference between the systolic and diastolic blood pressures) may be helpful; in patients with heart failure, the pulse pressure narrows. A pulse pressure of less than 25% of the systolic blood pressure generally correlates with a cardiac index of less than 2.2 L/min/m^2.

For patients in whom the hemodynamic profile needs to be more accurately defined or in whom initial therapy yields suboptimal results, direct measurement of hemodynamic parameters should be performed through the insertion of a Swan-Ganz catheter (Table 58-11). The information thus obtained may be used to guide the selection and titration of specific pharmacologic therapy. Such tailored therapy should be undertaken with the goal of manipulating medications to achieve optimal hemodynamics, including a right atrial pressure of less than 8 mm Hg, a pulmonary capillary wedge pressure of less than 18 mm Hg, a cardiac index above 2.2 L/min/m^2, and a systemic vascular resistance of 800 to 1200 dynes • cm • sec^{-5}.

Taken together, these findings can be used to classify the severity of hemodynamic impairment of a patient presenting with decompensated heart failure and to help make decisions about appropriate initial therapy (Fig. 58-6). Patients with left ventricular dysfunction who are well compensated generally have acceptable filling pressures and adequate cardiac outputs, do not have congestion, and appear well perfused. These patients require chronic heart failure therapy as outlined before for symptom control and mortality reduction. Patients with decompensated heart failure who have evidence of congestion without hypoperfusion have elevated filling pressures with adequate cardiac output. These patients may simply be volume overloaded and require aggressive diuresis. If the blood pressure is adequate, addition of a vasodilator (e.g., ACE inhibitor) may further augment cardiac output and facilitate diuresis. Patients with signs of hypoperfusion

Table 58-11
Potential Indications for Invasive Hemodynamic Assessment in Patients with Heart Failure

Assessment of volume status when clinical assessment is uncertain
Distinguishing heart failure from other causes of dyspnea (e.g., pulmonary disease)
Assessment of hemodynamic response to vasoactive medications
Guidance in achieving ideal hemodynamic goals (tailored therapy)
Assessment of filling pressure in patients with persistent symptoms of heart failure despite aggressive medical therapy
Determination of appropriate therapy in patients with persistent congestion and progressive renal insufficiency after diuretic therapy
Assessment of pulmonary vascular resistance during evaluation for cardiac transplantation
Perioperative monitoring of volume status in patients with severe left ventricular dysfunction undergoing prolonged procedures associated with significant volume shifts or in patients with decompensated heart failure on preoperative assessment

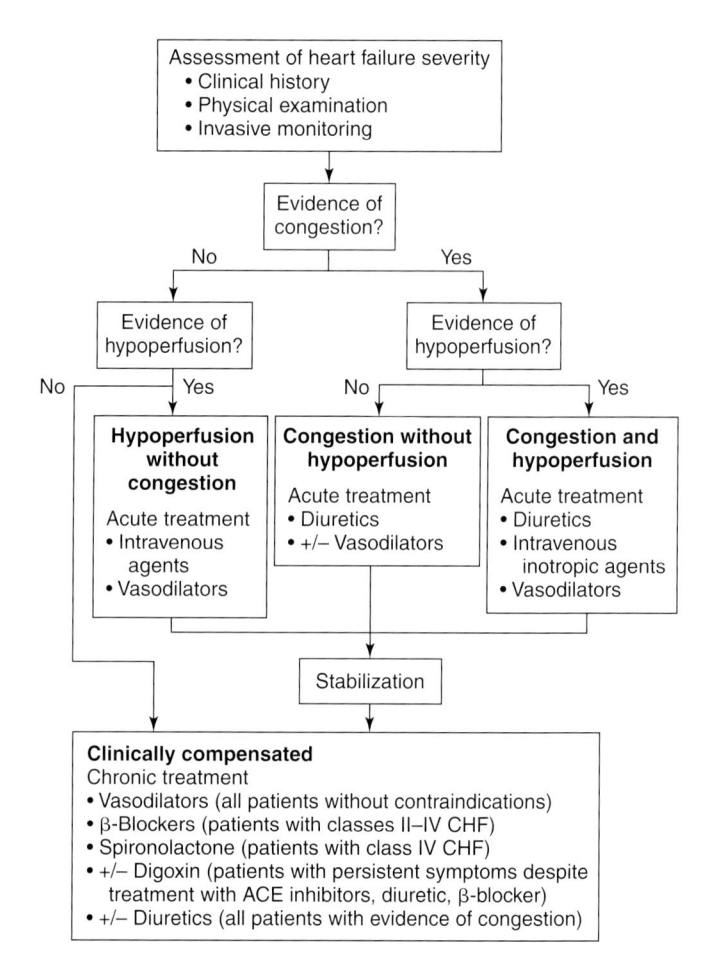

Assessment of heart failure severity
• Clinical history
• Physical examination
• Invasive monitoring

Evidence of congestion?

No → Evidence of hypoperfusion?
- No → (Stabilization / Clinically compensated)
- Yes → **Hypoperfusion without congestion**
  Acute treatment
  • Intravenous agents
  • Vasodilators

Yes → Evidence of hypoperfusion?
- No → **Congestion without hypoperfusion**
  Acute treatment
  • Diuretics
  • +/– Vasodilators
- Yes → **Congestion and hypoperfusion**
  Acute treatment
  • Diuretics
  • Intravenous inotropic agents
  • Vasodilators

Stabilization

Clinically compensated
Chronic treatment
• Vasodilators (all patients without contraindications)
• β-Blockers (patients with classes II–IV CHF)
• Spironolactone (patients with class IV CHF)
• +/– Digoxin (patients with persistent symptoms despite treatment with ACE inhibitors, diuretic, β-blocker)
• +/– Diuretics (all patients with evidence of congestion)

Figure 58-6
An approach to treatment of acute or decompensated heart failure. ACE, angiotensin-converting enzyme; CHF, congestive heart failure.

Table 58-12
Intravenous Agents Used in the Treatment of Decompensated Heart Failure

Medication	Hemodynamic Effects	Potential Adverse Clinical Effects
Dopamine		
Low dose	Splanchnic vasodilation, ↑GFR, ↑urine output	
Intermediate dose	↑HR, ↑contractility, ↑CO, ↑BP, ↑/–SVR	Myocardial ischemia, arrhythmias
High dose	↑HR, ↑↑contractility, ↑↑BP, ↑↑SVR, ↓CO, ↑PCW, ↓/–GFR	Myocardial ischemia, arrhythmias, ↑CHF, worsened renal function
Dobutamine	↑HR, ↑↑contractility, ↑CO, ↑/–BP, ↓SVR, ↓PCW	Myocardial ischemia, arrhythmias
Isoproterenol	↑↑HR, ↑contractility, ↑CO, ↓SVR	Myocardial ischemia
Epinephrine	↑HR, ↑contractility, ↑SVR, ↑BP	Myocardial ischemia, arrhythmias, ↑CHF, worsened renal function
Norepinephrine	↑HR, ↑contractility, ↑↑SVR, ↑↑BP	Myocardial ischemia, arrhythmias, ↑CHF, worsened renal function
Milrinone	↑Contractility, ↑↑CO, ↓↓SVR, ↓PVR, ↓↓PCW	Myocardial ischemia, arrhythmias, hypotension
Nitroprusside	↑↑CO, ↓↓SVR, ↓PVR, ↓↓PCW No effect on contractility	Hypotension, cyanide and thiocyanate toxicity
Nitroglycerin	↑CO, ↓SVR, ↓PVR, ↓↓PCW, coronary vasodilation No effect on contractility	Hypotension, headache, nitrate tolerance
Nesiritide	↑CO, ↓SVR, ↓↓PCW, ↑GFR Natriuresis, diuresis	Hypotension

BP, blood pressure; CHF, congestive heart failure; CO, cardiac output; GFR, glomerular filtration rate; HR, heart rate; PCW, pulmonary capillary wedge (pressure); PVR, pulmonary vascular resistance; SVR, systemic vascular resistance.

but without congestion have acceptable filling pressures but decreased cardiac output. Therapy in this setting should be guided by the patient's blood pressure; patients with hypotension require inotropic therapy, whereas patients with adequate systolic blood pressure (>100 mm Hg) should receive vasodilators with or without inotropic agents to augment cardiac output. These patients do not generally require aggressive diuresis and, in fact, may be volume depleted and require gentle hydration. Patients with evidence of both congestion and hypoperfusion have both elevated filling pressures and decreased cardiac output and are the most difficult to manage. These patients frequently require combination therapy with inotropic agents, intravenous vasodilator therapy, and use of diuretics. Invasive hemodynamic monitoring may be most helpful in guiding therapy in this group of patients, especially in patients with associated hypotension.

A variety of intravenous agents are available for use in the treatment of patients with decompensated heart failure (Table 58-12). Initial management should be guided by the patient's specific hemodynamic alterations. In patients with severe hypotension leading to organ dysfunction, stabilization of the blood pressure is the primary goal, and the initial drug of choice is usually dopamine at moderate to high doses. Epinephrine or norepinephrine may be added if high doses of dopamine are inadequate; however, these agents are rarely required in the absence of pathologic vasodilation (e.g., sepsis, after anesthesia). In general, vasoconstrictors should be avoided in patients with left ventricular dysfunction as they may lead to further depression of cardiac output. In patients with adequate blood pressure whose predominant manifestation of heart failure is congestion, initial treatment with nitroprusside (or nitroglycerin or nesiritide) is usually effective. In patients whose predominant manifestation is hypoperfusion, dobutamine, milrinone, nitroprusside, or nesiritide may be effective. The majority of patients with decompensated heart failure also require administration of intravenous diuretics and careful management of fluid balance.

Treatment of Diastolic Heart Failure

In contrast to the treatment of systolic heart failure, the treatment of diastolic heart failure has not been extensively studied, and there are no large-scale randomized trials by which to guide therapeutic recommendations. The general approach is aimed at treatment of the underlying cause and the relief of symptoms with medications that intuitively should reduce diastolic pressures. The impairment in diastolic filling results in an increase in atrial pressure early in the course of this disease, with resultant pulmonary and venous congestion. Diuretics therefore play an important role in the management of this syndrome and help control congestive symptoms. Care must be taken to avoid overdiuresis as these patients depend on an elevated filling pressure to maintain stroke volume. Calcium channel blockers (verapamil or diltiazem) and beta-blockers slow the heart rate, prolong diastole, and allow increased time for left ventricular filling. In addition, these agents may actually improve diastolic ventricular function (i.e., decrease left ventricular stiffness and improve left ventricular relaxation)

Table 58-13
Precipitants of Flash Pulmonary Edema and Their Therapeutic Implications

Acute	Specific Therapeutic Considerations
Ischemia or infarction	Cardiac catheterization and revascularization
Hypertension	Intravenous vasodilators (nitroprusside, enalaprilat) with 25% reduction in mean arterial pressure as initial goal
Renal artery stenosis	Percutaneous renal artery revascularization
Aortic stenosis	Aortic valve replacement after initial stabilization with diuretics, ± vasopressors, ± inotropic agents
Acute aortic insufficiency (endocarditis, aortic dissection)	Aortic valve replacement after initial stabilization with vasodilators ± inotropic agents
Acute mitral regurgitation (ischemia, endocarditis, ruptured chordae)	Consider intra-aortic balloon pump for hemodynamic stabilization before coronary revascularization for ischemic mitral regurgitation or mitral valve replacement for structural mitral regurgitation
Supraventricular tachyarrhythmias	Rate control or electrical cardioversion

by improvement in calcium homeostasis. In patients who are intolerant of these medications or who have continued symptoms despite their use, ACE inhibitors may offer further benefit. Data suggest that ventricular hypertrophy is associated with stimulation of the renin-angiotensin system and that chronic activation of this system results in fluid retention as well as myocardial fibrosis and increased ventricular stiffness. Inhibition of this system with ACE inhibitors or ARBs may therefore offer further treatment of the underlying pathophysiologic changes characteristic of diastolic heart failure. Inotropic therapy, including digoxin, should be avoided in diastolic heart failure; these agents are unlikely to be beneficial in the face of preserved systolic function and may worsen diastolic function, leading to further elevation of filling pressures and progressive heart failure.

Other therapies for diastolic heart failure are aimed at treating the underlying cause of the dysfunction and correcting associated abnormalities that may worsen this dysfunction. Hypertension is the most common condition that predisposes to diastolic heart failure. Small studies suggest that it is the extent of hypertension control, not the specific antihypertensive agent used, that results in improved diastolic function. Patients with secondary causes of hypertension (e.g., renal artery stenosis, hyperadrenalism) should undergo definitive therapy when possible. Patients with coronary artery disease should be aggressively treated with antianginal therapy, and coronary revascularization should be performed when appropriate. Aortic stenosis should be surgically corrected when it is associated with diastolic heart failure, even in the absence of systolic dysfunction. Patients with diastolic heart failure are highly preload dependent and may experience acute decompensation if they develop atrial fibrillation. This occurs in part because of the loss of the active atrial contribution to left ventricular filling and in part because the increased heart rate associated with the development of atrial fibrillation shortens diastole and allows less time for left ventricular filling. All efforts should be made to restore and to maintain sinus rhythm in these individuals.

Flash Pulmonary Edema

Decompensated heart failure that develops acutely in a previously asymptomatic or well-compensated patient is often the result of an abrupt change in cardiac structure or function (Table 58-13). The precipitous nature of the presentation of these patients accounts for the commonly used descriptive term *flash pulmonary edema*. In this setting, patients are often hemodynamically unstable and develop severe pulmonary congestion, although they frequently are not fluid overloaded. These patients are pharmacologically treated similarly to the decompensated patients described before; however, specific therapy should be guided by the underlying precipitating factor. Patients with ischemia precipitating acute heart failure frequently have severe coronary artery disease (i.e., three-vessel or left main coronary artery disease) or have papillary muscle dysfunction resulting in acute mitral regurgitation (most common with disease of the right coronary artery). In addition to heart failure therapy as dictated by their clinical presentation, these patients should receive aggressive antianginal therapy with intravenous nitrates and antiplatelet agents (i.e., aspirin, heparin, IIb/IIIa inhibitors), and urgent cardiac catheterization and coronary revascularization should be considered. For patients with refractory heart failure and ischemia, intra-aortic balloon pump counterpulsation may be a beneficial adjuvant therapy while awaiting definitive revascularization.

Severe hypertension may precipitate acute heart failure. Classically, this occurs with hypertension associated with pheochromocytomas, renal artery stenosis, and alcohol or cocaine use, but it can also be seen in patients with preexisting heart failure who are noncompliant with medications or dietary sodium restriction. Appropriate therapy in this setting is dependent on blood pressure control. Intravenous antihypertensive agents (e.g., nitroprusside, enalaprilat) should be started with the goal of lowering the mean arterial pressure by 25% in the first several hours and reducing the systolic blood pressure below 160 mm Hg within the first 24 hours. Acute severe aortic insufficiency as occurs with endocarditis or aortic dissection should be managed with intravenous inotropic agents or vasodilators (depending on systemic blood pressure) while preparing for emergent surgical therapy. Acute mitral regurgitation often responds to vasodilator therapy but may require intra-aortic balloon pump counterpulsation for stabilization before valve replacement.

Perioperative Heart Failure

For a variety of reasons, the incidence of heart failure is increased in the perioperative period. Many anesthetic agents have negative inotropic effects and can precipitate heart failure in patients with left ventricular systolic dysfunction, and the vasodilative effects of these agents may result in hypotension. Aggressive fluid resuscitation in this setting may lead to volume overload, elevated filling pressures, and pulmonary congestion. Similarly, appropriate replacement of blood products in the face of intraoperative blood loss may be poorly tolerated and may require the concomitant administration of diuretics. Mechanical ventilation produces beneficial hemodynamic effects in heart failure because of a reduction in venous return induced by the increased intrathoracic pressure. Conversely, the decrease in intrathoracic pressure associated with extubation may be followed by a sudden rise in preload and result in heart failure. Fluid that entered the extravascular space during the perioperative period reenters the vascular space several days postoperatively as patients begin to mobilize. This rise in circulating blood volume may similarly precipitate heart failure. These adverse effects are more likely to occur in patients with preexisting left ventricular dysfunction and in patients with overt heart failure preoperatively.

In the preoperative setting, the identification of decompensated heart failure is essential. The presence of pulmonary or systemic congestion or signs of hypoperfusion should prompt a thorough assessment of the patient's cardiac status, reevaluation of the patient's current therapy, and delay or cancellation of all but emergent procedures until the patient's status is stabilized. If the patient's ventricular function is not known, echocardiography should be performed to aid in determining the mechanism of heart failure and to guide appropriate therapy. In the postoperative period, heart failure may be mistaken for pneumonia, atelectasis, exacerbation of chronic obstructive pulmonary disease, or pulmonary embolism. Patients are often unable to communicate their symptoms to the treating physicians because of sedation and mechanical ventilation; thus, the physician's vigilance is essential. Identification of pulmonary rales, jugular venous distention, hepatojugular reflux, gallop rhythm, or peripheral edema should raise the concern of worsening heart failure, and close monitoring of the patient's weight and fluid balance should alert the physician to the possibility of volume overload.

In patients with more advanced heart failure (class III or IV) or with severely depressed left ventricular systolic function (<25%), placement of a pulmonary arterial catheter preoperatively should be strongly considered. In patients with decompensated heart failure, placement of this catheter the day before surgery allows time for maximization of their hemodynamic status, thereby potentially decreasing their overall perioperative risk. Continued invasive hemodynamic monitoring for 24 to 48 after surgery may be appropriate in some patients.

Patients with chronic heart failure are often dependent on medications to maintain their hemodynamic stability, and every effort should be made to continue these medications in the perioperative period. Although it may be appropriate to hold diuretics on the day of surgery, careful monitoring for evidence of volume retention is obligatory postoperatively, and intravenous diuretics should be administered at the first signs of congestion. Beta-blockers and ACE inhibitors should likewise be continued as the sudden withdrawal of these agents may result in neurohormonal activation and worsening of heart failure. Intravenous formulations may be substituted for many oral medications in patients who are unable to take oral agents postoperatively because of the nature of their surgery. However, well-compensated patients often tolerate withholding of their usual medications and can be managed for several days with intravenous diuretics and topical nitrates for preload reduction. If refractory congestion or signs of organ hypoperfusion develop, use of intravenous vasodilators or inotropes may become necessary. These agents may be transitioned to oral formulations as gut absorption improves. For patients who remain hemodynamically labile postoperatively, use of short-acting agents may be appropriate for several days; long-acting agents may be reinstituted when the volume shifts and hemodynamic derangements improve. Given the tenuous nature of these patients, it is often helpful to involve a cardiology consultant to help manage the complex hemodynamic changes that occur in the perioperative period.

SUGGESTED READING

Pathophysiology

Baig MK, Mahon N, McKenna WJ, et al. The pathophysiology of advanced heart failure. *Heart Lung* 1999;**28**:87-101.

Cohn JN, Ferrari R, Sharpe N. Cardiac remodeling—concepts and clinical implications: a consensus paper from an international forum on cardiac remodeling. *J Am Coll Cardiol* 2000;**35**:569-82.

Colucci WS, Braunwald E. Pathophysiology of heart failure. In: Braunwald E, Zipes DP, Libby P, editors. Heart disease—a textbook of cardiovascular medicine. 6th ed. Philadelphia: WB Saunders; 2001. P. 503–33.

Floras JS. Clinical aspects of sympathetic activation and parasympathetic withdrawal in heart failure. *J Am Coll Cardiol* 1993;**22**:72A.

Francis GS. Pathophysiology of chronic heart failure. *Am J Med* 2001;**110**: 37S-46S.

Grossman W, Jones D, McLaurin LP. Wall stress and patterns of hypertrophy in the human left ventricle. *J Clin Invest* 1975;**56**:56.

Konstam M, Dracup K, Baker D, et al. *Heart failure: evaluation and care of patients with left-ventricular systolic dysfunction. Clinical practice guideline number 11.* Rockville, MD: Agency for Health Care Policy and Research and the National Heart, Lung and Blood Institute, Public Health Service, U.S. Department of Health and Human Services; 1994.

Naunheim KS, Fiore AC, Wadley JJ, McBride LR, Kanter KR, Pennington DG, et al. The changing profile of the patient undergoing coronary artery bypass surgery. *J Am Coll Cardiol* 1988 Mar;**11**(3):494-8.

Packer M. Evolution of the neurohormonal hypothesis to explain the progression of chronic heart failure. *Eur Heart J* 1995;**16**(suppl F):4-6.

Zelis R, Sinoway LI, Musch TI, et al. Regional blood flow in congestive heart failure: concept of compensatory mechanisms with short and long term constants. *Am J Cardiol* 1988;**62**:2E.

Inotropic Agents

Adamopoulos S, Piepolo M, Qiang F, et al. Effects of pulsed beta-stimulant therapy on beta-adrenoceptors and chronotropic responsiveness in chronic heart failure. *Lancet* 1995;**345**:344.

Chanani NK, Cowan DB, Takeuchi K, Poutias DN, et al. Differential effects of amrinone and milrinone upon myocardial inflammatory signaling. *Circulation* 2002;**106**: I284-9.

Colucci WS, Wright RF, Jaski BE, Fifer MA, Braunwald E. Milrinone and dobutamine in severe heart failure: differing hemodynamic effects and individual patient responsiveness. *Circulation* 1986;**73**:III175-83.

Cuffe MS, Califf RM, Adams Jr KF, et al. Short-term intravenous milrinone for acute exacerbation of chronic heart failure: a randomized controlled trial. *JAMA* 2002;**287**:1541-7.

Maskin CS, Ocken S, Chadwick B, LeJemtel TH. Comparative systemic and renal effects of dopamine and angiotensin converting enzyme inhibition with enalaprilat in patients with heart failure. *Circulation* 1985;**72**:846.

Monrad ES, Baim DS, Smith HS, Lanoue AS. Milrinone, dobutamine, and nitroprusside: comparative effects on hemodynamics and myocardial energetics in patients with severe heart failure. *Circulation* 1986;**73**:III168-74.

Oliva F, Latini R, Politi A, et al. Intermittent 6-month low-dose dobutamine infusion in severe heart failure: DICE multicenter trial. *Am Heart J* 1999;**138**:247.

Packer M, Carver JR, Rodeheffer RJ, Ivanhoe RJ, DiBianco R, Zeldis SM, et al. Effect of oral milrinone on mortality in severe chronic heart failure. The PROMISE Study Research Group. *N Engl J Med* 1991; Nov 21(325):1468-75.

Ruffolo Jr RR. The pharmacology of dobutamine. *Am J Med Sci* 1987;**294**:244-8.

Seino Y, Momomura S, Takano T, et al. Multicenter, double-blind study of intravenous milrinone for patients with acute heart failure in Japan. *Crit Care Med* 1996;**24**:1490-7.

Stevenson LW, Colucci WS. Management of patients hospitalized with heart failure. In: Smith TW, editor. Cardiovascular therapeutics: a companion to Braunwald's heart disease. Philadelphia: WB Saunders; 1996. p. 199–209.

Diuretics

Brater DC. Diuretic therapy. *N Engl J Med* 1998;**339**:387-95.

Dormans TP, van Meyel JJ, Gerlag PG, Tan Y, Russel FG, Smits P. Diuretic efficacy of high dose furosemide in severe heart failure: bolus injection versus continuous infusion. *J Am Coll Cardiol* 1996;**28**:376-82.

Pitt B, Remme W, Zannad F, et al, for the Eplerenone Post-Acute Myocardial Infarction Heart Failure Efficacy and Survival Study Investigators. Eplerenone, a selective aldosterone blocker, in patients with left ventricular dysfunction after myocardial infarction. *N Engl J Med* 2003;**348**:1309-21.

Pitt B, Zannad F, Remme WJ, Cody R, Castaigne A, Perez A, et al. The effect of spironolactone on morbidity and mortality in patients with severe heart failure. Randomized Aldactone Evaluation Study Investigators. *N Engl J Med* 1999;**341**:709-17.

Zannad F, Alla F, Dousset B, Perez A, Pitt B. Limitation of excessive extracellular matrix turnover may contribute to survival benefit of spironolactone therapy in patients with congestive heart failure: insights from the Randomized Aldactone Valuation Study (RALES). Rales Investigators. *Circulation* 2000;**102**:2700-6.

Angiotensin-Converting Enzyme Inhibitors and Angiotensin Receptor Blocking Agents

Acute Infarction Ramipril Efficacy (AIRE) Study Investigators. Effects of ramipril on mortality and morbidity of survivors of acute myocardial infarction with clinical evidence of heart failure. *Lancet* 1993;**342**:821.

Annane D, Bellissant E, Pussard E, Asmar R, Lacombe F, Lanata E, et al. Placebo-controlled, randomized, double-blind study of intravenous enalaprilat efficacy and safety in acute cardiogenic pulmonary edema. *Circulation* 1996;**94**:1316-24.

Garg R, Yusef S. Overview of randomized trials of angiotensin converting enzyme inhibitors on mortality and morbidity of patients with heart failure. Collaborative Group on ACE Inhibitor Trials. *JAMA* 1995;**273**:1450-6.

Jong P, Demers C, McKelvie RS, Liu PP. Angiotensin receptor blockers in heart failure: meta-analysis of randomized controlled trials. *J Am Coll Cardiol* 2002;**39**:463-70.

Flather MD, Yusuf S, Kober L, et al. Long-term ACE-inhibitor therapy in patients with heart failure or left ventricular dysfunction: a systematic overview of data from individual patients. ACE-Inhibitor Myocardial Infarction Collaborative Group. *Lancet* 2000;**355**:1575-81.

Granger CB, McMurray JJV, Yusef S, et al. Effects of candesartan in patients with chronic heart failure and reduced left-ventricular systolic function intolerant to angiotensin-converting-enzyme inhibitors: the CHARM-Alternative trial. *Lancet* 2003;**362**:772-6.

McMurray JJV, Ostergren J, Swedburg K, et al. Effects of candesartan in patients with chronic heart failure and reduced left-ventricular systolic function taking angiotensin-converting-enzyme inhibitors: the CHARM-Added trial. *Lancet* 2003;**362**:767-71.

Pfeffer MA, Braunwald E, Moye LA, et al. Effect of captopril on mortality and morbidity in patients with left ventricular dysfunction after myocardial infarction. *N Engl J Med* 1992;**327**:669.

Pfeffer MA, Swedburg K, Granger CB, et al. Effects of candesartan on mortality and morbidity in patients with chronic heart failure: the CHARM-Overall programme. *Lancet* 2003;**362**:767-71.

Pitt B, Poole-Wilson PA, Segal R, et al. Effect of losartan compared with captopril on mortality in patients with symptomatic heart failure: randomised trial—the losartan heart failure survival study ELITE II. *Lancet* 2000;**355**:1582-7.

The CONSENSUS Trial Study Group. Effects of enalapril on mortality in severe congestive heart failure. *N Engl J Med* 1987;**316**:1429-35.

The SOLVD Investigators. Effect of enalapril on survival in patients with reduced left ventricular ejection fraction and congestive heart failure. *Circulation* 1991;**325**:293-302.

The SOLVD Investigators. Effect of enalapril on mortality and the development of heart failure in asymptomatic patients with reduced left ventricular ejection fraction. *N Engl J Med* 1992;**327**:685-91.

Yusef S, Pfeffer MA, Swedburg K, et al. Effects of candesartan in patients with chronic heart failure and preserved left-ventricular ejection fraction: the CHARM-Preserved trial. *Lancet* 2003;**362**:777-81.

Beta-Blockers

Bristow MR. β-Adrenergic receptor blockade in chronic heart failure. *Circulation* 2000;**101**:558-69.

CIBIS II, Investigators and Committees. The Cardiac Insufficiency Bisoprolol Study II (CIBIS II): a randomised trial. *Lancet* 1999;**353**:9-13.

Colucci WS, Packer M, Bristow MR, et al. Carvedilol inhibits clinical progression in patients with mild symptoms of heart failure. *Circulation* 1996;**94**:2800-6.

Lechat P, Packer M, Chalon S, et al. Clinical effects of beta-adrenergic blockade in chronic heart failure: a meta-analysis of double-blind, placebo-controlled, randomized trials. *Circulation* 1998;**98**:1184-91.

MERIT-HF Study Group. Effect of metoprolol CR/XL in chronic heart failure: Metoprolol CR/XL Randomized Intervention Trial in Congestive Heart Failure. *Lancet* 1999;**353**:2001-6.

Packer M, Bristow MR, Cohn JN, et al. Effect of carvedilol on morbidity and mortality in patients with chronic heart failure. *N Engl J Med* 1991;**325**:293-302.

Packer M, Colucci WS, Sacker-Bernstein JD, et al. Double-blind, placebo-controlled study of the effects of carvedilol in patients with moderate to severe heart failure: the PRECISE trial. *Circulation* 1996;**94**:2793-9.

Natriuretic Peptides

Colucci WS, Elkayam U, Horton DP, et al. Intravenous nesiritide, a natriuretic peptide, in the treatment of decompensated congestive heart failure. *N Engl J Med* 2000;**343**:246-53.

Marcus LS, Hart D, Packer M, et al. Hemodynamic and renal excretory effects of human brain natriuretic peptide infusion in patients with congestive heart failure. *Circulation* 1996;**94**:3184-9.

Mills RM, LeJemtel TH, Horton DP, et al. Sustained hemodynamic effects of an infusion of nesiritide (human b-type natriuretic peptide) in heart failure. *J Am Coll Cardiol* 1999;**34**:155-62.

Sackner-Bernstein JD, Kowalski M, Fox M, et al. Short-term risk of death after treatment with nesiritide for decompensated heart failure: a pooled analysis of randomized controlled trials. *JAMA* 2005;**293**:1900-5.

Sackner-Bernstein JD, Skopicki HA, Aaronson KD. Risk of worsening renal function with nesiritide in patients with acutely decompensated heart failure. *Circulation* 2005;**111**:1487-91.

VMAC Investigators Intravenous nesiritide vs nitroglycerine for treatment of decompensated congestive heart failure. *JAMA* 2002;**287**:1531-40.

Hydralazine

Cohn JN, Archibald DG, Ziesche S, et al. Effect of vasodilator therapy on mortality in chronic congestive heart failure. Results of a Veterans Administration Cooperative Study. *N EnglJMed* 1986;**314**:1547-52.

Cohn JN, Johnson G, Ziesche S, et al. A comparison of enalapril with hydralazine–isosorbide dinitrate in the treatment of chronic congestive heart failure. *N Engl J Med* 1991;**325**:303-10.

Digoxin

Hauptman PJ, Kelly RA. Digitalis. *Circulation* 1999;**99**:1265-70.

Packer M, Gheorghiade M, Young JB, et al. Withdrawal of digoxin from patients with chronic heart failure treated with angiotensin-converting enzyme inhibitors. *NEJM* 1993;**329**:1-7.

The Digitalis Investigation Group. The effect of digoxin on mortality and morbidity in patients with heart failure. *N Engl J Med* 1997;**336**:525-33.

Uretsky BF, Young JB, Shahidi, et al. Randomized study assessing the effect of digoxin withdrawal in patients with mild to moderate chronic congestive heart failure: results of the PROVED Trial. *J Am Coll Cardiol* 1993;**22**:955-62.

Reviews

Hunt SA, Abraham WT, Chin MH, et al. ACC/AHA 2005 guideline update for the diagnosis and management of chronic heart failure in the adult: a report of the American College of Cardiology/American Heart Association Task Force on Practice Guidelines. American College of Cardiology Web Site. Available at: http://www.acc.org/clinical/guidelines/failure//index.pdf.

Zile MR, Brutsaert DL. New concepts in diastolic dysfunction and diastolic heart failure: Part I. Diagnosis, prognosis, and measurements of diastolic function. *Circulation* 2002;**105**:1387-93.

Zile MR, Brutsaert DL. New concepts in diastolic dysfunction and diastolic heart failure: Part II. Causal mechanisms and treatment. *Circulation* 2002;**105**:1503-8.

D. Perioperative and Intraoperative Care of the Cardiac Surgical Patient

CHAPTER 59

The Coronary Circulation: Dietary and Pharmacologic Management of Atherosclerosis

John R. Guyton

Atherosclerosis
  Lesion Development
  Opportunities for Lesion Regression
    and Stabilization
Lipoprotein Metabolism
  Lipids
  Lipoproteins and Apolipoproteins
  Lipoprotein Pathways
  Triglyceride Metabolism

Cholesterol Metabolism
  Role of Lipoproteins in Atherogenesis
  Lipoprotein(a)
  The Metabolic Syndrome of Insulin
    Resistance and Cardiovascular Risk
Clinical Management
  Major Clinical Trials
  Guidelines for Lipid-Lowering Therapy
Diet in Prevention and Treatment

Body Weight
Dietary Components
**Drugs for Lipid Reduction
and Atherosclerosis Prevention**
Other Interventions
  Tobacco
  Antihypertensive Therapy
  Exercise
  Summary

Accumulating experience from epidemiology, research trials, and clinical practice indicates that it is possible to prevent atherosclerotic disease with a high expectation of success and also to achieve stabilization or regression of established disease in many if not most patients. Since 1980, mortality due to coronary heart disease has declined approximately 50% in the United States.[1] This may be attributed to number of factors—lower plasma cholesterol, improved treatment of hypertension, reduced smoking rates, intensive care for acute ischemia, and intervention by bypass surgery and angioplasty. Over the past 2 decades, more than 30 large randomized medical intervention trials have focused on clinical outcomes in patients with established coronary heart disease or with various levels of risk. The ability to alter the course of atherosclerotic disease by medical intervention has been proven beyond doubt. In smaller studies, usually employing combination therapy, event reductions exceeding 50% were suggested. Despite this progress, medical regimens for prevention and treatment of atherosclerosis remain underutilized. Thus, atherosclerotic vascular disease, which currently accounts for approximately one fourth of all deaths in the United States, is likely to remain a dominant clinical concern for decades to come. A cooperative interdisciplinary approach involving primary care physicians, midlevel providers, dietitians, cardiologists, endocrinologists, and surgeons will achieve the best results for individual patients. Physicians and allied health providers from a variety of subspecialties and specialties have gained expertise in lipid disorders and are able to provide consultative services on difficult patients. In the United States, clinical lipidologists may be located through the National Lipid Association (http://www.lipid.org), and comparable societies are forming throughout the world.

This chapter aims primarily to describe effective therapy to prevent, stabilize, or regress atherosclerosis. We begin with a brief review of lesion development. Because lipid-oriented therapy is so important to treatment of atherosclerosis, basic aspects of lipids and lipoproteins are described. A guide to practical decision making in atherosclerosis treatment is the largest section of the chapter.

ATHEROSCLEROSIS

Lesion Development

Fatty streaks are early atherosclerotic lesions that first appear normally in teenagers in the coronaries and the aorta (Fig. 59-1). These lesions do not disrupt the endothelial lining and have no clinical consequence in themselves. Histologically, fatty streaks are usually found to consist of lipid-filled macrophages with lesser numbers of lipid-bearing smooth muscle cells. The macrophages are derived from circulating monocytes that adhere to and migrate across arterial endothelium—an effect mediated by cellular adhesion molecules upregulated in states of hypercholesterolemia and inflammation.

Beginning at about age 20, especially in men, raised lesions are found in the proximal coronaries, in the iliac arteries, and in the carotid bulb. Progression of raised atherosclerosis extends from the iliac arteries proximally into the abdominal and later thoracic aorta, and distally toward the femoral arteries. The raised character of the lesions results from the proliferation of smooth muscle cells and macrophages, and from

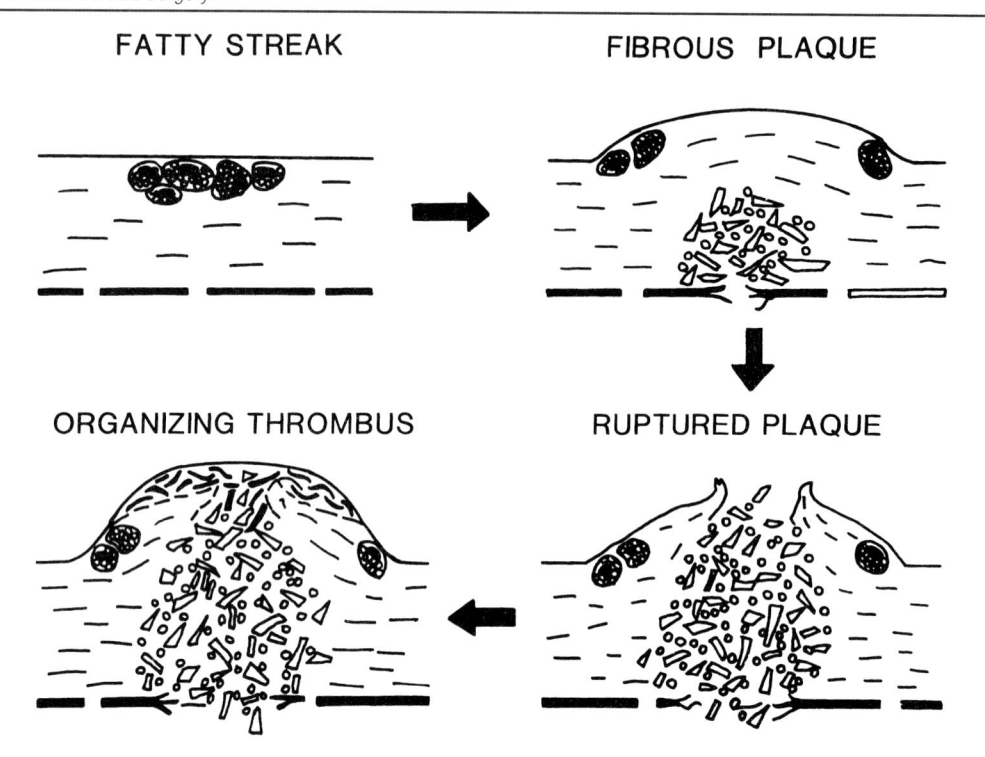

FATTY STREAK

FIBROUS PLAQUE

ORGANIZING THROMBUS

RUPTURED PLAQUE

Figure 59–1
Atherosclerotic lesion development. The fatty streak is a flat lesion in the artery wall, composed of foam cells. Fibrous plaques are raised lesions that usually, but not always, contain a cholesterol-rich, acellular core. Rupture of a fibrous plaque occurs after the expanding core weakens the support of the endothelial surface to the breaking point. The luminal thrombus resulting from plaque rupture is organized by ingrowth and proliferation of smooth muscle cells, leading to rapid, episodic growth of advanced lesions.

elaboration of large amounts of fibrous tissue, especially collagen. Raised lesions with an intact intimal surface are called *fibrous plaques*. The majority of raised lesions possess a lipid-rich, hypocellular or acellular core region. Early development of the lipid-rich core has also been described in flat aortic lesions resembling fatty streaks.[2] This finding is compatible with the hypothesis that most fibrous plaques are derived from preexisting fatty streaks (see Fig. 59-1).

As the fibrous plaque enlarges and begins to impinge on the arterial lumen, a compensatory enlargement of the entire artery occurs. This is probably a result of the physiologic regulation of arterial lumen diameter in response to blood velocity and shear rate. However, the compensatory enlargement eventually fails, perhaps when the collagenous lesion extends circumferentially almost all the way around the artery, leaving little normal wall to respond to blood flow.[3]

The most hazardous component of the atherosclerotic lesion is the lipid-rich core, which expands and erodes the fibrous cap of the lesion with time. When the fibrous cap finally ruptures, blood dissects rapidly into the core, and the thrombogenic contents of the core erupt into the vessel lumen, causing partial or complete thrombosis of the artery within a few minutes.[4]

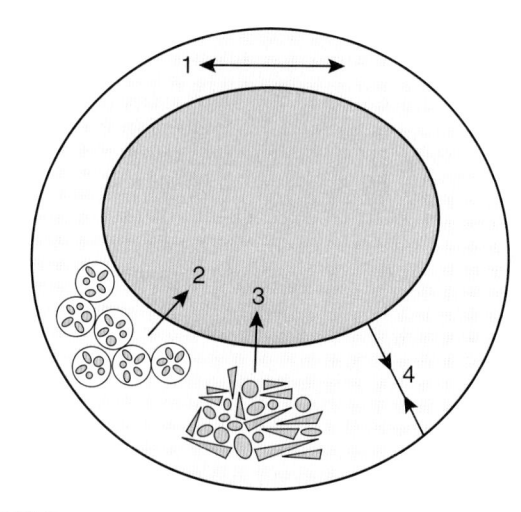

Figure 59–2
Four ways to lower the risk of an atherosclerotic lesion. *1*, Dilation of a normal segment of the arterial wall; *2*, regression of foam cells in the lesion cap or shoulder; *3*, removal of lipid from the core; *4*, regression of fibrous tissue. Of these potential processes, *1* and *2* seem most feasible.

Opportunities for Lesion Regression and Stabilization

Atherosclerotic regression is often conceived of as a diminution in the size of an atherosclerotic lesion that results in decreased stenosis. Such regression may occur, but other, more readily achievable goals should also be considered (Fig. 59-2). For example, hypercholesterolemia can interfere with normal vasorelaxant function of endothelium, and decreases in low-density-lipid (LDL) cholesterol can normalize endothelial-dependent relaxation.[5] The presence of macrophages in the fibrous cap of an atherosclerotic lesion predisposes the lesion to rupture.[6] Lipid lowering can cause relatively rapid regression of foam cells, which appears to stabilize the fibrous cap, prevent rupture, and forestall atherothrombotic events.

Table 59-1
Plasma Lipoproteins

Lipoprotein	Density (g/mL)	Diameter (nm)	Molecular Weight (kDa)	Electrophoretic Mobility	Most Abundant Chemical Constituents
Chylomicrons*	<0.93	75-1200	~400,000	Origin	Triglyceride
Very-low-density lipoprotein (VLDL)	0.93-1.006	30-80	10,000-80,000	Prebeta	Triglyceride
Intermediate-density lipoprotein (IDL)*	1.006-1.019	25-35	5000-10,000	Slow prebeta	Cholesteryl ester, triglyceride
Low-density lipoprotein (LDL)	1.019-1.063	18-25	2300	Beta	Cholesteryl ester
Lipoprotein(a)*	1.050-1.125	24-26	3000-5000	Slow prebeta	Cholesteryl ester
High-density lipoprotein 2 (HDL_2)	1.063-1.125	9-12	~360	Alpha	Protein, phospholipid, cholesteryl ester
High-density lipoprotein 3 (HDL_3)	1.125-1.210	5-9	~175	Alpha	Protein, phospholipid, cholesteryl ester

From references 7 to 10.
*These lipoproteins are usually not major components in fasting plasma. Chylomicrons normally circulate only postprandially. IDLs are formed continuously from VLDLs but are rapidly cleared or metabolized to LDL. Lipoprotein(a) is a minor lipoprotein in most individuals, but some persons are genetically predisposed to have substantial plasma lipoprotein(a) concentrations.

LIPOPROTEIN METABOLISM

Lipids

A high content of carbon and hydrogen makes all lipid molecules hydrophobic, so lipids tend to associate with other lipids in an aqueous environment, forming membranes, oily droplets, and micelles. Phospholipids are the broad, diverse class of phosphorus-containing lipids that form cell membranes and perform many other essential biologic functions. Phospholipid metabolism is not yet a target for antiatherosclerotic therapies, but exploratory investigations have begun.

Cholesterol is an essential component of most cell membranes. Fatty acids are the principal fuel used by muscle and most other body tissues. These lipids also serve as hormone precursors—steroids from cholesterol, prostaglandins and leukotrienes from arachidonic acid—but lipid-lowering treatment has never been shown to produce adverse endocrine effects.

Cholesteryl ester and triglyceride are lipid esters that provide efficient storage or transport of the corresponding active molecules, cholesterol and fatty acids. These lipid esters are so hydrophobic that they usually cannot enter or move across cell membranes. A recurring theme in lipoprotein metabolism is either formation or hydrolysis of lipid esters, accompanying the movement of cholesterol or fatty acids in and out of cells.

Lipoproteins and Apolipoproteins

Human plasma lipoproteins function to transport triglyceride and cholesterol/cholesteryl ester in plasma. They are spherical particles containing 100 to several million lipid molecules combined with one or more protein molecules. The oily core of lipoproteins is composed of triglycerides and cholesteryl esters, and lipoprotein classification is based on which of these species is predominant (Table 59-1).[7-10] The surface layer of lipoproteins is composed of phospholipids, free (unesterified) cholesterol, and protein.

The protein components, termed *apolipoproteins*, bear specific binding sites for lipoprotein receptors or for enzymes involved in lipoprotein metabolism and thus target the lipoproteins for tissue uptake or lipid delivery (Table 59-2).[8-10] All normal human lipoproteins contain either *apolipoprotein A-I* (apoA-I) or *apolipoprotein B* (apoB), or in the case of chylomicrons, both. Thus apoA-I and apoB appear to determine lipoprotein formation and structure as well as metabolic targeting. *High-density lipoproteins* (HDLs) characteristically contain apoA-I, whereas all lipoproteins of larger size and lower density contain apoB.

Lipoprotein Pathways

Chylomicrons are intestinally derived, triglyceride-rich lipoproteins of very large size, which appear transiently for several hours after the ingestion of fat in the diet. Chylomicrons are secreted into intestinal lymph and enter the bloodstream via the thoracic duct. From there, chylomicrons travel to peripheral capillaries, where they encounter an enzyme, lipoprotein lipase, which hydrolyzes triglyceride ester bonds to deliver free fatty acids to the tissues. After the lipoprotein lipase action, the chylomicron remnant is released and circulates back to the liver, where it is taken up very rapidly by a process that depends partly on apolipoprotein E present on the lipoprotein surface.

The metabolic pathways of apoB-containing lipoproteins originating in the liver are shown in Figure 59-3. A single molecule of apoB is incorporated into *very-low-density lipoprotein* (VLDL) before secretion from the liver, and this apoB molecule remains with the lipoprotein throughout all of its subsequent transformations, until the entire lipoprotein is taken

Table 59-2
Major Apolipoproteins

Apolipoprotein	Molecular Weight (kDa)	Distribution	Function
A-I	28,000	HDL, chylomicrons	Structural role in HDL; activates lecithin-cholesterol acyltransferase
A-II	17,000	HDL, chylomicrons	Structural role in HDL
B-48	264,000	Chylomicrons	Structural role in intestine-derived lipoproteins
B-100	550,000	LDL, IDL, VLDL, chylomicrons	Structural role; ligand for LDL receptor binding
C-II	9100	VLDL, IDL, HDL, chylomicrons	Activates lipoprotein lipase
C-III	8750	VLDL, IDL, HDL, chylomicrons	Inhibits hepatic uptake of lipoproteins
E	34,000	IDL, VLDL, chylomicrons, HDL	Ligand for LDL receptor binding of IDL; promotes hepatic uptake of chylomicron remnants
(a)	400,000-700,000	Lipoprotein(a), chylomicrons	Unknown

HDL, high-density lipoprotein; IDL, intermediate-density lipoprotein; LDL, low-density lipoprotein; VLDL, very-low-density lipoprotein.
From references 8-10.

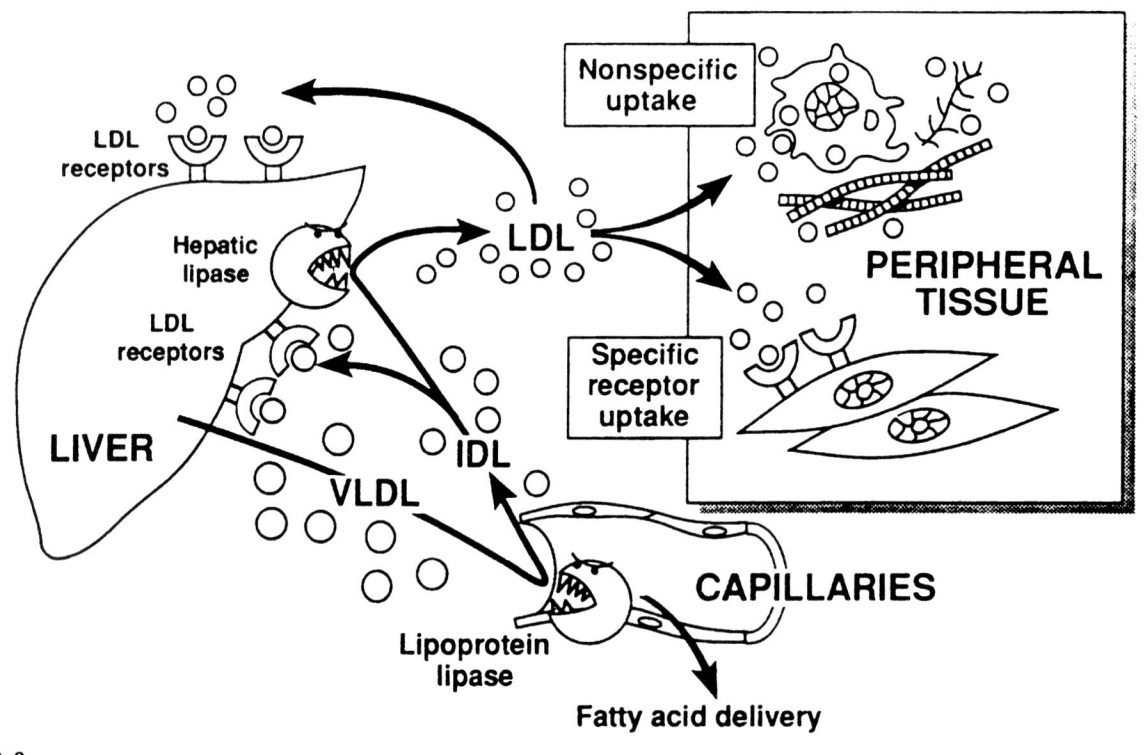

Figure 59-3
Pathways of apolipoprotein B (apoB)-containing lipoproteins derived from the liver. Triglyceride-rich very-low-density lipoproteins (VLDLs) encounter lipoprotein lipase, which hydrolyzes triglyceride, resulting in smaller, intermediate-density lipoproteins (IDLs, also called VLDL remnants). Some of the IDLs are taken up by the liver, and some are converted to low-density lipoprotein (LDL) by hepatic lipase. Three fates await LDL: uptake in the liver, uptake in peripheral cells via specific receptors, or nonspecific disposition in tissues via uptake in macrophages or adherence to collagen, elastin, or proteoglycans.

up and degraded by a cell. VLDLs, which are triglyceride rich, encounter lipoprotein lipase and deliver fatty acids to tissues in exactly the same manner as chylomicrons. As shown in Figure 59-3, some of the VLDL remnants (also known as *intermediate-density lipoproteins*, or IDL) are processed within the hepatic microcirculation to become *low-density lipoproteins*, the major cholesterol-carrying particles in plasma. Physiologic removal of LDL from plasma depends on the presence of LDL receptor molecules found on the surface of hepatocytes and peripheral cells.

Triglyceride Metabolism

The level of triglycerides in plasma depends on the balance of their entry in the form of VLDL and chylomicrons, and their exit via the action of lipoprotein lipase. Deficiency of lipoprotein lipase action can result from partial or complete genetic defects in the enzyme itself or in its cofactor, apoC-II, or from suppression by diabetes mellitus or ethanol abuse. Any of these factors can raise plasma triglyceride levels greatly. The most important regulator of VLDL production is body fat. Intracellular lipase activity in adipose tissue causes the release of fatty acids, which circulate as plasma free fatty acids to the liver. The liver re-esterifies the fatty acids, making triglyceride for secretion in VLDL. Thus excess body fat stimulates fatty acid–triglyceride cycling between liver and the periphery, marked clinically by high plasma levels of triglyceride in VLDL. Improved caloric balance—that is, reduced dietary calories or increased caloric expenditure with exercise—is the only way to reduce body fat and counter this stimulus to high plasma triglyceride. Another stimulus to high plasma triglyceride is a high percentage of carbohydrates in the diet.[11]

Cholesterol Metabolism

Between 30% and 60% of dietary cholesterol is absorbed, and it reaches the liver largely via chylomicron remnants. A more important source of cholesterol, however, is synthesis in the liver and other body tissues from acetyl coenzyme A (CoA). A rate-limiting step in synthesis is catalyzed by 3-hydroxy-3-methylglutaryl CoA reductase, which is potently inhibited by statins, a category of cholesterol-lowering drugs. The liver is also the site of exit for most of the cholesterol leaving the body's metabolic pools. Cholesterol cannot be broken down by mammalian cells to simple metabolic end-products such as carbon dioxide. The liver receives cholesterol by uptake of chylomicron and VLDL remnants, by uptake of a large percentage of LDL via the classic receptor expressed on hepatocytes, and by selective uptake of cholesteryl ester from HDL (see paragraph on reverse cholesterol transport, later). The liver converts cholesterol into bile acids; biliary secretion of these and of cholesterol itself account for the bulk of cholesterol removal from the body. More than 95% of bile acids are ordinarily reabsorbed in the terminal ileum.[12] Oral ingestion of nonabsorbable bile acid binders (cholestyramine, colestipol, colesevelam) can lead to far greater net excretion in the stool and thus effectively reduce body cholesterol via bile acid conversion. Inhibition of intestinal absorption of cholesterol itself (e.g., by ezetimibe or by plant sterol/stanol esters) also lowers cholesterol in liver and in plasma LDL. These strategies are particularly effective when combined with agents that block a compensatory increase in cholesterol synthesis. The profound role of the liver in cholesterol metabolism is the reason that liver transplantation can reverse the extreme hypercholesterolemia that occurs in patients with homozygous deficiency of LDL receptors.

Heterozygous LDL receptor deficiency leads to expression of half the normal numbers of functional cell surface receptors and to approximately twice the normal plasma LDL levels. This highly atherogenic condition occurs in 1 of 500 persons worldwide.[13] In a similar but much less frequent condition, heterozygous familial defective apoB, the binding site for the receptor is genetically dysfunctional on half of the circulating apoB molecules.[14] The most common genetic hyperlipidemia that leads to coronary artery disease is neither of these, however, but is familial combined hyperlipidemia, a multifactorial or polygenic condition characterized by oversecretion of VLDL. Among different members of a family or even in a single individual at different times, either LDL (plasma cholesterol) or VLDL (plasma triglyceride) or both may be elevated.[15]

Peripheral cells can incorporate cholesterol by endocytic uptake of LDL via LDL receptors. Macrophages, which have the function of clearing proteinaceous debris from body tissue, express other receptors such as CD36 and scavenger receptor A that bind chemically altered, oxidized, or aggregated LDL.[16]

Reverse cholesterol transport—that is, the movement of cholesterol from peripheral tissues back to the liver—has been clarified by the discovery of key facilitating molecules. Cholesterol loading of macrophages induces expression of the adenosine triphosphate–binding cassette A1 (ABC-A1) transporter, which transfers unesterified cholesterol to lipid-poor apoA-I and forms nascent HDL.[17] In disc-shaped nascent HDL, the enzyme lecithin-cholesterol acyltransferase (LCAT) functions to esterify cholesterol and thereby creates the oily lipid core of spherical HDL particles (which constitute almost all of the HDL in plasma). HDL can transport cholesterol to the liver by binding temporarily to scavenger receptor B1 on hepatocytes, which selectively removes cholesteryl ester from HDL and then releases the HDL particle for another round of reverse cholesterol transport. An alternative pathway for HDL cholesteryl ester is transfer via cholesteryl ester transfer protein (CETP) to LDL and VLDL, which are then taken up in the liver.[16] Overall, the system is complex, and its regulation remains incompletely understood. For example, deficiency or inhibition of CETP can raise HDL levels, but it remains unproved whether the effect is antiatherogenic.[18]

Role of Lipoproteins in Atherogenesis

The concentration of LDL in the arterial intima is approximately equal to the plasma LDL concentration, whereas interstitial fluid elsewhere in the body appears to have a concentration one-tenth that in the plasma. In other tissues, lymph vessels act as sumps to carry away excess tissue macromolecular species such as LDL, but lymph vessels are absent from arterial intima, perhaps because of high hydrostatic pressure in the intima. Furthermore, the tunica media is highly impermeable to LDL, so that slow diffusion or convection of LDL across the arterial endothelium leads to high LDL concentrations in the intima. The relatively high intimal LDL concentration probably explains why, with aging, pathologic deposits of cholesterol develop regularly only in the arterial intima and nowhere else.[19]

Intimal lipid deposits are found both intracellularly and extracellularly at various stages of atherosclerosis. In addition to cholesteryl ester in superficially located foam cells, extracellular lipid deposits rich in unesterified cholesterol are found in the deep intimal core of small fibrous plaques. The formation of these deposits is unexplained; their importance is emphasized by an association with the disappearance of cells and a weakening of tissue in the developing core.[20]

Oxidation of LDL may help to explain a number of pathogenic processes in atherosclerosis. Certain lipid oxidation products are inflammatory mediators, and mildly oxidized LDL stimulates endothelial cells to express cell surface adhesion molecules for attachment of monocytes. However, large clinical trials have not supported a role for antioxidants in the prevention of clinical atherosclerotic events (see Table 59-6).

Lipoprotein(a)

Lipoprotein(a) is an atherogenic lipoprotein whose role in lipid metabolism remains somewhat mysterious. It is essentially an LDL with an added large glycopeptide, apolipoprotein(a), attached to apoB via a cysteine-cysteine disulfide bond. Lipoprotein(a) particles self-aggregate easily, perhaps favoring their deposition in the arterial intima. The amino acid sequence of apolipoprotein(a) includes multiple repeats of a "kringle" sequence found in plasminogen and in tissue plasminogen activator. The kringle (named after a Danish pastry) fosters the attachment of these fibrinolytic enzymes to sites of clot formation. Lipoprotein(a) has been shown to interfere competitively with binding of the enzymes and thus with fibrinolysis. Clinically, a strong positive correlation has been found between lipoprotein(a) levels and various manifestations of atherosclerosis, including myocardial infarction and stroke. Lipoprotein(a) levels show a strong inheritance pattern and are largely unaffected by diet and medications, except that niacin and oral estrogen can give 20% to 30% reductions.[21]

The Metabolic Syndrome of Insulin Resistance and Cardiovascular Risk

The metabolic syndrome includes (1) disordered metabolism of body fuels—glucose and fat—featuring insulin resistance and abdominal obesity, (2) atherogenic dyslipidemia with high triglyceride, low HDL cholesterol (HDLC), and small dense LDL, (3) hypertension, and (4) abnormalities of coagulation and inflammation adding to high cardiovascular risk. In the industrialized world, this syndrome makes a greater contribution to atherosclerotic disease than any other condition. By criteria of the National Cholesterol Education Program (Table 59-3), more than 40% of U.S. adults older than 60 have the metabolic syndrome.[22]

In the metabolic syndrome, insulin resistance occurs in the phosphatidylinositol (PI) 3-kinase pathway of insulin signaling in cells, but not in the mitogen-activated protein (MAP) kinase pathway. The PI 3-kinase pathway is responsible for metabolic actions such as glucose uptake in peripheral cells and suppression of fatty acid release from adipocytes. The MAP kinase pathway, which may be overstimulated, leads to potentially atherogenic, mitogenic and proinflammatory effects.[23,24]

Fat overload and spillover can promote the metabolic syndrome.[25] Fat is the body's chief way of storing energy for future muscular activity. However, there is a finite capacity for the preferred site of energy storage in small peripheral adipocytes. Chronic energy imbalance—that is, too many calories in the diet or too few expended in exercise, or both—leads to spillover storage of triglyceride in skeletal myocytes, in hepatocytes, in excessive visceral adipocytes, and in abnormally large peripheral adipocytes. Excessive triglyceride in these sites leads to insulin resistance.[26] Patients with lipodystrophy, either genetically based or caused by protease inhibitor therapy for human immunodeficiency virus, have a striking lack of small peripheral adipocytes.[27] They develop central adiposity, hypertriglyceridemia, fatty liver, and insulin resistance or diabetes in an exaggerated form of the metabolic syndrome.

Table 59-3
Clinical Identification* of the Metabolic Syndrome

Risk Factor	Defining Level
Abdominal obesity	Waist circumference
Men	>40 inches (>102 cm)
Women	>35 inches (>88 cm)
Triglyceride	≥150 mg/dL
High-density lipoprotein cholesterol	
Men	<40 mg/dL
Women	<50 mg/dL
Blood pressure	≥130/≥85 mm Hg
Fasting glucose	≥110 mg/dL

*Diagnosis of the metabolic syndrome requires any three of these risk factors.

The dyslipidemic triad consists of high plasma triglyceride, low HDLC, and small dense LDL. In the metabolic syndrome, insulin resistance causes unsuppressed lipolysis of adipocyte triglyceride, which then leads excessive fatty acid delivery to the liver. The liver re-esterifies the fatty acids and exports them as VLDL triglyceride. Cholesteryl ester transfer protein mediates the exchange of VLDL triglyceride for cholesteryl ester in LDL and HDL. LDL and HDL thereby become enriched in triglyceride at the expense of core cholesteryl ester. The triglyceride-enriched LDL and HDL are subject to triglyceride hydrolysis by lipases that remove core lipids and make the lipoprotein particles smaller. Small dense LDLs appear to be more atherogenic than normal LDLs. Small dense HDLs are removed more rapidly from the circulation than normal HDLs, leading to reduced HDLC levels—another atherogenic situation.[28]

The adipocyte is now recognized as a source for multiple bioactive peptides, including angiotensinogen, tumor necrosis factor-alpha (TNF-α), leptin, and plasminogen activator inhibitor-1 (PAI-1).[29] Overproduction of angiotensinogen may help to explain the link between obesity and hypertension. PAI-1, which inhibits fibrinolysis, is itself a cardiovascular risk factor. The liver appears to overproduce C-reactive protein, an extraordinarily strong marker of cardiovascular risk, in response to inflammatory cytokines from excessive fat deposits.[30] Interestingly, low levels of cardiovascular fitness are independently associated with high C-reactive protein levels—another example of the relationship between energy metabolism and cardiovascular risk.[31]

CLINICAL MANAGEMENT
Major Clinical Trials

Medical treatment aimed at atherosclerosis can be classified as *primary* or *secondary prevention* depending on whether a person has previously presented clinically with symptomatic

Both viscous fiber and plant sterol/stanol esters are recommended as part of the NCEP TLC diet (see Box 59-2).

Many patients with symptomatic atherosclerosis are able to make dietary changes that go well beyond the TLC diet, and they should be encouraged to do so. Diligent and intensive dietary change may be just as effective, or more effective, than medication in producing relief of anginal symptoms, reversal of stenosis, and prevention of events in patients with coronary artery disease. Institution of a Mediterranean diet or even a vegetarian diet can be an appropriate therapeutic maneuver in motivated patients with advanced atherosclerosis.[45,62]

Most people in the world eat a diet high in complex carbohydrates and relatively low in fat and protein, compared with people in Western industrialized society. People on such a diet typically have low body weights and relatively low plasma total cholesterol levels averaging 140 to 160 mg/dL, with HDLC also low. In these populations, rates of coronary disease are only a small fraction of the rates in Western nations.

However, it has become apparent that a public health message of "low fat" prevents neither obesity nor cardiovascular disease in societies where food is abundant. The classic food pyramid with grains and starches (usually refined) providing the broad base of dietary calories was replaced in 2005 by a new one that reduces starches and allocates calories more equally among food groups.[65] The optimal diet for cardiovascular prevention may be low in refined grain products; high in whole grains, vegetables, fruits, and nuts; and adequate in omega-3 fatty acids, while substituting natural polyunsaturated and monounsaturated fats for saturated and trans-unsaturated (hydrogenated) fats.[66] Furthermore, some patients with hypertriglyceridemia may benefit from carbohydrate reduction even if body weight remains constant.[67]

Moderate intake of alcohol, in the range of one to three drinks per day in men and one-half to two drinks per day in women, can reduce the risk of coronary heart disease by as much as 50%.[68] Both HDL_2 and HDL_3 (Table 59-1) are increased by ethanol, but direct effects on the arterial wall may be postulated to play a role as well. Risk reduction is not likely to occur in patients with hypertriglyceridemia, as ethanol aggravates this condition. Furthermore, the blood pressure–raising effects of ethanol should be kept in mind. Because of risks of accidents and addiction, it is not appropriate to counsel persons to drink for cardiovascular health, but ethanol intake can be approved if already established as a stable part of a person's life.

A high intake of fish in the diet has long been associated with reduced coronary disease rates in epidemiologic studies. Five randomized trials involving omega-3 fatty acids showed improved clinical cardiovascular outcomes, especially reduction of sudden cardiac death.[69,70] However, one randomized trial in men with stable angina yielded significantly worse cardiac mortality (see Table 59-5).[43] It has been speculated that omega-3 fatty acids incorporated in cardiac phospholipids are released by phospholipase activity in ischemic or stressed myocardium, and that the free omega-3 fatty acids act on ion channels or signaling pathways to stabilize the cardiac rhythm, preventing ventricular fibrillation and death. Based on current data, either fish oil or omega-3 fatty acids from terrestrial sources can be favorably considered for cardiovascular risk reduction. However, conflicting results (including the study cited earlier) have appeared. A consensus guideline statement on secondary prevention notably omits any recommendation regarding omega-3 fatty acids.[71]

DRUGS FOR LIPID REDUCTION AND ATHEROSCLEROSIS PREVENTION

Drug therapy for prevention and treatment of atherosclerosis should begin with consideration of aspirin for every person at risk. Aspirin dosages between 30 and 325 mg per day appear to be equivalent in their ability to inhibit arterial thrombosis. In secondary prevention, the risk reduction is 30% for recurrent myocardial infarction and 15% for cardiac death.[72] Rates in primary prevention are probably similar. Because aspirin is thought to chiefly affect thrombosis and not to inhibit atherosclerosis development, there is no reason to recommend regular aspirin use until thrombosis risk is substantial—generally after age 50, or earlier if severe or multiple risk factors are present. In certain situations, other antiplatelet agents have been shown to give better protection than aspirin alone—for example, clopidogrel after coronary stenting or acute coronary syndrome, and dipyridamole-aspirin for high risk of thrombotic stroke.[71,73]

Some therapies previously thought beneficial have shown adverse results in large randomized trials (see Table 59-6). Oral estrogen replacement in postmenopausal women clearly increases stroke risk. Estrogen-progestin combination therapy used in women with intact uteri increases coronary heart disease risk as well.[49,50] Vitamin E, sometimes combined with other antioxidants, failed to protect from cardiovascular disease, instead showing mildly adverse effects.[74,75]

The most effective regimens for hyperlipidemia use, singly or in combination, drugs from six groups—inhibitors of hydroxymethylglutaryl coenzyme A reductase (reductase inhibitors or statins), niacin, fibric acid derivatives, bile acid sequestrants, cholesterol absorption inhibitor(s), and fish oil. Each of these drug classes has been shown to reduce clinical cardiovascular events in randomized clinical trials (see Tables 59-4 and 59-5), with the exception of the recently introduced cholesterol absorption inhibitor, ezetimibe.

The statins are the most effective single agents available for lowering LDLC, and their effectiveness in reducing cardiovascular events is the foundation of atherosclerosis treatment by lipid management. The safety of these agents has been confirmed in more than 100,000 adult patients followed prospectively, the first of whom began taking lovastatin in the early 1980s. Statins competitively block the synthesis of mevalonic acid, a precursor in the cholesterol synthetic pathway. Although mevalonic acid leads to several other metabolites as well, the clinically available statins do not ordinarily interfere with crucial cellular functions, nor with the synthesis of steroid and sex hormones that use cholesterol as a precursor. Statins reduce triglyceride and raise HDLC, but other agents have greater effects on these lipoproteins. Patients should be monitored for hepatic transaminase elevations. An interaction of statins with cyclosporine, fibric acid derivatives such as gemfibrozil, erythromycin, clarithromycin, nefazodone, or azole antifungals can lead to myopathy and sometimes rhabdomyolysis. Rarely, monotherapy wit statins leads to myopathy.[76] A fraction of patients, perhaps between 0.5% and 15%, may experience myalgia or fatigue on statins treatment. This symptom usually recurs with all statins attempted at the same effective dosage. It may respond to a fourfold reduction of the dosage of statins, perhaps coupled with switching to pharmacokinetically different statins or employing nonstatins therapy in combination.

Niacin, also known as nicotinic acid, is a form of vitamin B_3. Lipid-lowering dosages can be 50 to 100 times the vitamin dosage. Niacinamide (nicotinamide) also acts as a vitamin but has no lipid-lowering effect. Niacin acts to inhibit lipolysis and production of free fatty acids from adipose tissue and also to decrease the production of VLDL from the liver.[77] Immediate-release niacin is usually given 2 to 4 times per day, always with food or skim milk in the stomach, at a total daily dosage beginning as low as 100 mg and increasing over weeks to months to 1000 to 4000 mg. Sustained-released niacin, usually administered twice a day, is more likely to cause hepatotoxicity, and the total dosage should be limited to 2000 to 2250 mg daily. An extended-release prescription form of niacin, given once daily at bedtime, has well-documented hepatic safety in dosages up to 2000 mg.[78] Niacin is the most effective pharmacologic agent for raising HDLC; daily dosages of 1000 to 2000 mg raise HDLC by 10% to 25%.[79] Dosages in the range of 1500 to 3000 mg/day reduce triglyceride, LDLC, and lipoprotein(a) levels. Side effects of niacin include flushing (very common, but disappearing or diminishing with continued regular use), dyspepsia, hyperglycemia, transaminase elevations, atrial fibrillation, peptic ulcer, gout, skin dryness, and visual disturbances.

Bile acid sequestrants include cholestyramine and colestipol, which are therapeutically very similar, and colesevelam, which has better tolerability. These nonabsorbed polymers bind bile acids in the small intestine, preventing their reabsorption in the terminal ileum. The liver detects bile acid depletion and diverts cholesterol stores toward bile acid synthesis, establishing a drain on body stores of cholesterol. The bile acid sequestrants reduce LDLC by 10% to 30%, depending on dosage. Triglyceride levels tend to increase with use of bile acid sequestrants; therefore, hypertriglyceridemia is a relative contraindication. Because the bile acid sequestrants are not absorbed into the bloodstream, they have excellent theoretical and practical safety, sufficient to recommend them for reducing LDLC in pediatric cases and in women of childbearing potential. The major side effects of cholestyramine and colestipol are constipation (15% of cases) and abdominal bloating. Drug absorption may be inhibited, particularly warfarin, vitamin K (in warfarin-treated patients), digoxin, diuretics, and thyroxine. Colesevelam has much better gastrointestinal tolerability and minimal drug interactions.[80]

The fibric acid derivatives or fibrates generally employed in the United States are gemfibrozil and fenofibrate. The fibrates perform best at lowering triglyceride levels; reductions of 40% to 55% can be expected in hypertriglyceridemic patients. HDLC increases of 6% to 20% can occur. Fenofibrate reduces LDLC moderately in normotriglyceridemic patients. Gemfibrozil reduced cardiovascular events in a secondary prevention trial of patients with low HDLC (see Table 59-4).[37] Fenofibrate showed a similar trend toward fewer coronary events in diabetic subjects, but the primary endpoint was not statistically significant (see Table 59-4).[40] Further clinical outcome data on the addition of fenofibrate to statins therapy in diabetes is anticipated from a large trial sponsored by the National Institutes of Health (NIH) ending in 2010.[81] Because both gemfibrozil and fenofibrate are cleared from the circulation largely by the kidney, dosages should be decreased in patients with renal insufficiency. Side effects shared by these drugs include dyspepsia, hypersensitivity rash, hepatic transaminase elevations, increased warfarin effect, and increased lithogenicity of bile. Rarely, fenofibrate causes photosensitivity of the skin.[82]

Ezetimibe is the first member of a new pharmacologic class that inhibits cholesterol absorption by intestinal mucosa. Ordinarily, the intestine is exposed to 200 to 400 mg of dietary cholesterol and 1000 mg of biliary cholesterol daily, of which 30% to 60% may be absorbed. After ingestion, ezetimibe is concentrated in the intestinal mucosal brush border, where it appears to block the action of a sterol transport peptide. Ezetimibe at 10 mg daily gives 18% to 19% LDLC lowering. When ezetimibe is added to an existing statin regimen, LDLC is reduced 20% to 25% from the post-statins baseline. Side effects of ezetimibe have been minimal and not significantly different from those of placebo.[83]

In high dosages (at least 3.4 g daily), marine omega-3 fatty acids have the useful effect of lowering plasma triglyceride by 30% to 40%.[84] Marine omega-3 fatty acids from fish or algae have 20 or 22 carbon atoms, whereas alpha-linolenic acid is an 18-carbon omega-3 derived from terrestrial sources such as flaxseed, walnuts, canola oil, and soybean oil. Alpha-linolenic acid does not lower triglyceride at all.

Because an LDLC of less than 100 mg/dL is the goal in patients with atherosclerotic disease, combinations of the previously listed medications are often used. In combination therapy, moderate dosages can often be used to achieve excellent LDLC reduction. Niacin-statin combination therapy has shown promise for reducing cardiovascular events in small randomized trials.[85] This combination is being evaluated in two large clinical trials, with results expected between 2011 and 2013.[86,87] If gemfibrozil is used in combination with statins, up to 4% of patients may experience myopathy, unless the statin dosage is kept at or near the usual starting dosage. Fenofibrate can also potentiate statin myopathy, but at a much lower frequency (estimated to be 15-fold less). Ezetimibe, bile acid sequestrants, and fish oil can be added to statins therapy or to niacin and fibrates without an increased risk of myopathy or other synergistic adverse effects.[88]

OTHER INTERVENTIONS

Tobacco

Smoking one to two packs of cigarettes per day doubles the risk of coronary atherosclerotic events. The most important fact to communicate to patients is that the risk declines rapidly when smoking is stopped, such that coronary risk is almost normal within 1 or 2 years.[89] This fact, along with basic research results, suggests that a major effect of smoking is to enhance thrombus formation, perhaps via injurious effects of nicotine or other tobacco components on endothelium. Smoking also promotes atherogenesis, especially in the arterial supply to the lower extremities. Some, but not all, of the chronic atherogenic effects of smoking may be mediated by decreased plasma levels of HDLC. With smoking cessation, HDLC increase is commonly seen. Modest weight gain may accompany smoking cessation, but clinical benefits far outweigh any adverse effects of weight gain.

Antihypertensive Therapy

Medical therapy of hypertension reduces risk of stroke by 30% to 40% and myocardial infarction by 20%, according to a meta-analysis of clinical trials.[90] Initial treatment with a thiazide-type diuretic is superior to or at least as good as treatment with other classes of antihypertensive agents in routine cases.[91] However, patients with stable angina and hypertension are best treated first with a beta-blocker. During or after acute coronary syndromes, beta-blockers and angiotensin-converting enzyme inhibitors have been shown to be efficacious. In many cases, especially when initial systolic pressures exceed 160 mm Hg, two or more antihypertensive drugs may be needed to reach the goal of less than 140 systolic and less than 90 diastolic mm Hg. However, blood pressures measured by patients at home tend to be lower, and the goal then should be less than 135/85 mm Hg. In patients with diabetes or chronic kidney disease, the goal for office blood pressure is less than 130/80 mm Hg. The Seventh Report of the Joint National Committee provides an excellent, concise guideline for blood pressure control.[92]

Both thiazide and loop diuretics cause, on average, small increases in triglyceride and LDLC levels. Beta-blockers tend to raise triglyceride and reduce HDLC levels.[93] However, the proven benefits of these agents on clinical outcomes usually outweigh their impact on lipids, and adjustment of antihypertensive therapy to optimize the lipid profile is usually not appropriate.

Inhibition of angiotensin formation by a converting enzyme inhibitor was shown to reduce cardiovascular events in patients with vascular disease or diabetes, even in those who are normotensive (see HOPE trial in Table 59-5).[47] Subsequently, the use of an angiotensin receptor blocker was determined to work equally well in this broad group of patients.[94]

Exercise

Although myocardial infarction is more likely to occur at times of unaccustomed moderate-to-intense exercise, a steady pattern of exercise clearly reduces risk.[95] The lack of any large randomized trial may lead to an underappreciation of the cardiovascular benefit of exercise. In a large observational study, physical fitness determined by treadmill testing was the strongest determinant of future cardiovascular risk, eclipsing the effects of body mass index, blood pressure, cholesterol, and smoking.[96] Multiple studies support a strong role of cardiac rehabilitation programs in the treatment of coronary artery disease.

Summary

Although it is better to prevent atherosclerosis than to treat it, the presence of established disease should no longer be regarded as predictive of inexorable progression. In the treatment of atherosclerosis, smoking cessation is essential. Besides smoking cessation, modification of plasma lipoprotein levels, especially LDLC, is the most effective way to change the course of the disease. Recent evidence suggests that raising HDLC might add substantially to atherosclerosis treatment. Strong efforts in diet and exercise, as well as appropriate medication, are often needed together. Control of hypertension and diabetes should be maintained. In the majority of patients, a reasonable goal is more than 50% risk reduction, and highly motivated patients can do substantially better.

REFERENCES

1. Ford ES, Capewell S. Coronary heart disease mortality among young adults in the U.S. from 1980 through 2002: concealed leveling of mortality rates. *J Am Coll Cardiol* 2007;**50**:2128-32.
2. Guyton JR, Klemp KF. Transitional features in human atherosclerosis: intimal thickening, cholesterol clefts, and cell loss in human aortic fatty streaks. *Am J Pathol* 1993;**143**:1444-57.
3. Glagov S, Weisenberg E, Zarins CK, et al. Compensatory enlargement of human atherosclerotic coronary arteries. *N Engl J Med* 1987;**316**:1371-5.
4. Fuster V, Stein B, Ambrose JA, et al. Atherosclerotic plaque rupture and thrombosis. *Circulation* 1990;**82**(suppl. II):47-59.
5. Kinlay S, Libby P, Ganz P. Endothelial function and coronary artery disease. *Curr Opin Lipidol* 2001;**12**:383-9.
6. Lendon CL, Davies MJ, Born GV, et al. Atherosclerotic plaque caps are locally weakened when macrophages density is increased. *Atherosclerosis* 1991;**87**:87-90.
7. Gotto Jr AM, Pownall HJ, Havel RC. Introduction to the plasma lipoproteins. *Methods Enzymol* 1986;**128**:1-41.
8. Smith LC, Massey JB, Sparrow JT, et al. Structure and dynamics of human plasma lipoproteins. In: Pifat G, Herak JN, editors. *Supramolecular structure and function*. New York: Plenum Press; 1983. p. 205-31.
9. Havel RC, Goldstein JL, Brown MS. Lipoproteins and lipid transport. In: Bondy PK, Rosenberg LE, editors. *Metabolic control and disease*. Philadelphia: WB Saunders; 1980. p. 393-494.
10. Morrisett JD, Guyton JR, Gaubatz JW, et al. Lipoprotein(a): structure, metabolism and epidemiology. In: Gotto Jr AM, editor. *Plasma lipoproteins, new comprehensive biochemistry*. Amsterdam: Elsevier; 1987, *vol*. p. 14129–52.
11. Grundy SM, Denke MA. Dietary influences on serum lipids and lipoproteins. *J Lipid Res* 1990;**31**:1149-72.
12. Grundy SM. Cholesterol metabolism in man. *West J Med* 1978;**128**:13-25.
13. Goldstein JL, Brown MS. Familial hypercholesterolemia. In: Scriver CR, Beaudet AL, Sly WS, Valle D, editors. *The metabolic basis of inherited disease*. New York: McGraw-Hill; 1989. p. 1215-50.
14. Innerarity TL, Mahley RW, Weisgraber KH, et al. Familial defective apolipoprotein B-100: a mutation of apolipoprotein B that causes hypercholesterolemia. *J Lipid Res* 1990;**31**:1337-49.
15. Goldstein JL, Schrott HG, Hazzard WR, et al. Hyperlipidemia in coronary heart disease: II. Genetic analysis of lipid levels in 176 families and delineation of a new inherited disorder, combined hyperlipidemia. *J Clin Invest* 1973;**52**:1544-68.
16. Li AC, Glass CK. The macrophage foam cell as a target for therapeutic intervention. *Nat Med* 2002;**8**:1235-42.
17. Brewer Jr HB, Santamarina-Fojo S. New insights into the role of the adenosine triphosphate-binding cassette transporters in high-density lipoprotein metabolism and reverse cholesterol transport. *Am J Cardiol* 2003;**91**:3E-11.
18. Barter PJ, Rye KA. Cholesteryl ester transfer protein, high density lipoprotein and arterial disease. *Curr Opin Lipidol* 2001;**12**:377-82.
19. Guyton JR. Phospholipid hydrolytic enzymes in a "cesspool" of arterial intimal lipoproteins: a mechanism for atherogenic lipid accumulation. *Arterioscler Thromb Vasc Biol* 2001;**21**:884-6.
20. Guyton JR, Klemp KF. Development of the lipid-rich core in human atherosclerosis. *Arterioscler Thromb Vasc Biol* 1996;**16**:4-11.
21. Rader DJ, Brewer HB. Lipoprotein(a): clinical approach to a unique atherogenic lipoprotein. *JAMA* 1993;**267**:1109-12.
22. Ford ES, Giles WH, Dietz WH. Prevalence of the metabolic syndrome among US adults: findings from the third National Health and Nutrition Examination Survey. *JAMA* 2002;**287**:356-9.
23. Le Roith D, Zick Y. Recent advances in our understanding of insulin action and insulin resistance. *Diabetes Care* 2001;**24**:588-97.
24. Hsueh WA, Law RE. Insulin signaling in the arterial wall. *Am J Cardiol* 1999;**84**:21J-4J.
25. Danforth Jr E. Failure of adipocyte differentiation causes type II diabetes mellitus? *Nat Genet* 2000;**26**:13.
26. Kelley DE, Mandarino LJ. Fuel selection in human skeletal muscle in insulin resistance: a reexamination. *Diabetes* 2000;**49**:677-83.
27. Carr A, Samaras K, Burton S, et al. A syndrome of peripheral lipodystrophy, hyperlipidaemia and insulin resistance in patients receiving HIV protease inhibitors. *AIDS* 1998;**12**:F51-8.
28. Ginsberg HN. Insulin resistance and cardiovascular disease. *J Clin Invest* 2000;**106**:453-8.
29. Miranda PJ, DeFronzo RA, Califf RM, et al. Metabolic syndrome: definition, pathophysiology, and mechanisms. *Am Heart J* 2005;**149**:33-45.
30. Ridker PM, Buring JE, Cook NR, et al. C-reactive protein, the metabolic syndrome, and risk of incident cardiovascular events: an 8-year follow-up of 14 719 initially healthy American women. *Circulation* 2003;**107**:391-7.

31. LaMonte MJ, Durstine JL, Yanowitz FG, et al. Cardiorespiratory fitness and C-reactive protein among a tri-ethnic sample of women. *Circulation* 2002;**106**:403-6.
32. The Coronary Drug Project Research Group. Clofibrate and niacin in coronary heart disease. *JAMA* 1975;**231**:360-81.
33. Canner PL, Berge KG, Wenger NK, et al. Fifteen year mortality in Coronary Drug Project patients: long-term benefit with niacin. *J Am Coll Cardiol* 1986;**8**:1245-55.
34. Lipid Research Clinics Program. The Lipid Research Clinics Coronary Primary Prevention Trial results: I. Reduction in incidence of coronary heart disease. *JAMA* 1984;**251**:351-74.
35. Scandinavian Simvastatin Survival Study Group. Randomised trial of cholesterol lowering in 4444 patients with coronary heart disease: the Scandinavian Simvastatin Survival Study (4S). *Lancet* 1994;**344**:1383-9.
36. Downs JR, Clearfield M, Weis S, et al. Primary prevention of acute coronary events with lovastatin in men and women with average cholesterol levels: results of AFCAPS/TexCAPS. *JAMA* 1998;**279**:1615-22.
37. Rubins HB, Robins SJ, Collins D, et al. Gemfibrozil for the secondary prevention of coronary heart disease in men with low levels of high-density lipoprotein cholesterol Veterans Affairs High-Density Lipoprotein Cholesterol Intervention Trial Study Group. *N Engl J Med* 1999;**341**:410-8.
38. Heart Protection Study Collaborative Group. MRC/BHF Heart Protection Study of cholesterol lowering with simvastatin in 20,536 high-risk individuals: a randomised placebo-controlled trial. *Lancet* 2002;**360**:7-22.
39. Larosa JC, Grundy SM, Waters DD, et al. Intensive lipid lowering with atorvastatin in patients with stable coronary disease. *N Engl J Med* 2005;**352**:1425-35.
40. Keech A, Simes RJ, Barter P, et al. Effects of long-term fenofibrate therapy on cardiovascular events in 9795 people with type 2 diabetes mellitus (the FIELD study): randomised controlled trial. *Lancet* 2005;**366**:1849-61.
41. Med J. Physicians' Health Study Research Group. Preliminary report: findings from the aspirin component of the ongoing physicians' health study. *N Engl* 1988;**318**:262-4.
42. Burr ML, Fehily AM, Gilbert JF, et al. Effects of changes in fat, fish, and fibre intakes on death and myocardial reinfarction: Diet and Reinfarction Trial (DART). *Lancet* 1989;**2**:757-61.
43. Burr ML, Ashfield-Watt PA, Dunstan FD, et al. Lack of benefit of dietary advice to men with angina: results of a controlled trial. *Eur J Clin Nutr* 2003;**57**:193-200.
44. Investigators GISSI-Prevenzione. Dietary supplementation with n-3 polyunsaturated fatty acids and vitamin E after myocardial infarction: results of the GISSI-Prevenzione trial. *Lancet* 1999;**354**:447-55.
45. de Lorgeril M, Salen P, Martin JL, et al. Mediterranean diet, traditional risk factors, and the rate of cardiovascular complications after myocardial infarction: final report of the Lyon Diet Heart Study. *Circulation* 1999;**99**:779-85.
46. Yokoyama M, Origasa H, Matsuzaki M, et al. Effects of eicosapentaenoic acid on major coronary events in hypercholesterolaemic patients (JELIS): a randomised open-label, blinded endpoint analysis. *Lancet* 2007;**369**:1090-8.
47. Yusuf S, Sleight P, Pogue J, et al. Effects of an angiotensin-converting-enzyme inhibitor, ramipril, on cardiovascular events in high-risk patients. The Heart Outcomes Prevention Evaluation Study Investigators. *N Engl J Med* 2000;**342**:145-53.
48. Lindholm LH, Ibsen H, Dahlof B, et al. Cardiovascular morbidity and mortality in patients with diabetes in the Losartan Intervention for Endpoint Reduction in Hypertension study (LIFE): a randomised trial against atenolol. *Lancet* 2002;**359**:1004-10.
49. Rossouw JE, Anderson GL, Prentice RL, et al. Risks and benefits of estrogen plus progestin in healthy postmenopausal women: principal results from the Women's Health Initiative randomized controlled trial. *JAMA* 2002;**288**:321-33.
50. Anderson GL, Limacher M, Assaf AR, et al. Effects of conjugated equine estrogen in postmenopausal women with hysterectomy: the Women's Health Initiative randomized controlled trial. *JAMA* 2004;**291**:1701-12.
51. Executive Summary of the Third Report of the National Cholesterol Education Program (NCEP) Expert Panel on Detection, Evaluation, and Treatment of High Blood Cholesterol in Adults (Adult Treatment Panel III). *JAMA* 2001;**285**:2486-97.
52. Adult Treatment Panel III. *Third Report of the National Cholesterol Education Program (NCEP) expert panel on detection, evaluation, and treatment of high blood cholesterol in adults.* Bethesda, MD: National Institutes of Health; 2002, NIH Publication No. 02-5215.
53. Grundy SM, Cleeman JI, Merz CN, et al. Implications of recent clinical trials for the National Cholesterol Education Program Adult Treatment Panel III guidelines. *Circulation* 2004;**110**:227-39.
54. Ridker PM, Rifai N, Rose L, et al. Comparison of C-reactive protein and low-density lipoprotein cholesterol levels in the prediction of first cardiovascular events. *N Engl J Med* 2002;**347**:1557-65.
55. Guyton JR. Clinical assessment of atherosclerotic lesions: emerging from angiographic shadows. *Circulation* 2002;**106**:1308-9.
56. Lonn E. Homocysteine-lowering B vitamin therapy in cardiovascular prevention: wrong again? *JAMA* 2008;**299**:2086-7.
57. Dattilo AM, Kris-Etherton PM. Effects of weight reduction on blood lipids and lipoproteins: a meta-analysis. *Am J Clin Nutr* 1992;**56**:320-8.
58. Bantle JP, Wylie-Rosett J, Albright AL, et al. Nutrition recommendations and interventions for diabetes: a position statement of the American Diabetes Association. *Diabetes Care* 2008;**31**(Suppl. 1):S61-78.
59. Gardner CD, Kiazand A, Alhassan S, et al. Comparison of the Atkins, Zone, Ornish, and LEARN diets for change in weight and related risk factors among overweight premenopausal women: the A TO Z Weight Loss Study: a randomized trial. *JAMA* 2007;**297**:969-77.
60. Sjostrom L, Lindroos AK, Peltonen M, et al. Lifestyle, diabetes, and cardiovascular risk factors 10 years after bariatric surgery. *N Engl J Med* 2004;**351**:2683-93.
61. Keys A, Parlin RW. Serum cholesterol response to changes in dietary lipids. *Am J Clin Nutr* 1966;**19**:175-81.
62. Ornish D, Brown SE, Scherwitz LW, et al. Can lifestyle changes reverse coronary heart disease? The Lifestyle Heart Trial. *Lancet* 1990;**336**:129-33.
63. Wright JD, Wang CY, Kennedy-Stephenson J, et al. Dietary intake of ten key nutrients for public health, United States: 1999-2000. *Adv Data* 2003;**334**(1-4).
64. Jenkins DJA, Wolever TMS, Rao AV, et al. Effect on blood lipids of very high intakes of fiber in diets low in saturated fat and cholesterol. *N Engl J Med* 1993;**329**:21-6.
65. U.S. Department of Agriculture. Available at www.mypyramid.gov (accessed January 26, 2009).
66. Hu FB, Willett WC. Optimal diets for prevention of coronary heart disease. *JAMA* 2002;**288**:2569-78.
67. Reissell PK, Mandella PA, Poon-King TMW, et al. Treatment of hypertriglyceridemia. *Am J Clin Nutr* 1966;**19**:84-98.
68. Kreisberg RA. A votre santé: alcohol and coronary artery disease. *Arch Intern Med* 1992;**152**:263-5.
69. Investigators GISSI-HF. Effect of n-3 polyunsaturated fatty acids in patients with chronic heart failure (the GISSI-HF trial): a randomised, double-blind, placebo-controlled trial. *Lancet* 2008;**372**:1223-30.
70. Hooper L, Thompson RL, Harrison RA, et al. Risks and benefits of omega 3 fats for mortality, cardiovascular disease, and cancer: systematic review. *BMJ* 2006;**332**:752-60.
71. Smith Jr SC, Allen J, Blair SN, et al. AHA/ACC guidelines for secondary prevention for patients with coronary and other atherosclerotic vascular disease: 2006 update: endorsed by the National Heart, Lung, and Blood Institute. *Circulation* 2006;**113**:2363-72.
72. Antiplatelet Trialists' Collaboration. Secondary prevention of vascular disease by prolonged antiplatelet treatment. *BMJ* 1988;**296**:320-31.
73. Liao JK. Secondary prevention of stroke and transient ischemic attack: is more platelet inhibition the answer? *Circulation* 2007;**115**:1615-21.
74. Yusuf S, Dagenais G, Pogue J, et al. Vitamin E supplementation and cardiovascular events in high-risk patients. The Heart Outcomes Prevention Evaluation Study Investigators. *N Engl J Med* 2000;**342**:154-60.
75. Heart Protection Study Collaborative Group. MRC/BHF Heart Protection Study of antioxidant vitamin supplementation in 20,536 high-risk individuals: a randomised placebo-controlled trial. *Lancet* 2002;**360**:23-33.
76. Omar MA, Wilson JP, Cox TS. *Rhabdomyolysis and HMG-CoA reductase inhibitors.* *Ann Pharmacother* 2001;**35**:1096-107.
77. Guyton JR, Gotto Jr AM. Drug therapy of dyslipoproteinemias. In: Fruchart JC, Shepherd J, editors. *Human plasma lipoproteins. Clinical biochemistry series.* Berlin: Walter deGruyter; 1989, p. 335-61.
78. Guyton JR, Goldberg AC, Kreisberg RA, et al. Effectiveness of once nightly dosing of extended-release niacin alone and in combination for hypercholesterolemia. *Am J Cardiol* 1998;**82**:737-43.
79. Guyton JR, Blazing MA, Hagar J, et al. Extended-release niacin versus gemfibrozil for treatment of low levels of high density lipoprotein cholesterol. *Arch Intern Med* 2000;**160**:1177-84.
80. Bays H, Dujovne C. Colesevelam HCl: a non-systemic lipid-altering drug. *Expert Opin Pharmacother* 2003;**4**:779-90.
81. Action to Control Cardiovascular Risk in Diabetes (ACCORD, NCT00000620). Available at www.clinicaltrials.gov (accessed January 26, 2009).
82. Keating GM, Ormrod D. Micronised fenofibrate: an updated review of its clinical efficacy in the management of dyslipidaemia. *Drugs* 2002;**62**:1909-44.
83. Bays HE, Moore PB, Drehobl MA, et al. Effectiveness and tolerability of ezetimibe in patients with primary hypercholesterolemia: pooled analysis of two phase II studies. *Clin Ther* 2001;**23**:1209-30.
84. Goldberg RB, Sabharwal AK. Fish oil in the treatment of dyslipidemia. *Curr Opin Endocrinol Diabetes Obes* 2008;**15**:167-74.
85. Brown BG, Zhao XQ, Chait A, et al. Simvastatin and niacin, antioxidant vitamins, or the combination for the prevention of coronary disease. *N Engl J Med* 2001;**345**:1583-92.
86. Niacin Plus Statin to Prevent Vascular Events (AIM-HIGH, NCT00120289). Available at www.clinicaltrials.gov (accessed January 26, 2009).

87. Treatment of HDL to Reduce the Incidence of Vascular Events HPS2-THRIVE (NCT00461630). Available at www.clinicaltrials.gov (accessed January 26, 2009).
88. Guyton JR. Combination drug therapy for combined hyperlipidemia. *Curr Cardiol Rep* 1999;**1**:244-50.
89. Manson JE, Tosteson H, Ridker PM, et al. The primary prevention of myocardial infarction. *N Engl J Med* 1992;**326**:1406-16.
90. Neal B, MacMahon S, Chapman N. Effects of ACE inhibitors, calcium antagonists, and other blood-pressure-lowering drugs: results of prospectively designed overviews of randomised trials. Blood Pressure Lowering Treatment Trialists' Collaboration. *Lancet* 2000;**356**:1955-64.
91. Major outcomes in high-risk hypertensive patients randomized to angiotensin-converting enzyme inhibitor or calcium channel blocker vs diuretic: the Antihypertensive and Lipid-Lowering Treatment to Prevent Heart Attack Trial (ALLHAT). *JAMA* 2002;**288**:2981-97.
92. Chobanian AV, Bakris GL, Black HR, et al. The Seventh Report of the Joint National Committee on Prevention, Detection, Evaluation, and Treatment of High Blood Pressure: the JNC 7 report. *JAMA* 2003;**289**:2560-72.
93. Lardinois CK, Neumann SL. The effects of antihypertensive agents on serum lipids and lipoproteins. *Arch Intern Med* 1988;**148**:1280-8.
94. Yusuf S, Teo KK, Pogue J, et al. Telmisartan, ramipril, or both in patients at high risk for vascular events. *N Engl J Med* 2008;**358**:1547-59.
95. Mittleman MA, Maclure M, Tofler GH, et al. Triggering of acute myocardial infarction by heavy physical exertion. *N Engl J Med* 1993;**329**:1677-83.
96. Blair SN, Kohl III HW, Barlow CE, et al. Changes in physical fitness and all-cause mortality: a prospective study of healthy and unhealthy men. *JAMA* 1995;**273**:1093-8.

CHAPTER 60
Adult Cardiac Anesthesia
Feroze Mahmood, Xiaoqin Zhao, and Robina Matyal

Preoperative Evaluation
Intraoperative Management
  Monitoring
  Choice of Anesthetic Agents
  Regional Anesthesia and Analgesia
  Intraoperative Blood Glucose Control
  Acid–Base Management during Hypothermia

Anticoagulation for Cardiopulmonary
  Bypass
Use of Antifibrinolytics
Cerebral Protection during Deep
  Hypothermic Circulatory Arrest
Hemodynamic Support on Separation from
  Cardiopulmonary Bypass

Special Considerations
  Fast-Track Cardiac Surgery
  Off-Pump Coronary Artery Bypass
  Port-Access Minimally Invasive Cardiac
    Surgery
  Robotic-Assisted Cardiac Surgery

The first successful cardiac surgical procedure was in 1902, when Hill closed a stab wound to the heart of a 13-year-old boy. After the introduction of a cardiopulmonary bypass (CPB) machine in 1953 by Gibbon, the concept of a cardiac surgical team made up of a cardiac surgeon, a cardiac anesthesiologist, and a perfusionist gradually developed. Today, transesophageal echocardiography (TEE) plays an essential role in the cardiac patient's intraoperative diagnosis, monitoring, and even prognosis, and the anesthesiologist with competence in TEE is indispensable in the cardiac surgical suite. The discipline of cardiac anesthesia encompasses an expanding body of knowledge. This chapter provides a brief overview of preoperative anesthetic evaluation and intraoperative anesthetic management for adult cardiac surgery.

PREOPERATIVE EVALUATION

The preoperative anesthetic evaluation of the cardiac surgical patient includes the following: (1) review of the events that led to the indication for cardiac surgery, (2) identification and optimization of risk factors that could lead to mortality and morbidity resulting from cardiac surgery, and (3) gathering of information relevant to selecting monitoring modalities and management techniques during surgery. Higgins and colleagues[1] performed a retrospective logistic regression on data from more than 5000 patients who underwent coronary artery bypass grafts, and they then prospectively applied the retrospectively identified risk factors to a group of more than 4000 patients. They found that 30-day mortality was predicted by the emergency nature of the procedure, preoperative serum creatinine of more than 168 mmol/L, left ventricular ejection fraction of less than 35%, preoperative hematocrit level of less than 35, age greater than 70 years, chronic pulmonary disease, prior vascular surgery, reoperation, and mitral regurgitation. Emergency cases were transfers from the coronary care unit with unstable angina (48%), complications of percutaneous intervention (40%), and complications of routine cardiac catheterizations (12%). In addition to these risk factors, nonfatal morbidity was predicted by diabetes mellitus, body weight of 65 kg or less, aortic stenosis, and cerebrovascular disease. Presence of these risk factors needs to be ascertained when obtaining preoperative history prior to cardiac surgery.

Emergency patients from the catheterization laboratory may have taken inhibitors of platelet aggregation. Clopidogrel (Plavix) and ticlopidine (Ticlid) inhibit ADP-induced platelet aggregation by irreversibly modifying platelet P2 receptors for the life span of these cells. Abciximab (ReoPro) is a monoclonal antibody fragment against glycoprotein (GP) IIb/IIIa receptor, which allows platelet binding to von Willebrand factor and fibrinogen. Abciximab is administered intravenously with an initial bolus of 0.25 mg/kg, followed by an infusion of 0.25 mg/kg/min (up to 10 mg/min) for 12 hours. After discontinuance, platelet function recovers gradually over the next 48 hours.[2,3] Eptifibatide (Integrilin) is a peptide inhibitor of GP IIb/IIIa receptor with an elimination half-life of 1 to 2 hours. After discontinuance, platelet function (as measured by bleeding time) recovers in 2 to 4 hours.[4] Tirofiban (Aggrastat) is a peptidomimetic antagonist of GP IIb/IIIa receptor with an elimination half-life of about 2 hours; platelet function returns to normal within 4 to 8 hours after discontinuing the medication.[5,6] Whereas abciximab consistently prolongs the activated clotting time (ACT) used to monitor heparinization by 30 to 50 seconds and necessitates a reduction in the dosage of heparin used concurrently to decrease bleeding complications, eptifibatide does not have a similar effect on ACT.[7]

Additional historical information about anticoagulant use that needs to be gathered preoperatively includes duration of use of heparin, heparin resistance, heparin-induced thrombocytopenia, use of Coumadin, dosage and the time of the last dose, and the use of thrombolytics such as streptokinase. Additional historical information pertinent to cardiac surgery includes the presence of esophageal disease that may contraindicate the use of TEE, a history of cold agglutinin antibody (which may contraindicate hypothermic CPB), a history of antiphospholipid syndrome (which will adversely affect measurement of ACT), a history of previous thoracic surgery or radiation, and the presence of a pacemaker or an implantable cardioverter/defibrillator. Finally, a list of medications should be obtained. In general, all cardiovascular medications should be continued even on the day of surgery, except perhaps diuretics. Preoperative β-adrenergic blocker use has been associated with survival after coronary artery surgery.[8]

Physical examination of the patient should be focused on the airway and the cardiovascular system. The airway examination should include dentition: any evidence of infection or abscess must be discovered. Blood pressure should be measured on both arms, and any significant difference should be noted to rule out possible subclavian artery stenosis. Peripheral pulses should be palpated and graded. Allen's test may be performed in case a radial artery harvest is being considered to provide a conduit. Femoral pulsation should be palpated, and the presence of any peripheral vascular disease should be noted (this may make the placement of an intra-aortic balloon challenging). Carotid bruits should be listened for, and cardiac sounds should be auscultated. Hepatomegaly, jugular venous distention, and peripheral edema should be noted.

Preoperative laboratory tests should include hematocrit, platelet count, coagulation parameters, electrolytes, serum creatinine, glucose, 12-lead electrocardiogram, and a chest radiograph. An echocardiogram, if obtained, provides not only information about preoperative ventricular and valvular function and anatomy but also a baseline with which intraoperative TEE findings can be compared. The catheterization report should be reviewed for the distribution of coronary artery disease, ventricular systolic and diastolic dysfunction, valvular abnormalities, pulmonary hypertension, and intracardiac shunt.

INTRAOPERATIVE MANAGEMENT

Monitoring

The American Society of Anesthesiologists' standard monitoring protocol includes surface electrocardiography (ECG), pulse oximeter, capnography, (noninvasive) blood pressure monitoring, and temperature monitoring. On surface ECG, ST-segment analysis should be continuously performed. When ischemia is defined as greater than or equal to 0.1 mV (1 mm) horizontal or downsloping ST depression, greater than or equal to 0.15 mV (1.5 mm) upsloping ST depression, or greater than or equal to 0.15 mV (1.5 mm) ST elevation in a non-Q wave lead, the sensitivity of the V5 lead alone is 75%; that of V5 and V4 is 90%; that of V5 and II is 80%; and that of V5, V4, and II is 96%.[9] Use of the standard five-lead ECG system does not allow simultaneous monitoring of V5 and V4, and the most practical alternative is to monitor leads V5 and II, the latter of which is also useful for arrhythmia monitoring. When right-sided ischemia is of concern, the right shoulder lead (usually white) may be placed in the right precordial area, and then lead I becomes the right precordial lead (V_4R).[10] Simultaneous monitoring of V5, II, and V_4R allows for the detection of virtually 100% of all ischemic episodes that are detectable with full 12-lead ECG.[10]

In addition to the noninvasive monitors, invasive monitors are routinely employed in cardiac surgery. An arterial line is a must for continuous blood pressure monitoring and intermittent blood sampling. A radial artery is most commonly used—preferably one that is contralateral to the internal mammary artery to be used as a conduit—because of the theoretical concern of subclavian distortion by the retractor during conduit harvest. If the surgery involves the takeoff of the innominate artery or the left subclavian artery, or if the radial artery is to be harvested as a conduit, the corresponding radial artery should not be used for an arterial line, and an alternative site should be sought. For an operation of the descending thoracic aorta, two arterial lines with one proximal to the proximal clamp and one distal to the distal clamp are recommended. The proximal arterial line (usually in the right radial artery) provides information about the perfusion pressure of the myocardium and the brain. The distal arterial line (usually a femoral artery line or, in the absence of a peripheral vascular disease, a dorsalis pedis line), in conjunction with an intrathecal catheter, allows the calculation of the perfusion pressure of the spinal cord.

A central venous line (CVL) is routinely employed in cardiac surgery to allow the reliable administration of cardiovascular medications and heparin and to monitor central venous pressures. Whether the use of a pulmonary artery catheter (PAC) should be routine or used selectively in cardiac surgery has been a matter of debate. In a prospective comparison of a CVL with a PAC in 1094 patients undergoing coronary artery surgery (including the highest-risk patients), Tuman and colleagues[11] found that there was no difference in outcome. Likewise, Schwann and coworkers[12] reported that, in their experience with 2685 consecutive patients undergoing coronary artery bypass surgery, the use of a PAC was limited to 9% (2.4% unplanned—i.e., converted from a CVL) of the patients and predicted by ejection fraction, Society of Thoracic Surgeons risk score, intra-aortic balloon pump, congestive heart failure, re-do surgery, and New York Heart Association class IV. With such a selective use, their observed-to-expected ratio of mortality as compared with the Society of Thoracic Surgeons database was 0.73. Furthermore, the presence of a PAC has not been shown to influence anesthetic management during induction,[13] which is generally considered one of the most risky periods during anesthesia. These studies suggest that the surgeon should be highly selective when choosing coronary surgery patients in whom to use a PAC. However, a PAC, unlike a CVL, can provide information about cardiac output, systemic and pulmonary vascular resistance, and mixed venous saturation, and it can also be used to pace the heart. On the other hand, TEE may negate some of the potential advantages of a PAC over a CVL: cardiac output measured by TEE can be reliable and comparable with that measured by a PAC,[14] TEE-guided right and left ventricular oximetry may be feasible,[15] and pulmonary artery pressures can be estimated by TEE.[16]

A detailed review of the indications and capabilities of TEE is beyond the scope of this chapter, but several excellent books about TEE are available. The American Society of Echocardiography and the Society of Cardiovascular Anesthesiologists have published guidelines for the comprehensive intraoperative TEE examination[17] and how to be trained and certified for competence in perioperative TEE.[9,18] Current indications and use of perioperative TEE are expanding. In addition to serving as a monitor of myocardial function and ischemia and valvular function, TEE is an invaluable guide for the placement of coronary sinus and intra-aortic catheters, for the delineation of the anatomy and pathology of valve lesions, and for before-and-after comparison of myocardial perfusion and function and valvular anatomy and function (Figs. 60-1 and 60-2). In addition, TEE may be used to assess the delivery of cardioplegia,[19,20] and to predict changes in regional myocardial function after coronary artery bypass.[21]

In surgeries of the descending thoracic aorta, cerebrospinal fluid pressure (CSFP) may be measured with an intrathecal catheter. If such a catheter is placed, CSFP should be maintained at less than or equal to 10 cm H_2O, and CSF should be allowed to drain when CSFP is greater than 10 cm H_2O.[22] However, spinal cord perfusion depends not only on CSFP

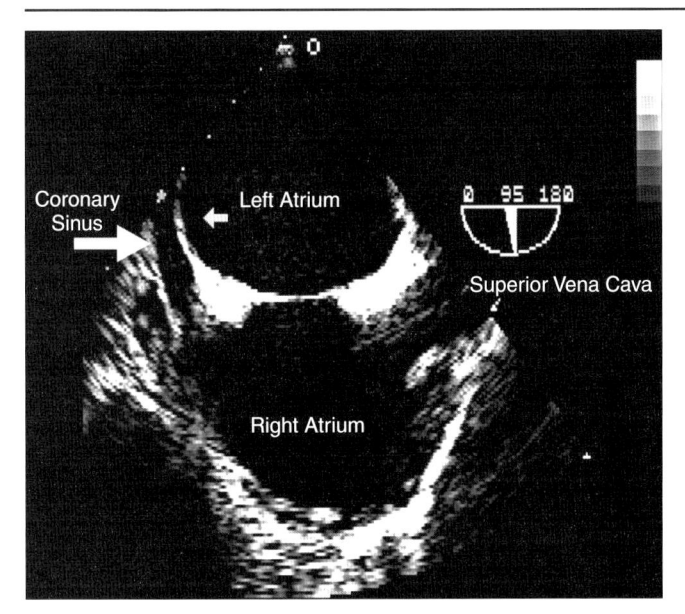

Figure 60-1
A modified midesophageal bicaval view demonstrating the left atrium.

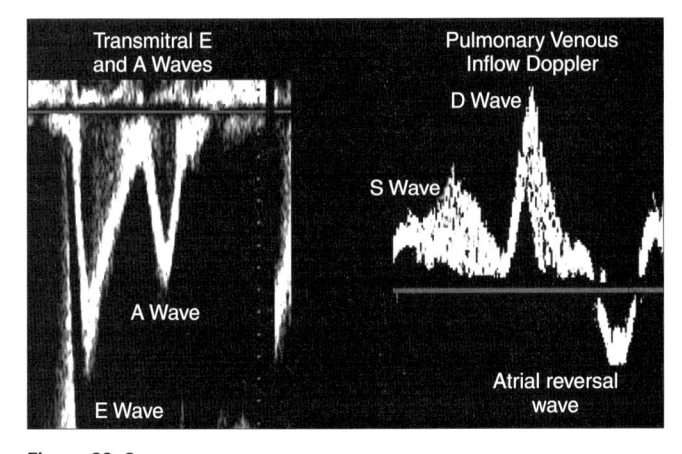

Figure 60-2
The left ventricular diastolic function may be assessed by examination of the mitral inflow into the ventricle and the pulmonary venous inflow. A wave, atrial filling phase; D wave, diastolic wave; E wave, rapid filling phase; S wave, systolic wave.

but also on the arterial pressure distal to the distal clamp, and maintenance of the distal arterial pressure may be just as important when using, for example, a partial bypass or a shunt. Whether monitoring of CSFP and drainage of CSF to maintain CSFP at less than 10 cm H_2O prevents paraplegia after descending thoracic aortic surgery is still being debated.[23]

Choice of Anesthetic Agents

High-dose opioid anesthesia was developed in the late 1960s, and it was based on the observation by Lowenstein and colleagues[24] that patients on mechanical ventilation after cardiac surgery tolerated large dosages of morphine (0.5 to 3 mg/kg) for sedation and analgesia with minimal hemodynamic effects. Such large dosages were then tried immediately before operation as an adjunct to anesthesia for cardiac surgery, with significant success.[25] Opioids by themselves do not ensure amnesia, and they require supplementation with an amnestic such as a benzodiazepine or scopolamine, the latter with unreliable effectiveness and declining popularity. Synthetic opioids such as fentanyl (50 to 100 mg/kg) or sufentanil (5 to 10 mg/kg) provide similar hemodynamic effects but without the fluid retention often seen with high-dose morphine anesthesia. Although highly successful and popular in the 1980s and early 1990s, high-dose opioid anesthesia has gradually given way to a balanced anesthetic technique that involves employing a modest dosage of opioids in conjunction with inhalational anesthetics and other intravenous adjuncts that have a faster onset and offset to facilitate early extubation and discharge from the intensive care unit (ICU).

Although the observation by Reiz and colleagues[26] in 1983 that isoflurane may cause coronary steal (a phenomenon in which coronary blood flow is diverted away from the collateral-dependent region of the myocardium) tended to discourage the use of the inhalational agent, subsequent investigators failed to duplicate the findings.[27-29] The newer agents sevoflurane and desflurane do not cause coronary steal, either.[30,31] In addition, animal studies suggested that isoflurane may preferentially dilate large coronary arteries rather than arterioles (thus mimicking the effect of nitroglycerin[32]) and normal coronary arterioles rather than arterioles from a collateral-dependent region of the myocardium.[33,34] Furthermore, there is mounting evidence that inhalational agents precondition the heart, thus protecting it from subsequent ischemic episodes in a fashion analogous to that of ischemic preconditioning, in which a brief period of ischemia protects the heart from subsequent prolonged ischemic episodes.[35-37] Anesthetic-induced preconditioning occurs via activation of ATP-sensitive potassium channels.[38] Currently, inhalational agents are the mainstay of anesthesia for cardiac surgery, and these are supplemented with muscle relaxants and a modest amount of opioids for analgesia.

Regional Anesthesia and Analgesia

The use of thoracic epidural anesthesia (TEA) as a supplement to general anesthesia carries several potential advantages. TEA attenuates the sympathetic stress response to surgical stimulation, reduces heart rate and myocardial oxygen consumption, and decreases the release of troponin T.[39,40] Postoperatively, TEA provides superior analgesia, thus enabling early extubation and vigorous pulmonary toilet and reducing the incidence of lower respiratory tract infections as compared with conventional intravenous analgesia.[41,42] Despite these advantages, TEA has not been widely accepted for cardiac surgery because of concern for a potential epidural hematoma in patients who are to be anticoagulated for CPB. The true incidence of an epidural hematoma in cardiac surgery is not known, because such a complication has not yet been reported in cardiac surgical settings. A mathematical model suggests that the risk ranges from 1:150,000 to 1:1500.[43] If TEA is to be used, it should be avoided in patients who are receiving preoperative anticoagulation, and catheter placement may be performed the day before surgery, with postponement of surgery and neurologic monitoring if the placement results in bleeding.

Recently, with the advent of off-pump, minimally invasive cardiac surgery, several European groups have reported using TEA as the sole anesthetic modality without endotracheal intubation in patients undergoing coronary artery bypass surgery,[44,45] and aortic valve replacement.[46] The authors state that potential advantages of avoiding general anesthesia might include the use of the patient's mental status as a monitor of cerebral ischemia and achievement of truly fast-track cardiac surgery. In a study of this modality by Karagoz and colleagues,[45] 8 out of 137 patients went home the day of surgery, and 58 of these 137 did not require any ICU stay, for an overall mean hospitalization of 1 day. However, 39 out of the 137 patients had a pneumothorax, and 4 of them had to be converted to general anesthesia because of pneumothorax-related respiratory difficulties. Potential disadvantages of an awake technique in cardiac surgery include the stress response of an awake patient to surgical maneuvers such as sternotomy, and a delay in surgical progress.[47] An awake TEA for cardiac surgery has not yet found acceptance in the United States.

Intraoperative Blood Glucose Control

Acute and chronic hyperglycemia increase the risk of myocardial ischemic injury through several mechanisms.[48] Hyperglycemia decreases coronary collateral blood flow, causes endothelial dysfunction, and compromises the salutary effect of ischemic preconditioning or anesthetic-induced pharmacologic preconditioning.[49,50] Among oral hypoglycemic agents, sulfonylureas and other insulin secretagogues impair K_{ATP} channel activation and may therefore hinder ischemic or pharmacologic preconditioning. Such agents should be discontinued for 24 to 48 hours before surgery and avoided perioperatively.[48]

Hyperglycemia occurs frequently in patients with and without diabetes during cardiac surgery.[51] Intraoperative hyperglycemia is associated with a higher morbidity and mortality in patients undergoing cardiac surgery,[52-54] which might suggest that tight intraoperative glycemic control would reduce postoperative complications. Although postoperative strict blood glucose control with insulin has been shown to definitely decrease mortality and morbidity in patients after cardiac surgery,[55,56] similar results have not been obtained when the control was initiated during the surgery.[57] Furnary and others[58] performed a prospective study of nearly 2500 consecutive diabetic patients undergoing cardiac surgery who were randomized to receive either intensive insulin therapy with continuous infusion to maintain blood glucose at less than 200 mg/dL or intermittent subcutaneous insulin injections on a sliding scale. Blood glucose was better controlled with intravenous infusion (85% of patients with blood glucose <200 mg/dL on postoperative day 1, with a mean level of 199 ± 1.4 mg/dL) than with subcutaneous injections (47% of patients with <200 mg/dL, with a mean level of 241 ± 1.9 mg/dL). The incidence of deep sternal wound infection was significantly reduced in the infusion group (0.8% versus 2.0%, $P = .01$) and approached that of the nondiabetic patients. Mortality was likewise reduced with intensive insulin therapy (3.0% versus 6.1%, $P = .03$). In a retrospective review of 3554 diabetic patients from the same group,[59] mortality was directly related to postoperative mean glucose; it was demonstrated to be 0.9% for those with a level of less than 150 mg/dL, 1.3% for those with 150 to 175 mg/dL, 2.3% for those with 175 to 200 mg/dL, 4.1% for those with 200 to 225 mg/dL, 6.0% for those with 225 to 250 mg/dL, and 14.5% for those with greater than 250 mg/dL.

Intensive insulin therapy to tightly control blood glucose should not be employed intraoperatively only but should be extended into the postoperative period in the ICU. In a prospective study of 1548 patients in the surgical ICU (about two thirds of whom had been through cardiac surgery), intensive insulin therapy to a maintain a glucose level between 80 and 110 mg/dL was associated with a lower mortality as compared with conventional therapy to maintain a glucose level between 180 and 200 mg/dL (4.6% versus 8.0%, $P < .04$).[55] For perioperative glycemic control in diabetes, Martinez and colleagues[60] have suggested that all patients, even those not on an oral diet, require a basal insulin infusion, and that exogenous insulin must be given for insulin-deficient patients. Their recommendation was to maintain the blood glucose level at less than 180 mg/mL at all times (between 80 and 110 mg/mL in the ICU), to avoid oral hypoglycemics until the patients are on an oral diet, to provide basal insulin to patients who are insulin deficient,[61] and to implement a hypoglycemia-prevention protocol.[60]

Acid–Base Management during Hypothermia

As the temperature decreases, the dissociation of water to H^+ and OH^- decreases. The pH at electroneutrality, where $[H^+] = [OH^-]$, therefore increases with a decrease in temperature. At 37° C, $[H^+]$ at electroneutrality is 40 nEq/L, which corresponds with a pH of 7.4. The two approaches currently in use for acid–base management during hypothermic CPB are pH-stat and alpha-stat management. With pH-stat management, the clinical objective is to maintain a pH of 7.4 at the patient's true core temperature. Blood gases and pH are measured with a correction for temperature. To maintain a pH of 7.4 at hypothermic temperatures requires the addition of exogenous CO_2 to maintain a temperature-corrected Pa_{CO_2} of 35 to 40 mm Hg. The objective of alpha-stat management is to maintain electroneutrality. With this approach, blood gases and pH are measured without temperature correction (i.e., as if the patient's temperature were always 37° C) and maintained at a Pa_{CO_2} of 40 mm Hg and a pH of 7.4. The actual pH is allowed to vary with body temperature.

With pH-stat measurement, the addition of CO_2 corrects the hypothermia-induced leftward shift of the oxyhemoglobin dissociation curve and may improve oxygen delivery to the tissues. On the other hand, because the cerebral blood flow response to CO_2 is preserved during hypothermia, pH-stat management may lead to excessive cerebral blood flow and interference with cerebral autoregulation and flow–metabolism coupling.[62,63] However, clinical neuropsychological outcome has not been shown to differ between pH-stat and alpha-stat management.[64]

Anticoagulation for Cardiopulmonary Bypass

Heparin sulfate, which is produced from porcine gut or bovine lung, is used to mimic the natural role of heparan sulfate on the vascular endothelial surface. Heparin—although it has no anticoagulant effect by itself—complexes with and enhances the activity of antithrombin-III (AT-III) in irreversibly neutralizing thrombin and factor Xa. Heparin also increases the activity of heparin cofactor II to inhibit the action of thrombin.[65] What constitutes a safe and effective level of heparinization for CPB has not been established, in part because of the inconsistent relationship between heparin dosage, plasma heparin concentration, and clinical effect (as measured by the ACT), and in part because the ACT is a nonspecific test affected not only by heparin but also by platelets and temperature.[66] Most currently accepted heparin regimens use an initial dosage of 250 to 400 IU/kg to maintain an ACT of greater than 400 to 480 seconds.[67] However, animal studies suggest that reduced heparin administration to maintain an ACT between 250 and 300 seconds may be just as adequate.[68]

Administration of heparin may be followed by hypotension in association with hyperkalemia[69]; part of the reason for hypotension may be the heparin-induced production of nitric oxide.[70] Heparin resistance may be defined as the failure of 500 IU/kg of heparin to prolong the ACT to 480 seconds or greater.[71] Factors that predict heparin resistance include AT-III levels of 60% or less, preoperative subcutaneous or intravenous heparin therapy, platelet count of 300,000 or more per milliliter, and age of 65 years or older.[72] AT-III levels may be low because of reduced synthesis related to genetic defects or from acquired causes such as liver disease, oral contraceptive use, and disseminated intravascular coagulation; from increased consumption related to disseminated intravascular coagulation, extensive deep vein thrombosis, sepsis, or preeclampsia; or from concomitant use of heparin, nitroglycerin, or the chemotherapeutic agent L-asparaginase. Treatment of heparin resistance with increasingly higher dosages of heparin is intended to maximally bind all available AT-III and may, at times, be effective. Alternatively, the patient may receive fresh frozen plasma[73] or AT-III concentrate. In vivo recovery of AT-III activity is about 1.4% per unit of administered AT-III concentrate,[74] and the therapeutic goal should be to maintain AT-III activity at more than 80%. After separation from CPB, heparin activity is neutralized by the administration of protamine. Protamine in dosages of up to 1 to 1.3 mg per milligram of heparin (i.e., 100 IU of heparin) may be used, taking into account the heparin activity half-life of 90 minutes. Just as incomplete reversal of heparinization may lead to excessive post-bypass bleeding, excessive protamine can decrease both platelet number and function,[75] can prolong ACT,[76] and can reduce the effect of thrombin.[77] Determining whether a prolonged ACT after an adequate dosage of protamine indicates incomplete heparin reversal or excessive protamine may require measurement of the thrombin time and the heparinase-ACT, as well as the low-level titration of heparin and protamine.

Another cause of postoperative bleeding is heparin rebound. Heparin that has bound nonspecifically to plasma proteins may induce the reappearance of anticoagulant activity after adequate neutralization with protamine and cause excessive post-bypass bleeding. Postoperative protamine infusion eliminates heparin rebound.[78]

Heparin can cause thrombocytopenia. Heparin-induced thrombocytopenia (HIT) is divided into type I (HIT-I) and type II (HIT-II). HIT-II is a serious adverse effect of heparin exposure that can progress to arterial or venous thrombosis; it has also been called heparin-associated immune thrombocytopenia, heparin-associated thrombocytopenia and thrombosis (HITT), and white clot syndrome.[79,80] HIT usually occurs within 4 to 10 days after heparin treatment,[79] but it may also occur after heparin has been withdrawn (delayed-onset HIT)[81] or rapidly after the start of heparin administration (median time, 10.5 hours for early-onset HIT).[82] It is useful to know the duration of the prior exposure to heparin and platelet count.

Unfractionated heparin (UFH), which is used for anticoagulation during CPB, is associated with a higher risk for HIT than low-molecular-weight heparin (LMWH).[83] The incidence of clinically significant HIT was low in cardiac surgery with CPB,[84] although the incidence of heparin-dependent immunoglobulin G (IgG) antibodies was 15% to 20% in patients undergoing cardiac surgery.[85] Patients who have a history of HIT but are negative for HIT antibodies at the time of surgery, and who require CPB, have been successfully anticoagulated with a brief course of treatment with UFH, without complications.[86] If perioperative HIT is diagnosed, all exposure to heparin should be immediately ceased, and argatroban, lepirudin, or bivalirudin should be considered for prophylactic therapy of thrombosis until the platelet count has recovered.

Five types of protamine-related adverse reactions have been recognized. First, rapid administration of protamine (>5 mg/min) may at times induce the release of histamine from mast cells and thus cause systemic hypotension.[87] Second, protamine may act like an antigen and initiate an immunoglobulin (Ig)G- or IgE-mediated anaphylactic reaction, especially in diabetic patients who take protamine-containing insulin preparations,[88-90] and possibly in those with a true fish (not shellfish) allergy or those who have just had a vasectomy.[87] Third, protamine-heparin complexes may activate the complement system, thereby leading to an anaphylactoid reaction.[91,92] Fourth, protamine-heparin–mediated complement activation may lead to thromboxane A_2 generation, precipitating catastrophic pulmonary hypertension[93]; this is in contrast to the low systemic and pulmonary pressures seen in classic anaphylactoid reactions. In a pig model, this reaction was preventable by prior administration of indomethacin or a thromboxane A_2 receptor antagonist.[94] Last, fulminant noncardiogenic pulmonary edema and systemic anasarca have been reported 15 minutes to more than 1 hour after the administration of protamine.[87] Treatment of a protamine reaction is supportive, and various agents (e.g., diphenhydramine, steroids) and hemodynamic support have been tried. In a patient with a history of prior adverse reaction to protamine, it should be determined whether the reaction was immunologically mediated. Levels of IgG, IgE, thromboxane, and C5a at the time of the reaction, if available, may be useful, but a skin test or enzyme-linked immunosorbent assay has not been found to be useful.[95] When the cause of the reaction is uncertain, some people advocate pretreatment of the patient with steroids and histamine blockers and the slow administration of protamine. If a true immunologically mediated protamine reaction occurred, it would be best to avoid it. Protamine alternatives that are being tested include recombinant platelet factor 4,[96] hexadimethrine,[97] heparinase,[98] and a heparin removal device that uses a venovenous circuit with a poly-L-lysine-agarose surface.[99]

Use of Antifibrinolytics

Despite adequate heparinization, CPB is usually accompanied by a low-level activation of coagulation and fibrinolysis,[100] which leads to the consumption of coagulation factors and increased bleeding postoperatively. Three antifibrinolytics in common use are ε-aminocaproic acid (EACA), tranexamic acid (TA), and aprotinin. EACA and TA are synthetic analogs of the amino acid lysine and competitively block the lysine binding sites between plasmin and fibrin or fibrinogen. They reduce fibrinolysis and, by reducing fibrin split products, indirectly prevent platelet dysfunction. No uniform dosage regimen has been established for either EACA or TA. For EACA, a plasma level of 130 mg/mL is needed for the complete inhibition of fibrinolysis,[101] and dosage regimens include three doses of 10 g (before the incision, on pump, and after bypass) or a weight-based initial loading of 150 mg/kg followed by an infusion of at least 15 mg/kg/hr. For TA, Horrow and colleagues[102] recommend a 10-mg/kg load followed by an infusion of 1 mg/kg/hr, but other regimens have also been published. Both EACA and TA are renally eliminated. In direct, head-to-head comparison, TA has been found to be as effective as, or more effective than, EACA for reducing blood loss, but both were better than placebo.[103,104] In patients requiring deep hypothermic circulatory arrest (DHCA), there have been reports of fatal thrombosis in association with EACA use.[105]

Aprotinin is a serine protease inhibitor that inhibits not only plasmin but also trypsin, kallikrein, and bradykinin-kinin. The activity of aprotinin is measured in kallikrein-inhibiting units (KIU), and 1 mg of aprotinin is equal to 7140 KIU. In addition to inhibiting fibrinolysis, aprotinin may reduce the consumption of coagulation factors and the activation of mediators of inflammation. Aprotinin is at least as effective as TA or EACA for reducing perioperative blood loss, but it is much more costly.[103] High-dose (also referred to as full-dose) aprotinin involves a loading dose of 2,000,000 KIU (280 mg) followed by an infusion dose of 500,000 KIU/hr, with an additional 2,000,000 KIU in the pump. Because of concern about the cost and side effects of the medication, a low-dose (half-dose) regimen, which consisted of a loading dose of 1,000,000 KIU (280 mg) followed by an infusion dose of 250,000 KIU/hr, with an additional 2,000,000 KIU in the pump, has been tried and appears to be equally effective.[106-108] Aprotinin is cleared renally and may cause thrombotic sludging in the renal tubules, thus leading to a risk-adjusted increase in serum creatinine level and renal dysfunction but not renal failure (thus, dialysis is not necessary).[109,110] A recent nonrandomized retrospective study by Mangano and coworkers demonstrated that aprotinin was associated a doubled risk of renal failure requiring dialysis.[111] However, other studies showed that aprotinin was not associated with clinically significant renal dysfunction.[112,113] It has also been suggested that the increased incidence of renal failure with aprotinin therapy could be attributed to the increased number of blood transfusions in patients who were administered aprotinin.[114] Aprotinin has been used safely even in patients with chronic renal failure or preexisting renal dysfunction.[115,116] In one report, renal dysfunction and thrombotic complications were noted with aprotinin use in patients requiring DHCA,[117] but other authors found aprotinin to be safe even with DHCA.[118-120] Although nonrandomized retrospective studies have shown that aprotinin was associated with higher mortality, myocardial infarction, and stroke,[109,111,121] another meta-analysis of 138 randomized controlled trials did not demonstrate any significant risks for mortality, stroke, or myocardial infarction with aprotinin use.[110] A recent multicenter randomized blinded trial with a head-to-head comparison of aprotinin, ε-aminocaproic acid, and tranexamic acid concluded that although aprotinin was a more effective hemostatic agent, it was associated with increased 30-day hospital mortality.[122] As a result of these findings, an aprotinin advisory was issued in 2008 by the U.S. Food and Drug Administration on the safety profile of the drug. Because aprotinin is isolated from bovine-lung mast cells, there is a risk of allergic reactions, with the incidence of anaphylaxis reported to be less than 0.6% on initial exposure but up to 5% with reexposure within 6 months,[123] although the incidence falls rapidly to 1.9% in the 6- to 12-month period, and 0.4% in the greater than 12-month period.[124] Before administration of the regular dose, a test dose of 10,000 KIU of aprotinin should be given, and histamine blockers and steroids may be considered if there is a history of previous exposure within 6 months.

Cerebral Protection during Deep Hypothermic Circulatory Arrest

Techniques that have been used to ameliorate ischemic injury of the brain during DHCA include selective cannulation and perfusion of cerebral vessels, retrograde cerebral perfusion, pharmacologic brain protection, and the achievement of deep hypothermia. At normothermia, roughly half of the oxygen consumed is used to maintain cellular integrity ("basal" cerebral metabolic rate [CMR]O_2), and the other half is used to maintain electrical activity ("functional" $CMRO_2$).[125] Hypothermia has a greater effect on the basal $CMRO_2$ than on the functional $CMRO_2$.[126] The electroencephalogram (EEG) becomes isoelectric at 18° C, and below this temperature, any further reduction in $CMRO_2$ is from a decrease in basal $CMRO_2$. Barbiturates, which reduce functional $CMRO_2$ without having much effect on basal $CMRO_2$, do not produce any additional metabolic suppression under conditions of deep hypothermia (15° C), and they are not likely to be of benefit.[127] On the other hand, barbiturates may be of benefit for ameliorating the effects of temporary focal ischemia (e.g., from an air embolus on normothermic bypass) by the suppression of functional $CMRO_2$.

Ischemic injury from DHCA may be temporally divided into four phases.[128,129] The first phase is marked by energy production failure and membrane depolarization. After ischemic depolarization occurs, detrimental neuro-excitatory transmitters such as glutamate are released. With the restoration of blood flow, the third phase ensues, marked by an increased release of oxygen free radicals and subsequent tissue damage. In the fourth phase, ischemia may also trigger apoptosis or programmed cell death over the ensuing weeks. Inhalational anesthetics lower the critical cerebral blood flow to a level below which the majority of patients develop ischemic EEG changes.[130,131] At normothermia, the critical cerebral blood flow is 10 mL/100 g/min for isoflurane, 11.5 mL/100 g/min for sevoflurane, 15 mL/100 g/min for enflurane, and 20 mL/100 g/min for halothane. This metabolic suppression effect of inhalational agents amounts to delaying the first phase of ischemic injury. In addition, isoflurane may inhibit excitotoxicity from the accumulation of glutamate during the second phase of ischemic injury. Isoflurane has been shown to reduce the release of glutamate during ischemia[132] and may also be an antagonist of glutamate receptors, thereby diminishing deleterious calcium influx.[133] Because of its effect on the first two phases of ischemic injury, isoflurane may buy time before irreversible neuronal damage sets in. However, in aortic surgery settings where DHCA is used, anesthetics have not been demonstrated to be of benefit. Similarly, although various other pharmacologic modalities (e.g., diuretics, steroids, calcium-channel blockers) have been used, none has been demonstrated to be of benefit in DHCA.

Hemodynamic Support on Separation from Cardiopulmonary Bypass

Separating a patient from CPB may be considered a form of cardiopulmonary resuscitation, and thus it should start with the confirmation of a patent airway (usually with an endotracheal tube) and the reestablishment of ventilation. For support of the circulation, the anesthesiologist needs to continually assess and treat the five elements of preload, afterload, contractility, rate, and rhythm and the metabolic parameters that affect myocardial function, such as pH, electrolytes (especially potassium, calcium, and magnesium), oxygen-carrying capacity (hemoglobin), and temperature. In addition, the anesthesiologist needs to be in communication with the surgeon, because certain surgical maneuvers may mechanically affect myocardial function, and TEE assessment of the adequacy of the surgery (e.g., valvular anatomy and function) and the patient's ability to remain separated from CPB needs to be communicated to the surgeon.

Usually, epicardial pacing wires are placed, and the pacing function is tested before separation. A rhythm (e.g., sinus rhythm, AV sequential pacing) that preserves the atrial augmentation of ventricular preload is preferred. If the pump flow is set at an adequate cardiac output, the vascular tone of the patient may be adjusted to the desired mean pressure while the patient is still on CPB; this way, the mean pressure will be in the desired range if the patient generates the desired cardiac output after separation. Then, the heart is filled, a process that is guided by the appearance of the heart in the surgical field and on TEE, as well as by the filling pressures (Fig. 60-3). Wall motion on TEE and cardiac output measurement then serve as practical surrogate measures of contractility. Further adjustment of preload may be made by additional filling or draining of the heart by the perfusionist, by adjustment of the operating table position, or by intravenous fluid administration. Adjustment of the afterload to maintain the systemic and pulmonary vascular resistance in the normal range may be made with vasopressors (e.g., phenylephrine, norepinephrine, dopamine) or dilators (e.g., nitroglycerin, nitroprusside). In cases of catecholamine-resistant refractory hypotension, vasopressin in dosages of 7 to 20 U/hr may be attempted.[134] Inotropic assistance to augment myocardial contractility may be provided by catecholaminergic agents (e.g., epinephrine, dopamine, dobutamine) or phosphodiesterase inhibitors (e.g., milrinone).[135] When pharmacologic and metabolic support prove insufficient, consideration should be given to mechanical support devices (e.g., an intra-aortic balloon pump, a ventricular assist device) or to returning the patient to CPB for further surgical remedies. Only when the patient is hemodynamically stable after separation from CPB should the reversal of heparinization be started.

SPECIAL CONSIDERATIONS

Fast-Track Cardiac Surgery

Fast-track cardiac surgery (FTCS) refers to a multidisciplinary approach to providing care to cardiac surgical patients, with emphasis placed on early tracheal extubation (within

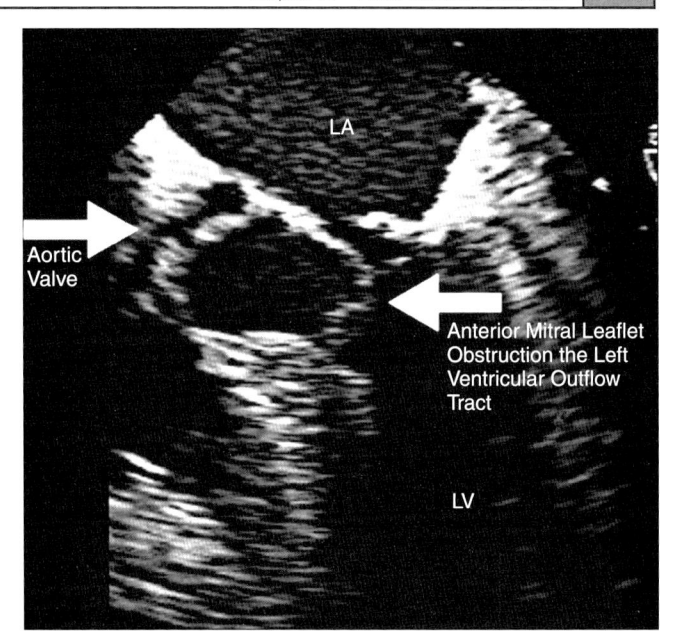

Figure 60-3
Transesophageal echocardiograph demonstrating systolic anterior motion of the anterior leaflet of the mitral valve. The presence of systolic anterior motion should alter the hemodynamic management strategy to avoid the use of an inotropic agent and a vasodilator, and to ensure adequate filling of the left ventricle (LV). LA, left atrium.

6 to 10 hours postoperatively) and expedited mobilization of the patient (with consequent reductions in ICU and hospital lengths of stay and cost).[136] Factors that predict the success or failure of this approach (other than age) are intraoperative and postoperative clinical process variables, such as intraoperative inotrope use, intraoperative placement of an intra-aortic balloon pump, and postoperative atrial arrhythmias; thus, there is no need to preselect patients for FTCS, and everyone may be considered a potential candidate for early extubation.[136] An important component of FTCS is an anesthetic technique that allows early extubation and mobilization of the patient.[137] Instead of a long-acting muscle relaxant (e.g., pancuronium), a shorter-acting agent (e.g., rocuronium, cisatracurium) may be used.[138-140] Any residual blockade at the end of surgery or during the initiation of weaning may be reversed with an acetylcholinesterase inhibitor (e.g., neostigmine) in combination with an antimuscarinic agent. Instead of a high-dose opioid technique, a low- or moderate-dose opioid technique in combination with inhalational anesthetics or neuraxial analgesia (or both) may facilitate early tracheal extubation.[141] Hypothermia at the end of surgery should be prevented.[142] Although early extubation is favored, there is no benefit of pushing for tracheal extubation in the operating room.[143] The cost of extended operating room time and the risk of cardiorespiratory instability during the period immediately after closure should also be considered. In both a retrospective review[144] and a prospective randomized controlled trial,[145] it has been demonstrated that FTCS is not associated with any increase in hospital mortality or morbidity. Rather, the rate of nosocomial pneumonia may be decreased with FTCS.[144] The reintubation rate is not significantly different between FTCS and the conventional approach, and both ICU and hospital length of stay are decreased with FTCS. In response

to concerns that FTCS may result in cost shifting rather than cost savings, Cheng and colleagues[146] examined the resource use of both FTCS and conventional patients for a year after hospital discharge. Although insurance claims for outpatient visits were not significantly different at 3 months and 12 months, insurance claims and costs for inpatient care were significantly lower for the FTCS group. The savings in inpatient care were 68% at 3 months and about 50% at 1 year. Thus, FTCS may lead to savings during both the initial hospitalization for the surgery and the subsequent follow-up period.

Off-Pump Coronary Artery Bypass

Off-pump coronary artery bypass (OPCAB) involves bypass grafting on a beating heart without usng CPB. Surgical techniques, complications, and success rates of OPCAB are covered elsewhere in this book. For an anesthesiologist, OPCAB involves more intensive hemodynamic management, with the potential for instability because of retraction and compression of the heart and consequent potential myocardial ischemia.[147] After sternotomy and exposure of the heart, each target vessel is identified, and a specialized retractor is applied to provide exposure of the target site. Test occlusion of the target vessel to assess its effect on myocardial function or to provide ischemic preconditioning (or both) is performed in some centers. The heart itself may be lifted and twisted to improve surgical exposure, and this maneuver may compromise the filling of the cardiac chambers. To maintain coronary perfusion pressure, the patient may be placed in the Trendelenburg position, given fluids, and supported with a vasopressor (e.g., phenylephrine). Constant communication between the anesthesiologist and the surgeon is the key to preventing unexpected hemodynamic compromise. With lifting of the heart, visualization by TEE is compromised, and the surgeon must rely on direct visualization of the surgical field and traditional hemodynamic monitors such as an arterial line and a PAC. Proximal anastomoses are performed with a side-biter clamp on the aorta. Systemic blood pressure and aortic wall tension need to be controlled for the application and removal of the side biter.

The level of heparinization required for OPCAB has not been standardized.[148,149] At some centers, "full" heparinization to maintain the ACT at more than 480 seconds is used, whereas others use limited heparinization to maintain the ACT in the 200- to 300-second range, as is done for vascular procedures. Neither approach has been demonstrated to be clearly better than the other.

Port-Access Minimally Invasive Cardiac Surgery

The port-access system is used for minimally invasive cardiac surgery (MICS) that requires the institution of CPB. Preoperative preparation of the patient requires discussion between the surgeon and the anesthesiologist about the exact nature of the surgery planned.[150,151] The usual intravenous access and monitoring modalities (i.e., those used for conventional cardiac surgery) need to be placed. TEE is an essential modality, and contraindications to the use of TEE would almost preclude port-access MICS. A modified lateral decubitus position is usually used, and this may have implications for line placement. To provide lung isolation, a double-lumen bronchocatheter or a bronchial blocker may be used. Position of the broncho-catheter should be confirmed with a fiberoptic bronchoscope upon placement and after final positioning of the patient. The bronchoscope should be readily available throughout the procedure, because any malposition of the tube can result in lung inflation and thus make the surgery almost impossible through the limited incision. Before positioning the patient, external cardioversion pads should be applied for urgent pacing or cardioversion, because the limited access means that internal paddles cannot be employed.

The mainstays of the port-access system are the coronary sinus catheter (CSC) for retrograde cardioplegia, the pulmonary artery vent (PAV), and the endovascular aortic cannula, which also acts as an endovascular clamp (see Fig. 60-1). Unlike the regular PAC, the CSCs are not heparin bonded by the manufacturers, so 5000 units of heparin is administered before placement of these catheters. Before CSC placement, a left-sided superior vena cava needs to be excluded by TEE. Under TEE guidance, the success rate of CSC placement has been reported to be 95% and to be superior to fluoroscopy.[152,153] After successful placement of the CSC, its position is further confirmed by balloon inflation and visualization of the arterialization of the pressure tracing. Although it is not essential, keeping the balloon inflated and the wire loaded into the catheter until immediately before administration of retrograde cardioplegia may help prevent catheter dislodgement. The PAV is also inserted through the right internal jugular vein and guided into the pulmonary artery in the same manner as a regular PAC. However, central venous pressure cannot be measured with the PAV. Venous access or a drainage line is placed through the femoral vein, and TEE is used to accurately position the cannula. Similarly, the endovascular aortic cannula can be very accurately placed under TEE guidance. The positions of the catheters should be confirmed after a change of position from supine to lateral and before commencement of CPB, because poor visibility makes it very difficult to reposition the catheters after commencement of CPB.

Regardless of the type of surgery, recognition of intracardiac air and monitoring the success of de-airing maneuvers is a crucial TEE function. The left ventricular apex, which may not be accessible to the surgeon for needle aspiration, needs to be carefully examined by TEE. TEE is the only monitor used to assess the completeness of de-airing.[153]

Other factors to consider during MICS include the possibility of urgent cardiac pacing and external cardioversion; suture placement in difficult sites, which can lead to bleeding; inadequate valve repair resulting in residual regurgitation; and air embolism. Even a small amount of bleeding in a minimally exposed place can result in tamponade after chest closure. The duration of anesthesia and surgery tends to be prolonged, and there is always the risk of a technically unsatisfactory result and conversion to an open conventional surgery. At the end of the surgery, the CSC is removed and, depending on the condition of the patient, the PAV may be replaced with a PAC for postoperative monitoring of the patient.

Recent developments in echocardiography have enabled cardiac surgeons and anesthesiologists to visualize the mitral valve dynamically in three dimensions, allowing a dynamic mitral valve assessment with an excellent spatial and temporal orientation. More important, it provides an en face surgical view of the mitral valve, with both leaflets and commissures visualized dynamically (Fig. 60-4). This technology provides information that was available only after direct surgical

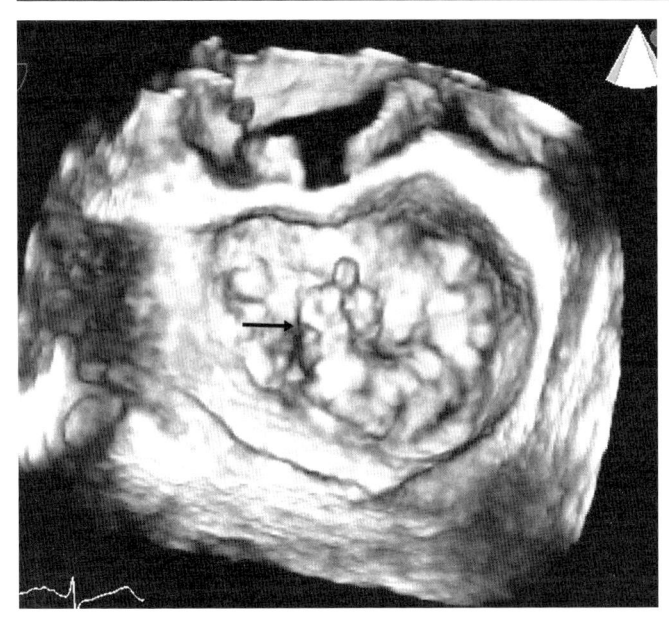

Figure 60–4
An en face, three-dimensional left atrial view of the mitral valve showing a flail P2 segment.

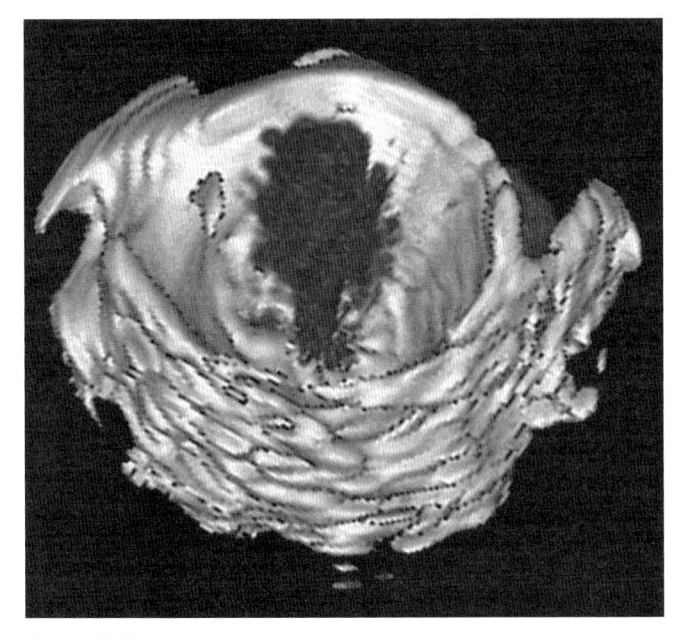

Figure 60–5
Three-dimensional view of the mitral valve with color-flow Doppler information showing a mitral regurgitation jet of moderate intensity.

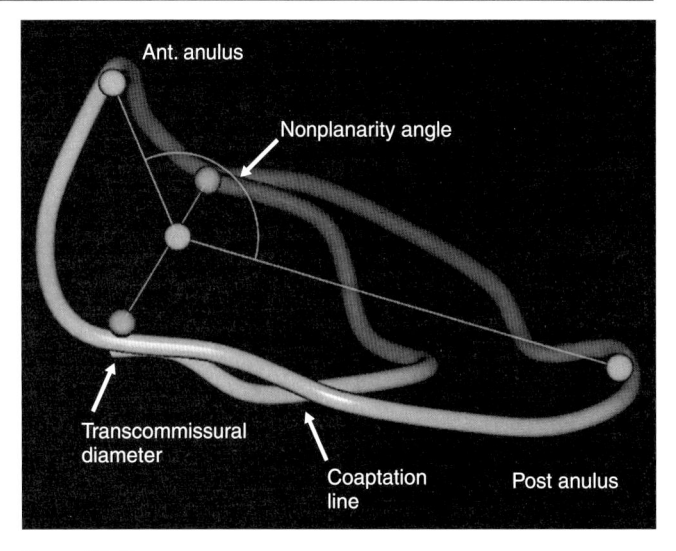

Figure 60–6
Three-dimensional reconstruction of the mitral anulus for geometric analysis before the repair.

examination of mitral valve. The ability to incorporate color-flow Doppler information into three-dimensional volume sets has further increased the diagnostic potential of perioperative TEE as well as its ability to be used in diagnosing and quantifying mitral regurgitation (Fig. 60-5). Recently, it has been demonstrated that three-dimensional echocardiography can be used to geometrically analyze the mitral valve and provide real-time information about the changes in mitral annular structure with repair (Fig. 60-6).[154] This has opened the door for the cardiac anesthesiologists to perform predictive geometric modeling of the mitral valve and hence aid in valve repairs. Similarly, advances in perioperative TEE have almost obviated the need for a direct surgical valve analysis to plan a repair.

Robotic-Assisted Cardiac Surgery

Robotic-assisted cardiac surgery (RACS), the next step in the evolution of MICS, is available in only a few places in the world. Its goal is to perform the procedure with as small an incision as possible, with an outcome that is equivalent or superior to that of the conventional procedure.[155,156] Anesthetic management for RACS requires all of the techniques outlined earlier for port-access MICS, and the possibility of significantly prolonged surgery and the potential for positional neurovascular injuries (e.g., to the brachial plexus) must be considered.[156] Preliminary reports indicate faster recovery and a reduction in complications,[157,158] but long-term results are still pending.

REFERENCES

1. Higgins TL, Estafanous FG, Loop FD, Beck GJ, Blum JM, Paranandi L. Stratification of morbidity and mortality outcome by preoperative risk factors in coronary artery bypass patients: a clinical severity score. *JAMA* 1992;**267**:2344-8.
2. Simoons ML, de Boer MJ, van den Brand MJ, van Miltenburg AJ, Hoorntje JC, Heyndrickx GR, et al. Randomized trial of a GPIIb/IIIa platelet receptor blocker in refractory unstable angina. European Cooperative Study Group. *Circulation* 1994;**89**:596-603.
3. Tcheng JE, Ellis SG, George BS, Kereiakes DJ, Kleiman NS, Talley JD, et al. Pharmacodynamics of chimeric glycoprotein IIb/IIIa integrin antiplatelet antibody Fab 7E3 in high-risk coronary angioplasty. *Circulation* 1994;**90**:1757-64.
4. Scarborough RM. Development of eptifibatide. *Am Heart J* 1999;**138**:1093-104.
5. Jennings LK, Jacoski MV, White MM. The pharmacodynamics of parenteral glycoprotein IIb/IIIa inhibitors. *J Interv Cardiol* 2002;**15**:45-60.
6. Kondo K, Umemura K. Clinical pharmacokinetics of tirofiban, a nonpeptide glycoprotein IIb/IIIa receptor antagonist: comparison with the monoclonal antibody abciximab. *Clin Pharmacokinet* 2002;**41**:187-95.
7. Dauerman HL, Ball SA, Goldberg RJ, Desourdy MA, Furman MI. Activated clotting times in the setting of eptifibatide use during percutaneous coronary intervention. *J Thromb Thrombolysis* 2002;**13**:127-32.

8. Weightman WM, Gibbs NM, Sheminant MR, Whitford EG, Mahon BD, Newman MA. Drug therapy before coronary artery surgery: nitrates are independent predictors of mortality and beta-adrenergic blockers predict survival. *Anesth Analg* 1999;**88**:286-91.
9. Aronson S, Butler A, Subhiyah R, Buckingham Jr RE, Cahalan MK, Konstandt S, et al. Development and analysis of a new certifying examination in perioperative transesophageal echocardiography. *Anesth Analg* 2002;**95**:1476-82.
10. De Hert SG, Moens MM, Vermeyen KM, Hageman MP. Use of the right-sided precordial lead V4R in the detection of intraoperative myocardial ischemia. *J Cardiothorac Vasc Anesth* 1993;**7**:659-67.
11. Tuman KJ, McCarthy RJ, Spiess BD, DaValle M, Hompland SJ, Dabir R, Ivankovich AD. Effect of pulmonary artery catheterization on outcome in patients undergoing coronary artery surgery. *Anesthesiology* 1989;**70**:199-206.
12. Schwann TA, Zacharias A, Riordan CJ, Durham SJ, Engoren M, Habib RH. Safe, highly selective use of pulmonary artery catheters in coronary artery bypass grafting: an objective patient selection method. *Ann Thorac Surg* 2002;**73**: 401-2:1394-401; discussion.
13. Wall MH, MacGregor DA, Kennedy DJ, James RL, Butterworth J, Mallak KF, Royster RL. Pulmonary artery catheter placement for elective coronary artery bypass grafting: before or after anesthetic induction? *Anesth Analg* 2002;**94**:1409-15; table of contents.
14. Zhao X, Mashikian JS, Panzica P, Lerner A, Park KW, Comunale ME. Comparison of thermodilution bolus cardiac output and Doppler cardiac output in the early post-cardiopulmonary bypass period. *J Cardiothorac Vasc Anesth* 2003;**17**: 193-8.
15. Margreiter J, Keller C, Brimacombe J. The feasibility of transesophageal echocardiograph-guided right and left ventricular oximetry in hemodynamically stable patients undergoing coronary artery bypass grafting. *Anesth Analg* 2002;**94**:794-8; table of contents.
16. Kawahito S, Kitahata H, Tanaka K, Nozaki J, Oshita S. Pulmonary arterial pressure can be estimated by transesophageal pulsed Doppler echocardiography. *Anesth Analg* 2001;**92**:1364-9.
17. Shanewise JS, Cheung AT, Aronson S, Stewart WJ, Weiss RL, Mark JB, et al. ASE/SCA guidelines for performing a comprehensive intraoperative multiplane transesophageal echocardiography examination: recommendations of the American Society of Echocardiography Council for Intraoperative Echocardiography and the Society of Cardiovascular Anesthesiologists Task Force for Certification in Perioperative Transesophageal Echocardiography. *Anesth Analg* 1999;**89**:870-84.
18. Cahalan MK, Abel M, Goldman M, Pearlman A, Sears-Rogan P, Russell I, et al. American Society of Echocardiography and Society of Cardiovascular Anesthesiologists task force guidelines for training in perioperative echocardiography. *Anesth Analg* 2002;**94**:1384-8.
19. Aronson S, Lee BK, Liddicoat JR, Wiencek JG, Feinstein SB, Ellis JE, et al. Assessment of retrograde cardioplegia distribution using contrast echocardiography. *Ann Thorac Surg* 1991;**52**:810-4.
20. Aronson S, Lee BK, Wiencek JG, Feinstein SB, Roizen MF, Karp RB, Ellis JE. Assessment of myocardial perfusion during CABG surgery with two-dimensional transesophageal contrast echocardiography. *Anesthesiology* 1991;**75**:433-40.
21. Aronson S, Dupont F, Savage R, Drum M, Gunnar W, Jeevanandam V. Changes in regional myocardial function after coronary artery bypass graft surgery are predicted by intraoperative low-dose dobutamine echocardiography. *Anesthesiology* 2000;**93**:685-92.
22. Svensson LG, Hess KR, D'Agostino RS, Entrup MH, Hreib K, Kimmel WA, et al. Reduction of neurologic injury after high-risk thoracoabdominal aortic operation. *Ann Thorac Surg* 1998;**66**:132-8.
23. Ling E, Arellano R. Systematic overview of the evidence supporting the use of cerebrospinal fluid drainage in thoracoabdominal aneurysm surgery for prevention of paraplegia. *Anesthesiology* 2000;**93**:1115-22.
24. Lowenstein E, Hallowell P, Levine FH, Daggett WM, Austen WG, Laver MB. Cardiovascular response to large doses of intravenous morphine in man. *N Engl J Med* 1969;**281**:1389-93.
25. Lowenstein E. Morphine "anesthesia": a perspective. *Anesthesiology* 1971;**35**:563-5.
26. Reiz S, Balfors E, Sorensen MB, Ariola Jr S, Friedman A, Truedsson H. Isoflurane: a powerful coronary vasodilator in patients with coronary artery disease. *Anesthesiology* 1983;**59**:91-7.
27. Cason BA, Verrier ED, London MJ, Mangano DT, Hickey RF. Effects of isoflurane and halothane on coronary vascular resistance and collateral myocardial blood flow: their capacity to induce coronary steal. *Anesthesiology* 1987;**67**: 665-75.
28. Hartman JC, Kampine JP, Schmeling WT, Warltier DC. Alterations in collateral blood flow produced by isoflurane in a chronically instrumented canine model of multivessel coronary artery disease. *Anesthesiology* 1991;**74**:120-33.
29. Moore PG, Kien ND, Reitan JA, White DA, Safwat AM. No evidence for blood flow redistribution with isoflurane or halothane during acute coronary artery occlusion in fentanyl-anesthetized dogs. *Anesthesiology* 1991;**75**:854-65.
30. Hartman JC, Pagel PS, Kampine JP, Schmeling WT, Warltier DC. Influence of desflurane on regional distribution of coronary blood flow in a chronically instrumented canine model of multivessel coronary artery obstruction. *Anesth Analg* 1991;**72**:289-99.
31. Kersten JR, Brayer AP, Pagel PS, Tessmer JP, Warltier DC. Perfusion of ischemic myocardium during anesthesia with sevoflurane. *Anesthesiology* 1994;**81**: 995-1004.
32. Sellke FW, Myers PR, Bates JN, Harrison DG. Influence of vessel size on the sensitivity of porcine coronary microvessels to nitroglycerin. *Am J Physiol* 1990;**258**:H515-20.
33. Park KW, Dai HB, Lowenstein E, Sellke FW. Vasomotor responses of rat coronary arteries to isoflurane and halothane depend on preexposure tone and vessel size. *Anesthesiology* 1995;**83**:1323-30.
34. Park KW, Lowenstein E, Dai HB, Lopez JJ, Stamler A, Simons M, Sellke FW. Direct vasomotor effects of isoflurane in subepicardial resistance vessels from collateral-dependent and normal coronary circulation of pigs. *Anesthesiology* 1996;**85**:584-91.
35. Cason BA, Gamperl AK, Slocum RE, Hickey RF. Anesthetic-induced preconditioning: previous administration of isoflurane decreases myocardial infarct size in rabbits. *Anesthesiology* 1997;**87**:1182-90.
36. Cope DK, Impastato WK, Cohen MV, Downey JM. Volatile anesthetics protect the ischemic rabbit myocardium from infarction. *Anesthesiology* 1997;**86**:699-709.
37. Toller WG, Kersten JR, Pagel PS, Hettrick DA, Warltier DC. Sevoflurane reduces myocardial infarct size and decreases the time threshold for ischemic preconditioning in dogs. *Anesthesiology* 1999;**91**:1437-46.
38. Kersten JR, Schmeling TJ, Pagel PS, Gross GJ, Warltier DC. Isoflurane mimics ischemic preconditioning via activation of K(ATP) channels: reduction of myocardial infarct size with an acute memory phase. *Anesthesiology* 1997;**87**:361-70.
39. Kirno K, Friberg P, Grzegorczyk A, Milocco I, Ricksten SE, Lundin S. Thoracic epidural anesthesia during coronary artery bypass surgery: effects on cardiac sympathetic activity, myocardial blood flow and metabolism, and central hemodynamics. *Anesth Analg* 1994;**79**:1075-81.
40. Loick HM, Schmidt C, Van Aken H, Junker R, Erren M, Berendes E, et al. High thoracic epidural anesthesia, but not clonidine, attenuates the perioperative stress response via sympatholysis and reduces the release of troponin T in patients undergoing coronary artery bypass grafting. *Anesth Analg* 1999;**88**:701-9.
41. Scott NB, Turfrey DJ, Ray DA, Nzewi O, Sutcliffe NP, Lal AB, et al. A prospective randomized study of the potential benefits of thoracic epidural anesthesia and analgesia in patients undergoing coronary artery bypass grafting. *Anesth Analg* 2001;**93**:528-35.
42. Tenling A, Joachimsson PO, Tyden H, Hedenstierna G. Thoracic epidural analgesia as an adjunct to general anaesthesia for cardiac surgery. Effects on pulmonary mechanics. *Acta Anaesthesiol Scand* 2000;**44**:1071-6.
43. Ho AM, Chung DC, Joynt GM. Neuraxial blockade and hematoma in cardiac surgery: estimating the risk of a rare adverse event that has not (yet) occurred. *Chest* 2000;**117**:551-5.
44. Aybek T, Kessler P, Khan MF, Dogan S, Neidhart G, Moritz A, Wimmer-Greinecker G. Operative techniques in awake coronary artery bypass grafting. *J Thorac Cardiovasc Surg* 2003;**125**:1394-400.
45. Karagoz HY, Kurtoglu M, Bakkaloglu B, Sonmez B, Cetintas T, Bayazit K. Coronary artery bypass grafting in the awake patient: three years' experience in 137 patients. *J Thorac Cardiovasc Surg* 2003;**125**:1401-4.
46. Schachner T, Bonatti J, Balogh D, Margreiter J, Mair P, Laufer G, Putz G. Aortic valve replacement in the conscious patient under regional anesthesia without endotracheal intubation. *J Thorac Cardiovasc Surg* 2003;**125**:1526-7.
47. Mangano CT. Risky business. *J Thorac Cardiovasc Surg* 2003;**125**:1204-7.
48. Gu W, Pagel PS, Warltier DC, Kersten JR. Modifying cardiovascular risk in diabetes mellitus. *Anesthesiology* 2003;**98**:774-9.
49. Kehl F, Krolikowski JG, Mraovic B, Pagel PS, Warltier DC, Kersten JR. Hyperglycemia prevents isoflurane-induced preconditioning against myocardial infarction. *Anesthesiology* 2002;**96**:183-8.
50. Kersten JR, Montgomery MW, Ghassemi T, Gross ER, Toller WG, Pagel PS, Warltier DC. Diabetes and hyperglycemia impair activation of mitochondrial K(ATP) channels. *Am J Physiol Heart Circ Physiol* 2001;**280**:H1744-50.
51. Carvalho G, Moore A, Qizilbash B, Lachapelle K, Schricker T. Maintenance of normoglycemia during cardiac surgery. *Anesth Analg* 2004;**99**:319-24.
52. Gandhi GY, Nuttall GA, Abel MD, Mullany CJ, Schaff HV, Williams BA, et al. Intraoperative hyperglycemia and perioperative outcomes in cardiac surgery patients. *Mayo Clin Proc* 2005;**80**:862-6.

53. Ouattara A, Lecomte P, Le Manach Y, Landi M, Jacqueminet S, Platonov I, et al. Poor intraoperative blood glucose control is associated with a worsened hospital outcome after cardiac surgery in diabetic patients. *Anesthesiology* 2005;**103**:687-94.
54. Doenst T, Wijeysundera D, Karkouti K, Zechner C, Maganti M, Rao V, Borger MA. Hyperglycemia during cardiopulmonary bypass is an independent risk factor for mortality in patients undergoing cardiac surgery. *J Thorac Cardiovasc Surg* 2005;**130**:1144.
55. van den Berghe G, Wouters P, Weekers F, Verwaest C, Bruyninckx F, Schetz M, et al. Intensive insulin therapy in the critically ill patients. *N Engl J Med* 2001;**345**:1359-67.
56. Ingels C, Debaveye Y, Milants I, Buelens E, Peeraer A, Devriendt Y, et al. Strict blood glucose control with insulin during intensive care after cardiac surgery: impact on 4-years survival, dependency on medical care. quality-of-life. *Eur Heart J* 2006;**27**:2716-24.
57. Gandhi GY, Nuttall GA, Abel MD, Mullany CJ, Schaff HV, O'Brien PC, et al. Intensive intraoperative insulin therapy versus conventional glucose management during cardiac surgery: a randomized trial. *Ann Intern Med* 2007;**146**:233-43.
58. Furnary AP, Zerr KJ, Grunkemeier GL, Starr A. Continuous intravenous insulin infusion reduces the incidence of deep sternal wound infection in diabetic patients after cardiac surgical procedures. *Ann Thorac Surg* 1999;**67**:60-2: 352-60; discussion.
59. Furnary AP, Gao G, Grunkemeier GL, Wu Y, Zerr KJ, Bookin SO, et al. Continuous insulin infusion reduces mortality in patients with diabetes undergoing coronary artery bypass grafting. *J Thorac Cardiovasc Surg* 2003;**125**:1007-21.
60. Martinez EA, Williams KA, Pronovost PJ. Thinking like a pancreas: perioperative glycemic control. *Anesth Analg* 2007;**104**:4-6.
61. Garber AJ, Moghissi ES, Bransome Jr ED, Clark NG, Clement S, Cobin RH, et al. American College of Endocrinology position statement on inpatient diabetes and metabolic control. *Endocr Pract* 2004;**10**(Suppl. 2):4-9.
62. Murkin JM, Farrar JK, Tweed WA, McKenzie FN, Guiraudon G. Cerebral autoregulation and flow/metabolism coupling during cardiopulmonary bypass: the influence of $PaCO_2$. *Anesth Analg* 1987;**66**:825-32.
63. Rogers AT, Stump DA, Gravlee GP, Prough DS, Angert KC, Wallenhaupt SL, et al. Response of cerebral blood flow to phenylephrine infusion during hypothermic cardiopulmonary bypass: influence of $PaCO_2$ management. *Anesthesiology* 1988;**69**:547-51.
64. Bashein G, Townes BD, Nessly ML, Bledsoe SW, Hornbein TF, Davis KB, et al. A randomized study of carbon dioxide management during hypothermic cardiopulmonary bypass. *Anesthesiology* 1990;**72**:7-15.
65. Tollefsen DM, Majerus DW, Blank MK. Heparin cofactor II: purification and properties of a heparin-dependent inhibitor of thrombin in human plasma. *J Biol Chem* 1982;**257**:2162-9.
66. Esposito RA, Culliford AT, Colvin SB, Thomas SJ, Lackner H, Spencer FC. The role of the activated clotting time in heparin administration and neutralization for cardiopulmonary bypass. *J Thorac Cardiovasc Surg* 1983;**85**:174-85.
67. Gravlee GP, Haddon WS, Rothberger HK, Mills SA, Rogers AT, Bean VE, et al. Heparin dosing and monitoring for cardiopulmonary bypass: a comparison of techniques with measurement of subclinical plasma coagulation. *J Thorac Cardiovasc Surg* 1990;**99**:518-27.
68. Cardoso PF, Yamazaki F, Keshavjee S, Schaefers HJ, Hsieh CM, Wang LS, et al. A reevaluation of heparin requirements for cardiopulmonary bypass. *J Thorac Cardiovasc Surg* 1991;**101**:153-60.
69. Jacka MJ, Clark AG. Cardiovascular instability requiring treatment after intravenous heparin for cardiopulmonary bypass. *Anesth Analg* 2000;**90**:42-4.
70. Li JM, Hajarizadeh H, La Rosa CA, Rohrer MJ, Vander Salm TJ, Cutler BS. Heparin and protamine stimulate the production of nitric oxide. *J Cardiovasc Surg (Torino)* 1996;**37**:445-52.
71. Staples MH, Dunton RF, Karlson KJ, Leonardi HK, Berger RL. Heparin resistance after preoperative heparin therapy or intraaortic balloon pumping. *Ann Thorac Surg* 1994;**57**:1211-6.
72. Ranucci M, Isgro G, Cazzaniga A, Soro G, Menicanti L, Frigiola A. Predictors for heparin resistance in patients undergoing coronary artery bypass grafting. *Perfusion* 1999;**14**:437-42.
73. Sabbagh AH, Chung GK, Shuttleworth P, Applegate BJ, Gabrhel W. Fresh frozen plasma: a solution to heparin resistance during cardiopulmonary bypass. *Ann Thorac Surg* 1984;**37**:466-8.
74. Schwartz RS, Bauer KA, Rosenberg RD, Kavanaugh EJ, Davies DC, Bogdanoff DA. Clinical experience with antithrombin III concentrate in treatment of congenital and acquired deficiency of antithrombin. The Antithrombin III Study Group. *Am J Med* 1989;**87**:53S-60S.
75. Velders AJ, Wildevuur CR. Platelet damage by protamine and the protective effect of prostacyclin: an experimental study in dogs. *Ann Thorac Surg* 1986;**42**:168-71.
76. Mochizuki T, Olson PJ, Szlam F, Ramsay JG, Levy JH. Protamine reversal of heparin affects platelet aggregation and activated clotting time after cardiopulmonary bypass. *Anesth Analg* 1998;**87**:781-5.
77. Cobel-Geard RJ, Hassouna HI. Interaction of protamine sulfate with thrombin. *Am J Hematol* 1983;**14**:227-33.
78. Teoh KH, Young E, Blackall MH, Roberts RS, Hirsh J. Can extra protamine eliminate heparin rebound following cardiopulmonary bypass surgery? *J Thorac Cardiovasc Surg* 2004;**128**:211-9.
79. Warkentin TE, Greinacher A. Heparin-induced thrombocytopenia: recognition, treatment, and prevention: the Seventh ACCP Conference on Antithrombotic and Thrombolytic Therapy. *Chest* 2004;**126**:311S-37.
80. Stanton Jr PE, Evans JR, Lefemine AA, Vo NM, Rannick GA, Morgan Jr CV, et al. White clot syndrome. *South Med J* 1988;**81**:616-20.
81. Warkentin TE, Kelton JG. Delayed-onset heparin-induced thrombocytopenia and thrombosis. *Ann Intern Med* 2001;**135**:502-6.
82. Warkentin TE, Kelton JG. Temporal aspects of heparin-induced thrombocytopenia. *N Engl J Med* 2001;**344**:1286-92.
83. Warkentin TE, Sheppard JA, Sigouin CS, Kohlmann T, Eichler P, Greinacher A. Gender imbalance and risk factor interactions in heparin-induced thrombocytopenia. *Blood* 2006;**108**:2937-41.
84. Cines DB, Rauova L, Arepally G, Reilly MP, McKenzie SE, Sachais BS, Poncz M. Heparin-induced thrombocytopenia: an autoimmune disorder regulated through dynamic autoantigen assembly/disassembly. *J Clin Apher* 2007;**22**:31-6.
85. Warkentin TE, Sheppard JA, Horsewood P, Simpson PJ, Moore JC, Kelton JG. Impact of the patient population on the risk for heparin-induced thrombocytopenia. *Blood* 2000;**96**:1703-8.
86. Potzsch B, Klovekorn WP, Madlener K. Use of heparin during cardiopulmonary bypass in patients with a history of heparin-induced thrombocytopenia. *N Engl J Med* 2000;**343**:515.
87. Horrow JC. Protamine allergy. *J Cardiothorac Anesth* 1988;**2**:225-42.
88. Gottschlich GM, Gravlee GP, Georgitis JW. Adverse reactions to protamine sulfate during cardiac surgery in diabetic and non-diabetic patients. *Ann Allergy* 1988;**61**:277-81.
89. Stewart WJ, McSweeney SM, Kellett MA, Faxon DP, Ryan TJ. Increased risk of severe protamine reactions in NPH insulin-dependent diabetics undergoing cardiac catheterization. *Circulation* 1984;**70**:788-92.
90. Weiss ME, Nyhan D, Peng ZK, Horrow JC, Lowenstein E, Hirshman C, Adkinson Jr NF. Association of protamine IgE and IgG antibodies with life-threatening reactions to intravenous protamine. *N Engl J Med* 1989;**320**:886-92.
91. Best N, Sinosich MJ, Teisner B, Grudzinskas JG, Fisher MM. Complement activation during cardiopulmonary bypass by heparin-protamine interaction. *Br J Anaesth* 1984;**56**:339-43.
92. Kirklin JK, Chenoweth DE, Naftel DC, Blackstone EH, Kirklin JW, Bitran DD, et al. Effects of protamine administration after cardiopulmonary bypass on complement, blood elements, and the hemodynamic state. *Ann Thorac Surg* 1986;**41**:193-9.
93. Morel DR, Zapol WM, Thomas SJ, Kitain EM, Robinson DR, Moss J, et al. C5a and thromboxane generation associated with pulmonary vaso- and broncho-constriction during protamine reversal of heparin. *Anesthesiology* 1987;**66**: 597-604.
94. Conzen PF, Habazettl H, Gutmann R, Hobbhahn J, Goetz AE, Peter K, Brendel W. Thromboxane mediation of pulmonary hemodynamic responses after neutralization of heparin by protamine in pigs. *Anesth Analg* 1989;**68**:25-31.
95. Horrow JC, Pharo GH, Levit LS, Freeland C. Neither skin tests nor serum enzyme-linked immunosorbent assay tests provide specificity for protamine allergy. *Anesth Analg* 1996;**82**:386-9.
96. Levy JH, Cormack JG, Morales A. Heparin neutralization by recombinant platelet factor 4 and protamine. *Anesth Analg* 1995;**81**:35-7.
97. Kikura M, Lee MK, Levy JH. Heparin neutralization with methylene blue, hexadimethrine, or vancomycin after cardiopulmonary bypass. *Anesth Analg* 1996;**83**:223-7.
98. Heres EK, Horrow JC, Gravlee GP, Tardiff BE, Luber Jr J, Schneider J, et al. A dose-determining trial of heparinase-I (Neutralase) for heparin neutralization in coronary artery surgery. *Anesth Analg* 2001;**93**:1446-52; table of contents.
99. Zwischenberger JB, Vertrees RA, Brunston Jr RL, Tao W, Alpard SK, Brown Jr PS. Application of a heparin removal device in patients with known protamine hypersensitivity. *J Thorac Cardiovasc Surg* 1998;**115**:729-31.
100. Kucuk O, Kwaan HC, Frederickson J, Wade L, Green D. Increased fibrinolytic activity in patients undergoing cardiopulmonary bypass operation. *Am J Hematol* 1986;**23**:223-9.
101. Bennett-Guerrero E, Sorohan JG, Canada AT, Ayuso L, Newman MF, Reves JG, Mythen MG. Epsilon-aminocaproic acid plasma levels during cardiopulmonary bypass. *Anesth Analg* 1997;**85**:248-51.
102. Horrow JC, Van Riper DF, Strong MD, Grunewald KE, Parmet JL. The dose-response relationship of tranexamic acid. *Anesthesiology* 1995;**82**:383-92.

103. Casati V, Guzzon D, Oppizzi M, Cossolini M, Torri G, Calori G, Alfieri O. Hemostatic effects of aprotinin, tranexamic acid and epsilon-aminocaproic acid in primary cardiac surgery. *Ann Thorac Surg* 1999;**68**:6-7:2252-6; discussion.
104. Hardy JF, Belisle S, Dupont C, Harel F, Robitaille D, Roy M, Gagnon L. Prophylactic tranexamic acid and epsilon-aminocaproic acid for primary myocardial revascularization. *Ann Thorac Surg* 1998;**65**:371-6.
105. Fanashawe MP, Shore-Lesserson L, Reich DL. Two cases of fatal thrombosis after aminocaproic acid therapy and deep hypothermic circulatory arrest. *Anesthesiology* 2001;**95**:1525-7.
106. Levy JH, Pifarre R, Schaff HV, Horrow JC, Albus R, Spiess B, et al. A multicenter, double-blind, placebo-controlled trial of aprotinin for reducing blood loss and the requirement for donor-blood transfusion in patients undergoing repeat coronary artery bypass grafting. *Circulation* 1995;**92**:2236-44.
107. Liu B, Tengborn L, Larson G, Radberg LO, Belboul A, Dernevik L, Roberts D. Half-dose aprotinin preserves hemostatic function in patients undergoing bypass operations. *Ann Thorac Surg* 1995;**59**:1534-40.
108. Schonberger JP, Everts PA, Ercan H, Bredee JJ, Bavinck JH, Berreklouw E, Wildevuur CR. Low-dose aprotinin in internal mammary artery bypass operations contributes to important blood saving. *Ann Thorac Surg* 1992;**54**:1172-6.
109. Shaw AD, Stafford-Smith M, White WD, Phillips-Bute B, Swaminathan M, Milano C, et al. The effect of aprotinin on outcome after coronary-artery bypass grafting. *N Engl J Med* 2008;**358**:784-93.
110. Brown JR, Birkmeyer NJ, O'Connor GT. Meta-analysis comparing the effectiveness and adverse outcomes of antifibrinolytic agents in cardiac surgery. *Circulation* 2007;**115**:2801-13.
111. Mangano DT, Tudor IC, Dietzel C. The risk associated with aprotinin in cardiac surgery. *N Engl J Med* 2006;**354**:353-65.
112. Lemmer Jr JH, Stanford W, Bonney SL, Chomka EV, Karp RB, Laub GW, et al. Aprotinin for coronary artery bypass grafting: effect on postoperative renal function. *Ann Thorac Surg* 1995;**59**:132-6.
113. Dietrich W, Busley R, Boulesteix AL. Effects of aprotinin dosage on renal function: an analysis of 8,548 cardiac surgical patients treated with different dosages of aprotinin. *Anesthesiology* 2008;**108**:189-98.
114. Furnary AP, Wu Y, Hiratzka LF, Grunkemeier GL, Page 3rd US. Aprotinin does not increase the risk of renal failure in cardiac surgery patients. *Circulation* 2007;**116**:I127-33.
115. Lemmer Jr JH, Metzdorff MT, Krause AH, Okies JE, Molloy TA, Hill JG, et al. Aprotinin use in patients with dialysis-dependent renal failure undergoing cardiac operations. *J Thorac Cardiovasc Surg* 1996;**112**:192-4.
116. Maslow AD, Chaudrey A, Bert A, Schwartz C, Singh A. Perioperative renal outcome in cardiac surgical patients with preoperative renal dysfunction: aprotinin versus epsilon aminocaproic acid. *J Cardiothorac Vasc Anesth* 2008;**22**:6-15.
117. Sundt 3rd TM, Kouchoukos NT, Saffitz JE, Murphy SF, Wareing TH, Stahl DJ. Renal dysfunction and intravascular coagulation with aprotinin and hypothermic circulatory arrest. *Ann Thorac Surg* 1993;**55**:1418-24.
118. Eaton MP, Deeb GM. Aprotinin versus epsilon-aminocaproic acid for aortic surgery using deep hypothermic circulatory arrest. *J Cardiothorac Vasc Anesth* 1998;**12**:548-52.
119. Okita Y, Takamoto S, Ando M, Morota T, Yamaki F, Kawashima Y. Is use of aprotinin safe with deep hypothermic circulatory arrest in aortic surgery? investigations on blood coagulation. *Circulation* 1996;**94**:II177-81.
120. Seigne PW, Shorten GD, Johnson RG, Comunale ME. The effects of aprotinin on blood product transfusion associated with thoracic aortic surgery requiring deep hypothermic circulatory arrest. *J Cardiothorac Vasc Anesth* 2000;**14**:676-81.
121. Schneeweiss S, Seeger JD, Landon J, Walker AM. Aprotinin during coronary-artery bypass grafting and risk of death. *N Engl J Med* 2008;**358**:771-83.
122. Fergusson DA, Hebert PC, Mazer CD, Fremes S, MacAdams C, Murkin JM, et al. A comparison of aprotinin and lysine analogues in high-risk cardiac surgery. *N Engl J Med* 2008;**358**:2319-31.
123. Dietrich W, Spath P, Ebell A, Richter JA. Prevalence of anaphylactic reactions to aprotinin: analysis of two hundred forty-eight reexposures to aprotinin in heart operations. *J Thorac Cardiovasc Surg* 1997;**113**:194-201.
124. Dietrich W, Ebell A, Busley R, Boulesteix AL. Aprotinin and anaphylaxis: analysis of 12,403 exposures to aprotinin in cardiac surgery. *Ann Thorac Surg* 2007;**84**:1144-50.
125. Nemoto EM, Klementavicius R, Melick JA, Yonas H. Suppression of cerebral metabolic rate for oxygen (CMRO2) by mild hypothermia compared with thiopental. *J Neurosurg Anesthesiol* 1996;**8**:52-9.
126. Nemoto EM, Klementavicius R, Melick JA, Yonas H. Effect of mild hypothermia on active and basal cerebral oxygen metabolism and blood flow. *Adv Exp Med Biol* 1994;**361**:469-73.
127. Steen PA, Newberg L, Milde JH, Michenfelder JD. Hypothermia and barbiturates: individual and combined effects on canine cerebral oxygen consumption. *Anesthesiology* 1983;**58**:527-32.
128. Todd MM, Warner DS. A comfortable hypothesis reevaluated: cerebral metabolic depression and brain protection during ischemia. *Anesthesiology* 1992;**76**:161-4.
129. Warner DS. Isoflurane neuroprotection: a passing fantasy, again? *Anesthesiology* 2000;**92**:1226-8.
130. Grady RE, Weglinski MR, Sharbrough FW, Perkins WJ. Correlation of regional cerebral blood flow with ischemic electroencephalographic changes during sevoflurane-nitrous oxide anesthesia for carotid endarterectomy. *Anesthesiology* 1998;**88**:892-7.
131. Michenfelder JD, Sundt TM, Fode N, Sharbrough FW. Isoflurane when compared to enflurane and halothane decreases the frequency of cerebral ischemia during carotid endarterectomy. *Anesthesiology* 1987;**67**:336-40.
132. Patel PM, Drummond JC, Cole DJ, Goskowicz RL. Isoflurane reduces ischemia-induced glutamate release in rats subjected to forebrain ischemia. *Anesthesiology* 1995;**82**:996-1003.
133. Miao N, Frazer MJ, Lynch 3rd C. Volatile anesthetics depress Ca^{2+} transients and glutamate release in isolated cerebral synaptosomes. *Anesthesiology* 1995;**83**:593-603.
134. Overand PT, Teply JF. Vasopressin for the treatment of refractory hypotension after cardiopulmonary bypass. *Anesth Analg* 1998;**86**:1207-9.
135. Butterworth 4th JF, Hines RL, Royster RL, James RL. A pharmacokinetic and pharmacodynamic evaluation of milrinone in adults undergoing cardiac surgery. *Anesth Analg* 1995;**81**:783-92.
136. Cheng DC. Fast track cardiac surgery pathways: early extubation, process of care, and cost containment. *Anesthesiology* 1998;**88**:1429-33.
137. Hickey RF, Cason BA. Timing of tracheal extubation in adult cardiac surgery patients. *J Card Surg* 1995;**10**:340-8.
138. Murphy GS, Szokol JW, Marymont JH, Avram MJ, Vender JS, Rosengart TK. Impact of shorter-acting neuromuscular blocking agents on fast-track recovery of the cardiac surgical patient. *Anesthesiology* 2002;**96**:600-6.
139. Ouattara A, Richard L, Charriere JM, Lanquetot H, Corbi P, Debaene B. Use of cisatracurium during fast-track cardiac surgery. *Br J Anaesth* 2001;**86**:130-2.
140. Thomas R, Smith D, Strike P. Prospective randomised double-blind comparative study of rocuronium and pancuronium in adult patients scheduled for elective "fast-track" cardiac surgery involving hypothermic cardiopulmonary bypass. *Anaesthesia* 2003;**58**:265-71.
141. Bettex DA, Schmidlin D, Chassot PG, Schmid ER. Intrathecal sufentanil-morphine shortens the duration of intubation and improves analgesia in fast-track cardiac surgery. *Can J Anaesth* 2002;**49**:711-7.
142. Leslie K, Sessler DI. The implications of hypothermia for early tracheal extubation following cardiac surgery. *J Cardiothorac Vasc Anesth* 1998;**12**:41-4:30-4; discussion.
143. Montes FR, Sanchez SI, Giraldo JC, Rincon JD, Rincon IE, Vanegas MV, Charris H. The lack of benefit of tracheal extubation in the operating room after coronary artery bypass surgery. *Anesth Analg* 2000;**91**:776-80.
144. London MJ, Shroyer AL, Jernigan V, Fullerton DA, Wilcox D, Baltz J, et al. Fast-track cardiac surgery in a Department of Veterans Affairs patient population. *Ann Thorac Surg* 1997;**64**:134-41.
145. Silbert BS, Santamaria JD, O'Brien JL, Blyth CM, Kelly WJ, Molnar RR. Early extubation following coronary artery bypass surgery: a prospective randomized controlled trial. The Fast Track Cardiac Care Team. *Chest* 1998;**113**:1481-8.
146. Cheng DC, Wall C, Djaiani G, Peragallo RA, Carroll J, Li C, Naylor D. Randomized assessment of resource use in fast-track cardiac surgery 1-year after hospital discharge. *Anesthesiology* 2003;**98**:651-7.
147. Michelsen LG, Horswell J. Anesthesia for off-pump coronary artery bypass grafting. *Semin Thorac Cardiovasc Surg* 2003;**15**:71-82.
148. Carrier M, Robitaille D, Perrault LP, Pellerin M, Page P, Cartier R, Bouchard D. Heparin versus danaparoid in off-pump coronary bypass grafting: results of a prospective randomized clinical trial. *J Thorac Cardiovasc Surg* 2003;**125**:325-9.
149. Donias HW, D'Ancona G, Pande RU, Schimpf D, Kawaguchi AT, Karamanoukian HL. Heparin dose, transfusion rates, and intraoperative graft patency in minimally invasive direct coronary artery bypass. *Heart Surg Forum* 2003;**6**:176-80.
150. Chaney MA. Anaesthetic management of port-access minimally invasive cardiac surgery. *J Indian Med Assoc* 1999;**97**:425-7:31.
151. Ganapathy S. Anaesthesia for minimally invasive cardiac surgery. *Best Pract Res Clin Anaesthesiol* 2002;**16**:63-80.
152. Applebaum RM, Cutler WM, Bhardwaj N, Colvin SB, Galloway AC, Ribakove GH, et al. Utility of transesophageal echocardiography during port-access minimally invasive cardiac surgery. *Am J Cardiol* 1998;**82**:183-8.
153. Mierdl S, Meininger D, Byhahn C, Aybek T, Kessler P, Westphal K. Transesophageal echocardiography or fluoroscopy during port-access surgery? *Ann Acad Med Singapore* 2002;**31**:520-4.

154. Mahmood F, Karthik S, Subramaniam B, Panzica PJ, Mitchell J, Lerner AB, et al. Intraoperative application of geometric three-dimensional mitral valve assessment package: a feasibility study. *J Cardiothorac Vasc Anesth* 2008;**22**:292-8.
155. Czibik G, D'Ancona G, Donias HW, Karamanoukian HL. Robotic cardiac surgery: present and future applications. *J Cardiothorac Vasc Anesth* 2002;**16**:495-501.
156. D'Attellis N, Loulmet D, Carpentier A, Berrebi A, Cardon C, Severac-Bastide R, et al. Robotic-assisted cardiac surgery: anesthetic and postoperative considerations. *J Cardiothorac Vasc Anesth* 2002;**16**:397-400.
157. Chitwood Jr WR, Nifong LW. Minimally invasive videoscopic mitral valve surgery: the current role of surgical robotics. *J Card Surg* 2000;**15**:61-75.
158. Reichenspurner H, Boehm DH, Gulbins H, Schulze C, Wildhirt S, Welz A, et al. Three-dimensional video and robot-assisted port-access mitral valve operation. *Ann Thorac Surg* 2000;**69**:81-2:1176-81; discussion.

CHAPTER 61
Critical Care for the Adult Cardiac Patient

Edward Cantu III, Carmelo A. Milano, and Peter K. Smith

Immediate Postoperative Care
  Initial Evaluation
    Airway and Ventilation
    Initial Electrocardiogram
    Peripheral Perfusion
    Abdominal Examination
    Genitourinary Examination
    Neurologic Examination
    Initial Cardiac Auscultation
    Body Temperature
    Hemodynamics
    Lines
    Chest Tubes
    Initial Chest Radiograph
  Cardiac Surgery with Cardiopulmonary Bypass
  Cardiac Surgery without Cardiopulmonary Bypass

Cardiac Dysfunction after Cardiac Surgery
  Low Cardiac Output State
    Output and Filling Pressure
    Oxygen Delivery
  Preload
  Afterload
    Postoperative Effects
    Therapeutic Approaches
  Heart Rate
  Inotropic State
  Cardiac Tamponade
  Vasoplegic Syndrome
  Right Heart Dysfunction
  Arrhythmias
    Atrial Flutter
    Atrial Fibrillation
    Ventricular Arrhythmias
Graft Occlusion

Intraoperative Injury and Graft Occlusion
Postoperative Bleeding
  Coagulopathy
    Heparin Effect
    Thrombocytopenia
    Thrombasthenia
    Specific Factor Deficiencies
  Management of Bleeding
  Blood Conservation
Pharmacologic Considerations
  Desmopressin
  Aprotinin
  ε-Aminocaproic Acid
  Recombinant Activated Factor VII
Neurologic Complications
Infection
  Fever
  Evaluation and Treatment

The purpose of this chapter is to familiarize the caregiver with the expected or normal course after adult cardiac surgery. The management of patients immediately after cardiac surgery is described, using a systematic approach. In addition, the common and important side effects or complications of cardiac surgery are described, and their managements are reviewed. The references provided support management strategies and approaches to common postoperative complications, and they give a more detailed analysis of particular problems. The chapter focuses on common management strategies and complications and is not meant to be comprehensive.

IMMEDIATE POSTOPERATIVE CARE

Initial Evaluation

A systematic evaluation of the patient should be performed immediately on arrival in the intensive care unit. Communication with the surgical and anesthesia team should provide an overview of the procedure performed, the response of the cardiovascular system to the procedure, intraoperative hemodynamic management, and current medications.

The patient's comorbid conditions and allergies should be ascertained and confirmed with the team members who have evaluated the awake and alert patient. Although attention may be focused initially on one aspect of the patient's condition (hypotension on arrival, e.g.), it is critical to develop a systematic approach to evaluation. The patient's outcome depends on the coordinated and efficient delivery of care, and dysfunction of any element of the support system can be rapidly fatal. Surgical dressings must be kept intact during the first 48 hours for infection control. If they must be disturbed for diagnostic purposes, strict aseptic technique should be followed.

Airway and Ventilation

Adequacy of ventilation and absence of tension pneumothorax should be confirmed. The trachea should be palpated and confirmed to be in the midline, and breath sounds should be auscultated bilaterally. The ventilator should be functioning normally and without alarms—if it is not, the patient should be immediately converted to hand-controlled ventilation. The peak inspiratory pressure should be noted so that changes in chest wall and pulmonary mechanics can be correctly interpreted later in the course of recovery. High inspiratory pressures may indicate a tension pneumothorax, inappropriate ventilator settings, or severe pulmonary or chest wall restriction. Pulse oximetry, mixed venous oximetry, and direct measurement of arterial gas tensions are used to confirm adequate oxygen delivery and CO_2 elimination.

Initial Electrocardiogram

The initial electrocardiogram (ECG) can be difficult to interpret because of lead placement changes related to surgical dressings, cardiac pacing, and the common presence of conduction abnormalities. Right bundle branch block and first-degree atrioventricular (AV) block occur frequently but usually resolve in the first few postoperative hours. Establishing and maintaining normal sinus rhythm with an adequate rate is particularly important in the early postoperative period, when cardiac function may be impaired because of intraoperative ischemia or because of temporary diastolic dysfunction resulting from myocardial edema.

First-degree AV block can result in substantial reduction in the instantaneous end-diastolic left ventricular volume, which determines stroke volume. The use of atrial or AV sequential pacing can overcome these transient derangements, and, in the latter instance, it is common to see improved cardiac function with normalization of the AV interval despite abnormal ventricular activation with the ventricular pacing component.

Atrial fibrillation is poorly tolerated in the first postoperative day, and every effort should be made to maintain sinus rhythm, even in patients who had chronic atrial fibrillation preoperatively. Immediate cardioversion is often required in the intensive care unit (ICU), although atrial fibrillation occurring on the third postoperative day or later is usually well tolerated.

Ventricular arrhythmias may result from early graft failure or coronary spasm, which should be ruled out. A malpositioned pulmonary artery catheter irritating the right ventricular (RV) outflow tract is more easily correctable. Arrhythmias may have many contributing factors (e.g., hypothermia, electrolyte derangement, acid–base imbalances, drug side effects), which must be considered and addressed.

Peripheral Perfusion

The adequacy of global and regional perfusion should be assessed by physical examination of the vascular system, including examination of accessible pulse character and the quality of skin and soft tissue perfusion. Intraoperative embolization, vascular injury, or low cardiac output in the setting of peripheral vascular disease may compromise limb viability.

Abdominal Examination

Abdominal examination will reveal the presence of bowel sounds and a well-positioned nasogastric tube. Exclusion of masses, unsuspected hepatomegaly, or generalized abdominal distention should be documented.

Genitourinary Examination

Correct placement of the indwelling urinary catheter should be confirmed and both phimosis and paraphimosis excluded. Urine should be clear, not concentrated, and free of hemoglobin or frank blood.

Neurologic Examination

Evaluation of the patient's neurologic status should be performed frequently until ensured to be unchanged. Uncontrollable hypertension or extreme variability of peripheral vascular resistance may result from severe neurologic injury initially ascribed to a residual anesthetic agent.

Initial Cardiac Auscultation

The cardiac examination should document normal heart sounds and the character of any murmurs. This is very important in patients who have had valve replacement.

Body Temperature

Initial hypothermia is the rule, and it is best avoided by expeditious surgery and adequate rewarming while the patient is on cardiopulmonary bypass. Hypothermia compromises cardiac function, causes shivering and excessive metabolic demand, interferes with normal coagulation, and can aggravate or cause rhythm disturbances.[1] Blankets and other auxiliary warming devices should be employed, particularly in the bleeding patient receiving cold intravenous solutions and blood products. Fever, particularly in the early postoperative period, is poorly tolerated. It should be treated aggressively with antipyretics and possibly with intravenous steroids if there is hemodynamic compromise.

Hemodynamics

With appropriate cardiac rhythm, the patient should have a cardiac index of greater than 2 L/min/m^2 with blood pressure adequate for the patient. This requires consideration of the patient's age, preoperative blood pressure, and renal function. The importance of generating adequate cardiac output has been established by several studies with mortality as the outcome variable. Acceptance of lower cardiac output occasionally results in good outcome when associated with reasonable mixed venous oxygen saturation (MV_{O_2}) (>55%), adequate urine output (>20 mL/hr without stimulation), and evidence of good peripheral and central perfusion (physical examination, maintenance of acid–base balance). There is no evidence that supranormal cardiac output is beneficial.

Elevated central venous pressure, especially when associated with facial edema or facial discoloration, must be aggressively evaluated. Possible causes include cardiac tamponade, general fluid overload, or technical errors that have compromised superior vena caval flow. Elevated pulmonary artery pressures may indicate left ventricular (LV) dysfunction or cardiac tamponade, or may be related to preoperative changes in pulmonary vascular resistance. All central pressures should be related to initial values obtained during preoperative invasive monitoring and to those obtained after completion of surgery but before transfer to the ICU. These measurements are also quite sensitive to afterload, which can vary widely and rapidly in the early postoperative course in patients who are often hypovolemic. Elevation of intrathoracic pressure can frequently mimic cardiac failure in the patient with chest wall rigidity because of emergence from anesthetic effect and shivering. The latter process can increase metabolic demand and reduce MV_{O_2} to very low levels.

Lines

All indwelling lines must be confirmed to be functional, particularly those delivering vasoactive drugs. Transport of the patient can partially or completely dislodge intravenous lines, many of which were outside the drape and unobserved during surgery. Hemodynamic instability resulting from failure of drug delivery and tissue injury resulting from drug infiltration must be avoided.

Chest Tubes

Mediastinal and pleural space tubes are always placed to underwater seal and are usually set to have -20 cm H_2O suction applied. Mediastinal tubes should be examined for the amount and nature of drainage. The initial amount of drained blood should be less than 100 mL, and larger amounts should be explained by the surgical team. The initial rate of drainage may reflect drainage of blood or irrigation fluid that has accumulated, particularly in the left thoracic gutter. Nonetheless, an initial assessment of the bleeding rate, quality of blood clotting in the tubes, correlation of drainage with intravascular volume replacement, and tube patency is critically important.

Initial Chest Radiograph

A portable chest radiograph should be obtained immediately on arrival and must be interpreted by the responsible physicians as soon as available. Critical aspects include (1) position of the endotracheal tube, (2) pneumothorax and mediastinal shift, (3) lobar atelectasis, (4) pleural and extrapleural fluid collections, (5) size of the mediastinal silhouette, (6) correct intravascular location of invasive lines and catheters, and (7) normal position of radiopaque markers, sternal wires, and drainage tubes.

Cardiac Surgery with Cardiopulmonary Bypass

Cardiopulmonary bypass (CPB) induces many of the physiologic changes apparent in the postoperative patient, and its duration is a primary determinant of the rapidity of recovery. CPB nonspecifically activates the inflammatory system.[2] This phenomenon begins with the interaction of heparinized blood and the bypass circuit.[3,4] Generalized complement activation is seen, with elevations in C3a and C5a anaphylatoxins after discontinuation of CPB.[3,5-9] This activation can lead to pulmonary sequestration of leukocytes[3,6,10] and the production of superoxides and other products of lipoxygenation. This causes further leukocyte activation and the generation of leukotactic circulating factors that increase the local inflammatory response.[11,12] Elevations in tumor necrosis factor, interleukin (IL)-1, and prostaglandin E_1 have been described.[13-15] The generalized inflammatory reaction seen after CPB may change vascular permeability and cause pulmonary hypertension as well as bronchial hyperreactivity.[16] Together with transient elevations in left atrial pressure, reduced oncotic pressure from hemodilution and increased vascular permeability also contribute to increased pulmonary shunt from the resultant extravascular water.[17]

Cellular components that play a significant role in inflammatory response to CPB include circulating cells (platelets, neutrophils, monocytes) and regulatory cells (endothelial cells).

Platelets are activated by shear forces, heparin, foreign surfaces, and activated thrombin. Thrombin is a potent platelet agonist. Despite full anticoagulation with heparin, thrombin continues to be generated.[18,19] The clinical consequences of platelet activation include generation of microemboli, thrombosis, and bleeding by diminution of platelet number and function.[20] Additionally, vasoactive substances may be liberated from platelets in response to CPB or protamine infusion, which can cause pulmonary hypertension and systemic hypotension.[21]

Neutrophil activation occurs consequent to the complex interaction of blood with the CPB circuit. Proinflammatory mediators (e.g., IL-1, -2, -6, and -8 and tumor necrosis factor alpha [TNFα]), complement anaphylatoxins (C3a and C5a), platelet-activating factor (PAF), and leukotriene-B4 (LTB4) increase the number of cell surface adhesion molecules and promote neutrophil adhesion to the pulmonary endothelium. Neutrophil adherence and transmigration into the lung occurs under the influence of IL-8. Proteolytic enzyme and oxygen free radical release from activated neutrophils promote further tissue injury and inflammatory activation of endothelial cells.[22]

Endothelial cells are a central player in inflammation and coagulation. Specific agonists responsible for endothelial activation have been characterized and include IL-1β, TNFα, C5a, and thrombin.[9,23] Endothelial cell activation results in a procoagulant, vasoconstrictive, and proinflammatory response. Once activated, the anticoagulant properties of the endothelial cell are dramatically reduced, with loss of heparan sulfate proteoglycan, conformational changes in the endothelial cell (which result in increased exposure to tissue factor and von Willebrand's factor in the cellular submatrix), increased expression of tissue factor and plasminogen activator inhibitor type 1, and loss of thrombomodulin. The vasoconstrictive effects occur through the production of endothelin-1 and thromboxane A2. Proinflammatory changes are seen with increased expression of P and E selectins and consequent recruitment and sequestration of inflammatory cells.[4]

A specific manifestation of the inflammatory response in cardiothoracic surgery is the post-pericardiotomy syndrome.[24] This syndrome, occurring in 10% to 30% of patients, is a self-limited condition beginning in the second or third week after surgery. It is associated with fever and pleuritic, precordial, or substernal chest pain.[25] Chest radiographs in patients with post-pericardiotomy syndrome commonly show pleural and pericardial effusions (Fig. 61-1). This syndrome has been associated with specific reactive antibodies and may be seen after any operation that violates the pericardium.[25,26] It is treated with nonsteroidal anti-inflammatory agents, although corticosteroids may be necessary in severe cases.[27,28]

Cardiac Surgery without Cardiopulmonary Bypass

On-pump coronary artery bypass surgery has been demonstrated to reduce symptoms and prolong life; however, this still comes at some cost. Neurocognitive dysfunction (50% to 75%), atrial fibrillation (30%), transfusion (30% to 90%), stroke (2%), and death (2% to 5%) continue to temper the success of conventional coronary artery bypass surgery.[29] Because CPB is perhaps the most invasive aspect of conventional coronary revascularization, and because morbidity of coronary revascularization can been attributed to the bypass circuit, hypothermic cardiac arrest, aortic cannulation, and cross-clamping,[30] surgeons are now using advanced stabilizing devices to perform coronary anastomoses on the beating heart without CPB. With this approach, through a standard sternotomy incision and with available stabilizing systems, complete revascularization of all three coronary distributions can be performed with the heart beating. The term *off-pump*

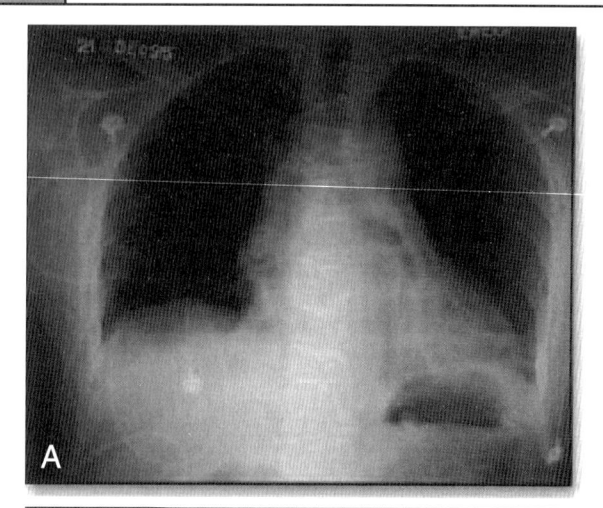

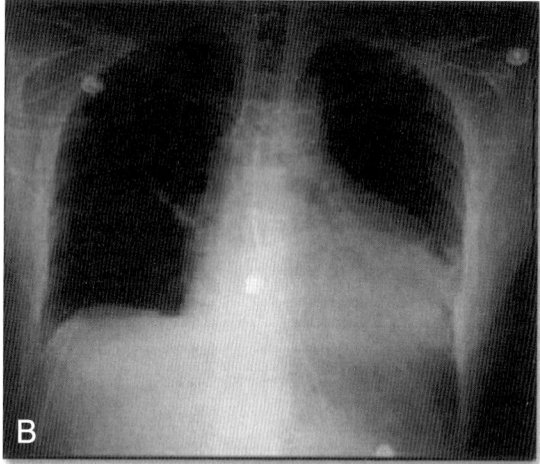

Figure 61-1
Post-pericardiotomy syndrome is commonly associated with pericardial and pleural effusions. **A,** Chest radiograph on a patient soon after aortic valve replacement shows expected postoperative findings. **B,** Chest radiograph 2 weeks later shows pericardial effusion compatible with the clinical symptoms of post-pericardiotomy syndrome.

coronary artery bypass (OPCAB) generally refers to multivessel coronary artery bypass performed off the CPB machine, through a standard sternotomy. This approach has achieved considerable support, with between 20% and 25% of coronary surgery in the United States being performed in this manner.[31] Some individual surgeons or institutions are now performing the majority of coronary revascularization procedures without CPB. Although initially a number of cases were considered inappropriate for OPCAB techniques, more and more of these have been successfully performed in this manner. For example, cases of re-do coronary grafting and complete arterial grafting have been successfully performed as OPCABs. Many surgeons, however, still view intramyocardial coronary arteries and severe LV dysfunction as strong contraindications to OPCAB.

There are specific differences between OPCAB and conventional on-pump revascularization procedures, which ultimately impact the patient's recovery. During OPCAB procedures, coronary arteries are individually snared proximally and occluded during the performance of the coronary anastomosis. Depending on whether intracoronary shunts are used, there may be periods of local ischemia without cardioplegic arrest. However, unlike in the conventional on-pump procedures, there are no periods of aortic cross-clamping and global cardiac arrest. For these reasons, the degree of myocardial stunting during OPCABs may be reduced relative to on-pump procedures. Furthermore, during OPCABs, normothermic pulsatile flow is maintained throughout the procedure, whereas conventional on-pump procedures include a period of nonpulsatile perfusion (while on CPB) and generally some degree of systemic cooling and rewarming. Finally, although both techniques require anticoagulation with heparin, many centers practice reduced-heparin dosing for OPCAB. Initially, OPCAB techniques resulted in longer total operating room (OR) times, but as these procedures have become more common, predictably OR times have been reduced and some surgeons now argue that OPCAB can be performed faster than equivalent on-pump procedures.

Although OPCAB procedures are ultimately focused on reduction of morbidity and mortality, initial studies have sought to confirm equivalent operative mortality and graft patency relative to conventional on-pump procedures. These early studies included low-risk, highly selected patients undergoing one- or two-vessel bypass.[30]

Despite many randomized controlled trials and three meta-analyses, the issue of off-pump versus on-pump myocardial revascularization has not been definitively addressed and remains an area of controversy. Proponents stress that OPCAB decreases the odds of postoperative atrial fibrillation by up to 42%, transfusions by up to 57%, need for inotropes by up to 52%, neurocognitive dysfunction at 2 to 6 months by up to 44%, and average hospital length of stay by up to 1 day at no measurable risk to the patient.[30] However, the concern that fewer grafts tend to be performed with OPCAB than with standard coronary artery bypass graft (CABG) surgery,[30] and that freedom from revascularization favors on-pump CABG has tempered global adoption of the OPCAB technique.[32,33] Given our current understanding, a consensus statement has been published by the International Society for Minimally Invasive Cardiothoracic Surgery to better define current practices. They suggest OPCAB is a safe alternative to conventional CABG and should be considered specifically in high-risk patients undergoing surgical revascularization and in patients with specifically identified risk factors to reduce perioperative mortality, morbidity, and resource utilization.[34]

As mentioned, conventional cardiac surgery results in a significant inflammatory response. This response appears to be a nonspecific response that includes complement and leukocyte activation.[2,3,5-7,10-12] Although the exact mechanism of activation is unclear, the strongest stimulant for the response is the blood–artificial surface contact that occurs with CPB. This response can be modified by coating the tubing and oxygenator surfaces with biological materials, and by improving the hemodynamic performance of the system. Theoretically, by eliminating the heart-lung machine entirely, this response could be significantly reduced.

At least two studies have now investigated the inflammatory response during heart surgery, comparing groups in which coronary revascularization is performed with and without CPB.[35,36] Angelini and colleagues[37] looked at four important inflammatory markers: neutrophil elastase (an endopeptidase released with neutrophil activation), IL-8 (a potent neutrophil chemotactic and activating factor), and C3a and C5a (fragments generated with activation of the common complement pathway). These markers were measured at four time-points within the first 24 hours postoperatively. Patients were randomized to two groups: coronary revascularization with CPB and standard cardioplegic arrest, and OPCAB. The OPCAB group demonstrated significantly lower levels of all four markers and had reduced leukocyte, neutrophil, and monocyte counts. Together, these findings strongly support a reduced inflammatory response with OPCAB. The clinical significance of this difference is unclear, because by 4 hours the activated complement components have decreased in the on-pump group to OPCAB levels, which interestingly are still higher than baseline.[38] Ideally, larger prospective randomized trials will help determine the clinical impact of reduced inflammatory response.

Coagulopathy and postoperative bleeding represent a major morbidity for cardiac surgery patients. Many surgeons believe that OPCAB procedures will help to reduce these problems. OPCAB requires less intraoperative anticoagulation and avoids blood–artificial surface contact, which should reduce platelet activation and destruction. Furthermore, systemic cooling that may further impact negatively on coagulation function can be avoided with OPCAB. Several studies have compared on-pump procedures to OPCAB and report significant reduction in postoperative bleeding, reduced need for perioperative transfusion, and reduced rate of take-back for bleeding.[39] Indeed, when coagulation and fibrinolysis variables have been studied, marked changes in fibrinolytic and coagulation variables occur within the first 24 hours. Conventional on-pump revascularization causes a transient decrease in the platelet count, fibrinogen level, and activation of plasminogen with increased D-dimer formation, which only after 24 hours approximate the levels seen in OPCAB.[40] Furthermore, a few studies[41,42] have compared the differences seen between OPCAB and conventional revascularization with respect to platelet activation and endothelial activation, and they have not demonstrated any significant differences in platelet function or endothelial activation markers.[38]

CARDIAC DYSFUNCTION AFTER CARDIAC SURGERY

Low Cardiac Output State

Output and Filling Pressure

Low cardiac output after CPB has historically been recognized as a cause of sudden death.[43] Low cardiac output resulting from ventricular dysfunction causes a series of adaptive neurohumoral responses, as well as, geometric changes (dilation and hypertrophy) in the heart. Acute loss of 20% to 25% of functioning myocardium[44] causes significant reduction in cardiac output and carries extremely poor short-term[45] and long-term prognoses.[46]

Measurement and therapeutic manipulation of both cardiac output and central filling pressures are critical to the postoperative care of cardiac surgical patients and are predictive of survival (Fig. 61-2).[47] Central pressures, cardiac output, and venous saturation are routinely measured by means of a flow-directed pulmonary artery catheter. The cardiac index (cardiac output expressed as liters per minute per meter squared) has a normal range of 2.1 to 4.9 L/min/m².[48] In adults, a cardiac index of at least 2.0 L/min/m² during the immediate postoperative period is required for normal convalescence.[47]

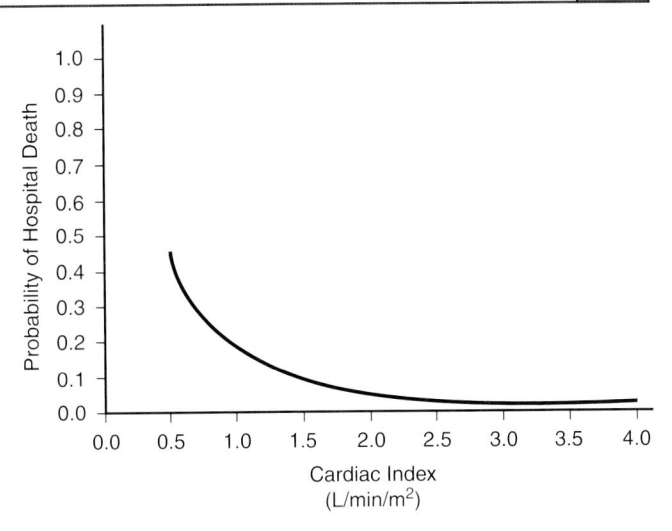

Figure 61-2
The graph shows the relationship between postoperative cardiac index and probability of death for adults after mitral valve replacement. (Reproduced with permission from Kouchoukos NT. Detection and treatment of impaired cardiac performance following cardiac surgery. In: Davila JC, editor. Henry Ford Hospital International Symposium on Cardiac Surgery. 2nd ed. New York: Appleton-Century-Crofts; 1977.)

Oxygen Delivery

Shock is currently conceptualized as a clinical syndrome resulting from an imbalance between tissue oxygen demand and tissue oxygen supply. The general goals of postoperative care are to prevent shock and provide adequate oxygen delivery. Oxygen delivery of less than 335 mL/min/m² has been associated with a decrease in oxygen consumption[49] and with the development of progressive lactic acidosis.[50]

Lactic acidosis has been suggested as a metabolic monitor to correlate with total oxygen debt, the magnitude of hypoperfusion, and the severity of shock.[51-53] However, a direct relationship to total oxygen delivery has been disputed.[54] MVO_2 provides a useful index of the adequacy of circulation and reflects to some extent mean tissue oxygen level.[55] MVO_2 is measured with specialized pulmonary artery catheters, and patients with a saturation of less than 60% or those who demonstrate a decrease of more than 5% suffer more frequent postoperative complications.[56] However, others have shown poor correlation between saturation, or trends in saturation, and outcome.[57] Rapid changes in whole-body oxygen consumption may reduce its overall predictive value.

Adequate regional oxygen delivery is even more difficult to determine. Organ requirements and hormonally activated reflex changes in regional blood supply may occur in the postoperative state. For example, the kidneys, skin, and resting muscles are blood-supply independent and maintain viability by increased oxygen extraction. The heart and brain, on the other hand, are blood-supply dependent, with near maximal oxygen extraction at rest. Sympathetically controlled reflexes compensate for these differences by a shift of blood flow from the skin and splanchnic region at low circulating volumes.[58] Increasingly, the effects of splanchnic hypoperfusion on postoperative complications and persistent acidosis are being recognized.[59] Acute changes in regional blood supply may be mediated by differing degrees of sympathetic innervation to precapillary sphincters and arterioles.[60] Alterations in the metabolic activity are common after

Illustrations for Pulmonary Artery Pressure

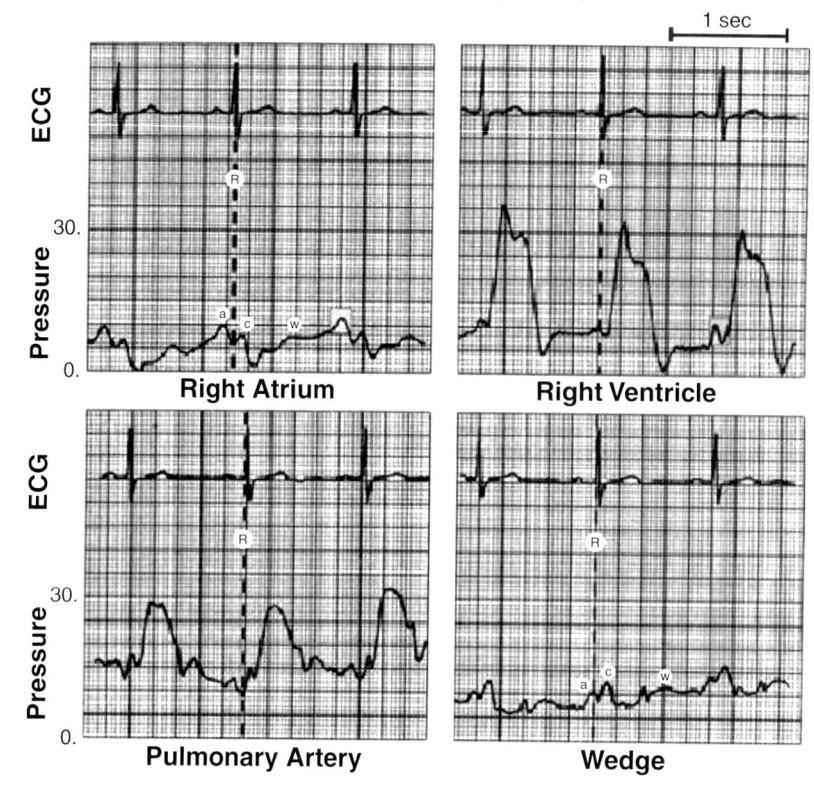

Figure 61-3
Pulmonary artery pressure waveforms recorded from a pulmonary artery catheter as it passes through the right atrium and right ventricle to the pulmonary artery and wedge positions. Right ventricular end-diastolic pressure is measured at the time of the electrocardiographic (ECG) R wave and is estimated best by the right atrial *a* wave pressure peak. The *a*, *c*, and *w* waves are recorded from both the right atrium and pulmonary artery wedge positions. *(Reproduced with permission from Mark JB. Atlas of cardiovascular monitoring. New York: Churchill Livingstone; 1998.)*

heart surgery. These can be monitored through capnography, which determines the partial pressure of CO_2 in expired gases.[61] Rewarming, with subsequent peripheral vasodilation, and shivering have been shown to increase metabolic and circulatory demands[62] and can be eliminated with paralysis and sedation. This promotes hemodynamic stability and decreases the need for inotropic support.[63] Thus, the actual definition of low cardiac output syndrome must include evidence of inadequate oxygen delivery relative to consumption. Clinical evidence of diminished peripheral perfusion and end-organ ischemia must be coupled with the objective measurements of cardiac output and MV_{O_2} to establish the diagnosis.

Preload

Maintenance of adequate preload is fundamental in the postoperative management of cardiac surgical patients (Fig. 61-3). The optimal pulmonary capillary wedge pressure in postoperative cardiac surgical patients is unknown, but a range of 14 to 18 mm Hg has been suggested, with increases in extravascular lung water occurring above this level.[64] Preload correlates directly with the force of ventricular contraction, and the result is a ventricular volume change from end diastole to end systole determined by transmural pressure and compliance of the ventricular wall. Pericardial pressure is normally reflected by the right atrial pressure (Fig. 61-4). However, tight closure of the pericardium may adversely affect transmural pressure and decrease stroke volume.[37,65] Pulmonary artery wedge pressures and the central venous pressure (CVP), indicating LV and RV volumes, respectively, accurately reflect reduced filling pressures, whereas high filling pressures may be determined by changes in transmural pressure or myocardial compliance rather than accurately reflecting preload. Most postoperative cardiac surgical patients are relatively hypovolemic and have a labile reactive vasculature.[66] In the immediate postoperative period, causes of hypovolemia include large urine volumes, ongoing blood loss, and a significant cross-sectional increase in vascular beds with rewarming.

The summation of these physiologic changes is a reduced preload, particularly in the left ventricle. This trend should be anticipated and managed with appropriate volume therapy to prevent precipitous hypotension and low cardiac output. Immediate preload augmentation may be achieved with passive straight leg raising, with transient 8% to 10% increase in cardiac output,[67] although this should be viewed as only a temporizing measure and should be quickly supplanted by appropriate volume administration.

Afterload

Postoperative Effects

After a cardiac operation, elevation in afterload is a well-recognized phenomenon. The incidence varies with cardiac pathology, operative procedure, and definition of the resulting

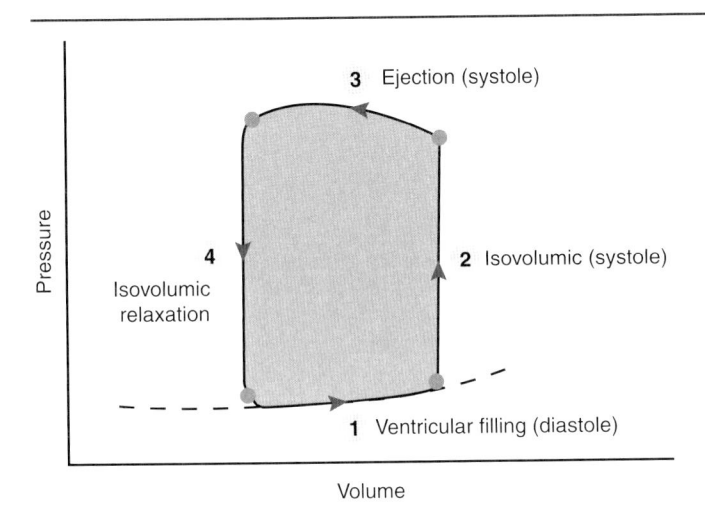

Figure 61-4
Idealized pressure–volume loop for the left ventricle represents a single cardiac cycle. *(Reproduced with permission from Chatterjee K, Parmley WW: The role of vasodilator therapy in heart failure. Prog Cardiovasc Dis 1977;**19**:301.)*

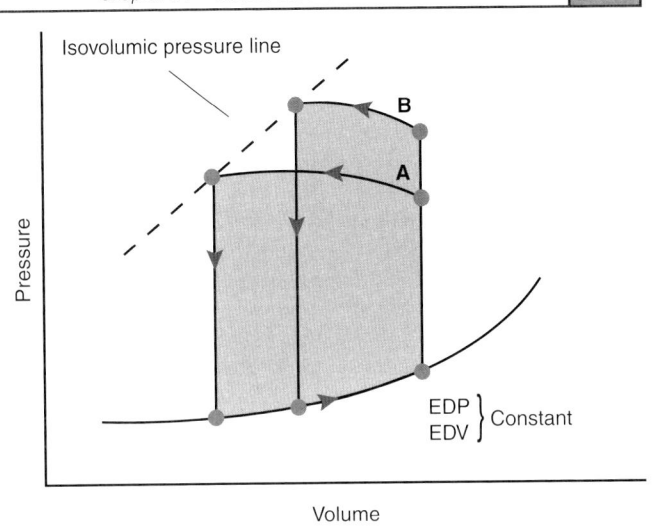

Figure 61-5
Acute postoperative afterload reduction. Two idealized pressure–volume loops are at the same level of contractility and end-diastolic volume (EDV), but with a reduction in arterial pressure from loop B to loop A, which results in an increase in stroke volume. EDP, end-diastolic pressure. *(Reproduced with permission from Chatterjee K, Parmley WW. The role of vasodilator therapy in heart failure. Prog Cardiovasc Dis 1977;**19**:301.)*

hypertension. After valve replacement, the reported incidence ranges between 8% and 12%.[68] After myocardial revascularization, afterload is elevated in 8% to 61% of patients.[69,70] Increased systemic vascular resistance at the arteriolar level appears to be the major determinant of arterial pressure after coronary artery surgery.[71] The etiology of postoperative hypertension remains unclear, but contributing factors include a decreased baroreceptor sensitivity[23,66] and an elevated renin-angiotensin activity.[72,73]

Sympathetic stimulation and elevated levels of catecholamines also have been identified in the early postoperative period.[70,74,75] Furthermore, postoperative pain may increase afterload and can be managed with the administration of morphine sulfate.[76] Alternatively, some patients develop hypotension postoperatively, which may be related to the systemic inflammatory response or the release of vasoactive substances.

Although pulmonary artery pressures are measured directly (RV afterload), the ascending aortic pressure is inferred by measurements made at a peripheral artery (usually the radial). Systolic amplification may occur, elevating the measured systolic radial artery pressure. However, mean pressures are similar between peripheral and central regions, and these should be considered when managing patients in the postoperative setting. In the control of afterload, autoregulation at various sites should be considered. The central nervous system autoregulates mean blood pressures of 50 to 150 mm Hg.[77] A reset lower limit for autoregulation may be higher in hypertensive patients.[78] Renal autoregulation requires a mean blood pressure of 70 mm Hg.[58] The heart with residual coronary disease also requires adequate mean arterial pressure (65 mm Hg), as do patients with pathologic concentric myocardial hypertrophy.[79]

Acute afterload reduction in the postoperative period is frequently beneficial (Fig. 61-5). Adequate preload must be achieved before the institution of vasodilating agents. Afterload reduction with low filling pressures often produces a compensatory tachycardia, which may be deleterious. When it is applied to patients with high filling pressures, there is usually no change or a slight reduction in heart rate. Additionally, experimental evidence suggests that afterload reduction, when applied to low or normally filled ventricles, may increase infarct size.[80] When applied in a setting of high preload, infarct size may be reduced.[81,82] This may have implications in patients after incomplete myocardial revascularization.

Therapeutic Approaches

The degree to which hemodynamic improvement can be obtained with afterload reduction is difficult to predict. Therapeutic results depend on the end-systolic pressure–volume relationship of each patient. However, afterload reduction generally improves cardiovascular function and diminishes preload. Preload augmentation coupled with afterload reduction has additional positive effects on overall cardiac function.[83] Afterload reduction also improves forward ejection in patients with residual mitral[84] and aortic insufficiency.[85]

Although various afterload-reducing agents are available, nitroglycerin and nitroprusside are the most frequently used agents in the immediate postoperative period. Nitroprusside may increase ST-segment elevation in perioperative ischemia and cause significant intracoronary shunt.[86] Nonetheless, it continues to be the agent of choice for the acute management of postoperative hypertension.[87] Nitroglycerin improves coronary collateral flow and may prevent coronary spasm, and it is frequently used for the first 12 to 24 hours after coronary revascularization.[86,88]

The frequent use of nitroprusside mandates a knowledge of its adverse effects. The lethal dose is approximately 7 mg/kg.[89] When high doses are used (greater than 7 μg/kg/min) for prolonged therapy, cyanogen, cyanide, and thiocyanate are potential toxic breakdown products. Signs of toxicity are subtle and include a narrowing of the arteriovenous oxygen difference and the development of metabolic acidosis.[90] Thiocyanate levels may be measured under these circumstances, with levels of 50 to 100 mg/L associated with cyanate toxicity, and 200 mg/L may be lethal. Discontinuance and dialysis are the mainstays of treatment, although prophylactic infusion of hydroxocobalamin (25 mg/hr) has been shown to decrease cyanate concentration.

Alternative parenteral agents should be considered when high-dose nitroprusside therapy is necessary: (1) Hydralazine, although longer acting, may also be effective.[91] (2) Beta-blockers are effective in the management of postoperative hypertension and are being used more commonly in patients with LV failure. Esmolol, a short-acting selective beta-blocker, may be particularly useful in this setting, although these agents may have a significant negative inotropic effect. (3) Intravenous nitroglycerin may achieve afterload reduction as well as coronary dilation.

Many patients require afterload reduction throughout their postoperative course. Patients with persistent hypertension and with reduced LV function will benefit from long-term afterload reduction and should be converted to oral medications. Chronic afterload reduction, in patients with significant congestive heart failure, has been shown to have a positive impact on survival.[92] In one large study of patients with symptomatic congestive heart failure (New York Heart Association [NYHA] class II and class III), a significant reduction in long-term morbidity and mortality was seen in those treated with enalapril, an angiotensin-converting enzyme (ACE) inhibitor.[93] Additional studies have confirmed that ACE inhibitors are particularly useful in the management of this problem.[94,95]

Patients with asymptomatic LV dysfunction (NYHA class I and class II) may benefit significantly from long-term therapy with ACE inhibitors. Although no significant difference in overall mortality was observed when compared with placebo, 37% and 36% decreases in development of symptomatic congestive heart failure and hospital admission for congestive heart failure, respectively, have been demonstrated.[96] Although the mechanism of this positive impact has not been completely defined, two-dimensional echocardiographic studies in post–myocardial infarction patients have shown that ACE inhibitors attenuate LV enlargement.[97] Nitrates[92] and hydralazine[98] have also been used but are less effective than ACE inhibitors.[99]

Heart Rate

The postoperative control of heart rate is important and mandates standard application of temporary, epicardial, bipolar atrial, and ventricular pacing wires in most patients. Normal sinus rhythm, through synchronized end-diastolic preload augmentation, is responsible for approximately 25% of cardiac output in the postoperative setting (Fig. 61-6).[100] Changes in heart rate are common after cardiac surgery and include sinus bradycardia, junctional rhythm, and first-, second-, or third-degree heart block. These phenomena are usually transient and may be related to perioperative beta-blockade, intraoperative antiarrhythmics, or metabolic damage during cardioplegic arrest (potassium or magnesium).[101,102] Inadequate myocardial protection may cause ischemia of the conduction system.[102,103] Permanent injury to the conduction system is most often the result of direct surgical injury during intracardiac procedures. Management of disturbances in heart rate must be individualized. Simple atrial pacing (in

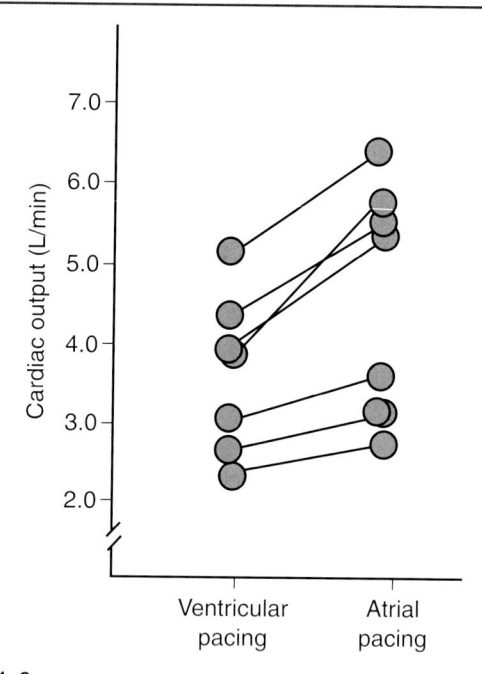

Figure 61-6
Synchronized end-diastolic preload augmentation. A comparison of cardiac output with ventricular pacing (without synchronous atrial systole) and with atrial pacing shows an overall increase in cardiac output with atrial pacing of approximately 26% in patients after cardiac surgery. *(Reproduced with permission from Hartzler GO, Maloney JD, Curtis JJ, Barnhorst DA. Hemodynamic effects of atrioventricular sequential pacing after cardiac surgery. Am J Cardiol 1977;**40**:232.)*

the range of 90 to 110 beats per minute) is optimal for sinus bradycardia. With AV nodal blocks, AV pacing with an interval in the range of 150 to 175 msec is usually optimal.[104,105] The AV interval also depends on selected heart rate (Fig. 61-7). The normalization of AV synchrony by these means is associated with a loss of the normal ventricular activation sequence, depressing ventricular function at constant preload and afterload by approximately 10% to 15%. Optimal heart rate determination must be individualized for each patient with reference to measurements of cardiac output. When in place, temporary pacing wires constitute a direct current pathway to the heart and must be insulated when not in use. Caution is needed when connecting a rapid-pacing device to the wires to ensure atrial connection. Temporary pacing wires are usually removed in the early postoperative period but may be left in place indefinitely. High pacing thresholds usually develop within 2 weeks, unlike permanent endocardial electrodes. When temporary pacing is not possible, bradyarrhythmias can be treated pharmacologically with atropine or isoproterenol. Alternatively, a pulmonary artery catheter with an additional pacing port or the Zoll transthoracic pacemaker may be employed.[106]

Inotropic State

Inotropic agents may be necessary to achieve adequate cardiac function (Fig. 61-8) and to maintain peripheral oxygen delivery. Improvement in cardiac function by pharmacologic intervention is generally achieved at the expense of increased myocardial oxygen consumption. Inotropic agents should be considered only after manipulations of heart rate, preload,

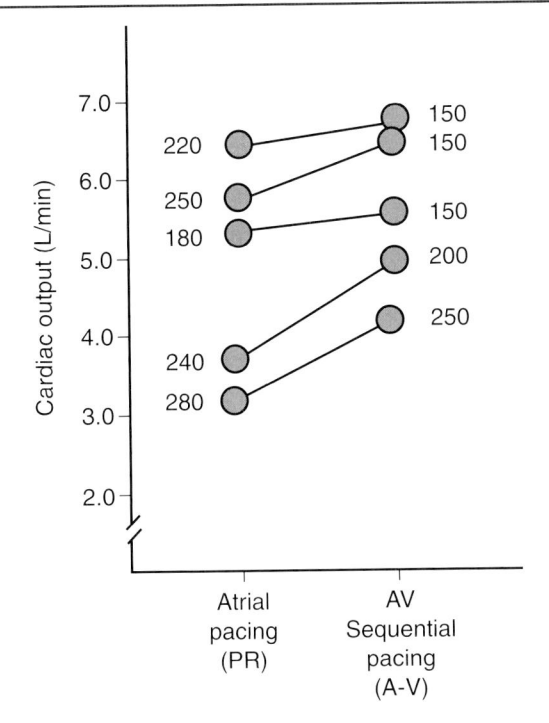

Figure 61-7
Cardiac output with AV sequential versus atrial pacing. A comparison of atrioventricular (AV) sequential pacing and atrial pacing in patients with a prolonged postoperative PR interval (intrinsic and paced PR intervals are shown in milliseconds to the left for atrial pacing and to the right for AV sequential pacing). Note the uniform increase in cardiac output that is induced by pacing, despite absolute differences in the shortening of the PR interval, and the overlap between paced PR intervals and intrinsic PR intervals between patients. *(Reproduced with permission from Hartzler GO, Maloney JD, Curtis JJ, Barnhorst DA. Hemodynamic effects of atrioventricular sequential pacing after cardiac surgery. Am J Cardiol 1977;**40**:232.)*

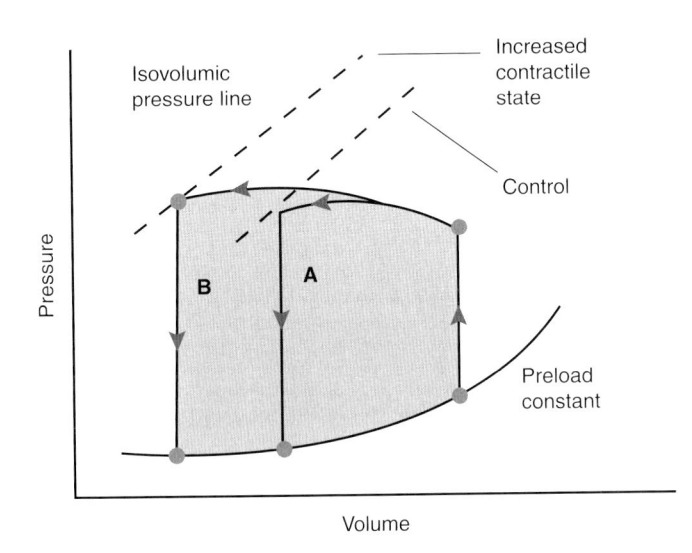

Figure 61-8
Pressure–volume loops inscribed under conditions of constant preload and afterload. An induced increase in inotropic state from loop A to loop B shifts the end-systolic pressure–volume relationship *(dashed lines)* and results in increased stroke volume in loop B. *(Reproduced with permission from Chatterjee K, Parmley WW. The role of vasodilator therapy in heart failure. Prog Cardiovasc Dis 1977;**19**:301.)*

and afterload have been maximized. In general, myocardial function improves throughout the postoperative course, allowing weaning from inotropic support.[107]

Various inotropic agents are available and all are administered by either intravenous bolus or continuous infusion. They should be administered through a central venous or pulmonary artery catheter whose intravascular position has been ascertained to prevent perivascular infiltration. Most inotropic agents act through stimulation of adrenergic receptors (Table 61-1). β-Adrenergic agonists mediate an increase in intracellular calcium concentration.[108] Clinical experience with multiple inotropic agents has demonstrated synergism[109] despite in vitro evidence that the maximal positive inotropic effect of one drug precludes augmentation by another. This may be because of alterations in the adenylate cyclase system in patients with heart failure, or because of alterations in beta-adrenoreceptor density.[108,110-114]

Nonadrenergic inotropes include digoxin, calcium chloride, phosphodiesterase inhibitors (amrinone, milrinone, and enoximone), and triiodothyronine. The presence of metabolic acidosis may interfere with the effectiveness of inotropic agents.[115,116] Notably, most inotropic agents (most importantly, β-adrenergic agonists) have proarrhythmic effects. Improved cardiac output must be balanced against risks of inducing either atrial or ventricular arrhythmias. Patients who require high doses of dopamine, epinephrine, or norepinephrine experience dangerous vasoconstrictive effects because of the α-adrenergic agonist effect of these agents at higher doses. This effect can result in limb, mesenteric, or renal ischemic injury.

Mechanical ventricular support should be considered before the patient suffers significant end-organ hypoperfusion, which may retard ultimate recovery. Insertion of an intra-aortic balloon pump (IABP) via a percutaneous femoral arterial approach is the initial step in mechanical ventricular support. A properly functioning IABP provides increased diastolic coronary perfusion and augmented cardiac output by reducing LV afterload (Fig. 61-9). Greater deterioration of ventricular function may warrant assist devices that provide complete support; these devices are used as bridges to either myocardial recovery or possible cardiac transplantation.

Cardiac Tamponade

Tamponade results from occupation of the mediastinal space by fluid or clotted blood, which restricts the end-diastolic volume of both ventricles. It has been reported to occur acutely in 3.4% to 5.8% of cases.[117-119] The constellation of findings associated with acute postoperative cardiac tamponade includes (1) increased variation in blood pressure with respiration (pulsus paradoxus); (2) equalization and elevation of the central venous pressure, pulmonary artery diastolic pressure, and left atrial pressure or pulmonary artery wedge pressure[120]; (3) a fall in urine output (often an early finding); (4) excessive chest tube drainage or, paradoxically, minimal or no chest tube drainage, especially with heavy clots noted within the chest tubes; (5) mediastinal widening on chest film; (6) low cardiac output (late); and (7) hypotension (late). No single finding or combination of findings is sufficient to establish the diagnosis, and a high index of clinical suspicion should be maintained. Early postoperative tamponade is treated by reoperation, ideally in the operating room. Patients in extremis may require reopening

Table 61-1
Inotropes

Vasoactive Drug	Dose (µg/kg/min)	AR Activation			Physiologic Response				
		α_1	β_1	β_2	SVR	MAP	CO	HR	PAWP
Dopamine	<5	−	++	−	↔	↑	↑	↑	↔
	>5	++	++	−	↑↑	↑↑	↑	↑	↑
Dobutamine	2-20	−	++	+	↓	↑	↑	↑	↓
Epinephrine	<0.05	−	++	+	↓	↑	↑	↑	↓
	>0.05	++	++	+	↑↑	↑↑	↑	↑	↑
Norepinephrine	0.03-1.0	++	+	−	↑↑	↑↑	↔	↑	↑
Phenylephrine	0.6-2.0	++	−	−	↑↑	↑↑	↓	↔	↑
Isoproterenol	0.03-0.15	−	++	++	↓	↔	↑	↑↑	↓
Milrinone	0.3-1.5	—	PDEI*	—	↓	↔	↑	↔	↓
Amrinone	5-20	—	PDEI*	—	↓	↔	↑	↔	↓

*Amrinone and milrinone are common phosphodiesterase inhibitors (PDEIs).
AR, adrenergic receptor activation; α_1, peripheral vasculature; β_1, myocardium; β_2, peripheral vasculature and myocardium; CO, cardiac output; HR, heart rate; MAP, mean arterial pressure; PAWP, pulmonary arterial wedge pressure; SVR, systemic vascular resistance.

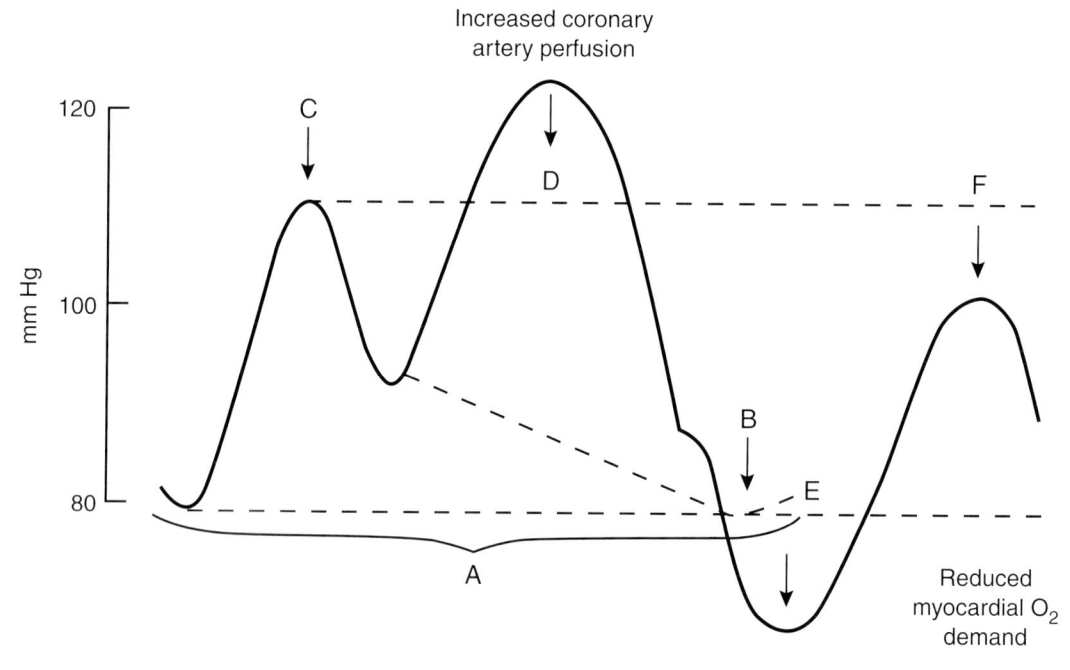

Figure 61-9
Intra-aortic balloon pump (IABP) timing: synchronization with the cardiac cycle. Arterial pressure waveform with correct IABP timing: A, one complete cardiac cycle; B, unassisted aortic end-diastolic pressure; C, unassisted systolic pressure; D, diastolic augmentation; E, reduced aortic end-diastolic pressure; F, reduced systolic pressure. (Reproduced with permission from Helman DN. Intracorporeal support: the intra-aortic balloon pump. In: Goldstein DJ, Oz MC, editors. Cardiac assist devices. New York: Futura; 2000, p. 298.)

of their sternotomy in the ICU. Temporizing management consists of (1) volume loading, (2) reduction of airway pressure (removal of positive end-expiratory pressure [PEEP], anesthetizing agents, diminishing tidal volume with increasing ventilatory rate), and (3) inotropic support.

Cardiac tamponade may be present with any amount of retained blood or fluid, which in most cases is circumferential but which may be loculated and still adversely affect cardiac function.[121,122] In patients with decreased ventricular function, smaller amounts of space occupation will result in tamponade physiology.[123] For patients with severe ventricular dysfunction, simple reapproximation of the sternum after cardiac surgery may not be possible. Delayed sternal closure may be necessary in 1% to 2% of high-risk patients, and subsequent closure is usually possible between 1 and 4 days after initial operation.[124]

To a certain extent, the pleural and mediastinal spaces are continuous, and resulting intrathoracic pressure is distributed to affect the lungs and cardiac chambers simultaneously. An open pericardium and pleural space can neither prevent nor minimize cardiac tamponade. Increases in airway pressure, which may result from changing lung compliance or the application of PEEP, or a change in chest wall compliance may be directly transmitted to the heart. Such increases in airway pressure cause additive space occupation and can make tamponade manifest at lower volumes of retained fluid.

Although cardiac tamponade usually presents within the first 24 hours after surgery, there is a definite incidence of late presentation.[122,125-127] Most cases occur in patients with large amounts of postoperative bleeding, those who require anticoagulation, or those with active inflammation (postpericardiotomy syndrome). Delayed diagnosis is attributed to the associated nonspecific symptoms of malaise, dyspnea, chest pain, and anorexia. Echocardiography is the mainstay in diagnosis of delayed cardiac tamponade.[128-130]

Vasoplegic Syndrome

Cardiopulmonary bypass induces a systemic inflammatory response that in some patients may manifest as vasodilatory shock. The clinical state of profound hypotension, low systemic vascular resistance, massive volume requirement, and increased use of vasopressors has been named vasoplegic syndrome (VS). This syndrome has generally been defined as an arterial pressure of less than 50 mm Hg, a cardiac index of greater than 2.5 L/min/m^2, a right atrial pressure of less than 5 mm Hg, a left atrial pressure of less than 10 mm Hg, and low systemic vascular resistance (<800 dyne•sec/cm^5).[131] The incidence of VS has been reported to range between 8.8% and 10% after cardiac surgery, and up to 42% after LVAD placement.[132,133]

Several factors are associated with VS, including preoperative intravenous heparin, ACE inhibitors, and calcium channel blockers, with reported incidences as high as 55.6%, 44.4%, and 47.2%, respectively. Other reported risk factors include the use of alcuronium, the presence of diabetes, the use of protamine, and preoperative heart failure.[133] The mortality associated with this condition is considerable.[134] Standard vasopressors such as norepinephrine, phenylephrine, or vasopressin have been used both intraoperatively and postoperatively to provide hemodynamic support. However, a small percentage of patients remain in vasodilatory shock despite aggressive treatment. In these patients, methylene blue has been demonstrated to be well tolerated, to significantly increase systemic vascular resistance, and to reduce mortality when given as an intravenous infusion (1.5 to 2 mg/kg over 20 to 60 min).[133] The side effects of methylene blue include arrhythmias; vasoconstriction of coronary, renal, mesenteric, and pulmonary vascular beds; reduced cardiac output; and angina. Most side effects, however, are dose dependent and do not occur with dosages of less than 2 mg/kg.[131] It should not be used in patients with severe renal insufficiency, with hypersensitivity to previous administration, or with gluscose-6-phosphate dehydrogenase (G6PD) deficiency. Also, it should be used with caution in patients receiving dapsone because of its potential to cause hemolytic anemia. Although preliminary data suggest that its use as a rescue agent is warranted, the data are not sufficient to support its use as a first-line agent.[133]

Right Heart Dysfunction

Although right heart dysfunction is most commonly secondary to left heart failure, it may occur as an isolated condition. In this setting, the left ventricle may display relatively preserved intrinsic function, but cardiac output remains low because of poor LV filling. Other important manifestations of isolated right heart failure include elevated CVP, poor right ventricular contractility, and elevated pulmonary vascular resistance. With severely impaired RV function, pulmonary artery pressures may not be elevated. Treatment strategies for isolated right heart dysfunction are similar to those used to manage a low cardiac output state caused by more conventional LV dysfunction. Preload, which consists of the CVP, may need to be increased to greater than 20 mm Hg. Heart rate and rhythm should be optimized (sinus rhythm, rate 90 to 100). β-Adrenergic receptor agonists may be helpful, but higher doses of epinephrine, norepinephrine, or dopamine may further increase pulmonary vascular resistance and exacerbate right heart failure. Milrinone is an important agent in these circumstances, as it provides a positive inotropic effect for the right ventricle but also reduces pulmonary artery pressures as well as pulmonary vascular resistance. Finally, inhaled nitric oxide represents the most specific pulmonary vasodilator; nitric oxide, unlike milrinone, does not induce systemic hypotension. The starting dose for inhaled nitric oxide should be between 20 and 40 parts per million. A final strategy for isolated right heart failure is a right ventricle assist device. In general, this invasive strategy should be used only after less invasive approaches have failed.

Arrhythmias

Atrial Flutter

Atrial flutter is generated by a macro-reentrant phenomenon[135] and can be treated rapidly and effectively with electrical stimulation. Although this arrhythmia may be interrupted by a single, appropriately timed atrial extrasystole, it is most commonly interrupted by one of the following methods: (1) Entrainment, which means determining the atrial rate and instituting atrial pacing at a slightly higher rate to capture the atria. Regularization of the ventricular response and an altered P-wave morphology are usually produced. Termination of pacing is ordinarily followed by normal sinus rhythm (Fig. 61-10). (2) Nonspecific rapid atrial stimulation.[136] Rapid atrial pacing is performed by introducing trains of atrial pacing at rates in the range of 450 to 600 beats per minute. Short trains (less than 1 second) effectively introduce single extra stimuli within the effective refractory period of the pacing site and thus can interrupt atrial flutter and reinstate the normal sinus rhythm. If the train of rapid atrial pacing is too long, it may induce atrial fibrillation, which cannot be treated with these pacing techniques. However, in the atrial fibrillation that may ensue, the ventricular response is usually slower and

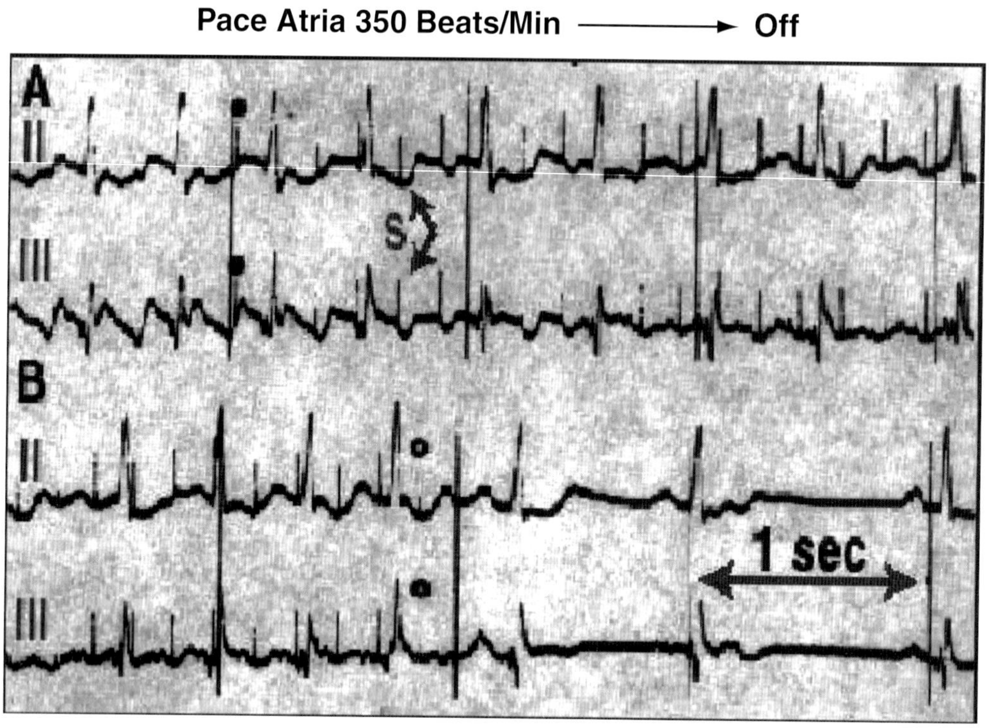

Figure 61-10
Atrial flutter in postoperative cardiac patients. Electrocardiograph leads II and III show atrial flutter with 2:1 AV block. **A** and **B** are not continuous. At the *black dot* in **A**, the P-wave morphology has changed from negative to positive, which indicates entrainment. In **B**, after 30 seconds of pacing at 350 beats/min, atrial pacing is terminated *(open circle)*. Sinus rhythm appears spontaneously. S, stimulus artifact. *(Reproduced with permission from Waldo AL, MacLean WAH. Diagnosis and treatment of cardiac arrhythmias following open-heart surgery. Mt. Kisco, NY: Futura; 1980.)*

thus better tolerated than that of atrial flutter.[137] It is common for atrial fibrillation induced in this manner to revert spontaneously to normal sinus rhythm.

Atrial Fibrillation

Incidence and Risk

Atrial fibrillation is the most common supraventricular arrhythmia after cardiac surgery. The incidence has varied from 28% to 54% of patients undergoing cardiac operations.[138-140] The etiology is unknown, but atrial fibrillation may result from (1) unprotected ischemia,[102,141] (2) multidose cardioplegic solution administration with high potassium concentration,[101] (3) atrial dilation or inadequate atrial protection,[142,143] or (4) postoperative pericarditis.[144]

The incidence of postoperative atrial fibrillation is higher in patients with echocardiographic evidence of pericardial effusion. Certain patients may also have an inherent propensity to develop supraventricular arrhythmias related to the preoperative accumulation of catecholamines in intramyocardial axons.[145] Additional risk factors predictive of an increased incidence of atrial fibrillation include advanced age, chronic obstructive pulmonary disease, prolonged cross-clamp periods,[146] and discontinuation of preoperative beta-blockers. Although this arrhythmia has not been shown to increase the 30-day mortality rate, it does prolong length of hospital stay in patients undergoing CABG. Furthermore, there is an increased incidence of malignant ventricular rhythms (both ventricular tachycardia and ventricular fibrillation) and a significant increase in the postoperative stroke rate.[146]

Diagnosis and Treatment

Although various diagnostic methods can be used, these have generally been supplanted by direct examination of atrial and ventricular bipolar ECGs.[136] The presence of chaotic and rapid atrial depolarization indicates atrial fibrillation, whereas a regular rapid atrial depolarization with an organized ventricular response (usually 2:1 or 3:1) indicates atrial flutter (Fig. 61-11). Therapeutic objectives in patients with atrial fibrillation, in order of importance, are (1) heart rate control, (2) conversion to sinus rhythm, and (3) prevention of embolic complications. Rapid supraventricular arrhythmias causing significant hemodynamic compromise should be treated by cardioversion or defibrillation. In hemodynamically stable patients, the drug of choice for controlling ventricular response is a calcium channel antagonist: either verapamil, administered in 2.5- to 5-mg boluses to a total of 20 mg, or diltiazem given as an intravenous load followed by a continuous infusion. These agents rapidly reduce the ventricular response by increasing AV block.[147] The salutary effect of reduction in ventricular rate is usually more important than the negative inotropic effect of these drugs.[148-150] Adverse effects of calcium channel antagonists may be treated with calcium infusion,[151] glucagon,[152] or inotropic agents.[153]

Alternatively, beta-blockers, especially those with short action (esmolol), have been studied for the acute management of atrial fibrillation. The response to beta-blockade varies considerably when it is used to treat atrial fibrillation in the post-CABG patient. In addition, hypotension may be a significant side effect in as many as 20% to 40% of patients treated. Digoxin has been similarly used, although immediate

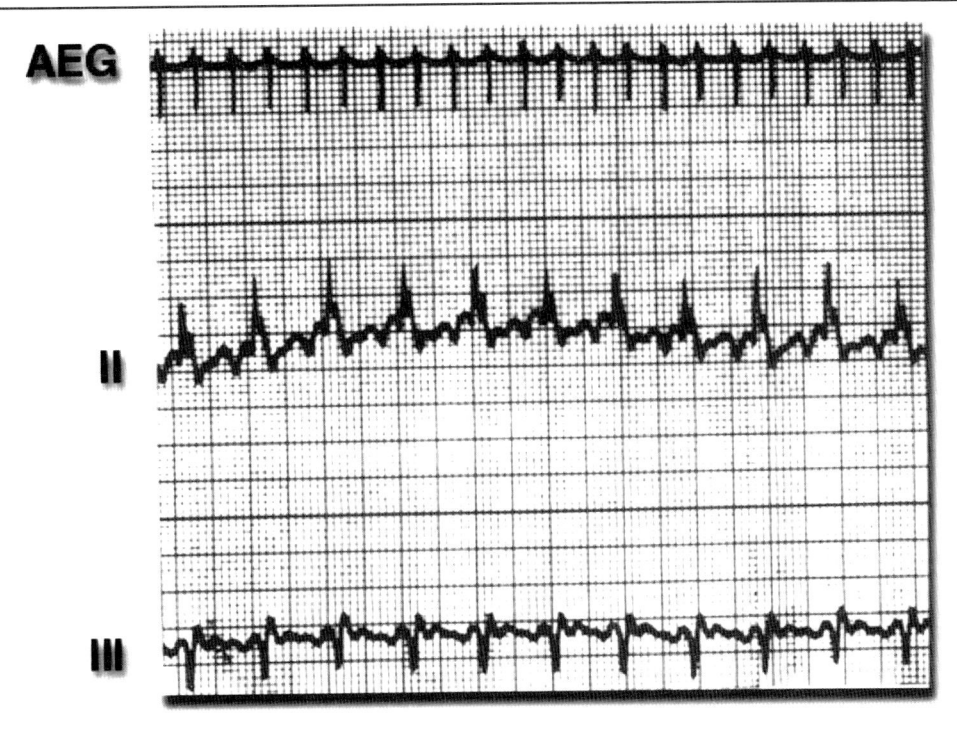

Figure 61-11
Bipolar atrial electrogram (AEG) showing atrial flutter is seen in the upper trace, with simultaneous electrocardiograph leads II and III that show atrial flutter with 2:1 AV block. Recording speed is 25 mm/sec. *(Reproduced with permission from Waldo AL, Cooper TB, MacLean WAH. Cardiac pacing in the treatment of cardiac arrhythmias following open heart surgery: use of temporarily placed atrial and ventricular wire electrodes. In: Samet P, El-Sherif N, editors. Cardiac pacing. 2nd ed. New York: Grune & Stratton; 1980.)*

heart rate control is rarely achieved.[154] Multidrug combinations can be hazardous in patients without temporary pacing wires. The combination of digoxin, verapamil, and a β-adrenergic antagonist can lead to complete heart block, and verapamil and a β-adrenergic antagonist may lead to sinus arrest.[155] Once heart rate control has been achieved, conversion to and maintenance of sinus rhythm with an antiarrhythmic agent may be necessary.

Two newer agents that have been used extensively for postoperative atrial fibrillation are amiodarone and sotalol. Relative to class IA agents, these drugs are felt to have equivalent efficacy and better side-effect profiles. These agents are very effective at converting atrial fibrillation, and both also retard AV nodal conduction, thereby reducing the ventricular response to atrial fibrillation. Amiodarone is typically administered as a 1-g intravenous infusion, which is given over a 24-hour period, with the initial 150 mg given over 20 minutes. Subsequent doses are given orally (400 mg, three times a day). Sotalol is available only as an oral preparation, 40 to 160 mg, twice a day. A common approach is to first attempt chemical cardioversion with these agents, and if this fails, to perform electrical cardioversion. Sotalol can induce significant bradycardia and probably should not be combined with other beta-blockers. In addition, harmful proarrhythmic effects including ventricular tachycardia have been described with sotalol. The incidence of these harmful rhythms has correlated with QT prolongation, and this should be monitored. Chronic amiodarone therapy can induce pulmonary fibrosis and hypothyroidism. In general, the risk of postoperative atrial fibrillation is considerably reduced after the first month, and antiarrhythmics initiated for isolated postoperative atrial fibrillation should be discontinued after this point. There has been much interest in the prophylactic use of antiarrhythmic agents to diminish the incidence of supraventricular arrhythmias (atrial fibrillation, in particular) after cardiac surgery. However, prophylactic use of antiarrhythmics in all patients may lead to unwanted side effects in patients who would otherwise convalesce normally. As attempts to identify perioperative risk factors continue, many cardiac surgeons prefer to treat arrhythmias only when they are present.[27]

Ventricular Arrhythmias

Sustained ventricular arrhythmias are an uncommon postoperative issue but are life-threatening and require a prompt and organized treatment strategy. Immediate electrical cardioversion should be followed by a thorough investigation for treatable causes, which may include electrolyte imbalance, hypoxia, malpositioned Swan-Ganz catheter, and proarrhythmic effects of inotropes or other agents. Myocardial ischemia should always be ruled out as the cause of the ventricular arrhythmias. A 12-lead ECG should be performed, and if ischemic changes are present, cardiac catheterization with coronary angiography should be considered. Persistent ventricular arrhythmias in the postoperative patient lead quickly to hypoperfusion and a dangerous spiral. For this reason, early placement of IABP for ventricular assistance is often helpful. Persistent arrhythmias also warrant initiation of either lidocaine or amiodarone intravenously. Formal electrophysiologic testing and an implantable defibrillator may be indicated.

GRAFT OCCLUSION

Intraoperative Injury and Graft Occlusion

Early graft failure usually results from technical factors, although it may be produced by scarring and is seen more frequently in patients with inflammatory pericardial syndromes. Early graft failure may manifest as ventricular arrhythmias or as hemodynamic compromise with evidence of ischemia; alternatively, the occurrence may be clinically silent. Factors that affect the presentation include the nature of the collateral blood supply from other grafts or from the native coronary circulation. Also important is the amount of viable myocardium at risk. Patients with ventricular arrhythmias, hemodynamic change, and evidence of ischemia warrant urgent coronary angiography. Graft failure can be addressed with percutaneous interventions, or the patient can be returned to the OR for graft revision. Perioperative myocardial infarction (MI) is defined by ECG changes, creatine phosphokinase and methylene blue measurements, and the development of new regional LV dysfunction. Perioperative MI does not result solely from graft or coronary occlusion; it may also result from compromised myocardial protection or atheroembolic events. Treatment is mainly supportive with intravenous nitroglycerin and afterload reduction. Inotropic agents or IABP may be required during a period of myocardial recovery.

Graft survival is enhanced by the perioperative administration of antiplatelet agents. Initially, aspirin and dipyridamole were used,[156] but subsequent work suggests that low-dose aspirin alone (325 mg/day) is as effective as a combination of agents.[157] Aspirin should be administered the morning after surgery. Clopidogrel bisulfate (Plavix) has also been considered for postoperative antiplatelet therapy. Plavix is an inhibitor of adenosine diphosphate (ADP)-induced platelet aggregation. It acts as a direct inhibitor of ADP by binding ADP receptors on platelets and preventing the subsequent ADP-mediated activation of the glycoprotein IIb/IIIa complex. The clinical evidence for the efficacy of Plavix is derived from the CAPRIE (Clopidogrel versus Aspirin in Patients at Risk of Ischemic Events) trial (Fig. 61-12).[158] A randomized double-blind placebo-controlled trial is currently accruing patients to clarify the role of Plavix in antiplatelet therapy after CABG surgery,[159] but until those results are made available, the results of the CAPRIE subgroup analysis support the use of Plavix antiplatelet therapy in place of aspirin for high-risk patients after coronary artery bypass. The recommended dose of Plavix in the postoperative setting is 75 mg/day. The most important side effect is bleeding: in CAPRIE, the incidence of gastrointestinal bleeding was 2.0% versus 2.7% with aspirin; intracranial hemorrhage was 0.4% for Plavix versus 0.5% for aspirin. Overall gastrointestinal complaints were similar for Plavix and aspirin.

POSTOPERATIVE BLEEDING

Postoperative bleeding is always present to some degree after cardiac surgery. Bleeding is related to a combination of mechanical factors that are surgically correctable, and also to coagulopathy. A surgically correctable cause predominates in fewer than 3% of cases and is indicated by brisk hemorrhage (>200 mL/hr), normal or near-normal coagulation studies, and the appearance of blood clots in the mediastinal drainage tubes. The amount of bleeding that occurs after surgery, the number of transfusions required, and the filtering of transfused components are related to outcome.[160]

Coagulopathy

Coagulopathy is a common feature of patients placed on CPB. Its effects are exacerbated by the preoperative use of antiplatelet agents, thrombolytic agents, and heparin. The predominant cause of abnormal bleeding after CPB is a fall in platelet number and impaired platelet function.[161,162] Hypothermia associated with CPB also contributes to decreased platelet function and postoperative coagulopathy and hemorrhage.[118,163,164] Platelet dysfunction is related to passage through the extracorporeal circuit, with resulting decrease in platelet membrane receptors for fibrinogen as well as for glycoprotein Ib and glycoprotein IIb/IIIa complex. A second mechanism for coagulopathy is progressive fibrinolytic state of variable intensity related to the length of time of the CPB. Coagulopathy may be associated with variable or no bleeding and is recognized by the presence of abnormal clotting parameters (prothrombin time [PT], partial thromboplastin time [PTT], fibrinogen level, platelet count) and the absence of solid clot formation in the mediastinal drainage tubes.

The management of patients with excessive mediastinal hemorrhage is complex and may be hazardous. Bleeding resulting predominantly from coagulopathy is treated by both specific and nonspecific means. Postoperative coagulopathy must be specifically diagnosed by laboratory and clinical evaluation of the coagulation system. Any or all of the following abnormalities may be present.

Heparin Effect

The heparin effect is demonstrated by a prolonged PTT or a prolonged activated clotting time (ACT), or both. ACT should be measured on admission to the ICU, as the heparin effect is usually seen early in the postoperative course (the half-life of heparin is approximately 1 hour).[165] The specific treatment is administration of protamine sulfate (25- to 50-mg doses are given, and the ACT is repeated).[166] Consideration of CPB time and dosages of heparin and protamine must guide decision making.

A randomized trial suggested that higher heparin dosages using point-of-care, patient-specific monitoring during CPB reduced transfusion by 50% as compared with empiric dosages (17% versus 33%, P = .005).[167] Higher stable heparin concentrations results in decreased thrombin generation,[168] inhibition of clot-bound thrombin,[19] and preserved platelet function after prolonged (>2 hr) CPB.[169,170] In addition, heparin reversal with empiric half-dose or protamine titration methods (protamine-to-heparin ratio, less than 1) may also decrease chest tube drainage and transfusion requirements.[170]

Thrombocytopenia

Thrombocytopenia results from destruction of platelets during CPB or from consumption.[171,172] In the absence of other abnormalities, treatment is platelet transfusion.[173] Notably, if a patient is not actively bleeding, thrombocytopenia is generally not corrected with transfusion, because the platelet level usually normalizes spontaneously over the next few days. As many patients are maintained preoperatively on heparin,

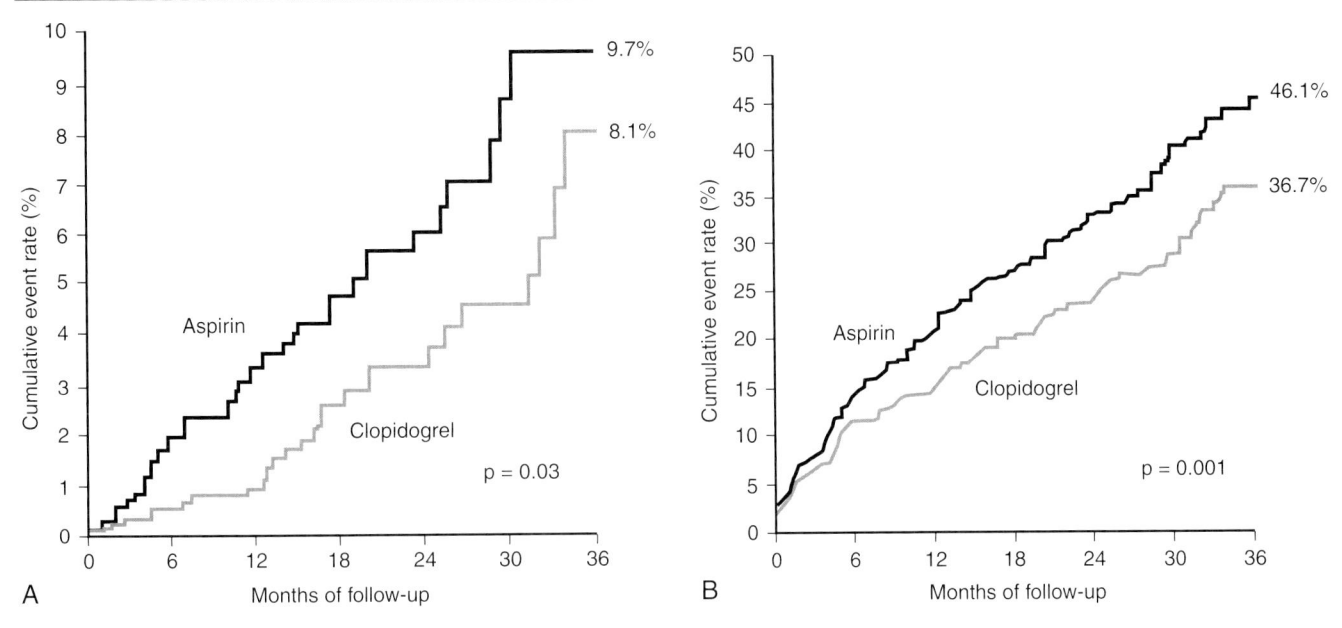

Figure 61-12
Superiority of clopidogrel versus aspirin in patients with prior cardiac surgery. Data from the CAPRIE trial, surgical subset analysis. **A,** Kaplan-Meier curves for clopidogrel versus aspirin for vascular death with cumulative event rates. **B,** Kaplan-Meier curves for clopidogrel versus aspirin for composite of vascular death, myocardial infarction, stroke, or rehospitalization for ischemia or bleeding with cumulative event rates. *(Reproduced with permission from Bhatt DL, Chew DP, Hirsch AT, Ringleb PA, Hacke W, Topol EJ. Superiority of clopidogrel versus aspirin in patients with prior cardiac surgery.* Circulation 2000;**103**:366.)

persistent postoperative thrombocytopenia may be induced by the presence of heparin-dependent antibodies. In this setting, resulting thromboembolic events as well as significant bleeding have been observed.[174] Diagnosis of heparin-induced thrombocytopenia can be made with heparin-platelet aggregation testing and a platelet factor intravenous assay to confirm the presence of antibodies in vitro. All heparin should be discontinued promptly in these patients.

Thrombasthenia

In patients with thrombasthenia, the platelet count is normal but clot formation is inadequate. This remains a significant problem in the postcardiac surgical patient.[162] It can be documented by measuring bleeding time using the Ivy method, or it is more accurately defined using the thromboelastogram (TEG).[175,176] Qualitative defects in platelet function result from CPB[162,177,178] or from antiplatelet therapy.[23,179] Aspirin and Plavix can irreversibly affect platelet function, the life span of which is 6 to 7 days. Therefore, a single dose administered within the 7 days before the operation diminishes platelet function, which can result in a significant increase in bleeding complication and transfusion requirements.[180,181] Current guidelines from the American College of Cardiology and American Heart Association (ACC/AHA) and Society of Thoracic Surgeons (STS) recommend discontinuing ADP inhibitors 5 to 7 days before cardiac surgery, if possible.[170,182,183]

Specific Factor Deficiencies

Specific factor deficiencies are usually manifested by elevation of the PT or the PTT. Abnormalities may result from a specific genetic disorder, liver disease, prior Coumadin therapy, hemodilution, or disseminated intravascular coagulation (DIC). These disorders are generally treated by specific factor therapy, fresh frozen plasma, or cryoprecipitate.

Management of Bleeding

Specific treatment consists of blood component therapy based on an accurate diagnosis and an understanding of the changes that occur during CPB. Guidelines for transfusion support as well as management of postoperative patients with significant hemorrhage have been suggested.[170,173] The observed rate of bleeding must be correlated with its character (the initial bleeding rate may reflect drainage of sequestered blood or irrigation fluid) and hemodynamic effect (ineffective drainage may lead to an underestimate of ongoing intravascular depletion). The quality of blood clotting may be effectively estimated by close observation of the drainage tube contents and manual manipulation of the tubes. Large amounts of clot that repeatedly obstruct the tubes indicate a surgical source of bleeding. Nonclotting, freely draining blood, or the presence of loosely organized clot, indicates that a state of coagulopathy exists.

Bleeding at a rate of more than 200 mL/hr requires immediate action to search for and correct the underlying cause. Delays in laboratory testing frequently preclude accurate and timely diagnosis. Algorithms outlining empiric treatment are usually developed with input from surgeons and blood bank directors.

The single most practical treatment is to administer platelet concentrate, which is often effective despite an apparently adequate platelet count when the platelets are dysfunctional. Fresh frozen plasma fraction is employed to replenish coagulation factors manifested as a prolongation of the PT for PTT. Cryoprecipitate is administered to replenish consumed fibrinogen. With appropriate treatment of coagulation deficiencies, coagulopathy usually resolves within a few hours. Bleeding usually diminishes to modest levels (50 to 100 mL/hr) within 4 hours, and rarely is the total amount drained more than 1 L.

Reoccurrence of high drainage rates should be addressed immediately, despite the fact that sudden drainage of sequestered blood is common when the patient is repositioned. It is not uncommon for a new bleeding site to develop with clot lysis or after a brief episode of severe hypertension. A common scenario is initial bleeding at rates of 150 to 250 mL/hr, followed by alternating periods of inconsequential drainage and substantial drainage. This often indicates surgically correctable bleeding, with a large burden of intramediastinal clot and ineffective tube drainage resulting from clot obstruction. When the bleeding issue is not resolved within a few hours, a second chest radiograph should be obtained to ensure that mediastinal and pleural drainage has been effective.

The major side effects of postoperative bleeding are volume loss and retention of clotted blood in the mediastinum. Nonspecific therapy consists of continuous, adequate volume replacement, maintenance of free drainage, and prevention of hypothermia. Hypothermia has a generalized anticoagulant effect that increases PT and PTT in direct accordance with the degree of temperature change.[184] Specific anticoagulant effects may be corrected by warming.

Volume replacement may be provided by continuous autotransfusion, but it also requires the infusion of nonspecific agents. Crystalloid solutions may be provided as normal saline or lactated Ringer's solution. Colloid solutions include the following: (1) Serum albumin as a 25% solution. Serum albumin in its 25% solution must recruit extravascular fluid to result in effective volume replacement. (2) Plasma protein fraction (Plasmanate) as a 5% protein solution containing both albumin and alpha and beta globulins. Plasmanate may cause a paradoxical hypotension attributed to the use of acetate, present as a buffer,[185] or may cause the presence of Hageman-factor fragments.[186] (3) Hydroxyethyl starch (Hetastarch). Hetastarch provides plasma volume expansion for greater than 24 hours and may be safely used to a total volume of 1.5 L. Because it has a chemical composition similar to that of dextran, associated urticarial and anaphylactoid reactions may occur. However, unlike with dextran, coagulation abnormalities associated with Hetastarch have generally been related to hemodilution rather than to a specific anticoagulant effect.

The choice of colloid versus crystalloid must be made on an individual basis. The largest randomized prospective clinical trial available comparing saline to albumin was unable to demonstrate any difference in numbers of days spent in the ICU (6.5 ± 6.6 in the albumin group and 6.2 ± 6.2 in the saline group, $P = .44$), days spent in the hospital (15.3 ± 9.6 and 15.6 ± 9.6, respectively; $P = .30$), days of mechanical ventilation (4.5 ± 6.1 and 4.3 ± 5.7, respectively; $P = .74$), or days of renal-replacement therapy (0.5 ± 2.3 and 0.4 ± 2.0, respectively; $P = .41$).[187]

Mechanical means should be used to maintain mediastinal chest tube patency, including (1) application of suction, (2) stripping and milking of chest tubes (mechanical stripping of chest tubes can create negative pressures as high as 1500 mm Hg and can be potentially damaging to entrapped tissues), and (3) occasionally, Fogarty catheter thrombectomy of the mediastinal tubes. Catheter thrombectomy usually precedes reoperation and may relieve significant tamponade.

Other nonspecific measures include strict control of blood pressure and induction of mild controlled hypotension, which can markedly diminish bleeding rate. However, afterload reduction can be particularly dangerous in the hypovolemic patient with ongoing blood loss and early cardiac tamponade. Levels of PEEP in the range of 10 to 12 cm H_2O have been suggested as a means to reduce postoperative bleeding.[188-190] The efficacy of PEEP in slowing postoperative bleeding remains controversial,[170,191] and acute reduction in preload with this level of PEEP is potentially dangerous.[192]

Blood Conservation

Blood conservation requires a programmatic approach but is essential to improving patient outcome. There is ample evidence that blood and blood products negatively influence outcome, expose patients to viral and bacterial infection, and may reduce host resistance to infection.[160] The tolerance of a reduced hematocrit in the postoperative cardiac patient is an important component in the avoidance of blood transfusion. Although classic teaching states that the optimal hematocrit is between 0.30 and 0.40,[58,193-195] this is no longer the case. In healthy individuals, tissue oxygenation is maintained at hematocrits of 15% to 20%. In mostly observational studies with Jehovah's Witnesses, significant mortality due to anemia is not generally seen until hemoglobin levels fall below 5 g/dL. Given these findings and a lack of high-level evidence to guide transfusion decisions, several guidelines have been published by the National Institutes of Health, and more recently by the STS, stating that it is reasonable to transfuse blood in postoperative patients with a hemoglobin of less than 7 g/dL.[196] Though not explicitly stated, it is reasonable to not transfuse a postoperative patient who has a hemoglobin of 7 g/dL or greater based on the patient's clinical situation and if end-organ ischemia is not demonstrated. Oral iron therapy, and occasionally folic acid, can restore normal hematocrit within 6 weeks of surgery.

PHARMACOLOGIC CONSIDERATIONS

Desmopressin

Desmopressin (1-deamino-8-D-arginine vasopressin, DDAVP), a synthetic analog of L-arginine vasopressin, has improved platelet function and reduced hemorrhage in a variety of clinical disorders. DDAVP appears to act by increasing the concentration of von Willebrands factor, an important mediator of platelet adhesion. No clear consensus exists regarding the prophylactic use of DDAVP.[142,197] However, patients who have ongoing hemorrhage should be considered for administration of 3 μg/kg given over 15 minutes.[173] Recent evidence has demonstrated that an acquired type 2A von Willebrand's syndrome is common in patients with severe aortic stenosis,[198] and DDAVP may help reduce perioperative blood loss in these patients.

Aprotinin

Aprotinin is a nonspecific protease inhibitor extracted from bovine lung, and it has been suggested as a method of reducing postoperative mediastinal bleeding. Administration of aprotinin before CPB can preserve platelet function otherwise lost during CPB.[199-201] It can be administered before CPB in a low dose (2×10^6 Kallikrein inhibitor units [KIU]) or as a continuing infusion during bypass in a high dose (6×10^6 KIU). The beneficial effects of aprotinin are mediated by its antifibrinolytic, antithrombotic, and anti-inflammatory effects. Despite nearly 20 years of use and several studies documenting the overall safety of full-dose aprotinin and the resultant reduction in stroke incidence,[200,201] the safety of its use has been repeatedly questioned with respect to its thrombotic potential. Three recent trials have called into question the safety of aprotinin,[202-204] and with the premature stoppage of the Blood Conservation Using Antifibrinolytics in a Randomized Trial (BART) because of an increase in all-cause 30-day mortality in patients receiving aprotinin, the marketing and distribution of aprotinin has been suspended.[205]

Previously, aprotinin use was advocated in the setting of reoperative cardiac surgery, aortic surgery, and recent Plavix exposure, and when bleeding risk is high in situations such as left ventricle assist device (LVAD) implantation. Given the 50% increase in mortality and modest decrease in postoperative hemorrhage seen in the aprotinin arm of the BART study, further use of aprotinin cannot be justified.[206]

ε-Aminocaproic Acid

Prophylactic antifibrinolytic therapy is common in modern cardiac surgery, with intraoperative and postoperative administration of ε-aminocaproic acid evolving into the standard of care in the United States. This should be continued at 1 g/hr. If it has not been used, a 5-g load followed by 1 g/hr may be beneficial.

Recombinant Activated Factor VII

Recombinant factor VIIa (rFVIIa) is a vitamin K–dependent glycoprotein that promotes hemostasis by activating the extrinsic pathway of the coagulation cascade. It replaces deficient activated coagulation factor VII, which complexes with tissue factor and may activate the conversion of coagulation factor X to factor Xa, and factor IX to IXa. When complexed with other factors, coagulation factor Xa converts prothrombin to thrombin, a key step in the formation of a fibrin–platelet hemostatic plug. As a new hemostatic agent, rFVIIa is increasingly being used off-label in cardiac surgery for treatment of severe coagulopathic bleeding that is not responsive to typical factor replacement. It is not currently approved for this indication, and its risk-to-benefit ratio has not been elucidated by any large-scale, placebo-controlled randomized clinical trial. Current recommendations suggest its use be limited to coagulopathic nonsurgical bleeding as rescue therapy, given at one to two doses of 35 to 70 μg/kg.[207]

NEUROLOGIC COMPLICATIONS

Neurologic dysfunction is a major cause of death and disability after cardiac surgery. Neurologic injury encompasses a spectrum of disorders such as stroke, encephalopathy, and cognitive dysfunction. Frank stroke occurs in as many as 10% of patients, but in most series the figure is between 1% and 3%.[208] Its occurrence is related to patient risk factors, identified in prospective studies that relate preoperative and intraoperative characteristics. Clinical variables found to increase risk include neurologic disease, age, hypertension, female sex, atherosclerosis of the ascending aorta, and diabetes.

The etiology of neurologic dysfunction is multifactorial, and it is the subject of much ongoing research. Causal factors include (1) particulate and gaseous emboli from the cardiopulmonary bypass apparatus, (2) macroemboli from aortic manipulation, (3) macroemboli from the extracranial cerebral vasculature, (4) regional malperfusion resulting from extracranial vascular obstruction, (5) regional malperfusion resulting from generalized hypoperfusion during CPB (watershed cerebral infarction), (6) regional malperfusion resulting from impaired cerebral autoregulation (more prevalent in diabetics), and (7) generalized central nervous system edema after CP.

Major stroke is often caused by atherosclerotic emboli originating in the aorta; more subtle neuropsychological deficits may be caused by microemboli.[209] Autopsy studies in patients who have undergone CPB have detected microscopic emboli, composed primarily of lipid, dispersed in the cerebral microvasculature.[210] The simple, initial approach has been the placement of an arterial line filter that has become standard equipment on most CPB circuits. Such filters, however, do not eliminate the microscopic lipid deposit that enters shed blood in the mediastinum (Fig. 61-13).[211] Furthermore, the use of cardiotomy suction to recover shed blood in combination with CPB results in significantly more microembolic events relative to CPB alone. Other studies have introduced the possibility that processing shed blood by washing and centrifugation (with a cell-saver device) before return to the CPB circuit may reduce these events.[212,213] This has led to increased use of cell saver in routine cardiac cases and more avoidance of conventional cardiotomy suction devices. Prospective randomized trials to determine whether these techniques will improve neurologic outcomes have not yet been performed.

Given the mechanism of neurocognitive injury with conventional cardiac surgery (i.e., emboli from cannulation and fatty or gaseous microemboli that are not filtered with standard CPB techniques), OPCAB has been suggested as a potential avenue to improve neurocognitive outcomes. There is clear evidence that there are fewer microemboli to the brain in patients having OPCAB than in those having conventional on-pump revascularization.[214,215] The significance of fewer microembolization events, however, is not entirely clear. A large prospective randomized clinical trial failed to show any difference in cognitive decline between off- and on-pump revascularization after 5 years of follow-up.[216] Furthermore, a recent nonrandomized four-arm prospective cohort study comparing (1) patients who had on-pump surgery, (2) patients who had off-pump surgery, (3) patients without surgery who had coronary disease that was medically managed, and (4) patients without coronary disease. Interestingly, there was no difference in cognitive outcome between all groups with coronary disease at 3 years, whether they had conventional CPB or OPCAB or medical management, but the patients without coronary disease had significantly higher cognitive performance than any of the other three groups at all time points. This suggests that coronary disease may be a surrogate marker for coincident occult cerebrovascular disease, and that cognitive decline may be consequent to the natural history of cerebrovascular disease itself.[217] A recent update on this cohort

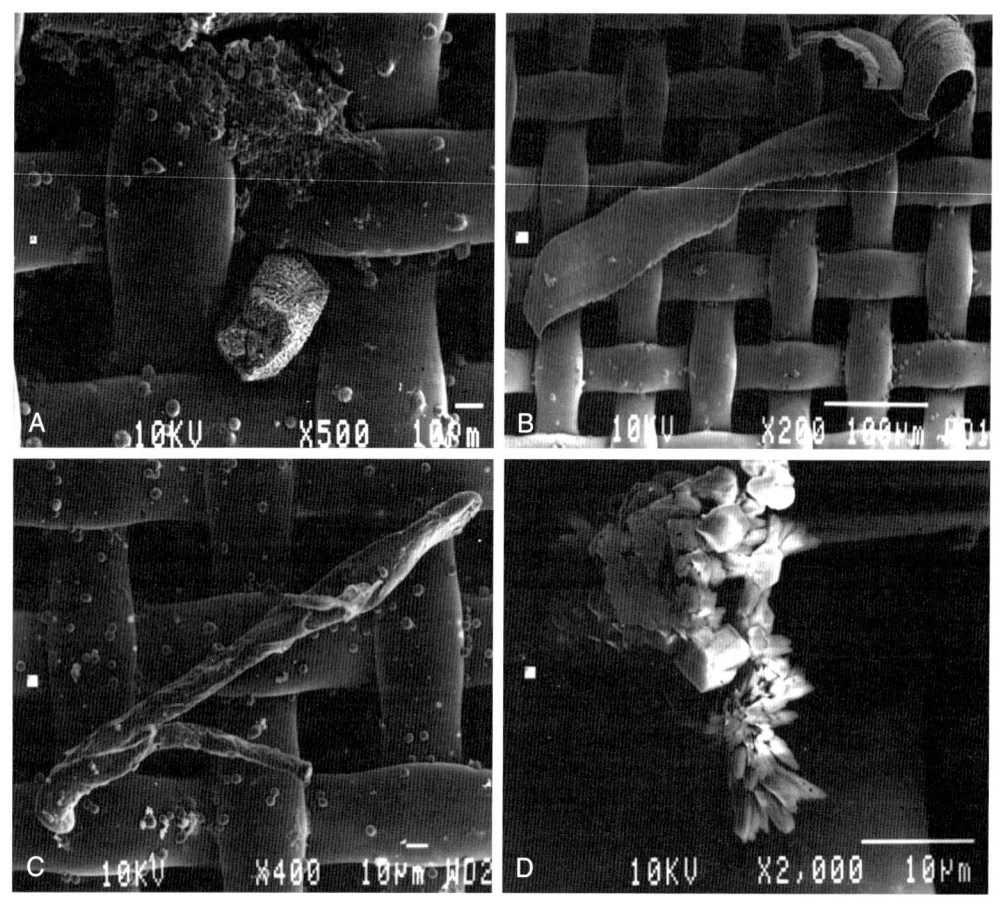

Figure 61-13
Debris commonly found on in-line arterial filters. Scanning electron micrographs of 40-micron arterial line filters after clinically uneventful cardiopulmonary bypass. **A,** Crystalline material can be seen embedded in the filter mesh with an adherent mass of fibrinous material incorporating erythrocytes. **B,** Particle measuring some 80 × 600 μm, thought to be spallated silicone rubber. **C,** Exogenous, organic fiber. **D,** Complex crystalline deposit. *(Reproduced with permission from Hogue CW. Cardiopulmonary bypass management and neurologic outcomes: an evidence-based appraisal of current practices.* Anesth Analg 2006;**103**:23.)

has demonstrated no difference in the long-term trajectory of cognitive function between groups at 6 years.[218] These results suggest that patients with coronary artery disease are at increased risk for neurologic dysfunction independent of CABG, and arguments suggesting that medical management can prevent or minimize neurologic dysfunction are false.

Other factors that contribute to neurologic dysfunction, particularly in older adults, include (1) "ICU psychosis" related to stress, environmental impact, and loss of ability to compensate to surroundings; (2) sleep deprivation; (3) adverse drug reactions; and (4) revelation of previously well-compensated mild dementia.

Often focal deficits are completely reversible if the patient is appropriately managed. The maintenance of adequate perfusion and oxygen delivery is critical to recovery. Cerebral blood flow is improved by head elevation to reduce edema and hyperventilation to provide moderate hypocapnia. General support includes protection of the patient's airway, management of pulmonary secretions, avoidance of pulmonary aspiration, and provision of nutrition. Because dramatic recovery is frequent, patient and family support should be aggressive in the first few days after surgery unless a definitive mortal injury can be defined.

INFECTION

Fever

The incidence of fever decreases exponentially throughout the postoperative course. Fevers not related to infectious causes are most commonly low grade (<38.9° C, rectal) and most resolve before the 15th postoperative day. A temperature higher than 38.9° C at any time in the postoperative course is more likely to be related to a specific infection. The presence or absence of leukocytosis has not been helpful in this differentiation.[219] For days 4 to 9 postoperatively, 25% of fevers may be related to serious infection.[220]

Evaluation and Treatment

When infection is suspected, aggressive evaluation is indicated. Aerobic and anaerobic cultures of blood, urine, sputum, and abnormal fluid collections are mandatory, and should precede broad-spectrum antibiotic coverage.

Indwelling catheters should be considered potential infectious sites; appropriate infection control practices help to prevent or at least limit serious infections stemming from catheter use.[190,221,222] When antibiotics have already been

Table 61-2
Univariate Logistic Regression Analysis*

Variable	Coefficient	χ^2	P
Obesity†	1.3	10.94	.009
NYHA congestive heart failure class†	0.32	9.34	.002
Diabetes mellitus (DM)	0.62	6.87	.009
Previous heart surgery†	0.85	6.83	.009
Duration of bypass†	0.005	5.48	.02
Comorbid condition	0.64	4.56	.03
Hemostasis at closure	1.2	2.94	.09
Peripheral vascular disease	0.37	1.55	.21
IMA graft (0, 1, or 2)	NA	0.95	.62
IMA graft (yes/no)	0.21	0.79	.37
Chronic obstructive pulmonary disease	0.39	0.61	.43
Sex	0.18	0.56	.45
Renal insufficiency	0.35	0.4	.53
Preoperative intra-aortic balloon pump	−0.3	0.38	.54
Coronary artery disease index	0.003	0.22	.64
Length of stay (before surgery)	−0.008	0.15	.71
Age	−0.003	0.1	.75
Ejection fraction	−0.002	0.05	.82
DM with bilateral IMA graft	NA	0.03	Diabetes, .01 Bilateral IMA, .30 Interaction, .28
Cardiac shock	0.07	0.01	.92
Operation type	−0.02	<0.0001	.96

*Univariate logistic regression analysis predicting mediastinitis; variables listed in order of significance. Variables with univariate P < .1 were included in the multivariate analysis.
†Significant predictions by multivariate analysis.
IMA, internal mammary artery; NYHA, New York Heart Association.
From Milano CA, Kesler K, Archibald N, et al. Mediastinitis after coronary artery bypass graft surgery: risk factors and long-term survival. Circulation 1995;22:45-51.

Figure 61-14
A, Unadjusted Kaplan-Meier survival plot is shown for patients with and without mediastinitis after coronary artery bypass graft (CABG) surgery. The numbers of surviving patients in each group at 0, 1, and 2 years after surgery are shown at the bottom of the graph. **B,** Variable-adjusted survival plot after CABG surgery. Kaplan-Meier survival plot is adjusted for age, ejection fraction, extent of coronary artery disease, peripheral vascular disease, cerebrovascular disease, recent myocardial infarction, angina status, and mitral insufficiency. *(Reproduced with permission from Milano CA, Kesler K, Archibald N, et al. Mediastinitis after coronary artery bypass graft surgery: risk factors and long-term survival. Circulation 1995;**92**:2245-51.)*

administered, cultures should be obtained using specific antimicrobial-absorbing resins.

Soft tissue infection is most commonly due to *Staphylococcus aureus*, although *Staphylococcus epidermidis* has emerged as an important pathogen. *Pseudomonas* and other gram-negative infections become more common when the intensive-care stay exceeds 7 days and in patients receiving broad-spectrum antibiotic therapy.[223]

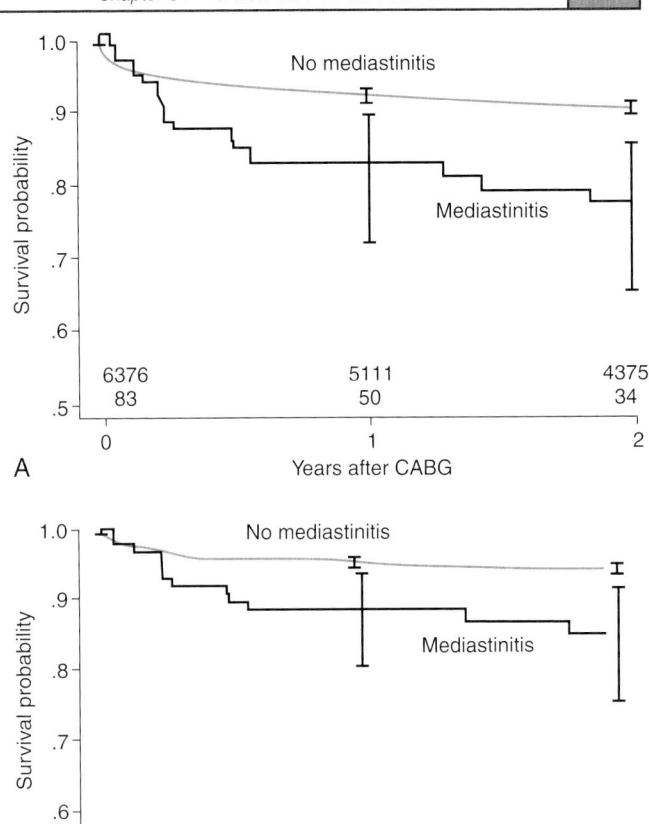

Prolonged intensive care and antibiotic use can also cause systemic fungal infections and loss of the gastric mucosal barrier.[224-226] These infections are particularly difficult to diagnose because of their protean manifestations.[126]

Mediastinitis is of particular concern in all cardiac surgical patients and can be cryptic in presentation. The incidence has been reported to range from 0.8% to 1.86%.[227-230] The risk factors associated with mediastinitis have been determined (Table 61-2), as has a negative impact on long-term survival independent of other preoperative risk factors (Fig. 61-14). Sternal and mediastinal infections must be differentiated from simple subcutaneous fat necrosis, sterile sternal dehiscence, and the post-pericardiotomy syndrome.

Deep sternal infections and mediastinitis are commonly associated with systemic symptoms (fever, leukocytosis), localized tenderness, severe persistent chest pain, and sternal instability.[196,229,231-235] Chest film, computed tomography, and indium-111 leucocyte scanning can be used to confirm the clinical diagnosis. Initial treatment consists of operative wound exploration, débridement, and drainage.[196] Although some infected patients can be treated with reclosure and irrigation,[236] diminished morbidity has been noted with bilateral pectoral flap or omental flap closure.[237] Flap closure may be performed as a primary procedure with accompanying sternal débridement[238] or as a staged procedure with sternal débridement followed by closure in 3 to 4 days.[237,239] A recent cohort study demonstrated similar survival rates of patients with mediastinitis treated with vacuum-assisted closure and patients without mediastinitis who underwent coronary revascularization alone, suggesting that vacuum-assisted closure may be as effective as flap closure.[240]

Soft tissue infections involving saphenous vein harvest, though usually minor, represent a significant source of morbidity after coronary revascularization. This complication has been reported to occur in 1% of patients[241] and is more common in the thigh harvest site. They are best prevented by careful selection of harvest sites and the use of meticulous surgical technique. Endoscopic vein harvest appears to have made a favorable impact on the rate of this complication. Most saphenous vein harvest site infections mat be treated effectively by simple drainage, dressing changes, and prescription of antibiotics. However, in severe cases, wide débridement and skin grafting may be necessary.

REFERENCES

1. Frank SM, Higgins MS, Fleisher LA, Sitzmann JV, Raff H, Breslow MJ. Adrenergic, respiratory, and cardiovascular effects of core cooling in humans. *Am J Physiol* 1997;**272**(2 Pt 2):R557-62.
2. Westaby S. Organ dysfunction after cardiopulmonary bypass: a systemic inflammatory reaction initiated by the extracorporeal circuit. *Intens Care Med* 1987;**13**(2):89-95.
3. Chenoweth DE, Cooper SW, Hugli TE, Stewart RW, Blackstone EH, Kirklin JW. Complement activation during cardiopulmonary bypass: evidence for generation of C3a and C5a anaphylatoxins. *N Engl J Med* 1981;**304**(9):497-503.
4. Wachtfogel YT, Kucich U, Greenplate J, et al. Human neutrophil degranulation during extracorporeal circulation. *Blood* 1987;**69**(1):324-30.
5. Kirklin JW, Archie Jr JP. The cardiovascular subsystem in surgical patients. *Surg Gynecol Obstet* 1974;**139**(1):17-23.
6. Moore Jr FD, Warner KG, Assousa S, Valeri CR, Khuri SF. The effects of complement activation during cardiopulmonary bypass: attenuation by hypothermia, heparin, and hemodilution. *Ann Surg* 1988;**208**(1):95-103.
7. Videm V, Fosse E, Mollnes TE, Garred P, Svennevig JL. Time for new concepts about measurement of complement activation by cardiopulmonary bypass? *Ann Thorac Surg* 1992;**54**(4):725-31.
8. Shabetai R. Pericardial and cardiac pressure. *Circulation* 1988;**77**(1):1-5.
9. Steinberg JB, Kapelanski DP, Olson JD, Weiler JM. Cytokine and complement levels in patients undergoing cardiopulmonary bypass. *J Thorac Cardiovasc Surg* 1993;**106**(6):1008-16.
10. Craddock PR, Fehr J, Dalmasso AP, Brighan KL, Jacob HS. Hemodialysis leukopenia: pulmonary vascular leukostasis resulting from complement activation by dialyzer cellophane membranes. *J Clin Invest* 1977;**59**(5):879-88.
11. Dinarello CA. Interleukin-1 and the pathogenesis of the acute-phase response. *N Engl J Med* 1984;**311**(22):1413-8.
12. McCord JM, Wong K, Stokes SH, Petrone WF, English D. Superoxide and inflammation: a mechanism for the anti-inflammatory activity of superoxide dismutase. *Acta Physiol Scand* 1980;**492**:25-30.
13. Butler J, Parker D, Pillai R, Westaby S, Shale DJ, Rocker GM. Effect of cardiopulmonary bypass on systemic release of neutrophil elastase and tumor necrosis factor. *J Thorac Cardiovasc Surg* 1993;**105**(1):25-30.
14. Jansen EW, Borst C, Lahpor JR, et al. Coronary artery bypass grafting without cardiopulmonary bypass using the octopus method: results in the first one hundred patients. *J Thorac Cardiovasc Surg* 1998;**116**(1):60-7.
15. Markewitz A, Faist E, Lang S, Endres S, Fuchs D, Reichart B. Successful restoration of cell-mediated immune response after cardiopulmonary bypass by immunomodulation. *J Thorac Cardiovasc Surg* 1993;**105**(1):15-24.
16. Klausner JM, Morel N, Paterson IS, et al. The rapid induction by interleukin-2 of pulmonary microvascular permeability. *Ann Surg* 1989;**209**(1):119-28.
17. Maggart M, Stewart S. The mechanisms and management of noncardiogenic pulmonary edema following cardiopulmonary bypass. *Ann Thorac Surg* 1987;**43**(2):231-6.
18. Boisclair MD, Lane DA, Philippou H, et al. Mechanisms of thrombin generation during surgery and cardiopulmonary bypass. *Blood* 1993;**82**(11):3350-7.
19. Weitz JI, Hudoba M, Massel D, Maraganore J, Hirsh J. Clot-bound thrombin is protected from inhibition by heparin-antithrombin III but is susceptible to inactivation by antithrombin III-independent inhibitors. *J Clin Invest* 1990;**86**(2):385-91.
20. Edmunds Jr LH, Colman RW. Thrombin during cardiopulmonary bypass. *Ann Thorac Surg* 2006;**82**(6):2315-22.
21. Jastrzebski J, Sykes MK, Woods DG. Cardiorespiratory effects of protamine after cardiopulmonary bypass in man. *Thorax* 1974;**29**(5):534-8.
22. Clark SC. Lung injury after cardiopulmonary bypass. *Perfusion* 2006;**21**(4):225-8.
23. Fouad FM, Estafanous FG, Bravo EL, Iyer KA, Maydak JH, Tarazi RC. Possible role of cardioaortic reflexes in postcoronary bypass hypertension. *Am J Cardiol* 1979;**44**(5):866-72.
24. Ito T, Engle MA, Goldberg HP. Postpericardiotomy syndrome following surgery for nonrheumatic heart disease. *Circulation* 1958;**17**(4 Pt 1):549-56.
25. Engle MA, Ito T. The postpericardiotomy syndrome. *Am J Cardiol* 1961;**7**:73-82.
26. Engle MA, Zabriskie JB, Senterfit LB, Tay DJ, Ebert PA. Immunologic and virologic studies in the postpericardiotomy syndrome. *J Pediatr* 1975;**87**(6 Pt 2):1103-8.
27. Horneffer PJ, Miller RH, Pearson TA, Rykiel MF, Reitz BA, Gardner TJ. The effective treatment of postpericardiotomy syndrome after cardiac operations: a randomized placebo-controlled trial. *J Thorac Cardiovasc Surg* 1990;**100**(2):292-6.
28. Kirsh MM, McIntosh K, Kahn DR, Sloan H. Postpericardiotomy syndromes. *Ann Thorac Surg* 1970;**9**(2):158-79.
29. Bainbridge D, Cheng D, Martin J, Novick R. Does off-pump or minimally invasive coronary artery bypass reduce mortality, morbidity, and resource utilization when compared with percutaneous coronary intervention? A meta-analysis of randomized trials. *J Thorac Cardiovasc Surg* 2007;**133**(3):623-31.
30. Cheng DC, Bainbridge D, Martin JE, Novick RJ. Does off-pump coronary artery bypass reduce mortality, morbidity, and resource utilization when compared with conventional coronary artery bypass? A meta-analysis of randomized trials. *Anesthesiology* 2005;**102**(1):188-203.
31. Lytle BW, Sabik JF. On-pump and off-pump bypass surgery: tools for revascularization. *Circulation* 2004;**109**(7):810-2.
32. Hannan EL, Wu C, Smith CR, et al. Off-pump versus on-pump coronary artery bypass graft surgery: differences in short-term outcomes and in long-term mortality and need for subsequent revascularization. *Circulation* 2007;**116**(10):1145-52.
33. Wijeysundera DN, Beattie WS, Djaiani G, et al. Off-pump coronary artery surgery for reducing mortality and morbidity: meta-analysis of randomized and observational studies. *J Am Coll Cardiol* 2005;**46**(5):872-82.
34. Puskas JD, Cheng D, Knight J, Angelini G, DeCannier D, Diegeler A, et al. Off-pump versus conventional coronary artery bypass grafting: a meta-analysis and consensus statement from the 2004 ISMICS consensus conference. *Innovations* 2005;1(1):3-27.
35. Ascione R, Lloyd CT, Underwood MJ, Lotto AA, Pitsis AA, Angelini GD. Inflammatory response after coronary revascularization with or without cardiopulmonary bypass. *Ann Thorac Surg* 2000;**69**(4):1198-204.
36. Gu YJ, Mariani MA, van Oeveren W, Grandjean JG, Boonstra PW. Reduction of the inflammatory response in patients undergoing minimally invasive coronary artery bypass grafting. *Ann Thorac Surg* 1998;**65**(2):420-4.
37. Angelini GD, Fraser AG, Koning MM, et al. Adverse hemodynamic effects and echocardiographic consequences of pericardial closure soon after sternotomy and pericardiotomy. *Circulation* 1990;**82**(Suppl. 5):IV397-406.
38. Elahi MM, Khan JS, Matata BM. Deleterious effects of cardiopulmonary bypass in coronary artery surgery and scientific interpretation of off-pump's logic. *Acute Card Care* 2006;**8**(4):196-209.
39. Kshettry VR, Flavin TF, Emery RW, Nicoloff DM, Arom KV, Petersen RJ. Does multivessel, off-pump coronary artery bypass reduce postoperative morbidity? *Ann Thorac Surg* 2000;**69**(6):1725-30, discussion 30-1.
40. Casati V, Gerli C, Franco A, et al. Activation of coagulation and fibrinolysis during coronary surgery: on-pump versus off-pump techniques. *Anesthesiology* 2001;**95**(5):1103-9.
41. Matata BM, Sosnowski AW, Galinanes M. Off-pump bypass graft operation significantly reduces oxidative stress and inflammation. *Ann Thorac Surg* 2000;**69**(3):785-91.
42. Czerny M, Baumer H, Kilo J, et al. Inflammatory response and myocardial injury following coronary artery bypass grafting with or without cardiopulmonary bypass. *Eur J Cardiothorac Surg* 2000;**17**(6):737-42.

43. Boyd AD, Tremblay RE, Spencer FC, Bahnson HT. Estimation of cardiac output soon after intracardiac surgery with cardiopulmonary bypass. *Ann Surg* 1959;**150**:613-26.
44. Swan HJ, Forrester JS, Diamond G, Chatterjee K, Parmley WW. Hemodynamic spectrum of myocardial infarction and cardiogenic shock: a conceptual model. *Circulation* 1972;**45**(5):1097-110.
45. Kumon K, Tanaka K, Hirata T, Naito Y, Fujita T. Organ failures due to low cardiac output syndrome following open heart surgery. *Jpn Circ J* 1986;**50**(4):329-35.
46. Massie B, Ports T, Chatterjee K, et al. Long-term vasodilator therapy for heart failure: clinical response and its relationship to hemodynamic measurements. *Circulation* 1981;**63**(2):269-78.
47. Appelbaum A, Kouchoukos NT, Blackstone EH, Kirklin JW. Early risks of open heart surgery for mitral valve disease. *Am J Cardiol* 1976;**37**(2):201-9.
48. Reeves JT, Grover RF, Filley GF, Blount Jr SG. Cardiac output in normal resting man. *J applied physiology* 1961;**16**:276-8.
49. Shibutani K, Komatsu T, Kubal K, Sanchala V, Kumar V, Bizzarri DV. Critical level of oxygen delivery in anesthetized man. *Crit Care Med* 1983;**11**(8):640-3.
50. Rashkin MC, Bosken C, Baughman RP. Oxygen delivery in critically ill patients: relationship to blood lactate and survival. *Chest* 1985;**87**(5):580-4.
51. Broder G, Weil MH. Excess lactate: an index of reversibility of shock in human patients. *Science* 1964;**143**:1457-9.
52. Mizock BA, Falk JL. Lactic acidosis in critical illness. *Crit Care Med* 1992;**20**(1):80-93.
53. Weil MH, Afifi AA. Experimental and clinical studies on lactate and pyruvate as indicators of the severity of acute circulatory failure (shock). *Circulation* 1970;**41**(6):989-1001.
54. Astiz ME, Rackow EC, Kaufman B, Falk JL, Weil MH. Relationship of oxygen delivery and mixed venous oxygenation to lactic acidosis in patients with sepsis and acute myocardial infarction. *Crit Care Med* 1988;**16**(7):655-8.
55. Kirklin JK, Westaby S, Blackstone EH, Kirklin JW, Chenoweth DE, Pacifico AD. Complement and the damaging effects of cardiopulmonary bypass. *J Thorac Cardiovasc Surg* 1983;**86**(6):845-57.
56. Krauss XH, Verdouw PD, Hughenholtz PG, Nauta J. On-line monitoring of mixed venous oxygen saturation after cardiothoracic surgery. *Thorax* 1975;**30**(6):636-43.
57. Vaughn S, Puri VK. Cardiac output changes and continuous mixed venous oxygen saturation measurement in the critically ill. *Crit Care Med* 1988;**16**(5):495-8.
58. Bryan-Brown CW. Blood flow to organs: parameters for function and survival in critical illness. *Crit Care Med* 1988;**16**(2):170-8.
59. Landow L. Splanchnic lactate production in cardiac surgery patients. *Crit Care Med* 1993;**21**(Suppl. 2):S84-91.
60. Mellander S, Johansson B. Control of resistance, exchange, and capacitance functions in the peripheral circulation. *Pharmacol Rev* 1968;**20**(3):117-96.
61. Chiara O, Giomarelli PP, Biagioli B, Rosi R, Gattinoni L. Hypermetabolic response after hypothermic cardiopulmonary bypass. *Crit Care Med* 1987;**15**(11):995-1000.
62. Rodriguez JL, Weissman C, Damask MC, Askanazi J, Hyman AI, Kinney JM. Physiologic requirements during rewarming: suppression of the shivering response. *Crit Care Med* 1983;**11**(7):490-7.
63. Zwischenberger JB, Kirsh MM, Dechert RE, Arnold DK, Bartlett RH. Suppression of shivering decreases oxygen consumption and improves hemodynamic stability during postoperative rewarming. *Ann Thorac Surg* 1987;**43**(4):428-31.
64. Crexells C, Chatterjee K, Forrester JS, Dikshit K, Swan HJ. Optimal level of filling pressure in the left side of the heart in acute myocardial infarction. *N Engl J Med* 1973;**289**(24):1263-6.
65. Tyberg JV, Taichman GC, Smith ER, Douglas NW, Smiseth OA, Keon WJ. The relationship between pericardial pressure and right atrial pressure: an intraoperative study. *Circulation* 1986;**73**(3):428-32.
66. Hanson EL, Kane PB, Askanazi J, Neville Jr JF, Webb WR. Comparison of patients with coronary artery or valve disease: intraoperative differences in blood volume and observations of vasomotor response. *Ann Thorac Surg* 1976;**22**(4):343-6.
67. Gaffney FA, Bastian BC, Thal ER, Atkins JM, Blomqvist CG. Passive leg raising does not produce a significant or sustained autotransfusion effect. *J Trauma* 1982;**22**(3):190-3.
68. Bolanowski PJ, Bauer J, Machiedo G, Neville WE. Prostaglandin influence on pulmonary intravascular leukocytic aggregation during cardiopulmonary bypass. *J Thorac Cardiovasc Surg* 1977;**73**(2):221-4.
69. Estafanous FG, Tarazi RC. Systemic arterial hypertension associated with cardiac surgery. *Am J Cardiol* 1980;**46**(4):685-94.
70. Weinstein GS, Zabetakis PM, Clavel A, et al. The renin-angiotensin system is not responsible for hypertension following coronary artery bypass grafting. *Ann Thorac Surg* 1987;**43**(1):74-7.
71. Gall WE, Clarke WR, Doty DB. Vasomotor dynamics associated with cardiac operations: I. Venous tone and the effects of vasodilators. *J Thorac Cardiovasc Surg* 1982;**83**(5):724-31.
72. Taylor KM, Brannan JJ, Bain WH, Caves PK, Morton IJ. Role of angiotensin II in the development of peripheral vasoconstriction during cardiopulmonary bypass. *Cardiovasc Res* 1979;**13**(5):269-73.
73. Taylor KM, Morton IJ, Brown JJ, Bain WH, Caves PK. Hypertension and the renin-angiotensin system following open-heart surgery. *J Thorac Cardiovasc Surg* 1977;**74**(6):840-5.
74. Packer M. Neurohormonal interactions and adaptations in congestive heart failure. *Circulation* 1988;**77**(4):721-30.
75. Whelton PK, Flaherty JT, MacAllister NP, et al. Hypertension following coronary artery bypass surgery: role of preoperative propranolol therapy. *Hypertension* 1980;**2**(3):291-8.
76. Zelis R, Mansour EJ, Capone RJ, Mason DT. The cardiovascular effects of morphine: the peripheral capacitance and resistance vessels in human subjects. *J Clin Invest* 1974;**54**(6):1247-58.
77. Johnson PC. *The peripheral circulation*. New York: Wiley; 1978.
78. Strandgaard S, Olesen J, Skinhoj E, Lassen NA. Autoregulation of brain circulation in severe arterial hypertension. *Br Med J* 1973;**1**(5852):507-10.
79. Marcus ML, Harrison DG, Chilian WM, et al. Alterations in the coronary circulation in hypertrophied ventricles. *Circulation* 1987;**75**(1 Pt 2):I19-25.
80. Redwood DR, Smith ER, Epstein SE. Coronary artery occlusion in the conscious dog: effects of alterations in heart rate and arterial pressure on the degree of myocardial ischemia. *Circulation* 1972;**46**(2):323-32.
81. Luz PL, Forrester JS, Wyatt HL, et al. Hemodynamic and metabolic effects of sodium nitroprusside on the performance and metabolism of regional ischemic myocardium. *Circulation* 1975;**52**(3):400-7.
82. Watanabe T, Covell JW, Maroko PR, Braunwald E, Ross Jr J. Effects of increased arterial pressure and positive inotropic agents on the severity of myocardial ischemia in the acutely depressed heart. *Am J Cardiol* 1972;**30**(4):371-7.
83. Stinson EB, Holloway EL, Derby G, et al. Comparative hemodynamic responses to chlorpromazine, nitroprusside, nitroglycerin, and trimethaphan immediately after open-heart operations. *Circulation* 1975;**52**(Suppl. 2):I26-33.
84. Chatterjee K, Parmley WW, Swan HJ, Berman G, Forrester J, Marcus HS. Beneficial effects of vasodilator agents in severe mitral regurgitation due to dysfunction of subvalvar apparatus. *Circulation* 1973;**48**(4):684-90.
85. Bolen JL, Alderman EL. Hemodynamic consequences of afterload reduction in patients with chronic aortic regurgitation. *Circulation* 1976;**53**(5):879-83.
86. Chiariello M, Gold HK, Leinbach RC, Davis MA, Maroko PR. Comparison between the effects of nitroprusside and nitroglycerin on ischemic injury during acute myocardial infarction. *Circulation* 1976;**54**(5):766-73.
87. Bixler TJ, Gardner TJ, Donahoo JS, Brawley RK, Potter A, Gott VL. Improved myocardial performance in postoperative cardiac surgical patients with sodium nitroprusside. *Ann Thorac Surg* 1978;**25**(5):444-8.
88. Goldstein RE, Stinson EB, Scherer JL, Seningen RP, Grehl TM, Epstein SE. Intraoperative coronary collateral function in patients with coronary occlusive disease: nitroglycerin responsiveness and angiographic correlations. *Circulation* 1974;**49**(2):298-308.
89. Davies DW, Kadar D, Steward DJ, Munro IR. A sudden death associated with the use of sodium nitroprusside for induction of hypotension during anaesthesia. *Can Anaesth Soc J* 1975;**22**(5):547-52.
90. Michenfelder JD, Tinker JH. Cyanide toxicity and thiosulfate protection during chronic administration of sodium nitroprusside in the dog: correlation with a human case. *Anesthesiology* 1977;**47**(5):441-8.
91. Sladen RN, Rosenthal MH. Specific afterload reduction with parenteral hydralazine following cardiac surgery. *J Thorac Cardiovasc Surg* 1979;**78**(2):195-202.
92. Massie BM, Conway M. Survival of patients with congestive heart failure: past, present, and future prospects. *Circulation* 1987;**75**(5 Pt 2):IV11-9.
93. Hood Jr WB. Role of converting enzyme inhibitors in the treatment of heart failure. *J Am Coll Cardiol* 1993;**22**(4 Suppl A):154A-7A.
94. Davis R, Ribner HS, Keung E, Sonnenblick EH, LeJemtel TH. Treatment of chronic congestive heart failure with captopril, an oral inhibitor of angiotensin-converting enzyme. *N Engl J Med* 1979;**301**(3):117-21.
95. Konstam MA, Kronenberg MW, Udelson JE, et al. Effect of acute angiotensin converting enzyme inhibition on left ventricular filling in patients with congestive heart failure: relation to right ventricular volumes. *Circulation* 1990;**81**(Suppl. 2):III115-22.
96. Pitt B. Use of converting enzyme inhibitors in patients with asymptomatic left ventricular dysfunction. *J Am Coll Cardiol* 1993;**22**(4 Suppl A):158A-61A.
97. St John Sutton M, Pfeffer MA, Plappert T, et al. Quantitative two-dimensional echocardiographic measurements are major predictors of adverse cardiovascular events after acute myocardial infarction: the protective effects of captopril. *Circulation* 1994;**89**(1):68-75.
98. Cohn JN, Archibald DG, Ziesche S, et al. Effect of vasodilator therapy on mortality in chronic congestive heart failure: results of a Veterans Administration Cooperative Study. *N Engl J Med* 1986;**314**(24):1547-52.

99. Cohn JN, Johnson G, Ziesche S, et al. A comparison of enalapril with hydralazine-isosorbide dinitrate in the treatment of chronic congestive heart failure. *N Engl J Med* 1991;**325**(5):303-10.
100. Skinner Jr NS, Mitchell JH, Wallace AG, Sarnoff SJ. Hemodynamic effects of altering the timing of atrial systole. *Am J Physiol* 1963;**205**:499-503.
101. Ellis RJ, Mavroudis C, Gardner C, Turley K, Ullyot D, Ebert PA. Relationship between atrioventricular arrhythmias and the concentration of K+ ion in cardioplegic solution. *J Thorac Cardiovasc Surg* 1980;**80**(4):517-26.
102. Smith PK, Muhlbaier LH. Aprotinin: safe and effective only with the full-dose regimen. *Ann Thorac Surg* 1996;**62**(6):1575-7.
103. Smith PK, Tyson Jr GS, Hammon Jr JW, et al. Cardiovascular effects of ventilation with positive expiratory airway pressure. *Ann Surg* 1982;**195**(2):121-30.
104. Guyton RA, Andrews MJ, Hickey PR, Michaelis LL, Morrow AG. The contribution of atrial contraction to right heart function before and after right ventriculotomy: experimental and clinical observations. *J Thorac Cardiovasc Surg* 1976;**71**(1):1-10.
105. Hartzler GO, Maloney JD, Curtis JJ, Barnhorst DA. Hemodynamic benefits of atrioventricular sequential pacing after cardiac surgery. *Am J Cardiol* 1977;**40**(2):232-6.
106. Zoll PM. Resuscitation of the heart in ventricular standstill by external electric stimulation. *N Engl J Med* 1952;**247**(20):768-71.
107. Van Trigt P, Spray TL, Pasque MK, et al. The influence of time on the response to dopamine after coronary artery bypass grafting: assessment of left ventricular performance and contractility using pressure/dimension analyses. *Ann Thorac Surg* 1983;**35**(1):3-13.
108. Erdmann E. The effectiveness of inotropic agents in isolated cardiac preparations from the human heart. *Klin Wochenschr* 1988;**66**(1):1-6.
109. Vernon DD, Garrett JS, Banner Jr W, Dean JM. Hemodynamic effects of dobutamine in an intact animal model. *Crit Care Med* 1992;**20**(9):1322-9.
110. Bristow MR, Ginsburg R, Minobe W, et al. Decreased catecholamine sensitivity and beta-adrenergic-receptor density in failing human hearts. *N Engl J Med* 1982;**307**(4):205-11.
111. DiSesa VJ. The rational selection of inotropic drugs in cardiac surgery. *J Card Surg* 1987;**2**(3):385-406.
112. Fowler MB, Laser JA, Hopkins GL, Minobe W, Bristow MR. Assessment of the beta-adrenergic receptor pathway in the intact failing human heart: progressive receptor down-regulation and subsensitivity to agonist response. *Circulation* 1986;**74**(6):1290-302.
113. Glaubiger G, Lefkowitz RJ. Elevated beta-adrenergic receptor number after chronic propranolol treatment. *Biochem Biophys Res Commun* 1977;**78**(2):720-5.
114. Lefkowitz RJ. Direct binding studies of adrenergic receptors: biochemical, physiologic, and clinical implications. *Ann Intern Med* 1979;**91**(3):450-8.
115. Kosugi I, Tajimi K. Effects of dopamine and dobutamine on hemodynamics and plasma catecholamine levels during severe lactic acid acidosis. *Circ Shock* 1985;**17**(2):95-102.
116. Tajimi K, Kosugi I, Hamamoto F, Kobayashi K. Plasma catecholamine levels and hemodynamic responses of severely acidotic dogs to dopamine infusion. *Crit Care Med* 1983;**11**(10):817-9.
117. Craddock DR, Logan A, Fadali A. Reoperation for haemorrhage following cardiopulmonary by-pass. *Br J Surg* 1968;**55**(1):17-20.
118. Engelman RM, Spencer FC, Reed GE, Tice DA. Cardiac tamponade following open-heart surgery. *Circulation* 1970;**41**(Suppl. 5):II165-71.
119. Nelson RM, Jenson CB, Smoot 3rd WM. Pericardial tamponade following open-heart surgery. *J Thorac Cardiovasc Surg* 1969;**58**(4):510-6.
120. Weeks KR, Chatterjee K, Block S, Matloff JM, Swan HJ. Bedside hemodynamic monitoring: its value in the diagnosis of tamponade complicating cardiac surgery. *J Thorac Cardiovasc Surg* 1976;**71**(2):250-2.
121. Fowler NO, Gabel M, Buncher CR. Cardiac tamponade: a comparison of right versus left heart compression. *J Am Coll Cardiol* 1988;**12**(1):187-93.
122. Russo AM, O'Connor WH, Waxman HL. Atypical presentations and echocardiographic findings in patients with cardiac tamponade occurring early and late after cardiac surgery. *Chest* 1993;**104**(1):71-8.
123. Shabetai R. Changing concepts of cardiac tamponade. *J Am Coll Cardiol* 1988;**12**(1):194-5.
124. Furnary AP, Magovern JA, Simpson KA, Magovern GJ. Prolonged open sternotomy and delayed sternal closure after cardiac operations. *Ann Thorac Surg* 1992;**54**(2):233-9.
125. Bortolotti U, Livi U, Frugoni C, et al. Delayed cardiac tamponade following open heart surgery: analysis of 12 patients. *Thorac Cardiovasc Surg* 1981;**29**(4):233-6.
126. Ellison N, Beatty CP, Blake DR, Wurzel HA, MacVaugh 3rd H. Heparin rebound. Studies in patients and volunteers. *J Thorac Cardiovasc Surg* 1974;**67**(5):723-9.
127. Hardesty RL, Thompson M, Lerberg DB, et al. Delayed postoperative cardiac tamponade: diagnosis and management. *Ann Thorac Surg* 1978;**26**(2):155-64.
128. Fyke 3rd FE, Tancredi RG, Shub C, Julsrud PR, Sheedy 2nd PF. Detection of intrapericardial hematoma after open heart surgery: the roles of echocardiography and computed tomography. *J Am Coll Cardiol* 1985;**5**(6):1496-9.
129. Kronzon I, Cohen ML, Winer HE. Diastolic atrial compression: a sensitive echocardiographic sign of cardiac tamponade. *J Am Coll Cardiol* 1983;**2**(4):770-5.
130. Singh BN, Nademanee K. Use of calcium antagonists for cardiac arrhythmias. *Am J Cardiol* 1987;**59**(3):153B-62B.
131. Ozal E, Kuralay E, Yildirim V, et al. Preoperative methylene blue administration in patients at high risk for vasoplegic syndrome during cardiac surgery. *Ann Thorac Surg* 2005;**79**(5):1615-9.
132. Levin RL, Degrange MA, Bruno GF, et al. Methylene blue reduces mortality and morbidity in vasoplegic patients after cardiac surgery. *Ann Thorac Surg* 2004;**77**(2):496-9.
133. Shanmugam G. Vasoplegic syndrome: the role of methylene blue. *Eur J Cardiothorac Surg* 2005;**28**(5):705-10.
134. Egi M, Bellomo R, Langenberg C, et al. Selecting a vasopressor drug for vasoplegic shock after adult cardiac surgery: a systematic literature review. *Ann Thorac Surg* 2007;**83**(2):715-23.
135. Manolis AS, Estes 3rd NA. Supraventricular tachycardia: mechanisms and therapy. *Arch Intern Med* 1987;**147**(10):1706-16.
136. Waldo AL, MacLean WA, Karp RB, Kouchoukos NT, James TN. Entrainment and interruption of atrial flutter with atrial pacing: studies in man following open heart surgery. *Circulation* 1977;**56**(5):737-45.
137. Lister JW, Cohen LS, Bernstein WH, Samet P. Treatment of supraventricular tachycardias by rapid atrial stimulation. *Circulation* 1968;**38**(6):1044-59.
138. Lauer MS, Eagle KA, Buckley MJ, DeSanctis RW. Atrial fibrillation following coronary artery bypass surgery. *Prog Cardiovasc Dis* 1989;**31**(5):367-78.
139. Rubin DA, Nieminski KE, Reed GE, Herman MV. Predictors, prevention, and long-term prognosis of atrial fibrillation after coronary artery bypass graft operations. *J Thorac Cardiovasc Surg* 1987;**94**(3):331-5.
140. Silverman NA, DuBrow I, Kohler J, Levitsky S. Etiology of atrioventricular-conduction abnormalities following cardiac surgery. *J Surg Res* 1984;**36**(3):198-204.
141. Silverman NA, Wright R, Levitsky S. Efficacy of low-dose propranolol in preventing postoperative supraventricular tachyarrhythmias: a prospective, randomized study. *Ann Surg* 1982;**196**(2):194-7.
142. Ansell J, Klassen V, Lew R, et al. Does desmopressin acetate prophylaxis reduce blood loss after valvular heart operations? A randomized, double-blind study. *J Thorac Cardiovasc Surg* 1992;**104**(1):117-23.
143. Cox JL. A perspective of postoperative atrial fibrillation in cardiac operations. *Ann Thorac Surg* 1993;**56**(3):405-9.
144. Page PL, Plumb VJ, Okumura K, Waldo AL. A new animal model of atrial flutter. *J Am Coll Cardiol* 1986;**8**(4):872-9.
145. Kyosola K, Mattila T, Harjula A, Kyosola H, Waris T. Life-threatening complications of cardiac operations and occurrence of myocardial catecholamine bombs. *J Thorac Cardiovasc Surg* 1988;**95**(2):334-9.
146. Creswell LL, Schuessler RB, Rosenbloom M, Cox JL. Hazards of postoperative atrial arrhythmias. *Ann Thorac Surg* 1993;**56**(3):539-49.
147. Singh BN. A fourth class of anti-dysrhythmic action? effect of verapamil on ouabain toxicity, on atrial and ventricular intracellular potentials, and on other features of cardiac function. *Cardiovasc Res* 1972;**6**(2):109-19.
148. Nayler WG, Szeto J. Effect of verapamil on contractility, oxygen utilization, and calcium exchangeability in mammalian heart muscle. *Cardiovasc Res* 1972;**6**(2):120-8.
149. Packer M, Kessler PD, Lee WH. Calcium-channel blockade in the management of severe chronic congestive heart failure: a bridge too far. *Circulation* 1987;**75**(6 Pt 2):V56-64.
150. Plumb VJ, Karp RB, Kouchoukos NT, Zorn Jr GL, James TN, Waldo AL. Verapamil therapy of atrial fibrillation and atrial flutter following cardiac operation. *J Thorac Cardiovasc Surg* 1982;**83**(4):590-6.
151. Perkins CM. Serious verapamil poisoning: treatment with intravenous calcium gluconate. *Br Med J* 1978;**2**(6145):1127.
152. Linden CH, Aghababian RV. Further uses of glucagon. *Crit Care Med* 1985;**13**(4):248.
153. Singh S, Wann LS, Schuchard GH, et al. Right ventricular and right atrial collapse in patients with cardiac tamponade: a combined echocardiographic and hemodynamic study. *Circulation* 1984;**70**(6):966-71.
154. Goldman S, Probst P, Selzer A, Cohn K. Inefficacy of "therapeutic" serum levels of digoxin in controlling the ventricular rate in atrial fibrillation. *Am J Cardiol* 1975;**35**(5):651-5.

155. Lee TH, Salomon DR, Rayment CM, Antman EM. Hypotension and sinus arrest with exercise-induced hyperkalemia and combined verapamil/propranolol therapy. *Am J Med* 1986;**80**(6):1203-4.
156. Chesebro JH, Clements IP, Fuster V, et al. A platelet-inhibitor-drug trial in coronary-artery bypass operations: benefit of perioperative dipyridamole and aspirin therapy on early postoperative vein-graft patency. *N Engl J Med* 1982;**307**(2):73-8.
157. Lorenz RL, Schacky CV, Weber M, et al. Improved aortocoronary bypass patency by low-dose aspirin (100 mg daily): effects on platelet aggregation and thromboxane formation. *Lancet* 1984;**1**(8389):1261-4.
158. Bhatt DL, Chew DP, Hirsch AT, Ringleb PA, Hacke W, Topol EJ. Superiority of clopidogrel versus aspirin in patients with prior cardiac surgery. *Circulation* 2000;**103**:363-8.
159. Kulik A, Le May M, Wells GA, Mesana TG, Ruel M. The clopidogrel after surgery for coronary artery disease (CASCADE) randomized controlled trial: clopidogrel and aspirin versus aspirin alone after coronary bypass surgery [NCT00228423]. *Curr Control Trials Cardiovasc Med* 2005;**6**:15.
160. van de Watering LM, Hermans J, Houbiers JG, et al. Beneficial effects of leukocyte depletion of transfused blood on postoperative complications in patients undergoing cardiac surgery: a randomized clinical trial. *Circulation* 1998;**97**(6):562-8.
161. Boldt J, Knothe C, Zickmann B, Bill S, Dapper F, Hempelmann G. Platelet function in cardiac surgery: influence of temperature and aprotinin. *Ann Thorac Surg* 1993;**55**(3):652-8.
162. Harker LA. Bleeding after cardiopulmonary bypass. *N Engl J Med* 1986;**314**(22):1446-8.
163. Valeri CR, Khabbaz K, Khuri SF, et al. Effect of skin temperature on platelet function in patients undergoing extracorporeal bypass. *J Thorac Cardiovasc Surg* 1992;**104**(1):108-16.
164. Despotis GJ, Filos KS, Zoys TN, Hogue Jr CW, Spitznagel E, Lappas DG. Factors associated with excessive postoperative blood loss and hemostatic transfusion requirements: a multivariate analysis in cardiac surgical patients: anesthesia and analgesia 1996;**82**(1):13-21.
165. Estes JW. Kinetics of the anticoagulant effect of heparin. *JAMA* 1970;**212**(9):1492-5.
166. Bull BS, Huse WM, Brauer FS, Korpman RA. Heparin therapy during extracorporeal circulation: II. The use of a dose-response curve to individualize heparin and protamine dosage. *J Thorac Cardiovasc Surg* 1975;**69**(5):685-9.
167. Despotis GJ, Hogue Jr CW, Santoro SA, Joist JH, Barnes PW, Lappas DG. Effect of heparin on whole blood activated partial thromboplastin time using a portable, whole blood coagulation monitor. *Crit Care Med* 1995;**23**(10):1674-9.
168. Gravlee GP, Haddon WS, Rothberger HK, et al. Heparin dosing and monitoring for cardiopulmonary bypass: a comparison of techniques with measurement of subclinical plasma coagulation. *J Thorac Cardiovasc Surg* 1990;**99**(3):518-27.
169. Okita Y, Takamoto S, Ando M, et al. Coagulation and fibrinolysis system in aortic surgery under deep hypothermic circulatory arrest with aprotinin: the importance of adequate heparinization. *Circulation* 1997;**96**(Suppl. 9):376-81:II.
170. Ferraris VA, Ferraris SP, Saha SP, et al. Perioperative blood transfusion and blood conservation in cardiac surgery: the Society of Thoracic Surgeons and the Society of Cardiovascular Anesthesiologists clinical practice guideline. *Ann Thorac Surg* 2007;**83**(Suppl. 5):S27-86.
171. Bachmann F, McKenna R, Cole ER, Najafi H. The hemostatic mechanism after open-heart surgery: I. Studies on plasma coagulation factors and fibrinolysis in 512 patients after extracorporeal circulation. *J Thorac Cardiovasc Surg* 1975;**70**(1):76-85.
172. Milam JD. Blood transfusion in heart surgery. *Surg Clin North Am* 1983;**63**(5):1127-47.
173. Goodnough LT, Johnston MF, Ramsey G, et al. Guidelines for transfusion support in patients undergoing coronary artery bypass grafting. Transfusion Practices Committee of the American Association of Blood Banks. *Ann Thorac Surg* 1990;**50**(4):675-83.
174. Walls JT, Curtis JJ, Silver D, Boley TM, Schmaltz RA, Nawarawong W. Heparin-induced thrombocytopenia in open heart surgical patients: sequelae of late recognition. *Ann Thorac Surg* 1992;**53**(5):787-91.
175. Kang YG, Martin DJ, Marquez J, et al. Intraoperative changes in blood coagulation and thrombelastographic monitoring in liver transplantation. *Anesth Analg* 1985;**64**(9):888-96.
176. Spiess BD, Tuman KJ, McCarthy RJ, DeLaria GA, Schillo R, Ivankovich AD. Thromboelastography as an indicator of post-cardiopulmonary bypass coagulopathies. *J Clin Monit* 1987;**3**(1):25-30.
177. Bagge L, Lilienberg G, Nystrom SO, Tyden H. Coagulation, fibrinolysis and bleeding after open-heart surgery. *Scand J Thorac Cardiovasc Surg* 1986;**20**(2):151-60.
178. Guidelines for transfusion for massive blood loss. a publication of the British Society for Haematology. British Committee for Standardization in Haematology Blood Transfusion Task Force. *Clin Lab Haematol* 1988;**10**(3):265-73.
179. Ferraris VA, Ferraris SP, Lough FC, Berry WR. Preoperative aspirin ingestion increases operative blood loss after coronary artery bypass grafting. *Ann Thorac Surg* 1988;**45**(1):71-4.
180. Sethi GK, Copeland JG, Goldman S, Moritz T, Zadina K, Henderson WG. Implications of preoperative administration of aspirin in patients undergoing coronary artery bypass grafting. Department of Veterans Affairs Cooperative Study on Antiplatelet Therapy. *J Am Coll Cardiol* 1990;**15**(1):15-20.
181. Taggart DP, Siddiqui A, Wheatley DJ. Low-dose preoperative aspirin therapy, postoperative blood loss, and transfusion requirements. *Ann Thorac Surg* 1990;**50**(3):424-8.
182. Ferraris VA, Ferraris SP, Moliterno DJ, et al. The Society of Thoracic Surgeons practice guideline series: aspirin and other antiplatelet agents during operative coronary revascularization (executive summary). *Ann Thorac Surg* 2005;**79**(4):1454-61.
183. Braunwald E, Antman EM, Beasley JW, et al. ACC/AHA 2002 guideline update for the management of patients with unstable angina and non-ST-segment elevation myocardial infarction—summary article: a report of the American College of Cardiology/American Heart Association task force on practice guidelines (Committee on the Management of Patients With Unstable Angina). *J Am Coll Cardiol* 2002;**40**(7):1366-74.
184. Rohrer MJ, Natale AM. Effect of hypothermia on the coagulation cascade. *Crit Care Med* 1992;**20**(10):1402-5.
185. Olinger GN, Werner PH, Bonchek LI, Boerboom LE. Vasodilator effects of the sodium acetate in pooled protein fraction. *Ann Surg* 1979;**190**(3):305-11.
186. Alving BM, Hojima Y, Pisano JJ, et al. Hypotension associated with prekallikrein activator (Hageman-factor fragments) in plasma protein fraction. *N Engl J Med* 1978;**299**(2):66-70.
187. Finfer S, Bellomo R, Boyce N, French J, Myburgh J, Norton R. A comparison of albumin and saline for fluid resuscitation in the intensive care unit. *N Engl J Med* 2004;**350**(22):2247-56.
188. Hoffman WS, Tomasello DN, MacVaugh H. Control of postcardiotomy bleeding with PEEP. *Ann Thorac Surg* 1982;**34**(1):71-3.
189. Ilabaca PA, Ochsner JL, Mills NL. Positive end-expiratory pressure in the management of the patient with a postoperative bleeding heart. *Ann Thorac Surg* 1980;**30**(3):281-4.
190. Mills NL, Ochsner JL. Experience with atrial pacemaker wires implanted during cardiac operations. *J Thorac Cardiovasc Surg* 1973;**66**(6):878-86.
191. Zurick AM, Urzua J, Ghattas M, Cosgrove DM, Estafanous FG, Greenstreet R. Failure of positive end-expiratory pressure to decrease postoperative bleeding after cardiac surgery. *Ann Thorac Surg* 1982;**34**(6):608-11.
192. Smith PK, Buhrman WC, Ferguson Jr TB, Levett JM, Cox JL. Conduction block after cardioplegic arrest: prevention by augmented atrial hypothermia. *Circulation* 1983;**68**(3 Pt 2):II41-8.
193. Asmundsson T, Kilburn KH. Survival after acute respiratory failure: 145 patients observed 5 to 8 and one-half years. *Ann Intern Med* 1974;**80**(1):54-7.
194. Czer LS, Shoemaker WC. Optimal hematocrit value in critically ill postoperative patients. *Surg Gynecol Obstet* 1978;**147**(3):363-8.
195. Wolfe JH, Waller DG, Chapman MB, Blackford HN, Prout WG. The effect of hemodilution upon patients with intermittent claudication. *Surg Gynecol Obstet* 1985;**160**(4):347-51.
196. Serry C, Bleck PC, Javid H, et al. Sternal wound complications: management and results. *J Thorac Cardiovasc Surg* 1980;**80**(6):861-7.
197. Lazenby WD, Russo I, Zadeh BJ, et al. Treatment with desmopressin acetate in routine coronary artery bypass surgery to improve postoperative hemostasis. *Circulation* 1990;**82**(Suppl. 5):IV413-9.
198. Vincentelli A, Susen S, Le Tourneau T, et al. Acquired von Willebrand syndrome in aortic stenosis. *N Engl J Med* 2003;**349**(4):343-9.
199. de Smet AA, Joen MC, van Oeveren W, et al. Increased anticoagulation during cardiopulmonary bypass by aprotinin. *J Thorac Cardiovasc Surg* 1990;**100**(4):520-7.
200. van Oeveren W, Harder MP, Roozendaal KJ, Eijsman L, Wildevuur CR. Aprotinin protects platelets against the initial effect of cardiopulmonary bypass. *J Thorac Cardiovasc Surg* 1990;**99**(5):788-96, discussion 96-117.
201. Kristeller JL, Roslund BP, Stahl RF. Benefits and risks of aprotinin use during cardiac surgery. *Pharmacotherapy* 2008;**28**(1):112-24.
202. Karkouti K, Beattie WS, Dattilo KM, et al. A propensity score case-control comparison of aprotinin and tranexamic acid in high-transfusion-risk cardiac surgery. *Transfusion* 2006;**46**(3):327-38.
203. Mangano DT, Miao Y, Vuylsteke A, et al. Mortality associated with aprotinin during 5 years following coronary artery bypass graft surgery. *JAMA* 2007;**297**(5):471-9.

204. Mangano DT, Tudor IC, Dietzel C. The risk associated with aprotinin in cardiac surgery. N Engl J Med 2006;354(4):353-65.
205. Fergusson DA, Hebert PC, Mazer CD, et al. A comparison of aprotinin and lysine analogues in high-risk cardiac surgery. N Engl J Med 2008;358(22):2319-31.
206. Ray WA, Stein CM. The aprotinin story: is BART the final chapter? N Engl J Med 2008;358(22):2398-400.
207. Karkouti K, Beattie WS, Crowther MA, et al. The role of recombinant factor VIIa in on-pump cardiac surgery: proceedings of the Canadian Consensus Conference. Can J Anaesth 2007;54(7):573-82.
208. Hogue Jr CW, Palin CA, Arrowsmith JE. Cardiopulmonary bypass management and neurologic outcomes: an evidence-based appraisal of current practices. Anesth Analg 2006;103(1):21-37.
209. Sylivris S, Levi C, Matalanis G, et al. Pattern and significance of cerebral microemboli during coronary artery bypass grafting. Ann Thorac Surg 1998;66(5):1674-8.
210. Moody DM, Bell MA, Challa VR, Johnston WE, Prough DS. Brain microemboli during cardiac surgery or aortography. Ann Neurol 1990;28(4):477-86.
211. Brown WR, Moody DM, Challa VR, Stump DA. Histologic studies of brain microemboli in humans and dogs after cardiopulmonary bypass. Echocardiography 1996;13(5):559-66.
212. Brooker RF, Brown WR, Moody DM, et al. Cardiotomy suction: a major source of brain lipid emboli during cardiopulmonary bypass. Ann Thorac Surg 1998;65(6):1651-5.
213. Kincaid EH, Jones TJ, Stump DA, et al. Processing scavenged blood with a cell saver reduces cerebral lipid microembolization. Ann Thorac Surg 2000;70(4):1296-300.
214. Bowles BJ, Lee JD, Dang CR, et al. Coronary artery bypass performed without the use of cardiopulmonary bypass is associated with reduced cerebral microemboli and improved clinical results. Chest 2001;119(1):25-30.
215. Lund C, Hol PK, Lundblad R, et al. Comparison of cerebral embolization during off-pump and on-pump coronary artery bypass surgery. Ann Thorac Surg 2003;76(3):765-70:discussion 70.
216. van Dijk D, Spoor M, Hijman R, et al. Cognitive and cardiac outcomes 5 years after off-pump vs on-pump coronary artery bypass graft surgery. JAMA 2007;297(7):701-8.
217. Selnes OA, Grega MA, Bailey MM, et al. Neurocognitive outcomes 3 years after coronary artery bypass graft surgery: a controlled study. Ann Thorac Surg 2007;84(6):1885-96.
218. Selnes OA, Grega MA, Bailey MM, et al. Cognition 6 years after surgical or medical therapy for coronary artery disease. Ann Neurol 2008;63(5):581-90.
219. Livelli Jr FD, Johnson RA, McEnany MT, et al. Unexplained in-hospital fever following cardiac surgery: natural history, relationship to postpericardiotomy syndrome, and a prospective study of therapy with indomethacin versus placebo. Circulation 1978;57(5):968-75.
220. Pien F, Ho PW, Fergusson DJ. Fever and infection after cardiac operation. Ann Thorac Surg 1982;33(4):382-4.
221. Norwood SH, Cormier B, McMahon NG, Moss A, Moore V. Prospective study of catheter-related infection during prolonged arterial catheterization. Crit Care Med 1988;16(9):836-9.
222. Wormser GP, Onorato IM, Preminger TJ, Culver D, Martone WJ. Sensitivity and specificity of blood cultures obtained through intravascular catheters. Crit Care Med 1990;18(2):152-6.
223. Freeman R, McPeake PK. Acquisition, spread, and control of Pseudomonas aeruginosa in a cardiothoracic intensive care unit. Thorax 1982;37(10):732-6.
224. Ford EG, Baisden CE, Matteson ML, Picone AL. Sepsis after coronary bypass grafting: evidence for loss of the gut mucosal barrier. Ann Thorac Surg 1991;52(3):514-7.
225. Marshall JC, Christou NV, Horn R, Meakins JL. The microbiology of multiple organ failure: the proximal gastrointestinal tract as an occult reservoir of pathogens. Arch Surg 1988;123(3):309-15.
226. Stoutenbeek CP, van Saene HK, Miranda DR, Zandstra DF. The effect of selective decontamination of the digestive tract on colonisation and infection rate in multiple trauma patients. Intens Care Med 1984;10(4):185-92.
227. Culliford AT, Girdwood RW, Isom OW, Krauss KR, Spencer FC. Angina following myocardial revascularization: does time of recurrence predict etiology and influence results of operation? J Thorac Cardiovasc Surg 1979;77(6):889-95.
228. Iberti TJ, Leibowitz AB, Papadakos PJ, Fischer EP. Low sensitivity of the anion gap as a screen to detect hyperlactatemia in critically ill patients. Crit Care Med 1990;18(3):275-7.
229. Loop FD, Lytle BW, Cosgrove DM, et al. J. Maxwell Chamberlain memorial paper. Sternal wound complications after isolated coronary artery bypass grafting: early and late mortality, morbidity, and cost of care. Ann Thorac Surg 1990;49(2):179-86:discussion 86-7.
230. Ottino G, De Paulis R, Pansini S, et al. Major sternal wound infection after open-heart surgery: a multivariate analysis of risk factors in 2,579 consecutive operative procedures. Ann Thorac Surg 1987;44(2):173-9.
231. Sanfelippo PM, Danielson GK. Complications associated with median sternotomy. J Thorac Cardiovasc Surg 1972;63(3):419-23.
232. Sarr MG, Gott VL, Townsend TR. Mediastinal infection after cardiac surgery. Ann Thorac Surg 1984;38(4):415-23.
233. Shafir R, Weiss J, Herman O, Cohen N, Stern D, Igra Y. Faulty sternotomy and complications after median sternotomy. J Thorac Cardiovasc Surg 1988;96(2):310-3.
234. Stoney WS, Alford Jr WC, Burrus GR, Frist RA, Thomas Jr CS. Median sternotomy dehiscence. Ann Thorac Surg 1978;26(5):421-6.
235. Ulicny Jr KS, Hiratzka LF. The risk factors of median sternotomy infection: a current review. J Card Surg 1991;6(2):338-51.
236. Thurer RJ, Bognolo D, Vargas A, Isch JH, Kaiser GA. The management of mediastinal infection following cardiac surgery: an experience utilizing continuous irrigation with povidone-iodine. J Thorac Cardiovasc Surg 1974;68(6):962-8.
237. Jurkiewicz MJ, Bostwick 3rd J, Hester TR, Bishop JB, Craver J. Infected median sternotomy wound: successful treatment by muscle flaps. Ann Surg 1980;191(6):738-44.
238. Jeevanandam V, Smith CR, Rose EA, Malm JR, Hugo NE. Single-stage management of sternal wound infections. J Thorac Cardiovasc Surg 1990;99(2):256-62, discussion 262-3.
239. Johnson RG, Thurer RL, Kruskall MS, et al. Comparison of two transfusion strategies after elective operations for myocardial revascularization. J Thorac Cardiovasc Surg 1992;104(2):307-14.
240. Sjogren J, Nilsson J, Gustafsson R, Malmsjo M, Ingemansson R. The impact of vacuum-assisted closure on long-term survival after post-sternotomy mediastinitis. Ann Thorac Surg 2005;80(4):1270-5.
241. DeLaria GA, Hunter JA, Goldin MD, Serry C, Javid H, Najafi H. Leg wound complications associated with coronary revascularization. J Thorac Cardiovasc Surg 1981;81(3):403-7.

CHAPTER 62
Cardiopulmonary Bypass: Technique and Pathophysiology
Fraser D. Rubens

Technical Aspects of Cardiopulmonary Bypass
  Device Overview
  Principles of Current Oxygenator Design and Function
  Hypothermia and Acid–Base Balance
  Hematocrit and Priming
  Flow Rates, Perfusion Pressure, and Autoregulation
  Pumps for CPB
  Cardiotomy
  Cardiac Venting for CPB
  Cannulation for CPB

Venous Cannulation
Arterial Cannulation
Pathophysiology of Cardiopulmonary Bypass
  Noncellular Response
  Cellular Activation during CPB: Platelets, Endothelial Cells, Leukocytes
  Nonbiomaterial-Related Activation during CPB
Heparin–Protamine Axis
  Heparin: Pharmacology, Dosage, and Complications
  Protamine: Pharmacology, Complications

Pharmacologic Adjuncts to Minimize the Consequences of CPB
Biomaterial-Dependent Strategies to Minimize Blood Activation from CPB
  Biomembrane Mimicry
  Heparin-Coated Circuits
  Surfaces with Modified Protein Adsorption
Organ Derangement Related to Cardiopulmonary Bypass
  Neuroendocrine Response to CPB
  CNS Injury with CPB
  Pulmonary Dysfunction with CPB
  Renal Dysfunction with CPB
The Future of Cardiopulmonary Bypass

Cardiopulmonary bypass (CPB) is one of the most important biomedical inventions in the history of health care, rivaling the development of roentgenography and hemodialysis in its clinical impact. The scope of its application is far reaching, as its birth paralleled the evolution of an entire surgical subspecialty, and without its use, surgeons would be cowed by the prospect of intracardiac repair.

Despite the belief that the need for CPB would be significantly diminished because of the surge in interest in off-pump coronary artery bypass grafting (CABG), the predictions have not materialized, and most institutions have reduced their use of off-pump CABG to only 10% to 15% of cases.[1] In many practices, complex multiple arterial reconstruction and minimal-access surgery such as mini-thoracotomy mitral valve surgery are more comfortably and accurately approached using longer periods of CPB and techniques of myocardial protection. Therefore, we must be able to assess the impact of CPB on our patients. The surgeon must have a comprehensive understanding of all aspects of CPB, from the physiology of gas exchange to the molecular mechanisms characteristic of biocompatibility.

The evolution of CPB reflects ingenuity bred of necessity. A parallel discovery that contributed to the feasibility of extracorporeal circulation was the isolation of the natural anticoagulant heparin. Dr. John H. Gibbon, Jr. (Fig. 62-1), a "receptive and talented surgeon with foresight . . . who could envision an intact surviving patient beyond the isolated organ studies,"[2] was the inventor of the Gibbons-IBM oxygenator. In 1953, this device was successfully used to correct an atrial septal defect. Although it was initially successful, three subsequent attempts at intracardiac repair were fatal, resulting in a self-imposed moratorium on its clinical use. Nevertheless, the feasibility of this approach had now been demonstrated.

The first clinically successful film and bubble oxygenators brought blood in direct contact with respiratory gases, to equilibrate with them. Complications related to blood trauma eventually led to a decline in their popularity, and they are rarely used today. Membrane oxygenators were introduced in the 1950s after the observation by Kolff and Berk[3] that venous blood was oxygenated while flowing through a cellophane dialysis tube in contact with O_2-containing dialysate. The first membranes were relatively impermeable to gases, requiring huge surface areas and massive priming volumes. Formed of silicone rubber, they were designed in either an extraluminal format (blood flowing on the outside of the tube with gas on the inside) or, less often, in an intraluminal format (the reverse). The refinements were subtle but significant, and we now have oxygenators with surface areas of 2.0 m^2. The resulting minimization of prime volume has contributed more than any other factor to blood conservation practice in modern-day cardiac surgery.

TECHNICAL ASPECTS OF CARDIOPULMONARY BYPASS

Device Overview

Gravity drainage usually allows collection of blood from the venous circulation into the venous reservoir. Through separate inflows on the reservoir, blood can also be returned from the pericardial well (cardiotomy blood) and from cardiac and aortic vents. A centrifugal or roller pump is used to divert the venous reservoir blood to the oxygenator. After the blood

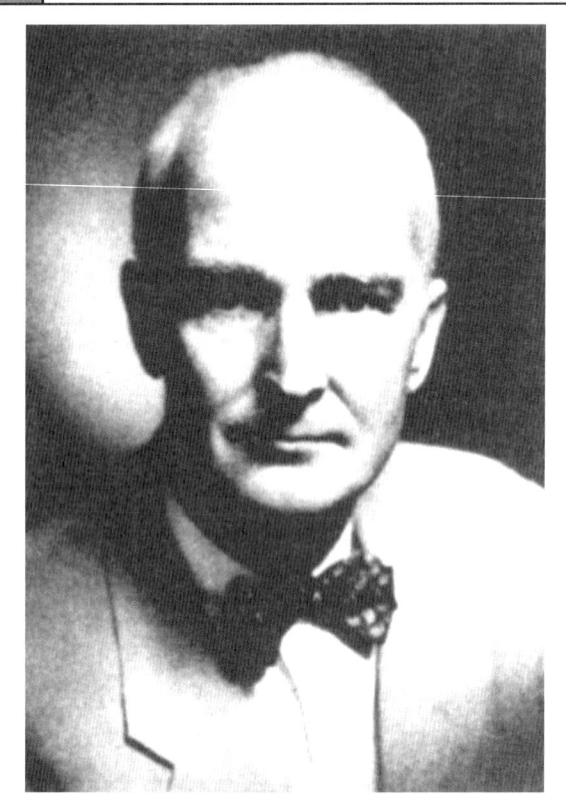

Figure 62–1
Dr. John H. Gibbon, Jr. (1903-1973).

passes through the integrated heat exchanger and oxygenator, it is circulated through an arterial filter and bubble trap and returned to the patient through the arterial cannula (Fig. 62-2). Cardioplegia setups are often intimately incorporated into the CPB circuit.

Principles of Current Oxygenator Design and Function

Diffusion of gases at the blood–membrane interface can be predicted by Fick's law, which says that the rate of diffusion is proportional to the partial pressure gradient of the gas in the direction of diffusion. The rate of gas transfer is also inversely proportional to the distance through which it must pass (the thickness of the membrane), and it depends on the property of *diffusivity* of the membrane biomaterial. Currently used membranes are very permeable to O_2, but they are often less permeable to CO_2. The problem of poor diffusion of CO_2 was solved by the introduction of microporous membranes. These surfaces allow transient direct blood–gas interfacing at pore structures smaller than blood cells; however, the hydrophobic nature of the membrane results in changes in blood surface tension, blocking direct contact between the two phases. As a result, the interface in microporous membranes behaves like a very thin stagnant film of plasma water that offers little resistance to gas exchange. Progressive protein accretion at the pores occurs over time, resulting in a finite functional capacity, detected by worsening efficiency in gas transfer, which is why oxygenators must be replaced with long CPB runs (Fig. 62-3).

As opposed to the relatively facile transfer of O_2 gas through a membrane, when the O_2 is dissolved in plasma or blood, its diffusivity is 25 times less than that of CO_2. Two modifications have been introduced to overcome this problem. First, the path length (the distance the blood travels as it passes the gas-exchange surface) has been maximized. This modification is limited by the parallel need to increase the priming volume. Second, disturbed flow patterns are used to promote mixing and to bring deoxygenated blood closer to the exchange surface. Mechanisms that interfere with the development of fully developed flow patterns enhance diffusion by keeping the boundary layer narrow. In an oxygenator, this can be accomplished by making the surface irregular or by positioning elements in the flow stream to disrupt smooth flow and to enhance mixing. This is the rationale for the extraluminal hollow fiber design.

Hypothermia and Acid–Base Balance

The feasibility and applicability of hypothermia for heart surgery was first suggested by Bigelow and colleagues in 1950.[4] They demonstrated the safety benefit of hypothermia as a means to decrease O_2 consumption during inflow occlusion in an animal model. O_2 consumption decreases by 50% for every 10° C drop in temperature (Fig. 62-4). Lower flows decrease collateral flow and rewarming of the heart from contact with adjacent tissues, and they provide a margin of safety if equipment fails.

Hypothermia is associated with marked changes in blood pH and $P\text{CO}_2$ levels. With a rise in temperature, CO_2 becomes less soluble in blood, and there is a greater tendency for the dissolved CO_2 to come out of solution (increased gaseous phase). Thus, CO_2 solubility increases with decreasing temperature. When blood from a hypothermic patient (e.g., at 24° C) is introduced into a CO_2 electrode for measurement, it is first warmed to 37° C (increasing the amount of CO_2 in the gaseous phase), and therefore the measured partial pressure of CO_2 is higher than it was in reality at the cooler temperature. The correction for $P\text{CO}_2$ is based on a calculated decrease of 4.5% per degree Celsius. On the other hand, the pH increases 0.015 units per degree Celsius drop in temperature. This shift in pH is partially related to the influence of buffers such as the imidazole moiety of histidine, but it is also related to the dynamics of the Henderson-Hasselbalch equation, $pH = pK + [HCO_3^-]/(0.03 \times P\text{CO}_2)$.

Because alkalosis and hypocarbia trigger a decrease in cerebral blood flow (CBF), some investigators have suggested the addition of CO_2 during hypothermia to compensate and to keep the pH unchanged (pH-stat strategy). In 1987, Murkin and coworkers[5] confirmed that pH-stat management results in a greater ratio of CBF to cerebral metabolic rate ($CMRO_2$) than alpha-stat management (i.e., no active correction of pH with hypothermia).[5] Most agree that a pH-stat strategy is probably preferable in children, where increased CBF does increase the rate of cooling and thus increases the chance of achieving uniform cerebral hypothermia.[6] The rate of brain oxygen depletion during deep hypothermic circulatory arrest is also considerably slower with pH-stat strategy. As a result, pH-stat substantially prolongs the interval between the onset of arrest and the exhaustion of brain oxygen stores and may be associated with better clinical outcomes in this group.[7]

In contrast, in adults, an alpha-stat strategy may provide greater cerebral protection during hypothermia on CPB. Alpha-stat management is certainly easier to accomplish, and

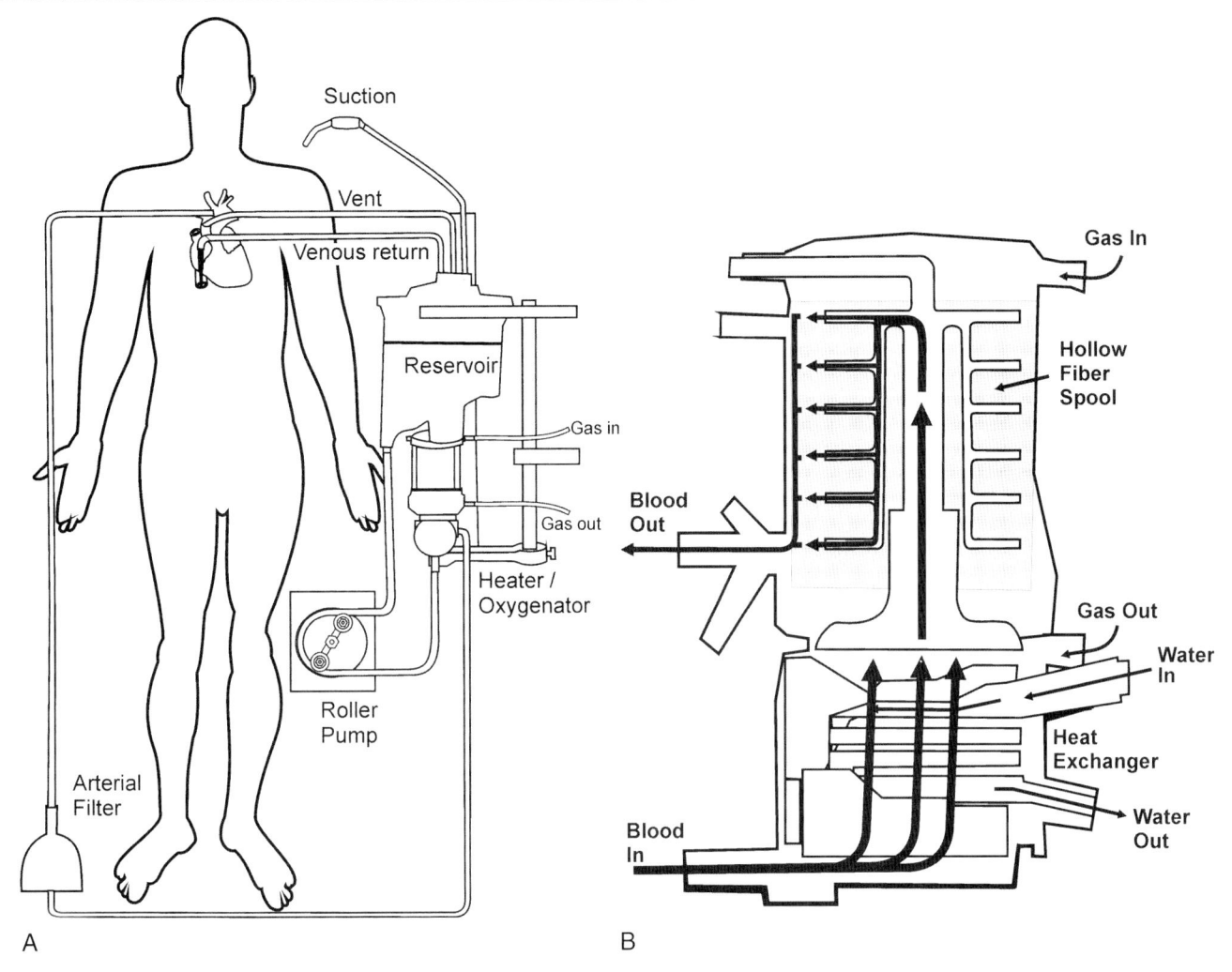

Figure 62–2
A, Overview of the cardiopulmonary bypass circuit. B, Typical integrated heat exchanger–membrane oxygenator.

a justification is that most cellular mechanisms are capable of maintaining intracellular pH despite fluctuations in extracellular conditions. Because excess CO_2 is added in a pH-stat strategy, brain acidosis may occur during rewarming, and, combined with decreased O_2 delivery after CPB, this may augment CNS injury in adults. Most importantly, as mentioned, a pH-stat strategy results in excessive CBF, which may increase embolic load. Finally, pH-stat strategy is associated with a decreased ability to maintain autoregulation at low pressures. Three randomized controlled trials have demonstrated a small but present benefit of alpha-stat strategy in terms of neurologic and neurocognitive outcome in adults, especially when CPB time exceeded 90 minutes.[8]

Hematocrit and Priming

The 1960s saw the introduction of crystalloid (dextrose 5% in water, or D5W) in prime as an alternative to routine whole blood prime. An increase in efficiency of oxygenation and a decrease in end-organ complications were seen with this approach.[9] Now hemodilution is commonly practiced in virtually all adult and pediatric cardiac surgeries, and the

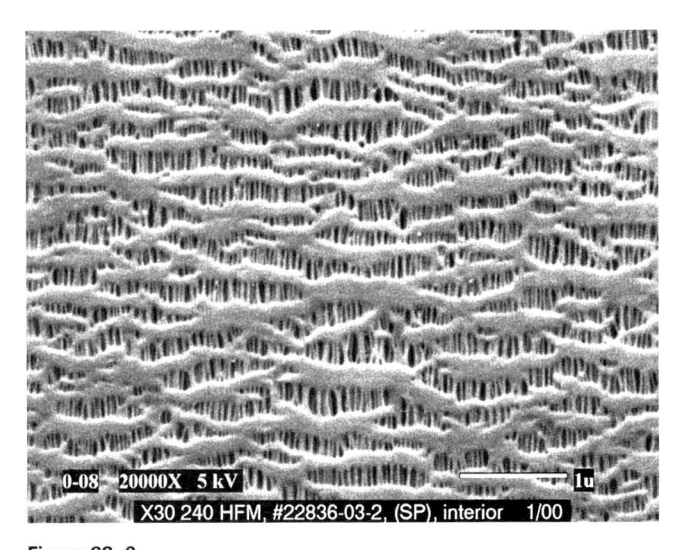

Figure 62–3
Scanning electron micrograph of a microporous membrane (Celgard) used in a membrane oxygenator (×20,000). *(Courtesy of Membrana GmbH, Germany.)*

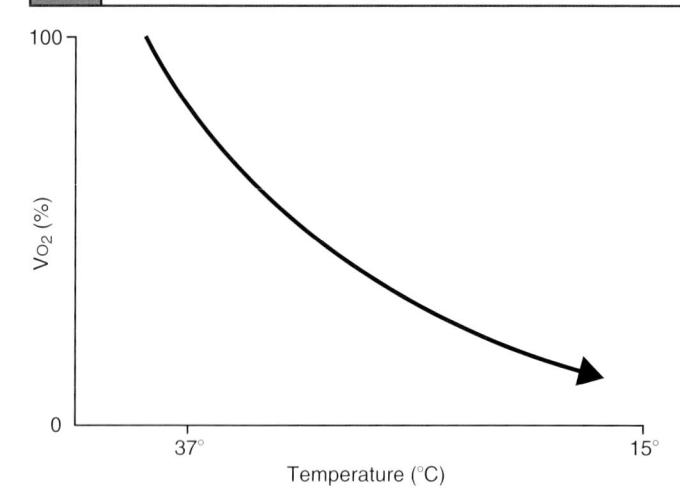

Figure 62–4
The effect of hypothermia on oxygen consumption (Vo_2).

hematocrit (Hct) is maintained between 20% and 25% during CPB. Hemodilution has a major effect on blood viscosity, primarily at the capillary level where the radius is small and the shear rate is low. Low flow at the capillary level increases viscosity of the blood, further increasing the resistance, but this effect is counter-balanced by the effect of hemodilution.

The drop in O_2 content at most levels of moderate hemodilution is more than compensated for by augmented cardiac output (CO), so total O_2 delivery (CO × O_2 content of blood) is increased; the optimal Hct is probably in the range of 30% for this effect. Hemodilution results in a significant increase in flow without a parallel increase in perfusion pressure. Hypothermia complicates the effects of hemodilution, as the decreased temperature causes increased viscosity and induces vasoconstriction.

The optimal Hct for CPB remains a topic of significant controversy. A post-hoc assessment of the impact of low Hct on admission of cardiac patients to the intensive care unit (ICU) by Spiess and colleagues[10] found an inverse correlation between admission Hct and the risk of Q-wave myocardial infarction (MI). On the other hand, studies have demonstrated that an Hct of less than 20% may be associated with abnormal distribution of blood flow to organs, and that an Hct of less than 15% may lead to maldistribution of coronary flow away from the subendocardium in the presence of residual coronary stenosis.[11] Retrospective observational studies of consecutive patients undergoing isolated CABG have demonstrated that a lower minimum Hct is associated with a significantly increased risk of renal injury[12] and mortality.[13,14] As excessive hemodilution also increases CBF, it may cause a parallel increase in microembolization and thus may theoretically be a contributor to neurologic damage after CPB and the increased risk of stroke observed with lower Hct on CPB.[15]

Most centers prime the CPB circuit with a solution of balanced salt with or without the addition of a colloid solution such as pentastarch. Infants and children often need blood added directly to the prime, depending on the anticipated Hct after initiation of bypass (calculated from standard nomograms). Other additives to the prime may include calcium, mannitol, and pharmacologic agents such as heparin and aprotinin. The minimum priming volume is mandated by the patient's circulating volume and the pump prime volume. Although the prime volume averages 1 L, experienced practitioners can achieve 200 mL in pediatric circuits.

Flow Rates, Perfusion Pressure, and Autoregulation

Flow is generally kept in the range of 2.2 to 2.5 L/min/m^2 to provide a margin of safety during CPB, as systemic blood flow distribution and O_2 consumption remain normal at this level. At normothermia, a target mean blood pressure of 50 to 70 mm Hg is generally used. The perfusionist can control the pressure by increasing or decreasing flow, or by the addition of vasoconstrictors or vasodilators (inhalational anesthetics). At lower temperatures, a mean pressure of 35 mm Hg is still generally accepted as safe. A number of investigators have recommended greater vigilance to prevent any hypotension (<45 to 50 mm Hg) during CPB,[16] but these findings are controversial.[17]

Although the brain comprises only 2% of body weight, its metabolic needs demand 15% of the CO, extracting as much as 25% of the delivered O_2. Temperature is the most important element influencing CBF during CPB. As the temperature is dropped, the $CMRO_2$ decreases exponentially and the CBF decreases linearly (Fig. 62-5). As a consequence, the ratio of CBF to $CMRO_2$ increases, resulting in "luxuriant" flow, further facilitated by hemodilution.

Autoregulation of CBF is also related to changes in perfusion pressure. At normothermia, a mean pressure of 50 mm Hg is the threshold at which the brain autoregulates flow, but with hypothermia (26° C), the threshold drops to 30 mm Hg (Fig. 62-6). At deep hypothermia (<20° C), there is a loss of pressure-flow autoregulation, as severe temperature reductions impair cerebral vascular relaxation,[18] and changes in cerebral perfusion pressure alone result in corresponding proportional changes in CBF. Other factors that influence CBF and $CMRO_2$ include blood viscosity, intracranial pressure and central venous pressure (CVP), and the blood gas status (pH, $Paco_2$, Pao_2). CBF varies linearly with the $Paco_2$, in the range of 20 to 80 mm Hg, whereas a Pao_2 of less than 50 causes cerebral vasodilation, which overrides pressure-flow autoregulation.

Pumps for CPB

The two commonly used types of pumps for CPB involve roller and centrifugal fluid propulsion. Noninterrupted contact of the rollers with the tubing in the track results in the nonpulsatile nature of the flow (Fig. 62-7A). A low compression will result in inadequate flow, whereas excessive compression may aggravate hemolysis and tubing wear. Other complications associated with the use of the roller pump include cavitation caused by excess pressure, and spallation (the release of particles from the inner surface).

Centrifugal pumps (see Fig. 62-7B) are a popular alternative to the roller pump, particularly in pediatric cardiac surgery and in cases with anticipated long CPB runs. The flow in a centrifugal pump is afterload dependent, and it is not predictable solely on the basis of the calculated revolutions per minute, so an in-line flowmeter is essential. Theoretically, its use should result in less blood trauma, particularly with prolonged CPB times, so this device is preferred for

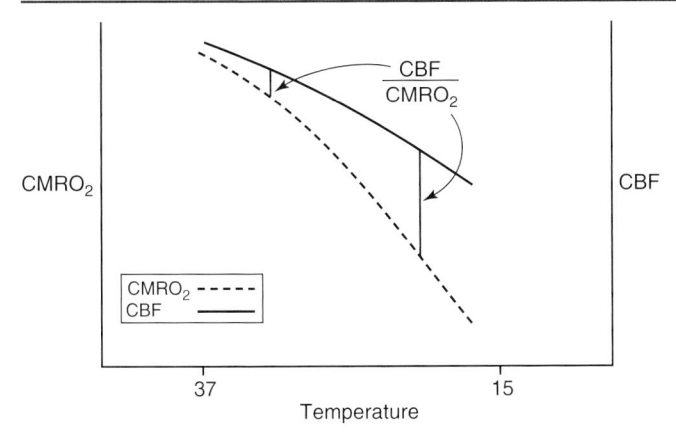

Figure 62–5
The effect of hypothermia on cerebral metabolic rate ($CMRO_2$) and cerebral blood flow (CBF).

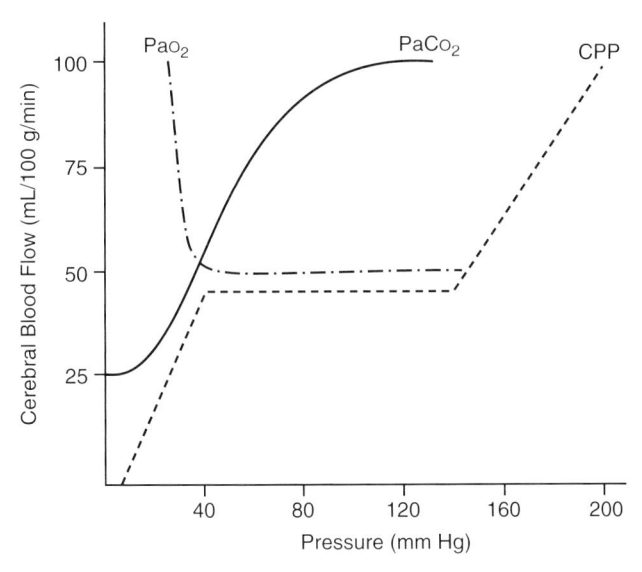

Figure 62–6
Through autoregulation, cerebral blood flow (CBF) is constant from cerebral perfusion pressure (CPP) 40 to 140 mm Hg. Other factors that independently affect CBF include $Paco_2$ and Pao_2. *(Modified with permission from Kelly BJ, Luce JM. Current concepts in cerebral protection. Chest 1993;103:1246-54. Copyright 1993, American College of Chest Physicians.)*

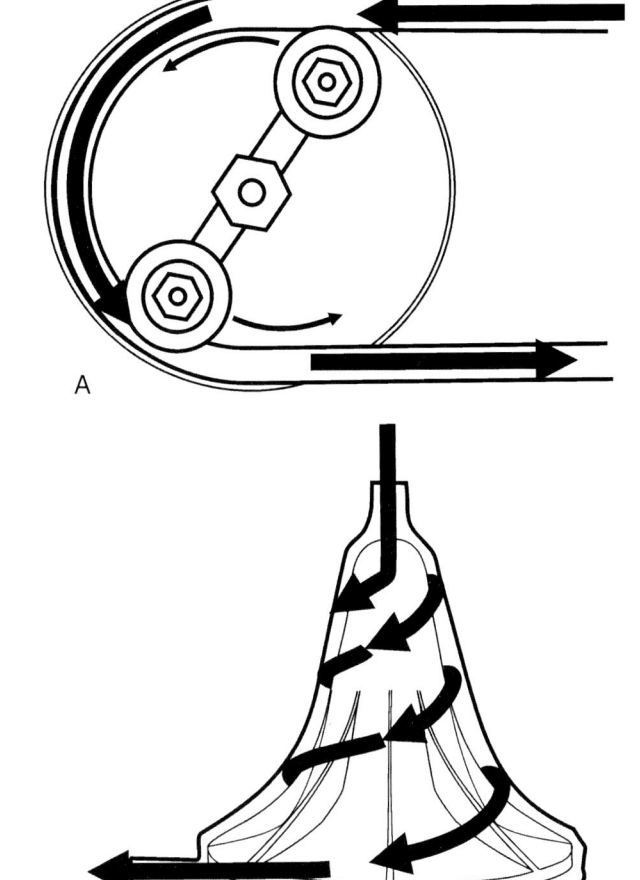

Figure 62–7
A, A double roller pump has rotating arms oriented at 180º like spokes on a wheel. Spool-shaped rollers are located at the ends of the arms. A length of tubing is locked inside a curved track at the outer circumference of a partial circle of 210 degrees. **B,** A typical centrifugal pump has a cone-shaped outer housing with an upper inlet and a single lower outlet. The inner chamber contains spinning concentric smooth cones or fins, mounted on a central impeller. *Arrows* indicate direction of blood flow.

extracorporeal membrane oxygenation (ECMO). In children, the use of the centrifugal pump has been associated with decreased hemolysis, platelet activation, and inflammation and bleeding,[19] although these findings have not been reproduced by other investigators.[20] Aside from their expense ($150 per case), these devices are susceptible to air locks, thus requiring extreme vigilance by the perfusionist. On the other hand, this may be protective, as there is less chance of pumping large volumes of air into the patient via an inadvertent leak, and the lines cannot be over-pressurized with distal obstruction, as occurs with roller pumps. These devices are not valved, and if rotation stops without clamping the outflow, rapid retrograde flow from the arterial line occurs in milliseconds, essentially exsanguinating the patient. Finally, roller pumps can be operated manually, but a power outage with a centrifugal pump can be a disaster.

Cardiotomy

Cardiotomy blood is the extravascular blood collected in the thoracic wound during CPB. In general, blood from the wound cavity is aspirated through a sucker device and transferred to a cardiotomy reservoir. Because of the close proximity of tissues in the wound and the potential for particulate matter to be collected, a filter and a defoaming chamber are incorporated into the cardiotomy reservoir. Mechanical injury, such as hemolysis, may result from the air–blood interface at the sucker, as well as from the compressive effects of the roller pump. Other mechanical complications from cardiotomy suction include the formation of particulate emboli including fibrin, macroaggregates of denatured proteins and lipoproteins, fat globules, platelet and leukocyte aggregates, calcium, cellular debris, talc, and suture material.

Cardiac Venting for CPB

Cardiac venting involves the active aspiration of blood from the heart, thus creating a bloodless field to facilitate visualization. Venting in some form is necessary in virtually all cardiac operations involving CPB, primarily to aid visualization but also to avoid chamber distension. When the aorta is cross-clamped and the native coronary circulation is stopped, a variable amount of noncoronary collateralization remains, particularly related to bronchial artery flow and return from the thebesian veins. Blood flow can also occur through the heart as a result of continued transit of blood through the right heart, through the lungs, and into the left heart. Potential sites for cardiac venting include the pulmonary artery, the superior pulmonary vein, the left atrium, the left ventricle, and the ascending aorta.

Cannulation for CPB

Venous Cannulation

Siphonage generates the negative pressure necessary to draw blood from the venous circulation. The determinants of drainage include the height of the patient above the venous reservoir, the patient's blood volume, the resistance of the tubing, and the cannula dimensions (as this is the narrowest part of the venous return). Augmented venous return refers to the use of either a pump (e.g., centrifugal) inserted in series between the venous line and the reservoir (kinetic-assisted venous drainage) or the application of a vacuum to a closed hard-shell venous reservoir (vacuum-assisted venous drainage).

In the majority of cases of cardiac surgery, cannulation is directly through the right atrium. Bicaval cannulation refers to the use of two single-stage cannulas introduced into the superior vena cava (SCV) and the inferior vena cava (IVC), usually through the right atrial wall. Cavoatrial cannulation involves the use of a two-stage venous cannula, inserted through the right atrium in the region of the atrial appendage, with the tip of the cannula directed into the IVC. The cannula is constructed with a fenestrated basket at the level of the right atrium to allow collection of blood from the coronary sinus and from the SVC. Bicaval cannulation is used when an "airless" right atrium is required, such as in tricuspid valve surgery. It is also preferred in mitral valve surgery, when distortion of the right atrium with retraction may lead to a compromise in SVC blood return and a rise in the CVP. Placing tourniquets around the SVC and IVC during bicaval cannulation allows the institution of *total* as opposed to *partial* bypass. With partial bypass, some return of venous blood still takes place through the tricuspid valve and subsequently through the pulmonary circulation. Occasionally in some pediatric cases or in complex adult or reoperative surgery, it is necessary to directly cannulate into the innominate vein or the SVC. Alternative sites for venous access include the femoral, iliac, and axillary veins.

Cannula size should be chosen so that the anticipated pressure drop across the cannula is equal to or less than the siphonage pressure that is applied on the basis of the height of the patient above the pump, and the patient's blood volume. If this principle is not followed, the CVP might increase, which could compromise cerebral perfusion pressure. Like aortic cannulas, venous cannulas are often wire reinforced, and the tips may be constructed of thin metal to optimize the inner-to-outer-diameter ratio.

Arterial Cannulation

Oxygenated blood is returned to the arterial circulation through specially designed arterial cannulas, which come in a variety of configurations. Cannula characteristics include their length, the orientation of the tip (straight or right angle), the presence of a flange, and distal tapering. The arterial cannula is the narrowest portion of the CPB circuit after the oxygenator, and thus it is the site of the highest potential gradient. It has been demonstrated that gradients in excess of 100 mm Hg can be associated with hemolysis.[21] There is no definite correlation between the French size of the cannula and the gradient, so investigators have derived alternative means to predict hemodynamics, such as the M number[22] and the performance index.[23] Finally, although the size and shape of the cannula have not been shown to influence the rate of transcranial Doppler-detected microemboli,[24] design concepts, such as tips to diffuse the sand-blasting effect of flow, differential flow to the arch vessels, and distal baskets to capture debris, have been introduced to minimize (at least theoretically) the potential that the cannula may contribute to atheroemboli.

Complications of ascending aortic cannulation include aortic intramural hematoma and dissection (0.01% to 0.09%), atheroemboli either directly from the cannula or from a jet effect, carotid hypoperfusion, air embolism, injury of the back wall of the aorta, and misdirection of the tip of the cannula either posteriorly across the aortic valve (causing severe aortic insufficiency) or anteriorly into the arch vessels or against the wall of the aorta. Femoral cannulation is most commonly used in situations of reoperative surgery and anticipated substernal adhesions. The dissection rate with femoral cannulation has been described between 0.2% and 3%. Retroperitoneal access to the iliac vessels by suprainguinal retroperitoneal dissection may also be necessary. Another attractive approach, particularly in cases of aortic dissection, involves the use of axillary cannulation. This artery is less likely to be involved with atherosclerosis than the lower extremities. There is exceptional collateral flow compared with the leg vessels, so the procedure is well tolerated and infrequently results in limb ischemia. The direction of flow during axillary cannulation also favors noncerebral embolization should there be atherosclerotic disease in the arch of the aorta. Complication rates of this procedure are minimized by cannulation through a short tube graft, anastomosed in an end-to-side manner to the axillary artery, as opposed to direct cannulation.

One of the most perplexing problems related to arterial cannulation is the management of patients with extensive aortic calcification. With bypass grafting, the use of off-pump surgery with a "no-touch" technique may be considered. Alternatively, femoral or axillary cannulation can be used with fibrillatory arrest, left heart venting, and arterial grafting. A third potential strategy involves the threading of a long cannula beyond the atheroma, into the descending thoracic aorta. Long cannulas are associated with a decreased peak, forward flow velocity, and turbulence compared with short cannulas.[25] Borger and Feindel[26] demonstrated that cannulation beyond the cerebral vessels with a long cannula decreased the count of cerebral emboli as detected by transcranial Doppler. Finally, in extreme cases, surgeons may cannulate the apex of the left ventricle with an armored venous cannula passed through the apex into the ascending aorta across the aortic valve. Epiaortic scanning has been advocated as a means to detect problems with the aorta and, when used consistently, may alter surgical management in terms of cannulation and clamp site as well as offering the option to proceed with off-pump surgery.[27] This modality is effective in trained hands and more sensitive than epiaortic scanning and digital palpation.

PATHOPHYSIOLOGY OF CARDIOPULMONARY BYPASS

Noncellular Response

The pathophysiology of CPB relates to the unique responses that occur when the blood contacts the biomaterial surface (biomaterial-dependent processes) and non–contact-related processes such as cardiotomy blood collection and the effect of nonpulsatile flow. Within milliseconds of the blood's contacting the synthetic surfaces of the CPB circuit, plasma proteins become adsorbed to the biomaterial. Although the amount, composition, and conformation of protein adsorption may differ between surfaces, there is no surface on which this process is completely inhibited, and each surface has a characteristic blood-adsorption pattern. Further exposure of the surface to blood results in activation of proteins of the contact-activation system (Fig. 62-8). This system comprises four primary plasma proteins: factors XII and XI, prekallikrein, and high-molecular-weight kininogen (HMWK). In the presence of the negatively charged biomaterial, a conformational change occurs in factor XII that permits its activation in the presence of prekallikrein and HMWK. Factor XIIa activates factor XI and initiates the intrinsic coagulation pathway, with the subsequent generation of thrombin and the cleavage of fibrinogen to produce fibrin, which is cross-linked by activated factor XIII. Factor XIIa also activates prekallikrein to form kallikrein within seconds of the start of bypass. Kallikrein catalyzes the conversion of HMWK to bradykinin and plays a role in the activation of the fibrinolytic system. Bradykinin has a very short half-life in the plasma because of its rapid metabolism by angiotensin-converting enzyme in the pulmonary circulation[28] and by the vascular endothelium.[29] It is believed to be a key mediator of increased capillary permeability and the development of tissue edema. Bradykinin mediates vasodilation by stimulating the release of endothelial nitric oxide,[29] and it may also be an important mediator of cerebral ischemia.[30]

Activation of the fibrinolytic system during CPB is evidenced by increased levels of tissue plasminogen activator (tPA) and plasmin–antiplasmin complexes. Thrombin and bradykinin contribute to fibrinolysis through the direct activation of endothelial cells and the release of tPA, which further increases plasmin generation.[31] Kallikrein-mediated activation of the fibrinolytic system includes its role in catalyzing the conversion of plasminogen to plasmin and the activation of pro-urokinase.[32] Despite these findings, the contribution of fibrinolysis to post-bypass bleeding is controversial, as clot lysis activity subsides within minutes of terminating bypass.[33] Another mechanism by which plasmin generation may contribute to bleeding is through its direct effect on platelet receptors during CPB.[34]

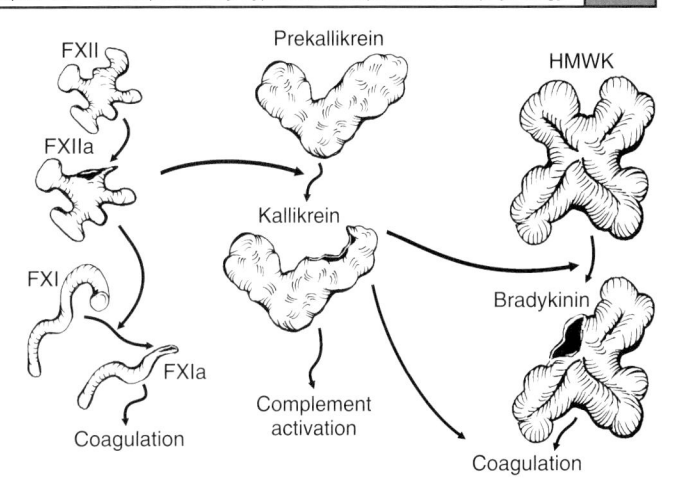

Figure 62–8
Proteins of the contact activation system. FXII and FXI, factors XII, XI; FXIIa and FXIa, activated factors XII and XI; HMWK, high-molecular-weight kininogen.

The complement system is activated through several mechanisms during CPB (Fig. 62-9). First, the third component of complement (C3), adsorbed to the CPB surface after releasing the potent chemoattractant C3a, is joined by the inactive factor B and properdin to produce the active proteolytic enzyme C3 convertase. C3 convertase cleaves the fifth component C5 to generate the active fragment C5a and the terminal complement complex C5b-9. Other mechanisms for complement generation through alternative pathways include the direct cleavage of C5 by kallikrein to produce C5a and the direct cleavage of C3 by plasmin. Complement generation has also been reported to be induced directly by endotoxin or directly by the cytokines tumor necrosis factor (TNF) and interleukin (IL)-6.[35] Heparin–protamine complexes formed at the end of CPB activate the classical complement pathway, as does immunoglobulin bound on the biomaterial surface, which complexes with C1q.[36]

The generation of complement plays a key role in the recruitment of leukocytes, the upregulation of neutrophil activation markers, and the production of cytokines. Studies by Kirklin's group[37] confirmed that the incidence and degree of deranged function of the heart, lung, and kidney after CPB could be related to the raised plasma concentration of the complement fragment C3a. Furthermore, inhibition of production of terminal complement complex by a protease inhibitor was associated with a significant reduction in the deleterious effects of ischemia-reperfusion to the myocardium after CPB.[38]

Nitric oxide (NO) is a potent inflammatory mediator whose production is increased after CPB. Endogenously produced NO may cause tissue injury through formation of toxic peroxynitrites, activation of cyclooxygenase, and DNA deamination. Studies have reported a significant increase in inducible nitric oxide synthase (iNOS) expression in human lung after CPB, which may be related to cytokine release (e.g., TNF, IL-1, IL-6).[39] This induction has also been shown to be associated with myocardial depression secondary to reperfusion injury.[40]

Finally, CPB initiates a cascade of events that results in cytokine release. This response may be triggered by changes in bowel mucosal blood flow and by bacterial translocation,

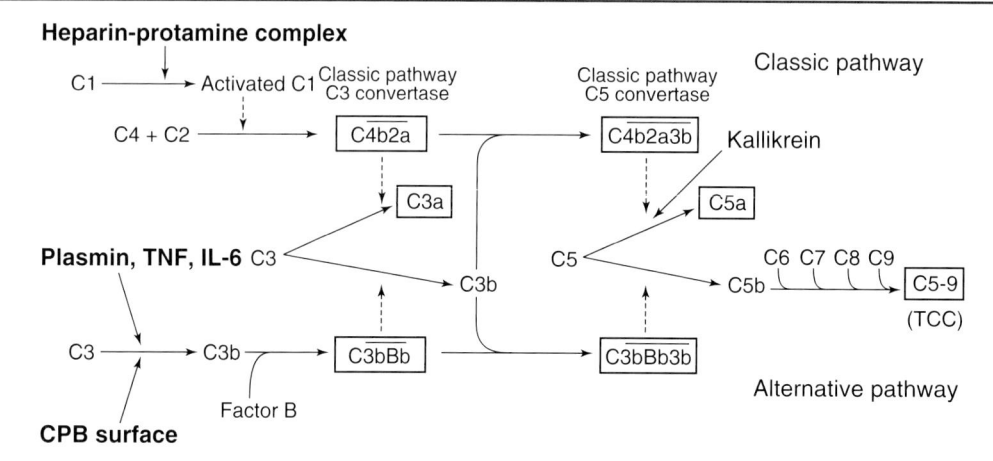

Figure 62-9
Mechanisms of complement activation during cardiopulmonary bypass (CPB). IL-6, interleukin 6; TNF, tumor necrosis factor; TCC, terminal complement complex.

as lipopolysaccharide (LPS) concentration increases by 100% immediately on CPB institution, with another significant increase seen after aortic cross-clamp release. LPS induces a broad range of immunologic effects and is considered the most potent stimulator of TNFα production from macrophages. TNF induces monocyte IL-1 production, and TNF and IL-1 in concert induce IL-6 production and release.[41] Whereas a rise in TNF and IL-1 as a result of CPB has not been regularly demonstrated in all studies, a marked increase in IL-6 levels appears consistently with CPB. Peak concentration of IL-6 occurs a few hours after the end of CPB, with a gradual decrease toward preoperative levels in the following 24 hours,[42] as seen in noncardiac surgery.[43]

Several investigators have demonstrated a correlation between the release of inflammatory mediators and myocardial dysfunction after coronary artery bypass surgery. Peak IL-6 and IL-8 levels correlate with the degree of myocardial dysfunction.[44] TNF may be released locally in the myocardium, and this may be related to postischemic myocardial stunning.[45] Jansen and coworkers[46] demonstrated that a rise in TNF can be detected after release of the aortic cross-clamp. TNF, IL-6,[47] and IL-8 levels correlated with the duration of the cross-clamping and the degree of myocardial injury as reflected by the creatine kinase (CK) MB isoenzyme levels.[47]

Cellular Activation during CPB: Platelets, Endothelial Cells, Leukocytes

Although the cellular events during CPB are influenced by the dynamic nature of the activation by the unique soluble products produced at the biomaterial, they are more significantly affected by the composition of proteins adsorbed on the non-endothelial surface. Surface-adsorbed fibrinogen is the key mediator of platelet accumulation on foreign materials. Platelet adhesion to artificial surfaces increases with increasing surface concentration of adsorbed fibrinogen if the bound fibrinogen maintains a conformation such that the functional domains of the molecule are recognizable by the activated platelet GP IIb/IIIa receptor. This latter interaction is probably the most important factor mediating platelet consumption during CPB. The three-dimensional conformation of adsorbed fibrinogen also influences the degree of platelet accumulation.

CPB is associated with a consistent increase in the proportion of activated circulating platelets. Agonists of platelet activation during CPB include thrombin, adenosine diphosphate (ADP), heparin, protamine, activated complement, and plasmin. Physical activators of platelets include hypothermia and the process of cardiotomy blood collection. The latter effect may be related to the air–blood interface, the blood–tissue interface, or the exposure to thrombin generation in cardiotomy blood.

The most consistently documented measure of CPB-related activation is an increase in the expression of guanosine monophosphate (GMP)-140 (P-selectin).[48] Platelet glycoprotein (GP) IIb/IIIa is also likely activated,[49] but it is controversial whether there is loss of other surface receptors such as GP Ib. Platelet microparticles, which may be highly procoagulant, can be consistently detected by flow cytometry after CPB.[50] Other platelet products increased after CPB include β-thromboglobulin and platelet factor 4 (PF4).[51]

In clinical CPB, thrombocytopenia is seen commonly, with platelet counts dropping more than 50%, resulting not only from platelet adhesion to surfaces but also from hemodilution, platelet aggregate formation, and the formation of platelet–leukocyte complexes. With these changes, it is not surprising that the most predictable alteration in hemostatic function observed after CPB is platelet dysfunction. Clinical reflectors of this process include a universal prolongation of the bleeding time that is directly related to postoperative blood loss.[52] Platelet aggregation to ADP and epinephrine is consistently abnormal,[53] and there is decreased response to thrombin agonist receptor peptide (TRAP), suggesting a decrease in receptor sensitivity.[54]

Because of the intense anti-inflammatory reaction related to CPB, it might be expected that the endothelial layer would be at the front line of many of the cellular changes related to CPB. It is now evident that it is the activation of this axis that mediates many of the injurious processes related to CPB, such as reperfusion injury. The generation of cytokines is a major contributor to endothelial cell activation, primarily because they upregulate receptors necessary for neutrophil–endothelial cell binding.[55] Endothelial cells undergo upregulation of intercellular adhesion molecule (ICAM) and E selectin. The latter binds to the integrin CD11a/CD18 present on resting polymorphonuclear leukocytes (PMN). PMN and monocytes may be activated with upregulation of the integrin CD11b/CD18 complex,[56] which also binds ICAM on endothelial cells.[57] The response to acute injury of the endothelium during CPB is evident by the acute rise in soluble P-selectin, with a concomitant fall in soluble E-selectin, and by increased elastase release.[58] Leukocytes interact with platelets during CPB as another means of systemic inflammation. Increased GMP140 on the platelet surface is essential to mediate complex formation of platelets and monocytes or PNMs.[57] Monocyte–platelet conjugates increased from 18% to 44%, whereas PMN–platelet conjugates increased only slightly.[57]

Nonbiomaterial-Related Activation during CPB

Exposure of cardiotomy blood well to wound surfaces is probably the most important source of thrombin generation during CPB, despite the large dosages of heparin given (Fig. 62-10). Several factors contribute to persistent thrombin generation in cardiotomy blood. First, heparin levels in the cardiotomy blood are well below those found in the systemic blood,[59] as heparin may be bound to nonplasma components such as platelets or debris and it may be consumed by PF4. Further, any heparin that is present is not capable of inhibiting thrombin completely; especially thrombin that is bound to fibrin.[60] Second, thrombin is generated via coagulation pathways other than the intrinsic pathway, and these are less effectively inhibited by heparin. Tissue factor on the wound surface and on the surface of activated monocytes contributes to coagulation,[61] as does the monocyte CD11b activation of factor X.[62] Finally, cardiotomy blood contributes to fibrinolysis induction[63] and this may enhance systemic fibrinolysis after cardiotomy blood re-administration.

HEPARIN–PROTAMINE AXIS

Heparin: Pharmacology, Dosage, and Complications

Heparin, derived from bovine or porcine intestinal mucosa, is a glycosaminoglycan composed of chains of alternating residues of D-glucosamine and uronic acid. It is commonly used in its unfractionated form (UFH) consisting of a spectrum of molecular weights between 1000 and 30,000 Da with a mean of 15,000. The anticoagulant activity of heparin is intimately associated with the protein biochemistry of antithrombin III (ATIII). ATIII is a natural inhibitor of thrombin, but the presence of heparin accelerates this action more than 4000-fold. Heparin's effect is accounted for by a unique pentasaccharide sequence with a high-affinity binding sequence to ATIII. The inhibition of thrombin is also dependent on the heparin fraction with a minimum of 18 pentasaccharide units, allowing simultaneous binding of ATIII and thrombin. Heparin is then able to dissociate from this ternary complex to be reused again in the circulation. UFH-ATIII complexes can catalyze the inhibition of factors IXa, Xa, and XIa,[64] but they have little effect on factor XIIa.[65] Heparin's other actions as an anticoagulant include the facilitation of thrombin inhibition by heparin cofactor II and its inhibition of the extrinsic pathway by heparin-mediated release of tissue factor pathway inhibitor. Finally, there is increasing evidence that heparin's principal inhibitory effect on coagulation is through the inhibition of thrombin-induced activation of factors V and VIII.[66]

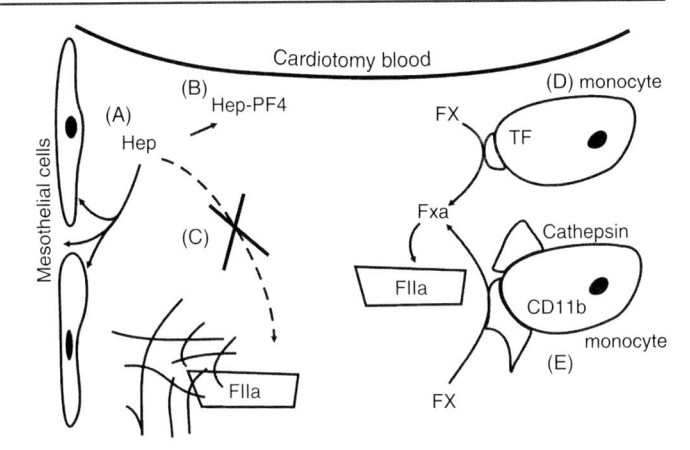

Figure 62–10
Mechanisms contributing to thrombin generation in cardiotomy blood. Heparin (Hep) levels are decreased as a result of (A) binding to wound surfaces and (B) binding to platelet factor 4 (PF4). Heparin is also ineffective because of (C) its inability to inhibit clot-bound thrombin. Thrombin generation occurs through other monocyte-dependent processes such as (D) tissue factor (TF) and (E) cathepsin/CD11b complex–mediated factor X (FX) activation.

The clearance of heparin is influenced by its molecular size, with higher-molecular-weight species being removed from the circulation more rapidly than the lower-molecular-weight species. UFH is cleared through two phases: a rapid saturable phase and a slower phase of first-order mechanism; thus, anticoagulant response is not linear but increases in intensity and duration with increasing dosage.[67] After injection, UFH is bound by a number of plasma proteins including histidine-rich glycoprotein, PF4, vitronectin, fibronectin, and von Willebrand's factor (vWF). This contributes to the variability of anticoagulant response to fixed-dosage heparin and the laboratory phenomenon of heparin resistance. The binding of UFH to endothelial cells and macrophages also contributes to its complicated pharmacokinetics.

During CPB, heparin is generally used in generous dosages of up to 300 U/kg, with an aim to achieve and maintain a target activated clotting time (ACT) of 400 to 480 seconds. This rather primitive test, although automated, involves the addition of an aliquot of whole blood to a test tube containing a blood activator (celite or kaolin). In the Hemochron ACT device (International Technidyne Corp., Edison, NJ), when a clot forms, resistance to movement of a small magnet in the tube is detected and the timer stops. The HemoTec ACT device (Medtronic HemoTec, Englewood, CO), which uses kaolin as an activator, uses a plastic plunger for continuous mixing. The absence of plunger fall after a clot forms is detected photo-optically and the counter ceases.

Heparin may contribute to the bleeding diathesis after surgery, independent of its action as an antithrombotic. UFH may contribute to platelet dysfunction directly[68] or through its ability to bind to vWF. Heparin-induced platelet activation may also result in clearance of platelets from the circulation, thus contributing to postoperative thrombocytopenia. Heparin has an independent role as a profibrinolytic agent[69] before the initiation of CPB, which may be related to its activation of the kallikrein system.

Two forms of thrombocytopenia are related to heparin administration independent of CPB. The first is a benign

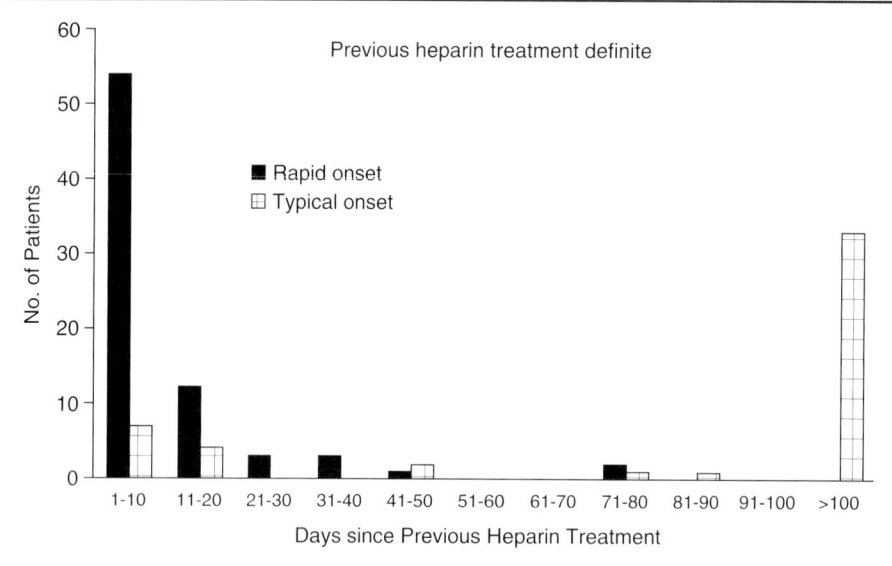

Figure 62-11
Temporal pattern of heparin-induced thrombocytopenia in relation to previous treatment with heparin. None of the patients whose prior heparin treatment had occurred more than 100 days earlier had rapid-onset thrombocytopenia. *(Reproduced with permission from Warkentin TE, Kelton JG. Temporal aspects of heparin-induced thrombocytopenia.* N Engl J Med *2001:344;1286-92. Copyright 2001, Massachusetts Medical Society.)*

reversible nonimmune thrombocytopenia, which immediately responds to the discontinuation of heparin and may be related to direct weak activation of platelets by heparin. The second, more serious reaction is an IgG-mediated immune thrombocytopenia referred to as heparin-induced thrombocytopenia and thrombosis (HITT). The syndrome is secondary to platelet activation from an IgG that binds the FcγII receptor.[70] The heparin–PF4 complex on the platelet surface is the responsible target antigen. A secondary thrombogenic diathesis may result from platelet activation related to microparticle release.[71]

HITT usually begins 5 to 15 days after the commencing of heparin therapy, but recent data have suggested that it can be detected within a mean of 10 hours of commencement of heparin in patients with previous exposure.[72] The incidence is lower with bovine heparin.[73] In general, 1% of heparinized patients will develop HITT at 7 days, and 3% at 14 days.[74] Although thrombocytopenia may be evident, the surgeon must be wary of a normal platelet count in the postoperative period in the presence of unexplained thrombosis, when reactive thrombocytosis should be evident.

HITT is diagnosed using an assay that measures the release of radiolabelled serotonin from donor platelets after patient serum exposure, or using an enzyme-linked immunosorbent assay for the PF4–heparin complex antigen. Surgical approaches to patients with HITT depend on the degree of urgency of the anticipated procedure. In elective situations, when patients with a history of HITT can be postponed (>100 days), they may not be at risk for thrombotic complications if heparin is used a second time (Fig. 62-11).[72] If the surgery cannot be postponed, avoidance of CPB with off-pump techniques may be considered, but some form of anticoagulation is still necessary during anastomosis. Each institution should develop a strategy for the emergency management of CPB in the presence of HITT. Traditionally, a platelet-"paralyzing" agent such as prostacyclin was used, but the attendant hypotension was often difficult to manage.[75] Of the alternatives to UFH,

LMWH is not suitable as there is greater than 90% immune cross-reactivity with UFH, and CPB with LMWH is associated with significant bleeding.[76] The heparinoid danaparoid (Orgaran, NV Organon, The Netherlands) has less than 10% antibody cross-reactivity and less than 5% clinical cross-reactivity[77] and thus may be useful, but no neutralizing agent is available and because of its long half-life, significant bleeding must be anticipated after its use.[78] Ancrod (Viprinex, Abbott Laboratories, Canada) is a defibrinogenating agent derived from snake venom. The clinical experience with this agent is limited, and its drawbacks include that it blocks neither thrombin generation nor platelet activation, it is antigenic, and a delay of 12 hours for the full effect is required.

ATIII-independent thrombin inhibitors such as hirudin, bivalirudin, and argatroban hold promise as the best alternatives for CPB management in these difficult situations. Recombinant hirudin (Refludan, Hoechst, Kansas City, MO) binds the catalytic and fibrinogen binding sites of thrombin. It has been successfully used in clinical CPB[79] and in deep hypothermic circulatory arrest.[80] This drug can be monitored using the ecarin clotting time.[81] Bivalirudin has been demonstrated as safe as heparin for on-pump surgery,[82] and it may be easier to use than hirudin because of its shorter half-life.[83] Argatroban also specifically binds the catalytic site of thrombin. Its potential benefit over hirudin relates to its shorter half-life (15 to 30 minutes, compared with 30 to 60 minutes for hirudin), which compensates for its lack of a reversing agent. This drug has been used in CPB,[84] but greater experience is needed before giving it a universal recommendation.

Protamine: Pharmacology, Complications

Protamine is a polycationic protein derived from salmon sperm. The positive charges on protamine combine ionically with the negative moieties of the heparin molecule, separating it from ATIII and producing a stable precipitate that is rapidly cleared from the circulation. The drug is given intravenously at a fixed ratio of 1 to 1.3 mg/100 U administered heparin. The most common problem related to protamine is heparin rebound, which is a frequent cause of postoperative bleeding. This phenomenon is related to the delayed desorption of heparin from plasma proteins and endothelium after the first dose of protamine has been cleared. It usually becomes evident 2 to 3 hours after arrival in the ICU, and its presence is reflected by increasing chest tube losses accompanied by a new prolongation of the ACT or thrombin time. The problem can be obviated by the routine addition of a protamine drip after surgery. Hypotension is another common consequence of protamine administration, particularly with rapid intravenous administration. The mechanism of this rate-related effect is not known, but its magnitude is greater in situations of low preload and afterload. Protamine may also be responsible for several idiosyncratic hypotensive reactions. Anaphylactoid reactions are mediated primarily by complement and histamine. Anaphylactic reactions involve the IgE-mediated release of histamine and other vasoactive mediators. Both reactions are characterized by edema, hives, and bronchospasm in the presence of low blood pressure, CVP, and pulmonary artery pressure, and decreased supraventricular rhythm. The most serious form of protamine-related hypotension is catastrophic pulmonary vasoconstriction. In contrast to the other two forms of idiosyncratic protamine reactions, this syndrome may be associated with bronchospasm, and with pulmonary hypertension with an elevated CVP. The mechanism is probably related to IgG release with activation of complement and PMN, and release of platelet thromboxane A_2.[85] Theoretically, patients at risk for protamine reactions include those with previous vasectomy, previous exposure to protamine, or previous exposure to protamine-containing insulin.[86]

Protamine may contribute to excessive postoperative bleeding because of a direct antiplatelet effect. It also has a direct anticoagulant effect, but this can be demonstrated in vitro only at dosages much higher than those required to neutralize heparin during clinical CPB.

When problems with protamine have been detected in advance, the cardiac surgeon can prepare alternative strategies to prevent anticipated problems after CPB. In minor cases with low risk, premedication with steroids (at least 12 to 24 hours in advance) and histamine blockers may be all that is required. A small test dose (5 mg) should also be given to ensure safety. Avoidance of neutralization after the massive dosages required for CPB may be difficult because of the prolonged half-life of heparin. Experimentally, recombinant PF4 has shown promise as an alternative to protamine.[87]

The rationale for heparinizing to an ACT of between 400 and 480 seconds during CPB is based on early work that demonstrated that at this level of ACTs, no gross evidence of thrombosis occurred in the reservoir. However, many researchers have expressed doubt about the validity of using ACT as gold standard for anticoagulation during CPB. In particular, there is clear evidence that the ACT does not reflect the heparin level accurately, particularly after a long duration of CPB, and that other factors, such as hypothermia, hemodilution, and drugs, may contribute (Fig. 62-12).[88] As CPB progresses, celite-based ACT values may be further influenced by the use of aprotinin. The Hepcon device (Medtronic HemoTec, Englewood, CO) is composed of a series of ACT cuvettes containing incrementally increased protamine dosages that can be used to precisely calculate the circulating heparin level. Patient-specific preoperative standard curves with target heparin concentrations can be precisely calculated. Interestingly, using this technique, overall heparin requirements are higher (25%). However, factor consumption during CPB is decreased, most likely related to an inhibition of low-grade coagulation. In clinical trials, this technique also resulted in a shorter bleeding time on arrival in the ICU that was associated with decreased blood product use.[89] These findings have been controversial[90]; although this form of heparin–protamine titration has significant potential, careful monitoring is necessary to compensate for aspects such as heparin rebound, which is intensified by the higher heparin dosage used.

PHARMACOLOGIC ADJUNCTS TO MINIMIZE THE CONSEQUENCES OF CPB

Steroids are widely used for the suppression of inflammation in chronic inflammatory diseases. During CPB, steroids blunt complement activation, upregulation of glycoprotein CD11b,[91] and the release of histamine,[92] TNF,[93] IL-6,[94] IL-8,[93] and neutrophil elastase.[95] Finally, steroids reduce airway NO concentrations during CPB,[96] compatible with inhibition of bronchial epithelial iNOS expression. Steroids have also been demonstrated to be associated with decreased CK MB.[97] The inhibition of these aspects of inflammation may explain the stabilizing effect of these drugs on hemodynamics after CPB. Contrary to expectations, steroid use has not been demonstrated to be associated with postoperative wound infection in cardiac surgery.[98]

Although the primary indication for the use of the serine protease inhibitor aprotinin is to reduce blood loss during and after CPB, a number of studies have shown that aprotinin reduces cytokine levels and cytokine-induced events when used during CPB.[99] However, this drug is very expensive when compared with steroid therapy, and it may not have as general an effect on the inflammatory system. Diego and colleagues[100] demonstrated that the anti-inflammatory effect of methylprednisolone (MPSS) exceeded that of aprotinin as reflected by a greater inhibition of IL-6 at all time points after CPB. On the other hand, steroids may augment the anti-inflammatory action of aprotinin. Tassani and coworkers[101] demonstrated that high-dose MPSS attenuates the systemic inflammatory response during coronary bypass grafting in aprotinin-treated patients. IL-6 and IL-8 were significantly less in the MPSS group, whereas the anti-inflammatory IL-10 was greater. These changes corresponded to augmented oxygenation, improved lung compliance, and improved cardiac index in the steroid-treated group. As a result of concerns of excessive mortality and complications with aprotinin, this drug is no longer available for use in cardiac surgery.

BIOMATERIAL-DEPENDENT STRATEGIES TO MINIMIZE BLOOD ACTIVATION FROM CPB

A biomaterial-dependent strategy involves the choice of a CPB circuit composed of a biomaterial with enhanced biocompatibility. The quest for an ideal biomaterial substrate for the construction of CPB circuits has culminated in three types of surface modifications that either have been tested in human trials or are on the verge of clinical evaluation.

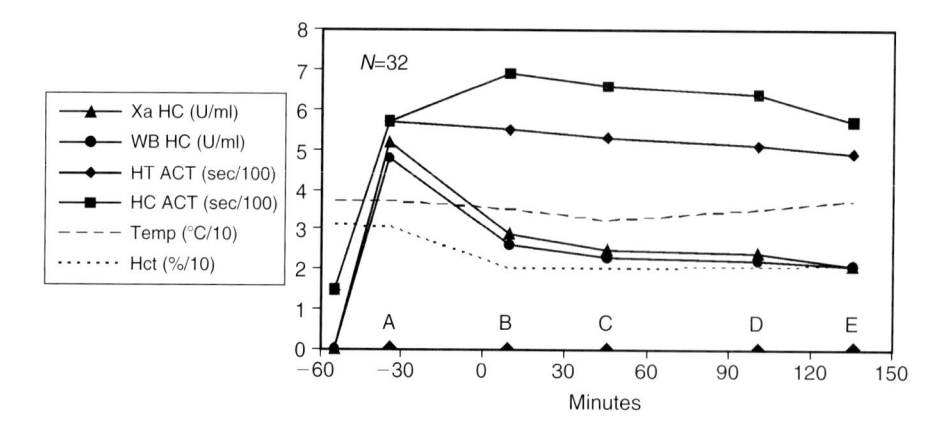

Figure 62–12
Time course of physiologic and hematologic mean values for patient with cardiopulmonary bypass (CPB). Mean values for activated clotting time (ACT) expressed in seconds per 100 for both Hemochron (HC ACT) and Hepcon (HT ACT) assays. Plasma-equivalent heparin concentration (WB HC) and anti-Xa plasma heparin concentration (Xa HC) expressed in units per milliliter. Hematocrit (Hct) values expressed as percent divided by 10 (%/10), and core body temperature (Temp) expressed in degrees centigrade divided by 10 (°C/10). Mean values for derived physiologic and hematologic variables are plotted as a function of time in minutes. Phase II time points begin before heparin administration, and then 10 minutes after each of the following: heparin administration (A), initiation of CPB (B), achievement of hypothermia (C), rewarming (D), and immediately before discontinuation of CPB (E). *(Reproduced with permission from Despotis GJ, Summerfield AL, Joist JH, et al. J Thorac Cardiovasc Surg 1994;108;1076-82. Copyright 1994 Mosby-Year Book Inc.).*

Biomembrane Mimicry

A biomaterial has been developed that mimics the antithrombotic behavior of natural cell membranes. It is coated with a derivative of phosphorylcholine, which is the major lipid headgroup component found on the outer surface of biologic cell membranes.[102] In vitro data have demonstrated the efficacy of this modified surface (Memsys, Sorin Biomedica) in inhibiting fibrinogen adsorption and platelet deposition.[102] Clinical experience in CPB with this device is limited, but in a recent pediatric trial, limited platelet activation was seen with this coating.[103]

Heparin-Coated Circuits

Two types of heparin-coated circuits are clinically relevant. In the first group, heparin is bound so that it may be slowly released into the circulation from the surface. The original ionic binding pioneered by Gott and colleagues[104] now exists as the DurofloII surface (Baxter Healthcare Corporation, Irvine, CA), in which the heparin is ionically bound to benzalkonium attached to the substrate polymer. In the second group, heparin is immobilized permanently on the biomaterial surface by covalent bonding. Polyethylene oxide is used as a spacer group, as its hydrophilic character and its dynamic motion further inhibit platelet interactions. The Carmeda product (Carmeda, Medtronic, Minneapolis, MN) is a commercial example of this technology for CPB, in which heparin is covalently bound via an end-point immobilization technique. The Trillium Biopassive Surface (Medtronic, Minneapolis, MN) is a similar coating process involving two polymers on the substrate surface. The first polymer functions as a primer, strongly bonding to the surface of the substrate. The second polymer, which is bound to the primer coat, is composed of sulfate and sulfonate groups, the latter providing a negative surface charge, as well as polyethylene oxide chains covalently bound to heparin. BioLine (Jostra, Germany) is a hybrid surface (i.e., a combination of heparin-releasing and heparin-immobilized) in which heparin is adsorbed onto a layer of immobilized polypeptides through a combination of ionic interactions and covalent bonds.

Convincing in vitro evidence of the thromboresistant behavior of heparin-coated surfaces led to the hypothesis that less intense anticoagulation would be required for CPB when heparin-coated circuits were used. Many of the early clinical trials compared outcomes after CPB in which heparin-coated circuits were combined with lower dosages of heparin (one third to one half) versus control (uncoated) circuits and standard heparin dosages (300 units/kg). Advantages included decreased perioperative bleeding and transfusion. In a large clinical trial reported by Aldea and colleagues,[105] an integrated blood conservation strategy that included heparin-coated circuits and decreased heparin dosing was applied. This approach resulted in decreased blood transfusion requirements and significantly improved clinical outcomes as measured by ICU and hospital lengths of stay, and by duration of ventilatory support. This translated into cost savings of approximately $1700 per patient,[105] similar to that found in a recent meta-analysis assessing this technology.[106]

Compelling as these clinical results are, neither thrombin generation nor fibrinolysis has been consistently demonstrated to be decreased during CPB with heparin-coated circuits in human trials, with either standard or decreased heparin dosages compared with standard (non–heparin-coated) circuits.[107] Therefore, it is difficult to justify decreasing the heparin dosage, given the potential risk of low-grade thrombosis. Also, any measured differences in a patient's clinical and biochemical outcomes may be related to differences in the amounts of administered heparin and not to the surface, as heparin itself can induce a myriad of cellular and biochemical changes such as fibrinolysis[69] and platelet dysfunction.[69] As the dosage of the protamine must also be increased, it is anticipated that changes such as complement activation must be proportionally increased. In the majority of clinical trials in which the same dosages of heparin are used with both heparin-coated circuits and standard circuits, little clinical benefit has been consistently demonstrated, except perhaps in high-risk patients.[108]

Beneficial clinical impacts of heparin-coated circuits are almost entirely related to their intrinsic anti-inflammatory effect. What has been consistently demonstrated is the capacity of heparin-coated surfaces to decrease complement activation[109] independent of the heparin dosage. Other demonstrated anti-inflammatory effects of heparin-coated surfaces include decreased leukocyte surface activation markers or receptors,[110] decreased cytokine production,[111] and decreased monocyte tissue factor.[112] The anti-inflammatory action of heparin-coated circuits in the absence of coagulation inhibition may be related to its action as a selective "protein sink" for such proteins as high-molecular-weight kininogen.[113] Surface-adsorbed HMWK may interact with antithrombin III in the presence of surface heparin to potentiate heparin-mediated inhibition of kallikrein.[107,114]

In summary, heparin-coated surfaces have been demonstrated to exhibit potent antithrombotic behavior in in vitro testing. Although there is no evidence of decreased thrombogenicity when used clinically, there is consistent evidence that inflammation related to complement activation is decreased, and this may be responsible for the improvement seen in some clinical outcomes after CPB.

Surfaces with Modified Protein Adsorption

Another biomaterial-dependent strategy involves surfaces whose biocompatibility has been predicted on the basis of protein adsorption characteristics. An example of this approach includes a new generation of biomaterials into which a surface-modifying additive (SMA) has been incorporated.[115] The additive is a triblock-copolymer with polar and nonpolar polymer chains.[115] During the manufacturing process, the SMA migrates to the surface of the base polymer, yielding a stable microdomain-like configuration. Although the mechanism of action by which SMA decreases blood protein and cellular activation is not precisely known, it is hypothesized that the alternating hydrophobic and hydrophilic regions of the microdomain surface lead to uniform adhesion of fibrinogen, so that all of the sites for potential platelet interaction with surface-bound fibrinogen are occupied. A randomized controlled trial in which patients underwent CPB using a standard control circuit or a circuit prepared "tip-to-tip" with the SMA copolymer (SMA-CPB)[116] showed striking changes in the effect of this surface on markers of coagulation, fibrinolysis, and platelet number and function. Thrombin generation was significantly decreased with SMA-CPB compared with controls, despite carefully matched heparin dosages in the two groups. Defraigne and coworkers[117] in a larger clinical trial confirmed the same degree of platelet preservation with SMA-CPB and a similar decreased release of β-thromboglobulin. In addition, there was evidence of a decreased need for the transfusion of platelets and fresh frozen plasma in the group with SMA-CPB circuits.

Terumo Corporation (Tokyo, Japan) developed a surface for CPB circuits with a biocompatibility profile similar to that of SMA, in that it was engineered to positively influence protein adsorption. Surfaces are coated with poly(2-methoxyethylacrylate) [PMEA]), which has a hydrophobic polyethylene backbone, and its residue has mild hydrophilicity with no chemical functional groups such as -OH or -NH_2. It was predicted that as the outer side of the PMEA molecule is inactive chemically, the surface would have little tendency to react with blood components. Although clinical studies in humans are not available, promising data from in vitro and in vivo models support the potential improved biocompatibility of PMEA-coated surfaces.[118] Analysis of the composition of the adsorbed protein layer on PMEA-coated surfaces demonstrated a striking decrease in the amount of adsorbed IgG. This finding correlated with platelet count preservation as compared with uncoated surfaces, as surface-bound IgG is a well-known platelet activator. The use of the PMEA circuit was also associated with a significant decrease in CD35-positive monocytes during CPB.[119] Decreased adsorption of immunoglobulin is again probably the causative mechanism for decreased complement activation. Plasma bradykinin levels are decreased with PMEA,[118] as are thrombin–antithrombin III levels.[118]

ORGAN DERANGEMENTS RELATED TO CARDIOPULMONARY BYPASS

Neuroendocrine Response to CPB

The changes in neuroendocrine response related to CPB are different from those observed in noncardiac surgery. Hormones under hypothalamic-pituitary control include growth hormone, vasopressin, the adrenal cortical axis, and the thyroid hormone system. Growth hormone increases significantly during and after CPB.[120] Vasopressin is a key regulator of renal water excretion and peripheral vascular resistance and it may contribute to endothelial activation through release of vWF.[121] Marked increases in vasopressin are seen after cardiac surgery with CPB, with the elevated levels persisting for hours.[122] This may be a protective effect, as depressed levels postoperatively are associated with vasodilatory shock.[123]

There is a definite increase in adrenocorticotropic hormone with CPB, although the adrenocorticotropic hormone response is blunted after administration of corticotrophin-releasing hormone during CPB.[124] Total plasma cortisol concentrations typically decrease immediately on initiation of CPB as a consequence of hemodilution, but later values return to normal or higher than baseline accompanied by parallel increases in unbound cortisol, suggesting that this increase is related to increased total secretion.[125] Thyroid hormone dysfunction may play a role in the unique clinical response seen after CPB. Investigators have demonstrated that although thyroid-stimulating hormone remains normal, total and free T3 drop and remains depressed for 24 hours after surgery, and reverse T3 shows a fourfold rise at 8 and 24 hours postoperatively thus producing a picture of sick euthyroid syndrome.[126]

The catecholamines epinephrine and norepinephrine are both increased after CPB, which may be a contributing cause of severe postoperative hypertension.[127] The sympathetic system regulates glucose control at the level of the pancreas by controlling the release of insulin and glucagon. After the onset of CPB, blood glucose concentrations rise steadily in parallel with a drop in insulin levels, and insulin resistance is seen with higher than average dosages.[128] During and after CPB, renin levels increase, and this is associated with a rise in measured angiotensin II and aldosterone.[129]

Among the locally released hormones, atrial natriuretic factor levels are probably reduced during CPB, especially in patients with preoperative elevations, but elevated levels may be seen in the presence of complications.[130] Other locally released factors include histamine and serotonin, related to leukocyte and platelet activation.[131] Histamine produces vasodilation and hypotension and may contribute to tPA release.[132] Its increase may be abolished by high-dose steroids and prostacyclin infusions.[133] Finally, CPB provides a consistent stimulus for prostacyclin and inflammatory eicosanoid formation, as evidenced by a marked increase in 6-keto-prostaglandin F_{1a} (a stable metabolite of prostacyclin),[134] thromboxane B_2,[135] and prostaglandin E_2 concentrations.[136]

Central Nervous System Injury with CPB

Cerebral damage during heart surgery may be the complication most feared and respected by cardiac surgeons. There are three major types of neurologic injury after CPB, but the distinction between them is blurred and they probably reflect a continuum of pathologic changes based on location, extent, and permanence of the injury. Stroke is the easiest injury to recognize after CPB. Its incidence is difficult to pinpoint, but the best estimate is around 3% of patients undergoing CABG.[137] Based on the information from the Society of Thoracic Surgeons database, this complication is increased in women and in older adults. The incidence rises to 8% after isolated valve surgery and 11% after CABG combined with other surgery.[138] The cause is probably macroemboli from an aortic source. Stroke is associated with a marked increase in 30-day mortality, and its occurrence doubles hospital stay and cost.[137]

Delirium, seen in up to 3% of patients, is a state characterized by confusion and disorientation in the presence of an altered state of consciousness,[139] a problem that may increase hospital stay fivefold.[139] Risk factors include increased age, hypertension, and a history of previous CABG, pulmonary disease, or alcohol abuse.[139]

Cognitive decline (postoperative cognitive deficit [POCD]) is defined as a change in memory, concentration, psychomotor speed, or dexterity. Although it may go unnoticed, sometimes the patient recognizes inability to complete previously facile tasks, or it may be recognized by the family. Quantitation depends on sensitive neuropsychological findings involving a reproducible battery of tests. A pooled analysis of six highly comparable studies by Van Dijk and colleagues[140] yielded a proportion of POCD after CPB of 22.5% (95% confidence interval, 18.7%-26.4%). Newman and colleagues,[141] Robinson and colleagues,[142] and Borowicz and colleagues[143] provide comprehensive reviews of studies of POCD after CABG; the reported incidences in larger studies range from 35% to 75% early postoperatively and 11% to 40% after more than 6 months. Sotaniemi and coworkers found that even if the early postoperative changes disappeared, affected individuals were more likely to show early dementia 5 years later,[144] as the underlying neuronal loss may make an individual more vulnerable to age-dependant cell loss in the future. Newman and coworkers[145] showed that patients demonstrating significant impairment early are impaired at 5 years, compared with patients not having early deficits.

Recently, however, the relationship of CPB to neurocognitive dysfunction has been called into question. First, several prospective randomized controlled trials failed to show a clear benefit of off-pump compared with on-pump surgery in terms of the incidence of neurocognitive dysfunction.[146] Second, it was shown that nonsurgical control populations with coronary disease undergoing medical therapy or percutaneous intervention have the same rate of neurocognitive decline as those patients undergoing on-pump CABG.[147] Finally, the model of neurocognitive testing is debatable, as these evaluations were never designed as a pre-post test.

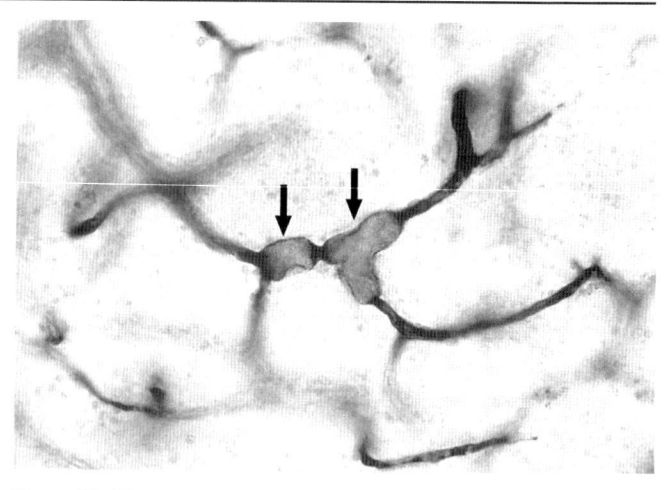

Figure 62-13
Postmortem specimen of brain section illustrating small capillary and arteriolar dilatation (SCAD) (arrows) after cardiopulmonary bypass (CPB). (Image courtesy of Dr. Dixon Moody, Wake Forest University.)

One characteristic pathologic finding in canine and human cerebral tissue after CPB is referred to as small capillary and arteriolar dilations (SCADs) (Fig. 62-13). These are believed to be the sites of fat, particulate, or gas emboli.[148] Transcranial Doppler studies of patients during CPB have confirmed the frequent occurrence of embolic material in the cerebral circulation. Furthermore, the cerebral embolic load was found to be directly proportional to the length of CPB in an autopsy study by Brown and colleagues.[149] There is a direct correlation between POCD and retinal microemboli on fluorescein angiography.[150] Magnetic resonance imaging immediately after CABG has identified global cerebral swelling even in low-risk patients.[151] Finally, there is strong experimental evidence that cardiotomy suction blood may be the most important source of lipid emboli.[152] Two recent clinical trials had different results as to whether processing cardiotomy blood has an impact on neurocognitive outcome,[153,154] but this intervention did result in a significant increase in postoperative bleeding[153,154] and transfusion,[154] and thus it is debatable whether cardiotomy blood processing is safe.

Pulmonary Dysfunction with CPB

After CPB, there is a documented incidence of pulmonary dysfunction—from 12% for mild lung injury to 1.3% for ARDS.[155] This problem is more common in older adults, the obese, and patients with low cardiac output or pulmonary hypertension, and after long CPB.[155] In the majority of cases of CPB-related lung injury, full recovery occurs, but severe lung injury has a mortality of greater than 50%.[156] Clinical findings of lung injury include an increase in the alveolar-arterial oxygen pressure difference and the pulmonary shunt fraction, together with a decrease in the functional residual capacity. There may be increased pulmonary vascular resistance as well as evidence of increased lung permeability.[157] The etiology of CPB-related lung injury does not appear to be related to hypoxia induced by partial CPB, as the bronchial circulation is adequate to prevent necrosis.[158] There is, however, definite evidence of increased pulmonary inflammation with increased bronchoalveolar lavage fluid–activated neutrophils,[159] increased matrix metalloproteinases and myeloperoxidase levels,[160] and increased IL-8 and elastase,[161] all of which may contribute to breakdown of the pulmonary ultrastructure.[162]

Off-pump techniques have not consistently minimized pulmonary insufficiency after cardiac surgery,[163] nor have steroids helped.[164] Leukocyte depletion may limit pulmonary reperfusion injury after CPB and result in improved lung function.[165] Heparin-coated circuits have been shown to improve lung compliance and pulmonary vascular resistance, with particular improvement seen when low heparin protocols are used.[105] Some authors have recommended maintaining mechanical ventilation during CPB, but most studies failed to show significant persistent benefit.[157] No impact of temperature management on pulmonary outcome could be demonstrated.[157] Maintaining lung perfusion during CPB (Drew-Anderson technique) refers to using the patient's own lungs as an oxygenator and supplying only biventricular pump function, and this may have some clinical benefits,[166] but its practicality is not universally accepted.

Renal Dysfunction with CPB

Data from the Multicenter Study of Perioperative Ischemia Research Group[167] demonstrated a 7.7% incidence of postoperative renal dysfunction, with 1.4% of all patients needing dialysis. Renal insufficiency is associated with increased hospital and ICU stay and mortality, emphasizing its clinical relevance. The contribution of CPB to renal damage during cardiac surgery is supported by clinical studies comparing outcomes with off-pump techniques. In high-risk patients (serum creatinine > 150 µmol/L), the use of CPB was associated with increased postoperative levels of serum creatinine and urea.[168] Glomerular filtration as assessed by creatinine clearance and urinary microalbumin-to-creatinine ratio was significantly worse in on-pump groups,[169] and there is a lower incidence of microalbuminuria, improved free water clearance and fractional excretion of sodium, and decreased N-acetyl-β-D-glucosaminidase (NAG) in the urine with off-pump surgery.[170] Although factors such as nonpulsatile flow and obstructive atheromatous microemboli may contribute, the diffuse inflammatory change related to CPB may have an independent toxic effect on the kidneys. Proximal tubular dysfunction has been demonstrated by increased urinary release of NAG and elevated urine levels of the cytokines IL-1 receptor antagonist and TNF soluble receptor 2.[171]

Numerous strategies have been advocated as potentially renal-protective during CPB. Leukodepletion resulted in decreased urinary microalbumin and retinol binding protein release.[172] Mannitol is a popular diuretic agent that can increase diuresis if added in dosages of 10 to 30 g. This drug has also been shown to preserve creatinine levels and lower urinary albumin excretion rates after pediatric cardiac surgery.[173] Renal-dosage dopamine (2 to 3 µg/kg/min) has been assessed in several randomized controlled trials of patients at high risk for renal failure, and the results have been controversial.[174] Fenoldopam, a selective dopamine receptor agonist, was shown in a randomized controlled trial to preserve renal function as demonstrated by maintained creatinine clearance postoperatively compared with placebo infusion.[175] Several trials have demonstrated that N-acetyl cysteine does not prevent acute renal injury after cardiac surgery.

THE FUTURE OF CARDIOPULMONARY BYPASS

There is great potential for continuing evolution of CPB circuit design and techniques that may enhance clinical outcomes with cardiac surgery. For example, newer devices have incorporated novel technology to integrate all CPB components to markedly minimize the pump prime and the surface area (COR_x, CardioVention, Inc., Santa Clara, CA). However, their application will necessitate marked acceptance of modified surgical techniques (e.g., retrograde autologous priming, absence of venous reservoir or cardiotomy), which will limit their generalized acceptance and facility.

An illustrative paper by Bartels and coworkers[176] demonstrated our previous naivety with regard to the means by which we conduct CPB. "On the basis of our scientific evaluation of the current literature on 48 principles of CPB, not a single condition was of sufficient scientific merit to conclude that we were dealing with a principle for which there is clear evidence, scientific agreement, or both, that a given procedure or treatment is useful and effective."[176] On the other hand, positive steps have now been taken to apply evidence-based guidelines to perfusion practice.[177] It is only through this contemplation of our everyday actions in the OR that we can hope to continue to minimize the effect of CPB on our patients.

REFERENCES

1. Guru V, Glasgow KW, Fremes SE, Austin PC, Teoh K, Tu JV. The real-world outcomes of off-pump coronary artery bypass surgery in a public health care system. *Can J Cardiol* 2007;**23**(4):281-6.
2. DeWall RA, Grage TB, McFee AS, Chiechi MA. Theme and variations on blood oxygenators: I. Bubble oxygenators. *Surgery* 1961;**50**:931-40.
3. Kolff WJ, Berk HTJ. Artificial kidney: dialyzer with great area. *Acta Med Scand* 1944;**117**:121-34.
4. Bigelow WG, Calaghan JC, Hopps JA. General hypothermia for experimental intra-cardiac surgery. *Ann Surg* 1950;**132**:531-9.
5. Murkin JM, Farrar JK, Tweed WA, McKenzie FN, Guiraudon G. Cerebral autoregulation and flow/metabolism coupling during cardiopulmonary bypass: the influence of PaCO2. *Anesth Analg* 1987;**66**(9):825-32.
6. Kurth CD, O'Rourke MM, O'Hara IB. Comparison of pH-stat and alpha-stat cardiopulmonary bypass on cerebral oxygenation and blood flow in relation to hypothermic circulatory arrest in piglets. *Anesthesiology* 1998;**89**(1):110-18.
7. Torii K, Iida K, Miyazaki Y, et al. Higher concentrations of matrix metalloproteinases in bronchoalveolar lavage fluid of patients with adult respiratory distress syndrome. *Am J Respir Crit Care Med* 1997;**155**(1):43-6.
8. Murkin JM, Martzke JS, Buchan AM, Bentley C. A randomized study of perfusion technique and pH management strategy in 316 patients undergoing coronary artery bypass surgery. *J Thorac Cardiovasc Surg* 1995;**110**:349-62.
9. Cooper Jr JR, Giesecke NM. Hemodilution and priming solutions. In: Gravlee GP, Davis RF, Kurusz M, Utley JR, editors. *Cardiopulmonary bypass: principles and practice*. 2nd ed. Philadelphia: Lippincott Williams & Wilkins; 2000, p. 186-96.
10. Spiess BD, Ley C, Body SC, et al. Hematocrit value on intensive care unit entry influences the frequency of q-wave myocardial infarction after coronary artery bypass grafting. *J Thorac Cardiovasc Surg* 1998;**116**:460-7.
11. Hagl S, Heimisch W, Meisner H, Erben R, Baum M, Mendler N. The effect of hemodilution on regional myocardial function in the presence of coronary stenosis. *Basic Res Cardiol* 1977;**72**:344-64.
12. Habib RH, Zacharias A, Schwann TA, et al. Role of hemodilutional anemia and transfusion during cardiopulmonary bypass in renal injury after coronary revascularization: implications on operative outcome. *Crit Care Med* 2005;**33**(8):1749-56.

13. DeFoe GR, Ross CS, Olmstead EM, et al. Lowest hematocrit on bypass and adverse outcomes associated with coronary artery bypass grafting. Northern New England Cardiovascular Disease Study Group. *Ann Thorac Surg* 2001;**71**(3):769-76.
14. Fang WC, Helm RE, Krieger KH, et al. Impact of minimum hematocrit during cardiopulmonary bypass on mortality in patients undergoing coronary artery surgery. *Circulation* 1997;**96**:194-9:II.
15. Karkouti K, Djaiani G, Borger MA, et al. Low hematocrit during cardiopulmonary bypass is associated with increased risk of perioperative stroke in cardiac surgery. *Ann Thorac Surg* 2005;**80**(4):1381-7.
16. Gold JP, Charlson ME, Williams-Russo P, et al. Improvement of outcomes after coronary artery bypass. A randomized trial comparing intraoperative high versus low mean arterial pressure. *J Thorac Cardiovasc Surg* 1995;**110**(5):1302-11.
17. Reves JG, White WD, Amory DW. Improvement of outcomes after coronary artery bypass. *J Thorac Cardiovasc Surg* 1997;**113**(6):1118-20.
18. Davies LK. Hypothermia: Physiology and clinical use. In: Gravlee GP, Davis RF, Kurusz M, Utley JR, editors. *Cardiopulmonary bypass: principles and practice*. 2nd ed. Philadelphia: Lippincott Williams & Wilkins; 2000, p. 197-213.
19. Klein M, Mahoney CB, Probst C, Schulte HD, Gams E. Blood product use during routine open heart surgery: the impact of the centrifugal pump. *Artif Organs* 2001;**25**(4):300-5.
20. Scott DA, Silbert BS, Blyth C, O'Brien J, Santamaria J. Blood loss in elective coronary artery surgery: a comparison of centrifugal versus roller pump heads during cardiopulmonary bypass. *J Cardiothorac Vasc Anesth* 2001;**15**(3):322-5.
21. Hessel EA, Hill AG. Circuitry and cannulation techniques. In: Gravlee GP, Davis RF, Kurusz M, Utley JR, editors. *Cardiopulmonary bypass: principles and practice*. 2nd ed. Philadelphia: Lippincott Williams & Wilkins; 2000, p. 69-97.
22. Sinard JM, Merz SI, Hatcher MD, Montoya JP, Bartlett RH. Evaluation of extracorporeal perfusion catheters using a standardized measurement technique: the M-number. *ASAIO Trans* 1991;**37**(2):60-4.
23. Hessel EAI, Hill AG. Circuitry and cannulation techniques. In: Gravlee GP, Davis RF, Kurusz M, Utley JR, editors. *Cardiopulmonary bypass: principles and practice*. 2nd ed. Philadelphia: Lippincott Williams & Wilkins; 2000, p. 69-97.
24. Benaroia M, Baker AJ, Mazer CD, Errett L. Effect of aortic cannula characteristics and blood velocity on transcranial Doppler-detected microemboli during cardiopulmonary bypass. *J Cardiothorac Vasc Anesth* 1998;**12**(3):266-9.
25. Grossi EA, Kanchuger MS, Schwartz DS, et al. Effect of cannula length on aortic arch flow: protection of the atheromatous aortic arch. *Ann Thorac Surg* 1995;**59**:710-2.
26. Borger MA, Feindel CM. Cerebral emboli during cardiopulmonary bypass: effect of perfusionist interventions and aortic cannulas. *J Extra Corpor Technol* 2002;**34**(1):29-33.
27. Rosenberger P, Shernan SK, Loffler M, et al. The influence of epiaortic ultrasonography on intraoperative surgical management in 6051 cardiac surgical patients. *Ann Thorac Surg* 2008;**85**(2):548-53.
28. Bakhle YS. Pulmonary metabolism of bradykinin analogues and the contribution of angiotensin converting enzyme to bradykinin inactivation in isolated lungs. *Br J Pharmacol* 1977;**59**(1):123-8.
29. Mombouli JV, Vanhoutte PM. Endothelial dysfunction: from physiology to therapy. *J Mol Cell Cardiol* 1999;**31**(1):61-74.
30. Kamitani T, Little MH, Ellis EF. Evidence for a possible role of the brain kallikrein-kinin system in the modulation of the cerebral circulation. *Circ Res* 1985;**57**(4):545-52.
31. Kitaguchi H, Hijikata A, Hirata M. Effect of thrombin on plasminogen activator release from isolated perfused dog leg. *Thromb Res* 1979;**16**:407-15.
32. Ichinose A, Kisiel W, Fujikawa K. Proteolytic activation of tissue plasminogen activator by plasma and tissue enzymes. *FEBS Lett* 1984;**175**(2):412-8.
33. Campbell FW. The contribution of platelet dysfunction to postbypass bleeding. *J Cardiothorac Vasc Anaesth* 1991;**5**:8-12.
34. Lu H, Soria C, Cramer EM, et al. Temperature dependence of plasmin-induced activation or inhibition of human platelets. *Blood* 1991;**77**(5):996-1005.
35. van Deventer SJ, Hack CE, Wolbink CE, et al. Endotoxin-induced neutrophil activation: the role of complement revisited. *Prog Clin Biol Res* 1991;**367**:101-9.
36. Tengvall P, Askendal A, Lundstrom I. Temporal studies on the deposition of complement on human colostrum IgA and serum IgG immobilized on methylated silicon. *J Biomed Mater Res* 1997;**35**(1):81-92.
37. Chenoweth DE, Cooper SW, Hugli TE, Stewart RW, Blackstone EH, Kirklin JW. Complement activation during cardiopulmonary bypass: evidence for generation of C3a and C5a anaphylatoxins. *N Engl J Med* 1981;**304**(9):497-503.
38. Homeister JW, Satoh P, Lucchesi BR. Effects of complement activation in the isolated heart. Role of the terminal complement components. *Circ Res* 1992;**71**(2):303-19.
39. Moncada S, Higgs A. The L-arginine-nitric oxide pathway. *N Engl J Med* 1993;**329**(27):2002-12.
40. Matheis G, Sherman MP, Buckberg GD, Haybron DM, Young HH, Ignarro LJ. Role of L-arginine-nitric oxide pathway in myocardial reoxygenation injury. *Am J Physiol* 1992;**262**(2 Pt 2):H616-20.
41. Schindler R, Mancilla J, Endres S, Ghorbani R, Clark SC, Dinarello CA. Correlations and interactions in the production of interleukin-6 (IL- 6), IL-1, and tumor necrosis factor (TNF) in human blood mononuclear cells: IL-6 suppresses IL-1 and TNF. *Blood* 1990;**75**(1):40-7.
42. Steinberg JB, Kapelanski DP, Olson JD, Weiler JM. Cytokine and complement levels in patients undergoing cardiopulmonary bypass. *J Thorac Cardiovasc Surg* 1993;**106**(6):1008-16.
43. Pullicino EA, Carli F, Poole S, Rafferty B, Malik ST, Elia M. The relationship between the circulating concentrations of interleukin 6 (IL-6), tumor necrosis factor (TNF) and the acute phase response to elective surgery and accidental injury. *Lymphokine Res* 1990;**9**(2):231-8.
44. Hennein HA, Ebba H, Rodriguez JL, et al. Relationship of the proinflammatory cytokines to myocardial ischemia and dysfunction after uncomplicated coronary revascularization. *J Thorac Cardiovasc Surg* 1994;**108**(4):626-35.
45. Finkel MS, Oddis CV, Jacob TD, Watkins SC, Hattler BG, Simmons RL. Negative inotropic effects of cytokines on the heart mediated by nitric oxide. *Science* 1992;**257**(5068):387-9.
46. Jansen NJ, van Oeveren W, van den BL, et al. Inhibition by dexamethasone of the reperfusion phenomena in cardiopulmonary bypass [see Comments]. *J Thorac Cardiovasc Surg* 1991;**102**(4):515-25.
47. Kawamura T, Wakusawa R, Okada K, Inada S. Elevation of cytokines during open heart surgery with cardiopulmonary bypass: participation of interleukin 8 and 6 in reperfusion injury [see comments]. *Can J Anaesth* 1993;**40**(11):1016-21.
48. Mazer CD, Hornstein A, Freedman J. Platelet activation in warm and cold heart surgery. *Ann Thorac Surg* 1995;**59**:1481-6.
49. Gluszko P, Rucinski B, Musial J, et al. Fibrinogen receptors in platelet adhesion to surfaces of extracorporeal circuit. *Am J Physiol* 1987;**252**(3 Pt 2):H615-21.
50. Abrams CS, Ellison N, Budzynski AZ, Shattil SJ. Direct detection of activated platelets and platelet-derived microparticles in humans. *Blood* 1990;**75**:128-38.
51. Zilla P, Fasol R, Groscurth P, Klepetko W, Reichensperner H, Wolner E. Blood platelets in cardiopulmonary bypass operations. Recovery occurs after initial stimulation, rather than continual activation. *J Thorac Cardiovasc Surg* 1989;**97**(3):379-88.
52. Khuri SF, Wolfe JA, Josa M, et al. Hematologic changes during and after cardiopulmonary bypass and their relationship to the bleeding time and nonsurgical blood loss. *J Thorac Cardiovasc Surg* 1992;**104**:94-107.
53. McKenna R, Bachmann F, Whittaker B, Gilson JR, Weinberg M. The hemostatic mechanism after open-heart surgery. II. Frequency of abnormal platelet functions during and after extracorporeal circulation. *J Thorac Cardiovasc Surg* 1975;**70**:298-308.
54. Ferraris VA, Ferraris SP, Singh A, et al. The platelet thrombin receptor and postoperative bleeding. *Ann Thorac Surg* 1998;**65**:352-8.
55. Osborn L. Leukocyte adhesion to endothelium in inflammation. *Cell* 1990;**62**(1):3-6.
56. Johnson D, Thomson D, Hurst T, et al. Neutrophil-mediated acute lung injury after extracorporeal perfusion. *J Thorac Cardiovasc Surg* 1994;**107**(5):1193-202.
57. Rinder CS, Bonan JL, Rinder HM, Hines R, Smith BR. Cardiopulmonary bypass induces leukocyte-platelet adhesion. *Blood* 1992;**79**:1201-5.
58. Menasche P, Peynet J, Haeffner-Cavaillon N, et al. Influence of temperature on neutrophil trafficking during clinical cardiopulmonary bypass. *Circulation* 1995;**92**(Suppl. 9):II334-40.
59. Tabuchi N, de Haan J, Boonstra PW, van Oeveren W. Activation of fibrinolysis in the pericardial cavity during cardiopulmonary bypass. *J Thorac Cardiovasc Surg* 1993;**106**:828-33.
60. Weitz JI, Hudoba M, Massel D, Maraganore J, Hirsh J. Clot-bound thrombin is protected from inhibition by heparin-antithrombin III but is susceptible to inactivation by antithrombin III-independent inhibitors. *J Clin Invest* 1990;**86**:385-91.
61. Ernofsson M, Thelin S, Siegbahn A. Monocyte tissue factor expression, cell activation, and thrombin formation during cardiopulmonary bypass: a clinical study. *J Thorac Cardiovasc Surg* 1997;**113**:576-84.
62. Parratt R, Hunt BJ. Direct activation of factor X by monocytes occurs during cardiopulmonary bypass. *Br J Haemat* 1998;**101**:40-6.
63. de Haan J, Boonstra PW, Monnink SHJ, Ebels T, van Oeveren W. Retransfusion of suctioned blood during cardiopulmonary bypass impairs hemostasis. *Ann Thorac Surg* 1995;**59**:901-7.
64. Badellino KO, Walsh PN. Localization of a heparin binding site in the catalytic domain of factor XIa. *Biochem* 2001;**40**(25):7569-80.
65. Pixley RA, Schapira M, Colman RW. *Effect of heparin on the inactivation rate of human activated factor XII by antithrombin III*. *Blood* 1985;**66**(1):198-203.

66. Ofosu FA, Hirsh J, Esmon CT, et al. Unfractionated heparin inhibits thrombin-catalysed amplification reactions of coagulation more efficiently than those catalysed by factor Xa. *Biochem J* 1989;**257**(1):143-50.
67. de Swart CA, Nijmeyer B, Roelofs JM, Sixma JJ. Kinetics of intravenously administered heparin in normal humans. *Blood* 1982;**60**(6):1251-8.
68. Muriithi EW, Belcher PR, Day SP, Menys VC, Wheatley DJ. Heparin-induced platelet dysfunction and cardiopulmonary bypass. *Ann Thorac Surg* 2000;**69**(6):1827-32.
69. Khuri S, Valeri CR, Loscalzo J, et al. Heparin causes platelet dysfunction and induces fibrinolysis before cardiopulmonary bypass. *Ann Thorac Surg* 1995;**60**:1008-14.
70. Kelton JG, Sheridan D, Santos A, et al. Heparin-induced thrombocytopenia: laboratory studies. *Blood* 1988;**72**:925-30.
71. Warkentin TE, Hayward CP, Boshkov LK, et al. Sera from patients with heparin-induced thrombocytopenia generate platelet-derived microparticles with procoagulant activity: an explanation for the thrombotic complications of heparin-induced thrombocytopenia. *Blood* 1994;**84**(11):3691-9.
72. Warkentin TE, Kelton JG. Temporal aspects of heparin-induced thrombocytopenia. *N Engl J Med* 2001;**344**(17):1286-92.
73. Warkentin TE, Levine MN, Hirsh J, et al. Heparin-induced thrombocytopenia in patients treated with low-molecular-weight heparin or unfractionated heparin. *N Engl J Med* 1995;**332**(20):1330-5.
74. Warkentin TE, Kelton JG. Heparin-induced thrombocytopenia. *Prog Hemost Thromb* 1991;**10**:1-34.
75. Kappa JR, Fisher CA, Todd B, et al. Intraoperative management of patients with heparin-induced thrombocytopenia. *Ann Thorac Surg* 1990;**49**:714-22;discussion 723.
76. Altes A, Martino R, Gari M, et al. Heparin-induced thrombocytopenia and heart operation: management with Tedelparin. *Ann Thorac Surg* 1995;**59**:508-9.
77. Magnani HN. Heparin-induced thrombocytopenia (HIT): an overview of 230 patients treated with Orgaran (Org 10172). *Thromb Haemost* 1993;**70**(4):554-61.
78. Wilhelm MJ, Schmid C, Kececioglu D, Mollhoff T, Ostermann H, Scheld HH. Cardiopulmonary bypass in patients with heparin-induced thrombocytopenia using Org 10172. *Ann Thorac Surg* 1996;**61**:920-4.
79. Koster A, Kuppe H, Hetzer R, Sodian R, Crystal GJ, Mertzlufft F. Emergent cardiopulmonary bypass in five patients with heparin-induced thrombocytopenia type II employing recombinant hirudin. *Anesthesiology* 1998;**89**:777-80.
80. Rubens FD, Sabloff M, Wells PS, Bourke M. Use of recombinant-hirudin in pulmonary thromboendarterectomy. *Ann Thorac Surg* 2000;**69**(6):1942-3.
81. Potzsch B, Madlener K, Seelig C, Riess CF, Greinacher A, Muller-Berghaus G. Monitoring of r-hirudin anticoagulation during cardiopulmonary bypass: assessment of the whole blood ecarin clotting time. *Thromb Haemostas* 1997;**77**(5):920-5.
82. Dyke CM, Smedira NG, Koster A, et al. A comparison of bivalirudin to heparin with protamine reversal in patients undergoing cardiac surgery with cardiopulmonary bypass: the EVOLUTION-ON study. *J Thorac Cardiovasc Surg* 2006;**131**(3):533-9.
83. Warkentin TE, Greinacher A. Heparin-induced thrombocytopenia and cardiac surgery. *Ann Thorac Surg* 2003;**76**(2):638-48.
84. Furukawa K, Ohteki H, Hirahara K, Narita Y, Koga S. The use of argatroban as an anticoagulant for cardiopulmonary bypass in cardiac operations. *J Thorac Cardiovasc Surg* 2001;**122**(6):1255-6.
85. Morel DR, Zapol WM, Thomas SJ, et al. C5a and thromboxane generation associated with pulmonary vaso- and broncho-constriction during protamine reversal of heparin. *Anesthesiology* 1987;**66**(5):597-604.
86. Horrow JC. Protamine: a review of its toxicity. *Anesth Analg* 1985;**64**(3):348-61.
87. Dehmer GJ, Fisher M, Tate DA, Teo S, Bonnem EM. Reversal of heparin anticoagulation by recombinant platelet factor 4 in humans. *Circulation* 1995;**91**:2188-94.
88. Despotis GJ, Summerfield AL, Joist JH, et al. Comparison of activated coagulation time and whole blood heparin measurements with laboratory plasma anti-Xa heparin concentration in patients having cardiac operations. *J Thorac Cardiovasc Surg* 1994;**108**(6):1076-82.
89. Despotis GJ, Joist JH, Hogue CW, et al. More effective suppression of hemostatic system activation in patients undergoing cardiac surgery by heparin dosing based on heparin blood concentrations rather than ACT. *Thromb Haemost* 1996;**76**:902-8.
90. Hardy JF, Belisle S, Robitaille D, Perrault J, Roy M, Gagnon L. Measurement of heparin concentration in whole blood with the hepcon/HMS device does not agree with laboratory determination of plasma heparin concentration using a chromogenic substrate for activated factor X. *J Thorac Cardiovasc Surg* 1996;**112**:154-61.
91. Hill GE, Alonso A, Thiele GM, Robbins RA. Glucocorticoids blunt neutrophil CD11b surface glycoprotein upregulation during cardiopulmonary bypass in humans. *Anesth Analg* 1994;**79**(1):23-7.
92. van Overveld FJ, De Jongh RF, Jorens PG, Walter P, Bossaert L, De Backer WA. Pretreatment with methylprednisolone in coronary artery bypass grafting influences the levels of histamine and tryptase in serum but not in bronchoalveolar lavage fluid. *Clin Sci (Lond)* 1994;**86**(1):49-53.
93. Teoh KH, Bradley CA, Gauldie J, Burrows H. Steroid inhibition of cytokine-mediated vasodilation after warm heart surgery. *Circulation* 1995;**92**(Suppl. 9):II347-53.
94. Inaba H, Kochi A, Yorozu S. Suppression by methylprednisolone of augmented plasma endotoxin-like activity and interleukin-6 during cardiopulmonary bypass [see Comments]. *Br J Anaesth* 1994;**72**(3):348-50.
95. Jansen NJ, van Oeveren W, van Vliet M, Stoutenbeek CP, Eysman L, Wildevuur CR. The role of different types of corticosteroids on the inflammatory mediators in cardiopulmonary bypass. *Eur J Cardiothorac Surg* 1991;**5**(4):211-7.
96. Hill GE, Snider S, Galbraith TA, Forst S, Robbins RA. Glucocorticoid reduction of bronchial epithelial inflammation during cardiopulmonary bypass. *Am J Respir Crit Care Med* 1995;**152**(6 Pt 1):1791-5.
97. Yilmaz M, Ener S, Akalin H, Sagdic K, Serdar OA, Cengiz M. Effect of low-dose methyl prednisolone on serum cytokine levels following extracorporeal circulation. *Perfusion* 1999;**14**(3):201-6.
98. Whitlock RP, Chan S, Devereaux PJ, et al. Clinical benefit of steroid use in patients undergoing cardiopulmonary bypass: a meta-analysis of randomized trials. *Eur Heart J* 2008;**29**(21):2592-2600.
99. Kim KU, Kwon OJ, Jue DM. Pro-tumour necrosis factor cleavage enzyme in macrophage membrane/particulate. *Immunology* 1993;**80**:134-9.
100. Diego RP, Mihalakakos PJ, Hexum TD, Hill GE. Methylprednisolone and full-dose aprotinin reduce reperfusion injury after cardiopulmonary bypass. *J Cardiothorac Vasc Anesth* 1997;**11**(1):29-31.
101. Tassani P, Richter JA, Barankay A, et al. Does high-dose methylprednisolone in aprotinin-treated patients attenuate the systemic inflammatory response during coronary artery bypass grafting procedures? *J Cardiothorac Vasc Anesth* 1999;**13**(2):165-72.
102. Campbell EJ, O'Byrne V, Stratford PW, et al. Biocompatible surfaces using methacryloylphosphorylcholine laurylmethacrylate copolymer. *ASAIO J* 1994;**40**(3):M853-7.
103. De Somer F, Francois K, van Oeveren W, et al. Phosphorylcholine coating of extracorporeal circuits provides natural protection against blood activation by the material surface. *Eur J Cardiothorac Surg* 2000;**18**(5):602-6.
104. Gott VL, Whiffen JD, Dutton RC. Heparin bonding on colloidal graphite surfaces. *Science* 1963;**14**:1297-8.
105. Aldea GS, Doursounian M, O'Gara P, et al. Heparin-bonded circuits with a reduced anticoagulation protocol in primary CABG: a prospective, randomized study. *Ann Thorac Surg* 1996;**62**:410-18.
106. Mahoney CB. Heparin-bonded circuits: clinical outcomes and costs. *Perfusion* 1988;**13**:192-204.
107. te Velthuis H, Baufreton C, Jansen PGM, et al. Heparin coating of extracorporeal circuits inhibits contact activation during cardiac operations. *J Thorac Cardiovasc Surg* 1997;**114**:117-22.
108. Ranucci M, Mazzucco A, Pessotto R, et al. Heparin-coated circuits for high-risk patients: a multicenter, prospective, randomial trial. *Ann Thorac Surg* 1999;**67**:994-1000.
109. Baufreton C, Jansen PG, Le Besnerais P, et al. Heparin coating with aprotinin reduces blood activation during coronary artery operations. *Ann Thorac Surg* 1997;**63**(1):50-6.
110. Moen O, Høgåsen K, Fosse E, et al. Attenuation of changes in leukocyte surface markers and complement activation with heparin-coated cardiopulmonary bypass. *Ann Thorac Surg* 1997;**63**:105-11.
111. Steinberg BM, Grossi EA, Schwartz DS, et al. Heparin bonding of bypass circuits reduces cytokine release during cardiopulmonary bypass. *Ann Thorac Surg* 1995;**60**(3):525-9.
112. Barstad RM, Ovrum E, Ringdal M-AL, et al. Induction of monocyte tissue factor procoagulant activity during coronary artery bypass surgery is reduced with heparin-coated extracorporeal circuit. *Br J Haematol* 1996;**94**:517-25.
113. Wendel HP, Weber N, Ziemer G. Increased adsorption of high molecular weight kininogen to heparin-coated artificial surfaces and correlation to hemocompatibility. *Immunopharmacology* 1999;**43**(2-3):149-53.
114. Olson ST, Sheffer R, Francis AM. High molecular weight kininogen potentiates the heparin-accelerated inhibition of plasma kallikrein by antithrombin: role for antithrombin in the regulation of kallikrein. *Biochem* 1993;**32**(45):12136-47.
115. Ward RS, Riffle JS. Polysiloxane-polylactone block copolymers. U.S. patent 1987;**4663413**.

116. Rubens FD, Labow RS, Lavallee GR, et al. Hematologic evaluation of cardiopulmonary bypass circuits prepared with a novel block copolymer. *Ann Thorac Surg* 1999;**67**:689-98.
117. Defraigne JO, Pincemail J, Dekoster G, et al. SMA circuits reduce platelet consumption and platelet factor release during cardiac surgery. *Ann Thorac Surg* 2000;**70**(6):2075-81.
118. Suhara H, Sawa Y, Nishimura M, et al. Efficacy of a new coating material, PMEA, for cardiopulmonary bypass circuits in a porcine model. *Ann Thorac Surg* 2001;**71**(5):1603-8.
119. Fearon DT. Identification of the membrane glycoprotein that is the C3b receptor of the human erythrocyte, polymorphonuclear leukocyte. B lymphocyte, and monocyte. *J Exp Med* 1980;**152**(1):20-30.
120. Powell H, Castell LM, Parry-Billings M, Desborough JP, Hall GM, Newsholme EA. Growth hormone suppression and glutamine flux associated with cardiac surgery. *Clin Physiol* 1994;**14**(5):569-80.
121. Hashemi S, Palmer DS, Aye MT, Ganz PR. Molecular mechanisms of cellular responses to DDAVP. In: Mariani G, editor. Desmopressin in bleeding disorders. 1st ed. New York: Plenum Press; 1992, p. 43-56.
122. Kaul TK, Swaminathan R, Chatrath RR, Watson DA. Vasoactive pressure hormones during and after cardiopulmonary bypass. *Int J Artif Organs* 1990;**13**(5):293-9.
123. Argenziano M, Chen JM, Choudhri AF, et al. Management of vasodilatory shock after cardiac surgery: identification of predisposing factors and use of a novel pressor agent. *J Thorac Cardiovasc Surg* 1998;**116**(6):973-80.
124. Amado JA, Diago MC. Delayed ACTH response to human corticotropin releasing hormone during cardiopulmonary bypass under diazepam-high dose fentanyl anaesthesia. *Anaesthesia* 1994;**49**(4):300-3.
125. Raff H, Norton AJ, Flemma RJ, Findling JW. Inhibition of the adrenocorticotropin response to surgery in humans: interaction between dexamethasone and fentanyl. *J Clin Endocrinol Metab* 1987;**65**(2):295-8.
126. Thrush DN, Austin D, Burdash N. Cardiopulmonary bypass temperature does not affect postoperative euthyroid sick syndrome? *Chest* 1995;**108**(6):1541-5.
127. Wallach R, Karp RB, Reves JG, Oparil S, Smith LR, James TN. Pathogenesis of paroxysmal hypertension developing during and after coronary bypass surgery: a study of hemodynamic and humoral factors. *Am J Cardiol* 1980;**46**(4):559-65.
128. Kuntschen FR, Galletti PM, Hahn C. Glucose-insulin interactions during cardiopulmonary bypass: hypothermia versus normothermia. *J Thorac Cardiovasc Surg* 1986;**91**(3):451-9.
129. Weinstein GS, Zabetakis PM, Clavel A, et al. The renin-angiotensin system is not responsible for hypertension following coronary artery bypass grafting. *Ann Thorac Surg* 1987;**43**(1):74-7.
130. Roth-Isigkeit A, Dibbelt L, Eichler W, Schumacher J, Schmucker P. Blood levels of atrial natriuretic peptide, endothelin, cortisol and ACTH in patients undergoing coronary artery bypass grafting surgery with cardiopulmonary bypass. *J Endocrinol Invest* 2001;**24**(10):777-85.
131. Valen G, Kaszaki J, Nagy S, Vaage J. Open heart surgery increases the levels of histamine in arterial and coronary sinus blood. *Agents Actions* 1994;**41**(1-2):11-6.
132. Smith D, Gilbert M, Owen WG. Tissue plasminogen activator release in vivo in response to vasoactive agents. *Blood* 1985;**66**(4):835-9.
133. Man WK, Brannan JJ, Fessatidis I, Beckett J, Taylor KM. Effect of prostacyclin on the circulatory histamine during cardiopulmonary bypass. *Agents Actions* 1986;**18**(1-2):182-5.
134. Denizot Y, Feiss P, Nathan N. Are lipid mediators implicated in the production of pro- and anti- inflammatory cytokines during cardiopulmonary bypass graft with extracorporeal circulation? *Cytokine* 1999;**11**(4):301-4.
135. Ylikorkala O, Saarela E, Viinikka L. Increased prostacyclin and thromboxane production in man during cardiopulmonary bypass. *J Thorac Cardiovasc Surg* 1981;**82**(2):245-7.
136. Faymonville ME, Deby-Dupont G, Larbuisson R, et al. Prostaglandin E2, prostacyclin, and thromboxane changes during nonpulsatile cardiopulmonary bypass in humans. *J Thorac Cardiovasc Surg* 1986;**91**(6):858-66.
137. Hogue Jr CW, Barzilai B, Pieper KS, et al. Sex differences in neurological outcomes and mortality after cardiac surgery: a society of thoracic surgery national database report. *Circulation* 2001;**103**(17):2133-7.
138. Wolman RL, Nussmeier NA, Aggarwal A, et al. Cerebral injury after cardiac surgery: identification of a group at extraordinary risk. Multicenter Study of Perioperative Ischemia Research Group (McSPI) and the Ischemia Research Education Foundation (IREF) Investigators. *Stroke* 1999;**30**(3):514-22.
139. Roach GW, Kanchuger M, Mangano CM, et al. Adverse cerebral outcomes after coronary bypass surgery. *N Engl J Med* 1996;**335**:1857-63.
140. Van Dijk D, Keizer AM, Diephuis JC, Durand C, Vos LJ, Hijman R. Neurocognitive dysfunction after coronary artery bypass surgery: a systematic review. *J Thorac Cardiovasc Surg* 2000;**120**(4):632-9.
141. Newman M, Frasco P, Kern F, Greeley WJ, Blumenthal JA, Reves JG. Central nervous system dysfunction after cardiac surgery. *Adv Card Surg* 1992;**3**:243-84.
142. Robinson M, Blumenthal J, Burker EJ. Coronary artery bypass grafting and cognitive function: a review. *J Cardiopulm Rehab* 1990;**10**:180-9.
143. Borowicz LM, Goldsborough MA, Seines OA, McKhann GM. Neuropsychologic change after cardiac surgery: a critical review. *J Cardiothorac Vasc Anesth* 1996;**10**:105-12.
144. Sotaniemi KA, Mononen H, Hokkanan TE. Long-term cerebral outcome after open heart surgery. A five year neuropsychological follow up study. *Stroke* 1986;**17**(3):410-6.
145. Newman MF, Kirchner JL, Phillips-Bute B, et al. Longitudinal assessment of neurocognitive function after coronary-artery bypass surgery. *N Engl J Med* 2001;**344**:395-402.
146. Marasco SF, Sharwood LN, Abramson MJ. No improvement in neurocognitive outcomes after off-pump versus on-pump coronary revascularisation: a meta-analysis. *Eur J Cardiothorac Surg* 2008;**33**(6):961-70.
147. Selnes OA, Grega MA, Bailey MM, et al. Neurocognitive outcomes 3 years after coronary artery bypass graft surgery: a controlled study. *Ann Thorac Surg* 2007;**84**(6):1885-96.
148. Moody DM, Bell MA, Challa VR, Johnston WE, Prough DS. Brain microemboli during cardiac surgery or aortography. *Ann Neurol* 1990;**28**:477-86.
149. Brown WR, Moody DM, Challa VR, Stump DA, Hammon JW. Longer duration of cardiopulmonary bypass is associated with greater numbers of cerebral microemboli. *Stroke* 2000;**31**:707-13.
150. Blauth C, Kohner EM, Arnold J, Taylor KM. Retinal microembolism during cardiopulmonary bypass demonstrated by fluorescein angiography. *Lancet* 1986;**2**:837-9.
151. Harris DNF, Bailey SM, Smith PLC, Taylor KM, Oatridge A, Bydder GM. Brain swelling in first hour after coronary artery bypass surgery. *Lancet* 1993;**342**:586-7.
152. Brooker RF, Brown WR, Moody DM, et al. Cardiotomy suction: a major source of brain lipid emboli during cardiopulmonary bypass. *Ann Thorac Surg* 1998;**65**:1651-5.
153. Rubens FD, Boodhwani M, Mesana T, Wozny D, Wells G, Nathan HJ. The cardiotomy trial: a randomized, double-blind study to assess the effect of processing of shed blood during cardiopulmonary bypass on transfusion and neurocognitive function. *Circulation* 2007;**116**:I89-I97.
154. Djaiani G, Fedorko L, Borger MA, et al. Continuous-flow cell saver reduces cognitive decline in elderly patients after coronary bypass surgery. *Circulation* 2007;**116**(17):1888-95.
155. Rady MY, Ryan T, Starr NJ. Early onset of acute pulmonary dysfunction after cardiovascular surgery: risk factors and clinical outcome. *Crit Care Med* 1997;**25**(11):1831-9.
156. Messent M, Sullivan K, Keogh BF, Morgan CJ, Evans TW. Adult respiratory distress syndrome following cardiopulmonary bypass: incidence and prediction. *Anaesthesia* 1992;**47**(3):267-8.
157. Ng CS, Wan S, Yim AP, Arifi AA. Pulmonary dysfunction after cardiac surgery. *Chest* 2002;**121**(4):1269-77.
158. Loer SA, Kalweit G, Tarnow J. Effects of ventilation and nonventilation on pulmonary venous blood gases and markers of lung hypoxia in humans undergoing total cardiopulmonary bypass [see Comments]. *Crit Care Med* 2000;**28**(5):1336-40.
159. Kotani N, Hashimoto H, Sessler DI, et al. Cardiopulmonary bypass produces greater pulmonary than systemic proinflammatory cytokines. *Anesth Analg* 2000;**90**(5):1039-45.
160. Zimmerman GA, Amory DW. Transpulmonary polymorphonuclear leukocyte number after cardiopulmonary bypass. *Am Rev Respir Dis* 1982;**126**(6):1097-8.
161. Kotani N, Hashimoto H, Sessler DI, et al. Neutrophil number and interleukin-8 and elastase concentrations in bronchoalveolar lavage fluid correlate with decreased arterial oxygenation after cardiopulmonary bypass. *Anesth Analg* 2000;**90**:1046-51.
162. Carney DE, Lutz CJ, Picone AL, et al. Matrix metalloproteinase inhibitor prevents acute lung injury after cardiopulmonary bypass. *Circulation* 1999;**100**(4):400-6.
163. Cox CM, Ascione R, Cohen AM, Davies IM, Ryder IG, Angelini GD. Effect of cardiopulmonary bypass on pulmonary gas exchange: a prospective randomized study. *Ann Thorac Surg* 2000;**69**(1):140-5.
164. Chaney MA, Nikolov MP, Blakeman B, Bakhos M, Slogoff S. Pulmonary effects of methylprednisolone in patients undergoing coronary artery bypass grafting and early tracheal extubation. *Anesth Analg* 1998;**87**(1):27-33.
165. Palanzo DA, Manley NJ, Montesano RM, Yeisley GL, Gordon D. Clinical evaluation of the LeukoGuard (LG-6) arterial line filter for routine open-heart surgery. *Perfusion* 1993;**8**:489-96.
166. Richter JA, Meisner H, Tassani P, Barankay A, Dietrich W, Braun SL. Drew-Anderson technique attenuates systemic inflammatory response syndrome and improves respiratory function after coronary artery bypass grafting. *Ann Thorac Surg* 2000;**69**(1):77-83.

167. Mangano CM, Diamondstone LS, Ramsay JG, Aggarwal A, Herskowitz A, Mangano DT. Renal dysfunction after myocardial revascularization: risk factors, adverse outcomes, and hospital resource utilization. The Multicenter Study of Perioperative Ischemia Research Group. *Ann Intern Med* 1998;**128**(3):194-203.
168. Ascione R, Nason G, Al Ruzzeh S, Ko C, Ciulli F, Angelini GD. Coronary revascularization with or without cardiopulmonary bypass in patients with preoperative nondialysis-dependent renal insufficiency. *Ann Thorac Surg* 2001;**72**(6):2020-5.
169. Ascione R, Lloyd CT, Underwood MJ, Gomes WJ, Angelini GD. On-pump versus off-pump coronary revascularization: evaluation of renal function. *Ann Thorac Surg* 1999;**68**(2):493-8.
170. Loef BG, Epema AH, Navis G, Ebels T, van Oeveren W, Henning RH. Off-pump coronary revascularization attenuates transient renal damage compared with on-pump coronary revascularization. *Chest* 2002;**121**(4):1190-4.
171. Gormley SM, McBride WT, Armstrong MA, et al. Plasma and urinary cytokine homeostasis and renal dysfunction during cardiac surgery. *Anesthesiology* 2000;**93**(5):1210-6.
172. Tang AT, Alexiou C, Hsu J, Sheppard SV, Haw MP, Ohri SK. Leukodepletion reduces renal injury in coronary revascularization: a prospective randomized study. *Ann Thorac Surg* 2002;**74**(2):372-7.
173. Rigden SP, Dillon MJ, Kind PR, de Leval M, Stark J, Barratt TM. The beneficial effect of mannitol on postoperative renal function in children undergoing cardiopulmonary bypass surgery. *Clin Nephrol* 1984;**21**(3):148-51.
174. Woo EB, Tang AT, El Gamel A, et al. Dopamine therapy for patients at risk of renal dysfunction following cardiac surgery: science or fiction? *Eur J Cardiothorac Surg* 2002;**22**(1):106-11.
175. Halpenny M, Lakshmi S, O'Donnell A, O'Callaghan-Enright S, Shorten GD. Fenoldopam: renal and splanchnic effects in patients undergoing coronary artery bypass grafting. *Anaesthesia* 2001;**56**(10):953-60.
176. Bartels C, Gerdes A, Babin-Ebell J, et al. Cardiopulmonary bypass: evidence or experience based? *J Thorac Cardiovasc Surg* 2002;**124**(1):20-7.
177. Shann KG, Likosky DS, Murkin JM, et al. An evidence-based review of the practice of cardiopulmonary bypass in adults: a focus on neurologic injury, glycemic control, hemodilution, and the inflammatory response. *J Thorac Cardiovasc Surg* 2006;**132**(2):283-90.

CHAPTER 63
Myocardial Protection
Sidney Levitsky and James D. McCully

Historical Development
  Fibrillatory Arrest
  Continuous Coronary Perfusion
  Hypothermia
  Reintroduction of Cardioplegia
Biology of Surgically Induced Myocardial Ischemia
  Myocardial Oxygen Consumption
  Biochemical Alterations
  Ischemia-Reperfusion Injury
  Irreversible Cell Injury
  Inflammation

Effects of Age
  Cyanosis
  Ventricular Hypertrophy
Cardioplegia: Basic Principles
  Rapid Cardiac Arrest
  Hypothermia
  Buffering of the Cardioplegic Solution
  Avoidance of Myocardial Edema
Alternative Arresting Agents and Additives
  Beta-Blockers
  Agents Affecting Calcium Transport
  Metabolic Substrates

Crystalloid (Acellular) and Blood Cardioplegia
  Crystalloid Cardioplegia
  Blood Cardioplegia
    Methodologies
Potential New Technologies
  Ischemic Preconditioning
  Remote Preconditioning
  Postconditioning
  Sodium-Hydrogen Exchangers
  Molecular Manipulation

The heart... moves of itself and does not stop unless forever.
  Leonardo da Vinci (Dell'Anatomia, Foglia B)

Despite meticulous adherence to presently known principles of myocardial protection, perioperative myocardial damage related to ischemia-reperfusion injury continues to occur after cardiac operations that have been performed in a technically adequate manner. Ischemia-reperfusion injury associated with surgically induced myocardial ischemia secondary to aortic cross-clamping results from the attenuation or cessation of coronary blood flow such that oxygen delivery to the myocardium is insufficient to meet basal myocardial requirements to preserve cellular membrane stability and viability. Recovery after surgically induced ischemic arrest involves (1) resumption of normal oxidative metabolism and the restoration of myocardial energy reserves; (2) reversal of ischemia-induced cell swelling, loss of ion gradients, and adenine nucleotide losses; and (3) repair of damaged cell organelles such as mitochondria and the sarcoplasmic reticulum.

HISTORICAL DEVELOPMENT

After the initiation of open heart surgery with use of extracorporeal circulation by Gibbon,[1] it soon became obvious that aortic cross-clamping was necessary to provide a bloodless field to facilitate the precise repair of intracardiac defects, to prevent air embolism when the left side of the heart was opened, and to avoid a turgid myocardium resistant to retraction. To overcome the difficulties of operating on a rheumatic mitral valve in a patient with aortic regurgitation, Melrose and colleagues[2] introduced the concept of "elective cardiac arrest" by rapidly injecting into the aortic root, after aortic cross-clamping, a 2.5% potassium citrate solution in warm blood to arrest the heart. Soon thereafter, experimental and clinical evidence[3] demonstrated the development of severe myocardial necrosis associated with the Melrose technique.

During the 1960s, two distinct technical pathways for management of ischemic arrest evolved. The "rapid operators" performing uncomplicated cases with short ischemic times adopted the use of normothermic ischemic arrest, until operative mortalities from the "stone heart" syndrome related to ischemic contracture of the myocardium[4] associated with low levels of high-energy phosphate moieties became apparent.[5] Intermittent aortic cross-clamping, involving reperfusion of the coronary circulation for 5 minutes after 15 minutes of ischemic arrest, is an empiric technique, still in use, and was based on the concept that after 15 minutes of ischemia, a sufficient concentration of high-energy phosphate moieties remained in the myocardium to allow replenishment of myocardial stores during the reperfusion period.[6] Later studies demonstrated that there was no functional or metabolic advantage to intermittent reperfusion for normothermic ischemic periods up to 60 minutes.[7,8] Nevertheless, intermittent cross-clamping accompanied by ventricular fibrillation continues to be used for coronary artery bypass surgery with results comparable to those of cardioplegic techniques.[9]

Fibrillatory Arrest

Electrically induced ventricular fibrillation with coronary perfusion was introduced by Glenn and Sewell[10] and Senning[11] as a means of avoiding air embolism. However, Buckberg and Hottenrott[12] and Hottenrott and coworkers[13] demonstrated subendocardial ischemia and necrosis with this technique, particularly in the hypertrophied ventricle. Later studies showed that if ventricular distention is avoided and coronary perfusion is maintained, postischemic fibrillation is not deleterious in the nonhypertrophied heart.[14] Further validation of this technique, modified by mild hypothermia and the avoidance of aortic cross-clamping, has produced comparable clinical results for coronary revascularization.[15,16]

Continuous Coronary Perfusion

In an attempt to mimic the physiologic state, continuous coronary perfusion with a beating heart at normothermia or mild hypothermia at 32°C to prevent the onset of ventricular fibrillation became the preferred technique of myocardial preservation in the late 1960s and early 1970s, particularly after the report by McGoon and colleagues[17] of 100 consecutive aortic valve replacements without a mortality. If aortic valve regurgitation was present or aortic root surgery was performed, the heart was kept beating by perfusing the individual coronary arteries with cannulas inserted into the ostia. However, in reality, continuous perfusion became intermittent as coronary perfusion was often discontinued to achieve better visualization of the operative field during critical portions of the procedure.[18] In addition, problems with the coronary cannula, such as poor fixation, leaking associated with calcified ostia, early division of the left main coronary artery resulting in high perfusion pressure necrosis, and damage to the coronary artery such as dissection and late stenosis, continued to occur.[19,20] Nevertheless, the technique of continuous coronary artery perfusion, either during the performance of complex aortic root surgery or for special situations such as re-do mitral valve surgery through a right thoracotomy incision after previous coronary artery revascularization with arterial conduits, continues to be used.[21]

Hypothermia

The earliest attempts to perform open heart surgery before the advent of the heart-lung machine used systemic hypothermia produced by surface cooling not only to protect the heart but to protect the brain and other organs during circulatory arrest.[22,23] Hypothermia protects the ischemic myocardium by decreasing heart rate, slows the rate of high-energy phosphate degradation,[24] and decreases myocardial oxygen consumption (Fig. 63-1).[25,26] However, uniform cardiac hypothermia is difficult to achieve solely by the introduction of cold intracoronary perfusates, and systemic hypothermia is necessary, particularly in the presence of coronary obstruction, ventricular hypertrophy, rewarming of the right ventricle by the liver's acting as a "heat sink," and environmental rewarming.[27] In an attempt to overcome this problem, Shumway and associates[28] introduced the concept of profound local (topical) hypothermia by filling the pericardial sac with ice-cold saline.[29] Although this technique is still used as an adjunct to other methods of myocardial protection, it is rarely used as the sole protective method because of the problem of warm bronchial collateral flow reaching the heart cavity, resulting in transmyocardial temperature gradients and resultant ischemia.[30,31]

Reintroduction of Cardioplegia

While cardioplegia had been abandoned for alternative techniques in the United States after the adverse experience with the Melrose potassium solution, Bretschneider,[32] in Germany, continued studying induced cardiac arrest with use of a sodium-poor, calcium-free, procaine-containing solution (Bretschneider solution). Clinical application soon followed by Kirsch and asssociates[33] using a magnesium aspartate–procaine solution. Hearse and coworkers[34] introduced the concept of using an extracellular rather than an intracellular solution (St. Thomas' solution), which was first applied clinically by Braimbridge and coworkers.[18] On the basis of improved clinical outcomes, North American investigators[35-38] initiated experimental studies using potassium cardioplegia followed by clinical reports[39,40] demonstrating the efficacy of cardioplegia. During the next 3 decades, numerous investigators have continued their "quest for ideal myocardial protection."[41-44]

BIOLOGY OF SURGICALLY INDUCED MYOCARDIAL ISCHEMIA

Global ischemia is not an all-or-nothing phenomenon; rather, it is heterogeneous in that at any moment of time, myocardial cells will have varying extents of damage.[45,46] These changes affect cellular metabolism, ion transport, electrical activity, contractile function, vascular responsiveness, tissue ultrastructure, changes in nuclear and mitochondrial DNA, release of free radical oxygen species, and activation of inflammatory components.

Myocardial Oxygen Consumption

Because the heart is an obligate aerobic organ, it depends on a continuous supply of oxygen to maintain normal function. Myocardial oxygen reserve is exhausted within 8 seconds after the onset of normothermic global ischemia.[47] Myocardial oxygen consumption $M\dot{V}O_2$ is compartmentalized into the oxygen needed for external work of contraction (80% to 90%) and the unloaded contraction, such as basal metabolism, excitation-contraction coupling, and heat production.[48] A unique aspect of myocardial energetics is that 75% of the coronary arterial oxygen presented to the myocardium is extracted during a single passage through the heart; thus, depressed coronary venous oxygen content persists despite a wide range of cardiac workloads. Therefore, the heart is susceptible to the limitations of oxygen delivery, whereby an increase in $M\dot{V}O_2$ can be met only by augmentation of coronary blood flow. This is diametrically opposite to skeletal muscle, in which increased oxygen demand can initially be met by an increase in oxygen extraction. Clinically, a marked increase in coronary blood flow is observed at the beginning of the reperfusion period, after the aortic clamp is removed.

Biochemical Alterations

Under aerobic conditions, the heart derives its energy primarily from mitochondrial oxidative processes, using a variety of substrates such as glucose, free fatty acids, lactate, pyruvate,

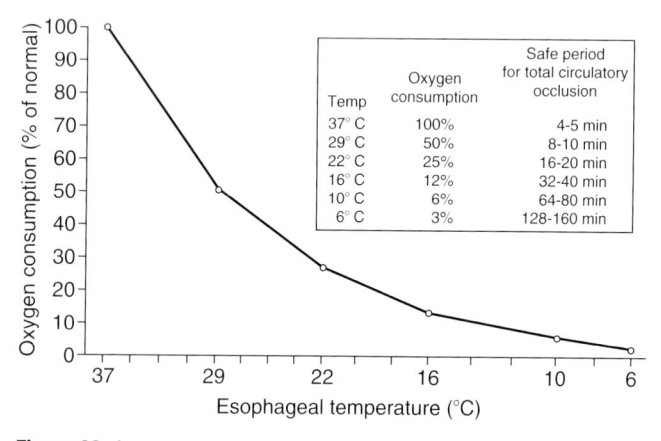

Figure 63-1
Relationship between body temperature and oxygen consumption in dogs cooled by means of an extracorporeal pump (mean value for 10 dogs). *(From Gordon AS, Meyer BW, Jones JC. Open heart surgery during deep hypothermia without an oxygenator[26].)*

Temp	Oxygen consumption	Safe period for total circulatory occlusion
37° C	100%	4-5 min
29° C	50%	8-10 min
22° C	25%	16-20 min
16° C	12%	32-40 min
10° C	6%	64-80 min
6° C	3%	128-160 min

acetate, ketone bodies, and amino acids.[49,50] However, oxidation of fatty acids provides the major source of energy production and is used in preference to carbohydrates. As tissue PO_2 falls, oxidative phosphorylation, electron transport, and mitochondrial adenosine triphosphate (ATP) production cease. Early in ischemia, the heart depends on the energy production of glycogenolysis and aerobic glycolysis (Pasteur effect). Reduced mitochondrial activity leads to the accumulation of glycolytic intermediaries, reduced NADH, and the reduction of pyruvate to lactate. The resultant severe intracellular acidosis impairs contractile function, enzyme transport, and cell membrane integrity. This results in a cellular loss of potassium and pathologic accumulation of sodium, calcium, and water (Fig. 63-2).[51]

Ischemia-Reperfusion Injury

Ischemia-reperfusion injury occurs as the result of attenuation or cessation of coronary blood flow such that oxygen delivery to the myocardium is insufficient to meet basal myocardial oxygen requirements to preserve cellular membrane stability and viability. The initiation of myocardial injury requires an ischemic episode that, by itself, may induce reversible or irreversible cellular injury.[52]

Reversible ischemia-reperfusion injury may be manifested as either stunning or hibernation. Stunning "describes the mechanical dysfunction that persists after reperfusion despite the absence of myocellular damage and despite the return of normal or near-normal perfusion."[53,54] A second form of reversible ischemia-reperfusion injury is hibernation, which is a syndrome of reversible, chronically reduced contractile function as a result of one or more recurrent episodes of acute or persistent ischemia, referred to as chronic stunning.

As in stunning, hibernating myocardium is viable but not functional and is reversible with coronary revascularization.[55,56] There is good clinical evidence that despite seemingly adequate application of modern methods of myocardial protection, all patients undergoing cardiac surgery have varying degrees of myocardial stunning.[57,58] Evidence to support this concept is based on the requirement of inotropic support for separation from bypass for hours or days after surgery in some patients who are eventually weaned from these drugs as the stunning abates, without objective evidence of a myocardial infarction.[59]

Two major theories have been proposed as possible mechanisms leading to ischemia-reperfusion injury (Fig. 63-3).

The calcium hypothesis suggests that the inability of the myocyte to modulate intracellular and intraorganellar calcium homeostasis induces a cascade of events culminating in cell injury and death (Fig. 63-4). Ischemia leads to the induction of metabolic acidosis and the activation of the sodium-proton exchanger, resulting in the transport of hydrogen ions to the extracellular space and the movement of sodium into the cytosol. As the sodium-calcium exchanger is activated, sodium is transported to the extracellular space and calcium is taken up into the cytosol, increasing cytosolic calcium concentration ($[Ca^{2+}]_i$). Increased $[Ca^{2+}]_i$ accumulation is also augmented by ischemia-induced depolarization of the membrane potential, which allows the opening of the L-type calcium channels and further calcium entry into the myocyte. Cellular and cytosolic calcium-dependent phospholipases and proteases are in turn activated, inducing membrane injury and the further entry of calcium into the cell. These processes

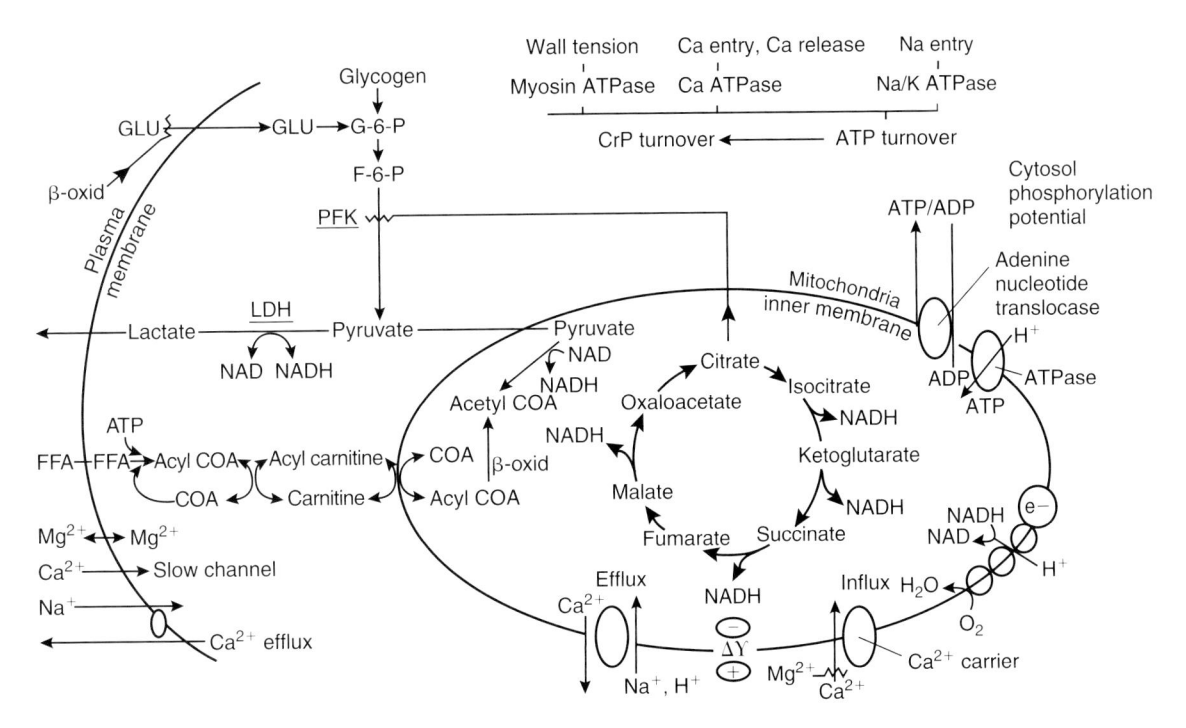

Figure 63–2
The biochemical anatomy of the normal functioning myocardial cell. The three main reactions using ATP are (1) myosin ATPase involved in the development of wall tension, (2) Ca^{2+}/Mg^{2+}-ATPase involved in sequestration of Ca^{2+} that enters the cell with each beat and as well as the Ca^{2+} that is liberated from sarcoplasmic reticulum in the activation of contractile protein, and (3) Na^+/K^+-ATPase involved in Na^+ efflux. The action of this vectorial ATPase establishes the monovalent cation gradient across the membrane that is used to maintain cell excitability and the efflux of Ca^{2+}. (From Feinberg H, Levitsky S. Biochemical rationale of cardioplegia. In: Engelman RM, Levitsky S, editors. A textbook of clinical cardioplegia. New York: Futura; 1982, p. 131-139.)

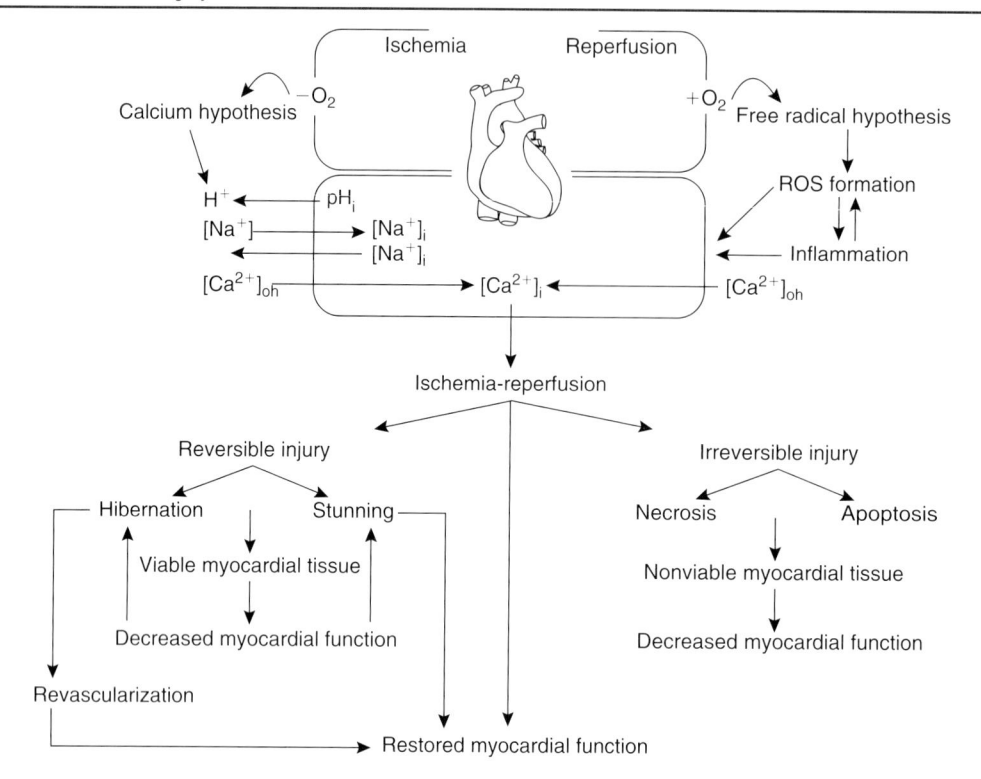

Figure 63–3
Mechanisms of ischemia-reperfusion injury. Putative mechanisms of the calcium and free radical hypotheses and inflammation in the generation of ischemia-reperfusion injury. ROS, reactive oxygen species.

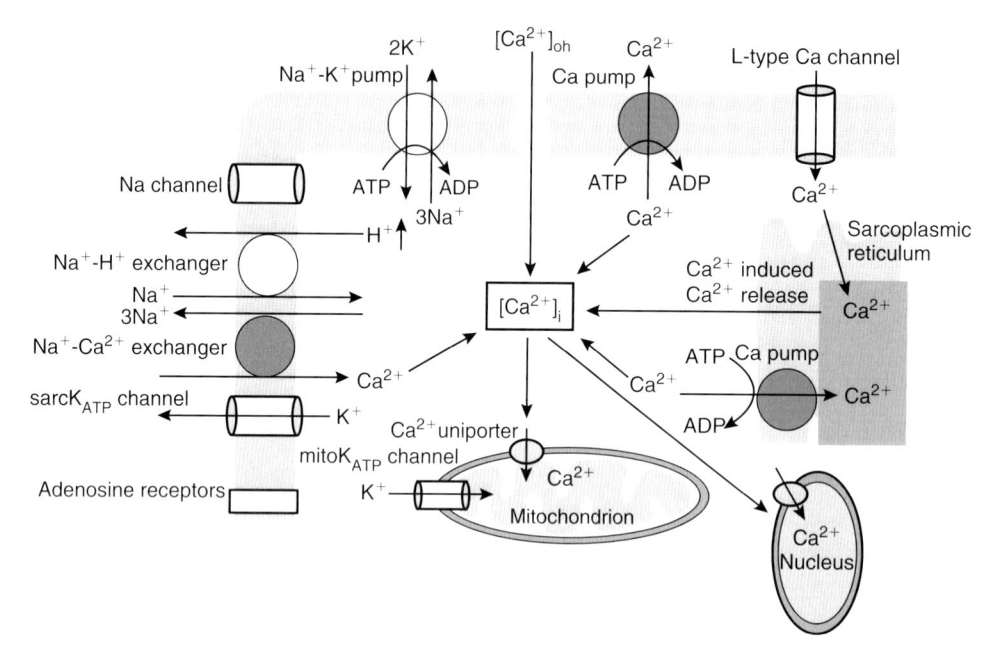

Figure 63–4
Sources of calcium regulation. The inability of the myocyte to modulate intracellular and intraorganellar calcium homeostasis during ischemia and during early reperfusion is the basis of the calcium hypothesis for ischemia-reperfusion injury. Increased intracellular calcium ($[Ca^{2+}]_i$) induces a cascade of events culminating in increased mitochondrial and nuclear calcium accumulation and cell injury and death.

alter myocardial cellular homeostasis, leading to cellular dysfunction or, if they are of sufficient duration or intensity, cell injury or death. Alternative explanations include the concept of reperfusion-induced myocardial contracture resulting from rapid re-energization of contractile cells with persistent calcium overload affecting myofibrillar calcium sensitivity.[60]

The free radical hypothesis suggests that the accumulation of partially reduced molecular oxygen collectively known as reactive oxygen species during the early stages of reperfusion causes myocardial cellular damage and cell death through microsomal peroxidation of the cellular phospholipid layer, leading to loss of cellular integrity and function (Fig. 63-5).[61]

Figure 63–5
Sources of reactive oxygen species generation. The free radical hypothesis suggests that accumulation of partially reduced molecular oxygen collectively known as reactive oxygen species (ROS) during the early stages of reperfusion causes myocardial cellular damage and cell death. Reactive oxygen species are formed by the acquisition of a single electron, making them highly reactive and cytotoxic. The major reactive oxygen species in order of production are superoxide ($^{\bullet}OH^-$), hydrogen peroxide (H_2O_2), hydroxy radical ($^{\bullet}OH$), and lipid peroxides. Reactive oxygen species formation has been shown to cause myocellular injury through microsomal peroxidation of the cellular phospholipid layer, leading to loss of cellular integrity and function.

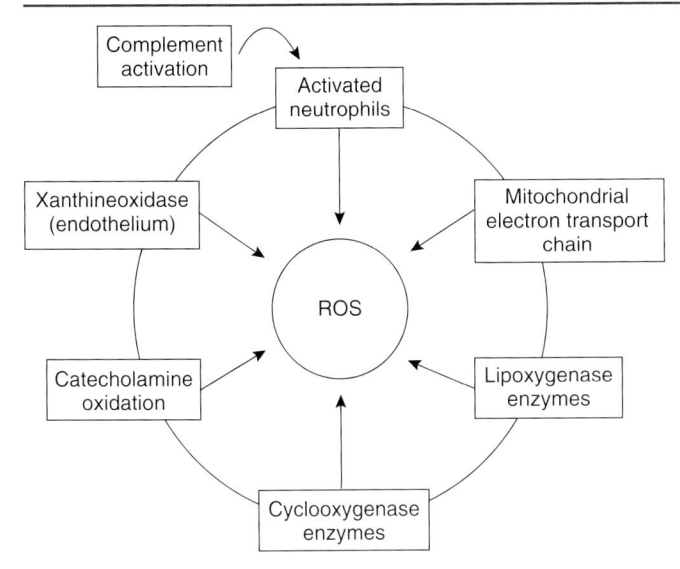

The generation of reactive oxygen species is believed to be mediated by xanthine oxidase, activation of neutrophils, or dysfunction of the mitochondrial electron transport chain. It has been suggested that the generation of reactive oxygen species may induce cellular membrane damage, thus facilitating calcium entry and the induction of cellular death. This hypothesis unifies both prevailing theories and is currently considered to be valid. However, therapeutic attempts to control calcium and reactive oxygen species overload have not yielded meaningful advantage.

Alternative explanations include the concept of lethal reperfusion injury, defined as death of myocardial cells that were viable immediately before reperfusion.[62] In an excellent review by Yellon and Hausenloy,[63] alternative cardioprotective strategies are suggested to manage this injury by reperfusion injury salvage kinase pathways and targeting mitochondrial permeability transition pores to avoid mitochondrial calcium overload. Cyclosporine, a potent inhibitor of mitochondrial permeability transition pores, has recently been shown to limit infarct size after percutaneous coronary intervention during acute myocardial infarction.[64]

Irreversible Cell Injury

Irreversible cell injury, described ultrastructurally by Schaper and coworkers,[46] occurs by two morphologically distinct pathways, necrosis and apoptosis. Necrosis is initiated by noncellular mechanisms with cell swelling, depletion of ATP stores, and disruption of the cellular membrane involving fluid and electrolyte alterations.[65] In contrast, apoptosis or programmed cell death[66] is an evolution-based mode of cell death characterized by a discrete set of biochemical and morphologic events involving the regulated action of catabolic enzymes (proteases and nucleases) that results in the ordered disassembly of the cell, distinct from cell death provoked by external injury.[67]

Inflammation

Inflammation has been implicated as a secondary mechanism contributing to injury after reperfusion. It is initiated through complement activation leading to the sequential formation of a membrane attack complex, which creates a cellular lesion and eventual cell lysis.[68] In addition, cytokines, vasoactive and chemotactic agents, adhesive molecule expression, and leukocyte and platelet activation participate in the inflammatory process, producing cytotoxic molecules that facilitate cell death.[69,70] Oxygen-derived free radical scavengers have also been used to limit reperfusion injury.[71] Tissue factor, an inflammatory and procoagulant mediator, initiates the extrinsic coagulation cascade, resulting in thrombin generation and fibrin deposition, and may be related to the no-reflow phenomenon.[72] Clinical applicability of anti-inflammatory agents awaits well-designed clinical trials because studies up until now have not shown any "meaningful cardioprotective effect."[63,73] Endothelium-dependent microvascular responses and coronary artery spasm may be related to reduced myocardial perfusion after reperfusion.[74]

Effects of Age

The vulnerability of the heart to ischemia-reperfusion injury is altered with temporal development. The newborn heart is more resistant to the effects of ischemia-reperfusion, which may be related to developmental differences in calcium transport and sequestration, and it is better able to restore myocardial function and myocardial high-energy phosphate stores after an ischemic event.[75-77] In the adult heart, functional recovery is significantly delayed, and the recovery of high-energy phosphate stores is slower in returning to preischemic levels.[78] As the heart ages, there are anatomic, mechanical, ultrastructural, and biochemical alterations that compromise the adaptive response of the heart.[79] As a result, the senescent myocardium is less tolerant than the mature myocardium to surgically induced ischemia.[80] The susceptibility of the aged myocardium to ischemia-induced injury is evident at many levels. Morphologically, with age, left ventricular mass is increased, as is a reduction in the size of the left ventricular cavity, accompanied by increased calcification of the valve anulus and coronary arteries.[81] Ultrastructurally, there is decreased mitochondria to myofibril ratio, cardiac myocyte enlargement, and loss of mitochondrial organization as well as alteration in myocardial contractile properties.[82] As a consequence of these changes, cardiac surgical operative mortality increases with age.[83]

Cyanosis

Cyanosis significantly increases the vulnerability of the myocardium to ischemia-reperfusion injury.[84,85] However, cyanotic myocardial cells exhibit normal metabolism when they are provided with adequate oxygen and substrate.[86] Mortality rates in patients undergoing elective repair for tetralogy

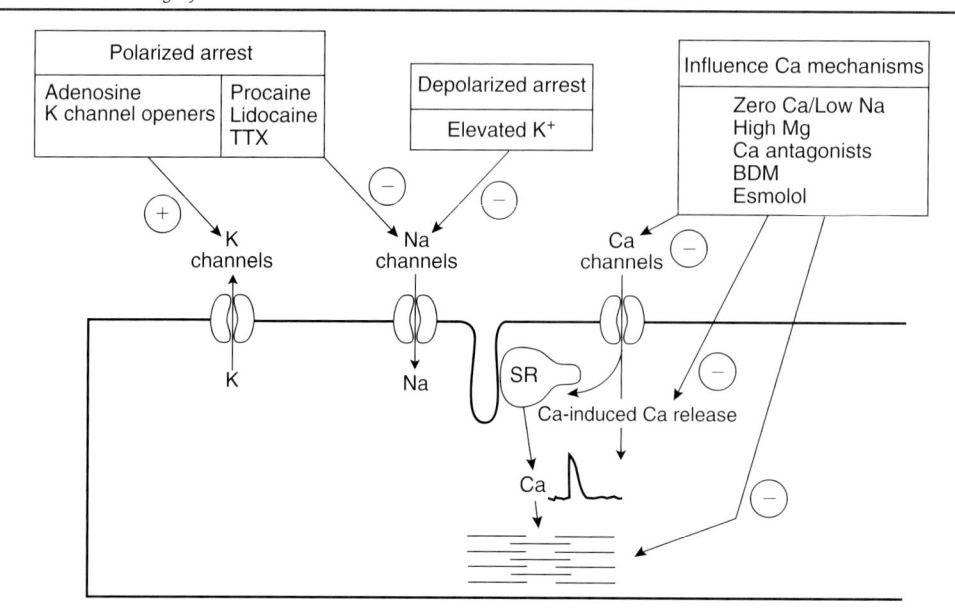

Figure 63–6
Excitation-contraction coupling in depolarized and polarized arrest. Excitation-contraction coupling and the targets within this pathway that are inhibited or activated by agents that induce depolarized arrest, polarized arrest, or arrest by influencing calcium mechanisms. BDM, 2,3-butanedione monoxime; SR, sarcoplasmic reticulum; TTX, tetrodotoxin. *(From Chambers DJ. Mechanisms and alternative methods of achieving cardiac arrest[98].)*

of Fallot are related to the method of myocardial protection as well as to the patient's age, duration and extent of cyanosis, and extent of hypertrophy.[87]

Ventricular Hypertrophy

Increased myocardial mass is an adaptive response to prolonged increases in myocardial workload due to pressure or volume overload. If it is untreated, progressive ventricular hypertrophy results in ventricular dilation and contractile dysfunction.[88] Hypertrophied hearts have an increased vulnerability to ischemic injury, which has been attributed to accelerated loss of high-energy phosphate moieties,[89] increased accumulation of lactate and hydrogen ions, earlier onset of ischemic contracture, and accelerated calcium overload after reperfusion.[78,90,91] With ventricular hypertrophy, epicardial coronary arteries dilate in response to increased oxygen demands, while there is a decreased capillary density and vascular dilation reserve in the subendocardial regions resulting in increased ischemic vulnerability.[92] Subendocardial ischemia leading to necrosis can occur during periods of hypotension, inadequate cardiopulmonary bypass, and ventricular fibrillation.[93] The hypertrophied heart is particularly susceptible to ischemic injury in the early postoperative period, when hypotension associated with surgically induced myocardial stunning, hypothermia, and vasoconstrictor agents are present.

CARDIOPLEGIA: BASIC PRINCIPLES

A rational approach for protecting the heart during surgically induced ischemia not only must focus on the requirements for sustaining the ischemic cell but also must be compatible with the technical aspects of the operative procedure. Operative procedures require a flaccid arrested heart, a bloodless operative field, and sufficient time for the satisfactory repair of complex cardiac defects. Moreover, the ability of the heart to assume normal electromechanical function adequate to support the systemic circulation must rapidly follow the ischemic interval. The need for inotropic support or mechanical support devices (e.g., intra-aortic balloon assist device, ventricular assist device) to wean the patient from cardiopulmonary bypass when support was not required preoperatively represents a failure of myocardial protection. Studies demonstrate that dopamine treatment of postischemic myocardial stunning induces apoptosis.[94] Nevertheless, despite meticulous adherence to known principles of protection, these events not infrequently and randomly occur and represent the limitations of present knowledge. Most investigators agree that the basic principles for adequate myocardial protection include (1) rapid induction of arrest, (2) mild or moderate hypothermia, (3) appropriate buffering of the cardioplegic solution, (4) avoidance of substrate depletion, and (5) attention to intracellular edema.[95-97]

Rapid Cardiac Arrest

Rapid cardiac arrest remains the mainstay of adequate myocardial protection and is "achieved by targeting various points in the excitation-contraction coupling pathway" (Fig. 63-6).[98] The induction of immediate cardiac arrest after the aorta has been clamped minimizes the depletion of high-energy phosphate moieties by useless mechanical work (Table 63-1). Potassium is the most common agent used for chemical cardioplegia and produces rapid diastolic arrest (Fig. 63-7). As the extracellular potassium concentration increases, the resting myocardial cell membrane becomes depolarized; the voltage-dependent fast sodium channel is inactivated, arresting the heart in diastole; and the slow calcium channel is activated, resulting in cytosolic calcium overload.[99,100] The optimum concentration of potassium is thought to vary between 15 and 40 mmol/L,[101] although it has been suggested that concentrations exceeding 20 mmol/L promote calcium overload and subsequent injury.[102] Because

Table 63-1
Cardioplegia Solutions in Common Use

		Buckberg			Depolarizing Cardioplegia Formulas						St. Thomas'	
	Adenosine	Induction	Maintenance	Reperfusion	Bretschneider HTK	CHB	DSA	GIK	St. Thomas' I	I Blood	St. Thomas' II
K+ (mmol/L)	16	16-20	8-10		9	5	12	80-100	20	20	16
NaCl (mmol/L)					15						
Mg2+ (mmol/L)	16			10	4	40	0.8		16	16	16
Na2+ (mmol/L)	117								144	142	117
Ca2+ (mmol/L)	1.2								2.2	1.7	1.2
HCO3− (mmol/L)	25					0.4				30-40	25
Citrate-phosphate-dextrose (mL)		225	50	50							
THAM (mmol/L)							2				
Tromethamine (300 mmol/L) (mL)		225	200	50							
Adenosine (mmol/L)	0.5						2.7				
Dextrose (50% in water) (mL)		40									
Dextrose (5% in water) (mL)		200	550								
Dextrose (5% in water; 1:isotonic saline) (mL)				1000							
Glucose (mmol/L)								30-50			
Mannitol (25%) (mL)				50							
Insulin (IU/L)								25-70			
Procaine (mmol/L)	1								1	1	1
Lidocaine (%)						0.8					

(Continued)

Table 63-1
Cardioplegia Solutions in Common Use—cont'd

		Buckberg			Depolarizing Cardioplegia Formulas						
	Adenosine	Induction	Maintenance	Reperfusion	Bretschneider HTK	CHB	DSA	GIK	St. Thomas' I	St. Thomas' I Blood	St. Thomas' II
Histadine (mmol/L)					180						
His-HCl (mmol/L)					18						
Tryptophan (mmol/L)					2						
∝-Ketoglutarate (mmol/L)					1						
L-Aspartate (mmol/L)		13									
L-Glutamate (mmol/L)		13									
Hematocrit (%)	10-12	20	20	20	10-12		10-12		0	10-12	10-12
pH	5.5-7.0	7.5-7.7	7.6-7.8	7.5-7.6	7.4		7.4		5.5-7.0	7.4	5.5-7.0
mOsm/L	294	380-400	340-360	340-360	310		310		300-320	310-330	294
Blood: crystalloid	4:1	4:1	4:1	4:1	4:1	1:4	4:1			4:1	4:1
Infusion interval			15 min								
Infusion rate (mL/kg/hr)								0.75-1.5			
Volume (mL)											

CHB, Children's Hospital, Boston; *DSA*, Deaconess Surgical Association; *GIK*, glucose-insulin-potassium.

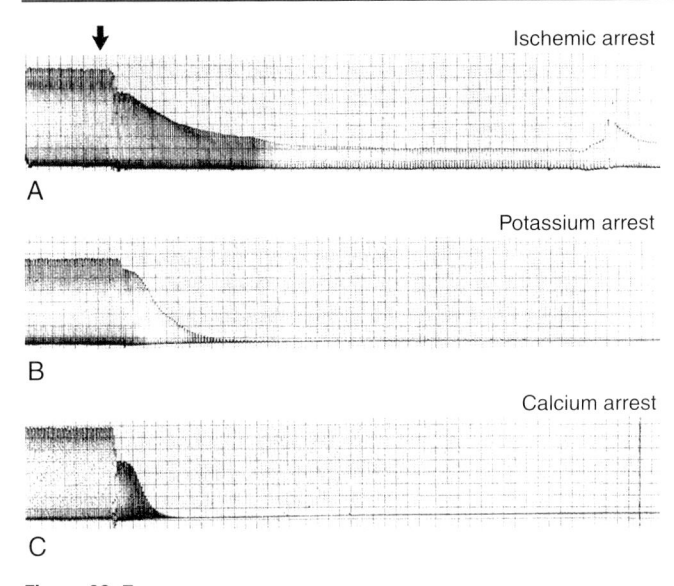

Figure 63-7
The induction of cardiac arrest: **A,** by unmodified ischemia; **B,** by potassium cardioplegia; **C,** by calcium depletion. *(From Hearse DJ, O'Brien K, Braimbridge MV. Protection of the myocardium during ischemic arrest. Dose-response curves for procaine and lignocaine in cardioplegic solutions[105].)*

the heart will remain arrested until the concentration of extracellular potassium or other cardioplegic ingredient is decreased by noncoronary collateral mediastinal blood flow, re-infusions of cardioplegia are necessary every 15 to 30 minutes.[103] Clinical studies indicate that despite the infusion of large volumes of hyperkalemic cardioplegic solution for complex procedures requiring prolonged ischemic times, serum potassium levels in patients with normal renal function rarely exceed 5.5 mEq/L, as increased urinary excretion of potassium rapidly compensates for the endogenous administration of potassium.[104]

Agents inducing polarized arrest, in which the cell membrane potential remains close to resting potential, have significant advantages by limiting ionic movement and thereby reducing myocardial energy use.[98] Sodium channel blockade, which arrests the heart by preventing the rapid sodium-induced depolarization of the action potential, includes procaine[105] and tetrodotoxin.[106] This class of drugs has been used successfully experimentally but is rarely used clinically at present. Potassium channel openers induce arrest by membrane hyperpolarization, couple the membrane potential to the cellular metabolic status, and afford cardioprotection by a similar mechanism associated with ischemic preconditioning.[107] Two potassium–adenosine triphosphate (K_{ATP}) channel subtypes have been shown to coexist in the myocardium; one subtype is located in the sarcolemma (sarcK_{ATP}) membrane and the other in the inner membrane of the mitochondria (mitoK_{ATP}), and they can be pharmacologically manipulated by openers and blockers.[96] Potassium channel openers have been used in conjunction with hyperkalemic and magnesium-containing cardioplegic solutions, although their clinical use remains controversial.[108,109] However, mitochondria-specific potassium channel openers, such as diazoxide, have been demonstrated to have potential benefits when they are used with magnesium-supplemented potassium cardioplegia.[110,111]

Adenosine is an endogenous nucleoside formed as a consequence of the breakdown of high-energy phosphate and is rapidly phosphorylated by adenosine kinase to adenosine monophosphate and incorporated into the high-energy phosphorus pool or deaminated by adenosine deaminase, present in erythrocytes, to inosine, which is transported from the cell.[112] Extracellular adenosine is cleared through cellular uptake, primarily by erythrocytes and vascular endothelial cells, and has a reported half-life of less than 10 seconds in whole blood, which limits its use during a prolonged period of surgically induced ischemia.[113] Adenosine induces hyperpolarized cardiac arrest by antagonizing calcium channels and has been shown to inhibit both the sinoatrial and the atrioventricular nodes and atrial myocardial contraction.[114] Adenosine, by its ability to antagonize the direct depressant effects on both the sinoatrial and atrioventricular nodes and atrial tissue, results in sinus slowing and arrest. Clinically, adenosine has been used as a pretreatment before the initiation of cardiopulmonary bypass, when it has been shown to increase postoperative cardiac index and to reduce creatine kinase release[115]; as an arresting agent by bolus infusion[116]; and as an additive to potassium cardioplegia, when it reduces the time to arrest[117] and reduces potassium-induced cytosolic calcium overload.[118] It may also improve functional recovery when it is infused during the reperfusion period.[119] Compared with the acellular St. Thomas cardioplegic solution, the addition of adenosine appeared to enhance postoperative cardiac function in a series of patients undergoing coronary revascularization.[120] Phase II studies suggest that adenosine may reduce postoperative complications,[121] although the results are open to question.[122] Nevertheless, additional clinical trials are suggested.[123]

Hypothermia

Hypothermia, whether it is mild (tepid at the room temperature range of 28°C to 32°C) or moderate (22°C to 25°C), continues to remain an indispensable adjunct for adequate myocardial protection. As noted in the Historical Development section, hypothermia decreases the rate of the metabolic degradation of energy stores during surgically induced ischemia. In addition, there is experimental evidence that there is a significant decrease of left ventricular myocardial oxygen consumption of the heart in the beating nonworking, fibrillating, and arrested states at 22°C compared with a myocardial temperature of 37°C (Fig. 63-8).[124] However, there is minimal advantage in reducing the myocardial temperature below 22°C in that the myocardial oxygen consumption is decreased by only a minimal amount, from 0.31 mL at 22°C to 0.27 mL at 15°C per 100 g of left ventricular tissue per minute.[125] Moreover, in the clinical setting, it is virtually impossible to maintain a uniform myocardial temperature below 22°C solely by the use of cold (4°C) intracoronary cardioplegia infusates accompanied by regional hypothermia, particularly in the presence of coronary obstructions, ventricular hypertrophy, and variations in mediastinal noncoronary collateral blood flow. In addition, the atrial and ventricular septa are warmed by systemic and pulmonary venous return, heat sinks such as the liver warm the base of the heart, and the anterior-situated right ventricle is warmed by the operative environment. Because of the lack of uniformity of myocardial temperatures in various myocardial segments, there is no correlation between myocardial tissue acidosis and temperature, leading to the recent abandonment by many surgeons of routine myocardial temperature monitoring during operative procedures.[126]

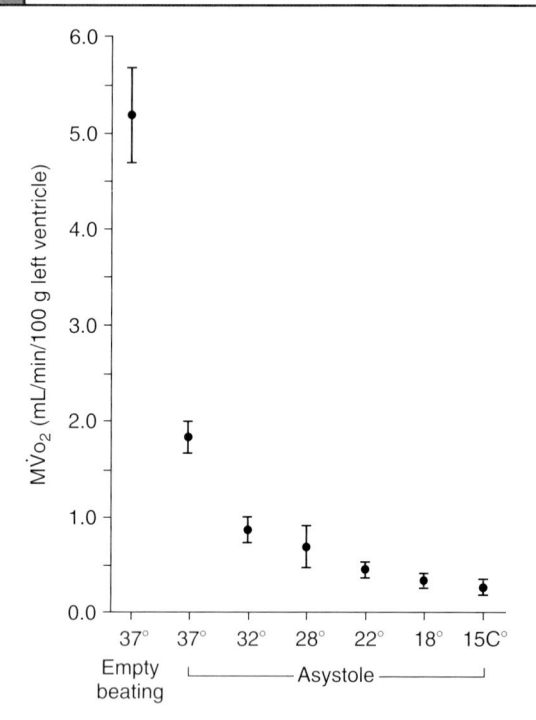

Figure 63–8
Effects of hypothermia on myocardial oxygen consumption in the potassium-arrested dog heart. *(From Chitwood WR, Sink JD, Hill RC, et al. The effects of hypothermia on myocardial oxygen consumption and transmural coronary blood flow in the potassium-arrested heart[25].)*

Buffering of the Cardioplegic Solution

Buffering of the cardioplegic solution is necessary to combat the unremitting intracellular acidosis associated with surgically induced myocardial ischemia. Because the myocardium has the highest oxygen use of any organ in the body related to its concentration of mitochondria, ischemia results in the rapid accumulation of hydrogen ions and the reduction of intracellular pH, which has been quantified by the measurement of tissue P_{CO_2} and hydrogen ion with phosphorus P 31 nuclear magnetic resonance spectroscopy in the laboratory and a pH probe in the operating room.[78,127] With the recent development of a myocardial tissue pH probe, there is clinical evidence that maintenance of the tissue pH of 6.8 or greater is associated with adequate myocardial protection (Fig. 63-9).[128] Thus, frequent infusions of cardioplegia, every 15 to 20 minutes, are necessary to prevent intracellular acidosis from reaching irreversible metabolic levels. In addition, hypothermia assists in the neutralization of acidosis because pH rises 0.0134 unit for each degree decrease in degree centigrade.[129] However, the infusion of hypothermic cardioplegia does not restore pH_i to prearrest levels but rather prevents further deterioration of the pH. When intermittent warm blood cardioplegia is used, lengthening of the ischemic period progressively increases intracellular metabolic acidosis and is probably associated with increased injury during repeated episodes of normothermic arrest.[130,131] Bicarbonate, phosphate, aminosulfonic acid, tris-hydroxymethylamino-methane

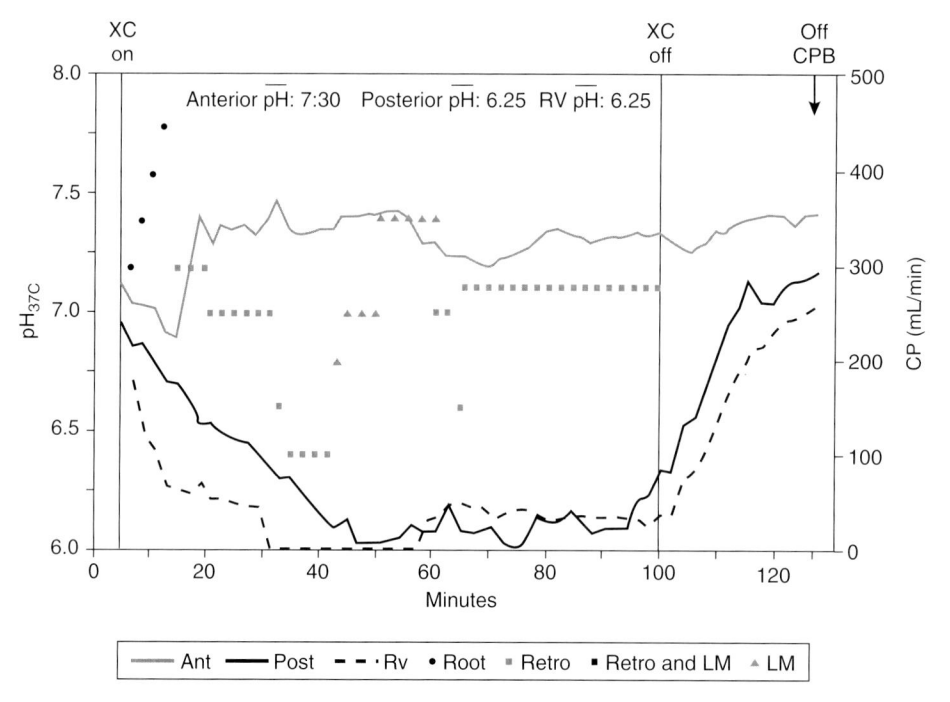

Figure 63–9
pH and myocardial protection. pH (37°C) tracing in the left ventricular wall in a 67-year-old man undergoing complex aortic valve replacement. Measurements were obtained from three sites: anterior left ventricular (LV) wall; posterior LV wall; and anterior right ventricular (RV) wall. pH_{37C} reached a low of 6.0 in the posterior LV wall and 5.8 in the RV wall. This marked discrepancy between anterior and posterior wall pH_{37C} occurred in the face of continuous delivery of blood cardioplegia at high rates, mostly through the coronary sinus. Delivery of cardioplegic solutions through the ostium of the left main alone, through the coronary sinus alone, or simultaneously through the left main and coronary sinus failed to reverse the fall in pH_{37C} in the posterior LV and anterior RV walls. Integrated mean pH_{37C} during the period of aortic clamping was 7.30 in the anterior LV wall, 6.2 in the posterior LV wall, and 6.05 in the anterior RV wall, indicating poor protection of the posterior LV wall and anterior RV wall. The patient had to be defibrillated three times and required significant inotropic support to be weaned from cardiopulmonary bypass (CPB). He continued to require inotropic support for 24 hours postoperatively. CP, cardioplegia; XC, cross-clamping. *(From Khuri SF, Josa M, Marston W, et al. First report of intramyocardial pH in man. II. Assessment of adequacy of myocardial preservation[128].)*

(THAM), and histidine buffers have all been used as cardioplegia additives to modulate pH.

Avoidance of Myocardial Edema

Avoidance of myocardial edema by controlling osmolarity is important to control volume regulation of the fluid compartments of the heart because myocardial edema is a known consequence of ischemia.[132] The extent of myocardial edema has been shown to be directly modulated by osmolarity and onconicity of cardioplegia, with decreases being directly associated with increased myocardial edema and impaired diastolic filling.[133] Hypotonic cardioplegic solutions cause myocardial edema[134]; hyperosmotic cardioplegia with an osmolarity in excess of 400 mOsm/L has been shown to cause myocardial dehydration.[135] Isotonic solutions in the range of 290 to 330 mOsm/L or slightly hyperosmolar solutions appear to have the greatest clinical use, which is of particular importance in dealing with acellular cardioplegic solutions.[40] Inert sugars including mannitol and sorbitol as well as metabolizable sugars such as glucose and dextrose have been used to increase osmolarity. However, when large volumes of continuous cardioplegia are administered, there is concern about producing hyperglycemia. Oncotic agents such as albumin and macromolecules, including dextrans and hydroxyethyl starches, have been used to prevent myocardial edema.[136] Besides cardioplegic infusions, the hemodilution from crystalloid priming of the extracorporeal circuit, the activation of humoral and cellular mediators that increase microvascular permeability, and the impairment of myocardial lymphatic function may play major roles in the development of myocardial edema. Myocardial lymphatic function is dependent on the beating heart to transport fluid and is significantly reduced or completely stopped during cardiac arrest. Experimental evidence has indicated that during normothermic continuous antegrade blood cardioplegia, myocardial lymph flow is reduced to less than 20% of that in the normal beating heart.[137]

ALTERNATIVE ARRESTING AGENTS AND ADDITIVES

Beta-Blockers

As the ascending aorta is clamped, there is the nonexocytotic release of norepinephrine from the cardiac sympathetic nerves acting on β-adrenergic receptors on the outer surface of the sarcolemma, causing an increase in cAMP-dependent protein kinase activity, phosphorylation of the calcium release channels, and increased Ca^{2+} influx, resulting in increased Ca^{2+}-dependent contractility and rapid depletion of glycogen stores.[138] Early studies suggested that long-acting beta-blockers improved myocardial protection during ischemia but unfortunately have a prolonged negative inotropic effect, which limits their clinical use.[139] For the most part, beta-blockers such as propranolol have been used as an adjunct to anesthesia to block β-adrenergic–stimulating episodes associated with coronary ischemia during the course of the operative procedure. Ultra-short-acting cardioselective beta-blockers such as landiolol and esmolol provide polarized cardiac arrest by maintaining the membrane potential at or near the resting membrane potential.[140] The cardioselectivity of these agents is 50 to 250 times that of propranolol, and the half-life of esmolol is only 9 minutes because it is rapidly hydrolyzed by red blood cell esterase.[141] Esmolol has been used to enhance myocardial protection during intermittent arrest[142] and has been shown to provide myocardial preservation equivalent to or better than cold crystalloid or blood cardioplegia.[143-145] With esmolol cardioplegia, there is a slow undulating ventricular contraction that may decrease myocardial edema but does not provide a quiescent operating field.

Agents Affecting Calcium Transport

The infusion of calcium-free cardioplegic solutions induces rapid diastolic cardiac arrest by inhibiting excitation-coupling and increases permeability of the sarcolemma.[146] When a calcium-containing perfusate is then re-infused, during reperfusion, there is a rapid influx of calcium into the cell, resulting in myocardial contracture and extensive ultrastructural damage, the "calcium paradox."[147,148] Nevertheless, hypocalcemic cardioplegic solutions have been used during hypothermic arrest to prevent ischemic contracture and necrosis.[149] Calcium antagonist agents administered before ischemia have been proposed as a possible mechanism to reduce ischemic cellular injury. Calcium channel blocking agents, including verapamil, diltiazem, and nifedipine, prevent calcium-induced calcium release in myocardial cells and as an adjunct to normothermic cardioplegia have been shown to improve postischemic systolic function.[150] Calcium blockers have no effect if they are administered before reperfusion, are temperature dependent, and have limited effect during hypothermia. Because high concentrations are required for cardioprotection, their prolonged membrane binding prevents rapid recovery, thus limiting their clinical usefulness.

Magnesium inhibits calcium entry into the cell by displacing calcium from its binding sites in the sarcolemmal membrane.[151] It has limited use as an arresting agent because high concentrations are required, cardiac arrest is delayed, and postischemic functional recovery is decreased in comparison to potassium cardioplegia.[2] The advantages of magnesium have been shown to be optimal when it is included with high-potassium cardioplegia, in which it has been demonstrated to ameliorate cytosolic, nuclear, and mitochondrial calcium accumulation and to preserve high-energy phosphate moieties and to enhance postischemic functional recovery.[152,153]

Metabolic Substrates

Metabolic substrates have been added to cardioplegic solutions to enhance anaerobic metabolism during ischemia or to provide citric acid cycle intermediaries to facilitate homeostasis during reperfusion. Agents used include glucose and insulin[154,155]; nucleosides,[156] such as adenosine,[157] aspartate, and glutamate[158]; and L-arginine to stimulate nitric oxide production.[159] Although metabolic substrate enhancement has been used in a variety of clinical situations, none has achieved universal adoption.

CRYSTALLOID (ACELLULAR) AND BLOOD CARDIOPLEGIA

Crystalloid Cardioplegia

With the advent of myocardial protection, asanguineous solutions composed of varying electrolyte compositions, but always featuring hyperkalemic diastolic arrest, were clinically

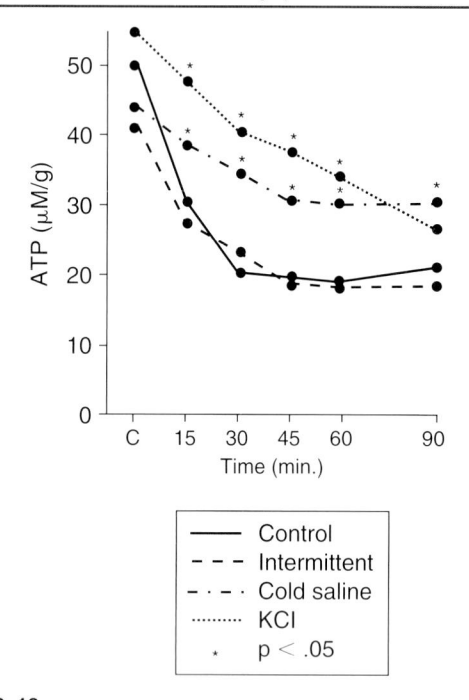

Figure 63-10
High-energy phosphates. Adenosine triphosphate (ATP) values during aortic cross-clamping (60 minutes) and reperfusion (30 minutes) for control (no treatment), intermittent reperfusion (15-minute cross-clamping and 5-minute reperfusion), regional hypothermia, and potassium cardioplegia. *(From Wright RN, Levitsky S, Rao KS, et al. Potassium cardioplegia: an alternative method of myocardial protection[38].)*

used in Europe[17,30,32] in the early 1970s and in the United States[38,39] in the late 1970s. However, these solutions contained minimal amounts (0.6 mL/100 mL at a P_{O_2} of 100 mm Hg at a temperature of 10°C) of dissolved oxygen, whereas the myocardium consumes 0.33 mL of oxygen per 100 g at 15°C. Because even a short period of ischemia results in the gradual accumulation of oxygen debt, moderate to severe myocardial hypothermia is necessary to prevent the rapid degradation of energy stores (Fig. 63-10).[38,160] To overcome the oxygen deficit issue, oxygenation of crystalloid cardioplegia has been clinically used and has demonstrated a decrease in creatine kinase MB levels in patients when the cross-clamping time exceeded 29 minutes compared with a group of patients who received unoxygenated cardioplegia.[161] Nevertheless, subsequent clinical studies with unoxygenated crystalloid documented significant decreases in operative mortality and perioperative myocardial infarction for coronary artery surgery, as demonstrated by the large Collaborative Study in Coronary Artery Surgery.[162] For the most part, most groups at that time, including our own, used Ringer's solution (sodium chloride, 147.3 mmol/L; potassium, 4.02 mmol/L; and calcium chloride, 2.25 mmol/L) to which was added 24 mmol/L of potassium chloride to effect a total dose of 28 mmol/L, 7 g/L of glucose, and 0.8 mL of THAM.[163] The resultant solution had an osmolarity of 375 mOsmol/L and a pH of 7.42 at 37°C. The classic St. Thomas' solution differed by having a lower concentration of potassium chloride, 19.59 mmol/L, and added 15.90 mmol/L of magnesium chloride and 1 mmol/L of procaine hydrochloride.[18]

Clinical steps for myocardial protection with use of crystalloid cardioplegia include the following.

1. Before the onset of surgery, the operating room temperature is cooled to 63°F to 65°F (17°C to 19°C) to avoid warming of the anterior surface of the heart by convection and radiation from high-intensity lighting.
2. Cardiopulmonary bypass is initiated at a temperature of 28°C. A cannula is placed in the ascending aorta proximal to the aortic root for the antegrade infusion of cardioplegic solution and for the removal of air after the clamp is removed from the ascending aorta and as the patient is weaned from bypass.
3. A myocardial electrocardiographic lead and temperature probe are placed on the anterior wall of the right ventricle because it constitutes two thirds of the anterior surface of the heart, and its rewarming during surgically induced ischemia may partially explain the occasional observation of selective right ventricular failure after the termination of bypass.[164] In addition, an insulation pad is placed in the posterior pericardial sac and along the left ventricular lateral wall to protect the left phrenic nerve from thermal injury associated with regional hypothermia and to prevent rewarming of the heart from heat sinks (i.e., liver).
4. The systemic perfusate temperature is temporarily decreased to 10°C to 15°C to "precool" the heart (infusion hypothermia), and iced saline slush is placed into the pericardial sac to achieve rapid myocardial cooling. Transient periods of ventricular fibrillation during this period of initial cooling appear to have no adverse effects.
5. When a myocardial temperature of 28°C is reached, the ascending aorta is cross-clamped, and cold crystalloid cardioplegia solution at a temperature of 5°C is infused into the aortic root at a pressure not exceeding 90 mm Hg. The initial volume has been empirically determined to be 10 mL/kg body weight. The myocardial temperature rapidly decreases to 10°C to 15°C, and asystole usually occurs within 10 to 15 seconds.
6. At the termination of the initial cardioplegic infusion, the systemic temperature is elevated to 20°C, and the systemic perfusion flow rate is decreased from 2.2 to 1.5 L/min/m². In this manner, the collateral aortocoronary and bronchopulmonary blood flow is kept cold, and the lowered systemic perfusion pressure prevents rapid dilution and washout of the cardioplegic solution. Every 15 to 20 minutes or earlier if there is an increase in myocardial temperature above 20°C or if there is any electrocardiographic activity or observed ventricular motion, the solution is re-infused at a volume of 5 mL/kg.
7. Five minutes before removal of the aortic clamp, the systemic perfusate temperature is raised to 30°C, and flow is increased to 2.2 L/min/m². After the aortic crossclamp is removed, the perfusate temperature is raised to 38°C and the room temperature is raised to 25°C to 30°C. Cardiopulmonary bypass is continued until the esophageal temperature is 37°C and the rectal temperature is in the range of 35°C to 37°C. Rewarming is usually necessary in the early postoperative period.

The major disadvantage of this technique is the extensive rewarming period, which may exceed 30 to 45 minutes. Nevertheless, this prolonged period on bypass allows the restabilization of metabolic inequities and the subsequent smooth weaning from bypass. Evidence includes clinical reports of the safe use of crystalloid cardioplegia for periods exceeding

150 minutes.[165] However, clinical studies evaluating myocardial metabolism and ventricular function indicate that cold crystalloid cardioplegia results in slow recovery of myocardial metabolism and a poor response to postoperative hemodynamic stress.[166] Although most surgeons in the United States have switched to blood cardioplegia techniques, many groups throughout the world continue to use crystalloid cardioplegia and to obtain excellent outcomes.

Blood Cardioplegia

In an attempt to avoid the oxygen deficits associated with crystalloid cardioplegia, blood was introduced as a suitable vehicle to obtain optimum oxygenation.[167,168] Alternative methods of increasing oxygenation, including oxygenated crystalloid,[161] fluorocarbons,[76] and stroma-free hemoglobin,[169] have never achieved significant clinical use. Moreover, experimentally, blood cardioplegia has been demonstrated to be superior to oxygenated crystalloid cardioplegia (Fig. 63-11).[48] Beside the enhanced ability to exchange oxygen and carbon dioxide, the physiologic advantages of blood include the buffering and reducing capacity, the presence of colloid to avoid adverse oncotic pressure gradients, and the presence of oxygen free radical scavengers.[170] In addition, blood and albumin-containing crystalloid cardioplegia solutions have been shown to preserve microvascular responses compared with crystalloid cardioplegia.[171] However, concerns associated with cold blood cardioplegia include (1) the hypothermic shift to the left of the oxyhemoglobin dissociation curve, thereby reducing the release of oxygen at the tissue level; (2) the experimental evidence that blood cardioplegia may not protect the myocardium at low temperatures[172]; and (3) the potential of hypothermia-induced sludging and red cell rouleau formation. Other studies have demonstrated that hypothermia at 5°C to 10°C does not affect capillary flow[173] and that the viscosity of blood is not significantly affected by hypothermia unless the hematocrit is greater than 50%,[174] which would be unlikely because during bypass, hemodilution maintains the hematocrit in the 20% to 25% range. There have been numerous experimental and clinical studies advocating the superiority of either crystalloid or blood cardioplegia, without arrival at a definitive conclusion.[175-178]

The ratio of blood to crystalloid in formulating the blood cardioplegic solution has undergone progressive change since the initial clinical introduction of this technique. The early blood cardioplegia solutions used a ratio of four parts blood to one part crystalloid (4:1) as hemodiluted blood was withdrawn from the perfusion circuit and mixed with a crystalloid solution containing citrate-phosphate-dextrose to lower ionic calcium, THAM for buffering, and potassium adjusted to produce a concentration of 20 to 30 mmol/L to induce diastolic arrest. Experimental studies demonstrated that a hematocrit as low as 9% provided sufficient oxygen transport at hypothermic levels of 5°C to 10°C (Fig. 63-12).[179-181] To avoid excessive hemodilution associated with administration of large volumes of cardioplegia solution, leading to dilutional coagulopathy, the blood to crystalloid ratio has been gradually increased from 4:1 to 8:1. This change has also been accompanied by increased use of tepid and warm cardioplegic techniques; the associated higher temperatures require a higher hematocrit to achieve oxygen transport to support myocardial metabolism. Miniplegia or whole blood cardioplegia using minimal

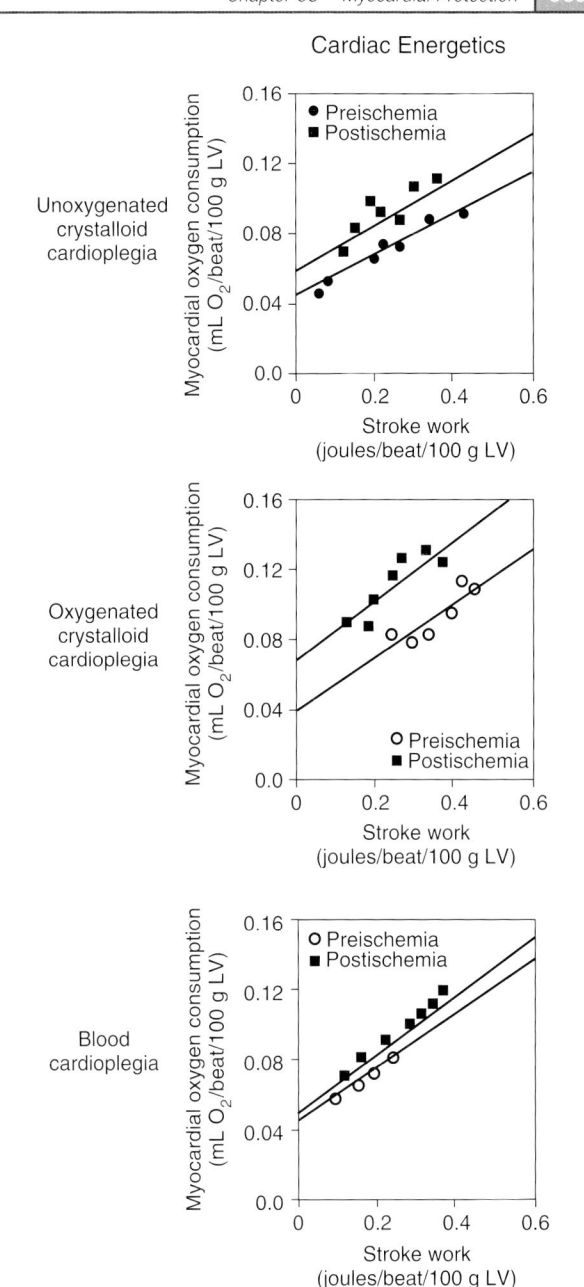

Figure 63-11
Myocardial oxygen consumption and stroke work. Energetic plots of myocardial oxygen consumption versus stroke work before (preischemia) and after (postischemia) unoxygenated crystalloid cardioplegia, oxygenated crystalloid cardioplegia, and blood cardioplegia. Postischemic myocardial oxygen consumption versus stroke work relationships were significantly increased with both unoxygenated crystalloid cardioplegia and oxygenated crystalloid cardioplegia arrest; in blood cardioplegia, the preischemia and postischemia myocardial oxygen consumption versus stroke work relationships were superimposable. LV, left ventricle. *(From Krukenkamp IB, Silverman NA, Levitsky S, et al. The effect of cardioplegic oxygenation on the correlation between linearized Frank-Starling relationship and myocardial energetics in the ejecting postischemic heart[48].)*

amounts of potassium and magnesium to achieve arrest avoids the problem of hemodilution, eliminates concerns about buffering, and avoids pharmaceutical costs.[182] Although experimental studies have not shown any significant advantage in reperfusion myocardial edema in comparing miniplegia with

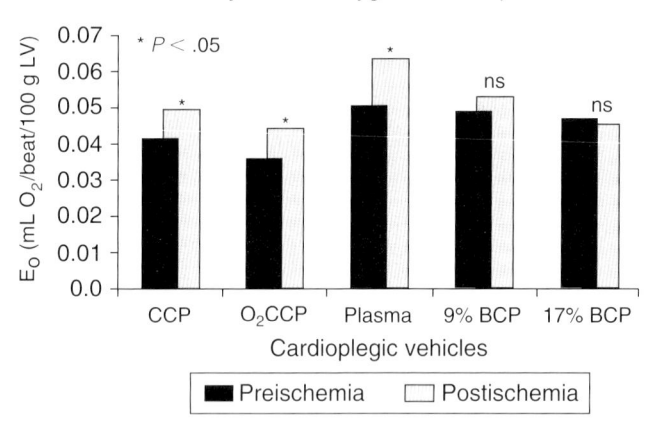

Myocardial Oxygen Consumption

Figure 63–12
Oxygen use and hematocrit concentration. The increased postischemic oxygen use for maximally unloaded contraction (E_O) can be prevented by having a critical red cell mass in cardioplegic solution. This salutary effect of red blood cells cannot be accounted for solely by their oxygen-carrying capacity, as oxygenated crystalloid and plasma solutions did not have similar efficacy. CCP, crystalloid cardioplegia; O_2CCP, oxygenated crystalloid cardioplegia; BCP, blood cardioplegia with hematocrit of 9% and 17% volume. (From Silverman NA, Del Nido P, Krukenkamp I, Levitsky S. Biologic rationale for formulation of antegrade cardioplegic solutions. In: Chitwood WR, editor. Cardiac surgery: state of the art reviews. Philadelphia: Hanley & Belfus; 1988, p. 181-195.)

4:1 blood cardioplegia, the comparative hematocrits of 12% ± 2% and 7% ± 1%, respectively, used in this study are not in the clinical range of 22% to 25% for miniplegia, which may have adversely affected the results.[183] However, in a clinical study comparing miniplegia with standard 4:1 blood cardioplegia, there was significantly greater myocardial oxygen consumption, lower lactate release, and better postoperative left ventricular function in the miniplegia group.[184] Others have demonstrated decreased postoperative inotropic use with miniplegia compared with 4:1 blood cardioplegia, suggesting a decrease in postoperative stunning.[185]

Methodologies

Cardioplegia Temperature

The debate regarding the appropriate cardioplegia temperature has shifted from the classic cold (5°C to 10°C) to warm (37°C) in the recent past and to tepid (28°C to 32°C) at present. Warm heart surgery assumes that aerobic arrest, whereby the heart is electromechanically arrested and continuously perfused with warm blood cardioplegia, is the ideal state for the performance of safe cardiac surgery.[186] The apparent advantages of this technique include the presumed elimination of anaerobic ischemic injury with crossclamp times safely extended up to 6.5 hours[187]; the early resumption of a normal sinus rhythm after removal of the aortic clamp; the avoidance of a prolonged rewarming and reperfusion time, thus decreasing total bypass time; and the elimination of systemic hypothermia and associated vasoconstriction in the early postoperative period. However, difficulties in visualization of the operative field, particularly in performing distal coronary anastomoses, mandated temporary discontinuation of the warm cardioplegic infusion, resulting in ischemic injury if the ischemia time exceeded 15 minutes.[131] Additional problems include (1) ischemic injury when antegrade warm blood cardioplegia cannot be delivered homogeneously in the presence of aortic insufficiency and left main coronary ostial stenosis,[188] (2) difficulties in maintaining complete electromechanical arrest, (3) the need for vasoconstrictive α-agonists during bypass to maintain adequate perfusion pressure because of severe systemic vasodilation,[189] and (4) the risk of neurologic events related to cardiopulmonary bypass and associated microemboli, which is exacerbated if the brain is not cooled.[190] Nevertheless, warm heart surgery offered the promise to resuscitate ischemically jeopardized myocardium during the course of the operative procedure.[191] In addition, late results of the Warm Heart Trial demonstrated that late survival at 6 years was nonsignificantly greater in the warm cardioplegia patients compared with the cold cardioplegia group and was significantly reduced in the group with nonfatal perioperative events.[192]

Tepid (29°C) cardioplegia was introduced as a means of overcoming the deficits of warm cardioplegia, without the adverse effects of cold cardioplegia. In a series of clinical studies, Hayashida and coworkers[193] demonstrated that reducing the cardioplegia temperature from 37°C to 29°C did not alter myocardial oxygen consumption, reduced anaerobic lactate and acid release during arrest, and preserved myocardial function. Further postoperative cardiac function enhancement was obtained with a combination of intermittent antegrade and continuous retrograde tepid cardioplegia.[194] In a series of low-risk patients undergoing coronary artery bypass, there was no difference in cardiac troponin release in comparing warm and tepid cardioplegia.[195] Further studies of high-risk patients with prolonged crossclamp times may allow differentiation of these methodologies.

Delivery Systems

Numerous clinical studies have documented the efficacy of a variety of cardioplegia delivery systems and perfusion intervals. All of these reports suffer from the variability in disease (e.g., extent of ischemic or fibrotic myocardium and the variation in segmental coronary disease) as well as the lack of prospective head-to-head comparisons of large numbers of patients. All of these issues contribute to the wide variety of empirical clinical choices. Antegrade administration of cardioplegia, by use of a catheter or needle, in the ascending aorta has been the initial, traditional approach. Difficulties include (1) rupture of an atherosclerotic plaque at the insertion site, resulting in either microemboli or aortic dissection; (2) aortic insufficiency, resulting in ventricular dilation and inadequate flow into the coronary arteries; (3) left main ostial, occlusive, and variable coronary artery obstructions, leading to cardioplegic maldistribution; and (4) enlargement of the catheter-induced aortic opening at the insertion site, particularly in association with a thin-walled aorta related to poststenotic aortic dilation.

Retrograde perfusion of the coronary sinus, initially described by Pratt,[196] was first used clinically by Lillehei and colleagues[197] during the early days of open heart surgery to protect the heart during aortic valve replacement. Interest was renewed with this technique after Menasché and associates[198] reported improved outcomes for aortic valve replacement, prompting numerous studies on the anatomy and physiology of the coronary sinus.[199] Although most clinicians employ direct cannulation of the coronary sinus with a balloon-tipped catheter, Fabiani and coworkers,[200] in a series of clinical

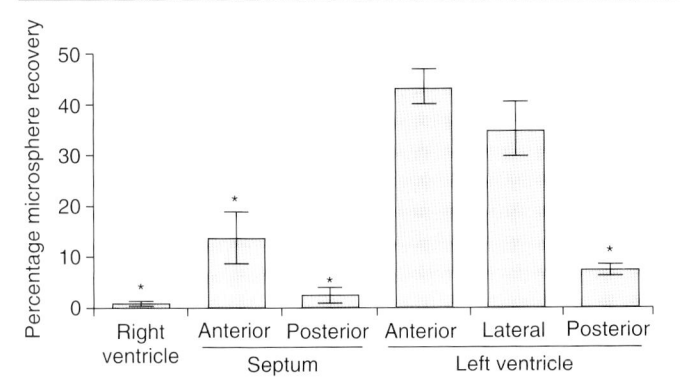

Figure 63-13
Warm retrograde cardioplegia distribution. Percentage microsphere recovery according to anatomic site. Data are presented as the mean ± the standard error of the mean. The asterisk denotes $P < .01$ versus the anterior left ventricle (post hoc Tukey test). (From Calderone CA, Krukenkamp IB, Misare BD, Levitsky S. Perfusion deficits with retrograde warm cardioplegia[202].)

studies, suggested infusion into the pressurized right atrium (obtained by occluding the vena cava and main pulmonary artery) to impede shunting of the cardioplegic solution into the right atrium through the thebesian veins. Major advantages of retrograde perfusion include (1) distribution of the cardioplegic solution to myocardial segments perfused by obstructed or occluded coronary arteries or the internal mammary artery during re-do coronary surgery; (2) avoidance of the need for direct coronary ostial cannulation, with its attendant traumatic injury and subsequent stenotic potential, in performing aortic root procedures; (3) ability to administer cardioplegia during mitral valve surgery without removal of the retractor; (4) ability to provide continuous cardioplegia; and (5) avoidance of debris and subsequent embolization from atheromatous vein graft material during re-do coronary surgery. However, problems associated with retrograde cardioplegia include (1) slowness in achieving diastolic arrest if it is used for the initial introduction of cardioplegia, (2) occasional difficulty in blind insertion of the catheter into the coronary sinus, (3) easy dislocation of the catheter into the right atrium despite the use of ribbed balloon-tipped catheters, (4) traumatic injury and perforation during insertion of the catheter and occasionally spontaneous rupture of the great cardiac vein in fragile elderly patients even with autoinflatable balloon-tipped catheters, and (5) inadequate perfusion of the right ventricle and posterior ventricular septum (Fig. 63-13).[201,202] Major technical issues include the requirement to measure coronary sinus pressure constantly to avoid infusion pressures exceeding 30 mm Hg and never to exceed an infusion rate greater than 200 mL/min because venovenous anastomoses and shunts at higher flows will direct more than 60% of the potential "nutrient flow" into the ventricular cavities through the thebesian channels.[203,204]

Descriptions of the simultaneous delivery of cardioplegia have been confused by variations in the definition of the methodology. Most authors have avoided delivery of cardioplegia solution simultaneously into the coronary sinus and the aortic root to avoid excessive pressurization with subsequent injury to the coronary microvasculature and to allow rapid egress of the solution.[205] Delivery of cardioplegia through the coronary sinus (retrograde) and concurrently antegrade through each completed vein graft by use of a manifold with multiple side arms and a single pump head, in association with venting of the aortic root, has been designated combination delivery.[206] This technique has been especially useful after completion of all the distal anastomoses during coronary revascularization as the proximal anastomoses are being performed or during closure of the left atrium or aortotomy during valve surgery; and if it is performed at 37°C for approximately 20 minutes, it is essentially the first stage of reperfusion and allows the restoration of postischemic oxygen uptake to return to baseline levels.[207] For the most part, most surgeons use all of these techniques, termed integrated cardioplegia, which involves antegrade, retrograde, and combination delivery systems in either a continuous or alternate manner, depending on the clinical circumstances.

Warm induction with warm oxygenated cardioplegia has been suggested as a means of achieving "active resuscitation" in energy-depleted hearts, before proceeding with maintenance cardioplegia by any means or temperature level.[208] Whether 5 minutes is sufficient time to reverse the adverse biochemical effects of depleted high-energy phosphate stores remains open to question, although functional experimental studies demonstrate improvement.[209]

Terminal warm blood cardioplegia ("hot shot") for 3 to 5 minutes before aortic unclamping has been experimentally and clinically demonstrated to improve post-bypass ventricular performance after cold maintenance blood cardioplegia.[210,211] However, a controlled trial of terminal warm cardioplegia for 5 minutes versus simple reperfusion did not demonstrate any advantage.[212] As with warm induction, the question of whether 3 to 5 minutes of warm blood reperfusion is sufficient to restore energy stores is open to question. To overcome this deficit, combination blood cardioplegia delivery may be the preferred approach with a better chance of restoring energy stores. On occasion, prolonged terminal warm cardioplegia may lead to intracellular potassium accumulation with resultant reperfusion asystole during the early reperfusion period and requires temporary ventricular pacing to wean the patient from bypass.[213] Secondary cardioplegia, which involves rearresting the heart for a prolonged period (more than 20 minutes) of warm cardioplegia, is an extension of the concept of terminal warm cardioplegia and may be useful in patients difficult to wean from bypass or with uncontrolled arrhythmias.[214,215]

Clinical steps for myocardial protection with use of blood cardioplegia include the following.

1. Hypothermia at the initiation of cardiopulmonary bypass is avoided, and both the perfusate and cardioplegia temperature are allowed to equilibrate with room temperature (tepid at approximately 29°C).
2. As the ascending aorta is cross-clamped, whole blood (miniplegia) antegrade cardioplegia is infused into the aortic root at a rate of 100 to 200 mL/min at an aortic root pressure of 90 mm Hg. A potassium concentration of 28 to 30 mmol/L is initially used until diastolic arrest occurs, and then the potassium concentration is gradually dialed down until the lowest concentration (usually 3 to 5 mmol/L) that will maintain arrest is achieved. After 5 mL/kg is administered antegrade, an additional 5 mL/kg is administered retrograde.
3. The occluded or most severely stenosed coronary vessel is bypassed first.
4. After each vessel is bypassed, cardioplegia, 5 mL/kg, is infused simultaneously down the conduits in an antegrade

direction and the retrograde cannula by use of a single pump head with a multiport manifold.
5. After completion of the last bypass graft, systemic perfusate and cardioplegia rewarming is initiated. The proximal bypass grafts are inserted on the ascending aorta as blood is aspirated from the aorta to maintain a level of blood just below the opening in the aorta to avoid obscuring the operative field.
6. As the last proximal anastomosis is completed, potassium is discontinued in the retrograde infusion, and whole blood is infused to wash out potassium. Air is evacuated from both the aorta and ventricles as the heart starts to contract, and the clamp is removed from the aorta.
7. After hemostasis is confirmed, cardiopulmonary bypass is discontinued. If the heart remains in asystole, temporary atrial and ventricular pacing is instituted.

POTENTIAL NEW TECHNOLOGIES

Ischemic Preconditioning

Ischemic preconditioning (IPC), first described by Murry and coworkers,[216] is an adaptive response of endogenous myocardial protection, in which the imposition of one or more brief periods of sublethal ischemia (3 to 5 minutes) followed by reperfusion protects the heart such that injury manifested by infarct size, apoptosis, and reperfusion-associated arrhythmias is significantly reduced during a subsequent period of sustained ischemia.[217] The mechanism by which preconditioning affords myocardial protection has yet to be elucidated, but numerous studies have indicated that IPC, in a species-dependent manner, is associated with the preservation of creatine phosphate, ATP, and intracellular pH; decreased ultrastructural abnormalities; induction of heat-shock proteins; increased release of adenosine and activation of the adenosine receptors; activation of G proteins; and activation of protein kinase C.[218] The effects of ischemic IPC are bimodal, occurring in two phases: an early phase and a delayed late phase or "second window" of cardioprotection. In the early phase, the protective effects of IPC are transitory, with infarct limitation being lost if the subsequent sustained ischemic insult is delayed beyond 30 to 120 minutes.[219] Approximately 24 to 96 hours after the induction of IPC, a second window of less potent cardioprotection occurs in which the infarct protection is reestablished.[220]

In humans, the applicability of IPC as an adjunct to conventional cardioplegia remains to be determined.[221] Collateral evidence exists to suggest that IPC may occur in patients undergoing balloon angioplasty[222] or may be elicited by the trauma associated with the onset of cardiopulmonary bypass.[223] Experiments using in vitro monolayer cultures of quiescent human ventricular cardiomyocytes have shown that cellular injury is significantly decreased in preconditioned cells.[224] Results from this study indicated that 20-minute ischemia and 20-minute reperfusion provided the best protection from the subsequent effects of 90-minute ischemia based on enzyme leakage, hydrogen ion release, and cellular viability. Yellon and coworkers[225] have shown that in patients on cardiopulmonary bypass, the use of IPC (two 3-minute periods of ischemia and 2 minutes of reperfusion) before 10 minutes of ischemia significantly preserved ATP measured during the initial reperfusion period. Additional studies also reported that the use of IPC in coronary artery bypass graft surgery significantly decreased troponin T levels at 72 hours compared with cold crystalloid St. Thomas' cardioplegia solution; no comparison with conventional blood cardioplegia was performed.[226] Others have reported that either IPC provided no benefit compared with cold blood cardioplegia, because cardiopulmonary bypass per se induces preconditioning,[223,227] or its use was deleterious in human cardiac surgery.[228,229]

The use of IPC in off-pump coronary artery bypass grafting is also, at present, controversial. Laurikka and colleagues,[230] in a randomized, controlled study, induced IPC by occluding the left anterior descending coronary artery with a silicon tape placed proximal to and distal to the site of the anastomosis for two cycles of 2 minutes of occlusion and 3 minutes of reperfusion; the IPC group had a significantly increased recovery of the mean stroke volume index with a significant decrease in mean heart rate on the first postoperative day and a significantly lower cardiac troponin I level compared with controls. Others,[231] using similar protocols, have found no statistically significant differences between the IPC and control groups. Whether induced pharmacologic preconditioning, by adenosine,[232] adenosine enhanced by a single cycle of IPC,[233] or a combination of adenosine and diazoxide[110] and a nitric oxide donor to enhance mitochondrial potassium ATP channel opening, an essential component of IPC, will enhance mechanical induced IPC remains to be determined.[234] Remote preconditioning—involving the activation of the preconditioning stimulus at a distant site, such as the leg or arm, with subsequent transfer of non-neuronal protein kinase C–dependent signal transduction to a secondary organ, such as the heart—appears to be transferred equally to the heart whether the initiating site of induction is interorgan or intraorgan and is currently under investigation.[235]

There is also controversy about the use of IPC in female patients and the aged. Previous studies have shown that young women have a greater resistance to myocardial ischemic injury and that this resistance is lost after menopause.[236,237] Others have shown in the rodent model that IPC is less effective in the female than in the male.[238] These differences are the result of differences in hormonal mediation of threshold stimulation, and the stimulus for IPC may need to be prolonged (i.e., prolonged initiating ischemic event) to achieve cardioprotection similar to that in males.[239] In aged hearts, IPC is less effective in ameliorating myocardial injury than in the mature heart.[237]

Remote Preconditioning

Remote ischemic preconditioning (RIPC), defined as transient ischemia and reperfusion in a tissue or organ remote from the heart, such as the extremities, has been demonstrated to protect the heart after surgically induced myocardial ischemia in both children and adults by decreasing postoperative serum troponin T release[240,241] by protecting mitochondrial integrity.[242] Similarly, remote ischemic postconditioning, instituted at the time of reperfusion, may have a similar effect.[243] The advantages of RIPC are that there is no need for involvement of the ischemic artery or arteries. RIPC can be achieved through brief ischemia-reperfusion induction at a remote limb or organ. The mechanisms through which RIPC provides cardioprotection are believed to involve possible neural and humoral pathways or systemic responses that interact with known IPC effectors.[244] The cardioprotection afforded by RIPC is limited and much reduced compared with IPC, and efficacy in the female patient and the aged has not been determined.

Postconditioning

The induction of postconditioning occurs during the initiation of reperfusion rather than before index sublethal ischemia, thus improving clinical utility.[245] Various algorithms involving different reperfusion-ischemia and reperfusion times and sublethal index ischemia and reperfusion times have been formulated. The postconditioning algorithm consists of repeated ischemia and reperfusion episodes, resulting in an interrupted or stuttering reperfusion that ameliorates the effects of reperfusion injury. The mechanisms of postconditioning are still under investigation and appear to be similar to those of IPC. The efficacy of postconditioning in the aged and in women has also been questioned.[246] In preliminary human studies using percutaneous coronary intervention for acute ST-segment elevation myocardial infarction, postconditioning has been shown to be efficacious in reducing myocardial cell injury.[247]

Sodium-Hydrogen Exchangers

Sodium-hydrogen exchangers (NHE) play a central role in the regulation of intracellular sodium and calcium concentrations, pH homeostasis, and volume regulation by facilitating the electroneutral exchange of intracellular hydrogen ions for extracellular sodium ions across the cell membrane.[248] Under basal conditions, the sodium-calcium exchanger extrudes calcium to maintain normal intracellular calcium concentration. However, during ischemia, intracellular sodium accumulates because of inactivation of the ATP-dependent sodium extrusion system. NHE-mediated sodium influx during ischemia reduces activity of the sodium-calcium exchanger, resulting in a net increase in intracellular calcium, which is exacerbated during reperfusion. Consequently, inhibition of the isoform NHE-1, located on the plasma membrane of the cardiac myocyte, is thought to inhibit calcium overload and to serve as a myoprotective agent.[249] The NHE isoforms can be nonspecifically inhibited by a variety of antagonists, including amiloride and its 5-amino–substituted analogs as well as the benzoylguanidine derivative cariporide (HOE-642). The use of cariporide has been shown to reduce myocardial infarct size and to improve postischemic functional recovery after ischemia and reperfusion.[250] The administration of NHE-1 antagonists before ischemia or both before ischemia and during reperfusion has been shown to provide significantly greater cardioprotection compared with administration during reperfusion alone.[251] Clinical trials in patients treated for an acute myocardial infarction by coronary angioplasty with cardiac enzyme release as a biological endpoint have resulted in conflicting results.[252,253] In an additional randomized clinical trial (GUARDIAN) of 11,590 patients with unstable angina and non–ST-segment elevation myocardial infarction undergoing either angioplasty or surgical revascularization, NHE inhibition with cariporide failed to reduce the incidence of myocardial infarction and death.[254] However, in a subgroup analysis of patients undergoing coronary artery bypass, there was a decrease in myocardial infarction or death 6 months postoperatively, provoking another trial (EXPEDITION) limited only to patients undergoing surgical revascularization, which demonstrated a decrease in myocardial infarction accompanied by an increase in the incidence of stroke.[255]

Molecular Manipulation

During the normal temporal development of the myocardium, there is the phenotypic induction, expression, and synthesis of a defined number of genes. Under pathophysiologic conditions including stress, disease, and induction resulting from intrinsic or extrinsic insult, there is an adaptive remodulation of gene synthesis that is often not initially apparent at the gross anatomic or histologic level. Recent advances in molecular, cellular, and genetically based technologies have allowed these events and altered genes and gene products to be identified, which may aid in the development of new therapeutic interventions. Apoptosis inhibitors represent a potential therapeutic approach to limit cell death. Apoptosis has been partially alleviated under experimental conditions through the use of synthetic cell-permeable tetrapeptide caspase inhibitors, which provide irreversible inhibition of caspase activity.[256] No human studies have been reported with these modalities.

REFERENCES

1. Gibbon JH. Application of mechanical heart and lung apparatus to cardiac surgery. *Minn Med* 1954;**37**:171-81.
2. Melrose DG, Dreyer B, Bentall HH, Baker JBE. Elective cardiac arrest. *Lancet* 1955;**2**:21-2.
3. McFarland JA, Thomas LB, Gilbert JW, et al. Myocardial necrosis following elective cardiac arrest induced with potassium citrate. *J Thorac Cardiovasc Surg* 1960;**64**:833-9.
4. Hearse DJ, Garlick PB, Humphrey SM. Ischemic contracture of the myocardium: mechanisms and prevention. *Am J Cardiol* 1977;**39**:986-93.
5. Cooley DA, Ruel GJ, Wukasch DC. Ischemic contracture of the heart: "Stone Heart." *Am J Cardiol* 1972;**29**:575-7.
6. Merchant F, Feinberg H, Levitsky S. Sequential analysis of altered myocardial metabolism and contractility induced by normothermic arrest and reperfusion. *J Surg Res* 1974;**16**:153-61.
7. Engelman RM, Adler S, Gouge TH, et al. The effect of normothermic anoxic arrest and ventricular fibrillation on coronary blood flow distribution of the pig. *J Thorac Cardiovasc Surg* 1975;**69**:858-69.
8. Levitsky S, Wright RN, Rao KS, et al. Does intermittent perfusion offer greater myocardial protection than continuous aortic cross clamping? *Surgery* 1977;**82**:51-9.
9. Liu Z, Valencia O, Treasure T, et al. Cold blood cardioplegia or intermittent cross-clamping in coronary artery bypass grafting. *Ann Thorac Surg* 1998;**66**:462-5.
10. Glenn WWL, Sewell WH. Experimental cardiac surgery. IV. The prevention of air embolism in open heart surgery; repair of interauricular septal defects. *Surgery* 1953;**34**:195-206.
11. Senning A. Ventricular fibrillation during extracorporeal circulation; used as a method to prevent air embolisms and to facilitate intracardiac operations. *Acta Chir Scand* 1952;**171**(Suppl.).
12. Buckberg GD, Hottenrott CE. Ventricular fibrillation: its effect on myocardial flow, distribution and performance. *Ann Thorac Surg* 1975;**20**:76-85.
13. Hottenrott CE, Towers B, Kurkji HJ, et al. The hazard of ventricular fibrillation in hypertrophied ventricles during cardiopulmonary bypass. *J Thorac Cardiovasc Surg* 1973;**66**:742-53.
14. Krukenkamp IB, Badellino M, Levitsky S. Effects of ischemic ventricular fibrillation on myocardial mechanics and energetics in the porcine heart. *Surg Forum* 1990;**41**:239-40.
15. Akins CW. Early and late results following emergency isolated myocardial revascularization during hypothvermic fibrillatory arrest. *Ann Thorac Surg* 1987;**43**:131-7.
16. Levitsky S. Is fibrillatory arrest a rational alternative to cardioplegic arrest? (editorial) *Ann Thorac Surg* 1987;**43**:127-8.
17. McGoon DW, Pestana C, Moffitt EA. Decreased risk of aortic valve surgery. *Arch Surg* 1965;**91**:779-86.

18. Braimbridge MV, Chayen J, Bitensky L, et al. Cold cardioplegia or continuous coronary perfusion? Report on preliminary clinical experience as assessed cytochemically. *J Thorac Cardiovasc Surg* 1977;**74**:900-6.
19. Reed GE, Spencer FC, Boyd AD, et al. Late complications of intraoperative coronary artery perfusion. *Circulation* 1973;**48**(Suppl. III):8-4.
20. Silver MD, Wigle ED, Trimble AS, et al. Iatrogenic coronary ostial stenosis. *Arch Pathol* 1969;**88**:73-7.
21. Holman WL, Goldberg SP, Early LJ, et al. Right thoracotomy for mitral reoperation: analysis of technique and outcome. *Ann Thorac Surg* 2000;**70**:1970-3.
22. Bigelow WG, Mustard WY, Evans JG. Some physiologic concepts of hypothermia and their applications to cardiac surgery. *J Thorac Cardiovasc Surg* 1954;**28**:463-80.
23. Swan H, Zeavin I. Cessation of circulation in general hypothermia. III. Technics of intracardiac surgery under direct vision. *Ann Surg* 1954;**139**:385-96.
24. Flaherty JT, Schaff HV, Goldman RA, Gott VL. Metabolic and functional effects of progressive degrees of hypothermia during global ischemia. *Am J Physiol* 1979;**236**:H839-845.
25. Chitwood WR, Sink JD, Hill RC, et al. The effects of hypothermia on myocardial oxygen consumption and transmural coronary blood flow in the potassium-arrested heart. *Ann Surg* 1979;**190**:106-16.
26. Gordon AS, Meyer BW, Jones JC. Open heart surgery during deep hypothermia without an oxygenator. *J Thorac Cardiovasc Surg* 1960;**40**:787-812.
27. Borst HG, Iversen SE. Myocardial temperature in clinical cardioplegia. *Thorac Cardiovasc Surg* 1980;**28**:29-33.
28. Shumway NE, Lower RR, Stofer RC. Selective hypothermia of the heart in anoxic cardiac arrest. *Surg Gynecol Obstet* 1959;**109**:750-4.
29. Griepp RB, Stinson EB, Shumway NE. Profound local hypothermia for myocardial protection during open heart surgery. *J Thorac Cardiovascular Surg* 1973;**55**:731-41.
30. Rao KS, Schutz R, Feinberg H, Levitsky S. Metabolic evidence that regional hypothermia induced by cold saline protects the heart during ischemic arrest. *J Surg Res* 1976;**20**:421-5.
31. Rosenfeldt FL, Watson II DA. Interference with local myocardial cooling by heat gain during aortic cross-clamping. *Ann Thorac Surg* 1979;**27**:13-6.
32. Bretschneider HJ. Überlebenszeit und Wiederbelebungzeit des Herzens bei Normo- und Hypothermie. *Verh Dtsch Ges Kreislaufforsch* 1964;**30**:11-34.
33. Kirsch U, Rodewald G, Kalmar P. Induced ischemic arrest. *J Thorac Cardiovasc Surg* 1972;**63**:121-30.
34. Hearse DJ, Stewart DA, Braimbridge MV. Cellular protection during myocardial ischemia: the development and characterization of a procedure for the induction of reversible ischemic arrest. *Circulation* 1976;**54**:193-202.
35. Gay WA, Ebert PA. Functional, metabolic and morphologic effects of potassium-induced cardioplegia. *Surgery* 1973;**74**:284-90.
36. Levitsky S, Merchant FJ, Feinberg H. Effects of KCl-induced cardiac arrest on energy metabolism and contractility of ischemic dog heart. *Fed Proc* 1974;**33**:3.
37. Todd GJ, Tyers GFO. Potassium-induced arrest of the heart: effect of low potassium concentrations. *Surg Forum* 1975;**26**:255-6.
38. Wright RN, Levitsky S, Rao KS, et al. Potassium cardioplegia: an alternate method of myocardial protection. *Arch Surg* 1978;**113**:976-80.
39. Roe BB, Hutchinson JC, Fishman NM, et al. Myocardial protection with cold, ischemic potassium-induced cardioplegia. *J Thorac Cardiovasc Surg* 1977;**73**:366-70.
40. Tyers GFO, Manley NJ, Williams EH, et al. Preliminary clinical experience with isotonic hypothermic potassium-induced arrest. *J Thorac Cardiovasc Surg* 1977;**74**:674-81.
41. Engelman RM, Levitsky S, editors. *A Textbook of Clinical Cardioplegia*. New York: Futura; 1982.
42. Engelman RM, Levitsky S. *A Textbook of Cardioplegia for Difficult Clinical Problems*. New York: Futura; 1992.
43. Levitsky S. Myocardial protection. *Ann Thorac Surg* 1987;**44**:328-9.
44. McGoon DC. The ongoing quest for ideal myocardial protection: a catalog of the recent English literature (editorial). *J Thorac Cardiovasc Surg* 1985;**89**:639.
45. Jennings RB, Ganote CE. Structural changes in myocardium during acute ischemia. *Circ Res* 1974;**34**(Suppl. 3):156-72.
46. Schaper J, Mulcj J, Wingler B, Schaper W. Ultrastructural, functional and biochemical criteria for estimation of reversibility of ischemic injury: a study on the effects of global ischemia on the isolated dog heart. *J Mol Cell Cardiol* 1979;**11**:521-41.
47. Kubler W, Spieckermann PG. Regulation of glycolysis in the ischemic and anoxic myocardium. *J Mol Cell Cardiol* 1970;**1**:351-77.
48. Krukenkamp IB, Silverman NA, Levitsky S. The effect of cardioplegic oxygenation on the correlation between linearized Frank-Starling relationship and myocardial energetics in the ejecting postischemic heart. *Circulation* 1987;**76**(Suppl. V):V122-8.
49. Feinberg H, Levitsky S. Biochemical rationale of cardioplegia. In: Engelman RM, Levitsky S, editors. *A Textbook of Clinical Cardioplegia*. New York: Futura; 1982. p. 131-9.
50. Myears DW, Sobel BE, Bergmann SR. Substrate use in ischemic and reperfused canine myocardium. *Am J Physiol* 1987;**22**:H107-14.
51. Pridjian A, Levitsky S, Krukenkamp I, et al. Intracellular sodium and calcium in the postischemic myocardium. *Ann Thorac Surg* 1987;**43**:416-9.
52. Piper HM, Garcia-Dorado D. Prime causes of rapid cardiomyocyte death during reperfusion. *Ann Thorac Surg* 1999;**68**:1913-9.
53. Braunwald E, Kloner RA. The stunned myocardium: prolonged, post-ischemic ventricular dysfunction. *Circulation* 1982;**66**:1146-9.
54. Kloner RA, Bolli R, Marban E, et al. Medical and cellular implications of stunning, hibernation and preconditioning. An NHLBI Workshop. *Circulation* 1998;**97**:1848-67.
55. Braunwald E, Rutherford JD. Reversible ischemic left ventricular dysfunction: evidence for the "hibernating myocardium" *J Am Cardiol* 1986;**8**:1467-70.
56. Camici PG, Rimoldi OE. Myocardial blood flow in patients with hibernating myocardium. *Cardiovasc Res* 2003;**57**:302-11.
57. Gray R, Maddhai J, Berman D, et al. Scintigraphic and hemodynamic demonstration of transient left ventricular dysfunction immediately after uncomplicated coronary artery bypass grafting. *J Thorac Cardiovasc Surg* 1979;**77**:504-10.
58. Kloner RA, Przyklenk K, Kay GL. Clinical evidence for stunned myocardium after coronary artery bypass surgery. *J Cardiac Surg* 1994;**9**(Suppl.):397-402.
59. Breisblatt WM, Stein KL, Wolfe CJ, et al. Acute myocardial dysfunction and recovery: a common occurrence after coronary bypass surgery. *J Am Coll Cardiol* 1990;**15**:1261-9.
60. Piper HM, Meuter K, Schafer C. Cellular mechanisms of ischemia-reperfusion injury. *Ann Thorac Surg* 2003;**75**:S644-8.
61. Bolli R. Causative role of oxyradicals in myocardial stunning: a proven hypothesis. A brief review of the evidence demonstrating a major role of reactive oxygen species in severe forms of postischemic dysfunction. *Basic Res Cardiol* 1998;**93**:156-62.
62. Piper HM, Garcia-Dorado D, Ovize M. A fresh look at reperfusion injury. *Cardiovasc Res* 1998;**38**:291-300.
63. Yellon DM, Hausenloy DJ. Myocardial reperfusion injury. *N Engl J Med* 2007;**357**:1121-35.
64. Piot C, Croisille P, Staat P, et al. Effect of cyclosporine on reperfusion injury in acute myocardial infarction. *N Engl J Med* 2008;**359**:473-81.
65. Kroemer G, Reed JC. Mitochondrial control of cell death. *Nat Med* 2000;**6**:513-9.
66. Valen G. The basic biology of apoptosis and its implications for cardiac function and viability. *Ann Thorac Surg* 2003;**75**:S656-60.
67. Veinot JP, Gattinger DA, Fliss H. Early apoptosis in human myocardial infarcts. *Hum Pathol* 1997;**28**:485-92.
68. Chakraborti T, Mandal A, Mandal M, et al. Complement activation in heart disease. *Cell Signal* 2000;**12**:607-17.
69. Matsumura K, Jeremy RW, Schaper J, et al. Progression of myocardial necrosis during reperfusion of ischemic myocardium. *Circulation* 1998;**97**:795-804.
70. Verrier ED, Morgan EN. Endothelial response to cardiopulmonary bypass surgery. *Ann Thorac Surg* 1998;**66**:S17-9.
71. Gardner TJ, Stewart JR, Casale AS, et al. Reduction of myocardial ischemic injury with oxygen-derived free radical scavengers. *Surgery* 1983;**94**:423-7.
72. Chung AJ, Pohlman TH, Hampton CR, et al. Tissue factor and thrombin mediate myocardial ischemia-reperfusion injury. *Ann Thorac Surg* 2003;**75**:S649-55.
73. Baxter GF. Leucocytes in myocardial ischemia/reperfusion. The neutrophil as a mediator of myocardial ischemia/reperfusion injury: time to move on. *Basic Res Cardiol* 2002;**97**:268-75.
74. Sellke FW, Boyle EM, Verrier ED. Endothelial cell injury in cardiovascular surgery: the pathophysiology of vasomotor dysfunction. *Ann Thorac Surg* 1996;**62**:1222-8.
75. Najm HK, Wallen WJ, Belanger MP, et al. Does the degree of cyanosis affect myocardial adenosine triphosphate levels and function in children undergoing procedures for congenital heart disease? *J Thorac Cardiovasc Surg* 2000;**119**:515-24.
76. Novick RJ, Stefaniszyn HJ, Michel RP, et al. Protection of the hypertrophied pig myocardium. A comparison of crystalloid, blood and Fluosol-DA cardioplegia during prolonged aortic clamping. *J Thorac Cardiovasc Surg* 1985;**89**:547-66.
77. Pridjian AK, Levitsky S, Krukenkamp I, et al. Developmental changes in reperfusion injury: a comparison of intracellular cation accumulation in the newborn, neonatal and adult heart. *J Thorac Cardiovasc Surg* 1987;**93**:428-33.
78. Walker CA, Crawford FA, Spinale FG. Myocyte contractile dysfunction with hypertrophy and failure: relevance to cardiac surgery. *J Thorac Cardiovasc Surg* 2000;**119**:388-400.

79. McCully JD, Levitsky S. Myocardial protection in the elderly: biology of the senescent heart. *Ann N Y Acad Sci* 1996;**793**:305-18.
80. Misare BD, Krukenkamp IB, Levitsky S. Age-dependent sensitivity to unprotected cardiac ischemia: the senescent myocardium. *J Thorac Cardiovasc Surg* 1992;**103**:60-5.
81. Lakatta EG, Mitchell JH, Pomerance A, Rowe GG. Human aging: changes in structure and function. *J Am Coll Cardiol* 1987;**10**:42-7.
82. Lakatta EG. Cardiovascular regulatory mechanisms in advanced age. *Physiol Rev* 1993;**73**:413-67.
83. Dalrymple-Hay MJ, Alzetani A, Aboel-Nazar S, et al. Cardiac surgery in the elderly. *Eur J Cardiothorac Surg* 1999;**15**:61-6.
84. Fujiwara T, Kurtts T, Anderson W, et al. Myocardial protection in cyanotic neonatal lambs. *J Thorac Cardiovasc Surg* 1988;**96**:700-10.
85. Silverman NA, Kohler J, Levitsky S, et al. Chronic hypoxemia depresses global ventricular function and predisposes to the depletion of high-energy phosphates during cardioplegic arrest: implications for surgical repair of cyanotic congenital heart defects. *Ann Thorac Surg* 1984;**37**:304-8.
86. Friedli B, Haenni B, Moret P. Myocardial metabolism in cyanotic congenital heart disease studied by arteriovenous differences of lactate, phosphate, and potassium at rest and during atrial pacing. *Circulation* 1977;**55**:647-52.
87. Del Nido P, Mickle DA, Wilson DA, et al. Inadequate myocardial protection with cold cardioplegic arrest during repair of tetralogy of Fallot. *J Thorac Cardiovasc Surg* 1988;**95**:223-9.
88. Meerson FZ. Contractile function of the heart in hyperfunction, hypertrophy, and heart failure. *Circ Res* 1969;**25**(Suppl. 2):9-25.
89. Coughlin TR, Levitsky S, O'Donoghue M, et al. Evaluation of hypothermic cardioplegia in ventricular hypertrophy. *Circulation* 1979;**60**(2 Pt. 2):164-9.
90. Friehs I, del Nido PJ. Increased susceptibility of hypertrophied hearts to ischemic injury. *Ann Thorac Surg* 2003;**75**:S678-684.
91. Sink JD, Pellom GL, Currie WD, et al. Response of hypertrophied myocardium to ischemia: correlation with biochemical and physiological parameters. *J Thorac Cardiovasc Surg* 1981;**81**:865-72.
92. Archie JP, Fixler DE, Ullyot DJ, et al. Regional myocardial blood flow in lambs with concentric right ventricular hypertrophy. *Circ Res* 1974;**34**:143-54.
93. Buckberg GD, Towers B, Paglia DE, et al. Subendocardial ischemia after cardiopulmonary bypass. *J Thorac Cardiovasc Surg* 1972;**64**:669-84.
94. Stamm C, Friehs I, Cowan DB, et al. Dopamine treatment of postischemic myocardial stunning rapidly induces calcium-dependant pro-apoptotic signaling. *Circulation* 2001;**104**(Suppl. II):II-522.
95. Buckberg GD. A proposed "solution" to the cardioplegic controversy. *J Thorac Cardiovasc Surg* 1979;**77**:803-15.
96. Grover G. Pharmacology of ATP-sensitive potassium channel openers in models of myocardial ischemia and reperfusion. *Can J Physiol Pharmacol* 1997;**75**:309-15.
97. Levitsky S. Intracoronary perfusates for myocardial protection (editorial). *Ann Thorac Surg* 1977;**24**:297-8.
98. Chambers DJ. Mechanisms and alternative methods of achieving cardiac arrest. *Ann Thorac Surg* 2003;**75**:S661-666.
99. Opie LH. Channels, pumps and exchangers. In: Opie LH, editor. *The Heart: Physiology and Metabolism*. New York: Raven Press; 1991. p. 67-101.
100. Sperelakis N, Sunagawa M, Nakamura M. Electrogenesis of the resting potential. In: Sperelakis N, Kurachi Y, Terezic A, Cohen MV, editors. *Heart Physiology and Pathophysiology*. San Diego: Academic Press; 2001. p. 175-98.
101. Rousou JH, Engelman RM, Dobbs WA, et al. The optimal potassium concentration in cardioplegic solutions. *Ann Thorac Surg* 1981;**32**:75-9.
102. Chambers DJ, Braimbridge MV. Cardioplegia with extracellular formulation. In: Piper HM, Preusse CJ, editors. *Ischemia-Reperfusion in Cardiac Surgery*. Dordrecht: Kluwer Academic Publishers; 1993. p. 135-79.
103. Brazier J, Hottenrott C, Buckberg GD. Noncoronary collateral myocardial blood flow. *Ann Thorac Surg* 1975;**19**:426-35.
104. Mammana RB, Levitsky S, Beckman CB, et al. Systemic effects of multidose hypothermic potassium cardioplegia. *Ann Thorac Surg* 1981;**31**:347-934.
105. Hearse DJ, O'Brien K, Braimbridge MV. Protection of the myocardium during ischemic arrest. Dose-response curves for procaine and lignocaine in cardioplegic solutions. *J Thorac Cardiovasc Surg* 1981;**81**:873-9.
106. Tyers GFO, Todd GJ, Niebauer IM, et al. Effect of intracoronary tetrodotoxin on recovery of the isolated working rat heart from sixty minutes of ischemia. *Circulation* 1974;**49/50**(Suppl. II):II175-9.
107. Cohen NM, Wise RM, Wechsler AS, et al. Elective cardiac arrest with a hyperpolarizing adenosine triphosphate–sensitive potassium channel opener: a novel form of myocardial protection? *J Thorac Cardiovasc Surg* 1993;**106**:317-28.
108. Ducko CT, Stephenson ER, Jayawant AM, et al. Potassium channel openers: are they effective as pretreatment or additives to cardioplegia? *Ann Thorac Surg* 2000;**69**:1363-8.
109. Lopez JR, Jahangir R, Shen WK, et al. Potassium channel openers prevent potassium-induced calcium loading of cardiac cells: possible implications in cardioplegia. *J Thorac Cardiovasc Surg* 1996;**112**:820-31.
110. McCully JD, Levitsky S. The mitochondrial K_{ATP} channel and cardioprotection. *Ann Thorac Surg* 2003;**75**:S667-73.
111. Toyoda Y, Levitsky S, McCully JD. Opening of mitochondrial ATP-sensitive potassium channels enhances cardioplegic protection. *Ann Thorac Surg* 2001;**71**:1281-9.
112. Oldenburg O, Cohen MV, Yellon DM, et al. Mitochondrial K channels: role in cardioprotection. *Cardiovasc Res* 2002;**55**:429-37.
113. Deussen A. Metabolic flux rates of adenosine in the heart. *Naunyn Schmiedebergs Arch Pharmacol* 2000;**362**:351-62.
114. Ely SW, Berne RM. Protective effects of adenosine in myocardial ischemia. *Circulation* 1992;**85**:893-904.
115. Lee HT, La Faro RJ, Reed GE. Pretreatment of human myocardium with adenosine during open heart surgery. *J Cardiac Surg* 1995;**10**:665-76.
116. Boehn DH, Human PA, von Oppell U, et al. Adenosine cardioplegia: reducing reperfusion injury of the ischaemic myocardium? *Eur J Cardiothorac Surg* 1991;**5**:542-5.
117. de Jong JW, van der Meer P, van Loon H, et al. Adenosine as an adjunct to potassium cardioplegia: effect on function, energy metabolism, and electrophysiology. *J Thorac Cardiovasc Surg* 1990;**100**:445-54.
118. Jovanovic A, Alekseev AE, Lopez JR, et al. Adenosine prevents hyperkalemic-induced calcium loading in cardiac cells: relevance for cardioplegia. *Ann Thorac Surg* 1997;**63**:153-61.
119. Ledingham S, Katayama O, Lachno D, et al. Beneficial effect of adenosine during reperfusion following prolonged cardioplegic arrest. *Cardiovasc Res* 1990;**24**:247-53.
120. Chauhan S, Wasir HS, Bhan A, et al. Adenosine for cardioplegic induction: a comparison with St. Thomas solution. *J Cardiothorac Vasc Anesth* 2000;**14**:21-4.
121. Mentzer RM, Birjiniuk V, Khuri S, et al. Adenosine myocardial protection: preliminary results of a phase II clinical trial. *Ann Surg* 1999;**229**:643-9.
122. Cohen G, Feder-Elituv R, Iazetta J, et al. Phase 2 studies of adenosine cardioplegia. *Circulation* 1998;**98**(Suppl. II):II225-233.
123. Bolli R, Becker L, Gross G, et al. Myocardial protection at a crossroads: the need for translation into clinical therapy. *Circ Res* 2004;**95**:125-34.
124. Buckberg GD, Brazier JR, Nelson RL, et al. Studies of the effects of hypothermia on regional myocardial blood flow and metabolism during cardiopulmonary bypass: I. The adequately perfused beating, fibrillating and arrested heart. *J Thorac Cardiovasc Surg* 1977;**73**:87-94.
125. Bretschneider JH, Hubner G, Knoll D, et al. Myocardial resistance and tolerance to ischemia, physiological and biochemical basis. *J Cardiovasc Surg (Torino)* 1975;**16**:241-60.
126. Dearani JA, Axford TA, Patel MA, et al. Role of temperature measurements in monitoring the adequacy of myocardial protection during cardiac surgery. *Ann Thorac Surg* 2001;**72**:S2235-44.
127. Khabbaz KR, Zankoul F, Warner KG. Operative metabolic monitoring of the heart: II. Online measurement of myocardial tissue pH. *Ann Thorac Surg* 2001;**72**:S2227-34.
128. Khuri SF, Josa M, Marston W, et al. First report of intramyocardial pH in man: II. Assessment of adequacy of myocardial preservation. *J Thorac Cardiovasc Surg* 1983;**86**:667-78.
129. Rosenthal TB. The effects of temperature on the pH of blood and plasma in vitro. *J Biol Chem* 1948;**173**:25-30.
130. Graffigna ACL, Nollo G, Pederzolli C, et al. Continuous monitoring of myocardial acid-base status during intermittent warm blood cardioplegia. *Eur J Cardiothorac Surg* 2002;**21**:995-1001.
131. Misare B, Krukenkamp IB, Calderone C, et al. Can continuous warm cardioplegia be safely interrupted? *Surg Forum* 1992;**43**:208-10.
132. Leaf A. Regulation of intracellular fluid volume and disease. *Am J Med* 1970;**49**:291-5.
133. Starr JP, Jia CX, Amirhamzeh MM, et al. Coronary perfusate composition influences diastolic properties, myocardial water content, and histological characteristics of the rat left ventricle. *Ann Thorac Surg* 1999;**68**:925-30.
134. Foglia RP, Steed DL, Follette DM, et al. Iatrogenic myocardial edema with potassium cardioplegia. *J Thorac Cardiovasc Surg* 1979;**78**:217-22.
135. Wildenthal K, Mierzwiak DS, Mitchell J. Acute effects of increased serum osmolarity on left ventricular performance. *Am J Physiol* 1969;**216**:898-904.
136. Bodenhamer RM, Johnson RG, Randolph JD, et al. The effect of adding mannitol or albumin to a crystalloid cardioplegic solution: a prospective, randomized clinical study. *Ann Thorac Surg* 1985;**40**:374-9.
137. Mehlhorn U, Geissler HJ, Laine GA, et al. Myocardial fluid balance. *Eur J Cardiothorac Surg* 2001;**20**:1220-30.

138. Kurz T, Richardt G, Halg S, et al. Two different mechanisms of noradrenaline release during normoxia and simulated ischemia in human cardiac tissue. *J Mol Cell Cardiol* 1995;**27**:1161-72.
139. Magee PG, Gardner TJ, Flaherty JT, et al. Improved myocardial protection with propranolol during induced ischemia. *Circulation* 1980;**62**(Suppl.):I49-56.
140. Gorczynske RJ. Basic pharmacology of esmolol. *Am J Cardiol* 1991;**56**:3F-13F.
141. Quon CY, Stampfli HF. Biochemical properties of blood esterase. *Drug Metab Dispos* 1985;**13**:420-34.
142. Bessho R, Chambers DJ. Myocardial protection:the efficacy of an ultra-short-acting beta-blocker, esmolol, as a cardioplegic agent. *J Thorac Cardiovasc Surg* 2001;**122**:993-1003.
143. Ede M, Ye J, Gregorash L, et al. Beyond hyperkalemia: beta-blocker–induced cardiac arrest for normothermic cardiac operations. *Ann Thorac Surg* 1997;**63**:721-7.
144. Kuhn-Regnier F, Natour E, Dhein S, et al. Beta-blockade versus Buckberg blood-cardioplegia in coronary bypass operation. *Eur J Cardiothorac Surg* 1999;**15**: 67-74.
145. Melhorn U. Improved myocardial protection using continuous coronary perfusion with normothermic blood and beta-blockade with esmolol. *Thorac Cardiovasc Surg* 1997;**45**:224-31.
146. Rich TL, Langer GA, Klassen MG. Two components of coupling calcium in single ventricular cell of rabbits and rats. *Am J Physiol* 1988;**254**:H937-46.
147. Jynge P. Protection of the ischemic myocardium: calcium-free cardioplegic infusates and additive effects of coronary infusion and ischemia in the induction of the calcium paradox. *Thorac Cardiovasc Surg* 1980;**28**:303-9.
148. Zimmerman ANE, Daems W, Hulsmann W, et al. Morphological changes of heart muscle caused by successive perfusion with calcium-free and calcium-containing solutions (calcium paradox). *Cardiovasc Res* 1967;**1**:201-9.
149. Robinson LA, Harwood DL. Lowering the calcium concentration in St. Thomas Hospital cardioplegic solution improves protection during hypothermic ischemia. *J Thorac Cardiovasc Surg* 1991;**101**:314-25.
150. Balderman SC, Schwartz K, Aldrich J, et al. Cardioplegic arrest of the myocardium with calcium blocking agents. *J Cardiovasc Pharmacol* 1992;**19**:1-9.
151. Meissner G, Henderson JS. Rapid calcium release from cardiac sarcoplasmic reticulum vesicles is dependent on calcium and is modulated by magnesium, adenine nucleotide, and calmodulin. *J Biol Chem* 1987;**262**:3065-73.
152. Hearse DJ, Stewart DA, Braimbridge MV. Myocardial protection during ischemic cardiac arrest: the importance of magnesium in cardioplegic infusates. *J Thorac Cardiovasc Surg* 1978;**75**:877-85.
153. Tsukube T, McCully JD, Faulk E, et al. Magnesium cardioplegia reduces cytosolic and nuclear calcium and DNA fragmentation in the senescent myocardium. *Ann Thorac Surg* 1994;**58**:1005-11.
154. Doenst T, Bothe W, Beyersdorf F. Therapy with insulin in cardiac surgery: controversies and possible solutions. *Ann Thorac Surg* 2003;**75**:S721-8.
155. Rao V, Borger MA, Weisel RD, et al. Insulin cardioplegia for elective coronary bypass surgery. *J Thorac Cardiovasc Surg* 2000;**119**:1176-84.
156. Silverman NA, Kohler J, Feinberg H, et al. Beneficial effects of nucleoside augmentation on reperfusion injury following cardioplegic arrest. *Chest* 1983;**83**:787-92.
157. Vinten-Johansen J, Zhao ZQ, Corvera JS, et al. Adenosine in myocardial protection in on-pump and off-pump cardiac surgery. *Ann Thorac Surg* 2003;**75**:S691-699.
158. Rosenkranz ER, Okamoto F, Buckberg GD, et al. Aspartate enrichment of glutamate blood cardioplegia in energy-depleted hearts after ischemic and reperfusion injury. safety of prolonged aortic clamping with blood cardioplegia. *J Thorac Cardiovasc Surg* 1986;**91**:428-35.
159. Carrier M, Khalil A, Tourigny A, et al. Effects of l-arginine on metabolic recovery of the myocardium. *Ann Thorac Surg* 1996;**61**:1651-7.
160. Engelman RM, Auvil J, O'Donoghue M, et al. The significance of multidose cardioplegia and hypothermia in myocardial preservation during hypothermic arrest. *J Thorac Cardiovasc Surg* 1978;**75**:555-63.
161. Guyton RA, Dorsey LMA, Craver JM, et al. Improved myocardial recovery after cardioplegic arrest with oxygenated crystalloid solution. *J Thorac Cardiovasc Surg* 1985;**89**:877-87.
162. Berger RI, Davis KB, Kaiser GC, et al. Preservation of the myocardium during coronary artery bypass grafting. *Circulation* 1981;**64**(Suppl. 2):61-6.
163. Silverman NA, Wright R, Levitsky S, et al. Efficacy of crystalloid cardioplegic solutions in patients undergoing myocardial revascularization. Effect of infusion route and regional wall motion on preservation of adenine nucleotide stores. *J Thorac Cardiovasc Surg* 1985;**89**:90-6.
164. Fisk RL, Ghaswalla D, Guilbeau EJ. Asymmetrical myocardial hypothermia during hypothermic cardioplegia. *Ann Thorac Surg* 1982;**34**:318-23.
165. Bleese N, Doring V, Kalmar P, et al. Clinical application of cardioplegia in aortic crossclamping periods longer than 150 minutes. *Thorac Cardiovasc Surg* 1979;**27**:390-2.
166. Fremes SE, Weisel RD, Mickle DAG, et al. Myocardial metabolism and ventricular function following cold potassium cardioplegia. *J Thorac Cardiovasc Surg* 1985;**89**:531-46.
167. Barner HB, Laks H, Codd JE, et al. Cold blood as a vehicle for potassium cardioplegia. *Ann Thorac Surg* 1979;**28**:509-21.
168. Follette DM, Mulder DG, Maloney JV, et al. Advantages of blood cardioplegia over continuous coronary perfusion to intermittent ischemia: experimental and clinical study. *J Thorac Cardiovasc Surg* 1978;**76**:604-19.
169. Elert O, Ottermann U. Cardioplegic hemoglobin perfusion for human myocardium. In: Isselhard K, editor. Myocardial Protection for Cardiovascular Surgery. International Symposium; Pharmazeutische Verlagsgesellschaft: 1979. p. 134-43.
170. Julia PL, Buckberg GD, Acar C, et al. XXI, Superiority of blood cardioplegia over crystalloid cardioplegia in limiting reperfusion damage: importance of endogenous free-radical scavengers in red blood cells. Reperfusion composition. *J Thorac Cardiovasc Surg* 1991;**101**:303-13.
171. Sellke FW, Shafique T, Johnson RG, et al. Blood and albumin cardioplegia preserve endothelial-dependent microvascular responses. *Ann Thorac Surg* 1993;**55**:977-85.
172. Magovern Jr GJ, Flaherty JT, Gott VL, et al. Failure of blood cardioplegia to protect the myocardium at lower temperature. *Circulation* 1982;**66**(Suppl. 2): 160-7.
173. Standeven JW, Jellinek M, Menz LJ, et al. Cold blood cardioplegia. Evaluation of glutathione and postischemic cardioplegia. *J Thorac Cardiovasc Surg* 1979;**78**:893-907.
174. Marty AT, Eraklis AJ, Pelletier GA, et al. The rheologic effects of hypothermia on blood with high hematocrit values. *J Thorac Cardiovasc Surg* 1971;**61**: 735-9.
175. Follette D, Fey K, Becker H. Superiority of blood cardioplegia over asanguinous cardioplegia: experimental and clinical study. *Circulation* 1979;**59-60**(Suppl. II): 11-36.
176. Fremes SE, Christakis GT, Weisel RD, et al. A clinical trial of blood and crystalloid cardioplegia. *J Thorac Cardiovasc Surg* 1984;**88**:726-41.
177. Nwaneri N, Levitsky S, Silverman NA, et al. Introduction of cardioplegia with blood and crystalloid potassium solutions during prolonged aortic cross clamping. *Surgery* 1983;**94**:836-41.
178. Young JN, Choy IO, Silva NK, et al. Antegrade cold blood cardioplegia is not demonstrably advantageous over cold crystalloid cardioplegia in surgery for congenital heart disease. *J Thorac Cardiovasc Surg* 1997;**114**:1002-8.
179. Illes RW, Silverman NA, Krukenkamp IB, et al. A critical cell volume is necessary in oxygenated cardioplegic vehicles. *Surg Forum* 1987;**38**:263-5.
180. Rousou JA, Engelman RM, Breyer RH, et al. The effects of temperature and hematocrit level of oxygenated cardioplegic solutions on myocardial preservation. *J Thorac Cardiovasc Surg* 1988;**95**:625-30.
181. Silverman NA, del Nido P, Krukenkamp I, et al. Biologic rationale for formulation of antegrade cardioplegic solutions. In: Chitwood WR, editor. *Cardiac Surgery: State of the Art Reviews*. Philadelphia: Hanley & Belfus; 1988. p. 181-95.
182. Menasché P. Blood cardioplegia: do we still need to dilute? *Ann Thorac Surg* 1993;**55**:177-8.
183. Velez DA, Morris CD, Budde JM, et al. All-blood (miniplegia) versus dilute cardioplegia in experimental surgical revascularization of evolving infarction. *Circulation* 2001;**104**(Suppl. I):I-296-I-302.
184. Hayashida N, Isomura T, Sato T, et al. Minimally diluted tepid blood cardioplegia. *Ann Thorac Surg* 1998;**65**:615-21.
185. Levitsky S. Protecting the myocardial cell during coronary revascularization. *Circulation* 2006;**114**:I-339-I-343.
186. Lichtenstein SV, Ashe KA, El Delati H, et al. Warm heart surgery. *J Thorac Cardiovasc Surg* 1991;**101**:269-74.
187. Lichtenstein SV, El Dalati H, Panos A, et al. Long cross-clamp times with warm heart surgery (letter). *Lancet* 1989;**1**:1443.
188. Misare BD, Krukenkamp IB, Lazar ZP, et al. Retrograde is superior to antegrade continuous warm cardioplegia for acute cardiac ischemia. *Circulation* 1992;**86** (Suppl. 5):II393-7.
189. Christakis GT, Koch JP, Deemar KA, et al. A randomized study of the effects of warm heart surgery. *Ann Thorac Surg* 1992;**54**:449-59.
190. Martin TD, Craver JM, Gott JP, et al. Prospective, randomized trial of retrograde warm blood cardioplegia: myocardial benefit and neurologic threat. *Ann Thorac Surg* 1994;**57**:298-304.
191. The Warm Heart Investigators. Randomized trial of normothermic versus hypothermic coronary bypass surgery. *Lancet* 1994;**343**:559-63.
192. Fremes SE, Tamariz MG, Abramov D, et al. Late results of the Warm Heart Trial: the influence of nonfatal cardiac events on late survival. *Circulation* 2000;**102**(Suppl. 3):III339-45.
193. Hayashida N, Ikonomidis JS, Weisel RD, et al. The optimal cardioplegic temperature. *Ann Thorac Surg* 1994;**58**:961-71.

194. Hayashida N, Weisel RD, Shirai T, et al. Tepid antegrade and retrograde cardioplegia. *Ann Thorac Surg* 1995;**59**:723-9.
195. Falcoz PE, Kaili H, Chocron S, et al. Warm and tepid cardioplegia: do they provide equal myocardial protection? *Ann Thorac Surg* 2002;**74**:2156-60.
196. Pratt FH. The nutrition of the heart through vessels of Thebesius and the coronary veins. *Am J Physiol* 1898;**1**:86.
197. Lillihei CW, Dewall RA, Gott VL, et al. The direct vision correction of calcification of calcific aortic stenosis by means of pump-oxygenator and retrograde sinus perfusion. *Dis Chest* 1956;**30**:123-32.
198. Menasché P, Kural S, Fauchet M, et al. Retrograde coronary sinus perfusion: a safe alternative for ensuring cardioplegic delivery in aortic valve surgery. *Ann Thorac Surg* 1982;**34**:647-58.
199. Mohl W, Wolner E, Glogar D, editors. *The Coronary Sinus*. New York: Springer-Verlag; 1984.
200. Fabiani J-N, Relland J, Carpentier AF. Myocardial protection via the coronary sinus in cardiac surgery: comparative evaluation of two techniques. In: Mohl W, Wolner E, Gloger D, editors. *The Coronary Sinus*. New York: Springer-Verlag; 1984. p. 305-11.
201. Borger MA, Wei KS, Weisel RD, et al. Myocardial perfusion during warm antegrade and retrograde cardioplegia: a contrast echo study. *Ann Thorac Surg* 1999;**68**:955-61.
202. Calderone CA, Krukenkamp IB, Misare BD, Levitsky S. Perfusion deficits with retrograde warm cardioplegia. *Ann Thorac Surg* 1994;**57**:403-6.
203. Ikonomidis JS, Yau TM, Weisel RD, et al. Optimal flow rates for retrograde warm cardioplegia. *J Thorac Cardiovasc Surg* 1994;**107**:510-9.
204. Ye TM, Sun J, Shen J, et al. Does retrograde warm cardioplegia provide equal protection to both ventricles? A magnetic resonance spectroscopy study in pigs. *Circulation* 1997;**96**(Suppl. 9):II-210-215.
205. Shirai T, Rao V, Weisel RD, et al. Antegrade and retrograde cardioplegia: alternate or simultaneous? *J Thorac Cardiovasc Surg* 1996;**112**:787-96.
206. Cohen G, Borger MA, Weisel RD, et al. Intraoperative myocardial protection: current trends and future perspectives. *Ann Thorac Surg* 1999;**68**:1995-2001.
207. Allen BS, Okamoto F, Buckberg GD, et al. XII. Considerations of reperfusion "duration" vs "dose" on regional functional, biochemical, and histochemical recovery. Studies of controlled reperfusion after ischemia: reperfusion conditions. *J Thorac Cardiovasc Surg* 1986;**92**:594-604.
208. Rosenkranz ER, Vinten-Johansen J, Buckberg GD, et al. Benefits of normothermic induction of cardioplegia in energy-depleted hearts, with maintenance of arrest by multidose cold blood cardioplegia infusions. *J Thorac Cardiovasc Surg* 1982;**84**:667-76.
209. Rosenkranz ER, Okamoto F, Buckberg GD. The safety of prolonged aortic clamping with blood cardioplegia. II. Glutamine enrichment in energy-depleted hearts. *J Thorac Cardiovasc Surg* 1984;**88**:401-10.
210. Follette DM, Steel DL, Foglia RP, et al. Reduction of post-ischemic myocardial damage by maintaining arrest during initial reperfusion. *Surg Forum* 1977;**28**:281-3.
211. Teoh KH, Christakis GT, Weisel RD, et al. Accelerated myocardial recovery with terminal blood cardioplegia. *J Thorac Cardiovasc Surg* 1986;**91**:888-95.
212. Edwards R, Treasure T, Hossein-Nia M, et al. A controlled trial of substrate-enhanced, warm reperfusion ("hot shot") versus simple reperfusion. *Ann Thorac Surg* 2000;**69**:334-5.
213. Levitsky S. Another look at reperfusion asystole (editorial). *Ann Thorac Surg* 1988;**45**:471.
214. Lazar HL, Buckberg GD, Manganaro AJ, et al. Reversal of ischemic damage with secondary blood cardioplegia. *J Thorac Cardiovasc Surg* 1979;**78**:688-97.
215. Robicsek F. Biochemical termination of sustained fibrillation occurring after artificially induced ischemic arrest. *J Thorac Cardiovasc Surg* 1984;**87**:143-5.
216. Murry CE, Jennings RB, Reimer KA. Preconditioning with ischemia: a delay of lethal cell injury in ischemic myocardium. *Circulation* 1986;**74**:1124-36.
217. Qiu Y, Tang XL, Park SW, et al. The early and late phases of ischemic preconditioning: a comparative analysis of the effects on infarct size, myocardial stunning and arrhythmias in conscious pigs undergoing a 40-minute coronary occlusion. *Circ Res* 1997;**80**:730-42.
218. Yellon DM, Dana A. The preconditioning phenomenon: a tool for the scientist or clinical reality? *Circ Res* 2000;**87**:543-50.
219. Schwartz LM, Sebbag L, Jennings RB, et al. Duration and reinstatement of myocardial protection against infarction in open chest dogs. *J Mol Cell Cardiol* 2001;**32**:1561-70.
220. Pagliaro P, Gattullo D, Rastaldo R, et al. Ischemic preconditioning: from the first to the second window of protection. *Life Sci* 2001;**69**:1-5.
221. Kolocassides KG, Galinanes M, Hearse DJ. Ischemic preconditioning, cardioplegia or both? Differing approaches to myocardial and vascular protection. *J Mol Cell Cardiol* 1996;**28**:623-34.
222. Deutsch E, Berger M, Kussmaul WG, et al. Adaptation to ischemia during percutaneous transluminal coronary angioplasty. Clinical, hemodynamic, and metabolic features. *Circulation* 1990;**82**:2044-51.
223. Burns PG, Krukenkamp IB, Calderone CA, et al. Does cardiopulmonary bypass alone elicit myoprotective conditioning? *Circulation* 1995;**92**:II447-51.
224. Ikonomidis JS, Tumiati LC, Weisel RD, et al. Preconditioning of human ventricular cardiomyocytes with brief periods of simulated ischemia. *Cardiovasc Res* 1994;**28**:1285-91.
225. Yellon DM, Alkulaifi AM, Pugsley WB. Preconditioning the human myocardium. *Lancet* 1993;**342**:276-7.
226. Teoh LK, Grant R, Hulf JA, et al. A comparison between ischemic preconditioning, intermittent cross-clamp fibrillation and cold crystalloid cardioplegia for myocardial protection during coronary artery bypass graft surgery. *Cardiovasc Surg* 2002;**10**:251-5.
227. Ghosh S, Galinanes M. Protection of the human heart with ischemic preconditioning during cardiac surgery: role of cardiopulmonary bypass. *J Thorac Cardiovasc Surg* 2003;**126**:133-42.
228. Perrault LP, Menasché P, Bel A, et al. Ischemic preconditioning in cardiac surgery: a word of caution. *J Thorac Cardiovasc Surg* 1996;**112**:1378-86.
229. Valen G, Takeshima S, Vaage J. Preconditioning improves cardiac function after global ischemia, but not after cold cardioplegia. *Ann Thorac Surg* 1996;**62**:1397-403.
230. Laurikka J, Wu Z-K, Iisalo P, et al. Regional ischemic preconditioning enhances myocardial performance in off-pump coronary artery bypass grafting. *Chest* 2002;**121**:1183-9.
231. Penttila HJ, Lepojarvi MVK, Kaukoranta PK, et al. Ischemic preconditioning does not improve myocardial preservation during off-pump multivessel coronary operation. *Ann Thorac Surg* 2003;**75**:1246-52.
232. Lasley RD, Konyn PJ, Hegge JO, et al. The effects of ischemic and adenosine preconditioning on interstitial fluid adenosine and myocardial infarct size. *Am J Physiol* 1995;**269**:H1460.
233. McCully JD, Ueumatsu M, Levitsky S. Adenosine enhanced ischemic preconditioning provides myocardial protection equal to that of cold blood cardioplegia. *Ann Thorac Surg* 1999;**67**:699-704.
234. Uchiyama Y, Otani H, Okada Y, et al. Integrated pharmacological preconditioning in combination with adenosine, a mitochondrial K_{ATP} channel opener and a nitric oxide donor. *J Thorac Cardiovasc Surg* 2003;**126**:148-59.
235. Przyklenk L, Darling CE, Dickson EW, et al. Cardioprotection outside the box. The evolving paradigm of remote preconditioning. *Basic Res Cardiol* 2003;**98**:149-57.
236. Willems L, Zatta A, Holmgren K, et al. Age-related changes in ischemic tolerance in male and female mouse hearts. *J Mol Cell Cardiol* 2005;**38**:245-56.
237. McCully JD, Toyoda Y, Wakiyama H, et al. Age and gender related differences in ischemia/reperfusion injury and cardioprotection: effects of diazoxide. *Ann Thorac Surg* 2006;**82**:117-23.
238. Pitcher JM, Nagy RD, Tsai BM, et al. Is the preconditioning threshold different in females? *J Surg Res* 2005;**125**:168-72.
239. Nelson NT, Mahomed AJ, Pitcher JM, et al. Does endogenous testosterone mediate the lower preconditioning threshold in males? *J Surg Res* 2006;**131**:86-90.
240. Cheung MM, Kharbanda RK, Konstantinov IE, et al. Randomized controlled trial of the effects of remote ischemic preconditioning on children undergoing cardiac surgery: first clinical application in humans. *J Am Coll Cardiol* 2006;**47**:2277-82.
241. Hausenloy DJ, Mwamure PK, Venugopal V, et al. Effect of remote ischemic preconditioning on myocardial injury in patients undergoing coronary artery bypass graft surgery: a randomized controlled trial. *Lancet* 2007;**370**:575-9.
242. Wang L, Oka N, Tropak M, et al. Remote ischemic preconditioning elaborates a transferable blood-borne effector that protects mitochondrial structure and function and preserves myocardial performance after neonatal cardioplegic arrest. *J Thorac Cardiovasc Surg* 2008;**136**:335-42.
243. Kerendi F, Kin H, Halkos ME, et al. Remote post conditioning: brief renal ischemia and reperfusion applied before coronary artery reperfusion reduces myocardial infarct size via endogenous activation of adenosine receptors. *Basic Res Cardiol* 2005;**100**:404-12.
244. Hausenloy DJ, Yellon DM. Remote ischaemic preconditioning: underlying mechanisms and clinical application. *Cardiovasc Res* 2008;**79**:377-86.
245. Vinten-Johansen J, Zhao ZQ, Zatta AJ, et al. Postconditioning—a new link in nature's armor against myocardial ischemia-reperfusion injury. *Basic Res Cardiol* 2005;**100**:295-310.
246. Przyklenk K, Maynard M, Darling CE, et al. Aging mouse hearts are refractory to infarct size reduction with post-conditioning. *J Am Coll Cardiol* 2008;**51**:1393-8.
247. Laskey WK, Yoon S, Calzada N, et al. Concordant improvements in coronary flow reserve and ST-segment resolution during percutaneous coronary intervention for acute myocardial infarction: a benefit of postconditioning. *Catheter Cardiovasc Interv* 2008;**72**:212-20.
248. Karmazyn M, Gan XT, Humphreys RA, et al. The Na^+-H^+ exchange: structure, regulation, and its role in heart disease. *Circ Res* 1999;**85**:777-86.
249. Mentzer RM, Lasley RD, Jessel A, et al. Intracellular sodium hydrogen exchange inhibition and clinical myocardial protection. *Ann Thorac Surg* 2003;**75**:S700-8.

250. Scholz W, Albus U, Counillon L, et al. Protective effects of HOE642, a selective sodium-hydrogen exchange subtype 1 inhibitor, on cardiac ischaemia and reperfusion. *Cardiovasc Res* 1995;**29**:260-8.
251. Toyoda Y, Khan S, Chen W-M, et al. Effects of NHE-1 inhibition on cardioprotection and impact on protection by K/Mg cardioplegia. *Ann Thorac Surg* 2001;**72**:836-43.
252. Rupprecht H, vom Dahl J, Terres W, et al. Cardioprotective effects of the Na+/H+ exchange inhibitor cariporide in patients with acute anterior myocardial infarction undergoing direct PTCA. *Circulation* 2000;**101**:2902-8.
253. Zeymer U, Suryapranata H, Monassier JP, et al. The Na+/H+ exchange inhibitor eniporide as an adjunct to early reperfusion therapy for acute myocardial infarction: results of the evaluation of the safety and cardioprotective effects of eniporide in acute myocardial infarction (ESCAMI) trial. *J Am Coll Cardiol* 2001;**38**:1644-50.
254. Theroux P, Chaitman BR, Danchin N, et al. Inhibition of sodium-hydrogen exchanger with cariporide to prevent myocardial infarction in high-risk ischemic situations; results of the GUARDIAN trial. Guard During Necrosis (GUARDIAN) investigators. *Circulation* 2000;**102**:3032-8.
255. Mentzer RM, Bartels C, Bolli R, et al. Sodium-hydrogen exchange inhibition by cariporide to reduce the risk of ischemic cardiac events in patients undergoing coronary artery bypass grafting: results of the EXPEDITION study. *Ann Thorac Surg* 2008;**85**:1261-70.
256. Yaoita H, Ogawa K, Maehara K, et al. Attenuation of ischemia/reperfusion injury in rats by caspase inhibitor. *Circulation* 1998;**97**:276-81.

CHAPTER 64
Deep Sternal Wound Infection
Pierre Voisine, Richard Baillot, and François Dagenais

Definition
Incidence and Etiology
Risk Factors
Diagnosis
Prevention
Surgical Management
Primary Closure and Irrigation
Soft Tissue Flaps
  Omental Flaps
  Pectoralis Major Muscle Flaps
Rectus Abdominis Muscle
  Flaps
Fixation
Vacuum-Assisted Closure Therapy
Treatment Algorithm

Most cardiac surgery procedures are performed through a median sternotomy, an approach pioneered by Milton in 1897.[1] Although fairly uncommon, infective complications for this type of incision remain a difficult challenge for cardiac surgeons.

DEFINITION

Sternal wound complications have been classified by El Oakley and Wright[2] as follows:

1. *mediastinal dehiscence:* median sternotomy wound breakdown in the absence of clinical or microbiologic evidence of infection; and
2. *mediastinal wound infection:* clinical or microbiologic evidence of infected presternal tissue and sternal osteomyelitis, with or without mediastinal sepsis and with or without unstable sternum. Subtypes include *superficial wound infection,* wound infection confined to the subcutaneous tissue; and *deep wound infection (mediastinitis),* wound infection associated with sternal osteomyelitis with or without infected retrosternal space.

It is the deep wound infection subtype that is the focus of this chapter.
According to the guidelines from the Centers for Disease Control and Prevention in the United States,[3] deep sternal wound infection (DSWI) can be defined by one of the following: (1) the presence of an organism isolated from culture of mediastinal tissue or fluid; (2) evidence of mediastinitis seen during operation; and (3) one of the following conditions: chest pain, sternal instability, or fever (>38° C) *in combination* with either purulent discharge from the mediastinum or an organism isolated from blood culture or culture of mediastinal drainage.

INCIDENCE AND ETIOLOGY

The incidence of DSWI in most recent series ranges from 0.75% to 2.4%.[4-7] In our institution, prospectively collected results for 23,499 sternotomies performed between 1992 and 2007 were retrospectively reviewed. A total of 267 patients presented with DSWI, accounting for 1.1% of the surgical population. *Staphylococcus aureus* and coagulase-negative staphylococci are the most commonly found microorganisms.[8] In their review of 30,102 consecutive patients undergoing sternotomy for cardiac surgery between 1990 and 2003, Tang and collaborators[9] found them to be respectively responsible for 42% and 24% of DSWI. Gram-negative bacteria and fungi are less commonly encountered. These offending organisms have been associated with different predisposing factors and modes of presentation.[10,11] Coagulase-negative staphylococci colonize the wound from the normal skin flora and proliferate within a self-contained pocket protected by an extracellular polysaccharide biofilm. The infection is mostly seen in obese patients and those affected by chronic obstructive pulmonary disease; it is associated with a slow and late onset with resulting sternal instability but fewer systemic signs. *S. aureus* infections are more aggressive in nature and more often associated with classic systemic signs and bacteremia. Perioperative contamination but also nasopharyngeal colonization are important sources for this type of infection. Gram-negative bacteria are more commonly associated with a more complicated postoperative course and concomitant nosocomial infections such as pneumonia, urinary tract infections, and abdominal sepsis.

RISK FACTORS

Host predispositions as well as a large number of perioperative environmental and technical aspects can play a significant role in the development of DSWI. There is a vast body of literature concerning the most important of these factors that have commonly been associated with a higher incidence of DSWI.[4,5,12-22] Obesity, diabetes mellitus, chronic obstructive pulmonary disease, heart failure, renal failure, smoking, older age, and male gender have consistently been identified in patients more prone to DSWI. Preoperative considerations include prolonged hospital stay and the use of an intra-aortic balloon pump. The use of both internal thoracic arteries, re-do surgeries, excessive use of bone wax, and prolonged procedural times have all been described as perioperative contributing factors. Reexploration for bleeding, transfusions, prolonged intensive care unit stay, and prolonged intubation time are commonly associated in the postoperative period. Specific mechanisms have been proposed to account for the increased risk seen in patients affected by these conditions. Poor distribution of antibiotics in adipose tissue and inadequate skin preparation in obese patients, impaired wound healing by elevated blood glucose concentration in diabetes mellitus, improper sternal vascularization associated with the use of both internal thoracic arteries, and heart failure–induced low cardiac output are common examples. In our series, prolonged intubation was the strongest predictor of DSWI with an odds ratio of 5.7, probably reflecting composite indices of risk and patient fragility.

DIAGNOSIS

DSWI diagnosis should be suspected whenever sternal tenderness or instability, erythema, fluid collection, wound dehiscence, or purulent discharge is found, especially in the presence of fever or leukocytosis. The diagnosis is essentially clinical and based on the criteria listed in the Definition section. Blood cultures should be done when patients present with pyrexia. Any fluid discharge from the wound should also be cultured. Chest radiography is of limited interest for diagnostic purposes but may reveal ruptured or malpositioned wires as well as sternal fractures or dehiscence as indirect signs of DSWI. Computed tomography can help determine the extent, depth, and localization of the infectious process. It has been associated with 95.3% sensitivity and 81.7% specificity.[23] Computed tomography is also useful to guide needle aspiration and culture. Nuclear imaging has not been used extensively, but labeling of leukocytes with ^{99m}Tc-HMPAO has shown promise as a reliable method for the early diagnosis of sternal infections in a small cohort of 41 patients.[24]

PREVENTION

Modifiable preoperative risk factors are intuitive targets for DSWI prevention. Smoking cessation and weight loss should be sought whenever possible. Perioperative strategies to reduce DSWI are numerous, but overall attention to these multiple details is of utmost importance.

The incidence of nasal colonization with *S. aureus* ranges from 10% to 15% in the normal population and increases the risk of sternal wound infection.[11] Perioperative intranasal application of mupirocin is a safe and inexpensive method to significantly reduce DSWI.[25] Skin preparation should be performed immediately before surgery, and hair is removed preferably by clipping rather than by shaving.[3] Prophylactic antibiotics before surgery are recommended and should be administered to reach therapeutic concentrations before the initial incision and maintained throughout the procedure and for several hours after closure. The intravenous administration of cefazolin (1 g) or cefuroxime (1.5 g) is recommended within 30 to 60 minutes before the procedure; vancomycin should be used, in a dose adjusted to renal function, for patients with a history of penicillin allergy or at risk for methicillin-resistant *S. aureus*.[3] Unless there is evidence of ongoing sepsis, prophylactic use of antibiotics should not be extended beyond 36 to 48 hours.

Blood glucose levels should be controlled, as maintenance at or below 110 mg/dL has been shown to decrease morbidity and mortality among critically ill patients, regardless of a presurgical history of diabetes.[26] Furnary and coworkers[27] have demonstrated that maintenance of blood glucose concentration between 150 and 200 mg/dL through continuous insulin infusion compared with intermittent subcutaneous insulin led to a significant reduction in the incidence of DSWI (0.8% versus 2%).

During surgery, caution to perform a precise midline sternotomy and discriminate use of the electrocautery and bone wax are simple methods that can contribute to DSWI prevention. The use of both internal thoracic arteries should also be weighed against potential risks of infection and tailored for each patient. Diabetic patients are particularly at risk, especially when other factors such as obesity and chronic obstructive pulmonary disease are present.[28] Skeletonized bilateral internal thoracic artery grafting can contribute to lowering of the risk of DSWI in these patients.[29] A closure technique that affords sternal stability should be adopted.[30] A review of a variety of primary closure techniques designed to further stabilize the sternum and to lower the risks of dehiscence and infection is provided by Losanoff and coworkers.[31]

SURGICAL MANAGEMENT

Like any surgical wound infection, DSWI requires appropriate assessment of the underlying causes. This includes identification of the causative pathogens and usually involves surgical revision, thorough débridement, and wound preparation for reconstruction, with or without soft tissue flaps or plate fixation. Poststernotomy mediastinitis was initially approached by surgical revision with frequent dressing changes to promote granulation leading to sternal rewiring or secondary wound closure. The method was flawed by long hospital stays and mortality rates as high as 45%.[32]

PRIMARY CLOSURE AND IRRIGATION

An important contribution to the treatment of DSWI came in 1963 from Shumacker and Mandelbaum,[33] who first described the technique of débridement, sternal reclosure, and mediastinal antibiotic irrigation. The technique offers the advantages of a closed wound and a stable sternum but is associated with limitations in patient mobility and slower rehabilitation, and high rates of failure are still being reported.[34] Nonetheless, this approach is still used and a viable option. Poncelet and coworkers[7] recently proposed an algorithm including primary closure for most patients with DSWI. Multiple procedures eventually including the use of muscle flaps were necessary in more than a third of the patients, and 90-day mortality for DSWI remained high at 14.5%. With multiperforated (Redon) catheters that are used for irrigation and progressively removed during the course of several days, another group reported an overall in-hospital mortality of 23.6%.[35] These results contrast with those reported by Molina and coworkers,[36] who have used a single approach for 24 years consisting of débridement, lateral reinforcement of the sternum, and placement of a combination of irrigation catheters and suction tubes both anterior and posterior to the closed sternum. The skin is closed, the irrigation catheters are kept in place for 1 week, and then the suction tubes are progressively taken out during 5 to 7 additional days. The authors reported a 98% cure rate and no mortality in 114 patients.

SOFT TISSUE FLAPS

Omental Flaps

Based on the rich blood supply of the greater omentum and its potential capacity to nourish infected tissue and to improve wound healing, Lee introduced the idea of omental flaps to treat DSWI in 1976.[37] Despite good flap viability and interesting protection afforded by the technique, with a reported 16% mortality in a cohort of 47 patients, of whom more than 50% had methicillin-resistant *S. aureus* infection,[38] donor site complications resulting from omental flap transposition remain high[39] and include abdominal wall herniation (20%), hematoma (8%), and seroma (4%). Omental flaps are now mostly used as an adjunct to other therapeutic modalities or as a second resort when previous techniques have failed, and it is thus difficult to fully appreciate the intrinsic benefits of the approach. A study[40] reviewing their use in 52 patients during a 15-year period demonstrated a 60-day mortality of 11% for primary reconstruction compared with 29% as a salvage procedure. Flap-related complications occurred in 23% of cases, with complete flap loss in 3.8%. Donor site complications were seen in 27% of cases.

Pectoralis Major Muscle Flaps

Flaps derived from the pectoralis major are dependent on its primary and secondary blood supplies, respectively the thoracoacromial neurovascular bundle and the perforators from the internal thoracic arteries.[41] Complete transposition by folding of the muscle over on itself requires transection of the thoracoacromial artery and can obviously not be done on the side where an internal mammary artery has been harvested; however, partial flaps can be created by preserving the primary blood supply and advancing part of the muscles to cover the sternum. In most instances, both muscles are prepared by this approach, detached from their insertions on the humeri, and advanced into the wound, perfused by the thoracoacromial arteries. One of the muscles can also be folded with use of the secondary blood supply for the pedicle if the ipsilateral internal thoracic artery is intact. This can allow splitting of the muscle along its midline, extending the surface that can be covered. When the entire sternum cannot be covered, concomitant use of the rectus abdominis is sometimes required. However, by skeletonizing the vascular pedicle back to near the origin of the thoracoacromial axis to create an extended island flap of the pectoralis major, as recently described by Hallock,[42] the need for additional muscle flap preparation can be virtually eliminated. In a review of their 20-year experience with mediastinitis management with pectoralis major flaps in 76.6% of their last 186 patients, Jones and coworkers[43] reported a 9.1% mortality with 18.8% flap closure complications.

Rectus Abdominis Muscle Flaps

The rectus abdominis can be harvested as a muscular or myocutaneous vertical flap, with use of the superior epigastric artery and vein for blood supply, assuming integrity of the arteriovenous arcade connecting the inferior and superior epigastric vessels.[41] This approach is mostly used when pectoralis major flap transposition does not provide adequate coverage of the wound or has failed. Oh and coworkers[44] reported 12% mortality with 29% flap complications in 34 patients operated on during a 10-year period. A more recent report from Jacobs and Ghersi[45] using at least one intercostal artery as additional blood supply to the superior gastric artery in 72 patients for 15 years demonstrated 7% mortality and 7% morbidity. Retrospectively comparing the results of 41 patients and 56 patients, respectively, undergoing pectoralis

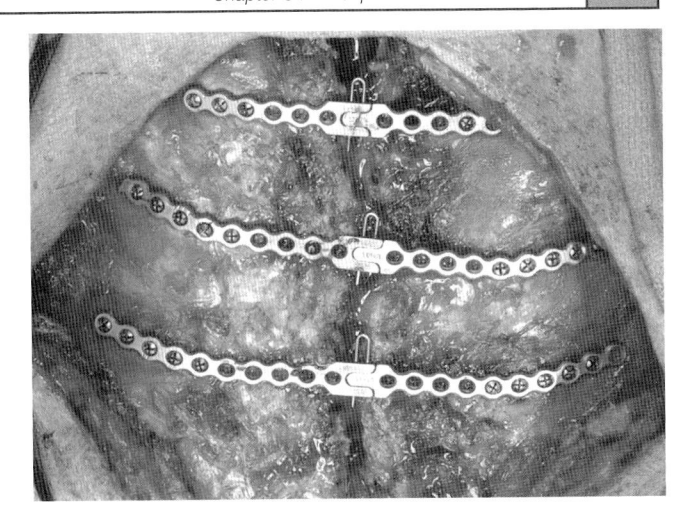

Figure 64-1
Titanium fixation plates fixed with locking screws on the cartilaginous portions of the ribs.

and rectus abdominis reconstruction, Davison and coworkers[46] showed similar success rates (defined as a healed wound and discharged patient at 30 days) of 85% and 86%, 34% morbidity for both approaches, and 5% and 7% respective mortality rates. Rectus abdominis transposition proved more efficient at preventing dehiscence of the inferior third of the sternum, whereas an advantage was found for pectoralis transposition in preventing superior third complications.

FIXATION

Rigid plates can be used for the apposition of sternal edges to promote bone union in complicated sternal closures. Plates are transversely placed across the sternal halves at separate levels (Fig. 64-1). Plate fixation was used in 50 such cases in conjunction with simple bilateral pectoralis advancement flaps for repair of sternal wound dehiscence, osteomyelitis, and nonunion after median sternotomy. Complete bone union was achieved in 98% of cases, with only 2% recurrences.[47] The technique has also been used in prophylaxis for 326 patients between 2000 and 2005 and results compared with those of 215 patients with similar risk profiles treated with a standard approach.[48] Fixation plates were associated with a reduction in mediastinitis complications from 13% to none and in mortality from 8.6% to 3.8%. It remains unclear whether the presence of foreign material could translate to a higher incidence of recurrences, but the approach is promising at least as an adjunct to conventional closure techniques.

VACUUM-ASSISTED CLOSURE THERAPY

Vacuum-assisted closure (VAC) therapy for wound healing is based on the application of local negative pressure through an open-pore polyurethane foam covered with an adhesive drape and connected to a vacuum source (Fig. 64-2). Continuous drainage in an otherwise moist environment increases blood flow in the wound and favors granulation tissue formation while providing sternal stabilization to allow physiotherapeutic mobilization of the patient.[12] This technique can be used as a single-line treatment modality followed

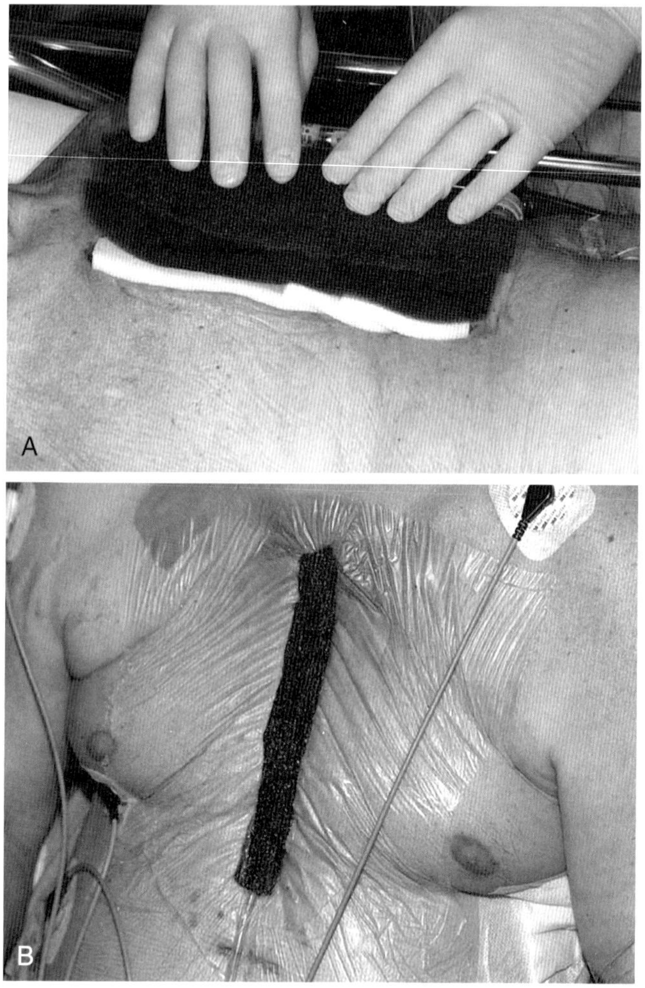

Figure 64-2
Installation of the VAC system. **A,** Open-pore foam sponges used to fill the space between sternal halves. **B,** Complete system with adhesive drape and suction tubing connected to vacuum source.

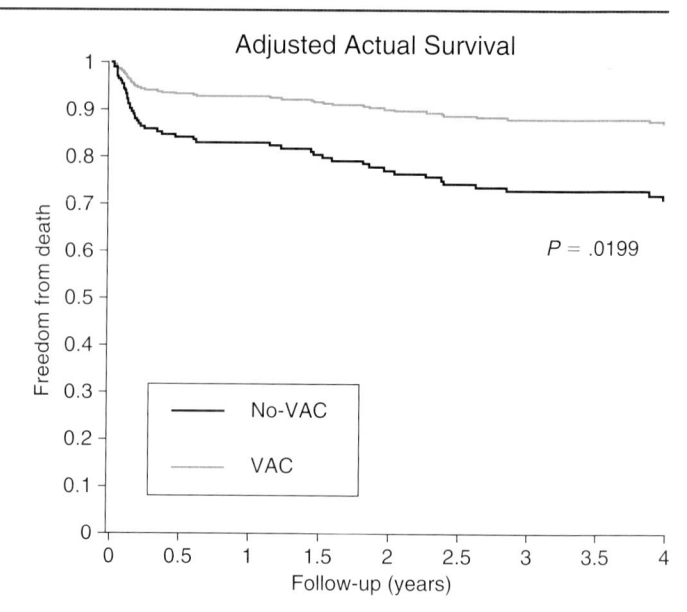

by reclosure or as a temporary means of providing optimal conditions for second-line procedures, such as flap transposition and plate fixation. It has been successfully applied by several groups[18,49,50] and shown to improve survival in patients with DSWI.[12] Based on the demonstration that C-reactive protein levels can guide the optimal timing for VAC cessation,[51] an algorithm for treatment has been proposed by Sjögren and coworkers.[12]

TREATMENT ALGORITHM

A similar algorithm has been concomitantly developed at our institution starting in January 2002. Of 10,319 patients undergoing cardiac surgery, 149 presented with DSWI (1.4%) during that period. Patients were systematically brought to the operating room for débridement, removal of all foreign material including sternal wires, and wound culture at different levels. Appropriate antibiotherapy was instituted and a VAC system installed with negative pressure ranging from −75 mm Hg to −125 mm Hg. Wound care with additional débridement was performed as needed every 2 to 3 days, with return to the operating room when necessary, until the wound was clean, repeated cultures were negative, and C-reactive protein levels were below 60 mg/L. Thick paraffin gauzes were sometimes used under the foam sponges to protect the right ventricle. Most patients were then treated with bilateral pectoralis major muscle flap advancement and titanium plate fixation (62%); 22% had VAC therapy followed by pectoralis major transposition only, and 16% were closed by rewiring only. In comparison to the remaining 13,180 who were treated without VAC therapy as a first-line approach, in-hospital mortality was lowered from 14.1% to 4.8% ($P = .009$). After adjustment for risk factors, early survival was also better after VAC therapy at 1, 2, and 3 years versus the non-VAC groups (respectively 93% versus 83%, 90% versus 76%, and 88% versus 61%; $P = .02$; Fig. 64-3). In our experience, more complex muscle flap transpositions have been limited to those extremely rare instances in which bone union could not be achieved, mostly for mediastinal protection purposes.

Deep sternal wound infection remains an important problem after median sternotomy, associated with significant morbidity and mortality. Good clinical practice based on appropriate preventive measures, early recognition, and treatment are mandatory as they have been shown to provide significant improvement in outcome.

Figure 64-3
Adjusted survival for patients treated with multimodal therapy including rewiring with or without pectoralis major flap advancement with or without plate fixation, either with (VAC) or without (No-VAC) preparation with vacuum-assisted closure therapy.

REFERENCES

1. Milton H. Mediastinal Surgery. *Lancet* 1897;**1**:872-5.
2. El Oakley RM, Wright JE. Postoperative mediastinitis: classification and management. *Ann Thorac Surg* 1996;**61**:1030-6.
3. Mangram AJ, Horan TC, Pearson ML, Silver LC, Jarvis WR. Guideline for Prevention of Surgical Site Infection, Centers for Disease Control and Prevention (CDC) Hospital Infection Control Practices Advisory Committee. *Am J Infect Control* 1999;**27**:97-132.
4. Borger MA, Rao V, Weisel RD, Ivanov J, Cohen G, Scully HE, David TE. Deep sternal wound infection: risk factors and outcomes. *Ann Thorac Surg* 1998;**65**:1050-6.

5. Crabtree TD, Codd JE, Fraser VJ, Bailey MS, Olsen MA, Damiano Jr RJ. Multivariate analysis of risk factors for deep and superficial sternal infection after coronary artery bypass grafting in a tertiary care medical center. *Semin Thorac Cardiovasc Surg* 2004;**16**:53-61.
6. Eklund AM, Lyytikäinen O, Klemets P, Huotari K, Anttila VJ, Werkkala KA, Valtonen M. Mediastinitis after more than 10,000 cardiac surgical procedures. *Ann Thorac Surg* 2006;**82**:1784-9.
7. Poncelet AJ, Langele B, Delaere B, Zech F, Glineur D, Funken JC, et al. Algorithm for primary closure in sternal wound infection: a single institution 10-year experience. *Eur J Cardiothorac Surg* 2007;**33**:232-8.
8. Mangram AJ, Horan TC, Pearson ML, Silver LC, Jarvis WR. Guidelines for prevention of surgical site infections 1999. Hospital Infection Control Practices Advisory Committee. *Infect Control Hosp Epidemiol* 1999;**20**:250-78.
9. Tang GHL, Maganti M, Weisel RD, Borger MA. Prevention and management of deep sternal wound infection. *Semin Thorac Cardiovasc Surg* 2004;**16**:62-9.
10. Gradlund B, Bikover CY, Vaage J. Postoperative mediastinitis in cardiac surgery—microbiology and pathogenesis. *Eur J Cardiothorac Surg* 2002;**21**:825-30.
11. Fynn-Thompson F, Vander Salm TJ. Methods for reduction of sternal wound infection. *Semin Thorac Cardiovasc Surg* 2004;**16**:77-80.
12. Sjögren J, Malmsjö M, Gustafsson R, Ingemansson R. Poststernotomy mediastinitis: a review of conventional surgical treatments, vacuum-assisted closure therapy and presentation of the Lund University Hospital mediastinitis algorithm. *Eur J Cardiothorac Surg* 2006;**30**:898-905.
13. Milano CA, Kesler K, Archibald N, Sexton DJ, Jones RH. Mediastinitis after coronary artery bypass surgery. Risk factors and long-term survival. *Circulation* 1995;**92**:2245-51.
14. Ottino G, De Paulis R, Pansini S, Rocca G, Tallone MV, Comoglio C, et al. Major sternal wound infection after open-heart surgery: a multivariate analysis of risk factors in 2,579 consecutive operative procedures. *Ann Thorac Surg* 1987;**44**:173-9.
15. Loop FD, Lytle BW, Cosgrove DM, Mahfood S, McHenry MC, Goormastic M, et al. Maxwell Chamberlain Memorial Paper. Sternal wound complications after isolated coronary artery bypass grafting: early and late mortality, morbidity and cost of care. *Ann Thorac Surg* 1990;**49**:179-86.
16. Ridderstolpe L, Gill H, Granfeldt H, Ahlfeldt H, Rutberg H. Superficial and deep sternal wound complications: incidence, risk factors and mortality. *Eur J Cardiothorac Surg* 2001;**20**:1168-75.
17. The Parisian Mediastinitis Study Group. Risk factors for deep sternal wound infection after sternotomy: a prospective, multicenter study. *J Thorac Cardiovasc Surg* 1996;**111**:1200-7.
18. Sjögren J, Gustafsson R, Nilsson J, Malmsjö M, Ingemansson R. Clinical outcome after poststernotomy mediastinitis: vacuum-assisted closure versus conventional treatment. *Ann Thorac Surg* 2005;**79**:2049-55.
19. Abboud CS, Wey SB, Baltar VT. Risk factors for mediastinitis after cardiac surgery. *Ann Thorac Surg* 2004;**77**:676-83.
20. Demmy TL, Park SB, Liebler GA, Burkholder JA, Maher TD, Benckart DH, et al. Recent experience with major sternal wound complications. *Ann Thorac Surg* 1990;**49**:458-62.
21. Nagachita T, Stephens M, Reitz B, Polk BF. Risk factors for surgical-wound infection following cardiac surgery. *J Infect Dis* 1987;**156**:867-973.
22. Munoz P, Menaslavas A. Bernaldo de Quiros JC, Desco M, Vallejo JL, Bouza E. Postsurgical mediastinitis: a case-control study. *Clin Infect Dis* 1997;**25**:1060-4.
23. Gur E, Stern D, Weiss J, Herman O, Wertheym E, Cohen M, Shafir R. Clinical-radiological evaluation of poststernotomy wound infection. *Plast Reconstr Surg* 1998;**101**:348-55.
24. Quirce R, Carril JM, Gutierrez-Mendiguchia C, Serrano J, Rabasa JM, Bernal JM. Assessment of the diagnostic capacity of planar scintigraphy and SPECT With 99mTc-HMPAO–labelled leukocytes in superficial and deep sternal infections after median sternotomy. *Nucl Med Commun* 2002;**23**:453-9.
25. Cimochowski G, Harostock M, Brown R, Bernardi M, Alonzo N, Coyle K. Intranasal mupirocin reduces sternal wound infection after open heart surgery in diabetics and nondiabetics. *Ann Thorac Surg* 2001;**71**:1572-9.
26. Van Den Berghe G, Wouters P, Weekers F, Verwaest C, Bruyninckx F, Schetz M, et al. Intensive insulin therapy in critically ill patients. *N Engl J Med* 2001;**345**:1359-67.
27. Furnary AP, Zerr KJ, Grunkemeier GL, Starr A. Continuous intravenous insulin infusion reduces the incidence of deep sternal wound infection in diabetic patients after cardiac surgical procedures. *Ann Thorac Surg* 1999;**67**:352-62.
28. Tavolacci MP, Merle V, Josset V, Bouchart F, Litzler PY, Tabley A, et al. Mediastinitis after coronary artery bypass graft surgery: influence of the mammary grafting for diabetic patients. *J Hosp Infect* 2003;**55**:21-5.
29. Peterson MD, Borger MA, Rao V, Peniston CM, Feindel CM. Skeletonization of bilateral internal thoracic artery graft lowers the risk of sternal infection in patients with diabetes. *J Thorac Cardiovasc Surg* 2003;**126**:1314-9.
30. Losanoff J, Jones J, Richman B. Primary closure of median sternotomy: techniques and principles. *Cardiovasc Surg* 2002;**10**:102-10.
31. Losanoff JE, Richman BW, Jones JW. Disruption and infection of median sternotomy: a comprehensive review. *Eur J Cardiothorac Surg* 2002;**21**:831-9.
32. Sarr MG, Gott VL, Townsend TR. Mediastinal infection after cardiac surgery. *Ann Thorac Surg* 1984;**38**:415-23.
33. Shumacker Jr HB, Mandelbaum I. Continuous antibiotic irrigation in the treatment of infection. *Arch Surg* 1963;**86**:384-7.
34. Catarino PA, Chamberlain MH, Wright NC, Black E, Campbell K, Robson D, Pillai RG. High-pressure suction drainage via a polyurethane foam in the management of poststernotomy mediastinitis. *Ann Thorac Surg* 2000;**70**:1891-5.
35. Kirsch M, Mekontso-Dessap A, Houël R, Giroud E, Hillion ML, Loisance DY. Closed drainage using Redon catheters for poststernotomy mediastinitis: results and risk factors for adverse outcome. *Ann Thorac Surg* 2001;**71**:1580-6.
36. Molina JE, Nelson EC, Smith RRA. Treatment of postoperative sternal dehiscence with mediastinitis: twenty-four-year use of a single method. *J Thorac Cardiovasc Surg* 2006;**132**:782-7.
37. Lee Jr AB, Schimert G, Shaktin S, Seigel JH. Total excision of the sternum and thoracic pedicle transposition of the greater omentum; useful stratagem in managing severe mediastinal infection following open heart surgery. *Surgery* 1976;**80**:433-6.
38. Weinzweig N, Yetman R. Transposition of the greater omentum for recalcitrant median sternotomy wound infections. *Ann Plast Surg* 1995;**34**:471-7.
39. Yasuura K, Okamoto H, Morita S, Ogawa Y, Sawazaki M, Seki A, et al. Results of omental flap transposition for deep sternal wound infection after cardiovascular surgery. *Ann Surg* 1998;**3**:455-9.
40. Ghazi BH, Carlson GW, Losken A. Use of the greater omentum for reconstruction of infected sternotomy wounds. *Ann Plast Surg* 2008;**60**:169-73.
41. Graeber GM, McClelland WT. Current concepts in the management and reconstruction of the dehisced median sternotomy. *Semin Thorac Cardiovasc Surg* 2004;**16**:92-107.
42. Hallock GG. The pectoralis major muscle extended island flap for complete obliteration of the median sternotomy wound. *Ann Plast Surg* 2007;**59**:655-8.
43. Jones G, Jurkiewicz MJ, Bostwick J, Wood R, Bried JT, Culbertson J, et al. Management of the infected median sternotomy wound with muscle flaps: the Emory 20-year experience. *Ann Surg* 1997;**6**:766-78.
44. Oh AK, Lechtman AN, Whetzel TP, Stevenson TR. The infected sternotomy wound: management with the rectus abdominis musculocutaneous flap. *Ann Plast Surg* 2004;**52**:367-70.
45. Jacobs B, Ghersi MM. Intercostal artery–based rectus abdominis transposition flap for sternal wound reconstruction: fifteen-year experience and literature review. *Ann Plast Surg* 2008;**60**:410-5.
46. Davison SP, Clemens MW, Armstrong D, Newton ED, Swartz W. Sternotomy wounds: rectus flap versus modified pectoral reconstruction. *Plast Reconstr Surg* 2007;**120**:929-34.
47. Cicilioni OJ, Stieg III FH, Papanicolaou G. Sternal wound reconstruction with transverse plate fixation. *Plast Reconstr Surg* 2005;**115**:1297-303.
48. Raman J, Song DH, Bolotin G, Jeevanandam V. Sternal closure with titanium plate fixation—a paradigm shift in preventing mediastinitis. *Interact Cardiovasc Thorac Surg* 2006;**5**:336-9.
49. Agarwal JP, Ogilvie M, Wu LC, Lohman RF, Gottlieb LJ, Franczyk M, Song DH. Vacuum-assisted closure for sternal wounds: a first-line therapeutic management approach. *Plast Reconstr Surg* 2005;**116**:1035-40.
50. Fleck TM, Koller R, Giovanoli P, Moidl R, Czerny M, Fleck M, et al. Primary or delayed closure for the treatment of post-sternotomy wound infections? *Ann Plast Surg* 2004;**52**:310-4.
51. Gustafsson R, Johnsson P, Algotsson L, Blomquist S, Ingemansson R. Vacuum-assisted closure therapy guided by C-reactive protein level in patients with deep sternal wound infection. *J Thorac Cardiovasc Surg* 2002;**123**:895-900.

CHAPTER 65
Neuropsychological Deficits and Stroke
John W. Hammon and David A. Stump

Assessment
Populations at Risk

Mechanisms of Injury
Strategies for Reducing Injury

Neuroprotective Strategies
Prognosis

The brain is the effector organ for all behavior, innate and learned. It is the monarch of blood flow and will shut down all other vascular systems to preserve its own supply. Conversely, dysfunction in other organs can adversely affect brain function. It monitors other organ systems and is acutely sensitive and responsive to both the external and internal environment. Thus, even small injuries to the brain may produce symptomatic, functional losses that would not be detectable or important in other organs. Regional hypoperfusion, edema, microemboli, circulating cytotoxins, and subtle changes in blood glucose, insulin, or calcium concentration may result in changes in cognitive function ranging from subtle to profound. A small 2-mm infarct may cause a disruption of behavioral patterns; physiologic and physical function changes can pass unnoticed, be accepted and dismissed, or profoundly compromise the patient's quality of life. Move the lesion half a centimeter, and the same volume lesion may result in a catastrophic stroke. Thus, the brain is the most sensitive organ exposed to damage by cardiopulmonary bypass (CPB) and also the organ that, with the heart, is most important to protect.

ASSESSMENT

Routine assessment of neurologic injury that occurs in the setting of cardiac surgery is not done for most patients because of the priority of the cardiac lesion and because of costs in time and money. General neurologic examinations by members of the surgical team or individuals lacking specialized training are not adequate to rule out subtle neurologic injuries, and this is the principal reason that the incidence of stroke and neurologic or neuropsychological injury varies widely in the surgical literature.[1-3]

For studies designed to assess or to reduce neurologic injury in the setting of cardiac surgery, nonroutine preoperative and postoperative tests are required. These special tests include a complete neurologic examination by a neurologist or a well-trained surrogate. To improve accuracy, a single neurologist should ideally conduct all serial examinations. A standardized protocol of examination should be followed, with uniform reporting of results. The basic, structured examination includes a mental state examination; cranial nerve, motor, sensory, and cerebellar examinations; and examination of gait, station, and deep tendon and primitive reflexes.

The most obvious neurologic abnormalities are paresis, loss of vital brain functions (such as speech, vision, or comprehension), and coma. These are commonly lumped under the general heading of stroke. Disorders of awareness or consciousness can include coma, delirium, and confusion, but transitory episodes of delirium and confusion are often dismissed as due to anesthesia or medications. More subtle losses are determined by comparison of preoperative and postoperative performances with a standard battery of neuropsychological tests prepared by a group of neuropsychologists.[4] A neuropsychological examination is basically an extension of the neurologic examination with a much greater emphasis on higher cortical function. Dysfunction is objectively defined as a deviation from the expected, relative to a large population. For example, although performing at a 95 IQ level is in the normal range, it is low for a physician, and a search for a neurologic impairment would be triggered by such a poor performance. A 20% decline in two or more of these test results, compared with the patient's baseline, suggests a neuropsychological deficit that should be followed until it is resolved or not resolved.[5] In studies involving long-term follow-up, the inclusion of a control group of nonsurgical patients with the same disease and of similar demographics helps define the causes of neuropsychological decline that occurs later than 3 to 6 months after surgery.[6]

Computed axial tomograms or magnetic resonance imaging (MRI) scans are essential for the definitive diagnosis of stroke, delirium, or coma. Preoperative imaging is usually not necessary when new techniques such as diffusion-weighted MRI imaging, MRI spectroscopy, and MRI angiography are used to assess possible new lesions after operation.[7-9] However, studies demonstrate that patients with dementia have a loss in cell volume due to microinfarctions that are not detectable with current radiologic techniques.[64] Histologic studies performed on patients who did not survive cardiac surgery have demonstrated millions of small lipid microemboli that may result in massive cell loss and increased volume of ventricles (Fig. 65-1).

Biochemical markers of neurologic injury after cardiac surgery are relatively nonspecific and inconclusive. Neuron-specific enolase is an intracellular enzyme found in neurons, normal neuroendocrine cells, platelets, and erythrocytes.[10] S-100 is an acidic calcium-binding protein found in the brain.[11,12]

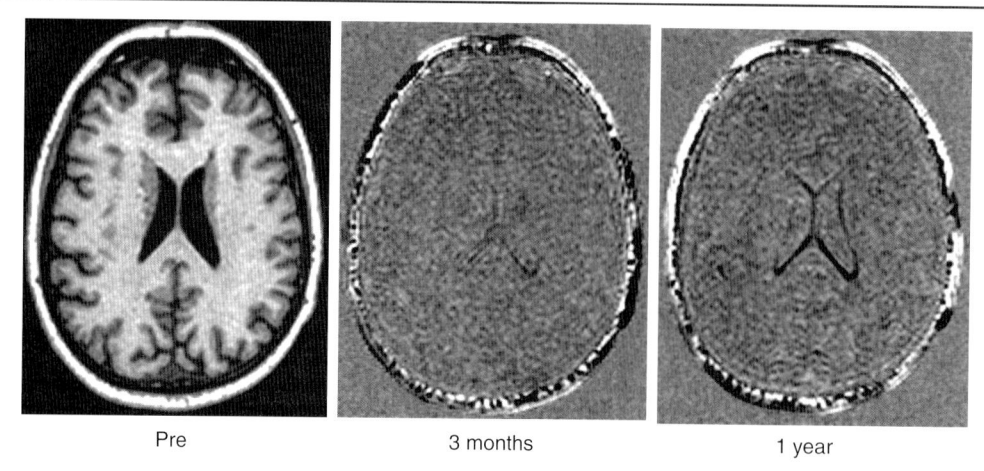

Figure 65-1
Preoperative magnetic resonance image of the brain from a patient undergoing extensive cardiac surgery superimposed on identical images taken at 3 months and 1 year postoperatively. The appearance of the ventricles at 1 year indicates brain shrinkage, presumably from apoptosis of neurons. *(Modified with permission from Kohn A. Magnetic resonance imaging registration and quantification of the brain before and after coronary artery bypass grafting surgery.* Ann Thorac Surg *2002;73:S363-5.)*

The beta dimer resides in glial and Schwann cells. Both S-100 and neuron-specific enolase increase in spinal fluid with neuronal death[11,12] and may correlate with stroke or spinal cord injury after CPB.[13] However, plasma levels are contaminated by aspiration of wound blood into the pump and hemolysis and are often elevated after prolonged CPB in patients without otherwise detectable neurologic injury.[14] Newer blood-borne biochemical markers are being identified but as yet have not been shown to be diagnostic for subtle neurologic injury.

POPULATIONS AT RISK

Advancing age increases the risk of stroke or cognitive impairment in the general population, and surgery, regardless of type, increases the risk still higher.[15] In 1985, Gardner and colleagues[16] reported the risk of stroke during coronary artery bypass graft surgery to be directly related to age. A European study compared 321 elderly patients without surgery to 1218 patients who had noncardiac surgery and found a 26% incidence of cognitive dysfunction 1 week after operation and a 10% incidence at 3 months.[17] Between 1974 and 1990, the number of patients older than 60 years and older than 70 years undergoing cardiac surgery increased twofold and sevenfold, respectively.[18] Genetic factors also influence the incidence of cognitive dysfunction after cardiac surgery.[19] The incidence of cognitive dysfunction at 1 week after cardiac surgery is approximately double that of noncardiac surgery.

As the age of cardiac surgical patients increases, the number with multiple risk factors for neurologic injury also increases. Risk factors for adverse cerebral outcomes are listed in Table 65-1.[20] These factors are divided into stroke with a permanent fixed neurologic deficit (type I) and coma or delirium (type II). Hypertension and diabetes occur in approximately 55% and 25% of cardiac surgical patients, respectively.[21] Fifteen percent have carotid stenosis of 50% or greater, and up to 13% have had a transient ischemic attack or prior stroke. The total number of MRI atherosclerotic lesions in the brachiocephalic vessels adds to the risk of stroke or cognitive dysfunction,[22] as does the severity of atherosclerosis in the ascending aorta as detected by epiaortic ultrasound scanning.[23] Palpable ascending aortic atherosclerotic plaques markedly increase the risk of right carotid arterial emboli as detected by Doppler ultrasound examination.[24] The incidence of severe aortic atherosclerosis is 1% in cardiac surgical patients younger than 50 years and 10% in those aged 75 to 80 years.[25]

MECHANISMS OF INJURY

The three major causes of neurologic dysfunction and injury during cardiac surgery are microemboli, hypoperfusion, and a generalized inflammatory reaction that can occur in the same patient at the same time for different reasons. The majority of intraoperative strokes are due to the embolization of atherosclerotic material from the aorta and brachiocephalic vessels. This results from manipulation of the heart and major thoracic vasculature as well as from dislodgement of atheromas by shearing forces directed at the walls of vessels from inflow CPB cannulas.[26] Microemboli are distributed in proportion to blood flow[27]; thus, reduced cerebral blood flow reduces microembolic injury but increases the risk of hypoperfusion.[28] During CPB, both alpha-stat acid-base management and phenylephrine reduce cerebral injury in adults, probably by causing cerebral vessel vasoconstriction and reducing the number of microemboli.[28,29] Air,[30] atherosclerotic debris,[31] and fat are the major types of microemboli causing brain injury in clinical practice, and all cause neuronal necrosis by blocking cerebral vessels.[32] Massive air embolism causes a large ischemic injury, but gaseous cerebral microemboli may directly damage endothelium in addition to blocking blood flow.[33] The identification of unique small capillary arteriolar dilations in the brain associated with fat emboli (Fig. 65-2)[34] raises the possibility that these emboli not only block small vessels but also release cytotoxic free radicals, which may significantly increase the damage to lipid-rich neurons.

Anemia and elevated cerebral temperature increase cerebral blood flow but may cause inadequate oxygen delivery to the brain[35]; however, these conditions are easily avoided during clinical cardiac surgery. Although some investigators speculate that normothermic or hyperthermic CPB causes cerebral hypoperfusion,[36] experimental studies indicate that

Table 65–1

Adjusted Odds Ratios for Type I and Type II Cerebral Outcomes Associated with Selected Risk Factors

Factor	Model for Type I Cerebral Outcome	Model for Type II Cerebral Outcome
Significant factors, P < .05		
Proximal aortic atherosclerosis	4.52	
History of neurologic disease	3.19	
Use of intra-aortic balloon pump	2.60	
Diabetes mellitus	2.59	
History of hypertension	2.31	
History of pulmonary disease	2.09	2.37
History of unstable angina	1.83	
Age (per additional decade)	1.75	2.20
Systolic blood pessure > 180 mm Hg at admission		3.47
History of excessive alcohol consumption		2.64
History of CABG		2.18
Dysrhythmia on day of surgery		1.97
Antihypertensive therapy		1.78
Other factors (P not significant)		
Perioperative hypotension	1.92	1.88
Ventricular venting	1.83	
Congestive heart failure on day of surgery		2.46
History of peripheral vascular disease		1.64

Modified from Roach GW, Kanchuger M, Mangano CM, et al. Adverse cerebral outcomes after coronary bypass surgery. Multicenter Study of Perioperative Ishemia Research Group and the Ischemia Research and Education Foundation Investigators.

cerebral blood flow increases with temperature.[37] Brain injuries associated with this practice are more likely due to increased cerebral microemboli, which produce larger lesions at higher cerebral temperatures.[38] Reduced brain temperature is protective against neural cell injury and remains an important neuroprotective strategy (Fig. 65-3).

All surgery, like accidental trauma, triggers an acute inflammatory response that can result in neurologic injury, but the continuous exposure of heparinized blood to non–endothelial cell surfaces followed by reinfusion of wound blood and recirculation within the body greatly magnifies this response in operations in which CPB is used. Although it is far from fully described and understood, this primary "blood injury" produces a unique response, which is different in detail from that caused by other threats to homeostasis.

The principal blood elements involved in this acute defense reaction are contact and complement plasma protein systems, neutrophils, monocytes, endothelial cells, and, to a lesser extent, platelets. When activated during CPB, the principal blood elements release vasoactive and cytotoxic substances, produce cell signaling inflammatory and inhibitory cytokines, express complementary cellular receptors that interact with specific cell signaling substances and other cells, and generate a host of vasoactive and cytotoxic substances that circulate.[39] Normally, these reactive blood elements mediate and regulate the defense reaction,[40-42] but during CPB, an orderly, targeted response is overwhelmed by the massive activation and circulation of these reactive blood elements. This massive attack damages the endothelium, increases the size of ischemic lesions, and causes organ dysfunction.

STRATEGIES FOR REDUCING INJURY

Important methods for reducing emboli deserve emphasis (Table 65-2). Principles include adequate anticoagulation, washing of blood aspirated from the surgical wound, filtering of arterial inflow and venous outflow, strict control of all air entry sites within the perfusion circuit, removal of residual air from the heart and great vessels, and avoidance of atherosclerotic emboli.[43-45]

Many intraoperative strategies are available to reduce cerebral atherosclerotic embolization. These include routine epicardial echocardiography of the ascending aorta to detect both anterior and posterior atherosclerotic plaques and to find sites free of atherosclerosis for placement of the aortic cannula.[46] Recently, special catheters with or without baffles or screens have been developed to reduce the number of atherosclerotic emboli that reach the cerebral circulation.[44-47] In patients with moderate or severe ascending aortic atherosclerosis, a single application of the aortic clamp as opposed to partial or multiple applications is strongly recommended and has been shown to reduce postoperative neurocognitive deficits in a large clinical series.[48] Retrograde cardioplegia is preferred to antegrade cardioplegia in these patients to avoid a sandblasting effect of the cardioplegic solution.[49] No aortic clamp may be safe or even possible in some patients with severe atherosclerosis or porcelain aorta. If intracardiac surgery is required in these patients, deep hypothermia may be used with or without graft replacement of the ascending aorta. If only revascularization is needed, pedicled single or sequential arterial grafts,[50] T or Y grafts from a pedicled mammary artery,[51] or vein grafts anastomosed to arch vessels can be used. Patients with intracardiac thrombus or vegetations require aortic cross-clamping before cardiac manipulation to avoid dislodgement of embolic material.

In-depth or screen filters are essential for cardiotomy reservoirs and are usually used in arterial lines. The efficacy of arterial line filters is controversial; screen filters with a pore size of less than 20 μm cannot be used because of flow resistance across the filter. However, air and fat emboli can pass through filters, although 20-μm screen filters more effectively trap microemboli than larger sizes do.[52]

NEUROPROTECTIVE STRATEGIES

Recommended conditions for protecting the brain during CPB include mild hypothermia (32° C to 34° C; see Fig. 65-3) and hematocrit above 25%.[37] Temporary increases in cerebral venous pressure caused by superior vena cava obstruction

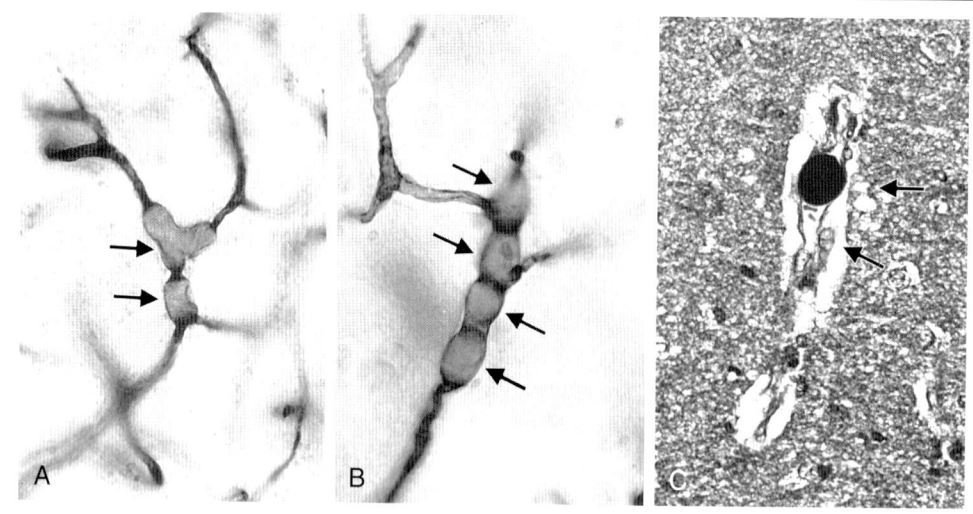

Figure 65–2
High-magnification photomicrograph showing small capillary arteriolar dilatations from the brain of a patient dying soon after cardiac surgery. A and B, Small capillary arteriolar dilations in arterioles *(dark arrows)*. (Alkaline phosphatase stained, celloidin imbedded; magnification ×50.) C, Small capillary arteriolar dilations stained black with osmium, indicating fat. Arrows indicate tissue edema and vacuoles from injury. (Osmium stained, paraffin embedded; 5-μm-thick section.)

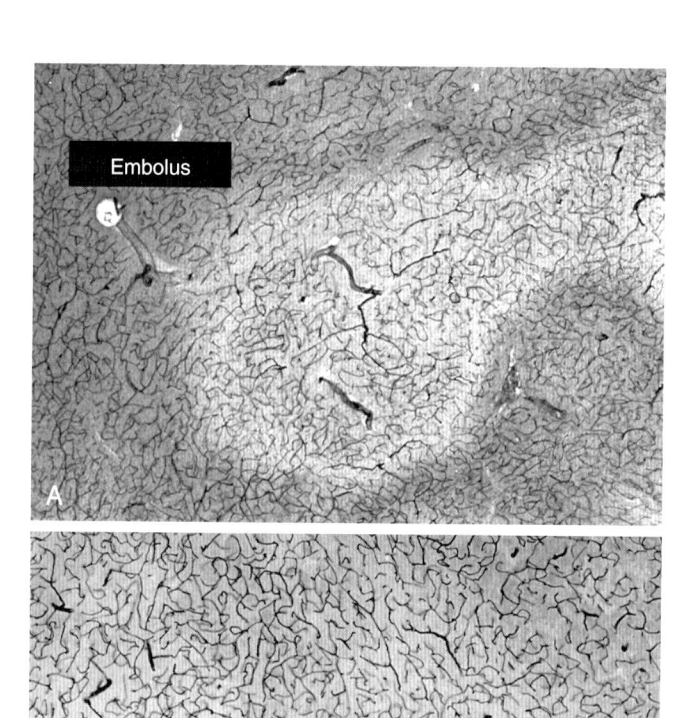

Table 65–2
Strategies for Emboli Protection During Cardiac Surgery

Proven
Adequate anticoagulation
Membrane oxygenator
Closed-system CPB
Washing of blood aspirated from surgical wound (no need to wash blood from cardiac chambers)
Filtering of arterial inflow and venous outflow
Control of all sites of air entry into CPB
Removal of residual air from heart and great vessels
Epiaortic ultrasound mapping of ascending aorta
Minimal aortic manipulation (single aortic crossclamp)
Retrograde cardioplegia
Experimental
Off-pump surgery
Selective filtration of brachiocephalic vessels
Ultrasonic venous and arterial embolus detection
Pharmacologic brain protection

Figure 65–3
Experimental brain ischemia from glass bead embolization.
A demonstrates a large area of ischemia in an animal at normothermia.
B is from an animal embolized at 32° C with no evident ischemia.
(Paraffin embedded, stained for heat shock protein.)

and excessive rewarming above blood temperatures of 37° C should be avoided.[38,53] A randomized study in which patients were mildly rewarmed to 35° C core temperature demonstrated improved neurocognitive outcomes over patients rewarmed to 37° C.[53] Either jugular venous bulb oxygen saturation or near-infrared cerebral oximetry is recommended for monitoring of cerebral perfusion in patients who may be at high risk for cerebral injury.[54]

Persistent Neurobehavioral Deficits at 6 Months
Fisher's Exact Text, P = .061

[Bar graph showing: Multi: No Deficit 68.2%, Persistent Deficit 31.8%; OPCAB: No Deficit 69.6%, Persistent Deficit 30.4%; Single: No Deficit 88.9%, Persistent Deficit 11.1%]

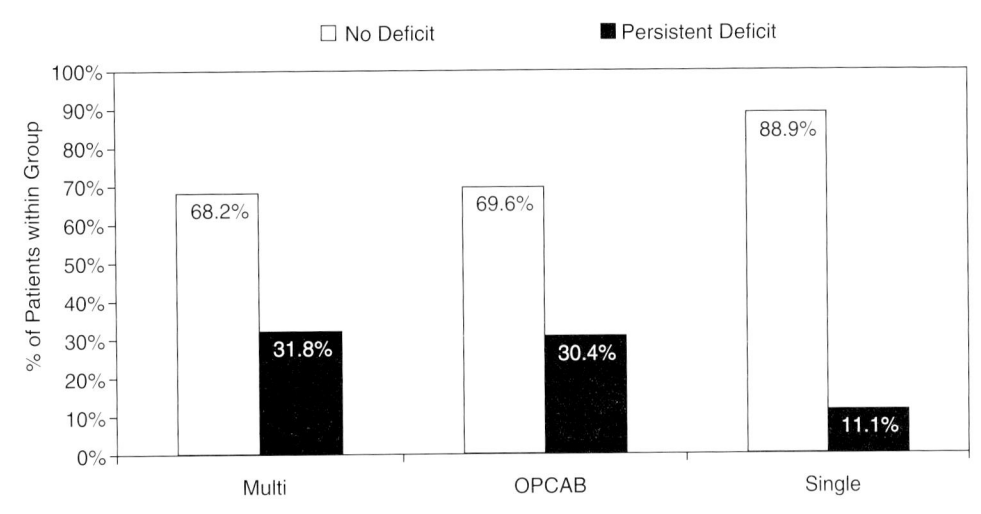

Figure 65–4
Bar graph with results of neuropsychological testing at 6 months after coronary artery bypass grafting by three different techniques. Note that patients with single aortic clamping have many fewer persistent neuropsychological deficits than did patients with multiple aortic clamping or off-pump coronary artery bypass grafting (OPCAB). *(Reproduced with permission from Hammon JW, Stump DA, Butterworth JF, et al. Coronary artery bypass grafting with single cross-clamp results in fewer persistent neuropsychological deficits than multiple clamp or off-pump coronary artery bypass grafting.)*

Barbiturates reduce cerebral metabolism by decreasing spontaneous synaptic activity[55] and provide a definite neuroprotective effect during clinical cardiac surgery with CPB.[56] Unfortunately, these agents delay emergence from anesthesia and prolong intensive care unit stays. A study of high-risk patients randomized to aprotinin or placebo found a powerful protective effect against stroke for full-dose aprotinin in patients undergoing coronary artery bypass graft surgery.[57] However, renal and cardiac toxic side effects limit effectiveness. NMDA (N-methyl-D-aspartate) antagonists, which are effective in animals, provide mild protection compared with control patients but have a high incidence of neurologic side effects.[58] A small study demonstrated a neuroprotective effect of lidocaine, but this beneficial effect has not been reproduced.[59] Currently, no pharmacologic agent is recommended for protection of the central nervous system during CPB.

Off-pump myocardial revascularization theoretically avoids many of the causes of cerebral injury due to CPB, but as noted before, many causes of neuronal injury are independent of CPB and related to atherosclerosis and air entry sites into the circulation. Nonrandomized measurements of carotid emboli by Doppler ultrasonography indicate fewer emboli and slightly improved neurocognitive outcomes in high-risk patients who have off-pump surgery.[60] Clinical trials of off-pump versus on-pump patients failed to show a significant difference in neurologic outcome between methods.[61]

PROGNOSIS

Patients with intraoperative stroke or who develop stroke symptoms in the first week after surgery often improve in direct relation to the lesion size and location on imaging studies. Neuropsychological deficits that are present after 3 months are almost always permanent.[62] Assessments after that time are confounded by development of new deficits, particularly in aged patients.[63,64]

The difficulty of separating intraoperative brain injury from that which occurs in the early or late postoperative period has been recently addressed by a reanalysis of data published earlier. The authors tracked specific neuropsychological deficits that persisted unchanged for 6 months (persistent deficits) and separated them from new deficits that appeared after surgery (Fig. 65-4).[65] By use of this technique, it is possible to accurately measure surgical brain injury and to design techniques to eliminate this important cause of morbidity. Late follow-up studies should include a control group with similar risk factors but not having cardiac operations.[66] This technique demonstrated similar outcomes in surgical and nonsurgical controls at 3 years, putting to rest the previous fear that surgical patients had recurrent neurocognitive deficits and were thus at greater risk for poor long-term outcomes.[62] In one study, a group of surgical patients who were evaluated with preoperative and postoperative neuropsychological studies had rigid control of cardiovascular risk factors.[67] They demonstrated no delayed or late cognitive decline, offering hope that aggressive medical therapy can complement skillful surgery in preventing neurologic injury.

REFERENCES

1. Shaw PJ, Bates D, Cartlidge NE, French JM, Heaviside D, Julian DG, Shaw DA. Long-term intellectual dysfunction following coronary artery bypass surgery: a six month follow-up study. *Q J Med* 1987;**62**:259-68.
2. Newman S. The incidence and nature of neuropsychological morbidity following cardiac surgery. *Perfusion* 1989;**4**:93-100.
3. Svensson LG, Nadolny EM, Kimmel WA. Multimodal protocol influence on stroke and neurocognitive deficit prevention after ascending/arch aortic operations. *Ann Thorac Surg* 2002;**74**:2040-6.
4. Newman S, Smith P, Treasure T, et al. Acute neuropsychological consequences of coronary artery bypass surgery. *Curr Psychol Res Rev* 1987;**6**:115-24.

5. Murkin JM, Stump DA, Blumenthal JA, et al. Defining dysfunction: group means versus incidence analysis—a statement of consensus. *Ann Thorac Surg* 1997;**64**:904-5.
6. Selnes OA, Grega MA, Bailey MM, et al. Neurocognitive outcomes 3 years after coronary artery bypass graft surgery: a controlled study. *Ann Thorac Surg* 2007;**84**:1885-96.
7. Baird A, Benfield A, Schlaug G, et al. Enlargement of human cerebral ischemic lesion volumes measured by diffusion-weighted magnetic resonance imaging. *Ann Neurol* 1997;**41**:581-9.
8. Bendszus M, Reents W, Franke D, et al. Brain damage after coronary artery bypass grafting. *Arch Neurol* 2002;**59**:1090-5.
9. Rosen B, Belliveau J, Vevea J, et al. Perfusion imaging with NMR contrast agents. *Magn Reson Med* 1990;**14**:249-65.
10. Maragos PJ, Schmechel DE. Neuron-specific enolase, a clinically useful marker for neurons and neuroendocrine cells. *Annu Rev Neuro Sci* 1987;**10**:269-95.
11. Persson L, Hardemark HG, Gustafsson J, et al. S-100 protein and neuron-specific enolase in cerebrospinal fluid and serum: markers of cell damage in human central nervous system. *Stroke* 1987;**18**:911-8.
12. Zimmer DB, Cornwall EH, Landar A, Song W. The S-100 protein family: history, function, and expression. *Brain Res Bull* 1995;**37**:417-29.
13. Johnsson P, Blomquist S, Luhrs C, et al. Neuron-specific enolase increases in plasma during and immediately after extracorporeal circulation. *Ann Thorac Surg* 2000;**69**:750-4.
14. Anderson RE, Hansson LO, Liska J, et al. The effect of cardiotomy suction on the brain injury marker S100 beta after cardiopulmonary bypass. *Ann Thorac Surg* 2000;**69**:847-50.
15. Shaw PJ, Bates D, Cartlidge NE, et al. Neurologic and neuropsychological morbidity following major surgery: comparison of coronary artery bypass and peripheral vascular surgery. *Stroke* 1987;**18**:700-7.
16. Gardner TJ, Horneffer PJ, Manolio TA, et al. Stroke following coronary artery bypass surgery: a ten-year study. *Ann Thorac Surg* 1985;**40**:574-81.
17. Moller JT, Cluitmans P, Rasmussen LS, et al. Long-term postoperative cognitive dysfunction in the elderly ISPOCD study. ISPOCD investigators. International Study of Post-Operative Cognitive Dysfunction. *Lancet* 1998;**351**:857-61.
18. Jones EL, Weintraub WS, Craver JM, et al. Coronary bypass surgery: is the operation different today? *J Thorac Cardiovasc Surg* 1991;**101**:108-15.
19. Tardiff BE, Newman MF, Saunders AM, et al. Preliminary report of a genetic basis for cognitive decline after cardiac operations. *Ann Thorac Surg* 1997;**64**:715-20.
20. Roach GW, Kanchuger M, Mangano CM, et al. Adverse cerebral outcomes after coronary bypass surgery. Multicenter Study of Perioperative Ischemia Research Group and the Ischemia Research and Education Foundation Investigators. *N Engl J Med* 1996;**335**:1857-63.
21. Weintraub WS, Wenger NK, Jones EL, et al. Changing clinical characteristics of coronary surgery patients: differences between men and women. *Circulation* 1993;**88**:79-86.
22. Goto T, Baba T, Yoshitake A, et al. Craniocervical and aortic atherosclerosis as neurologic risk factors in coronary surgery. *Ann Thorac Surg* 2000;**69**:834-40.
23. Wareing TH, Davila-Roman VG, Daily BB, et al. Strategy for the reduction of stroke incidence in cardiac surgical patients. *Ann Thorac Surg* 1993;**55**:1400-8.
24. Stump DA, Kon NA, Rogers AT, et al. Emboli neuropsychologic outcome following cardiopulmonary bypass. *Echocardiography* 1996;**13**:555-8.
25. Tuman KJ, McCarthy RJ, Najafi H, et al. Differential effects of advanced age on neurologic and cardiac risks of coronary operations. *J Thorac Cardiovasc Surg* 1992;**104**:1510-7.
26. Lata A, Stump D, Deal D, et al. Cannula design reduces particulate and gaseous emboli during cardiopulmonary bypass for coronary artery bypass grafting. Ann Thoracic Surg (in press).
27. Jones TJ, Stump DA, Deal D, et al. Hypothermia protects the brain from embolization by reducing and redirecting the embolic load. *Ann Thorac Surg* 1999;**68**:1465.
28. Gold JP, Charlson ME, Williams-Russo P. Improvement of outcomes after coronary artery bypass; a randomized trial comparing high versus low mean arterial pressure. *J Thorac Cardiovasc Surg* 1995;**110**:1302-14.
29. Murkin JM, Farrar JK, Tweed WA, et al. Cerebral autoregulation and flow/metabolism coupling during cardiopulmonary bypass: the role of Paco$_2$. *Anesth Analg* 1987;**66**:665-72.
30. Hill AG, Groom RC, Tewksbury L, et al. Sources of gaseous microemboli during cardiopulmonary bypass. *Proc Am Acad Cardiovasc Perfus* 1998;**9**:122-30.
31. Blauth Cl. Macroemboli and microemboli during cardiopulmonary bypass. *Ann Thorac Surg* 1995;**59**:1300-3.
32. Stump DA, Brown WR, Moody DM, et al. Microemboli and neurologic dysfunction after cardiovascular surgery. *Semin Cardiothorac Vasc Anesth* 1999;**3**:47-54.
33. Helps SC, Parsons DW, Reilly PL, et al. The effect of gas emboli on rabbit cerebral blood flow. *Stroke* 1990;**21**:94-9.
34. Moody DM, Brown WR, Challa VR, et al. Efforts to characterize the nature and chronicle the occurrence of brain emboli during cardiopulmonary bypass. *Perfusion* 1995;**9**:316-9.
35. Cook DJ, Oliver WC, Orsulak TA, et al. Cardiopulmonary bypass temperature, hematocrit, and cerebral oxygen delivery in humans. *Ann Thorac Surg* 1995;**60**:1671-7.
36. Martin TC, Craver JM, Gott MP, et al. Prospective, randomized trial of retrograde warm-blood cardioplegia: myocardial benefit and neurological threat. *Ann Thorac Surg* 1994;**59**:298-304.
37. Engelman RM, Pleet AB, Rouson JA, et al. What is the best perfusion temperature for coronary revascularization? *J Thorac Cardiovasc Surg* 1996;**112**:1622-33.
38. Avraamides EJ, Murkin JM. The effect of surgical dislocation of the heart on cerebral blood flow in the presence of a single, two-stage venous cannula during cardiopulmonary bypass. *Can J Anaesth* 1996;**43**:A36.
39. Downing SW, Edmunds Jr LH. Release of vasoactive substances during cardiopulmonary bypass. *Ann Thorac Surg* 1992;**54**:1236-43.
40. Warren JS, Ward PA, et al. The inflammatory response. In: Beutler E, Coller BS, Lichtman MA, editors. *Williams Hematology*. 6th ed. New York: McGraw-Hill; 2001. p. 67.
41. Wewers MD. Cytokines and macrophages. In: Remick DG, Friedland JS, editors. Cytokines in health and disease. 2nd ed. New York: Marcel Dekker; 1997, p. 339.
42. Fantone JC. Cytokines and neutrophils: neutrophil-derived cytokines and the inflammatory response. In: Remick DG, Friedland JS, editors. Cytokines in health and disease. 2nd ed. New York: Marcel Dekker; 1997, p. 373.
43. Kincaid EH, Jones TJ, Stump DA, et al. Processing scavenged blood with a cell saver reduces cerebral lipid microembolization. *Ann Thorac Surg* 2000;**70**:1296-300.
44. Reichenspurner H, Navia JA, Benny G, et al. Particulate embolic capture by an intra-aortic filter device during cardiac surgery. *J Thorac Cardiovasc Surg* 2000;**119**:233-44.
45. Cook DJ, Zehr KJ, Orszulak TA, Slater JM. Profound reduction in brain embolization using an endoaortic baffle during bypass in swine. *Ann Thorac Surg* 2002;**73**:198-202.
46. Barzilai B, Marshall Jr WG, Saffitz JE, et al. Avoidance of embolic complications by ultrasonic characterization of the ascending aorta. *Circulation* 1989;**80**:1275-9.
47. Macoviak JA, Hwang J, Boerjan KL, Deal DD. Comparing dual-stream and standard cardiopulmonary bypass in pigs. *Ann Thorac Surg* 2002;**73**:203-8.
48. Hammon JW, Stump DA, Butterworth JE, et al. Single cross clamp improves six month cognitive outcome in high risk coronary bypass patients. *J Thorac Cardiovasc Surg* 2006;**131**:114-21.
49. Loop FD, Higgins TL, Panda R, et al. Myocardial protection during cardiac operations: decreased morbidity and lower cost with blood cardioplegia and coronary sinus perfusion. *J Cardiovasc Surg* 1992;**104**:608-18.
50. Sundt TM, Barner HB, Camillo CJ, et al. Total arterial revascularization with an internal thoracic artery and radial artery T graft. *Ann Thorac Surg* 1999;**68**:399-405.
51. Tector AJ, Amundsen S, Schmahl TM, et al. Total revascularization with T grafts. *Ann Thorac Surg* 1994;**57**:33-9.
52. Jones TJ, Deal DD, Vernon JC, et al. The propagation of entrained air during cardiopulmonary bypass is affected by circuit design but not by vacuum assisted venous drainage. *Ann Thorac Surg* 2002;**74**:2132-7.
53. Nathan HJ, Wells GA, Munson JL, Wozny D. Neuroprotective effect of mild hypothermia in patients undergoing coronary artery surgery with cardiopulmonary bypass. *Circulation* 2001;**104**(suppl. I):I85-95.
54. Brown R, Wright G, Royston D. A comparison of two systems for assessing cerebral venous oxyhaemoglobin saturation during cardiopulmonary bypass in humans. *Anaesthesia* 1993;**48**:697-700.
55. Michenfelder JD. The interdependency of cerebral functional and metabolic effects following massive doses of thiopental in the dog. *Anesthesiology* 1974;**41**:231-6.
56. Nussmeier N, Arlund C, Slogoff S. Neuropsychiatric complications after cardiopulmonary bypass: cerebral protection by a barbiturate. *Anesthesiology* 1986;**64**:165-70.
57. Frumento RJ, O'Malley CM, Bennett-Guerrero E. Stroke after cardiac surgery: a retrospective analysis of the effects of aprotinin dosing regimens. *Ann Thorac Surg* 2003;**75**:479-83.
58. Arrowsmith JE, Harrison MJ, Newman SP, et al. Neuroprotection of the brain during cardiopulmonary bypass: a randomized trial of remacemide during coronary artery bypass in 171 patients. *Stroke* 1998;**29**:2357-62.
59. Mitchell SJ, Pellet O, Gorman DF, et al. Cerebral protection by lidocaine during cardiac operations. *Ann Thorac Surg* 1999;**67**:1117-24.
60. Diegeler A, Hirsch R, Schneider F, et al. Neuromonitoring and neurocognitive outcome in off-pump versus conventional coronary bypass operation. *Ann Thorac Surg* 2000;**69**:1162-6.

61. Puskas J, Cheng D, Knight J, et al. Off-pump versus conventional coronary artery bypass grafting: a meta-analysis and consensus statement from the 2004 ISMICS consensus conference. *Innov Cardiothorac Surg* 2005;**1**:3-27.
62. Newman MF, Kirchner JL, Phillips-Bute B, et al. Longitudinal assessment of neurocognitive function after coronary artery bypass grafting. *N Engl J Med* 2001;**344**:395-402.
63. Sotaniemi KA. Cerebral outcome after extracorporeal circulation: comparison between prospective and retrospective evaluations. *Arch Neurol* 1983;**40**:75-7.
64. Vermeer SE, Longstreth Jr WT, Koudstaal PJ. Silent brain infarcts: a systematic review. *Lancet Neurol* 2007;**6**:611-9.
65. Hammon JW, Stump DA, Butterworth JF, et al. Coronary artery bypass grafting with single cross-clamp results in fewer persistent neuropsychological deficits than multiple clamp or off-pump coronary artery bypass grafting. *Ann Thorac Surg* 2007;**84**:1174-9.
66. Selnes OA, Grega MA, Borowicz LM, et al. Cognitive outcomes three years after coronary bypass surgery: a comparison of on-pump coronary bypass surgery and nonsurgical controls. *Ann Thorac Surg* 2005;**79**:1201-9.
67. Mullges W, Babin-Ebell J, Reents W, Toyka KV. Cognitive performance after coronary bypass grafting: a follow-up study. *Neurology* 2002;**59**:741-3.

CHAPTER 66
Clinical Quality and Safety in Cardiac Surgery
Justine M. Carr

National Landscape for Quality and Safety
Evolving Landscape of Quality and Safety in Cardiac Surgery
Safe and Effective Care of Cardiac Surgery Patients
  Perioperative Care
    Pre-procedure Verification, Marking, and Time Out
    Antibiotic Administration
    Preoperative Beta-Blockade
    Postoperative Glucose Control
  Postoperative Morbidity
    Ventilator-Associated Pneumonia
    Central Line Infections
    Deep Sternal Wound Infections
    Response to Changes in a Patient's Condition
  Medication Safety
    Medication Reconciliation
    Active Involvement of Patients in Their Own Care
    Communication among Caregivers
  Measurement of Care
Conclusion

At the turn of the 20th century, Dr. Ernest A. Codman (1869-1940) was rejected by the Boston medical community for his maverick ideas supporting the evaluation and publication of surgical outcomes. Codman eventually founded his own hospital dedicated to the study of "end results" and published his outcomes.[1] His work was seminal in the establishment of the American College of Surgeons and the Joint Commission. A half-century later, the Boston medical community redeemed itself with the landmark report by Beecher and Todd, "A Study of the Deaths Associated with Anesthesia and Surgery."[2] Death was the designated outcome, as it was the one that could be agreed on by all investigators.[3] Two decades later, the focus shifted to the application of the critical incident technique and identification of remediable factors that contribute to anesthesia-related morbidity and mortality, and the eventual creation of the Anesthesia Patient Safety Foundation.[4-6]

In the spirit of Codman's focus on end results and the Anesthesia Patient Safety Foundation's focus on remediation, cardiac surgeons have played a major role in the study of outcomes and the implementation of quality improvement techniques. The relative uniformity and limited types of cardiac operations, together with their case volume, aggregate cost, and high public profile, impelled interested stakeholders to quantify outcomes. In 1972, the Department of Veterans Affairs (VA) created a Cardiac Surgery Consultants Committee Advisory Group, which resulted in the first multi-institutional cardiac surgery outcomes database. Until 1988, the main outcomes were volume and unadjusted mortality.[7] In 1987, the Health Care Financing Administration (HCFA) published raw institution-specific mortality rates for Medicare patients.[8] Mortality rates were generated for entire hospitals in aggregate, as well as for specific diagnosis-related groups (DRGs), including coronary artery bypass grafting (CABG). With growing concern over the confusion developing from raw mortality rates, the VA introduced a risk-adjustment model and created what is now known as the VA Continuous Improvement in Cardiac Surgery Program.[9] Motivated by both clinical and statistical imperatives, in 1989 the Society of Thoracic Surgeons (STS) developed its own voluntary, risk-adjusted database for cardiac surgery. Also in 1989, Parsonnet and colleagues pioneered a predictive model that classified patients into five groups of increasing operative risk according to 14 preoperative risk factors.[10] The model proved to be highly predictive when applied to a large number of patients in three hospitals. The 1990s saw the development of various statistical methods to adjust for preoperative risk hazard as well as social and geographic differences.[11,12] In 1987 in New England, a consortium of hospitals, the Northern New England Cardiovascular Disease Study Group, began to collect data uniformly in a common registry.[13] The Alabama Coronary Artery Bypass Grafting Cooperative project gathered data beginning in 1995.[14] However, among these and other registries established in the early and mid-1990s, the universal finding was that operative mortality varied widely among institutions, even after risk adjustment.[14-16] This observation presaged complementary movements: (1) public reporting of statewide outcomes and (2) strategic interventions to improve outcomes. Hannan and coworkers' studies of CABG mortality in New York State led to the first statewide reporting of operative mortality.[17,18] Statutory requirement for public reporting was subsequently adopted in Pennsylvania, New Jersey, and Massachusetts.[19-21]

An equally important result has been the cooperative analysis of outcomes with a focus on performance improvement. The Northern New England Cardiovascular Disease Study Group became a leader in this movement, in which surgeons, cardiologists, anesthesiologists, nurses, and perfusionists collaborated to review data and current practice, target key variables that drive outcomes, and organize improvement projects, such as inter-institutional site visits and study protocols, with resultant decline in CABG mortality.[15] A number of regional, national, and even international groups have followed this registry and quality improvement model, establishing benchmarks for the cardiac surgical "industry."[22-24]

Around the turn of the 21st century, national specialty societies began establishing guidelines for the application of interventional and surgical technologies. The American College

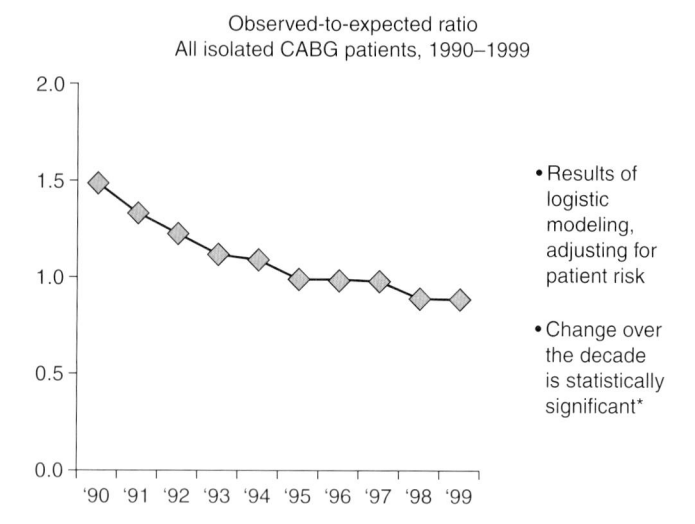

Figure 66-1
Observed-to-expected ratio for all isolated coronary artery bypass graft patients) from 1990 to 1999. Graph shows the results of logistic modeling for patient risk. The decline over the decade is statistically significant ($P < .0001$) for the trend (1990-1999). *(From Grover FL. The bright future of cardiothoracic surgery. Ann Thorac Surg 2008;**85**:8-24.)*

Box 66–1
Types of Medical Errors

Diagnostic
- Error or delay in diagnosis
- Failure to employ indicated tests
- Use of outmoded tests or therapy
- Failure to act on results of monitoring or testing

Treatment
- Error in the performance of an operation, procedure, or test
- Error in administering the treatment
- Error in the dosage or method of using a drug
- Avoidable delay in treatment or in responding to an abnormal test
- Inappropriate (not indicated) care

Preventive
- Failure to provide prophylactic treatment
- Inadequate monitoring or follow-up of treatment

Other
- Failure of communication
- Equipment failure
- Other system failure

*Adapted from Leape L, Lawthers AG, Brennan TA, et al. Preventing medical injury. Qual Rev Bull 1993;**19**:144-9.*

---

of Cardiology (ACC) and American Heart Association (AHA) published their first Guidelines for Coronary Bypass Surgery in 1999, with an update in 2005.[25,26] These include class I, useful and effective; class IIa, evidence favors usefulness; class IIb, evidence less well established; class III, not useful or effective, and in some cases harmful. Similar guidelines have been established for valvular surgery.[27,28]

The net impact of all these activities is dramatically apparent when viewing the decline in the ratio of observed (O) to expected (E) CABG mortality of patients, as measured by the STS database. In 1990 the O-to-E ratio was 1.49, and by 1999 it was 0.88, $P < .0001$ (Fig. 66-1).[29]

NATIONAL LANDSCAPE FOR QUALITY AND SAFETY

In addition to quality and safety initiatives specific to cardiac surgery, there has been a major cultural change nationally over the past decade. Leadership in the prioritization of quality and safety has come from the Institute of Medicine (IOM). In a groundbreaking publication in 1999, "To Err Is Human," the IOM made several important contributions.[30] First, the report estimated that up to 98,000 patients per year may have died as a result of medical error. They identified that errors are often caused by faulty systems, processes, and conditions. They cited the work of Lucian Leape and colleagues, who codified four types of errors: diagnostic, treatment, preventive, and other (Box 6-1).[31]

To achieve a better safety record, the IOM report recommended a four-tiered approach:

1. Establishing a national focus to create leadership, research, tools, and protocols to enhance the knowledge base about safety.
2. Identifying and learning from errors by developing a nationwide public mandatory reporting system and by encouraging health-care organizations and practitioners to develop and participate in voluntary reporting systems.
3. Raising performance standards and expectations of improvements in safety through the actions of oversight organizations, professional groups, and group purchasers of health care.
4. Implementing safety systems in health-care organizations to ensure safe practices at the delivery level (i.e., a culture of safety).

Two years later, the IOM published another landmark report, "Crossing the Quality Chasm,"[32] which set a national agenda aimed at narrowing differences in quality among providers of medical care. Instead of attention to a single outcome, the IOM focused on the quality of the entire patient experience, defining it in six key dimensions as being *"safe, effective, efficient, timely, patient-centered, and equitable."* The model promulgated a balanced approach to assessment of quality, incorporating clinical outcomes with patient experience and the appropriate allocation of resources. Furthermore, the report identified key redesign imperatives for care delivery:

- Reengineered care processes
- Effective use of information technologies
- Knowledge and skills management
- Development of effective teams
- Coordination of care across patients—conditions, services, sites of care—over time

These two IOM reports raised the bar to a new level of excellence that transcended the expertise of a single care provider. In 2006, a third IOM report, "Performance Measurement: Accelerating Improvement," laid the groundwork for performance measurement.[33] Achieving excellence now required a careful orchestration of care delivery, incorporating evidence-based care processes, as well as coordinated care infrastructure across the care delivery continuum—both inpatient and outpatient. Hardwiring for excellence became a priority, leading the Joint Commission (formerly known as JCAHO) to begin requiring demonstration of evidence-based and safe practices in the delivery of care. Payers and purchasers followed suit. The Centers for Medicare and Medicaid Services (CMS) instituted the requirement for submission of "core measures," evidence-based practices in the care of patients with acute myocardial infarction, heart failure, pneumonia, and selected surgeries (including cardiac surgery).

Another key player has been the National Quality Forum (NQF), a public–private partnership created to develop and implement a national strategy for health-care quality measurement and reporting. NQF member organizations have worked together to promote a common approach to measuring health-care quality and fostering system-wide capacity for quality improvement. Yet another influence has come from the Leapfrog Group, an association of private and public sector group purchasers, who have created a market-based strategy to improve safety and quality. Their public ranking includes recognition for the use of computerized provider order entry, evidence-based hospital referrals, and the staffing of intensive care units with physicians credentialed in critical care medicine.

An outcome of these various national initiatives is the standardization of surgical care. Postoperative complications have a significant impact on mortality, length of stay (3 to 11 days), and cost.[34] Increased costs of complications are estimated to be $1398 per patient for infectious complications, $7789 per patient for cardiovascular complications, $52,466 per patient for respiratory complications, and $1810 per patient for thromboembolic complications.[35] In 2002, CMS, in collaboration with the Centers for Disease Control and Prevention, implemented the National Surgical Infection Prevention Project with the goal of decreasing the morbidity and mortality associated with postoperative surgical site infections by promoting appropriate selection and timing of prophylactic antimicrobials.[36] In April 2003, this group joined with representatives of the VA, the American College of Surgeons, the American Society of Anesthesiologists, the Agency for Healthcare Research and Quality, the American Hospital Association, and the Institute for Healthcare Improvement, to align efforts to reduce surgical complications and mortality. This collaboration resulted in the development of the Surgical Care Improvement Project (SCIP), a national quality partnership of organizations committed to improving the safety of surgical care through the reduction of postoperative complications.[36] The SCIP steering committee established a national goal of reducing preventable surgical morbidity and mortality by 25% by 2010. The rapid rate of adoption of the SCIP measures can be tracked on the CMS website Hospital Compare (www.hospitalcompare.hhs.gov), showing percent compliance with these measures in hospitals across the country.

EVOLVING LANDSCAPE OF QUALITY AND SAFETY IN CARDIAC SURGERY

From 1989 to 2007, the STS database grew to become the largest and most comprehensive single-specialty clinical database in health care in the world.[37] In view of the increasing interest of payers and regulators to compare cardiac surgery quality, the STS established a Quality Measurement Task Force (QMTF). Their goal was to develop a methodology for comprehensive assessment of adult cardiac surgery quality of care. The assessment was to include both individual measures and a composite quality score. Guiding principles included the following[38]:

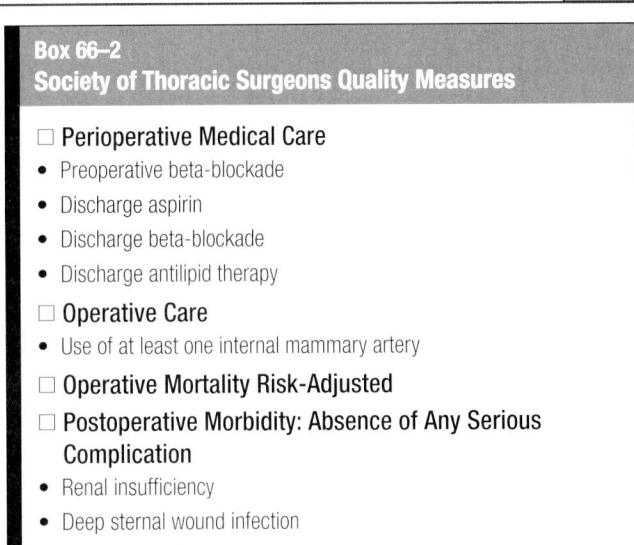

- Quality assessment should be at the level of the program or hospital, rather than the individual surgeon.
- Initial quality reports should focus on coronary artery bypass grafting surgery.
- Quality measures should be chosen from among those endorsed by the National Quality Forum.
- Quality measure selection should be consistent with the principles and criteria recommended in the 2006 Institute of Medicine report "Performance Measurement: Accelerating Improvement."
- Quality measures should be available as data elements in the STS National Adult Cardiac Surgery Database.
- Quality scores should take into account structure, process, and outcomes.
- Quality scores should assess three temporal domains—preoperative, operative, and postoperative.
- Quality scores should satisfy multiple criteria for validity.
- Quality scores should be interpretable and actionable by providers.

In 2007, the STS QMTF created 11 measures within four domains: perioperative medical care, intraoperative care, risk-adjusted operative mortality, and postoperative morbidity.[39] Statistical analysis was based on actual 2004 STS data, representing 133,149 coronary artery bypass procedures.[38] The STS QMTF measures are listed in Box 66-2. Table 66-1 summarizes the impressive array of measure from the Leapfrog Group, CMS, and the Joint Commission that have been

---

Box 66–2
Society of Thoracic Surgeons Quality Measures

☐ **Perioperative Medical Care**
- Preoperative beta-blockade
- Discharge aspirin
- Discharge beta-blockade
- Discharge antilipid therapy

☐ **Operative Care**
- Use of at least one internal mammary artery

☐ **Operative Mortality Risk-Adjusted**

☐ **Postoperative Morbidity: Absence of Any Serious Complication**
- Renal insufficiency
- Deep sternal wound infection
- Reexploration for any cause
- Stroke
- Prolonged ventilation/intubation

Adapted from Shahian DM, Edwards FH, Ferraris VA, et. al. Quality measurement in adult cardiac surgery. Part 1: conceptual framework and measure selection. Ann Thorac Surg 2007;**83** (Suppl):S3-12.

Table 66-1

Summary of Cardiac Surgery Quality Measures

Category	Measure	NQF	CMS	STS (CABG)	Joint Commission
Measurement	Participation in a systematic database for cardiac surgery	X	P	NA	
Volume	Surgical volume for isolated coronary artery bypass graft (CABG) surgery, valve surgery, and CABG + valve surgery	X			
Perioperative care	Conduct a pre-procedure verification process, making the procedure site, performing time out				NPSG
	Timing of antibiotic administration for cardiac surgery patients	X	R		R
	Selection of antibiotic administration for cardiac surgery patients	X	R		R
	Preoperative beta-blockade	X	P	X	
	Duration of prophylaxis for cardiac surgery patients	X	R		R
	Antiplatelet medications at discharge	X		X	
	Beta-blockade at discharge	X		X	
	Antilipid treatment at discharge	X		X	
	Glucose control postoperatively		R		
Operative care	Use of internal mammary artery	X		X	
Postoperative morbidity	Prolonged intubation	X		X	
	Ventilator-associated pneumonia				NPSG
	Central line infection				NPSG
	Deep sternal wound infection rate	X		X	NPSG
	Stroke/cerebrovascular accident rate	X		X	
	Postoperative renal insufficiency rate	X		X	
	Surgical reexploration rate	X		X	
	Improve recognition and response to changes in a patient's condition				NPSG
Mortality	Risk-adjusted inpatient operative mortality for CABG	X			
	Risk-adjusted operative mortality for CABG 30 day	X		X	
	Risk-adjusted operative mortality for aortic valve replacement (AVR)	X			
	Risk-adjusted operative mortality for mitral valve replacement (MVR)	X			
	Risk-adjusted operative mortality for MVR + CABG	X			
	Risk-adjusted operative mortality for AVR + CABG	X			
Effective communication	Improve effectiveness of communication among caregivers				NPSG
	Encourage patients' active involvement in their own care as a patient safety strategy				NPSG
Medications	Improve safety of using medications				NPSG
	Accurately and completely reconcile medications across the continuum of care				NPSG

CMS, Centers for Medicare and Medicaid Services; NA, not measured because measurements are only reported on STS participants; NPSG, Joint Commission National Patient Safety Goal; NQF, National Quality Forum; P, pending; R, reporting required; STS, Society of Thoracic Surgeons; X, measured.

developed and endorsed, and that are in use 10 years after the first IOM report.

SAFE AND EFFECTIVE CARE OF CARDIAC SURGERY PATIENTS

Defining best practice through quality and safety measures has been a major accomplishment. Implementing these measures has proved to be a challenge because it has required a reengineering of workflow and, in some cases, a redesigning of care delivery. Successful implementation of best practices depends on teamwork across medical specialties and across disciplines, as well as with the patients and their families. The interventions that can contribute to the quality and safety of care delivered to cardiac surgery patients follow.

Perioperative Care

Pre-procedure Verification, Marking, and Time Out

Much has been written about the importance of the Universal Protocol for Preventing Wrong Site, Wrong Procedure, and Wrong Person Surgery, and few would dispute the value of this pre-procedure checking.[40-43] Although a major focus was initially on operating room (OR) procedures, the Universal Protocol applies to most other procedures that involve puncture or incision of the skin, or insertion of an instrument or foreign material into the body—for example, peripherally inserted central catheter lines, percutaneous aspirations, biopsies, cardiac and vascular catheterizations, and endoscopies. Growing experience has demonstrated the value of hardwiring the Universal Protocol with specific rules and clear accountability. Who is the person who is accountable for each of these steps—doing and signing off? When do these steps occur? Who must be present for the verification? The marking? The time out (i.e., to conduct a final check for correct patient, procedure, site)? Workflow must be reengineered to ensure the availability of critical parties. Introduction of stopgap measures is helpful (e.g., the blade is not put on the scalpel until the time out is completed). Most important is the culture of safety that ensures that every member of the team is empowered to speak up with any concern at any time.

Antibiotic Administration

The goal of antibiotic prophylaxis is to use an agent that is safe and cost-effective, and that has a spectrum of action that covers most of the probable intraoperative organisms. Antibiotic administration must be completed before incision and should not be given more than 1 hour before excision (except for vancomycin, which can be 2 hours). Antibiotic selection should align with evidence-based recommendations. There should be coordination between anesthesiologist and surgeon. Communication from surgeon to anesthesiologist about antibiotic selection is most effective when it occurs in a standardized fashion. Reasons for exceptions to standard antibiotic protocol need to be documented and communicated. Pharmacy staff also needs to be in the communication loop to ensure that drug preparations are available for timely infusion and completion before surgery. Postoperative orders need to be clear about the number of postoperative antibiotic doses due, and by what time the last dose should be completed to stay within the 48-hour postoperative window. Although there is some evidence that single-dose prophylaxis or 24-hour prophylaxis may be as effective as 48-hour prophylaxis, the STS published a practice guideline recommending 48 hours of prophylaxis, because few studies have directly compared 24 hours of prophylaxis with 48 hours of prophylaxis.[44] However, prophylaxis should be concluded at 48 hours, because administration for longer periods has been associated with an increased risk of infection with drug-resistant organisms.[45]

Preoperative Beta-Blockade

An observational analysis of 629,877 patients undergoing CABG between 1996 and 1999 demonstrated that preoperative beta-blocker therapy was associated with a small but consistent survival benefit, except among patients with a left ventricular ejection fraction of less than 30%.[46] Furthermore, many studies have demonstrated the benefit of preoperative beta-blockers in reducing the incidence of postoperative atrial fibrillation.[47] Atrial fibrillation occurs in up to one third of patients after open heart surgery. In an analysis of 52 published studies representing nearly 10,000 patients undergoing open heart surgery, supraventricular tachycardias, including atrial fibrillation, occurred in 29% of patients who did not receive prophylactic drugs and in 19% of patients given beta-blockers.[47]

Postoperative Glucose Control

Glucose control through continuous infusion of insulin has been shown to reduce mortality and surgical site infections in both diabetic and nondiabetic patients.[48-51] Intraoperatively, several factors contribute to hyperglycemia, including cardiopulmonary bypass (CPB) pump prime fluid composition, temperature while on CPB, and medications such as catecholamines and glucocorticoids.[52] The current measure of glucose control is based on the value identified at 6 AM postoperatively, with a goal of less than or equal to 200 mg/dL. During the first 24 postoperative hours, glucose control is best achieved through intravenous insulin titrated on a sliding scale, based on fingerstick glucose levels measured every 1 to 2 hours, and this requires effective nursing leadership. Protocols should incorporate mechanisms to recognize when the patient's endogenous glucose regulation begins to normalize, so as to avoid hypoglycemia. Full implementation of these interventions requires careful orchestration of critical care staff members, including nursing, respiratory therapy, midlevel practitioners, and physicians, with clear designation of accountability for tracking and reporting.

Postoperative Morbidity

Ventilator-Associated Pneumonia

Most cardiac surgery patients are extubated within a day of surgery. However, for those who remain intubated for longer, meticulous attention to prevention of ventilator-associated pneumonia (VAP) is critical. VAP is an airway infection that develops more than 48 hours after intubation. Ventilated patients with VAP have a mortality of 46% as compared with 32% for ventilated patients without VAP.[53] On the basis of a growing body of literature, the Institute for Health Care Improvement identified four best practices that can decrease the incidence of VAP: (1) elevation of the head of the bed, (2) daily "sedation vacations" and assessment of readiness to extubate, (3) peptic ulcer disease prophylaxis, and (4) deep venous thrombosis prophylaxis.[54,55]

Central Line Infections

Central line infections are another source of morbidity and mortality, with mortality estimates ranging from 4% to 20%.[56] The Institute for Health Care Improvement recommends five key interventions to decrease central line infections: (1) hand hygiene; (2) maximal barrier precautions on insertion; (3) chlorhexidine skin antisepsis; (4) optimal catheter site selection, with subclavian vein as the preferred site for nontunneled catheters; (5) daily review of line necessity, with prompt removal of unnecessary lines. As with VAP, reduction in central line infection is a shared responsibility of all of the critical care staff.[57,58]

Deep Sternal Wound Infections

Deep sternal wound infections are estimated to occur in 1% to 3% of cardiac surgery patients; they result in an in-hospital mortality of up to 20%, and, in some studies, an increase in long-term mortality as well.[59,60] Risk factors include obesity, malnutrition, diabetes mellitus, smoking, preoperative hemodynamic instability, preoperative renal failure on dialysis, use of bilateral internal thoracic arteries, and sepsis or endocarditis after CABG.[59-62] *Staphylococcus aureus* is a common pathogen.[63] Infection-reduction strategies include glucose control for diabetic as well as nondiabetic patients, reduction of colonization through a chlorhexidine scrub the night before surgery, mupirocin to the nares preoperatively and postoperatively, appropriate antibiotic selection, optimal administration time and duration of administration, and minimizing traffic in and out of the OR during surgery.[49,60-62] Surgical interventions include standardized preparation and draping, hair clipping instead of shaving, and meticulous wound closure.[60-62,64] Postoperatively, there is evidence for the benefit of sports-bra support for large-breasted patients.[62] Deep sternal wound infection (mediastinitis) is viewed as a preventable condition by CMS. Therefore, patients who develop a deep sternal wound infection during the admission for cardiac surgery no longer receive the incremental payment for this condition.

Response to Changes in a Patient's Condition

Most patients who experience a cardiac arrest in the hospital demonstrate identifiable signs of deterioration before the arrest. The most common signs are abnormal vital signs and hypoxia.[65-67] A rapid response team (RRT) is a group of clinicians who deliver emergency care to a patient at the bedside. The RRT does not replace the patient's care team but ensures that immediate assistance is available when there is a sudden deterioration. The RRT may include the critical care nurse or physician as well as a respiratory therapist. The RRT may be called at any time by anyone in the hospital to assist in the care of a patient who appears acutely ill, so as to avoid a cardiac arrest or other adverse event. Facilities that have implemented RRTs have reported a reduction in cardiac arrests and deaths, as well as a reduction in intensive care unit and hospital length of stay among survivors of cardiac arrest.[67] On surgical services, implementation of RRTs has been associated with a reduction in the incidence of respiratory failure, stroke, severe sepsis, acute renal failure, and postoperative mortality.[68]

Medication Safety

The IOM estimated that medication errors have accounted for 7000 deaths each year.[30] Injuries attributable to the use of medications are designated as adverse drug events (ADEs). Hospitalized patients who experience an ADE have a mortality rate that is nearly twice that of patients without an ADE.[69] Prevention of ADEs has been designated a national priority.[70] The Joint Commission has identified four categories of high-risk medications: anticoagulants, insulin, sedatives, and opioids. Most cardiac surgery patients receive most or all of these types of medications. Attention to administration is critical during the hospital stay, during transfers in and out of critical care or recovery units, and at discharge.

Anticoagulation errors can be reduced with the implementation of standardized protocols for initiation and dosage adjustment of warfarin and heparin. Anticoagulation protocols should specify target laboratory values and frequency of monitoring, as well as designated accountability for dose adjustments. Insulin administration protocols should also specify target glucose values and frequency of monitoring. Protocols for administration of intravenous insulin infusion outside a critical care setting should address nursing staff ratios to ensure timely and frequent glucose monitoring. Sedation and opioid protocols should address the management of sleep apnea, identifying high-risk patients in advance of surgery.[71] Timely pain assessment and control is a priority of the Joint Commission. Designating target pain scale values may be beneficial (e.g., a target of 1 to 4), noting, however, that a pain level of 0 may be a sign of overmedication and thus a risk for respiratory depression.

Medication Reconciliation

Of all medication errors, 46% occur at transition points (e.g., admission to hospital, transfer between units, discharge from hospital).[72] Medication reconciliation across the continuum of care ensures that patients receive all intended medications and no unintended medications after transitions in care locations. The Joint Commission has defined medication reconciliation as the process of comparing a patient's medication orders to all of the medications that the patient has been taking. The purpose is to avoid medication errors such as omissions, duplications, dosing errors, or drug interactions. Medication reconciliation should be performed at every transition of care in which new medications are ordered or existing orders are rewritten. The process has five steps: (1) develop a list of current medications, (2) develop a list of medications to be prescribed, (3) compare the medications on the two lists, (4) make clinical decisions based on the comparison, and (5) communicate the new list to appropriate caregivers and to the patient. Medication reconciliation has been shown to significantly decrease medication errors.[72]

Active Involvement of Patients in Their Own Care

Patients and their families play an active role in the medication reconciliation process. They should review all medications and understand both generic and proprietary names. For cardiac surgery patients being discharged on warfarin, the patient and family should receive instructions on how to take the medication, the foods and medications that can affect warfarin effectiveness, and how to recognize and what to do for signs and symptoms of bleeding. The clinician responsible for monitoring and dose adjustments should be clearly designated, and an appointment for the postdischarge blood level monitoring made.

Communication among Caregivers

Transitions across units and in and out of the hospital are periods of risk. Standardized handoffs by clinical staff are a way of ensuring that each caregiver has complete information. There must be timely and complete communication with the primary care physician who will be caring for the patient after discharge.

Measurement of Care

The IOM has provided clinicians with a clear roadmap for improvement, focusing on safety and quality and the assessment of outcomes. Regular and frequent measurement is essential to achieving and maintaining excellence. Participation in national and state databases affords the opportunity to compare performance with that achieved in benchmark institutions. However, these reports may lag by months to years, and performance measures must be tracked in real time for early detection of variances. In addition to looking at databases that are populated by manual data abstraction (e.g., that of the STS), some vendors and payers may calculate and publicize mortality rates based on proprietary risk-adjustment models derived from International Statistical Classification of Diseases and Related Health Problems (ICD)-9 codes. ICD-9 codes are assigned by coders at the time of discharge and are based on documentation in the chart from physicians, nurse practitioners, and physician assistants. The precision of the documentation has an impact on the level of detail of the ICD-9 codes assigned. Complete capture of all relevant ICD-9 codes ensures that risk-adjustment models accurately depict a patient's risk. Notable is the fact that coders cannot code from laboratory results, only from the notes of a physician or mid-level practitioner. For example, a patient who has a creatinine of 2.5 is not assigned a diagnosis of renal failure or renal insufficiency unless those words appear in the documentation. Furthermore, clinicians should review terminology definitions. "Renal failure" is major comorbidity or complication reflecting an acute rise in creatinine from baseline. "Renal insufficiency," in contrast, is a chronic steady-state condition and does not contribute to the coded risk profile.

In addition to reported measures, areas of focus or changes in practice should be accompanied by tracking measures of change. Such measures might include "time since last infection," "percent of time a patient's glucose is less than 150 mg/dL," "percent of patients extubated within target timeframe," or "percentage of CABG patients receiving red cell transfusions." Sharing these results routinely with the entire clinical team can demonstrate progress or trigger inquiry into opportunities for improvement.

Finally, a great advance in the measurement of care is the availability of the patient's own assessment of the care delivered. In 2006, CMS introduced the Hospital Consumer Assessment of Healthcare Provider Survey. The survey is administered, usually by mail, to a statistically significant subset of discharged patients. It includes questions about the treatment of pain, the communication by physicians and nurses, and the clarity of discharge instructions. Although these are publicly reported in aggregate (with a delay of months), it is possible and important to review them close to real time and stratify by surgeon.

CONCLUSION

Cardiac surgery outcomes have continued to improve over the past decade, despite the fact that the patients are sicker. Quality of care has increased as performance improvement initiatives have expanded. Initially, the focus was on the technical expertise and experience of the surgeon; this has expanded to care outside the operating room, with evidence-based processes for quality care as well as safety initiatives for prevention of complications and adverse events. The latest advance is the active involvement of patients and families in medication reconciliation and other care processes, which rounds out the care delivery team. Furthermore, measuring the patient's assessment of communication and care ensures that interventions by caregivers were effective for the patient, the most important person in the care delivery.

REFERENCES

1. *A study in hospital efficiency: as demonstrated by the first five years of a private hospital.* Boston, MA: Private publisher; 1916.
2. Beecher HK, Todd DP. A study of the deaths associated with anesthesia and surgery. *Ann Surg* 1954;**140**:2-34.
3. Todd DP. Personal communication, 1986.
4. Cooper JB, Newbower RS, Long CD, et al. Preventable anesthesia mishaps: a study of human factors. *Anesthesiology* 1978;**49**:399-406.
5. Cooper JB, Long CD, Newbower RS, et al. Critical incidents associated with intraoperative exchanges of anesthesia personnel. *Anesthesiology* 1982;**56**: 456-46.
6. Cooper JB, Newbower RS, Kitz RJ. An analysis of major errors and equipment failures in anesthesia management: considerations for prevention and detection. *Anesthesiology* 1984;**60**:34-42.
7. Database Grover F. In: Kaiser LR, Kron IL, Spray TL, editors. Mastery of cardiothoracic surgery. Philadelphia: Lippincott Williams & Wilkins; 2006. p. 326.
8. Health Care Financing Administration. *Mortality rates.* Baltimore: Department of Health and Human Resources; 1987.
9. Grover FL, Johnson RR, Shroyer AL, et al. The Veterans Affairs Continuous Improvement in Cardiac Surgery Study. *Ann Thorac Surg* 1994;**58**:1845-51.
10. Parsonnet V, Dean D, Bernstein AD. A method of uniform stratification of risk for evaluating the results of surgery in acquired adult heart disease. *Circulation* 1989;**79**(6 Pt 2):I3-12.
11. Ivanov J, Tu JV, Naylor CD. Ready-made, recalibrated, or remodeled? Issues in the use of risk indexes for assessing mortality after coronary bypass graft surgery. *Circulation* 1999;**99**:2098-104.
12. Jones RH, Hannan EL, Hammermeister KE, et al. Identification of preoperative variables needed for risk adjustment of short-term mortality after coronary artery bypass graft surgery. The Working Group Panel on the Cooperative CABG Database Project. *J Am Coll Cardiol* 1996;**28**:1478-87.
13. O'Connor GT, Plume SK, Olmstead EM, et al. A regional prospective study of in-hospital mortality associated with coronary artery bypass surgery. The Northern New England Cardiovascular Disease Study Group. *JAMA* 1991;**266**:803-9.
14. Holman WL, Peterson ED, Athanasuleas CL, et al. Alabama CABG Cooperative Project Study Group. *Ann Thorac Surg* 1999;**68**:1592-8.
15. O'Connor GT, Plume SK, Olmstead EM, et al. A regional intervention to improve the hospital mortality associated with coronary artery bypass graft surgery. The Northern New England Cardiovascular Disease Study Group. *JAMA* 1996;**275**:841-6.
16. Williams SV, Nash DB, Goldfarb N. Differences in mortality from coronary bypass graft surgery at five teaching hospitals. *JAMA* 1991;**266**:810-5.
17. Hannan EL, Kilburn H, O'Donnell JF, et al. Adult open heart surgery in New York State: an analysis of risk factors and hospital mortality rates. *JAMA* 1990;**264**:2768-74.
18. Hannan EL, Kumar D, Racz M, et al. New York State's Cardiac Surgery Reporting System: four years later. *Ann Thorac Surg* 1994;**58**:1852-7.
19. A consumer guide to coronary artery bypass graft surgery. Vol I-IF. Harrisburg: Pennsylvania Health Care Cost Containment Council, 1992-1995.
20. *Coronary artery bypass graft surgery in New Jersey.* Trenton: New Jersey Department of Health and Senior Services; 1998, 1999.
21. 105 Commonwealth of Massachusetts Regulations 130.020 (Regulations to implement the recommendations of the Cardiac Care Quality Commission created by Section 248 of Chapter 159 of the Acts of 2000).
22. Page US, Washburn T. Using tracking data to find complications that physicians miss: the case of renal failure in cardiac surgery. *Jt Comm J Qual Improv* 1997;**23**:511-20.
23. Ferguson Jr TB, Dziuban Jr SW, Edwards FH, et al. The STS national database: current changes and challenges for the new millennium. *Ann Thorac Surg* 2000;**69**:680-91.
24. Hammermeister KE, Daley J, Grover FL. Using outcomes data to improve clinical practice; what we have learned. *Ann Thorac Surg* 1994;**58**:1809-11.
25. Eagle KA, Guyton RA, Davidoff R, et al. ACC/AHA Guidelines for Coronary Artery Bypass Graft Surgery: A Report of the American College of Cardiology/American Heart Association Task Force on Practice Guidelines Committee to Revise the 1991 Guidelines for Coronary Artery Bypass Graft Surgery. American College of Cardiology/American Heart Association. *J Am Coll Cardiol* 1999;**34**:1262-347.
26. Eagle KA, Guyton RA, Davidoff R, et al. ACC/AHA Guideline Update for Coronary Artery Bypass Graft Surgery. *J Am Coll Cardiol* 2004;**44**:1146-54.
27. Bonow RO, Carabello B, de Leon AC, et al. ACC/AHA guidelines for the management of patients with valvular heart disease. A report of the American College of Cardiology/American Heart Association. Task Force on Practice Guidelines Committee on Management of Patients with Valvular Heart Disease. *J Am Coll Cardiol* 1998;**325**:1486-588.
28. Bonow RO, Carabello BA, Chatterjee K, et al. ACC/AHA 2006 Guidelines for the Management of Patients with Valvular Heart Disease. *Circulation* 2006;**114**:e84-231.
29. Grover FL. The bright future of cardiothoracic surgery in the era of changing health care delivery: an update. *Ann Thorac Surg* 2008;**85**:8-24.
30. Kohn LT, Corrigan JM, Donaldson MS, editors. Institute of Medicine Committee on Quality of Health Care in America. To err is human: building a safer health system. Washington, DC: National Academies Press; 1999.

31. Leape L, Lawthers AG, Brennan TA, et al. Preventing medical injury. *Qual Rev Bull* 1993;**19**:144-9.
32. Institute of Medicine Committee on Quality of Health Care in America. *Crossing the quality chasm: a new health system for the 21st century Institute of Medicine.* Washington, DC: National Academies Press; 2001.
33. Institute of Medicine Committee on Redesigning Health Insurance Performance Measures. *Payment, and Performance Improvement Programs. Performance measurement: accelerating improvement.* Washington, DC: National Academies Press; 2006.
34. Bratzler DW, Hunt DR. The Surgical Infection Prevention and Surgical Care Improvement Projects: national initiatives to improve outcomes for patients having surgery. *Clin Infect Dis* 2006;**43**:322-30.
35. Dimick JB, Chen SL, Taheri PA, et al. Hospital costs associated with surgical complications: a report from the private-sector National Surgical Quality Improvement Program. *J Am Coll Surg* 2004;**99**:531-7.
36. Bratzler DW, Houck PM. Antimicrobial prophylaxis for surgery: an advisory statement from the National Surgical Infection Prevention Project. *Clin Infect Dis* 2004;**38**:1706-15.
37. Grover FL. An innovative new concept for quality measurement in adult cardiac surgery. *Ann Thorac Surg* 2007;**83**:1237-9.
38. Shahian DM, Edwards FH, Ferraris VA, et al. Quality measurement in adult cardiac surgery. Part 1: conceptual framework and measure selection. *Ann Thorac Surg* 2007;**83**(Suppl.):S3-12.
39. O'Brien SM, Shahian DM, DeLong ER, et al. Quality measurement in adult cardiac surgery. Part 2: statistical considerations in composite measure scoring and provider rating. *Ann Thorac Surg* 2007;**83**(Suppl.):S13-26.
40. Carayon P, Schultz K, Hundt AS. Right wrong site surgery. *Jt Comm J Qual Safety* 2004;**30**:405-10.
41. Knight R, Galvin M, Davoren K, et al. The evolution of universal protocol in interventional radiology. *J Radiol Nursing* 2006;**25**:106-15.
42. Saufl NM. Universal protocol for preventing wrong site, wrong procedure, wrong person surgery. *J Perianesthesia Nurs* 2004;**19**:348-51.
43. Siddiqui MT. Pathologist performed fine needle aspirations & implementation of JCAHO Universal Protocol and "Time out." *Cytojournal* 2007;**4**:19.
44. Edwards FH, Engelman RM, Houck P, et al. The Society of Thoracic Surgeons practice guideline series: antibiotic prophylaxis in cardiac surgery. Part I: duration. *Ann Thorac Surg* 2006;**1**:397-404.
45. Harbarth S, Samore MH, Lichtenberg D, et al. Prolonged antibiotic prophylaxis after cardiovascular surgery and its effect on surgical site infections and antimicrobial resistance. *Circulation* 2000;**101**:2916-21.
46. Ferguson TB, Coombs LP, Peterson ED. Preoperative beta-blocker use and mortality and morbidity following CABG surgery in North America. *JAMA* 2002;**287**:2221-7.
47. DiDomenico RJ, Massad MG. Pharmacologic strategies for prevention of atrial fibrillation after open heart surgery. *Ann Thorac Surg* 2005;**79**:728-40.
48. Furnary AP, Gao G, Grunkemeier GL, et al. Continuous insulin infusion reduces mortality in patients with diabetes undergoing coronary artery bypass grafting. *J Thorac Cardiovasc Surg* 2003;**125**:1007-21.
49. Kramer R, Groom R, Weldner D, et al. Glycemic control and reduction of deep sternal wound infection rates: a multidisciplinary approach. *Arch Surg* 143 2008:451-6.
50. Latham R, Lancaster AD, Covington, et al. The association of diabetes and glucose control with surgical site infections among cardiothoracic surgery patients. *Infect Control Hosp Epidemiol* 2001;**22**:607-12.
51. Carr JM, Sellke F, Fey M, et al. Implementing tight glucose control after coronary artery bypass surgery. *Ann Thorac Surg* 2005;**80**:902-9.
52. Rassias AJ. Intraoperative management of hyperglycemia in the cardiac surgical patient. *Sem Thorac Cardiovasc Surg* 2006;**18**:330-8.
53. Ibrahim EH, Tracy L, Hill C, et al. The occurrence of ventilator-associated pneumonia in a community hospital: risk factors and clinical outcomes. *Chest* 2001;**120**:555-61.
54. Resar R, Pronovost P, Haraden C, et al. Using a bundle approach to improve ventilator care and reduce ventilator-associated pneumonia. *Jt Comm J Qual Patient Saf* 2005;**31**:243-8.
55. American Thoracic Society. Guidelines for the management of adults with hospital acquired, ventilator-associated, and healthcare-associated pneumonia. *Am J Respir Crit Care Med* 2005;**171**:388-416.
56. Soufir L, Timsit JF, Mahe C, et al. Attributable morbidity and mortality of catheter-related septicemia in critically ill patients: a matched, risk-adjusted, cohort study. *Infect Control Hosp Epidemiol* 1999;**6**:396-401.
57. Berenholtz SM, Pronovost PJ, Lipsett PA, et al. Eliminating catheter-related bloodstream infections in the intensive care unit. *Crit Care Med* 2004;**32**:2014-20.
58. Pronovost P, Needham D, Berenholtz S, et al. An intervention to decrease catheter-related bloodstream infections in the ICU. *N Engl J Med* 2006;**355**:2725-32.
59. Eklund AM, Lyytikäinen O, Klemets P, et al. Mediastinitis after more than 10,000 cardiac surgical procedures. *Ann Thorac Surg* 2006;**82**:1784-9.
60. Toumpoulis IK, Anagnostopoulos CE, DeRose JJ, et al. The impact of deep sternal wound infection on long-term survival after coronary artery bypass grafting. *Chest* 2005;**127**:464-71.
61. Mangram AJ, Horan TC, Pearson ML, et al. Guideline for prevention of surgical site infection. *Infect Control Hosp Epidemiol* 1999;**20**:247-79.
62. Lutarewych M, Morgan SP, Hall M. Improving outcomes of coronary artery bypass graft infections with multiple interventions: putting science and data to the test. *Infect Control Hosp Epidemiol* 2004;**25**:517-9.
63. Sharma M, Berriel-Cass D, Baran J. Sternal surgical-site infection following coronary artery bypass graft: prevalence, microbiology, and complications during a 42-month period. *Infect Control Hosp Epidemiol* 2004;**25**:468-71.
64. Ko W, Lazenby WD, Zelano JA, et al. Effects of shaving methods and intraoperative irrigation on suppurative mediastinitis after bypass operations. *Ann Thorac Surg* 1992;**53**:301-5.
65. Schein RM, Hazday N, Pena M, et al. Clinical antecedents to in-hospital cardiopulmonary arrest. *Chest* 1990;**98**:1388-92.
66. Buist M, Bernard S, Nguyen TV, et al. Association between clinically abnormal observations and subsequent in-hospital mortality: a prospective study. *Resuscitation* 2004;**62**:137-41.
67. Franklin C, Mathew J. Developing strategies to prevent in-hospital cardiac arrest: analyzing responses of physicians and nurses in the hours before the event. *Crit Care Med* 1994;**22**:244-7.
68. Bellomo R, Goldsmith D, Uchino S, et al. Prospective controlled trial of effect of medical emergency team on postoperative morbidity and mortality rates. *Crit Care Med* 2004;**32**:916-21.
69. Classen DC, Pestotnik SL, Evans RS, et al. Adverse drug events in hospitalized patients: excess length of stay, extra costs, and attributable mortality. *JAMA* 1997;**277**:301-6.
70. Adams K, Corrigan JM, editors. Priority areas for national action: transforming health care quality. Washington, DC: National Academies Press; 2003.
71. Meoli AL, Rosen CL, Kristo D, et al. Upper airway management of the adult patient with obstructive sleep apnea in the perioperative period: avoiding complications. *Sleep* 2003;**26**:1080-5.
72. Pronovost P, Weast B, Schwarz M, et al. Medication reconciliation: a practical tool to reduce the risk of medication errors. *J Crit Care* 2003;**18**:201-5.

E. Surgical Management of Aortic Disease

CHAPTER 67

Surgery of the Aortic Root and Ascending Aorta

Tirone E. David

Functional Anatomy of the Aortic Root
Pathology of the Aortic Root and Ascending Aorta
  Degenerative Aneurysm of the Ascending Aorta
  Marfan Syndrome
  Loeys-Dietz Syndrome
  Ehlers-Danlos Syndrome
  Bicuspid Aortic Valve Disease
  Atherosclerosis
  Infectious Aneurysms

Aortitis
Aortic Dissection
Ascending Aorta Tumors
Ascending Aorta Trauma
Surgical Treatment of Ascending Aortic Aneurysms
  Operative Techniques
  Clinical Outcomes
Surgical Treatment of Aortic Root Aneurysms
  Operative Techniques

Remodeling of the Aortic Root
Reimplantation of the Aortic Valve
Aortic Root Replacement
Clinical Outcomes
Ross Procedure
  Operative Techniques
  Subcoronary Implantation
  Aortic Root Replacement
  Aortic Root Inclusion
  Clinical Outcomes

FUNCTIONAL ANATOMY OF THE AORTIC ROOT

The aortic root is the anatomic segment between the left ventricle and the ascending aorta. It contains the aortic valve and other anatomic elements, which function as a unit. The aortic root has several anatomic components: the subcommissural triangles, the aortic anulus, the aortic cusps, the aortic sinuses or sinuses of Valsalva, and the sinotubular junction.

The subcommissural triangles are part of the left ventricular outflow tract, but they play an important role in the function of the aortic valve. The subcommissural triangles of the noncoronary aortic cusp are fibrous extension of the intervalvular fibrous body and membranous septum, whereas the subcommissural triangle beneath the left and the right aortic cusps is an extension of the muscular interventricular septum (Fig. 67-1). The aortic anulus, a fibrous structure with a scalloped shape, attaches the aortic valve to the left ventricle. It is attached directly to the myocardium in approximately 45% of its circumference, and to fibrous structures in the remaining 55%. Histologic examination of the aortic anulus reveals that the aortic root has a fibrous continuity with the anterior leaflet of the mitral valve and membranous septum, and it is attached to the muscular interventricular septum by fibrous strands (Fig. 67-2). An important structure immediately below the membranous septum is the bundle of His. The atrioventricular node lies in the floor of the right atrium between the tricuspid anulus and the coronary sinus orifice. This node gives origin to the bundle of His, which travels through the right fibrous trigone along the posterior edge of the membranous septum to the muscular interventricular septum. At this point, the bundle of His divides into left and right bundle branches, which run subendocardially along both sides of the interventricular septum.

The normal aortic valve has three cusps. Each cusp has a semilunar shape and has a base and a free margin. The base is attached to the aortic annulus in a crescent fashion. The point at which the free margin of a cusp joins its base is the commissure, and the ridge in the aortic wall that lies immediately above the commissures is the sinotubular junction. The spaces contained between the aortic annulus and the sinotubular junction are the aortic sinuses, or sinuses of Valsalva. There are three cusps and three sinuses: left cusp and sinus, right cusp and sinus, and noncoronary cusp and sinus. The left main coronary artery arises from the left aortic sinus, and the right coronary artery from the right aortic sinus.

The normal aortic root has a fairly consistent shape, and the sizes of the cusps, the aortic anulus, the aortic sinuses, and the sinotubular junction are somewhat interdependent.[1-4] Thus, large cusps have a proportionally large anulus, sinus, and sinotubular junction. The three aortic cusps often have different sizes in a person, and the right and noncoronary cusps are usually larger than the left cusp.[3] The same cusp may have different sizes in individuals with the same body surface area.[3,4] There are, however, certain geometric parameters that are fairly constant among the various components of the aortic root, and this knowledge is indispensable to understanding the principles of aortic valve repair or replacement with stentless biological valves.

The free margin of an aortic cusp extends from one of its commissures to the other. The length of the free margin of an aortic cusp is approximately 1.5 times the length of its base (Fig. 67-3). During diastole, the free margins and part of the body of the three cusps touch each other approximately in the center of the aortic root to seal the aortic orifice. Thus, the average length of the free margins of three aortic cusps must exceed the diameter of the sinotubular junction to allow

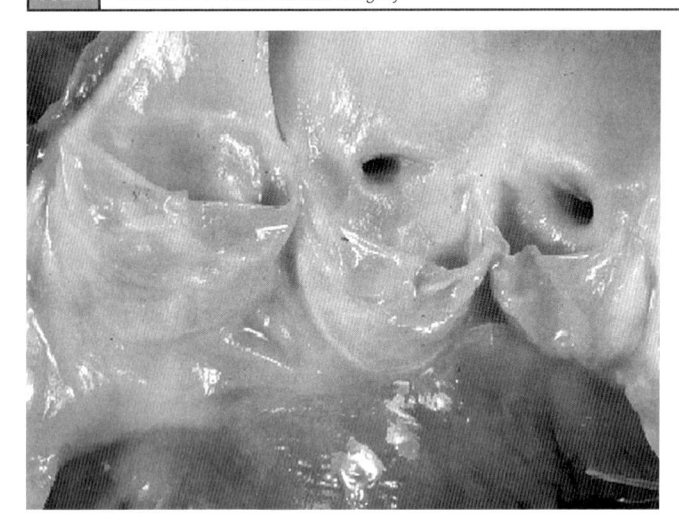

Figure 67-1
The inside of the aortic root.

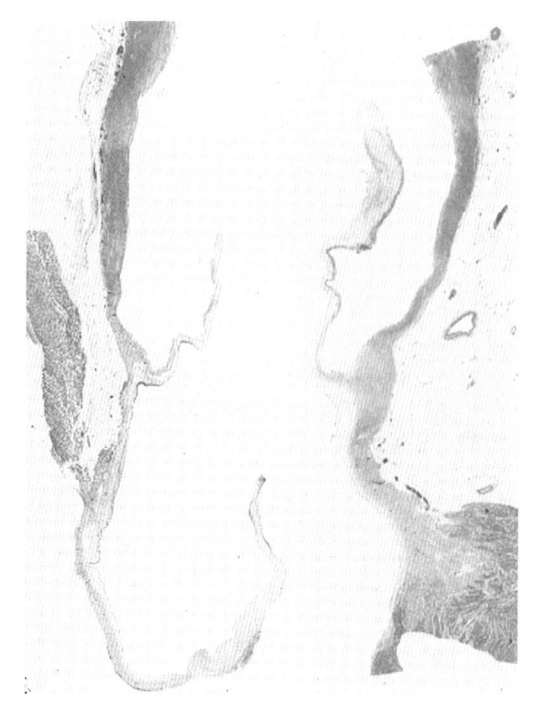

Figure 67-2
Microphotograph of the aortic anulus, cusps, and sinuses.

the cusps to coapt centrally and render the aortic valve competent. If a pathologic process causes shortening of the length of the free margin of a cusp, or if the sinotubular junction dilates, the cusps cannot coapt centrally, resulting in aortic insufficiency (Fig. 67-4). If the length of a free margin is elongated, the cusp prolapses, and depending on the degree of prolapse, aortic insufficiency ensues (Fig. 67-5).

The diameter of the aortic anulus is 10% to 20% larger than the diameter of the sinotubular junction of the aortic root in young patients (see Fig. 67-3). As the number of elastic fibers in the arterial wall decreases with age, the sinotubular junction dilates, and its diameter tends to become equal to that of the aortic anulus in older patients.

Dilation of the aortic anulus pulls the belly of the aortic cusps apart, decreasing the coaptation area, and it eventually causes aortic insufficiency (Fig. 67-6). With dilation of the aortic anulus, the subcommissural triangles of the noncoronary cusp tend to become more obtuse as the crescent shape of the aortic anulus along its fibrous insertion flattens (see Fig. 67-6). The subcommissural triangle beneath the right and left cusps does not change much in patients with annuloaortic ectasia because it is part of the muscular interventricular septum and is not affected by the connective tissue disorder that causes dilation of the fibrous skeleton of the heart.

The aortic sinuses facilitate closure of the aortic valve by creating eddies and currents between the cusps and arterial wall (Fig. 67-7). They also prevent the cusps from occluding the coronary artery orifices during systole, thus guaranteeing myocardial perfusion during the entire cardiac cycle. Isolated dilation of the aortic sinuses does not cause aortic insufficiency.[5]

The aortic root of young individuals is elastic and very compliant. It expands and contracts during the cardiac cycle. Expansion and contraction of the aortic anulus are heterogeneous, probably because of its attachments to contractile myocardium and to fibrous structures such as the membranous septum and intervalvular fibrous body. On the other hand, the expansion and contraction of the sinotubular junction are more uniform. The aortic root also displays some degree of torsion during isovolumic contraction and ejection of the left ventricle.[6] Compliance decreases with aging because of loss of elastic fibers, and the movements of the aortic anulus, cusps, sinuses, and sinotubular junction also change.

PATHOLOGY OF THE AORTIC ROOT AND ASCENDING AORTA

The wall of the aorta is composed of three layers: intima, media, and adventitia. The intima is a thin layer of ground substance lined by endothelium, and it is easily traumatized. The media is the thickest of the three layers, and it is made of elastic fibers arranged in spiral fashion to increase the tensile strength. The adventitia is a thin fibrous layer and contains the vasa vasorum, which carry the nutrients to the media. The aorta is very compliant and expands and contracts during the cardiac cycle because of the elastic fibers in the media. Compliance decreases with aging because of fragmentation of the elastic fibers and an increase in the amount of fibrous tissue in the media. Hypertension, hypercholesterolemia, and coronary artery disease cause premature aging of the aorta.[7-9] Exercise seems to protect the elasticity of the aorta.[8]

Degenerative diseases of the media with aneurysm formation are the most common disorders of the aortic root and ascending aorta. A broad spectrum of pathologic and clinical entities is grouped under degenerative disorders, ranging from severe degeneration of the media, which can become clinically important early in life in cases such as Marfan syndrome in children, to cases of the not so important mild dilation of the ascending aorta in older adults. Bicuspid and unicusp aortic valve diseases are often associated with dilation of the aorta. Atherosclerosis, infectious and noninfectious aortitis, and trauma are other pathologic entities with which the cardiac surgeon must be familiar. Primary tumors of the aortic root and ascending aorta are very rare. False aneurysms and aortic root abscess are problems commonly encountered in clinical practice.

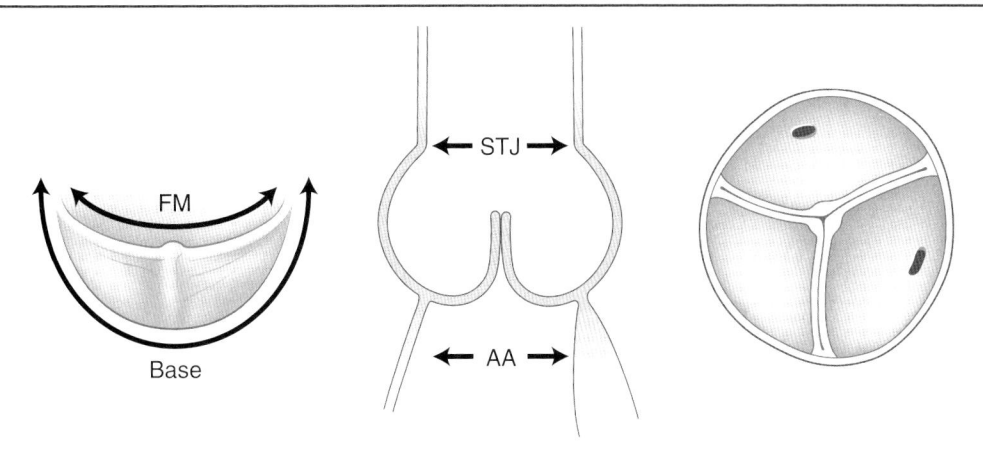

Figure 67–3
Geometric relationship between the free margin (FM) and base of the aortic cusps, sinotubular junction (STJ), and aortic anulus (AA).

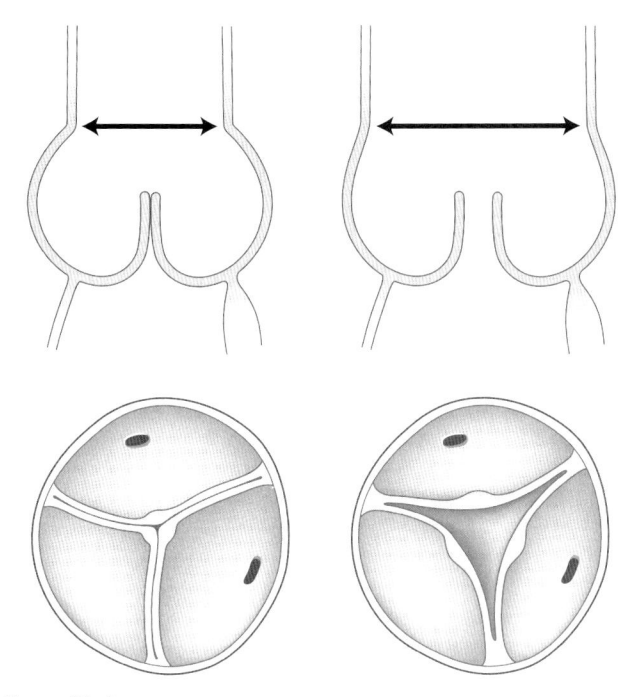

Figure 67–4
Dilation of the sinotubular junction causes aortic insufficiency.

Degenerative Aneurysm of the Ascending Aorta

Aneurysms of the ascending aorta are often caused by cystic medial degeneration (cystic medial necrosis). Histologically, necrosis and disappearance of muscle cells in the elastic lamina, and cystic spaces filled with mucoid material are often observed. Although these changes occur more often in the ascending aorta, they may affect any portion or the entire aorta. These changes weaken the arterial wall, which dilates and forms a fusiform aneurysm. The aortic root may be involved in this pathologic process, and in patients with Marfan syndrome, the aneurysm usually begins in the aortic sinuses. A large proportion of patients with aortic root aneurysms do not fulfill the criteria of diagnosis of Marfan syndrome, but the gross appearance of the aneurysm and the histology of the arterial wall may be indistinguishable from that of Marfan syndrome. These cases are referred to as forma frusta of Marfan syndrome. Patients with aortic root aneurysms are usually in their second or third decade of life when the diagnosis is made. Other patients have relatively normal aortic roots but develop ascending aortic aneurysms. These patients are usually in their fifth or sixth decade of life. Finally, certain patients have extensive degenerative disease of the entire aorta and develop the so-called mega-aorta syndrome with dilation of the thoracic and abdominal aorta.

Ascending aortic aneurysms tend to increase in size and eventually rupture or cause aortic dissection. The transverse diameter of the aneurysm is the most important predictor of rupture or dissection. In a study by Coady and associates[10] of 370 patients with thoracic aneurysms (201 ascending aortic aneurysms), during a mean follow-up of 29.4 months, the incidence of acute dissection or rupture was 8.8% for aneurysms less than 4 cm, 9.5% for aneurysms of 4 to 4.9 cm, 17.8% for 5 to 5.9 cm, and 27.9% for those greater than 6 cm. The median size of the ascending aortic aneurysm at the time of rupture or dissection was 5.9 cm.

The growth rates of thoracic aneurysms are exponential.[10] In the Coady study, the growth rate ranged from 0.08 cm/yr for small (<4-cm) aneurysms to 0.16 cm/yr for large (8-cm) aneurysms.[10] The growth rates for chronic dissecting aneurysms were much higher than for chronic nondissecting aneurysms. Other studies found greater annual growth rates than the Coady group.[11,12] In addition, the growth rates for aortic root aneurysms may be different from those of ascending aortic aneurysms.

Most patients with aortic root or ascending aortic aneurysms are asymptomatic, and the aneurysm is usually found during routine chest radiographs, which show a widened mediastinum.[13] Tracheal and esophageal displacement may be observed in the posterolateral view of the chest radiographs. Approximately one third of the patients complain of vague chest pain.[13] In patients with a massive ascending aortic aneurysm, signs of superior vena cava obstruction may be present. If aortic insufficiency is present, there may be cardiac enlargement and the physical findings associated with it. The diagnoses of aortic root and ascending aortic aneurysm can be confirmed by echocardiography.

Transesophageal echocardiography is the best diagnostic tool to study aortic root aneurysm and the mechanism

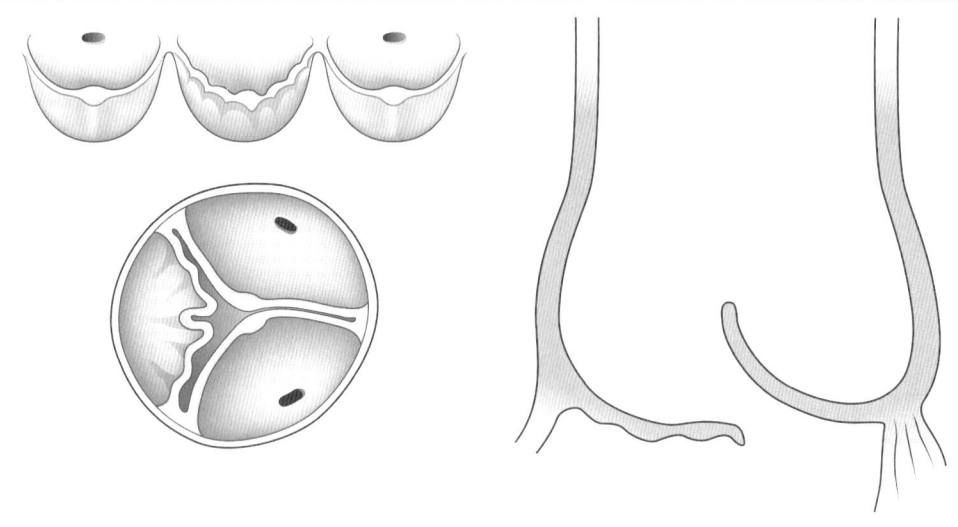

Figure 67–5
Elongation of the free margin of an aortic cusp causes prolapse with resulting aortic insufficiency.

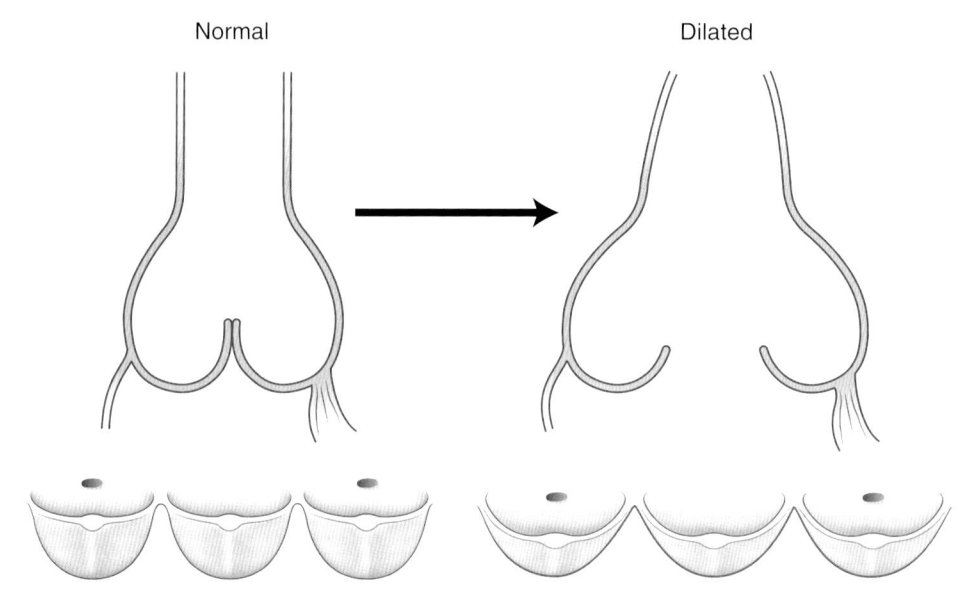

Normal   Dilated

Figure 67–6
Dilation of the aortic anulus. The subcommissural triangles of the noncoronary cusp become more obtuse.

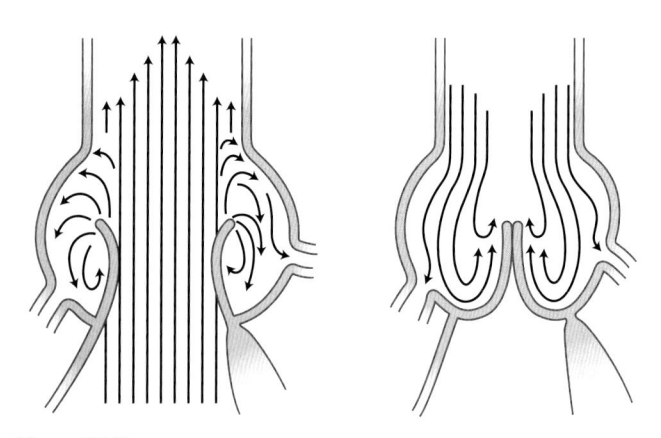

Figure 67–7
The aortic sinuses create eddies and currents and facilitate aortic valve closure.

of aortic insufficiency. The echocardiographer should obtain information on each component of the aortic root, and particularly the aortic cusps. The number of cusps, their thickness, the appearance of free margins, and the excursion of each cusp during the cardiac cycle must be carefully observed. The coaptation areas of the cusps should also be investigated in multiple views and Doppler imaging recorded. Information regarding the morphologic features of the aortic sinuses, sinotubular junction, and ascending aorta is also important. The diameters of the aortic anulus, aortic sinuses, sinotubular junction, and ascending aorta should be obtained in multiple views. The lengths of the free margins of the cusps should be estimated if possible. The mechanism of aortic insufficiency can often be determined by transesophageal echocardiography. Dilation of the sinotubular junction is a common cause of aortic insufficiency in patients with ascending aortic aneurysm and normal aortic cusps. Dilation of the aortic anulus

Table 67–1
Diagnostic Criteria* for Marfan Syndrome (See text)

System	Major Criteria	Minor Criteria
Family history	Independent diagnosis in parent, child, sibling	None
Genetics	Mutation in FBN1	None
Cardiovascular	Aortic root dilation Dissection of ascending aorta	Mitral valve prolapse Calcification of the mitral valve (age < 40 yr) Dilation of the pulmonary artery Dilation or dissection of the descending aorta

Ocular	Ectopia lentis	Two needed:
		  Flat cornea
		  Myopia
		  Elongated globe

Skeletal	Pectus excavatum needing surgery
	Pectus carinatum
	Pes planus
	Wrist and thumb sign
	Scoliosis > 20 degrees or spondylolisthesis
	Arm span–height ratio > 1.05
	Protrusio acetabula (radiograph, MRI)
	Diminished extension elbows (<170 degrees)
		Two major or one major and two minor signs:
		  Moderate pectus excavatum
		  High, narrowly arched palate
		  Typical facies
		  Joint hypermobility

Pulmonary	—	Spontaneous pneumothorax Apical bulla
Skin	—	Unexplained stretch marks (striae) Recurrent or incisional herniae
Central nervous	Lumbosacral dural ectasia (CT or MRI)	—

*The presence of major criteria in two separate systems and involvement of a third (minor or major) are needed to establish the diagnosis of Marfan syndrome.

and of the sinotubular junction is usually the cause of aortic insufficiency in patients with aortic root aneurysm. Although fenestrations in the cusps are not easily seen with echocardiography, a regurgitant jet in a commissural area is suggestive of fenestration.

Computed tomography (CT) with intravenous contrast enhancement permits accurate evaluation of the extent and size of the aneurysm. Three-dimensional imaging techniques can provide additional information on the extensiveness and type of aneurysm (e.g., fusiform or saccular).

Magnetic resonance imaging (MRI) provides even more information than CT scanning because it visualizes the arterial wall and surrounding structures with greater contrast. In addition, it has been increasingly used in the diagnosis and management of patients with heart diseases.[14] Magnetic resonance angiography (MRA) is replacing contrast angiography.[15]

Marfan Syndrome

Marfan syndrome is an autosomal dominant, variably penetrant, inherited disorder of the connective tissue in which cardiovascular, skeletal, ocular, and other abnormalities may be present to variable degrees. The prevalence is estimated to be around 1 in 5000 individuals. It is caused by mutations in the gene that encodes fibrillin-1 (FBN1) on chromosome 15. This is a large gene (approximately 10,000 nucleotides in the mRNA), and identification of the mutation is a complex task. More than 1000 mutations in FBN1 have been identified. The phenotype is highly variable because of varying genotype expression.

The clinical features of Marfan syndrome were thought to be caused by weaker connective tissues resulting from defects in fibrillin-1, a glycoprotein and principal component of the extracellular matrix microfibril. This concept was inadequate to explain the overgrowth of long bones, osteopenia, reduced muscular mass and adiposity and craniofacial abnormalities often seen in Marfan syndrome.[16] Dietz and colleagues[16,17] showed in experimental mice with Marfan syndrome that many findings are the result of abnormal levels of activation of transforming growth factor β (TGF-β), a potent stimulator of inflammation, fibrosis, and activation of certain matrix metalloproteinases, especially matrix metalloproteinases 2 and 9. Excess TGF-β activation in tissues correlates with failure of lung septation, development of a myxomatous mitral valve, and aortic root dilation in mice.[18] This combination of structural microfibril matrix abnormality, dysregulation of matrix homeostasis mediated by excess TGF-β, and abnormal cell–matrix interactions is responsible for the phenotypic features of Marfan syndrome.[16-18] Ongoing destruction of the elastic and collagen lamellae and medial degeneration result in progressive dilation of the aortic root, as well as in a predisposition to aortic dissection from the loss of appropriate medial layer support. Loss of elasticity in the media causes increased aortic stiffness and decreased distensibility.[19]

The diagnosis of Marfan syndrome is made on clinical grounds, and it is not always simple because of the variability in clinical expression (Table 67-1). A multidisciplinary approach is needed to diagnose and manage patients afflicted with this syndrome. The presence of major criteria in two separate systems and involvement of a third (minor or major) are needed to establish the diagnosis.[20]

The most common cardiovascular features are aortic root aneurysm and mitral valve prolapse. These anatomic abnormalities may cause aortic rupture, aortic dissection, aortic insufficiency, and mitral insufficiency.

Mitral valve prolapse is age dependent and more common in women. It is caused by myxomatous degeneration of the mitral valve apparatus, which is present in up to 80% of patients with Marfan syndrome, but only 25% of them develop mitral insufficiency. The posterior mitral anulus is grossly dilated in patients with mitral insufficiency, and it is often displaced posteriorly.[21] The mitral anulus may also become heavily calcified and display a horseshoe appearance on radiographs.

The dilation of the aortic root is often progressive, and the rate of expansion, which varies somewhat, is usually less than 1 or 2 mm/yr. Shores and colleagues[12] randomized 70 patients with Marfan syndrome into propranolol-treated and placebo groups. The growth rates of the aortic root aneurysms in untreated patients were slightly more than three times those of patients who received β-adrenergic blockage. This study has been the scientific basis to treat these patients with a beta-blocker agent. Calcium antagonists and angiotension-converting enzymes have also been reported as effective in delaying aortic dilation, but at present, beta-blocker remains the drug of choice.[22]

Aortic dissection is rare in patients with aortic root aneurysm of less than 50 mm, unless they have a family history of aortic dissection. The dissection in most patients starts at the level of the sinotubular junction (Stanford type A aortic dissection). In approximately 10% of patients, it starts just beyond the left subclavian artery (Stanford type B aortic dissection). Without surgery, most patients with Marfan syndrome die in their third decade, from complications of aortic root aneurysm such as rupture, aortic dissection, or aortic insufficiency.[23,24]

Patients with Marfan syndrome should be followed at regular time intervals. Doppler echocardiography is the best diagnostic tool for monitoring changes in the mitral valve and aortic root. Patients with an aortic root greater than 40 mm should be followed with echocardiographic measurements twice yearly. MR images of the remaining thoracic and abdominal aorta should also be obtained when indicated.

Pregnancy in women with Marfan syndrome has two potential problems: the risk of having a child who will inherit the disorder and the risk of acute aortic dissection during the third trimester, parturition, or the first postpartum month. Offspring have a 50% risk of inheriting the syndrome. The risk of aortic dissection is less known, but it appears to be low in patients with normal aortic root and cardiac function.[25]

Loeys-Dietz syndrome

Mutations in the genes encoding TGF-β receptors 1 and 2 have been found in association with a continuum of clinical features. On the mild end is a presentation similar to that of the Marfan syndrome, or familial thoracic aneurysm and dissection,[26,27] and on the severe end, there is a complex phenotype in which aortic dissection or rupture commonly occurs in childhood.[28] This complex phenotype is characterized by the triad of hypertelorism, bifid uvula (or cleft palate), and generalized arterial tortuosity with widespread vascular aneurysm and dissection. This phenotype has been classified as Loeys-Dietz syndrome.[29] Affected patients have a high risk of aortic dissection or rupture at an early age and at relatively small aortic diameters. CT angiograms should be obtained from the head to the pelvis. Surgery is recommended for adults when the aortic root exceeds 4 cm or the descending thoracic aorta exceeds 5 cm. If the craniofacial features are severe in children, surgery is recommended when the aortic root Z-score is greater than 3, or when the expansion is greater than 0.5 cm in 1 year.[30]

Ehlers-Danlos Syndrome

The Ehlers-Danlos syndrome encompasses a group of heterogeneous connective tissue disorders that involve the skin and joints and cause hyperelasticity and fragility of the former and hypermobility of the latter. It may also involve the cardiovascular system. Vascular Ehlers-Danlos syndrome is a rare autosomal dominant inherited disorder of the connective tissue resulting from mutation of the COL3A1 gene encoding type III collagen.[31] Affected individuals are prone to serious vascular, intestinal, and obstetric complications. These problems are rare during infancy but occur in up to 25% of affected persons before the age of 20 years and in 80% before the age of 40. Median survival is 48 years. Spontaneous rupture without dissection of large- and medium-caliber arteries such as the abdominal aorta and its branches, the branches of the aortic arch, and the large arteries of the limbs accounts for most deaths. Intestinal perforation, usually involving the colon, is less often fatal. Pregnancy is a high risk for women with this syndrome. Aortic root dilation was present in 28% in a series of 71 patients with Ehlers-Danlos syndrome.[32] Aortic dissection is uncommon.

As with many rare diseases, delayed or incorrect diagnosis can lead to inadequate or inappropriate management. Diagnosis is based on clinical findings including specific facial features, thin translucent skin, propensity to bleeding, and rupture of vessels or viscera. Diagnosis can be confirmed by biochemical assays showing qualitative or quantitative abnormalities in type III collagen secretion, or by molecular biology studies demonstrating mutation of the COL3A1 gene. Varied molecular mechanisms have been observed with different mutations in each family. No correlation has been established between genotype and phenotype. Diagnosis should be suspected in any young person presenting with arterial or visceral rupture or colonic perforation. There is currently no specific treatment for this syndrome.

Bicuspid Aortic Valve Disease

Congenital aortic valve malformations include a phenotypic continuum of unicuspid valves (severe form), the various types of bicuspid aortic valves (moderate form), tricuspid valves (normal), and the rare quadricuspid valves.[33]

Bicuspid aortic valve, the most common of these malformations, occurs in 1% to 2% of the population. Movahed and colleagues[34] recently reviewed 24,265 patients who had echocardiograms performed for various clinical reasons, and 1742 echocardiograms obtained by screening teenage athletes in Southern California, and found a prevalence of bicuspid aortic valves of 0.6% in the large cohort and 0.5% in the smaller one. Males are affected more than females at a ratio of 4:1. There is a relatively high incidence of familial clustering, which suggests an autosomal dominant inheritance with reduced penetrance.[35,36] However, it remains unproved that bicuspid aortic valve is an inherited disorder. Patients with bicuspid aortic valve usually have three aortic sinuses and two cusps of different sizes. The larger cusp, usually the one attached to the interventricular septum, contains a raphe, which probably represents an incomplete commissure. Bicuspid aortic valves with two cusps and two sinuses are far less common than bicuspid aortic valves with two cusps and three sinuses. Most patients with bicuspid aortic valves have a dominant circumflex artery and a small right coronary artery. Normally functioning bicuspid aortic valves may last the patient's lifetime. Others become stenotic by the fourth or fifth decade of life. Aortic insufficiency may also occur, and it is often associated with dilated aortic anulus.[37] It is more common in younger patients, and it results from the prolapse of one cusp, usually the one that contains the raphe.

Both bicuspid and unicuspid aortic valves are often associated with premature degenerative changes in the media of the wall of the aortic root and ascending aorta.[38,39] These patients are at risk of developing chronic degenerative aneurysms of the ascending aorta and type A aortic dissection.[40]

Atherosclerosis

Atherosclerosis of the ascending aorta and transverse arch is a common cause of stroke.[41,42] Sometimes, atherosclerosis can cause extensive calcification of the aortic root, ascending aorta, and transverse arch, which is often associated with coronary artery disease, stenosis of one or both coronary arteries orifices, and aortic valve stenosis. Extensive calcification of the ascending aorta is clinically described as "porcelain" aorta.[43,44]

Atherosclerotic aneurysms of the ascending aorta are uncommon. They are more common in the abdominal aorta and to a lesser degree in the descending thoracic aorta. Atherosclerosis often causes irregular and saccular aneurysms of the ascending aorta rather than the more fusiform shape of those caused by degenerative disease of the media.

Infectious Aneurysms

Syphilis was a common cause of aneurysm of the ascending aorta, but it is now rare. The spirochetal infection destroys the muscular and elastic fibers of the media, which are replaced by fibrous and other inflammatory tissues. The ascending aorta is the most common site of involvement, and the aneurysm is usually saccular.[45] The wall of the ascending aorta is frequently calcified. Syphilitic aortitis also causes coronary ostial stenosis and aortic valve insufficiency.[46] Although it is rare, other bacteria can also cause aneurysm of the ascending aorta.

Aortitis

Various types of aortitis may involve the ascending aorta.[46-51] Giant cell arteritis is among the more common and it involves medium-sized arteries, but the aorta and its branches are involved in approximately 15% of the cases.[50] The etiology of aortitis, also called temporal arteritis, is unknown. The characteristic lesion is a granulomatous inflammation of the media of large- and medium-caliber arteries such as the temporal artery. Narrowing of the aorta is rare. Occasionally the inflammatory process weakens the aorta, leading to aneurysm formation, aortoannular ectasia, and aortic insufficiency.[49] Patients are usually older than 50 years, with a mean age of 67 years, and most are women. Diagnosis is established by biopsy of the involved artery, usually the temporal artery.

Takayasu's arteritis is a chronic inflammatory disease that often involves the aortic arch and its major branches. The pulmonary artery may also be involved. The lesions are purely stenotic in 85% of patients, aneurysmal in 2%, and mixed in 13%.[47,48] Aortic insufficiency occurs in approximately 25% of the cases. It has been classified as type I when the aortic arch is involved, type II when the arch is free of disease but the thoracoabdominal aorta and its branches are affected, type III when both areas are affected, and type IV when the pulmonary artery is involved.[48,51] The etiology is unknown but it is probably an autoimmune disorder. It occurs worldwide, but most cases are seen in Asia and Africa. The disease affects women more than men at a ratio of 8:1.[47,48] The mean age at the time of the diagnosis is 29 years.

Ankylosing spondylitis, Reiter's syndrome, psoriatic arthritis, and polyarteritis nodosa can cause aortic insufficiency because of annuloaortic ectasia. Behçet's disease can cause aneurysm of the ascending aorta.

Aortic Dissection

Aortic dissections are discussed in Chapters 70 and 71.

Ascending Aorta Tumors

Primary tumors of the ascending aorta are extremely rare. Most aortic tumors are located in the descending thoracic or abdominal aorta, and they are usually sarcomas.[52,53]

Ascending Aorta Trauma

Nonpenetrating traumatic injuries of the ascending aorta are often fatal and diagnosed at autopsy.[54] The penetrating trauma is usually a bullet or stab wound, and it causes cardiac tamponade when the intrapericardial portion of the aorta is involved. These injuries are frequently fatal.

SURGICAL TREATMENT OF ASCENDING AORTIC ANEURYSMS

Although ascending aortic aneurysms may be isolated lesions, more often they are associated with aortic valve disease. Both bicuspid and tricuspid aortic valve diseases may be associated with degenerative aneurysms of the ascending aorta, but bicuspid aortic valve disease appears to be associated with premature degeneration of the media of the aorta.

Ascending aortic aneurysm may cause aortic insufficiency in patients with anatomically normal aortic valve cusps if the sinotubular junction becomes dilated (see Fig. 67-4). These patients may develop symptoms related to the aortic insufficiency, but more often the aneurysm is asymptomatic and discovered during a routine chest radiograph or echocardiogram done as part of the workup for an unrelated problem. Surgery is recommended when the transverse diameter of the ascending aorta exceeds 55 mm.[10] If there is moderate or severe aortic insufficiency, the aortic valve cusps are normal by echocardiography, and the valve is judged to be repairable, operation is justifiable when the ascending aorta reaches 50 mm in diameter.[55-57]

Operative Techniques

Surgery for ascending aortic aneurysm is performed using cardiopulmonary bypass, which is established by cannulating the transverse aortic arch, right axillary artery or femoral artery, and the right atrium. Because the aneurysm frequently extends up to the origin of the innominate artery, a brief period of circulatory arrest is necessary to resect the arch aneurysm and perform the distal anastomosis. The proximal anastomosis should be performed at the level of the sinotubular junction. The Dacron graft used to replace the ascending

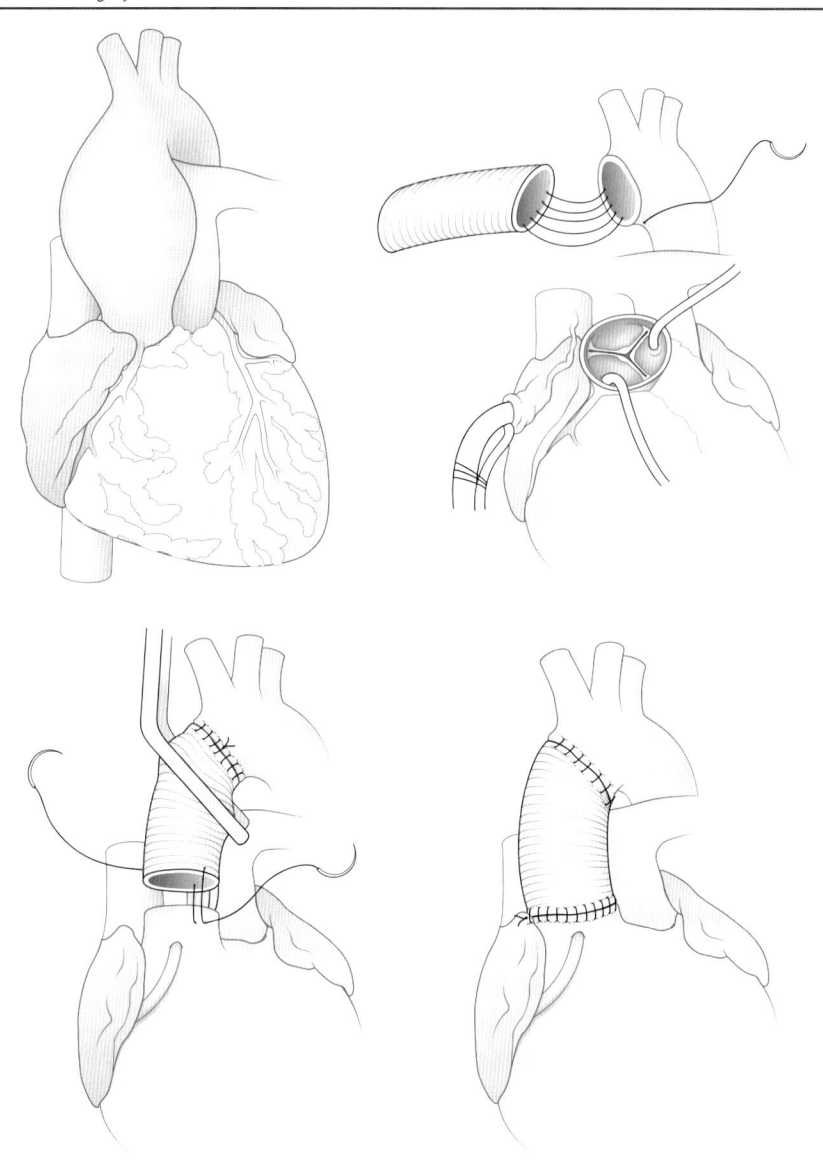

Figure 67-8
Replacement of the ascending aorta for aneurysm.

aorta should not be too long or too large. When the ascending aorta expands to develop an aneurysm, it also becomes elongated. Thus, during its replacement, the graft should be much shorter than the aneurysm. In fact, a graft of 5 or 6 cm in length is all that is needed to replace the entire ascending aorta from sinotubular junction to the level of the innominate artery. Longer grafts may kink and cause partial obstruction and even hemolysis. A single graft can be used, but it should be beveled at the distal anastomosis, and its shorter side should be aligned with the medial part of the arch (Fig. 67-8). The diameter of the graft should be between 24 and 30 mm, depending on the patient's body surface area. When the diameter of the graft used is larger than the diameter of the sinotubular junction by more than a couple of millimeters, its caliber should be reduced to that of the sinotubular junction at the level of the anastomosis. This is easily done by plication of that end of the graft. Matching the diameter of the graft to that of the sinotubular junction is important to prevent late development of aortic insufficiency.

If the aortic valve is incompetent but the aortic cusps are normal and the sinotubular junction is dilated, all that is needed to reestablish valve competence is to reduce the diameter of the sinotubular junction to allow the cusps to coapt again. The ascending aorta is transected 5 mm above the sinotubular junction. All three commissures are pulled upward and approximate to each other until the cusps coapt centrally. The diameter of an imaginary circle that contains all three commissures is the correct diameter of the sinotubular junction. A graft of that diameter is then sutured to the remnants of ascending aorta wall at the level of the sinotubular junction. Because the aortic cusps are frequently of different sizes, the spaces between the commissures should reflect that during performance of the proximal anastomosis. Aortic valve competence can be assessed by injecting cardioplegia solution under pressure in the graft and observing the left ventricle for distention. In our group, we prefer to use two separate segments of grafts when aortic valve repair is necessary and the entire ascending aorta or transverse arch, or both, need replacement. We usually do the distal anastomosis first (under hypothermic circulatory arrest) and work on the aortic valve during rewarming of the patient. The distal and proximal grafts are trimmed and sutured to one another (Fig. 67-9).

If the noncoronary aortic sinus is aneurysmal, it should be replaced along with the ascending aorta. This is accomplished by selecting a graft of an appropriate diameter, as previously described, and then creating a neoaortic sinus in one of its ends. The width of the neoaortic sinus is equal to the distance between the commissures of the cusp, and the height is approximately equal to the diameter of the graft. This neoaortic sinus is sutured directly to the remnant of arterial wall and aortic anulus (Fig. 67-10).

Sometimes one aortic cusp is slightly elongated and its free margin coapts at a level lower than the other two cusps. The free margin can be shortened by plication of the central portion (Fig. 67-11). If the free margin is elongated and thinned or has a fenestration near a commissure, it can be reinforced with a double layer of a 6-0 expanded polytetrafluoroethylene suture (Fig. 67-12).

Patients with a normally functioning bicuspid aortic valve, normal aortic root, and ascending aortic aneurysm can be treated by simple replacement of the ascending aorta.

Patients with aortic valve disease not amenable to repair and an ascending aortic aneurysm are treated by aortic valve replacement and supracoronary replacement of the ascending aorta. If only the noncoronary aortic sinus is dilated, aortic valve replacement of the ascending aorta with a graft extension into the noncoronary sinus (see Fig. 67-10) is preferable to composite replacement of the aortic valve and ascending aorta with reimplantation of the coronary arteries. If two aortic sinuses are dilated, composite replacement of the aortic valve and ascending aorta with reimplantation of the coronary arteries should be performed as described for aortic root aneurysm.

Clinical Outcomes

Isolated replacement of the ascending aorta for chronic aneurysm is uncommon.[58,59] Patients with ascending aortic aneurysm often have aortic insufficiency or aortic valve disease that may also need surgical attention. Whether the operation is done in isolation or combined with other procedures, the operative mortality for elective surgery is low.[57,60] In our experience with 103 patients who had aortic valve–sparing operations for ascending aortic aneurysm and aortic insufficiency, only one patient died perioperatively.[57] We reviewed our experience with aortic valve replacement

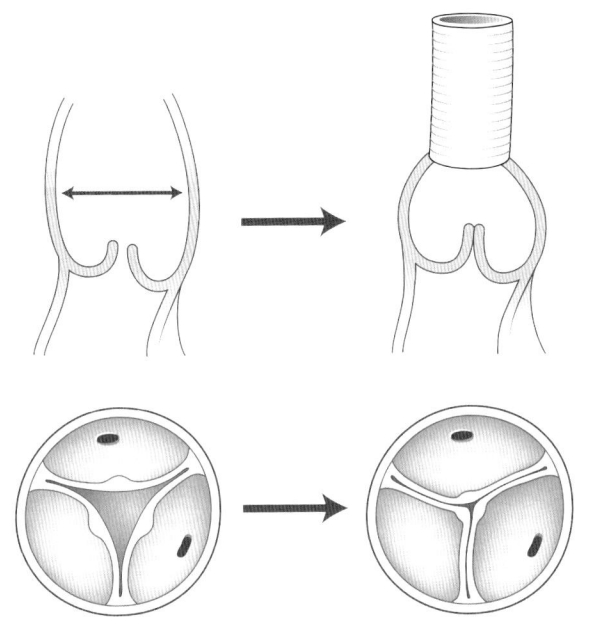

Figure 67-9
Replacement of the ascending aorta with adjustment of the diameter of the sinotubular junction.

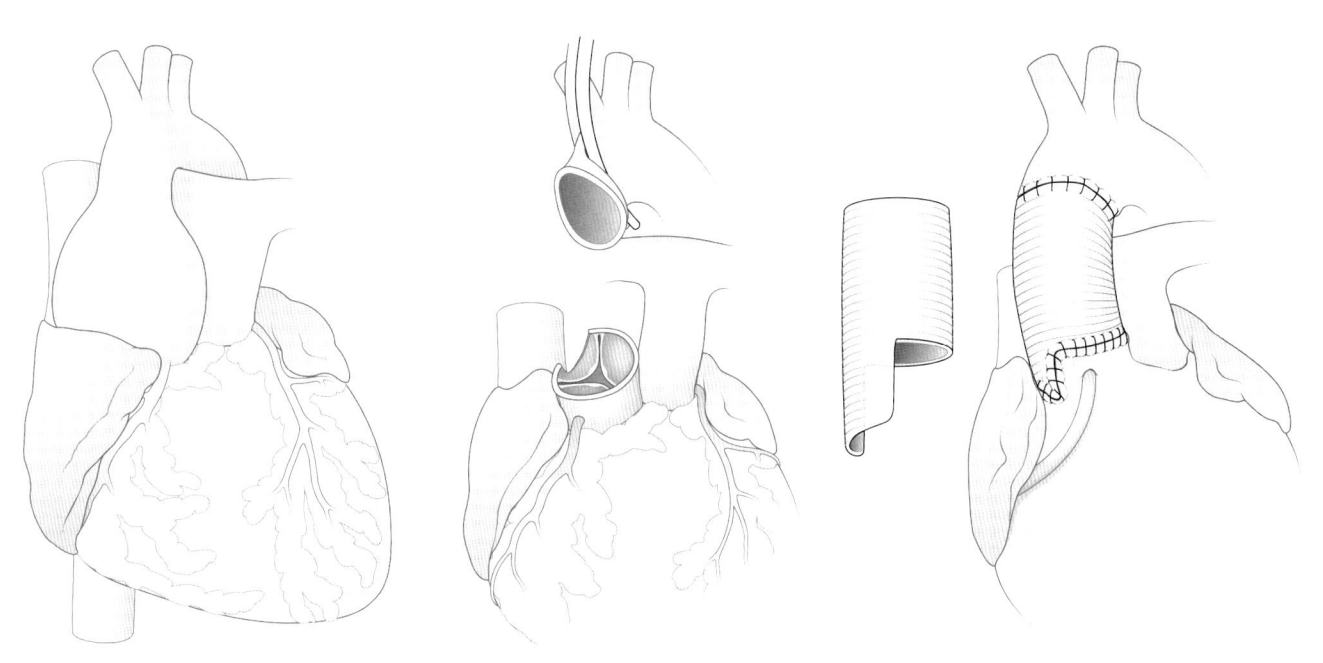

Figure 67-10
Replacement of the ascending aorta and noncoronary aortic sinus.

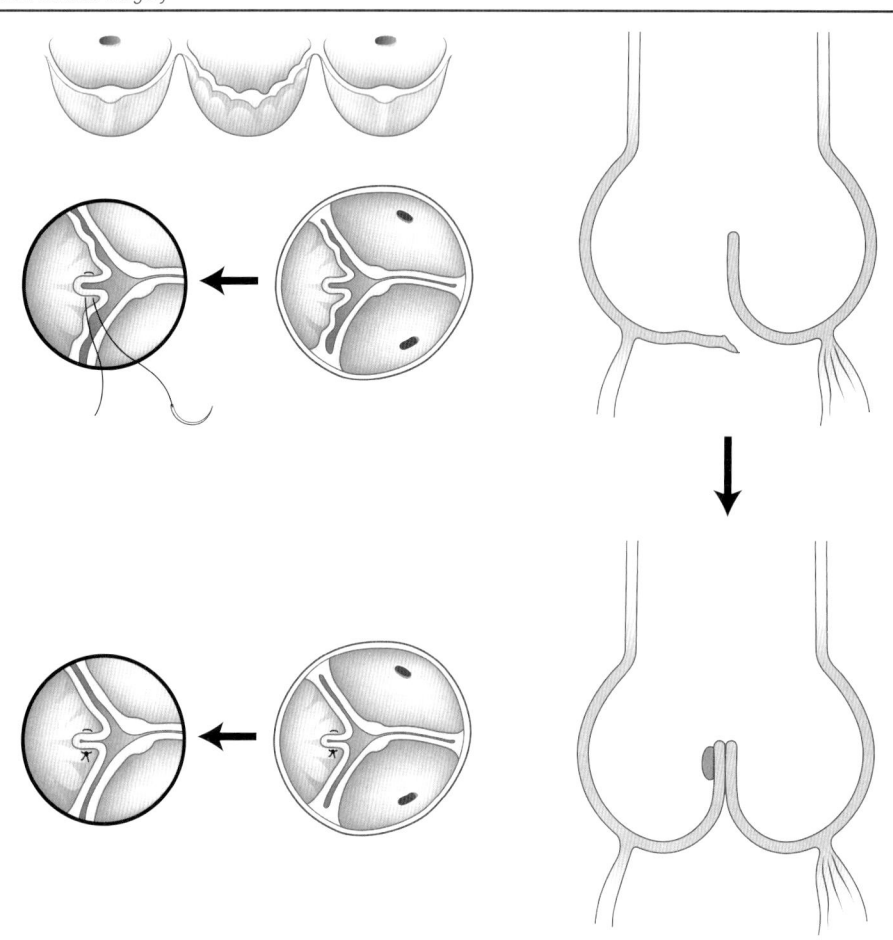

Figure 67–11
Repair of aortic cusp prolapse by shortening its free margin.

and supracoronary replacement of the ascending aorta at Toronto General Hospital during a 12-year interval and identified 132 patients.[61] There were six operative deaths, and the series included acute aortic dissections, acute infective endocarditis, and reoperations.[61] Cohn and colleagues[60] also reported a low operative mortality for replacement of the ascending aorta. The operative mortality for ascending aortic surgery has decreased over the past 4 decades.[62] Age, functional class, and associated diseases play an important role in the operative risk.

The long-term survival of our 103 patients who had aortic valve–sparing operations for ascending aortic aneurysm and aortic insufficiency was only 54% at 10 years, but most of them had extensive vascular disease including transverse aortic arch disease or mega-aorta syndrome.[57] Our patients who had aortic valve replacement and supracoronary replacement of the ascending aorta had a 10-year survival of 70%, but they were younger than those who had aortic valve repair and had less extensive vascular disease.[61]

Patients who had replacement of the ascending aorta with or without aortic valve surgery must be evaluated annually with echocardiography to assess the size of the retained aortic root and the function of the aortic valve; they should also have CT scans or MRI of the remaining thoracic and abdominal aorta. Aneurysms of the aortic root, false aneurysms, valve dysfunction, and infections in the graft or aortic valve are problems that may develop and need surgical treatment.[62]

Patients who had aortic valve repair or replacement with bioprosthetic valves do not need anticoagulation if they are in sinus rhythm. Those with mechanical valves should be anticoagulated with warfarin sodium. Other systemic disorders are common among these patients, particularly hypertension and coronary artery disease, which should also be treated.

SURGICAL TREATMENT OF AORTIC ROOT ANEURYSMS

Aortic root aneurysm may or may not be associated with the Marfan syndrome. Composite replacement of the aortic valve and ascending aorta with reimplantation of the coronary arteries has been the standard operation for patients with aortic root aneurysm with or without aortic insufficiency.[58,59,63-65] Patients with normal or near-normal aortic cusps can safely have the aortic valve preserved during repair of the aortic root aneurysm.[55,56] Because of very favorable mid-term results with aortic valve–sparing procedures in patients with Marfan syndrome, we recommended surgery when the transverse diameter of the aortic root nears 50 mm.[66] If a patient has a family history of aortic dissection, surgery should probably be done when the aortic root reaches 45 mm in diameter. The 2006 guidelines from the American College of Cardiology and American Heart Association suggest that surgery should be considered when the transverse diameter of the aortic root or ascending aorta reaches 50 mm.[67] Unless surgery can be done with very low operative

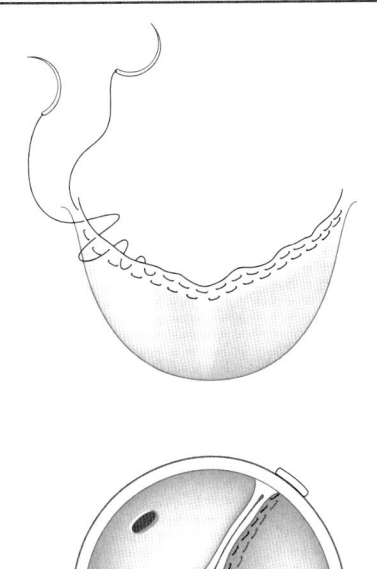

Figure 67-12
Reinforcement of the free margin of the aortic cusp with a double layer of a 6-0 expanded polytetrafluoroethylene suture.

mortality (about 1%), we find it difficult to justify surgery this early in the course of the disease, because the risk of dissection or rupture is probably lower than the operative mortality.

Operative Techniques

The two basic types of aortic valve–sparing operations for patients with aortic root aneurysms are remodeling of the aortic root and reimplantation of the aortic valve.[62,63]

Remodeling of the Aortic Root

The aortic root is dissected circumferentially down to the level of the aortic anulus, and the three aortic sinuses are excised, leaving approximately 5 mm of tissue attached to the aortic anulus and around the coronary artery orifices. The three commissures are gently suspended upward and approximated until the three cusps coapt. The diameter of an imaginary circle that includes all three commissures is approximately the diameter of the tubular Dacron graft to be used for reconstruction of the aortic sinuses (Fig. 67-13). One of the ends of this graft is tailored to create neoaortic sinuses. The widths of the neoaortic sinuses are based on the distance between commissures of each cusp when they are pulled upward to determine the diameter of the graft. The heights of the neoaortic sinuses should be approximately equal to their width. The three commissures are secured on the outside of the graft immediately above the neoaortic sinuses, and the remnants of aortic wall and aortic anulus are sutured to the neoaortic sinuses with a continuous 4-0 polypropylene (see Fig. 67-13). The coronary arteries are reimplanted into their respective sinuses. If an aortic cusp coapts at a level lower than the other two, shortening of the free margin corrects the problem (see Figs. 67-11 and 67-12).

Reimplantation of the Aortic Valve

The aortic root is dissected circumferentially and prepared as just described. Next, multiple 3-0 or 4-0 polyester sutures are passed from the inside to the outside of the left ventricular outflow tract through a single horizontal plane corresponding to the lowest portion of the aortic anulus along its fibrous components and following the scalloped shape of the anulus along its muscular component (Fig. 67-14). If the fibrous portion of the left ventricular outflow tract is thin, Teflon felt pledgets should be used in those sutures. The diameter of the sinotubular junction is estimated by pulling the three commissures upward until the cusps coapt. A tubular Dacron graft 4 to 6 mm larger than the diameter of the sinotubular junction is selected, and a small triangular excision is made in one of its ends and the remaining portion is plicated in two or three places to reduce its diameter by 3 to 4 mm. Most grafts we currently use are 30 to 34 mm in diameter, depending on the size of the patient and the aortic cusps. The sutures passed through the left ventricular outflow tract are then passed from the inside to the outside of the tailored end of the graft. If reduction in diameter of the aortic anulus is desirable, it is done beneath the commissures of the noncoronary cusp. This is accomplished by placing the sutures closer in the graft than they are beneath the commissures of the noncoronary cusp. The aortic valve is placed inside the graft and all sutures are tied on the outside. The three commissures are suspended inside the graft and secured to it with 4-0 polypropylene sutures. These sutures are then used to secure the aortic anulus and remnants of the aortic sinuses to the graft. The coronary arteries are reimplanted into their respective sinuses. The spaces between commissures are plicated to create a slight bulge in the neoaortic sinuses and to reduce the diameter of the graft to that of the desirable sinotubular junction. Cusp prolapse or reinforcement can be done if needed (see Figs. 67-11 and 67-12).

Patients with a normally functioning bicuspid aortic valve and aortic root aneurysm are also candidates for aortic valve–sparing operations.

There is a commercially available Dacron graft with neo–sinuses of Valsalva.[68] Some surgeons who have wide experience with aortic valve–sparing procedures have used the "Valsalva graft" for aortic valve reimplantation.[69] We have not used it because we believe it deforms the aortic anulus, which normally evolves along a single horizontal plane. If the aortic anulus is correctly resuspended into the Valsalva graft, the anulus plane changes from a horizontal to a curved shape. This may compromise the durability of the repair.

Aortic Root Replacement

Replacement of the aortic root is performed when the aortic cusps are abnormal and cannot be safely repaired.[56,70] The aortic cusps are excised and the coronary arteries detached from their sinuses with 5 or 6 mm of aortic sinus wall around them. A valved conduit is then used to replace the aortic root. This conduit can be a commercially available Dacron tube with a mechanical valve already attached to one of its ends. The valved conduit is sutured to the aortic anulus and the coronary arteries are reimplanted into the graft (Fig. 67-15).

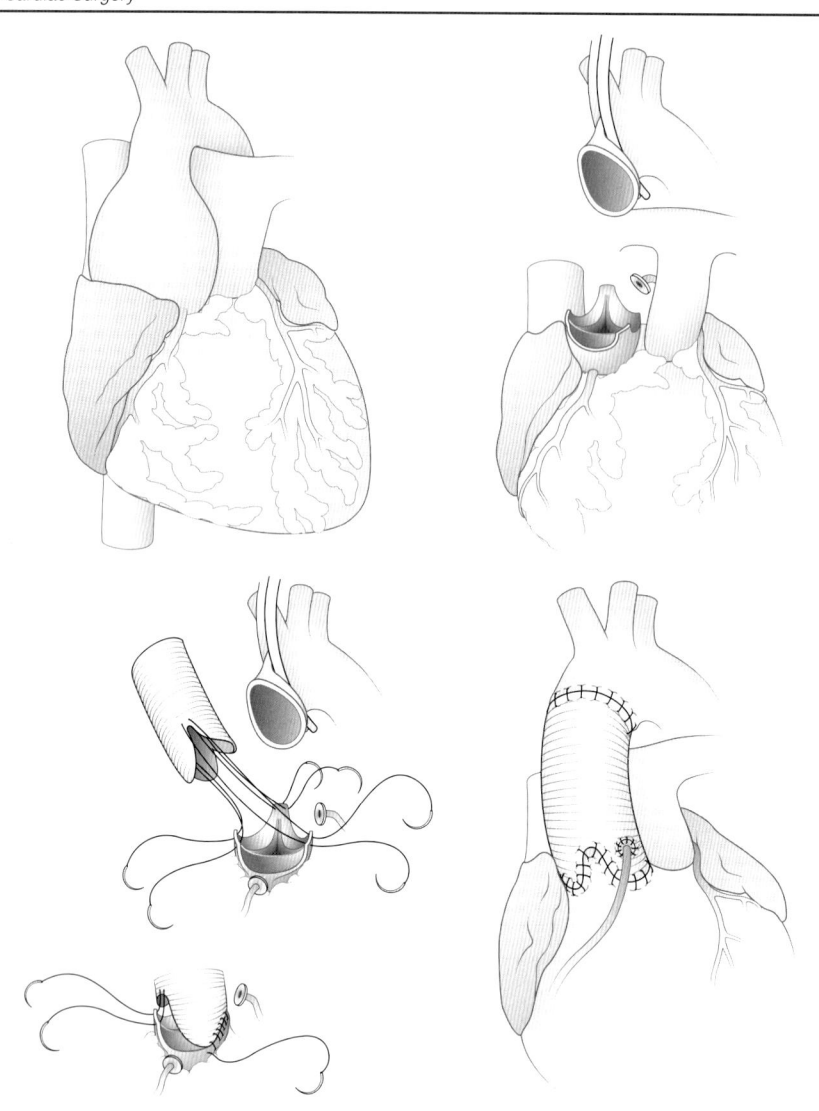

Figure 67–13
Aortic valve–sparing operation: remodeling of the aortic root.

An aortic homograft or a xenograft can also be used for aortic root replacement. It is not wise to use a pulmonary autograft for replacement of the aortic root in patients with aortic root aneurysms, because the pulmonary autograft may become aneurysmal when subjected to systemic pressures. Finally, aortic root replacement also can be performed with a conduit prepared in the operating room. When a stented bioprosthetic valve is desirable, the bioprosthesis and the Dacron tube can be secured to the aortic anulus using the same sutures. Another method is to secure the bioprosthetic valve inside a tubular Dacron graft 1 cm from one of its ends and secure the Dacron graft alone to the anulus (Fig. 67-16). This approach allows aortic valve re-replacement without taking down the original graft or the coronary arteries when the bioprosthetic valve fails. The technique of securing a tubular Dacron graft in the left ventricular outflow tract before implanting a prosthetic valve into it is very useful when there is, for example, a narrow or destroyed aortic anulus resulting from multiple previous operations, calcification, or endocarditis. The Dacron graft can be tailored to conform to the anatomy of the left ventricular outflow tract before it is sutured to it.[71]

In the original description of aortic root replacement by Bentall and DeBono in 1968, the aneurysm was opened and a tubular Teflon graft containing a mechanical valve was sutured to the aortic anulus, to the coronary arteries (by suturing the graft to the aortic sinus wall around their orifices), and to the distal aorta.[63] The aneurysm wall was wrapped around the graft and closed tightly for hemostasis. Pseudoaneurysm formation at the coronary artery and the aortic anastomoses was a complication of this technique.[59] To decompress the space between the graft and aneurysm wall, Cabrol and colleagues described the creation of a shunt between that space and the right atrium.[72] Kouchoukos and coworkers[59] stressed the importance of not wrapping the graft with the aneurysm wall to avoid tension on the anastomoses when accumulation of blood occurs between the aneurysmal wall and the graft. They recommended an open technique in which the coronary arteries are detached from the aortic sinuses and sutured to the tubular Dacron graft.[59] Cabrol and colleagues[73] described a technique whereby the two coronary arteries were connected to each other with a smaller graft and anastomosed side to side with the valved conduit. This technique, however,

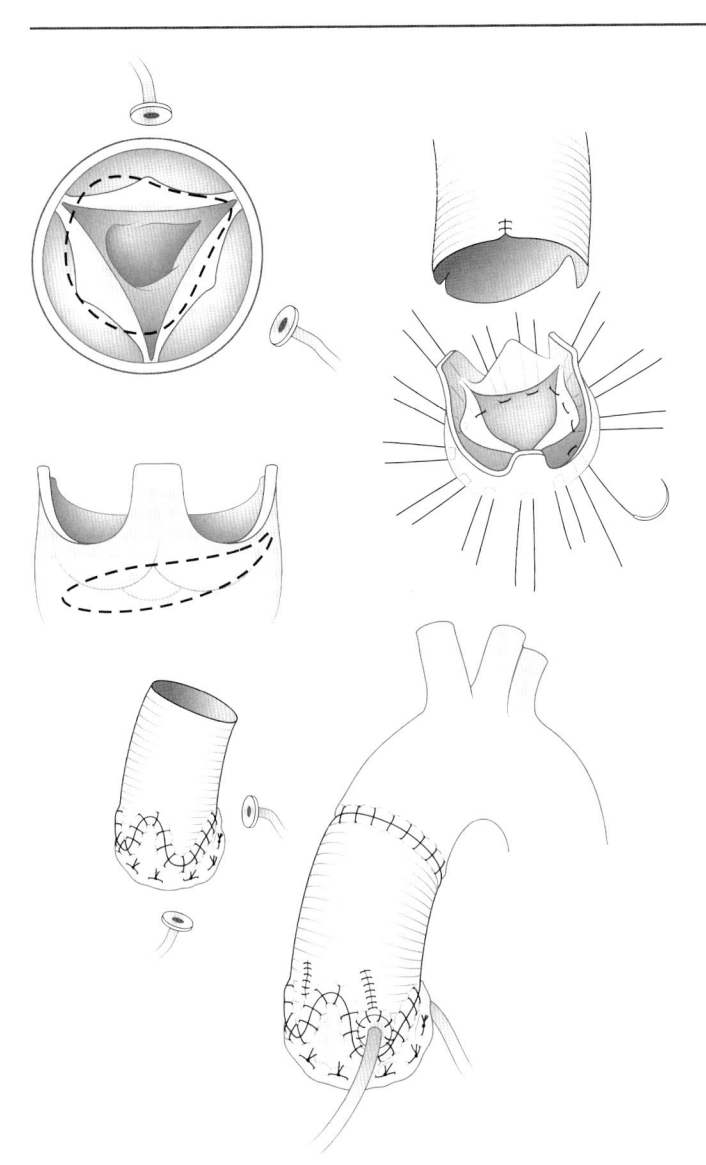

Figure 67-14
Aortic valve–sparing operation: reimplantation of the aortic valve.

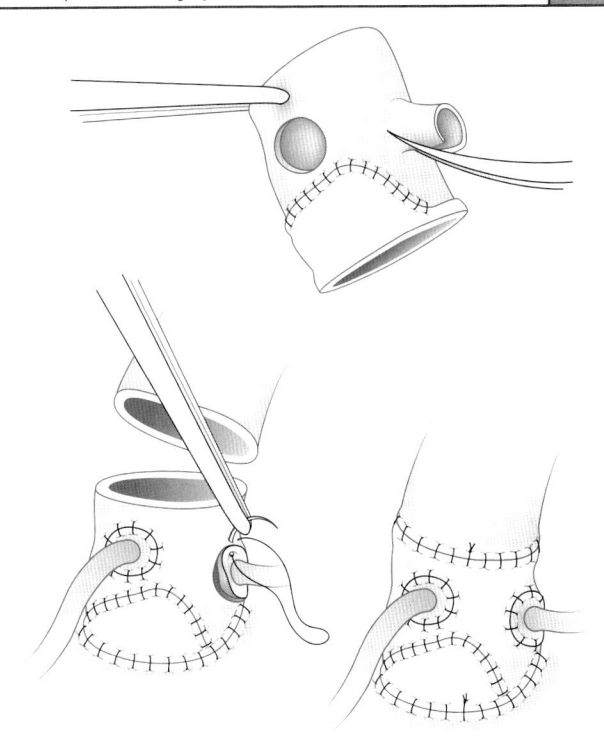

Figure 67-15
Composite replacement of the ascending aorta and aortic valve with a stentless porcine aortic root.

has not provided long-term results that were as good as direct coronary artery reimplantation.[74]

Clinical Outcomes

Surgery for aortic root aneurysm is associated with low operative mortality and morbidity, particularly when performed electively. In a recent report of our experience with aortic valve sparing operations, there were only three operative deaths among 220 patients operated for aortic root aneurysms, including 24 with acute type A aortic dissection.[75] Other investigators reported similarly low operative mortality with aortic valve–sparing operations.[70,75-78] The long-term survival of these patients is excellent. In our experience, the survival at 10 years was 88% and that of a general population of Ontario matched for age and sex was 91%.[75] Yacoub and colleagues[78] reported an 80% 10-year survival for all patients. Birks and coworkers[76] from the same group reported an 84% 10-year survival for those with Marfan syndrome. Most late deaths result from dissection or complications of aortic dissection. Aortic valve insufficiency is also a potential problem after aortic valve–sparing operations. Although 95% of our patients were free from reoperations at 10 years, the freedom from moderate or severe aortic insufficiency was 85%.[75]

The freedom from moderate or severe aortic insufficiency was higher in patients who had the reimplantation of the aortic valve than in those who had remodeling of the aortic root (94% versus 75%).[75] Increased experience, better operative techniques, and perfect aortic cusps coaptation by shortening of the free margins of the cusps when needed are expected to improve the long-term results of these operations. The principal advantages of aortic valve–sparing operations over aortic valve replacement are the low risks of thromboembolism, hemorrhage, and infective endocarditis.[66]

In a report by Gott and coworkers[64] on the outcomes of aortic root surgery in patients with Marfan syndrome operated on at 10 experienced surgical centers, the operative mortality was 1.5% among 455 patients who had elective surgery, 2.6% among 117 who had urgent surgery, and 11.7% among 103 who had emergency surgery, mostly for acute aortic dissection. However, in the experience of Gott and colleagues at the Johns Hopkins Hospital,[65] there was no operative death among 235 patients who had elective surgery and only two deaths among 36 who had urgent or emergent surgery. In our personal experience with 105 patients with Marfan syndrome in whom 44 had root replacement and 61 had aortic valve sparing, there was only one operative death, which occurred in a patient who was in preoperative cardiogenic shock because of end-stage aortic insufficiency.[66] Patients with Marfan syndrome are usually young when they require aortic root surgery,

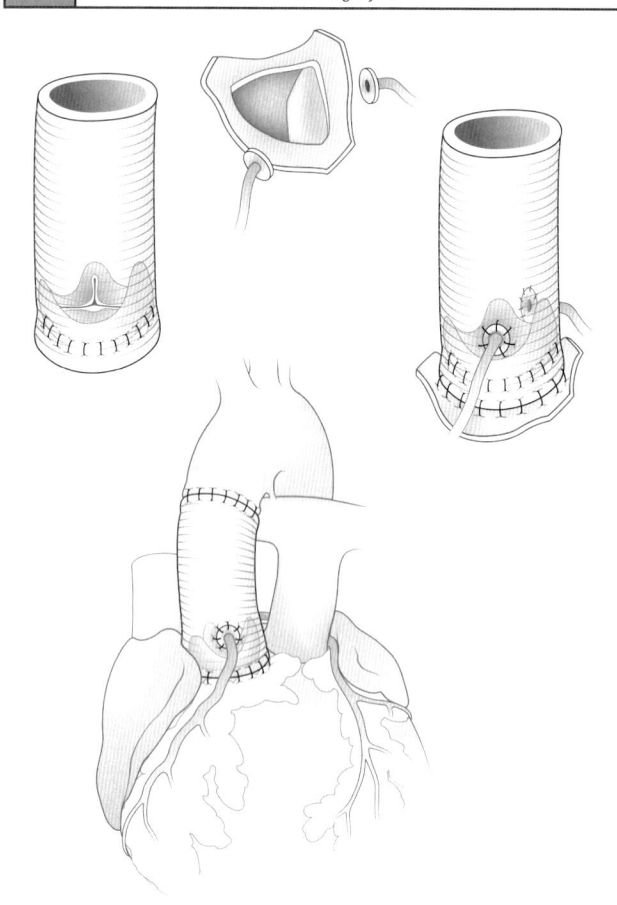

Figure 67–16
Composite replacement of the ascending aorta and aortic valve with a bioprosthetic valve.

which is one reason the operative mortality is low. Surgery in older patients is associated with higher risk.[74,79] Not only age but also the clinical presentation is an important determinant of outcome.[58,74,79,80] Surgery in patients with acute type A aortic dissection is associated with higher operative and late mortality (see Chapter 70). Overall, the operative mortality for aortic root replacement is around 5% to 10%.[58,74,70-80]

The long-term survival after aortic root replacement in patients with Marfan syndrome is very good. Gott and associates[64] reported from multiple institutions that the 10-year survival after aortic root surgery ranged from 60% to 80%, depending on the clinical presentation, but in their experience at Johns Hopkins, the 10-year survival was 81%.[65] Dissection or rupture of the residual aorta and dysrhythmias were the leading causes of late death.

Thromboembolism, hemorrhage, and endocarditis remain problems for patients who had aortic root replacement with mechanical valves,[64,66,74,79] and tissue degeneration and reoperation are problems for those who had biological aortic valve.[66]

Patients who had aortic root replacement require periodical checkups including a transthoracic echocardiogram and CT scans or MRI of the residual aorta. Patients with Marfan syndrome should take a beta-blocker if tolerated.

Reoperations in the aortic root after replacement with valved conduits can be difficult, but in the hands of experts it can be done with relatively low operative mortality.[71,81,82]

When the problem is graft infection, the use of an aortic homograft is believed to offer the patient the best chance of cure.[83,84] We and others have obtained similar results by using an approach of radical resection of infected tissues and reconstruction with synthetic grafts.[85-87]

ROSS PROCEDURE

The Ross procedure is a type of aortic valve replacement. It is a complex operation whereby the diseased aortic valve is replaced with the patient's own normal pulmonary valve, and a biological valve, usually a pulmonary homograft, is used to replace the pulmonary valve. This operation was first described in the experimental laboratory by Lower and colleagues in 1960[88] and clinically performed by Ross in 1967.[89] The original technique consisted of implanting the pulmonary autograft into the aortic root in a subcoronary position. For the next 2 decades, Donald Ross was practically the only surgeon performing this procedure.[90] Interest in this operation increased after the initial report by Stelzer and colleagues in late 1980s, who performed it using the technique of aortic root replacement, a more reproducible method.[91]

The Ross procedure is ideal for children because the pulmonary autograft grows with the child.[91,92] Although the Ross procedure can be used in patients of any age,[93,94] most surgeons prefer to use it in children and young adults.[95,96] Some surgeons consider it ideal for treating patients with active infective endocarditis.[97] The Ross procedure also has been performed in patients with dilated ascending aorta or even aneurysms.[98] It should not be used in patients with Marfan syndrome or in others with connective tissue disorders.

Although the Ross procedure was developed more than 4 decades ago, it gained popularity only in the 1990s. However, according to the Society of Thoracic Surgeons database, the number of these operations performed presently is very small.

Operative Techniques

The three basic methods to transfer the pulmonary autograft into the aortic position are subcoronary implantation, aortic root replacement, and aortic root inclusion.

Subcoronary Implantation

The aortic valve should be exposed through a transverse aortotomy 1 cm above the sinotubular junction. The diseased aortic valve is excised and all calcified tissues are completely débrided from the aortic anulus, membranous septum, and anterior leaflet of the mitral valve. The diameters of the aortic anulus and sinotubular junction are measured with a metric sizer. The pulmonary artery is opened just before its bifurcation, and the valve cusps are inspected. If they are normal, the pulmonary root is excised. The incision in the right ventricular outflow tract is made along a single horizontal plane approximately 3 mm below the lowest level of the pulmonary anulus. Care must be exercised to prevent damage to the left anterior descending artery and the first septal perforator branch. It is difficult to measure the diameter of the pulmonary anulus because it is entirely attached to distensible muscle, but it can be estimated by measuring the diameter of the sinotubular junction of the pulmonary root. The diameter of the pulmonary anulus is 15% to 20% larger than the diameter

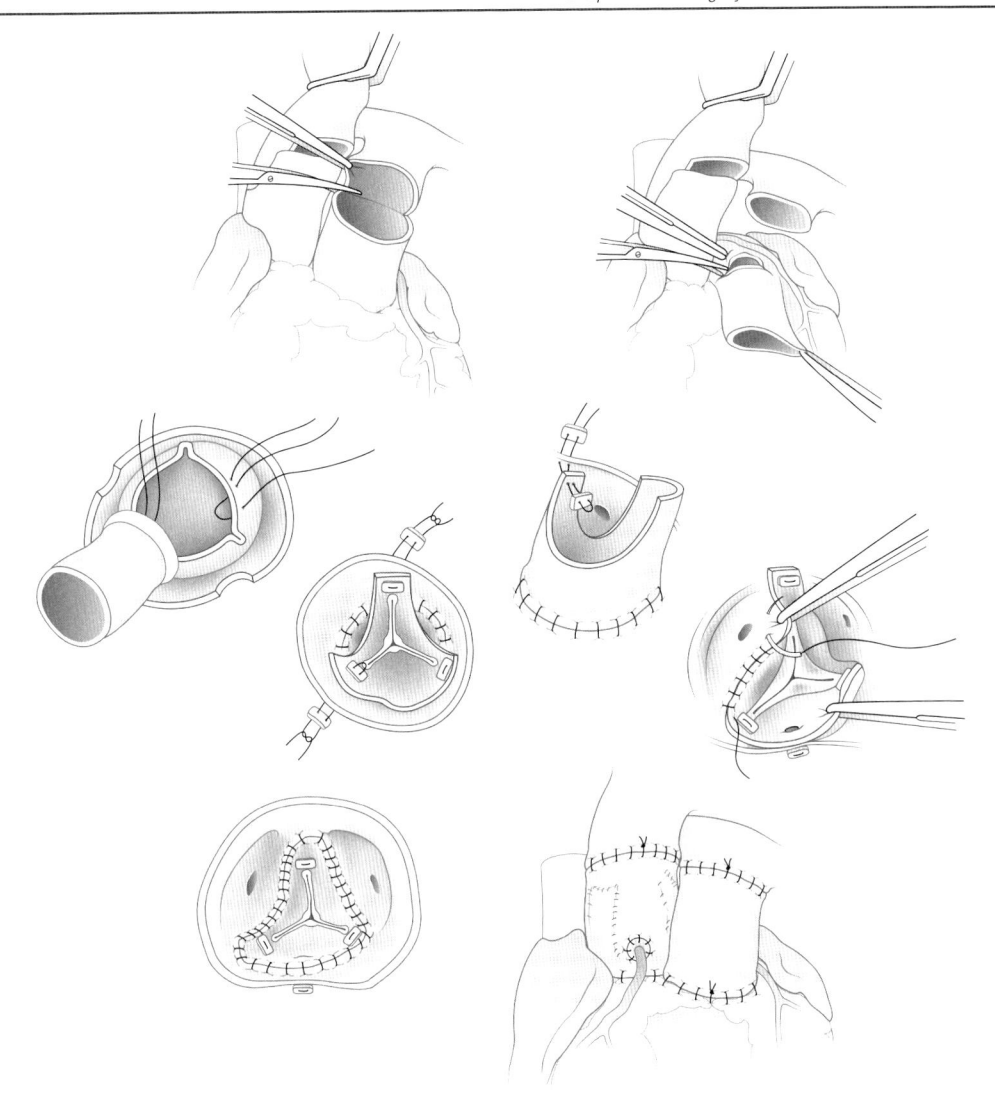

Figure 67–17
The Ross procedure: subcoronary implantation.

of the sinotubular junction. If the diameters of the aortic anulus and sinotubular junction of the two roots are similar, the technique of subcoronary implantation will work well. If there is mismatch in size, an alternative technique should be used and the difference in diameters corrected.[99] When the pulmonary anulus is slightly larger than the aortic anulus, it can be reduced by placing the sutures beneath the subcommissural triangles close together in the left ventricular outflow tract rather than in the pulmonary autograft. The smallest pulmonary sinus (usually the posterior sinus) should be oriented toward the left aortic sinus. The pulmonary autograft is secured to the left ventricular outflow tract and aortic anulus with multiple interrupted 4-0 polyester sutures. It is very important that all sutures be precisely distributed along a single horizontal plane at the level where the pulmonary anulus coincides with the level of the aortic anulus. Yacoub and colleagues[100] scallop the inflow of the pulmonary autograft before implanting it into the left ventricular outflow tract. If this technique is used, one has to be very meticulous about the spatial distribution of the three subcommissural spaces and maintenance of the normal scallop-shaped pulmonary anulus. Once the inflow suture line is completed, the three commissures are precisely suspended in the aortic root, and stay sutures through both arterial walls are placed immediately above the commissures. The sinuses of the pulmonary autograft that face the left and right coronary arteries are partially excised and sutured to the aortic sinuses around the coronary artery orifices with a continuous 6-0 or 5-0 polypropylene suture. The sinus of the pulmonary autograft that faces the noncoronary aortic sinus need not be excised, and it is sutured to the aortic root. It is important not to alter the diameter of the sinotubular junction of the pulmonary autograft when it is being sutured to the aortic root or when the aortotomy is closed. The right side of the heart is reconstructed with a pulmonary homograft. This homograft should be larger than the pulmonary autograft. Figure 67-17 illustrates the technique of subcoronary implantation.

Aortic Root Replacement

Aortic root replacement with a pulmonary autograft is done as previously described for aortic root aneurysm. The aortic valve is excised and so are the sinuses, leaving 5 mm of arterial wall around the coronary artery orifices. The same steps described previously are used to harvest the pulmonary autograft and measure it. If the aortic anulus is larger than the pulmonary anulus, a reduction anuloplasty is necessary. This can be accomplished by closing the subcommissural triangles of the noncoronary sinus of the aortic root (Fig. 67-18). The pulmonary autograft is secured to the left ventricular outflow tract with simple multiple interrupted 4-0 polyester sutures along a single horizontal plane. A strip of Teflon felt in this suture line improves hemostasis and may prevent annular dilation. The coronary arteries are reimplanted into the respective sinuses. The pulmonary autograft is sutured to the ascending aorta. If the ascending aorta is dilated, it may need replacement or plication (see Fig. 67-19). A strip of Dacron fabric or Teflon felt along this anastomosis prevents late dilation of the sinotubular junction.[101]

Aortic Root Inclusion

Another method of implanting the pulmonary autograft is the aortic root inclusion technique. The noncoronary aortic sinus should be incised vertically toward the aortic anulus to enhance exposure of the aortic root. The pulmonary autograft is secured to the aortic anulus using the technique described previously. After suturing the pulmonary autograft in the left ventricular outflow tract, the three commissures are pulled gently upward to determine the positions of the right and left coronary artery orifices in the pulmonary autograft. Small openings (5 or 6 mm in diameter) are made in the pulmonary autograft sinuses that correspond to the coronary artery orifices. The arterial wall of the pulmonary sinus is then sutured to the aortic sinus around the coronary artery orifices with a continuous 6-0 polypropylene suture. The three commissures of the pulmonary autograft are also sutured to the aortic wall, and the aortotomy is closed, including the aortic and pulmonary arterial walls. The incision made in the noncoronary sinus of the aortic root should be closed only if there is no bleeding between the two roots and if closure causes no distortion of the pulmonary autograft after unclamping the aorta. Figure 67-19 illustrates the technique of aortic root inclusion.

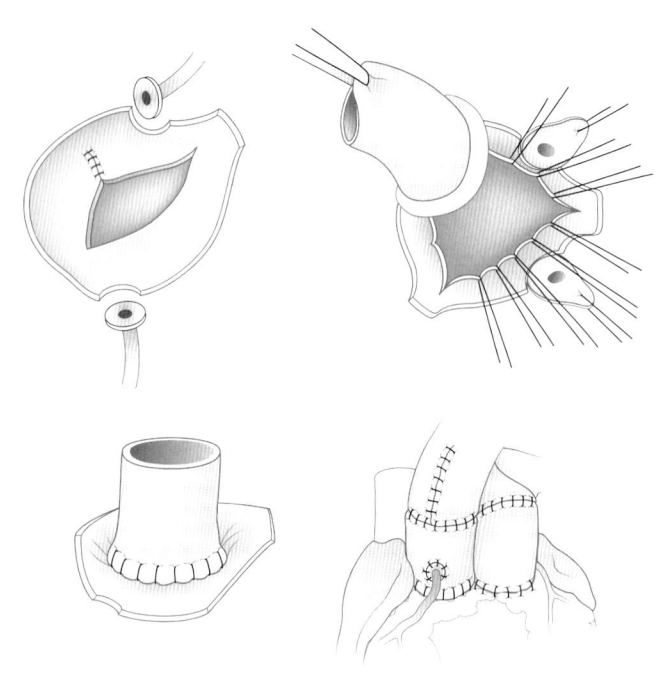

Figure 67–18
The Ross procedure: aortic root replacement.

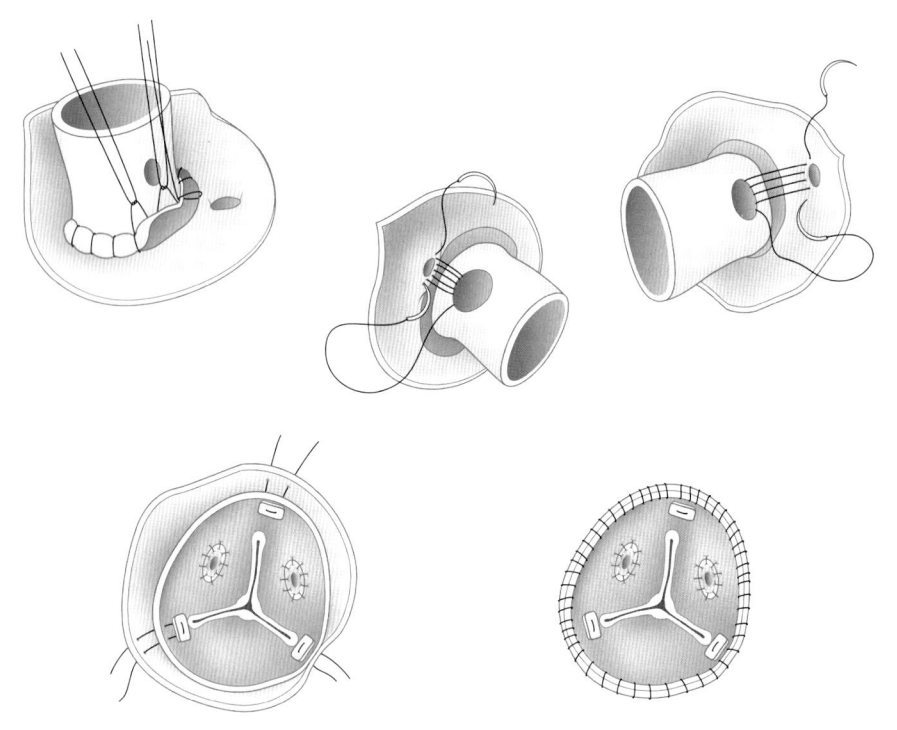

Figure 67–19
The Ross procedure: aortic root inclusion.

Clinical Outcomes

Despite its technical complexity, the operative mortality associated with the Ross procedure is reportedly low. It ranges from 0% to 5%, and this variation is largely the result of associated procedures.[93-96,100,101] A serious problem is aortic insufficiency due to technical errors.[99] Thromboembolic complications are rare because of the nature of the valves used and the patients' ages. Once the autograft is healed in the aortic root, it should not be thrombogenic. We have documented a few episodes of transient ischemic attacks during the first few weeks after surgery but never after the first couple of months. The risk of infective endocarditis is also very low. Subaortic false aneurysm is rare, but it may occur during the first postoperative year.[102,103]

Patients who had the Ross procedure should have annual Doppler echocardiography to assess the function of the neoaortic and pulmonary homograft, and to measure the size of the aortic root. Long-term survival after the Ross procedure is excellent.[96,100] Early development of aortic insufficiency is usually the result of technical problems,[99] and late aortic insufficiency is caused by dilation of the pulmonary autograft (aortic anulus or sinotubular junction, or both).[100,101,104] This problem is less likely to occur among patients who had the aortic root inclusion technique.[101] Aneurysms of the sinuses of the pulmonary autograft have been described.[101,105,106] If the pulmonary cusps remain normal, an aortic root reconstruction with preservation of the pulmonary valve is feasible; otherwise, the patient needs replacement of the entire pulmonary autograft.[75,105,106] In the original experience of Ross, who used almost exclusively the subcoronary implantation technique, the freedom from autograft failure that needed reoperation was 75% at 20 years.[95] Sievers and associates[107] reported very low rates of aortic insufficiency and reoperation using the subcoronary implantation and argued that this technique of implantation may be more appropriate for this operation. In a report by Yacoub and colleagues[100] that described the experience from Harefield, United Kingdom, and Rotterdam, The Netherlands, the freedom from any reoperation was 89.7% at 10 years, but at Harefield it was 94%, and only the aortic root replacement technique was used. It remains unknown if the differences in outcomes result from the operative techniques or patient selection, or both. Many surgeons believe patients who had aortic root replacement with pulmonary autograft should be treated with a β-blocker or angiotensin-converting enzyme inhibitor, or both, during the first postoperative year to prevent dilation during the adaptation of the graft to systemic pressures, but there are no scientific data to support this treatment.

Another problem with the Ross procedure is dysfunction of the biological valve used to reconstruct the right ventricular outflow tract.[95,96,108] A pulmonary homograft is probably the best conduit to use, but it is not free from complications, and a number of patients develop stenosis of the graft.[95,96,108] Stenosis of the pulmonary artery rather than the valve is usually the case. When the peak gradient reaches 50 mm Hg or the patient develops symptoms, percutaneous balloon dilation with stenting or pulmonary valve re-replacement is indicated. In the series by Elkins and colleagues, freedom from reoperation on the pulmonary homograft was 94% at 8 years.[96] Percutaneous implantation of bioprosthetic valves into failed pulmonary homograft is now feasible, and the results are very good.[109]

REFERENCES

1. Brewer R, Deck JD, Capati B, Nolan SP. The dynamic aortic root: its role in aortic valve function. *J Thorac Cardiovasc Surg* 1976;**72**:413-7.
2. Kunzelman KS, Grande J, David TE, et al. Aortic root and valve relationships: impact on surgical repair. *J Thorac Cardiovasc Surg* 1994;**107**:162-70.
3. Sands MP, Rittenhouse EA, Mohri H, Merendino K. An anatomical comparison of human, pig, calf and sheep aortic valves. *Ann Thorac Surg* 1969;**8**:407-14.
4. Swanson WM, Clark RE. Dimensions and geometric relationships of the human aortic valve as a function of pressure. *Circ Res* 1974;**35**:871-82.
5. Furukawa K, Ohteki H, Cao ZL, et al. Does dilatation of the sinotubular junction cause aortic insufficiency? *Ann Thorac Surg* 1989;**68**:949-53.
6. Dagum P, Green GR, Nistal FJ, et al. Deformational dynamics of the aortic root: modes and physiologic determinants. *Circulation* 1999;**100**(Suppl. II):II-54-II-62.
7. Dart AM, Lacombe F, Yeoh JK, et al. Aortic distensibility in patients with isolated hypercholesterolemia, coronary artery disease, or cardiac transplant. *Lancet* 1991;**338**:270-3.
8. Mohiaddin RH, Underwood SR, Bogren HG, et al. Regional aortic compliance studied by magnetic resonance imaging: the effects of age, training, and coronary artery disease. *Br Heart J* 1989;**62**:90-6.
9. Shimojo M, Tsuda N, Iwasaka T, Inuda M. Age-related changes in aortic elasticity determined by gated radionuclide angiography in patients with systemic hypertension or healed myocardial infarcts and in normal subjects. *Am J Cardiol* 1991;**68**:950-3.
10. Coady MA, Rizzo JA, Hammond GL, et al. Surgical intervention criteria for thoracic aortic aneurysms: a study of growth rates and complications. *Ann Thorac Surg* 1999;**67**:1922-6.
11. Hirose Y, Hamada S, Takamiya M, et al. Aortic aneurysms: growth rates measured with CT. *Radiology* 1992;**185**:249-52.
12. Shores J, Berger KR, Murphy EA, et al. Progression of aortic dilatation and the benefit of long-term b-adrenergic blockage in Marfan's syndrome. *N Engl J Med* 1994;**330**:1335-41.
13. Pressler V, McNamara JJ. Aneurysm of the thoracic aorta: review of 260 cases. *J Thorac Cardiovasc Surg* 1985;**89**:50-4.
14. Paelinck BP, Lasbm HJ, Bax JJ, et al. Assessment of diastolic function by cardiovascular magnetic resonance. *Am Heart J* 2002;**144**:198-205.
15. Blankenship J, Iliadis L. Coronary magnetic resonance angiography. *N Engl J Med* 2002;**346**:1413-4.
16. Dietz HC, Loeys BL, Carta L, Ramirez F. Recent progress towards a molecular understanding of Marfan syndrome. *Am J Med Genet* 2005;**139C**:4-9.
17. Bee KJ, Wilkes D, Devereux RB, Lerman BB, Dietz HC, Basson CT. Structural and functional genetic disorders of the great vessels and outflow tracts. *Ann N Y Acad Sci* 2006;**1085**:256-69.
18. Ng C, Cheng A, Myers L, Martinez-Murillo F, Jie C, Bedja D, et al. TGF-β-dependent pathogenesis of mitral valve prolapse in a mouse model of Marfan syndrome. *J Clin Invest* 2004;**114**:1586-92.
19. Hirata K, Tripsokiadis F, Sparks E, Bowen J, Wooley CF, Boudoulas H. The Marfan syndrome: abnormal aortic properties. *J Am Coll Cardiol* 1991;**18**:57-63.
20. De Paepe A, Devereux RB, Dietz HC, et al. Revised diagnostic criteria for the Marfan syndrome. *Am J Med Genet* 1996;**62**:417-26.
21. Hutchins GM, Moore GW, Skoog DK. The association of floppy mitral valve with disjunction of the mitral annulus fibrosus. *N Engl J Med* 1996;**14**:535-40.
22. Williams A, Davies S, Stuart AG, Wilson DG, Frase AG. Medical treatment of Marfan syndrome: a time for change. *Heart* 2008;**94**:414-21.
23. Murdoch JL, Walker BA, Halpern BL. Life expectancy and causes of death in the Marfan syndrome. *N Engl J Med* 1972;**286**:804-8.
24. Silverman DI, Burton KJ, Gray J. Life expectancy in the Marfan syndrome. *Am J Cardiol* 1995;**75**:157-60.
25. Rossiter JP, Morales AJ, Repke JT, et al. A prospective longitudinal evaluation of pregnancy in the Marfan syndrome. *Am J Obstet Gynecol* 1995;**173**:1599-604.
26. Mizuguchi T, Collod-Beroud G, Akiyama T, Abifadel M, Harada N, Morisaki T, et al. Heterozygous TGFBR2 mutations in Marfan syndrome. *Nat Genet* 2004;**36**:855-60.
27. Pannu H, Fadulu VT, Chang J, Lafont A, Hasham SN, Sparks E, et al. Mutations in transforming growth factor-beta receptor type II cause familial thoracic aortic aneurysms and dissections. *Circulation* 2005;**112**:513-20.
28. Loeys BL, Chen J, Neptune ER, Judge DP, Podowski M, Holm T, et al. A syndrome of altered cardiovascular, craniofacial, neurocognitive and skeletal development caused by mutations in TGFBR1 or TGFBR2. *Nat Genet* 2005;**37**:275-81.
29. Loeys BL, Schwarze U, Holm T, Callewaert BL, Thomas GH, Pannu H, et al. Aneurysm syndromes caused by mutations in the TGF-beta receptor. *N Engl J Med* 2006;**355**:788-98.
30. Williams JA, Loeys BL, Nwakanma LU, Dietz HC, Spevak PJ, Patel ND, et al. Early surgical experience with Loeys-Dietz: a new syndrome of aggressive thoracic aortic aneurysm disease. *Ann Thorac Surg* 2007;**83**:S757-63.

31. Germain DP. Clinical and genetic features of vascular Ehlers-Danlos syndrome. Ann Vasc Surg 2002;16(3):391-7.
32. Wenstrup RJ, Meyer RA, Lyle JS, et al. Prevalence of aortic root dilation in the Ehlers-Danlos syndrome. Genet Med 2002;4:112-7.
33. Fernandez MC, Duran AC, Real R, et al. Coronary artery anomalies and aortic valve morphology in the Syrian hamster. Lab Anim 2000;34:145-54.
34. Movahed MR, Hepner AD, Ahmadi-Kashani M. Echocardiographic prevalence of bicuspid aortic valve in the population. Heart Lung Circ 2006;15:297-9.
35. Clementi M, Notari L, Gorghi A, et al. Familial congenital bicuspid aortic valve: a disorder of uncertain inheritance. Am J Med Genet 1996;62:336-8.
36. Huntington K, Hunter AG, Char KL. A prospective study to assess the frequency of familial clustering of congenital bicuspid aortic valve. J Am Coll Cardiol 1997;30:1809-12.
37. Sadee A, Becker AE, Verheul HA, et al. Aortic valve regurgitation and the congenitally bicuspid aortic valve: a clinico-pathological correlation. Br Heart J 1992;67:439-41.
38. de Sa M, Moshkovitz Y, Butany J, et al. Histologic abnormalities of the ascending aorta and pulmonary trunk in patient with bicuspid aortic valve disease: clinical relevance to the Ross procedure. J Thorac Cardiovasc Surg 1999;118:588-94.
39. Niwa K, Perloff JK, Bhuta SM, et al. Structural abnormalities of great arterial walls in congenital heart disease: light and electron microscopic analyses. Circulation 2001;103:393-400.
40. Edwards WD, Leaf DS, Edwards JE. Dissecting aortic aneurysm associated with congenital bicuspid aortic valve. Circulation 1978;57:1022-5.
41. Amarenco P, Cohen A, Tzourio C, et al. Atherosclerotic disease of the aortic arch and the risk of ischemic stroke. N Engl J Med 1994;331:1474-9.
42. Matsumura Y, Osaki Y, Fukui T, et al. Protruding atherosclerotic aortic plaques and dyslipidaemia: correlation to subtypes of ischaemic stroke. Eur J Echocardiogr 2002;3:1-2.
43. Byrne JG, Aranki SF, Cohn LH. aortic valve operations under deep hypothermic circulatory arrest for the porcelain aorta: "no touch" technique. Ann Thorac Surg 1998;65:1313-5.
44. Yasuda T, Kawasuji M, Sakakibara N, Watanabe Y. Aortic valve replacement for calcified ascending aorta in homozygous familial hypercholesterolemia. Eur J Cardiothorac Surg 2000;18:249-50.
45. Heggtveit HA. Syphilitic aortitis: a clinicopathologic autopsy study of 100 cases, 1950 to 1960. Circulation 1994;29:346-52.
46. Kerr LD, Chang YJ, Spiera H, Fallon JT. Occult active giant cell aortitis necessitating surgical repair. J Thorac Cardiovasc Surg 2000;120:813-5.
47. Klein RG, Hunder GG, Stanson AW, Sheps SG. Larger artery involvement in giant cell (temporal) arteritis. Ann Intern Med 1975;83:806-12.
48. Lupi-Herrera E, Sanches-Torres G, Marcushamer J, et al. Takayasu's arteritis: clinical study of 107 cases. Am Heart J 1977;93:94-103.
49. Nesi G, Anichini C, Pedemonte E, et al. Giant cell arteritis presenting with annuloaortic ectasia. Chest 2002;121:1365-7.
50. Rojo-Leyva F, Ratliff NB, Cosgrove 3rd DM, Hoffman GS. Study of 52 patients with idiopathic aortitis from a cohort of 1,204 surgical cases. Arthritis Rheum 2000;43:901-7.
51. Ueno A, Awane G, Wakabayachi A. Successfully operated obliterative brachiocephalic arteritis (Takayasu) associated with elongated coarctation. Jpn Heart 1967;8:538-44.
52. Fyfe BS, Quintana CS, Kaneka M, Griepp RB. Aortic sarcoma four years after Dacron graft insertion. Ann Thorac Surg 1994;58:1752-4.
53. Wright EP, Glick AD, Virmani R, Page DL. Aortic intimal sarcoma with embolic metastases. Am J Surg Pathol 1985;9:950-7.
54. Feczko JD, Lynch L, Pless JE, et al. An autopsy case review of 142 nonpenetrating (blunt) injuries to the aorta. J Trauma 1992;33:846-9.
55. David TE. Remodeling of the aortic root and preservation of the native aortic valve. Oper Tech Cardiovasc Thorac Surg 1996;1:44-56.
56. David TE. Surgery of the aortic valve. Curr Probl Surg 1999;36:421-504.
57. David TE, Feindel CM, Armstrong S, Maganti M. Replacement of the ascending aorta with reduction of the diameter of the sinotubular junction to treat aortic insufficiency in patients with ascending aortic aneurysm. J Thorac Cardiovasc Surg 2007;133:414-8.
58. Kouchoukos NT, Marshall Jr WG, Wedige-Stecher TA. Eleven-year experience with composite graft replacement of the ascending aorta and aortic valve. J Thorac Cardiovasc Surg 1986;92:691-705.
59. Kouchoukos NT, Wareing TH, Murphy SF, Perrillo JB. Sixteen-year experience with aortic root replacement. Ann Surg 1991;214:308-20.
60. Cohn LH, Rizzo RJ, Adams DH, et al. Reduced mortality and morbidity for ascending aortic aneurysm resection regardless of cause. Ann Thorac Surg 1996;62:463-8.
61. Sioris T, David TE, Ivanov J, Armstrong S, Feindel CM. Clinical outcomes after separate and composite replacement of the aortic valve and ascending aorta. J Thorac Cardiovasc Surg 2004;128:260-5.
62. Lawrie GM, Earle N, DeBakey ME. Long-term fate of the aortic root and aortic valve after ascending aneurysm surgery. Ann Surg 1993;217:711-20.
63. Bentall HH, DeBono A. A technique of complete replacement of the ascending aorta. Thorax 1968;23:338-9.
64. Gott VL, Greene PS, Alejo DE, et al. Replacement of the aortic root in patients with Marfan's syndrome. N Engl J Med 1999;340:1307-13.
65. Gott VL, Cameron DE, Alejo DE, et al. Aortic root replacement in 271 Marfan patients: a 24-year experience. Ann Thorac Surg 2002;73:438-43.
66. de Oliveira NC, David TE, Ivanov J, et al. Results of surgery for aortic root aneurysm in patients with the Marfan syndrome. J Thorac Cardiovasc Surg 2003;125:1143-52.
67. Bonow RO, Carabello BA, Kanu C, de Leon Jr AC, Faxon DP, Freed MD, et al. ACC/AHA 2006 guidelines for the management of patients with valvular heart disease: a report of the American College of Cardiology/American Heart Association Task Force on Practice Guidelines. Circulation 2006;114:84-231.
68. De Paulis R, De Matteis GM, Nardi P, Scaffa R, Colella DF, Bassano C, et al. One-year appraisal of a new aortic root conduit with sinuses of Valsalva. J Thorac Cardiovasc Surg 2002;123:33-9.
69. Patel ND, Weiss ES, Alejo DE, Nwakanma LU, Williams JA, Dietz HC, et al. Aortic root operations for Marfan syndrome: a comparison of the Bentall and valve-sparing procedures. Ann Thorac Surg 2008;85:2003-10.
70. Schäfers HJ, Aicher D, Langer F. Correction of leaflet prolapse in valve-preserving aortic replacement: pushing the limits? Ann Thorac Surg 2002;74:S1762-4.
71. Krasopoulos G, David TE, Armstrong S. Custom-tailored valved conduit for complex aortic root disease. J Thorac Cardiovasc Surg 2008;135:3-7.
72. Cabrol C, Pavie A, Gandjbakhch I, et al. Complete replacement of the ascending aorta with reimplantation of the coronary arteries: new surgical approach. J Thorac Cardiovasc Surg 1981;81:309-15.
73. Cabrol C, Pavie A, Gandjbakhch I, et al. Complete replacement of the ascending aorta with reimplantation of the coronary arteries: new surgical approach. J Thorac Cardiovasc Surg 1986;91:17-25.
74. Bachet K, Termignon JL, Goudot B, et al. Aortic root replacement with a composite graft: factors influencing immediate and long-term results. Eur J Cardiothorac Surg 1996;10:207-13.
75. David TE, Feindel CM, Webb GD, Colman JM, Armstrong S, Maganti M. Long-term results of aortic valve-sparing operations for aortic root aneurysm. J Thorac Cardiovasc Surg 2006;132:347-54.
76. Birks EJ, Webb C, Child A, et al. Early and long-term results of a valve-sparing operation for Marfan syndrome. Circulation 1999;100(Suppl. II):II29-35.
77. Kallenback K, Karck M, Leyh RG, et al. Valve-sparing aortic root reconstruction in patients with significant aortic insufficiency. Ann Thorac Surg 2002;74:S1765-8.
78. Yacoub MH, Gehle P, Chandrasekaran V, et al. Late results of a valve-preserving operation in patients with aneurysms of the aorta and root. J Thorac Cardiovasc Surg 1998;115:1080-90.
79. Mingke D, Dresler C, Stone CD, Borst HG. Composite graft replacement of the aortic root in 335 patients with aneurysm or dissection. Thorac Cardiovasc Surg 1998;46:12-9.
80. Dossche KM, Schepens MA, Morshuis WJ, et al. A 23-year experience with composite valve graft replacement of the aortic root. Ann Thorac Surg 1999;67:1070-7.
81. LeMaire SA, DiBardino DJ, Koksoy C, Coselli JS. Proximal aortic reoperations in patients with composite valve grafts. Ann Thorac Surg 2002;74:S1777-80.
82. Raanani E, David TE, Dellgren G, et al. Redo aortic root replacement: experience with 31 patients. Ann Thorac Surg 2001;71:1460-3.
83. Lytle BW, Sabik JF, Blackstone EH, et al. Reoperative cryopreserved root and ascending aorta replacement for acute aortic prosthetic valve endocarditis. Ann Thorac Surg 2002;74:S1754-7.
84. Vogt PR, Brunner-LaRocca HP, Carrel T, et al. Cryopreserved arterial allografts in the treatment of major vascular infection: a comparison with conventional surgical techniques. J Thorac Cardiovasc Surg 1998;116:965-72.
85. Hagl C, Galla JD, Lansman SL, et al. Replacing the ascending aorta and aortic valve for acute prosthetic valve endocarditis: is using prosthetic material contraindicated? Ann Thorac Surg 2002;74:S1781-5.
86. Ralph-Edwards A, David TE, Bos J. Infective endocarditis in patients who had replacement of the aortic root. Ann Thorac Surg 1994;35:429-33.
87. David TE, Regesta T, Gavra G, Armstrong S, Maganti MD. Surgical treatment of paravalvular abscess: long-term results. Eur J Cardiothorac Surg 2007;31:43-8.
88. Lower RR, Stoffer RC, Shumway NE. Autotransplantation of the pulmonic valve into the aorta. J Thorac Cardiovasc Surg 1960;39:680-7.
89. Ross DN. Replacement of aortic and mitral valves with a pulmonary autograft. Lancet 1967;2:956-8.
90. Matsuki O, Okita Y, Almeida RS, et al. Two decades' experience with aortic valve replacement with pulmonary autograft. J Thorac Cardiovasc Surg 1988;95:705-11.

91. Stelzer P, Jones DJ, Elkins RC. Aortic root replacement with pulmonary autograft. *Circulation* 1988;**80**(Suppl. III):III209-13.
92. Elkins RC, Knott-Craig CJ, Ward KE, et al. Pulmonary autograft in children: realized growth potential. *Ann Thorac Surg* 1994;**57**:1387-94.
93. Böhm JO, Botha CA, Hemmer WB, et al. Older patients fare better with the Ross operation. *Ann Thorac Surg* 2003;**75**:769-801.
94. Chemidtke C, Bechtel MF, Noetzold A, et al. Up to seven years experience with the Ross procedure in patients >60 years of age. *J Am Coll Cardiol* 2000;**36**:1173-7.
95. Chambers CC, Sommerville J, Stone S, et al. Pulmonary autograft procedure for aortic valve disease: long term results of the pioneer series. *Circulation* 1997;**96**:2206-14.
96. Elkins RC. The Ross operation: a 12-year experience. *Ann Thorac Surg* 1999;**68**:S14-8.
97. Oswalt JD, Dewan SJ, Mueller MC, Nelson S. Highlights of a ten-year experience with the Ross procedure. *Ann Thorac Surg* 2001;**71**:S332-5.
98. Elkins RC, Lane MM, McCue C. Ross procedure for ascending aortic replacement. *Ann Thorac Surg* 1999;**67**:1843-5.
99. David TE, Omran A, Webb G, et al. Geometric mismatch of the aortic and pulmonary roots causes aortic insufficiency after the Ross procedure. *J Thorac Cardiovasc Surg* 1996;**112**:1231-9.
100. Yacoub MH, Klieverik LM, Melina G, Edwards SE, Sarathchandra P, Bogers AJ, et al. An evaluation of the Ross operation in adults. *J Heart Valve Dis* 2006;**15**:531-9.
101. David TE, Omran A, Ivanov J, et al. Dilation of the pulmonary autograft after the Ross procedure. *J Thorac Cardiovasc Surg* 2000;**119**:210-20.
102. Kouchoukos NT, Masetti P, Nickerson NJ, Castner CF, Shannon WD, Dávila-Román VG. The Ross procedure: long-term clinical and echocardiographic follow-up. *Ann Thorac Surg* 2004;**78**:773-81.
103. Ozaslan F, Wittlinger T, Monsefi N, Bouhmidi T, Theres S, Doss M, et al. Long-term follow-up of supra-annular pulmonary autograft aortic root replacement in patients with bicuspid aortic valve. *Eur J Cardiothorac Surg* 2008;**34**(3):583-8:discussion 588.
104. Luciani GB, Casali G, Favaro A, Prioli MA, Barozzi L, Santini F, Mazzucco A. Fate of the aortic root late after Ross operation. *Circulation* 2003;**108**(Suppl. 1):II61–167.
105. Schmidtke C, Stierle U, Sievers HH. Valve-sparing aortic root remodeling for pulmonary autograft aneurysm. *J Heart Valve Dis* 2002;**123**:437-41.
106. Sundt TM, Moon MR, Xu R. Reoperation for dilatation of the pulmonary autograft after the Ross procedure. *J Thorac Cardiovasc Surg* 2001;**122**:1249-52.
107. Sievers HH, Hanke T, Stierle U, Bechtel MF, Graf B, Robinson DR, Ross DN. A critical reappraisal of the Ross operation: renaissance of the subcoronary implantation technique?. *Circulation* 2006;**114**(Suppl. 1):I504-11.
108. Raanani E, Yau TM, David TE, et al. Risk factors for late pulmonary homograft stenosis after the Ross procedure. *Ann Thorac Surg* 2000;**70**:1953-7.
109. Lurz P, Coats L, Khambadkone S, Nordmeyer J, Boudjemline Y, Schievano S, et al. Percutaneous pulmonary valve implantation: impact of evolving technology and learning curve on clinical outcome. *Circulation* 2008;**117**:1964-72.

Index

Note: Page numbers followed by f refer to figures; page numbers followed by t refer to tables; page numbers followed by b refer to boxed text.

A

Abciximab, 760
  bleeding with, 1284
  in coronary artery bypass grafting, 1378
  preoperative evaluation of, 919
Abdominal aorta
  aneurysm of. See Aortic aneurysm, thoracoabdominal
  angiography of, 1159–1160, 1161f
  atherosclerosis of, 1165, 1166f
Abdominal esophagus, 517f–519f, 518–519, 549, 549f
  lymphatic drainage of, 520, 520f
Abdominal examination, after cardiac surgery, 934
Abdominal wall defects, ectopia cordis and, 380, 381f
AbioCor heart, 1525–1527, 1526f
Abiomed AB5000 device, 1512, 1512f
Abiomed BVS 5000 device, 1511–1512, 1512f
Abiomed Impella device, 1512, 1513f
Ablation therapy. See Catheter ablation; Laser therapy; Radiofrequency ablation
Abscess
  mediastinal, 658–659, 659f
  mitral anulus, 1227
  paraspinous, 659, 659f
  paravalvular, 843
  pulmonary, 181–182
    clinical features of, 181
    etiology of, 181, 182t
    imaging in, 31, 181–182, 182f, 183f
    location of, 181
    after lung transplantation, 221
    pathogens in, 181
    treatment of, 31, 182, 183f
Accessory pathway, in adult congenital heart disease, 2092–2094
Accessory pathway–mediated tachycardia, 1334–1335, 1335t, 1336f
Achalasia, 561–563, 562f
  barium esophagography in, 552f, 562
  botulinum toxin injection in, 562
  Heller myotomy in, 562–563
  manometry in, 562, 562f
  pneumatic dilation in, 562
Acid-base balance
  in cardiac surgery, 922
  in cardiopulmonary bypass, 922, 958–959
Acid injury, esophageal, 571–572
Activated clotting time, in cardiopulmonary bypass, 922–923, 946, 967, 968f
Acute coronary syndromes, 867. See also Angina; Coronary artery disease; Myocardial infarction (MI)
  ACC/AHA guidelines for, 867
  definition of, 867
  diagnosis of, 868–869, 869f, 869t
  inflammation in, 867–868
  management of, 871–873, 872t
  myocardial perfusion imaging in, 816–817
    resting, 816, 817f
  non–ST-segment elevation, 873–878, 873t, 875t, 876f
    angiotensin-converting enzyme inhibitors in, 877–878
    antiischemic agents in, 873
    antithrombotic therapy in, 873–874, 875t, 876f
    beta-blockers in, 877
    fibrinolytic agents in, 878–879, 878t
    intravenous glycoprotein IIb/IIIa inhibitors in, 875–877
    morphine in, 873
    statins in, 878
  pathophysiology of, 867–868, 868f

Acute coronary syndromes (Continued)
  plaque rupture in, 868, 868f
  platelets in, 868, 869f
  previous bypass surgery and, 879
  risk stratification in, 869–871, 870f–871f, 879
  ST-segment elevation, 878–879, 878t. See also Myocardial infarction (MI), ST-segment elevation
Acute lung injury
  transfusion-related, 764
  trauma-related, 107
Acute myocardial infarction. See Myocardial infarction (MI)
Acute respiratory distress syndrome
  postoperative, 54
  trauma-related, 107, 107b
Acyclovir, after lung transplantation, 219
Adenoid cystic carcinoma
  pulmonary, 329–331, 330f, 330t
  tracheal, 116, 118f
Adenoma
  alveolar, 156
  mucous gland, 154, 154f
  parathyroid, 640
Adenomatoid tumor, 455
Adenosine, in myocardial protection, 983t–984t, 985
Adipose tissue–derived cells, in regenerative cell-based therapy, 1600t, 1601f, 1603–1604
Adrenal gland, metastatic disease of, 30, 269–270
Adrenal insufficiency, in congenital diaphragmatic hernia, 494
β-Adrenergic agonist, after cardiac surgery, 941, 942t
β-Adrenergic antagonists
  in acute coronary syndromes, 877
  in afterload reduction, 940
  after coronary artery bypass grafting, 1382
  in heart failure, 891t, 892–893, 892f, 897, 897t
  in myocardial protection, 987
  in postoperative atrial fibrillation, 54, 944–945
  preoperative, 1017
  in tetralogy of Fallot, 1883
  in type B aortic dissection, 1120–1121
β-Adrenergic receptors, 717
Adrenocorticotropic hormone
  in bronchopulmonary carcinoid tumor, 325
  after cardiopulmonary bypass, 969
Adriamycin, in malignant pleural effusion, 441
Adson test, 393, 394f
Adult congenital heart disease. See Congenital heart disease, adult
Adverse drug event, 1018
Aerophagia, gastroesophageal reflux disease and, 524–525
AESOP system, 1296
Afterload
  after cardiac surgery, 938–940, 939f
  cellular biology of, 729, 729f, 733–734
  ejection fraction and, 745
  after pediatric cardiac surgery, 1759
  sarcomeric correlates of, 729, 729f
  ventricular coupling and, 748
Age. See also Children
  aorta changes with, 1022
  aortic root changes with, 1022
  cardiac surgery–related neurologic disorders and, 1006, 1007t
  esophagectomy and, 40
  ischemic preconditioning and, 992
  lung cancer treatment and, 40
  myocardium changes with, 981
  perioperative complications and, 44

Age (Continued)
  surgical complications and, 44, 44t
  surgically induced myocardial ischemia and, 981
  thoracic trauma and, 86
Agenesis
  diaphragmatic, 509
  pulmonary, 139–140, 140f
  tracheal, 130–131, 131f
Air embolism, 102–103
Air leak
  after chest wall resection/reconstruction, 307, 307f
  postoperative, 55
  traumatic, 93
Airway
  heart-lung transplantation–related complications of, 1568
  imaging of
    in nontraumatic lesions, 26, 29f
    in trauma, 26
  lung transplantation–related complications of, 223
  malignant obstruction of, laser therapy in, 74, 75t
  management of
    bronchoscopy in, 64
    after cardiac surgery, 933
    surgical, 50
    in tracheobronchial injury, 93
  stenting of, 71–74
    in benign stricture, 72–73
    in emphysema, 204
    indications for, 72
    in malignant stricture, 73
    metal stent for, 71–72, 72t
    silicone-based stent for, 71–72, 72t
    technique for, 71–72
  stricture of
    benign, 72–73
    malignant, 73
Albuterol, 52–53
Alcohol consumption, 913
Alcohol septal ablation
  in hypertrophic cardiomyopathy, 860
  vs. septal myectomy, 1501, 1504f
Aldosterone inhibitors, in heart failure, 887t, 888, 897, 897t
Alfentanil, in congenital heart disease, 1757
Alkali injury, esophageal, 571–572
Allen test, 1372–1374
Alpha-fetoprotein
  in anterior mediastinal mass, 637, 639
  in pleural effusion, 435t
Alpha-stat strategy, in cardiopulmonary bypass, 922, 958–959
Aluminum chloride hexahydrate 20% anhydrous ethyl alcohol solution, in hyperhidrosis, 663
Aluminum toxicity, sucralfate-related, 48–49
Alveolar adenoma, 156
Amebiasis, pericardial, 1485
Amiloride, 887t, 888, 993
ε-Aminocaproic acid
  in cardiac surgery, 765–766, 949
  in cardiopulmonary bypass, 923–924, 1724
  in children, 765–766
  in congenital diaphragmatic hernia, 502, 504
  in postinfarction ventricular septal defect repair, 1454
Amiodarone
  in postoperative atrial fibrillation, 54, 945
  pulmonary toxicity of, 165
Amlodipine, 890, 891t
Amplatzer VSD device, 1454

Index

Amrinone
  after cardiac surgery, 940–941, 942t
  in heart failure, 895
  in pediatric pulmonary hypertension, 1752
Amylase, pleural fluid, 433
Amyloid, pulmonary deposition of, 156
Analgesia, 52
  in children, 1756
  after thoracotomy, 56
Anaphylactoid reaction
  after percutaneous coronary intervention, 854–855
  protamine-related, 923
Anaphylaxis
  aprotinin-related, 767
  protamine-related, 923
Anasarca, protamine-related, 923
Anastomosis, leak from, 56
Anatomy, 3. *See also at specific structures and disorders*
  esophageal, 20–23, 22f
  mediastinal, 12, 13t, 14f
  neural, 23–24
  pulmonary, 14–20, 15f–16f, 17t–18t, 19f–21f
  surface, 10–12, 11f, 12t, 13f
  thoracic cage, 3–6, 3f–4f
  thoracic muscle, 6–10, 7f, 8t, 9f
  tracheobronchial tree, 12–14
  vessel, 23
Anesthesia
  for cardiac surgery. *See* Cardiac surgery, anesthesia in
  for congenital heart disease surgery. *See* Congenital heart disease, surgical treatment of, anesthesia in
  for lung transplantation, 214
  for pediatric cardiac catheterization, 1693
  physiologic effects of, 39
  for tracheal resection, 117–119
Aneurysm
  aortic. *See* Aortic aneurysm
  aortic arch. *See* Aortic arch aneurysm
  aortic root. *See* Aortic root, aneurysm of
  atrial septum, 1799
  coronary artery, 1472
  left ventricular, 1576–1577, 1577f
    resection of, 1577–1578
  pulmonary artery, 145
  sinus of Valsalva, 793, 794f
Angina. *See also* Acute coronary syndromes; Myocardial infarction (MI)
  asymptomatic/mild, coronary artery bypass grafting in, 1369, 1370t, 1385–1386
  refractory, transmyocardial laser therapy for. *See* Transmyocardial laser revascularization
  stable
    coronary artery bypass grafting in, 1369, 1370t
    percutaneous coronary intervention for, 849–852
    single-photon emission computed tomography in, 813–814, 814b
  vs. thoracic outlet syndrome, 397
  unstable, 868
    classification of, 869, 869t
    coronary artery bypass grafting in, 1369, 1370t
    diagnosis of, 868–869, 869f, 869t
    percutaneous coronary intervention for, 848–849
Angioedema, ACE inhibitor–related, 891–892
Angiogenesis, 719, 720f
  in myocardial cell-based regenerative therapy, 1607, 1608f
  nitric oxide in, 719, 720f
  with transmyocardial laser therapy, 1463
Angiography. *See also* Aortography
  in atrioventricular canal defects, 1836
  in chronic thromboembolic pulmonary hypertension, 1622
  coronary. *See* Coronary angiography
  in Pancoast tumor, 315f
  in pectus excavatum, 363
  peripheral. *See* Peripheral angiography
  in postinfarction ventricular septal defect, 1449
  in pulmonary arteriovenous malformation, 146f
  in thoracic aortic aneurysm, 1068, 1073
  in thoracic outlet syndrome, 396, 399f
  in trauma, 87–88, 88f, 89b
  in vascular ring, 1791
Angiosarcoma
  cardiac, 1635t, 1637, 1637f
  pulmonary, 332

Angioscopy, pulmonary, in chronic thromboembolic pulmonary hypertension, 1622
Angiotensin-converting enzyme (ACE) inhibitors
  in aortic stenosis, 1197
  in asymptomatic left ventricular dysfunction, 940
  before coronary artery bypass grafting, 1374
  in heart failure, 890–892, 890f, 891t, 897t
  in NSTE acute coronary syndromes, 877–878
Angiotensin receptor blocking agents, in heart failure, 891t, 892
Ankle-brachial index, 1163
Anomalous aorta–pulmonary artery course of coronary arteries, 1971–1975
  anatomy of, 1971–1972
  clinical presentation of, 1973
  diagnosis of, 1973
  pathophysiology of, 1972
  surgical management in, 1973–1975
    indications for, 1973
    neo-ostium creation for, 1973–1974
    results of, 1974–1975
    unroofing procedure for, 1973, 1974f
Anomalous origin of coronary artery from aorta, 1467
Anomalous origin of coronary artery from contralateral sinus of Valsalva, 802, 805f, 1467–1469, 1469f
Anomalous origin of coronary artery from pulmonary artery, 1470, 1963–1971, 1964b
  anatomy of, 1963–1964, 1964f–1965f
  clinical presentation of, 1965
  diagnosis of, 1965–1966
  pathophysiology of, 1964–1965
  surgical management of, 1966–1969
    in adult, 1966, 1971
    bypass grafts in, 1966
    care after, 1969
    coronary artery bypass grafting in, 1966
    direct reimplantation in, 1966–1970, 1966f–1968f
    indications for, 1966
    ligation in, 1966, 1969
    mitral regurgitation and, 1970–1971
    modified Takeuchi operation in, 1968–1969, 1969f–1972f
    results of, 1969–1970
Anomalous pulmonary venous drainage/connection
  partial, 1817–1819
    anatomy of, 1817, 1818f
    clinical presentation of, 1817–1818
    pathophysiology of, 1818
    repair of, 1818–1819, 1820f
    scimitar syndrome and, 1819–1821, 1821f
  total, 1821–1826
    anatomy of, 1822
      cardiac, 1822
      infracardiac, 1822
      mixed, 1822
      supracardiac, 1822
    clinical presentation of, 1822–1823, 1822f
    diagnosis of, 1823–1824, 1823f
    in heterotaxy, 1826–1827
    pathophysiology of, 1823
    prognosis for, 1826
    repair of, 1824–1825, 1825f–1826f
      pulmonary vein stenosis after, 1827
      results of, 1826
    in single ventricle, 2043
Antecubital vein, for temporary pacemaker insertion, 1306, 1307b
Anti-CD3 monoclonal antibody
  in heart-lung transplantation, 1564–1565
  in heart transplantation, 1546
Antiangiogenic therapy, in mesothelioma, 465–466
Antibiotics
  in aortic graft infection, 1078
  in aspiration pneumonia, 179
  in community-acquired pneumonia, 176–178, 178f
  in empyema, 417–419
  in native valve endocarditis, 1260
  in post-traumatic pneumonia, 108
  postoperative, 49, 52
  prophylactic
    in cardiac surgery, 1017
    for dental procedures, 1269, 1269t
    postoperative, 49
    in sternal wound infection prevention, 1000
  in prosthetic valve endocarditis, 1271, 1273

Antibodies, in heparin-induced thrombocytopenia, 759–760
Anticoagulation, 758–760. *See also specific anticoagulants*
  with cardiopulmonary bypass, 922–923, 965–967, 966f, 968f, 1283, 1286–1287
  coronary artery bypass grafting and, 858
  errors with, 1018
  after Fontan procedure, 2049–2050
  in heart transplantation, 1531
  with intra-aortic balloon assist device, 1286
  postoperative, 52
  pregnancy and, 1959
  preoperative evaluation of, 919
  with prosthetic heart valves, 50, 1280–1284, 1281f–1282f. *See also specific anticoagulants*
  in prosthetic valve endocarditis, 1271–1272
  reversal of, 770
  with ventricular assist devices, 1283, 1521
Antiemetics, 52
Antifibrinolytics
  in cardiac surgery, 765–771, 765b
  in cardiopulmonary bypass, 923–924
  in coronary artery bypass grafting, 1378
  in postinfarction ventricular septal defect repair, 1454
Antihypertensives, in atherosclerosis management, 914–915
Antineutrophil cytoplasmic antibodies, in Wegener's granulomatosis, 163
Antiplatelet agents
  in coronary artery bypass grafting, 1378
  in NSTE acute coronary syndromes, 873–874
  in prosthetic heart valve anticoagulation, 1280–1281, 1282f, 1284
Antithrombin therapy, in NSTE acute coronary syndromes, 874–875, 875t, 876f
Antithymocyte globulin
  in heart-lung transplantation, 1564–1565, 1564t
  in heart transplantation, 1546
Anuloplasty
  mitral, 1221, 1223f. *See also* Mitral valve repair
    in chronic ischemic regurgitation, 1433, 1439f, 1439t, 1442–1445, 1443f–1444f
    in regurgitation, 1221, 1223f, 1227
    in type I congenital mitral anomaly, 2021, 2021f
  tricuspid, 1251–1252, 1252f–1253f
Aorta. *See also at* Aortic
  abdominal
    aneurysm of. *See* Aortic aneurysm, thoracoabdominal
    angiography of, 1159–1160, 1161f
    atherosclerosis of, percutaneous intervention for, 1165, 1166f
  adventitia of, 1022
  age-related changes in, 1022
  anatomy of, 706, 706f–707f, 1042
  aneurysm of. *See* Aortic aneurysm; Aortic arch aneurysm
  anomalous coronary artery origin from, 1467
  ascending
    anatomy of, 706
    aneurysm of. *See* Aortic aneurysm, ascending
    atherosclerosis of, 1027
      coronary artery bypass grafting and, 1377–1378, 1378f
    calcification of, 1027
    dissection of. *See* Aortic dissection
    inflammation of, 1027
    in Loeys-Dietz syndrome, 1026
    in off-pump coronary artery bypass grafting, 1403–1404, 1404f
    porcelain, 1027, 1077–1078
    trauma to, 1027, 1179, 1179f
      penetrating, 103
    tumors of, 1027
  atherosclerosis of, 1027
    coronary artery bypass grafting and, 1377–1378, 1378f
    imaging of, 793–794
    percutaneous intervention for, 1165, 1166f
  coarctation of. *See* Coarctation of aorta
  compliance of, 1022
  coronary artery reimplantation into, 1966–1970, 1966f–1968f
  cross-clamping of
    duration of, 1065, 1065f
    spinal cord injury and, 1065, 1065f, 1069–1075, 1070f, 1074f

Aorta (Continued)
    dissection of. See Aortic dissection
    with double-outlet right ventricle, 1861
    giant cell arteritis of, 1066
    intima of, 1022
    media of, 1022
    pressure in, 780t, 781
    retroesophageal, circumflex, 1788–1789, 1788f, 1791
    Takayasu's disease of, 1066–1067
    thoracic, 23
        anatomy of, 706
        aneurysm of. See Aortic aneurysm, thoracic
        angiography of, 1159, 1160f
        dissection of. See Aortic dissection
        echocardiography of, 843–844, 844f
        false aneurysm of, 1097–1098
        injury to, 93–94, 1065–1066, 1066f, 1178–1181, 1179f–1180f
            assessment of, 1178–1181, 1179f
            diagnosis of, 1178
            imaging in, 25–26, 26f–27f, 93–94, 94f
            management of, 94, 102, 1077, 1178–1181, 1179f–1180f
            stent graft for, 94
            mechanism of, 1178
            natural history of, 1178
            penetrating, 103
        intramural hematoma of, 793, 1139–1140
        penetrating atherosclerotic ulcer of, 1139–1140
        prosthetic vascular graft for, thrombosis with, 1288–1289, 1289f
        transection of, 87–88, 88f
    transposition of. See Transposition of great arteries
    ulcers of
        atherosclerotic, 1139–1140
        imaging of, 794
        in type B aortic dissection, 1115–1117, 1120
Aortic aneurysm
    ascending
        atherosclerotic, 1027
        degenerative, 1023–1025
        dissection of, 1023
        growth of, 1023
        infectious, 1027
        rupture of, 1023
        surgical treatment of, 1027–1030, 1028f–1031f
        syphilitic, 1027
    thoracic, 1063, 1129–1136
        angiography in, 1068, 1073
        aortitis and, 1066–1067
        cardiac catheterization in, 1068
        classification of, 1063, 1064f
        clinical manifestations of, 1067–1068
        congenital lesions and, 1063–1064
        creatinine levels in, 1069
        endovascular treatment of, 1082, 1082t
            access for, 1132–1133, 1132f–1133f, 1135
            anatomic considerations in, 1132–1134
            complications of, 1135–1136, 1135t
            endoleak with, 1135–1136, 1135t
            European registries of, 1135
            Gore TAG device for, 1130, 1131f, 1134
            historical perspective on, 1129
            indications for, 1130, 1130f
            landing zones in, 1133–1134, 1133f
            multicenter clinical trials of, 1134–1135
            neurologic complications of, 1136
            results of, 1134–1135
            Talent device for, 1130–1131, 1131f, 1134–1135
            Valiant device for, 1131
            Zenith TX2 device for, 1131–1132, 1132f, 1134–1135
        hydrogen mapping in, 1073
        imaging of, 791–792, 792f–793f
        incidence of, 1129
        medial degenerative, 1064
        mycotic, 1064–1065, 1065f
        natural history of, 1129–1130
        patient history in, 1067–1068
        physical examination in, 1067–1068
        preoperative testing in, 1068–1069
        pulmonary function testing in, 1068–1069
        reoperation in, 1067, 1078
        rupture of, 1129–1130
        saccular, 1064–1065, 1065f, 1077

Aortic aneurysm (Continued)
    surgical treatment of, 1075–1079, 1076f
        artery of Adamkiewicz in, 1072–1073
        care after, 1074
        cerebrospinal fluid drainage in, 1074–1075, 1074f–1075f
        cross-clamping in, 1069–1075, 1070f, 1074f
        entire aorta repair in, 1086f
        entire aorta replacement in, 1078–1079, 1082–1085, 1083f
        infection and, 1078
        intercostal vessels in, 1072–1073
        motor evoked potentials in, 1073–1074
        outcomes of, 1085–1086, 1086f
        reoperative, 1067, 1078
        segmental sequential technique in, 1069–1071
        spinal cord anatomy in, 1071, 1072f
        spinal cord protection for, 1069–1075, 1070f, 1072f, 1074f–1075f
        trauma and, 1065–1066, 1065f–1066f
        tumors and, 1067
        twenty-four-hour Holter examination in, 1068
    thoracoabdominal
        angiography in, 1068
        aortitis and, 1066–1067
        cardiac catheterization in, 1068
        classification of, 1063, 1064f
        clinical manifestations of, 1067–1068
        creatinine levels in, 1069
        endovascular treatment of, 1082, 1082t
            outcomes of, 1086
        medial degenerative, 1064
        mycotic, 1064–1065
        patient history in, 1067–1068
        physical examination in, 1067–1068
        preoperative testing in, 1068–1069
        pulmonary function testing in, 1068–1069
        reoperation in, 1067
        surgical treatment of, 1076f, 1079–1082, 1080f–1081f
            care after, 1074
            cerebrospinal fluid drainage in, 1074–1075, 1074f–1075f
            motor evoked potentials in, 1073–1074
            outcomes of, 1085–1086, 1086f
            segmental sequential technique in, 1069–1071
            spinal cord anatomy in, 1071, 1072f
            spinal cord protection in, 1069–1075
            trauma and, 1065–1066
            tumors and, 1067
            twenty-four-hour Holter examination, 1068
Aortic anulus, 1021, 1022f
    diameter of, 1022
    dilation of, 1022, 1024f
Aortic arch, 706, 706f–707f, 1041. See also Brachiocephalic artery (arteries)
    aneurysm of. See Aortic arch aneurysm
    angiography of, 1159, 1160f
    atresia of, 1928–1929. See also Aortic arch, interrupted
    bovine, 1159
    in coarctation of aorta, 1785
    in congenitally corrected transposition of great arteries, 2004
    definition of, 1041
    dissection of, 1042, 1046f, 1102, 1105, 1159, 1160f. See also Aortic dissection
    double, 1787, 1787f, 1790f, 1791
    in hypoplastic left heart syndrome, 2032, 2034f
    inflammation of, 1027, 1043–1044, 1046f
    injury to, 1044, 1178–1181
        diagnosis of, 1178
        management of, 1178–1181, 1180f
        mechanism of, 1178
        natural history of, 1178
    interrupted, 1927
        anatomy of, 1927–1929, 1928f
        cardiac catheterization in, 1930
        clinical presentation of, 1929–1930
        echocardiography in, 1930
        historical perspective on, 1927
        left ventricular outflow tract obstruction and, 1931–1934, 1932f
        nomenclature for, 1927–1929
        preoperative management of, 1929–1930
        surgical management of, 1930–1937

Aortic arch (Continued)
        cardiopulmonary bypass support in, 1934–1937, 1935f
        continuous cerebral perfusion in, 1936–1937, 1936f–1937f
        direct end-to-side anastomosis in, 1935–1936, 1935f
        historical aspects of, 1930–1931
        homograft vascular patch augmentation in, 1935–1936, 1936f
        indications for, 1930
        left main-stem bronchus compression after, 1939–1940
        left ventricular outflow tract obstruction and, 1931–1934, 1932f–1933f, 1938–1939, 1938f–1939f
        results of, 1931, 1931f, 1937–1940, 1938f–1939f
        technique of, 1931, 1934–1937, 1935f–1937f
        timing of, 1930
        ventricular septal defect closure in, 1930–1931, 1931f
    in truncus arteriosus, 1913, 1916–1917, 1917f
    type A, 1928–1929, 1928f
    type B, 1928–1929, 1928f
    type C, 1928–1929, 1928f
    ventricular septal defect and, 1929
    left
        with anomalous right subclavian artery, 1789, 1789f, 1791–1792
        with left descending aorta, 1788–1789
        with right descending aorta, 1788–1789, 1788f
    reoperation on, 1044–1046, 1047f, 1057–1058
    right, 1042, 1044f–1045f
        with left ligamentum arteriosum, 1787–1788, 1788f, 1791
        in tetralogy of Fallot, 1881
    in transposition of great arteries, 1994, 1998–1999
    tumors of, 1044
Aortic arch aneurysm, 1041
    classification of, 1041–1042
    clinical manifestations of, 1046–1048, 1067
    congenital, 1042, 1043f–1045f
    degenerative, 1042
    evaluation of, 1046–1048
    fusiform, 1042
    in genetic disease, 1046
    mycotic, 1042–1043
    pathology of, 1042
    preoperative evaluation of, 1047–1048
    reoperation for, 1044–1046
    saccular, 1042, 1077
    surgical treatment of, 1053–1058, 1077
        arterial inflow for, 1048
        bifurcated graft technique in, 1057–1058, 1059f
        brain protection in, 1049–1053, 1050f
        branch graft technique in, 1057
        carbon dioxide in, 1050
        cardiopulmonary perfusion in, 1048–1049, 1048f
        elephant trunk procedure in, 1054–1056, 1055f, 1057f
        endarterectomy in, 1057
        femoral artery for, 1048–1049
        hemiarch replacement in, 1053–1054
        historical perspective on, 1041
        long tongue hemiarch replacement in, 1054
        neurocognitive deficit prevention in, 1051–1053, 1052f
        outcomes of, 1041, 1058–1059
        patch technique in, 1057
        reoperative, 1044–1046
        S-100 after, 1051, 1052f
        stroke prevention in, 1050–1051, 1051t
        subclavian artery for, 1048–1049, 1048f
        thiopental in, 1050–1051
        total arch replacement in, 1053–1056, 1055f, 1057f–1058f
        valved conduit technique in, 1058, 1060f
Aortic autograft translocation, in transposition of great arteries, 1996, 1997f–1998f
Aortic dissection, 1136–1139
    aortic valve insufficiency and, 1096, 1199, 1202
    classification of, 1042, 1046f, 1090–1091, 1090f, 1136–1137
    computed tomography in, 25, 26f, 792–793, 792f
    echocardiography in, 25, 844, 844f, 1099–1100

Aortic dissection (Continued)
  in Ehlers-Danlos syndrome, 1092–1093
  endovascular treatment of, 1137–1138, 1138f
    indications for, 1137
    results of, 1138–1139
    technical considerations in, 1137–1138, 1138f
    in type B dissection, 1122, 1138–1139
  epidemiology of, 1091–1092
  in Loeys-Dietz syndrome, 1093
  magnetic resonance imaging in, 25, 792–793, 792f–793f
  in Marfan syndrome, 1092, 1955
  medical treatment of, 1137
  mortality with, 1090, 1091f
  natural history of, 1136–1137
  retro-A, 1090, 1090f, 1105
  risk of, 1129–1130
  surgical treatment of, 1137
  type A, 1089, 1137
    acute, 1090, 1096–1098
      management of, 1100–1106
        aortic arch in, 1102–1105, 1104f
        aortic root in, 1104–1105
        BioGlue in, 1101–1102
        coarctation in, 1105
        follow-up in, 1109
        gelatin-resorcin-formalin glue in, 1101–1102
        malperfusion after, 1105–1106
        operative technique in, 1102–1104, 1103f–1104f
        principles of, 1101
        reoperation in, 1108–1109, 1109f
        results of, 1106–1109, 1108f
        retrograde extension in, 1105
        technical considerations in, 1101–1102
    angiography in, 1100
    aortic branch compromise with, 1095–1096, 1095f
    aortography in, 1098
    arterial hypertension and, 1092
    biomarkers in, 1100
    cardiovascular manifestations of, 1096
    chest radiography in, 1098
    chronic, 1090, 1097–1098
      management of, 1106
    classification of, 1090–1091, 1090f–1091f
    clinical manifestations of, 1096–1098
    cocaine use and, 1093
    computed tomography in, 25, 26f, 1098–1099, 1116
    congenital heart disease and, 1093
    connective tissue disease and, 1092–1093
    diagnosis of, 1098–1100
    echocardiography in, 1099–1100
    epidemiology of, 1091–1092
    historical perspective on, 1089–1090
    iatrogenic injury and, 1093
    intimal tear in, 1094, 1094f
    intramural hematoma in, 1090–1091, 1095, 1095f, 1100–1101
    magnetic resonance imaging in, 1099
    management of, 1100–1106
      in acute disease, 1100–1106, 1103f–1104f, 1108f
      in chronic disease, 1106
    medial degeneration in, 1093–1094
    natural history of, 1092
    pain in, 1096
    pathophysiology of, 1093–1096
    peripheral vascular manifestations of, 1096–1097, 1097t
    pregnancy and, 1093
    propagation of, 1094–1095
    subacute, 1090
    syndromic associations of, 1093
    systemic manifestations of, 1096
  type B, 25, 1090f, 1115
    aortic branch vessels in, 1117
    blood pressure in, 1117
    chronic, 1119, 1122–1123
    classification of, 1090–1091, 1115–1116
    clinical manifestations of, 1117–1119
    complicated, 1137, 1139
    computed tomography in, 1116, 1119
    contrast aortography in, 1119–1120, 1120f
    diagnosis of, 1116, 1119–1121
    echocardiography in, 1119
    epidemiology of, 1116

Aortic dissection (Continued)
    historical perspective on, 1123
    intramural hematoma in, 1090–1091, 1115–1117, 1120
    magnetic resonance angiography in, 1119
    management of, 1120, 1115
      in acute disease, 1121–1122
      in chronic disease, 1122–1123
      early survival with, 1123–1124, 1124f
      endovascular, 1122, 1138–1139
      follow-up in, 1126
      historical perspective on, 1123
      late survival with, 1124, 1125f
      medical, 1120–1121, 1123, 1124f, 1137
      peripheral vascular disease treatment in, 1122
      reintervention, 1124–1125, 1125f
      results of, 1123–1125
      surgical, 1121–1123
    natural history of, 1116
    pain in, 1117
    pathophysiology of, 1116–1117
    penetrating ulcers and, 1115–1117, 1120
    peripheral vascular complications in, 1117–1118, 1118t, 1122
    tamponade in, 1117
    uncomplicated, 1137–1139
Aortic regurgitation, 1199–1200
  in aortic dissection, 1096, 1199, 1202
  catheterization in, 784
  clinical findings in, 1200
  diagnosis of, 1200
  echocardiography in, 827f–828f, 829, 830f, 838–839, 839f, 1200
  etiology of, 1199
  magnetic resonance imaging in, 799, 801f
  management of, 1200. See also Aortic valve replacement
  natural history of, 1200
  pathophysiology of, 1199–1200
  pediatric, 1954–1959
    aortic valve reconstruction in, 1955, 1956f
    aortic valve replacement in, 1955–1957, 1956f–1957f
    leaflet extension for, 1955
    after neonatal valvuloplasty, 1695, 1954
    Ross operation in, 1958–1959
    ventricular septal defect and, 1857, 1955
Aortic root
  age-related changes in, 1022
  anatomy of, 1021–1022, 1022f–1024f
  aneurysm of, 1023–1025, 1042
    in Marfan syndrome, 1025–1026
    surgical treatment of, 1030–1034, 1032f–1034f
  dilatation of, 845, 845f
  in Ehlers-Danlos syndrome, 1026
  elasticity of, 1022
  in Loeys-Dietz syndrome, 1026
  remodeling of, 1031, 1032f
    outcomes of, 1033–1034
  replacement of, 1031–1033, 1033f–1034f
    outcomes of, 1033–1034
  in type A aortic dissection, 1104–1105
Aortic sinuses, 1022, 1024f, 1944
  neo-ostium creation in, 1973–1974
Aortic stenosis, 1195–1199
  catheterization in, 783–784
  clinical findings in, 1197
  compensatory changes in, 1196–1197
  computed tomography in, 799, 801f, 1197, 1198f
  congenital, 1944–1947
    cardiac catheterization in, 1945
    clinical presentation of, 1944
    diagnosis of, 1944–1945
    echocardiography in, 1944
    mild, 1945
    moderate, 1945
    natural history of, 1945
    in neonate, 1945–1946, 1945f
    in older child, 1946–1947
    prevalence of, 1944
    severe, 1945
    stress testing in, 1944–1945
    subvalvular, 1947–1951, 1947f
      membranous, 1947–1948, 1948f
      tunnel-like, 1948–1951, 1949f–1952f
    supravalvular, 1952–1954

Aortic stenosis (Continued)
    clinical presentation of, 1952, 1953f
    treatment of, 1952–1954, 1953f–1955f
    treatment of, 1694–1695, 1945–1947, 1945f
      in infant, 1946
      in neonate, 1695, 1945–1946, 1945f
      in older child, 1946–1947
  diagnosis of, 1197, 1198f
  diastolic dysfunction in, 744
  echocardiography in, 828f, 838
  grading of, 1197, 1197t
  hypoplastic left heart syndrome with, prenatal intervention for, 1701–1702, 1702t–1703t
  left ventricular hypertrophy with, 1196–1197
  low-gradient, low-flow, 1198–1199, 1199f
  magnetic resonance imaging in, 799, 801f
  management of, 1199f. See also Aortic valve replacement
    balloon valvuloplasty in, 858, 1198, 1199f
    in low-gradient, low-flow disease, 1198–1199, 1199f
    medical, 1197
  mortality with, 1197–1199, 1204–1205
  natural history of, 1197
  pathophysiology of, 1195–1196, 1196f
  prenatal intervention for, 1701–1702, 1702t–1703t
Aortic valve
  anatomy of, 705–706, 1195, 1196f, 1943–1944, 1944f
  bicuspid, 1026–1027, 1195, 1196f, 1199
    echocardiography of, 845, 845f
    repair of, 1202, 1202f
    Ross operation and, 1958–1959
  blunt injury to, 1174
  on cardiac catheterization, 783–786
  cross-sectional area of, 1196
  cusps of, 1021–1022, 1024f
  diameter of, 1672, 1673f
  endocarditis of
    native valve, 1259–1262, 1262f, 1264
    prosthetic valve, 1204, 1273–1275, 1274f–1275f
  in hypertrophic cardiomyopathy, 1495
  leaflets of, 1944
    augmentation surgery for, 1955
  pressure across, 1195–1196
  reimplantation of, 1031, 1033f
  repair of, 858–859, 1198, 1199f, 1202, 1202f–1203f. See also Aortic valve replacement
    in children, 1695, 1955, 1956f
    in fetus, 1696f–1697f, 1701–1702
  stenosis of. See Aortic stenosis
  tricuspid, 1196f
    repair of, 1202, 1203f
Aortic valve replacement, 1029–1030, 1029f, 1199f, 1200–1202, 1201f. See also Prosthetic heart valves
  approach in, 1200–1201, 1201f
  complications of, 1204
  effective orifice area in, 1186
  endocarditis with, 1204, 1273–1275, 1274f–1275f
  hemodynamic assessment in, 1186
  hemolysis after, 1204
  incision for, 1200–1201, 1201f
  in low-gradient, low-flow aortic stenosis, 1198–1199, 1199f
  mortality with, 1204
  outcomes of, 1204–1205
  paravalvular leak with, 1204
  pediatric, 1286, 1955–1957
    autograft vs. homograft in, 1957
    mechanical vs. tissue valve in, 1955–1957, 1956f–1957f
  prosthesis implantation in, 1201–1202, 1202f
  prosthesis selection for, 1201
  reoperation after, infection and, 1046, 1047f
  Ross operation for, 1034–1037, 1035f–1036f. See also Ross operation
  survival after, 1204–1205
  thromboembolism with, 1204, 1285
  timing of, 1197–1198
  transcatheter, 1203–1204, 1203f
  valve dysfunction with, 1204, 1205f
  ventricular recovery after, 1205
Aortic valvotomy, in neonatal aortic stenosis, 1945–1946
Aortic valvuloplasty, 858–859, 1198, 1199f
  fetal, 1696f–1697f, 1701–1702
  pediatric, 1695, 1955, 1956f

Aortitis
  aortic arch, 1043–1044, 1046f
  ascending, 1027
  descending, 1066–1067
  syphilitic, 1027
Aorto-apical conduit, in tunnel-like subaortic stenosis, 1952
Aortography
  abdominal, 1159–1160, 1161f
  before aortic arch surgery, 1048
  in aortic transection, 27f
  thoracic, 1159, 1160f
  in type A aortic dissection, 1098
  in type B aortic dissection, 1119–1120, 1120f
Aortopexy, in tracheomalacia, 133, 133f, 542, 543f
Aortopulmonary window, 1919–1924
  anatomy of, 1919–1920, 1920f
  associated anomalies of, 1920
  cardiac catheterization in, 1921
  chest radiography in, 1920
  clinical features of, 1920
  diagnosis of, 1920–1921
  echocardiography in, 1920–1921, 1921f
  embryology of, 1919
  natural history of, 1921
  pathophysiology of, 1920
  surgical treatment of, 1921–1923, 1922f–1923f
    management after, 1924
    pulmonary flap technique in, 1922
    residual defect after, 1924
    results of, 1924
    transwindow (sandwich-type) repair in, 1922, 1923f
AP-1, in mesothelioma, 452
Apical suction retractors, in off-pump coronary artery bypass grafting, 1402, 1402f–1403f
Apixaban, 759
Apolipoproteins, 905, 906f, 906t
Apoptosis
  inhibitors of, in myocardial protection, 993
  in mesothelioma, 453
Aprotinin
  anaphylactic reaction with, 767
  in cardiac surgery, 766–768, 1009
  in cardiopulmonary bypass, 923–924, 967
  in children, 766–767
  in coronary artery bypass surgery, 1283, 1378
  in patent foramen ovale, 1804
  in postinfarction ventricular septal defect repair, 1454
  in postoperative bleeding, 948–949
  renal effects of, 767
  risk-benefit characteristics of, 767–768
Argatroban
  in cardiopulmonary bypass, 966
  in NSTE acute coronary syndromes, 875
Arrhythmias. *See also specific arrhythmias*
  in adult congenital heart disease, 2071, 2088–2094, 2090t–2092t
  after atrial septal defect closure, 1808–1809
  after atrial switch procedures, 1986
  in blunt cardiac injury, 95
  after cardiac surgery, 943–945
  catheter ablation for, 1329. *See also* Catheter ablation
    electrophysiology study for, 1329–1330
    technique of, 1330–1331
  cryoablation therapy in, 1331
  in Ebstein's anomaly, 2059, 2065–2066
  after esophagectomy, 611
  fetal, 1672
  after Fontan procedure, 2049, 2088–2091, 2090t–2091t
  implantable cardioverter-defibrillator for. *See* Implantable cardioverter-defibrillator
  pacemakers for. *See* Pacemaker
  surgical ventricular restoration and, 1591–1593
  after tetralogy of Fallot repair, 1891
Arterial switch operation, 1987–1992, 1989f
  care after, 1988
  in complex transposition, 1996
  late follow-up of, 1991, 1992f
  after left ventricular retraining, 1999
  outcomes of, 1988–1992
  reoperation after, 1991–1992
Arterioles. *See* Microvessels
Arteriovenous fistula, 108
Arteriovenous malformation, 145–147, 146f
  in single ventricle, 2044
Arteritis, Takayasu's. *See* Takayasu's arteritis

Artery (arteries). *See also* Microvessels *and specific arteries*
  anatomy of, 711
  flow-induced dilation of, 716–717, 717f
  tone of. *See* Vascular tone
Artificial heart, 1525
  CardioWest, 1527f
    vs. AbioCor heart, 1525–1527, 1526f–1527f
    cigarette smoking and, 1529
    complications of, 1528
    consoles for, 1526–1527, 1527f
    explantation of, 1531
    FDA study of, 1527–1528, 1528f
    implantation of, 1529–1530, 1529f–1531f
    patient selection for, 1528–1529
    survival with, 1528, 1528f, 1531
  historical perspective on, 1525–1527, 1526t
Asbestos fibers
  clastogenic properties of, 451
  exposure to, 450–451
  mesothelioma and, 450–451. *See also* Mesothelioma
  oncogenic potential of, 450
  pathogenic effects of, 451–453
  types of, 449
Askin tumor, 456–457
Aspergilloma, 188–189, 189f
Aspergillosis, 188–190, 188f–189f
  bronchopulmonary, allergic, 190, 190f
  diagnosis of, 28f, 185–186
  invasive, 189–190
  after lung transplantation, 221–222, 222f
Asphyxia, traumatic, 92
Asphyxiating thoracic dystrophy, 382–383, 383f
Aspiration, after heart-lung transplantation, 1568
Aspiration pneumonia, 179
Aspiration therapy, in spontaneous pneumothorax, 410
Aspirin
  in atherosclerosis management, 913
  bleeding with, 1284
  in cardiopulmonary bypass, 1287
  after coronary artery bypass grafting, 946, 947f, 1382
  before coronary artery bypass grafting, 1374
  in NSTE acute coronary syndromes, 873–874
  in patent foramen ovale, 1804
  platelet dysfunction and, 760
  preoperative, 946, 947f
  in prosthetic heart valve anticoagulation, 1280–1281
Asthma, chest wall deformities and, 359
Atelectasis
  after Pancoast tumor treatment, 319
  postoperative, 53
  with pulmonary metastases, 339
Atherectomy devices, 856, 856f
Atherosclerosis, 867–868, 868f, 903–904. *See also* Acute coronary syndromes; Coronary artery disease; Myocardial infarction (MI)
  aortic, 1027
    coronary artery bypass grafting and, 1377–1378, 1378f
    imaging of, 793–794
    percutaneous intervention for, 1165, 1166f
  brachiocephalic artery. *See* Brachiocephalic artery (arteries), occlusive disease of
  coronary artery. *See* Coronary artery disease
  development of, 903–904, 904f
  dyslipidemic triad in, 908
  familial apoB defect and, 907
  familial combined hyperlipidemia and, 907
  fatty streaks in, 903
  LDL receptor deficiency and, 907
  lipoprotein(a) in, 908
  lipoproteins in, 907–908
  management of, 908–911, 909t–910t
    alcohol in, 913
    antihypertensive therapy in, 914–915
    aspirin in, 913
    bile acid sequestrants in, 914
    clinical trials of, 908–909
    combination niacin-statin in, 914
    diet in, 910t, 912b, 911–913
    estrogen in, 910t, 913
    exercise in, 915
    ezetimibe in, 914
    fiber in, 912–913
    fibrates in, 909t, 914
    fish consumption in, 910t, 913

Atherosclerosis (Continued)
    guidelines for, 909–911, 911b, 911t
    lipid-lowering therapy in, 909–911, 911t, 913–914
    niacin in, 914
    omega-3 fatty acids in, 914
    smoking cessation in, 914
    statins in, 908–909, 909t, 913–914
    weight loss in, 911–912
  metabolic syndrome and, 908, 908t
  regression of, 904, 904f
  risk factors for, 911b
  stabilization of, 904
Atresia
  aortic arch, 1928–1929. *See also* Aortic arch, interrupted
  bronchial, 133–134
  esophageal, 535–543. *See also* Esophageal atresia
  pulmonary. *See* Pulmonary atresia with intact ventricular septum; Pulmonary atresia with ventricular septal defect
  tracheal, 130–131
Atrial-arterial switch, in congenitally corrected transposition of great arteries, 2006–2007, 2009–2010, 2011f, 2012
Atrial cuff, in lung transplantation, 212–213, 213f
Atrial fibrillation, 1345–1357
  in adult congenital heart disease, 2091
  antiarrhythmic agents in, 1346–1347
  atrial transection procedure in, 1347–1348
  after cardiac surgery, 934
  catheter ablation in, 1338–1340, 1340f
    circumferential left atrial strategy for, 1339
    complications of, 1339
    indications for, 1351
    pulmonary vein isolation strategy for, 1339
    stepwise technique for, 1339
  classification of, 1345
  after coronary artery bypass grafting, 1384
  corridor procedure in, 1347
  Cox-Maze procedure in, 1348–1351, 1348f
    ablation technology for, 1348–1349
    cryothermal sources for, 1349–1350
    high-intensity focused ultrasound in, 1350–1351
    indications for, 1351
    left-sided lesions in, 1352–1353, 1353f
    pulmonary vein lesions in, 1354, 1354f
    radiofrequency energy for, 1350
    results of, 1353–1354, 1354f, 1357
    right-sided lesions in, 1352, 1352f
    stroke and, 1354
    technique of, 1351–1353, 1351f–1353f
  electrocardiography in, 1346
  electrophysiology of, 1345–1346
  epidemiology of, 1345
  His bundle ablation in, 1347
  historical perspective on, 1347–1348
  left atrial isolation procedure in, 1347
  long-standing, 1345
  medical treatment of, 1346–1347
  mitral regurgitation and, 1218
  mortality rate and, 1345
  pacemaker in, 1311b. *See also* Pacemaker, permanent
  paroxysmal, 1345–1346
  persistent, 1345
  postoperative, 944–945
    diagnosis of, 944–945
    incidence of, 944
    prevention of, 48, 1017
    risk for, 48, 944
    treatment of, 54, 944–945
  pulmonary vein in, 1346
  pulmonary vein isolation in, 1346, 1354–1355, 1354f–1355f
    results of, 1356–1357
  stroke risk and, 1345
  after thoracoscopic lobectomy, 284
Atrial flutter
  in adult congenital heart disease, 2088–2091
  after cardiac surgery, 943–944, 944f, 1356
  catheter ablation in, 1334
Atrial natriuretic peptide
  after cardiopulmonary bypass, 969–970
  in heart failure, 895
  in myocardial infarction, 871

Atrial pacing, after cardiac surgery, 940, 940f–941f
Atrial septal aneurysm, 1799
Atrial septal defect, 1797–1809. *See also* Atrioventricular canal defects; Patent foramen ovale
  adult, 1808, 2073–2074, 2074f
  associated defects with, 1801
  clinical presentation of, 1802
  closure of, 1803–1808
    in adult, 1808, 2074, 2074f
    arrhythmias and, 1808–1809
    complications of, 1805, 1808
    contraindications to, 1803
    exercise capacity and, 1809
    indications for, 1803
    minimally invasive, 1807–1808
    outcomes of, 1808
    physiology of, 1808–1809
    surgical, 1805–1807, 1805f–1807f
    transcatheter, 783f, 860–861, 1698–1699, 1804–1805
  conduction abnormalities with, 1801
  coronary sinus–type, 1799–1800, 1800f
  cyanosis in, 1802
  diagnosis of, 1802, 1802f
  echocardiography in, 834–835, 834f
  embryology of, 1797–1800, 1799f
  genetics of, 1798
  hemodynamics of, 1801–1802
  historical perspective on, 1797, 1798f
  iatrogenic, 1800
  incidence of, 1800–1801
  left-to-right shunt in, 781–782, 782f, 1801
  left ventricular assist device implantation and, 1509
  mitral valve abnormalities with, 1801
  natural history of, 1800–1801
  pathophysiology of, 1801–1802
  primum, 1798, 1800f
    treatment of, 1806–1807
  pulmonary hypertension and, 1801–1802
  pulmonary vascular disease in, 1801–1802
  secundum, 1798, 1800f
    treatment of, 1805, 1805f
  sinus venosus, 1798–1799, 1800f
    adult, 2074–2075
    treatment of, 1805–1806, 1806f–1807f
  syndromic associations of, 1801
  traumatic, 1800
  tricuspid abnormalities with, 1801
  ventricular septal defect with, 1801
Atrial septoplasty, fetal, 1702–1704, 1703f
Atrial septum. *See also* Atrial septal defect
  anatomy of, 700, 701f
  aneurysm of, 1799
  blunt injury to, 1174
  embryology of, 1644, 1645f, 1797–1798, 1799f
  lipomatous hypertrophy of, 796, 798f, 1637
  primum, 1644, 1645f, 1647
  secundum, 700, 701f, 1644, 1645f
Atrial tachycardia, catheter ablation in, 1332–1334, 1333f
Atrial transection procedure, in atrial fibrillation, 1347–1348
Atrioventricular block
  acquired, 1329
  in adult congenital heart disease, 2093–2094
  after cardiac surgery, 933–934
  in endocarditis, 1271
  pacemaker in, 1308b. *See also* Pacemaker, permanent
Atrioventricular canal defects, 1646–1647, 1831
  anatomy of, 1831–1834, 1832f
  angiography in, 1836
  aortic valve in, 1832
  associated cardiac lesions with, 1841–1844
  atrioventricular node in, 1832–1833, 1833f
  atrioventricular valve in, 1832–1833
  atrioventricular valve regurgitation in, 1834, 1845
  bundle of His in, 1832–1833, 1833f
  classification of, 1832–1833, 1833f
  coarctation of aorta and, 1842
  complete, 1831, 1832f–1833f
    prognosis for, 1846
    treatment of, 1835, 1837–1840, 1837f–1841f
  conduction tissue in, 1832–1833, 1833f
  coronary sinus in, 1832–1833, 1833f
  double-orifice mitral valve and, 1843, 1845
  double-outlet right ventricle and, 1842

Atrioventricular canal defects (*Continued*)
  in Down syndrome, 1834
  echocardiography in, 1836
  electrocardiography in, 1836
  embryology of, 1831–1834, 1832f
  inlet deficiency in, 1832
  left-to-right shunt in, 1834
  left ventricular outflow tract in, 1832, 1842–1843
  murmur in, 1836
  parachute mitral valve and, 1843
  partial, 1831
    prognosis for, 1846
    treatment of, 1835, 1841, 1841f
  pathophysiology of, 1834
  pulmonary hypertension and, 1835
  pulmonary vascular obstructive disease and, 1834
  Rastelli A, 1832, 1833f
  Rastelli B, 1832, 1833f
  Rastelli C, 1832, 1833f
  recurrent mitral regurgitation and, 1844–1846
  surgical treatment of, 1836–1841
    age and, 1845
    care after, 1844–1845
    coarctation of aorta and, 1842
    in complete defects, 1835, 1837–1840, 1837f–1841f
    double-orifice mitral valve and, 1843, 1845
    double-outlet right ventricle and, 1842
    double-patch technique in, 1837–1838, 1838f–1839f
    evaluation before, 1835–1836
    left ventricular outflow tract obstruction and, 1842–1843
    low cardiac output after, 1845
    modified single-patch technique in, 1840, 1841f
    outcomes of, 1845–1846
    parachute mitral valve and, 1843
    in partial defects, 1835, 1841, 1841f
    pulmonary hypertension after, 1845
    regurgitation after, 2018
    single-patch technique in, 1838–1840, 1840f
    sternotomy for, 1836, 1836f
    technique of, 1836–1841, 1836f
    tetralogy of Fallot and, 1841–1842
    timing of, 1834–1835
    transesophageal echocardiography during, 1844–1845
    in transitional defects, 1835, 1840–1841, 1841f
    transposition of great arteries and, 1843
    unbalanced canal in, 1843–1844
  tetralogy of Fallot and, 1841–1842, 1892
  transitional, 1835
    surgical treatment of, 1835, 1840–1841, 1841f
  transposition of great arteries and, 1843
  unbalanced atrioventricular canal and, 1843–1844
Atrioventricular junction
  catheter ablation of, 1338–1339
  embryology of, 1645, 1645f
Atrioventricular nodal reentrant tachycardia, 1331–1332, 1332f
  catheter ablation in, 1331–1332
Atrioventricular node, 1021
  anatomy of, 700–701, 701f, 1850, 1850f
  catheter ablation of, 1347
  in congenitally corrected transposition of great arteries, 2004–2005, 2005f
Atrioventricular pacing, after cardiac surgery, 940, 941f
Atrioventricular septal defect. *See* Atrioventricular canal defects
Atrium (atria). *See also* Ventricle(s)
  left, 702–703
    anatomy of, 702–703, 702f, 1655f
    appendage of, 702, 702f
    contraction of, ventricular filling and, 743
    incision of, 702, 702f
    venous component of, 702, 702f
  right, 699–701
    anatomy of, 699–701, 700f–701f, 1654f
    appendage of, 697, 698f, 699–700, 700f
    atrioventricular node of, 700–701, 701f
    Bachmann's bundle of, 699–700, 700f
    central fibrous body of, 701, 701f–702f
    penetrating injury to, 1177
    pressure in, 779, 780f, 780t, 828–829, 829f, 829t
    septum secundum of, 700, 701f
    sinus node of, 699–700
    vestibule of, 699–701, 700f

Atropine, in congenital heart disease, 1754
ATS Medical, 3f, 1191–1192, 1192f
ATS Medical Open Pivot heart valve, 1189
Austin Flint murmur, 1200
Autofluorescence bronchoscopy, 247–248
Autoimmune disease, thymoma and, 635–636, 636b
Autoimmune pericarditis, 1485–1486
Automated distal anastomotic devices, in coronary artery bypass grafting, 1407, 1407f
Autonomic nervous system
  anatomy of, 662, 662f
  in cardiac contractility, 747
  function of, 662, 663f
  in heart rate, 746–747
  in myocardial excitation-contraction coupling, 731–732, 732f
  in vascular tone, 717–718
Autoregulation, vascular, 716
Axillary hyperhidrosis, 661–662. *See also* Hyperhidrosis
Axillary vein
  effort thrombosis of, 392–393, 398–400
  for permanent pacemaker insertion, 1320, 1320f
Azathioprine
  in heart transplantation, 1545
  in lung transplantation, 219
Azygos lobe, 137, 138f
Azygos vein, 23

B

B-19, in pleural effusion, 435t
Bachmann's bundle, 699–700, 700f
Bacteremia, prosthetic valve endocarditis and, 1268
Bacterial infection. *See* Infection
Bainbridge reflexes, 747
Balloon valvuloplasty
  aortic, 858–859, 1198, 1199f
  mitral, 858, 859f, 1211, 1212f
  pulmonary, 1694, 1883–1884
Barbiturates
  in cardiac surgery, 1009
  in congenital heart disease, 1754
Bare area, diaphragmatic, 475, 477f
Barium esophagography, 550
  in achalasia, 552f
  before/after Heller myotomy, 553f
  in diffuse esophageal spasm, 551f, 563
  in epiphrenic diverticulum, 565, 566f
  in esophageal granular cell tumor, 567–568, 567f
  in histoplasmosis, 187f
  in perforation, 572, 572f
  in Schatzki's ring, 552f
  in stricture, 551f–552f, 569
  in Zenker's diverticulum, 564f, 565
Barium examination
  in hiatal hernia, 655
  in retrocardiac mass, 655
Barlow's disease, 1213–1214, 1214f
Baroreceptor, heart rate and, 747
Barotrauma, in congenital diaphragmatic hernia, 500
Barrett's esophagus
  photodynamic therapy in, 69–71
  radiofrequency ablation in, 70–71
Batista procedure, 1578, 1579f
BCA-225, in pleural effusion, 435t
Beck's triad, 1176
Behçet's syndrome, pulmonary artery aneurysm in, 145
Benzodiazepines, in congenital heart disease, 1757
BER-EP4, in pleural effusion, 435t
Berlin Heart, 1517, 1744–1745, 1744f–1745f
  in single ventricle, 2050
Bernoulli equation, 1675
Bevacizumab, in mesothelioma, 465–466
Bicuspid aortic valve, 1026–1027, 1195, 1196f, 1199
  echocardiography of, 845, 845f
  repair of, 1202, 1202f
  Ross operation and, 1958–1959
Bidirectional cavopulmonary anastomosis
  bilateral, in single ventricle, 2044
  in single ventricle, 2043–2044, 2043f
Bile, esophageal probe for, 532
Bile acid sequestrants, 914
Bilitec 2000 fiberoptic spectrophotometer, 556

Biopsy
  esophageal, 61
  lung
    in cancer, 64–65, 246–248, 247f
    in desquamative interstitial pneumonia, 167
    in interstitial disease, 169–170, 169f
    in metastatic disease, 340
    navigational bronchoscopy for, 64–65
    in nodule evaluation, 152, 237
    in nonspecific interstitial pneumonia, 167
  mediastinal, 630–631, 638, 640–641, 646. See also Mediastinal lymph node dissection
  pericardial, 1484
  pleural, 433
  thymic tumor, 638
Bisoprolol, in heart failure, 891t, 892–893
Bivalirudin
  in cardiopulmonary bypass, 966
  in NSTE acute coronary syndromes, 875
Bladder catheter, 53
Blastoma, pleuropulmonary, 456
Blastomycosis, 185, 188
  treatment of, 188
Bleeding
  in adult congenital heart disease surgery, 2072–2073
  aspirin-related, 1284
  after cardiopulmonary bypass, 1287
  after coronary artery bypass grafting, 858
  gastrointestinal, 61
  glycoprotein IIb/IIIa agent–related, 1284
  after heart transplantation, 1544–1545
  heparin-related, 1283–1284
  after left ventricular assist device implantation, 1521
  with mediastinoscopy, 631
  after pediatric cardiopulmonary bypass, 1723–1724
  postoperative, 54
    after cardiac surgery, 946–948. See also Cardiac surgery, bleeding after
    after esophagectomy, 610
    management of, 947–948
    volume replacement in, 948
  with prosthetic heart valves, 1187
  pulmonary, idiopathic, vs. Goodpasture's syndrome, 165
  thoracic, trauma-related, thoracotomy in, 100
  warfarin-related, 1283–1284
Bleomycin, for pleurodesis, 438, 441t–442t
Blood flow
  in cardiopulmonary bypass, 960
  cerebral
    in cardiopulmonary bypass, 960, 961f
    temperature and, 1006–1007
  pulmonary, 1692
    in hypoplastic left heart syndrome, 2031
  systemic, 1692
  vessel dilation with, 716–717, 717f
Blood gases
  in pediatric cardiopulmonary bypass, 1720, 1722–1723
  preoperative, 44
Blood patch, in postoperative air leak, 55
Blood pressure
  ethanol effects on, 913
  in hypoplastic left heart syndrome, 2031–2032
  intraoperative monitoring of, 920
  in type A aortic dissection, 1096
  in type B aortic dissection, 1117
Blood transfusion, 761–763
  acute lung injury with, 764
  adverse effects of, 763–765
  autologous donation for, 764
  cell salvage for, 764–765
  guidelines for, 762b
  hemoglobin level and, 762
  leukoreduction for, 763
  massive, 763
  normovolemic hemodilution for, 764
  postoperative, 49–51
  preoperative, 49–50
  red blood cells for, 762
Blunt trauma. See Cardiac injury, blunt; Trauma, blunt
Bochdalek's hernia. See also Congenital diaphragmatic hernia
  in adult, 481
Body temperature
  after cardiac surgery, 934
  intraoperative, 50

Bone marrow, tumor cell detection in, 673
Bone morphogenetic proteins, in cardiac embryology, 1641
Bone scan, in lung cancer, 246
Botulinum toxin
  in achalasia, 562
  in diffuse esophageal spasm, 563
  in hyperhidrosis, 663
Brachial plexus, 4, 4f
Brachiocephalic artery (arteries). See also specific brachiocephalic arteries
  occlusive disease of, 1143–1152
    anatomic considerations in, 1146
    clinical presentation of, 1144–1145, 1144f
    diagnosis of, 1145–1146
    embolic, 1144–1145
    imaging of, 1145–1146
    multivessel, 1151
    neurologic examination in, 1145
    pathophysiology of, 1143–1144
    stenotic, 1144–1145
    surgical treatment of, 1146–1152, 1147f–1150f
      cerebral protection in, 1146
      neural structures in, 1146
      sternotomy for, 1146
      thymus in, 1146
  radiation-induced stenosis of, 1144
  surface anatomy of, 12
  Takayasu's arteritis of, 1144–1145, 1151–1152
Brachiocephalic vein, 3–4
Brachytherapy, endoscopic, 75
  in adenoid cystic carcinoma, 330
Brain, 1005
  air in, after chest wall resection/reconstruction, 307, 307f
  injury to. See Neurologic disorders
  ischemia of. See also Stroke
    deep hypothermic circulatory arrest and, 924–925
  metastatic tumor of, 30, 270, 583–584
  protection of. See Brain protection
Brain natriuretic peptide, in heart failure, 895
Brain protection
  in aortic arch aneurysm treatment, 1049–1053, 1050f
  in brachiocephalic artery occlusive disease, 1146
  in cardiac surgery, 924–925
  in cardiopulmonary bypass, 958–959, 1007–1009
  in pediatric cardiopulmonary bypass, 1721
Breast cancer
  chest wall invasion in, 380, 381
  pleural effusion in, 433, 441
  pulmonary metastases in, 169f, 345–346
Breathing. See also Respiration
  postoperative, 39
Bronchial artery, 17, 19f, 519, 519f, 706, 707f
Bronchial atresia, 133–134
Bronchial fistula, 55
Bronchial valve placement, in emphysema, 204
Bronchial vein, 17
Bronchiectasis, 179–181, 181f
  congenital, 134
  diffuse, 180
  etiology of, 180, 180t
  focal, 180
  imaging in, 180, 181f
  treatment of, 180–181
Bronchiolitis obliterans organizing pneumonia, 168
Bronchiolitis obliterans syndrome, 223–224, 224f, 1566–1567, 1567b
Bronchioloalveolar carcinoma, 271–272
  treatment of, 271–272
Bronchitis, plastic, 2050
Bronchoalveolar lavage
  in cryptogenic organizing pneumonitis, 168
  in desquamative interstitial pneumonia, 167
  in hypersensitivity pneumonitis, 161
  in interstitial lung disease, 169
  in lymphocytic interstitial pneumonia, 168
Bronchobiliary fistula, 135–136, 136f
Bronchogenic cyst, 138–139, 139f, 647
  computed tomography in, 27
  differential diagnosis of, 138
  excision of, 138–139
Bronchopleural fistula, 414–415
  bronchoscopy in, 64
  after chest wall resection/reconstruction, 306
  post-traumatic, 108

Bronchopleural fistula (Continued)
  postoperative, 55, 423
    clinical presentation of, 423
    diagnosis of, 423
    management of, 423
Bronchopulmonary dysplasia, congenital diaphragmatic hernia and, 505
Bronchopulmonary foregut malformations, 136, 137f–138f
Bronchoscopy, 63–66
  in bronchopulmonary carcinoid tumor, 326
  flexible, 63b, 65
    complications of, 65
    indications for, 63–64
    in lung cancer, 246–247
    morbidity of, 65
    in pneumonia, 64
    technique of, 65
    in tracheobronchial injury, 93, 99
  fluorescence, in lung cancer, 235, 247–248
  navigational, 64–65
  rigid, 65–66
    complications of, 66
    in congenital tracheal disease, 1766
    in esophageal atresia, 538
    in lung cancer, 246–247
    technique of, 66
  toilet, 64
  in tracheal disorders, 117–119, 126
  in vascular ring, 1791
Bronchovascular fistula, 55
Bronchus (bronchi)
  anatomy of, 14, 14f
    variations in, 14
  atresia of, 133–134
  congenital anomalies of, in lung transplantation, 214
  left mainstem, compression of, interrupted aortic arch treatment and, 1939–1940
  trauma to
    blunt, 93
    penetrating, 98–99
Brugada syndrome, 1330
Bullectomy, 195–196, 204
Bullet embolism, 102–103
Bumetanide, 887, 887t
Bundle branch block, right
  after cardiac surgery, 933–934
  after ventricular septal defect closure, 1857–1858
Bundle of His, 1021
  in atrioventricular canal defects, 1832–1833, 1833f
  catheter ablation of, 1347
  in tetralogy of Fallot, 1880–1881
Burns, chemical, of esophagus, 571–572
Bypass grafting
  carotid artery, 1149–1150
  coronary artery. See Coronary artery bypass grafting
  innominate artery, 1148–1149
  subclavian artery, 1150–1151

C

C-reactive protein
  cardiovascular fitness and, 908
  in community-acquired pneumonia, 177
  in myocardial infarction, 871
  with pediatric cardiopulmonary bypass, 1727
CA 15.3, in pleural effusion, 435t
CA19-9, in pleural effusion, 435t
N-Cadherin, in pleural effusion, 435t
Calcification
  of aortic valve. See Aortic stenosis
  of ascending aorta, 1069
  of mitral anulus, 1215, 1227, 1231–1232
  in pulmonary metastases, 340
Calcifying fibrous tumor, 455
Calcineurin inhibitors
  in heart transplantation, 1545
  in lung transplantation, 219
Calcium, in myocardial excitation-contraction coupling, 730–733, 731f
Calcium channel blocking agents
  in heart failure, 890, 891t
  in myocardial protection, 987

Calories, neonatal requirement for, 1750
Calretinin, in pleural effusion, 435t
Cancer
　breast
　　chest wall invasion in, 380, 381
　　pleural effusion in, 433, 441
　　pulmonary metastases in, 169f, 345–346
　cardiac. See Heart, tumors of
　chylothorax with, 427–428
　esophageal. See Esophageal cancer
　after heart transplantation, 1551
　lung. See Lung cancer
　metastatic. See Lung(s), metastases to; Lung cancer, non–small cell, metastatic; Metastasectomy, pulmonary
　pericardial effusion in. See Pericardial effusion, malignant
　pericarditis with, 1486
　pleural. See Mesothelioma and at Pleura
　pleural effusion in. See Pleural effusion, malignant
Candesartan, 891t
Candida albicans infection, after lung transplantation, 221
Cantrell's pentalogy, 380–382, 381f, 382t–383t
Capillaries, 711
Captopril, 890–892, 891t
CarboMedics
　Mitroflow aortic pericardial valve, 1191
　prosthetic heart valve, 1189, 1189f
Carbon dioxide, in hypoplastic left heart syndrome, 2027
Carbon monoxide, diffusing capacity for (DL_{CO}), 41–42
Carcinoembryonic antigen (CEA)
　in lung cancer, 674–675
　in pleural effusion, 435t
Carcinogenesis, 669
Carcinoid syndrome, 325
Carcinoid tumor, 323–329
　atypical, 324, 324f, 324t, 327–329, 328t
　biochemistry of, 324–325
　bronchoscopy in, 326
　β-catenins in, 324–325
　chemotherapy in, 327
　clinical presentation of, 325
　diagnosis of, 325–326, 325f–326f
　E-cadherin in, 324–325
　endobronchial management in, 327
　endocrinopathy in, 325
　epidemiology of, 323
　genetics of, 324–325
　imaging of, 325–326, 325f–326f
　location of, 323–324, 324t
　lymph node dissection in, 327
　in multiple endocrine neoplasia 1, 324
　p53 protein in, 324
　pathology of, 323–324, 324f, 324t
　prognosis for, 327–329, 328t
　radiation in, 327
　serotonin in, 326
　staging of, 326
　surgery in, 326–327, 327f
　tumor markers in, 326
　typical, 323–324, 324f, 324t, 327–329, 328t
　urinary 5-hydroxyindoleacetic acid in, 326
　WHO classification of, 323
Carcinoid tumorlets, 329
Carcinosarcoma, 334
Cardiac allograft vasculopathy, 1550–1551
Cardiac arrest
　electrophysiology study in, 1330
　in-hospital, 1018
　for myocardial protection. See Cardioplegia
Cardiac catheterization. See also Coronary angiography
　in adult congenital heart disease, 2071
　in anomalous origin of coronary artery from pulmonary artery, 1965
　before aortic arch surgery, 1047–1048
　aortic dissection with, 1093
　in aortic regurgitation, 784
　in aortic stenosis, 783–784
　in atrial septal defect, 781–782, 782f, 1802
　in bidirectional shunt, 783
　in chronic thromboembolic pulmonary hypertension, 1622
　coronary artery trauma during, 1474
　hemodynamics on, 779–781, 780f, 780t–781t
　　aortic pressure in, 780t, 781
　　cardiac output in, 781, 781t

Cardiac catheterization (Continued)
　　left ventricle pressure in, 780t
　　pediatric, 1692–1693
　　pulmonary artery pressure in, 780f, 780t, 781
　　pulmonary capillary wedge pressure in, 780f, 780t, 781
　　right atrium pressure in, 779, 780f, 780t
　　right ventricle pressure in, 779–781, 780f, 780t
　　systemic arterial pressure in, 781
　in hypertrophic cardiomyopathy, 1498
　left-to-right shunt on, 781–782, 782f–783f
　in mitral regurgitation, 785, 1216
　in mitral stenosis, 784, 1211
　pediatric, 776, 1692f
　　anesthesia for, 1693
　　for angioplasty, 1695–1698, 1697f
　　in aortopulmonary window, 1921
　　in atrial septal defect, 1802
　　in atrioventricular canal defects, 1836
　　in congenital aortic stenosis, 1945
　　in cor triatriatum, 1810
　　in Ebstein's anomaly, 2059
　　hemodynamic data on, 1692–1693
　　in hypoplastic left heart syndrome, 2026
　　vs. imaging, 1691–1692
　　in interrupted aortic arch, 1930
　　premedication for, 1693
　　pressure data on, 1692–1693
　　in pulmonary atresia with ventricular septal defect, 1899–1900, 1900f, 1904
　　roles of, 1691
　　sedation for, 1693
　　for septal defect closure, 1698–1699
　　in single-ventricle disease, 1692
　　in tetralogy of Fallot, 1883
　　in total anomalous pulmonary venous drainage, 1824
　　in transposition of great arteries, 1984, 1994
　　in truncus arteriosus, 1914
　　for valvuloplasty, 1694–1695
　　vascular access for, 1693–1694
　in pericardial disease, 785–786, 786f–787f, 1483–1484
　right heart, 779
　in right-to-left shunt, 782
　in thoracic aortic aneurysm, 1068
　in valve assessment, 783–786
Cardiac cycle, 740–741
　electrocardiography of, 740–741, 741f
　electromechanical activation of, 740
　pressure-volume analysis of, 741
Cardiac function curve, 734–737, 736f–737f
Cardiac index
　after cardiac surgery, 934, 937, 937f
　definition of, 745, 779, 781, 1692
　normal value for, 781t
　in pectus excavatum, 363
Cardiac injury, 1173
　blunt, 94–96, 95t, 1173–1175
　　arterial, 1174–1175
　　chamber rupture with, 1175
　　clinical presentation of, 1173–1174
　　contusion with, 1175
　　diagnosis of, 1173–1174
　　echocardiography in, 1174
　　electrocardiography in, 1174
　　enzyme levels in, 1174
　　historical perspective on, 1173
　　incidence of, 1173
　　management of, 1174–1175, 1175f
　　mechanism of, 1173
　　pathophysiology of, 1173
　　pericardial, 1174
　　radionuclide imaging in, 1174
　　septal, 1174
　　troponins in, 95, 1174
　　valvular, 1174
　penetrating, 100–102, 102f, 1175–1178
　　arterial, 1177
　　atrial, 1177
　　clinical presentation of, 1176
　　complex, 1177
　　diagnosis of, 1176
　　echocardiography in, 1176
　　historical perspective on, 1175
　　incidence of, 1175–1176

Cardiac injury (Continued)
　　management of, 1176–1177
　　mechanism of, 1175–1176
　　pathophysiology of, 1175–1176
　　ventricular, 1177
Cardiac output, 744–745
　after cardiac surgery, 934, 937–938, 937f
　after coronary artery bypass grafting, 1383
　exercise-related, 725–726, 726f
　extrinsic regulation of, 746–747
　intrinsic regulation of, 746, 747f
　measurement of, 745, 779, 781, 781t
　after pediatric cardiac surgery, 1757–1759, 1758t
　Starling curves of, 734–737, 735f–736f, 746, 747f
　time–ventricular volume relationship and, 725–726, 726f
　ventricular pressure–ventricular volume relationship and, 730, 730f
Cardiac pacing. See also Pacemaker
　after cardiac surgery, 940, 940f–941f
Cardiac resynchronization therapy, 1588–1591
　pediatric, 2085
Cardiac surgery. See also Cardiopulmonary bypass; Coronary artery bypass grafting; Percutaneous coronary interventions and at specific congenital heart diseases
　acid-base management during, 922
　afterload after, 938–940
　　reduction in, 939–940, 939f, 948
　anesthesia in, 919
　　agents for, 921
　　evaluation for, 919–920
　　intraoperative management of, 920–925, 921f
　　monitoring of, 920–921
　　thoracic epidural, 921–922
　antifibrinolytic agents in, 765–771
　aortic clamp application in, 1007, 1009f
　arrhythmias after, 943–945, 944f–945f
　arterial line filters in, 1007
　arterial line for, 920
　atrial fibrillation after, 944–945
　atrial flutter after, 943–944, 944f–945f
　auscultation after, 934
　barbiturates during, 1009
　bleeding after, 946–948
　　ε-aminocaproic acid in, 765–766, 949
　　aprotinin in, 948–949
　　desmopressin in, 948–949
　　drug-related risk factors in, 761
　　management of, 757, 761–763, 947–948. See also Blood transfusion
　　patient-related risk factors in, 761
　　physician-related risk factors in, 761
　　procedure-related risk factors in, 761
　　recombinant activated factor VII in, 949
　　risk for, 757, 757b, 761
　blood glucose control and, 922
　blood pressure monitoring during, 920
　blood transfusion after, 948
　cardiac dysfunction after, 937–945
　　afterload, 938–940, 939f
　　arrhythmic, 943–945, 944f
　　heart rate, 940, 940f–941f
　　inotropic agents in, 940–941, 941f–942f, 942f
　　low output, 937–938, 937f
　　preload, 938, 938f–939f
　　right heart, 943
　　tamponade, 941–943
　　treatment of, 939–940
　cardiac index after, 934, 937, 937f
　cardiac output after, 934, 937–938, 937f
　care after, 933
　　abdominal examination in, 934
　　airway evaluation in, 933
　　body temperature in, 934
　　cardiac auscultation in, 934
　　chest radiography in, 935
　　chest tube assessment in, 935, 948
　　electrocardiography in, 933–934
　　genitourinary examination in, 934
　　hemodynamic assessment in, 934
　　indwelling line assessment in, 934–935
　　neurologic examination in, 934
　　patient evaluation in, 933–935
　　peripheral perfusion assessment in, 934
　　ventilation evaluation in, 933

Cardiac surgery (Continued)
  central venous line for, 920
  central venous pressure after, 934
  cerebral ischemia in, 924–925
  cerebral protection during, 924–925
  cerebrospinal fluid pressure in, 920–921
  coagulopathy after, 946–947
  electrocardiographic monitoring during, 920
  evaluation for, 919–920
  fast-track, 925–926
  fever after, 950
  hematocrit after, 948
  historical perspective on, 919
  infectious complications of, 950–952, 951f, 951t
  inflammatory reaction after, 935–937, 1007
  intra-aortic balloon pump after, 941, 942f
  laboratory testing before, 920
  lactic acidosis after, 937
  magnetic resonance imaging after, 1005, 1006f
  microemboli with, 1006, 1008f
    prevention of, 1007, 1008t
  minimally invasive, 926–927, 927f
  morbidity with, 919
  mortality with, 919
  myocardial protection in. See Myocardial protection
  neurologic disorders after, 949–950, 950f, 1005
    assessment of, 1005–1006, 1006f
    mechanisms of, 1006–1007, 1008f
    prevention of, 1007–1009, 1008t
    prognosis for, 1009, 1009f
    risk for, 1006, 1007t
  oxygen delivery after, 937–938
  pericardial pressure after, 938
  pericarditis after, 1486
  physical examination before, 919–920
  port-access, 926–927
  post-pericardiotomy syndrome after, 935, 936f
  preload after, 938, 938f–939f
  prohemostatic agents in, 765–771
  pulmonary artery catheter for, 920
  pulmonary artery pressure after, 938, 938f
  quality and safety of, 1013
    antibiotic prophylaxis in, 1017
    central line infection prevention in, 1017
    communication in, 1016t, 1018
    historical perspective on, 1013–1014, 1014f
    medication measures in, 1016t, 1018
    medication reconciliation in, 1018
    national perspective on, 1014–1015, 1014b
    patient assessments in, 1019
    perioperative care in, 1016–1017, 1016t
    postoperative care in, 1016t, 1017–1018
    postoperative glucose control in, 1017
    pre-procedure checking in, 1016t, 1016–1017
    preoperative beta-blocker in, 1017
    rapid response team in, 1018
    sternal wound infection prevention in, 1017–1018
    STS Quality Measurement Task Force for, 1015–1016, 1015b, 1016t
    tracking measures for, 1016t, 1018–1019
    ventilator-associated pneumonia prevention in, 1017
  robot-assisted. See Robot-assisted cardiac surgery
  sternal wound infection with. See Sternal wound infection
  thrombasthenia after, 947
  transesophageal echocardiography in, 920, 921f
  vasoplegic syndrome after, 943
  ventricular arrhythmias after, 945
Cardiac tamponade, 1481b, 1487
  after cardiac surgery, 941–943
  catheterization in, 785, 786f, 1483–1484
  diagnosis of, 1487
  echocardiography in, 837, 1483f
  etiology of, 1487
  pathophysiology of, 1481
  pericardiocentesis in, 1484, 1484f
  pulsus paradoxus in, 1481
  treatment of, 1487
  in type A aortic dissection, 1096
  in type B aortic dissection, 1117
Cardiac tumors. See Heart, tumors of
Cardiac valves. See Aortic valve; Mitral valve; Prosthetic heart valves; Pulmonary valve; Tricuspid valve
Cardiac veins, 710, 710f
Cardiac venting, in cardiopulmonary bypass, 962

Cardiomyopathy
  dilated, 1578–1579, 1579f
    diastolic dysfunction in, 743
    echocardiography in, 826f, 836–837, 836f
    heart transplantation for, 1535, 1535t
    left ventricular dyssynchrony in, 1588–1591
    left ventricular geometry in, 1575, 1575f, 1575t
    left ventricular remodeling in, 1573–1574, 1574b
    left ventricular restoration in. See Heart failure, surgical ventricular restoration in
    mitral regurgitation in, 1215, 1231
  histiocytoid, 1634t
  hypertrophic, 1493
    aortic valve in, 1495
    cardiac catheterization in, 1498
    chest radiography in, 1497–1498
    classification of, 1494–1496
    clinical presentation of, 1497–1498
    coronary arteries in, 1495–1496
    definition of, 1493
    diastolic dysfunction in, 1496–1497
    echocardiography in, 836–837, 836f, 1498
    electrocardiography in, 1497–1498
    ethanol septal ablation in, 860
    genetics of, 1496
    histopathology of, 1496
    historical perspective on, 1493–1494
    imaging of, 799, 802f
    implantable cardioverter-defibrillator in, 1499
    interstitial fibrosis in, 1496
    left ventricular outflow obstruction in, 1497–1499, 1499f
    magnetic resonance imaging in, 1498
    mitral valve in, 1495, 1495f
    mitral valve regurgitation in, 1497
    morphology of, 1494–1496, 1494f
    myocardial fiber disarray in, 1496
    natural history of, 1498–1499
    obstructed vs. nonobstructed, 1498–1499, 1499f
    pacemaker in, 1311b. See also Pacemaker, permanent
    pathophysiology of, 1496–1497
    right ventricle in, 1495
    signs of, 1497
    surgical treatment of, 1499–1501
      care after, 1500–1501
      indications for, 1499
      morbidity after, 1502
      mortality after, 1501, 1502f
      outcomes of, 1501–1503
      vs. septal artery ablation, 1503–1504, 1504f
      symptom relief after, 1502–1503, 1502f
      technique of, 1499–1500, 1500f–1501f
    survival in, 1498, 1503, 1503f
    symptoms of, 1497
  imaging of, 799–800, 802f–803f
  ischemic, 1574–1575, 1577f–1578f. See also Heart failure, surgical ventricular restoration in
    coronary artery bypass grafting for, 1593–1594
    heart transplantation for, 1535, 1535t
    vs. left ventricular aneurysm, 1576–1577
    mitral regurgitation with, 1214–1215. See also Mitral regurgitation, ischemic
    surgical ventricular restoration for, 1582–1585, 1582f–1585f, 1583b
  obstructive, hypertrophic, congenital, 1951–1952
  restrictive
    echocardiography in, 837–838
    mitral regurgitation in, 1215
Cardioplegia, 978, 982–987
  antegrade administration of, 990
  blood, 989–992, 989f–990f
  crystalloid, 987–989, 988f
  delivery systems in, 990–992, 991f
  hypothermia with, 985, 986f
  metabolic substrates in, 987
  in mitral valve surgery, 1219
  myocardial edema with, 987
  rapid cardiac arrest with, 982, 982–985, 982f, 985f
  retrograde administration of, 990–991, 991f
  solutions for, 983t–984t
    buffering in, 986–987, 986f
    crystalloid, 987–989, 988f
    hypocalcemic, 987
    metabolic substrates in, 987
    osmolarity of, 987
  temperature in, 990

Cardiopulmonary bypass, 957, 1397–1398
  acid-base balance in, 958–959
  activated clotting time in, 922–923, 946, 967, 968f
  alpha-stat strategy in, 922, 958–959
  ε-aminocaproic acid in, 923–924
  anticoagulation for, 1283, 1286–1287
  antifibrinolytics in, 923–924
  aprotinin in, 923–924, 967
  argatroban in, 966
  arterial cannulation in, 962–963
  barbiturates during, 1009
  bivalirudin in, 966
  cannulation for, 962–963
    arterial, 962–963
    venous, 962
  cardiac venting for, 962
  cardiotomy reservoir for, 961
  care after, 935, 936f
  central nervous system injury with, 970, 970f
  cerebral blood flow in, 960, 961f
  cerebral perfusion pressure in, 960, 961f
  circuit for, 957–958, 959f, 967–969
    biomembrane mimicry for, 968
    heparin-coated, 968–969
    surface-modifying additives for, 969
  coagulopathy after, 946–947
  complement system in, 963, 964f
  complications of, 1286–1287
  in congenitally corrected transposition of great arteries, 2007–2009
  contact-activation system in, 963, 963f
  corticosteroids in, 967
  cytokines in, 963–965, 964f
  dopamine in, 971
  Drew-Anderson technique in, 971
  endothelial cells in, 935, 964–965
  fibrinolytic system activation in, 923–924, 963
  flow rate for, 960
  glucose control after, 1017
  hematocrit in, 959–960
  heparin-induced thrombocytopenia in, 923, 946–947, 965–966, 966f
  heparin-protamine axis in, 922–923, 946, 965–967, 966f, 968f
  heparin rebound in, 923, 966–967
  hirudin in, 966
  historical perspective on, 957, 958f
  hypothermia for, 958–959, 960f–961f, 1006–1007, 1008f
  inflammatory reaction after, 935–937, 1007
  leukocytes in, 964–965
  leukodepletion in, 971
  with lung transplantation, 216–217, 217f
  mannitol in, 971
  methylprednisolone in, 967
  neuroendocrine response to, 969–970
  neurologic disorders after, 949–950, 950f, 1005
    assessment of, 1005–1006, 1006f
    mechanisms of, 1006–1007, 1008f
    prevention of, 1007–1009, 1008t
    prognosis for, 1009, 1009f
    risk for, 1006, 1007t
  neuroprotection in, 958–959, 1007–1009
  neutrophil activation with, 935
  nitric oxide in, 963
  oxygenator for, 958, 959f
  pathophysiology of, 963–965
    cellular, 964–965
    nonbiomaterial-related activation in, 965, 965f
    noncellular, 963–964, 963f–964f
  pediatric, 1712–1728
    vs. adult, 1713–1719
    arterial blood gases during, 1720, 1722–1723
    arterial cannulas for, 1715–1716, 1715t
    bleeding after, 1723–1724
    blood glucose in, 1720–1721
    brain injury during, 1725–1726
    circuit components in, 1713–1719, 1714t
    circuit monitoring in, 1719–1720
    discontinuation of, 1756–1762
    filters for, 1716–1717
    hematocrit in, 1717–1718
    hemodilution in, 1717–1718
    heparin reversal in, 1719
    heparinization in, 1718–1719

Cardiopulmonary bypass (Continued)
　　historical perspective on, 1712–1713
　　hypothermic, 1721
　　　　deep, 1713, 1721–1722
　　　　low-flow, 1721
　　initiation of, 1719
　　in interrupted aortic arch repair, 1934–1937, 1935f
　　low-flow, 1721
　　monitoring of, 1719–1722, 1753
　　organ injury during, 1713, 1724–1727
　　oxygenators for, 1713–1714
　　packed red cells in, 1717
　　patient factors in, 1713
　　patient monitoring in, 1720–1721
　　pH-stat strategy in, 1723
　　pulmonary injury during, 1725
　　pump flow rates in, 1718, 1718t
　　pump for, 1714
　　pump prime for, 1717
　　renal injury during, 1725
　　steroids before, 1727–1728
　　stress response to, 1726
　　systemic inflammatory response to, 1726–1727
　　in tetralogy of Fallot, 1884
　　tubing for, 1714, 1715t
　　ultrafiltration with, 1728
　　venous cannulas for, 1716, 1716t
　　venous drainage for, 1714–1715
　　venous oxygen saturation in, 1720
　　weaning from, extracorporeal membrane oxygenation and, 1737
　　whole blood in, 1717
　pH-stat strategy in, 922, 958
　platelets in, 964–965, 1287
　post-pericardiotomy syndrome after, 935, 936f
　priming in, 959–960
　protamine-related hypotension in, 966–967
　in pulmonary atresia with ventricular septal defect, 1902
　pulmonary dysfunction with, 970–971
　pumps for, 960–961, 961f
　renal dysfunction with, 924, 971
　separation from, 925, 925f
　small capillary and arteriolar dilatations after, 970, 970f
　technical aspects of, 957–963, 959f
　thrombin in, 935, 965, 965f
　tranexamic acid in, 923–924
　valirudin in, 966
　vascular complications of, 1286–1287
　vasoplegic syndrome after, 943
　venous cannulation in, 962
　weaning from, 1381–1382
Cardiopulmonary resuscitation, pediatric, extracorporeal membrane oxygenation in, 1738–1739, 1739t
CardioSEAL device, in postinfarction ventricular septal defect repair, 1454
Cardiotomy
　left ventricular assist device after, 1508, 1519–1520
　pediatric, extracorporeal membrane oxygenation after, 1737
Cardiotomy reservoir, in cardiopulmonary bypass, 961
Cardiovascular system
　imaging of, 789. See also Computed tomography (CT), cardiovascular; Magnetic resonance imaging (MRI), cardiovascular
　preoperative assessment of, 42–43, 43f, 47, 816, 852–853
Cardioverter-defibrillator, implantable. See Implantable cardioverter-defibrillator
CardioWest artificial heart, 1527f
　vs. AbioCor heart, 1525–1527, 1526f–1527f
　cigarette smoking and, 1529
　complications of, 1528
　consoles for, 1526–1527, 1527f
　explantation of, 1531
　FDA study of, 1527–1528, 1528f
　implantation of, 1529–1530, 1529f–1531f
　patient selection for, 1528–1529
　survival with, 1528, 1528f, 1531
Carinal dissection, 629–630, 629f–630f
Cariporide, 993
Carney complex/triad, 154, 1633

Carotid artery
　anatomy of, 1161–1162, 1162f
　angiography of, 1158, 1161–1162, 1162f
　occlusive disease of, 1149–1150, 1162
　　bypass for, 1149–1150, 1149f
　　coronary artery bypass grafting and, 1374
　　coronary artery disease and, 1152–1154
　　endarterectomy for. See Carotid endarterectomy
　　stenting for, 1150, 1150f
　stenting of, 1150, 1150f, 1165–1167
　　coronary artery bypass graft after, 1154
　　coronary artery bypass graft with, 1374
　　distal protection devices for, 1167, 1167f
　surface anatomy of, 12
Carotid endarterectomy, 1150, 1150f, 1165–1167
　coronary artery bypass graft after, 1153
　coronary artery bypass graft before, 1153–1154
　coronary artery bypass graft with, 1153, 1374
　off-pump coronary artery bypass graft with, 1154
Carpentier-Edwards prosthetic valves
　PERIMOUNT, 1190–1191, 1191f
　porcine, 1190
CARTO electro-anatomic mapping system, 1331
Carvedilol, 891t, 892–893, 1535
Castleman's disease, 647, 656–657
　localized, 657
　lymphoma progression in, 657, 658f
　multicentric, 657
CATCH-22 syndrome, 1648, 1882
β-Catenin
　in bronchopulmonary carcinoid tumor, 324–325
　in mesothelioma, 452
Catheter(s)
　coronary. See Cardiac catheterization; Percutaneous coronary interventions
　coronary sinus, 926
　intraoperative, 50–51
　pericardial, in malignant pericardial effusion, 443–444
　pleural, in effusion, 436
　postoperative, 53
　Swan-Ganz, 745
　thrombosis with, 1289–1290
Catheter ablation, 1329
　in accessory pathway–mediated tachycardia, 1334–1335, 1335t, 1336f
　in atrial fibrillation, 1338–1340, 1340f
　in atrial flutter, 1334
　in atrial tachycardia, 1332–1334, 1333f
　of atrioventricular junction, 1338–1339
　in atrioventricular nodal tachycardia, 1331–1332, 1332f
　electrophysiology study for, 1329–1330
　in idiopathic ventricular tachycardia, 1338
　radiofrequency current for, 1331
　technique of, 1330–1331
　in ventricular tachycardia, 1335–1337, 1337f–1338f
Caustic agent injury, esophageal, 571–572
Cavopulmonary anastomosis, in single ventricle, 2043–2044, 2043f
CD44, in pleural effusion, 435t
CDK inhibitor, in mesothelioma, 452
Cell-based therapy. See Regenerative cell-based therapy
Central fibrous body, 701, 701f–702f
Central venous catheterization
　in cardiac surgery, 920, 1017
　thrombosis with, 1289–1290
Central venous pressure
　after cardiac surgery, 934
　in children, 1753
Cephalic vein
　in coronary artery bypass grafting, 1412
　for permanent pacemaker insertion, 1319–1320, 1320f
Cerebral blood flow
　in cardiopulmonary bypass, 960, 961f
　temperature and, 1006–1007
Cerebral metabolic rate, hypothermia effect on, 924
Cerebrospinal fluid (CSF)
　drainage of, in aortic aneurysm repair, 1074–1075, 1074f–1075f
　leak of
　　after chest wall resection/reconstruction, 306–307
　　postoperative, 58
　pressure of, in cardiac surgery, 920–921
Cervical cancer, pulmonary metastases in, 346
Cervical esophagus, 517f–518f, 518, 549, 549f
　lymphatic drainage of, 520, 520f

Cervical ganglia, 23
Cervical mediastinoscopy, 248, 249t, 646
　extended, 248–249, 641
Cervical mediastinotomy, for biopsy, 640
Cervical rib, in thoracic outlet syndrome, 391, 392f, 393, 396f
Cervical spondylosis, vs. thoracic outlet syndrome, 397
Cervicothoracic junction. See Thoracic inlet
Chamberlain procedure, 646
Charlson Comorbidity Index, 39–40
Chemical injury, esophageal, 571–572
Chemoperfusion, in non–small cell lung cancer, 690–691
Chemoradiotherapy
　adjuvant, in esophageal cancer, 621
　in esophageal cancer, 579, 582, 582f, 619–621, 619t
　induction (neoadjuvant)
　　in esophageal cancer, 619–620, 619t
　　in non–small cell lung cancer, 289–290
　　in Pancoast tumor, 290–291
Chemotherapy
　adjuvant
　　in esophageal cancer, 620–621
　　in non–small cell lung cancer, 287–288
　in bronchopulmonary carcinoid tumor, 327
　in esophageal cancer, 582f, 618–621, 619t
　induction (neoadjuvant)
　　in esophageal cancer, 618–619, 619t
　　in non–small cell lung cancer, 288–291
　in malignant pericardial effusion, 446
　in malignant pleural effusion, 441
　in mesothelioma, 461, 464–465, 464b, 466t
　perfusion, in metastatic lung cancer, 347
　for pleurodesis, 442t
　in thymoma, 638
Chest. See also Chest wall
　flail, 90–91, 91f
Chest physiotherapy
　after lung transplantation, 218
　postoperative, 52–53
Chest radiography
　in acute interstitial pneumonitis, 167
　in acute lung rejection, 1565, 1565f
　in acute pulmonary embolism, 1616
　anatomy on, 10, 12, 13f
　in anomalous origin of coronary artery from pulmonary artery, 1965
　in aortic arch injury, 1178
　in aortic injury, 25–26, 26f, 93–94, 94f
　in aortic stenosis, 1197
　in aortopulmonary window, 1920
　in aspergilloma, 189, 189f
　in asphyxiating thoracic dystrophy, 383f
　in atrial septal defect, 1802
　in azygos lobe, 137, 138f
　in bronchogenic cyst, 138, 139f
　in bronchopulmonary carcinoid tumor, 325
　after cardiac surgery, 935
　of cervical rib, 393, 396f
　in chronic thromboembolic pulmonary hypertension, 1621–1622
　in congenital aortic stenosis, 1944
　in congenital diaphragmatic hernia, 495–496, 496f, 499
　in congenital lobar emphysema, 140–141, 141f
　in congenital mitral anomalies, 2019
　in congenital tracheal disease, 1765–1766
　in constrictive pericarditis, 1482f
　in coronary artery fistula, 1975–1976
　in cryptogenic organizing pneumonitis, 168
　in cystic adenomatoid malformation, 142, 142f
　in desquamative interstitial pneumonia, 167
　in diaphragmatic injury, 96, 96f, 478
　in Ebstein's anomaly, 2057, 2057f
　in empyema, 416–417
　in eosinophilic pneumonia, 164
　in esophageal atresia, 536–537, 537f–538f
　in esophageal cancer, 655
　in esophageal duplication, 543
　of esophageal physiology, 525–526
　in esophageal trauma, 26
　in giant lymph node hyperplasia, 657f
　in hamartoma, 153, 153f
　in histiocytosis X, 164
　in histoplasmosis, 187f

Chest radiography (Continued)
  in hypersensitivity pneumonitis, 161
  in hypertrophic cardiomyopathy, 1497–1498
  in idiopathic pulmonary fibrosis, 166–167
  in interstitial lung disease, 168–169
  in lung cancer, 244
  in lymphocytic interstitial pneumonia, 168
  in malignant mesothelioma, 33f, 457–458
  in mediastinal mass, 26–27, 29f, 637f
  of middle mediastinum, 645, 646f
  in mucormycosis, 190–191, 191f
  in non–small cell lung cancer, 31f
  in Pancoast tumor, 320f
  in paraspinous abscess, 659f
  in patent ductus arteriosus, 1782
  in pectus carinatum, 374f
  in pericardial cyst, 655f, 1488f
  in pericardial effusion, 443
  in pleural effusion, 431, 432f, 434
  in post-pericardiotomy syndrome, 935, 936f
  in posterior mediastinal neurofibroma, 652f
  postoperative, 34
  in pulmonary abscess, 181–182, 182f–183f
  in pulmonary agenesis, 140, 140f
  in pulmonary atresia with ventricular septal defect, 1899–1900
  in pulmonary leiomyoma, 157f
  in pulmonary lymphangiectasia, 143–144, 143f
  in pulmonary metastases, 339–340, 339f
  in pulmonary thymoma, 158f
  in scimitar syndrome, 145–147, 146f
  soap bubble appearance on, 143–144, 143f
  in spondylothoracic dysplasia, 384f
  in spontaneous pneumothorax, 409–410
  in sternal wound infection, 1385f
  in tetralogy of Fallot, 1882
  in thoracic aorta injury, 1178, 1179f
  in thoracic outlet syndrome, 393
  in total anomalous pulmonary venous drainage, 1823
  in tracheal disorders, 117
  in tracheal trauma, 26
  in trauma, 86–87
  in truncus arteriosus, 1914
  in type A aortic dissection, 1098
  in vascular ring, 1790
  in ventricular septal defect, 1853, 1853f
  in Wegener's granulomatosis, 163
Chest tube
  after cardiac surgery, 935, 948
  management of, 53
  in postoperative air leak, 55
Chest wall
  chondroma of, 384
  chondrosarcoma of, 385, 386f
  congenital deformities of, 359. See also specific deformities
  in congenital diaphragmatic hernia, 505
  desmoid of, 385
  fibrous histiocytoma of, 385
  imaging of, 34
  osteochondroma of, 384
  pectus carinatum of. See Pectus carinatum
  pectus excavatum of. See Pectus excavatum
  reconstruction of, 303–306, 305f, 380, 382
    in children, 305–306
    complications of, 306–307, 307f
    historical perspective on, 381
    indications for, 381, 383
    methods of, 382
    seroma with, 383
    soft tissue coverage in, 383, 384f
    sutures for, 383
    synthetic materials for, 381f, 382
  rhabdomyosarcoma of, 385, 386f
  trauma to. See also Cardiac injury; Trauma
    asphyxia with, 92
    clavicular fracture with, 91
    flail chest with, 90–91, 91f
    penetrating, 98
    pulmonary contusion with, 92
    rib fracture with, 90
    scapular fracture with, 92
    sternal fracture with, 91
  tumors of
    invasive, 295
      clinical presentation of, 296–297, 296f, 297t

Chest wall (Continued)
    diagnosis of, 297–298, 298f
    historical perspective on, 295–296
    pathology of, 307–308
    staging of, 298–300
    treatment of, 300, 301f, 303f. See also Chest wall, reconstruction of
      care after, 306
      complications of, 306–307
      results of, 308–309
  primary, 379
    benign, 384
    in children, 379
    clinical presentation of, 379–380
    incidence of, 379
    malignant, 385
    treatment of, 379, 380, 380f. See also Chest wall, reconstruction of
      historical perspective on, 381
      indications for, 381–382, 382f
      resection margin in, 380, 382t
      results of, 385–386, 386f
Children
  antifibrinolytic agents in, 765–766
  aprotinin in, 766–767
  arteriovenous malformations in, 145–147, 146f
  asphyxiating thoracic dystrophy in, 382–383, 383f
  atrioventricular canal defects in. See Atrioventricular canal defects
  bronchial atresia in, 133–134
  bronchiectasis in, 134
  bronchobiliary fistula in, 135–136, 136f
  bronchopulmonary foregut malformations in, 136, 137f–138f
  cardiac resynchronization therapy for, 2085
  cardiac sympathetic denervation for, 2085–2088, 2087f, 2088f
  cardiopulmonary bypass in. See Cardiopulmonary bypass, pediatric
  congenital chest wall deformities in, 359. See also specific deformities
  congenital chylothorax in, 427
  congenital diaphragmatic hernia in. See also Congenital diaphragmatic hernia, 489
  congenital esophageal disease in, 535. See specific diseases
  congenital heart disease in. See Congenital heart disease; Heart, embryology of; and specific congenital cardiac disorders
  congenital lung disease in, 129. See also specific abnormalities and diseases
  congenital sternal defects in, 374–382, 379f, 379t–380t
  congenital tracheal disease in, 1765. See Trachea, congenital disease of; Tracheal stenosis, congenital; Tracheomalacia
  coronary artery fibrosis in, 1476
  cystic adenomatoid malformation in, 142–143, 142f
  diaphragmatic elevation in, 479
  diaphragmatic hernia in. See Congenital diaphragmatic hernia
  disc battery ingestion by, 571
  double-outlet right ventricle in, 1858–1863. See also Double-outlet right ventricle
  echocardiography in. See Echocardiography, pediatric
  ectopia cordis in, 376–382, 380f–381f, 380t–383t
  extracorporeal membrane oxygenation in. See Extracorporeal membrane oxygenation, pediatric
  hyperlucent lung syndrome in, 144
  implantable cardiac defibrillator for, 2085, 2086f, 2086b
  intra-aortic balloon counterpulsation for, 1742
  Kawasaki's disease in, 1475
  laryngotracheoesophageal cleft in, 135
  left ventricular assist devices in, 1742–1745, 1743f
  lobar emphysema in, 140–141, 141f
  lung bud anomalies in, 139–144
  lung resection in, 130
  lung transplantation in, 227
  magnetic resonance imaging in. See Magnetic resonance imaging (MRI), pediatric
  malignant mesothelioma in, 451
  neurogenic tumors in, 651–655
  pacemaker for, 1312b, 2083–2085, 2084b
  pectus carinatum in. See Pectus carinatum
  pectus excavatum in. See Pectus excavatum
  Poland's syndrome in, 373–374, 376f–378f

Children (Continued)
  postintubation tracheal stenosis in, 1777–1778
  pulmonary artery aneurysm in, 145
  pulmonary artery sling in, 1773–1776, 1775f–1776f
  pulmonary atresia with intact ventricular septum in, 1865. See also Pulmonary atresia with intact ventricular septum
  pulmonary atresia with ventricular septal defect in, 1897. See also Pulmonary atresia with ventricular septal defect
  pulmonary emphysema in, 143
  robot-assisted surgery for, 1712, 1712f
  Ross procedure for, 1034–1037, 1035f–1036f
  spondylothoracic dysplasia in, 383–384, 384f
  sternotomy in. See Sternotomy, pediatric
  tetralogy of Fallot in, 1877. See also Tetralogy of Fallot
  thoracoscopy in, 1712, 1712f
  tracheal stenosis in, 1765. See also Tracheal stenosis
  tracheal web in, 1778
  tracheobronchial-esophageal fistula in, 135
  tracheomalacia in, 132–133, 1776–1777. See also Tracheomalacia
  vascular ring in, 1787–1793. See also Vascular rings
  ventricular septal defect in, 1849–1858. See also Ventricular septal defect
Chirality, cardiac, 1653–1654, 1658f–1659f
Chlamydia, in community-acquired pneumonia, 175
Chloral hydrate, in congenital heart disease, 1756–1757
Chlorothiazide, 887t
Chlorthalidone, 887t
Cholesterol, 905
  guidelines for, 909–911
  metabolism of, 907
  reverse transport of, 907
Cholesteryl ester, 905
Cholestyramine, 914
Chondroma
  chest wall, 384–385
  pulmonary, 156
Chondrosarcoma, 34, 34f, 385–386, 386f
Chordae tendineae
  mitral, 1209–1210, 1210f
    artificial, 1224–1225, 1226f, 1232
    shortening of, 1226
    transfer of, 1223, 1225f
    transposition of, 1223–1224
  tricuspid, 1243
Chordoplasty, mitral, 1224–1225, 1226f, 1232
Chromogranin staining, in thymoma, 634
Chromosome abnormalities, in mesothelioma, 451–452
Chromosome 22q11 deletion, 1648
Chronic obstructive pulmonary disease, 40
Churg-Strauss syndrome, 163
Chyle, 428
  leakage of. See Chylothorax
Chylomicrons, 905, 905t
Chylopericardium, 1486
Chylothorax, 427
  anatomy of, 427
  cancer-related, 427–428
  classification of, 427
  congenital, 144, 427
  definition of, 427
  diagnosis of, 428
  esophagectomy-related, 427–429, 610–611
  lymphography in, 428
  pathophysiology of, 427–428
  pneumonectomy-related, 427, 429
  postoperative, 56–57, 427
  traumatic, 427–428
  treatment of, 428–429, 429t, 611
Cigarette smoking, 39–40
  aortic aneurysm and, 1064, 1067–1068
  CardioWest artificial heart and, 1529
  cessation of, 47
  in atherosclerosis management, 914
CircuLite device, 1519, 1519f
Circumflex retroesophageal aorta, 1788–1789, 1788f, 1791
CKMNF 116, in pleural effusion, 435t
Clagett procedure, 420–422
Clamshell incision, in lung transplantation, 214, 215f

Claudication
  lower extremity, 1157, 1158t, 1163, 1163f
  upper extremity, 1158, 1160
Clavicle, 11
  fracture of, 91
Clear cell tumor, 157
Cleft sternum, 375, 379f, 379t
Clipping procedure, in hyperhidrosis, 666
Clopidogrel
  after carotid artery stenting, 1154
  after coronary artery bypass grafting, 946, 947f
  in NSTE acute coronary syndromes, 874
  platelet dysfunction and, 760
  preoperative, 919, 946, 947f
  in prosthetic heart valve anticoagulation, 1280
Coagulation, 1279–1280, 1280f
Coagulopathy
  after cardiac surgery, 947
  after cardiopulmonary bypass, 946–947
Coarctation of aorta, 1783–1787
  anatomy of, 1783–1784
  atrioventricular canal defect and, 1842
  clinical presentation of, 1784
  diagnosis of, 1784–1785, 1784f
  imaging of, 794, 794f
  magnetic resonance angiography in, 1157
  natural history of, 1784
  pathophysiology of, 1783–1784
  prognosis for, 1786–1787
  recurrent, 1695–1696, 1786
  restenosis in, 1695–1696
  treatment of, 1785–1786
    in adults, 1164–1165, 1165f
    complications of, 1786
    medical, 1785
    stent placement in, 1696, 1786
    surgical, 706, 1785–1786, 1785f
    transcatheter, 1695–1696, 1786
  type A aortic dissection and, 1105
  ventricular septal defect and, 1786, 1852, 1857
Cocaine use/abuse
  aortic dissection with, 1093
  coronary artery effects of, 1476–1477
Coccidioidomycosis, 185–188, 187f
  diagnosis of, 185–188
  treatment of, 188
Coeur en sabot, 1882
Cognitive function. See also Neurologic disorders
  after aortic arch surgery, 1051–1053, 1052f
  after cardiac surgery, 1006
  after cardiopulmonary bypass, 970
  congenital diaphragmatic hernia and, 505
  after off-pump coronary artery bypass grafting, 1404–1405
  after pediatric deep hypothermic circulatory arrest, 1725–1726
Colchicine, in idiopathic pericarditis, 1485
Colestipol, 914
Collagen-based hemostatic agents, 770–771
Colon, postesophagectomy conduit creation with, 604–605, 605f–606f
  contraindications to, 605
  indications for, 604–605
  left colon for, 605, 605f–606f
  preparation for, 605
  right colon for, 605–606
Colorectal cancer, pulmonary metastases in, 345
Coma, in type A aortic dissection, 1096–1097
Commissurotomy
  mitral, 1221, 1222f, 1228–1229
  tricuspid, 1249, 1250f
Common atrioventricular canal. See Atrioventricular canal defects
Commotio cordis, 1173
Communication, caregiver, 1018
Community-acquired pneumonia. See Pneumonia, community-acquired
Complement system, in cardiopulmonary bypass, 963, 964f
Compression stockings, in pulmonary embolism prophylaxis, 1617
Computed tomography (CT)
  in allergic bronchopulmonary aspergillosis, 190, 190f
  in anomalous aorta–pulmonary artery coronary artery course, 1973

Computed tomography (Continued)
  in anomalous origin of coronary artery from pulmonary artery, 1965–1966
  in aortic aneurysm, 791–792, 792f, 1064
  in aortic arch aneurysm, 1043f–1044f
  in aortic arch injury, 1178
  before aortic arch surgery, 1046–1048
  in aortic atherosclerotic plaque, 793–794
  in aortic coarctation, 794, 794f
  in aortic dissection, 25, 26f, 792–793, 792f
  in aortic injury, 103
  in aortic intramural hematoma, 793
  in aortic stenosis, 799, 801f, 1197, 1198f
  in aortic trauma, 25–26, 27f
  in ascending aortic aneurysm, 1025
  in aspergilloma, 189f
  in brachiocephalic artery disease, 1145
  in bronchiectasis, 180, 181f
  in bronchogenic cyst, 27
  in bronchopulmonary carcinoid tumor, 325, 325f–326f
  in cardiac mass, 796
  in cardiac trauma, 101
  in cardiomyopathy, 799–800
  cardiovascular, 789
    clinical applications of, 791–802
    contrast in, 790
    image acquisition in, 790
    instrumentation for, 789–790
    vs. magnetic resonance imaging, 790
    precautions for, 791
    radiation exposure with, 791
    resolution in, 790
  in chondrosarcoma, 34f
  in chronic thromboembolic pulmonary hypertension, 1622
  in coarctation of aorta, 1785
  in coccidioidomycosis, 187, 187f
  in congenital disease, 795–796
  in congenital tracheal disease, 1765–1766, 1768f
  in constrictive pericarditis, 1482f, 1487
  in coronary artery disease, 800–802, 804f
  in cryptogenic organizing pneumonitis, 168
  in cystic adenomatoid malformation, 142
  in desquamative interstitial pneumonia, 167
  in diaphragmatic elevation, 479f
  in diaphragmatic injury, 478
  in esophageal cancer, 580, 617, 618f
  in esophageal duplication, 543
  in ganglioneuroblastoma, 653f
  in giant lymph node hyperplasia, 656–657, 657f
  in hamartoma, 152f–153f
  in histoplasmosis, 187f
  in hypersensitivity pneumonitis, 161
  in idiopathic pulmonary fibrosis, 166–167, 167f, 217f
  in inflammatory pseudotumor, 155f
  in interstitial lung disease, 33f, 168–169
  in interstitial pneumonitis, 33f, 167
  in intrapulmonary fibrous tumor, 154f
  in invasive aspergillosis, 190
  in lung cancer, 245, 247f
  in lung cancer screening, 233–237, 234t
  in lymphocytic interstitial pneumonia, 168
  in malignant mesothelioma, 33, 33f, 457–458
  in mediastinal tumors, 26–27, 29f
  of middle mediastinum, 645, 646f
  in Morgagni hernia, 479f
  in myocardial infarction, 795
  in neurofibroma, 654f
  in non–small cell lung cancer, 29f, 30, 31f, 297–298, 298f
  in Pancoast tumor, 314f
  in paraspinous abscess, 659, 659f
  in patent ductus arteriosus, 794
  in pericardial cyst, 655f, 1488f
  in pericardial disease, 797–799, 799f–800f, 1483
  in pericardial effusion, 443, 443f
  in pleural effusion, 431–432, 432f
  in post-transplant lymphoproliferative disorders, 225f–226f
  of posterior mediastinum, 650
  postoperative, 34
  in pulmonary abscess, 181–182
  in pulmonary embolism, 34–35, 35f
  in pulmonary leiomyoma, 157f
  in pulmonary leiomyosarcoma, 331, 331f

Computed tomography (Continued)
  in pulmonary metastases, 169f, 339–340, 339f
  in pulmonary nodule, 13f, 28–29, 151–152, 235–237
  in pulmonary thymoma, 158f
  in sarcoidosis, 162f
  in sinus of Valsalva aneurysm, 793
  in spontaneous pneumothorax, 410
  in sternal wound infection, 1000
  in substernal thyroid, 640
  in Takayasu's arteritis, 794
  in tetralogy of Fallot, 1878f
  in thoracic aorta injury, 1178
  in thoracic aortic aneurysm, 1132, 1132f
  in thoracic trauma, 794–795
  in thymoma, 636–637, 636f
  in tracheal trauma, 26, 28f
  in tracheal tumors, 117, 118f
  in tracheobronchomegaly, 134–135, 134f
  in trauma, 87
  in tuberculosis, 162f
  in type A aortic dissection, 1098–1099
  in valvular heart disease, 799, 801f
  in vascular ring, 1790
  in ventricular assessment, 741, 795
  in Wegener's granulomatosis, 163f
Computed tomography angiography (CTA)
  in aortic transection, 88, 88f
  in coarctation of aorta, 1785
  in pulmonary embolism, 34–35
  in trauma, 87
  in type B aortic dissection, 1116, 1119
Computed tomography–positron emission tomography (CT-PET)
  in esophageal cancer, 581–583, 581f
  in lung cancer, 30, 30f, 32f, 250, 299–300
  in malignant mesothelioma, 34, 457–458
  in pleural effusion, 432
Conal septum, 1992–1993
  deviation of, in transposition of great arteries, 1992–1993, 1994f, 1995, 1996f
Congenital diaphragmatic hernia, 5, 489
  adrenal insufficiency in, 494
  aminocaproic acid in, 502, 504
  associated anomalies in, 496
  bronchopulmonary dysplasia and, 505
  cardiac anomalies in, 496, 497t
  chest radiography in, 495–496, 496f, 499
  chest wall development in, 505
  chromosomal anomalies in, 497t
  clinical manifestations of, 495
  CNS anomalies in, 497t
  cognitive development and, 505
  vs. cystic adenomatoid malformation, 142
  diagnosis of, 495–496, 496f
  differential diagnosis of, 495–496
  emphysematous changes in, 505
  epidemiology of, 490
  etiology of, 491
  experimental, 506–507, 506f
  familial, 490
  fluid therapy in, 504
  follow-up for, 505–506
  gastroesophageal reflux and, 505
  gastrointestinal anomalies in, 497t
  gastrointestinal obstruction in, 495, 504–506
  genitourinary anomalies in, 497t
  hearing deficits in, 505
  historical perspective on, 489–490
  late-presentation, 496, 504
  mediastinal deviation in, 494
  microscopy in, 493
  Morgagni, 5, 481, 491t, 508f, 509
  mortality in, 498–499
  musculoskeletal anomalies in, 497t
  pathogenesis of, 491–492
  pathologic anatomy of, 492–493, 492f–493f
  pathophysiology of, 493–495
  prenatal diagnosis of, 495, 498–499
  prognosis for, 498–499
  pulmonary anomalies in, 497t
  pulmonary hypoplasia in, 492–493, 493f
  pulmonary vascular resistance in, 494
  recurrence of, 506
  respiratory distress in, 495, 504
  smooth muscle hypothesis of, 492

Congenital diaphragmatic hernia (Continued)
    treatment of, 499–504
        barotrauma and, 500
        care after, 504
        care before, 499–502
        diaphragmatic reconstruction in, 507
        extracorporeal membrane oxygenation in, 502
        guidelines for, 500
        high-frequency oscillatory ventilation in, 501
        intratracheal pulmonary ventilation in, 501
        laparoscopic, 503–504
        liquid ventilation in, 501
        lung transplantation in, 507
        mechanical ventilation in, 501
        nitric oxide in, 501
        PFC-based lung distention in, 506–507, 507f
        pulmonary vasodilators in, 500–501
        results of, 504–505
        surfactant in, 501
        surgery in, 502–504, 503f
        thoracoscopic, 503–504
        in utero, 506
    vena cava syndrome in, 504
Congenital disease
    cardiac. See Congenital heart disease; Heart, embryology of; and specific congenital cardiac disorders
    chest wall, 359. See also specific deformities
    diaphragmatic, 489. See also Congenital diaphragmatic hernia
    esophageal, 535. See also specific abnormalities and diseases
    pulmonary, 129. See also specific abnormalities and diseases
    sternal, 374–382, 379f, 379t–380t
    tracheal, 1765. See also specific abnormalities and diseases
Congenital heart disease. See also Heart, embryology of, and specific congenital disorders
    adult, 2069. See also specific diseases
    arrhythmias in, 2071, 2088–2094, 2090t–2092t. See also specific arrhythmias
        center-based care for, 2069–2070
        epidemiology of, 2069, 2071f
        evaluation of, 2071, 2071f
        magnetic resonance imaging in, 2071f, 2072, 2077, 2078f
        perioperative management in, 2071–2073
        surgical treatment of, 2070–2071
            bleeding in, 2072–2073
            management after, 2073
            sternal reentry protocol in, 2072
    aortic dissection and, 1093
    aortopulmonary collateral vessel closure in, 1698
    balloon angioplasty in, 1695–1698, 1697f
    cardiac catheterization in. See Cardiac catheterization, pediatric
    diaphragmatic hernia and, 496, 497t
    echocardiography in, 844–845, 845f, 1665–1676. See also Echocardiography, pediatric
    etiology of, 1648. See also Heart, embryology of
    fetal intervention for, 1699–1700. See also Prenatal intervention
    magnetic resonance imaging in, 796f–797f, 1676–1685, 1691–1692 See also Magnetic resonance imaging (MRI), pediatric, 795–796
    pacemaker in, 1312b. See also Pacemaker, permanent
    pathophysiology of, 1749–1750
        altered blood flow patterns and, 1700
        decreased ventricular loading and, 1700
        increased ventricular loading and, 1700
    physiologic classification of, 1750–1752, 1750t
        complex shunts in, 1751
        mixing defects in, 1750
        outflow obstruction in, 1751
        pulmonary hypertension in, 1751–1752, 1751b
        simple shunts in, 1750–1751, 1750t, 1751b
    prenatal diagnosis of, 1666f, 1671–1672, 1672f
    surgical treatment of. See also specific at congenital heart diseases
        analgesia after, 1756
        anesthesia in, 1753–1756
            induction of, 1754
            maintenance of, 1754
            pathophysiologic factors and, 1749–1750
            risk of, 1753–1754
            stress response and, 1754–1756, 1755b
        cardiac output after, 1757–1759, 1758t
        cardiopulmonary bypass for. See Cardiopulmonary bypass, pediatric

Congenital heart disease (Continued)
    discharge after, 1762, 1762b
    echocardiography during, 1753
    evaluation before, 1752
    extubation after, 1761–1762, 1761b
    fluid management after, 1759
    management after, 1756
    mechanical ventilation after, 1759–1761, 1760b
    monitoring during, 1752–1753
    neurologic monitoring during, 1753
    outcome assessment of, 2105
        Aristotle complexity score for, 2110–2111, 2110t, 2111f
        complexity stratification for, 2107–2109, 2109t
        data verification for, 2112–2113
        database standards for, 2106, 2106t, 2107f, 2109t
        follow-up protocols for, 2113–2114
        multidisciplinary participation for, 2113
        nomenclature for, 2105–2106
        RACHS-1 complexity stratification for, 2109–2110, 2110f
        risk adjustment for, 2109–2110, 2110f
    preoperative evaluation for, 1752
    pulmonary function after, 1759–1760
    quality assessment and improvement for, 2114–2120, 2115f–2117f
    quality indicators for, 2114–2120, 2117b, 2118b, 2122
    sedation for, 1756–1757
Congenitally corrected transposition of great arteries See Transposition of great arteries, congenitally corrected
Congestive heart failure. See Heart failure
Connective tissue disease. See Ehlers-Danlos syndrome; Loeys-Dietz syndrome; Marfan syndrome
Conoventricular (membranous) ventricular septal defect, 1850–1851, 1851f, 1853–1855, 1854f
Constrictive pericarditis. See Pericarditis, constrictive
Continuous coronary perfusion, 977–978
Continuous venovenous hemofiltration, after pediatric cardiac surgery, 1759
Contrast agents
    anaphylactoid reaction to, 854–855
    in angiography, 776
    in computed tomography, 790
    in echocardiography, 826, 827f–828f
    in magnetic resonance imaging, 790–791
    nephropathy with, 854
Contusion
    cardiac. See Cardiac injury
    pulmonary, 92
Cor bovinum, 1199–1200
Cor triatriatum, 1809–1811, 1809f
    associated abnormalities of, 1810
    clinical presentation of, 1810
    embryology of, 1810
    pathophysiology of, 1810
    treatment of, 1810–1811
Coronary angiography, 775. See also Cardiac catheterization
    access for, 776
    in aortic regurgitation, 1200
    catheter for, 776
        complications of, 776, 776t
    complications of, 775–776, 776t, 1474
    in congenital anomalies, 776, 777f
    contraindications to, 775, 775b
    contrast injection for, 776
    before coronary artery bypass grafting, 1374, 1375f
    in coronary artery fistula, 1976
    diagonal arteries on, 778
    of graft, 778–779, 779f
    hemodynamic assessment with, 779–781
        aortic pressure in, 780t
        cardiac output in, 781, 781t
        left ventricle pressure in, 780t
        pulmonary artery pressure in, 780f, 780t, 781
        pulmonary capillary wedge pressure in, 780f, 780t, 781
        right atrium pressure in, 779, 780f, 780t
        right ventricle pressure in, 779–781, 780f, 780t
        systemic arterial pressure in, 781
    indications for, 775
    internal mammary artery for, 778–779, 779f
    left, 776, 777f–778f
    left anterior descending artery on, 776, 777f, 778
        intramyocardial, 1374, 1375f

Coronary angiography (Continued)
    left circumflex artery on, 776, 777f, 778
    left main coronary artery on, 776–777, 777f
    projections for, 777–778, 778f
    right coronary artery on, 776, 777f–778f, 778
    in type A aortic dissection, 1100
Coronary artery (arteries)
    adipose encasement of, 709–710
    β-adrenergic receptors of, 717
    anatomy of, 707–710, 708f–710f, 1963
    aneurysm of, 1472
    angiography of. See Coronary angiography
    anomalies of, 1467–1472, 1468f–1469f
        in transposition of great arteries, 1982, 1983f, 1993–1994
        in truncus arteriosus, 1913
    anomalous aorta–pulmonary artery course of, 1971–1975
        anatomy of, 1971–1972, 1972f
        cardiac catheterization in, 1973
        clinical presentation of, 1973
        computed tomography in, 1973
        diagnosis of, 1973
        echocardiography in, 1973
        electrocardiography in, 1973
        magnetic resonance imaging in, 1973
        pathophysiology of, 1972
        stress testing in, 1973
        surgical management in, 1973–1975
            coronary artery bypass grafting for, 1974
            indications for, 1973
            neo-ostium creation for, 1973–1974
            results of, 1974–1975
            translocation and reimplantation for, 1974
            unroofing procedure for, 1973, 1974f
    anomalous origin of
        from aorta, 1467
        from contralateral sinus of Valsalva, 802, 805f, 1467–1469, 1469f
        from pulmonary artery, 1470, 1963–1971. See also Anomalous origin of coronary artery from pulmonary artery
    blood flow in, 718
    blunt injury to, 1174–1175
    bypass grafting of. See Coronary artery bypass grafting
    circulatory assist devices for, 861, 861f–862f
    cocaine effects on, 1476–1477
    computed tomography of, 800–802, 804f
    in congenitally corrected transposition of great arteries, 2004, 2005f
    diameter of, myocardial perfusion and, 721
    disease of. See Coronary artery disease
    dissection of, 1473–1474
    with double-outlet right ventricle, 1861
    embolization of, 1472–1473
    endarterectomy of, 1380, 1380f
    extravascular forces on, 718
    extrinsic compression of, 1476
    fibrous hyperplasia of, 1476
    fistula of, 1470–1471. See also Coronary artery fistula
    high takeoff ostia of, 1469, 1470f
    humoral forces on, 718
    in hypertrophic cardiomyopathy, 1495–1496
    infection of, 1475
    intermural course of, 707–708
    in Kawasaki's disease, 1475, 1476f
    left
        angiography of, 776–778, 777f
        anterior descending
            angiography of, 776, 777f, 778
            intramyocardial, 1374, 1375f
        circumflex branch of, 709, 709f
            angiography of, 776, 777f, 778
        dominant, 709, 709f
        epicardial course of, 709, 709f
        origin of, 708, 1467–1470, 1468f
    magnetic resonance imaging of, 800–802, 803f
    mechanical injury to, 1472–1474
    in metabolic disease, 1476
    myocardial bridge over, 709–710
    nonatherosclerotic occlusive disease of, 1474–1476
    occlusion of. See Myocardial infarction (MI)
    origins of, 707–708, 1467, 1468f
    ostial atresia of, 1469
    penetrating injury to, 1177

Coronary artery (Continued)
    percutaneous procedures for. See Percutaneous coronary interventions
    polyarteritis nodosa of, 1474
    post-transplantation disease of, 1476
    pressure losses in, 712, 713f
    pseudoaneurysm of, 1472, 1473f
    radiation injury to, 1476
    right
        angiography of, 776, 777f, 778
        epicardial course of, 708–709, 708f–709f
        origin of, 708, 1467, 1468f, 1469, 1470f
        to sinus node, 699–700
    single, 1469
    in systemic lupus erythematosus, 1475
    Takayasu's disease of, 1475
    in tetralogy of Fallot, 1881, 1881f, 1886–1887, 1889f
    thrombosis of, 1474. See also Myocardial infarction (MI)
    tone of. See Vascular tone
    translocation and reimplantation of, in anomalous aorta–pulmonary artery coronary artery course, 1974
    trauma to, 101–102, 1173–1174, 1474
        iatrogenic, 1474
        nonpenetrating, 1474
        penetrating, 1474
    tunneled, 1471–1472, 1471f
    vasculitis of, 1474–1475
    in Wegener's granulomatosis, 1475
Coronary artery bypass grafting, 1367
    in acute coronary syndromes, 1369–1371, 1370t
    acute coronary syndromes after, 879
    in advanced-age patient, 1385
    anastomoses for
        assessment of, 1381
        automated connectors for, 1380–1381
        distal, 1378–1380, 1379f
        proximal, 1380–1381
        self-closing devices for, 1380
    anatomic considerations in, 1368–1369
    angiography of, 778–779, 779f
    in anomalous origin of coronary artery from pulmonary artery, 1966
    anticoagulation and, 858
    aortic dissection with, 1093
    aprotinin in, 1283
    in asymptomatic/mild angina, 1369, 1370t, 1385–1386
    atrial arrhythmias after, 1384
    automated distal anastomotic devices in, 1407, 1407f
    bleeding and, 858, 1383
    cardioplegia for, 1377. See also Cardioplegia
    cardiopulmonary bypass for, 1377–1378. See also Cardiopulmonary bypass
        weaning from, 1381–1382
    care after, 935–937
    carotid artery stenting before, 1154
    carotid artery stenting with, 1374
    carotid endarterectomy after, 1153–1154
    carotid endarterectomy before, 1153
    carotid endarterectomy with, 1153, 1374
    in chronic mitral valve regurgitation, 1433–1439, 1441
    in chronic stable angina, 1369, 1370t
    coagulation impairment and, 1378
    conduit for, 1375–1376, 1411
        biological, 1418
        cephalic vein, 1412
        gastroepiploic artery, 1376, 1376f, 1386t, 1387, 1413t, 1416–1417
            contraindications to, 1372–1374
            grafting strategy for, 1417, 1417f
            harvesting of, 1416–1417
            patency of, 1375f, 1386–1387
        inferior epigastric artery, 1376, 1413t, 1417
            grafting strategy for, 1417
            harvesting of, 1417
        lateral femoral circumflex artery, 1418
        left internal thoracic artery, 1375, 1386t, 1387, 1412–1414, 1413t
            bilateral, 1375, 1385
            contraindications to, 1372
            free vs. in situ, 1375
            grafting strategy for, 1414
            harvesting of, 1377, 1414
            occlusion of, 1421, 1422f

Coronary artery bypass grafting (Continued)
        patency of, 1414
        pharmacology for, 1414
        skeletonization of, 1375
        spasm of, 1414
    lesser saphenous vein, 1376, 1412
        patency of, 1386–1387, 1386t
    radial artery, 1375–1376, 1386t, 1387, 1413t, 1415–1416
        contraindications to, 1372–1374, 1376
        grafting strategy for, 1416, 1416f
        harvesting of, 1415
        neurologic complications of, 1376
        patency of, 1375, 1375f, 1386–1387, 1416
        pharmacology for, 1415–1416
        phenoxybenzamine flush for, 1376
    right internal thoracic artery, 1413t, 1414–1415
        grafting strategy for, 1415
    saphenous vein, 1376, 1386–1387, 1386t, 1411–1412, 1413t
        grafting strategy for, 1412
        harvesting of, 1411–1412
        infection and, 952
        patency of, 1386–1387, 1386t, 1412, 1418
    synthetic, 1418
    ulnar artery, 1418
    coronary endarterectomy with, 1380, 1380f
    Cox-Maze procedure in, 1357
    diffuse aortic disease and, 1377–1378, 1378f
    emergency, 853–854
    in failed percutaneous coronary intervention, 1371, 1371f
    fluorescent imaging during, 1381
    functional status after, 1386
    graft occlusion after, 946
    historical perspective on, 1367–1368, 1368f, 1397, 1411
    hybrid minimally invasive, 1406
    incomplete revascularization with, 1457. See also Transmyocardial laser revascularization
    indications for, 1369–1371, 1369t
    intramural thrombus after, 1368
    intramyocardial left anterior descending artery in, 1374, 1375f
    intraoperative assessment in, 1381
    in ischemic cardiomyopathy, 1593–1594
    in left ventricular dysfunction, 1371, 1386
    limited access, 1405
    low cardiac output syndrome after, 1383
    minimally invasive, 1405, 1405f–1406f
    mitral regurgitation after, 1436
    morbidity of, 1383–1384
    mortality of, 1384–1385
    myocardial infarction after, 1383
    neurologic complications of, 949–950, 1384. See also Neurologic disorders, cardiac surgery–related
    in non-ST-segment-elevation myocardial infarction, 1369, 1370t
    off-pump, 926, 1398–1405
        aortic manipulation during, 1403–1404, 1404f
        apical suction devices in, 1402, 1402f–1403f
        capture-type coronary stabilizers in, 1398–1399, 1399f
        care after, 935–937
        carotid endarterectomy with, 1154
        coagulation function and, 937
        compression-type coronary stabilizers in, 1398, 1398f
        deep pericardial sutures in, 1400, 1400f–1401f
        exposure techniques for, 1399–1402
        hemodynamic stability during, 1399
        ischemic preconditioning in, 992
        left ventricle function during, 1399
        mitral regurgitation during, 1399
        myocardial ischemia during, 1399, 1400f
        neurocognitive complications of, 949–950, 1009, 1404–1405
        vs. on-pump procedures, 936, 1402–1403, 1405–1406
        reoperative, 1403
        results of, 1402–1403
        right hemisternal elevation in, 1401–1402, 1402f
        right pleurotomy in, 1400–1401
        right ventricle function during, 1399
        right vertical pericardiotomy in, 1400–1401, 1401f
        self-retaining coronary stabilizers in, 1398–1399, 1398f–1399f
        suction-type coronary stabilizers in, 1398, 1398f

Coronary artery bypass grafting (Continued)
    operative preparation for, 1377–1381
    vs. percutaneous coronary intervention, 849–852, 849b, 850f, 851t, 853f, 1387–1389, 1388t
    percutaneous coronary interventions after, 857, 857b
    port-access, 1407
    postoperative care after, 1382–1383
    preoperative cardiogenic shock and, 1378
    preoperative preparation for, 1372–1374
        angiography in, 1374, 1375f
        laboratory tests in, 1374
        medication history in, 1374
        patient history in, 1372–1374, 1373t
        physical examination in, 1372–1374, 1373t
    quality of life after, 1386
    renal dysfunction after, 1383
    reoperative, 1370t, 1371, 1372f, 1421
        assessment for, 1424
        cannulation for, 1424–1425
        conduit preparation for, 1424–1425
        graft selection for, 1425–1427, 1426f
        indications for, 1422–1423
        left thoracotomy for, 1426, 1426f
        median sternotomy for, 1424–1425, 1424f
        multiple, 1427
        off-pump, 1426, 1426f
        vs. percutaneous treatment, 1421, 1423
        results of, 1423f, 1427
        stenotic vein grafts and, 1425–1426, 1426f
        technical aspects of, 1423–1424
        transmyocardial laser revascularization in, 1427
    results of, 1383–1389
    robot-assisted, 1405–1406, 1406f
    Short Form Health Survey score after, 1386
    SPECT imaging after, 821
    in ST-segment-elevation myocardial infarction, 1369–1371, 1370t
    sternal wound infection after, 1384, 1385f
    stroke and, 1152–1153
    sutureless distal connectors in, 1380
    sutureless proximal connectors in, 1380–1381
    totally endoscopic, 1299
    tracheostomy and, 1378
    transcranial Doppler scanning in, 1377
    transit-time flow measurement after, 1381
    transmyocardial laser revascularization with, 1461
    in unstable angina, 1369
    in ventricular arrhythmias, 1359, 1371
Coronary artery disease. See also Acute coronary syndromes; Angina; Myocardial infarction (MI)
    anatomic considerations in, 1368–1369
    angiogenic growth factor treatment of, 721
    aortic aneurysm and, 1068
    arterial location of, 1368
    carotid artery disease and, 1152–1154
    circulatory effects of, 720–721, 721f
    collateral vessels in, 721, 1368
    computed tomography in, 800–802, 804f
    demand ischemia in, 1368
    echocardiography in, 832–834
    exercise stress testing in, 810
    graft, 1567, 1567f
    left ventricular assist device implantation and, 1509
    left ventricular ejection fraction in, 817–818
    magnetic resonance imaging in, 800–802, 803f
    myocardial bridging in, 1368
    myocardial perfusion imaging in
        pharmacologic, 812–813
        SPECT, 810–811
        treatment-related, 814–815, 815f
    postinfarction ventricular septal defect and, 1453
    preoperative evaluation of, 816
    recurrent, after percutaneous coronary intervention, 855, 855t
    SPECT myocardial perfusion imaging in, 810–811
    stress testing in, 810–813
        prognostic value of, 813–816, 814b
    supply ischemia in, 1368
    in systemic lupus erythematosus, 1475
    treatment of
        coronary artery bypass in. See Coronary artery bypass grafting
        percutaneous interventions in. See Percutaneous coronary interventions
        stress myocardial perfusion imaging in, 814–815, 815f

Coronary artery disease (Continued)
    transmyocardial laser revascularization in. See Transmyocardial laser revascularization
    ventricular tachycardia with, catheter ablation in, 1335–1337
Coronary artery fistula, 1470–1471, 1975–1978
    anatomy of, 1975
    clinical presentation of, 1975
    diagnosis of, 1975–1976
    natural history of, 1975
    pathophysiology of, 1975
    surgical management of, 1976–1978
        indications for, 1976
        results of, 1978
        technique of, 1976–1977, 1976f–1978f
Coronary endarterectomy, 1380, 1380f
Coronary perfusion, continuous, 977–978
Coronary sinus, 710, 710f
    left, 707, 708f
    right, 707, 708f
Coronary sinus catheter, 926
Coronary sinus–type atrial septal defect, 1799–1800, 1800f
Coronary steal syndrome, 921, 1144f, 1152
Coronary–subclavian steal syndrome, 921, 1144f, 1152
Coronary veins, 710, 710f
Corridor procedure, in atrial fibrillation, 1347
Corticosteroids
    in cardiopulmonary bypass, 967
    in community-acquired pneumonia, 177
    after lung transplantation, 219
    with pediatric cardiopulmonary bypass, 1727–1728
Cortisol, serum, after pediatric cardiac surgery, 1758
Corynebacterium parvum, for pleurodesis, 438–439
Costal cartilages, 12t
Costoclavicular ligament, 399, 402f
Costoclavicular test, 393, 394f
Cough
    ACE inhibitor–related, 891–892
    postoperative, 52–53
Coumadin, in patent foramen ovale, 1804
COX inhibitors, in patent ductus arteriosus, 1782
Cox-Maze procedure. See Atrial fibrillation, Cox-Maze procedure in
Creatinine
    after cardiopulmonary bypass, 971
    preoperative, 919
    in thoracic aortic aneurysm, 1069
Creatinine kinase–myocardial bands, in blunt cardiac injury, 95, 1174
Cribriform diaphragm, 510
Cricopharyngeal myotomy, in Zenker's diverticulum, 75–76
Cross-bridges, 728f, 732
Cross-clamping, aortic
    duration of, 1065
    spinal cord injury and, 1065, 1065f, 1069–1075, 1070f, 1074f
"Crossing the Quality Chasm" (Institute of Medicine), 1014
Cryoablation therapy, in arrhythmias, 1331
Cryoplasty, in femoral artery disease, 1169
Cryoprecipitate, 762b, 763
Cryptococcosis, 190
Cryptogenic organizing pneumonitis, 168
Crystalloid solutions, for cardioplegia, 987–989, 988f
CT. See Computed tomography (CT)
Culture
    in empyema, 416
    in endocarditis, 1260, 1271
CURB-65, in community-acquired pneumonia, 176
Cushing syndrome, in bronchopulmonary carcinoid tumor, 325
Cyanide toxicity, 889
Cyanosis
    in atrial septal defect, 1802
    in congenitally corrected transposition of great arteries, 2005–2006
    after Fontan procedure, 2049
    in myocardial ischemia-reperfusion injury, 981–982
    in tetralogy of Fallot, 1882–1883
    in transposition of great arteries, 1983
Cyclosporine
    in heart transplantation, 1545–1546
    in lung transplantation, 219

Cyst(s)
    bronchogenic, 138–139, 139f, 647, 655–656, 1634t
    esophageal, 565–568, 566b, 569f
    gastroenteric, 656
    mediastinal, 655–656, 655f
    mesothelial
        multilocular, 455
        simple, 455
    neuroenteric, 656
    pericardial, 648, 655, 655f, 1487–1488, 1488f
    pulmonary, parenchymal, congenital, 141–142
    thymic, 639
Cystadenoma, mucinous, 156
Cystic adenomatoid malformation, congenital, 142–143, 142f
Cystic fibrosis
    bronchiectasis in, 180
    lung transplantation in, 209
Cytokeratin
    in lung cancer, 673, 675
    in sarcoma, 334
    in thymoma, 634
Cytokines
    in cardiopulmonary bypass, 963–965, 964f
    in malignant pleural effusion, 441
    in myocardial cell-based regenerative therapy, 1607–1608
    with pediatric cardiopulmonary bypass, 1727
Cytolytic induction therapy, in heart transplantation, 1546
Cytomegalovirus (CMV) infection
    after heart-lung transplantation, 1566
    after heart transplantation, 1549–1550, 1550t
    after lung transplantation, 219, 221f

D

Da Vinci system, 1295–1296, 1296f. See also Robot-assisted cardiac surgery
Dalteparin, in NSTE acute coronary syndromes, 874–875
Damus-Stansel-Kaye procedure, 2043
Darbepoetin, preoperative/postoperative, 49
Decompression illness, patent foramen ovale and, 1804
Decortication, in empyema, 422
Deep hypothermic circulatory rest. See also Hypothermia
    brain ischemia and, 924–925
    pediatric, 1713, 1721–1722
        brain injury with, 1725–1726
Deep pericardial sutures, in off-pump coronary artery bypass grafting, 1400, 1400f–1401f
Deep venous thrombosis
    prevention of, 48, 48b, 49t
    risk for, 48, 48b, 49t
Delirium, after cardiopulmonary bypass, 970
Deltoid muscle, 8t
Dental procedures, antibiotic prophylaxis for, 1269, 1269t
Denver pleuroperitoneal shunt, in malignant pericardial effusion, 445
Deoxyribonucleic acid, hypermethylation of, in mesothelioma, 452
Desert fever, 187
Desmin, in pleural effusion, 435t
Desmoid tumor
    chest wall, 385
    pleural, 455
Desmoplastic small round cell tumor, 457
Desmopressin
    in cardiac surgery, 769
    in postoperative bleeding, 948–949
Dexmedetomidine, in congenital heart disease, 1757
Diabetes mellitus
    coronary circulation in, 720–721, 721f
    preoperative assessment of, 48
    sternal wound infection and, 1000
Dialysis, after pediatric cardiac surgery, 1759
Diaphragm, 473
    agenesis of, 509
    anatomy of, 4–5, 473–474
        arterial, 475–476, 477f
        lymphatic, 476
        neural, 476–477
        venous, 475–476
    aortic opening of, 4, 474
    blood supply of, 4

Diaphragm (Continued)
    congenital hernia of. See Congenital diaphragmatic hernia
    cribriform, 510
    duplication of, 509–510
    elevation of, 478–480, 479f. See also Diaphragm, eventration of
        acquired, 478–479
    embryology of, 473, 474f, 490–491, 490f, 491t
    esophageal opening of, 4, 474
    eventration of, 478–480, 507–509, 508f
        in adults, 479–480, 481f
        central tendon plication for, 479–480, 480f
        plication for, 479–480, 480f–481f
        pulmonary failure with, 479
        subcostal radial plication for, 480, 480f
        thoracoscopic plication for, 480, 481f
        transthoracic radial plication for, 480, 481f
    function of, 473–474
    hernia of, 480–482
        congenital. See Congenital diaphragmatic hernia
    incisions for, 477, 478f
        central tendon, 477
        circumferential, 477, 478f
        radial, 477
    inferior vena cava opening of, 474
    innervation of, 476–477
    in inspiration, 474
    lung cancer invasion of, 485
    neonatal, 1749
    openings in, 4, 474, 475f
    pericardial hernia of, 491t, 508f, 509
    peritoneal attachments of, 474–475
    pleural attachments of, 474–475, 477f
    postoperative function of, 39
    reconstruction of, in congenital diaphragmatic hernia, 507
    resection of, 485–486, 485f
        prosthetic patch in, 486, 486f
    respiration-related movement of, 4, 10, 474
    trauma to, 96–97, 96f, 478
        imaging in, 478
        laparoscopy in, 97, 478
        laparotomy in, 97, 478
        left-sided, 96, 96f
        mortality from, 97
        penetrating, 103–105
        repair of, 478
        right-sided, 96
        rupture with, 478
        thoracoscopy in, 478
        thoracotomy in, 97
    tumors of, 484–485
        resection of, 485–486, 485f
Diaphragmatic pacing, 483–484, 484f
Diaphragmatic patch, 486, 486f
Diastole, 741–744, 741f–742f. See also Ventricle(s), left, diastolic function of
Diazoxide, in myocardial protection, 985
Diet
    alcohol intake in, 913
    in atherosclerosis prevention, 910t, 912b, 911–913
    carbohydrates in, 913
    cholesterol in, 912
    fiber in, 912–913
    Mediterranean, 913
    saturated fat in, 912
    vegetarian, 913
    for weight reduction, 912
Diffuse esophageal spasm, 563
Diffuse idiopathic pulmonary neuroendocrine cell hyperplasia, 329
Diffusing capacity for carbon monoxide (DL_{CO}), 41–42
DiGeorge syndrome, 1648, 1882, 1927
Digital subtraction angiography
    of abdominal aorta, 1161f
    in brachiocephalic artery disease, 1145
    of femoral artery, 1164f
    of iliac artery, 1163f
    of popliteal artery, 1159, 1159f
    of subclavian artery, 1161f
Digoxin
    before coronary artery bypass grafting, 1374
    in heart failure, 891t, 893, 893t, 897, 897t
    toxicity of, 893, 893t

Dilated cardiomyopathy. *See also* Cardiomyopathy, dilated
Diltiazem
    in heart failure, 890, 891t
    in postoperative atrial fibrillation, 944
Dipyridamole
    in prosthetic heart valve anticoagulation, 1280–1281
    vasodilatory effects of, 711, 712f
Disc battery ingestion, 571
Discharge, 58
    after congenital heart disease treatment, 1762, 1762b
Dissection
    aortic. *See* Aortic dissection
    coronary artery, 1473–1474
Diuretics
    in heart failure, 887–888, 887t, 897, 897t
    after lung transplantation, 218
    in tetralogy of Fallot, 1883
Diver, decompression illness in, patent foramen ovale and, 1804
Diverticulum (diverticula)
    esophageal, 563–565
        epiphrenic, 565, 566f
        midthoracic, 551f, 565
        pulsion, 563–564
        Zenker's. *See* Zenker's diverticulum
    pericardial, 1487–1488
DNA hypermethylation, in mesothelioma, 452
DNA microarray analysis, 670–673, 671f
Dobutamine
    after cardiac surgery, 940–941, 942t
    in heart failure, 894, 899, 899t
Doege-Potter syndrome, 454
Dopamine
    after cardiac surgery, 940–941, 942t
    in cardiopulmonary bypass, 971
    in heart failure, 893–894, 899, 899t
    after pediatric cardiac surgery, 1758
Doppler echocardiography, 748–749, 827–829, 828f–830f, 829t
    pediatric, 1666–1667, 1667f
        myocardial motion on, 1675, 1675f
        pressure gradients on, 1675–1676
Dor procedure, 1360–1361
Dorsal sympathectomy, 400–404
    complications of, 403
    neuralgia after, 403
    pathophysiology of, 402–403
    recurrent symptoms after, 403
    results of, 404
    surgical approaches for, 403
    technique of, 404
    transaxillary approach for, 404
    transaxillary first rib resection with, 404
    variations of, 403–404
Double-orifice mitral valve, 1843, 1845, 2016–2017
Double-outlet left ventricle, 1652f, 1662–1663
Double-outlet right ventricle, 1652f, 1662–1663, 1858–1863. *See also* Ventricular septal defect
    atrioventricular canal defect and, 1842
    classification of, 1858–1859, 1858f
    conal septum with, 1860, 1860f
    coronary artery anatomy and, 1861
    with doubly committed ventricular septal defect, 1859, 1859t, 1861, 1862f
    evaluation of, 1861
    great artery relationship and, 1861
    with noncommitted ventricular septal defect, 1859, 1859t, 1861–1862
    pulmonary outflow tract obstruction with, 1860–1861
    with subaortic ventricular septal defect, 1858–1859, 1859f, 1859t, 1861, 1862f
    with subpulmonary ventricular septal defect, 1859, 1859f, 1859t, 1862
    surgical treatment of, 1861–1862, 1862f
        evaluation for, 1861
        results of, 1862–1863
    in transposition of great arteries, 1993, 1994f, 1997–1999
    tricuspid–pulmonary valve distance and, 1859–1860
Down syndrome
    atrial septal defect in, 1801
    atrioventricular canal defects in, 1834
Drainage
    intraoperative, 50–51
    postoperative, 53

Dressings, for surgical wound, 53
Dressler's syndrome, 1486
Drug(s). *See specific drugs*
    alveolar injury with, 165
    in atherosclerosis management, 909t–911t, 913–914
    errors with, 1018
    patient instructions for, 1018
    postoperative, 51–52
    pulmonary injury with, 165
    reconciliation of, 1018
Drug-eluting stents, 848, 855–856
    recurrent disease and, 855
Ductal stenting and bilateral pulmonary artery banding, in hypoplastic left heart syndrome, 2036–2037
Ductus arteriosus
    patent. *See* Patent ductus arteriosus
    spontaneous closure of, 1781–1782
Duke Activity Status Index, 40, 41t
Duke criteria
    in native valve endocarditis, 1260, 1261b
    in prosthetic valve endocarditis, 1271, 1272b
Dumping syndrome, postoperative, 57
Duplication
    diaphragmatic, 509–510
    esophageal, 543–544. *See also* Esophageal duplication
Duplication cyst, foregut, 543–544, 568, 569f, 656
Dusts, pulmonary deposition of, 161, 161t
Dyslipidemic triad, 908
Dysphagia
    aortic arch aneurysm and, 1046
    cancer-related
        photodynamic therapy in, 71
        stent therapy in, 73–74
    esophagoscopy in, 61
    fundoplication-related, 52
    postoperative, 56
Dysphonia, traumatic, 92
Dyspnea, in pulmonary metastases, 339

E

E-cadherin, in bronchopulmonary carcinoid tumor, 324–325
Ebstein's anomaly, 2055
    adult, 2076–2078, 2077f–2078f. *See also* Ebstein's anomaly, pediatric
        accessory pathways in, 2092–2094
    anatomy of, 2055
    classification of, 2055–2056, 2056t
    embryology of, 2055
    fetal, 2056
    historical perspective on, 2055
    infant, 2056–2058, 2057f, 2057t
    neonatal, 2056–2058
    pediatric, 2058–2066
        clinical presentation of, 2058–2059
        diagnosis of, 2058–2059, 2059f
        GOSE score in, 2057, 2057t
        natural history of, 2059–2060
        surgical management of, 2060–2066
            atrialized right ventricle plication in, 2065, 2065f
            heart transplantation in, 2058, 2066
            indications for, 2060
            outcomes of, 2066
            right reduction atrioplasty in, 2065–2066
            valve repair in, 2060–2062, 2061f–2062f
            valve replacement in, 2062–2063, 2064f
            1.5-ventricle repair in, 2064
    physiology of, 2056–2066
Echinococcosis, pericardial, 1485
Echocardiography, 825
    in acute pulmonary embolism, 1616–1617
    in anomalous aorta–pulmonary artery coronary artery course, 1973
    in anomalous origin of coronary artery from pulmonary artery, 1965
    in aortic disease, 843–844, 844f
    in aortic dissection, 25, 844, 844f, 1099–1100
    in aortic regurgitation, 827f–828f, 829, 830f, 838–839, 839f, 1200
    in aortic root dilatation, 845, 845f
    in aortic stenosis, 828f, 838
    in aortopulmonary window, 1920–1921

Echocardiography (*Continued*)
    in atrial septal defect, 1802
    in atrioventricular canal defects, 1836
    in bicuspid aortic valve, 845, 845f
    in cardiac masses, 834–836, 834f–835f
    in cardiac trauma, 95, 101
    in cardiomyopathy, 836–837, 836f
    in coarctation of aorta, 1784, 1784f
    in congenital aortic stenosis, 1944
    in congenital diaphragmatic hernia, 500
    in congenital heart disease, 844–845, 845f
    in congenital mitral anomalies, 2019–2020
    contrast, 826, 827f–828f
    in coronary artery disease, 832–834
    in diastolic function study, 831–832, 831f–832f
    Doppler, 748–749, 827–829, 828f–830f, 829t
    in Ebstein's anomaly, 2057, 2059, 2059f, 2077, 2077f
    in embolism, 835, 836f
    in endocarditis, 842–843, 843f
    epicardial, 826–827
    in esophageal atresia, 537
    in extracorporeal membrane oxygenation, 1741
    fetal, 1671–1672
        in arrhythmia, 1672
        clinical implications of, 1672
        in congenital heart disease, 1672
        in Ebstein's anomaly, 2056
        indications for, 1671, 1671b
        technique of, 1671, 1672f
        in tetralogy of Fallot, 1882–1883, 1883f
    in heart failure, 836
    in hypertrophic cardiomyopathy, 836–837, 836f, 1498
    in hypoplastic left heart syndrome, 2025–2026
    of inferior vena cava, 829f, 829t
    in interrupted aortic arch, 1930
    in intracardiac shunt, 826, 827f
    intraoperative, 826–827, 2099–2100, 2100f
        in children, 1753
    in ischemia, 832–834
    in lung transplantation, 214
    M-mode, 825, 827f
    in mitral regurgitation, 829, 830f, 840–841, 840f–841f, 1215–1216, 1216t
    in mitral stenosis, 839–840, 839f–840f, 1211
    modalities of, 825–827
    in myocardial infarction complications, 833–834, 834f
    in myxoma, 1634
    in patent ductus arteriosus, 1782, 1782f
    in patent foramen ovale, 835, 836f
    pediatric, 1665–1676
        anatomic analysis for, 1668–1669
        aortic valve diameter on, 1672, 1673f
        body surface area in, 1672, 1673f
        complications of, 1676
        contrast, 1667
        Doppler, 1666–1667, 1667f
            Bernoulli equation for, 1675
            myocardial motion on, 1675, 1675f
            pressure gradients on, 1675–1676
        examination technique for, 1667–1668, 1668f
        left ventricular volume on, 1673–1674, 1674f
        M-mode, 1666, 1666f
        objectives of, 1667–1669
        quantitative analysis of, 1672–1676, 1673f–1674f
        safety of, 1676
        speckle tracking in, 1675, 1675f
        technique of, 1665–1667
        three-dimensional, 1666, 1667f
        transesophageal, 1669–1671, 1670f
        two-dimensional, 1666, 1666f
        ventricular function on, 1674–1675, 1675f
        z score in, 1672–1673
    in penetrating cardiac injury, 1176
    in pericardial disease, 785, 837–838, 1483, 1483f
    in pericardial effusion, 443f, 444, 832, 832f, 837, 837f
    in pericarditis, 837–838
    principles of, 825
    in prosthetic valve endocarditis, 1271
    in prosthetic valve evaluation, 842, 842f
    in pulmonary atresia with intact ventricular septum, 1866–1867
    in pulmonary atresia with ventricular septal defect, 1899, 1904
    stress, 828f, 833
    in systolic function study, 829–831, 830f–831f

Echocardiography (Continued)
  in tetralogy of Fallot, 845, 1878f–1880f, 1882–1883, 1883f
  in total anomalous pulmonary venous drainage, 1823–1824, 1823f
  transesophageal, 825–826
    in atrioventricular canal defect repair, 1845
    in blunt cardiac injury, 1174
    in brachiocephalic artery disease, 1145
    in cardiac surgery, 920, 921f
    in cardiopulmonary bypass separation, 925, 925f
    in endocarditis, 842–843, 1260
    in mediastinal evaluation, 655
    in minimally invasive cardiac surgery, 926
    in mitral regurgitation, 1215–1216, 1436–1439, 1437f
    before mitral valve surgery, 1218, 1219f
    pediatric, 1669–1671, 1670f
    in type A aortic dissection, 1098–1100
    in type B aortic dissection, 1119
  in transplantation, 837
  in transposition of great arteries, 1984, 1994
  transthoracic, 825, 826f
    in atrial septal defect, 1802
    in blunt cardiac injury, 1174
    in chronic thromboembolic pulmonary hypertension, 1622
  in trauma, 87
  in tricuspid valve disease, 841–842, 841f
  in truncus arteriosus, 1914, 1914f
  in valvular disease, 838–843
  in ventricular function study, 829–832, 830f–832f
ECMO. See Extracorporeal membrane oxygenation (ECMO)
Ectopia cordis, 376–382
  etiology of, 376–377
  thoracic, 377–380, 380f–381f, 380t–381t
  thoracoabdominal, 380–382, 381f, 382t–383t
Effective orifice area, of prosthetic heart valves, 1186
Effet de mouette deformity, 1433
Effort thrombosis, 392–393, 398–400, 402f
Effusion. See Pericardial effusion; Pleural effusion
Ehlers-Danlos syndrome, 1026, 1092–1093, 2018
Eisenmenger's syndrome, 1556
Ejection fraction, 745
Electrocardiography
  in accessory pathway–mediated tachycardia, 1335, 1335t
  in acute pulmonary embolism, 1616
  in anomalous aorta–pulmonary artery course of coronary arteries, 1973
  in anomalous origin of coronary artery from pulmonary artery, 1965
  in aortic stenosis, 1197
  in atrial fibrillation, 1346
  in atrial flutter, 944f–945f, 1334
  in atrial septal defect, 1802
  in atrioventricular canal defects, 1836
  in blunt cardiac injury, 95, 1174
  of cardiac cycle, 740–741, 741f
  after cardiac surgery, 933–934
  in congenital aortic stenosis, 1944
  in congenital mitral anomalies, 2019
  in constrictive pericarditis, 1482f
  in cor triatriatum, 1810
  before coronary artery bypass grafting, 1374
  in coronary artery fistula, 1975–1976
  in Ebstein's anomaly, 2058
  in hypertrophic cardiomyopathy, 1497–1498
  intraoperative, 920, 1752
  in mitral regurgitation, 1215
  in pectus excavatum, 361
  after pediatric cardiac surgery, 1759
  in pericardial disease, 785, 1483
  in postinfarction ventricular septal defect, 1450
  with pre-procedure endoscopy, 62
  in tetralogy of Fallot, 1882
  in transposition of great arteries, 1984
  twenty-four-hour Holter, in thoracic aortic aneurysm, 1068
  in ventricular septal defect, 1853
Electrogram, 1331
Electrophysiology study
  indications for, 1329–1330
  technique of, 1330
Elephant trunk procedure, 1054–1056, 1055f, 1057f
Eloesser flap, 55, 414, 414f, 420, 421f–422f

Embolectomy
  in coronary artery embolism, 1472–1473
  in pulmonary embolism, 1618–1620, 1620t
Embolism
  air, 102–103
  bullet, 102–103
  coronary artery, 1472–1473
  with prosthetic heart valve, 1186–1187, 1204, 1285
  pulmonary. See Pulmonary embolism
Embryology
  cardiac. See Heart, embryology of
  diaphragmatic, 473, 474f, 490–491, 490f, 491t
  esophageal, 517–520, 535
  pleural, 449
  pulmonary, 129–130, 1817, 1818f
Embryonic stem cells, 1600, 1600t, 1601f
Emphysema, 195
  airway bypass stents for, 204
  bronchoscopic treatment for, 204
  bullectomy for, 195–196, 204
  historical perspective on, 195
  infantile, 143
  lobar
    acquired, 140–141
    congenital, 140–141, 141f
  lung transplantation for, 196–199, 204–205
    bilateral vs. unilateral, 197–198, 198f
    disadvantages of, 196–197
    indications for, 199b
    vs. medical therapy, 197, 198f
    patient selection for, 196
    results of, 196, 197f
    technique of, 198–199
  lung volume reduction for, 199–204
    as bridge procedure, 203–204, 203f
    indications for, 199b, 201t
    perfusion scintigraphy for, 200, 200f
    results of, 200–201, 201f–202f
    technique of, 201–203
  one-way valve placement for, 204
  pathogenesis of, 195
  pulmonary rehabilitation program for, 195
Empyema, 413
  acute, 417–420
  antibiotics in, 419
  bacteriology of, 416
  bronchopleural fistula and, 423
  chronic, 420–423, 421f
  complications of, 414–415
  culture in, 416
  decortication in, 422
  definition of, 413
  diagnosis of, 416–417
  drainage of, 418–419, 419t
  Eloesser flap in, 414, 414f, 420, 421f–422f
  empyemectomy in, 422
  historical perspective on, 413–414, 414f–415f
  intrapleural enzyme treatment in, 419–420
  management of, 417–423
  mortality rate with, 423
  muscle transposition procedure in, 422
  open thoracic window in, 420
  pathogenesis of, 415–416
  pleural fluid analysis in, 417
  pleuropneumonectomy in, 422
  post-traumatic, 108, 415
  postoperative, 56, 415–416
  rib resection drainage in, 420
  space-filling procedures in, 422–423
  space sterilization in, 420–422
  stages of, 414
  supportive measures in, 420
  talc treatment in, 420
  thoracoplasty in, 422–423
Empyema necessitatis, 414–415
Empyemectomy, 422
Enalapril
  for afterload reduction, 940
  in heart failure, 890–892, 891t
End-diastolic pressure
  cardiac output and, 734–737, 735f
  stroke volume and, 746, 747f. See also Frank-Starling curve/relationship
End-diastolic pressure–volume relationship, 741–744, 743f, 743b

End-diastolic volume
  cardiac output and, 734–737, 736f
  exercise-related, 725–726, 726f
  stroke work and, 746, 747f
  ventricle cross-section and, 730, 730f
End-systolic pressure, 730, 730f
  cardiac output and, 734–737, 735f
End-systolic pressure–volume relationship, 745, 746f, 748, 748f
End-systolic volume
  exercise-related, 725–726, 726f
  ventricle cross-section and, 730, 730f
Endarterectomy
  in aortic arch aneurysm, 1057
  carotid. See Carotid endarterectomy
  coronary, 1380, 1380f
  in innominate artery disease, 1147, 1148f
  pulmonary, 1622–1623
    principles of, 1623
    results of, 1625–1628, 1627t–1628t
    technique of, 1623–1624
Endobronchial ultrasound–transbronchial needle aspiration, 247, 247f, 631–632, 632f
Endocardial cushions
  defect of. See Atrioventricular canal defects
  embryology of, 1645, 1645f
Endocarditis
  native valve, 1259
    aortic valve, 1199, 1259–1262, 1262f, 1264
    clinical presentation of, 1260
    complications of, 843, 843f
    culture negative, 1260
    diagnosis of, 1260
    Duke criteria for, 1260, 1261b
    echocardiography in, 835, 842–843, 843f
    in hypertrophic cardiomyopathy, 1498
    imaging in, 842–843, 843f, 1260
    incidence of, 1259
    Libman-Sacks, 1475
    management of, 1260–1261, 1261b
    microbiology of, 1259–1260
    mitral valve, 1214, 1259–1264, 1263f
      surgical treatment of, 1218, 1227, 1231
    neurologic examination in, 1261
    pathology of, 1259
    surgical treatment of, 1262–1264, 1262f–1263f
      results of, 1264
      timing of, 1260
    systemic manifestations of, 1259
    tricuspid valve, 1244, 1248, 1259, 1263–1264
    vegetations in, 835, 842, 843f
  prosthetic valve, 1187, 1267
    antibiotic prophylaxis for, 1269, 1269t
    anticoagulation in, 1271–1272
    aortic valve, 1204, 1273–1275, 1274f–1275f
    bacteremia and, 1268
    blood culture in, 1271
    clinical manifestations of, 1271
    conduction abnormalities in, 1271
    diagnosis of, 1271
    Duke criteria in, 1271, 1272b
    early, 1268
    echocardiography in, 842–843, 843f, 1271
    fungal, 1268
    health care–associated, 1268–1269
    hemodialysis and, 1268
    historical perspective on, 1267
    intraoperative contamination and, 1268
    late, 1268
    mechanical vs. bioprosthetic valve and, 1269–1271
    medical management of, 1271–1273
    microbiology of, 1270, 1270t
    mitral valve, 1269, 1275, 1276f
    native valve endocarditis and, 1268–1270
    neurologic complications with, 1275
    nosocomial, 1268–1269
    pathology of, 1270–1271
    prosthesis type and, 1269
    risk for, 1267–1270
    sewing ring in, 1270
    surgical management of, 1267, 1272–1275, 1273b
      indications for, 1272
      mortality rate with, 1273
      prognosis for, 1273, 1273b
    S. aureus and, 1273

EndoCinch device, in gastroesophageal reflux, 80
Endoleak, in thoracic endovascular aortic repair, 1135–1136, 1135t
Endomyocardial fibrosis, 1215
Endoscopic ultrasonography, 62–63, 63b, 555–556, 557f
　in esophageal cancer, 577–580, 579f, 579t, 584f
　after neoadjuvant chemoradiation, 579
Endoscopy
　diagnostic, of esophagus, 526, 526f
　therapeutic, 67
　　in brachytherapy, 75, 77t
　　in gastroesophageal reflux, 78–80. *See also* Gastroesophageal reflux
　　laser, 74–75, 74t–75t, 77t
　　in malignant airway obstruction, 75, 76f
　　photodynamic, 67–71, 77t. *See also* Photodynamic therapy
　　in stent placement, 71–74, 72t, 77t
　　in Zenker's diverticulum, 75–78. *See also* Zenker's diverticulum
Endothelial progenitor cells, in regenerative cell-based therapy, 1600t, 1601–1603, 1601f, 1603f, 1608f
Endothelin-1, 718
Endothelin receptor antagonists, in hypoxic pulmonary vasoconstriction, 722, 722f
Endothelium
　in cardiopulmonary bypass, 935, 964–965
　in vasomotor tone regulation, 711, 712f, 713–716, 714f, 716f
Endothelium-derived hyperpolarizing factor, 715–716, 715f–716f
Endotoxin, with pediatric cardiopulmonary bypass, 1727
Endotracheal intubation
　in flail chest, 90–91
　injury with, 114–115, 114f
Energy
　myocardial consumption of, 747–748, 747f, 978–979, 979f
　neonatal requirement for, 1750
Enoxaparin, in NSTE acute coronary syndromes, 874–875, 875t, 876f
Enteryx injection, in gastroesophageal reflux, 79
Enzymes, therapeutic, in empyema, 419–420
Eosinophilic esophagitis, 570
Eosinophilic granuloma, 164
Eosinophilic pneumonia, 163–164
　acute, 164
　chronic, 164
　simple, 164
Epidermal growth factor receptor, in mesothelioma, 452–453
Epinephrine
　in cardiac contractility, 747
　after cardiac surgery, 940–941, 942t
　after cardiopulmonary bypass, 969
　in heart failure, 899, 899t
　after pediatric cardiac surgery, 1758
Epithelial membrane antigen, in pleural effusion, 435t
Epithelioid hemangioendothelioma, 332
Eplerenone, 887t
Eptifibatide, 760, 919
Erdheim deformity, 1042
Erlotinib, 678–679
Erythromycin, postoperative, 52
Erythropoietin, 49
Esmolol, for afterload reduction, 940
Esophageal artery, 519, 519f
Esophageal atresia, 535–543
　anatomy of, 536, 536f
　classification of, 536, 536f, 536t
　embryology of, 535
　epidemiology of, 536
　evaluation of, 536–537, 537f–538f
　historical perspective on, 535–536
　malnutrition with, 542
　management of
　　adult quality of life after, 542
　　bronchoscopy in, 538, 539f
　　circular myotomy in, 540
　　complications of, 541–543, 543f
　　delayed primary anastomosis in, 540
　　foreign body impaction after, 542
　　gastroesophageal reflux after, 542
　　initial, 537–538
　　long-term effects of, 541–543

Esophageal atresia (*Continued*)
　　manometric evaluation after, 542–543
　　operative, 538–541, 539f–542f
　　stricture after, 541
　　suction/drainage in, 537–538
　　timing of, 538
　murine model of, 535
　presentation of, 536, 537f
　tracheoesophageal fistula with, 536, 536f, 536t
　　emergent management of, 538
　　operative management of, 538–539, 539f
　　recurrence of, 542
　tracheomalacia and, 542, 543f
Esophageal cancer
　chemoradiotherapy in
　　adjuvant, 621
　　endoscopic ultrasonography after, 579
　　neoadjuvant, 579, 619–620, 619t
　　primary, 621
　　prognosis after, 582
　chemotherapy in
　　adjuvant, 620–621
　　neoadjuvant, 618–619, 619t
　　prognosis after, 582
　circulating tumor cell detection in, 677
　DNA microarray analysis in, 672–673
　dysphagia with
　　photodynamic therapy in, 71
　　stent therapy in, 73–74
　epidemiology of, 577
　imaging in, 27, 655
　laser therapy in, 74–75
　lymph nodes in, 621
　metastases from
　　brain, 583–584
　　endoscopic ultrasonography in, 580
　　lymphatic, 604, 621
　　molecular markers in, 584
　palliative treatment of
　　photodynamic therapy in, 71
　　stenting in, 73–74
　photodynamic therapy in, 69–71
　　palliative, 71
　polymerase chain reaction in, 675–676
　radiotherapy in
　　adjuvant, 620, 620t
　　neoadjuvant, 618
　　primary, 621
　recurrence of, 612
　resection of. *See* Esophagectomy
　staging of, 577, 584f, 617–618, 618f
　　computed tomography in, 580, 584f, 617, 618f
　　endoscopic ultrasonography in, 577–580, 579f, 579t, 584f, 617, 618f, 655
　　　accuracy of, 579
　　　in metastatic disease, 580
　　　after neoadjuvant chemoradiation, 579
　　laparoscopic, 618
　　molecular, 584
　　positron emission tomography in, 577, 580–581, 617, 618f
　　positron emission tomography–computed tomography in, 577, 581–583, 581f, 584f
　　　for initial staging, 581–582
　　　for interval staging, 582
　　　for restaging, 582–583, 582f
　　surgical, 583, 618
　　thoracoscopic, 618
　　TNM, 578, 578t
　survival rates in, 385, 577, 617
Esophageal duplication, 543–544
　anatomy of, 543
　diagnosis of, 543
　embryology of, 543
　incidence of, 543
　presentation of, 543
　treatment of, 543–544
Esophageal manometry, 527–528, 527f, 552, 553t, 554f
　after atresia repair, 542–543
　body motility on, 528, 528f–530f
　high-resolution, 528–529, 552, 553t, 554f
　lower sphincter on, 527, 527f, 552, 553t
　twenty-four–hour, 532
　upper sphincter on, 528, 530f

Esophageal sphincter
　lower, 522–525
　　anatomy of, 517f, 518–519
　　cardia anatomy and, 524
　　failure of, 522, 524–525, 524f. *See also* Gastroesophageal reflux disease
　　in fasting state, 524–525
　　high-pressure zone of, 522–524, 522f–523f
　　length of, 522–524, 523f
　　inflammation-related loss of, 525
　　manometric evaluation of, 527, 527f, 552, 553t, 554f
　　in swallowing, 550, 552, 554f
　upper, 548, 548f
　　radiographic evaluation of, 525
　　relaxation of, 521
　　in swallowing, 549–550, 552, 554f
Esophageal stricture, 568–571, 569b, 570f
　allergy-related, 570
　anastomotic, 571
　atresia repair and, 541
　barium esophagography in, 552f, 569
　benign, 73
　caustic, 572
　malignant, 73–74
　nasogastric tube–induced, 570, 571f
　peptic, 569–570
　photodynamic therapy–related, 71
　pill-induced, 570
　radiation-induced, 571
　treatment algorithm for, 569, 570f
Esophagectomy, 589
　age and, 40
　anastomotic leak after, 608–609
　anastomotic stricture after, 611
　arrhythmias after, 611
　bleeding with, 610
　cardiovascular morbidity after, 611
　cervical anastomotic leak after, 609
　chylothorax after, 56–57, 427–429, 610–611
　complications of
　　anastomotic, 608–609, 611
　　bleeding, 610
　　cardiovascular, 611
　　comparative studies of, 597–599
　　conduit-related, 57, 612
　　neural, 610
　　reflux, 612
　　respiratory, 609–610
　　thoracic duct, 610–611
　conduit creation in, 604–607
　　colon for, 604–605, 605f–606f
　　impaired emptying of, 612
　　jejunum for, 606–607, 607f–609f
　　stomach for, 592, 592f–594f, 612
　en bloc, 603–604
　　results of, 603–604
　　technique of, 603
　fluid therapy after, 50
　historical perspective on, 589
　intrathoracic anastomotic leak after, 608–609
　Ivor Lewis, 593–594
　　contraindications to, 594
　　indications for, 593
　　minimally invasive, 600–601
　　technique of, 594, 596f, 612
　　vs. transhiatal esophagectomy, 597–599, 599t
　left thoracoabdominal, 602–603
　　contraindications to, 602
　　indications for, 602
　　technique of, 602–603, 603f
　local recurrence after, 612
　margins in, 612
　minimally invasive, 599–602
　　conduit creation in, 600
　　Ivor Lewis, 600–601
　　laparoscopy in, 600
　　results of, 601–602
　　transhiatal, 601
　　tri-incisional, 599–600
　　video-assisted thoracoscopic esophageal mobilization in, 600
　modified McKeown (tri-incisional), 589–593
　　contraindications to, 590
　　indications for, 589–590
　　minimally invasive, 599–600

Esophagectomy (Continued)
    contraindications to, 599–600
    indications for, 599
    technique of, 600
  preparation for, 590
  technique of, 590–593
    blunt dissection in, 590–591, 591f
    cervical anastomosis in, 592–593, 594f–595f
    diaphragmatic rim resection in, 591–592, 591f
    esophagogastroduodenoscopy in, 590
    gastric tube creation in, 592–593, 593f
    gastric vessel division in, 592, 592f
    Penrose drain in, 590–592, 591f, 593f
    phrenoesophageal ligament division in, 591–592, 592f
    posterolateral thoracotomy in, 590, 590f
  mortality with, 608
  myocardial infarction after, 611
  nasogastric tube in, 53
  oral intake after, 52
  recurrent laryngeal nerve injury with, 610
  reflux after, 612
  respiratory complications of, 609–610
  results of, 621
  survival after, 612–613
  thoracic duct injury with, 610–611
  three-field lymph node dissection in, 604
  transhiatal, 594–597
    contraindications to, 596
    indications for, 594
    minimally invasive, 601
    preparation for, 596
    technique of, 596–597, 597f–599f
    vs. transthoracic, 597–599, 599t
Esophagitis, eosinophilic, 570
Esophagogastroduodenoscopy, 590
Esophagography
  barium. See Barium esophagography
  in esophageal atresia, 536–537, 538f
  in vascular ring, 1790, 1790f
Esophagoscopy, 61–62, 550–552
  flexible, 62
    complications of, 62
    technique of, 62
  indications for, 61–62, 62b
  pre-procedure, 62
  rigid, 62
Esophagus
  abdominal, 517f–519f, 518–519, 549, 549f
    lymphatic drainage of, 520, 520f
  abdominal herniation in, 551f, 556–557, 559f–561f
  acid injury to, 571–572
  adventitia of, 548
  alkali injury to, 571–572
  anatomy of, 20–23, 517–520, 517f–518f, 547–549, 547f–549f
  atresia of. See Esophageal atresia
  Barrett's. See Barrett's esophagus
  benign tumors of, 565–568, 566b
    mucosal, 566, 566b, 567f
    muscularis propria, 566b, 568, 568f
    submucosal, 566–568, 566b
  biopsy of, 61
  blood supply of, 21–23, 519–520, 519f
  blood supply to, 548
  cancer of. See Esophageal cancer
  cervical, 517f–518f, 518, 549, 549f
    lymphatic drainage of, 520, 520f
  congenital stenosis of, 544
  constrictions of, 21
  corrosive injury to, 571–572
    esophagoscopy for, 62
  cysts of, 565–568, 566b, 569f
  diffuse spasm of, 563
  diverticula of, 563–565
    epiphrenic, 565, 566f
    midthoracic, 551f, 565
    Zenker's. See Zenker's diverticulum
  duplication of, 543–544
  echogenic layers of, 63
  embryology of, 517–520, 535
  endoscopy of. See Esophagoscopy
  evaluation of, 550–556
    barium esophagography in, 550, 551f–553f

Esophagus (Continued)
  Bilitec 2000 fiberoptic spectrophotometer in, 556
  biopsy in, 61
  endoscopic ultrasound in, 555–556, 557f
  esophagoscopy in, 550–552
  impedance-manometry in, 556, 558f
  manometry in. See Esophageal manometry
  pH monitoring in, 552–555, 555f–556f, 555t
fibroma of, 567
fibrovascular polyps of, 566, 567f
foreign body in, 571–573
function of, 525–532, 549–550
  ambulatory 24-hour pH monitoring of, 529–532, 531f, 531t
  endoscopic evaluation of, 526, 526f
  manometric evaluation of, 527–528, 527f
    24-hour, 532
    body motility on, 528, 528f–530f
    high-resolution, 528–529
    lower sphincter on, 527, 527f
    upper sphincter on, 528, 530f
  radiographic evaluation of, 525–526
granular cell tumor of, 567–568, 567f
hemangioma of, 568
hypomotility disorders of, 563
ineffective motility of, 563
innervation of, 520, 520f, 549
leiomyoma of, 568, 568f
leiomyosarcoma of, 568
lipoma of, 566
lymphatics of, 519–520, 520f, 547f, 548
mucosa of, 21
muscularis propria of, 547f, 548
necrosis of, 98
neurofibroma of, 567
notch indentation of, 21
nutcracker, 563, 564f
perforation of, 572, 572f
  laser therapy–related, 74–75
  mediastinal infection with, 648
  photodynamic therapy–related, 71
peristalsis of, 521–522, 522f
pH of
  ambulatory monitoring of, 529–532, 531f, 531t, 552–553, 555t
  wireless monitoring of, 553, 555f
physiology of, 520–525, 521f–522f
resection of. See Esophagectomy
Schatzki's ring of, 552f, 570
scleroderma of, 563, 570
sphincters of. See Esophageal sphincter
squamous papilloma of, 566
stenting of, 71–74
  in benign stricture, 73
  in malignant stricture, 73–74
  metal stent for, 71–72, 72t
  silicone-based stent for, 71–72, 72t
  technique for, 71–72
stricture of. See Esophageal stricture
submucosa of, 547, 547f
in systemic disease, 550, 550b
thoracic, 517f, 518, 549, 549f
  lymphatic drainage of, 520, 520f
trauma to
  blunt, 97–98
  esophagoscopy for, 61–62
  penetrating, 105–107
venous drainage of, 519, 519f, 548–549
wall of, 547–549, 547f–548f
Zenker's diverticulum of. See Zenker's diverticulum
Esophyx device, in gastroesophageal reflux, 79
Estrogen, cardiovascular disease and, 910t, 913
Ethacrynic acid, 887, 887t
Ethanol septal ablation, in hypertrophic cardiomyopathy, 860
Etomidate, in congenital heart disease, 1754
Everolimus, 1545
Exercise
  in atherosclerosis management, 915
  after atrial septal defect closure, 1809
  cardiac output and, 725–726, 726f
  end-diastolic volume with, 725–726, 726f
  end-systolic volume with, 725–726, 726f
  heart rate with, 725–726, 726f

Exercise (Continued)
  left ventricular volume with, 725–726, 726f
  in pectus excavatum, 363
  postoperative, 53
  stroke volume with, 725–726, 726f
  after sympathicotomy, 666
  after transmyocardial laser therapy, 1460
Exercise testing. See Stress testing
External oblique muscle, 6, 7f, 8t
Extracellular matrix, ventricular, 739–740, 740f
Extracorporeal life support, in acute pulmonary embolism, 1619
Extracorporeal membrane oxygenation (ECMO), 1510–1512, 1511f
  anticoagulation for, 1283, 1287–1288
  in coarctation of aorta, 1785
  in congenital diaphragmatic hernia, 502, 504
  in hypoplastic left heart syndrome, 2031
  after lung transplantation, 220
  pediatric, 1735–1742
    applications of, 1735–1736, 1736f, 1736t
    cannula for, 1739–1741, 1740t
    circuit for, 1736, 1739–1741, 1740t–1741t
    after heart transplantation, 1738
    before heart transplantation, 1738
    after in-hospital cardiac arrest, 1738–1739, 1739t
    indications for, 1736–1739, 1737t
    in myocarditis, 1738
    outcomes of, 1735–1736, 1736f, 1736t
      longer-term, 1745–1746
    postcardiotomy, 1737
    postoperative, 1737
    preoperative, 1737
    in respiratory insufficiency, 1736
    weaning from, 1741–1742
  in pulmonary aplasia, 140
  vascular complications of, 1287–1288
Extubation, after pediatric cardiac surgery, 1761–1762, 1761b
Ezetimibe
  in aortic stenosis, 1197
  in atherosclerosis, 914

F

Factor VII, 949
Factor VIIa, 769–770, 769f, 770b
Factor Xa inhibitors, 1284
Factor XI, in cardiopulmonary bypass, 963, 963f
Factor XII, in cardiopulmonary bypass, 963, 963f
Failure to thrive, 1751b, 1752
Fallen lung sign of Kumpe, 99
Familial apoB defect, 907
Felodipine, 890
Femoral artery
  angiography of, 1164, 1164f
  for pediatric cardiac catheterization, 1693
  for percutaneous coronary interventions, 848
  superficial
    atherectomy of, 1169
    cryotherapy for, 1169
    laser therapy for, 1169
    paclitaxel-coated balloon therapy for, 1169
    stenting of, 1168–1169
Femoral vein
  for pediatric cardiac catheterization, 1693
  for temporary pacemaker insertion, 1307b
Fentanyl, in congenital heart disease, 1754, 1757
Fetus
  cystic adenomatoid malformation in, 143
  echocardiography in, 1671–1672
    in arrhythmia, 1672
    clinical implications of, 1672
    in congenital heart disease, 1672
    in Ebstein's anomaly, 2056
    indications for, 1671, 1671b
    technique of, 1671, 1672f
  warfarin effects on, 1959
Fever, after cardiac surgery, 950
Fiberoptic infrared endoscopy, 2100
Fibrates, 914
Fibric acid derivatives, 914
Fibrillin-1, 1025

Index

Fibrinogen
  in cardiac surgery, 769, 769f
  prosthetic surface deposition of, 1279
Fibrinolysis
  in cardiopulmonary bypass, 963, 1287
  in pediatric cardiopulmonary bypass, 1724
Fibrinolytic therapy
  in prosthetic heart valve anticoagulation, 1280, 1283
  in ST-segment elevation myocardial infarction, 878–879, 878t
Fibroelastoma, papillary, 1637
Fibroma
  cardiac, 1634t, 1636
  esophageal, 567
  myocardial, 798f
Fibrosing mediastinitis, 186, 187f, 648
Fibrosis
  coronary artery, 1476
  interstitial, in hypertrophic cardiomyopathy, 1496
Fibrous histiocytoma
  cardiac, 1635t
  chest wall, 385
  endobronchial, 154–155
Fibrous tumor
  intrapulmonary, 154, 154f
  pleural
    benign, 454–455
    calcifying, 455
    malignant, 456–457
Fibrovascular polyps, of esophagus, 566, 567f
Fick's law, 958
Finite-element model, of ventricle, 749–752, 750f–752f
Firearm injury, 98, 1175–1178. See also Cardiac injury, penetrating; Trauma, penetrating
Fish, dietary, 910t, 913
Fistula
  arteriovenous, traumatic, 108
  bronchial, postoperative, 55
  bronchobiliary, 135–136, 136f
  bronchopleural, 414–415
    bronchoscopy in, 64
    after chest wall resection/reconstruction, 306
    post-traumatic, 108
    postoperative, 55, 423
      clinical presentation of, 423
      diagnosis of, 423
      management of, 423
  bronchovascular, 55
  coronary artery, 1470–1471
    anatomy of, 1975
    clinical presentation of, 1975
    diagnosis of, 1975–1976
    natural history of, 1975
    pathophysiology of, 1975
    surgical management of, 1976–1978
      indications for, 1976
      results of, 1978
      technique of, 1976–1977, 1976f–1978f
  gastropericardial, 482–483, 483f
  tracheobronchial-esophageal, 135
  tracheoesophageal, 114f–115f, 115
    clinical presentation of, 117
    repair of, 121–123, 123f–124f, 125
  tracheoinnominate, 114f
    clinical presentation of, 117
    repair of, 121–123
Flail chest, 90–91, 91f
Flaps
  Eloesser, in empyema, 414, 414f, 420, 421f–422f
  latissimus dorsi, in chest wall reconstruction, 383–384, 385f
  myocutaneous, in chest wall reconstruction, 383–384, 385f
  omental, in sternal wound infection, 1000–1001
  pectoralis major
    in chest wall reconstruction, 383, 385f
    in sternal wound infection, 1001
  rectus abdominis
    in chest wall reconstruction, 384
    in sternal wound infection, 1001
  serratus anterior, in chest wall reconstruction, 385, 385f
  in sternal wound infection, 1000–1001
Fleischner line, in acute pulmonary embolism, 1616
Flow cytometry, in pleural effusion, 433

Fluid therapy
  in congenital diaphragmatic hernia, 504
  intraoperative, 50
  after lung transplantation, 218
  after pediatric cardiac surgery, 1759
  postoperative, 51
Fluorescence bronchoscopy, 235, 247–248
Fluoroscopy
  in aortic regurgitation, 1200
  intraoperative, 2100
Fondaparinux, 759, 1284
  contraindication to, 1284
  in NSTE acute coronary syndromes, 875
Fontan procedure. See also Single ventricle, Fontan procedure in
  in adult, 2078–2080, 2079f
  atrioventricular valve insufficiency and, 2046
  in biventricular hearts, 2048
  catheterization before, 1692
  extubation after, 1761–1762
  in hypoplastic left heart syndrome, 2035, 2036f
  intra-atrial reentrant tachycardia after, 2088–2091, 2090t
  in pulmonary atresia with intact ventricular septum, 1871, 1871f
Foramen ovale, patent. See Patent foramen ovale
Forced expiratory volume in 1 second (FEV_1)
  after lung transplantation, 224, 224t
  postoperative, 42, 42t
  preoperative, 41–42
Foregut duplication cysts, 543–544, 568, 569f, 656
Foreign body
  airway, 65
  cardiac, 102
  esophageal, 571–573
    after atresia repair, 542
  pulmonary, 161, 161t
Fosinopril, 891t
Fracture(s)
  clavicular, 91
  rib, 90
  scapular, 92
  sternal, 91
Frank-Starling curve/relationship, 734–737, 736f–737f, 746, 747f
  in acute heart failure, 885, 886f
Fresh-frozen plasma
  in anticoagulant reversal, 770
  transfusion of, 762–763, 762b
Functional capacity, preoperative assessment of, 43–44
Fundoplication
  dysphagia after, 52
  endoscopic, in gastroesophageal reflux, 79–80
  gas-bloat syndrome after, 57
  gastropericardial fistula and, 482–483, 483f
  in hiatal hernia, 482
  Nissen, 482–483
Fungal infection. See also specific infections
  aortic arch, 1042–1043
  after heart-lung transplantation, 1566
  after heart transplantation, 1550
  after lung transplantation, 219, 221–222, 222f
  mediastinal, 647–648
  in prosthetic valve endocarditis, 1268
  pulmonary, 185–191
    diagnosis of, 185–186
  thoracic aorta, 1065f
  thoracoabdominal aorta, 1064–1065
Furosemide
  in heart failure, 887–888, 887t
  after pediatric cardiac surgery, 1759

G

Ganglia
  cervical, 23
  thoracic, 23–24
Ganglioneuroblastoma, 651–652, 653f, 654
Ganglioneuroma, 651–652
Gas, diffusion of, 958
Gas-bloat syndrome, 57
Gastric artery, 519, 519f
Gastric emptying, after esophagectomy, 612

Gastric ulcers, prevention of, 48–49
Gastritis, prevention of, 48–49
Gastroenteric cyst, 656
Gastroepiploic artery conduit, 1372–1374, 1376, 1376f, 1386t, 1387, 1413t, 1416–1417, 1426–1427
  contraindications to, 1372–1374
  grafting strategy for, 1417, 1417f
  harvesting of, 1416–1417
  patency of, 1375f, 1386–1387
Gastroesophageal junction
  anatomy of, 20–21
  biopolymer injection at, 79
  endoscopic plication of, 79–80
  radiofrequency therapy to, 78–79
Gastroesophageal reflux. See also Gastroesophageal reflux disease (GERD)
  congenital diaphragmatic hernia and, 505
  after esophageal atresia treatment, 542
  postoperative, 57
Gastroesophageal reflux disease (GERD), 78–80, 558–561
  24-hour esophageal bile probe in, 532
  aerophagia in, 524–525
  ambulatory 24-hour esophageal manometry in, 532
  ambulatory 24-hour pH monitoring in, 529–532, 531f, 531t
  biopolymer injection in, 79
  body mass index in, 560–561
  causes of, 524–525
  complicated, 558–559
  defective lower esophageal sphincter in, 524–525, 524f
  definition of, 78
  EndoCinch device in, 80
  endoscopic plication in, 79–80
  esophagoscopy in, 61
  Esophyx device in, 79
  hiatal hernia and, 524–526, 557–558
  impedance-pH monitoring in, 553–555, 556f
  NDO plicator in, 80
  overeating and, 524–525
  progression of, 524f
  proton pump inhibitors in, 558
  radiofrequency therapy in, 78–79
  surgical management of, 558–560
Gastroesophageal valve, 526, 526f
Gastrointestinal bleeding, esophagoscopy in, 61
Gastrointestinal tract
  obstruction of, congenital diaphragmatic hernia and, 495, 504–506
  post-transplant disorders of, 225, 226f
Gastroparesis, after heart-lung transplantation, 1568
Gastropericardial fistula, fundoplication herniation and, 482–483, 483f
Gastrostomy tube, 51
GATA-4, 1647
Gefitinib, 678–679
Gelfoam, 770–771
Gene therapy
  in congenital diaphragmatic hernia, 507
  in mesothelioma, 467
Genitourinary examination, after cardiac surgery, 934
GERD. See Gastroesophageal reflux disease (GERD)
Germ cell tumor
  mediastinal, 639
  pulmonary metastases in, 346
Giant cell aortitis, 1027, 1044
Giant lymph node hyperplasia, 647, 656–657, 657f
Gibbon, John H., Jr., 957, 958f
Gladiolus, 5
Glenn procedure
  bidirectional, in hypoplastic left heart syndrome, 2034
  catheterization before, 1692
  extubation after, 1761
  in single ventricle, 2044
Glomerular filtration, after cardiopulmonary bypass, 971
Glucocorticoids, in interstitial lung disease, 170
Glucose
  blood
    intraoperative, 922
    in pediatric cardiopulmonary bypass, 1720–1721
    sternal wound infection and, 1000
  myocardial utilization of, 819
  pleural fluid, 433
  postoperative control of, 1017
GLUT1, in pleural effusion, 435t

Glycerol trinitrate, in pediatric pulmonary hypertension, 1752
Glycoprotein IIb/IIIa antagonists, 760
  bleeding with, 1284
  in NSTE acute coronary syndromes, 875–877
Glycopyrrolate, in hyperhidrosis, 663
Goodpasture's syndrome, 165
Gore TAG device, 1130, 1131f, 1134
GOSE score, in Ebstein's anomaly, 2057, 2057t
Granular cell tumor
  esophageal, 567–568, 567f
  pulmonary, 155
Granuloma(s), 159–164
  eosinophilic, 163–164
  foreign body, 161
  hypersensitivity, 161, 161t
  infectious, 154, 161, 162f
  inorganic dust, 161
  pathogenesis of, 159–161, 160f
  sarcoid, 162–163
  vasculitic, 163, 163f
Granulomatosis
  infectious, 154
  Wegener's, 163, 163f
Great arteries. See also Aorta; Pulmonary artery
  anatomically corrected malposition of, 1652f, 1662–1663
  rings of. See Vascular rings
  transposition of. See Transposition of great arteries
Greenfield filter, in acute pulmonary embolism, 1619
Growth factors
  in mesothelioma, 451–453
  in myocardial cell-based regenerative therapy, 1607–1608
Growth hormone, after cardiopulmonary bypass, 969
GuardWire, 1167, 1167f
Gunshot injury, 98, 1175–1178. See also Cardiac injury, penetrating; Trauma, penetrating

H

Hamartoma, 152–154
  cardiac, 1634t
  computed tomography of, 152f–153f
  gross examination of, 152–153, 153f
  malignant transformation of, 154
  radiography of, 153, 153f
Hancock porcine bioprosthesis, 1189
HAND1, 1644
HAND2, 1644
Hand-Schüller-Christian disease, 164
Head and neck cancer, pulmonary metastases in, 346
Health Insurance Portability and Accountability Act, 2113
Hearing loss, congenital diaphragmatic hernia and, 505
Heart. See also at Atrium (atria); Cardiac; Myocardium; Ventricle(s)
  anatomy of, 697, 1651. See also Atrium (atria); Ventricle(s)
    alignment, 1654–1661, 1660f
    atrioventricular alignment, 1652f, 1654–1661
    central fibrous body, 701, 701f–702f
    chiral, 1653–1654, 1658f–1659f
    crisscross, 1658f–1659f, 1661
    infundibuloarterial inversion, 1662
    inverted, 1661–1662
    isomeric, 1651
    left atrial, 702–703, 702f, 1655f
    left atrial appendage, 697, 698f
    left ventricle, 705–706, 705f, 1651–1653, 1652f, 1657f
    morphologic, 1651–1653, 1652f, 1654f–1657f
    right atrial, 699–701, 700f–701f, 1654f
    right atrial appendage, 697, 698f, 699–700
    right ventricle, 703–704, 703f–704f, 1651–1654, 1652f, 1656f, 1658f–1659f
    situs ambiguus, 1651
    situs inversus, 1651
    situs solitus, 1651, 1661
    superoinferior ventricle, 1661
    surface, 697–699, 697f–699f
    surgical relevance of, 1661–1663
    terminal groove (sulcus terminalis), 698–700, 699f
    ventricular mass, 697–698, 699f
    ventriculoarterial alignment, 1652f, 1660
    Waterston's groove, 698–699, 699f

Heart (Continued)
  angiosarcoma of, 1635t, 1637, 1637f
  artificial. See Artificial heart
  cell-based regenerative therapy for. See Regenerative cell-based therapy
  conduction system of, 1850, 1850f
  embryology of, 1641
    abnormalities of. See also specific congenital abnormalities
      etiology of, 1648
      laterality, 1642–1643
      outflow tract, 1648
      septal, 1646–1647
    anterior heart field in, 1647
    anterior heart–forming field in, 1641, 1647
    chamber specification in, 1643–1644
    mesoderm precursors in, 1641–1642, 1642f
    neural crest in, 1641, 1645–1648, 1646f
    outflow tract development in, 1647–1648
    retinoic acid in, 1648
    rightward looping in, 1642–1643, 1642f–1643f
    septation in, 1644–1647, 1645f–1646f
  fibroma of, 798f, 1634t
  foreign body in, 102
  hemangioma of, 1634t, 1637
  imaging of, 748–749, 789. See also Computed tomography (CT), cardiovascular; Echocardiography; Magnetic resonance imaging (MRI), cardiovascular; Single-photon emission computed tomography (SPECT), cardiac
  infection of. See Endocarditis
  injury to. See Cardiac injury
  lipoma of, 1634t–1635t, 1636–1637
  lipomatous hypertrophy of, 796, 798f, 1637
  metastatic tumors of, 1636t, 1637–1638
  myxoma of, 1633–1635, 1636f
  papillary fibroelastoma of, 1637
  in pectus excavatum, 362
  preoperative assessment of, 42–43, 43f, 47
  regeneration of. See Regenerative cell-based therapy
  rhabdomyoma of, 1634t, 1635, 1637f
  rupture of, 1175
  shunt of. See Shunt, cardiac
  thrombus of, 796
  transplantation of. See Heart-lung transplantation; Heart transplantation
  trauma to. See Cardiac injury
  tumors of, 1633
    benign, 1633–1637, 1634t, 1636f–1637f
    in children, 1682, 1684f
    echocardiography in, 835–836
    imaging of, 796, 798f
    malignant, 1635t, 1637, 1637f
    metastatic, 1636t, 1637–1638
  valves of. See Aortic valve; Mitral valve; Prosthetic heart valves; Pulmonary valve; Tricuspid valve
Heart block, bifascicular, pacemaker in, 1309b. See also Pacemaker, permanent
Heart failure, 883
  acute, 884–885
    compensatory mechanisms in, 885, 885t
    Frank-Starling curve in, 885, 886f
    hypertension and, 900
    preload in, 885, 886f
  backward, 884
  chronic, 885–886
    left ventricular assist device in, 1508–1509, 1520
    myocyte reduction in, 886
    perioperative, 900–901
    pharmacologic treatment of, 896–897, 897t
    renal dysfunction in, 886
    ventricular remodeling in, 885–886, 886t
  classification of, 884, 884t
  coronary artery bypass grafting and, 1372, 1593–1594
  decompensation in, 896, 896t, 898–899, 898f, 898t–899t
  diastolic, 883, 899–900
  echocardiography in, 836
  end-stage, 1533. See also Heart transplantation
  epidemiology of, 883
  evaluation of, 896, 896t
  flash pulmonary edema in, 900, 900t
  forward, 884
  high-output, 884
  in interrupted aortic arch, 1929
  intra-aortic balloon pump counterpulsation in, 1537–1538

Heart failure (Continued)
  left-sided, 883
  lifestyle modifications in, 896
  low-output, 884
  magnetic resonance imaging in, 1580–1581, 1580f–1581f
  mechanical assist devices in, 1537–1538
  mediastinal adenopathy in, 647
  mitral regurgitation and, 1216, 1229, 1230f, 1434
  mitral valve repair in, 1583–1584, 1585f–1587f, 1586t, 1594–1595
  mortality in, 1573, 1574t
  pacemaker in, 1307–1309, 1313f
  pathophysiology of, 883–886, 884t, 1573–1578
    left ventricular geometric abnormalities in, 1574–1575, 1575f, 1575t
    left ventricular remodeling in, 1573–1574, 1574b
  perioperative, 900–901
  pharmacologic treatment of, 886–895, 887t
    β-adrenergic antagonists in, 891t, 892–893, 892f
    aldosterone inhibitors in, 887t
    angiotensin-converting enzyme inhibitors in, 890–892, 890f, 891t
    angiotensin receptor blocking agents in, 891t, 892
    calcium channel blocking agents in, 890, 891t
    digoxin in, 893, 893t
    diuretics in, 887–888, 887t
    dobutamine in, 894
    dopamine in, 893–894
    before heart transplantation, 1537
    vs. heart transplantation, 1535
    hydralazine in, 889–890
    inotropic agents in, 891t, 893–895
    natriuretic peptides in, 895
    nitrovasodilators in, 888–889, 889f, 891t
    phosphodiesterase inhibitors in, 894–895, 895f
    vasodilators in, 888–890
  regenerative cell-based therapy in, 1610
  right-sided
    in acute pulmonary embolism, 1616
    after cardiac surgery, 943
    after heart transplantation, 1544–1545
    after left ventricular assist device implantation, 1509, 1522
  surgical ventricular restoration in, 1573
    anterior, 1582–1583, 1582f–1585f, 1583b
    asynergic area evaluation for, 1579–1581, 1580f
    diastolic function after, 1587–1588, 1591f
    in ischemic cardiomyopathy, 1582–1585, 1582f–1585f, 1583b
    left ventricular dyssynchrony and, 1588–1591, 1592f
    mitral valve repair during, 1583–1584, 1585f–1587f, 1586t, 1594–1595
    in nonischemic cardiomyopathy, 1578–1579, 1579f
    outcomes of, 1586–1595, 1589t, 1590f
    patient selection for, 1578–1581, 1580b
    posterior, 1584–1585, 1587f–1588f
    rationale for, 1575–1576, 1576f
    remote region evaluation for, 1581
    ventricular arrhythmias and, 1591–1593, 1593f
  systolic, 883, 898–899, 898f, 898t–899t
    pacemaker in, 1311b. See also Pacemaker, permanent
  in transposition of great arteries, 1983
  tricuspid regurgitation and, 1245
  tricuspid valve disease and, 1248
Heart Failure Survival Score index, 1535
Heart-lung transplantation, 1555. See also Heart transplantation
  abdominal complications after, 1568
  airway complications after, 1568
  cardiopulmonary physiology after, 1568
  complications of, 1565–1568, 1565f
  donor operative technique in, 1560–1562, 1561f
  donor-recipient matching in, 1557–1558
  donor selection in, 1559–1560, 1559b
  historical perspective on, 1555, 1555f
  indications for, 1555–1558, 1556f
  infection after, 1566
  lymphoproliferative disorder after, 1568
  organ preservation in, 1560
  percent reactive antibody titer in, 1558
  in pulmonary atresia with ventricular septal defect, 1902

Heart-lung transplantation (Continued)
  recipient diagnosis in, 1555–1557, 1556f
  recipient management in
    immunosuppression in, 1564–1565, 1564t, 1568
    intensive care unit for, 1564
    operative, 1562–1564, 1563f
    postoperative, 1564–1565, 1564t
    preoperative, 1558–1559, 1558b
  recipient selection for, 1557–1558
  rejection of
    acute, 1565–1566, 1565f
    bronchiolitis obliterans and, 1566–1567
    chronic, 1566–1567, 1567f
    graft coronary artery disease and, 1567
  results of, 1568–1569, 1568f–1569f
Heart murmur
  in aortic regurgitation, 1200
  in aortic stenosis, 1197
  in atrial septal defect, 1802
  in atrioventricular canal defects, 1836
  in congenital aortic stenosis, 1944
  in coronary artery fistula, 1975
  in Ebstein's anomaly, 2058
  in hypertrophic cardiomyopathy, 1497
  in pectus excavatum, 361
  in tetralogy of Fallot, 1882
  in truncus arteriosus, 1914
Heart rate
  autonomic nervous system effects on, 746–747
  after cardiac surgery, 940, 940f–941f
  exercise-related, 725–726, 726f
  force frequency relationship and, 746
  after sympathicotomy, 666
Heart transplantation, 1533
  anticoagulation in, 1531
  bridge to. See Artificial heart
  cardiac allograft vasculopathy after, 1550–1551
  complications of, 1546–1551
  contraindications to, 1535–1536, 1536b
  coronary artery disease after, 1476
  cytolytic induction therapy in, 1546
  cytomegalovirus infection after, 1549–1550, 1550t
  domino, 1556–1557
  donor management in, 1538–1539
  donor operative technique in, 1539–1540
  donor-recipient matching in, 1539
  donor selection in, 1538, 1538b
  dysrhythmias after, 1544
  in Ebstein's anomaly, 2058, 2066
  echocardiography in, 837
  evaluation for, 1534–1538, 1542f
    percent reactive antibody titer in, 1536–1537
  after Fontan procedure, 2050
  fungal infection after, 1550
  hemorrhage after, 1544–1545
  historical perspective on, 1533–1534
  in hypoplastic left heart syndrome, 2036
  immunosuppressive therapy in, 1536–1537, 1537b, 1545–1546, 1545b
  indications for, 1534–1538
  infection after, 1549–1550
  intravenous immune globulin in, 1536–1537, 1537b
  neoplasia after, 1551
  organ allocation in, 1539, 1539t
  organ preservation in, 1540
  pacemaker after, 1310b. See also Pacemaker, permanent
  pediatric
    extracorporeal membrane oxygenation after, 1738
    extracorporeal membrane oxygenation before, 1738
    in pulmonary atresia with intact ventricular septum, 1874–1875
  plasmapheresis in, 1536–1537, 1537b
  protozoal infection after, 1550
  recipient age limit for, 1536
  recipient management in
    postoperative, 1544–1546
    preoperative, 1537–1538
  recipient operative technique in, 1540–1543
    heterotopic, 1543, 1544f
    orthotopic bicaval, 1541, 1543f
    orthotopic standard, 1541, 1542f
    orthotopic total, 1541–1543
  recipient selection for, 1534–1536, 1535t

Heart transplantation (Continued)
  rejection of
    acute, 1547–1549, 1548t, 1549f
    antibody-mediated, 1546–1547, 1547b, 1548f
    hyperacute, 1546
  results of, 1551, 1551f
  retransplant, 1535, 1535t
  in single ventricle, 2050
  tricuspid valve disease after, 1248
  in ventricular arrhythmias, 1361
HeartWare device, 1518, 1519f
Heimlich valve, 55
Heller myotomy, 553f, 562–563
Hemangioendothelioma, epithelioid
  cardiac, 1634t
  pulmonary, 332
Hemangioma
  cardiac, 1634t, 1637
  esophageal, 568
Hematocrit
  in cardiopulmonary bypass, 959–960
  in pediatric cardiopulmonary bypass, 1717–1718
Hematoma, intramural
  of thoracic aorta, 793, 1139–1140
  in type A aortic dissection, 1090–1091, 1095, 1095f, 1100–1101
  in type B aortic dissection, 1090–1091, 1115–1117, 1120
Hemi-Fontan operation
  in hypoplastic left heart syndrome, 2034–2035, 2035f
  in single ventricle, 2044
Hemisternum, right, in off-pump coronary artery bypass grafting, 1401–1402, 1402f
Hemodialysis, after pediatric cardiac surgery, 1759
Hemodilution
  normovolemic, 764
  in pediatric cardiopulmonary bypass, 1717–1718
Hemodynamics. See Cardiac catheterization, hemodynamics on
Hemolysis, after aortic valve replacement, 1204
Hemopericardium, 1486
Hemoptysis, 65
Hemorrhage
  after heart transplantation, 1544–1545
  pulmonary, idiopathic, vs. Goodpasture's syndrome, 165
  thoracic, trauma-related, thoracotomy in, 100
Hemostasis, 757–758, 758f
  inhibition of. See Anticoagulation
Hemothorax
  after Pancoast tumor treatment, 318–319
  vs. post-traumatic empyema, 415
Hensen's node, 1642
Heparin, 758
  in acute pulmonary embolism, 1617–1618, 1617f
  bleeding with, 1283–1284
  in cardiopulmonary bypass, 922–923, 946, 965–967, 966f, 968f, 1287
  low-molecular-weight, 758–759
    in NSTE acute coronary syndromes, 874–875, 875t, 876f
  in NSTE acute coronary syndromes, 874–875, 875t, 876f
  in pediatric cardiopulmonary bypass, 1718–1719
  postoperative, 52
  preoperative, 919
  in prosthetic heart valve anticoagulation, 1280, 1284
  protamine reversal of, 758, 759f. See also Protamine
  resistance to, 923
  thrombocytopenia with, 759–760
Heparin-coated circuit, in cardiopulmonary bypass, 968–969
Heparin rebound, 923, 966–967
Hereditary hemorrhagic telangiectasia, 145
Hernia
  diaphragmatic
    congenital. See Congenital diaphragmatic hernia
  hiatal. See Hiatal hernia
  pericardial, 491t, 508f, 509
Heterotaxy syndrome, 1642–1643
  total anomalous pulmonary venous drainage in, 1826–1827
Hiatal hernia, 5, 508f, 509, 556–557
  barium examination in, 655
  esophagography in, 551f

Hiatal hernia (Continued)
  gastroesophageal reflux disease and, 524–526, 557–558
  repair of, 482
    esophageal length and, 482–483
  type I, 481, 556–557, 559f
  type II, 481, 556–557, 559f
  type III, 481–482, 556–557, 560f–561f
  type IV, 482, 556–557
High-frequency oscillatory ventilation, in congenital diaphragmatic hernia, 501
High-molecular-weight kininogen, in cardiopulmonary bypass, 963, 963f
Hirudin, in cardiopulmonary bypass, 966
Histamine-2 receptor blockers
  postoperative, 52
  preoperative, 48–49
Histiocytoma, fibrous
  cardiac, 1634t
  chest wall, 385
  endobronchial, 154–155
Histiocytosis X, 164
Histoplasmoma, 186
Histoplasmosis, 185–186, 187f
  diagnosis of, 185–186
  mediastinal, 647–648
  treatment of, 186
HLA antigens
  in heart-lung transplantation, 1558
  in heart transplantation, 1537, 1537b
Hoarseness, with aortic arch aneurysm, 1046
Holt-Oram syndrome, 1647, 1801
Holter electrocardiography, in thoracic aortic aneurysm, 1068
Hormones
  in cardiac contractility, 747
  after cardiopulmonary bypass, 969–970
Horner's syndrome
  dorsal sympathectomy and, 403
  after Pancoast tumor treatment, 318
  after sympathicotomy, 665
Horseshoe lung, 138
Hospital Consumer Assessment of Healthcare Provider Survey, 1019
Hughes-Stovin syndrome, 145
β-Human chorionic gonadotropin, in anterior mediastinal mass, 637, 639
Hybrid minimally invasive coronary artery bypass grafting, 1406
Hybrid procedures, 2099
  echocardiography for, 2099–2100, 2100f
  fiberoptic infrared endoscopy for, 2100
  multimodality imaging for, 2100–2101, 2101f
  for pulmonary artery stenting, 2103
  for single-ventricle palliation, 2101–2102, 2102t
  surgical simulation and, 2103
  for ventricular septal defect, 2102, 2102f
  video-assisted cardioscopy for, 2100
  X-ray fluoroscopy for, 2100
Hydralazine
  for afterload reduction, 940
  in heart failure, 889–890, 891t, 897t
Hydrochlorothiazide, 887t, 888
Hydrocortisone, after pediatric cardiac surgery, 1758
Hydropneumothorax, thoracentesis-related, 436
20-Hydroxyeicosatetraenoic acid (20-HETE), 718, 719f
5-Hydroxyindoleacetic acid, urinary, 326
Hyperabduction test, 393, 395f
Hyperbaric oxygen therapy, in wound healing, 53
Hyperglycemia
  intraoperative, 922
  postoperative, 1017
Hyperhidrosis, 661
  clinical presentation of, 661–662, 661f
  definition of, 662
  epidemiology of, 662
  family history of, 662
  nerve clipping procedure in, 666
  nonoperative treatment of, 663
  pathophysiology of, 662, 663f
  surgical treatment of, 663–665, 664f–665f
    cardiopulmonary complications of, 666
    compensatory sweating after, 665–666
    complications of, 665–666
    historical perspective on, 661
  sympathectomy in, 661, 663
  treatment of, 663–665

Hyperlipidemia, 720–721, 721f, 907. *See also* Atherosclerosis
Hyperlucent lung syndrome, 144
Hypersensitive carotid sinus syndrome, pacemaker in, 1310b. *See also* Pacemaker, permanent
Hypersensitivity pneumonitis, 161, 161t
Hypertension. *See also* Vascular tone
 acute heart failure and, 900
 aortic dissection and, 1092
 in atherosclerosis management, 914–915
 autoregulation in, 716
 pulmonary. *See* Pulmonary hypertension
Hyperthermic chemoperfusion, in non–small cell lung cancer, 690–691
Hypertrophic cardiomyopathy. *See* Cardiomyopathy, hypertrophic
Hypertrophic obstructive cardiomyopathy, congenital, 1951–1952
Hypoplastic left heart syndrome, 2025
 aortic atresia and mitral stenosis subtype of, 2028–2030, 2030f
 cardiac catheterization in, 2026
 clinical presentation of, 2025
 definition of, 2025
 diagnosis of, 2025–2026
 epidemiology of, 2025
 etiology of, 2026
 inspired carbon dioxide in, 2027
 inspired oxygen in, 2027
 pathophysiology of, 2026, 2026f
 prenatal diagnosis of, 2026
 prenatal intervention for, 2037–2038, 2037f
  aortic stenosis and, 1701–1702, 1702t–1703t
  intact/highly restrictive atrial septum and, 1702–1704, 1703f
 pulmonary vascular resistance in, 2027
 surgical management of, 2027
  fetal, 1701–1704, 1702t–1703t, 1703f, 2037–2038, 2037f
  Fontan operation in, 2035, 2036f
  hybrid procedure in, 2036–2037, 2101–2102, 2102t
  neurodevelopmental outcomes after, 2036
  stage I (Norwood operation), 1762, 2028–2033
   age and, 2030
   in anatomic subtypes, 2028–2033, 2030f–2033f, 2031b
   coronary circulation and, 2031–2032
   extracorporeal membrane oxygenation after, 2031
   interstage death after, 2030, 2033
   low birth weight and, 2030
   modifications of, 2031–2033, 2034f
   neo-aortic arch obstruction after, 2032, 2034f
   perfusion management in, 2032–2033, 2034f
   pulmonary blood flow control and, 2031
   recoarctation after, 2032
   results of, 2028–2030, 2029f
   standard, 2028, 2029f
  stage II, 2033–2035
   bidirectional Glenn operation in, 2034
   hemi-Fontan operation in, 2034–2035, 2035f
   results of, 2035
  transplantation in, 2036
 systemic vascular resistance in, 2027–2028
Hypotension
 ACE inhibitor–related, 891–892
 protamine-related, 966–967
Hypothermia. *See also* Deep hypothermic circulatory rest
 in cardiopulmonary bypass, 958–960, 960f–961f
 intraoperative, 50
 for myocardial protection, 978, 978f, 985, 986f
 in pediatric cardiopulmonary bypass, 1721–1722
Hypothyroidism, after pediatric cardiac surgery, 1759
Hypoventilation, diaphragmatic pacing in, 483–484, 484f
Hypoxia, pulmonary artery response to, 722, 722f

I

Ibuprofen
 in idiopathic pericarditis, 1485
 in patent ductus arteriosus, 1782
Idiopathic interstitial pneumonia, 165–168, 165b, 166t
Idiopathic pericarditis, 1485

Idiopathic pulmonary fibrosis, 165–167, 167f
 lung transplantation in, 167, 209, 217f
Idiopathic pulmonary hemorrhage, vs. Goodpasture's syndrome, 165
Idiopathic tracheal stenosis, 115–116
Iliac artery
 angiography of, 1162–1164, 1163f
 pressure gradient in, 1168
 revascularization procedures for, 1168
 stenting of, 1168
 for thoracic aortic endovascular repair, 1133, 1133f
Imaging, 25. *See also* Chest radiography; Computed tomography (CT); Echocardiography; Magnetic resonance imaging (MRI); Radionuclide imaging; Single-photon emission computed tomography (SPECT)
Imatinib, in adenoid cystic carcinoma, 330
Immune globulin, intravenous, in heart transplantation, 1536–1537, 1537b
Immune system
 in alveolitic interstitial lung disease, 164–165, 164f
 in granulomatous interstitial lung disease, 159–161, 160f
 in idiopathic pulmonary fibrosis, 166
Immunohistochemistry, in lung cancer, 673–674, 674f, 676t
Immunosuppression
 in heart-lung transplantation, 1564–1565, 1564t, 1568
 in heart transplantation, 1536–1537, 1537b, 1545–1546, 1545b
 in lung transplantation, 218–219
 in thoracoscopic lobectomy, 284
Immunotherapy, in mesothelioma, 467
Implantable cardioverter-defibrillator, 1309–1312, 1316–1318
 in adult congenital heart disease, 2094, 2095f
 antitachycardia pacing with, 1318, 1318f
 complications of, 1322–1323, 1322b
 contraindications to, 1311–1312
 high-energy defibrillation with, 1317, 1318f
 historical perspective on, 1305–1306, 1306f
 in hypertrophic cardiomyopathy, 1499
 implantation of, 1321–1322, 1321f
  care after, 1322
 indications for, 1309–1311, 1314b–1315b
 leads for, 1317
 low-energy synchronized cardioversion with, 1317
 pediatric, 1315b, 2085, 2086f, 2086b
 preoperative evaluation for, 1319
 pulse generator for, 1316–1317
 during surgery, 1325–1326
 tachyarrhythmias detection by, 1317
Inamrinone, 895
Inappropriate sinus tachycardia, 1357–1358
 superior right atrial isolation for, 1357–1358, 1357f
 results of, 1358
Incisional tachycardia, in adult congenital heart disease, 2088–2091
Indomethacin, in patent ductus arteriosus, 1782
Inducible pluripotent cells, 1600t, 1604
Infant. *See at* Children; Congenital
Infantile pulmonary emphysema, 143
Infantile syndrome, 1470
Infarct exclusion and endocardial patch repair, in postinfarction ventricular septal defect, 1452–1453
Infarctectomy and patch repair
 in anterior postinfarction ventricular septal defect, 1451–1452, 1452f
 in posteroinferior postinfarction ventricular septal defect, 1452, 1453f
Infection
 aortic graft, 1046, 1047f
 after cardiac surgery, 950–952
 catheter-related, 950–951
  prevention of, 1017
 after chest wall resection/reconstruction, 306
 coronary artery, 1475
 endocardial. *See* Endocarditis
 fungal. *See* Fungal infection
 after heart-lung transplantation, 1566
 after heart transplantation, 1549–1550
 after left ventricular assist device implantation, 1509, 1521
 after lung transplantation, 221–222, 221f–222f

Infection (*Continued*)
 mediastinal, 648, 658–659, 659f
 National Surgical Infection Prevention Project on, 1015
 pericardial, 1485
 prevention of, 49
 sternotomy-related. *See* Sternal wound infection
Inferior epigastric artery, in coronary artery bypass grafting, 1376, 1413t, 1417
Inferior vena cava, 829f, 829t
Inferior vena cava hiatus, 4
Inferior vena caval filter, 1619
Inflammation
 in acute coronary syndromes, 867–868
 after cardiac surgery, 935–937, 1007
 with cardiopulmonary bypass, 935–937, 1007, 1726–1727
 in myocardial reperfusion injury, 981
 after thoracoscopic lobectomy, 284
Inflammatory pseudotumor, 155, 155f, 454
Infraspinatus muscle, 8t
Infundibular septum, displacement of, 1877, 1878f. *See also* Tetralogy of Fallot
Injury. *See* Cardiac injury, blunt; Trauma, blunt
Innominate artery, 3–4
 injury to, 104f, 1180–1181, 1180f
 occlusive disease of, 1147–1149
  bypass grafting for, 1148–1149
  endarterectomy for, 1147, 1148f
  endovascular stenting for, 1149–1150, 1150f
Innominate artery compression syndrome, 1789, 1792
Innominate vein injury, 103
Inotropic agents
 after cardiac surgery, 940–941, 941f, 942t
 in heart failure, 891t, 893–895
Inspiration, diaphragm in, 474
Institute of Medicine, on quality and safety, 1014–1015, 1014b
Insulin
 errors with, 1018
 postoperative, 922
Insulin resistance, 908, 908t
Intercostal artery, 9f, 10
Intercostal muscles, 6–10
 anterolateral, 6–7
 anteromedial (transversus thoracis), 6–7
 external, 6
 internal, 6
 subcostal, 6–7
Intercostal nerves, 8–10, 9f
Intercostal vein, 9f, 10
Interferon-β, in malignant pleural effusion, 438–439
Interleukin-1, with pediatric cardiopulmonary bypass, 1727
Interleukin-2
 in malignant pleural effusion, 441
 in mesothelioma, 467
Interleukin-2 receptor antagonists, in heart transplantation, 1546
Interleukin-6, with pediatric cardiopulmonary bypass, 1727
Interleukin-8, with pediatric cardiopulmonary bypass, 1727
Interleukin-10, with pediatric cardiopulmonary bypass, 1727
Intermittent pneumatic compression devices, in pulmonary embolism prophylaxis, 1617
Internal mammary artery, for coronary angiography, 778–779, 779f
Internal thoracic artery
 left, in coronary artery bypass grafting, 1375, 1386t, 1387, 1412–1414, 1413t, 1426–1427
 right, in coronary artery bypass grafting, 1413t, 1414–1415, 1426
International Normalized Ratio, 1280–1281
Interrupted aortic arch. *See* Aortic arch, interrupted
Intersitital fibrosis, in hypertrophic cardiomyopathy, 1496
Interstitial lung disease, 159, 159b. *See also specific diseases*
 alveolitic, 159b, 164–168, 164f, 166t
 clinical presentation of, 159
 evaluation of, 168–170, 168f–169f
 granulomatous, 159–164, 159b, 160f, 166t
 imaging in, 31, 33f, 168–169
 respiratory bronchiolitis–associated, 167–168
 treatment of, 170

Interstitial pneumonitis, 33f, 167
Intervertebral disc herniation, cervical, vs. thoracic outlet syndrome, 396–397
Intra-aortic balloon pump, 861, 1510
　anticoagulation with, 1286
　after cardiac surgery, 941, 942f
　in heart failure, 1537–1538
　pediatric, 1742
　vascular complications of, 1286
Intra-atrial reentrant tachycardia, in adult congenital heart disease, 2088–2091
Intracoronary injection, in myocardial cell-based regenerative therapy, 1605–1606, 1605f, 1605t
Intramural hematoma. See Hematoma, intramural
Intramyocardial injection, in myocardial cell-based regenerative therapy, 1605f, 1605t, 1606
Intratracheal pulmonary ventilation, in congenital diaphragmatic hernia, 501
Intravenous injection, in myocardial cell-based regenerative therapy, 1605, 1605f, 1605t
Intraventricular conduction delay, 1329
Iontophoresis, in hyperhidrosis, 663
Irx4, 1644
Ischemia
　conduit, 57
　mesenteric, 1165
　myocardial. See Myocardial ischemia
　spinal cord
　　with thoracic endovascular aortic repair, 1136
　　with thoracic surgical aortic repair, 1069–1075, 1070f, 1072f, 1074f
Ischemia-reperfusion injury, 979–981, 980f
　age and, 981
　calcium hypothesis of, 979–980, 980f
　cyanosis and, 981–982
　free radical hypothesis of, 980–981, 980f–981f
　inflammation and, 981
　after lung transplantation, 220, 220f, 220t
Ischemic preconditioning, 992
　remote, 992–993
Isoproterenol
　after cardiac surgery, 940–941, 942t
　in heart failure, 899t
　in pediatric pulmonary hypertension, 1752
iv gene, 1643
Ivor Lewis esophagectomy, 593–594
　contraindications to, 594
　indications for, 593
　minimally invasive, 600–601
　technique of, 594, 596f, 612
　vs. transhiatal esophagectomy, 597–599, 599t

J

Jarcho-Levin syndrome, 383–384, 384f
Jarvik 2000 device, 1516–1517, 1517f
Jehovah's Witnesses, 948
Jejunostomy tube, postoperative, 51–52
Jejunum, postesophagectomy conduit creation with, 606–607, 607f–609f
　contraindications to, 606
　free interposition in, 607, 609f
　indications for, 606
　pedicled interposition in, 607, 609f
　preparation for, 606
　Roux-en-Y replacement in, 606–607, 607f
Jeune's disease, 382–383, 383f
　acquired, 369–371, 371f
Jugular vein
　internal, 3–4
　　for temporary pacemaker insertion, 1306, 1307b
　　for pediatric cardiac catheterization, 1693
Junctional ectopic tachycardia, after tetralogy of Fallot repair, 1890

K

Kawasaki's disease, 1475, 1476f
Kawashima operation, 2044
Keratin, in pleural effusion, 435t
Ketamine, in congenital heart disease, 1754

Ki-67, in pleural effusion, 433, 435t
Kidneys
　ACE inhibitor effects on, 891–892
　aprotinin effects on, 767
　disease of, aortic aneurysm and, 1068
　dysfunction of
　　after cardiopulmonary bypass, 924, 971, 1725
　　after coronary artery bypass grafting, 1383
　failure of, left ventricular assist device implantation and, 1509
　neonatal, 1750
Killian's triangle, 548, 548f
Klumpke-Déjérine syndrome, 318
Koch, triangle of, 700–701, 701f
Konno operation, modified, 1948–1950, 1949f
　results of, 1950–1951, 1951f
Konno-Rastan aortoventriculoplasty, 1950, 1950f
KS1/4, in lung cancer, 675
Kulchitsky cells, 329
Kumpe, fallen lung sign of, 99
Kuntz, nerve of, 24
Kussmaul's sign, 786, 787f, 1176, 1482, 1482f

L

Lactic acidosis, after cardiac surgery, 937
Lactic dehydrogenase, in anterior mediastinal mass, 637, 639
Laimer's triangle, 548, 548f
Langerhans cell histiocytosis, 164
Laparoscopy
　in diaphragmatic trauma, 97, 478
　in minimally invasive esophagectomy, 600
Laparotomy, in diaphragmatic trauma, 97, 478
LaPlace, law of, 750
Laryngotracheal stenosis. See also Tracheal stenosis
　bronchoscopy in, 117
　idiopathic, 115–116
　resection of, 120–121, 122f
Laryngotracheoesophageal cleft, 135, 544
Larynx, trauma to, 92–93
Laser therapy
　endoscopic, 74–75, 74t–75t
　　in adenoid cystic carcinoma, 330
　　in malignant airway obstruction, 74
　　in malignant esophageal tumors, 74–75
　in femoral artery disease, 1169
　in malignant pleural effusion, 440
　myocardial, percutaneous, 1461–1462
　transmyocardial. See Transmyocardial laser revascularization
Lateral femoral circumflex artery, in coronary artery bypass grafting, 1418
Latissimus dorsi flap, in chest wall reconstruction, 383–384
Latissimus dorsi muscle, 6, 7f, 8t
Law of LaPlace, 750
LDL receptor deficiency, 907
Left aortic arch
　with anomalous right subclavian artery, 1789, 1789f, 1791–1792
　with left descending aorta, 1788–1789
　with right descending aorta, 1788–1789, 1788f
Left atrial isolation procedure, 1347
Left atrioventricular valve regurgitation, recurrent, 2018, 2022–2023, 2023f
Left atrium. See Atrium (atria), left
Left cardiac sympathetic denervation, pediatric, 2085–2088, 2087f, 2088f
Left ligamentum arteriosum, right aortic arch with, 1787–1788, 1788f, 1791
Left main-stem bronchus compression, after interrupted aortic arch treatment, 1939–1940
Left ventricle. See Ventricle(s), left
Left ventricular assist device, 861, 861f–862f, 1507, 1528–1529
　anticoagulation for, 1283
　biomaterials for, 1288
　after cardiotomy, 1508, 1519–1520
　complications of, 1288, 1529
　in heart failure, 1508–1509, 1520
　before heart transplantation, 1508, 1520, 1537–1538
　historical perspective on, 1507
　implantation of, 1520–1521

Left ventricular assist device (*Continued*)
　　atrial septal defect and, 1509
　　bleeding after, 1521
　　complications of, 1521–1522
　　contraindications to, 1509–1510
　　coronary artery disease and, 1509
　　infection and, 1509, 1521
　　liver function and, 1509–1510
　　malfunction after, 1521
　　management after, 1521
　　multisystem organ failure after, 1522
　　patent foramen ovale and, 1509
　　renal failure and, 1509
　　right heart failure after, 1509, 1522
　　screening scale for, 1510
　　thromboembolism after, 1521
　　tricuspid regurgitation and, 1509
　indications for, 1507–1509
　after infarction, 1454, 1508, 1519–1520
　in myocarditis, 1508
　patient selection for, 1509–1510
　　cardiac factors in, 1509
　　noncardiac factors in, 1509–1510
　pediatric, 1742–1745, 1743f
　　Berlin Heart Excor, 1744–1745, 1744f–1745f
　　development of, 1745, 1745t
　　nonpulsatile, 1743–1744
　　pulsatile, 1744
　in refractory arrhythmias, 1361, 1508
　selection of, 1519–1520
　stroke with, 1529
　types of, 1510–1519
　　long-term, 1513–1519
　　　Berlin Heart Incor, 1517
　　　CircuLite, 1519, 1519f
　　　HeartWare, 1518, 1519f
　　　Jarvik 2000, 1516–1517, 1517f
　　　MicroMed DeBakey, 1517, 1517f
　　　Terumo DuraHeart, 1518, 1518f
　　　Thoratec HeartMate II, 1516, 1516f
　　　Thoratec HeartMate III, 1518
　　　Thoratec HeartMate XVE, 1513–1514, 1515f
　　　Thoratec intracorporeal device, 1515, 1516f
　　　Thoratec paracorporeal device, 1514–1515, 1515f
　　　VentraCor VentrAssist, 1517–1518, 1518f
　　　WorldHeart LevaCor, 1518, 1518f
　　short-term, 1510–1513
　　　Abiomed AB5000, 1512, 1512f
　　　Abiomed BVS5000, 1511–1512, 1512f
　　　Abiomed Impella, 1512, 1513f
　　　extracorporeal membrane oxygenation, 1510–1512, 1511f
　　　intra-aortic balloon pump, 1510
　　　Levitronix CentriMag, 1508, 1510–1511, 1511f
　　　TandemHeart, 1512–1513, 1514f
　vascular complications of, 1288
Left ventricular dysfunction. See also Heart failure
　coronary artery bypass grafting in, 1371, 1386
　implantable cardioverter-defibrillator for, 1314b. See also Implantable cardioverter-defibrillator
Left ventricular ejection fraction
　in coronary artery disease, 817–818
　in mitral regurgitation, 1216, 1217f
　preoperative, 919
Left ventricular hypertrophy
　aortic stenosis and, 1196–1197
　circulatory effects of, 721
　diastolic dysfunction in, 744
　ischemia and, 982
　vascular resistance in, 712, 713f
Left ventricular outflow tract obstruction, 1751
　atrioventricular canal defect and, 1842–1843
　in congenital aortic stenosis, 1945
　in congenitally corrected transposition of great arteries, 2004
　interrupted aortic arch and, 1931–1934, 1932f–1933f, 1938–1939, 1938f–1939f
　right ventricle–to–pulmonary artery conduit for, 1905. See also Right ventricle–to–pulmonary artery conduit
　in transposition of great arteries, 1993–1996, 1999
　ventricular septal defect and, 1852
Left ventricular restoration. See Heart failure, surgical ventricular restoration in

Left ventricular training
  in complex transposition of great arteries, 1999
  in congenitally corrected transposition of great arteries, 2007
Left ventricular volume
  echocardiographic analysis of, 1673–1674, 1674f
  exercise-related, 725–726, 726f
Legionella, in community-acquired pneumonia, 175, 176f
Leiomyoma
  cardiac, 1635t
  esophageal, 568, 568f
  pulmonary, 156–157, 157f
Leiomyosarcoma
  esophageal, 568
  pulmonary, 331–332, 331f
Lepirudin, in NSTE acute coronary syndromes, 875
Leriche syndrome, 1372
Lesser saphenous vein, in coronary artery bypass grafting, 1376, 1412
Letterer-Siwe disease, 164
Leu MI, in pleural effusion, 435t
Leukemia, Poland's syndrome and, 373–374
Leukocytes, in cardiopulmonary bypass, 964–965
Leukodepletion, in cardiopulmonary bypass, 971
Leukoreduction, for transfusion, 763
Levator scapulae, 8t
Levitronix CentriMag device, 1508, 1510–1511, 1511f
Libman-Sacks endocarditis, 1475
Lidocaine, in cardiac surgery, 1009
Lipid-lowering therapy, 909–911, 911t, 913–914
Lipids, 905
Lipoblastoma, 455
Lipoma
  cardiac, 1634t–1635t, 1636–1637
  esophageal, 566
  pleural, 455
  thymic, 639
Lipomatous hypertrophy, of interatrial septum, 796, 798f, 1637
Lipoprotein(a), 908
Lipoprotein(s), 905–908, 905t
  in atherogenesis, 907–908
  high-density, 905, 905t, 907
    cardiovascular risk and, 909–910
    oxidation of, 907–908
  intermediate-density, 905–906, 905t, 906f
  low-density, 905t, 907
    cardiovascular risk and, 909–910
    receptor for, deficiency of, 907
  very-low-density, 905–906, 905t, 906f
Liposarcoma, 456
Liquid ventilation, in congenital diaphragmatic hernia, 501
Lisinopril, 890–892, 891t
Liver
  function of, left ventricular assist device and, 1509–1510
  neonatal, 1750
Lobectomy, 254–255
  age and, 40
  blood vessel management in, 254–255
  bronchial management in, 255
  chest tube placement in, 255
  historical perspective on, 253
  incisions in, 254
  mobilization and dissection in, 254, 254f–255f
  positioning in, 254
  thoracoscopic, 279
    complications of, 284
    contraindications to, 280
    cost-effectiveness of, 284
    definition of, 279
    historical perspective on, 279, 280t
    indications for, 280
    inflammation after, 284
    instrumentation for, 281
    left lower, 282–283
    left upper, 281, 281f–282f
    mediastinal lymph node dissection in, 281
    oncologic effectiveness of, 284
    pain after, 283
    preparation for, 280–281
    pulmonary function after, 283–284
    results of, 283–284
    right lower, 282–283
    right middle, 282
    right upper, 282

Loeffler's syndrome, 164
Loeys-Dietz syndrome, 1026, 1093
Losartan, 891t
Louis, sternal angle of, 10, 12t
Low cardiac output syndrome, after coronary artery bypass grafting, 1383
Lower esophageal sphincter. *See* Esophageal sphincter, lower
Lung(s)
  abscess of, 181–182
    clinical features of, 181
    etiology of, 181, 182t
    imaging in, 31, 181–182, 182f–183f
    location of, 181
    after lung transplantation, 221
    pathogens in, 181
    treatment of, 31, 182, 183f
  acute injury to
    transfusion-related, 764
    trauma-related, 107
  adenoid cystic carcinoma of, 329–331, 330f, 330t
  agenesis of, 139–140, 140f
  alveolar adenoma of, 156
  anatomy of, 14–20, 15f
  angiosarcoma of, 332
  aplasia of, 139–140
  arteriovenous malformation of, 145–147, 146f, 2044
  azygos lobe of, 15, 137, 138f
  benign lesions of, 151. *See also specific lesions*
    definition of, 151, 151b
    evaluation of, 151–152, 152b
    incidence of, 151
  biopsy of. *See* Biopsy, lung
  blastoma of, 456
  cancer of. *See* Lung cancer
  carcinoid tumor of, 323–329. *See also* Carcinoid tumor
  carcinoid tumorlets of, 329
  carcinosarcoma of, 334
  chondroma of, 156
  chronic disease of, congenital diaphragmatic hernia and, 505
  clear cell tumor of, 157
  congenital disease of, 129. *See also specific abnormalities and diseases*
    historical perspective on, 129
  contusion of, 92
  cystic adenomatoid malformation of, 142–143, 142f
  drug-induced injury of, 165
  dysfunction of
    after cardiopulmonary bypass, 970–971
    after congenital heart disease treatment, 1759–1760
    after pediatric cardiopulmonary bypass, 1725
  embryology of, 129–130, 1817, 1818f
    abnormalities of, 129. *See also specific congenital abnormalities*
    canalicular phase of, 130
    embryonic phase of, 129–130
    pseudoglandular phase of, 130
    terminal sac phase of, 130
  emphysematous changes in, in congenital diaphragmatic hernia, 505
  epithelioid hemangioendothelioma of, 332
  fibrous histiocytoma of, 154–155
  fibrous tumor of, 154, 154f
  fissures of, 15, 19f–20f
  foreign particles in, 161, 161t
  granular cell tumor of, 155
  hamartoma of, 152–154, 152f–153f
  hila of, 15, 20f–21f
  horseshoe, 138
  hypoplasia of, 139–140
    in congenital diaphragmatic hernia, 492–493, 493f
  imaging of, 27–31
    in metastatic disease, 339–340, 339f
    in non–small cell cancer, 30–31, 31f, 244–246, 249–250
  infection of, 173
    bacterial, 173–182
      community-acquired, 173–178, 174t, 175f–178f
      health care–associated, 179
      hospital-acquired, 178–179
      ventilator-associated, 178–179
    mycobacterial, 182–185, 184f–185f
    mycotic, 185–191
  infectious granulomatosis of, 154
  inflammation of. *See* Interstitial lung disease
  inflammatory pseudotumor of, 155, 155f, 454

Lung(s) (*Continued*)
  interstitial disease of, 159, 159b. *See also* Interstitial lung disease
  interstitium of, 159
  leiomyoma of, 156–157, 157f
  lobes of, 15, 15f–16f, 17t–18t
    azygos, 15, 137, 138f
  lymphoma of, 333
  MALT lymphoma of, 333
  melanoma of, 333–334
  metastases to, 337, 338b. *See also* Lung cancer, non–small cell, metastatic
    from breast cancer, 169f, 345–346
    from cervical cancer, 346
    clinical presentation of, 339
    from colorectal cancer, 345
    from endocrine tumors, 347
    evaluation of, 339–340, 339f
    from germ cell tumor, 346
    from gynecologic tumors, 346
    from head and neck cancer, 346
    imaging of, 339–340, 339f
    from melanoma, 346–347
    from osteosarcoma, 345
    from ovarian cancer, 346
    palliative therapy in, 347
    pathophysiology of, 337–339
    perfusion chemotherapy in, 347
    radiofrequency ablation in, 347
    from renal cell carcinoma, 346
    from soft tissue sarcoma, 344–345
    spread of, 338
    surgical treatment of, 342–343
      historical perspective on, 337
      indications for, 340–342, 341t, 342b
      lymph node dissection in, 343
      results of, 343–344, 343t–344t, 344b
    tissue diagnosis of, 340
    unresectability of, 341
    from uterine cancer, 346
  mucinous cystadenoma of, 156
  mucoepidermoid carcinoma of, 329–331, 330f, 330t
  mucous gland adenoma of, 154, 154f
  myoepithelioma of, 156
  neuroendocrine cell hyperplasia of, 329
  nodular amyloid lesion of, 156
  nodules of. *See* Pulmonary nodule(s)
  parenchymal cyst of, congenital, 141–142
  plasmacytoma of, 332–333
  polyalveolar lobe of, 143
  postnatal development of, 130
  salivary gland–type tumors of, 329–331, 330f, 330t
  sarcoidosis of, 162–163, 162f
  sarcoma of, 331–332, 331f
  segments of, 15, 15f–16f, 17t–18t
  squamous papilloma of, 155–156
  surface anatomy of, 11–12, 11f
  thymoma of, 157, 158f
  transfusion-related injury to, 764
  transplantation of. *See* Heart-lung transplantation; Lung transplantation
  trauma to. *See also* Trauma
    air embolus with, 102
    penetrating, 99–100
    respiratory distress syndrome and, 107
  tuberculosis of, 161, 162f
Lung cancer
  biopsy in, 64–65, 246–248, 247f
  brachytherapy in, 75
  diaphragmatic invasion in, 485
  mediastinal lymph node dissection for, 257–258, 259f. *See also* Mediastinal lymph node dissection
  non–small cell
    adjuvant chemotherapy in, 287–288
    adjuvant radiotherapy in, 288
    autofluorescence bronchoscopy in, 247–248
    bone scan in, 246
    bronchioloalveolar subtype of, 271–272
    bronchoscopy in, 246–247
    cervical mediastinoscopy in, 248
    chemoperfusion in, 690–691
    chest radiography in, 31f, 244
    chest wall invasion with, 295
    chemotherapy in, 300
    clinical presentation of, 296–297, 296f, 297t

Lung cancer (Continued)
  diagnosis of, 297–298, 298f
  mortality in, 308–309
  pathology of, 307–308
  pulmonary function testing in, 300
  staging of, 298–300
  surgical treatment of, 262, 300
    assessment before, 300
    bronchoscopy before, 299
    care after, 306
    complications of, 306–307, 307f
    historical perspective on, 295–296
    reconstruction after, 303–306, 305f
    results of, 308–309
    techniques of, 300–303, 303f
  circulating tumor cell detection in, 676–677
  computed tomography in, 29f, 30, 31f, 245
  diagnosis of. See Lung cancer, non–small cell, staging of
  DNA microarray analysis in, 670–673, 671f
  endobronchial ultrasound–guided needle aspiration in, 247, 247f, 631–632, 632f
  epidemiology of, 241
  extended cervical mediastinoscopy in, 248–249
  genetic abnormalities in, 669
  immunohistochemistry in, 673–674, 674f
  individualized therapy in, 678–679
  induction (neoadjuvant) therapy in, 288–291
    chemoradiotherapy for, 289–290
    chemotherapy for, 289
    in early-stage tumors, 289
    in stage IIIA/B tumors, 289–290
    in superior sulcus tumors, 290–291
  inoperable, photodynamic therapy in, 69
  left anterior mediastinotomy in, 248–249
  lung metagene model of, 679
  M1a, 269
    ipsilateral lung nodules in, 269
    pleural effusion in, 269
  magnetic resonance imaging in, 30, 31f, 246
  M1b, 269–270
  metastatic, 338–339
    adrenal, 30, 269–270
    CNS, 30, 270
    evaluation of, 249–250, 249t–250t
    genetic abnormalities in, 669
    imaging in, 30–31, 32f, 249–250
    nodal, 30, 32f, 248–249, 249t
    occult, 673–676, 674f–675f, 676t
    positron emission tomography in, 245–246, 245f
    skeletal, 30–31
  microwave ablation in, 689–690, 692
  minimally invasive surgical treatment of, 279
    complications of, 284
    contraindications to, 280
    cost-effectiveness of, 284
    definition of, 279
    historical perspective on, 279, 280t
    indications for, 280
    inflammation after, 284
    left lower, 282–283
    left upper, 281, 281f–282f
    oncologic effectiveness of, 284
    pain after, 283
    preparation for, 280–281
    pulmonary function after, 283–284
    results of, 283–284
    right lower, 282–283
    right middle, 282
    right upper, 282
    segmental, 283
    technique of, 281–283
    wedge resection, 283
  molecular markers in, 670
  multimodal therapy in, 287
    adjuvant, 287–288
    neoadjuvant (induction), 288–291
    recommendations for, 291
  N2, 265–269, 266f
    on pretreatment staging, 267–268, 267f–268f
    at thoracotomy, 268–269, 268t
  N3, 269
  N0 and N1, 265
  p53 in, 677
  patient history in, 243–244
  percutaneous transthoracic needle biopsy in, 248

Lung cancer (Continued)
  photodynamic therapy in, 68–69
    complications of, 69
    palliative, 68–69, 69f–70f
  physical examination in, 243–244
  polymerase chain reaction in, 673–675, 675f
  positron emission tomography in, 30, 32f, 245–246, 245f, 299–300
  prognosis for
    personalized therapy and, 678–679
    proteomic study in, 677–678
    tumor marker panels in, 678
  proteomic study in, 677–678
  radiofrequency ablation in, 683–687, 683f
    animal models of, 684
    devices for, 684, 684f–685f
    patient selection for, 685, 685t
    results of, 686–687, 686f, 687f, 692
    technique of, 685–686, 689, 691–692
    timing of, 684
  scalene node biopsy in, 249
  sputum cytology in, 244–245
  staging of, 242–244, 242f, 243t–244t, 259f, 260t, 291, 298–300
    accuracy of, 270–271
    autofluorescence bronchoscopy in, 247–248
    bone scan in, 246
    bronchoscopy in, 246–247
    cervical mediastinoscopy in, 248, 249t
    chest radiography in, 244
    computed tomography in, 245
    endobronchial ultrasound–guided needle biopsy in, 247, 247f
    imaging in, 30–31, 32f, 299, 626t
    left anterior mediastinotomy in, 248–249
    lymph node stations for, 241–242
    magnetic resonance imaging in, 246
    mediastinal lymph nodes in, 624–625, 625f–626f, 626t. See also Mediastinal lymph node dissection
    patient history in, 243–244
    percutaneous transthoracic needle biopsy in, 248
    physical examination in, 244
    positron emission tomography in, 245–246, 245f
    scalene node biopsy in, 249
    sputum cytology in, 244–245
    thoracotomy in, 249
    transbronchial needle aspiration in, 246–247
    video-assisted thoracic surgery in, 249
  stereotactic radiosurgery in, 687–689
    patient selection for, 688
    results of, 688–689, 692
    technique of, 687–688, 688f, 691–692
  surgical treatment of, 258–270. See also Lung cancer, non–small cell, minimally invasive surgical treatment of
    induction (neoadjuvant) therapy before, 288–291
      chemoradiotherapy for, 289–290
      chemotherapy for, 289
      in early-stage tumors, 289
      in stage IIIA/B tumors, 289–290
    in M1a disease, 269
    in M1b disease, 269–270
    mediastinal lymph node dissection in, 270–271, 272t
    in N0 and N1 disease, 265
    in N2 disease, 265–269, 266f–268f, 268t
    in N3 disease, 269
    in T1 and T2 disease, 259–262, 260t–261t
    in T3 disease, 262–263
    in T4 disease, 263–264, 264t
  T3, 262–263
    carinal proximity, 262–263
    chest wall invasion, 262. See also Lung cancer, non–small cell, chest wall invasion with
    diaphragmatic invasion, 263
    mediastinal invasion, 263
    satellite lesions, 263
    superior sulcus, 262, 313. See also Pancoast tumor
  T4, 263–264
    cardiac invasion, 263
    carinal invasion, 263–264, 264t
    esophageal invasion, 264
    ipsilateral lobar metastasis, 264
    tracheal invasion, 263–264
    vertebral invasion, 264, 265f, 266t

Lung cancer (Continued)
  T1 and T2, 259–262
    sublobar resection in, 260–262, 261t
    surgical treatment of, 260–262, 261t. See also Lobectomy
  thoracotomy in, 249
  tumor markers in, 670, 676–678
  video-assisted thoracic surgery in, 249
  photodynamic therapy in, 68–69
  screening for, 231
    fluorescence bronchoscopy in, 235
    historical perspective on, 231–233, 232t
    low-dose computed tomography in, 233–234, 234t
    molecular diagnostics in, 235
    National Lung Screening Trial of, 233
    overdiagnosis bias and, 232–233
    PLCO (Prostate, Lung, Colorectal and Ovarian) trial of, 233
    regimen for, 235–236
    sputum evaluation in, 234–235
  small cell
    proteomic study in, 677–678
    surgical treatment of, 272–274
      local control after, 273
      in mixed-histology disease, 273
      randomized trials of, 273–274, 274t
      rationale for, 273
      salvage, 273
  sublobar resection for, 257, 258f
  surgical treatment of, 253. See also Lobectomy; Mediastinal lymph node dissection; Pneumonectomy
    age and, 40
    historical perspective on, 253
Lung infection, 173
  bacterial, 173–182
    community-acquired, 173–178, 174t, 175f–178f
    health care–associated, 179
    hospital-acquired, 178–179
    ventilator-associated, 178–179
  mycobacterial, 182–185, 184f–185f
  mycotic, 185–191
Lung metagene model, in lung cancer, 679
Lung perfusion scan, in pulmonary atresia with ventricular septal defect, 1900, 1904
Lung transplantation, 207. See also Heart-lung transplantation
  in α_1-antitrypsin deficiency, 209
  complications of, 219–225
    acute rejection, 222, 222f
    airway, 223
    anastomotic, 219, 223
    bacterial, 221
    chronic rejection, 223–224, 224f, 224t, 224b
    dehiscence-related, 223
    fungal, 221–222, 222f
    gastrointestinal, 225, 226f
    hemorrhagic, 219
    infectious, 221–222
    lymphoproliferative, 225, 225f
    necrosis-related, 223
    primary graft dysfunction, 220, 220f, 220t
    technical, 219–220
    viral, 221, 221f
  in congenital diaphragmatic hernia, 507
  in cystic fibrosis, 209
  disease-specific guidelines for, 209
  donor selection for, 209–210, 210b
  donor shortage for, 217
  donor surgery for, 210–214
    atrial cuff injury with, 212–213, 213f
    in brain-dead donor, 210–212, 211f–212f
    congenital bronchial anomalies and, 214
    lung separation with, 212
    in non-heart-beating donor, 212
    pulmonary artery injury with, 213–214
    pulmonary vein injury with, 212–213
  in emphysema, 196–199, 197f–198f, 199b, 203–205, 203f, 209
  ex vivo donor lung reconditioning for, 217, 218f
  historical perspective on, 207–208
  in idiopathic pulmonary fibrosis, 167, 209
  living donor for, 217
  lung allocation score in, 208
  management after, 218
    chest physiotherapy in, 218

Lung transplantation (*Continued*)
  fluids in, 218
  immunosuppression in, 218-219
  infection prophylaxis in, 219
  ventilation in, 218
non–heart-beating donor for, 210, 212, 217
pediatric, 227
in pulmonary atresia with ventricular septal defect, 1902
pulmonary function testing in, 209
in pulmonary hypertension, 209
recipient selection for, 208, 208b, 209b
recipient surgery for, 214-217
  anesthesia for, 214
  anterolateral thoracotomy in, 214
  bilateral anterolateral thoracotomy in, 214, 214f
  cardiopulmonary bypass in, 216-217, 217f
  clamshell incision in, 214, 215f
  implantation in, 215-216, 215f-216f
  incisions in, 214, 214f-215f
  median sternotomy in, 214
  monitoring during, 214
  pneumonectomy in, 214-215
  posterolateral thoracotomy in, 214
results of, 225-227, 226f
size matching/mismatched lungs in, 210, 217
split-lung, 210, 217
in tracheobronchomegaly, 135
volume reduction bridge to, 203-204, 203f
Lung volume, postoperative, 39
Lung volume reduction surgery, 199-204
  as bridge procedure, 203-204, 203f
  indications for, 199b, 201t
  perfusion scintigraphy for, 200, 200f
  results of, 200-201, 201f-202f
  technique of, 201-203
Lutembacher's syndrome, 1801
Lymph nodes
  delphian, 17
  esophageal, 23
  mediastinal. *See* Mediastinal lymph node(s)
  paratracheal, 17
  pulmonary, 17
Lymphadenectomy, mediastinal. *See* Mediastinal lymph node dissection
Lymphangiectasia, 143-144, 143f
Lymphangiomyomatosis, 156-157
Lymphatic system
  diaphragmatic, 476
  esophageal, 23
  pulmonary, 17
Lymphedema-distichiasis syndrome, 144
Lymphography, in chylothorax, 428
Lymphoma
  cardiac, 1635t
  mediastinal, 640, 647
    Castleman's disease and, 657, 658f
  pulmonary, 333
Lymphoproliferative disorders, post-transplantation, 225, 225f-226f

M

Macleod's syndrome, 144
Magnesium
  in myocardial protection, 987
  in postoperative atrial fibrillation, 54
Magnet, magnetic resonance imaging and, 1685
Magnetic resonance angiography (MRA)
  in acute pulmonary embolism, 1616-1617
  in chronic thromboembolic pulmonary hypertension, 1622
  in coarctation of aorta, 1157
  pediatric, 1681-1682, 1683f
  in scimitar syndrome, 1821f
  in total anomalous pulmonary venous drainage, 1822f
  in type B aortic dissection, 1119
Magnetic resonance imaging (MRI)
  in adult congenital heart disease, 2071f, 2072
  in anomalous aorta–pulmonary artery coronary artery course, 1973
  in anomalous origin of coronary artery from pulmonary artery, 1965-1966
  in aortic aneurysm, 791-792

Magnetic resonance imaging (*Continued*)
  before aortic arch surgery, 1046-1048
  in aortic atherosclerotic plaque, 793-794
  in aortic coarctation, 794
  in aortic dissection, 792-793, 792f-793f
  in aortic intramural hematoma, 793
  in aortic stenosis, 799, 801f
  in ascending aortic aneurysm, 1025
  in atrial septal defect, 795-796, 797f, 1802, 1802f
  in brachiocephalic artery disease, 1145-1146
  in cardiac mass, 796, 798f
  after cardiac surgery, 1005, 1006f
  in cardiomyopathy, 799-800, 802f-803f
  cardiovascular, 789
    clinical applications of, 791-802
    vs. computed tomography, 790
    contrast in, 790-791
    image acquisition in, 790
    precautions for, 791
    resolution in, 790
  in chest wall tumor, 379-380
  in chondrosarcoma, 34f
  in coarctation of aorta, 1785
  in congenital disease, 795-796, 796f-797f
  in congenital heart disease, 1683-1684
  in congenital tracheal disease, 1765-1766
  in coronary artery disease, 800-802, 803f, 805f
  in coronary artery fistula, 1975-1976
  in Ebstein's anomaly, 2059, 2077, 2078f
  in esophageal duplication, 543
  in esophageal fibrovascular polyp, 567f
  in heart failure, 1580-1581, 1580f-1581f
  in hypertrophic cardiomyopathy, 1498
  in lung cancer, 30, 31f, 246, 297-299
  in malignant pleural mesothelioma, 33
  in mediastinal tumors, 26-27
  of middle mediastinum, 645
  in myocardial infarction, 795, 795f
  in Pancoast tumor, 314, 314f-315f, 319f
  in patent ductus arteriosus, 794
  pediatric, 1676-1685
    blood flow analysis with, 1679-1681, 1681f-1682f
    cine sequences for, 1677-1678, 1679f
    complications of, 1685
    in congenital heart disease, 1683-1684
    contraindications to, 1685
    gadolinium contrast for, 1682, 1683f-1684f
    gating in, 1676-1677, 1677t
    indications for, 1682
    magnets and, 1685
    metal hazards in, 1685
    in myocardial ischemia, 1682, 1684f
    myocardial tagging in, 1678-1679, 1680f
    in myocardial viability assessment, 1682, 1684f
    safety of, 1685
    sedation for, 1684
    technique of, 1676-1682, 1677t
    tissue characteristics on, 1677, 1677t, 1678f
    in truncus arteriosus, 1914
    ventricular function on, 1678-1679, 1680f
  in pericardial disease, 797-799, 799f-800f, 1483
  in pleural effusion, 431-432
  pregnancy and, 1685
  in pulmonary atresia with ventricular septal defect, 1900
  in pulmonary embolism, 35
  in sinus of Valsalva aneurysm, 793, 794f
  in Takayasu's arteritis, 794
  in thoracic trauma, 794-795
  in total anomalous pulmonary venous drainage, 1824
  in truncus arteriosus, 1914
  in type A aortic dissection, 1098-1099
  in valvular heart disease, 799, 801f
  in vascular ring, 1790, 1790f
  of ventricle, 749
  in ventricular assessment, 795
Malignant fibrous histiocytoma, 385
Malignant mesothelioma. *See* Mesothelioma, malignant
Malignant pericardial effusion. *See* Pericardial effusion, malignant
Malignant pleural effusion. *See* Pleural effusion, malignant
Malnutrition, after esophageal atresia repair, 542
MALT lymphoma, 333
Mannitol, in cardiopulmonary bypass, 971

Manubrium, 3f, 5, 12t
Marfan syndrome, 1025-1026, 1954-1955, 2018
  aortic arch aneurysm in, 1042
  aortic dissection in, 1092, 1955
  aortic reoperation in, 1045
  aortic root aneurysm in, 1025-1026
  aortic root surgery in, 1033-1034, 1955
  diagnosis of, 1025, 1025t, 1041
  Erdheim deformity in, 1042
  mitral regurgitation in, 1214
  mitral valve prolapse in, 1025
  pectus excavatum in, 360
  pregnancy and, 1026
Maze procedure. *See* Atrial fibrillation, Cox-Maze procedure in
MCA, in pleural effusion, 435t
Mechanical ventilation
  after cardiac surgery, 933
  in congenital diaphragmatic hernia, 501
  after lung transplantation, 218
  after pediatric cardiac surgery, 1759-1761, 1760b
  pneumonia with, 178-179
  prevention of, 1017
  weaning from, after pediatric cardiac surgery, 1760-1761, 1760b
Median sternotomy. *See* Sternotomy, median
Mediastinal lymph node(s), 17, 22f, 624, 624f-625f
  enlargement of, 646-647, 647t
Mediastinal lymph node dissection, 257-258, 259f, 270-271, 626-627, 627f
  algorithm for, 626f
  anatomy for, 624, 625f
  biopsy technique with, 630-631
  bleeding with, 631
  in carcinoid tumor, 327
  carinal dissection for, 629-630, 630f
  complications of, 631
  evaluation for, 625-626
  extended, 631
  high paratracheal dissection for, 627-628, 627f-628f
  indications for, 624-625
  lower paratracheal dissection for, 628-629, 628f-629f
  thoracoscopic, 281
Mediastinitis
  after cardiac surgery, 951-952, 951f, 951t
  fibrosing, 186, 187f, 648
  necrotizing, 648, 658
Mediastinoscopy, 626-627, 626t, 627f. *See also* Mediastinal lymph node dissection
  bleeding with, 631
  cervical, 248, 249t, 646
    extended, 248-249, 641
  complications of, 631
  evaluation for, 625-626
  extended, 631
Mediastinotomy
  anterior, 646
    for biopsy, 640
  cervical, for biopsy, 640
  left anterior, in lung cancer, 248-249
Mediastinum
  anatomy of, 12, 623-624, 623f-624f
  anterior, 12, 13t, 623-624, 623f-624f, 633f, 634t, 645
    tumors of, 633, 634t. *See also specific tumors and disorders*
    biopsy of, 640-641
      Chamberlain procedure in, 640
      extended mediastinoscopy in, 641
    germ cell, 639
    imaging of, 26-27, 29f
    lymphoma, 640
    surgical treatment of, 641-642, 642f, 642t
    thoracoscopic biopsy in, 640-641
    thymic, 633-639. *See also* Thymoma
    transcervical biopsy in, 640
  deviation of, congenital diaphragmatic hernia, 492-494, 493f
  four-compartment model of, 623, 623f
  metastatic cancer of, 340
  middle, 12, 13t, 623-624, 623f-624f, 633f, 634t, 645
    computed tomography of, 27, 645
    endobronchial ultrasound–assisted biopsy of, 646
    endoscopic ultrasound–assisted biopsy of, 646
    infection of, 648
    lymph node disease of, 646-647, 647t
    lymphatics of, 645

Mediastinum (Continued)
    magnetic resonance imaging of, 645
    mediastinotomy of, 646
    percutaneous biopsy of, 646
    pericardial disorders of, 647–648. See also specific disorders
    pericardium of, 645
    positron emission tomography in, 645–646
    radiography of, 645, 646f
    trachea of, 645
    tracheal disorders of, 647. See also specific disorders
    ultrasonography of, 646
    video-assisted thoracoscopy surgery in, 646
  posterior, 12, 13t, 623–624, 624f, 633f, 634t, 645, 649
    abscess of, 658–659, 659f
    anatomy of, 649, 649f
    biopsy of, 650, 652–653
    bronchogenic cyst of, 655–656
    in children, 649
    computed tomography of, 650
    cysts of, 655–656, 655f
    dumbbell tumor of, 652
    esophagus-related masses of, 655
    evaluation of, 649–650
    gastroenteric cysts of, 656
    giant lymph node hyperplasia of, 656–657, 657f–658f
    infection of, 658–659, 659f
    neuroenteric cysts of, 656
    neurogenic tumors of, 651–655, 651b, 652f–654f
    paravertebral mass of, 656
    pericardial cyst of, 655, 655f
    surgery on, 650–651, 650f
    thoracoscopic surgery on, 650, 650f
    tumors of, 649f, 651–658
      epidemiology of, 649
      imaging of, 27, 649–650
      resection of, 650–651, 650f
  potential spaces in, 624
  superior, 623, 623f, 645
  three-compartment model of, 623–624, 624f
  widened, in aortic injury, 93–94, 94f
Medications. See Drug(s) and specific drugs
Medtronic-Hall tilting disc valve, 1187–1188, 1187f
Medtronic prosthetic valves
  Freestyle, 1191, 1191f
  Mosaic, 1189–1190, 1190f
Melanoma
  metastatic, 346–347
  primary, 333–334
Membranous subaortic stenosis, 1947–1948, 1947f–1948f
  surgical treatment of, 1947–1948
    results of, 1948
Mendelson's syndrome, 179
Menstruation, spontaneous pneumothorax with, 411
Mental retardation, in hypoplastic left heart syndrome, 2036
Merlin, in mesothelioma, 452
Mesenteric artery ischemia, 1165
  in type A aortic dissection, 1097, 1097t
Mesothelioma, 449–453
  fibrous, intrapulmonary, 154, 154f
  malignant, 457–464, 464b, 466t
    apoptotic processes in, 453
    asbestos fibers in, 449–453
    CDK inhibitor loss in, 452
    in children, 451
    chromosomal abnormalities in, 451–452
    clinical presentation of, 457–459
    computed tomography in, 457
    diagnosis of, 458–459
    differential diagnosis of, 458–459
    DNA microarray analysis in, 673
    epidemiology of, 450
    growth factors in, 451–453
    hypermethylation in, 452
    imaging in, 33–34, 33f
    localized, 456
    merlin protein in, 452
    oncogene activation in, 452
    papillary, 455–456
      well-differentiated, 455–456
    pericardial, 1488
    positron emission tomography–computed tomography in, 457–458
    prognosis for, 459

Mesothelioma (Continued)
    radiography in, 457
    RAS-ERK pathway in, 452
    staging of, 459, 460b, 461t
    subtypes of, 457–458, 458f
    SV40 in, 453
    treatment of, 459–463
      antiangiogenic therapy in, 465–466
      chemotherapy in, 461
      gene therapy in, 467
      immunotherapy in, 467
      intraoperative heated chemotherapy in, 465, 466t
      multimodality, 464–465, 464b
      photodynamic therapy in, 466–467
      radiation therapy in, 460–463
      surgery in, 461–463, 461b, 462f–463f
        care after, 463–464
        results of, 464
    tumor suppressor genes in, 452–453
Mesothelium
  benign reactive hyperplasia of, 454
  cysts of, 455
  malignant tumor of. See Mesothelioma
Metabolic disease
  coronary artery effects of, 1476
  pericarditis with, 1486
Metabolic equivalent (MET), 42
Metabolic syndrome, 908, 908t
Metal dusts, pulmonary deposition of, 161
Metal hazards, magnetic resonance imaging and, 1685
Metastasectomy, pulmonary. See also Lung(s), metastases to; Lung cancer, non–small cell, metastatic
  approach to, 342–343
  in breast cancer, 345–346
  in colorectal cancer, 345
  in endocrine tumors, 347
  in germ cell tumor, 346
  in gynecologic cancers, 346
  in head and neck cancer, 346
  historical perspective on, 337
  indications for, 340–342, 341t, 342b
  lymph node dissection with, 343
  in melanoma, 346–347
  in osteosarcoma, 345
  in renal cell carcinoma, 346
  results of, 343–344, 343t–344t, 344b
  in soft tissue sarcoma, 344–345
Metastases, 669
  cardiac, 1636t, 1637–1638
  pulmonary. See Lung(s), metastases to; Metastasectomy, pulmonary
Methylene blue, in vasodilatory shock, 943
Methylprednisolone
  in cardiopulmonary bypass, 967
  in heart-lung transplantation, 1564t, 1565
  in lung transplantation, 219
Methysergide maleate, coronary artery fibrosis and, 1476
Metoclopramide, 52
Metolazone, 887t, 888
Metoprolol, 891t, 892–893
MI. See Myocardial infarction (MI)
Micro-electromechanical systems, 1300
Microarray analysis, 670–673, 671f
Microemboli
  during aortic arch surgery, 1050–1052, 1051t
  during cardiac surgery, 1006–1007, 1008f, 1009
MicroMed DeBakey device, 1517, 1517f
Micrometastases, 673–676, 674f–675f, 676t
Microvessels, 711
  classification of, 713
  disease effects on, 720–721, 721f
  injury response of, 719, 720f
  intrinsic myogenic tone of, 718
  metabolic stimulation of, 713
  resistance in, 711–712. See also Vascular tone
Microwave ablation, in non–small cell lung cancer, 689–690
Migraine, patent foramen ovale and, 1804
Milrinone
  after cardiac surgery, 940–941, 942t
  in heart failure, 894–895, 895f, 899, 899t
  in pediatric pulmonary hypertension, 1752
  in right heart failure, 943
Milroy syndrome, 144

Minimally invasive direct coronary artery bypass grafting, 1405, 1405f–1406f
Minimally invasive esophagectomy. See Esophagectomy, minimally invasive
Mitral anuloplasty, 1221, 1223f. See also Mitral valve repair
  in chronic ischemic regurgitation, 1433, 1439f, 1439t, 1442–1445, 1443f–1444f
  in regurgitation, 1221, 1223f, 1227
  in type I congenital mitral anomaly, 2021, 2021f
Mitral anulus
  abscess of, 1227
  anatomy of, 1209, 1209f
  calcification of, 1215
    surgical treatment of, 1227, 1231–1232
  dilatation of, 1212, 1213f, 1221, 2017
  reconstruction of
    in chronic regurgitaton. See Mitral regurgitation, ischemic, chronic, surgical treatment of
    in endocarditis, 1263, 1263f
    in regurgitation, 1221, 1223f, 1227
    in type I congenital mitral anomaly, 2021, 2021f
Mitral-aortic intervalvular fibrosa, pseudoaneurysm of, 843, 843f
Mitral commissure
  anatomy of, 1208, 1209f
  incision of, 1221, 1222f, 1228–1229
  prolapse of, 1226
Mitral regurgitation, 1212–1218
  in anomalous origin of coronary artery from pulmonary artery, 1970–1971
  anulus calcification and, 1215
  atrial septal defect and, 1801
  after atrioventricular canal defect treatment, 1844–1846
  Carpentier's classification of, 1213, 1214t
  catheterization in, 785, 1216
  chronic, 1212–1213, 1213f
    treatment of. See Mitral regurgitation, surgical treatment of
  congenital, 2019, 2023. See also Mitral valve, congenital anomalies of
  degenerative, 1213–1214, 1214f
    Barlow's disease and, 1213–1214, 1214f
    fibroelastic deficiency and, 1213, 1214f
    Marfan syndrome and, 1214
    surgical treatment of, 1229–1230, 1230t–1231t, 1232f
  diagnosis of, 1215–1216, 1216t, 1221
  dilated cardiomyopathy and, 1215
  echocardiography in, 829, 830f, 840–841, 840f–841f, 1215–1216, 1216t, 1436–1439, 1437f
  endocarditis and, 1214
    surgical treatment of, 1218, 1227, 1231
  endomyocardial fibrosis and, 1215
  etiology of, 1213–1215, 1214f
  functional, 1429–1430
  historical perspective on, 1207–1208
  hypertrophic cardiomyopathy and, 1497
  ischemic, 1214–1215
    acute, 1430
      sheep model of, 1431
    chronic, 1424
      anular abnormalities in, 1431, 1433
      Carpentier type I, 1429–1431
      Carpentier type II, 1429
      Carpentier type IIIa, 1429
      Carpentier type IIIb, 1429–1431, 1430f
      clinical implications of, 1436
      clinical presentation of, 1430, 1430f
      after coronary artery bypass grafting, 1434, 1436
      coronary artery bypass grafting and, 1434–1439, 1437f
      definition of, 1429–1430
      effet de mouette deformity in, 1433
      heart failure and, 1434, 1583–1584, 1585f–1587f, 1586t, 1594–1595
      leaflet dysfunction in, 1433–1434, 1444–1445
      left ventricular abnormalities in, 1432, 1432f, 1434
      after myocardial infarction, 1435, 1436f
      myocardial infarction and, 1430
      papillary muscle displacement in, 1431–1433, 1433f, 1443–1444, 1444f
      papillary muscle dysfunction and, 1431

Mitral regurgitation (Continued)
　　pathophysiology of, 1430–1434, 1431f
　　after percutaneous coronary intervention, 1435, 1436f
　　prognosis for, 1435–1436
　　quantification of, 1430
　　subvalvar abnormalities in, 1431–1433, 1433f
　　surgical treatment of, 1433–1434, 1433f
　　　coronary artery revascularization in, 1433, 1433f, 1437–1438, 1441
　　　decision making in, 1434–1435, 1440–1441
　　　leaflet procedures in, 1434
　　　left ventricular procedures in, 1434
　　　mitral anuloplasty in, 1433, 1439f, 1439t, 1442–1445, 1443f–1444f
　　　　adjunctive procedures in, 1443
　　　　cordal cutting in, 1444
　　　　vs. coronary artery bypass grafting, 1435
　　　　mitral stenosis after, 1445
　　　　papillary muscle repositioning in, 1443–1444, 1444f
　　　　principles of, 1441–1442
　　　　residual regurgitation after, 1440–1441, 1440f
　　　　results of, 1438–1439, 1439f, 1439t, 1445
　　　　ring selection in, 1443, 1443f
　　　　risk of, 1440–1441
　　　　suture placement in, 1443
　　　　valve analysis in, 1442–1443
　　　　valve exposure in, 1442
　　　　vs. valve replacement, 1441
　　　principles of, 1441–1445
　　　residual regurgitation after, 1439–1440, 1440f
　　　subvalvar procedures in, 1433, 1433f
　　　valve replacement in, 1441
　　　transesophageal echocardiography in, 1436–1439, 1437f
　magnetic resonance imaging in, 799
　myocardial infarction and, 833, 1435, 1436f
　in off-pump coronary artery bypass grafting, 1399
　pathophysiology of, 1212–1213, 1213f, 1214t
　vs. postinfarction ventricular septal defect, 1450
　rheumatic disease and, 1214
　　surgical treatment of, 1230–1231
　surgical treatment of, 1217f, 1218–1228. See also Mitral valve repair; Mitral valve replacement
　　atrial fibrillation and, 1218
　　in congestive heart failure, 1216, 1229, 1230f
　　de-airing process in, 1221
　　endocarditis and, 1218
　　horizontal biatrial trans-septal approach to, 1220, 1220f
　　indications for, 1216–1218, 1217f
　　interatrial approach to, 1220, 1220f
　　left ventricular ejection fraction and, 1216, 1217f
　　left ventricular end-systolic diameter and, 1216–1218
　　median sternotomy in, 1218, 1220f
　　minimally invasive, 1219, 1235–1236
　　monitoring in, 1218, 1219f
　　myocardial protection in, 1219–1220
　　pulmonary artery pressure and, 1218
　　right anterolateral thoracotomy in, 1219, 1220f
　　superior biatrial trans-septal approach to, 1220–1221
　　valve exposure in, 1220–1221, 1220f
　traumatic, 1214
Mitral stenosis, 1210–1212
　atrial septal defect and, 1801
　auscultation in, 1211
　catheterization in, 784, 1211
　congenital, 2019–2020, 2023. See also Mitral valve, congenital anomalies of
　　valvuloplasty in, 1695
　diagnosis of, 1210–1211
　echocardiography in, 839–840, 839f–840f, 1211
　etiology of, 1210, 1211f
　historical perspective on, 1207–1208
　after mitral anuloplasty, 1445
　pathophysiology of, 1210
　percutaneous balloon valvuloplasty in, 858, 859f, 1211, 1212f
　percutaneous balloon valvulotomy in, 1211
　surgical treatment of, 1211–1212, 1212f. See also Mitral valve repair
　　commissurotomy in, 1221, 1222f, 1228–1229

Mitral valve
　accessory tissue of, 2017, 2018f, 2022
　anatomy of, 1208–1210
　　anulus, 1209, 1209f. See also Mitral anulus
　　commissure, 1208, 1209f. See also Mitral commissure
　　leaflet, 1209, 1209f
　aortic leaflet of, 705, 705f, 1209, 1209f
　arcade, 2017
　atresia of, in single ventricle, 2043
　blunt injury to, 1174
　on cardiac catheterization, 783–786
　cleft, 2016
　congenital anomalies of, 2015
　　accessory tissue, 2017, 2018f, 2022
　　anulus dilation, 2017
　　arcade valve, 2017
　　chest radiography in, 2019
　　classification of, 2019t, 2018
　　cleft valve, 2016
　　clinical examination in, 2019
　　diagnosis of, 2019–2020
　　echocardiography in, 2019–2020
　　electrocardiography in, 2019
　　hammock valve, 2017
　　leaflet excess, 2017–2018
　　leaflet hypoplasia, 2017
　　medical treatment of, 2020
　　papillary-muscle-to-commissure fusion, 2017, 2017f
　　parachute valve, 2016–2017, 2016f
　　pathologic features of, 2015–2018
　　prolapse syndrome, 2017–2018
　　supravalvular ring, 2016, 2015–2016, 2022
　　surgical treatment of, 2020–2023
　　　atrioventricular valve repair in, 2022–2023, 2023f
　　　leaflet augmentation in, 2022
　　　papillary muscle mobilization in, 2022, 2022f
　　　results of, 2023
　　　tissue resection in, 2022
　　　in type I anomalies, 2018, 2019t, 2021, 2021f
　　　in type II anomalies, 2018, 2019t, 2021–2022, 2022f
　　　in type III anomalies, 2018, 2019t, 2022–2023, 2022f, 2023f
　　　valve repair in, 2020–2023, 2021f–2022f
　　　valve replacement in, 2020
　in congenitally corrected transposition of great arteries, 2004
　cord elongation of, 2017
　double-orifice, 2016–2017
　　atrioventricular canal defect and, 1843, 1845
　echocardiography of, 926–927, 927f
　embryology of, 2015
　endocarditis of, 1214, 1259–1264, 1263f
　　prosthetic valve, 1269, 1275, 1276f
　　surgical treatment of, 1218, 1227, 1231
　hammock, 2017
　in hypertrophic cardiomyopathy, 1495, 1495f
　leaflets of, 705, 705f, 1209, 1209f
　　enlargement of, 2022
　　excess tissue of, 2017–2018
　　isolated hypoplasia of, 2017
　mural leaflet of, 705, 705f, 1209, 1209f
　papillary muscle elongation of, 2017
　papillary-muscle-to-commissure fusion of, 2017, 2017f
　parachute, 2016–2017, 2016f
　　atrioventricular canal defect and, 1843
　prolapse of
　　congenital, 2017–2018
　　in Marfan syndrome, 1025
　　in pectus excavatum, 363
　repair of. See Mitral anuloplasty; Mitral valve repair
　replacement of. See Mitral valve replacement
　robot-assisted surgery on, 1298–1299
　stenosis of. See Mitral stenosis
　supravalvular ring of, 2015–2016, 2022
　surgical exposure of, 1220–1221, 1220f
　transcatheter balloon dilation of, 1695
　vestibule of, 702–703, 702f
Mitral valve repair, 1221–1227. See also Mitral anuloplasty
　in anterior leaflet prolapse, 1223–1226, 1225f–1226f
　anular calcification and, 1227, 1231–1232
　artificial chordoplasty in, 1224–1225, 1226f, 1232
　assessment of, 1221–1222, 1224f
　chordal shortening in, 1226
　chordal transfer in, 1223, 1225f

Mitral valve repair (Continued)
　chordal transposition in, 1223–1224
　in commissural prolapse, 1226
　in congenital anomalies, 2020–2023, 2021f–2023f
　in degenerative valve disease, 1229–1230, 1230t–1231t, 1232f
　in dilated cardiomyopathy, 1231
　edge-to-edge, 1233–1234
　endocarditis and, 1227, 1231
　failure of, 1232–1234, 1233t, 1234f
　historical perspective on, 1207–1208
　morbidity after, 1229
　mortality after, 1229, 1229f–1230f
　papillary muscle shortening in, 1225–1226
　papillary muscle sliding plasty in, 1225
　in posterior leaflet prolapse, 1222–1223, 1224f–1225f
　remodeling ring anuloplasty in, 1221, 1223f
　reoperative, 1219–1220, 1234
　vs. replacement, 1234
　results of, 1229–1234, 1229f, 1230f–1231t, 1233t
　in rheumatic disease, 1230–1231
　saline test in, 1221–1222, 1224f
　systolic anterior motion after, 1234
　thromboembolic events after, 1234
　triangular resection in, 1223
　in type I dysfunction, 1222
　in type II dysfunction, 1222–1226, 1224f–1226f
　in type IIIa dysfunction, 1227
　in type IIIb dysfunction, 1227
　valve analysis for, 1221, 1223f
Mitral valve replacement, 1227–1228, 1228f. See also Prosthetic heart valves
　after atrioventricular canal defect treatment, 1844
　in chronic ischemic regurgitation, 1441, 1444–1445
　complications of, 1235, 1285
　in congenital anomalies, 2020
　endocarditis with, 1275, 1276f
　historical perspective on, 1207–1208
　left ventricular rupture after, 1235
　mortality after, 1234–1235
　results of, 1234–1235
　thrombotic complications of, 1285
Mitral valvuloplasty, 858, 859f, 1211, 1212f
Möbius syndrome, 373–374
MOC31, in pleural effusion, 435t
Modified Konno operation. See Konno operation, modified
Modified McKeown (tri-incisional) esophagectomy. See Esophagectomy, modified McKeown (tri-incisional)
Monitoring, intraoperative, 50
　in children, 1752–1753
Monoclonal antibody, in pleural effusion, 435t
Monostrut cardiac valve prosthesis, 1188
Morgagni hernia, 5, 481, 491f, 508f, 509
Morphine
　in congenital heart disease, 1757
　in NSTE acute coronary syndromes, 873
Mosaic bioprosthesis, 1189–1190, 1190f
Mounier-Kuhn syndrome, 134–135, 134f
MRI. See Magnetic resonance imaging (MRI)
Mucicarmine, in pleural effusion, 435t
Mucin, in pleural effusion, 435t
Mucinous cystadenoma, 156
Mucoepidermoid carcinoma, 329–331, 330f, 330t
Mucormycosis, 190–191, 191f
Mucous gland adenoma, 154, 154f
Multimodality imaging, intraoperative, 2100–2101, 2101f
Multiple endocrine neoplasia1, bronchopulmonary carcinoid tumor in, 324
Mupirocin, in sternal wound infection prevention, 1000
Murmur. See Heart murmur
Muscle(s), 6–10. See also specific muscles
Muscle bridge, myocardial, 1471–1472, 1471f
Mustard operation, 1985–1987, 1987f, 2011
Myasthenia gravis
　preoperative assessment of, 48
　thymectomy in, 641, 642t
　thymoma and, 635, 637
Myasthenic crisis, 57–58
MYBPC3, 1496
Mycobacterium avium infection, 183–184, 185f
Mycobacterium chelonae infection, 183–184, 184f

Mycobacterium tuberculosis infection, 161, 162f, 182–185. *See also* Nontuberculous mycobacterial infection
  aortic, 1066
  pericardial, 1485
Mycophenolate mofetil
  in heart-lung transplantation, 1564t, 1565
  in heart transplantation, 1545
Mycoplasma, in community-acquired pneumonia, 175, 175f
Mycotic aortic aneurysm
  arch, 1042–1043
  thoracic, 1065f
  thoracoabdominal, 1064–1065
Mycotic lung infection, 185–191
Myectomy. *See* Septal myectomy
MYH7, 1496
Myoblasts, 1599–1600, 1600t, 1601f
Myocardial contusion, 1173–1175
Myocardial fiber disarray, in hypertrophic cardiomyopathy, 1496
Myocardial infarction (MI)
  biomarkers in, 871
  C-reactive protein in, 871
  after coronary artery bypass grafting, 1383
  echocardiography after, 833–834, 834f
  electrophysiology study after, 1330
  after esophagectomy, 611
  left ventricular assist device after, 1454, 1508, 1519–1520
  left ventricular remodeling after, 1576–1577, 1577f–1578f
  magnetic resonance imaging in, 795, 795f
  mitral regurgitation after, 833, 1435, 1436f
  myocardial perfusion imaging after, 816–817
  myocardial viability after, 818
    blood flow quantification in, 819–820
    definition of, 818
    flow reserve in, 820
    glucose utilization quantification in, 819
    left ventricular ejection fraction in, 817–818
    positron emission tomography for, 818–820, 819f
    prognostic implications of, 820–821
    single-photon emission computed tomography in, 820
  non–ST-segment elevation, 868
    atrial natriuretic peptide in, 871
    coronary artery bypass grafting in, 1369, 1370t
    diagnosis of, 868–869, 869f
    management of, 873–878, 873t, 875t, 876f
      angiotensin-converting enzyme inhibitors in, 877–878
      antiischemic agents in, 873
      antithrombotic therapy in, 873–874
      beta-blockers in, 877
      fibrinolytic agents in, 878–879, 878t
      guidelines for, 871–878, 872t–873t
      intravenous antithrombin therapy in, 874–875, 875t, 876f
      morphine in, 873
      previous bypass surgery and, 879
      statins in, 878
    percutaneous coronary intervention in, 848–849
    risk stratification of, 869–871, 870f–871f
    troponins in, 871
  pacemaker after, 1309b. *See also* Pacemaker, permanent
  after percutaneous coronary intervention, 854
  pericarditis after, 1486
  postoperative, 54
  pseudoaneurysm and, 833
  regenerative cell-based therapy in, 1609
  ST-segment elevation, 868
    coronary artery bypass grafting in, 1369–1371, 1370t
    diagnosis of, 868–869, 869f
    management of, 878–879, 878t
      guidelines for, 871–873, 872t
      previous bypass surgery and, 879
    percutaneous coronary intervention in, 849
    risk stratification of, 869–871, 870f–871f
    troponins in, 871
  in systemic lupus erythematosus, 1475
  systolic function in, 746
  thrombectomy in, 856–857
  thrombi after, 834–835, 834f–835f
  ventricular septal defect after. *See* Ventricular septal defect, postinfarction

Myocardial ischemia. *See also* Acute coronary syndromes; Angina; Myocardial infarction (MI)
  in coronary–subclavian steal syndrome, 1144f, 1152
  diastolic dysfunction in, 743–744
  echocardiography in, 832–834
  in hypoplastic left heart syndrome, 2031–2032
  magnetic resonance imaging in, 1682, 1684f
  during off-pump coronary artery bypass grafting, 1399
  regenerative cell-based therapy in, 1609
  surgically induced, 978–982
    age and, 981
    biochemical alterations and, 978–979, 979f
    cyanosis and, 981–982
    inflammation and, 981
    irreversible cell injury and, 981
    ischemia-reperfusion injury and, 979–981, 980f–981f
    oxygen consumption and, 978
    ventricular hypertrophy and, 982
Myocardial laser revascularization, percutaneous, 1461–1462
Myocardial perfusion
  radionuclide imaging of, 809. *See also* Single-photon emission computed tomography (SPECT)
    equipment for, 810
    procedure for, 810
    tracers for, 809–810
  after transmyocardial laser therapy, 1461
Myocardial protection, 977
  β-adrenergic antagonists for, 987
  calcium channel blockers for, 987
  cardioplegia for, 978, 982–987
    antegrade administration of, 990
    blood, 989–992, 989f–990f
    crystalloid, 987–989, 988f
    delivery systems in, 990–992, 991f
    hypothermia with, 985, 986f
    metabolic substrates in, 987
    myocardial edema with, 987
    rapid cardiac arrest with, 982–985, 982f, 983t–984t, 985f
    retrograde administration of, 990–991, 991f
    secondary, 991
    solutions for, 983t–984t
      blood, 989–992, 989f–990f
      buffering of, 986–987, 986f
      crystalloid, 987–989, 988f
      hypocalcemic, 987
      osmolarity of, 987
    temperature in, 990
    tepid, 990
  cariporide for, 993
  continuous coronary perfusion for, 977–978
  fibrillatory arrest for, 977
  historical perspective on, 977–978
  hypothermia for, 978, 978f, 985, 986f
  ischemic preconditioning for, 992
  magnesium for, 987
  in mitral valve surgery, 1219–1220
  molecular manipulation for, 993
  postconditioning for, 993
  remote preconditioning for, 992–993
  sodium-hydrogen exchanger inhibitors for, 993
Myocardial regenerative therapy. *See* Regenerative cell-based therapy
Myocardial tagging, in magnetic resonance imaging, 1678–1679, 1680f
Myocardial viability
  pediatric, 1682, 1684f
  postinfarction, 818
    blood flow quantification in, 819–820
    definition of, 818
    flow reserve in, 820
    glucose utilization quantification in, 819
    left ventricular ejection fraction in, 817–818
    positron emission tomography for, 818–820, 819f
    prognostic implications of, 820–821
    single-photon emission computed tomography in, 820
Myocarditis
  left ventricular assist device in, 1508
  pediatric, extracorporeal membrane oxygenation after, 1738
  in systemic lupus erythematosus, 1475

Myocardium, 725. *See also at* Atrium (atria); Cardiac; Heart; Ventricle(s)
  age-related changes in, 981
  cell-based regenerative therapy for. *See* Regenerative cell-based therapy
  cellular biology of, 726, 727f
  contractility of, 732–733, 733f
  cross-bridges of, 732
  energy expenditure by, 747–748, 747f, 978–979, 979f
  excitation-contraction coupling of, 727f, 730–731, 731f
    phosphorylation modulation of, 731–732, 732f
  exercise effects on, 725–726, 726f
  force-velocity relationship of, 733–734, 734f
  function of, 725
  hibernating, 1368–1369
  infarction of. *See* Myocardial infarction (MI)
  intrinsic myogenic tone of, 718, 719f
  ischemia-reperfusion injury to, 979–981, 980f
    age and, 981
    calcium hypothesis of, 979–980, 980f
    cyanosis and, 981–982
    free radical hypothesis of, 980–981, 980f–981f
    inflammation and, 981
  long-term regulation of, 725
  neonatal, 1749
  oxygen consumption of, 716, 747–748, 747f, 978
  protection of. *See* Myocardial protection
  sarcomere mechanics of, 726–730, 727f–730f, 733, 734f–735f
  scar tissue of, 1368–1369
  stunned, 818, 1368–1369
Myocutaneous flaps, in chest wall reconstruction, 383–384, 384f
Myocytes, in hypertrophic cardiomyopathy, 1496
Myoepithelioma, 156
Myxoma, 1633–1635
  asymptomatic, 1634
  clinical manifestations of, 1633–1634
  diagnosis of, 1634, 1634t
  epidemiology of, 1633
  morphology of, 1633, 1636f
  resection of, 1634–1635

N

Nadroparin, in NSTE acute coronary syndromes, 874–875
Nasogastric tube
  esophageal stricture with, 570, 571f
  management of, 53
National Lung Screening Trial, 233
National Quality Forum, 1015
National Surgical Infection Prevention Project, 1015
Natriuretic peptides, in heart failure, 895
Nausea, postoperative, 52
Nd-YAG laser, 74. *See also* Laser therapy
NDO plicator, in gastroesophageal reflux, 80
Necrotizing mediastinitis, 648, 658
Neonate. *See at* Children; Congenital
Nephropathy, contrast, 854
Nerve clipping procedure, in hyperhidrosis, 666
Nerve of Kuntz, 24
Nesiritide, 895, 899, 899t
Neuralgia, postsympathectomy, 403
Neurilemoma (schwannoma), 651–655
Neuroblastoma, 651–652, 654–655
Neuroendocrine tumor. *See also* Carcinoid tumor
  thymic, 638–639
Neuroenteric cyst, 656
Neurofibroma
  esophageal, 567
  mediastinal, 651–655, 652f, 654f
Neurogenic tumors, 27, 651–655, 651b, 652f–654f
Neurologic disorders
  cardiac surgery–related, 949–950, 1005
    assessment of, 1005–1006, 1006f
    biochemical markers in, 1005–1006
    imaging in, 1005, 1006f
    mechanisms of, 1006–1007, 1008f
    prevention of, 1007–1009, 1008t
    prognosis for, 1009, 1009f
    risk for, 1006, 1007t

Neurologic disorders (Continued)
    after cardiopulmonary bypass, 970, 970f, 1725–1726
    after coronary artery bypass grafting, 1384
    in hypoplastic left heart syndrome, 2036
    after pediatric cardiopulmonary bypass, 1725–1726
    with thoracic endovascular aortic repair, 1136
Neurologic examination
    after cardiac surgery, 934, 1005–1006, 1006f
    in native valve endocarditis, 1261
Neuron-specific enolase, after cardiac surgery, 1005–1006
Neuropeptide Y, 718
Neuroprotection. See Brain protection; Spinal cord, protection of
Neuropsychological examination, 1005
Neurotransmitters
    in myocardial excitation-contraction coupling, 731–732, 732f
    in vascular tone, 717–718
Neutrophils, in cardiopulmonary bypass, 935, 1727
Niacin, in atherosclerosis management, 914
Nifedipine, in heart failure, 890
Nitric oxide
    in cardiopulmonary bypass, 963
    in congenital diaphragmatic hernia, 501
    in coronary artery disease, 720, 721f
    in hypoxic pulmonary vasoconstriction, 722, 722f
    inhibition of, 719
    in neonate, 1288
    in pediatric pulmonary hypertension, 1752
    in right heart failure, 943
    in vascular development, 719, 720f
    in vascular tone, 713–715, 715f–716f
Nitric oxide synthase, 713–715, 715f
Nitroglycerin
    for afterload reduction, 939
    after coronary artery bypass grafting, 1382
    in heart failure, 889, 899t
Nitroprusside
    for afterload reduction, 939–940
    in heart failure, 888–889, 889f, 899, 899t
    in pediatric pulmonary hypertension, 1752
Nitrovasodilators, in heart failure, 888–889
Nkx2.5, 1643–1644, 1647
NMDA (N-methyl-D-aspartate) antagonists, in cardiac surgery, 1009
Nodal, 1642–1643
Non–small cell lung cancer. See Lung cancer, non–small cell
Non–ST-segment elevation myocardial infarction. See Myocardial infarction (MI), non–ST-segment elevation
Nontuberculous mycobacterial infection, 183–184, 184f
    resection for, 185
    in women, 183–185, 185f
Noonan's syndrome, 1801
Norepinephrine
    after cardiac surgery, 940–941, 942t
    after cardiopulmonary bypass, 969
    in decompensated heart failure, 899, 899t
    after pediatric cardiac surgery, 1758
Normovolemic hemodilution, 764
Norwood operation, 2028–2033, 2029f. See also Hypoplastic left heart syndrome, surgical management of, stage I (Norwood operation)
NSTE syndromes. See Acute coronary syndromes, non–ST-segment elevation
Nutcracker esophagus, 563, 564f
Nutrition
    after esophageal atresia repair, 542
    postoperative, 52

O

Octreotide, in chylothorax, 56–57
Off-pump coronary artery bypass grafting. See Coronary artery bypass grafting, off-pump
Okihiro syndrome, 1801
Omega-3 fatty acids, 914
Omentum
    in chest wall reconstruction, 384, 384f
    in sternal wound infection treatment, 1000–1001
Omicarbon valve prosthesis, 1188
On-X prosthetic heart valve, 1189

Oncogenes, in mesothelioma, 452
One-and-a-half ventricle repair
    in Ebstein's anomaly, 2064
    in single ventricle, 2044–2045
Opioids
    in congenital heart disease, 1755, 1757
    errors with, 1018
Osler-Weber-Rendu syndrome, 145
Osteochondroma, 384
Osteosarcoma
    cardiac, 1635t
    pulmonary metastases in, 345
Ovarian cancer, pulmonary metastases in, 346
Overeating, gastroesophageal reflux disease and, 524–525
Oximetry, in left-to-right shunt, 782
Oxybutynin, in hyperhidrosis, 663
Oxycel, 770–771
Oxygen, myocardial consumption of, 716, 747–748, 747f, 978
Oxygen therapy. See also Extracorporeal membrane oxygenation
    in acute pulmonary embolism, 1618
    in hypoplastic left heart syndrome, 2027
    after pediatric cardiac surgery, 1758
Oxygenator, for cardiopulmonary bypass, 958, 959f, 1713–1714

P

p53
    in bronchopulmonary carcinoid tumor, 324
    in lung cancer, 677
    in mesothelioma, 451–452
    in pleural effusion, 433, 435t
Pace mapping, 1330–1331
    in atrial tachycardia, 1333
    in ventricular tachycardia, 1337
Pacemaker
    in adult congenital heart disease, 2094
    pediatric, 1312b, 2083–2085, 2084b
    permanent, 1307–1309, 1312–1316
        in atrial fibrillation, 1311b
        in atrioventricular block, 1308b
        capture in, 1313
        after cardiac transplantation, 1310b
        in children, 1312b
        in chronic bifascicular block, 1309b
        codes for, 1315–1316, 1316t
        complications of, 1322–1323, 1322b, 1323f
        in congenital heart failure, 1312b
        in congestive heart failure, 1307–1309, 1313f
        contraindications to, 1309
        historical perspective on, 1305–1306
        in hypersensitive carotid sinus syndrome, 1310b
        in hypertrophic cardiomyopathy, 1311b
        implantation of, 1319–1321
            axillary vein approach to, 1320
            care after, 1322
            cephalic vein (cutdown) approach to, 1319–1320
            subclavian vein approach to, 1320
            technique of, 1320–1321, 1320f–1321f
        indications for, 1307
        lead extraction for, 1323–1325, 1323b, 1325b
            angiographic catheter in, 1324
            Byrd dilator sheath in, 1324
            complications of, 1325, 1325b
            electrosurgical dissection system in, 1324
            excimer laser sheath in, 1324
            forceps in, 1324
            snares in, 1324
            through femoral vein, 1325
            through implant vein, 1324–1325
        leads for, 1313, 1315f
        modes for, 1315–1316, 1316f, 1316t
        after myocardial infarction, 1309b
        in neurocardiogenic syncope, 1310b
        pacing in, 1313, 1315–1316
        preoperative evaluation for, 1319
        pulse generator for, 1312–1313
        sensing in, 1313–1316
        in sinus node dysfunction, 1307b
        during surgery, 1325

Pacemaker (Continued)
    in systolic heart failure, 1311b
    in tachycardia, 1310b
    temporary, 1306
        complications of, 1322–1323, 1322b
        duration of, 1319
        implantation of, 1319
            care after, 1322
        indications for, 1306
        preoperative evaluation for, 1319
        during surgery, 1325
        venous access for, 1306, 1306t
Pacing wire, echocardiography of, 834–835, 834f
Paclitaxel-coated balloon, in femoral artery disease, 1169
Paget-Schroetter syndrome, 392–393, 398–400, 402f
Pain
    with aortic arch aneurysm, 1046
    sympathetically maintained, 403
    in thoracic outlet syndrome, 391–392, 396–397
    after thoracoscopic lobectomy, 283
    after thoracotomy, 56, 283
    with type A aortic dissection, 1096
    with type B aortic dissection, 1117
Palliative therapy
    in esophageal cancer, 621
    in metastatic lung cancer, 347
    in non–small cell lung cancer, 68–69, 69f–70f
Palm, sweating on. See Hyperhidrosis
Palmaz stent, in tracheomalacia, 1777, 1777f
Palpitations, 1330
Pancoast tumor, 262
    angiography in, 315f
    clinical presentation of, 313
    computed tomography of, 314f
    evaluation of, 313–314, 314f–315f
    magnetic resonance imaging of, 314, 314f–315f, 319f
    surgical treatment of, 314–315
        anterior transcervical approach to, 315–318, 315f, 319f–320f
        chest wall resection in, 317, 319f
        neurolysis in, 316–317, 318f
        prevertebral muscle resection in, 316–317, 318f
        subclavian artery dissection in, 316, 317f
        subclavian artery exposure in, 316, 316f
        subclavian vein exposure in, 316, 316f
        atelectasis after, 319
        chemotherapy before, 290–291
        hemothorax after, 318–319
        Horner's syndrome after, 318
        Klumpke-Déjérine syndrome after, 318
        morbidity of, 318–319
        prognosis for, 319–321
        results of, 319–321, 320t, 320b
Pancoast's syndrome, 313, 314
Pancuronium, in congenital heart disease, 1754
Papaverine, after aortic aneurysm repair, 1074–1075, 1075f
Papillary fibroelastoma, 1637
Papillary mesothelioma, 455–456
Papillary muscles
    mitral, 1210
        shortening of, 1225–1226
        sliding plasty of, 1225
    tricuspid, 1243
Papilloma, squamous
    endobronchial, 155–156
    esophageal, 566
Parachute mitral valve, 2016–2017, 2016f
    atrioventricular canal defect and, 1843
Paracrine effects, in myocardial cell-based regenerative therapy, 1607–1608
Paraganglioma, 1634t
Paraplegia
    after aortic repair, 94
    after chest wall resection/reconstruction, 307
    in type A aortic dissection, 1096–1097, 1097t
Parapneumonic effusion, 415
Parathyroid adenoma, mediastinal, 640
Paratracheal dissection
    high, 627–628, 627f–628f
    lower, 628–629, 628f–629f
Paravertebral mass, 656
Paroxysmal atrial fibrillation, 1345–1346
Partial anomalous pulmonary venous drainage. See Anomalous pulmonary venous drainage/connection, partial

Partial atrioventricular canal defects. *See* Atrioventricular canal defects, partial
Partial transposition of great arteries, 1662. *See also* Double-outlet right ventricle
Patent ductus arteriosus, 1781–1783
  clinical presentation of, 1782
  diagnosis of, 1782, 1782f
  imaging of, 794
  left-to-right shunt in, 781–782
  natural history of, 1781–1782
  pathophysiology of, 1781–1782
  prognosis for, 1783
  treatment of, 1782–1783
    in adults, 1782–1783
    in children, 1782–1783
    medical, 1782
    in premature infant, 1782, 1783f
    surgical, 1782–1783
    transcatheter, 1698, 1782–1783
      historical perspective on, 1698
    video-assisted thoracoscopic surgery in, 1793, 1793f
  ventricular septal defect and, 1852
Patent foramen ovale, 1798, 1800f
  closure of, 783f, 860f, 1803, 1805
    percutaneous, 860–861
  decompression illness and, 1804
  echocardiography in, 835, 836f
  left-to-right shunt in, 781–782
  left ventricular assist device implantation and, 1509
  migraine and, 1804
  in pulmonary atresia with ventricular septal defect, 1901
  stroke and, 1803–1804
  in tetralogy of Fallot, 1881
  in truncus arteriosus, 1913
Patient-controlled analgesia, 52
Pectoralis major, 6, 7f, 8t
  congenital absence of. *See* Poland's syndrome
Pectoralis major flap
  in chest wall reconstruction, 383, 384f
  in sternal wound infection, 1001
Pectoralis minor, 7f, 8t
Pectus carinatum, 371–373, 371t, 374f
  asymmetric, 371, 372f
  chondrogladiolar, 371, 372f
  chondromanubrial, 371–372, 373f–375f
  etiology of, 371–372
  musculoskeletal abnormalities with, 371, 373t
  pulmonary function testing in, 361–362
  repair of, 372–373, 374f–375f, 375f
Pectus excavatum, 359–371, 360f
  cardiovascular evaluation in, 362–363
  echocardiographic evaluation in, 363
  electrocardiography in, 361
  etiology of, 359–360
  genetics of, 360
  heart disease with, 359, 360t
  incidence of, 359–360
  in Marfan's syndrome, 360
  mitral valve prolapse in, 363
  murmur in, 361
  musculoskeletal abnormalities in, 360, 361t
  pathophysiology of, 361–363
  in prune-belly syndrome, 360
  pulmonary function testing in, 361–362
  repair of, 363–371
    cardiopulmonary function after, 361
    cardiovascular function after, 363
    hemorrhage with, 367
    minimally invasive, 364–367, 365f
    open, 367–371, 368f, 370f–371f, 370t
    overcorrection in, 367
    Silastic mold implantation in, 364
    sternal turnover in, 364
    tripod fixation in, 364
  symptoms of, 360
Penetrating trauma. *See* Cardiac injury, penetrating; Trauma, penetrating
Percent reactive antibody (PRA) titer
  in heart-lung transplantation, 1558
  in heart transplantation, 1536–1537, 1537b
PercuSurge GuardWire, 856
Percutaneous circulatory assist devices, 861, 861f–862f

Percutaneous coronary interventions, 847
  anaphylactoid reactions with, 854–855
  arterial access for, 848, 848f
  atherectomy devices in, 856, 856f
  benefits of, 849b
  in chronic stable angina, 849–852
  complications of, 853–855
  contrast nephropathy with, 854
  after coronary artery bypass grafting, 857, 857b
  vs. coronary artery bypass grafting, 849–852, 849b, 850f, 851t, 853f, 1387–1389, 1388f
  coronary artery bypass grafting with, 857
  drug-eluting stents in, 848, 855–856
    recurrent disease and, 855
  elective, 852–853
  facilitated, 849
  failed, coronary artery bypass grafting in, 1369–1371, 1371f
  hemorrhagic complications of, 854
  historical perspective on, 847–848, 847f
  in left main-stem disease, 852
  mitral regurgitation after, 1435, 1436f
  mortality during, 853
  multivessel, 849–852, 850f, 851t, 853f
  myocardial infarction after, 854
  in non-ST-segment myocardial infarction, 848–849
  noncardiac surgery and, 852–853
  in postinfarction ventricular septal defect repair, 1454
  vs. reoperative coronary artery bypass grafting, 1421, 1423
  restenosis after, 855, 855t
  SPECT imaging after, 821
  in ST-segment myocardial infarction, 849
  stents in, 848
    bypass grafting with, 857
    in left main-stem disease, 852
    noncardiac surgery after, 853
    recurrent disease and, 855
    thrombosis and, 855–856
  surgical backup for, 853–854
  thrombectomy with, 856–857
  ultrasound in, 857
  in unstable angina, 848–849
  vascular complications of, 854
Percutaneous endovascular valve replacement, 859–860, 859f
Percutaneous myocardial laser revascularization, 1461–1462
Percutaneous peripheral interventionsat, 1164–1169. *See also* Aorta *and at specific arteries*
  in aortic disease, 1164–1165, 1165f–1166f
  in head and neck vessels, 1165–1167, 1167f
  in lower extremity, 1168–1169
  in renal vessels, 1167–1168
Percutaneous transluminal coronary angioplasty, 847–848, 847f. *See also* Percutaneous coronary interventions
Perfluorocarbons, in congenital diaphragmatic hernia, 501, 506–507, 507f
"Performance Measurement: Accelerating Improvement" (Institute of Medicine), 1014–1015
Pericardial cavity
  anatomy of, 697, 697f–698f
  oblique sinus of, 697, 698f
  transverse sinus of, 697, 698f
Pericardial cyst, 648, 1487–1488, 1488f
Pericardial diverticula, 1487–1488
Pericardial effusion, 647
  catheterization in, 785, 786f
  echocardiography in, 443f, 444, 832, 832f, 837, 837f, 1483f
  imaging of, 797–799, 799f
  malignant, 442–446
    evaluation of, 443, 443f
    mechanism of, 442
    treatment of, 443–446, 444f–445f
  pathophysiology of, 1480–1481
  pericardiocentesis in, 1484, 1484f
Pericardial fluid, 1480
Pericardial hernia, 491t, 508f, 509
Pericardial pressure, 1480
  after cardiac surgery, 938
Pericardial rub, in pulmonary metastases, 339

Pericardial window
  in cardiac trauma, 101, 101f
  in malignant pericardial effusion, 444–445, 444f–445f
  subxiphoid, 101, 101f, 1175–1176, 1175f, 1485, 1489, 1489f
  transdiaphragmatic, 1490
  transpleural, 1490, 1490f
Pericardiectomy, 1487, 1490–1491, 1491f
  in malignant pericardial effusion, 444
Pericardiocentesis, 1484, 1484f
  in malignant pericardial effusion, 443
  in penetrating cardiac injury, 1176, 1176f
Pericardioperitoneal shunt, in malignant pericardial effusion, 445
Pericardioscopy, 1489
Pericardiotomy, in off-pump coronary artery bypass grafting, 1400–1401, 1401f
Pericarditis, 647
  catheterization in, 785–786, 786f–787f
  constrictive, 1481b, 1482f, 1487–1489
    diagnosis of, 1482f, 1483, 1487
    differential diagnosis of, 1482
    etiology of, 1487
    imaging of, 797–799, 800f
    pathophysiology of, 1481–1482
    treatment of, 1487–1489
  echocardiography in, 837–838
  magnetic resonance imaging of, 797–799, 799f–800f
  nonconstrictive, 1484–1487
    autoimmune, 1485–1486
    diagnosis of, 1484–1485
    etiology of, 1485–1487, 1485t
    idiopathic, 1485
    infectious, 1485
    malignant, 1486
    metabolic, 1486
    after myocardial infarction, 1486
    postoperative, 1486
    radiation-induced, 1486
    traumatic, 1486
  in systemic lupus erythematosus, 1475
Pericardium, 1479–1484
  absence of, 1488
  anatomy of, 697, 697f, 1479–1480, 1480f
  biopsy of, 1484
  blood supply of, 1480
  blunt injury to, 1174
  in cardiac function, 752
  congenital defects of, 1488–1489
  evaluation of, 1483–1484, 1483f–1484f
  historical descriptions of, 1479
  lipoma of, 1636–1637
  pathophysiology of, 1480–1482
  physiology of, 1480
  rupture of, 1489
  surgical procedures on, 1489–1491, 1489f
  tumors of, 1488
Perimysial fibers, 739–740, 740f
Peripheral angiography, 1157–1159
  of abdominal aorta, 1159–1160, 1161f
  of aorta, 1159–1160
  of carotid arteries, 1161–1162, 1162f
  complications of, 1158–1159, 1158t
  contraindications to, 1158, 1158t
  of head and neck, 1160–1162, 1161f
  of iliac artery, 1162–1164, 1163f
  indications for, 1157–1158, 1158t
  of infrainguinal vessels, 1164, 1164f
  of lower extremity, 1162–1164, 1163f
  of renal arteries, 1162
  of subclavian artery, 1160–1161, 1161f
  technical aspects of, 1159, 1159f
  of thoracic aorta, 1159, 1160f
Peripheral arterial disease, 1157
  angiography in. *See* Peripheral angiography
  grading of, 1157, 1158t
  percutaneous interventions for, 1164–1169. *See also specific arteries*
  in type B aortic dissection, 1117–1118, 1118t
Peristalsis, esophageal, 521–522, 522f
Peritoneum, diaphragmatic attachment of, 474–475
Permanent pacemaker. *See* Pacemaker, permanent

Neurologic disorders (Continued)
　　after cardiopulmonary bypass, 970, 970f, 1725–1726
　　after coronary artery bypass grafting, 1384
　　in hypoplastic left heart syndrome, 2036
　　after pediatric cardiopulmonary bypass, 1725–1726
　　with thoracic endovascular aortic repair, 1136
Neurologic examination
　　after cardiac surgery, 934, 1005–1006, 1006f
　　in native valve endocarditis, 1261
Neuron-specific enolase, after cardiac surgery, 1005–1006
Neuropeptide Y, 718
Neuroprotection. See Brain protection; Spinal cord, protection of
Neuropsychological examination, 1005
Neurotransmitters
　　in myocardial excitation-contraction coupling, 731–732, 732f
　　in vascular tone, 717–718
Neutrophils, in cardiopulmonary bypass, 935, 1727
Niacin, in atherosclerosis management, 914
Nifedipine, in heart failure, 890
Nitric oxide
　　in cardiopulmonary bypass, 963
　　in congenital diaphragmatic hernia, 501
　　in coronary artery disease, 720, 721f
　　in hypoxic pulmonary vasoconstriction, 722, 722f
　　inhibition of, 719
　　in neonate, 1288
　　in pediatric pulmonary hypertension, 1752
　　in right heart failure, 943
　　in vascular development, 719, 720f
　　in vascular tone, 713–715, 715f–716f
Nitric oxide synthase, 713–715, 715f
Nitroglycerin
　　for afterload reduction, 939
　　after coronary artery bypass grafting, 1382
　　in heart failure, 889, 899t
Nitroprusside
　　for afterload reduction, 939–940
　　in heart failure, 888–889, 889f, 899, 899t
　　in pediatric pulmonary hypertension, 1752
Nitrovasodilators, in heart failure, 888–889
Nkx2.5, 1643–1644, 1647
NMDA (N-methyl-D-aspartate) antagonists, in cardiac surgery, 1009
Nodal, 1642–1643
Non–small cell lung cancer. See Lung cancer, non–small cell
Non–ST-segment elevation myocardial infarction. See Myocardial infarction (MI), non–ST-segment elevation
Nontuberculous mycobacterial infection, 183–184, 184f
　　resection for, 185
　　in women, 183–185, 185f
Noonan's syndrome, 1801
Norepinephrine
　　after cardiac surgery, 940–941, 942t
　　after cardiopulmonary bypass, 969
　　in decompensated heart failure, 899, 899t
　　after pediatric cardiac surgery, 1758
Normovolemic hemodilution, 764
Norwood operation, 2028–2033, 2029f. See also Hypoplastic left heart syndrome, surgical management of, stage I (Norwood operation)
NSTE syndromes. See Acute coronary syndromes, non–ST-segment elevation
Nutcracker esophagus, 563, 564f
Nutrition
　　after esophageal atresia repair, 542
　　postoperative, 52

O

Octreotide, in chylothorax, 56–57
Off-pump coronary artery bypass grafting. See Coronary artery bypass grafting, off-pump
Okihiro syndrome, 1801
Omega-3 fatty acids, 914
Omentum
　　in chest wall reconstruction, 384, 384f
　　in sternal wound infection treatment, 1000–1001
Omicarbon valve prosthesis, 1188
On-X prosthetic heart valve, 1189

Oncogenes, in mesothelioma, 452
One-and-a-half ventricle repair
　　in Ebstein's anomaly, 2064
　　in single ventricle, 2044–2045
Opioids
　　in congenital heart disease, 1755, 1757
　　errors with, 1018
Osler-Weber-Rendu syndrome, 145
Osteochondroma, 384
Osteosarcoma
　　cardiac, 1635t
　　pulmonary metastases in, 345
Ovarian cancer, pulmonary metastases in, 346
Overeating, gastroesophageal reflux disease and, 524–525
Oximetry, in left-to-right shunt, 782
Oxybutynin, in hyperhidrosis, 663
Oxycel, 770–771
Oxygen, myocardial consumption of, 716, 747–748, 747f, 978
Oxygen therapy. See also Extracorporeal membrane oxygenation
　　in acute pulmonary embolism, 1618
　　in hypoplastic left heart syndrome, 2027
　　after pediatric cardiac surgery, 1758
Oxygenator, for cardiopulmonary bypass, 958, 959f, 1713–1714

P

p53
　　in bronchopulmonary carcinoid tumor, 324
　　in lung cancer, 677
　　in mesothelioma, 451–452
　　in pleural effusion, 433, 435t
Pace mapping, 1330–1331
　　in atrial tachycardia, 1333
　　in ventricular tachycardia, 1337
Pacemaker
　　in adult congenital heart disease, 2094
　　pediatric, 1312b, 2083–2085, 2084b
　　permanent, 1307–1309, 1312–1316
　　　in atrial fibrillation, 1311b
　　　in atrioventricular block, 1308b
　　　capture in, 1313
　　　after cardiac transplantation, 1310b
　　　in children, 1312b
　　　in chronic bifascicular block, 1309b
　　　codes for, 1315–1316, 1316t
　　　complications of, 1322–1323, 1322b, 1323f
　　　in congenital heart failure, 1312b
　　　in congestive heart failure, 1307–1309, 1313f
　　　contraindications to, 1309
　　　historical perspective on, 1305–1306
　　　in hypersensitive carotid sinus syndrome, 1310b
　　　in hypertrophic cardiomyopathy, 1311b
　　　implantation of, 1319–1321
　　　　axillary vein approach to, 1320
　　　　care after, 1322
　　　　cephalic vein (cutdown) approach to, 1319–1320
　　　　subclavian vein approach to, 1320
　　　　technique of, 1320–1321, 1320f–1321f
　　　indications for, 1307
　　　lead extraction for, 1323–1325, 1323b, 1325b
　　　　angiographic catheter in, 1324
　　　　Byrd dilator sheath in, 1324
　　　　complications of, 1325, 1325b
　　　　electrosurgical dissection system in, 1324
　　　　excimer laser sheath in, 1324
　　　　forceps in, 1324
　　　　snares in, 1324
　　　　through femoral vein, 1325
　　　　through implant vein, 1324–1325
　　　leads for, 1313, 1315f
　　　modes for, 1315–1316, 1316f, 1316t
　　　after myocardial infarction, 1309b
　　　in neurocardiogenic syncope, 1310b
　　　pacing in, 1313, 1315–1316
　　　preoperative evaluation for, 1319
　　　pulse generator for, 1312–1313
　　　sensing in, 1313–1316
　　　in sinus node dysfunction, 1307b
　　　during surgery, 1325

Pacemaker (Continued)
　　　in systolic heart failure, 1311b
　　　in tachycardia, 1310b
　　temporary, 1306
　　　complications of, 1322–1323, 1322b
　　　duration of, 1319
　　　implantation of, 1319
　　　　care after, 1322
　　　indications for, 1306
　　　preoperative evaluation for, 1319
　　　during surgery, 1325
　　　venous access for, 1306, 1306t
Pacing wire, echocardiography of, 834–835, 834f
Paclitaxel-coated balloon, in femoral artery disease, 1169
Paget-Schroetter syndrome, 392–393, 398–400, 402f
Pain
　　with aortic arch aneurysm, 1046
　　sympathetically maintained, 403
　　in thoracic outlet syndrome, 391–392, 396–397
　　after thoracoscopic lobectomy, 283
　　after thoracotomy, 56, 283
　　with type A aortic dissection, 1096
　　with type B aortic dissection, 1117
Palliative therapy
　　in esophageal cancer, 621
　　in metastatic lung cancer, 347
　　in non–small cell lung cancer, 68–69, 69f–70f
Palm, sweating on. See Hyperhidrosis
Palmaz stent, in tracheomalacia, 1777, 1777f
Palpitations, 1330
Pancoast tumor, 262
　　angiography in, 315f
　　clinical presentation of, 313
　　computed tomography of, 314f
　　evaluation of, 313–314, 314f–315f
　　magnetic resonance imaging of, 314, 314f–315f, 319f
　　surgical treatment of, 314–315
　　　anterior transcervical approach to, 315–318, 315f, 319f–320f
　　　　chest wall resection in, 317, 319f
　　　　neurolysis in, 316–317, 318f
　　　　prevertebral muscle resection in, 316–317, 318f
　　　　subclavian artery dissection in, 316, 317f
　　　　subclavian artery exposure in, 316, 316f
　　　　subclavian vein exposure in, 316, 316f
　　　atelectasis after, 319
　　　chemotherapy before, 290–291
　　　hemothorax after, 318–319
　　　Horner's syndrome after, 318
　　　Klumpke-Déjérine syndrome after, 318
　　　morbidity of, 318–319
　　　prognosis for, 319–321
　　　results of, 319–321, 320t, 320b
Pancoast's syndrome, 313, 314
Pancuronium, in congenital heart disease, 1754
Papaverine, after aortic aneurysm repair, 1074–1075, 1075f
Papillary fibroelastoma, 1637
Papillary mesothelioma, 455–456
Papillary muscles
　　mitral, 1210
　　　shortening of, 1225–1226
　　　sliding plasty of, 1225
　　tricuspid, 1243
Papilloma, squamous
　　endobronchial, 155–156
　　esophageal, 566
Parachute mitral valve, 2016–2017, 2016f
　　atrioventricular canal defect and, 1843
Paracrine effects, in myocardial cell-based regenerative therapy, 1607–1608
Paraganglioma, 1634t
Paraplegia
　　after aortic repair, 94
　　after chest wall resection/reconstruction, 307
　　in type A aortic dissection, 1096–1097, 1097t
Parapneumonic effusion, 415
Parathyroid adenoma, mediastinal, 640
Paratracheal dissection
　　high, 627–628, 627f–628f
　　lower, 628–629, 628f–629f
Paravertebral mass, 656
Paroxysmal atrial fibrillation, 1345–1346
Partial anomalous pulmonary venous drainage. See Anomalous pulmonary venous drainage/connection, partial

Partial atrioventricular canal defects. *See* Atrioventricular canal defects, partial
Partial transposition of great arteries, 1662. *See also* Double-outlet right ventricle
Patent ductus arteriosus, 1781–1783
　clinical presentation of, 1782
　diagnosis of, 1782, 1782f
　imaging of, 794
　left-to-right shunt in, 781–782
　natural history of, 1781–1782
　pathophysiology of, 1781–1782
　prognosis for, 1783
　treatment of, 1782–1783
　　in adults, 1782–1783
　　in children, 1782–1783
　　medical, 1782
　　in premature infant, 1782, 1783f
　　surgical, 1782–1783
　　transcatheter, 1698, 1782–1783
　　　historical perspective on, 1698
　　video-assisted thoracoscopic surgery in, 1793, 1793f
　ventricular septal defect and, 1852
Patent foramen ovale, 1798, 1800f
　closure of, 783t, 860f, 1803, 1805
　　percutaneous, 860–861
　decompression illness and, 1804
　echocardiography in, 835, 836f
　left-to-right shunt in, 781–782
　left ventricular assist device implantation and, 1509
　migraine and, 1804
　in pulmonary atresia with ventricular septal defect, 1901
　stroke and, 1803–1804
　in tetralogy of Fallot, 1881
　in truncus arteriosus, 1913
Patient-controlled analgesia, 52
Pectoralis major, 6, 7f, 8t
　congenital absence of. *See* Poland's syndrome
Pectoralis major flap
　in chest wall reconstruction, 383, 384f
　in sternal wound infection, 1001
Pectoralis minor, 7f, 8t
Pectus carinatum, 371–373, 371t, 374f
　asymmetric, 371, 372f
　chondrogladiolar, 371, 372f
　chondromanubrial, 371–372, 373f–375f
　etiology of, 371–372
　musculoskeletal abnormalities with, 371, 373t
　pulmonary function testing in, 361–362
　repair of, 372–373, 374f–375f, 375f
Pectus excavatum, 359–371, 360f
　cardiovascular evaluation in, 362–363
　echocardiographic evaluation in, 363
　electrocardiography in, 361
　etiology of, 359–360
　genetics of, 360
　heart disease with, 359, 360t
　incidence of, 359–360
　in Marfan's syndrome, 360
　mitral valve prolapse in, 363
　murmur in, 361
　musculoskeletal abnormalities in, 360, 361t
　pathophysiology of, 361–363
　in prune-belly syndrome, 360
　pulmonary function testing in, 361–362
　repair of, 363–371
　　cardiopulmonary function after, 361
　　cardiovascular function after, 363
　　hemorrhage with, 367
　　minimally invasive, 364–367, 365f
　　open, 367–371, 368f, 370f–371f, 370t
　　overcorrection in, 367
　　Silastic mold implantation in, 364
　　sternal turnover in, 364
　　tripod fixation in, 364
　symptoms of, 360
Penetrating trauma. *See* Cardiac injury, penetrating; Trauma, penetrating
Percent reactive antibody (PRA) titer
　in heart-lung transplantation, 1558
　in heart transplantation, 1536–1537, 1537b
PercuSurge GuardWire, 856
Percutaneous circulatory assist devices, 861, 861f–862f

Percutaneous coronary interventions, 847
　anaphylactoid reactions with, 854–855
　arterial access for, 848, 848f
　atherectomy devices in, 856, 856f
　benefits of, 849b
　in chronic stable angina, 849–852
　complications of, 853–855
　contrast nephropathy with, 854
　after coronary artery bypass grafting, 857, 857b
　vs. coronary artery bypass grafting, 849–852, 849b, 850f, 851f, 853f, 1387–1389, 1388t
　coronary artery bypass grafting with, 857
　drug-eluting stents in, 848, 855–856
　　recurrent disease and, 855
　elective, 852–853
　facilitated, 849
　failed, coronary artery bypass grafting in, 1369–1371, 1371f
　hemorrhagic complications of, 854
　historical perspective on, 847–848, 847f
　in left main-stem disease, 852
　mitral regurgitation after, 1435, 1436f
　mortality during, 853
　multivessel, 849–852, 850f, 851f, 853f
　myocardial infarction after, 854
　in non-ST-segment myocardial infarction, 848–849
　noncardiac surgery and, 852–853
　in postinfarction ventricular septal defect repair, 1454
　vs. reoperative coronary artery bypass grafting, 1421, 1423
　restenosis after, 855, 855t
　SPECT imaging after, 821
　in ST-segment myocardial infarction, 849
　stents in, 848
　　bypass grafting with, 857
　　in left main-stem disease, 852
　　noncardiac surgery after, 853
　　recurrent disease and, 855
　　thrombosis and, 855–856
　surgical backup for, 853–854
　thrombectomy with, 856–857
　ultrasound in, 857
　in unstable angina, 848–849
　vascular complications of, 854
Percutaneous endovascular valve replacement, 859–860, 859f
Percutaneous myocardial laser revascularization, 1461–1462
Percutaneous peripheral interventionsat, 1164–1169. *See also* Aorta *and at specific arteries*
　in aortic disease, 1164–1165, 1165f–1166f
　in head and neck vessels, 1165–1167, 1167f
　in lower extremity, 1168–1169
　in renal vessels, 1167–1168
Percutaneous transluminal coronary angioplasty, 847–848, 847f. *See also* Percutaneous coronary interventions
Perfluorocarbons, in congenital diaphragmatic hernia, 501, 506–507, 507f
"Performance Measurement: Accelerating Improvement" (Institute of Medicine), 1014–1015
Pericardial cavity
　anatomy of, 697, 697f–698f
　oblique sinus of, 697, 698f
　transverse sinus of, 697, 698f
Pericardial cyst, 648, 1487–1488, 1488f
Pericardial diverticula, 1487–1488
Pericardial effusion, 647
　catheterization in, 785, 786f
　echocardiography in, 443f, 444, 832, 832f, 837, 837f, 1483f
　imaging of, 797–799, 799f
　malignant, 442–446
　　evaluation of, 443, 443f
　　mechanism of, 442
　　treatment of, 443–446, 444f–445f
　pathophysiology of, 1480–1481
　pericardiocentesis in, 1484, 1484f
Pericardial fluid, 1480
Pericardial hernia, 491t, 508f, 509
Pericardial pressure, 1480
　after cardiac surgery, 938
Pericardial rub, in pulmonary metastases, 339

Pericardial window
　in cardiac trauma, 101, 101f
　in malignant pericardial effusion, 444–445, 444f–445f
　subxiphoid, 101, 101f, 1175–1176, 1175f, 1485, 1489, 1489f
　transdiaphragmatic, 1490
　transpleural, 1490, 1490f
Pericardiectomy, 1487, 1490–1491, 1491f
　in malignant pericardial effusion, 444
Pericardiocentesis, 1484, 1484f
　in malignant pericardial effusion, 443
　in penetrating cardiac injury, 1176, 1176f
Pericardioperitoneal shunt, in malignant pericardial effusion, 445
Pericardioscopy, 1489
Pericardiotomy, in off-pump coronary artery bypass grafting, 1400–1401, 1401f
Pericarditis, 647
　catheterization in, 785–786, 786f–787f
　constrictive, 1481b, 1482f, 1487–1489
　　diagnosis of, 1482f, 1483, 1487
　　differential diagnosis of, 1482
　　etiology of, 1487
　　imaging of, 797–799, 800f
　　pathophysiology of, 1481–1482
　　treatment of, 1487–1489
　echocardiography in, 837–838
　magnetic resonance imaging of, 797–799, 799f–800f
　nonconstrictive, 1484–1487
　　autoimmune, 1485–1486
　　diagnosis of, 1484–1485
　　etiology of, 1485–1487, 1485t
　　idiopathic, 1485
　　infectious, 1485
　　malignant, 1486
　　metabolic, 1486
　　after myocardial infarction, 1486
　　postoperative, 1486
　　radiation-induced, 1486
　　traumatic, 1486
　in systemic lupus erythematosus, 1475
Pericardium, 1479–1484
　absence of, 1488
　anatomy of, 697, 697f, 1479–1480, 1480f
　biopsy of, 1484
　blood supply of, 1480
　blunt injury to, 1174
　in cardiac function, 752
　congenital defects of, 1488–1489
　evaluation of, 1483–1484, 1483f–1484f
　historical descriptions of, 1479
　lipoma of, 1636–1637
　pathophysiology of, 1480–1482
　physiology of, 1480
　rupture of, 1489
　surgical procedures on, 1489–1491, 1489f
　tumors of, 1488
Perimysial fibers, 739–740, 740f
Peripheral angiography, 1157–1159
　of abdominal aorta, 1159–1160, 1161f
　of aorta, 1159–1160
　of carotid arteries, 1161–1162, 1162f
　complications of, 1158–1159, 1158t
　contraindications to, 1158, 1158t
　of head and neck, 1160–1162, 1161f
　of iliac artery, 1162–1164, 1163f
　indications for, 1157–1158, 1158t
　of infrainguinal vessels, 1164, 1164f
　of lower extremity, 1162–1164, 1163f
　of renal arteries, 1162
　of subclavian artery, 1160–1161, 1161f
　technical aspects of, 1159, 1159f
　of thoracic aorta, 1159, 1160f
Peripheral arterial disease, 1157
　angiography in. *See* Peripheral angiography
　grading of, 1157, 1158t
　percutaneous interventions for, 1164–1169. *See also specific arteries*
　in type B aortic dissection, 1117–1118, 1118t
Peristalsis, esophageal, 521–522, 522f
Peritoneum, diaphragmatic attachment of, 474–475
Permanent pacemaker. *See* Pacemaker, permanent

pH
  in cardiopulmonary bypass, 922, 958–959, 1722–1723
  esophageal
    24-hour monitoring of, 529–532, 531f, 531t, 552–553, 555t
    wireless monitoring of, 553, 555f
pH-stat strategy
  in adult cardiopulmonary bypass, 922, 958
  in pediatric cardiopulmonary bypass, 1723
Phenylephrine, after cardiac surgery, 940–941, 942t
Phosphodiesterase inhibitors, in heart failure, 894–895, 895f
Phospholipids, 905
Phosphorus-32, for malignant pleural effusion, 439–440
Phosphorylcholine coating, in cardiopulmonary bypass, 968
Photodynamic therapy, 67–71, 77t
  in Barrett's esophagus, 69–71
  contraindications to, 68
  definition of, 67
  diffuser fiber for, 68, 68f
  in esophageal cancer, 69–71
  in lung cancer, 68–69, 69f–70f
  mechanism of action of, 67
  in mesothelioma, 466–467
  photosensitivity reaction with, 69
  photosensitizers for, 67
  technique of, 67–68, 68f
Photosensitivity reaction, photodynamic therapy and, 69
Phrenic artery, 4, 475–476, 477f
Phrenic nerve, 475f
  anatomy of, 4, 19f, 24, 475f, 476–477
  embryology of, 491
  injury to, 478–479, 507–509
    phrenic nerve pacing in, 483
Phrenic nerve pacemaker, 483–484, 484f
Phrenic vein, 476
Physical opioid dependence, in children, 1757
Physical therapy, postoperative, 53
Pill, esophageal stricture with, 570
Pitx2, 1642–1643
Plantar hyperhidrosis, 661–662. See also Hyperhidrosis
Plaque, atherosclerotic, 868, 868f
Plasmacytoma, 332–333
Plasmapheresis
  in heart transplantation, 1536–1537, 1537b
  platelet, 764
Plastic bronchitis, 2050
Plate fixation, in sternal wound infection, 1001, 1001f
Platelet(s)
  activation of, 757–758, 758f
  in acute coronary syndromes, 868, 869f
  in cardiopulmonary bypass, 964–965
  dysfunction of
    acquired, 760
    cardiopulmonary bypass and, 1287, 1724
  prosthetic surface deposition of, 1279
  transfusion of
    in coronary artery bypass grafting, 1378
    guidelines for, 762b
    storage lesion and, 763–764
Platelet-derived growth factor, in mesothelioma, 452–453
Platelet plasmapheresis, 764
Pleura, 449
  adenomatoid tumor of, 455
  anatomy of, 449
  asbestos-associated pathology of, 449–453. See also Mesothelioma, malignant
  blastoma of, 456
  blood supply to, 449
  calcifying fibrous tumor of, 455
  desmoid tumor of, 455
  desmoplastic small round cell tumor of, 457
  diaphragmatic attachment of, 474–475, 477f
  effusion of. See Pleural effusion
  embryology of, 449
  inflammatory reactions of, 453–454, 453b
  injury response of, 449, 453–454, 453b
  intermediate lesions of, 454
  lipoblastoma of, 455
  lipoma of, 455
  liposarcoma of, 456
  mechanical abrasion of, 440

Pleura (Continued)
  mesothelial cyst of, 455
  mesothelioma of. See Mesothelioma
  metastatic tumors of, 457
  parietal, 449
  plaques of, 451
  primitive neuroectodermal tumor of, 456–457
  schwannoma of, 455
  solitary fibrous tumor of
    benign, 454–455
    malignant, 456–457
  surface anatomy of, 11
  synovial sarcoma of, 456
  thymoma of, 455–456
  tumors of
    benign, 454–455, 454b
    malignant, 454b, 455–467. See also Mesothelioma, malignant
    metastatic, 457
  vascular sarcoma of, 456
  visceral, 449
Pleural cavity chemoperfusion, in non–small cell lung cancer, 690–691
Pleural cupola, 4
Pleural effusion
  vs. chylothorax, 428
  imaging in, 34, 431–432, 433f
  malignant, 431–442, 457
    biopsy in, 433–434
    catheter drainage of, 436, 438f
    chemistry in, 433, 436t
    cytogenetics in, 433
    cytology in, 433–434
    demographics of, 431
    etiology of, 431
    evaluation of, 431–434
    imaging in, 431–432, 433f
    immunocytochemistry in, 433, 435t
    laboratory tests in, 432–433
    laser therapy in, 440
    in lung cancer, 269
    mechanical abrasion in, 440
    physical findings in, 431
    pleurectomy in, 440–441, 443f
    pleuroperitoneal shunting of, 436, 439f
    prognosis for, 440–442
    radiopharmaceutical interventions in, 439–440
    sclerosis-based management of, 436–439
      bleomycin for, 438, 441t–442t
      chest radiography after, 434
      Corynebacterium parvum for, 438–439
      cycline drugs for, 438, 441t–442t
      results of, 441t–442t
      talc for, 437–438, 440f, 441t–442t
    thoracentesis in, 432, 434f
    thoracoscopy in, 433, 437f
    treatment of, 434–440
Pleural fluid
  in empyema, 417
  triglycerides in, 428
Pleural membrane, 449
Pleural space sterilization, in empyema, 420–422
Pleural tent, 55
Pleurectomy
  in malignant pleural effusion, 440–441, 443f
  in mesothelioma, 463–464
Pleurodesis
  sclerosant, 436–439
    bleomycin for, 438
    chest radiography after, 434
    Corynebacterium parvum for, 438–439
    cycline drugs for, 438
    results of, 441t–442t
    talc for, 437–438, 440f, 441t
  in spontaneous pneumothorax, 410–411, 411f
Pleuroperitoneal shunting, in malignant pleural effusion, 436, 439f
Pleuropulmonary synovial sarcoma, 456
Pleurotomy, right, in off-pump coronary artery bypass grafting, 1400–1401
Pneumatic compression devices, in pulmonary embolism prophylaxis, 1617
Pneumocystis carinii infection
  after heart-lung transplantation, 1566
  after lung transplantation, 219

Pneumonectomy, 255–256. See also Lung cancer, non–small cell, surgical treatment of
  age and, 40
  bronchial management in, 256
  chest tube placement in, 256–257
  in children, 130
  chylothorax after, 427, 429
  drainage tube after, 51
  extrapleural
    in diaphragmatic disease, 485–486, 485f–486f
    in mesothelioma, 455–456, 461–462, 462f–463f, 464
  fluid therapy after, 50
  hilar dissection in, 254f, 256, 256f
  incision in, 255–256
  in lung transplantation, 214–215
  pulmonary edema after, 53–54
Pneumonia
  aspiration, 179
  community-acquired, 173–178
    atypical pathogens in, 173, 175, 175f–176f
    chest radiography in, 174, 175f–176f
    Chlamydia in, 175
    clinical presentation of, 174–175, 175f–177f
    definition of, 173
    drug-resistant, 177–178
    laboratory studies in, 174
    Legionella in, 175, 176f
    mortality with, 173
    Mycoplasma in, 175, 175f
    pathogens in, 173, 174t
    risk factors for, 173–174, 174t
    severity of, 175–176, 177f
    treatment of, 176–178, 178f
  eosinophilic, 163–164
  after esophagectomy, 609–610
  flexible diagnostic bronchoscopy, 64
  health care–associated, 179
  hospital-acquired, 178–179
    risk factors for, 178
  interstitial
    desquamative, 167
    idiopathic, 165–168, 165b, 166t
    lymphocytic, 168
    nonspecific, 167
    usual, 165–167
  pleural effusion with, 415
  post-traumatic, 107–108
  postoperative, 53, 56
    prevention of, 49
  ventilator-associated, 178–179
    prevention of, 1017
Pneumonia Severity Index, 175–176, 177f
Pneumonitis
  hypersensitivity, 161, 161t
  interstitial, 33f, 167
  organizing, cryptogenic, 167–168
Pneumopericardium, 1486–1487
Pneumothorax, 409
  aspiration of, 410
  catamenial, 411
  clinical presentation of, 409
  epidemiology of, 409
  etiology of, 409
  historical perspective on, 409
  imaging in, 409–410
  management of, 410–411
  observation for, 410
  pleurodesis for, 410–411, 411f
  secondary, 409, 411
  surgery for, 410–411, 411f
  tube thoracostomy for, 410
Poland's syndrome, 373–374, 376f–377f
  repair of, 374, 378f
Poly(2-methoxyethylacrylate), in cardiopulmonary bypass, 969
Polyalveolar lobe, 143
Polyarteritis nodosa, 1474
Polycythemia, in tetralogy of Fallot, 1882
Polymerase chain reaction
  in esophageal cancer, 675–676
  in lung cancer, 235, 673–675, 675f
  real-time, 674–675
Polyp(s)
  endobronchial, 155–156
  esophageal, 566, 567f

Polypropylene mesh, in chest wall reconstruction, 304, 382
Polypropylene mesh with methylmethacrylate, in chest wall reconstruction, 304, 306, 307f, 382–383
Polytetrafluoroethylene aortic graft, thrombotic complications of, 1288–1289, 1289f
Polytetrafluoroethylene patch, in chest wall reconstruction, 304, 382, 383f
Popliteal artery, digital subtraction angiography of, 1159, 1159f
Porcelain aorta, 1027, 1077–1078
Port-access coronary artery bypass grafting, 1407
Port-access minimally invasive cardiac surgery, 926–927, 927f
Positron emission tomography (PET)
  in bronchopulmonary carcinoid tumor, 325–326
  before coronary artery bypass grafting, 1372f, 1374
  in esophageal cancer, 580–581, 617
  in lung cancer, 30, 32f, 245–246, 245f, 299–300
  in malignant pleural mesothelioma, 33f, 34
  of middle mediastinum, 645–646
  in myocardial viability assessment, 818–820, 819f
  in pleural effusion, 432, 433f
  in pulmonary metastases, 340
  in pulmonary nodule, 29, 151–152, 236–237
Positron emission tomography–computed tomography (PET-CT)
  in esophageal cancer, 581–583, 581f
  in lung cancer, 30, 30f, 32f, 250, 299–300
  in malignant mesothelioma, 34, 457–458
  in pleural effusion, 432
Post-pericardiotomy syndrome, 935, 936f
Post-transplant lymphoproliferative disorder, 225, 225f–226f, 1568
Postoperative care, 51–58. See also Cardiac surgery, care after
  for acute respiratory distress syndrome, 54
  analgesia in, 52
  for anastomotic leak, 56
  for atelectasis, 53
  for atrial fibrillation, 54
  for bleeding, 54
  blood transfusion in, 51
  for bronchial fistula, 55
  for bronchopleural fistula, 55
  for bronchovascular fistula, 55
  for cerebrospinal fluid leak, 58
  for chylothorax, 56–57
  for conduit ischemia, 57
  drainage tubes in, 53
  for dysphagia, 56
  for empyema, 56
  fluids in, 51
  medications in, 51–52
  for myasthenic crisis, 57–58
  for myocardial infarction, 54
  nutrition in, 52
  physical therapy in, 53
  for pneumonia, 53
  for post-thoracotomy pain, 56
  for postpneumonectomy syndrome, 55–56
  for pulmonary complications, 55–56
  for pulmonary edema, 53–54
  for recurrent laryngeal nerve injury, 57
  for reflux, 57
  for respiratory failure, 53–54
  respiratory therapy in, 52–53
  for stricture, 57
  wound care in, 53
  for wound infection, 56
Postpneumonectomy syndrome, 55–56
Postpneumonic effusion, 415
Potassium channel activators, in hypoxic pulmonary vasoconstriction, 722, 722f
Potassium channel openers, in myocardial protection, 985
Pre-procedure verification, 1016–1017
Preconditioning, ischemic, 992
  remote, 992–993
Prednisone, in heart transplantation, 1545–1546
Pregnancy
  anticoagulation and, 1959
  aortic dissection during, 1093
  magnetic resonance imaging and, 1685
  in Marfan syndrome, 1026
  prosthetic heart valves and, 1959
  after Ross operation, 1959

Prekallikrein, in cardiopulmonary bypass, 963, 963f
Preload
  in acute heart failure, 885, 886f
  after cardiac surgery, 938, 938f–939f
  sarcomeric correlates of, 729, 729f
Premature ventricular complex, 1329
Prenatal diagnosis
  of congenital diaphragmatic hernia, 495, 498–499
  of congenital heart disease, 1666f, 1671–1672, 1672f
  of Ebstein's anomaly, 2056
  of hypoplastic left heart syndrome, 2026
  of transposition of great arteries, 1984
Prenatal intervention, 1699–1700
  in aortic stenosis with hypoplastic left heart syndrome, 1701–1702, 1702f–1703f
  historical perspective on, 1700–1701
  in hypoplastic left heart syndrome, 1701–1702, 1702t–1703t, 2037–2038, 2037f
  in hypoplastic left heart syndrome with intact/highly restrictive atrial septum, 1702–1704, 1703f
  indications for, 1699–1700, 1700t
  preparation for, 1701
  in pulmonary atresia with intact ventricular septum, 1704
  rationale for, 1699–1700
Preoperative evaluation, 39
  age in, 44
  arterial blood gas measurements in, 44
  cardiac assessment in, 42–43, 43f
  functional capacity assessment in, 43–44, 44f
  goals of, 40
  history in, 40–41, 40t–41t
  imaging studies in, 41
  laboratory studies in, 41
  physical examination in, 41
  postoperative lung function prediction in, 42, 42t
  pulmonary function testing in, 41–42
  pulmonary hemodynamics in, 44
  risk stratification in, 44–45, 44t
Pressure-volume analysis, of left ventricle, 741
Pressure-volume loop, of left ventricle, 730, 730f, 741, 742f
Prima Plus stentless bioprosthesis, 1191
Primitive neuroectodermal tumor, 456–457
Procaine, in myocardial protection, 985
Procalcitonin, in community-acquired pneumonia, 177
Progressive systemic sclerosis, esophageal, 563, 570
Prohemostatic agents, 765–771, 765b
Propofol, in congenital heart disease, 1754, 1757
Propranolol, in tetralogy of Fallot, 1883
Prostacyclin
  in congenital diaphragmatic hernia, 500–501
  in hypoxic pulmonary vasoconstriction, 722, 722f
  in vascular tone, 715–716
Prostaglandin(s)
  in pulmonary atresia with ventricular septal defect, 1900
  in vascular tone, 715–716, 716f
Prostaglandin E_1
  in coarctation of aorta, 1785
  in pediatric pulmonary hypertension, 1752
  in pulmonary atresia with intact ventricular septum, 1866–1867
  in transposition of great arteries, 1984
Prostaglandin I_2, in pediatric pulmonary hypertension, 1752
Prostanoids, in cardiopulmonary bypass, 1287
Prostate, Lung, Colorectal and Ovarian Cancer (PLCO) Screening trial, 233
Prosthetic heart valves, 1185
  anticoagulation for, 50, 1280–1284, 1281f–1282f
    antiplatelet agents for, 1280–1281, 1282f, 1284
    complications of, 1283–1284
    fibrinolytics for, 1280, 1283
    heparin for, 1280, 1284
    International Normalized Ratio in, 1280–1281
    pregnancy and, 1959
    warfarin for, 1280–1281, 1281f, 1283–1284
  bioprosthetic, 1189–1192
    anticoagulation with, 1281–1283
    ATS Medical, 3f, 1191–1192, 1192f
    Carpentier-Edwards, 1190
    Edwards, 1191
    fixation of, 1189
    Hancock, 1189
    Medtronic, 1189–1191, 1190f–1191f

Prosthetic heart valves (Continued)
    Mosaic, 1189–1190, 1190f
    pericardial, 1190–1191, 1191f
    St. Jude, 1190, 1190f
    stented, 1189–1190
      dysfunction of, 1204
    stentless, 1191–1192, 1191f, 1285
    Toronto SPV, 1191
  bleeding with, 1187
  coagulation cascade and, 1279–1280, 1280f
  echocardiographic evaluation of, 842, 842f
  effective orifice area of, 1186
  embolism with, 1186–1187
  endocarditis of. See Endocarditis, prosthetic valve
  endovascular placement of, 859–860, 859f
  hemodynamic assessment of, 1186
  historical perspective on, 1185–1186
  homograft, 1192
  ideal of, 1185
  mechanical, 1187–1192
    ATS Medical Open Pivot, 1189
    bileaflet, 1188–1189, 1188f
    caged ball, 1187, 1187f
    CarboMedics, 1189, 1189f
    Medtronic-Hall, 1187–1188, 1187f
    Monostrut, 1188
    Omnicarbon, 1188
    On-X, 1189
    St. Jude, 842f, 1188–1189, 1188f
    Starr-Edwards, 1187, 1187f
    tilting disc, 1187–1188, 1187f
  mortality with, 1186–1187
  selection of, 1192
  thromboresistant surfaces for, 1290, 1290f
  thrombosis with, 1186, 1284–1286
    anticoagulation for, 1280–1284, 1281f–1282f
    clinical presentation of, 1285
    incidence of, 1285
Protamine, 758, 768–769
  adverse reactions to, 768–769, 923
  in cardiopulmonary bypass, 923, 966–967, 1382
  overdosage of, 758, 759f
  in pediatric cardiopulmonary bypass, 1719
Protected health information, 2113
Protein C, activated, in community-acquired pneumonia, 177
Protein kinase C inhibitors, in hypoxic pulmonary vasoconstriction, 722, 722f
Protein-losing enteropathy, after Fontan procedure, 2050
Proteomics, 670, 677–678
Prothrombin complex concentrates, in anticoagulant reversal, 770
Proton pump inhibitors
  postoperative, 52
  preoperative, 48–49
Protozoan infection, after heart transplantation, 1550
Prune-belly syndrome, pectus excavatum in, 360
Pseudoaneurysm
  coronary artery, 1472, 1473f
  mitral-aortic intervalvular fibrosa, 843, 843f
  myocardial infarction and, 833
  after percutaneous coronary intervention, 854
Pseudochylothorax, 428
Pseudotumor, inflammatory, 155, 155f, 454
Pulmonary angiography, in chronic thromboembolic pulmonary hypertension, 1622
Pulmonary angioscopy, in chronic thromboembolic pulmonary hypertension, 1622
Pulmonary arteriovenous malformation, 145–147, 146f, 2044
Pulmonary artery (arteries)
  anatomy of, 15–17, 19f–20f, 706–707
    variations in, 16
  anomalous origin of coronary artery from. See Anomalous origin of coronary artery from pulmonary artery
  balloon dilation of, 1696–1697
    in pulmonary atresia with ventricular septal defect, 1902
  banding of, 1849, 1857
    in hypoplastic left heart syndrome, 2036–2037
    in transposition of great arteries, 1985
  branch, in truncus arteriosus, 1912
  congenital aneurysm of, 145
  coronary artery origin from, 1470

Pulmonary artery (arteries) (Continued)
  with double-outlet right ventricle, 1861
  hypoxia-induced constriction of, 722, 722f
  inflammation of, 1027
  injury to, 103
    in lung transplantation, 213–214
  intraoperative ballooning and stenting of, 2103
  left
    anomalous origin of, 144–145, 144f
    in tetralogy of Fallot, 1878, 1879f
  physiology of, 721–722, 722f
  preoperative assessment of, 44
  right, in tetralogy of Fallot, 1878, 1879f
  stenting of, 1696–1697, 1697f
  in tetralogy of Fallot, 1878
  transposition of. See Transposition of great arteries
  unilateral absence of, 144
Pulmonary artery pressure, 780f, 780t, 781, 828–829
  in cardiac surgery, 920, 938, 938f
  mitral regurgitation and, 1218
  in ventricular septal defect, 1852–1853
Pulmonary artery sling, 144–145, 144f, 1773–1776, 1775f–1776f, 1789, 1789f
  repair of, 1792
Pulmonary artery stenosis, in tetralogy of Fallot, 1885–1886, 1885f–1889f
Pulmonary atresia with intact ventricular septum, 1865
  anatomy of, 1865–1866, 1865f–1866f
  angiography in, 1691, 1692f
  classification of, 1867, 1867t
  clinical presentation of, 1866–1867
  echocardiography in, 1866–1867
  historical perspective on, 1865
  mortality with, 1865
  pathophysiology of, 1866
  prenatal intervention in, 1704
  prostaglandin E$_1$ in, 1866–1867
  right ventricle–dependent coronary circulation in, 1866, 1869, 1871, 1871f
  sinusoids in, 1866
  surgical management of, 1867–1871, 1867t
    one-and-one-half, 1869–1870, 1870f
    one-ventricle, 1870–1871, 1871f
    palliative, 1867–1869, 1868f–1870f
    results of, 1871–1873, 1872f–1874f, 1873t
    right ventricular decompression in, 1873–1874
    two-ventricle, 1869
  transcatheter pulmonary valvotomy in, 1874
  transplantation in, 1874–1875
  tricuspid valve Z-value in, 1867, 1867t, 1868f, 1870f
Pulmonary atresia with ventricular septal defect, 1897
  anatomy of, 1897–1898, 1898f
  cardiac catheterization in, 1899–1900, 1900f, 1904
  chest radiography in, 1899–1900
  classification of, 1898, 1899f
  clinical presentation of, 1899
  diagnosis of, 1899–1900
  ductal stenting in, 1902
  echocardiography in, 1899, 1904
  genetic factors in, 1897
  magnetic resonance imaging in, 1900
  major aortopulmonary collaterals in, 1897–1898, 1898f–1899f, 1903–1904
    coiling/stenting of, 1902
  MAPCA coiling/stenting in, 1902
  medical treatment of, 1900
  natural history of, 1899
  pathophysiology of, 1897–1898
  pulmonary artery balloon dilation in, 1902
  pulmonary hypertension in, 1899
  radiofrequency perforation and balloon dilation in, 1902
  radionuclide lung perfusion scan in, 1900, 1904
  subclavian-to-pulmonary artery shunt in, 1902
  surgical treatment of, 1900–1902
    cardiopulmonary bypass strategy in, 1902
    evaluation after, 1904
    multiple-stage, 1903–1904
    patent foramen ovale in, 1901
    results of, 1904
    right ventricle–to–pulmonary artery conduit in, 1901, 1905–1908, 1906t
    right ventricular pressure after, 1904
    single-stage, 1903, 1903f
    strategies for, 1903–1904, 1903f
    systemic-to-pulmonary artery shunt in, 1902

Pulmonary atresia with ventricular septal defect (Continued)
    transanular patch in, 1901
    transplantation in, 1902
    unifocalization in, 1900–1901, 1903, 1903f
    ventricular septal defect closure in, 1901
  transcatheter treatment of, 1902
  ventricular septal defect closure in, 1902
  without major aortopulmonary collaterals, 1898, 1903
Pulmonary blood flow
  in hypoplastic left heart syndrome, 2031
  in single ventricle, 2042–2044
Pulmonary capillary wedge pressure, 780f, 780t, 781
  after cardiac surgery, 938
Pulmonary contusion, 92
Pulmonary edema
  in heart failure, 900, 900t
  postoperative, 53–54
  protamine-related, 923
Pulmonary embolism, 1615
  acute, 1615–1620
    catheter-assisted thrombectomy in, 1618
    chest radiography in, 1616
    classification of, 1616
    clinical features of, 1615–1617
    electrocardiography in, 1616
    hormonal factors in, 1616
    incidence of, 1615
    magnetic resonance angiography in, 1616–1617
    major, 1616
    massive, 1616
    minor, 1616
    prevention of, 1617
    pulmonary hypertension after, 1615
    right ventricular failure in, 1616
    treatment of, 1617f
      embolectomy in, 1618–1620, 1620t
      extracorporeal life support in, 1619
      thrombolytic therapy in, 1617–1618
    ventilation-perfusion scan in, 1616–1617
  chronic, 1620–1628
    classification of, 1625, 1625f–1626f
    clinical manifestations of, 1621
    endarterectomy in, 1622–1623
      principles of, 1623
      results of, 1625–1628, 1627t–1628t
      technique of, 1623–1624
    evaluation of, 1621–1622
    incidence of, 1620–1621
    natural history of, 1620–1621
  historical perspective on, 1615
  imaging of, 34–35, 35f
Pulmonary function testing
  in aortic aneurysm, 1068–1069
  in bronchiolitis obliterans syndrome, 224, 224t
  in interstitial lung disease, 168–169
  in lung cancer with chest wall invasion, 300
  in lung transplantation, 209, 224, 224t
  in pectus carinatum, 361–362
  in pectus excavatum, 361–362
  postoperative, 42, 42t
  preoperative, 41–42
  after sympathicotomy, 666
  in thoracic aortic aneurysm, 1068–1069
  after thoracoscopic lobectomy, 283–284
Pulmonary hypertension
  heart-lung transplantation in, 1555–1556. See also Heart-lung transplantation
  lung transplantation in, 209
  in mitral regurgitation, 1215
  pediatric, 1751–1752, 1751b
    atrial septal defect and, 1801–1802
    atrioventricular canal defect and, 1835, 1845
    postoperative, 1751–1752
      after ventricular septal defect closure, 1857–1858
    in pulmonary atresia with ventricular septal defect, 1899
  thromboembolic, 1615, 1620–1621. See also Pulmonary embolism, chronic
    classification of, 1625, 1625f–1626f
    clinical manifestations of, 1621
    evaluation of, 1621–1622
    type 1, 1625, 1625f
    type 2, 1625, 1625f
    type 3, 1625, 1626f
    type 4, 1625

Pulmonary lymphangiectasia, 143–144, 143f
Pulmonary nodule(s)
  biopsy of, 237
  in breast cancer, 346
  computed tomography of, 13f, 235–237
  evaluation of, 151–152, 151b–152b, 157, 340
  fine needle aspiration of, 236–237
  imaging of, 28–29, 29f–30f
  positron emission tomography of, 236–237
  screen-detected, 236–237
Pulmonary regurgitation, stent-mounted bovine jugular valve placement in, 1695, 1696f
Pulmonary salivary gland–type tumors. See Salivary gland–type tumors
Pulmonary trunk, 706–707, 707f–708f
Pulmonary valve
  absence of, tetralogy of Fallot with, 1892
  anatomy of, 703, 703f
  on cardiac catheterization, 783–786
  stenosis of, 1694–1695
    in tetralogy of Fallot, 1877–1878, 1879f
Pulmonary valve replacement
  periventricular, 2103
  after tetralogy of Fallot repair, 1890–1891, 2076
  transcatheter, 1695, 1696f
Pulmonary valvotomy, in pulmonary atresia with intact ventricular septum, 1868, 1868f, 1874
Pulmonary valvuloplasty
  balloon, 1694
    in tetralogy of Fallot, 1883–1884
  fetal, 1704
Pulmonary varix, 145
Pulmonary vascular obstructive disease, atrioventricular canal defect and, 1834
Pulmonary vascular resistance
  congenital diaphragmatic hernia and, 494
  ventricular septal defect and, 1852–1853
Pulmonary vein
  anatomy of, 16–17, 19f
  aneurysmal dilation of, 145
  anomalous drainage of. See Anomalous pulmonary venous drainage/connection
  embryology of, 1817, 1818f
  injury to, 103
    in lung transplantation, 212–213
  stenosis of, 1697–1698
    congenital, 1828
    after total anomalous pulmonary venous drainage repair, 1827
Pulmonary vein isolation, 1346, 1354–1355, 1354f–1355f
  results of, 1356–1357
Pulmonectomy. See Pneumonectomy
Pulse oximetry, 1752–1753
Pulse pressure, in aortic regurgitation, 1200
Pulseless disease. See Takayasu's arteritis
Pulses, in type A aortic dissection, 1097, 1097t
Pulsus paradoxus, 786f, 1481
Pumps, in cardiopulmonary bypass, 960–961, 961f

Q

QRS tachycardia
  narrow, 1329
  wide, 1329
QT interval, prolonged, 1329
Quality Indicators for Congenital and Pediatric Cardiac Surgery, 2113, 2114
Quinapril, in heart failure, 891t

R

Radial artery
  cannulation-related thrombosis of, 1289
  in coronary artery bypass grafting, 1372–1376, 1386–1387, 1386f, 1413t, 1415–1416, 1416f
Radiation therapy
  in adenoid cystic carcinoma, 330
  brachiocephalic artery stenosis with, 1144
  in bronchopulmonary carcinoid tumor, 327
  coronary artery effects of, 1476
  in esophageal cancer, 618, 620–621, 620t

Radiation therapy (Continued)
    esophageal stricture with, 571
    in mesothelioma, 460–461, 464–465, 464b
    in non–small cell lung cancer, 288
    palliative, in esophageal cancer, 621
    pericarditis, 1486
    in thymoma, 638
Radiofrequency ablation
    in arrhythmias. See Catheter ablation
    in Barrett's esophagus, 70–71
    in metastatic lung cancer, 347
    in non–small cell lung cancer, 683–687, 683f–686f, 685t, 687t, 691–692
Radiofrequency perforation and balloon dilation, in pulmonary atresia with ventricular septal defect, 1902
Radiography. See Chest radiography
Radionuclide imaging
    in blunt cardiac injury, 95, 1174
    in bronchopulmonary carcinoid tumor, 325
    in emphysema, 200, 200f
    lung perfusion, in pulmonary atresia with ventricular septal defect, 1900, 1904
    myocardial perfusion, 810. See also Single-photon emission computed tomography (SPECT)
        equipment for, 810
        procedure for, 810
        tracers for, 809–810
Ramipril, 890–892, 891t
Rapamycin, 1545
Rapid response team, 1018
RAS-ERK pathway, in mesothelioma, 452
Rashkind atrial septostomy, in transposition of great arteries, 1984
Rastelli operation, 1995–1996, 1996f, 2010–2011, 2011f
Raynaud's phenomenon, in thoracic outlet syndrome, 392
Rb protein, in mesothelioma, 451–452
Rectus abdominis flap
    in chest wall reconstruction, 384
    in sternal wound infection, 1001
Rectus abdominis muscle, 6, 8t
Recurrent laryngeal nerve
    anatomy of, 23–24
    injury to, 57, 610
Red blood cell transfusion. See Blood transfusion
Reflex, Bainbridge, 747
Reflex sympathetic dystrophy, 403
Reflux. See Gastroesophageal reflux disease (GERD)
    after heart-lung transplantation, 1568
    postesophagectomy, 612
Regenerative cell-based therapy, 1599
    in acute myocardial infarction, 1609
        adipose tissue–derived cells for, 1600t, 1601f, 1603–1604
        angiogenesis in, 1607, 1609f, 1610–1611
        bone marrow–derived stem cells for, 1600–1603, 1600t, 1601f
        cardiac stem cells for, 1600t, 1601f, 1604
        cell differentiation in, 1607, 1609f
        cell fusion in, 1607, 1609f
        cell homing in, 1606–1607, 1609f
        in chronic myocardial ischemia, 1609–1610
        clinical applications of, 1602t, 1609–1610
        in congestive heart failure, 1610
        delivery methods for, 1604–1606, 1610, 1611f
            direct injection, 1606
            intracoronary, 1605–1606, 1605f, 1605t
            intramyocardial, 1605f, 1605t, 1606
            intravenous, 1605, 1605f, 1605t
        embryonic stem cells for, 1600, 1600t, 1601f
        endothelial progenitor cells for, 1600t, 1601–1603, 1601f, 1603f, 1608f
        hematopoietic stem cells for, 1600t, 1601, 1601f
        inducible pluripotent cells for, 1600t, 1604
        limitations of, 1610–1611
        mesenchymal stem cells for, 1600t, 1601f, 1603, 1603f, 1608f
        paracrine effects in, 1607–1608, 1609f
        side population cells for, 1600t, 1604
        skeletal myoblasts for, 1599–1600, 1600t, 1601f
        vasculogenesis in, 1607, 1609f
        ventricular remodeling in, 1608–1609, 1609f
Remodeling ring anuloplasty, 1221, 1223f
Remote ischemic preconditioning, 992–993

Renal artery (arteries)
    angiography of, 1158, 1162
    angioplasty for, 1167–1168
    ischemia of, in type A aortic dissection, 1097, 1097t
    pressure gradient in, 1168, 1168f
    stenting for, 1167–1168
Renal cell carcinoma, pulmonary metastases in, 346
Respiration
    after chest wall resection/reconstruction, 306, 308
    diaphragmatic movement with, 4, 10, 474
    neonatal, 1749–1750
    after pediatric cardiac surgery, 1759–1760
Respiratory bronchiolitis–associated interstitial lung disease, 167–168
Respiratory distress
    in congenital diaphragmatic hernia, 495, 504
    postoperative, 54
    trauma-related, 107, 107b
Respiratory failure
    after esophagectomy, 609–610
    postoperative, 53–54
    after thymectomy, 57–58
Respiratory therapy, postoperative, 52–53
Retinoic acid, in cardiac embryology, 1648
Retroesophageal aorta, circumflex, 1788–1789, 1788f, 1791
Rewarming, after cardiac surgery, 934, 937–938, 1722
Rhabdomyoma, 1634t, 1635, 1637f
Rhabdomyosarcoma
    cardiac, 1637
    chest wall, 385, 386f
Rheumatic disease, 1195, 1199, 1210, 1214, 1244. See also Aortic regurgitation Aortic stenosis; Mitral regurgitation; Mitral stenosis
Rhomboid muscle, 8t
Rib(s)
    anatomy of, 3f, 5–6, 6f
    cervical, in thoracic outlet syndrome, 391, 392f, 393, 396f
    chondrosarcoma of, 34, 34f
    first, 6
        fracture of, 90
        neurovascular bundle compression against. See Thoracic outlet syndrome
        transaxillary resection of, 397–398, 401f–402f
            dorsal sympathectomy with, 404
    fracture of, 90
    free-floating (vertebral), 5
    head of, 5, 6f
    neck of, 5, 6f
    shaft of, 5–6, 6f
    surface anatomy of, 11
    tubercle of, 5–6, 6f
    vertebrocostal, 5
    vertebrosternal, 5
Right atrium. See Atrium (atria), right
Right reduction atrioplasty, in Ebstein's anomaly, 2065–2066
Right-sided heart failure
    in acute pulmonary embolism, 1616
    after cardiac surgery, 943
    after heart transplantation, 1544–1545
    after left ventricular assist device implantation, 1509, 1522
Right ventricle. See Ventricle(s), right
Right ventricle–to–pulmonary artery conduit, 1901, 1905–1908, 1906t
    allograft (homograft), 1905, 1906t
    autologous, 1907
    durability of, 1906t, 1907–1908
    dysfunction of, 1908
    indications for, 1905
    pericardial, 1907
    replacement/reconstruction of, 1908
    results with, 1907–1908
    selection of, 1905–1907
    stenting of, 1908
    synthetic, 1906t, 1907
        nonvalved, 1907
        valved, 1906t, 1907
    xenograft, 1905–1907, 1906t
Right ventricular assist device, 1528–1529
Right ventricular outflow tract obstruction
    after tetralogy of Fallot treatment, 1890
    in transposition of great arteries, 1993
Right ventricular outflow tract reconstruction, in tetralogy of Fallot, 1884–1886, 1884f–1885f

Rivaroxaban, 759
Robot-assisted cardiac surgery, 927, 1295
    clinical applications of, 1297
    in coronary artery bypass grafting, 1299, 1405–1406, 1406f
    evolution of, 1296–1297
    haptics in, 1301, 1301f
    imaging in, 1301
    instruments for, 1300, 1300f
    limitations of, 1300
    miniaturization of, 1300
    in mitral valve disorders, 1298–1299
    mobile, 1300
    operative set-up for, 1297–1298, 1298f
    patient selection for, 1297, 1297b
    planning/simulation for, 1301, 1302f–1303f
    technique of, 1297–1298, 1297f–1298f
    technological advances in, 1300–1303
    telemanipulation systems for, 1295–1296, 1296f
    three-dimensional guidance system for, 1301
    training for, 1303
    virtual reality technology and, 1302–1303
    working port incision for, 1297–1298, 1297f
Ross-Konno operation, 1951, 1952f
Ross operation, 1034–1037, 1035f–1036f, 1958–1959
    bicuspid aortic valve disease and, 1958–1959
    contraindications to, 1958–1959
    outcomes of, 1037, 1958
    pregnancy after, 1959
    in prosthetic valve endocarditis, 1274
Rotational atherectomy catheter, 856, 856f
Rubinstein-Taybi syndrome, 1801

S

S-100
    after aortic arch surgery, 1051, 1052f
    after cardiac surgery, 1005–1006
St. Jude Medical prosthetic valve, 1188–1189, 1188f
    Biocor, 1190, 1190f
    Toronto Stentless, 1191
Saline test, in mitral valve repair, 1221–1222, 1224f
Salivary gland–type tumors, 329–331
    adjuvant therapy in, 330
    diagnosis of, 329–330
    endobronchial treatment in, 330
    imatinib in, 330
    pathology of, 329, 330t
    prognosis for, 330–331
    radiation therapy in, 330
    surgery in, 330
Saphenous vein, in coronary artery bypass grafting, 952, 1376, 1386–1387, 1386f, 1411, 1411–1412, 1413t
Sarcoidosis, 162–163, 162f
    mediastinal adenopathy in, 647
Sarcoma
    cardiac, 1635t
    pleural, 456
    pulmonary
        metastatic, 344–345
        primary, 331–332, 331f
Sarcomere, 726–730
    afterload and, 729, 729f
    contraction-relaxation cycle and, 729–730, 729f
    cross-bridges of, 726–728, 728f
    length-tension properties of, pressure-volume relationship and, 733, 734f–735f
    preload and, 729, 729f
    titin of, 727f–728f, 728–729, 742, 744f
    troponin of, 727–728, 728f
SAVE (septal anterior ventricular exclusion) procedure, 1578–1579, 1579f
Scalene node biopsy, 249
Scalene test, 393, 394f
Scalene triangle, 390, 391f
Scapula
    fracture of, 92
    surface anatomy of, 11, 12t
Schatzki's ring, 552f, 570
Schwannoma
    cardiac, 1635t
    pleural, 455

Scimitar syndrome, 145–147, 146f, 795–796, 796f, 1819–1821, 1821f
 surgical management of, 1819–1821
  complications of, 1821
Scleroderma, esophageal, 563, 570
Sclerosant therapy
 pericardial, 443–444
 pleural. See Pleurodesis, sclerosant
Screening, lung cancer, 231. See also Lung cancer, screening for
Sedation. See also Cardiac surgery, anesthesia in; Congenital heart disease, surgical treatment of, anesthesia in
 in congenital heart disease, 1756–1757
 errors with, 1018
 for pediatric cardiac catheterization, 1693
 for pediatric magnetic resonance imaging, 1684
Seminoma, 639
Senning operation, 1985–1987, 1986f, 2011
Septal artery ablation, vs. septal myectomy, 1501, 1504f
Septal myectomy, 1499–1501
 care after, 1500–1501
 indications for, 1499
 morbidity after, 1502
 mortality after, 1501, 1502f
 outcomes of, 1501–1503
 vs. septal artery ablation, 1503–1504, 1504f
 symptom relief after, 1502–1503, 1502f
 technique of, 1499–1500, 1500f–1501f
Septum. See Atrial septum; Conal septum; Ventricular septum
Septum secundum, 700, 701f, 1644, 1645f, 1647
Sequestration, pulmonary, 136–137, 137f–138f
Seroma, in chest wall reconstruction, 383
Serotonin
 in bronchopulmonary carcinoid tumor, 326
 vascular effects of, 718
Serratus anterior, 6, 7f, 8t
Serratus anterior flap, in chest wall reconstruction, 384, 385f
Serratus posterior, 8t
Shock
 after cardiac surgery, 937
 cardiogenic
  coronary artery bypass grafting and, 1378
  left ventricular assist device in, 1508, 1519–1520
  in postinfarction ventricular septal defect, 1450
 vasodilatory, after cardiopulmonary bypass, 943
Shone syndrome, 2016
Short chordae syndrome, 2017, 2017f
Shprintzen syndrome, 1648
Shunt
 cardiac
  bidirectional, 783
  echocardiography of, 826, 827f
  left-to-right, 781–782, 783f, 1750–1751, 1750t
   in anomalous origin of coronary artery from pulmonary artery, 1964–1965
   atrial septal defect and, 781–782, 782f, 1801, 1808
   in atrioventricular canal defects, 1834
   ventricular septal defect and, 781–782, 782f, 1852
  right-to-left, 782, 826, 827f
 cavopulmonary, in single ventricle, 2043–2044, 2043f
 systemic-to-pulmonary artery
  in pulmonary atresia with intact ventricular septum, 1868–1869, 1869f–1870f
  in pulmonary atresia with ventricular septal defect, 1902
  in tetralogy of Fallot, 1888–1889
Sibson's fascia, 4
Side population cells, 1600t, 1604
Sildenafil, in congenital diaphragmatic hernia, 501
SilverHawk device, in femoral artery disease, 1169
Simvastatin, in aortic stenosis, 1197
Single-lung ventilation, 50
Single-photon emission computed tomography (SPECT)
 cardiac, 810, 811f, 814f
  in acute coronary syndrome, 816–817, 817f
  in coronary artery disease detection, 810–813
  in exercise stress testing, 810–811, 814b
  in myocardial viability assessment, 820
  in pharmacologic stress testing, 812–813
  preoperative, 816
  prognostic use of, 813–816, 814b, 815f

Single-photon emission computed tomography (Continued)
  after revascularization, 821
  in stable angina, 813–814, 814b
  in stable coronary artery disease, 810–816
 in chronic thromboembolic pulmonary hypertension, 1622
Single ventricle, 2041
 adult, 2078–2080, 2079f
 anatomy of, 2041
 atrioventricular canal defect and, 1844
 bidirectional cavopulmonary anastomosis in, 2043–2044, 2043f
 bilateral bidirectional cavopulmonary anastomosis in, 2044
 cardiac catheterization in, 1692
 clinical presentation of, 2042
 Damus-Stansel-Kaye procedure in, 2043
 evaluation of, 2042
 excessive pulmonary blood flow in, 2042–2043
 Fontan procedure in, 2045–2046
  atrial arrhythmias after, 2049, 2088–2091, 2090t–2091t
  atrioventricular valve insufficiency and, 2046
  excessive pulmonary blood flow and, 2042–2043
  extracardiac conduit in, 2046–2047
  failure of, 2050
  fenestration for, 2046
  historical perspective on, 2046–2048
  inadequate pulmonary blood flow and, 2042
  late outcomes of, 2049
  lateral tunnel, 2046, 2047f
  McGoon ratio and, 2045
  modified Blalock-Taussig shunt before, 2042
  morbidity after, 2048–2049
  mortality after, 2048–2049
  nonoperative, 2047–2048
  obstructed pulmonary venous return and, 2043
  outcome of, 2048–2050
  plastic bronchitis after, 2050
  preparation for, 2042–2043
  prophylactic anticoagulation for, 2049–2050
  protein-losing enteropathy after, 2050
  pulmonary vasculature and, 2045
  selection criteria of, 2045–2046, 2045b
  sinus rhythm and, 2045
  systemic outflow obstruction and, 2043
  thromboembolism after, 2049–2050
  total cavopulmonary connection conversion of, 2050
  venovenous collaterals after, 2049
  ventricular function and, 2045–2046
 Glenn anastomosis in, 2044
 heart transplantation in, 2050
 hemi-Fontan procedure in, 2044
 hybrid procedure palliation in, 2101–2102, 2102t
 Kawashima operation in, 2044
 mechanical circulatory support in, 2050
 natural history of, 2041–2042
 obstructed pulmonary venous return and, 2043
 persistent left superior vena cava in, 2044
 pulmonary arteriovenous malformations in, 2044
 pulmonary blood flow in, 2042–2044
 systemic outflow obstruction and, 2043
 terminology for, 2041
 total anomalous pulmonary venous connection in, 2043
 1.5-ventricle repair in, 2044–2045
Sinoatrial node
 dysfunction of, in adult congenital heart disease, 2093
 surgical isolation of, 1357–1358, 1357f
  results of, 1358
Sinoatrial node reentrant tachycardia, 1333–1334
Sinus node, 699–700
 dysfunction of, 1329
 pacemaker in, 1307b. See also Pacemaker, permanent
Sinus of Valsalva
 aneurysm of, 793, 794f
 contralateral, coronary artery from, 802, 805f, 1467–1469, 1469f
Sinus tachycardia, inappropriate, 1357–1358
 superior right atrial isolation for, 1357–1358, 1357f
 results of, 1358
Sinus venosus defect, 1798–1799, 1800f
 adult, 2074–2075
 treatment of, 1805–1806, 1806f–1807f

Sirolimus
 in heart transplantation, 1545
 in lung transplantation, 219
Situs ambiguus, 1651
Situs inversus, 1651
Situs solitus, 1651, 1661
Slide tracheoplasty, 1768, 1769f–1770f
Small capillary and arteriolar dilatations, after cardiopulmonary bypass, 970, 970f
Smoking. See Cigarette smoking
Society of Thoracic Surgeons, Quality Measurement Task Force of, 1015–1016, 1015b, 1016t
Sodium-hydrogen exchangers, 993
 inhibitors of, 993
Solitary pulmonary nodule. See Pulmonary nodule(s)
Sonic hedgehog, 1642, 1643f
Sotalol, in postoperative atrial fibrillation, 54, 945
Spasm
 esophageal, 563
 left internal thoracic artery, 1414
Specimen, intraoperative management of, 51
Speckle tracing, in echocardiography, 1675, 1675f
SPECT. See Single-photon emission computed tomography (SPECT)
Spinal cord
 anatomy of, 1071, 1072f
 ischemia of
  with thoracic endovascular aortic repair, 1136
  with thoracic surgical aortic repair, 1069–1075, 1070f, 1072f, 1074f
 protection of, in aortic aneurysm treatment, 1069–1075, 1070f, 1072f, 1074f–1075f
Spinal nerve, 8–10
Spirometry, incentive, postoperative, 52–53
Spironolactone, 887t, 888, 897, 897t
Splanchnic nerve, 4–5
Split pleura sign, 181–182
Spondylothoracic dysplasia, 383–384, 384f
Sprengel's deformity, 373
Sputum examination, in lung cancer, 234–235, 244–245
Squamous cell carcinoma, tracheal, 116, 116f
Squamous papilloma, endobronchial, 155–156
Square-root sign, 1481, 1482f
ST-segment elevation myocardial infarction. See Myocardial infarction (MI), ST-segment elevation
Stabbing injury, 98. See also Trauma, penetrating
 cardiac, 1175–1178. See also Cardiac injury, penetrating
Staircase phenomenon, 746
Staphylococcus aureus, in prosthetic valve endocarditis, 1270t, 1273
Stapling, endoscopic, in Zenker's diverticulum. See Zenker's diverticulum, transoral endoscopic stapling in
Starr-Edwards ball valve prosthesis, 1187, 1187f
Statins
 in aortic stenosis, 1197
 in atherosclerosis, 908–909, 909t, 913–914
 in NSTE acute coronary syndromes, 878
Stem cells. See also Regenerative cell-based therapy
 bone marrow–derived, 1600–1603, 1600t, 1601f
 cardiac, 1600t, 1601f, 1604
 embryonic, 1600, 1600t, 1601f
 endothelial, 1600t, 1601f, 1603f, 1608f
 hematopoietic, 1600t, 1601, 1601f
 mesenchymal, 1600t, 1601f, 1603, 1603f, 1608f
Stenosis
 aortic. See Aortic stenosis
 esophageal, congenital, 544
 laryngotracheal. See Laryngotracheal stenosis
 mitral. See Mitral stenosis
 pulmonary artery, in tetralogy of Fallot, 1885–1886, 1885f–1889f
 pulmonary valve
  in tetralogy of Fallot, 1877–1878, 1879f
  transcatheter balloon dilation for, 1694
  valvuloplasty in, 1694–1695
 pulmonary vein, 1697–1698
  congenital, 1828
  after total anomalous pulmonary venous drainage repair, 1827
 subaortic. See Subaortic stenosis
 subclavian artery, 1372
 tracheal. See Tracheal stenosis

Stent(s)
  airway, 71–74
    in benign stricture, 72–73
    in emphysema, 204
    indications for, 72
    in malignant stricture, 73
    metal, 71–72, 72t
    silicone-based, 71–72, 72t
    technique for, 71–72
  aortic, in traumatic lesions, 94, 103
  carotid artery, 1150
    coronary artery bypass graft after, 1154
  coronary artery, 848
    bypass grafting with, 857
    drug-eluting, 848, 855–856
      recurrent disease and, 855
    in left main-stem disease, 852
    noncardiac surgery after, 853
    recurrent disease and, 855
    thrombosis and, 855–856
  ductal, in pulmonary atresia with ventricular septal defect, 1902
  esophageal, 71–74
    in benign stricture, 73
    in malignant stricture, 73–74
    metal, 71–72, 72t
    silicone-based, 71–72, 72t
    technique for, 71–72
  femoral artery, 1168–1169
  iliac artery, 1168
  innominate artery, 1149, 1150f
  right ventricle–to–pulmonary artery conduit, 1908
  subclavian artery, 1151
Stereotactic radiosurgery, in non–small cell lung cancer, 687–689, 688f, 691–692
Sternal angle of Louis, 10, 12t
Sternal reentry protocol, in adult congenital heart disease, 2072
Sternal wound infection, 999
  after coronary artery bypass grafting, 1384, 1385f
  definition of, 999
  diagnosis of, 1000
  etiology of, 999
  incidence of, 999
  management of, 1000
    algorithm for, 1002, 1002f
    omental flaps in, 1000–1001
    pectoralis major flaps in, 1001
    plate fixation in, 1001, 1001f
    primary closure in, 1000
    rectus abdominis flaps in, 1001
    soft tissue flaps in, 1000–1001
    vacuum-assisted closure in, 1001–1002, 1002f
  patient factors in, 999–1000
  prevention of, 1000, 1017–1018
  risk factors for, 999–1000
Sternocleidomastoid muscle, 7f, 12t
Sternothoracotomy, in lung transplantation, 214, 215f
Sternotomy
  infection with. See Sternal wound infection
  median
    in atrioventricular canal defect repair, 1836, 1836f
    in heart-lung transplantation, 1560–1562, 1561f, 1563f
    in lung transplantation, 214
    in mitral valve surgery, 1218, 1220f
    in penetrating cardiac injury, 1177
    in reoperative coronary artery bypass grafting, 1424–1425, 1424f
    in thymectomy, 641
  mediastinal infection after, 648
  pediatric
    full, 1709–1710
    limited, 1710
    midsternal mini, 1710
    trans-xiyphoid mini, 1710, 1710f–1711f
Sternum
  anatomy of, 3f, 5
  cleft, 375, 379f, 379t
  congenital defects of, 374–382, 379t
  repair of, 375, 379f, 380t
  fracture of, 91

Stomach
  cardia of, 524
  postesophagectomy conduit creation with, 592, 592f–594f
    complications of, 612
Streptokinase
  in empyema, 419
  in prosthetic heart valve anticoagulation, 1280
Stress response
  pediatric anesthesia and, 1754–1756, 1755b
  pediatric cardiopulmonary bypass and, 1726
Stress testing
  in anomalous aorta–pulmonary artery coronary artery course, 1973
  in aortic stenosis, 1197–1198
  in congenital aortic stenosis, 1944–1945
  in coronary artery disease, 810–816, 814b, 833
  preoperative, 43–44, 44f
Stress ulceration, prevention of, 48–49
Stretta procedure, 78–79
Stricture
  airway
    benign, 72–73
    malignant, 73
  esophageal. See Esophageal stricture
Stroke. See also Neurologic disorders
  aortic arch surgery and, 1049–1051, 1050f, 1058–1059
  atrial fibrillation and, 1345, 1354
  cardiac surgery and, 949–950, 1005, 1009
  cardiopulmonary bypass and, 970
  carotid artery stenting and, 1154
  coronary artery bypass grafting and, 1152–1153, 1374
  left ventricular assist device and, 1529
  patent foramen ovale and, 1803–1804
  prosthetic valve endocarditis and, 1275
  thoracic endovascular aortic repair and, 1136
  type A aortic dissection and, 1096–1097, 1097t
Stroke volume
  exercise-related, 725–726, 726f
  formula for, 827
  in pectus excavatum, 363
Stroke work, 748, 748f
  end-diastolic volume and, 746, 747f
SU5416, in mesothelioma, 465–466
Subaortic stenosis, 1947–1951
  membranous, 1947–1948, 1947f–1948f
    surgical treatment of, 1947–1948
    results of, 1948
  in single ventricle, 2043
  tunnel-like, 1947f, 1948–1951
    aorto-apical conduit for, 1952
    Konno-Rastan operation for, 1950, 1950f
    modified Konno operation for, 1948–1951, 1949f, 1951f
    Ross-Konno operation for, 1951, 1952f
Subclavian artery
  anatomy of, 4, 4f
  angiography of, 1158, 1160, 1161f
  false aneurysm of, 404–406, 405f
  injury to, 103, 104f–106f
  occlusive disease of, 1150–1151, 1160
    bypass for, 1150–1151
    endovascular stenting for, 1151
  right, aberrant
    aortic arch aneurysm with, 1042, 1043f–1044f, 1077
    interrupted aortic arch and, 1928
    left aortic arch with, 1789, 1789f, 1791–1792
  stenosis of, 1372
  surface anatomy of, 12
Subclavian steal syndrome, 921, 1144f, 1152
Subclavian-to-pulmonary artery shunt, in pulmonary atresia with ventricular septal defect, 1902
Subclavian vein
  anatomy of, 3–4, 4f
  effort thrombosis of, 392–393, 398–400
  injury to, 103
  for pediatric cardiac catheterization, 1693
  for permanent pacemaker insertion, 1320, 1320f
  for temporary pacemaker insertion, 1306, 1307b
Subclavius muscle, 8t
Subscapularis muscle, 8t
Substance abuse
  aortic dissection with, 1093
  coronary artery effects of, 1476–1477

Subvalvular aortic stenosis, 1947–1951, 1947f
  membranous, 1947–1948, 1948f
  tunnel-like, 1948–1951, 1949f–1952f
Subxiphoid window, 101, 101f, 1175–1176, 1175f, 1485, 1489, 1489f
Sucralfate, preoperative, 48–49
Suction retractors, in off-pump coronary artery bypass grafting, 1402, 1402f–1403f
Sufentanil, in congenital heart disease, 1757
Sugar tumor, 157
Sulfinpyrazone, in prosthetic heart valve anticoagulation, 1280–1281
Superior sulcus, lesions of, 313, 314. See also Pancoast tumor
Supraspinatus muscle, 8t
Suprasternal notch, 10
Supravalvular aortic stenosis, 1952–1954
  clinical presentation of, 1952, 1953f
  surgical treatment of, 1952–1954, 1953f
    results of, 1954, 1954f–1955f
Supraventricular arrhythmias
  digoxin in, 893
  after tetralogy of Fallot repair, 1891
Surface anatomy, 10–12, 11f, 12t, 13f
Surface-modifying additives, in cardiopulmonary bypass, 969
Surfactant, in congenital diaphragmatic hernia, 501
Surgery. See also at specific disorders and procedures
  body temperature during, 50
  care after, 51–58. See also Cardiac surgery, care after; Postoperative care
  care during, 50–51
  cigarette smoking cessation before, 47
  complications of, 40. See also at Postoperative care
    age and, 44, 44t
    risk for, 44–45, 44t
  discharge planning after, 58
  drainage during, 50–51
  evaluation before. See Preoperative evaluation
  fluid administration during, 50
  monitoring during, 50
  patient positioning during, 50
  physiologic effects of, 39
  preparation for, 47–50. See also Preoperative evaluation
  specimen management during, 51
  ventilation for, 50
  video-assisted. See Video-assisted thoracoscopic surgery (VATS)
Surgical Care Improvement Project, 1015
Surgicel, 770–771
Suture, deep pericardial, in off-pump coronary artery bypass grafting, 1400, 1400f–1401f
SV40 virus, in mesothelioma, 453
Swallowing
  air, gastroesophageal reflux disease and, 524–525
  barium esophagography of, 551f
  impedance-manometric evaluation of, 556, 558f
  manometric evaluation of, 527–528, 527f
    body motility on, 528, 528f–530f
    high-resolution, 528–529
    lower sphincter on, 527, 527f, 552, 554f
    upper sphincter on, 528, 530f, 552, 554f
  phases of, 549–550
  physiology of, 520–522, 521f–522f
  radiographic evaluation of, 525–526
Swan-Ganz catheter, 745
  heparin bonding for, 1290
Sweating, increase in. See Hyperhidrosis
Swyer-James syndrome, 144
Sympathectomy
  dorsal. See Dorsal sympathectomy
  failure of, 24
  in hyperhidrosis, 661, 663
Sympathetically maintained pain syndrome, 403
Sympathicotomy, in hyperhidrosis, 663–666, 664f
Syncope, 1329
  neurocardiogenic, 1310b pacemaker in. See also Pacemaker, permanent
Synovial sarcoma, 331–332
Syphilis
  aortic, 1027
  coronary artery, 1475
Systemic inflammatory response, 107
Systemic lupus erythematosus, 1475

Systemic-to-pulmonary artery shunt
　　in pulmonary atresia with intact ventricular septum, 1868–1869, 1869f–1870f
　　in pulmonary atresia with ventricular septal defect, 1902
　　in tetralogy of Fallot, 1888–1889
Systole, 741, 741f–742f, 744–746. *See also* Ventricle(s), left, systolic function of

T

Tachycardia
　　accessory pathway–mediated, catheter ablation in, 1334–1335, 1335t, 1336f
　　atrial, 1332–1334, 1333f
　　implantable cardioverter-defibrillator for, 1318, 1318f. *See also* Implantable cardioverter-defibrillator
　　incisional, 2088–2091
　　pacemaker in, 1310b. *See also* Pacemaker, permanent
　　sinus. *See* Sinus tachycardia
　　ventricular. *See* Ventricular tachycardia
Tacrolimus
　　in heart-lung transplantation, 1564t, 1565
　　in heart transplantation, 1545–1546
　　in lung transplantation, 219
Takao syndrome, 1648
Takayasu's aortitis, 1043–1044, 1046f, 1066–1067
Takayasu's arteritis, 1027, 1043–1044, 1046f
　　brachiocephalic artery, 1144–1145, 1151–1152
　　coronary artery, 1475
　　imaging of, 794
Takeuchi operation, 1968–1969, 1969f–1972f
Talc sclerosis
　　in empyema, 420
　　in malignant pleural effusion, 437–438, 440f, 441t–442t
　　in postoperative air leak, 55
Talent device, 1130–1131, 1131f, 1134–1135
Tamponade. *See* Cardiac tamponade
TandemHeart, 861, 862f, 1512–1513, 1514f
Tbx5, 1647
Temperature. *See also* Hypothermia
　　body
　　　after cardiac surgery, 934
　　　intraoperative, 50
　　cerebral, 1006–1007
Temporary pacemaker. *See* Pacemaker, temporary
Tendon of Todaro, 700–701, 701f
Teratoma
　　cardiac, 1634t
　　mediastinal, 29f, 636, 637f, 639
Teres major muscle, 8t
Teres minor muscle, 8t
Terumo DuraHeart device, 1518, 1518f
Tet spells, 1882–1883
Tetracycline, for pleurodesis, 438, 441t–442t
Tetralogy of Fallot, 1877
　　with absent pulmonary valve, 1892
　　acyanotic, 1881–1882
　　adult, 2075–2076, 2075f–2076f
　　　echocardiography in, 845
　　　ventricular tachycardia in, 2092–2093
　　anatomy of, 1877–1881, 1878f
　　atrioventricular canal defects and, 1841–1842, 1892
　　balloon pulmonary valvuloplasty in, 1883–1884
　　beta-blockers in, 1883
　　branch pulmonary arteries in, 1878
　　bundle of His in, 1880–1881
　　cardiac catheterization in, 1883
　　chest radiography in, 1882
　　clinical features of, 1881–1883
　　conduction system in, 1880–1881
　　coronary arteries in, 1881, 1881f, 1886–1887, 1889f
　　cyanosis in, 1882–1883
　　diagnosis of, 1881–1883
　　echocardiography in, 845, 1878f–1880f, 1882–1883, 1883f
　　electrocardiography in, 1882
　　genetic tests in, 1882
　　historical perspective on, 1877
　　hypercyanotic episodes in, 1882–1883
　　infundibular septum in, 1877, 1878f
　　laboratory studies in, 1882

Tetralogy of Fallot (*Continued*)
　　main pulmonary artery in, 1878, 1879f
　　medical management of, 1883–1884
　　murmur in, 1882
　　outpatient management of, 1883
　　patent foramen ovale in, 1881
　　physical examination in, 1882
　　pulmonary artery stenosis in, 1885–1886, 1885f–1889f
　　pulmonary atresia with. *See* Pulmonary atresia with ventricular septal defect
　　pulmonary valve stenosis in, 1877–1878, 1879f
　　right aortic arch in, 1881
　　surgical management of, 1884–1886
　　　in adult, 2075–2076, 2075f–2076f
　　　anomalous coronary arteries in, 1886–1887, 1889f
　　　arrhythmias after, 1891
　　　cardiopulmonary bypass in, 1884
　　　care after, 1889–1890
　　　functional status after, 1890
　　　intracardiac portion of, 1884–1885, 1884f
　　　junctional ectopic tachycardia after, 1890
　　　late pulmonary valve replacement after, 1890–1891
　　　long-term followup after, 1890–1891
　　　monocusp valve in, 1886
　　　pulmonary artery portion of, 1885–1886, 1885f–1889f
　　　right ventricular outflow tract obstruction after, 1890
　　　right ventricular outflow tract reconstruction in, 1884–1886, 1884f–1885f
　　　right ventricular performance after, 1889–1890
　　　timing of, 1887–1889
　　　ventricular septal defect after, 1890
　　　ventriculotomy vs. transatrial-transpulmonary approach in, 1887
　　systemic-to-pulmonary artery shunt in, 1888–1889
　　ventricular septal defect in, 1878–1880, 1880f
　　viral infection in, 1883
Tetrodotoxin, in myocardial protection, 985
Thalidomide, in mesothelioma, 465–466
Thebesian valve, 710
Thoracentesis, 432, 434f, 436
Thoracic aorta. *See* Aorta, thoracic
Thoracic artery, 10. *See also* Internal thoracic artery
Thoracic duct, 23, 427
　　injury to, chylothorax with. *See* Chylothorax
　　ligation of, 428–429, 429t, 611
　　percutaneous embolization of, 611
Thoracic epidural anesthesia, 921–922
Thoracic inlet, 3–4, 3f
Thoracic outlet, anatomy of, 3f–4f, 4
　　functional, 390, 391f
　　surgical, 389–390, 390f
Thoracic outlet syndrome, 5t, 389
　　Adson test in, 393, 394f
　　anatomy of
　　　functional, 390, 391f
　　　surgical, 389–390, 390f
　　angiography in, 396, 399f
　　cervical rib in, 391, 392f, 393, 396f
　　clinical manifestations of, 391–393, 392f–393f
　　computed tomography in, 397, 401f
　　costoclavicular test in, 393, 394f
　　definition of, 389, 390f
　　diagnosis of, 393–396, 394f–396f
　　　delayed, 391–392
　　differential diagnosis of, 396–397, 400b, 401f
　　etiology of, 391, 391b
　　historical perspective on, 389
　　hyperabduction test in, 393, 395f
　　nerve conduction velocity in, 393
　　　calculations for, 395, 399f
　　　equipment for, 393–395, 397f–398f
　　　grading with, 396
　　　normal values and, 395–396
　　　technique of, 395, 398f
　　Paget-Schroetter syndrome with, 392–393, 398–400, 402f
　　pain in, 391–392, 396–397
　　pseudorecurrence of, 405
　　radiography in, 393, 396f
　　Raynaud's phenomenon in, 392
　　recurrence of, 404–406, 405f–406f
　　scalene test in, 393, 394f

Thoracic outlet syndrome (*Continued*)
　　subclavian artery dilation in, 392, 392f
　　treatment of, 397–398
　　　dorsal sympathectomy in, 400–404
　　　　complications of, 403
　　　　neuralgia after, 403
　　　　pathophysiology of, 402–403
　　　　recurrent symptoms after, 403
　　　　results of, 404
　　　　surgical approaches for, 403
　　　　technique of, 404
　　　　transaxillary approach for, 404
　　　　transaxillary first rib resection with, 404
　　　　variations of, 403–404
　　　physiotherapy in, 397
　　　reoperation in, 404–406, 405f–406f
　　　transaxillary first rib resection in, 397–398, 401f–402f
　　　　dorsal sympathectomy with, 404
Thoracoabdominal aortic aneurysm. *See* Aortic aneurysm, thoracoabdominal
Thoracoplasty, in empyema, 422–423
Thoracostomy
　　open-window, in empyema, 420, 421f
　　tube
　　　in pulmonary injury, 99–100
　　　in spontaneous pneumothorax, 410
Thoracotomy
　　in air embolus, 102–103
　　anterolateral
　　　in mitral valve surgery, 1219, 1220f
　　　in penetrating cardiac injury, 1177
　　emergency department, 88–90, 89b
　　　CPR duration and, 89
　　　results of, 89–90
　　　technique of, 89
　　in empyema, 418–419
　　historical perspective on, 86
　　infection after, 56
　　in lung cancer evaluation, 249
　　in lung transplantation, 214, 214f
　　pain after, 56, 283
　　pediatric, 1793
　　　anterior, 1710–1711
　　　anterolateral, 1710–1711
　　　posterolateral, 1711, 1711f
　　　transaxillary, 1711–1712
　　in pulmonary injury, 100
　　in reoperative coronary artery bypass grafting, 1426, 1426f
Thoratec HeartMate II device, 1516, 1516f
Thoratec HeartMate III device, 1518
Thoratec HeartMate XVE device, 1513–1514, 1515f
Thoratec intracorporeal device, 1515, 1516f
Thoratec paracorporeal device, 1514–1515, 1515f
Thorax
　　anatomy of, 3–6, 3f
　　trauma to. *See* Trauma
Threshold testing, preoperative, 43–44, 44f
Thrombasthenia, after cardiac surgery, 947
Thrombectomy, 856–857, 1618
Thrombin
　　in acute coronary syndromes, 868
　　in cardiopulmonary bypass, 935, 965, 965f
　　direct inhibitors of, in NSTE acute coronary syndromes, 875
Thrombocytopenia
　　in cardiopulmonary bypass, 964
　　heparin-induced, 759–760, 923, 946–947, 1284
　　　in cardiopulmonary bypass, 923, 946–947, 965–966, 966f
Thromboembolism
　　after Fontan procedure, 2049–2050
　　after left ventricular assist device implantation, 1521
　　pulmonary. *See* Pulmonary embolism
Thrombolytic therapy
　　in acute pulmonary embolism, 1617–1618, 1617f
　　in Paget-Schroetter syndrome, 400
Thrombosis
　　with cardiopulmonary bypass circuits, 1286–1287
　　catheter-related, 1289–1290
　　coronary. *See* Myocardial infarction (MI), 1474
　　effort, 392–393, 398–400, 402f
　　with extracorporeal membrane oxygenation, 1287–1288

Thrombosis (Continued)
  with intra-aortic balloon assist device, 1286
  with prosthetic heart valves, 1186, 1279–1280, 1284–1286
  stent, 855–856
  with thoracic aortic graft, 1288–1289, 1289f
  with ventricular assist devices, 1288
Thymectomy, 641–642
  maximal, 641
  median sternotomy in, 641
  myasthenic crisis after, 57–58
  thoracoscopic, 642
  transcervical, 641, 642f
Thymolipoma, 639
Thymoma, 633–638
  classification of, 634–635, 635t
  computed tomography in, 636–637, 636f
  encapsulated, 633
  invasive, 633
  Masaoka classification of, 634–635, 635t
  Muller-Hermelink classification of, 635
  myasthenia gravis and, 635, 637
  pathology of, 634
  pleural, 455–456
  presentation of, 635
  prognosis for, 638
  pulmonary, 157, 158f
  surgical treatment of, 641–642
  systemic diseases and, 635–636, 636b
  treatment of, 638
  WHO classification of, 635, 635t
Thymus
  carcinoid tumor of, 639
  carcinoma of, 638
  cyst of, 639
  hyperplasia of, 639
  lipoma of, 639
  neuroendocrine tumor of, 638–639
  small cell carcinoma of, 639
  tumors of, 633–639, 635b. See also Thymoma
    biopsy of, 638
Thyroid artery, inferior, 519, 519f
Thyroid carcinoma, tracheal invasion of, 116, 117f, 126
Thyroid gland
  ectopic, 640
  substernal, 640
Ticlopidine
  preoperative evaluation of, 919
  in prosthetic heart valve anticoagulation, 1280
TIMP-2, in pleural effusion, 435t
Tirofiban, 760
  preoperative evaluation of, 919
Titin, 727f–728f, 728–729, 742, 744f
TNNT2, 1496
"To Err Is Human" (Institute of Medicine), 1014, 1014b
Todaro, tendon of, 700–701, 701f
Tolazoline
  in congenital diaphragmatic hernia, 500–501
  in pediatric pulmonary hypertension, 1752
Tolerance, opioid, in children, 1757
Torsemide, 887, 887t
Total anomalous pulmonary venous drainage. See Anomalous pulmonary venous drainage/connection, total
Total artificial heart. See Artificial heart
Townes-Brocks syndrome, 1801
TPM1, 1496
Trachea
  adenoid cystic carcinoma of, 116
  agenesis of, 130–131, 131f
  anatomy of, 12–14, 113, 114f, 647
  atresia of, 130–131
  blood supply of, 13, 113, 114f
  burn injury to, 113–114
  congenital disease of, 1765. See also Tracheal stenosis; Tracheomalacia
    diagnosis of, 1765, 1766f–1768f, 1767b
    historical perspective on, 1765
    surgery for, 1766–1773, 1769f, 1769t. See also Tracheoplasty
  injury to, 93
    burn-related, 113–114
    imaging in, 26, 28f
    penetrating, 98–99
    postintubation, 114–115, 114f–115f
    surgical management of, 99, 99f

Trachea (Continued)
  length of, 113
  reconstruction of. See Tracheoplasty
  resection of, 119–121, 119f, 121f–122f
    anastomotic complications of, 126
    anesthesia for, 117–119
    in children, 1766–1768, 1769f, 1769t
    complications of, 126
    historical perspective on, 113
    management after, 124
    vs. nonsurgical management, 126
    release procedures with, 121, 122f–123f
    results of, 124–126
  squamous cell carcinoma of, 116, 116f
  stenosis of. See Tracheal stenosis
  thyroid carcinoma invasion of, 116, 117f, 126
  tumors of, 116, 116f–117f, 647
    bronchoscopic removal of, 117
    clinical presentation of, 116–117
    imaging of, 117, 118f
    resection with, 120
      results of, 125–126
  webs of, 1778
Tracheal stenosis
  congenital, 131–132, 131f–132f
    cartilage tracheoplasty for, 1769–1771, 1771f–1772f
    diagnosis of, 1765, 1766f–1768f, 1767b
    historical perspective on, 1765
    homograft tracheoplasty for, 1773
    pericardial tracheoplasty for, 1771–1773, 1773f
    resection and reanastomosis for, 131–132, 132f, 1766–1768, 1769f, 1769t
    slide tracheoplasty for, 1768, 1769f–1770f
    surgery for, 1766–1773, 1769f, 1769t. See also Tracheoplasty
    tracheal autograft technique for, 1773, 1774f–1775f
    type I, 131
    type II, 131
    type III, 131
  dilatation of, 117
  idiopathic, 115–116
  postintubation, 114–115, 114f–115f
    in children, 1777–1778
  resection of, 119–121, 119f, 121f–122f
    in children, 1766–1768, 1769f, 1769t
    results of, 124–126
Tracheobronchial-esophageal fistula, 135
Tracheobronchial tree, 12–14, 13t, 14f
Tracheobronchomalacia, 116. See also Tracheomalacia
Tracheobronchomegaly, 134–135, 134f
Tracheobronchoscopy, 63–66
  indications for, 63–64, 63b
Tracheoesophageal fistula, 114f–115f, 115
  clinical presentation of, 117
  esophageal atresia and, 536, 536f, 536t
    operative management of, 538–539, 539f
  H-type, 536, 536f, 536t
    operative management of, 541, 541f–542f
  repair of, 121–123, 123f–124f, 125
Tracheoinnominate fistula, 114f
  clinical presentation of, 117
  repair of, 121–123
Tracheomalacia, 132–133, 133f, 647, 1776–1777
  aortopexy in, 133, 133f, 542, 543f
  diagnosis of, 133, 1765
  external stabilization procedure in, 1777, 1778f
  Palmaz stent in, 1777, 1777f
Tracheoplasty
  autograft, 1773, 1774f–1775f
  cartilage, 1769–1771, 1771f–1772f
  homograft, 1773
  pericardial, 1771–1773, 1773f
  slide, 1768, 1769f–1770f, 1771t
Tracheostomy
  bronchoscopy for, 64
  coronary artery bypass grafting and, 1378
  postoperative, 52–53
Trandolapril, 891t
Tranexamic acid
  in cardiac surgery, 765–766
  in cardiopulmonary bypass, 923–924, 1724
  in children, 765–766
Trans-xiphoid mini-sternotomy, 1710, 1710f–1711f
Transanular patch, in pulmonary atresia with ventricular septal defect, 1901

Transcervical extended mediastinal lymphadenectomy, 631
Transesophageal echocardiography. See also Echocardiography, transesophageal
Transforming growth factor β, in Marfan syndrome, 1025
Transhiatal esophagectomy. See also Esophagectomy, transhiatal
Transmyocardial laser revascularization, 1427, 1457
  angina class and, 1460, 1460t
  angiogenesis with, 1463
  channel patency with, 1462, 1463f
  coronary artery bypass grafting with, 1461
  denervation with, 1462–1463
  endpoints for, 1459
  exercise tolerance after, 1460
  historical perspective on, 1457
  hospitalization rate after, 1460
  mechanisms of, 1462–1463, 1462f
  vs. medical management, 1460, 1460t
  medical therapy and, 1460
  morbidity with, 1460
  mortality with, 1459–1460
  myocardial function and, 1460
  myocardial perfusion after, 1461
  patient selection for, 1458, 1458t
  vs. percutaneous myocardial laser revascularization, 1461–1462
  quality of life and, 1460
  results of, 1457–1462, 1460t
    long-term, 1461
  technique of, 1458, 1459f
  in transplant graft disease, 1463
Transplantation
  heart. See Heart-lung transplantation; Heart transplantation
  lung. See Lung transplantation
  stem cell. See Regenerative cell-based therapy
Transposition of great arteries, 1652f, 1662, 1981
  anatomy of, 1652f, 1658f–1660f, 1661, 1982, 1983f
  atrioventricular canal defect and, 1843
  balloon atrial septostomy in, 1694
  cardiac catheterization in, 1984, 1994
  classification of, 1981–1982
  clinical features of, 1982–1983, 1984f
  complete, 1662
  complex, 1992–1999
    aortic arch abnormalities in, 1994, 1998–1999
    cardiac catheterization in, 1994
    conal septum deviation in, 1992–1993, 1994f, 1995, 1996f
    coronary artery variation in, 1993–1994
    diagnosis of, 1994
    double-outlet right ventricle in, 1993, 1994f, 1997–1999
    echocardiography in, 1994
    left ventricular outflow tract obstruction in, 1993–1996, 1999
    noncommitted ventricular septal defect in, 1998
    right ventricular outflow tract obstruction in, 1993
    subpulmonary ventricular septal defect in, 1997–1998
    surgical management of
      with aortic arch obstruction, 1998–1999
      aortic autograft translocation in, 1996, 1997f–1998f
      with conal septum deviation, 1995, 1996f
      with double-outlet right ventricle, 1997–1999
      with left ventricular outflow tract obstruction, 1994–1996, 1999
      left ventricular retraining in, 1999
      Rastelli operation in, 1995–1996, 1996f
      results of, 1999
  congenitally corrected, 1652f, 1662, 2003
    aortic arch in, 2004
    clinical presentation of, 2005–2006
    conduction system in, 2004–2005, 2005f
    coronary arteries in, 2004, 2005f
    evaluation of, 2007
    left ventricle training in, 2007
    left ventricular outflow tract obstruction in, 2004
    mitral valve in, 2004
    morphologic right ventricle in, 2006–2007
    morphology of, 2003–2005, 2004f
    surgical management of, 2007–2011, 2008f
      anatomic, 2009–2012, 2011f

Transposition of great arteries (Continued)
  atrial-arterial switch in, 2006–2007, 2009–2010, 2011f, 2012
  cardiopulmonary bypass in, 2007–2008
  care after, 2011
  Mustard procedure in, 2011
  one-and-a-half operation in, 2011
  palliative, 2009
  physiologic, 2007–2009, 2009f, 2011–2012
  Rastelli-Senning procedure in, 2010–2011, 2011f
  results of, 2011–2012
  right ventricular dysfunction and, 2006
  Senning procedure in, 2011
  tricuspid valve repair/replacement in, 2008–2009
  valved conduit placement in, 2008
  ventricular septal defect closure in, 2008
 tricuspid valve in, 2004, 2006–2009
 ventricular septal defect in, 2004, 2008
congestive heart failure in, 1983
coronary artery variation in, 1982, 1983f, 1993–1994
cyanosis in, 1983
diagnosis of, 1983–1984
echocardiography in, 1984
electrocardiography in, 1984
embryology of, 1981–1982
epidemiology of, 1981
historical perspective on, 1981
medical management in, 1984
oxygen saturation in, 1983
partial, 1662. See also Double-outlet right ventricle
physical examination in, 1983–1984
pulmonary arterial banding in, 1985
pulmonary vascular disease in, 1983
Rashkind atrial septostomy in, 1984
surgical management in, 1985–1992
 arrhythmias after, 1986
 arterial switch operation in, 1987–1992, 1989f
  care after, 1988
  late followup after, 1991, 1992f
  outcome of, 1988–1992
  reoperation after, 1991–1992
 historical perspective on, 1985–1987
 Mustard operation for, 1985–1987, 1987f
 palliative, 1985
 right ventricular dysfunction after, 1986–1987
 Senning operation for, 1985–1987, 1986f
ventricular septal defect with, 1982–1983
Transpulmonary pressure gradient, 1693
Transthoracic echocardiography. See Echocardiography, transthoracic
Transvenous pacing. See Pacemaker
Trapezius muscle, 6, 7f, 8t
Trauma, 85
 acute lung injury with, 107
 age and, 86
 blunt, 90–98
  asphyxia with, 92
  cardiac injury with, 94–96, 95t, 1474
  chest wall, 90–92
  clavicular fracture with, 91
  diaphragmatic injury with, 96–97, 96f–97f
  esophageal injury with, 97–98
  flail chest with, 90–91, 91f
  great vessel injury with, 93–94, 94f, 1027
  laryngeal injury with, 92–93
  pulmonary contusion with, 92
  rib fracture with, 90
  scapular fracture with, 92
  sternal fracture with, 91
  tracheobronchial injury with, 93
 bronchopleural fistula after, 108
 cardiac. See Cardiac injury
 complications of, 107–108, 107b
 evaluation of, 86–88
  angiography in, 87–88, 88f, 89b
  chest radiography in, 86–87
  computed angiography in, 88, 88f
  echocardiography in, 87
  primary survey in, 86, 86t
  ultrasonography in, 87, 87f
 great vessel fistula after, 108
 historical perspective on, 85–86, 85f
 imaging in, 25–26, 26f–27f, 794–795
 mortality from, 86
 penetrating, 98–107

Trauma (Continued)
 air embolism with, 102–103
 bronchial injury with, 98–99
 bullet embolism with, 102–103
 cardiac injury with, 100–102, 101f–102f, 1474
 chest wall injury with, 98
 diaphragmatic injury with, 103–105
 esophageal injury with, 105–107
 great vessel injury with, 103, 104f–106f, 1027
 hemothorax injury with, 99–100
 pulmonary injury with, 99–100
 stabbing vs. firearm, 98
 tracheal injury with, 98–99, 99f
 VATS in, 104, 106b
pericarditis with, 1486
pleural space problems after, 108
pneumonia after, 107–108
respiratory distress syndrome with, 107, 107b
thoracotomy in, 88–90, 89b
Treppe phenomenon, 746
Tri-incisional (modified McKeown) esophagectomy. See Esophagectomy, modified McKeown (tri-incisional)
Triamterene, 887t, 888
Triangle of Koch, 700–701, 701f
Tricuspid anulus
 anatomy of, 1241–1242, 1242f, 1245f
 diameter of, 1246, 1247f
 reconstruction of, 1251–1252, 1252f–1253f
Tricuspid regurgitation, 1247f. See also Tricuspid valve, surgery on
 atrial septal defect and, 1801
 in congenitally corrected transposition of great arteries, 2005–2007
 conservative treatment of, 1246–1247
 degenerative, 1244–1245
 diagnosis of, 1245–1246
 echocardiography in, 841–842
 functional, 1245, 1248
 left ventricular assist device implantation and, 1509
 severity of, 1246
 traumatic, 1244
Tricuspid valve, 703, 703f
 anatomy of, 1241–1244, 1849
  anulus, 1241–1242, 1242f–1243f
  chordae tendineae, 1243
  leaflet, 1243, 1243f
  surgical implications of, 1243–1244, 1244f
  terminology for, 1243
 on cardiac catheterization, 783–786
 in congenitally corrected transposition of great arteries, 2004
 diameter of, in pulmonary atresia with intact ventricular septum, 1867, 1867f, 1868f, 1870f
 disease of, 1244–1245
  congestive heart failure and, 1248
  conservative approach to, 1246–1247
  diagnosis of, 1245–1246
  functional, 1245, 1245f, 1248
  after heart transplantation, 1248
  infective, 1248
  with left-sided valvular lesions, 1248
  organic, 1244–1245, 1244t, 1248
  trauma-related, 1248
 Ebstein's anomaly of. See Ebstein's anomaly
 echocardiography of, 841–842, 841f
 endocarditis of, 1244, 1248, 1259, 1263–1264
 repair of, 1250–1251, 1250f–1251f
  in congenitally corrected transposition of great arteries, 2008–2009
  in Ebstein's anomaly, 2060–2062, 2061f–2062f
  results of, 1254
 replacement of, 1252–1253
  in congenitally corrected transposition of great arteries, 2008–2009
  in Ebstein's anomaly, 2062–2063, 2064f
  results of, 1254–1255
 surgery on, 1248–1253
  anuloplasty for, 1251–1252, 1252f–1253f
  approaches in, 1249, 1249f
  commissurotomy for, 1249, 1250f
  indications for, 1246–1248
  repair for, 1250–1251, 1250f–1251f, 1254
  replacement for, 1252–1255
  results of, 1253–1255

Tricuspid valve (Continued)
 Z-values for, in pulmonary atresia with intact ventricular septum, 1867, 1867f, 1868f, 1870f
Triglycerides, 905, 907
 chyle, 610–611
 levels of, 910–911
 pleural fluid, 428
Triiodothyronine, after pediatric cardiac surgery, 1759
Troponins, 727–728, 728f
 in blunt cardiac injury, 95, 1174
 in myocardial infarction, 871
Truncus arteriosus, 1911–1919
 anatomy of, 1911–1913, 1912f–1913f, 1912t
 associated anomalies of, 1913
 branch pulmonary arteries in, 1912
 chest radiography in, 1914
 classification of, 1911, 1912t
 clinical features of, 1913–1914
 coronary artery variations in, 1913
 diagnosis of, 1913–1914
 echocardiography in, 1914, 1914f
 embryology of, 1911
 extracardiac anomalies in, 1913
 interrupted aortic arch in, 1913, 1916–1917, 1917f
 mortality with, 1915
 murmur in, 1914
 natural history of, 1915
 patent foramen ovale in, 1913
 pathophysiology of, 1913
 regurgitation in, 1913–1914, 1917
 stenosis in, 1913, 1917
 surgical treatment of, 1915–1916, 1915f–1916f
  care after, 1918–1919
  interrupted aortic arch in, 1916–1917, 1917f
  pulmonary outflow tract reconstruction in, 1917–1918
  results of, 1919
  truncal valve regurgitation and, 1917
  truncal valve stenosis and, 1917
 ventricular septal defect in, 1912, 1913f, 1915–1916, 1916f
Tube thoracostomy
 in pulmonary injury, 99–100
 in spontaneous pneumothorax, 410
Tuberculosis, 161, 162f, 182–185
 aortic, 1066
 collapse therapy in, 183
 extensively drug-resistant, 183
 incidence of, 182
 multidrug-resistant, 183
 pericardial, 1485
 resectional surgery in, 183
Tumors. See also specific sites and tumors
Tumor markers, 670
 blood detection of, 676–677
 panels of, 678
 in pleural effusion, 435t
 targeted cancer therapy and, 678–679
Tumor suppressor genes, in mesothelioma, 452
Type A aortic dissection. See Aortic dissection, type A
Type B aortic dissection. See Aortic dissection, type B

U

Ulcer(s)
 aortic
  atherosclerotic, 1139–1140
  imaging of, 794
  in type B aortic dissection, 1115–1117, 1120
 gastric, prevention of, 48–49
Ulex europaeus agglutinin, in pleural effusion, 435t
Ulnar artery, in coronary artery bypass grafting, 1418
Ulnar nerve, conduction velocity of, 393
 abnormal, 396
 calculations for, 395, 399f
 equipment for, 393–395, 397f–398f
 normal, 395–396
 technique of, 395, 398f
Ultrafiltration, in pediatric cardiac surgery, 1728
Ultrasonography
 cardiovascular. See Echocardiography
 E-FAST, in trauma, 87, 87f
 in empyema, 417
 endobronchial, 64

Ultrasonography (*Continued*)
of middle mediastinum, 646
for transbronchial needle aspiration, 247, 247f, 631–632, 632f
endoscopic, 62–63, 63b, 555–556, 557f
in esophageal cancer, 577–580, 579f, 579t, 584f, 617–618, 618f, 655
in metastatic disease, 580
after neoadjuvant chemoradiation, 579
of middle mediastinum, 646
esophageal
in foregut cyst, 568, 569f
in leiomyoma, 568, 568f
intravascular, 857
of middle mediastinum, 646
in non–small cell lung cancer, 298
in trauma, 87, 87f
Umbilical artery, cannulation-related thrombosis of, 1289
Umbilical vein, for pediatric cardiac catheterization, 1693
Unifocalization procedure, in pulmonary atresia with ventricular septal defect, 1900–1901, 1903, 1903f
Unroofing procedure, in anomalous aorta–pulmonary artery coronary artery course, 1973, 1974f
Upper esophageal sphincter. *See* Esophageal sphincter, upper
Urea, after cardiopulmonary bypass, 971
Uremic pericarditis, 1486
Urokinase
in empyema, 419
in prosthetic heart valve anticoagulation, 1280
Usual interstitial pneumonia, 165–167
Uterine cancer, pulmonary metastases in, 346

V

Vacuum-assisted closure therapy, in sternal wound infection, 1001–1002, 1002f
Vagus nerve, 17–20, 19f, 23–24, 520, 520f
Valiant device, 1131
Valirudin, in cardiopulmonary bypass, 966
Valley fever, 187
Valsartan, in heart failure, 891t
Valvuloplasty, balloon. *See also* Aortic valve, repair of; Mitral valve repair
aortic, 858–859, 1198, 1199f
mitral, 858, 859f, 1211, 1212f
pulmonary, 1694, 1883–1884
Varices, pulmonary, 145
Vascular endothelial growth factor, in pleural effusion, 433
Vascular resistance, 711–712. *See also* Vascular tone
assessment of, 781t, 783, 1693
dipyridamole effects on, 711, 712f
pulmonary, 781t, 783
in hypoplastic left heart syndrome, 2027
systemic, 781t, 783
in hypoplastic left heart syndrome, 2027–2028
venules in, 718
Vascular rings, 1787–1793
anatomy of, 1787–1789, 1787f–1789f
classification of, 1787
clinical presentation of, 1789–1790
complications of, 1792
diagnosis of, 1790–1791, 1790f
pathophysiology of, 1787–1789
prognosis for, 1792
treatment of, 1791–1792
approaches to, 1792–1793, 1793f
video-assisted thoracoscopic surgery for, 1793
Vascular tone, 711–718, 712f
autoregulation of, 716
endothelium effects on, 713–716, 714f–716f
extravascular factors in, 718
extrinsic regulation of, 712–713, 714f
flow-induced dilation in, 716–717, 717f
humoral factors in, 718
intrinsic myogenic tone and, 718, 719f
intrinsic regulation of, 712–713, 714f
microdomains in, 713
neurohumoral factors in, 717–718
Vasculitis, coronary artery, 1474–1475
Vasculogenesis, in myocardial cell-based regenerative therapy, 1607

Vasodilators
in congenital diaphragmatic hernia, 500–501
in heart failure, 888–890
Vasodilatory shock, after cardiopulmonary bypass, 943
Vasoplegic syndrome, after cardiopulmonary bypass, 943
Vasopressin
after cardiopulmonary bypass, 969
vascular effects of, 718
VATER association, 536, 537f
VATS. *See* Video-assisted thoracoscopic surgery (VATS)
Vegetations, in endocarditis, 835, 842, 843f
Velocardiofacial syndrome, 1882
Vena cava
inferior
injury to, 102–103
for pediatric cardiac catheterization, 1693
superior, injury to, 102–103
Vena cava syndrome, in congenital diaphragmatic hernia, 504
Vena caval filter, in acute pulmonary embolism, 1619
Ventilation
mechanical
after cardiac surgery, 933
in congenital diaphragmatic hernia, 501
after lung transplantation, 218
after pediatric cardiac surgery, 1759–1761, 1760b
pneumonia with, 178–179
prevention of, 1017
weaning from, after pediatric cardiac surgery, 1760–1761, 1760b
single-lung, 50
Ventilation-perfusion scan
in acute pulmonary embolism, 1616–1617
in chronic thromboembolic pulmonary hypertension, 1622
in pulmonary embolism, 35
Ventilator-associated pneumonia, 178–179
prevention of, 1017
VentraCor Ventr, 1517–1518, 1518f. *See also* Assist device
Ventricle(s). *See also* Atrium (atria)
left, 739. *See also at* Left ventricular
anatomy of, 705–706, 705f, 1651–1653, 1652f, 1657f
aneurysm of, 1576–1577, 1577f
resection of, 1577–1578
in chronic mitral regurgitation, 1432, 1432f, 1434
computed tomography of, 741
concentric hypertrophy of, 744
diastolic function of, 741–744, 741f–742f
atrial contraction and, 743
concentric hypertrophy and, 744
in dilated cardiomyopathy, 743
E-to-A ratio and, 743
echocardiographic evaluation of, 743, 745f, 831f–832f
end-diastolic pressure–volume relationship and, 741–744, 743f, 743b
extracellular matrix and, 739–740, 740f
in hypertrophic cardiomyopathy, 1496–1497
measurement of, 743, 745f
mitral flow patterns in, 743, 745f
myocardial ischemia and, 743–744
myocardial stiffness and, 742
myocyte relaxation and, 742, 743f
pressure-volume analysis of, 741
suction and, 743
torsion and, 742–743
after ventricular restoration, 1590f–1591f
Doppler imaging of, 748–749
double-outlet, 1652f, 1663
dysfunction of
coronary artery bypass grafting in, 1371, 1386
implantable cardioverter-defibrillator for, 1314b. *See also* Implantable cardioverter-defibrillator
dyssynchrony in, 1588–1591
echocardiography of, 743, 745f, 831–832, 831f–832f
pediatric, 1674–1675, 1675f
end-diastolic pressure of
cardiac output and, 734–737, 735f
stroke volume and, 746, 747f. *See also* Frank-Starling curve/relationship
end-diastolic pressure–volume relationship of, 740f, 742, 743f
myocardial ischemia and, 743–744

Ventricle(s) (*Continued*)
end-systolic diameter of, mitral regurgitation and, 1216–1218
end-systolic pressure–volume relationship of, 745, 746f
extracellular matrix of, 739–740
finite-element model of, 749–752, 750f–752f
force frequency relationship of, 746
geometry of, 1574–1575, 1575f, 1575t
hypertrophy of
aortic stenosis and, 1196–1197
circulatory effects of, 721
diastolic dysfunction in, 744
ischemia and, 982
vascular resistance in, 712, 713f
hypoplasia of. *See* Hypoplastic left heart syndrome
imaging of, 748–749. *See also* Computed tomography (CT), cardiovascular; Echocardiography; Magnetic resonance imaging (MRI), cardiovascular
inlet component of, 705, 705f
laminar organization of, 739, 740f
magnetic resonance imaging of, 739, 741, 749, 795
pediatric, 1678–1679, 1680f
myocyte orientation of, 739, 740f
myocyte relaxation in, 742, 743f
myocyte stiffness in, 742, 744f
in off-pump coronary artery bypass grafting, 1399
outlet component of, 705–706, 705f
perforation of, 705–706
pressure in, 780t
pressure-volume analysis of, 741
pressure-volume loop of, 730, 730f, 741, 742f
recoil of, 742–743
relaxation curve of, 742, 743f
remodeling of, 1573–1574, 1574b
in regenerative cell-based therapy, 1608–1609
right ventricle interaction with, 752
rupture of, mitral valve replacement and, 1235
suction in, 743, 744f
surgical restoration of. *See* Heart failure, surgical ventricular restoration in
in ventricular arrhythmias, 1360–1361, 1591–1593, 1593f
systolic function of, 741, 741f–742f, 744–746
cardiac index and, 744–745
cardiac output and, 744–745
echocardiographic evaluation of, 829–831, 830f
ejection fraction and, 745
end-systolic pressure–volume relationship and, 745, 746f
myocardial ischemia and, 746
torsion of, 742–743
trabecular component of, 705f
wall of, 1210
penetrating injury to, 1177
right, 703–704, 704f
anatomy of, 703–704, 703f–704f, 1651–1654, 1652f, 1656f, 1658f–1659f
atrialized, 2055. *See also* Ebstein's anomaly
plication of, 2065, 2065f
congenital malformation of, 704
decompression of, in pulmonary atresia with intact ventricular septum, 1873–1874
double-outlet. *See* Double-outlet right ventricle
dysfunction of
in congenitally corrected transposition of great arteries, 2006–2007
after transposition of great arteries correction, 1986
in hypertrophic cardiomyopathy, 1495
hypertrophy of, ischemia and, 982
inlet component of, 703, 703f
left ventricle interaction with, 752
magnetic resonance imaging of, 795
in off-pump coronary artery bypass grafting, 1399
outlet component of, 703, 703f
pressure in, 779–781, 780f, 780t
septomarginal trabeculation of, 703–704, 704f
septoparietal trabeculation of, 703–704, 704f
supraventricular crest of, 703–704, 704f
trabecular component of, 703, 703f
single. *See* Single ventricle
1.5-Ventricle repair
in Ebstein's anomaly, 2064
in single ventricle, 2044–2045

Ventricular arrhythmias. *See also* Ventricular tachycardia
 after cardiac surgery, 934, 945
  coronary artery bypass grafting in, 1371
  surgical ventricular restoration and, 1360–1361, 1591–1593, 1593f
 after tetralogy of Fallot repair, 1891
Ventricular assist devices, 1288. *See also* Artificial heart; Left ventricular assist device
Ventricular fibrillation
 electrically induced, 977
 implantable cardioverter-defibrillator for, 1314b, 1317, 1318f. *See also* Implantable cardioverter-defibrillator
Ventricular septal defect, 782f, 1849–1858. *See also* Atrioventricular canal defects; Double-outlet right ventricle
 anatomy of, 1849–1851, 1850f
 aortic cusp prolapse with, 1853
 aortic insufficiency and, 1857, 1955
 atrial septal defect and, 1801
 cardiopulmonary sequelae of, 1852
 classification of, 1850–1851, 1851f
 closure of, 1853–1858, 1854f–1856f
  care after, 1857
  in congenitally corrected transposition of great arteries, 2008
  historical perspective on, 1849
  hybrid procedure for, 2102, 2102f–2103f
  indications for, 1852–1853
  in interrupted aortic arch treatment, 1930–1931, 1931f
  in pulmonary atresia with ventricular septal defect, 1901–1902
  results of, 1857–1858
  in tetralogy of Fallot, 1884–1885, 1884f
  transcatheter, 861, 1699
  in truncus arteriosus, 1915–1916, 1916f
 coarctation of aorta and, 1786, 1852, 1857
 conal, 1851f, 1851f, 1856–1857, 1856f
 in congenitally corrected transposition of great arteries, 2004–2005
 conoventricular (membranous), 1850–1851, 1851f, 1853–1855, 1854f
 definition of, 1849
 diagnosis of, 1853, 1853f
 inlet (atrioventricular canal), 1851, 1851f, 1855–1856, 1855f
 in interrupted aortic arch, 1929–1931, 1931f, 1937–1938
 left ventricular outflow tract obstruction and, 1852
 muscular, 1851, 1851f, 1857, 2102
 natural history of, 1852–1853
 nonrestrictive, 1852
 patent ductus arteriosus and, 1852
 pathophysiology of, 1852
 postinfarction, 1449
  vs. acute mitral regurgitation, 1450
  clinical presentation of, 1450
  diagnosis of, 1450–1451
  etiology of, 1449–1450
  heart failure with, 1450
  historical perspective on, 1449
  incidence of, 1449
  location of, 1449, 1450f, 1451
  mortality with, 1450
  natural history of, 1450
  pathogenesis of, 1449–1450
  pathophysiology of, 1450
  percutaneous closure of, 1454
  preoperative management of, 1451
  recurrent, 1454–1455
  surgical management of, 1451–1454

Ventricular septal defect *(Continued)*
  in anterior septal rupture, 1451–1452, 1452f
  antifibrinolytic therapy in, 1454
  apical amputation in, 1451
  cardiopulmonary bypass weaning in, 1453–1454
  care after, 1454
  coronary artery disease and, 1453
  delayed, 1450, 1454
  indications for, 1451
  infarct exclusion with endocardial patch in, 1452–1453
  infarctectomy in, 1451–1452
  mortality with, 1454, 1455t
  outcomes of, 1454–1455, 1455f, 1455t
  percutaneous, 1454
  in posteroinferior septal rupture, 1452, 1453f
  recurrent defect after, 1454–1455
  risk predictors in, 1451, 1451t
  SHOCK study of, 1450
  ventricular assist devices in, 1454
 with prior pulmonary artery banding, 1857
 pulmonary atresia with. *See* Pulmonary atresia with ventricular septal defect
 pulmonary vascular disease and, 1852
 restrictive, 1852
 shunt in, 781–782, 782f, 1852
 subpulmonary, in transposition of great arteries, 1997–1998
 in tetralogy of Fallot, 1878–1880, 1880f
 after tetralogy of Fallot repair, 1890
 in transposition of great arteries, 1997–1998
 in truncus arteriosus, 1912, 1915–1916, 1916f
Ventricular septum
 blunt injury to, 1174
 defects of. *See* Ventricular septal defect
 embryology of, 1644–1646
 pulmonary atresia with. *See* Pulmonary atresia with intact ventricular septum
 right, 1849–1850, 1850f
Ventricular tachycardia, 1358–1361
 in adult congenital heart disease, 2092–2093
 cardiac assist device in, 1361
 catheter ablation in, 1335–1337, 1337f
 heart transplantation in, 1361
 idiopathic, catheter ablation in, 1338
 implantable cardioverter-defibrillator for, 1314b–1315b, 1317–1318, 1318f. *See also* Implantable cardioverter-defibrillator
 surgical management of
  endocardial resection in, 1360, 1360f
  historical perspective on, 1358–1359, 1358f–1359f
  indications for, 1359
  revascularization in, 1359
  ventricular reconstruction in, 1360–1361, 1591–1593, 1593f
 in tetralogy of Fallot, 2092–2093
Ventriculography, in tetralogy of Fallot, 1880f
Venules, in vascular resistance, 718
Verapamil
 in heart failure, 890, 891t
 in postoperative atrial fibrillation, 944
Vertebral artery, atherosclerosis of, 1161
Vicryl mesh, in chest wall reconstruction, 304
Video-assisted cardioscopy, intraoperative, 2100
Video-assisted mediastinoscopic lymphadenectomy, 631
Video-assisted thoracoscopic surgery (VATS). *See also* Lobectomy, thoracoscopic
 in anterior mediastinal mass, 640–641
 in children, 1712, 1712f
 in empyema, 418, 419t

Video-assisted thoracoscopic surgery (VATS) *(Continued)*
 in lung biopsy, 169–170, 169f, 237
 in lung cancer evaluation, 249
 in middle mediastinal disease, 646
 in patent ductus arteriosus, 1793, 1793f
 in pleural biopsy, 433
 in solitary pleural fibrous tumor, 455
 in spontaneous pneumothorax, 410–411, 411f
 in thoracic outlet syndrome, 400–404. *See also* Dorsal sympathectomy
 in vascular rings, 1793, 1793f
Vieussens, valve of, 710
Vimentin
 in pleural effusion, 435t
 in sarcoma, 334
Viral infection
 coronary artery, 1475
 after lung transplantation, 221, 221f
 pericardial, 1485
 in tetralogy of Fallot, 1883
Vitamin K, in anticoagulation reversal, 770

W

Warden procedure, 1806, 1807f
Warfarin, 759
 bleeding with, 1283–1284
 complications of, 1283–1284
 before coronary artery bypass grafting, 1374
 pregnancy and, 1959
 preoperative cessation of, 50
 in prosthetic heart valve anticoagulation, 1280–1281, 1281f, 1283–1284
 reversal of, 770
Web, tracheal, 1778
Wegener's granulomatosis, 163, 163f, 1475
Weight loss, in atherosclerosis prevention, 911–912
Westermark's sign, 1616
Wheezing, in pulmonary metastases, 339
Williams syndrome, 1952
Wolff-Parkinson-White syndrome, 1329
 catheter ablation in, 1334–1335, 1336f
WorldHeart LevaCor device, 1518, 1518f
Wound (surgical)
 infection of, 56. *See also* Sternal wound infection
 postoperative care of, 53

X

Ximelagatran, 759
Xiphisternal joint, 10
Xiphoid, 3f, 5
Xiphosternoplexy, 372

Z

Zenith TX2 device, 1131–1132, 1132f, 1134–1135
Zenker's diverticulum, 75–78, 564–565, 564f
 cricopharyngeal myotomy in, 75–76
 diverticulopexy and myotomy in, 76
 transoral endoscopic stapling in, 76–78, 565
  positioning for, 76
  preparation for, 76–77, 77f
  results of, 77–78
  technique of, 77, 78f